Eleventh Edition
Global Edition

Kozier & Erb's Fundamentals of Nursing

Concepts, Process, and Practice

Audrey Berman, PhD, RN
Professor, School of Nursing
Samuel Merritt University
Oakland, California

Shirlee J. Snyder, EdD, RN
Retired Dean and Professor, Nursing
Nevada State College
Henderson, Nevada

Geralyn Frandsen, EdD, RN
Professor of Nursing
Maryville University
St. Louis, Missouri

Please contact https://support.pearson.com/getsupport/s/contactsupport with any queries on this content.

Pearson Education Limited
KAO Two
KAO Park
Hockham Way
Harlow
Essex
CM17 9SR
United Kingdom

and Associated Companies throughout the world

Visit us on the World Wide Web at: www.pearsonglobaleditions.com

Authorized adaptation from the United States edition, entitled Kozier & Erb's Fundamentals of Nursing: Concepts, Process, and Practice, *11th Edition, ISBN 9780135428733, by Audrey Berman, Shirlee J. Snyder, and Geralyn Frandsen, published by Pearson Education © 2021.*

ISBN 10: 1-292-35979-X
ISBN 13: 978-1-292-35979-3

British Library Cataloguing-in-Publication Data
A catalogue record for this book is available from the British Library

1 21

Cover Photo Credit: Daxiao Productions/Shutterstock

Typeset by SPi Global
Printed and bound by L.E.G.O. S.p.A. Lavis (TN)

Dedication

Audrey Berman dedicates this eleventh edition to her mother, Lotte Henrietta Julia Sarah Rosenberg Berman Isaacs (1926–2017), who raised two strong daughters and served as a role model to each of them and also to her grandchildren, Brian and Jordanna, and great-grandsons, Benjamin and Adam. May her memory be a blessing.

Shirlee Snyder dedicates this eleventh edition in memory of her older brother, Ted Snyder, whose legacy is his loving and caring family; to her younger brother, Dan Snyder, who enjoys his retirement with his wife, children, and grandchildren; to Kelly Bishop, the best daughter ever and her first great-grandchild, Oliver; to her stepson, Steven Schnitter; to all the nurses who contribute to the nursing profession; and always, to her husband, Terry J. Schnitter, for his continual love and support.

Geralyn Frandsen dedicates this eleventh edition to her loving husband and fellow nursing colleague, Gary. He is always willing to answer questions and provide editorial support. She also dedicates this edition to her children, Claire and Joe; son-in-law, John Conroy; and daughter-in-law, Allyson Angelos.

About the Authors

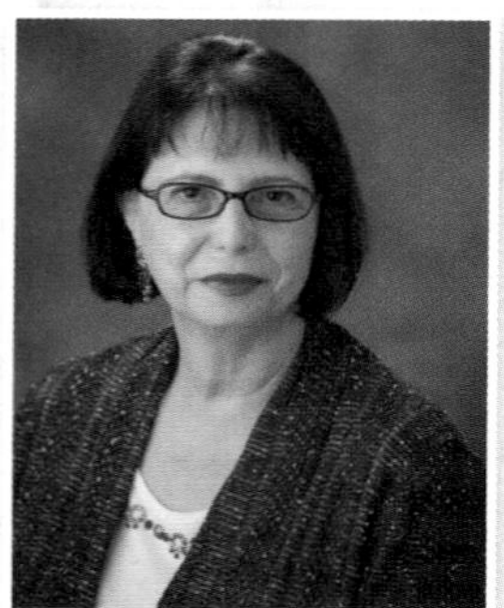

Audrey Berman, PhD, RN

A San Francisco Bay Area native, Audrey Berman received her BSN from the University of California–San Francisco and later returned to that campus to obtain her MS in physiologic nursing and her PhD in nursing. Her dissertation was entitled *Sailing a Course Through Chemotherapy: The Experience of Women with Breast Cancer*. She worked in oncology at Samuel Merritt Hospital prior to beginning her teaching career in the diploma program at Samuel Merritt Hospital School of Nursing in 1976. As a faculty member, she participated in the transition of that program into a baccalaureate degree and in the development of the master of science and doctor of nursing practice programs. Over the years, she has taught a variety of medical–surgical nursing courses in the prelicensure programs on three campuses. She served as the dean of nursing at Samuel Merritt University from 2004 to 2019 and was the 2014–2016 president of the California Association of Colleges of Nursing.

Dr. Berman has traveled extensively, visiting nursing and healthcare institutions in Australia, Botswana, Brazil, Finland, Germany, Israel, Japan, Korea, the Philippines, the Soviet Union, and Spain. She is a senior director of the Bay Area Tumor Institute and served 3 years as director on the Council on Accreditation of Nurse Anesthesia Educational Programs. She is a member of the American Nurses Association and Sigma Theta Tau and is a site visitor for the Commission on Collegiate Nursing Education. She has twice participated as an NCLEX-RN item writer for the National Council of State Boards of Nursing. She has presented locally, nationally, and internationally on topics related to nursing education, breast cancer, and technology in healthcare.

Dr. Berman authored the scripts for more than 35 nursing skills videotapes in the 1990s. She was a coauthor of the sixth, seventh, eighth, ninth, tenth, and eleventh editions of *Fundamentals of Nursing* and the fifth, sixth, seventh, eighth, and ninth editions of *Skills in Clinical Nursing*.

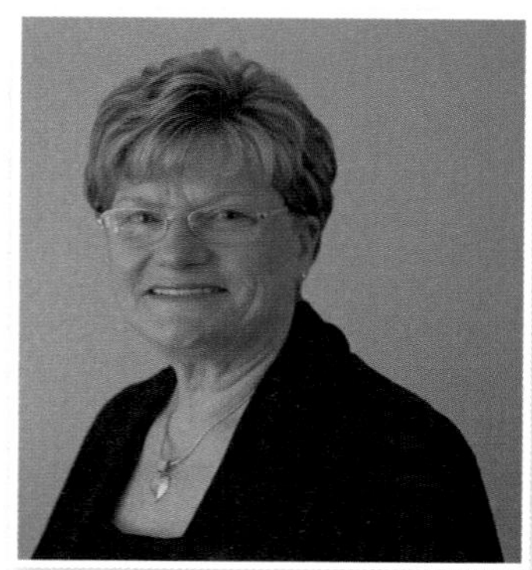

Shirlee J. Snyder, EdD, RN

Shirlee J. Snyder graduated from Columbia Hospital School of Nursing in Milwaukee, Wisconsin, and subsequently received a bachelor of science in nursing from the University of Wisconsin–Milwaukee. Because of an interest in cardiac nursing and teaching, she earned a master of science in nursing with a minor in cardiovascular clinical specialist and teaching from the University of Alabama in Birmingham. A move to California resulted in becoming a faculty member at Samuel Merritt Hospital School of Nursing in Oakland, California. Shirlee was fortunate to be involved in the phasing out of the diploma and ADN programs and development of a baccalaureate intercollegiate nursing program. She held numerous positions during her 15-year tenure at Samuel Merritt College, including curriculum coordinator, assistant director–instruction, dean of instruction, and associate dean of the Intercollegiate Nursing Program. She is an associate professor alumnus at Samuel Merritt College. Her interest and experiences in nursing education resulted in Shirlee obtaining a doctorate of education focused on curriculum and instruction from the University of San Francisco.

Dr. Snyder moved to Portland, Oregon, in 1990 and taught in the ADN program at Portland Community College for 8 years. During this teaching experience she presented locally and nationally on topics related to using multimedia in the classroom and promoting the success of students of diverse ethnic backgrounds and communities of color.

Another career opportunity in 1998 led her to the Community College of Southern Nevada in Las Vegas, Nevada, where Dr. Snyder was the nursing program director with responsibilities for the associate degree and practical nursing programs for 5 years. During this time she coauthored the fifth edition of *Kozier & Erb's Techniques in Clinical Nursing* with Audrey Berman.

In 2003, Dr. Snyder returned to baccalaureate nursing education. She embraced the opportunity to be one of the nursing faculty teaching the first nursing class in the baccalaureate nursing program at the first state college in Nevada, which opened in 2002. From 2008 to 2012, she was the dean of the School of Nursing at Nevada State College in Henderson, Nevada. She is currently retired.

Dr. Snyder enjoyed traveling to the Philippines (Manila and Cebu) in 2009 to present all-day seminars to approximately 5000 nursing students and 200 nursing faculty. She is a member of the American Nurses Association. She has been a site visitor for the National League for Nursing Accrediting Commission and the Northwest Association of Schools and Colleges.

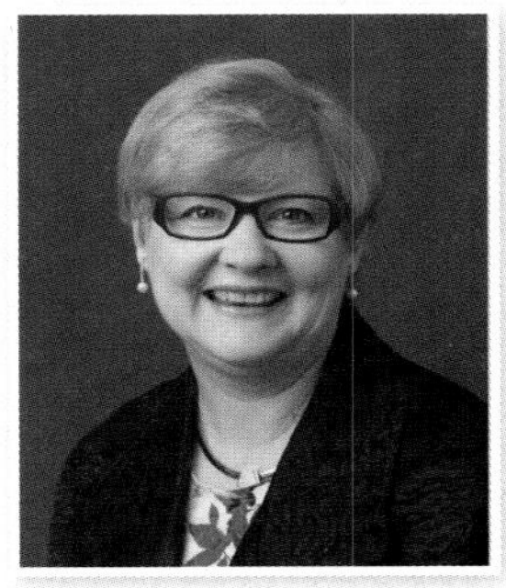

Geralyn Frandsen, EdD, RN

Geralyn Frandsen graduated in the last class from DePaul Hospital School of Nursing in St. Louis, Missouri. She earned a bachelor of science in nursing from Maryville College. She attended Southern Illinois University at Edwardsville, earning a master of science degree in nursing with specializations in community health and nursing education. Upon completion, she accepted a faculty position at her alma mater Maryville College, which has since been renamed Maryville University. In 2003 she completed her doctorate in higher education and leadership at Saint Louis University. Her dissertation was *Mentoring Nursing Faculty in Higher Education*.

She is a tenured full professor and currently serves as assistant director of the Catherine McAuley School of Nursing at Maryville. Her administrative responsibilities include the oversight of three pre-licensure tracks and the online Baccalaureate Completion program in the Robert E. and Joan Luttig Schoor Undergraduate Nursing Program. When educating undergraduate and graduate students, she utilizes a variety of teaching strategies to engage her students. When teaching undergraduate pharmacology she utilizes a team teaching approach, placing students in groups to review content. Each student is also required to bring a completed ticket to class covering the content to be taught. The practice of bringing a ticket to class was introduced to her by Dr. Em Bevis, who is famous for the *Toward a Caring Curriculum*.

Dr. Frandsen has authored textbooks in pharmacology and nursing fundamentals. In 2013 she was the fundamentals contributor for *Ready Point* and *My Nursing Lab*. These are online resources to assist students in reviewing content in their nursing fundamentals course. She has authored both *Nursing Fundamentals: Pearson Reviews and Rationales* and, in 2007, *Pharmacology Reviews and Rationales*.

Dr. Frandsen has completed the End-of-Life Nursing Education Consortium train-the-trainer courses for advanced practice nurses and the doctorate of nursing practice. She is passionate about end-of-life care and teaches a course to her undergraduate students. Dr. Frandsen is a member of Sigma Theta Tau International and the American Nurses Association, and serves as a site visitor for the Commission on Collegiate Nursing Education.

Acknowledgments

We wish to extend a sincere thank you to the talented team involved in the eleventh edition of this book: the contributors and reviewers who provide content and very helpful feedback; the nursing students, for their questioning minds and motivation; and the nurses and nursing instructors, who provided many valuable suggestions for this edition.

We would like to thank the editorial team, especially John Goucher, for his continual support; Melissa Bashe, Managing Producer, Health Science and Career and Student Success; and most of all Teri Zak, development editor, for keeping our noses to the grindstone and especially for her dedication and attention to detail that promoted an excellent outcome once again. Many thanks to the production team of Michael Giaccobe, Content Producer, and Meghan DeMaio and Patty Donovan, editorial project managers, for producing this book with precision.

Audrey Berman
Shirlee Snyder
Geralyn Frandsen

Thank You

We would like to extend our heartfelt thanks to our colleagues across the country who have given their time generously to help us create this learning package. These individuals helped us develop this textbook and supplements by reviewing chapters, art, and media, and by answering a myriad of questions right up until the time of publication. *Kozier & Erb's Fundamentals of Nursing, Eleventh Edition*, has benefited immeasurably from their efforts, insights, suggestions, objections, encouragement, and inspiration, as well as from their vast experience as teachers and nurses. Thank you again for helping us set the foundation for nursing excellence.

CONTRIBUTORS TO THE ELEVENTH EDITION

Sherrilyn Coffman, PhD, RN, COI
Professor Nevada State College
Chapter 15: Caring

Elizabeth Johnston Taylor, PhD, RN, FAAN
Associate Professor, Loma Linda University
Research Director, Mary Potter Hospice
Wellington South, New Zealand
Chapter 41: Spirituality

REVIEWERS OF THE ELEVENTH EDITION

Joy Borrero, MSN, RN
Suffolk County Community College
Selden, NY

Staci Boruff, PhD, RN
Walters State Community College
Morristown, TN

Rebecca Byrnes, MSN, RN
Viterbo University
La Crosse, WI

Maria Cho, PhD, RN, AOCNS, FNP
California State University East Bay
Hayward, CA

Darlene Clark, MS, RN
Penn State University
State College, PA

Carol Della Ratta, PhD, RN, CCRN
Stony Brook University
Stony Brook, NY

Ann Denney, MSN, RN
Thomas More University
Crestview Hills, KY

Marci Dial, DNP, MSN, BSN, ARNP, NP-C, RN-BC, CHSE, LNC
Valencia College
Orlando, FL

Michelle Edmonds, PhD, MSN, BSN
Jacksonville University
Jacksonville, FL

Laura Fowler, MSN, RN
Luzerne County Community College
Nanticoke, PA

Kathleen Fraley, MSN, BSN, RN, ADN
St. Clair County Community College
Port Huron, MI

Jennifer Fritzges, DNP, RN, CNE
Carroll Community College
Westminster, MD

Catherine Gabster, MSN, RN, CNL, CNS
University of California Los Angeles
Los Angeles, CA

Kelli Hand, DNP, MBA, RN
University of Tennessee Chattanooga
Chattanooga, TN

Jim Hunter, MSN, RN
British Columbia Institute of Technology
Burnaby, British Columbia, CA

Christine Kleckner, MA, MAN, RN
Minneapolis Community and Technical College
Minneapolis, MN

Carole McKenzie, PhD, CNM, RN
Texas A&M University Commerce
Commerce, TX

Susan Mullaney, EdD, MS, MA, RN, CNE
Framingham State University
Framingham, MA

Rebecca Otten, EdD, RN
California State University Fullerton
Fullerton, CA

Connie Pattison, DNP, MSN, RN-B
Montana State University

Anita Reed, MSN, RN
Saint Elizabeth School of Nursing
Lafayette, IN

Annette Ries, MSNEd, RN
Alverno College
Milwaukee, WI

Nita Slater, MSN, CMSRN, PHN
California State University Fullerton
Fullerton, CA

Carmen Stokes, PhD, FNP-BC, RN, CNE
University of Detroit Mercy
Detroit, MI

Susan Tucker, DNP, MSN, RN, CNE
Gadsden State Community College
Gadsden, AL

Amanda Veesart, PhD, RN, CNE
Texas Tech University
Lubbock, TX

Jean Yockey, FNP-BC, CNE
University of South Dakota
Vermillion, SD

Danielle Yocom, MSN, FNP-BC
Massachusetts College of Pharmacy and Health Sciences
Worcester, PA

Beth Zieman, MSN, RN
Delta College
University Center, MI

Pearson would like to thank and acknowledge the following people for their work on this Global Edition.

CONTRIBUTORS TO THE ELEVENTH EDITION

Josanne Drago Bason, MSN, BSN, RN
Visiting Senior Lecturer, University of Malta
Malta, Europe

Mary Grace Anne P. Batalla, MA, RN, RNA
Guy's and St. Thomas' NHS Foundation Trust
London, United Kingdom

Athina Karavasopoulou, MSc, RN, ANP, NINMP
Lecturer, King's College London
London, United Kingdom

REVIEWERS OF THE ELEVENTH EDITION

Peter James B. Abad, MSc, RN
University of the Philippines Manila
Manila, Philippines

Victoria Adebola, MSc, RN, SCPHP
University of West London
London, United Kingdom

Mary Grace Anne P. Batalla, MA, RN, RNA
Guy's and St. Thomas' NHS Foundation Trust
London, United Kingdom

Richard Brooksbank, MSc, PhD
University of the Witwatersrand
Johannesburg, South Africa

Petra Brysiewicz, PhD, MN, *f*ANSA, FAAN, ASSAf
University of KwaZulu-Natal
Durban, South Africa

Isabel Coetzee, PhD
University of Pretoria
Hatfield, South Africa

Rita Debnath, MSc, BSc (Hons), RN
University of Leeds
Leeds, United Kingdom

Claire Donnellan, PhD, MSc, MA, PG Dip Stats, BSc, CPsychol, RGN
Trinity College Dublin
Dublin, Ireland

Charlene Downing, DCur
University of Johannesburg
Johannesburg, South Africa

David Fisher, PhD
University of the Western Cape
Bellville, South Africa

Margaret Mc Adam, PhD, MA, BNS, RGN, RSCN
Trinity College Dublin
Dublin, Ireland

Gugu Mchunu, RN, MN, PhD
University of KwaZulu-Natal
Durban, South Africa

Ntombifikile Gloria Mtshali, PhD
University of KwaZulu-Natal
Durban, South Africa

John Joseph B. Posadas, MSAHP, RN
University of the Philippines
Manila City, NCR

Shelley Schmollgruber, PhD
University of the Witwatersrand
Johannesburg, South Africa

Preface

The practice of nursing continues to evolve . . . *the practice of caring is timeless.*

Nurses today must grow and evolve to meet the demands of a dramatically changing healthcare system. They need skills in science, technology, communication, and interpersonal relations to be effective members of the collaborative healthcare team. They need to think critically and be creative in implementing nursing strategies to provide safe and competent nursing care for clients of diverse cultural backgrounds in increasingly varied settings. They need skills in teaching, leading, managing, and the process of change. They need to be prepared to provide home- and community-based nursing care to clients across the lifespan—especially to the increasing numbers of older adults. They need to understand legal and ethical principles, holistic healing modalities, and complementary therapies. And, they need to continue their unique client advocacy role, which demands a blend of nurturance, sensitivity, caring, empathy, commitment, and skill founded on a broad base of knowledge.

Kozier & Erb's Fundamentals of Nursing, Eleventh Edition, addresses the concepts of contemporary professional nursing. These concepts include but are not limited to caring, wellness, health promotion, disease prevention, holistic care, critical thinking and clinical reasoning, multiculturalism, nursing theories, nursing informatics, nursing research, ethics, and advocacy. In this edition, every chapter has been reviewed and revised. The content has been updated to reflect the latest nursing evidence and the increasing emphasis on aging, wellness, safety, and home- and community-based care.

ORGANIZATION

The detailed table of contents at the beginning of the book makes its clear organization easy to follow. Continuing with a strong focus on nursing care, the eleventh edition of this book is divided into 10 units.

Unit 1, *The Nature of Nursing*, clusters four chapters that provide comprehensive coverage of introductory concepts of nursing.

In Unit 2, *Contemporary Healthcare*, four chapters include contemporary healthcare topics such as healthcare delivery systems, community-based care, home care, and informatics.

In Unit 3, *The Nursing Process*, six chapters introduce students to this important framework with each chapter dedicated to a specific step of the nursing process. Chapter 9 applies critical thinking, clinical reasoning, and the nursing process. A Nursing in Action case study is used as the frame of reference for applying content in all phases of the nursing process in Chapter 10, *Assessing*; Chapter 11, *Diagnosing*; Chapter 12, *Planning*; and Chapter 13, *Implementing and Evaluating*. Chapter 14 covers documenting and reporting.

Unit 4, *Integral Aspects of Nursing*, discusses topics such as caring; communicating; teaching; and leading, managing, and delegating. These topics are all crucial elements for providing safe, competent nursing care.

In Unit 5, *Health Beliefs and Practices*, four chapters include health-related beliefs and practices for individuals and families from a variety of cultural backgrounds.

Unit 6, *Lifespan Development*, consists of five chapters that discuss lifespan and development from conception to older adults.

Unit 7, *Assessing Health*, addresses vital signs, health assessment, and pain assessment and management skills in three separate chapters, to allow beginning students to understand normal assessment techniques and findings.

In Unit 8, *Integral Components of Client Care*, the focus shifts to those components of client care that are universal to all clients, including asepsis, safety, hygiene, diagnostic testing, medications, wound care, and perioperative care.

Unit 9, *Promoting Psychosocial Health*, includes six chapters that cover a wide range of areas that affect the individual's health. Sensory perception, self-concept, sexuality, spirituality, stress, and loss are all aspects that a nurse needs to consider to properly care for a client.

Unit 10, *Promoting Physiologic Health*, discusses a variety of physiologic concepts that provide the foundations for nursing care. These include activity and exercise; sleep; nutrition; elimination; oxygenation; circulation; and fluid, electrolyte, and acid–base balance.

HIGHLIGHTS OF THE ELEVENTH EDITION

- **QSEN linkages**. The delivery of high-quality and safe nursing practice is imperative for every nurse. The QSEN competencies were developed to address the gap between nursing education and practice. There are expectations for each of the six QSEN competencies and these expectations relate to knowledge, skills, and attitudes. Nursing students are expected to achieve these competencies during nursing school and use them in their professional role as RNs. This edition has incorporated QSEN competencies and specified expectations in most chapters. This QSEN content will guide students to learn and maintain safety and quality in their provision of nursing care.

- **Assignment:** Recognition of the evolving legal aspects of assigning and delegating nursing care, especially to assistive personnel.
- Current examples of nursing literature guiding evidence-based practice.
- Up-to-date samples of electronic health records that support nursing care.
- Updated and additional photos to assist the visual learner.
- **Standards of care.** This edition continues to value and update standards of care as evidenced by incorporating the latest National Patient Safety Goals; Infusion Nursing Society *Standards of Practice*; American Nurses Association (ANA) *Scope and Standards of Practice*; National Council of State Boards of Nursing *National Guidelines for Nursing Delegation*; current hypertension guidelines; pressure injury prevention guidelines; ANA *Safe Patient Handling and Mobility: Interprofessional National Standards Across the Care Continuum*; Occupational Safety and Health Administration and Centers for Disease Control and Prevention bloodborne pathogens and infection prevention standards; and cancer screening guidelines.

FEATURES

For years, *Kozier & Erb's Fundamentals of Nursing* has been a gold standard that helps students embark on their careers in nursing. This new edition retains many of the features that have made this textbook the number-one choice of nursing students and faculty. The walk-through at the beginning of the textbook illustrates these features.

Supplements That Inspire Success for the Student and the Instructor

Pearson is pleased to offer a complete suite of resources to support teaching and learning, including:

- TestGen Test Bank
- Lecture Note PowerPoints
- Instructor's Manual
- Image Library.
- Additional material on global standards and practices related to nursing available at www.pearsonglobaleditions.com
- A supplement on COVID-19 available on MyLab Nursing to help nurses cope with the rapidly evolving pandemic

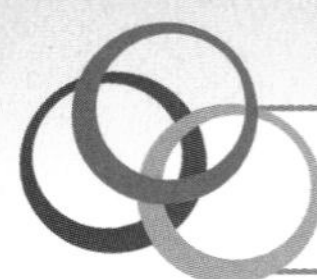

Features of the Eleventh Edition

SPECIAL FEATURES

provide the opportunity to link QSEN competencies and to think critically to make a connection to nursing practice. These features provide guidance on maintaining safety and quality of nursing care.

EVIDENCE-BASED PRACTICE

Evidence-Based Practice

What Is the Impact of Chlorhexidine Bathing on Healthcare-Associated Infections?

According to Denny and Munro (2017), approximately 4% of hospitalized clients contract a healthcare-associated infection (HAI) during their hospitalizations. These infections frequently result in increased morbidity, mortality, and length of hospital stay. Skin bacterial colonization aids in the transmission and development of HAIs. Nurses frequently use bathing with chlorhexidine gluconate (CHG) to reduce bacterial colonization on the client's skin. Studies have shown that bathing with CHG products has had mixed results in the prevention of HAIs. As a result, the authors performed a literature review to examine the current evidence on the impact of CHG bathing on HAIs. The literature search identified peer-reviewed studies and meta-analyses that examined the impact of CHG bathing in preventing HAIs, specifically surgical site infections (SSIs), central line–associated bloodstream infections (CLABSIs), ventilator-associated pneumonias (VAP), catheter-associated urinary-tract infections (CAUTIs), and *Clostridium difficile*–associated disease. The search resulted in 23 articles for review.

The findings concluded that there was good evidence to support using a CHG bathing regimen to reduce the incidence of CLABSIs, SSIs, vancomycin-resistant enterococci (VRE), and methicillin-resistant *Staphylococcus aureus* (MRSA) HAIs.

The authors, based on the literature search, raised questions for further research, including the value of using CHG liquid soap versus CHG-impregnated washcloths. Research has shown that application of CHG on the client's body without rinsing has greater impact than applying CHG followed by rinsing the body. Do CHG-impregnated washcloths have an advantage because the CHG in the wipes is not rinsed from the skin? Another issue raised by the authors was that most studies were conducted in targeted populations (e.g., intensive care units). They suggest that more research is needed on the benefits of bathing all clients versus a targeted (bathing only at-risk clients) approach.

IMPLICATIONS

Hospitals are beginning to replace the traditional soap and water bathing with CHG bathing in order to prevent HAIs. As the authors suggested, nurses need to assess for adverse reactions to the use of CHG and increase their awareness that, with the increasing use of CHG, organisms may develop resistance to the antiseptic.

Safety Alert! **SAFETY**

Side rail entrapment, injuries, and death do occur. When side rails are used, the nurse must assess the client's physical and mental status and closely monitor high-risk (frail, older, or confused) clients.

LIFESPAN CONSIDERATIONS Diagnosing

CHILDREN

Many developmental issues in pediatrics are not considered problems or illnesses, yet can benefit from nursing intervention. When applied to children and families, nursing diagnoses may reflect a condition or state of health. For example, parents of a newborn infant may be excited to learn all they can about infant care and child growth and development. Assessment of the family system might lead the nurse to conclude that the family is ready and able, even eager, to take on the new roles and responsibilities of being parents. An appropriate diagnosis for such a family could be willingness for improved family dynamics, and nursing care could be directed to educating and providing encouragement and support to the parents.

OLDER ADULTS

Older adults tend to have multiple problems with complex physical and psychosocial needs when they are ill. If the nurse has done a thorough and accurate assessment, nursing diagnoses can be selected to cover all problems and, at the same time, prioritize the special needs. For example, if a client is admitted with severe congestive heart fa... cardiac status a... to improve the... other nursing di... knowledge relat... attention. They... tive heart failure... outcomes and... be an essential...

CLIENT TEACHING Developing Written Teaching Aids

- Keep language level at a fifth- to sixth-grade level.
- Use active, not passive, voice (e.g., "take your medicine before breakfast" [active] versus "medicine should be taken before breakfast" [passive]).
- Use plain language; that is, easy, common words of one or two syllables (e.g., *use* instead of *utilize*, or *give* instead of *administer*).
- Use the second person (*you*) rather than the third person (*the client*).
- Use a large type size (14 to 16 point).
- Write short sentences.
- Avoid using all capital letters.
- Place priority information first and repeat it more than once.
- Use bold for emphasis.
- Use simple pictures, drawings, or cartoons, if appropriate.
- Leave plenty of white space.
- Focus material on desired behavior rather than on medical facts.
- Make it look easy to read.

ENHANCED PHOTO PROGRAM

shows procedural steps and the latest equipment.

The nursing process is a systematic, rational method of planning and providing nursing care. Its purpose is to identify a client's healthcare status, and actual or potential health problems, to establish plans to meet the identified needs, and to deliver specific nursing interventions to address those needs. The nursing process is cyclical; that is, its components follow a logical sequence, but more than one component may be involved at one time. At the end of the first cycle, care may be terminated if goals are achieved, or the cycle may continue with reassessment, or the plan of care may be modified.

ASSESSING
ASSESSING
- Collect data
- Organize data
- Validate data
- Document data

DIAGNOSING
DIAGNOSING
- Analyze data
- Identify health problems, risks, and strengths
- Formulate diagnostic statements

PLANNING
PLANNING
- Prioritize problems/diagnoses
- Formulate goals/desired outcomes
- Select nursing interventions
- Write nursing interventions

IMPLEMENTING
IMPLEMENTING
- Reassess the client
- Determine the nurse's need for assistance
- Implement the nursing interventions
- Supervise delegated care
- Document nursing activities

EVALUATING
EVALUATING
- Collect data related to outcomes
- Compare data with outcomes
- Relate nursing actions to client goals/outcomes
- Draw conclusions about problem status
- Continue, modify, or terminate the client's care plan

Figure 10.1 ■ The nursing process in action.

HALLMARK FEATURES

This eleventh edition maintains the best aspects of previous editions to provide the most valuable learning experience.

LEARNING OUTCOMES help identify critical concepts.

KEY TERMS provide a study tool for learning new vocabulary. Page numbers are included for easy reference.

20 Health, Wellness, and Illness

LEARNING OUTCOMES

After completing this chapter, you will be able to:

1. Identify influences on clients' definitions of health, wellness, and well-being.
2. Describe five components of wellness.
3. Compare various models of health.
4. Identify variables affecting health status, beliefs, and practices.
5. Describe factors affecting healthcare adherence.
6. Differentiate illness from disease and acute illness from chronic illness.
7. Identify Parsons's four aspects of the sick role.
8. Explain Suchman's stages of illness.
9. Describe the effects of illness on clients' and family members' roles and functions.

KEY TERMS

acute illness, *391*
adherence, *389*
chronic illness, *391*
disease, *390*
etiology, *390*
exacerbation, *391*
health, *382*
health behaviors, *386*
health beliefs, *386*
health status, *386*
illness, *390*
illness behavior, *391*
lifestyle, *387*
locus of control, *388*
remission, *391*
risk factors, *387*
well-being, *384*
wellness, *384*

Introduction

Nurses' understanding of health and wellness largely determines the scope and nature of nursing practice. Clients' health beliefs influence their health practices. Some "nts think of health and wellness (or well-being) as the ıe thing or, at the very least, as accompanying one ıther. However, health may not always accompany ll-being: A client who has a terminal illness may have ense of well-being; conversely, another client may lack ense of well-being yet be in a state of good health. For ny years, the concept of disease was the yardstick by ich health was measured. In the late 19th century, the ıw" of disease (pathogenesis) was the major concern ıealth professionals. The 20th century focused on find- cures for diseases. Currently, healthcare providers are reasing their emphasis on preventing illness and pro- ting health and wellness in individuals, families, and ımunities.

ɔncepts of Health, Wellness, ıd Well-Being

ılth, wellness, and well-being have many definitions l interpretations. The nurse should be familiar with the st common aspects of the concepts and consider how y may be individualized with specific clients.

Health

Traditionally, **health** was defined in terms of the presence or absence of disease. Florence Nightingale (1860/1969) defined health as a state of being well and using every power the individual possesses to the fullest extent. The World Health Organization (WHO, 1948) takes a more holistic view of health. Its constitution defines health as "a state of complete physical, mental, and social well-being, and not merely the absence of disease or infirmity." This definition reflects concern for the individual as a total person, functioning physically, psychologically, and socially. Mental processes determine individuals' relationships with their physical and social surroundings, their attitudes about life, and their interaction with others. Individuals' lives, and therefore their health, are affected by everything they interact with—not only environmental influences such as climate and the availability of food, shelter, clean air, and water to drink but also other individuals, including family, lovers, employers, coworkers, friends, and associates.

Health has also been defined in terms of role and performance. Talcott Parsons (1951), an eminent American sociologist and creator of the concept of "sick role," conceptualized health as the ability to maintain normal roles.

In 1953, the U.S. President's Commission on Health Needs of the Nation (1953) made the following statement about health: "Health is not a condition; it is an adjustment. It is not a state but a process. The process adapts the individual not only to our physical but also our social

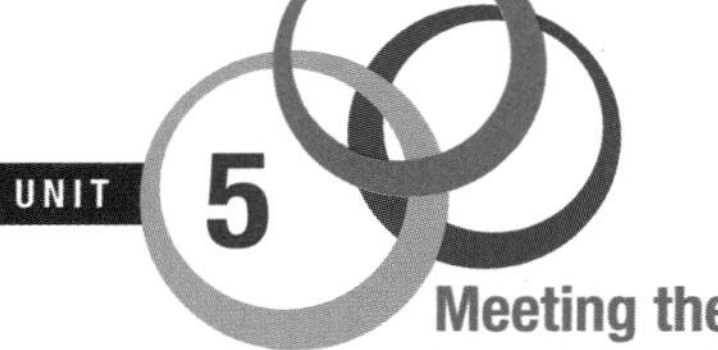

UNIT 5 Meeting the Standards

In this unit, we have explored concepts related to health, health promotion, wellness, illness, culture and heritage, and complementary and alternative healing modalities. These topics heighten awareness of the individualistic nature of the relationship between the nurse and the client and the importance of assessing the breadth of factors that affect health decisions and behaviors. In the case described here, you will see how one client demonstrates complicated, interrelated, personal definitions of health and illness influenced by her medical condition, her heritage, and her demographic characteristics (e.g., age and family structure). These definitions and perspectives in turn influence her choices for care and support—including the role of her nurses.

CLIENT: Manuela AGE: 55
CURRENT MEDICAL DIAGNOSIS: Still's Disease

Medical History: Manuela has experienced some type of health challenge for most of her adult life. She was diagnosed with adult-onset Still's disease (AOSD) at about age 35 after several years of tests to try to determine exactly what syndrome her symptoms reflected. She complained of joint pain, rash, and fevers, which came and went, and she had an enlarged spleen and liver. This disease shares many similarities with rheumatoid and autoimmune diseases, but those conditions were all removed from consideration because the tests were negative. AOSD is a chronic condition for which there is no known cure. In addition to joint deterioration, it can progress to affect the lungs and heart. Initial treatment consists of steroids and nonsteroidal anti-inflammatory drugs (NSAIDs). If those are ineffective, other medications, such as gold and chemotherapeutics are used; however, they have severe side effects, such as kidney damage and bone marrow suppression. The condition worsens when the individual is under physical or emotional stress. Manuela underwent a hip replacement about 4 years ago and recently has had several hospitalizations for respiratory failure.

Personal and Social History: Manuela has never married and has lived near or with her parents or siblings for all her life. She has many friends, drives, and has an active social life when she is feeling well. She uses the computer extensively for communication, especially when having visitors or talking by phone is too exhausting. She must follow a strict diet of food and liquids that are easy to swallow and digest. She is a spiritual individual but not overly religious. She is quick to laugh and generally has an optimistic outlook, but she expresses awareness that her life could end at any time—certainly long before her full life expectancy.

Manuela is a college graduate but has been able to work only part time for most of her life. Recently, she was declared permanently disabled, which allows her access to financial and other support systems. She is creative in adapting her living situation to her disabilities and unwilling to give up her beloved pet dog.

Questions

American Nurses Association Standard of Practice #3 *is Outcomes Identification: The nurse collaborates with the healthcare consumer to define expected outcomes integrating the healthcare consumer's culture, values, and ethical considerations. As you learned in Chapter 19* ⚭, Manuela's needs fall into the category of tertiary prevention in which rehabilitation and movement toward optimal levels of functionality within the individual's constraints are the focus.

1. What are some outcomes for Manuela that would reflect this focus?
2. Do you need to know her personal definitions of health and health beliefs (Chapter 20 ⚭) before you can work with her to set expected outcomes?

American Nurses Association Standard of Practice #5b *is Health Teaching and Health Promotion: The nurse employs strategies to promote health and a safe environment.*

3. What are some aspects of Manuela's situation that you would consider incorporating into a teaching plan t environment for her?

American Nurses Association Standard of P formance #10 *is Collaboration: Nurses partner to create, implement, and evaluate a compreher*

4. Which healthcare team members other than p would likely be important to include in Manuel

American Nurses Association Standard of P formance #13 *is Evidence-Based Practice and*

5. What evidence might you have or seek to sup tive or complementary treatment modalities in

American Nurses Association. (2015). *Nursing: Scope and star* Silver Spring, MD: Author.

Answers to Meeting the Standards questions are available on t Please consult with your instructor.

MEETING THE STANDARDS end-of-unit activities provide the opportunity to think through themes and competencies presented across chapters in a unit and think critically to link theory to nursing practice.

NURSING CARE PLAN Margaret O'Brien

Nursing Diagnosis: Altered respiratory status related to viscous secretions secondary to alteration in fluid volume and shallow chest expansion secondary to pain and fatigue

DESIRED OUTCOMES*/INDICATORS	NURSING INTERVENTIONS	RATIONALE
Respiratory Status: Gas Exchange [0402], as evidenced by • Absence of pallor and cyanosis (skin and mucous membranes) • Use of correct breathing/coughing technique after instruction	Monitor respiratory status q4h: rate, depth, effort, skin color, mucous membranes, amount and color of sputum. Monitor results of blood gases, chest x-ray studies, and incentive spirometer volume as available. Monitor level of consciousness.	*To identify progress toward or deviations from goal.* Altered repiratory status *leads to poor oxygenation, as evidenced by pallor, cyanosis, lethargy, and drowsiness.*
• Productive cough • Symmetric chest excursion of at least 4 cm	Auscultate lungs q4h. Vital signs q4h (TPR, BP, pulse oximetry, pain).	*Inadequate oxygenation and pain cause increased pulse rate. Respiratory rate may be decreased by narcotic analgesics. Shallow breathing further compromises oxygenation.*

NURSING CARE PLANS help you approach care from the nursing perspective.

APPLYING CRITICAL THINKING

1. What assumptions does the nurse make when deciding that using a standardized care plan for impaired fluid volume is appropriate for this client?
2. Identify an outcome in the care plan and its nursing intervention that contribute to discharge care planning. What evidence supports your choice?
3. Consider how the nurse shares the development of the care plan and outcomes with the client.
4. Not every intervention has a time frame or interval specified. It may be implied. Under what circumstances is this acceptable practice?
5. In Table 12.1, altered respiratory status is Margaret's highest priority nursing diagnosis. Under what conditions might this diagnosis be of only moderate priority in Margaret's case?

Answers to Applying Critical Thinking questions are available on the faculty resources site. Please consult with your instructor.

APPLYING CRITICAL THINKING questions come at the end of select sample Nursing Care Plans to encourage further reflection and analysis.

CONCEPT MAPS provide visual representations of the nursing process, nursing care plans, and the relationships between difficult concepts.

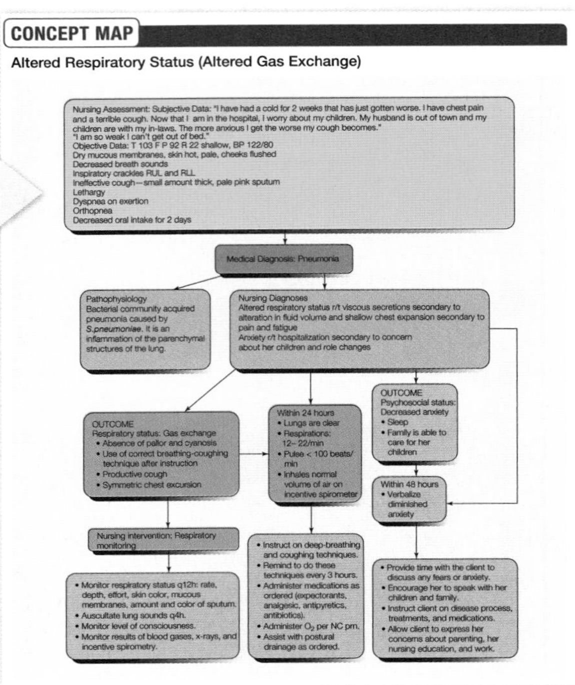

CONCEPT MAP
Altered Respiratory Status (Altered Gas Exchange)
Nursing Assessment: Subjective Data: "I have had a cold for 2 weeks that has just gotten worse. I have chest pain and a terrible cough. Now that I am in the hospital, I worry about my children. My husband is out of town and my children are with my in-laws. The more anxious I get the worse my cough becomes."
"I am so weak I can't get out of bed."
Objective Data: T 103 F P 92 R 22 shallow, BP 122/80
Dry mucous membranes, skin hot, pale, cheeks flushed
Decreased breath sounds
Inspiratory crackles RUL and RLL
Ineffective cough—small amount thick, pale pink sputum
Lethargy
Dyspnea on exertion
Orthopnea
Decreased oral intake for 2 days
Medical Diagnosis: Pneumonia
Pathophysiology
Bacterial community acquired pneumonia caused by S.pneumoniae. It is an inflammation of the parenchymal structures of the lung.
Nursing Diagnoses
Altered respiratory status r/t viscous secretions secondary to alteration in fluid volume and shallow chest expansion secondary to pain and fatigue
Anxiety r/t hospitalization secondary to concern about her children and role changes
OUTCOME
Respiratory status: Gas exchange
• Absence of pallor and cyanosis
• Use of correct breathing-coughing technique after instruction
• Productive cough
• Symmetric chest excursion
Within 24 hours
• Lungs are clear
• Respirations: 12–22/min
• Pulse < 100 beats/min
• Inhales normal volume of air on incentive spirometer
OUTCOME
Psychosocial status: Decreased anxiety
• Sleep
• Family is able to care for her children
Within 48 hours
• Verbalize diminished anxiety
Nursing intervention: Respiratory monitoring
• Monitor respiratory status q12h: rate, depth, effort, skin color, mucous membranes, amount and color of sputum.
• Auscultate lung sounds q4h.
• Monitor level of consciousness.
• Monitor results of blood gases, x-rays, and incentive spirometry.
• Instruct on deep-breathing and coughing techniques.
• Remind to do these techniques every 3 hours.
• Administer medications as ordered (expectorants, analgesic, antipyretics, antibiotics).
• Administer O2 per NC prn.
• Assist with postural drainage as ordered.
• Provide time with the client to discuss any fears or anxiety.
• Encourage her to speak with her children and family.
• Instruct client on disease process, treatments, and medications.
• Allow client to express her concerns about parenting, her nursing education, and work.

SETTING THE FOUNDATION FOR CLINICAL COMPETENCE!

STEP-BY-STEP SKILLS provide an easy-to-follow format that helps you to understand techniques and practice sequences.

- Includes a complete **Equipment** list for easy preparation.
- Clearly labeled **Assignment** boxes assist you in assigning tasks appropriately.
- Easy-to-find **rationales** give you a better understanding of why things are done.
- Critical steps are visually represented with **full-color photos** and **illustrations**.

SKILL 31.2

Applying and Removing Personal Protective Equipment (Gloves, Gown, Mask, Eyewear)

PURPOSE

- To protect healthcare workers and clients from transmission of potentially infective materials

ASSESSMENT

Consider which activities will be required while the nurse is in the client's room at this time. **Rationale:** *This will determine which equipment is required.*

PLANNING

- Application and removal of PPE can be time consuming. Prioritize care and arrange for personnel to care for your other clients if indicated.
- Determine which supplies are present within the client's room and which must be brought to the room.
- Consider if special handling is indicated for removal of any specimens or other materials from the room.

Assignment

Use of PPE is identical for all healthcare providers. Clients whose care requires use of PPE may be assigned to AP. Healthcare team members are accountable for proper implementation of these procedures by themselves and others.

Equipment

As indicated according to which activities will be performed, ensure that extra supplies are easily available.

- Gown
- Mask
- Eyewear
- Clean gloves

IMPLEMENTATION

Preparation

Remove or secure all loose items such as name tags or jewelry.

Performance

1. Prior to performing the procedure, introduce self and verify the client's identity using agency protocol. Explain to the client what you are going to do, why it is necessary, and how to participate.
2. Perform hand hygiene.
3. Apply a clean gown.
   - Pick up a clean gown, and allow it to unfold in front of you without allowing it to touch any area soiled with body substances.
   - Slide the arms and the hands through the sleeves.
   - Fasten the ties at the neck to keep the gown in place.
   - Overlap the gown at the back as much as possible, and fasten the waist ties or belt. ❶ **Rationale:** *Overlapping securely covers the uniform at the back. Waist ties keep the gown from falling away from the body, which can cause inadvertent soiling of the uniform.*
4. Apply the face mask.
   - Locate the top edge of the mask. The mask usually has a narrow metal strip along the edge.
   - Hold the mask by the top two strings or loops.
   - Place the upper edge of the mask over the bridge of the nose, and tie the upper ties at the back of the head or secure the loops around the ears. If glasses are worn, fit the upper edge of the mask under the glasses. ❷ **Rationale:** *With the edge of the mask under the glasses, clouding of the glasses is less likely to occur.*
   - Secure the lower edge of the mask under the chin, and tie the lower ties at the nape of the neck. **Rationale:** *To be effective, a mask must cover both the nose and the mouth, because air moves in and out of both.*
   - If the mask has a metal strip, adjust this firmly over the bridge of the nose. **Rationale:** *A secure fit prevents both the escape and the inhalation of microorganisms around the edges of the mask and the fogging of eyeglasses.*

❶ Overlapping the gown at the back to cover the nurse's uniform.

❷ A face mask tucked under eye protection.
Andresr/Shutterstock

Clinical Alert!

Older adults may not show the classic signs of infection (e.g., fever, tachycardia, increased WBC count); instead there may be an abrupt change in their mental status.

CLINICAL ALERTS highlight special information useful for clinical settings.

PRACTICE GUIDELINES provide instant-access summaries of clinical dos and don'ts.

PRACTICE GUIDELINES Long-Term Care Documentation

- Complete the assessment and screening forms (MDS) and plan of care within the time period specified by regulatory bodies.
- Keep a record of any visits and of phone calls from family, friends, and others regarding the client.
- Write nursing summaries and progress notes that comply with the frequency and standards required by regulatory bodies.
- Review and revise the plan of care every 3 months or whenever the client's health status changes.
- Document and report any change in the client's condition to the primary care provider and the client's family within 24 hours.
- Document all measures implemented in response to a change in the client's condition.
- Make sure that progress notes address the client's progress in relation to the goals or outcomes defined in the plan of care.

DRUG CAPSULE boxes provide a brief overview of drug information, nursing responsibilities, and client teaching to help you understand implications of pharmacotherapy in different situations.

DRUG CAPSULE

Benzodiazepine: midazolam hydrochloride (Versed)

THE CLIENT UNDERGOING ANESTHESIA

IV anesthetic agent used to induce general anesthesia.

Commonly used prior to conscious sedation to produce anxiolytic, hypnotic, anticonvulsant, muscle relaxant, and amnesic effects.

NURSING RESPONSIBILITIES

- Obtain baseline vital signs and level of consciousness before administration.
- Monitor vital signs, level of consciousness, and oxygen saturation q3–5min intraoperatively and postoperatively. Notify primary care provider or CRNA if there are any changes.
- Have resuscitative equipment readily available.
- A too rapid IV administration or excessive dose increases the risk of respiratory depression or arrest.
- Dosage must be individualized based on age, underlying disease, and desired effect. Too much or too little a dosage or improper administration may result in cerebral hypoxia, agitation, involuntary movement, hyperactivity, and combativeness.

Note: Prior to administering any medication, review all aspects with a current drug handbook or other reliable source.

ANATOMY & PHYSIOLOGY REVIEW

ANATOMY & PHYSIOLOGY REVIEW

Client Positioning

The most common position for a client during a surgical procedure is the supine position. This position provides approaches to the cranial, thoracic, and peritoneal body cavities as well as to all four extremities and the perineum. Proper body alignment and padding of potential pressure areas are essential to preventing client risk for injury during surgery.

The potential pressure areas are the occiput, scapulae, olecranon, thoracic vertebrae, sacrum, coccyx, and calcaneus. The nursing intervention is to pad and protect bony prominences, pressure sites, and vulnerable nerves with pressure-reducing devices made of foam or gel. Proper positioning must provide optimal exposure to the surgical site as well as provide for client comfort and safety.

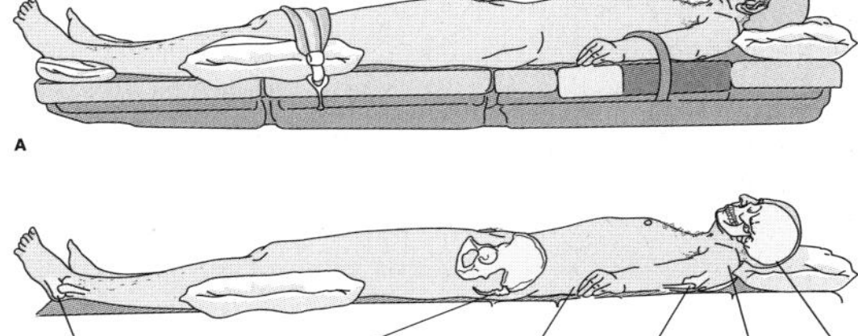

A, Supine position during a surgical procedure; *B*, potential pressure points noted.

QUESTIONS

A 78-year-old male client scheduled for a colon resection is brought to the operating room. He weighs 82 kg (180 lb), has type 2 diabetes, and has a history of arthritis in his hips and shoulders.

1. What baseline assessments would you gather before taking this client to the operating room?
2. What areas on this client are most likely to be injured as a result of poor positioning or inadequate padding?
3. What is the priority nursing diagnosis and outcome for this client?

Answers to Anatomy & Physiology Review Questions are available on the faculty resources site. Please consult with your instructor.

CRITICAL THINKING CHECKPOINTS provide a brief case study followed by questions that encourage you to analyze, compare, contemplate, interpret, and evaluate information.

Critical Thinking Checkpoint

Mr. Teng is a 77-year-old client with a history of COPD. Currently his respiratory condition is being controlled with medications and he is free of infection. He has just been transferred to the PACU following a hernia repair performed under spinal anesthesia. His blood pressure is 132/88 mmHg, pulse 84 beats/min, respirations 28/min, and tympanic temperature 36.5°C (97.8°F). He is awake and stable.

1. What factors place Mr. Teng at increased risk for the development of complications during and after surgery?
2. Speculate about why Mr. Teng's surgeon and anesthesiologist decided to perform Mr. Teng's surgery under regional anesthesia as opposed to general anesthesia.
3. What preparations were taken during the preoperative period to protect Mr. Teng from possible complications during and after his surgery?
4. How will Mr. Teng's postoperative assessments differ from those of a client who received general anesthesia?
5. What postoperative precautions are especially important to Mr. Teng in view of his chronic lung condition?

Answers to Critical Thinking Checkpoint questions are available on the faculty resources site. Please consult with your instructor.

EXTENSIVE END-OF-CHAPTER REVIEW

CHAPTER HIGHLIGHTS focus your attention and review critical concepts.

TEST YOUR KNOWLEDGE helps you prepare for the NCLEX® exam. Alternative-style questions are included. Answers and rationales are in Appendix A.

Chapter 28 Review

CHAPTER HIGHLIGHTS

- Vital signs reflect changes in body function that otherwise might not be observed.
- Body temperature is the balance between heat produced by and heat lost from the body.
- Factors affecting body temperature include age, diurnal variations, exercise, hormones, stress, and environmental temperatures.
- Four common types of fever are intermittent, remittent, relapsing, and constant.
- During a fever, the set point of the hypothalamic thermostat changes suddenly from the normal level to a higher than normal level, but several hours elapse before the core temperature reaches the new set point.
- Hypothermia involves three mechanisms: excessive heat loss, inadequate heat production by body cells, and increasing impairment of hypothalamic thermoregulation.
- The nurse selects the most appropriate site to measure temperature according to the client's age and condition.
- Pulse rate and volume reflect the stroke volume output, the compliance of the client's arteries, and the adequacy of blood flow.
- Normally a peripheral pulse reflects the client's heartbeat, but it may differ from the heartbeat in clients with certain cardiovascular diseases; in these instances, the nurse takes an apical pulse and compares it to the peripheral pulse.
- Many factors may affect an individual's pulse rate: age, sex, exercise, presence of fever, certain medications, hypovolemia, dehydration, stress (in some situations), position changes, and pathology.
- Although the radial pulse is the site most commonly used, eight other sites may be used in certain situations.
- The difference between the apical and radial pulses is called the pulse deficit.
- Respirations are assessed by observing respiratory rate, depth, rhythm, quality, and effectiveness.
- Blood pressure reflects the pumping action of the heart, peripheral vascular resistance, blood volume, and blood viscosity.
- Among the factors influencing blood pressure are age, exercise, stress, race, sex, medications, obesity, diurnal variations, medical conditions, and temperature.
- Orthostatic hypotension occurs when the blood pressure falls as the client assumes an upright position.
- A blood pressure cuff that is too narrow or too wide will give false readings.
- During blood pressure measurement, the artery must be held at heart level.
- A pulse oximeter measures the percent of hemoglobin saturated with oxygen. A normal result is 95% to 100%.
- Pulse oximeter sensors may be placed on the finger, toes, nose, earlobe, or forehead, or around the hand or foot of the neonate.

TEST YOUR KNOWLEDGE

1. Which of the following sites would be the most appropriate choice to use to measure the temperature of a client who has a history of heart disease and has eaten a bowl of vegetable soup 45 minutes ago?
1. Axilla
2. Oral
3. Popliteal
4. Rectal

2. Which client meets the criteria for selection of the apical site for assessment of the pulse rather than a radial pulse?
1. A client who is in shock
2. A client whose pulse changes with body position changes
3. A client with an arrhythmia
4. A client who had surgery less than 24 hours ago

READINGS AND REFERENCES give you a source for evidence-based material and additional information.

READINGS AND REFERENCES

Suggested Reading

Fuchs, V. R. (2018). Is US medical care inefficient? *JAMA, 320*(10), 971–972. doi:10.1001/jama.2018.10779
The author of this commentary proposes the challenges of comparing American health and mortality statistics and efficiencies with those of other countries.

Related Research

Kaissi, A., Shay, P., & Roscoe, C. (2016). Hospital systems, convenient care strategies, and healthcare reform. *Journal of Healthcare Management, 61*, 148–163.

References

Centers for Medicare and Medicaid Services. (2016). *National health expenditure fact sheet*. Retrieved from https://www.cms.gov/research-statistics-data-and-systems/statistics-trends-and-reports/nationalhealthexpenddata/nhe-fact-sheet.html

Centers for Medicare and Medicaid Services. (2018). *National health expenditure projections 2017–2026*. Retrieved from http://www.cms.gov/Research-Statistics-Data-and-Systems/Statistics-Trends-and-Reports/NationalHealthExpendData/NationalHealthAccountsProjected.html

Garfield, R., Damico, A., & Orgera, K. (2018). *The coverage gap: Uninsured poor adults in states that do not expand Medicaid*. Retrieved from https://www.kff.org/medicaid/issue-brief/the-coverage-gap-uninsured-poor-adults-in-states-that-do-not-expand-medicaid

Kaiser Family Foundation. (2019). *Primary care health professional shortage areas*. Retrieved from http://kff.org/other/state-indicator/primary-care-health-professional-shortage-areas-hpsas

Livingston, G. (2018). *The changing profile of unmarried parents*. Retrieved from http://www.pewsocialtrends.org/2018/04/25/the-changing-profile-of-unmarried-parents

Meyers, D., Miller, T., Genevro, J., Zhan, C., De La Mare, J., Fournier, A., . . . McNellis, R. J. (2018). EvidenceNOW: Balancing primary care implementation and implementation research. *Annals of Family Medicine, 16*(Suppl. 1), S5–S11. doi:10.1370/afm.2196

Roberts, A. W., Ogunwole, S. U., Blakeslee, L., & Rabe, M. A. (2018). *The population 65 years and older in the United States: 2016*. Retrieved from https://www.census.gov/content/dam/Census/library/publications/2018/acs/ACS-38.pdf

Shi, L., & Singh, D. A. (2017). *Essentials of the U.S. health care system* (4th ed.). Burlington, ME: Jones & Bartlett.

Stein, P. N., & Smoller, A. H. (2018). The united state of medicine: Healing identity confusion. *The American Journal of Medicine, 131*, 1141–1142. doi:10.1016/j.amjmed.2018.05.011

U.S. Census Bureau. (2018). *An aging nation: Projected number of children and older adults*. Retrieved from https://www.census.gov/library/visualizations/2018/comm/historic-first.html

U.S. Department of Health and Human Services. (n.d.). *Healthy people 2030 framework*. Retrieved from http://healthypeople.gov/2020/About-Healthy-People/Development-Healthy-People-2030/Framework

Selected Bibliography

Administration on Aging, Administration for Community Living, U.S. Department of Health and Human Services. (2018). *2017 profile of older Americans*. Retrieved from https://acl.gov/sites/default/files/Aging%20and%20Disability%20in%20America/2017OlderAmericansProfile.pdf

American Association of Colleges of Nursing. (1995). *A model for differentiated nursing practice*. Washington, DC: Author.

Austin, A., & Wetle, V. (2017). *The United States health care system: Combining business, health, and delivery* (3rd ed.). Boston, MA: Pearson.

Duston, P. S. (2016). *Analyzing form, function, and financing of the U.S. health care system*. Boca Raton, FL: CRC.

Herman, B. (2016). Health systems with insurance operations have tough 2015. *Modern Healthcare, 46*(26), 12.

Knickman, J. R., & Elbel, B. (Eds.). (2019). *Jonas & Kovner's health care delivery in the United States* (12th ed.). New York, NY: Springer.

Niles, N. J. (2018). *Basics of the U.S. health care system* (3rd ed.). Burlington, ME: Jones & Bartlett.

Shi, L., & Singh, D. A. (2017). *Essentials of the U.S. health care system* (4th ed.). Burlington, ME: Jones & Bartlett.

Contents

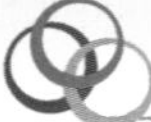

UNIT 2 Contemporary Healthcare 112

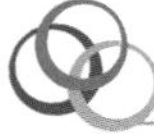

UNIT 3 The Nursing Process 176

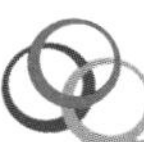

UNIT 1

The Nature of Nursing

1 Historical and Contemporary Nursing Practice

LEARNING OUTCOMES

After completing this chapter, you will be able to:

1. Discuss historical factors and nursing leaders, female and male, who influenced the development of nursing.
2. Discuss the evolution of nursing education and entry into professional nursing practice.
3. Describe the different types of educational programs for nurses.
4. Describe the major purpose of theory in the sciences and practice disciplines.
5. Identify the components of the metaparadigm for nursing.
6. Identify the role of nursing theory in nursing education, research, and clinical practice.
7. Explain the importance of continuing nursing education.
8. Describe how the definition of nursing has evolved since Florence Nightingale.
9. Identify the four major areas of nursing practice.
10. Identify the purposes of nurse practice acts and standards of professional nursing practice.
11. Describe the roles of nurses.
12. Describe the expanded career roles of nurses and their functions.
13. Discuss the criteria of a profession and professional identity formation.
14. Discuss Benner's levels of nursing proficiency.
15. Describe factors influencing contemporary nursing practice.
16. Explain the functions of national and international nurses' associations.

KEY TERMS

Alexian Brothers, *30*
caregiver, *43*
case manager, *44*
change agent, *43*
Clara Barton, *34*
client, *41*
client advocate, *43*
communicator, *43*
consumer, *41*
continuing education (CE), *40*
counseling, *43*
Dorothea Dix, *30*
environment, *40*
Ernest Grant, *35*
Fabiola, *30*
Florence Nightingale, *33*
governance, *45*
Harriet Tubman, *30*
health, *40*
in-service education, *40*
Knights of Saint Lazarus, *30*
Lavinia L. Dock, *35*
leader, *43*
Lillian Wald, *34*
Linda Richards, *34*
Luther Christman, *35*
manager, *43*
Margaret Higgins Sanger, *35*
Mary Breckinridge, *35*
Mary Mahoney, *34*
metaparadigm, *40*
nursing, *40*
patient, *41*
Patient Self-Determination Act (PSDA), *49*
practice discipline, *39*
profession, *45*
professional identity, *46*
Sairey Gamp, *32*
Sojourner Truth, *30*
Standards of Practice, *43*
Standards of Professional Performance, *43*
teacher, *43*
telehealth, *48*
telenursing, *49*
theory, *39*

Introduction

Nursing today is far different from nursing as it was practiced years ago, and it is expected to continue changing during the 21st century. To comprehend present-day nursing and at the same time prepare for the future, one must understand not only past events but also contemporary nursing practice and the sociologic and historical factors that affect it.

Historical Perspectives

Nursing has undergone dramatic change in response to societal needs and influences. A look at nursing's beginnings reveals its continuing struggle for autonomy and professionalization. In recent decades, a renewed interest in nursing history has produced a growing amount of related literature. This section highlights only selected aspects of events that have influenced nursing practice. Recurring themes of women's and men's roles and status, religious (Christian) values, war, societal attitudes, and visionary nursing leadership have influenced nursing practice in the past. Many of these factors still exert their influence today.

Women's Roles

Traditional female roles of wife, mother, daughter, and sister have always included the care and nurturing of other family members. From the beginning of time, women have cared for infants and children; thus, nursing could be said to have its roots in the home. Additionally, women, who in general occupied a subservient and dependent role, were called on to care for others in the community who were ill. Generally, the care provided was related to physical maintenance and comfort. Thus, the traditional nursing role has always entailed humanistic caring, nurturing, comforting, and supporting.

Men's Roles

Men have worked as nurses as far back as before the Crusades. Although the history of nursing primarily focuses on the female figures in nursing, schools of nursing for men existed in the United States from the late 1880s until 1969. Male nurses were denied admission to the Military Nurse Corps during World War II based on gender. It was believed at that time that nursing was women's work and combat was men's work. During the 20th century, men were denied admission to most nursing programs.

In 1971, registered nurse Steve Miller formed an organization called Men in Nursing, and in 1974, Luther Christman organized a group of male nurses. The two groups reorganized into the National Male Nurses Association with the primary focus of recruiting more men into nursing. In 1981, the organization was renamed the American Assembly for Men in Nursing (AAMN). The purpose of the AAMN is to "provide a framework for nurses, as a group, to meet, to discuss and influence factors, which affect men as nurses" (AAMN, n.d., "Vision," para. 2).

The percentage of men included in the nation's nursing workforce does vary. For example, a survey by the National Council of State Boards of Nursing (Smiley et al., 2018) indicated a total of 9.1% male nurses in the workforce, an increase of 2.5% compared to the previous 2013 report. In 2017, the Health Resources and Services Administration (HRSA) reported 9.6%, which is less than the 12% male RNs as reported by Buerhaus, Skinner, Auerbach, and Staiger (2017b, p. 231).

Men do experience barriers to becoming nurses. For example, the nursing image is one of femininity, and nursing has been slow to adopt a gender-neutral image. As a result, people may believe that men who choose the profession of nursing are emasculated, gay, or sexually deviant, which is not true (Hodges et al., 2017). Other barriers and challenges for male nursing students include the lack of male role models in nursing, stereotyping, and differences in caring styles between men and women (Zhang & Liu, 2016).

Improved recruitment and retention of men and other minorities into nursing continues to be needed to strengthen the profession. This is illustrated by professional surveys. A 2016 National League for Nursing (NLN, 2017a) survey found that men in basic registered nursing programs represented 14% of the total enrollment, a 1% decrease compared to the 2012 survey. In comparison, bachelor of science in nursing (BSN) programs enrolled 15% male students, a 2% increase from 2012. In addition, a 2016 survey by the American Association of Colleges of Nursing (AACN, 2017) reflected that only 12% of students in baccalaureate and graduate programs were male.

EVIDENCE-BASED PRACTICE

Evidence-Based Practice

What Motivates Men to Choose Nursing?

Yi and Keogh (2016) state that "knowledge of the factors that motivate men to choose nursing will assist in the development of evidence-based recruitment strategies to increase the number of men entering the nursing profession" (p. 96). As a result, they conducted a systematic literature review of data from qualitative studies that described male nurses' motivations for choosing nursing. A comprehensive search of over 11,000 citations and screening for inclusion criteria resulted in six studies being included in the review. Analytic processes resulted in four themes.

The first theme described how early exposure to nursing and other healthcare professionals influenced the male nurses' decision to become nurses. Examples consisted of where the men received encouragement from female and male friends and relatives who were nurses. Some men were exposed to nursing through experiences of caring for a sick or dying loved one, which became a factor in their decision-making process. The second theme described how the men chose nursing by chance, based on their circumstances at the time of the decision. For example, some men were looking for work and had friends who were nurses and thus decided to try nursing. Some chose nursing because they were not accepted into their preferred program. The third theme described extrinsic motivating factors such as job opportunity and salary. The fourth theme described intrinsic motivating factors such as personal satisfaction and enjoyment with helping people. Other intrinsic motivating factors included a sense of altruism and caring and their perception of nursing as a vocation.

Implications

A limitation expressed by the researchers was that the review would have provided a more comprehensive description if both quantitative and qualitative studies had been included. Three of the themes were congruent with previous literature reviews. However, the theme of entering nursing by chance, depending on the men's circumstances, was new. As a result, the authors recommended that strategies to enhance retention within the nursing program be developed for those males who pursued nursing by chance. Examples could include providing male role models during clinical experiences and supporting male nurses' caring abilities in a welcoming environment to promote intrinsic motivating factors during the program.

Religion

Religion has also played a significant role in the development of nursing. Although many of the world's religions encourage benevolence, it was the Christian value of "love thy neighbor as thyself" and Christ's parable of the Good Samaritan that had a significant impact on the development of Western nursing. During the third and fourth centuries, several wealthy matrons of the Roman Empire, such as **Fabiola**, converted to Christianity and used their wealth to provide houses of care and healing (the forerunner of hospitals) for the poor, the sick, and the homeless. Women were not, however, the sole providers of nursing services.

The Crusades saw the formation of several orders of knights, including the Knights of Saint John of Jerusalem (also known as the Knights Hospitalers), the Teutonic Knights, and the Knights of Saint Lazarus (Figure 1.1 ■). These brothers in arms provided nursing care to their sick and injured comrades. These orders also built hospitals, the organization and management of which set a standard for the administration of hospitals throughout Europe at that time. The **Knights of Saint Lazarus** dedicated themselves to the care of people with leprosy, syphilis, and chronic skin conditions.

During medieval times, there were many religious orders of men in nursing. For example, the **Alexian Brothers** organized care for victims of the Black Plague in the 14th century in Germany. In the 19th century, they followed the same traditions as women's religious nursing orders and established hospitals and provided nursing care.

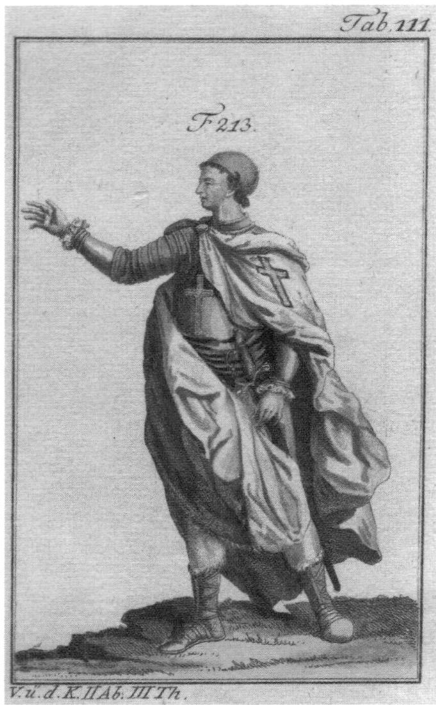

Figure 1.1 ■ The Knights of Saint Lazarus (established circa 1200) dedicated themselves to the care of people with leprosy, syphilis, and chronic skin conditions. From the time of Christ to the mid-13th century, leprosy was viewed as an incurable and terminal disease.
Florilegius/Alamy Stock Photo.

The deaconess groups, which had their origins in the Roman Empire of the third and fourth centuries, were suppressed during the Middle Ages by the Western churches. However, these groups of nursing providers resurfaced occasionally throughout the centuries, most notably in 1836 when Theodor Fliedner reinstituted the Order of Deaconesses and opened a small hospital and training school in Kaiserswerth, Germany. Florence Nightingale received her training in nursing at the Kaiserswerth School.

Early religious values, such as self-denial, spiritual calling, and devotion to duty and hard work, have dominated nursing throughout its history. Nurses' commitment to these values often resulted in exploitation and few monetary rewards. For some time, nurses themselves believed it was inappropriate to expect economic gain from their "calling."

War

Throughout history, wars have accentuated the need for nurses. During the Crimean War (1854–1856), the inadequacy of care given to soldiers led to a public outcry in Great Britain. The role Florence Nightingale played in addressing this problem is well known. Nightingale and her nurses transformed the military hospitals by setting up sanitation practices, such as hand washing. Nightingale is credited with performing miracles; the mortality rate, for example, was reduced from 42% to 2% in 6 months (Donahue, 2011, p. 118).

During the American Civil War (1861–1865), several nurses emerged who were notable for their contributions to a country torn by internal conflict. **Harriet Tubman** and **Sojourner Truth** (Figures 1.2 ■ and 1.3 ■) provided care and safety to slaves fleeing to the North on the Underground Railroad. Mother Biekerdyke and Clara Barton searched the battlefields and gave care to injured and dying soldiers. Noted authors Walt Whitman and Louisa May Alcott volunteered as nurses to give care to injured soldiers in military hospitals. Another female leader who provided nursing care during the Civil War was **Dorothea Dix**

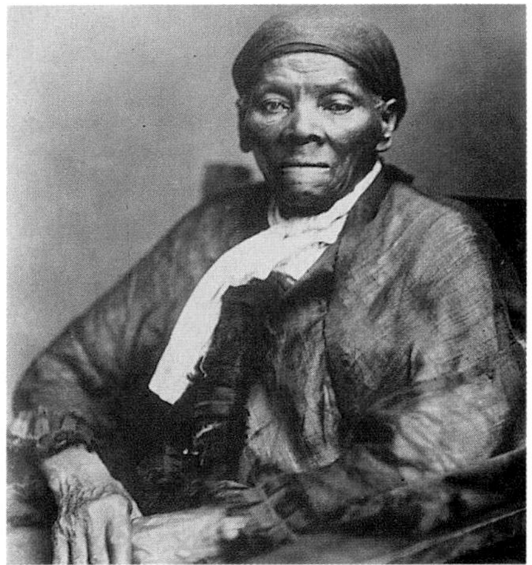

Figure 1.2 ■ Harriet Tubman (1820–1913) was known as "The Moses of Her People" for her work with the Underground Railroad. During the Civil War she nursed the sick and suffering of her own race.
Universal Images Group/Getty Images.

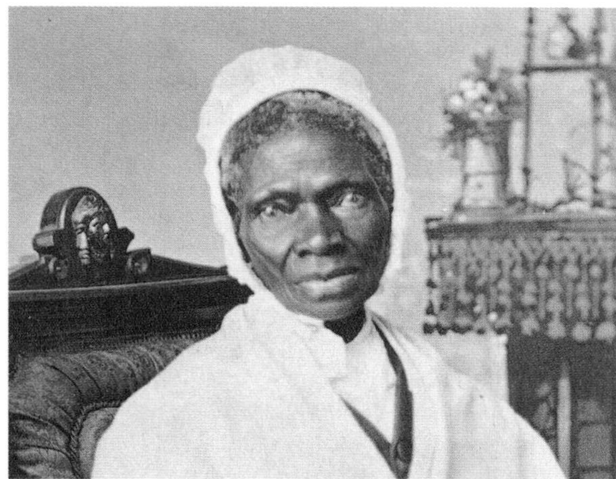

Figure 1.3 ■ Sojourner Truth (1797–1883), abolitionist, Underground Railroad agent, preacher, and women's rights advocate, was a nurse for more than 4 years during the Civil War and worked as a nurse and counselor for the Freedmen's Relief Association after the war.
National Portrait Gallery, Smithsonian Institution/Art Resources, NY.

(Figure 1.4 ■). She became the Union's superintendent of female nurses responsible for recruiting nurses and supervising the nursing care of all women nurses working in the army hospitals.

The arrival of World War I resulted in American, British, and French women rushing to volunteer their nursing services. These nurses endured harsh environments and treated injuries not seen before. A monument entitled "The Spirit of Nursing" stands in Arlington National Cemetery (Figure 1.5 ■). It honors the nurses who served in the U.S. armed services in World War I, many of whom are buried in Section 21, which is also called the "Nurses Section" (Arlington National Cemetery, n.d.). Progress in healthcare occurred

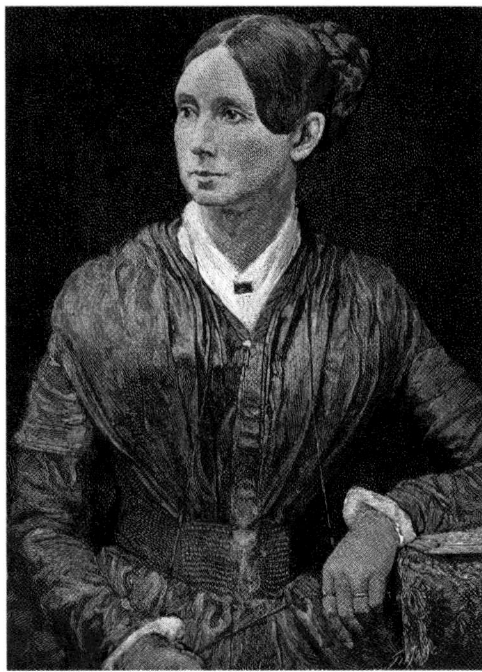

Figure 1.4 ■ Dorothea Dix (1802–1887) was the Union's superintendent of female nurses during the Civil War.
North Wind Picture Archives/Alamy Stock Photo.

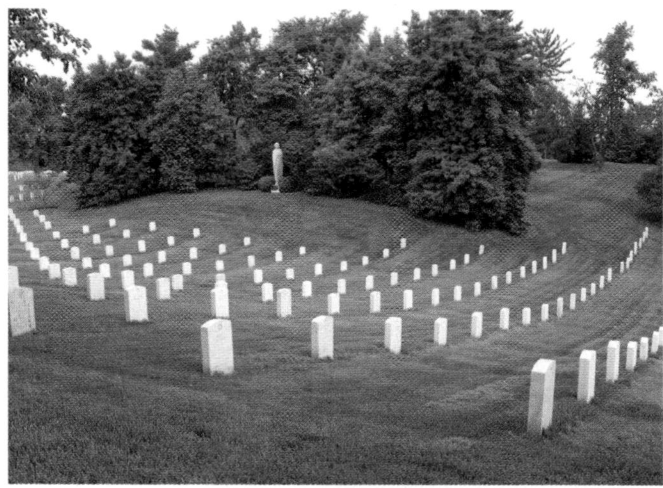

A

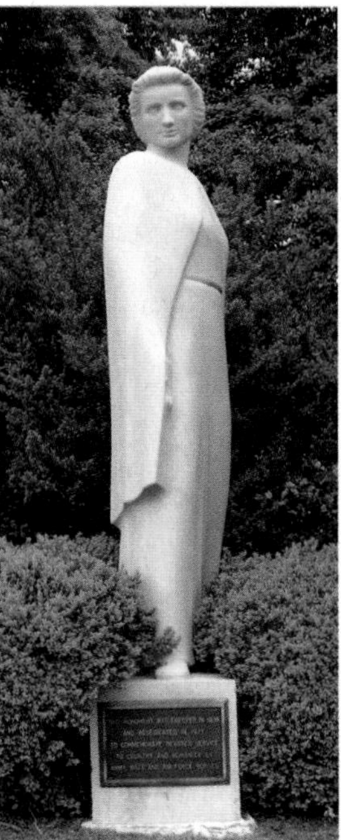

B

THIS MONUMENT WAS ERECTED IN 1938
AND REDEDICATED IN 1971
TO COMMEMORATE DEVOTED SERVICE
TO COUNTRY AND HUMANITY BY
ARMY, NAVY AND AIR FORCE NURSES

C

Figure 1.5 ■ *A*, Section 21 in Arlington National Cemetery honors the nurses who served in the Armed Services in World War I. *B*, "The Spirit of Nursing" monument that stands in Section 21. *C*, Monument plaque.
Photos by Sherrilyn Coffman, PhD, RN.

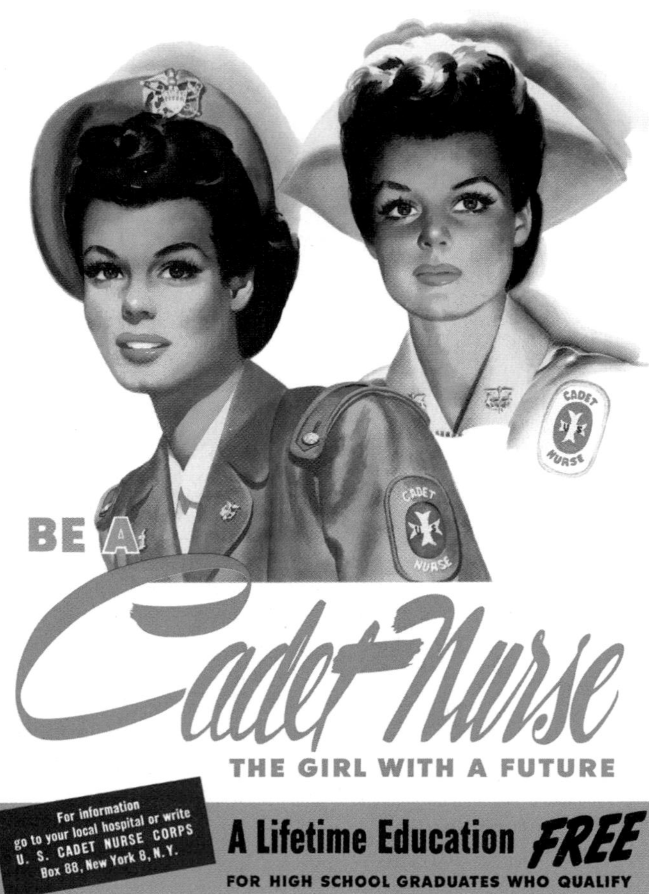
BE A
Cadet Nurse
THE GIRL WITH A FUTURE
For information go to your local hospital or write U. S. CADET NURSE CORPS Box 88, New York 8, N. Y.
A Lifetime Education FREE
FOR HIGH SCHOOL GRADUATES WHO QUALIFY

Figure 1.6 ■ Recruiting poster for the Cadet Nurse Corps during World War II.
John Parrot/Stocktrek Images, Inc./Alamy Stock Photo.

during World War I, particularly in the field of surgery. For example, advancements were made in the use of anesthetic agents, infection control, blood typing, and prosthetics.

World War II casualties created an acute shortage of caregivers, and the Cadet Nurse Corps was established in response to a marked shortage of nurses (Figure 1.6 ■). Also at that time, auxiliary healthcare workers became prominent. "Practical" nurses, aides, and technicians provided much of the actual nursing care under the instruction and supervision of better prepared nurses. Medical specialties also arose at that time to meet the needs of hospitalized clients.

During the Vietnam War, approximately 11,000 American military women stationed in Vietnam were nurses. Most of them volunteered to go to Vietnam right after they graduated from nursing school, making them the youngest group of medical personnel ever to serve in wartime (Vietnam Women's Memorial Foundation, n.d.). Near the Vietnam Veterans Memorial ("The Wall") stands the Vietnam Women's Memorial (Figure 1.7 ■).

Nurses served in the Afghanistan and Iraq wars. A total of 6,326 nurses deployed to Afghanistan, Iraq, or both between September 1, 2001 and July 31, 2015. Of these deployed nurses, 55% were male. During this time six army nurses were killed, four in Afghanistan and two in Iraq (Berry-Caban, Rivers, Beltran, & Anderson, 2018).

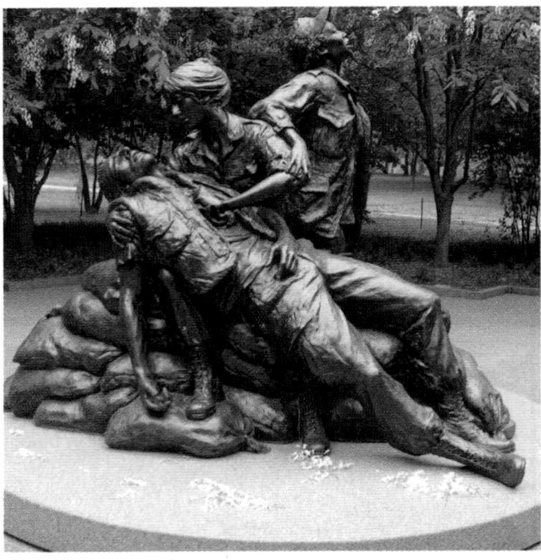

Figure 1.7 ■ Vietnam Women's Memorial. Four figures include a nurse tending to the chest wound of a soldier, another woman looking for a helicopter for assistance, and a third woman (behind the other figures) kneeling while staring at an empty helmet in grief.
Courtesy of Sherrilyn Coffman, PhD, RN.

Societal Attitudes

Society's attitudes about nurses and nursing have significantly influenced professional nursing.

Before the mid-1800s, nursing was without organization, education, or social status; the prevailing attitude was that a woman's place was in the home and that no respectable woman should have a career. The role for the Victorian middle-class woman was that of wife and mother, and any education she obtained was for the purpose of making her a pleasant companion to her husband and a responsible mother to her children. Nurses in hospitals during this period were poorly educated; some were even incarcerated criminals. Society's attitudes about nursing during this period are reflected in the writings of Charles Dickens. In his book *Martin Chuzzlewit* (1844), Dickens reflected his attitude toward nurses through his character **Sairey Gamp** (Figure 1.8 ■). Mrs. Gamp was portrayed as a drunk, disreputable nurse who neglected, stole from, and physically abused the sick. This literary portrayal of nurses greatly influenced the negative image and attitude toward nurses in the 19th century.

In contrast, the *guardian angel* or *angel of mercy* image arose in the latter part of the 19th century, largely because of the work of Florence Nightingale during the Crimean War. After Nightingale brought respectability to the nursing profession, nurses were viewed as noble, compassionate, moral, religious, dedicated, and self-sacrificing.

Another image arising in the early 19th century that has affected subsequent generations of nurses and the public and other professionals working with nurses is that of the *doctor's handmaiden*. This image evolved when women had yet to obtain the right to vote, when family structures were largely paternalistic, and when the medical profession increasingly applied scientific knowledge that, at that time, was viewed as a male domain. Since that time, several images of nursing have been portrayed. The *heroine* portrayal evolved from nurses' acts of bravery in World

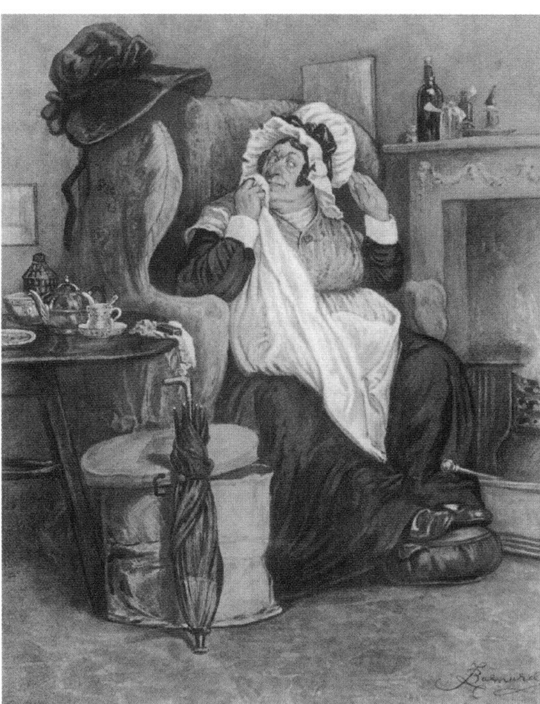

Figure 1.8 ■ Sairey Gamp, a character in Dickens' book *Martin Chuzzlewit*, represented the negative image of nurses in the 1800s.
Historia/Shutterstock.

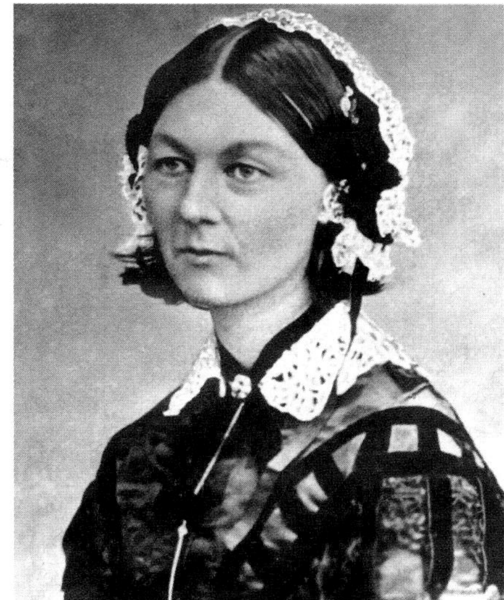

Figure 1.9 ■ Considered the founder of modern nursing, Florence Nightingale (1820–1910) was influential in developing nursing education, practice, and administration. Her publication *Notes on Nursing: What It Is, and What It Is Not*, first published in England in 1859 and in the United States in 1860, was intended for all women.
David Cole/Alamy Stock Photo.

War II and their contributions in fighting poliomyelitis—in particular, the work of the Australian nurse Elizabeth Kenney. Other images in the late 1900s include the nurse as sex object, surrogate mother, and tyrannical mother.

The nursing profession has taken steps to improve the image of the nurse. In the early 1990s, the Tri-Council for Nursing (the American Association of Colleges of Nursing, the American Nurses Association [ANA], the American Organization of Nurse Executives, and the National League for Nursing [NLN]) initiated a national effort, titled "Nurses of America," to improve the image of nursing. Launched in 2002, Johnson & Johnson corporation's "Campaign for Nursing's Future" promotes nursing as a positive career choice. Through various outreach programs, this campaign increases exposure to the nursing profession, raises awareness about its challenges, and encourages people of all ages to consider a career in nursing.

Nursing Leaders

Florence Nightingale, Clara Barton, Linda Richards, Mary Mahoney, Lillian Wald, Lavinia Dock, Margaret Sanger, Mary Breckinridge, Luther Christman, and Ernest Grant are among the leaders who have made notable contributions both to nursing's history and to American history. These nurses were all politically astute pioneers. Their skills at influencing others and bringing about change remain models for political nurse activists today.

Nightingale (1820–1910)

The contributions of **Florence Nightingale** to nursing are well documented. Her achievements in improving the standards for the care of war casualties in the Crimea earned her the title "Lady with the Lamp." Her efforts in reforming hospitals and in producing and implementing public health policies also made her an accomplished political nurse: She was the first nurse to exert political pressure on government. Through her contributions to nursing education—perhaps her greatest achievement—she is also recognized as nursing's first scientist-theorist for her work *Notes on Nursing: What It Is, and What It Is Not* (1860/1969).

Nightingale (Figure 1.9 ■) was born to a wealthy and intellectual family. She believed she was "called by God to help others . . . [and] to improve the well-being of mankind" (Schuyler, 1992, p. 4). She was determined to become a nurse in spite of opposition from her family and the restrictive societal code for affluent young English women. As a well-traveled young woman of the day, she visited Kaiserswerth in 1847, where she received 3 months' training in nursing. In 1853 she studied in Paris with the Sisters of Charity, after which she returned to England to assume the position of superintendent of a charity hospital for ill governesses.

When she returned to England from the Crimea, a grateful English public gave Nightingale an honorarium of £4500. She later used this money to develop the Nightingale Training School for Nurses, which opened in 1860. The school served as a model for other training schools. Its graduates traveled to other countries to manage hospitals and institute nurse training programs. These training schools, at the time, accepted only females because Nightingale viewed nursing as being unsuitable for men. It is believed, unfortunately, that this perception has played a role in the invisibility of male nurses (Yi & Keogh, 2016, p. 95).

Despite poor health that left her an invalid, Florence Nightingale worked tirelessly until her death at age 90. As a passionate statistician, she conducted extensive research and analysis. Nightingale is often referred to as the first nurse researcher. For example, her record keeping proved

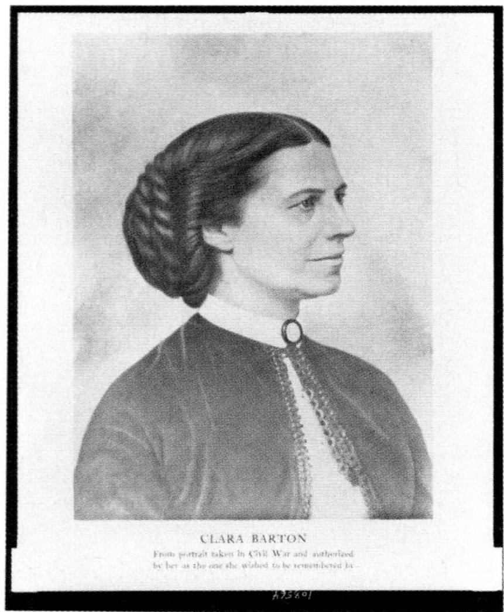

Figure 1.10 ■ Clara Barton (1821–1912) organized the American Red Cross, which linked with the International Red Cross when the U.S. Congress ratified the Geneva Convention in 1882.
Library of Congress.

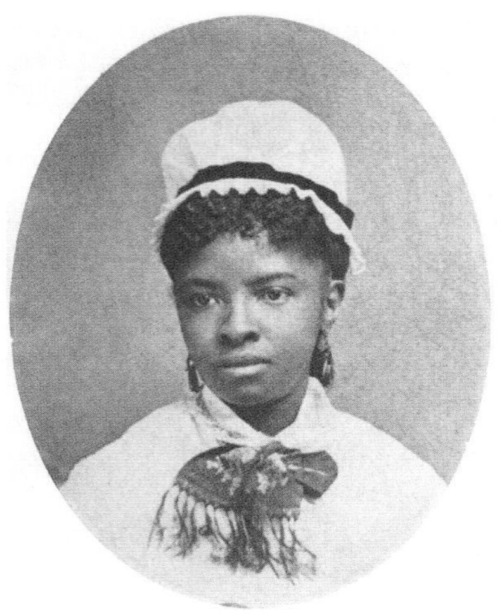

Figure 1.12 ■ Mary Mahoney (1845–1926) was the first African American trained nurse.
Schomberg Center for Research in Black Culture/NYPL/Art Resource.

that her interventions dramatically reduced mortality rates among soldiers during the Crimean War.

Nightingale's vision of nursing changed society's view of nursing. She believed in personalized and holistic client care. Her vision also included public health and health promotion roles for nurses.

Barton (1821–1912)

Clara Barton (Figure 1.10 ■) was a schoolteacher who volunteered as a nurse during the American Civil War. Her responsibility was to organize the nursing services. Barton is noted for her role in establishing the American Red Cross, which linked with the International Red Cross when the U.S. Congress ratified the Treaty of Geneva (Geneva Convention). It was Barton who persuaded Congress in 1882 to ratify this treaty so that the Red Cross could perform humanitarian efforts in times of peace.

Richards (1841–1930)

Linda Richards (Figure 1.11 ■) was America's first trained nurse. She graduated from the New England Hospital for Women and Children in 1873. Richards is known for introducing nurse's notes and doctor's orders. She also initiated the practice of nurses wearing uniforms (ANA, n.d.c). She is credited for her pioneering work in psychiatric and industrial nursing.

Mahoney (1845–1926)

Mary Mahoney (Figure 1.12 ■) was the first African American professional nurse. She graduated from the New England Hospital for Women and Children in 1879. She constantly worked for the acceptance of African Americans in nursing and for the promotion of equal opportunities (Donahue, 2011, p. 144). The ANA (n.d.e) gives a Mary Mahoney Award biennially in recognition of significant contributions in interracial relationships.

Wald (1867–1940)

Lillian Wald (Figure 1.13 ■) is considered the founder of public health nursing. Wald and Mary Brewster were

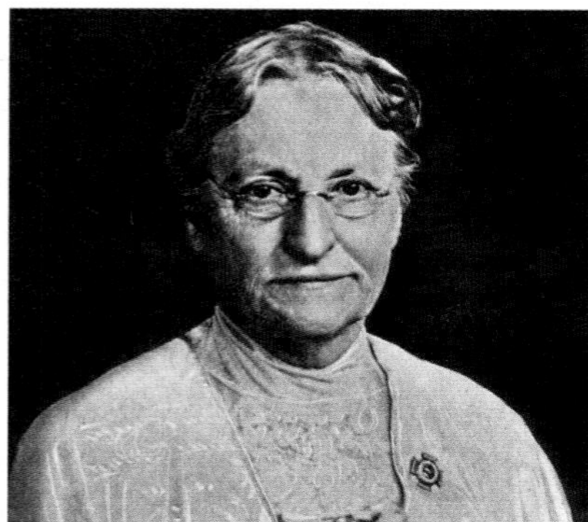

Figure 1.11 ■ Linda Richards (1841–1930) was America's first trained nurse.
National League for Nursing. National League for Nursing Records. 1894–1952. Located in: Archives and Modern Manuscripts Collection, History of Medicine Division, National Library of Medicine, Bethesda, MD; MS C 274.

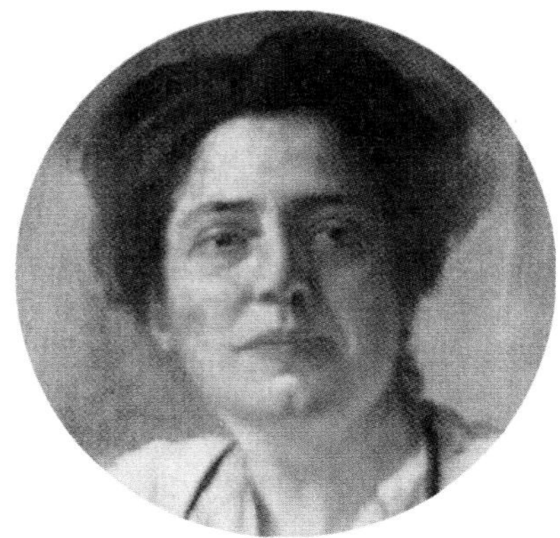

Figure 1.13 ■ Lillian Wald (1867–1940) founded the Henry Street Settlement and Visiting Nurse Service (circa 1893), which provided nursing and social services and organized educational and cultural activities. She is considered the founder of public health nursing.
National Portrait Gallery, Smithsonian Institution/Art Resources, NY.

the first to offer trained nursing services to the poor in the New York slums. Their home among the poor on the upper floor of a tenement, called the Henry Street Settlement and Visiting Nurse Service, provided nursing services and social services, and organized educational and cultural activities. Soon after the founding of the Henry Street Settlement, school nursing was established as an adjunct to visiting nursing.

Dock (1858–1956)

Lavinia L. Dock was a feminist, prolific writer, political activist, suffragette, and friend of Wald. She participated in protest movements for women's rights that resulted in the 1920 passage of the 19th Amendment to the U.S. Constitution, which granted women the right to vote. In addition, Dock campaigned for legislation to allow nurses rather than physicians to control their profession. In 1893, Dock, with the assistance of Mary Adelaide Nutting and Isabel Hampton Robb, founded the American Society of Superintendents of Training Schools for Nurses of the United States, a precursor to the current National League for Nursing.

Sanger (1879–1966)

Margaret Higgins Sanger (Figure 1.14 ■), a public health nurse in New York, has had a lasting impact on women's healthcare. Imprisoned for opening the first birth control information clinic in America, she is considered the founder of Planned Parenthood. Her experience with the large number of unwanted pregnancies among the working poor was instrumental in addressing this problem.

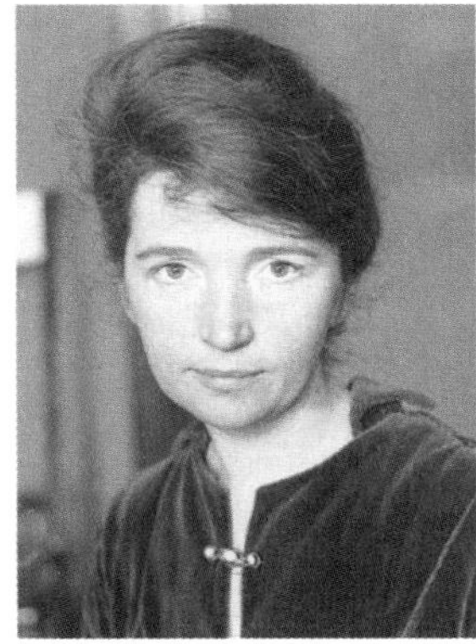

Figure 1.14 ■ Nurse activist Margaret Sanger (1879–1966), considered the founder of Planned Parenthood, was imprisoned for opening the first birth control information clinic in Baltimore in 1916.

Breckinridge (1881–1965)

After World War I, **Mary Breckinridge** (Figure 1.15 ■), a notable pioneer nurse, established the Frontier Nursing Service (FNS). In 1918, she worked with the American Committee for Devastated France, distributing food, clothing, and supplies to rural villages and taking care of sick children. In 1921, Breckinridge returned to the United States with plans to provide healthcare to the people of rural America. In 1925, Breckinridge and two other nurses began the FNS in Leslie County, Kentucky. Within this organization, Breckinridge started one of the first midwifery training schools in the United States.

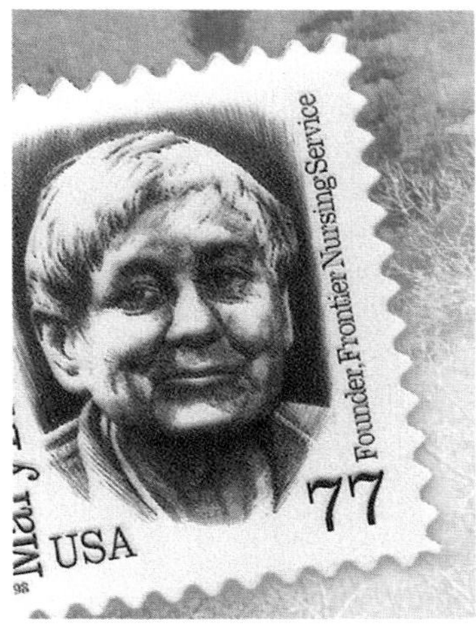

Figure 1.15 ■ Mary Breckinridge (1881–1965), a nurse who practiced midwifery in England, Australia, and New Zealand, founded the Frontier Nursing Service in Kentucky in 1925 to provide family-centered primary healthcare to rural populations.
T. Tso KRT/Newscom.

Christman (1915–2011)

Luther Christman, one of the founders of the AAMN, graduated from the Pennsylvania Hospital School of Nursing for Men in 1939 and experienced discrimination while in nursing school. For example, he was not allowed a maternity clinical experience, yet he was expected to know the information related to that clinical experience for the licensing exam. After becoming licensed, he wanted to earn a baccalaureate degree in nursing but was denied access to two universities because of his gender. After receiving his doctorate, he accepted the position as dean of nursing at Vanderbilt University, making him the first man to be a dean at a university school of nursing. He accomplished many firsts: (a) the first man nominated for president of the ANA; (b) the first man elected to the American Academy of Nursing (AAN), which presented him with its highest honor by naming him a "Living Legend"; and (c) the first man inducted into ANA's Hall of Fame for his extraordinary contributions to nursing. The ANA currently bestows the Luther Christman Award, which acknowledges the valuable role of men in nursing (ANA, n.d.d).

Grant (1958–)

Ernest Grant made professional nursing history when he became the first male president of the American Nurses Association in January 2019. He is also the first African American man to serve as ANA vice president (Trossman,

2018). Grant began his distinguished nursing career as a student in a licensed practical nurse (LPN) program and progressed through baccalaureate and graduate nursing programs to earning a PhD in nursing from the University of North Carolina–Greensboro. After working early in his career at a burn center, he made this work his mission and is now recognized as an internationally known expert on burn care and fire safety. In 2002, President George W. Bush gave Grant a Nurse of the Year Award for his work treating burn victims from the 2001 terrorist attack on the World Trade Center in New York. His top priorities include ensuring that nurses have the educational opportunities and tools needed for the best client outcomes, encouraging nurses to become more politically involved, and encouraging young nurses to become involved with their national and state nursing associations (Nelson, 2019, p. 66).

Political Nurse Activists Today

The nursing profession continues to provide dynamic challenges to all nurses to keep current with the needs of the public and the role of the nurse. Current nursing leaders include presidents of national professional organizations; members of national foundations that contribute to high-quality, safe, client-centered care; and nurses who serve in public office. For example, in 2017 three nurses served in Congress (ANA, n.d.f) and a nurse, Dr. Trent-Adams, became the first individual who is not a physician to serve as surgeon general (NLN, 2017b). Nursing leader Linda Burnes Bolton was vice chair of the Institute of Medicine Commission on the Future of Nursing and in 2011 was named one of the top 25 women in healthcare. Dr. Linda Cronenwett led the Quality and Safety Education in Nursing (QSEN) project, which identified the knowledge, skills, and attitudes (KSAs) that nurses must possess to deliver safe, effective care (AACN, n.d.b). In the 2018 midterm elections, Eddie Bernice Johnson (D-Texas), a former psychiatric nurse and the first nurse elected to Congress, was re-elected to a 14th term, and Lauren Underwood (D-Illinois), an RN who specializes in public health nursing and is a health policy expert, won the race for Illinois' 14th Congressional District. These are just a few examples of contemporary nursing leaders.

Nursing Education

The practice of nursing is controlled from within the profession through state boards of nursing and professional nursing organizations. These groups also determine the content and type of education that is required for different levels or scopes of nursing practice. Originally, the focus of nursing education was to teach the knowledge and skills that would enable a nurse to practice in a hospital setting. However, as nursing roles have evolved in response to new scientific knowledge; advances in technology; and cultural, political, and socioeconomic changes in society, nursing education curricula have been revised to enable nurses to work in more diverse settings and assume more diverse roles. Nursing programs are based on a broad knowledge of biological, social, and physical sciences, as well as the liberal arts and humanities. Current nursing curricula emphasize critical thinking and the application of nursing and supporting knowledge to health promotion, health maintenance, and health restoration as provided in both community and hospital settings (Figure 1.16 ■).

There are two types of entry-level generalist nurses: the registered nurse (RN) and the licensed practical or vocational nurse (LPN or LVN). Responsibilities and licensure requirements differ for these two levels. The majority of new RNs are graduates of associate degree or baccalaureate degree nursing programs. In some states, an individual can be eligible to take the licensure exam through other qualifications such as completing a diploma nursing program or challenging the exam as a military corps person or LVN after completing specified coursework. The U.S. Navy and Marine Corps have a pathway to a commission in the Nurse Corps. Qualified enlisted men and women serving on active duty can apply to participate in the Medical Enlisted Commissioning Program (MECP). This program has been successful in increasing the diversity of nursing within the military. There are also "generic" master's and doctoral programs that lead to eligibility for RN licensure. These latter programs are for students who already have a baccalaureate degree in a discipline other than nursing. On completion of the program, which may be from 1 to 3 years in length, graduates obtain their initial professional degree in nursing. Graduates of these programs are eligible to take the licensure examination to become an RN and may continue into specialty roles such as nurse practitioner or nurse educator.

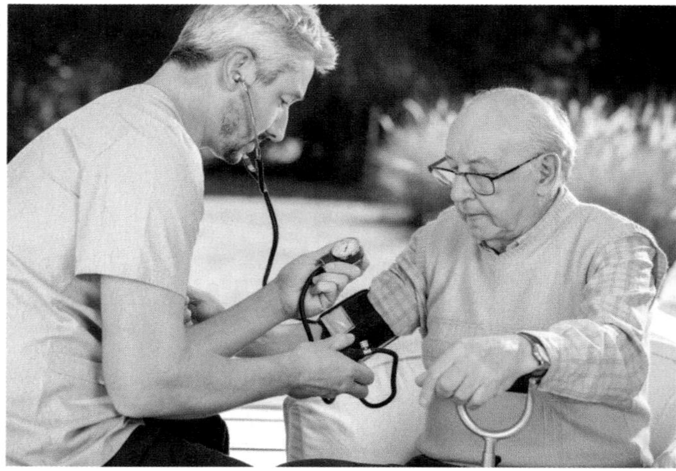

Figure 1.16 ■ Nursing students learn to care for clients in community settings.
Tyler Olson/123RF.

Although educational preparation varies considerably, all RNs in the United States take the same licensure examination, the National Council Licensure Examination (NCLEX-RN). This examination is administered in each state, and the successful candidate becomes licensed in that particular state, even though the examination is of national origin. To practice nursing in another state, the nurse must receive reciprocal licensure by applying to that state's board of nursing. Some state legislatures have created a regulatory model called *mutual recognition* that allows for multistate licensure under one license. Nurses who have received their training in other countries may be granted registration after successfully completing the NCLEX. Both licensure and registration must be renewed regularly in order to remain valid. For additional information about licensure and registration, see Chapter 3 ∞.

The legal right to practice nursing requires not only passing the licensing examination, but also verification that the candidate has completed a prescribed course of study in nursing. Some states may have additional requirements. All U.S. nursing programs must be approved by their state board of nursing. In addition to state approval, the Accreditation Commission for Education in Nursing (ACEN) provides accreditation for all levels of nursing programs, and the Commission on Collegiate Nursing Education (CCNE) accredits baccalaureate and higher degree programs. Accreditation is a voluntary, peer review process. Accredited programs meet standard requirements that are evaluated periodically through written self-studies and on-site visitation by peer examiners.

Types of Education Programs

Education programs available for nurses include practical or vocational nursing, registered nursing, graduate nursing, and continuing education. All levels of nursing are needed in healthcare today. Each has a unique scope of practice and by working collaboratively can help meet the often complex needs of clients.

Licensed Practical (Vocational) Nursing Programs

Practical or vocational nursing programs are housed in community colleges, vocational schools, hospitals, or other independent health agencies. These programs generally last 9 to 12 months and include both classroom and clinical experience. At the end of the program, graduates take the NCLEX-PN to obtain licensure as a practical or vocational nurse. Some LPN and LVN programs articulate with associate degree programs. In these *ladder programs*, the practical or vocational education component constitutes the first year of an associate degree program for registered nursing, and, if successful in passing the NCLEX-PN, students can work while continuing their registered nurse education.

Practical nurses work under the supervision of an RN in numerous settings, including hospitals, nursing homes, rehabilitation centers, home health agencies, ambulatory care, and hospice. Although the scope of practice varies by state regulation and agency policy, LPNs usually provide basic direct technical care to clients. Employment of LPNs has shifted away from acute care settings to care of older adults in community-based settings, including long-term care.

Registered Nursing Programs

Currently, three major routes lead to eligibility for RN licensure: completion of a diploma, associate degree, or baccalaureate program.

DIPLOMA PROGRAMS

After Florence Nightingale established the Nightingale Training School for Nurses at St. Thomas Hospital in England in 1860, the concept traveled quickly to North America. Hospital administrators welcomed the idea of training schools as a source of nursing staff for free or inexpensive staffing for the hospital. In early years, nursing education largely took the form of apprenticeship programs. With little formal classroom instruction, students learned by doing—that is, by providing direct care to clients. There was no standardization of curriculum and no accreditation. Programs were designed to meet the service needs of the hospital, not the educational needs of the students.

Three-year diploma programs were the dominant nursing programs and the major source of nursing graduates from the late 1800s until the mid-1960s. Today's diploma programs are hospital-based educational programs that provide rich clinical experiences for nursing students. These programs often are associated with colleges or universities. Approximately 12% of RNs obtained their initial nursing education in diploma programs in 2017, which is a decrease of 5.4% since 2013 (Smiley et al., 2018, p. S15).

ASSOCIATE DEGREE PROGRAMS

Associate degree nursing programs, which originated in the early 1950s, were the first and only educational programs for nursing that were systematically developed from planned research and controlled experimentation. Most of these programs take place in community colleges. The graduating student receives an associate degree in nursing (ADN) or an associate of arts (AA), associate of science (AS), or associate in applied science (AAS) degree with a major in nursing. Several trends and events prompted the development of these programs: (a) the Cadet Nurse Corps, (b) the community college movement, (c) earlier nursing studies, and (d) Dr. Mildred Montag's proposal for an associate degree.

The Cadet Nurse Corps of the United States was legislated and financed during World War II to provide nurses to meet both military and civilian needs. The corps demonstrated that qualified nurses could be educated in less time than the traditional 3 years of most diploma programs.

After World War II, the number of community colleges in the United States increased rapidly. The low tuition and open-door admission policy of these colleges, as well as their location in towns and cities lacking 4-year colleges and universities, made higher education accessible to more individuals by offering the first 2 years of a 4-year college program, as well as vocational programs that addressed community needs.

Studies of nursing education, such as the Goldmark Report in 1923, the Committee on the Grading of Nursing Schools in 1934, and the Brown Report in 1948, also had a significant influence on the development of 2-year nursing programs. The recommendations in these reports supported the idea of independent schools of nursing in institutions of higher learning separate from hospitals.

In the United States, associate degree nursing programs were started after Mildred Montag published her doctoral dissertation, *The Education of Nursing Technicians*, in 1951. This study proposed a 2-year education program for RNs in community colleges as a solution to the acute shortage of nurses that came about because of World War II. Dr. Montag conceptualized a "nursing technician" or "bedside nurse" able to perform nursing functions broader than those of a practical nurse, but lesser in scope than those of the professional nurse. At the end of the 2 years, the student was to be awarded an ADN and be eligible to take the state board examination for RN licensure. The first ADN program was established at Columbia University Teachers College in 1952 under the direction of Dr. Montag. Currently, 36.3% of all new RNs each year are initially educated in associate degree programs, which is a decrease of 1.9% since 2013 (Smiley et al., 2018, p. S15).

Dr. Montag's original idea that these graduates be nursing technicians and that the degree become a terminal one did not last. In 1978, the ANA proposed that associate degree programs no longer be considered terminal, but part of a career upward-mobility plan. Today many students enter an associate degree program with the intention of continuing their education to the baccalaureate or higher level. Many community colleges have articulation agreements with college and university bachelor of science in nursing (BSN) programs to facilitate the upward mobility toward the BSN. RN to master of science in nursing (MSN) programs are also available to the associate degree nurse.

BACCALAUREATE DEGREE PROGRAMS

The first school of nursing in a university setting was established at the University of Minnesota in 1909. This program's curriculum, however, differed little from that of a 3-year diploma program. It was not until 1919 that the University of Minnesota established its undergraduate baccalaureate degree in nursing. Most of the early baccalaureate programs were 5 years in length. They consisted of the basic 3-year diploma program plus 2 years of liberal arts education. In the 1960s, the number of students enrolled in baccalaureate programs increased markedly.

Almost 42% of RNs in the United States are initially educated in baccalaureate programs (Smiley et al., 2018, p. S15). Baccalaureate programs are located in senior colleges and universities and are generally 4 years in length. Programs include courses in the liberal arts, sciences, humanities, and nursing, including nursing leadership, nursing research, and community health nursing. Graduates must complete both the degree requirements of the college or university and the nursing program before being awarded a baccalaureate degree. The usual degree awarded is a BSN. Partially in response to the significant shortage of RNs, some schools have established accelerated BSN programs. These programs may include summer coursework in order to shorten the length of time required to complete the curriculum or may be a modified curriculum designed for students who already have a baccalaureate degree in another field. These "second degree" or "fast track" BSN programs can be completed in as little as 12 to 18 months of study.

Many baccalaureate programs also admit RNs who have a diploma or associate degree. These programs typically are referred to as BSN completion, BSN transition, 2 + 2, or RN-BSN programs. Most RN-BSN programs have a special curriculum designed to meet the needs of these students. Many accept transfer credits from other accredited colleges or universities and award academic credit for the nursing coursework completed previously in a diploma or associate degree program. An increasing number of RN-BSN programs are offered online. In the four years between 2007 to 2011, there was an 86% increase in RN to BSN graduates (HRSA, 2013, p. 48).

Because of changes in the practice environment, the nurse who holds a baccalaureate degree generally experiences more autonomy, responsibility, participation in institutional decision making, and career advancement than the nurse prepared with a diploma or associate degree. Some employers have different salary scales for nurses with a baccalaureate degree, as opposed to an associate degree or diploma. In addition, the American Nurses Credentialing Center (ANCC) requires a baccalaureate degree for initial basic certification in most nursing specialties, and certification often is rewarded with a salary increase. The Magnet Recognition Program, developed by the ANCC to recognize healthcare organizations that provide nursing excellence, requires that 75% of nurse managers hold at least a baccalaureate degree. Also, the Institute of Medicine's (IOM) publication *The Future of Nursing* (2010) recommended that 80% of RNs be baccalaureate prepared by 2020. All of these points provide an incentive for nurses with diplomas and associate degrees to continue their formal preparation in baccalaureate completion programs. This is reflected in the increasing enrollment in RN to BSN programs.

Graduate Nursing Programs

Although graduate schools differ, typical requirements for admission to a graduate program in nursing include the following:

- Licensure as an RN or eligibility for licensure.
- A baccalaureate degree in nursing from an approved college or university. Some graduate programs accept individuals with a diploma or associate degree in nursing and a baccalaureate degree in another field of study. Some accept individuals with an associate degree in nursing as their only postsecondary education.
- Evidence of scholastic ability (usually a minimum grade point average of 3.0 on a 4.0 scale).
- Satisfactory achievement on a standard qualifying examination such as the Graduate Record Examination (GRE) or Miller Analogies Test (MAT).
- Letters of recommendation from supervisors, nursing faculty, or nursing colleagues indicating the applicant's ability to do graduate study.

MASTER'S DEGREE PROGRAMS

The growth of baccalaureate nursing programs encouraged the development of graduate study in nursing. Approximately 18.9% of licensed RNs hold a master's or higher degree in nursing (Smiley et al., 2018, p. S17). Master's prepared nurses work in a variety of roles, including clinical nurse specialist (CNS), nurse practitioner (NP, also called advanced practice registered nurse [APRN]), nurse midwife (CNM), and nurse anesthetist (CRNA). The emphasis of master's degree programs is on preparing nurses for advanced leadership roles in administration, clinical practice, or teaching (Figure 1.17 ■).

A nursing role developed by the AACN is the clinical nurse leader (CNL). The CNL is a master's degree–prepared clinician who oversees the integration of care for a specific group of clients. CNLs are prepared for practice across the continuum of care in any healthcare setting (AACN, n.d.a).

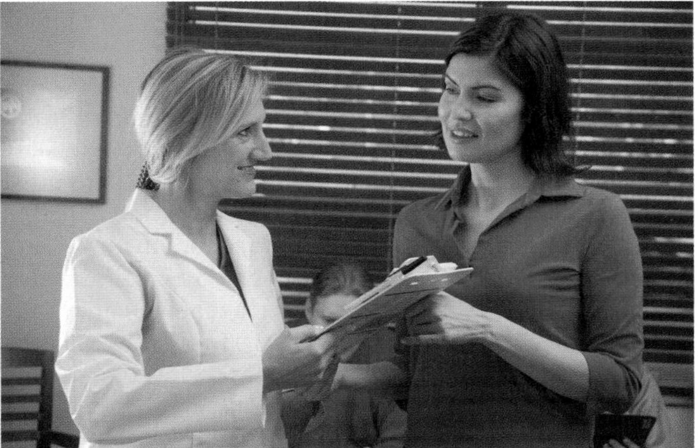

Figure 1.17 ■ A nurse practitioner holds a master's degree and assumes an advanced practice role.
Custom Medical Stock Photo/Alamy.

DOCTORAL PROGRAMS

Doctoral programs in nursing began in the 1960s in the United States. Before 1960, nurses who pursued doctoral degrees chose related fields such as education, psychology, sociology, and physiology. The two primary doctoral degrees in nursing are the PhD and DNP (doctor of nursing practice). Nurses who earn a PhD in nursing generally assume faculty roles in nursing education programs or work in research programs. The DNP, a practice-focused doctorate, has been increasing in popularity and is the highest degree for nurse clinicians. Nurses with a DNP received additional education in evidence-based practice, quality improvement, and systems leadership to promote improved client outcomes. Doctorates in related fields such as education or public health are still highly relevant for nurses depending on their practice role.

Nursing Theories

As a profession, nursing is involved in identifying its own unique body of knowledge essential to nursing practice—nursing science. To identify this knowledge base, nurses must develop and recognize concepts and theories specific to nursing. Because theories in some other disciplines were developed and used long before nursing theories, it is helpful to explore briefly how theory has been used by those disciplines before considering theory in nursing.

A **theory** may be defined as a system of ideas that is presumed to explain a given phenomenon. For now, think of a theory as a major, very well-articulated idea about something important. Theories are used to describe, predict, and control phenomena.

Most undergraduate students are introduced to the major theories in their disciplines. For example, psychology majors study Freud and Jung's theories of the unconscious; sociology majors study Marx's theory of alienation; biology majors are introduced to Darwin's theory of evolution; and physics majors are introduced to a historical progression of theorists including Copernicus, Newton, Einstein, and newer theorists in quantum mechanics.

The extent to which theories build on or modify previous theories varies with the discipline, as does the importance of theory in the discipline. Students in nursing, teaching, and management often take some courses in theory, but these students generally focus on learning their practice. The term **practice discipline** is used for fields of study in which the central focus is performance of a professional role (e.g., nursing, teaching, management, music). Practice disciplines are differentiated from the disciplines that have research and theory development as their central focus, for example, the natural sciences. In the practice disciplines, the main function of theory (and research) is to provide new possibilities for understanding the discipline's practice.

Context for Theory Development in American Universities

In the 19th century, Florence Nightingale thought that the people of Great Britain needed to know more about how to maintain healthy homes and how to care for sick family members. *Nightingale's Notes on Nursing: What It Is, and What It Is Not* (1860/1969) was nursing's first textbook on home care and community health. However, the audience for that text was the public at large, not a separate discipline or profession.

In the 20th century, nursing education in the United States took a different path from nursing education in Great Britain and Europe. The drive to establish nursing departments in colleges and universities exposed American nursing to the dominant ideas and pressures in American higher education at the time. During the latter half of the 20th century, disciplines seeking to establish themselves in universities had to demonstrate something that Nightingale had not envisioned for nursing: a unique body of theoretical knowledge.

The Metaparadigm for Nursing

In the late 20th century, much of the theoretical work in nursing focused on articulating relationships among four major concepts: person, environment, health, and nursing. Because these four concepts can be superimposed on almost any work in nursing, they are collectively referred to as the **metaparadigm** for nursing. The term originates from two Greek words: *meta*, meaning "with," and *paradigm*, meaning "pattern." Many consider the following four concepts to be central to nursing:

1. The individuals or clients are the recipients of nursing care (includes individuals, families, groups, and communities).
2. The **environment** is the internal and external surroundings that affect the client.
3. **Health** is the degree of wellness or well-being that the client experiences.
4. **Nursing** is the attributes, characteristics, and actions of the nurse providing care on behalf of, or in conjunction with, the client.

During this time, a number of nurse theorists developed their own theoretical definitions of nursing. Theoretical definitions are important because they go beyond simplistic common definitions. They describe what nursing is and the interrelationship among nurses, nursing, the client, the environment, and the intended client outcome: health.

Certain themes are common to many of these definitions:

- Nursing is caring.
- Nursing is an art.
- Nursing is a science.
- Nursing is client centered.
- Nursing is holistic.
- Nursing is adaptive.
- Nursing is concerned with health promotion, health maintenance, and health restoration.
- Nursing is a helping profession.

Role of Nursing Theory

Direct links exist among nursing theory, education, research, and clinical practice. In many cases, nursing theory guides knowledge development and directs education, research, and practice, although each influences the others. The interface between nursing experts in each area helps to ensure that work in the other areas remains relevant, current, and useful and ultimately influences health. Some nursing programs and healthcare delivery systems use a theoretical framework. Examples include Orem's General Theory of Nursing, Leininger's Cultural Care Diversity and Universality Theory, Neuman's Systems Model, and Roy's Adaptation Model. Nursing theory remains an important focus of nurses' work.

Continuing Education

The term **continuing education (CE)** refers to formalized experiences designed to enhance the knowledge or skills of practicing professionals. Compared to advanced educational programs, which result in an academic degree, CE courses tend to be more specific and shorter. Participants may receive certificates of completion or specialization.

CE is the responsibility of all practicing nurses. For example, one of ANA's Standards of Professional Performance is education, which states, "The registered nurse seeks knowledge and competence that reflects current nursing practice and promotes futuristic thinking," with one of the competencies describing a commitment to lifelong learning through self-reflection and inquiry for learning and personal growth (ANA, 2015b, p. 76). Constant updating and growth are essential to keep abreast of scientific and technologic changes and changes within healthcare and the nursing profession. A variety of educational and healthcare institutions conduct CE programs on site, via home study, and online.

CE programs usually are designed to meet one or more of the following needs: (a) to inform nurses of new techniques and knowledge; (b) to help nurses attain expertise in a specialized area of practice, such as critical care nursing; and (c) to provide nurses with information essential to nursing practice, such as knowledge about legal and ethical aspects of nursing. Some states require nurses to obtain a certain number of CE credits to renew their license. Required contact hours typically range from 15 to 30 hours per 2-year license renewal period. A few states also require a certain number of hours of practice, either independently or in lieu of study hours, before licensure renewal.

An **in-service education** program is a specific type of CE program that is offered by an employer. It is designed to upgrade the knowledge or skills of employees, as well as to validate continuing competence in selected procedures and areas of practice. For example, an employer might offer an in-service program to inform nurses about a new piece of equipment or a new surgical procedure, new documentation procedures, or methods of implementing a nurse theorist's conceptual framework for nursing. Some in-service programs are mandatory on a regular basis, such as cardiopulmonary resuscitation and fire safety programs.

Contemporary Nursing Practice

An understanding of contemporary nursing practice includes a look at definitions of nursing, recipients of nursing, scope of nursing, settings for nursing practice, nurse practice acts, and current standards of clinical nursing practice.

Definitions of Nursing

Professional nursing associations have examined nursing and developed their definitions of it. In 1973, the ANA described nursing practice as "direct, goal oriented, and adaptable to the needs of the individual, the family, and community during health and illness" (ANA, 1973, p. 2). In 1980, the ANA changed this definition of nursing to this: "Nursing is the diagnosis and treatment of human responses to actual or potential health problems" (ANA, 1980, p. 9). In 1995, the ANA recognized the influence and contribution of the science of caring to nursing philosophy and practice. Research to explore the meaning of caring in nursing has been increasing. Details about caring are discussed in Chapter 15 ∞. The current definition of nursing remains unchanged from the 2003 edition of *Nursing's Social Policy Statement*: "Nursing is the protection, promotion, and optimization of health and abilities, preventions of illness and injury, alleviation of suffering through the diagnosis and treatment of human response, and advocacy in the care of individuals, families, communities, and populations" (ANA, 2010, p. 10; ANA, 2015b, p. 7).

Recipients of Nursing

The recipients of nursing are sometimes called consumers, sometimes patients, and sometimes clients. A **consumer** is an individual, a group of people, or a community that uses a service or commodity. People who use healthcare products or services are consumers of healthcare.

A **patient** is an individual who is waiting for or undergoing medical treatment and care. The word *patient* comes from a Latin word meaning "to suffer" or "to bear." Traditionally, the individual receiving healthcare has been called a patient. Usually, people become patients when they seek assistance because of illness or for surgery. Some nurses believe that the word *patient* implies passive acceptance of the decisions and care of health professionals. Additionally, with the emphasis on health promotion and prevention of illness, many recipients of nursing care are not ill. Moreover, nurses interact with family members and significant others to provide support, information, and comfort in addition to caring for the patient.

For these reasons, nurses increasingly refer to recipients of healthcare as *clients*. A **client** is an individual who engages the advice or services of another who is qualified to provide this service. The term *client* presents the receivers of healthcare as collaborators in the care, that is, as people who are also responsible for their own health. Thus, the health status of a client is the responsibility of the individual in collaboration with health professionals. In this book, *client* is the preferred term, although *consumer* and *patient* are used in some instances.

Scope of Nursing

Nurses provide care for three types of clients: individuals, families, and communities. Theoretical frameworks applicable to these client types, as well as assessments of individual, family, and community health, are discussed in Chapters 6 and 27 ∞.

Nursing practice involves four areas: promoting health and wellness, preventing illness, restoring health, and caring for the dying.

Promoting Health and Wellness

When health is defined broadly as actualization of human potential, it has been called wellness (Murdaugh, Parsons, & Pender, 2019, p. 12). Nurses promote wellness in clients who are both healthy and ill. This may involve individual and community activities to enhance healthy lifestyles, such as improving nutrition and physical fitness, preventing drug and alcohol misuse, restricting smoking, and preventing accidents and injury in the home and workplace. See Chapter 19 ∞ for details.

Preventing Illness

The goal of illness prevention programs is to maintain optimal health by preventing disease. Nursing activities that prevent illness include immunizations, prenatal and infant care, and prevention of sexually transmitted infections.

Restoring Health

Restoring health focuses on the ill client, and it extends from early detection of disease through helping the client during the recovery period. Nursing activities include the following:

- Providing direct care to the ill individual, such as administering medications, baths, and specific procedures and treatments
- Performing diagnostic and assessment procedures, such as measuring blood pressure and examining feces for occult blood

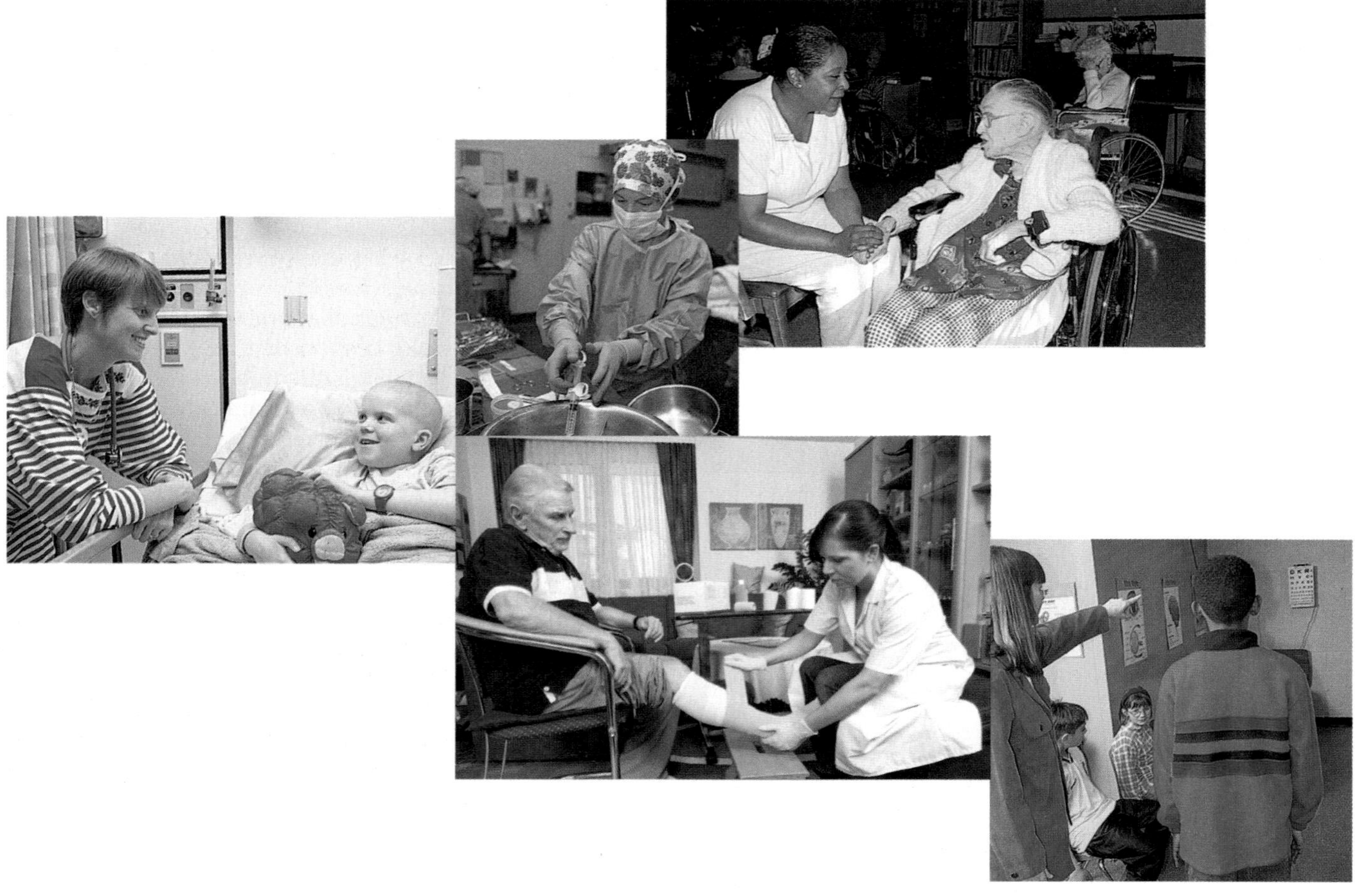

Figure 1.18 ■ Nurses practice in a variety of settings.
(Bottom middle) Lisa S./Shutterstock.

- Consulting with other healthcare professionals about client problems
- Teaching clients about recovery activities, such as exercises that will accelerate recovery after a stroke
- Rehabilitating clients to their optimal functional level following physical or mental illness, injury, or chemical addiction.

Caring for the Dying

This area of nursing practice involves comforting and caring for people of all ages who are dying. Palliative care nurses are part of a medical team that focuses on providing relief from the symptoms and stress of a serious illness (e.g., cancer). The goal is to improve the quality of life for both the client and the family. A hospice nurse provides end-of-life care by giving medical, psychologic, and spiritual support. The goal is to help people who are dying have peace, comfort, and dignity. Nurses carrying out these activities work in homes, hospitals, and extended care facilities.

Settings for Nursing

In the past, the acute care hospital was the main practice setting open to most nurses. Today many nurses work in hospitals, but increasingly they work in clients' homes, community agencies, ambulatory clinics, long-term care facilities, health maintenance organizations (HMOs), and nursing practice centers (Figure 1.18 ■).

Nurses have different degrees of nursing autonomy and nursing responsibility in the various settings. They may provide direct care, teach and support clients, serve as nursing advocates and agents of change, and help determine health policies affecting consumers in the community and in hospitals. For information about the models for delivery of nursing, see Chapter 5 ∞.

Nurse Practice Acts

Nurse practice acts, or legal acts for professional nursing practice, regulate the practice of nursing in the United States, with each state having its own act. Although nurse practice acts differ in various jurisdictions, they all have a common purpose: to protect the public. Nurses are responsible for knowing their state's nurse practice act as it governs their practice. For additional information, see Chapter 3 ∞.

Standards of Nursing Practice

Establishing and implementing standards of practice are major functions of a professional organization. The purpose of the ANA **Standards of Practice** is to describe the responsibilities for which nurses are accountable. The ANA developed standards of nursing practice that are generic in nature, by using the nursing process as a foundation, and provide for the practice of nursing regardless of area of specialization. Various specialty nursing organizations have further developed specific standards of nursing practice for their area. The ANA **Standards of Professional Performance** describe behaviors expected in the professional nursing role.

Roles and Functions of the Nurse

Nurses assume a number of roles when they provide care to clients. Nurses often carry out these roles concurrently, not exclusively of one another. For example, the nurse may act as a counselor while providing physical care and teaching aspects of that care. The roles required at a specific time depend on the needs of the client and aspects of the particular environment.

Caregiver

The **caregiver** role has traditionally included those activities that assist the client physically and psychologically while preserving the client's dignity. The required nursing actions may involve full care for the completely dependent client, partial care for the partially dependent client, and supportive-educative care to assist clients in attaining their highest possible level of health and wellness. Caregiving encompasses the physical, psychosocial, developmental, cultural, and spiritual levels. The nursing process provides nurses with a framework for providing care (see Chapters 9 through 13 ∞). A nurse may provide care directly or assign it to other caregivers.

Communicator

Communication is integral to all nursing roles. Nurses communicate with the client, support individuals, other health professionals, and people in the community.

In the role of **communicator**, nurses identify client problems and then communicate these verbally or in writing to other members of the healthcare team. The quality of a nurse's communication is an important factor in nursing care. The nurse must be able to communicate clearly and accurately in order for a client's healthcare needs to be met (see Chapters 14 and 16 ∞).

Teacher

As a **teacher**, the nurse helps clients learn about their health and the healthcare procedures they need to perform to restore or maintain their health. The nurse assesses the client's learning needs and readiness to learn, sets specific learning goals in conjunction with the client, enacts teaching strategies, and measures learning. Nurses also teach assistive personnel (AP) to whom they assign care, and they share their expertise with other nurses and health professionals. See Chapter 17 ∞ for additional details about the teaching–learning process.

Client Advocate

A **client advocate** acts to protect the client. In this role the nurse may represent the client's needs and wishes to other health professionals, such as relaying the client's request for information to the healthcare provider. They also assist clients in exercising their rights and help them speak up for themselves (see Chapter 4 ∞).

Counselor

Counseling is the process of helping a client to recognize and cope with stressful psychologic or social problems, to develop improved interpersonal relationships, and to promote personal growth. It involves providing emotional, intellectual, and psychologic support. The nurse counsels primarily healthy individuals with normal adjustment difficulties and focuses on helping the individual develop new attitudes, feelings, and behaviors by encouraging the client to look at alternative behaviors, recognize the choices, and develop a sense of control.

Change Agent

The nurse acts as a **change agent** when assisting clients to make modifications in their behavior. Nurses also often act to make changes in a system, such as clinical care, if it is not helping a client return to health. Nurses are continually dealing with change in the healthcare system. Technologic change, change in the age of the client population, and changes in medications are just a few of the changes nurses deal with daily. See Chapter 18 ∞ for additional information about change.

Leader

A **leader** influences others to work together to accomplish a specific goal. The leader role can be employed at different levels: individual client, family, groups of clients, colleagues, or the community. Effective leadership is a learned process requiring an understanding of the needs and goals that motivate people, the knowledge to apply the leadership skills, and the interpersonal skills to influence others. The leadership role of the nurse is discussed in Chapter 18 ∞.

Manager

The nurse manages the nursing care of individuals, families, and communities. The nurse **manager** also assigns and delegates nursing activities to ancillary workers and other nurses, and supervises and evaluates their performance. Managing requires knowledge about organizational structure and dynamics, authority and accountability, leadership, change theory, advocacy, assignment, delegation, and supervision and evaluation. See Chapter 18 for additional details.

Case Manager

Nurse case managers work with the multidisciplinary healthcare team to measure the effectiveness of the case management plan and to monitor outcomes. Each agency or unit specifies the role of the nurse **case manager**. In some institutions, the case manager works with primary or staff nurses to oversee the care of a specific caseload. In other agencies, the case manager is the primary nurse or provides some level of direct care to the client and family. Insurance companies have also developed a number of roles for nurse case managers, and responsibilities may vary from managing acute hospitalizations to managing high-cost clients or case types. Regardless of the setting, case managers help ensure that care is oriented to the client, while controlling costs.

Research Consumer

Nurses often use research to improve client care. In a clinical area, nurses need to (a) have some awareness of the process and language of research, (b) be sensitive to issues related to protecting the rights of human subjects, (c) participate in the identification of significant researchable problems, and (d) be a discriminating consumer of research findings.

Expanded Career Roles

Nurses are fulfilling expanded career roles. APRNs are RNs who have advanced practice training and have completed a master's or higher education degree and certification in their specialty of advanced practice roles. APRN roles include certified nurse practitioner (CNP), certified nurse midwife (CNM), certified registered nurse anesthetist (CRNA), and clinical nurse specialist (CNS). Other expanded roles include nurse educator, nurse researcher, and informatics nurse specialist (INS). Expanded nursing roles allow greater independence and autonomy (see Box 1.1).

BOX 1.1 Selected Expanded Career Roles for Nurses

ADVANCED PRACTICE REGISTERED NURSE (APRN)

APRNs have a master's degree, post-master's certificate, or practice-focused DNP degree in one of four specific roles:

- Certified Nurse Practitioner (CNP)
  CNPs provide care, independently, in a range of settings and in one of six defined client populations: family and individual across the lifespan; adult-gerontology (acute care or primary care); women's health and gender-related health; neonatal; pediatrics (acute care or primary care); and psychiatric or mental health.
- Clinical Nurse Specialist (CNS)
  CNSs usually work in a specialized area of nursing practice defined by parameters such as disease or medical specialty (e.g., oncology, diabetes); population (e.g., children, seniors, women); setting (e.g., critical care, emergency department); type of care (e.g., rehabilitation, mental health); and type of problem (e.g., pain, eating disorders). CNSs may serve as educators or outcome managers, conduct research, supervise staff, or manage cases to ensure the best possible client treatment.
- Certified Registered Nurse Anesthetist (CRNA)
  CRNAs administer anesthesia for surgical and other procedures and provide pre- and postanesthesia care for individuals across the lifespan. This care is provided in diverse settings, including hospital surgical suites.
- Certified Nurse Midwife (CNM)
  CNMs provide primary healthcare for women from adolescence throughout the lifespan. In addition to general primary care, they also provide the following: gynecological and family planning services; pregnancy, childbirth, and postpartum care; healthy newborn baby care; and treatment of male partners for sexually transmitted diseases. It is a misconception that CNMs are primarily used in at-home births. More than half of CNMs are employed by hospitals (GraduateNursingEDU.org, n.d.).

OTHER EXPANDED NURSING ROLES

Nurse Researcher

Nurse researchers investigate nursing problems to improve nursing care and to refine and expand nursing knowledge. They are employed in academic institutions, teaching hospitals, and research centers such as the National Institute for Nursing Research in Bethesda, Maryland. Nurse researchers usually have advanced education at the doctoral level.

Nurse Administrator

The nurse administrator manages client care, including the delivery of nursing services. The administrator may have a middle management position, such as head nurse or supervisor, or a more senior management position, such as director of nursing services. The functions of nurse administrators include budgeting, staffing, and planning programs. The educational preparation for nurse administrator positions is at least a baccalaureate degree in nursing and frequently a master's or doctoral degree.

Nurse Educator

Nurse educators are employed in nursing programs, at educational institutions, and in hospital staff education. The nurse educator usually has a baccalaureate degree or more advanced preparation and frequently has expertise in a particular area of practice. The nurse educator is responsible for classroom and, often, clinical teaching. There is now a process to become a certified nurse educator (CNE).

Nurse Entrepreneur

A nurse entrepreneur usually has an advanced degree and manages a health-related business. The nurse may be involved in education, consultation, or research, for example.

Forensic Nurse

The forensic nurse provides specialized care for individuals who are victims or perpetrators of trauma. Forensic nurses have knowledge of the legal system and skills in injury identification, evaluation, and documentation. After tending to the client's medical needs, the forensic nurse collects evidence, provides medical testimony in court, and consults with legal authorities. Forensic nurses work in a variety of fields including sexual assault, domestic violence, child abuse and neglect, mistreatment of older adults, death investigation, and corrections. They may be called on in mass disasters or community crisis situations (International Association of Forensic Nurses, n.d.). Nurses complete a certification process to become a forensic nurse.

Informatics Nurse Specialist (INS)

The INS is an RN with formal graduate-level education in informatics or an informatics-related field. The INS is responsible for implementing or coordinating projects involving multiple professions and specialties. They support other RNs to use data, information, knowledge, and technology in their practice (ANA, 2015a, p. 7).

Criteria of a Profession

Nursing is gaining recognition as a profession. A **profession** has been defined as an occupation that requires extensive education or a calling that requires special knowledge, skill, and preparation. A profession is generally distinguished from other kinds of occupations by (a) its requirement of prolonged, specialized training to acquire a body of knowledge pertinent to the role to be performed; (b) an orientation of the individual toward service, either to a community or to an organization; (c) ongoing research; (d) a code of ethics; (e) autonomy; and (f) a professional organization.

Specialized Education

Specialized education is an important aspect of professional status. Education for the professions has shifted toward programs in colleges and universities. Many nursing educators believe that the undergraduate nursing curriculum should include liberal arts education in addition to the biological and social sciences and the nursing discipline.

In the United States today, there are five means of entry into registered nursing: hospital diploma, associate degree, baccalaureate degree, master's degree, and doctoral degree.

Body of Knowledge

As a profession, nursing is establishing a well-defined body of knowledge and expertise. A number of nursing theories and conceptual frameworks contribute to the knowledge base of nursing and give direction to nursing practice, education, and ongoing research.

Service Orientation

A service orientation differentiates nursing from an occupation pursued primarily for profit. Many consider altruism (selfless concern for others) the hallmark of the profession. Nursing has a tradition of service to others. This service, however, must be guided by certain rules, policies, or codes of ethics. Today, nursing is also an important component of the healthcare delivery system.

Ongoing Research

Research in nursing is contributing to nursing practice. In the 1940s, nursing research was at a very early stage of development. In the 1950s, increased federal funding and professional support helped establish centers for nursing research. Most early research was directed at the study of nursing education. In the 1960s, studies were often related to the nature of the knowledge base underlying nursing practice. Since the 1970s, nursing research has focused on practice-related issues. Nursing research as a dimension of the nurse's role is discussed further in Chapter 2 ∞.

Code of Ethics

Nurses have traditionally placed a high value on the worth and dignity of others. The nursing profession requires integrity of its members; that is, a member is expected to do what is considered right regardless of the personal cost.

Ethical codes change as the needs and values of society change. Nursing has developed its own codes of ethics and in most instances has set up means to monitor the professional behavior of its members. See Chapter 4 ∞ for additional information on ethics.

Autonomy

A profession is autonomous if it regulates itself and sets standards for its members. Providing autonomy is one of the purposes of a professional association. If nursing is to have professional status, it must function autonomously in the formation of policy and in the control of its activity. To be autonomous, a professional group must be granted legal authority to define the scope of its practice, describe its particular functions and roles, and determine its goals and responsibilities in delivery of its services.

To practitioners of nursing, autonomy means independence at work, responsibility, and accountability for one's actions. Autonomy is more easily achieved and maintained from a position of authority. For example, all states have passed legislation granting CNPs supervisory, collaborative, or independent authority to practice, and currently, 26 states do not require physician oversight of NPs to practice (American Association of Nurse Practitioners [AANP], 2018).

Professional Organization

Operation under the umbrella of a professional organization differentiates a profession from an occupation. **Governance** is the establishment and maintenance of social, political, and economic arrangements by which practitioners control their practice, their self-discipline, their working conditions, and their professional affairs. Nurses, therefore, need to work within their professional organizations.

The ANA is a professional organization that adopts high nursing practice standards, supports a safe work environment for nurses, encourages a healthy lifestyle of nurses, and calls attention to healthcare issues that affect the public and nurses (ANA, n.d.a).

Professional Identity Formation

The standards of education and practice for the profession are determined by the members of the profession, rather than by outsiders. The development of professional identity begins during one's nursing education. **Professional identity** is a "sense of oneself that is influenced by characteristics, norms, and values of the nursing discipline, resulting in an individual thinking, acting, and feeling like a nurse" (Godfrey & Crigger, 2017, p. 1260). The term *professional identity* is replacing terminology such as *professional role* and *professionalism*.

Benner (2001) was the first to describe the development of professional expertise with the five levels of proficiency in nursing based on the Dreyfus general model of skill acquisition. The five stages, which have implications for teaching and learning, are novice, advanced beginner, competent, proficient, and expert. Benner writes that experience is essential for the development of professional expertise (see Box 1.2).

BOX 1.2 Benner's Stages of Nursing Expertise

STAGE I: NOVICE
No experience (e.g., nursing student). Performance is limited, inflexible, and governed by context-free rules and regulations rather than experience.

STAGE II: ADVANCED BEGINNER
Demonstrates marginally acceptable performance. Recognizes the meaningful "aspects" of a real situation. Has experienced enough real situations to make judgments about them.

STAGE III: COMPETENT
Has 2 or 3 years of experience. Demonstrates organizational and planning abilities. Differentiates important factors from less important aspects of care. Coordinates multiple complex care demands.

STAGE IV: PROFICIENT
Has 3 to 5 years of experience. Perceives situations as wholes rather than in terms of parts, as in Stage II. Uses maxims as guides for what to consider in a situation. Has holistic understanding of the client, which improves decision making. Focuses on long-term goals.

STAGE V: EXPERT
Performance is fluid, flexible, and highly proficient; no longer requires rules, guidelines, or maxims to connect an understanding of the situation to appropriate action. Demonstrates highly skilled intuitive and analytic ability in new situations. Is inclined to take a certain action because "it felt right."

From *Novice to Expert: Excellence and Power in Clinical Nursing Practice, Commemorative Edition*, by P. Benner, 2001. Electronically reproduced by permission of Pearson Education, Inc., Upper Saddle River, New Jersey.

As stated previously, it is within the nursing educational program that the student nurse develops, clarifies, and internalizes professional values as part of professional identity formation. Specific professional nursing values are stated in nursing codes of ethics (see Chapter 4 ∞), in standards of nursing practice (discussed earlier in this chapter), and in the legal system itself (see Chapter 3 ∞). Additionally, the National Student Nurses' Association (NSNA) has a code of ethics that includes a code of academic and clinical conduct (see Box 1.3).

BOX 1.3 NSNA Code of Academic and Clinical Conduct

Students of nursing have a responsibility to society in learning the academic theory and clinical skills needed to provide nursing care. The clinical setting presents unique challenges and responsibilities while caring for human beings in a variety of healthcare environments.

The *Code of Academic and Clinical Conduct* is based on an understanding that to practice nursing as a student is an agreement to uphold the trust with which society has placed in us. The statements of the code provide guidance for nursing students in their personal development of an ethical foundation and need not be limited strictly to the academic or clinical environment but can assist in the holistic development of the client.

As students are involved in the clinical and academic environments we believe that ethical principles are a necessary guide to professional development. Therefore, within these environments we:

1. Advocate for the rights of all clients.
2. Maintain client confidentiality.
3. Take appropriate action to ensure the safety of clients, self, and others.
4. Provide care for the client in a timely, compassionate, and professional manner.
5. Communicate client care in a truthful, timely, and accurate manner.
6. Actively promote the highest level of moral and ethical principles and accept responsibility for our actions.
7. Promote excellence in nursing by encouraging lifelong learning and professional development.
8. Treat others with respect and promote an environment that respects human rights, values, and choice of cultural and spiritual beliefs.
9. Collaborate in every reasonable manner with the academic faculty and clinical staff to ensure the highest quality of client care.
10. Use every opportunity to improve faculty and clinical staff understanding of the learning needs of nursing students.
11. Encourage faculty, clinical staff, and peers to mentor nursing students.
12. Refrain from performing any technique or procedure for which the student has not been adequately trained.
13. Refrain from any deliberate action or omission of care in the academic or clinical setting that creates unnecessary risk of injury to the client, self, or others.
14. Assist the staff nurse or preceptor in ensuring that there is full disclosure and that proper authorizations are obtained from clients regarding any form of treatment or research.
15. Abstain from the use of alcoholic beverages or any substances in the academic and clinical setting that impair judgment.
16. Strive to achieve and maintain an optimal level of personal health.
17. Support access to treatment and rehabilitation for students who are experiencing impairments related to substance abuse and mental or physical health issues.
18. Uphold school policies and regulations related to academic and clinical performance, reserving the right to challenge and critique rules and regulations as per school grievance policy.

From *Code of Ethics*, (pp. 6–16) by National Student Nurses' Association, Inc., 2018. New York, NY: Author.

Factors Influencing Contemporary Nursing Practice

To understand nursing as it is practiced today and as it will be practiced tomorrow requires an understanding of some of the social forces currently influencing this profession. These forces usually affect the entire healthcare system, and nursing, as a major component of that system, cannot avoid the effects.

Nursing Workforce Issues and Challenges

Registered nurses are the largest segment of the healthcare workforce. A historical perspective of the healthcare workforce reflects a cyclical pattern of nursing shortages and surpluses (Snavely, 2016). For example, nursing shortages in the hospital setting persist in good times and disappear during economic recessions (Johnson, Butler, Harootunian, Wilson, & Linan, 2016, p. 387).

One challenge to the nursing workforce is the expected retirement of one million RNs between 2017 and 2030. As these RNs exit the workforce, their years of nursing knowledge and experience will not be available to the nursing workforce (Buerhaus et al., 2017a). From an optimistic perspective, recent studies indicate that growth in the nursing workforce up to 2030 will be sufficient to replace the retiring RNs. The growth, however, will be uneven among the states, resulting in local shortages versus a national shortage (Buerhaus et al., 2017b).

Another challenge for nursing is the aging of the nation's baby boom generation. Baby boomers (individuals born between 1946 and 1964) will be 66 years and older by 2030. As a result, Medicare enrollment is projected to grow and lead to a big increase in demand for healthcare. This means an increasing demand for nurses *and* an increase in intensity and complexity of the required nursing care (Buerhaus et al., 2017a, pp. 40–41).

The 2017 National Nursing Workforce Survey (Smiley et al., 2018) concluded that "the workforce of tomorrow will be slightly younger, highly educated, with higher numbers working in the community providing primary healthcare and using technology and telehealth as a means to deliver healthcare" (p. S5). New environments and settings for the nursing workforce include microhospitals and pop-up clinics. The popularity of microhospitals (facilities of 8 to 15 beds) is increasing. They are part of a larger health system and found in communities that do not have a larger community hospital. The goal of the microhospital is to bring pre-acute care into neighborhoods with a higher level of service than found at an urgent care facility, such as scaled-down emergency departments, imaging and diagnostic suites, and dietary services (National Council of State Boards of Nursing [NCSBN], 2018, pp. S13–14).

Health insurance is either unavailable or unaffordable for many people. Pop-up clinics help provide healthcare access, often in regions with large uninsured populations. The clinics are usually held in convention centers and last for 1 to 2 days. They offer a wide variety of free services such as dental, vision, medical, and dietary counseling. Pop-up clinics are funded by donors and rely on volunteer providers (NCSBN, 2018). Healthcare delivery and the role of the nurse are constantly changing. As a result, the supply and demand for nurses will vary.

Healthcare System Reform

The ANA believes that all individuals have a right to quality healthcare and as an organization fights for meaningful healthcare reform. Since 2016 there have been many attempts to repeal the Affordable Care Act (ACA), and ANA had a part in stopping the proposed legislation that would have weakened the healthcare delivery system. The future of the ACA is uncertain and the discussions about healthcare will continue. The ANA will remain dedicated to informing the public about the relevant issues involved in future healthcare reform (ANA, n.d.b).

In 2010, an IOM report, *The Future of Nursing: Leading Change, Advancing Health*, provided recommendations on what nursing needed to do to provide better client care in the new systems that would be part of health reform. This report identified four key areas: nurses practicing to the fullest extent of their skills and knowledge; nurses achieving higher levels of education; nurses being full partners with physicians and other healthcare professionals; and improving data collection and information infrastructure (IOM, 2010, p. 4). The IOM evaluated the progress made from 2010 to 2015 and found that significant progress was made over the five years. The 2016 report, however, recommended future additional work in specific areas (see Box 1.4).

BOX 1.4 Assessing Progress on the Institute of Medicine Report *The Future of Nursing*

The following address the challenges that require additional focus and attention for continued progress in achieving the IOM landmark report on *The Future of Nursing* recommendations:

1. Remove scope-of-practice barriers for APRNs.
2. Expand opportunities for nurses to lead and increase interprofessional collaborative efforts to improve healthcare practice.
3. Explore funds to increase transition-to-practice nurse residency programs.
4. Increase the proportion of nurses with a baccalaureate degree to 80 percent by 2020.
5. Double the number of nurses with a doctorate by 2020.
6. Ensure that nurses engage in lifelong learning.
7. Prepare and enable nurses to lead change to advance health.
8. Build an infrastructure for the collection and analysis of interprofessional healthcare workforce data.
9. Increase the diversity of the nursing workforce.

Quality and Safety in Healthcare

Quality and safety are essential universal values on which healthcare is based. However, the report *To Err Is Human,* published by the IOM in 2000, revealed a gap between the status of American healthcare and the quality of care Americans should receive. The 2003 IOM report, *Health Professions Education: A Bridge to Quality,* called for a redesign of the education for healthcare professions and described six core competencies needed to improve 21st-century healthcare: patient-centered care, teamwork and collaboration, evidence-based practice, quality improvement, safety, and informatics. In 2005, the Robert Wood Johnson Foundation funded a project called Quality and Safety Education for Nurses (QSEN). The goal for the QSEN project was to "meet the challenge of preparing future nurses who will have the knowledge, skills and attitudes (KSAs) necessary to continuously improve the quality and safety of the healthcare systems within which they work" (QSEN Institute, n.d.). This project used the IOM's six competencies, along with the knowledge and experiences of QSEN faculty and a national advisory board, to define quality and safety competencies for nursing. The project also proposed KSAs for each competency that could be used as guides for curriculum development in prelicensure nursing programs (see the table at the QSEN website).

Consumer Demands

Consumers of nursing services (the public) have become an increasingly effective force in changing nursing practice. On the whole, people are better educated and have more knowledge about health and illness than in the past. Consumers also have become more aware of others' needs for care. The ethical and moral issues raised by poverty and neglect have made people more vocal about the needs of minority groups and the poor.

The public's concepts of health and nursing have also changed. Most now believe that health is a right of all people, not just a privilege of the rich. The media emphasize the message that individuals must assume responsibility for their own health by obtaining a physical examination regularly, checking for the seven danger signals of cancer, and maintaining their mental well-being by balancing work and recreation. Interest in health and nursing services is therefore greater than ever. Furthermore, many people now want more than freedom from disease—they want energy, vitality, and a feeling of wellness.

Increasingly, the consumer has become an active participant in making decisions about health and nursing care. Planning committees concerned with providing nursing services to a community usually have active consumer membership. Recognizing the validity of public input, many state nursing associations and regulatory agencies have consumer representatives on their governing boards.

Family Structure

Family structures influence the need for and provision of nursing services. More people are living away from the extended family and the nuclear family, and the family breadwinner is no longer necessarily the husband. Today, many single men and women rear children, and in many two-parent families both parents work. It is also common for young parents to live at great distances from their own parents. These young families need support services, such as daycare centers. For additional information about the family, see Chapter 27 ∞.

Adolescent mothers also need specialized nursing services, both while they are pregnant and after their babies are born. These young mothers usually have the normal needs of teenagers as well as those of new mothers. Many teenage mothers are raising their children alone with little, if any, assistance from the child's father. This type of single-parent family is especially vulnerable because motherhood compounds the difficulties of adolescence. Also, because many of these families may live in poverty, the children often do not receive preventive immunizations and are at increased risk for nutritional and other health problems.

Science and Technology

Advances in science and technology affect nursing practice. Biotechnology is affecting healthcare. For example, research in genetics and genomics has led to the development of precision medicine that aims to discover the right treatment for the right client at the right time. Prevention, diagnosis, and treatment are based on the client's genome, lifestyle, environment, and other personal characteristics to allow health professionals to focus their efforts on the individual (NCSBN, 2018, p. 58). This requires nurses to learn new skills and knowledge, such as genetics, pharmacogenomics, and use of new technology. As technologies change, nursing education changes, and nurses require increasing education to provide effective, safe nursing practice.

Internet, Telehealth, and Telenursing

The internet has affected healthcare, with more and more clients becoming well informed about their health concerns. As a result, nurses may need to interpret information from internet sources for clients and their families. Because not all internet-based information is accurate, nurses need to help clients access high-quality, valid websites; interpret the information; and evaluate the information and determine if it is useful to them.

The prefix *tele* means "distance" and is used to describe the many healthcare services provided via technology. **Telehealth** is the "delivery of health-related services and information via telecommunication technologies" (Lee & Billings, 2016, p. 252). The words *telemedicine* and *telehealth* are often used interchangeably. Telemedicine is often associated with direct client clinical services, whereas telehealth has a broader definition of remote healthcare services. **Telenursing** is the use of technology to provide nursing practice at a distance (Asiri & Househ, 2016). The delivery of telehealthcare, however, is not limited to physicians and nurses; it includes other health disciplines such as radiology, pathology, and pharmacology. These disciplines also deliver care using electronic information and telecommunications technologies and are accordingly called *teleradiology*, *telepathology*, and *telepharmacy*. Nurses engaged in telenursing practice continue to use the nursing process to provide care to clients, but they do so using technologies such as the internet, computers, telephones, video teleconferencing, and telemonitoring equipment. Telenursing continues to grow, especially in home healthcare and in rural communities.

Telehealth recognizes no state boundaries and, subsequently, licensure issues have been raised. For example, if a nurse licensed in one state provides health information to a client in another state, does the nurse need to maintain licensure in both states? The National Council of State Boards of Nursing (NCSBN) endorses a change from single-state licensure to a mutual recognition model. Many state legislatures have adopted mutual recognition language into statutes and are currently implementing it (NCSBN, n.d.b). See Chapter 3 ∞.

Legislation

Legislation about nursing practice and health matters affects both the public and nursing. Legislation related to nursing is discussed in Chapter 3 ∞. Changes in legislation relating to health also affect nursing. For example, the **Patient Self-Determination Act (PSDA)** requires that all competent adults be informed in writing on admission to a healthcare institution about their rights to accept or refuse medical care and to use advance directives. See Chapter 3 ∞ for more information about the PSDA and advance directives.

Healthcare reform and the shortage of physicians calls for an increase in APRNs such as CNPs. APRN regulations are determined at the state level through legislation. This causes wide variations in state regulation of nurse practitioner practice (Lugo, 2016). As a result, CNPs cannot easily move from state to state, which decreases access to care for clients. The APRN Compact, approved in 2015, allows an APRN to hold one multistate license with a privilege to practice in other compact states. The APRN Compact will be implemented when 10 states have enacted the legislation. As of January 2019, three states have enacted the legislation (NCSBN, n.d.a). The American Medical Association and the American Society of Anesthesiologists oppose the APRN Compact (NCSBN, 2018).

Collective Bargaining

The ANA participates in collective bargaining on behalf of nurses through its economic and general welfare programs. Today, some nurses are joining other labor organizations that represent them at the bargaining table. Nurses have gone on strike over economic concerns and over issues about safe care for clients and safety for themselves.

Nursing Associations

Professional nursing associations have provided leadership that affects many areas of nursing. Voluntary accreditation of nursing education programs by the Accreditation Commission for Education in Nursing (ACEN) and Commission on Collegiate Nursing Education (CCNE) has also influenced nursing. Many nursing programs have steadily improved to meet the standards for accreditation over the years. As a result, nurse graduates are better prepared to meet the demands of society.

To influence policymaking for healthcare, a group of professional nurses organized formally to promote political action in the nursing and healthcare arenas. Nurses for Political Action (NPA) formed in 1971 and became an arm of the ANA in 1974, when its name changed to Nurses' Coalition for Action in Politics (N-CAP). In 1986, the name was changed to American Nurses Association—Political Action Committee (ANA-PAC). Through this group, nurses have lobbied actively for legislation affecting healthcare. A number of nursing leaders hold positions of authority in government. Attaining such positions is essential if nurses hope to exert ongoing political influence.

Nursing Organizations

As nursing has developed, an increasing number of nursing organizations have formed. These organizations are at the local, state, national, and international levels. The organizations that involve most North American nurses are the ANA, the National League for Nursing, the International Council of Nurses, and the National Student Nurses' Association. The number of nursing specialty organizations is also increasing, for example, the Academy of Medical Surgical Nursing, the National Association of Hispanic Nurses, the National Black Nurses Association, Philippine Nurses Association of America, and the American Assembly for Men in Nursing. Participation in the activities of nursing associations enhances the growth of involved individuals and helps nurses collectively influence policies affecting nursing practice. See Table 1.1 for examples of major nursing organizations.

TABLE 1.1 Examples of Major Nursing Organizations

Organization	Description
American Nurses Association (ANA)	• The national professional organization for nursing in the United States. • The purposes are to foster high standards of nursing practice and to promote the educational and professional advancement of nurses so that all people may have better nursing care. • In 1982, the organization became a federation of state nurses' associations. Individuals participate in the ANA by joining their state nurses' associations. • The official journal of the ANA is *American Nurse Today*, and *The American Nurse* is the official newspaper.
National League for Nursing (NLN)	• The NLN is an organization of both individuals and agencies. • Its objective is to foster the development and improvement of all nursing services and nursing education. • People who are not nurses but have an interest in nursing services, for example, hospital administrators, can be members of the league. This feature of the NLN—involving non-nurse members, consumers, and nurses from all levels of practice—is unique. • The official journal of the NLN is *Nursing and Health Care Perspectives*.
International Council of Nurses (ICN)	• The council is a federation of national nurses' associations, such as the ANA and Canada Nursing Association. • The ICN provides an organization through which member national associations can work together for the mission of representing nursing worldwide, advancing the profession, and influencing health policy. • The official journal of the ICN is *International Nursing Review*.
National Student Nurses' Association (NSNA)	• The official preprofessional organization for nursing students. • Exposes student nurses to issues impacting the nursing profession while promoting collegiality and leadership qualities. • To qualify for membership in the NSNA, a student must be enrolled in a state-approved nursing education program. • The official journal of the NSNA is *Imprint* magazine.
International Honor Society: Sigma Theta Tau	• The international honor society in nursing. • The Greek letters stand for the Greek words *storga*, *tharos*, and *tima*, meaning "love," "courage," and "honor." • The society's purpose is professional rather than social. Membership is attained through academic achievement. Students in baccalaureate programs in nursing and nurses in master's, doctoral, and postdoctoral programs are eligible to be selected for membership. • Potential members, who hold a minimum of a bachelor's degree and have demonstrated achievement in nursing, can apply for membership as a nurse leader in the community. • The official journal is the *Journal of Nursing Scholarship*. • The society also publishes *Reflections*, a quarterly newsletter that provides information about the organization and its various chapters.

Chapter 1 Review

CHAPTER HIGHLIGHTS

- Historical perspectives of nursing practice reveal recurring themes or influencing factors. For example, women have traditionally cared for others, but often in subservient roles. Religious orders left an imprint on nursing by instilling such values as compassion, devotion to duty, and hard work. Wars created an increased need for nurses and medical specialties. Societal attitudes have influenced nursing's image. Visionary leaders have made notable contributions to improve the status of nursing.
- Although the history of nursing primarily focuses on female figures, men have worked as nurses as far back as before the Crusades. During the 20th century, men were denied admission to most nursing programs. There has been a gradual increase in the number of male nursing students and male nurses in the workforce. Improved recruitment and retention of men and other minorities continues to be needed to strengthen the profession.
- Originally, the focus of nursing education was to teach the knowledge and skills that would enable a nurse to practice in a hospital setting. Today, nursing education curricula are continually undergoing revisions in response to new scientific knowledge and technologic, cultural, political, and socioeconomic changes in society to enable nurses to work in more diverse settings and assume more diverse roles.

- In the practice disciplines, the main function of theory (and research) is to provide new possibilities for understanding the discipline's focus.
- During the latter half of the 20th century, disciplines seeking to establish themselves in universities had to demonstrate something that Nightingale had not envisioned for nursing—a unique body of theoretical knowledge.
- In the late 20th century, much of the theoretical work in nursing focused on articulating relationships between four major concepts: person, environment, health, and nursing. Because these four concepts can be superimposed on almost any work in nursing, they are sometimes collectively referred to as a *metaparadigm* for nursing.
- Continuing education is the responsibility of each practicing nurse to keep abreast of scientific and technologic change and changes within the nursing profession.
- The scope of nursing practice includes promoting health and wellness, preventing illness, restoring health, and caring for the dying.
- Although traditionally the majority of nurses were employed in hospital settings, today the numbers of nurses working in home healthcare, ambulatory care, and community health settings are increasing.
- Nurse practice acts vary among states, and nurses are responsible for knowing the act that governs their practice.
- Standards of nursing practice provide criteria against which the effectiveness of nursing care and professional performance behaviors can be evaluated.
- Every nurse may function in a variety of roles that are not exclusive of one another; in reality, they often occur together and serve to clarify the nurse's activities. These roles include caregiver, communicator, teacher, client advocate, counselor, change agent, leader, manager, case manager, and research consumer.
- With advanced education and experience, nurses can fulfill advanced practice roles such as clinical nurse specialist (CNS), certified nurse midwife (CNM), certified registered nurse anesthetist (CRNA), certified nurse educator (CNE), administrator, informatics nurse specialist (INS), and researcher.
- The nursing profession requires specialized education; a unique body of knowledge, including specific skills and abilities; a service orientation; ongoing research; a code of ethics; autonomy; and a professional organization.
- Professional identity formation begins during one's nursing education. It is the process whereby the values and norms of the nursing discipline are internalized into the nurse's own behavior and self-concept.
- Contemporary nursing practice is influenced by nursing workforce issues and challenges; healthcare reform; quality and safety in healthcare; consumer demands; family structure; science and technology; the internet, telehealth, and telenursing; legislation; collective bargaining; and the work of nursing associations.
- Participation in the activities of nursing associations enhances the growth of involved individuals and helps nurses collectively influence policies that affect nursing practice.

TEST YOUR KNOWLEDGE

1. Which of the following nurse leaders envisioned public health and health promotion roles for nurses?
   1. Clara Barton
   2. Lillian Wald
   3. Mary Brewster
   4. Florence Nightingale

2. Which of the following kind of nurse can provide consultation, education, and support and can manage a client's chemotherapy regimen?
   1. Nurse practitioner
   2. Clinical nurse specialist
   3. Nurse educator
   4. Nurse entrepreneur

3. Individuals or clients, environment, health, and nursing constitute the metaparadigm for nursing because they do which of the following?
   1. Provide a framework for implementing the nursing process
   2. Can be used in any setting when caring for a client
   3. Can be used to determine applicability of a research study
   4. Focus on the needs of a group of clients

4. Which is an example of continuing education for nurses?
   1. Attending the hospital's orientation program
   2. Completing a workshop on ethical aspects of nursing
   3. Obtaining information about the facility's new computer charting system
   4. Talking with a company representative about a new piece of equipment

5. Health promotion is best represented by which activity?
   1. Administering immunizations
   2. Giving a bath
   3. Preventing accidents in the home
   4. Performing diagnostic procedures

6. Who were America's first two trained nurses?
   1. Barton and Wald
   2. Dock and Sanger
   3. Richards and Mahoney
   4. Henderson and Breckinridge

7. A nurse with 2 to 3 years of experience who has the ability to coordinate multiple complex nursing care demands is at which stage of Benner's stages of nursing expertise?
   1. Advanced beginner
   2. Competent
   3. Proficient
   4. Expert

8. Which professional organization developed a code for nursing students?
   1. ANA
   2. NLN
   3. AACN
   4. NSNA

9. Which social force is most likely to significantly impact the future supply and demand for nurses?
   1. Aging
   2. Economics
   3. Science/technology
   4. Telecommunications

10. A registered nurse is interested in functioning as a healthcare advocate for individuals whose lives are affected by violence. This nurse will be investigating which expanded career role?
   1. Clinical nurse specialist
   2. Forensic nurse
   3. Nurse practitioner
   4. Nurse educator

See Answers to Test Your Knowledge in Appendix A.

READINGS AND REFERENCES

Suggested Readings

Pollitt, P. (2018). Nurses fight for the right to vote. *American Journal of Nursing*, *118*(11), 46–54. doi:10.1097/01.NAJ.0000547639.70037.cd

The author provides a look at the lives of four nurse suffragists—Lavinia Lloyd Dock, Mary Bartlett Dixon, Sarah Tarleton Colvin, and Hattie Frances Kruger—who were arrested for their involvement in the women's suffrage movement.

Strickler, J. (2018). Clara Barton: Angel of the battlefield. *Nursing*, *48*(3), 43–45. doi:10.1097/01.NURSE.0000529805.60418.26

This article, a part of the Pioneers in Nursing series, celebrates the life and accomplishments of Clara Barton.

Strickler, J., & Farmer, T. (2019). Dorothea Dix: Crusader for patients with mental illness. *Nursing*, *49*(1), 49–51. doi:10.1097/01.NURSE.0000549724.14939.d8

Another part of the Pioneers in Nursing series, this article describes how Dix, who was not formally trained as a nurse, influenced mental health nursing.

References

American Assembly for Men in Nursing. (n.d.). *About us*. Retrieved from https://www.aamn.org

American Association of Colleges of Nursing. (n.d.a). *Clinical nurse leader (CNL)*. Retrieved from https://www.aacnnursing.org/CNL

American Association of Colleges of Nursing. (n.d.b). *QSEN learning module series*. Retrieved from https://www.aacnnursing.org/Faculty/Teaching-Resources/QSEN/QSEN-Learning-Module-Series

American Association of Colleges of Nursing. (2017). *Policy brief: The changing landscape: Nursing student diversity on the rise*. Retrieved from https://www.aacnnursing.org/Portals/42/Diversity/Student-Diversity.pdf

American Association of Nurse Practitioners. (2018). *State practice environment*. Retrieved from https://www.aanp.org/legislation-regulation/state-legislation/state-practice-environment

American Nurses Association. (n.d.a). *About ANA*. Retrieved from https://www.nursingworld.org/ana/about-ana

American Nurses Association. (n.d.b). *Health system reform*. Retrieved from https://www.nursingworld.org/practice-policy/health-policy/health-system-reform

American Nurses Association. (n.d.c). *Linda Anne Judson Richards*. Retrieved from https://www.nursingworld.org/ana/about-ana/history/hall-of-fame/inductees-listed-alphabetically

American Nurses Association. (n.d.d). *Luther Christman award*. Retrieved from https://www.nursingworld.org/ana/national-awards-program/luther-christman-award

American Nurses Association. (n.d.e). *Mary Eliza Mahoney*. Retrieved from https://www.nursingworld.org/ana/about-ana/history/hall-of-fame/inductees-listed-alphabetically

American Nurses Association. (n.d.f). *Nurses serving in Congress*. Retrieved from http://www.nursingworld.org/MainMenuCategories/Policy-Advocacy/Federal/Nurses-in-Congress

American Nurses Association. (1973). *Standards of nursing practice*. Kansas City, MO: Author.

American Nurses Association. (1980). *Nursing: A social policy statement*. Kansas City, MO: Author.

American Nurses Association. (2010). *Nursing's social policy statement: The essence of the profession*. Washington, DC: Author.

American Nurses Association. (2015a). *Nursing informatics: Scope and standards of practice* (2nd ed.). Silver Spring, MD: Author.

American Nurses Association. (2015b). *Nursing scope and standards of practice* (3rd ed.). Silver Spring, MD: Author.

Arlington National Cemetery. (n.d.). *Nurses memorial*. Retrieved from https://www.arlingtoncemetery.mil/Explore/Monuments-and-Memorials/Nurses-Memorial

Asiri, H., & Househ, M. (2016). The impact of telenursing on nursing practice and education: A systematic literature review. *Studies in Health Technology and Informatics*, *226*, 105–108.

Benner, P. (2001). *From novice to expert: Excellence and power in clinical nursing practice* (Commemorative ed.). Upper Saddle River, NJ: Prentice Hall Health.

Berry-Caban, C., Rivers, F., Beltran, T. A., & Anderson, L. (2018). Description of United States military nurses deployed to Afghanistan & Iraq, 2001-2015. *Open Journal of Nursing*, *8*, 93–101. doi:10.4236/ojn.2018.81008

Buerhaus, P. I., Skinner, L. E., Auerbach, D. I., & Staiger, D. O. (2017a). Four challenges facing the nursing workforce in the United States. *Journal of Nursing Regulation*, *8*(2), 40–46. doi:10.1016/S2155-8256(17)30097-2

Buerhaus, P. I., Skinner, L. E., Auerbach, D. I., & Staiger, D. O. (2017b). State of the registered nurse workforce as a new era of health reform emerges. *Nursing Economic$*, *35*(5), 229–237.

Donahue, M. P. (2011). *Nursing: The finest art. An illustrated history* (3rd ed.). St. Louis, MO: Mosby.

Godfrey, N., & Crigger, N. (2017). Professional identity. In J. Giddens (Ed.), *Concepts of nursing practice* (2nd ed., pp. 1259–1283). St. Louis, MO: Elsevier.

GraduateNursingEDU.org. (n.d.). *APRN definition: Advanced practice registered nursing defined*. Retrieved from http://www.graduatenursingedu.org/aprn-definition

Health Resources and Services Administration. (2013). *The U.S. nursing workforce: Trends in supply and education*. Retrieved from https://bhw.hrsa.gov/sites/default/files/bhw/nchwa/projections/nursingworkforcetrendsoct2013.pdf

Health Resources and Services Administration. (2017). *Sex, race, and ethnic diversity of U.S. health occupations (2011–2015)*. Retrieved from https://bhw.hrsa.gov/sites/default/files/bhw/nchwa/diversityushealthoccupations.pdf

Hodges, E. A., Rowsey, P. J., Gray, T. F., Kneipp, S. M., Giscombe, C. W., Foster, B. B., . . . Kowlowitz, V. (2017). Bridging the gender divide: Facilitating the educational path for men in nursing. *Journal of Nursing Education*, *56*(5), 295–299. doi:10.3928/01484834-20170421-08

Institute of Medicine. (2000). *To err is human: Building a safer health system*. Washington, DC: The National Academies.

Institute of Medicine. (2003). *Health professions education: A bridge to quality*. Washington, DC: The National Academies.

Institute of Medicine. (2010, October 5). *The future of nursing: Leading change, advancing health*. Washington, DC: National Academies.

International Association of Forensic Nurses. (n.d.). *What is forensic nursing?* Retrieved from http://www.forensicnurses.org/?page=WhatisFN

Johnson, W. G., Butler, R., Harootunian, G., Wilson, B., & Linan, M. (2016). Registered nurses: The curious case of a persistent shortage. *Journal of Nursing Scholarship*, *48*(4), 387–396. doi:10.1111/jnu.12218

Lee, A. W., & Billings, M. (2016). Telehealth implementation in a skilled nursing facility: Case report for physical therapist practice in Washington. *Physical Therapy*, *96*(2), 252–259. doi:10.2522/ptj.20150079

Lugo, N. R. (2016). Full practice authority for advanced practice registered nurses is a gender issue. *Online Journal of Issues in Nursing*, *21*(2), 1. doi:10.3912/OJIN.Vol21No02PPT54

Murdaugh, C., Parsons, M. A., & Pender, N. (2019). *Health promotion in nursing practice* (8th ed.). New York, NY: Pearson.

National Academies of Sciences, Engineering, and Medicine. (2016). *Assessing progress on the Institute of Medicine report* The future of nursing. Washington, DC: National Academies.

National Council of State Boards of Nursing. (n.d.a). *APRN compact*. Retrieved from https://www.ncsbn.org/aprn-compact.htm

National Council of State Boards of Nursing. (n.d.b). *Nurse licensure compact*. Retrieved from https://www.ncsbn.org/nurse-licensure-compact.htm

National Council of State Boards of Nursing. (2018). The nursing regulatory environment in 2018: Issues and challenges. *Journal of Nursing Regulation*, *9*(1), 52–65. doi:10.1016/S2155-8256(18)30055-3

National League for Nursing. (2017a). *Findings from the 2016 NLN Biennial survey of schools of nursing academic year 2015–2016: Executive summary*. Retrieved from http://www.nln.org/docs/default-source/newsroom/nursing-education-statistics/biennial-survey-executive-summary-(pdf).pdf?sfvrsn=0

National League for Nursing. (2017b). *NLN congratulates Rear Adm. Sylvia Trent-Adams, acting U.S. Surgeon General* [Press release]. Retrieved from http://www.nln.org/newsroom/news-releases/news-release/2017/04/25/nln-congratulates-rear-adm.-sylvia-trent-adams-acting-u.s.-surgeon-general

National Student Nurses' Association. (2018). *Code of ethics*. New York, NY: Author.

Nelson, R. (2019). Ernest Grant breaks barriers. *American Journal of Nursing*, *119*(1), 65–66. doi:10.1097/01.NAJ.0000552617.90814.d5

Nightingale, F. (1969). *Notes on nursing: What it is, and what it is not*. New York, NY: Dover. (Original work published 1860)

QSEN Institute. (n.d.). *Definitions and pre-licensure KSAs*. Retrieved from http://qsen.org/competencies/pre-licensure-ksas

Schuyler, C. B. (1992). Florence Nightingale. In F. Nightingale, *Notes on nursing: What it is, and what it is not* (Commemorative ed., pp. 3–17). Philadelphia, PA: Lippincott.

Smiley, R. A., Lauer, P., Bienemy, C., Berg, J. G., Shireman, E., Reneau, K. A., & Alexander, M. (2018). The 2017 National Nursing Workforce Survey. *Journal of Nursing Regulation*, 9(3, Suppl.), S11–S45. doi:10.1016/S2155-8256(18)30131-5

Snavely, T. M. (2016). Data watch. A brief economic analysis of the looming nursing shortage in the United States. *Nursing Economic$*, *34*(2), 98–100.

Trossman, S. (2018). Getting to know incoming ANA president Ernest Grant. *American Nurse Today*, *13*(9), 79–80.

Vietnam Women's Memorial Foundation. (n.d.). *During the Vietnam era . . .* Retrieved from http://www.vietnamwomensmemorial.org/vwmf.php

Yi, M., & Keogh, B. (2016). What motivates men to choose nursing as a profession? A systematic review of qualitative studies. *Contemporary Nurse*, *52*, 95–105. doi:10.1080/10376178.2016.1192952

Zhang, W., & Liu, Y. (2016). Demonstration of caring by males in clinical practice: A literature review. *International Journal of Nursing Sciences*, *3*(3), 323–327. doi:10.1016/j.ijnss.2016.07.006

Selected Bibliography

American Association of Colleges of Nursing. (2017). *The impact of education on nursing practice*. Retrieved from https://www.aacnnursing.org/News-Information/Fact-Sheets/Impact-of-Education

American Association of Colleges of Nursing. (2017). *Nursing faculty shortage*. Retrieved from https://www.aacnnursing.org/News-Information/Fact-Sheets/Nursing-Faculty-Shortage

Arzouman, J. (2016). The future of nursing 5 years later—Where are we now? *MEDSURG Nursing*, *25*(1), 5, 43.

Collins, B. L., & Saylor, J. (2018). The Affordable Care Act: Where are we now? *Nursing*, *48*(5), 43–47. doi:10.1097/01.NURSE.0000531892.08687.b7

Fathi, J. T., Modin, H. E., & Scott, J. D. (2017). Nurses advancing telehealth services in the era of healthcare reform. *Online Journal of Issues in Nursing*, *22*(2). doi:10.3912/OJIN.Vol22No02Man02

Herman, B. (2016). Virtual reality: More insurers are embracing telehealth. *Modern Healthcare*, *46*(8), 16–19.

Kleinpell, R., Barden, C., Rincon, T., McCarthy, M., & Zapatochny, R. (2016). Assessing the impact of telemedicine on nursing care in intensive care units. *American Journal of Critical Care*, *25*(1), e14–e20. doi:10.4037/ajcc2016808

Potera, C. (2018). The AACN drafts proposal for BSN as the entry level for RNs, gets pushback. *American Journal of Nursing*, *118*(9), 14.

Rosenkoetter, M. M. (2016). Overview and summary: Organizational outcomes for providers and patients. *Online Journal of Issues in Nursing*, *21*(2), 1–1. doi:10.3912/OJIN.Vol21No02ManOS

Evidence-Based Practice and Research in Nursing

2

LEARNING OUTCOMES

After completing this chapter, you will be able to:

1. Explain the relationship between research and evidence-based nursing practice.
2. Apply the steps of change used in implementing evidence-based practice.
3. Describe limitations in relying on research as the primary source of evidence for practice.
4. Differentiate the quantitative approach from the qualitative approach in nursing research.
5. Outline the steps of the research process.
6. Describe research-related roles and responsibilities for nurses.
7. Describe the nurse's role in protecting the rights of human participants in research.

KEY TERMS

comparative analysis, *59*
confidentiality, *63*
content analysis, *59*
cost–benefit analysis, *59*
critique, *61*
dependent variable, *57*
descriptive statistics, *58*
ethnography, *56*
evidence-based practice (EBP), *53*
extraneous variables, *56*
grounded theory, *56*
hypothesis, *57*
independent variable, *57*
inferential statistics, *58*
logical positivism, *56*
measures of central tendency, *58*
measures of variability, *58*
methodology, *57*
naturalism, *56*
phenomenology, *56*
pilot study, *58*
protocols, *58*
qualitative research, *56*
quantitative research, *56*
reliability, *58*
research, *54*
research design, *58*
research process, *57*
sample, *58*
scientific validation, *59*
statistically significant, *58*
target population, *58*
validity, *58*

Introduction

All nurses need a basic understanding of the research process and its relationship to evidence-based practice. Current standards of professional performance for nurses include using evidence and research findings in practice. At the minimum, all nurses are expected to use evidence and research to determine proper nursing actions, to engage in research activities as appropriate to their abilities, and to share knowledge with other nurses (American Nurses Association, 2015). Additionally, nurses today are actively involved in generating and publishing evidence in order to improve client care and expand nursing's knowledge base. These activities support the current emphasis on practice that is based on evidence and on all nurses needing to be able to locate, understand, and evaluate both research findings and nonresearch evidence.

Evidence-Based Practice

Evidence-based practice (EBP), or evidence-based nursing, occurs when the nurse can "integrate best current evidence with clinical expertise and patient/family preferences and values for delivery of optimal healthcare" (Cronenwett et al., 2007). See Figure 2.1 ■. Thus, as evidence changes, so must practice. One model for changing practice as a result of evidence (Melnyk & Fineout-Overholt, 2019) uses the following seven steps:

- ***Cultivate a spirit of inquiry.*** Nurses need to be curious and willing to investigate how various practices compare and which might be best for a specific client.
- ***Ask clinical questions.*** For consistency and efficiency, nurses should state the question in a standard format such as PICOT (see page 57).
- ***Search for the best evidence.*** In the previous step, key terms are identified that facilitate identifying relevant evidence in the literature.
- ***Critically appraise the evidence.*** Several toolkits or schema are available to assist the nurse in determining the most valid, reliable, and applicable evidence. In some cases, relevant studies may already have been synthesized (see Box 2.1).
- ***Integrate the evidence with clinical expertise and client/family preferences and values.*** Evidence must not be automatically applied to the care of individual clients. Each nurse must determine how the evidence fits with

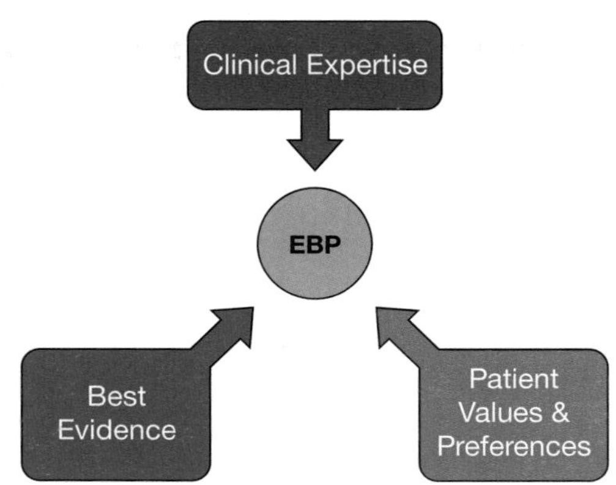

Figure 2.1 ■ Components of evidence-based practice.

the clinical condition of the client, available resources, institutional policies, and the client's wishes. Only then can an appropriate intervention be established.

- ***Implement and evaluate the outcomes of the intervention.*** The nurse gathers all relevant data that may indicate whether or not the intervention was successful. If the outcomes varied from those reported in the evidence, this evaluation can help determine the reasons for the variable responses and will contribute to improving the evidence available for future situations.
- ***Disseminate the outcomes.*** Nurses need to share the results of their work with others. This can be done locally with colleagues or more formally through publications, posters, or conference presentations.

See Chapter 18 ∞ for further description of the nurse's role in managing change.

Some scholars contend that, while evidence includes theories, opinions of recognized experts, clinical expertise, clinical experiences, and findings from client assessments, findings from research studies are often given the most weight in the decision-making process. This emphasis is because **research** entails using formal and systematic processes to solve problems and answer questions. The disciplined thinking and the careful planning and execution that characterize research mean that the resulting findings should be accurate, dependable, and free from bias.

Other scholars and practitioners express concerns about the current prominence and conception of EBP as primarily using research as the source of evidence. Some believe that the best evidence for EBP is theory rather than research. Reasons for concerns about reliance solely on research for EBP include the following:

1. Research is often done under controlled circumstances, which is very different from the real world of healthcare delivery.
2. Research evidence suggests that there is one best solution to a problem for all clients, and this limited perspective stifles creativity.
3. Research may ignore the significance of life events to the individual. Nursing care should consider feasibility, appropriateness, meaningfulness, and effectiveness of interventions and plans.
4. Not all published research is robust and flawless.
5. EBP should promote cost-effective care, but cost is often not included in traditional research studies.

A variety of models are available to assist nurses in using EBP. These include the ACE Star Model (Stevens, 2012), Iowa Model (Buckwalter et al., 2017), Johns Hopkins EBP Model (Dang & Dearholt, 2017), and Stetler Model (Stetler, 2010).

BOX 2.1 Sources of Synthesized Knowledge

Cochrane Library
Evidence-Based Nursing Journal
Joanna Briggs Institute
National Guidelines Clearinghouse
Essential Evidence Plus/Patient-Oriented Evidence That Matters (POEMS)
U.S. National Library of Medicine Health Information Databases
Worldviews on Evidence-Based Nursing

Nursing Research

Using research findings to guide decisions about client care is nothing new. As early as 1854, Florence Nightingale demonstrated how research findings could be used to improve nursing care. When Nightingale arrived in the Crimea in 1854, she found the military hospital barracks overcrowded, filthy, infested with fleas and rats, and lacking in food, drugs, and essential medical supplies. By systematically collecting, organizing, and reporting data, Nightingale was able to institute sanitary reforms and significantly reduce mortality rates from contagious diseases and infection. Although the Nightingale tradition influenced the establishment of American nursing schools, her ideas about the importance of research did not take hold in nursing until early in the 20th century.

Currently, accrediting organizations require all baccalaureate and higher degree programs to include coursework in research and EBP. Many associate degree and diploma programs also include content in these important areas. Research-related role expectations for nurses with different levels of educational preparation were reaffirmed by the American Association of Colleges of Nursing (AACN) in 2006 and are presented in Table 2.1. All nurses, however, have a responsibility to identify nursing issues that require research and to participate in research studies to the extent they are able.

The journal *Nursing Research* was first published in 1952 to serve as a vehicle for communicating nurses' research findings. The publication of many other nursing research journals followed, some dedicated to research and others combining clinical and research articles. The breadth and diversity of nursing research is reflected in the examples of recent nursing studies shown in Box 2.2.

TABLE 2.1 Research-Related Role Expectations for Nurses with Different Levels of Educational Preparation

Educational Preparation	Identified Expectations
Baccalaureate degree	Basic understanding of the research process. Able to understand and apply research findings from nursing and other disciplines in clinical practice. Understand the basic elements of EBP. Work with others to identify potential research problems. Collaborate on research teams.
Master's degree	Evaluate research findings. Implement EBP guidelines. Form and lead research teams in work settings and professional groups. Identify practice and systems problems that require study. Work with scientists to initiate research.
Practice-focused doctoral (DNP) degree	Focus on the evaluation and use of research rather than the conduct of research. Translate scientific knowledge into complex clinical interventions tailored to meet individual, family, and community health and illness needs. Use leadership skills to evaluate the translation of research into practice. Collaborate with scientists on new health policy research opportunities that evolve from the translation and evaluation processes. Complete a clinical scholarly project.
Research-focused doctoral (PhD) degree	Conduct independent research. Seek needed support for the initial phases of a research program. Involve others in research projects. Publish a dissertation.
Postdoctoral preparation	Establish and pursue a focused research agenda.

From *AACN Position Statement on Nursing Research*, by American Association of Colleges of Nursing, 2006, Washington, DC: Author.

BOX 2.2 Examples of Current Nursing Research Studies

- The effectiveness of interventions needs to be determined not just at the completion of the study period but over longer times. Allen et al. (2018) used both quantitative and qualitative methods to evaluate the status of practice improvements and the role of pain resource nurses that had been created in a study conducted 8 years previously.
- Pressure injuries and incontinence-associated dermatitis are challenging problems. Avşar and Karadağ (2018) studied 154 clients in two intensive care units. The intervention group had nurses trained in data collection tools and in evidence-based practices to improve tissue tolerance. Routine nursing care was given to the clients in the control group. The cost of the evidence-based preventive initiatives was higher compared to the control group, but the former provided a significant reduction in the prevalence of tissue integrity deterioration.
- Using evidence-based improvement plans in long-term care settings can be difficult due to the shortage of staff qualified to design, implement, and evaluate the plans. Using a qualitative descriptive design, Edwards and Higuchi (2018) interviewed staff at 12 long-term care facilities and implemented a 9-month intervention focused on topics such as team functioning and communication. Factors that enhanced the success of the intervention were identified and formed the beginnings of a model that could be used in diverse settings.
- An increasing number of residents of nursing homes have diabetes mellitus. Hurley et al. (2017) used survey, interview, and focus group strategies to explore resident care issues with nurse managers. The authors determined that there was a need for the development of clinical guidelines and standards of care for this population.

In 1985, after intense lobbying by the American Nurses Association (ANA), the U.S. Congress passed a bill creating the National Center for Nursing Research as a part of the National Institutes of Health. The center was elevated to institute status in 1993 and became the National Institute of Nursing Research (NINR). The establishment of NINR puts nursing research on an equal footing with research by other health-related professions by supporting research training and research related to client care. The budget of the NINR reflects a steady increase in federal funding for nursing research. Current priority areas for research funding by NINR are health promotion and disease prevention, symptom management, self-management of chronic illness, innovation, developing nurse scientists, and palliative/end-of-life care (NINR, 2016). Many nursing specialty organizations also regularly identify priority areas for research funding.

Approaches to Nursing Research

Nurse researchers use two major approaches to investigating clients' responses to health alterations and nursing interventions. These approaches, quantitative and qualitative research, originate from different philosophical perspectives and generate different types of data. Both approaches make valuable contributions to EBP.

Additional examples of research are found in the more than 50 Evidence-Based Practice boxes featured throughout this textbook.

Quantitative Research

Quantitative research entails the systematic collection, statistical analysis, and interpretation of numerical data. Quantitative research is characterized by planned and fixed study processes, careful attention to **extraneous variables** (any variables that could influence the results of the study other than the specific variable[s] being studied for their influence) or contaminating factors in the study environment, and an objective and distanced relationship between the researcher and what is being studied. Reports of quantitative research are characterized by statistical information, tables, and graphs, which can make them intimidating to read. The quantitative approach to research is linked to the philosophical perspective of **logical positivism**, which maintains that "truth" is absolute and can be discovered by careful measurement. This perspective proposes that phenomena are best understood by examining their component parts; this is referred to as a reductionistic perspective. Positivism is the philosophical perspective of natural sciences such as biology and chemistry. It focuses on the who, what, where, when, why, and how questions.

A quantitative approach to research is useful for research questions such as the following:

- What causes ___________?
- Which treatment for a condition is more effective?
- What factors are associated with a specific condition or outcome?
- If I know *X*, to what extent can I predict the occurrence of *Y*?

Qualitative Research

Qualitative research is the systematic collection and thematic analysis of narrative data. In other words, the research collects and analyzes words, rather than numbers. The qualitative approach to research is rooted in the philosophical perspective of **naturalism** (sometimes referred to as constructivism), which maintains that reality is relative or contextual and constructed by individuals who are experiencing a phenomenon. This philosophical perspective is reflected in the human sciences, such as anthropology, sociology, and existential psychology.

A qualitative approach to research is characterized by flexible and evolving study processes and by minimized "distancing" between the researcher and study informant. In contrast to a quantitative study, where objectivity is sought and valued, in a qualitative study, the researcher's subjectivity and values are seen as inevitable and even desirable. Qualitative research has a holistic perspective and results in a report that may read like a story. Nurse researchers tend to use one of three distinct qualitative traditions: phenomenology, ethnography, or grounded theory. **Phenomenology** focuses on lived experiences, **ethnography** focuses on cultural patterns of thoughts and behaviors, and **grounded theory** focuses on social processes. Additional qualitative types include historical and case study research.

A qualitative approach to research is useful for research questions such as the following:

- What is the experience of receiving diagnosis *X* or undergoing treatment *Y*? (phenomenology)
- What are typical behaviors of certain groups of clients (who may be defined by a diagnosis or membership in a cultural or ethnic group)? (ethnography)
- How do individuals cope with *X*? (grounded theory)

Individual qualitative research studies are not designed with the intent to change nursing practice directly. In addition, compared to quantitative research, there are few publications that summarize the findings and implications from groups of qualitative studies on related topics. However, the nurse must still be able to evaluate qualitative research in order to determine its relevance to the questions and problems central to nursing.

Table 2.2 compares the quantitative and qualitative approaches to research.

TABLE 2.2 Comparison of Quantitative and Qualitative Research Approaches

Characteristic	Quantitative Research	Qualitative Research
Meaning	Logical conclusions	Understanding, describing
Reality	Stable	Personal, contextual
Data	Numbers, "hard" data	Words, "soft" data
Perspective	Outsider	Insider
Approach to knowing	Reductionistic, deductive	Contextual, holistic, inductive
Research approach	Objective, structured, rational, empirical, conclusive	Subjective, artistic, intuitive, exploratory, discovery
Sampling	Random	Purposive
Research conditions	Controlled, laboratory	Naturalistic, fieldwork
Hypothesis/theory	Tested	Generated
Methods	Measurement (e.g., survey, observation)	Thick description (e.g., interview)
Data analyses	Deductive, statistics/mathematical	Inductive, intuitive, themes
Findings/results	Replicable, reliable, generalizable	Valid, credible, transferable

Overview of the Research Process

The **research process** is a method in which decisions are made that result in a detailed plan or proposal for a study, as well as the actual implementation of the plan. Nurses who are reading research reports to inform their practice need a basic understanding of the research process in order to judge the credibility of a study's findings and their usefulness for EBP. Nurses who are assisting with a study as a member of a research team need to understand the research process in order to provide meaningful input into a study and help ensure that it results in credible and useful information. Although the research process unfolds somewhat differently for quantitative and qualitative studies, the same general steps are involved: formulating the research problem and purpose, determining study methods, collecting research data, analyzing research data, communicating research findings, and using research findings in practice.

Formulating the Research Problem and Purpose

The researcher's first task is to narrow a broad area of interest into a more specific problem that indicates the issue of concern behind the study. Ideas for research problems may arise from recurrent problems encountered in practice, questions that are difficult to resolve because of contradictions in the literature, or areas in which minimal or no research has been done. Because conducting a study requires resources and the time and effort of study participants, a research problem should be significant to nursing and offer the potential to improve client care. The problem must also be feasible to study in light of the resources (including time and skill) that are available to conduct the study. Taking shortcuts because of insufficient resources can compromise the quality of study findings. A research problem also must be something that can be answered by scientific investigation. Questions that deal with moral or ethical issues such as "Should assisted suicide be allowed in this hospital?" are timely and relevant, but cannot be answered through research. Finally, because conducting a study requires a lot of time and energy, a research problem should be of interest to the researcher. The researcher's enthusiasm and commitment to the problem can be a factor in the successful completion of the study.

In addition to determining the specific problem that will be the focus of the study, the researcher must also decide on the purpose of the study or on the nature of information that it will provide. A study's purpose statement is characterized by an action verb that indicates whether the study will provide descriptive information, explanatory information, cause-and-effect information, or information that will allow prediction and control. A study's purpose statement has important implications for how the study will be conducted and how the data collected will be analyzed.

One strategy for stating the problem you wish to explore is to use the PICO format:

P – Patient, population, participant, or problem of interest
I – Intervention or therapy to consider for the subject of interest
C – Comparison of interventions, such as no treatment, or control
O – Outcome of the intervention.

For example, you have clients with migraine headaches who do not respond to conventional treatment and want to know if some alternative treatments such as biofeedback can help them. The PICO is as follows:

P – Patients with migraines nonresponsive to conventional therapy
I – Biofeedback
C – No biofeedback (and/or other alternative treatments such as music therapy)
O – Reduction in migraines.

Based on these components, one version of the final PICO question would be "Is biofeedback for clients with migraines nonresponsive to conventional therapy more effective at reducing headaches than no biofeedback?"

In some cases, additional components are added to make PICO into PICOD by adding study Design, PICOS by adding Setting, PICOC by adding Context, and PICOT by adding Time frame. Several other frameworks are available and are not limited to asking nursing questions.

Formulating the research problem and purpose is facilitated by conducting a review of the relevant literature. This literature review helps the researcher become familiar with the current state of knowledge in regard to the problem area and build on that knowledge when designing the current study. Reviewing the literature can also help the researcher identify strategies that have been used successfully (and unsuccessfully) in the past to investigate the problem and to measure the variables of interest. A **dependent variable** is a behavior, characteristic, or outcome that the researcher wishes to explain or predict. An **independent variable** is the presumed cause of or influence on the dependent variable. In some studies, the researcher may develop a **hypothesis** or a predictive statement about the relationship between two or more variables.

Determining Study Methods

A study's **methodology** can be thought of as its logistics or mechanics. The methodological elements of the research process deal with how the study is organized, who or what will be the sources of information for the study, and data collection details such as what data will be collected, how data will be collected, and the timing of data collection. The first methodological decision made by a researcher is whether the study will use a quantitative or qualitative research approach. This decision has implications for subsequent methodological decisions about research design, sampling, and data collection, as well as data analysis.

Research design refers to the overall structure or blueprint or the general layout of a study. The research design indicates how many times data will be collected in a study, the timing of data collection relative to other study events, the types of relationships between variables that are being examined, the number of groups being compared in the study, and how extraneous variables will be controlled so that study findings are more reliable and accurate. There are two major types of research designs. With an *experimental design*, the researcher controls the independent variable by administering an experimental treatment to some participants while withholding it from others. Experimental designs are used to determine cause-and-effect relationships. With a *nonexperimental design*, there is no manipulation of the independent variable; in fact, there may be no identifiable independent and dependent variables in the study. Nonexperimental designs are used for descriptive research studies.

Another key methodological decision is determining who (or what) will provide the data for the study. The **sample** or sources of information for a study may be humans, events, behaviors, documents, or biological specimens. Samples are carefully selected so that they are as accurate a representation as possible of the **target population**, or the universe of elements to which the researcher wishes to be able to apply the study's findings. The sample is a carefully chosen segment of the target population. Sampling decisions are also a key factor in the usefulness of a study's findings for EBP, since similar results are more likely to be found in practice settings when there is a close match between the characteristics of the study sample and the characteristics of the client population to which the study findings will be applied.

Nurse researchers use a wide variety of data collection strategies, including questionnaires, interviews, observation, record reviews, and biophysical measures. Data collection decisions spell out how any intervention that is going to be administered to study participants will be implemented. Data collection decisions interface closely with sampling decisions. For example, if a researcher is going to distribute a questionnaire to collect data, study participants must be able to read it!

One quality control strategy in research is to conduct a pilot study. A **pilot study** is a "rehearsal" before the actual study begins, consisting of testing the study with a small sample or over a short period of time. Pilot studies are helpful for detecting problems such as instructions or questionnaire items that can be misunderstood and for providing a chance to correct these problems before formal data collection procedures get under way.

Collecting Research Data

During the actual data collection phase of a research study, all the methodological decisions that have been made are implemented. Researchers expend great effort to ensure that data collection occurs in a consistent manner throughout the course of the study. Detailed data collection **protocols** or instructions and careful training of research assistants are strategies that can be used to ensure the consistency and integrity of data collection procedures.

Various procedures are available for establishing the reliability and validity of research data. **Reliability** refers to the consistency of measures. **Validity** refers to the completeness and conceptual accuracy of measures. The way in which reliability and validity are established depends on the data collection procedure being used and the nature of the data being collected. Conducting a pilot test allows a researcher to do a preliminary estimate of reliability and validity.

Analyzing Research Data

During the data analysis stage of the research process, the collected data are organized and analyzed to answer the research question(s) or test the study's hypothesis. If a study has used a quantitative approach, data analysis involves the application of a variety of statistical procedures. **Descriptive statistics** are procedures that organize and summarize large volumes of data including measures of central tendency and measures of variability. **Measures of central tendency** provide a single numerical value that denotes the "average" value for a variable. **Measures of variability** describe how values for a variable are dispersed or spread out. Specific measures of central tendency and variability are defined in Box 2.3.

BOX 2.3 Descriptive Statistics: Measures of Central Tendency and Variability

MEASURES OF CENTRAL TENDENCY

Mean—the arithmetic average for a set of scores. The mean is calculated by summing all scores and dividing by the number of scores.

Median—the middle value in a distribution of scores or the value above and below which 50% of the scores lie.

Mode—the most common or frequently occurring value.

MEASURES OF VARIABILITY

Range—the difference or span between the lowest and highest value for a variable.

Standard deviation—the average amount by which a single score in a distribution deviates or differs from the mean score.

The use of **inferential statistics** allows researchers to test hypotheses about relationships between variables or differences between groups. Inferential statistics are particularly useful when a researcher wants to establish the effectiveness of an intervention. Commonly used inferential statistics are defined in Box 2.4.

After inferential statistics have been computed, the results are inspected for statistical significance. If results are **statistically significant**, it means that they are not likely to have occurred only by chance. The notion of statistical significance is linked to probability. By convention, probability (a p value) of less than .05 is considered to indicate statistical significance. A p value of .05 means that the observed statistical results are likely to occur solely by chance only 5% of the time. Another measure of the

BOX 2.4 Commonly Used Inferential Statistics

Independent *t*-test—used to compare the mean performance of two independent groups (such as men and women).
Dependent (or paired) *t*-tests—used to compare the mean performance of two dependent or related groups (such as a before and after test given to the same individuals).
Analysis of variance (ANOVA)—used to compare the mean performance of three or more groups.
Pearson's product-moment correlation coefficient (Pearson's *r*)—used to describe and test the relationship between two continuous variables (such as age and weight).
Chi-squared—used to compare the distribution of a condition across two or more groups.

significance of findings is the confidence interval (CI). The CI indicates the range within which the true value lies, with a specific level of confidence. For example, if a study indicates that something occurs, on average, 2.5 times more often in one group than in another, with a 95% CI of 1.9–3.2, this means that there is a 95% likelihood that it occurs between 1.9 and 3.2 times more often. As long as zero does not fall within the CI, the findings are statistically significant. It is important to keep in mind that just because results are statistically significant does not automatically mean that they are clinically significant.

Statistical significance is not the same concept as clinical significance. Nurses need to help answer the question "Does it matter?"—especially from the client's perspective. For example, if research has shown statistically that a medication lowers blood pressure by 3 mmHg, the nurse, using the principles in EBP, helps determine if the clinical impact is more beneficial than the negative aspects of the treatment, such as cost and side effects. Clinical significance may vary dramatically from one client or context to another. For example, whereas one client considering the pros and cons of undergoing a cancer treatment shown, statistically, to extend life for four months might decide in favor, another client might decide against.

If a research study uses a qualitative approach, data analysis involves searching for themes and patterns. This procedure is sometimes referred to as **content analysis** because the content of narrative materials is being analyzed. Qualitative researchers may synthesize their findings to develop a theory or conceptual framework of the phenomenon being studied.

Communicating Research Findings

Research findings must be disseminated if they are to become accessible and used to guide practice decisions. Research findings can be communicated through publication in journals or at conferences. Even small-scale research projects that are carried out in a clinical setting should be communicated. Newsletter articles and research posters are ideally suited for this purpose.

Sometimes, readers only need to read a short summary of the research in order to determine whether the details are important for their own knowledge. In this case, the abstract section of the publication is extremely useful. Usually, the abstract is presented on the first page of the article, is about 400 words long, and includes the study objectives, design, data sources, review methods, results, and conclusions. See Figure 2.2 ■.

Using Research Findings in Practice

As described earlier, EBP entails using research findings and other sources of evidence to guide decisions about client care. Before a study's findings are used to guide practice, they should undergo three types of evaluation: scientific validation, comparative analysis, and cost–benefit analysis.

Scientific validation is a thorough critique of a study for its conceptual and methodological integrity. This means scrutinizing how the study was conceptualized, designed, and conducted in order to make a judgment about the overall quality of its findings. **Comparative analysis** involves assessing study findings for their implementation potential. Three factors are considered: (1) how the study's findings compare to findings from other studies about the problem, (2) how the study's findings will transfer from the research conditions to the clinical practice conditions in which they will be used, and (3) practical or feasibility considerations that need to be addressed when applying the findings in practice. The closer the fit between the characteristics of the setting and sample of the study and the conditions and clients with which the findings will be used, the more likely it is that the desired outcomes will be achieved. **Cost–benefit analysis** involves consideration of the potential risks and benefits of both implementing a change based on a study's findings and not implementing a change. Both immediate and delayed potential costs and benefits to clients, nursing staff, and the organization as a whole should be considered. With the evaluation of an EBP innovation, the research process begins again.

Research-Related Roles and Responsibilities for Nurses

In today's EBP environment, all nurses, regardless of their educational preparation, need to be able to assume two research-related roles: that of research consumer and research team member.

Research Consumer

Being a research consumer means routinely searching and reading the current research literature in order to stay current with new insights in client experiences and nursing and medical interventions. Two skills are fundamental to this role: locating relevant literature and critiquing research reports.

LOCATING RESEARCH LITERATURE

Increasingly, policies and procedures used in hospitals and other healthcare settings are evidence based, meaning that nurses who develop such documents must be familiar

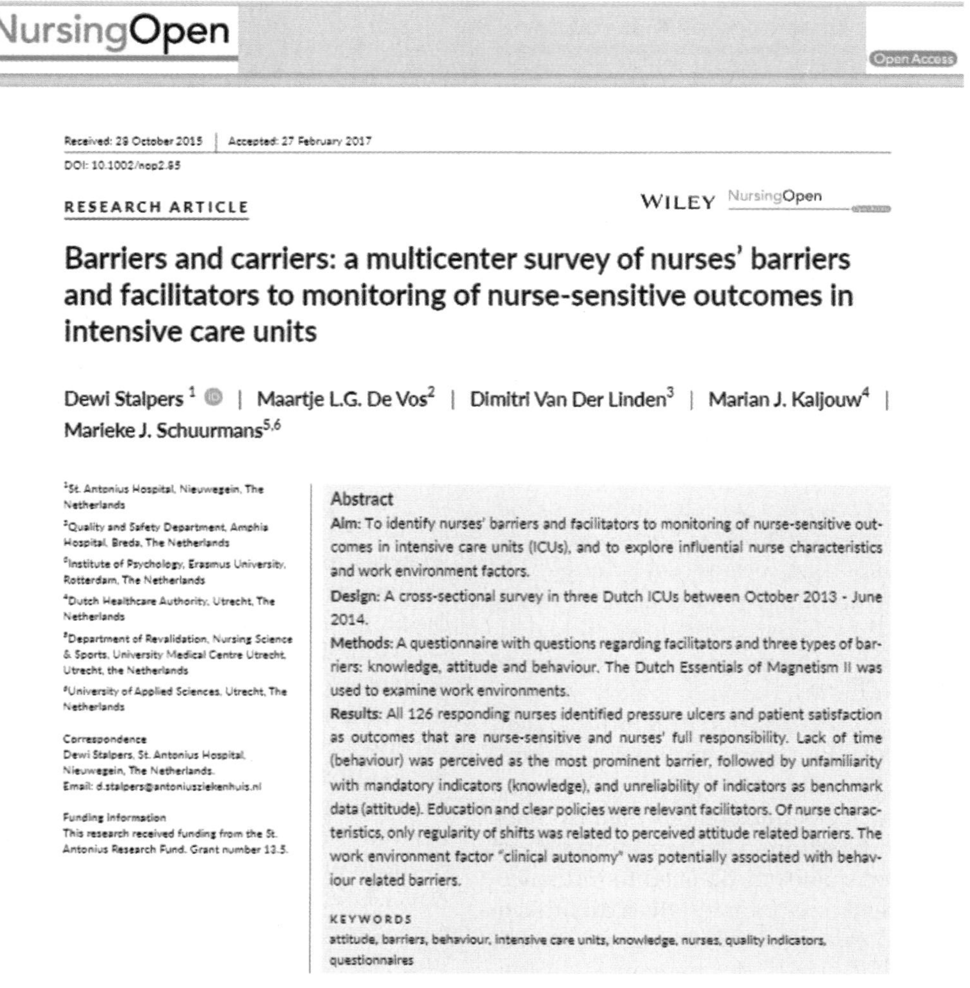

NursingOpen
Open Access

Received: 29 October 2015 | Accepted: 27 February 2017
DOI: 10.1002/nop2.85

RESEARCH ARTICLE

WILEY NursingOpen

Barriers and carriers: a multicenter survey of nurses' barriers and facilitators to monitoring of nurse-sensitive outcomes in intensive care units

Dewi Stalpers [1] | Maartje L.G. De Vos[2] | Dimitri Van Der Linden[3] | Marian J. Kaljouw[4] | Marieke J. Schuurmans[5,6]

[1]St. Antonius Hospital, Nieuwegein, The Netherlands
[2]Quality and Safety Department, Amphia Hospital, Breda, The Netherlands
[3]Institute of Psychology, Erasmus University, Rotterdam, The Netherlands
[4]Dutch Healthcare Authority, Utrecht, The Netherlands
[5]Department of Revalidation, Nursing Science & Sports, University Medical Centre Utrecht, Utrecht, the Netherlands
[6]University of Applied Sciences, Utrecht, The Netherlands

Correspondence
Dewi Stalpers, St. Antonius Hospital, Nieuwegein, The Netherlands.
Email: d.stalpers@antoniusziekenhuis.nl

Funding Information
This research received funding from the St. Antonius Research Fund. Grant number 13.5.

Abstract

Aim: To identify nurses' barriers and facilitators to monitoring of nurse-sensitive outcomes in intensive care units (ICUs), and to explore influential nurse characteristics and work environment factors.

Design: A cross-sectional survey in three Dutch ICUs between October 2013 - June 2014.

Methods: A questionnaire with questions regarding facilitators and three types of barriers: knowledge, attitude and behaviour. The Dutch Essentials of Magnetism II was used to examine work environments.

Results: All 126 responding nurses identified pressure ulcers and patient satisfaction as outcomes that are nurse-sensitive and nurses' full responsibility. Lack of time (behaviour) was perceived as the most prominent barrier, followed by unfamiliarity with mandatory indicators (knowledge), and unreliability of indicators as benchmark data (attitude). Education and clear policies were relevant facilitators. Of nurse characteristics, only regularity of shifts was related to perceived attitude related barriers. The work environment factor "clinical autonomy" was potentially associated with behaviour related barriers.

KEYWORDS
attitude, barriers, behaviour, intensive care units, knowledge, nurses, quality indicators, questionnaires

Figure 2.2 ■ Example of a structured abstract for a nursing research article.
Research article abstract from Nursing Open © 2017 The Authors. Nursing Open published by John Wiley & Sons Ltd. http://onlinelibrary.wiley.com/doi/10.1002/nop2.85/epdf

with the current evidence as it is presented in a variety of information sources. Searching the current information on a specific topic can be overwhelming. Because most literature searches are conducted by using key terms to locate information sources that are available through an electronic database, careful planning is important so that the sources identified stand the best chance of being relevant.

Once key terms have been identified, this information can be entered into one of the many health-related electronic databases that are available. The most comprehensive electronic database for nurses is CINAHL (Cumulative Index to Nursing and Allied Health Literature). CINAHL and other useful databases and the type of information they include are listed in Box 2.5. Although many

BOX 2.5 Useful Electronic Databases

Academic Search Premier: An academic multidisciplinary database that provides abstracts and other information for more than 13,600 publications, including full-text access to over 4700 scholarly publications.

CINAHL (Cumulative Index to Nursing and Allied Health Literature): Indexes current nursing and allied health journals and publications dating back to 1937.

ERIC: Provides citations and abstracts from more than 1180 educational and education-related journals.

Health Source: Nursing/Academic Edition: Provides access to full-text scholarly journals focusing on nursing and allied health.

MEDLINE: The U.S. National Library of Medicine's bibliographic database consists of more than 11 million articles from over 4800 indexed titles.

ProQuest: Provides an interdisciplinary index of magazines, newspapers, and scholarly journals.

PsycINFO: Published by the American Psychological Association. Contains more than 2 million citations and summaries of journal articles, book chapters, books, and dissertations, all in the field of psychology, dating as far back as 1840.

PubMed: Provides access to MEDLINE and additional biomedical information resources.

Social Services Abstracts: Abstracts and indexes more than 1300 journals, dissertations, and citations in social work, human services, social welfare, social policy, and community development.

Virginia Henderson Global Nursing e-Repository (Henderson Repository): The only repository solely dedicated to sharing works created by nurses. Open-access, digital academic and clinical scholarship service that freely collects, preserves, and disseminates full-text nursing research and EBP materials.

BOX 2.6 Tips for Conducting a Literature Search

1. Consider the purpose of the review. Is it for your own knowledge, to write a scholarly paper, or to inform a clinical practice change? The answer may influence how many sources you need, whether they need to be peer-reviewed or researched, if you need full text, how recent the sources should be, and other similar variables.
2. Identify keywords you will use to guide your search. Some journals, databases, and search engines identify keywords associated with particular articles.
3. Develop a system to keep track of references you locate so you can find them again when you need them.
4. Consult the reference lists in useful articles.
5. Be flexible and creative. If a keyword does not give many results, consider its synonyms.
6. Ask for help from a librarian!

of these databases are fee based, authors and publishers are moving toward open-access (free full-text) scholarly journals. Tips for conducting a literature search are shared in Box 2.6.

CRITIQUING RESEARCH REPORTS

In addition to locating research literature about current clinical topics and identified clinical problems, nurses must be able to **critique** or critically read and evaluate research articles. A research critique enables the nurse, as a research consumer, to determine whether the findings of a study are of sufficient quality to be used to influence practice decisions. A research critique involves dissecting a study to determine its strengths and weaknesses, its statistical and clinical significance, and the generalizability and applicability of its results. Conducting an effective critique of a research study entails reading it several times. First, scan the article from start to finish to get a general sense of how the study was conducted. Next, focus on the results and discussion sections of the article. A key question that guides the research critique process is "Do the study findings and the researcher's interpretation of these findings make sense in view of how the study was conducted?" This is true for both quantitative and qualitative research studies.

WRITING A REVIEW OF THE LITERATURE

After reading and critiquing the relevant documents, you likely will need to write a summary review of the literature. The length of the review depends on the purpose, such as whether it is part of a manuscript being submitted for publication or it is required for an academic course in school. The review will include an introduction describing the purpose of the review, the issue or problem being investigated, and the method of obtaining the documents reviewed. The main section is the critique of the documents, written logically and objectively so the reader can understand the value of the literature reviewed. The conclusion summarizes the findings, identifies gaps in the literature, and provides direction for further research or use of the findings.

Research Team Member

In addition to being well-informed research consumers, in today's EBP environment, nurses need to be able to function as a member of a research team. This role is particularly important in hospitals that are seeking or wishing to maintain magnet recognition status. Nurses in hospitals with this designation are expected to be involved in research and EBP activities on an ongoing basis. Research priorities were established by the Magnet National Research Agenda Study and include items in the categories of clinical outcomes, client and nurse satisfaction, practice environment, human resources, and financial and material resources (American Nurses Credentialing Center, n.d.). Depending on their individual experience with research, nurses who are working directly with clients can make particularly valuable contributions to research projects, including the following:

- Identifying clinically relevant problems that need to be studied
- Reviewing the literature to provide background information for a study
- Recruiting study participants
- Securing clients' consent to participate in a study
- Designing data collection instruments
- Pilot-testing data collection procedures
- Collecting research data
- Monitoring for adverse effects of study participation
- Implementing research interventions
- Assisting with interpretation of study findings.

A chief responsibility in all of these activities is serving as a client advocate and protecting the rights of clients who are involved in a research study. Unfortunately, there are many historical instances of our failure to advocate for ethical treatment of clients in the conduct of research. Examples include the 40-year-long study of Black men in Alabama in the mid-1900s who were allowed to go untreated for syphilis in order to investigate the progression of the disease, commonly referred to as the Tuskegee study; the 1992 Kennedy Krieger Institute study in which young children were knowingly exposed to lead in their homes; the Havasupai Arizona Indian tribe study where blood drawn to study diabetes was used for additional research regarding genetic tendencies in the population without their permission; and Henrietta Lacks, whose cervical cancer cells were harvested without authorization in 1951 and used to create the first human immortal cell line. The nurse's responsibility to protect clients' rights is discussed in more depth in the following section.

PROTECTING THE RIGHTS OF STUDY PARTICIPANTS

Because nursing research usually involves humans, a major nursing responsibility is to be aware of and to advocate on behalf of clients' rights. Before any research can be started, the researcher must obtain approval from the relevant committee designated to protect human subjects' rights. This includes research that does not require direct participation of the client, involving only access to data about the client. This committee is often called the Institutional Review Board (IRB). The IRB ensures that all clients are informed of and understand the consequences of consenting to serve as research participants (Figure 2.3 ■). The participants' rights to be included in consent are listed in Box 2.7.

The client needs to have enough information to be able to assess whether an appropriate balance exists between the risks and inconvenience of participating in a study and the potential benefits, either to the client or to the development of knowledge that may benefit others.

For many years, adults have been the focus of much healthcare research conducted on human participants. The American Academy of Pediatrics has identified the need to conduct pediatric research so that children can benefit from advances in medical science. At the same time, because children are so vulnerable, extra precautions must be taken to ensure their rights are upheld and they are not harmed. It is critical to have pediatric expertise on panels that review prospective research studies and in research development. All nurses who practice in settings where research is being conducted with humans or who participate in such research play an important role in safeguarding the values discussed next.

Do No Harm The risk of harm to a research subject is exposure to the possibility of injury going beyond everyday situations. The risk can be immediate or delayed and can be physical, emotional, legal, financial, or social in nature. For instance, withholding standard care from a client in labor for the purpose of studying the course of natural childbirth clearly poses a potential physical danger. Risks can also involve psychologic factors such as exposure to stress or anxiety, or social factors, such as loss of confidentiality or loss of privacy.

Full Disclosure Even though it may be possible to collect research data about a client as part of everyday care without the client's particular knowledge or consent, to do so is considered unethical. Full disclosure, the act of making clear the client's role in a research situation, is a basic right. This means that deception, by either withholding information about a client's participation in a study or giving the client false or misleading information about what participating in the study will involve, must not occur.

Self-Determination Many clients feel pressured to participate in studies. They believe that they must please the physicians and nurses who are responsible for their treatment and care. The right to self-determination means that participants should feel free from constraints, coercion, or any undue influence to participate in a study. Hidden inducements—for instance, suggesting to potential participants that by taking part in the study they might become famous, make an important contribution to science, or receive special attention—must be strictly avoided.

Privacy Privacy enables a client to participate without worrying about later embarrassment. The anonymity of a study participant must be ensured even if the investigator cannot link a specific person to the information reported.

BOX 2.7 Sample Medical Research Patient's Bill of Rights

California law, under Health and Safety Code 24172, requires that any person asked to serve as a participant in research involving a medical experiment, or any person asked to consent to such participation on behalf of another, is entitled to receive the following list of rights written in a language in which the individual is fluent. This list includes the right to:

a. Be informed of the nature and purpose of the experiment.
b. Be given an explanation of the procedures to be followed in the medical experiment, and any drug or device to be utilized.
c. Be given a description of any attendant discomforts and risks reasonably to be expected from the experiment.
d. Be given an explanation of any benefits to the subject reasonably to be expected from the experiment, if applicable.
e. Be given a disclosure of any appropriate alternative procedures, drugs, or devices that might be advantageous to the subject, and their relative risks and benefits.
f. Be informed of the avenues of medical treatment, if any, available to the subject after the experiment if complications should arise.
g. Be given an opportunity to ask any questions concerning the experiment or the procedures involved.
h. Be instructed that consent to participate in the medical experiment may be withdrawn at any time and the subject may discontinue participation in the medical experiment without prejudice.
i. Be given a copy of the signed and dated written consent form.
j. Be given the opportunity to decide to consent or not to consent to a medical experiment without the intervention of any element of force, fraud, deceit, duress, coercion, or undue influence on the subject's decision.

California Health & Safety Code 24172. Retrieved from https://oag.ca.gov/sites/all/files/agweb/pdfs/research/safety_24172.pdf?

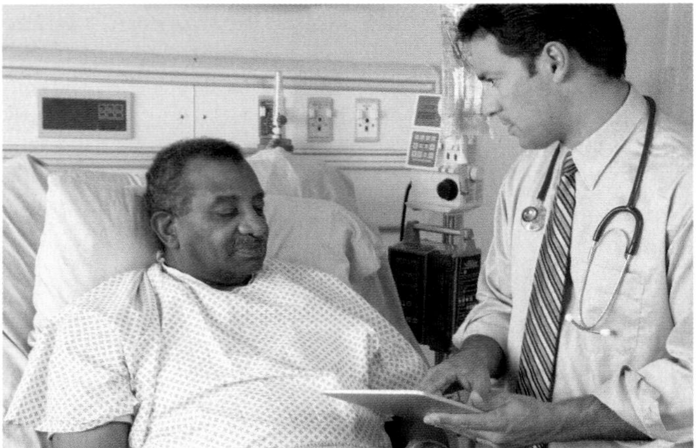

Figure 2.3 ■ It is important for clients to be fully informed before they participate in a research study.
Shutterstock.

Confidentiality means that any information a participant relates will not be made public or available to others without the participant's consent. Investigators must inform research participants about the laws (such as the Privacy and Security Rules of the Health Insurance Portability and Accountability Act of 1996 [HIPAA]) and measures that provide for these rights. Such measures may include the use of pseudonyms or code numbers or reporting only aggregate or group data in published research.

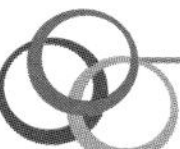

Critical Thinking Checkpoint

Imagine that you have read a research report that found a new type of mattress overlay reduced the incidence of skin breakdown by 25%. Before you recommend that your agency purchase these overlays:

1. What other aspects of the research study should be carefully examined?
2. How would other aspects of EBP be brought into this situation?
3. What additional aspects would you take into consideration?

Answers to Critical Thinking Checkpoint questions are available on the faculty resources site. Please consult with your instructor.

Chapter 2 Review

CHAPTER HIGHLIGHTS

- Evidence-based practice, or evidence-based nursing, involves clinical decision making using a variety of sources of evidence modified for use in specific settings and for individual clients.
- Change in practice requires assessing the need for change; locating and analyzing the best evidence; designing, implementing, and evaluating the practice change; and integrating and maintaining the change.
- Some nurses believe that research should not be the sole or primary source of evidence for practice because it may differ greatly from the real world of practice, limits creativity, does not adequately consider meaning and significance to clients, and has not been demonstrated to be cost effective.
- Nursing research began in North America in the early 1900s. Since that time, the concept of research has been introduced into nursing education programs, research journals in nursing have been developed, and the National Institute for Nursing Research has been established.
- Nurses use both quantitative and qualitative approaches to address issues of concern for client care. Quantitative studies are reported using descriptive and analytical statistics, and qualitative studies are reported in narrative format.
- In today's EBP environment, all nurses need to be well-informed consumers of research and able to serve as effective research team members.
- A key responsibility for nurses who are assisting on a research team is to protect the rights of clients who are participating in the study.

TEST YOUR KNOWLEDGE

1. Which of the following is the lowest level of "best evidence" for evidence-based practice?
   1. Clinical experiences
   2. Opinions of experts
   3. Client values and preferences
   4. Trial and error

2. A nurse researcher is testing the effects of a new dressing preparation on certain participants while continuing to use older and more familiar products on others. Which type of research design is this an example of?
   1. Quasi-experimental
   2. Experimental
   3. Nonexperimental
   4. Pilot study

3. A qualitative research approach is most appropriate for which study?
   1. A study measuring nutrition and weight loss or gain in clients with cancer
   2. A study examining oxygen levels after endotracheal suctioning
   3. A study examining client reactions to stress after open heart surgery
   4. A study measuring differences in blood pressure before, during, and after a procedure

4. A key function of a study's methodology is to
   1. Determine the hypotheses that will be tested in the study.
   2. Exercise control over contaminating factors in the study environment.
   3. Identify grants and other funding sources for conducting the study.
   4. Protect the rights of the study's participants.

5. In the PICO format for phrasing research questions and identifying key terms for a literature search, what does the *P* stand for?
1. Patterns
2. Population
3. Probability
4. Purpose

6. A nurse practitioner believes it is important to participate in nursing research. Which activity is most appropriate for this nurse's level of education and position?
1. Helping to identify clinical problems in direct client care
2. Using research findings to develop policies and procedures
3. Critically analyzing and interpreting research for application to practice
4. Participating in data collection

7. A nurse researcher is considering the use of various nonpharmacological distraction techniques that have shown success for behavior control in troubled adolescents. Which of the following criterion is this researcher considering?
1. Significance
2. Researchability
3. Feasibility
4. Interest

8. An 85-year-old client in a nursing home tells a nurse, "Because the doctor was so insistent, I signed the papers for that research study. Also, I was afraid he would not continue taking care of me." Which client right is being violated?
1. Right not to be harmed
2. Right to full disclosure
3. Right to privacy and confidentiality
4. Right to self-determination

9. Place each of the following steps of evidence-based practice change in their usual sequence.
1. _____ Locate the best evidence.
2. _____ Ask the clinical question.
3. _____ Assess the need for change.
4. _____ Integrate the change with client preferences.
5. _____ Analyze the evidence.
6. _____ Implement and evaluate the change.

10. A nurse proposes that the hospital apply the findings from a recent research study that shows that clients appreciate classical orchestra music and playing it frequently lowers clients' blood pressure. Which aspect of research suggests that it may not be appropriate to implement this as evidence-based practice?
1. All research is flawed.
2. The research would not have taken into consideration the cost of acquiring and playing the music in a hospital.
3. One study would not be sufficient to show that all clients would find orchestral music pleasing.
4. Research cannot demonstrate clients' appreciation of music since research is only appropriate for physiologic problems.

See Answers to Test Your Knowledge in Appendix A.

READINGS AND REFERENCES

Suggested Reading

DiNapoli, P. P. (2016). Implementation science: A framework for integrating evidence-based practice. *American Nurse Today*, *11*(7), 40–41.
This article defines implementation science and describes the stages of the implementation process. Understanding the drivers that support or inhibit application of evidence to practice is essential if change is to be successful.

Related Research

Scala, E., Price, C., & Day, J. (2016). An integrative review of engaging clinical nurses in nursing research. *Journal of Nursing Scholarship*, *48*, 423–430. doi:10.1111/jnu.12223

Tam, W. W. S., Lo, K. K. H., Khalechelvam, P., Seah, J., & Goh, S. Y. S. (2017). Is the information of systematic reviews published in nursing journals up-to-date? A cross-sectional study. *BMC Medical Research Methodology*, *17*, 1–9. doi:10.1186/s12874-017-0432-3

References

Allen, E., Williams, A., Jennings, J., Stomski, N., Goucke, R., Toye, C., . . . McCullough, K. (2018). Revisiting the pain resource nurse role in sustaining evidence-based practice changes for pain assessment and management. *Worldviews on Evidence-Based Nursing*, *15*, 368–376. doi:10.1111/wvn.12318

American Association of Colleges of Nursing. (2006). *AACN position statement on nursing research*. Washington, DC: Author.

American Nurses Association. (2015). *Nursing: Scope and standards of practice* (3rd ed.). Silver Spring, MD: Author.

American Nurses Credentialing Center. (n.d.). *National magnet research priorities*. Retrieved from https://www.nursingworld.org/organizational-programs/magnet/program-resources/research-materials/

Avşar, P., & Karadağ, A. (2018). Efficacy and cost-effectiveness analysis of evidence-based nursing interventions to maintain tissue integrity to prevent pressure ulcers and incontinence-associated dermatitis. *Worldviews on Evidence-Based Nursing*, *15*, 54–61. doi:10.1111/wvn.12264

Buckwalter, K. C., Cullen, L., Hanrahan, K., Kleiber, C., McCarthy, A. M., Rakel, B., . . . Tucker, S. (2017). Iowa Model of evidence-based practice: Revisions and validation. *Worldviews on Evidence-Based Nursing*, *14*, 175–182. doi:10.1111/wvn.12223

Cronenwett, L., Sherwood, G., Barnsteiner, J., Disch, J., Johnson, J., Mitchell, P., . . . Warren, J. (2007). Quality and safety education for nurses. *Nursing Outlook*, *55*, 122–131. doi:10.1016/j.outlook.2007.02.006

Dang, D., & Dearholt, S. L. (2017). *Johns Hopkins nursing evidence-based practice: Model and guidelines* (3rd ed.). Indianapolis, IN: Sigma Theta Tau International.

Edwards, N. C., & Higuchi, K. S. (2018). Process evaluation of a participatory, multimodal intervention to improve evidence-based care in long-term care settings. *Worldviews on Evidence-Based Nursing*, *15*, 361–367. doi:10.1111/wvn.12313

Hurley, L., O'Donnell, M., O'Caoimh, R., Dinneen, S. F. (2017). Investigating the management of diabetes in nursing homes using a mixed methods approach. *Diabetes Research and Clinical Practice*, *127*, 156–162. doi:10.1016/j.diabres.2017.03.010

Melnyk, B. M., & Fineout-Overholt, B. (2019). *Evidence-based practice in nursing and healthcare: A guide to best practice* (4th ed.). Philadelphia, PA: Wolters Kluwer.

National Institute of Nursing Research, National Institutes of Health. (2016). *The NINR strategic plan: Advancing science, improving lives* (NIH Publication No. 16-NR-7783). Retrieved from https://www.ninr.nih.gov/sites/files/docs/NINR_StratPlan2016_reduced.pdf

Stetler, C. B. (2010). Stetler model. In J. Rycroft-Malone & T. Bucknall (Eds.). *Models and frameworks for implementing evidence-based practice: Linking evidence to action*. Oxford, United Kingdom: Wiley-Blackwell.

Stevens, K. R. (2012). *Star model of EBP: Knowledge transformation*. Academic Center for Evidence-based Practice. The University of Texas Health Science Center at San Antonio. Retrieved from http://nursing.uthscsa.edu/onrs/starmodel/star-model.asp

Selected Bibliography

Boswell, C., & Cannon, S. (2020). *Introduction to nursing research: Incorporating evidence-based practice* (5th ed.). Burlington, MA: Jones & Bartlett.

Brown, S. J. (2017). *Evidence-based nursing: The research–practice connection* (4th ed.). Burlington, MA: Jones & Bartlett.

Cronin, P., Coughlan, M., & Smith, V. (2015). *Understanding nursing and healthcare research*. Los Angeles, CA: Sage.

Gray, J. R., Grove, S. K., & Sutherland, S. (2017). *Burns & Grove's the practice of nursing research: Appraisal, synthesis, and generation of evidence* (8th ed.). St. Louis, MO: Elsevier.

Polit, D. F., & Beck, C. T. (2016). *Nursing research: Generating and assessing evidence for nursing practice* (10th ed.). Philadelphia, PA: Wolters Kluwer.

Schmidt, N. A., & Brown, J. M. (2018). *Evidence-based practice for nurses: Appraisal and application of research* (4th ed.). Sudbury, MA: Jones & Bartlett.

Sherwood, G., & Barnsteiner, J. (Eds.). (2017). *Quality and safety in nursing: A competency approach to improving outcomes* (2nd ed.). Hoboken, NJ: John Wiley & Sons.

Surbhi, S. (2016). *Difference between qualitative and quantitative research.* Retrieved from http://keydifferences.com/difference-between-qualitative-and-quantitative-research.html

Legal Aspects of Nursing 3

LEARNING OUTCOMES

After completing this chapter, you will be able to:

1. List sources of law and types of laws.
2. Describe ways nurse practice acts, credentialing, standards of care, and agency policies and procedures affect the scope of nursing practice.
3. Compare and contrast the state-based licensure model and the enhanced nurse licensure compact for multistate licensure.
4. Describe the purpose and essential elements of informed consent.
5. Describe the purpose of the Americans with Disabilities Act.
6. Discuss substance use disorder in nursing and available alternative-to-discipline or peer assistance programs.
7. Recognize the nurse's legal responsibilities with selected aspects of nursing practice.
8. Discriminate between negligence and professional negligence or malpractice.
9. Delineate the elements of professional negligence.
10. Compare and contrast intentional torts (assault and battery, false imprisonment, invasion of privacy, defamation) and unintentional torts (professional negligence).
11. Describe the four specific areas of the Health Insurance Portability and Accountability Act and their impact on nursing practice.
12. Discuss the benefits and consequences of participating in social media.
13. Describe the laws and strategies that protect the nurse from litigation.
14. Discuss the legal responsibilities of nursing students.

KEY TERMS

advance healthcare directives, *79*
answer, *67*
assault, *85*
autopsy, *81*
battery, *85*
breach of duty, *83*
burden of proof, *67*
causation, *83*
civil actions, *67*
civil law, *66*
common law, *66*
complaint, *67*
contract, *70*
contract law, *67*
contractual obligations, *71*
contractual relationships, *71*
coroner, *82*
credentialing, *69*
crime, *83*
criminal actions, *67*
criminal law, *66*
damages, *83*
decision, *67*
defamation, *86*
defendants, *67*
delegation, *76*
discovery, *67*
do not resuscitate (DNR), *81*
duty, *83*
Enhanced Nurse Licensure Compact (eNLC), *69*
euthanasia, *81*
expert witness, *67*
express consent, *73*
false imprisonment, *86*
felony, *83*
foreseeability, *83*
gross negligence, *83*
harm, *83*
healthcare proxy, *79*
implied consent, *73*
implied contract, *71*
informed consent, *72*
injury, *83*
inquest, *82*
invasion of privacy, *86*
law, *65*
liability, *71*
libel, *86*
license, *69*
litigation, *67*
living will, *79*
malpractice, *83*
mandated reporters, *77*
manslaughter, *83*
medical examiner, *82*
misdemeanor, *83*
mutual recognition model, *69*
negligence, *83*
Nurse Licensure Compact (NLC), *69*
plaintiff, *67*
postmortem examination, *81*
private law, *66*
public law, *66*
res ipsa loquitur, *84*
respondeat superior, *71*
responsibility, *72*
right, *72*
shared medical decision making, *73*
slander, *86*
standards of care, *70*
statutory laws, *66*
strike, *72*
substance use disorder (SUD), *77*
tort, *83*
tort law, *67*
trial, *67*
unprofessional conduct, *88*
verdict, *67*

Introduction

Nursing practice is governed by many legal concepts. It is important for nurses to know the basics of legal concepts, because nurses are accountable for their professional judgments and actions. Accountability is an essential concept of professional nursing practice and the law. Knowledge of laws that regulate and affect nursing practice is needed for two reasons:

1. To ensure that the nurse's decisions and actions are consistent with current legal principles
2. To protect the nurse from liability.

General Legal Concepts

Law can be defined as "the sum total of rules and regulations by which a society is governed. As such, law is created by people and exists to regulate all persons" (Guido, 2020, p. 2).

Functions of the Law in Nursing

The law serves a number of functions in nursing:

- It provides a framework for establishing which nursing actions in the care of clients are legal.
- It differentiates the nurse's responsibilities from those of other health professionals.
- It helps establish the boundaries of independent nursing action.
- It assists in maintaining a standard of nursing practice by making nurses accountable under the law.

Sources of Law

Nursing derives its legal basis from several sources. This legal basis differs among countries, mostly depending on the nature and structure of their laws. Regardless of the differences, legal frameworks regulate the practice of the profession. Figure 3.1 ■ provides an overview of the primary sources of law (i.e., how laws are created): constitutions, statutes, administrative agencies, and decisions of courts (common law).

Constitutional Law

A constitution is a collection of statements that embodies the fundamental principles and ideals of a country. It defines the basic rights of its citizens, describes the structures and processes of government organizations, and guides social order. Countries that have a constitution (e.g., the United States, India, the Philippines, South Africa, Italy, and France) consider it the highest set of laws. All legislation, including those governing the practice of nursing, should align with the principles of that country's constitution for them to possess a legal basis.

Legislation (Statutory Law)

Laws enacted by any legislative body are called **statutory laws**. Statutory laws are superior to local or administrative laws. In some countries, such as the United States and the Philippines, nursing practices are regulated by state laws. In other countries, nursing practices are regulated by secondary legislative bodies authorized by other legislative bodies. For example, in the United Kingdom, the Nursing and Midwifery Council, mandated by the Parliament's Health Act 1999, regulates nursing practices.

Clinical Alert!

It is important for nurses to keep their legislators informed about nursing because it is the legislature that passes laws that affect nursing practice.

Administrative Law

When a state legislature passes a statute, an administrative agency is given the authority to create rules and regulations to enforce the statutory laws. For example, state boards of nursing write rules and regulations to implement and enforce a nurse practice act, which was created through statutory law.

Common Law

Laws evolving from court decisions are referred to as **common law**. In addition to interpreting and applying constitutional or statutory law, courts also are asked to resolve disputes between two parties. Common law is continually being adapted and expanded. In deciding specific controversies, courts generally adhere to the doctrine of *stare decisis*—"to stand by things decided"—usually referred to as "following precedent." In other words, to arrive at a ruling in a particular case, the court applies the same rules and principles applied in previous, similar cases.

Types of Laws

Laws can be further classified into different types. The two main types are public law and private or civil law.

Public law refers to the body of law that deals with relationships between individuals and the government and governmental agencies. An important segment of public law is **criminal law**, which deals with actions against the safety and welfare of the public. Examples are homicide, manslaughter, and theft. Crimes can be classified as either felonies or misdemeanors, which are described in more detail later in this chapter.

Private law, or **civil law**, is the body of law that deals with relationships among private individuals. It can be

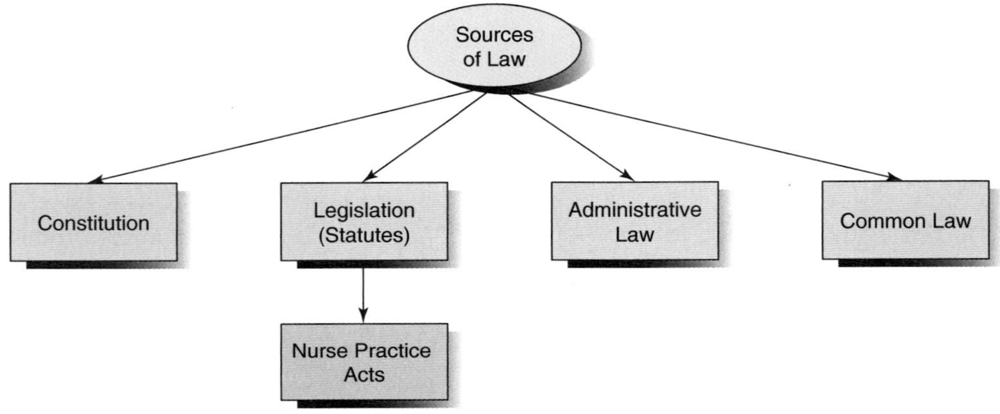

Figure 3.1 ■ Overview of sources of law.

categorized into a variety of legal specialties such as contract law and tort law. **Contract law** involves the enforcement of agreements among private individuals or the payment of compensation for failure to fulfill agreements. **Tort law** defines and enforces duties and rights among private individuals that are not based on contractual agreements. Some examples of tort laws applicable to nurses are professional negligence, invasion of privacy, and assault and battery, which are discussed in more detail later in this chapter. See Table 3.1 for selected categories of law affecting nurses in the United States.

Kinds of Legal Actions

There are two kinds of legal actions: civil or private actions and criminal actions. **Civil actions** deal with the relationships among individuals in society; for example, a man may file a suit against an individual who he believes cheated him. Civil actions that are of concern to nurses in the United States include the torts and contracts listed in Table 3.1. **Criminal actions** deal with disputes between an individual and society as a whole; for example, if a man shoots an individual, society brings him to trial. The major difference between civil and criminal law is the potential outcome for the defendant. If found guilty in a civil action, such as professional negligence, the defendant will have to pay a sum of money. If found guilty in a criminal action, the defendant may lose money, be jailed, or be executed and, if a nurse, could lose his or her license. The action of a lawsuit is called **litigation**, and lawyers who participate in lawsuits may be referred to as litigators.

TABLE 3.1 Selected Categories of Laws Affecting Nurses

Category	Examples
Constitutional	Due process Equal protection
Statutory (legislative)	Nurse practice acts Good Samaritan acts Child and adult abuse laws Living wills Sexual harassment laws Americans with Disabilities Act
Criminal (public)	Homicide, manslaughter Theft Arson Active euthanasia Sexual assault Illegal possession of controlled drugs
Contracts (private/civil)	Nurse and client Nurse and employer Nurse and insurance Client and agency
Torts (private/civil)	Professional negligence or malpractice Libel and slander Invasion of privacy Assault and battery False imprisonment Abandonment

The Civil Judicial Process

The judicial process primarily functions to settle disputes peacefully and in accordance with the law. A lawsuit has strict procedural rules. There are generally five steps:

1. A document, called a **complaint**, is filed by an individual referred to as the **plaintiff**, who claims that his or her legal rights have been infringed on by one or more other individuals or entities, referred to as **defendants**.
2. A written response, called an **answer**, is made by the defendants.
3. Both parties engage in pretrial activities, referred to as **discovery**, in an effort to obtain all the facts of the situation.
4. In the **trial** of the case, all relevant facts are presented to a judge or to a jury.
5. The judge renders a **decision**, or the jury renders a **verdict**. If the outcome is not acceptable to one of the parties, an appeal can be made for another trial.

During a trial, a plaintiff must offer evidence of the defendant's wrongdoing. This duty to prove an assertion of wrongdoing is called the **burden of proof**. See Figure 3.2 ■ for a diagram of the judicial process in the United States.

Nurses as Witnesses

A nurse may be called to testify in a legal action. It is advisable that any nurse who is asked to testify in such a situation seek the advice of an attorney before providing testimony. In most cases, the attorney for the nurse's employer will provide support and counsel during the legal case. If the nurse is the defendant, however, the nurse should retain his or her own attorney to protect the nurse's interests.

A nurse may also be asked to provide testimony as an expert witness. An **expert witness** has special training, experience, or skill in a relevant area and is allowed by the court to offer an opinion on some issue within his or her area of expertise. The nurse's credentials and expertise help a judge or jury understand the appropriate standard of care. The nurse expert, thus, has the ability to analyze the facts or evidence and draw inferences. For example, the nurse expert may offer an opinion on whether or not a particular standard of care was met.

Regulation of Nursing Practice

Protection of the public is the legal purpose for defining the scope of nursing practice, licensing requirements, and standards of care. Nurses who know and follow their nurse practice act and standards of care provide safe, competent nursing care.

Nurse Practice Acts

In the United States, each state has a nurse practice act, which protects the public by legally defining and

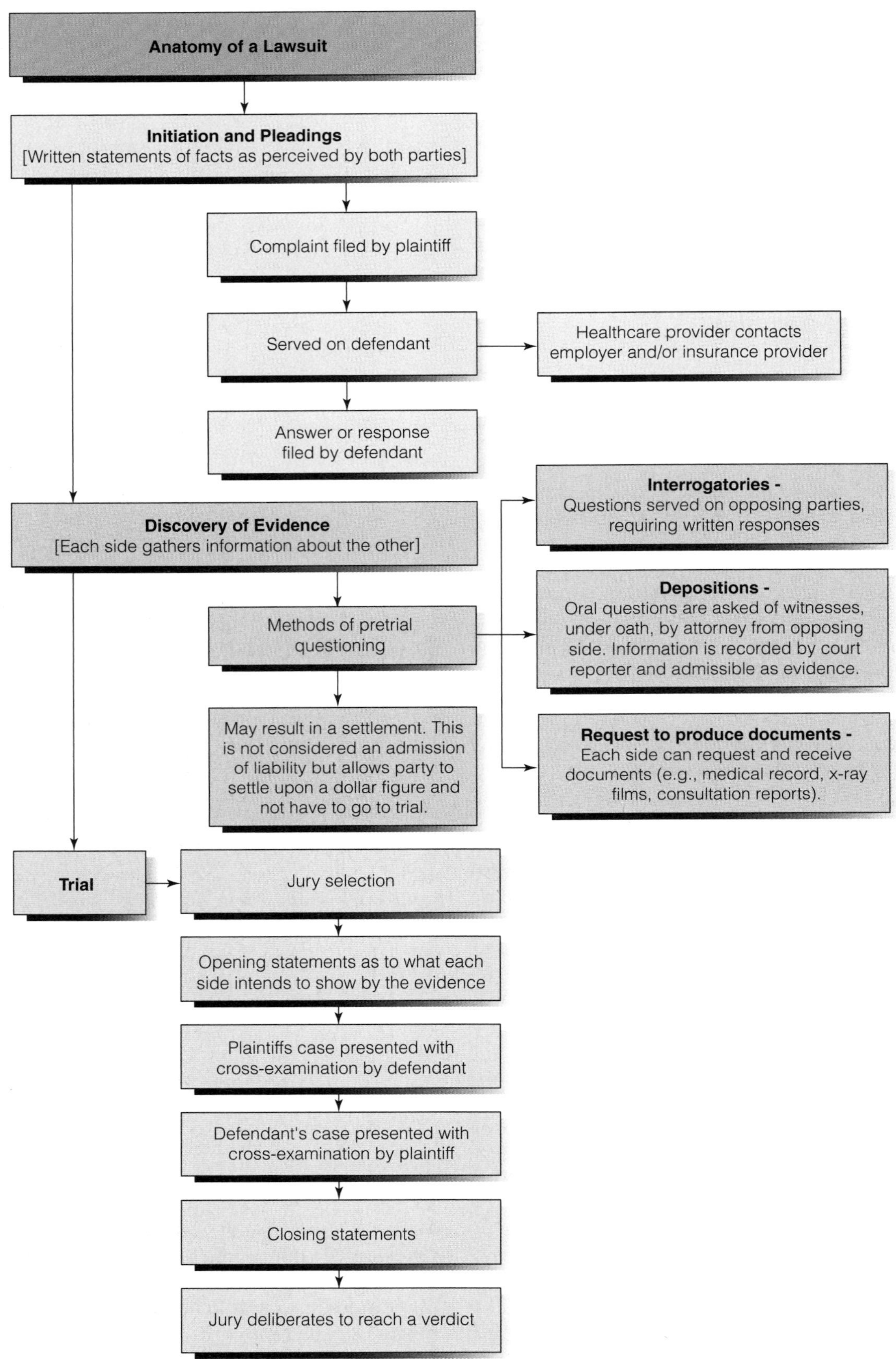

Figure 3.2 ■ Anatomy of a lawsuit.
Adapted from *Legal and Ethical Issues in Nursing*, 7th ed. (pp. 16–24), by G. W. Guido, 2020, Upper Saddle River, NJ: Pearson Education, Inc.

describing the *scope of nursing practice*. State nurse practice acts also legally control nursing practice through licensing requirements. For advanced nursing practice, many states require a different license or have an additional clause that pertains to actions that may be performed only by nurses with advanced education. For example, an additional license may be required to practice as a nurse midwife, nurse anesthetist, or nurse practitioner. The advanced practice nurse also requires a license to prescribe medication or order treatments from physical therapists or other health professionals.

Nurse practice acts, although similar, do differ from state to state. For example, they may differ in their scope of practice definition and in licensing and license renewal requirements. It is the nurse's responsibility to know the nurse practice act of the state in which he or she practices nursing. A state's nurse practice act is easily accessed at the specific state board of nursing's website.

Credentialing

Credentialing is the process of determining and maintaining competence in nursing practice. The credentialing process is one way in which the nursing profession maintains standards of practice and accountability for the educational preparation of its members. Credentialing includes licensure, certification, and accreditation.

Licensure

A **license** is a legal permit that a government agency grants to individuals to engage in the practice of a profession and to use a particular title. Licensure is the process by which this permit is granted. The methods by which individuals gain a license differ across countries. In Australia, Canada, and the United States, applicants need to qualify in an examination that aims to assess whether applicants' levels of knowledge and competence meet the standards required to obtain the license. In other countries, such as Nepal, Mexico, and the United Kingdom, where there are no licensure examinations, student nurses are supervised and assessed during their clinical placements, and they gain the permit to practice nursing upon graduating.

Regardless of the method of licensure, all nurses who obtain a license are included in a register. In the United Kingdom, the "license" is more commonly known as registration. Professional bodies that maintain the register of licensed nurses, such as the Nursing and Midwifery Council, nursing state boards, and the Board of Nursing, stipulate and enforce the standards required for obtaining and retaining the place in the register. This is to ensure that only those nurses who are found to be competent to apply for or hold a license are allowed to practice nursing.

Licensures exist primarily to protect the public's welfare. Nurses can lose their license if, for example, they become criminally liable, they engage in immoral and illegal activities, they falsify documents that enabled them to apply for the license, or their behavior and competence drop below nationally accepted standards. In the United Kingdom, a process called fitness to practice (Box 3.1) exists to hear cases of nurses who are found to be remiss in maintaining the standards required for their continued registration.

Nurses have the option of working wherever their license is valid. Most licenses are valid at a national level (i.e., a nurse with a license in the Philippines can work anywhere in the Philippines). However, the practice can be different in some countries where licensure for nurses is state based; that is, the state's board of nursing has licensed all nurses practicing in the state. For instance, previously in the United States, each state had autonomy in setting nursing practice standards for registration within their jurisdictions, and nurses wishing to practice in multiple states had to apply for separate licenses. Later, the National Council of State Boards of Nursing (NCSBN) developed a new regulatory model named the **mutual recognition model**, which allows for multistate licensure. With mutual recognition, a nurse who is not under any disciplinary action can practice in person or electronically across state lines under one license. For example, a nurse who lives on the border of a state can practice in both states under one license if the adjoining states have an interstate compact.

An interstate compact called the **Nurse Licensure Compact (NLC)** (an agreement between two or more states) is the mechanism used to create mutual recognition among states in the United States. However, the NCSBN, influenced by the growing need for clarification of practice for all nurses engaged in telenursing, had previously been working to revise the NLC. As a result, in May 2015, significant revisions were made to the original NLC resulting in new model legislation. The **Enhanced Nurse Licensure Compact (eNLC)** is an updated version of the original NLC. The major difference between the NLC and the eNLC is the addition of the Uniform Licensure Requirements, which includes licensure qualifications, education qualifications, English proficiency, successful NCLEX-RN or NCLEX-PN examination, criminal background check, no misdemeanor or felony offense, not enrolled in an alternative program, and a valid U.S. social security number. The eNLC allows all RNs and LPNs to have one multistate license, with the ability to practice in both their home state and all other compact states. As of January 2019, 31 state legislatures have adopted eNLC.

Nurses can also work in other territories and countries in addition to their usual place of residence. However, because of the differences in qualifications required by each country, nurses have to fulfil all criteria stated by that country in order to obtain a license to practice there. Some countries like the United States, Canada, the United Kingdom, Australia, and Saudi Arabia may require overseas nurses to complete a course, pass a structured examination, pass a clinical examination, and meet equivalent minimum educational requirements. On top of this, a nurse intending to work in another country or territory will have to meet the immigration requirements of that country in order to obtain and keep the license. Such variations impact the ways in which national nursing boards and councils regulate the nursing profession within and across borders.

BOX 3.1 Fitness to Practice

Fitness to Practice (FtP) is the process by which the Nursing and Midwifery Council (NMC) in the United Kingdom ensures that nurses and midwives remain competent and have the right knowledge, skills, and character to practice within their roles without endangering public health and safety. Negligent nurses are brought before an FtP panel to assess whether their fitness to practice is impaired or not. Allegations investigated by the FtP panel are

- Misconduct
- Lack of competence
- Insufficient knowledge of English
- Criminal behavior
- Serious ill health

From https://www.nmc.org.uk/concerns-nurses-midwives/dealing-concerns/what-is-fitness-to-practise/.

Certification

Certification is the voluntary practice of validating that an individual nurse has met minimum standards of nursing competence in specialty areas such as maternal–child health, pediatrics, mental health, gerontology, and school nursing. In the United States, national certification may be required to become licensed as an advanced practice nurse. Certification programs are conducted by the American Nurses Association (ANA) and by specialty nursing organizations.

Accreditation and Approval of Basic Nursing Education Programs

Approval of nursing education programs offered by colleges and universities entails ensuring that the contents, methods of teaching, methods of assessing and evaluating students' progress, and overall curricular design meet nationally set standards. Accreditation, on the other hand, is a process to evaluate whether a nursing education program maintains the level of quality, determined by current evidence and policies, set by the accrediting body.

In countries like Denmark, Ireland, and Taiwan, the professional body that sets the standards for competence is separate from the regulatory authority, but in principle, the two institutions work in agreement with each other. In some other countries, the professional body that sets the standards for licensure also regulates the standards required to approve nursing education programs. This is to ensure that the way in which the program is run and the standards by which students are evaluated upon completing the program align with the legally and socially acceptable requirements to grant nurses licenses.

Standards of Care

The purpose of standards of care is to protect the public. **Standards of care** are the "skills and learning commonly possessed by members of a profession" (Guido, 2020, p. 53). These standards are used to evaluate the quality of care nurses provide and, therefore, become legal guidelines for nursing practice in the United States (Box 3.2).

BOX 3.2 Court Case Example: Expert Witnesses on Standards of Care

An emergency department (ED) nurse administered an injection of Demerol and Vistaril, per MD order, to a client complaining of chest pain. The client claimed inability to work for several weeks after the injection because of hip pain and a lump at the injection site. Two months later, a neurologist diagnosed cutaneous gluteal neuropathy. The client sued the ED nurse who gave the injection and her employer, the hospital alleging the nurse injured the client by administering the injection in a substandard manner.

The nurse admitted to failing to chart the site and mode of the injection she administered. The nurse's testimony of her usual practice for giving an IM reflected correct understanding of how and where to administer an injection. Two physicians testified the client's injury could have been caused by a faulty subcutaneous injection of the drug Vistaril, and a third physician stated that the needle could have hit a nerve due to inaccurate site location for the injection. According to the court, critical testimony came from two nurse expert witnesses who stated that not charting information about the injection was not the professional standard of care. This charting omission convinced the court that the nurse did not administer the IM injection correctly (Pellerin vs. Humedicenters, Inc., 969 So. 2d 590 [La. App., 1997]) (Snyder, 1997, p. 7).

Nursing standards of care can be classified into two categories: internal and external standards. Internal standards of care include "the nurse's job description, education, and expertise as well as an institution's policies and procedures" (Guido, 2020, p. 54).

External standards consist of the following:

- Nurse practice acts
- Professional organizations (e.g., ANA)
- Nursing specialty-practice organizations (e.g., Emergency Nurses Association, Oncology Nursing Society)
- Federal organizations and federal guidelines (e.g., The Joint Commission and Medicare).

It is important, therefore, for nurses to know their institution's policies and procedures and nurse practice act. They also need to remain competent through reading professional journals and attending continuing education and in-service programs. Again, the purpose of knowing and practicing nursing's standards of care is to protect the client and consumer.

Contractual Arrangements in Nursing

A contract is the basis of the relationship between a nurse and an employer—for example, a nurse and a hospital or a nurse and a primary care provider. A **contract** is an agreement between two or more competent individuals, on sufficient consideration (compensation), to do or not to do some lawful act. A contract may be written or oral.

An oral contract is as equally binding as a written contract. The terms of the oral contract, however, may be more difficult to prove in a court of law. A written contract cannot be changed legally by an oral agreement. If two people wish to change some aspect of a written contract, the change must be written into the contract, because one party cannot hold the other to an oral agreement that differs from the written one.

A contract is considered to be *expressed* when the two parties discuss and agree, orally or in writing, to terms and conditions during the creation of the contract. For example, a nurse will work at a hospital for a stated length of time and under stated conditions. An **implied contract** is one that has not been explicitly agreed to by the parties but that the law nevertheless considers to exist. For example, the nurse is expected to be competent and to follow hospital policies and procedures even though these expectations were not written or discussed. Likewise, the hospital is expected to provide the necessary supplies and equipment needed to provide competent nursing care.

A lawful contract requires the following four features (Guido, 2020, p. 306):

1. Promise or agreement between two or more individuals for the performance of an action or restraint from certain actions
2. Mutual understanding of the terms and meaning of the contract
3. A lawful purpose (i.e., the activity must be legal)
4. Compensation in the form of something of value—in most cases, compensation is monetary.

Legal Roles of Nurses

Nurses have three separate, interdependent legal roles, each with rights and associated responsibilities: provider of service, employee or contractor for service, and citizen.

Provider of Service

The nurse is expected to provide safe and competent care. Implicit in this role are several legal concepts: liability, standards of care, and contractual obligations.

Liability is the quality or state of being legally responsible for one's obligations and actions and for making financial restitution for wrongful acts. A nurse, for example, has an obligation to practice and direct the practice of others under the nurse's supervision so that harm or injury to the client is prevented and standards of care are maintained. Even when a nurse carries out treatments ordered by the primary care provider, the responsibility for the nursing activity belongs to the nurse. When a nurse is asked to carry out an activity that the nurse believes will be injurious to the client, the nurse's responsibility is to refuse to carry out the order and report this to the nurse's supervisor.

The standards of care by which a nurse acts or fails to act are legally defined by nurse practice acts and by the rule of reasonable and prudent action—what a reasonable and prudent professional with similar preparation and experience would do in similar circumstances. **Contractual obligations** refer to the nurse's duty of care, that is, duty to render care, established by the presence of an expressed or implied contract.

Employee or Contractor for Service

A nurse who is employed by an agency works as a representative of the agency, and the nurse's contract with clients is an implied one. However, a nurse who is employed directly by a client, for example, a private nurse, may have a written contract with that client in which the nurse agrees to provide professional services for a certain fee. A nurse might be prevented from carrying out the terms of the contract because of illness or death. However, personal inconvenience and personal problems, such as the nurse's car failure, are not legitimate reasons for failing to fulfill a contract.

Contractual relationships vary among practice settings. An independent nurse practitioner is a contractor for service whose contractual relationship with the client is an independent one. The nurse employed by a hospital functions within an employer–employee relationship in which the nurse represents and acts for the hospital and therefore must function within the policies of the employing agency. This type of legal relationship creates the ancient legal doctrine known as ***respondeat superior*** ("let the master answer"). In other words, the master (employer) assumes responsibility for the conduct of the servant (employee) and can also be held responsible for professional negligence by the employee. By virtue of the employee role, therefore, the nurse's conduct is the hospital's responsibility.

This doctrine does not imply that the nurse cannot be held liable as an individual. Nor does it imply that the doctrine will prevail if the employee's actions are extraordinarily inappropriate, that is, beyond those expected or foreseen by the employer. For example, if the nurse hits a client, the employer could disclaim responsibility because this behavior is beyond the bounds of expected behavior. Criminal acts, such as assisting with criminal abortions or taking tranquilizers from a client's supply for personal use, would also be considered extraordinarily inappropriate behavior. Nurses can be held liable for *failure* to act as well. For example, a nurse who sees another nurse consistently performing in an incompetent manner and fails to do anything to protect the client may be considered negligent.

The nurse in the role of employee or contractor for service has obligations to the employer, the client, and other personnel. The nursing care provided must be within the limitations and terms specified. The nurse has an obligation to contract only for those responsibilities that the nurse is competent to discharge. For example, the nurse must practice according to the state's nurse practice act and the policies and procedures of the facility or organization.

The nurse is expected to respect the rights and responsibilities of other healthcare participants. For example, although the nurse has a responsibility to explain nursing activities to a client, the nurse does not have the right to comment on medical practice in a way that disturbs the client or accuses the primary care provider. At the same time, the nurse has the right to expect reasonable and prudent conduct from other health professionals.

Citizen

The rights and responsibilities of the nurse in the role of citizen are the same as those of any individual under the legal system. Rights of citizenship protect clients from harm and ensure consideration for their personal property rights, rights to privacy, confidentiality, and other rights discussed later in this chapter. These same rights apply to nurses.

Nurses move in and out of these roles when carrying out professional and personal responsibilities. An understanding of these roles and the rights and responsibilities associated with them promotes legally responsible conduct and practice by nurses. A **right** is a privilege or fundamental power to which an individual is entitled unless it is revoked by law or given up voluntarily; a **responsibility** is the obligation associated with a right. See Table 3.2 for examples of the responsibilities and rights associated with each role.

Collective Bargaining

Collective bargaining is the formalized decision-making process between representatives of management (employer) and representatives of labor (employee) to negotiate wages and conditions of employment, including work hours, working environment, and fringe benefits of employment (e.g., vacation time, sick leave, and personal leave). Through a written agreement, both management and employees legally commit themselves to observe the terms and conditions of employment.

The collective bargaining process involves the recognition of a certified bargaining agent for the employees. This agent can be a union, a trade association, or a professional organization. The agent represents the employees in negotiating a contract with management. The ANA, through its state constituent associations (e.g., MNA—Michigan Nurses Association), has represented the interests of nurses within individual states in the United States.

When collective bargaining breaks down because an agreement cannot be reached, the employees usually call a strike. A **strike** is an organized work stoppage by a group of employees to express a grievance, enforce a demand for changes in conditions of employment, or solve a dispute with management.

Because nursing practice is a service to people who are often ill or vulnerable, striking presents a moral dilemma to many nurses. Actions taken by nurses can affect the safety of people. When faced with a strike, each nurse must make an individual decision to cross or not to cross a picket line. Nursing students may also be faced with decisions about crossing picket lines in the event of a strike at a clinical agency used for learning experiences. The ANA supports striking as a means of achieving economic and general welfare.

Selected Legal Aspects of Nursing Practice

Nurses need to know and apply legal aspects in their many different roles. For example, as client advocates, nurses ensure the client's right to informed consent or refusal, and they identify and report violent behavior and neglect of vulnerable clients. Legal aspects also include the duty to report the nurse suspected of chemical impairment.

Informed Consent

Informed consent is an agreement by a client to accept a course of treatment or a procedure after being provided complete information, including the benefits and risks of

TABLE 3.2 Legal Roles, Responsibilities, and Rights

Role	Responsibilities	Rights
Provider of service	To provide safe and competent care commensurate with the nurse's preparation, experience, and circumstances To inform clients of the consequences of various alternatives and outcomes of care To provide adequate supervision and evaluation of others for whom the nurse is responsible To remain competent	Right to adequate and qualified assistance as necessary Right to reasonable and prudent conduct from clients (e.g., provision of accurate information as required)
Employee or contractor for service	To fulfill the obligations of contracted service with the employer To respect the employer To respect the rights and responsibilities of other healthcare providers	Right to adequate working conditions (e.g., safe equipment and facilities) Right to compensation for services rendered Right to reasonable and prudent conduct by other healthcare providers
Citizen	To protect the rights of the recipients of care	Right to respect by others of the nurse's own rights and responsibilities Right to physical safety

treatment, alternatives to the treatment, and prognosis if not treated by a healthcare provider (Box 3.3). A new standard for informed consent, which has emerged over the past several years, is called **shared medical decision making**. This is a process where the primary healthcare provider gives the client the relevant information for all treatment alternatives, and the client provides the primary healthcare provider relevant personal information that might make one treatment or therapy more appropriate for the individual client. Supporters of shared medical decision making believe the process increases client autonomy and comprehension. Usually the client signs a form provided by the agency. The form is a *record* of the informed consent, *not* the informed consent itself.

BOX 3.3 Court Case Example: Informed Consent

A client with a neck mass and persistent sore throat was diagnosed with metastatic cancer. The physician wrote a detailed note about the office visit when he explained to the client about the plan for a comprehensive neck dissection including the goals, rationale, risks, and treatment recommendations about the procedure. The client did not sign a surgical consent form at the physician's office or at the hospital. After the procedure, the client sued the physician, claiming the absence of his signature made the procedure a case of medical battery. The court, after reading the nursing record, found the following: on the day of surgery a checked box next to the statement "Patient verbalizes understanding of perioperative instructions"; a nurse's initials next to the statement "Planned procedure and physician confirmed with patient"; and a note from the circulating nurse stating, "Client could state surg procedure to neck & purpose."

The court ruled that the nursing documentation was sufficient confirmation that the client understood and agreed to have the procedure performed (Studnicka v. Pinheiro, 2008 WL 4717471 [D. Minn., October 24, 2008]) (Snyder, 2008, p. 6).

There are two types of consent: express and implied. **Express consent** may take the form of either an oral or a written agreement. Usually, the more invasive a procedure or the greater the potential for risk to the client, the greater the need for written permission. **Implied consent** exists when the individual's nonverbal behavior indicates agreement. For example, clients who position their bodies for an injection or cooperate with the taking of vital signs infer implied consent. Consent is also implied in a medical emergency when an individual cannot provide express consent because of physical condition.

Obtaining informed consent for specific medical and surgical treatments is the responsibility of the individual who is going to perform the procedure. Generally this individual is the primary care provider; however, it could also be a nurse practitioner, nurse anesthetist, nurse midwife, clinical nurse specialist, or physician assistant who is performing procedures in their advanced practices.

Informed consent also applies to nurses who are not independent practitioners and are performing direct nursing care for such procedures as nasogastric tube insertion or medication administration. The nurse relies on orally expressed consent or implied consent for most nursing interventions. It is necessary to remember the importance of communicating with the client by explaining nursing procedures, ensuring the client understands, and obtaining permission.

The law says that a "reasonable amount" of information required for the client to make an informed decision is what any other reasonable healthcare practitioner would disclose under similar circumstances. General guidelines include the following:

- The diagnosis or condition that requires treatment
- The purposes of the treatment
- What the client can expect to feel or experience
- The intended benefits of the treatment
- Possible risks or negative outcomes of the treatment
- Advantages and disadvantages of possible alternatives to the treatment (including no treatment).

Informed consent has three major elements:

1. The consent must be given voluntarily.
2. The consent must be given by a client or individual with the capacity and competence to understand.
3. The client or individual must be given enough information to be the ultimate decision maker.

To give informed consent voluntarily, the client must not feel pressured. Sometimes fear of disapproval by a health professional can be the motivation for giving consent; such consent is not voluntarily given. Pressure cancels the consent. It is important, therefore, for the individual obtaining the consent to invite and answer client questions.

Cultural perspective also needs to be considered when clients are asked to make decisions about a procedure or treatment. For example, informed consent in the United States is based on the principle of autonomy. That is, each individual has the right to decide what can or cannot be done to his or her person. The competent adult client is expected to have the autonomy to make his or her own healthcare decisions. In contrast to this individual perspective, some people may apply a group perspective to decision making. They may believe that another member of their family, group, or tribe should make the decision. The nurse can provide culturally responsive care by asking clients if there is someone they would like to be present when information or discussion of their healthcare treatment occurs.

It is also important for the client to understand the written material. Illiteracy continues to present a challenge as it pertains to recognizing and understanding words commonly used in consent forms. Technical words and language barriers inhibit understanding and may encourage a signature without discussion of its actual meaning when the client has a lower literacy level. See Chapter 17 for literacy definitions.

Clinical Alert!

Consent forms often consist of language that exceeds the average reading level of clients. As a result, many clients do not read the form before signing it.

EVIDENCE-BASED PRACTICE

Evidence-Based Practice

What Is the Prevalence of Health Literacy Education in BSN Programs?

Over 75 million Americans have low health literacy, which causes negative health outcomes. Knowledge about health literacy is important for nurses, yet studies show that many nurses have never heard of the concept before attending a training session. In addition, nurse faculty who have not received formal training in their own undergraduate programs are less likely to include health literacy in the curriculum. While national nursing organizations agree on the importance of health literacy education (HLE), there are no established guidelines about what HLE should be included in the curriculum. The research in the area of HLE in nursing programs has primarily focused on evaluation of health literacy knowledge among nursing students.

As a result, Scott (2016) conducted a descriptive study using an online survey to ask the following questions: (a) What is the prevalence of HLE in the curricula of BSN programs in the United States? and (b) In BSN programs that offer HLE, what content is included and what teaching strategies are used to facilitate learning? The researcher used a modified version of the Health Literacy Survey, a tool originally created to obtain information about health literacy content in U.S. medical schools. The modifications involved changing wording from medical school terms to terms used in nursing programs. The survey was sent electronically to the directors of 150 randomly chosen BSN programs, and 57 (38%) of the nursing programs responded to the survey. The settings of the respondents were evenly distributed: 17 from urban, 16 from suburban, and 17 from rural settings. The types of programs were also equally distributed with 26 from state and 25 from private programs.

Despite the low response rate, findings showed that the majority of participating programs did include HLE in the curriculum. The number of hours, however, varied from 1 hour to 45 hours. Another positive finding was that programs that did include HLE in the curriculum addressed recommended topics such as the impact of health literacy on client outcomes and the importance of using plain language skills for oral and written communication.

Implications

Although this study had a small response rate, it is worthy of attention. The importance of health literacy and its impact on client outcomes cannot be denied, and faculty need to be aware of this crucial issue. The study found that nursing programs primarily used written exams and clinical observation to evaluate student learning about health literacy. Nursing programs should consider using more hands-on activities (e.g., simulation and role playing) to teach and evaluate students' knowledge about health literacy. As the researcher suggested, additional studies with both ADN and BSN programs should be conducted to obtain a larger response rate, which would provide a more representative sample of the current state of HLE in nursing programs.

QSEN Patient-Centered Care: Providing Culturally and Linguistically Appropriate Services

Health institutions have a legal and ethical responsibility to provide language access services to clients who do not speak English as their primary language and who have limited ability to speak, read, write, or understand the English language (limited English proficiency [LEP]). Appropriate communication between provider and client is essential for ensuring quality and safety in healthcare. The Office of Minority Health developed 15 national standards for culturally and linguistically appropriate services (CLAS). The National CLAS Standards aim to improve healthcare quality and advance health equity by establishing a framework for organizations to serve the increasingly diverse communities in the United States. Four of the standards address communication and language assistance:

- Offer language assistance to individuals who have LEP or other communication needs, at no cost to them, to facilitate timely access to all healthcare and services.
- Inform all individuals of the availability of language assistance services clearly and in their preferred language, verbally and in writing.
- Ensure the competence of individuals providing language assistance, recognizing that the use of untrained individuals or minors as interpreters should be avoided.
- Provide easy-to-understand print and multimedia materials and signage in the languages commonly used by the populations in the service area (U.S. Department of Health and Human Services, Office of Minority Health, 2018).

Health organizations need to address the communication needs of clients who have language and cultural barriers. For example, if a client cannot read, the consent form must be read to the client, and the client must state understanding before the form is signed. If the client does not speak the same language as the health professional who is providing the information, an interpreter must be present. However, even with an interpreter, it is important to remember that potential interpretation errors can occur.

QSEN Patient-Centered Care: Working with a Healthcare Interpreter

The interpreter's primary task is to transmit verbatim the message expressed by the health professional and the client, that is, to bridge the communication gap between individuals who do not speak the same language. This encounter is a highly interactive process in which the nurse uses language that can be understood and provides teaching. The interpreter also serves as a cultural broker by providing a cultural framework for both the healthcare provider and the client to understand the message being interpreted given the subtle differences and hidden sociocultural assumptions embedded in each other's language.

Following are helpful guidelines when working with an interpreter (U.S. Department of Health and Human Services, n.d.a):

BEFORE THE INTERVIEW

- Use qualified interpreters. Have access to experienced and qualified interpreters who know their role, limitations, and responsibilities. Refrain from using children, relatives, and friends of clients, because they are not qualified for health-related interpretation and may compromise the client's health outcomes and right to confidentiality.
- Have a brief pre-interview meeting with the interpreter to explain the situation and purpose of the interview.
- Plan extra time for the interview.
- Arrange chairs to facilitate communication between the client and the healthcare provider.
- Insist on sentence-by-sentence interpretation.

DURING THE INTERVIEW

- Talk to the client directly, not the interpreter. Watch the client, not the interpreter.
- Ask only one question at a time. Keep your sentences short.
- Use words, not gestures, to convey your meaning. This makes it easier for the interpreter.
- Speak in a normal voice, clearly, and not too fast.
- Avoid jargon and technical terms.
- Expect the interpreter to interrupt when necessary for clarification.
- Be prepared to repeat yourself in different words if your message is not understood.
- Ask the client to repeat instructions.

AFTER THE INTERVIEW

- Have a brief post-interview meeting with the interpreter to address any questions or concerns about the process of communication.
- Document in the client's chart that the client gave consent to use an interpreter, the process used, the client's verbal and nonverbal responses, the full name and title of the professional medical language interpreter, the translation service, and the names of all those present during the interaction.

If given sufficient information, a competent adult can make decisions regarding health. A competent adult is an individual over 18 years of age who is conscious and oriented. A client who is confused, disoriented, or sedated is not considered functionally competent. A legal guardian or representative can provide or refuse consent for the incompetent adult.

Informed consent regulations were originally written with acute care settings in mind. Nonetheless, ensuring informed consent is equally important in providing nursing care in the home. Because the provision of home care often occurs over an extended period of time, the nurse has multiple opportunities to ensure that the client agrees to the plan of treatment. A challenge to informed consent in the home, however, is that the plan may affect other members of the family and, if so, they need to be consulted.

Exceptions

In the United States, three groups of people cannot provide consent. The first is minors. In most areas, a parent or guardian must give consent before minors can obtain treatment. The same is true of an adult who has the mental capacity of a child and who has an appointed guardian. In some states, however, minors are allowed to give consent for such procedures as blood donations, treatment for substance abuse, treatment for mental health problems, and treatment for reproductive health concerns such as sexually transmitted infections or pregnancy. In addition, certain groups of minors are often legally permitted to provide their own consent. These include those who are married, pregnant, parents, members of the military, or emancipated (living on their own). These statutes may vary by state.

The second group is individuals who are unconscious or injured in such a way that they are unable to give consent. In these situations, consent is usually obtained from the closest adult relative if existing statutes permit. In a life-threatening emergency, if consent cannot be obtained from the client or a relative, then the law generally agrees that consent is implied to provide necessary care for the client's emergency condition.

The third group is people with mental illnesses who have been judged by professionals to be incompetent. State mental health acts or similar statutes generally provide definitions of mental illness and specify the rights of those who have mental illnesses under the law as well as the rights of the staff caring for such clients.

Nurse's Role

Nurses are often asked to obtain a signed consent form. The nurse is not responsible for explaining the procedure but for witnessing the client's signature on the form (Figure 3.3 ■). The nurse's signature confirms three things:

- The client gave consent voluntarily.
- The signature is authentic.
- The client appears competent to give consent.

The nurse advocates for the client by verifying that the client received enough information to give consent. Therefore, it is important for the nurse to assess the client's understanding and identify any misconceptions. If clients are just asked if they understand, most will answer "yes." To prevent this, the nurse can ask clients to restate in their own words what the individual who is going to perform the procedure explained to them. If the client has questions or if the nurse has doubts about the client's understanding, the nurse must notify the healthcare provider. Again, the nurse is not responsible for explaining the medical or surgical procedure. In fact, the nurse could be liable for giving incorrect or incomplete information or interfering with the client–provider relationship.

Safety Alert! SAFETY

Ask clients to state in their own words what they have been told about the procedure or treatment.

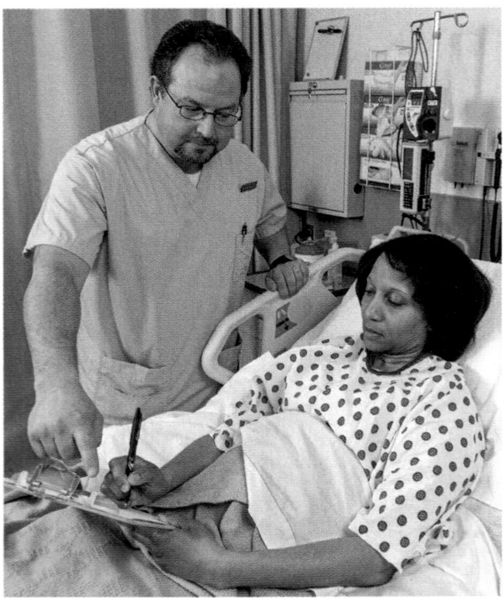

Figure 3.3 ■ Obtaining informed consent is the responsibility of the individual performing the procedure. The nurse may be asked to witness the client's signature on the consent form.

The right of consent also involves the right of refusal (Guido, 2020). Remind clients that they can change their minds and cancel the procedure at any time because the right to refuse continues even after signing the consent. Similar to informed consent, it is important to verify that the client is aware of the pros and cons of refusal and is making an informed decision. The nurse needs to notify the healthcare provider of the client's refusal and document the refusal in the chart.

Documentation is an important aspect of informed consent. A client's concerns or questions must be documented along with the notification of the healthcare provider. Equally important is documenting when the client states understanding. Record any teaching as a result of nursing-related questions by the client. Any special circumstances, such as use of an interpreter, should be documented. When documenting the use of an interpreter, include the interpreter's full name and title.

Delegation

Delegation is "allowing a delegatee to perform a specific nursing activity, skill, or procedure that is *beyond the delegatee's traditional role and not routinely performed*. A delegatee may be an RN, LPN/VN or assistive personnel (ANA & NCSBN, 2019, p. 2). To perform the delegated care, the delegatee must have acquired the additional knowledge and training and validated competence to perform the delegated responsibility (Box 3.4). The licensed nurse delegating the responsibility is accountable for the client while the delegatee is responsible for the delegated activity, procedure, or skill. The professional functions of nursing judgment, clinical reasoning, or critical decision making cannot be delegated.

BOX 3.4 Court Case Example: Improper Delegation

A nurse had the responsibility of administering specific oral medications before the client was transported from a tuberculosis (TB) isolation unit to another department for a diagnostic procedure. Rather than getting the required mask to enter the isolation unit, the nurse asked the transport individual, who was wearing the required mask, to take the medications into the isolation unit and administer them to the client. The transporter was reluctant but the nurse insisted. The nurse watched on a closed-circuit monitor while the transporter administered the medications. Afterwards, the transporter reported the incident to a supervisor. Management terminated the nurse. The nurse sued for age and national origin discrimination. At the time, she was 59 and from India. The US District Court for the Eastern District of Michigan dismissed her case (Varughese v. William Beaumont Hosp., 2014 WL 3361897 [E.D. Mich., July 8, 2014]).

State nursing regulations on delegation of nursing responsibilities require the nurse to determine that the individual to whom a task is delegated has the necessary knowledge and skills for the task. When the nurse was asked how this was determined, the nurse responded that "anyone can give a couple of pills . . . ." The nurse also stated familiarity with the hospital's policies for medication administration, which included verbally confirming the client's identity, checking information against the client's wrist band, educating the client about any possible adverse reactions, and remaining with the client until the medication was taken. The court determined that a client transporter did not have the required knowledge and skills for medication administration (Snyder, 2014, p. 4).

It is important to know the difference between delegation and assignment. When performing a fundamental skill learned in the delegatee's basic educational program and within his scope of practice, the delegatee is carrying out an *assignment*. The licensed nurse is still responsible for ensuring an assignment given to a delegatee is carried out completely and correctly (ANA & NCSBN, 2019, p. 2).

Competent assistive personnel (AP) can be of assistance to the nurse, which allows the nurse to perform those functions appropriate to the nurse's scope of practice. From a legal perspective, however, the nurse's authority to delegate or assign is based on state laws and regulations. Therefore, nurses must be familiar with their nurse practice act.

Nurses must know not only their own scope of practice but also the scope of practice of the AP and the LVN or LPN, which may vary depending on a facility's policies and procedures. Thus, the nurse must know the employer's policies and procedures for delegation and the job descriptions and skill levels of the AP and LVN or LPN. Is the AP or the LVN or LPN competent to perform the delegated task? The NCSBN has provided "five rights of delegation" to help nurses make delegation decisions (see Chapter 18 ∞).

Violence, Abuse, and Neglect

Violent behavior can include domestic violence, child abuse, abuse of older adults, and sexual abuse. Neglect is the absence of care necessary to maintain the health and safety of a vulnerable individual such as a child or older adult. Nurses, in their many roles (e.g., home health nurse, pediatric nurse, ED nurse), can often identify and assess cases of violence against others. As a result, they are often considered **mandated reporters**, meaning that law requires them to report suspected abuse, neglect, or exploitation. Mandated reporting is designed to detect cases of abuse and neglect at an early stage, protect children, and facilitate the provision of services to children and families. Healthcare providers are protected when they, in good faith, report suspected abuse even if subsequent investigation shows the report to be groundless (Guido, 2020). See Chapter 24 ∞ for additional information about child abuse and Chapter 26 ∞ for information about abuse of older adults.

Discrimination

Discrimination is the prejudicial or unfair treatment of an individual or a group of people. In the United Kingdom, the Equality Act 2010 protects people from discrimination based on age, disability, marriage and civil partnership, pregnancy and maternity, race and ethnicity, religion or belief, sex, sexual orientation, and gender reassignment. Similarly, other countries have legal frameworks that protect individuals against discrimination and penalize any discriminatory actions.

In the United States the U.S. Congress passed the Americans with Disabilities Act (ADA) in 1990, and fully implemented it in 1994. The act prohibits discrimination on the basis of disability in employment, public services, and public accommodations. The purposes of the act are as follows:

- To provide a clear and comprehensive national mandate for eliminating discrimination against individuals with disabilities
- To provide clear, strong, consistent, enforceable standards addressing discrimination against individuals with disabilities
- To ensure that the federal government plays a central role in enforcing standards established under the act

The ADA is about productivity, economic independence, and the ability to move about freely in society. Box 3.5 lists the criteria for ADA eligibility.

Nurses can play a significant role in preventing discrimination in the workplace and discrimination against the ability to access healthcare services. In recent years, the nursing workforce has been marked with increasing diversity, consisting of nurses from varied cultural and racial backgrounds. Nurses can protect each other from possible discrimination by increasing awareness of each other's prejudices and ensuring that their rights as employees are upheld by their employers and labor organizations.

BOX 3.5 Meeting ADA Eligibility

The employee or applicant for employment must show:

- A physical or mental impairment that substantially limits one or more major life activities of such individual;
- A record of such an impairment; or
- Being regarded as having such an impairment.

From *Legal and Ethical Issues in Nursing*, 7th ed. (p. 273), by G. W. Guido, 2020, Upper Saddle River, NJ: Pearson Education, Inc. Reprinted with permission.

Controlled Substances

U.S. laws regulate the distribution and use of controlled substances such as opioids, depressants, stimulants, and hallucinogens. Misuse of controlled substances leads to criminal penalties.

Substance Use Disorder in Nursing

Substance use disorder (SUD) "encompasses a pattern of behaviors that range from misuse to dependency or addiction to alcohol or (legal and/or illegal) drugs. SUD is a treatable, chronic brain disease" (NCSBN, 2019, slide 7). Nurses may be at an increased risk because of easy access to medications, the stressors of nursing, and lack of education on the addictive process and its signs and symptoms. Nurses administer medications for all purposes (e.g., to relieve pain, prevent infections, decrease anxiety and depression). The availability of drugs is an occupational hazard, especially if the administration of controlled substances in the healthcare agency is poorly managed. Increased client acuity, variable working hours, staffing shortages, fatigue, and isolation can cause stress. Substance use may be a way of coping with the stress. To help identify SUD, there are three things nurses should focus their attention on: behavior changes, physical signs of the disease, and drug diversion (NCSBN, 2019, slide 42).

Evidence has shown that the frequency of SUD among nurses is similar to that of the general population, approximately 10% (Stewart & Mueller, 2018). The American Nurses Association estimates that 6 to 8% of nurses use alcohol or drugs to an extent that it impairs professional performance (Brent, 2019, p. 15). Nurses with SUD place the client *and* themselves at risk for serious injury or death. As a result, professional nursing organizations have passed resolutions to ensure that nurses and student nurses with SUD receive treatment and support, not discipline and disrespect.

The mission of any board of nursing is to protect the health and well-being of the public. For nurses with SUD, boards of nursing in the United States can take two different regulatory options: disciplinary action or entry into an alternative-to-discipline program (ADP) (NCSBN, 2019). A variety of ADP programs have been developed to assist nurses with SUD to recover. In many states, nurses who voluntarily enter an ADP (sometimes called a peer assistance program) do not have their nursing license revoked if they follow treatment requirements. Their practice, however, is closely supervised within specific guidelines (e.g., working on a general nursing unit versus critical care area, no overtime, work only day shift, not allowed to administer or have access to controlled substances). The programs require counseling and ongoing participation in support groups with periodic progress reports that may include random drug screening. The nurse may petition the state board of nursing for reinstatement of full licensure after a specified amount of time and evidence of recovery as determined by the state board. ADPs allow for rehabilitation of the nurse while still being able to work in the profession. They also allow the state board to protect the public while complying with the ADA.

Employers must have sound policies and procedures for identifying and intervening in situations involving a nurse with possible SUD. The primary concern is for the protection of clients, but it is also critically important that the nurse's problem be identified quickly so that appropriate treatment may be instituted. Box 3.6 lists possible signs of substance use disorders and psychiatric disorders.

BOX 3.6 Possible Signs and Symptoms of Substance Use Disorder

BEHAVIORAL CHANGES
- Frequent absence from unit
- Frequent trips to the bathroom
- Arriving late or leaving early
- Increasing number of mistakes, including medication errors

PHYSICAL CHANGES
- Increasing isolation from others
- Slight changes in appearance that increase over time
- Decreased alertness, confusion, or memory lapses
- Inappropriate verbal or emotional responses

POSSIBLE DRUG DIVERSION
- Incorrect controlled substance counts
- Excessive wastage or breakage of controlled substances
- Often volunteers to medicate other nurses' clients
- Altered verbal or phone medication orders
- Client complains that pain medication is not effective.

From "A Nurse's Guide to Substance Use Disorder in Nursing," 2018a, p. 5, 7, by National Council of State Boards of Nursing. Reprinted with permission.

Clinical Alert!

It is important for student nurses and nurses to become knowledgeable about the risk factors of substance use disorder and its early identification and interventions.

Nurses usually avoid dealing with impaired colleagues. Nurses work as a team, and the friendships that develop can be barriers to reporting problems. Although the reporting of unsafe or suspicious behavior may be difficult, it is important to remember that nurses have a professional and ethical responsibility to report a colleague's unsafe practice or suspected drug use to their nurse manager or supervisor, and in some states, to the board of nursing. Reporting a nurse may save the nurse's license and possibly his or her life. The Practice Guidelines later in this chapter can be used to report the nurse suspected of SUD.

The updated version of the ANA *Code of Ethics for Nurses with Interpretive Statements* (2015) states that the "nurse promotes, advocates for, and protects the rights, health, and safety of the patient." (p. 35). It also includes the responsibility that nurses have to their colleagues. For example, the code states: "The nurse's duty is to take action to protect patients and to ensure that the impaired individual receives assistance," "The nurse should extend compassion and caring to colleagues," and "Advocacy includes supporting the return to practice of individuals who have sought assistance and, after recovery, are ready to resume professional duties" (p. 39).

Sexual Harassment

Sexual harassment is a violation of an individual's rights and a form of discrimination. In 1987, the law prohibiting sexual discrimination was clarified to apply to all educational and employing institutions receiving federal funding in the United States. The Equal Employment Opportunity Commission (EEOC) defines sexual harassment as "unwelcome sexual advances, requests for sexual favors, and other verbal or physical conduct of a sexual nature" occurring in the following circumstances (Guidelines on Discrimination Because of Sex, 2016, section 1604.11):

- "When submission to such conduct is considered, either explicitly or implicitly, a condition of an individual's employment
- When submission to or rejection of such conduct is used as the basis for employment decisions affecting the individual
- When such conduct interferes with an individual's work performance or creates an intimidating, hostile, or offensive working environment."

The victim or the harasser may be male or female. The victim does not have to be of the opposite sex. Nurses must develop skills of assertiveness to prevent sexual harassment in the workplace. In addition, nurses must be familiar with the sexual harassment policies and procedures that must be in place in every institution. These will include information regarding the reporting procedure, to whom incidents should be reported, the investigative process, and how confidentiality will be protected to the extent possible.

Abortions

Abortion laws provide specific guidelines for nurses about what is legally permissible. In 1973, when the *Roe v. Wade* and *Doe v. Bolton* cases were decided, the Supreme Court of the United States held that the constitutional rights of privacy give a woman the right to control her own body to the extent that she can abort her fetus in the early stages of pregnancy.

In 1989, the Supreme Court's decision in *Webster v. Reproductive Health Services* upheld a Missouri law banning the use of public funds or facilities for performing or assisting with abortions. In 1992, President Clinton rescinded the 1991 *Rust v. Sullivan* decision, dubbed the "gag rule," that prevented healthcare providers from discussing abortion services with clients in not-for-profit agencies. The Supreme Court and state legislatures continue to struggle with the issue of abortion.

Many statutes also include conscience clauses, upheld by the Supreme Court, designed to protect nurses and hospitals. These clauses give hospitals the right to deny admission to abortion clients and give healthcare personnel, including nurses, the right to refuse to participate in abortions. When these rights are exercised, the statutes also protect the agency and employee from discrimination or retaliation.

Countries across the world have different legal, ethical, and moral views regarding abortion. Such variation stems from the unique religious, social, and cultural contexts of each country. Nurses should be aware about the laws regarding abortion in the country where they practice and assess the impact of such laws on their own ethical and moral values.

Death and Related Issues

The nurse's role in legal issues related to death is prescribed by the laws of the region and the policies of the healthcare institution. For example, in some states, a feeding tube cannot be removed from an individual in a persistent vegetative state without a prior directive from the client, but in other states the removal is allowed at the family's request or a primary care provider's order. Some facilities permit do-not-resuscitate orders or protocols that specify the extent of invasive life-sustaining measures. Caring for dying clients who have agreed to organ donation can also be complex in terms of determining which medications, treatments, or equipment must be continued until the time for harvesting the organs has arrived. Many of these legal issues stimulate strong ethical concerns. It is important for the nurse to have support from other team members in understanding and providing appropriate care to clients facing death.

Advance Healthcare Directives

Advance healthcare directives include a variety of legal and lay documents that allow individuals to specify aspects of care they wish to receive should they become unable to make or communicate their preferences. The Patient Self-Determination Act implemented in 1991 requires all healthcare facilities receiving Medicare and Medicaid reimbursement to (a) recognize advance directives, (b) ask clients whether they have advance directives, and (c) provide educational materials advising clients of their rights to declare their personal wishes regarding treatment decisions, including the right to refuse medical treatment. Clients and families often have difficulty making advance treatment decisions for end-of-life matters. They need to be reassured that even if they make a decision and have an advance directive, they will always have the option to change their decision. For example, clients who are terminally ill may have decided not to have ventilator support, but if and when the actual situation occurs, they have the right to change their mind or take more time to make the decision.

Nurses need to assess if clients and families have an accurate understanding of life-sustaining measures. They may misunderstand what actually sustains life and base their decisions on that. Nurses need to incorporate teaching in this area and continue to be supportive of clients' decisions.

In the United States, the two types of advance healthcare directives are the living will and the healthcare proxy or surrogate. The **living will** provides specific instructions about what medical treatment the client chooses to omit or refuse (e.g., ventilator support) in the event that the client is unable to make those decisions.

The **healthcare proxy**, also referred to as a *durable power of attorney for healthcare*, is a notarized or witnessed statement appointing someone else (e.g., a relative or trusted friend) to manage healthcare treatment decisions when the client is unable to do so. Figure 3.4 ■ shows an example of an advance healthcare directive that combines a living will declaration and a durable power of attorney for healthcare. A form specific to each U.S. state can be obtained from the National Hospice and Palliative Care Organization.

Clinical Alert!

What should you do if asked to witness a client's private financial or healthcare decision-making determination? Politely decline because it may be viewed as a conflict of interest. Ask your supervisor if there is someone else in the facility that may be able to appropriately assist the client (Starr, 2016).

Nurses should learn the law regarding client self-determination for the state in which they practice, as well as the policies and procedures for implementation in the institution where they work. The legally binding nature and specific requirements of advance medical directives are determined by individual state legislation. In most U.S. states, advance directives must be witnessed by two people but do not require review by an attorney.

POWER OF ATTORNEY FOR HEALTH CARE

(1) **DESIGNATION OF AGENT:** I designate the following individual as my agent to make health care decisions for me: ______________________

____
(Name of individual you choose as agent)

____
(address) (city) (state) (zip code)

____
(home phone) (work phone)

OPTIONAL: If I revoke my agent's authority or if my agent is not willing, able, or reasonably available to make a health care decision for me, I designate as my first alternate agent:

____
(Name of individual you choose as first alternate agent)

____
(address) (city) (state) (zip code)

____
(home phone) (work phone)

OPTIONAL: If I revoke the authority of my agent and first alternate agent or if neither is willing, able, or reasonably available to make a health care decision for me, I designate as my second alternate agent:

____
(Name of individual you choose as second alternate agent)

____
(address) (city) (state) (zip code)

____
(home phone) (work phone)

(2) **AGENT'S AUTHORITY:** My agent is authorized to make all health care decisions for me, including decisions to provide, withhold, or withdraw artificial nutrition and hydration, and all other forms of health care to keep me alive, **except** as I state here:

(3) **WHEN AGENT'S AUTHORITY BECOMES EFFECTIVE:** My agent's authority becomes effective when my primary physician determines that I am unable to make my own health care decisions unless I mark the following box. If I mark this box [ ], my agent's authority to make health care decisions for me takes effect immediately.

(4) **AGENT'S OBLIGATION:** My agent shall make health care decisions for me in accordance with this power of attorney for health care, any instructions I give below, and my other wishes to the extent known to my agent. To the extent my wishes are unknown, my agent shall make health care decisions for me in accordance with what my agent determines to be in my best interest. In determining my best interest, my agent shall consider my personal values to the extent known to my agent.

(5) **AGENT'S POSTDEATH AUTHORITY:** My agent is authorized to make anatomical gifts, authorize an autopsy, and direct disposition of my remains, except as I state here or elsewhere in this form:

INSTRUCTIONS FOR HEALTH CARE

Strike any wording you do not want.

(6) **END-OF-LIFE DECISIONS:** I direct that my health care providers and others involved in my care provide, withhold, or withdraw treatment in accordance with the choice I have marked below: **(Initial only one box)**
[ ] (a) **Choice NOT to Prolong Life**
I do not want my life to be prolonged if (1) I have an incurable and irreversible condition that will result in my death within a relatively short time, (2) I become unconscious and, to a reasonable degree of medical certainty, I will not regain consciousness, or (3) the likely risks and burdens of treatment would outweigh the expected benefits, **OR**
[ ] (b) **Choice to Prolong Life**
I want my life to be prolonged as long as possible within the limits of generally accepted health care standards.

(7) **RELIEF FROM PAIN:** Except as I state in the following space, I direct that treatment for alleviation of pain or discomfort should be provided at all times even if it hastens my death:

DONATION OF ORGANS AT DEATH

(8) Upon my death: (mark applicable box)
[ ] (a) I give any needed organs, tissues, or parts,
OR
[ ] (b) I give the following organs, tissues, or parts only: ______________________
[ ] (c) My gift is for the following purposes:
(strike any of the following you do not want)
(1) Transplant
(2) Therapy
(3) Research
(4) Education

(9) **EFFECT OF COPY:** A copy of this form has the same effect as the original.

(10) **SIGNATURE:** Sign and date the form here:

______________________	______________________
(date)	(sign your name)
______________________	______________________
(address)	(print your name)
______________________	______________________
(city)	(state)

(11) **WITNESSES:** This advance health care directive will not be valid for making health care decisions unless it is either: (1) signed by two (2) qualified adult witnesses who are personally known to you and who are present when you sign or acknowledge your signature; or (2) acknowledged before a notary public.

Figure 3.4 ■ Sample advance healthcare directive.

Some states do not permit relatives, heirs, or primary care providers to witness advance directives. As a client advocate, it is important for the nurse to facilitate family discussion about end-of-life concerns and decisions.

Autopsy

An **autopsy** or **postmortem examination** is an examination of the body after death. It is performed only in certain cases. The law describes under what circumstances an autopsy must be performed, for example, when death is sudden or occurs within 48 hours of admission to a hospital. The organs and tissues of the body are examined to establish the exact cause of death, to learn more about a disease, and to assist in the accumulation of statistical data.

The primary care provider or, in some instances, a designated individual in the hospital is responsible for obtaining consent for an autopsy. Consent must be given by the decedent (before death) or by the next of kin. Laws in many states prioritize the family members who can provide consent as follows: surviving spouse, adult children, parents, and siblings. After an autopsy, hospitals cannot retain any tissues or organs without the permission of the individual who consented to the autopsy.

Certification of Death

The formal determination of death, or pronouncement, must be performed by a primary care provider, a coroner, or a nurse. The granting of the authority to nurses to pronounce death is regulated by the state. It may be limited to nurses in long-term care, home health, and hospice agencies or to advanced practice nurses. By law, a death certificate must be made out when an individual dies. It is usually signed by the attending primary care provider and filed with a local health or other government office. The family is usually given a copy to use for legal matters, such as insurance claims.

Do-Not-Resuscitate Orders

Primary care providers may order "no code" or **"do not resuscitate" (DNR)** for clients who are in a stage of terminal, irreversible illness or expected death. A DNR order is generally written when the client or proxy has expressed the wish for no resuscitation in the event of a respiratory or cardiac arrest. Many primary care providers are reluctant to write such an order if there is any conflict between the client and family members or among family members. A DNR order is written to indicate that the goal of treatment is a comfortable, dignified death and that further life-sustaining measures are not indicated. If it is contrary to the nurse's personal beliefs to carry out a DNR order, the nurse should consult the nurse manager for a change in assignment. Family members may think that DNR means giving permission to terminate an individual's life. The term *allow natural death* (AND) is clear, more descriptive, and perhaps less threatening (ANA, 2012, p. 8).

The ANA (2012) makes the following recommendations for clinical nurses:

- Clinical nurses actively participate in timely and frequent discussions on changing goals of care and initiate DNR-AND discussions with patients and their families and significant others.
- Clinical nurses ensure that DNR orders are clearly documented, reviewed, and updated periodically to reflect changes in the patient's condition.
- All nurses ensure that, whenever possible, the DNR decision is a subject of explicit discussion between the healthcare team, patient, and family (or designated surrogate), and that actions taken are in accordance with the patient's wishes.
- All nurses facilitate and participate in interdisciplinary mechanisms for the resolution of disputes among patients, families, and clinicians' DNR orders.
- All nurses actively participate in developing DNR policies within the institutions where they work. (pp. 35–36)

Many states (but not all) permit clients living at home to arrange special orders so that emergency technicians called to the home in the event of a cardiopulmonary arrest will respect the client's wish not to be resuscitated. Some emergency medical services have written policies specifying that staff may withhold CPR if the client has a signed order or approved form or wears a medical alert DNR medallion. Nurses should be familiar with the federal and state laws and the policies of their agency concerning withholding life-sustaining measures (Box 3.7).

BOX 3.7 Court Case Example: DNR

A client in a skilled nursing facility began choking and gasping for breath. Her son called for a nurse. When the nurse entered the room the client was gasping for breath and had no palpable pulse. The nurse asked the son if his mother had a DNR. The son replied that he did not know what the nurse meant. The nurse left to look through the client's paperwork to determine if there was a DNR. Eight minutes later, the nurse verified that there was no DNR order and CPR was started. The client was transported to a hospital where a neurologic consultation diagnosed brain death. The family withdrew life support and the client expired. The family sued the nursing home for the nurse's negligence (IHS Acquisition v. Crowson, 351 S.W.3d 368, 2010 WL 636964 [Tex. App., February 24, 2010]).

In Texas, as in other states, a qualified expert's report must be filed with the court along with any civil lawsuit alleging professional negligence. The expert's testimony correctly stated the standard of care: If the client's DNR status is unknown, CPR and a full code must begin immediately. The 8-minute delay while the nurse was looking for DNR documentation was inexcusable (Snyder, 2010, p. 1).

Euthanasia

Euthanasia is the act of painlessly putting to death people suffering from incurable or distressing disease. It is sometimes referred to as "mercy killing." Regardless of compassion and good intentions or moral convictions, euthanasia is legally wrong in the United States and can lead to criminal charges of homicide or to a civil lawsuit for withholding treatment or providing an unacceptable standard of care. Because advanced technology has enabled the medical profession to sustain life almost indefinitely, people are increasingly considering the meaning of quality of life. For some people, the withholding of artificial life-support measures or even the withdrawal of life support is a desired and acceptable practice for clients who are terminally ill or who are incurably disabled and believed unable to live their lives with some happiness and meaning.

Voluntary euthanasia refers to situations in which the dying individual desires some control over the time and manner of death. All forms of euthanasia are illegal except in states where right-to-die statutes and living wills exist. In 1994, the state of Oregon approved the first U.S. physician-assisted suicide law, the Death with Dignity Act (DWDA), which permits primary care providers to prescribe lethal doses of medications. Since the law was passed in 1997, and as of January 2018, a total of 1967 people have had DWDA prescriptions written, and 1275 clients have died from ingesting medications prescribed under the DWDA. Of the 218 clients for whom prescriptions were written during 2017, 130 (59.6%) ingested the medication, 129 died from ingesting the medication, and one individual ingested the medication but regained consciousness before dying from the underlying illness. An additional 44 individuals (20.2%) did not take the medications and subsequently died of other causes (Oregon Public Health Division, 2018, p. 5). As of January 2019, the following states have a death with dignity statute: California, Colorado, District of Columbia, Oregon, Vermont, Washington, and Hawaii. Death with dignity is legal in Montana by way of a state Supreme Court ruling (Death with Dignity National Center, n.d.).

Inquest

An **inquest** is a legal inquiry into the cause or manner of a death. When a death is the result of an accident, for example, an inquest is held into the circumstances of the accident to determine any blame. The inquest is conducted under the jurisdiction of a coroner or medical examiner. A **coroner** is a public official, not necessarily a physician, appointed or elected to inquire into the causes of death, when appropriate. A **medical examiner** is a physician and usually has advanced education in pathology or forensic medicine. Agency policy dictates who is responsible for reporting deaths to the coroner or medical examiner.

Organ Donation

Under the Uniform Anatomical Gift Act and the National Organ Transplant Act (NOTA in the United States), people 18 years or older and of sound mind may make a gift of all or any part of their own bodies for the following purposes: for medical or dental education, research, advancement of medical or dental science, therapy, or transplantation. The donation can be made by registering with the National Donate Life Registry, which ensures that your donor registration travels with you, no matter where you live or move; designating your choice on your driver's license; or telling your family your wishes about donation. A living will can also state your wishes; however, that might not be available at the time of death. In most states, the individual can revoke the gift, either by destroying the card or by revoking the gift orally in the presence of two witnesses. Nurses may serve as witnesses for people consenting to donate organs.

The NOTA created the national Organ Procurement and Transplantation Network (OPTN). This network is a public–private partnership consisting of organ procurement organizations (OPOs) around the country. It links professionals involved in the U.S. donation and transplantation system to match donor organs to waiting recipients (U.S. Department of Health and Human Services, n.d.b). One of the goals is to increase the number of and access to transplants. Unfortunately, there is a greater need for transplantation than there are available organs.

The donation process begins when individuals make the decision to donate their organs when they die. See Box 3.8 for the basic steps in donation from deceased

BOX 3.8 The Basic Path of Organ Donation

The following describes the basic steps in organ donation from deceased donors (U.S. Department of Health and Human Services, n.d.c):

- *Transport*. EMTs and paramedics begin life-saving efforts at the scene.
- *Treatment*. ED doctors and nurses use advanced life-support equipment to continue life-saving measures.
- *Intensive care*. After being stabilized, the client is transferred to the ICU. Tests are performed to determine the extent of damage to the brain and organs. Medical treatment continues.
- *Brain death declared*. After brain death is determined, the donor's body is kept functioning by artificial means (e.g., ventilator).
- *Evaluation*. A specially trained nurse from the OPO goes to the hospital to determine if the client is medically suitable.
- *Consent*. The doctor discusses the client's death with the family. Someone from the OPO or specially trained hospital staff talk with the family about donation and answer any questions.
- *Placement*. Data enters the United Network for Organ Sharing national computer system to begin the organ allocation process. Candidates are found that best match the data of the donor.
- *Organ recovery*. The donor is taken to the OR and organs are surgically removed and sent to the hospital where the candidate is waiting for them.
- *Funeral*. The donor is taken to a funeral home. The OPO works with the funeral home to avoid delays. The family can have an open casket if desired because organ donation is rarely disfiguring.
- *Follow-up*. A few weeks later, the OPO sends a letter to the donor's family informing them which organs were transplanted. The names of the recipients are confidential. Most OPOs continue to provide support to donor families (e.g., bereavement counseling).

donors. The details regarding this process of requesting donation from family members and other legal aspects of organ donation vary by state. The nurse needs to be familiar with the appropriate legislation.

Areas of Potential Liability in Nursing

Nursing liability is usually involved with tort law. It is important for the nurse to know the differences between professional negligence (an unintentional tort) and intentional torts. Nurses must also recognize those nursing situations in which negligent actions are most likely to occur and take measures to prevent them.

Crimes and Torts

A **crime** is an act committed in violation of public (criminal) law and punishable by a fine or imprisonment. A crime does *not* have to be intentional in order to be a crime. For example, a nurse may accidentally give a client an additional and lethal dose of a controlled substance to relieve discomfort.

Crimes are classified as either felonies or misdemeanors. A **felony** is a crime of a serious nature, such as murder, punishable by a term in prison. In some areas, second-degree murder is called **manslaughter**. A nurse who accidentally gives an additional and lethal dose of a narcotic can be accused of manslaughter.

Crimes are punished through criminal action by the state against an individual. A **misdemeanor** is an offense of a less serious nature and is usually punishable by a fine or short-term jail sentence, or both.

A **tort** is a civil wrong committed against an individual or an individual's property. Torts are usually litigated in court by civil action between individuals. In other words, the individual or individuals claimed to be responsible for the tort are sued for damages. Tort liability almost always is based on fault, which is something that was done incorrectly (an unreasonable act of commission) or something that should have been done but was not (an act of omission).

Torts are classified as unintentional or intentional.

Unintentional Torts

Negligence and professional negligence are examples of unintentional torts that may occur in the healthcare setting. **Negligence** is misconduct or practice that is below the standard expected of an ordinary, reasonable, and prudent individual. Such conduct places another individual at risk for harm. Both nonmedical and professional individuals can be liable for negligent acts. **Gross negligence** involves extreme lack of knowledge, skill, or decision making that the individual clearly should have known would put others at risk for harm. **Malpractice** is "professional negligence," that is, negligence that occurred while the individual was performing as a professional. Malpractice applies to primary care providers, dentists, and lawyers, and generally includes nurses. In some states nurses cannot be sued for malpractice, only professional negligence. The terms *malpractice* and *professional negligence* are often used interchangeably. Six elements must be present for a case of nursing professional negligence to be proven:

- **Duty**. The nurse must have (or should have had) a relationship with the client that involves providing care and following an acceptable standard of care. Such duty, for example, is evident when the nurse has been assigned to care for a client in the home or hospital. A nurse also has a general duty of care, even if not specifically assigned to a client, if the client needs help.

Clinical Alert!

It is a nurse's duty to respond to all clients' call lights, not just those of assigned clients.

- **Breach of duty**. There must be a standard of care that is expected in the specific situation but that the nurse did not observe. For example, something was done that should not have been done or nothing was done when it should have been done. This is the failure to act as a reasonable, prudent nurse under the circumstances. The standard can come from documents published by national or professional organizations, boards of nursing, institutional policies and procedures, or textbooks or journals, or it may be stated by expert witnesses. Current trends in professional liability suggest that the gold standard is evidence-based practice.
- **Foreseeability**. A link must exist between the nurse's act and the injury suffered.
- **Causation**. It must be proved that the harm occurred as a direct result of the nurse's failure to follow the standard of care and that the nurse could have (or should have) known that failure to follow the standard of care could result in such harm.
- **Harm** or **injury**. The client or plaintiff must demonstrate some type of harm or injury (physical, financial, or emotional) as a result of the breach of duty owed the client. The plaintiff will be asked to document physical injury, medical costs, loss of wages, "pain and suffering," and any other damages.
- **Damages**. If professional negligence caused the injury, the nurse is held liable for damages that may be compensated. The goal of awarding damages is to assist the injured party to his or her original position as far as financially possible.

Clinical Alert!

The best defense against a professional negligence claim is to know your nursing responsibilities and the scope of practice of members of your health team (e.g., LPN or LVN, AP).

Several legal doctrines or principles are related to negligence. One such doctrine is *respondeat superior*. A lawsuit for a negligent act performed by a nurse will also name the nurse's employer. In addition, employers may be held liable for negligence if they fail to provide adequate human and material resources for nursing care, fail to properly educate nurses on the use of new equipment or procedures, or fail to orient nurses to the facility. Another doctrine or principle is ***res ipsa loquitur*** ("the thing speaks for itself"). In some cases, the harm cannot be traced to a specific healthcare provider or standard but does not normally occur unless there has been a negligent act. An example is harm that results when surgical instruments or bandages are accidentally left in a client during surgery.

To defend against a professional negligence lawsuit, the nurse must prove that one or more of the six required elements is not met. There is also a limit to the amount of time that can pass between recognition of harm and the bringing of a suit. This is referred to as the statute of limitations. The exact time limitation varies by type of suit and state.

To avoid charges of professional negligence, nurses must recognize those nursing situations in which negligent actions are most likely to occur, and take measures to prevent them. The most common situation is the *medication error*. Because of the large number of medications on the market today and the variety of methods of administration, these errors may be on the increase. Nursing errors include failing to read the medication label, misreading or incorrectly calculating the dosage, failing to correctly identify the client, preparing the wrong concentration, or administering a medication by the wrong route (e.g., intravenously instead of intramuscularly). Some medication errors are very serious and can result in death. For example, administering dicumarol, an anticoagulant, to a client recently returned from surgery could cause the client to hemorrhage. Nurses always must check medications very carefully. Even after checking, the nurse is wise to recheck the medication order and the medication before administering it if the client states, for example, "I did not have a green pill before."

Clinical Alert!

To be a client advocate, you must know about the medications being administered. Know why the client is receiving the medication, the dosage range, possible adverse effects, toxicity levels, and contraindications.

Clients often fall unintentionally, sometimes with resultant injury. Some falls can be prevented by elevating the side rails on the cribs, beds, and stretchers of babies and small children and, when necessary, of adults. If a nurse leaves the rails down or leaves a baby unattended on a bath table, that nurse is guilty of professional negligence if the client falls and is injured as a direct result. Most hospitals and nursing homes have policies regarding the use of safety devices. The nurse needs to be familiar with these policies and to take indicated precautions to prevent injuries (see Chapter 32 ∞).

Safety Alert! SAFETY

Assess clients for fall potential. Document all nursing measures taken to protect the client (e.g., "Instructed client how to use the call light").

In some instances, ignoring a client's complaints can constitute professional negligence. This type of professional negligence is termed *failure to observe and take appropriate action*. The nurse who does not report a client's complaint of acute abdominal pain is negligent and may be found guilty of professional negligence if resulting in appendix rupture and death. By failing to take the blood pressure and pulse and to check the dressing of a client who has just had abdominal surgery, a nurse omits important assessments. If the client hemorrhages and dies, the nurse may be held responsible for the death because of this professional negligence. Base your observations and monitoring on orders *and* professional judgment. For example, if the client is to have neurologic checks every 2 hours and develops cognitive changes, perform a complete neurologic assessment (Flynn, 2016, p. 16).

Clinical Alert!

Monitor both the physical and psychosocial status of the client. Document observations and interventions.

Incorrectly identifying clients is a problem, particularly in busy hospital units. Unfortunate occurrences, such as removal of a healthy gallbladder from the wrong individual, have resulted from nurses preparing the wrong client for surgery. Cases of *mistaken identity* are costly to the client and make the nurse liable for professional negligence.

Another reason for professional negligence is *failure to communicate*. Nurses have been found to be negligent when they did not communicate concerns to colleagues, charge nurses, and physicians. Do not assume that the client's healthcare provider is aware of changes in status. Changes in laboratory values, vital signs, and complaints or any new problem must be reported immediately to the appropriate practitioner (Brown, 2016). It is also important to document these changes and efforts to notify the healthcare provider.

The number of nurses being named in professional negligence suits is increasing. The most common causes of nursing professional negligence include failure to communicate, failure to perform assessment and notify healthcare provider, and failure to document and report a deteriorating condition (Flynn, 2016; Brown, 2016). See Practice Guidelines later in this chapter for steps to help nurses reduce potential liability.

Intentional Torts

Several differences distinguish unintentional torts from intentional torts. Unintentional torts (e.g., professional negligence) do not require intent but do require the element of harm. In contrast, with intentional torts, the defendant executed the act on purpose or with intent. No harm need be caused by intentional torts for liability to exist. Also, since no standard is involved, no expert witnesses are needed. Four intentional torts related to nursing are discussed here: assault/battery, false imprisonment, invasion of privacy, and defamation (libel or slander). Figure 3.5 ■ provides an overview of the types of law in nursing.

The terms *assault* and *battery* are often heard together, but each has its own meaning. **Assault** can be described as an attempt or threat to touch another individual unjustifiably. Assault precedes battery; it is the act that causes the individual to believe a battery is about to occur. For example, the individual who threatens someone by making a menacing gesture with a club or a closed fist is guilty of assault. A nurse who threatens a client with an injection after the client refuses to take the medication orally would be committing assault.

Battery is the willful touching of an individual (or the individual's clothes or even something the individual is carrying) that may or may not cause harm. To be actionable at law, however, the touching must be wrong in some way; for example, touching done without permission, that is embarrassing, or that causes injury. In the previous example, if the nurse followed through on the threat and gave the injection without the client's consent, the nurse would be committing battery. Liability applies even though the primary care provider ordered the medication

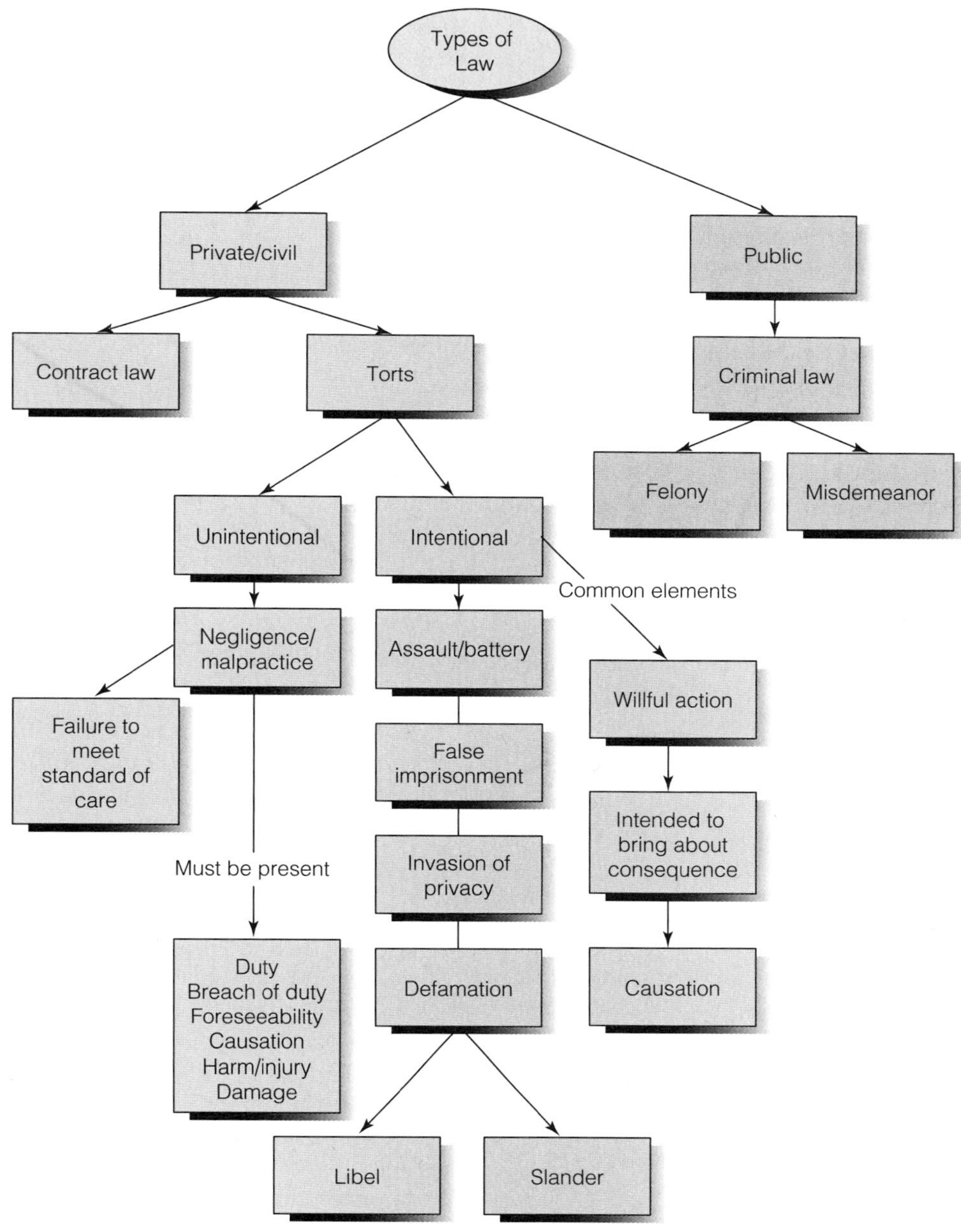

Figure 3.5 ■ An overview of the types of law in nursing practice.

or the activity and even if the client benefits from the nurse's action.

Consent is required before procedures are performed. Battery exists when there is no consent, even if the plaintiff was not asked for consent. Unless there is implied consent, such as in life-threatening emergencies, a procedure performed on an unconscious client without informed consent is battery. Another requirement for consent is that the client be competent to give consent. It can be very difficult to determine if clients who are older, who have specific mental disorders, or who take particular medications are competent to agree to treatments. If the nurse is uncertain whether a client refusing a treatment is competent, the supervisor and primary care provider should be consulted so that ethical treatment that does not constitute battery can be provided. Determination of competency is not a medical decision; it is one made through court hearings.

False imprisonment is the "unjustifiable detention of a person without legal warrant to confine the person" (Guido, 2020, p. 86). False imprisonment accompanied by forceful restraint or threat of restraint is battery.

Although nurses may suggest under certain circumstances that a client remain in the hospital room or in bed, the client must not be detained against the client's will. The client has a right to insist on leaving even though it may be detrimental to health. In this instance, the client can leave by signing an AWA (absence without authority) or AMA (against medical advice) form. As with assault or battery, client competency is a factor in determining whether there is a case of false imprisonment or a situation of protecting a client from injury. To guide nurses in such dilemmas, agencies usually have clear policies regarding the application of restraints (see Chapter 32 ∞).

Invasion of privacy is a direct wrong of a personal nature. It injures the feelings of the individual and does not take into account the effect of revealed information on the reputation of the individual in the community. The right to privacy is the right of individuals to withhold themselves and their lives from public scrutiny. It can also be described as the right to be left alone. Liability can result if the nurse breaches confidentiality by passing along confidential client information to others or intrudes into the client's private domain (Box 3.9).

BOX 3.9 Court Case Example: Invasion of Privacy

A client was scheduled to have surgery for removal of excess skin after major weight loss. Before the surgery, she signed a consent form allowing the plastic surgery clinic to take "before and after" photos of her only to document in her own medical chart. She specifically declined to initial the boxes allowing use of the photos for anything else.

The clinic's office nurse gave a local reporter a computer disc containing the photos. Two of the client's photos appeared in print and online versions of the reporter's story. The photos did not reveal the client's face or her name. The court ("Jane Doe" v. Young, 2009 WL 3680988 [ED. Mo., October 30, 2009]) ruled that the client could sue the clinic for negligence, invasion of privacy, and wrongful commercial appropriation (Snyder, 2009, p. 5).

In this context, a delicate balance must be maintained between the need of a number of people to contribute to the diagnosis and treatment of a client and the client's right to confidentiality. In most situations, necessary discussion about a client's medical condition is considered appropriate, but unnecessary discussions and gossip are considered breaches of confidentiality. Necessary discussion involves only those people engaged in the client's care.

Clinical Alert!

Never discuss client situations in the elevator, cafeteria, or other public areas.

Most jurisdictions of the country have a variety of statutes that impose a duty to report certain confidential client information. Four major categories are (a) vital statistics, such as births and deaths; (b) infections and communicable diseases, such as diphtheria, syphilis, and typhoid fever; (c) child abuse or abuse of older adults; and (d) violent incidents, such as gunshot wounds and knife wounds.

The client must be protected from four types of invasion:

- ***Use of the client's name or likeness for profit, without consent.*** This refers to use of identifiable photographs or names such as advertising for the healthcare agency or provider without the client's permission.
- ***Unreasonable intrusion.*** This involves observation of client care (such as by nursing students) or taking of photographs for any purpose without the client's consent.
- ***Public disclosure of private facts.*** This occurs when private information is given to others who have no legitimate need for that information.
- ***Putting a client in a false light.*** This type of invasion involves publishing information that is normally considered offensive and is not true.

Defamation is communication that is false, or made with a careless disregard for the truth, and results in injury to the reputation of an individual. Both libel and slander are wrongful actions that come under the heading of defamation. **Libel** is defamation by means of print, writing, or pictures. Writing in the nurse's notes that a primary care provider is incompetent because he did not respond immediately to a call is an example of libel. **Slander** is defamation by the spoken word, stating unprivileged (not legally protected) or false words by which a reputation is damaged. An example of slander would be for the nurse to tell a client that another nurse is incompetent.

Only the client defamed may bring the lawsuit. The defamatory material must be communicated to a third party such that the client's reputation may be harmed. For example, a comment made in private criticizing that client's competence is not defamation since a third party did not hear it.

Nurses have a qualified privilege to make statements that could be considered defamatory, but only as a part of nursing practice and only to a primary care provider or another health team member caring directly for the client. The communication must be made in good faith with the intent to protect the quality of client care—for example, when a nurse manager provides a prospective employer with information about a nurse's professional practice (Box 3.10).

BOX 3.10 Court Case Example: Defamation Dismissed

The mother of an adult daughter with chronic brain and nervous system damage filed a civil lawsuit for defamation against a hospital and several physicians. The mother, who took care of the daughter in her home, thought her daughter had pneumonia and called an ambulance to take the daughter to the hospital. While in the hospital, hospital personnel became concerned about the advanced decubitus ulcer on the daughter's back. Adult protective services was called, and after an investigation, the daughter was removed from the home.

The lawsuit was dismissed (Kirby v. Prime Healthcare, 2012 WL 946309 [Cal. App., March 21, 2012]). The daughter was a dependent adult and her mother was the caretaker. By law, healthcare personnel are mandatory reporters of suspected abuse or neglect of dependent adults by their caretakers. Failure to report is a criminal offense for a mandatory reporter (Snyder, 2012, p. 6).

Privacy of Clients' Health Information

Protecting clients' confidentiality has always been an important responsibility of nursing. Recent changes in the laws regarding privacy have implications for healthcare providers and organizations. The Health Insurance Portability and Accountability Act of 1996 (HIPAA) is the first nationwide legislation to protect privacy for health information in the United States. It is important to be aware of identifying information that is protected under HIPAA but may not be initially perceived as health information. Examples include Social Security number, name, address, phone number, email address, and fingerprints. Age should also be a consideration because age can become an identifier in the population older than age 89.

HIPAA includes four specific areas:

1. *Electronic transfer of information* among organizations. Instead of each health provider using its own electronic format to transact claims, HIPAA implements a national uniform standard to simplify such transactions.
2. *Standardized numbers* for identifying providers, employers, and health plans. Instead of each healthcare organization using different formats for identification, HIPAA published standard identifiers. For example, an employer's tax ID number or employer identification number is the standard for electronic transactions.
3. The *security rule* provides for a uniform level of protection of all health information. This rule requires healthcare organizations and providers to ensure the confidentiality, integrity, and availability of all electronic protected health information (ePHI).
4. The *privacy rule* sets standards defining appropriate disclosure of protected health information. This rule also gives clients new rights to understand and control how their health information is used (i.e., how to access their medical records, restrict access by others, request changes, and learn how they have been accessed).

See Box 3.11 for examples of how HIPAA compliance affects nursing practice.

BOX 3.11 Examples of HIPAA Compliance and Nursing Practice

- Store charts in a secure, nonpublic location to prevent the public from viewing or accessing confidential health information.
- Place clipboards face down.
- Do not leave printed copies of protected health information unattended at a printer or fax machine.
- Verify the number dialed before faxing personal health information.
- Encrypt personal health information when transmitting by email.
- Limit access to protected health information to those authorized to obtain the information.
- Require healthcare providers to have passwords to access a client's electronic chart.
- Post or provide a notice informing clients of their rights to privacy regarding their health information.
- Lower voice levels to minimize disclosure of information when, for example, discussing a client's condition over the telephone, giving a report, or reading information aloud from a computer screen or chart.
- Ensure that healthcare providers stay current with HIPAA regulations.

Social Media

The use of social media and other types of electronic communication is rapidly growing. Social media is a valuable tool when used wisely. Nurses and nursing students must understand the benefits and consequences of participating in social networking of all types. Many nurses assume their employer or the nursing board has no authority over them when they are not working, at home, or using their personal devices (Brous & Olsen, 2017, p. 51). This is not true. Inappropriate use of social networking by nurses has resulted in nurses losing their jobs and being disciplined by the board of nursing. Both the NCSBN and ANA have published social media guidelines for nurses.

Comments made on social media are considered public information. Identifying oneself as a nurse carries serious responsibility. Public communication by nurses needs to meet professional standards by being accurate and respectful and following ethical practice.

Healthcare organizations have policies about the use of electronic and social media in the workplace. Therefore, it is usually the nurse's use of social media *outside* of the workplace where the nurse may face serious consequences for inappropriate use of social media. Here are guidelines from the ANA (2011) and NCSBN (2018a) for avoiding the inappropriate use of social media:

- Remember that the standards of professionalism (e.g., an ethical and legal obligation to maintain client privacy and confidentiality at all times) are the same online as in any other circumstance.
- Do not take photos or videos of clients on personal devices, including cell phones.
- Maintain professional boundaries when using electronic media.
- Do not transmit or place online individually identifiable client information.
- Report any identified breach of confidentiality or privacy.

Loss of Client Property

Loss of client property, such as jewelry, money, eyeglasses, and dentures, is a constant concern for hospital personnel. Today, agencies are taking less responsibility for property and are generally requesting clients to sign a waiver on admission relieving the hospital and its employees of any responsibility for property. Situations arise, however, in which the client cannot sign a waiver and the nursing staff must follow prescribed policies for safeguarding the client's property. Nurses are expected to take reasonable precautions to safeguard a client's property, and they can be held liable for its loss or damage if they do not exercise reasonable care.

Unprofessional Conduct

According to most nurse practice acts, unprofessional conduct is considered one of the grounds for action against a nurse's license. **Unprofessional conduct** includes incompetence or gross negligence, conviction for practicing without a license, falsification of client records, and illegally obtaining, using, or possessing controlled substances. Having a personal relationship with a client, especially a vulnerable client, may be considered unprofessional conduct because the *Code of Ethics for Nurses* states that nurses are responsible for maintaining their professional boundaries (ANA, 2015, p. 7). Certain acts may constitute a tort or crime in addition to being unprofessional conduct.

Unethical conduct may also be addressed in nurse practice acts. Unethical conduct includes violation of professional ethical codes, breach of confidentiality, fraud, or refusing to care for clients of specific socioeconomic or cultural origins (see Chapter 4 ∞).

Nurses at all levels of nursing practice can be reported to national data banks. The Healthcare Integrity and Protection Data Bank (HIPDB) was created for the reporting of civil judgments or criminal convictions related to healthcare and licensure or certification actions. Another data bank, the National Practitioner Data Bank (NPDB), was established to identify incompetent and unprofessional healthcare practitioners. The information in these two data banks is not accessible by the public. It can be accessed, however, by state licensing boards, HMOs, hospitals, and professional organizations. The data banks are examples of a nationwide effort to protect the public and to identify and track professionals found liable of professional negligence or actions taken against their license. NPDB annual reports of group data are available at their website.

Legal Protections in Nursing Practice

Laws and strategies are in place to protect the nurse against litigation. Good Samaritan acts are an example of laws designed to help protect nurses when assisting at the scene of an emergency. Providing safe, competent practice by following the nurse practice act and standards of practice is a major legal safeguard for nurses. Accurate and complete documentation is also a critical component of legal protection for the nurse.

Good Samaritan Acts

Good Samaritan acts are laws designed to protect healthcare providers who provide assistance at the scene of an emergency against claims of professional negligence unless it can be shown that there was a gross departure from the normal standard of care or willful wrongdoing on their part. Gross negligence usually involves further injury or harm to the individual. For example, an automobile may strike an injured child left on the side of the road when the nurse leaves to obtain help.

In the United States, most state statutes do not require citizens to render aid to people in distress. Such assistance is considered more of an ethical than a legal duty. To encourage citizens to be Good Samaritans, most states have now enacted legislation releasing a Good Samaritan from legal liability for injuries caused under such circumstances, even if the injuries resulted from negligence of the individual offering emergency aid. It is important, however, to check your state's statute since some states (e.g., Vermont) require people to stop and aid individuals in danger.

It is generally believed that an individual who renders help in an emergency, at a level that would be provided by any reasonably prudent individual under similar circumstances, cannot be held liable. The same reasoning applies to nurses, who are among the people best prepared to help at the scene of an accident. If the level of care a nurse provides is of the caliber that would have been provided by any other nurse, then the nurse will not be held liable.

Guidelines for nurses who choose to render emergency care are as follows:

- Limit actions to those normally considered first aid, if possible.

- Do not perform actions that you do not know how to do.
- Offer assistance, but do not insist.
- Have someone call or go for additional help.
- Do not leave the scene until the injured individual leaves or another qualified individual takes over.
- Do not accept any compensation.

Professional Liability Insurance

Because of the increase in the number of professional negligence lawsuits against health professionals, nurses are advised to carry their own liability insurance. Most hospitals have liability insurance that covers all employees, including all nurses. However, some smaller facilities, such as walk-in clinics, may not. Thus, the nurse should always check with the employer at the time of hiring to see what coverage the facility provides. A primary care provider or a hospital can be sued because of the negligent conduct of a nurse, and the nurse can also be sued and held liable for professional negligence. Because hospitals have been known to countersue nurses when they have been found negligent and the hospital was required to pay, nurses are advised to provide their own insurance coverage and not rely on hospital-provided insurance.

Additionally, nurses often provide nursing services outside of employment-related activities, such as being available for first aid at children's sport or social activities or providing health screening and education at health fairs. Neighbors or friends may seek advice about illnesses or treatment for themselves or family members. In the latter situation, the nurse may be tempted to give advice; however, it is always advisable for the nurse to refer friends or neighbors to their family primary care provider. The nurse may be protected from liability under Good Samaritan acts when nursing service is volunteered; however, if the nurse receives any compensation or if there is a written or verbal agreement outlining the nurse's responsibility to the group, the nurse needs liability coverage for legal expenses in the event that the nurse is sued.

Liability insurance coverage usually defrays all costs of defending a nurse, including the costs of retaining an attorney. The insurance also covers all costs incurred by the nurse up to the face value of the policy, including a settlement made out of court. In return, the insurance company may have the right to make the decisions about the claim and the settlement.

Nursing faculty and nursing students are also vulnerable to lawsuits. Students and teachers of nursing employed by community colleges and universities are not likely to be covered by the insurance carried by hospitals and health agencies. It is advisable for nursing students to check with their school about the coverage that applies to them. Increasingly, faculty carry their own professional liability insurance. Liability insurance can be obtained through the ANA or private insurance companies. Nursing students can also obtain insurance through the National Student Nurses' Association. In some states, hospitals do not allow nursing students to provide nursing care without liability insurance or a signed disclaimer placing the responsibility of the student's actions while in the clinical setting on the student.

Carrying Out a Physician's Orders

Nurses are expected to analyze procedures and medications ordered by the physician or primary care provider. It is the nurse's responsibility to seek clarification of ambiguous or seemingly erroneous orders from the prescriber. Clarification from any other source is unacceptable and regarded as a departure from competent nursing practice.

If the order is neither ambiguous nor apparently erroneous, the nurse is responsible for carrying it out. For example, if the order is for oxygen to be administered at 4 liters per minute, the nurse must administer oxygen at that rate, and not at 2 or 6 liters per minute. If the orders state that the client is not to have solid food after a bowel resection, the nurse must ensure that no solid food is given to the client.

There are several categories of orders that nurses must question to protect themselves legally:

- ***Question any order a client questions.*** For example, if a client who has been receiving an intramuscular injection tells the nurse that the healthcare provider changed the order from an injectable to an oral medication, the nurse must recheck the order before giving the medication.
- ***Question any order if the client's condition has changed.*** The nurse is considered responsible for notifying the primary care provider of any significant changes in the client's condition, whether the primary care provider requests notification or not. For example, if a client who is receiving an intravenous infusion suddenly develops a rapid pulse, chest pain, and a cough, the nurse must notify the primary care provider immediately and question continuance of the ordered rate of infusion. If a client who is receiving morphine for pain develops severely depressed respirations, the nurse must withhold the medication and notify the primary care provider.
- ***Question and record verbal orders to avoid miscommunications.*** In addition to recording the time, the date, the primary care provider's name, and the orders, the nurse documents the circumstances that occasioned the call to the primary care provider, reads the orders back to the primary care provider, and documents that the primary care provider confirmed the orders as the nurse read them back.
- ***Question any order that is illegible, unclear, or incomplete.*** Misinterpretations in the name of a drug or in dose, for example, can easily occur with handwritten orders. The nurse is responsible for ensuring that the order is interpreted the way it was intended and that it is a safe and appropriate order.

Providing Competent Nursing Care

Competent practice is a major legal safeguard for nurses. Nurses need to provide care that is within the legal boundaries of their practice and within the boundaries of agency policies and procedures. Nurses therefore must be familiar with their various job descriptions, which may differ from agency to agency. All nurses are responsible for ensuring that their education and experience are adequate to meet the responsibilities delineated in the job description.

Competency also involves care that protects clients from harm. Nurses need to anticipate sources of client injury, educate clients about hazards, and implement measures to prevent injury.

Application of the nursing process is another essential aspect of providing safe and effective client care. Clients need to be assessed and monitored appropriately and involved in care decisions. All assessments and care must be documented accurately. Effective communication can also protect the nurse from negligence claims. Nurses need to approach every client with sincere concern and include the client in conversations. In addition, nurses should always acknowledge when they do not know the answer to a client's questions, telling the client they will find out the answer and then follow through.

Methods of legal protection are summarized in the accompanying Practice Guidelines.

Documentation

The client's medical chart is a legal document and can be produced in court as evidence. Often, the chart is used to remind a witness of events surrounding a lawsuit, because several months or years usually pass by before a suit goes to trial. The effectiveness of a witness's testimony can depend on the accuracy of the nurse's documentation of nursing care. Nurses, therefore, need to provide accurate and complete documentation of the nursing care provided to clients. Failure to properly document can constitute negligence and be the basis for tort liability. Insufficient or inaccurate assessments and documentation can hinder proper diagnosis and treatment and result in injury to the client (Figure 3.6 ■). See Chapter 14 ∞ for types of records and facts about recording.

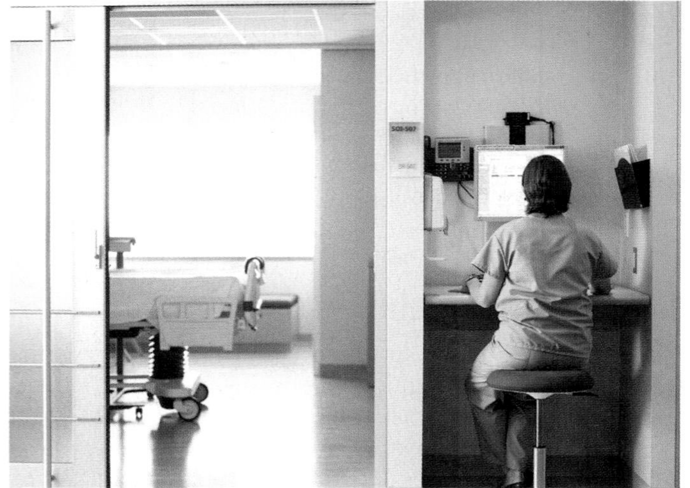

Figure 3.6 ■ Clear and accurate documentation is the nurse's best defense against potential liability.
Ryan McVay/Getty Images.

The Incident Report

An incident report (also called an unusual occurrence report) is an agency record of an accident or unusual occurrence. Incident reports are used to make all facts available to agency personnel, to contribute to statistical data about accidents or incidents, and to help health personnel prevent future incidents or accidents. All accidents are usually reported on incident forms.

Some agencies also report a "near miss," "close call," or "good catch." These terms refer to when an error was committed but the client experienced no harm because of an intervention by healthcare staff, or the client or family, or luck. The situation did not harm the client but the potential existed. For example, a nurse administers medication to the wrong client. The client realizes that the medication is intended for the client in the next bed and informs the nurse. Depending on the type of medication, the client could have been injured through administration of the wrong medication. Obtaining this type of data helps organizations to promote client safety and prevent errors.

The nurse completes the following tasks when completing an incident report:

- Identify the client by name, initials, and hospital or identification number.
- Give the date, time, and place of the incident.
- Describe the facts of the incident. Avoid any conclusions or blame. Describe the incident as you saw it even if your impressions differ from those of others.
- Incorporate the client's account of the incident. State the client's comments by using direct quotes.
- Identify all witnesses to the incident.
- Identify any equipment by number and any medication by name and dosage.

The report should be completed as soon as possible and filed according to agency policy. Because incident reports are not part of the client's medical record, the facts of the incident should also be noted in the medical record. Do not record in the client record that an incident report has been completed because the facts are already documented in the chart. The purpose of the report form is to alert the risk manager to the event.

The individual who identifies that the incident occurred should complete the incident report. This may not be the same individual actually involved with the incident. For example, the nurse who discovers that an incorrect medication has been administered completes the form even if it was another nurse who administered the medication. In addition, all witnesses to an incident, such

PRACTICE GUIDELINES Legal Protection for Nurses

- Function within the scope of your education, job description, and nurse practice act.
- Follow the policies and procedures of the employing agency.
- Build and maintain good rapport with clients.
- Always check the identity of a client to make sure it is the right client.
- Observe and monitor the client accurately. Communicate and record significant changes in the client's condition to the primary care provider.
- Promptly and accurately document all assessments and care given.
- Be alert when implementing nursing interventions, and give each task your full attention and skill.
- Perform procedures correctly and appropriately.
- Make sure the correct medications are given in the correct dose, by the right route, at the scheduled time, and to the right client.
- When delegating or assigning nursing responsibilities, make sure that the individual who is assigned or delegated a task understands what to do and has the required knowledge and skill.
- Protect clients from injury.
- Report all incidents involving clients.
- Always check any order that a client questions.
- Know your own strengths and weaknesses. Ask for assistance and supervision in situations for which you feel inadequately prepared.
- Maintain your clinical competence. For students, this demands study and practice before caring for clients. For graduate nurses, it means continued study to maintain and update clinical knowledge and skills.

as a client fall, are listed on the incident form even if they were not directly involved.

Incident reports are often reviewed by an agency risk management committee, which decides whether to investigate the incident further. Nurses may be required to answer such questions as what they believe precipitated the accident, how it could have been prevented, and whether any equipment should be adjusted.

When an accident occurs, the nurse should first assess the client and intervene to prevent injury. If a client is injured, nurses must take steps to protect the client, themselves, and their employer. Most agencies have policies regarding accidents. It is important to follow these policies and not to assume one is negligent. Although negligence may be involved, accidents can and do happen even when every precaution has been taken to prevent them.

Reporting Crimes, Torts, and Unsafe Practices

Nurses may need to report nursing colleagues or other health professionals for practices that endanger the health and safety of clients. For instance, alcohol and drug use, theft from a client or agency, and unsafe nursing practice should be reported. Reporting a colleague is not easy. The individual reporting may feel disloyal, encounter the disapproval of others, or perceive that chances for promotion are at risk. When reporting an incident or series of incidents, the nurse must be careful to describe observed behavior only and not make inferences as to what might be happening. The accompanying Practice Guidelines can be used for reporting a crime, tort, or unsafe practice.

In some states, it is mandatory for a nurse with knowledge of unprofessional conduct to report that behavior to the state board of nursing. In addition, reporting illegal, unethical, or incompetent performance is an expectation found in the ANA *Code of Ethics*.

Legal Responsibilities of Students

Nursing students are responsible for their own actions and liable for their own acts of negligence committed during the course of clinical experiences. When they perform duties that are within the scope of professional nursing, such as administering an injection, they are legally held to the same standard of skill and competence as a registered professional nurse. Lower standards are not applied to the actions of nursing students. A student does not work under another nurse's license (Brooks, 2017).

PRACTICE GUIDELINES Reporting a Crime, Tort, or Unsafe Practice

- Write a clear description of the situation you believe you should report.
- Make sure that your statements are factual and complete.
- Make sure you are credible.
- Obtain support from at least one trustworthy individual before filing the report.
- Report the matter starting at the lowest possible level in the agency hierarchy.
- Assume responsibility for reporting the individual by being open about it. Sign your name to the letter.
- See the problem through once you have reported it.

Clinical Alert!

Each nurse and nursing student is responsible and accountable for providing safe client care.

Nursing students are not considered employees of the agencies in which they receive clinical experience because these nursing programs contract with agencies to provide clinical experiences for students. In cases of negligence involving such students, the hospital or agency (e.g., public health agency) and the educational institution will be held potentially liable. Some nursing schools require students to carry individual professional liability insurance.

Nursing students need to be aware that most state boards of nursing in the United States require a reporting of prior criminal history when applying for licensure. An individual with past felony and some misdemeanor offenses may be denied licensure even though that individual graduated from an approved nursing program. Nursing students who are unsure of their personal situation are advised to contact their state board of nursing for more information. Many nursing schools currently require a background check of students before they can attend their clinical practicum. The purpose of this requirement is to protect the public.

Students in clinical situations must be assigned learning experiences within their capabilities and be given reasonable guidance and supervision. The nursing instructor and nursing preceptor (nurse responsible for the client's care) are accountable for assigning students to the care of clients and for providing reasonable supervision. Failure to provide reasonable supervision or the assignment of a client to a student who is not prepared and competent can be a basis for liability.

To fulfill responsibilities to clients and to minimize chances for liability, nursing students need to:

- Make sure they are prepared to carry out the necessary care for assigned clients.
- Ask for additional help or supervision in situations for which they feel inadequately prepared.
- Comply with the policies of the agency in which they obtain their clinical experience.
- Comply with the policies and definitions of responsibility supplied by the school of nursing.

Students who work as part-time or temporary nursing assistants or aides must also remember that legally they can perform only those tasks that appear in the job description of a nurse's aide or assistant. Even though a student may have received instruction and acquired competence in administering injections or suctioning a tracheostomy tube, the student cannot legally perform these tasks while employed as an aide or assistant. While acting as a paid employee, the student is covered for negligent acts by the employer, not the school of nursing.

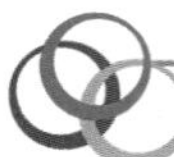

Critical Thinking Checkpoint

A female adult client who has been blind since birth is admitted to the surgical unit. She is to have surgery the next morning. The primary care provider has written an order for the client to sign the surgical consent form. The husband is in the client's room when the nurse approaches the client to sign the consent form. The husband says that he will sign for his wife.

1. What question(s) should the nurse ask before addressing the signing of the form?
2. Can someone who is blind give consent?
3. How can the nurse ensure that the client is aware of what she is signing?
4. What else should the nurse consider when obtaining a signature?
5. What would the nurse include in the documentation?

Answers to Critical Thinking Checkpoint questions are available on the faculty resources site. Please consult with your instructor.

Chapter 3 Review

CHAPTER HIGHLIGHTS

- Accountability is an essential concept of professional nursing practice under the law.
- Nurses need to understand laws that regulate and affect nursing practice to ensure that nurses' actions are consistent with current legal principles and to protect themselves from liability.
- Nurse practice acts legally define and describe the scope of nursing practice that the law seeks to regulate.
- Competence in nursing practice is determined and maintained by various credentialing methods, such as licensure, certification, and accreditation, to protect the public's welfare and safety.
- Standards of practice published by national and state nursing associations, agency policies and procedures, and job descriptions further delineate the scope of a nurse's practice.
- The nurse has specific legal obligations and responsibilities to clients and employers. As a citizen, the nurse has the rights and responsibilities shared by all individuals in the society.
- Collective bargaining is one way nurses can improve their working conditions and economic welfare.
- Informed consent implies that (a) the consent was given voluntarily, (b) the client was of age and had the capacity and competency to

understand, and (c) the client was given enough information on which to make an informed decision.

- The Americans with Disabilities Act of 1990 prohibits discrimination on the basis of disability in employment, public services, and public accommodations. Nurses need to know how the ADA affects nursing practice.
- Substance use disorder (SUD) involves a pattern of behaviors ranging from misuse to dependency or addiction to alcohol or drugs. Nurses can be at increased risk because of the high levels of stress involved in many healthcare settings and the easy access to drugs. The nurse needs to know the proper reporting procedures for nurses whose practice is affected by SUD.
- Nurses must be knowledgeable of their responsibilities about legal issues surrounding death: advance directives, autopsies, certification of death, DNR orders, euthanasia, inquests, and organ donation.
- Nurse professional negligence, an unintentional tort, can be established when the following criteria are met: (a) the nurse (defendant) owed a duty to the client, (b) the nurse failed to carry out that duty according to standards, (c) there was foreseeability of harm, (d) the client's injury was caused by the nurse's failure to follow the standard, and (e) the client (plaintiff) was injured. The nurse is liable for damages that may be compensated.
- Nurses can be held liable for intentional torts, such as assault and battery, false imprisonment, invasion of privacy, and defamation.
- The Health Insurance Portability and Accountability Act of 1996 (HIPAA) was the first nationwide legislation to protect the privacy of health information. HIPAA includes four specific areas: a uniform standard for electronic transfer of information among organizations; standardized numbers for identifying providers, employers, and health plans; a security rule; and a privacy rule.
- Nurses and nursing students must understand the benefits and consequences of participating in social networking of all types. Both the ANA and NCSBN have published social media guidelines for nurses.
- Good Samaritan acts protect health professionals from claims of professional negligence when they offer assistance at the scene of an emergency, provided that there is no willful wrongdoing or gross departure from normal standards of care.
- Nursing students and practicing nurses can obtain professional liability insurance through professional nursing associations.
- When a client is accidentally injured or involved in an unusual situation, the nurse's first responsibility is to take steps to protect the client and then to notify appropriate agency personnel.
- Nursing students are held to the same standard as licensed nurses and, therefore, need to make certain that they are prepared to provide the necessary care to assigned clients. It is important that students ask for help or supervision in situations for which they feel inadequately prepared.

TEST YOUR KNOWLEDGE

1. A physician is to perform an invasive procedure on a client. The client is questioning the meaning of some of the terminology in the consent form. Which of the following is an appropriate response by the nurse?
1. "Just sign the form, and I'll make sure your physician talks to you before he begins the procedure."
2. "I'll explain whatever you don't understand."
3. "You should have asked your physician when he was here."
4. "I'll call your physician back in the room to answer your questions."

2. Although the client refused the procedure, the nurse insisted and inserted a nasogastric tube in the right nostril. The administrator of the hospital decides to settle the lawsuit because the nurse is most likely to be found guilty of which of the following?
1. An unintentional tort
2. Assault
3. Invasion of privacy
4. Battery

3. A nurse discovers that a primary care provider has prescribed an unusually large dosage of a medication. Which is the most appropriate action?
1. Administer the medication.
2. Notify the prescriber.
3. Call the pharmacist.
4. Refuse to administer the medication.

4. A client woke in the middle of the night, confused and unaware of the surroundings. Although the call light was within reach, the client got out of bed unassisted, tripped on the bedside chair, and fell. Which of the following elements of malpractice is missing in this case?
1. Foreseeability
2. Damages
3. Injury
4. Duty

5. A nurse has delegated the task of obtaining a client's vital signs to a UAP (unlicensed assistive personnel). The task is completed, but the vitals were not recorded accurately. Who is fully responsible for this action?
1. The UAP
2. The nurse
3. Both the UAP and the nurse
4. The nurse manager on the unit

6. The primary care provider wrote a do-not-resuscitate (DNR) order. The nurse recognizes that which applies in the planning of nursing care for this client?
1. The client may no longer make decisions regarding his or her own healthcare.
2. The client and family know that the client will most likely die within the next 48 hours.
3. The nurses will continue to implement all treatments focused on comfort and symptom management.
4. A DNR order from a previous admission is valid for the current admission.

7. The nurse's partner undergoes exploratory surgery at the hospital where the nurse is employed. Which practice is most appropriate?
1. Because the nurse is an employee, access to the chart is allowed.
2. The relationship with the client provides the nurse special access to the chart.
3. Access to the chart requires a signed release form.
4. The nurse can ask the surgeon to discuss the outcome of the surgery.

8. Following a motor vehicle crash, a nurse stops and offers assistance. Which of the following actions is/are most appropriate? Select all that apply.
1. The nurse needs to know the Good Samaritan Act for the state.
2. The nurse is not held liable unless there is gross negligence.
3. After assessing the situation, the nurse can leave to obtain help.
4. The nurse can expect compensation for helping.
5. The nurse offers to help but cannot insist on helping.

9. The nurse notices that a colleague's behaviors have changed during the past month. Which behaviors could indicate signs of SUD? Select all that apply.
1. Is increasingly absent from the nursing unit during the shift
2. Interacts well with others
3. "Forgets" to sign out for administration of controlled substances
4. Offers to administer prn opioids for other nurses' clients
5. Is able to say no to requests to work more shifts

10. Which nursing actions could result in professional negligence? Select all that apply.
1. Learns about a new piece of equipment
2. Forgets to complete the assessment of a client
3. Does not follow up on client's complaints
4. Charts client's drug allergies
5. Questions primary care provider about an illegible order

See Answers to Test Your Knowledge in Appendix A.

READINGS AND REFERENCES

Suggested Readings

Flynn, J. (2018). Medical malpractice 101. *Imprint*, *65*(3), 24–27.

The author provides an overview of professional negligence, including the elements that must occur, the importance of good documentation, knowing the facility's policies and procedures, and key points for protecting your career.

Lilly, L. L. (2016). Risky business: Your personal conduct outside of work can lead to discipline from the nursing boards. *Alaska Nurse*, *67*(3), 3–5.

This article, written by a nurse attorney, describes how certain behaviors in nurses' private lives or involving only their personal conduct can result in disciplinary action. Examples are given regarding off-the-job behavior, on-the-job behavior, and social media.

U.S. Department of Health and Human Services, Office of Minority Health. (n.d.). *Think cultural health. Culturally competent nursing care: A cornerstone of caring*. Retrieved from https://ccnm.thinkculturalhealth.hhs.gov/Content/Introduction/Introduction1.asp?

Culturally Competent Nursing Care is an e-learning program designed to help nurses deliver culturally and linguistically competent care. This program offers the opportunity to gain the awareness, knowledge, and skills to improve the quality of care nurses provide to their clients.

Related Research

Mumba, M. N. (2018). Employment implications of nurses going through peer assistance programs for substance use disorders. *Archives of Psychiatric Nursing*, *32*, 561–567. doi:10.1016/j.apnu.2018.03.001

References

American Nurses Association. (2011). *Principles for social networking and the nurse*. Silver Spring, MD: Author.

American Nurses Association. (2012). *Nursing care and do not resuscitate (DNR) and allow natural death (AND) decisions. Revised position statement*. Retrieved from https://www.nursingworld.org/~4af287/globalassets/docs/ana/ethics/ps_nursing-care-and-do-not-resuscitate--allow-natural-death.pdf

American Nurses Association. (2015). *Code of ethics for nurses with interpretive statements*. Silver Spring, MD: Author.

American Nurses Association & National Council of State Boards of Nursing. (2019). *Joint statement on delegation: American Nurses Association and National Council of State Boards of Nursing Position Statement*. Retrieved from https://www.nursingworld.org/practice-policy/nursing-excellence/official-position-statements/id/joint-statement-on-delegation-by-ANA-and-NCSBN

Brent, N. J. (2019). When a BON disciplinary process is based on substance misuse disorder. *American Nurse Today*, *14*(3), 14–16.

Brooks K. L. (2017). Issues of liability: The myth of another working under the nurse's license. *New Mexico Nurse*, *62*(3), 5.

Brous, E., & Olsen, D. P. (2017). Lessons learned from litigation: Legal and ethical consequences of social media. *American Journal of Nursing*, *117*(9), 50–54. doi:10.1097/01.NAJ.0000524546.50943.9e

Brown, G. (2016). Averting malpractice issues in today's nursing practice. *ABNF Journal*, *27*(2), 25–27.

Death with Dignity National Center. (n.d.). *Frequently asked questions*. Retrieved from https://www.deathwithdignity.org/faqs/

Flynn, J. (2016). If you see something, say something. *New Hampshire Nursing News*, *40*(3), 16.

Guidelines on Discrimination Because of Sex, 29 C.F.R. § 1604.11 (2016). Retrieved from https://www.gpo.gov/fdsys/pkg/CFR-2016-title29-vol4/xml/CFR-2016-title29-vol4-part1604.xml

Guido, G. W. (2020). *Legal and ethical issues in nursing* (7th ed.). Upper Saddle River, NJ: Pearson.

Lee, A. W., & Billings, M. (2016). Telehealth implementation in a skilled nursing facility: Case report for physical therapist practice in Washington. *Physical Therapy*, *96*, 252–259. doi:10.2522/ptj.20150079

National Council of State Boards of Nursing. (n.d.a). *APRN compact*. Retrieved from https://www.aprncompact.com/stay-informed.htm

National Council of State Boards of Nursing. (n.d.b). *eNLC fast facts*. Retrieved from https://www.ncsbn.org/NLC_Fast_Facts.pdf

National Council of State Boards of Nursing. (n.d.c). *NLC member states*. Retrieved from https://www.ncsbn.org/listofmemberstatesanddates111618.pdf

National Council of State Boards of Nursing. (n.d.d). *Uniform licensure requirements for a multistate license*. Retrieved from https://www.ncsbn.org/ULR_Updated_Jan_2018.pdf

National Council of State Boards of Nursing. (2018a). *A Nurse's Guide to Substance Use Disorder in Nursing*. Retrieved from https://ncsbn.org/3718.htm

National Council of State Boards of Nursing. (2018b). *A nurse's guide to the use of social media*. Retrieved from https://www.ncsbn.org/3739.htm

National Council of State Boards of Nursing. (2018c). The nursing regulatory environment in 2018: Issues and challenges. *Journal of Nursing Regulation*, *9*(1), 52–65. doi:10.1016/S2155-8256(18)30055-3

National Council of State Boards of Nursing. (2019). *Understanding substance use disorder in nursing*. Retrieved from https://www.learningext.com/#/online-courses/0fcf5dc0-03f2-4f95-b604-db8d095bb09b

Oregon Public Health Division. (2018). *Oregon Death with Dignity Act: 2017 data summary*. Retrieved from https://www.oregon.gov/oha/PH/PROVIDERPARTNERRESOURCES/EVALUATIONRESEARCH/DEATHWITHDIGNITYACT/Documents/year20.pdf

Scott, S. A. (2016). Health literacy education in baccalaureate nursing programs in the United States. *Nursing Education Perspectives*, *37*, 153–158. doi:10.1097/01.NEP.0000000000000005

Snyder, E. K. (1997, October). Injection site and mode not charted: Nurse found guilty of substandard practice. *Legal Eagle Eye Newsletter for the Nursing Profession*, 7.

Snyder, E. K. (2008, December). Informed consent: Nursing notes compel dismissal of medical-battery lawsuit. *Legal Eagle Eye Newsletter for the Nursing Profession*, 7.

Snyder, E. K. (2009, December). Invasion of privacy: Plastic surgery patient's photos published. *Legal Eagle Eye Newsletter for the Nursing Profession*, 5.

Snyder, E. K. (2010, April). Do not resuscitate: Nurse faulted for delay while looking for patient's code paperwork. *Legal Eagle Eye Newsletter for the Nursing Profession*, 1.

Snyder, E. K. (2012, April). Abuse reporting: Defamation suit dismissed. *Legal Eagle Eye Newsletter for the Nursing Profession*, 6.

Snyder, E. K. (2014, August). Improper delegation of nursing responsibility: Discrimination lawsuit dismissed. *Legal Eagle Eye Newsletter for the Nursing Profession*, 4.

Starr, K. T. (2016). Should you witness a signature on a patient's personal legal document? *Nursing*, *46*(12), 14. doi:10.1097/01.NURSE.0000504688.51378.eb

Stewart, D. M., & Mueller, C. A. (2018). Substance use disorder among nurses. A curriculum improvement initiative. *Nurse Educator*, *43*(3), 132–135. doi:10.1097/NNE.0000000000000466

U.S. Department of Health and Human Services. (n.d.a). *Culturally competent nursing care: A cornerstone of caring*. Retrieved from https://www.thinkculturalhealth.hhs.gov/education/nurses

U.S. Department of Health and Human Services. (n.d.b). *Organ procurement and transplantation network: About the OPTN*. Retrieved from https://optn.transplant.hrsa.gov/governance/about-the-optn

U.S. Department of Health and Human Services. (n.d.c). *Organ procurement and transplantation network: The basic path of donation*. Retrieved from https://optn.transplant.hrsa.gov/learn/about-donation/the-basic-path-of-donation

U.S. Department of Health and Human Services, Office of Minority Health. (2018). *The national CLAS standards*. Retrieved from http://minorityhealth.hhs.gov/omh/browse.aspx?lvl=2&lvlid=53

Weinberg, K. (2018). The eNLC—What you need to know. *Iowa Board of Nursing Newsletter*, *37*(3), 1.

Selected Bibliography

American Nurses Association. (n.d.). *Substance use among nurses and nursing students*. Retrieved from https://www.nursingworld.org/practice-policy/work-environment/health-safety/healthy-nurse-healthy-nation/substance-abuse

American Nurses Association. (2016). *Nurses' roles and responsibilities in providing care and support at the end of life: Position statement*. Retrieved from https://www.nursingworld.org/practice-policy/nursing-excellence/official-position-statements/id/nurses-roles-and-responsibilities-in-providing-care-and-support-at-the-end-of-life

Balestra, M. (2018). Social media missteps could put your nursing license at risk. *American Nurse Today*, *13*(3), 20–21, 63.

Brous, E. (2016). Legal considerations in telehealth and telemedicine. *American Journal of Nursing*, *116*(9), 64–67. doi:10.1097/01.NAJ.0000494700.7816.d3

Brown, L. A. (2016). Substance abuse and the law: A case study. *Nursing*, *46*(6), 58–61. doi:10.1097/01.NURSE.0000482872.32838.b6

Emergency Nurses Association (ENA) & International Nurses Society on Addictions (IntNSA). (2017). *Substance use among nurses and nursing students: Joint position statement*. Retrieved from https://www.nursingworld.org/practice-policy/nursing-excellence/official-position-statements/id/substance-use-among-nurses-and-nursing-students

Freedman, L. F., & Rattigan, K. M. (2018). The intersection between medicine and law: Legal nurse consultants' roles and responsibilities under HIPAA. *Journal of Legal Nurse Consulting*, *29*(2), 14–17. doi:10.30710/JLNC.29.2.2018.14

Kerr, L. (2016). Low health literacy is common, but can be addressed. *Urology Times*, *44*(5), 20.

Lockhart, L., & Davis, C. (2017). Spotting impairment in the healthcare workplace. *Nursing Made Incredibly Easy!*, *15*(3), 38–44. doi:10.1097/01.NME.0000514209.85144.4b

Loughran, M. (2017). The enhanced nursing compact and its implications. *Journal of Legal Nurse Consulting*, *28*(4), 10–13.

McCulloh, K., & Marks, B. (2016). Challenges and strategies of nursing students and nurses with disabilities. *Nursing News*, *40*(1), 6–7.

New Enhanced Nurse Licensure Compact (eNLC) expands access to care: Changes to revise Nurse Licensure Compact. (2018). *Virginia Nurses Today*, *26*(3), 6.

Olsen, D. P., & Brous, E. (2018). The ethical and legal implications of a nurse's arrest in Utah. *American Journal of Nursing*, *118*(3), 47–53. doi:10.1097/01.NAJ.0000530938.88865.7f

Pate, J. M. (2016). Professional liability insurance: Fact or fiction? *AAACN Viewpoint*, *38*(5), 9–11.

Simmons, K. (2016). Authority to give informed consent for minors. *AORN Journal*, *104*(2), 18–19. doi:10.1016/S0001-2092(16)30395-7

Starr, K. T. (2018). You've been served: Responding to a malpractice summons. *Nursing*, *48*(8), 11–12. doi:10.1097/01.NURSE.0000541395.59728.a4

Stockwell, S. (2018). What nurses need to know about cybersecurity. *American Journal of Nursing*, *118*(12), 17–18. doi:10.1097/01.NAJ.0000549682.13264.dc

Truglio-Londrigan, M. (2016). Shared decision making through reflective practice: Part I. *MEDSURG Nursing*, *25*(4), 260–264.

4 Values, Ethics, and Advocacy

LEARNING OUTCOMES

After completing this chapter, you will be able to:

1. Explain how values, moral frameworks, and codes of ethics affect moral decisions.
2. Explain how nurses use knowledge of values to make ethical decisions and to assist clients in clarifying their values.
3. When presented with an ethical situation, identify the moral issues and principles involved.
4. Discuss common ethical issues currently facing healthcare professionals.
5. Discuss the advocacy role of the nurse.

KEY TERMS

Introduction

In their daily work, nurses deal with intimate and fundamental human events such as birth, death, and suffering. They must decide the **morality** (standards of right and wrong) of their own actions when they face the many ethical issues that surround such sensitive areas. Because of the special nurse–client relationship, nurses are the ones who are there to support and advocate for clients and families who are facing difficult choices, and for those who are living the results of choices that others make for and about them.

The present environment of cost containment and the nursing shortage tends to emphasize business values. This creates new moral problems and intensifies old ones, making it more critical than ever for nurses to make sound moral decisions. Therefore, nurses need to (a) develop sensitivity to the ethical dimensions of nursing practice, (b) examine their own and clients' values, (c) understand how values influence their decisions, and (d) think ahead about the kinds of moral problems they are likely to face. This chapter explores the influences of values and moral frameworks on the ethical dimensions of nursing practice and on the nurse's role as a client advocate.

Values

Values are enduring beliefs or attitudes about the worth of an individual, object, idea, or action. Values are important because they influence decisions and actions, including nurses' ethical decision making. Questions of value underlie all moral dilemmas, even though they may be unspoken and perhaps even unconsciously held. Not all values are moral values. For example, people hold values about work, family, religion, politics, money, and relationships. Values are often taken for granted. In the same way that people are not aware of their breathing, they usually do not think about their values; they simply accept them and act on them.

People organize their values internally along a continuum from most important to least important, forming a **value system**. Value systems give direction to life and form the basis of behavior—especially behavior that is based on decisions or choices.

Beliefs and attitudes are related, but not identical, to values. People have many different beliefs and attitudes, but a smaller number of values. **Beliefs** (or opinions) are interpretations or conclusions that people accept as true. They are based more on faith than fact. Beliefs do not necessarily involve values. For example, the statement

"If I study hard I will get a good grade" expresses a belief that does not involve a value. By contrast, the statement "Good grades are really important to me and I must study hard to obtain good grades" involves both a value and a belief.

Attitudes are mental positions or feelings toward an individual, object, or idea (e.g., acceptance, compassion, openness). Typically, an attitude lasts over time, whereas a belief may last only briefly. Attitudes are often judged as bad or good, positive or negative, whereas beliefs are judged as correct or incorrect. Attitudes have thinking and behavioral aspects and vary greatly among individuals. For example, some clients may feel strongly about their need for privacy, whereas others may dismiss it as unimportant.

Values Transmission

Values are learned through observation and experience. As a result, they are heavily influenced by an individual's sociocultural environment—that is, by societal traditions; by cultural, ethnic, and religious groups; and by family and peer groups. For example, if a parent consistently demonstrates honesty in dealing with others, the child will probably begin to value honesty. Historically, American values reflected the influence of original settlers, who originated from a limited number of countries. In a classic essay, members of the Washington International Center described 13 U.S. values in an attempt to assist immigrants from other countries to understand Americans (Kohls, 1984). Some of those values persist, such as an emphasis on the productive use of time.

Nurses should keep in mind the influence of values on health (see Chapter 20 ∞). For example, some cultures value treatment by a folk healer over that by a physician. For additional information about cultural values related to health and illness, see Chapter 21 ∞.

Personal Values

Although people derive values from society and their individual subgroups, they internalize some or all of these values as **personal values**. People need societal values to feel accepted, and they need personal values to have a sense of individuality.

Professional Values

Nurses' **professional values** are acquired during socialization into nursing from codes of ethics, nursing experiences, teachers, and peers. The American Association of Colleges of Nursing (2008) identified five values essential for the professional nurse: altruism, autonomy, human dignity, integrity, and social justice (Box 4.1).

BOX 4.1 Essential Nursing Values

Altruism is a concern for the welfare and well-being of others. In professional practice, altruism is reflected by the nurse's concern for the welfare of patients, other nurses, and other healthcare providers.

Autonomy is the right to self-determination. Professional practice reflects autonomy when the nurse respects patients' rights to make decisions about their healthcare.

Human dignity is respect for the inherent worth and uniqueness of individuals and populations. In professional practice, human dignity is reflected when the nurse values and respects all patients and colleagues.

Integrity is acting in accordance with an appropriate code of ethics and accepted standards of practice. Integrity is reflected in professional practice when the nurse is honest and provides care based on an ethical framework that is accepted within the profession.

Social justice is acting in accordance with fair treatment regardless of economic status, race, ethnicity, age, citizenship, disability, or sexual orientation.

From *The Essentials of Baccalaureate Education for Professional Nursing Practice* (pp. 27–28), American Association of Colleges of Nursing, 2008, Washington, DC: Author. Reprinted with permission.

Values Clarification

Values clarification is a process by which people identify, examine, and develop their own individual values. A principle of values clarification is that no one set of values is right for everyone. When people can identify their values, they can retain or change them and thus act based on freely chosen, rather than unconscious, values. Values clarification promotes personal growth by fostering awareness, empathy, and insight. Therefore, it is an important step for nurses to take in dealing with ethical problems.

One widely used theory of values clarification was developed by Raths, Harmin, and Simon (1978). They described a "valuing process" of thinking, feeling, and behavior that they termed "choosing," "prizing," and "acting" (Box 4.2). In some cases, a values clarification

BOX 4.2 Values Clarification

Choosing (Cognitive) Beliefs are chosen

- Freely, without outside pressure
- From among alternatives
- After reflecting and considering consequences.

Example: A person learns about energy resources, production, and consumption; the greenhouse effect; and other environmental issues, including ways to minimize use of and to recycle limited resources.

Prizing (Affective) Chosen beliefs are prized and cherished.

Example: The person is proud of the belief that he or she has an obligation to participate in some way in reducing environmental waste.

Acting (Behavioral) Chosen beliefs are

- Affirmed to others
- Incorporated into one's behavior
- Repeated consistently in one's life.

Example: The person participates in the city recycling program for household waste, uses public transportation rather than driving a personal car when possible, helps organize recycling in the workplace, and is active in legislative and political activities related to environmental issues.

From *Values and Teaching: Working with Values in the Classroom*, 2nd ed., by L. Raths, J. Harmin, and S. Simon. Published by C. E. Merrill Publishing Company, 1978. Used by permission of James Raths.

exercise can be useful in helping individuals or groups to become more aware of their values and how they may influence their actions. For example, asking a client to agree or disagree with a list of statements or to rank in order of importance a list of beliefs can assist the nurse and client to make the client's values more open so they can be considered in planning the client's care.

Clarifying the Nurse's Values

Nurses and nursing students need to reflect on the values they hold about life, death, health, and illness. Nurses hold both personal and professional values. One strategy for gaining awareness of personal values is to consider attitudes about specific issues such as abortion or euthanasia, asking: "Can I accept this, or live with this?" "What would I do or want done in this situation?" As is true with all people, nurses' values are influenced by culture, education, and age. Although there may be some variation in perspectives of nurses from different generations, fundamental professional nursing values are caring, integrity, diversity, and excellence (National League for Nursing, 2018).

Clarifying Client Values

To plan effective client-centered care, nurses need to identify clients' values as they influence and relate to a particular health problem. For example, a client with failing eyesight will probably place a high value on the ability to see, and a client with chronic pain will value comfort. Normally, people take such things for granted. For information about health beliefs and practices, see Chapter 20 ∞. The nurse should never assume that the client has any particular values. Rather, the nurse explores client values through discussion. As described in the QSEN competencies, clients' values, and thus their preferences, are assessed and used in each step of nursing care, including the communication of these values to other members of the healthcare team (Cronenwett et al., 2007). When it seems as if clients hold unclear or conflicting values that are detrimental to their health, the nurse should use values clarification as an intervention. Examples of behaviors that may indicate the need for clarification of health values are listed in Table 4.1.

The following process may help clients clarify their values:

1. ***List alternatives.*** Make sure that the client is aware of all alternative actions. Ask "Are you considering other courses of action?" "Tell me about them."
2. ***Examine possible consequences of choices.*** Make sure the client has thought about possible results of each action. Ask "What do you think you will gain from doing that?" "What benefits do you foresee from doing that?"
3. ***Choose freely.*** To determine whether the client chose freely, ask "Did you have any say in that decision?" "Do you have a choice?"
4. ***Describe feelings about the choice.*** Some clients may not feel satisfied with their decision. A sensitive question may be "Some people feel good after a decision is made; others feel bad. How do you feel?"
5. ***Affirm the choice.*** Ask "How will you discuss this with others (family, friends)?"
6. ***Act with a pattern.*** To determine whether the client consistently behaves in a certain way, ask "How many times have you done that before?" or "Would you act that way again?"

When implementing these steps to clarify values, the nurse assists the client to think each question through, but does not impose personal values. The nurse rarely, if ever, offers an opinion when the client asks for it—and then only with great care or when the nurse is an expert in the content area. Because each situation is different, what the nurse would choose in his or her own life may not be relevant to the client's circumstances. Thus, if the client asks the nurse "What would you have done in my situation?" it is best to redirect the question back to the client rather than answering from the nurse's personal view.

Ethics and Morality

The term **ethics** has several meanings in common use. It refers to (a) a method of inquiry that helps people to understand the morality of human behavior (i.e., it is the study of morality), (b) the practices or beliefs of a certain group (e.g., medical ethics, nursing ethics), and (c) the expected standards of moral behavior of a particular group as described in the group's formal code of professional ethics. Nurses have been viewed as the most honest and ethical professionals in U.S. Gallup polls every year since 1999 except when firefighters ranked first shortly after the September 11, 2001, terrorist attacks (Brenan, 2018). **Bioethics** is ethics as applied

TABLE 4.1 Behaviors That May Indicate Unclear Values

Behavior	Example
Ignoring a health professional's advice	A client with heart disease who values hard work ignores advice to exercise regularly.
Inconsistent communication or behavior	A pregnant woman says she wants a healthy baby but continues to drink alcohol and smoke tobacco.
Numerous admissions to a health agency for the same problem	A middle-aged obese woman repeatedly seeks help for back pain but does not lose weight.
Confusion or uncertainty about which course of action to take	A woman wants to obtain a job to meet financial obligations but also wants to stay at home to care for an ailing husband.

to human life or health (e.g., to decisions about abortion or euthanasia). **Nursing ethics** refers to ethical issues that occur in nursing practice. The American Nurses Association's (ANA) *Nursing: Scope and Standards of Practice* (2015a) holds nurses accountable for their ethical conduct. Professional Performance Standard 7 relates to ethics. The current edition of this standard was significantly expanded to include greater emphasis on nurse advocacy and professional responsibility.

Morality (or morals) is similar to ethics, and many people use the terms interchangeably. Morality usually refers to private, personal standards of what is right and wrong in conduct, character, and attitude. Sometimes the first clue to the moral nature of a situation is an active conscience or an awareness of feelings such as guilt, hope, or shame. Another indicator is the tendency to respond to the situation with words such as *ought*, *should*, *right*, *wrong*, *good*, and *bad*. Moral issues are concerned with important social values and norms; they are not about trivial things.

Nurses should distinguish between morality and law. Laws reflect the moral values of a society, and they offer guidance in determining what is moral. However, an action can be legal but not moral. For example, an order for full resuscitation of a dying client is legal, but one could still question whether the act is moral. On the other hand, an action can be moral but illegal. For example, in a medical emergency it may be moral but not legal to exceed the speed limit when driving to the hospital. Legal aspects of nursing practice are covered in Chapter 3 ∞.

Nurses should also distinguish between morality and religion as they relate to health practices, although the two concepts are related. For example, according to some religious beliefs, women should undergo procedures such as female circumcision that may cause physical mutilation. Other religions or groups may consider this practice to be an ethical violation of the human right to self-determination. Additional common instances of differences in moral perspectives on health involving religious beliefs include blood transfusions, abortion, sterilization, and contraceptive and safer sex counseling.

QSEN Patient-Centered Care: Religious Beliefs

Many people are members of either the Confucian or the Buddhist religion. Confucian religious beliefs do not consider a fetus a human being. However, Buddhists believe the fetus is a form of human life. As a result, people may vary in their views on abortion, depending on their religious affiliation.

Moral Development

Ethical decisions require individuals to think and reason. Reasoning is a cognitive function and is, therefore, developmental. **Moral development** is the process of learning to tell the difference between right and wrong and of learning what ought and ought not to be done. It is a complex process that begins in childhood and continues throughout life.

Theories of moral development attempt to answer questions such as these: How does an individual become moral? What factors influence the way an individual behaves in a moral situation? Two well-known theorists of moral development are Lawrence Kohlberg (1969) and Carol Gilligan (1982). Kohlberg's theory emphasizes rights and formal reasoning; Gilligan's theory emphasizes care and responsibility, although it points out that people use the concepts of both theorists in their moral reasoning. For a full discussion of these two theories, see Chapter 23 ∞.

Moral Frameworks

Moral theories provide different frameworks through which nurses can view and clarify disturbing client care situations. Nurses can use moral theories in developing explanations for their ethical decisions and actions and in discussing problem situations with others. Three types of moral theories are widely used, and they can be differentiated by their emphasis on (a) consequences, (b) principles and duties, or (c) relationships.

Consequence-based (teleological) theories look to the outcomes (consequences) of an action in judging whether that action is right or wrong. **Utilitarianism**, one form of consequentialist theory, views a good act as one that is the most useful—that is, one that brings the most good and the least harm to the greatest number of people. This is called the principle of **utility**. This approach is often used in making decisions about the funding and delivery of healthcare. Teleological theories focus on issues of fairness.

Principles-based (deontological) theories involve logical and formal processes and emphasize individual rights, duties, and obligations. The morality of an action is determined not by its consequences but by whether it is done according to an impartial, objective principle. For example, following the rule "Do not lie," a nurse might believe he or she should tell the truth to a dying client, even though the physician has given instructions not to do so. There are many deontological theories; each justifies the rules of acceptable behavior differently.

Relationships-based (caring) theories emphasize courage, generosity, commitment, and the need to nurture and maintain relationships. Unlike the two preceding theories, which frame problems in terms of justice (fairness) and formal reasoning, caring theories (see Chapter 15 ∞) judge actions according to a perspective of caring and responsibility. Principles-based theories stress individual rights, but caring theories promote the common good or the welfare of the group.

A moral framework guides moral decisions, but it does not determine the outcome. Imagine a situation in which a frail, older adult client has made it clear that he does not want further surgery, but the family insists. Three nurses have each decided that they will not help with preparations for surgery and that they will work through proper channels to try to prevent it. Using consequence-based reasoning, Nurse A thinks, "Surgery will cause him more suffering; he probably will not survive it anyway, and the family may even feel guilty later." Using principles-based reasoning, Nurse B thinks, "This violates the principle of autonomy. This man has a right to decide what happens to his body." Using caring-based reasoning, Nurse C thinks, "My relationship to this client commits me to protecting him and meeting his needs, and I feel such compassion for him. I must try to help the family understand that he needs their support." Each of these perspectives is based on the nurse's moral framework.

Moral Principles

Moral principles are statements about broad, general, philosophical concepts such as autonomy and justice. They provide the foundation for **moral rules**, which are specific prescriptions for actions. For example, the rule "Do not lie" is based on the moral principle of respect for individuals (autonomy). Principles are useful in ethical discussions because even if people disagree about which action is right in a situation, they may be able to agree on the principles that apply. Such an agreement can serve as the basis for a solution that is acceptable to all parties. For example, most people would agree to the principle that nurses are obligated to respect their clients, even if they disagree as to whether the nurse should deceive a particular client about his or her prognosis.

Autonomy refers to the right to make one's own decisions. Nurses who follow this principle recognize that each client is unique, has the right to be him- or herself, and has the right to choose personal goals. People have "inward autonomy" if they have the ability to make choices; they have "outward autonomy" if their choices are not limited or imposed by others.

Honoring the principle of autonomy means that the nurse respects a client's right to make decisions even when those choices seem to the nurse not to be in the client's best interest. It also means treating others with consideration. In a healthcare setting, this principle is violated, for example, when a nurse disregards clients' subjective accounts of their symptoms (e.g., pain). Finally, respect for autonomy means that people should not be treated as impersonal sources of knowledge or training. This principle comes into play, for example, in the requirement that clients provide informed consent before tests, procedures, or participation in a research project can be carried out. See the discussion of informed consent in Chapter 3 ∞.

Nonmaleficence is the duty to "do no harm." Although this would seem to be a simple principle to follow, in reality it is complex. Harm can mean intentionally causing harm, placing someone at risk of harm, and unintentionally causing harm. In nursing, intentional harm is never acceptable. However, placing someone at risk of harm has many facets. A client may be at risk of harm as a known consequence of a nursing intervention that is intended to be helpful. For example, a client may react adversely to a medication. Unintentional harm occurs when the risk could not have been anticipated. For example, while catching a client who is falling, the nurse grips the client tightly enough to cause bruises to the client's arm. Caregivers do not always agree on the degree of risk that is morally permissible in order to attempt the beneficial result.

Beneficence means "doing good." Nurses are obligated to do good, that is, to implement actions that benefit clients and their support individuals. However, doing good can also pose a risk of doing harm. For example, a nurse may advise a client about a strenuous exercise program to improve general health, but should not do so if the client is at risk of a heart attack.

Justice is frequently referred to as fairness. Nurses often face decisions in which a sense of justice should prevail. For example, a nurse making home visits finds one client tearful and depressed, and knows she could help by staying for 30 more minutes to talk. However, that would take time from her next client, who has diabetes and needs a great deal of teaching and observation. The nurse will need to weigh the facts carefully in order to divide her time justly among her clients.

Fidelity means to be faithful to agreements and promises. By virtue of their standing as professional caregivers, nurses have responsibilities to clients, employers, government, and society, as well as to themselves. Nurses often make promises such as "I'll be right back with your pain medication" or "I'll find out for you." Clients take such promises seriously, and so should nurses.

Veracity refers to telling the truth. Although this seems straightforward, in practice, choices are not always clear. Should a nurse tell the truth when it is known that it will cause harm? Does a nurse tell a lie when it is known that the lie will relieve anxiety and fear? Lying to sick or dying people is rarely justified. The loss of trust in the nurse and the anxiety caused by not knowing the truth, for example, usually outweigh any benefits derived from lying.

Nurses must also have professional accountability and responsibility. According to the *Code of Ethics for Nurses* (Fowler, 2015), **accountability** means "answerable, or to give an account or defense to oneself and others for one's own choices, decisions and actions as measured against a standard" (p. 59), whereas **responsibility** refers to "the blameworthiness or praiseworthiness that one bears for one's conduct or the performance of duties" (p. 59). Thus, the ethical nurse is able to explain the rationale behind every action and recognize the standards to which he or she will be held.

QSEN Patient-Centered Care: Moral Principles

Moral principles are commonly accepted as universal. However, the principles that guide bioethics are rooted in a secular Western European perspective. Thus, there is often conflict in creating a fit between these principles and the guiding moral principles of various cultural groups. Religious groups (such as Catholics, Jehovah's Witnesses, and Muslims) and ethnic groups (such as African, Asian, and Latin American) may hold different views from those of healthcare providers. Nurses must be familiar with each of these principles as it relates to ethical decision making, in addition to gaining an understanding of the client's moral principles.

Autonomy. The client and family may expect the healthcare provider to respect their right to refuse a treatment. Primary responsibility for decision making may rest with others, such as the family, elders, or religious community. The family and community are viewed as affected by the client's condition and decisions as much as the client is affected.

Veracity. Clients may not value truth-telling for life-threatening conditions, because this may eliminate hope and, therefore, hasten death. Family members may request that the client not be told of his or her diagnosis.

Nonmaleficence. Discussion of advance directives and issues such as cardiopulmonary resuscitation may be viewed as physically and emotionally harmful to the client. Withdrawal of life support or withdrawal of futile or damaging treatments may be seen as decreasing length of life or hastening death.

Beneficence. The client and family may expect healthcare providers to promote client well-being and hope, and provide treatment that will help prolong life.

Nursing Ethics

In the past, nurses looked on ethical decision making as the physician's responsibility. However, no one profession is responsible for ethical decisions, nor does expertise in one discipline such as medicine or nursing necessarily make someone an expert in ethics. As situations become more complex, input from all caregivers becomes increasingly important.

Ethical standards of The Joint Commission mandate that healthcare institutions provide ethics committees or a similar structure to write guidelines and policies and to provide education, counseling, and support on ethical issues (Chaet, 2016). These multidisciplinary committees include nurses and can be asked to review a case and provide guidance to a competent client, an incompetent client's family, or healthcare providers. They ensure that the relevant facts of a case are brought out, provide a forum in which diverse views can be expressed, provide support for caregivers, and can reduce the institution's legal risks. In some settings, ethics rounds are held. In these meetings, ethical dilemmas from real or simulated cases are presented from a theoretical perspective, introducing those present to the issues and processes used in analyzing such dilemmas (Figure 4.1 ■).

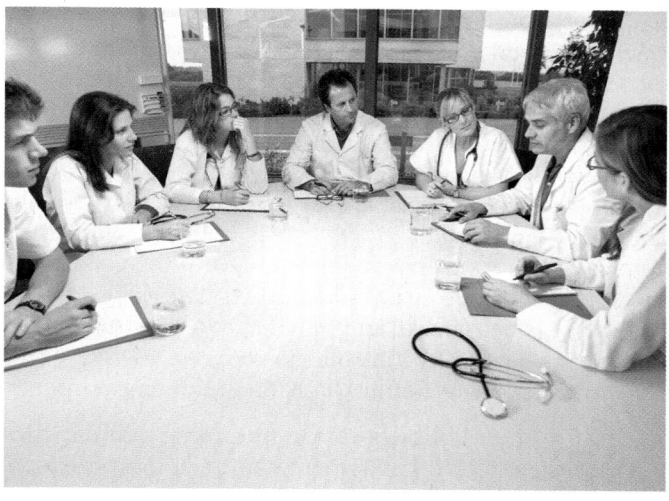

Figure 4.1 ■ An ethics committee contemplates all aspects of the case being considered.
Ghislain & Marie David de Lossy/Image Source/Alamy Stock photo.

Nursing Codes of Ethics

A **code of ethics** is a formal statement of a group's ideals and values. It is a set of ethical principles that (a) is shared by members of the group, (b) reflects their moral judgments over time, and (c) serves as a standard for their professional actions. Codes of ethics usually have higher requirements

EVIDENCE-BASED PRACTICE

Evidence-Based Practice

Do Nurses' and Physicians' Feelings About End-of-Life Care Allow Them to Act Ethically?

End-of-life care and ethical decisions are often made in the intensive care unit. In spite of this being a common situation, the emotional connections and reactions of physicians and nurses influence the experience for everyone involved. In this study, 10 physicians and 10 nurses were interviewed about the decision-making process and the impact of the process on their relationships with the client and family and on their relationships with other health professional colleagues (Laurent, Bonnet, Capellier, Aslanian, & Hebert, 2017).

Thematic analysis revealed that most often nurses felt they were only following physician orders and not necessarily acting on what they believed to be in the client's best interests. Physicians acknowledged their decision-making role but also expressed frustration and distress that life-saving measures were no longer a possibility. Thus, some degree of conflict between nurses and physicians arose, and neither professional group felt they were as sensitive to client and family needs as they would have liked to be.

Implications

Clients and their families trust that their healthcare providers act in their best interests and will carry out their expressed approach to end-of-life care. This research suggests that the ethical and moral beliefs of the providers can interfere with their ability to truly advocate for the clients. The authors recommend that these findings be shared with the staff in efforts to resolve at least some of the conflict.

than legal standards, and they are never lower than the legal standards of the profession. Nurses are responsible for being familiar with the code that governs their practice.

International, national, and state nursing associations have established codes of ethics. The International Council of Nurses (ICN) first adopted a code of ethics in 1953, and the most recent revision (2012) is shown in Box 4.3. The ANA first adopted a *Code for Nurses* in 1950. The current version reflects several major changes in the code (now called the *Code of Ethics for Nurses*). A statement on compassion has been added, and the duty to protect clients has been broadened to include all client rights.

Nursing codes of ethics have the following purposes:

1. Inform the public about the minimum standards of the profession and help them understand professional nursing conduct.
2. Provide a sign of the profession's commitment to the public it serves.
3. Outline the major ethical considerations of the profession.
4. Provide ethical standards for professional behavior.
5. Guide the profession in self-regulation.
6. Remind nurses of the special responsibility they assume when caring for the sick.

Origins of Ethical Problems in Nursing

Nurses' growing awareness of ethical problems has occurred largely because of (a) social and technologic changes and (b) nurses' conflicting loyalties and obligations.

Social and Technologic Changes

Social changes, such as the women's movement and growing consumerism, expose problems. The number of people without health insurance, the high cost of healthcare, and workplace redesign under managed care all raise issues of fairness and allocation of resources.

Technology creates new issues. Before monitors, respirators, and parenteral feedings, there was no question about whether to "allow" an 800-gram premature infant to

BOX 4.3 International Council of Nurses Code of Ethics Preamble

Nurses have four fundamental responsibilities: to promote health, to prevent illness, to restore health and to alleviate suffering. The need for nursing is universal.

Inherent in nursing is respect for human rights, including cultural rights, the right to life and choice, to dignity and to be treated with respect. Nursing care is respectful of and unrestricted by considerations of age, colour, creed, culture, disability or illness, gender, sexual orientation, nationality, politics, race or social status.

Nurses render health services to the individual, the family and the community and coordinate their services with those of related groups.

THE ICN CODE

The *ICN Code of Ethics for Nurses* has four principal elements that outline the standards of ethical conduct.

Elements of the Code

1. Nurses and People

The nurse's primary professional responsibility is to people requiring nursing care.

In providing care, the nurse promotes an environment in which the human rights, values, customs and spiritual beliefs of the individual, family and community are respected.

The nurse ensures that the individual receives accurate, sufficient and timely information in a culturally appropriate manner on which to base consent for care and related treatment. The nurse holds in confidence personal information and uses judgement in sharing this information.

The nurse shares with society the responsibility for initiating and supporting action to meet the health and social needs of the public, in particular those of vulnerable populations.

The nurse advocates for equity and social justice in resource allocation, access to healthcare, and other social and economic services.

The nurse demonstrates professional values such as respectfulness, responsiveness, compassion, trustworthiness, and integrity.

2. Nurses and Practice

The nurse carries personal responsibility and accountability for nursing practice, and for maintaining competence by continual learning.

The nurse maintains a standard of personal health such that the ability to provide care is not compromised.

The nurse uses judgement regarding individual competence when accepting and delegating responsibility.

The nurse at all times maintains standards of personal conduct which reflect well on the profession and enhance public confidence.

The nurse, in providing care, ensures that use of technology and scientific advances are compatible with the safety, dignity and rights of people.

The nurse strives to foster and maintain a practice culture promoting ethical behaviour and open dialogue.

3. Nurses and the Profession

The nurse assumes the major role in determining and implementing acceptable standards of clinical nursing practice, management, research and education.

The nurse is active in developing a core of research-based professional knowledge.

The nurse is active in developing and sustaining a core of professional values.

The nurse, acting through the professional organisation, participates in creating and maintaining safe, equitable social and economic working conditions in nursing.

The nurse practices to sustain and protect the natural environment and is aware of its consequences on health.

The nurse contributes to an ethical organisational environment and challenges unethical practices and settings.

4. Nurses and Co-workers

The nurse sustains a co-operative and respectful relationship with co-workers in nursing and other fields.

The nurse takes appropriate action to safeguard individuals, families and communities when their health is endangered by a co-worker or any other person.

The nurse takes appropriate action to support and guide co-workers to advance ethical conduct.

die. Before organ transplantation, death did not require a legal definition that permits viable tissues to be removed and given to other living people. Advances in the ability to decode and control the growth of tissues through gene manipulation present new potential ethical dilemmas related to cloning organisms and altering the course of hereditary diseases and biological characteristics. Today, with treatments that can prolong and enhance biological life, these questions arise: Should we do what we know we can? Who should be treated—everyone, only those who can pay, only those who have a chance to improve?

Conflicting Loyalties and Obligations

Because of their unique position in the healthcare system, nurses experience conflicts among their loyalties and obligations to clients, families, primary care providers, employing institutions, and licensing bodies. Client needs may conflict with institutional policies, primary care provider preferences, needs of the client's family, or even laws of the state. According to the nursing code of ethics, the nurse's first loyalty is to the client. However, it is not always easy to determine which action best serves the client's needs. For instance, the nurse may be aware that marijuana has been shown to be effective for a condition a client has that has not responded to mainstream therapies. Although legal issues are involved, the nurse must determine if, ethically, the client should be made aware of a potentially effective alternative. Another example is individual nurses' decisions regarding honoring picket lines during employee strikes. The nurse may experience conflict among feeling the need to support coworkers in their efforts to improve working conditions, feeling the need to ensure clients receive care and are not abandoned, and feeling loyalty to the hospital employer.

Making Ethical Decisions

Many nursing problems are not moral problems at all, but simply questions of good nursing practice. An important first step in ethical decision making is to determine whether a moral situation exists. The following criteria may be used:

- A difficult choice exists between actions that conflict with the needs of one or more people.
- Moral principles or frameworks exist that can be used to provide some justification for the action.
- The choice is guided by a process of weighing reasons.
- The decision must be freely and consciously chosen.
- The choice is affected by personal feelings and by the particular context of the situation.

Responsible ethical reasoning is rational and systematic. It should be based on ethical principles and codes rather than on emotions, intuition, fixed policies, or precedent (that is, an earlier similar occurrence). A variety of decision-making models are available that are compatible with the nursing process. Each institution adopts its own set of steps for making formal ethical decisions, but each nurse also benefits from having an organizing framework for analyzing ethical issues.

A good decision is one that is in the client's best interest and at the same time preserves the integrity of all involved. Nurses have ethical obligations to their clients, to the agency that employs them, and to primary care providers. Therefore, nurses must weigh competing factors when making ethical decisions. See Box 4.4 for examples.

BOX 4.4 Examples of Nurses' Obligations in Ethical Decision Making

- Maximize the client's well-being.
- Balance the client's need for autonomy with family members' responsibilities for the client's well-being.
- Support each family member and enhance the family support system.
- Carry out hospital policies.
- Protect other clients' well-being.
- Protect the nurse's own standards of care.

Although ethical reasoning is principle based and has the client's well-being at the center, being involved in ethical problems and dilemmas is stressful for the nurse. The nurse may feel torn between obligations to the client, the family, and the employer. What is in the client's best interest may be contrary to the nurse's personal belief system. This conflict is referred to as **moral distress** and is considered a serious issue in the workplace. For example, moral distress is cited as a driving factor in the ANA draft position statement on managing pain and suffering (ANA, 2018). Researchers have used a variety of questionnaires and tools to measure moral distress in nurses, many using a modified version of an existing moral distress scale (Mealer & Moss, 2016). One method to assist nurses in coping with moral distress is using the four steps of *The 4 A's to Rise Above Moral Distress*: ask, affirm, assess, act (American Association of Critical-Care Nurses, 2004). Using this model, the nurse *asks* whether signs of moral distress are present, *affirms* a commitment to addressing the distress, *assesses* the sources and severity of the distress plus readiness to act, and *acts* to implement a plan to reduce the distress. In settings in which ethical issues arise frequently, nurses should establish support systems such as team conferences and use of counseling professionals to allow expression of their feelings.

Safety Alert! SAFETY

Addressing moral distress is consistent with the Quality and Safety Education for Nurses patient-centered care attitude competencies: "Acknowledge the tension that may exist between patient rights and the organizational responsibility for professional, ethical care. Appreciate shared decision making with empowered patients and families, even when conflicts occur" (Cronenwett et al., 2007, p. 124).

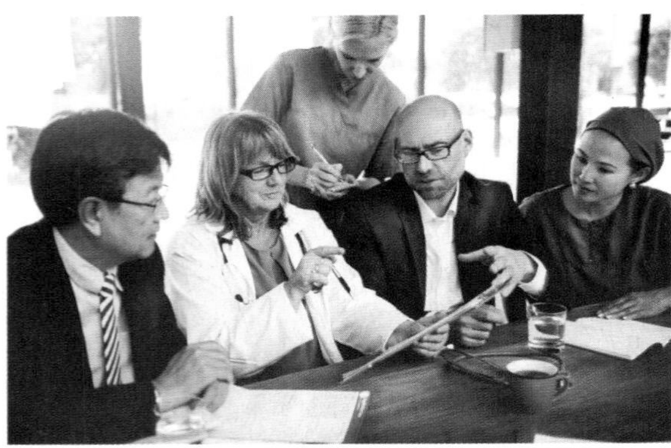

Figure 4.2 ■ When there is a need for ethical decisions or client advocacy, many different individuals contribute to the final outcome.
Rawpixel.com/Shutterstock.

One structure that may be useful to nurses in ethical decision making is the Four Boxes method (Fowler, 2015). This structure provides questions that guide the nurse in gathering all relevant information in the four boxes: medical indications, patient preferences, quality of life, and contextual features. Once the data have been collected, ethical principles such as autonomy, nonmaleficence, beneficence, and justice are reviewed against the data to reach a decision or resolution.

Although the nurse's input is important, in reality several people are usually involved in making an ethical decision. The client, family, spiritual support persons, and other members of the healthcare team work together in reaching ethical decisions (Figure 4.2 ■). Therefore, collaboration, communication, and compromise are important skills for health professionals. When nurses do not have the autonomy to act on their moral or ethical choices, compromise becomes essential.

Box 4.5 presents an example of an approach to ethical decision making for a specific clinical case.

Strategies to Enhance Ethical Decisions and Practice

Several strategies help nurses overcome possible organizational and social constraints that may hinder the ethical practice of nursing and create moral distress for nurses. You as a nurse should do the following:

- Become aware of your own values and the ethical aspects of nursing.
- Be familiar with nursing codes of ethics.
- Seek continuing education opportunities to stay knowledgeable about ethical issues in nursing.
- Respect the values, opinions, and responsibilities of other healthcare professionals that may be different from your own.
- Participate in or establish ethics rounds. Ethics rounds use hypothetical or real cases that focus on the ethical dimensions of client care rather than the client's clinical diagnosis and treatment.
- Serve on institutional ethics committees.
- Strive for collaborative practice in which nurses function effectively in cooperation with other healthcare professionals.

Specific Ethical Issues

Some of the ethical problems nurses encounter most frequently are issues in the care of clients with HIV infection, AIDS, abortion, organ or tissue transplantation, end-of-life decisions, cost-containment issues that jeopardize client welfare and access to healthcare (resource allocation), and breaches of client confidentiality (e.g., computerized information management).

BOX 4.5 Application of a Bioethical Decision-Making Model

SITUATION

Mrs. L., a 67-year-old woman, is hospitalized with multiple fractures and lacerations caused by an automobile collision. Her husband, who was killed in the collision, was taken to the same hospital. Mrs. L., who had been driving the automobile, constantly questions her nurse about her husband. The surgeon has told the nurse not to tell Mrs. L. about the death of her husband; however, the surgeon does not give the nurse any reason for these instructions. The nurse expresses concern to the charge nurse, who says the surgeon's orders must be followed—that the surgeon will decide when Mrs. L. should be told. However, the nurse is not comfortable with this and wonders what should be done.

Nursing Actions	Considerations
1. Identify the moral aspects. See the criteria provided on page 103 to determine whether a moral situation exists.	Alternative actions are to tell the truth or withhold it. The moral principles involved are honesty and loyalty. These principles conflict because the nurse wants to be honest with Mrs. L. without being disloyal to the surgeon and the charge nurse. The nurse weighs reasons in making a freely and consciously chosen choice. The choice will be affected by feelings of concern for Mrs. L. and a context that includes the surgeon's incomplete communication with the client and the nurse.
2. Gather relevant facts that relate to the issue.	Data should include information about the client's health problems. Determine who is involved, the nature of their involvement, and their motives for acting. In this case, the people involved are the client (who is concerned about her husband), the husband (who is deceased), the surgeon, the charge nurse, and the primary nurse. Motives are not known. Perhaps the nurse wishes to protect the therapeutic relationship with Mrs. L.; possibly the surgeon believes this action protects Mrs. L. from psychological trauma and consequent physical deterioration.

BOX 4.5 Application of a Bioethical Decision-Making Model—*continued*

Nursing Actions	Considerations
3. Determine ownership of the decision. For example, for whom is the decision being made? Who should decide and why?	In this case, the decision is being made for Mrs. L. The surgeon obviously believes that a physician should be the one to decide, and the charge nurse agrees. It would be helpful if caregivers agreed on criteria for deciding who the decision maker should be.
4. Clarify and apply personal values.	We can infer from this situation that Mrs. L. values her husband's welfare, that the charge nurse values policy and procedure, and that the nurse seems to value a client's right to have information. The nurse needs to clarify his or her own and the surgeon's values, as well as confirm the values of Mrs. L. and the charge nurse.
5. Identify ethical theories and principles.	For example, failing to tell Mrs. L. the truth can negate her autonomy. The nurse would uphold the principle of honesty by telling Mrs. L. The principles of beneficence and nonmaleficence are also involved because of the possible effects of the alternative actions on Mrs. L.'s physical and psychological well-being.
6. Identify applicable laws or agency policies.	Because the surgeon simply "gave instructions" rather than an actual order, agency policies might not require the nurse to follow the instructions. The nurse should clarify this with the charge nurse and be familiar with the nurse practice act in that state.
7. Use competent interdisciplinary resources.	In this case, the nurse might consult the literature to find out whether clients are harmed by receiving bad news when they are injured and might also consult with the chaplain.
8. Develop alternative actions and project their outcomes on the client and family. Possibly because of the limited time available for ethical deliberations in the clinical setting, nurses tend to identify two opposing, either–or alternatives (e.g., to tell or not to tell) instead of generating multiple options. This creates a dilemma even when none exists.	Two alternative actions, with possible outcomes, follow (others may also be appropriate): 1. Follow the charge nurse's advice and do as the surgeon says. Possible outcomes: (a) Mrs. L. might become anxious and angry when she finds out that information has been withheld from her; or (b) by waiting until Mrs. L. is stronger to give her the bad news, the healthcare team may avoid harming Mrs. L.'s health. 2. Discuss the situation further with the charge nurse and surgeon, pointing out Mrs. L.'s right to autonomy and information. Possible outcomes: (a) The surgeon acknowledges Mrs. L.'s right to be informed, or (b) the surgeon states that Mrs. L.'s health is at risk and insists that she not be informed until a later time. Regardless of whether the action is congruent with the nurse's personal value system, Mrs. L.'s best interests take precedence.
9. Apply nursing codes of ethics to help guide actions. (Codes of nursing usually support autonomy and nursing advocacy.)	If the nurse believes strongly that Mrs. L. should hear the truth, then as a client advocate, the nurse should choose to confer again with the charge nurse and surgeon.
10. For each alternative action, identify the risk and seriousness of consequences for the nurse. (Some employers may not support nursing autonomy and advocacy in ethical situations.)	If the nurse tells Mrs. L. the truth without the agreement of the charge nurse and surgeon, the nurse risks the surgeon's anger and a reprimand from the charge nurse. If the nurse follows the charge nurse's advice, the nurse will receive approval from the charge nurse and surgeon; however, the nurse risks being seen as unassertive, and the nurse violates a personal value of truthfulness. If the nurse requests a conference, the nurse may gain respect for assertiveness and professionalism, but the nurse risks the surgeon's annoyance at having the instructions questioned.
11. Participate actively in resolving the issue. Recommend actions that can be ethically supported, recognizing that all actions have positive and negative aspects.	The appropriate degree of nursing input varies with the situation. Sometimes nurses participate in choosing what will be done; sometimes they merely support a client who is making the decision. In this situation, if an action cannot be agreed on, the nurse must decide whether this issue is important enough to merit the personal risks involved.
12. Implement the action.	The nurse will carry out one of the actions developed in step 8.
13. Evaluate the action taken. Involve the client, family, and other healthcare members in the evaluation, if possible.	The nurse can begin by asking, "Did I do the right thing?" Would the nurse make the same decisions again if the situation were repeated? If the nurse is not satisfied, the nurse can review other alternatives and work through the process again.

AIDS

Because of its association with sexual behavior, illicit drug use, and physical decline and death, AIDS bears a social stigma. According to an ANA position statement, the moral obligation to care for a client cannot be set aside unless the risk to the caregiver exceeds the responsibility (ANA, 2015b).

Other ethical issues center on testing for HIV infection status and for the presence of AIDS in health professionals and clients. Questions arise as to whether testing of all providers and clients should be mandatory or voluntary and whether test results should be released to insurance companies, sexual partners, or caregivers. As with all ethical dilemmas, each possibility has both positive and negative implications for specific individuals.

Abortion

Abortion is a highly publicized issue about which many people feel very strongly. Debate continues, pitting the principle of sanctity of life against the principle of autonomy and a woman's right to control her own body. This is an especially volatile issue because no public consensus has yet been reached.

Most state laws have provisions known as conscience clauses that permit individual primary care providers and nurses, as well as institutions, to refuse to assist with an abortion if doing so violates their religious or moral principles. However, nurses have no right to impose their values on a client. Nursing codes of ethics support clients' rights to information and counseling in making decisions.

Organ and Tissue Transplantation

Organs or tissue for transplantation may come from living donors or from donors who have just died. Many living people choose to become donors by giving consent under the Uniform Anatomical Gift Act (see Chapter 43 ∞). Ethical issues related to organ transplantation include allocation of organs, selling of body parts, involvement of children as potential donors, consent, clear definition of death, and conflicts of interest between potential donors and recipients. In some situations, an individual's religious beliefs may also present conflict. For example, certain religions forbid the mutilation of the body, even for the benefit of another individual.

Individuals' spiritual beliefs and views on when human life begins have an impact on their opinions about stem cell research. Stem cell research is the foundation for cell-based therapies in which stem cells are induced to differentiate into the specific cell type required to repair damaged or destroyed cells or tissues. Both embryonic and adult cells are used in this research. Embryonic cells are derived from a 5-day preimplantation embryo. Adult cells are undifferentiated cells found in differentiated tissue. There are many moral, ethical, and legal debates regarding the use of and research about stem cells (Warren, 2016).

End-of-Life Issues

The increase in technologic advances and the growing number of older adults have expanded ethical dilemmas. Providing information and professional assistance, as well as the highest quality of care and caring, is of the utmost importance during the end-of-life period. Some of the most frequent disturbing ethical problems for nurses involve issues that arise around death and dying. These include euthanasia, assisted suicide, termination of life-sustaining treatment, and withdrawing or withholding of food and fluids.

Advance Directives

Many moral problems surrounding the end of life can be resolved if clients complete advance directives. Presently, all 50 of the United States have enacted advance directive legislation. Advance directives direct caregivers as to the client's wishes about treatments, providing an ongoing voice for clients when they have lost the capacity to make or communicate their decisions. See Chapter 43 ∞ for a full discussion of advance directives.

Euthanasia and Assisted Suicide

Euthanasia, a Greek word meaning "good death," is popularly known as "mercy killing." **Active euthanasia** involves actions to bring about the client's death directly, with or without client consent. An example of this would be the administration of a lethal medication to end the client's suffering. Regardless of the caregiver's intent, active euthanasia is forbidden by law and can result in criminal charges of murder.

A variation of active euthanasia is **assisted suicide**, or giving clients the means to kill themselves if they request it (e.g., providing lethal doses of pills). Some countries or states have laws permitting assisted suicide for clients who are severely ill, who are near death, and who wish to commit suicide. Although some people may disagree with the concept, assisted suicide is currently legal in the states of California, Montana, Oregon, Vermont, and Washington, whereas it is specifically prohibited in many other states. In any case, the nurse should recall that legality and morality are not the same thing. Determining whether an action is legal is only one aspect of deciding whether it is ethical. The questions of suicide and assisted suicide are still controversial in Western society. The ANA's position statement on assisted suicide and active euthanasia (2013) states that both active euthanasia and assisted suicide are in violation of the *Code of Ethics for Nurses*.

Passive euthanasia, more commonly referred to now as withdrawing or withholding life-sustaining therapy (WWLST), involves the withdrawal of extraordinary means of life support, such as removing a ventilator or withholding special attempts to revive a client (e.g., giving the client "no code" status) and allowing the client to die of the underlying medical condition. WWLST may be both legally and ethically more acceptable to most people than assisted suicide.

Termination of Life-Sustaining Treatment

Antibiotics, organ transplants, and technologic advances (e.g., ventilators) help to prolong life, but not necessarily to restore health. Clients may specify that they wish to have life-sustaining measures withdrawn, they may have advance directives on this matter, or they may appoint a surrogate decision maker. However, it is usually more troubling for healthcare professionals to withdraw a treatment than to decide initially not to begin it. Nurses must understand that a decision to withdraw treatment is not a decision to withdraw care. Nurses must ensure that sensitive care and comfort measures are given as the client's illness progresses. When the client is at home, nurses often provide this type of education and support through hospice services (see Chapter 43 ∞ for more information regarding hospice and end-of-life care).

It is difficult for families to withdraw treatment, which makes it very important that they fully understand the treatment. They often have misunderstandings about which treatments are life sustaining. Keeping clients and families well informed is an ongoing process, allowing them time to ask questions and discuss the situation. It is also essential that they understand that they can reevaluate and change their decision if they wish.

Withdrawing or Withholding Food and Fluids

It is generally accepted that providing food and fluids is part of ordinary nursing practice and, therefore, a moral duty. However, when food and fluids are administered by tube to a dying client, or are given over a long period to an unconscious client who is not expected to improve, then some consider it to be an extraordinary, or heroic, measure. A nurse is morally obligated to withhold food and fluids (or any treatment) if it is determined to be more harmful to administer them than to withhold them. The nurse must also honor competent and informed clients' refusal of food and fluids (ANA, 2017). The ANA *Code of Ethics for Nurses* (Fowler, 2015) supports this position through the nurse's role as a client advocate and through the moral principle of autonomy. However, the debate on ethical, legal, personal, and religious grounds continues—especially as it relates to the care of children who are unable to speak for themselves. In addition, client views on the acceptability of these actions vary according to culture (Fang, Sixsmith, Sinclair, & Horst, 2016).

Allocation of Scarce Health Resources

Allocation of limited supplies of healthcare goods and services, including organ transplants, artificial joints, and the services of specialists, has become an especially urgent issue as medical costs continue to rise and more stringent cost-containment measures are implemented. The moral principle of autonomy cannot be applied if it is not possible to give each client what he or she chooses. In this situation, healthcare providers may use the principle of justice—attempting to choose what is most fair to all.

Nursing care is also a health resource. Institutions have been implementing "workplace redesign" to cut costs. Some nurses are concerned that staffing in their institutions is not adequate to give the level of care they value. California is the first state to enact legislation mandating specific nurse-to-client ratios in hospitals and other healthcare settings. With a nationwide shortage of nurses, an ethical dilemma arises when, in order to provide adequate staffing, facilities must turn away needy clients. Nurses must continue to look for ways to balance economics and caring in the allocation of health resources.

Management of Personal Health Information

In keeping with the principle of autonomy, nurses are obligated to respect clients' privacy and confidentiality. Privacy is both a legal and ethical mandate. The Health Insurance Portability and Accountability Act of 1996 (HIPAA) includes standards protecting the confidentiality, integrity, and availability of data, and standards defining appropriate disclosures of identifiable health information and client rights protection. Clients must be able to trust that nurses will reveal details of their situations only as appropriate and will communicate only the information necessary to provide for their healthcare. Computerized client records make sensitive data accessible to more people and accent issues of confidentiality. Nurses should help develop and follow security measures and policies to ensure appropriate use of client data.

Advocacy

When people are ill, they are frequently unable to assert their rights as they would if they were healthy. An **advocate** is one who expresses and defends the cause of another. The healthcare system is complex, and many clients are too ill to deal with it. If they are to keep from "falling through the cracks," clients need an advocate to cut through the layers of bureaucracy and help them get what they require. Values basic to client advocacy are shown in Box 4.6. Clients may also advocate for themselves. Today, clients are seeking more self-determination and control over their own bodies.

BOX 4.6 Values Basic to Client Advocacy

- The client is a holistic, autonomous being who has the right to make choices and decisions.
- Clients have the right to expect a nurse–client relationship that is based on shared respect, trust, collaboration in solving problems related to health and healthcare needs, and consideration of their thoughts and feelings.
- It is the nurse's responsibility to ensure the client has access to healthcare services that meet health needs.

If a client lacks decision-making capacity, is legally incompetent, or is a minor, these rights can be exercised on the client's behalf by a designated surrogate or proxy decision maker. It is important, however, for the nurse to remember that client control over health decisions is a Western view. In other societies, such decisions may normally be made by the head of the family or another member of the community. The nurse must ascertain the client's and family's views and honor their traditions regarding the locus of decision making.

To help make clients' rights more explicit to both the client and the healthcare provider, several versions of a patient's bill of rights have been published by consumer organizations. The most commonly used, the Patient Care Partnership, was last revised in 2003 by the American Hospital Association.

The Advocate's Role

The overall goal of the client advocate is to protect clients' rights. An advocate informs clients about their rights and provides them with the information they need to make informed decisions.

An advocate supports clients in their decisions, giving them full or at least mutual responsibility in decision making when they are capable of it. The advocate must be careful to remain objective and not convey approval or disapproval of the client's choices. Advocacy requires accepting and respecting the client's right to decide, even if the nurse believes the decision to be wrong.

In mediating, the advocate directly intervenes on the client's behalf, often by influencing others. An example of acting on behalf of a client is asking a primary care provider to review with the client the reasons for and the expected duration of therapy because the client says he always forgets to ask the primary care provider.

Advocacy in Home Care

Although the goals of advocacy remain the same, home care poses unique concerns for the nurse advocate. For example, while in the hospital, people may operate from the values of the nurses and primary care providers. When they are at home, they tend to operate from their own personal values and may revert to old habits and ways of doing things that may not be beneficial to their health. The nurse may see this as nonadherence; nevertheless, client autonomy must be respected.

In home care, limited resources and a lack of client care services may shift the focus from client welfare to concerns about resource allocation. Financial considerations can limit the availability of services and materials, making it difficult to ensure that client needs are met.

Professional and Public Advocacy

Advocacy is needed for the nursing profession as well as for the public. Gains that nursing makes in developing and improving health policy at the institutional and government levels help to achieve better healthcare for the public.

Nurses who function responsibly as professional and public advocates are in a position to effect change. To act as an advocate in this arena, the nurse needs an understanding of the ethical issues in nursing and healthcare, as well as knowledge of the laws and regulations that affect nursing practice and the health of society (see Chapter 3 ∞).

Being an effective client advocate involves the following:

- Being assertive
- Recognizing that the rights and values of clients and families must take precedence when they conflict with those of healthcare providers
- Being aware that conflicts may arise over issues that require consultation, confrontation, or negotiation between the nurse and administrative personnel or between the nurse and a primary care provider
- Working with community agencies and lay practitioners
- Staying knowledgeable about the legislation relevant to the client population. Local, regional, state, and federal laws and regulations change frequently.
- Knowing that advocacy may require political action—communicating a client's healthcare needs to government and other officials who have the authority to do something about these needs.

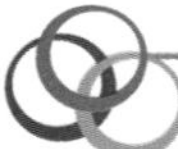

Critical Thinking Checkpoint

A 79-year-old man with severe peripheral vascular disease has been told that a nonhealing lesion on his foot must be treated with either vascular bypass surgery or amputation of the foot. Although the surgeon believes the foot can be saved with bypass, the man elects to have the amputation. His main reason is that the site will heal more quickly and allow him to resume normal activities sooner. He asks for the nurse's opinion.

1. What values and beliefs does the client seem to embrace?
2. What additional information might the nurse need to gather from the client or the surgeon?
3. What are the nurse's ethical and moral responsibilities in this instance?
4. What conflicting loyalties and obligations does the nurse face?
5. Of what value is the *Code of Ethics for Nurses* to the nurse in solving this dilemma?

Answers to Critical Thinking Checkpoint questions are available on the faculty resources site. Please consult with your instructor.

Chapter 4 Review

CHAPTER HIGHLIGHTS

- Values are enduring beliefs that give direction and meaning to life and guide an individual's behavior.
- Values clarification is a process in which people identify, examine, and develop their own values.
- Nursing ethics refers to the ethical problems that occur in nursing practice and to ethical decisions that nurses make.
- Morality refers to private, personal standards of what is right and wrong in conduct, character, and attitude.
- Moral issues are those that arouse the conscience or awareness of feelings such as guilt, hope, or shame; are concerned with important social values and norms; and evoke words such as *good*, *bad*, *right*, *wrong*, *should*, and *ought*.

- Three common moral frameworks (approaches) are consequence-based (teleological), principles-based (deontological), and relationships-based (caring-based) theories.
- Moral principles (e.g., autonomy, nonmaleficence, beneficence, justice, fidelity, and veracity) are broad, general philosophical concepts that can be used to make and explain moral choices.
- A professional code of ethics is a formal statement of a group's ideals and values that serves as a standard and guideline for the group's professional actions and informs the public of its commitment.
- Ethical problems are created as a result of changes in society, advances in technology, conflicts within nursing itself, and nurses' conflicting loyalties and obligations (e.g., to clients, families, employers, primary care providers, and other nurses).
- The goal of ethical reasoning, in the context of nursing, is to reach a mutual, peaceful agreement that is in the best interests of the client; reaching the agreement may require compromise.
- Nurses are responsible for determining their own actions and for supporting clients who are making moral decisions or for whom decisions are being made by others.
- Nurses can enhance their ethical practice and client advocacy by clarifying their own values, understanding the values of other healthcare professionals, becoming familiar with nursing codes of ethics, and participating in ethics committees and rounds.
- Client advocacy involves concern for and actions on behalf of another individual or organization in order to bring about change.
- The functions of the advocacy role are to inform, support, and mediate.

TEST YOUR KNOWLEDGE

1. When an ethical issue arises, one of the most important nursing responsibilities in managing client care situations is which of the following?
   1. Be able to defend the morality of one's own actions.
   2. Remain neutral and detached when making ethical decisions.
   3. Ensure that a team is responsible for deciding ethical questions.
   4. Follow the client and family's wishes exactly.

2. Which situation is most clearly a violation of the underlying principles associated with professional nursing ethics?
   1. A hospital's policy permits use of internal fetal monitoring during labor. However, there is literature to both support and refute the value of this practice.
   2. When asked about the purpose of a medication, a nurse colleague responds, "Oh, I never look them up. I just give what is prescribed."
   3. The nurses on the unit agree to sponsor a fundraising event to support a labor strike proposed by fellow nurses at another facility.
   4. A client reports that he didn't quite tell the doctor the truth when asked if he was following his therapeutic diet at home.

3. Following a motor vehicle crash, the parents of a child with no apparent brain function refuse to permit withdrawal of life support from the child. Although the nurse believes the child should be allowed to die and organ donation considered, the nurse supports their decision. Which moral principle provides the basis for the nurse's actions?
   1. Respect for autonomy
   2. Nonmaleficence
   3. Beneficence
   4. Justice

4. Which statement would be *most* helpful when a nurse is assisting clients in clarifying their values?
   1. "That was not a good decision. Why did you think it would work?"
   2. "The most important thing is to follow the plan of care. Did you follow all your doctor's orders?"
   3. "Some people might have made a different decision. What led you to make your decision?"
   4. "If you had asked me, I would have given you my opinion about what to do. Now, how do you feel about your choice?"

5. A home health client has been prescribed nutritional supplements three times a day. The formula is expensive, and the client tells the home health nurse that she is taking them three times a day but is diluting them so she can use only one can instead of three, per day. As a client advocate, the nurse should:
   1. Help the client look for available community resources that may be of assistance.
   2. Tell the client that she needs to take the prescribed amount.
   3. Report the situation to the physician.
   4. Weigh the client on a weekly basis to monitor weight gain or loss.

6. A nurse manager has a staff nurse who observes certain religious holidays. The manager tries to make sure that these observances can be met if possible. Which of the following values is the manager practicing?
   1. Human dignity
   2. Social justice
   3. Autonomy
   4. Altruism

See Answers to *Test Your Knowledge* in Appendix A.

READINGS AND REFERENCES

Suggested Reading

Aulisio, M. P. (2016). Why did hospital ethics committees emerge in the US? *AMA Journal of Ethics, 18*, 546–553. doi:10.1001/journalofethics.2016.18.05.mhst1-1605

This article describes the creation of hospital ethics committees beginning in the 1960s. In some cases, the ethical dilemmas arose from a shortage of resources, whereas in other situations the driving factors were autonomy or privacy. Some issues were particularly emotional, having to do with infants, reproductive rights, or end-of-life situations, and others were more practical, technologic, or even financial. A driving force has been accreditation requirements.

Related Research

Robinson, R. (2016). Moral distress: A qualitative study of emergency nurses. *Dimensions of Critical Care Nursing, 35*, 235–240. doi:10.1097/DCC.0000000000000185

References

American Association of Colleges of Nursing. (2008). *The essentials of baccalaureate education for professional nursing practice*. Washington, DC: Author.

American Association of Critical-Care Nurses. (2004). *The 4 A's to rise above moral distress*. Aliso Viejo, CA: Author. Retrieved from http://www.emergingrnleader.com/wp-content/uploads/2012/06/4As_to_Rise_Above_Moral_Distress.pdf

American Hospital Association. (2003). *The patient care partnership: Understanding expectations, rights and responsibilities*. Retrieved from http://www.aha.org/advocacy-issues/communicatingpts/pt-care-partnership.shtml

American Nurses Association. (2013). *Euthanasia, assisted suicide, and aid in dying: Position statement*. Retrieved from https://www.nursingworld.org/practice-policy/nursing-excellence/official-position-statements/id/euthanasia-assisted-suicide-and-aid-in-dying/

American Nurses Association. (2015a). *Nursing: Scope and standards of practice* (2nd ed.). Silver Spring, MD: Author.

American Nurses Association. (2015b). *Risk and responsibility in providing nursing care: Position statement*. Retrieved from https://www.nursingworld.org/~4af23e/globalassets/docs/ana/ethics/riskandresponsibilitypositionstatement2015.pdf

American Nurses Association. (2017). *Nutrition and hydration at the end of life: Position statement*. Retrieved from https://www.nursingworld.org/practice-policy/nursing-excellence/official-position-statements/id/nutrition-and-hydration-at-the-end-of-life

American Nurses Association. (2018). *The ethical responsibility to manage pain and suffering: Position statement*. Retrieved from https://www.nursingworld.org/practice-policy/nursing-excellence/official-position-statements/id/the-ethical-responsibility-to-manage-pain-and-the-suffering-it-causes/

Brenan, M. (2018). *Nurses again outpace other professions for honesty, ethics*. Retrieved from https://news.gallup.com/poll/245597/nurses-again-outpace-professions-honesty-ethics.aspx

Chaet, D. (2016). The AMA Code of Medical Ethics' opinions on ethics committees and consultations. *AMA Journal of Ethics*, *18*, 499–500. doi:10.1001/journalofethics.2016.18.05.coet1-1605

Cronenwett, L., Sherwood, G., Barnsteiner, J., Disch, J., Johnson, J., Mitchell, P., . . . Warren, J. (2007). Quality and safety education for nurses. *Nursing Outlook*, *55*, 122–131. doi:10.1016/j.outlook.2007.02.006

Fang, M. L., Sixsmith, J., Sinclair, S., & Horst, G. (2016). A knowledge synthesis of culturally- and spiritually-sensitive end-of-life care: Findings from a scoping review. *BMC Geriatrics*, *16*, 107. doi:10.1186/s12877-016-0282-6

Fowler, M. D. M. (2015). *Guide to the code of ethics for nurses with interpretative statements: Development, interpretation, and application* (2nd ed.). Silver Spring, MD: American Nurses Association.

Gilligan, C. (1982). *In a different voice*. Cambridge, MA: Harvard University.

International Council of Nurses. (2012). *The ICN code of ethics for nurses*. Geneva, Switzerland: Imprimerie Fornara.

Kohlberg, L. (1969). Stage and sequence: The cognitive-developmental approach to socialization. In D. A. Goslin (Ed.), *Handbook of socialization theory and research* (pp. 347–480). Chicago, IL: Rand McNally.

Kohls, L. R. (1984). *The values Americans live by*. Retrieved from https://careercenter.lehigh.edu/sites/careercenter.lehigh.edu/files/AmericanValues.pdf

Laurent, A., Bonnet, M., Capellier, G., Aslanian, P., & Hebert, P. (2017). Emotional impact of end-of-life decisions on professional relationships in the ICU: An obstacle to collegiality? *Critical Care Medicine*, *45*, 2023–2030. doi:10.1097/CCM.0000000000002710

National League for Nursing. (2018). *Core values*. Retrieved from http://www.nln.org/about/core-values

Mealer, M., & Moss, M. (2016). Moral distress in ICU nurses. *Intensive Care Medicine*, *42*, 1615–1617. doi:10.1007/s00134-016-4441-1

Raths, L., Harmin, M., & Simon, S. (1978). *Values and teaching: Working with values in the classroom* (2nd ed.). Columbus, OH: Merrill.

Warren, H. (2016). Embryonic stem cell research: A policy analysis. *Plastic Surgical Nursing*, *36*, 157–161. doi:10.1097/PSN.0000000000000156

Selected Bibliography

Annas, G., & Grodin, M. (2016). Hospital ethics committees, consultants, and courts. *AMA Journal of Ethics*, *18*, 554–559. doi:10.1001/journalofethics.2016.18.05.sect1-1605

Beauchamp, T., & Childress, J. (1979). *Principles of biomedical ethics*. New York, NY: Oxford University Press.

Butts, J. B., & Rich, K. L. (2016). *Nursing ethics: Across the curriculum and into practice* (4th ed.). Burlington, MA: Jones & Bartlett.

Courtwright, A., & Jurchak, M. (2016). The evolution of American hospital ethics committees: A systematic review. *Journal of Clinical Ethics*, *27*, 322–340.

Dewey, A., & Holecek, A. (2019). *The nurse's healthcare ethics committee handbook: Use of leadership, advocacy, and empowerment to develop a nurse-led ethics committee*. Indianapolis, IN: Sigma Theta Tau International.

Ellis, P. (2017). *Understanding ethics for nursing students* (2nd ed.). Thousand Oaks, CA: Sage.

Geppert, C. M. A., & Shelton, W. (2016). Health care ethics committees as mediators of social values and the culture of medicine. *AMA Journal of Ethics*, *18*, 534–539. doi:10.1001/journalofethics.2016.18.05.msoc1-1605

Johnston, C., & Bradbury, P. (2016). *100 cases in clinical ethics and law* (2nd ed.). Boca Raton, FL: CRC Press.

Traudt, T., Liaschenko, J., & Peden-McAlpine, C. (2016). Moral agency, moral imagination, and moral community: Antidotes to moral distress. *Journal of Clinical Ethics*, *27*, 201–213.

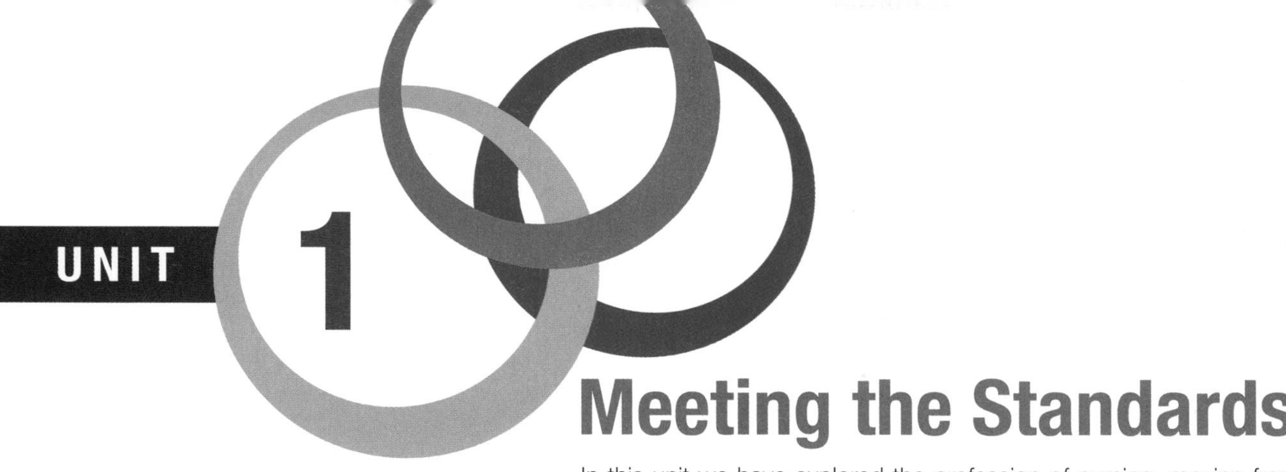

Meeting the Standards

In this unit we have explored the profession of nursing, moving from the history of nursing to the contemporary issues facing nurses today. Nurses must consider legal and ethical issues and the increasing need to develop and maintain an evidence-based practice to provide optimal care to clients. This is occurring at a time when there is a rapidly evolving body of knowledge resulting from research both within nursing and in other disciplines included in nursing practice. In the case study described below, you will explore how the nurse responds to client and family needs while upholding the standards essential to the nursing profession.

CLIENT: Megan AGE: 19
CURRENT MEDICAL DIAGNOSIS: Cystic Fibrosis, Pneumonia

Medical History: Megan was diagnosed with cystic fibrosis when she was 3 months old. Her parents were very protective and home schooled her during cold and flu seasons to reduce her exposure to viruses. She has been hospitalized several times throughout her life, mostly for pulmonary infections, but has remained fairly healthy compared to others with cystic fibrosis. This is largely due to her parents' vigilance in meeting her healthcare needs. Megan contracted influenza approximately 5 days ago and became increasingly short of breath. She has been unable to adequately clear pulmonary secretions, and has not been able to meet her caloric needs due to severe coughing episodes that cause vomiting, resulting in a 3.6-kg (8-lb) weight loss. Her temperature is 38.8°C (101.8°F) tympanically. Breath sounds reveal course crackles throughout, and her x-ray shows dense concentrations of fluid in the bases of both lungs.

Personal and Social History: After graduating from high school last year, Megan entered a college located approximately 100 miles from her parents and is currently living in the dormitory. She has relished her independence but recognizes her parents' concerns. Her mother calls frequently to make sure she is eating properly, taking her medications, and doing her breathing exercises as prescribed. In order not to worry her mother, Megan did not tell her when her roommate contracted the flu. Then Megan dreaded having to call and tell her parents she herself had the flu and had been admitted to the hospital near her college. Her parents arrived at the hospital within 2 hours of learning their daughter had been admitted, and her mother sought out the nurse assigned to her care shortly after greeting her daughter.

Questions

American Nurses Association Standard of Professional Performance #7 is Ethics: *The registered nurse delivers care in a manner that preserves and protects healthcare consumer autonomy, dignity, rights, values, and beliefs while upholding the client's confidentiality within legal and regulatory parameters.*

1. Megan's mother asks the nurse to call Megan's doctor so she can speak with him and asks what the x-ray and diagnostic studies have indicated about her daughter's condition. What information can the nurse legally share with Megan's mother about Megan's condition?
2. Megan's doctor explains to Megan and her parents that her condition has worsened, and recommends intubation and placement on a mechanical ventilator. Megan says, "No, I do not want to be placed on a ventilator," but her mother urges compliance with the recommended treatment. Megan's mother turns to the nurse and says, "Tell her she must agree to follow the doctor's recommendations!" What is the nurse's best response?
3. The doctor suggests Megan be included in a research study for people with cystic fibrosis who want to avoid mechanical ventilation. What are the nurse's responsibilities in protecting Megan's rights based on your reading in Chapter 2 ∞?

American Nurses Association Standard of Practice #1 is Assessment: *The registered nurse collects comprehensive data pertinent to the client's health and/or the situation by using appropriate evidence-based assessment techniques, instruments, and tools.*

4. What is the nurse's responsibility when caring for Megan once she is enrolled in the research study?
5. If the nurse questions the currency of an assessment technique found in the hospital's policy and procedure manual, what steps can the nurse take to ensure that evidence-based practice is used?

American Nurses Association. (2015). *Nursing: Scope and standards of practice* (2nd ed.). Silver Spring, MD: Author.

Answers to Meeting the Standards questions are available on the faculty resources site. Please consult with your instructor.

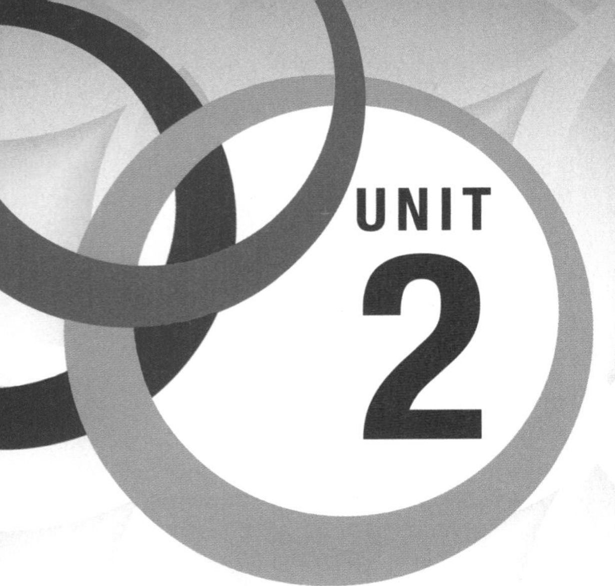

UNIT 2

Contemporary Healthcare

Healthcare Delivery Systems 5

LEARNING OUTCOMES

After completing this chapter, you will be able to:

1. Differentiate healthcare services based on primary, secondary, and tertiary disease prevention categories.
2. Describe the functions and purposes of the healthcare agencies outlined in this chapter.
3. Identify the roles of various healthcare professionals.
4. Describe the factors that affect healthcare delivery.
5. Describe frameworks for the delivery of nursing care.
6. Compare various systems of payment for healthcare services.

KEY TERMS

accountable care organizations (ACOs), *128*
assistive personnel (AP), *119*
case management, *125*
coinsurance, *127*
critical pathways, *125*
diagnosis-related groups (DRGs), *127*
differentiated practice, *125*
healthcare system, *113*
health maintenance organization (HMO), *128*
independent practice associations (IPAs), *129*
integrated delivery system (IDS), *129*
licensed practical nurse (LPN), *119*
licensed vocational nurse (LVN), *119*
managed care, *124*
Medicaid, *127*
Medicare, *126*
preferred provider arrangements (PPAs), *128*
preferred provider organization (PPO), *128*
safety-net hospitals, *116*
Supplemental Security Income (SSI) benefits, *127*
team nursing, *126*

Introduction

A **healthcare system** is the totality of services offered by all health disciplines. It is one of the largest industries in the United States. Previously, the major purpose of a healthcare system was to provide care to individuals who were ill or injured. However, with increasing awareness of health promotion, illness prevention, and levels of wellness, healthcare systems are changing, as are the roles of nurses in these areas. The services provided by a healthcare system are commonly categorized according to type and level.

Types of Healthcare Services

Healthcare services are often described in terms of how they are correlated with levels of disease prevention: (a) primary prevention, which consists of health promotion and illness prevention; (b) secondary prevention, which consists of diagnosis and treatment; and (c) tertiary prevention, which consists of rehabilitation, health restoration, and palliative care.

Primary Prevention: Health Promotion and Illness Prevention

Based on the notion of maintaining an optimum level of wellness, the World Health Organization (WHO) developed a project called Healthy People. The U.S. Department of Health and Human Services (n.d.) project that evolved from the original work is called *Healthy People 2020*. *Healthy People 2030* is already designed and has the same four overarching goals as the 2020 initiative plus a fifth goal focused on the role of leaders: (1) Attain healthy, thriving lives and well-being, free of preventable disease, disability, injury, and premature death. (2) Eliminate health disparities, achieve health equity, and attain health literacy to improve the health and well-being of all. (3) Create social, physical, and economic environments that promote attaining full potential for health and well-being for all. (4) Promote healthy development, healthy behaviors, and well-being across all life stages. (5) Engage leadership, key constituents, and the public across multiple sectors to take action and design policies that improve the health and well-being of all.

Health promotion was slow to develop until the 1980s. Since that time, more and more people have recognized the advantages of staying healthy and avoiding illness. Primary prevention programs address areas such as adequate and proper nutrition, weight control and exercise, and stress reduction. Health promotion activities emphasize the important role clients play in maintaining their own health and encourage them to maintain the highest level of wellness they can achieve.

Clinical Alert!

As insurance companies have realized that keeping individuals healthy is less expensive than treating illnesses, their insurance plans have begun to pay for preventive healthcare activities.

Illness prevention programs may be directed at the client or the community and involve such practices as providing immunizations, identifying risk factors for illnesses, and helping individuals take measures to prevent these illnesses from occurring. Significant examples are the smoking cessation campaigns that both assist individuals to stop smoking and protect the public from ill effects of secondhand smoke by regulating where people are permitted to smoke. Illness prevention also includes environmental programs that can reduce the incidence of illness or disability. For example, to decrease air pollution, automobile exhaust systems are inspected to ensure acceptable levels of fumes. Environmental protective measures are frequently legislated by governments and lobbied for by citizens groups.

Secondary Prevention: Diagnosis and Treatment

In the past, the largest segment of healthcare services was dedicated to the diagnosis and treatment of illness. Hospitals and physicians' offices have been the major agencies offering these complex secondary prevention services. Hospitals continue to focus significant resources on clients who require emergency, intensive, and around-the-clock acute care.

Freestanding diagnostic and treatment facilities have evolved and serve ever-growing numbers of clients. For example, MRI and related radiologic diagnostic procedures are commonly performed at physician- or corporate-owned centers. Similar structures exist in outpatient surgical units (surgi-centers). Urgent care centers and independent emergency rooms are also more common than in previous years.

Also included as a health promotion service is early detection of disease. This is accomplished through routine screening of the population and focused screening of those at increased risk of developing certain conditions. Examples of early detection services include regular dental exams from childhood throughout life and bone density studies for women at menopause to evaluate for early osteoporosis. Community-based agencies have become instrumental in providing these services. For example, clinics in some communities provide mammograms and education regarding the early detection of cancer of the breast. Voluntary HIV testing and counseling is another example of the shift in services to community-based agencies. Some malls and shopping centers have walk-in clinics that provide diagnostic tests, such as screening for cholesterol and high blood pressure.

Tertiary Prevention: Rehabilitation, Health Restoration, and Palliative Care

The goal of tertiary prevention is to help individuals move to their previous level of health (i.e., to their previous capabilities) or to the highest level they are capable of given their current health status. Rehabilitative care emphasizes the importance of assisting clients to function adequately in the physical, mental, social, economic, and vocational areas of their lives. For example, someone with an injured neck or back from an automobile crash may have restrictions in the ability to perform work or daily activities. If the injury is temporary, rehabilitation can assist in return to former function. If the injury is permanent, rehabilitation assists the client in adjusting the way activities are performed in order to maximize the client's abilities. Rehabilitation may begin in the hospital, but will eventually lead clients back into the community for further treatment and follow-up once health has been restored.

An example of tertiary mental health prevention is an outreach program that follows individuals with mental disorders in the community to ensure that they adhere to their medication regimens. These programs can reduce acute psychiatric hospital admissions and long-term institutionalization and enable individuals with mental disorders to live independently.

Sometimes, individuals cannot be returned to health. A growing field of nursing and tertiary prevention services is that of palliative care—providing comfort and treatment for symptoms. End-of-life care may be conducted in many settings, including the home.

Types of Healthcare Agencies and Services

Healthcare agencies and services in the United States are both varied and numerous. Some healthcare agencies or systems provide services in different settings; for example, a hospital may provide acute inpatient services, outpatient clinic or ambulatory care services, and emergency department services. Hospice services may be provided in the hospital, in the home, or in another agency within the community. Because the array of healthcare agencies and services is so great, nurses often need to help clients choose that which best suits their needs. Clients may be seen by any number and type of nurses and other providers, depending on their care requirements and ability to pay for the services.

Public Health

Government (official) agencies are established at the local, state, and federal levels to provide public health services. Health agencies at the state, county, or city level vary according to the needs of the area. Their funds, usually generated from taxes, are administered by elected or appointed officials. Local health departments are responsible for developing programs to meet the health needs of the individuals, providing the necessary nursing and other staff and facilities to carry out these programs, continually evaluating the effectiveness of the programs, and monitoring changing needs (Figure 5.1 ■). State health

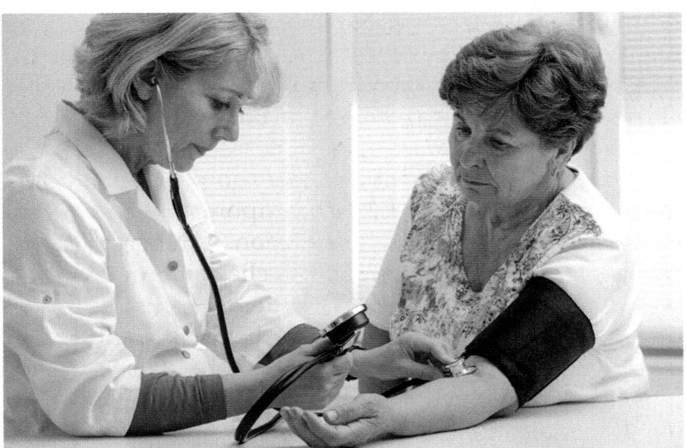

Figure 5.1 ■ Health departments may provide screening services for all age groups.
Michelle Bridwell/PhotoEdit.

organizations are responsible for assisting the local health departments. In some remote areas, state departments also provide direct services to individuals.

The Public Health Service of the U.S. Department of Health and Human Services is an official agency at the federal level. Its functions include conducting research and providing training in the health field, assisting communities in planning and developing health facilities, and assisting states and local communities through financing and provision of trained personnel. Also at the national level in the United States are research institutions such as the National Institutes of Health (NIH). The NIH has 27 institutes and centers, for instance the National Institute on Drug Abuse, the National Institute on Alcohol Abuse and Alcoholism, and the NIH Clinical Center. The Centers for Disease Control and Prevention (CDC) in Atlanta, Georgia, administers a broad program related to surveillance of diseases and behaviors that lead to disease and disability. By means of laboratory and epidemiologic investigations, data are made available to the appropriate authorities. The CDC also publishes recommendations about the prevention and control of infections and administers a national health program. The federal government also administers a number of Veterans Affairs (VA) services in the United States.

Physicians' Offices

In North America, the physician's office is a significant care setting. The majority of physicians either have their own offices or work with several other physicians in a group practice. Clients usually go to a physician's office for routine health screening, illness diagnosis, and treatment. Individuals seek consultation from physicians when they are experiencing symptoms of illness or when a significant other considers the individual to be ill.

In some medical office practices, such as those of family practice physicians or specialists such as dermatologists or surgeons, nurse practitioners (NPs) practice alongside physicians. Often, physicians' offices do not require the expertise of registered nurses (RNs). In offices that do have RNs, the RNs have a variety of roles and responsibilities, including preparing the client for an examination, obtaining health information, and providing information. Other functions may include obtaining specimens, assisting with procedures, and providing some treatments. In offices without RNs, some of these tasks may be performed by medical assistants.

Ambulatory Care Centers

Ambulatory care centers, one type of outpatient setting, are used in many communities. Most ambulatory care centers have diagnostic and treatment facilities that provide medical, nursing, laboratory, and radiologic services, and they may or may not be associated with an acute care hospital. Depending on regulations, advanced practice RNs may be able to provide services in these settings without physician oversight. Some ambulatory care centers provide services to individuals who require minor surgical procedures that can be performed outside the hospital. After surgery, the client returns home, often the same day. These centers offer two advantages: They permit the client to live at home while obtaining necessary healthcare, and they free up costly hospital beds for seriously ill clients. The term *ambulatory care center* has replaced the term *clinic* in many places.

Occupational Health Clinics

The industrial (occupational) clinic is gaining importance as a setting for employee healthcare. The importance of employee health to productivity has long been recognized. Today, more companies recognize the value of healthy employees and encourage healthy lifestyles by providing exercise facilities and coordinating health promotion activities.

Community health nurses in the occupational setting have a variety of roles. Worker safety has always been a concern of occupational nurses. Today, nursing functions in industrial healthcare include work safety and health education, annual employee health screening for tuberculosis, and maintaining immunization information. Other functions may include screening for such health problems as hypertension and obesity, caring for employees following injury, and counseling (Figure 5.2 ■).

Hospitals

Hospitals vary in size from the 12-bed rural hospital to the 1500-bed metropolitan hospital. Hospitals can be classified according to their ownership or control as governmental (public) or nongovernmental (private). In the United States, governmental hospitals are either federal, state, county, or city hospitals. The federal government provides hospital facilities for veterans and merchant mariners (VA hospitals). Military hospitals provide care to military personnel and their families. Private hospitals are often operated by churches, corporations, communities, and charitable

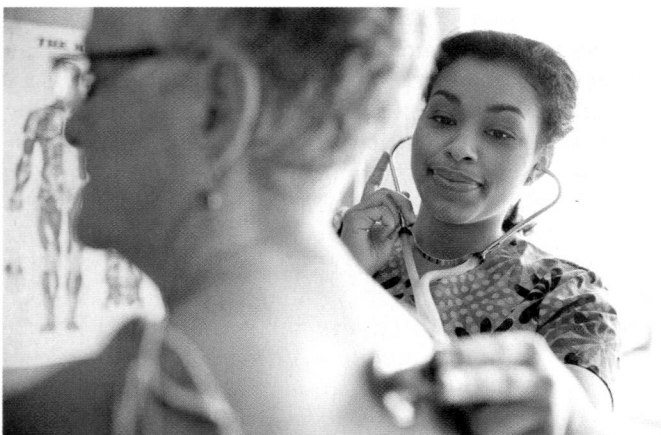

Figure 5.2 ■ In occupational health clinics, primary care providers may examine clients with occasional symptoms.
Hero Images/Getty Images.

organizations. Private hospitals may be for-profit or not-for-profit institutions. Although hospitals are chiefly viewed as institutions that provide care, they have other functions, such as providing sources for health-related research and teaching. Academic medical centers are hospitals that are directly associated with a medical school.

Hospitals are also classified by the services they provide. General hospitals admit clients requiring a variety of services, such as medical, surgical, obstetric, pediatric, and psychiatric services (Figure 5.3 ■). Other hospitals offer only specialty services, such as psychiatric or pediatric care. An acute care hospital provides assistance to clients whose illness and need for hospitalization are relatively short term, for example, several days.

The variety of healthcare services that hospitals provide usually depends on their size and location. Large urban hospitals usually have inpatient beds, emergency services, diagnostic facilities, ambulatory surgery centers, pharmacy services, intensive and coronary care services, and multiple outpatient services provided by clinics. Some large hospitals have other specialized services such as spinal cord injury and burn units, oncology services, and infusion and dialysis units. In addition, some hospitals have substance abuse treatment units and health promotion units. Emergency departments may be designated a specific level of trauma capability. A level I trauma center can handle the most complex cases, while a level V center can perform initial evaluation, stabilization, diagnostic capabilities, and transfer to a higher level of care. Small rural hospitals often are limited to inpatient beds, radiology and laboratory services, and basic emergency services. The number of services a rural hospital provides is usually directly related to its size and its distance from an urban center.

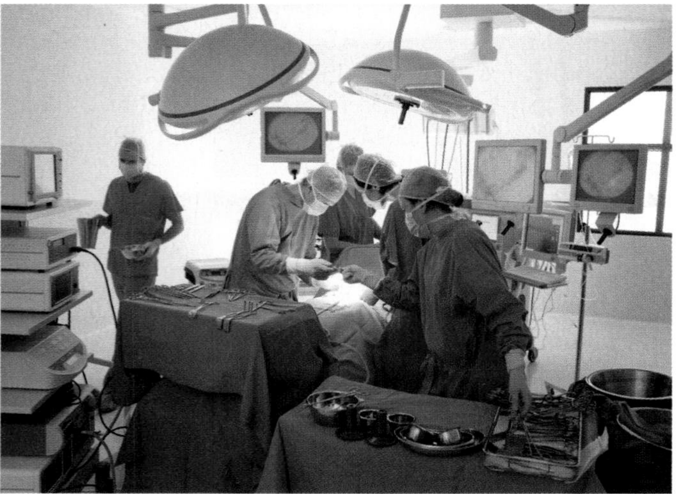

Figure 5.3 ■ Most acute care hospitals have active operating room services.
Chris Ryan/OJO Images/Getty Images.

Hospitals in the United States have undergone organizational changes in order to contain costs or to attract clients. Some hospitals have merged with other hospitals or have been purchased by large multihospital corporations (e.g., Ascension, Community Health Systems, Hospital Corporation of America, Tenet Healthcare, and Trinity Health). Other hospitals are providing innovative outpatient services, such as fitness classes, day care for older adults, nutrition classes, and alternative birth centers. Hospitals that provide a significant level of care to low-income, uninsured, and vulnerable populations are referred to as **safety-net hospitals**.

Subacute Care Facilities

Subacute care is a variation of inpatient care designed for someone who has an acute illness, injury, or exacerbation of a disease process. Clients may be admitted after, or instead of, acute hospitalization or to administer one or more technically complex treatments. Generally, the individual's condition is such that the care does not depend heavily on high-technology monitoring or complex diagnostic procedures. Subacute care requires the coordinated services of an interprofessional team including physicians, nurses, and other relevant professional disciplines. Subacute care may be delivered in a long-term care facility, skilled nursing facility, or long-term care hospital and often lasts 20–90 days (Shi & Singh, 2017).

Extended (Long-Term) Care Facilities

Extended care facilities, formerly called nursing homes, are now often multilevel campuses that include independent living quarters for older adults, assisted living facilities, skilled nursing facilities (intermediate care), and extended care (long-term care) facilities that provide levels of personal care for those who are chronically ill or are unable to care for themselves without assistance (Figure 5.4 ■). Traditionally, extended care facilities provided care only for older adult clients, but they now provide care to clients of all ages who require rehabilitation or custodial care. Because clients are being discharged earlier from acute care hospitals, some clients may still require supplemental care in a skilled nursing or extended care facility before they return home.

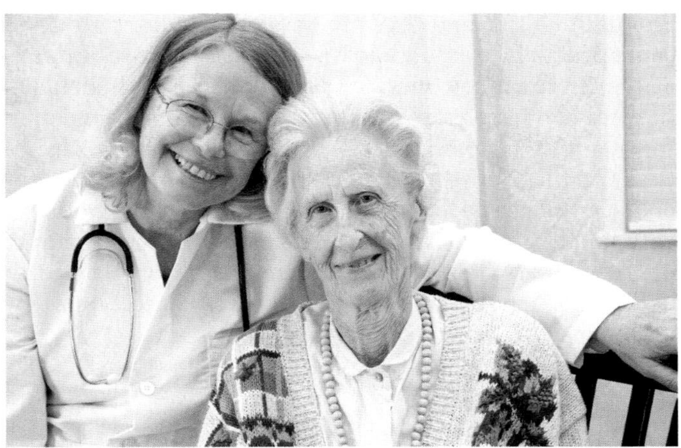

Figure 5.4 ■ Nurses in long-term care facilities develop strong relationships with clients.
fstop123/E+/Getty Images.

Because chronic illness occurs most often in older adults, long-term care facilities have programs that are oriented to the needs of this age group. Facilities are intended for individuals who require not only personal services (bathing, hygiene, eating) but also some regular nursing care and occasional medical attention. However, the type of care provided varies considerably. Some facilities admit and retain only residents who are able to dress themselves and are ambulatory. Other extended care facilities provide bed care for clients who are more incapacitated. These facilities can, in effect, become the client's home, and consequently the individuals who live there are frequently referred to as residents rather than patients or clients.

Specific guidelines govern the admission procedures for clients admitted to an extended care facility. Insurance criteria, treatment needs, and nursing care requirements must all be assessed beforehand. Extended care and skilled nursing facilities are becoming increasingly popular means for managing the healthcare needs of clients who do not meet the criteria for remaining in the hospital. Nurses in extended care facilities assist clients with their daily activities, provide care when necessary, and coordinate rehabilitation activities.

Clinical Alert!

Older adults may move among levels of care several times—from independent living, to a hospital, to a rehabilitation center, to long-term care, and hopefully back to independent or assisted living. The sequence varies, as will the length of time in each setting.

Retirement and Assisted Living Centers

Retirement or assisted living centers consist of separate houses, condominiums, or apartments for residents. Residents live relatively independently; however, many of these facilities offer meals, laundry services, nursing care, transportation, and social activities. Some centers have an affiliated hospital to care for residents with short-term or long-term illnesses. Often these centers also work collaboratively with other community services including case managers, social services, and a hospice agency to meet the needs of the residents who live there. The retirement or assisted living center is intended to meet the needs of individuals who are unable to remain at home but do not require hospital or nursing home care. Nurses in retirement and assisted living centers provide limited care to residents, usually related to the administration of medications and minor treatments, but conduct significant care coordination and health promotion activities.

Rehabilitation Centers

Rehabilitation centers usually are independent community centers or special units. However, because rehabilitation ideally starts the moment the client enters the healthcare system, nurses who are employed on orthopedic, pediatric, psychiatric, stroke, or surgical units of hospitals also help to rehabilitate clients. Rehabilitation centers play an important role in assisting clients to restore their health and recuperate. Drug and alcohol rehabilitation centers, for example, help free clients of drug and alcohol dependence and assist them to re-enter the community and function to the best of their ability. Today, the concept of rehabilitation is applied to all illness and injury (physical and mental) (Figure 5.5 ■). Nurses in the rehabilitation setting coordinate client activities and ensure that clients are complying with their treatments. This type of nursing often requires specialized skills and knowledge.

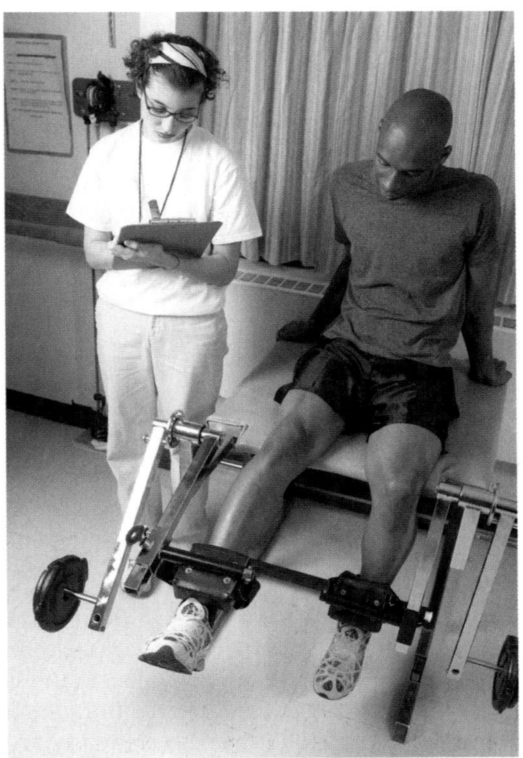

Figure 5.5 ■ Physical therapy services are an integral service in rehabilitation centers.
Ingram Publishing/Alamy.

Home Healthcare Agencies

The implementation of prospective payment programs (discussed later in this chapter) and the resulting earlier discharge of clients from hospitals have made home care an essential aspect of the healthcare delivery system. As concerns about the cost of healthcare have escalated, the use of the home as a care delivery site has increased. In addition, the scope of services offered in the home has broadened. Home healthcare nurses and other staff offer education to clients and families and also provide comprehensive care to clients who are acutely, chronically, or terminally ill.

Day Care Centers

Day care centers serve many functions and many age groups. Some day care centers provide care for infants and children while parents work. Other centers provide care and nutrition for adults who cannot be left at home alone but do not need to be in an institution. Older adult care centers often provide care involving socializing, exercise programs, and stimulation. Some centers provide counseling and physical therapy. Nurses who are employed in day care centers may provide medications, treatments, and counseling, thereby facilitating continuity between day care and home care.

Rural Care

Rural primary care hospitals were created as a result of the 1987 Omnibus Budget Reconciliation Act to provide emergency care to clients in rural areas. In 1997, the Balanced Budget Act authorized the Medicare Rural Hospital Flexibility Program in order to continue to make available primary care access and improve emergency care for rural residents. This program established a new classification called critical access hospitals, which receive federal funding to remain open and provide the breadth of services needed for rural residents, including interfaces with regional tertiary care centers. Each state has an Office of Rural Health Programs that assesses and identifies interventions for the healthcare needs of the local population. Nurses in rural settings must be generalists who are able to manage a wide variety of clients and healthcare problems. Due to their training in providing comprehensive primary care across the lifespan, NPs are particularly suited to these roles.

Hospice Services

Originally, a *hospice* was a place for travelers to rest. Recently the term has come to mean interprofessional healthcare service for the dying, provided in the home or another healthcare setting. The hospice movement subsumes a variety of services given to clients who are terminally ill, their families, and support individuals. The central concept of the hospice movement, as distinct from the acute care model, is not saving life but improving or maintaining the quality of life until death. Hospice nurses serve primarily as case managers and supervise the delivery of direct care by other members of the team. Clients in hospice programs are cared for at home, in hospitals, in freestanding hospice facilities, or in skilled nursing facilities. The place of healthcare delivery may vary as the client's condition declines or as the ability of the family to care for the client changes. The hospice nurse performs ongoing assessments of needs of the client and family and helps to find the appropriate resources and additional services for them as needed.

Crisis Centers

Crisis centers provide emergency services to clients experiencing life crises. These centers may operate out of a hospital or in the community, and most provide 24-hour telephone service. Some also provide direct counseling to individuals at the center or in their homes. The primary purpose of the center is to help individuals cope with an immediate crisis and then provide guidance and support for long-term therapy.

Nurses working in crisis centers need well-developed communication and counseling skills. The nurse must immediately identify the individual's problem, offer assistance to help the individual cope, and perhaps later direct the individual to resources for long-term support.

Mutual Support and Self-Help Groups

In North America today, there are more than 500 mutual support or self-help groups that focus on nearly every major health problem or life crisis individuals experience. These groups may be for the client or for the friends and family of the client, who also need education, guidance, and support. Such groups arose largely because individuals felt their needs were not being met by the existing healthcare system. Alcoholics Anonymous, which formed in 1935, served as the model for many of these groups. The American Self-Help Group Clearinghouse provides information on current support groups and guidelines about how to start a self-help group. The nurse's role in self-help groups is discussed in Chapter 17 ∞.

Providers of Healthcare

The providers of healthcare, also referred to as the healthcare team or health professionals, are nurses and health personnel from different disciplines who coordinate their skills to assist clients and their support individuals. Their mutual goal is to restore a client's health and promote wellness. The choice of personnel for a particular client depends on the needs of the client. Health teams commonly include the nurse and several different personnel (Figure 5.6 ■). Nurses' roles are described in Chapter 1 ∞ and throughout this text. The following sections on the nonnurse providers are in alphabetical order and do not represent an all-inclusive list of possible

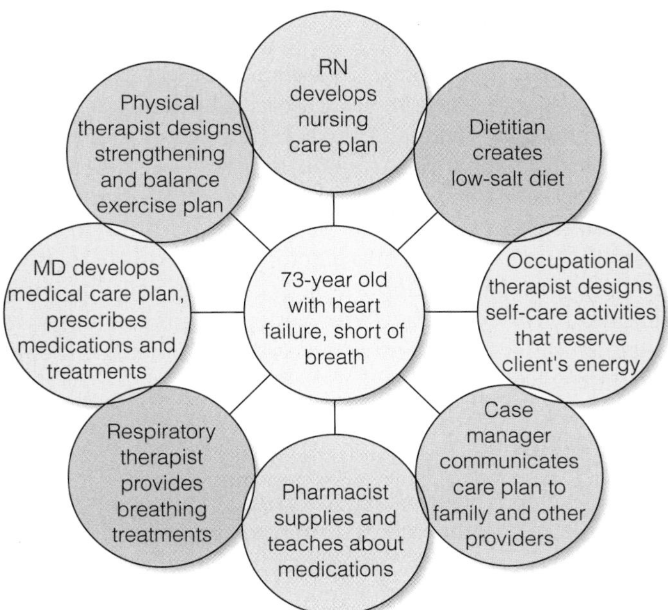

Figure 5.6 ■ Although all members of the healthcare team individualize care for the client based on their expertise in their own discipline, there are areas of overlap facilitated through teamwork.

providers. The scope of practice, qualifications, education, licensure, certification, and accreditation of these providers is determined by the regulations of the state in which they practice.

Nurse

The role of the nurse varies with the needs of the client, the nurse's credentials, and the type of employment setting. An RN assesses a client's health status, identifies health problems, and develops and coordinates care. A **licensed vocational nurse (LVN)**, in some states known as a **licensed practical nurse (LPN)**, provides direct client care under the direction of an RN, physician, or other licensed practitioner. As nursing roles have expanded, new dimensions for nursing practice have been established. Nurses can pursue a variety of practice specialties (e.g., critical care, mental health, oncology). Advanced practice registered nurses (APRNs) provide direct client care as NPs, nurse midwives, certified registered nurse anesthetists, and clinical nurse specialists. These nurses have education and certifications that—depending on state regulations—may allow them to provide primary care, prescribe medications, and receive third-party (insurance) reimbursement directly for their services.

Alternative (Complementary) Care Provider

Alternative or complementary healthcare refers to those practices not commonly considered part of Western medicine. See Chapter 22 ∞ for detailed descriptions of these. Chiropractors, herbalists, acupuncturists, massage therapists, reflexologists, holistic health healers, and other healthcare providers are playing increasing roles in the contemporary healthcare system. These providers may practice alongside Western healthcare providers, or clients may use their services in conjunction with, or in lieu of, Western therapies.

Assistive Personnel

Assistive personnel (AP) are healthcare staff who assume delegated aspects of basic client care. These tasks include bathing, assisting with feeding, and collecting specimens. AP titles include nurse's aides, hospital attendants, nurse technicians, client care technicians, and orderlies. Some of these categories of provider may have standardized education and job duties (e.g., certified nurse assistants), whereas others do not. The parameters regarding when a nurse can delegate to AP are delineated by state boards of nursing.

Case Manager

The case manager's role is to ensure that clients receive fiscally sound, appropriate care in the best setting. This role is often filled by the member of the healthcare team who is most involved in the client's care. Depending on the nature of the client's concerns, the case manager may be a nurse, a social worker, an occupational therapist, a physical therapist, or any other member of the healthcare team.

Dentist

Dentists diagnose and treat mouth, jaw, and dental problems. Dentists (and their dental hygienists) are also actively involved in preventive measures to maintain healthy oral structures (e.g., teeth and gums).

Dietitian or Nutritionist

A dietitian has special knowledge about the diets required to maintain health and to treat disease. Dietitians in hospitals generally are concerned with therapeutic diets, supervise the preparation of meals to ensure that clients receive the proper diet, and may design special diets to meet the nutritional needs of individual clients.

A nutritionist is an individual who has special knowledge about nutrition and food. The nutritionist in a community setting recommends healthy diets and provides broad advisory services about the purchase and preparation of foods. Community nutritionists often function at the preventive level. They promote health and prevent disease, for example, by advising families about balanced diets for growing children and pregnant women.

Emergency Medical Personnel

Several different categories of providers are associated with ambulance or emergency medical services agencies (e.g., fire departments) that provide first-responder care in the community. Titles, education, and certification vary for emergency medical technicians (EMTs) and paramedics. In general, however, these personnel are trained to assess, treat, and transport clients experiencing a medical emergency, accident, or trauma.

Occupational Therapist

An occupational therapist (OT) assists clients with impaired function to gain the skills to perform activities of daily living (ADLs). For example, an OT might teach a man with severe arthritis in his arms and hands how to adjust his kitchen utensils so that he can continue to cook. The OT teaches skills that are therapeutic and at the same time provide some fulfillment. For example, weaving is a recreational activity but also exercises the arthritic man's arms and hands.

Paramedical Technologist

Laboratory technologists, radiologic technologists, and nuclear medicine technologists are just three kinds of paramedical technologists in the expanding field of medical technology. *Paramedical* means having some connection with medicine. Laboratory technologists examine specimens such as urine, feces, blood, and discharges from wounds to provide exact information that facilitates the medical diagnosis and the prescription of a therapeutic regimen. The radiologic technologist assists with a wide variety of x-ray film procedures, from simple chest radiography to more complex fluoroscopy. The nuclear medicine technologist uses radioactive substances to provide diagnostic information and can administer radioactive materials as part of a therapeutic regimen.

Pharmacist

A pharmacist prepares and dispenses pharmaceuticals in hospital and community settings. The role of the pharmacist in monitoring and evaluating the actions and effects of medications on clients is becoming increasingly prominent. A clinical pharmacist is a specialist who guides primary care providers in prescribing medications. Pharmacists also work directly with clients and with other healthcare team members to ensure safe integration of medications into the client's comprehensive health plan.

Clinical Alert!

Significant overlap may occur among those providers who can perform certain healthcare activities. For example, an anesthesiologist (MD), a neonatal care nurse, or a respiratory therapist may be responsible for assisting a newborn baby with breathing problems. All providers perform client teaching.

Physical Therapist

The physical therapist (PT) assists clients with musculoskeletal problems. Physical therapists treat movement dysfunctions by means of heat, water, exercise, massage, and electric current. The functions of a PT include assessing client mobility and strength, providing therapeutic measures (e.g., exercises and heat applications to improve mobility and strength), and teaching new skills (e.g., how to walk with an artificial leg). Some PTs provide their services in hospitals; however, independent practitioners establish offices in communities and serve clients either at the office or in the home.

Physician

The physician is responsible for medical diagnosis and for determining the therapy required by an individual who has a disease or injury. The physician's role has traditionally been the treatment of disease and trauma (injury); however, many physicians include health promotion and disease prevention in their practice. Some physicians are primary care practitioners (also known as general or family practitioners); others are specialists such as dermatologists, neurologists, oncologists, orthopedists, pediatricians, psychiatrists, radiologists, or surgeons—to name a few. Physicians who specialize in the care of clients in hospitals are referred to as hospitalists, and hospitalists who specialize in critical care are called intensivists. Primary care physicians are those who provide the first point of contact for most clients and can include allopathic (Western) medical doctors (MDs) trained in areas such as internal medicine, gynecology, and geriatrics, and doctors of osteopathy (DOs), a branch of medicine traditionally focused on primary care. Differences between allopathic and osteopathic physicians are becoming fewer (Stein & Smoller, 2018).

Physician Assistant

Physician assistants (PAs) perform certain tasks under the direction of a physician and are increasingly positioned to provide primary care. They treat various diseases, conditions, and injuries. In many states, nurses are not legally permitted to follow a PA's orders unless they are co-signed by a physician. In some settings, PAs and NPs have similar job descriptions.

Podiatrist

Doctors of podiatric medicine (DPM) diagnose and treat foot and ankle conditions. They are licensed to perform surgery and prescribe medications.

Respiratory Therapist

A respiratory therapist is skilled in therapeutic measures used in the care of clients with respiratory problems.

These therapists are knowledgeable about oxygen therapy devices, respirators, mechanical ventilators, and accessory devices used in inhalation therapy. Respiratory therapists administer many of the pulmonary function tests.

Social Worker

A social worker counsels clients and their support individuals regarding problems such as finances, marital difficulties, and adoption of children. They are particularly familiar with both public and private resources available to clients according to their socioeconomic qualifications. It is not unusual for health problems to produce problems in day-to-day living and vice versa. For example, an elderly woman who lives alone and has a stroke resulting in impaired walking may find it impossible to continue to live in her third-floor apartment. Finding a more suitable living arrangement can be the responsibility of the social worker if the client has no support network in place.

Spiritual Support Personnel

Chaplains, pastors, rabbis, priests, and other religious or spiritual advisers serve as part of the healthcare team by attending to the spiritual needs of clients. In most facilities, local clergy volunteer their services on a regular or on-call basis. Hospitals affiliated with specific religions, as well as many large medical centers, have full-time chaplains on staff. The nurse is often instrumental in identifying the client's desire for spiritual support and notifying the appropriate individual.

Factors Affecting Healthcare Delivery

Today's healthcare consumers have greater knowledge about their health than in previous years, and they are increasingly influencing healthcare delivery. Formerly, consumers expected a primary care provider to make decisions about their care; today, however, they expect to be involved in making any decisions. Consumers have also become aware of how lifestyle affects health. As a result, they desire more information and services related to health promotion and illness prevention. A number of other factors affect the ability of the healthcare delivery system to meet the needs of the population.

Increasing Number of Older Adults

By the year 2035, it is estimated that the number of U.S. adults over the age of 65 years will be more than 78 million—21.4% of the population—and for the first time, will exceed the U.S. population under age 18 (U.S. Census Bureau, 2018). Long-term illnesses are prevalent among this group, and older adults frequently require special housing, treatment services, financial support, and social networks. The frail elderly, considered to be individuals over age 85, are projected to be the fastest growing population in the United States and will number more than 9 million by 2030 and 11 million by 2035 (U.S. Census Bureau, 2018). Because less than 4% of older adults are institutionalized with health problems (Roberts, Ogunwole, Blakeslee, & Rabe, 2018), substantial home management and nursing support services are required to assist those living in their homes and communities.

Older adults also need to feel they are part of a community even though they are approaching the end of their lives. The feeling of being a useful, wanted, and productive citizen is essential to every individual's health. Special programs are being designed in communities so that the talents and skills of this group will be used and not lost to society.

Advances in Technology

Scientific knowledge and technology related to healthcare are rapidly increasing. Improved diagnostic procedures and sophisticated equipment permit early recognition of diseases that might otherwise have remained undetected. New medications are continually being manufactured to treat infections and multidrug-resistant organisms. Surgical procedures involving the heart, lungs, and liver that were nonexistent years ago are common today. Laser and microscopic procedures streamline the less invasive treatment of diseases that required surgery in the past.

Computers, bedside charting, and the ability to store and retrieve large volumes of information in databases are becoming required of healthcare organizations. In addition, as a result of the availability of internet access from numerous public and private locations, clients now have access to medical information similar to that of healthcare providers (although not all websites provide accurate information). One example of a reliable source of healthcare information for clients is the U.S. Department of Health and Human Services' Agency for Healthcare Research and Quality (AHRQ) website.

Clients are increasingly likely to be treated in the community, utilizing resources, technology, and treatments outside the hospital. For example, years ago an individual having cataract surgery had to remain in bed in the hospital for 10 days; today, most cataract removals are performed in outpatient surgery centers.

Technologic advances and specialized treatments and procedures may come, unfortunately, with a high price tag. Some diagnostic equipment may cost millions of dollars. Due to this expenditure plus the expense of training specialized personnel to perform the tests, each procedure can cost consumers hundreds or thousands of dollars.

Economics

Paying for healthcare services is becoming a greater problem. The healthcare delivery system is very much affected by a country's total economic status. According to the Centers for Medicare and Medicaid Services (CMS, 2018), health spending in 2016 was estimated at $3.3 trillion in the United States and projected to reach $5.7 trillion by 2026. This is currently equal to over $10,000 per year for every man, woman, and child and will increase to almost $16,000 by 2025. About 32% are inpatient hospital expenses, 20% provider office and clinic expenses, 10% prescription drug expenses, 13% residential and home care, and the remainder emergency department, administrative and insurance overhead costs, and related services. Approximately 33% of these costs are paid through private insurance, 37% through public programs, 10.5% out of pocket (paid directly by the individual), and 15% from other insurance or third-party payors. The trend over the past 10 years, and projected to continue, is a decrease in the percentages paid by private insurance and out of pocket and an increase from Medicare sources.

The major reasons for cost increases are as follows:

- Existing equipment and facilities continually become obsolete as research uncovers new and better methods in healthcare. Healthcare providers and clients want the newest and the best, and replacing equipment costs more each year.
- Inflation increases all costs.
- The total population is growing, especially the segment of older adults who tend to have greater healthcare needs than younger individuals. Children account for about 25% of the population and 13% of healthcare spending. Adults over age 85 are the smallest population group at about 13% (but increasing rapidly) and account for 34% of spending (CMS, 2016).
- As more individuals recognize that health is everyone's right, large numbers of individuals are seeking assistance in health matters. The average American sees a doctor three times per year.
- The relative number of individuals who provide healthcare services has increased.
- The cost of prescription drugs is increasing. Medicare recipients are eligible for prescription drug coverage to help cover some basic and catastrophic medication costs.

Women's Health

The women's movement has been instrumental in changing healthcare practices. Examples are the provision of childbirth services in more relaxed settings such as birthing centers, and the provision of overnight facilities for parents in children's hospitals. Until recently, women's health issues focused on the reproductive aspects of health, disregarding many healthcare concerns that are unique to women. Investigators are beginning to recognize the need for research that examines women equally to men in health issues such as osteoporosis, heart disease, and responses to various treatment modalities. Current provision of healthcare shows an increased emphasis on the psychosocial aspects of women's health, including the impact of career, delayed childbearing, role of caregiver to older family members, and extended lifespan.

Uneven Distribution of Services

Serious problems in the distribution of health services exist in the United States. Two facets of this problem are (a) uneven distribution and (b) increased specialization. In some areas, particularly remote and rural locations, the number of healthcare professionals and services available to meet the healthcare needs of individuals is insufficient. One measure of this disparity is the number of health professional shortage areas (HPSAs) designated by the government. Uneven distribution is evidenced by the relatively higher number of providers who would be needed to remove the HPSA designation in states such as California, Florida, and New Mexico (Figure 5.7 ■). One response to insufficient numbers of physicians qualified to provide hospital services has been the creation of hospitalist and intensivist specialties. Funding to increase the number of primary care providers, including nurse practitioners and physician assistants, is intended to help ease the provider shortage.

An increasing number of healthcare personnel provide specialized services. Specialization can lead to fragmentation of care and, often, increased cost of care. To clients, it may mean receiving care from 5 to 30 individuals during their hospital experience. This seemingly endless stream of personnel and required paperwork is often confusing and frightening.

Access to Health Insurance

Another problem plaguing individuals is access to health insurance. Without health insurance, individuals receive less preventive care, delay or avoid care and medications, are diagnosed later in their illnesses, and have higher mortality. In addition, because of low or absent reimbursement for services, primary care providers may hesitate to provide care.

The number of uninsured individuals is changing. Due primarily to the Patient Protection and Affordable Care Act (referred to as the ACA), almost 9 million more Americans were insured in 2014 than in 2013. As part of the ACA, states were encouraged to expand Medicaid enrollment. However, several million adults

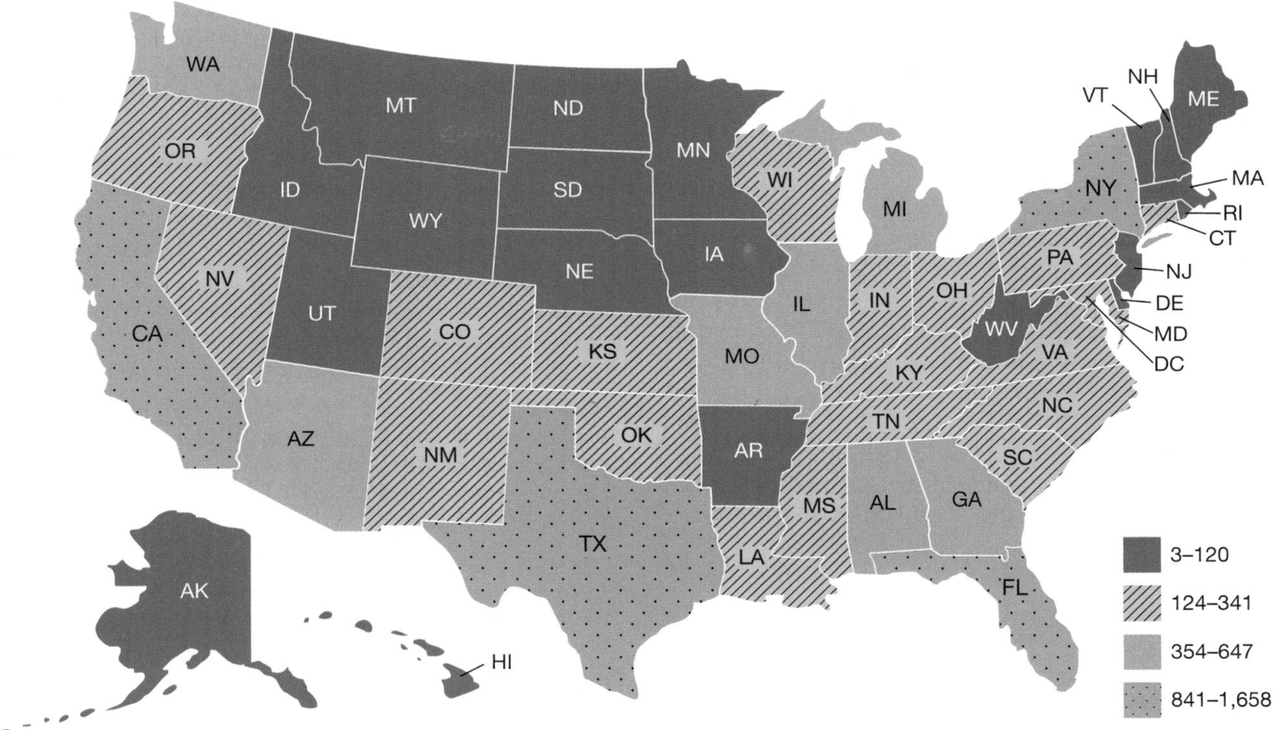

Figure 5.7 ■ Number of practitioners needed to remove HPSA designation, as of December 31, 2018.
KKF's State Health Facts, Date Source: Bureau of Health Workforce, Health Resources & Services Administration, HHS, Designated Health Professional Shortage Area Statistics: Designated HPSA Quarterly Summary, as of December 31, 2018.

fall into the insurance coverage gap due to their state's decision not to expand (Garfield, Damico, & Orgera, 2018). The insured share of the population is projected to decline slightly from 91.1% in 2016 to 89.3% in 2026 (CMS, 2018). Lack of health insurance is related to income. Low income has been associated with relatively higher rates of infectious diseases (e.g., tuberculosis, AIDS), problems with substance abuse, rape, violence, and chronic diseases. Thus, those with the greatest need for healthcare are often those least able to pay for it.

Governmental sources of health insurance cover individuals at both ends of the age spectrum. Medicare covers those who are disabled or over age 65, and Medicaid and public children's insurance programs cover those under age 18. Even though some government assistance is available, eligibility for government insurance programs and benefits varies considerably from state to state and is continually being re-evaluated.

The Homeless and the Poor

Because of the conditions in which homeless individuals live (in shelters, on the streets, in parks, in tents, under temporary covers and dwellings, in transportation terminals, or in cars), their health problems are often exacerbated and sometimes become chronic. Physical, mental, social, and emotional factors create healthcare challenges for the homeless and the poor (Box 5.1). These individuals may lack convenient or timely transportation to healthcare facilities, especially if repeated visits are necessary. Limited access to healthcare services significantly contributes to the general

BOX 5.1 Factors Contributing to Health Problems of the Homeless and the Poor

- Poor physical environment resulting in increased susceptibility to infections
- Inadequate rest and privacy
- Improper nutrition
- Poor access to facilities for personal hygiene
- Exposure to the elements
- Lack of social support
- Few personal resources
- Questionable personal safety (physical assault is a constant threat for the homeless)
- Inconsistent healthcare
- Difficulty with adherence to treatment plans

poor health of individuals who are homeless and poor in the United States.

Health Insurance Portability and Accountability Act

One of the major alterations in how healthcare is practiced in this country may be attributed to the Health Insurance Portability and Accountability Act of 1996 (HIPAA). The HIPAA regulations were instituted to protect the privacy of individuals by safeguarding individually identifiable healthcare records, including those housed in electronic media (Box 5.2). Protection of individual medical records extends not only to clinical healthcare sites but also to all ancillary healthcare providers such as pharmacies, laboratories, and third-party payers. Each healthcare provider dealing with client healthcare information must, by HIPAA regulations, provide for secure, limited access to that information. This is accomplished by restricting access to only those individuals who truly need to possess the information to aid the client, by locking documents in file cabinets, and by limiting access to computerized healthcare files.

The regulated privacy has altered the way healthcare providers share information. Each client is provided a notice of privacy practices for each type of healthcare provider. These notices clearly state how and under what conditions individual healthcare records will be shared with other individuals or agencies. Violation of HIPAA regulations by healthcare providers or agencies can result in heavy fines for this breach of trust.

BOX 5.2 Intent of HIPAA Regulation

- Provides individuals with more control over their health information
- Establishes limits for appropriate use and release of healthcare information
- Requires healthcare providers and their agents to comply with safeguards to protect individual privacy related to healthcare information
- Delineates a set of civil and criminal penalties holding HIPAA regulation transgressors accountable for actions if a client's healthcare privacy is violated.

Nurses must protect their own health and private information just as clients do. Be sure your personal healthcare team provides you with the appropriate HIPAA documents and safeguards your privacy. And remember, privacy regulations apply to care of all clients—even those who happen to be friends, family, or coworkers.

Demographic Changes

The characteristics of the North American family have changed considerably in the past few decades. The numbers of single-parent families and alternative family structures have increased markedly. In 2017, 32% of parents with children under age 18 were unmarried: 53% of those families were headed by single mothers, 12% were headed by single fathers, and 35% were unmarried partners (Livingston, 2018).

Recognition of the cultural and ethnic diversity of the United States is also increasing. Healthcare professionals and agencies are aware of this diversity and are employing means to meet the challenges it presents. For example, more agencies are employing nurses who are bilingual and who can communicate with clients whose primary language is not English.

Frameworks for Care

A number of configurations for the delivery of nursing care support continuity of care and cost effectiveness. These include managed care, case management, differentiated practice, the case method, the functional method, team nursing, and primary nursing. These have evolved, some from each other, for reasons such as the need to decrease healthcare costs and to improve the utilization of limited human and physical resources. Some configurations are more suited for inpatient (hospital and long-term care) settings, whereas others are better suited to community or ambulatory settings. A particular agency may use more than one configuration—for example, a hospital may have team nursing on the medical–surgical units and primary nursing on the cardiac surgery unit.

Managed Care

Managed care describes a healthcare system whose goals are to provide cost-effective, quality care that focuses on decreased costs and improved outcomes for groups of clients. In managed care, healthcare providers and agencies collaborate to render the most appropriate, fiscally responsible care possible. Managed care denotes an emphasis on cost controls, customer satisfaction, health promotion, and preventive services. Health maintenance organizations and preferred provider organizations are examples of provider systems committed to managed care.

Managed care can be used with primary, team, functional, and alternative nursing care delivery systems. Although managed care has been embraced as a model for healthcare reform, many question the application of this business approach to a commodity as precious as health.

EVIDENCE-BASED PRACTICE

Evidence-Based Practice

How Can Evidence-Based Practice Improvement Projects Provide Meaningful Outcomes Data Across Diverse Settings?

The Agency for Healthcare Research and Quality (AHRQ) generates knowledge about how America's healthcare delivery system provides high-quality care and disseminates this evidence to healthcare professionals. EvidenceNOW is a national $112 million effort by AHRQ to disseminate and implement client-centered outcomes research evidence in more than 1500 small and medium-sized primary care practices, and to study how quality-improvement support can build the capacity of the practices to understand and apply evidence related to cardiovascular care (Meyers et al., 2018).

The challenge in this effort is to sufficiently standardize approaches, data collection, and evaluation across the seven funded projects such that outcome measures and pooled data provide useful results. In addition, the effectiveness of the quality-improvement support strategies provided to the diverse practice settings needs to be evaluated.

Implications

Federally funded improvement projects must be designed to provide cost-effective, timely, and useful results. Understanding the process and decisions of a federal agency in designing a large clinical practice transformation initiative may provide researchers, policymakers, and clinicians with insights into future implementation research, and decrease time from dissemination of findings to the implementation of evidence in routine clinical care.

Case Management

Case management describes a range of models for integrating healthcare services for individuals or groups. Generally, case management involves multidisciplinary teams that assume collaborative responsibility for planning, assessing needs, and coordinating, implementing, and evaluating care for groups of clients from preadmission to discharge or transfer and recuperation. In some areas of the United States, case managers may be called discharge planners.

Case management may be used as a cost-containment strategy in managed care. Both case management and managed care systems often use **critical pathways** to track the client's progress. A critical pathway is a plan or tool that specifies interprofessional assessments, interventions, treatments, and outcomes for health-related conditions across a time line. Critical pathways are also called critical paths, interprofessional plans, anticipated recovery plans, and action plans.

Differentiated Practice

Differentiated practice is a system in which the best possible use of nursing personnel is based on their educational preparation and resultant skill sets. Thus, differentiated practice models consist of specific job descriptions for nurses according to their education or training, for example, LVN, associate degree RN, bachelor's degree RN, master's degree RN, APRN, or doctor of nursing practice RN. The model is customized within each healthcare institution by the nurses employed there. The institution must first identify the nursing competencies required by the clients within the specific practice environment. This model further requires the delineation of roles between both licensed nursing personnel and AP. This enables nurses to progress and assume roles and responsibilities appropriate to their level of experience, capability, and education. As with managed care and case management, differentiated nursing practice seeks to provide quality care at an affordable cost.

Case Method

The case method, also referred to as total care, is one of the earliest nursing models developed. In this client-centered method, one nurse is assigned to and is responsible for the comprehensive care of a group of clients during a shift. For each client, the nurse assesses needs, makes nursing plans, formulates nursing diagnoses, implements care, and evaluates the effectiveness of care. In this method, a client has consistent contact with one nurse during a shift but may have different nurses on other shifts. The case method, considered the precursor of primary nursing, continues to be used in a variety of practice settings such as intensive care nursing.

Functional Method

The functional nursing method focuses on the jobs to be completed (e.g., bedmaking, temperature measurement). In this task-oriented approach, personnel with less preparation than the professional nurse perform less complex care requirements. It is based on a production and efficiency model that gives authority and responsibility to the individual assigning the work, for example, the head nurse. Clearly defined job descriptions, procedures, policies, and lines of communication are required. The functional approach to nursing is economical and efficient and permits centralized direction and control. Its disadvantages are fragmentation of care and the possibility that nonquantifiable aspects of care, such as meeting the client's emotional needs, may be overlooked.

Team Nursing

Team nursing is the delivery of nursing care to individual clients by a group of providers led by a professional nurse. A nursing team consists of RNs, LPNs, and AP. This team is responsible for providing coordinated nursing care to a set of clients for a specific period of time, for example, one shift. The RN retains responsibility and authority for client care but delegates appropriate tasks to the other team members.

Primary Nursing

Primary nursing is a system in which one nurse is responsible for overseeing the total care of a number of hospitalized clients 24 hours a day, 7 days a week, even if he or she does not deliver all of the care personally. It is a method of providing comprehensive, individualized, and consistent care.

Primary nursing uses the nurse's technical knowledge and management skills. The primary nurse assesses and prioritizes each client's needs, identifies nursing diagnoses, develops a plan of care with the client, and evaluates the effectiveness of care. Associates provide some care, but the primary nurse coordinates it and communicates information about the client's health to other nurses and other health professionals. Primary nursing encompasses all aspects of the professional role, including teaching, advocacy, decision making, and continuity of care. The primary nurse is the first-line manager of the client's care with all its inherent accountabilities and responsibilities. Primary nurses should be those who work consistently on the nursing unit. Thus, one of the challenges with primary nursing is the variable number of part-time nurses who may not be appropriate for the primary nurse role.

Financing Healthcare

Although efforts have been made to control the costs of healthcare, these costs continue to increase. Employers, legislators, insurers, and healthcare providers continue to collaborate in efforts to resolve issues surrounding how to best finance healthcare costs. Among these efforts, the United States has implemented some cost-containment strategies including health promotion and illness prevention activities, managed care systems, and alternative insurance delivery systems. The U.S. Center for Evidence and Practice Improvement (CEPI) conducts and supports studies on the outcomes and effectiveness of diagnostic, therapeutic, and preventive healthcare services and procedures, including cost.

The primary purpose of the ACA is to require most Americans and legal residents to have some form of health insurance. The legalities and practicalities of the ACA have caused much controversy, and its full impact will not be known for many years. Some key features of the very complex ACA are as follows:

- Individuals will be fined if they do not have health insurance (the individual mandate).
- Employers must offer insurance coverage if they meet specific requirements.
- Eligibility for Medicaid can be significantly expanded.
- State-based American Health Benefit Exchanges and Small Business Health Options Program (SHOP) Exchanges were created. They are administered by a governmental agency or not-for-profit organization, through which individuals and small businesses can purchase insurance.
- Modified private health insurance plans allow extended coverage for children and options for individuals with preexisting health problems.
- A not-for-profit Patient-Centered Outcomes Research Institute was established to identify research priorities and conduct research that compares the clinical effectiveness of medical treatments.
- The National Prevention Council was established to coordinate federal prevention, wellness, and public health activities.

Payment Sources in the United States

In most situations, a healthcare agency receives funding from several of the available payment sources. For example, an older adult client may have Medicare coverage and supplement Medicare with private insurance plus the need to pay some out-of-pocket expenses (Figure 5.8 ■). Almost all insurance plans include a per-visit or per-prescription co-payment.

Medicare and Medicaid

In the United States, the 1965 **Medicare** amendments (Title 18) to the Social Security Act provided a national and state health insurance program for older adults. By the mid-1970s, virtually everyone over 65 years of age was

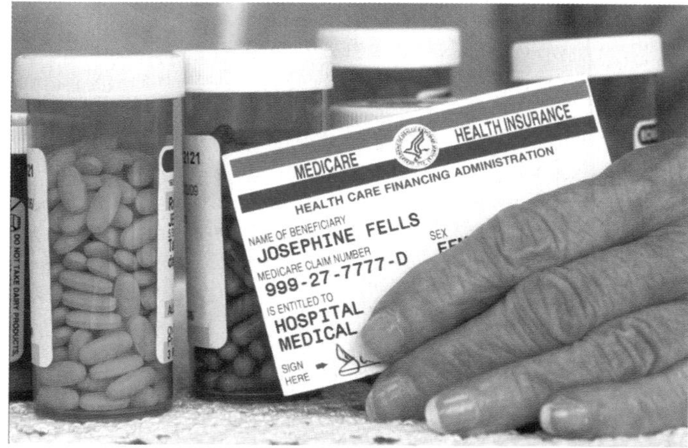

Figure 5.8 ■ Medicare helps defray the costs of healthcare.
Photo Researchers/Science Source/Getty Images.

protected by hospital insurance under Part A, which also includes post-hospital extended care and home health benefits. In 1972, its coverage was broadened to include workers with permanent disabilities and their dependents who are eligible for disability insurance under Social Security. In 1988, Congress expanded Medicare to include extremely expensive hospital care, "catastrophic care," and expensive drugs.

The Medicare plan is divided into parts: Part A is available to individuals with disabilities and individuals age 65 years and older. It provides insurance toward hospitalization, home care, and hospice care. Part B is voluntary and provides partial coverage of outpatient and physician services to individuals eligible for Part A. Part D is the voluntary prescription drug plan begun in January 2006. Most clients pay a monthly premium for Parts B and D coverage.

All Medicare clients pay a deductible and coinsurance. **Coinsurance** is the percentage share (usually 20%) of a government-approved charge that is paid by the client; the remaining percentage is paid by the plan.

Medicare does not cover dental care, dentures, eyeglasses, hearing aids, or examinations to prescribe and fit hearing aids. Most preventive care, including routine physical examinations and associated diagnostic tests, is also not included. However, as part of the 1997 Balanced Budget Act, annual screening mammograms for women over age 40 are a fully covered cost under Medicare. Medicare also does not cover long-term care.

Medicaid was also established in 1965 under Title 19 of the Social Security Act. Medicaid is a federal public assistance program paid out of general taxes to individuals who require financial assistance, such as those with low incomes. Medicaid is paid by federal and state governments. Each state program is distinct. Some states provide very limited coverage, whereas others pay for dental care, eyeglasses, and prescription drugs.

In 1972, Congress directed the U.S. Department of Health, Education, and Welfare to create professional standards review organizations to monitor the appropriateness of hospital use under the Medicare and Medicaid programs. In 1974, the National Health Planning and Resources Development Act established health systems agencies throughout the United States for comprehensive health planning. In 1978, the Rural Health Clinics Act provided for the development of healthcare in medically underserved rural areas. This act opened the door for NPs to provide primary care.

Supplemental Security Income

Individuals with disabilities or those who are blind may be eligible for special payments called **Supplemental Security Income (SSI) benefits**. These benefits are also available to individuals not eligible for Social Security, and payments are not restricted to healthcare costs. Clients often use this money to purchase medicines or to cover costs of extended healthcare.

Children's Health Insurance Program (CHIP)

The CHIP was established by the U.S. government to provide insurance coverage for poor and working-class children. The program expands coverage for children under Medicaid and subsidizes low-cost state insurance alternatives. Coverage includes visits to primary healthcare providers, prescription medicines, and hospitalization. State eligibility requirements vary, but generally, those with family incomes of less than twice the federal poverty line are eligible.

Women, Infants, and Children Program

The Special Supplemental Nutrition Program for Women, Infants, and Children, popularly known as WIC, provides nutritious foods to supplement diets, information on healthy eating, and referrals to healthcare for mothers and for children up to age 5. WIC provides federal grants to states for low-income pregnant, breastfeeding, and non-breastfeeding postpartum women, and to infants and children who are found to be at nutritional risk. It is administered by the Food and Nutrition Service of the U.S. Department of Agriculture.

Prospective Payment System

To curtail healthcare costs in the United States, Congress passed legislation putting the prospective payment system into effect. This legislation limits the amount paid to hospitals that are reimbursed by Medicare. Reimbursement is made according to a classification system known as **diagnosis-related groups (DRGs)**. The system has categories that establish pretreatment diagnosis billing categories.

Under this system, the hospital is paid a predetermined amount for clients with a specific diagnosis. For example, a hospital that admits a client with a diagnosis of uncomplicated asthma is reimbursed a specified amount, regardless of the cost of services, the length of stay, or the acuity or complexity of the client's illness. Prospective payment or billing is formulated before the client is even admitted to the hospital; thus, the record of admission, rather than the record of treatment, now governs payment. DRG rates are set in advance of the prospective year during which they apply and are considered fixed except for major, uncontrollable occurrences.

In efforts to decrease costs and encourage attention to preventable conditions, hospitals no longer receive additional payment for cases in which one of several identified preventable conditions was not present on admission. That is, the case would be paid as though the secondary diagnosis were not present. Examples of hospital-acquired conditions (HACs) are pressure ulcers and urinary tract infections following catheterization. In addition, certain HAC "never events" have been identified that can result in fines to the healthcare provider on top of the missed reimbursement. Examples of never events are objects accidentally left in the body during surgery or incorrect blood type transfusions. Hospitals also receive reduced payments from Medicare for certain outcomes or excesses that can be prevented, such as readmission to the hospital within 30 days of discharge.

Insurance Plans

A variety of plans have come into existence to finance healthcare in the United States. These include private insurance and group insurance. Each individual and group plan offers different options for consumers to consider.

Commonly, healthcare providers bill the insurance company directly for their services, and the consumer may be responsible for a co-payment or deductible. In some situations, the consumer must pay the provider fees and then submit a claim to the insurance company for eligible reimbursements. Another type of insurance that is usually a reimbursed plan is long-term care insurance. This covers a portion of the cost of care in the home or at assisted living, adult day care, respite care, hospice care, nursing home, and Alzheimer's facilities.

Private Insurance

In the United States, numerous commercial health insurance carriers offer a wide range of coverage plans. The two types of private insurance are not-for-profit (e.g., AARP) and for-profit (e.g., Aetna and Anthem Blue Cross/Blue Shield) insurance. Private health insurance pays either the entire bill or, more often, 80% of the costs of healthcare services. With private insurance health plans, the insurance company reimburses the healthcare provider a fee for each service provided (fee-for-service). The term *third-party reimbursement* refers to the insurance company that pays the client's (first party) bill to the provider (second party).

These insurance plans may be purchased either as an individual plan or as part of a group plan through an individual's employer, union, student association, or similar organization. For private insurance not covered by an employer, the individual usually pays a monthly premium for healthcare insurance. Group plans offer lower premiums that may be paid for completely by the employer, completely by group members, or by some combination of the two.

Group Plans

Healthcare group plans provide blanket medical service in exchange for a predetermined monthly payment. A variety of group plans have come into existence to finance healthcare in the United States. These include health maintenance organizations, accountable care organizations, preferred provider organizations, preferred provider arrangements, independent practice associations, and physician-hospital organizations. Each group plan offers different options for consumers to consider when choosing a prepaid healthcare program.

HEALTH MAINTENANCE ORGANIZATIONS

A **health maintenance organization (HMO)** is a group healthcare agency that provides health maintenance and treatment services to voluntary enrollees. A fee is set without regard to the amount or kind of services provided.

The HMO plan emphasizes client wellness; the better the health of the individual, the fewer the HMO services that are needed and the greater the agency's profit. Members of HMOs choose a primary care provider (PCP) such as an internal medicine physician, general practitioner, or NP who evaluates their health status and coordinates their care. If the primary care provider cannot treat a particular problem because of its special nature, he or she may make a referral to a specialist provider. To reduce costs, HMOs will pay for specialty services only if the PCP has made a referral to the specialist. It is an expectation between the HMO and PCPs being reimbursed under their plans that PCPs will treat clients and reduce costs whenever possible.

Thus, under HMO plans, clients are limited in their ability to select healthcare providers and services, but available services are at a reduced and predetermined cost to the client. Because health promotion and illness prevention are highly emphasized in HMOs, nurses in HMOs focus on these aspects of care. Companies that provide HMO plans such as Kaiser Permanente and UnitedHealthcare have been established across the United States, although not in every community. HMOs can be for-profit or not-for-profit.

ACCOUNTABLE CARE ORGANIZATIONS

Accountable care organizations (ACOs) are characterized by a payment and care delivery model that ties provider reimbursements to quality metrics and reductions in the total cost of care for an assigned population of clients. In many ways, they are similar to HMOs. There are incentives to hospitals, physicians, post–acute care facilities, and other providers to facilitate coordination of care delivery. ACOs are able to contract to provide services for clients covered under Medicare.

PREFERRED PROVIDER ORGANIZATIONS

The **preferred provider organization (PPO)** consists of a group of providers and perhaps a healthcare agency (often a hospital) that provide an insurance company or employer with health services at a discounted rate. One advantage of the PPO is that it offers clients a choice of healthcare providers and services. Providers can belong to one or several PPOs, and the client can choose among the providers belonging to the PPO. A disadvantage of PPOs is that they tend to be more expensive than HMO plans, and if individuals wish to join a PPO, they might have to pay more for the additional choices. Some companies offer both HMO and PPO plans.

PREFERRED PROVIDER ARRANGEMENTS

Preferred provider arrangements (PPAs) are similar to PPOs. The main difference is that the PPAs can be contracted with individual healthcare providers, whereas PPOs involve an organization of healthcare providers.

A PPA plan can be limited or unlimited. A limited PPA restricts the client to using only preferred providers of healthcare; an unlimited PPA permits the client to use any healthcare provider in the area who accepts the contractual agreement of the plan. Again, with PPAs, more choices in healthcare providers may mean more cost to the enrollee.

INDEPENDENT PRACTICE ASSOCIATIONS

Independent practice associations (IPAs) are somewhat like HMOs and PPOs. The IPA provides care in offices, just as the providers belonging to a PPO do. The difference is that clients pay a fixed prospective payment to the IPA, and the IPA pays the provider. In some instances, the healthcare provider bills the IPA for services; in others, the provider receives a fixed fee for services given. At the end of the fiscal year, any surplus money is divided among the providers; any loss is assumed by the IPA.

PHYSICIAN-HOSPITAL ORGANIZATIONS

Physician-hospital organizations (PHOs) are joint ventures between a group of private practice physicians and a hospital. PHOs combine both resources and personnel to provide managed care alternatives and medical services. PHOs work with a variety of insurers to provide services. A typical PHO will include primary care providers and specialists.

A PHO may be part of an **integrated delivery system (IDS)**. Such a system incorporates acute care services, home healthcare, extended and skilled care facilities, and outpatient services. Most integrated delivery systems provide care throughout the lifespan. Insurers can contract with IDSs to provide all required services, rather than the insurer contracting with multiple agencies for the same services. Ideally, an IDS enhances continuity of care and communication between professionals and various agencies providing managed care.

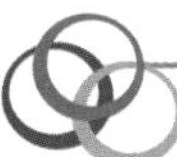

Critical Thinking Checkpoint

Mr. Mendel is an 83-year-old married man. He has a history of severe osteoarthritis leading to bilateral hip replacements and one knee replacement. He has mild hypertension controlled by oral medication. His last orthopedic surgery was done to replace a hip component that failed due to repeated dislocations. At that time, he developed a severe urinary tract infection resulting in weight loss, fatigue, and weakness. After stabilizing, he was sent to the skilled nursing unit of the hospital for 2 weeks until ready to go back home. Occupational therapists consulted with him and his wife during his hospitalization.

He lives in a three-story house with the bedrooms on the top floor, kitchen and living room on the middle floor, and family room on the bottom floor. He has not driven since the last operation, but would like to. He has smoked cigars for years and sits on the front porch to smoke. Physical therapists have come to the house three times a week for several months. A home health nurse has also been consulted periodically to assist with nutrition and elimination difficulties.

1. In what ways has Mr. Mendel used (a) health promotion and illness prevention (primary prevention), (b) diagnosis and treatment (secondary prevention), and (c) rehabilitation and health restoration (tertiary prevention) healthcare services?
2. Name three types of healthcare agencies he has used. What are the strengths of each of these?
3. Mr. Mendel's insurance company has assigned him a case manager. What would this individual's responsibilities be in his particular case?
4. What other members of the healthcare profession would most likely be on the case manager's team and why?

Answers to Critical Thinking Checkpoint questions are available on the faculty resources site. Please consult with your instructor.

Chapter 5 Review

CHAPTER HIGHLIGHTS

- Healthcare delivery services can be categorized by the type of service: (a) primary prevention: health promotion and illness prevention, (b) secondary prevention: diagnosis and treatment, and (c) tertiary prevention: rehabilitation, health restoration, and palliative care.
- Hospitals provide a wide variety of services on an inpatient and outpatient basis. Hospitals can be categorized as public or private, for-profit or not-for-profit, and acute care or long-term care. Many other settings, such as clinics, offices, and day care centers, also provide care.
- Various providers of healthcare coordinate their skills to assist a client. Their mutual goal is to restore a client's health and promote wellness.
- The role of the nurse in providing care to clients will vary depending on the employment setting, the nurse's credentials, and the needs of the client.
- The many factors affecting healthcare delivery include the increasing number of older adults, advances in knowledge and technology, economics, increased emphasis on women's health, uneven distribution of health services, access to health insurance, healthcare for the homeless and poor, HIPAA, and demographic changes.
- Delivery of nursing care that supports continuity of client-focused care and is cost effective may be implemented by any of the following methods: managed care, case management, differentiated practice, the case method, the functional method, team nursing, and primary nursing.

- In the United States, healthcare is financed largely through government agencies and private organizations that provide healthcare insurance, prepaid plans, and federally funded programs. Government-financed plans include Medicare and Medicaid. Private plans include Blue Cross and Blue Shield. Prepaid group plans include HMOs, ACOs, PPOs, PPAs, IPAs, and PHOs.

TEST YOUR KNOWLEDGE

1. Which of the following is an example of a primary prevention activity?
   1. Antibiotic treatment of a suspected urinary tract infection
   2. Occupational therapy to assist a client in adapting his or her home environment following a stroke
   3. Nutrition counseling for young adults with a strong family history of high cholesterol
   4. Removal of tonsils for a client with recurrent tonsillitis

2. The manager of a small clinic has cross-trained the nurses to not only provide basic nursing care but also perform ECG testing, phlebotomy, and some respiratory therapy interventions. Which delivery model is this clinic an example of?
   1. Managed care
   2. Case management
   3. Patient-focused care
   4. Critical pathways

3. A new graduate nurse is looking for employment and is hoping to find a facility that utilizes nursing personnel based on their educational preparation and skill set. Which of the following systems implements this practice?
   1. Patient-focused care
   2. Shared governance
   3. Differentiated practice
   4. Managed care

4. Which of the following factors have an effect on health care delivery? Select all that apply.
   1. Increased use of complementary and alternative medicine
   2. More knowledgeable consumers
   3. Increase in the number of the elderly
   4. Decrease in chronic disease
   5. Technological advances
   6. Economics

5. A client is seeking to control healthcare costs for both preventive and illness care. Although no system guarantees exact out-of-pocket expenditures, the most prepaid and predictable client contribution would be seen with
   1. Medicare
   2. An individual fee-for-service insurance
   3. A preferred provider organization (PPO)
   4. A health maintenance organization (HMO)

See Answers to Test Your Knowledge in Appendix A.

READINGS AND REFERENCES

Suggested Reading

Fuchs, V. R. (2018). Is US medical care inefficient? *JAMA, 320*(10), 971–972. doi:10.1001/jama.2018.10779

The author of this commentary proposes the challenges of comparing American health and mortality statistics and efficiencies with those of other countries.

Related Research

Kaissi, A., Shay, P., & Roscoe, C. (2016). Hospital systems, convenient care strategies, and healthcare reform. *Journal of Healthcare Management, 61*, 148–163.

References

Centers for Medicare and Medicaid Services. (2016). *National health expenditure fact sheet*. Retrieved from https://www.cms.gov/research-statistics-data-and-systems/statistics-trends-and-reports/nationalhealthexpenddata/nhe-fact-sheet.html

Centers for Medicare and Medicaid Services. (2018). *National health expenditure projections 2017–2026*. Retrieved from http://www.cms.gov/Research-Statistics-Data-and-Systems/Statistics-Trends-and-Reports/NationalHealthExpendData/NationalHealthAccountsProjected.html

Garfield, R., Damico, A., & Orgera, K. (2018). *The coverage gap: Uninsured poor adults in states that do not expand Medicaid*. Retrieved from https://www.kff.org/medicaid/issue-brief/the-coverage-gap-uninsured-poor-adults-in-states-that-do-not-expand-medicaid

Kaiser Family Foundation. (2019). *Primary care health professional shortage areas*. Retrieved from http://kff.org/other/state-indicator/primary-care-health-professional-shortage-areas-hpsas

Livingston, G. (2018). *The changing profile of unmarried parents*. Retrieved from http://www.pewsocialtrends.org/2018/04/25/the-changing-profile-of-unmarried-parents

Meyers, D., Miller, T., Genevro, J., Zhan, C., De La Mare, J., Fournier, A., . . . McNellis, R. J. (2018). EvidenceNOW: Balancing primary care implementation and implementation research. *Annals of Family Medicine, 16*(Suppl. 1), S5–S11. doi:10.1370/afm.2196

Roberts, A. W., Ogunwole, S. U., Blakeslee, L., & Rabe, M. A. (2018). *The population 65 years and older in the United States: 2016*. Retrieved from https://www.census.gov/content/dam/Census/library/publications/2018/acs/ACS-38.pdf

Shi, L., & Singh, D. A. (2017). *Essentials of the U.S. health care system* (4th ed.). Burlington, ME: Jones & Bartlett.

Stein, P. N., & Smoller, A. H. (2018). The united state of medicine: Healing identity confusion. *The American Journal of Medicine, 131*, 1141–1142. doi:10.1016/j.amjmed.2018.05.011

U.S. Census Bureau. (2018). *An aging nation: Projected number of children and older adults*. Retrieved from https://www.census.gov/library/visualizations/2018/comm/historic-first.html

U.S. Department of Health and Human Services. (n.d.). *Healthy people 2030 framework*. Retrieved from http://healthypeople.gov/2020/About-Healthy-People/Development-Healthy-People-2030/Framework

Selected Bibliography

Administration on Aging, Administration for Community Living, U.S. Department of Health and Human Services. (2018). *2017 profile of older Americans*. Retrieved from https://acl.gov/sites/default/files/Aging%20and%20Disability%20in%20America/2017OlderAmericansProfile.pdf

American Association of Colleges of Nursing. (1995). *A model for differentiated nursing practice*. Washington, DC: Author.

Austin, A., & Wetle, V. (2017). *The United States health care system: Combining business, health, and delivery* (3rd ed.). Boston, MA: Pearson.

Duston, P. S. (2016). *Analyzing form, function, and financing of the U.S. health care system*. Boca Raton, FL: CRC.

Herman, B. (2016). Health systems with insurance operations have tough 2015. *Modern Healthcare, 46*(26), 12.

Knickman, J. R., & Elbel, B. (Eds.). (2019). *Jonas & Kovner's health care delivery in the United States* (12th ed.). New York, NY: Springer.

Niles, N. J. (2018). *Basics of the U.S. health care system* (3rd ed.). Burlington, ME: Jones & Bartlett.

Shi, L., & Singh, D. A. (2017). *Essentials of the U.S. health care system* (4th ed.). Burlington, ME: Jones & Bartlett.

Community Nursing and Care Continuity 6

LEARNING OUTCOMES

After completing this chapter, you will be able to:

1. Discuss factors influencing healthcare reform.
2. Describe various community-based healthcare frameworks, including integrated healthcare systems, community initiatives and conditions, and case management.
3. Differentiate community healthcare settings from traditional settings.
4. Differentiate community-based nursing from traditional institutional-based nursing.
5. Discuss competencies community-based nurses need for practice, including the Pew Health Professions Commission recommendations for health competencies for future health practitioners.
6. Explain essential aspects of collaborative healthcare: definitions, objectives, benefits, and the nurse's role.
7. Describe the role of the nurse in providing continuity of care.

KEY TERMS

collaboration, *138*
community, *134*
community-based healthcare (CBHC), *133*
community-based nursing (CBN), *137*
community health nursing, *134*
community nursing centers, *137*
continuity of care, *140*
discharge planning, *140*
integrated healthcare system, *135*
population, *134*
primary care (PC), *133*
primary healthcare (PHC), *132*

Introduction

The healthcare system is continuously undergoing change. Escalating healthcare costs, advancements in technology, changing patterns of demographics, shorter hospital stays, increased client acuity, and limited access to healthcare are some of the factors motivating change. The location of client care is expanding out of traditional settings into the community and neighborhoods. For example, healthcare activities such as intravenous fluid administration or mechanical ventilation, once considered safe only in hospital settings, are now available for clients in their homes (see Chapter 7 ∞) and in ambulatory surgical, rehabilitation, and dialysis centers.

One resource to track the shifting of care from hospitals to the community is the annual survey of healthcare dollar expenditures conducted by the U.S. government. The most recent data show that about 38% of total healthcare dollars spent are for hospital care (National Center for Health Statistics, 2018). Although hospitals and other healthcare institutions remain key components of the healthcare system, the trend is toward an integrated healthcare system—one that is community based. The shift from institutional to community care also brings changes in the roles and responsibilities of healthcare professionals.

Many things influence whether clients select to have their care in hospitals or in community settings. Some variables include clients' knowledge and awareness of community resources, cost, availability of home care, and perceived safety of home care. More research is needed to show differences in health outcomes based on location of care.

The Movement of Healthcare to the Community

Healthcare professionals, consumers, and legislators have expressed major dissatisfaction with the current healthcare system, which focuses on expensive, acute, hospital-based care. Nurses, professional organizations, and consumers influence healthcare reform. Nurses provide a unique perspective on the healthcare system because of their constant presence in a variety of settings and their contact both with consumers who receive the benefits of the system's most complex services and with those who have problems with the system's inefficiencies. The increased numbers of advanced practice nurses in recent years (Fang, Li, Turinetti, & Trautman, 2018) have resulted in the provision of primary care to many consumers who had previously been neglected—those living in rural areas, the poor, undocumented immigrants, older adults, and women and infants.

Through nurses' major organizations, nursing has presented a strong voice in describing what a new system should include and what nursing's contributions should be. In 1991, the American Nurses Association (ANA) published *Nursing's Agenda for Health Care Reform*, which set forth the ANA's recommendations for healthcare reform. Although the agenda called for "immediate" changes, the majority of the recommendations have still not been implemented more than 25 years later. The ANA continues to advocate for system reform and to respond to proposed legislation (2017).

Consumers are also effecting major changes in healthcare delivery systems. They are adopting health-related values that include the following:

- Health means more than the absence of disease; it encompasses well-being and quality of life.
- Quality of life is related to a healthy community, which includes healthy families and a healthy environment.
- Individuals can actively participate in promoting and maintaining their health through behavior and lifestyle changes.
- Disease prevention is important.

These values indicate that consumers support an increased emphasis on healthcare services and programs that promote wellness and restoration and prevent disease.

After significant debate and negotiation, former President Obama signed the most significant change in healthcare legislation in American history on March 23, 2010: the Patient Protection and Affordable Care Act (Public Law 111-148) (ACA). The ANA (2014), in response to the ACA, stated:

> As the largest single group of clinical healthcare professionals within the health system, registered nurses are educated and practice within a holistic framework that views the individual, family and community as an interconnected system that can keep us well and help us heal. Registered nurses are fundamental to the critical shift needed in health services delivery, with the goal of transforming the current "sick care" system into a *true* "health care" system. The ANA is actively engaging with federal policymakers and regulators to advocate for system transformation that includes the valuable contributions of nursing and nurses. (p. 1)

Two of the key components of the ACA are preventing insurance companies from denying coverage to individuals with previous health conditions and expansion of the criteria for individuals to be eligible for federal and state health insurance. Increasing numbers of young adults have health insurance and are receiving routine healthcare under the system (McClellan, 2017).

This legislation assists the Health Resources and Services Administration (HRSA) to meet its goals. The HRSA focuses on uninsured, underserved, and special needs populations and aims to:

1. Improve access to healthcare
2. Improve health outcomes
3. Improve the quality of healthcare
4. Eliminate health disparities
5. Improve the public health and healthcare systems
6. Enhance the ability of the healthcare system to respond to public health emergencies
7. Achieve excellence in management practices.

For nurses, the ACA means:

- Expanded scholarships and loan forgiveness programs for nurses at both entry-level and advanced practice levels who are willing to work with underserved populations
- Increased funding for nurses wishing to become faculty
- Support for programs that allow diploma and associate-degree nurses to obtain their BSN degrees
- Grants to programs preparing nurses to work with older adults and in long-term care settings
- A grant program for states to establish community-based interprofessional teams to support primary care practices
- Grants for nurse-managed clinics and school-based health centers
- A Public Health Workforce Loan Repayment Program to ensure an adequate supply of public health professionals. Under this program, the U.S. Department of Health and Human Services (HHS) will help repay loans incurred by a public health or health professions student in exchange for that student's agreement to accept employment with a public health agency.

Primary Healthcare and Primary Care

Another major influence promoting healthcare reform has been the work on *Healthy People 2020* and *2030* (HHS, 2018). This project presents health-related objectives that provide a framework for national health promotion, health protection, and disease prevention. Details of *Healthy People 2020* are discussed in Chapter 19 ∞.

The forerunner of *Healthy People* and *Nursing's Agenda for Health Care Reform* was the 1978 World Health Organization (WHO) report *Primary Health Care*. The term *primary healthcare* (PHC) was coined in the World Health Assembly by WHO and the United Nations International Children's Emergency Fund (UNICEF). **Primary healthcare (PHC)** is defined as follows:

> . . . essential healthcare based on practical, scientifically sound and socially acceptable methods and technology made universally accessible to individuals and families in the community through their full participation and at a cost that the community and country can afford to maintain at every stage of their development in the spirit of self-reliance and self-determination. (WHO, 1978, p. 35)

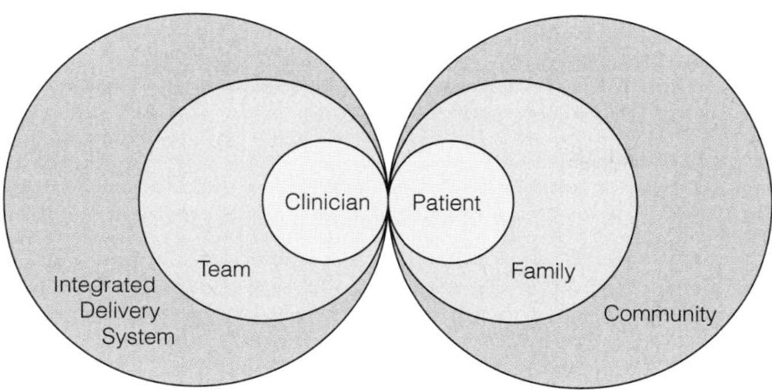

Figure 6.1 ■ The interdependence of the constituents of primary care showing the centrality of the clinician–patient relationship in the context of family and community and as furthered by teams and integrated delivery systems.
From *Primary Care: America's Health in a New Era* (p. 34), by M. S. Donaldson, K. D. Yordy, K. N. Lohr, & N. A. Vanselow (Eds.), 1996, Washington, DC: National Academies Press. Retrieved from http://books.nap.edu/catalog.php?record_id=5152.

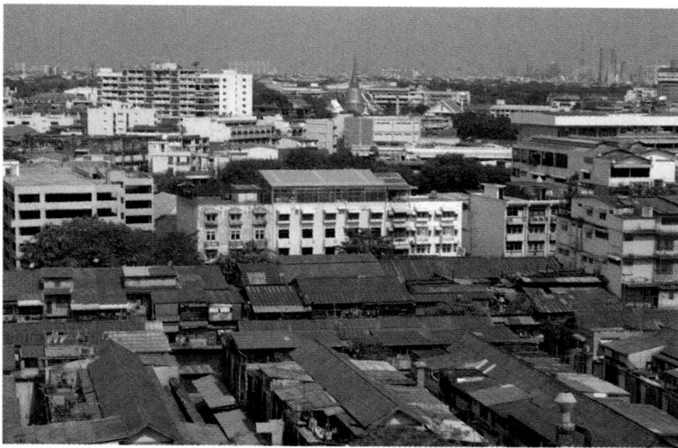

Figure 6.2 ■ Communities may consist of several types of neighborhoods.
Valery Shanin/Shutterstock.

Deep concern about healthcare for the majority of the world's population, specifically low life expectancies and high mortality rates among children, led to the global health strategy of primary healthcare. The WHO declaration emphasized health or well-being as a fundamental right and a worldwide social goal. It attempted to address inequality in health status of individuals in all countries and to target government responsibility for policies that would promote economic, social, and health development. Both economic and social development were considered basic to the achievement of health for all. Thus, PHC extends beyond the boundaries of traditional healthcare services. It involves issues of the environment, agriculture, housing, and other social, economic, and political issues such as poverty, transportation, unemployment, and economic development to sustain the population. A major feature of PHC is that consumers, governments, and public institutions such as public health departments and city councils should be involved in the planning and delivery of healthcare.

PHC differs from primary care (PC). Primary care addresses personal health services and not population-based public health services. **Primary care (PC)**, according to the Institute of Medicine (IOM), is "the provision of integrated, accessible healthcare services by clinicians who are accountable for addressing a large majority of personal health services, developing a sustained partnership with clients, and practicing in the context of family and community" (Donaldson, Yordy, Lohr, & Vanselow, 1996, p. 1). The constituents of PC are shown in Figure 6.1 ■.

PHC is community based and driven and requires active community involvement in making decisions to improve health. PC, on the other hand, is expert driven and involves health professionals who advise individuals and communities about what is best for their health. Other differences are shown in Table 6.1.

PHC and PC also have similarities. Both acknowledge the prevention and promotion components of health and well-being. Both strive for universal access to and affordability of healthcare, support empowerment of the client, and target those at risk for preventable health problems.

Community-Based Healthcare

Community-based healthcare (CBHC) is a PHC system that provides health-related services within the context of individuals' daily lives—that is, in places where individuals spend their time, for example, in the home, in shelters, in long-term care residences, at work, in schools, in senior citizens' centers, in ambulatory settings, and in hospitals. The care is directed toward a specific group within the geographic neighborhood (Figure 6.2 ■). The group may be established by a physical boundary, an employer, a school district, a managed care insurance provider, or a

TABLE 6.1 Differences Between Primary Care and Primary Healthcare

Primary Care	Primary Healthcare
• Community participation is provider directed. • The professional's role is expert, provider, authority, and team leader. • Collaboration occurs among members of the healthcare team. • The individual or family is the focus. • Access is limited. • Healthcare is available within given healthcare institutions. • Empowerment is a provider-assisted process.	• Community participation is client directed. • The professional's role is that of facilitator, consultant, and resource. • Collaboration goes beyond the healthcare sector. • The community or some aggregate is the focus. • Access is universal. • Healthcare is available where individuals live and work. • Empowerment is a collaborative, enabling process.

specific medical need or category. In contrast to the traditional healthcare system that focuses primarily on those who are ill or injured, community-based care is holistic. It involves a broad range of services designed not only to restore health but also to promote health, prevent illness, and protect the public.

To be truly effective, a CBHC system needs to (a) provide easy access to care, (b) be flexible in responding to the care needs that individuals and families identify, (c) promote care between and among healthcare agencies through improved communication mechanisms, (d) provide appropriate support for family caregivers, and (e) be affordable. With the ACA, a key task is to create sustainable implementation of community-based models of primary care integrated with public health (IOM, 2016).

Community Health

A **community** is a collection of individuals who share some attribute of their lives and interact with one another in some way. They may live in the same locale, attend a particular church, or even share a particular interest such as art. Groups that constitute a community because of common member interests are often referred to as *communities of interest* (e.g., religious and cultural groups). A community can also be defined as a social system in which the members interact formally or informally and form networks that operate for the benefit of all individuals in the community. Five of the main functions of a community are described in Box 6.1. In community health, the community may be viewed as having a common health problem, such as a high incidence of infant mortality or of tuberculosis, HIV infection, or another communicable disease. Box 6.2 lists the characteristics of a healthy community. A **population** is composed of individuals who share some common characteristic but who do not necessarily interact with one another. **Community health nursing** focuses on promoting and preserving the health of population groups.

Communities, like individuals and families, are living entities. As such, the nurse will need to carry out an assessment of this community as the client. Several community assessment frameworks have been devised. Students who enroll in a community health nursing course will study these in some detail. In one framework, Anderson and McFarlane (2019) identified eight subsystems of the community for analysis. The subsystems are illustrated around a core, which consists of the individuals and their characteristics, values, history, and beliefs. The first stage in assessment is to learn about the individuals in the community. These community-level subsystems may be thought of as analogous to the physiologic subsystems of an individual. Box 6.3 shows major aspects of a community subsystems assessment. Box 6.4 shows sources of community data that the nurse may draw on to help identify healthcare concerns and to aid in intervention planning for any acknowledged community health issues.

Planning community health may be oriented toward improved crisis management, disease prevention, health maintenance, or health promotion. The responsibility for planning at the community level is usually broadly based and needs to include as many of the community partners as possible. The exact resources and skills of members of the community often depend on the size of the community. A broadly based planning group is most likely to create a plan that is acceptable to members of the community.

BOX 6.1 Five Main Functions of a Community

1. *Production, distribution, and consumption of goods and services.* These are the means by which the community provides for the economic needs of its members. This function includes not only the supplying of food and clothing but also the provision of water, electricity, and police and fire protection and the disposal of refuse.
2. *Socialization.* Socialization refers to the process of transmitting values, knowledge, culture, and skills to others. Communities usually contain a number of established institutions for socialization: families, places of worship, schools, media, voluntary and social organizations, and so on.
3. *Social control.* Social control refers to the way in which order is maintained in a community. Laws are enforced by the police; public health regulations are implemented to protect individuals from certain diseases. Social control is also exerted through the family, religious institutions, and schools.
4. *Social interparticipation.* Social interparticipation refers to community activities that are designed to meet individuals' needs for companionship. Families have traditionally met this need; however, many public and private organizations also serve this function.
5. *Mutual support.* Mutual support refers to the community's ability to provide resources at a time of illness or disaster. Although the family is usually relied on to fulfill this function, health and social services may be necessary to augment the family's assistance if help is required over an extended period.

BOX 6.2 Ten Characteristics of a Healthy Community

A HEALTHY COMMUNITY

- Is one in which members have a high degree of awareness of being a community.
- Uses its natural resources while taking steps to conserve them for future generations.
- Openly recognizes the existence of subgroups and welcomes their participation in community affairs.
- Is prepared to meet crises.
- Is a problem-solving community; it identifies, analyzes, and organizes to meet its own needs.
- Possesses open channels of communication that allow information to flow among all subgroups of citizens in all directions.
- Seeks to make each of its systems' resources available to all members.
- Has legitimate and effective ways to settle disputes that arise within the community.
- Encourages maximum citizen participation in decision making.
- Promotes a high level of wellness among all its members.

BOX 6.3 Major Aspects of a Community Subsystems Assessment

PHYSICAL ENVIRONMENT
Consider the natural boundaries, size, and population density; types of dwellings; and incidence of crime, vandalism, and substance abuse.

EDUCATION
Consider educational facilities; existing school health facilities; type and amount of health services handled by the school; school lunch programs; extracurricular sports, libraries, and counseling services; continuing education or extended education programs; and extent of parental involvement in the schools.

SAFETY AND TRANSPORTATION
Consider fire, police, and sanitation services; sources of water and its treatment; quality of the air; garbage disposal service; availability and safety of public transportation; and availability of ambulance services.

POLITICS AND GOVERNMENT
Consider kind of government; organizations active in the community; influential individuals in the community; issues that have recently appeared on local ballots; and the average election turnout.

HEALTH AND SOCIAL SERVICES
Consider existing hospitals, healthcare facilities, and healthcare services; number, type, and routine caseloads of community health professionals; geographic, economic, and cultural accessibility to healthcare services; sources of health information; level of immunization among children and adults; life expectancy in the community; availability of home healthcare and long-term care services; and availability of transportation service to all major health facilities.

COMMUNICATION
Consider local newspapers; radio and TV stations, postal services, Internet access, and telephone services; frequency of public forums; and presence of informal bulletin boards.

ECONOMICS
Consider the main industries and occupations; percentage of the population employed or attending school; income levels and quality and type of housing; occupational health programs; and major employers in the community.

RECREATION
Consider recreational facilities in the community and outside the community; theaters and movie houses; number and types of church and religious services; number and utilization of playgrounds, pools, parks, and sports facilities; level of participation in various church programs; and number and types of social committees, organizations, and clubs available.

From *Community as Partner: Theory and Practice in Nursing* (8th ed., p. 178), by E. T. Anderson and J. McFarlane, 2019, Philadelphia, PA: Lippincott Williams & Wilkins.

BOX 6.4 Sources of Community Assessment Data

- City maps to locate community boundaries, roads, churches, schools, parks, hospitals, and so on
- State census data for population composition and characteristics
- Chamber of commerce for employment statistics, major industries, and primary occupations
- County or state health departments for location of health facilities, occupational health programs, numbers of health professionals, numbers of welfare recipients, and so on
- City or regional health planning boards for health needs and practices
- Telephone book for location of social, recreational, and health organizations, committees, and facilities
- Public and university libraries for district social and cultural research reports
- Health facility administrators for information about employee caseloads, prevalent types of problems, and dominant needs
- Recreational directors for programs provided and participation levels
- Police department for incidence of crime, vandalism, and drug addiction
- Teachers and school nurses for incidence of children's health problems and information on facilities and services to maintain and promote health
- Local newspapers for community activities related to health and wellness, such as health lectures or health fairs
- Online computer services that may provide access to public documents related to community health

Also, individuals who are involved in planning become educated about the problems, the resources, and the interrelationships within the system.

When setting priorities, health planners must work with consumers, interest groups, or other involved individuals to prioritize health problems. It is important to take into consideration the values and interests of community members, the severity of the problems, and the resources available to identify and act on the problems. Because any plan is likely to result in change, members of the planning group should understand and use planned change theory.

In community health, evaluation determines whether the planned interventions have led to the achievement of the established goals and objectives; for example, was the immunization rate of preschool children improved? Because community health is usually a collaborative process among health providers, community leaders, politicians, and consumers, all may be involved in the evaluation process. Often the community health nurse is the agent of evaluation, collecting and assessing the data that determine the effectiveness of implemented programs.

Community-Based Frameworks

Various approaches are emerging to address community health. Some of these are an integrated healthcare system, community initiatives, community coalitions, managed care, case management, and outreach programs using lay health workers.

An **integrated healthcare system** makes all levels of care available in an integrated form—primary care, secondary care, and tertiary care (Figure 6.3 ■). Its goals are to facilitate care across settings, recovery, positive health outcomes, and the long-term benefits of modifying harmful

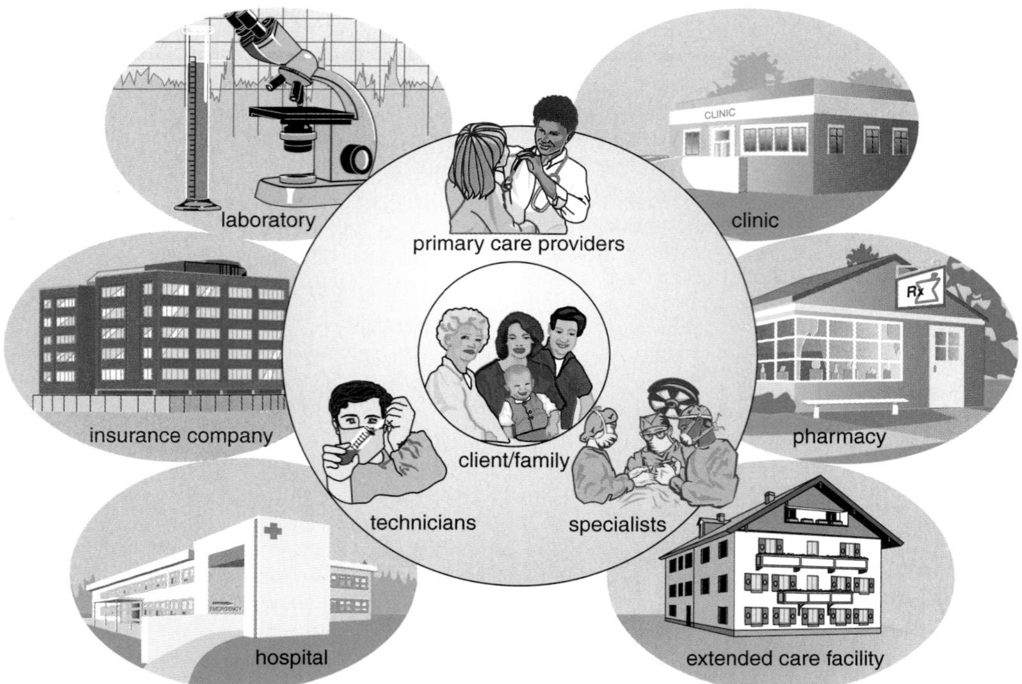

Figure 6.3 ■ Model of an integrated healthcare delivery system.

lifestyles through health promotion and disease prevention. In many parts of the country, hospitals are reflecting this concept by changing their names to *healthcare organization* or *integrated healthcare system*. This type of system is sometimes referred to as *seamless care*.

Community initiatives are being sponsored by some hospitals or local community agencies. These initiatives, called *healthy cities* and *healthier communities*, involve members of the community in establishing health priorities, setting measurable goals, and determining actions to reach these goals. If a community agency is initiating this project, the associated hospital generally contributes human resources to assist in this endeavor.

Community coalitions bring together individuals and groups for the shared purpose of improving the community's health. Nurses are major participants and contributors in these coalitions and often assume leadership positions. Community coalitions may focus on a single or multifaceted problem. Examples include establishment of an abuse program, a gang prevention program, an older adult assessment program, or an immunization program for a high-risk group.

In managed care, which is a common model in healthcare restructuring, healthcare providers (hospitals, physicians, nurse practitioners, insurance carriers, and so on) join to meet health needs across the care continuum. The managed care organization serves as a "go-between" or "gatekeeper" with the client, provider, and payer. Providers are organized into groups, and the client must select one from the group to which he or she belongs. Managed care aims in this way to enhance the quality and cost effectiveness of healthcare.

Case management is an integrative healthcare model that tracks clients' needs and services through a variety of care settings to ensure continuity. The case manager is familiar with the clients' health needs and resources available through their insurance coverage so they can receive cost-effective care. Another important aspect of case management is assisting the client and family to understand and navigate their way through the healthcare system.

Outreach programs using lay health workers are one method of linking underserved or high-risk populations with the formal healthcare system. They can minimize or reduce barriers to healthcare, increase access to services, and thus improve the health status of the community. They involve partnerships between nurses and members of the community. Interested and committed lay health workers are identified who will assist their neighbors through outreach networks. Nurses provide training, consultation, and support to these individuals.

Community-Based Settings

Traditionally, community nursing services have been provided in county and state health departments (public health nursing), in schools (school nursing), in workplaces (occupational nursing), and in homes (home healthcare and hospice nursing). Over the years, numerous other settings have been established, including day care centers, senior centers, storefront clinics, homeless shelters, mental health centers, crisis centers, drug rehabilitation programs, and ambulatory care centers. More recent settings for community nursing practice include nurse-managed community nursing centers, parish nursing, corrections nursing, and telehealth projects.

Community Nursing Centers

Community nursing centers provide primary care to specific populations and are staffed by nurse practitioners and community health nurses. Although the nurses are the primary providers of care to clients visiting the center, a physician's consultation is available as needed. Nursing centers may be located in schools, workplaces, or other community agencies, or be freestanding. Nursing centers must interface with nurse-managed services in other settings across the healthcare continuum, that is, services being provided to clients in their home, hospital, or long-term care facility. There are various categories of community nursing centers:

- ***Community outreach centers.*** Relatively small freestanding clinics providing services similar to those traditionally provided by large public health clinics but focused on a narrower population. Services focus on hard-to-reach clients such as homebound older adults.
- ***Institution-based centers.*** Associated with a large parent organization such as a hospital, corporation, or university or college.
- ***School-based centers.*** Placed within school facilities from kindergarten through college level to provide services such as emergency first aid, diagnosis of acute illnesses, health promotion and maintenance programs, and health education of school-age populations.
- ***Wellness centers.*** Provide services such as health promotion, health maintenance, education, counseling, and screening. In some settings, wellness centers are staffed by members of the healthcare team other than nurses (e.g., physical therapists or occupational therapists).

Parish or Faith Community Nursing

Parish nursing was founded in the United States in Illinois in the mid-1980s by Reverend Granger Westberg (O'Brien, 2018) and became a specialty recognized by the ANA in 1998. The roles of the parish nurse include the following:

- Personal health counselor who discusses health issues and problems with individuals and makes home, hospital, and nursing home visits as needed
- Health educator who educates and supports individuals through health education activities that promote an understanding of the relationship between values, attitudes, lifestyle, faith, and well-being
- Referral source who acts as a liaison to other congregational and community resources
- Facilitator who recruits and coordinates volunteers within the congregation and develops support groups
- Integrator of faith and health.

An estimated 15,000 nurses serve churches, synagogues, and temples in the United States. The role of a parish or faith community nurse is governed by the ANA's *Faith Community Nursing: Scope and Standards of Practice* (2017), co-published by the Health Ministries Association. Most nurses are volunteers, but about one-third are employees paid by the congregation or an affiliated institution such as a health system or community agency. Parish or faith community nursing is nondenominational and includes nurses of all religious faiths. This is one of the few community-based nursing roles found with a similar structure and focus in nations around the world.

Correctional Nursing

Correctional nursing includes the care of clients placed in jails, prisons, group homes, detention centers, and other correctional facilities. Correctional nursing is a subset of the broader category of forensic nursing, which encompasses criminal investigations (including those for assault, rape, or suspected abuse), death investigations, and expert legal testimony. Correctional nursing is the "practice of nursing and the delivery of patient care within the unique and distinct environment of the criminal justice system" (ANA, 2013, p. 1). One example of the work of correctional nurses is to assist with implementation of the standards for compliance with the Prison Rape Elimination Act of 2003. In addition to this example of work specific to the care of incarcerated clients, the more than 25,000 correctional nurses encompass the full range of nursing—from health promotion through illness and end-of-life care.

Telehealth

Telehealth projects use communication and information technology to provide health information and healthcare services to individuals in rural, remote, or underserved areas. The Office for the Advancement of Telehealth (OAT) in the Federal Office of Rural Health Policy (FORHP) promotes the use of telehealth technologies for healthcare delivery, education, and health information services. Video conferences or "video clinics" enable healthcare workers to provide distant consultation to assess and treat ambulatory clients who have a variety of healthcare needs. These video conferences are similar to any outpatient clinic visit except that the client and healthcare specialist are miles apart. A related development to telehealth is telenursing, in which nurses provide client teaching and health promotion to distant clients. Telemonitoring allows transmittal of data from client to healthcare providers and immediate responses. The literature describes the use of telehealth in a wide variety of clinical conditions. With clients who have chronic conditions such as lung disease or heart failure, a telehealth nurse may be better able to prioritize which clients to see in person and, thus, manage many times more clients than without the technology (Fathi, Modin, & Scott, 2017).

Community-Based Nursing

Community-based nursing (CBN) is nursing care directed toward specific individuals. However, community-based nursing involves nursing care that is not confined to one practice setting. It extends beyond institutional boundaries and involves a network of nursing services: nursing wellness centers, ambulatory care, acute care, long-term care nursing services, telephone advice, home health, school health, and hospice services. For example, a nurse case manager may be involved in (a) visiting a newly admitted client in the hospital to take a detailed nursing history, confer with the primary nurse, and begin discharge planning; (b) making several home visits to monitor a client recently transferred from a hospital to a long-term care agency to discuss the client's progress with the nursing staff; or (c) making consultative telephone calls to other health professionals (physicians, social workers, respiratory therapists, and so on) and to clients who are managing self-care independently but who may need support.

Other nurses who work in community-based settings, such as case managers, occupational health nurses, school nurses, and public health department nurses, need to be prepared to make home visits. Home visits can provide information that is not obtainable in other ways.

Clinical Alert!

Community-based nursing and community health nursing are not the same concept. Community-based nursing focuses on care of individuals in geographically local settings, whereas community health nursing emphasizes the promotion and preservation of the health of groups (populations or aggregates).

Competencies Required for Community-Based Care

Nurses practicing in community-based integrated healthcare systems need to have specialized knowledge and skills. In 1998, the Pew Health Professions Commission (O'Neil & Pew Health Professions Commission, 1998) identified 21 competencies that future health professionals would require (Box 6.5). Note that the competencies include the need for knowledge and skills in the areas of primary care, preventive care, population-based care, healthcare access, community partnerships, interprofessional teams, and public policy—all essential for effective community-based nursing. Although nurses educated at the diploma and associate degree levels are introduced to concepts and experiences of caring for clients in the community, coursework addressing the breadth and depth of knowledge and skills for community health nursing is usually taught in baccalaureate and higher degree programs.

Collaborative Healthcare

Collaboration among healthcare professionals becomes increasingly important as more practitioners specialize in progressively more narrow areas of expertise while others take on the generalist role. Over time, the boundaries and legal scope of practice of each healthcare profession may change. To deliver optimal healthcare to the client, nurses must work as a member of the team providing comprehensive healthcare.

In 1992, the ANA Congress on Nursing Practice adopted the following operational definition of the concept of collaboration:

> **Collaboration** means a collegial working relationship with another healthcare provider in the provision of (to supply) patient care. Collaborative practice requires (may include) the discussion of patient diagnosis and cooperation in the management and delivery of care. (ANA, 1992)

A number of different organizations have issued standards and guidelines for collaboration among healthcare providers. Of the six Quality and Safety Education for Nurses competencies, one is Teamwork and Collaboration, defined as the ability to "function effectively within nursing and inter-professional teams, fostering open communication, mutual respect, and shared decision-making to achieve quality patient care" (Cronenwett et al., 2007, p. 125).

BOX 6.5 Pew Commission Competencies for Future Practitioners

1. Embrace a personal ethic of social responsibility and service.
2. Exhibit ethical behavior in all professional activities.
3. Provide evidence-based, clinically competent care.
4. Incorporate the multiple determinants of health in clinical care.
5. Apply knowledge of the new sciences.
6. Demonstrate critical thinking, reflection, and problem-solving skills.
7. Understand the role of primary care.
8. Rigorously practice preventive healthcare.
9. Integrate population-based care and services into practice.
10. Improve access to healthcare for those with unmet health needs.
11. Practice relationship-centered care with individuals and families.
12. Provide culturally sensitive care to a diverse society.
13. Partner with communities in healthcare decisions.
14. Use communication and information technology effectively and appropriately.
15. Work in interdisciplinary teams.
16. Ensure care that balances individual, professional, system, and societal needs.
17. Practice leadership.
18. Take responsibility for quality of care and health outcomes at all levels.
19. Contribute to continuous improvement of the healthcare system.
20. Advocate for public policy that promotes and protects the health of the public.
21. Continue to learn and help others learn.

From *Recreating Health Professional Practice for a New Century*, by E. H. O'Neil and the Pew Health Professions Commission, 1998, San Francisco, CA: Pew Health Professions Commission.

EVIDENCE-BASED PRACTICE

Evidence-Based Practice

Is Care Improved if Provided by an Interprofessional Team in the ICU?

Clients in the intensive care unit (ICU) receive care from a wide variety of healthcare professionals. Sometimes, the providers function almost independently, but in other situations, members of different disciplines must work as a team. This teamwork and interprofessional approach may consist of different providers performing the same function (e.g., nurses and respiratory therapists trade off suctioning endotracheal airways) or performing separate aspects leading to a single goal (e.g., physicians, pharmacists, and spiritual care professionals providing unique expertise in end-of-life care). Donovan et al. (2018) conducted an extensive review of the literature to identify the evidence supporting interprofessional care models and examples of efforts that require an interprofessional model of care for successful outcomes. The authors describe one example in detail: how the individual contributions of seven professionals are essential in achieving optimal success of early exercise or mobility programs in the ICU.

Implications

It is essential that nurses learn the roles of various members of the healthcare team, including those for which the scope of practice is unique and those that overlap nursing. No one individual or profession can accomplish the destined outcomes of a care plan. If nurses can identify those goals that are particularly enhanced by a team of providers, those efforts can be established early in the client's care situation.

One ANA Standard of Professional Performance (2015) is collaboration. The standard is "the registered nurse collaborates with the healthcare consumer and other key stakeholders in the conduct of nursing practice" (p. 73). Key words in the competencies for that standard include that the nurse partners, communicates, cooperates, participates, and engages with other members of the team. In 2011, six organizations representing nursing, medicine, pharmacy, dentistry, and public health issued Core Competencies for Interprofessional Collaborative Practice, and in 2016, the collaborative updated the competencies (IPEC Interprofessional Education Collaborative, 2016) and expanded them to include 14 additional organizations, including podiatric medicine, physical therapy, occupational therapy, psychology, veterinary medicine, optometry, allied health professions, social work, and physician assistants.

The Nurse as a Collaborator

Nurses collaborate with nurse colleagues and other healthcare professionals. They frequently collaborate about client care but may also be involved, for example, in collaborating on bioethical issues, on legislation, on health-related research, and with professional organizations. Box 6.6 outlines selected aspects of the nurse's role as a collaborator.

To fulfill a collaborative role, nurses need to assume accountability and increased authority in practice areas. Education is integral to ensuring that the members of each professional group understand the collaborative nature of their roles, specific contributions, and the importance of working together. Each professional needs to understand how an integrated delivery system centers on the client's healthcare needs rather than on the particular care given by one group.

Competencies Basic to Collaboration

Key elements necessary for collaboration include effective communication skills, mutual respect, trust, and a decision-making process.

COMMUNICATION

Collaborating to solve complex problems requires effective communication skills. Effective communication can occur only if the involved parties are committed to understanding

BOX 6.6 The Nurse as a Collaborator

WITH NURSE COLLEAGUES

- Shares personal expertise with other nurses and elicits the expertise of others to ensure quality client care.
- Develops a sense of trust and mutual respect with peers that recognizes their unique contributions.

WITH OTHER HEALTHCARE PROFESSIONALS

- Recognizes the contribution that each member of the interprofessional team can make by virtue of his or her expertise and view of the situation.
- Listens to each individual's views.
- Shares healthcare responsibilities in exploring options, setting goals, and making decisions with clients and families.
- Participates in collaborative interprofessional research to increase knowledge of a clinical problem or situation.

WITH PROFESSIONAL NURSING ORGANIZATIONS

- Seeks opportunities to collaborate with and within professional organizations.
- Serves on committees in state and national nursing organizations or specialty groups.
- Supports professional organizations in political action to create solutions for professional and healthcare concerns.

WITH LEGISLATORS

- Offers expert opinions on legislative initiatives related to healthcare.
- Collaborates with other healthcare providers and consumers on healthcare legislation to best serve the needs of the public.

one another's professional roles and appreciating one another as individuals. Additionally, they must be sensitive to differences among communication styles. Instead of focusing on distinctions, a group of professionals needs to center on their common ground: the client's needs.

MUTUAL RESPECT AND TRUST

Mutual respect occurs when two or more individuals show or feel honor or esteem toward one another. Trust occurs when an individual is confident in the actions of another individual. Both mutual respect and trust imply a mutual process and outcome. They must be expressed both verbally and nonverbally.

DECISION MAKING

The decision-making process at the team level involves shared responsibility for the outcome. To create a solution, the team must follow each step of the decision-making process, beginning with a clear definition of the problem. Team decision making must be directed at the objectives of the specific effort. It requires full consideration and respect for diverse viewpoints. Members must be able to verbalize their perspectives in a nonthreatening environment.

An important aspect of decision making is satisfied when the interprofessional team focuses on the client's priority needs and organizes interventions accordingly. The discipline best able to address the client's needs is given priority in planning and is responsible for providing its interventions in a timely manner. For example, a social worker may first direct attention to a client's social needs when these needs interfere with the client's ability to respond to therapy. Nurses, by the nature of their holistic practice, are often able to help the team identify priorities and areas requiring further attention.

Continuity of Care

A major responsibility of the nurse is to ensure continuity of care. **Continuity of care** is the coordination of healthcare services by healthcare providers for clients moving from one healthcare setting to another and between and among healthcare professionals. Continuity ensures uninterrupted and consistent services for the client from one level of care to another. When coordinated appropriately, it maintains client-focused individualized care and helps optimize the client's health status based on the client's needs and preferences (Agency for Healthcare Research and Quality, 2018). In 2012, the ANA issued a position statement on the registered nurse's role in care coordination. This statement promotes the responsibility of the nurse to be prepared to partner with the client to provide quality and access to appropriate healthcare resources across a variety of settings (ANA 2012).

To provide continuity of care, nurses need to accomplish the following:

- Initiate discharge planning for all clients when they are admitted to any healthcare setting.
- Involve the client and the client's family or support individuals in the planning process.
- Collaborate with other healthcare professionals as needed to ensure that biopsychosocial, cultural, and spiritual needs are met.

Achieving continuity, however, assumes that needed client data are shared with other providers while implementing strategies to protect client privacy. The Health Insurance Portability and Accountability Act of 1996 (HIPAA) requires that health information about clients be secured in such a way that only those with the right and need to acquire the information are able to do so.

The privacy aspect of HIPAA results in a balance between protecting disclosure of confidential client information and the need for certain data to be released to specific agencies. Ultimately, clients have increased control over their own information, and those who violate the rule face significant penalties. Community nursing practice has altered in the face of the HIPAA regulations. Case managers and public health nurses need to maintain vigilance to protect the privacy of client healthcare information when sending and receiving telephone messages, faxes, and electronic documentation when in field settings as well as within healthcare facilities.

Care Across the Lifespan

The majority of children and older adults receive their healthcare in their communities rather than in hospitals. From home births, to school-based childhood immunization programs, to sex education for teens, to chronic disease management in adults, to hospice care, the nurse works with clients and a wide variety of community health organizations to provide wellness and illness care. A wide variety of initiatives focused on care provided in the community for children is found at the American Academy of Pediatrics website.

Discharge Planning

Discharge planning is the process of preparing a client to leave one level of care for another within or outside the current healthcare agency. Usually, discharge planning refers to the client leaving the hospital for home. However, discharges occur among many other settings. Within a facility, it can occur from one unit to another. For example, a client with a stroke may move from a medical unit to a rehabilitation unit, or a client with trauma may move from the emergency department to an intensive care unit. Clients may move from a hospital to a long-term care agency, from a rehabilitation center to home, from a home healthcare setting to a hospital, and so on.

Each agency generally has its own policies and procedures related to discharge. Many agencies have case managers or discharge planners, a health or social services professional who coordinates the transition and acts as a link between the discharging agency and the receiving facility. Often, a nurse assumes this responsibility of providing continuity of care.

Discharge planning needs to begin as soon as a client is admitted to the agency, especially in hospitals where stays are relatively short. Effective discharge planning involves ongoing assessment to obtain comprehensive information about the client's ongoing needs and nursing care plans to ensure that the client's and receiving agency caregivers' needs are met. In some situations discharge planning necessitates health team conferences and family conferences. At a health team conference, healthcare professionals focus on ways to individualize care for the client. At a family conference, both health professionals and the family discuss family issues related to the client. Both types of conferences give the client, family, and healthcare professionals the opportunity to mutually plan care and set goals.

Preparing Clients to Go Home

Nurses preparing to send clients home from the hospital need to assess their clients' personal and health data; ability to perform activities of daily living; any physical, cognitive, or other functional limitations; caregivers' responses and abilities; adequacy of financial resources; community supports; hazards or barriers that the home environment presents; and need for healthcare assistance in the home. Box 6.7 outlines details for each of these parameters.

The data are used to establish which nursing activities are required before the client can be discharged. These activities most often include teaching the client to cope with continuing self-care at home and a home care referral.

Medication Reconciliation

When a client moves from one location or level of care to another, current information regarding medications must be communicated within the healthcare team to prevent errors and unintended consequences. The Joint Commission (2019) continues to emphasize medication reconciliation as one of the National Patient Safety Goals for hospitals, ambulatory and behavioral healthcare, and home care settings. Medication reconciliation is the process of comparing all the medications a client is taking (and should be taking) with newly ordered or changed medications. The comparison addresses duplications, omissions, and interactions. Reconciliation must occur during transitions in care both within and outside of the organization and include client education on safe medication use and communications with other providers. The organization obtains the client's medication information at the beginning of an episode of care. The information is updated when the client's medications change. Often, clients—especially older adults—do not recall their medication names or even the conditions for which they are taking them. The responsibility for conducting medication reconciliation often falls to the nurse.

Home Healthcare Teaching

Clients need help to understand their health condition, to make healthcare decisions, and to learn new health behaviors. Because of today's shortened hospital stays, it is often unrealistic to teach clients everything they need to know prior to discharge. Referral to a home health agency for follow-up teaching may be necessary. Essential information before discharge includes information about medications, dietary and activity restrictions, signs of complications that need to be reported to the primary care provider, follow-up appointments and telephone numbers, and where supplies can be obtained. Clients or caregivers also need to demonstrate safe performance of any necessary treatments. Information needs to be provided

BOX 6.7 Discharge Planning: Home Assessment Parameters

PERSONAL AND HEALTH DATA

Age; sex; height and weight; cultural beliefs and practices; medical history; current health status; prognosis; surgery

ABILITY TO PERFORM ACTIVITIES OF DAILY LIVING

Abilities for dressing; eating; toileting; bathing (tub, shower, sponge); ambulating (with or without aids such as a cane, crutches, walker, wheelchair); transferring (from bed to chair, in and out of bath, in and out of car); meal preparation; transportation; shopping

DISABILITIES/LIMITATIONS

Sensory losses (auditory, visual); motor losses (paralysis, amputation); communication disorder; mental confusion or depression; incontinence

CAREGIVERS' RESPONSES AND ABILITIES

Principal caregiver's relationship to client; thoughts and feelings about client's discharge; expectations for recovery; health and coping abilities; comfort with performing needed care

FINANCIAL RESOURCES

Financial resources and needs (note equipment, supplies, medications, special foods required)

COMMUNITY SUPPORTS

Family members, friends, neighbors, volunteers; resources such as Medicaid; food stamps; nutrition services; health centers; community health nurses; day programs; legal assistance; home care; respite care

HOME HAZARD APPRAISAL

Safety precautions (stairs with or without handrails; lighting in rooms, hallways, stairways; night-lights in hallways or bathroom; grab bars near toilet and tub; firmly attached carpets and rugs); self-care barriers (lack of running water, lack of wheelchair access to bathroom or home, lack of space for required equipment, lack of elevator) (Note: A detailed home hazard appraisal is provided in Chapter 7).

NEED FOR HEALTHCARE ASSISTANCE

Home-delivered meals; special dietary needs; volunteers for telephone reassurance, friendly visiting, transportation, shopping; assistance with bathing; assistance with housekeeping; assistance with wound care, ostomies, tubes, intravenous medications

LIFESPAN CONSIDERATIONS Healthcare Delivery

CHILDREN

The Search Institute has identified evidence-based assets characteristic of healthy communities and of different age groups of children. These assets are both external and internal to the individual, and if promoted in communities, will contribute to the healthy development of children and families and the positive life of the community. The impact of these assets has been studied in children from birth through adolescence, and many communities across the United States are using them to structure programs for children and youth. Among the assets are such things as family support, family values of equality and social justice, involvement of children and youth with adults and community organizations, constructive use of young individual's time, and engagement in learning. The institute also has five action strategies for transforming communities for the betterment of youth: engaging adults, mobilizing youth, activating organizations, expanding programs, and influencing policy.

OLDER ADULTS

Due to the changes caused by aging and the increase of chronic illnesses in older adults, various levels of healthcare delivery are often required. Clients may go back and forth between these levels as their needs fluctuate. At various times and situations, they might need care from hospitals, home care, extended care facilities, ambulatory care, and assisted living. Maintaining communications and providing continuity of care during these changes are essential.

Caregivers of older adults are often older themselves and may have health problems of their own. Attention should be given to signs of emotional and physical fatigue and other problems that might arise for them. Community health nurses have the opportunity to do ongoing assessments of this as they see clients and caregivers in their home environment. They can then provide support and resources as needed.

verbally and in writing. Details about effective teaching strategies are provided in Chapter 17 ∞. Reinforcement of acute care discharge information will often fall in the domain of the community-oriented nurse. Client issues related to health literacy, language barriers, and access to resources to carry out the provided healthcare instruction are major concerns of community nurses.

Referrals

The referral process is a systematic problem-solving approach that helps clients to use resources that meet their healthcare needs. The process involves knowledge of community resources and an ability to solve problems, set priorities, coordinate, and collaborate. Home care referrals are often made before discharge for the following clients:

- Older adults
- Children with complex conditions
- Frail individuals who live alone
- Those who lack or have a limited support system
- Those who have a caregiver whose abilities are limited
- Those whose home presents barriers to their safety (e.g., stairs).

Referrals need to present as much information as possible about the client and the hospitalization to the agency. Most agencies have well-established protocols and detailed referral forms. The assessment parameters in Box 6.7 may also be used as a guide. The nurse caring for the hospital client is responsible for confirming and documenting that the relevant referrals have been made. To identify and recommend referrals, the nurse must already be familiar with the resources that are available in the community. Using this knowledge, plus information regarding the client's previous awareness and choice of community resources, hospital nurses play a key role in maintaining effective continuity of healthcare.

To ensure appropriate reimbursement to the home health agency, the primary care provider must provide a written order for a home care referral and subsequent home visits. Clients must meet specific criteria to have Medicare or other third-party payers reimburse them for home care services. Chapter 7 ∞ provides details about home health nursing.

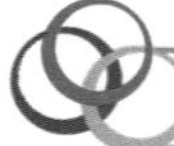

Critical Thinking Checkpoint

Nurses are, and should be, taking an active role in influencing the direction of healthcare. Recognizing that there are finite limits to the amount of money and healthcare providers available, desirable outcomes often compete for resources. Consider a clinical situation such as the "drive-through (or 24-hour) mastectomies" in which clients are moved through the acute care (hospital) system extremely quickly compared to previously. *ANA's Principles for Health System Transformation* (ANA, 2016) states that the system must (a) ensure universal access to a standard package of essential healthcare services for all citizens and residents; (b) optimize primary, community-based, and preventive services while supporting the cost-effective use of innovative, technology-driven, acute, hospital-based services; and (c) encourage mechanisms to stimulate economical use of healthcare services while supporting those who do not have the means to share in costs.

1. How does the mastectomy clinical example reflect or not reflect the principles?
2. Which of the three principles listed do you consider the most important and why?
3. How might different community-based frameworks manage the clinical example?
4. How would the nurse use collaboration with insurance payers, clients, or surgeons to resolve any concerns with the clinical example?

Answers to Critical Thinking Checkpoint questions are available on the faculty resources site. Please consult with your instructor.

Chapter 6 Review

CHAPTER HIGHLIGHTS

- Consumers support an increased emphasis on healthcare measures that promote wellness.
- *ANA's Principles for Health System Transformation* (2016) and *Healthy People 2020* and *2030* by the HHS (2018) have set forth recommendations for healthcare reform. These focus on accessibility of healthcare services, health promotion and disease prevention, and steps to consider how healthcare costs can be reduced.
- Healthcare costs, access to healthcare, and the quality of healthcare are major areas of concern surrounding the current healthcare system.
- Community-based healthcare, akin to primary healthcare, provides health-related services in places where individuals spend their time—in homes, in shelters, in long-term care residences, at work, in schools, in senior citizens' centers, and so on.
- A community is a collection of individuals who share some attribute of their lives.
- For community assessment, eight subsystems proposed by Anderson and McFarlane (2019) can be used: physical environment, education, safety and transportation, politics and government, health and social services, communication, economics, and recreation.
- Approaches are emerging to address community-based care. These include an integrated healthcare system, community initiatives, community coalitions, managed care, case management, and outreach programs using lay health workers.
- Numerous community settings have been established. Ones that are more recent include nurse-managed community nursing centers, parish nursing, corrections nursing, and telehealth projects.
- Community-based nursing directs nursing care toward specific individuals. It is not confined to one practice setting; it extends beyond institutional boundaries involving a network of nursing services: nursing wellness centers, ambulatory care, long-term care, telephone advice, home health, school health, and hospice care.
- To practice in community healthcare systems, nurses need knowledge and skills in primary care, preventive care, population-based care, healthcare access, community partnerships, interprofessional teams, and public policy.
- Collaboration among healthcare providers is key to providing comprehensive healthcare.
- A major responsibility of the nurse is to ensure continuity of care as clients move from one level of care to another.
- Continuity of care involves (a) discharge planning that begins when clients are admitted to an agency, (b) cooperation with the client and support individuals, and (c) interprofessional collaboration.
- Nurses need to ensure that clients have essential information and skills to manage self-care before being discharged to their homes. In some situations, referral to a home health agency is necessary.

TEST YOUR KNOWLEDGE

1. A nurse educator is explaining primary healthcare (PHC) and the extension of its boundaries beyond traditional health care services. Which of the following includes issues related to PHC?
   1. Distribution and participation
   2. Environment, agriculture, and housing
   3. Consumerism and governmental subsidies
   4. Low life expectancies and high mortality rates among children

2. Which of the following is characteristic of nursing care provided in community-based health?
   1. Clients are primarily those with identified illnesses.
   2. Clients are individuals in groups according to their geographic commonalities.
   3. Care is paid for by the community as a whole rather than by individuals.
   4. All clients are case managed.

3. A nurse is helping to set up an elder social group at a local senior center where residents can come to play cards or participate in structured activities three times a week. Which function of community is this nurse facilitating?
   1. Socialization
   2. Social control
   3. Social interparticipation
   4. Mutual support

4. The nurse concludes that effective discharge planning (hospital to home) has been conducted when the client states which of the following?
   1. "As soon as I get home, the nurse will come out, look at where I live, and see what kind of care I will need."
   2. "All I need are my medications and a ride home. Then I'm all ready for discharge."
   3. "When I visit my doctor in 10 days, they will show me how to change my bandages."
   4. "I have the phone numbers of the home care nurse and the therapist who will visit me at home tomorrow."

5. After a community was hit by a tornado, the nurses of the local Red Cross Chapter helped to make sure that people had adequate food and clothing. Which function of community were these nurses focused on restoring?
   1. Social control
   2. Social interparticipation
   3. Mutual support
   4. Distribution of goods and services

See Answers to Test Your Knowledge in Appendix A.

READINGS AND REFERENCES

Suggested Reading

Berish, D., Nelson, I., Mehdizadeh, S., & Applebaum, R. (2019). Is there a woodwork effect? Addressing a 200-year debate on the impacts of expanding community-based services. *Journal of Aging & Social Policy*, *31*, 85–98. doi: 10.1080/08959420.2018.1528115

If services and benefits are increased, will more consumers move to these, thus increasing cost? One state investigated the effects of expanding home- and community-based services (HCBS) on use of its long-term services and support (LTSS) system. The article describes the lack of impact on LTSS cost in moving from 80% nursing home (NH), 20% HCBS to 49% NH, 51% HCBS.

Related Research

De Keyser Ganz, F., Engelberg, R., Torres, N., & Curtis, J. R. (2016). Development of a model of interprofessional shared clinical decision making in the ICU: A mixed-methods study. *Critical Care Medicine*, *44*, 680–689. doi:10.1097/CCM.0000000000001467

Romanelli, R. J., Ikeda, L. I., Lynch, B., Craig, T., Cappelleri, J. C., Jukes, T., & Ishisaka, D. Y. (2017). Opioid prescribing for chronic pain in a community-based healthcare system. *American Journal of Managed Care*, *23*, e138–e145.

References

Agency for Healthcare Research and Quality. (2018). *Care coordination*. Retrieved from https://www.ahrq.gov/professionals/prevention-chronic-care/improve/coordination/index.html

American Nurses Association. (1991). *Nursing's agenda for health care reform*. Kansas City, MO: Author.

American Nurses Association. (1992). *House of Delegates report: 1992 convention, Las Vegas, Nevada* (pp. 104–120). Kansas City, MO: Author.

American Nurses Association. (2012). *Care coordination and registered nurses' essential role*. Retrieved from https://www.nursingworld.org/practice-policy/nursing-excellence/official-position-statements/id/care-coordination-and-registered-nurses-essential-role/

American Nurses Association. (2013). *Correctional nursing: Scope and standards of practice* (2nd ed.). Silver Spring, MD: Author.

American Nurses Association. (2014). *Health care transformation: The Affordable Care Act and more*. Retrieved from https://www.nursingworld.org/~4afc9b/globalassets/practiceandpolicy/health-policy/healthcare-reform-document.pdf

American Nurses Association. (2015). *Nursing: Scope and standards of practice* (3rd ed.). Silver Spring, MD: Author.

American Nurses Association. (2016). *ANA's principles for health system transformation 2016*. Retrieved from https://www.nursingworld.org/~4afd6b/globalassets/practiceandpolicy/health-policy/principles-healthsystemtransformation.pdf

American Nurses Association. (2017). *ANA and health care reform: A history*. Retrieved from https://www.nursingworld.org/~4afd6b/globalassets/practiceandpolicy/health-policy/ana-health-care-reform-infographic_2017mar23.pdf

American Nurses Association & Health Ministries Association. (2017). *Faith community nursing: Scope and standards of practice* (3rd ed.). Silver Spring, MD: Author.

Anderson, E. T., & McFarlane, J. (2019). *Community as partner: Theory and practice in nursing* (8th ed.). Philadelphia, PA: Wolters Kluwer Health/Lippincott Williams & Wilkins.

Cronenwett, L., Sherwood, G., Barnsteiner J., Disch, J., Johnson, J., Mitchell, P., . . . Warren, J. (2007). Quality and safety education for nurses. *Nursing Outlook*, *55*, 122–131. doi:10.1016/j.outlook.2007.02.006

Donaldson, M. S., Yordy, K. D., Lohr, K. N., & Vanselow, N. A. (Eds.). (1996). *Primary care: America's health in a new era*. Washington, DC: National Academies. Retrieved from http://books.nap.edu/catalog.php?record_id=5152

Donovan, A. L., Aldrich, J. M., Gross, A. K., Barchas, D. M., Thornton, K. C., Schell-Chaple, H. M., . . . Pathak, C. (2018). Interprofessional care and teamwork in the ICU. *Critical Care Medicine*, *46*, 980–990. doi:10.1097/CCM.0000000000003067

Fang, D., Li, Y., Turinetti, M. D., & Trautman, D. E. (2018). *2017–2019 enrollment and graduations in baccalaureate and graduate programs in nursing*. Washington, DC: American Association of Colleges of Nursing.

Fathi, J. T., Modin, H. E., & Scott, J. D. (2017). Nurses advancing telehealth services in the era of healthcare reform. *OJIN: The Online Journal of Issues in Nursing*, *22*(2), Manuscript 2. doi:10.3912/OJIN.Vol22No02Man02

Institute of Medicine. (2016). *Collaboration between health care and public health: Workshop summary*. Washington, DC: National Academies. doi:10.17226/21755

IPEC Interprofessional Education Collaborative. (2016). *Core competencies for interprofessional collaborative practice: 2016 update*. Retrieved from https://www.ipecollaborative.org/resources.html

The Joint Commission. (2019). *2019 National patient safety goals*. Retrieved from https://www.jointcommission.org/standards_information/npsgs.aspx

McClellan, C. (2017). The Affordable Care Act's dependent care coverage and mortality. *Medical Care*, *55*, 514–519. doi:10.1097/MLR.0000000000000711

National Center for Health Statistics. (2018). *Health: United States, 2017*. Hyattsville, MD: Author. Retrieved from http://www.cdc.gov/nchs/data/hus/hus17.pdf

O'Brien, M. E. (2018). *Spirituality in nursing* (6th ed.). Burlington, MA: Jones & Bartlett.

O'Neil, E. H., & Pew Health Professions Commission. (1998). *Recreating health professional practice for a new century*. San Francisco, CA: Pew Health Professions Commission.

U.S. Department of Health and Human Services. (2018). *Healthy people 2020*. Retrieved from https://www.healthypeople.gov

World Health Organization. (1978). *Primary health care: Report of the International Conference on Primary Health Care*. Geneva, Switzerland: Author.

Selected Bibliography

American Nurses Association. (2013). *Public health nursing: Scope and standards of practice* (2nd ed.). Washington, DC: Author.

Clark, M. J. (2015). *Population and community health nursing* (6th ed.). Boston, MA: Pearson.

Denham, N., & Matthews, B. (2018). Nurses underscore value of collaboration when implementing health technology. *Biomedical Instrumentation & Technology*, *52*(1), 32–36. doi:10.2345/0899-8205-52.1.32

Devideo, J. A., Doswell, W. M., Braxter, B. J., Terry, M. A., & Charron-Prochownik, D. (2018). Exploring the experiences, challenges, and approaches of parish nurses in their community practice. *Journal of Holistic Nursing*, *20*, 1–9. doi:10.1177/0898010118801414

Eren, H., & Webster, J. G. (2018). *Telemedicine and electronic medicine*. Boca Raton, FL: CRC.

Harkness, G. A., & DeMarco, R. F. (2016). *Community and public health nursing: Evidence for practice* (2nd ed.). Philadelphia, PA: Lippincott Williams & Wilkins.

Institute of Medicine, Committee on Quality of Health Care in America. (2001). *Crossing the quality chasm: A new health system for the 21st century*. Washington, DC: National Academies.

Interprofessional Education Collaborative Expert Panel. (2011). *Core competencies for interprofessional collaborative practice: Report of an expert panel*. Washington, DC: Interprofessional Education Collaborative. https://www.aacom.org/docs/default-source/insideome/ccrpt05-10-11.pdf?sfvrsn=77937f97_2

McHugh, C., Krinsky, R., & Sharma, R. (2018). Innovations in emergency nursing: Transforming emergency care through a novel nurse-driven ED telehealth express care service. *Journal of Emergency Nursing*, *44*, 472–477. doi:10.1016/j.jen.2018.03.001

Nies, M. A., & McEwen, M. (2019). *Community/public health nursing* (7th ed.). St. Louis, MO: Elsevier.

Peart, D. (2016). Overcoming barriers to access, one community support at a time. *Canadian Nurse*, *112*(3), 24–25.

Schroepfer, E. (2016). Professional Issues. A renewed look at faith community nursing. *MEDSURG Nursing*, *25*(1), 62–66.

Stanhope, M., & Lancaster, J. (2018). *Foundations for population health in community/public health nursing* (5th ed.). St. Louis, MO: Elsevier.

Wordsworth, H., Moore, R., & Woodhouse, D. (2016). Parish nursing: A unique resource for community and district nurses. *British Journal of Community Nursing*, *21*(2), 66–74. doi:10.12968/bjcn.2016.21.2.66

Home Health Nursing Care 7

LEARNING OUTCOMES

After completing this chapter, you will be able to:

1. Define home healthcare.
2. Compare the characteristics of home healthcare nursing to those of institutional nursing care.
3. Describe the types of home health agencies, including referral and reimbursement sources.
4. Describe the roles of the home healthcare nurse.
5. Identify the essential aspects of the home visit.
6. Discuss the safety and infection control dimensions applicable to the home care setting.
7. Identify ways the home healthcare nurse can recognize and minimize caregiver role strain.

KEY TERMS

caregiver role strain, *151*
durable medical equipment (DME) company, *147*
home healthcare, *145*
home health nursing care, *145*
hospice nursing, *145*
registry, *147*
visiting nursing, *145*

Introduction

Historically, home healthcare consisted primarily of nurses providing private duty care in clients' homes and care of the ill by their own family members. However, the delivery of professional nursing services in home settings has increased in frequency, scope, and complexity in the past decades. **Home healthcare** today involves a wide range of healthcare professionals providing services in the home setting to individuals recovering from an acute illness or injury or those with a disability or a chronic condition. A number of factors have contributed to this trend. Among them are rising healthcare costs, an aging population, and a growing emphasis on managing chronic illness and stress, preventing illness, and enhancing the quality of life. In the not-too-distant past, home healthcare occurred at the end of the client care continuum—that is, after discharge from an acute care facility. Today the trend is changing to use of home healthcare services to avoid hospitalization. In 2015, approximately 3.5 million individuals on Medicare received home care. The provision of home care cost Medicare approximately $18.1 billion (MedPAC, 2017).

Direct nursing care may be provided by nurses from different educational backgrounds. Although associate degree and diploma prepared nurses usually do not work in community health (see Chapter 6 ∞), they may be employed by home healthcare agencies. Because home healthcare nurses must function independently in a variety of home settings and situations, some employers prefer that the nurse be prepared at the baccalaureate level or above.

Home Health Nursing Care

The delivery of nursing services in the home has been called a variety of terms, including *home health nursing care* and *visiting nursing*. For example, the mission of the Visiting Nurse Associations of America (VNAA) is to assist both individual visiting nurses' associations and home healthcare agencies in their work. **Home health nursing care** or **visiting nursing** includes the nursing services and products provided to clients in their homes that are needed to maintain, restore, or promote their physical, psychologic, and social well-being. The focus of home health nursing care is individuals and their families. This differs somewhat from the focus of community health nursing, which focuses on individuals, families, and aggregate groups (see Chapter 6 ∞). Of course, a home may consist of a wide variety of settings from individual dwellings to group housing. Even those who are considered homeless may require care from a home health nurse, and this could occur in a shelter, a mobile care unit, or wherever the individuals have their belongings.

Hospice nursing focuses on caring and supportive nursing and medical interventions to promote a good death. It is often considered a subspecialty of home health nursing care because hospice services are frequently delivered to clients who are terminally ill in their residence. However, there is also funding for its provision of care in nursing homes. See Chapter 43 ∞ for further information about hospice care.

Home health nursing care is one of the growing sectors of the healthcare system. Expenditures for home healthcare are significantly influenced by increasing or decreasing Medicare payment policies, but they increase approximately 10% each year. Hospice care is provided in extended care facilities, residential care communities, adult day care centers, and home health agencies. Adult day care service agencies provide 12.4% of the total long-term care for hospice clients. The greatest provision of hospice care is noted in nursing homes or extended care facilities at a rate of 79.5%. In many instances hospice agencies provide hospice services in long-term care facilities. The percentage of home health agencies that also provide hospice services is 5.4% (Harris-Kojetin et al., 2016).

Factors that have contributed to the growth of home health nursing care include (a) the increase in the older population, who are frequent recipients of home care services; (b) third-party payers who favor home healthcare to control costs; (c) the ability of agencies and institutions to successfully deliver high-technology services in the home; and (d) consumers who prefer to receive care in the home rather than in an institution. A common misperception by the general public is that home health nursing is only custodial in its scope of practice. However, health promotion is used by home health nurses to promote client self-care. Home healthcare nurses are actively engaged in providing support and education for family caregivers as well as clients.

Unique Aspects of Home Health Nursing Care

Home healthcare nurses must function independently in a variety of unfamiliar home settings and situations. Because the home is the family's territory, power and control issues in delivering nursing care differ from those in the hospital. For example, entry into a home is granted, not assumed; the nurse must therefore establish trust and rapport with the client and family. Home healthcare nurses must remember that they are invited into the home as a stranger, and it is important to honor and respect the homes they enter (Marrelli, 2017). Medicare and insurance companies may limit the number of visits a client can have per week. The limited time between visits can result in less progress toward recovery for clients in the home than those in residential care facilities.

Healthcare that is provided in the home is often given with other family members present. Families may feel freer to question advice, to ignore directions, to do things differently, and to set their own priorities and schedules. Home healthcare nurses implement every step of the nursing process, using critical thinking and clinical reasoning skills in designing, implementing, and evaluating the plan of care.

Home healthcare nurses have identified significant advantages in caring for individuals and families in the home. The home setting is intimate; this intimacy fosters familiarity, sharing, connections, and caring among clients, families, and their nurse. Behaviors are more natural, cultural beliefs and practices are more visible, and multigenerational interactions tend to be displayed. Nurses often get to know the client and family well because they may care for clients over weeks or months.

Home healthcare nurses have also identified issues that negatively affect care in the home. More than any other care providers, these nurses have firsthand knowledge and experience of the burden of caregiving and the role of family dynamics in healthcare practices. In the interest of cutting healthcare costs, policymakers, third-party payers, and medical providers are placing increasingly complex responsibilities on clients' families and significant other(s). Family caregiving demands may go on for months or years, placing the caregivers themselves (many of whom are older adults) at risk for physiologic and psychosocial problems. Additionally, nurses may enter homes where the living conditions and support systems are inadequate.

Nurses caring for clients in rural home settings have challenges different from those in urban or suburban environments. These include the need for flexibility (since clients may live far distances from the nurse and require care in the evening or at night), creativity, the ability to practice independently because fewer resources (including other nurses) are available, and the ability to work in an environment over which the nurse has little control. Thus, those nurses who require a high degree of certainty, structure, and consistency are less likely to be successful in rural home health locations.

The Home Healthcare System

The need for home healthcare may be identified by any individual involved with the client. Clients are referred to a home health agency or private-duty nursing agency. Individuals with extremely complex needs, beyond those that direct nursing care alone can provide, may benefit from the services of an agency with direct connections to a medical equipment company. Payment for home healthcare is accomplished through private-pay sources, third-party reimbursement, or a combination of sources.

Referral Process

Clients may be referred to home healthcare providers by a physician, nurse, social worker, therapist (e.g., physical therapist), case manager, or family member. Families often initiate the process by approaching one of these referral sources or by directly contacting the home health agency to make inquiries. Home healthcare cannot begin, however, without a physician's order and a physician-approved treatment plan. This is a legal and reimbursement requirement.

Hospital nurses may be responsible for assisting with the transition to home health by obtaining consent for transfer of confidential records, establishing the initial communication between home care and client, and completing a thorough set of transfer documents. These documents must include a detailed description of the changes in medications from prehospitalization, throughout hospitalization, and to home orders. This is Goal 3 of the National Patient Safety Goals established by The Joint Commission to help accredited organizations address specific areas of concern in regards to client safety. In addition, client and family teaching, along with a description of their understanding of potential complications and whom and when to contact should those occur, must be included.

After an initial set of physician's orders is obtained, a nursing evaluation visit is scheduled to enroll the client and identify the client's needs. The initial visit, often referred to as "opening the case," should include the client and the immediate family involved with the client's care. At this visit, the nurse develops a plan of care, which must be reviewed, approved, authorized, and signed by the attending physician before home health agency providers can continue with services.

Safety Alert! SAFETY

2019 The Joint Commission National Patient Safety Goals

Goal 3: Improve the Safety of Using Medications

1. Obtain information on the medications the patient currently takes.
2. Define the types of medication information (for example, name, dose, route, frequency, purpose) to be collected in different settings and patient circumstances.
3. Compare the medication information the patient is currently taking with the medications ordered for the patient in order to identify and resolve discrepancies.
4. Provide the patient (or family as needed) with written information on the medications the patient should be taking when he or she leaves the organization's care (for example, name, dose, route, frequency, purpose).
5. Explain the importance of managing medication information to the patient.

The Joint Commission. (2019). National patient safety goalshospital. Retrieved from https://www.jointcommission.org/assets/1/6/NPSG_Chapter_HAP_Jan2019.pdf

Home Healthcare Agencies

Home healthcare agencies offer coordinated professional, skilled, and paraprofessional services. Because clients often require the services of several professionals, case coordination (case management) is essential. This responsibility generally rests with the registered nurse. Depending on the agency, additional providers may include nurse practitioners, practical nurses, nursing assistants, home healthcare aides, physical therapists, occupational therapists, respiratory therapists, speech therapists, social workers, dietitians, and a pastoral care minister or chaplain. In addition, it is not unusual for home healthcare agencies to offer the services of specialized nurses such as wound-ostomy-continence nurses or diabetes educators. The care plan implemented by the home healthcare agency may require services by additional providers once or twice a day, up to 7 days a week. The minimum time of each period of care, or visit, is usually 1 hour.

There are several different types of home healthcare agencies:

- Official or public agencies are operated by state or local governments and financed primarily by tax funds.
- Voluntary or private not-for-profit agencies are supported by donations, endowments, charities such as the United Way, and third-party reimbursement.
- Private, proprietary agencies are for-profit organizations and are governed by either individual owners or national corporations. Some of these agencies participate in third-party reimbursement; others rely on private-pay sources.
- Institution-based agencies operate under a parent organization, such as a hospital, and are funded by the same sources as the parent.

Regardless of the type of agency, all home healthcare agencies must meet specific standards for licensing, certification, and accreditation.

Private Duty Agencies

This type of agency may be referred to as a **registry**, which contracts with individual practitioners (e.g., nurses, home health aides) to care for the client in the home. The client may require care coverage from the agency for 4 to 24 hours a day. Private duty agencies also supply staff to hospitals, clinics, and other care settings, so they do not afford the coordinated focus of a home care agency. Private duty care is expensive. Commercial insurance generally provides limited reimbursement. Otherwise, the client must pay privately.

Durable Medical Equipment Companies

A **durable medical equipment (DME) company** provides healthcare equipment for the client at home. The types of equipment can range from hospital beds and bedside commodes to ventilators, oxygen units, and apnea monitors. Because of the cost associated with medical equipment, the nurse needs to ensure that clients have a primary care provider's order and either Medicare, Medicaid, or a DME benefit within their commercial insurance, or that they are able to pay privately. Before billing Medicare for any DME, the nurse should consult the list of equipment for which Medicare will reimburse the client. Most DME companies today seek accreditation from The Joint Commission to ensure compliance with quality standards for equipment and services.

Reimbursement

Home healthcare agencies in the United States receive reimbursement for services they provide from various sources: Medicare, Medicaid, private insurance companies, and private pay. The Medicare and Medicaid programs have strict guidelines governing reimbursement for home healthcare. For example, the client must (a) need reasonable and necessary home care including skilled care; (b) be homebound, that is, confined to the home except for occasional outings for medical treatment, for a trip to the barber, or for a drive, and require the use of supportive devices, special transportation, or the escort of another individual; (c) have a plan of care that includes all of Medicare's or Medicaid's criteria; and (d) need nursing care on an intermittent basis (Centers for Medicare and Medicaid Services, 2017). The agency too must meet specific conditions.

Payers other than Medicare or Medicaid, such as Blue Cross, Blue Shield, and Health Net, typically negotiate reimbursement rates for home healthcare services. Not-for-profit agencies, like the VNA or hospital-based home healthcare agencies, are reimbursed by public and private insurance plus charitable donations to the agency. Most long-term care insurance plans include coverage for care in the home.

All healthcare agencies need to adhere to established guidelines and provide care within the predetermined reimbursement levels. Treatment plans (developed by the home healthcare agency providers and authorized by the physician) are used by the reimbursement source. Only interventions identified on the treatment plan are paid for. Periodically the reimbursement source may request the home healthcare provider's notes to substantiate what is being done in the home. This is a major reason why accurate documentation is critical.

Roles of the Home Healthcare Nurse

Historically, nurses who provided direct services in the home were strong generalists who focused on long-term preventive, educational, and rehabilitative outcomes. Today many home healthcare nurses possess high-technology skills that were formerly used only in acute care settings. For example, nurses provide a variety of intravenous (IV) therapies in the home setting and monitor clients who are dependent on technologically complex medical equipment, such as ventilators. These nurses collaborate with physicians and other healthcare professionals in providing care. They play a key role in facilitating an effective plan of care as clients move among hospitals, home, school, work, and other care settings such as clinics or long-term care.

The major roles of the home healthcare nurse are those of advocate, caregiver (provider of direct care), educator, and case manager or coordinator.

Advocate

Advocacy begins on the first visit. The nurse explores and supports the client's choices in healthcare; all viable options are considered. Advocacy includes having discussions about the client's rights, advance medical directives, living wills, and durable power of attorney for healthcare. It also usually involves providing assistance to access community resources, to make informed decisions, to recognize and cope with necessary changes in lifestyle, to negotiate medical insurance, and to understand ways to effectively use the complex medical system.

The home healthcare nurse provides indirect care to the client each time the nurse consults with other healthcare providers about ways to improve nursing care for the client. This consultation about client care issues often manifests itself in multidisciplinary care conferences where the role of the home healthcare nurse is as client advocate. Advocacy can be a particular challenge when family members' or other caregivers' views differ from those of the client. In the event of conflict, the nurse, being the client's primary advocate, ensures that the client's rights and desires are upheld.

Caregiver

The home healthcare nurse's major role as caregiver is to assess and diagnose the client's actual and potential health problems, plan care, and evaluate the client's outcomes. Home healthcare nurses routinely perform physical assessments, change wound dressings, insert and maintain IV access for various therapies, establish and monitor indwelling urinary catheters, and monitor exercise or nutritional therapies (Figure 7.1 ■). Direct personal care activities such as bathing, changing linens, feeding, and light housekeeping activities to maintain a clean and safe home environment are usually provided by a family member or a home health aide arranged by the nurse.

Educator

The educator role of the home healthcare nurse focuses on teaching illness care, the prevention of problems, and the promotion of optimal wellness or well-being to the

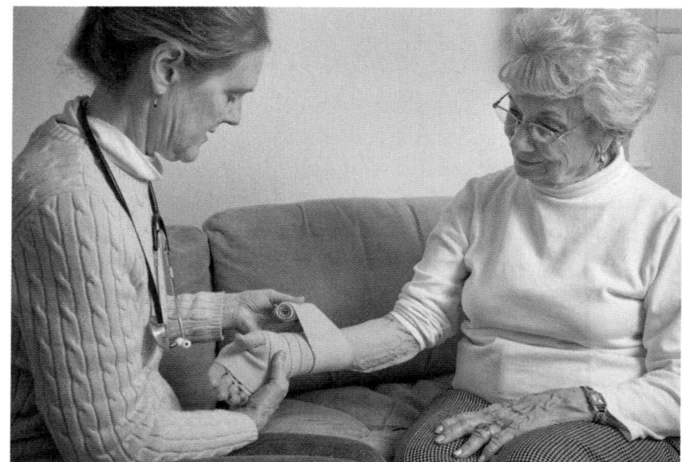

Figure 7.1 ■ Home healthcare nurses perform skilled direct care such as changing dressings.
dszc/E+/Getty Images.

client, the family, caregivers, and other support individuals. A common example is that of guiding the health and development of newborns. Some clients of all ages have acute illnesses that will resolve, while others have chronic conditions that will last the lifetime. The nurse's teaching and learning methods will vary based on the need of these clients. Nurses clarify misconceptions about the course of the illness, the treatment plan, and medications and potential interactions with over-the-counter drugs. They also educate the client and family on how to access the healthcare system appropriately.

The nurse may also be involved in teaching others with whom the client interacts such as the schoolteachers of children with special needs. Education is ongoing and can be considered the crux of home healthcare practice; its goal is to help clients learn to manage as independently as possible. All home healthcare nurses need to be skilled in teaching and learning principles and strategies that facilitate learning. (See Chapter 17 ∞ for detailed information.)

Case Manager or Coordinator

The home healthcare nurse coordinates the activities of all other home healthcare team members involved in the client's treatment plan. Coordination can occur individually, in person, or by telephone, with a specific team member such as the dietitian or respiratory therapist, or during a team conference where each team member provides information about the client's health status. The nurse is the main contact to report any changes in the client's condition and to bring about a revision in the plan of care as needed. Documentation of care coordination is a legal and reimbursement requirement and must be recorded on the client's medical record.

Perspectives of Home Healthcare Clients

Home healthcare clients include a diverse population that encompasses all ages, a variety of health problems, and families of different structures and cultural backgrounds. Home healthcare clients have a wide range of health problems, including disabilities, perinatal problems, mental illnesses, and acute and chronic illnesses. The nurse should not assume that the client understands the various personnel and their roles in providing home healthcare.

Although the individual receiving care is considered the primary client in home healthcare, the client's family can be considered secondary clients because often they are associated with caregiving and have a major impact on the client's wellness status. The home healthcare nurse will encounter many different family structures ranging from single families to extended families and dwellings that house multiple families. In the home setting, family members may include not only individuals related by birth and marriage, but also friends, other significant individuals, and animals.

Various cultural influences also affect the client's healthcare beliefs and practices. The home healthcare nurse needs to be culturally sensitive, that is, to be aware of the client's culture and form a nursing care plan with the client that incorporates his or her culture. See Chapter 21 ∞ for detailed information about making cultural assessments and providing culturally competent and responsive care.

Selected Dimensions of Home Healthcare Nursing

Selected dimensions of home healthcare nursing include assessing the home for safety features, infection control, and caregiver support.

Client Safety

Hazards in the home are major causes of falls, fire, poisoning, and other accidents, such as those caused by improper use of household equipment (e.g., tools and cooking utensils). The appraisal of such hazards and suggestions for remedies is an essential nursing function.

Obviously home healthcare nurses cannot expect to change a family's living space and lifestyle. However, they can express their concern and react appropriately when a situation suggests that an injury is imminent. Nurses must document information they provide and the family's response to instruction, and make ongoing assessments about the family's use of safety precautions. During the home healthcare visit the home healthcare nurse must address specific areas of the home that may result in an unsafe environment.

QSEN Patient-Centered Care: Home Hazard Appraisal for Adults

The following areas may lead to falls or injury:

- *Walkways and stairways (inside and outside)*: Note uneven sidewalks or paths, broken or loose steps, absence of handrails or placement on only one side of stairways, insecure handrails, congested hallways or other traffic areas, and adequacy of lighting at night.
- *Floors*: Note uneven and highly polished or slippery floors and any unanchored rugs or mats.
- *Furniture*: Note hazardous placement of furniture with sharp corners. Note chairs or stools that are too low to get into and out of or that provide inadequate support.
- *Bathroom(s)*: Note presence of grab bars around tubs and toilets, nonslip surfaces in tubs and shower stalls, handheld showerhead, adequacy of night lighting, need for raised toilet seat or bath chair in tub or shower, ease of access to shelves, and water temperature regulated at a maximum of 49°C (120°F).

- *Kitchen*: Note pilot lights (gas stove) in need of repair, inaccessible storage areas, and hazardous furniture.
- *Bedrooms*: Note adequacy of lighting, in particular the availability of night lights and accessibility of light switches; ease of access to commode, urinal, or bedpan; and need for hospital bed or bedrails.
- *Electrical*: Note unanchored or frayed electrical cords and outlets that are overloaded or near water.
- *Fire protection*: Note presence or absence of smoke detectors, fire extinguisher, and fire escape plan, and improper storage of combustibles (e.g., gasoline) or corrosives (e.g., rust remover).
- *Toxic substances*: Note improperly labeled cleaning solutions.
- *Communication devices*: Note presence of method to call for help, such as a telephone or intercom in the bedroom and elsewhere (e.g., kitchen), and access to emergency telephone numbers.
- *Medications*: Note medications kept beyond date of expiration, adequacy of lighting for medication cabinet or storage, and method of disposal of sharp objects such as needles used for injections.

Other aspects of client safety relate to emergency situations. The home healthcare nurse can assist the client and caregivers as follows:

- Post a list of all emergency telephone numbers (ambulance, fire, police, primary care provider) at each land line and cell phone.
- Post a list of all the client's medications and potential side effects in a central location, such as on the refrigerator.
- Help the client and family apply for a medical alert system such as a bracelet or necklace (Figure 7.2 ■). Information on the MedicAlert system can be obtained by contacting MedicAlert Foundation International.

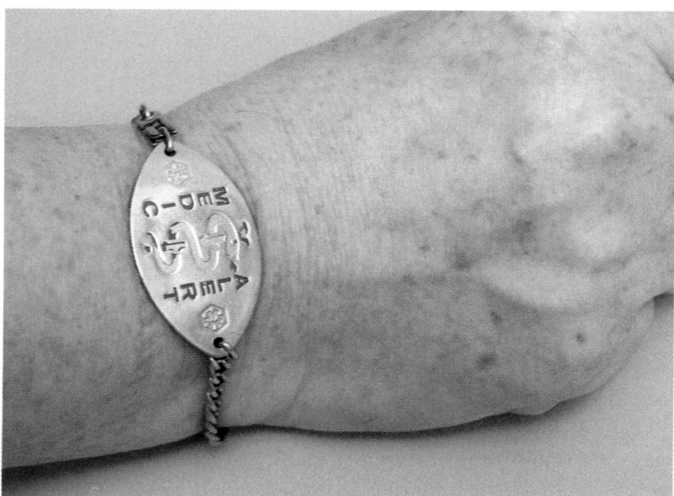

Figure 7.2 ■ MedicAlert emblem.
John T. Fowler/Alamy Stock Photo.

- Enroll the client in a program that places all the client's vital medical information in one place for emergency personnel to have in the event of a life-threatening situation. The program can be joined through a pharmacy, a primary care provider's office, a VNA, or other community support groups. The kit contains a plastic vial, a medical information form, a decal, and an instruction sheet. The information form is filled out, rolled, and placed in the vial. The vial is placed in the refrigerator, and emergency personnel are trained to routinely check there. The decal is placed on the refrigerator as a signal that the vial is inside.
- Recommend that the client purchase an emergency response system. These systems provide a small device with a help button that attaches to a wrist or neck chain. The home base station can require the client to send a signal daily that indicates that he or she is okay. If the signal is not sent or if the portable device is activated, the system automatically calls the client and then dials a previously established list of emergency contacts. This system is particularly useful for clients who are alone because if they should fall, for instance, and be unable to reach a telephone, they might be left helpless for extended periods of time.

Home Healthcare Nurse Safety

Some less desirable living locations can pose personal safety concerns for the nurse. Many home healthcare agencies have contracts with security firms to escort nurses needing to see clients in potentially unsafe neighborhoods. The nurse should avoid taking any personal belongings during these visits and have a pre-established mechanism to signal for help. Home healthcare agencies provide training for nurses in ways to decrease personal risk. Little has been published on this important topic of safety.

Home healthcare nurses may also be susceptible to occupational injuries—especially musculoskeletal ones—due to limited resources available in the home. The nurse's safety is influenced by the functionality and availability of assistive personnel and devices, number of clients who are obese or dependent, presence of pets, and varying house and yard arrangements. When the client is at risk in the home environment so is the home healthcare nurse. Falls are one of the most common accidents noted for home healthcare nurses. The nurse sees clients in all seasons of the year and is at risk for falls, particularly in the winter months. Many clients are immobile, are obese, or have functional disabilities. Home healthcare nurses see clients alone, and the need to move the client and provide care increases the nurse's risk for occupational health injuries (Marrelli, 2017). Both the nurse and the employing agency must assume responsibility for protecting the nurse.

Infection Prevention

The goal of infection prevention in the home is to protect clients, caregivers, and the general community from the transmission of disease. This is particularly important for clients who are immunocompromised, who have infectious or communicable diseases, or who have wounds, drainage tubes, or invasive access devices. The nurse's major role in infection prevention is health teaching. Clients and caregivers need to learn about effective hand washing, use of gloves, handling of linens, and disposal of wastes and soiled dressings. Infection prevention can present a challenge to the home healthcare nurse, especially if the home care facilities are not conducive to basic aseptic requirements such as running water for hand washing.

An important aspect of infection prevention involves handling the home healthcare nurse's equipment and supplies. Supplies may include materials for hand cleansing; assessment equipment such as a stethoscope, blood pressure cuff and manometer, thermometer, and tape measure; infection control items such as gowns, goggles, masks, gloves, and blood spill kit; and antimicrobial cleaning agents.

The same organizations that accredit hospitals evaluate home healthcare nurses' practice. Although some modifications in technique may be indicated in the home setting, such as the use of clean rather than sterile technique in caring for chronic wounds, all the basic principles still apply. Nurses need to follow agency protocol about aseptic practice in the home.

Caregiver Support

Caregiving may be requested for individuals of any age and varies from short term to long term according to the physical or mental disabilities of the care receivers. For example, some children who have permanent disabilities and adults who experience progressive deterioration such as those with Alzheimer's disease or multiple sclerosis require care on a permanent basis. Others who are recovering from a surgical procedure require only temporary care. Most caregivers have close relationships with the care receiver, that is, a spouse, partner, parent, child, friend, or other significant relationship. Many caregiving relationships, therefore, represent a change from the caring and caregiving intrinsic to all close relationships to an extraordinary and unequal burden for the caregiver. Caregivers may experience **caregiver role strain** when they have physical, emotional, social, and financial burdens that can seriously jeopardize their own health and well-being.

The home healthcare nurse needs to recognize signs of caregiver role strain and suggest ways to minimize or alleviate this problem. Signs of caregiver overload include the following:

- Difficulty performing routine tasks for the client
- Reports of declining physical energy and insufficient time for caregiving
- Concern that caregiving responsibilities interfere with other roles such as those of parent, spouse, worker, friend
- Anxiety about ability to meet future care needs of the client
- Feelings of anger and depression
- Dramatic change in the home environment's appearance.

The nurse needs to encourage caregivers to express their feelings and at the same time convey understanding about the difficulties associated with caregiving and acknowledge the caregivers' competence. The nurse can obtain a realistic appraisal of the situation by asking a caregiver to describe a typical day and daily or weekly leisure and social activities. It is also helpful to identify activities for which assistance is desired. These activities may include client care needs such as hygiene, mobility, feeding, or treatments; house cleaning; laundry; shopping; house repairs; yard work; transportation; doctor's or hairdresser's appointments; or respite.

Activities that are commonly done by nurses and aides, such as changing an occupied bed and transferring a client from bed to chair, may be overwhelming to a caregiver who has not performed them before. Demonstrating them in the home and allowing caregivers to perform them with the nurse's supervision increases their confidence and increases the likelihood of them asking for assistance in other situations.

When activities for which assistance is required are identified, the nurse and caregiver need to identify possible sources of help. Both volunteer and agency sources need to be explored. Volunteer sources of help may include family members (cousins, siblings), neighbors, friends, church associates, or caregiver support groups in the community. Other sources include, for example, a home health aide for light housekeeping and grocery shopping, Meals on Wheels, day care, transportation, and counseling and social services. Families with a member who is chronically ill may benefit from a weekend respite—a program some hospitals provide in which the client is admitted to a skilled unit for observation and care, enabling the caregiver to take a break from providing ongoing healthcare needs.

Caregivers need to be reminded of the importance of caring for themselves by getting adequate sleep, eating nutritious meals, asking for help, delegating household chores, and making time for leisure activities or simply some time alone. Family members other than the caregiver also may need help to learn ways to support the caregiver. The nurse can discuss with the caregiver the importance of maintaining interests outside of the caregiver environment, such as connecting with friends and family by phone, social media, or email. The nurse should listen intently to the needs of the caregiver and offer encouragement without providing advice. It is important to convey to the caregiver acceptance and appreciation of the care that is being provided. In addition, the nurse should acknowledge the burden of caregiving.

A particular challenge exists when the nurse is in a position to be a caregiver to a family member. Although the nurse's clinical expertise and familiarity with the client and setting can be especially useful, negotiating the professional distancing that is sometimes needed when providing care to clients can be difficult with family. The nurse may feel obligated to provide care, even when this is over and above regular employment responsibilities. The nurse must have the opportunity to step back and experience the role and emotions of being a family member—not only those of being a nurse.

The Practice of Home Health Nursing Care

The home healthcare nurse assesses the healthcare demands of the client and family and the home and community environment. This process actually begins when the nurse contacts the client for the initial home health visit and reviews documents received from the referral agency. The goal of the initial visit is to obtain a comprehensive clinical picture of the client's needs.

Most agencies have a packet or electronic health record that includes forms for consent to treatment; physical, psychosocial, and spiritual assessment; medications; pain assessment; family data; financial assessment including insurance verification; client's bill of rights; care plan; and daily visit notes. During the initial home health visit, the home healthcare nurse obtains a health history from the client (Figure 7.3 ■), examines the client, observes the relationship of the client and caregiver, and assesses the home and community environment. Parameters for assessment of the home environment include client and caregiver mobility, client ability to perform self-care, the cleanliness of the environment, the availability of caregiver support, safety, food preparation, financial supports, and the emotional status of the client and caregiver.

Following this initial client examination, the nurse determines whether further consults and support personnel are needed. For example, is a home health aide needed to assist with activities of daily living (ADLs) and homemaker tasks? Is a social worker needed to help with financial resources or future care needs such as placement in a nursing home? What additional supplies does the client need?

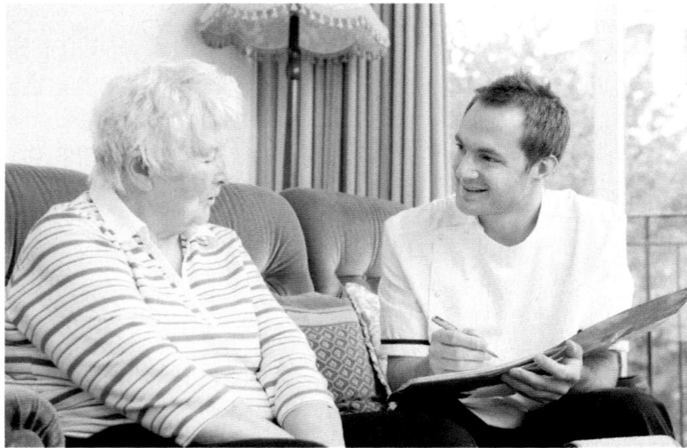

Figure 7.3 ■ Interviewing the home healthcare client.
SarahlWard/E+/Getty Images.

Before completing the initial interview, the nurse also discusses what the client and family can expect from home care, what other healthcare providers may be needed to help the client achieve independence, and the frequency of home visits.

Establishing Health Issues

As in other care environments, the nurse identifies both actual and potential client problems. One of the most common examples of health issues that nurses address with clients in home care settings is lack of knowledge related to health conditions and self-care. Because client education is considered a skill reimbursed by Medicare and other commercial insurance carriers, it is important for the nurse to include knowledge deficits within the plan of care.

Planning and Delivering Care

In planning care, the nurse needs to encourage and permit clients to make their own decisions regarding goals. Alternatives may need to be suggested if the nurse identifies potential harm from a chosen course of action. Strategies to meet goals include teaching the client and family techniques of care and identifying appropriate resources to assist the client and family in maintaining self-sufficiency. Box 7.1 lists the data required by Medicare for the nursing plan of care.

BOX 7.1 Medicare's Required Data for the Nursing Plan of Care

1. All pertinent diagnoses
2. A notation of the beneficiary's mental status
3. Types of services, supplies, and equipment ordered
4. Frequency of visits to be made
5. Client's prognosis
6. Client's rehabilitation potential
7. Client's functional limitations
8. Activities permitted
9. Client's nutritional requirements
10. Client's medications and treatments
11. Safety measures to protect against injuries
12. Discharge plans
13. Any other items the home health agency or physician wishes to include

From *Medicare Benefit Policy Manual: Chapter 7, Home Health Services* (CMS Publication 233, 02-24-17, Section 30.2.1), by Centers for Medicare & Medicaid Services, 2017. Retrieved from https://www.cms.gov/Regulations-and-Guidance/Guidance/Manuals/downloads/bp102c07.pdf

To implement the plan, the home healthcare nurse performs nursing interventions, including teaching; coordinates and uses referrals and resources; provides and monitors all levels of technical care; collaborates with other disciplines and providers; identifies clinical problems and solutions from research and other health literature; supervises ancillary personnel; and advocates for the client's right to self-determination.

Even though the client and family may become independent in self-care skills, the home healthcare nurse still has the ultimate responsibility for evaluating the effectiveness of the plan. Ongoing communication with the primary care provider about the client's progress is critical, and the nurse must make ongoing assessments to determine if modifications in the care plan are required (Figure 7.4 ■).

On subsequent home visits, the nurse observes the same parameters assessed on the initial home visit and relates findings to the expected outcomes or goals (Figure 7.5 ■). The nurse can also teach caregivers parameters of evaluation so that they can obtain professional intervention if needed. Documentation of care given and the client's progress toward goal achievement at each visit is essential. Notes must also reflect plans for subsequent visits and when the client may be sufficiently prepared for self-care and discharge from the agency.

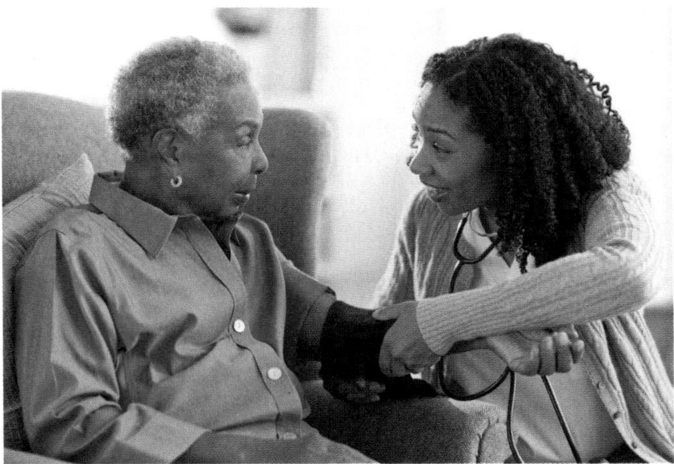

Figure 7.4 ■ The nurse monitors the client's response to treatments and therapy.
Blend Images - JGI/Tom Grill/Getty Images.

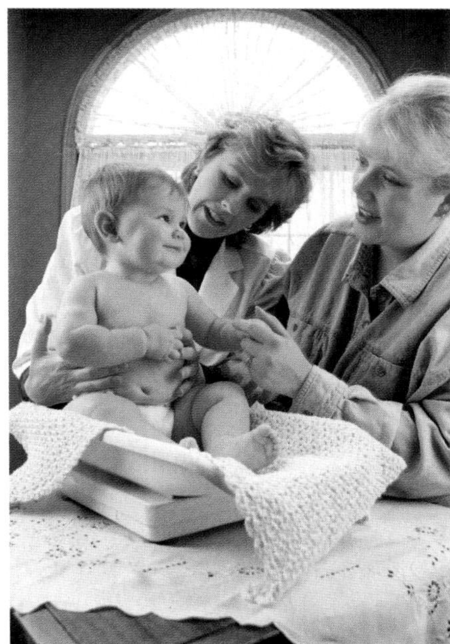

Figure 7.5 ■ Determining the success of the care plan includes comparing assessment findings to previous values. Comparing this baby's weight to previous values can determine if changes are occurring in the desired direction.
Barros & Barros/The Image Bank/Getty Images.

Resources for Home Healthcare Nursing

With the expansion and increasing complexity of home care nursing, the nurse must remain aware of the various sources of regulations, tools, and supports available for both nurse and client. The Centers for Medicare and Medicaid Services' (CMS) Home Health Quality Improvement

EVIDENCE-BASED PRACTICE

Evidence-Based Practice

What Is the Impact of Home Healthcare on the Older Adult Refugee Population?

Every year, approximately 70,000 refugees from war-torn countries seek asylum or an opportunity to improve their lives in the United States. In the pilot study the investigators assessed the impact of home healthcare on the older adult refugee population (Miner et al., 2017). They examined 40 refugee clients' charts and analyzed each client's health outcomes using the OASIS-C data. The OASIS-C is a tool designed by the CMS to rate the outcomes of home healthcare from the start of care until discharge. The analysis of the health outcomes for the clients included the clients' level of pain and anxiety, their ability to manage their ADLs, and their ability to manage their medications. The review of charts revealed that the clients' pain and anxiety levels improved, as did their ability to manage medications and perform ADLs. They also used emergency department and hospital services less often compared to other clients in the home healthcare agency.

Implications

Based on the results of this small pilot study a larger study is needed to confirm the success of home healthcare for the refugee population. The population of older refugees in the United States is rising given the unrest in other countries globally. The need for home healthcare will have a potential to improve the health of all citizens, particularly refugees who may have lacked access to healthcare.

(HHQI) National Campaign provides free evidence-based educational resources, individualized data reports, networking opportunities, and assistance for home health and cross-setting providers to reduce avoidable hospitalizations and improve care quality. The foundational information includes the underserved, those with health disparities, and resources for small not-for-profit home healthcare agencies. Specific best practices for the underserved populations can be found at the Home Health Quality Improvement website.

Collaboration for Homecare Advances in Management and Practice (CHAMP), based at the Center for Home Care Policy and Research of the Visiting Nurse Service of New York, is the first national initiative to advance home care excellence for older individuals. CHAMP makes the latest evidence-based tools, e-learning, and expert advice easily accessible to home care clinicians, from any computer.

For Medicare-approved home healthcare agencies, the Outcome and Assessment Information Set (OASIS) is a group of data elements that represent core items of a comprehensive assessment for an adult home care client and form the basis for measuring client outcomes for the purposes of outcome-based quality improvement. For example, OASIS standardizes definitions and coding for pressure ulcers and surgical wounds.

The Program of All-Inclusive Care for the Elderly (PACE) is another CMS program. PACE supports individuals ages 55 and older with chronic care needs who wish to reside at home. Participants are screened by a team of physicians, nurses, and other health professionals. PACE provides medical and supportive services along the entire continuum of care, including adult day care with nursing; physical, occupational, and recreational therapies; meals; nutritional counseling; social work; personal care; and respite care. Care is coordinated by a PACE physician familiar with the history, needs, and preferences of each participant. All necessary prescription drugs are provided, as well as medical specialty services including audiology, dentistry, optometry, podiatry, and speech therapy.

The Future of Home Healthcare

What is the future for home healthcare? More studies are needed to determine the practicality, safety, effectiveness, cost, and satisfaction with home care—especially new models of "hospital-at-home" care. However, there is no question that home health nursing care will be an expanding area of practice. Trends in the home healthcare industry include the following:

1. Ethics committees to handle ethical issues that arise in the home. These committees may be necessary for agencies to receive accreditation.
2. Third-party reimbursement for community clinical nurse specialists and psychiatric nurse specialists. These advanced practice nurses can provide education, support, counseling, and therapy for clients and their families.
3. Third-party reimbursement for social workers. Social workers can assist clients and their families in the home with financial and household problems, freeing the nurse to focus on nursing care.
4. Nurse pain specialists to assess and manage pain in the home, thus avoiding costly hospitalizations and procedures.
5. Pet care for clients who may become too ill to care for them. Clients can make arrangements for the care of a pet if they are hospitalized or die.
6. Telehealth is a tool in the provision of care for chronically ill clients. The client must not require invasive procedures to be provided. This form of home care is used to obtain blood pressure readings or support population health initiatives (Marrelli, 2017).

LIFESPAN CONSIDERATIONS Home Care

CHILDREN

One goal of *Healthy People 2020* is to reduce the number of children and youth with disabilities (21 years and under) living in congregate care facilities with 16 beds or more (U.S. Department of Health and Human Services, 2010). Ideally, all children with disabilities would live in a secure, "permanent" family environment. Such an environment is one that supports family strengths, connects families to their community, and fosters ongoing, secure relationships. At times, children with disabilities may need to be placed in adoptive or medical foster homes. Home healthcare nurses can strengthen family functioning by:

- Providing information, advice, and instruction on care of the child
- Identifying natural support systems (e.g., extended family, neighbors, friends)
- Helping families find community resources to meet their needs (e.g., respite care, technical and equipment services)
- Assisting families with alternative placement options as needed (e.g., medical foster care)
- Advocating for families with other healthcare providers and policymakers.

OLDER ADULTS

Clients who have been hospitalized are often discharged after short stays and may still be acutely ill. This becomes a challenge for home healthcare nurses when planning and implementing care. Special areas of concern for older adults in this situation include the following:

- Healing time is slower due to changes that normally occur in aging, such as impaired circulation and alteration in immune response.
- Changes in medications or lingering traces of anesthesia may alter cognitive status, even though it is usually temporary.
- Weakness and fatigue create safety issues, such as risk for falling.

LIFESPAN CONSIDERATIONS Home Care—*continued*

- Chronic diseases already present may have been complicated by other conditions acquired while hospitalized.
- Assessment should be initiated while the client is in the hospital to determine the need for assistive devices or environmental changes when the client returns home. Some examples of these devices are walkers, raised toilet seats, safety bars in the bathroom, and better lighting. Good planning eases the transition to home care for the client and caregiver.

In the future, although the number of older adults will increase, fewer family caregivers may be available. However, older adults usually appreciate receiving care from family members, and nurses should facilitate this when possible.

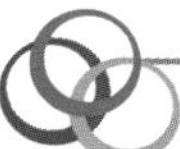

Critical Thinking Checkpoint

Mr. Madden is a 67-year-old African American male with a 20-year history of hypertension and diabetes mellitus. He has recently undergone amputation of three toes due to poor circulation.

Because he is progressing well and his diabetes is under control, he is being discharged from the acute care setting to go home. He has been referred to a hospital-based home health agency, which will assign a nurse to change his foot dressings, administer IV antibiotics, and monitor his blood glucose levels.

1. When delivering care in the home environment, how will the nurse's role be similar to and different from that of the nurse's role in the acute care environment?
2. What rights does the client have when being cared for at home that may not be afforded him while institutionalized?
3. What factors could negatively affect the care of Mr. Madden in his own home?
4. Speculate about personal and financial savings derived by clients being cared for at home rather than in a hospital or other institution.

Answers to Critical Thinking Checkpoint questions are available on the faculty resources site. Please consult with your instructor.

Chapter 7 Review

CHAPTER HIGHLIGHTS

- Home healthcare is an alternative to provision of care in acute and subacute healthcare facilities. The trend has changed from using home healthcare after hospitalization to using it to avoid hospitalization.
- Hospice nursing, often considered a subspecialty of home nursing, supports clients who are terminally ill and their families during the last stages of life and bereavement.
- Referrals for home healthcare services may be made by the client's physician, nurse, social worker, therapist, discharge planner, or family member. Home healthcare, however, requires a physician's order and an approved treatment plan in order for insurance to provide reimbursement.
- Home healthcare agencies offer skilled professional and paraprofessional services. Because clients often require the services of several professionals simultaneously, case coordination is essential.
- There are several types of home healthcare agencies: official or public agencies, voluntary or private not-for-profit agencies, private proprietary agencies, and institution-based agencies. All home healthcare agencies must meet specific standards for licensing, certification, and accreditation.
- Private duty agencies provide professional nursing and home healthcare aide.
- Healthcare agencies in the United States receive reimbursement for services they provide from various sources: Medicare and Medicaid, private insurance companies, and private-pay sources. The Medicare and Medicaid programs have strict guidelines for reimbursement.
- The major roles of the home healthcare nurse are those of advocate, caregiver, educator, and case manager.
- Home healthcare clients include a diverse population that encompasses all ages, a variety of health problems, and families of different structures and cultural backgrounds. The home healthcare nurse needs to be culturally sensitive, that is, be aware of the client's culture, and form a nursing care plan with the client that incorporates the client's culture.
- Important dimensions of home health nursing care include assessing the home for safety features, infection prevention, and caregiver support.
- The home healthcare nurse assesses the care needs of clients in their home; plans, implements, and supervises that care; teaches clients and their families self-care; and mobilizes the resources of hospitals, primary care providers, and community agencies in meeting the needs of the clients and their families.
- Resources for the nurse and client regarding home healthcare are available from the Centers for Medicare and Medicaid Services.

TEST YOUR KNOWLEDGE

1. Care in the home is an alternative to hospital placement. Which of the following is one major difference associated with in-home care?
   1. Does not focus on curative and lifesaving approaches.
   2. Is less able to manage complex symptoms.
   3. Facilitates extensive involvement of significant others and family.
   4. Permits use of pain medication regimens not allowed in the hospital.

2. A home health client is having difficulty with the medication regimen that is prescribed by the physician. The nurse helps with this situation by consulting the pharmacist for ideas on how to improve the situation. This is an example of which of the following?
   1. Hands-on care
   2. Direct care
   3. Advocacy
   4. Indirect care

3. The home health nurse is assessing the client's environment for safety concerns and finds that most of the rooms in the house have only one outlet with various cords entering the outlet. The nurse shares this concern with the client and the client's spouse. They inform the nurse that "this is the way we've lived for years." What should the nurse do?
   1. Provide telephone numbers for local electricians.
   2. Continue to persuade the client to have the home rewired.
   3. Not bring the subject up again.
   4. Document the findings and the client and spouse's response to the concern.

4. A home healthcare nurse is providing care for a client who has paralysis on one side and whose spouse provides most of the care. Which of the following may be a sign of caregiver role strain?
   1. The caregiver loses weight and has insomnia.
   2. The caregiver asks other family and friends for help.
   3. The caregiver asks the nurse what other ways he or she can help the client.
   4. The caregiver seems sad whenever the client's prognosis is discussed.

5. A client is scheduled to be discharged from the hospital. Which should the discharge planner at the hospital acquire first before home nursing care can be initiated?
   1. Insurance coverage
   2. An in-home caregiver
   3. A curable health problem
   4. A physician's authorization

6. The nurse doing home healthcare recognizes that the practice includes which of the following? Select all that apply.
   1. Hospice care
   2. Visiting home health clients living in skilled nursing facilities
   3. Care of both the client and the family
   4. Absence of high-tech equipment and procedures
   5. Care of clients who cannot afford to go to the doctor's office or clinic
   6. Performing physical, psychosocial, and emotional interventions

7. Which of the following indicates the client and family require some added health-related teaching?
   1. Client wears a medical alert bracelet at all times.
   2. A list of medications is posted on the refrigerator.
   3. Area rugs have been removed.
   4. Client puts on an emergency response necklace whenever leaving home.

See Answers to Test Your Knowledge in Appendix A.

READINGS AND REFERENCES

Suggested Reading

Burden, M., & Thornton, M. (2018). Reducing the risks of surgical site infection: The importance of the multidisciplinary team. *British Journal of Nursing, 27*(17), 976–979. doi:10.12968/bjon.2018.27.17.976

The implementation of effective communication and cooperation between the members of the multidisciplinary healthcare team is important in the prevention of surgical site infection. Many surgical site infections are preventable. In the preoperative phase, information is gathered on the patient's health, which can identify potential risks for postoperative infection. In surgery, the team is responsible for sterility and cleanliness. In the postoperative phase, attention to nutrition, pain control, and prevention of skin breakdown is imperative.

Schaffer, M. A., Anderson, L. J. W., & Rising, S. (2016) Public health interventions for school nursing practice. *The Journal of School Nursing, 32*, 195–208. doi:10.1177/1059840515605361

The Public Health Intervention Wheel explains interventions utilized by school nurses to facilitate communication with other healthcare professionals. The knowledge gained from the Public Health Intervention Wheel can contribute to reforming healthcare goals and providing care to a greater number of students.

Related Research

Lewis, A., Kitson, A., & Harvey, G. (2016). Improving oral health for older people in the home care setting: An exploratory implementation study. *Australasian Journal on Ageing, 35*, 273–280. doi:10.1111/ajag.12326

References

Centers for Medicare and Medicaid Services. (2017). *Medicare benefit policy manual, chapter 7—home health services* (CMS Publication 233, 02-24-17). Retrieved from https://www.cms.gov/Regulations-and-Guidance/Guidance/Manuals/downloads/bp102c07.pdf

Harris-Kojetin, L., Sengupta, M., Park-Lee, E., Valverde, R., Caffrey, C., Rome, V., & Lenden, J. (2016). *Long-term care providers and services users in the United States: Data from the National Study of Long-Term Care Providers, 2013–2014*. Retrieved from https://www.cdc.gov/nchs/data/series/sr_03/sr03_038.pdf

The Joint Commission. (2019). *National patient safety goals-hospital*. Retrieved from https://www.jointcommission.org/assets/1/6/NPSG_Chapter_HAP_Jan2019.pdf

Marrelli, T. M. (2017). *Home care nursing: Surviving in an ever-changing care environment*. Indianapolis, IN: Sigma Theta Tau International.

MedPAC. (2017). *Report to the Congress: Medicare payment policy*. Retrieved from http://medpac.gov/docs/default-source/reports/mar17_entirereport.pdf

Miner, S. M., Liebel, D., Wilde, M. H., Carroll, J. K., Zicari, E., & Chalupa, S. (2017). Meeting the needs of older adult refugee populations with home health services. *Journal of Transcultural Nursing, 28*, 128–136. doi:10.1177/1043659615623327

U.S. Department of Health and Human Services. (2010). *Healthy people 2020*. Retrieved from http://www.healthypeople.gov/2020/default.aspx

Selected Bibliography

Anderson, E. T., & McFarlane, J. (2019). *Community as partner: Theory and practice in nursing* (8th ed.). Philadelphia, PA: Wolters Kluwer.

Harkness, G. A., & DeMarco, R. F. (2016). *Community and public health nursing: Evidence for practice* (2nd ed.). Philadelphia, PA: Lippincott Williams & Wilkins.

Home Health Quality Improvement. (n.d.). *Underserved populations BPIP*. Retrieved from http://www.homehealthquality.org/Education/Best-Practices/BPIPs/Underserved-Populations-BPIP.aspx

Hunt, R. (2013). *Introduction to community-based nursing* (5th ed.). Philadelphia, PA: Lippincott Williams & Wilkins.

Lippert, M., Semmens, S., Tacey, L., Rent, T., Defoe, K., Bucsis, M., . . . Lafay-Cousin, L. (2017). The hospital at home program: No place like home. *Current Oncology, 24*(1), 23–27. doi:10.3747/co.24.3326

Maurer, F. A., & Smith, C. M. (2013). *Community/public health nursing practice: Health for families and populations* (5th ed.). St. Louis, MO: Elsevier.

Simpser, E., & Hudak, M. L. (2017). Financing of pediatric home health care. *Pediatrics, 139*(3), e20164202. doi:10.1542/peds.2016-4202

U.S. Department of Health and Human Services (n.d.). *U.S. Department of Health and Human Services report to Congress: Plan to implement a Medicare home health agency value-based purchasing program*. Retrieved from https://www.cms.gov/Medicare/Medicare-Fee-for-Service-Payment/HomeHealthPPS/Downloads/Stage-2-NPRM.pdf

Electronic Health Records and Information Technology 8

LEARNING OUTCOMES

After completing this chapter, you will be able to:

1. Describe the uses of computers and technology in nursing.
2. Discuss the advantages of and concerns about computerized clinical documentation systems.
3. Identify computer applications used in client assessment and care.
4. List ways technology may be used by nurse administrators in the areas of human resources, facilities management, finance, quality improvement, and accreditation.
5. Identify the role of technology in each step of the research process.

KEY TERMS

clinical decision support systems, *165*
computer-based patient records (CPRs), *163*
computer literacy, *157*
data warehousing, *162*
distance learning, *161*
electronic health records (EHRs), *163*
health informatics, *157*
hospital information system (HIS), *159*
informatics, *157*
information technology (IT), *157*
management information system (MIS), *159*
nurse informaticist, *164*
nursing informatics, *157*
telemedicine, *168*

Introduction

Computers have become a part of everyday life for many individuals, including nurses. Computers are used for educating nursing students and clients; assessing, documenting, and testing clients' health conditions; managing medical records; communicating among healthcare providers and with clients; and conducting nursing research. All nurses must have a basic level of **computer literacy** (the knowledge and ability to use computers or technology) in order to perform their jobs.

General Concepts

Informatics refers to the science of computer information systems. It is a Quality and Safety Education in Nursing (QSEN) competency defined as "use information and technology to communicate, manage knowledge, mitigate error, and support decision-making" (Cronenwett et al., 2007, p. 129). **Health informatics**, or health information technology, then, is the management of healthcare information, using computers. **Nursing informatics** is the science of using computer information systems in the practice of nursing. It is defined by the American Nurses Association (ANA, 2014) as "the specialty that integrates nursing science with multiple information and analytical sciences to identify, define, manage, and communicate data, information, knowledge, and wisdom in nursing practice . . . [to support] nurses, consumers, patients, the interprofessional healthcare team, and other stakeholders in their decision-making in all roles and settings to achieve desired outcomes" (p. 1).

The first nursing information systems conference was held in the United States in 1977. Nurses have taken significant strides since then to design and adapt computer processes to enhance client care, education, administration and management, and nursing research. Advanced practice in nursing informatics is a growing specialty. The first ANA certification examination in nursing informatics was given in October 1995. Nursing informaticists or nursing informatics specialists are currently in much demand. Job descriptions for these practitioners often include the important roles of interfacing between the client care and information technology departments and assisting with the development, implementation, and evaluation of initiatives in clinical information systems.

The use of computers to systematically solve problems is referred to as **information technology (IT)**. In nursing, the Technology Informatics Guiding Education Reform (TIGER) Initiative began in 2006 to identify information and knowledge management best practices and effective technology capabilities for nurses. TIGER is focused on clinician education through the integration of IT, information literacy, informatics and technologies, developing and implementing learning innovations, and increasing

TABLE 8.1 Common Computer-Related Acronyms

Acronym	Meaning
CAI	Computer-assisted instruction
CPOE	Computerized provider (or physician) order entry
CPR	Computer-based patient record
EHR	Electronic health record
HIS	Hospital information system
LAN; WAN	Local-area network; wide-area network
MB; GB; TB	Megabyte; gigabyte; terabyte
MIS	Management information system
PDA	Personal digital assistant
PHI	Protected health information
PHR	Personal health record
URL	Universal resource locator (web address)
VPN	Virtual private network

faculty and student acceptance and understanding of health IT through education and training, incentives, and supports (Healthcare Information and Management Systems Society, 2019).

The terminology used to describe the parts and functions of computer technology can be confusing. New terms emerge daily and it is a challenge to keep up with them. See Tables 8.1 and 8.2 for lists of common computer-related acronyms and definitions.

Clinical Alert!

Nurses increasingly use smartphones or PDAs as calendars, address books, drug and disease database storage devices, and data entry and retrieval devices.

Computers have significantly expanded access to information from around the globe for both healthcare team members and consumers. Nurses should evaluate health websites as they access them and assist clients in doing the same. Tools for doing this include (as of this publication) the *HONcode Site Evaluation Form* from the Health on the Net Foundation, *Find Good Health Information* from the Medical Library Association, and the *Evaluating Internet Health Information* tutorial from the National Library of Medicine. Criteria should always include those described in Box 8.1.

Computer Systems

A computer system—not in the sense of one machine but of a network of computers, users, programs, and procedures in an organization—assists the healthcare team with decision making and communication. The two most common types of computer systems used by nurses are management information systems and hospital information systems.

TABLE 8.2 Computer Terminology

Term	Definition
App	Application; a small computer program that performs useful tasks
Blog/weblog	Website that contains dated text entries in reverse chronologic order (most recent first) about a particular topic
Database	Groups of computer-accessible information records made up of variables or fields
Internet	Worldwide computer network
Ethernet	A group of technologies that allow computers to share information over a LAN
Network	System of interconnected computers
Online	Computer-to-computer or computer-to-network connection
Phishing	A link in an email or text message that attempts to make the user enter sensitive personal information
Podcast	Syndicated digital audio or video that is downloaded onto a computer or portable media player
RSS feed	Rich site summary or really simple syndication. Frequently updated information published on a website, accessed manually or through subscription
Smartphone	Mobile phone with computer-like capability such as email, internet access, audiovisual players, camera, and computer programs optimized for mobile use with apps
Social media networks	Online directories of members that allow posts, blogs, photo sharing (e.g., Facebook, Flickr, Flipboard, LinkedIn, Pinterest)
Spreadsheet	Data in rows and columns that can be mathematically manipulated
Tablet PC	Portable computer that uses a touchscreen as its primary input device (e.g., iPad, Kindle Fire)
Twitter	Social networking and news service in which short text messages called *tweets* are posted to multiple individuals who have chosen to follow another individual
Virus	Replicating computer code that acts as a malicious program (malware) causing varying types of harm to hardware and data
Widget	Small onscreen tool or application that displays dynamic content (e.g., clock, games)
Wiki	Collaborative websites that can be edited by multiple individuals

BOX 8.1 Sample Criteria for Evaluating Internet Health Information

- *Author or sponsor*: Who created and updates the site? Are their credentials listed and appropriate?
- *Purpose*: Is it clear whether the site is informational or commercial? Who is the intended audience? Sometimes, the website URL provides some of this information, for example, .gov for government sites, .org for professional organizations, .edu for educational institutions, and .com for companies.
- *Recency*: When was the information in the site last updated?
- *Accuracy and sourcing*: Where does the site get its information? Are factual statements cited?

The complexity and breadth of computer applications are expanding exponentially. Computer access is rapidly increasing, while computer costs have decreased over time. Technology is evolving in the areas of virtual reality, remote access, task automation, robotics, and bioengineering. Simultaneously, however, concerns regarding privacy, access by individuals with disabilities and in underdeveloped countries, piracy, intellectual property debates (who owns web content), destructive programs (computer viruses), and ergonomic injuries continue to arise.

Management Information Systems

A **management information system (MIS)** is designed to facilitate the structure and application of data used to manage an organization or department. The system provides analyses used for strategic planning, decision making, and evaluation of management activities. All levels of management benefit from the ability to access accumulated data.

Hospital Information Systems

A **hospital information system (HIS)** is an MIS that focuses on the types of data needed to manage client care activities and healthcare organizations. As with any system, the goal is to provide individuals with the data they need to determine appropriate actions and control them. Typically, an HIS will have subsystems in the areas of admissions, medical records (Figure 8.1 ■), clinical laboratory, pharmacy, order entry, and finance. The personnel in these areas record the data needed to allow management of billing, quality improvement, scheduling, and inventory both within their own areas and across the institution.

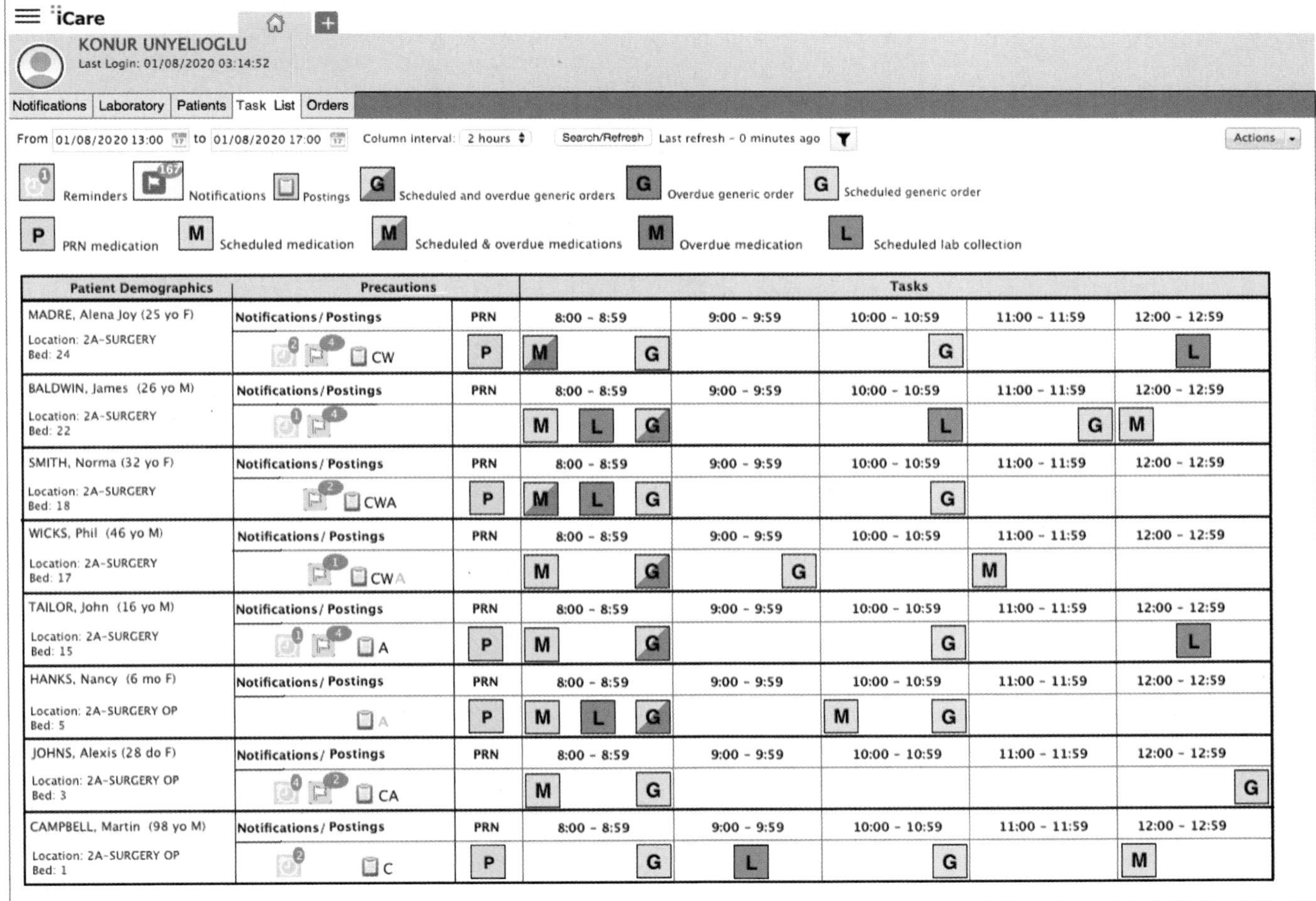

Figure 8.1 ■ Client Dashboard. This is an example of a view the nurse sees when logging into the EHR. This view shows the current clients, their status, and any alerts, activities, reminders, and notifications. From here, the nurse can link to the full client chart.
iCare.

Increasingly, accrediting organizations mandate the use of an HIS and require that reports be submitted using computerized formats. Eventually, integrated HISs—those that allow access and exchange of information among all end users—will form the center of all record keeping and analysis for interdisciplinary healthcare. Integrated systems allow nurses to communicate care plans across the healthcare continuum without needing to regather or repeat information.

The Health Insurance Portability and Accountability Act of 1996 (HIPAA) established legal requirements for the protection, security, and appropriate sharing of client personal health information (referred to as protected health information or PHI). Because PHI is now stored electronically, HIPAA regulations have mandated strict control over access and communication of HIS data. Each healthcare agency in which students and nurses work will orient them to the specific technologic controls in place. Violations of HIPAA are extremely serious and can result in significant fines. Nurses' jobs are in jeopardy if they violate HIPAA and purposely or unintentionally disclose PHI such as by having a computer, tablet, or phone stolen, or posting confidential information on social media.

Technology in Nursing Education

Computers are used extensively in all aspects of nursing education. Nursing programs require computerized access to library resources; faculty members use technologic teaching strategies in the classroom and for outside assignments, as well as for demonstrating and using applications in clinical rotations; and academic record keeping is facilitated by database programs.

Teaching and Learning

Computers enhance academics for both students and faculty in at least four ways. These include access to literature, computer-assisted instruction, classroom technologies, and strategies for learning at a distance.

Literature Access and Retrieval

It is a challenge to keep abreast of the information on any subject. Computers have significantly improved our abilities in this by presenting materials in a way that can be searched systematically. Continuously updated cumulative indexes of related materials can be searched electronically. Searchers can specify the recency, language, document type, and other characteristics as they look for desired materials. Once a list of search matches is displayed on the computer screen, users can select all or certain citations and either print them or store them on their own local computers. Box 8.2 lists commonly used bibliographic systems and databases.

BOX 8.2 Common Health-Related Bibliographic Systems and Databases

AIDS information (AIDS*info*)
Alt HealthWatch
Cochrane Library
Cumulative Index to Nursing and Allied Health Literature (CINAHL)
Educational Resources Information Center (ERIC)
National Library of Medicine's bibliographic database (MEDLINE)
National Guideline Clearinghouse (AHRQ)
Nursing & Allied Health Source (ProQuest)
Psychological Abstracts (PsycINFO)

In addition to searching lists of documents, actual complete publications and materials are available in computerized formats. These include medical textbooks, the full texts of journals, drug references, digitized x-rays or scans, and graphics including clip art (Figure 8.2 ■). Through the internet, both classic and current information can be found on any topic. Users can access statistics from the Centers for Disease Control and Prevention, census data, the National Institutes of Health, and the National Library of Medicine, among others.

Computer-Assisted Instruction

Nursing has benefited from the computer revolution in the form of computer-assisted instruction (CAI). Dozens of software programs help nursing students and nurses learn and demonstrate learning. Programs cover topics from drug dosage calculations to ethical decision making and are classified according to format: tutorial, drill and practice, simulation, or testing.

Tutorials on electrocardiogram (ECG) interpretation, drug interactions, and legal aspects of nursing are examples of CAI programs. Students who become familiar with CAI will also find that they have an easier time adjusting to the software programs many employers require them to complete for annual competency testing mandated by accrediting bodies in certain areas (e.g., bloodborne

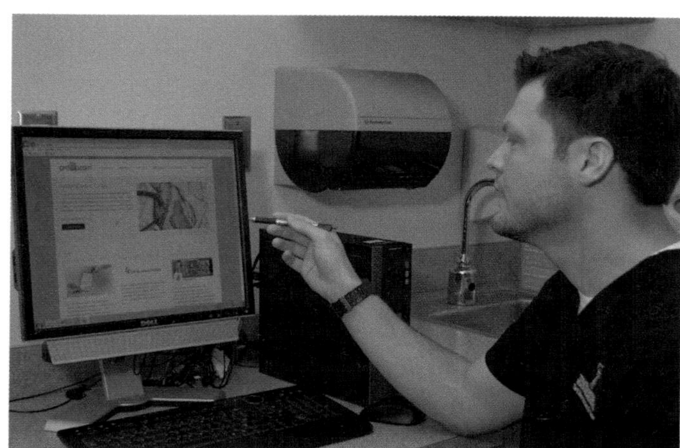

Figure 8.2 ■ Computerized reference resources are available to nurses at the point of care.

pathogens, HIPAA, and fire safety). Completion of CAI programs may also be an acceptable means of demonstrating continuing education activities required for registered nurse license renewal.

Classroom Technology

Most new educational buildings are wired to accommodate technology. "Smart" classrooms with projectors that display computer screens and document cameras that display objects and print materials for the entire classroom to view are becoming standard. Other classroom technology includes the use of individual audience response systems (often referred to as "clickers") and class-capture systems that record and post lectures and visuals to the internet. Mobile phones are also used in class to search for literature, videos, and websites, and to gather data from students using a variety of survey applications.

SIMULATION

Computer technology has significantly enhanced the realism provided in the traditional nursing skills laboratory. Mannequins, models, task trainers, and other tools can simulate realistic healthcare of clients. These tools range from systems that use computers and small devices to provide skills practice, such as learning to insert an IV catheter, to full-sized adults, children, and infants (referred to as high-fidelity human patient simulators) with the ability to breathe, speak, and display digital readouts that reflect the impact of nursing interventions.

Case scenarios can be authored in which one or more care providers interact with the simulated client(s) to role-play a specific situation. Even when all the actors in a scenario are live individuals, such as with standardized clients, technology is used to record the interactions, mark and categorize events in the recording that depict specific learning objectives, and allow replay of the scenario during debriefing.

Clinical Simulation in Nursing, the official journal of the International Nursing Association for Clinical Simulation and Learning (INACSL), is one resource for more information about nursing and healthcare education and practice using simulation and technology.

Distance Learning

There are several different models of **distance learning**—educational opportunities delivered under situations in which the teacher and the learner are not physically in the same place at the same time. Distance learning may be categorized as *asynchronous* when the individuals involved are not interacting at the same "real" time or as *synchronous* when teachers and students are communicating simultaneously. In one model of asynchronous distance learning, the student receives course materials, communicates with the faculty and other students, and submits assignments completely by mail, phone, fax, email, website, or remote storage service, often referred to as "in the cloud." Another type of computerized delivery of knowledge is through ebooks. Textbooks are available on a mobile device and can be annotated and searched. In addition, lectures can be delivered through podcasts.

Many schools use a learning management system such as Blackboard, Canvas, eCollege, or Moodle to make course documents and activities available through internet access. Faculty can post syllabi, handouts, assignments, and examinations in individual course shells, and students can submit papers and hold discussions online. In general, a course that never requires students to come to a campus is considered *online* and one in which no more than 50% of the coursework is on technology and the remainder is conducted on campus is considered *hybrid*.

Technology even allows us to create virtual communities. In these interactive web-based environments, faculty and students create a virtual self, known as an avatar. Using an avatar, you can navigate through simulated worlds and communicate using audio-video lectures, discussions, and posters. One example of such interactive virtual communities in healthcare and education is the three-dimensional simulated world of Second Life.

A model of synchronous distance learning involves groups of students in classrooms at different sites participating in a class session using two-way videoconferencing. Students who are not at the site where the faculty member is located can communicate via voice-activated microphones or response pads. These pads have buttons that permit the students to indicate that they wish to ask a question or even to respond to multiple-choice test questions. Synchronous distance learning can also be accomplished through the use of chat, instant messaging, and one-to-one video chat.

Testing

The computer is ideal for conducting certain types of learning evaluations. Surveys can be completed online, including anonymous questionnaires. Large banks of potential test items can be written that allow the computer to generate different exams for each student depending on the selection criteria designated by the faculty. Students' answers can be scored electronically and the overall exam results analyzed quickly. Some schools subscribe to a service that provides testing and customized instruction, for example, ATI Nursing Education, Health Education Systems Incorporated (HESI), and Kaplan Nursing. Since 1994, the National Council Licensure Examination for RNs (NCLEX-RN) in the United States has been taken on computer. The computer determines if the applicant passed the examination by using a scoring algorithm that ensures all required competencies have been evaluated fairly.

Student and Course Record Management

Computers are also very useful for maintaining results of students' grades or attendance. Often student answer sheets are imported directly into a gradebook on the computer. The program can then calculate percentages, assign letter grades, and make results available to both students and faculty.

Students are frequently asked to evaluate faculty and courses online or using machine-readable forms. These data are also stored in the computer, allowing cumulative results to be calculated. This is an example of what is called **data warehousing**—the accumulation of large amounts of data that are stored over time and can be examined for output in different types of reports (charts and tables).

Technology in Nursing Practice

Many activities of the registered nurse involve collecting, recording, and using data. Computers are well suited to assist the nurse in these functions. Specifically, the nurse records client information in computer records, accesses other departments' information from centralized computers, uses computers to manage client scheduling, and uses programs for unique applications such as home health nursing and case management. Improvement in both clinical and nonclinical processes can occur through technology in biomedical monitoring, communication, client safety systems, decision support, and education. As a component of accreditation of schools of nursing as well as health organizations, nurses are expected to have knowledge about the benefits and limitations of technology, skills in using technology for communication and decision making, and attitudes needed to value technology and use informatics to both support and protect clients.

Documentation of Client Status and Medical Record Keeping

How do computers assist individual nurses with their daily activities? In the typical day of a nurse providing direct client care, as much as one-third of the time may be spent recording in the client's chart (Weaver & O'Brien, 2016). Additional time is spent trying to access data about the client that may be somewhere in the medical record or elsewhere in the healthcare agency. Nurses access standardized forms, policies, and procedures. Also, nurses gather broader client information such as length of stay for specific diagnoses. Computers can assist with each of these tasks.

Bedside Data Entry

There are several different types of computerized bedside data entry systems. These allow safety checks and recording of medication administration (Figures 8.3 ■ and 8.4 ■), client assessments, progress notes, care plan updating, and client acuity (Figure 8.5 ■). The terminal can be fixed or handheld, and hardwired to the central system or wireless with the ability to transmit the data to distant sites, such as from the client's home to the agency office. When using bedside terminals, the nurse must remain sensitive to client concerns related to the technology. Learn how to navigate and troubleshoot the device before using it at

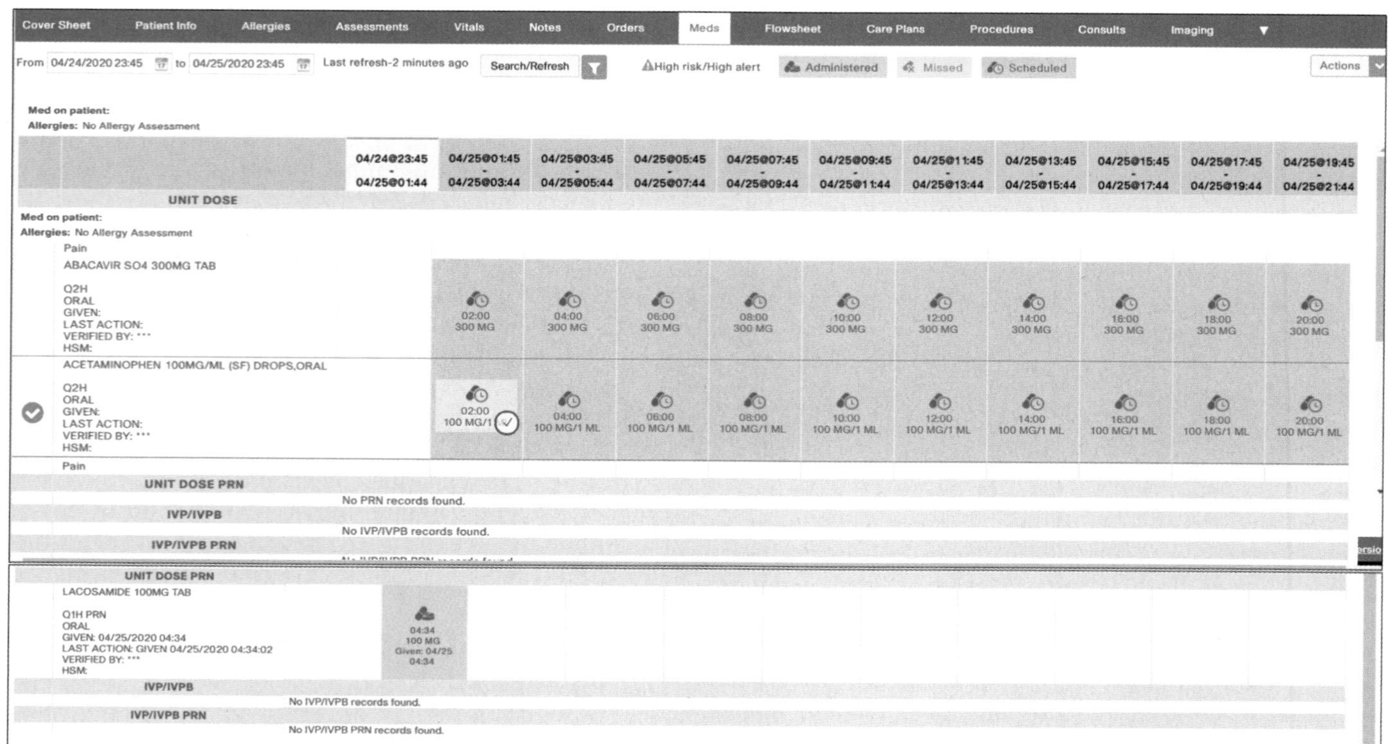

Figure 8.3 ■ This screen shows a MAR (medication administration record) for several regularly scheduled and prn medications. The worksheet displays the next time the medications may be administered.
iCare.

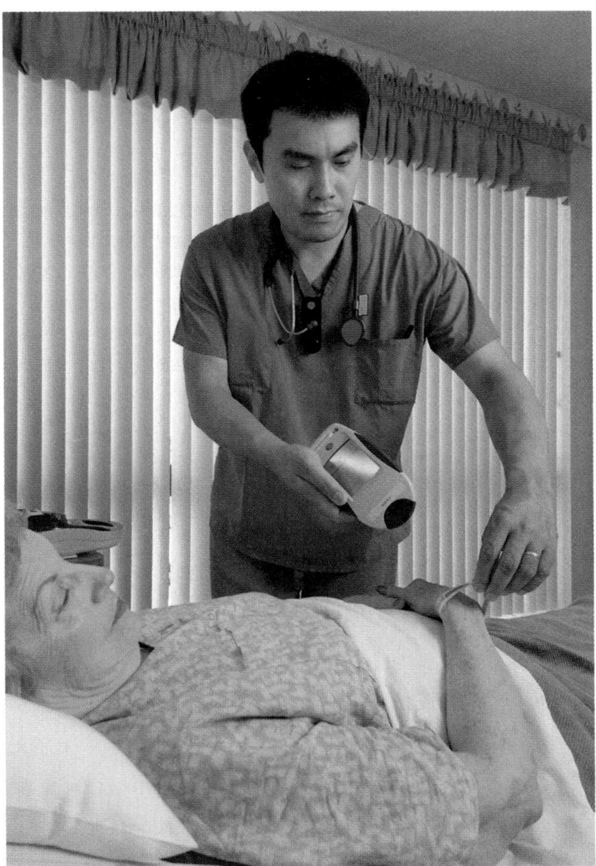

Figure 8.4 ■ The nurse uses a handheld reader to scan the bar code on the client's identification band prior to administering medications and other treatments.
David Joel/Photographer's Choice RF/Getty Images.

the bedside so the client does not observe any frustration if you experience difficulties. Always address the client before using the computer. Explain what the computer is for and how the client's confidentiality is assured.

Computer-Based Client Records

Electronic health records (EHRs) or **computer-based patient records (CPRs)** permit electronic client data entry and retrieval by caregivers, administrators, accreditors, and other individuals who require the data. An EHR can improve healthcare in at least four ways: (1) constant availability of client health information across the lifespan, (2) ability to monitor quality, (3) access to warehoused (stored) data, and (4) ability for clients to share in knowledge and activities influencing their own health. The Centers for Medicare and Medicaid Services (CMS) Electronic Health Record Incentive Program provides financial incentives to providers who demonstrate that they have made "meaningful use" of EHR technology. The program established core required objectives such as to maintain an active medication allergy list for clients. In this example, the objective will be met if review of the provider's electronic system shows that more than 80% of all clients seen have at least one entry in the category of allergies (or an indication that the client has no known medication allergies). In 2019, meaningful use requirements were replaced with the value-based program Medicare Access and CHIP Reauthorization Act (MACRA), which modifies how healthcare providers will be reimbursed based on their use of healthcare technology (Fathi, Modin, & Scott, 2017).

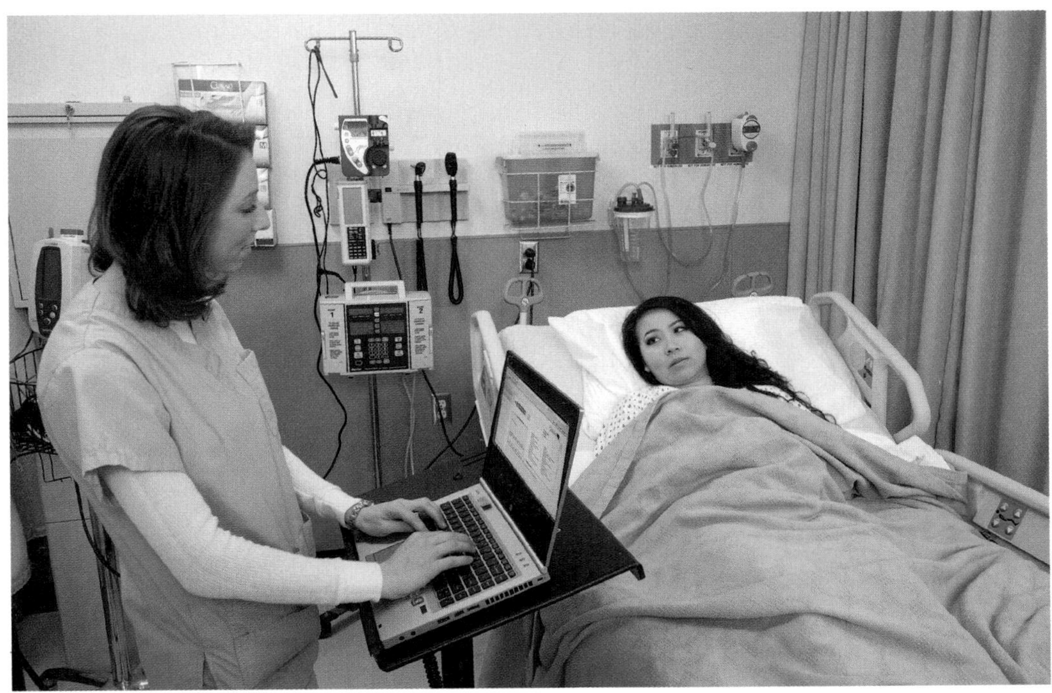

Figure 8.5 ■ The nurse is using a laptop computer to record data at the client's bedside.

Because of the way computers provide access to EHRs, providers can easily retrieve specific data such as trends in vital signs (Figure 8.6 ■), immunization records, and current problems. The system can be designed to warn providers about conflicting medications or client parameters that indicate dangerous conditions (Figure 8.7 ■). Sophisticated systems allow replay of audio, graphic, or video data for comparison with current status. Challenges with reading handwriting are eliminated and all text is searchable.

There are several areas of concern with EHRs. Maintaining the privacy and security of data is a significant issue. One way in which computers can protect data is by user authentication via passwords or biometric identifiers (e.g., fingerprint, palm vein, or retinal scans)—only those individuals who have a legitimate need to access the data receive the password. Additional policies and procedures for protecting the confidentiality of EHRs are evolving as the use of computer records becomes more widespread. One role of the **nurse informaticist**, an expert who combines computer, information, and nursing sciences, is to develop policies and procedures that promote effective and secure use of computerized records by nurses and other healthcare professionals. Other concerns involving

Temperature | Entered in Error | Enter Vitals

Vitals	04-23-20 14:00:00	04-23-20 12:00:00	04-23-20 10:00:00
Temp.	97.6	98	100
Pulse	76	86	88
Resp.	22*	20*	22*
B/P	120/80	130/80	110/60*
P Ox%	98	99	98
Pain	0	0	0
Ht (in)	68.8980	68.8980	68.8980
Wt (lbs.)	171.96	171.96	154.32
BMI	25.52	25.52	22.90
C/G	68	68	60
CVP (cmH20)			
Location	CARDIOLOGY	CARDIOLOGY	CARDIOLOGY
Entered By	GEORGE,ROSILY	GEORGE,ROSILY	GEORGE,ROSILY
Data Source	Vitals	Vitals	Vitals

Figure 8.6 ■ This screen displays the client's vital signs. They can be entered by the nurse (or anyone with the security rights to do so) at the bedside, and then displayed wherever needed.
iCare.

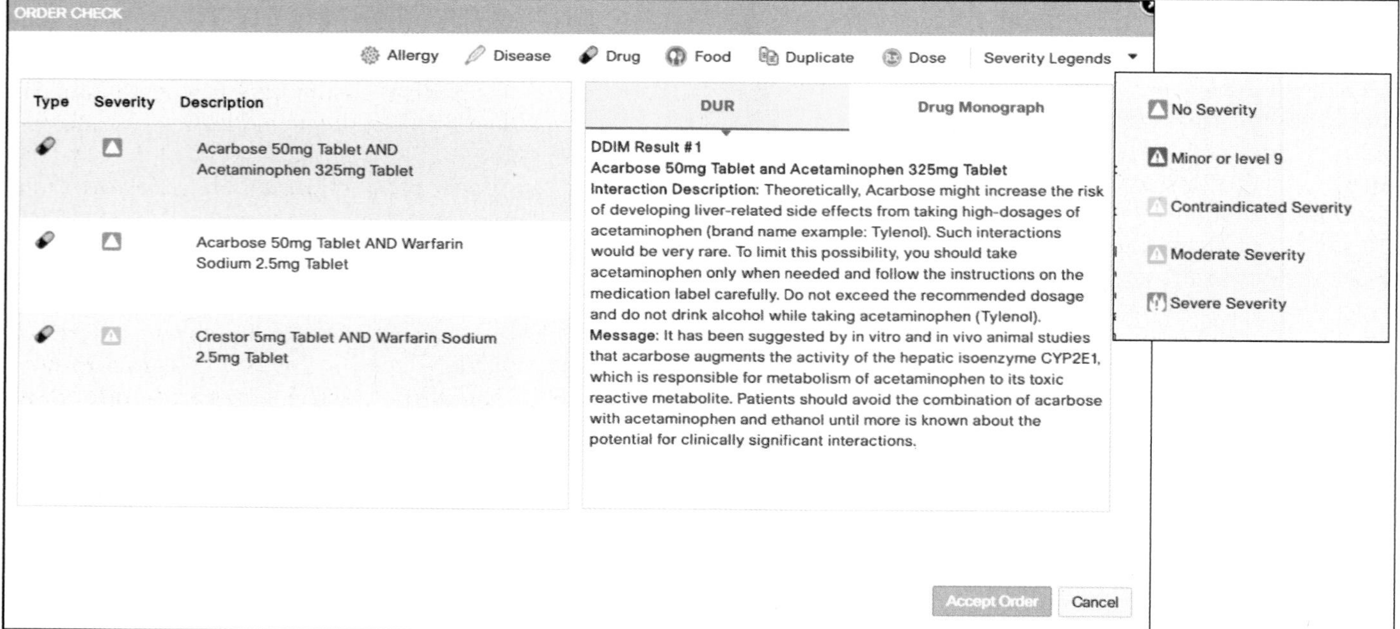

Figure 8.7 ■ One of the strengths of an electronic health record is its ability to alert the clinician to potential adverse drug interactions, providing warnings like the one displayed.
iCare.

EHRs include errors such as wrong-site surgery, medication errors, and delays in treatment that result from improper data entry.

Different from an EHR is a personal health record (PHR), which is an electronic document that contains the client's medical, personal, and health information but is controlled by the client, rather than the healthcare provider. The PHR can be stored on a computer database, in an electronic computer file, or on a portable "smart card" similar to a credit card. A significant advantage of a PHR stored in a commonly accessible format (e.g., word processor document or portable document format [pdf]) is that clients can transport and give the information to any care provider they wish, whenever necessary. A challenge is to keep the information current, however. Ideally, the PHR interfaces with the EHR, but this requires the use of a unique electronic identifier for each individual, and these standards are not yet in place (Sewell, 2019).

Clinical Decision Support Systems

For many years, nurses have used charts, templates, algorithms, and other tools to assist in reaching decisions regarding client care. **Clinical decision support systems** are electronic forms of these tools, which incorporate evidence from the literature into particular client situations in order to guide care planning. In particular, with these systems, characteristics of individual clients are used to generate client-specific assessments or recommendations that are then presented to clinicians for consideration. Such systems' usefulness in nursing relates, in part, to the inability of humans to retain or recall sufficient quantities of the immense amount of knowledge needed to provide safe care. Decision support includes (1) alerts and reminders (e.g., medication due, client has an allergy, potassium level abnormal), (2) clinical guidelines (e.g., best practice for prevention of skin breakdown), (3) online information retrieval (e.g., database searches, drug information), (4) clinical order sets and protocols, and (5) online access to organizational policies and procedures (Barey, Mastrian, & McGonigle, 2018). An ideal decision support system is available at the point of care, responds quickly to input, is integrated into other systems and practices, and is user friendly. In addition, a well-defined, intuitive, and comprehensive system can streamline communication, reduce errors, improve efficiency, and ultimately impact patient outcomes (Clarke, Wilson, & Terhaar, 2016).

Many different computer systems exist. Some are simple alarms that appear when medical orders conflict with another aspect of the client's situation (e.g., allergies, contraindicated treatments). Other systems provide step-by-step online tools to assist emergency department nurses in determining which clients should receive the most immediate attention or are comprehensive programs integrated with a system-wide EHR. As EHRs become more prevalent, clinical decision support systems for nursing practice are likely to become more common also.

Data Standardization and Classifications

There are many reasons why nursing benefits from the use of standard classifications and terms to describe and measure clinical, disease, procedure, and outcomes data. One reason is that, for nursing to be recognized for the value it adds to client well-being, research that shows client improvement must be based on accepted standards. This necessitates the use of common, consistent, clear, and rule-based standards.

Standards for clinical data such as laboratory test results and their documentation in the EHR have been proposed by the American National Standards Institute Healthcare Information Technology Standards Panel, the American Society for Testing and Materials, the European Technical Committee for Standardization, the International Standards Organization, and the Workgroup for Electronic Data Interchange. Disease classification standards are in use in a variety of forms. The most common are the World Health Organization's *International Classification of Diseases* (ICD), the World Organization of National Colleges' *International Classification of Primary Care* (ICPC), and the American Psychiatric Association's *Diagnostic and Statistical Manual of Mental Disorders* (DSM).

Nursing classifications or taxonomies have also been developed. The Nursing Minimum Data Set (NMDS) contains 16 elements of nursing data, along with their definitions, in three categories: nursing care, client demographics, and service. The NMDS can be used for data collection and documentation and allows sharing of information regarding the quality, cost, and effectiveness of nursing. Other classification systems include the NANDA International nursing diagnosis taxonomy, the Omaha System, the Home Health Care Classification (HHCC), the Nursing Interventions Classification (NIC), the Nursing Outcomes Classification (NOC), the International Council of Nurses' International Classification for Nursing Practice, and the International Health Terminology Standards Development Organization's Systematized Nomenclature of Medicine—Clinical Terms (SNOMED CT). It may take years to determine which standards will allow optimal access to and manipulation of computerized records and who will be the determining body.

Tracking Client Status

Once an EHR has been established, the nurse can retrieve and display a client's physiological parameters across time (Figure 8.8 ■). In addition to the rather straightforward viewing of trends in vital signs, for example, the nurse can also track more global client progress. Standardized nursing care plans, care maps, critical pathways, or other prewritten treatment protocols can be stored in the computer and easily placed in the EHR electronically. Then the nurse and other healthcare personnel can examine progress toward and variance from the expected plan directly on the computer. EHR vendors often include components for authoring nursing care plans and tracking care delivery and outcomes (Figure 8.9 ■).

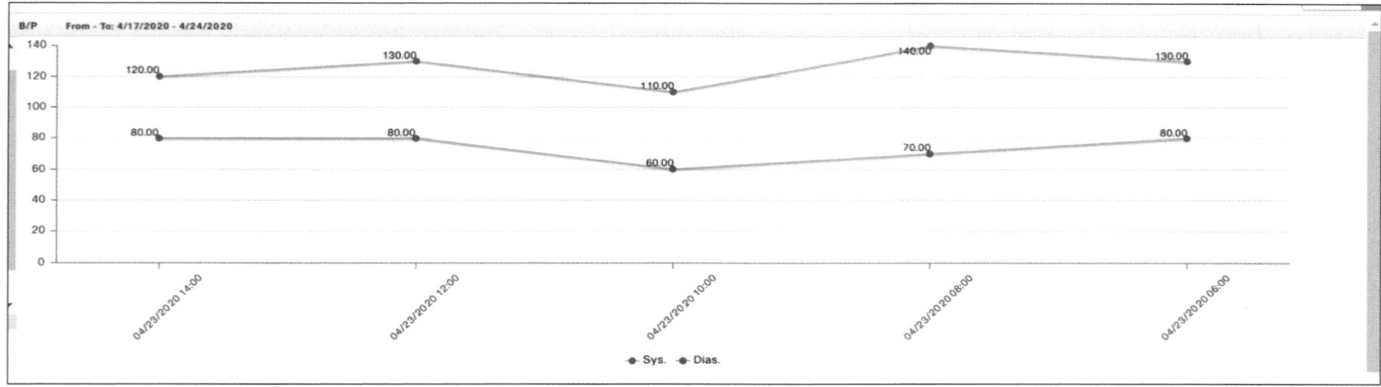

Figure 8.8 ■ Numerical results can be graphed to show trends.
iCare.

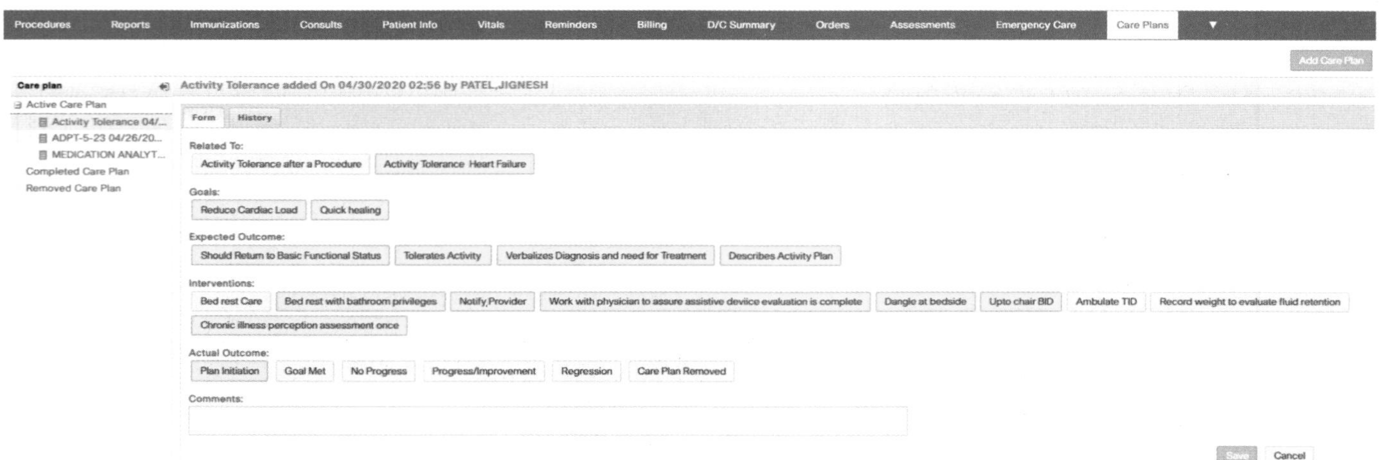

Figure 8.9 ■ In this screen, the nurse selects goals, expected outcomes, and interventions in an evidence-based plan of care for activity tolerance in a client with heart failure.
iCare.

Electronic Access to Client Data

Besides computers designed for record keeping, other computers are used extensively in healthcare to assess and monitor clients' conditions. The data accumulated from various electronic devices can be part of the EHR and also stored for research purposes. Electronic records take up much less space than paper records and may be stored more securely. Copies can be made easily on various types of electronic media that tend to be more compact and durable than paper. Data can also be transmitted electronically to a consulting specialist in another location.

Client Monitoring and Computerized Diagnostics

Nursing has benefited greatly from the myriad of client monitors. Medical devices, with their powerful computer chips, make it possible to extend the nurse's observations and provide valid and reliable data. In everyday practice, nurses use digital or tympanic thermometers, digital scales, pulse oximetry, ECG/telemetry/hemodynamic monitoring, apnea monitors, fetal heart monitors, blood glucose analyzers, ventilators, and IV pumps. Most of these monitors are applied externally, implanted, or even ingested (swallowed), and are proving to have great value. For example, a surgically placed wireless sensor can measure the pressure inside a bulging weakened blood vessel (aneurysm) and warn of potential rupture. These instruments can be used in any care setting, from intensive care to the home. Most keep a record of the most recent values. Some can transmit their data to a more sophisticated computer or print out a paper record. Some have digital displays that "talk" to the user, giving instructions or results. Although these devices are extremely useful, they also raise concerns about cost and privacy. Most devices have error detection or alarms to indicate either that the instrument is malfunctioning or that the assessed value is outside predetermined parameters. Although alarms are essential, they also carry the risk of leading to *alarm fatigue*, when nurses become less sensitive to the alarms because

EVIDENCE-BASED PRACTICE

Evidence-Based Practice

Do Older Adults and Caregivers Differ in Their Views on Technology?

Wang, Carroll, Peck, Myneni, and Gong (2016) studied 29 residents of a retirement community and 6 of their caregivers on the interest in and usefulness of mobile and wearable technology. Older adult participants were interviewed regarding their views on their safety, social support, and experience and interest in technology. Caregivers were asked about the usefulness of devices that could track the residents' activity, sleep, vital signs, and blood glucose, and the usefulness of EHRs. Half the older adults used a computer, tablet, or cell phone, but only 14% had ever used or were interested in wearable technology. All the caregivers were interested in technology to track the residents' conditions and health status.

Implications

Even the most accurate and informative technology may not be useful if unacceptable to the client. Even if they were aware of the potential of technology, the older adults in this study preferred to have a "real person" measure their health status indicators directly. The study has limited applicability due to the small sample and inability to generalize characteristics from this particular set of older adults to different individuals. However, as the generations of digital natives age, nurses should expect that clients will become much more knowledgeable about and accepting of technology for health monitoring. In the meantime, nurses should assess the acceptability of technology to the client and adjust the care plan accordingly.

of their frequency and incidence of false alarms (Robert Wood Johnson Foundation, 2016). Nurses must always balance the data from technologic instruments with their own judgment. Some practitioners trust their technology over their own analysis (known as automation bias), while others ignore or overlook data from computers (known as automation complacency) (Institute for Safe Medication Practices [ISMP] Canada, 2016).

In various specialty areas of healthcare, clients undergo diagnostic procedures in which computers play a major role. Computerized axial tomography (CAT) scans, magnetic resonance imaging (MRI), and positron emission tomography (PET) scans use computers extensively to perform tests and analyze the findings. Blood gas analyzers, pulmonary function test machines, and intracranial pressure monitors all use computer processing (Figure 8.10 ■). All of these can be linked directly to an EHR, which stores the test results (Figure 8.11 ■). There are many more

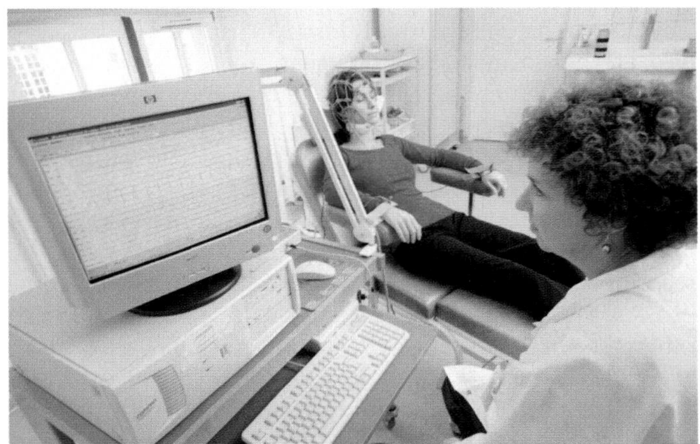

Figure 8.10 ■ Client undergoing an electroencephalogram (EEG), a graphic record of a brain's electrical activity.
Phanie/Science Source.

Flowsheet View(s)

Rosily George :

Add Data | Time Interval: 1 hour | Previous Next

	04/24/2020 13:00 04/24/2020 13:56	04/24/2020 12:00 04/24/2020 12:59	04/24/2020 11:00 04/24/2020 11:59	04/24/2020 10:00 04/24/2020 10:59	04/24/2020 09:00 04/24/2020 09:59
1. CHEST TUBE DRAINAGE	NONE [13:00]	SCANT [12:00]	NONE [11:00]	SMALL [10:00]	MODERATE [09:00]
Temperature	98.4 (DEGREES F) [13:00]	98.4 (DEGREES F) [12:00]	99 (DEGREES F) [11:00]	100 (DEGREES F) [10:00]	100 (DEGREES F) [09:00]
RESPIRATIONS	20 (BPM) [13:00]	22 (BPM) [12:30] ~~22 (BPM)~~ [12:00]	22 (BPM) [11:00]	22 (BPM) [10:00]	24 (BPM) [09:00]
Total Score					

Figure 8.11 ■ This screen displays a flowsheet view of available results for a particular client. The information can be reported from most summarized to most detailed so that the user gets an overview first and can then "drill down" to see the details.
iCare.

examples of ways in which computers assist nurses in monitoring and diagnosing client conditions.

Telemedicine or Telehealth

One of the most exciting areas being developed in computer-assisted healthcare is telemedicine. **Telemedicine** or telehealth uses technology to transmit electronic data about clients to healthcare providers at distant locations. In one example, two-way audiovisual communication allows an international expert to examine and consult on a client's case from thousands of miles away. X-rays, scans, stored computer data, and almost anything imaginable can be "sent" using computers. Another example is the ability for a few healthcare providers to provide primary healthcare to clients living in remote areas using the kinds of monitors described previously plus telephone, fax, and other relatively simple equipment in the client's home.

Concerns regarding telemedicine relate to legal and ethical issues. Who has responsibility for the client when a teleconsult is used? Does the care provider need to be licensed in the state or province where the client's primary care is given? The National Council of State Boards of Nursing has declared that the applicable regulations are those for where the client resides and not where the provider is located. This is also one of the reasons for the initiation of the mutual recognition compact that boards of nursing are promulgating to facilitate nurse licensure in several states (see Chapter 3 ∞). How is the client's privacy protected? For example, if a provider in state A was teleconsulting with providers in states B, C, and D, which state's privacy laws should take precedence over others? What if they conflict? HIPAA and several other projects are under way to answer these questions and to determine the most effective designs for telemedicine programs.

Practice Management

Beyond direct client care, computers also assist nurses in many ways in the management of their work. In hospitals, data terminals are commonly used to order supplies, tests, meals, and services from other departments, a process called computerized provider order entry (CPOE). Tracking of these orders allows the nursing service to determine the most frequent or most costly items used by a particular nursing unit. This information may lead to decisions to modify a budget, provide different staffing, move supplies to a different location, or make other changes for more efficient and higher quality care.

Computers are used extensively for scheduling. Client appointments can be easily entered or changed. Special notes or tags can be applied to the appointment as a reminder to the provider to perform particular services. The schedule for a single day can be printed so that all personnel have a copy. Staffing patterns must also be coordinated. Special requests for days off or continuing education classes can be entered, and the schedule can be viewed for a day, week, month, or year.

Each practice needs to keep track of procedures healthcare workers perform, client diagnoses, and time spent with clients so that billing can be accurate. Medicare and most other insurance companies require electronic submission of healthcare billing. In keeping with HIPAA regulations, electronic data interchange (EDI) protocols are used to maximize privacy and minimize the chances of inappropriate sharing of confidential client data. With managed care, information tracking is also aimed at determining trends in health problems and the need for providers with specific skills. The use of computerized databases filled with unique codes for each medication, medical and nursing diagnosis, treatment, and supply allows for accurate and timely management of these data.

Specific Applications of Computers in Nursing Practice

As previously described, numerous systems are in use for collecting and classifying the various types of data used in nursing practice. Some of these systems have been found particularly useful in specific settings.

Community and Home Health

Computer networks are being used in innovative ways in home settings. A computer placed in a high-risk client's or family's home allows them to access information on a variety of topics, search the internet, or email a healthcare provider with questions or concerns. Clients can also record data about their health status that can be transmitted to the healthcare provider at the central network computer. Examples that have been successful using this approach include monitoring women at risk for preterm labor, individuals with AIDS, and clients in very rural settings who are far from their providers. Digital cameras connected to the computer, often referred to as webcams, permit the healthcare provider to actually examine the client to some degree (Figure 8.12 ■). Home alert systems that allow the client to signal the base station in an emergency are also widely used.

Nurses who visit clients in their homes are using laptop or tablet computer systems to record assessments and transmit data to the main office. Similar systems have been developed so that nursing students in community health courses can communicate with their faculty.

Case Management

Case managers must be able to track a group of clients—the caseload. Software programs allow the case manager to enter client data and integrate this with predesigned care-tracking templates. In addition, the case manager must keep abreast of the latest regulations affecting

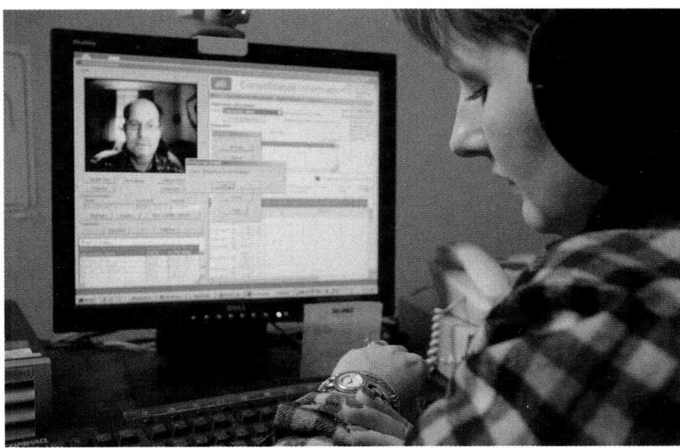

Figure 8.12 ■ The nurse wears headphones as she listens to and records a client's heart rate using a home telecare device. A growing number of healthcare providers are using video monitoring to check in on clients.
Jim McKnight/AP images.

eligibility for healthcare benefits, the reporting requirements of the payer agencies, and detailed facts about the variety of service providers the client may need to access. All of these data can be placed in integrated computer software programs. Finally, the case manager must document quality, that is, demonstrate client outcomes related to dollars spent.

Technology in Nursing Administration

As indicated in the section of this chapter on computers in nursing practice, the volume of data that nurses need to have available and the additional volume of data generated by nurses can and must be managed electronically. Nursing administrators require these data to develop strategic plans for the organization.

Human Resources

All employers must maintain a database on each employee. In addition to the usual demographic and salary data, the database for licensed or certified healthcare personnel has unique fields for areas such as life support certification, health requirements (e.g., tuberculosis testing, hepatitis immunization, rubella titers), and performance appraisals. Administrators can use this human resources database to communicate with employees, examine staffing patterns, and create budget projections.

Medical Records Management

Medical records must be maintained for many years in case the data are needed for client care or research. Storage of paper documentation can be cumbersome and costly. Although it is expensive to store records, the cost of human time and energy plus inefficiency in accessing the contents is even more expensive. Therefore, nurses require computer programs that allow client records to be searched for data such as the most common diagnoses, number of cases by diagnosis-related groups, most expensive cases, length of stay or total number of days the case was open, client outcomes, and so on. Nurse informaticists can assist with the design and implementation of systems that allow such searches to be generated, analyzed, printed, and distributed. Computerized records increase the ability to demonstrate the value of nursing care.

Facilities Management

Many aspects of managing buildings and nonnursing services can be facilitated by computer. Heating, air conditioning, ventilation, and alarm systems are computer controlled. Security devices such as readers that scan identification cards, bar codes, or magnetic strips permit only authorized personnel to enter client or private areas. Computers also manage and report inventory, tracking everything from pillowcases to syringes.

Budget and Finance

Advantages of computerized billing are that claims are transmitted much more quickly and have a greater likelihood of being complete and accurate compared to handwritten documents. If this is the case, claims will be paid sooner and the agency will have better control over its financial status. Computers can also affect cost savings by reducing the clerical services time needed for accounts payable and receivable. In cases where nursing can directly bill and be reimbursed by payers, the same benefits of computerized accounting apply.

The budget itself is generally a spreadsheet program. This software allows tracking as well as forecasting and planning. In uncertain times, the ability to perform "what if" calculations is especially valuable.

Quality Improvement and Utilization Review

Both internal and external stakeholders in healthcare organizations need to know that the services and activities of the organization have positive results. Once standards, pathways, key indicators, and other vital data have been identified and described, computers can facilitate the accumulation and analysis of data for individuals and groups of clients. Quality is considered a process and not an end point. Applying this perspective, computerized systems are ideal for taking a snapshot view of the institution's quality indices at any time.

Utilization review consists of examining trends and proposing advantageous use of resources (specifically, length of stay). For example, might clients who have had a fractured hip repaired have equivalent outcomes at lesser cost if transferred from the hospital to a skilled nursing facility sooner? Studies can be conducted with computer analyses to answer such questions.

Accreditation

The Joint Commission has mandated that hospitals have online mechanisms to monitor quality indicators, so as to reduce the difficulty and time involved in the accreditation process. Healthcare agencies must maintain databases of policies and procedures, standards of care, and employee accomplishment of The Joint Commission requirements such as continuing education and in-service trainings. The Joint Commission has also required a move to computer systems that assess outcomes rather than processes.

Another aspect of accreditation review is demonstrating adequate staffing for the number and acuity of clients. Each agency, whether hospital, outpatient, or home care, must use a method of determining the number of hours of nursing care required for its current clients. Computers used to implement this method can incorporate the severity of the clients' illnesses, length of time needed to perform certain procedures, training and expertise of the nursing staff, and any other parameters desired into the calculations. Computers facilitate review of required hours across time.

Data Mining

The use of computers in healthcare allows the collection and analysis of immense amounts of data. The term *big data* is used to describe the amount of data accumulated from digital sources such as sensors, social media, and monitoring devices in addition to traditional digital data from EHRs, diagnostic tests, and images (Alexander, Ramachandran, & Hankey-Underwood, 2019). Because of the sheer amount of data, special techniques are needed to locate and analyze what is needed to answer nursing questions. These techniques are referred to as *big data science* or *data mining*. Nurses can play a significant role in data mining by working on the standardization of data into formats that can be compiled and compared (Matney et al., 2017; Pruinelli, 2016).

Technology in Nursing Research

Computers are valuable assistants when conducting both quantitative and qualitative nursing research. In each step of the research process, computers facilitate generation, refinement, analysis, and output of data. Computer resources are an important component of the planning phase of any research project. The speed and processing power of the computer and its storage capacity must be adequate for the amount and type of data that will be collected, and the proper software programs must be in place to manage and analyze the data. Computerized word processing is also an integral component in the publication and dissemination of research.

Problem Identification

The first step of the research process is to identify and describe the problem of interest. The computer can be useful in locating current literature about the problem and related concepts. Perhaps, unknown to the researcher, a solution to the problem has already been found and reported. A search of existing documents and websites and emails to colleagues may help define the problem.

Literature Review

An exhaustive review of the literature can be time consuming. Without computer access to bibliographic databases, the researcher must wade through huge volumes of publications. The software programs that facilitate searches contain thesauruses so that the most appropriate terms can be selected. If the researcher determines that little has been published on the topic of interest, closely related terms and topics must also be searched. The increase in availability of full-text journal articles online has made the electronic literature search process even more productive.

Research Design

The design of a research study, including the choice of specific research method, is always driven by the research question. At the design stage, the investigator determines whether the study will use a qualitative or quantitative approach, what instruments will be used to collect data, and the types of analyses that will be carried out on the data to answer the research questions. Computers may be used during this step to search the literature for instruments that have already been established or to design and test instruments that need to be developed for the particular study. In addition, the investigator would not likely select an instrument or design that requires extensive computer or mathematical analysis if such resources are not available.

Data Collection and Analysis

Once the types of data to be collected have been determined, the investigator will create forms on the computer for collecting the data. These may include the informed consent document, a tool to collect demographic data, and recording forms for research variables. If possible, computer-readable forms are created so that the data can be scanned into the computer or the participant can key responses directly into the computer (e.g., an online survey). This eliminates the errors that can occur if the researcher must enter the data into the computer manually.

It is particularly important for all variables that will be computer analyzed to be identified in a way that the computer can recognize and manipulate. This may mean determining how to code the data for optimal manipulation. For example, will age be recorded in specific years or by categories such as 1–10, 11–15, 16–20, and so on? Software programs can assist with the analysis and coding of qualitative data. Such programs assist the researcher in finding and coding sections of text and organizing coded material.

When the variables have been coded, other programs can be used to calculate descriptive and analytic statistics. Calculations that formerly were extremely time consuming and complex can now be done by computer programs quickly and accurately. Commonly used software programs for quantitative data analysis include SPSS (Statistical Package for the Social Sciences), SAS (Statistical Analysis System), and SYSTAT. These programs perform analyses and display output in tables, charts, lists, and other easily read formats.

Research Dissemination

Research is of limited value if the findings are not widely dispersed to the practitioners who can use the findings to improve their practice. Computer word processing programs are used to author the final research reports and send them to various readerships. Most journals require that manuscripts be submitted for publication electronically. As noted earlier in this chapter, the number of electronic journals is increasing. With the rapid growth of email, authors can also send an article or data to interested individuals instantaneously. Computers speed completion of a research project and the availability of the findings to the public.

Computers are frequently used to present research at meetings. Using computer projectors to display screens of data and findings allows the researcher to highlight, modify, and manipulate content in an instant. In addition, companies and universities often post research papers and projects on their organizations' websites. There is also computer conferencing where researchers collaborate on a study from distant locations and can examine and analyze the data simultaneously onscreen.

Research Grants

Funds are available from a variety of resources to support the conduct of nursing research. The budget in a grant application may include a request to purchase computers or software needed to carry out the proposed study. Funds may also be requested to pay individuals to enter data into the computer and to run the statistical analyses.

Information about available grant funding is most easily found online. The U.S. federal government makes all the grant applications for nursing projects available only by downloading them from internet sites. Forms to be completed are computer generated and often must be submitted to the funding agency in electronic format.

LIFESPAN CONSIDERATIONS Computer Use

CHILDREN AND ADULTS

Computer programs are available for children and adults to learn everything from a foreign language to algebra. Many concerns are raised about the frequent and extended use of computers by all ages. In particular, repetitive motion injuries (especially of the hand) can occur with extensive typing, texting, and use of the computer mouse. Eye strain can occur from computer monitor viewing, and musculoskeletal damage is related to inadequate ergonomic arrangement of desk chairs, surface height, and monitor placement. Students and adults who use computers daily should be thoroughly evaluated and instructed in the prevention of these conditions.

Parents need to be reminded of potential risks to children from internet contact with strangers and adult-only websites. They also need to monitor schoolchildren's use of computers to ensure they are not being sidetracked from homework into computer games and messaging.

All individuals should be wary about protecting their financial and personal information when conducting business via computer.

OLDER ADULTS

Increasing numbers of older adults use computers as an avenue of communication and exposure to a vast amount of healthcare information. It is important to teach clients and the general public to evaluate information from the site and to be aware that misinformation can also be presented. Important guidelines that increase the validity of a site are as follows:

- The article or information lists the author and credentials or the institution from which the information came.
- A date is listed that states when information was updated.
- If healthcare information is presented, a disclaimer should be included. The disclaimer presents limitations of the information and should say that it is not medical advice.

Computer-assisted programs can be very effective teaching aids for older adults. They may provide audio and visual instruction and may be interactive. They are useful for teaching about medical conditions and medications and for providing information about procedures and surgeries to be performed.

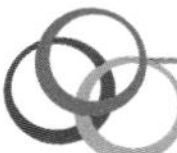

Critical Thinking Checkpoint

As a nurse working for a home care agency in a small, rural town, you would like your clients to receive up-to-date and accurate health information and care. High-speed computer access is available in your office, and many of the residents have computers in their homes since it provides a low-cost way of communicating with friends and relatives who are far away (for example, using email and sending digitized photos).

1. You have a difficult clinical case and want to investigate possible interventions. What are some of the ways computers could assist in this endeavor?
2. You decide that sending photos of the client would be useful to your colleagues in providing input. Because time is an issue, you determine that sending them electronically would be most expeditious. The client agrees to the photos but is worried about privacy in sending them through the computer. How would you handle this?
3. A client shares with you a website that states it can guarantee a cure to the client's illness. How would you respond?
4. Since you are in a rural town and not near an on-campus nursing program, you are considering enrolling in an advanced degree program that is offered online. What would be some of the advantages and disadvantages of such a program?

Answers to Critical Thinking Checkpoint questions are available on the faculty resources site. Please consult with your instructor.

Chapter 8 Review

CHAPTER HIGHLIGHTS

- Nursing informatics is the science of using computer information systems in the practice of nursing.
- A hospital information system (HIS) organizes data from various areas in the hospital such as admissions, medical records, clinical laboratory, pharmacy, order entry, and finance.
- Concerns regarding privacy and confidentiality of health records have arisen as electronic databases and communications have proliferated.
- Computers are used extensively to locate and access data through online databases and internet searching. Many nursing journals are electronic.
- Computer-assisted instruction programs include tutorial, drill and practice, simulation, or testing.
- In distance learning, the faculty and student may be located far apart and communicate via computer, phone, fax, and video technologies.
- Electronic health records (EHRs) enable data to be collected on a client and made available to all healthcare providers who require it. Such data warehousing also enables research to be conducted on quality of care, client outcomes, and a variety of other parameters. However, no national standards exist for the structure or content of these records.
- Nurses need to participate in the creation of classifications for electronic data. Existing models include the World Health Organization's *International Classification of Diseases* (ICD), the World Organization of National Colleges' *International Classification of Primary Care* (ICPC), the American Psychiatric Association's *Diagnostic and Statistical Manual of Mental Disorders* (DSM), the NANDA International nursing diagnosis taxonomy, the Omaha System, the Home Health Care Classification (HHCC), the Nursing Interventions Classification (NIC), the Nursing Outcomes Classification (NOC), the International Council of Nurses' International Classification for Nursing Practice, the Nursing Minimum Data Set (NMDS), and the Systematized Nomenclature of Medicine—Clinical Terms (SNOMED CT).
- Computer monitoring and diagnosing of client conditions is widespread. Examples include digital or tympanic thermometers, digital scales, pulse oximetry, ECG, telemetry, hemodynamic monitoring, apnea monitors, fetal heart monitors, blood glucose analyzers, ventilators, IV pumps, CAT scans, and MRI.
- Telemedicine or telehealth, which allows healthcare professionals to provide care via electronic means of communication, is a growing area that generates both excitement and concerns.
- Data terminals in healthcare settings allow placing of order requests and retrieval of client data and accounts. Appointments can be scheduled using computers.
- Computers are used by home health nurses to record client data and to communicate with the main office. Clients can also have computers in the home that allow them to monitor their own health status and send information about their condition to the nurse.
- Specialized computer software programs enable case managers to track clients' needs, resources, and healthcare outcomes.
- Computers are used in nursing administration to manage human resources, medical records, facilities, budgets, quality improvement, utilization review, and accreditation.
- Each step of the nursing research process makes use of computer technology. In particular, computers are used to access literature, analyze data, and report findings.

TEST YOUR KNOWLEDGE

1. A client in a health care facility asks the nurse about the facility's computerized system for keeping client information, especially confidentiality issues. Which is the best response by the nurse?
   1. "Don't worry, your information is always safe."
   2. "Information in our system requires a password to retrieve."
   3. "Our system was designed with a lot of input from the nursing staff."
   4. "I can see why you're worried with all the computer hackers out there these days."

2. What is the challenge most associated with the utilization of an electronic client record system?
   1. Cost
   2. Accuracy
   3. Privacy
   4. Durability

3. What is one disadvantage associated with electronic (e.g., internet-based) courses?
   1. They take longer.
   2. Interpersonal communication is not possible.
   3. Everyone has to "log on" at the same time.
   4. It is harder to establish a sense of community.

4. Nursing students are participating in an online delivery course in their nursing program. For their next assignment, they are to evaluate nursing research articles for credibility and reliability. Which of the following would be the best database to search for these articles?
   1. CINAHL
   2. Google
   3. ERIC
   4. PsycINFO

5. A nurse manager is responsible for scheduling the staff of all units in a critical-care hospital. Which of the following programs would work best for computer scheduling?
   1. Database
   2. Word processing
   3. Graphics program
   4. Spreadsheet

See Answers to Test Your Knowledge in Appendix A.

READINGS AND REFERENCES

Suggested Reading

Office of the National Coordinator for Health Information Technology, Office of the Secretary, United States Department of Health and Human Services. (2015). *Federal health IT strategic plan, 2015–2020.* Retrieved from https://www.healthit.gov/sites/default/files/9-5-federalhealthitstratplanfinal_0.pdf *This document describes how the U.S. federal government plans to use information and technology to achieve four goals: advance person-centered and self-managed health; transform healthcare delivery and community health; foster research, scientific knowledge, and innovation; and enhance the nation's health IT infrastructure. Vision, mission, and principles statements are also included.*

Related Research

Wang, P., Zhang, H., Li, P., & Lin, K. (2016). Making patient risk visible: Implementation of a nursing document information system to improve patient safety. In W. Sermeus, P. M. Procter, & P. Weber (Eds.), *Nursing informatics 2016* (pp. 8–12). Amsterdam, the Netherlands: IOS Press. doi:10.3233/978-1-61499-658-3-8

References

Alexander, S., Ramachandran, R., & Hankey-Underwood, D. (2019). Using big data analytics to answer questions in health care. In S. Alexander, K. H. Frith, & H. M. Hoy (Eds.), *Applied clinical informatics for nurses* (2nd ed., pp. 110–123). Burlington, MA: Jones & Bartlett.

American Nurses Association. (2014). *Nursing informatics: Scope and standards of practice* (2nd ed.). Washington, DC: Author.

Barey, E. B., Mastrian, K., & McGonigle, D. (2018). The electronic health record and clinical informatics. In D. Mc Gonigle & K. Mastrian, *Nursing informatics and the foundation of knowledge* (4th ed., pp. 266–290). Burlington, MA: Jones & Bartlett.

Clarke, S., Wilson, M. L., & Terhaar, M. (2016). Using dashboard technology and clinical decision support systems to improve heart team efficiency and accuracy: Review of the literature. In W. Sermeus, P. M. Procter, & P. Weber (Eds.), *Nursing informatics 2016* (pp. 364–366). Amsterdam, the Netherlands: IOS Press. doi:10.3233/978-1-61499-658-3-364

Cronenwett, L., Sherwood, G., Barnsteiner, J., Disch, J., Johnson, J., Mitchell, P., . . . Warren, J. (2007). Quality and safety education for nurses. *Nursing Outlook*, *55*, 122–131. doi:10.1016/j.outlook.2007.02.006

Fathi, J. T., Modin, H. E., & Scott, J. D. (2017). Nurses advancing telehealth services in the era of healthcare reform. *The Online Journal of Issues in Nursing*, *22*, Manuscript 2. doi:10.3912/OJIN.Vol22No02Man02

Healthcare Information and Management Systems Society. (2019). *The TIGER Initiative*. Retrieved from https://www.himss.org/professionaldevelopment/tiger-initiative?utm_source=commnews&utm_medium=email&utm_campaign=tiger

Institute for Safe Medication Practices Canada. (2016). Understanding human over-reliance on technology. *ISMP Canada Safety Bulletin*, *16*(5), 1–4.

Matney, S. A., Settergren, T., Carrington, J. M., Richesson, R. L., Sheide, A., & Westra, B. L. (2017). Standardizing physiologic assessment data to enable big data analytics. *Western Journal of Nursing Research*, *39*, 63–77. doi:10.1177/0193945916659471

Pruinelli, L. (2016). Nursing management minimum data set: Cost-effective tool to demonstrate the value of nurse staffing in the big data science era. *Nursing Economic$*, *34*(2), 66–89.

Robert Wood Johnson Foundation. (2016). Boon or bane? Making sure technologies improve (not impede) nursing care. *Charting Nursing's Future*, *29*, 1. Retrieved from http://www.rwjf.org/content/dam/farm/reports/issue_briefs/2016/rwjf433148

Sewell, J. (2019). *Informatics and nursing: Opportunities and challenges* (6th ed.). Philadelphia, PA: Wolters Kluwer.

Wang, J., Carroll, D., Peck, M., Myneni, S., & Gong, Y. (2016). Mobile and wearable technology needs for aging in place: Perspectives from older adults and their caregivers and providers. In W. Sermeus, P. M. Procter, & P. Weber (Eds.), *Nursing informatics 2016* (pp. 486–490). Amsterdam, the Netherlands: IOS Press. doi:10.3233/978-1-61499-658-3-486

Weaver, C., & O'Brien, A. (2016). Transforming clinical documentation in EHRs for 2020: Recommendations from University of Minnesota's Big Data Conference Working Group. In W. Sermeus, P. M. Procter, & P. Weber (Eds.), *Nursing informatics 2016* (pp. 18–22). Amsterdam, the Netherlands: IOS Press. doi:10.3233/978-1-61499-658-3-18

Selected Bibliography

Baker, K., Rasmussen, K., & Shimp, K. (2018). The imperative for an electronic nurse scheduling system: Prioritize the need and make a positive impact. *American Nurse Today*, *13*(9), 90–92.

Botin, L., & Nøhr, C. (2016). Nursing telehealth: Caring from a distance. In W. Sermeus, P. M. Procter, & P. Weber (Eds.), *Nursing informatics 2016* (pp. 188–192). Amsterdam, the Netherlands: IOS Press. doi:10.3233/978-1-61499-658-3-188

Clarke, S., Wilson, M. L., & Terhaar, M. (2016). Using clinical decision support and dashboard technology to improve heart team efficiency and accuracy in a transcatheter aortic valve implantation (TAVI) program. In W. Sermeus, P. M. Procter, & P. Weber (Eds.), *Nursing informatics 2016* (pp. 98–102). Amsterdam, the Netherlands: IOS Press. doi:10.3233/978-1-61499-658-3-98

Gartee, R. (2017). *Electronic health records: Understanding and using computerized medical records* (3rd ed.). New York, NY: Pearson.

Healthcare Information and Management Systems Society. (2017). *HIMSS 2017 nursing informatics workforce survey*. Retrieved from http://www.himss.org/sites/himssorg/files/2017-nursing-informatics-workforce-full-report.pdf

Lopez, K. D., Gephart, S. M., Raszewski, R., Sousa, V., Shehorn, L. E., & Abraham, J. (2017). Integrative review of clinical decision support for registered nurses in acute care settings. *Journal of the American Medical Informatics Association*, *24*, 441–450. doi:10.1093/jamia/ocw084

Marien, S., Krug, B., & Spinewine, A. (2017). Electronic tools to support medication reconciliation: A systematic review. *Journal of the American Medical Informatics Association*, *24*, 227–240. doi:10.1093/jamia/ocw068

Pagulayan, J., Eltair, S., & Faber, K. (2018). Nurse documentation and the electronic health record: Use the nursing process to take advantage of EHRs' capabilities and optimize patient care. *American Nurse Today*, *13*(9), 48–54.

Tacy, J. (2016). Technostress: A concept analysis. *Online Journal of Nursing Informatics*, *20*(2). Retrieved from http://www.himss.org/library/technostress-concept-analysis

Weiner, E., Trangenstein, P., McNew, R., & Gordon, J. (2016). Using the virtual reality world of Second Life to promote patient engagement. In W. Sermeus, P. M. Procter, & P. Weber (Eds.), *Nursing informatics 2016* (pp. 198–202). Amsterdam, the Netherlands: IOS Press. doi:10.3233/978-1-61499-658-3-198

Wentz, B., & Bowles, M. J. (2018). Mobile devices and health-care-associated infections: Nursing research—a win for nurses and patients. *American Nurse Today*, *13*(9), 56–59.

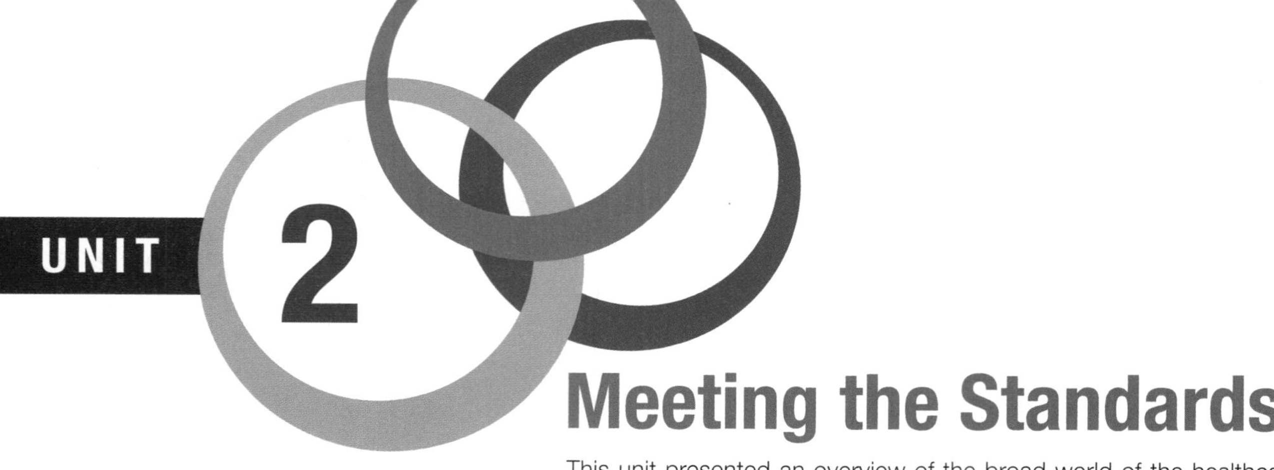

Meeting the Standards

This unit presented an overview of the broad world of the healthcare system and described care provided outside the hospital—including in cyberspace. In order for nurses to be effective members of the healthcare team, we must be knowledgeable about the variety of methods of delivering and paying for healthcare, the diverse members of the healthcare team, the unique aspects of nursing care delivered in the community and clients' homes, and the uses of information technology in clients' lives and in healthcare. To provide the best possible nursing care under all of these different circumstances, nurses must demonstrate critical thinking using evidence-based strategies and theoretical underpinnings.

In the case described below, a client uses one method of healthcare delivery and financing and accesses care outside of the hospital. The nurse remains an integral part of the client's health experience.

CLIENT: Rhett AGE: 66
CURRENT MEDICAL DIAGNOSIS: Prehypertension

Medical History: Rhett had many of the usual childhood diseases and several of the rarer ones including polio and rickets. He recovered almost completely from each, with only slight residual weakness in the upper extremities. He has borderline diabetes mellitus that is controlled by diet, weight management, and exercise. His most recent blood analyses showed all values within normal limits except for a slightly elevated fasting blood sugar. He takes 81 mg of aspirin daily. His only prescription medications are simvastatin for high cholesterol and, since his last primary care provider visit 1 month ago, a very low dose of the angiotensin-converting enzyme (ACE) inhibitor medication lisinopril for blood pressure. The primary care provider recommended that Rhett measure his blood pressure at home twice each day and send that information to the office every 2 weeks.

Personal and Social History: Rhett is divorced with one grown daughter. He moved to the United States at age 30 from a European country. He has several college degrees and now works as a translator. His work is computer based so he works from his home. He loves all forms of technology, from smartphones, to tablet personal computers, to web-based games. He is diligent about doing physical exercise daily, alternating cardiovascular with weight-training routines.

Rhett's diet leans toward high carbohydrate foods and he takes a variety of vitamin supplements including fish oils. He has 2 glasses of wine daily and does not smoke. There are no known genetic or inherited diseases in the family. He has health insurance through a health maintenance organization (HMO).

Questions

American Nurses Association Standard of Practice #5 is Implementation: *The competencies include that the nurse integrates critical thinking and technology solutions to implement the nursing process to collect, measure, record, retrieve, trend, and analyze data and information in order to enhance nursing practice and healthcare consumer outcomes.*

As you learned in Chapter 8, technology plays an important role in modern healthcare. During a visit to the clinic at the HMO, Rhett asks you if he can track his blood pressures online and send the measurements in electronically.

1. What would be the advantages and disadvantages of using technology for the purposes Rhett suggested? Include both general considerations and those unique to this client.

American Nurses Association Standard of Practice #5A is Coordination of Care: *The nurse is expected to coordinate and document care delivery and assist the client to identify options for care.*

2. In coordinating care to meet the competency, the nurse must consider if the client requires primary, secondary, or tertiary prevention as described in Chapter 5. How would you describe Rhett's needs? Is an HMO an effective insurance plan based on his history and current health status?
3. Chapter 6 discusses community-based health resources. What are some categories of community resources that may be appropriate for Rhett?
4. Chapter 7 describes home health. If Rhett requests that a nurse come to his home to check his blood pressure, how might you respond?

American Nurses Association Standard of Professional Performance #9 is Communication: *The nurse communicates effectively in all areas of practice, and in ways that are appropriate for the client's preferred style. In addition, the nurse questions processes and decisions that do not seem to support the best interests of the client.*

5. Rhett's knowledge and skill in technology may be greater than your own. How might you answer his question about online submission of blood pressure information?
6. The clinic has a policy that requires all reports of client data to be submitted in hard copy with an original signature. Does this policy meet the expected competency? If not, what action would you take next?

American Nurses Association. (2015). *Nursing: Scope and standards of practice* (3rd ed.). Silver Spring, MD: Author.

Answers to Meeting the Standards questions are available on the faculty resources site. Please consult with your instructor.

UNIT

3

The Nursing Process

Critical Thinking and Clinical Reasoning

9

LEARNING OUTCOMES

After completing this chapter, you will be able to:

1. Describe the significance of developing critical thinking abilities in order to practice safe, effective, and professional nursing care.
2. Describe the actions of clinical reasoning in the implementation of the nursing process.
3. Discuss the attitudes and skills needed to develop critical thinking and clinical reasoning.
4. Describe the components of clinical reasoning.
5. Integrate strategies to enhance critical thinking and clinical reasoning as the provider of nursing care.
6. Integrate strategies to implement clinical reasoning while caring for clients during clinical.
7. Describe the process of concept mapping to enhance critical thinking and clinical reasoning for the provision of nursing care.

KEY TERMS

clinical judgment, *181*
clinical reasoning, *177*
cognitive processes, *183*
concept mapping, *186*
creativity, *178*
critical analysis, *179*
critical thinking, *177*
deductive reasoning, *180*
inductive reasoning, *179*
intuition, *181*
metacognitive processes, *183*
nursing process, *180*
problem-solving, *181*
Socratic questioning, *179*
trial and error, *181*

Introduction

The term "thinking like a nurse" was introduced by Dr. Christine Tanner in 2006. To think like a nurse, critical thinking and clinical reasoning must be defined and understood. This chapter examines the influence of critical thinking and clinical reasoning on the care of clients. Both these terms describe the mental processes nurses use to ensure that they are doing their best thinking and decision-making. Nursing students in the clinical setting must begin to implement critical thinking and clinical reasoning to provide the most effective nursing care. Clinical experiences allow nursing students the ability to translate classroom theory and the skills learned in the nursing learning laboratory and the simulation environment. In New Zealand, Cook (2016) developed a toolkit for clinical educators to assist nursing students in the development of clinical reasoning and skill acquisition. Educating students on clinical skills in the hospital, skilled nursing facility, or the home increases their confidence and expertise.

The practice of nursing requires critical thinking and clinical reasoning. **Critical thinking** is the process of intentional higher level thinking to define a client's problem, examine the evidence-based practice in caring for the client, and make choices in the delivery of care. **Clinical reasoning** is the cognitive process that uses thinking strategies to gather and analyze client information, evaluate the relevance of the information, and decide on possible nursing actions to improve the client's physiologic and psychosocial outcomes. Clinical reasoning requires the integration of critical thinking in the identification of the most appropriate interventions that will improve the client's condition. Clinical reasoning combines both thinking and decision-making in the clinical setting. "Clinical reasoning comprises the set of reasoning strategies that permit us to combine and synthesize diverse data into one or more diagnostic hypotheses, make the complex trade-offs between the benefits and risks of tests and treatments, and formulate plans for patient management" (Cooper & Frain, 2017, p. 1). Clinical reasoning focuses on thinking processes that advance cognitive psychology for the promotion of decision-making when delivering client care. Clinical reasoning is utilized by all health-related professions.

Purpose of Critical Thinking

Critical thinking involves the differentiation of statements of fact, judgment, and opinion. The process of critical thinking requires the nurse to think ahead, to apply thinking while acting, and to think back, known as reflective thinking (Alfaro-LeFevre, 2017). Alfaro-LeFevre's 4-Circle Critical Thinking Model provides a visual representation

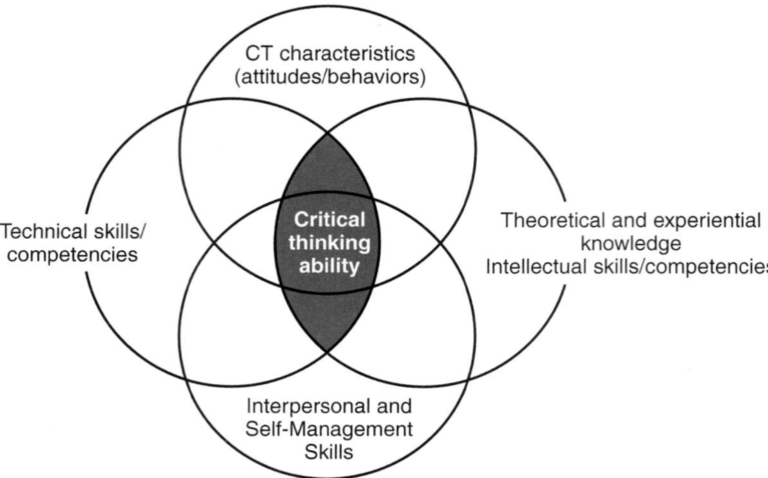

Figure 9.1 ■ Alfaro-LeFevre's 4-Circle Critical Thinking Model.
Reprinted with permission from Evidence-Based Critical Thinking Indicators available at www.alfaroteachsmart.com

of critical thinking abilities and promotes making meaningful connections between nursing research and critical thinking and practice (Figure 9.1 ■). According to Bowell and Kemp (2015), critical thinking is an evaluation of one's beliefs and actions. In critical thinking, a nurse critiques his or her thoughts to ascertain an appropriate outcome. This critique allows the nurse to make judgments, arrive at conclusions, and offer hypotheses.

Nurses use critical thinking skills in a variety of ways:

- *Nurses use knowledge from other subjects and fields.* Nurses use critical thinking skills when they reflect on knowledge derived from other interdisciplinary subject areas such as the biophysical and behavioral sciences and the humanities in order to provide holistic nursing care. For example, when providing care to a client at the end of life, it is important to have knowledge of culture and religion to enhance the delivery of culturally sensitive care and enhance the client's spiritual well-being to promote a good death.
- *Nurses deal with change in stressful environments.* A client's condition may rapidly change and routine protocol may not be adequate to cover every unexpected situation. Critical thinking enables the nurse to recognize important cues, respond quickly, and adapt interventions to meet specific client needs at the right time. Box 9.1 lists some personal critical thinking indicators.
- *Nurses make important decisions.* Every day, and every moment during the day, nurses use critical thinking skills and clinical reasoning to make judgments about a client's care. For example, determining which observations must be reported to the primary care provider immediately and which can be noted in the electronic medical record for later consultation with the primary care provider requires critical thinking. Also, clients have different health needs simultaneously. For example, a client who is experiencing an acute asthma attack with air hunger will also experience anxiety. The nurse must administer a medication to improve breathing before addressing the client's anxiety.

Critical thinking cognitively fuels the intellectual, artistic activity of creativity. When nurses incorporate creativity, they are able to find unique solutions to unique problems. **Creativity** is thinking that results in the development of new ideas and products. Creativity in problem-solving and decision-making is the ability to develop and implement new and better solutions for healthcare outcomes.

Creativity is required when the nurse encounters a new situation or a client situation in which traditional interventions are not effective. Creative thinkers must assess a problem and be knowledgeable about the underlying facts and principles that apply. An example would be a 4-year-old child who has sustained a severe burn and has been discharged from the hospital. The home care nurse has orders to soak and cleanse the wound in the bathtub. After arriving at the child's home, the nurse determines the family does not have hot water service due to an inability to pay the gas bill. The nurse warms water on the electric stove so the wound can be cleansed in the bathtub as ordered by the primary care provider. Next the nurse contacts the social worker to help the family obtain financial assistance so the gas bill can be paid and the hot water restored.

In this clinical scenario the nurse has utilized creativity by warming the water on the stove. The nurse has also utilized knowledge of the role the social worker plays in providing care to the child and family. The use of creativity provides the nurse with the ability to:

- Generate many ideas rapidly.
- Be generally flexible and natural; that is, able to change viewpoints or directions in thinking rapidly and easily.

BOX 9.1 Personal Critical Thinking Indicators: Behaviors, Attitudes, and Characteristics

- *Self-aware:* Identifies own learning, personality, and communication style preferences; clarifies biases, inclinations, strengths, and limitations; acknowledges when thinking may be influenced by emotions or self-interest.
- *Genuine/authentic:* Shows true self; demonstrates behaviors that indicate stated values.
- *Effective communicator:* Listens well (shows deep understanding of others' thoughts, feelings, and circumstances); speaks and writes with clarity (gets key points across to others).
- *Curious and inquisitive:* Asks questions; looks for reasons, explanations, and meaning; seeks new information to broaden understanding.
- *Alert to context:* Looks for changes in circumstances that warrant a need to modify approaches; investigates thoroughly when situations warrant precise, in-depth thinking.
- *Reflective and self-corrective:* Carefully considers meaning of data and interpersonal interactions, asks for feedback; corrects own thinking, is alert to potential errors by self and others, finds ways to avoid future mistakes.
- *Analytical and insightful:* Identifies relationships; expresses deep understanding.
- *Logical and intuitive:* Draws reasonable conclusions (if this is so, then it follows that . . . because . . .); uses intuition as a guide and acts on intuition only with knowledge of risks involved.
- *Confident and resilient:* Expresses faith in ability to reason and learn; overcomes problems and disappointments.
- *Honest and upright:* Looks for the truth, even if it sheds unwanted light; demonstrates integrity (adheres to moral and ethical standards; admits flaws in thinking).
- *Autonomous and responsible:* Self-directed, self-disciplined, and accepts accountability.
- *Careful and prudent:* Knows own limits—seeks help as needed; suspends or revises judgment as indicated by new or incomplete data.
- *Open and fair-minded:* Shows tolerance for different viewpoints; questions how own viewpoints are influencing thinking.
- *Sensitive to diversity:* Expresses appreciation of human differences related to values, culture, personality, or learning style preferences; adapts to preferences when feasible.
- *Creative:* Offers alternative solutions and approaches; comes up with useful ideas.
- *Realistic and practical:* Admits when things are not feasible; looks for useful solutions.
- *Proactive:* Anticipates consequences, plans ahead, acts on opportunities.
- *Courageous:* Stands up for beliefs, advocates for others, does not hide from challenges.
- *Patient and persistent:* Waits for the right moment; perseveres to achieve best results.
- *Flexible:* Changes approaches as needed to get the best results.
- *Health-oriented:* Promotes a healthy lifestyle; uses healthy behaviors to manage stress.
- *Empathetic:* Listens well; shows ability to imagine others' feelings and difficulties.
- *Improvement-oriented (self, patients, systems):* Self—identifies learning needs; finds ways to overcome limitations, seeks out new knowledge. Patients—Promotes healthcare systems; maximizes function, comfort, and convenience. Systems—Identifies risks and problems with healthcare systems; promotes safety, quality, satisfaction, and cost-containment.

Reprinted with permission from Evidence-Based Critical Thinking Indicators available at www.alfaroteachsmart.com

- Create original solutions to problems.
- Be independent and self-confident, even when under pressure.
- Demonstrate individuality.

Techniques of Critical Thinking

The techniques used to ensure effective problem-solving and decision-making include critical analysis, inductive and deductive reasoning, making valid inferences, differentiating facts from opinions, evaluating the credibility of information sources, clarifying concepts, and recognizing assumptions.

Critical analysis is the application of a set of questions to a particular situation or idea to determine essential information and ideas and discard unimportant information and ideas. The questions are not sequential steps; rather they are a set of criteria for judging an idea. Not all questions will need to be applied to every situation, but one should be aware of all of the questions in order to choose those questions appropriate to a given situation.

Socrates was a Greek philosopher who developed the method of posing questions and seeking an answer. **Socratic questioning** is a technique one can use to look beneath the surface, recognize and examine assumptions, search for inconsistencies, examine multiple points of view, and differentiate what one knows from what one merely believes. Box 9.2 lists Socratic questions to use in critical analysis. Nurses should employ Socratic questioning when reporting about a client's condition and current status, reviewing a client's history and progress notes, and planning care.

Two other critical thinking skills are inductive and deductive reasoning. In **inductive reasoning**, generalizations are formed from a set of facts or observations. When viewed together, certain bits of information suggest a particular interpretation. Inductive reasoning moves from specific examples (premises) to a generalized conclusion—for example, after touching several hot flames (premise), we conclude that *all* flames are hot. A nurse who observes a client who has dry skin, poor turgor, sunken eyes, and dark amber urine and who is determined to be dehydrated (premise) concludes that the presence of those signs in other clients indicates that they are dehydrated.

BOX 9.2 Socratic Questions

QUESTIONS ABOUT THE DECISION (OR PROBLEM)
- Is this question clear, understandable, and correctly identified?
- Is this question important?
- Could this question be broken down into smaller parts?
- How might ____________ state this question?

QUESTIONS ABOUT ASSUMPTIONS
- You seem to be assuming ____________; is that so?
- What could you assume instead? Why?
- Does this assumption always hold true?

QUESTIONS ABOUT POINT OF VIEW
- You seem to be using the perspective of ____________. Why?
- What would someone who disagrees with your perspective say?
- Can you see this any other way?

QUESTIONS ABOUT EVIDENCE AND REASONS
- What evidence do you have for that?
- Is there any reason to doubt the evidence?
- How do you know?
- What would change your mind?

QUESTIONS ABOUT IMPLICATIONS AND CONSEQUENCES
- What effect would that have?
- What is the probability that will actually happen?
- What are the alternatives?

Deductive reasoning, by contrast, is reasoning from general premise to the specific conclusion. If you begin with the premise that the sum of the angles in any triangle is always 180 degrees, you can conclude that the sum of the angles in the triangle you happen to have is also 180 degrees. A nurse might start with a premise that all children love peanut butter sandwiches. Thus, if the nurse is trying to encourage a child to eat, then the nurse should offer the child a peanut butter sandwich. This is an example in which the premise is not always valid and, thus, the conclusion also may not be valid. Nurses use critical thinking to help analyze situations and establish which premises are valid.

In critical thinking, the nurse also differentiates statements of fact, inference, judgment, and opinion. Table 9.1 shows how these statements may be applied to nursing care. Evaluating the credibility of information sources is an important step in critical thinking. Unfortunately, we cannot always believe what we read or are told. The nurse must ascertain the accuracy of information by checking other documents or with other informants. Hence, the expanding need for evidence-based nursing practice. To comprehend a client situation clearly, the nurse and the client must agree on the meaning of terms. For example, if the client says to the nurse, "I think I have a tumor," the nurse needs to clarify what the word means to the client—the medical definition of a tumor (a solid mass) or the common lay meaning of cancer—before responding. People also live their lives under certain assumptions. Some people view humans as having a basically generous nature, whereas others believe that the human tendency is to act in their own best interest. The nurse may believe that life should be considered worth living no matter what the condition, whereas the client may believe that quality of life is more important than quantity of life. If the nurse and client recognize that they make choices based on these assumptions, they can still work together toward an acceptable plan of care. Difficulty arises when people do not take the time to consider what assumptions underlie their beliefs and actions.

Applying Critical Thinking to Nursing Practice

When a nurse uses intentional thinking, a relationship develops among the knowledge, skills, and attitudes that are ascribed to critical thinking and clinical reasoning, the nursing process, and the problem-solving process.

Implementation of the nursing process provides nurses with a creative approach to thinking and doing to obtain, categorize, and analyze client data and plan actions that will meet the client's needs. The **nursing process** is a systematic, rational method of planning and providing individualized nursing care. It begins with assessment of the client and use of clinical reasoning to identify client problems. The phases of the nursing process are assessing, diagnosing, planning, implementing, and evaluating. These phases are described in detail in Chapters 10 through 14 ∞.

TABLE 9.1 Differentiating Types of Statements

Statement	Description	Example
Facts	Can be verified through investigation	Blood pressure is affected by blood volume.
Inferences	Conclusions drawn from the facts; going beyond facts to make a statement about something not currently known	If blood volume is decreased (e.g., in hemorrhagic shock), the blood pressure will drop.
Judgments	Evaluation of facts or information that reflects values or other criteria; a type of opinion	It is harmful to the client's health if the blood pressure drops too low.
Opinions	Beliefs formed over time; include judgments that may fit facts or be erroneous	Nursing interventions can assist in maintaining the client's blood pressure within normal limits.

Problem-Solving

Problem-solving is a mental activity in which a problem is identified that represents an unsteady state. It requires the nurse to obtain information that clarifies the nature of the problem and suggests possible solutions. Throughout the problem-solving process, the implementation of critical thought may or may not be required in working toward a solution (Wilkinson, 2012). The nurse carefully evaluates the possible solutions and chooses the best one to implement. The situation is carefully monitored over time to ensure that its initial and continued effectiveness returns the client to a steady state. The nurse does not discard the other solutions, but holds them in reserve in the event that the first solution is not effective. Therefore, problem-solving for one situation contributes to the nurse's body of knowledge for problem-solving in similar situations. Commonly used approaches to problem-solving include trial and error, intuition, and the research process.

Trial and Error

One way to solve problems is through **trial and error**, in which a number of approaches are tried until a solution is found. However, without considering alternatives systematically, one cannot know why the solution works. The use of trial-and-error methods in nursing care can be dangerous because the client might suffer harm if an approach is inappropriate. However, nurses often use trial and error in the home setting due to logistics, equipment, and client lifestyle. For example, when teaching a client to perform a colostomy irrigation, a bent coat hanger hung on the shower curtain rod provides an appropriate height to perform the irrigation. In the hospital setting a lowered IV pole is more likely utilized.

Intuition

Intuition is a problem-solving approach that relies on a nurse's inner sense. It is a legitimate aspect of a nursing judgment in the implementation of care (Wilkinson, 2012). Intuition is the understanding or learning of things without the conscious use of reasoning. It is also known as sixth sense, hunch, instinct, feeling, or suspicion. As a problem-solving approach, intuition is viewed by some people as a form of guessing and, as such, an inappropriate basis for nursing decisions. However, others view intuition as an essential and legitimate aspect of clinical judgment acquired through knowledge and experience. **Clinical judgment** in nursing is a decision-making process to ascertain the right nursing action to be implemented at the appropriate time in the client's care. The nurse must first have the knowledge base necessary to practice in the clinical area and then use that knowledge in clinical practice. Clinical experience allows the nurse to recognize cues and patterns and begin to reach correct conclusions.

Experience is important in improving intuition because the rapidity of the judgment depends on the nurse having seen similar client situations many times before. Sometimes nurses use the words "I had a feeling" to describe the critical thinking element of considering evidence. These nurses are able to judge quickly which evidence is most important and to act on that limited evidence. Nurses in critical care often pay closer attention than usual to a client when they sense that the client's condition could change suddenly.

Although the intuitive method of problem-solving is gaining recognition as part of nursing practice, it is not recommended for novices or students, because they usually lack the knowledge base and clinical experience on which to make a valid judgment.

Research Process

The research process, discussed in Chapter 2 ∞, is a formalized, logical, systematic approach to problem-solving. The classic quantitative research process is most useful when the researcher is working in a controlled situation. Health professionals, often working with people in uncontrolled situations, require a modified approach for solving problems. For example, unlike many experiments with animals in which the environment can be strictly regulated, the effects of diet on health in humans are complicated by an individual's genetic variations, lifestyle, and personal preferences. However, it is becoming increasingly important for nurses to identify evidence that supports effective nursing care. One critical source of this evidence is research.

Attitudes That Foster Critical Thinking

Certain attitudes are crucial to critical thinking. These attitudes are based on the assumption that a rational individual is motivated to develop, learn, grow, and be concerned with what to do or believe. A critical thinker works to develop the following nine attitudes or traits: independence, fair-mindedness, insight, intellectual humility, intellectual courage, integrity, perseverance, confidence, and curiosity.

Independence

Critical thinking requires that individuals think for themselves. People acquire many beliefs as children, not necessarily based on reason but in order to have an explanation they comprehend. As they mature and acquire knowledge and experience, critical thinkers examine their beliefs in the light of new evidence. Critical thinkers consider seriously a wide range of ideas, learn from them, and then make their own judgments about them. Nurses are open-minded about considering different methods of performing technical skills—not just the single way they may have been taught in school. Nurses should not ignore what other people think, but they should consider a wide range of ideas, learn from them, and then take the time to build their own judgments (Wilkinson, 2012).

Fair-Mindedness

Critical thinkers are fair-minded and make impartial judgments. They assess all viewpoints with the same standards and do not base their judgments on personal or group bias or prejudice (Wilkinson, 2012). Fair-mindedness helps one to consider opposing points of view and to try to understand new ideas fully before rejecting or accepting them. Critical thinkers strive to be open to the possibility that new evidence could change their minds. The nurse listens to the opinions of all members of a family, young and old. Sometimes the traditional approach will emerge as the most effective strategy, whereas at other times a new and possibly unproven approach should be tried. In every case, the nurse must be able to provide the rationale for any action taken.

Insight into Egocentricity

Critical thinkers are open to the possibility that their personal biases or social pressures and customs could unduly affect their thinking. They actively try to examine their own biases and bring them to awareness each time they think or make a decision. By failing to reflect on personal biases, the nurse may reach inappropriate conclusions for the individual client. For example, a nurse spends extensive time teaching a client who is obese about nutrition and weight loss to prevent recurrence of back pain, but is mystified when the client appears uninterested and does not follow the nurse's advice. The nurse's bias of assuming that all clients will incorporate preventive care (just because the nurse would do this) resulted in an inaccurate assessment of the client's motivation; both the nurse's and the client's time was wasted. Possibly, the client's cultural views of weight are different from those of the nurse. Had the nurse assessed the client's background and beliefs about weight and collected sufficient evidence, the nurse might have identified a problem more relevant to the client's priorities and, thus, developed a better care plan.

Intellectual Humility

Intellectual humility means having an awareness of the limits of one's own knowledge. Critical thinkers are willing to admit what they do not know; they are willing to seek new information and to rethink their conclusions in light of new knowledge. They never assume that what everybody believes to be right will always be right, because new evidence may emerge. A hospital nurse might be unable to imagine how an older adult's wife will care for her husband who has recently had a stroke. However, the nurse also recognizes that it is not really possible to know what the couple can achieve.

Intellectual Courage to Challenge the Status Quo and Rituals

With an attitude of courage, a nurse is willing to consider and examine fairly his or her own ideas or views, especially those to which the nurse may have a strongly negative reaction. This type of courage comes from recognizing that beliefs are sometimes false or misleading. Values and beliefs are not always acquired rationally. Rational beliefs are those that have been examined and found to be supported by solid reasons and data. After such examination, it is inevitable that some beliefs previously held to be true will be found to contain questionable elements and that some truth will emerge from ideas considered dangerous or false. Courage is needed to be true to new thinking in such cases, especially if social penalties for nonconformity are severe. For example, many nurses previously believed that allowing family members to observe emergency procedures (such as cardiopulmonary resuscitation) would be psychologically harmful to the family and that members would get in the healthcare team's way. Others felt that blanket exclusion of family members was unnecessary and extremely stressful for some of them. As a result, nurses initiated research that has demonstrated that family presence can be accomplished without detrimental effects to the nurse, the client, or the family. This is also an example of how evidence, rather than just tradition, guides our nursing practice.

Integrity

Intellectual integrity requires that individuals apply the same rigorous standards of proof to their own knowledge and beliefs as they apply to the knowledge and beliefs of others. Critical thinkers question their own knowledge and beliefs as quickly and thoroughly as they challenge those of another. They are readily able to admit and evaluate inconsistencies within their own beliefs and between their own beliefs and those of another. A nurse might believe that wound care always requires sterile technique. Reading a new article on the use and outcomes of clean technique for some wounds leads the critically thinking nurse to reconsider.

Perseverance

Because critical thinking is a lifelong endeavor, nurses who are critical thinkers show perseverance in finding effective solutions to client and nursing problems. This determination enables them to clarify concepts and sort out related issues, in spite of difficulties and frustrations. Confusion and frustration are uncomfortable, but critical thinkers resist the temptation to find a quick and easy answer. Important questions tend to be complex and confusing and therefore often require a great deal of thought and research to arrive at an answer. The nurse needs to continue to address the issue until it is resolved. For example, the nurses on a unit have tried to establish a policy for selected clients to leave the hospital on a pass rather than have to be discharged and readmitted in the same day. The need for involvement of nursing, medical, administrative, and accounting staff gradually generates solutions to obstacles. The development of the policy moves forward, although very slowly.

Confidence

Critical thinkers believe that well-reasoned thinking will lead to trustworthy conclusions. Therefore, they cultivate an attitude of confidence in the reasoning process and examine emotion-laden arguments using the standards for evaluating thought, by asking questions such as these: Is that argument fair? Is it based on sufficient evidence? Consider nurses attempting to determine the best way to allocate holiday time off for staff. Should they go by seniority, use random selection (lottery), give preference to those who have children, use "first-come, first-served," or use another method?

The critical thinker develops skill in both inductive reasoning and deductive reasoning. As the nurse gains greater awareness of the thinking process and more experience in improving such thinking, confidence in the process will grow. This nurse will not be afraid of disagreement and indeed will be concerned when others agree too quickly. Such a nurse can serve as a role model to colleagues, inspiring and encouraging them to think critically as well.

Curiosity

The mind of a critical thinker is filled with questions: Why do we believe this? What causes that? Does it have to be this way? Could something else work? What would happen if we did it another way? Who says that is so? The curious nurse may value tradition but is not afraid to examine traditions to be sure they are still valid. The nurse may, for example, apply these questions to the issue of moving responsibility for a procedure such as the drawing of arterial blood samples among the nursing, respiratory therapy, or laboratory department staff.

Components of Clinical Reasoning

"Clinical reasoning describes the thinking and decision-making processes associated with clinical practice" (Cooper & Frain, 2017, p. 1). Clinical reasoning is the analysis of a clinical situation as it unfolds or develops. It requires the nurse to use cognitive and metacognitive processes. **Cognitive processes** are the thinking processes based on the knowledge of aspects of client care. Cognitive skills are learned through reading and applying health-related literature. Cognitive skills are enhanced through the use of critical thought to understand and apply content the nurse has previously learned. **Metacognitive processes** include reflective thinking and awareness of the skills learned by the nurse in caring for the client. The nurse reflects on the client's status, and through the use of critical thinking skills determines the most effective plan of care.

Benner, Sutphen, Leonard, and Day (2010) state that thinking like a nurse requires clinical reasoning (p. 85). They identify clinical reasoning as the ability to reason about a clinical situation as it unfolds (p. 46). It is important for the nurse to be "tuned in" to the client's experiences and concerns. As the client's condition changes, the nurse must assess the client and then identify the interventions that will lead to the improvement of the client's health-related outcomes. Changes in a client's condition can occur in an instant. It is the responsibility of the nurse to detect these changes, implement nursing assessments and interventions, notify members of the healthcare team, and evaluate the client's response. Benner et al. (2010) describe the components of clinical reasoning to include setting priorities, developing rationales, learning how to act, clinical reasoning-in-transition, and responding to changes in the client's condition. It is also important to reflect on the care provided and the client's response.

Setting Priorities

In the current nursing world, nurses have to think quickly to resolve problems. As a nursing student entering clinical, it is important to organize the care to be provided by organizing the clinical day. The nursing student sets priorities, is flexible, and understands the day may be subject to change (Berman & Snyder, 2012). In the often fast-paced clinical environment, the nurse must know what assessments, tasks, requests, and concerns need to be completed first. Priority setting needs to be dynamic or flexible, because the clinical environment can change quickly, requiring changes in priorities. Beginning nursing students often view everything as being of equal importance. They are often task oriented and focused on what needs to be done and not necessarily on what is most important. As they gain more clinical experience, they start to determine which data are most relevant and important to each client's situation. Most nursing programs require beginning students to complete preclinical preparation. This is a strategy to help them set their priorities based on information they gathered before the actual clinical experience. It is important for students to remember that, once they begin providing client care, the priorities they set in the preclinical preparation may change based on the *current* client situation. See Box 9.3 for a case analysis linking the knowledge gained in fundamentals of nursing and pathophysiology to increase clinical reasoning skills in the provision of care to the client.

Clinical reasoning was initially introduced to the healthcare disciplines by medicine, physical therapy, and occupational therapy. Since that time, the nursing profession has applied these strategies to enhance client care. Michele Wojciechowski wrote the article "How to Improve Clinical Reasoning Skills" in 2016. Contributors to this article provided strategies to build healthcare practitioners' clinical reasoning skills. Gail Jansen is the graduate dean and professor of physical therapy at Creighton University. According to Jansen, clinical reasoning involves the knowledge acquired during the healthcare professional's education. Clinical reasoning and knowledge development go hand in hand. With clinical reasoning, the nurse must analyze nursing actions through critical thought. The nurse critiques his or her actions. This process allows the nurse to critically think about the care provided and

BOX 9.3 Development of Clinical Reasoning Skills

How does your knowledge of fundamental nursing care lead to clinical reasoning?

- The knowledge gained in fundamentals of nursing allows you to provide safe and effective nursing care.

CASE ONE

Case Analysis: Rosalind Meyer is 87 years old and resides in a nursing home. Three years ago she suffered a stroke, which left her paralyzed on the right side. She has since sustained contractures of her left hand and left foot. During her bath you notice a distinct foul-smelling odor that is most notable near her left hand. While cleaning her left hand yellow drainage is noted on the washcloth.

How does your knowledge of nursing fundamentals lead to clinical reasoning?

Nursing Action:

- Reflect on the nursing care implemented for a client with contractures of paralyzed hands.
- Determine the assessments to be implemented.
- Reflect on the interventions to implement when there is an alteration of skin integrity.

Implementation of Interventions:

- Inspect the right hand for a wound.
- You note a wound on the client's palm. You culture, measure, and cleanse the wound and notify the primary care provider.
- The primary care provider has ordered polyurethane foam applied to the wound with a secondary dressing applied over the foam. You dress the wound.
- Assess wound healing with every dressing change.
- Apply a rolled washcloth in the hand to prevent pressure.
- Consult with the occupational therapist to construct a splint to prevent pressure from the contracted hand.

How does your knowledge of pathophysiology lead to clinical reasoning?

- Knowledge of the client's diagnosis and the pathophysiology of the client's disease will assist you in knowing the progression of the disease and interventions implemented to assist the client to a resolution of symptoms.

CASE TWO

Case Analysis: Elijah Gastopolis is admitted to the telemetry division with a diagnosis of heart failure. He has fluid volume excess, shortness of breath, and a rapid heart rate.

Nursing Action:

- Reflect on the interventions that should be implemented to improve the client's cardiac output.
- Reflect on the care provided to other clients with similar symptoms.
- Review pharmacologic agents that will improve the client's heart failure.
- Reflect on the health assessments to be implemented.

Implementation of Interventions:

- Assess the cardiac rate and rhythm, peripheral vascular pulses, pedal edema, increased abdominal girth, respiratory rate, lung sounds, and signs and symptoms of dyspnea.
- Administer a low-sodium diet.
- Consult with the primary care provider to determine pharmacologic therapy.
- Administer furosemide (a potassium-depleting diuretic).
- Administer cardioglycosides to improve cardiac output.

develop conclusions as to why it was or was not effective in relieving symptoms. Through the analysis of nursing actions and the outcomes of care, the nurse can identify errors in care and make changes as necessary in delivering care to future clients in similar circumstances. When caring for a future client with similar issues, the nurse is then able to reflect and reason to provide the best possible nursing action to benefit client outcomes. Box 9.3 enables you to apply the knowledge you are gaining in your education toward the development of clinical reasoning skills.

When caring for a client in the home, it is important to apply the following clinical reasoning skills.

- Interview the home care client in a nonthreatening and relaxing setting.
- When describing the client's chief complaint, utilize the client's own words.
- Inform the primary care provider of the client's physiologic and psychologic status.
- Consult with other healthcare team members to determine if they have experience with clients who have had similar health problems whose conditions changed. In collaboration with the healthcare team, determine the priority interventions to be implemented.
- Evaluate the outcome of the interventions implemented.
- If the client's status has not improved, consult the healthcare team and implement clinical reasoning strategies to address the client's health-related outcomes.

Developing Rationales

After assessing the data and determining what is relevant to the client's condition and concerns, the nurse identifies interventions and sets priorities for the most urgent needs (Benner et al., 2010). This is when the nurse transfers nursing knowledge to the clinical situation to justify the plan of care. Nursing students are often asked to explain the "why" of their priority setting and subsequent interventions. Being able to state the rationale, based on nursing knowledge, acts as a check for potential errors, justifies the nurse's actions, contributes to client safety, and helps the beginning nursing student learn how a nurse thinks in practice.

Learning How to Act

The nurse must know how and when to respond in a clinical situation by recognizing what is most urgent or significant. To take action, the nurse needs to understand the

EVIDENCE-BASED PRACTICE

Evidence-Based Practice

How Do Prelicensure Nursing Students Perceive Their Development of Clinical Reasoning?

Herron, Sudia, Kimble, and Davis (2016) conducted a qualitative study with prelicensure nursing students. They interviewed nursing students to collect data related to their perceptions of their development of clinical reasoning skills. Three themes emerged from this study: the characteristics of clinical reasoning, the importance of clinical reasoning, and the best place to learn their clinical reasoning skills. The students understood the importance of clinical reasoning and its connection to maintaining safe and effective clinical practice. They also reported that their clinical experiences were most beneficial in developing clinical reasoning skills.

Implications

As students understand the reason for the development of clinical reasoning skills, they can then reflect on care they have provided to clients and ascertain ways to improve care based on past experiences. In addition, faculty members can implement teaching strategies that improve students' clinical reasoning skills.

relevant medical and nursing information and translate this knowledge into a plan of care (Benner et al., 2010). An example is thinking about potential complications given the client's current problems. Applying this knowledge increases the nurse's ability to quickly identify assessment data that indicate a potential complication. Thus, the nurse can initiate nursing interventions or actions quickly because he or she prepared for the possibility. Avoiding potential complications promotes client safety.

Clinical Reasoning-in-Transition

It is important to realize that clinical situations are complex and always changing, especially given the acuity level of clients in today's hospital settings. Clinical reasoning-in-transition is the ability to recognize subtle changes in a client's condition over time. It includes the evaluation of nursing interventions and the trending of relevant assessment data. Nurses need to develop a sense of what is most important in each changing clinical situation and remember that the primary focus is on the client's well-being.

Responding to Changes in the Client's Condition

Nurses spend more time with clients than do other healthcare providers. As a result, an important aspect of nursing practice and the nurse's responsibility is to detect changes in the client's condition, recognize a need to change priorities, adjust nursing care, and alert the primary care provider when appropriate.

Clinical reasoning involves an understanding and assessment of the client's relevant history and current condition and how it may be changing. By closely monitoring and comparing any changes from previous assessment data, the nurse is able to recognize a change in status that may prevent an adverse outcome.

Reflection

Reflection is a key to the success of clinical reasoning. Through reflection the nurse identifies factors that improved client care and those that required changing or elimination. It is important to reflect on whether the client was assessed accurately and in a timely manner. The nurse thinks back on the interventions implemented and whether they were effective. Most importantly, reflection includes information on the outcome of care. The nurse also reflects on previous clinical experiences similar to this one to determine if the outcomes of care improved the clients' conditions.

Integration of Critical Thinking and Clinical Reasoning

Nurses use critical thinking and clinical reasoning skills when making decisions about client care. The decision-making process includes prioritizing care not only with one client but when providing care to many clients. Nurses must make decisions and also assist clients to make decisions. When faced with several client needs at the same time, the nurse must prioritize and decide which client to assist first.

In the home care setting, the nurse must decide if the client's condition can be managed in the home or requires hospitalization. The nurse must assess the ability of the caregiver and client to understand and follow all aspects of the healthcare teaching the nurse has provided.

The nurse must consider the client's cultural and religious background because both influence the outcomes of care. For example, in some cultures, it is traditional for female relatives to care for a new baby, thus allowing the new mother time to rest. If the nurse fails to review cultural practices and insists that the new mother provide the parenting, then the nurse has not utilized critical thought in the process of clinical reasoning during the implementation of care.

Logical reasoning is a critical thinking skill that closely aligns with clinical reasoning. In the planning of care, nurses must question whether knowledge they possess about the care of the client is consistent with the most current evidence-based practice. The nurse must review the most current nursing and health-related literature prior to implementing care.

Dalton, Gee, and Levett-Jones (2015) utilized a flipped curriculum approach to develop and extend students' clinical reasoning skills through the implementation of simulated clinical learning environments. The use of simulation allows the nursing student to think like a nurse. Laboratory simulations also enhance safe client care. A nurse's ability to accurately implement and integrate critical thinking, clinical judgment, and clinical reasoning is enhanced with a commitment to lifelong learning.

Concept Mapping

Concept mapping is a technique that uses a graphic depiction of nonlinear and linear relationships to represent critical thinking. Also known as *mind mapping*, concept maps are context dependent and can be used to develop analytical skills. The attributes of the concept are linked, making meaning of the concept they represent. Concept maps provide an opportunity to visualize things in your own way (Alfaro-LeFevre, 2016). The concept map allows the nurse to map words on a page and focus on concepts and relationships. A general benefit of these maps is that they are quicker than note taking and highlight key ideas (Alfaro-LeFevre, 2016). This text contains more than a dozen concept maps that demonstrate care planning and physiologic processes.

Concept Mapping and Enhancing Critical Thinking and Clinical Reasoning

In planning the care delivered to clients and their families, it is important to plan and organize nursing care (Schuster, 2016). Concept mapping provides nurses with a link between existing nursing knowledge and new information. This learning strategy requires critical thinking and can assist the nursing student in understanding complex concepts (Schuster, 2016). Concept maps often begin with the client's principle physiologic or psychosocial problem. The nursing student learns to establish a diagram of signs and symptoms that interrelate to those physiologic and psychosocial problems. The assessment data gathered by the nurse or nursing student also are interrelated concepts that contribute to the development of the concept map. Shapes as seen in Figure 9.2 ■ show the interrelationship of the concepts. Rather than address one single client problem, the concept map can incorporate multiple problems. This allows the nurse to demonstrate interrelationships among a client's problems and determine care based on the complexity of those problems (Billings & Halstead, 2016). Thus, concept mapping may be a valuable tool to improve critical thinking. Four basic types of maps are described in Box 9.4 and Figure 9.2 ■. Figure 9.3 ■ provides a concept map for preparation of the clinical day.

BOX 9.4 Types of Concept Maps

- Hierarchical maps—concept and attributes arranged in a hierarchical pattern and typically constructed in a descending order of importance. Relationships are identified between and among a concept and its attributes (see Figure 9.2A)
- Spider maps—depict the interrelatedness of the concept and its attributes in the map (see Figure 9.2B)
- Flowchart maps—linear diagrams demonstrating sequence or cause-and-effect relations (see Figure 9.2C)
- Systems maps—inputs and outputs illustrate relationships among the concept and its attributes (see Figure 9.2D)

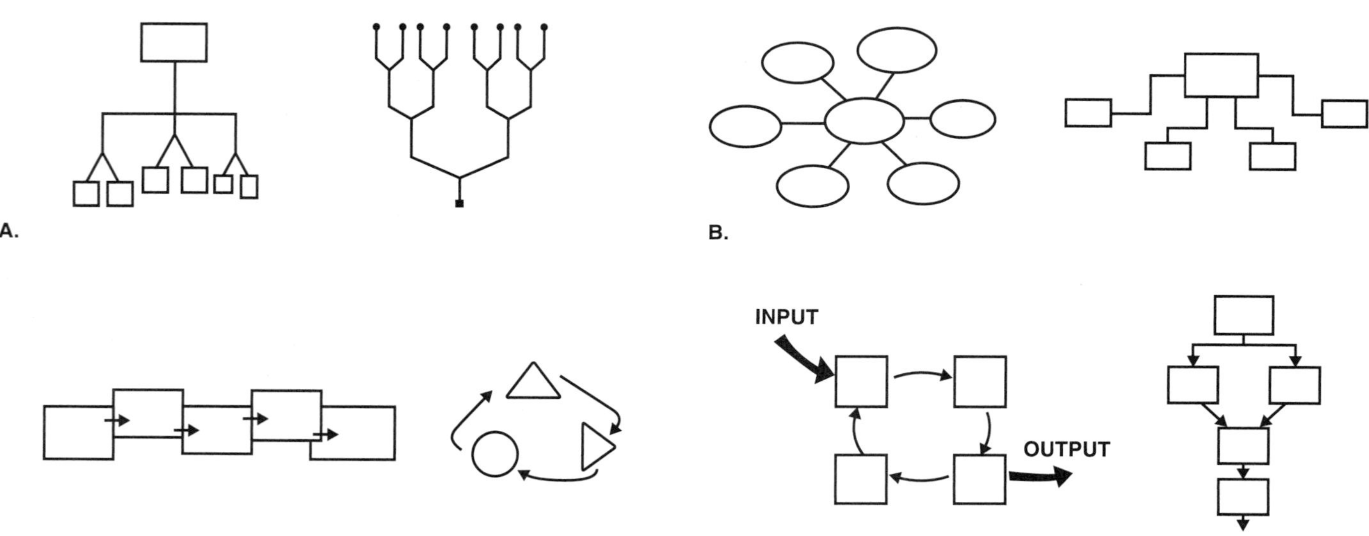

Figure 9.2 ■ Types of concept maps: *A*, hierarchical, *B*, spider, *C*, flowchart, *D*, systems.

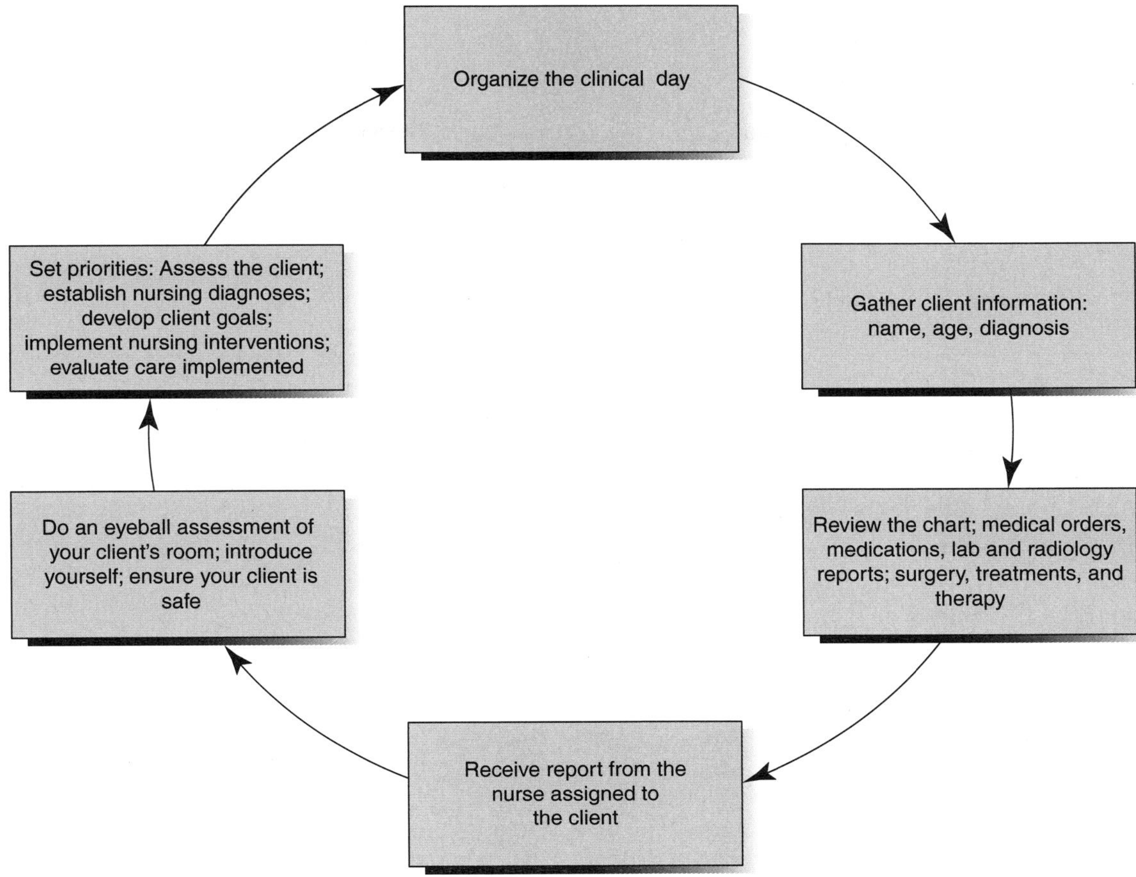

Figure 9.3 ■ Concept map: planning for the clinical day.

LIFESPAN CONSIDERATIONS Healthcare Decisions

CHILDREN

Parents most often make decisions about the healthcare of children. Growing children, however, can participate in those decisions in age-appropriate ways. As described by Piaget, the ability of children to reason and think critically about themselves and their situation develops gradually (see Chapter 24 ∞). At each stage, nurses should be aware of the ways children think and be sensitive to how they can be involved in healthcare decisions:

- Infants progress from reflexive behavior to simple, repetitive behavior and then to imitative behaviors, learning the concepts of cause and effect and object permanence. Though not involved in making decisions, they need to be comforted and secure as care is given.
- Toddlers and preschoolers are very egocentric and engage in magical thinking. They cannot reason out the implications of care, but need explanations in language they can understand. Play therapy and use of dolls and toys can help them adjust to care, and they can sometimes be given options (e.g., do you want your dressing changed before breakfast or after?).
- School-age children tend to be concrete thinkers. They benefit from simple, direct explanations; hands-on exploration of equipment and materials; and helping the care provider as appropriate during procedures. Involving these children in care can increase cooperation and decrease anxiety.
- Adolescents are increasingly able to think abstractly and may make many of their own healthcare decisions. They should be actively consulted as a part of the family system.

OLDER ADULTS

It is important to include all adult clients in decision making and planning nursing care. However, it is especially difficult to do this when working with older adults who have impaired cognitive abilities as is seen with, for example, Alzheimer disease. The nurse should allow them as much control and input as possible, keeping things simple and direct so they understand. Older adults with impairments are usually unable to perform multiple tasks or even to think of more than one step at a time. The nurse must have patience and be willing to calmly repeat instructions if necessary. Presenting and discussing issues in basic terms helps to maintain respect and dignity and allows older adults to participate in their own care for as long as possible. If the older adult is unable to perform self-care activities such as bathing or health-related activities such as a dressing change, the nurse should seek appropriate alternative methods for assisting the older adult with these.

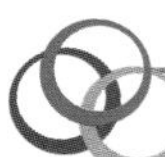

Critical Thinking Checkpoint

Mr. W. is a 63-year-old recently retired engineer with a history of irritable bowel syndrome that causes frequent diarrhea and rectal bleeding. His wife is a schoolteacher. In mid-December he comes to the acute care clinic complaining about "not feeling good." You conclude he is having a recurrence of his intestinal problem.

1. What questions would you ask yourself to check this assumption?
2. How would you demonstrate that you are using the critical thinking attitude of "confidence in reasoning"?
3. Socrates might ask you about the consequences of your conclusion by posing the question "What are the implications of your thinking?" How would you answer? Consider the implications if you are correct and if you are incorrect in your assumption.
4. Critical thinkers look for subtle cues. Which cues in this situation require follow-up?

Answers to Critical Thinking Checkpoint questions are available on the faculty resources site. Please consult with your instructor.

Chapter 9 Review

CHAPTER HIGHLIGHTS

- Nurses need critical thinking skills and attitudes to be safe, competent, skillful practitioners.
- Nurses use clinical reasoning skills to assess each client's condition and identify interventions that improve clients' physiologic and psychosocial outcomes.
- Creativity enhances critical thinking. Creative nurses generate many ideas rapidly, are flexible and natural, create original solutions to problems, tend to be independent and self-confident, and demonstrate individuality.
- Critical thinking skills include the ability to do critical analysis, perform inductive and deductive reasoning, make valid inferences, differentiate facts and opinions, evaluate the credibility of information sources, clarify concepts, and recognize assumptions.
- Critical thinkers have certain attitudes: independence, fair-mindedness, insight, intellectual humility, intellectual courage to challenge the status quo and rituals, integrity, perseverance, confidence, and curiosity.
- Nurses utilize cognitive processes in clinical reasoning, and their thinking is based on the knowledge of the aspects of client care.
- Nurses also utilize metacognitive processes in clinical reasoning through the knowledge they gain in the care of clients.
- Clinical reasoning-in-transition is the ability to recognize subtle changes in a client's condition over time.
- Reflection is the identification of factors that improve clients' care.

TEST YOUR KNOWLEDGE

1. Nurses must use critical thinking in their day-to-day practice, especially in circumstances surrounding client care and wise use of resources. In which of the following situations would critical thinking be most beneficial?
   1. Administering IV push meds to critically ill clients
   2. Educating a home health client about treatment options
   3. Teaching new parents car seat safety
   4. Assisting an orthopedic client with the proper use of crutches
2. A client reports feeling hungry, but does not eat when food is served. Using clinical reasoning skills, the nurse should perform which of the following?
   1. Assess why the client is not ingesting the food provided.
   2. Continue to leave the food at the bedside until the client is hungry enough to eat.
   3. Notify the primary care provider that tube feeding may be indicated soon.
   4. Believe the client is not really hungry.
3. A client complains of shortness of breath. During assessment the nurse observes that the client has edema of the left leg only. The nurse reviews evidence-based practice literature and reflects on a previous client with the same clinical manifestations. What do these actions represent?
   1. Clinical judgment
   2. Clinical reasoning
   3. Reflection
   4. Intuition
4. The client who is short of breath benefits from the head of the bed being elevated. Because this position can result in skin breakdown in the sacral area, the nurse decides to study the amount of sacral pressure occurring in other positions. What decision-making is the nurse engaging in?
   1. The research method
   2. The trial-and-error method
   3. Intuition
   4. The nursing process

5. A nurse enters the room of a critically ill child and has a sense that "something" isn't right. After performing an initial physical assessment and finding that the child is stable, the nurse continues to perform a check of all the lines and equipment in the room and finds that the last IV solution hung by the previous nurse was not the correct solution. This nurse was utilizing which method of problem solving?
1. Trial and error
2. Intuition
3. Judgment
4. Scientific method

6. The nurse is concerned about a client who begins to breathe very rapidly. Which action by the nurse reflects clinical reasoning?
1. Notify the primary care provider.
2. Obtain vital signs and oxygen saturation.
3. Request a chest x-ray.
4. Call the rapid response team.

7. The nurse is teaching a client about wound care during a follow-up visit in the client's home. Which critical thinking attitude causes the nurse to reconsider the plan and supports evidence-based practice when the client states, "I just don't know how I can afford these dressings"?
1. Integrity
2. Intellectual humility
3. Confidence
4. Independence

8. In which of the following responses does a nurse's understanding of the importance of critical thinking in today's nursing profession come through? Select all that apply.
1. "Patient acuity is so much greater than it was even 10 years ago."
2. "Care delivery systems are only as good as the nurses delivering care."
3. "Nurses have always relied on common sense thinking to provide quality, appropriate nursing care."
4. "With health care being so expensive, nursing has to take on responsibility to keep the costs controlled."
5. "My practice involves caring for clients who require care that didn't even exist when I went to school."

9. A client in a cardiac rehabilitation program says to the nurse, "I have to eat a low-sodium diet for the rest of my life, and I hate it!" Which is the most appropriate response by the nurse?
1. "I will get a dietary consult to talk to you before next week."
2. "What do you think is so difficult about following a low-sodium diet?"
3. "At least you survived a heart attack and are able to return to work."
4. "You may not need to follow a low-sodium diet for as long as you think."

10. Which reasoning process describes the nurse's actions when the nurse evaluates possible solutions for care of an infected wound for optimal client outcomes?
1. Intuition
2. Research process
3. Trial and error
4. Problem-solving

See Answers to Test Your Knowledge in Appendix A.

READINGS AND REFERENCES

Suggested Reading

Georg, C., Karlgren, K., Ulfvarson, J., Jirwe, M., & Welin, E. (2018). A rubric to assess students' clinical reasoning when encountering virtual patients. *Journal of Nursing Education*, *57*(7), 408–415. doi:10.3928/01484834-20180618-05
This research article utilized deductive and abductive analyses with the Lasater Clinical Judgement Rubric to assess the clinical reasoning skills of nursing students during virtual patient simulation. The adapted rubric can be used to assess students' clinical reasoning process and provide feedback for learning when encountering virtual patients during simulation.

Related Research

Huhn, K. (2017). Effectiveness of clinical reasoning course on willingness to think critically and skills of self-reflection. *Journal of Physical Therapy Education*, *31*(4), 59–63. doi:10.1097/JTE.0000000000000007

References

Alfaro-LeFevre, R. (2016). *Critical thinking indicators (CTIs): 2016 evidence-based version*. Retrieved from http://www.alfaroteachsmart.com/2016CTIsRich.pdf

Alfaro-LeFevre, R. (2017). *Critical thinking, clinical reasoning, and clinical judgment: A practical approach* (6th ed.). Philadelphia, PA: Elsevier.

Benner, P., Sutphen, M., Leonard, V., & Day, L. (2010). *Educating nurses: A call for radical transformation*. San Francisco, CA: Jossey-Bass.

Berman, A., & Snyder, S. (2012). *Clinical handbook: Kozier & Erb's fundamentals of nursing concepts, process, and practice* (9th ed.). Upper Saddle River, NJ: Pearson.

Billings, D., & Halstead, J. (2016). *Teaching in nursing* (5th ed.). St. Louis, MO: Elsevier.

Bowell, T., & Kemp, G. (2015). *Critical thinking: A concise guide* (4th ed.). New York, NY: Routledge.

Cook, C. (2016). A "toolkit" for clinical educators to foster learners' clinical reasoning and skills acquisition. *Nursing Praxis in New Zealand*, *32*(1), 28–37.

Cooper, N., & Frain, J. (2017). *ABC of clinical reasoning*. West Sussex, United Kingdom: John Wiley & Sons.

Dalton, L., Gee, T., & Levett-Jones, T. (2015). Using clinical reasoning and simulation-based education to "flip" the enrolled nurse. *Australian Journal of Advanced Nursing*, *32*(1), 28–37.

Herron, E. K., Sudia, T., Kimble, L. P., & Davis, A. H. (2016). Prelicensure baccalaureate nursing students: Perceptions of their development of clinical reasoning. *Journal of Nursing Education*, *55*(6), 329–335. doi:10.3928/01484834-20160516-05

Schuster, P. M. (2016). *Concept mapping: A critical thinking approach to care planning* (4th ed.). Philadelphia, PA: F.A. Davis.

Tanner, C. A. (2006). Thinking like a nurse: A research-based model of clinical judgment in nursing. *Journal of Nursing Education*, *45*, 204–211.

Wilkinson, J. M. (2012). *Nursing process and critical thinking* (5th ed.). Upper Saddle River, NJ: Pearson.

Wojciechowski, M. (2016, July). How to improve clinical reasoning skills. *PTinMOTION*, 32–36.

Selected Bibliography

Dickinson, P., Haerling, K. A., & Lasater, K. (2019). Integrating the National Council of State Boards of Nursing Clinical Judgement Model into nursing educational frameworks. *Journal of Nursing Education*. *58*(2), 72–78. doi:10.3928/01484834-20190122-03

Hagell, P., Edfors, E., Hedin, G., Westergren, A., & Hamarlund, C. S. (2016). Group concept mapping for evaluation and development in nursing education. *Nurse Education in Practice*, *20*, 147–153. doi:10.1016/j.nepr.2016.08.006

Wilson, J., Mandich, A., & Magalhaes, L. (2016). Concept mapping: A dynamic individualized and qualitative method for eliciting meaning. *Qualitative Health Research*, *26*(8), 1151–1161. doi:10.1177/1049732315616623

Young, K. J., & Jung, K. E. (2015). Effects of simulation on students' knowledge, clinical reasoning, and self-confidence: A quasi-experimental study. *Korean Journal of Adult Nursing*, *27*(5), 604–611. doi:10.7475/kjan.2015.27.5.604

10 Assessing

LEARNING OUTCOMES

After completing this chapter, you will be able to:

1. Describe the phases of the nursing process.
2. Identify major characteristics of the nursing process.
3. Identify the purpose of assessing.
4. Identify the four major activities associated with the assessing phase.
5. Differentiate objective and subjective data and primary and secondary data.
6. Identify three methods of data collection, and give examples of how each is useful.
7. Compare directive and nondirective approaches to interviewing.
8. Compare closed and open-ended questions, providing examples and listing advantages and disadvantages of each.
9. Describe important aspects of the interview setting.
10. Contrast various frameworks used for nursing assessment.

KEY TERMS

assessing, *195*
cephalocaudal, *204*
closed questions, *200*
cues, *208*
data, *195*
database, *196*
directive interview, *200*
focused interview, *200*
inferences, *208*
interview, *200*
leading question, *201*
neutral question, *201*
nondirective interview, *200*
nursing process, *190*
objective data, *198*
open-ended questions, *201*
rapport, *200*
review of systems, *204*
screening examination, *204*
signs, *198*
subjective data, *198*
symptoms, *198*
validation, *208*

Introduction

The **nursing process** is a systematic, rational method of planning and providing individualized nursing care. Its purposes are to identify a client's health status and actual or potential healthcare problems or needs, to establish plans to meet the identified needs, and to deliver specific nursing interventions to meet those needs. The client may be an individual, a family, a community, or a group.

Hall originated the term *nursing process* in 1955, and Johnson (1959), Orlando (1961), and Wiedenbach (1963) were among the first to use it to refer to a series of phases describing the practice of nursing. Since then, various nurses have described the process of nursing and organized the phases in different ways.

Overview of the Nursing Process

The use of the nursing process in clinical practice gained additional legitimacy in 1973 when the phases were included in the American Nurses Association (ANA) *Standards of Nursing Practice*. Figure 10.1 ■ illustrates the nursing process in action.

Phases of the Nursing Process

The Standards of Practice within the most current *Scope and Standards of Nursing Practice* include six phases of the nursing process: assessment, diagnosis, outcomes identification, planning, implementation, and evaluation (ANA, 2015). The national licensure examination for registered nurses (NCLEX) uses five phases: assessment, analysis, planning, implementing, and evaluation. This text, and most others, uses five phases: assessing, diagnosing (which includes outcomes identification and analysis), planning, implementing, and evaluating. Although nurses may use different terms to describe the phases (or steps) of the nursing process, the activities of the nurse using the process are similar. For example, *implementing* may be called *implementation*, *intervention*, or *intervening*.

An overview of the five-phase nursing process is shown in Table 10.1. Each of the five phases is discussed in depth in this and subsequent chapters of this unit. The phases of the nursing process are not separate entities but overlapping, continuing subprocesses (Figure 10.2 ■). For example, assessing, which may be considered the first phase of the nursing process, is also carried out during the implementing and evaluating phases. For instance, while actually administering medications (implementing), the nurse continuously notes the client's skin color, level of consciousness, and so on.

TABLE 10.1 Overview of the Nursing Process

Phase and Description	Purpose	Activities
ASSESSING Collecting, organizing, validating, and documenting client data	To establish a database about the client's response to health concerns or illness and the ability to manage healthcare needs	Establish a database: • Obtain a nursing health history. • Conduct a physical assessment. • Review client records. • Review nursing literature. • Consult support persons. • Consult health professionals. Update data as needed. Organize data. Validate data. Communicate and document data.
DIAGNOSING Analyzing and synthesizing data	To identify client strengths and health problems that can be prevented or resolved by collaborative and independent nursing interventions To develop a list of nursing and collaborative problems	Interpret and analyze data: • Compare data against standards. • Cluster or group data (generate tentative hypotheses). • Identify gaps and inconsistencies. Determine client's strengths, risks, and problems. Formulate nursing diagnoses and collaborative problem statements. Document nursing diagnoses on the care plan.
PLANNING Determining how to prevent, reduce, or resolve the identified priority client problems; how to support client strengths; and how to implement nursing interventions in an organized, individualized, and goal-directed manner	To develop an individualized care plan that specifies client goals or desired outcomes and related nursing interventions	Set priorities and goals or desired outcomes in collaboration with client. Write goals or desired outcomes. Select nursing strategies and interventions. Consult other health professionals. Write nursing interventions and nursing care plan. Communicate care plan to relevant healthcare providers.
IMPLEMENTING Carrying out (or delegating) and documenting the planned nursing interventions	To assist the client to meet desired goals or outcomes; promote wellness; prevent illness and disease; restore health; and facilitate coping with altered functioning	Reassess the client to update the database. Determine the nurse's need for assistance. Perform planned nursing interventions. Communicate what nursing actions were implemented: • Document care and client responses to care. • Give verbal reports as necessary.
EVALUATING Measuring the degree to which goals or outcomes have been achieved and identifying factors that positively or negatively influence goal achievement	To determine whether to continue, modify, or terminate the plan of care	Collaborate with client and collect data related to desired outcomes. Judge whether goals or outcomes have been achieved. Relate nursing actions to client goals or outcomes. Make decisions about problem status. Review and modify the care plan as indicated or terminate nursing care. Document achievement of outcomes and modification of the care plan.

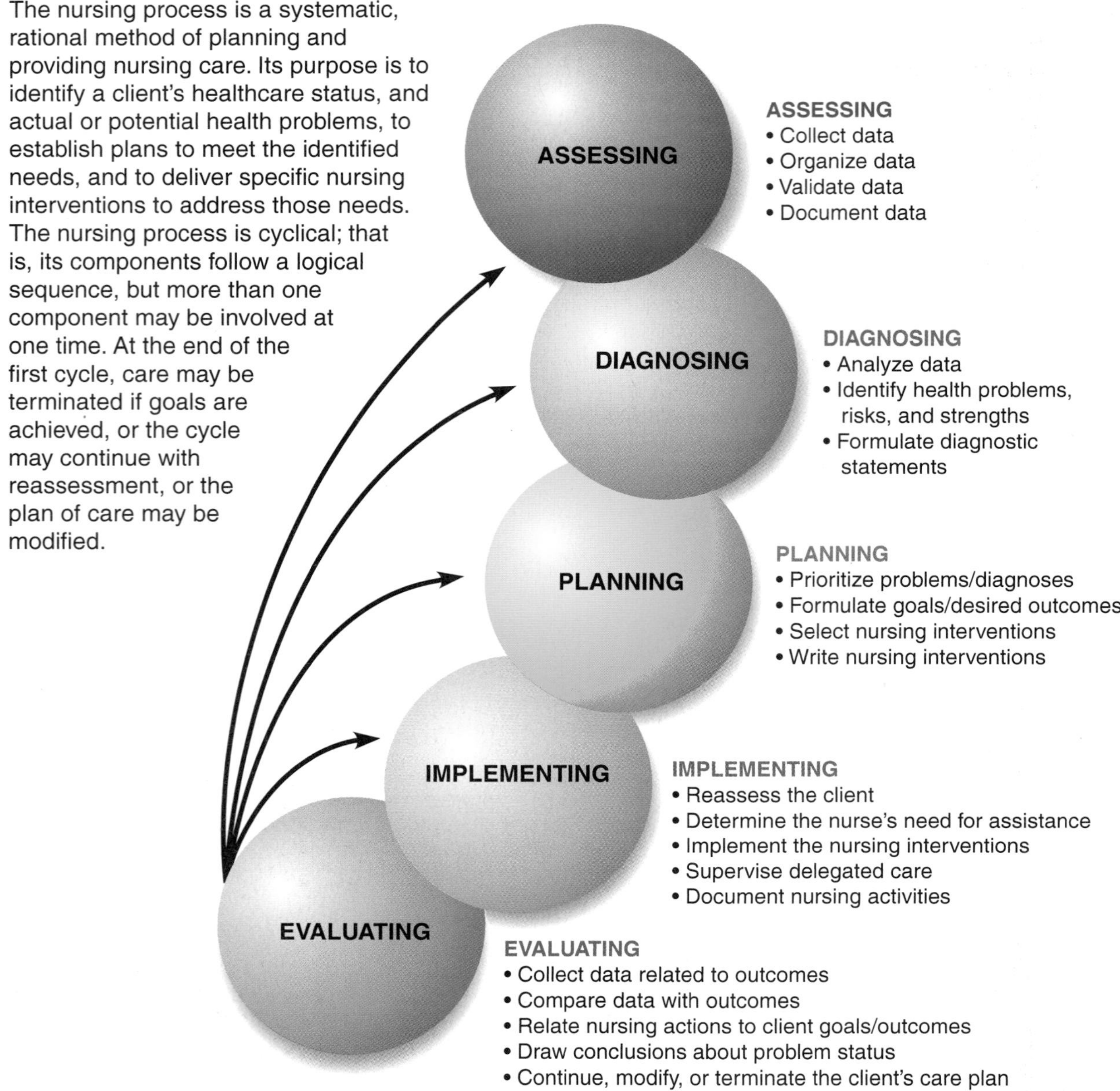
The nursing process is a systematic, rational method of planning and providing nursing care. Its purpose is to identify a client's healthcare status, and actual or potential health problems, to establish plans to meet the identified needs, and to deliver specific nursing interventions to address those needs. The nursing process is cyclical; that is, its components follow a logical sequence, but more than one component may be involved at one time. At the end of the first cycle, care may be terminated if goals are achieved, or the cycle may continue with reassessment, or the plan of care may be modified.
ASSESSING
ASSESSING
• Collect data
• Organize data
• Validate data
• Document data
DIAGNOSING
DIAGNOSING
• Analyze data
• Identify health problems, risks, and strengths
• Formulate diagnostic statements
PLANNING
PLANNING
• Prioritize problems/diagnoses
• Formulate goals/desired outcomes
• Select nursing interventions
• Write nursing interventions
IMPLEMENTING
IMPLEMENTING
• Reassess the client
• Determine the nurse's need for assistance
• Implement the nursing interventions
• Supervise delegated care
• Document nursing activities
EVALUATING
EVALUATING
• Collect data related to outcomes
• Compare data with outcomes
• Relate nursing actions to client goals/outcomes
• Draw conclusions about problem status
• Continue, modify, or terminate the client's care plan

Figure 10.1 ■ The nursing process in action.

Each phase of the nursing process affects the others; they are closely interrelated. For example, if inadequate data are obtained during assessing, the nursing diagnoses will be incomplete or incorrect; inaccuracy will also be reflected in the planning, implementing, and evaluating phases.

Characteristics of the Nursing Process

The nursing process has distinctive characteristics that enable the nurse to respond to the changing health status of the client. These characteristics include its cyclic and dynamic nature, client centeredness, focus on problem-solving and decision-making, interpersonal and collaborative style, universal applicability, and use of critical thinking and clinical reasoning.

- Data from each phase provide input into the next phase. Findings from the evaluation phase feed back into assessment. Hence, the nursing process is a regularly repeated event or sequence of events (a cycle) that is continuously changing (dynamic) rather than staying the same (static).

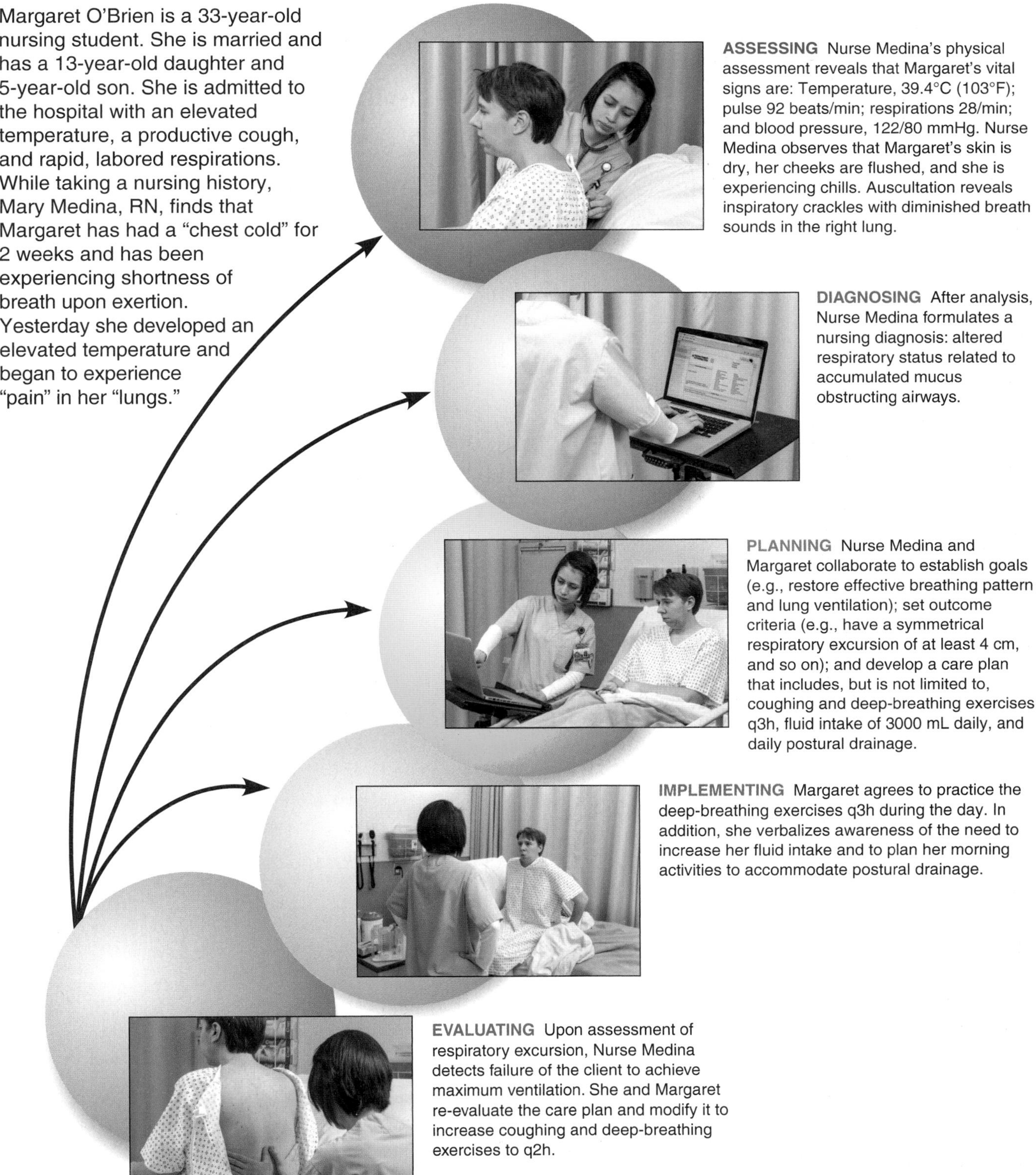

Margaret O'Brien is a 33-year-old nursing student. She is married and has a 13-year-old daughter and 5-year-old son. She is admitted to the hospital with an elevated temperature, a productive cough, and rapid, labored respirations. While taking a nursing history, Mary Medina, RN, finds that Margaret has had a "chest cold" for 2 weeks and has been experiencing shortness of breath upon exertion. Yesterday she developed an elevated temperature and began to experience "pain" in her "lungs."
ASSESSING Nurse Medina's physical assessment reveals that Margaret's vital signs are: Temperature, 39.4°C (103°F); pulse 92 beats/min; respirations 28/min; and blood pressure, 122/80 mmHg. Nurse Medina observes that Margaret's skin is dry, her cheeks are flushed, and she is experiencing chills. Auscultation reveals inspiratory crackles with diminished breath sounds in the right lung.
DIAGNOSING After analysis, Nurse Medina formulates a nursing diagnosis: altered respiratory status related to accumulated mucus obstructing airways.
PLANNING Nurse Medina and Margaret collaborate to establish goals (e.g., restore effective breathing pattern and lung ventilation); set outcome criteria (e.g., have a symmetrical respiratory excursion of at least 4 cm, and so on); and develop a care plan that includes, but is not limited to, coughing and deep-breathing exercises q3h, fluid intake of 3000 mL daily, and daily postural drainage.
IMPLEMENTING Margaret agrees to practice the deep-breathing exercises q3h during the day. In addition, she verbalizes awareness of the need to increase her fluid intake and to plan her morning activities to accommodate postural drainage.
EVALUATING Upon assessment of respiratory excursion, Nurse Medina detects failure of the client to achieve maximum ventilation. She and Margaret re-evaluate the care plan and modify it to increase coughing and deep-breathing exercises to q2h.

Figure 10.1 ■ *Continued*

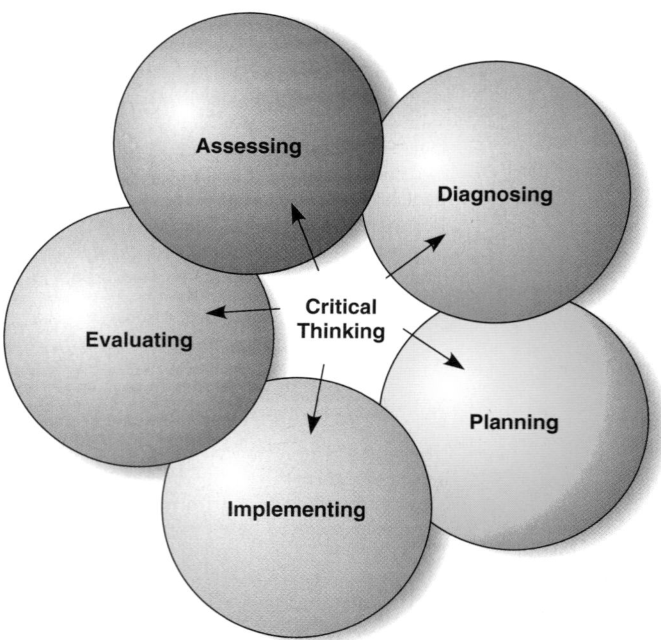

Figure 10.2 ■ The five overlapping phases of the nursing process. Each phase depends on the accuracy of the other phases. Each phase involves critical thinking.

- The nursing process is client centered. The nurse organizes the plan of care according to client problems rather than nursing goals. In the assessment phase, the nurse collects data to determine the client's habits, routines, and needs, enabling the nurse to incorporate client routines into the care plan as much as possible.
- The nursing process is an adaptation of problem-solving (see Chapter 9 ∞) and systems theory (see Chapter 27 ∞). It can be viewed as parallel to but separate from the process used by physicians (the medical model). Both processes (a) begin with data gathering and analysis, (b) base action (intervention or treatment) on a problem statement (nursing diagnosis or medical diagnosis), and (c) include an evaluative component. However, the medical model focuses on physiologic systems and the disease process, whereas the nursing process is directed toward a client's responses to real or potential disease and illness.
- Decision-making is involved in every phase of the nursing process. Nurses can be highly creative in determining when and how to use data to make decisions. They are not bound by standard responses and may apply their repertoire of skills and knowledge to assist clients. This facilitates the individualization of the nurse's plan of care.
- The nursing process is interpersonal and collaborative. It requires the nurse to communicate directly and consistently with clients and families to meet their needs. It also requires that nurses collaborate, as members of the healthcare team, in a joint effort to provide quality client care.
- The universally applicable characteristic of the nursing process means that it is used as a framework for nursing care in all types of healthcare settings, with clients of all age groups.
- Nurses must use a variety of critical thinking skills to carry out the nursing process (see Chapter 9 ∞). Table 10.2 provides examples of critical thinking in the nursing process.
- Nurses must utilize clinical reasoning throughout the delivery of nursing care. By reflecting, the nurse determines whether the outcome of care was appropriate. Figure 10.3 ■ provides an overview of the nursing process and reflection questions to be asked by the nurse while providing and evaluating care.

TABLE 10.2 Examples of Critical Thinking in the Nursing Process

Nursing Process Phase	Critical Thinking Activities
Assessing	Making reliable observations
	Distinguishing relevant from irrelevant data
	Distinguishing important from unimportant data
	Validating data
	Organizing data
	Categorizing data according to a framework
	Recognizing assumptions
	Identifying gaps in the data
Diagnosing	Finding patterns and relationships among cues
	Making inferences
	Suspending judgment when lacking data
	Stating the problem
	Examining assumptions
	Comparing patterns with norms
	Identifying factors contributing to the problem
Planning	Forming valid generalizations
	Transferring knowledge from one situation to another
	Developing evaluative criteria
	Hypothesizing
	Making interdisciplinary connections
	Prioritizing client problems
	Generalizing principles from other sciences
Implementing	Applying knowledge to perform interventions
	Testing hypotheses
Evaluating	Deciding whether hypotheses are correct
	Making criterion-based evaluations

From *Nursing Process and Critical Thinking*, 5th ed. (pp. 59–61), by J. M. Wilkinson, 2012, Upper Saddle River, NJ: Pearson.

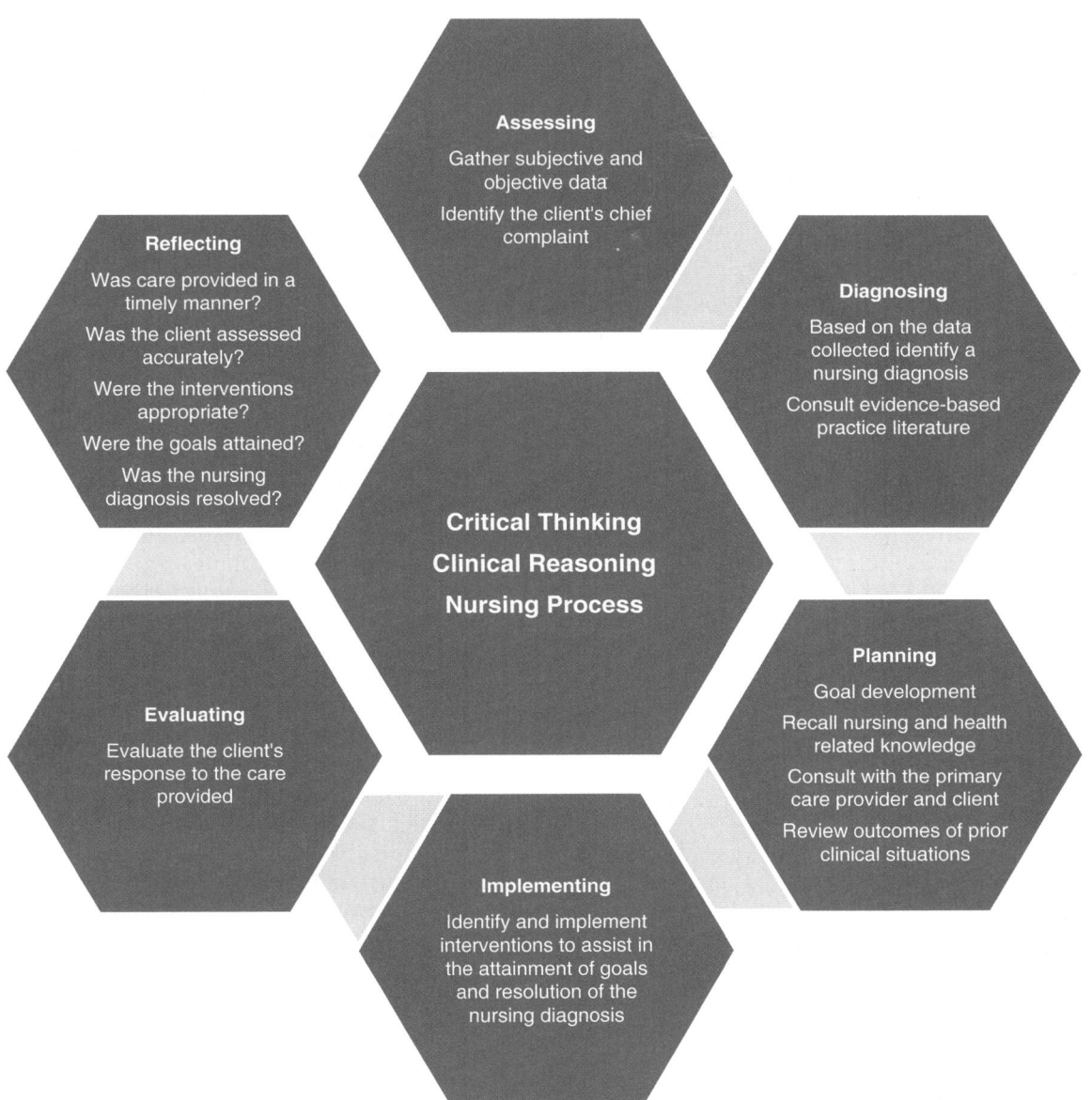

Figure 10.3 ■ Critical thinking, clinical reasoning, and the nursing process.

Assessing

Assessing is the systematic and continuous collection, organization, validation, and documentation of **data** (information) (Figure 10.4 ■). In effect, assessing is a continuous process carried out during all phases of the nursing process. For example, in the evaluation phase, the client is reassessed to determine the outcomes of the nursing strategies and to evaluate goal achievement. All phases of the nursing process depend on the accurate and complete collection of data. The four different types of assessments are the initial nursing assessment, problem-focused assessment, emergency assessment, and time-lapsed reassessment (Table 10.3). Assessments vary according to their purpose, timing, time available, and client status.

Nursing assessments focus on a client's responses to a health problem. A nursing assessment should include the client's perceived needs, health problems, related experience, health practices, values, and lifestyle. To be most useful, the data collected should be relevant to a particular health problem. Therefore, nurses should think critically about what to assess. In 2008, The Joint Commission established a nursing practice guideline stating that each client should have an initial nursing assessment consisting of a history and physical examination performed and documented within 24 hours of admission as an inpatient. This assessment guideline remains in effect today. The guideline states further that a licensed practical nurse (LPN) may gather the data but the registered nurse (RN) is responsible for care and must assess the data determining the needs of the client. The RN also has the responsibility for developing

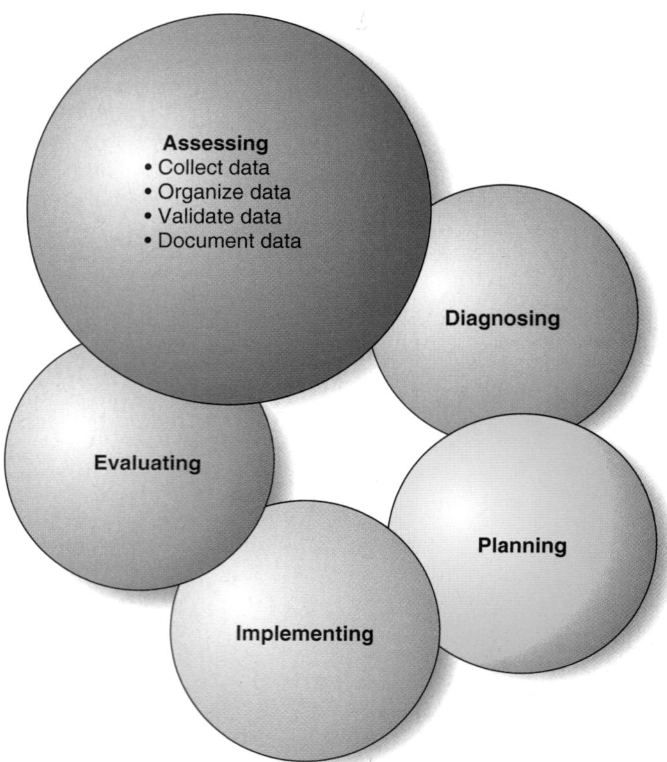

Figure 10.4 ■ Assessing. The assessment process involves four closely related activities.

the client's plan of care. In regards to the use of scribes to gather subjective data, The Joint Commission (2019) does not endorse or prohibit scribes. However, there must be a sufficient orientation and training that is specific to the scribe's role and the organization. The licensed practitioner or physician must authenticate the information, and it must be signed and dated by the practitioner.

The ANA Standard 1: Assessment (2015) states the RN is responsible for the collection of pertinent data, including demographics, social determinants of health, health disparities, and physical, functional, psychosocial, emotional, cognitive, sexual, cultural, age-related, environmental, spiritual, transpersonal, and economic assessments. Data should be collected in a systematic way and be ongoing with compassion and respect for the inherent dignity, worth, and unique attributes of every individual (ANA, 2015, p. 52). ANA also recognizes the importance of the assessment of clients based on the parameters outlined by *Healthy People 2020*. It is also important to assess the client's values, attitudes, beliefs, and family dynamics.

Collecting Data

Data collection is the process of gathering information about a client's health status. Data collection must be both systematic and continuous to prevent the omission of significant data and reflect a client's changing health status.

A **database** contains all the information about a client; it includes the nursing health history (Box 10.1), physical assessment, primary care provider's history and physical examination, results of laboratory and diagnostic tests, and material contributed by other health personnel.

Client data should include past history as well as current problems. For example, a history of an allergic reaction to penicillin is a vital piece of historical data. Past surgical procedures, folk healing practices, and chronic diseases are also examples of historical data. Current data relate to present circumstances, such as pain, nausea, sleep patterns, and religious practices. To collect data accurately, both the client and nurse must actively participate. Data can be of the subjective or objective and constant or

TABLE 10.3 Types of Assessment

Type	Time Performed	Purpose	Example
Initial assessment	Performed within specified time after admission to a healthcare agency	To establish a complete database for problem identification, reference, and future comparison	Nursing admission assessment
Problem-focused assessment	Ongoing process integrated with nursing care	To determine the status of a specific problem identified in an earlier assessment	Hourly assessment of client's fluid intake and urinary output in an intensive care unit (ICU)
			Assessment of client's ability to perform self-care while assisting a client to bathe
Emergency assessment	During any physiologic or psychologic crisis of the client	To identify life-threatening problems To identify new or overlooked problems	Rapid assessment of an individual's airway, breathing status, and circulation during a cardiac arrest Assessment of suicidal tendencies or potential for violence
Time-lapsed reassessment	Several months after initial assessment	To compare the client's current status to baseline data previously obtained	Reassessment of a client's functional health patterns in a home care or outpatient setting or, in a hospital, at shift change

BOX 10.1 Components of a Nursing Health History

BIOGRAPHIC DATA

Client's name, address, age, sex, marital status, occupation, religious preference, healthcare financing, and usual source of medical care.

CHIEF COMPLAINT OR REASON FOR VISIT

The answer given to the question "What is troubling you?" or "Describe the reason you came to the hospital or clinic today." The chief complaint should be recorded in the client's own words.

History of Present Illness

- When the symptoms started
- Whether the onset of symptoms was sudden or gradual
- How often the problem occurs
- Exact location of the distress
- Character of the complaint (e.g., intensity of pain or quality of sputum, emesis, or discharge)
- Activity in which the client was involved when the problem occurred
- Phenomena or symptoms associated with the chief complaint
- Factors that aggravate or alleviate the problem

PAST HISTORY

- *Illnesses*, such as chickenpox, mumps, measles, rubella (German measles), rubeola (red measles), streptococcal infections, scarlet fever, rheumatic fever, hepatitis, polio, and other significant illnesses
- *Immunizations* and the date of the last tetanus shot
- *Allergies* to drugs, animals, insects, or other environmental agents, the type of reaction that occurs, and how the reaction is treated
- *Accidents and injuries*: how, when, and where the incident occurred, type of injury, treatment received, and any complications
- *Hospitalization for serious illnesses*: reasons for the hospitalization, dates, surgery performed, course of recovery, and any complications
- *Medications*: all currently used prescription and over-the-counter medications, such as aspirin, nasal spray, vitamins, laxatives, and herbal supplements

FAMILY HISTORY OF ILLNESS

To ascertain risk factors for certain diseases, the ages of siblings, parents, and grandparents and their current state of health, or, if they are deceased, the cause of death, are obtained. Particular attention should be given to disorders such as heart disease, cancer, diabetes, hypertension, obesity, allergies, arthritis, tuberculosis, bleeding, alcoholism, and any mental health disorders.

LIFESTYLE

- *Personal habits:* the amount, frequency, and duration of substance use (tobacco, alcohol, coffee, cola, tea, and illegal or recreational drugs)
- *Diet:* description of a typical diet on a normal day or any special diet, number of meals and snacks per day, who cooks and shops for food, ethnic food patterns, and allergies
- *Sleep patterns:* usual daily sleep and wake times, difficulties sleeping, and remedies used for difficulties
- *Activities of daily living (ADLs):* any difficulties experienced in the basic activities of eating, grooming, dressing, elimination, and locomotion
- *Instrumental ADLs:* any difficulties experienced in food preparation, shopping, transportation, housekeeping, laundry, and ability to use the telephone, handle finances, and manage medications
- *Recreation and hobbies:* exercise activity and tolerance, hobbies and other interests, and vacations

SOCIAL DATA

- *Family relationships and friendships:* the client's support system in times of stress (who helps in time of need?), what effect the client's illness has on the family, and whether any family problems are affecting the client (see also the discussion of family assessment in Chapter 27 ∞)
- *Ethnic affiliation:* health customs and beliefs; cultural practices that may affect healthcare and recovery (see also the detailed ethnic and cultural assessment guide in Chapter 21 ∞)
- *Educational history:* data about the client's highest level of education attained and any past difficulties with learning
- *Occupational history:* current employment status, the number of days missed from work because of illness, any history of accidents on the job, any occupational hazards with a potential for future disease or accident, the client's need to change jobs because of past illness, the employment status of spouses or partners and the way child care is handled, and the client's overall satisfaction with the work
- *Economic status:* information about how the client is paying for medical care (including what kind of medical and hospitalization coverage the client has) and whether the client's illness presents financial concerns
- *Home and neighborhood conditions:* home safety measures and adjustments in physical facilities that may be required to help the client manage a physical disability, activity intolerance, and activities of daily living; the availability of neighborhood and community services to meet the client's needs

PSYCHOLOGIC DATA

- *Major stressors* experienced and the client's perception of them
- *Usual coping pattern* for a serious problem or a high level of stress
- *Communication style*: ability to verbalize appropriate emotion; nonverbal communication—such as eye movements, gestures, use of touch, and posture; interactions with support persons; and the congruence of nonverbal behavior and verbal expression

PATTERNS OF HEALTHCARE

All healthcare resources the client is currently using and has used in the past. These include the primary care provider, specialists (e.g., ophthalmologist or gynecologist), dentist, folk practitioners (e.g., herbalist or *curandero*), health clinic, or health center; whether the client considers the care being provided adequate; and whether access to healthcare is a problem.

TABLE 10.4 Examples of Subjective and Objective Data

Subjective	Objective
"I feel weak all over when I exert myself."	Blood pressure 90/50 mmHg* Apical pulse 104 beats/min Skin pale and diaphoretic
Client states he has a cramping pain in his abdomen. States, "I feel sick to my stomach."	Vomited 100 mL green-tinged fluid Abdomen firm and slightly distended Active bowel sounds auscultated in all four quadrants
"I'm short of breath."	Lung sounds clear bilaterally; diminished in right lower lobe
Wife states: "He doesn't seem so sad today." (This is subjective and secondary source data.)	Client cried during interview
"I would like to see the chaplain before surgery."	Holding open Bible Has small silver cross on bedside table

*Blood pressure obtained using an external cuff and manometer may be considered secondary or indirect data since it does not directly measure the pressure within the arteries.

variable types, and from a primary or secondary source. The collection of data allows the nurse, client, and healthcare team to identify health-related problems or risk factors that could cause changes in a client's health status.

Types of Data

Subjective data, also referred to as **symptoms** or covert data, are apparent only to the individual affected and can be described or verified only by that individual. Itching, pain, and feelings of worry are examples of subjective data. Subjective data include the client's sensations, feelings, values, beliefs, attitudes, and perception of personal health status and life situation.

Objective data, also referred to as **signs** or overt data, are detectable by an observer or can be measured or tested against an accepted standard. They can be seen, heard, felt, or smelled, and they are obtained by observation or physical examination. For example, a discoloration of the skin or a blood pressure reading is objective data. During the physical examination, the nurse obtains objective data to validate subjective data and to complete the assessment phase of the nursing process.

Constant data is information that does not change over time such as race or blood type. Variable data can change quickly, frequently, or rarely and include such data as blood pressure, level of pain, and age.

A complete database provides a baseline for comparing the client's responses to nursing and medical interventions. Examples of subjective and objective data are shown in Table 10.4.

Sources of Data

Sources of data are primary or secondary. The client is the primary source of data. Family members or other support persons, other health professionals, records and reports, laboratory and diagnostic analyses, and relevant literature are secondary or indirect sources. In fact, all sources other than the client are considered secondary sources. All data from secondary sources should be validated if possible.

Client

The best source of data is usually the client, unless the client is too ill, young, or confused to communicate clearly. The nurse is often much closer to the client than other members of the healthcare team. In community and acute care settings, the nurse has the closest relationship with the client and family. It is important to develop strategies to build therapeutic relationships with the client and family. When establishing a rapport with the client it is important to share that, by gathering a thorough assessment, the nurse will be able to meet the needs of the client to ensure better health outcomes. When developing a therapeutic relationship, Feo, Rasmussen, Wiechula, Conroy, and Kitson (2017) have identified the following factors when focusing on providing client care. The nurse should give the client undivided attention. The nurse should anticipate the client's needs. The nurse should inform the client of healthcare decisions and evaluate the quality of the relationship. The client can provide subjective data that no one else can offer. Most often, primary data consist of statements made by the client but also include the objective data that can be directly obtained from the client, such as gender. Some clients cannot or do not wish to provide accurate data. Family members or significant others can be secondary sources of data if the client cannot participate, is a poor historian, or is a young child. If the client is hesitant to provide data, remind the client that the privacy of all data collected is protected and data can be shared only with individuals who have legitimate health-related needs to know it. If necessary, review for yourself the mandates of the Health Insurance Portability and Accountability Act of 1996 (HIPAA) so you can explain this in a way that the client can understand. Summarized information about HIPAA in terms understandable to both nurses and clients is available on the U.S. Department of Health and Human Services website.

Support People

Family members, friends, and caregivers who know the client well often can supplement or verify information provided by the client. They might convey information about the client's response to illness, the stresses the client was experiencing before the illness, family attitudes on illness and health, and the client's home environment.

Support people are an especially important source of data for a client who is very young, unconscious, or confused. In some cases—a client who is physically or emotionally abused, for example—the individual giving information may wish to remain anonymous. Before eliciting data from support people, the nurse should ensure that the client, if mentally able, authorizes such input. The nurse should also indicate on the nursing history that the data were obtained from a support person.

Information supplied by family members, significant others, or other health professionals is considered subjective if it is not based on fact. If the client's daughter says, "Dad is very confused today," that is secondary subjective data because it is an interpretation of the client's behavior by the daughter. The nurse should attempt to verify the reported confusion by interviewing the client directly. However, if the daughter says, "Dad said he thought it was the year 1941 today," that may be considered secondary objective data since the daughter heard her father state this directly.

Client Records

Client records include information documented by various healthcare professionals. Client records also contain data regarding the client's occupation, religion, and marital status. By reviewing such records before interviewing the client, the nurse can avoid asking questions for which answers have already been supplied. Repeated questioning can be stressful and annoying to clients and cause concern about the lack of communication among health professionals. Types of client records include medical records, records of therapies, and laboratory records.

Medical records (e.g., medical history, physical examination, operative report, progress notes, and consultations done by primary care providers) are often a source of a client's present and past health and illness patterns. These records can provide nurses with information about the client's coping behaviors, health practices, previous illnesses, and allergies.

Records of therapies provided by other health professionals, such as social workers, nutritionists, dietitians, or physical therapists, help the nurse obtain relevant data not expressed by the client. For example, a social agency's report on a client's living conditions or a home healthcare agency's report on a client's ability to cope at home help the nurse conducting an assessment.

Laboratory records also provide pertinent health information. For example, the determination of blood glucose level allows health professionals to monitor the administration of oral hypoglycemic medications. Any laboratory data about a client must be compared to the agency or performing laboratory's norms for that particular test and for the client's age, gender, and other characteristics. Commonly ordered diagnostic studies are discussed in Chapter 34 ∞.

The nurse must always consider the information in client records in light of the current situation. For example, if the most recent medical record is 10 years old, the client's health practices and coping behaviors are likely to have changed. Older clients may have numerous previous records. These are very useful and contribute to a full understanding of the health history, especially if the client's memory is impaired.

Healthcare Professionals

Because assessment is an ongoing process, verbal reports from other healthcare professionals serve as other potential sources of information about a client's health. Nurses, social workers, primary care providers, and physiotherapists, for example, may have information from either previous or current contact with the client. Sharing of information among professionals is especially important to ensure continuity of care when clients are transferred to and from home and healthcare agencies.

Literature

The review of nursing and related literature, such as professional journals and reference texts, can provide additional information for the database. A literature review includes but is not limited to the following information:

- Standards or norms against which to compare findings (e.g., height and weight tables, normal developmental tasks for an age group)
- Cultural and social health practices
- Spiritual beliefs
- Assessment data needed for specific client conditions
- Nursing interventions and evaluation criteria relevant to a client's health problems
- Information about medical diagnoses, treatment, and prognoses
- Current methodologies and research findings.

Data Collection Methods

The principal methods used to collect data are observing, interviewing, and examining. Observing occurs whenever the nurse is in contact with the client or support persons. Interviewing is used mainly while taking the nursing health history. Examining is the major method used in the physical health assessment.

In reality, the nurse uses all three methods simultaneously when assessing clients. For example, during the client interview the nurse observes, listens, asks questions, and mentally retains information to explore in the physical examination.

Observing

To *observe* is to gather data by using the senses. Observing is a conscious, deliberate skill that is developed through effort and with an organized approach. Although nurses observe mainly through sight, most of the senses are engaged during careful observations. Examples of client data observed through the senses are shown in Table 10.5.

Observing has two aspects: (a) noticing the data and (b) selecting, organizing, and interpreting the data. A nurse who observes that a client's face is flushed must relate that observation to findings such as body temperature, activity, environmental temperature, and blood pressure. Errors can occur in selecting, organizing, and interpreting data. For example, a nurse might not notice certain signs, either because they are unexpected or because they do not conform to preconceptions about a client's illness. Nurses often need to focus on specific data in order not to be overwhelmed by a multitude of data. Observing, therefore, involves distinguishing data in a meaningful manner. For example, nurses caring for newborns learn to ignore the usual sounds of machines in the nursery but respond quickly to an infant's cry or movement.

The experienced nurse is often able to attend to an intervention (e.g., give a bed bath or monitor an IV infusion) and at the same time make important observations (e.g., note a change in respiratory status or skin color). The beginning student must learn to make observations and complete tasks simultaneously.

TABLE 10.5 Using the Senses to Observe Client Data

Sense	Example of Client Data
Vision	Overall appearance (e.g., body size, general weight, posture, grooming); signs of distress or discomfort; facial and body gestures; skin color and lesions; abnormalities of movement; nonverbal demeanor (e.g., signs of anger or anxiety); religious or cultural artifacts (e.g., books, icons, candles, beads)
Smell	Body or breath odors
Hearing	Lung and heart sounds; bowel sounds; ability to communicate; language spoken; ability to initiate conversation; ability to respond when spoken to; orientation to time, person, and place; thoughts and feelings about self, others, and health status
Touch	Skin temperature and moisture; muscle strength (e.g., hand grip); pulse rate, rhythm, and volume; palpable lesions (e.g., lumps, masses, nodules)

Nursing observations must be organized so that nothing significant is missed. Most nurses develop a particular sequence for observing events, usually focusing on the client first. For example, a nurse walks into a client's room and observes, in the following order:

1. Clinical signs of client distress (e.g., pallor or flushing, labored breathing, and behavior indicating pain or emotional distress)
2. Threats to the client's safety, real or anticipated (e.g., a lowered side rail)
3. The presence and functioning of associated equipment (e.g., IV equipment and oxygen)
4. The immediate environment, including the people in it.

Interviewing

An **interview** is a planned communication or a conversation with a purpose, for example, to get or give information, identify problems of mutual concern, evaluate change, teach, provide support, or provide counseling or therapy. One example of the interview is the nursing health history, which is a part of the nursing admission assessment. In a **focused interview** the nurse asks the client specific questions to collect information related to the client's problem. This allows the nurse to collect information that may have previously been missed and yields more in-depth information (D'Amico & Barbarito, 2016).

There are two approaches to interviewing: directive and nondirective. The **directive interview** is highly structured and elicits specific information. The nurse establishes the purpose of the interview and controls the interview, at least at the outset. The client responds to questions but may have limited opportunity to ask questions or discuss concerns. Nurses frequently use directive interviews to gather and to give information when time is limited (e.g., in an emergency situation).

By contrast, during a **nondirective interview**, or rapport-building interview, the nurse allows the client to control the purpose, subject matter, and pacing. **Rapport** is an understanding between two or more people.

A combination of directive and nondirective approaches is usually appropriate during the information-gathering interview. The nurse begins by determining areas of concern for the client. If, for example, a client expresses worry about surgery, the nurse pauses to explore the client's worry and to provide support. Simply noting the worry, without dealing with it, can leave the impression that the nurse does not care about the client's concerns or dismisses them as unimportant.

TYPES OF INTERVIEW QUESTIONS

Questions are often classified as closed or open ended, and neutral or leading. **Closed questions**, used in the directive interview, are restrictive and generally require only "yes" or "no" or short factual answers that provide specific information. Closed questions often begin with "when," "where," "who," "what," "do (did, does)," or "is (are, was)." Examples of closed questions are "What medication did you take?" "Are you having pain now? Show me where it is." "How old are you?" "When did you fall?" Closed questions are often used when information is needed quickly, such as in an emergency situation. Individuals who are highly stressed or have difficulty communicating will find closed questions easier to answer than open-ended questions.

Open-ended questions, associated with the nondirective interview, invite clients to discover and explore, elaborate, clarify, or illustrate their thoughts or feelings. An open-ended question specifies only the broad topic to be discussed and invites answers longer than one or two words. Such questions give clients the freedom to divulge only the information that they are ready to disclose. The open-ended question is useful at the beginning of an interview or to change topics and to elicit attitudes.

Open-ended questions may begin with "what" or "how." Examples of open-ended questions are "How have you been feeling lately?" "What brought you to the hospital?" "How did you feel in that situation?" "Would you describe more about how you relate to your child?" "What would you like to talk about today?"

The type of question a nurse chooses depends on the needs of the client at the time. Nurses often find it necessary to use a combination of closed and open-ended questions throughout an interview to accomplish the goals of the interview and obtain needed information. See Table 10.6 for advantages and disadvantages of open-ended and closed questions.

A **neutral question** is a question the client can answer without direction or pressure from the nurse, is open ended, and is used in nondirective interviews. Examples are "How do you feel about that?" "What do you think led to the operation?" A **leading question**, by contrast, is usually closed, used in a directive interview, and thus directs the client's answer. Examples are "You're stressed about surgery tomorrow, aren't you?" "You will take your medicine, won't you?" The leading question gives the client less opportunity to decide whether the answer is true or not. Leading questions create problems if the client, in an effort to please the nurse, gives inaccurate responses. This can result in inaccurate data.

Try to avoid asking "why" questions. These questions can be perceived as a form of interrogation by the client (Kneisl & Trigoboff, 2013). Because the goal of questioning is to elicit as much purposeful information as possible, anything that puts the client on the defensive will interfere with reaching that goal. However, in an emergency situation the use of probing and direct questioning may be appropriate to gain a greater volume of data in a shorter period of time (Kneisl & Trigoboff, 2013).

PLANNING THE INTERVIEW AND SETTING

Before beginning an interview, the nurse reviews available information, for example, the operative report,

TABLE 10.6 Selected Advantages and Disadvantages of Open-Ended and Closed Questions

Advantages	Disadvantages
OPEN-ENDED QUESTIONS	
1. They let the interviewee do the talking. 2. The interviewer is able to listen and observe. 3. They reveal what the interviewee thinks is important. 4. They may reveal the interviewee's lack of information, misunderstanding of words, frame of reference, prejudices, or stereotypes. 5. They can provide information the interviewer may not ask for. 6. They can reveal the interviewee's degree of feeling about an issue. 7. They can convey interest and trust because of the freedom they provide.	1. They take more time. 2. Only brief answers may be given. 3. Valuable information may be withheld. 4. They often elicit more information than necessary. 5. Responses are difficult to document and require skill in recording. 6. The interviewer requires skill in controlling an open-ended interview. 7. Responses require insight and sensitivity from the interviewer.
CLOSED QUESTIONS	
1. Questions and answers can be controlled more effectively. 2. They require less effort from the interviewee. 3. They may be less threatening, since they do not require explanations or justifications. 4. They take less time. 5. Information can be asked for sooner than it would be volunteered. 6. Responses are easily documented. 7. Questions are easy to use and can be handled by unskilled interviewers.	1. They may provide too little information and require follow-up questions. 2. They may not reveal how the interviewee feels. 3. They do not allow the interviewee to volunteer possibly valuable information. 4. They may inhibit communication and convey lack of interest by the interviewer. 5. The interviewer may dominate the interview with questions.

information about the current illness, or literature about the client's health problem. The nurse also reviews the agency's data collection form to identify which data must be collected and which data are within the nurse's discretion to collect based on the specific client. If a form is not available, most nurses prepare an interview guide to help them remember areas of information and determine what questions to ask. The guide includes a list of topics and subtopics rather than a series of questions.

Both nurses and clients are made comfortable in order to encourage an effective interview by balancing several factors. Each interview is influenced by time, place, seating arrangement or distance, and language.

Time Nurses need to plan interviews with clients when the client is physically comfortable and free of pain, and when interruptions by friends, family, and other health professionals are minimal. Nurses should schedule interviews with clients in their homes at a time selected by the client.

Place A well-lit, well-ventilated room that is relatively free of noise, movements, and distractions encourages communication. In addition, a place where others cannot overhear or see the client is desirable.

Seating Arrangement By standing and looking down at a client who is in bed or in a chair, the nurse risks intimidating the client. When a client is in bed, the nurse can sit at a 45-degree angle to the bed. This position is less formal than sitting behind a table or standing at the foot of the bed. During an initial admission interview, a client may feel less confronted if there is an overbed table between the client and the nurse. Sitting on a client's bed hems the client in and makes staring difficult to avoid.

A seating arrangement with the nurse behind a desk and the client seated across creates a formal setting that suggests a business meeting between a superior and a subordinate. In contrast, a seating arrangement in which the parties sit on two chairs placed at right angles to a desk or table or a few feet apart, with no table between, creates a less formal atmosphere, and the nurse and client tend to feel on equal terms. In groups, a horseshoe or circular chair arrangement can avoid a superior or head-of-the-table position.

Distance The distance between the interviewer and interviewee should be neither too small nor too great, because people feel uncomfortable when talking to someone who is too close or too far away. *Proxemics* is the study of use of space. As a species, humans are highly territorial but we are rarely aware of it unless our space is somehow violated. Most people feel comfortable maintaining a distance of 2 to 3 feet during an interview. Some clients require more or less personal space, depending on their cultural and personal needs. For additional information, see Chapter 21 ∞.

QSEN Patient-Centered Care: Personal Space

The accepted distance between individuals in a conversation varies. Some individuals are comfortable with less distance than others. Anxiety and direct eye contact increase the need for space. Physical contact is used only if it has a therapeutic purpose. It is important to note that touch, even a simple hand on the shoulder, can be misinterpreted, especially between individuals of the opposite gender.

Language Failure to communicate in language the client can understand is a form of discrimination. The nurse must convert complicated medical terminology into common English usage, and interpreters or translators are needed if the client and the nurse do not speak the same language or dialect (a variation in a language spoken in a particular geographic region). Translating medical terminology is a specialized skill because not everyone who is fluent in the conversational form of a language is familiar with anatomic or other health terms. Interpreters, however, may make judgments about precise wording but also about subtle meanings that require additional explanation or clarification according to the specific language and ethnicity. They may edit the original source to make the meaning clearer or more culturally appropriate.

If giving written documents to clients, the nurse must determine that the client can read in his or her native language. Live translation is preferred since the client can then ask questions for clarification. Nurses must be cautious when asking family members, client visitors, or agency nonprofessional staff to assist with translation. Issues of confidentiality or gender mismatch can interfere with effective communication. Services such as AT&T Language Line are available 24 hours a day in about 170 languages, for a fee paid by the healthcare provider. Many large agencies possess their own on-call translator services for the languages or dialects commonly spoken in their area.

Even among clients who speak English, there may be differences in understanding terminology. Clients from different parts of the country may have strong accents, or clients less well educated and teen clients may ascribe different meanings to words. For example, "cool" may imply something good to one client and something not warm to another. The nurse must always confirm accurate understandings.

STAGES OF AN INTERVIEW

An interview has three major stages: the opening or introduction, the body or development, and the closing.

The Opening The opening can be the most important part of the interview because what is said and done at that time sets the tone for the remainder of the interview.

The purposes of the opening are to establish rapport and orient the interviewee.

Establishing rapport is a process of creating goodwill and trust. It can begin with a greeting ("Good morning, Mr. Johnson") or a self-introduction ("Good morning. I'm Becky James, a nursing student") accompanied by nonverbal gestures such as a smile, a handshake, and a friendly manner. The nurse must be careful not to overdo this stage; too much superficial talk can arouse anxiety about what is to follow and may appear insincere.

In orientation, the nurse explains the purpose and nature of the interview, for example, what information is needed, how long it will take, and what is expected of the client. The nurse tells the client how the information will be used and usually states that the client has the right not to provide data.

The following is an example of an interview introduction:

Step 1. Establish Rapport

Nurse: Hello, Ms. Goodwin, I'm Ms. Fellows. I'm a nursing student, and I'll be assisting with your care here today.
Client: Hi. Are you a student from the college?
Nurse: Yes, I'm in my final year. Are you familiar with the campus?
Client: Oh, yes! I'm an avid football fan. My nephew graduated in 2017, and I often attend football games with him.
Nurse: That's great! Sounds like fun.
Client: Yes, I enjoy it very much.

Step 2. Orientation

Nurse: May I sit down with you here for about ten minutes to talk about your care while you're here?
Client: All right. What do you want to know?
Nurse: Well, to plan your care after your operation, I'd like to get some information about your usual daily activities and what you expect here in the hospital. I'll take notes while we talk to get the important points and have them available to the other staff who will also look after you.
Client: OK. That's all right with me.
Nurse: If there is anything you don't want to talk about, please feel free to say so. Everything you tell me will be confidential and shared only with others who have the legal right to know it.
Client: Sure, that will be fine.

The Body In the body of the interview, the client communicates what he or she thinks, feels, knows, and perceives in response to questions from the nurse. Effective development of the interview demands that the nurse use communication techniques that make both parties feel comfortable and serve the purpose of the interview (see Chapter 16 ∞). For communicating during an interview, see the Practice Guidelines.

The Closing The nurse terminates the interview when the needed information has been obtained. In some cases, however, a client terminates it, for example, when deciding not to give any more information or when unable to offer more information for some other reason—fatigue, for example. The closing is important for maintaining rapport and trust and for facilitating future interactions. The following techniques are commonly used to close an interview:

1. Offer to answer questions: "Do you have any questions?" "I would be glad to answer any questions you have." Be sure to allow time for the individual to answer, or the offer will be regarded as insincere.
2. Conclude by saying, "Well, that's all I need to know for now" or "Well, those are all the questions I have for now." Preceding a remark with the word "well" generally signals that the end of the interaction is near.
3. Thank the client: "Thank you for your time and help. The questions you have answered will be helpful in planning your nursing care." You may also shake the client's hand.
4. Express concern for the client's welfare and future: "I hope all goes well for you."

PRACTICE GUIDELINES Communication During an Interview

- Listen attentively, using all your senses, and speak slowly and clearly.
- Use language the client understands, and clarify points that are not understood.
- Plan questions to follow a logical sequence.
- Ask only one question at a time. Multiple questions limit the client to one choice and may confuse the client.
- Acknowledge the client's right to look at things the way they appear to him or her and not the way they appear to the nurse or someone else.
- Do not impose your own values on the client.
- Avoid using personal examples, such as saying, "If I were you. . . ."
- Nonverbally convey respect, concern, interest, and acceptance.
- Be aware of the client's and your own body language.
- Be conscious of the client's and your own voice inflection, tone, and affect.
- Sit down to talk with the client (be at an even level).
- Use and accept silence to help the client search for more thoughts or to organize them.
- Use eye contact and be calm, unhurried, and sympathetic.

5. Plan for the next meeting, if there is to be one, or state what will happen next. Include the day, time, place, topic, and purpose: "Let's get together again here on the fifteenth at nine a.m. to see how you are managing." Or "Ms. Goodwin, I will be responsible for giving you care three mornings per week while you are here. I will be here each Monday, Tuesday, and Wednesday between eight o'clock and noon. At those times, we can adjust your care as needed."
6. Provide a summary to verify accuracy and agreement. Summarizing serves several purposes: It helps to terminate the interview, it reassures the client that the nurse has listened, it checks the accuracy of the nurse's perceptions, it clears the way for new ideas, and it helps the client to note progress and a forward direction. "Let's review what we have just covered in this interview." Summaries are particularly helpful for clients who are anxious or who have difficulty staying with the topic. "Well, it seems to me that you are especially worried about your hospitalization and chest pain because your father died of a heart attack five years ago. Is that correct? I'll discuss this with you again tomorrow, and we'll decide what plans need to be made to help you."

Examining

The physical examination or physical assessment is a systematic data collection method that uses observation (i.e., the senses of sight, hearing, smell, and touch) to detect health problems. To conduct the examination, the nurse uses techniques of inspection, auscultation, palpation, and percussion (see Chapter 29 ∞).

The physical examination is carried out systematically. It may be organized according to the examiner's preference, in a head-to-toe approach or a body systems approach. Usually, the nurse first records a general impression about the client's overall appearance and health status: for example, age, body size, mental and nutritional status, speech, and behavior. Then the nurse takes such measurements as vital signs, height, and weight. The **cephalocaudal** or head-to-toe approach begins the examination at the head; progresses to the neck, thorax, abdomen, and extremities; and ends at the toes. The nurse using a body systems approach investigates each system individually, that is, the respiratory system, the circulatory system, the nervous system, and so on. During the physical examination, the nurse assesses all body parts and compares findings on each side of the body (e.g., lungs). These techniques are discussed in detail in Chapters 28 and 29 ∞.

Instead of giving a complete examination, the nurse may focus on a specific problem area noted from the nursing assessment, such as the inability to urinate. On occasion, the nurse may find it necessary to resolve a client complaint or problem (e.g., shortness of breath) before completing the examination. Alternatively, the nurse may perform a screening examination. A **screening examination**, also called a **review of systems**, is a brief review of essential functioning of various body parts or systems. An example of a screening examination is the nursing admission assessment form shown in Figure 10.5. Data obtained from this examination are measured against norms or standards, such as ideal height and weight standards or norms for body temperature or blood pressure levels.

Organizing Data

The nurse uses a written (or electronic) format that organizes the assessment data systematically. This is often referred to as a nursing health history, nursing assessment, or nursing database form. The format may be modified according to the client's physical status such as one focused on musculoskeletal data for orthopedic clients.

Conceptual Models and Frameworks

Most schools of nursing and health care agencies have developed their own structured assessment format. Many of these are based on selected nursing models or frameworks (see Chapter 1 ∞). Three examples are Gordon's functional health pattern framework, Orem's self-care model, and Roy's adaptation model.

LIFESPAN CONSIDERATIONS Assessment

CHILDREN

Consider this example: A 4-year-old girl is admitted following emergency surgery for a ruptured appendix. She is awake and alert, but refuses to talk. Her parents have had little sleep for more than 24 hours and are extremely anxious.

- Gathering assessment data in this situation requires the nurse to be sensitive to the parents' needs for sleep and assurance. At the same time, the nurse must collect information to compile an adequate database for appropriate nursing care decisions. Assessment will involve monitoring the condition of the child as she recovers from surgery and being alert to potential problems.
- The parents become the major source of subjective data, although the child should be encouraged to tell the nurse how she is feeling.
- Objective data collected include vital signs including level of and response to pain; bleeding or discharge from the incision; mobility; integrity of dressings, IV lines, catheters, nasogastric tubes or other medical devices; and mental status.
- Since children are a part of families, assessment will include observation of family dynamics and questions that could lead to care of the family system.

Gordon (2016) provides a framework of 11 functional health patterns. The 11 functional health patterns are health perception and management, nutritional-metabolic, elimination, activity, sleep, cognitive, self-perception and self-concept, role relationship, sexuality, coping and stress, and value belief systems. Gordon uses the word *pattern* to signify a sequence of recurring behavior. The nurse collects data about dysfunctional as well as functional behavior. Thus, by using Gordon's framework to organize data, nurses are able to discern emerging patterns.

Orem's self-care model (2001) delineates eight universal self-care requisites of humans. The model describes the client's need for adequate nutrition, normal elimination, and adequate rest to promote normal human functioning and development. Roy (2009) outlines the data to be collected according to the Roy adaptation model and classifies observable behavior into four categories: physiologic, self-concept, role function, and interdependence (Box 10.2).

BOX 10.2 Roy's Adaptation Model

ADAPTIVE MODES

1. Physiologic needs
   - Activity and rest
   - Nutrition
   - Elimination
   - Fluid and electrolytes
   - Oxygenation
   - Protection
   - Regulation: temperature
   - Regulation: the senses
   - Regulation: endocrine system
2. Self-concept
   - Physical self
   - Personal self
3. Role function
4. Interdependence

Figure 10.5 ■ is a concise data collection tool that is organized according to body systems and specific nursing concerns (e.g., screening for falls and allergies); it does not use one particular nursing model. In Box 10.3, the data for the case study client Margaret O'Brien from Figure 10.5 are shown after being organized according to Gordon's 11 functional health patterns. Note how the categories in the box differ somewhat from those in Figure 10.5. As a rule, the nurse organizes the data using the same model on which the data collection tool is based. However, different models are provided here to demonstrate differences in organizing frameworks, and to show that the nurse is not limited to the exact framework provided by the data collection tool.

No Associated Problem.

Form | Data | History

CARDIOVASCULAR ASSESSMENT

Heart Rythm		Nail Bed Color	Edema
☑ Regular	☐ S 1	◉ Normal Ethnicity	☑ None
☐ Irregular		○ Dark	☐ Anasarca
☐ Bradycardia		○ Dusky	☐ Generalised
☐ Tachycardia		○ Pale	☐ Localized

Antiembolism Device	Antiembolism Device Removal Reason
☐ Foot Pumps	☐ Activity
☐ Graduated compression stocking knee High	☐ ADL Care
☐ Graduated compression stocking thigh High	☐ Patient Refused
☐ Intermittent pneumatic compression devices knee high	☐ Procedure Treatment
☐ Intermittent pneumatic compression devices thigh high	☐ Skin Care

NOTES

Figure 10.5 ■ Assessment for Margaret O'Brien.
iCare.

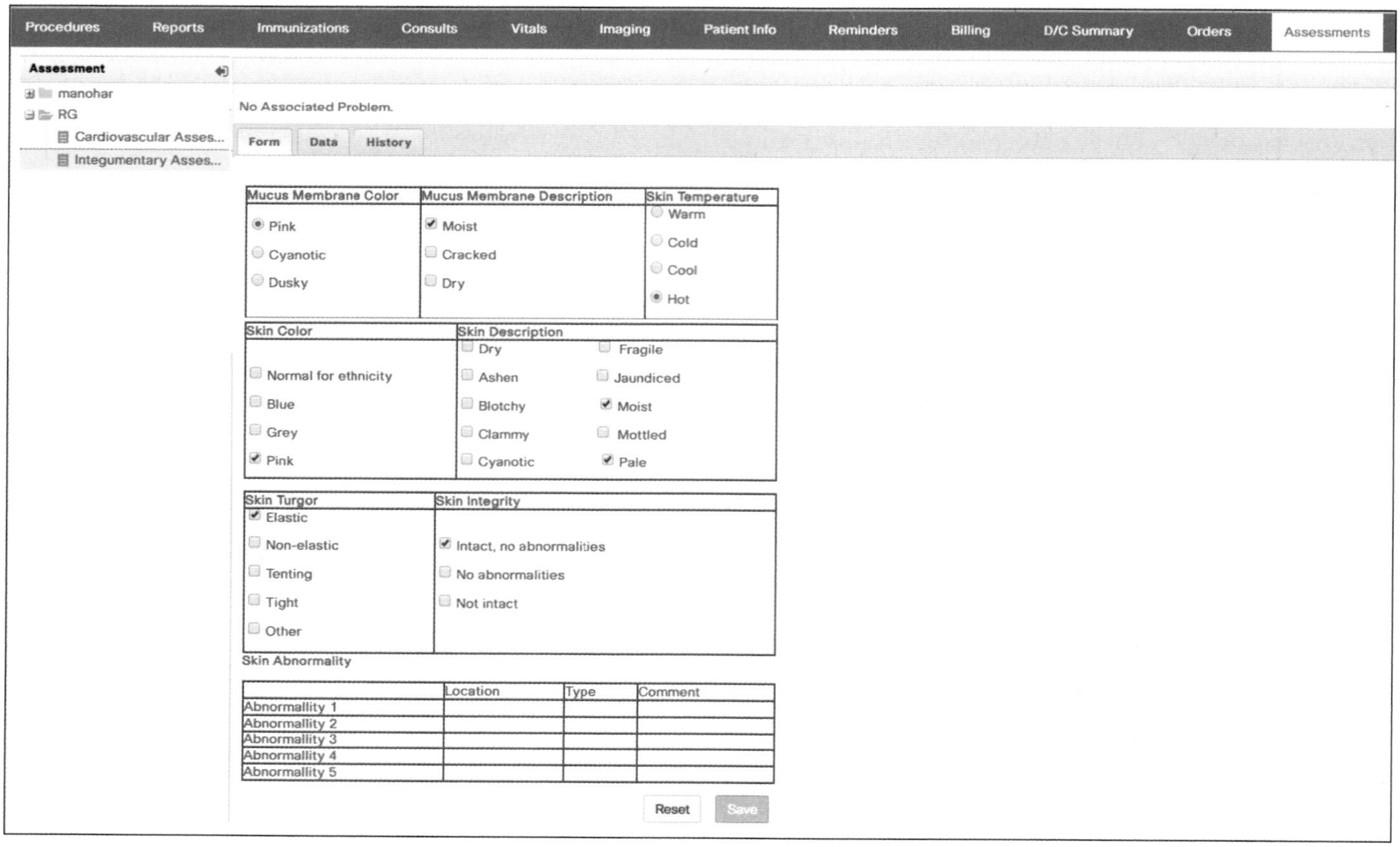

Procedures | Reports | Immunizations | Consults | Vitals | Imaging | Patient Info | Reminders | Billing | D/C Summary | Orders | Assessments

Assessment

- manohar
- RG
  - Cardiovascular Asses...
  - Integumentary Asses...

No Associated Problem.

Form | Data | History

Mucus Membrane Color	Mucus Membrane Description	Skin Temperature
(●) Pink ( ) Cyanotic ( ) Dusky	[✓] Moist [ ] Cracked [ ] Dry	( ) Warm ( ) Cold ( ) Cool (●) Hot

Skin Color	Skin Description	
[ ] Normal for ethnicity [ ] Blue [ ] Grey [✓] Pink	[ ] Dry [ ] Ashen [ ] Blotchy [ ] Clammy [ ] Cyanotic	[ ] Fragile [ ] Jaundiced [✓] Moist [ ] Mottled [✓] Pale

Skin Turgor	Skin Integrity
[✓] Elastic [ ] Non-elastic [ ] Tenting [ ] Tight [ ] Other	[✓] Intact, no abnormalities [ ] No abnormalities [ ] Not intact

Skin Abnormality

	Location	Type	Comment
Abnormallity 1			
Abnormallity 2			
Abnormallity 3			
Abnormallity 4			
Abnormallity 5			

Reset | Save

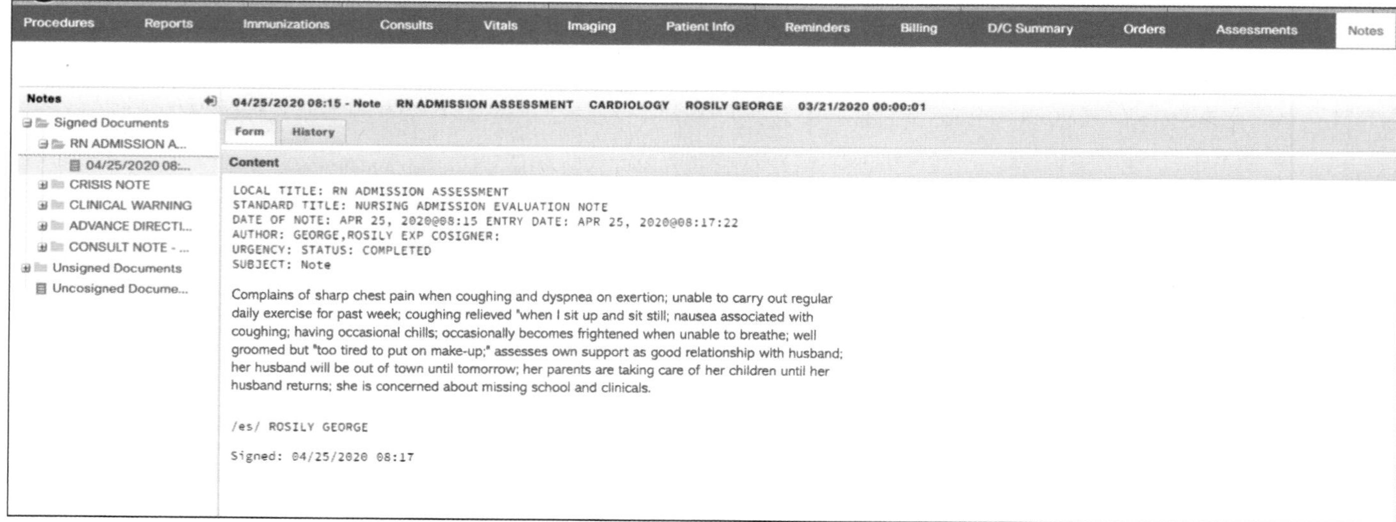

Procedures | Reports | Immunizations | Consults | Vitals | Imaging | Patient Info | Reminders | Billing | D/C Summary | Orders | Assessments | Notes

Notes

- Signed Documents
  - RN ADMISSION A...
    - 04/25/2020 08:...
  - CRISIS NOTE
  - CLINICAL WARNING
  - ADVANCE DIRECTI...
  - CONSULT NOTE - ...
- Unsigned Documents
- Uncosigned Docume...

04/25/2020 08:15 - Note RN ADMISSION ASSESSMENT CARDIOLOGY ROSILY GEORGE 03/21/2020 00:00:01

Form | History

Content

```
LOCAL TITLE: RN ADMISSION ASSESSMENT
STANDARD TITLE: NURSING ADMISSION EVALUATION NOTE
DATE OF NOTE: APR 25, 2020@08:15 ENTRY DATE: APR 25, 2020@08:17:22
AUTHOR: GEORGE,ROSILY EXP COSIGNER:
URGENCY: STATUS: COMPLETED
SUBJECT: Note
```

Complains of sharp chest pain when coughing and dyspnea on exertion; unable to carry out regular daily exercise for past week; coughing relieved "when I sit up and sit still; nausea associated with coughing; having occasional chills; occasionally becomes frightened when unable to breathe; well groomed but "too tired to put on make-up;" assesses own support as good relationship with husband; her husband will be out of town until tomorrow; her parents are taking care of her children until her husband returns; she is concerned about missing school and clinicals.

```
/es/ ROSILY GEORGE

Signed: 04/25/2020 08:17
```

Figure 10.5 ■ *Continued*

Wellness Models

Nurses use wellness models to assist clients to identify health risks and to explore lifestyle habits and health behaviors, beliefs, values, and attitudes that influence levels of wellness. Such models generally include the following:

- Health history
- Physical fitness evaluation
- Nutritional assessment
- Life-stress analysis
- Lifestyle and health habits
- Health beliefs
- Sexual health
- Spiritual health
- Relationships
- Health risk appraisal.

See Chapter 20 ∞ for details.

BOX 10.3 Data for Margaret O'Brien, Organized According to Functional Health Patterns

HEALTH PERCEPTION AND HEALTH MANAGEMENT

- Aware/understands medical diagnosis
- Gives thorough history of illnesses and surgeries
- Complies with Synthroid regimen
- Relates progression of illness in detail
- Expects to have antibiotic therapy and "go home in a day or two"
- States usual eating pattern "three meals a day"

NUTRITIONAL-METABOLIC

- 158 cm (5 ft, 2 in.) tall; weighs 56 kg (125 lb)
- Usual eating pattern "three meals a day"
- "No appetite" since having "cold"
- Has not eaten today; last fluids at noon
- Nauseated
- Oral temperature 39.4°C (103°F)
- Decreased skin turgor

ELIMINATION

- Usually no problem
- Decreased urinary frequency and amount × 2 days
- Last bowel movement yesterday, formed, states was "normal"

ACTIVITY-EXERCISE

- No musculoskeletal impairment
- Difficulty sleeping because of cough
- "Can't breathe lying down"
- States "I feel weak"
- Short of breath on exertion
- Exercises daily

COGNITIVE-PERCEPTUAL

- No sensory deficits
- Pupils 3 mm, equal, brisk reaction
- Oriented to time, place, and person
- Responsive, but fatigued
- Responds appropriately to verbal and physical stimuli
- Recent and remote memory intact
- States "short of breath" on exertion
- Reports "pain in lungs," especially when coughing
- Experiencing chills
- Reports nausea

ROLES-RELATIONSHIPS

- Lives with husband, 13-year-old daughter, and 5-year-old son
- Husband out of town; will be back tomorrow afternoon
- Children are with their grandparents until husband returns
- States "good" relationships with friends and coworkers
- Nursing student and part-time home health aid

SELF-PERCEPTION OR SELF-CONCEPT

- Expresses "concern" and "worry" over leaving her children with their grandparents until husband returns
- Anxiety related to missing her nursing classes, missing her medical–surgical clinical day, and inability to study
- Well-groomed; says, "Too tired to put on makeup"

COPING-STRESS

- Anxious: "I can't breathe"
- Facial muscles tense; trembling
- Expresses concerns about work: "I'll never get caught up"

VALUE-BELIEF

- Catholic
- No special practices desired except anointing of the sick
- Middle-class, professional orientation
- No wish to see chaplain or priest at present

MEDICATION AND HISTORY

- Synthroid 0.1 mg per day
- Client has history of appendectomy, partial thyroidectomy

NURSING PHYSICAL ASSESSMENT

- 33 years old
- Height 158 cm (5 ft, 2 in.); weight 56 kg (125 lb)
- TPR 39.4°C (103°F), 92 beats/min, 28/min
- Radial pulses weak, regular
- Blood pressure 122/80 mmHg sitting
- Skin hot and pale, cheeks flushed
- Mucous membranes dry and pale
- Respirations shallow; chest expansion less than 3 cm
- Cough productive of small amounts of pale pink sputum
- Inspiratory crackles auscultated throughout right upper and lower chest
- Diminished breath sounds on right side
- Abdomen soft, not distended
- Old surgical scars: anterior neck, RLQ abdomen
- Diaphoretic

Nonnursing Models

Frameworks and models from other disciplines may also be helpful for organizing data. These frameworks are narrower than the model required in nursing; therefore, the nurse usually needs to combine these with other approaches to obtain a complete history.

Body Systems Model

The body systems model focuses on abnormalities of the following anatomic systems:

- Integumentary system
- Respiratory system
- Cardiovascular system
- Nervous system
- Musculoskeletal system
- Gastrointestinal system
- Genitourinary system
- Reproductive system
- Immune system.

Maslow's Hierarchy of Needs

Maslow's hierarchy of needs clusters data pertaining to the following:

- Physiologic needs (survival needs)
- Safety and security needs
- Love and belonging needs

- Self-esteem needs
- Self-actualization needs.

See Chapter 19 for details.

Developmental Theories

Several physical, psychosocial, cognitive, and moral developmental theories may be used by the nurse in specific situations. Examples include the following:

- Havighurst's age periods and developmental tasks
- Freud's five stages of development
- Erikson's eight stages of development
- Piaget's phases of cognitive development
- Kohlberg's stages of moral development.

See Chapter 23 for additional information.

Validating Data

The information gathered during the assessment phase must be complete, factual, and accurate because the nursing diagnoses and interventions are based on this information. **Validation** is the act of "double-checking" or verifying data to confirm that it is accurate and factual. Validating data helps the nurse complete these tasks:

- Ensure that assessment information is complete.
- Ensure that objective and related subjective data agree.
- Obtain additional information that may have been overlooked.
- Differentiate between cues and inferences. **Cues** are subjective or objective data that can be directly observed by the nurse; that is, what the client says or what the nurse can see, hear, feel, smell, or measure. **Inferences** are the nurse's interpretation or conclusions made based on the cues (e.g., a nurse observes the cues that an incision is red, hot, and swollen; the nurse makes the inference that the incision is infected).
- Avoid jumping to conclusions and focusing in the wrong direction to identify problems.

Not all data require validation. For example, data such as height, weight, birth date, and most laboratory studies that can be measured with an accurate scale can be accepted as factual. As a rule, the nurse validates data when there are discrepancies between data obtained in the nursing interview (subjective data) and the physical examination (objective data), or when the client's statements vary at different times in the assessment. Guidelines for validating data are shown in Table 10.7.

To collect data accurately, nurses need to be aware of their own biases, values, and beliefs and to separate fact from inference, interpretation, and assumption (see Chapter 9). For example, a nurse seeing a man holding his arm to his chest might assume that he is experiencing chest pain, when in fact it is his hand that hurts.

To build an accurate database, nurses must validate assumptions regarding the client's physical or emotional behavior. In the previous example, the nurse should ask the client why he is holding his arm to his chest. The client's response may validate the nurse's assumptions

TABLE 10.7 Validating Assessment Data

Guidelines	Example
Compare subjective and objective data to verify the client's statements with your observations.	Client's perceptions of "feeling hot" need to be compared with measurement of the body temperature.
Clarify any ambiguous or vague statements.	*Client:* "I've felt sick on and off for 6 weeks."
	Nurse: "Describe what your sickness is like. Tell me what you mean by 'on and off.'"
Be sure your data consist of cues and not inferences.	*Observation:* Dry skin and reduced tissue turgor
	Inference: Dehydration
	Action: Collect additional data that are needed to make the inference in the diagnosing phase. For example, determine the client's fluid intake, amount and appearance of urine, and blood pressure.
Double-check data that are extremely abnormal.	*Observation:* A resting pulse of 30 beats/min or a blood pressure of 210/95 mmHg
	Action: Repeat the measurement. Use another piece of equipment as needed to confirm abnormalities, or ask someone else to collect the same data.
Determine the presence of factors that may interfere with accurate measurement.	A crying infant will have an abnormal respiratory rate and will need quieting before accurate assessment can be made.
Use references (textbooks, journals, research reports) to explain phenomena.	A nurse considers tiny purple or bluish-black swollen areas under the tongue of an older adult client to be abnormal until reading about physical changes of aging. Such varicosities are common.

or prompt further questioning. Figure 10.5 indicates that the nurse auscultated Margaret O'Brien's heart and lungs to validate her statement that she had "lung pain" and "shortness of breath" on exertion. Failure to validate assumptions can lead to an inaccurate or incomplete nursing assessment and could compromise client safety.

Documenting Data

To complete the assessment phase, the nurse records client data. Accurate documentation is essential and should include all data collected about the client's health status. Data are recorded in a factual manner and not interpreted by the nurse. For example, the nurse records the client's breakfast intake (objective data) as "coffee 240 mL, juice 120 mL, 1 egg, and 1 slice of toast," rather than as "appetite good" (a judgment). A judgment or conclusion such as "appetite good" or "normal appetite" may have different meanings for different people. To increase accuracy, the nurse records subjective data in the client's own words, using quotation marks. Restating in other words what someone says increases the chance of changing the original meaning (see Chapter 14 ∞).

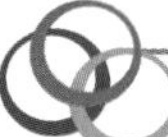

Critical Thinking Checkpoint

Eighty-two-year-old Ms. T. is in the hospital for hip replacement surgery.

1. What are the key areas of information to obtain regarding her past history?
2. Which physiologic systems are the most important for data collection before her surgery?
3. What exactly would you say to her to determine if someone will be at home to assist her after discharge?
4. Which other sources of data might be appropriate to access in her case?

Answers to Critical Thinking Checkpoint questions are available on the faculty resources site. Please consult with your instructor.

Chapter 10 Review

CHAPTER HIGHLIGHTS

- The nursing process is a systematic, rational method of planning and providing individualized nursing care for individuals, families, communities, and groups.
- The goals of the nursing process are to identify a client's health status and actual or potential healthcare needs, to establish plans to meet the identified needs, and to deliver and evaluate specific nursing interventions to meet those needs.
- The nursing process is organized into five interrelated, interdependent phases: assessing, diagnosing, planning, implementing, and evaluating.
- The nursing process can be used in all healthcare settings. It is cyclic and dynamic, client centered, focused on problem-solving and decision-making, interpersonal and collaborative, and universally applicable, and requires critical thinking and clinical reasoning.
- Clinical reasoning allows the nurse to reflect on the care delivered throughout the phases of the nursing process.
- Assessing involves collecting, organizing, validating, and documenting data.
- Diagnosing is analyzing data, identifying a client's potential or actual health problems, and formulating diagnostic statements.
- Planning involves setting priorities, formulating goals or desired outcomes, and selecting nursing interventions.
- Implementing is carrying out the nursing interventions. It includes reassessing the client, determining the nurse's need for assistance, supervising delegated care, and documenting nursing activities.
- Evaluating is the process of comparing data to outcomes to determine the status of the problem. It includes review and modification of the care plan.
- Assessment involves active participation by the client and nurse in obtaining subjective and objective data about the client's health status.
- Subjective data are the client's personal perceptions, often gathered during the nursing health history.
- Objective data (e.g., data observed and collected during the physical examination) are detectable by an observer.
- The client is the primary source of data. Secondary sources are family members and other support persons, other health professionals, records and reports, laboratory and diagnostic analyses, and relevant literature.

- The primary methods of data collection are observing, interviewing, and examining.
- Observation is a conscious, deliberate skill involving use of the senses.
- The nurse uses a combination of directive and nondirective interviewing (including closed and open-ended questions) to obtain the nursing health history.
- Nursing models provide formats for collecting and organizing client data.
- The nursing assessment must be complete and accurate because nursing diagnoses and interventions are based on this information.
- Some data must be validated. Subjective data can be used to validate objective data, and vice versa.

TEST YOUR KNOWLEDGE

1. When learning how to implement the nursing process into a plan of care for a client, the student nurse realizes that part of the purpose of the nursing process is to do which of the following?
   1. Deliver care to a client in an organized way
   2. Implement a plan that is close to the medical model
   3. Identify client needs and deliver care to meet those needs
   4. Make sure that standardized care is available to clients

2. A nursing student is learning how to implement the nursing process in the clinical area. Which of the following does the purpose of the diagnosis phase include?
   1. Develop a list of problems
   2. Identify client strengths
   3. Develop a plan
   4. Specify goals and outcomes
   5. Identify problems that can be prevented

3. Which element is best categorized as secondary subjective data?
   1. The nurse measures a weight loss of 10 pounds since the last clinic visit.
   2. Spouse states the client has lost all appetite.
   3. The nurse palpates edema in lower extremities.
   4. Client states severe pain when walking up stairs.

4. During an initial interview, the client makes this statement: "I don't understand why I have to have surgery, I'm really not that sick or in pain right now." What is the nurse's best response?
   1. "It's OK to be worried. Surgery is a big step."
   2. "What kind of questions do you have about your surgery?"
   3. "I think these are things you should be asking your doctor."
   4. "Have you had surgery before?"

5. The use of a conceptual or theoretical framework for collecting and organizing assessment data ensures which of the following?
   1. Correlation of the data with other members of the healthcare team
   2. Demonstration of cost-effective care
   3. Utilization of creativity and intuition in creating a plan of care
   4. Collection of all necessary information for a thorough appraisal

6. Which of the following is the purpose of assessing?
   1. Establish a database of client responses to his or her health status.
   2. Identify client strengths and problems.
   3. Develop an individualized plan of care.
   4. Implement care, prevent illness, and promote wellness.

7. In the validating activity of the assessing phase of the nursing process, the nurse performs which of the following?
   1. Collects subjective data.
   2. Applies a framework to the collected data.
   3. Confirms data are complete and accurate.
   4. Records data in the client record.

8. A major characteristic of the nursing process is which of the following?
   1. A focus on client needs
   2. Its static nature
   3. An emphasis on physiology and illness
   4. Its exclusive use by and with nurses

9. Which statement would be true regarding use of the observing method of data collection?
   1. When observing, the nurse uses only the visual sense.
   2. Observing is done only when no other nursing interventions are being performed at the same time.
   3. Data should be gathered as they occur, rather than in any particular order.
   4. Observed data should be interpreted in relation to other sources of collected data.

10. Which of the following represent effective planning of the interview setting? Select all that apply.
   1. Keep the lighting dimmed so as not to stress the client's eyes.
   2. Ensure that no one can overhear the interview conversation.
   3. Stand near the client's head while he or she is in the bed or chair.
   4. Keep approximately 3 feet from the client during the interview.
   5. Use a standard form to be sure all relevant data are covered in the interview.

See Answers to Test Your Knowledge in Appendix A.

READINGS AND REFERENCES

Suggested Reading

Aria, A., Sander, R., & Siek, T. (2018). Simulations as an assessment strategy to assist with unit placement for new graduate nurses. *Journal for Nurses in Professional Development*, *34*(2), 78–83. doi:10.1097/NND.0000000000000424

The nurse residency program in the healthcare facility where this study was conducted revised the onboarding of new graduate nurses with the use of simulation and lecture, along with critical thinking case studies and active learning experiences. The education team utilized simulation and a simulation assessment score for formative and summative evaluation. The addition of simulation resulted in increased readiness for nursing practice and increased safety.

Related Research

Colla, L., Fuller-Tyszkiewicz, M., Tomyn, A., Richardson, B., & Tomyn, J. (2016). Use of weekly assessment data to enhance evaluation of a subjective wellbeing intervention. *Quality of Life Research*, *25*, 517–524. doi:10.1007/s11136-015-1150-0

Kohtz, C., Brown, S. C., Williams, R., & O'Connor, P. A. (2017). Physical assessment techniques in nursing education: A replicated study. *Journal of Nursing Education*, *56*(5), 287–291. doi:10.3928/01484834-20170421-06

References

American Nurses Association. (2015). *Nursing: Scope and standards of nursing practice* (3rd ed.). Silver Spring, MD: Author.

D'Amico, D., & Barbarito, C. (2016). *Health & physical assessment in nursing* (3rd ed.). Upper Saddle River, NJ: Pearson Prentice Hall.

Feo, R., Rasmussen, P., Wiechula, R., Conroy, T., & Kitson, A. (2017). Developing effective and caring nurse-patient relationships. *Nursing Standard*, *31*(28), 54–62. doi:107748/ns.2017.e10735

Gordon, M. (2016). *Manual of nursing diagnosis* (13th ed.). Boston, MA: Jones & Bartlett.

Hall, L. (1955, June). Quality of nursing care. *Public Health News*. Newark, NJ: State Department of Health.

Johnson, D. E. (1959). A philosophy of nursing. *Nursing Outlook*, *7*, 198–200.

The Joint Commission. (2019). *Documentation assistance provided by scribes*. Retrieved from https://www.jointcommission.org/standards_information/jcfaqdetails.aspx?StandardsFAQId=1809

Kneisl, C. R., & Trigoboff, E. (2013). *Contemporary psychiatric–mental health nursing* (3rd ed.). Upper Saddle River, NJ: Prentice Hall.

Orem, D. E. (2001). *Nursing: Concepts of practice* (6th ed.). St. Louis, MO: Mosby.

Orlando, I. (1961). *The dynamic nurse–patient relationship*. New York, NY: Putnam.

Roy, C. (2009). *The Roy adaptation model* (3rd ed.). Upper Saddle River, NJ: Prentice Hall.

Wiedenbach, E. (1963). The helping art of nursing. *American Journal of Nursing*, *63*(11), 54–57. doi:10.2307/3453018

Wilkinson, J. M. (2012). *Nursing process and critical thinking* (5th ed.). Upper Saddle River, NJ: Pearson.

Selected Bibliography

Alfaro-LeFevre, R. (2017). *Critical thinking, clinical reasoning, and clinical judgment: A practical approach* (6th ed.). Philadelphia, PA: Elsevier.

Frank, C. A., Schroeter, K., & Shaw, C. (2017). Addressing traumatic stress in the acute traumatically injured patient. *Journal of Trauma Nursing*, *24*(2), 78–84. doi:10.1097/JTN.0000000000000270

The Joint Commission. (2019). *Nursing assessments—Licensed Practical Nurse*. Retrieved from https://www.jointcommission.org/standards_information/jcfaqdetails.aspx?StandardsFaqId=1590&ProgramId=46

Vaughn, J., & Parry, A. (2016). Assessment and management of the septic patient: Part 2. *British Journal of Nursing*, *25*(21), 1196–1200. doi:10.12968/bjon.2016.25.21.1196

11 Diagnosing

LEARNING OUTCOMES

After completing this chapter, you will be able to:

1. Differentiate nursing diagnoses according to status.
2. Identify the components of a nursing diagnosis.
3. Compare nursing diagnoses, medical diagnoses, and collaborative problems.
4. Identify the basic steps in the diagnostic process.
5. Describe various formats for writing nursing diagnoses.
6. List guidelines for writing a nursing diagnosis statement.
7. Describe the evolution of the nursing diagnosis movement, including work currently in progress.

KEY TERMS

defining characteristics, *214*
dependent functions, *215*
diagnosis, *212*
health promotion diagnosis, *213*
independent functions, *215*
norm, *216*
nursing diagnosis, *212*
PES format, *219*
qualifiers, *213*
risk factors, *213*
risk nursing diagnosis, *213*
standard, *216*
syndrome diagnosis, *213*

Introduction

Diagnosing is the second phase of the nursing process. In this phase, nurses use critical thinking skills to interpret assessment data and identify client strengths and problems. Diagnosing is a pivotal step in the nursing process. Activities preceding this phase are directed toward formulating the nursing diagnoses; the care planning activities following this phase are based on the nursing diagnoses (Figure 11.1 ■).

The identification and development of nursing diagnoses began formally in 1973, when two faculty members of Saint Louis University, Kristine Gebbie and Mary Ann Lavin, perceived a need to identify nurses' roles in an ambulatory care setting. The first national conference to identify nursing diagnoses was sponsored by the Saint Louis University School of Nursing and Allied Health Professions in 1973. Subsequent national conferences occurred in 1975, in 1980, and every 2 years thereafter.

International recognition came with the First Canadian Conference in Toronto in 1977 and the International Nursing Conference in May 1987 in Calgary, Alberta, Canada. In 1982, the conference group accepted the name North American Nursing Diagnosis Association (NANDA), recognizing the participation and contributions of nurses in the United States and Canada. In 2002, the organization changed its name to NANDA International to further reflect the worldwide interest in nursing diagnosis.

Nursing Diagnoses

To use the concept of nursing diagnoses effectively in generating and completing a nursing care plan, the nurse must be familiar with the definitions of terms used and the components of nursing diagnoses.

Definitions

The term *diagnosing* refers to the reasoning process, whereas the term **diagnosis** is a statement or conclusion regarding the nature of a phenomenon. The **nursing diagnosis** contains a diagnostic phrase or diagnostic label followed by an etiology phrase. The diagnostic phrase or label is a statement of the client's problem. The etiology is the causal relationship betweent he client's problem or risk factors.

Wilkinson & Barcus (2017) identifies the growing need for a standardized nursing language to describe client problems. "Nursing diagnosis fulfills that need and helps define the scope of nursing practice by descrbing conditions the nurse can independently treat. Nursing diagnosis highlights crticial thinking and decision-making and provides consistent and universally understood terminology among nurses working in various settings, including hospitals, ambulatory care clinics, extended care facilities, occupational health facilities, and private practice" (Wilkinson & Barcus, 2017, p. 1).

- Professional nurses (registered nurses) are responsible for making nursing diagnoses, even though other nursing personnel may contribute data to the process of

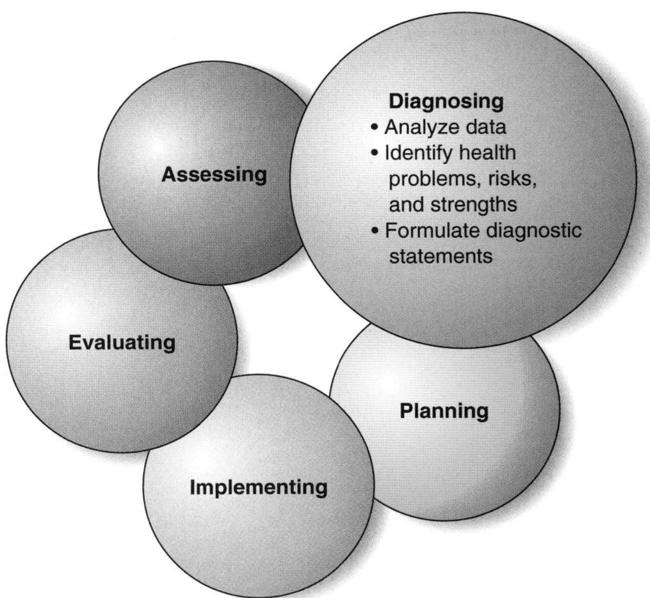

Figure 11.1 ■ Diagnosing—the pivotal second phase of the nursing process.

diagnosing and may implement specified nursing care. The American Nurses Association's *Nursing: Scope and Standards of Practice* (2015) states that nurses are accountable for analyzing data to determine diagnoses or issues. The standard also specifies that nurses should use standardized classification systems when naming diagnoses.

- The domain of nursing diagnosis includes only those health states that nurses are educated and licensed to treat. For example, generalist nurses are not educated to diagnose or treat diseases such as diabetes mellitus; this task is defined legally as within the practice of medicine. Yet nurses can diagnose and treat a client's insufficient knowledge of the disease process, a lack of the ability to cope with the medical diagnosis, and inadequate dietary nutrition, all of which are the human responses to the medical diagnosis of diabetes mellitus.
- A nursing diagnosis is a judgment made only after thorough, systematic data collection.
- Nursing diagnoses describe a continuum of health states: deviations from health, presence of risk factors, and areas of enhanced personal growth.

Status of the Nursing Diagnoses

Nurses develop nursing diagnoses based on the client's actual or potential health problems and related needs. There are four types of nursing diagnoses: actual, health promotion, risk, and syndrome diagnoses.

1. An *actual nursing diagnosis* is also known as a problem-based diagnosis. This nursing diagnosis is a client problem that is present at the time of the nursing assessment. Examples are altered respiratory status or impaired ability to cope. An actual or problem-based nursing diagnosis is based on the presence of associated signs and symptoms.
2. A **health promotion diagnosis** relates to clients' preparedness to implement behaviors to improve their health condition. These diagnosis labels begin with the phrase *willingness to learn* about the health maintenance or *willingness to change* health practices.
3. A **risk nursing diagnosis** is a clinical judgment that a problem does not exist, but the presence of **risk factors** indicates that a problem is likely to develop unless nurses intervene. For example, all people admitted to a hospital have some possibility of acquiring an infection; however, a client with diabetes or a compromised immune system is at higher risk than others. Therefore, the nurse would appropriately use the label risk for or potential for impaired breathing patterns to describe the client's health status.
4. A **syndrome diagnosis** is a clinical nursing judgement when a client has several similar nursing diagnoses such as impaired respiratory status related to increased secretions and restricted pulmonary airflow related to a lack of alveoli elasticity.

Components of a Nursing Diagnosis

A nursing diagnosis has three components: (1) the problem and its definition, (2) the etiology, and (3) the defining characteristics. Each component serves a specific purpose.

Problem (Diagnostic Label) and Definition

The problem statement, or diagnostic label, describes the client's health problem or response for which nursing therapy is given. It describes the client's health status clearly and concisely in a few words. The purpose of the diagnostic label is to direct the formation of client goals and desired outcomes. It may also suggest some nursing interventions.

Qualifiers are words that are added to the nursing diagnosis to provide additional meaning to the diagnostic statement, for example:

- inadequate in amount, quality, or degree; not sufficient; incomplete
- made worse, weakened, damaged, reduced, deteriorated
- lesser in size, amount, or degree
- not producing the desired effect
- vulnerable to threat.

Etiology (Related Factors and Risk Factors)

The etiology component of a nursing diagnosis identifies one or more probable causes of the health problem, gives direction to the required nursing therapy, and enables the nurse to individualize the client's care. As shown in

EVIDENCE-BASED PRACTICE

Evidence-Based Practice

What Nursing Diagnoses, Outcomes, and Interventions Are Measures of Client Complexity in the Delivery of Care in the Intensive Care Unit?

Castellan, Sluga, Spina, and Sanson (2016) sought to describe the complexity of nursing care in the intensive care unit (ICU). This prospective study examined the pattern and frequency of nursing diagnoses, nursing outcome classifications, and nursing intervention classifications. This examination is known as the NNN taxonomy. Seventy-one nursing diagnoses were selected at least one time. Of these diagnoses, 47 were actual nursing diagnoses and 24 were risk diagnoses. On average, 24 nursing outcomes and 60 nursing interventions classifications were noted. The plans of care most commonly identified in the ICU support self-care deficits and impaired family processes. The most common outcomes were the prevention of infection, prevention of disease, and prevention of impaired skin integrity. The study results indicated that nursing diagnoses, outcomes, and interventions have activity with regards to a broad spectrum of client needs.

Implications

The authors suggest that the prevalence of nursing diagnoses, outcomes, and interventions in the care of clients in the ICU allows for the measurement and evaluation of the outcome of client care.

TABLE 11.1 Components of a Nursing Diagnosis

Diagnosis and Definition	Related Factors	Defining Characteristics
Impaired acitivity: decreased physical or emotional ability to engage in activities of daily living.	Shortness of breath Immobility Physical disability	Fatigue or weakness Tachycardia with activity Heart rhythm changes Dyspnea

Table 11.1, the probable causes of impaired activity include generalized weakness, sedentary lifestyle, and so on. Differentiating among possible causes in the nursing diagnosis is essential because each may require different nursing interventions. Table 11.2 provides an example of a problem that has different etiologies and therefore requires different interventions.

Each diagnostic label such as, ineffective breathing clarifies the meaning of the diagnosis. For example, the definition of the diagnostic label impaired activity is shown in Table 11.1.

Defining Characteristics

Defining characteristics are the cluster of signs and symptoms that indicate the presence of a particular diagnostic label. For actual nursing diagnoses, the defining characteristics are the client's signs and symptoms. For risk nursing diagnoses, no subjective and objective signs are present. Thus, the factors that cause the client to be more vulnerable to the problem form the etiology of a risk nursing diagnosis.

TABLE 11.2 Examples of Nursing Diagnoses with Different Etiologies

Diagnostic Label (Problem)	Client	Etiology
Constipation	Al Martinez	Long-term laxative use
	Jerry Wong	Inactivity and insufficient fluid intake
	Tanya Brown	Threat to physiologic integrity: possible cancer diagnosis
	Caitlin Shea	Effects of aging (reduced hearing, vision, mobility)

Differentiating Nursing Diagnoses from Medical Diagnoses

Both the nursing diagnoses and medical diagnoses provide each profession with a common language to describe and code its knowledge. The nursing diagnosis provides a way to describe the client's area of concern. A nursing diagnosis is a statement of clinical judgment that concerns a human response to a health condition that nurses, by virtue of their education, experience, and expertise, are licensed to treat. A medical diagnosis is made by a physician and refers to a condition that only a physician can treat. Medical diagnoses refer to disease processes—specific pathophysiologic responses that are fairly uniform from one client to another. In contrast, nursing diagnoses describe the human response, a client's physical, sociocultural, psychologic, and spiritual responses to an illness or a health problem. See how these responses vary among individuals:

> Seventy-year-old Mary Cain and 20-year-old Kristi Vidan both have rheumatoid arthritis. Their disease processes are much the same. X-ray studies show that in both clients, the extent of inflammation and the number of joints involved are similar, and both clients experience almost constant pain. Ms. Cain views her condition as part of the aging process and is responding with acceptance. Ms. Vidan, however, is responding with anger and hostility because she views her disease as a threat to her personal identity, role performance, and self-esteem.

A client's medical diagnosis remains the same for as long as the disease process is present, but nursing diagnoses change as the client's responses change. Ms. Vidan's response to her illness may change over time to become more similar to that of Ms. Cain.

Nurses have responsibilities related to both medical and nursing diagnoses. Nursing diagnoses relate primarily to the nurse's **independent functions**, that is, the areas of healthcare that are unique to nursing and separate and distinct from medical management. However, the nurse is still responsible for identifying and responding to data that indicate real or potential medical problems.

A nurse may not be able to prescribe all of the care for a nursing diagnosis, but the nurse can prescribe most of the interventions needed for prevention or resolution. For example, most clients with a nursing diagnosis of *Pain* have medical orders for analgesics, but many independent nursing interventions can also alleviate pain (e.g., guided imagery or teaching a client to "splint" an incision). With regard to medical diagnoses, nurses are obligated to carry out physician-prescribed therapies and treatments, that is, **dependent functions**. See Chapter 12 ∞ for a discussion of independent and dependent nursing interventions.

Differentiating Nursing Diagnoses from Collaborative Problems

A collaborative problem is a type of potential problem that nurses manage using both independent and physician-prescribed interventions. Independent nursing interventions for a collaborative problem focus mainly on monitoring the client's condition and preventing development of the potential complication. Definitive treatment of the condition requires both medical and nursing interventions.

Collaborative problems are present when a particular disease or treatment is present; that is, each disease or treatment has specific complications that are always associated with it. For example, a statement of collaborative problems is "Potential complications of pneumonia: atelectasis, respiratory failure, pleural effusion, pericarditis, and meningitis."

Nursing diagnoses, by contrast, involve human responses, which vary greatly from one individual to the next. Therefore, the same set of nursing diagnoses cannot be expected to occur with all clients who have a particular disease or condition; moreover, a single nursing diagnosis may occur as a response to any number of diseases. For example, all postpartum clients have similar collaborative problems, such as "Potential complication of childbearing: postpartum hemorrhage," but not all new mothers have the same nursing diagnoses. Some might experience altered parenting (delayed bonding), but most will not; some might have a knowledge deficit, whereas others will not. Thus, the nurse uses nursing diagnoses rather than collaborative problems whenever possible, since nursing diagnoses are more individualized to a specific client and emphasize human responses to which the nurse can independently take action. Table 11.3 provides a comparison of nursing diagnoses, medical diagnoses, and collaborative problems.

TABLE 11.3 Comparison of Nursing Diagnoses, Medical Diagnoses, and Collaborative Problems

	Nursing Diagnoses	Medical Diagnoses	Collaborative Problems
Example	Impaired activity related to decreased cardiac output	Myocardial infarction	Potential complication of myocardial infarction: congestive heart failure
Description	Describe human responses to disease process or health problem; consist of a one-, two-, or three-part statement, usually including problem and etiology	Describe disease and pathology; do not consider other human responses; usually consist of not more than three words	Involve human responses—mainly physiologic complications of disease, tests, or treatments; consist of a two-part statement of situation or pathophysiology and the potential complication
Orientation and responsibility for diagnosing	Oriented to the individual; nurses responsible for diagnosing	Oriented to pathology; physician responsible for diagnosing; diagnosis not within the scope of nursing practice	Oriented to pathophysiology; nurses responsible for diagnosing
Nursing focus	Treat and prevent	Implement medical orders for treatment and monitor status of condition	Prevent and monitor for onset or status of condition
Nursing actions	Independent	Dependent (primarily)	Some independent actions, but primarily for monitoring and preventing
Duration	Can change frequently	Remains the same while disease is present	Present when disease or situation is present
Classification system	Classification system is developed and being used but is not universally accepted	Well-developed classification system accepted by the medical profession	No universally accepted classification system

The Diagnostic Process

The diagnostic process uses the critical thinking skills of analysis and synthesis. In critical thinking, an individual reviews data and considers explanations before forming an opinion. Analysis is the separation into components, that is, the breaking down of the whole into its parts (deductive reasoning). Synthesis is the opposite, that is, the putting together of parts into the whole (inductive reasoning). See Chapter 9 ∞ to review the concepts of deductive and inductive reasoning.

The diagnostic process is used continuously by most nurses. An experienced nurse may enter a client's room and immediately observe significant data and draw conclusions about the client. As a result of attaining knowledge, skill, and expertise in the practice setting, the expert nurse may seem to perform these mental processes automatically. Novice nurses, however, need guidelines to understand and formulate nursing diagnoses. The diagnostic process has three steps:

- Analyzing data
- Identifying health problems, risks, and strengths
- Formulating diagnostic statements.

For experienced nurses, these activities occur continuously rather than sequentially.

Analyzing Data

In the diagnostic process, analyzing involves the following steps:

1. Compare data against standards (identify significant cues).
2. Cluster the cues (generate tentative hypotheses).
3. Identify gaps and inconsistencies.

Comparing Data with Standards

Nurses draw on knowledge and experience to compare client data to standards and norms and identify significant and relevant cues. A **standard** or **norm** is a generally accepted measure, rule, model, or pattern. The nurse uses a wide range of standards, such as growth and development patterns, normal vital signs, and laboratory values. A cue is considered significant if it does any of the following:

- Points to negative or positive change in a client's health status or pattern. For example, the client states: "I have recently experienced shortness of breath while climbing stairs" or "I have not smoked for 3 months."
- Varies from norms of the client population. The client may consider a pattern—for example, eating very small meals and having little appetite—to be normal. This pattern, however, may not be healthy and may require further exploration.
- Indicates a developmental delay. To identify significant cues, the nurse must be aware of the normal patterns and changes that occur as the individual grows and develops. For example, by age 9 months an infant is usually able to sit alone without support. The infant who has not accomplished this task needs further assessment for possible developmental delays.

Table 11.4 lists specific examples of client cues and norms to which they may be compared.

Clustering Cues

Data clustering or grouping of cues is a process of determining the relatedness of facts and determining whether

TABLE 11.4 Comparing Cues to Standards and Norms

Type of Cue	Client Cues	Standard/Norm
Deviation from population norms	Height is 158 cm (5 ft, 2 in.). Woman with small frame. Weighs 109 kg (240 lb).	Height and weight tables indicate that the "ideal" weight for a woman 158 cm (5 ft, 2 in.) with a small frame is 49–53 kg (108–121 lb).
Developmental delay	Child is 17 months old. Parents state child has not yet attempted to speak. Child laughs aloud and makes cooing sounds.	Children usually speak their first word by 10–12 months of age.
Changes in client's usual health status	States, "I'm just not hungry these days." Ate only 15% of food on breakfast tray. Has lost 13 kg (30 lb) in past 3 months.	Client usually eats three balanced meals per day. Adults typically maintain stable weight.
Dysfunctional behavior	Amy's mother reports that Amy has not left her room for 2 days. Amy is age 16. Amy has stopped attending school and has withdrawn from social contact.	Adolescents usually like to be with their peers; social group very important. Functional behavior includes school attendance.
Changes in client's usual behavior	Mrs. Stuart reports that lately her husband angers easily. "Yesterday he even yelled at the dog." "He just seems so tense."	Mr. Stuart is usually relaxed and easygoing. He is friendly and kind to animals.

any patterns are present, whether the data represent isolated incidents, and whether the data are significant. This is the beginning of synthesis.

The nurse may cluster data inductively (as in Table 11.5) by combining data from different assessment areas to form a pattern; or the nurse may begin with a framework, such as Gordon's functional health patterns, and organize the subjective and objective data into the appropriate categories (see Box 10.3 and Table 10.4, pages 207 and 198). The latter is a deductive approach to data clustering (see Chapter 9 ∞).

Experienced nurses may cluster data as they collect and interpret it, as evidenced in remarks or thoughts such as "I'm getting a sense of . . . " or "This cue doesn't fit the picture." The novice nurse does not have the knowledge base or the clinical experience that aids in recognizing cues. Thus, the novice must take careful assessment notes, search data for abnormal cues, and use textbook resources for comparing the client's cues with the defining characteristics and etiologic factors of the accepted nursing diagnoses.

Data clustering involves making inferences about the data. The nurse interprets the possible meaning of the cues, and labels the cue clusters with tentative diagnostic hypotheses. Data clustering or grouping for Margaret O'Brien is illustrated in Table 11.5, in which data are clustered according to standardized diagnostic labels.

TABLE 11.5 Formulating Nursing Diagnoses for Margaret O'Brien

Functional Health Pattern	Client Cue Clusters	Inferences (Tentative Identification of Problems)	Diagnostic Statements
Nutritional-metabolic (includes hydration)	"No appetite" since having "cold"; has not eaten today; last fluids at noon today Nauseated × 2 days	Impaired nutritional status	Impaired nutritional status: decreased caloric intake related to decreased appetite and nausea and increased metabolism (secondary to disease process) *Strength:* normal weight for height
	Last fluids at noon today Oral temp 39.4°C (103°F) Skin hot and pale, cheeks flushed Mucous membranes dry Poor skin turgor *Cues from elimination pattern:* Decreased urinary frequency and amount × 2 days	Alteration in fluid volume	Alteration in fluid volume related to intake insufficient to replace fluid loss secondary to fever, diaphoresis, anorexia
Activity-exercise	Difficulty sleeping because of cough "Can't breathe lying down"	Impaired sleep	Impaired sleep related to cough, pain, orthopnea, fever, and diaphoresis
	States "I feel weak" Short of breath on exertion *Cues from cognitive-perceptual pattern:* Responsive but fatigued "I can think OK, just weak." *Cues from cardiovascular pattern:* Radial pulses weak, regular Pulse rate 92 beats/min	Impaired activity	Impaired activity related to general weakness, imbalance between oxygen supply and demand *Strength:* no musculoskeletal impairment, normal energy level is satisfactory, exercises regularly
Cognitive-perceptual	Reports pain in chest, especially when coughing	Pain	Pain related to cough secondary to pneumonia
	Responsive but fatigued "I can think OK, just weak."	These are cognitive-perceptual data, but they reflect symptoms of problems in the activity-exercise pattern	*Strength:* no cognitive or sensory deficits
Roles-relationships	Husband out of town; will be back tomorrow afternoon Children with grandparents until husband returns	Impaired family dynamics related to mother's illness and temporary unavailability of father to provide child care	Impaired family dynamics related to mother's illness and temporary unavailability of father to provide child care *Strength:* in-laws available and willing to help
Self-perception or self-concept	Expresses "concern" and "worry" over leaving daughter and son with their grandparents until husband returns	Cue is a symptom of a problem in the coping-stress pattern	No self-perception or self-concept problem

Continued on page 218

TABLE 11.5 Formulating Nursing Diagnoses for Margaret O'Brien—*continued*

Functional Health Pattern	Client Cue Clusters	Inferences (Tentative Identification of Problems)	Diagnostic Statements
Coping-stress	Anxious: "I can't breathe." Facial muscles tense; trembling Expresses concerns about her nursing classes: "I'll never get caught up." *Cues from role-relationship pattern:* Husband out of town; will be back tomorrow afternoon Children with in-laws until husband returns *Cues from self-perception or self-concept patterns:* Expresses "concern" and "worry" over leaving children with in-laws	Anxiety related to difficulty breathing, inability to attend nursing classes and to study, and child care	Anxiety related to difficulty breathing and concerns over work and parenting roles
Medication and history	No significant cues	No problem	No problem
PHYSICAL ASSESSMENT			
• Cardiovascular	Radial pulses weak, regular Pulse rate 92 beats/min	Cues are symptoms only; symptoms of exercise-rest and oxygenation problems	No cardiovascular problem
• Oxygenation	Skin hot, pale, and moist Respirations shallow; chest expansion, 3 cm Cough productive of small amounts of thick pale pink sputum Inspiratory crackles auscultated throughout right upper and lower lungs Diminished breath sounds on right side Mucous membranes pale, dry	Altered respiratory status related to disease process	Altered respiratory status related to viscous secretions and shallow chest expansion secondary to pain, fluid volume deficit, and fatigue

Identifying Gaps and Inconsistencies in Data

Skillful assessment minimizes gaps and inconsistencies in data. However, data analysis should include a final check to ensure that data are complete and correct.

Inconsistencies are conflicting data. Possible sources of conflicting data include measurement error, expectations, and inconsistent or unreliable reports. For example, a nurse may learn from the nursing history that the client reports not having seen a healthcare provider in 15 years, yet during the physical health examination he states, "My doctor takes my blood pressure every year." All inconsistencies must be clarified before a valid pattern can be established. See the Validating Data section in Chapter 10 ∞.

Identifying Health Problems, Risks, and Strengths

After data are analyzed, the nurse and client can together identify strengths and problems. This is primarily a decision-making process (see Chapter 9 ∞).

Determining Problems and Risks

After grouping and clustering the data, the nurse and client together identify problems that support tentative actual, risk, and potential diagnoses. In addition, the nurse must determine whether the client's problem is a nursing diagnosis, medical diagnosis, or collaborative problem. See Figure 11.2 ■ and Table 11.5.

Significant cues and data clusters for Margaret O'Brien that were extracted from Figure 10.5 on pages 205–206 and Box 10.3 on page 207 are shown in Table 11.5. In this example, the nurse and client identified eight tentative problems: impaired nutritional status: decreased caloric intake, alteration in fluid volume, impaired sleep, impaired activity, pain, impaired family dynamics, anxiety, and altered respiratoty status.

Note that some data may indicate a possible problem but when clustered with other data, the possible problem disappears. For example, the following data for Margaret O'Brien, "Decreased urinary frequency and amount × 2 days," suggests a possible urinary elimination problem. However, when these data are considered along with data associated with alteration in fluid volume, the nurse eliminates urinary elimination as a problem.

Determining Strengths

At this stage, the nurse and client also establish the client's strengths, resources, and abilities to cope. Most people have a clearer perception of their problems or weaknesses

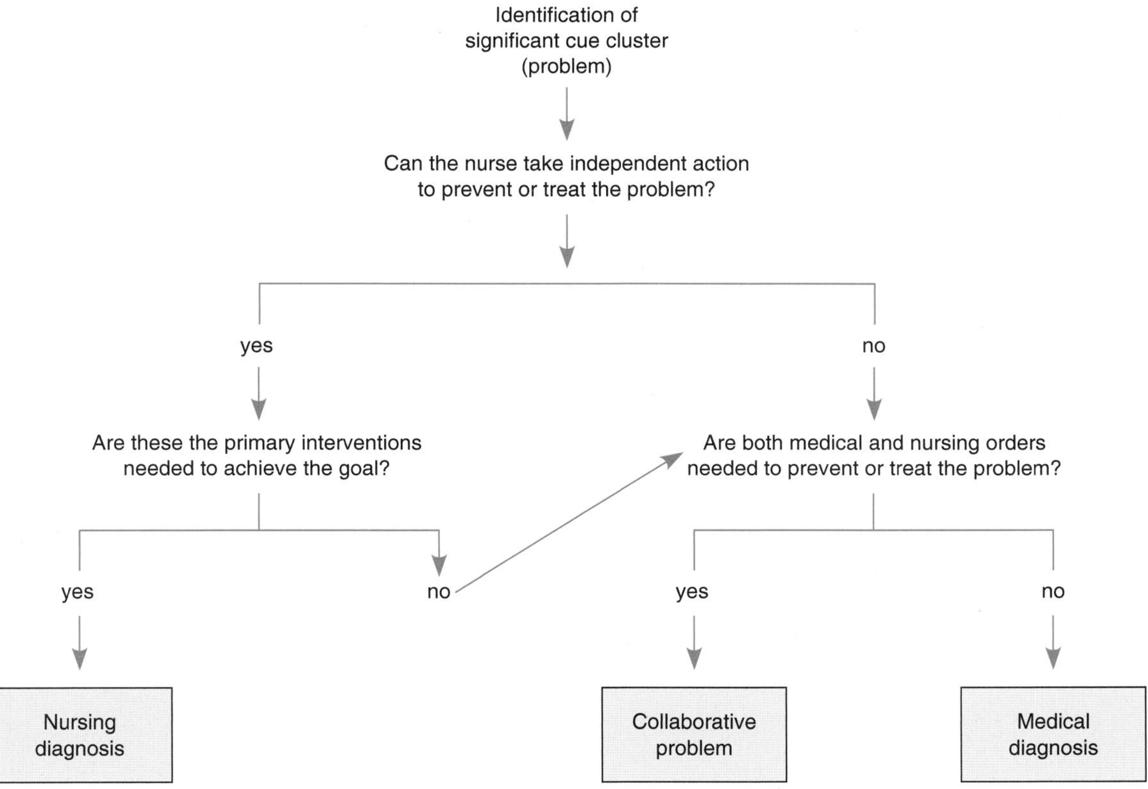

Figure 11.2 ■ Decision tree for differentiating among nursing diagnoses, collaborative problems, and medical diagnoses.

than of their strengths and assets, which they often take for granted. By taking an inventory of strengths, the client can develop a more well-rounded self-concept and self-image. Strengths can be an aid to mobilizing health and regenerative processes.

A client's strength might be weight that is within the normal range for age and height, thus enabling the client to cope better with surgery. In another instance, a client's strengths might be absence of allergies and being a nonsmoker.

A client's strengths can be found in the nursing assessment record (health, home life, education, recreation, exercise, work, family and friends, religious beliefs, and sense of humor, for example), the health examination, and the client's records. See Table 11.5 for the strengths identified for Margaret O'Brien.

Formulating Diagnostic Statements

Most nursing diagnoses are written as two-part or three-part statements, but there are variations of these.

Basic Two-Part Statements

The basic two-part statement includes the following:

1. ***Problem (P):*** statement of the client's response
2. ***Etiology (E):*** factors contributing to or probable causes of the responses.

The two parts are joined by the words *related to* rather than *due to*. The phrase *due to* implies that one part causes or is responsible for the other part. By contrast, the phrase *related to* merely implies a relationship. Some examples of two-part nursing diagnoses are shown in Box 11.1.

For a nursing diagnosis that contains the word "specify", the nurse must add words to indicate the problem more specifically. The format is still a two-part statement. For example, nonadherence (specify) would be nonadherence (diabetic diet) related to denial of having disease. For ease in alphabetizing, many nursing diagnosis lists are arranged with qualifying words after the main word (e.g., infection, potential for). Avoid writing diagnostic statements in that manner; instead, write them as they would be stated in normal conversation (e.g., potential for infection).

Basic Three-Part Statements

The basic three-part nursing diagnosis statement is called the **PES format** and includes the following:

1. ***Problem (P):*** statement of the client's response (nursing diagnosis label)

BOX 11.1 Basic Two-Part Diagnostic Statement

Problem	Related to	Etiology
Constipation	related to	prolonged laxative use
Anxiety	related to	threat to physiologic integrity: possible cancer diagnosis

BOX 11.2 Basic Three-Part Diagnostic Statement

Problem	Related to	Etiology	As Manifested by	Signs and Symptoms
Impaired self-esteem	related to (r/t)	feelings of rejection by husband	as manifested by (a.m.b.)	hypersensitivity to criticism; states "I don't know if I can manage by myself" and rejects positive feedback

2. *Etiology (E):* factors contributing to or probable causes of the response
3. *Signs and symptoms (S):* defining characteristics manifested by the client.

Actual nursing diagnoses can be documented by using the three-part statement (see Box 11.2) because the signs and symptoms have been identified. This format cannot be used for risk diagnoses because the client does not have signs and symptoms of the diagnosis.

The PES format is especially recommended for beginning diagnosticians because the signs and symptoms validate why the diagnosis was chosen and make the problem statement more descriptive. The PES format can create very long problem statements, sometimes making the problem and etiology unclear. To minimize long problem statements, the nurse can record the signs and symptoms in the nursing notes instead of on the care plan. Another possibility, recommended for students, is to list the signs and symptoms on the care plan below the nursing diagnosis, grouping the subjective (S) and objective (O) data. The signs and symptoms are easily accessible, and the problem and etiology stand out clearly. For example:

Nonadherence (diabetic diet) related to unresolved anger about diagnosis as manifested by

S— "I forget to take my pills."
"I can't live without sugar in my food."

O— Weight 98 kg (215 lb) (gain of 4.5 kg [10 lb])
Blood pressure 190/100 mmHg

One-Part Statements

Some diagnostic statements, such as health promotion diagnoses and syndrome nursing diagnoses, consist of a nursing diagnosis label only. As the diagnostic labels are refined, they tend to become more specific, so that nursing interventions can be derived from the label itself. Therefore, an etiology may not be needed.

Health promotion diagnoses will be developed as one-part statements beginning with the words *willingness for improved* followed by the desired higher level of wellness (for example, willingness for improved parenting). A syndrome diagnosis is a diagnosis that is associated with a cluster of other diagnoses (Alfaro-LeFevre, 2017). An example of a syndrome diagnosis is potential for disuse syndrome. It may be experienced by long-term bedridden clients. Clusters of diagnoses associated with this syndrome include imapired activity, potential for skin breakdown, potential for infection, potential for constipation, potential for injury, and impaired respiratory status.

Variations of Basic Formats

Variations of the basic one-, two-, and three-part statements include the following:

1. Writing *unknown etiology* when the defining characteristics are present but the nurse does not know the cause or contributing factors. One example is nonadherence to medical regimen related to unknown etiology.
2. Using the phrase *complex factors* when there are too many etiologic factors or when they are too complex to state in a brief phrase. The actual causes of chronic low self-esteem, for instance, may be long term and complex, as in the following nursing diagnosis: Chronic pain related to complex factors.
3. Using the word *possible* to describe either the problem or the etiology. When the nurse believes more data are needed about the client's problem or the etiology, the word *possible* is inserted. Examples are possible low self-esteem related to loss of job and rejection by family; alteration in thought processes possibly related to unfamiliar surroundings.
4. Using *secondary to* to divide the etiology into two parts, thereby making the statement more descriptive and useful. The part following *secondary to* is often a pathophysiologic or disease process or a medical diagnosis, as in potential for impaired skin integrity related to decreased peripheral circulation secondary to diabetes.
5. Adding a second part to the general response or nursing diagnosis label to make it more precise. For example, the diagnosis altered skin integrity does not indicate the location of the problem. To make this label more specific, the nurse can add a descriptor as follows: altered skin integrity (left lateral ankle) related to decreased peripheral circulation.

Collaborative Problems

Carpenito (2017) has suggested that all collaborative (multidisciplinary) problems begin with the diagnostic label *Potential Complication* (PC). Nurses should include in the diagnostic statement both the possible complication they are monitoring and the disease or treatment that is present to produce it. For example, if the client has a head injury and could develop increased intracranial pressure, the nurse should write the following:

Potential Complication of Head Injury:
increased intracranial pressure

BOX 11.3 Collaborative Problems

Disease/Situation	Complication	Related to	Etiology
Potential complication of childbirth:	hemorrhage	related to	uterine atony
			retained placental fragments
			bladder distention
Potential complication of diuretic therapy:	arrhythmia	related to	low serum potassium

When monitoring for a group of complications associated with a disease or pathology, the nurse states the disease and follows it with a list of the complications:

> *Potential Complication of Pregnancy-Induced Hypertension:* seizures, fetal distress, pulmonary edema, hepatic or renal failure, premature labor, central nervous system (CNS) hemorrhage

In some situations, an etiology might be helpful in suggesting interventions. Nurses should write the etiology when (a) it clarifies the problem statement, (b) it can be concisely stated, and (c) it helps to suggest nursing actions. See the examples in Box 11.3.

Evaluating the Quality of the Diagnostic Statement

In addition to using the correct format, nurses must consider the content of their diagnostic statements. The statements should, for example, be accurate, concise, descriptive, and specific. The nurse must always validate the diagnostic statements with the client and compare the client's signs and symptoms to the nursing diagnosis defining characteristics. The nurse should identify the client's risk factors in formulating the nursing diagnosis. See guidelines for writing nursing diagnoses, in Table 11.6.

Avoiding Errors in Diagnostic Reasoning

Some error is inherent in any human undertaking, and diagnosis is no exception. However, it is important for nurses to make nursing diagnoses with a high level of accuracy. Nurses can avoid some common errors of reasoning by recognizing them and applying the appropriate critical thinking skills. Error can occur at any point in the diagnostic process: data collection, data interpretation, and data clustering.

The following suggestions help to minimize diagnostic error:

- ***Verify.*** Hypothesize possible explanations of the data, but realize that all diagnoses are only tentative until

TABLE 11.6 Guidelines for Writing a Nursing Diagnostic Statement

Guideline	Correct Statement	Incorrect or Ambiguous Statement
1. State in terms of a problem, not a need.	Alteration in fluid volume (problem) related to fever	Fluid replacement (need) related to fever
2. Word the statement so that it is legally advisable.	Altered skin integrity related to immobility (legally acceptable)	Altered skin integrity related to improper positioning (implies legal liability)
3. Use nonjudgmental statements.	Impaired spirituality related to inability to attend church services secondary to immobility (nonjudgmental)	Impaired spirituality related to strict rules necessitating church attendance (judgmental)
4. Make sure that both elements of the statement do not say the same thing.	Potential for altered skin integrity related to immobility	Altered skin integrity related to ulceration of sacral area (response and probable cause are the same)
5. Be sure that cause and effect are correctly stated (i.e., the etiology causes the problem or puts the client at risk for the problem).	Pain: Severe headache related to avoidance of narcotics due to fear of addiction	Pain related to headache
6. Word the diagnosis specifically and precisely to provide direction for planning nursing intervention.	Alteration in mucous membrane integrity related to decreased salivation secondary to radiation of neck (specific)	Alteration in mucous membrane integrity related to noxious agent (vague)
7. Use nursing terminology rather than medical terminology to describe the client's response.	Potential for altered respiratory status related to accumulation of secretions in lungs (nursing terminology)	Potential for pneumonia (medical terminology)
8. Use nursing terminology rather than medical terminology to describe the probable cause of the client's response.	Potential for altered respiratory status related to accumulation of secretions in lungs (nursing terminology)	Potential for altered respiratory status related to emphysema (medical terminology)

LIFESPAN CONSIDERATIONS Diagnosing

CHILDREN

Many developmental issues in pediatrics are not considered problems or illnesses, yet can benefit from nursing intervention. When applied to children and families, nursing diagnoses may reflect a condition or state of health. For example, parents of a newborn infant may be excited to learn all they can about infant care and child growth and development. Assessment of the family system might lead the nurse to conclude that the family is ready and able, even eager, to take on the new roles and responsibilities of being parents. An appropriate diagnosis for such a family could be willingness for improved family dynamics, and nursing care could be directed to educating and providing encouragement and support to the parents.

OLDER ADULTS

Older adults tend to have multiple problems with complex physical and psychosocial needs when they are ill. If the nurse has done a thorough and accurate assessment, nursing diagnoses can be selected to cover all problems and, at the same time, prioritize the special needs. For example, if a client is admitted with severe congestive heart failure, prompt attention will be focused on impaired cardiac status and increased fluid volume, with interventions selected to improve these areas quickly. As these conditions improve, then other nursing diagnoses, such as decreased activity and decreased knowledge related to a new medication regimen, might require more attention. They are all part of the same medical problem of congestive heart failure, but each nursing diagnosis has specific expected outcomes and nursing interventions. The client's strengths should be an essential consideration in all phases of the nursing process.

they are verified. Begin and end the diagnostic process by talking with the client and family. When collecting data, ask them what their health problems are and what they believe the causes to be. At the end of the process, ask them to confirm the accuracy and relevance of your diagnoses.

- ***Build a good knowledge base and acquire clinical experience.*** Nurses must apply knowledge from many different areas to recognize significant cues and patterns and generate hypotheses about the data. To name only a few, principles from chemistry, anatomy, and pharmacology each help the nurse understand client data in a different way.
- ***Have a working knowledge of what is normal.*** Nurses need to know the population norms for vital signs, laboratory tests, speech development, breath sounds, and so on. In addition, nurses must determine what is usual for a particular client, taking into account age, physical makeup, lifestyle, culture, and the client's own perception of what his or her normal status is. For example, normal blood pressure for adults is less than 120 mmHg systolic and less than 80 mmHg diastolic. The nurse should compare actual findings to the client's baseline when possible.
- ***Consult resources.*** Both novices and experienced nurses should consult appropriate resources whenever in doubt about a diagnosis. Professional literature, nursing colleagues, and other professionals are all appropriate resources.
- ***Base diagnoses on patterns—that is, on behavior over time—rather than on an isolated incident.*** For example, even though Margaret O'Brien is concerned today about needing to leave her children with her in-laws, it is likely that this concern will be resolved without intervention by the next day. Therefore, the admitting nurse should not diagnose alterations in family processes but, rather, impaired family dynamics.
- ***Improve critical thinking skills.*** These skills help the nurse to be aware of and avoid errors in thinking, such as overgeneralizing, stereotyping, and making unwarranted assumptions. See Chapter 9 ∞.

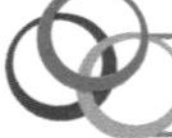

Critical Thinking Checkpoint

A client has recently been diagnosed with lung cancer. Someone has written the nursing diagnosis of anxiety on the care plan.

1. What data and defining characteristics would support this nursing diagnosis?
2. Which related factors might exist in this situation?
3. Which other nursing diagnoses might you expect to find in this case?
4. Another nursing diagnosis on the care plan reads "Lung cancer related to smoking." Is this diagnosis written in an acceptable format? If not, why not?

Answers to Critical Thinking Checkpoint questions are available on the faculty resources site. Please consult with your instructor.

Chapter 11 Review

CHAPTER HIGHLIGHTS

- A diagnosis is a statement or conclusion regarding the nature of a phenomenon.
- Professional standards of care hold that registered nurses are responsible for making nursing diagnoses, even though others may contribute data or implement care.
- A nursing diagnosis is a clinical judgment about the client's responses to actual and potential health problems or life processes.
- A nursing diagnosis provides the basis for selecting independent nursing interventions to achieve outcomes for which the nurse is accountable.
- Nursing diagnoses have a status of actual, health promotion, risk, and wellness.
- A nursing diagnosis has three components: the problem (and its definition), the etiology, and the defining characteristics. Each component serves a specific purpose.
- Nursing diagnoses differ from medical diagnoses and collaborative problems in orientation, duration, and nursing focus.
- A collaborative problem is a type of potential problem that nurses manage using both independent and physician-prescribed interventions.
- The three phases of the diagnostic process are data analysis; identification of the client's health problems, health risks, and strengths; and formulation of diagnostic statements.
- In data analysis and processing, the nurse compares data against standards to identify significant cues, clusters the data, and identifies gaps and inconsistencies.
- Significant cues are those that (a) point to change in a client's health status or pattern, (b) vary from norms of the client population, or (c) indicate a developmental delay.
- It is important to identify client strengths as well as problems.
- The basic format for a nursing diagnostic statement is "*Problem* related to *etiology*." However, there are several variations of this format.

TEST YOUR KNOWLEDGE

1. A student nurse understands that clustering data comes with experience and recognizing cues. What is the best way for this student to recognize patterns or cues in the data?
   1. Depend on knowledge gained from peers' experiences
   2. Work with seasoned and experienced nurses and learn from them
   3. Take assessment notes and utilize information from textbooks for comparison
   4. Know that this will take time, and experience is the best teacher

2. In the diagnostic statement "increased fluid volume related to decreased venous return as manifested by lower extremity edema (swelling)," the etiology of the problem is which of the following?
   1. Increased fluid volume
   2. Decreased venous return
   3. Edema
   4. Unknown

3. Which nursing diagnosis contains the proper components?
   1. Potential for impairment in caregiver role related to unpredictable illness course
   2. Potential for falls related to tendency to collapse when having difficulty breathing
   3. Altered communication related to stroke
   4. Altered sleep secondary to fatigue and a noisy environment

4. One of the primary advantages of using a three-part diagnostic statement such as the problem–etiology–signs and symptoms (PES) format includes which of the following?
   1. Decreases the cost of healthcare.
   2. Improves communication between nurse and client.
   3. Helps the nurse focus on health and wellness elements.
   4. Standardizes organization of client data.

5. A collaborative (multidisciplinary) problem is indicated instead of a nursing or medical diagnosis
   1. If both medical and nursing interventions are required to treat the problem.
   2. When independent nursing actions can be utilized to treat the problem.
   3. In cases where nursing interventions are the primary actions required to treat the problem.
   4. When no medical diagnosis (disease) can be determined.

6. A client who has been in a wheelchair for several years is currently experiencing problems with skin breakdown and urinary retention in addition to depression. When formulating a nursing diagnosis, which of the following would be an appropriate selection?
   1. Syndrome diagnosis
   2. Risk nursing diagnosis
   3. Actual diagnosis
   4. Wellness diagnosis

7. Which statement is true regarding the state of the science in regard to nursing diagnosis?
1. The original taxonomy has proven to be adequate in scope.
2. The organizing framework of the taxonomy is based on the work of Florence Nightingale.
3. More research is needed to validate and refine the diagnostic labels.
4. New diagnostic labels are approved by means of a vote of registered nurses.

8. Which of the following would indicate a significant cue when comparing data to standards? Select all that apply.
1. The client has moved partway toward a set goal (e.g., weight loss).
2. The client's vision is within normal range only when wearing glasses.
3. A child is able to control bladder and bowels at age 18 months.
4. A recently widowed woman states she is "unable to cry."
5. A 16-year-old high school student reports spending 6 hours doing homework 5 nights per week.

See Answers to Test Your Knowledge in Appendix A.

READINGS AND REFERENCES

Suggested Reading

Hasemann, W., Tolson, D., Godwin, J., Spirig, R., Frei, I. A., & Kressig, R. W. (2018). Nurses' recognition of hospitalized older patients with delirium and cognitive impairment using the delirium observation screening scale: A prospective comparison study. *Journal of Gerontological Nursing*, *44*(12), 35–43. doi:10.3928/00989134-20181018-02

This study reported findings regarding delirium detection when nurses screened for delirium in patients with cognitive impairment using the Delirium Observation Screening Scale compared to the Confusion Assessment Method. Of 138 patients in the study, 44 developed delirium within 3 days. The nurses correctly identified delirium in 56% of the clients.

Related Research

Diniz, C. M., Ferreira, G., & Martins, M. C. (2017). Nursing diagnoses associated with the national policy for health. *Investigación y Educación Enfermería*, *35*(1), 78–85. doi:10.17533/udea.iee.v35n1a09

References

Alfaro-LeFevre, R. A. (2017). *Applying the nursing process: The foundation for clinical reasoning* (8th ed.). Philadelphia, PA: Lippincott Williams & Wilkins.

American Nurses Association. (2015). *Nursing: Scope and standards of practice* (3rd ed.). Silver Spring, MD: Author.

Carpenito, L. J. (2017). *Nursing diagnosis: Application to clinical practice* (15th ed.). Philadelphia, PA: Lippincott Williams & Wilkins.

Castellan, C., Sluga, S., Spina, E., & Sanson, G. (2016). Nursing diagnoses, outcome, and interventions as measures of patient complexity and nursing care requirement in intensive care unit. *Journal of Advanced Nursing*, *72*(6), 1273–1286. doi:101111/jan.12913

Kim, M. J., McFarland, G. K., & McLane, A. M. (Eds.). (1984). *Classification of nursing diagnoses: Proceedings of the fifth national conference.* St. Louis, MO: Mosby.

Wilkinson, J. M., & Barcus, L. (2017). *Pearson nursing diagnosis handbook.* (11th ed.). Boston, MA: Pearson.

Selected Bibliography

Ackley, B. J., & Ladwig, G. B. (2017). *Nursing diagnosis handbook* (11th ed.). St. Louis, MO: Elsevier.

Gordon, M. (1982). Historical perspective: The National Group for Classification of Nursing Diagnoses. In M. J. Kim & D. A. Moritz (Eds.), *Classification of nursing diagnoses: Proceedings of the fourth national conference*. New York, NY: McGraw-Hill.

Gordon, M. (2016). *Manual of nursing diagnosis* (13th ed.). Sudbury, MA: Jones & Bartlett.

Wilkinson, J. M. (2012). *Nursing process and critical thinking* (5th ed.). Upper Saddle River, NJ: Prentice Hall.

Planning 12

LEARNING OUTCOMES

After completing this chapter, you will be able to:

1. Identify activities that occur in the planning process.
2. Compare and contrast initial planning, ongoing planning, and discharge planning.
3. Explain how standards of care and predeveloped care plans can be individualized and used in creating a comprehensive nursing care plan.
4. Identify essential guidelines for writing nursing care plans.
5. Identify factors that the nurse must consider when setting priorities.
6. Discuss the Nursing Outcomes Classification, including an explanation of how to use the outcomes and indicators in care planning.
7. State the purposes of establishing client goals or desired outcomes.
8. Identify guidelines for writing goals or desired outcomes.
9. Describe the process of selecting and choosing nursing interventions.
10. Discuss the Nursing Interventions Classification, including an explanation of how to use the interventions and activities in care planning.

KEY TERMS

collaborative care plans, *229*
collaborative interventions, *237*
concept map, *229*
critical pathways, *229*
dependent interventions, *237*
discharge planning, *226*
formal nursing care plan, *226*
goals or desired outcomes, *233*
independent interventions, *237*
indicators, *234*
individualized care plan, *226*
informal nursing care plan, *226*
multidisciplinary care plan, *229*
nursing intervention, *225*
Nursing Interventions Classification (NIC), *239*
Nursing Outcomes Classification (NOC), *233*
policies, *227*
priority setting, *231*
procedures, *227*
protocols, *227*
rationale, *229*
standardized care plan, *226*
standing order, *229*

Introduction

Planning is an intentional, systematic phase of the nursing process that involves decision-making and problem-solving. In planning, the nurse refers to the client's assessment data and diagnostic statements for direction in formulating client goals and designing the nursing interventions required to prevent, reduce, or eliminate the client's health problems (Figure 12.1 ■). A **nursing intervention** is "any treatment, based upon clinical judgment and knowledge, that a nurse performs to enhance patient/client outcomes" (Butcher, Bulechek, Dochterman, & Wagner, 2018, p. xii). The end product of the planning phase is a client care plan.

Although planning is basically the nurse's responsibility, input from the client and support persons is essential if a plan is to be effective. Nurses do not plan for the client but encourage the client to participate actively to the extent possible. In a home setting, the client's support people and caregivers are the ones who implement the plan of care; thus, its effectiveness depends largely on them.

Types of Planning

Planning begins with the first client contact and continues until the nurse–client relationship ends, usually when the client is discharged from the healthcare agency. All planning is multidisciplinary (involves all healthcare providers interacting with the client) and includes the client and family to the fullest extent possible in every step.

Initial Planning

The nurse who performs the admission assessment usually develops the initial comprehensive plan of care. This nurse has the benefit of seeing the client's body language and can also gather some intuitive kinds of information that are not available solely from the written database. Planning should be initiated as soon as possible after the initial assessment.

Ongoing Planning

All nurses who work with the client do ongoing planning. As nurses obtain new information and evaluate the

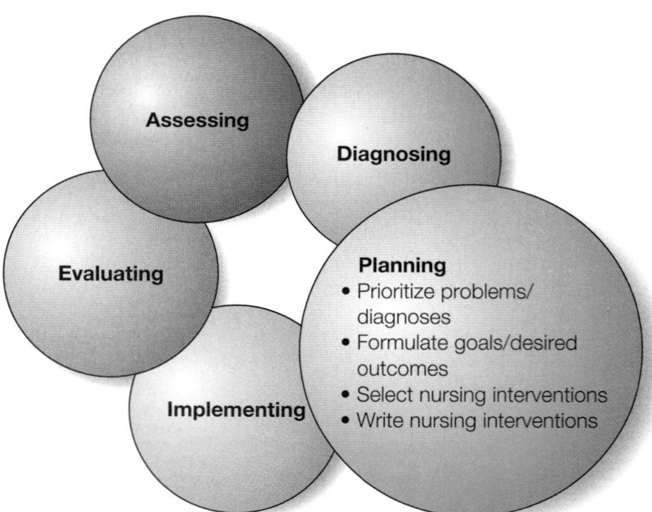

Figure 12.1 ■ Planning—the third phase of the nursing process. In this phase the nurse and client develop client goals or desired outcomes and nursing interventions to prevent, reduce, or alleviate the client's health problems.

client's responses to care, they can individualize the initial care plan further. Ongoing planning also occurs at the beginning of a shift as the nurse plans the care to be given that day. Using ongoing assessment data, the nurse carries out daily planning for the following purposes:

1. To determine whether the client's health status has changed
2. To set priorities for the client's care during the shift
3. To decide which problems to focus on during the shift
4. To coordinate the nurse's activities so that more than one problem can be addressed at each client contact.

Discharge Planning

Discharge planning, the process of anticipating and planning for needs after discharge, is a crucial part of a comprehensive healthcare plan and should be addressed in each client's care plan. Because the average stay of clients in acute care hospitals has become shorter, people are sometimes discharged still needing care. Although many clients are discharged to other agencies (e.g., long-term care facilities), such care is increasingly being delivered in the home. Effective discharge planning begins at first client contact and involves comprehensive and ongoing assessment to obtain information about the client's ongoing needs. For details about discharge planning, see the Continuity of Care section in Chapter 6 ∞.

Developing Nursing Care Plans

The end product of the planning phase of the nursing process is a formal or informal plan of care. An **informal nursing care plan** is a strategy for action that exists in the nurse's mind. For example, the nurse may think, "Mrs. Phan is very tired. I will need to reinforce her teaching after she is rested." A **formal nursing care plan** is a written or computerized guide that organizes information about the client's care. The most obvious benefit of a formal written care plan is that it provides for continuity of care.

A **standardized care plan** is a formal plan that specifies the nursing care for groups of clients with common needs (e.g., all clients with myocardial infarction). An **individualized care plan** is tailored to meet the unique needs of a specific client—needs that are not addressed by the standardized plan. It is important for all caregivers to work toward the same outcomes and, if available, use approaches shown to be effective with a particular client. Nurses also use the formal care plan for direction about what needs to be documented in client progress notes and as a guide for delegating and assigning staff to care for clients. When nurses use the client's nursing diagnoses to develop goals and nursing interventions, the result is a holistic, individualized plan of care that will meet the client's unique needs.

Care plans include the actions nurses must take to address the client's nursing diagnoses and produce the desired outcomes. The nurse begins the plan when the client is admitted to the agency and updates it throughout the client's stay in response to changes in the client's condition and evaluations of goal achievement. During the planning phase, the nurse must (a) decide which of the client's problems need individualized plans and which problems can be addressed by standardized plans and routine care, and (b) write individualized desired outcomes and nursing interventions for client problems that require nursing attention beyond preplanned, routine care.

The complete plan of care for a client is made up of several different documents. Some documents describe the routine care needed to meet basic needs (e.g., bathing, nutrition), and others address the client's nursing diagnoses and collaborative problems. There may also be documents that specify the nurse's responsibilities in carrying out the medical plan of care (e.g., keeping the client from eating or drinking before surgery; scheduling a laboratory test). A complete plan of care integrates dependent and independent nursing functions into a meaningful whole and provides a central source of client information. Figure 12.2 ■ illustrates the various types of documents that may be included in a nursing care plan.

Standardized Approaches to Care Planning

Most healthcare agencies have devised a variety of standardized plans for providing essential nursing care to specified groups of clients who have certain needs in

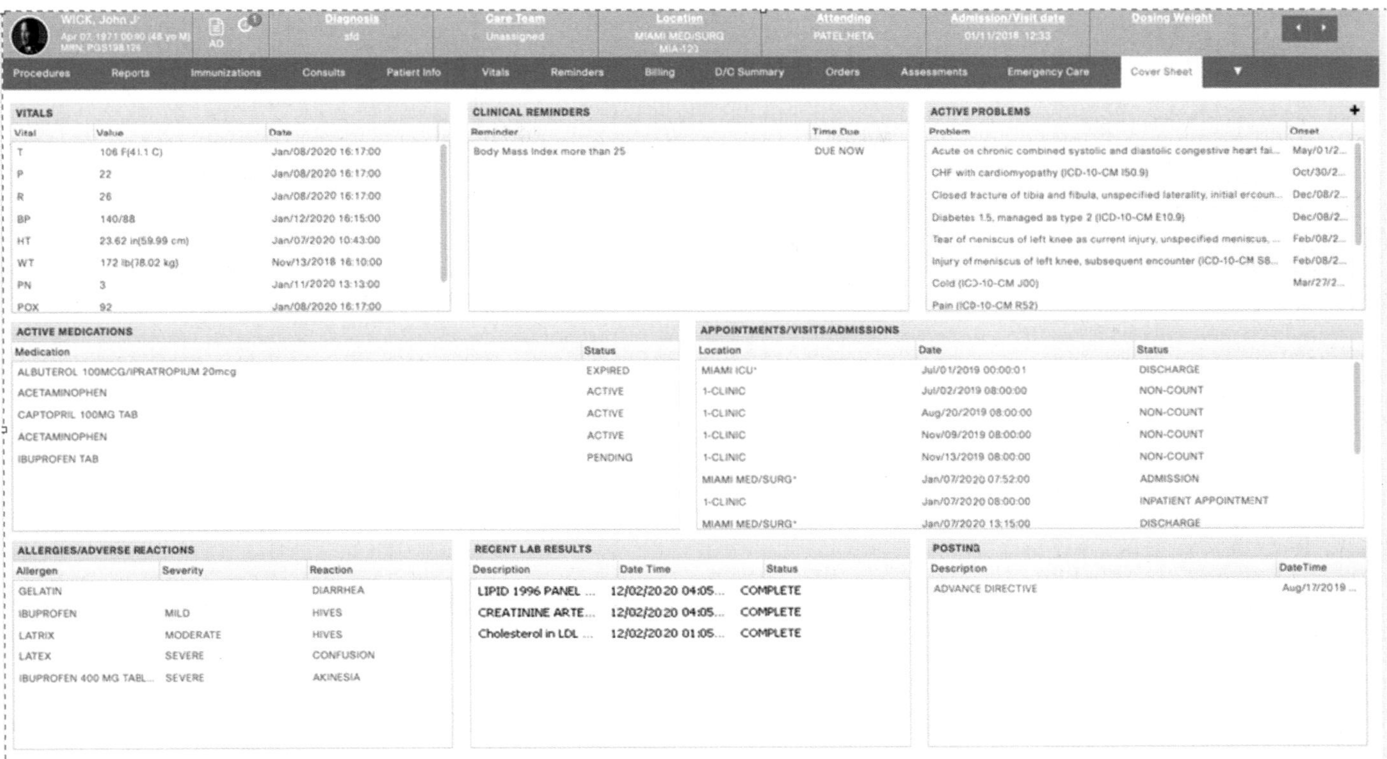

Figure 12.2 ■ Electronic health record containing client information and a summary of care.
iCare.

common (e.g., all clients with pneumonia). Standards of care, standardized care plans, protocols, policies, and procedures are developed and accepted by the nursing staff in order to (a) ensure that minimally acceptable criteria are met and (b) promote efficient use of nurses' time by removing the need to author common activities that are done repeatedly for many of the clients on a nursing unit.

Standards of care describe nursing actions for clients with similar medical conditions rather than individuals, and they describe achievable rather than ideal nursing care. They define the interventions for which nurses are held accountable; they do not contain medical interventions. Standards of care are usually agency records and not part of the client's care plan, but they may be referred to in the plan (e.g., a nurse might write "See unit standards of care for cardiac catheterization"). Standards of care may or may not be organized according to problems or nursing diagnoses. They are written from the perspective of the nurse's responsibilities. Figure 12.3 ■ shows unit standards of care for the client with thrombophlebitis.

Standardized care plans are predeveloped guides for the nursing care of a client who has a need that arises frequently in the agency (e.g., a specific nursing diagnosis or all nursing diagnoses associated with a particular medical condition). They are written from the perspective of what care the client can expect. They should not be confused with standards of care. Although the two have some similarities, they have important differences. Figure 12.4 ■ shows a standardized care plan for alteration in fluid volume. Standardized care plans:

- Are kept with the client's individualized care plan on the nursing unit. When the client is discharged, they become part of the permanent medical record.
- Provide detailed interventions and contain additions or deletions from the standards of care of the agency.
- Typically are written in the nursing process format:

  Problem → Goals/Desired Outcomes →
  Nursing Interventions → Evaluation.
- Frequently include checklists, blank lines, or empty spaces to allow the nurse to individualize goals and nursing interventions.

Like standards of care and standardized care plans, **protocols** are predeveloped to indicate the actions commonly required for a particular group of clients. For example, an agency may have a protocol for admitting a client to the intensive care unit or for caring for a client receiving continuous epidural analgesia. Protocols may include both the primary care provider's orders and nursing interventions. Depending on the agency, protocols may or may not be included in the client's permanent record.

Policies and **procedures** are developed to govern the handling of frequently occurring situations. For example, a hospital may have a policy specifying the number of

STANDARDS OF CARE: Client with Thrombophlebitis.

Goal:
1. To monitor for early signs and symptoms of compromised respiratory status.
2. To report any abnormal signs and/or symptoms promptly to the medical staff.
3. To initiate appropriate nursing actions when signs and/or symptoms of compromised respiratory status occur.
4. To institute protocol for emergency intervention should the client develop cardiopulmonary dysfunction.

SUPPORTIVE DATA: The purpose of these standards of care is to prevent, monitor, report, and record the client's response to a diagnosis of thrombophlebitis. Thrombophlebitis places the client at risk for pulmonary embolism. The hemodynamic consequences of embolic obstruction to pulmonary blood flow involve increased pulmonary vascular resistance,increased right ventricular workload,decreased cardiac output,and development of shock and pulmonary arrest.

CLINICAL MANIFESTATIONS: Nursing assessments performed q3–4h should monitor for the following signs/symptoms:

- Dyspnea: generally consistently present
- Sudden substernal pain
- Rapid/weak pulse
- Syncope
- Anxiety
- Fever
- Cough/hemoptysis
- Accelerated respiratory rate
- Pleuritic type chest pain
- Cyanosis

PREVENTIVE NURSING MEASURES:

- Encourage increased fluid intake to prevent dehydration.
- Maintain anticoagulant intravenous therapy as prescribed (See Protocol for Anticoagulant Administration).
- Maintain prescribed bed rest.
- Prevent venous stasis from improperly fitting elastic stockings;check q3–4h.
- Encourage dorsiflexion exercises of the lower extremities while on bed rest.

INDIVIDUALIZED PLANS/ADDITIONAL NURSING/MEDICAL ORDERS

Do not massage lower extremities.

Intake and output q8h.

Initiated by: *S. Ibarra, RN* Date: *04-09-20*

Figure 12.3 ■ Standards of care for the client with thrombophlebitis.

From *Nursing Process and Critical Thinking*, 5th ed. (p. 351), by J. M. Wilkinson, 2012, Upper Saddle River NJ: Pearson. Adapted with permission.

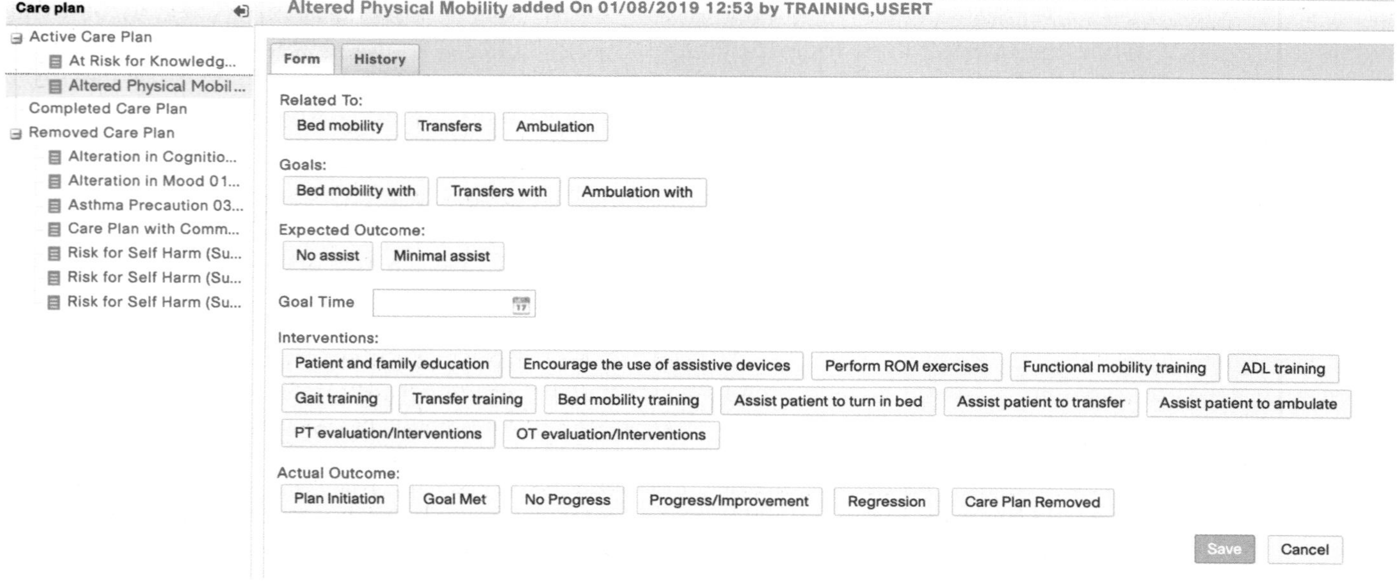

Figure 12.4 ■ A standardized care plan for the nursing diagnosis of altered physical mobility.

visitors a client may have. Some policies and procedures are similar to protocols and specify what is to be done, for example, in the case of cardiac arrest. If a policy covers a situation pertinent to client care, it is usually noted on the care plan (e.g., "Make social service referral according to Policy Manual"). Policies are institutional records and do not become a part of the care plan or permanent record.

A **standing order** is a written document about policies, rules, regulations, or orders regarding client care. Standing orders give nurses the authority to carry out specific actions under certain circumstances, often when a primary care provider is not immediately available. In a hospital critical care unit, a common example is the administration of emergency antiarrhythmic medications when a client's cardiac monitoring pattern changes. In a home care setting, a primary care provider may write a standing order for the nurse to obtain blood tests for a client who has been on a certain therapy for a prescribed amount of time.

Regardless of whether care plans are handwritten, computerized, or standardized, nursing care must be individualized to fit the unique needs of each client. In practice, a care plan usually consists of both preauthored and nurse-created sections. The nurse uses standardized care plans for predictable, commonly occurring problems, and creates an individual plan for unusual problems or problems needing special attention. For example, a standardized care plan for clients with a medical diagnosis of pneumonia would probably include a nursing diagnosis of alteration in fluid volume and direct the nurse to assess the client's hydration status. On a respiratory or medical unit, this would be a common nursing diagnosis; therefore, Margaret O'Brien's nurse was able to obtain a standardized plan directing care commonly needed by clients with alteration in fluid volume (see Figure 12.4). However, the nursing diagnosis impaired family dynamics would not be common to all clients with pneumonia; it is specific to Margaret. Therefore, the goals and nursing interventions for that diagnosis would need to be created by the nurse.

Formats for Nursing Care Plans

Although formats differ from agency to agency, the care plan is often organized into four sections: (1) problem or nursing diagnoses, (2) goals or desired outcomes, (3) nursing interventions, and (4) evaluation. Some agencies use a three-section plan in which evaluation is done with the goals or in the nursing notes; others have five sections that add assessment data preceding the problem or nursing diagnosis.

Student Care Plans

Because student care plans are a learning activity as well as a plan of care, they may be lengthier and more detailed than care plans used by working nurses. To help students learn to write care plans, educators may require that more of the plan be original work. They may also modify the plan by adding "Rationale" after the nursing interventions. A **rationale** is the evidence-based principle given as the reason for selecting a particular nursing intervention. Students may also be required to cite supporting literature for their stated rationale. For an example of a Nursing Care Plan, see pages 240–241.

Another method of organizing and representing care plan information is to use a concept map. A **concept map** is a visual tool in which ideas or data are enclosed in circles or boxes of some shape, and relationships between these are indicated by connecting lines or arrows (Figure 12.5 ■). Concept maps are creative endeavors. They can take many different forms and encompass various categories of data, according to the creator's interpretation of the client or health condition. The concept map for Margaret O'Brien later in this chapter is another way of depicting her nursing care plan and includes unique boxes that enclose assessment, nursing diagnosis, goals or desired outcomes, and interventions. The arrows represent the flow of the phases of the nursing process. (See the Concept Map on page 242.) Concept maps other than care plans are often used to depict complex relationships among ideas, processes, actions, and so on. Some are referred to as mind maps (see Chapter 9 ∞). Students are often asked to complete pathophysiology flow sheets or concept maps as a method of learning and demonstrating the linkages among disease processes, laboratory data, medications, signs and symptoms, risk factors, and other relevant data.

Computerized Care Plans

Computers are increasingly being used to create and store nursing care plans. The computer can generate both standardized and individualized care plans. Nurses access the client's stored care plan from a centrally located terminal at the nurses' station or from terminals in client rooms. For an individualized plan, the nurse chooses the appropriate diagnoses from a menu suggested by the computer. The computer then lists possible goals and nursing interventions for those diagnoses; the nurse chooses those appropriate for the client and types in any additional goals and interventions or nursing actions not listed on the menu. The nurse can read the plan on the computer screen or print out an updated working copy.

Multidisciplinary (Collaborative) Care Plans

A **multidisciplinary care plan** is a standardized plan that outlines the care required for clients with common, predictable—usually medical—conditions. Such plans, also referred to as **collaborative care plans** and **critical pathways**, sequence the care that must be given on each day during the projected length of stay for the specific type of condition. Like the traditional nursing care plan, a

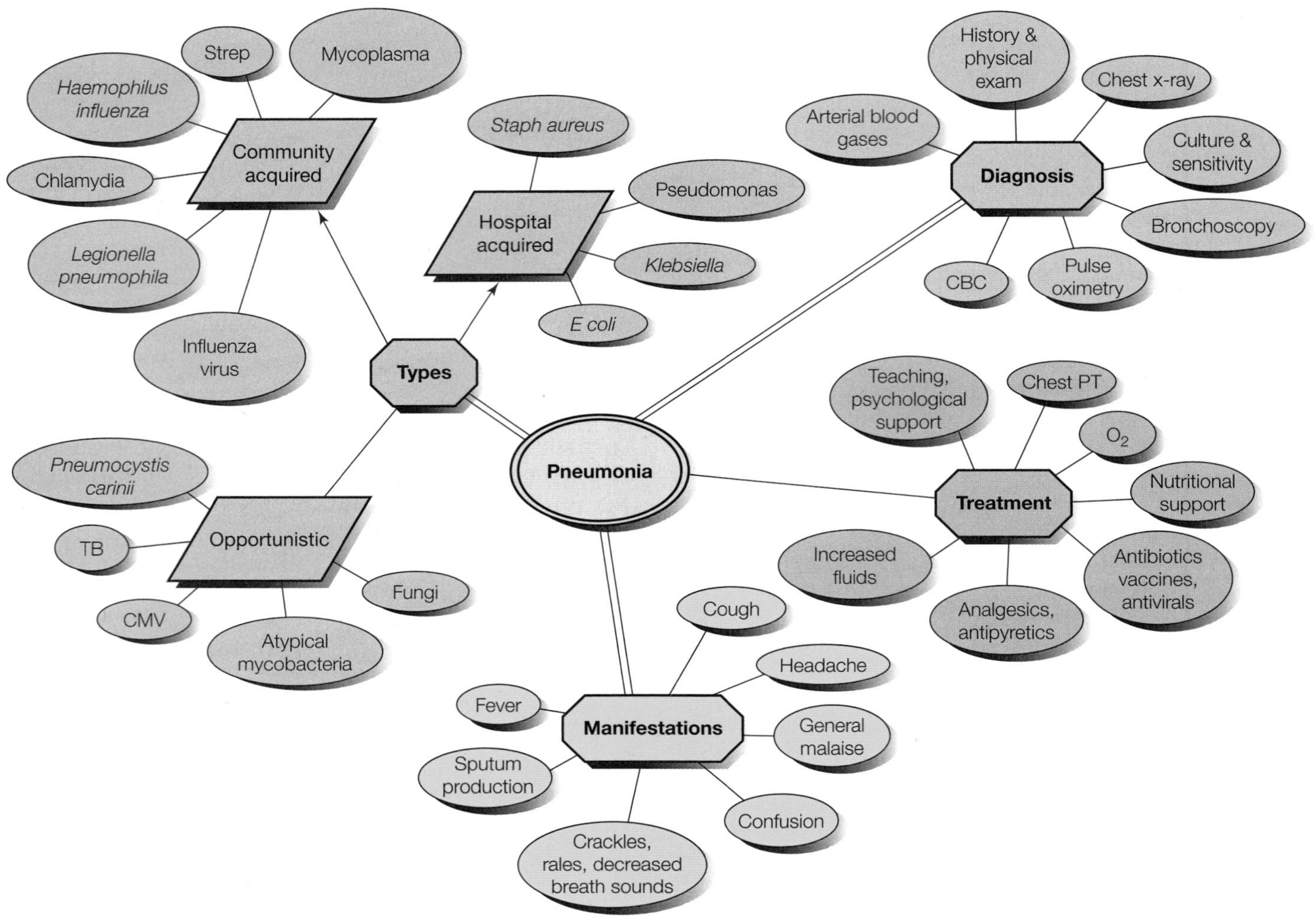

Figure 12.5 ■ A sample pathophysiology concept map.

multidisciplinary care plan can specify outcomes and nursing interventions to address client problems (including nursing diagnoses). However, it includes medical treatments to be performed by other healthcare providers as well.

The plan is usually organized with a column for each day, listing the interventions that should be carried out and the client outcomes that should be achieved on that day. There are as many columns on the multidisciplinary care plan as the preset number of days allowed for the client's diagnosis-related group (DRG). For further information, see Chapter 5 ∞. Multidisciplinary care plans do not include detailed nursing activities. They should be drawn from but do not replace standards of care and standardized care plans.

Guidelines for Writing Nursing Care Plans

The nurse should use the following guidelines when writing nursing care plans:

1. ***Date and sign the plan.*** The date the plan is written is essential for evaluation, review, and future planning. The nurse's signature demonstrates accountability to the client and to the nursing profession, since the effectiveness of nursing actions can be evaluated.
2. ***Use category headings.*** "Nursing Diagnoses," "Goals/Desired Outcomes," "Nursing Interventions," and "Evaluation" are the common headings. Include a date for the evaluation of each goal.
3. ***Use standardized, approved medical or English symbols and key words rather than complete sentences to communicate your ideas unless agency policy dictates otherwise.*** For example, write "Turn and reposition q2h" rather than "Turn and reposition the client every two hours." Or, write "Clean wound $\bar{c}$ H_2O_2 bid" rather than "Clean the client's wound with hydrogen peroxide twice a day, morning and evening." See Table 14.4 on page 273 for a list of standard medical abbreviations.
4. ***Be specific.*** Because nurses are now working shifts of different lengths, with some working 12-hour shifts and some working 8-hour shifts, it is even more important to be specific about expected timing of an intervention. If the intervention reads "change incisional dressing q shift," it could mean either twice in

24 hours, or three times in 24 hours, depending on the shift time. This miscommunication becomes even more serious when medications are ordered to be given "q shift." Writing down specific times during the 24-hour period will help clarify.

5. ***Refer to procedure books or other sources of information rather than including all the steps on a written plan.*** For example, write "See unit procedure book for tracheostomy care," or attach a standard nursing plan about such procedures as radiation-implantation care and preoperative or postoperative care.
6. ***Tailor the plan to the unique characteristics of the client by ensuring that the client's choices, such as preferences about the times of care and the methods used, are included.*** This reinforces the client's individuality and sense of control. For example, the written nursing intervention "Provide prune juice at breakfast rather than other juice" should indicate that the client was given a choice of beverages.
7. ***Ensure that the nursing plan incorporates preventive and health maintenance aspects as well as restorative ones.*** For example, carrying out the intervention "Provide active-assistance ROM (range-of-motion) exercises to affected limbs q2h" addresses the goal of preventing joint contractures and maintaining muscle strength and joint mobility.
8. ***Ensure that the plan contains ongoing assessment of the client*** (e.g., "Inspect incision q8h").
9. ***Include collaborative and coordination activities in the plan.*** For example, the nurse may write interventions to ask a nutritionist or physical therapist about specific aspects of the client's care.
10. ***Include plans for the client's discharge and home care needs.*** The nurse begins discharge planning as soon as the client has been admitted. It is often necessary to consult and make arrangements with the community health nurse, social worker, and specific agencies that supply client information and needed equipment. Add teaching and discharge plans as addenda if they are lengthy and complex.

The Planning Process

In the process of developing client care plans, the nurse engages in the following activities:

- Setting priorities
- Establishing client goals or desired outcomes
- Selecting nursing interventions and activities
- Writing individualized nursing interventions on care plans.

Setting Priorities

Priority setting is the process of establishing a preferential sequence for addressing nursing diagnoses and interventions. The nurse and client begin planning by deciding which nursing diagnosis requires attention first, which second, and so on. Instead of rank-ordering diagnoses, nurses can group them as having high, medium, or low priority. Life-threatening problems, such as impaired respiratory or cardiac function, are designated as high priority. Health-threatening problems, such as acute illness and decreased coping ability, are assigned medium priority because they may result in delayed development or cause destructive physical or emotional changes. A low-priority problem is one that arises from normal developmental needs or that requires only minimal nursing support.

Nurses frequently use Maslow's hierarchy of needs when setting priorities (see Figure 19.3 on page 365). In Maslow's hierarchy, physiologic needs such as air, food, and water are basic to life and receive higher priority than the need for security or activity. Growth needs, such as self-esteem, are not perceived as "basic" in this framework. Thus, nursing diagnosis of altered respiratory status would take priority over nursing diagnoses such as anxiety or impaired coping.

It is not necessary to resolve all high-priority diagnoses before addressing others. The nurse may partially address a high-priority diagnosis and then deal with a diagnosis of lesser priority. Furthermore, because the client may have several problems, the nurse often deals with more than one diagnosis at a time. Table 12.1 lists the priorities assigned to Margaret O'Brien's nursing diagnoses, which were identified in Chapter 11 ∞.

Priorities change as the client's responses, problems, and therapies change. The nurse must consider a variety of factors when assigning priorities, including the following:

1. ***Client's health values and beliefs.*** Values concerning health may be more important to the nurse than to the client. For example, a client may believe that being home for the children is more urgent than a health problem. When such a difference of opinion arises, the client and nurse should discuss it openly to resolve any conflict.
2. ***Client's priorities.*** Involving the client in prioritizing and care planning enhances cooperation. Sometimes, however, the client's perception of what is important conflicts with the nurse's knowledge of potential problems or complications. For example, an older client may not regard turning and repositioning in bed as important, preferring to be undisturbed. The nurse, however, aware of the potential complications of prolonged bedrest (e.g., muscle weakness and pressure injuries), needs to inform and work with the client to carry out these necessary interventions.
3. ***Resources available to the nurse and client.*** If finances, equipment, or personnel are scarce in a healthcare agency, then a problem may be given a lower priority than usual. Nurses in a home setting, for example, do not have the resources of a hospital. If the necessary resources are not available, the solution to that problem might need to be postponed, or the client may

TABLE 12.1 Assigning Priorities to Nursing Diagnoses for Margaret O'Brien

Nursing Diagnosis	Priority	Rationale
Altered respiratory status related to (1) viscous secretions secondary to impaired fluid volume and (2) shallow chest expansion secondary to pain and fatigue	High priority	Loss of respiratory functioning is a life-threatening problem. The nurse's primary concern must be to promote Margaret's oxygenation by addressing the etiologies of this problem.
Alteration in fluid volume: intake insufficient to replace fluid loss related to fever and diaphoresis	High priority	Severe alteration in fluid volume is life-threatening. Although not that severe for Margaret, it is a high-priority problem because it is also a contributing factor for altered respiratory status. Collaborative efforts to improve her hydration have already begun (intravenous fluids). The nurse must immediately and continuously assess and promote Margaret's hydration.
Anxiety related to (1) difficulty breathing and (2) concerns over work and parenting roles	Medium priority	Although Margaret is concerned about school and parenting roles, these are not a threat to life. Also, treatment of her high-priority problem, impaired respiratory status, will relieve one of the etiologies of this problem (dyspnea). Meanwhile, the nurse must provide symptomatic relief of Margaret's anxiety during periods of dyspnea because extreme anxiety could further compromise her oxygenation by causing her to breathe ineffectively and increase the rate at which she uses oxygen.
Impaired family dynamics related to mother's illness and potential temporary unavailability of father to provide child care	Low priority	Margaret's children are currently being cared for by their grandparents until Margaret's husband returns as planned, so this potential problem will not develop into an actual problem. No interventions are needed at present, except for continued assessment and reassurance.
Impaired nutritonal status related to decreased appetite, nausea, and increased metabolism secondary to disease process	Low priority	This problem is not currently health threatening, but it could be if it were to persist. It will almost certainly resolve in a day or two as the medical problem is treated. If the medical problem does not resolve quickly, this will change to a medium priority.
Alteration in the ability to perform self-care related to weakness secondary to altered respiratory status and sleep pattern disturbance	Low priority	This problem is caused by the other higher priority problems; therefore, it will resolve as they resolve. Meanwhile, the nurse merely needs to assist Margaret with bathing and so on to support and conserve her energy until she is strong enough to resume her own care.
Impaired sleep related to cough, pain, orthopnea, fever, and diaphoresis	Low priority	Lack of sleep is health threatening. At the moment (until night), the nurse does not need to address this problem. Impaired sleep does contribute to Margaret's altered respiratory status, but it is not the main cause. Therefore, measures to promote sleep will be low priority until evening. After the nurse has attended to Margaret's oxygenation and hydration needs, this problem priority will change.
Acute pain (chest) related to cough secondary to pneumonia	Not on care plan	The nurse did not write pain as a problem on the care plan because pain is to be addressed as the etiology of impaired sleep and altered respiratory status. The pain etiologies (cough and pneumonia) will be treated by medications (collaborative interventions). Independent nursing actions would address the problem rather than the etiology and would be the same as the nursing actions for altered respiratory status.

need a referral. Client resources, such as finances or coping ability, may also influence the setting of priorities. For example, a client who is unemployed may defer dental treatment; a client whose husband is terminally ill and dependent on her may feel unable to cope with nutritional guidance directed toward losing weight.

4. ***Urgency of the health problem.*** Regardless of the framework used, life-threatening situations require that the nurse assign them a high priority. For example, in Table 12.1, although Margaret O'Brien is anxious about child care, her altered respiratory status has higher priority. Situations that affect the integrity of the client, that is, those that could have a negative or destructive effect on the client, also have high priority. Such health problems as drug abuse and radical alteration of self-concept due to amputation can be destructive both to the individual and to the family.

5. *Medical treatment plan.* The priorities for treating health problems must be congruent with treatment by other health professionals. For example, a high priority for the client might be to become ambulatory; however, if the primary care provider's therapeutic regimen calls for extended bedrest, then ambulation must assume a lower priority in the nursing care plan. The nurse can provide or teach exercises to facilitate ambulation later, provided the client's health permits. The nursing diagnosis related to ambulation is not ignored; it is merely deferred.

Establishing Client Goals or Desired Outcomes

After establishing priorities, the nurse and client set goals for each nursing diagnosis (Figure 12.6 ■). On a care plan, the **goals or desired outcomes** describe, in terms of observable client responses, what the nurse hopes to achieve by implementing the nursing interventions. The terms *goal* and *desired outcome* are used interchangeably in this text, except when discussing and using standardized language. Some references also use the terms *expected outcome, predicted outcome, outcome criterion,* and *objective*.

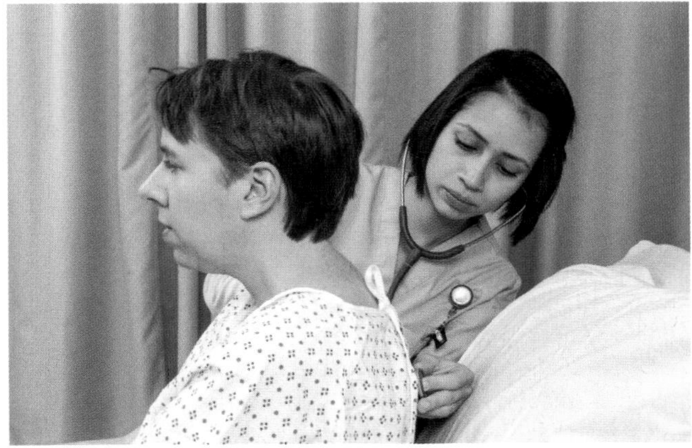

Figure 12.6 ■ Nurse Medina and Margaret collaborate to set goals and outcome criteria and develop a care plan.

Some nursing literature differentiates the terms by defining goals as broad statements about the client's status and desired outcomes as the more specific, observable criteria used to evaluate whether the goals have been met. For example:

Goal (broad):	Improved nutritional status.
Desired outcome (specific):	Gain 5 lb by April 25.

When goals are stated broadly, as in this example, the care plan must include both goals and desired outcomes. They are sometimes combined into one statement linked by the words "as evidenced by," as follows:

> Improved nutritional status as evidenced by weight gain of 5 lb by April 25.

Writing the broad, general goal first may help students to think of the specific outcomes that are needed, but the broad goal is just a starting point for planning. It is the specific, observable outcomes that must be written on the care plan and used to evaluate client progress. Table 12.2 shows both broad goals and specific outcomes.

The Nursing Outcomes Classification

Standardized or common nursing language is required in all phases of the nursing process if nursing data are to be included in computerized databases that are analyzed and used in nursing practice. Nurse leaders and researchers have been working since 1991 to develop a taxonomy, the **Nursing Outcomes Classification (NOC)**, for describing client outcomes that respond to nursing interventions. In the taxonomy, over 385 outcomes belong to one of seven domains (e.g., physiologic health or family health) and a class within the domain (e.g., nutrition under physiologic health or family well-being under family health). Each NOC outcome is assigned a four-digit identifier, indicated in this text by square brackets, and a definition.

"A nursing-sensitive client outcome is an individual, family, or community state, behavior, or perception that is measured along a continuum in response to a nursing intervention(s)" (Moorhead, Johnson, Maas, & Swanson, 2018, p. 2). The NOC outcomes are broadly stated and

TABLE 12.2 Deriving Desired Outcomes from Nursing Diagnoses

Nursing Diagnosis	Opposite Healthy Responses (Goals)	Desired Outcomes: The Client Will
Alteration in mobility: inability to bear weight on left leg, related to inflammation of knee joint	Improved mobility Ability to bear weight on left leg	Ambulate with crutches by end of the week. Stand without assistance by end of the month.
Altered respiratory status related to poor cough effort, secondary to incision pain and fear of damaging sutures	Effective airway clearance	Have lungs clear to auscultation during entire postoperative period. Have no skin pallor or cyanosis by 12 hours postoperation. Demonstrate good cough effort within 24 hours after surgery.

conceptual. They are variable concepts, meaning that the client's responses to interventions can be evaluated over time. This is different from a goal, which is either met or not met. To be measured, an outcome must be made more specific by identifying the indicators that apply to a particular client. It is important to note the nursing-sensitive outcome indicators assess the effectiveness of nursing interventions. Broadly written outcomes will have interventions from a variety of healthcare-related disciplines. **Indicators** are stated in neutral terms, and each outcome includes a five-point scale (a measure) that is used to rate the client's status on each indicator. (See Appendix B.) When using the NOC taxonomy to write a desired outcome on a care plan, the nurse writes the label, the indicators that apply to the particular client, the NOC rating at initiation (initial client status), and the outcome target (location on the measuring scale that is desired for each indicator). For example, using the NOC outcome for the client diagnosed in Table 12.2, the individualized desired outcomes would read as follows:

Mobility Level:
Indicators: Walking (independent with assistive device), moves with ease
NOC Rating at Initiation: 2 (substantially compromised)
Outcome Target Rating: 4 (mildly compromised)

Stated in traditional language, that goal would read: "Client will have improved mobility, as evidenced by ability to walk with assistive device (walker) and move easily."

Purpose of Goals or Desired Outcomes

Although goals and outcomes are not necessarily the same concept, the terms are used by some people interchangeably. If referenced to NOC, goals are considered to be met or not met, while progress toward outcomes can be described along a continuum and in comparison to previous status (Moorhead et al., 2018). Goals/desired outcomes serve the following purposes:

1. ***Provide direction for planning nursing interventions.*** Ideas for interventions come more easily if the desired outcomes state clearly and specifically what the nurse hopes to achieve.
2. ***Serve as criteria for evaluating client progress.*** Although developed in the planning step of the nursing process, desired outcomes serve as the criteria for judging the effectiveness of nursing interventions and client progress in the evaluation step (see Chapter 13 ∞).
3. ***Enable the client and nurse to determine when the problem has been resolved.***
4. ***Help motivate the client and nurse by providing a sense of achievement.*** As goals are met, both client and nurse can see that their efforts have been worthwhile. This provides motivation to continue following the plan, especially when difficult lifestyle changes need to be made.

Short-Term and Long-Term Goals

Goals may be short term or long term. A short-term goal might be "Client will raise right arm to shoulder height by Friday." In the same context, a long-term goal or outcome might be "Client will regain full use of right arm in 6 weeks." Short-term goals are useful for clients who (a) require healthcare for a short time or (b) are frustrated by long-term goals that seem difficult to attain and who need the satisfaction of achieving a short-term goal. In an acute care setting, much of the nurse's time is spent on the client's immediate needs, so most goals are short term. However, clients in acute care settings also need long-term goals or outcomes to guide planning for their discharge to long-term agencies or home care, especially in a managed care environment. Outcomes are often set for clients who live at home and have chronic health problems and for clients in nursing homes, extended care facilities, and rehabilitation centers.

Relationship of Goals or Desired Outcomes to Nursing Diagnoses

Goals and outcomes are derived from the client's nursing diagnoses—primarily from the diagnostic label. The diagnostic label contains the unhealthy response; it states what should change. For example, if the nursing diagnosis is alteration in fluid volume related to diarrhea and inadequate intake secondary to nausea, the essential goal statement might be:

> The client will re-establish fluid balance, as evidenced by urinary and stool output in balance with fluid intake, normal skin turgor, and moist mucous membranes.

In this example, a general goal (fluid balance) is stated as the opposite of the problem (alteration in fluid volume) and then followed by a list of observable desired outcomes. If achieved, the outcomes would be evidence that the problem, alteration in fluid volume, has been prevented.

For every nursing diagnosis, the nurse must write the desired outcome(s) that, when achieved, directly demonstrates resolution of the problem. When developing goals or desired outcomes, ask the following questions:

1. What is the client's problem?
2. What is the opposite, healthy response?
3. How will the client look or behave if the healthy response is achieved? (What will I be able to see, hear, measure, palpate, smell, or otherwise observe with my senses?)
4. What must the client do and how well must the client do it to demonstrate problem resolution or to demonstrate the capability of resolving the problem?

Components of Goal or Desired Outcome Statements

Goal or desired outcome statements should have the following four components:

1. ***Subject.*** The subject, a noun, is the client, any part of the client, or some attribute of the client, such as the

client's pulse or urinary output. The subject is often omitted in goals; it is assumed that the subject is the client unless indicated otherwise.

2. ***Verb.*** The verb specifies an action the client is to perform, for example, what the client is to do, learn, or experience. Verbs that denote directly observable behaviors, such as *administer*, *show*, or *walk*, must be used. See Box 12.1 for some examples.

BOX 12.1 Examples of Action Verbs

Apply	Drink	Select
Assemble	Explain	Share
Breathe	Help	Sit
Choose	Identify	Sleep
Compare	Inject	State
Define	List	Talk
Demonstrate	Move	Transfer
Describe	Name	Turn
Differentiate	Prepare	Verbalize
Discuss	Report	

3. ***Conditions or modifiers.*** Conditions or modifiers may be added to the verb to explain the circumstances under which the behavior is to be performed. They explain what, where, when, or how. For example:
   Walks with the help of a cane (how).
   After attending two group diabetes classes, lists signs and symptoms of diabetes (when).
   When at home, maintains weight at existing level (where).
   Discusses *food pyramid and recommended daily servings* (what).
   Conditions need not be included if the criterion of performance clearly indicates what is expected.

4. ***Criterion of desired performance.*** The criterion indicates the standard by which a performance is evaluated or the level at which the client will perform the specified behavior. These criteria may specify time or speed, accuracy, distance, and quality. To establish a time-achievement criterion, the nurse needs to ask "How long?" To establish an accuracy criterion, the nurse asks "How well?" Similarly, the nurse asks "How far?" and "What is the expected standard?" to establish distance and quality criteria, respectively. Examples are:
   Weighs 75 kg *by April* (time).
   Lists *five out of six* signs of diabetes (accuracy).
   Walks *one block per day* (distance and time).
   Administers insulin *using aseptic technique* (quality).

Table 12.3 illustrates the format that should be used to write outcomes. Table 12.4 lists desired outcomes that were developed for Margaret O'Brien.

Guidelines for Writing Goals or Desired Outcomes

The following guidelines can help nurses write useful goals or desired outcomes:

1. Write goals and outcomes in terms of client responses, not nursing activities. Beginning each goal statement with *The client will* may help focus the goal on client behaviors and responses. Avoid statements that start with *enable, facilitate, allow, let, permit,* or similar verbs followed by the word *client.* These verbs indicate what the nurse hopes to accomplish, not what the client will do.
   Correct: The client will drink 100 mL of water per hour (client behavior).
   Incorrect: Maintain client hydration (nursing action).
2. Be sure that desired outcomes are realistic for the client's capabilities, limitations, and designated time span, if it is indicated. Limitations refers to finances, equipment, family support, social services, physical and mental condition, and time. For example, the outcome "Measures insulin accurately" may be unrealistic for a client who has poor vision due to cataracts.

TABLE 12.3 Components of Goals/Desired Outcomes

Subject	Verb	Conditions/Modifiers	Criterion of Desired Performance
Client	drinks	2500 mL of fluid	daily (time)
Client	administers	correct insulin dose	using aseptic technique (quality standard)
Client	lists	three hazards of smoking	(accuracy indicated by "three hazards")
Client	recalls	five symptoms of diabetes	(accuracy indicated by "five symptoms") before discharge (time)
Client	walks	the length of the hall without a cane	by date of discharge (time)
Client's ankle	measures	less than 25 cm (10 in.) in circumference	in 48 hours (time)
Client	performs	leg ROM exercises as taught	every 8 hours (time)
Client	identifies	foods high in salt from a prepared list	before discharge (time)
Client	states	the purposes of his medications	before discharge (time)

TABLE 12.4 Desired Outcomes for Margaret O'Brien

Nursing Diagnosis*	Goal Statements [NOC]/Desired Outcomes
Altered respiratory status related to viscous secretions secondary to alteration in fluid volume and shallow chest expansion secondary to pain and fatigue	Respiratory Status: Gas Exchange [0402], as evidenced by • Absence of pallor and cyanosis (skin and mucous membranes) • Use of correct breathing/coughing technique after instruction • Productive cough • Symmetric chest excursion of at least 4 cm (1.6 in.) Within 48–72 h: • Lungs clear to auscultation • Respirations 12–22/min, pulse less than 100 beats/min • Inhales normal volume of air on incentive spirometer
Alteration in fluid volume: intake insufficient to replace fluid loss related to vomiting, fever, and diaphoresis	Fluid Balance [0601], as evidenced by • Urine output greater than 30 mL/h • Urine specific gravity 1.005–1.025 • Good skin turgor • Moist mucous membranes • Stating the need for oral fluid intake
Anxiety related to difficulty breathing and concerns about school and parenting roles	Anxiety Control [1402], as evidenced by • Listening to and following instructions for correct breathing and coughing technique, even during periods of dyspnea • Verbalizing understanding of condition, diagnostic tests, and treatments (by end of day) • Decrease in reports of fear and anxiety; none within 12 h • Voice steady, not shaky • Respiratory rate of 12–22/min • Freely expressing concerns and possible solutions about work and parenting roles
Impaired family dynamics related to mother's illness and temporary unavailability of father to provide child care	Family Coping [2600], as evidenced by • Report of satisfactory child care arrangements having been made • Client and husband communicating effectively and working together to solve problems • Family members expressing feelings and providing mutual support
Impaired nutritonal status related to decreased appetite, nausea, and increased metabolism secondary to disease process	Nutritional Status: Nutrient Intake [1009], as evidenced by • Eating at least 85% of each meal • Maintaining present weight • Verbalizing importance of adequate nutrition • Verbalizing improved appetite
Inability to perform self care related to activity intolerance secondary to airway clearance and sleep pattern disturbance	Self-Care: Activities of Daily Living [0300], as evidenced by • Ambulates to bathroom without dyspnea, fatigue, ineffective or shortness of breath • Within 24 h, bathes with assistance in bed; within 48 h, bathes with assistance at sink; within 72 h, bathes in shower without dyspnea • Reports satisfaction and comfort with hygiene needs
Impaired sleep related to cough, pain, orthopnea, and diaphoresis	Sleep [0004], as evidenced by • Observed sleeping at night rounds • Reports feeling rested • Does not experience orthopnea

*The nursing diagnoses are listed in priority order.

3. Ensure that the goals or desired outcomes are compatible with the therapies of other professionals. For example, the outcome "The client will increase the time spent out of bed by 15 minutes each day" is not compatible with a primary care provider's prescribed therapy of bedrest.
4. Make sure that each goal is derived from only one nursing diagnosis. For example, the goal "The client will increase the amount of nutrients ingested and show progress in the ability to feed self" is derived from two nursing diagnoses: impaired nutritional status and inability to eat independently. Keeping the goal statement related to only one diagnosis facilitates evaluation of care by ensuring that planned nursing interventions are clearly related to the diagnosis.
5. Use observable, measurable terms for outcomes. Avoid words that are vague and require interpretation or judgment by the observer. For example, phrases such as *increase daily exercise* and *improve knowledge of nutrition* can mean different things to different

people. If used in outcomes, these phrases can lead to disagreements about whether the outcome was met. These phrases may be suitable for a broad client goal but are not sufficiently clear and specific to guide the nurse when evaluating client responses.

6. Make sure the client considers the goals or desired outcomes important and values them. Some outcomes, such as those for problems related to self-esteem, parenting, and communication, involve choices that are best made by the client or in collaboration with the client.

Some clients may know what they wish to accomplish with regard to their health problem; others may not know all the possibilities. The nurse must actively listen to the client to determine personal values, goals, and desired outcomes in relation to current health concerns. Clients are usually motivated and will expend the necessary energy to reach goals they consider important. See the Nursing Care Plan on pages 240–241 for desired outcomes for three of Margaret O'Brien's nursing diagnoses.

Selecting Nursing Interventions and Activities

Nursing interventions and activities are the actions that a nurse performs to achieve client goals. The specific interventions chosen should focus on eliminating or reducing the etiology of the nursing diagnosis, which is the second clause of the diagnostic statement.

When it is not possible to change the etiologic factors, the nurse chooses interventions to treat the signs and symptoms. Examples of this situation would be pain related to surgical incision and anxiety related to unknown etiology.

Interventions for risk nursing diagnoses should focus on measures to reduce the client's risk factors, which are also found in the second clause. Correct identification of the etiology during the diagnosing phase provides the framework for choosing successful nursing interventions. For example, the diagnostic label impaired activity may have several etiologies: pain, weakness, sedentary lifestyle, anxiety, or cardiac arrhythmias. Interventions will vary according to the cause of the problem.

Types of Nursing Interventions

Nursing interventions are identified and written during the planning step of the nursing process; however, they are actually performed during the implementing step. Nursing interventions include both direct and indirect care, as well as nurse-initiated, physician-initiated, and other provider-initiated treatments. Direct care is an intervention performed by the nurse through interaction with the client. Indirect care is an intervention delegated by the nurse to another provider or performed away from but on behalf of the client, such as interdisciplinary collaboration or management of the care environment.

Independent interventions are those activities that nurses are licensed to initiate on the basis of their knowledge and skills. They include physical care, ongoing assessment, emotional support and comfort, teaching, counseling, environmental management, and making referrals to other healthcare professionals. Recall from Chapter 11 ∞ that nursing diagnoses are client problems that can be treated primarily by independent nursing interventions. In performing an autonomous activity, the nurse determines that the client requires certain nursing interventions, either carries these out or delegates them to other nursing personnel, and is accountable or answerable for the decision and the actions. An example of an independent action is planning and providing special mouth care for a client after diagnosing alteration in mucous membrane integrity.

Dependent interventions are activities carried out under the orders or supervision of a licensed physician or other healthcare provider authorized to write orders to nurses. Primary care providers' orders commonly direct the nurse to provide medications, intravenous therapy, diagnostic tests, treatments, diet, and activity. With the client, the nurse is responsible for assessing the need for, explaining, and administering the medical orders. Nursing interventions may be written for the purpose of individualizing the medical order based on the client's status. For example, for a medical order of "Progressive ambulation, as tolerated," a nurse might write the following:

1. Dangle for 5 min, 12 hours postop.
2. Stand at bedside 24 hours postop; observe for pallor, dizziness, and weakness.
3. Check pulse before and after ambulating. Do not progress if pulse is greater than 110.

Collaborative interventions are actions the nurse carries out in collaboration with other health team members, such as physical therapists, social workers, dietitians, and primary care providers. Collaborative nursing activities reflect the overlapping responsibilities of, and collegial relationships among, health personnel. For example, the primary care provider might order physical therapy to teach the client crutch-walking. The nurse would be responsible for informing the physical therapy department and for coordinating the client's care to include the physical therapy sessions. The nurse may assist with crutch-walking and collaborate with the physical therapist to evaluate the client's progress.

The amount of time the nurse spends in an independent versus a collaborative or dependent role varies according to the clinical area, type of institution, and specific position of the nurse.

Considering the Consequences of Each Intervention

Usually several possible interventions can be identified for each nursing goal. The nurse's task is to choose those that are most likely to achieve the desired client outcomes. The nurse begins by considering the risks and benefits of each intervention. An intervention may have more than one consequence. For example, "Provide accurate information" could result in the following client behaviors:

- Increased anxiety
- Decreased anxiety
- Wish to talk with the primary care provider
- Cooperation
- Relaxation.

Determining the consequences of each intervention requires nursing knowledge and experience. For example, the nurse's experience may suggest that providing information the night before the client's surgery may increase the client's worry and tension, whereas maintaining the usual rituals before sleep is more effective. The nurse might then consider providing information several days before surgery.

Criteria for Choosing Nursing Interventions

After considering the consequences of the alternative nursing interventions, the nurse chooses one or more that are likely to be most effective. Although the nurse bases this decision on knowledge and experience, the client's input is important.

The following criteria can help the nurse choose the best nursing interventions. The plan must be:

- Safe and appropriate for the individual's age, health, and condition.
- Achievable with the resources available. For example, a home care nurse might wish to include an intervention for an older client to "Check blood glucose daily." In order for that to occur, the client must have intact sight, cognition, and memory to carry this out independently, family who can assist with this task, or available and affordable daily visits from a home care nurse.
- Congruent with the client's values, beliefs, and culture.
- Congruent with other therapies (e.g., if the client is not permitted food, the strategy of an evening snack must be deferred until health permits).
- Based on nursing knowledge and experience or knowledge from relevant sciences (i.e., based on a rationale). For examples of rationales, refer to the Nursing Care Plan for Margaret O'Brien on pages 240–241.
- Within established standards of care as determined by state laws, professional organizations (e.g., American Nurses Association), accrediting organizations (e.g., The Joint Commission), and the policies of the institution. Many agencies have policies to guide the activities of health professionals and to safeguard clients. Rules for visiting hours and procedures to follow when a client has cardiac arrest are examples. If a policy does not benefit clients, nurses have a responsibility to bring this to the attention of the appropriate people and facilitate a modification of the policy.

Writing Individualized Nursing Interventions

After choosing the appropriate nursing interventions, the nurse writes them on the care plan. See examples of nursing interventions for Margaret O'Brien in the accompanying Nursing Care Plan on pages 240–241.

Date nursing interventions on the care plan when they are written and review regularly at intervals that depend on the individual's needs. In an intensive care unit, for example, the plan of care will be continually monitored and revised. In a community clinic, weekly or biweekly reviews may be indicated.

The format of written interventions is similar to that of outcomes: verb, conditions, and modifiers, plus a time element. The action verb starts the intervention and must be precise. For example, "Explain (to the client) the actions of insulin" is a more precise statement than "Teach (the client) about insulin." "Measure and record ankle circumference daily at 0900" is more precise than "Assess edema of left ankle daily." Sometimes a modifier for the verb can make the nursing intervention more precise. For example, "Apply spiral bandage firmly to left lower leg" is more precise than "Apply spiral bandage to left leg."

The time element answers when, how long, or how often the nursing action is to occur. Examples are "Assist client with tub bath at 0700 daily" and "Administer analgesic 30 minutes prior to physical therapy."

In some settings, the intervention (and other segments of the nursing care plan) is signed. The signature of the nurse prescribing the intervention shows the nurse's accountability and has legal significance.

Relationship of Nursing Interventions to Problem Status

Depending on the type of client problem, the nurse writes interventions for observation, prevention, treatment, and health promotion.

Observations include assessments made to determine whether a complication is developing, as well as observation of the client's responses to nursing and other therapies. The nurse should write observations for both real problems and those for which the client is at risk. Some examples are "Auscultate lungs q8h," "Observe for redness over sacrum q2h," and "Record intake and output hourly."

Prevention interventions prescribe the care needed to avoid complications or reduce risk factors. They are needed mainly for potential nursing diagnoses and collaborative problems. Examples are "Turn, cough, and deep breathe q2h" (prevents respiratory complications) and "Keep bedrails raised and bed in low position" (minimizes chances of clients falling out of bed or injuring themselves should they fall over the rails).

Treatments include teaching, referrals, physical care, and other care needed for an actual nursing diagnosis. Some interventions may accomplish either prevention or treatment functions, depending on the status of the problem. In the preceding examples, "Turn, cough, and deep breathe q2h" can also be intended to treat an existing respiratory problem.

Enhancement or promotion interventions are appropriate when the client has no health problems or when the nurse makes a health promotion nursing diagnosis. Such nursing interventions focus on helping the client identify areas for improvement that will lead to a higher level of wellness and actualize the client's overall health potential. Examples are "Discuss the importance of daily exercise" and "Explore infant stimulation techniques."

Delegating Implementation

Determining whether delegation is indicated is another activity that occurs during the planning phase of the nursing process. While choosing and writing nursing interventions on the client's care plan, the nurse must also determine who should actually perform the activity. In 2015 the National Council of State Boards of Nursing (NCSBN) convened two panels of experts to develop national guidelines based on the current literature and research to provide a standardized nursing delegation process (NCSBN, 2016). It is important that delegation not be confused with the assignment of routine care, activities, and procedures that are in the scope of the nurse's practice or a routine function of unlicensed assistive personnel. A licensed nurse has the responsibility to maintain accountability for a client when care has been delegated to a licensed practical or vocational nurse or to a certified nursing assistant or medication aid. To delegate appropriately, the nurse must match the needs of the client and family with the skills and knowledge of the available caregivers. This requires knowing the background, experience, knowledge, skills, and strengths of each individual, and understanding which tasks are and are not within their legal scope of practice.

The nurse has several responsibilities in delegating. These include appropriate delegation of duties (that is, giving individuals duties within their scope of practice and abilities and under the right circumstances) and adequate direction, communication, and supervision of personnel to whom work is delegated or assigned. The RN can delegate certain tasks to unlicensed personnel but cannot assign responsibility for total nursing care. The RN is responsible for seeing that delegated tasks are carried out properly. Assistive personnel may perform tasks such as measuring intake and output, but the RN is still responsible for analyzing data, planning care, and evaluating outcomes. Because there are no universal standards for the training of unlicensed personnel, nurses often must assume responsibility for supplementing the training those staff members have received (see also Chapter 18 ∞).

The Nursing Interventions Classification

A taxonomy of nursing interventions referred to as the **Nursing Interventions Classification (NIC)** taxonomy, developed by the Iowa Intervention Project, was first published in 1992 and has been updated every 4 years since then. This taxonomy consists of three levels: level 1, domains; level 2, classes; and level 3, interventions. (Butcher et al., 2018).

When planning and documenting care in an agency that uses the NIC taxonomy, the nurse chooses the broad intervention label (e.g., Touch). Not all activities suggested for the intervention would be needed for every client, so the nurse chooses the activities appropriate for the client and individualizes them to fit the supplies, equipment, and other resources available in the agency. When writing individualized nursing interventions on a care plan, the nurse should record customized activities rather than the broad intervention labels. In domain 1, for example, the nurse is caring for the client's physiologic needs. The care provided should support physical functioning. In regards to the client's elimination, the interventions promote regular bowel and urinary elimination (Moorhead et al., 2018).

The NIC taxonomy provides many benefits to nurse practitioners, nurse educators, nurse administrators, and the nursing profession as a whole (Box 12.2).

BOX 12.2 Benefits of Standardized Interventions

- Enhances communication among nurses and among nurses and nonnurses.
- Makes it possible for researchers to determine the effectiveness and cost of nursing treatments.
- Helps communicate the nature of nursing to the public.
- Helps demonstrate the impact that nurses have on healthcare.
- Makes it easier for nurses to select appropriate interventions by reducing the need for memorization and recall.
- Facilitates the teaching of clinical decision-making.
- Contributes to the development and use of computerized clinical records.
- Assists in effective planning for staff and equipment needs.
- Aids in development of a system of payment for nursing services.
- Promotes full and meaningful participation of nurses in the multidisciplinary team.

From *Nursing Process and Critical Thinking*, 5th ed. (p. 253), by J. M. Wilkinson, 2012, Upper Saddle River, NJ: Pearson. Adapted with permission.

LIFESPAN CONSIDERATIONS Nursing Care Plan

OLDER ADULTS

When a client is in an extended care facility or a long-term care facility, interventions and medications often remain the same day after day. It is important to review the care plan on a regular basis, because changes in the condition of older adults may be subtle and go unnoticed. This applies to both changes of improvement and deterioration. Either one should receive attention so that appropriate revisions can be made in expected outcomes and interventions. Outcomes need to be realistic with consideration given to the client's physical condition, emotional condition, support systems, and mental status. Outcomes often have to be stated and expected to be completed in very small steps. For instance, clients who have had a cerebrovascular accident may spend weeks learning to brush their own teeth or dress themselves. When these small steps are successfully completed, it gives the client a sense of accomplishment and motivation to continue working toward increasing self-care. This particular example also demonstrates the need to work collaboratively with other departments, such as physical and occupational therapy, to develop the nursing care plan.

NURSING CARE PLAN Margaret O'Brien

Nursing Diagnosis: Altered respiratory status related to viscous secretions secondary to alteration in fluid volume and shallow chest expansion secondary to pain and fatigue

DESIRED OUTCOMES*/INDICATORS	NURSING INTERVENTIONS	RATIONALE
Respiratory Status: Gas Exchange [0402], as evidenced by • Absence of pallor and cyanosis (skin and mucous membranes) • Use of correct breathing/coughing technique after instruction	Monitor respiratory status q4h: rate, depth, effort, skin color, mucous membranes, amount and color of sputum. Monitor results of blood gases, chest x-ray studies, and incentive spirometer volume as available. Monitor level of consciousness.	*To identify progress toward or deviations from goal.* Altered repiratory status *leads to poor oxygenation, as evidenced by pallor, cyanosis, lethargy, and drowsiness.*
• Productive cough • Symmetric chest excursion of at least 4 cm	Auscultate lungs q4h. Vital signs q4h (TPR, BP, pulse oximetry, pain).	*Inadequate oxygenation and pain cause increased pulse rate. Respiratory rate may be decreased by narcotic analgesics. Shallow breathing further compromises oxygenation.*
Within 48–72 hours: • Lungs clear to auscultation • Respirations 12–22/min; pulse, less than 100 beats/min	Instruct in breathing and coughing techniques. Remind to perform, and assist q3h.	*To enable client to cough up secretions. May need encouragement and support because of fatigue and pain.*
• Inhales normal volume of air on incentive spirometer	Administer prescribed expectorant; schedule for maximum effectiveness. Maintain Fowler's or semi-Fowler's position. Administer prescribed analgesics. Notify primary care provider if pain not relieved.	*Helps loosen secretions so they can be coughed up and expelled.* *Gravity allows for fuller lung expansion by decreasing pressure of abdomen on diaphragm.* *Controls pleuritic pain by blocking pain pathways and altering perception of pain, enabling client to increase thoracic expansion. Unrelieved pain may signal impending complication.*
	Administer oxygen by nasal cannula as prescribed. Provide portable oxygen if client goes off unit (e.g., for x-ray examination).	*Supplemental oxygen makes more oxygen available to the cells, even though less air is being moved by the client, thereby reducing the work of breathing.*

NURSING CARE PLAN Margaret O'Brien—*continued*

Nursing Diagnosis: Altered respiratory status related to viscous secretions secondary to alteration in fluid volume and shallow chest expansion secondary to pain and fatigue

DESIRED OUTCOMES*/INDICATORS	NURSING INTERVENTIONS	RATIONALE
	Assist with postural drainage daily at 0930.	*Gravity facilitates movement of secretions upward through the respiratory passage.*
	Administer prescribed antibiotic to maintain constant blood level. Observe for rash and GI or other side effects.	*Resolves infection by bacteriostatic or bactericidal effect, depending on type of antibiotic used. Constant level required to prevent pathogens from multiplying. Allergies to antibiotics are common.*

Nursing Diagnosis: Alteration in fluid volume: intake insufficient to replace fluid (Figure 12.4)
Nursing Diagnosis: Anxiety related to difficulty breathing and concern about school and parenting roles

DESIRED OUTCOMES*/INDICATORS	NURSING INTERVENTIONS	RATIONALE
Anxiety Control [1402], as evidenced by	When client is dyspneic, stay with her; reassure her you will stay.	*Presence of a competent caregiver reduces fear of being unable to breathe.*
• Listening to and following instructions for correct breathing and coughing technique, even during periods of dyspnea	Remain calm; appear confident. Encourage slow, deep breathing.	*Control of anxiety will help client to maintain effective breathing pattern.*
• Verbalizing understanding of condition, diagnostic tests, and treatments (by end of day)	When client is dyspneic, give brief explanations of treatments and procedures.	*Reassures client the nurse can help her. Focusing on breathing may help client feel in control and decrease anxiety.*
• Decrease in reports of fear and anxiety • Voice steady, not shaky • Respiratory rate of 12–22/min	When acute episode is over, give detailed information about nature of condition, treatments, and tests.	*Anxiety and pain interfere with learning. Knowing what to expect reduces anxiety.*
• Freely expressing concerns and possible solutions about work and parenting roles	As client can tolerate, encourage to express and expand on her concerns about her child and her work. Explore alternatives as needed.	*Awareness of source of anxiety enables client to gain control over it. Husband's continued absence would constitute a sign or symptom for this nursing diagnosis.*
Note whether husband returns as scheduled. If not, institute care plan for actual impaired family dynamics.		

APPLYING CRITICAL THINKING

1. What assumptions does the nurse make when deciding that using a standardized care plan for impaired fluid volume is appropriate for this client?
2. Identify an outcome in the care plan and its nursing intervention that contribute to discharge care planning. What evidence supports your choice?
3. Consider how the nurse shares the development of the care plan and outcomes with the client.
4. Not every intervention has a time frame or interval specified. It may be implied. Under what circumstances is this acceptable practice?
5. In Table 12.1, altered respiratory status is Margaret's highest priority nursing diagnosis. Under what conditions might this diagnosis be of only moderate priority in Margaret's case?

Answers to Applying Critical Thinking questions are available on the faculty resources site. Please consult with your instructor.

*The NOC # for desired outcomes is listed in brackets following the appropriate outcome.

CONCEPT MAP

Altered Respiratory Status (Altered Gas Exchange)

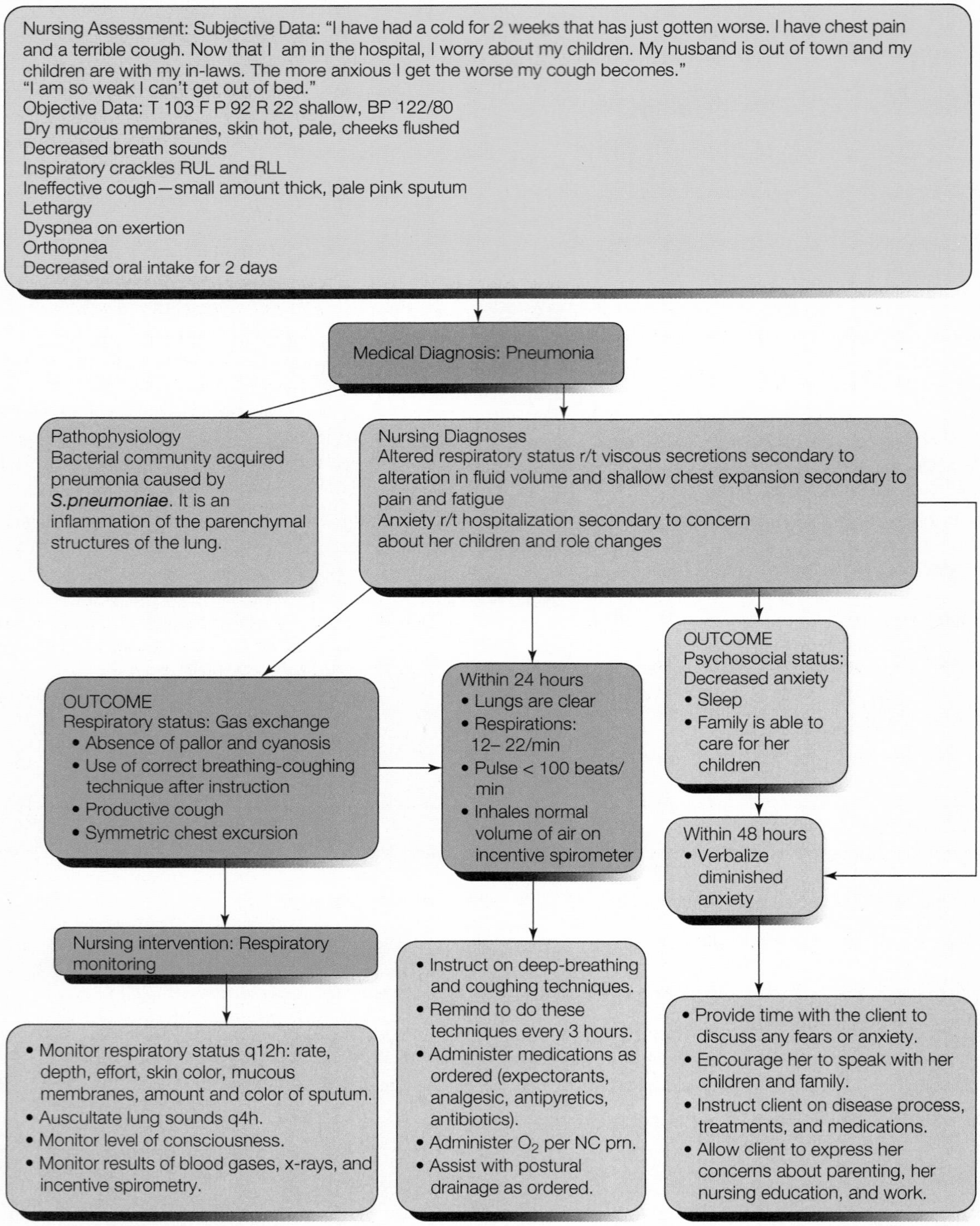

Nursing Assessment: Subjective Data: "I have had a cold for 2 weeks that has just gotten worse. I have chest pain and a terrible cough. Now that I am in the hospital, I worry about my children. My husband is out of town and my children are with my in-laws. The more anxious I get the worse my cough becomes."
"I am so weak I can't get out of bed."
Objective Data: T 103 F P 92 R 22 shallow, BP 122/80
Dry mucous membranes, skin hot, pale, cheeks flushed
Decreased breath sounds
Inspiratory crackles RUL and RLL
Ineffective cough—small amount thick, pale pink sputum
Lethargy
Dyspnea on exertion
Orthopnea
Decreased oral intake for 2 days

Medical Diagnosis: Pneumonia

Pathophysiology
Bacterial community acquired pneumonia caused by *S.pneumoniae*. It is an inflammation of the parenchymal structures of the lung.

Nursing Diagnoses
Altered respiratory status r/t viscous secretions secondary to alteration in fluid volume and shallow chest expansion secondary to pain and fatigue
Anxiety r/t hospitalization secondary to concern about her children and role changes

OUTCOME
Respiratory status: Gas exchange
- Absence of pallor and cyanosis
- Use of correct breathing-coughing technique after instruction
- Productive cough
- Symmetric chest excursion

Within 24 hours
- Lungs are clear
- Respirations: 12– 22/min
- Pulse < 100 beats/min
- Inhales normal volume of air on incentive spirometer

OUTCOME
Psychosocial status: Decreased anxiety
- Sleep
- Family is able to care for her children

Within 48 hours
- Verbalize diminished anxiety

Nursing intervention: Respiratory monitoring

- Monitor respiratory status q12h: rate, depth, effort, skin color, mucous membranes, amount and color of sputum.
- Auscultate lung sounds q4h.
- Monitor level of consciousness.
- Monitor results of blood gases, x-rays, and incentive spirometry.

- Instruct on deep-breathing and coughing techniques.
- Remind to do these techniques every 3 hours.
- Administer medications as ordered (expectorants, analgesic, antipyretics, antibiotics).
- Administer O_2 per NC prn.
- Assist with postural drainage as ordered.

- Provide time with the client to discuss any fears or anxiety.
- Encourage her to speak with her children and family.
- Instruct client on disease process, treatments, and medications.
- Allow client to express her concerns about parenting, her nursing education, and work.

Chapter 12 Review

CHAPTER HIGHLIGHTS

- Planning is the process of designing nursing activities required to prevent, reduce, or eliminate a client's health problems.
- Planning involves the nurse, the client, support people, and other caregivers.
- Shorter acute care hospitalization stays necessitate careful discharge planning.
- Standardized care plans should be adapted and used with individualized plans to meet individual client needs.
- The nursing care plan provides direction for individualized care of the client.
- The planning process includes setting diagnostic priorities, establishing client goals or desired outcomes, selecting nursing interventions and activities, and writing individualized nursing interventions on the care plan.
- Nursing diagnoses are assigned high, medium, and low priorities in consultation with the client, if health permits.
- Client goals or desired outcomes are used to plan nursing interventions that will achieve anticipated changes in the client.
- A taxonomy of nursing outcome statements, the Nursing Outcomes Classification (NOC), has been developed to describe measurable states, behaviors, or perceptions that respond to nursing interventions. Each outcome has a definition, a measuring scale, and an indicator.
- Desired outcomes describe specific and measurable client responses and help the nurse evaluate the effectiveness of the nursing interventions.
- Client goals or desired outcomes are derived from the first clause of the nursing diagnosis.
- Nursing interventions are focused on the etiology or second clause of the nursing diagnosis.
- Independent nursing interventions are those the nurse is licensed to prescribe or delegate.
- Determining the consequences of each nursing strategy requires nursing knowledge and experience.
- A taxonomy of nursing interventions referred to as the Nursing Interventions Classification (NIC) taxonomy has been developed.

TEST YOUR KNOWLEDGE

1. After being admitted directly to the surgery unit, a 75-year-old client who had elective surgery to replace an arthritic hip was discharged from the postanesthesia recovery unit. The client has been on the orthopedic floor for several hours. Which type of planning will be *least* useful during the first shift on the orthopedic unit?
   1. Initial
   2. Ongoing
   3. Discharge
   4. Strategic

2. According to a care plan, a client is to receive chest physiotherapy twice daily. The client lives alone in a rural area, does not drive, and is 40 miles away from the hospital. Which of the following will the home health nurse do when setting priorities?
   1. Make sure that he or she is able to get to the client's home.
   2. Assist the client in finding an alternative plan for achieving the therapy's outcomes.
   3. Tell the client that this therapy will be impossible to receive.
   4. Make arrangements to have the client moved to a long-term care facility.

3. The nurse assesses a postoperative client with an abdominal wound and finds the client drowsy when not aroused. The client's pain is ranked 2 on a scale of 0 to 10, vital signs are within preoperative range, extremities are warm with good pulses but skin is very dry. The client declines oral fluids due to nausea, and reports no bowel movement in the past 2 days. Hip dressing is dry with drains intact. Which element is most likely to be considered of high priority for a change in the current care plan?
   1. Pain
   2. Nausea
   3. Constipation
   4. Potential for wound infection

4. One of the discharge goals for a client is that they will have improved mobility. Which one of the following is an appropriately written desired outcome statement?
   1. Client will ambulate without a walker by 6 weeks.
   2. Client will ambulate freely in the house.
   3. Client will not fall.
   4. Client will have freer movement in daily activities.

5. The care plan includes a nursing intervention "4/2/15 Measure client's fluid intake and output. F. Jenkins, RN." What element of a proper nursing intervention has been omitted?
   1. Action verb
   2. Content
   3. Time
   4. None

6. Place the following activities of planning in the correct order of their use.
   1. Establish goals or outcomes.
   2. Write the care plan.
   3. Set priorities.
   4. Choose interventions.

7. A client is admitted for complications following a routine diagnostic procedure of the colon. Which is the type of care plan that will most likely be implemented for this client?
   1. Informal nursing care plan
   2. Formal nursing care plan
   3. Standardized care plan
   4. Individualized care plan

8. Which of the following is likely to occur if a goal statement is poorly written?
   1. There is no standard against which to compare outcomes.
   2. The nursing diagnoses cannot be prioritized.
   3. Only dependent nursing interventions can be used.
   4. It is difficult to determine which nursing interventions can be delegated.

9. When written properly, Nursing Outcome Classification (NOC) outcomes and indicators
   1. Do not require customization.
   2. Address several nursing diagnoses.
   3. Are broad statements of desired end points.
   4. Reflect both the nurse's and the client's values.

10. Which principle does the nurse use in selecting interventions for the care plan?
   1. Actions should address the etiology of the nursing diagnosis.
   2. Always select independent interventions when possible.
   3. There is one best intervention for each goal or outcome.
   4. Interventions should be "doing," not just "monitoring."

See Answers to Test Your Knowledge in Appendix A.

READINGS AND REFERENCES

Suggested Reading

Sandoval, C. P. (2017). Nonpharmacological interventions for sleep promotion in the intensive care unit. *Critical Care Nurse*, *37*, 100–102. doi:10.4037/ccn2017855

This study assessed the effectiveness of nonpharmacologic interventions to improve sleep in critically ill clients. In their review of nonpharmacologic interventions, the researchers reported that the use of earplugs or eye masks improved total sleep quality.

Related Research

Weldam, S. W., Lammers, J., Awakman, M., & Schuurmans, M. J. (2017). Nurses' perspectives of a new individualized nursing care intervention for COPD patients in primary care settings: A mixed method study. *Applied Nursing Research*, *33*, 85–92. doi:10.1016/j. apnr.2016.10.010

References

Butcher, H. K., Bulechek, G. M., Dochterman, J. C., & Wagner, C. M. (Eds.). (2018). *Nursing interventions classification (NIC)* (7th ed.). St. Louis, MO: Elsevier.

Moorhead, S., Johnson, M., Maas, M. L., & Swanson, E. (Eds.). (2018). *Nursing outcomes classification (NOC)* (6th ed.). St. Louis, MO: Elsevier.

National Council of State Boards of Nursing. (2016). National guidelines for nursing delegation. *Journal of Nursing Regulation*, *7*(1), 5–14. Retrieved from https://www.ncsbn.org/NCSBN_Delegation_Guidelines.pdf

Wilkinson, J. M. (2012). *Nursing process and critical thinking* (5th ed.). Upper Saddle River, NJ: Pearson.

Selected Bibliography

Alfaro-LeFevre, R. A. (2017). *Applying the nursing process: The foundation for clinical reasoning* (9th ed.). Philadelphia, PA: Lippincott Williams & Wilkins.

Carpenito, L. J. (2016). *Nursing diagnosis: Application to clinical practice* (15th ed.). Philadelphia, PA: Lippincott Williams & Wilkins.

Wilkinson, J. M., & Barcus, L. (2017). *Nursing diagnosis handbook* (11th ed.). Hoboken, NJ: Pearson.

Implementing and Evaluating 13

LEARNING OUTCOMES

After completing this chapter, you will be able to:

1. Explain how implementing relates to other phases of the nursing process.
2. Describe three categories of skills used to implement nursing interventions.
3. Discuss the five activities of the implementing phase.
4. Identify guidelines for implementing nursing interventions.
5. Explain how evaluating relates to other phases of the nursing process.
6. Describe five components of the evaluation process.
7. Describe the steps involved in reviewing and modifying the client's care plan.
8. Describe three components of quality evaluation: structure, process, and outcomes.
9. Differentiate quality improvement from quality assurance.

KEY TERMS

audit, *254*
cognitive skills, *246*
concurrent audit, *254*
evaluating, *248*
evaluation statement, *249*
implementing, *245*
interpersonal skills, *246*
outcome evaluation, *252*
process evaluation, *252*
quality assurance (QA) program, *252*
quality improvement (QI), *253*
retrospective audit, *254*
root cause analysis, *253*
sentinel event, *252*
structure evaluation, *252*
technical skills, *246*

Introduction

The nursing process is action oriented, client centered, and outcome directed. After developing a plan of care based on the assessing and diagnosing phases, the nurse implements the interventions and evaluates the desired outcomes. On the basis of this evaluation, the plan of care is either continued, modified, or terminated. As in all phases of the nursing process, clients and support persons are encouraged to participate as much as possible.

Implementing

In the nursing process, implementing is the action phase in which the nurse performs the nursing interventions. Using Nursing Interventions Classification (NIC) terminology (Butcher, Bulechek, Dochterman, & Wagner 2018), **implementing** consists of doing and documenting the activities that are the specific nursing actions needed to carry out the interventions. The nurse performs or assigns the nursing activities for the interventions that were developed in the planning step and then concludes the implementing step by recording nursing activities and the resulting client responses.

The fifth standard of the American Nurses Association (ANA) Standards of Practice is implementation. Three of the implementation substandards apply to all registered nurses: coordination of care, health teaching and health promotion, and consultation. The fourth substandard, prescriptive authority and treatment, applies only to advanced practice nurses (ANA, 2015).

Relationship of Implementing to Other Nursing Process Phases

The first three nursing process phases—assessing, diagnosing, and planning—provide the basis for the nursing actions performed during the implementing step. In turn, the implementing phase provides the actual nursing activities and client responses that are examined in the final phase, the evaluating phase. Using data acquired during assessment, the nurse can individualize the care given in the implementing phase, tailoring the interventions to fit a specific client rather than applying them routinely to categories of clients (e.g., all clients with pneumonia).

While implementing nursing care, the nurse continues to reassess the client at every contact, gathering data about the client's responses to the nursing activities and about any new problems that may develop. A nursing activity on the client's care plan for the NIC intervention Airway Management might read "Auscultate breath sounds q4h." When performing this activity, the nurse is both carrying out the intervention (implementing) and performing an assessment. Some routine nursing activities are, themselves, assessments. For example, while bathing an older client, the nurse observes a reddened area on the client's sacrum. Or, when emptying a urinary catheter bag, the nurse measures 200 mL of offensively smelling, brown urine.

Implementing Skills

To implement the care plan successfully, nurses need cognitive, interpersonal, and technical skills. These skills are distinct from one another; in practice, however, nurses use them in various combinations and with different emphasis, depending on the activity. The nurse must supervise all aspects of care as documented in the care plan. For example, when inserting a urinary catheter, the nurse needs cognitive knowledge of the principles and steps of the procedure, interpersonal skills to inform and reassure the client, and technical skill in draping the client and manipulating the equipment. In addition, the care plan must reflect all aspects of care implemented and evaluated for a client with a urinary catheter (see Chapter 47). The nurse also uses cognitive knowledge to educate the client on the health promotion and disease management needs.

The **cognitive skills** (intellectual skills) include problem-solving, decision-making, critical thinking, clinical reasoning, and creativity. They are crucial to safe, intelligent nursing care (see Chapter 9).

Interpersonal skills are all of the activities, verbal and nonverbal, people use when interacting directly with one another. The effectiveness of a nursing action often depends largely on the nurse's ability to communicate with others. The nurse uses therapeutic communication to understand the client and in turn be understood. A nurse also needs to work effectively with others as a member of the healthcare team.

Interpersonal skills are necessary for all nursing activities: caring, comforting, advocating, referring, counseling, and supporting are just a few. Interpersonal skills include conveying knowledge, attitudes, feelings, interest, and appreciation of the client's cultural values and lifestyle. Before nurses can be highly skilled in interpersonal relations, they must have self-awareness and sensitivity to others (see Chapters 15 and 39).

Technical skills are purposeful "hands-on" skills such as manipulating equipment, giving injections, bandaging, moving, lifting, and repositioning clients. These skills are also called tasks, procedures, or psychomotor skills. The term *psychomotor* refers to physical actions that are controlled by the mind, not by reflexes.

Technical skills require knowledge and, frequently, manual dexterity. The number of technical skills expected of a nurse has greatly increased in recent years because of the pervasive use of technology, especially in acute care hospitals.

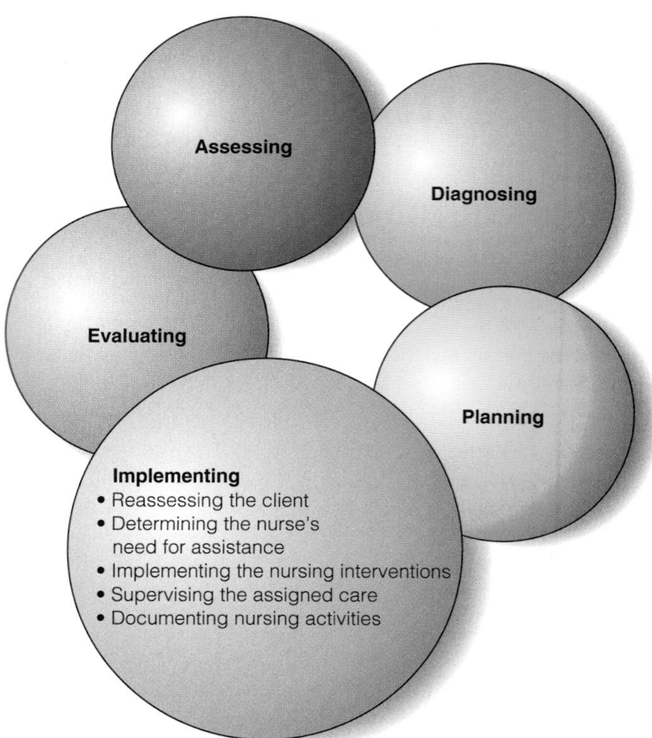

Figure 13.1 ■ Implementing—the fourth phase of the nursing process. In this phase the nurse implements the nursing interventions and documents the care provided.

Process of Implementing

The process of implementing (Figure 13.1 ■) normally includes the following:

- Reassessing the client
- Determining the nurse's need for assistance
- Implementing the nursing interventions
- Supervising the assigned care
- Documenting nursing activities.

Reassessing the Client

Just before implementing an intervention, the nurse must reassess the client to make sure the intervention is still needed. Even though an order is written on the care plan, the client's condition may have changed. For example, a client has a nursing diagnosis of Impaired sleep related to anxiety and unfamiliar surroundings. During rounds, the nurse discovers that the client is sleeping and therefore defers the back massage that had been planned as a relaxation strategy.

New data may indicate a need to change the priorities of care or the nursing activities. For example, a nurse begins to teach a client who has diabetes how to give himself insulin injections. Shortly after beginning the teaching, the nurse realizes that he is not concentrating on the lesson. Subsequent discussion reveals that he is worried about his eyesight and fears he is going blind. Realizing that the client's level of stress is interfering with his learning, the nurse ends the lesson and arranges for a primary care provider to examine the client's eyes. The nurse also provides supportive communication to help alleviate the client's stress.

Determining the Nurse's Need for Assistance

When implementing some nursing interventions, the nurse may require assistance for one or more of the following reasons:

- The nurse is unable to implement the nursing activity safely or efficiently alone (e.g., ambulating an unsteady obese client).
- Assistance would reduce stress on the client (e.g., turning a client who experiences acute pain when moved).
- The nurse lacks the knowledge or skills to implement a particular nursing activity (e.g., a nurse who is not familiar with a particular model of traction equipment needs assistance the first time it is applied).

Implementing the Nursing Interventions

It is important to explain to the client what interventions will be done, what sensations to expect, what the client is expected to do, and what the expected outcome is. For many nursing activities it is also important to ensure the client's privacy, for example, by closing doors, pulling curtains, or draping the client. The number and kind of direct nursing interventions are almost unlimited. Nurses also coordinate client care. This activity involves scheduling client contacts with other departments (e.g., laboratory and x-ray technicians, physical and respiratory therapists) and serving as a liaison among the members of the health-care team.

When implementing interventions, nurses should follow these guidelines:

- Base nursing interventions on scientific knowledge, nursing research, and professional standards of care (evidence-based practice) when these exist. The nurse must be aware of the scientific rationale, as well as possible side effects or complications, of all interventions. For example, a client has been taking an oral medication after meals; however, this medication is not absorbed well in the presence of food. Therefore, the nurse will need to explain why this practice needs to be altered.
- Clearly understand the interventions to be implemented and question any that are not understood. The nurse is responsible for intelligent implementation of medical and nursing plans of care. This requires knowledge of each intervention, its purpose in the client's plan of care, any contraindications (e.g., allergies), and changes in the client's condition that may affect the order.
- Adapt activities to the individual client. A client's beliefs, values, age, health status, and environment are factors that can affect the success of a nursing action. For example, the nurse determines that a client chokes when swallowing pills. The nurse consults with the primary care provider to change the order to a liquid form of the medication. Or, the nurse observes that some clients prefer to drink hot water rather than ice water and, after confirming this preference with a specific client, supplies this at the bedside.
- Implement safe care. For example, when changing a sterile dressing, the nurse practices sterile technique to prevent infection; when giving a medication, the nurse administers the correct dosage by the ordered route.
- Provide teaching, support, and comfort. See Chapter 17 for details on client teaching and Box 17.4 for examples of verbs used in writing learning outcomes. The nurse should always explain the purpose of interventions, what the client will experience, and how the client can participate. The client must have sufficient knowledge to agree to the plan of care and to be able to assume responsibility for as much self-care as desirable. These independent nursing activities enhance the effectiveness of nursing care plans (Figure 13.2 ■).
- Be holistic. The nurse must always view the client as a whole and consider the client's responses in that context. For example, whenever possible, the nurse honors the client's expressed preference that interventions be planned for times that fit with the client's usual schedule of visitors, work, sleep, or eating.
- Respect the dignity of the client and enhance the client's self-esteem. Providing privacy and encouraging clients to make their own decisions are ways of respecting dignity and enhancing self-esteem.
- Encourage clients to actively participate in implementing the nursing interventions. Active participation enhances the client's sense of independence and control. However, clients vary in the degree of participation they desire. Some want total involvement in their care, whereas others prefer little involvement. The amount of desired involvement may be related to the severity of the illness; the client's culture; or the client's

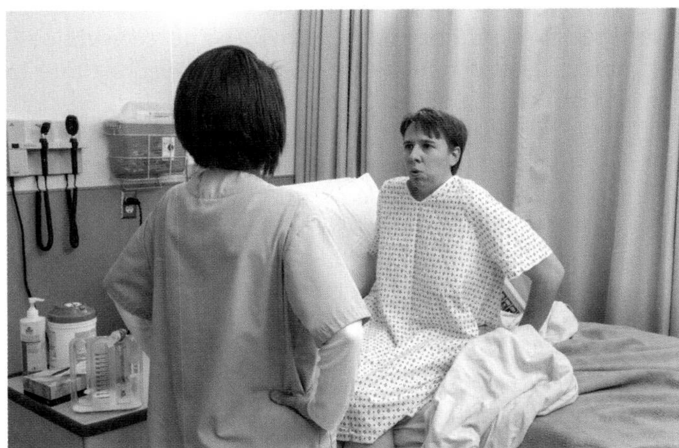

Figure 13.2 ■ Margaret agrees to practice deep-breathing exercises q3h during the day. In addition, she verbalizes awareness of the need to increase her fluid intake.

fear, understanding of the illness, and understanding of the intervention.

Supervising Delegated or Assigned Care

If care has been assigned or delegated to other healthcare personnel, the nurse responsible for the client's overall care must ensure that the activities have been implemented according to the care plan. Other caregivers may be required to communicate their activities to the nurse by documenting them on the client record, reporting verbally, or filling out a written form. The nurse validates and responds to any adverse findings or client responses. This may involve modifying the nursing care plan.

According to the National Council of State Boards of Nursing (2017), delegation involves another individual completing a specific nursing activity, skill, or procedure that is routinely out of his or her traditional role. Unlicensed assistive personnel are assigned nursing care that is deemed as routine functions of that individual. This activity applies to both licensed and unlicensed assistive personnel. The nurse is accountable for any delegation of care and for evaluation of the care that has been implemented.

Clinical Alert!

Do not confuse delegation with an assignment. Routine functions of an unlicensed healthcare provider or licensed nurse is an assignment.

Documenting Nursing Activities

After carrying out the nursing activities, the nurse completes the implementing phase by recording the interventions and client responses in the nursing progress notes. These are a part of the agency's permanent record for the client. Nursing care must not be recorded in advance because the nurse may determine on reassessment of the client that the intervention should not or cannot be implemented. For example, a nurse is authorized to inject 10 mg of morphine sulfate subcutaneously to a client, but the nurse finds that the client's respiratory rate is 8 breaths per minute. This finding contraindicates the administration of morphine (a respiratory depressant). The nurse withholds the morphine and reports the client's respiratory rate to the nurse in charge or the primary care provider.

The nurse may record routine or recurring activities (e.g., mouth care) in the client record at the end of a shift. In the meantime, the nurse maintains a personal record of these interventions on a worksheet. In some instances, it is important to record a nursing intervention immediately after it is implemented. This is particularly true of the administration of medications and treatments because recorded data about a client must be up to date, accurate, and available to other nurses and healthcare professionals. Immediate recording helps safeguard the client, for example, from receiving a duplicate dose of medication.

Nursing activities are communicated verbally as well as in writing. When a client's health is changing rapidly, the charge nurse and the primary care provider may want to be kept up to date with verbal reports. Nurses also report client status at a change of shift and on a client's discharge to another unit or health agency in person, via a voice recording, or in writing. For information on documenting and reporting, see Chapter 14.

Evaluating

To evaluate is to judge or to appraise. Evaluating is the fifth phase of the nursing process. In this context, **evaluating** is a planned, ongoing, purposeful activity in which clients and healthcare professionals determine (a) the client's progress toward achievement of goals or outcomes and (b) the effectiveness of the nursing care plan. Evaluation is an important aspect of the nursing process because conclusions drawn from the evaluation determine whether the nursing interventions should be terminated, continued, or changed. Evaluation is the sixth standard of the ANA Standards of Practice and states that "the registered nurse evaluates progress towards attainment of outcomes" (ANA, 2015, p. 66).

Evaluation is continuous. Evaluation done while or immediately after implementing a nursing order enables the nurse to make on-the-spot modifications in an intervention. Evaluation performed at specified intervals (e.g., once a week for the home care client) shows the extent of progress toward achievement of goals or outcomes and enables the nurse to correct any deficiencies and modify the care plan as needed. Evaluation continues until the client achieves the health goals or is discharged from nursing care. Evaluation at discharge includes the status of goal achievement and the client's self-care abilities with regard to follow-up care. Most agencies have a special discharge record for this evaluation.

Through evaluating, nurses demonstrate responsibility and accountability for their actions, indicate interest in the results of the nursing activities, and demonstrate a desire not to perpetuate ineffective actions and instead to adopt more effective ones.

Relationship of Evaluating to Other Nursing Process Phases

Successful evaluation depends on the effectiveness of the steps that precede it. Assessment data must be accurate and complete so that the nurse can formulate appropriate nursing diagnoses and desired outcomes. The desired outcomes must be stated concretely in behavioral terms if they are to be useful for evaluating client responses. Finally, without the implementing phase in which the plan is put into action, there would be nothing to evaluate.

The evaluating and assessing phases overlap. As previously stated, assessment is ongoing and continuous at every client contact. However, data are collected for different purposes at different points in the nursing process. During the assessment phase the nurse collects data for the purpose of making diagnoses. During the evaluation step the nurse collects data for the purpose of comparing it to preselected goals or outcomes and judging the effectiveness of the nursing care. The act of assessing is the same; the differences lie in (a) when the data are collected and (b) how the data are used.

Process of Evaluating Client Responses

Before evaluation, the nurse identifies the desired outcomes (indicators) that will be used to measure client goal achievement. (This is done in the planning step.) Desired outcomes serve two purposes: They establish the kind of evaluative data that need to be collected and provide a standard against which the data are judged. For example, given the following expected outcomes, any nurse caring for the client would know what data to collect:

- Daily fluid intake will not be less than 2500 mL.
- Urinary output will balance with fluid intake.
- Residual urine will be less than 100 mL.

The evaluation phase has five components (Figure 13.3 ■):

- Collecting data related to the desired outcomes (NOC indicators): Did the client improve or deteriorate compared to the previous evaluation?
- Comparing the data with desired outcomes: What improvements have been made in client care?
- Relating nursing activities to outcomes: Have the nursing interventions resulted in the attainment of outcomes?
- Drawing conclusions about problem status: What outcomes have been attained?
- Continuing, modifying, or terminating the nursing care plan: What changes are needed in the plan of care to attain outcomes?

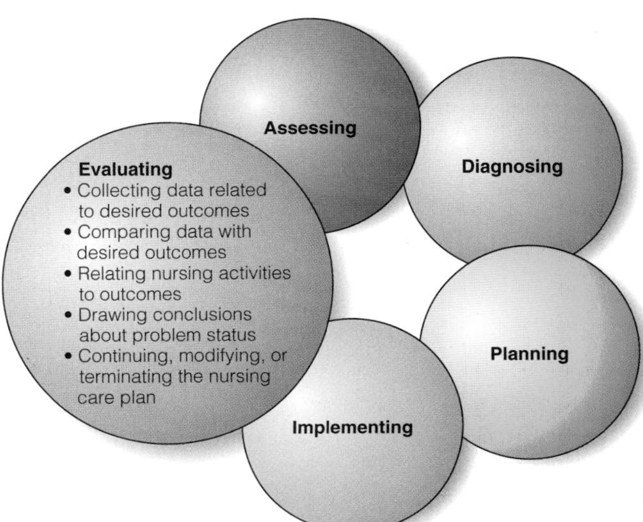

Figure 13.3 ■ Evaluating—the final phase of the nursing process. In this phase the nurse determines the client's progress toward goal achievement and the effectiveness of the nursing care plan. The plan may be continued, modified, or terminated.

Collecting Data

Using the clearly stated, precise, and measurable desired outcomes as a guide, the nurse collects data so that conclusions can be drawn about whether goals have been met. It is usually necessary to collect both objective and subjective data.

Some data may require interpretation. Examples of objective data requiring interpretation are the degree of tissue turgor of a dehydrated client or the degree of restlessness of a client with pain. Examples of subjective data needing interpretation include complaints of nausea or pain by the client. When interpreting subjective data, the nurse must rely on either (a) the client's statements (e.g., "My pain is worse now than it was after breakfast") or (b) objective indicators of the subjective data, even though these indicators may require further interpretation (e.g., decreased restlessness, decreased pulse and respiratory rates, and relaxed facial muscles as indicators of pain relief). Data must be recorded concisely and accurately to facilitate the next part of the evaluating process.

Comparing Data with Desired Outcomes

If the first two parts of the evaluating process have been carried out effectively, it is relatively simple to determine whether a desired outcome has been met. Both the nurse and client play an active role in comparing the client's actual responses with the desired outcomes. Did the client drink 3000 mL of fluid in 24 hours? Did the client walk unassisted the specified distance per day? When determining whether a goal has been achieved, the nurse can draw one of three possible conclusions:

1. The goal was met; that is, the client response is the same as the desired outcome.
2. The goal was partially met; that is, either a short-term outcome was achieved but the long-term goal was not, or the desired goal was incompletely attained.
3. The goal was not met.

After determining whether or not a goal has been met, the nurse writes an evaluation statement (either on the care plan or in the nurse's notes). An **evaluation statement** consists of two parts: a conclusion and supporting data. The conclusion is a statement that the goal or desired outcome was met, partially met, or not met. The supporting data are the list of client responses that support the conclusion, for example:

> Goal met: Oral intake 300 mL more than output; skin turgor resilient; mucous membranes moist.

See the Nursing Care Plan at the end of the chapter for evaluation statements for Margaret O'Brien. Data in the Evaluation Statements column on this table represent Margaret's responses to care as observed by the night nurse on the morning after her admission to the unit. In practice, care plans usually do not have a column for evaluation statements; rather, these are recorded in the nurse's notes. If NOC indicators are being used with the outcomes, scores on the scales after intervention would be compared with those measured at baseline to determine improvement.

Relating Nursing Activities to Outcomes

The third phase of the evaluating process is determining whether the nursing activities had any relation to the outcomes. It should never be assumed that a nursing activity was the cause of or the only factor in meeting, partially meeting, or not meeting a goal.

For example, a client was obese and needed to lose 14 kg (30 lb). When the nurse and client drew up a care plan, one goal was "Lose 1.4 kg (3 lb) in 4 weeks." A nursing strategy in the care plan was "Explain how to plan and prepare a 1200-calorie diet." Four weeks later, the client weighed herself and had lost 1.8 kg (4 lb). The goal had been met—in fact, exceeded. It is easy to assume that the nursing strategy was highly effective. However, it is important to collect more data before drawing that conclusion. On questioning the client, the nurse might find any of the following: (a) The client planned a 1200-calorie diet and prepared and ate the food; (b) the client planned a 1200-calorie diet but did not prepare the correct food; (c) the client did not understand how to plan a 1200-calorie diet, so she did not bother with it.

If the first possibility is found to be true, the nurse can safely judge that the nursing strategy "Explain how to plan and prepare a 1200-calorie diet" was effective in helping the client lose weight. However, if the nurse learns that either the second or third possibility actually happened, then it must be assumed that the nursing strategy did not affect the outcome. The next step for the nurse is to collect data about what the client actually did to lose weight. It is important to establish the relationship (or lack thereof) of the nursing actions to the client responses.

Drawing Conclusions About Problem Status

The nurse uses the judgments about goal achievement to determine whether the care plan was effective in resolving, reducing, or preventing client problems. When goals have been met, the nurse can draw one of the following conclusions about the status of the client's problem:

- The actual problem stated in the nursing diagnosis has been resolved, or the potential problem is being prevented and the risk factors no longer exist. In these instances, the nurse documents that the goals have been met and discontinues the care for the problem.
- The potential problem stated in the nursing diagnosis is being prevented, but the risk factors are still present. In this case, the nurse keeps the problem on the care plan.
- The actual problem still exists even though some goals are being met. For example, a desired outcome on a client's care plan is "Will drink 3000 mL of fluid daily." Even though the data may show this outcome has been achieved, other data (dry oral mucous membranes) may indicate that the nursing diagnosis of alteration in fluid volume is applicable. Therefore, the nursing interventions must be continued even though this one goal was met.

When goals have been partially met or when goals have not been met, two conclusions may be drawn:

- The care plan may need to be revised, since the problem is only partially resolved. The revisions may need to occur during the assessing, diagnosing, or planning phases, as well as during implementing.

OR

- The care plan does not need revision, because the client merely needs more time to achieve the previously established goal(s). To make this decision, the nurse must assess why the goals are being only partially achieved, including whether the evaluation was conducted too soon (Figure 13.4 ■).

Continuing, Modifying, or Terminating the Nursing Care Plan

After drawing conclusions about the status of the client's problems, the nurse modifies the care plan as indicated. Depending on the agency, modifications may be made by drawing a line through portions of the care plan, marking portions using a highlighting pen, or indicating revisions as appropriate for electronic charting systems. The nurse may also write "discontinued" ("dc'd"), "goal met," or "problem resolved" and the date.

Whether or not goals were met, a number of decisions need to be made about continuing, modifying, or terminating nursing care for each problem. See Table 13.1 for a checklist to use when reviewing a care plan. Although the checklist uses a closed-ended yes–no format, its only intent is to identify areas that require the nurse's further examination.

Before making modifications, the nurse must determine the effectiveness of the plan as a whole. This requires a review of the entire care plan and a critique of each step of the nursing process involved in its development.

ASSESSING

An incomplete or incorrect database influences all subsequent steps of the nursing process and care plan. If data

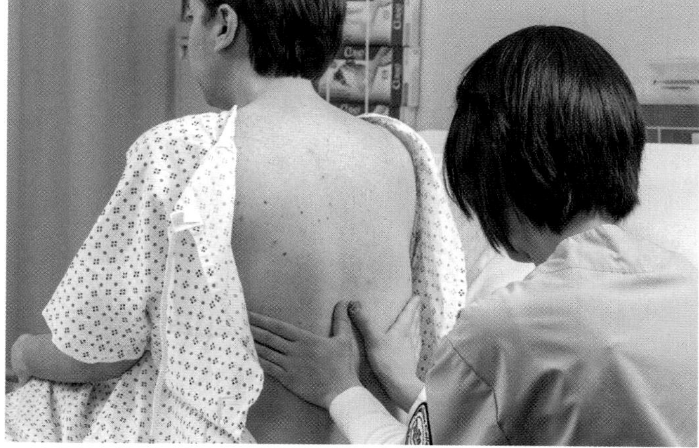

Figure 13.4 ■ Upon assessment of respiratory excursion, Nurse Medina detects failure of the client to achieve maximum ventilation. She and Margaret re-evaluate the care plan and modify it to increase coughing and deep-breathing exercises to q2h.

TABLE 13.1 Evaluation Checklist

Assessing	Diagnosing	Planning	Implementing
— Are data complete, accurate, and validated? — Do new data require changes in the care plan?	— Are nursing diagnoses relevant and accurate? — Are nursing diagnoses supported by the data? — Has problem status changed (i.e., potential, actual, risk)? — Are the diagnoses stated clearly and in correct format? — Have any nursing diagnoses been resolved?	**Desired Outcomes** — Do new nursing diagnoses require new goals? — Are goals realistic? — Was enough time allowed for goal achievement? — Do the goals address all aspects of the problem? — Does the client still concur with the goals? — Have client priorities changed?	— Was client input obtained at each step of the nursing process? — Were goals and nursing interventions acceptable to the client? — Did the caregivers have the knowledge and skill to perform the interventions correctly? — Were explanations given to the client prior to implementing?
		Nursing Interventions — Do nursing interventions need to be written for new nursing diagnoses or new goals? — Do the nursing interventions seem to be related to the stated goals? — Is there a rationale to justify each nursing order? — Are the nursing interventions clear, specific, and detailed? — Are new resources available? — Do the nursing interventions address all aspects of the client's goals? — Were the nursing interventions actually carried out?	

are incomplete, the nurse needs to reassess the client and record the new data. In some instances, new data may indicate the need for new nursing diagnoses, new goals or outcomes, and new nursing interventions.

DIAGNOSING

If the database was incomplete, new diagnostic statements may be required. If the database was complete, the nurse needs to analyze whether the problems were identified correctly and whether the nursing diagnoses were relevant to that database. After making judgments about problem status, the nurse revises or adds new diagnoses as needed to reflect the most recent client data.

PLANNING: DESIRED OUTCOMES

If a nursing diagnosis was inaccurate, obviously the goal or outcome statement will need revision. If the nursing diagnosis was appropriate, the nurse then checks if the goals were realistic and attainable. Unrealistic goals require correction. The nurse should also determine whether priorities have changed and whether the client still agrees with the priorities. For example, maybe the amount of time delineated for a specific amount of weight loss was too short and should be extended. Goals or desired outcomes must also be written for any new nursing diagnoses.

PLANNING: NURSING INTERVENTIONS

The nurse investigates whether the nursing interventions were related to goal achievement and whether the best nursing interventions were selected. Even when diagnoses and goals or outcomes were appropriate, the nursing interventions selected may not have been the best ones to achieve the goal. New nursing interventions may reflect changes in the amount of nursing care the client needs, scheduling changes, or rearrangement of nursing activities to group similar activities or to permit longer rest or activity periods for the client. For example, for a client who wishes to stop smoking, there are many potential interventions. If medication was prescribed but the client is still smoking, possibly a behavioral intervention such as group counseling needs to be added. If new nursing diagnoses have been written, then new nursing interventions will also be necessary.

IMPLEMENTING

Even if all sections of the care plan appear to be satisfactory, the manner in which the plan was implemented may have interfered with goal achievement. Before selecting new interventions, the nurse should check whether they were carried out. Other personnel may not have carried them out, either because the interventions were unclear or because they were unreasonable in terms of external constraints such as money, staff, time, and equipment.

After making the necessary modifications to the care plan, the nurse implements the modified plan and begins the nursing process cycle again. Refer to the Nursing Care Plan at the end of this chapter to see how the plan for Margaret O'Brien was modified after evaluation of goal achievement and review of the nursing process. A line has been drawn through portions the nurse wished to delete; additions to the care plan are shown in italics.

Evaluating the Quality of Nursing Care

In addition to evaluating goal achievement for individual clients, nurses are also involved in evaluating and modifying the overall quality of care given to groups of clients. This is an essential part of professional accountability. In each of the processes described in the following sections, nurses and all other healthcare providers work together as an interprofessional team focused on improving client care. The activities both use and contribute to evidence-based practice.

Quality Assurance

A **quality assurance (QA) program** is an ongoing, systematic process designed to evaluate and promote excellence in the healthcare provided to clients. Quality assurance frequently refers to evaluation of the level of care provided in a healthcare agency, but it may be limited to the evaluation of the performance of one nurse or more broadly involve the evaluation of the quality of the care in an agency, or even in a country.

Quality assurance requires evaluation of three components of care: structure, process, and outcome. Each type of evaluation requires different criteria and methods, and each has a different focus.

Structure evaluation focuses on the setting in which care is given. It answers this question: What effect does the setting have on the quality of care? Structural standards describe desirable environmental and organizational characteristics that influence care, such as equipment and staffing.

Process evaluation focuses on how the care was given. It answers questions such as these: Is the care relevant to the client's needs? Is the care appropriate, complete, and timely? Process standards focus on the manner in which the nurse uses the nursing process. Some examples of process criteria are "Checks client's identification band before giving medication" and "Performs and records chest assessment, including auscultation, once per shift."

Outcome evaluation focuses on demonstrable changes in the client's health status as a result of nursing care. Outcome criteria are written in terms of client responses or health status, just as they are for evaluation within the nursing process. For example, "How many clients undergoing hip repairs develop pneumonia?" or "How many clients who have a colostomy experience an infection that delays discharge?"

Quality Improvement

Serious national efforts are currently under way to evaluate and improve the quality of healthcare based on internal assessment by healthcare providers and increasing awareness by the public that medical errors are not uncommon and can be lethal. In 2000 the Committee on Quality of Health Care in America of the Institute of Medicine (IOM) issued a landmark report, *To Err Is Human: Building a Safer Health System* (Kohn, Corrigan, & Donaldson, 2000). The emphases of the report are increasing knowledge related to medical errors and establishing systems for enhancing safe care. The IOM followed with another report in 2001, *Crossing the Quality Chasm: A New Health System for the 21st Century*, which delineated that care should be safe, effective, client centered, timely, efficient, and equitable. The entire reports are available at the National Academies Press website. Since the reports were issued, improved attention to these issues has come from a variety of sources.

Clinical Alert!

Bad systems—not bad people—lead to most errors.

The Center for Improvement in Healthcare Quality (CIHQ, n.d.) has a mission "to create a regulatory environment that enables healthcare organizations to effectively deliver safe, quality patient care" (para. 2). The organization advocates for the development of standards and regulations to shape the accreditation and regulation of healthcare. It also provides education on standards, regulations, and the survey process to individuals who are involved in the accreditation of healthcare facilities. CIHQ assists it members to determine compliance with accreditation standards and successfully meet the demands of the regulatory environment.

The International Society for Quality in Health Care is a global organization established in 1985. Its mission is "to inspire and drive improvement in the quality and safety of health care worldwide through education and knowledge sharing, external evaluation, supporting health systems, and connecting people through global networks" (Source: https://www.isqua.org/about.html).

The mission of The Joint Commission (2018) is "to continuously improve healthcare for the public, in collaboration with other stakeholders, by evaluating healthcare organizations and inspiring them to excel in providing safe and effective care of the highest quality and value" (para. 2). The Joint Commission places great emphasis on the importance of sentinel events. A **sentinel event** is an unexpected occurrence involving death, permanent harm, or severe temporary harm and intervention required to sustain life (The Joint Commission, 2017). Sentinel events provide the impetus for immediate investigation as to the cause and determine the appropriate response. The Joint Commission has developed sentinel event policies for all types of agencies that are accredited by the Joint Commission. Organizations must respond to their sentinel events by assessing the cause, identifying a plan for intervention, and evaluating the results of the plan. Often, assessment involves a root cause analysis. **Root cause analysis** is a process for identifying the factors that bring about deviations in practices that lead to the event. It focuses primarily on systems and processes, not individual performance. It begins with examination of the single event with the purpose of determining which organizational improvements are needed to decrease the likelihood of such events occurring again.

Unlike quality assurance, **quality improvement (QI)** follows client care rather than organizational structure, focuses on process rather than individuals, and uses a systematic approach with the intention of *improving* the quality of care rather than *ensuring* the quality of care. QI studies often focus on identifying and correcting a system's problems, such as duplication of services in a hospital. QI is also known as continuous quality improvement (CQI), total quality management (TQM), performance improvement (PI), or persistent quality improvement (PQI).

Quality improvement is one of the six competencies in the Quality and Safety Education for Nurses (QSEN) project. In this context, QI is defined as "Use data to monitor the outcomes of care processes and use improvement methods to design and test changes to continuously improve the quality and safety of healthcare systems" (Cronenwett et al., 2007, p. 127). Johnson (2012) states:

> To improve care, nurses must first know how well they are doing. Data reflecting the important elements of care is the only credible way of demonstrating the quality of care nurses provide. Thus, it is essential that nurses be taught a systematic process of defining problems, identifying potential causes of those problems, and methods for testing possible solutions to improve care. (p. 113)

As with all QSEN competencies, QI involves knowledge, skills, and attitudes important for every registered nurse to use in understanding and improving variations in the outcomes of nursing care. A second QSEN competency related to QI is safety, in which the nurse "minimize[s] risk of harm to patients and providers through both system effectiveness and individual performance" (Cronenwett et al., 2007, p. 128).

Nursing-Sensitive Indicators

The purpose of nursing-sensitive indicators is to promote client safety. The National Quality Forum (NQF) is a not-for-profit organization focused on improving healthcare. The NQF identified and endorsed national voluntary standards for nursing-sensitive care, including evidence-based performance measures, a framework for measuring nursing-sensitive care, and related research recommendations. The Joint Commission (2010) tested and revised the measures and released a final set of 12 nursing-sensitive care measures in 2009. This work allows nurses to consistently gather data in a manner that allows them to be used to evaluate the quality of nursing care. Examples of these measures are the prevalence of healthcare-associated pressure injuries and client falls.

In addition to the lists of nursing-sensitive care indicators, NQF also publishes a list of serious reportable events (SREs), often referred to as "never events" since they should not occur if individuals act appropriately. Many states require healthcare facilities to report SREs, and many insurance companies will not reimburse facilities for the care of clients who experience a never event. The 28 events are grouped into the categories of surgical, product or device, client protection, care management, environmental, and criminal events.

The National Database of Nursing Quality Indicators (NDNQI) is a proprietary database of the ANA. The ANA has partnered with Press Ganey, a not-for-profit organization that combines the NDNQI quality indicators with client experience and nurse engagement survey data. Approximately 2000 U.S. hospitals and healthcare systems participate in the NDNQI program. The surveys measure nursing quality, assess staffing levels, improve student engagement, and strengthen the nursing work environment (Press Ganey, n.d.). The database evaluates unit-specific nurse-sensitive data from hospitals in the United States. Some of the NDNQI indicators are the same as the NQF measures. NDNQI also surveys nurses annually regarding the practice environment and nurse satisfaction.

EVIDENCE-BASED PRACTICE

Evidence-Based Practice

Will the Implementation of a QI Project Utilizing a Civility Training Program Increase the Staff Nurses' Ability to Recognize and Reduce Incivility on a Nursing Unit?

The objective of this QI project, conducted by Dr. Nancy Armstrong (2017), was to determine if the implementation of a workplace civility training program would increase staff nurses' ability to recognize incivility, reduce incivility, and have the confidence to respond in situations where incivility has occurred. This project was implemented in a rural Kentucky hospital with nine registered nurses. Incivility in nursing has been well documented by Dr. Cynthia Clark and Dr. Susan Luparell. The project included team-building exercises, discussion about the workplace, and other learning activities. As a result of this project, the nurses reported the ability to recognize and respond to workplace incivility. They also stated that they were more confident in their ability to respond to incivility.

Implications

This study provides evidence that nurses can be educated on incivility and that a positive workplace environment will result.

Nursing Audit

An **audit** refers to the examination or review of records. A **retrospective audit** is the evaluation of a client's record after discharge from an agency. *Retrospective* means "relating to past events." A **concurrent audit** is the evaluation of a client's healthcare while the client is still receiving care from the agency. These evaluations use interviewing, direct observation of nursing care, and review of clinical records to determine whether specific evaluative criteria have been met.

LIFESPAN CONSIDERATIONS Evaluating

Evaluation of goals, selected outcomes, and interventions needs to be continuous, with ongoing assessment and reassessment of the situation. Needs can change quickly and must be reprioritized when problems occur. Infants and young children are vulnerable to rapid change in their condition due to their small body size, disproportionate size of organs, and immaturity of body systems. Also, they may not be able to verbalize how they are feeling. Older adults may have conditions that impair communication, such as aphasia from a cerebrovascular accident, dementia, multiple sclerosis, or other neurologic conditions. In such cases, the nurse needs to be even more astute in performing nonverbal assessments, being alert to potential problems, and detecting changes in the client's condition. If evaluations are done often and thoroughly, changes can be made quickly to intervene more effectively and improve outcomes. Constant assessment, communication, and interpersonal skills are as essential in the evaluation phase as they are during the initial assessment.

Another type of evaluation of care is the *peer review*. In a nurse peer review, nurses functioning in the same capacity, that is, peers, appraise the quality of care or practice performed by other equally qualified nurses. The peer review is based on pre-established standards or criteria.

There are two types of peer reviews: individual and nursing audits. The individual peer review focuses on the performance of an individual nurse. The nursing audit focuses on evaluating nursing care through the review of records. The success of these audits depends on accurate documentation.

NURSING CARE PLAN For Margaret O'Brien Modified Following Implementation and Evaluation

Nursing Diagnosis: Altered respiratory status related to viscous secretions secondary to alteration in fluid volume and shallow chest expansion secondary to pain and fatigue

DESIRED OUTCOMES*/ INDICATORS	EVALUATION STATEMENTS	NURSING INTERVENTIONS**	EXPLANATION FOR CONTINUING OR MODIFYING NURSING INTERVENTIONS
Respiratory status: gas exchange [0402], as evidenced by			
• Absence of pallor and cyanosis (skin and mucous membranes)	Partially met. Skin and mucous membranes not cyanotic, but still pale.	Monitor respiratory status q4h; rate, depth, effort, skin color, mucous membranes, amount and color of sputum.	*Retain nursing interventions to continue to identify progress. Goal status indicates problem not resolved.*
• Use of correct breathing/ coughing technique after instruction	Partially met. Uses correct technique when pain well controlled by narcotic analgesics.	Monitor results of blood gases, chest x-ray studies, pulse oximetry, and incentive spirometer volume as available.	
• Productive cough	Met. Cough productive of moderate amounts of thick, yellow, pink-tinged sputum.	Monitor level of consciousness.	
• Symmetric chest excursion of at least 4 cm	Not met. Chest excursion = 3 cm.	Auscultate lungs q4h.	
• Lungs clear to auscultation within 48–72 h	Not met. Scattered inspiratory crackles auscultated throughout right anterior and posterior chest.	Vital signs q4h (TPR, BP, pulse oximetry, pain).	*Does not need to be reinstructed as client demonstrates correct techniques. May still need support and encouragement because of fatigue and pain of breathing.*
• Respirations 12–22/min, pulse, less than 100 beats/min	Partially met. Respirations 26/min, pulse 96 beats/min.	Instruct in breathing and coughing techniques. Remind to perform and assist q3h. *Support and encourage. (8/27/20, JW)*	

NURSING CARE PLAN **For Margaret O'Brien Modified Following Implementation and Evaluation—*continued***

Nursing Diagnosis: Altered respiratory status related to viscous secretions secondary to alteration in fluid volume and shallow chest expansion secondary to pain and fatigue

DESIRED OUTCOMES*/ INDICATORS	EVALUATION STATEMENTS	NURSING INTERVENTIONS**	EXPLANATION FOR CONTINUING OR MODIFYING NURSING INTERVENTIONS
• Inhaling normal volume of air on incentive spirometer	Not met. Tidal volume only 350 mL *(Evaluated 8/27/20, JW)*	Administer prescribed expectorant; schedule for maximum effectiveness. Maintain Fowler's or semi-Fowler's position. Administer prescribed analgesics. Notify primary care provider if pain not relieved.	*As soon as client is hydrated and fever is controlled, she will probably be discharged to self-care at home.*
Respiratory status: gas exchange [0402], as evidenced by			
• Absence of pallor and cyanosis (skin and mucous membranes)	Partially met. Skin and mucous membranes not cyanotic, but still pale.	Monitor respiratory status q4h; rate, depth, effort, skin color, mucous membranes, amount and color of sputum.	*Retain nursing interventions to continue to identify progress. Goal status indicates problem not resolved.*
• Use of correct breathing/coughing technique after instruction	Partially met. Uses correct technique when pain well controlled by narcotic analgesics.	Monitor results of blood gases, chest x-ray studies, pulse oximetry, and incentive spirometer volume as available.	
• Productive cough	Met. Cough productive of moderate amounts of thick, yellow, pink-tinged sputum.	Monitor level of consciousness.	
• Symmetric chest excursion of at least 4 cm	Not met. Chest excursion = 3 cm.	Auscultate lungs q4h.	
• Lungs clear to auscultation within 48–72 h	Not met. Scattered inspiratory crackles auscultated throughout right anterior and posterior chest.	Vital signs q4h (TPR, BP, pulse oximetry, pain).	*Does not need to be reinstructed as client demonstrates correct techniques. May still need support and encouragement because of fatigue and pain of breathing.*
• Respirations 12–22/min, pulse, less than 100 beats/min	Partially met. Respirations 26/min, pulse 96 beats/min.	Instruct in breathing and coughing techniques. Remind to perform and assist q3h. *Support and encourage. (8/27/20, JW)*	
• Inhaling normal volume of air on incentive spirometer	Not met. Tidal volume only 350 mL *(Evaluated 8/27/20, JW)*	Administer prescribed expectorant; schedule for maximum effectiveness. Maintain Fowler's or semi-Fowler's position. Administer prescribed analgesics. Notify primary care provider if pain not relieved. Administer oxygen by nasal cannula as prescribed. Provide portable oxygen if client goes off unit (e.g., for x-ray examination). Assist with postural drainage daily at 0930. *On 8/27 teach to continue prn at home. (8/27/20, JW)* Administer prescribed antibiotic to maintain constant blood level. Observe for rash and GI or other side effects.	*As soon as client is hydrated and fever is controlled, she will probably be discharged to self-care at home.*

Continued on page 256

NURSING CARE PLAN **For Margaret O'Brien Modified Following Implementation and Evaluation—*continued***

Nursing Diagnosis: Altered respiratory status related to viscous secretions secondary to alteration in fluid volume and shallow chest expansion secondary to pain and fatigue

DESIRED OUTCOMES*/ INDICATORS	EVALUATION STATEMENTS	NURSING INTERVENTIONS**	EXPLANATION FOR CONTINUING OR MODIFYING NURSING INTERVENTIONS
Anxiety control [1402], as evidenced by			
• Listening to and following instructions for correct breathing and coughing technique, even during periods of dyspnea	Met. Performed coughing techniques as instructed during periods of dyspnea.	When client is dyspneic, stay with her; reassure her you will stay. Remain calm, appear confident.	
• Verbalizing understanding of condition, diagnostic tests, and treatments (by end of day)	Met. See nurse's notes for 3–11 shift. Stated, "I know I need to try to breathe deeply even when it hurts." Demonstrated correct use of incentive spirometer and stated understanding of the need to use it. Understands IV is for hydration and antibiotics. *(Evaluated 8/27/20, JW)*	Encourage slow, deep breathing. When client is dyspneic, give brief explanations of treatments and procedures.	
• Decrease in reports of fear and anxiety	Met. Stated, "I know I can get enough air, but it still hurts to breathe."		
• Voice steady, not shaky	Met. Speaks in steady voice.		
• Respiratory rate of 12–22/min	Not met. Rate 26–36/min.	~~When acute episode is over, give detailed information about nature of condition, treatments, and tests.~~ *Reassess whether client needs any information on condition, treatments, or tests. (8/27/20, JW)*	*Detailed information has been given. Because client shows understanding, there is no need to repeat information.*
• Freely expresses concerns and possible solutions about work and parenting roles	Partially met. Discussed only briefly on 3–11 shift. Not done on 11–7 shift because of client's need to rest. *(Evaluated 8/27/20, JW)*	As client can tolerate, encourage to express and expand on her concerns about her children and her work. Explore alternatives as needed. Note whether husband returns as scheduled. If he does not, institute care plan for actual Impaired Family Dynamics *(Do on 8/27, day shift) (8/27/20, JW)*	It is important that this assessment be made right away, so child care can be arranged if needed.

*The NOC # for desired outcomes is listed in brackets following the appropriate outcome.

**In this care plan, a line has been drawn through portions the nurse wished to delete; additions to the care plan are shown in italics.

APPLYING CRITICAL THINKING

1. From reviewing Margaret O'Brien's nursing care plan, what general conclusions can you make about the desired outcomes for altered respiratory status and anxiety?
2. Despite some of the outcomes being only partially met or not met, no new interventions were written for several outcomes. What reasons might there be for this?
3. For the nursing diagnosis of anxiety, most of the outcomes are fully met. Would you delete this diagnosis from the care plan at this time? Why or why not?
4. Since the Evaluation Statements column is generally not used on written care plans, where would auditors or individuals conducting quality assessments find these data?

Answers to Applying Critical Thinking questions are available on the faculty resources site. Please consult with your instructor.

Chapter 13 Review

CHAPTER HIGHLIGHTS

- Implementing is putting planned nursing interventions into action.
- Successful implementing and evaluating depend in part on the quality of the preceding phases of assessing, diagnosing, and planning.
- Reassessing occurs simultaneously with the implementing phase of the nursing process.
- Cognitive, interpersonal, and technical skills are used to implement nursing strategies.
- Before implementing an order, the nurse reassesses the client to be sure that the order is still appropriate.
- The nurse must determine whether assistance is needed to perform a nursing intervention knowledgeably, safely, and comfortably for the client.
- The implementing phase terminates with the documentation of the nursing activities and client responses.
- After the care plan has been implemented, the nurse evaluates the client's health status and the effectiveness of the care plan in achieving client goals.
- The desired outcomes formulated during the planning phase serve as criteria for evaluating client progress and improved health status.
- The desired outcomes determine the data that must be collected to evaluate the client's health status.
- Re-examining the client care plan is a process of making decisions about problem status and critiquing each phase of the nursing process.
- Professional standards of care hold that nurses are responsible and accountable for implementing and evaluating the plan of care.
- Quality assurance evaluation includes consideration of the structures, processes, and outcomes of nursing care.
- Quality improvement is a philosophy and process internal to the institution and does not rely on inspections by an external agency.

TEST YOUR KNOWLEDGE

1. When initiating the implementation phase of the nursing process, the nurse performs which phase first?
   1. Carrying out nursing interventions
   2. Determining the need for assistance
   3. Reassessing the client
   4. Documenting interventions

2. Under what circumstances is it considered acceptable practice for the nurse to document a nursing activity *before* it is carried out?
   1. When the activity is routine (e.g., raising the bedrails)
   2. When the activity occurs at regular intervals (e.g., turning the client in bed)
   3. When the activity is to be carried out immediately (e.g., a stat medication)
   4. It is never acceptable.

3. What should students remember in order to differentiate between evaluation and assessment?
   1. Assessment is done at the beginning of the process.
   2. Evaluation is completed at the end of the process.
   3. They are the same and there is no need to differentiate.
   4. The difference is in how the data are used.

4. The client has a high-priority nursing diagnosis of potential for altered skin integrity related to the need for several weeks of imposed bedrest. The nurse evaluates the client after 1 week and finds the skin integrity is not impaired. When the care plan is reviewed, the nurse should perform which of the following?
   1. Delete the diagnosis since the problem has not occurred.
   2. Keep the diagnosis since the risk factors are still present.
   3. Modify the nursing diagnosis to alteration in mobility.
   4. Demote the nursing diagnosis to a lower priority.

5. If the nurse planned to evaluate the length of time clients must wait for a nurse to respond to a client need reported over the intercom system on each shift, which process does this reflect?
   1. Structure evaluation
   2. Process evaluation
   3. Outcome evaluation
   4. Audit

6. When does the nurse show an understanding of the relationship of evaluation with the other phases of the nursing process? Select all that apply.
   1. Being careful to effectively assess the client's needs
   2. Selecting the appropriate nursing diagnosis related to the client's needs
   3. Collecting client-focused data with a specific need in mind
   4. Evaluating by using assessment data to determine effective achievement of goals and outcomes
   5. Basing evaluation on assessment data collected during the admission phase.

7. The care plan calls for administration of a medication plus client education on diet and exercise for high blood pressure. The nurse finds the blood pressure extremely elevated. The client is very distressed with this finding. Which nursing skill of implementing would be needed most?
   1. Cognitive
   2. Intellectual
   3. Interpersonal
   4. Psychomotor

8. Which of the following demonstrates appropriate use of guidelines in implementing nursing interventions? Select all that apply.
   1. No interventions should be carried out without the nurse having clear rationales.
   2. Always follow the primary care provider's orders exactly, without variation.
   3. Encourage all clients to be as dependent as desired and allow the nurse to perform care for them.
   4. When possible, give the client options in how interventions will be implemented.
   5. Each intervention should be accompanied by client teaching.
9. Which of the following represents application of the components of evaluating?
   1. Goal achievement must be written as either completely met or unmet.
   2. Data related to expected outcomes must be collected.
   3. If the outcome was achieved, conclude that the plan was effective.
   4. After determining that the outcome was not met, start over with a new nursing care plan.
10. An element of quality improvement, rather than quality assurance, is which of the following?
   1. Focus is on individual outcomes.
   2. Evaluates organizational structures.
   3. Aims to confirm that quality exists.
   4. Plans corrective actions for problems.

See Answers to Test Your Knowledge in Appendix A.

READINGS AND REFERENCES

Suggested Reading

Dizon, M. L., & Reinking, C. (2017). Reducing readmissions: Nurse-driven interventions in the transitions of care from the hospital. *Worldviews on Evidence-Based Nursing, 14*(6), 432–439. doi:10.1111/wvn.12260

The goal of this study was to establish transition of care interventions for clients to reduce readmissions to the acute care settings. The interventions were a multifaceted approach with efforts on admission, predischarge, and postdischarge.

Related Research

Laflamme, L. L. (2017). Enhancing perioperative patient safety: A collective responsibility. *Operating Room Nurses Association, 35*(4), 13–33.

References

American Nurses Association. (2015). *Nursing: Scope and standards of practice* (3rd ed.). Silver Spring, MD: Author.

Armstrong, N. E. (2017). A quality improvement project measuring the effect of an evidence-based civility training program on nursing workplace incivility in a rural hospital using quantitative methods. *Online Journal of Rural Nursing and Health Care, 17*(1), 100–137. doi:10.14574/ojrnhc.v17i1.438

Butcher, H. K., Bulechek, G. M., Dochterman, J. C., & Wagner, C. (Eds.). (2018). *Nursing interventions classification (NIC)* (7th ed.). St. Louis, MO: Mosby Elsevier.

Center for Improvement in Healthcare Quality. (n.d.). *About our organization*. Retrieved from https://cihq.org/about_our_organization.asp

Cronenwett, L., Sherwood, G., Barnsteiner J., Disch, J., Johnson, J., Mitchell, P., . . . Warren, J. (2007). Quality and safety education for nurses. *Nursing Outlook, 55*, 122–131. doi:10.1016/j.outlook.2007.02.006

Institute of Medicine, Committee on Quality of Health Care in America. (2001). *Crossing the quality chasm: A new health system for the 21st century*. Retrieved from http://www.nap.edu/books/0309072808/html

The International Society for Quality in Health Care. (n.d.). *Who we are*. Retrieved from https://isqua.org/who-we-are/who-we-are

Johnson, J. (2012). Quality improvement. In G. Sherwood & G. Barnsteiner (Eds.), *Quality and safety in nursing: A competency approach to outcomes* (pp. 113–132). Oxford, United Kingdom: Wiley Blackwell.

The Joint Commission. (2010). *Implementation guide for the NQF endorsed nursing-sensitive care measure set 2009*. Retrieved from http://www.jointcommission.org/assets/1/6/NSC%20Manual.pdf

The Joint Commission. (2017). *Sentinel event policy and procedures*. Retrieved from https://www.jointcommission.org/sentinel_event_policy_and_procedures

The Joint Commission. (2018). *About The Joint Commission*. Retrieved from https://www.jointcommission.org/about_us/about_the_joint_commission_main.aspx

Kohn, L. T., Corrigan, J. M., & Donaldson, M. S. (Eds.). (2000). *To err is human: Building a safer health system*. Retrieved from http://books.nap.edu/books/0309068371/html/index.html

Moorhead, S., Johnson, M., Maas, M. L., & Swanson, E. (Eds.). (2018). *Nursing outcomes classification (NOC): Measurement of health outcomes* (6th ed.). St. Louis, MO: Elsevier.

National Council of State Boards of Nursing. (2017). National guidelines for nursing delegation. *Journal of Nursing Regulation, 7*(1), 5–14. doi:10.1016/S2155-8256(16)31035-3

Press Ganey. (n.d.). *Nursing quality (NDNQI): Improve care quality, prevent adverse events with deep nursing quality insights*. Retrieved from http://www.pressganey.com/solutions/clinical-quality/nursing-quality

Selected Bibliography

Carpenito, L. J. (2016). *Nursing diagnosis: Application to clinical practice* (3rd ed.). Philadelphia, PA: Lippincott Williams & Wilkins.

Doenges, M. E., & Moorhouse, M. F. (2013). *Application of nursing process and nursing diagnosis: An interactive text for diagnostic reasoning* (6th ed.). Philadelphia, PA: F.A. Davis.

Wilkinson, J. M. (2012). *Nursing process and critical thinking* (6th ed.). Upper Saddle River, NJ: Prentice Hall.

Documenting and Reporting 14

LEARNING OUTCOMES

After completing this chapter, you will be able to:

1. List the measures used to maintain confidentiality and security of computerized client records.
2. Discuss purposes for client records.
3. Compare and contrast different documentation methods: source-oriented and problem-oriented medical records, PIE, focus charting, charting by exception, computerized records, and the case management model.
4. Explain how various forms in the client record (e.g., critical pathways care plans, Kardexes, flow sheets, progress notes, discharge and transfer forms) are used to document steps of the nursing process (assessing, diagnosing, planning, implementing, and evaluating).
5. Compare and contrast the documentation needed for clients in acute care, long-term care, and home healthcare settings.
6. Discuss guidelines for effective recording that meet legal and ethical standards.
7. Identify prohibited abbreviations, acronyms, and symbols that cannot be used in any form of clinical documentation.
8. Identify essential guidelines for reporting client data.

KEY TERMS

Introduction

Effective communication among health professionals is vital to the quality of client care. Generally, health personnel communicate through discussion, reports, and records. A **discussion** is an informal oral consideration of a subject by two or more healthcare personnel to identify a problem or establish strategies to resolve a problem. A **report** is oral, written, or computer-based communication intended to convey information to others. For instance, nurses always report on clients at the end of a hospital work shift.

A **record**, also called a **chart** or **client record**, is a formal, legal document that provides evidence of a client's care and can be written or computer based. Although healthcare organizations use different systems and forms for documentation, all client records have similar information. The process of making an entry on a client record is called **recording, charting**, or **documenting**.

Each healthcare organization has policies about recording and reporting client data, and each nurse is accountable for practicing according to these standards. Agencies also indicate which nursing assessments and interventions can be recorded by RNs and which can be charted by unlicensed personnel. In addition, The Joint Commission requires client record documentation to be timely, complete, accurate, confidential, and specific to the client. Healthcare reform has been pivotal in the process of increasing the use of the electronic health record (EHR).

Ethical and Legal Considerations

The American Nurses Association Code of Ethics was revised in 2015. Provision 3 states, "The nurse promotes, advocates for, and protects the rights, health, and safety of the patient" (ANA, 2015). This provision focuses on confidentiality. It is imperative in nursing that any client information be maintained as an obligatory secret. The client's record is also protected legally as a private record of the client's care. Access to the record is restricted to health professionals involved in giving care to the client. The institution or agency is the rightful owner of the client's record. This does not, however, exclude the client's rights to the same records.

Changes in the laws regarding client privacy became effective on April 14, 2003. The new HIPAA regulations maintain the privacy and confidentiality of protected health information (PHI). HIPAA refers to the Health Insurance Portability and Accountability Act of 1996.

PHI is identifiable health information that is transmitted or maintained in any form or medium, including verbal discussions, electronic communications with or about clients, and written communications (Hebda, Hunter, & Czar, 2019).

For purposes of education and research, most agencies allow student and graduate health professionals access to client records. The records are used in client conferences, clinics, rounds, client studies, and written papers. The student or graduate is bound by a strict ethical code and legal responsibility to hold all information in confidence. It is the responsibility of the student or health professional to protect the client's privacy by not using a name or any statements in the notations that would identify the client.

Safety Alert! SAFETY

Take safety measures before faxing confidential information. A fax cover sheet should contain instructions that the faxed material is to be given only to the named recipient. Consent is needed from the client to fax information. Make sure that personally identifiable information (e.g., client name, Social Security number) has been removed. Finally, check that the fax number is correct, check the number on the display of the machine after dialing, and check the number a third time before pressing the "send" button.

Ensuring Confidentiality of Computer Records

Because of the increased use of EHRs (see Chapter 8), healthcare agencies have developed policies and procedures to ensure the privacy and confidentiality of client information stored in computers. In addition, the Security Rule of HIPAA became mandatory in 2005. This rule governs the security of electronic PHI. The following are some suggestions for ensuring the confidentiality and security of computerized records:

1. A personal password is required to enter and sign off computer files. Do not share this password with anyone, including other health team members.
2. After logging on, never leave a computer terminal unattended.
3. Do not leave client information displayed on the monitor where others may see it.
4. Shred all unneeded computer-generated worksheets.
5. Know the facility's policy and procedure for correcting an entry error.
6. Follow agency procedures for documenting sensitive material, such as a diagnosis of AIDS.
7. Information technology (IT) personnel must install a firewall to protect the server from unauthorized access.

Purposes of Client Records

Client records are kept for a number of purposes including communication, planning client care, auditing health agencies, research, education, reimbursement, legal documentation, and healthcare analysis.

Clinical Alert!

Documentation in healthcare has primarily changed to the electronic health record (EHR). The EHR has also been known as the electronic medical record (EMR). The EHR has allowed hospitals and healthcare systems to evaluate the quality of care, promote client safety, and assist in the regulation of staffing needs. In 2015 the Nursing Practice Committee of the Missouri Nurses Association documented the views of nurses regarding the use of the EHR. Based on this study it is recommended that nurses should share any concerns about the EHR with the IT staff and EHR vendors. Issues identified include medication safety, documentation and standards of practice, and EHR efficiency. The study also identified IT concerns, such as interoperability, vendors, innovation, nursing voice, education, and collaboration (Lavin, Harper, & Barr, 2015).

Communication

The record serves as the vehicle by which different health professionals who interact with a client communicate with each other. This prevents fragmentation, repetition, and delays in client care.

Planning Client Care

Each health professional uses data from the client's record to plan care for that client. A primary care provider, for example, may order a specific antibiotic after establishing that the client's temperature is steadily rising and that laboratory tests reveal the presence of a certain microorganism. Nurses use baseline and ongoing data to evaluate the effectiveness of the nursing care plan.

Auditing Health Agencies

An audit is a review of client records for quality assurance purposes (see Chapter 13). Accrediting agencies such as The Joint Commission may review client records to determine if a particular health agency is meeting its stated standards.

Research

The information contained in a record can be a valuable source of data for research. The treatment plans for a number of clients with the same health problems can yield information helpful in treating other clients.

Education

Students in health disciplines often use client records as educational tools. A record can frequently provide a comprehensive view of the client, the illness, effective

Clinical Alert!

Confidentiality in nursing and other healthcare-related fields has taken on a greater urgency in light of the increasing use of social media. It is against the policies of some institutions to communicate with a client or family on social media. There is also a potential for cyberbullying. Nurses need to be aware of the institutional social media policies. In addition, nursing students must be aware of the school of nursing social media policy, as well as with similar policies at the institutions where they are attending their clinical rotations. Nurses and nursing students need to be vigilant of professional boundaries and cognizant of their clients' and families' privacy (Green, 2017).

treatment strategies, and factors that affect the outcome of the illness.

Reimbursement

Documentation also helps a facility receive reimbursement from the federal government. For a facility to obtain payment through Medicare, the client's clinical record must contain the correct diagnosis-related group (DRG) codes and reveal that the appropriate care has been given.

Codable diagnoses, such as DRGs, are supported by accurate, thorough recording by nurses. This not only facilitates reimbursement from the federal government, but also facilitates reimbursement from insurance companies and other third-party payers. If additional care, treatment, or length of stay becomes necessary for the client's welfare, thorough charting will help justify these needs.

Legal Documentation

The client's record is a legal document and is usually admissible in court as evidence. In some jurisdictions, however, the record is considered inadmissible as evidence when the client objects, because information the client gives to the primary care provider is confidential.

Healthcare Analysis

Information from records may assist healthcare planners to identify agency needs, such as overutilized and underutilized hospital services. Records can be used to establish the costs of various services and to identify those services that cost the agency money and those that generate revenue.

Documentation Systems

A number of documentation systems are in current use: the source-oriented record; the problem-oriented medical record; the problems, interventions, evaluation (PIE) model; focus charting; charting by exception (CBE); computerized documentation; and case management. These documentation systems can be implemented using the traditional paper forms or with EHRs.

Source-Oriented Record

The traditional client record is a **source-oriented record**. Each healthcare provider or department makes notations in a separate section or sections of the client's chart. For example, the admissions department has an admission sheet; the primary care provider has a physician's order form, a physician's history sheet, and progress notes; nurses use the nurse's notes; and other departments or personnel have their own records. In this type of record, information about a particular problem is distributed throughout the record. For example, if a client had left hemiplegia (paralysis of the left side of the body), data about this problem might be found in the physician's history sheet, on the physician's order form, in the nurse's notes, in the physical therapist's record, and in the social service record. Table 14.1 lists the components of a source-oriented record.

Narrative charting is a traditional part of the source-oriented record (Figure 14.1 ■). It consists of written notes that include routine care, normal findings, and client problems. There is no right or wrong order to the information, although chronologic order is frequently used. Today, few institutions use only narrative charting. Narrative recording is being replaced by other systems, such as charting by exception and focus charting. Many agencies combine narrative charting with another system. For example, an agency using a charting-by-exception system (discussed later) may use narrative charting when describing abnormal findings. When using narrative charting, it is important to organize the information in a clear, coherent manner. Using the nursing process as a framework is one way to do this. See Box 14.1.

Source-oriented records are convenient because care providers from each discipline can easily locate the forms on which to record data and it is easy to trace the information specific to one's discipline. The disadvantage is that information about a particular client problem is scattered throughout the chart, so it is difficult to find chronologic information on a client's problems and progress. When using this form of charting it is important to maintain a high level of communication among all healthcare disciplines.

Problem-Oriented Medical Record

In the **problem-oriented medical record (POMR)**, or **problem-oriented record (POR)**, established by Lawrence Weed in the 1960s, the data are arranged according to the problems the client has rather than the source of the information. Members of the healthcare team contribute to the problem list, plan of care, and progress notes. Plans for each active or potential problem are drawn up, and progress notes are recorded for each problem.

The advantage of POMR is that (a) it encourages collaboration and (b) the problem list in the front of the chart alerts caregivers to the client's needs and makes it easier

TABLE 14.1 **Components of the Source-Oriented Record**

Form	Information
Admission (face) sheet	Legal name, birth date, age, gender Social Security number Address Marital status; closest relatives or individual to notify in case of emergency Date, time, and admitting diagnosis Food or drug allergies Name of admitting (attending) primary care provider Insurance information Any assigned diagnosis-related group (DRG)
Initial nursing assessment	Findings from the initial nursing history and physical health assessment
Graphic record	Body temperature, pulse rate, respiratory rate, blood pressure, daily weight, and special measurements such as fluid intake and output and oxygen saturation
Daily care record	Activity, diet, bathing, and elimination records
Special flow sheets	Examples: fluid balance record, skin assessment
Medication record	Name, dosage, route, time, date of regularly administered medications Name or initials of individual administering the medication
Nurse's notes	Pertinent assessment of client Specific nursing care including teaching and client's responses Client's complaints and how client is coping
Medical history and physical examination	Past and family medical history, present medical problems, differential or current diagnoses, findings of physical examination by the primary care provider
Physician's order form	Medical orders for medications, treatments, and so on
Physician's progress notes	Medical observations, treatments, client progress, and so on
Consultation records	Reports by medical and clinical specialists
Diagnostic reports	Examples: laboratory reports, x-ray reports, CT scan reports
Consultation reports	Physical therapy, respiratory therapy
Client discharge plan and referral summary	Started on admission and completed on discharge; includes nursing problems, general information, and referral data

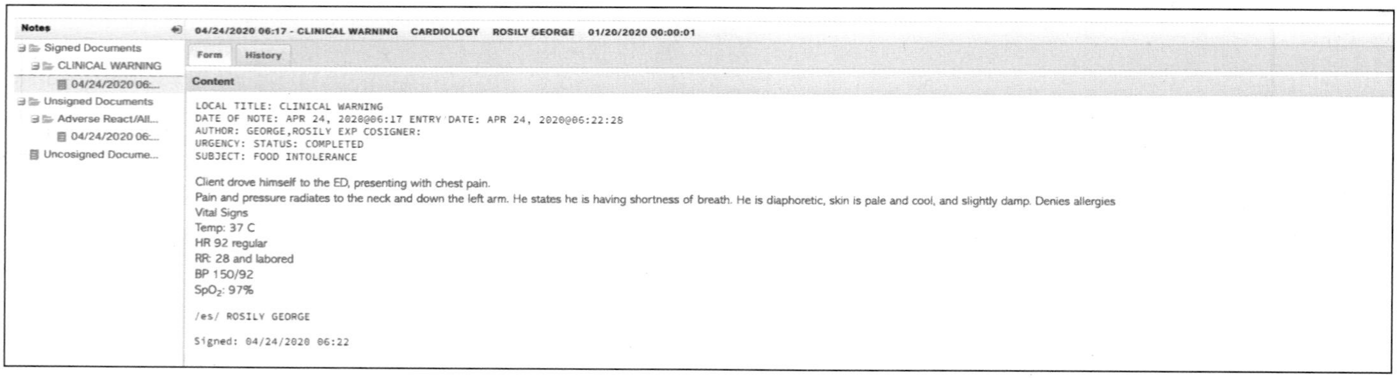

Notes
Signed Documents
CLINICAL WARNING
04/24/2020 06:...
Unsigned Documents
Adverse React/All...
04/24/2020 06:...
Uncosigned Docume...

04/24/2020 06:17 - CLINICAL WARNING CARDIOLOGY ROSILY GEORGE 01/20/2020 00:00:01

Form History

Content

LOCAL TITLE: CLINICAL WARNING
DATE OF NOTE: APR 24, 2020@06:17 ENTRY DATE: APR 24, 2020@06:22:28
AUTHOR: GEORGE,ROSILY EXP COSIGNER:
URGENCY: STATUS: COMPLETED
SUBJECT: FOOD INTOLERANCE

Client drove himself to the ED, presenting with chest pain.
Pain and pressure radiates to the neck and down the left arm. He states he is having shortness of breath. He is diaphoretic, skin is pale and cool, and slightly damp. Denies allergies
Vital Signs
Temp: 37 C
HR 92 regular
RR: 28 and labored
BP 150/92
SpO_2: 97%

/es/ ROSILY GEORGE

Signed: 04/24/2020 06:22

Figure 14.1 ■ A narrative note in an EHR.
iCare.

to track the status of each problem. Its disadvantages are that (a) caregivers differ in their ability to use the required charting format, (b) it takes constant vigilance to maintain an up-to-date problem list, and (c) it is somewhat inefficient because assessments and interventions that apply to more than one problem must be repeated.

The POMR has four basic components:

- Database
- Problem list
- Plan of care
- Progress notes.

BOX 14.1 Example of Organizing Narrative Charting

Situation: Client is postoperative day 2 after abdominal surgery.
Questions to ask yourself:

- What assessment data are relevant?
- What nursing interventions have I completed?
- What is my evaluation of the result of the interventions and/or what is the client's response to the interventions?

EXAMPLE

1000 Diminished breath sounds in all lung fields with crackles in LLL. Not using incentive spirometer (IS). Stated he's "not sure how to use it." Temperature 99.6. Instructed how to use IS. Discussed the importance of deep breathing and coughing after surgery. Administered analgesic for c/o abdominal pain rating of 5/10. After pain relief (1/10), able to demonstrate correct use of IS. ——— S. Martin, RN

1400 Using IS each hour. Lungs less diminished with fewer LLL crackles. Temp 99. ——— S. Martin, RN

In addition, flow sheets and discharge notes are added to the record as needed.

Database

The database consists of all information known about the client when the client first enters the healthcare agency. It includes the nursing assessment, the primary care provider's history, social and family data, and the results of the physical examination and baseline diagnostic tests. Data are constantly updated as the client's health status changes.

Problem List

The problem list (Figure 14.2 ■) is derived from the database. It is usually kept at the front of the chart and serves as an index to the numbered entries in the progress notes. Problems are listed in the order in which they are identified, and the list is continually updated as new problems are identified and others resolved. All caregivers may contribute to the problem list, which includes the client's physiologic, psychologic, social, cultural, spiritual, developmental, and environmental needs. Primary care providers write problems as medical diagnoses, surgical procedures, or symptoms; nurses write problems as nursing diagnoses.

As the client's condition changes or more data are obtained, it may be necessary to "redefine" problems. Figure 14.2 illustrates the client's problem of alteration in mobility, which was confirmed by the nursing staff. The second problem, altered urinary status, was identified by the medical staff. The lower portion of Figure 14.2 illustrates how problems are added to the client's EHR.

Plan of Care

The initial list of orders or plan of care is made with reference to the active problems. Care plans are generated by the individual who lists the problems. Primary care providers write physician's orders or medical care plans; nurses write nursing orders or nursing care plans. The written plan in the record is listed under each problem in the progress notes and is not isolated as a separate list of orders.

Progress Notes

A **progress note** in the POMR is a chart entry made by all health professionals involved in a client's care; they all use the same type of sheet for notes. Progress notes are numbered to correspond to the problems on the problem list and may be lettered for the type of data. For example, the SOAP format is frequently used. **SOAP** is

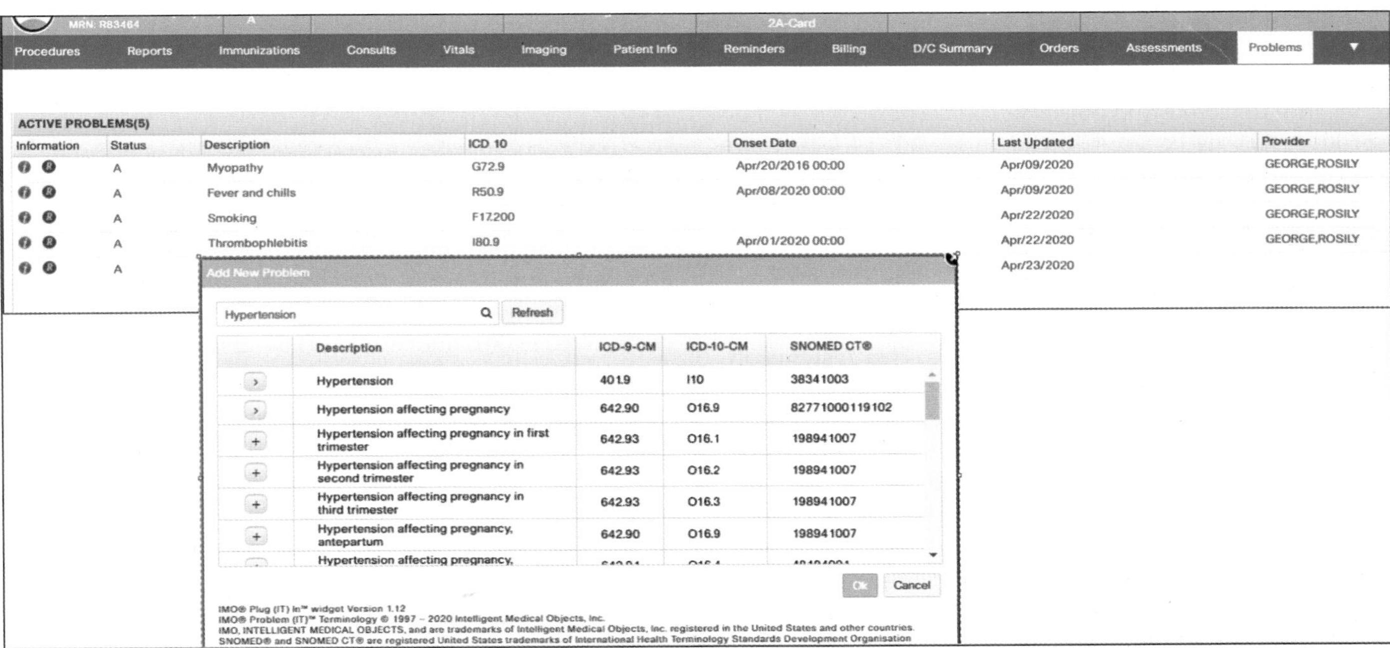

Figure 14.2 ■ An example of a problem list in the POMR in an EHR. In this record the nurse clicks on the problem to obtain more information. The lower screen allows the nurse or other healthcare provider to add problems to the problem list.
iCare.

an acronym for subjective data, objective data, assessment, and planning.

S—*Subjective data* consist of information obtained from what the client says. It describes the client's perceptions of and experience with the problem (see Chapter 10 ∞). When possible, the nurse quotes the client's words; otherwise, they are summarized. Subjective data are included only when it is important and relevant to the problem.

O—*Objective data* consist of information that is measured or observed by use of the senses (e.g., vital signs, laboratory and x-ray results).

A—*Assessment* is the interpretation or conclusions drawn about the subjective and objective data. During the initial assessment, the problem list is created from the database, so the "A" entry should be a statement of the problem. In all subsequent SOAP notes for that problem, the "A" should describe the client's condition and level of progress rather than merely restating the diagnosis or problem.

P—The *plan* is the plan of care designed to resolve the stated problem. The initial plan is written by the staff member who enters the problem into the record. All subsequent plans, including revisions, are entered into the progress notes.

Over the years, the SOAP format has been modified. The acronyms *SOAPIE* and *SOAPIER* refer to formats that add interventions, evaluation, and revision:

I—*Interventions* refer to the specific interventions that have actually been performed by the caregiver.

E—*Evaluation* includes client responses to nursing interventions and medical treatments. This is primarily reassessment data.

R—*Revision* reflects care plan modifications suggested by the evaluation. Changes may be made in desired outcomes, interventions, or target dates.

Newer versions of this format eliminate the subjective and objective data and start with *assessment*, which combines the subjective and objective data. The acronym then becomes *AP*, *APIE*, or *APIER*. See Figure 14.3 ■ for an example of a SOAP note.

PIE

The **PIE** documentation model groups information into three categories. *PIE* is an acronym for problems, interventions, and evaluation of nursing care. This system consists of a client care assessment flow sheet and progress notes. The **flow sheet** uses specific assessment criteria in a particular format, such as human needs or functional health patterns. The time parameters for a flow sheet can vary from minutes to months. In a hospital intensive care unit, for example, a client's blood pressure may be monitored by the minute, whereas in an ambulatory clinic a client's blood glucose level may be recorded once a month.

After the assessment, the nurse establishes and records specific problems on the progress notes, often using nursing diagnoses to word the problem. If there is no approved nursing diagnosis for a problem, the nurse develops a problem statement using a three-part format: client's response, contributing or probable causes of the response, and characteristics manifested by the client (see Chapter 11 ∞). The *problem statement* is labeled "P" and referred to by number (e.g., P #5). The *interventions* employed to manage the problem are labeled "I" and numbered according to the problem (e.g., I #5). The *evaluation* of the effectiveness of the interventions is also labeled and numbered according to the problem (e.g., E #5).

The PIE system eliminates the traditional care plan and incorporates an ongoing care plan into the progress notes. Therefore, the nurse does not have to create and update a separate plan. A disadvantage is that the nurse must review all the nursing notes before giving care to determine which problems are current and which interventions were effective.

Focus Charting

Focus charting is intended to make the client and client concerns and strengths the focus of care. Three columns for recording are usually used: date and time, focus, and progress notes. The *focus* may be a condition, a nursing diagnosis, a behavior, a sign or symptom, an acute change in the client's condition, or a client strength. The progress notes are organized into (D) data, (A) action, and (R) response, referred to as DAR. The *data* category reflects the assessment phase of the nursing process and consists of observations of client status and behaviors, including data from flow sheets (e.g., vital signs, pupil reactivity). The nurse records both subjective and objective data in this section.

The *action* category reflects planning and implementation and includes immediate and future nursing actions. It may also include any changes to the plan of care. The *response category* reflects the evaluation phase of the nursing process and describes the client's response to any nursing and medical care.

The focus charting system provides a holistic perspective of the client and the client's needs. It also provides a nursing process framework for the progress notes (DAR). The three components do not need to be recorded in order, and each note does not need to have all three categories. Flow sheets and checklists are frequently used on the client's chart to record routine nursing tasks and assessment data.

Date/Hour	Focus	Progress Notes
2/11/20 0900	Pain	**D:** Guarding abdominal incision. Facial grimacing. Rates pain at "8" on scale of 0–10.
		A: Administered morphine sulfate 4 mg IV.
0930		**R:** Rates pain at "1." States willing to ambulate.

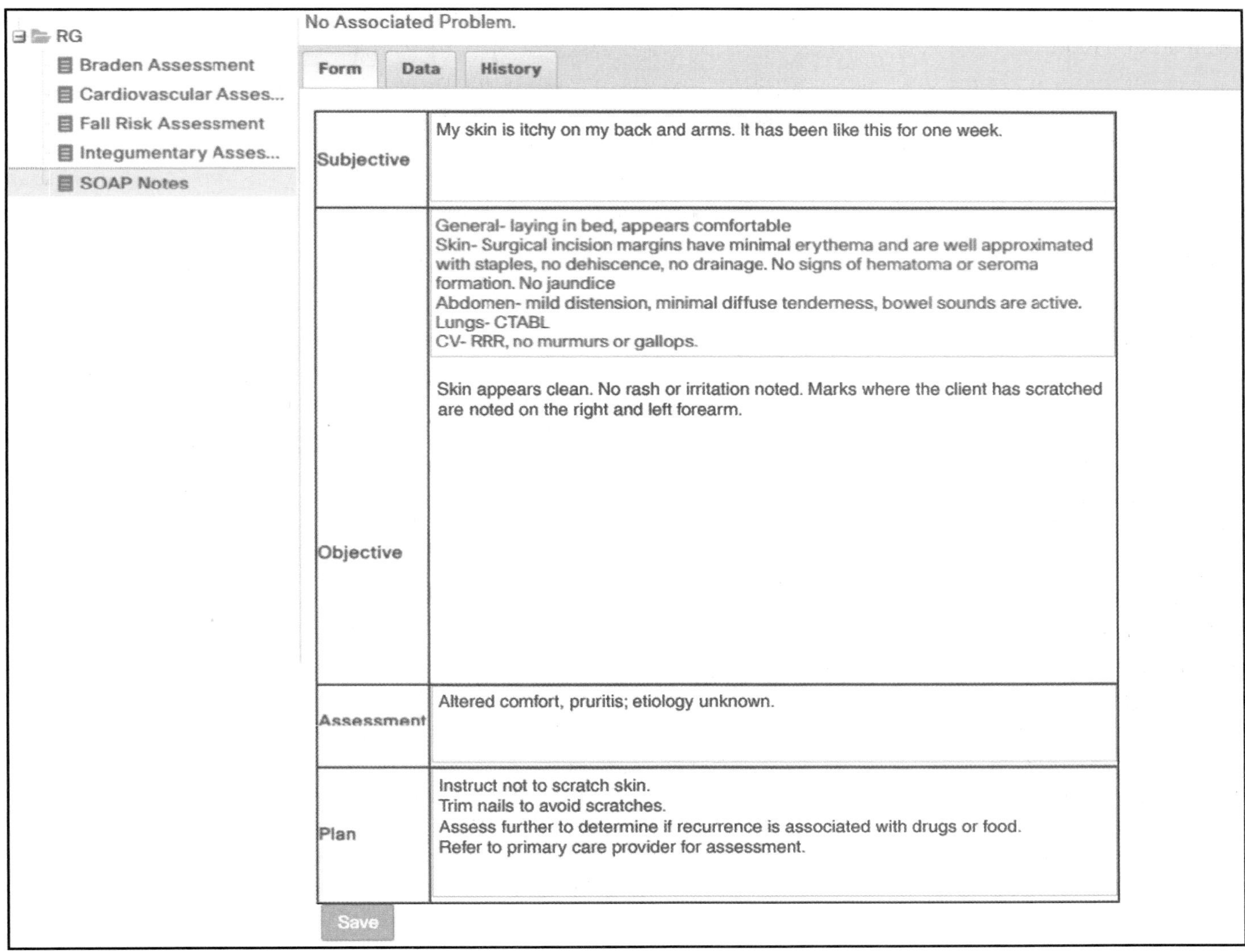

Figure 14.3 ■ An example of a SOAP note in an EHR.
iCare.

Charting by Exception

Charting by exception (CBE) is a documentation system in which only abnormal or significant findings or exceptions to norms are recorded. CBE incorporates three key elements (Guido, 2020):

1. ***Flow sheets.*** Examples of flow sheets include table or graphic records of a vital sign sheet, as shown in Figure 14.4 ■; a head and face assessment in a daily nursing assessments record (Figure 14.5 ■); and a fall risk assessment of the skin (Figure 14.6 ■).
2. ***Standards of nursing care.*** Documentation by reference to the agency's printed standards of nursing practice eliminates much of the repetitive charting of routine care. An agency using CBE must develop its own specific standards of nursing practice that identify the minimum criteria for client care regardless of clinical area. Some units may also have unit-specific standards unique to their type of client. For example, "The nurse must ensure that the unconscious client has oral care at least q4h." Documentation of care according to these specified standards involves only a check mark in the routine standards box on the graphic record. If all the standards are not implemented, an asterisk on the flow sheet is made with reference to the nursing notes. All exceptions to the standards are fully described in narrative form on the nursing notes.
3. ***Bedside access to chart forms.*** In the CBE system, all flow sheets are kept at the client's bedside to allow immediate recording and to eliminate the need to transcribe data from the nurse's worksheet to the permanent record.

Pulse | Entered in Error | Enter Vitals

Vitals	04-23-20 14:00:00	04-23-20 12:00:00	04-23-20 10:00:00	04-23-20 08:00:00	04-23-20 06:00:00
Temp.	97.6	98	100	99	98.4
Pulse	76	86	88	86	86
Resp.	22*	20*	22*	24*	22*
B/P	120/80	130/80	110/60*	140/70	130/80
P Ox%	98	99	98	99	99
Pain	0	0	0	0	0
Ht (in)	68.8980	68.8980	68.8980	68.8980	68.8980
Wt (lbs.)	171.96	171.96	154.32	171.96	180.78
BMI	25.52	25.52	22.90	25.52	26.83
C/G	68	68	60	76	80
CVP (cmH20)					
Location	CARDIOLOGY	CARDIOLOGY	CARDIOLOGY	CARDIOLOGY	CARDIOLOGY
Entered By	GEORGE,ROSILY	GEORGE,ROSILY	GEORGE,ROSILY	GEORGE,ROSILY	GEORGE,ROSILY
Data Source	Vitals	Vitals	Vitals	Vitals	Vitals

Figure 14.4 ■ Table of vital signs and SpO_2. The normal range can be set and abnormal values can be highlighted.
iCare.

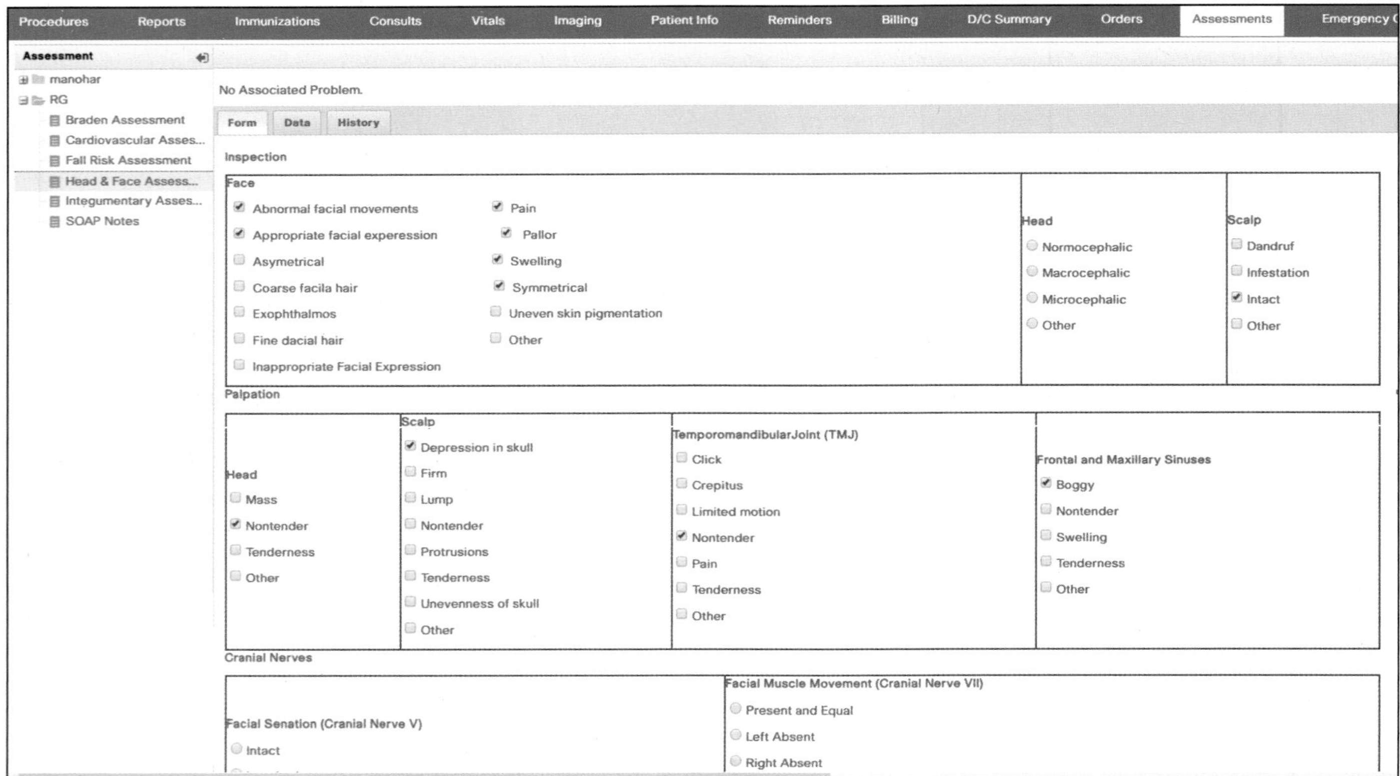

Figure 14.5 ■ Sample of a head and face assessment on a daily nursing CBE assessment form in an EHR.
iCare.

The advantages to this system are that it eliminates lengthy, repetitive notes and it makes client changes in condition more obvious. Inherent in CBE is the presumption that the nurse did assess the client and determined what responses were normal and abnormal. Many nurses believe in the saying "not charted, not done" and subsequently may feel uncomfortable with the CBE documentation system. One suggestion is to type or key in N/A on flow sheets where the items are not applicable and to not leave blank spaces. This would then avoid the possible misinterpretation that the assessment or intervention was not done by the nurse.

The disadvantages of this form of charting can place the nurse and hospital or healthcare system at risk of malpractice or negligence litigation. Due to the lack of extensive documentation it fails to provide a full picture of the client's health-related needs. The most prominent case according to Guido (2020) is *Lama v. Borras* in 1994. In this case the client's surgical dressing was soiled, and the client complained of severe incisional pain, which was later diagnosed as diskitis requiring antibiotic therapy. During litigation the jury determined that the lack of extensive documentation compromised the client's care.

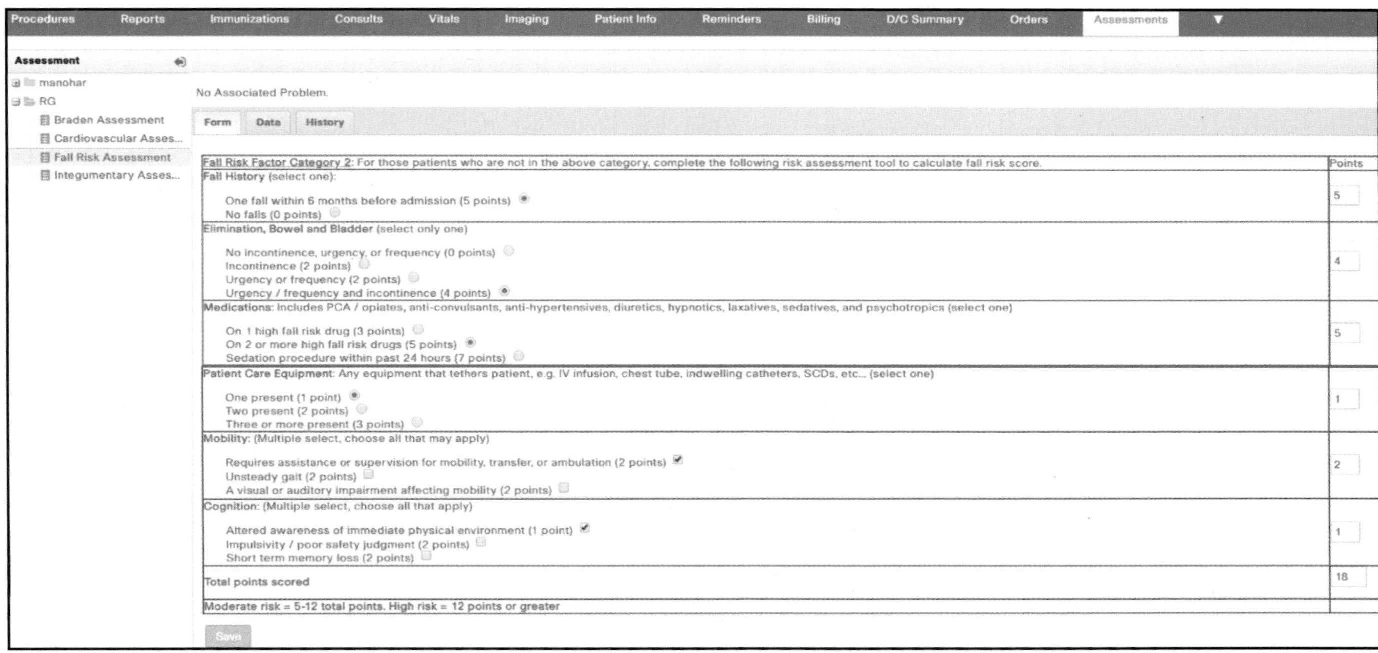

Procedures | Reports | Immunizations | Consults | Vitals | Imaging | Patient Info | Reminders | Billing | D/C Summary | Orders | Assessments

Assessment

manohar

RG

Braden Assessment

Cardiovascular Asses...

Fall Risk Assessment

Integumentary Asses...

No Associated Problem.

Form | Data | History

Fall Risk Factor Category 2: For those patients who are not in the above category, complete the following risk assessment tool to calculate fall risk score.	Points
Fall History (select one): One fall within 6 months before admission (5 points); No falls (0 points)	5
Elimination, Bowel and Bladder (select only one): No incontinence, urgency, or frequency (0 points); Incontinence (2 points); Urgency or frequency (2 points); Urgency / frequency and incontinence (4 points)	4
Medications: Includes PCA / opiates, anti-convulsants, anti-hypertensives, diuretics, hypnotics, laxatives, sedatives, and psychotropics (select one): On 1 high fall risk drug (3 points); On 2 or more high fall risk drugs (5 points); Sedation procedure within past 24 hours (7 points)	5
Patient Care Equipment: Any equipment that tethers patient, e.g. IV infusion, chest tube, indwelling catheters, SCDs, etc... (select one): One present (1 point); Two present (2 points); Three or more present (3 points)	1
Mobility: (Multiple select, choose all that may apply): Requires assistance or supervision for mobility, transfer, or ambulation (2 points); Unsteady gait (2 points); A visual or auditory impairment affecting mobility (2 points)	2
Cognition: (Multiple select, choose all that apply): Altered awareness of immediate physical environment (1 point); Impulsivity / poor safety judgment (2 points); Short term memory loss (2 points)	1
Total points scored	18
Moderate risk = 5-12 total points. High risk = 12 points or greater	

Save

Figure 14.6 ■ A fall risk assessment form in an EHR.
iCare.

Computerized Documentation

EHRs are used to manage the huge volume of information required in contemporary healthcare. That is, the EHR can integrate all pertinent client information into one record. Nurses use computers to store the client's database, add new data, create and revise care plans, and document client progress (Figure 14.7 ■). Some institutions have a computer terminal at each client's bedside, or nurses carry a small handheld terminal, enabling the nurse to document care immediately after it is given.

Multiple flow sheets are not needed in computerized record systems because information can be easily retrieved in a variety of formats. For example, the nurse can obtain results of a client's blood test, a schedule of all clients on the unit who are to have surgery during the day, a suggested list of interventions for a nursing diagnosis, a graphic chart of a client's vital signs, or a printout of all progress notes for a client. Many systems can generate a work list for the shift, with a list of all treatments, procedures, and medications needed by the client.

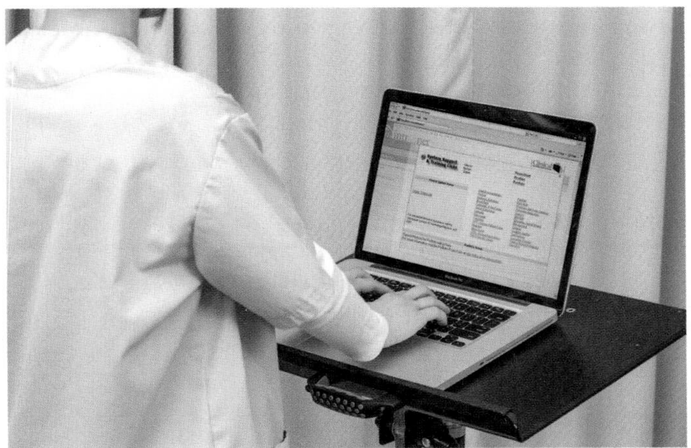

Figure 14.7 ■ A bedside computer.

Computers make care planning and documentation relatively easy. To record nursing actions and client responses, the nurse either chooses from standardized lists of terms or types narrative information into the computer. Automated speech-recognition technology now allows nurses to enter data by voice for conversion to written documentation. Again, according to HIPAA, if the spoken word is used to create PHI, the nurse must be alert and aware of others who might hear the dictation.

The computerization of clinical records has made it possible to transmit information from one care setting to another. The Nursing Minimum Data Set (NMDS) is an effort to establish uniform definitions and categories (e.g., nursing diagnoses) for collecting essential nursing data for inclusion in computer databases. Selected pros and cons of computer documentation are shown in Box 14.2.

Case Management

The case management model emphasizes quality, cost-effective care delivered within an established length of stay. This model uses a multidisciplinary approach to planning and documenting client care, using *critical pathways*. These forms identify the outcomes that certain

BOX 14.2 Selected Pros and Cons of Computer Documentation

PROS

- Computer records can facilitate a focus on client outcomes.
- Bedside terminals can synthesize information from monitoring equipment.
- Such systems allow nurses to use their time more efficiently.
- The system links various sources of client information.
- Client information, requests, and results are sent and received quickly.
- Links to monitors improve accuracy of documentation.
- Bedside terminals eliminate the need to take notes on a worksheet before recording.
- Bedside terminals permit the nurse to check an order immediately before administering a treatment or medication.
- Information is legible.
- The system incorporates and reinforces standards of care.
- Standard terminology improves communication.

CONS

- Client's privacy may be infringed on if security measures are not used.
- Breakdowns make information temporarily unavailable.
- The system is expensive.
- Extended training periods may be required when a new or updated system is installed.

CRITICAL PATHWAY: TOTAL HIP REPLACEMENT

	DOS/Day 1	Days 2–3
Pain Management	Outcome: • Verbalizes comfort or tolerance of pain Circle: V NV Variance:	Outcome: • Verbalizes comfort with pain control measures Circle: V NV Variance:
Respiratory	Outcomes: • Breath sounds clear to auscultation • Achieves 50% of volume goal on incentive spirometer Circle: V NV Variance:	Outcomes: • Breath sounds clear to auscultation • Achieves 100% of volume goal on incentive spirometer Circle: V NV Variance:
Key: V = Variance	NV = No Variance	
Signature:	Initials:	
Signature:	Initials:	

Figure 14.8 ■ Excerpt from a critical pathway documentation form.

groups of clients are expected to achieve on each day of care, along with the interventions necessary for each day. See Figure 14.8 ■ and Chapter 5 ∞ for more information about critical pathways.

Along with critical pathways, the case management model incorporates graphics and flow sheets. Progress notes typically use some type of CBE. For example, if goals are met, no further charting is required. A goal that is not met is called a **variance**. A variance is a deviation from what was planned on the critical pathway—unexpected occurrences that affect the planned care or the client's responses to care. When a variance occurs, the nurse writes a note documenting the unexpected event, the cause, and actions taken to correct the situation or justify the actions. See Table 14.2 for an example of how a variance might be documented.

The case management model promotes collaboration and teamwork among caregivers, helps to decrease length of stay, and makes efficient use of time. Because care is goal focused, the quality may improve. However, critical pathways work best for clients with one or two diagnoses and few individualized needs. Clients with multiple diagnoses (e.g., a client with a hip fracture, pneumonia, diabetes, and a pressure sore) or those with an unpredictable course of symptoms (e.g., a neurologic client with seizures) are difficult to document on a critical path.

Documenting Nursing Activities

The client record should describe the client's ongoing status and reflect the full range of the nursing process. Regardless of the records system used in an agency, nurses document evidence of the nursing process on a variety of forms throughout the clinical record (Table 14.3).

TABLE 14.2 Example of Variance Documentation (Critical Pathway)

A client has had a below-the-knee amputation. On the third postoperative day he has a temperature of 38.8°C (102°F). Lung sounds are clear and he is not coughing. The nurse notices redness and skin breakdown over the client's sacrum. The critical pathway outcomes specified for day 3 are "Oral temperature 37.7°C (100°F)" and "Skin intact over bony prominences." The nurse should chart the following variances:

Date/Time	Variance	Cause	Action Taken/Plans
4/16/20 0900	Elevated temperature (38.9°C [102°F])	Possible sepsis	4/16—Blood cultures × 3 per order. Monitor temp q1h. Monitor I&O, hydration, and mental status.
4/16/20 1130	Impaired skin integrity: stage 1 redness, 5-cm (2-in.) circular area on sacrum	Client does not move about in bed unless reminded	4/16—Positioned on L side. Turn side-to-side q2h while awake. On every client contact, remind client to move about in bed. Apply Duoderm after bath.

TABLE 14.3 Documentation for the Nursing Process

Step*	Documentation Forms
Assessment	Initial assessment form, various flow sheets
Nursing diagnosis	Nursing care plan, critical pathway, progress notes, problem list
Planning	Nursing care plan, critical pathway
Implementing	Progress notes, flow sheets
Evaluating	Progress notes

*All steps are recorded on discharge and referral summaries.

Admission Nursing Assessment

A comprehensive admission assessment, also referred to as an initial database, nursing history, or nursing assessment, is completed when the client is admitted to the nursing unit. As discussed in Chapter 10 ∞, these forms can be organized according to health patterns, body systems, functional abilities, health problems and risks, nursing model, or type of healthcare setting (e.g., labor and delivery, pediatrics, mental health). The nurse generally records ongoing assessments or reassessments on flow sheets or on nursing progress notes.

Nursing Care Plans

The Joint Commission requires that the clinical record include evidence of client assessments, nursing diagnoses and client needs, nursing interventions, client outcomes, and evidence of a current nursing care plan. Depending on the records system being used, the nursing care plan may be separate from the client's chart, recorded in progress notes and other forms in the client record, or incorporated into a multidisciplinary plan of care.

There are two types of nursing care plans: traditional and standardized. The *traditional care plan* is written for each client. The form varies from agency to agency according to the needs of the client and the department. Most forms have three columns: one for nursing diagnoses, a second for expected outcomes, and a third for nursing interventions. See Chapter 12 ∞ for additional information.

Standardized care plans were developed to save documentation time. These plans may be based on an institution's standards of practice, thereby helping to provide a high quality of nursing care. For further information, see Chapter 12 ∞. Standardized plans must be individualized by the nurse in order to adequately address individual client needs.

Kardexes

The **Kardex** is a widely used, concise method of organizing and recording data about a client, making information quickly accessible to all health professionals. The system consists of a series of cards kept in a portable index file or on computer-generated forms. The card for a particular client can be quickly accessed to reveal specific data. The Kardex may or may not become a part of the client's permanent record. In some organizations it is a temporary worksheet written in pencil for ease in recording frequent changes in details of a client's care. The information on Kardexes may be organized into sections, for example:

- Pertinent information about the client, such as name, room number, age, admission date, primary care provider's name, diagnosis, and type of surgery and date
- Allergies
- List of medications, with the date of order and the times of administration for each
- List of intravenous fluids, with dates of infusions
- List of daily treatments and procedures, such as irrigations, dressing changes, postural drainage, or measurement of vital signs
- List of diagnostic procedures ordered, such as x-ray or laboratory tests
- Specific data on how the client's physical needs are to be met, such as type of diet, assistance needed with feeding, elimination devices, activity, hygienic needs, and safety precautions (e.g., one-person assist)
- A problem list, stated goals, and a list of nursing approaches to meet the goals and relieve the problems.

Although much of the information on the Kardex may be recorded by the nurse in charge or a delegate (e.g., the nursing unit clerk), any nurse who cares for the client plays a key role in initiating the record and keeping the data current. Whether the Kardex is a written paper or computerized, it is important to have a place on it to record dates and the initials of the nurse reviewing or revising it. It is a quick visual guide to ensure that information is current and updated on a regular basis.

Flow Sheets

A flow sheet enables nurses to record nursing data quickly and concisely and provides an easy-to-read record of the client's condition over time.

Graphic Record

This record typically indicates body temperature, pulse, respiratory rate, blood pressure, weight, and, in some agencies, other significant clinical data such as admission or postoperative day, bowel movements, appetite, and activity.

Intake and Output Record

All routes of fluid intake and all routes of fluid loss or output are measured and recorded on this form. See Chapter 51 ∞ for more information.

Medication Administration Record

Medication flow sheets usually include designated areas for the date of the medication order, the expiration date, the medication name and dose, the frequency of administration and route, and the nurse's signature. Some records also include a place to document the client's allergies (see Chapter 35 ∞).

Skin Assessment Record

A skin or wound assessment is often recorded on a flow sheet such as the one shown earlier in Figure 14.6. This EHR specifically utilizes the Braden Assessment. EHRs may include categories related to stage of skin injury, drainage, odor, culture information, and treatments.

Progress Notes

Progress notes made by nurses provide information about the progress a client is making toward achieving desired outcomes. Therefore, in addition to assessment and reassessment data, progress notes include information about client problems and nursing interventions. The format used depends on the documentation system in place in the institution. Various kinds of nursing progress notes are discussed in the Documentation Systems section earlier in this chapter.

Nursing Discharge and Referral Summaries

A discharge note and referral summary are completed when the client is being discharged and transferred to another institution or to a home setting where a visit by a community health nurse is required. See the discussion of discharge planning in Chapter 6 ∞ and the assessment parameters suggested when preparing clients to go home. Many institutions provide forms for these summaries. Some records combine the discharge plan, including instructions for care, and the final progress note. Many are designed with checklists to facilitate data recording.

If the discharge plan is given directly to the client and family, it is imperative that instructions be written in terms that can be readily understood. For example, medications, treatments, and activities should be written in layman's terms, and use of medical abbreviations (such as ad lib) should be avoided.

If a client is transferred within the facility or from a long-term facility to a hospital, a report needs to accompany the client to ensure continuity of care in the new area. It should include all components of the discharge instructions, but also describe the condition of the client before the transfer. Any teaching or client instruction that has been done should also be described and recorded.

If the client is being transferred to another institution or to a home setting where a visit by a home health nurse is required, the discharge note takes the form of a referral summary. Regardless of format, discharge and referral summaries usually include some or all of the following:

- Description of client's physical, mental, and emotional status at discharge or transfer
- Resolved health problems
- Unresolved continuing health problems and continuing care needs; may include a review-of-systems checklist that considers integumentary, respiratory, cardiovascular, neurologic, musculoskeletal, gastrointestinal, elimination, and reproductive problems
- Treatments that are to be continued (e.g., wound care, oxygen therapy)
- Current medications
- Restrictions that relate to (a) activity such as lifting, stair climbing, walking, driving, work; (b) diet; and (c) bathing such as sponge bath, tub, or shower
- Functional and self-care abilities in terms of vision, hearing, speech, mobility with or without aids, meal preparation and eating, preparing and administering medications, and so on
- Comfort level
- Support networks including family, significant others, religious adviser, community self-help groups, home care and other community agencies available, and so on
- Client education provided in relation to disease process, activities and exercise, special diet, medications, specialized care or treatments, follow-up appointments, and so on
- Discharge destination (e.g., home, nursing home) and mode of discharge (e.g., walking, wheelchair, ambulance)
- Referral services (e.g., social worker, home health nurse).

Long-Term Care Documentation

Long-term facilities usually provide two types of care: skilled or intermediate. Clients needing skilled care require more extensive nursing care and specialized nursing skills. In contrast, an intermediate care focus is needed for clients who usually have chronic illnesses and may only need assistance with activities of daily living (such as bathing and dressing).

Requirements for documentation in long-term care settings are based on professional standards, federal and state regulations, and the policies of the healthcare agency. Laws influencing the kind and frequency of documentation required are the Health Care Financing Administration and the Omnibus Budget Reconciliation Act (OBRA) of 1987. The OBRA law, for example, requires that (a) a comprehensive assessment (the Minimum Data Set [MDS] for Resident Assessment and Care Screening) be performed within 4 days of a client's admission to a long-term

LIFESPAN CONSIDERATIONS **Long-Term Care**

OLDER ADULTS

Older adults in long-term care facilities tend to have chronic conditions and generally experience subtle, small changes in their condition. However, when problems do occur, such as a hip fracture, cardiovascular accident, or pneumonia, they are serious and require prompt attention. This points out the importance of keeping Kardexes and charting in long-term facilities current and up to date in the event that the client needs to be transferred for more skilled care and further treatment. A thorough transfer summary will facilitate communication and promote continuity of care in these situations.

PRACTICE GUIDELINES Long-Term Care Documentation

- Complete the assessment and screening forms (MDS) and plan of care within the time period specified by regulatory bodies.
- Keep a record of any visits and of phone calls from family, friends, and others regarding the client.
- Write nursing summaries and progress notes that comply with the frequency and standards required by regulatory bodies.
- Review and revise the plan of care every 3 months or whenever the client's health status changes.
- Document and report any change in the client's condition to the primary care provider and the client's family within 24 hours.
- Document all measures implemented in response to a change in the client's condition.
- Make sure that progress notes address the client's progress in relation to the goals or outcomes defined in the plan of care.

care facility, (b) a formulated plan of care must be completed within 7 days of admission, and (c) the assessment and care screening process must be reviewed every 3 months.

Accurate completion of the MDS is required for reimbursement from Medicare and Medicaid. These requirements vary with the level of service provided and other factors. For example, Medicare provides little reimbursement for services provided in long-term care facilities except for services that require skilled care such as chemotherapy, tube feedings, ventilators, and so on. For such Medicare clients, the nurse must provide daily documentation to verify the need for service and reimbursement.

Nurses need to familiarize themselves with regulations influencing the kind and frequency of documentation required in long-term care facilities. Usually the nurse completes a nursing care *summary* at least once a week for clients requiring skilled care and every 2 weeks for those requiring intermediate care. Summaries should address the following:

- Specific problems noted in the care plan
- Mental status
- Activities of daily living
- Hydration and nutrition status
- Safety measures needed
- Medications
- Treatments
- Preventive measures
- Behavioral modification assessments, if pertinent (if client is taking psychotropic medications or demonstrates behavioral problems).

See the Practice Guidelines for documentation in long-term care facilities.

Home Care Documentation

In 1985, the Health Care Financing Administration, a branch of the U.S. Department of Health and Human Services, mandated that home healthcare agencies standardize their documentation methods to meet requirements for Medicare and Medicaid and other third-party disbursements. Two records are required: (a) a home health certification and plan of treatment form and (b) a medical update and client information form. The nurse assigned to the home care client usually completes the forms, which must be signed by both the nurse and the attending primary care provider. See the Practice Guidelines for home healthcare documentation.

Some home health agencies provide nurses with laptop or handheld computers to make records available in multiple locations. With the use of a modem, the nurse can add new client information to records at the agency without traveling to the office.

General Guidelines for Recording

Because the client's record is a legal document and may be used to provide evidence in court, many factors are considered in recording. Healthcare personnel must not only

PRACTICE GUIDELINES Home Healthcare Documentation

- Complete a comprehensive nursing assessment and develop a plan of care to meet Medicare and other third-party payer requirements. Some agencies use the certification and plan of treatment form as the client's official plan of care.
- Write a progress note at each client visit, noting any changes in the client's condition, nursing interventions performed (including education and instructional brochures and materials provided to the client and home caregiver), client responses to nursing care, and vital signs as indicated.
- Provide a monthly progress nursing summary to the attending primary care provider and to the reimburser to confirm the need to continue services.
- Keep a copy of the care plan in the client's home and update it as the client's condition changes.
- Report changes in the plan of care to the primary care provider and document that these were reported. Medicare and Medicaid will reimburse only for the skilled services provided that are reported to the primary care provider.
- Encourage the client or home caregiver to record data when appropriate.
- Write a discharge summary for the primary care provider to approve the discharge and to notify the reimbursers that services have been discontinued. Include all services provided, the client's health status at discharge, outcomes achieved, and recommendations for further care.

maintain the confidentiality of the client's record but also meet legal standards in the process of recording.

Date and Time

Document the date and time of each recording. This is essential not only for legal reasons but also for client safety. Record the time in the conventional manner (e.g., 9:00 a.m. or 3:15 p.m.) or according to the 24-hour clock (military clock), which avoids confusion about whether a time was a.m. or p.m. (Figure 14.9 ■).

Timing

Follow the agency's policy about the frequency of documenting, and adjust the frequency as a client's condition indicates; for example, a client whose blood pressure is changing requires more frequent documentation than a client whose blood pressure is constant. As a rule, documenting should be done as soon as possible after an assessment or intervention. No recording should be done *before* providing nursing care.

Legibility

All entries must be legible and easy to read to prevent interpretation errors. Hand printing or easily understood handwriting is usually permissible. Follow the agency's policies about handwritten recording.

Permanence

All entries on the client's record are made in dark ink so that the record is permanent and changes can be identified. Dark ink reproduces well on microfilm and in duplication processes. Follow the agency's policies about

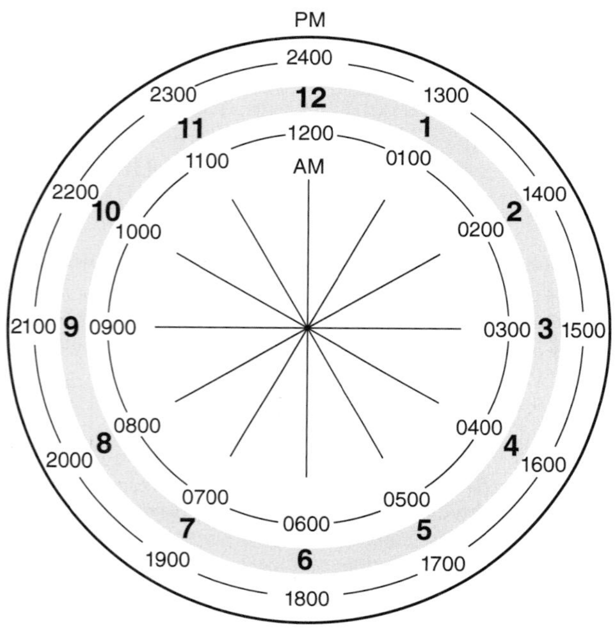

Figure 14.9 ■ The 24-hour clock.

the type of pen and ink used for recording. In regards to EHRs, changes are made in accordance with the software guidelines. It is important for the nurse to understand the policies and procedures of the healthcare institution regarding documentation.

Accepted Terminology

Abbreviations are used because they are short, convenient, and easy to use. People are often in a hurry and use abbreviations when texting or text paging. Abbreviations are convenient; however, they are often ambiguous. Ambiguity occurs when an abbreviation can stand for more than one term, leading to misinterpretation. For example, a client was being treated for a viral infection and died as a result of the use of the abbreviation HD for an order of "acyclovir unknown dose with HD." HD was to represent hemodialysis, and the dosage (unknown) needed to be adjusted due to the client's renal impairment. The order was misunderstood and the dosage of acyclovir was not adjusted in consideration of the client's renal impairment.

Therefore, it is important to use only commonly accepted abbreviations, symbols, and terms that are specified by the agency. Many abbreviations are standard and used universally; others are used only in certain geographic areas. Many healthcare facilities supply an approved list of abbreviations and symbols to prevent confusion. When in doubt about whether to use an abbreviation, write the term out in full until certain about the abbreviation. Table 14.4 lists some common abbreviations (except those used for medications, which are described in Chapter 35 ∞).

In 2004, The Joint Commission developed National Patient Safety Goals (NPSGs) to reduce communication errors. These goals are required to be implemented by all organizations accredited by the commission. As a result, the accredited organizations must develop a do-not-use list of abbreviations, acronyms, and symbols. This list must include those banned by The Joint Commission (Table 14.5).

Correct Spelling

Correct spelling is essential for accuracy in recording. If unsure how to spell a word, look it up in a dictionary or other resource book. Two decidedly different medications may have similar spellings, for example, Fosamax and Flomax.

Clinical Alert!

Incorrect spelling gives a negative impression to the reader and thereby decreases the nurse's credibility.

Signature

Each recording on the nursing notes is signed by the nurse making it. The signature includes the name and title, for example, "Susan J. Green, RN" or "SJ Green, RN." Some

TABLE 14.4 Commonly Used Abbreviations*

Abbreviation	Term	Abbreviation	Term
Abd	Abdomen	MEDS	Medications
ABO	The main blood group system	mL	Milliliter
ac	Before meals	mod	Moderate
ad lib	As desired	neg	Negative
ADL	Activities of daily living	∅	None
Adm	Admitted or admission	#	Number or pounds
am	Morning	NPO (NBM)	Nothing by mouth
amb	Ambulatory	NS (N/S)	Normal saline
amt	Amount	O_2	Oxygen
approx	Approximately	OD	Right eye or overdose
bid	Twice daily	OOB	Out of bed
BM (bm)	Bowel movement	OS	Left eye
BP	Blood pressure	$\bar{p}$	After
BRP	Bathroom privileges	pc	After meals
$\bar{c}$	With	PE (PX)	Physical examination
C	Celsius (centigrade)	per	By or through
CBC	Complete blood count	pm	Afternoon
c/o	Complains of	po	By mouth
DAT	Diet as tolerated	postop	Postoperatively
Dc	Discontinue	preop	Preoperatively
drsg	Dressing	prep	Preparation
Dx	Diagnosis	prn	When necessary
ECG (EKG)	Electrocardiogram	qid	Four times a day
F	Fahrenheit	(R)	Right
fld	Fluid	$\bar{s}$	Without
GI	Gastrointestinal	stat	At once, immediately
gtt	Drop	tid	Three times a day
h (hr)	Hour	TO	Telephone order
H_2O	Water	TPR	Temperature, pulse, respirations
I&O	Intake and output	VO	Verbal order
IV	Intravenous	VS	Vital signs
(L)	Left	WNL	Within normal limits
LMP	Last menstrual period	WT	Weight

*Institutions may elect to include some of these abbreviations on their "do-not-use" list. Check the agency's policy.

agencies have a signature sheet and after signing it, nurses can use their initials. With computerized charting, each nurse has his or her own code, which allows the documentation to be identified.

The following title abbreviations are often used, but nurses need to follow agency policy about how to sign their names:

RN	registered nurse
LVN	licensed vocational nurse
LPN	licensed practical nurse
NA	nursing assistant
NS	nursing student
PCA	patient care associate
SN	student nurse

Accuracy

The client's name and identifying information should be stamped or written on each page of the clinical record. Before making an entry, check that the chart is the correct one. Do not identify charts by room number only; check the client's name. Special care is needed when caring for clients with the same last name.

Notations on records must be accurate and correct. Accurate notations consist of facts or observations rather than opinions or interpretations. It is more accurate, for example, to write that the client "refused medication" (fact) than to write that the client "was uncooperative" (opinion); to write that a client "was crying" (observation) is preferable to noting that the client "was depressed" (interpretation). Similarly, when a client expresses worry

TABLE 14.5 Official "Do Not Use" List*

Do Not Use	Potential Problem	Use Instead
U, u (unit)	Mistaken for "0" (zero), the number "4" (four), or cc	Write "unit"
IU (for International Unit)	Mistaken for IV (intravenous) or the number 10 (ten)	Write "International Unit"
Q.D. QD, q.d., qd (daily) Q.O.D., QOD, q.o.d., qod (every other day)	Mistaken for each other Period after the Q mistaken for "I" and "O" mistaken for "I"	Write "daily" Write "every other day"
Trailing zero (X.0 mg)** Lack of leading zero (.X mg)	Decimal point is missed.	Write X mg Write 0.X mg
MS MSO_4 and $MGSO_4$	Can mean morphine sulfate or magnesium sulfate. Confused for one another	Write "morphine sulfate" Write "magnesium sulfate"

*Applies to all orders and all medication-related documentation that is handwritten (including free-text computer entry) or on preprinted forms.

**A "trailing zero" may be used only where required to demonstrate the level of precision of the value being reported, such as for laboratory results, imaging studies that report the size of lesions, or catheter/tube sizes. It may not be used in medication orders or other medication-related documentation.

about the diagnosis or problem, this should be quoted directly on the record: "Stated: 'I'm worried about my leg.'" When describing something, avoid general words, such as *large*, *good*, or *normal*, which can be interpreted differently. For example, chart specific data such as "2 cm × 3 cm bruise" rather than "large bruise."

When a recording mistake is made, draw a single line through it to identify it as erroneous with your initials or name above or near the line (depending on agency policy). Do not erase, blot out, or use correction fluid. The original entry must remain visible. When using computerized charting, the nurse needs to be aware of the agency's policy and process for correcting documentation mistakes. See Figure 14.10 ■ for an example.

Write on every line but never between lines. If a blank appears in a notation, draw a line through the blank space so that no additional information can be recorded at any other time or by any other personnel, and sign the notation.

Clinical Alert!

Avoid writing the word *error* when a recording mistake has been made. Some believe that the word *error* is a "red flag" for juries and can lead to the assumption that a clinical error has caused a client injury.

Sequence

Document events in the order in which they occur; for example, record assessments, then the nursing interventions, and then the client's responses. Update or delete problems as needed.

Appropriateness

Record only information that pertains to the client's health problems and care. Any other personal information that the client conveys is inappropriate for the record. Recording irrelevant information may be considered an invasion of the client's privacy or libelous. A client's disclosure that she was addicted to heroin 15 years ago, for example, would *not* be recorded on the client's medical record unless it had a direct bearing on the client's health problem.

Completeness

Not all data that a nurse obtains about a client can be recorded. However, the information that is recorded needs to be complete and helpful to the client and healthcare professionals.

Nursing notes need to reflect the nursing process. Record all assessments, dependent and independent nursing interventions, client problems, client comments and responses to interventions and tests, progress toward goals, and communication with other members of the health team.

Care that is *omitted* because of the client's condition or refusal of treatment must also be recorded. Document what was omitted, why it was omitted, and who was notified.

Date	Time	Progress Notes
9/12/2020	0800	~~Breath sounds diminished throughout all lung fields. C/O "shortness of breath".~~ N. Smith, RN.

Figure 14.10 ■ Correcting a charting error.

Clinical Alert!

Do not assume that the individual reading your charting will know that a common intervention (e.g., turning) has occurred because you believe it to be an "obvious" component of care.

Conciseness

Recordings need to be brief as well as complete to save time in communication. The client's name and the word *client* are omitted. For example, write "Perspiring profusely. Respirations shallow, 28/min." End each thought or sentence with a period.

Legal Prudence

Accurate, complete documentation should give legal protection to the nurse, the client's other caregivers, the healthcare facility, and the client. Admissible in court as a legal document, the clinical record provides proof of the quality of care given to a client. Documentation is usually viewed by juries and attorneys as the best evidence of what really happened to the client.

Clinical Alert!

Complete charting, for example, by using the steps of the nursing process as a framework, is the best defense against malpractice.

For the best legal protection, the nurse should not only adhere to professional standards of nursing care but also follow agency policy and procedures for intervention and documentation in all situations—especially high-risk situations. For example:

> 1100—c/o of feeling dizzy. Raised top two side rails and instructed to stay in bed and ring call bell if requiring assistance. 1130—found lying on floor beside the bed. Stated, "I climbed out of bed all by myself." When asked about pain, replied, "I feel fine but a little dizzy." Helped into bed. BP 100/60 P90 R24. Dr. RJ Naden notified. RS Woo RN

Reporting

The purpose of reporting is to communicate specific information to an individual or group of people. A report, whether oral or written, should be concise, including pertinent information but no extraneous detail. In addition to change-of-shift reports and telephone reports, reporting can also include the sharing of information or ideas with colleagues and other health professionals about some aspect of a client's care. Examples include the care plan conference and nursing rounds.

Change-of-Shift Reports

Various forms of the change-of-shift report have been used over the years. Most recently a standardized form of handoff communication has been implemented. An incomplete handoff communication is associated with sentinel events that will result in adverse healthcare outcomes or death. Healthcare institutions must clearly define the elements to be included in handoff communication, thus preventing these adverse health outcomes. Every hospital and healthcare system is required to implement a standardized approach to **handoff communication**, which is defined as a process in which information about client care is communicated. The standardized approach to handoff in the transition of care is imperative for the safety of the client. The handoff of a client to another healthcare provider occurs at many levels in the healthcare setting. For example, the admission of the client to the emergency department and then to intensive care or other hospital division requires a handoff from nurse to nurse, nurse to physician, physician to physician, and ultimately to other healthcare providers.

PRACTICE GUIDELINES Documentation

DO

- Chart a change in a client's condition *and* show that follow-up actions were taken.
- Read the nurse's notes prior to care to determine if there has been a change in the client's condition.
- Be timely. A late entry is better than no entry; however, the longer the period of time between actual care and charting, the greater the suspicion.
- Use objective, specific, and factual descriptions.
- Correct charting errors.
- Chart all teaching.
- Record the client's actual words by putting quotes around the words.
- Chart the client's response to interventions.
- Review your notes—are they clear and do they reflect what you want to say?

DON'T

- Leave a blank space for a colleague to chart later.
- Chart in advance of the event (e.g., procedure, medication).
- Use vague terms (e.g., "appears to be comfortable," "had a good night").
- Chart for someone else.
- Record "patient" or "client" because it is their chart.
- Alter a record even if requested by a superior or a primary care provider.
- Record assumptions or words reflecting bias (e.g., "complainer," "disagreeable").

Box 14.3 lists the elements of performance required for effective handoff communication.

BOX 14.3 Key Elements for Effective Handoff Communication

The communication should include the following:

- Up-to-date information
- Interactive communication allowing for questions between the giver and receiver of client information
- Method for verifying the information (e.g., repeat-back, read-back techniques)
- Minimal interruptions
- Opportunity for receiver of information to review relevant client data (e.g., previous care and treatment).

The handoff communication or **change-of-shift report** is given to all nurses on the next shift. Face-to-face communication allows the oncoming nurse the ability to ask questions and gain confidence to care for the client. The incoming and departing nurses establish priorities for the care of the client in the upcoming hours by reviewing checklists and the client's medical record. Content of the handoff, which captures intention, includes client problems and interventions to care for the client's problems. The nurse must focus on the needs of the client and not become distracted by irrelevant information (Box 14.4).

Change-of-shift reports may be written or given orally, either in a face-to-face exchange or by audiotape recording. The face-to-face report at the client's bedside permits the nurse to introduce the oncoming nurse to the client and family. The oncoming nurse has the ability to ask questions during the report and address concerns. This allows clients to be involved in their care. Face-to-face report may also take place in a designated room, at the nurses' station, or at the client's bedside. Written and tape-recorded reports are often briefer and less time consuming; however, verbal updates may be needed. A variety of handoff communication tools have been developed to facilitate consistency in communication. Examples include, but are not limited to, I PASS, I-SBAR, PSYCH, or I PUT PATIENTS FIRST (psychiatric nursing hand off communication) (The Joint Commission, 2017.). Each tool is unique and specific to the needs of the environment. Box 14.5 provides specifics for each mnemonic.

BOX 14.5 Sample Handoff Communication Tools

- I PASS the BATON: Introduction, Patient, Assessment, Situation, Safety Concerns, Background, Actions, Timing, Ownership, Next
- I-SBAR: Introduction, Situation, Background, Assessment, Recommendation
- PACE: Patient/Problem, Assessment/Actions, Continuing (treatments)/Changes, Evaluation
- Five-P's: Patient, Plan, Purpose, Problem, Precautions, Physician (assigned to coordinate)

From *Essentials of perioperative nursing* (6th ed.), by T. Goodman and C Spry, 2017. Burlington, MA: Jones and Bartlett.

Many hospitals use the SBAR tool along with a verbal report for handoffs for change-of-shift reports. The tools may vary among institutions regarding the information to include in the report; however, all provide a printed standardized form for the nurse to use during a handoff. The Institute for Healthcare Improvement (2017) states that "the SBAR allows for an easy and focused way to set expectations for what will be communicated and how between members of the team, which is essential for developing teamwork and fostering a culture of patient safety" (para. 1).

In recent years electronic handoff tools have been developed to improve communication, thus increasing client safety and improving nurse satisfaction. iCare is a

BOX 14.4 Focusing on Relevant Information During a Change-of-Shift Report

- Follow a particular order (e.g., follow room numbers in a hospital).
- Provide basic identifying information for each client (e.g., name, room number, bed designation). Report information in the same order every time.
- For new clients, provide the reason for admission or medical diagnosis (or diagnoses), surgery (date), diagnostic tests, and therapies in the past 24 hours.
- Include significant changes in the client's condition and present information in order (i.e., assessment, nursing diagnoses, interventions, outcomes, and evaluation). For example, "Mr. Ronald Oakes said he had an aching pain in his left calf at 1400 hours. Inspection revealed no other signs. Calf pain is related to altered blood circulation. Rest and elevation of his legs on a footstool for 30 minutes provided relief. Notified Dr. S.M. of the client's complaint of calf pain."
- Provide exact information, such as "Ms. Jessie Jones received morphine 6 mg IV at 1500 hours," not "Ms. Jessie Jones received some morphine during the evening."
- Report clients' need for special emotional support. For example, a client who has just learned that his biopsy results revealed malignancy and who is now scheduled for a laryngectomy needs time to discuss his feelings before preoperative teaching is begun.
- Include current nurse-prescribed and primary care provider–prescribed orders.
- Clearly state priorities of care and care that is due after the shift begins. For example, in a 7 A.M. report the nurse might say, "Mr. Li's vital signs are due at 0730, and his IV bag will need to be replaced by 0800." Give this information at the end of that client's report, because memory is best for the first and last information given.
- Be concise. Don't elaborate on background data or routine care (e.g., do not report "Vital signs at 0800 and 1150" when that is the unit standard). Do not report coming and going of visitors unless there is a problem or concern, or visitors are involved in teaching and care. Social support and visits are the norm.
- Incorporate a verification process (e.g., opportunity to ask and respond) to ensure that information is both received and understood.

company that provides an inpatient EHR for hospitals and health systems. The automated transitions continuity of care communication is an integrated communication system and document repository to allow all users a complete view of the client record within one screen. This system enhances the transitions of care (iCARE, 2019).

Box 14.6 provides a sample SBAR communication tool.

BOX 14.6 Sample SBAR Communication Tool

S = Situation
- State your name, unit, and client name.
- Briefly state the problem.

B = Background
- State client admission diagnosis and date of admission.
- State pertinent medical history.
- Provide brief summary of treatment to date.
- Code status (if appropriate).

A = Assessment
- Vital signs
- Pain scale
- Is there a change from prior assessments?

R = Recommendation
- State what you would like to see done *or* specify that the care provider needs to assess the client.
- Ask if healthcare provider wants to order any tests or medications.
- Ask healthcare provider if he or she wants to be notified for any reason.
- Ask, if no improvement, when you should call again.

Telephone Reports

Health professionals frequently report about a client by telephone. Nurses inform primary care providers about a change in a client's condition; a radiologist reports the results of an x-ray study; a nurse may report to a nurse on another unit about a transferred client.

The nurse receiving a telephone report should document the date and time, the name of the individual giving the information, and the subject of the information received, and sign the notation. For example:

> 6/6/20 1035 G Messina, laboratory technician, reported by telephone that Mrs. Sara Ames's hematocrit is 39%. B. Ireland RN

The individual receiving the information should *repeat it back* to the sender to ensure accuracy.

When giving a telephone report to a primary care provider, it is important that the nurse be concise and accurate. The SBAR communication tool is often used for telephone reports. Begin with name and relationship to the client (e.g., "This is Jana Gomez, RN; I'm calling about your client, Dorothy Mendes. I'm her nurse on the 7 p.m. to 7 a.m. shift").

Telephone reports usually include the client's name and medical diagnosis, changes in nursing assessment, vital signs related to baseline vital signs, significant laboratory data, and related nursing interventions. The nurse should have the client's chart ready to give the primary care provider any further information.

After reporting, the nurse should document the date, time, and content of the call. For example:

> 1200—Admitted from ED. c/o burning upper right quadrant abdominal pain. Rates pain at 6/10. BP 115/80, P100, R15.Morphine 5 mg given IM per order. 1300—BP 100/40, P115, R30. Pain unchanged. Color pale and diaphoretic. Reported by telephone to Dr. Burns at 1305. T.S. Jones RN

Telephone and Verbal Orders

Primary care providers often order a therapy (e.g., a medication) for a client by telephone or verbally (face-to-face). Most agencies have specific policies about telephone and verbal orders. Many agencies allow only registered nurses to take these orders.

While the primary care provider gives the order, *write* the complete order down on the physician's order form and *read it back* to the primary care provider to ensure accuracy. Question the primary care provider about any order that is ambiguous, unusual (e.g., an abnormally high dosage of a medication), or contraindicated by the client's condition. Have the primary care provider verbally acknowledge the read-back of the telephone or verbal order. Then indicate on the physician's order form that it is a telephone order (TO) or a verbal order (VO). See Box 14.7 for selected guidelines.

BOX 14.7 Guidelines for Telephone and Verbal Orders

1. Know the state nursing board's position on who can give and accept verbal and phone orders.
2. Know the agency's policy regarding phone orders (e.g., colleague listens on extension and cosigns order sheet).
3. Ask the prescriber to speak slowly and clearly.
4. Ask the prescriber to spell out the medication if you are not familiar with it.
5. Question the drug, dosage, or changes if they seem inappropriate for this client.
6. Write the order down or enter into a computer on the physician's order form.
7. Read the order back to the prescriber. Use words instead of abbreviations (i.e., "3 times a day" instead of "tid").
8. Have the prescriber verbally acknowledge the read-back (i.e., "Yes, that is correct").
9. Record date and time and indicate it was a TO or VO. Sign name and credentials.
10. When writing a dosage always put a number before a decimal (i.e., 0.3 mL) but never after a decimal (i.e., 6 mg).
11. Write out units (i.e., 15 units of insulin, not 15 u of insulin).
12. Transcribe the order.
13. Follow agency protocol about the prescriber's protocol for signing telephone orders (i.e., within 24 hours).
14. Never follow a voice-mail order. Call the prescriber for a client order. Write it down and read it back for confirmation.

Once the order is written on the physician's order form, the order must be countersigned by the primary care provider within a time period described by agency

EVIDENCE-BASED PRACTICE

Evidence-Based Practice

How Does an Electronic Checklist Improve the Clinician's Performance in Medical Emergencies?

Sevilla-Berrios et al. (2018) conducted a study that examined the use of a checklist during a high-fidelity simulation. The researchers developed an electronic tool, the Checklist for Early Recognition and Treatment of Acute Illness (CERTAIN). In the medical emergency simulation, the response team had a prompter who reviewed the checklist with the emergency response team. Eighteen clinicians completed the baseline and posteducation sessions. The implementation of CERTAIN prompting reduced the omission of critical tasks, and assessment tasks were completed in a timely manner with most participants feeling better about the performance of the tasks implemented in the medical emergency simulation.

Implications

The implementation of the CERTAIN checklist during the medical emergency simulation improved the clinicians' performance and satisfaction when engaged in medical emergencies during a high-fidelity simulation.

policy. Many acute care hospitals require that this be done within 24 hours.

Care Plan Conference

A care plan conference is a meeting of a group of nurses to discuss possible solutions to certain problems of a client, such as inability to cope with an event or lack of progress toward goal attainment. The care plan conference allows each nurse an opportunity to offer an opinion about possible solutions to the problem. Other health professionals may be invited to attend the conference to offer their expertise; for example, a social worker may discuss the family problems of a child with severe burns, or a dietitian may discuss the dietary problems of a client who has diabetes.

Care plan conferences are most effective when there is a climate of respect—that is, nonjudgmental acceptance of others even though their values, opinions, and beliefs may seem different. Nurses need to accept and respect each individual's contributions, listening with an open mind to what others are saying even when there is disagreement.

Nursing Rounds

Nursing rounds are procedures in which two or more nurses visit selected clients at each client's bedside to:

- Obtain information that will help plan nursing care.
- Provide clients the opportunity to discuss their care.
- Evaluate the nursing care the client has received.

During rounds, the nurse assigned to the client provides a brief summary of the client's nursing needs and the interventions being implemented. Nursing rounds offer advantages to both clients and nurses: Clients can participate in the discussions, and nurses can see the client and the equipment being used. To facilitate client participation in nursing rounds, nurses need to use terms that the client can understand. Medical terminology excludes the client from the discussion.

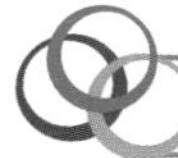

Critical Thinking Checkpoint

Mr. Anderson, an 80-year-old male, was admitted for back pain. He has a past medical history of hypertension. He told the admitting nurse that he has lost interest in many of his normal activities because of the constant pain.

You read the following documentation entry by a previous nurse:

8—Client is a complainer. I listened to him for 15 minutes with no success. BP 210/90 and 180/70. P 72, R 18.

12—Refused lunch.

2—Client fell out of bed.

1. What guidelines were *not* used in this documentation?
2. The nursing diagnosis for Mr. Anderson is acute pain. What would you expect to document?
3. Sort the following pieces of data for Mr. Anderson into a SOAP note:
   a. "I didn't sleep last night"
   b. Positioned on side with pillows behind back
   c. Continues to need narcotic medication to progress toward goal of pain relief
   d. States pain is 8 out of 10
   e. "I feel better" (after interventions)
   f. Last medicated 5 hours previously
   g. Heating pad applied to lower back
   h. BP 210/90, P 72, R 18
   i. Add to plan of care to offer analgesic around the clock q4h versus prn
   j. 6/6/20 #1 Pain
   k. "Sharp, stabbing pain in lower back that radiates to left leg"
   l. Medicated with ordered analgesic
4. Sort the pieces of data from question 3 into a DAR note.

Answers to Critical Thinking Checkpoint questions are available on the faculty resources site. Please consult with your instructor.

Chapter 14 Review

CHAPTER HIGHLIGHTS

- Client records are legal documents that provide evidence of a client's care.
- The nurse has a legal and ethical duty to maintain confidentiality of the client's record; this includes special measures to protect client information stored in computers.
- Client records are kept for a number of purposes, including communication, planning client care, auditing health agencies, research, education, reimbursement, legal documentation, and healthcare analysis.
- Examples of documentation systems include source oriented, problem oriented, PIE, focus charting, charting by exception, computerized documentation, and case management.
- In source-oriented clinical records, each healthcare professional group provides its own record. Recording is oriented around the source of the information.
- In problem-oriented clinical records, recording is organized around client problems.
- Computers make care planning and documentation relatively easy. The use of computer terminals at the bedside allows immediate documentation of nursing actions.
- The case management model emphasizes quality, cost-effective care delivered within an established length of stay.
- The Kardex is used to organize client data, making information quick to access for health professionals.
- Nursing progress notes provide information about the progress the client is making toward desired outcomes. The format for the progress note depends on the documentation system at the facility.
- Long-term documentation varies depending on the level of care provided and requirements set by Medicare and Medicaid.
- Home health agencies must standardize their documentation methods to meet requirements for Medicare and Medicaid and other third-party disbursements.
- Legal guidelines for the process of recording in a client record include documenting date and time, legible entries, using dark ink, using accepted terminology and spelling, accuracy, sequence, appropriateness, completeness, conciseness, and including an appropriate signature.
- The purpose of reporting is to communicate specific information for the goal of improving quality of care. Examples include change-of-shift reports, telephone reports, telephone orders, care plan conferences, and nursing rounds.
- A change-of-shift report and a telephone report are considered handoff communications. The Joint Commission requires hospitals to implement a standardized approach for handing off communications, including an opportunity to ask and respond to questions.

TEST YOUR KNOWLEDGE

1. Which action by a nurse ensures confidentiality of a client's computer record?
   1. The nurse logs on to the client's file and leaves the computer to answer the client's call light.
   2. The nurse shares her computer password.
   3. The nurse closes a client's computer file and logs off.
   4. The nurse leaves client computer worksheets at the computer workstation.

2. A client states: "I really don't want anyone who has not been cleared by me first to visit me." If utilizing the SOAP format, this statement would be documented under which category?
   1. Subjective data
   2. Objective data
   3. Assessment
   4. Planning

3. After completing client care and documenting it in the progress notes, the nursing student discovered he had written in the wrong chart. What is the correct action?
   1. Use white-out over the mistake.
   2. Take a wide permanent marker and blacken out all the documentation.
   3. Put an "X" through the entire page, identify it as an "error," initial, and move on to the correct chart.
   4. Draw a single line through the documentation, write "mistaken entry" next to the original entry, and initial it.

4. Which charting entry would be the most defensible in court?
   1. Client fell out of bed
   2. Client drunk on admission
   3. Large bruise on left thigh
   4. Notified Dr. Jones of BP of 90/40

5. The client's VS are WNL. He has BRP and he receives his pain pill prn. His nutrition is DAT. Interpret the commonly used abbreviations.
   1. WNL: ________________
   2. BRP: ________________
   3. prn: ________________
   4. DAT: ________________

6. During the first day a nurse is caring for a client who has been in the hospital for 2 days, the nurse thinks that the client's blood pressure seems high. What is the next step?
   1. Ask the client about past blood pressure ranges.
   2. Review the graphic record on the client's record.
   3. Examine the medication record for antihypertensive medications.
   4. Review the progress notes included in the client's record.

7. A student nurse observes the change-of-shift report. Which behavior(s) by the reporting nurse represents effective nursing practice? Select all that apply.
   1. Provides the medical diagnosis or reason for admission.
   2. States the time the client last received pain medication.
   3. Speaks loudly when giving report.
   4. States priorities of care that are due shortly after the report.
   5. Reports on number of visitors for each client.

8. Which charting entries are written correctly? Select all that apply.
1. MS 5 gr given IV for c/o abdominal pain
2. Lanoxin 0.25 mg given orally per Dr. Smith's stat order
3. KCl 15 mL given orally for K^+ level of 2.9
4. Regular insulin 10.0 u given SQ for capillary blood glucose of 180
5. Ambien 5 mg given orally at bedtime per request

9. A nurse responds to a client's call light. On entering the room, the nurse sees that the client is lying on the floor, with the bed linens around the legs. What is the most correctly written chart entry?
1. Client fell out of bed but did push the call button for assistance.
2. Client became tangled in the bed linens, then called for assistance after falling out of bed.
3. Recorder responded to client's call light, upon entering the room, found client on floor.
4. Client found on floor, appeared to have fallen out of bed as a result of getting tangled in bed linens.

10. Which charting rule(s) will keep the nurse legally safe? Select all that apply.
1. Use military time.
2. Document worries or concerns expressed by the client.
3. Perform most of the charting at the end of the shift.
4. Record only information that pertains to the client's health problems.

See Answers to Test Your Knowledge in Appendix A.

READINGS AND REFERENCES

Suggested Reading

Zou, X., & Zhang, Y. (2016). Rates of nursing errors in a medical unit following implementation of a standardized nursing handoff form. *Journal of Nursing Care Quality*, *31*(1), 61–67. doi:10.1097/NCQ0000000000000133

In this prospective intervention study, the researchers utilized a standard nursing handoff form. The use of this form resulted in a significant reduction in total nursing errors and handoff-related errors.

Related Research

Schaar, G. L., & Wilson, G. M. (2015). Evaluating senior baccalaureate nursing students' documentation accuracy through an interprofessional activity. *Nurse Educator*, *40*(1), 7–9. doi:10.1097/NNE.0000000000000079

References

American Nurses Association. (2015). *Code of ethics for nurses with interpretive statements*. Silver Spring, MD: Author.

Association of Operating Room Nurses. (2017). *Five ways to improve hand-off communication*. Retrieved from: https://www.aorn.org/about-aorn/aorn-newsroom/or-exec-newsletter/2017/2017-articles/hand-off-communication-5-areas-of-focus-for-safer-care

Goodman, T., & Spry, C. (2017). *Essentials of perioperative nursing* (6th ed.). Burlington, MA: Jones & Bartlett Learning.

Green, J. (2017). Nurses' online behavior: Lessons for the nursing profession. *Contemporary Nursing*, *53*(3), 355–367. https://doi.org/10.1080/10376178.2017.1381749

Guido, G. W. (2020). *Legal and ethical issues in nursing* (7th ed.). Upper Saddle River, NJ: Pearson.

Hebda, T. L., Hunter, K., & Czar, P. (2019). *Handbook of informatics for nurses and healthcare professionals* (5th ed.). Upper Saddle River, NJ: Pearson.

iCARE. (2019). *Automated transitions continuity of care communication*. Retrieved from https://www.icare.com/hospitals-health-systems-inpatient-ehr

Institute for Healthcare Improvement. (2017). *SBAR tool: Situation-background-assessment-recommendation.*

Retrieved from http://www.ihi.org/resources/Pages/Tools/sbartoolkit.aspx

The Joint Commission. (2017) *Inadequate hand-off communication.* Retrieved from https://www.jointcommission.org/assets/1/18/SEA_58_Hand_off_Comms_9_6_17_FINAL_(1).pdf

The Joint Commission. (2018). *Facts about the official "do not use" list*. Retrieved from https://www.jointcommission.org/facts_about_do_not_use_list

Lavin, M. A., Harper, E., & Barr, N. (2015). Health information technology, patient safety, and professional nursing care documentation in acute care settings. *Online Journal of Issues in Nursing*, *20*(2). doi:10.3912/OJIN.Vol20No02PPT03

Sevilla-Berrios, R., O'Horo, J. C., Schmickl, C. N., Erdogan, A., Chen, X., Garcia Arguello, L. Y., . . . Gajic, O. (2018). Prompting with electronic checklist improves clinical performance in medical emergencies: A high-fidelity simulation study. *International Journal of Emergency Nursing*, *11*(26), 1–6. doi:10.1186/s12245-018-0185-8

Selected Bibliography

Abrahamson, K., DeCrane, S., Mueller, S., Davila, H. W., & Arling, G. (2015). Implementation of a nursing home quality improvement project to reduce resident pain: A qualitative case study. *Journal of Nursing Care Quality*, *30*(3), 261–268. doi:10.1097/NCQ.0000000000000099

Cutugno, C., Hozak, M., Fitzsimmons, D., & Hulya, E. (2015). Documentation of preventive nursing measures in the elderly trauma patient: Potential financial impact and the health record. *Nursing Economics*, *33*(4), 219–226.

Sodhi, J. K., Sharma, K., & Kaur, J. (2015). Development of patient handover documentation tool for staff nurses using Modified Delphi Technique. *International Journal of Nursing Education*, *7*(2), 165–169. doi:10.5958/0974-9357.2015.00096.3

Tubaishat, A., Tawalbeh, L. I., AlAzzam, M., AlBashtawy, M., & Batiha, A. (2015). Electronic versus paper records: Documentation of pressure ulcer data. *British Journal of Nursing*, *24*(Suppl 6), S30–S37. doi:10.12968/bjon.2015.24.Sup6.S30

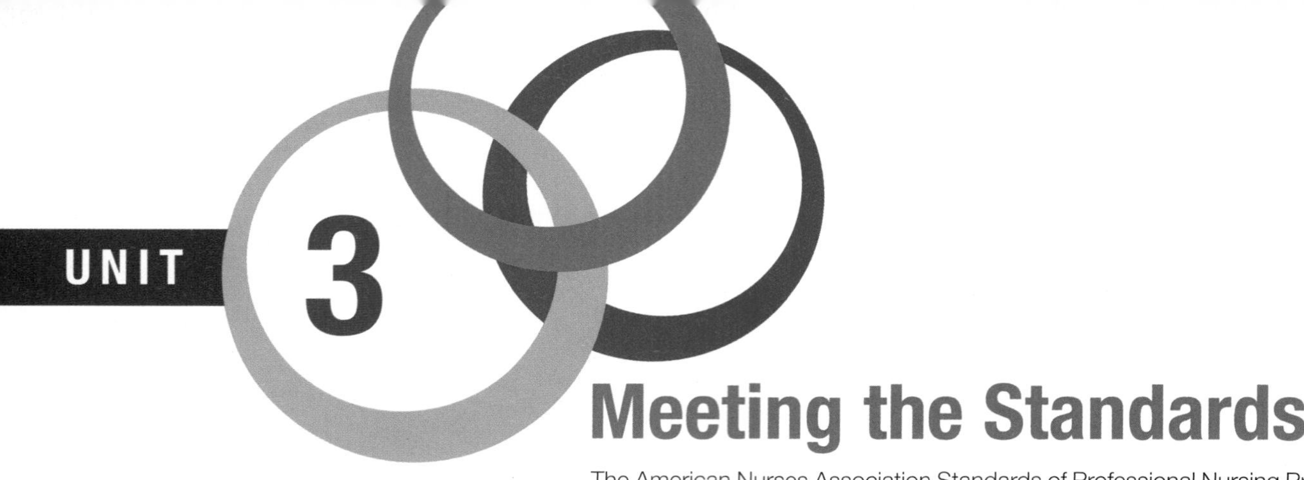

Meeting the Standards

The American Nurses Association Standards of Professional Nursing Practice consists of 6 Standards of Practice and 10 Standards of Professional Performance. The Standards of Practice are the components of the nursing process. The chapters in this unit of *Fundamentals* are Critical Thinking and Clinical Reasoning, Assessing, Diagnosing, Planning, Implementing and Evaluating, and Documenting and Reporting. They provide details about the steps of applying critical thinking to nursing practice and using a systematic approach in nursing care. Possibly no other structure is as universally applicable in organizing the nurse's thinking and guiding the nurse's actions.

CLIENT: Benjamin AGE: 35 CURRENT MEDICAL DIAGNOSIS: Torn Anterior Cruciate Ligament (ACL) Left Knee STATUS: Presurgical

Medical History: Benjamin is a well-nourished, well-developed man with no history of chronic illnesses. He has had the usual childhood diseases, and medical care has been limited to occasional sports-related trauma.

Personal and Social History: Benjamin is a married computer technician with three children ages 16, 6, and 2. He plays many sports including basketball, softball, and golf. He drives to work approximately 20 miles each way. His job is primarily desk work with some standing, walking, lifting, and bending. He has a baccalaureate degree in business.

Questions

American Nurses Association Standard of Practice #1 is Assessment: *The registered nurse collects comprehensive data pertinent to the patient's health and/or the situation.*

The nurse will care for many clients who do not have an acute illness. These clients may require health promotion, health maintenance, or wellness care. Others, like Benjamin, have health issues for which treatment is considered at least partially elective—meaning that it is not urgent and can probably be managed according to his preferred schedule. In assessing this client, the nurse focuses on gathering those data from all systems that provide information useful to the nurse and the healthcare team in planning his care and recovery.

1. As discussed in Chapter 10 ∞, the standard states that the nurse "collects pertinent data, including but not limited to demographics, social determinants of health, health disparities, and physical, functional, psychosocial, emotional, cognitive, sexual, cultural, age-related, environmental, spiritual/transpersonal, and economic assessments in a systematic ongoing process with compassion and respect for inherent dignity, worth, and unique attributes of every person" (ANA, 2015, p. 53). How would you determine the best way to conduct Benjamin's assessment that will provide the most useful findings?

American Nurses Association Standard of Practice #2 is Diagnosis: *The registered nurse analyzes the assessment data to determine the diagnoses or issues. Competencies for this step of the nursing process as delineated in the standard include that the nurse validates the nursing diagnosis with the client and that both actual and potential problems are identified.*

Another nurse has written the following nursing diagnosis on Benjamin's medical record: potential for altered parenting related to physical illness, manifested by pain and postoperative immobility.

2. Describe the thinking process you would use to seek validation that this diagnosis is appropriate. What data would you use? What questions would you ask, and of whom?

American Nurses Association Standard of Practice #4 is Planning: *The registered nurse develops a plan that prescribes strategies and alternatives to attain expected outcomes.*

Planning may involve the use of standardized care plans that have desired outcomes and interventions already written for common medical diagnoses. The standardized care plan for repair of a torn ACL emphasizes mobility, pain control, and wound care. Planning also includes competencies related to documenting the plan of care using standardized language and terminology understood by everyone using the documentation.

3. How might you individualize and add to the care plan to address the psychosocial needs identified for Benjamin that are related to his family and employment?
4. If you were caring for Benjamin on the evening of the day he had surgery, describe at least three different places in the medical record where you would document his care and what you might record there.

American Nurses Association. (2015). *Nursing: Scope and standards of practice* (3rd ed.). Silver Spring, MD: Author.

Answers to Meeting the Standards questions are available on the faculty resources site. Please consult with your instructor.

UNIT

4

Integral Aspects of Nursing

15 Caring

LEARNING OUTCOMES

After completing this chapter, you will be able to:

1. Discuss the meaning of caring.
2. Analyze the importance of different types of knowledge in nursing.
3. Describe the nursing theories of Roach, Watson, and Swanson.
4. Describe how nurses demonstrate caring in practice.
5. Evaluate the importance of self-care for the professional nurse.
6. Identify the value of reflective practice in nursing.

KEY TERMS

aesthetic knowing, *285*
caring, *284*
caring practice, *284*
empirical knowing, *285*
ethical knowing, *285*
personal knowing, *285*
reflection, *291*

Introduction

In this age of technologic competence and efficiency, the knowledge and skills embedded in caring practices are often overlooked. Technology does not negate caring. Rather, the thoughtful, knowledgeable use of caring theory by the nurse profoundly influences the nurse's expression of compassion in the technologic environment (Locsin, 2016). Caring is a dimension of human relating and is often referred to as the art of nursing. It is central to all helping professions, and it enables people to create meaning in their lives. **Caring** is sharing deep and genuine concern about the welfare of another individual.

Professionalization of Caring

Caring practice involves connection, mutual recognition, and involvement between nurse and client. Consider the following examples of caring, emerging from nursing situations:

- A client experiencing postoperative pain is given medication to control her symptoms, and then the nurse talks quietly and holds her hand for a few minutes as the pain lessens. The nurse's presence provides comfort for the client.
- After the student nurse washes the hair of an older woman who is immobilized and applies her makeup, she helps the woman into a wheelchair to greet her daughter and grandchildren. The woman is extremely grateful and her sense of dignity is enhanced by this personal care.

Just as clients benefit from caring practices, the nurses involved in these situations experience caring through knowing that they have made a difference in their clients' lives. The ability to give clients focused attention means leaving the egocentric self behind. Students of nursing can develop this ability by studying the meaning of caring in nursing.

Caring as "Helping the Other Grow"

Milton Mayeroff (1990), a noted philosopher, proposes that to care for others is to help them grow and actualize themselves. Caring is a process that develops over time, resulting in a deepening and transformation of the relationship. Recognizing the other as having potential and the need to grow, the caregiver does not impose direction, but allows the direction of the other individual's growth to help determine how to respond.

Mayeroff (1990) also proposes that the caring process has benefits for the one giving care. By helping the other individual grow, the caregiver moves toward self-actualization. By caring and being cared for, each individual finds his or her "place" in the world. By serving others through caring, individuals live the meaning of their own lives.

Types of Knowledge in Nursing

Nursing involves different types of knowledge that are integrated to guide nursing practice. Nurses require scientific competence (empirical knowledge), therapeutic use of self (personal knowing), moral or ethical awareness (ethical knowing), and creative action (aesthetic knowing). Carper (2012) identified these four types of knowledge from her observations of nurses' activities. An understanding of each type of knowledge is important for the student of nursing because only by integrating all ways

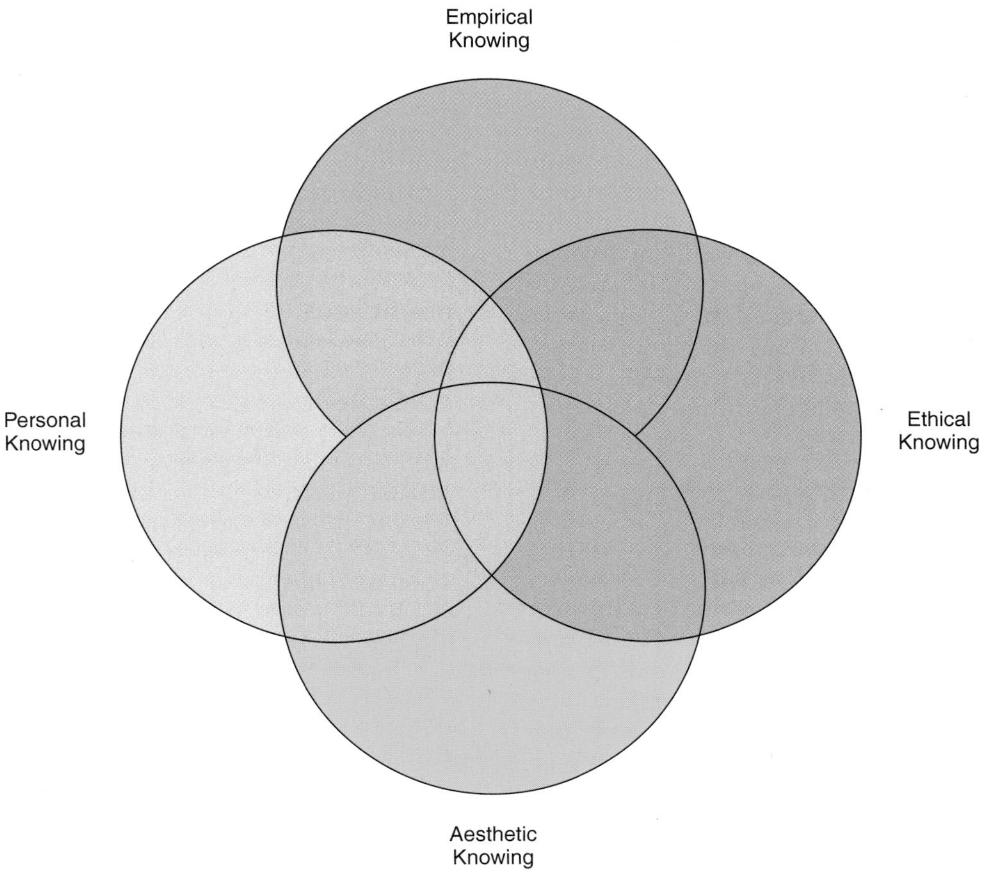

Figure 15.1 ■ The four ways of knowing.

of knowing can the nurse develop a professional practice. Figure 15.1 ■ illustrates the interconnection of these different types of knowledge.

Empirical Knowing: The Science of Nursing

Knowledge about the empirical world is systematically organized into laws and theories for the purpose of describing, explaining, and predicting phenomena of special concern to the discipline of nursing. **Empirical knowing** ranges from factual, observable phenomena (e.g., anatomy, physiology, chemistry) to theoretical analysis (e.g., developmental theory, adaptation theory).

Personal Knowing: The Therapeutic Use of Self

Personal knowledge is concerned with the knowing, encountering, and actualizing of the concrete, individual self. Because nursing is an interpersonal process, the nurse's view of self, as well as the client, is a critical factor in the therapeutic relationship. The nurse is aware of his or her own attitudes and behavior and views the client as a unique individual who is free to choose and create her or his own life. **Personal knowing** promotes wholeness and integrity in the personal encounter, achieves engagement rather than detachment, and denies the manipulative or impersonal approach.

Ethical Knowing: The Moral Component

Goals of nursing include the conservation of life, alleviation of suffering, and promotion of health. **Ethical knowing** focuses on "matters of obligation or what ought to be done" (Carper, 2012, p. 204) and goes beyond simply observing the nursing code of ethics. Nursing care involves a series of deliberate actions or choices that are subject to the judgment of right or wrong. Occasionally, the principles and norms that guide choices may be in conflict. The more sensitive and knowledgeable the nurse is to these issues, the more ethical the nurse will be.

Aesthetic Knowing: The Art of Nursing

Aesthetic knowing is the art of nursing and is expressed by the individual nurse through his or her creativity and style in meeting the needs of clients. The nurse uses aesthetic knowing to provide care that is both effective and satisfying. Empathy, compassion, holism, and sensitivity are important modes in the aesthetic pattern of knowing.

Developing Ways of Knowing

Different methods are used for developing each type of knowledge. For example, personal knowing is developed through critical reflection on one's own actions and feelings in practice. Empirical knowing is gained from studying scientific models and theories and from making objective observations. Ethical knowing involves confronting and resolving conflicting values and beliefs. Aesthetic knowing arises from a deep appreciation of the uniqueness of each individual and the meanings that individual ascribes to a given situation. The nurse who practices effectively can integrate all types of knowledge to understand situations more holistically.

Nursing Theories of Caring

The focus of any professional discipline is derived from its belief and value system, the nature of its service, and its area of knowledge development. Caring is at the heart of nursing's identity; indeed, the root of the word *nursing* means "nurturance" or "care." Nurse scholars have reviewed the literature, conducted research, and analyzed nurses' experiences, resulting in the development of theories and models of caring. These theories and models are grounded in humanism and the idea that caring is the basis for human science. Each theory develops different aspects of caring, describing how caring is unique in nursing. Several nursing theorists focus on caring. This chapter will address the theories of Roach, Watson, and Swanson.

Caring, the Human Mode of Being (Roach)

Roach (2013) focuses on caring as a philosophical concept and proposes that caring is the human mode of being. All individuals are caring and develop their caring abilities by being true to self, being real, and being who they truly are. Thus, caring is not unique to nursing.

Roach (2013) visualizes caring to be unique in nursing, however, because caring is the center of all attributes she uses to describe nursing. Roach defines these attributes as the six C's of caring: compassion, competence, confidence, conscience, commitment, and comportment. See Box 15.1 for definitions of each characteristic. The six C's are used as a broad framework, suggesting categories of behavior that describe professional caring. Each category reflects specific values and includes virtuous actions by which a nurse can demonstrate caring.

Theory of Human Care (Watson)

Watson's theory of human care views caring as the essence and the moral ideal of nursing. Human care is the basis for nursing's role in society; indeed, nursing's contribution to society lies in its moral commitment to human care.

BOX 15.1 The Six C's of Caring in Nursing

COMPASSION
Awareness of one's relationship to others, sharing their joys, sorrows, pain, and accomplishments. Participation in the experience of another.

COMPETENCE
Having the "knowledge, judgment, skills, energy, experience and motivation required to respond adequately to the demands of one's professional responsibilities" (Roach, 2013, p. 172).

CONFIDENCE
Comfort with self, client, and others that allows one to build trusting relationships.

CONSCIENCE
Morals, ethics, and an informed sense of right and wrong. Awareness of personal responsibility.

COMMITMENT
The deliberate choice to act in accordance with one's desires as well as obligations, resulting in investment of self in a task or cause.

COMPORTMENT
Appropriate bearing, demeanor, dress, and language that are in harmony with a caring presence. Presenting oneself as someone who respects others and demands respect.

From "Caring: The Human Mode of Being," by M. S. Roach, 2013. In M. Smith, M. Turkel, & Z. Wolf, *Caring in nursing classics: An essential resource* (pp. 165–179), New York, NY: Springer.

Nursing as human care goes beyond the realm of ethics (Willis & Leone-Sheehan, 2018).

Watson emphasizes nursing's commitment to care of the whole individual as well as a concern for the health of individuals and groups (Box 15.2). The nurse and client are coparticipants in the client's movement toward health and wholeness. This human connection is labeled *transpersonal human caring*, through which the nurse enters the experience of the client, and the client enters the nurse's experience. By identifying with each other, the nurse and client gain self-knowledge and, in doing so, keep alive their common humanity and avoid reducing the other to an object.

BOX 15.2 Social and Ethical Responsibilities of Nurses in Relation to Caring

- The nurse must care for the self in order to care for others.
- Nurses must remain committed to human care ideals.
- Cultivation of a higher/deeper self and a higher consciousness leads to caring.
- Human care can only be demonstrated through interpersonal relationships.
- Honoring the connectedness of all (unitary consciousness) leads to transpersonal caring-healing.
- Education and practice systems must be based on human values and concern for the welfare of others.

From "Watson's Philosophy and Theory of Transpersonal Caring," by D. G. Willis & D. M. Leone-Sheehan, 2018. In M. Alligood (Ed.), *Nursing theorists and their work* (9th ed., pp. 66–79), St. Louis, MO: Elsevier.

Watson emphasizes that the practice of nursing is both transpersonal and metaphysical. While the nurse maintains professional objectivity as a scientist, scholar, clinician, and moral agent, the nurse is also subjectively engaged in the interpersonal relationship with the client. Within the actual caring situation, each individual (nurse and client) seeks a sense of harmony within the mind, body, and soul, thereby actualizing the real self. This transpersonal contact has the potential to touch the higher, spiritual sense of self, or the soul. Such contact, which touches the soul, has the power to generate the self-healing process.

Theory of Caring (Swanson)

Swanson defines caring as "a nurturing way of relating to a valued 'other,' toward whom one feels a personal sense of commitment and responsibility" (Wojnar, 2018, p. 554). An assumption of her theory is that a client's well-being should be enhanced through the caring of a nurse who understands the common human responses to a specific health problem. Swanson's theory was developed through interactions with parents at the time of pregnancy, miscarriage, and birth. Further research will test the applicability of these caring dimensions to other client populations.

The theory focuses on caring processes as nursing interventions. The five caring processes are described as: (1) *Knowing*, which is defined as "striving to understand an event as it has meaning in the life of the other"; (2) *Being With*, which is "being emotionally present to the other"; (3) *Doing For*, or "doing for the other as he or she would do for the self if it were at all possible"; (4) *Enabling*, which is defined as "facilitating the other's passage through life transitions and unfamiliar events"; and (5) *Maintaining Belief*, or "sustaining faith in the other's capacity to get through an event or transition and face a future with meaning" (Wojnar, 2018, p. 554).

Caring Encounters

How does a nurse demonstrate caring? Given similar situations, why is one nurse judged to be "caring" while another is said to be "uncaring"? Nurse theorists and researchers have studied this question and identified caring attributes and behaviors. Consider, for example, Roach's six C's and Swanson's structure of caring. Because caring is contextual, a nursing approach used with a client in one situation may be ineffective in another. Caring responses are as varied as clients' needs, environmental resources, and nurses' imaginations. When clients perceive the encounter to be caring, their sense of dignity and self-worth is increased, and feelings of connectedness are expressed. Common caring patterns include knowing the client, nursing presence, empowering the client, compassion, and competence.

Knowing the Client

Caring attends to the totality of the client's experience. The nurse asks: Who is this individual? What is the client's history? Needs? Desires? Dreams? Spiritual beliefs? Who loves and cares for this client at home? Where is home and what resources are there? What does this client need today, from me, right now? Can this client tell me what is needed? Personal knowledge of the client is a key in the caring relationship between nurse and client. The nurse aims to know who the client is, in his or her *uniqueness*. The nurse gains this knowledge by observing and talking with the client and family while using effective listening and communication skills. By being actively engaged with the client, the nurse cannot remain detached.

Knowing the client and family ultimately involves the nurse and client in a caring transaction. By attending broadly to personal, ethical, aesthetic, and empirical knowledge, the nurse understands events as they have meaning in the life of the client. The nurse's *knowing the client* ultimately increases the possibilities for therapeutic interventions to be perceived as relevant.

Nursing Presence

Caring in nursing always takes place in a relationship. Mutuality within this relationship involves a partnership between the nurse and client. Watson describes the transpersonal caring relationship, in which the nurse enters the life space of another individual (Willis & Leone-Sheehan, 2018). Establishment of a caring relationship depends on a moral commitment by the nurse and the nurse's ability to assess and realize another individual's state of being. As nurses and student nurses increase their self-awareness and commitment to nursing, the ability to be authentically present to the other grows (see Box 15.2).

Healing presence requires an openness and consciousness of the self and the client. The nurse must create some space for awareness by being truly present and focused on the moment. The nurse is aware of his or her own thoughts and feelings, while also aware of an interconnectedness with the client. Authentic presence involves empathy and openness to positive or negative feelings, nonpossessive warmth, a relaxed posture, and facial expressions that are congruent with other communications (Willis & Leone-Sheehan, 2018).

Swanson's caring process of *being with* provides a description of nursing presence. By being emotionally present to the client and family, the nurse conveys that they and their experiences matter. Being present is a way of sharing in the meanings, feelings, and lived experiences of the client. Physical presence is combined with the promise of availability, especially during a time of need. This may be as simple as responding promptly to a call light on a hospital unit or as complex as sitting with a parent who has just lost a child in a neonatal intensive care unit.

Empowering the Client

Through knowing the client and engaging in a mutual relationship, the nurse can identify and build on client and family strengths. This empowering relationship includes mutual respect, trust, and confidence in the other's abilities and motives. Swanson's caring process of *enabling* includes coaching, informing, explaining, supporting, assisting, guiding, focusing, and validating. There are times when enabling involves substitutive care (doing for the client who is unable to do for him- or herself), but doing no more than is needed at the time. At other times, enabling involves providing an environment in which the client can function safely and effectively. The nurse should remain mindful of professional boundaries and responsibilities to avoid enabling pathologic or undesirable choices by the client. The goal is always to promote healthy growth and development.

Nurses both *advocate for* (verb) and are *advocates* (noun) for clients and families. Through advocacy, nurses are champions for their clients. They empower clients and families through activities that enhance well-being, understanding, and self-care.

Compassion

Universally, clients equate compassion with caring. The caring nurse is described as warm and empathetic, compassionate and concerned. Compassion involves participating in the client's experience, with sensitivity to the client's pain or discomfort, and a willingness to share in his or her experience. Compassion is given as part of the caring relationship, as the nurse shares the client's joys, sorrows, pain, and accomplishments. Compassion requires courage and openness, as the nurse experiences his or her own humanness and interconnectedness with the client (Boykin & Schoenhofer, 2013). Compassion is a gift from the heart, rather than an advanced skill or technique.

Attention to spiritual needs is part of compassionate care particularly in the face of death and bereavement. The nurse is aware that spiritual and religious beliefs are important coping mechanisms in dealing with issues of mortality (see Chapter 41 ∞). The nurse does not impose his or her own spiritual beliefs, but rather assists the client and family in drawing on their own beliefs as spiritual resources.

Comfort is often associated with compassionate care and many nursing interventions are carried out to provide comfort. For example, bathing, positioning, talking, touching, and listening are often performed to increase the client's comfort level. Just like pain or discomfort, comfort is subjective and is defined as "whatever the client says it is," based on the individual's perceptions. Despite this subjectivity, comfort care is often the basis for nursing in settings ranging from intensive care to hospice, and serves as a motivator for nursing interventions. Nurses are challenged to be creative and innovative, basing interventions on knowledge of the client's preferences, to provide comfort care.

Competence

The competent nurse employs the necessary knowledge, judgment, skills, and motivation to respond adequately to the client's needs. Just as competence without compassion is cold and inhumane, compassion without competence is meaningless and dangerous. The competent nurse, as described by Roach (2013), understands the client's condition, treatment, and associated care. The nurse provides the necessary care while guiding the client and family through the process. The nurse's abilities to assess, plan, implement, and evaluate a plan of care are focused on meeting the client and family needs. Practice of these skills requires a high level of cognitive, affective, technical, and administrative skills.

Maintaining Caring Practice

The concept of caring for self seems almost foreign to many nurses and student nurses because of the professional emphasis on meeting others' needs. Yet, as nurses take on multiple commitments to family, work, school, and community, they risk exhaustion, burnout, and stress. Obstacles to self-care may be professional, related to the demands of a work setting, or may be personal, such as poor health habits or unrealistic expectations of self. (See Chapter 42 ∞ for more information on stress and coping.) Despite these challenges, it is imperative that nurses attend to their own needs, because caring for self is central to caring for others.

The American Nurses Association (ANA, n.d.a) defines a healthy nurse as one who "takes care of his or her personal health, safety, and wellness and lives life to their fullest capacity" (para. 1). To emphasize the importance of being a healthy nurse, the ANA Enterprise launched the Healthy Nurse, Healthy Nation™ Grand Challenge in January 2017. This Grand Challenge is a national social movement that uses the concept that the health of America can be improved by improving the health of the nation's 4 million registered nurses (ANA, n.d.b). When nurses are healthy, they are more likely to counsel clients about healthy behaviors. The ANA website has an entire section dedicated to Healthy Nurse. Healthy Nurse resources focus on nurse fatigue, nutrition, work environment, tobacco-free nurses, safe client handling, and more (Schaeffer, 2016).

Caring for Self

Mayeroff (1990) describes caring for self as helping yourself grow and actualize your possibilities. Caring for self means taking the time to nurture yourself. This involves initiating and maintaining behaviors that promote healthy living and well-being. Although different activities may be helpful to different people, some examples of these activities include:

- A healthy lifestyle (e.g., nutrition, activity and exercise, recreation)
- Mind–body therapies (e.g., guided imagery, meditation, yoga).

Self-care focuses on care of the self in the deepest sense. Self-awareness and self-esteem are connected to self-care. Each individual is unique and possesses specific strengths and weaknesses. Self-care practices are intentionally created by the self and carefully maintained. This is a lifelong unfolding process, leading to wholeness that comes from and contributes to self-esteem. In its core values, the American Holistic Nurses Association (2013) states that the nurse has a responsibility to model healthcare behaviors. "Holistic nurses strive to achieve harmony and balance in their own lives and to assist others to do the same. They create healing environments for themselves by attending to their own well-being, letting go of self-destructive behaviors and attitudes, and practicing centering and stress reduction techniques" (p. 21).

A Healthy Lifestyle

Everyone needs to pay attention to nutrition and exercise, and to avoid unhealthy lifestyle practices. Key words for a healthy lifestyle are *balance* and *moderation*. These lifestyle practices are supplemented by regular physical examinations and health screenings.

NUTRITION

Healthy eating is important for everyone. A nutritionally balanced eating plan provides energy, builds endurance to carry out daily activities, and reduces the risk for certain health problems. Healthy eating means learning to make good choices in the foods eaten, preparing foods appropriately, and eating in moderation. It is important to select a variety of foods, to eat regular meals, and to eat the correct amount to maintain a healthy weight. Dietary guidelines and standards for a healthy diet are included in Chapter 46 ∞.

ACTIVITY AND EXERCISE

Exercise is recognized as a lifetime endeavor that is essential for healthy living (Figure 15.2 ■). The benefits of exercise have been linked to many physiologic and psychologic responses, from a reduced feeling of stress to an increased sense of well-being. Exercise strengthens the heart, lungs, and blood vessels to prevent heart disease; keeps the joints flexible; and helps many individuals deal with sad or unhappy feelings. For individuals who are overweight, exercise has the added benefit of burning calories, resulting in weight loss or maintenance. American Heart Association (2017) guidelines recommend that healthy adults, ages 18 to 65 years, engage in the following activities to promote and maintain health:

- At least 30 minutes of moderate-intensity aerobic activity at least 5 days per week for a total of 150 minutes

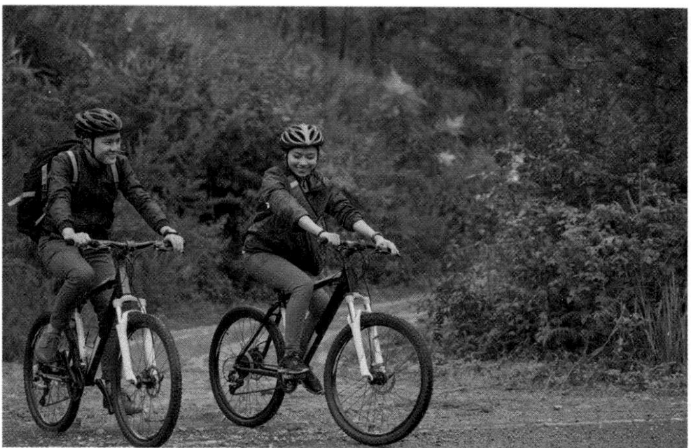

Figure 15.2 ■ Regular exercise is an effective self-care practice.
Dragon Images/Shutterstock.

  OR
- At least 25 minutes of vigorous aerobic activity at least 3 days per week for a total of 75 minutes; or a combination of the two
  AND
- Moderate to high intensity muscle-strengthening activity at least 2 or more days per week for additional health benefits.

Nurses participate in activities that call for knowledge to prevent self-injuries. Self-care practices are based on competence and compliance with use of assistive devices, such as the different types of hydraulic lifts and assistive transfer equipment. An in-depth discussion of these devices is included in Chapter 44 ∞.

RECREATION

Self-care also includes taking time to do the things that bring joy and stimulate creativity. Nurses need to reward themselves, to experience spontaneity, and even to take downtime or time to do nothing. Defending the right to this time may take courage and conviction in the face of others' demands. "Twelve Things You Would Love to Do" in Box 15.3 is intended to help an individual recapture a sense of joy, fun, and self-reward.

AVOIDING UNHEALTHY PATTERNS

Part of staying healthy is avoiding unhealthy life patterns. This means avoiding activities or thought patterns that contribute to negative health outcomes. Negative thinking can create a stress response with all its physiologic, mental, and emotional outcomes. It is not what happens, but how events are perceived, that determines an individual's reaction. Practices such as identifying negative feelings, refocusing on the positive, and using humor are helpful to avert the stress response by changing thought patterns. Using positive affirmations, as listed in Box 15.4, can lead to greater self-esteem and control self-doubt. It is also important to avoid destructive lifestyle choices such as smoking, abuse of alcohol or drugs, and misuse of medications.

BOX 15.3 Twelve Things You Would Love to Do

We often put off doing the simple things that bring us joy and happiness. Make a list of 12 things you would love to do after reviewing the list on the left. Post your list where you can see it. Resolve to carry out one activity by a specified time. Enjoy!

Some Ideas	Your List
1. Go out for ice cream.	1. ____________
2. Take a nap.	2. ____________
3. Dance a samba.	3. ____________
4. Make a campfire.	4. ____________
5. Roast marshmallows.	5. ____________
6. Ride a bike.	6. ____________
7. Shop for new shoes.	7. ____________
8. Watch a favorite movie.	8. ____________
9. Rearrange your furniture.	9. ____________
10. Take a ceramics class.	10. ____________
11. Read a mystery novel.	11. ____________
12. Walk in the park.	12. ____________

BOX 15.4 Positive Affirmations

Begin the day with positive statements about how you want to think and act:

I am an individual of worth and goodness.
I am happy to be alive.
I am in the right place at the right time.
I am prepared to do a good job today.
I am surrounded by people that I love, who love me.
I am doing what brings me joy.
This is an opportunity to grow.

Mind–Body Therapies

The interconnectedness of the mind and body is the basis for the complementary therapies. Imagery, meditation, storytelling, music therapy, and yoga are examples of complementary therapies that bring balance to thoughts and emotions. Practice of one or more mind–body therapies is an effective self-care strategy to help restore peace and balance. More in-depth information on different types of complementary therapies is included in Chapter 22 ∞.

GUIDED IMAGERY

Imagery is a mind–body intervention that uses the power of the imagination as a therapeutic tool. Imagery is used to promote relaxation, decrease anxiety, and enhance psychologic or spiritual insight. Through forming mental images of an object, event, or situation, the individual can reframe negative responses into positive images, enhancing healing and emotional well-being.

MEDITATION

Through quieting the mind and focusing it on the present, meditation assists the individual in releasing fears, worries, and doubts. The technique involves both relaxation and focused attention. Guidelines for mindful meditation include choosing a quiet space, sitting comfortably, achieving progressive relaxation through deep breathing, and focusing attention on breathing or a mental image.

STORYTELLING

As expressions of human consciousness, stories help individuals gain a greater understanding of life. Stories communicate life experience and are often shared with clients and others to inspire and comfort. The language of stories allows nurses to begin to understand the deeper meaning of clinical situations. Edwards (2016) proposes that when experience is converted to story, it becomes more organized and can be used to promote analysis, critique, and learning. Stories are also a mechanism to deal with stress and move toward wholeness.

MUSIC THERAPY

Using music as therapy includes listening, singing, rhythm, and body movement. Quiet, soothing music is often used to induce relaxation. Active rhythms can awaken feelings of power and control. Familiar music allows the listener to recall past events or feelings. Music can also serve as an effective distraction technique. Each individual's likes and dislikes are considered in order to achieve the desired emotional response.

YOGA

The practice of yoga unites the body, mind, and spirit (Figure 15.3 ■). Through daily practice of the various postures and breathing practices of yoga, an individual can achieve increased balance and flexibility, mental alertness, and calmness. The bending, stretching, and holding properties of the postures help to relax and tone the muscles and improve function of the internal organs. Breath control is designed to still the mind and enhance awareness. The American Heart Association (2016)

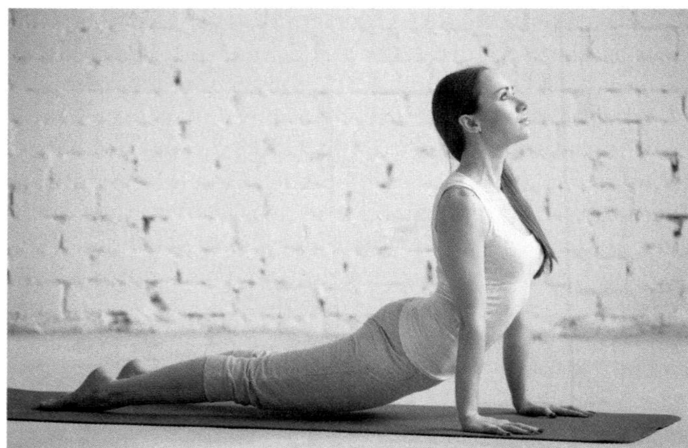

Figure 15.3 ■ Yoga is a mind–body self-care strategy to help restore peace and balance.
Russell Sadur/Getty Images.

promotes long-term, sustained yoga as part of an overall healthy lifestyle, helping to lower blood pressure, increase lung capacity, improve respiratory function and heart rate, and enhance circulation and muscle tone.

Reflection on Practice

Critical thinking, self-analysis, and reflection are required to learn from your experience. The student develops as a practitioner by thinking about how values and standards guide practical experience. **Reflection** is thinking from a critical point of view, analyzing why you acted in a certain way, and assessing the results of your actions. To develop as a caring practitioner, reflection on practice must be personal and meaningful.

Reflective practice is a method of self-examination that involves thinking back over what happened in a nursing situation. It also includes becoming aware of how you feel about yourself and recognizing how you think and act. Reflective practice requires discipline, action, openness, and trust. It is a form of self-evaluation.

Reflective journaling, as a tool for learning, is usually shared with a mentor or teacher, who works in partnership with the student. A framework, such as the one in Box 15.5, provides structure for the journaling process. Writing reflections in a journal provides a space for the student to look at and acknowledge the deeper self. Guidance from a mentor or teacher can help the student view a nursing situation from many different perspectives. It helps the student find meaning in the event, understand and learn through it, and emerge at a higher level of understanding.

Box 15.6 provides an example of a beginning nursing student's experience. See how it compares to your own. Think about the questions and use them for your own reflection.

BOX 15.5 A Framework for Reflective Journaling

Using a framework is especially helpful to the beginner who is establishing the process of reflection. The framework listed below includes suggestions from several different models on reflection, and can be further developed by the individual practitioner. The goal of any reflective framework is to encourage description and self-awareness as well as critical thinking and analysis.

1. *What happened?* Describe the situation or event, including who was involved and the associated events. Avoid making judgments; simply describe.
2. *What did you do and think?* Describe your role in the situation, what you did, and your thoughts at the time. Again, focus on description only.
3. *What did it mean?* Analyze the meaning of the event to those involved. How did the environment or context of the event influence the participants? Bring in ideas from outside of the experience to enlighten and compare.
4. *How do you evaluate the situation?* What was good or bad about the experience, in light of your own values and feelings?
5. *What did you learn?* What conclusions did you reach about the situation, in a general sense? More specifically, what did you learn about yourself and your own way of working?
6. *Now what?* What are you going to do differently (or the same) based on what you learned from this experience? Where can you get more information to improve your understanding and approach to practice?

BOX 15.6 Nursing Student Reflection Checkpoint

Debbie started nursing school in September, and by October felt overwhelmed by the amount of reading and studying that was required. Her anxiety level began to rise, but at the same time, she became more aware of her feelings and reactions to situations. In her nursing courses she was studying nursing as caring, and in the clinical setting she focused on applying these ideas in her practice with clients. She was surprised how genuinely her clients responded to a kind word of encouragement, the attention of personal care, and her concern for their well-being. Her clients' responses boosted her confidence and motivated her to learn more about their conditions and needs.

Each week Debbie analyzed and described the clinical situations encountered in practice in a reflective journal. Through reflecting on her clinical experiences and feedback from her clinical instructor, she identified her personal strengths and areas for growth. She began to think about how she could better organize her study schedule, plan time with her family, and provide the same level of caring for herself that she desired to give her clients.

1. Being in nursing school is often an overwhelming experience. How do you relate to Debbie's situation?
2. As you study caring in nursing, what ideas interest you most? How have you implemented these ideas in your own practice as a student nurse?
3. According to Carper's four ways of knowing, give examples of how you practiced each of these ways of knowing in your care of clients.
4. What value do you see in keeping a reflective journal? As you reflect on practice situations, have you written down your thoughts?
5. What changes can you make in your weekly schedule to be more efficient with studying and plan time for self-care?
6. What self-care activities would be most helpful to you right now? Changes in diet? Scheduled exercise or recreation? Meditation, yoga, or another mind–body therapy?
7. Do you have unhealthy patterns, such as smoking or negative thinking, that you need to work on? Develop an action plan to change these behaviors.

EVIDENCE-BASED PRACTICE

Evidence-Based Practice

Can Nursing Faculty Infuse Caring Science into Simulation Learning?

Because of the strong reliance on technologic learning in the high-fidelity simulation laboratory, research on caring in this setting is relatively new. While scenarios tend to disregard caring, simulation has the potential to influence student self-worth and, therefore, caring practice. Scenarios include interactions among staff and live actors, which provide opportunities for teaching, supporting, and witnessing human reactions. During the post-scenario debriefing, learners create the meaning of experience by reflecting on behaviors and feelings. The new knowledge gained through reflection is conceptualized and incorporated into the learner's knowledge base.

Reflecting on how caring science can be taught in the simulation laboratory, one nursing faculty developed a framework focusing on three concepts: *knowing*, *being*, and *doing* (Coffman, 2016). The concept of *knowing* addresses the question, "What does the nurse need to know in order to practice from a caring perspective?" Learners are encouraged to explore multiple ways of knowing, including empirical, personal, ethical, and aesthetic. This means understanding the client's disease process and treatment plan as well as client and family perceptions, fears, and understandings. The concept of *being* focuses on inner consciousness and addresses the question, "What state of mind and intentions should be held by the nurse, in order to care for others?" Important aspects of this component are maintaining a nonjudgmental, respectful attitude toward others in the nursing situation; being mindful of the other individual's reality; and accepting positive and negative feelings. The concept of *doing* addresses the question, "What activities are required to implement caring in this situation?" These include implementing a safe and effective treatment plan; providing information to the client, family, and staff; and using therapeutic communication that acknowledges the other's illness experience (Coffman, 2016).

Application of the know-be-do learning framework is exemplified in the scenario of a 5-year-old girl hospitalized with asthma:

- *Knowing*: Appreciate the stress involved in parenting a hospitalized child. Understand the effect of secondhand smoke on a child's asthma. Know community resources for smoking cessation.
- *Being*: Practice authentic presence to develop a transpersonal relationship with parent and child. Maintain a nonjudgmental, respectful attitude toward the parent. Accept both positive and negative feelings.
- *Doing*: Acknowledge the parent's and child's illness experiences. Provide information to explain nursing actions, asthma signs and symptoms, and how to access community resources.

The author conducted a phenomenologic study, working with nursing faculty as they taught baccalaureate students in the simulation laboratory. The aim of the study was to describe how faculty introduced caring science into simulation learning. The nine faculty members in the study reflected on how they taught caring concepts to students in the laboratory. Faculty found that the know-be-do learning framework provided a helpful structure for teaching students about caring practice. Also important was using scenarios that were well written and well executed by faculty, and undertaking simulation learning in a safe, nonjudgmental environment. The debriefing phase was seen to be particularly important for learning, because the process of human caring came to life as students focused in more depth on relationship issues and recognized their personal intentions (Coffman, 2016). The study concluded that using the know-be-do learning framework helped students discover more of the whole of the nursing situation, revealing more aspects of caring in the simulation scenario.

Implications

Development of caring by nursing students can be enhanced when students focus on the components of *knowing* (e.g., knowledge needed for safe practice), *being* (e.g., setting your intentions to do good for the client), and *doing* (e.g., therapeutic communication). Students' development of caring is facilitated when the debriefing reflection is structured around these components. Other factors that facilitate learning are well-developed scenarios carried out in a safe learning environment.

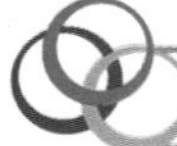

Critical Thinking Checkpoint

After morning report, the nurse, Megan, approaches Robbie James, a 10-year-old boy lying quietly in his hospital bed. She introduces herself and writes her name on the whiteboard in the room, so that when Robbie's mother arrives, she will know the name of Robbie's nurse. Megan's client assignment today consists of four acutely ill children of different ages. As Megan makes her initial rounds, she assesses the immediate needs of each child and begins to prioritize her nursing activities.

Megan has her own needs. She is tired from the night before when her own daughter was up late with coughing and fever. She is comfortable with her arrangements for child care, however, and is able to focus on her care of the clients on the pediatric unit.

When Megan returns with intravenous morphine, Robbie barely speaks, a pinched look of discomfort on his face. Using the FACES pain scale, Robbie has identified his pain as the "worst possible pain." This is his first day postop after surgery for a ruptured appendix, and he has a nasogastric (NG) tube in place, draining to wall suction. Megan administers the medication according to unit protocol and continues her assessment. She checks patency and placement of the NG tube and measures Robbie's vital signs.

Megan notes a "walking chart" on the wall beside Robbie's bed. The walking chart includes spaces to place a sticker each time Robbie walks in the hall. Robbie knows that after three stickers, he can choose a prize from the treasure box. Before Megan leaves the room, she suggests to Robbie, "When you feel better from this medicine, I'll help you walk, and we'll put another sticker on that chart!"

1. Describe which aspect of the nurse's approach relates to each of the following six C's of caring in nursing as outlined by Roach: compassion, competence, confidence, conscience, commitment, and comportment.
2. In analyzing this case study and reflecting on the four ways of knowing (personal, empirical, aesthetic, and ethical), describe how each type of knowing prepared the nurse, Megan, for her caring approach.

Answers to Critical Thinking Checkpoint questions are available on the faculty resources site. Please consult with your instructor.

Chapter 15 Review

CHAPTER HIGHLIGHTS

- Caring practice involves connection, mutual recognition, and involvement between nurse and client. Caring is central to nursing practice.
- To care for another is to help the individual grow and actualize him or herself. By helping the other individual grow, the caregiver moves toward self-actualization.
- Nursing involves different types of knowledge that are integrated to guide nursing practice. Empirical knowing includes scientific competence, personal knowing focuses on the self, ethical knowing requires moral or ethical awareness, and aesthetic knowing is the creative art of nursing.
- Various theorists have focused on caring as the essence of nursing. Each theory develops different aspects of caring, describing how caring is unique in nursing.
- Caring encounters are influenced by the diversity of human responses. Common caring patterns include knowing the client, nursing presence, empowering the client, compassion, and competence.
- Caring for self is central to caring for others. Nurse self-care includes a healthy lifestyle (e.g., nutrition, activity and exercise, recreation) and mind–body therapies (e.g., guided imagery, meditation, yoga).
- The student nurse matures as a practitioner by reflecting on practice. Through reflection, nurses can grow and participate more fully in caring-healing relationships.

TEST YOUR KNOWLEDGE

1. A nurse is emulating the characteristics of caring, as described by Mayeroff. Which of the following is an example of *knowing* in relationship to caring?
   1. Seeing that a client is withdrawn and sullen, and spending extra time when providing care or treatments
   2. Understanding the reason behind a client's elevated lab values
   3. Seeing the connection between the pathophysiology of the cardiac condition and treatment, and giving the rationale for certain medications when the client asks
   4. Getting an extra blanket when the client says he is cold

2. The nurse teaches a client with diabetes how to make decisions about insulin management after discharge. This teaching most clearly reflects which caring activity?
   1. Empowering the client
   2. Compassion
   3. Knowing the client
   4. Nursing presence

3. The six C's of caring framework was developed by which theorist?
   1. Swanson
   2. Mayeroff
   3. Roach
   4. Watson

4. A nursing student is writing a paper about his first day providing nursing care for a client. He described his initial anxiety and how he learned that when he focused on the client he remembered helpful information from his classes and labs. This description reflects which of the four ways of knowing?
   1. Personal
   2. Aesthetic
   3. Empirical
   4. Ethical

5. A nurse has been asked to be a member of a hospital's internal review board and evaluate research studies. Which of the following does this nurse most likely possess?
   1. Sound empirical knowledge
   2. Sound personal knowledge
   3. Sound aesthetic knowledge
   4. Sound ethical knowledge

6. A student nurse is following a preceptor on the assigned clinical shift. Which of the following behaviors of the nurse would the student interpret as caring?
   1. Making sure that all medications and treatments are provided on time
   2. Using aseptic technique when performing a dressing change
   3. Advising the physician that the client wants to speak to him or her prior to a procedure
   4. Explaining an invasive procedure to the client, then asking if it is all right to begin the procedure

7. Three nursing students have formed a study group. They are discussing activities they can do after a study session to help decrease stress. Which activities focus on the concept of caring for self? Choose all that apply.
   1. Take a walk and window shop.
   2. Meet at a restaurant or bar for a glass of wine.
   3. Go to a new movie they all want to see.
   4. Eat a meal of health foods.
   5. Gossip about their teachers.

8. The nursing student reviews the pathophysiology of myocardial infarction in preparation for the next day's clinical experience. This activity is an example of which type of knowledge development?
   1. Empirical knowing
   2. Aesthetic knowing
   3. Personal knowing
   4. Ethical knowing

9. A nurse sitting quietly in a chair, breathing deeply, and focusing on the mental image of a crystal is using which mind–body therapy?
1. Storytelling
2. Yoga
3. Music therapy
4. Meditation

10. A 40-year-old client who comes to the clinic for a routine physical exam asks the nurse how much exercise is recommended for a healthy lifestyle. Which answer is most appropriate?
1. Moderate activity for 10 minutes daily
2. Moderate activity for 20 minutes two to three times a week
3. Vigorous activity for 25 minutes three days a week
4. Vigorous activity for 30 minutes daily

See Answers to Test Your Knowledge in Appendix A.

READINGS AND REFERENCES

Suggested Readings

Alligood, M. A. (2018). *Nursing theorists and their work* (9th ed.). St. Louis, MO: Elsevier.
This book summarizes the major nursing theories, including credentials of the theorist, components of each theory, and a critique of clarity and simplicity of each work. Use of each theory in practice, research, administration, and education is discussed, with references for additional information.

Costello, M. (2018). Watson's caritas processes® as a framework for spiritual end of life care for oncology patients. *International Journal of Caring Sciences*, *11*(2), 639–644.
Spirituality is an important aspect of nursing care for individuals at the end of life. The author describes how Watson's theory of caring science can provide a framework for the development of caring and healing practices to facilitate spiritual care.

Nguyen, J. (2016). New grad connection: Healthy nurse healthy nation. *Arizona Nurse*, *69*(3), 8.
The author describes how, as a new graduate RN, she wasn't prepared for the mental and physical stress of the job. She reviews how she stayed healthy when the job focused on keeping others healthy. Her main points are: find a support system, find an outlet for stress, make work fun, take a deep breath, and stay active.

Related Research

Adimando, A. (2018). Preventing and alleviating compassion fatigue through self-care: An educational workshop for nurses. *Journal of Holistic Nursing*, *36*(4), 304–317. doi:10.1177/0898010117721581

Nurse-Clarke, N., DiCicco-Bloom, B., & Limbo, R. (2019). Application of caring theory to nursing care of women experiencing stillbirth. *MCN The American Journal of Maternal/Child Nursing*, *44*(1), 27–32. doi:10.1097/NMC.0000000000000494

Perkins, J. B., & Aquino-Russell, C. (2017). Graduate nurses experience the sacred during transcendental meditation. *International Journal for Human Caring*, *21*(4), 163–171. doi:10.20467/HumanCaring-D-17-00034

Sitzman, K. (2017). Evolution of Watson's human caring science in the digital age. *International Journal for Human Caring*, *21*(1), 46–52. doi:10.20467/1091-5710-21.1.46

References

American Heart Association. (2016). *Exercise mind and body with yoga and mindful movement.* Retrieved from https://www.heart.org/en/healthy-living/healthy-lifestyle/mental-health-and-wellbeing/exercise-mind-and-body-with-yoga-and-mindful-movement

American Heart Association. (2017). *American Heart Association recommendations for physical activity in adults.* Retrieved from https://www.heart.org/HEARTORG/GettingHealthy/PhysicalActivity/StartWalking/American-Heart-Association-Recommendations-for-Physical-Activity-in-Adults_UCM_307976_Article.jsp#.WBZZVaLzM8A

American Holistic Nurses Association & American Nurses Association. (2013). *Holistic nursing: Scope and standards of practice* (2nd ed.). Silver Spring, MD: Nursebooks.org.

American Nurses Association. (n.d.a). *Healthy nurse.* Retrieved from http://www.nursingworld.org/healthynurse

American Nurses Association. (n.d.b). *What is the Healthy Nurse Healthy Nation Grand Challenge?* Retrieved from http://www.healthynursehealthynation.org

Boykin, A., & Schoenhofer, S. (2013). Caring in nursing: Analysis of extant theory. In M. Smith, M. Turkel, & Z. Wolf (Eds.), *Caring in nursing classics: An essential resource* (pp. 33–57). New York, NY: Springer.

Carper, B. (2012). Fundamental patterns of knowing in nursing. In P. Reed & N. Shearer (Eds.), *Perspectives on nursing theory* (6th ed., pp. 377–384). Philadelphia, PA: Wolters Kluwer.

Coffman, S. (2016). Faculty experiences teaching caring in the simulation lab. *International Journal for Human Caring*, *20*, 197–201. doi:10.20467/1091-5710-20.4.197

Edwards, S. L. (2016). Narrative analysis: How students learn from stories of practice. *Nurse Researcher*, *23*(3), 18. doi:10.7748/nr.23.3.18.s5

Locsin, R. C. (2016). Technological competency as caring in nursing: Co-creating moments in nursing occurring within the universal technological domain. *Journal of Theory Construction & Testing*, *10*(1), 5–11.

Mayeroff, M. (1990). *On caring*. New York, NY: HarperCollins.

Roach, M. S. (2013). Caring: The human mode of being. In M. Smith, M. Turkel, & Z. Wolf (Eds.), *Caring in nursing classics: An essential resource* (pp. 165–179). New York, NY: Springer.

Schaeffer, R. (2016). Healthy Nurse, Healthy Nation™ Grand Challenge: Arizona nurses chosen as betasite. *Arizona Nurse*, *69*(3), 3.

Willis, D. G., & Leone-Sheehan, D. M. (2018). Watson's philosophy and theory of transpersonal caring. In M. Alligood (Ed.), *Nursing theorists and their work* (9th ed., pp. 66–79). St. Louis, MO: Elsevier.

Wojnar, D. (2018). Kristen M. Swanson: Theory of caring. In M. Alligood (Ed.), *Nursing theorists and their work* (9th ed., pp. 553–563). St. Louis, MO: Elsevier.

Selected Bibliography

American Nurses Association. (2017). *Executive summary: American Nurses Association health risk appraisal.* Retrieved from https://www.nursingworld.org/~4aeeeb/globalassets/practiceandpolicy/work-environment/health--safety/ana-healthriskappraisalsummary_2013-2016.pdf

Cettina, L. A. (2018). Meditation, not medication, to relieve anxiety. *Nursing*, *48*(9), 44–47. doi:10.1097/01.NURSE.0000541390.29234.0b

Dean, P. J. (2016). Nursing considerations for an emerging and enlarging symbiosis between technology and integrative human health: Need for a systematized base for caring science. *International Journal for Human Caring*, *20*(4), 171–175. doi:10.20467/1091-5710-20.4.171

Fuller, W. (2018). Technology and bureaucracy: Are these CARING words? *Florida Nurse*, *66*(4), 2.

Henson, S. J. (2017). When compassion is lost. *MEDSURG Nursing*, *26*(2), 139–142.

Savel, R. H., & Munro, C. L. (2017). Quiet the mind: Mindfulness, meditation, and the search for inner peace. *American Journal of Critical Care*, *26*(6), 433–436. doi:10.4037/ajcc2017914

Watson, J. (2018). *Unitary caring science: The philosophy and praxis of nursing*. Louisville, CO: University Press of Colorado.

Woodley, L. K. (2018). The reciprocity of touch. *Nursing*, *48*(7), 54–55. doi:10.1097/01.NURSE.0000534091.41368.08

Communicating 16

LEARNING OUTCOMES

After completing this chapter, you will be able to:

1. Describe the components of the communication process.
2. Discuss the various aspects that nurses need to consider when using the different forms of communication.
3. Describe factors influencing the communication process.
4. Compare therapeutic communication techniques that facilitate communication and focus on client concerns.
5. Recognize barriers to communication.
6. Describe the four phases of the helping relationship.
7. Discuss how nurses use communication skills in each phase of the nursing process.
8. State why effective communication is imperative among health professionals.
9. Describe the following disruptive behaviors and how they affect the healthcare environment and client safety: incivility, bullying, and workplace violence.
10. Discuss the differences between nurse and physician communication and how to address these differences.
11. Differentiate the major characteristics of assertive and nonassertive communication.

KEY TERMS

attentive listening, *304*
boundaries, *304*
bullying, *314*
communication, *295*
congruent communication, *302*
decode, *297*
elderspeak, *304*
electronic communication, *296*
email, *300*
emotional intelligence (EI), *316*
empathy, *309*
encoding, *296*
feedback, *297*
helping relationships, *308*
incivility, *314*
nonverbal communication, *297*
personal space, *301*
process recording, *313*
proxemics, *301*
territoriality, *302*
therapeutic communication, *304*
verbal communication, *297*

Introduction

Communication is a critical skill for nursing. It is the process by which humans meet their survival needs, build relationships, and experience emotions. In nursing, communication is a dynamic process used to gather assessment data, to teach and persuade, and to express caring and comfort. It is an integral part of the helping relationship.

Communicating

The term *communication* has various meanings, depending on the context in which it is used. To some, communication is the interchange of information between two or more people; in other words, the exchange of ideas or thoughts. This kind of communication uses methods such as talking and listening or writing and reading. However, painting, dancing, and storytelling are also methods of communication. In addition, thoughts are expressed to others not only by spoken or written words but also by gestures or body actions.

Communication may have a more personal meaning than the interchange of ideas or thoughts. It can be a transmission of feelings or a more personal and social interaction between individuals. Frequently, one member of a couple comments that the other is not communicating. Some teenagers complain about a generation gap—being unable to communicate with understanding or feeling to a parent or authority figure. Sometimes a client may say that a nurse is efficient but lacking in something called *bedside manner*. In this text, **communication** is any means of exchanging information or feelings between two or more individuals. It is a basic component of human relationships, including nursing.

The intent of any communication is to obtain a response. Thus, communication is a process. It has two main purposes: to influence others and to gain information. Communication can be described as helpful or unhelpful. The former encourages a sharing of information, thoughts, or feelings between two or more individuals. The latter hinders or blocks the transfer of information and feelings.

Nurses who communicate effectively are better able to collect assessment data, initiate interventions, evaluate outcomes of interventions, initiate change that promotes health, and prevent the safety and legal problems associated with nursing practice. The communication process is built on a trusting relationship with a client and the client's support people. Effective communication is essential for the establishment of a nurse–client relationship.

Communication can occur on an intrapersonal level within a single individual as well as on interpersonal and group levels. Intrapersonal communication is the communication that you have with yourself; another name is *self-talk*. Both the sender and the receiver of a message usually engage in self-talk. It involves thinking about the message before it is sent, while it is being sent, and after it is sent, and it occurs constantly. Consequently, intrapersonal communication can interfere with an individual's ability to hear a message as the sender intended (Figure 16.1 ■).

The Communication Process

Face-to-face communication involves a sender, a message, a receiver, and a response, or feedback (Figure 16.2 ■). In its simplest form, communication is a two-way process involving the sending and the receiving of a message. Because the intent of communication is to elicit a response, the process is ongoing; the receiver of the message then becomes the sender of a response, and the original sender then becomes the receiver.

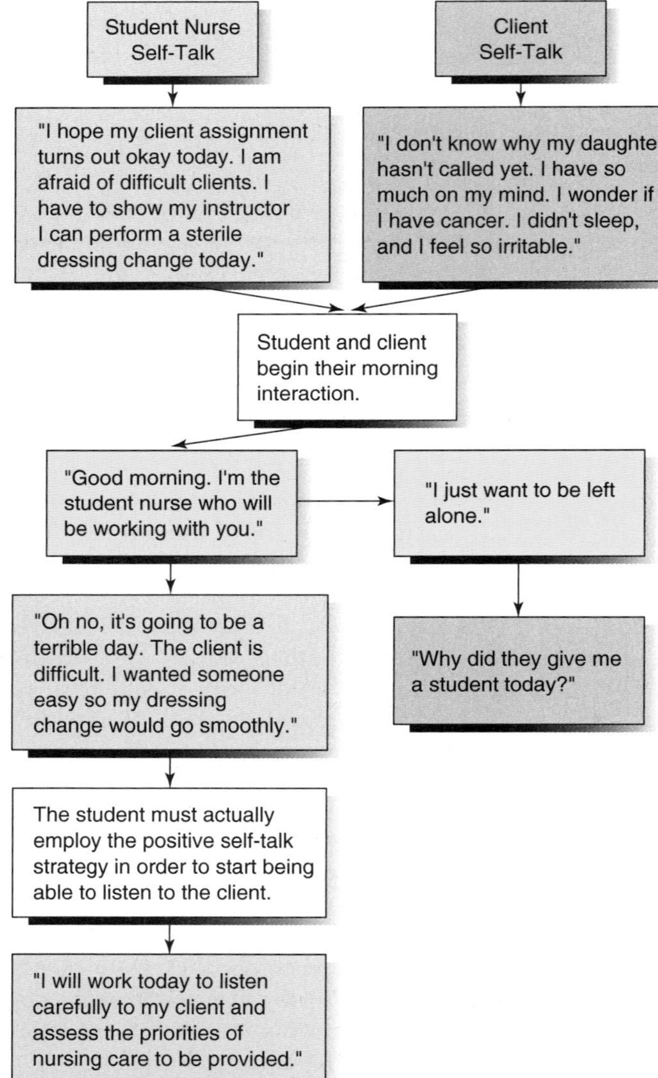

Figure 16.1 ■ Student nurse self-talk.

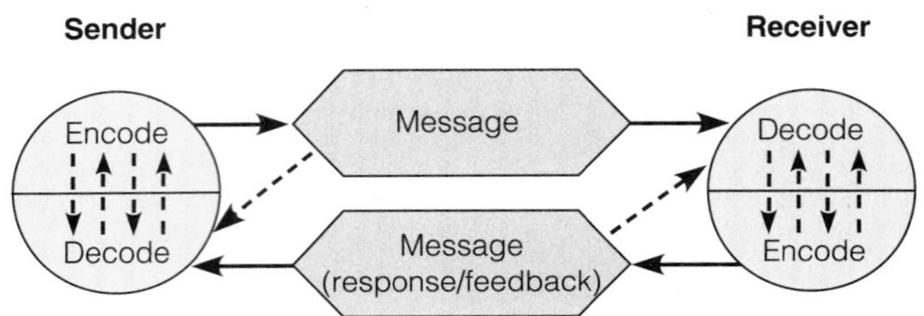

Figure 16.2 ■ The communication process. The dashed arrows indicate intrapersonal communication (self-talk). The solid lines indicate interpersonal communication.

Sender

The *sender*, an individual or group wishing to communicate a message to another, can be considered the *source-encoder*. This term suggests that the individual or group sending the message must have an idea or reason for communicating (source) and must put the idea or feeling into a form that can be transmitted. **Encoding** involves the selection of specific signs or symbols (codes) to transmit the message, such as which language and words to use, how to arrange the words, and what tone of voice and gestures to use. For example, if the receiver speaks English, the sender usually selects English words. If the message is "Mr. Johnson, you have to wait another hour for your pain medication," the tone of voice selected and a shake of the head can reinforce it. The nurse must not only deal with dialects and foreign languages but also cope with two language levels—the layperson's and the health professional's.

Message

The second component of the communication process is the *message* itself—what is actually said or written, the body language that accompanies the words, and how the message is transmitted. The method used to convey the message can target any of the receiver's senses. It is important for the method to be appropriate for the message, and it should help make the intent of the message clearer. For example, talking face to face with an individual may be more effective in some instances than telephoning, emailing, or texting a message. Written communication is often appropriate for long explanations or for a communication that needs to be preserved.

Another form of communication has evolved with technology—**electronic communication**. Common forms of electronic communication are email and texting, in which an individual can send a message, by computer or smartphone, to another individual or group of people. The use of email and texting has become prevalent as a primary form of *personal* communication. It is important to know the rules of etiquette for each. For example, emails should be short and to the point, and punctuation matters. Acronyms should be used sparingly, and do not write in all caps because it implies you are shouting. Texting is even more concise, and if the information is complex, consider using email or telephone or speaking with the individual in person. Communicating by email and text does not provide the sender relevant information, such as if the receiver is confused, upset, or needs clarification. Therefore, it is important to reread what you email or text before pressing the send button. Nurses need to know when it is and when it is not appropriate to use email for communicating with clients, which is discussed later in the chapter.

The nonverbal channel of touch is often highly effective (Figure 16.3 ■). Nurses use touch in two key circumstances. For example, touch is used frequently when completing a physical task while providing nursing care of a client (e.g., taking blood pressure, administering medications, changing a dressing). The other circumstance is driven by an emotional response to a client's distress (e.g., holding a hand, stroking a shoulder, providing a comforting embrace).

Receiver

The *receiver*, the third component of the communication process, is the listener, who must listen, observe, and attend. This individual is the *decoder*, who must perceive what the sender intended (interpretation). Perception uses all the senses to receive verbal and nonverbal messages. To **decode** means to translate the message sent via the receiver's knowledge and experiences to sort out the meaning of the message. Whether the message is decoded accurately by the receiver, according to the sender's intent, depends largely on their similarities in knowledge and experience and sociocultural background. If the meaning of the decoded message matches the intent of the sender, then the communication has been effective. Ineffective communication occurs when the receiver misinterprets the sent message. For example, Mr. Johnson may perceive the message accurately—"No pain medication for another hour." However, if experience has taught him that he can receive the pain medication early if a certain nurse is on duty, he will interpret the intent of the message differently.

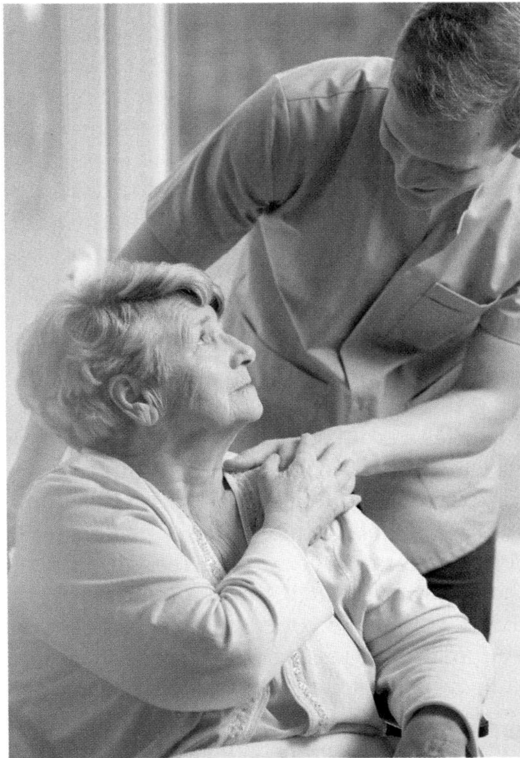

Figure 16.3 ■ Appropriate forms of touch can communicate caring.
Katarzyna Bialasiewicz/123RF.

Response

The fourth component of the communication process, the *response*, is the message that the receiver returns to the sender. It is also called **feedback**. Feedback can be either verbal, nonverbal, or both. Nonverbal examples are a nod of the head or a yawn. Either way, feedback allows the sender to correct or reword a message. In the case of Mr. Johnson, the receiver may appear irritated or say, "Well, the nurse on the other shift gives me my pain medication early if I need it." The sender then knows the message was interpreted accurately. However, now the original sender becomes the receiver, who is required to decode and respond.

Modes of Communication

Communication is generally carried out in two different modes: verbal and nonverbal. **Verbal communication** uses the spoken or written word; **nonverbal communication** uses other forms, such as gestures, facial expressions, and touch. Although both kinds of communication occur concurrently, most communication is nonverbal. Learning about nonverbal communication is important for nurses in developing effective communication patterns and relationships with clients.

Verbal Communication

Verbal communication is largely conscious because people choose the words they use. The words used vary among individuals according to culture, socioeconomic background, age, and education. As a result, countless possibilities exist for the way ideas are exchanged. An abundance of words can be used to form messages. In addition, a wide variety of feelings can be transmitted when people talk.

Nurses need to consider the following when choosing words to say or write: pace and intonation, simplicity, clarity and brevity, timing and relevance, adaptability, credibility, and humor.

PACE AND INTONATION

The manner of speech, as in the rate or rhythm and tone, will modify the feeling and impact of a message. The tone of words can express enthusiasm, sadness, anger, or amusement. The rate of speech may indicate interest, anxiety, boredom, or fear. For example, speaking slowly and softly to an excited client may help calm the client.

SIMPLICITY

Simplicity includes the use of commonly understood words, brevity, and completeness. The use of complex technical terms becomes natural to nurses. However, clients often misunderstand these terms. Words such as *vasoconstriction* or *cholecystectomy* are meaningful to the nurse and easy to use but not advised when communicating with clients. Nurses need to select appropriate, understandable, and simple terms based on the client's age, knowledge, culture, and education. For example, instead of saying to a client, "I will be catheterizing you for a urine analysis," it may be more appropriate and understandable to say, "I need to get a sample of your urine, so I will collect it by putting a small tube into your bladder." The latter statement is more likely to elicit a response from the client asking why it is needed and whether it will be uncomfortable because the client understands the message being conveyed by the nurse.

CLARITY AND BREVITY

A message that is direct and simple will be effective. Clarity is saying precisely what is meant, and brevity is using the fewest words necessary. The result is a message that is simple and clear. An aspect of this is congruence, or consistency, where the nurse's behavior or nonverbal communication matches the words spoken. When the nurse tells the client, "I am interested in hearing what you have to say," the nonverbal behavior would include the nurse facing the client, making eye contact, and leaning forward. The goal is to communicate clearly so that all aspects of a situation or circumstance are understood. To ensure clarity in communication, nurses also need to enunciate (pronounce) words carefully.

TIMING AND RELEVANCE

Nurses need to be aware of both relevance and timing when communicating with clients. No matter how clearly or simply words are stated or written, the timing needs to be appropriate to ensure that words are heard. Furthermore, the messages need to relate to the client or to the client's interests and concerns.

This involves sensitivity to the client's needs and concerns. For example, a client who is fearful of the possibility of cancer may not hear the nurse's explanations about the expected procedures before and after gallbladder surgery. In this situation, it is better for the nurse first to encourage the client to express concerns and then to deal with those concerns. The necessary explanations can be provided at another time when the client is better able to listen.

Another problem in timing is asking several questions at once. For example, a nurse enters a client's room and says in one breath, "Good morning, Mrs. Brody. How are you this morning? Did you sleep well last night? Your husband is coming to see you before your surgery, isn't he?" The client no doubt wonders which question to answer first, if any. A related pattern of poor timing is to ask a question and then not wait for an answer before making another comment. Conversely, by allowing the client to respond to the social talk or chat, the nurse develops a rapport with the client that can help facilitate effective therapeutic communication.

ADAPTABILITY

The nurse needs to alter spoken messages in accordance with behavioral cues from the client. This adjustment is referred to as *adaptability*. What the nurse says and how it is said must be individualized and carefully considered. This requires smart assessment and sensitivity on the part of the nurse. For example, a nurse who usually smiles, appears cheerful, and greets the client with an enthusiastic "Hi, Mrs. Brown!" notices that the client is not smiling and appears distressed. It is important for the nurse to then modify his or her tone of speech and express concern by facial expression while moving toward the client.

CREDIBILITY

Credibility means worthiness of belief, trustworthiness, and reliability. Credibility may be the most important criterion for effective communication. Nurses foster credibility by being consistent, dependable, and honest. The nurse needs to be knowledgeable about what is being discussed and to have accurate information. Nurses should convey confidence and certainty in what they are saying while being able to acknowledge their limitations (e.g., "I don't know the answer to that, but I will find someone who does").

HUMOR

The use of humor can be a positive and powerful tool in the nurse–client relationship, but it must be used with care. Humor can be used to help clients adjust to difficult and painful situations. The physical act of laughter can be an emotional and physical release, reducing tension by providing a different perspective and promoting a sense of well-being.

When using humor, it is important to consider the client's perception of what is considered humorous. Timing is also important to consider. Although humor and laughter can help reduce stress and anxiety, the feelings of the client need to be considered.

Nonverbal Communication

Nonverbal communication, sometimes called *body language*, includes gestures, body movements, use of touch, and physical appearance, including adornment. Nonverbal communication often tells others more about what an individual is feeling than what is being said because nonverbal behavior is controlled less consciously than verbal behavior (Figure 16.4 ■). Nonverbal communication either reinforces or contradicts what is said verbally. For example, if a nurse says to a client, "I'd be happy to sit here and talk to you for a while," yet glances nervously at a watch every few seconds, the actions contradict the verbal message. The client is more likely to believe the nonverbal behavior, which conveys "I am very busy and need to leave."

Observing and interpreting the client's nonverbal behavior is an essential skill for nurses to develop. To observe nonverbal behavior efficiently requires a systematic assessment of the client's overall physical appearance, posture, gait, facial expressions, and gestures. The nurse, however, needs to exercise caution in interpretation, always clarifying any observation with the client.

Clients who have altered thought processes, such as in schizophrenia or dementia, may experience times when expressing themselves verbally is difficult or impossible. During these times, the nurse needs to be able to interpret the feeling or emotion that the client is expressing nonverbally. An attentive nurse who clarifies observations very often portrays caring and acceptance to the client. This can be a beginning for establishing a trusting relationship between the nurse and the client, even in clients who have difficulty communicating appropriately.

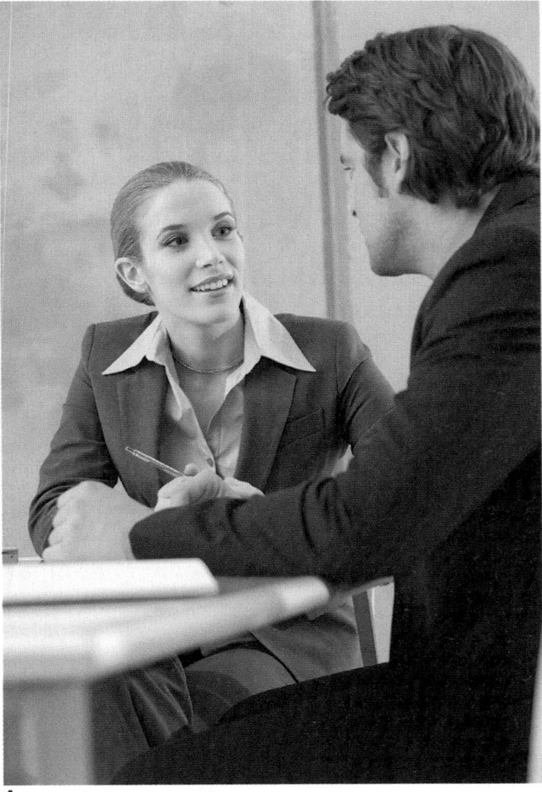

A

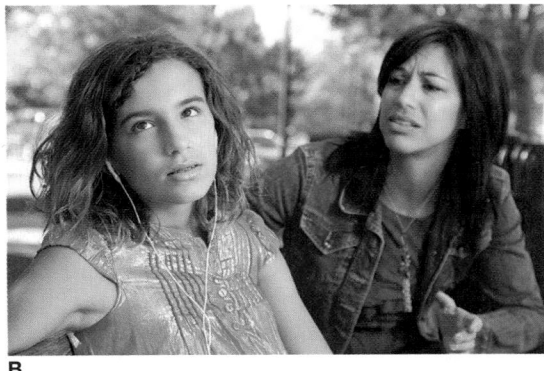

B

Figure 16.4 ■ Nonverbal communication sometimes conveys meaning more effectively than words. *A*, The postures of these individuals indicate openness to communication. *B*, The listener's posture and nonverbal demeanor suggest resistance to communication.
A, Westend61/Getty Images; *B*, SDI Productions/E+/Getty Images.

Transculturally, nonverbal communication varies widely (Seiler, Beall, & Mazer, 2017). Even for behaviors such as smiling and handshaking, cultures differ. For example, to some individuals, smiling and handshaking are an integral part of an interaction and essential to establishing trust. The same behavior might be perceived by others as insolent and frivolous.

The nurse cannot always be sure of the correct interpretation of feelings that are expressed nonverbally. The same feeling can be expressed nonverbally in more than one way, even within the same cultural group. For example, anger may be communicated by aggressive or excessive body motion, or it may be communicated by frozen stillness. In some cultures, a smile may be used to conceal anger. Therefore, the interpretation of such observations requires validation with the client. For example, the nurse might say, "You look like you have been crying. Is something upsetting you?"

PERSONAL APPEARANCE

Clothing and adornments can be sources of information about an individual. Although the choice of apparel is highly personal, it may convey social and financial status, culture, religion, group association, and self-concept. Charms and amulets may be worn for decorative or for health protection purposes. When the symbolic meaning of an object is unfamiliar, the nurse can inquire about its significance, which may foster rapport with the client.

How an individual dresses is often an indicator of how the individual feels. People who are tired or ill may not have the energy or the desire to maintain their normal grooming. When a client known for immaculate grooming becomes careless about appearance, the nurse may suspect a loss of self-esteem or a physical illness. The nurse must validate these observed nonverbal data by asking the client. For acutely ill clients in hospital or home care settings, a change in grooming habits may signal that the client is feeling better. For example, a man may request a shave, or a woman may request shampoo and some makeup.

POSTURE AND GAIT

The ways people walk and carry themselves are often reliable indicators of self-concept, current mood, and health. Erect posture and an active, purposeful stride suggest a feeling of well-being. Slouched posture and a slow, shuffling gait suggest depression or physical discomfort. Tense posture and a rapid, determined gait suggest anxiety or anger. The posture of people when they are sitting or lying down can also indicate feelings or mood. Again, the nurse clarifies the meaning of the observed behavior by describing to the client what the nurse sees and then asking what it means or whether the nurse's interpretation is correct. For example, "You look like it really hurts you to move.

I'm wondering how your pain is and if you might need something to make you more comfortable?"

FACIAL EXPRESSION

No part of the body is as expressive as the face (Figure 16.5 ■). Feelings of surprise, fear, anger, disgust, happiness, and sadness can be conveyed by facial expressions. Although the face may express the individual's genuine emotions, it is also possible to control these muscles so that the emotion expressed does not reflect what the individual is feeling. When the message is not clear, it is important to get feedback to be sure of the intent of the expression. Many facial expressions convey a universal meaning. The smile expresses happiness. Disapproval is conveyed by the mouth turned down, the head tilted back, and the eyes directed down the nose. No single expression can be interpreted accurately, however, without considering other reinforcing physical cues, the setting in which it occurs, the expression of others in the same setting, and the background of the client.

Nurses need to be aware of their own expressions and what they are communicating to others. Clients are quick to notice the nurse's facial expression, particularly when they feel unsure or uncomfortable. The client who questions the nurse about a feared diagnostic result will watch whether the nurse maintains eye contact or looks away when answering. The client who has had disfiguring surgery will examine the nurse's face for signs of disgust. It is impossible to control all facial expression, but the nurse must learn to control expressions of feelings such as fear or disgust in some circumstances.

Eye contact is another essential element of facial communication. In many cultures, mutual eye contact acknowledges recognition of the other individual and a willingness to maintain communication. Often, an individual initiates contact with another individual with a glance, capturing the individual's attention prior to communicating. An individual who feels weak or defenseless often averts the eyes or avoids eye contact; the communication received may be too embarrassing or too dominating.

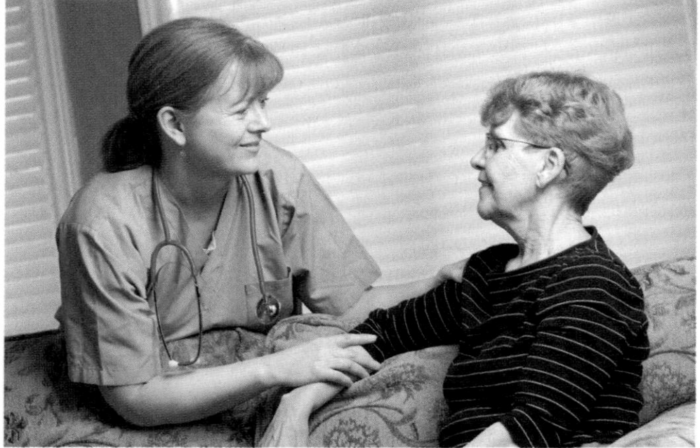

Figure 16.5 ■ The nurse's facial expression communicates warmth and caring.
eyetoeyePIX/E+/Getty images.

GESTURES

Hand and body gestures may emphasize and clarify the spoken word, or they may occur without words to indicate a feeling or to give a sign. A father awaiting information about his daughter in surgery may wring his hands, tap his foot, pick at his nails, or pace back and forth. A gesture may more clearly indicate the size or shape of an object. A wave goodbye and the motioning of a visitor toward a chair are gestures that have relatively universal meanings. Some gestures, however, are culture specific. The gesture meaning "shoo" or "go away" in some cultures means "come here" or "come back" in other cultures.

For individuals with special communication challenges, such as those with hearing impairments, the hands are invaluable in communication. Many people who are deaf learn sign language. Ill individuals who are unable to reply verbally can similarly devise a communication system using the hands. The client may be able to raise an index finger once for "yes" and twice for "no." Other signals can often be devised by the client and the nurse to denote other meanings.

Electronic Communication

Computers play an increasing role in nursing practice. Many healthcare agencies are moving toward electronic medical records where nurses document their assessments and nursing care. Email can be used in healthcare facilities for many purposes: to schedule and confirm appointments, to report normal laboratory results, to conduct client education, and for follow-up with discharged clients.

EMAIL

Email is the most common form of electronic communication. It is important for the nurse to know the advantages and disadvantages of email and other guidelines to ensure client confidentiality.

Advantages Email has many positive advantages. It is a fast, efficient way to communicate, and it is legible. It provides a record of the date and time of the message that was sent or received. Some health facilities provide their clients with a portal to schedule appointments, refill prescriptions, and send secure email messages to their healthcare providers. This improves communication and continuity of client care. Email promises better access, and evidence has shown that clients who communicated with their healthcare providers were found to have improved healthcare measures (Industry Watch, 2016).

Disadvantages One disadvantage or negative aspect of email is concern by both clients and primary care providers regarding privacy, confidentiality, and potential misuse of information, such as cyberattacks and hacking aimed at healthcare organizations (Biddle & Milstead, 2016). Protection of client privacy remains an issue when transferring information electronically. The healthcare agency needs to have an email encryption system to ensure security. An agency may have its own system or outsource it to an encryption service.

Another disadvantage is one of socioeconomics. Not everyone has a computer, and even if people have access to computers at, say, a public library, not everyone has the necessary computer skills. Email may enhance communication with some clients but not all clients. Other forms of communication will be needed for clients who have limited abilities with speaking English, reading, writing, or using a computer.

Other Guidelines Agencies usually develop standards and guidelines for the use of email in healthcare. Nurses need to know their agency's guidelines about what can be sent to clients by email. The client usually signs an email consent form. This form provides information about the risks of email and authorizes the health agency to communicate with the client at a specified email address.

Information sent to a client via email is considered part of the client's medical record. Therefore, a copy of the email needs to be put in the client's chart. Emails, like other documentation in the client's record, may be used as evidence during litigation.

The use of email can enhance effective relationships with clients. It is not, however, a substitute for effective verbal and nonverbal communication. Nurses need to use their professional judgment about what form of communication(s) will best meet their clients' health needs.

Factors Influencing the Communication Process

Many factors influence the communication process. Some of these are development, gender, values and perceptions, personal space, territoriality, roles and relationships, environment, congruence, interpersonal attitudes, and boundaries.

Development

Language, psychosocial, and intellectual development move through stages across the lifespan. Knowledge of a client's developmental stage will allow the nurse to modify the message accordingly. The use of dolls and games coupled with simple language may help explain a procedure to an 8-year-old. With adolescents who have developed more abstract thinking skills, a more detailed explanation can be given, whereas a well-educated, middle-aged business executive may wish to have detailed technical information provided. Older clients are apt to have had a wider range of experiences with the healthcare system, which may influence their response or understanding. With aging also come changes in vision and hearing acuity that can affect nurse–client interactions.

Gender

From an early age, females and males communicate differently. Girls tend to use language to seek confirmation, minimize differences, and establish intimacy. Boys use language to establish independence and negotiate status within a group. These differences can continue into adulthood, so a man and a woman may interpret the same communication differently.

Values and Perceptions

Values are the standards that influence behavior, and *perceptions* are the personal view of an event. Because each individual has unique personality traits, values, and life experiences, each will perceive and interpret messages and experiences differently. For example, if the nurse draws the curtains around a crying woman and leaves her alone, the woman may interpret this as "The nurse thinks that I will upset others and that I shouldn't cry" or "The nurse respects my need to be alone." It is important for the nurse to be aware of a client's values and to validate or correct perceptions to avoid creating barriers in the nurse–client relationship.

Personal Space

Personal space is the distance people prefer in interactions with others. **Proxemics** is the study of distances that people allow between themselves and objects or other people. Communication thus varies in accordance with four distances, each with a close and a far phase. Beebe, Beebe, and Ivy (2019, pp. 83–84) list the following examples:

1. ***Intimate:*** 0 to $1\frac{1}{2}$ feet
2. ***Personal:*** $1\frac{1}{2}$ to 4 feet
3. ***Social:*** 4 to 12 feet
4. ***Public:*** 12 feet and beyond.

Intimate distance communication is characterized by body contact, heightened sensations of body heat and smell, and vocalizations that are low. Vision is intense, is restricted to a small body part, and may be distorted. Nurses frequently use intimate distance. Examples include cuddling a baby, touching a client who is blind, positioning clients, assessing an incision, and restraining a toddler for an injection.

It is a natural protective instinct for people to maintain a certain amount of space immediately around them, and the amount varies with individuals and cultures. When someone who wants to communicate steps into another individual's personal space, the receiver unconsciously responds by stepping back a pace or two. In their therapeutic roles, nurses often are required to violate this personal space. However, it is important for them to be aware of when this will occur and to alert the client. In many instances, the nurse can respect (not come as close as) a client's intimate distance. In other instances, the nurse may come within intimate distance to communicate warmth and caring.

Personal distance is less overwhelming than intimate distance. Voice tones are moderate, and body heat and smell are noticed less. Physical contact such as a handshake or touching a shoulder is possible. More of the individual is perceived at a personal distance, so nonverbal behaviors such as body stance or full facial expressions are seen with less distortion. Much communication between nurses and clients occurs at this distance. Examples occur when nurses are sitting with a client, giving medications, or establishing an intravenous infusion. Communication at a close personal distance can convey involvement by facilitating the sharing of thoughts and feelings. On the other hand, it can also create tension if the distance encroaches on the other individual's personal space (Figure 16.6 ■). At the outer extreme of 4 feet, however, less involvement is expressed. Bantering and some social conversations usually take place at this distance.

Social distance is characterized by a clear visual perception of the whole individual. Body heat and odor are imperceptible, eye contact is increased, and vocalizations are loud enough to be overheard by others. Communication is therefore more formal and is limited to seeing and hearing. The individual may feel protected and out of reach for touch or personal sharing of thoughts or feelings. Social distance allows more activity and movement back and forth. It is expedient for communicating with several people at the same time or within a short time. Examples occur when nurses make rounds or wave a greeting to someone. Social distance is important in accomplishing the business of the day. However, it is frequently misused. For example, the nurse who stands in the doorway and asks a client "How are you today?" will receive a more noncommittal reply than the nurse who moves to a personal distance to make the same inquiry.

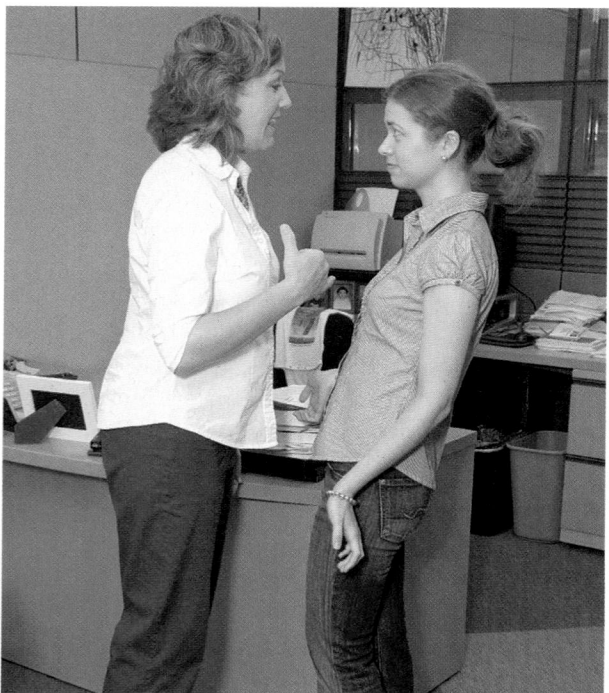

Figure 16.6 ■ Personal space influences communication in social and professional interactions. Encroachment into another individual's personal space creates tension.

Public distance requires loud, clear vocalizations with careful enunciation. Although the faces and forms of people are seen at a public distance, individuality is lost. Instead, the perception is of the group of people or the community.

Territoriality

Territoriality is a concept of the space and things that an individual considers as belonging to the self. Territories marked off by people may be visible to others. For example, clients in a hospital often consider their territory as bounded by the curtains around the bed unit or by the walls of a private room. Healthcare workers must recognize this human tendency to claim territory. Clients often feel the need to defend their territory when others invade it; for example, when a visitor or nurse removes a chair to use at another bed, the visitor has inadvertently violated the territoriality of the client whose chair was removed. Nurses need to obtain permission from clients to remove, rearrange, or borrow objects in their hospital area.

Roles and Relationships

The roles and the relationships between the sender and receiver affect the communication process. Roles such as nursing student and instructor, client and primary care provider, or parent and child affect the content and responses in the communication process. Choice of words, sentence structure, and tone of voice vary considerably from role to role. In addition, the specific relationship between the communicators is significant. The nurse who meets with a client for the first time communicates differently from the nurse who has previously developed a relationship with that client.

Environment

People usually communicate most effectively in a comfortable environment. Temperature extremes, excessive noise, and a poorly ventilated environment can all interfere with communication. Also, lack of privacy may interfere with a client's communication about matters the client considers private. For example, a client who is worried about the ability of his wife to care for him after discharge from the hospital may not wish to discuss this concern with a nurse within the hearing range of other clients in the room. Environmental distraction can impair and distort communication.

Congruence

In **congruent communication**, the verbal and nonverbal aspects of the message match. Clients more readily trust the nurse when they perceive the nurse's communication

LIFESPAN CONSIDERATIONS Communication with Children

The ability to communicate is directly related to the development of thought processes, the presence of intact sensory and motor systems, and the extent and nature of an individual's opportunities to practice communication skills. As children grow, their communication abilities change markedly.

INFANTS

- Infants communicate nonverbally, often in response to body feelings rather than in a conscious effort to be expressive.
- Infants' perceptions are related to sensory stimuli, so a gentle voice is soothing, for example, while tension and anger around them create distress.

TODDLERS AND PRESCHOOLERS

- Toddlers and young children gain skills in both expressive (i.e., telling others what they feel, think, want, care about) and receptive (hearing and understanding what others are communicating to them) language.
- Allow time for them to complete verbalizing their thoughts without interruption.
- Provide a simple response to questions because they have short attention spans.
- Drawing a picture can provide another way for the child to communicate.

SCHOOL-AGE CHILDREN

- Talk to the child at his or her eye level to help decrease intimidation.
- Include the child in the conversation when communicating with the parents.

ADOLESCENTS

- Take time to build rapport with the adolescent.
- Use active listening skills.
- Project a nonjudgmental attitude and nonreactive behaviors, even when the adolescent makes disturbing remarks.

Nurses can use the following communication techniques to work effectively with children and their families:

- Play, the universal language, allows children to use other symbols, not just words, to express themselves.
- Nonverbal children may be able to use drawing, painting, and other art forms to communicate.
- Storytelling, in which the nurse and child take turns adding to a story or putting words to pictures, can help the child feel safer in expressing emotions and feelings.
- Word games that pose hypothetical situations or put the child in control, such as "What if . . . ?" "If you could . . . ," "If a genie came and gave you a wish . . . ," can help a child feel more powerful or explore ideas about how to manage the illness.
- Read books with a theme similar to the child's condition or problem, and then discuss the meaning, characters, and feelings generated by the book. Movies or videos can also be used in this way.
- Writing can be used by older children to reflect on their situation, develop meaning, and gain a sense of control.

In all interactions with children, it is important to give them opportunities to be expressive, listen openly, and respond honestly, using words and concepts they understand.

as congruent. This will also help to prevent miscommunication. Both nurse and client can easily determine if there is congruence between verbal expression and nonverbal expression. Nurses are taught to assess clients, but clients are often just as adept at reading a nurse's expression or body language. If there is incongruence between verbal and nonverbal expression, the body language or nonverbal communication is usually the one with the true meaning. For example, when teaching a client how to care for a colostomy, the nurse might say, "You won't have any problem with this." However, if the nurse looks worried while saying this, the client is less likely to trust the nurse's words.

Interpersonal Attitudes

Attitudes convey beliefs, thoughts, and feelings about people and events. Attitudes are communicated convincingly and rapidly to others. Attitudes such as caring, warmth, respect, and acceptance facilitate communication, whereas condescension, lack of interest, and coldness inhibit communication.

Caring and *warmth* convey a feeling of emotional closeness, in contrast to an impersonal approach. Caring is more enduring and intense than warmth. It conveys deep and genuine concern for the individual, whereas warmth conveys friendliness and consideration, shown by acts of smiling and attention to physical comforts. Caring involves giving feelings, thoughts, skill, and knowledge. It requires psychologic energy and poses the risk of gaining little in return; yet by caring, people usually reap the benefits of greater communication and understanding.

Respect is an attitude that emphasizes the other individual's worth and individuality. It conveys that the individual's hopes and feelings are special and unique even though they are like others in many ways. People have a need to be different from—and at the same time similar to—others. Being too different can be isolating and threatening. A nurse conveys respect by listening with an open mind to what the other individual is saying, even if the nurse disagrees. Nurses can learn new ways of approaching situations when they conscientiously listen to another individual's perspective.

Healthcare providers may unknowingly use speech that they believe shows caring but the client perceives as demeaning or patronizing. This frequently happens in settings that provide healthcare to older adults and individuals with obvious physical or mental disabilities. **Elderspeak** is a speech style similar to baby talk that gives the message of dependence and incompetence and is viewed as patronizing by older adults. It does not communicate respect. Many healthcare providers are not aware that they use elderspeak or that it can have negative meanings to the client. The characteristics of elderspeak include inappropriate terms of endearment (e.g., "honey," "grandma"); inappropriate plural pronoun use (e.g., "Are *we* ready for *our* bath?"); tag questions (e.g., "You want to wear this dress, don't you?"); and slow, loud speech. Although elderspeak is often used by well-intentioned care providers, the literature suggests that elderspeak can negatively affect the overall social and psychologic health of older adults (Corwin, 2018; Williams et al., 2017).

Acceptance emphasizes neither approval nor disapproval. The nurse willingly receives the client's honest feelings. An accepting attitude allows clients to express personal feelings freely and to be themselves. The nurse may need to restrict acceptance in situations where clients' behaviors are harmful to themselves or to others. Helping the client to find appropriate behaviors for feelings is often part of client teaching.

Boundaries

Boundaries are the "defining limits of individuals, objects, or relationships" (Boyd, 2017, "Boundaries and Body Space Zones" section, para 1). For nurses, professional boundaries are crucial in the context of the nurse–client relationship. To maintain clear boundaries, the nurse keeps the focus on the client and avoids sharing personal information or meeting his or her own needs through the nurse–client relationship. If the client seeks friendship with the nurse or a relationship outside the work environment, the nurse affirms his or her professional role and declines the invitation. Some indicators that boundary issues need to be addressed include gift-giving by the nurse or client, spending more time than necessary with a client, or the nurse believing only he or she understands the client (Boyd, 2017).

Web-based social networks such as Facebook, Myspace, and Twitter are experiencing increased usage. Unfortunately, online sites such as these have brought new hazards to nursing professionalism. Unprofessional uses of social networking tools are common; thus, the nurse needs to be diligent about not crossing nurse–client boundaries in an online setting. The American Nurses Association (ANA) Code of Ethics for Nurses (2015a) states that the nurse is responsible for maintaining professional boundaries in all communications and actions (p. 7). It is important to remember that the need for nurses to behave professionally is constant, even when off duty, including social media or any other means of communication (p. 9).

Therapeutic Communication

Therapeutic communication promotes understanding and can help establish a constructive relationship between the nurse and the client. Unlike a social relationship, where there may not be a specific purpose or direction, the therapeutic helping relationship is client and goal directed.

Nurses need to respond not only to the content of a client's verbal message but also to the feelings expressed. It is important to understand how the client views the situation and feels about it before responding. The content of the client's communication is the words or thoughts, as distinct from the feelings. Sometimes people can convey a thought in words while their emotions contradict the words; that is, words and feelings are incongruent. For example, a client says, "I am glad he has left me; he was very cruel." However, the nurse observes that the client has tears in her eyes as she says this. To respond to the client's *words*, the nurse might simply rephrase, saying, "You are pleased that he has left you." To respond to the client's *feelings*, the nurse would need to acknowledge the tears in the client's eyes, saying, for example, "You seem saddened by all this." Such a response helps the client to focus on her feelings. In some instances, the nurse may need to know more about the client and her resources for coping with these feelings.

Sometimes clients need time to deal with their feelings. Strong emotions are often draining. People usually need to deal with feelings before they can cope with other matters, such as learning new skills or planning for the future. This is most evident in hospitals when clients learn that they have a terminal illness. Some require hours, days, or even weeks before they are ready to start other tasks. Some need only time to themselves, others need someone to listen, others need assistance identifying and verbalizing feelings, and others need assistance making decisions about future courses of action.

Attentive Listening

Attentive listening is listening actively and with mindfulness, using all the senses, and paying attention to what the client says, does, and feels as opposed to listening passively with just the ear. It is probably the most important technique in nursing and is basic to all other techniques. Attentive listening is an active process that requires energy and concentration. It involves paying attention to the total message, both verbal and nonverbal, and noting whether these communications are congruent. Attentive listening means absorbing both the content and the feeling the client is conveying while putting aside your own judgments and ideas to really hear and focus on the client's needs. Attentive listening conveys an attitude of caring and interest, thereby encouraging the client to trust you, open up, and talk (Figure 16.7 ■).

Attentive listening also involves listening for key themes in the communication. The nurse must be careful

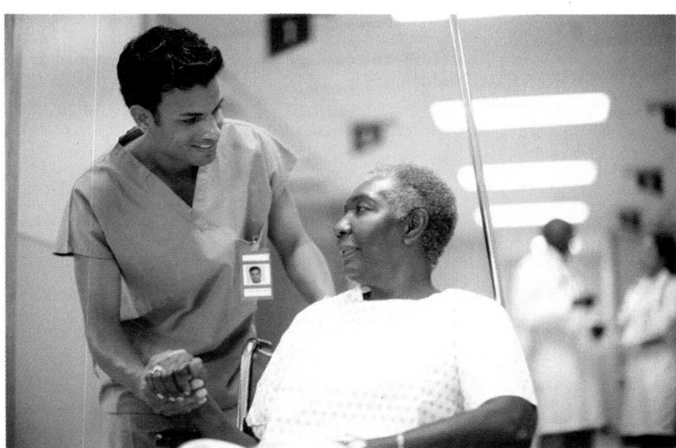

Figure 16.7 ■ The nurse conveys attentive listening through a posture of involvement.
Thomas M Jackson/Redferns/Getty Images.

not to react quickly to the message. The nurse should not interrupt the speaker, and the nurse (the responder) should take time to think about the message before responding. As a listener, the nurse also should ask questions either to obtain additional information or to clarify. The message sender (i.e., the client) should decide when to close a conversation. When the nurse closes the conversation, the client may assume that the nurse considers the message unimportant. It is also important for nurses to be aware of their own biases. A message from a client that reflects different values or beliefs should not be discredited for that reason.

In summary, attentive listening is a highly developed skill, and it can be learned with practice. A nurse can communicate attentive listening to clients in various ways. Common responses are nodding the head, uttering "Uh huh" or "Mmm," repeating the words that the client has used, or saying "I see what you mean." Each nurse has characteristic ways of responding, and the nurse must take care not to sound insincere or phony.

Visibly Tuning In

At times, your nonverbal behavior may be as important, or more important, than your words. Active learners are engaged physically and mentally in the listening process. They have good eye contact with the client and communicate their interest with an intent facial expression, a natural forward lean, and appropriate head nods (Beebe et al., 2019).

Therapeutic communication techniques facilitate communication and focus on the client's concerns (Table 16.1).

Barriers to Communication

Nurses need to recognize barriers or nontherapeutic responses to effective communication (Table 16.2). Failing to listen, improperly decoding the client's intended message, and placing the nurse's needs above the client's needs are major barriers to communication.

TABLE 16.1 Therapeutic Communication Techniques

Technique	Description	Examples
Using silence	Accepting pauses or silences that may extend for several seconds or minutes without interjecting any verbal response	Sitting quietly (or walking with the client) and waiting attentively until the client is able to put thoughts and feelings into words
Providing general leads	Using statements or questions that (a) encourage the client to verbalize, (b) choose a topic of conversation, and (c) facilitate continued verbalization	"Can you tell me how it is for you?" "Perhaps you would like to talk about . . . " "Would it help to discuss your feelings?" "Where would you like to begin?" "And then what?"
Being specific and tentative	Making statements that are specific rather than general and tentative rather than absolute	"Rate your pain on a scale of 0 to 10." (specific statement) "Are you in pain?" (general statement) "You seem unconcerned about your diabetes." (tentative statement)
Using open-ended questions	Asking broad questions that lead or invite the client to explore (elaborate, clarify, describe, compare, or illustrate) thoughts or feelings. Open-ended questions specify only the topic to be discussed and invite answers that are longer than one or two words.	"I'd like to hear more about that." "Tell me more . . . " "How have you been feeling lately?" "What brought you to the hospital?" "What is your opinion?" "You said you were frightened yesterday. How do you feel now?"

Continued on page 306

TABLE 16.1 Therapeutic Communication Techniques—*continued*

Technique	Description	Examples
Using touch	Providing appropriate forms of touch to reinforce caring feelings. Because tactile contacts vary considerably among individuals, families, and cultures, the nurse must be sensitive to the differences in attitudes and practices of clients and self.	Putting an arm over the client's shoulder. Placing your hand over the client's hand.
Restating or paraphrasing	Actively listening for the client's basic message and then repeating those thoughts or feelings in similar words. This conveys that the nurse has listened and understood the client's basic message and also offers clients a clearer idea of what they have said.	*Client:* "I couldn't manage to eat any dinner last night—not even the dessert." *Nurse:* "You had difficulty eating yesterday." *Client:* "Yes, I was very upset after my family left."
Seeking clarification	A method of making the client's broad overall meaning of the message more understandable. It is used when paraphrasing is difficult or when the communication is rambling or garbled. To clarify the message, the nurse can restate the basic message or confess confusion and ask the client to repeat or restate the message. Nurses can also clarify their own message with statements.	"I'm puzzled." "I'm not sure I understand that." "Would you please say that again?" "Would you tell me more?" "I meant this rather than that." "I'm sorry that wasn't very clear. Let me try to explain another way."
Perception checking or seeking consensual validation	A method similar to clarifying that verifies the meaning of specific words rather than the overall meaning of a message	*Client:* "My husband never gives me any presents." *Nurse:* "You mean he has never given you a present for your birthday or Christmas?" *Client:* "Well—not never. He does get me something for my birthday and Christmas, but he never thinks of giving me anything at any other time."
Offering self	Suggesting one's presence, interest, or wish to understand the client without making any demands or attaching conditions that the client must comply with to receive the nurse's attention	"I'll stay with you until your daughter arrives." "We can sit here quietly for a while; we don't need to talk unless you would like to." "I'll help you to dress to go home, if you like."
Giving information	Providing, in a simple and direct manner, specific factual information the client may or may not request. When information is not known, the nurse states this and indicates who has it or when the nurse will obtain it.	"Your surgery is scheduled for 11 a.m. tomorrow." "You will feel a pulling sensation when the tube is removed from your abdomen." "I do not know the answer to that, but I will find out from Mrs. King, the nurse in charge."
Acknowledging	Giving recognition, in a nonjudgmental way, of a change in behavior, an effort the client has made, or a contribution to a communication. Acknowledgment may be with or without understanding, verbal or nonverbal.	"You trimmed your beard and mustache and washed your hair." "I notice you keep squinting your eyes. Are you having difficulty seeing?" "You walked twice as far today with your walker."
Clarifying time or sequence	Helping the client clarify an event, situation, or happening in relation to time	*Client:* "I vomited this morning." *Nurse:* "Was that after breakfast?" *Client:* "I feel that I have been asleep for weeks." *Nurse:* "You had your operation Monday, and today is Tuesday."
Presenting reality	Helping the client to differentiate the real from the unreal	"That telephone ring came from the program on television." "Your magazine is here in the drawer. It has not been stolen."

TABLE 16.1 Therapeutic Communication Techniques—*continued*

Technique	Description	Examples
Focusing	Helping the client expand on and develop a topic of importance. It is important for the nurse to wait until the client finishes stating the main concerns before attempting to focus. The focus may be an idea or a feeling; however, the nurse often emphasizes a feeling to help the client recognize an emotion disguised behind words.	*Client:* "My wife says she will look after me, but I don't think she can, what with the children to take care of, and they're always after her about something—clothes, homework, what's for dinner that night." *Nurse:* "Sounds like you are worried about how well she can manage."
Reflecting	Directing ideas, feelings, questions, or content back to clients to enable them to explore their own ideas and feelings about a situation	*Client:* "What can I do?" *Nurse:* "What do you think would be helpful?" *Client:* "Do you think I should tell my husband?" *Nurse:* "You seem unsure about telling your husband."
Summarizing and planning	Stating the main points of a discussion to clarify the relevant points discussed. This technique is useful at the end of an interview or to review a health teaching session. It often acts as an introduction to future care planning.	"During the past half hour, we have talked about . . . " "Tomorrow afternoon, we may explore this further." "In a few days, I'll review what you have learned about the actions and effects of your insulin." "Tomorrow, I will look at your feeling journal."

TABLE 16.2 Barriers to Communication

Technique	Description	Examples
Stereotyping	Offering generalized and oversimplified beliefs about groups of people that are based on experiences too limited to be valid. These responses categorize clients and negate their uniqueness as individuals.	"Two-year-olds are brats." "Women are complainers." "Men don't cry." "Most people don't have any pain after this type of surgery."
Agreeing and disagreeing	Similar to judgmental responses, agreeing and disagreeing imply that the client is either right or wrong and that the nurse is in a position to judge this. These responses deter clients from thinking through their position and may cause a client to become defensive.	*Client:* "I don't think Dr. Broad is a very good doctor. He doesn't seem interested in his clients." *Nurse:* "Dr. Broad is head of the department of surgery and is an excellent surgeon."
Being defensive	Attempting to protect an individual or healthcare services from negative comments. These responses prevent the client from expressing true concerns. The nurse is saying, "You have no right to complain." Defensive responses protect the nurse from admitting weaknesses in healthcare services, including personal weaknesses.	*Client:* "Those night nurses must just sit around and talk all night. They didn't answer my light for over an hour." *Nurse:* "I'll have you know we literally run around on nights. You're not the only client, you know."
Challenging	Giving a response that makes clients prove their statement or point of view. These responses indicate that the nurse is failing to consider the client's feelings, making the client feel it is necessary to defend a position.	*Client:* "I felt nauseated after that red pill." *Nurse:* "Surely you don't think I gave you the wrong pill?" *Client:* "I feel as if I am dying." *Nurse:* "How can you feel that way when your pulse is 60?" *Client:* "I believe my husband doesn't love me." *Nurse:* "You can't say that; why, he visits you every day."
Probing	Asking for information chiefly out of curiosity rather than with the intent to assist the client. These responses are considered prying and violate the client's privacy. Asking "why" is often probing and places the client in a defensive position.	*Client:* "I was speeding along the street and didn't see the stop sign." *Nurse:* "Why were you speeding?" *Client:* "I didn't ask the doctor when he was here." *Nurse:* "Why didn't you?"

Continued on page 308

TABLE 16.2 Barriers to Communication—*continued*

Technique	Description	Examples
Testing	Asking questions that make the client admit to something. These responses permit the client only limited answers and often meet the nurse's need rather than the client's.	"Who do you think you are?" (forces people to admit their status is only that of client) "Do you think I am not busy?" (forces the client to admit that the nurse really is busy)
Rejecting	Refusing to discuss certain topics with the client. These responses often make clients feel that the nurse is rejecting not only their communication but also the clients themselves.	"I don't want to discuss that. Let's talk about . . . " "Let's discuss other areas of interest to you rather than the two problems you keep mentioning."
Changing topics and subjects	Directing the communication into areas of self-interest rather than considering the client's concerns is often a self-protective response to a topic that causes anxiety. These responses imply that what the nurse considers important will be discussed and that clients should not discuss certain topics.	"I can't talk now. I'm on my way for a coffee break." *Client:* "I'm separated from my wife. Do you think I should have sexual relations with another woman?" *Nurse:* "I see that you're 36 and that you like gardening. This sunshine is good for my roses. I have a beautiful rose garden."
Unwarranted reassurance	Using clichés or comforting statements of advice as a means to reassure the client. These responses block the fears, feelings, and other thoughts of the client.	"You'll feel better soon." "I'm sure everything will turn out all right." "Don't worry."
Passing judgment	Giving opinions and approving or disapproving responses, moralizing, or implying one's own values. These responses imply that the client must think as the nurse thinks, fostering client dependence.	"That's good (bad)." "You shouldn't do that." "That's not good enough." "What you did was wrong (right)."
Giving common advice	Telling the client what to do. These responses deny the client's right to be an equal partner. Note that giving expert rather than common advice is therapeutic.	*Client:* "Should I move from my home to a nursing home?" *Nurse:* "If I were you, I'd go to a nursing home, where you'll get your meals cooked for you."

The Helping Relationship

Nurse–client relationships are referred to by some as *interpersonal relationships*, by others as *therapeutic relationships*, and by still others as **helping relationships**. Helping is a growth-facilitating process that strives to achieve three basic goals (Egan & Reese, 2019, pp. 14–17):

1. Help clients manage their problems in living more effectively and develop unused or underused opportunities more fully.
2. Help clients become better at helping themselves in their everyday lives.
3. Help clients develop an action-oriented prevention mentality in their lives.

A helping relationship may develop over weeks of working with a client, or within minutes. The keys to the helping relationship are (a) the development of trust and acceptance between the nurse and the client and (b) an underlying belief that the nurse cares about and wants to help the client.

The personal and professional characteristics of the nurse and the client influence the helping relationship. Age, gender, appearance, diagnosis, education, values, ethnic and cultural background, personality, expectations, and setting can all affect the development of the nurse–client relationship. Consideration of all these factors, combined with good communication skills and sincere interest in the client's welfare, will enable the nurse to create a helping relationship. Characteristics of helping relationships are listed in Box 16.1.

Phases of the Helping Relationship

The helping relationship process can be described in terms of four sequential phases, each characterized by

BOX 16.1 Characteristics of a Helping Relationship

A helping relationship:

- Is an intellectual and emotional bond between the nurse and the client and is focused on the client.
- Respects the client as an individual, including
  - Maximizing the client's abilities to participate in decision-making and treatments
  - Considering ethnic and cultural aspects
  - Considering family relationships and values.
- Respects client confidentiality.
- Focuses on the client's well-being.
- Is based on mutual trust, respect, and acceptance.

identifiable tasks and skills. The relationship must progress through the stages in succession because each builds on the one before. Nurses can identify the progress of a relationship by understanding these phases: preinteraction phase, introductory phase, working (maintaining) phase, and resolution phase.

Preinteraction Phase

The preinteraction phase is like the planning stage before an interview. In most situations, the nurse has information about the client before the first face-to-face meeting. Such information may include the client's name, address, age, medical history, and social history. Planning for the initial visit may generate some anxious feelings in the nurse. If the nurse recognizes these feelings and identifies specific information to be discussed, positive outcomes can evolve.

Introductory Phase

The introductory phase, also referred to as the *orientation phase* or the *prehelping phase*, is important because it sets the tone for the rest of the relationship. During this initial encounter, the client and the nurse closely observe each other and form judgments about the other's behavior. The goal of the nurse in this phase is to develop trust and security within the nurse–client relationship (Boyd, 2017). Other important tasks of the introductory phase include getting to know each other and developing a degree of trust.

By the end of the introductory phase, clients should begin to:

- Develop trust in the nurse.
- View the nurse as a competent professional capable of helping.
- View the nurse as honest, open, and concerned about their welfare.
- Believe the nurse will try to understand and respect their cultural values and beliefs.
- Believe the nurse will respect client confidentiality.
- Feel comfortable talking with the nurse about feelings and other sensitive issues.
- Understand the purpose of the relationship and the roles.
- Feel that they are active participants in developing a mutually agreeable plan of care.

Working Phase

During the working phase of a helping relationship, the nurse and the client begin to view each other as unique individuals. They begin to appreciate this uniqueness and care about each other. Caring is sharing deep and genuine concern about the welfare of another individual. Once caring develops, the potential for empathy increases.

The working phase has two major stages: exploring and understanding thoughts and feelings, and facilitating and acting. The nurse helps the client to explore thoughts, feelings, and actions and helps the client plan a program of action to meet preestablished goals.

EXPLORING AND UNDERSTANDING THOUGHTS AND FEELINGS

The nurse must have the following skills for this phase of the helping relationship:

- ***Empathetic listening and responding.*** Nurses must listen attentively and communicate (respond) in ways that indicate they have listened to what was said and understand how the client feels. The nurse responds to content or feelings or both, as appropriate. The nurse's nonverbal behaviors are also important. Nonverbal behaviors indicating empathy include moderate head nodding, a steady gaze, moderate gesturing, and little activity or body movement. According to Boyd (2017), **empathy** is the ability to experience, in the present, a situation as another did at some time in the past, the ability to put oneself in another individual's circumstances and imagine what it would be like to share their feelings. Empathetic listening focuses on "being with" clients to develop an understanding of them and their world. This understanding, however, must also be communicated effectively to the client in the form of an empathetic response. The result of empathy is comforting and caring for the client and a helping, healing relationship.
- ***Respect.*** The nurse must show respect for the client's willingness to be available, a desire to work with the client, and a manner that conveys the idea of taking the client's point of view seriously.
- ***Genuineness.*** The ability to be real or honest with another is genuineness. To be effective, genuineness must be based on a solid relationship that is empathic and not phony. Phoniness can be expressed in a variety of ways, such as pretending to like someone when you do not or overstressing your professional role (e.g., I am the expert, the one with all the answers). The nurse who is genuine is more likely to help the client.
- ***Concreteness.*** The nurse must assist the client to be concrete and specific rather than to speak in generalities. When the client says, "I'm stupid and clumsy," the nurse narrows the topic to the specific by pointing out, "You tripped on the rug."
- ***Confrontation.*** The nurse points out discrepancies between thoughts, feelings, and actions that inhibit the client's self-understanding or exploration of specific areas. This is done empathetically, not judgmentally.

During this first stage of the working phase, the intensity of interaction increases, and feelings such as anger, shame, or self-consciousness may be expressed. If the nurse is skilled in this stage and if the client is willing to pursue self-exploration, the outcome is a beginning understanding on the part of the client about behavior and feelings.

FACILITATING AND TAKING ACTION

Ultimately, the client must make decisions and take action to become more effective. The responsibility for action belongs to the client. The nurse, however, collaborates in these decisions, provides support, and may offer options or information.

Resolution Phase

The final phase of the relationship is resolution, which begins when the actual problems are resolved and ends with the termination of the relationship (Boyd, 2017).

Many methods can be used to terminate relationships. Summarizing or reviewing the process can produce a sense of accomplishment. This may include sharing reminiscences of how things were at the beginning of the relationship and comparing them to how they are now. It is also helpful for both the nurse and the client to express their feelings about termination openly and honestly. Thus, termination discussions need to start in advance of the termination interview. This allows time for the client to adjust to independence. In some situations, referrals are necessary, or it may be appropriate to offer an occasional standby meeting to give support as needed. Follow-up phone calls and emails are other interventions that ease the client's transition to independence.

Developing Helping Relationships

Whatever the practice setting, the nurse establishes some type of helping relationship in which mutual goals (outcomes) are set with the client or, if the client is unable to participate, with support people. Although special training in counseling techniques is advantageous, there are many ways of helping clients that do not require special training:

- Listen actively.
- Help to identify what the client is feeling. Clients who are troubled are often unable to identify or label their feelings and consequently have difficulty working them out or talking about them. Responses such as "You seem angry about taking orders from your boss" or "You sound as if you've been lonely since your wife died" can help clients recognize what they are feeling and talk about it.
- Put yourself in the client's shoes (i.e., empathize). Communicate to the client in a way that shows an understanding of the client's feelings and the behavior and experience underlying these feelings.
- Be honest. In effective relationships, nurses honestly recognize any lack of knowledge by saying "I don't know the answer to that right now"; openly discuss their own discomfort by saying, for example, "I feel uncomfortable about this discussion"; and admit tactfully that problems do exist, for instance, when a client says "I'm a mess, aren't I?"
- Be genuine and credible. Clients will sense whether you are truly concerned.
- Use your resourcefulness. There are always many courses of action to consider in handling problems. Whatever course is chosen needs to further the achievement of the client's goals (outcomes), be compatible with the client's value system, and offer the probability of success.
- Be aware of cultural differences that may affect meaning and understanding (see Chapter 21 ∞). To facilitate nurse–client interaction, recognize the language(s) and dialect(s) the client uses. Provide a bilingual interpreter as needed for clients who have limited English language skills.
- Maintain client confidentiality. To maintain the client's right to privacy, share information only with other healthcare professionals as needed for effective care and treatment.
- Know your role and your limitations. Every client has unique strengths and problems. When you feel unable to handle some problems, the client should be informed and referred to the appropriate health professional. Clarify functions and roles, specifically what is expected of the client, the nurse, and the primary care provider.

Communication and the Nursing Process

Communication is an integral part of the nursing process. Nurses use communication skills in each phase of the nursing process. Communication skills are also important when caring for clients who have communication problems. They are even more important when the client has sensory, language, or cognitive deficits.

●○● NURSING MANAGEMENT

Assessing

To assess the client's communication abilities, the nurse determines communication impairments or barriers and communication style. Remember that culture may influence when and how a client speaks. Obviously, language varies according to age and development. With children, the nurse observes sounds, gestures, and vocabulary.

Impairments to Communication

Various barriers may alter a client's ability to send, receive, or comprehend messages. These include language deficits, sensory deficits, cognitive impairments, structural deficits, and paralysis. The nurse must assess each to determine their presence.

Language Deficits

Determine the client's primary language for communicating and whether a fluent interpreter is required. The language skills of some clients who use English as a second language may be inadequate to meet their needs.

Sensory Deficits

The ability to hear, see, feel, and smell are important adjuncts to communication. Deafness can significantly alter the message the client receives; impaired vision alters the ability to observe nonverbal behavior, such as a smile or a gesture; inability to feel and smell can impair the client's abilities to report injuries or detect the smoke from a fire. For clients with severe hearing impairments, follow these steps:

- Look for a medical alert bracelet (or necklace or tag) indicating hearing loss.
- Determine whether the client wears a hearing aid and whether it is functioning.
- Observe whether the client is attempting to see your face to read lips.
- Observe whether the client is attempting to communicate with sign language.

Cognitive Impairments

Any disorder that impairs cognitive functioning (e.g., cerebrovascular disease, Alzheimer's disease, and brain tumors or injuries) may affect a client's ability to use and understand language. These clients may develop total loss of speech, impaired speech or pronunciation, or the inability to find or name words. Certain medications, such as sedatives, antidepressants, and neuroleptics, may also impair speech, causing the client to use incomplete sentences or to slur words.

The nurse assesses whether these clients respond when asked a question and, if so, assesses the following: Is the client's speech fluent or hesitant? Does the client use words correctly? Can the client comprehend instructions as evidenced by following directions? Can the client repeat words or phrases? In addition, the nurse assesses the client's ability to understand written words: Can the client follow written directions? Can the client respond correctly by pointing to a written word? Can the client read aloud? Can the client recognize words or letters if unable to read whole sentences? The nurse uses large, clearly written words when trying to establish abilities in this area.

When the client is unconscious, the nurse looks for any indication that suggests comprehension of what is communicated (e.g., tries to arouse the client verbally and through touch). Ask a closed question like "Can you hear me?" and watch for a nonverbal response such as a nod of the head for yes or a shake for no; or ask for a hand squeeze or blink of the eye, once for yes or twice for no.

Structural Deficits

Structural deficits of the oral and nasal cavities and respiratory system can alter an individual's ability to speak clearly and spontaneously. Examples include cleft palate, artificial airways such as an endotracheal tube or tracheostomy, and laryngectomy (removal of the larynx). Extreme dyspnea (shortness of breath) can also impair speech patterns.

Paralysis

If verbal impairment is combined with paralysis of the upper extremities that impairs the client's ability to write, the nurse should determine whether the client can point, nod, shrug, blink, or squeeze a hand. Any of these gestures could be used to devise a beginning communication system.

Style of Communication

In assessing communication style, the nurse considers both verbal and nonverbal communication. In addition to physical barriers, some psychologic illnesses (e.g., depression or psychosis) influence the ability to communicate. The client may demonstrate constant verbalization of the same words or phrases, a loose association of ideas, or flight of ideas.

LIFESPAN CONSIDERATIONS Communication with Older Adults

Older adults may have physical or cognitive problems that necessitate nursing interventions for the improvement of communication skills. Some of the common ones are as follows:

- Sensory deficits, such as vision and hearing
- Cognitive impairment, as in dementia
- Neurologic deficits from strokes or other neurologic conditions, such as aphasia (expressive or receptive) and lack of movement
- Psychosocial problems, such as depression.

Recognition of specific needs and obtaining appropriate resources for clients can greatly increase their socialization and quality of life. Interventions directed toward improving communication in clients with these special needs are as follows:

- Make sure that assistive devices, glasses, and hearing aids are being used and are in good working order.
- Make referrals to appropriate resources, such as speech therapy.
- Make use of communications aids, such as communication boards, computers, or pictures, when possible.
- Keep environmental distractions to a minimum.
- Speak in short, simple sentences, one subject at a time—reinforce or repeat what is said when necessary.
- Always face the client when speaking—coming up behind someone may be frightening.
- Include family and friends in conversation.
- Use reminiscing, either in individual conversations or in groups, to maintain memory connections and to enhance self-identity and self-esteem in the older adult.
- When verbal expression and nonverbal expression are incongruent, believe the nonverbal. Clarification of this and attentiveness to client feelings will help promote a feeling of caring and acceptance.
- Find out what has been important and has meaning to the client, and try to maintain these things as much as possible. Even simple things such as bedtime rituals become important if clients are in a hospital or extended care setting.

Verbal Communication

When assessing verbal communication, the nurse focuses on three areas: the content of the message, the themes, and verbalized emotions. In addition, the nurse considers the following:

- Whether the communication pattern is slow, rapid, quiet, spontaneous, hesitant, evasive, and so on
- The vocabulary of the individual, particularly any changes from the vocabulary normally used (For example, a client who normally never swears may indicate increased stress or illness by an uncharacteristic use of profanity.)
- The presence of hostility, aggression, assertiveness, reticence, hesitance, anxiety, or loquaciousness (incessant verbalization) in communication
- Difficulties with verbal communication, such as slurring, stuttering, inability to pronounce a sound, lack of clarity in enunciation, inability to speak in sentences, loose association of ideas, flight of ideas, or the inability to find or name words or identify objects
- Refusal or inability to speak.

Nonverbal Communication

Consider nonverbal communication in relation to the client's culture. Pay attention to facial expression, gestures, body movements, affect, tone of voice, posture, and eye contact.

Diagnosing

An example of a nursing diagnosis for clients with communication problems can include altered verbal communication. Communication problems may be receptive (e.g., difficulty hearing) or expressive (e.g., difficulty speaking).

This nursing diagnosis is *not* useful when a client's communication problems are caused by a psychiatric illness. For example, a client with depression may have difficulty expressing feelings or have slowed thinking or responses time.

Other nursing diagnoses used for clients experiencing communication problems that involve altered verbal communication as the *etiology* could include the following: anxiety related to altered verbal communication; social seclusion related to altered verbal communication; potential for reduced social interaction related to altered verbal communication

Planning

When a nursing diagnosis related to altered verbal communication has been made, the nurse and client determine outcomes and begin planning ways to promote effective communication. The overall client outcome for individuals with altered verbal communication is to reduce or resolve the factors impairing the communication. Specific nursing interventions will be planned from the stated etiology. Examples of outcome criteria to evaluate the effectiveness of nursing interventions and the achievement of client goals follow.

The client:

- Communicates that needs are being met.
- Begins to establish a method of communication:
  - Signals yes or no to direct questions using vocalization or agreed-on physical cue (i.e., eye blink, hand squeeze).
  - Uses verbal or nonverbal techniques to indicate needs.
- Perceives the message accurately, as evidenced by appropriate verbal or nonverbal responses.
- Communicates effectively:
  - Using his or her dominant language
  - Using a translator or an interpreter
  - Using sign language
  - Using a word board or a picture board
  - Using a computer.
- Regains maximum communication abilities.
- Expresses minimum fear, anxiety, frustration, and depression.
- Uses resources appropriately.

Implementing

Nursing interventions to facilitate communication with clients who have problems with speech or language include manipulating the environment, providing support, employing measures to enhance communication, and educating the client and support person.

Manipulate the Environment

A quiet environment with limited distractions will make the most of the communication efforts of both the client and the nurse and increase the possibility of effective communication. Sufficient light will help in conveying nonverbal messages, which is especially important if visual or auditory acuity is impaired. Initially, the nurse needs to provide a calm, relaxed environment, which will help reduce any anxiety the client may have. Remember that any factor that affects communication can create feelings of frustration, anxiety, depression, or hostility in the client. Communication normally contributes to a client's sense of security and feelings that he or she is not alone, so communication problems may cause some clients to feel isolated and confused. To further reduce these emotions, the nurse should acknowledge and praise the client's attempts at communication.

Provide Support

The nurse should convey encouragement to the client and provide nonverbal reassurance, perhaps by touch if appropriate. If the nurse does not understand, it is critical to let the client know so that he or she can provide clarification with other words or through some other means of communication. When speaking with a client who will have difficulty understanding, the nurse should check frequently to determine what the client has heard and understood. Using open-ended questions will assist the nurse in obtaining accurate information about the effectiveness of communication. For example, a female client who has limited English skills is being taught about diet related to her Crohn disease. If the nurse asks, "Do you understand what to eat?" the client may nod her head yes. However, this does not give the nurse confirmation that the client received the message given. Rather, the nurse needs to say, "What do you think will be good for you to eat when you go home?" The nurse's body language (e.g., gestures, posture, facial expression, and eye contact) should convey acceptance and approval.

Employ Measures to Enhance Communication

First determine how the client can best receive messages: by listening, by looking, through touch, or through an interpreter. Ways to help communication include keeping words simple and concrete and discussing topics of interest to the client. It is often helpful to use alternative communication strategies such as word boards, pictures, or paper and pencil.

Interpreters can often assist a client and nurse to communicate when the client lacks fluency in the dominant language. Some hospitals have a list of interpreters for various languages who can assist at the bedside. If the client's support person offers to interpret, it is important to ask the client's permission, for the sake of confidentiality. Then instruct the individual interpreting to translate as precisely as possible, without interruption (see Chapter 3 ∞ for working with a healthcare interpreter).

Educate the Client and Support People

Sometimes clients and support people can be prepared in advance for communication problems, for example, before an intubation or throat surgery. When the nurse explains anticipated problems, the client is often less anxious when problems arise.

Evaluating

Evaluation is useful for both client and nurse communication.

Client Communication

To establish whether client outcomes have been met in relation to communication, the nurse must listen actively, observe nonverbal cues, and use therapeutic communication skills to determine that communication was effective. Examples of statements indicating outcome achievement include "Using picture board effectively to indicate needs" or "The client stated, 'I listened more closely to my daughter yesterday and found out how she feels about our divorce.'"

Nurse Communication

For nursing students to evaluate the effectiveness of their own communication with clients, process recordings are frequently used. A **process recording** is a verbatim (word-for-word) account of a conversation. It can be taped or written and includes all verbal and nonverbal interactions of both the client and nurse.

One method of writing a process recording is to make two columns on a page. The first column lists what the nurse and the client said along with the associated nonverbal behavior. The second column contains an analysis of the nurse's responses.

Once a process recording has been completed, it should be analyzed in terms of the content and meaning of the interaction based on communication theory. Each of the nursing student's statements is interpreted in terms of the communication skill used, with the rationale for and effectiveness of its use. Any barriers to effective communication can be identified, with a possible alternative response noted. The outcome should be increased awareness and insight regarding one's communication strengths, as well as the identification of areas for future skills development.

Communication Among Health Professionals

Effective communication among the health professions is as important as the promotion of therapeutic communication between the nurse and the client. Communication problems among healthcare personnel threaten client well-being and safety. For example, victims of incivility or bullying often fear being near the uncivil individuals. This can lead to important client information not being shared and jeopardizing client safety. Besides undermining client care, disruptive behaviors also negatively affect staff morale.

Many nurses report being victims of incivility and bullying, with even more reporting witnessing abusive behavior in healthcare (Chu & Evans, 2016; Sauer & McCoy, 2018). These disruptive behaviors have a negative impact on the work environment and are one of the reasons nurses leave the profession.

The Joint Commission recognizes workplace intimidation as a threat to client safety and requires healthcare facilities to design and implement a system-wide approach for ensuring employee awareness of disruptive and bullying behaviors (The Joint Commission, 2016). Nevertheless, the literature reflects that the disruptive behaviors of incivility and bullying persist.

Disruptive Behaviors

Incivility, bullying, and workplace violence have touched too many members of the nursing profession for nearly a century. They affect every nursing specialty (ANA, 2015b).

Incivility

Incivility consists of behaviors that are disrespectful, rude, impolite, and promote conflict while increasing stress (ANA, 2015b; Danza, 2018, p. 49). Examples include, but are not limited to, rolling of the eyes, gossiping, spreading rumors, name calling, using a condescending tone, sarcastic comments, interrupting others when they are speaking, and using public criticism. Marshall (2017) states, "Nursing students are no different from other people who find themselves affected by incivility—sometimes as the target, sometimes as the perpetrator, and sometimes as an observer" (p. 5).

Research literature supports a relationship between workplace incivility and negative health consequences, such as emotional exhaustion. The literature also describes a relationship between incivility and nurse productivity. Examples include absenteeism, decreased commitment to the organization, decreased effort at work, incivility toward others, decreased communication, decreased reporting of problems, and leaving the organization.

Incivility and its consequences destroy the ideal organizational climate of mutual respect. Moreover, incivility may become a precursor to bullying and workplace violence.

Bullying

Bullying is "repeated, health-harming mistreatment of one or more persons by one or more perpetrators" (The Joint Commission, 2016, para 2). Central to all bullying behavior in nursing is the *consistent* demonstration of inappropriate behavior. An *occasional* angry outburst or rude comment constitutes poor judgment but is generally not bullying behavior (Meires, 2018, p. 150).

The Joint Commission (2016) states that bullying is "abusive conduct that takes one or more of the following forms: verbal abuse; threatening, intimidating or humiliating behaviors (including nonverbal); work interference—sabotage—which prevents work from getting done" (para 2). Examples of bullying actions include those that harm, undermine, and degrade. These include behaviors such as persistent hostility, intimidation, isolation, exclusion, regular verbal attacks, refusal to assist with duties, and taunting the nurse in front of others (ANA, 2015b; Keller, Budin, & Allie, 2016). These actions can cause physical and psychologic effects on victims, such as headaches, anxiety, insomnia, gastrointestinal disorders, poor concentration, depression, helplessness, and loss of confidence and self-esteem (Danza, 2018).

Bullying often involves an abuse or misuse of power. It may be directed from the top down (employers against employees), from the bottom up (employees against employers), or laterally or horizontally (colleagues against colleagues; ANA, 2015b, p. 3). There is the saying in nursing that nurses "eat their young," meaning that experienced nurses bully newly licensed nurses (NLNs). Unfortunately, many NLNs believe this is a rite of passage, and they will eventually mimic the bullying behavior with future NLNs (Chu & Evans, 2016). Bullying, however, also occurs in novice nurses against experienced nurses. For example, NLNs may be critical of or impatient with the experienced nurses because they may not be as technologically proficient in the use of electronic health records, or they may think the experienced nurse's practice is outdated. Bullying causes health problems for the target, a hostile work environment that hinders effective communication, and nurse-retention problems for the organization.

Workplace Violence

The Occupational Safety and Health Administration (OSHA) defines workplace violence as "any act or threat of physical violence, harassment, intimidation, or other threatening disruptive behavior that occurs at the work site. It ranges from threats and verbal abuse to physical assaults and even homicide" (OSHA, n.d., para 1). There are four types of violence that nurses may come upon in the work setting, with types 2 and 3 being the most common in healthcare:

1. ***Criminal intent.*** The perpetrator has no relationship with the victim, and the violence is carried out in conjunction with a crime.
2. ***Customer or client.*** This is the most common healthcare environment–based assault, in which the perpetrator is a member of the public with whom the nurse is interacting during the course of the nurse's regular duties.
3. ***Worker-on-worker.*** Commonly perceived as bullying, in these instances, the perpetrator and victim work together, although not necessarily in the same role or at the same level.
4. ***Personal relationship.*** In these incidents, the victim has been targeted as a result of an existing exterior relationship with the perpetrator, with the violence taking place in the workplace (ANA, n.d.; ANA, 2017).

The highest risk for workplace violence is found in the following settings: emergency departments, intensive care units, behavioral health units, and long-term care facilities (ANA, 2015b; Chu & Evans, 2016; The Joint Commission, 2016). The nursing literature provides evidence of the attitude that workplace violence is a culturally accepted and expected part of the healthcare occupation. Unfortunately, too often, client safety is given priority over employee safety when both are needed for quality, safe care.

Responding to Disruptive Behaviors

Several organizations have issued statements regarding the harmful effect of disruptive behaviors on both nurses and client safety. The Joint Commission (n.d.) provides an online portal to share information and resources regarding the prevention of workplace violence in healthcare

EVIDENCE-BASED PRACTICE

Evidence-Based Practice

What Are the Experiences of Bullying Encountered by Nursing Students in the Clinical Setting?

Research studies reflect that nursing students experience bullying behaviors. Smith, Gillespie, Brown, and Grubb (2016), however, found that little is known about nursing students' beliefs about and responses to bullying. They conducted a descriptive qualitative study to describe the experiences of bullying encountered by nursing students in the clinical setting. They believe that understanding these aspects may provide important information from which interventions can be developed. Fifty-six senior baccalaureate nursing students from four college campuses in the midwestern United States completed the study. The nursing students attended a focus-group session held at their college. They were asked to describe their personal experiences of bullying while a nursing student in the clinical setting, the impact bullying had on achieving their learning objectives while in the clinical setting, and recommendations for future nursing students who may encounter bullying in the clinical setting. Focus-group data were coded and analyzed, resulting in four categories identified as bullying behaviors, rationale for bullying, response to bullying, and recommendations to address bullying. Each category had corresponding themes. The category of bullying behaviors had six themes: being ignored, avoided, or isolated; witnessing nonverbal behaviors; experiencing negative interactions; being denied an opportunity to learn; being hazed; and being intimidated. The category of rationale for bullying included five unique themes: rite of passage, unpreventable, students not welcome, other stressors, and not a nice person. The category of response to bullying included seven distinct themes: physical, emotional, psychologic, avoidance, productivity and performance, learning, and view of healthcare. The final category, recommendations to address bullying, identified eight specific areas of focus: Educate and prepare students, student responses to bullying, support, faculty responses, facility-organization responses, qualifications of preceptors, making student assignments, and clarifying the role of nursing students.

Implications

The researchers state that the findings from this study indicate that nursing students do experience bullying behaviors in the clinical setting. Interventions based on these findings and implemented by nurse educators could assist nursing students with recognizing and responding to bullying behaviors in ways that promote a positive and ethical work culture. Nurse educators must work collaboratively with clinical nurses and leaders in the healthcare agencies where clinical experiences are held to support a culture of safety and zero tolerance for bullying and other types of workplace aggression.

settings. Although The Joint Commission does not have standards specific to workplace violence, several standards relate directly or indirectly to its prevention (The Joint Commission, 2018).

The ANA issued a zero-tolerance position statement entitled *Incivility, Bullying, and Workplace Violence* (ANA, 2015b). This statement emphasizes the shared roles and responsibilities of RNs and employers to create and sustain healthy workplaces. The ANA *Code of Ethics for Nurses with Interpretive Statements* reinforces that nurses have an ethical, moral, and legal responsibility to create a healthy and safe work environment by stating that nurses are required to "create an ethical environment and culture of civility and kindness, treating colleagues, coworkers, employees, students, and others with dignity and respect" (ANA, 2015a, p. 4).

Efforts at both state and national levels are being proposed to help organizations prevent the occurrence of workplace violence. For example, California and eight other states (Connecticut, Illinois, Maine, Maryland, New Jersey, New York, Oregon, and Washington) have created laws mandating plans for workplace violence prevention within healthcare facilities (Kopp, 2018, p. 13).

Interventions for promoting and creating a culture of health and safety (e.g., a safe environment) are needed at the individual, administrative, and educational levels (Box 16.2). The goal is to create a respectful work environment that empowers nurses and enhances the well-being of their clients.

Nurse and Physician Communication

There are guidelines for written documentation and for nurses communicating with clients. However, few guidelines exist for the frequent verbal communication that occurs between nurses and physicians. This lack of guidelines or format may contribute to medical errors because of communication problems.

Communication Styles

In general, nurses have been taught to be descriptive in verbal and written communication. Conversely, physicians are trained to be concise, to the point, and focused on a problem. These differences in communication styles may hinder physician–nurse collaboration. Communication errors in the healthcare setting often have severe consequences that can lead to negative client outcomes, such as increased length of stay, client dissatisfaction, and even death. Thus, The Joint Commission and the Institute for Healthcare Improvement have mandated that healthcare organizations improve professional communication. One model, called SBAR (situation, background, assessment, recommendations), provides a standardized framework

BOX 16.2 Interventions to Promote a Safe Work Environment

INDIVIDUAL

- Be respectful of others.
- Raise awareness of disruptive behaviors in self and others.
- Increase communication skills to intervene when others display disruptive behaviors.
- Create norms for a civil workplace.
- Establish an agreed-upon code word or signal to seek support when feeling threatened.
- Become familiar with the employer's incivility and bullying prevention policies and procedures.
- Understand policies and procedures related to workplace violence prevention and response.

ADMINISTRATIVE

- Develop a position statement that supports zero tolerance for incivility, bullying, and workplace violence.
- Develop a violence prevention program.
- Clearly define the disruptive behavior that is not allowed.
- Orient employees to strategies available for conflict resolution and respectful communication.
- Develop an emotionally safe work environment.
- Develop and implement a strong code of conduct.
- Assess the culture of the work unit(s) for the presence of disruptive behavior.
- Intervene when disruptive behaviors occur.
- Model professional ethical behavior.

NURSING ACADEMIC PROGRAMS AND NURSING CONTINUING EDUCATION

- Develop and implement curricula that educate nursing students on the incidence of disruptive behaviors along with steps to stop the behavior.
- Model desired actions to promote both a culture of civility and a healthy workplace.
- Provide training in conflict management.
- Develop educational programs regarding strategies on how to recognize and address disruptive behaviors.

for communicating important information. The SBAR format can be used by nurses in almost all forms of communication, including when calling a primary care provider about a change in a client's condition, providing shift reports, giving reports on clients being transferred within or outside the health facility, and sending clients for procedures. Box 16.3 contains more details on this communication framework.

Clinical Alert!

Prepare before calling the primary care provider to report a client problem. You will be using the SBAR method. However, you also need to think about what information may be asked of you and be prepared to answer those questions. This means knowing the most recent client assessment data, including vital signs, laboratory data, and other tests, if appropriate. Have the client's medical record, medication administration record, and other flow sheets as needed available to you.

Emotional Intelligence

Emotional intelligence (EI) is the ability to form work relationships with colleagues, display maturity in a variety of situations, and resolve conflicts while taking into consideration the emotions of others. In work environments, professionals can demonstrate EI by accurately identifying their own emotions and the emotions of others, managing those emotions, and then deciding how to interact with colleagues constructively to achieve a positive outcome.

EI is accepted as an essential quality of successful leaders, and there is growing recognition that it is also an important characteristic of nurses. For example, Fitzpatrick (2016) proposes using the Emotional Competence Framework to develop EI skills in nursing students as part of their basic nursing programs. This framework outlines the personal skills (self-awareness, self-control, and self-motivation) and the social competence skills (including social awareness and social skills) necessary for EI.

BOX 16.3 SBAR: Situation, Background, Assessment, Recommendation Model

A FRAMEWORK FOR NURSE–HEALTHCARE PROVIDER COMMUNICATION

S = Situation: What is the situation you are calling about? Provide your name, health agency, client name, and *brief* information about the problem.

B = Background: Provide information pertinent to the current situation, such as admitting diagnosis, date of admission, and important clinical information that relates to the call.

A = Assessment: This refers to the current condition of the client (e.g., vital signs, oxygen saturation, pain scale, level of consciousness) and any change in the assessment since the previous communication. Indicate the severity of the problem.

R = Recommendation: What is your recommendation for resolving the problem, or what do you need from the healthcare provider (e.g., come see the client, transfer to another unit, or an order for a medication)?

EXAMPLE OF USING SBAR WHEN CALLING A HEALTHCARE PROVIDER ABOUT A CLIENT PROBLEM

S: Healthcare provider called. Nurse has given name and unit of healthcare agency. "I'm calling about Sally Somers, a 19-year-old admitted this morning with a ruptured appendix. She is now 6 hours postop and has not voided.

B: Her bladder is distended. She is complaining of urgency to void but unable to do so even with sitting on commode, running water. Everything else is stable.

A: She is very uncomfortable and crying because of her urinary retention.

R: "Could you give an order for a straight urinary catheterization?"

Assertive Communication

Assertive communication promotes client safety by minimizing miscommunication with colleagues. People who use assertive communication are honest, direct, and appropriate while being open to ideas and respecting the rights of others.

An important characteristic of assertive communication includes the use of "I" statements versus "you" statements. The "you" statement places blame and puts the listener in a defensive position, whereas the "I" statement encourages discussion. For example, a nurse who states "I am concerned about . . . " will be gaining the attention of the primary care provider while also giving a message about the importance of working together for the benefit of the client. It is then important for the nurse to be clear, concise, organized, and fully informed when verbally presenting the client concern.

Nonassertive Communication

Two types of interpersonal behaviors are considered nonassertive: passive and aggressive.

PASSIVE

When people use a passive or submissive communication style, they say nothing even when they have been wronged. This is also known as self-silencing (Beebe et al., 2019). Individuals who use passive communication tend to internalize their frustrations, which may build into rage that explodes later.

AGGRESSIVE

There is a fine line between assertive and aggressive communication. Assertive communication is an open expression of ideas and opinions while respecting the rights, opinions, and ideas of others. Aggressive communication is self-serving in that it is directed toward what one wants without considering the feelings of others (Beebe et al., 2019). This type of communication is ineffective and leads to frustration for the nurse and the primary care provider.

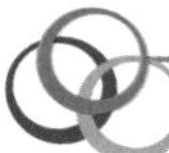

Critical Thinking Checkpoint

You are the nursing student assigned to care for Mr. Manasovitz, a 45-year-old man who will be returning from the recovery room after undergoing the removal of a mass from his abdomen. While you are preparing his room for his return, the nurse and primary care provider arrive to talk with Mrs. Manasovitz about her husband's surgery. The primary care provider explains that the mass was malignant and invasive. Mr. Manasovitz is a candidate for chemotherapy, but his prognosis is guarded because of the extent of the tumor growth. Mrs. Manasovitz looks away, closes her eyes, and only nods her head "yes." As the primary care provider leaves, the nurse approaches Mrs. Manasovitz, sits next to her, and puts her arm around Mrs. Manasovitz, who begins to cry. The nurse uses a soothing voice to tell Mrs. Manasovitz that it is okay to cry and assures her she will remain with her. The two of them sit in silence until Mrs. Manasovitz is able to express her feelings. The nurse listens attentively. Later, the nurse offers to get a cup of coffee for Mrs. Manasovitz and asks if there is anything she can do to assist Mrs. Manasovitz at this difficult time.

1. Interpret Mrs. Manasovitz's nonverbal behavior in response to the news about her husband's surgery.
2. Evaluate the nurse's response toward Mrs. Manasovitz based on the concepts of caring and comforting.
3. Why is it important for the nurse to effectively communicate with Mrs. Manasovitz at this time?
4. The nurse was described as listening attentively to Mrs. Manasovitz. Cite actions that portray attentive listening.

Answers to Critical Thinking Checkpoint questions are available on the faculty resources site. Please consult with your instructor.

Chapter 16 Review

CHAPTER HIGHLIGHTS

- Communication is a critical nursing skill used to gather assessment data for nursing diagnoses, to teach and persuade, and to express caring and comfort.
- Communication is a two-way interpersonal process involving the sender of the message and the receiver of the message. It also involves intrapersonal messages, or self-talk, which can affect the message, the interpretation of the message, and the response.
- The communication process includes four elements: sender, message, receiver, and response or feedback. The sender must encode the message and determine the appropriate form for transmitting it. The receiver must perceive the message, decode it, and then respond.
- Verbal communication is effective when the criteria of pace and intonation, simplicity, clarity and brevity, timing and relevance, adaptability, credibility, and humor are met.
- Nonverbal communication often reveals more about an individual's thoughts and feelings than verbal communication; it includes personal appearance, posture, gait, facial expressions, and gestures.
- When assessing verbal and nonverbal communication, the nurse needs to consider cultural influences and be aware that a single

nonverbal expression can indicate any of a variety of feelings and that words can have various meanings.

- The use of electronic communication in nursing practice is increasing. Although email provides positive advantages for improving communication and the continuity of client care, the nurse needs to be aware of the risk to client confidentiality.
- Many factors influence the communication process: development, gender, values and perceptions, personal space (intimate, personal, social, and public distances), territoriality, roles and relationships, environment, congruence, interpersonal attitudes, and boundaries.
- Many techniques facilitate therapeutic communication: using silence, providing general leads, being specific and tentative, using open-ended questions, using touch, restating or paraphrasing, seeking clarification, perception checking or seeking consensual validation, offering self, giving information, acknowledging, clarifying time or sequence, presenting reality, focusing, reflecting, summarizing, and planning.
- Techniques that inhibit communication include stereotyping, being defensive, challenging, testing, rejecting, changing topics and subjects, unwarranted reassurance, passing judgment, and giving common advice.
- The effective nurse–client relationship is a helping relationship that facilitates the growth of the client.
- Four phases of the helping relationship include the preinteraction phase, the introductory phase, the working phase, and the resolution phase; each has specific tasks and skills.
- To help clients with communication problems, the nurse manipulates the environment, provides support, employs measures to enhance communication, and educates the client and support people.
- Process recordings are frequently made by nursing students to evaluate the effectiveness of their own communication. With them, students can analyze both the process and the content of the communication.
- Effective communication between health professionals is vital for client safety.
- Many nurses report disruptive behaviors from physicians and other nurses. Disruptive behavior is defined as behavior that interferes with effective communication among healthcare providers and negatively impacts performance and outcomes. Three common disruptive behaviors are incivility, bullying, and workplace violence.
- Several organizations have issued statements regarding the harmful effects of disruptive behaviors on both nurses and client safety. Nurses must be as proficient in communication skills as they are in clinical skills.
- Communication styles can differ between nurses and physicians. Nurses tend to be more narrative and descriptive and strive for consensus. Physicians focus on a need or problem and are trained to give and want information in bullet points. The SBAR model is one approach aimed at addressing these differences in communication style and approach. Studies have shown that interdisciplinary simulations can also enhance communication between nurses and physicians.
- Assertive communication promotes client safety by minimizing miscommunication with colleagues. An important characteristic of assertive communication is to use "I" statements.
- Nonassertive communication includes two types of interpersonal behaviors: passive and aggressive.

TEST YOUR KNOWLEDGE

1. A student nurse is caring for a 72-year-old client with Alzheimer's disease who is very confused. Which is the most appropriate communication strategy to be used by the student nurse?
   1. Written directions for bathing
   2. Speaking very loudly
   3. Gentle touch while providing activities of daily living
   4. Flat facial expression

2. Place the following descriptions of the helping relationship phases in the correct sequence.
   1. _____ After introductions, the nurse asks, "What plans do you have for the upcoming holiday weekend?"
   2. _____ The nurse states, "It sounds like you are concerned about the possible complications of having diabetes. What would be the most helpful for you at this time?"
   3. _____ The nurse reads in the medical history that the client was diagnosed with diabetes 1 week ago.
   4. _____ The nurse states, "When we met, you knew very little about diabetes, and now you are able to use your new information and apply it to your own personal situations."

3. A client is nonverbal, and the assigned nurse is implementing strategies to promote communication. Which of the following would be appropriate for the client in this situation?
   1. Using a picture board to facilitate communication
   2. Facing the client when speaking
   3. Employing an interpreter
   4. Making sure that the language spoken is the client's dominant language

4. A nurse tells a client who is struggling with cancer pain, "It is normal to feel frustrated about the discomfort." Which is most representative of the skills associated with the working phase of the helping relationship?
   1. Respect
   2. Genuineness
   3. Concreteness
   4. Confrontation

5. The nurse will need to assess which of the following clients for the possible nursing diagnosis of altered verbal communication? Select all that apply.
   1. A client who uses sign language
   2. A client with a psychiatric illness
   3. A client with the medical diagnosis of cerebral vascular accident (stroke)
   4. A client having a problem coping with a cancer diagnosis
   5. A client experiencing extreme dyspnea (shortness of breath)

6. After being admitted for emergency surgery, an 80-year-old client has just returned to the hospital room from the postanesthesia room. Which nursing interventions are most likely to facilitate effective communication with this client? Select all that apply.
   1. Ask the client, "Do you know where you are?"
   2. Ask the client or support person(s) about visual or learning problems.
   3. Inform the client and support person(s) about events likely to occur during the next 2 hours.
   4. Provide the client with instructions about discharge.
   5. Tell the client, "You will feel better soon."
7. A nurse enters a client's room and finds that the telephone is lying on the client's lap, tissues are wadded up on the bed, and the client's eyes are red and watery. What is the best response by the nurse?
   1. "Can I hang that phone up for you?"
   2. "Well, it's a beautiful day outside. Let's open the blinds."
   3. "Has your doctor been in to talk to you yet?"
   4. "You look upset. Is there anything you'd like to talk about?"
8. The client made the following statement to the nurse, "My doctor just told me that he cannot save my leg and that I need to have an above-the-knee amputation." Which response by the nurse is most appropriate?
   1. "Dr. Jones is an excellent surgeon."
   2. "Are you in pain?"
   3. "If I were you, I'd get a second opinion."
   4. "Tell me more . . . "
9. Assertive communication is an appropriate approach for nurses to use in the clinical area. Which of the following would be an example of this type of communication technique when a nurse is addressing a physician?
   1. "You need to check the laboratory results of the client in room 423."
   2. "You should visit with the client's family about the upcoming procedure."
   3. "We need to be more aware of the situation among the client and the client's family."
   4. "I am concerned that the client does not have adequate pain management."
10. The nurse asks the client, "What do you fear most about your surgery tomorrow?" This is an example of which communication technique?
   1. Providing general leads
   2. Seeking clarification
   3. Presenting reality
   4. Summarizing

See Answers to Test Your Knowledge in Appendix A.

READINGS AND REFERENCES

Suggested Readings

Ciocco, M. (2018). Speaking to the bully within. *Imprint, 65*(5), 24–27.

The author writes about bullying among nursing students. Find out if you could be considered a bully. Do not become a "wounded healer."

Malone, B. R. (2016). Intimidating behavior among healthcare workers is still jeopardizing medication safety. *Nephrology Nursing Journal*, *43*(2), 157–159.

The author presents data from the Institute for Safe Medication Practices (ISMP). The data reflect that many healthcare providers have encountered instances of intimidation and disrespectful behavior in their practice, which may have led to a larger incidence of medication errors.

Squires, A. (2017). Evidence-based approaches to breaking down language barriers. *Nursing*, *47*(9), 34–40. doi:10.1097/01.NURSE.0000522002.60278.ca

This article provides background information about language barriers between nurses and clients and strategies for addressing these gaps.

Related Research

Corwin, A. I. (2018). Overcoming elderspeak: A qualitative study of three alternatives. *The Gerontologist*, *58*, 724–729. doi:10.1093/geront/gnx009

Funk, A., Garcia, C., & Mullen, T. (2018). Understanding the hospital experience of older adults with hearing impairment. Findings from a qualitative study. *American Journal of Nursing*, *118*(6), 28–34. doi:10.1097/01.NAJ.0000534821.03997.7b

Sauer, P. A., & McCoy, T. P. (2018). Nurse bullying and intent to leave. *Nursing Economic$*, *36*(5), 219–224, 245.

References

American Nurses Association. (n.d.). *Violence, incivility, & bullying*. Retrieved from https://www.nursingworld.org/practice-policy/work-environment/violence-incivility-bullying

American Nurses Association. (2015a). *Code of ethics for nurses with interpretive statements*. Silver Spring, MD: Author.

American Nurses Association. (2015b). *Position statement on incivility, bullying, and workplace violence*. Retrieved from https://www.nursingworld.org/~49d6e3/globalassets/practiceandpolicy/nursing-excellence/incivility-bullying-and-workplace-violence-ana-position-statement.pdf

American Nurses Association. (2017). *Workplace violence*. Retrieved from https://www.nursingworld.org/practice-policy/advocacy/state/workplace-violence2

Beebe, S. A., Beebe, S. J., & Ivy, D. K. (2019). *Communication: Principles for a lifetime* (7th ed.). Boston, MA: Pearson.

Biddle, S., & Milstead, A. J. (2016). The intersection of policy and informatics. *Nursing Management*, *47*(2), 12–13. doi:10.1097/01.NUMA.0000479453.73651.89

Boyd, M. (2017). *Essentials of psychiatric nursing*. Philadelphia, PA: Wolters Kluwer.

Chu, R. Z., & Evans, M. M. (2016). Lateral violence in nursing. *Med-Surg Matters*, *25*(6), 4–6.

Danza, P. (2018). On the line: Confronting isolation and bullying in the workplace. *Nursing*, *48*(11), 48–53. doi:10.1097/01.NURSE.0000546460.41768.aa

Egan, G., & Reese, R. J. (2019). *The skilled helper: A problem-management & opportunity-development approach to helping* (11th ed.). Boston, MA: Cengage.

Fitzpatrick, J. J. (2016). Helping nursing students develop and expand their emotional intelligence. *Nursing Education Perspectives*, *37*, 124. doi:10.1097/01.NEP.0000000000000020

Industry Watch. (2016). Doctor/patient communications. Can email improve patient outcomes? *Health Management Technology*, *37*(4), 6.

The Joint Commission. (n.d.). *Workplace violence prevention resources for health care*. Retrieved from https://www.jointcommission.org/workplace_violence.aspx

The Joint Commission. (2016). *Quick safety 24: Bullying has no place in health care*. Retrieved from https://www.jointcommission.org/issues/article.aspx?Article=rFhOFvmOhideyaeaXWHwdF7ilsdGP+TcEobEhA7d2RU=

The Joint Commission. (2018). *Questions & answers: Hospital accreditation standards & workplace violence*. Retrieved from https://www.jointcommission.org/questions_answers_hospital_accreditation_standards_workplace_violence

Keller, R., Budin, W., & Allie, T. (2016). A task force to address bullying. *American Journal of Nursing*, *116*(2), 52–58. doi:10.1097/01.NAJ.0000480497.63846.d0

Kneisl, C. R. *Sample process recording material*. Orange Beach, AL: Author.

Kopp, G. S. (2018). Workplace violence: Understanding and dealing with it. *AAACN Viewpoint*, *40*(4), 12–14.

Marshall, L. S. (2017). Incivility is not normal, and it's certainly not acceptable! *Reflections on Nursing Leadership*, *43*(1), 31–37.

Meires, J. (2018). Workplace incivility. The essentials: Using emotional intelligence to curtail bullying in the workplace. *Urologic Nursing*, *38*, 150–153. doi:10.7257/1053-816X.2018.38.3.150

Occupational Safety and Health Administration. (n.d.). *Workplace violence*. Retrieved from https://www.osha.gov/SLTC/workplaceviolence

Seiler, W. J., Beall, M., & Mazer, J. P. (2017). *Communication: Making connections* (10th ed.). Boston, MA: Pearson.

Smith, C. R., Gillespie, G. L., Brown, K. C., & Grubb, P. L. (2016). Seeing students squirm: Nursing students' experiences of bullying behaviors during clinical rotations. *Journal of Nursing Education*, *55*(9), 505–513. doi:10.3928/01484834-20160816-04

Williams, K., Shaw, C., Lee, A., Kim, S., & Dinneen, E., Turk, M., . . . Liu, W. (2017). Voicing ageism in nursing home dementia care. *Journal of Gerontological Nursing*, *43*(9), 16–20. doi:10.3928/00989134-20170523-02

Selected Bibliography

Anderson, A. (2018). Getting and giving report. *American Journal of Nursing*, *118*(6), 56–60. doi:10.1097/01.NAJ.0000534853.43008.d6

Beebe, S. A., & Masterson, J. T. (2016). *Communicating in small groups: Principles and practices* (11th ed.). Upper Saddle River, NJ: Pearson.

Breiten, K., Condie, E., Vaillancourt, S., Walker, J., & Moore, G. (2018). Successfully managing challenging patient encounters. *American Nurse Today*, *13*(10), 6–9.

Choudhary, L. (2018). Educational strategies for conflict management. *Nursing*, *48*(12), 14–15. doi:10.1097/01.NURSE.0000547734.74555.3c

Civility best practices for nurses. (2018). *Kentucky Nurse*, *66*(4), 12–13.

Flood, T. (2018). Promoting patient- and family-centered care with virtual rounding. *American Nurse Today*, *13*(9), 84–85.

Germann, S., & Moore, S. (2017). Lateral violence, a nursing epidemic? *Reflections on Nursing Leadership*, *43*(1), 39–43.

Institute for Healthcare Improvement. (2016). *SBAR toolkit*. Retrieved from http://www.ihi.org/resources/Pages/Tools/SBARToolkit.aspx

Judd, M. (2017). Communication strategies for patients with dementia. *Nursing*, *47*(12), 58–61. doi:10.1097/01.NURSE.0000524758.05259.f7

Meires, J. (2018a). Workplace incivility. The essentials: Here's what you need to know about bullying in nursing. *Urologic Nursing*, *38*(2), 95–98. doi:10.7257/1053-816X.2018.38.2.95

Meires, J. (2018b). Workplace incivility: When students bully faculty. *Urologic Nursing*, *38*(5), 251–254. doi:10.7257/1053-816X.2018.38.5.251

Neil, H. P. (2018). Incivility in the workplace. *Med-Surg Matters*, *27*(6), 8–9.

Nelson, R. (2018). Sexual harassment in nursing. *American Journal of Nursing*, *118*(5), 19–20. doi:10.1097/01.NAJ.0000532826.47647.42

Nolte, J. A. (2018). Physician-nurse relationships after participation in a shadowing program. *Nursing*, *48*(12), 66–69. doi:10.1097/01.NURSE.0000547726.15352.ac

Perry, V. (2016). CNE SERIES. A daily goals tool to facilitate indirect nurse-physician communication during morning rounds on a medical-surgical unit. *MEDSURG Nursing*, *25*(2), 83–87.

Singleton, C. (2016). Sticks and stones. *Journal of Community Nursing*, *30*(1), 12–13.

Streeton, A. (2016). Improving nurse-physician teamwork: A multidisciplinary collaboration. *MEDSURG Nursing*, *25*(1), 31–66.

Tapper, M. L. (2016). Radical acceptance. *MEDSURG Nursing*, *25*(1), 1–3.

Trossman, S. (2018). On unsafe ground. A call for real change and policies to prevent violence against nurses. *American Nurse Today*, *13*(1), 36–38.

Wilson, J. L. (2016). An exploration of bullying behaviours in nursing: A review of the literature. *British Journal of Nursing*, *25*(6), 303–306. doi:10.12968/bjon.2016.25.6.303

Teaching 17

LEARNING OUTCOMES

After completing this chapter, you will be able to:

1. Discuss the importance of the teaching role of the nurse.
2. Compare and contrast andragogy, pedagogy, and geragogy.
3. Describe the three learning domains.
4. Discuss the learning theories of behaviorism, cognitivism, and humanism and how nurses can use each of these theories.
5. Identify factors that affect learning.
6. Discuss the implications of using the internet as a source of health information.
7. Assess learning needs of learners and the learning environment.
8. Discuss the implications of low health literacy skills.
9. Identify nursing diagnoses, outcomes, and interventions that reflect the learning needs of clients.
10. Describe the essential aspects of a teaching plan.
11. Discuss guidelines for effective teaching.
12. Discuss strategies to use when teaching clients of different cultures.
13. Identify methods to evaluate learning.
14. Describe effective documentation of teaching–learning activities.

KEY TERMS

adherence, *323*
affective domain, *323*
andragogy, *323*
behaviorist theory, *324*
cognitive domain, *323*
cognitive theory, *324*
compliance, *323*
geragogy, *323*
health literacy, *331*
humanistic learning theory, *324*
imitation, *324*
learning, *323*
learning need, *323*
modeling, *324*
motivation, *325*
pedagogy, *323*
positive reinforcement, *324*
psychomotor domain, *323*
readiness, *325*
teaching, *321*

Introduction

Teaching client education is a major aspect of nursing practice and an important independent nursing function. In 1992, the American Hospital Association initiated *A Patient's Bill of Rights*, mandating client education as a right of all clients. State nurse practice acts include client teaching as a function of nursing, thereby making teaching a legal and professional responsibility. In addition, the American Nurses Association (ANA, 2015) has regularly issued statements on the scope and standards of professional nursing practice, of which client teaching is a key element.

Client education is multifaceted, involving promoting, protecting, and maintaining health. It involves teaching about reducing health risk factors, increasing aclient's level of wellness, and taking specific protective health measures. Box 17.1 lists specific areas of health teaching.

Teaching

Teaching is a system of activities intended to produce learning. The teaching process is intentionally designed to produce specific learning.

The teaching–learning process involves dynamic interaction between teacher and learner. Each participant in the process communicates information, emotions, perceptions, and attitudes to the other. The teaching process and the nursing process are much alike (Table 17.1).

Nurses teach a variety of learners in various settings. They teach clients and their families or significant others in the hospital, primary care clinics, urgent care, managed care, the home, and assisted living and long-term care facilities. Nurses teach large and small groups of learners in community health education programs.

Nurses also teach professional colleagues and other healthcare personnel in academic institutions such as vocational schools, colleges, and universities and in healthcare facilities such as hospitals or nursing homes.

Teaching Clients and Their Families

Nurses may teach individual clients in one-to-one teaching episodes. For example, the nurse may teach about wound care while changing a client's dressing or may teach about diet, exercise, and other lifestyle behaviors that minimize the risk of a heart attack for a client who has a cardiac problem. The nurse may also be involved in teaching family members or other support people who are caring for the client. Nurses working in obstetric and pediatric areas teach parents and sometimes grandparents how to care for children.

BOX 17.1 Areas for Client Education

PROMOTION OF HEALTH

- Increasing a client's level of wellness
- Growth and development topics
- Fertility control
- Hygiene
- Nutrition
- Exercise
- Stress management
- Lifestyle modification
- Resources within the community

PREVENTION OF ILLNESS OR INJURY

- Health screening (e.g., blood glucose levels, blood pressure, blood cholesterol, Pap test, mammograms, vision, hearing, routine physical examinations)
- Reducing health risk factors (e.g., lowering cholesterol level)
- Specific protective health measures (e.g., immunizations, use of condoms, use of sunscreen, use of medication, umbilical cord care)
- First aid
- Safety (e.g., using seat belts, helmets, walkers)

RESTORATION OF HEALTH

- Information about tests, diagnosis, treatment, medications
- Self-care skills or skills needed to care for family member
- Resources within healthcare setting and community

ADAPTING TO ALTERED HEALTH AND FUNCTION

- Adaptations in lifestyle
- Problem-solving skills
- Adaptation to changing health status
- Strategies to deal with current problems (e.g., home intravenous [IV] line skills, medications, diet, activity limits, prostheses)
- Strategies to deal with future problems (e.g., fear of pain with terminal cancer, future surgeries, or treatments)
- Information about treatments and likely outcomes
- Referrals to other healthcare facilities or services
- Facilitation of strong self-image
- Grief and bereavement counseling

TABLE 17.1 Comparison of the Teaching Process and the Nursing Process

Step	Teaching Process	Nursing Process
1	Collect data; analyze client's learning strengths and deficits.	Collect data; analyze client's strengths and deficits.
2	Make educational diagnoses.	Make nursing diagnoses.
3	Develop teaching plan based on mutually determined outcomes: • Write learning outcomes. • Select content and time frame. • Select teaching strategies.	Plan nursing goals and desired outcomes and select interventions.
4	Implement teaching plan.	Implement nursing strategies.
5	Evaluate client learning based on achievement of learning outcomes.	Evaluate client outcomes based on achievement of goal criteria.

Because of decreased length of hospital stays, time constraints on client education may occur. Nurses need to provide client education that will ensure the client's safe transition from one level of care to another and make appropriate plans for follow-up education in the client's home. Discharge plans must include information about what the client has been taught before transfer or discharge and what remains for the client to learn to perform self-care in the home or another residence (see Chapter 7 ∞).

Teaching in the Community

Nurses are often involved in community health education programs. Such teaching activities may be voluntary as part of the nurse's involvement in an organization such as the Red Cross or Planned Parenthood, or they may be compensated as part of the nurse's work role, such as school nurses. Community teaching activities may be aimed at large groups of individuals who have an interest in some aspect of health, such as nutrition classes, classes on cardiopulmonary resuscitation (CPR) or the reduction of cardiac risk factors, and bicycle or swimming safety programs. Community education programs can also be designed for small groups or individual learners, such as childbirth classes or family planning classes.

Teaching Health Personnel

Nurses are also involved in the instruction of professional colleagues through continuing education, in-service programs, and staff development. For example, experienced nurses may function as preceptors for new graduate nurses or for newly employed nurses. Nurses with specialized knowledge and experience share that knowledge and experience with nurses who are new to that practice area. Examples of such specialized courses include critical care nursing, perioperative nursing, and quality improvement and quality assurance. In addition, nurses in nursing practice settings are often involved in the clinical instruction of nursing students.

Nurses are also involved in teaching other health professionals. Nurses may participate in the education of medical students or allied health students. In this capacity, the nurse educator clarifies the role of the nurse for other health professionals and how nurses can assist them in their care of clients.

Learning

Like all individuals, clients have a variety of learning needs. A **learning need** is a desire or a requirement to know something that is presently unknown to the learner. Learning needs include new knowledge or information but can also include a new or different skill or physical ability, a new behavior, or a need to change an old behavior. **Learning** is a change in human disposition or capability that persists and that cannot be solely accounted for by growth. Learning is represented by a change in behavior. See Client Teaching for attributes of learning.

CLIENT TEACHING Attributes of Learning

Learning is:

- An experience that occurs inside the learner
- The discovery of the personal meaning and relevance of ideas
- A consequence of experience
- A collaborative and cooperative process
- An evolutionary process that builds on past learning and experiences
- A process that is both intellectual and emotional.

An important aspect of learning is the individual's desire to learn and to act on the learning, referred to as **compliance**. In the healthcare context, compliance is the extent to which a client's behavior coincides with medical or health advice. Compliance is best illustrated when the client recognizes and accepts the need to learn, then follows through with the appropriate behaviors that reflect the learning. For example, a client diagnosed as having diabetes willingly learns about the needed special diet and then plans and follows the learned diet. Many clients, however, view the term *compliance* in a negative light because the term implies the teacher as the authority and the learner in a submissive role, and this conflicts with the learner's right to determine his or her own healthcare decisions rather than be told what to do by a healthcare professional. In addition, it is important not to label a client as noncompliant without obtaining further information. For example, the client intended to comply but was unable to do so because the client could not afford the cost of the medications.

Another term seen in healthcare literature is **adherence**, which is the degree to which clients follow the agreed-on recommendations of healthcare providers. *Adherence* is viewed as being a more client-centered term because it supports the client's right to choose whether to follow treatment recommendations (Bastable, 2017, pp. 158–159). Adherence implies a collaborative and cooperative relationship between nurses and clients that is based on shared responsibility. Nurses view clients as active participants in promoting, maintaining, and restoring their health.

Andragogy is the art and science of teaching adults, in contrast to **pedagogy**, the discipline concerned with helping children learn. **Geragogy** is the term used to describe the process involved in helping older adults to learn (Bastable, 2017). An individual's developmental stage influences the learning abilities of children, adults, and older adults.

Nurses can use the following andragogical principles and assumptions about adult learners as a guide for client teaching (Knowles, Holton, & Swanson, 2015, p. 88):

- Adults need to know why they need to learn something before learning it.
- The self-concept of adults is heavily dependent on a move toward self-direction.
- The prior experiences of the learner provide a rich resource for learning.
- Adults typically become ready to learn when they experience a need to cope with a life situation or perform a task.
- Adults have a life-centered orientation to learning; education is a process of developing increased competency levels to achieve their full potential.
- The motivation for adult learners is internal rather than external.

Learning Domains

Bloom (1956) identified three domains or areas of learning: cognitive, affective, and psychomotor. The *updated* **cognitive domain**, the "thinking" domain, includes six intellectual abilities and thinking processes: "remembering, understanding, applying, analyzing, evaluating, and creating" (Miller & Stoeckel, 2016, p. 228). The **affective domain**, known as the "feeling" domain, relates to the client's attitudes, interests, attention, awareness, and values (Miller & Stoeckel, 2016, p. 228). The **psychomotor domain**, the "skill" domain, includes physical movement and coordination, such as giving an injection.

Nurses should include *each* of Bloom's three domains in client teaching plans. For example, teaching a client how to self-administer insulin is in the psychomotor domain. But an important part of a teaching plan for a client with diabetes is to teach why insulin is needed and what to do when not feeling well; this is in the cognitive domain. Helping the client accept the chronic implications of diabetes and maintain self-esteem is in the affective domain.

Learning Theories

There are many different theories relating to the way individuals learn. Following are three main theories of behaviorism, cognitivism, and humanism.

Behaviorism

The major behaviorism theorists include Thorndike, Pavlov, Skinner, and Bandura. In the behaviorist school of thought, an act is called a *response* when it can be traced to the effects of a stimulus. Behaviorists closely observe responses and then manipulate the environment to bring about the intended change.

Skinner's and Pavlov's work focused on conditioning behavioral responses to a stimulus that causes the response or behavior. To increase the probability of a response, Skinner introduced the importance of **positive reinforcement** (e.g., a pleasant experience such as praise and encouragement) in fostering the repetition of an action. Bandura's research, however, focuses on **imitation**, the process by which individuals copy or reproduce what they have observed, and **modeling**, the process by which an individual learns by observing the behavior of others.

Nurses using the **behaviorist theory** identify what is to be taught and shape behavior through positive or negative reinforcement. However, the theory is not easily applied to complex learning situations and limits the learner's role in the teaching process (e.g., being a passive learner). In summary, nurses applying behavioristic theory will:

- Provide sufficient practice time, including both immediate and repeat testing and return demonstration.
- Provide opportunities for learners to solve problems by trial and error.
- Select teaching strategies that avoid distracting information and that evoke the desired response.
- Praise the learner for correct behavior and provide positive feedback at intervals throughout the learning experience.
- Provide role models of desired behavior.

Cognitivism

Cognitivism depicts learning as a complex cognitive activity. In other words, it focuses on what happens in the mind, such as thinking and problem-solving. New knowledge is built on previous information, and learners actively participate in the learning process. Cognitivists also emphasize the importance of the social, emotional, and physical contexts in which learning occurs, such as the teacher–learner relationship and the environment. Developmental readiness and individual readiness (i.e., motivation) are other key factors associated with cognitive approaches.

Major cognitive theorists include Piaget, Lewin, and Bloom. Piaget's five major phases of cognitive development are discussed in Chapter 23 ∞. According to Lewin, learning involves four different types of changes: cognitive structure, motivation, one's sense of belonging to the group, and gain in voluntary muscle control. As previously mentioned, Bloom identified the three domains of learning. Users of **cognitive theory** recognize the developmental level of the learner and acknowledge the learner's motivation and environment. However, some or many of the motivational and environmental factors may be beyond the teacher's control.

Nurses applying cognitive theory will:

- Provide a social, emotional, and physical environment conducive to an active learning process.
- Encourage a positive teacher–learner relationship.
- Select multisensory teaching strategies because perception is influenced by the senses.
- Recognize that personal characteristics have an impact on how cues are perceived and develop appropriate teaching approaches to target different learning styles.
- Assess a learner's developmental and personal readiness to learn and adapt teaching strategies to the learner's developmental level.
- Select behavioral objectives and teaching strategies that encompass the cognitive, affective, and psychomotor domains of learning.

Humanism

Humanistic learning theory focuses on both the cognitive and affective qualities of the learner. Prominent members of this school of thought include Abraham Maslow and Carl Rogers. According to humanistic theory, learning is believed to be self-motivated, self-initiated, and self-evaluated. Everyone is viewed as unique. Learning focuses on self-development and achieving full potential; it is best when it is relevant to the learner. Autonomy and self-determination are important; the learner identifies the learning needs and takes the initiative to meet these needs. The learner is an active participant and takes responsibility for meeting individual learning needs.

Nurses applying humanistic theory will:

- Communicate empathy in the nurse–client relationship.
- Encourage the learner to establish goals and promote self-directed learning.
- Encourage active learning by serving as a facilitator, mentor, or resource for the learner.
- Use active learning strategies to assist the client's adoption of new behavior.
- Expose the learner to new, relevant information and ask appropriate questions to encourage the learner to seek answers, learn from any mistakes, and not be threatened by external factors.

Being aware of the focus and limitations of the various learning theories allows the nurse to use one or more of them when developing a teaching plan for a client. Knowing what is important (e.g., knowledge, motivation, feelings, attitudes) assists the nurse in choosing the appropriate learning theory or theories. The nurse also needs to be aware of the different factors that can affect the client's learning.

Factors Affecting Learning

Many factors can facilitate or hinder learning by a client. The nurse should be aware of these factors, particularly when available teaching time is limited.

Age and Developmental Stage

The nurse needs to consider the age and developmental stage of the learner because they influence the client's ability to learn. Three major factors that influence a client's learning needs across the lifespan are biological characteristics, developmental tasks, and psychosocial stages. These factors must be considered at each developmental period throughout the lifecycle (Miller & Stoeckel, 2016, p. 144). Furthermore, The Joint Commission mandates that healthcare agencies provide teaching plans that address developmental stage–specific competencies of the learner.

Motivation

Motivation to learn is the desire to learn. It greatly influences how quickly and how much an individual learns. Motivation is generally greatest when an individual recognizes a need and believes the need will be met through learning. It is not enough for the need to be identified and verbalized by the nurse; it must be experienced by the client. Often, the nurse's task is to help the client personally work through the problem and identify the need. Sometimes clients or support people need help identifying information relevant to their situation before they can see a need. For instance, clients with heart disease may need to know the effects of smoking before they recognize the need to stop smoking. Adolescents may need to know the consequences of an untreated sexually transmitted infection before they see the need for treatment.

Readiness

Readiness to learn is the demonstration of behaviors or cues that reflect the learner's motivation to learn at a specific time. Readiness reflects not only the desire or willingness to learn but also the ability to learn at a specific time. For example, a client may want to learn self-care during a dressing change, but if the client experiences pain or discomfort, the client may not be able to learn. The nurse can provide pain medication to make the client more comfortable and more able to learn. The nurse's role is often to encourage the development of readiness.

Active Involvement

When the learner is actively involved, learning becomes more meaningful. If the learner actively participates in planning and discussion, learning is faster, and retention is better (Figure 17.1 ■). Active learning promotes critical thinking, enabling learners to solve problems more effectively. Clients who are actively involved in learning about their healthcare may be more able to apply the learning to their own situation. For example, clients who are actively involved in learning about their therapeutic diets may be more able to apply the principles being taught to their cultural food preferences and their usual eating habits. Passive learning, such as listening to a lecture or watching a film, does not foster optimal learning.

Relevance

The knowledge or skill to be learned must be personally relevant to the learner. Clients learn more easily if they can connect the new knowledge to that which they already know or have experienced. For example, if a client is diagnosed with hypertension, is overweight, and has symptoms of headaches and fatigue, he is more likely to understand the need to lose weight if he remembers having more energy when he weighed less. The nurse needs to validate the relevance of learning with the client throughout the learning process.

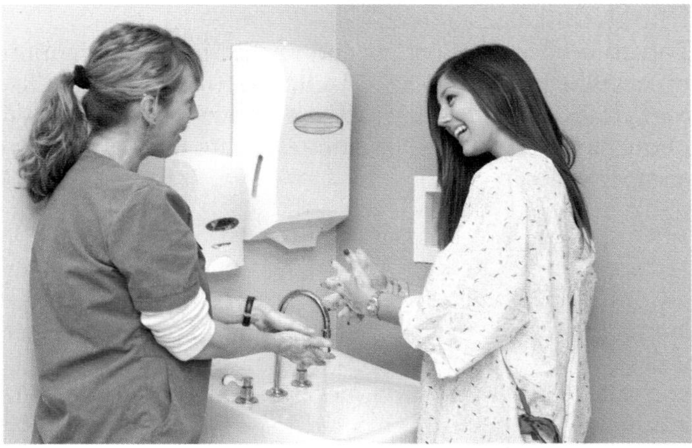

Figure 17.1 ■ Learning is facilitated when the client is interested and actively involved.
nano/E+/Getty Images.

Feedback

Feedback is information regarding a client's performance in reaching a desired goal. It must be meaningful to the learner. Feedback that accompanies the practice of psychomotor skills helps the client to learn those skills. Support of desired behavior through praise, positively worded corrections, and suggestions of alternative methods are ways of providing positive feedback. Negative feedback, such as ridicule, anger, or sarcasm, can lead clients to withdraw from learning. Such feedback, viewed as a type of punishment, may cause the client to avoid the teacher to avoid punishment.

Nonjudgmental Support

Individuals learn best when they believe they are accepted and will not be judged. The individual who expects to be judged as a "poor" or "good" client will not learn as well as the client who feels no such threat. Once learners have succeeded in accomplishing a task or understanding a concept, they gain self-confidence in their ability to learn. This reduces their anxiety about failure and can motivate greater learning. Successful learners have increased confidence with which to accept failure.

Simple to Complex Learning

Learning is facilitated by material that is logically organized and proceeds from the simple to the complex. Such organization enables the learner to comprehend new information, assimilate it with previous learning, and form new understandings. Of course, *simple* and *complex* are relative terms, depending on the level at which the client is learning. What is simple for one client may be complex for another.

Repetition

Repetition of key concepts and facts facilitates retention of newly learned material. Practice of psychomotor skills, particularly with feedback from the nurse, improves the performance of those skills and facilitates their transfer to another setting.

Timing

Individuals retain information and psychomotor skills best when the time between learning and active use of the learning is short; the longer the time interval, the easier it is to forget the learning. For example, a client who is only shown literature and videotapes about administering insulin but is not permitted to administer his or her own insulin until discharge from the hospital is unlikely to remember what was learned. However, giving his or her own injections while in the hospital enhances the client's learning.

Environment

An optimal learning environment facilitates learning by reducing distraction and providing physical and psychologic comfort. It has adequate lighting that is free from glare, a comfortable room temperature, and good ventilation. Most students know what it is like to try to learn in a hot, stuffy room; the consequent drowsiness interferes with concentration. Noise can also distract the student and interfere with listening and thinking. To facilitate learning in a hospital setting, nurses should choose a time when no visitors are present and interruptions are unlikely.

Privacy is essential for some learning. For example, when a client is learning to change a colostomy bag, the presence of others can be embarrassing and thus interfere with learning. However, when a client is particularly anxious, having a support person present may give the client confidence.

Many factors inhibit learning. Some of the most common barriers to learning are described next and in Table 17.2.

Emotions

Emotions such as fear, anger, and depression can impede learning. A high level of anxiety resulting in agitation and the inability to focus or concentrate can also inhibit learning. Clients or families who are experiencing extreme emotional states may not hear spoken words or may retain only part of the communication. Emotional responses such as fear and anxiety decrease with information that relieves uncertainty. Medications may be prescribed for extremely distraught clients or families to reduce their anxiety and put them in an emotional state in which understanding or learning can occur.

TABLE 17.2 Barriers to Learning

Barrier	Explanation	Nursing Implications
Acute illness	Client requires all resources and energy to cope with illness.	Defer teaching until client is less ill.
Pain	Pain decreases ability to concentrate.	Conduct pain assessment before teaching.
Prognosis	Client can be preoccupied with illness and unable to concentrate on new information.	Defer teaching to a better time.
Biorhythms	Mental and physical performances have a circadian rhythm.	Adapt time of teaching to suit client.
Emotion (e.g., anxiety, denial, depression, grief)	Emotions require energy and distract from learning.	Deal with emotions and possible misinformation first.
Language	Client may not be fluent in the nurse's language.	Obtain services of an interpreter or nurse with appropriate language skills.
Age		
• Older adults	Vision, hearing, and motor control can be impaired in older adults.	Consider sensory and motor deficits, and adapt teaching plan as needed.
• Children	Children have a shorter attention span and vocabulary differences.	Plan shorter and more active learning episodes.
Culture/religion	A client's culture or religion may place restrictions on certain types of knowledge, for example, birth control information.	Assess the client's cultural and religious needs when planning learning activities.
Physical disability	Visual, hearing, sensory, or motor impairments may interfere with a client's ability to learn.	Plan teaching activities appropriate to the learner's physical abilities. For example, provide audio learning tools for the client who is blind or large-print materials for the client whose vision is impaired.
Mental disability	Impaired cognitive ability may affect the client's capacity for learning.	Assess the client's capacity for learning, and plan teaching activities to complement the client's ability while planning more complex learning for the client's caregivers.

Physiologic Events

Physiologic events such as a critical illness, pain, or sensory deficits inhibit learning. Because the client cannot concentrate and apply energy to learning, the learning itself is impaired. The nurse should try to reduce the physiologic barriers to learning as much as possible before teaching. For example, providing analgesics and rest before teaching is often helpful.

Cultural Aspects

Cultural barriers to learning include language and values. The client who does not understand the nurse's language may learn little. Western medicine may conflict with a client's cultural healing beliefs and practices. To be effective, nurses must be culturally sensitive and competent; otherwise, the client may be partially or totally noncompliant with recommended treatments. Another impediment to learning is differing values held by the client and the health team. For example, if a client comes from a culture that views being overweight or "plump" as positive, the nurse should present information in the client's cultural context. Then the nurse and the client should together determine an acceptable weight and develop a plan for achieving that weight (Bastable, 2017; Miller & Stoeckel, 2016).

Psychomotor Ability

It is important for the nurse to be aware of a client's psychomotor skills when planning teaching. Psychomotor skills can be affected by health. For example, an older client who has severe osteoarthritis of the hands may not be able to self-administer insulin. The following physical abilities are important for learning psychomotor skills:

1. *Muscle strength.* For example, an older client who cannot rise from a chair because of insufficient leg and muscle strength cannot be expected to learn to lift herself out of a bathtub.
2. *Motor coordination.* Gross motor coordination is required for movements such as walking, and fine motor coordination is needed when using utensils, such as a fork for eating. For example, a client who has advanced amyotrophic lateral sclerosis (ALS) involving the lower limbs will probably be unable to use a walker.
3. *Energy.* Energy is required for most psychomotor skills, and learning these skills uses more energy. Older adults and clients who are ill often have limited energy resources; learning and carrying out these skills must be timed for when the client's energy sources are at their peak.
4. *Sensory acuity.* Sight is used for most learning (i.e., walking with crutches, changing a dressing, drawing a medication into a syringe). Clients who have a visual impairment often need the assistance of a support person to carry out such tasks.

Technology and Health Information

The internet has become part of the lives of many Americans, allowing them to communicate and obtain information quickly. Internet technology has dramatically changed the activities of business, including healthcare. Two terms, *telemedicine* and *telehealth*, are often used interchangeably to describe the use of technology to provide healthcare services. Telehealth is usually used to refer to a broader scope of healthcare services. These may include services to identify and meet client care needs, online appointment access, electronic prescriptions, billing review, email access between the client and healthcare provider, and online health information (Schramm, 2016).

There are three traditional modalities of telehealth. One is *real-time*, a live, two-way interaction between the client and healthcare provider using audiovisual technology (e.g., telephone or smartphone and video conferencing). *Store-and-forward* technology is another means of interacting with a client; it combines the use of a camera, computer, microphone, and image management software to transmit a client's health information (e.g., x-rays). The third, *remote client monitoring*, involves continuous tracking of a client's personal health and medical data via electronic communication technologies such as a Holter monitor (Fronczek & Rouhana, 2018, p. 234). In addition, there are a growing number of mobile health, or mHealth, technologies. For example, individuals can maintain or improve their health through applications and online services sold directly to them, such as wearable devices to track health and wellness (Davis et al., 2017).

Online Health Information

Findings from a national survey found that 65% of U.S. consumers who go online for health information follow up with a healthcare provider, whereas the remaining 35% use the information to treat themselves at home (Bastable, 2017, p. 465). In addition, a Pew Research Center report analyzed the ownership of smartphones, which has significantly increased. For example, nearly 95% of Americans own a cell phone of some kind. Of that group, one in five adults is a "smartphone-only" internet user, meaning the adult owns a smartphone but does not have traditional home broadband service. Reliance on smartphones for online access is common among younger adults, non-White Americans, and lower-income Americans (Pew Research Center, 2018).

This increasing use of information technology decreases the gap between the teacher and the learner. In the past, the nurse had the primary responsibility for informing clients about their medical condition. Now, nurses are facilitators, rather than providers of information. Thus, it is necessary for the nurse to provide a collaborative environment when in a teaching–learning client situation. The numbers of clients entering a healthcare agency who have already accessed online information about their health concerns demonstrate this need. They are prepared to discuss this information with their healthcare providers. Bastable (2017) states that part of a preteaching assessment should include asking clients about their computer use and interest in using online information regarding their healthcare.

The teaching role of the nurse remains important but has changed. Nurses need to be prepared to use technology in their teaching, help clients to access online information, evaluate the online information clients find, and then discuss the information with the client. See Box 17.2 for guidelines to evaluate online health information.

Older Adults and Use of the Internet

Older adults are increasingly adopting technology, with about 42% reporting that they own a smartphone. Internet use among this group has also risen substantially to 67%. In spite of these gains, many older adults remain disconnected, with 33% saying they never use the internet and about 49% not having home broadband services (Anderson & Perrin, 2017).

Although the number of health information resources available online for older adults has exploded, the quality of online information and readability level of this information are concerns. Additionally, age-related physical changes can interfere with computer use. For example, motor skill decreases with age, and arthritis can affect typing, manipulation of the mouse, and scrolling down a page. The visual changes that accompany aging may also impact the older adult, especially if the website uses a small type size or fancy fonts. Making adjustments to the computer can help to overcome these challenges.

Older adults with low incomes, lower education levels, or from rural areas often do not own a computer or have internet access. As a result, these groups do not benefit from internet health resources, resulting in a gap between older Americans who have the privilege of internet access and those who do not. Older adults often learn about computer use at public libraries and learning centers that provide access to computer use and education. Community partnerships can facilitate activities to bridge the gap of older adult computer usage.

BOX 17.2 Guidelines for Evaluating Online Health Information

- What is the source of the information?
  You want a trusted source. Click on the "About Us" link. It should say who is running the website and why and the organization's mission or purpose. Look at the letters at the end of the URL. An address that ends in ".gov" means it is a government-sponsored site, ".edu" indicates an educational institution, ".org" is a noncommercial organization, and ".com" is a commercial organization.
- Is the source of the documents identified?
  The distinction between health information and advertisements should be clear. A website selling a product or recommending a certain treatment is not considered an objective source of information.
- What is the quality of the information?
  Look at where the information comes from or who writes it. The writers of the information should be identified. Are they recognized experts? Good sites should rely on medical research, not opinion. Look for claims that sound too good to be true.
- Is the information reviewed?
  The site has more credibility if individuals with trustworthy professional and scientific qualifications review the information before it is posted. Some websites have an editorial board that reviews the content, whereas others may list the names and credentials of those who reviewed the content.
- How current is the information?
  Check the date the information was posted and the last time the page was updated. Does the site provide references and maintain hyperlinks to other credible sites? If there are no dates on the site's pages, you do not know if the information is current.
- Is the website secure? Does it protect your privacy?
  Does the site require you to share your name and email address? Check for a privacy policy that explains how this information will be used. A credible site will tell you what it will and will not do with the information. Many commercial sites sell the collected data to other companies.

Adapted from *Client Education: Theory and Practice*, 2nd ed., by M. A. Miller and P. R. Stoeckel, 2016, Boston, MA: Jones & Bartlett; "Evaluating Internet Health Information: A Tutorial from the National Library of Medicine," by MedlinePlus, n.d. Retrieved from https://medlineplus.gov/webeval/webeval_start.html; and "Finding and Evaluating Online Resources," by National Institute of Health, 2018. Retrieved from https://nccih.nih.gov/health/webresources

Implications

Technology provides an important source of health information for many adult clients in the United States. Therefore, nurses need to know and be able to integrate this technology into the teaching plans for those clients who use online resources. Nurses involved in the provision of online information can advocate for website designs that provide accessibility accommodations for older adults. On the other hand, nurses also need to apply effective teaching strategies for those clients who do not use online technology.

Nurse as Educator

Being an educator or teacher is an important and primary role for the nurse. Clients and families have the right to health education to make informed decisions about their health. The nurse is able to promote healthy lifestyles in clients and their families through the application of health knowledge, the change process, learning theories, and the nursing and teaching roles.

●○● NURSING MANAGEMENT

Assessing

A comprehensive assessment of learning needs combines data from the nursing health history and physical assessment and addresses the client's support system. It also considers client characteristics that may influence the learning process: readiness to learn, motivation to learn, and reading

EVIDENCE-BASED PRACTICE

Evidence-Based Practice

What Are the Issues with Older Adults Accessing Health Information Online?

Online information can help meet the healthcare needs of a growing older population, particularly for those living in isolated rural communities. Waterworth and Honey (2018) believe there is a need to understand how older adults (age 65 and older) use the internet for accessing healthcare information and the possible barriers and facilitators for them seeking online health information. They used an integrated literature review methodology. That is, they identified over 3000 studies from three databases, reviewed these studies for their inclusion criteria (adults 65 years or older, published between 2006 and 2016, and reasons for using the internet for accessing health information), and concluded with a final number of eight articles.

It is expected that the acceptance rate of older adults using the internet for seeking health information will increase as baby boomers transition into the over-65 age group. Education showed the strongest influence on older adults accessing online health information. Another determining factor was socioeconomic status, and using the internet for information seeking was significantly higher among older adults with higher incomes.

Older adults, however, still have barriers to adopting the internet for seeking health information. These barriers include low trust in the credibility of the information, financial barriers, lack of knowledge of the internet and skills needed to seek information, and low health literacy levels.

Implications

The researchers emphasize that education and support are needed to promote older adults' use of valuable online resources in an effective, safe, and efficient way. Technologic features need to be made familiar, easier, and more usable for older adults and for those with disabilities. Nurses can intervene by acting as information advisors to identify credible internet sites and as translators to assist older adults and their families in understanding the health information they find. This begins by the nurse incorporating an assessment of the older adult's use of online health information.

and comprehension level, for example. Assessing a client's stage of change and any barriers to change is also important and is often overlooked (see Chapter 19 ∞).

The nurse's knowledge of common learning needs required by clients experiencing similar health problems is another source of information. Learning needs change as the client's health status changes, so nurses must constantly reassess them.

Nursing History

Several elements in the nursing health history provide clues to learning needs. These elements include (a) age, (b) the client's understanding and perceptions of the health problem, (c) health beliefs and practices, (d) cultural factors, (e) economic factors, (f) learning style, and (g) the client's support systems. Examples of interview questions to elicit this information are in the accompanying Assessment Interview. Note the number of open-ended questions.

ASSESSMENT INTERVIEW Learning Needs and Characteristics

PRIMARY HEALTH PROBLEM

- Tell me what you know about your current health problem. What do you think caused it?
- What concerns do you have about it?
- How has the problem affected what you can or cannot do during your usual activities (e.g., work, recreation, shopping, housework)?
- What do you or did you do at home to relieve the problem? How helpful was it?
- How have the treatments you have started helped your problem?
- What, if any, difficulties have the treatments caused you (e.g., inconvenience, cost, discomfort)?
- Tell me about the tests, surgery, or treatments you are going to have.

HEALTH BELIEFS

- How would you describe your health generally?
- What things do you usually do to keep healthy?
- What health problems do you think you may be at risk for because of family history, age, diet, occupation, inadequate exercise, or other habits, such as smoking?
- What changes would you be willing to make to decrease your risk for these problems or to improve your health?

CULTURAL FACTORS

- What language do you use most often when speaking and writing?
- Do you seek the advice of another health practitioner?
- Do you use herbs or other medications or treatments commonly used in your cultural group? Does your current primary care provider know about these?
- What advice or treatments given previously by your primary care provider conflicted with values or beliefs you consider important?
- When a conflict arose, what did you do?

LEARNING STYLE

- Note the client's age and developmental level.
- What level of education have you received?
- Do you like to read?
- Where do you obtain health information (e.g., primary care provider, nurse, internet, magazines, books, pharmacist)?
- How do you best learn new things?
  a. By reading about them
  b. By talking about them
  c. By watching a movie or demonstration
  d. By computer
  e. By listening to the teacher
  f. By first being shown how something works and then doing it
  g. On your own or in a group.

CLIENT SUPPORT SYSTEM

- Would you like a family member or friend to help you learn about things you need to do to take care of yourself?
- Who do you think would be interested in learning with you?

Age

Age provides information on the client's developmental status that may indicate distinctive health teaching content and teaching approaches. Simple questions to school-age children and adolescents will elicit information on what they know. Observing children at play provides information about their motor and intellectual development as well as relationships with other children. For older clients, conversation and questioning may reveal slow recall or limited psychomotor skills, sensory deficits, and learning difficulties (see Lifespan Considerations).

Client's Understanding of Health Problem

A client's perception of a current health problem and concerns may indicate poor knowledge or misinformation. In addition, the effects of the problem on the client's usual activities can alert the nurse to other areas requiring instruction. For example, clients who cannot manage self-care at home often need information about community resources and services.

Health Beliefs and Practices

A client's health beliefs and practices are important to consider in any teaching plan. The health belief model described in Chapter 20 ∞ provides a predictor of preventive health behavior. However, even if a nurse is convinced that a client's health beliefs should be changed, doing so may not be possible because so many factors are involved in an individual's health beliefs.

Cultural Factors

Cultural groups often have their own folk beliefs and practices, with many of these being related to diet, health, illness, and lifestyle. It is therefore important to discuss the client's cultural perspective on illness and therapy. The cultural practices and values held by clients will affect their learning needs. For example, the client may understand the healthcare information being taught, but this learning may not be used if the client primarily believes in folk medical practices (see Chapter 21 ∞).

LIFESPAN CONSIDERATIONS Special Teaching Considerations

OLDER ADULTS

Older adults often have chronic illnesses that require multiple treatments or medications. Health teaching will focus on the same areas as with other ages—health and wellness promotion and prevention of illness and injury—but often the client needs are greatest in learning to manage their lives to live with chronic health conditions and maintain optimal health and functioning. For older adults to be motivated to learn, the material must be practical and have meaning for them individually, especially if the information is new to them. Special considerations in teaching older adults include the following:

- Health promotion is a priority need and should include these areas:
  - Exercise
  - Nutrition
  - Safety habits
  - Having regular health checkups
  - Understanding medications.
- Set achievable goals—involve the client and family in doing this.
- If developing written materials:
  - Use large print (e.g., at least 14-point type size) in bulleted format.
  - Use buff-colored paper or white paper that has a matte (dull) finish (to avoid glare).
  - Present the information at a sixth- to eighth-grade reading level.
- Increase time for teaching and allow for rest periods because processing of information is slower in older adults.
  - Verbal presentation of material should be well organized.
  - Ensure that there is minimal distraction.
- Repeat information if necessary.
- Use return demonstrations with psychomotor skills (show back), such as teaching someone how to do insulin injections.
- Determine where clients obtain most of their health information (e.g., newspapers, magazines, television, computer).
- Use examples to which clients can relate in their daily lives.
- Be aware of sensory deficits, such as hearing and vision.
- Use the setting with which the individual is most comfortable—either a group or one-on-one setting.
- If noncompliance is a problem, investigate the cause. It could be due to lack of finances, transportation problems, poor access to medical care, and so on.

Older adults come with a lifetime of experiences and learned knowledge of their own. Respect this, and always have them use their strengths to work with any problems. Positive reinforcement and ongoing evaluation of what has been taught are important factors in effective health teaching with older adults.

CHILDREN

It has often been said that the parent is a child's first and most important teacher. Every interaction between a child and parent (or other adults and children) is a moment in which teaching and learning occur, often unconsciously. Sometimes the results are ones parents desire and strive for; sometimes they are not what the parent would have wished.

Nurses need to take every opportunity to teach parents about health promotion and disease prevention and to provide guidelines regarding normal growth and development. Considerations in teaching children include the following:

PRESCHOOL CHILDREN (3–5 YEARS OF AGE)

- Concerned about fear of pain and bodily harm. Reassure them and allow them to tell you about these fears. Use words carefully; for example, use "fix" instead of "cut."
- Allow the child to play with replicas or dolls to learn about body parts.
- Give praise and approval to motivate learning.

MIDDLE AND LATE CHILDHOOD (6–11 YEARS OF AGE)

- Able to think logically and developing ability to think abstractly.
- Like to be actively involved in the learning process.
- Teaching for health promotion often occurs through the school nurse.

ADOLESCENT (12–19 YEARS OF AGE)

- Have a strong need to belong to a group and a need for friendships and peer support.
- Need to develop a mutually respectful and trusting relationship with them.

Economic Factors

Economic factors can also affect a client's learning. For example, a client who cannot afford to obtain a new sterile syringe for each injection of insulin may find it difficult to learn to administer the insulin when the nurse teaches that a new syringe should be used each time.

Learning Style

Considerable research has been done on individual learning styles. The best way to learn varies with the individual. Some individuals are visual learners and learn best by watching. Other individuals do not visualize an activity well; they learn best by handling equipment and discovering how it works. Others can learn well from reading things presented in an orderly fashion. Still others learn best in groups where they can relate to other individuals. For some, stressing the thinking part of a skill and its logic will promote learning. For others, stressing the feeling part or interpersonal aspect motivates and promotes learning.

A client's learning style may be based in his or her cultural background. For example, clients from cultures that have a strong oral tradition may prefer educational videos presented in their language.

The nurse seldom has the time or skills to assess each learner, identify the client's learning style, and then adapt teaching accordingly. What the nurse can do, however, is ask clients how they have learned things best in the past or how they like to learn. Many clients know what helps them learn, and the nurse can use this information in planning the teaching. Using a variety of teaching techniques and varying activities during teaching are good ways to match learners with learning styles. One technique will be most effective for some clients, whereas other techniques will be suited to clients with different learning styles.

Client's Support System

The nurse explores the client's support system to determine the extent to which others may enhance learning and offer support. Family members or a close friend may help the client perform the required skills at home and maintain required lifestyle changes.

Physical Examination

The general survey part of the physical examination provides useful clues to the client's learning needs, such as mental status, energy level, and nutritional status. Other parts of the physical examination reveal data about the client's physical capacity to learn and perform self-care activities. For example, visual ability, hearing ability, and muscle coordination affect the selection of content and approaches to teaching.

Readiness to Learn

Clients who are ready to learn often behave differently from those who are not. A client who is ready may search out information, for instance, by asking questions, researching online resources, reading books or articles, talking to others, and generally showing interest. The client who is not ready to learn is more likely to avoid the subject or situation. In addition, the unready client may change the subject when the nurse brings it up. For example, the nurse might say, "I was wondering about when would be a good time to show you how to change your dressing," and the client responds, "Oh, my wife will take care of everything."

The nurse assesses for these readiness characteristics:

- ***Physical readiness.*** Is the client able to focus on things other than physical status, or are pain, fatigue, and immobility using all the client's time and energy? How much coordination and energy will be needed to complete the task?
- ***Emotional readiness.*** Is the client emotionally ready to learn self-care activities? Clients who are extremely anxious, depressed, or grieving over their health status are not ready. An available and strong support system can positively influence emotional readiness.
- ***Cognitive readiness.*** Can the client think clearly at this point? Are the effects of anesthesia and analgesia altering the client's level of consciousness? What is the client's knowledge base, cognitive ability, and preferred learning style?

Nurses can promote readiness to learn by providing physical and emotional support during the critical stage of recovery. As the client stabilizes physically and emotionally, the nurse can provide opportunities to learn.

Motivation

Motivation relates to whether the client wants to learn and is usually greatest when the client is ready, the learning need is recognized, and the information being offered is meaningful to the client. Assessment of motivation, however, may be difficult. Communication skills used by the nurse can obtain helpful information indicating readiness for change, such as "I'm really ready to lose weight this time." On the other hand, nonverbal behaviors such as indifference, lack of attention, and missed appointments can indicate a decreased motivation to learn.

Nurses can increase a client's motivation in several ways:

- By relating the learning to something the client values and helping the client see the relevance of the learning
- By helping the client make the learning situation pleasant and nonthreatening
- By encouraging self-direction and independence
- By demonstrating a positive attitude about the client's ability to learn
- By offering continuing support and encouragement as the client attempts to learn (i.e., positive reinforcement)
- By creating a learning situation in which the client is likely to succeed (Succeeding in small tasks motivates the client to continue learning.)
- By assisting the client to identify the benefits of changing behavior.

Health Literacy

The World Health Organization (Reprinted from 'Health literacy and health behaviour', World Health Organization) defines **health literacy** as "the cognitive and social skills which determine the motivation and ability of individuals to gain access to, understand, and use information in ways which promote and maintain good health" (para 1). The Patient Protection and Affordable Care Act of 2010, Title V, defines health literacy as "the degree to which an individual has the capacity to obtain, communicate, process, and understand basic health information and services to make appropriate health decisions" (Centers for Disease Control and Prevention [CDC], 2016, para 1). Health literacy includes such tasks as comprehending prescription labels, interpreting appointment slips, completing health insurance forms, and following instructions for diagnostic tests. According to the Agency for Healthcare Research and Quality (AHRQ), only 12% of U.S. adults have the health literacy skills needed to manage the demands of the healthcare system, and their ability to understand and use health information can be further compromised by stress or illness (Brega et al., 2015). In addition, more than 36% of the population has low health literacy, which means they do not understand important warnings on the label of an over-the-counter medication (Scott, 2016). An individual with low or limited literacy skills is not illiterate. See Box 17.3 for literacy definitions.

BOX 17.3 Literacy Definitions

- *Literacy:* an individual's ability to read, write, and speak in English and compute and solve problems at levels of proficiency necessary to function on the job and in society, achieve one's goals, and develop one's knowledge and potential
- *Low literacy:* a *limited* ability to do what is defined as literacy (previous definition)
- *Illiteracy:* being unable to read or write
- *Health literacy:* the degree to which individuals have the capacity to obtain, process, and understand basic health information and services needed to make appropriate health decisions.

From "Plain Language: A Promising Strategy for Clearly Communicating Health Information and Improving Health Literacy," by U.S. Department of Health and Human Services, n.d. Retrieved from http://www.health.gov/communication/literacy/plainlanguage/PlainLanguage.htm

There is a link between literacy, health, and client safety. Adverse and even potentially life-threatening errors can occur if a client cannot read a pill bottle label or an educational brochure. For example, a client may not be able to read a prescription to know how many pills to take or may take the wrong number of pills (e.g., *once* means "eleven" in Spanish). Clients with low literacy skills have less information about health promotion and management of a disease process for themselves and their families because they are unable to read the educational materials, and they often fail to seek preventive care (e.g., vaccinations, mammograms).

Communication is critical for client safety and quality nursing care. The increasing diversity of the client population means that nurses are treating individuals with limited English proficiency (LEP) because of language, literacy, or cultural barriers. It is common for clients who do not understand health information to become embarrassed and not ask questions.

Low health literacy is a silent epidemic, and there is no physical examination, blood test, or diagnostic imaging procedure that can tell you who is at risk. Research has shown that healthcare providers are poor predictors of client health literacy and nurses often overestimate a consumer's health literacy. As a result, the AHRQ developed a health literacy universal precautions toolkit. Universal precautions for health literacy are the steps that the members of the healthcare team take when they assume that *all* clients may have difficulty comprehending health information and accessing health service (Brega et al., 2015; Watts, Stevenson, & Adams, 2017). That means using clear communication and plain language that creates a foundation for *all* clients to be able to understand and act on health information. The toolkit provides evidence-based guidance that addresses improving spoken and written communication.

Clinical Alert!

Many clients are embarrassed about their reading level or will conceal that they cannot read. Instead, they may say things like "I forgot my glasses," "The form is too long," "I want my family to read it first," or "There are too many medical and legal terms." Most clients at the lowest reading levels, if asked, will report that they "read well."

The National Patient Safety Foundation (2016) developed an educational tool titled "Ask Me 3™." This tool promotes three simple questions that clients should ask all healthcare providers in all healthcare interactions:

- What is my main problem?
- What do I need to do?
- Why is it important for me to do this?

When verbally teaching clients, it is important to use communication techniques that will enhance their understanding. The Health Literacy Universal Precautions Toolkit (Brega et al., 2015) suggests the following techniques:

- Use plain, nonmedical language.
- Speak clearly and at a moderate pace.
- Limit information to two or three important points at a time.
- Repeat key points.
- Use graphics such as drawings or models.
- Encourage questions (i.e., "What questions do you still have?" and "That was a lot of information; what do I need to go over again?").
- Use "teach-back" and "show-back" techniques. "Teach-back" is when the nurse has clients say in their own words what is important that they know and do. The "show-back" technique is when the nurse demonstrates a skill and asks the client to perform a return demonstration.

Clinical Alert!

When using the "teach-back" technique, you do not want clients to feel that you are testing them. Place the responsibility on yourself. For example, tell the client that you want to be sure that you did a good job of explaining (topic) because it can be confusing. Ask: "What information was most helpful to you, or what will you now do differently?"

Nurses involved in developing written health teaching materials should write for lower reading levels (see Client Teaching: Developing Written Teaching Aids). The goal is for the educational materials to be at a third- to sixth-grade readability level (Brega et al., 2015, p. 35). Readability formulas (e.g., simplified measure of gobbledygook [SMOG]) can be used to assess the readability of educational materials by grade level. Clients with good reading skills do not take offense with simple reading material and prefer easy-to-read information. Even the simplest written directions, however, will not be helpful for the client with low or no reading skills. See the Client Teaching: Teaching Clients with Low Literacy Levels box for suggestions on how to teach clients with low literacy levels.

Diagnosing

Nursing diagnoses for clients with learning needs can be designated in two ways: as the client's primary concern or problem or as the etiology of a nursing diagnosis associated with the client's response to health alterations or dysfunction.

Learning Need as the Diagnostic Label

Examples of nursing diagnoses for clients with learning needs can include lack of knowledge (specify). Whenever this nursing diagnosis is used, either the client is seeking health information or the nurse has identified a learning need. The area of deficiency should always be included in the diagnosis. The following examples use the nursing diagnosis, lack of knowledge, as the primary concern: lack of knowledge (low-calorie diet) related to inexperience with newly ordered therapy; lack of knowledge (home safety hazards) related to denial of declining health and living alone.

Wilkinson and Barcus (2017) propose that if lack of knowledge is used as the primary concern or problem, one client goal must be "client will acquire knowledge about" (Wilkinson and Barcus, 2017, p. 490). The nurse needs to provide information that has the potential to change the client's behavior rather than focus on the behaviors caused by the client's lack of knowledge.

A second nursing diagnosis where a learning need may be the primary concern is willingness for knowledge enhancement. This is a health promotion diagnosis in which the client's behaviors are congruent with the client's knowledge. When using this nursing diagnosis, the client may or may not have an altered response or dysfunction at the time but may be seeking information to improve health or prevent illness. In the following examples, the nursing diagnosis, willingness for knowledge enhancement, is used as the primary concern:

- Willingness for knowledge enhancement (exercise and activity) related to a desire to improve health behaviors

CLIENT TEACHING Developing Written Teaching Aids

- Keep language level at a fifth- to sixth-grade level.
- Use active, not passive, voice (e.g., "take your medicine before breakfast" [active] versus "medicine should be taken before breakfast" [passive]).
- Use plain language; that is, easy, common words of one or two syllables (e.g., *use* instead of *utilize*, or *give* instead of *administer*).
- Use the second person (*you*) rather than the third person (*the client*).
- Use a large type size (14 to 16 point).
- Write short sentences.
- Avoid using all capital letters.
- Place priority information first and repeat it more than once.
- Use bold for emphasis.
- Use simple pictures, drawings, or cartoons, if appropriate.
- Leave plenty of white space.
- Focus material on desired behavior rather than on medical facts.
- Make it look easy to read.

CLIENT TEACHING Teaching Clients with Low Literacy Levels

- Use multiple teaching methods: Show pictures. Read important information. Lead a small-group discussion. Role play. Demonstrate a skill. Provide hands-on practice.
- Emphasize key points in simple terms, and provide examples.
- Avoid acronyms (e.g., CAT scan, HDL).
- Limit the amount of information in a single teaching session. Instead of one long session with a great deal of information, it is better to have more frequent sessions with a major point at each session.
- Associate new information with something the client already knows or associates with his or her job or lifestyle.
- Reinforce information through repetition.
- Involve the client in the teaching.
- Use the "teach-back" method by asking clients to repeat *in their own words* what they need to know. This will help you assess clients' understanding of your instructions.
- Avoid handouts with many pages and the classroom lecture format with a large group.

and decrease the risk of heart disease. This nursing diagnosis may be appropriate for the client who has knowledge of cardiac risk factors, has identified a personal health risk for a cardiac condition, and wants more information to minimize that risk through exercise.

- Willingness for knowledge enhancement (home safety hazards) related to a desire to minimize the risk of injury. This nursing diagnosis may be appropriate for parents who are seeking additional information to ensure that their home is safe for their toddler child. The diagnosis might also be used when an adult child seeks information to ensure that the home of an aging parent is free of risk factors for falls or other injuries common to the older adult.

Lack of Knowledge as the Etiology

Another way to deal with the identified learning needs of clients is to write "lack of knowledge" as the etiology, or second part, of the nursing diagnosis statement. Such nursing diagnoses can be written in the following format: potential for (specify) related to lack of knowledge (specify).

Examples include the following: potential for impaired parenting related to lack of knowledge (skills in infant care and feeding); anxiety related to lack of knowledge (bone marrow aspiration). Note also that most nursing diagnoses imply a teaching or learning need. For example, the nursing diagnosis potential for constipation suggests the need for a review of bowel hygiene practices, including diet, hydration, exercise, and activity.

Planning

Developing a teaching plan is accomplished in a series of steps. Involving the client promotes the formation of a meaningful plan and stimulates client motivation. The client who helps develop the teaching plan is more likely to achieve the desired outcomes (see Client Teaching).

Clinical Alert!

Knowing the client's stage of change helps determine which interventions will help the client change.

CLIENT TEACHING Sample Teaching Plan for Wound Care

Assessment of Learner: A 24-year-old male college student had a 7-cm (2.5-in.) laceration on the left lower anterior leg after being injured during a hockey game. The laceration was cleaned, sutured, and bandaged. The client was given an appointment to return to the health clinic in 10 days for suture removal. Client states that he lives in the college dormitory and can do wound care if given instructions. Client understands and reads English. Assessed to be in the "preparation" and "action" stages of change.

Nursing Diagnosis: Lack of knowledge (care of sutured wound) related to no prior experience.

Long-Term Goal: Client's wound will heal completely without infection or other complications.

Intermediate Goal: At clinic appointment, client's wound will be healing without signs of infection, loss of function, or other complication.

Short-Term Goals: Client will acquire knowledge about (a) correctly list three signs and symptoms of wound infection and (b) correctly perform a return demonstration of wound cleansing and bandaging.

Learning Outcomes	Content Outline	Teaching Methods
Upon completion of the instructional session, the client will:		
1. Describe normal wound healing.	**i.** Normal wound healing	Describe normal wound healing with the use of audiovisuals.
2. Describe signs and symptoms of wound infection.	**ii.** Infection Signs and symptoms include wound warm to touch, misalignment of wound edges, and purulent wound drainage. Signs of systemic infection include fever and malaise.	Discuss the mechanism of wound infection. Use audiovisuals to demonstrate infected wound appearance. Provide handout describing signs and symptoms of wound infection.
3. Identify equipment needed for wound care.	**iii.** Wound care equipment a. Cleansing solution as prescribed by primary care provider (e.g., clear water, mild soap and water, or antimicrobial solution) b. Bandaging material: Telfa, gauze wrap, adhesive tape	Demonstrate equipment needed for cleansing and bandaging wound. Provide handout listing equipment needed.
4. Demonstrate wound cleansing and bandaging.	**iv.** Demonstration of wound cleansing and bandaging on the client's wound or a mannequin	Demonstrate wound cleansing and bandaging on the client's wound or a mannequin. Provide handout describing procedure for cleansing and bandaging wound.
5. Describe appropriate action if questions or complications arise.	**v.** Resources available for client questions include health clinic, emergency department.	Discuss available resources. Provide handout listing available resources and follow-up treatment plan.

CLIENT TEACHING Sample Teaching Plan for Wound Care—*continued*

Learning Outcomes	Content Outline	Teaching Methods
6. Identify date, time, and location of follow-up appointment for suture removal.	**vi.** Follow-up treatment plan; where and when	Provide written instructions.

Evaluation: The client will:

1. Respond to questions regarding self-care of wound.
2. Demonstrate appropriate wound cleansing and bandaging.
3. State contact individual and telephone number to obtain assistance.
4. State date, time, and location of follow-up appointment.

Determining Teaching Priorities

The client's learning needs must be ranked according to priority. The client and the nurse should do this together, with the client's priorities always being considered. Once a client's priorities have been addressed, the client is generally more motivated to concentrate on other identified learning needs. For example, a man who wants to know all about coronary artery disease may not be ready to learn how to change his lifestyle until he meets his own need to learn more about the disease. Nurses can also use theoretical frameworks, such as Maslow's hierarchy of needs, to establish priorities.

Setting Learning Outcomes

Learning outcomes can be considered the same as the desired outcomes for other nursing diagnoses. They are written in the same way. Like client outcomes, learning outcomes:

- State the client (learner) behavior or performance, not nurse behavior. For example, "Identify personal risk factors for heart disease" (client behavior), *not* "Teach the client about cardiac risk factors" (nurse behavior).
- Reflect an observable, measurable activity. The performance may be visible (e.g., walking) or invisible (e.g., adding numbers). It is necessary, however, to be able to evaluate whether an unobservable activity has been mastered from some performance that represents the activity. For example, the performance of an outcome might be written: "Selects low-fat foods from a menu" (observable), *not* "Understands low-fat diet" (unobservable). Examples of measurable verbs used for learning outcomes are shown in Box 17.4. Avoid using words such as *knows*, *understands*, *believes*, and *appreciates* because they are neither observable nor measurable.
- May add conditions or modifiers as required to clarify what, where, when, or how the behavior will be performed. Examples are "Demonstrates four-point crutch gait *correctly*" (condition), "Administers own insulin *independently* (condition) as taught," or "States *three* (condition) factors that affect blood sugar level."
- Include criteria specifying the time by which learning should have occurred. For example, "The client will state three things that affect blood sugar level *by end of second diabetes management class.*"

Learning outcomes can reflect the learner's command of simple to complex concepts. For example, the learning outcome "The client will list cardiac risk factors" is a low-level knowledge outcome that simply requires the learner to identify all cardiac risk factors; it does not suggest application of the knowledge to the learner's own behaviors. The learning outcome "The client will list personal cardiac risk factors" requires that the learner not only know cardiac risk factors in general but also know his own behaviors that place him at risk for cardiac disease.

BOX 17.4 Examples of Verbs for Writing Learning Outcomes

Cognitive Domain	Affective Domain	Psychomotor Domain
Compares	Accepts	Assembles
Describes	Attends	Calculates
Evaluates	Chooses	Changes
Explains	Discusses	Demonstrates
Identifies	Displays	Measures
Labels	Initiates	Moves
Lists	Joins	Organizes
Names	Participates	Shows
Plans	Shares	
Selects	Uses	
States		
Writes		

In writing learning outcomes, the nurse must be specific about what behaviors and knowledge (cognitive, psychomotor, and affective) learners must have to be able to positively influence their health state. In most cases, the learning needs are more complex than simple acquisition of knowledge and include the application of that knowledge to oneself.

Choosing Content

The content, or what is to be taught, is determined by learning outcomes. For instance, "Identify appropriate sites for insulin injection" means the nurse must include content about the body sites suitable for insulin injections. Nurses can select among many sources of information, including books, nursing journals, the internet, and other nurses and primary care providers. Whatever sources the nurse chooses, content should be:

- Accurate
- Current
- Based on learning outcomes

- Adjusted for the learner's age, culture, and ability
- Consistent with information the nurse is teaching
- Selected with consideration of how much time and what resources are available for teaching.

Selecting Teaching Strategies

The method of teaching that the nurse chooses should be suited to the individual and to the material to be learned (Figure 17.2 ■). For example, the client who cannot read needs material presented in other ways, a discussion is usually not the best strategy for teaching how to give an injection, and a nurse using group discussion for teaching should be a competent group leader. As stated earlier, some clients are visually oriented and learn best through seeing; others learn best through hearing and having the skill explained. Table 17.3 lists selected teaching strategies.

Organizing Learning Experiences

To save nurses time in constructing their own teaching guides, some health agencies have developed guides for teaching sessions that nurses commonly give. These guides standardize content and teaching methods and make it easier for the nurse to plan and implement client teaching. Standardized teaching plans also ensure consistency of content for the learner, thereby decreasing the risk of confusion if different practices are taught. For example, when teaching infant bathing, the nurse on the unit should be consistent about which soaps are appropriate for the infant's bath and distinguish those that are not. Whether the nurse is implementing a plan devised by another or developing an individualized teaching plan, some guidelines can help the nurse sequence the learning experience:

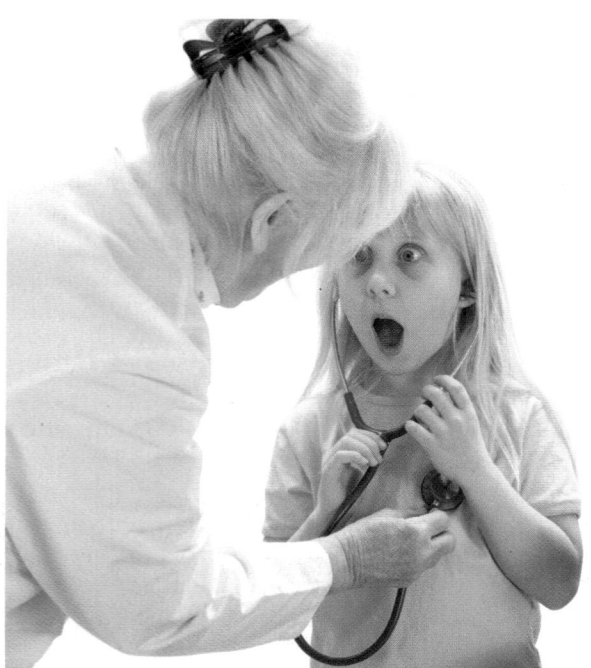

Figure 17.2 ■ Teaching materials and strategies should be suited to the client's age and learning abilities.
GaryAlvis/E+/Getty Images.

- Start with something the learner is concerned about; for example, before learning how to administer insulin to himself, an adolescent wants to know how to adjust his lifestyle and yet still play football.

Clinical Alert!

Leave a notepad and pen at the client's bedside, and encourage the client to write down questions for the nurse or the primary care provider.

- Discover what the learner knows, and then proceed to the unknown. This gives the learner confidence. Sometimes you will not know the client's knowledge or skill base and will need to elicit this information, either by asking questions or by having the client fill out a form, such as a pretest.
- Address early on any area that is causing the client anxiety. A high level of anxiety can impair concentration in other areas. For example, a woman highly anxious about her fear of the needle breaking off into the skin may not be able to learn how to self-administer an insulin injection until her fear is resolved.
- Teach the basics before proceeding to the variations or adjustments (e.g., simple to complex). It is confusing for learners to have to consider possible adjustments and variations before they master the basic concepts. For example, when teaching a client how to perform intermittent self-catheterization, it is best to teach the basic procedure before teaching any adjustments that might be needed if the catheter stops draining after insertion.
- Schedule time for review of content and questions the client(s) may have to clarify information.

Clinical Alert!

If the client has no questions, you can help introduce questions by beginning with, "A few frequently asked questions are," then providing examples.

Implementing

The nurse needs to be flexible in implementing any teaching plan because the plan may need revising. The client may become tired sooner than anticipated or be faced with too much information too quickly, the client's needs may change, or external factors may intervene. For instance, the nurse and the client plan to change his dressing at 10 a.m., but when the time comes, the client wants to observe the nurse once more before doing it himself.

In this case, the nurse alters the teaching plan and discusses any desired information, provides another demonstration, and defers teaching the psychomotor skill until the next day. It is also important for nurses to use teaching techniques that enhance learning and reduce or eliminate any barrier to learning, such as pain or fatigue (see Table 17.2 earlier in this chapter).

TABLE 17.3 Selected Teaching Strategies

Strategy	Major Type of Learning	Characteristics
Explanation or description (e.g., lecture)	Cognitive	Teacher controls content and pace. Learner is passive and therefore retains less information than when actively participating. Feedback is determined by the teacher. May be given to individual or group.
One-on-one discussion	Affective, cognitive	Encourages participation by learner. Permits reinforcement and repetition at the learner's level. Permits introduction of sensitive subjects.
Answering questions	Cognitive	Teacher controls most of content and pace. Teacher must understand question and what it means to the learner. Learner may need to overcome cultural perception that asking questions is impolite and may embarrass the teacher. Can be used with individuals and groups. Teacher sometimes needs to confirm whether the question has been answered by asking the learner, for example, "Does that answer your question?"
Demonstration	Psychomotor	Often used with explanation. Can be used with individuals and small or large groups. Does not permit use of equipment by learner; learner is passive.
Discovery	Cognitive, affective	Teacher guides problem-solving situation. Learner is active participant; therefore, retention of information is high.
Group discussions	Affective, cognitive	Learner can obtain assistance from supportive group. Group members learn from one another. Teacher needs to keep the discussion focused and prevent monopolization by one or two learners.
Practice	Psychomotor	Allows repetition and immediate feedback. Permits hands-on experience.
Printed and audiovisual materials	Cognitive	Types include books, pamphlets, films, programmed instruction, and computer learning. Learners can proceed at their own speed. Nurse can act as resource, need not be present during learning. Potentially ineffective if reading level of the materials is too high. Teacher needs to select language of materials that meets learner needs if English is a second language.
Role playing	Affective, cognitive	Permits expression of attitudes, values, and emotions. Can assist in development of communication skills. Involves active participation by learner. Teacher must create supportive, safe environment for learners to minimize anxiety.
Modeling	Affective, psychomotor	Nurse sets example by attitude, psychomotor skill.
Computer learning resources	All types of learning	Learner is active. Learner controls pace. Provides immediate reinforcement and review. Use with individuals or groups.

Clinical Alert!

Many nurses find that they teach while performing nursing care (e.g., giving medication). Remember to document this informal teaching.

Guidelines for Teaching

Knowledge alone is not enough to motivate a client to change a behavior. Do not assume that providing information will automatically result in clients changing their behavior. Learning what needs to be done to change behavior and acting on that knowledge are two different processes. The stages of change, the client's willingness and perceived need to change, and barriers to change are important elements to reflect on when implementing a teaching plan (see Chapter 19 ∞). When a client is ready to change a health behavior and when implementing a teaching plan, the nurse may find the following guidelines helpful:

- A respectful relationship between teacher and learner is essential. A relationship that is accepting, friendly, and positive will best assist learning. The following attitudes are important for the nurse to exhibit: Value seeing the healthcare situation "through the client's eyes"; respect and encourage individual expression of the client's values, preferences, and expressed needs; value the client's expertise with his or her own health and symptoms (QSEN Institute, n.d.). Knowing the learner and the previously described factors that affect learning should be established before planning the teaching.

- The teacher who uses the client's previous learning in the present situation encourages the client and facilitates learning new skills. For instance, a client who already knows how to cook can use this knowledge when learning to prepare food for a special diet.
- The optimal time for each session depends largely on the learner. Whenever possible, ask the client for help to choose the best time, for example, when she feels most rested or when no other activities are scheduled. Look for "teachable moments" that may occur during normal routine care. For example, if a client asks why a certain medication (e.g., Coumadin) is needed, it is an opportunity ("teachable moment") to explain the reason for the medication, signs to watch for, and if follow-up laboratory work is needed.
- The nurse teacher must be able to communicate clearly and concisely. The words used need to have the same meaning to the client as to the teacher. A client who is taught not to put water on an area of skin may think a wet washcloth is permissible for washing the area. In effect, the nurse needs to explain that no water or moisture should touch the area.
- Using a layperson's vocabulary enhances communication. Nurses often use terms and abbreviations that have meaning to other health professionals but make little sense to clients. Even words such as *urine* or *feces* may be unfamiliar to clients, and abbreviations such as ICU (intensive care unit) or PACU (postanesthesia care unit) are often misunderstood.
- The pace of each teaching session also affects learning. Nurses should be sensitive to any signs that the pace is too fast or too slow. A client who appears confused or does not comprehend material when questioned may be finding the pace too fast. When the client appears bored and loses interest, the pace may be too slow, the learning period may be too long, or the client may be tired.
- An environment can detract from or assist learning; for example, noise or interruptions usually interfere with concentration, whereas a comfortable environment promotes learning. If possible, the client should be out of bed for learning activities. Most clients associate lying in bed with rest and sleep, not with learning. Placing the client in a position and location associated with activity or learning may influence the amount of learning that takes place. For instance, a client who is shown a videotape while in bed may be more likely to become drowsy during instruction than a client who is sitting in a bedside chair.
- Teaching aids can foster learning and help focus a learner's attention. To ensure the transfer of learning, the nurse should use the type of supplies or equipment the client will eventually use. Before the teaching session, the nurse needs to assemble all equipment and visual aids and ensure that all audiovisual equipment is functioning effectively. See Client Teaching for teaching tools for children.
- Teaching that involves several of the learner's senses often enhances learning. For instance, when teaching about changing a surgical dressing, the nurse can tell the client about the procedure (hearing), show how to change the dressing (sight), and show how to manipulate the equipment (touch).
- Learning is more effective when the learners discover the content for themselves. Ways to increase learning include stimulating motivation and self-direction, for example, (a) by providing specific, realistic, achievable outcomes; (b) by giving feedback; and (c) by helping the learner derive satisfaction from learning. The nurse may also encourage self-directed, independent learning by encouraging the client to explore sources of information required. If certain activities do not assist the learner in attaining outcomes, these need to be reassessed; perhaps other activities can replace them. Explanation alone may not be sufficient to teach a client to handle a syringe. Handling the syringe may be more effective (Figure 17.3 ■).
- Repetition reinforces learning. Summarizing content, rephrasing (using other words), and approaching the material from another point of view are ways of repeating and clarifying content. For instance, after discussing the kinds of foods that can be included in a diet, the nurse describes the foods again, but in the context of the three meals eaten during one day.
- It is helpful to employ "organizers" to introduce material to be learned. Advanced organizers provide a means of connecting unknown material to known material and generating logical relationships. The following statement can be an advanced organizer: "You understand how urine flows down a catheter from the

CLIENT TEACHING Teaching Tools for Children

- *Visits.* Visiting the hospital and treatment rooms; seeing individuals dressed in uniforms, scrubs, protective gear.
- *Dress-up.* Touching and dressing in the clothing they will see and wear.
- *Coloring books.* Using coloring books to prepare for treatments, surgery, or hospitalization; show what rooms, people, and equipment will look like.
- *Storybooks.* Storybooks describe how the child will feel, what will be done, and what the place will look like. Parents can read these stories to children several times before the experience. Younger children like this repetition.
- *Dolls.* Practicing procedures on dolls or teddy bears that they will later experience; gives a sense of mastery of the situation. Custom dolls are often available for inserting tubes and giving injections, for example.
- *Puppet play.* Puppets can be used in role-play situations to provide information and show the child what the experience will be like; they help the child express emotions.
- *Health fairs.* Health fairs can educate children about their bodies and ways to stay healthy. Fairs can focus on high-risk problems children face, such as injury prevention, poison control, and other topics identified in the community as a concern.

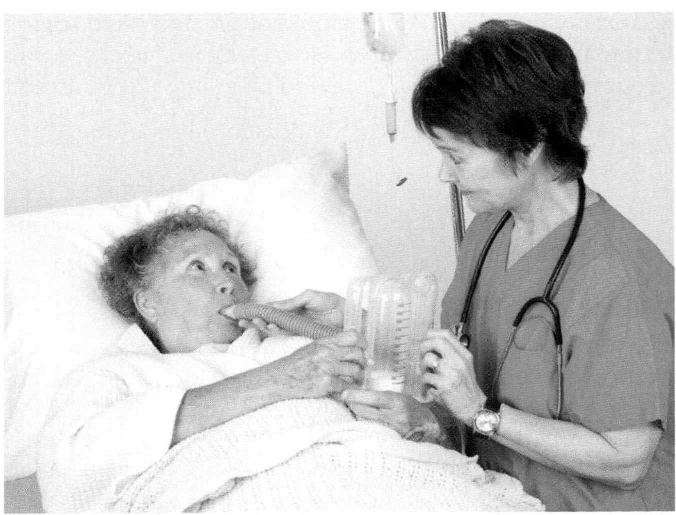

Figure 17.3 ■ Teaching activities may need to include hands-on client participation.
Lisa Young/123RF.

bladder. Now I will show you how to inject fluid so that it flows up the catheter into the bladder." The details that follow are then seen within a framework that adds meaning.

- The anticipated behavioral changes that indicate learning has taken place must always be within the context of the client's lifestyle and resources. It would be unreasonable to expect a woman to soak in a tub of hot water 2 times a day if she did not have a bathtub or had to heat water on a stove.

Special Teaching Strategies

One-on-one discussion is the most common method of teaching used by nurses. However, nurses can choose from several special teaching strategies: client contracting, group teaching, computer learning resources, discovery by problem-solving, and behavior modification. Any strategy the nurse selects must be appropriate for the learner and the learning objectives.

Client Contracting

Client contracting involves establishing a learning contract with a client that specifies certain outcomes and when they are to be met. Here is an example of a self-contract:

> I, Amy Martin, will exercise strenuously for 20 minutes 3 times per week for a period of 2 weeks and will then buy myself six yellow roses.
>
> Amy Martin — A. Ward, RN
>
> July 30, 2020

The contract, drawn up and signed by the client and the nurse, may specify the learning outcomes, the responsibilities of the client and the nurse, and the methods of follow-up and evaluation. The contract can be changed in two ways: if the client meets the contract outcomes and wants to negotiate new learning outcomes and if the client decides that he or she is unable to meet the existing learning outcomes and wants to revise them. The learning contract allows for freedom, mutual respect, and mutual responsibility.

Group Teaching

Group instruction is economical, and it provides members with an opportunity to share with and learn from others. A small group allows for discussion in which everyone can participate. A large group often necessitates a lecture technique or use of films, videos, slides, or role playing by teachers.

All members involved in group instruction should have a common need (e.g., prenatal health or preoperative instruction), and sociocultural factors should be considered in the formation of a group.

Computer Learning Resources

Using computers for instruction is common. Computers were initially used primarily for the learning of facts. Now, however, computers can also be used to teach the following:

- Application and retention of information (e.g., answering questions after reading the information about a health subject)
- Psychomotor skills (e.g., filling a syringe on the computer screen to the correct dosage line on the syringe)
- Complex problem-solving skills (e.g., responding to questions based on a client situation).

Computers can be used in a variety of ways:

- Individual healthcare professionals or clients using one computer
- Families or small groups of three to five clients gathered around one computer taking turns reading the information and answering questions together
- Large groups with the computer display screen projected onto an overhead screen and a teacher or one learner using the keyboard
- Individuals or small groups at computers using programs through shared network platforms or through internet websites.

Individuals using a computer can set the pace that meets their learning needs. Small groups are less able to do this, and large groups progress through the program at a pace that may be too slow for some learners and too fast for others. It is therefore helpful to group learners of similar needs and abilities together. Whether using the computer alone or in large groups, learners read and view informational material, answer questions, and receive immediate feedback. The correct answer is usually indicated by colors, flashing signs, or written praise. When the learner selects an incorrect answer, the computer may respond with an explanation of why that was not the best answer and encouragement to try again. Many programs ask learners whether they want to review the material on which the question and answer were based. Some computer programs feature simulated situations that allow learners to manipulate objects on the screen to learn psychomotor skills. When used to teach such skills, computer instruction must be followed up with practice on actual equipment supervised by the teacher.

Some clients may have a negative attitude about computers that could act as a barrier to learning. The nurse helps these clients by explaining how the computer can help meet their needs. Matching a computer program or website to the client's individual health circumstances may encourage computer use. Providing a resource list of free community sites for training and access may also help.

Most media catalogs, professional journals, and healthcare libraries contain information about computer software programs available to the nurse for client education. The media specialist or librarian in a healthcare facility or educational institution is an excellent resource to help the nurse locate appropriate computer programs. Computer educational material is also available for clients with different language needs, for clients with special visual needs, and for clients at different growth and development levels.

The internet is an important source of health information, particularly for clients with chronic illnesses. It is important for the nurse to teach the client who uses the internet how to evaluate if the site is a relevant and credible source for health information.

Discovery by Problem-Solving

In using the discovery by problem-solving technique, the nurse presents some initial information and then asks the learners a question or presents a situation related to the information. The learner applies the new information to the situation and decides what to do. Learners can work alone or in groups. This technique is well suited to family learning. The teacher guides the learners through the thinking process necessary to reach the best solution to the question or the best action to take in the situation. This may also be referred to as *anticipatory problem-solving*. For example, the nurse educator might present information on diabetes and glucose management. Then the nurse might ask the learners how they think their insulin or diet should be adjusted if their morning glucose was too low. In this way, clients learn what critical components they need to consider to reach the best solution to the problem.

Behavior Modification

The behavior modification system for changing behavior has as its basic assumptions (a) that human behaviors are learned and can be selectively strengthened, weakened, eliminated, or replaced and (b) that an individual's behavior is under conscious control. Under this system, desirable behavior is rewarded, and undesirable behavior is ignored. The client's response is the key to behavior change. For example, clients trying to quit smoking are not criticized when they smoke, but they are praised or rewarded when they go without a cigarette for a certain period of time. For some clients, a learning contract is combined with behavior modification and includes the following pertinent features:

- Positive reinforcement (e.g., praise) is used.
- The client participates in the development of the learning plan.
- Undesirable behavior is ignored, not criticized.
- The expectation of the client and the nurse is that the task will be mastered (i.e., the behavior will change).

Transcultural Teaching

The nurse and clients of different cultural and ethnic backgrounds have additional barriers to overcome in the teaching–learning process. These barriers include language and communication challenges, differing concepts of time, conflicting cultural healing practices, beliefs that may positively or negatively influence compliance with health teaching, and unique high-risk or high-frequency health problems that can be addressed with health promotion instruction (see Chapter 19 ∞). Nurses should consider the following guidelines when teaching clients from various ethnic backgrounds:

- ***Obtain teaching materials, pamphlets, and instructions in languages used by clients.*** Nurses who are unable to read the foreign-language material for themselves can have the translator read the material to them. The nurse can then evaluate the quality of the information and update it with the translator's help as needed.
- ***Use visual aids, such as pictures, charts, or diagrams, to communicate meaning.*** Audiovisual material may be helpful if the English is spoken clearly and slowly. Even if understanding the verbal message is a problem for the client, seeing a skill or procedure may be helpful. In some instances, a translator can be asked to clarify the video. Alternatively, the video may be available in several languages, and the nurse can request the necessary version from the company.
- ***Use concrete rather than abstract words.*** Use simple language (short sentences, short words), and present only one idea at a time.
- ***Allow time for questions.*** This helps the client mentally separate one idea or skill from another.
- ***Avoid the use of medical terminology or healthcare language,*** such as "taking your vital signs" or "apical pulse." Rather, nurses should say they are going to take a blood pressure or listen to the client's heart.
- ***If understanding another's pronunciation is a problem, validate brief information in writing.*** For example, during assessments, write down numbers, words, or phrases and have the client read them to verify accuracy.
- ***Use humor very cautiously.*** Meaning can change in the translation process.
- ***Do not use slang words or colloquialisms.*** These may be interpreted literally.
- ***Do not assume that a client who nods, uses eye contact, or smiles is indicating an understanding of what is being taught.*** These responses may simply be

the client's way of indicating respect. The client may feel that asking the nurse questions or stating a lack of understanding is inappropriate because it might embarrass or cause the nurse to "lose face."

- ***Invite and encourage questions during teaching.*** Urge clients to ask questions and be involved in making information clearer. When asking questions to evaluate client understanding, avoid asking negative questions, which can be interpreted differently by clients for whom English is a second language. "Do you understand how far you can bend your hip after surgery?" is better than the negative question "You don't understand how far you can bend your hip after surgery, do you?" Even better is the question, "What do you remember about how far you can bend your hip after surgery?" With particularly difficult information or skills teaching, the nurse might say, "This is a lot of information. Can I please review the key points one more time?"

  In some cultures, expressing a need is not appropriate, and expressing confusion or asking to be shown something again is considered rude. For example, some clients may want to "save face" for themselves and others. As a result, they may agree to what is being said or nod their heads in agreement to avoid being considered offensive or disruptive by disagreeing with the nurse or physician. They may need to be given permission to ask questions. Care must also be taken to not interpret nods as gestures of informed consent.
- ***When explaining procedures or functioning related to personal areas of the body, it may be appropriate to have a nurse of the same gender do the teaching.*** Because of modesty concerns in many cultures and beliefs about what is considered appropriate and inappropriate male–female interaction, it is wise to have a female nurse teach a female client about personal care, birth control, sexually transmitted infections, and other potentially sensitive areas. If a translator is needed during the explanation of procedures or teaching, the translator should also be female.
- ***Include the family in planning and teaching. This promotes trust and mutual respect.*** Identify a respected family member and incorporate that individual into the planning and teaching to promote and support the health teaching. In some cultures, the male head of household is the critical family member to include in health teaching; in other cultures, it is the oldest female member; and in some cultures, it is important for the nurse to direct teaching to include all interested family members.
- ***Consider the client's time orientation.*** The client may be more oriented to the present (what is currently occurring) than the nurse, who may be focused on preventing future health problems. For example, schedules may be very flexible in present-oriented societies, with sleeping and eating patterns varying greatly. Teaching clients to take medications at bedtime or with a meal does not necessarily mean that these activities will occur at the same time each day. For this reason, the nurse should assess the client's daily routine before teaching the client to pair a treatment or medication with an event the nurse assumes occurs at the same time every day. When teaching a client when to take medication, the nurse should determine whether a clock or watch is available to the client and whether the client can tell time.

  Preventing future problems may not be as important for the client oriented to the present. In such instances, the nurse can emphasize preventing short-term rather than long-term problems. Failure to keep clinic appointments or to arrive on time is common in clients who have a present-time orientation. The nurse can help by accommodating these clients when they arrive for their appointments.
- ***Identify cultural health practices and beliefs.*** Nonadherence with health teaching may be related to a conflict with folk medicine beliefs. It may also be related to lack of understanding or fatalism, a belief that life events are predestined or fixed in advance and that the client is powerless to change them. To encourage adherence, the nurse needs to learn the client's explanation of why the illness developed and how it might be treated.

The nurse should treat the client's cultural healing beliefs with respect and identify whether any agree or are in conflict with what is being taught. The nurse can then focus on the ones in agreement to promote the integration of new learning with the familiar health practices. The goal is to arrive at a mutually agreeable plan: Decide which instructions must be followed for client safety, and negotiate less crucial folk healing practices.

Evaluating

Evaluating is both an ongoing and a final process in which the client, the nurse, and often the support people determine what has been learned.

Evaluating Learning

The process of evaluating learning is the same as evaluating client achievement of desired outcomes for other nursing diagnoses. Learning is measured against the predetermined learning outcomes selected in the planning phase of the teaching process. Thus, the outcomes serve not only to direct the teaching plan but also to provide outcome criteria for evaluation. For example, the outcome "Selects foods that are low in carbohydrates" can be evaluated by asking the client to name such foods or to select low-carbohydrate foods from a list.

The best method for evaluating depends on the type of learning. In *cognitive learning*, the client demonstrates the acquisition of knowledge. Examples of evaluation tools for cognitive learning include the following:

- Direct observation of behavior (e.g., observing the client selecting the solution to a problem using the new knowledge)
- Written measurements (e.g., tests)
- Oral questioning (e.g., asking the client to restate information or correct verbal responses to questions)

- Self-reports and self-monitoring. These can be useful during follow-up phone calls and home visits. Evaluating individual self-paced learning, as might occur with computer instruction, often incorporates self-monitoring.

The acquisition of *psychomotor skills* is best evaluated by observing how well the client carries out a procedure, such as self-administration of insulin.

Affective learning is more difficult to evaluate. Whether attitudes or values have been learned may be inferred by listening to the client's responses to questions, noting how the client speaks about relevant subjects, and observing the client's behavior that expresses feelings and values. For example, have parents learned to value health sufficiently to have their children immunized? Do clients who state that they value health use condoms every time they have sex with a new partner?

Following evaluation, the nurse may find it necessary to modify or repeat the teaching plan if the objectives have not been met or have been met only partially. Follow-up teaching in the home or by phone may be needed for the client discharged from a health facility.

Behavior change does not always take place immediately after learning. Clients often accept change intellectually first and then change their behavior only periodically (e.g., a client knows that she must lose weight but diets and exercises off and on). If the new behavior is to replace the old behavior, it must emerge gradually; otherwise, the old behavior may prevail. The nurse can assist clients with behavior change by allowing for client vacillation and by providing encouragement.

Evaluating Teaching

It is important for nurses to evaluate their own teaching and the content of the teaching program just as they evaluate the effectiveness of nursing interventions for other nursing diagnoses. Evaluation should include a consideration of all factors—the timing, the teaching strategies, the amount of information, whether the teaching was helpful, and so on. The nurse may find, for example, that the client was overwhelmed with too much information, was bored, or was motivated to learn more.

Both the client and the nurse should evaluate the learning experience. The client may tell the nurse what was helpful, interesting, and so on. Feedback questionnaires and videotapes of the learning sessions can also be helpful.

The nurse should not feel ineffective as a teacher if the client forgets some of what is taught. Forgetting is normal and should be anticipated. Having the client write down information, repeating information during teaching, giving handouts on the information, and having the client be active in the learning process all promote retention.

Documenting

Documentation of the teaching process is essential because it provides a legal record that the teaching took place and communicates the teaching to other health professionals. If teaching is not documented, then legally, it did not occur.

It is also important to document the responses of the client and support people to teaching activities. What did the client or support person say or do to indicate that learning occurred? Has the client demonstrated mastery of a skill or the acquisition of knowledge? The nurse records this in the client's chart as evidence of learning. A sample documentation of teaching follows:

6/8/2020 1130 Learning to use glucometer to check her own capillary blood glucose levels. Noted a slight hesitation with each step. Demonstrated correct technique. Stated that she is "feeling more comfortable" each time she does it but still "needs to stop and think about the process." Will continue to monitor client's progress. S. Brown, RN

The parts of the teaching process that should be documented in the client's chart include the following:

- Diagnosed learning needs
- Learning outcomes
- Topics taught
- Client outcomes
- Need for additional teaching
- Resources provided.

The written teaching plan that the nurse uses as a resource to guide future teaching sessions might also include these elements:

- Actual information and skills taught
- Teaching strategies used
- Time framework and content for each class
- Teaching outcomes and methods of evaluation.

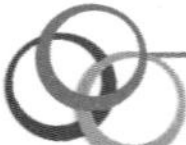

Critical Thinking Checkpoint

Mrs. Yorty is a 59-year-old bank vice president who is heavily relied on by her boss and coworkers. Three days ago, she was admitted to the hospital with complaints of shortness of breath and mild chest pain. A diagnostic evaluation indicates that she has significant coronary artery disease but has not yet had a heart attack. Her primary care provider has indicated that Mrs. Yorty will need to make significant lifestyle changes to reduce her heart attack risk. As her nurse, you have been requested to teach Mrs. Yorty about her disease process, diet, exercise, and stress reduction. As you begin teaching Mrs. Yorty, you note that she is very pleasant and frequently nods her head, but she also seems preoccupied and is easily distracted.

1. How would you evaluate Mrs. Yorty's readiness to learn?
2. Of what benefit would a learning needs assessment be because Mrs. Yorty is obviously a well-educated client?
3. You recognize that you have a great deal of information to deliver to Mrs. Yorty, and you are concerned that you will not be able to teach it all. What can you do to help Mrs. Yorty and still accomplish the learning outcomes?
4. How will you know if your teaching is effective?
5. How might your teaching differ if you were instructing Mrs. Yorty at home rather than in a hospital or acute care setting?

Answers to Critical Thinking Checkpoint questions are available on the faculty resources site. Please consult with your instructor.

Chapter 17 Review

CHAPTER HIGHLIGHTS

- Teaching clients and families about their health needs is a major role of the nurse. Nurses also teach colleagues, subordinates, nursing and other healthcare students, and groups in community education programs.
- Learning is represented by a change in behavior.
- Bloom identified three learning domains: cognitive, affective, and psychomotor.
- Three main theories of learning are behaviorism, cognitivism, and humanism.
- Several factors affect learning, including age and developmental stage, motivation, readiness, active involvement, relevance, feedback, nonjudgmental support, simple to complex learning, repetition, timing, environment, emotions, physiologic events, cultural aspects, and psychomotor ability.
- Many adults in the United States use technology to access health information. Nurses need to know and integrate this technology into their teaching plans.
- Low health literacy is a silent epidemic. It is associated with poor health outcomes and higher healthcare costs. Using the "teach-back" technique helps the nurse assess the client's understanding of what was taught.
- Teaching, like the nursing process, consists of six activities: assessing the learner, diagnosing learning needs, developing a teaching plan, implementing the plan, evaluating learning outcomes and teaching effectiveness, and documenting instructional activities.
- The teaching strategies chosen by the nurse should be suited to the client and to the material to be learned.
- A teaching plan is a written plan consisting of learning outcomes, content to teach, and strategies to use in teaching the content. The plan must be revised when the client's needs change or the teaching strategies prove ineffective.
- Evaluating the teaching–learning process is both an ongoing and a final process in which the client, nurse, and support people determine what has been learned.
- Documentation of client teaching is essential to communicate the teaching to other health professionals and to provide a record for legal purposes.

TEST YOUR KNOWLEDGE

1. Which learning activity reflects Bloom's affective domain?
   1. Administering an injection
   2. Accepting the loss of a limb
   3. Inserting a catheter
   4. Learning how to read

2. Which is the best method of helping a client newly diagnosed with diabetes to learn the dietary requirements associated with the disease?
   1. Provide a videotape that addresses the dietary requirements associated with the disease.
   2. Ask a nutritionist to visit the client to present information and handouts about the diabetic diet.
   3. Ask the client to make a list of her favorite foods and how to work them into her diet.
   4. Have the client attend a group meeting for clients with diabetes to discuss their adaptation to this chronic health condition.

3. A nurse is presenting teaching sessions to a group of residents in a home for long-term physical rehabilitation. Which client exhibits the highest motivation?
   1. An individual who has been struggling to follow nursing directives regarding discharge goals
   2. The client who has just moved in and is already waiting for discharge
   3. A client who is excited to learn about his new prosthesis
   4. A client who has been there the longest and is a great "coach" for newcomers

4. How can the nurse best assess a client's style of learning?
   1. Ask the client how he or she learns best.
   2. Use a variety of teaching strategies.
   3. Observe the client's interactions with others.
   4. Ask family members.

5. A 74-year-old client who takes multiple medications tells the nurse, "I have no idea what that little yellow pill is for." What is the best nursing diagnosis for this client?
   1. Lack of knowledge
   2. Willingness for knowledge enhancement
   3. Lack of knowledge (medication information)
   4. Potential for lack of knowledge

6. A client is scheduled to have a diagnostic procedure. Which questions by the nurse will most likely produce a "teachable moment"? Select all that apply.
   1. "Have you ever had this procedure before?"
   2. "What are your concerns about this procedure?"
   3. "What would you like to know about the procedure?"
   4. "Are you prepared for this procedure?"
   5. "What have you heard or read about the procedure?"

7. The nurse instructs a client on self-care for a new ostomy. Which client behaviors demonstrate that instruction has been effective? Select all that apply.
   1. Client provides skin care and changes ostomy device.
   2. Client states what items are needed to perform ostomy care.
   3. Client is unable to identify changes in skin around the stoma.
   4. Client tells the nurse that he does not want to do the care.
   5. Client asks his wife to learn how to perform the care so he will not have to do it.

8. A primary care provider admitted a client experiencing hypertensive crisis because of the failure to take his prescribed medications. To determine learning needs, which client assessment by the nurse would have the highest priority?
   1. Age
   2. Perception of the effects of hypertension
   3. Ability to purchase needed medications
   4. Support system

9. A client has a learning outcome of "Select foods that are low in fat content." Which statement reflects that the client has met this learning outcome?
1. "I understand the importance of maintaining a low-fat diet."
2. "I feel better about myself now."
3. "I revised my favorite recipe to be lower in fat."
4. "Since changing my diet, my husband is also losing weight."

10. A client's learning outcome is "Client will verbalize medication name, purpose, and appropriate precautions." Which documented statement reflects evidence of learning?
1. Taught name, purpose, and precautions for the new cardiac medication; seemed to understand.
2. Provided and reviewed written information about the medication; correct responses were given to follow-up questions.
3. Written information read to client; client stated he would read it when he got home.
4. Asked questions about the new cardiac medication; satisfied with the information.

See Answers to Test Your Knowledge in Appendix A.

READINGS AND REFERENCES

Suggested Readings

Brega, A. G., Barnard, J., Mabachi, N. M., Weiss, B. D., DeWalt, D. A., Brach, C., . . . West, D. R. (2015). *AHRQ health literacy universal precautions toolkit* (2nd ed.). Retrieved from http://www.ahrq.gov/sites/default/files/publications/files/healthlittoolkit2_4.pdf

This toolkit includes valuable information, including brochures, posters, and videos (e.g., a 6-minute video on the importance of health literacy by showing a client's misunderstanding of health information and a short video demonstrating "teach-back"). Many tools are available for improving spoken and written health communication and a client's self-management and empowerment.

Ethnomed.org

The objective of this website is to make information about culture, language, health, illness, and community resources directly accessible to healthcare providers who see clients from different ethnic groups.

Polster, D. S. (2018). Confronting barriers to improve healthcare literacy and cultural competency in disparate populations. *Nursing*, *48*(12), 28–33. doi:10.1097/01.NURSE.0000547717.61986.25

The author emphasizes how clear communication and understanding are important for positive client outcomes. The article reviews the need for understanding healthcare literacy, cultural competency, and health disparities/inequalities to provide empathetic care to clients and their families.

Related Research

Davis, D. W., Logsdon, M. C., Vogt, K., Rushton, J., Myers, J., Lauf, A., & Hogan, F. (2017). Parent education is changing: A review of smartphone apps. *The American Journal of Maternal/Child Nursing*, *42*(5), 248–256. doi:10.1097/NMC.0000000000000353

Hobbs, J. K. (2016). Reducing hospital readmission rates in patients with heart failure. *MEDSURG Nursing*, *25*(3), 145–152.

Price-Haywood, E. G., Harden-Barrios, J., Ulep, R., & Luo, Q. (2017). eHealth literacy: Patient engagement in identifying strategies to encourage use of patient portals among older adults. *Population Health Management*, *20*, 486–494. doi:10.1089/pop.2016.0164

References

American Nurses Association. (2015). *Scope and standards of practice* (3rd ed.). Silver Spring, MD: Nursebooks.org.

Anderson, M., & Perrin, A. (2017). *Tech adoption climbs among older adults.* Retrieved from http://www.pewinternet.org/2017/05/17/tech-adoption-climbs-among-older-adults

Bastable, S. B. (2017). *Essentials of patient education* (2nd ed.). Burlington, MA: Jones & Bartlett.

Bloom, B. S. (Ed.). (1956). *Taxonomy of education objectives. Book 1, cognitive domain.* New York, NY: Longman.

Centers for Disease Control and Prevention. (2016). *What is health literacy?* Retrieved from https://www.cdc.gov/healthliteracy/learn

Fronczek, A. E., & Rouhana, N. A. (2018). Attaining mutual goals in telehealth encounters: Utilizing King's framework for telenursing practice. *Nursing Science Quarterly, 31*(3), 233–236. doi:10.1177/0894318418774884

Knowles, M. S., Holton, E. F., & Swanson, R. A. (2015). *The adult learner. The definitive classic in adult education and human resource development* (8th ed.). New York, NY: Routledge.

MedlinePlus. (n.d.). *Evaluating internet health information: A tutorial from the National Library of Medicine*. Retrieved from https://medlineplus.gov/webeval/webeval_start.html

Miller, M. A., & Stoeckel, P. R. (2016). *Client education: Theory and practice* (2nd ed.). Boston, MA: Jones & Bartlett.

National Institutes of Health. (2018). *Finding and evaluating online resources*. Retrieved from https://nccih.nih.gov/health/webresources

National Patient Safety Foundation. (2016). *Leveling the challenges of health literacy with Ask Me 3*. Retrieved from http://c.ymcdn.com/sites/www.npsf.org/resource/resmgr/AskMe3/AskMe3_HealthLiteracyTrainin.pdf?hhSearchTerms=%22Ask%22

Pew Research Center. (2018). *Mobile fact sheet*. Retrieved from http://www.pewinternet.org/fact-sheet/mobile

QSEN Institute. (n.d.). *QSEN competencies*. Retrieved from http://qsen.org/competencies/pre-licensure-ksas

Schramm, M. A. (2016). Home telehealth: A tool for diabetic self-management. *AAACN Viewpoint*, *38*(1), 4–7.

Scott, S. A. (2016). Health literacy education in baccalaureate nursing programs in the United States. *Nursing Education Perspectives*, *37*, 153–158. doi:10.1097/01.NEP.0000000000000005

U.S. Department of Health and Human Services. (n.d.). *Plain language: A promising strategy for clearly communicating health information and improving health literacy*. Retrieved from https://health.gov/communication/literacy/plainlanguage/PlainLanguage.htm

Waterworth, S., & Honey, M. (2018). On-line health seeking activity of older adults: An integrative review of the literature. *Geriatric Nursing*, *39*(3), 310–317. doi:10.1016/j.gerinurse.2017.10.016

Watts, S. A., Stevenson, C., & Adams, M. (2017). Improving health literacy in patients with diabetes. *Nursing*, *47*(1), 24–31. doi:10.1097/01.NURSE.0000510739.60928.a9

Wilkinson, J. M., & Barcus, L. (2017). *Pearson nursing diagnosis handbook* (11th ed.). Boston, MA: Pearson.

World Health Organization. (n.d.). *Health literacy and health behaviour*. Retrieved from http://www.who.int/healthpromotion/conferences/7gchp/track2/en

Selected Bibliography

Blakely, M. D. (2018). Level connections: Educating patients more effectively. *Med-Surg Matters*, *27*(5), 13–15.

Brous, E. (2016). Legal considerations in telehealth and telemedicine. *American Journal of Nursing*, *116*(9), 64–67. doi:10.1097/01.NAJ.0000494700.78616.d3

deCastro, M., & Sawatzky, J. (2018). Mobile health interventions for primary prevention of cardiovascular disease. *Journal for Nurse Practitioners*, *14*(8), e165–e168. doi:10.1016/j.nurpra.2018.06.001

Hayes, C. (2016). Approaches to continuing professional development: Putting theory into practice. *British Journal of Nursing*, *25*(15), 860–864. doi:10.12968/bjon.2016.25.15.860

Ingram, R. R., & Kautz, D. D. (2018). Creating "win-win" outcomes for patients with low health literacy: A nursing case study. *MEDSURG Nursing*, *27*(2), 132–134.

Jaimet, K. (2016). Ready to embrace the future? Two experts look at where health care is headed, how patients' expectations are changing and what nurses can do to adapt and lead. *Canadian Nurse*, *112*(3), 20–21.

Jiang, J. (2018). *Millennials stand out for their technology use, but older generations also embrace digital life*. Retrieved from http://www.pewresearch.org/fact-tank/2018/05/02/millennials-stand-out-for-their-technology-use-but-older-generations-also-embrace-digital-life

Kerr, L. (2016). Low health literacy is common, but can be addressed. *Urology Times*, *44*(5), 20.

Marshall, L. C. (2016). *Mastering patient & family education. A healthcare handbook for success*. Indianapolis, IN: Sigma Theta Tau.

Meetoo, D., Rylance, R., & Abuhaimid, H. A. (2018). Health care in a technological world. *British Journal of Nursing*, *27*(20), 1172–1177. doi:10.12968/bjon.2018.27.20.1172

Miller, S., Lattanzio, M., & Cohen, S. (2016). "Teach-back" from a patient's perspective. *Nursing 46*(2), 63–64. doi:10.1097/01.NURSE.0000476249.18503.f5

Pavlov, I. P. (1927). *Conditioned reflexes* (G. V. Anrep, trans.). London, United Kingdom: Oxford University.

Piaget, J. (1966). *Origins of intelligence in children*. New York, NY: W. W. Norton.

Prabhu, S. R. (2016). The real value of IoT at home. *Health Management Technology*, *37*(6), 17.

Rogers, C. R. (1961). *On becoming a person*. Boston, MA: Houghton-Mifflin.

Rogers, C. R. (1969). *Freedom to learn*. Columbus, OH: Chas. E. Merrill.

Sanchez, L. M., & Cooknell, L. E. (2017). The power of 3: Using adult learning principles to facilitate patient education. *Nursing*, *47*(2), 17–19. doi:10.1097/01.NURSE.0000511819.18774.85

Shustack, L. (2019). Going digital with patient teaching. *Nursing*, *49*(1), 65–66. doi:10.1097/01.NURSE.0000549742.35131.e4

Skinner, B. F. (1953). *Science and human behavior*. New York, NY: Macmillan.

Teitelman, A. M. (2018). Using mobile technologies to improve women's health. *Journal of Obstetric, Gynecologic, & Neonatal Nursing*, *47*, 830–832. doi:10.1016/j.jogn.2018.09.004

18 Leading, Managing, and Delegating

LEARNING OUTCOMES

After completing this chapter, you will be able to:

1. Compare and contrast leadership and management.
2. Compare and contrast different leadership styles.
3. Identify characteristics of an effective leader.
4. Compare and contrast the levels of management.
5. Describe the four functions of management.
6. Discuss the roles and functions of nurse managers.
7. Identify the skills and competencies needed by a nurse manager.
8. Describe the characteristics of tasks appropriate to assign or delegate to licensed nurses or assistive personnel.
9. List the five rights of delegation.
10. Describe the role of the leader or manager in planning for and implementing change.

KEY TERMS

accountability, *351*
autocratic (authoritarian) leader, *346*
authority, *351*
bureaucratic leader, *348*
change, *352*
change agents, *352*
charismatic leader, *348*
coordinating, *351*
delegation, *354*
democratic leader, *346*
directing, *351*
effectiveness, *352*
efficiency, *352*
first-level managers, *350*
formal leader, *346*
influence, *349*
informal leader, *346*
laissez-faire (permissive) leader, *348*
leader, *345*
leadership style, *346*
manager, *345*
mentor, *352*
middle-level managers, *350*
networking, *351*
organizing, *351*
planned change, *353*
planning, *350*
preceptor, *352*
productivity, *352*
responsibility, *351*
risk management, *350*
role model, *349*
shared governance, *349*
shared leadership, *349*
situational leader, *348*
transactional leader, *348*
transformational leader, *349*
unplanned change, *353*
upper-level (top-level) managers, *350*
vision, *349*

Introduction

Although aspects of the individual nurse's role vary according to practice location and type, leadership, management, delegation, and change are consistent aspects of the role. Nurses function within healthcare systems, working with multiple clients and other healthcare providers. As a part of multidisciplinary teams, the nurse is often in a leadership position and frequently delegates aspects of care to others. There are opportunities in nursing to become leaders at various levels and also many situations in which the nurse functions as a manager and as a change agent.

The Nurse as Leader and Manager

The professional nurse frequently assumes the roles of leader and manager. These two roles are linked—that is, managers must have leadership abilities, and leaders often manage—but the two roles differ.

A **leader** influences others to work together to accomplish a specific goal. Leaders are often visionary; they are informed, articulate, confident, and self-aware. Leaders also usually have outstanding interpersonal skills and are excellent listeners and communicators. They have initiative and the ability and confidence to innovate change, motivate, facilitate, and mentor others. Within their organizations, nurse leaders participate in and guide teams that assess the effectiveness of care, implement evidence-based practice, and construct process-improvement strategies. They may be employed in a variety of positions—from shift team leader to institutional president. Leaders may also hold volunteer positions, such as chairperson of a professional organization, or be a member of a community board of directors.

A **manager** is an employee of an organization who is given authority, power, and responsibility for planning, organizing, coordinating, and directing the work of others and for establishing and evaluating standards. Managers understand organizational structure and culture. They control human, financial, and material resources. Managers set goals, make decisions, and solve problems. They initiate and implement change.

TABLE 18.1 Comparison of Leader and Manager Roles

Leaders	Managers
May or may not be officially appointed to the position	Are appointed officially to the position
Have power and authority to enforce decisions only as long as followers are willing to be led	Have power and authority to enforce decisions
Influence others toward goal setting, either formally or informally	Carry out policies, rules, and regulations
Are interested in risk taking and exploring new ideas	Maintain an orderly, controlled, rational, and equitable structure
Relate to individuals personally in an intuitive and empathetic manner	Relate to individuals according to their roles
Feel rewarded by personal achievements	Feel rewarded when fulfilling organizational mission or goals
May or may not be successful as managers	Are managers as long as the appointment holds
Manage relationships	Manage resources
Focus on individuals	Focus on systems

Nurses are responsible for managing client care. Some nurses assume a position within the organization as unit manager, supervisor, or executive. As a manager, the nurse is responsible for (a) efficiently accomplishing the goals of the organization; (b) efficiently using the organization's resources; (c) ensuring effective client care; and (d) ensuring compliance with institutional, professional, regulatory, and governmental standards. Managers are also responsible for the development of licensed and unlicensed personnel within their work group. Table 18.1 further compares the leader and manager roles. Figure 18.1 ■ illustrates some of the leading and managing roles.

Leadership

Leadership may be formal or informal. The **formal leader**, or appointed leader, is selected by an organization and given official authority to make decisions and act. An **informal leader** is not officially appointed to direct the activities of others, but because of seniority, age, or special abilities, the individual is recognized by the group as its leader and plays an important role in influencing colleagues, coworkers, or other group members to achieve the group's goals.

Leadership Theory

Early leadership theories focused on what leaders are (trait theories), what leaders do (behavioral theories), and how leaders adapt their leadership style according to the situation (contingency theories). Theories about **leadership style** describe the traits, behaviors, motivations, and choices used by individuals to effectively influence others.

Classic Leadership Theories

The trait theorists found that leaders often possess specific qualities and abilities, including good judgment, decisiveness, knowledge, adaptability, integrity, tact, self-confidence, and cooperativeness. The behaviorists believed that through education, training, and life experiences, leaders develop a particular leadership style. These styles have been characterized as autocratic, democratic, laissez-faire, and bureaucratic.

An **autocratic (authoritarian) leader** makes decisions for the group. The leader believes individuals are externally motivated (their driving force is extrinsic; they desire rewards from others) and are incapable of independent decision-making. Likened to a dictator, the autocratic leader determines policies, giving orders and directions to the group. Under this leadership style, the group may feel secure because procedures are well defined and activities are predictable. Productivity may also be high. However, the group's needs for creativity, autonomy, and self-motivation are not met, and the degree of openness and trust between the leader and the group members is minimal or absent. Members are often dissatisfied with this leadership style; however, at times, an autocratic style is the most effective. When urgent decisions are necessary (e.g., a cardiac arrest, a unit fire, or a terrorist attack), one person must assume the responsibility for making decisions without being challenged by other team members. When group members are unable to or do not wish to participate in making a decision, the authoritarian style solves the problem and enables the individual or group to move on. This style can also be effective when a project must be completed quickly and efficiently.

A **democratic leader** encourages group discussion and decision-making. This type of leader acts as a catalyst or facilitator, actively guiding a group toward achieving the group's goals. Group productivity and satisfaction are high as group members contribute to the work effort. The democratic leader assumes individuals are internally motivated (their driving force is intrinsic, they desire self-satisfaction), are capable of making decisions, and

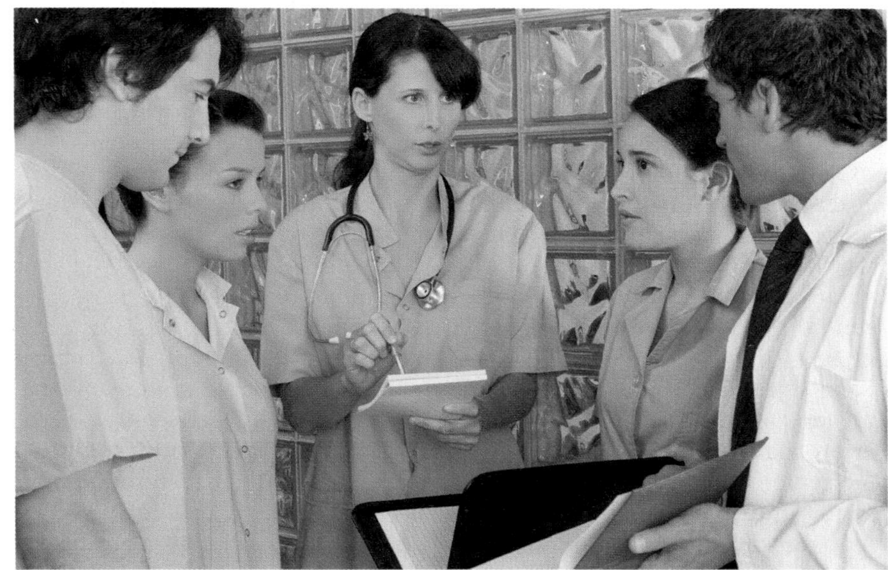

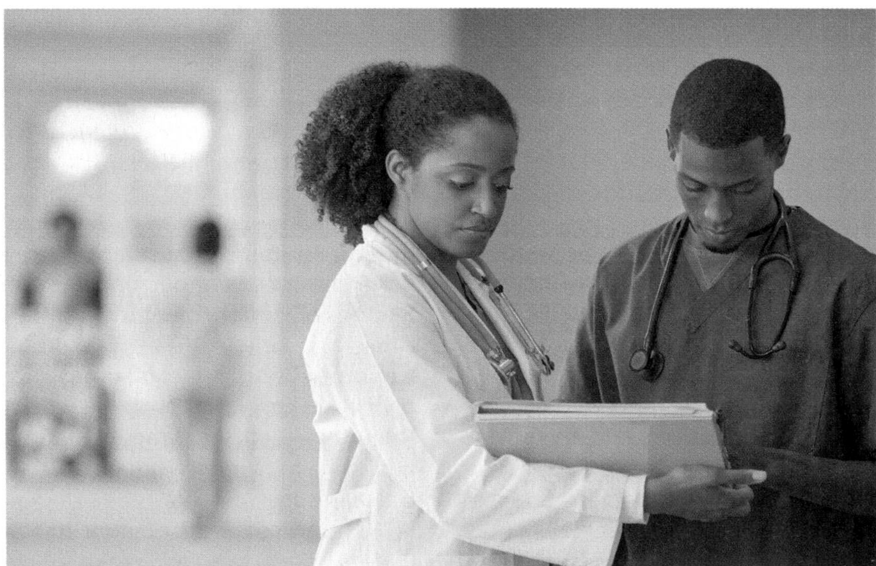

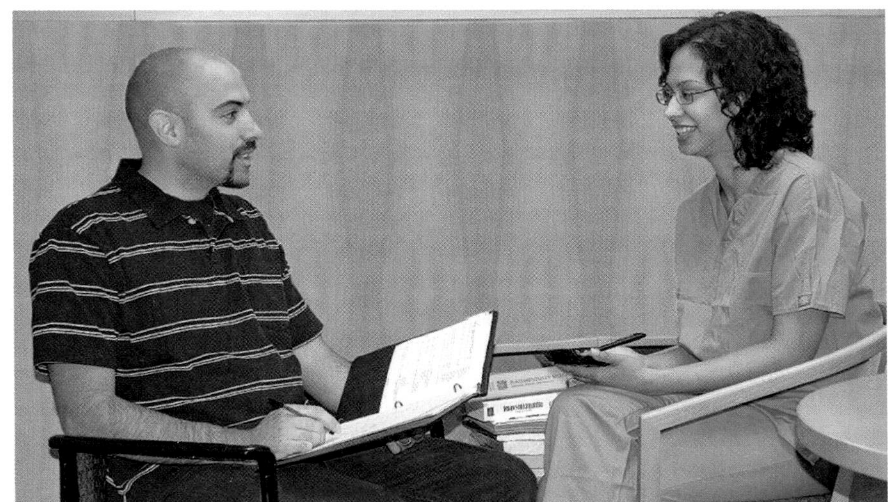

Figure 18.1 ■ Nurses as leaders and managers. *A*, The nurse manager discusses work assignments during change-of-shift report. *B*, The nurse delegates basic client care activities to the nursing assistant. *C*, The nurse consults the social worker during discharge planning.

A, Glow Images/Getty Images; *B*, Terry Vine/DigitalVision/Getty Images.

value independence. Providing constructive feedback, offering information, making suggestions, and asking questions become the focus of the democratic leader. This leadership style demands that the leader have faith in the group members to accomplish the goals. Although democratic leadership has been shown to be less efficient and more cumbersome than authoritarian leadership, it allows for more self-motivation and more creativity among group members. It also calls for a great deal of cooperation and coordination among group members. This leadership style can be extremely effective in the healthcare setting.

The **laissez-faire (permissive) leader** recognizes the group's need for autonomy and self-regulation. The leader assumes a "hands-off" approach. The leader presupposes the group is internally motivated. However, group members may act independently and at opposing purposes because of a lack of cooperation and coordination. A laissez-faire style is most effective for groups whose members have both personal and professional maturity. When the group has made a decision, the members become committed to it. Individual group members then perform tasks in their area of expertise while the leader acts as resource person.

The **bureaucratic leader** does not trust self or others to make decisions. Instead, this type of leader relies on the organization's rules, policies, and procedures to direct the group's work efforts. Group members are usually dissatisfied with the leader's inflexibility and impersonal relations with them. Table 18.2 compares the autocratic, democratic, laissez-faire, and bureaucratic leadership styles.

According to contingency theorists, effective leaders adapt their leadership style to the situation. A popular contingency theory describes the situational leader. The **situational leader** (a) flexes task and relationship behaviors, (b) considers the staff members' abilities, (c) knows the nature of the task to be done, and (d) is sensitive to the context or environment in which the task takes place. The task-orientation style focuses the leader on activities that encourage group productivity to get the work done. The relationship-orientation style is concerned with interpersonal relationships and focuses on activities that meet group members' needs.

Situational leaders adapt their leadership style to the readiness and willingness of the individual or group to perform the assigned task. When employees are insecure or unable or unwilling to perform the task, the leader uses a highly directive style, providing specific instructions and close supervision. If the group is motivated and willing but unable to perform the task, the leader again uses a highly directive style, but in this case, the leader explains decisions and provides the opportunity for clarification. When the group is able but unwilling or lacking in confidence, the leader shares ideas and facilitates decision-making. For a group that is willing, able, and confident to perform the task, the leader delegates, turning responsibility for decision-making and implementation over to the group.

Contemporary Leadership Theories

Contemporary theorists have described charismatic leaders, transactional leaders, transformational leaders, and shared leadership.

A **charismatic leader** is rare and is characterized by having an emotional relationship with the group members. The charming personality of the leader evokes strong feelings of commitment to both the leader and the leader's cause and beliefs. When this type of nurse leader speaks to a group, nurses feel inspired and motivated to do whatever they can to meet the leader's expectations. The followers of a charismatic leader often overcome extreme hardship to achieve the group's goals because of faith in the leader.

The **transactional leader** has a relationship with followers based on an exchange for some resource valued by

TABLE 18.2 Comparison of Autocratic, Democratic, Laissez-Faire, and Bureaucratic Leadership Styles

	Autocratic	Democratic	Laissez-Faire	Bureaucratic
Degree of control	Makes decisions alone	Collaborative	No control	Strict reliance on policy
Leader activity level	High	High	Minimal	High
Assumption of responsibility	Primarily the leader	Shared	Relinquished	Leader
Output of the group	High quantity, good quality	Creative, high quality	Variable, may be of poor quality	Good quality through following standard procedures
Efficiency	Very efficient	Less efficient than autocratic	Inefficient	Efficient

the follower. These incentives are used to promote loyalty and performance. For example, to ensure adequate staffing on the night shift, the nurse manager entices a staff nurse to work the night shift in exchange for a weekend shift off. The transactional leader represents the traditional manager, focused on the day-to-day tasks of achieving organizational goals and on understanding and meeting the needs of the group.

In contrast, a **transformational leader** fosters creativity, risk taking, commitment, and collaboration by empowering the group to share in the organization's vision. The leader inspires others with a clear, attractive, and attainable goal and enlists the group to participate in attaining the goal. The group is empowered because members and leader share values, honesty, trust, and continual learning. Independence, individual growth, and change are facilitated. For example, the nurses working with this type of leader to implement a major change in the model of nursing care delivered to a group of clients will each accept responsibility for a segment of the project, keep all members informed of their progress, and consider the impact of their actions on the larger group.

One subtype of transformational leadership is servant leadership, based on the concept that leaders serve their constituencies. Members of an organization act as both servants and leaders within a work environment of mutual respect, trust, and collaboration. As is true in many situations, servant leadership can be effectively demonstrated by both formal and informal leaders (Fahlberg, 2016; Hunt, 2016). In nursing, this concept is internally consistent with a focus on caring.

Shared leadership recognizes that a professional workforce is made up of many leaders. No one person is considered to have knowledge or ability beyond that of other members of the work group. Appropriate leadership is thought to emerge in relation to the challenges that confront the work group. Examples of shared leadership in nursing are self-directed work teams, co-leadership, and shared governance. **Shared governance** distributes decision-making among a group of individuals. It provides structure by articulating a mechanism for advocacy and influence of the staff nurse through all levels of nursing. It focuses on nurses controlling their professional practice through formal organization in which nurses make decisions about clinical practice standards, quality improvement, staff and professional development, and research. The practicing nurse has not only the right but the power to make decisions through participatory scheduling, joint staffing decisions, or shared unit responsibilities to achieve the best patient care outcomes (Motacki & Burke, 2017).

Effective Leadership

Much has been written about effective leadership and style; some descriptive statements about effective leaders are listed in Box 18.1. Leadership is a learned process. To be an effective leader requires an understanding of factors such as the needs, goals, and rewards that motivate individuals; knowledge of leadership skills and of the group's activities; and possession of the interpersonal skills to influence others. Principles of effective leadership include vision, influence, and acting as a role model.

Vision is a mental image of a possible and desirable future state. Leaders transform visions into realistic goals and communicate their visions to others who accept them as their own.

Influence is an informal strategy used to gain the cooperation of others without exercising formal authority. Influence is exercised through persuasion and excellent communication skills; it is based on a trusting relationship with the followers.

An effective leader needs to show sensitivity to being a positive **role model**, someone who sets the example for

EVIDENCE-BASED PRACTICE

Evidence-Based Practice

Can a Shared Governance Structure Empower Nurses to Design and Implement Change?

Although nurses usually rise to leadership positions from the role of direct client care, those nurses at the "bedside" are the most knowledgeable about what policies, procedures, and practices are the most effective at creating a safe and effective environment. Gordon (2016) describes the process of making a major change in the organizational structure of the oncology infusion units at a large cancer center prompted by significant increases in the number of clients. The nurse leader, in consultation with human resources and the organizational development staff, implemented a shared governance project to allow the nurses to participate in the design of the new structure. The project team of nurses formed to set a goal and implementation strategy. The project was successful in many ways even though the first specific goal was not completely met. Two subsequent teams were formed to continue the work.

Implications

The author reports many benefits of using shared governance as a method to design and implement aspects of the new structure combining several nursing units. There was a statistically significant decrease in the amount of time clients had to wait to receive their chemotherapy. The nurses learned new management skills, became more confident, and reported increased satisfaction from working together to set goals and meet challenges.

BOX 18.1 Characteristics of Effective Leaders

Effective leaders:

- Use a leadership style that is natural to them.
- Use a leadership style appropriate to the task and the members.
- Assess the effects of their behavior on others and the effects of others' behavior on themselves.
- Are sensitive to forces acting for and against change.
- Express an optimistic view of human nature.
- Are energetic.
- Are open and encourage openness, so that real issues are confronted.
- Facilitate personal relationships.
- Plan and organize activities of the group.
- Are consistent in behavior toward group members.
- Delegate tasks and responsibilities to develop members' abilities, not merely to get tasks performed.
- Involve members in all decisions.
- Value and use group members' contributions.
- Encourage creativity.
- Encourage feedback about their leadership style.
- Assess for and promote the use of current technology.

others to follow. As is appropriate for any health and caring profession, leadership should also be humanistic; that is, leaders should act in ways that stress individuals' dignity and worth. Being a good leader takes thought, care, insight, commitment, and energy. The leader demonstrates caring toward coworkers and clients.

Management

The manager's job is to accomplish the work of the organization. To this end, managers perform roles and functions that vary with the type of organization and the level of management.

Levels of Management

Traditional management is divided into three levels of responsibility. The reporting relationship among staff and managers is often referred to as the chain of command. **First-level managers** are responsible for managing the work of nonmanagerial personnel and the day-to-day activities of a specific work group or groups. Their primary responsibility is to motivate staff to achieve the organization's goals. This level of manager communicates staff issues to upper administration and reports administrative messages back to staff. Titles may include team leader or charge nurse.

Middle-level managers supervise a number of first-level managers and are responsible for the activities in the departments they supervise. Middle-level managers serve as liaisons between first-level managers and upper-level managers. They may be called supervisors, nurse managers, or head nurses.

Upper-level (top-level) managers are organizational executives who are primarily responsible for establishing goals and developing strategic plans. Nurse executives are registered nurses who are responsible for the management of nursing within the organization and the practice of nursing. Some nurse executives are also responsible for auxiliary units such as the pharmacy, laboratory, and dietary departments. Nurses in these positions may be called vice president for client care services, vice president for nursing, director of nursing, or chief nurse.

Clinical Alert!

Nurses generally move from first- to middle- to upper-level management positions through promotion. In addition, nursing administration graduate academic programs are available at some nursing schools.

Management Functions

Four management functions are planning, organizing, directing, and coordinating. These four functions help to achieve the broad goal of quality client care.

Planning

Planning is an ongoing process that involves (a) assessing a situation, (b) establishing goals and objectives based on assessment of a situation or future trends, and (c) developing a plan of action that identifies priorities, delineates who is responsible, determines deadlines, and describes how the intended outcome is to be achieved and evaluated. In short, it involves deciding what, when, where, and how to do it; by whom; and with what resources. The distribution of money, personnel, equipment, and physical space is included in the planning for resource allocation. An upper-level manager spends considerable time planning goals and services and determining the numbers and types of nurses and other personnel needed to provide these services. On the other hand, a first-level manager such as a staff nurse spends less time planning but manages individual clients by use of the nursing process.

An example of the planning function is **risk management**, having in place a system to reduce danger to clients and staff. The steps of risk management include anticipating and seeking sources of risk; analyzing, classifying, and prioritizing risks; developing a plan to avoid and manage risk; gathering data that indicate success at avoiding or minimizing risk; and evaluating and modifying risk reduction programs. Central to the process of risk management is communication among all involved individuals.

Organizing

Organizing is also an ongoing process of coordinating work. After identifying the work and evaluating human and material resources, the manager arranges the work into smaller units. Organizing involves determining responsibilities, communicating expectations, and establishing the chain of command for authority and communication. Although upper-level managers delegate much of the work and responsibility and accountability for the work to others, they need to ensure that department objectives, priorities, job descriptions, lines of communication, policies, and procedures clearly describe the expectations.

Directing

Directing is the process of getting the organization's work accomplished. Directing involves assigning and communicating expectations about the task to be completed, providing instruction and guidance, and ongoing decision-making. Upper-level managers devote less time to directing than to planning, organizing, and coordinating. Directing at this level of management generally involves supervision of the next level of managers, such as those in middle management. Unit managers (charge nurses) and staff nurses devote more time to directing. For example, charge nurses direct shift work by assigning clients and scheduling meal and break times. Staff nurses direct the care of clients by organizing nursing care, communicating care in written care plans and shift reports, and supervising care that is given by others.

Coordinating

Coordinating is the process of ensuring that plans are carried out and evaluating outcomes. The manager measures results or actions against standards or desired outcomes and then reinforces effective actions or changes ineffective ones. For example, an upper-level manager evaluates the effectiveness of recruitment, staff turnover, and budget performance. The charge nurse appraises staff performance. The staff nurse determines whether nursing interventions have helped the client achieve desired outcomes.

Principles of Management

A manager has authority, accountability, and responsibility. **Authority** is defined as the legitimate right to direct the work of others. It is an integral component of managing. Authority is conveyed through leadership actions; it is determined largely by the situation, and it is always associated with responsibility and accountability. The manager must accept the authority granted.

Accountability is the ability and willingness to assume ownership for one's actions and to accept the consequences of one's behavior. Accountability can be viewed as hierarchic, starting at the individual level, then the institutional or professional level, and finally the societal level. At the individual or client level, accountability is reflected in the nurse's ethical integrity. At the institutional level, it is reflected in the statement of philosophy and objectives of the nursing department and nursing audits. At the professional level, it is reflected in standards of practice developed by national nursing associations. At the societal level, it is reflected in legislated nurse practice acts.

Responsibility is an obligation to perform a task. Managers are responsible for effective utilization of resources, communication to subordinates, and implementation of organizational goals and objectives. Responsibility for nursing actions can be transferred to another practitioner, but accountability is always shared.

Skills and Competencies of Nurse Managers

To be effective managers, nurses need to think critically, communicate well, manage resources effectively and efficiently, enhance employee performance, build and manage teams, manage conflict, manage time, and initiate and manage change. Change is discussed on pages 351–353.

Critical Thinking

Critical thinking is a creative cognitive process that includes problem-solving and decision-making. The nurse manager reasons with logic and explores assumptions, alternatives, and the consequences of actions. See Chapter 9 ∞ for further discussion of critical thinking.

Communicating

Managers report spending much of their day communicating. Good communication is essential and often determines the manager's success. Managers use both verbal and written communication. Effective managers communicate assertively, expressing their ideas clearly, accurately, and honestly.

Managers use **networking**, a process whereby professional links are established through which individuals can share ideas, knowledge, and information; offer support and direction to each other; and facilitate accomplishment of professional goals.

Managing Resources

One of the greatest responsibilities of managers is their accountability for human, fiscal, and material resources. Budgeting and determining variances between the actual and budgeted resources are crucial skills for any manager.

Enhancing Employee Performance

Several ways of enhancing employee performance are available to managers. Managers are responsible for ensuring that employees develop by providing appropriate learning opportunities, such as in-service education; by facilitating attendance at professional workshops and conventions; and by encouraging achievement of advanced education, such as higher degrees or certifications. The nurse manager who empowers the staff by providing information, support, resources, and opportunities to participate will find that employees have greater commitment to the institution, are more effective in their role, have increased self-esteem, and are better able to meet their goals.

In addition, the manager may provide day-to-day coaching or serve as a mentor or preceptor. A **mentor** voluntarily assists the mentee to develop values, attitudes, ethical comportment, and critical thinking and role models appropriate behavior (Marquis & Huston, 2017). Having a mentor is recognized as important for career development.

In the clinical area, the term **preceptor** is used to describe an experienced nurse who assists the "new" nurse in improving clinical nursing skill and judgment. The preceptor also instills an understanding of the routines, policies, and procedures of the institution and the unit.

Building and Managing Teams

In addition to personnel development, managers are responsible for building and managing work teams. Familiarity with group processes facilitates a manager's ability to lead a group and enhances the development of that group into a work team. Groups develop in stages, during which roles and relationships are established. The purposes of the team as a whole and the role of each member must be clear. Each member must feel that the manager and the other members recognize his or her contributions. In healthcare, the team may consist of any healthcare providers: nurses, therapists, assistive personnel, clergy, and so on. All members of the team need to use effective communication skills.

Evaluating the group's work is another responsibility of the manager. Effectiveness, efficiency, and productivity are three outcome measures that are frequently used. In healthcare, **effectiveness** is a measure of the quality or quantity of services provided. **Efficiency** is a measure of the resources used in the provision of nursing services. In nursing, **productivity** is a performance measure of both the effectiveness and efficiency of nursing care. Productivity is frequently measured by the amount of nursing resources used per client or in terms of required versus actual hours of care provided.

Managing Conflict

Nurse managers are frequently in a position to manage conflict among individuals, groups, or teams. The conflict may arise from differing values, philosophies, or personalities. For example, employees may have strong disagreements about whether each member of the nursing team is doing a fair share of the work. In healthcare, conflict can also arise due to competition for resources, especially funding for staff positions or equipment.

There are many methods the nurse can use to manage conflict, and each has its advantages and disadvantages. Among the most common are compromise, negotiation, and collaboration. The new nurse manager may require training to become proficient in the use of these methods. Basic principles for all types of conflict management include demonstrating respect for all parties, avoiding blame, allowing full discussion, using ground rules during meetings to promote fairness, encouraging active listening, identifying the themes in the discussion, and exploring alternative solutions. An effective manager recognizes that if the problem is significant to any of the individuals involved, avoiding or failing to handle the conflict is likely to result in the problem becoming larger and more difficult (Finkelman, 2016).

Managing Time

The effective nurse manager uses time effectively and assists others in doing the same. Many factors inhibit good use of time, such as a preference for doing things the nurse likes to do before things the nurse prefers not to do, emergencies or crises that divert the nurse's attention, and unrealistic demands from others. Strategies that the manager—and all nurses—can use in order to use time well involve setting goals and priorities, delegating appropriately, examining how time is used, minimizing paperwork (automating whenever possible), and using regular schedules that avoid interruptions and set time limits on activities.

Managing Change

Change is the process of making something different from what it was. Change can involve gaining new knowledge or adapting what is currently known in the light of new information. It can also involve obtaining new skills. Change is an integral aspect of nursing, and nurses are often **change agents**, that is, individuals who initiate, motivate, and implement change. Change that is viewed as a threat by one nurse may be viewed as an opportunity by another nurse.

Change agents:

- Have excellent communication and interpersonal skills with individuals, groups, and all levels of the organization involved in change

- Have knowledge of available resources and how to use them: people, time, money, facilities, and information
- Are skilled in problem-solving
- Are skilled in teaching
- Are respected by those involved in the change
- Have the ability to encourage and nurture those going through change
- Are self-confident, are able to take risks, and inspire trust in themselves and others
- Are able to make decisions
- Have a broad base of knowledge
- Have a good sense of timing.

TYPES OF CHANGE

Planned change is an intended, purposeful attempt by an individual, group, organization, or larger social system to influence its own current status. Problem-solving skills, decision-making skills, and interpersonal skills are important factors in planned change.

Unplanned change is an alteration imposed by external events or individuals. It occurs when unexpected events force a reaction. It is usually haphazard, and the results can be unpredictable. Situational, or natural, change may be considered unplanned and occurs without any control by the person or group impacted. An example is the change that occurs because of a war or a natural disaster. Not all situational changes are negative. For example, as agencies open or close units, the nurse may have the opportunity to change to a new workplace.

Change may be considered covert or overt. A *covert change* is hidden or occurs without the individual's awareness. An example is the gradual, subtle increase in the severity of the clients' conditions on a nursing unit. *Overt change* is change of which a person is aware. An example might be that a piece of equipment will no longer be available because the agency has changed suppliers. Individuals who experience overt unplanned change may experience anxiety. Overt change often necessitates behavioral changes that create conflict with the person's needs or goals.

THE NURSE'S ROLE IN CHANGE

In his classic work, Lewin (1951) described change as involving three stages: unfreezing, moving, and refreezing. During the unfreezing stage, the need for change is recognized, driving and restraining forces are identified, alternative solutions are generated, and participants are motivated to change. In the second stage, moving, participants agree the status quo is undesirable, and the actual change is planned in detail and implemented. In the final stage, refreezing, the change is integrated and stabilized.

An important aspect of planning change is establishing the likelihood of the acceptance of the change and then determining the criteria by which that acceptance can be identified. Accepting change often takes time, particularly when it does not fit into a person's attitudinal framework. The course of acceptance is easier for individuals if they are involved in the process. If possible, change should be instituted on a small or pilot scale before full implementation. To facilitate acceptance of the change, the change agent needs to identify common driving and restraining forces (Box 18.2). Guidelines for dealing with resistance to change are given in Box 18.3.

Change requires energy, much of which comes from those who have power. To access optimal power, use the following strategies:

1. Analyze the organizational chart; know the formal lines of authority. Identify informal lines as well.
2. Identify key persons who will be affected by the change. Pay attention to those in the chain of command immediately above and below the point of change.
3. Find out as much as possible about these key individuals. What are their "tickle points"? What interests them, gets them excited, turns them off? What is on

BOX 18.2 Common Driving and Restraining Forces for Change

DRIVING FORCES

- Perception that the change is challenging
- Economic gain
- Perception that the change will improve the situation
- Visualization of the future impact of change
- Potential for self-growth, recognition, achievement, and improved relationships

RESTRAINING FORCES

- Fear that something of personal value will be lost (e.g., threat to job security or self-esteem)
- Misunderstanding of the change and its implications
- Low tolerance for change related to intellectual or emotional insecurity
- Perception that the change will not achieve goals; failure to see the big picture
- Lack of time or energy
- Perceived loss of freedom to engage in particular behaviors

BOX 18.3 Guidelines for Dealing with Resistance to Change

1. Talk with those who oppose the change. Get to the root of their reasons for opposition.
2. Clarify information, and provide accurate information.
3. Be open to revisions but clear about what must remain.
4. Present the negative consequences of resistance (e.g., threats to organizational survival, compromised client care).
5. Emphasize the positive consequences of the change and how the individual or group will benefit. However, do not spend too much energy on rational analysis of why the change is good and why the arguments against it do not hold up. Individuals' resistance frequently flows from feelings that are not rational.
6. Keep resisters involved in face-to-face contact with supporters. Encourage proponents to empathize with opponents, recognize valid objections, and relieve unnecessary fears.
7. Maintain a climate of trust, support, and confidence.
8. Divert attention by creating a different disturbance. Energy can shift to a more important problem inside the system, thereby redirecting resistance. Alternately, attention can be brought to an external threat to create a bully phenomenon. When members perceive a greater environmental threat (e.g., competition or restrictive governmental policies), they tend to unify internally.

their personal and organizational agendas? Who typically aligns with whom on important decisions?

4. Begin to build a coalition of support before you start the change process. Identify the key individuals who will most likely support your idea and those who are most likely to be persuaded easily. Talk informally with them to flush out possible objections to your idea and potential opponents. What will be the costs and benefits to them—especially in political terms? Can your idea be modified in ways that retain your objectives but appeal to more key individuals?
5. Follow the organizational chain of command when communicating with administrators. Do not bypass anyone to avoid having an excellent proposal undermined. (Sullivan, 2018, p. 70)

All nurses are affected by change; nobody can avoid it. Nurses knowledgeable about the historical and current trends in nursing and current political, social, technologic, and economic issues make rational plans to deal with opportunities to initiate and guide needed change and to respond to change that affects them in the workplace, government, organizations, and the community.

The Nurse as Delegator

Delegation is "allowing a delegatee to perform a specific nursing activity, skill, or procedure that is beyond the delegatee's traditional role and not routinely performed" (National Council of State Boards of Nursing [NCSBN], 2016, p. 6). Delegation is differentiated from *assignment*, which consists of those duties that are already within the scope of practice of the member of the nursing team (NCSBN, 2016). Thus, the majority of care provided by nursing personnel falls within the personnel's legal scope of practice and education or training and is done through an assignment. Care is only delegated when it falls outside of the caregiver's usual scope and the delegator has determined that such care can be safely delivered by a delegatee who meets specific requirements. The delegatee assumes responsibility for the actual performance of the task or procedure. The delegator retains accountability for the outcome. Delegation is a tool that allows the delegator to devote more time to tasks that cannot be delegated. It also enhances the skills and abilities of the delegatee, which builds self-esteem, promotes morale, and enhances teamwork and attainment of the organization's goals. In nursing, delegation refers to indirect care—the intended outcome is achieved through the work of someone supervised by the nurse—and involves defining the task, determining who can perform the task, describing the expectation, seeking agreement, monitoring performance, and providing feedback to the delegatee regarding performance.

Registered nurses delegate components of nursing care to other members of the nursing team: other RNs, licensed vocational or practical nurses, and assistive personnel (AP). An RN who delegates a task is accountable for selecting an appropriately skilled caregiver and for continued evaluation of the client's care. AP may be identified by a variety of titles, including certified nursing aides or assistants, home health aides, medication assistants, patient care technicians, orderlies, or surgical technicians. They have had diverse degrees of training and experience. They are employees and do not include family members or friends who provide some client care.

Each state nursing practice act specifies which actions constitute the legal practice of nursing, which actions are the purview only of nurses, and which may be assigned or delegated to others. The model state nursing practice act authored by the NCSBN (2012) states that both the RN (including advanced practice nurses) and the licensed vocational or practical nurse (LVN/LPN) may assign or delegate nursing interventions to implement the plan of care.

The NCSBN (1996) published five "rights" of delegation: The nurse delegates the *right task*, under the *right circumstances*, to the *right person*, with the *right directions and communication*, and the *right supervision and evaluation*. "The steps of the delegation process include assessment of the client, the staff and the context of the situation; communication to provide direction and opportunity for interaction during the completion of the delegated task; surveillance and monitoring to assure compliance with standards of practice, policies and procedures; and evaluation to consider the effectiveness of the delegation and whether the desired client outcome was attained" (NCSBN, 2005, p. 1).

It is not possible to generate an exhaustive list of exactly which actions can be delegated to AP, especially since these actions vary by state and the type of employment setting (e.g., long-term care facility versus acute care hospital). Even if an action can be delegated by law, it may be prohibited by agency policy. Examples of tasks that are commonly assigned and those that may and may not be delegated are given in Box 18.4.

The unlicensed individual may not delegate tasks to another individual. Principles guiding the nurse's decision to delegate ensure the safety and quality of outcomes. These principles are listed in Box 18.5. Even if the task is one that may legally be delegated, the individual nurse must still determine if the task can be delegated to a particular AP for a specific client. Once the decision has been made to delegate, the nurse must communicate clearly to the AP and verify that the AP understands:

- The specific tasks to be done for each client
- When each task is to be done
- The expected outcomes for each task, including parameters outside of which the AP must immediately report to the nurse (and any action that must urgently be taken)
- Who is available to serve as a resource if needed
- When and in what format (written or verbal) a report on the tasks is expected.

A specific task that can be delegated to one AP may not be appropriate for another AP, depending on each AP's experience and individual skill sets. Also, a task that is appropriate for the AP to perform with one client may not be appropriate with a different client or the same client under altered circumstances. For example, the taking of routine vital signs may be delegated to AP for a client in stable condition but would not be delegated for the same client who has become unstable. It is important to note that the nurse is not held legally responsible for the acts of the AP but is accountable for the quality of the act of delegation and has the ultimate responsibility for ensuring that proper care is provided.

Safety Alert! **SAFETY**

Each nurse or other licensed or unlicensed healthcare provider is responsible for his or her own actions. Anyone who feels unqualified to perform an assigned or delegated task must decline to perform it.

In addition to delegating to AP, the RN also delegates to LVN/LPNs. Because LVN/LPNs are licensed, the nurse must know their state-specific scope of practice in order to delegate effectively. When delegating to this nurse, the RN retains primary responsibility and accountability for the implementation of the nursing process. LVN/LPNs require less direct supervision than APs. In some regions and some agencies, LVN/LPNs may perform tasks generally considered the role of the RN if they have received special training. For example, in most U.S. states they may assess intravenous (IV) infusion sites, but in only some states can LVN/LPNs administer IV fluids or medications, initiate IV lines, administer parenteral nutrition, or delegate to others. The process of delegating to these LVN/LPNs is the same as it is in delegating to AP. For example, LVN/LPNs may be authorized to provide client teaching from a standard teaching plan, but the RN must still confirm that the particular LVN/LPN's job description, education, and competency meet the needs of the specific situation. In addition, LVN/LPNs can delegate to other LVN/LPNs or AP (Weberg, Mangold, O'Grady, & Malloch, 2019).

The RN also assigns or delegates to other RNs. This is part of the daily routine of determining which of the available nurses should care for which clients or when specific additional assistance is required for one client. When delegating to RNs who are new to a particular setting—such as when the nurse from one unit in a hospital is temporarily assigned to a different unit (called "floating")—the delegating nurse must confirm that the five rights are still met.

Delegation can be an extremely useful strategy in providing thorough and effective nursing care. Skill in delegation, however, must be learned and developed over time. The nurse should not hesitate to consult with others regarding the appropriateness of delegation.

BOX 18.4 Examples of Tasks That Are Commonly Assigned and Tasks That May and May Not Be Delegated to Assistive Personnel

TASKS THAT ARE COMMONLY ASSIGNED TO ASSISTIVE PERSONNEL

- Taking of vital signs on stable clients
- Basic hygiene techniques
- Bedmaking
- Client transfers and ambulation
- Personal care
- Food service
- Documentation
- Safety measures (including fire, safety, and disaster preparedness, and infection control)
- Performing basic life support (cardiopulmonary resuscitation [CPR])
- Basic preventative and restorative care and procedures
- Basic observation procedures such as weighing and measuring

TASKS THAT MAY BE DELEGATED TO ASSISTIVE PERSONNEL

- Postmortem care
- Gastrostomy feedings in established systems
- Administering nonparenteral medications
- Administering injections
- Performing simple dressing changes
- Suctioning of chronic tracheostomies

TASKS THAT MAY NOT BE DELEGATED TO ASSISTIVE PERSONNEL

- Assessment
- Interpretation of data
- Making a nursing diagnosis
- Creation of a nursing care plan
- Evaluation of care effectiveness
- Care of invasive lines
- Administering intravenous medications
- Insertion of nasogastric tubes
- Client education
- Performing triage
- Giving telephone advice
- Tasks requiring sterile technique
- Obtaining orders from physicians

BOX 18.5 Principles Used by the Nurse to Determine Delegation to Assistive Personnel

1. The nurse must assess the individual client prior to delegating tasks.
2. The client must be medically stable or in a chronic condition and not fragile.
3. The task must be considered routine for this client.
4. The task must not require a substantial amount of scientific knowledge or technical skill.
5. The task must be considered safe for this client.
6. The task must have a predictable outcome.
7. Learn the agency's procedures and policies about delegation.
8. Know the scope of practice and the customary knowledge, skills, and job description for each member of your team.
9. Be aware of individual variations in work abilities. Each individual caregiver has different experiences and may not be capable of performing every task cited in the job description.
10. When unsure about an assistant's abilities to perform a task, observe while the individual performs it, or demonstrate it to the individual and get a return demonstration before allowing the individual to perform it independently.
11. Clarify reporting expectations to ensure the task is accomplished.
12. Create an atmosphere that fosters communication, teaching, and learning. For example, encourage staff members to ask questions, listen carefully to their concerns, and make use of every opportunity to teach.

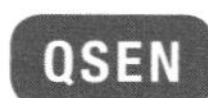

Patient-Centered Care: Cultural Considerations in Leadership, Management, and Delegation

In the same way that nurses consider how care is influenced by the client's culture, the nurse must consider how leading, managing, delegating, and promoting change are influenced by the culture of the caregivers. Specific examples include:

- *Communication:* Volume, tone, and choice of words plus nonverbal behavior used in communicating ideas and instructions may be interpreted differently in different cultures.
- *Space:* The distance between two individuals or the seating arrangement in a group may either promote or impede effective teamwork.
- *Time:* There are culturally defined perspectives on what situations are considered emergencies as well as how much time is meant by words such as *now, soon,* or *immediately*. Also, a specific culture may be more focused on the present, past, or future than on the other time frames.
- *Power and control:* Cultures vary in their views of whether events are internally or externally controlled, and this may influence personnel initiative. Some individuals may always wait to be told when to perform activities, whereas others may do so independently. Beliefs also vary related to luck, fate, destiny, and personal choice.

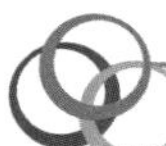

Critical Thinking Checkpoint

You have just interviewed for two nursing positions and are trying to decide which job to pursue. During your first interview, the nurse manager, Mr. Caruso, was cheerful, spoke highly of his current staff and complimented them for their ability to set goals and participate in decision-making, listened to your ideas, and explored ways in which you could contribute to this team's effectiveness. The second nurse manager, Mrs. Turner, was also cheerful and talkative. She provided you with a job description, explained her expectations of you as a new employee, and spoke of new programs she was attempting to implement. Both nurse managers talked about changes taking place in their facilities and the need for employees to remain flexible.

1. Based on the brief data provided, speculate about the leadership style of each of these nurse managers.
2. Both nurse managers spoke of changes that were taking place in their facility. As a nurse, how can you assist your peers who are unhappy and seem to resist change even when it is positive?
3. How might the delegation of tasks to other nurses or unlicensed assistive personnel be different in the two settings?
4. Think about managers (or leaders) you have known and admired. What characteristics did they have that you would like to integrate into your own management style should you become a nurse manager?

Answers to Critical Thinking Checkpoint questions are available on the faculty resources site. Please consult with your instructor.

Chapter 18 Review

CHAPTER HIGHLIGHTS

- The professional nurse frequently assumes the roles of leader and manager. Leaders, as employees or volunteers, influence others to accomplish a specific goal, whereas managers have responsibility and accountability for accomplishing the tasks of an organization.
- Several leadership styles have been described, including autocratic, democratic, laissez-faire, and bureaucratic. These styles are often blended to fit the situation. Nurses need to know which style is most consistent with their behavior and learn to incorporate aspects of other styles into their practice.
- Four major management functions are planning, organizing, directing, and coordinating.

- Nurse managers work within the organizational framework of the employing agency. Principles of management include authority, accountability, and responsibility.
- Effective managers need to be skilled at critical thinking; communication; resource management; enhancing employee performance; building and managing teams; and managing conflict, time, and change.
- Nurses function as change agents to initiate, motivate, and implement change.
- Delegation is a tool that allows the nurse delegator to devote more time to tasks that cannot be delegated. The nurse transfers responsibility and authority to another but retains accountability for the task.

TEST YOUR KNOWLEDGE

1. The nurse leader informs staff members about a local emergency and instructs them to stay at the hospital to prepare for major casualties. The staff members display high levels of anxiety and disorganization. Which is the most appropriate leadership style at this time?
   1. Autocratic
   2. Democratic
   3. Laissez-faire
   4. Bureaucratic

2. During client rounds, a client tells the nurse manager that he has not received his medications all shift. In using the skills and competencies of a manager, what will be the nurse's first action?
   1. Communicate: Discuss the client's statement with the assigned nurse.
   2. Manage resources: Assign another nurse to administer the client's medications.
   3. Enhance employee performance: Provide the client's nurse with a mentor to review proper medication procedures.
   4. Manage conflict: Call the nurse into the client's room and mediate a discussion between them.

3. An RN delegates the task of taking a newly admitted client's vital signs to a nurse's aide. The client's blood pressure was 182/98 but did not get reported to the physician for several hours. Who is responsible for the lapse in time between discovery and action?
   1. Nurse manager
   2. Aide
   3. Client
   4. RN

4. A nurse is determining whether an activity can be delegated to an unlicensed assistant (UAP). What will the nurse use to make this determination? Select all that apply.
   1. Determine whether it is the right task.
   2. Determine whether it is under the right circumstances.
   3. Determine whether it is to the right person.
   4. Determine the type of communication.
   5. Determine whether there is enough time.

5. The nurse manager plans to implement a new method for scheduling staff vacations. Senior staff members oppose the change, whereas newer staff members are more accepting. Which is the most effective strategy for resolving this difference?
   1. Provide an extensive and detailed rationale for the proposed change, then implement it.
   2. Explain that the change will occur as designed, regardless of the staff's preference.
   3. Withdraw the proposal to prevent a decrease in staff morale.
   4. Encourage interaction between the opposing sides to attempt resolution.

6. Which is more commonly a characteristic of a manager rather than a leader?
   1. Is visionary
   2. Has been given legitimate power by the organization
   3. Primary effectiveness is through influencing others
   4. Often takes risks and explores new solutions to problems

7. A nurse is identified as being an effective leader. With this designation, the nurse will most likely demonstrate which characteristics? Select all that apply.
   1. Self-aware
   2. Focus on people
   3. Excellent communicator
   4. Mentor to others
   5. Focus on systems

8. When economic conditions are tight, a hospital may reduce the number of middle-level nurse managers. This can potentially disrupt nursing care because middle-level managers are responsible for which of the following?
   1. Supervision of nonmanagerial staff
   2. Reporting institutional changes to direct-care staff
   3. The productivity and effectiveness of a group of managers
   4. Creating institutional goals and strategic plans

9. A management function of bedside direct-care nurses includes determining whether the client has reached the intended outcomes designated in the care plan. This is an example of which of the four management functions?
   1. Planning
   2. Organizing
   3. Directing
   4. Coordinating

10. The nurse asks an assistant (AP) to weigh a client. The AP carefully assists the client out of bed to stand on the scale, weighs the client, and safely returns the client to bed. Later, when the AP reports the weight to the nurse, it is discovered that the client had been placed on bedrest and should not have been allowed out of bed. This situation violates which of the following five rights of delegation?
   1. Right task
   2. Right person
   3. Right direction and communication
   4. Right supervision and evaluation

See Answers to Test Your Knowledge in Appendix A.

READINGS AND REFERENCES

Suggested Reading

Adams, J. M., Djukic, M., Gregas, M., & Fryer, A.-K. (2018). Influence of nurse leader practice characteristics on patient outcomes: Results from a multi-state study. *Nursing Economic$, 36*, 259–267.

This article describes a research study examining the relationship between more than 750 nurse leaders' self-reported personal and practice characteristics and selected client outcomes such as urinary catheter infections and client falls. The most influential characteristic for improving client outcomes was found to be the leader's expectations of the staff.

Related Research

Elliott, L., Persaud, M., Nielsen, L. S., & Boscart, V. (2018). A focused ethnography of nursing team culture and leadership on a transitional care unit. *Perspectives: The Journal of the Gerontological Nursing Association*, *40*(2), 6–14.

References

Fahlberg, B. (2016). Servant leadership: A model for emerging nurse leaders. *Nursing*, *46*(10), 49–52. doi:10.1097/01.NURSE.0000494644.77680.2a

Finkelman, A. W. (2016). *Leadership and management for nurses: Core competencies for quality care* (3rd ed.). Boston, MA: Pearson.

Gordon, J. N. (2016). Empowering oncology nurses to lead change through a shared governance project. *Oncology Nursing Forum*, *43*, 688–690. doi:10.1188/16.ONF.688-690

Hunt, K. (2016). Leading the way in nursing through servant leadership. *Imprint*, *63*(2), 30–33.

Lewin, K. (1951). *Field theory in social science*. New York, NY: Harper & Row.

Marquis, B. L., & Huston, C. J. (2017). *Leadership roles and management functions in nursing: Theory and application* (9th ed.). Philadelphia, PA: Wolters Kluwer.

Motacki, K., & Burke, K. (2017). *Nursing delegation and management of patient care* (2nd ed.). St. Louis, MO: Elsevier.

National Council of State Boards of Nursing. (1996). *Delegation: Concepts and decision-making process*. Chicago, IL: Author.

National Council of State Boards of Nursing. (2005). *Working with others: A position paper*. Retrieved from https://www.ncsbn.org/Working_with_Others.pdf

National Council of State Boards of Nursing. (2012). *NCSBN model act*. Retrieved from https://www.ncsbn.org/14_Model_Act_0914.pdf

National Council of State Boards of Nursing. (2016). National guidelines for nursing delegation. *Journal of Nursing Regulation*, *7*, 5–14. Retrieved from https://www.ncsbn.org/NCSBN_Delegation_Guidelines.pdf

Sullivan, E. J. (2018). *Effective leadership and management in nursing* (9th ed.). New York, NY: Pearson.

Weberg, D., Mangold, K., O'Grady, T. P., & Malloch. K. (2019). *Leadership in nursing practice: Changing the landscape of health care* (3rd ed.). Burlington, MA: Jones & Bartlett.

Selected Bibliography

Catalano, J. T. (2019). Leadership, followership, and management. In J. T. Catalano (Ed.), *Nursing now! Today's issues, tomorrow's trends* (8th ed., pp. 257–284). Philadelphia, PA: F. A. Davis.

Davidson, S., Weberg, D. R., Porter-O'Grady, T., & Malloch, K. (Eds.). (2017). *Leadership for evidence-based innovation in nursing and health professions*. Burlington, MA: Jones & Bartlett.

Grossman, S. C., & Valiga, T. M. (2017). *New leadership challenge: Creating the future of nursing* (5th ed.). Philadelphia, PA: F. A. Davis.

Kelly, P., & Quesnelle, H. (2016). *Nursing leadership and management* (3rd Canadian ed.). Clifton Park, NY: Delmar.

Nelson, K. E. (2017). Nurse manager perceptions of work overload and strategies to address it. *Nurse Leader*, *15*, 406–408. doi:10.1016/j.mnl.2017.09.009

Nelson-Brantley, H. V., Ford, D. J., Miller, K. L., & Bott, M. J. (2018). Nurse executives leading change to improve critical access hospital outcomes: A literature review with research-informed recommendations. *Online Journal of Rural Nursing & Health Care*, *18*(1), 148–179. doi:10.14574/ojrnhc.v18i1.510

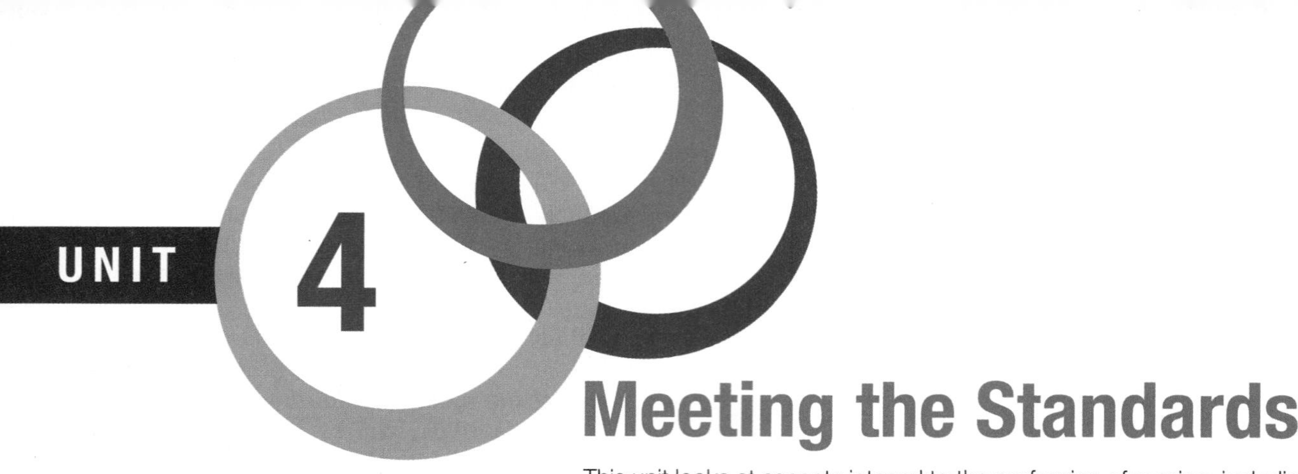

Meeting the Standards

This unit looks at aspects integral to the profession of nursing, including caring; communicating; teaching; and leading, managing, and delegating. In order for nurses to provide high-quality care, they must demonstrate caring, communicate effectively with both the client and the healthcare team, teach clients and their family members, act as leaders of the nursing team, and delegate tasks to others. Only when the nurse incorporates all of these aspects into the care of the client can optimal care be delivered.

CLIENT: Michael AGE: 62
CURRENT MEDICAL DIAGNOSIS: Lung Cancer

Medical History: Michael was diagnosed with an advanced stage of lung cancer 2 months ago following a lung biopsy that revealed oat cell carcinoma, one of the fastest-growing forms of lung cancer. His oncologist recommended treatment with chemotherapy and radiation therapy but informed him that the prognosis was poor and his condition was most likely terminal. Since that time, Michael has undergone four chemotherapy treatments and 6 weeks of radiation therapy, but additional chemotherapy treatments needed to be held until his platelet count improved. Diagnostic tests revealed metastasis to the brain and the bone. He has decided to discontinue all treatments and was admitted to hospice home care.

Personal and Social History: Michael lives with his wife of 40 years. They have two sons who are grown and live out of state with their wives and families. Michael's wife accompanies him to all of his doctor's appointments and therapies, and they are frequently seen in the waiting room or examination room holding hands and laughing together. Michael works as an architect, and his wife owns her own business selling children's clothing. They have a comfortable life together and were looking forward to spending their retirement years together traveling. Michael says he can't stop apologizing to his wife because "I would never have developed lung cancer if I had quit smoking, and now she has to live alone because of my stupid habit." Whenever he apologizes, his wife tells him that it is not his fault and that she loves him, but she tells the nurse privately that she feels angry that he is dying so young.

Questions

American Nurses Association Standard of Practice #5 is Implementation: *The registered nurse demonstrates caring behaviors to develop therapeutic relationships.*

1. Using Roach's six C's of caring discussed in Chapter 15 ∞, how would you demonstrate caring to Michael and his wife?
2. Using the nonverbal communication methods discussed in Chapter 16 ∞, how can the nurse communicate caring to this family?

American Nurses Association Standard of Practice #5B is Health Teaching and Health Promotion: *The registered nurse uses health promotion and health teaching methods, in collaboration with the healthcare consumer's values, beliefs, health practices, developmental level, learning needs, readiness and ability to learn, language preference, spirituality, culture, and socioeconomic status.*

3. The hospice nurse sees that Michael's death is imminent within the next few hours or days and wants to teach his wife about what to expect. Based on what you learned in Chapter 17, what factors would the nurse interpret as indicating his wife's readiness to learn?

American Nurses Association Standard of Professional Performance #11 is Leadership: *The registered nurse leads within the professional practice setting and the profession and retains accountability for delegated nursing care.*

4. The hospice nurse arranges for 24-hour care during Michael's final days. What types of care will the nurse assign to the assistive personnel (AP)? What care will only the registered nurse perform?
5. What instructions will the nurse provide the AP related to things to report immediately if they occur?

American Nurses Association Standard of Professional Performance #11 is Leadership: Another competency for this standard is that *the nurse mentors colleagues for the advancement of nursing practice and the profession to enhance safe, quality healthcare.*

6. On the next visit to the family, the nurse reviews the AP's care of the client and notes that the client is not being repositioned and is developing signs of a pressure ulcer. What should the nurse do?

American Nurses Association. (2015). *Nursing: Scope and standards of practice* (3rd ed.). Silver Spring, MD: Author.

Answers to Meeting the Standards questions are available on the faculty resources website. Please consult with your instructor.

UNIT

5

Health Beliefs and Practices

19 Health Promotion

LEARNING OUTCOMES

After completing this chapter, you will be able to:

1. Explain the relationship of individuality and holism to nursing practice.
2. List four main characteristics of homeostatic mechanisms.
3. Identify theoretical frameworks used in individual health promotion.
4. Describe the vision, mission, and goals of *Healthy People 2020* to help improve the health of a community.
5. Differentiate health promotion from health protection or illness prevention.
6. Identify various types and sites of health promotion programs.
7. Discuss the Health Promotion Model.
8. Explain the stages of health behavior change.
9. Discuss the nurse's role in health promotion.
10. Describe components of health assessment that pertain to health promotion.
11. Discuss nursing diagnosing, planning, implementing, and evaluating as they relate to health promotion.

KEY TERMS

action stage, *372*
boundary, *363*
closed system, *363*
compensatory, *363*
contemplation stage, *372*
equilibrium, *363*
feedback, *364*
health promotion, *362*
health risk assessment (HRA), *375*
holism, *363*
homeostasis, *363*
input, *363*
maintenance stage, *372*
negative feedback, *364*
open system, *363*
output, *364*
positive feedback, *364*
precontemplation stage, *371*
preparation stage, *372*
primary prevention, *367*
psychologic homeostasis, *365*
secondary prevention, *367*
self-regulation, *363*
system, *363*
termination stage, *372*
tertiary prevention, *367*
throughput, *363*

Introduction

Health promotion is an important component of nursing practice. It is a way of thinking that revolves around a philosophy of wholeness, wellness, and well-being. In the past 2 decades, the public has become increasingly aware of and interested in health promotion. Many people are aware of the relationship between lifestyle and illness and the development of health-promoting habits, such as getting adequate exercise, rest, and relaxation; maintaining good nutrition; and controlling the use of tobacco, alcohol, and other drugs. Murdaugh, Parsons, and Pender (2019) consider **health promotion** to be different from disease prevention or health protection:

> Health promotion has moved from being considered a goal or desired end point to a process to facilitate movement toward accomplishment of health goals. It is both the art and science of supporting people to make lifestyle changes and create an environment conducive to health. A combination of health promotion strategies is needed to address multiple determinants of health. Ecologic strategies address the social, economic, and physical environments that influence health. Health promotion spans from the prevention of disease to empowering individuals, to promoting environmental and policy change. (Murdaugh et al., 2019, p. 23)

Assessing and planning the healthcare of the individual client is enhanced when the nurse understands the concepts of individuality, holism, homeostasis, and human needs. The beliefs and values of each client and the support he or she receives come in large part from the family and are reinforced by the community. The reverse is also true—the health of a community is affected by the beliefs, attitudes, and behaviors of the individuals in the community.

Individual Health

Dimensions of individuality include the person's total character, self-identity, and perceptions. The individual's total character encompasses behaviors, emotional state, attitudes, values, motives, abilities, habits, and appearances. The individual's self-identity encompasses the perception of self as a separate and distinct entity alone and in interactions with others. The individual's perceptions encompass the way the individual interprets the environment or situation, directly affecting how he or she thinks, feels, and acts in any given situation.

Concept of Individuality

To help clients attain, maintain, or regain an optimal level of health, nurses need to understand clients as individuals. Each individual is a unique being who is different from every other human being, with a different combination of genetics, life experiences, and environmental interactions.

When providing care, nurses need to focus on the client within the contexts of both total care and individualized care. In the total-care context, the nurse considers all the principles and areas that apply when taking care of any client of that age and condition. In the individualized-care context, the nurse becomes acquainted with the client as an individual, using the total-care principles that apply to this person at this time. For example, a nurse who is advising the mother of a preschooler understands that the child's desire to explore his or her world is a developmental stage that all preschoolers experience. However, the preschooler diagnosed with attention-deficit/hyperactivity disorder may have an increased risk of injuries when interacting with the environment, due to his or her impulsivity and poor self-control.

Concept of Holism

Nurses are concerned with the individual as a whole, complete, or holistic person, not as an assembly of parts and processes. When applied in nursing, the concept of **holism** emphasizes that nurses must keep the whole person in mind and strive to understand how one area of concern relates to the whole person. The nurse must also consider the relationship of the individual to the external environment and to others. For example, in helping a man who is grieving over the death of his spouse, the nurse explores the impact of the loss on the whole person (i.e., on the man's appetite, rest and sleep pattern, energy level, sense of well-being, mood, usual activities, family relationships, and relationships with others). Nursing interventions are directed toward restoring overall harmony, so they depend on the man's sense of purpose and meaning of his life. For additional information about holistic practices, see Chapter 22 ∞.

Concept of Homeostasis

The concept of **homeostasis** was first introduced by Cannon (1939) to describe the relative constancy of the internal processes of the body, such as blood oxygen and carbon dioxide levels, blood pressure, body temperature, blood glucose, and fluid and electrolyte balance. To Cannon, the word *homeostasis* did not imply something stagnant, set, or immobile; it meant a condition that might vary but remained relatively constant. Cannon viewed the human being as separate from the external environment and constantly endeavoring to maintain physiologic **equilibrium**, or balance, through adaptation to that environment. Homeostasis, then, is the tendency of the body to maintain a state of balance or equilibrium while continually changing.

Physiologic Homeostasis

Physiologic homeostasis means that the internal environment of the body is relatively stable and constant. All cells of the body require a relatively constant environment to function; thus, the body's internal environment must be maintained within narrow limits. Homeostatic mechanisms have four main characteristics:

1. They are self-regulating.
2. They are compensatory.
3. They tend to be regulated by negative feedback systems.
4. They may require several feedback mechanisms to correct only one physiologic imbalance.

Self-regulation means that homeostatic mechanisms come into play automatically in the healthy person. However, if a person is ill, or if an organ such as a lung is injured, the homeostatic mechanisms may not be able to respond to the stimulus as they would normally. Homeostatic mechanisms are **compensatory** (counterbalancing) because they tend to counteract conditions that are abnormal for the person. An example is a sudden drop in air temperature. The compensatory mechanisms are that the peripheral blood vessels constrict, thereby diverting most of the blood internally, and increased muscular activity and shivering occur to create heat. Through these mechanisms, the body temperature remains stable despite the cold.

Homeostasis occurs within the physiologic **system**, a set of interacting identifiable parts or components. The fundamental components of a system are matter, energy, and communication. Without any one of these, a system does not exist. The individual is a human system with matter (the body), energy (chemical or thermal), and communication (e.g., the nervous system). The **boundary** of a system, such as the skin in the human system, is a real or imaginary line that differentiates one system from another system or a system from its environment.

There are two general types of systems: closed and open. A **closed system** does not exchange energy, matter, or information with its environment; it receives no input from the environment and gives no output to the environment. An example of a closed system is a chemical reaction that takes place in a test tube. In reality, outside the laboratory, no closed systems exist. In an **open system**, energy, matter, and information move into and out of the system through the system's boundary. All living systems, such as plants, animals, people, families, and communities, are open systems because their survival depends on a continuous exchange of energy. They are, therefore, in a constant state of change.

An open system depends on the quality and quantity of its input, output, and feedback. **Input** consists of information, material, or energy that enters the system. After the input is absorbed by the system, it is processed in a way useful to the system. This transformation is called **throughput**. For example, food is input to the digestive system; it is digested (throughput) so that it can be used by

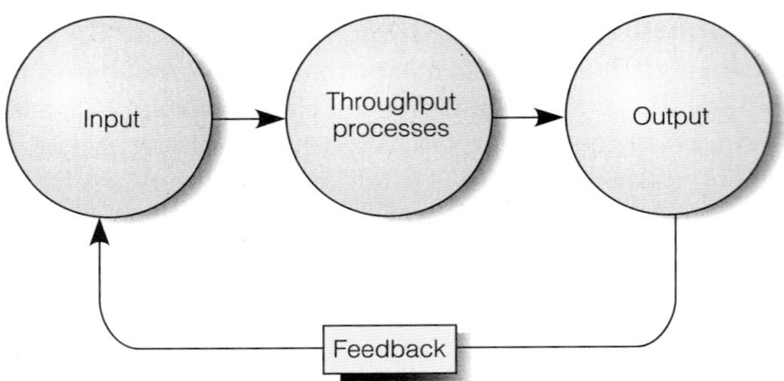

Figure 19.1 ■ An open system with a feedback mechanism.

the body. **Output** from a system is energy, matter, or information given out by the system as a result of its processes. Output from the digestive system includes caloric energy, nutrients, urine, and feces.

Feedback is the mechanism by which some of the output of a system is returned to the system as input. Feedback enables a system to regulate itself by redirecting the output back into the system, thus forming a feedback loop (Figure 19.1 ■). This input influences the behavior of the system and its future output. **Negative feedback** inhibits change; **positive feedback** stimulates change. Most biological systems are controlled by negative feedback to bring the system back to stability. This type of feedback system senses and counteracts any deviations from normal. The deviations may be greater or less than the normal level or range. For example, an increase in the production of parathyroid hormone is stimulated by a drop in blood calcium, but when additional parathyroid hormone raises the level of blood calcium, the hormone's production is then inhibited (Figure 19.2 ■). With hypoxia (shortage of oxygen), the concentration of red blood cells increases, and the heart rate becomes faster to transport the blood and available oxygen around the body adequately. People interact with the environment by adjusting themselves to it or adjusting it to themselves. This premise directs the nurse to look at environmental factors influencing the system and to plan nursing interventions to help the client maintain homeostasis. For example, the individual who is experiencing severe anxiety may be taught a variety of stress management techniques.

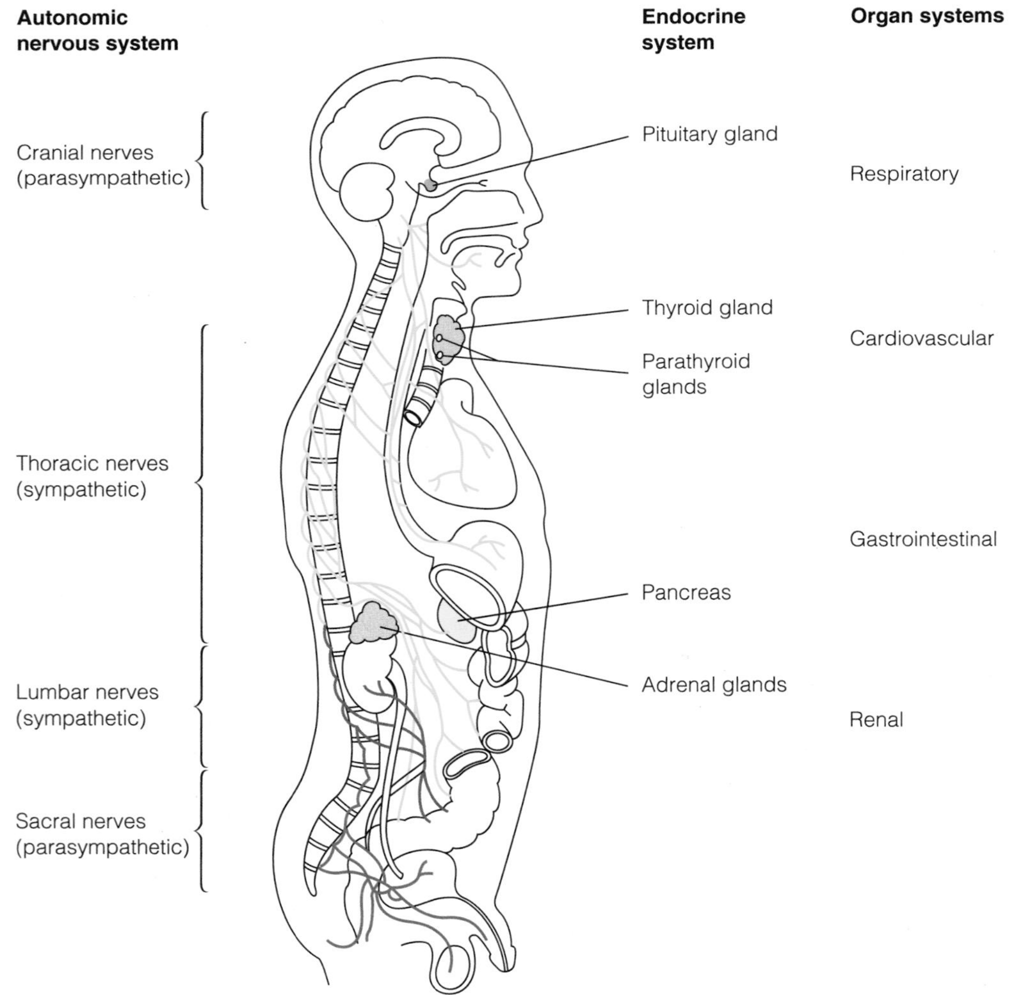

Figure 19.2 ■ The homeostatic regulations of the body: autonomic nervous system, endocrine system, and specific organ systems.

Psychologic Homeostasis

The term **psychologic homeostasis** refers to emotional or psychologic balance or a state of mental well-being. It is maintained by a variety of mechanisms. Each individual has certain psychologic needs, such as the need for love, security, and self-esteem, which must be met to maintain psychologic homeostasis. When one or more of these needs is not met or is threatened, certain coping mechanisms are activated to provide protection and psychologic homeostasis.

Psychologic homeostasis is acquired or learned through the experience of living and interacting with others. In addition, societal norms and culture influence behavior. Some prerequisites for a person to develop psychologic homeostasis can be summarized as follows:

- A stable physical environment in which the person feels safe and secure. For example, the basic needs for food, shelter, and clothing must be met consistently from birth onward.
- A stable psychologic environment from infancy onward, so that feelings of trust and love develop. Growing children and adolescents need kind but firm and consistent discipline, encouragement, and support to be their own unique selves.
- A social environment that includes adults who are healthy role models. Children learn the customs and values of society from these individuals.
- A life experience that provides satisfaction. Throughout life, people encounter many frustrations. People deal with these better if enough satisfying experiences have occurred to counterbalance the frustrating ones.

Assessing the Health of Individuals

A thorough assessment of an individual's health status is basic to health promotion. Components of this assessment are the health history and physical examination, physical fitness assessment, lifestyle assessment, health risk appraisal, health beliefs review, and life-stress review. Details about these assessments are discussed in Chapters 10 and 29.

Applying Theoretical Frameworks

Various theoretical frameworks provide the nurse with a holistic overview of health promotion for the individual and families across the lifespan. Two major theoretical frameworks that nurses use in promoting the health of the individual are needs theories and developmental stage theories.

Needs Theories

In needs theories, human needs are ranked on an ascending scale according to how essential the needs are for survival. Abraham Maslow (1970), perhaps the most renowned needs theorist, ranks human needs on five levels (Figure 19.3). The five levels in ascending order are as follows:

- ***Physiologic needs.*** Needs such as air, food, water, shelter, rest, sleep, activity, and temperature maintenance are crucial for survival.
- ***Safety and security needs.*** The need for safety has both physical and psychologic aspects. The person needs to feel safe, both in the physical environment and in relationships.
- ***Love and belonging needs.*** The third level of needs includes giving and receiving affection, attaining a place in a group, and maintaining the feeling of belonging.
- ***Self-esteem needs.*** The individual needs both self-esteem (i.e., feelings of independence, competence, and self-respect) and esteem from others (i.e., recognition, respect, and appreciation).
- ***Self-actualization.*** When the need for self-esteem is satisfied, the individual strives for self-actualization, the innate need to develop one's maximum potential and realize one's abilities and qualities.

Kalish's Hierarchy of Needs

Richard Kalish (1983) adapted Maslow's hierarchy of needs into six levels rather than five. He suggests an additional category between the physiologic needs and the safety and security needs. This category, referred to as *stimulation needs*, includes sex, activity, exploration, manipulation, and novelty (see Figure 19.3). Kalish

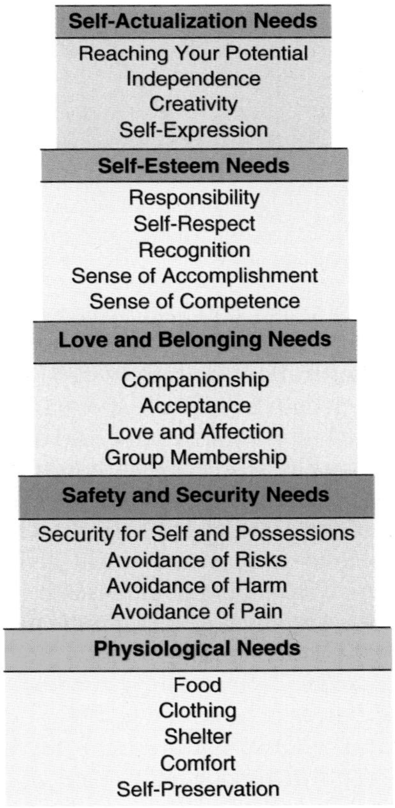

Self-Actualization Needs
Reaching Your Potential
Independence
Creativity
Self-Expression

Self-Esteem Needs
Responsibility
Self-Respect
Recognition
Sense of Accomplishment
Sense of Competence

Love and Belonging Needs
Companionship
Acceptance
Love and Affection
Group Membership

Safety and Security Needs
Security for Self and Possessions
Avoidance of Risks
Avoidance of Harm
Avoidance of Pain

Physiological Needs
Food
Clothing
Shelter
Comfort
Self-Preservation

Figure 19.3 Maslow's needs.

emphasizes that children need to explore and manipulate their environments to achieve optimal growth and development. He notes that adults, too, often seek novel adventures or stimulating experiences before considering their safety or security needs.

Characteristics of Basic Needs

All people have the same basic needs; however, each individual's needs and reactions to those needs are influenced by the culture with which the individual identifies. For example, professional achievement, independent functioning, and privacy may be important in one culture or subculture and unimportant in another.

- People meet their own needs relative to their own priorities. For example, a poor mother might give up her share of food so that her child might have sufficient food to live.
- Although basic needs generally must be met, some needs can be deferred. An example is the need for independence, which an ill individual can defer until well.
- Failure to meet needs results in one or more homeostatic imbalances, which can eventually result in illness.
- A need can make itself felt by either external or internal stimuli. An example is the need for food. A person may experience hunger as a result of physiologic processes (internal stimulation) or as a result of seeing a beautiful cake (external stimulation).
- An individual who perceives a need can respond in several ways to meet it. The choice of response is largely a result of learned experiences, lifestyle, and the values of the culture. For example, many people's food choices at mealtimes and snack times are based on past experiences, lifestyle, and culture.
- Needs are interrelated. Some needs cannot be met unless related needs are also met. The need for hydration can be influenced by the need for the elimination of urine. Likewise, the need for security can be markedly altered if the need for oxygen is threatened by a respiratory obstruction.

Needs can be satisfied in healthy and unhealthy ways. Ways of meeting basic needs are considered healthy when they are not harmful to others or to self, conform to the individual's sociocultural values, and are within the law. Conversely, unhealthy behavior may be harmful to others or to self, does not conform to the individual's sociocultural values, or is not within the law. People who satisfy their basic needs appropriately are healthier, happier, and more effective than those whose needs are frustrated.

Knowledge of the theoretical bases of human needs assists nurses in responding therapeutically to a client's behaviors and in understanding themselves and their own responses to needs. Human needs serve as a framework for assessing behaviors, assigning priorities to desired outcomes, and planning nursing interventions. For example, an adult with poor self-esteem would have difficulty accomplishing self-actualization. Therefore, nursing interventions would focus on increasing the client's self-esteem.

Developmental Stage Theories

Developmental stage theories categorize a person's behaviors or tasks into approximate age ranges or in terms that describe the features of an age group. The age ranges of the stages do not take into account individual differences; however, the categories do describe characteristics associated with the majority of individuals at periods when distinctive developmental changes occur and with the specific tasks that must be accomplished. See Chapter 23 ∞ for further information about developmental stages.

Developmental stage theories allow nurses to describe typical behaviors of an individual within a certain age group, explain the significance of those behaviors, predict behaviors that might occur in a given situation, and provide a rationale to control behavioral manifestations. Individuals can be compared with a representative group of people at the same point in time or at different points in time. The nurse's knowledge of developmental stage theories can be used in parental and client education, counseling, and anticipatory guidance.

Healthy People 2020

The vision of health promotion was initially expressed in 1979 with the surgeon general's report *Healthy People*, which emphasized health promotion and disease prevention. *Healthy People 2000* followed in 1990 and provided a framework for national health promotion, health protection, and preventive service strategy. The *Healthy People* initiative is updated and changed every 10 years. *Healthy People 2020* (U.S. Department of Health and Human Services, 2010) presents the current vision, mission, and overarching goals (Box 19.1). Specific objectives and strategies were developed to achieve them. The *Healthy People 2020* objectives, which are organized by topic areas, reflect public comments and the deliberation of work groups such as the Federal Interagency Workgroup on Healthy People 2020 and the Secretary's Advisory Committee on National Health Promotion and Disease Prevention Objectives for 2020. In 2014, a progress update on the leading health indicators was released (U.S. Department of Health and Human Services, 2014). Box 19.1 addresses the updates published by the U.S. government.

The foundation for *Healthy People 2020* is the belief that individual health is closely linked to community health, and the reverse. For example, community health is affected by the beliefs, attitudes, and behaviors of the individuals who live in the community. As a result, partnerships are important to improve individual and community health. Businesses, local government, and civic, professional, and religious organizations can all participate. Examples include sponsoring a health fair, establishing fitness programs, beginning community recycling programs, and printing immunization schedules.

Healthy People 2030

Healthy People 2030 is currently being developed. On June 22, 2017, an informational webinar was conducted to outline the programmatic priorities beginning in January

BOX 19.1 ***Healthy People 2020* Update on the Progress of Leading Health Indicators**

- Access to health services—little to no detectable change
- Clinical preventive services—improvement for adults with hypertension and colorectal cancer; improvement in children being immunized; no detectable change in hemoglobin A1C values
- Environmental quality—air quality index and children exposed to second-hand smoke: target met
- Injury and violence—injury deaths (age adjusted per 100,000): improving; homicides (age-adjusted per 100,000): target met
- Maternal, infant, and child health: target met
- Mental health—suicide and adolescents with major depressive disorders: getting worse
- Nutrition, physical activity, and obesity—adults meeting physical activity guidelines: target met; obesity: little or no detectable change
- Oral health—persons who visited the dentist in the past 2 years: getting worse
- Reproductive and sexual health; knowledge of serostatus: improving
- Social determinants—students graduating from high school: improving
- Substance abuse—adolescents using alcohol or illicit drugs: improving
- Tobacco—adults using cigarettes: improving; adolescents: little change

Adapted from *Healthy People 2020* Leading Health Indicators: Progress Update. Retrieved from https://www.healthypeople.gov/sites/default/files/LHI-ProgressReport-ExecSum_0.pdf

2030 (Office of Disease Prevention and Health Promotion, 2017). There will be a three-pronged approach to the development of *Healthy People 2030*. The three prongs include the Secretary's Advisory Committee on National Health Promotion and Disease Prevention Objectives for 2030. The second prong is public comment, and the third prong is the Healthy People Federal Interagency Workgroup (HPFIW). The Secretary's Advisory Committee develops recommendations to the Health and Human Services secretary for the development and implementation of *Healthy People 2030*. There is ongoing commentary from both the public and key stakeholders. The HPFIW develops guidance from key agencies to create recommendations for the *Healthy People 2030* framework and objectives. The charge to the committee is to ensure the selection criteria address the public health issues shown to be high-impact priorities by current national data, to identify the leading health indicators, and to implement *Healthy People 2030* (Office of Disease Prevention and Health Promotion, 2018).

Defining Health Promotion

Considerable differences appear in the literature regarding the use of the terms *health promotion*, *primary prevention*, *health protection*, and *illness prevention*. Edelman and Kudzma (2018) state that "prevention, in a narrow sense, means avoiding the development of disease in the future, and, in the broader sense, consists of all interventions to limit progression of a disease" (p. 9). The levels of prevention occur at various points in the course of disease progression. Leavell and Clark (1965) defined three levels of prevention: primary, secondary, and tertiary. Five steps describe these levels: **Primary prevention** focuses on (a) health promotion and (b) protection against specific health problems (e.g., immunization against hepatitis B). The purpose of primary prevention is to decrease the risk or exposure of the individual or community to disease. **Secondary prevention** focuses on (a) early identification of health problems and (b) prompt intervention to alleviate health problems. Its goal is to identify individuals in an early stage of a disease process and to limit future disability. **Tertiary prevention** focuses on restoration and rehabilitation, with the goal of returning the individual to an optimal level of functioning. Table 19.1 provides examples of activities for each level of prevention. The three levels of prevention may overlap in practice. For example, a client may have experienced a heart attack, and a goal of secondary prevention is to limit disability. The teaching (e.g., lifestyle changes) for the client's rehabilitation will be similar to the health education activities used for primary prevention teaching.

Murdaugh et al. (2019) consider health promotion to be different from disease prevention or health protection. Health promotion must address physical and social situations that cause poor health. The individual's underlying motivation for the behavior is the major difference.

The difficulty in separating the terms *health promotion* and *disease prevention* or *health protection* lies in the fact that an activity may be carried out for numerous reasons. For example, a 40-year-old male may begin a program of walking 3 miles each day. If the goal of his program were to "decrease the risk of cardiovascular disease," then the activity would be considered disease prevention or health protection. By contrast, if the motivation for his walking regimen were to "increase his overall health and feeling of well-being," then the activity would be considered a health promotion behavior. It is most helpful to think of health promotion and health protection as being complementary processes because both affect the quality of health. Murdaugh et al. (2019) identified the changing landscape of health promotion. There are multilevel interventions and strategies that address health issues on many levels. These levels include individuals, families, schools, communities, worksites, and diverse populations. The health promotion interventions to be implemented at any level should be based on evidence and address the social determinants of health.

The ever-changing world of technology and technologic advances is another area that has changed the landscape of health promotion and disease prevention. The expansion of mobile wireless computer technologies and social media applications, including telemedicine and telecare, has had a major influence on health promotion and prevention, unlike any in recent history. E-health (electronic health) or Mhealth (mobile health) includes a diverse set of informatics tools that have been embraced as a promising new way to prevent health problems and promote healthy behaviors at all levels and that play a

TABLE 19.1 Levels of Prevention

Level and Description	Examples
Primary prevention: Generalized health promotion and specific protection against disease. It precedes disease or dysfunction and is applied to generally healthy individuals or groups.	• Health education about injury and poisoning prevention, standards of nutrition and of growth and development for each stage of life, exercise requirements, stress management, protection against occupational hazards, and so on • Immunizations • Risk assessments for specific disease • Family planning services • Environmental sanitation and provision of adequate housing, recreation, and work conditions
Secondary prevention: Emphasizes early detection of disease, prompt intervention, and health maintenance for individuals experiencing health problems. Includes prevention of complications and disabilities.	• Screening surveys and procedures of any type (e.g., Denver Developmental Screening Test, hypertension screening) • Encouraging regular medical and dental checkups • Teaching self-examination for breast and testicular cancer • Assessing the growth and development of children • Nursing assessments and care provided in home, hospital, or other agency to prevent complications (e.g., maintaining skin integrity; turning, positioning, and exercising clients; ensuring adequate rest, food, and fluid intake; promoting fecal and urinary elimination; administering medical therapies such as medications; and so on)
Tertiary prevention: Begins after an illness, when a defect or disability is fixed, stabilized, or determined to be irreversible. Its focus is to help rehabilitate individuals and restore them to an optimal level of functioning within the constraints of the disability.	• Referring a client who has had a colostomy to a support group • Teaching a client who has diabetes to identify and prevent complications • Referring a client with a spinal cord injury to a rehabilitation center to receive training that will maximize use of remaining abilities

significant role in promoting the health of all individuals and communities (Murdaugh et al., 2019, p. 4).

In a recent article, Adams, Liguori, and Lofgren (2017) proposed the use of technology as a tool to encourage young adults to maintain healthy sleep and eating habits. Because young adults require approximately 8 hours of sleep per night, the use of SleepBot can be beneficial. SleepBot is a smartphone app that integrates a smart alarm and a sleep-cycle tracker. By tracking the sleep cycle, it allows the adolescent or young adult to wake gently during the lightest cycle of sleep. The MyFitnessPal is a free diet and exercise app that tracks the daily intake of calories, vitamins, and minerals. It identifies and analyzes diet patterns and exercise. These features can influence a client's dietary choices.

Health promotion can be offered to all clients regardless of their health and illness status or age. For example, weight-control measures can benefit clients with obesity who are without disease and clients with cardiac or joint disease. Age-specific health promotion activities are discussed in Chapters 24, 25, and 26 ∞. See Lifespan Considerations for examples of health promotion topics.

LIFESPAN CONSIDERATIONS Health Promotion Topics

INFANTS
Infant-parent attachment and bonding
Breastfeeding
Sleep patterns
Playful activity to stimulate development
Immunizations
Safety promotion and injury control

CHILDREN
Nutrition
Dental checkups
Rest and exercise
Immunizations
Safety promotion and injury control

ADOLESCENTS
Communicating with the teen
Hormonal changes
Nutrition
Exercise and rest
Peer group influences
Self-concept and body image
Sexuality
Safety promotion and injury prevention

OLDER ADULTS
Adequate sleep
Appropriate use of alcohol
Dental and oral health
Drug management
Exercise
Foot health
Health screening recommendations
Hearing aid use
Immunizations
Medication instruction
Mental health
Nutrition
Physical fitness
Preventive health services
Safety precautions
Smoking cessation
Weight control

Sites for Health Promotion Activities

Health promotion programs exist in many settings. Programs and activities may be offered to individuals and families in the home or in the community setting and at schools, hospitals, or worksites. Some individuals may feel more comfortable having a nurse, diet counselor, or fitness expert come to their home for teaching and follow-up on individual needs. This type of program, however, is not cost effective for most individuals. Many people prefer the group approach, find it more motivating, and enjoy the socializing and support. Most programs offered in the community are group oriented.

Cities and towns frequently offer community programs. The type of program depends on the current concerns and the expertise of the sponsoring department or group. Program offerings may include health promotion, specific protection, and screening for early detection of disease. The local health department may offer a town-wide immunization program because immunization provides one of the most cost-effective means of protecting infants and children. Other examples include the fire department distributing fire prevention information or the police offering a bicycle safety program for children or a safe-driving campaign for young adults.

Hospitals began the emphasis on health promotion and prevention by focusing on the health of their employees. Because of the stress involved in caring for the sick and the various shifts that nurses and other healthcare workers must work, the lifestyles and health habits of healthcare employees were given priority.

Programs offered by healthcare organizations initially began with a specific focus on prevention. Examples include infection control, fire prevention and fire drills, limiting exposure to x-rays, and the prevention of back injuries. Gradually, issues related to the health and lifestyle of the employee were addressed with programs on topics such as smoking cessation, exercise and fitness, stress reduction, and time management. Increasingly, hospitals have offered a variety of these programs and others (e.g., women's health) to the community as well as to their employees. Such community activities enhance the public image of the hospital, increase the health of the surrounding population, and generate some additional income.

School health promotion programs may serve as a foundation for children of all ages to gain basic knowledge about personal hygiene and issues in the health sciences. Because school is the focus of a child's life for so many years, the school provides a cost-effective and convenient setting for health-focused programs. The school nurse may teach programs about basic nutrition, dental care, activity and play, drug and alcohol abuse, domestic violence, child abuse, and issues related to sexuality and pregnancy. Classroom teachers may include health-related topics in their lesson plans, for example, the way the normal heart functions or the need for clean air and water in the environment.

Worksite programs for health promotion have developed out of the need for businesses to control the rising costs of healthcare and employee absenteeism. Many industries feel that both employers and employees benefit from healthy lifestyles and behaviors. The convenience of the worksite setting makes these programs particularly attractive to many adults who would otherwise not be aware of them or motivated to attend them. Health promotion programs may be held in the company cafeteria so that employees can watch a film or attend a discussion group during their lunch break. Worksite programs may include programs that address air quality standards for the office, classroom, or plant; programs aimed at specific populations, such as injury prevention for the machine worker or back-saver programs for the individual involved in heavy lifting; programs to screen for high blood pressure; or health enhancement programs, such as fitness information and relaxation techniques. Benefits to the worker may include an increased feeling of well-being, fitness, weight control, and decreased stress. Benefits to the employer may include an increase in employee motivation and productivity, an increase in employee morale, a decrease in absenteeism, and a lower rate of employee turnover, all of which may decrease business and healthcare costs.

Older adults who have retired often have more time for health promotion activities than they did before retirement. The nurse can inform older adults of available community resources such as walking groups. Nurses can address the need for health protection and health promotion through teaching classes at retirement communities and other community resource centers for older adults.

Health Promotion Model

The initial version of the Health Promotion Model (HPM) appeared in the nursing literature in the early 1980s and focused on health-promoting behaviors rather than health protection or illness prevention behaviors. The initial model has been replaced by the Health Promotion Model (Revised) as shown in Figure 19.4 ■. The HPM is a competence- or approach-oriented model in which the motivational source for behavior change is based on the individual's subjective value of the change—that is, how the client perceives the benefits of changing the given health behavior. The HPM does not include "fear" or "threat" as a motivating source for changing health behavior (Murdaugh et al., 2019, p. 40).

Individual Characteristics and Experiences

The importance of an individual's unique personal factors or characteristics and experiences will depend on the target behavior for health promotion. There is flexibility in the HPM to select those characteristics that are relevant to the particular health behavior. Personal factors are categorized as biological (e.g., age, strength, balance), psychologic (e.g., self-esteem, self-motivation), and sociocultural

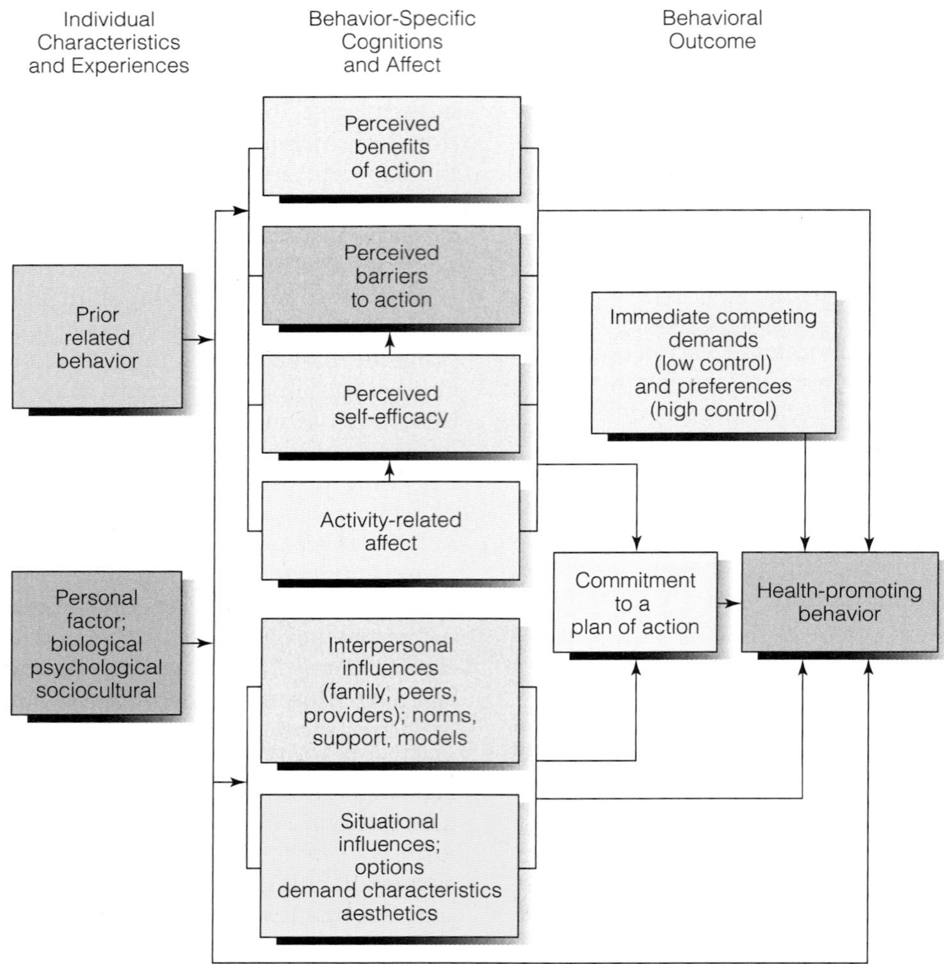

Figure 19.4 ■ The Health Promotion Model (Revised).
PENDER, NOLA J.; MURDAUGH, CAROLYN L.; PARSONS, MARY ANN, HEALTH PROMOTION IN NURSING PRACTICE (SUBSCRIPTION), 8th Ed., © 2019. Reprinted and Electronically reproduced by permission of Pearson Education, Inc., New York, NY.

(e.g., race, ethnicity, education, socioeconomic status). Some personal factors can influence health behaviors, whereas others, such as age, cannot be changed. Prior related behavior includes previous experience, knowledge, and skill in health-promoting actions. Individuals who made a habit of a previous health-promoting behavior and received a positive benefit as a result will probably engage in future health-promoting behaviors. In contrast, an individual with a history of barriers to achieving the behavior remembers the "hurdles," which creates a negative effect. The nurse can assist by focusing on the positive benefits of the behavior, teaching how to overcome the hurdles, and providing positive feedback for the client's successes.

Nursing interventions usually focus on factors that can be modified. It is just as important, however, to also focus on factors that cannot be changed, such as family history. For instance, if a woman has a strong family history of breast cancer, she may neglect self-care practices such as performing breast self-exams and having regular mammograms or may even opt for extreme clinical measures such as a mastectomy. She may do this out of fear of finding a lump or just a feeling that with her family history, it is inevitable that she will have breast cancer. Nurses should recognize this and direct more support and information to this group of women, reinforcing the idea that even with a strong family history, early detection and treatment are especially important and offer more hope for a cure. Helping to transform that fear into hope for early detection can make a difference in health attitudes and behaviors. The *Healthy People 2020* objective to increase the proportion of women with a family history of breast or ovarian cancer who receive genetic counseling supports the need for early detection, support, and information.

Behavior-Specific Cognitions and Affect

This set of variables is of major motivational significance for acquiring and maintaining health-promoting behaviors. Behavior-specific cognitions constitute a critical "core" for intervention because nursing interventions can modify them. They include the following:

- ***Perceived benefits of action.*** Anticipated benefits or outcomes (e.g., physical fitness, stress reduction) affect the client's plan to participate in health-promoting behaviors and may facilitate continued practice. Prior positive experience with the behavior or observations of others engaged in the behavior can be a motivational factor.

- ***Perceived barriers to action.*** A client's perceptions about available time, inconvenience, expense, and difficulty performing the activity may act as barriers (imagined or real). Perceived barriers to action affect health-promoting behaviors by decreasing the individual's commitment to a plan of action.
- ***Perceived self-efficacy.*** This concept refers to the conviction that a client can successfully carry out the behavior necessary to achieve a desired outcome, such as maintaining an exercise program to lose weight. Clients who have serious doubts about their capabilities often decrease their efforts and give up, whereas those with a strong sense of efficacy exert greater effort to master problems or challenges.
- ***Activity-related affect.*** The subjective feelings that occur before, during, and following an activity can influence whether a client will repeat the behavior again or maintain the behavior. What is the client's reaction to the thought of the behavior? Is it perceived as fun, enjoyable, or unpleasant? A behavior associated with a positive affect or emotional response is likely to be repeated, and behaviors associated with a negative affect are usually avoided.
- ***Interpersonal influences.*** Interpersonal influences are a person's perceptions concerning the behaviors, beliefs, or attitudes of others. Family, peers, and health professionals are sources of interpersonal influences that can affect a client's health-promoting behaviors. Interpersonal influences include expectations of significant others, social support (e.g., emotional encouragement), and learning through observing others or modeling.
- ***Situational influences.*** Situational influences are direct and indirect influences on health-promoting behaviors and include perceptions of available options, demand characteristics, and the aesthetic features of the environment. An example of a client's perception of available options can include easy access to healthy alternatives, such as vending machines and restaurants that provide healthful menu options. Demand characteristics can directly affect healthy behaviors through policies such as a company regulation that demands safety equipment to be worn or that establishes a nonsmoking environment. Individuals are more apt to perform health promotion behaviors if they are comfortable in the environment versus feeling alienated. Environments that are considered safe as well as interesting are also desirable aesthetic features that facilitate health promotion behaviors.

Commitment to a Plan of Action

Commitment to a plan of action involves two processes: commitment and identifying specific strategies for carrying out and reinforcing the behavior. Strategies are important because commitment alone often results in "good intentions" and not the actual performance of the behavior.

Immediate Competing Demands and Preferences

Competing demands are those behaviors over which an individual has a low level of control. For example, an unexpected work or family responsibility may compete with a planned visit to the health club, and not responding to this responsibility may cause a more negative outcome than missing the exercise routine. Competing preferences are behaviors over which an individual has a high level of control; however, this control depends on the individual's ability to be self-regulating or to not "give in." For example, a person who chooses a high-fat food over a low-fat food because it tastes better has "given in" to an urge based on a competing preference.

Behavioral Outcome

Health-promoting behavior, the outcome of the HPM, proposes a framework that integrates nursing and behavioral science perspectives with factors influencing health behaviors. Health-promoting behaviors should result in improved health, enhanced functional ability, and better quality of life at all stages of development (Murdaugh et al., 2019, p. 44).

Stages of Health Behavior Change

Health behavior change is a cyclic phenomenon in which clients progress through several stages. In the first stage, the client does not think seriously about changing a behavior; by the time the client reaches the final stage, he or she is successfully maintaining the change in behavior. Several models of behavior change have been proposed. The Transtheoretical Model (TTM), proposed by Prochaska, Redding, and Evers (2009), is discussed here. The stages are (a) precontemplation, (b) contemplation, (c) preparation, (d) action, (e) maintenance, and (f) termination. If the person does not succeed in changing behavior, relapse occurs.

Precontemplation Stage

In the **precontemplation stage**, the client does not think about changing his or her behavior in the next 6 months. The client may be uninformed or underinformed about the consequences of the risk behavior(s). The client who has tried changing previously and was unsuccessful may now see the behavior as his or her "fate" or believe that change is hopeless. Clients in this stage tend to avoid reading, talking, or thinking about their high-risk behaviors (Prochaska et al., 2009, p. 100).

Contemplation Stage

During the **contemplation stage**, the client acknowledges having a problem, seriously considers changing a specific behavior, actively gathers information, and verbalizes plans to change the behavior in the near future (e.g., next 6 months). The client, however, may not be ready to commit to action. Some people may stay in the contemplative stage for months or years before taking action.

Preparation Stage

The **preparation stage** occurs when the client intends to take action in the immediate future (e.g., within the next month). Some client in this stage may have already started making small behavioral changes, such as buying a self-help book. At this stage, the client makes the final specific plans to accomplish the change.

Action Stage

The **action stage** occurs when the client actively implements behavioral and cognitive strategies of the action plan to interrupt previous health risk behaviors and adopt new ones. This stage requires the greatest commitment of time and energy.

Maintenance Stage

During the **maintenance stage**, the client strives to prevent relapse by integrating newly adopted behaviors into his or her lifestyle. This stage lasts until the client no longer experiences temptation to return to previous unhealthy behaviors. It is estimated that maintenance lasts from 6 months to 5 years (Prochaska et al., 2009, p. 100). The relapse is usually to the precontemplation or contemplation stage.

Termination Stage

The **termination stage** is the ultimate goal; it is the point at which the client has complete confidence that the problem is no longer a temptation or threat. It is as if the client never acquired the habit in the first place or the new behavior has become automatic (Prochaska et al., 2009, p. 102). Experts debate whether some behaviors can be terminated versus requiring continual maintenance. For example, adults who automatically buckle their seat belts when getting in their vehicle may reach the termination stage. Other behaviors, such as smoking or overeating, may never reach the termination stage because relapse temptations are too strong. The goal of maintenance may be more appropriate for those clients.

These six stages are cyclical; client generally move through one stage before progressing to the next. However, at any point, a client may relapse or recycle to any previous stage. In fact, the average successful self-changer recycles through the stages several times before making it to the top and exiting the cycle (Prochaska, Norcross, & DiClemente, 1994, pp. 47–48). The majority of clients who relapse return to the contemplation stage. During this time, they can think about what they learned and plan for the next action attempt.

The Nurse's Role in Health Promotion

Individuals and communities seeking to increase their responsibility for personal health and self-care require health education. The trend toward health promotion has created the opportunity for nurses to strengthen the profession's influence on health promotion, disseminate information that promotes an educated public, and assist individuals and communities in changing long-standing health behaviors.

A variety of programs can be used for the promotion of health, including (a) information dissemination, (b) health risk appraisal and wellness assessment, (c) lifestyle and behavior change, and (d) environmental control programs.

Information dissemination is the most basic type of health promotion program. This method makes use of a variety of media to offer information to the public about the risk of particular lifestyle choices and personal behavior, as well as the benefits of changing that behavior and improving the quality of life. Billboards, posters, brochures, newspaper features, books, and health fairs all offer opportunities for the dissemination of health promotion information. Alcohol and drug abuse, driving under the influence of alcohol, hypertension, and the need for immunizations are some of the topics frequently discussed. Information dissemination is a useful strategy for raising the level of knowledge and awareness of individuals and groups about health habits.

When planning information dissemination, it is important to consider factors such as cultural influences and different age groups. Knowing the best place and method to distribute information will increase the effectiveness. For example, older adults usually have strong ties to their churches for social support as well as religious practices. Knowing this, the church can often be the appropriate place to hold health fairs or even small-group discussions on various health topics. It acts as a stepping-stone for providing information and suggesting resources for special needs—all done in a comfortable, nonthreatening environment for individuals in that age group and culture.

It is just as critical to know where people get "misinformation." Multiple mailings and TV infomercials have become a marketing ploy for advertising "miracle" vitamins, herbs, and food supplements. These are heavily directed toward older adults who may choose this route of purchasing items if they have transportation problems.

Health risk appraisals and wellness assessment programs explain to individuals the risk factors that are inherent in their lives in order to motivate them to reduce specific risks and develop positive health habits. Wellness assessment programs focus on more positive methods of enhancement, in contrast to the risk-factor approach used in the health appraisal. Various tools are available to facilitate these assessments. Some of these tools are computer based and can therefore be offered to educational institutions and industries at a reasonable cost.

Lifestyle and behavior-change programs require the participation of the individual and are geared toward enhancing the quality of life and extending the lifespan. Individuals generally consider lifestyle changes after they learn of the need to change their health behavior and become aware of the potential benefits of the process. Many programs are available to the public, both on a group and individual basis, some of which address stress management, nutrition awareness, weight control, smoking cessation, and exercise.

Environmental control programs have been developed in response to the continuing increase of contaminants of human origin that have been introduced into our environment. The amounts of contaminants that are already present in the air, food, and water will affect the health of our descendants for several generations. The most common concerns of community groups are toxic and nuclear wastes, nuclear power plants, air and water pollution, and herbicide and pesticide use.

Health promotion activities, such as the variety of programs previously discussed, involve collaborative relationships with both clients and primary care providers. The role of the nurse is to work *with* people, not *for* them—that is, to act as a facilitator of the process of assessing, evaluating, and understanding health. The nurse may act as advocate, consultant, teacher, or coordinator of services. For examples of the nurse's role in health promotion, see Box 19.2.

In these roles, the nurse may work with individuals of all age groups and diverse family units or concentrate on a specific population, such as new parents, school-age children, or older adults. In any case, the nursing process is a basic tool for the nurse in a health promotion role. Although the process is the same, the nurse emphasizes teaching the client (who can be either an individual or a family unit) self-care responsibility. Adult clients decide the goals, determine the health promotion plans, and take responsibility for the success of the plans.

BOX 19.2 The Nurse's Role in Health Promotion

- Model healthy lifestyle behaviors and attitudes.
- Facilitate client involvement in the assessment, implementation, and evaluation of health goals.
- Teach clients self-care strategies to enhance fitness, improve nutrition, manage stress, and enhance relationships.
- Assist individuals, families, and communities to increase their levels of health.
- Educate clients to be effective healthcare consumers.
- Assist clients, families, and communities in developing and choosing health-promoting options.
- Guide clients' development in effective problem-solving and decision-making.
- Reinforce clients' personal and family health-promoting behaviors.
- Advocate in the community for changes that promote a healthy environment.

The Nursing Process and Health Promotion

A thorough assessment of client's health status is basic to health promotion. As nurses move toward greater autonomy in providing client care, expanded assessment skills are essential to provide the meaningful data needed for health planning.

●○● NURSING MANAGEMENT

Assessing

Components of this assessment are the health history and physical examination, physical fitness assessment, lifestyle assessment, spiritual health assessment, social support systems review, health risk assessment, health beliefs review, and life-stress review.

Health History and Physical Examination

The health history and physical examination discussed in Chapter 29 ∞ provide a means for detecting any existing problems. The age of the individual must be considered when collecting data. For example, an environmental safety assessment and immunization history must be appropriate to the client's age. A nutritional assessment is an important part of the health history. The nurse must consider both the age and the body build of the client when gathering information on dietary patterns. See Chapter 46 ∞ for more information about nutritional assessment.

Physical Fitness Assessment

During an evaluation of physical fitness, the nurse assesses several components of the body's physical functioning: muscle endurance, flexibility, body composition, and cardiorespiratory endurance. Aerobic and bone-strengthening activities for children and adolescents are given in Table 19.2. Adults and older adults require 2 hours and 30 minutes of moderate aerobic exercise per week. Older adults need to be monitored carefully for fatigue during strength and endurance tests.

Lifestyle Assessment

Lifestyle assessment focuses on the personal lifestyle and habits of the client as they affect health. Categories of lifestyle generally assessed are physical activity, nutritional practices, stress management, and such habits as smoking, alcohol consumption, and drug use. Other categories may be included. Several tools are available to assess lifestyle.

TABLE 19.2 Aerobic and Muscle- and Bone-Strengthening Activities: What Counts

	Age Group	
Type of Physical Activity	**Children**	**Adolescents**
Moderate-intensity aerobic	• Active recreation such as hiking, skateboarding, rollerblading • Bicycle riding • Walking to school	• Active recreation, such as canoeing, hiking, cross-country skiing, skateboarding, rollerblading • Brisk walking • Bicycle riding (stationary or road bike) • House and yard work such as sweeping or pushing a lawn mower • Playing games that require catching and throwing, such as baseball, softball, basketball, and volleyball
Vigorous-intensity aerobic	• Active games involving running and chasing, such as tag • Bicycle riding • Jumping rope • Martial arts, such as karate • Running • Sports such as ice or field hockey, basketball, swimming, tennis, or gymnastics	• Active games involving running and chasing, such as flag football, soccer • Bicycle riding • Jumping rope • Martial arts such as karate • Running • Sports such as tennis, ice or field hockey, basketball, swimming • Vigorous dancing • Aerobics • Cheerleading or gymnastics
Muscle strengthening	• Games such as tug-of-war • Modified push-ups (with knees on the floor) • Resistance exercises using body weight or resistance bands • Rope or tree climbing • Sit-ups • Swinging on playground equipment/bars • Gymnastics	• Games such as tug-of-war • Push-ups • Resistance exercises with exercise bands, weight machines, handheld weights • Rock climbing • Sit-ups • Cheerleading or gymnastics
Bone strengthening	• Games such as hopscotch • Hopping, skipping, jumping • Jumping rope • Running • Sports such as gymnastics, basketball, volleyball, tennis	• Hopping, skipping, jumping • Jumping rope • Running • Sports such as gymnastics, basketball, volleyball, tennis

Centers for Disease Control and Prevention. (2015). *Physical activity for a healthy weight*. Retrieved from

The goals of lifestyle assessment tools are to provide the following:

1. An opportunity for clients to assess the impact of their present lifestyle on their health
2. A basis for decisions related to desired behavior and lifestyle changes.

Spiritual Health Assessment

Spiritual health is the ability to develop one's inner nature to its fullest potential, including the ability to discover and articulate one's basic purpose in life; to learn how to experience love, joy, peace, and fulfillment; and to learn how to help ourselves and others achieve their fullest potential (Murdaugh et al., 2019, p. 101). Spiritual beliefs can affect a client's interpretation of the events in his or her life, and therefore an assessment of spiritual well-being is a part of evaluating the client's overall health. See Chapter 41 ∞ for more information.

Social Support Systems Review

Understanding the social context in which a client lives and works is important in health promotion. Individuals and groups, through interpersonal relationships, can provide comfort, assistance, encouragement, and information. Social support fosters successful coping and promotes satisfying and effective living.

Social support systems contribute to health by creating an environment that encourages healthy behaviors, promotes self-esteem and wellness, and provides feedback that the client's actions will lead to desirable outcomes. Examples of social support systems include family, peer support groups (including computer-based support groups), community-organized religious support systems (e.g., churches), and self-help groups (e.g., Mended Hearts, Weight Watchers).

The nurse can begin a social support system review by asking the client to do the following:

- List individuals who provide personal support.
- Indicate the relationship of each family member, fellow worker or colleague, or social acquaintance on the list.
- Identify which individuals have been a source of support for 5 or more years.

This assessment allows the nurse and client to discuss and evaluate the adequacy of the support system together and, if necessary, plan options for enhancing the support system.

Health Risk Assessment

A **health risk assessment (HRA)** is an assessment and educational tool that indicates a client's risk for disease or injury during the next 10 years by comparing the client's risk with the mortality risk of the corresponding age, gender, and racial group. The client's general health, lifestyle behaviors, and demographic data are compared to data from a large national sample. Individual risk reports are based on statistics for the population group that matches the individual's surveyed characteristics. The HRA includes a summary of the client's health risks and lifestyle behaviors with educational suggestions on how to reduce the risk.

Many HRA instruments are available today in paper-and-pencil formats or as computerized forms. Recently, HRAs have begun to reflect a broader approach to health as companies use the HRA as a means to begin a health promotion and risk reduction program. Occupational health nurses can identify risk factors and subsequently plan interventions aimed at decreasing illness, absenteeism, and disability.

HRAs are helpful for assessing individual and group health risks. They are not, however, substitutes for medical care and are not appropriate for all clients. For example, clients with chronic illnesses such as cancer or heart disease may not obtain accurate risk assessments. Certain populations (e.g., very young, older adults, some sociocultural groups) may not be fully represented in the population databases, and therefore the HRA may not project an accurate risk assessment.

Health Beliefs Review

Clients' health beliefs need to be clarified, particularly those beliefs that determine how they perceive control of their own healthcare status. Locus of control is a measurable concept that can be used to predict which clients are most likely to change their behavior (see Chapter 20 ∞). Several instruments are available that assess a client's health beliefs. Assessment of clients' health beliefs provides the nurse with an indication of how much they believe they can influence or control health through personal behaviors. Some people have a strong belief in fate: "Whatever will be, will be." They do not feel that they can do anything to change the course of their disease. An example is adhering to instructions about diabetes, which often requires lifestyle changes in diet and exercise and close control of glucose to prevent complications. If clients believe they have no control over the outcome, it is difficult to provide motivation for them to make the necessary changes. These differences in health beliefs can provide a better indication of readiness and motivation on the part of the client to engage in healthy behaviors. See Lifespan Considerations for factors that might indicate a need for additional information or resources for older adults.

QSEN Patient-Centered Care: Social Support

In American cultures, there are many similarities in social support. The client's social structure reinforces the client's social support and the individual's sense of belonging. Nurses need to understand culturally sensitive theoretical views in order to understand the role of social support for the person or population receiving nursing care. For example, the client's family and friends are important sources of social support (Murdaugh et al., 2019, p. 194).

Life-Stress Review

There is abundant literature about the impact of stress on mental and physical well-being. A variety of stress-related instruments can be found in the literature. For example, Holmes and Rahe (1967) developed a Life-Change Index, a tool that assigns numerical values to life events. For example, life changes (e.g., death of a spouse, divorce, marital separation, pregnancy) have an impact score. The individual adds up all of the current life events and compares the total life-changes score to the likelihood of illness in the near future. Studies have shown that a high score is associated with an increased possibility of illness. Nursing school is stressful. A few guidelines for dealing with the stress include good time management, setting priorities, establishing realistic expectations, and taking time to exercise and relax.

Validating Assessment Data

Following the collection of assessment data, the nurse and client need to review, validate, and summarize the

EVIDENCE-BASED PRACTICE

Evidence-Based Practice

How Does Youth Exposure to Alcohol Advertising in National Magazines Affect Health Risk Assessments?

Ross, Henehan, and Jerrigan (2017) investigated youth exposure to alcohol advertising in US national magazines from 2001–2011. In 2010, underage drinking cost the US economy $24.3 billion. A public health goal is to reduce underage drinking. Magazines that have a large underage following must reduce alcohol advertising. The results of this study confirmed that magazine alcohol advertising was reduced by 62.9%. Although the exposure declined, it was found that 168 magazines exceeded the recommended exposure.

Implications

It is important for school nurses to educate adolescents on the health risks of ingesting alcohol. In addition, adolescents should be educated on the risk of injury or death with the abuse of alcohol.

LIFESPAN CONSIDERATIONS **Factors Affecting Health Promotion and Illness Prevention**

CHILDREN

Childhood obesity is becoming a serious health problem. According to the Centers for Disease Control and Prevention (2018), data from 2015–2016 show that nearly 1 in 5 school-age children and young people aged 6 to 19 is obese. Obesity and being overweight as children contribute to long-term health problems, such as heart disease and diabetes mellitus. Factors that contribute to obesity include genetics, metabolism, diminished sleep, decreased physical activity, and the design or safety of a community. Children may limit outside play in areas with increased crime or lack of recreational parks.

Although specific causes of obesity and appropriate management to reduce weight will vary from child to child, healthy eating habits and adequate exercise patterns form the basis for healthy growth and prevention of obesity in children. It is the responsibility of parents and caregivers to provide children with healthy food choices and an environment that makes eating a pleasure. It is the responsibility of children to decide how much and what foods to eat. Adults must be role models for their children, eating well and exercising regularly themselves.

OLDER ADULTS

In older adults, health promotion and illness prevention are important, but the focus is often on learning to adapt to and live with increasing changes and limitations. Maximizing strengths continues to be of prime importance in maintaining optimal function and quality of life. Factors to be aware of that might indicate a need for additional information or resources include these:

- An increase in physical limitations
- Presence of one or more chronic illnesses
- Change in cognitive status
- Difficulty in accessing healthcare services due to transportation problems
- Poor support system
- Need for environmental modifications for safety and to maintain independence
- Attitude of hopelessness and depression, which decreases the motivation to use resources or learn new information.

information. The nurse and the client carry this step out together. During this process, the nurse verbally reviews the current practices and attitudes of the client. This allows validation of the information by the client and may increase awareness of the need to change behavior. The nurse and client need to consider the following:

- Any existing health problems
- The client's perceived degree of control over health status
- Key health beliefs
- Level of physical fitness and nutritional status
- Illnesses for which the client is at risk
- Current positive health practices
- Spirituality
- Sources of life stress and ability to handle stress
- Social support systems
- Information needed to enhance healthcare practices
- Client strengths.

Diagnosing

The development and application of the nursing diagnosis for health promotion is to maintain or exceed the individual's level of health promotion activities and function. It is important for the individual to maintain a responsiveness to health promoting behaviors and the continuation of health related interventions. When the nurse and client conclude that the client has positive functioning in a certain pattern area, such as adequate nutrition or effective coping, the nurse can use this information to help the client reach a higher level of functioning. Examples of health promotion nursing diagnoses that may be appropriate for health promotion include: willingness to engage in health promotion education; willingness to engage in health promotion lifestyle changes; willingness to engage in health management; increased activity to promote health; adequate nutrition to promote health.

Planning

Health promotion plans need to be developed according to the needs, desires, and priorities of the client. The client decides on health promotion goals, the activities or interventions to achieve those goals, the frequency and duration of the activities, and the method of evaluation. During the planning process, the nurse acts as a resource person rather than as an adviser or counselor. The nurse provides information when asked, emphasizes the importance of small steps to behavioral change, and reviews the client's goals and plans to make sure they are realistic, measurable, and acceptable to the client.

Steps in Planning

Murdaugh et al. (2019, pp. 115–126) outline several steps in the process of developing a joint health promotion and prevention plan (Box 19.3). These steps actively involve both the nurse and the client:

1. ***Review and summarize data from assessment.*** The nurse shares with the client a summary of the data collected from the various assessments (e.g., physical health and fitness, nutrition, sources of stress, spirituality, health practices).
2. ***Emphasize strengths and competencies of the client.*** The nurse and the client come to a consensus about areas in which the client is doing well and areas that need further development.
3. ***Identify health goals and related behavior-change options.*** The client selects two or three top-priority personal health goals, prioritizes them, and reviews behavior-change options.
4. ***Identify desired behavioral health outcomes.*** For each of the selected goals or areas in step 3, the nurse and client determine what specific behavioral changes are needed to bring about the desired outcome. For example, to reduce the risk of cardiovascular disease,

BOX 19.3 Example of an Individual Health Promotion and Prevention Plan

Designed for: James Moore
Home Address: 714 George
Home Telephone Number: 222-3333
Occupation (if employed): Building services supervisor
Work Telephone Number: 445-6666
Cultural Identification: African American
Birth Date: 3/14/68
Date of Initial Plan: 1/15/2020

Client strengths	Satisfactory peer relationships, spiritual strength, adequate sleep pattern
Major risk factors	Elevated cholesterol, mild obesity, sedentary lifestyle, moderate life change, multiple daily hassles, few reported uplifts
Nursing diagnoses (derived from assessment of functional health patterns)	Impaired deviation in activity and engagement Overweight Increased role strain in caregiving (older adult mother)
Medical diagnoses (if any)	Mild hypertension
Age-specific screening recommendations:	Blood pressure, cholesterol, fecal occult blood, malignant skin lesions, depression
Desired behavioral and health outcomes	Become a regular exerciser (3×/week), lower my blood pressure, weigh 165 lb

Personal Health Goals (1 = Highest Priority)	Selected Behaviors to Accomplish Goals	Stage of Change	Strategies/Interventions for Change
1. Achieve desired body weight.	Begin a progressive walking program.	Planning	Counterconditioning Reinforcement management Client contracting
	Decrease caloric intake while maintaining good nutrition.	Action (eating two fruits and two vegetables daily; using low-fat dairy products for past 2 months)	Stimulus control Cognitive restructuring
2. Decrease risk for hypertension-related disorders.	Change from high- to low-sodium snacks.	Contemplation	Consciousness raising Learning facilitation
3. Learn to manage stress effectively.	Attend relaxation classes and use home relaxation tapes.	Contemplation	Consciousness raising Self-reevaluation Simple relaxation therapy
4. Increase leisure-time activities.	Join a local bowling league.	Contemplation	Support system enhancement

the client may need to stop smoking, lose weight, and increase his or her activity level.

5. ***Develop a behavior-change plan based on the client's preferences.*** A constructive program of change is based on client "ownership" of those behavior changes selected for implementation within everyday life (Murdaugh et al., 2019, p. 118). Clients may need to be assisted in examining value–behavior inconsistencies and in selecting behavioral options that are most appealing and that they are most willing to try. Clients' priorities will reflect personal values, activity preferences, and expectations for success.
6. ***Reinforce benefits of change.*** The positive benefits will probably need to be reiterated by both the nurse and the client even though the client is committed to the change. The health-related and non–health-related benefits should be kept before the client as central motivating factors.
7. ***Address environmental and interpersonal facilitators and barriers to change.*** Environmental and interpersonal factors that support positive change should be used to reinforce the client's efforts to change their lifestyle. All people experience barriers, some of which can be anticipated and planned for, thereby making the change more likely to occur.
8. ***Determine a time frame for implementation.*** By developing a time frame, the appropriate knowledge and skills can be developed before a new behavior is implemented. The time frame may be several weeks or months. Scheduling short-term goals and rewards can offer encouragement to achieve long-term objectives. Clients may need help to be realistic and to deal with one behavior at a time.
9. ***Formalize commitment to behavior-change plan.*** Commitments to changing behaviors have usually been verbal. Increasingly, a formal, written behavioral

contract is being used to motivate the client to follow through with selected actions (see Chapter 17 ∞). Motivation to follow through is provided by a positive reinforcement or reward stated in the contract. Contracting is based on the belief that all people have the potential for growth and the right of self-determination, even though their choices may be different from the norm. (Murdaugh et al., 2019, p. 115).

Exploring Available Resources

Another essential aspect of planning is identifying support resources available to the client. These may be community resources, such as a fitness program at a local gymnasium, or educational programs, such as stress management, breast self-examination, nutrition, smoking cessation, and health lectures.

Implementing

Implementing is the "doing" part of behavior change. Self-responsibility is emphasized for implementing the plan. Depending on the client's needs, the nursing interventions may include supporting, counseling, facilitating, teaching, enhancing the behavior change, and modeling.

Providing and Facilitating Support

A major nursing role is to support the client. A vital component of lifestyle change is ongoing support that focuses on the desired behavior change and is provided in a nonjudgmental manner. Support can be offered by the nurse on an individual basis or in a group setting. The nurse can also facilitate the development of support networks for the client, such as family members and friends.

Individual Counseling Sessions

Counseling sessions may be routinely scheduled as part of the plan or may be provided if the client encounters difficulty in carrying out interventions or meets insurmountable barriers to change. In a counseling relationship, the nurse and client share ideas. In this sharing relationship, the nurse acts as a facilitator, promoting the client's decision-making with regard to the health promotion plan.

Telephone or Internet Counseling

Regular telephone sessions or online computer interaction with the client may be provided to help answer questions, review goals and strategies, and reinforce progress. The client may find that scheduling a weekly interaction is helpful or may wish to initiate a call if a problem occurs. The client is asked, "Is your plan working?" If the plan is not working, the nurse asks, "What would you like to do?" The client may wish to continue or may wish to change the plan to a more realistic one. Telephone support is efficient for the busy client who may not have the time for in-person sessions.

Mental health issues among all ages are increasing in the United States and other countries. In the adolescent and young adult population, this is particularly evident. This population is utilizing the internet for mental health interventions. Online counseling is emerging as a delivery mode for mental healthcare. Roddy, Nowlan, and Doss (2017) conducted a study to assess an online psychotherapy intervention for distressed couples. They found that the use of online self-help interventions decreased the barriers to treatment and provided couples with high-quality, research-based counseling programs. The couples in the study produced significant gains in the functioning of their relationships. It is important to note that the use of online counseling provides all individuals with greater access to mental health services.

Group Support

Group sessions provide an opportunity for participants to learn the experiences of others in changing behavior. Group contact gives individuals a renewed commitment to their goals. Groups can be scheduled at monthly or less frequent intervals for over a year.

Facilitating Social Support

Social networks, such as family and friends, can facilitate or impede the efforts directed toward health promotion and prevention. The nurse's role is to assist the client to assess, modify, and develop the social support necessary to achieve the desired change. To provide the necessary support, families must communicate effectively, be aware of and support each other's needs and goals, and provide help and assistance to one another to achieve those goals. The client may wish the nurse to meet with the family or significant others and help enlist their understanding and support.

Providing Health Education

Health education programs on a variety of topics discussed earlier can be provided to groups, individuals, or communities. Group programs need to be planned carefully before they are implemented. The decision to establish a health promotion program must be based on the health needs of the people; also, specific health promotion goals must be set. After the program is implemented, outcomes must be evaluated.

Enhancing Behavior Change

Whether people will make and maintain changes to improve health or prevent disease depends on many interrelated factors. To help clients succeed in implementing behavior changes, the nurse needs to understand the stages of change and effective interventions that focus on progressing the individual through the stages of change. Figure 19.5 ■ provides suggested strategies to assist clients depending on their stage of change. Nurses can use the stages of change to recognize a client's readiness to change and assist the client to the next stage of change.

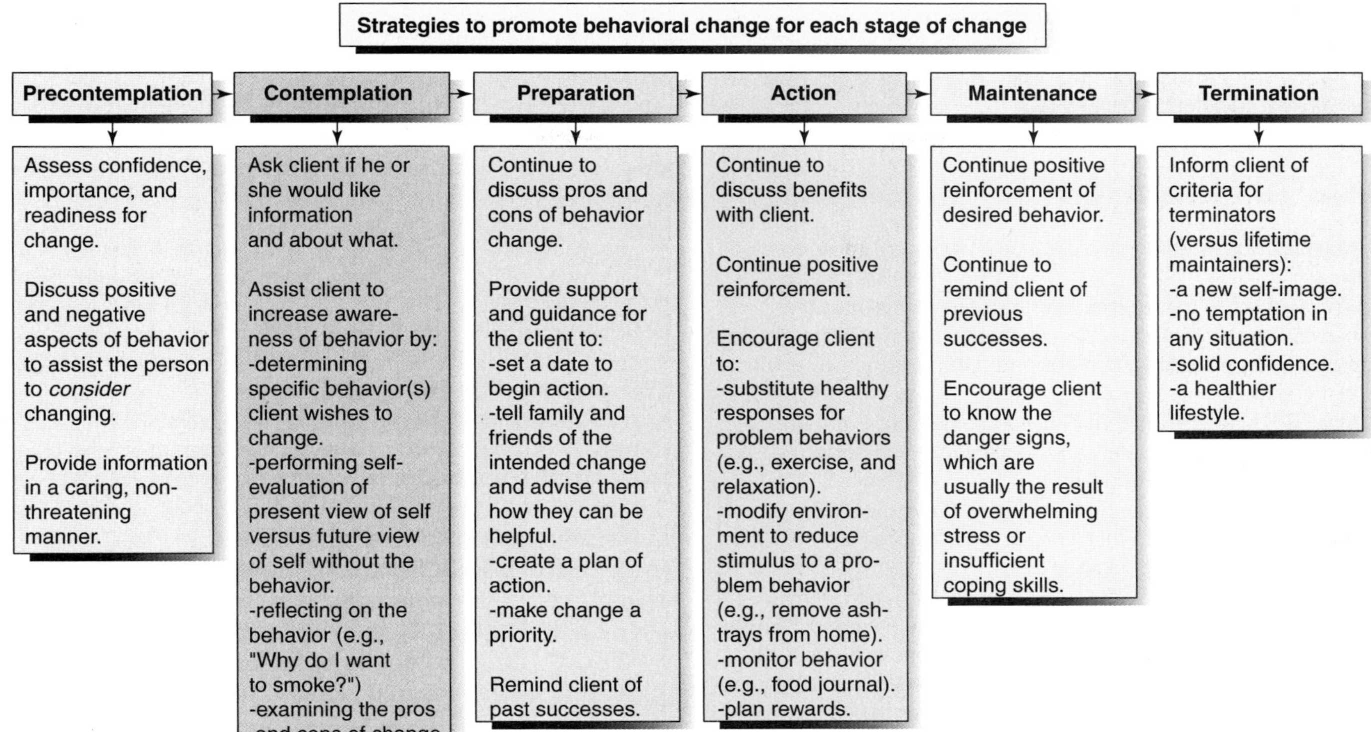

Figure 19.5 ■ Strategies to promote behavioral change for each stage of change.

Modeling

Through observing a model, the client acquires ideas for behavior and coping strategies that can be used with specific problems. The client is not expected to mimic the sequence of actions or behavior patterns of the model. The nurse and client should mutually select models with whom the client can identify because the cultural and ethnic backgrounds and age of the nurse and client often differ. Models should be people the client respects. Nurses should also serve as models of wellness. To model effectively, nurses need to have a philosophy and lifestyle that demonstrate good health habits.

Evaluating

Evaluation takes place on an ongoing basis, both during the attainment of short-term goals and after the completion of long-term goals. Goals are written during the planning phase, and a date is determined for attaining the specific results or behaviors that are desired to promote health or prevent illness. During evaluation, the client may decide to continue with the plan, reorder priorities, change strategies, or revise the health promotion and prevention contract. Evaluation of the plan is a collaborative effort between the nurse and the client.

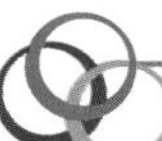

Critical Thinking Checkpoint

Mr. W., a 50-year-old professional man, has pneumonia and is currently being treated with antibiotics. He smokes two packs of cigarettes a day. Since this bout of pneumonia, he voices concern about his smoking and wonders if he should try to quit again. He states, "I've tried everything, and nothing works. The longest I last is about 1 month." He admits to being 30 pounds overweight and states that he and his wife have started walking for 30 minutes every evening. His wife has also started making low-fat meals. He is concerned that if he quits smoking, he will gain more weight.

1. What information and knowledge are important for the nurse to remember when assisting a client in advancing to the next stage of change?
2. Each contact between a nurse and a client is an opportunity for health promotion. Based on the knowledge or key concepts listed previously, what question(s) would you ask Mr. W.?
3. Mr. W. is in which stage of change relating to his cigarette smoking? What strategies could you, the nurse, consider?

Answers to Critical Thinking Checkpoint questions are available on the faculty resources site. Please consult with your instructor.

Chapter 19 Review

CHAPTER HIGHLIGHTS

- Nursing involves viewing the client as an individual and in a holistic way.
- Homeostasis is the tendency of the body to maintain a state of balance or equilibrium while constantly changing. Both physiologic and psychologic homeostasis are maintained by a variety of mechanisms.
- Maslow's hierarchy of human needs consists of five categories: physiologic (survival), safety and security, love and belonging, self-esteem, and self-actualization.
- All people have the same basic needs; however, each person's needs and reactions to those needs are influenced by the culture with which the person identifies.
- *Healthy People 2020* (U.S. Department of Health and Human Services, 2010) states the leading health indicators that reflect 12 high-priority health issues and communicates actions to address them.
- Health promotion is defined as client behavior directed toward developing well-being and actualizing human health potential. Health protection is client behavior geared toward preventing illness, detecting it early, or maintaining function.
- The Health Promotion Model (Murdaugh et al., 2019) is a competence- or approach-oriented model that depicts the multidimensional nature of individuals interacting with their interpersonal and physical environments as they pursue health. It includes major motivational variables that can be modified through nursing interventions.
- Prochaska et al. (2009) describe a six-stage model for health behavior change. The stages are precontemplation, contemplation, preparation, action, maintenance, and termination. An understanding of these stages enables the nurse to provide appropriate nursing interventions.
- The nurse's role in health promotion is to act as a facilitator of the process of assessing, evaluating, and understanding health. It is the opportunity for nurses to strengthen the profession's influence on health promotion, disseminate information that promotes an educated public, and assist individuals and communities in changing long-standing adverse health behaviors.
- A complete and accurate assessment of a client's health status is basic to health promotion. Lifestyle assessment tools give clients the opportunity to assess the impact of their present lifestyle behaviors on their health and to make decisions about specific lifestyle changes. Health risk appraisals provide data that may influence the individual to adopt healthier lifestyles and behaviors. Assessments or reviews of a client's spiritual health, social support, health beliefs, and life stress are also important because they impact a client's health.
- Health promotion plans need to be developed according to the needs, desires, and priorities of the client.
- The nurse acts as a resource person, provides ongoing support, and supplies additional information and education in a nonjudgmental manner to help clients change their lifestyles or health behaviors.
- Organizing assessment data from individual and family assessments enable the nurse to make health promotion nursing diagnoses that identify client strengths, recognize self-care abilities, and enhance health promotion goals to help the client reach a higher level of functioning.
- As role models for their clients, nurses should have a philosophy and lifestyle that demonstrate good health habits.
- During the evaluation phase of the health promotion process, the nurse assists clients in determining whether they will continue with the plan, reorder priorities, or revise the plan.

TEST YOUR KNOWLEDGE

1. A nurse is practicing the concept of holism to the client. Which of the following is the best example of this?
   1. The nurse considers how the loss of a client's job will affect the regulation of the client's diabetes.
   2. The nurse makes sure to do complete teaching regarding pharmacological interventions.
   3. The nurse is careful to follow physician treatments on schedule.
   4. The nurse is able to prioritize the needs of the client assigned according to Maslow's hierarchy.

2. A nurse is planning a workshop on health promotion for older adults. Which topic will be included?
   1. Prevention of falls
   2. Cardiovascular risk factors
   3. Adequate sleep
   4. How to stop smoking

3. While hospitalized, a client is very worried about business activities. The client spends a great deal of time on the phone and with colleagues instead of resting. Which principle of need therapy applies to this client?
   1. His higher-level need cannot be met unless the lower-level physiologic need is met.
   2. His lower-level physiologic needs are being deferred while higher needs are addressed.
   3. The higher need takes precedence, and the lower need no longer must be met.
   4. It is necessary for someone else to meet his higher-level needs so that he can focus on the lower-level needs.

4. Which statement by the client best represents the contemplation stage of the stages of behavior change?
   1. "I currently do not need to exercise and do not intend to start in the next 6 months."
   2. "I have tried several times to exercise 30 minutes three times a week but am seriously thinking of trying again in the next month."
   3. "I currently do not exercise 30 minutes three times a week, but I am thinking about starting to do so within the next 6 months."
   4. "I have exercised 30 minutes three times a week regularly for more than 6 months."
5. A nurse in charge of an assisted living complex that includes independent living apartments understands the unique needs of individuals of this age group. In planning health promotion strategies, which of the following factors would the nurse take into consideration?
   1. Rest and exercise
   2. Adjusting to physiologic changes and limitations
   3. High obesity percentages
   4. Safety promotion and injury prevention
6. Which of the following are overarching goals of *Healthy People 2020?* Select all that apply.
   1. Raise the education and literacy level.
   2. Increase quality and years of healthy life.
   3. Eliminate health disparities.
   4. Distribute health-related information.
   5. Promote healthy behaviors.
7. The nurse who is assisting a client in the action stage of change would use which strategy?
   1. Reinforce the importance of providing rewards for positive behavior.
   2. Ask the client if he or she would like information.
   3. Guide the client to create a plan of action.
   4. Remind the client of previous successes.
8. Which is the best response by the nurse if a client fails to follow the information or teaching provided?
   1. Give up because the client doesn't want to change.
   2. Develop a tough approach.
   3. Reteach the information because the nurse is the expert.
   4. Reassess the importance the client gives to the behavior and the client's readiness to change it.
9. Which of the following does the nurse identify as a homeostatic mechanism? Select all that apply.
   1. The client's heart rate increases when walking up a flight of stairs.
   2. Shivering when core body temperature drops.
   3. A child's bone growth occurs in spurts.
   4. Decreased secretion of insulin when food is not ingested.
   5. Lactation in a pregnant woman.
10. Using Maslow's framework, which statement characterizes the highest level of need?
   1. "Nurse, my pain is severe . . . is it time for my shot?"
   2. "I felt welcomed when I first joined the group, and I look forward to the monthly meetings."
   3. "I'm very proud of receiving the Employee of the Month award."
   4. "There have been home break-ins with burglary in our neighborhood. We are thinking of moving."

See Answers to Test Your Knowledge in Appendix A.

READINGS AND REFERENCES

Suggested Readings

Darch, J., Baillie, L., & Gillison, F. (2017). Nurses as role models in health promotion: A concept analysis. *British Journal of Nursing, 26*(17), 982–988. doi:10.12968/bjon.2017.26.17.982

The researchers in this study surveyed 39 nursing students, registered nurses, and nurse lecturers in London and South East London. They reported that being a role model in health-promoting behaviors and being an exemplar in portraying a healthy image had positive effects in caring for clients.

Related Research

Hasanpour-Dehkordi, A., Solati, K., Tali, S. S., & Dayani, M. A. (2019). Effect of progressive muscle relaxation with analgesic on anxiety status and pain in surgical patients. *British Journal of Nursing, 28*(3), 174–178. doi:10.12968/bjon.2019.28.3.174

References

Adams, S. K., Ligouri, G., & Lofgren, I. E. (2017). Technology as a tool to encourage young adults to sleep and eat healthy. *ACSM's Health and Fitness Journal, 21*(4), 4–6. doi:10.1249/FIT.0000000000000303

Cannon, W. B. (1939). *The wisdom of the body* (2nd ed.). New York, NY: Norton.

Centers for Disease Control and Prevention. (2015). *Physical activity for a healthy weight*. Retrieved from https://www.cdc.gov/healthyweight/physical_activity/index.html#physicalActivity

Centers for Disease Control and Prevention. (2018). *Childhood obesity facts*. Retrieved from https://www.cdc.gov/healthyschools/obesity/facts.htm

Edelman, C. L., & Kudzma, E. (2018). *Health promotion throughout the lifespan* (9th ed.). St. Louis, MO: Mosby.

Holmes, T. H., & Rahe, R. H. (1967). The social readjustment rating scale. *Journal of Psychosomatic Research, 11*, 213–218. doi:10.1016/0022-3999(67)90010-4

Kalish, R. A. (1983). *The psychology of human behavior* (5th ed.). Monterey, CA: Brooks Cole.

Leavell, H. R., & Clark, E. G. (1965). *Preventive medicine for the doctor in the community* (3rd ed.). New York, NY: McGraw-Hill.

Maslow, A. H. (1970). *Motivation and personality* (2nd ed.). New York, NY: Harper & Row.

Murdaugh, C. L., Parsons, M. A., & Pender, N. J. (2019). *Health promotion in nursing practice* (8th ed.). New York, NY: Pearson.

Office of Disease Prevention and Health Promotion. (2017). *Healthy People 2030 development: An informational webinar*. Retrieved from https://apha.org/-/media/files/pdf/webinars/2017/healthy_people_2030.ashx?la=en&hash=A7C219FBA84552464655F274837DBC6C87F02059

Office of Disease Prevention and Health Promotion. (2018). *Development of the national health promotion and disease prevention objectives for 2030*. Retrieved from https://www.healthypeople.gov/2020/About-Healthy-People/Development-Healthy-People-2030

Prochaska, J. O., Norcross, J. C., & DiClemente, C. C. (1994). *Changing for good: A revolutionary six-stage program for overcoming bad habits and moving your life positively forward*. New York, NY: HarperCollins.

Prochaska, J. O., Redding, C. A., & Evers, K. E. (2009). The transtheoretical model and stages of change. In K. Glanz, B. Rimer, & K. Viswanath (Eds.), *Health behavior and health education: Theory, research, and practice* (4th ed., pp. 97–121). San Francisco, CA: Jossey-Bass.

Roddy, M. K., Nowlan, K. M., & Doss, B. D. (2017). A randomized controlled trial of coach contact during a brief online intervention for distressed couples. *Family Process, 56*, 835–851. doi:10.1111/famp.12262

Ross, C. S., Henehan, E. R., & Jernigan, D. H. (2017). Youth exposure to alcohol advertising in national magazines in the United States, 2001–2011. *American Journal of Public Health, 107*, 136–142. doi:10.2105/AJPH.2016.303514

U.S. Department of Health and Human Services. (2010). *Healthy people 2020*. Retrieved from https://www.hhs.gov/opa/title-x-family-planning/preventive-services/healthy-people-2020/index.html

U.S. Department of Health and Human Services. (2014). *Healthy People 2020 leading health indicators: Progress update*. Retrieved from https://www.healthypeople.gov/sites/default/files/LHI-ProgressReport-ExecSum_0.pdf

Selected Bibliography

Dworatzek, P., & Stier, J. (2016). Dietitians' attitudes and beliefs regarding peer education in nutrition. *Canadian Journal of Dietetic Practice and Research, 77*, 170–176. doi:10.3148/cjdpr-2016-009

Eliopoulos, C. (2018). *Invitation to holistic health. A guide to living a balanced life* (4th ed.). Sudbury, MA: Jones & Bartlett.

Maslow, A. H. (1968). *Toward a psychology of being* (2nd ed.). New York, NY: John Wiley & Sons.

Tilsen, J., & Nylund, D. (2016). Cultural studies methodologies and narrative family therapy: Therapeutic conversations about pop culture. *Family Process, 55*, 225–337. doi:10.1111/famp.12204

Varghese, J. (2017). Effect of family focused intervention on perceived stress, quality of life, and relapse rate of clients with alcohol dependence syndrome. *International Journal of Nursing Education, 9*(1), 91–96. doi:10.5958/0974-9357.2017.00018.6

20 Health, Wellness, and Illness

LEARNING OUTCOMES

After completing this chapter, you will be able to:

1. Identify influences on clients' definitions of health, wellness, and well-being.
2. Describe five components of wellness.
3. Compare various models of health.
4. Identify variables affecting health status, beliefs, and practices.
5. Describe factors affecting healthcare adherence.
6. Differentiate illness from disease and acute illness from chronic illness.
7. Identify Parsons's four aspects of the sick role.
8. Explain Suchman's stages of illness.
9. Describe the effects of illness on clients' and family members' roles and functions.

KEY TERMS

Introduction

Nurses' understanding of health and wellness largely determines the scope and nature of nursing practice. Clients' health beliefs influence their health practices. Some clients think of health and wellness (or well-being) as the same thing or, at the very least, as accompanying one another. However, health may not always accompany well-being: A client who has a terminal illness may have a sense of well-being; conversely, another client may lack a sense of well-being yet be in a state of good health. For many years, the concept of disease was the yardstick by which health was measured. In the late 19th century, the "how" of disease (pathogenesis) was the major concern of health professionals. The 20th century focused on finding cures for diseases. Currently, healthcare providers are increasing their emphasis on preventing illness and promoting health and wellness in individuals, families, and communities.

Concepts of Health, Wellness, and Well-Being

Health, wellness, and well-being have many definitions and interpretations. The nurse should be familiar with the most common aspects of the concepts and consider how they may be individualized with specific clients.

Health

Traditionally, **health** was defined in terms of the presence or absence of disease. Florence Nightingale (1860/1969) defined health as a state of being well and using every power the individual possesses to the fullest extent. The World Health Organization (WHO, 1948) takes a more holistic view of health. Its constitution defines health as "a state of complete physical, mental, and social well-being, and not merely the absence of disease or infirmity." This definition reflects concern for the individual as a total person, functioning physically, psychologically, and socially. Mental processes determine individuals' relationships with their physical and social surroundings, their attitudes about life, and their interaction with others. Individuals' lives, and therefore their health, are affected by everything they interact with—not only environmental influences such as climate and the availability of food, shelter, clean air, and water to drink but also other individuals, including family, lovers, employers, coworkers, friends, and associates.

Health has also been defined in terms of role and performance. Talcott Parsons (1951), an eminent American sociologist and creator of the concept of "sick role," conceptualized health as the ability to maintain normal roles.

In 1953, the U.S. President's Commission on Health Needs of the Nation (1953) made the following statement about health: "Health is not a condition; it is an adjustment. It is not a state but a process. The process adapts the individual not only to our physical but also our social environments" (p. 4). In its 2010 social policy statement, the American Nurses Association (ANA) states, "Health and illness are human experiences. The presence of illness does not preclude health, nor does optimal health preclude illness" (ANA, 2010, p. 6).

Personal Definitions of Health

Health is a highly individual perception. Consider the following examples of individuals who would probably say they are healthy even though they have physical impairments that some would consider an illness:

- A 15-year-old with diabetes takes injectable insulin each morning. He plays on the school soccer team and is editor of the high school newspaper.
- A 32-year-old is paralyzed from the waist down and needs a wheelchair for mobility. He is taking an accounting course at a nearby college and uses a specially designed automobile for transportation.
- A 72-year-old takes antihypertensive medications to treat high blood pressure. She is a member of the neighborhood golf club, makes handicrafts for a local charity, and travels 2 months each year.

Many people describe health as the following:

- Being free from symptoms of disease and pain
- Being able to be active and to do what they want or must
- Being in good spirits most of the time.

These characteristics indicate that health is not something that an individual achieves suddenly at a specific time. It is an ongoing process—a way of life—through which an individual develops and encourages every aspect of the body, mind, and feelings to interrelate harmoniously as much as possible (Figure 20.1 ■).

Nurses' definitions of health largely determine the scope and nature of nursing practice. For example, when health is defined narrowly as a physiologic phenomenon, nurses confine themselves to assisting clients in regaining normal physiologic functioning. When health is defined more broadly, the scope of nursing practice enlarges correspondingly.

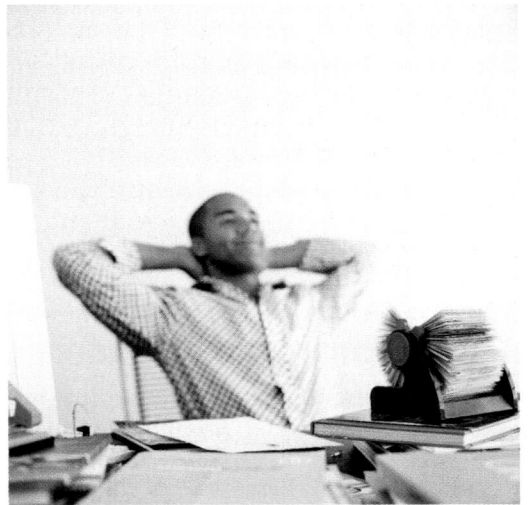

Figure 20.1 ■ Satisfaction with work enhances a sense of well-being and contributes to health.
George Doyle/Stockbyte/Getty Images.

A nurse's health values and practices may differ from those of a client. The nurse needs to develop a plan of care that relates to the client's concept of health rather than the nurse's belief system. Otherwise, the client may fail to respond to the healthcare regimen.

Nurses can ask the following questions to explore their personal definition of health. In what way:

- Is a person more than a biophysiologic system?
- Is health more than the absence of disease symptoms?
- Is health the ability of an individual to perform work?
- Is health the ability of an individual to adapt to the environment?
- Is health a state or a process?
- Is health the ability to perform self-care activities?
- Is health static or changing?
- Are health and wellness the same?
- Are disease and illness different?
- Are there levels of health?
- Are wellness, health, and illness separate entities or points along a continuum?
- Is health socially determined?
- Do you rate your health, and why?

Population Health

Populations may be determined by geography, familial relationships, or other common characteristics. These characteristics include the social, structural, physical, and behavioral determinants of health. The term *population health* has many definitions, but most include the concept of the health of a group of individuals linked to but different from epidemiology, public health, and community health. Fawcett and Ellenbecker (2015) describe the Conceptual Model of Nursing and Population Health, which is similar to some other models of population health but emphasizes the centrality of nursing over other health disciplines. In this model, "population health is defined as lifespan wellness and disease experiences of aggregate groups of people residing in local, state, national, or international geographic regions or those populations with common characteristics. Population health includes aspects of public health, healthcare delivery systems, and determinants of wellness and illness, emphasizing promotion, restoration, and maintenance of wellness and prevention of disease" (p. 294).

There is increasing awareness of the importance and influence of the social determinants of health on disparities in health outcomes among populations. WHO (n.d.) defines the social determinants of health as the "conditions in which people are born, grow, work, live, and age, and the wider set of forces and systems shaping the conditions of daily life. These forces and systems include economic policies and systems, development agendas, social norms, social policies and political systems." Poverty, unemployment, transportation, stress, social exclusion, lack of social support, substance use, and lack of adequate healthcare are among the most significant determinants (Artiga & Hinton, 2018). Upstream determinants refer to macro-level factors, such as culture, housing, education, and government policies. Midstream factors refer to social influences and individuals' health behaviors and also the nature of health systems. Downstream factors relate to biology and physiology at the individual level.

Wellness and Well-Being

Wellness is a state of well-being. Basic aspects of wellness include self-responsibility; an ultimate goal; a dynamic, growing process; daily decision-making in the areas of nutrition, stress management, physical fitness, preventive healthcare, and emotional health; and most importantly, the whole being of the individual. **Well-being** has many definitions but is commonly viewed as a "function of life opportunities and achievements. It is multidimensional, reflecting people's functioning . . . such as consumption and personal security—and their capabilities—the objective conditions in which choices are made and that shape people's abilities to transform resources into given ends, such as health" (WHO, 2013, p. 89). Well-being also appears in the 2018–2022 strategic plan of the U.S. Department of Health and Human Services (2018) in the form of Goal 3: Strengthen the Economic and Social Well-Being of Americans Across the Lifespan.

Models of Health and Wellness

Because health is such a complex concept, various researchers have developed models or paradigms to explain health and, in some instances, its relationship to illness or injury. Models can be helpful in assisting health professionals in meeting the health and wellness needs of individuals. Models of health include the clinical model, the role performance model, the adaptive model, the eudaimonistic model, the agent–host–environment model, and health–illness scales.

Clinical Model

The narrowest interpretation of health occurs in the clinical model. Individuals are viewed as physiologic systems with related functions, and health is identified by the absence of signs and symptoms of disease or injury. It is considered the state of not being "sick." In this model, the opposite of health is disease or injury.

Many practitioners have used the clinical model in their focus on the relief of signs and symptoms of disease and elimination of malfunction and pain. When these signs and symptoms are no longer present, the practitioner considers the individual's health restored.

Role Performance Model

Health is defined in terms of an individual's ability to fulfill societal roles, that is, to perform his or her work. Individuals usually fulfill several roles (e.g., mother, daughter, friend), and certain individuals may consider nonwork roles the most important ones in their lives. According to this model, individuals who can fulfill their roles are healthy even if they have health problems. For example, a man who works all day at his job as expected is healthy even though he has migraines. It is assumed in this model that sickness is the inability to perform one's work role.

Adaptive Model

In the adaptive model, health is a creative process; disease is a failure in adaptation, or maladaptation. The aim of treatment is to restore the ability of the individual to adapt, that is, to cope. According to this model, extreme good health is flexible adaptation to the environment and interaction with the environment to maximum advantage. The famous Roy adaptation model of nursing (Murdaugh, Parsons, & Pender, 2019) views the individual as an adaptive system. The focus of this model is stability, although there is also an element of growth and change.

Eudaimonistic Model

The eudaimonistic model incorporates a comprehensive view of health. Health is seen as a condition of actualization or realization of an individual's potential. Actualization is the apex of the fully developed personality, described by Abraham Maslow (see Chapter 19 ∞). In this model, the highest aspiration of individuals is fulfillment and complete development, which is actualization. Illness, in this model, is a condition that prevents self-actualization.

Murdaugh et al. (2019) include stabilizing and actualizing tendencies in their definition of health: "the realization of human potential through goal-directed behavior, competent self-care, and satisfying relationships with others while adapting to maintain structural integrity and harmony with the social and physical environments" (p. 14).

Agent–Host–Environment Model

The agent–host–environment model of health and illness, also called the ecologic model, originated in the community health work of Leavell and Clark (1965) and has been expanded into a general theory of the multiple causes of disease. The model is used primarily in predicting illness rather than in promoting wellness, although identification of risk factors that result from the interactions of agent, host, and environment are helpful in promoting

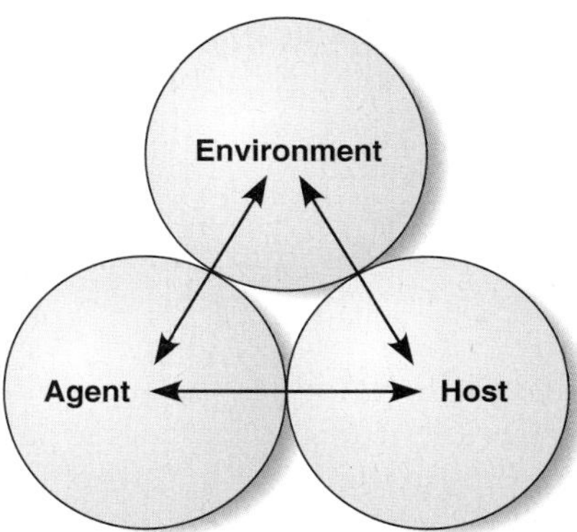

Figure 20.2 ■ The agent–host–environment model.

and maintaining health. The model has three dynamic, interactive elements (Figure 20.2 ■):

1. Agent. Any environmental factor or stressor (biological, chemical, mechanical, physical, or psychosocial) that by its presence or absence (e.g., lack of essential nutrients) can lead to illness or disease.
2. Host. Individual(s) who may or may not be at risk of acquiring a disease. Family history, age, and lifestyle habits influence the host's reaction.
3. Environment. All factors external to the host that may or may not predispose the individual to the development of disease. The physical environment includes climate, living conditions, sound (noise) levels, and economic level. Social environment includes interactions with others and life events, such as the death of a spouse.

Because each of the agent–host–environment factors constantly interacts with the others, health is an ever-changing state. When the variables are in balance, health is maintained; when the variables are not in balance, disease occurs.

Health–Illness Scales

Health–illness scales (grids or continua) can be used to measure an individual's perceived level of wellness. Health or wellness and illness or disease can be viewed as the opposite ends of a health continuum. From a high level of health, an individual's condition can move through good health, normal health, poor health, and extremely poor health, eventually to death. Individuals move back and forth day by day. There is no distinct boundary across which individuals move from health to illness or from illness back to health. How individuals perceive themselves and how others see them in terms of health and illness will also affect their placement on the continuum. The ranges in which individuals can be thought of as healthy or ill are considerable.

Dunn's High-Level Wellness Grid

Dunn (1959) described a health grid in which a health axis and an environmental axis intersect. The health axis ranges from wellness to death and the environmental axis from a very favorable environment to a very unfavorable one. The optimal quadrant is when individuals have both peak wellness and a favorable environment but individuals with poor health can be protected if they are in a favorable environment in which social institutions provide support.

Illness–Wellness Continuum

Various authors have proposed illness–wellness or illness–health continua. Many models illustrate arrows pointing in opposite directions and joined at a neutral point. Movement to one side of the neutral point indicates increasing levels of health and wellness for an individual. This is achieved through health knowledge, disease prevention, health promotion, and positive attitude. In contrast, movement to the opposite side of the neutral point indicates progressively decreasing levels of health. Some people believe that a health continuum is overly simplistic when the real concepts are more complex than a linear diagram suggests. An alternative depiction shows multiple levels of health in interaction with episodic illness (Figure 20.3 ■).

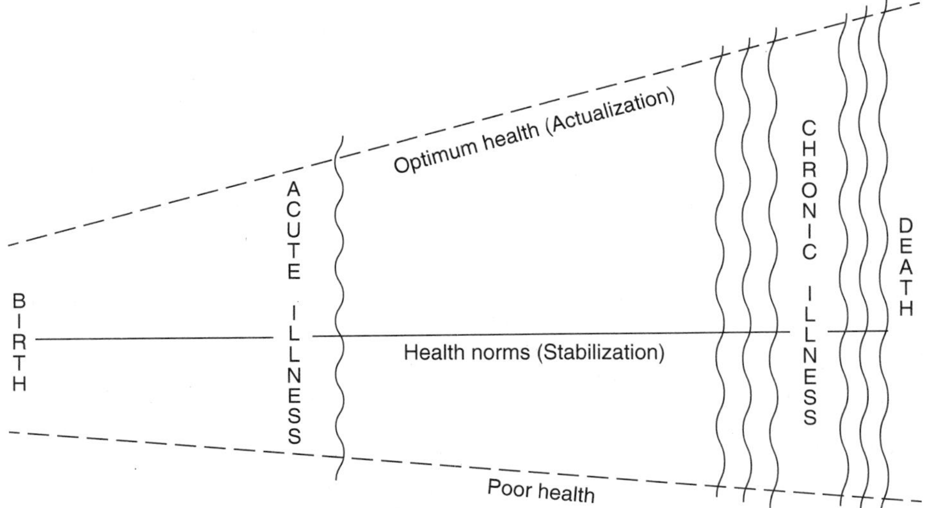

Figure 20.3 ■ The health continuum throughout the lifespan.
PENDER, NOLA J.; MURDAUGH, CAROLYN L.; PARSONS, MARY ANN, HEALTH PROMOTION IN NURSING PRACTICE (SUBSCRIPTION), 8th Ed., ©2019. Reprinted and Electronically reproduced by permission of Pearson Education, Inc., New York, NY.

Variables Influencing Health Status, Beliefs, and Behaviors

Many variables influence an individual's health status, beliefs, and behaviors or practices. These factors may or may not be under conscious control. Individuals can usually control their health behaviors and can choose healthy or unhealthy activities. In contrast, individuals have little or no choice over their genetic makeup, age, sex, culture, and sometimes their geographic environments. Box 20.1 differentiates health status, beliefs, and behaviors.

BOX 20.1 Health Status, Beliefs, and Behaviors

- **Health status**. State of health of an individual at a given time. A report of health status may include anxiety, depression, or acute illness and thus describe the individual's problem in general. Health status can also describe such specifics as pulse rate and body temperature.
- **Health beliefs**. Concepts about health that an individual believes are true. Such beliefs may or may not be founded on fact. Some of these are influenced by culture, such as the "hot–cold" belief system of some Asian, Hispanic, Filipino, and other groups. In this context, hot and cold do not denote temperature or spiciness but innate qualities of the food. For additional information about cultural views of health and illness, see Chapter 21 ∞.
- **Health behaviors**. The actions individuals take to understand their health state, maintain an optimal state of health, prevent illness and injury, and reach their maximum physical and mental potential. Behaviors such as eating wisely, exercising, paying attention to signs of illness, following treatment advice, avoiding known health hazards such as smoking, taking time for rest and relaxation, and managing one's time effectively are all examples.

Health behavior is intended to influence health status. Nurses preparing a plan of care need to consider the client's health beliefs before they suggest a change in health behaviors.

Internal Variables

Internal variables include biological, psychologic, and cognitive dimensions. They are often described as nonmodifiable variables because, for the most part, they cannot be changed. However, when internal variables are linked to health problems, the nurse must be even more diligent about working with the client to influence external variables (e.g., exercise and diet) that may assist in health promotion and prevention of illness. Regular health exams and appropriate screening for early detection of health problems become even more important.

Biological Dimension

Genetic makeup, sex, age, and developmental level all significantly influence an individual's health.

Genetic makeup influences biological characteristics, innate temperament, activity level, and intellectual potential. It has been related to susceptibility to specific disease, such as diabetes and breast cancer. For example, individuals of African heritage have a higher incidence of sickle cell disorder and hypertension than the general population but may be less susceptible to malaria. Nurses are expected to incorporate knowledge of genetics and genomics (how genetics interacts with the environment and other personal factors in influencing health) in their care and teaching of clients. See Chapter 10 ∞ for information on including items regarding genetic background when taking a client history.

Sex influences the distribution of disease. Certain acquired and genetic diseases are more common in one sex than in the other. Disorders more common among females include osteoporosis and autoimmune diseases such as rheumatoid arthritis. Those more common among males are stomach ulcers, abdominal hernias, and respiratory diseases.

Age is also a significant factor. The distribution of disease varies with age. For example, arteriosclerotic heart disease is common in middle-aged males but occurs infrequently in younger individuals; such communicable diseases as whooping cough and measles are common in children but rare in older adults, who often have acquired immunity to them.

Developmental level has a major impact on health status. Consider these examples:

- Infants lack physiologic and psychologic maturity, so their defenses against disease are lower during the first years of life.
- Toddlers who are learning to walk are more prone to falls and injury than are older children.
- Adolescents who strive to conform to peers are more prone to risk-taking behavior and subsequent injury than adults are.
- Declining physical and sensory-perceptual abilities limit the ability of older adults to respond to environmental hazards and stressors.

Psychologic Dimension

Psychologic (emotional) factors influencing health include mind–body interactions and self-concept.

Mind–body interactions can affect health status positively or negatively. Emotional responses to stress affect body function. For example, a student who is extremely anxious before a test may experience urinary frequency and diarrhea. Prolonged emotional distress may increase susceptibility to organic disease or precipitate it. Emotional distress may influence the immune system through central nervous system and endocrine alterations. Alterations in the immune system are related to the incidence of infections, cancer, and autoimmune diseases.

Increasing attention is being given to the mind's ability to direct the body's functioning. Relaxation, meditation, and biofeedback techniques are gaining wider recognition by individuals and healthcare professionals. For example, women often use relaxation techniques to decrease pain during childbirth. Other individuals may learn biofeedback skills to reduce hypertension.

Emotional reactions also occur in response to body conditions. For example, an individual diagnosed with a terminal illness may experience fear and depression. *Self-concept* is how an individual feels about self and perceives the physical self, needs, roles, and abilities. An example is a woman with anorexia who deprives herself of needed nutrients because she believes she is too fat even though she is well below an acceptable weight level. Self-concept is discussed in detail in Chapter 39 ∞. Self-perceptions are also associated with an individual's definition of health. For example, a 75-year-old man who feels he should be able to move large objects just as he did when he was younger may need to examine and redefine his concept of health in view of his age and abilities.

Cognitive Dimension

Cognitive or intellectual factors influencing health include lifestyle choices and spiritual and religious beliefs.

Lifestyle refers to an individual's general way of living, including those living conditions and individual patterns of behavior that are influenced by sociocultural factors and personal characteristics. Lifestyle choices may have positive or negative effects on health. Practices that have potentially negative effects on health are often referred to as **risk factors**. For example, overeating, getting insufficient exercise, and being overweight are closely related to the incidence of heart disease, arteriosclerosis, diabetes, and hypertension. Excessive use of tobacco is clearly implicated in lung cancer, emphysema, and cardiovascular diseases. See Box 20.2 for examples of healthy lifestyle choices.

BOX 20.2 Examples of Healthy Lifestyle Choices

- Regular exercise
- Weight control
- Avoidance of saturated fats
- Avoidance of excessive alcohol
- Abstaining from the use of tobacco and recreational drug products
- Seat belt use
- Bike helmet use
- Immunization updates
- Regular dental checkups
- Regular health maintenance visits for screening examinations or tests

Spiritual and religious beliefs can significantly affect health behavior. For example, Jehovah's Witnesses oppose blood transfusions; some fundamentalists believe that a serious illness is a punishment from God; some religious groups are strict vegetarians; and religious Jews perform circumcision on the eighth day of a male baby's life. The influence of spirituality and religion is discussed further in Chapter 41 ∞.

Knowledge of health behaviors does not always translate into action. The nurse should be self-reflective and consider both the personal and professional advantages of examining and minimizing barriers to becoming a positive role model.

External Variables

External variables affecting health include the physical environment, standards of living, family and cultural beliefs, and social support networks.

Environment

People are becoming increasingly aware of their environment and how it affects their health and level of wellness. Geographic location determines climate, and climate affects health. For instance, malaria and malaria-related conditions occur more frequently in tropical rather than temperate climates. Pollution of the water, air, and soil affects the health of cells. Some man-made substances in the environment, such as asbestos, are considered carcinogenic (i.e., they cause cancer). Tobacco is "hazardous to one's health," with rates of cancer higher among both smokers themselves and those who live or work near individuals who smoke in their environment.

An environmental hazard is radiation. The improper or excessive use of medical x-rays, for example, can harm many of the body's organs. Another common source of radiation is the sun's ultraviolet rays. Light-skinned individuals are more susceptible to the harmful effects of the sun than are dark-skinned individuals.

Sulfur dioxide and nitrogen oxides are produced by ore smelters and related industries. These emissions, brought down by the air when it rains (known as acid rain), are thought to damage forests, lakes, and rivers.

An environmental hazard that is receiving more attention is an increase in the "greenhouse effect." The glass roof of a greenhouse permits the sun's radiation to penetrate, but the resulting heat does not escape back through the glass. Carbon dioxide in the earth's atmosphere acts like the glass roof of a greenhouse, and as carbon dioxide levels increase due to industrial and automobile emissions, the surface temperature of the earth may also be increasing.

Other sources of environmental contamination are pesticides and chemicals used to control weeds and plant diseases. These contaminants can be found in some animals and plants that are subsequently eaten by humans. In excessive levels, they are harmful to health.

Standards of Living

An individual's standard of living (reflecting occupation, income, and education) is related to health, morbidity, and mortality. Hygiene, food habits, and the ability to seek healthcare advice and follow health regimens vary by income level.

Low income families must prioritize the use of their finances, often choosing food and housing over healthcare. They may have difficulty obtaining time off from work and transportation to healthcare facilities. Because their present problems are so great and all efforts are exerted toward survival, they may lack an orientation toward actions that help promote wellness.

The environmental conditions of impoverished areas have a bearing on overall health. Slum neighborhoods are overcrowded and in a state of deterioration. Sanitation services tend to be inadequate, streets are strewn with garbage, and pests are common. Fires and violence may be frequent. Recreational facilities are limited, forcing children to play in streets and alleys.

Occupational roles also predispose individuals to certain illnesses. For instance, some industrial workers may be exposed to carcinogenic agents. High-pressure social or occupational roles predispose to stress-related diseases. Such roles may also encourage overeating or social use of drugs or excessive alcohol.

Family and Cultural Beliefs

The family passes on patterns of daily living and lifestyles to offspring. For example, a man who was abused as a child may physically abuse his own children. Physical or emotional abuse may cause long-term health problems. Emotional health depends on a social environment that is free of excessive tension and does not isolate the individual from others. A climate of open communication, sharing, and love fosters the fulfillment of the individual's optimal potential.

Culture also influences how an individual perceives, experiences, and copes with health and illness. Each culture has ideas about health, and these are often transmitted from parents to children. Individuals of certain cultures may perceive home remedies or tribal health customs as superior to and more dependable than the healthcare practices of North American society. An example is the use of herbal remedies and acupuncture to treat pain rather than analgesic medications. Cultural rules, values, and beliefs give individuals a sense of being stable and able to predict outcomes. The challenging of old beliefs and values by second-generation cultural groups may give rise to conflict, instability, and insecurity, in turn contributing to illness. Heritage and cultural influences on health are discussed in detail in Chapter 21 ∞.

Language also plays an important role in health behaviors. Clients who are not fluent in the dominant language may misinterpret information they are given or be unsuccessful in communicating their beliefs and preferences.

Social Support Networks

Having a support network (family, friends, or a confidant) and job satisfaction can facilitate healthy behaviors. Support persons can help the individual confirm that illness exists. Individuals with inadequate support networks sometimes become increasingly ill before confirming the illness and seeking therapy. Support persons also provide the motivation for an ill individual to become well again.

Health Belief Models

Several theories or models of health beliefs and behaviors have been developed to help determine whether an individual is likely to participate in disease prevention and health promotion activities. These models can be useful tools in developing programs for helping individuals with healthier lifestyles and more positive attitudes toward preventive health measures (see also Chapter 19 ∞).

Health Locus of Control Model

Locus of control is a concept from social learning theory that nurses can use to determine whether clients are likely to take action regarding health, that is, whether clients believe that their health status is under their own or others' control. Individuals who believe that they have a major influence on their own health status—that health is largely self-determined—are called *internals*. Individuals who exercise internal control are more likely than others to take the initiative for their own healthcare, be more knowledgeable about their health, make and keep appointments with healthcare providers, maintain diets, and give up smoking. By contrast, individuals who believe their health is largely controlled by outside forces (e.g., chance or powerful others) are referred to as *externals*. Externals may doubt that changing their behavior will do good or that it is only important if someone important tells them to make the change.

Research has shown that locus of control plays a role in clients' choices about health behaviors and in their health experiences. A high external health locus of control has been related to greater information seeking in clients with cancer (Keinki et al., 2016). In one study, parents with a stronger internal locus of control believed that their parenting skills had a significant influence on their children's health behaviors more than did parents with an external locus of control (Puff & Renk, 2016).

Locus of control is a measurable concept that can be used to predict which individuals are most likely to change their behavior. Many measurement instruments are available to assess locus of control. One widely used example is the Multidimensional Health Locus of Control (MHLC) scale, most recently expanded to Form C (Wallston, Stein, & Smith, 1994).

EVIDENCE-BASED PRACTICE

Evidence-Based Practice

What Are the Health Locus of Control Profiles of Hispanic Americans?

Champagne, Fox, Mills, Sadler, and Malcarne (2016) applied complex statistical analysis to the MHLC scale and other cultural perspective tool data collected on 436 English and Spanish-speaking Hispanic American adults. The intent of the research was to examine profiles of sociocultural and demographic characteristics, health beliefs and behaviors, and physical and mental health outcomes. Instead of finding two health locus of control groups, the results indicated four groups: internally oriented—weak, internally oriented—moderate, internally oriented—strong, and externally oriented. Several differences and similarities among the MHLC data and health views were supported (e.g., the internally oriented—strong group was less fatalistic about cancer), but there were no differences among the groups in terms of anxiety, depression, or general physical health status.

Implications

The authors recognize the need for replication of their study, although the design and analysis were robust. In addition, the statistical analysis had not previously been applied to the MHLC using Hispanic respondents, and this is a growing population group in the United States. Nurses should reflect on these findings when considering clients' health locus of control and consider that there are variations even within the internal and external loci. It is premature to draw direct correlations between locus of control and the behaviors or decisions of any group or individual.

Rosenstock and Becker's Health Belief Model

Rosenstock and Becker's health belief model (Rosenstock, Strecher, & Becker, 1988) is based on the assumption that health-related action depends on the simultaneous occurrence of three factors: (1) sufficient motivation to make health issues be viewed as important, (2) belief that one is vulnerable to a serious health problem or its consequences, and (3) belief that following a particular health recommendation would be beneficial. The model includes individual perceptions, modifying factors, and variables likely to affect initiating action.

Nurses play a major role in helping clients implement healthy behaviors. They help clients monitor health, they supply anticipatory guidance, and they impart knowledge about health. Nurses can also reduce barriers to action (e.g., by minimizing inconvenience or discomfort) and can support positive actions.

Murdaugh et al. (2019) have modified this health belief model to develop a health promotion model because the health belief model explains health-protecting or preventive behaviors but does not emphasize health-promoting behaviors. See the discussion of Pender's Health Promotion Model in Chapter 19 ∞.

In addition to applying these models, the nurse uses other resources to evaluate options in planning interventions to maximize wellness. Two very useful sources developed by federal agencies are the Guide to Community Preventive Services website from the Centers for Disease Control and Prevention and the *Guide to Clinical Preventive Services* from the Agency for Healthcare Research and Quality (AHRQ, 2014) with recommendations from the U.S. Preventive Services Task Force (USPSTF). The electronic Preventive Services Selector (ePSS) allows users to download the USPSTF recommendations to mobile or tablet devices, receive notifications of updates, and search and browse recommendations online. Users can search the ePSS for recommendations by age, sex, and pregnancy status. A major emphasis in both resources is providing evidence-based recommendations for practices and policies aimed at improving health. Both resources are updated as the data become available and can be retrieved from their respective websites.

Healthcare Adherence

Adherence is the extent to which an individual's behavior (e.g., taking medications, following diets, or making lifestyle changes) coincides with medical or health advice. Another term used synonymously with *adherence* is *conformance*. The degree of adherence may range from disregarding every aspect of the recommendations to following the total therapeutic plan. There are many reasons why some individuals adhere and others do not (Box 20.3).

BOX 20.3 Factors Influencing Adherence

- Client motivation to become well
- Degree of lifestyle change necessary
- Perceived severity of the healthcare problem
- Value placed on reducing the threat of illness
- Ability to understand and perform specific behaviors
- Degree of inconvenience of the illness itself or of the regimens
- Beliefs that the prescribed therapy or regimen will or will not help
- Complexity, side effects, and duration of the proposed therapy
- Cultural heritage, beliefs, or practices that support or conflict with the regimen
- Degree of satisfaction and quality and type of relationship with the healthcare providers
- Overall cost of therapy or lifestyle change

ASSESSMENT INTERVIEW **Determining the Risk for Medication Nonadherence**

- Are you having side effects from any of your medications?
- Do you think your medications are helping?
- Do you have "tools" to remind you to take your medication? Examples could be an alarm or environmental cues (e.g., 6:00 news).
- Is there someone at home who helps you with your medications?
- How many times per day are your medications prescribed?
- How many pills do you take every day?
- Are there any special storage requirements for your medications?
- How much do your medication requirements interfere with your lifestyle?
- How well are you able to follow special dosing requirements?
- How many doses of your medications have you missed during the past 3 days?
- Does the cost of the medications influence how often you take them?

To enhance adherence, nurses need to ensure that the client is able to perform the activities, understands the necessary instructions, is a willing participant in establishing goals of therapy, and values the planned outcomes of behavior changes. Examples of questions to be included in the assessment of medication adherence are found in the Assessment Interview.

When a nurse identifies nonadherence, it is important to take the following steps:

- Establish why the client is not following the regimen. Depending on the reason, the nurse can provide information, correct misconceptions, attempt to decrease expense, or suggest counseling if psychologic problems are interfering with adherence. It is also essential for the nurse to reevaluate the suitability of the health advice provided. In situations where the client's cultural beliefs or age conflict with planned therapies, the nurse needs to consider ways to repattern and restructure care that will preserve and accommodate the client's practices. See the Providing Culturally Responsive Care section in Chapter 21 ∞.
- Demonstrate caring. Show sincere concern about the client's problems and decisions, and at the same time, accept the client's right to choose a course of action. For example, a nurse might tell a client who is not taking his heart medication, "I can appreciate how you feel about this, but I am very concerned about your heart."
- Encourage healthy behaviors through positive reinforcement. If the man who is not taking his heart medication is walking every day, the nurse might say, "You are really doing well with your walking."
- Use aids to reinforce teaching. For instance, the nurse can leave pamphlets for the client to read later or make a poster with pictures of low-salt foods the client prefers.
- Establish a therapeutic relationship of freedom, mutual understanding, and mutual responsibility with the client and support persons. By providing knowledge, skills, and information, the nurse gives clients control over their health and establishes a cooperative relationship, which results in greater adherence.

For influences on medication adherence according to age, see Lifespan Considerations.

Clinical Alert!

Chronic illness often requires complicated treatment regimens for lengthy periods that may include significant adverse reactions and be very costly. Thus, clients with chronic illnesses may be at increased risk for treatment nonadherence.

Illness and Disease

Illness is a highly personal state in which the individual's physical, emotional, intellectual, social, developmental, or spiritual functioning is thought to be diminished. It is not synonymous with disease and may or may not be related to disease. An individual could have a disease and not feel ill. Similarly, an individual can feel ill, that is, feel uncomfortable, and yet have no discernible disease.

Disease can be described as an alteration in body functions resulting in a reduction of capacities or a shortening of the normal lifespan. Traditionally, intervention by primary care providers has the goal of eliminating or ameliorating disease processes. Primitive people thought "forces" or spirits caused disease. Multiple factors are considered to interact in causing disease and determining an individual's response to treatment.

The causation of a disease or condition is called its **etiology**. A description of the etiology of a disease includes the identification of all causal factors that act together to bring about the particular disease. For example, the tubercle bacillus is designated as the biological agent of tuberculosis. However, other etiologic factors, such as age, nutritional status, and even occupation, are involved in the development of tuberculosis and influence the course of infection.

LIFESPAN CONSIDERATIONS **Medication Nonadherence**

CHILDREN

Microbial resistance to antibiotics has increased significantly in recent years, making it critical that antibiotics given to children are necessary, administered correctly by parents in the home, and taken as prescribed. Providers, parents, and children must work together in order to increase the adherence rate in taking antibiotics.

Adherence is influenced by:

- Attitudes toward medications. Some parents may think that when their child is feeling better, the medication is no longer necessary.
- Past experience. Children may remember a bad experience with taking a medication and resist parents' efforts to give them an antibiotic.
- Cost of medication. Generic drugs are less costly than trade-name drugs and can be equally effective.
- Cultural issues. Providers must work with families who have language or cultural differences to make sure they understand the family's needs and communicate the provider's recommendations.
- Number of doses necessary. Adherence improves if fewer doses per day are required and if the antibiotic can be taken over fewer days.
- Taste and palatability. Pharmaceutical companies continue to develop liquid medication that is more acceptable to young children.

ADOLESCENTS

Several causes of nonadherence are specific to teenagers. It is important for the nurse to consider these when working with adolescents because they:

- Less often consider the consequences of their actions
- Are in the early stages of demonstrating effective problem-solving
- Assert independence by rejecting adult values
- Conform to their peers and don't like being "different"
- Focus on self-concept and body image
- Live in the "here and now"
- May regress developmentally at times of stress or illness
- May be unable to distinguish benefits from disadvantages.

OLDER ADULTS

Issues that influence medication adherence in older adults include the following:

- Long-term lifestyle choices
- Limited or fixed income
- Availability of home and community-based services to maximize independence
- Available, acceptable, and cost-effective alternative or complementary therapies
- Housing and home modifications needed to accommodate the physical aspects of aging
- Affordable and accessible transportation to obtain the medication
- Beliefs about the value of preventive nursing and medical care
- Caregiving needs that overburden some family and informal caregivers
- Forgetfulness
- Dementia
- Feeling that they have lived their lives and it is time for life to end.

There are many diseases for which the specific cause is unknown (e.g., multiple sclerosis). Nurses have traditionally taken a holistic view of clients and base their practice on the multiple-causation theory of health problems.

There are many ways to classify illness and disease; one of the most common is as acute or chronic. **Acute illness** is typically characterized by symptoms of relatively short duration. The symptoms often appear abruptly and subside quickly and, depending on the cause, may or may not require intervention by healthcare professionals. Some acute illnesses are serious (e.g., appendicitis may require surgical intervention), but many acute illnesses, such as colds, subside without medical intervention or with the help of over-the-counter medications. Following an acute illness, most individuals return to their normal level of wellness.

A **chronic illness** is one that lasts for an extended period, usually 6 months or longer, and often for the individual's life. Chronic illnesses usually have a slow onset and often have periods of **remission**, when the symptoms disappear, and **exacerbation**, when the symptoms reappear.

Examples of chronic illnesses are arthritis, heart and lung diseases, and diabetes mellitus. Nurses are involved in caring for chronically ill individuals of all ages in all types of settings—homes, nursing homes, hospitals, clinics, and other institutions. Care needs to be focused on promoting the highest level possible of independence, sense of control, and wellness. Clients often need to modify their activities of daily living, social relationships, and perception of self and body image. In addition, many must learn how to live with increasing physical limitations and discomfort.

Illness Behaviors

When individuals become ill, they behave in certain ways that sociologists refer to as illness behavior. **Illness behavior**, a coping mechanism, involves the ways individuals describe, monitor, and interpret their symptoms; take remedial actions; and use the healthcare system. How individuals behave when they are ill is highly individualized and affected by many variables, such as age, sex, occupation, socioeconomic status, religion, ethnic origin, psychologic stability, personality, education, and modes of coping.

Parsons (1979) described four aspects of the sick role.

Rights:

1. Clients are not held responsible for their condition. Even if the illness was partially caused by a client's behavior (e.g., lung cancer from smoking), the individual is not capable of reversing the condition on his or her own.
2. Clients are excused from certain social roles and tasks. For example, an ill parent would not be expected to prepare meals for the family.

Obligations:

3. Clients are obliged to try to get well as quickly as possible. The ill client should follow legitimate advice regarding a specialized diet or activity restrictions that could help with recovery.
4. Clients or their families are obliged to seek competent help. For example, the ill client should contact the primary care provider rather than relying solely on his or her own ideas of how to recover.

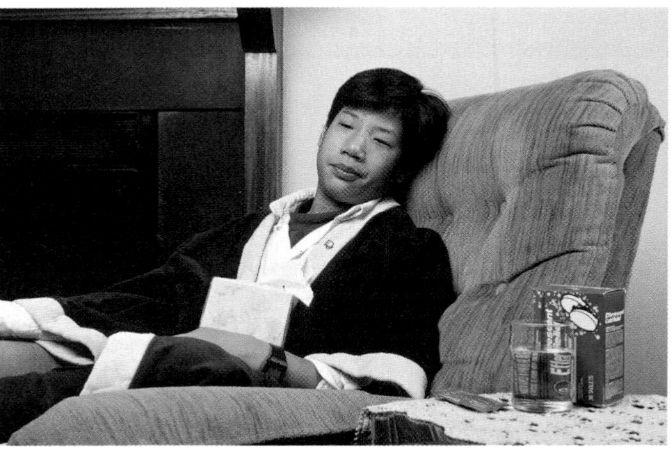

Figure 20.4 ■ In assuming the sick role for simple illnesses such as a cold, individuals are expected to rest and treat themselves with common remedies.
Matt Meadows/Photolibrary/Getty Images.

Suchman (1965) described five stages of illness: symptom experiences, assumption of the sick role, medical care contact, dependent client role, and recovery or rehabilitation. Not all clients progress through each stage. For example, the client who experiences a sudden heart attack is taken to the emergency department and immediately enters stages 3 and 4, medical care contact and dependent client role. Other clients may progress through only the first two stages and then recover. Details of Suchman's five stages follow.

Stage 1: Symptom Experiences

At this stage, the individual comes to believe something is wrong. Either someone significant mentions that the individual looks unwell, or the individual experiences some symptoms, such as pain, rash, cough, fever, or bleeding. Stage 1 has three aspects:

- The physical experience of symptoms
- The cognitive aspect (the interpretation of the symptoms in terms that have some meaning to the individual)
- The emotional response (e.g., fear or anxiety).

During this stage, the unwell individual usually consults others about the symptoms or feelings, validating with support people that the symptoms are real. At this stage, the sick individual may try home remedies. If self-management is ineffective, the individual enters the next stage.

Stage 2: Assumption of the Sick Role

The individual now accepts the sick role and seeks confirmation from family and friends. Individuals often continue with self-treatment and delay contact with healthcare professionals as long as possible. During this stage, individuals may be excused from normal duties and role expectations (Figure 20.4 ■). Emotional responses such as withdrawal, anxiety, fear, and depression are not uncommon depending on the severity of the illness, perceived degree of disability, and anticipated duration of the illness. When symptoms of illness persist or increase, the individual is motivated to seek professional help.

Stage 3: Medical Care Contact

Sick individuals seek the advice of a health professional either on their own initiative or at the urging of significant others. When individuals seek professional advice, they are really asking for three types of information:

- Validation of real illness
- Explanation of the symptoms in understandable terms
- Reassurance that they will be all right or a prediction of what the outcome will be.

The health professional may determine that the client does not have an illness or that an illness is present and may even be life threatening. The client may accept or deny the diagnosis. If the diagnosis is accepted, the client usually follows the prescribed treatment plan. If the diagnosis is not accepted, the client may seek the advice of others who will provide a diagnosis that fits the client's perceptions.

Stage 4: Dependent Client Role

After accepting the illness and seeking treatment, the client becomes dependent on the professional for help. Clients vary greatly in the degree of ease with which they can give up their independence, particularly in relation to life and death. Role obligations—such as those of wage earner, parent, student, sports team member, or choir member—complicate the decision to give up independence.

Most clients accept their dependence on the primary care provider, although they retain varying degrees of control over their own lives. For example, some clients request precise information about their disease, their treatment, and the cost of treatment and may delay the decision to accept treatment until they have all this information. Others prefer that the primary care provider proceed with treatment and do not request additional information.

For some clients, illness may meet dependence needs that have never been met and thus provide satisfaction. Other clients have minimal dependence needs and do everything possible to return to independent functioning. A few may even try to maintain independence to the detriment of their recovery.

Stage 5: Recovery or Rehabilitation

During this stage, the client is expected to relinquish the dependent role and resume former roles and responsibilities. For clients with acute illness, the time as an ill client is generally short, and recovery is usually rapid. Thus, most find it relatively easy to return to their former lifestyles. Clients who have long-term illnesses and must adjust their lifestyles may find recovery more difficult. For clients with a permanent disability, this final stage may require therapy to learn how to make major adjustments in functioning.

Effects of Illness

Illness brings about changes in both the involved client and in the family. The changes vary depending on the nature, severity, and duration of the illness; attitudes associated with the illness by the client and others; the financial demands; the lifestyle changes incurred; adjustments to usual roles; and so on.

Impact on the Client

Ill clients may experience behavioral and emotional changes, changes in self-concept and body image, and lifestyle changes. Behavioral and emotional changes associated with short-term illness are generally mild and short-lived. The client, for example, may become irritable and lack the energy or desire to interact in the usual fashion with family members or friends. More acute responses are likely with severe, life-threatening, chronic, or disabling illness. Anxiety, fear, anger, withdrawal, denial, a sense of hopelessness, and feelings of powerlessness are all common responses to severe or disabling illness. For example, a client experiencing a heart attack fears for his life and the financial burden it may place on his family. Another client informed about a diagnosis of a crippling neurologic disease may, over time, experience episodes of denial, anger, fear, and hopelessness.

Certain illnesses can also change the client's body image or physical appearance, especially if there is severe scarring or loss of a limb or sense organ. The client's self-esteem and self-concept may also be affected. Many factors can play a part in low self-esteem and a disturbance in self-concept: loss of body parts and function, pain, disfigurement, dependence on others, unemployment, financial problems, inability to participate in social functions, strained relationships with others, and spiritual distress. Nurses need to help clients express their thoughts and feelings and need to provide care that helps the client effectively cope with change.

Ill clients are also vulnerable to loss of *autonomy*, the state of being independent and self-directed, without outside control. Family interactions may change so that clients are no longer involved in making family decisions or even decisions about their own healthcare. Nurses need to support clients' right to self-determination and autonomy as much as possible by providing them with sufficient information to participate in decision-making processes and to maintain a feeling of being in control.

Illness also often necessitates a change in lifestyle. In addition to participating in treatments and taking medications, ill clients may need to change their diet, activity and exercise, and rest and sleep patterns.

Nurses can help clients adjust their lifestyles by these means:

- Provide explanations about necessary adjustments.
- Make arrangements wherever possible to accommodate the client's lifestyle.
- Encourage other health professionals to become aware of the client's lifestyle practices and to support healthy aspects of that lifestyle.
- Reinforce desirable changes in practices with a view to making them a permanent part of the client's lifestyle.

Impact on the Family

Illness affects not only the client who is ill but also the family or significant others. The kind of effect and its extent depend chiefly on three factors: (1) the member of the family who is ill, (2) the seriousness and length of the illness, and (3) the cultural and social customs the family follows.

The changes that can occur in the family include the following:

- Role changes
- Task reassignments and increased demands on time
- Increased stress due to anxiety about the outcome of the illness for the client and conflict about unaccustomed responsibilities
- Financial problems
- Loneliness as a result of separation and pending loss
- Change in social customs.

See Chapter 27 ∞ for further information about the effects of illness on the family.

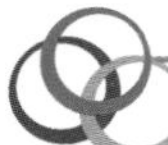

Critical Thinking Checkpoint

Both Jerry and Joe have had heart attacks. Jerry, upon advice from his primary care provider, started exercising, changed his dietary intake, entered stress reduction classes, and returned to work 6 weeks after his heart attack. He has a positive outlook, is doing well, and talks about being "well." Joe also changed his dietary habits and started exercising. However, Joe has been unable to quit smoking even though he wants to and has been advised to do so. Joe is frequently despondent, is very fearful of having another heart attack, has not yet returned to work, and frequently talks about being "ill."

1. How does Jerry's psychologic dimension of health status differ from Joe's?
2. Both Jerry and Joe have heart disease. Jerry considers himself "well," whereas Joe considers himself "ill." Explain this phenomenon based on the health locus of control model.
3. What external factors may have influenced Jerry's decision to implement positive health behaviors?
4. What factors may have prevented Joe from developing the same positive outlook and actions that Jerry was able to take in regard to his illness?
5. What nursing interventions would be most beneficial to Joe concerning his smoking problem?

Answers to Critical Thinking Checkpoint questions are available on the faculty resources site. Please consult with your instructor.

Chapter 20 Review

CHAPTER HIGHLIGHTS

- Nurses need to clarify their understanding of health because their definitions of health largely determine the scope and nature of nursing practice. Likewise, clients' health beliefs influence their health practices.
- The perspective from which health is viewed has changed; instead of the absence of disease, health has come to mean a high level of wellness or the fulfillment of one's maximum potential for physical, psychosocial, and spiritual functioning.
- Most people describe health as freedom from symptoms of disease, the ability to be active, and a state of being in good spirits.
- Nurses should be aware of their own personal definitions of health and appreciate that other people have their own individual definitions as well. By understanding clients' perceptions of health and illness, nurses can provide more meaningful assistance to help them maintain, regain, or attain a state of health.
- Wellness is an active, multidimensional process of becoming aware of and making choices toward a higher level of well-being.
- Well-being is also multidimensional, focusing on function and capability—the conditions in which choices are made and that shape clients' abilities to transform resources into given ends, such as health.
- Various models have been developed to explain health: the clinical, role-performance, adaptive, and eudaimonistic models; Leavell and Clark's agent–host–environment model; Dunn's high-level wellness grid; and the illness–wellness continuum.
- The health status of a client is affected by many internal and external variables over which the client has varying degrees of control.
- Internal variables include biological, psychologic, and cognitive dimensions. The biological dimension includes genetic makeup, gender, age, and developmental level. The psychologic dimension includes mind–body interactions and self-concept. The cognitive dimension includes lifestyle choices and spiritual and religious beliefs.
- External variables influencing health are the physical environment, standards of living, family and cultural beliefs, and social support networks.
- Health belief and behavior models have been developed to help determine whether an individual is likely to participate in disease prevention and health promotion activities. Examples of these are the locus of control model and Rosenstock and Becker's health belief model.
- A decision to implement health behaviors or to take action to improve health depends on such factors as the client's motivation to become well, perceived severity of the health problem, perceived benefits of preventive or therapeutic actions, inconvenience and unpleasantness involved, degree of lifestyle change necessary, cultural ramifications, and cost.
- Nurses can enhance healthcare adherence by identifying the reasons for nonadherence if it occurs; demonstrating caring; using positive reinforcement to encourage healthy behaviors; using aids to reinforce teaching; and establishing a therapeutic relationship of freedom, mutual understanding, and mutual responsibility with the client and support persons.
- Illness is usually associated with disease but may occur independently of it. Illness is a highly personal state in which the individual feels unhealthy or ill. Disease alters body functions and results in a reduction of capacities or a shortened lifespan.
- Various theorists have described stages and aspects of illness. Parsons describes four aspects of the sick role. Suchman outlines five stages of illness: symptom experiences, assumption of the sick role, medical care contact, dependent client role, and recovery or rehabilitation.
- A client's usual pattern of behavior changes with illness and hospitalization, which disrupt the client's privacy, autonomy, lifestyle, roles, and finances.
- Nurses need to be aware that the illness of one member of a family affects all other members.

TEST YOUR KNOWLEDGE

1. A client is attending classes on building positive relationships with significant others as well as learning skills to be open-minded and respectful to those whose opinions are different. Which component of wellness is this client focusing on?
   1. Physical
   2. Social
   3. Emotional
   4. Environment

2. Which individual appears to have "taken on" the sick role?
   1. A client who is obese states, "I deserve to have a heart attack."
   2. A mother is ill and says, "I won't be able to make your lunch today."
   3. A man with low back pain misses several physical therapy appointments.
   4. An older adult states, "My horoscope says I will be well again."

3. A community health nurse is testing the theory of locus of control (LOC). Which of the following clients demonstrates the internal control concept of this theory?
   1. A client who takes an active role in all health decisions
   2. A client who allows the primary care provider to make all the decisions
   3. A client who does not make any decisions without his or her spouse's input
   4. A client who relies on information from the local hospital for his or her health needs

4. Because a client with an infection is scheduled to begin several medications, the nurse will need to provide client education. Which client characteristics are most likely to predict adherence to the treatment program? Select all that apply.
   1. Educational level
   2. A trusting relationship with the healthcare provider
   3. An expectation that the medications will be helpful
   4. Being able to take the medications twice daily instead of 4 times daily
   5. Sex

5. Which one of the following might be the *best* way to measure adherence to a prescribed medication regime?
   1. Direct observation of medication administration
   2. Evidence of illness complications or exacerbations
   3. Monitoring laboratory values of elements influenced by the medication
   4. Questioning the client about his or her medication routine

6. Which of the following is *least* likely to influence a client's personal definition of health and wellness?
   1. The client's ability to perform his or her usual activities
   2. The cultural traditions the client uses in everyday life
   3. The availability and accessibility of healthcare services appropriate for the client's health condition
   4. The medical diagnostic terminology used to describe the client's signs and symptoms

7. Which of the following is an *internal* variable affecting health status, beliefs, or practices?
   1. Living situation
   2. Socioeconomic status
   3. Family structure
   4. Genetics

8. A client recently diagnosed with a chronic illness asks for help in understanding the term *chronic*. It would be correct for the nurse to say which of the following?
   1. Symptoms are always less severe than with an acute illness.
   2. Chronic illnesses are considered incurable.
   3. Signs and symptoms of chronic illnesses tend to be stable for many years.
   4. Chronic illnesses have no effective treatments.

9. Although not every client progresses in order through each stage, what is the usual sequence in Suchman's stages of illness?
   1. The client makes contact with medical care.
   2. The client goes into rehabilitation and recovery.
   3. Signs and symptoms appear.
   4. The client takes on the dependent role.
   5. The client takes on the sick role.

10. A married mother of three small children has frequent immobilizing headaches of unknown cause. The nurse anticipates that the woman may have which of the following possible reactions? Select all that apply.
   1. She feels guilty when unable to perform her usual activities.
   2. She is angry and acting out.
   3. She shifts some responsibilities to the spouse.
   4. She takes on a job to help pay for the medical expenses.
   5. She has fewer social interactions with her friends.

See Answers to Test Your Knowledge in Appendix A.

READINGS AND REFERENCES

Suggested Readings

Andermann, A., Pang, T., Newton, J. N., Davis, A., & Panisset, U. (2016). Evidence for health I: Producing evidence for improving health and reducing inequities. *Health Research Policy and Systems, 14*(18), 1–7. doi:10.1186/s12961-016-0087-2

Part I of this three-part series describes the first step in improving the health of individuals and populations: gaining a better understanding of what the main health problems are and which are the most urgent priorities. Data provide a health portrait perspective on why the local population believes that certain health challenges should be prioritized.

Andermann, A., Pang, T., Newton, J. N., Davis, A., & Panisset, U. (2016). Evidence for health II: Overcoming barriers to using evidence in policy and practice. *Health Research Policy and Systems, 14*(17), 1–7. doi:10.1186/s12961-016-0086-3

Part II of the three-part series identifies four barriers to using evidence to make decisions: (1) missing the window of opportunity, (2) knowledge gaps and uncertainty, (3) controversy, irrelevant and conflicting evidence, and (4) vested interests and conflicts of interest.

Andermann, A., Pang, T., Newton, J. N., Davis, A., & Panisset, U. (2016). Evidence for health III: Making evidence-informed decisions that integrate values and context. *Health Research Policy and Systems, 14*(16), 1–8. doi:10.1186/s12961-016-0085-4

Part III of this three-part series describes each of the 10 steps of an algorithm that addresses the key issues involved in making evidence-based decisions in healthcare.

Related Research

Moody's Analytics. (2017). *Understanding health conditions across the U.S.* Retrieved from https://www.bcbs.com/sites/default/files/file-attachments/health-of-america-report/BCBS.HealthOfAmericaReport.Moodys_02.pdf

References

Agency for Healthcare Research and Quality, U.S. Public Health Service. (2014). *Guide to clinical preventive services, 2014*. Retrieved from http://www.ahrq.gov/professionals/clinicians-providers/guidelines-recommendations/guide/index.html

American Nurses Association. (2010). *Nursing's social policy statement: The essence of the profession.* Silver Spring, MD: Author.

Artiga, S., & Hinton, E. (2018). *Beyond health care: The role of social determinants in promoting health and health equity.* Kaiser Family Foundation. Retrieved from http://files.kff.org/attachment/issue-brief-beyond-health-care

Champagne, B. R., Fox, R. S., Mills, S. D., Sadler, G. R., & Malcarne, V. L. (2016). Multidimensional profiles of health locus of control in Hispanic Americans. *Journal of Health Psychology, 21,* 2376–2385. doi:10.1177/1359105315577117

Dunn, H. L. (1959). High-level wellness for man and society. *American Journal of Public Health, 49,* 786–792. doi:10.2105/AJPH.49.6.786

Fawcett, J., & Ellenbecker, C. H. (2015). A proposed conceptual model of nursing and population health. *Nursing Outlook, 63,* 288–298. doi:10.1016/j.outlook.2015.01.009

Keinki, C., Seilacher, E., Ebel, M., Ruetters, D., Kessler, I., Stellamanns, J., . . . Huebner, J. (2016). Information needs of cancer patients and perception of impact of the disease, of self-efficacy, and locus of control. *Journal of Cancer Education, 31*, 610–616. doi:10.1007/s13187-015-0860-x

Leavell, H. R., & Clark, E. G. (1965). *Preventive medicine for the doctor in his community* (3rd ed.). New York, NY: McGraw-Hill.

Murdaugh, C. L., Parsons, M. J., & Pender, N. J. (2019). *Health promotion in nursing practice* (8th ed.). New York, NY: Pearson.

Nightingale, F. (1969). *Notes on nursing: What it is, and what it is not.* New York, NY: Dover Books. (Original work published 1860)

Parsons, T. (1951). *The social system.* Glencoe, IL: Free Press.

Parsons, T. (1979). Definitions of health and illness in the light of American values and social structure. In E. G. Jaco (Ed.), *Patients, physicians, and illness* (3rd ed., pp. 120–144). New York, NY: Free Press.

President's Commission on Health Needs of the Nation. (1953). *Building Americans' health* (Vol. 2). Washington, DC: U.S. Government Printing Office.

Puff, J., & Renk, K. (2016). Mothers' temperament and personality: Their relationship to parenting behaviors, locus of control, and young children's functioning. *Child Psychiatry & Human Development, 47,* 799–818. doi:10.1007/s10578-015-0613-4

Rosenstock, I. M., Strecher, V. J., & Becker, M. H. (1988). Social learning theory and the health belief model. *Health Education Quarterly, 12,* 175–183.

Suchman, E. A. (1965). Stages of illness and medical care. *Journal of Health and Human Behavior, 6*, 114–128. doi:10.2307/2948694.

U.S. Department of Health and Human Services. (2018). *Strategic plan 2018–2022*. Retrieved from https://www.hhs.gov/about/strategic-plan/index.html

Wallston, K. A., Stein, M. J., & Smith, C. A. (1994). Form C of the MHLC scales: A condition-specific measure of locus of control. *Journal of Personality Assessment, 63,* 534–553. doi:10.1207/s15327752jpa6303_10

World Health Organization. (n.d.). *Social determinants of health*. Retrieved from https://www.who.int/social_determinants/en

World Health Organization. (1948). *Preamble to the constitution of the World Health Organization as adopted by the International Health Conference.* New York, 19–22 June 1946; signed on 22 July 1946 by the representatives of 61 States (Official Records of the World Health Organization, no. 2, p. 100) and entered into force on 7 April 1948.

World Health Organization. (2013). *The European health report 2012: Charting the way to well-being*. Retrieved from http://www.euro.who.int/__data/assets/pdf_file/0004/197113/EHR2012-Eng.pdf

Selected Bibliography

Centers for Disease Control and Prevention. (n.d.). *About the community guide*. Retrieved from https://www.thecommunityguide.org/about/about-community-guide

Fawcett, J., & AbuFannouneh, A. M. (2017). Thoughts about population health nursing research methods: Questions about participants and informed consent. *Nursing Science Quarterly, 30,* 353–355. doi:10.1177/0894318417724461

Fawcett, J., Amweg, L. N., Legor, K., Kim, B. R., & Maghrabi, S. (2018). More thoughts about conceptual models and literature reviews: Focus on population health. *Nursing Science Quarterly, 31,* 384–389. doi:10.1177/0894318418792878

Handmaker, K. (2017). Incorporating social determinants into population health management. *hfm (Healthcare Financial Management), 71*(3), 60–64.

Hausman, J., & Odum, M. (2018). *Alters & Schiff essential concepts for healthy living* (8th ed.). Burlington, MA: Jones & Bartlett.

HealthITAnalytics, Xtelligent Healthcare Media. (2017). *What are the social determinants of population health?* Retrieved from https://healthitanalytics.com/features/what-are-the-social-determinants-of-population-health

Hood, L. J. (2017). *Leddy & Pepper's conceptual bases of professional nursing* (9th ed.). Philadelphia, PA: Lippincott Williams & Wilkins.

Mariner, W. K. (2016). Beyond lifestyle: Governing the social determinants of health. *American Journal of Law & Medicine, 42*(2–3), 284–309. doi:10.1177/0098858816658268

Raingruber, B. (2017). *Contemporary health promotion in nursing practice* (2nd ed.). Burlington, MA: Jones & Bartlett.

Stanhope, M., & Lancaster, J. (2018). *Foundations for population health in community/public health nursing* (5th ed.). St. Louis, MO: Elsevier.

Culturally Responsive Nursing Care 21

LEARNING OUTCOMES

After completing this chapter, you will be able to:

1. Describe concepts related to culture, such as race, ethnicity, and acculturation.
2. Examine factors that contribute to health disparities among racial and ethnic groups.
3. Describe the role of federal agencies and initiatives regarding the provision of culturally responsive healthcare.
4. Describe cultural models of care, such as cultural competency.
5. Describe health views from culturally diverse perspectives.
6. Differentiate culturally influenced approaches to healing and treatment.
7. Describe ways culture influences communication patterns and how to provide linguistically appropriate care.
8. Create self-awareness of your own culture, beliefs, biases, and assumptions.
9. Identify methods of cultural assessment.
10. Create a culturally responsive nursing care plan.

KEY TERMS

acculturation, *401*
assimilation, *402*
biomedical health belief, *404*
cultural broker, *407*
cultural competence, *403*
culturally responsive care, *397*
culture, *398*
discrimination, *399*
diversity, *398*
ethnicity, *398*
ethnocentrism, *399*
folk medicine, *405*
generalizations, *399*
health disparities, *399*
health equity, *400*
heritage, *398*
heritage consistent, *411*
heritage inconsistent, *411*
holistic health belief, *404*
interpreter, *407*
magico-religious health belief, *404*
multicultural, *398*
nationality, *399*
prejudice, *399*
race, *398*
racism, *399*
religion, *399*
scientific health belief, *404*
stereotyping, *399*
subculture, *398*
traditional, *403*
transcultural nursing, *402*
translator, *407*

Introduction

Nursing care is holistic and encompasses the client's perspectives on health, which are greatly influenced by the client's culture. Each individual is born into a culture influenced by place of birth and family of origin. A child learns the family's customs and beliefs, which shape his or her worldview. An individual's culture is dynamic and shifts over the course of a lifetime, influenced by many other factors, such as communities, schools, migration patterns, career choices, and religion. Similarly, a nurse's worldview is influenced by the culture of the nursing profession and the culture of the organization that he or she represents. Therefore, every nurse–client interaction is a cultural encounter. A nurse cannot assume sameness of values, even if the client appears to resemble the nurse in outward appearance. It is the nurse's responsibility to recognize the client's cultural perspectives.

Culturally responsive care is care that is centered on the client's cultural point of view and integrates the client's values and beliefs into the plan of care. To deliver such care, the nurse must first develop self-awareness of personal culture, attitudes, and beliefs and examine the biases and assumptions about different cultures. Next, the nurse needs to gain the necessary knowledge and skills to create an environment where trust can be developed with the client. This knowledge must include an understanding of health disparities as well as the historical and current portrayals of racial and ethnic groups in society. Additionally, cultural knowledge can help the nurse to better understand different perspectives while recognizing that cultural generalizations may not hold true at the individual level. Cultural assessment skills are essential in understanding the client's viewpoint more fully and learning what the client values as important. The nurse must partner with the client in a caring and respectful relationship that honors the client's differences and perspectives. In culturally responsive care, the nurse must respond to the client's needs, not vice versa. Only through self-awareness, deliberate cultural assessment, and incorporation of the client's culture into the plan of care can a nurse optimally care for a client.

Cultural Concepts

Culture is complex, with multiple definitions, and the term *culture* may be used interchangeably with other terms such as *race*, *ethnicity*, and *nationality* depending on the circumstances.

- **Culture** has many definitions, but concepts common to most include the thoughts, communications, actions, customs, beliefs, values, and institutions of racial, ethnic, religious, or social groups. It has been described as the learned and shared patterns of information that a group uses to generate meaning among its members. These patterns include nonverbal language and material goods. Within macro-cultures (national, ethnic, or racial groups) are micro-cultures (gender, age, or religious beliefs) in which members share a belief in certain rules, roles, behaviors, and values. Macro- and micro-cultures combine to shape the individual's worldview and influence interaction with others.
- A **subculture** is usually composed of individuals who have a distinct identity and yet are related to a larger cultural group. A subcultural group generally shares ethnic origin or physical characteristics with the larger cultural group. Examples of cultural subgroups include occupational groups (e.g., nurses), societal groups (e.g., feminists), and ethnic groups – (e.g., Sudanese, who migrate to European countries like Malta and Italy and settle there, either temporarily or permanently).
- **Multicultural** is used to describe an individual who has multiple patterns of identification or crosses several cultures, lifestyles, and sets of values. For example, a man whose father is Maltese and whose mother is Filipino may honor his Filipino **heritage** (things passed down from previous generations) while also being influenced by his father's cultural values. Another example exists in Australia where many Europeans migrated after the second world war, thereby strongly influencing the overall Australian culture. The term *multicultural* is often used interchangeably with *bicultural*, *biracial*, *multiracial*, and *multiethnic*.
- **Diversity** refers to the fact or state of being different. Many factors account for diversity: sex, age, culture, ethnicity, socioeconomic status, educational attainment, religious affiliation, and so on. Diversity, therefore, occurs not only *between* cultural groups but also *within* a cultural group.
- **Race** is a term with many definitions, often used interchangeably with the terms *ethnicity* and *culture*. The Office of Management and Budget (OMB, 1997), which determines U.S. federal standards for reporting race, stated that racial categories "should not be interpreted as being primarily biological or genetic in reference. Race and ethnicity may be thought of in terms of social and cultural characteristics as well as ancestry" (p. 36, 881).

The American Anthropological Association (1998) statement on race defines it as an idea created by Western Europeans following exploration across the world to account for differences among individuals and justify colonization, conquest, enslavement, and social hierarchy among humans. It has been used to refer to groupings of individuals according to common origin or background and associated with perceived biological markers. Ideas about race are culturally and socially transmitted and form the basis of racism, racial classification, and often complex racial identities.

The Human Genome Project has discovered that humans are 99.9% genetically alike and that the genetic variations related to geographic ancestry do not correlate with the socially constructed racial classifications; that is, there are no genetically discrete races. In fact, there is greater genetic variability within the racial categories than among them (Figure 21.1 ■). The official U.S. classification of race has varied throughout history. The 2010 U.S. Census racial classifications were White, Black/African American/Negro, American Indian or Alaska Native, Asian Indian, Chinese, Filipino, Japanese, Korean, Vietnamese, Other Asian, Native Hawaiian, Guamanian or Chamorro, Samoan, Other Pacific Islander, and Some Other Race. It does not classify Hispanic as a race. In addition to the question about race, respondents were asked if they were of Hispanic, Latino, or Spanish origin. For example, of the 50 million respondents to the 2010 U.S. Census who indicated they were Hispanic or Latino, 53% indicated their race as White; less than 3% as Black, Asian, Native Hawaiian/Pacific Islander, or American Indian or Alaska Native; 36.7% as Some Other Race; and 6% as Two or More Races (Humes, Jones, & Ramirez, 2011). As a result of the large number of respondents choosing "Some Other Race," the Census Bureau piloted modified categories for use in the 2020 census survey, including options to indicate a specific country of origin within each race or ethnicity (Matthews et al., 2017).

Although there are plans to reconsider some categories as related to research, the categories currently used by the National Institutes of Health (NIH, 2015) are American Indian or Alaska Native, Asian, Black or African American, Hispanic or Latino, Native Hawaiian or Other Pacific Islander, and White.

Although it is now recognized that there is no scientific merit to the concept of race, race remains an important social construct, whereby social meanings are attached to perceived physical differences, resulting in inequality among racial groups.

- **Ethnicity** is a term often used interchangeably used with *race*. Ethnicity may be viewed as a relationship among individuals who believe that they have distinctive

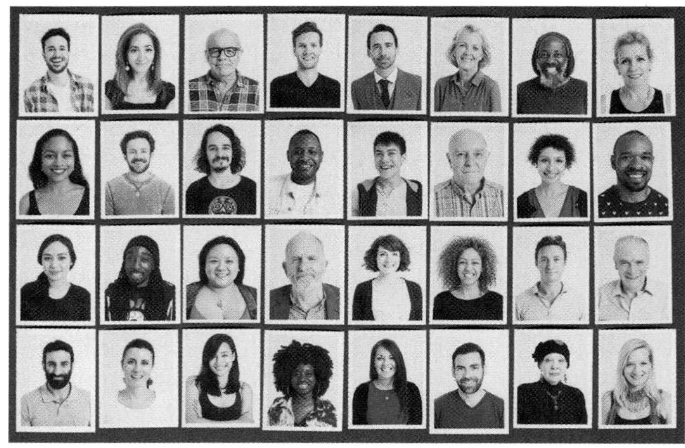

Figure 21.1 ■ Although differing in outward appearance, humans are biologically more similar to each other than they are different.
Plume Creative/DigitalVision/Getty Images.

characteristics that make them a group. Ethnicity is not a fixed concept. Much like culture, ethnicity may shift over time. Migration, intermarriage, and intermating patterns show that individuals move into another ethnic group and become participants in that ethnicity, sharing the language, religion, values, beliefs, and customs. Latino people, for instance, represent multiple geographic areas and multiple races and often share a common language. Ethnic groups may be self-defined, and labeling can become problematic.

- **Nationality** is sometimes used interchangeably with *ethnicity* or *citizenship*. It generally refers to the sovereign state or country where an individual has membership, which may be through birth, through inheritance (parents), or through naturalization. It is also possible to be a member of a nation where no such country is officially recognized, for instance, Native Americans. An individual may also be multinational, holding citizenship in two or more countries. Ethnic groups may have territories to which they have national affiliation. This was particularly evident in Eastern Europe, where group tensions led to divisions of multiethnic states along territorial lines. For instance, Czechoslovakia became two countries: the Czech Republic and Slovakia. Yugoslavia became six countries: Bosnia and Herzegovina, Croatia, Macedonia, Montenegro, Serbia, and Slovenia.
- **Religion** may be considered a system of beliefs, practices, and ethical values about divine or superhuman power(s) worshipped as the creator(s) and ruler(s) of the universe. The practice of religion is revealed in numerous denominations, organizations, sects, and cults. Ethnicity and religion are related, and one's religion is often determined by one's ethnic group. Religion gives an individual a frame of reference and a perspective with which to organize information. Religious teachings about health help to present a meaningful philosophy and system of practices within a system of social controls having specific values, norms, and ethics. Illness is sometimes seen as punishment for the violation of religious codes and morals. See Chapter 41 ∞ for more information on spirituality.
- **Ethnocentrism** is the belief in the superiority of one's own culture and lifestyle. Other viewpoints are not only considered different but also wrong or of lesser importance. A related concept is *xenophobia*—the fear or dislike of individuals different from oneself.
- **Prejudice** is a preconceived notion or judgment that is not based on sufficient knowledge; it may be favorable or unfavorable. Unfavorable prejudice may lead to stereotyping and discriminatory behavior toward groups of individuals. There are many types of prejudice, including racial prejudice.
- **Racism** refers to assumptions held about racial groups. Assumptions include the belief that races are biologically discrete and exclusive groups that are inherently unequal and ranked hierarchically. Cultural behaviors are viewed as inherited and exclusive to each group and form the basis of judging individuals based on their racial classification. *Institutional racism* or *institutional discrimination* is the denial of opportunities and equal rights based on race. Examples include standards for assessing credit risks that disadvantage African American and Hispanic individuals who may lack conventional credit references, higher insurance costs in low income areas, school testing that favors White middle-class children because of the types of questions included, and hiring practices that require experience at jobs not historically open to members of subordinate groups (Schaefer, 2019). In a system that advantages White people over other races, the advantages are often referred to as "White privilege."
- **Discrimination** refers to the negative treatment of individuals or groups on the basis of their race, ethnicity, gender, or other group membership. It occurs when rights and opportunities are denied for arbitrary or prejudicial reasons.
- **Generalizations** are statements about common cultural patterns. Generalizations may not hold true at the individual level and should serve only as openings for individuals to better understand each other. Unfortunately, generalizations are often interpreted as statements describing every individual in a group, which leads to stereotyping.
- **Stereotyping** refers to making the assumption that an individual reflects all characteristics associated with being a member of a group. For instance, a nurse may assume that a Latino client speaks limited English and comes from a large family. Rather than asking the client, the nurse immediately calls for an interpreter, speaks loudly and very slowly to the client, and tells the client that the visitor policy allows for only two visitors at a time and that the client's entire family cannot visit at the same time. Stereotyping serves as a barrier to communication and understanding and propagates discriminatory behavior. One type of stereotyping is racial profiling, in which police-initiated action is based on race, ethnicity, or national origin rather than the individual's behavior.

Health Disparities

Health disparities are the differences in care experienced by one population compared with another population. Dimensions of health disparities include health insurance coverage, access to healthcare, quality of care provided, inability of providers to recognize and address disparities, levels of health, data collection, and resources allocated to address disparities, such as research into the causes of disparities and solutions to differences in health outcomes (Orgera & Artiga, 2018). Just like the *National Healthcare Disparities Report* (2017) that shows how in the US some individuals receive inferior healthcare compared with others, the European Commission published a report about inequalities in the ability to access healthcare both within and across European member states (Baeten, Spasova, Vanhercke, & Coster, 2018).

This report concludes that there is a huge difference in the amount of money spent on healthcare by each EU member state. In some countries, healthcare and some medicines are provided for free, while in others they are not. However, in the former case, asylum seekers reported having limited access to care. There are EU member states that report an inadequate supply of healthcare services due to a shortage of healthcare staff and their unattractive work conditions.

The following are examples of health disparities in countries across the world.

Quality of care:

- Although the health of Europeans has improved over the years, one can still find persistent inequalities as a result of varying income levels in European countries, which in turn reflect each country's development. Forster, Kentikelenis, & Bambra (2018) observed differences in life expectancy within the European Union member states, and Eurostat (2018) linked a higher life expectancy to a higher GDP per unit of population, signifying that more affluent countries can provide better quality of care than less wealthy countries.
- In Wayanad, India, health inequalities persist in marginalized social groups. Between 2013 and 2014, tribal populations had a higher rate of infant mortality compared to Hindu and Muslim populations (Directorate of Health Services Kerala, 2015). Thresia (2017) attributed this to the fact that tribal populations are discriminated against and have constrained access to health care.

Access to care:

- According to the Australian Institute of Health and Welfare (2018), indigenous Australians affirm that they find it harder to access affordable health care services than non-indigenous Australians.
- Data suggests that within the EU member states, migrants do not access health care services as much as the EU nationals. Of specific significance is the low utilization rate of antenatal and pediatric services. Potential obstacles that hinder access to healthcare services are language barriers, differences in education and culture, and lack of complementary voluntary health insurance and legal issues. (Mladovski, 2007: p.1)

The following are examples of measures taken within the European Union member states and other countries to achieve **health equity**—the highest possible standard of health for all individuals, especially those at greatest risk for poor health.

- In Scotland, one can find all-embracing health inequality reduction strategies. Their Health Inequalities Action Framework establishes a link between social factors and disparities in health outcomes and encourages considering the steps that might be taken to mitigate these inequalities. Then, their Health Inequalities Policy Review highlights methods that effectively reduce health inequalities. Moreover, Public Health Scotland (2021) asserts the importance of supporting people working within NHS Scotland and Health and Social Care Partnerships (HSCPs) to equip them with the knowledge and skill required to provide quality service that helps to diminish health inequalities.
- There are also programs that focus on specific groups. One ethnic group of main concern in Europe is Roma. It poses some of the greatest health needs as there is a high prevalence of communicable and non-communicable diseases and noticeable lower life expectancies within this group than the rest of the population. (Parekh & Rose, 2011). Thus, In Central, Southern, and Eastern Europe, Roma Inclusion Strategies were formulated (Brown, Harrison, Ziglio, & Burns, 2014). Unfortunately, due to several reasons, including the absence of legal regulations, these strategies, up to 2020, did not accomplish any noteworthy improvement in bridging the gap between Roma and non-Roma populations. Thus, Roma remain the most underprivileged and socially excluded ethnic minority across the European Union, facing severe inequalities at a social and economic level (Zaharieva, 2020).
- Within the Commonwealth of Independent States (CIS) countries, health improvement goals and objectives are included in strategies aimed at reducing poverty at a national level (Brown et al, 2014). In the long run, these helped improve the circumstances of countries like Armenia, Azerbaijan, Albania, and Georgia (UNDP, 2015). On analyzing Tajikistan's Living Standards Survey (2007), it was found that the country's poverty had decreased considerably as a result of the government's adopting strategies and programs for socioeconomic development (International Monetary Fund, 2010).
- Moreover, as highlighted by Brown et al (2014), Latvia and Slovenia included specific health equity targets in their national development plans. The Ministry of Health works together with other sectors to track common equity goals, and over the last few years, methods of managing inequities have been scaled up both at local and national levels.
- In 2008, the member states of the World Health Organization (WHO) in the European Region embraced the Tallinn Charter, the purpose of which was to work on strengthening health systems to enhance people's health while keeping in mind the social, cultural, and economic diversity across the European Region. It also aimed to make health systems more amenable to people's requirements, preferences, and expectations (World Health Organization, Europe, 2008: 2). Thus, the member states committed themselves to provide suitable and acceptable services to meet the needs of all users, ensuring the preparedness of health systems in dealing with crises.

Only through training can providers begin to recognize and change the discriminatory practices that perpetuate health disparities. The efforts described in the following list are evidence of the increased emphasis on providing culturally appropriate healthcare in the United States:

- The NPA (National Partnership for Action to End Health Disparities) was established to mobilize a nationwide, comprehensive, community-driven, and sustained approach to combating health disparities and to move the nation toward achieving health equity. The mission of the NPA is to increase the effectiveness of programs that target the elimination of health disparities through the coordination of partners, leaders, and stakeholders committed to action.

- The NPA released the *National Stakeholder Strategy for Achieving Health Equity* in 2011, a common set of goals and objectives for public- and private-sector initiatives and partnerships to help racial and ethnic minorities and other underserved groups reach their full health potential.
- The U.S. Department of Health and Human Services (USDHHS) 2011 *HHS Action Plan to Reduce Racial and Ethnic Health Disparities* was written to operationalize the national strategy and the Affordable Care Act (USDHHS, 2011).
- The AHRQ, Centers for Disease Control and Prevention (CDC), Centers for Medicare and Medicaid Services (CMS), Food and Drug Administration (FDA), Health Resources and Services Administration (HRSA), and Substance Abuse and Mental Health Services Administration (SAMHSA) each created an Office of Minority Health within their agency as required by the Affordable Care Act.
- The Office of Minority Health (OMH) within the USDHHS, established in 1986, "addresses disease prevention, health promotion, risk reduction, healthier lifestyle choices, use of healthcare services, and barriers to healthcare for racial and ethnic minorities" (USDHHS OMH, 2018b). In collaboration with other organizations, it developed the *National Standards for Culturally and Linguistically Appropriate Services in Health Care* (CLAS), which were enhanced in 2012. "The National CLAS Standards are a set of 15 action steps intended to advance health equity, improve quality, and help eliminate healthcare disparities by establishing a blueprint for individuals and health and healthcare organizations to implement culturally and linguistically appropriate services" (USDHHS OMH, 2018a). Culture and language have a considerable impact on how clients access and respond to healthcare services.
- The CDC (2018) Office of Minority Health and Health Equity aims to "advance health equity and women's health issues across the nation through CDC's science and programs, and increase CDC's capacity to leverage its diverse workforce and engage stakeholders toward this end."
- The Affordable Care Act redesignated the National Center on Minority Health and Health Disparities within the NIH to the National Institute on Minority Health and Health Disparities (NIMHD), which coordinates all research and activities conducted or supported by the NIH on the health of specific populations and health disparities.
- The nursing profession plays a major role in a CDC program titled Racial and Ethnic Approaches to Community Health Across the United States (REACH U.S.). REACH U.S. strives to eliminate racial and ethnic disparities (inequalities) in infant mortality; in screening and management of breast and cervical cancer, cardiovascular diseases, diabetes, hepatitis, tuberculosis, asthma, HIV infections, and AIDS; and in infant mortality and child and adult immunizations. This program has achieved significant results, which are profiled on the agency's website.
- One of the major goals of *Healthy People* is to eliminate health disparities by gender, race or ethnicity, education, income, disability, geographic location, and sexual orientation (details of *Healthy People 2020* are discussed in Chapter 19 ∞). To achieve these goals, the HRSA aims to increase the number of underrepresented racial and ethnic groups entering the nursing profession through grants and scholarships provided by the Nurse Corps scholarship and loan-repayment programs.

Demographics

Statistics about the ethnicity of the population can be complicated to interpret. The U.S. Census Bureau (2017) revealed that in 2017, 96.7% of U.S. residents identified themselves as belonging to a single race. Of the total claiming a single race, 74.8% identified themselves as White people, 13.1% as Black or African American people, 5.8% as Asian people, 0.9% as American Indian or Alaska Native people, and 5.4% as some other race. Hispanic or Latino origin is considered an ethnicity, not a race, by the U.S. Census Bureau. The U.S. Census Bureau (2018b) estimated that 21% of the U.S. population was of Hispanic or Latino origin in 2017 and that by 2060, Hispanics or Latinos people of any race will increase to represent 27.5% of the total population, whereas the percentage of White non-Hispanic people will decrease from 61% to 44% of the total (U.S. Census Bureau, 2018c). The 2020 U.S. Census has two separate questions: one asking about Hispanic, Latino, or Spanish origin (including identification of the county of origin) and a second question about race that provides 13 options plus identification of country of origin (U.S. Census Bureau, 2018a).

Nurses' race or ethnicity is somewhat disproportionate to the demographic profile of the United States. Exact data vary according to the method used to collect the data. Census Bureau surveys reported that of all U.S. employed RNs in 2018, 75.5% self-reported as White, 13.1% of RNs as Black or African American, 9% as Asian, and 7.2% as Hispanic or Latino (U.S. Department of Labor, Bureau of Labor Statistics, 2019).

Immigration

Australia has a rich migration history. The foreign-born population in Australia numbered 7.5 million in 2019. Of these, the largest group consisted of people who were born in England. In the first half of 2019, 538,000 people arrived to live in Australia, and 298,000 persons left Australia to live in other countries (Australian Bureau of Statistics, ABS, 2020).

As immigrants become participants in the dominant culture, two important processes occur. They may continue to identify as members of the culture from which they originate. Individuals immigrating to Australia from any country will be associated with their native countries for many years, if not for all of their lives. The involuntary process of **acculturation** occurs when individuals incorporate traits from another culture. The members of the immigrant cultural group are often forced to adopt the new culture to survive. Acculturation can also be defined as the changes

LIFESPAN CONSIDERATIONS How Culture Affects Parenting

The influence of social diversity on human relationships has been the focus of several literature (Bhugun, 2017; Singla, 2015). Crippen and Brew (2007) highlighted that marriages between people from different cultures are on the increase, and Owen (2002) claimed that this could be one of the consequences of immigration. Parenting within intercultural marriages can pose several challenges for the couples as well as their children (Bhugun, 2017). However, it can also provide the children with a wealth of knowledge and an experience of the development of the multicultural world (Crippen, 2008). The difficulties of parents and children arise from varying views regarding values, religious convictions, and rituals (Bornstein, 2015). In an example, Bornstein discusses how the role of play may take different forms in different cultures. In some cultures, parents play with their children as they believe it to be an interactive, learning experience, but parents in other cultures who believe play to be only fun do not play with their children at all.

Bhugun's study participants revealed that culture should not be imposed on children. The concept of culture should be discussed and explained, and the children should be given choices in order to avoid confusion and to enhance the mitigation of cultural differences. Children raised by intercultural couples should be encouraged to have an open mind about cultures and embrace diversity. However, just like monocultural families, intercultural parents value communication, consistent parenting, and the teaching of moral values.

of one's cultural patterns to those of the host society. This is a two-way process in which the host society may also pick up certain traits from the immigrant group. An example of this was given by Terry, Ali, & Lê (2011). They found that upon arrival to Australia, all their Asian participants used traditional medicine to deal with health problems. However, this practice was lost by the time of the interviews. Yet, the use of traditional Chinese medicine has also been adopted in some areas of healthcare in Australia (Ferro et al., 2007). Even healthcare professionals can be migrants, thereby contributing to the cultural group they work with. **Assimiliation** is the process by which an individual develops a new cultural identity. Assimilation means becoming like the members of the local culture. The process of assimilation encompasses various aspects, such as behavioral, marital, identification, and civic aspects. The underlying assumption is that the individual from a given cultural group loses his or her original cultural identity to acquire the new one. In fact, because this is a conscious effort, it is not always possible or desirable to the individual, and the process may cause severe stress and anxiety. For example, in the late 18th century in New Zealand, European settlers adopted Maori words, while affecting the indigenous Maori population's vocabulary and phonology (Thomason, 2001). Moreover, by the late 20th century, the Maori population, influenced by European settlers, rapidly adopted the use of metals as opposed to stone to make tools (Neich, 2001). The use of European-style clothing was adopted more slowly (King, 2003).

The concepts of acculturation and assimilation are sensitive and complex. As we live in a society with many cultures, many variations of health beliefs and practices exist. Therefore, in order to provide culturally competent care, nurses have to be open minded and never assume that their clients are accultured and assimilated in the host society.

Cultural Models of Nursing Care

All members of the healthcare team have responsibility for supporting cultural competence. Culturally responsive care takes into account the context in which the client lives as well as the situations in which the client's health problems arise. Nurses must be able to assess and interpret a given client's health beliefs, practices, and cultural needs. Countless conflicts in the healthcare delivery arenas result from cultural misunderstandings. Although many of these misunderstandings are related to universal situations, such as verbal and nonverbal language misunderstandings, the conventions of courtesy, sequencing of interactions, phasing of interactions, and objectivity, many cultural misunderstandings are unique to the delivery of nursing and healthcare. Culturally responsive care alters the perspective of nursing care delivery because it enables the nurse to understand, from a cultural perspective, the manifestations of the client's healthcare beliefs and practices. Several cultural models are used to guide nursing care of the client.

The term *transcultural nursing* was promulgated by nurse Madeleine Leininger beginning in the 1950s. **Transcultural nursing** focuses on providing care within the differences and similarities of the beliefs, values, and patterns of cultures (McFarland & Wehbe-Alamah, 2018). Leininger created the theory of culture care diversity and universality.

American Association of Colleges of Nursing Competencies

In 2008, the American Association of Colleges of Nursing (AACN) published end-of-program cultural competencies for baccalaureate nursing education. These five competencies should be used to guide nursing practice:

1. Apply knowledge of social and cultural factors that affect nursing and healthcare across multiple contexts.
2. Use relevant data sources and best evidence in providing culturally competent care.
3. Promote achievement of safe and quality outcomes of care for diverse populations.
4. Advocate for social justice, including commitment to the health of vulnerable populations and the elimination of health disparities.
5. Participate in continuous cultural competency development. (AACN, 2008)

Cultural Competence

Cultural competence has been used as a goal for nurses over the past several decades but has different definitions depending on the author. One definition of **cultural competence** is the "provision of healthcare across cultural boundaries and takes into account the context in which the patient lives, as well as the situations in which the patient's health problems arise" (Spector, 2017, p. 8). Another definition is "an ongoing, multidimensional learning process that integrates transcultural nursing skills in all three dimensions (cognitive, practical, and affective), involves transcultural self-efficacy (confidence) as a major influencing factor, and aims to achieve culturally congruent care" (Jeffreys, 2016, p. 45). The Joint Commission (2010), the accrediting body for hospitals and other healthcare institutions, defines it as "the ability of health care providers and health care organizations to understand and respond effectively to the cultural and language needs brought by the patient to the health care encounter" (p. 1).

Many individuals believe it is not possible to be truly competent culturally and prefer the term *culturally congruent*, which implies that the care provided is consistent with the client's values, beliefs, and practices. In 2015, the American Nurses Association (ANA) revised the Scope and Standards of Practice and added Standard 8: Culturally Congruent Practice "The registered nurse practices in a manner that is congruent with cultural diversity and inclusion principles" (ANA, 2015).

HEALTH Traditions Model

In the United States, another model for providing culturally responsive care is to view health holistically, as a complex, interrelated, threefold phenomenon, that is, as the balance of all aspects of the individual—the body, mind, and spirit. The HEALTH traditions model (Spector, 2017) is predicated on the concept of holistic health and describes what individuals do from a traditional perspective to maintain, protect, and restore health. In this context, the term **traditional** refers to those customs, beliefs, or practices that have existed for many generations without changing.

- The body includes all physical aspects, such as genetic inheritance, body chemistry, gender, age, nutrition, and physical condition.
- The mind includes cognitive processes, such as thoughts, memories, and knowledge of such emotional processes as feelings, defenses, and self-esteem.
- The spirit includes both positive and negative learned spiritual practices and teachings, dreams, symbols, stories, protecting forces, and metaphysical or native forces.

These aspects are in constant flux and change over time, yet each is completely related to the others and also related to the context of the individual. The context includes the individual's family, culture, work, community, history, and environment.

The HEALTH traditions model, shown in Table 21.1, consists of nine interrelated facets, represented by the following:

1. Traditional methods of maintaining HEALTH—physical, mental, and spiritual—may include following a proper diet and wearing proper clothing, concentrating and using the mind, and practicing one's religion.
2. Traditional methods of protecting HEALTH—physical, mental, and spiritual—may include wearing protective objects, such as amulets; avoiding individuals who may cause trouble; and placing religious objects in the home.
3. Traditional methods of restoring HEALTH—physical, mental, and spiritual—may include the use of herbal remedies, exorcism, and healing rituals.

Symbolic Examples

Figure 21.2 ■ depicts symbolic HEALTH-related images that may be used by individuals of different heritages to maintain, protect, or restore physical, mental, or spiritual HEALTH.

1. Thousand-year-old eggs represent traditional foods that may be eaten daily to maintain physical HEALTH (China).

TABLE 21.1 The Nine Interrelated Facets of Health (Physical, Mental, and Spiritual) and Personal Methods of Maintaining Health, Protecting Health, and Restoring Health

	Physical	Mental	Spiritual
Maintain Health	Proper clothing Proper diet Exercise/rest	Concentration Social and family support systems Hobbies	Religious worship Prayer Meditation
Protect Health	Special foods and food combination Symbolic clothing	Avoid certain individuals who can cause illness Family activities	Religious customs Superstitions Wearing amulets and other symbolic objects to prevent the "evil eye" or defray other sources of harm
Restore Health	Homeopathic remedies Liniments Herbal teas Special foods Massage Acupuncture Moxibustion	Relaxation Exorcism Curanderos and other traditional healers Nerve teas	Religious rituals, special prayers Meditation Traditional healings Exorcism

From *Cultural Diversity in Health and Illness*, 9th ed. (p. 76), by R. E. Spector, 2017, New York, NY: Pearson. Reprinted with permission.

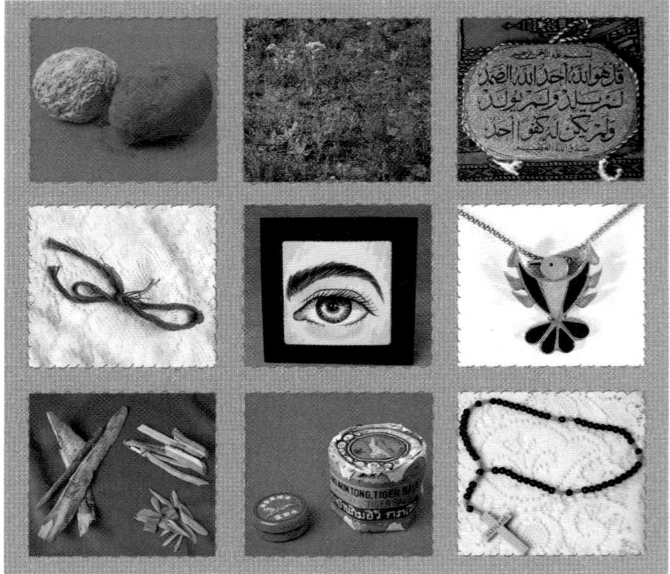

Figure 21.2 ■ Symbols of the HEALTH traditions model and themes.

2. The enjoyment of nature, the natural environment, may be a universal way of maintaining mental HEALTH.
3. The Islamic prayer represents a way of maintaining spiritual HEALTH (East Jerusalem).
4. Red string may be worn to protect physical HEALTH (Tomb of Rachel in Bethlehem, Israel).
5. The eye represents the plethora of eye-related objects that may be worn or hung in the home to protect the mental HEALTH of individuals by shielding them from the envy and bad wishes of others (Cuba).
6. The thunderbird may be worn for spiritual protection and good luck (Hopi Nation).
7. The herbal remedy represents aromatic plants that may be used by individuals from all ethnocultural traditional backgrounds as one method of restoring physical HEALTH (Africa).
8. Tiger balm represents substances that are used in massage therapy as a way of restoring mental HEALTH (Singapore).
9. Rosary beads symbolize prayer and meditation methods used in the spiritual restoration of HEALTH (Italy).

There is an infinite number of examples one could present, and many of these symbols are used across many cultures. A major aspect of conducting the heritage assessment of a client is to determine what items are used by a specific individual and their meaning to the individual.

Providing Culturally Responsive Care

In addition to the new ANA (2015) standard on culturally congruent care, other standards also emphasize culture. Standard 3: Outcomes Identification states "Formulates culturally sensitive expected outcomes derived from assessments and diagnoses" and "Collaborates with the healthcare consumer to define expected outcomes integrating the healthcare consumer's culture, values, and ethical considerations." Standard 5: Implementation states "Provides culturally congruent, holistic care that focuses on the healthcare consumer and addresses and advocates for the needs of diverse populations across the lifespan." Also Standard 9: Communication states "Demonstrates cultural empathy when communicating."

The nurse must gain cultural knowledge regarding clients' various worldviews in order to provide care. The nurse must then use this knowledge by acquiring the awareness, attitudes, and skills to care for diverse populations. Although nurses cannot possibly learn every cultural perspective, they can, at a minimum, become familiar with the cultures within the communities that they serve and be receptive to differing viewpoints. The cultural perspectives in the following sections provide examples and should not serve as the nurse's only cultural knowledge base.

Health Beliefs and Practices

Three commonly held views of health beliefs include magico-religious, scientific, and holistic. In the **magico-religious health belief** view, health and illness are controlled by supernatural forces. The client may believe that illness is the result of "being bad" or opposing the will of the creator(s). Getting well is also viewed as dependent on the will of the creator(s). The client may make statements such as "If it is God's will, I will recover" or "What did I do wrong to be punished with cancer?" Some cultures believe that magic can cause illness. Some individuals view illness as possession by an evil spirit. Others believe a sorcerer or witch may have placed a spell or hex on the client. Although these beliefs are not supported by empirical evidence, clients who hold these beliefs may in fact become ill as a result. Such illnesses may require magical treatments in addition to scientific treatments. For example, a man who experiences headaches after being told that a spell has been placed on him may recover only if the spell is removed by the culture's healer, and he may, in fact, not need a scientific intervention.

The **scientific health belief** or **biomedical health belief** view is based on the belief that life is controlled by physical and biochemical processes that can be manipulated by humans. The client with this view will believe that illness is caused by germs, viruses, bacteria, or a breakdown of the body. This client will expect a pill, treatment, or surgery to cure health problems.

The **holistic health belief** view holds that the forces of nature must be maintained in balance or harmony. Human life is one aspect of nature that must be in harmony with the rest of nature. When the natural balance or harmony is disturbed, illness results. The medicine wheel (Figure 21.3 ■) is an ancient symbol used by Native Americans of North and South America to express many concepts. For health and wellness, the medicine wheel teaches the four aspects of the individual's nature: the physical, the mental, the emotional, and the spiritual. The four dimensions must be in balance to be healthy. The medicine wheel can also

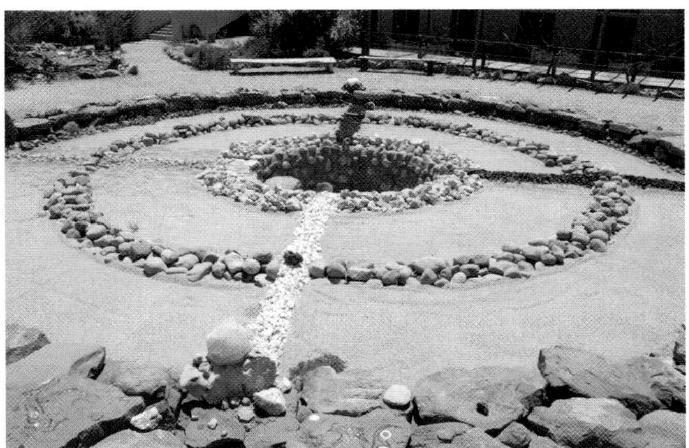

Figure 21.3 ■ A medicine wheel in Arizona.
Nick Hanna/Alamy.

be used to express the individual's relationship with the environment as a dimension of wellness.

The concept of yin and yang (in the Chinese culture) and the hot–cold theory of illness in many cultures (such as Middle Eastern, Spanish, and Asian) are examples of holistic health beliefs. When a Chinese client has a yin illness or a "cold" illness such as cancer, the treatment may include a yang or "hot" food (e.g., hot tea).

What is considered hot or cold varies considerably across cultures. In many cultures, the mother who has just delivered a baby is offered warm or hot foods and kept warm with blankets because childbirth is seen as a "cold" condition. To reduce a fever, conventional scientific thought recommends cooling the body. The primary care provider may order liquids for the client and cool compresses to be applied to the forehead, the axillae, or the groin. In contrast, many cultures believe that the best way to treat a fever is to increase the elimination of toxins through sweat baths. Clients from these cultures may want to cover up with several blankets, take hot baths, and drink hot beverages.

The nurse must keep in mind that a treatment strategy that is consistent with the client's beliefs may have a better chance of being successful. For example, the client who avoids "hot" foods when experiencing a stomach disturbance may be eating foods consistent with the bland diet that is normally prescribed by primary care providers. Even when a practice is different from what would be prescribed, the nurse should consider whether any harm is resulting from the practice and take caution to not judge *different* as *wrong*.

Sociocultural forces, such as politics, economics, geography, religion, and the predominant healthcare system, influence the client's health status and healthcare behavior. For example, someone who has limited access to scientific healthcare may turn to folk medicine or folk healing. **Folk medicine** is defined as those beliefs and practices relating to illness prevention and healing that derive from cultural traditions rather than from modern medicine's scientific base. Many individuals have family members who use special teas or "cures" (e.g., chicken soup) to prevent or treat colds, fevers, indigestion, and other common health problems. Why do individuals use traditional healing methods? Folk medicine is thought to be more humanistic than biomedical healthcare. The consultation and treatment take place in the community of the recipient, frequently in the home of the healer. It may be less expensive than scientific or biomedical care. The healer often prepares the treatments, for example, herbs to be ingested, poultices to be applied, or charms or amulets to be worn. A frequent component of treatment is some ritual practice on the part of the healer or the client to cause healing to occur. Because folk healing is more culturally based than conventional medicine as practiced in the United States, it is often more comfortable and less frightening for the client.

It is important for the nurse to obtain information about folk or family healing practices that may have been used before or while the client used conventional medical treatment. Often clients are reluctant to disclose the use of home remedies to healthcare professionals for fear of being laughed at or rebuked. However, a study on complementary and alternative medicine (CAM) use among adults in 2017 indicated that increasing numbers of adults in the United States had used meditation, yoga, or chiropractic during the previous 12 months (Clarke, Barnes, Black, Stussman, & Nahin, 2018). The increased use of traditional, alternative, and complementary healing practices in the United States represents an opportunity for nurses to inform clients about what the nursing profession offers in this regard (see Chapter 22 ∞).

Clinical Alert!

Treatments once considered to be folk treatments, including acupuncture, therapeutic touch, and massage, are now being investigated for their therapeutic effect. The National Center for Complementary and Integrative Health at the National Institutes of Health provides up-to-date information on this line of research.

Family Patterns

The family is considered the basic unit of society; however, the concept of family is complex and influenced by personal and social values. There is no agreed-on definition of family, and there is great diversity in family types and structures (see Chapter 27 ∞). Cultural values greatly influence communication patterns within the family group, the norm for family size, and the roles of specific family members. In some families, the male is considered the provider and decision maker. The female may need to consult her male partner before making decisions about her or her children's medical treatment. Some families are matriarchal; that is, the mother or grandmother is viewed as the leader of the family and is usually the decision maker. The nurse needs to identify who has the "authority" to make decisions in a client's family. If the decision maker is someone other than the client, the nurse needs to obtain the client's permission and then include that individual in healthcare discussions.

There are other forms of family, including same-sex families. These involve same-sex couples living together (either married or in civil partnership). There are countries like Malta, Iceland, and Norway where same-sex couples can opt to adopt or have children of their own (ILGA-Europe, 2014).

The value placed on children and older adults within a society is culturally derived. In some cultures, children are not disciplined by spanking or other forms of physical punishment. Rather, children are allowed to interact with their environment while caregivers provide subtle direction to prevent harm or injury. Responsibility for caring for older relatives and neighbors is also determined by cultural practices.

Cultural gender-role behavior may also affect nurse–client interactions. In some countries, males dominate and females have little status. Males from these countries may not accept instruction from a female nurse or primary care provider but will be receptive to the same instruction given by a male nurse or primary care provider. Some cultures have a prevailing concept of machismo, or male superiority. The positive aspects of machismo require the adult male provide for and protect his family, including extended family members. The female is expected to maintain the home and raise the children. Thus, female nurses may experience a negative aspect of machismo if it results in challenges in caring for dominant males or for females for whom a dominant male makes health decisions. One approach in this situation is to discuss the challenges with the client and family as they arise and, if appropriate, consult with others knowledgeable about similar situations.

Cultural family values may also dictate the extent of the family's involvement in the hospitalized client's care. In some cultures, only the nuclear and the extended family will want to visit for long periods and participate in care. In other cultures, the entire community may want to visit and participate in the client's care. The nurse should evaluate the positive benefits of family participation in the client's care and adapt visiting policies as appropriate. The nurse must also recognize that family roles often shift during hospitalization.

Cultures that value the needs of the extended family as much as those of the individual may believe that personal and family information must stay within the family. Some cultural groups are very reluctant to disclose family information to outsiders, including healthcare professionals. This attitude can present difficulties for healthcare professionals who require knowledge of family interaction patterns to help clients with emotional problems.

Naming systems in many cultures differ from those common in North America. In some cultures (e.g., Vietnamese), the family name comes first and the given name second. One or two names may be added between the family and given names. Other nomenclature may be used to delineate sex, child, or adult status. For example, in traditional Japanese culture, adults address other adults by their surname followed by *san*, meaning *Mr.*, *Mrs.*, or *Miss*. An example is *Maurakami san*. The children are often referred to by their first names followed by *kun* for boys and *chan* for girls. Sikhs and Hindus traditionally have three names. Sikhs have a personal name, then the title *Singh* for men and *Kaur* for women, and lastly the family name. Hindus usually have a personal name, a complimentary name, and then a family name. Names by marriage also vary. In Central America, a woman who marries often retains her father's name and takes her husband's. For example, if Louisa Viccario marries Carlos Gonzales, she becomes Louisa Viccario de Gonzales. The connecting *de* means "belonging to." Their son is Pedro Gonzales Viccario. Not all members of a specific culture will follow the traditional approach to naming. Nurses need to become familiar with a variety of appropriate ways to address clients and should ask clients about their preferences.

Communication Style

Communication and culture are closely interconnected. Through communication, the culture is transmitted from one generation to the next, and knowledge about the culture is transmitted within the group and to those outside the group. Communicating effectively with clients of various ethnic and cultural backgrounds is critical to providing culturally competent nursing care. Cultural variations are seen in both verbal and nonverbal communication.

There are 15 CLAS standards in three categories: Governance, Leadership, and Workforce; Communication and Language Assistance; and Engagement, Continuous Improvement, and Accountability. Under the category of Communication and Language Assistance, healthcare agencies are required to:

- Offer language assistance to individuals who have limited English proficiency or other communication needs, at no cost to them, to facilitate timely access to all healthcare and services.
- Inform all individuals of the availability of language assistance services clearly and in their preferred language, verbally and in writing.
- Ensure the competence of individuals providing language assistance, recognizing that the use of untrained individuals or minors as interpreters should be avoided.
- Provide easy-to-understand print and multimedia materials and signage in the languages commonly used by the populations in the service area (USDHHS, n.d.).

Verbal Communication

The most obvious cultural difference is in verbal communication: vocabulary, grammatical structure, voice qualities, intonation, rhythm, speed, pronunciation, and silence. In North America, the dominant language is English; however, immigrant groups who speak English still encounter language differences because English words can have different meanings in different English-speaking cultures. For example, in the United States, a *boot* is a type of footwear that comes to the ankle or higher; in England, a boot can also be the trunk of a car. Spanish is spoken by individuals throughout the world. It is the second most commonly spoken language in the United States. Nevertheless, each cultural group that speaks Spanish may speak with different accents and dialects, using different vocabulary, rules of grammar, and pronunciation, so that often two Spanish-speaking individuals of different cultures may not completely understand each other.

PRACTICE GUIDELINES Verbal Communication with Clients Who Have Limited English Proficiency (LEP)

- Avoid slang words, medical terminology, and abbreviations.
- Enhance spoken conversation with congruent gestures or pictures to increase the client's understanding.
- Speak slowly, in a respectful manner, and at a normal volume. Speaking loudly does not help the client understand and may be offensive.
- Frequently validate the client's understanding of what is being communicated. Do not automatically interpret a client's smiling and nodding to mean that the client understands; the client may only be trying to please the nurse and not understand what is being said.
- Use print resources that have been designed especially for clients with LEP.
- Offer clients the opportunity to express themselves through an interpreter's service.
- Keep in mind that certain words and expressions may not have exact English translations.

Initiating verbal communication may be influenced by cultural values. The busy nurse may want to complete nursing admission assessments quickly. The client, however, may be offended when the nurse immediately asks personal questions. In some cultures, social courtesies should be established before business or personal topics are discussed. Discussing general topics can convey that the nurse is interested and has time for the client. This enables the nurse to develop a rapport with the client before progressing to discussion that is more personal.

Verbal communication becomes even more difficult when an interaction involves clients who do not speak a common language. Both clients and health professionals experience frustration when they are unable to communicate verbally with each other. Techniques for therapeutic communication with clients who have limited English are listed in the accompanying Practice Guidelines.

For the client whose language is not the same as that of the healthcare provider, an intermediary may be necessary. A **translator** converts written material (e.g., client education pamphlets) from one language into another. Interpretation moves beyond translation. An **interpreter** is able to transform the message expressed in a spoken or signed source language into its equivalent in a target language so that the interpreted message has the potential of eliciting the same response in the listener as the original message. The clinical encounter is a highly interactive process in which the nurse uses language to understand, evaluate, and provide teaching. Healthcare facilities accredited by The Joint Commission are required to have qualified and competent interpreters available for clients who require them. The interpreter may be on-site, available by telephone, or accessed through videoconferencing. Studies have shown that fewer errors occur when professional (trained) interpreters are used with clients who have limited English proficiency (LEP) (Hu, 2018; Jacobs, Ryan, Henrichs, & Weiss, 2018; Karliner, Pérez-Stable, & Gregorich, 2017). The first U.S. standards for certification of medical interpreters were implemented in 2010 by the National Board of Certification for Medical Interpreters. Many institutions that are located in culturally diverse communities have interpreters available on staff or maintain a list of employees who are fluent in other languages. However, fluency alone in a language does not qualify the individual to be an interpreter—especially about healthcare issues. Embassies, consulates, ethnic churches (e.g., Russian Orthodox, Greek Orthodox), ethnic clubs (e.g., Polish American Club, Italian American Club), or telephone companies may also be able to provide qualified interpreters. Asking a family member or other nonprofessional to interpret can create difficulties. Cultural rules often dictate who can discuss what with whom.

The interpreter must also serve as a **cultural broker** and engage both provider and client effectively and efficiently in accessing the nuances and hidden sociocultural assumptions embedded in each other's language. The cultural broker serves four roles: (1) liaison between the clients or consumers and the providers in the healthcare agency, (2) guide to the healthcare setting on culture-related issues, (3) mediator between the community and the healthcare setting to establish a trusting relationship, and (4) catalyst for positive change (National Center for Cultural Competence, 2004). Guidelines for using an interpreter are listed in the Practice Guidelines.

PRACTICE GUIDELINES Using an Interpreter

- Avoid asking a member of the client's family, especially a child or spouse, to act as interpreter. The client, not wishing family members to know about his or her problem, may not provide complete or accurate information. A child who is used as an interpreter may be exposed to language and concepts that the child is not developmentally ready for.
- Be aware of gender and age differences; it is preferable to use an interpreter of the same gender as the client to avoid embarrassment and faulty translation of sexual matters.
- Choose an interpreter who is politically or socially compatible with the client. For example, a Bosnian Serb may not be the best interpreter for a Muslim, even if he speaks the language, because of possible ethnic, religious, or historical conflicts between the two groups.
- Address the questions to the client, not to the interpreter.
- Ask the interpreter to interpret as closely as possible the words used by the nurse.
- Speak slowly and distinctly. Do not use metaphors, for example, "Does it swell like a grapefruit?" or "Is the pain stabbing like a knife?"
- Observe the facial expressions and body language that the client assumes when listening and talking to the interpreter.
- Become aware of the individual expressions and colloquial words used in specific regions and acknowledge them when using interpreting services.

Nurses and other healthcare providers must remember that clients for whom English is a second language may lose command of their English when they are in stressful situations. Clients who have used English comfortably for years in social and business communication may forget and revert back to their primary language when they are ill or distressed. It is important for the nurse to assure the client that this is normal and to promote behaviors to facilitate verbal communication.

Multilingual nurses may provide nursing care in any language they speak. Nurses who speak more than one language may be asked to interpret for others. However, nursing schools and healthcare institutions may prohibit nurses or nursing students from interpreting for other healthcare providers unless they have received specialized training and are approved as language assistants or medical interpreters. Check the institution's policy before agreeing to interpret for institutional staff and primary care providers.

Nonverbal Communication

To communicate effectively with culturally diverse clients, the nurse needs to be aware of two aspects of nonverbal communication behaviors: what nonverbal behaviors mean to the client and what specific nonverbal behaviors mean in the client's culture. Before assigning meaning to nonverbal behavior, the nurse must consider the possibility that the behavior may have a different meaning for the client and the family. To provide safe and effective care, nurses who work with specific cultural groups should learn more about cultural behavior and communication patterns within these cultures.

Nonverbal communication can include the use of silence, touch, eye movement, facial expressions, and body posture. Some cultures are quite comfortable with long periods of silence, whereas others consider it appropriate to speak before the other individual has finished talking. Many individuals value silence and view it as essential to understanding an individual's needs or use silence to preserve privacy. Some cultures view silence as a sign of respect, whereas to other individuals, silence may indicate agreement.

Touching involves learned behaviors that can have both positive and negative meanings. In the American culture, a firm handshake is a recognized form of greeting that conveys character and strength. In some European cultures, greetings may include a kiss on one or both cheeks. In some societies, because of the belief that the soul can leave the body on physical contact, casual touching is forbidden. In some cultures, only certain older adults are permitted to touch the heads of others, and children are never patted on the head. Nurses should therefore touch a client's head only with permission. Cultures dictate what forms of touch are appropriate for individuals of the same and opposite gender. In many cultures, for example, a kiss is not appropriate for a public greeting between individuals of the opposite sex, even those who are family members; however, a kiss on the cheek is acceptable as a greeting among individuals of the same sex. The nurse should watch interaction among clients and families for cues to the appropriate degree of touch in that culture. The nurse can also assess the client's response to touch when providing nursing care, for example, by noting the client's reaction to the physical examination or the bath. The nurse should also inquire about clients' preferences, inform clients before touching them, and whenever possible, proceed after obtaining permission. For example, "I would like to check your pulse, and I will need to hold your wrist. Is that okay?"

Facial expression can also vary among cultures. In some cultures, individuals are more likely to smile readily and use facial expressions to communicate feelings, whereas in others, individuals may use fewer facial expressions and may be less open in their response, especially to strangers. Facial expressions can also convey a meaning opposite to what is felt or understood.

Eye movement during communication has cultural foundations. In many Western cultures, direct eye contact is regarded as important and generally shows that the other is attentive and listening. It is assumed to convey self-confidence, openness, interest, and honesty. Lack of eye contact may be interpreted as secretiveness, shyness, guilt, lack of interest, or even a sign of mental illness. However, other cultures may view direct eye contact as impolite or an invasion of privacy. In the Hmong culture, for example, continuous direct eye contact is considered rude, but intermittent eye contact is acceptable. The nurse must consider the cultural context to avoid misinterpreting avoidance of eye contact.

Body posture and hand gestures are also culturally learned. For example, the V sign means victory in some cultures, but it is an offensive gesture in other cultures. Giving someone a thumbs up may mean "right" or "great job" in the United States, but is an obscene gesture in many Middle Eastern countries, equivalent to a raised middle finger in the United States. Tapping the index finger on one's temple may mean someone is intelligent in the United States but "crazy" in the Netherlands.

Space Orientation

Space is a relative concept that includes the individual, the body, the surrounding environment, and objects within that environment. The relationship between the individual's own body and objects and individuals within that space is learned and is influenced by culture. For example, in nomadic societies, space is not owned; it is occupied temporarily until the tribe moves on. In many Western societies, individuals tend to be more territorial, as reflected in phrases such as "This is my space" or "Get out of my space." Spatial distances may be defined as the intimate zone, the personal zone, and the social and public zones. The size of these areas may vary with the specific culture. Nurses move through all three zones as they provide care for clients. The nurse needs to be aware of the client's response to movement toward the client. The client may physically withdraw or back away if the nurse is perceived as being too close. The nurse will need to explain to the client why there is a need to be close.

To assess the lungs with a stethoscope, for example, the nurse needs to move into the client's intimate space. The nurse should first explain the procedure and, when possible, await permission to continue.

Clients who reside in long-term care facilities or who are hospitalized for an extended time may want to personalize their space. They may want to arrange the room differently or control the placement of objects on the bedside cabinet. The nurse should be responsive to clients' needs to have some control over their space. When there are no medical contraindications, clients should be permitted and encouraged to have objects of personal significance. Having personal and cultural items in one's environment can increase self-esteem by promoting not only one's individuality but also one's cultural identity. Of course, the nurse should caution the client about the risk for loss or damage of personal items in the healthcare setting.

Time Orientation

Time orientation refers to an individual's focus on the past, the present, or the future. Most cultures include all three time orientations, but one orientation is more likely to dominate. The European American focus on time tends to be directed to the future, emphasizing time and schedules. European Americans often plan for next week, their vacation, or their retirement. Other cultures may have a different concept of time. For example, the Navajo Indians are present and past oriented and do not have a word for "late." A Navajo mother may view her child's development differently from European Americans and might not measure her child's milestones, such as toileting and walking, by the same targeted schedule as other cultures. African Americans are often generalized as present oriented as well, with a focus on current health status rather than the anticipation of what may happen in the future. Socioeconomic status may also influence time orientation. The middle class is generally future oriented; however, lower socioeconomic classes are generally present oriented because of the focus on daily survival, which may not allow for the luxury of being able to plan for the future.

The culture of nursing and healthcare values punctuality and is future oriented. Appointments are scheduled, and treatments are prescribed with time parameters (e.g., changing a dressing once a day). Medication orders include how often a medicine is to be taken and when (e.g., digoxin 0.25 mg, once a day, in the morning). Nurses need to be aware of the meaning of time for clients. When caring for clients who are "present oriented," it is important to avoid fixed schedules. The nurse can offer a time range for activities and treatments. For example, instead of telling the client to take digoxin every day at 10:00 A.M., the nurse might tell the client to take it every day in the morning or every day after getting out of bed.

Nutritional Patterns

Most cultures have staple foods that are plentiful or readily accessible in the environment. For example, the staple food of Asians is usually rice, and for Europeans, it may be bread or pasta. Even clients who have been in the United States for several generations often continue to eat the foods of their cultural homeland.

The way food is prepared and served is also related to cultural practices. For example, in the United States, a traditional food served for the Thanksgiving holiday is stuffed turkey; however, in different regions of the country, the contents of the stuffing may vary. In Southern states, the stuffing may be made of cornbread; in New England, it may be made of seasoned bread and chestnuts.

The way in which staple foods are prepared also varies. For example, some Asian cultures prefer steamed rice; others prefer boiled rice. Southern Asians from India prepare unleavened bread from wheat flour rather than the leavened bread of European Americans.

Food-related cultural behaviors can include whether to breastfeed or bottle-feed infants and when to introduce solid foods to infants. Food can also be considered either the cause or part of the remedy for illness. In some cultures, nutrients such as calcium, iron, potassium, or zinc, which are lacking in the usual diet, are supplemented by eating clay or dirt (Giger, 2017).

The religious practices associated with specific cultures also affect diet. Some Roman Catholics avoid meat on certain days, such as Ash Wednesday and Good Friday, and some Protestant faiths prohibit meat, tea, coffee, or alcohol. Both Orthodox Judaism and Islam prohibit the ingestion of pork or pork products. Orthodox Jews observe kosher customs, eating certain foods only if they have been inspected by a rabbi and prepared according to certain dietary laws. For example, the eating of milk products and meat products at the same meal is prohibited. Some Buddhists, Hindus, and Sikhs are strict vegetarians. The nurse must be sensitive to such religious dietary practices.

●○● NURSING MANAGEMENT

All phases of the nursing process are affected by the client's and the nurse's cultural values, beliefs, and behaviors. As the client's culture and the nurse's culture come together in the nurse–client relationship, a unique cultural environment is created that can improve or impair the client's outcome. Self-awareness of personal biases can enable nurses to develop modifying behaviors or (if they are unable to do so) to remove themselves from situations where care may be compromised. Nurses can become more aware of their own culture through values clarification (see Chapter 4 ∞). The nurse must also consider the cultural values dominant in the healthcare setting because those, too, may influence the client's outcome.

Developing Self-Awareness

In learning how to provide culturally responsive care, the nurse must first understand his or her own culture, beliefs, and assumptions. Many models have been documented in the literature to deepen this self-exploration (Albougami,

Pounds, & Alotaibi, 2016). Campinha-Bacote (2007) offers the ASKED mnemonic model to develop cultural consciousness: Awareness, Skill, Knowledge, Encounters, Desire. Using this model, nurses reflect on questions that focus on how well prepared they are to acknowledge their own biases, their openness to embracing differences in individuals, and their willingness to learn appropriate means of communicating and caring for diverse populations.

Other self-identity questions may include the following (Tochluk, 2016):

- When did you first realize you were a member of your culture/race/ethnicity? What did it mean to you at that time?
- How did your culture/race/ethnicity play a role in your childhood and adolescence?
- What important events changed your relationship to culture/race/ethnicity? What happened?
- What significant individuals and relationships shaped the way you experience being a member of your culture/race/ethnicity?
- How do you understand what it means to be a member of your culture/race/ethnicity at this time in your life?

Health-related questions may include:

- How does your ethnic/racial group view health and illness?
- What are the common healing practices in your cultural/ethnic/racial group?
- What are examples of your family's traditional health and illness beliefs and practices?
- Do they value stoic behavior in relation to pain, or is it permissible to state that you are in pain? Are the rights of the individual valued over and above the rights of the family?
- What is your view on health? How does it compare to your family's view of health?
- What beliefs do you hold about healthcare providers?

Conveying Cultural Sensitivity

Box 21.1 lists texts authored by nurses that may be helpful in developing cultural knowledge. The process of cultural assessment is important. How and when questions are asked requires sensitivity and clinical judgment. The timing and phrasing of questions need to be adapted to the individual. Timing is important in introducing questions. Sensitivity is needed in phrasing questions. Trust must be established before clients can be expected to volunteer and share sensitive information. The nurse therefore needs to spend time with clients and convey a genuine desire to understand their values and beliefs.

Before conducting a cultural assessment, determine what language the client speaks and the client's degree of fluency in the English language. It is also important to learn about the client's communication patterns and space orientation. This is accomplished by observing both verbal and nonverbal communication. For example, does the client do the speaking or defer to another? What nonverbal communication behaviors does the client exhibit (e.g., touching, eye contact)? What significance do these behaviors have for the nurse–client interaction? What is the client's proximity to other individuals and objects within the environment? How does the client react to the nurse's movement toward the client? What cultural objects within the environment have importance for health promotion or health maintenance?

It is vital for nurses to be culturally sensitive and to convey this sensitivity to clients, support people, and other healthcare personnel. Some ways to do so follow:

- Always address clients, support people, and other healthcare personnel by their last names (e.g., Mrs. Aylia, Dr. Rush) until they give you permission to use other names. In some cultures, the more formal style of address is a sign of respect, whereas the informal use of first names may be considered disrespectful. It is important to ask individuals how they wish to be addressed.
- When meeting an individual for the first time, introduce yourself by your full name, and then explain your role (e.g., "My name is Alicia Bernett, and I am a nursing student at Nightingale School of Nursing"). This helps establish a relationship and provides an opportunity for clients, others, and nurses to learn the pronunciation of one another's names and their roles.
- Be authentic with individuals, and be honest about your knowledge about their culture. When you do not understand an individual's actions, politely and respectfully seek information.
- Use language that is culturally sensitive; for example, say "gay," "lesbian," or "bisexual" rather than "homosexual"; do not use "man" or "mankind" when referring to a woman.

BOX 21.1 Selected Nurse-Authored Texts

Andrews, J. D., & Boyle, J. S. (2016). *Transcultural concepts in nursing care* (7th ed.). Philadelphia, PA: Wolters Kluwer.
Giger, J. N. (2017). *Transcultural nursing: Assessment and intervention* (7th ed.). St. Louis, MO: Mosby.
Holland, K. (2018). *Cultural awareness in nursing and health care: An introductory text* (3rd ed.). New York, NY: Routledge.
Jeffreys, M. R. (2016). *Teaching cultural competence in nursing and health care: Inquiry, action, and innovation* (3rd ed.). New York, NY: Springer.
McFarland, M. R., & Wehbe-Alamah, H. B. (2018). *Leininger's culture care diversity and universality: A worldwide nursing theory* (4th ed.). New York, NY: McGraw Hill.
Papadopoulos, I. (2018). *Culturally competent compassion: A guide for healthcare students and practitioners*. New York, NY: Routledge.
Ray, M. (2016). *Transcultural caring dynamics in nursing and health care* (2nd ed.). Philadelphia, PA: F. A. Davis.
Skemp, L. E. &. Dreher, M. C., Lehman, S. P. (2016). *Healthy places, healthy people* (3rd ed.). Indianapolis, IN: Sigma Theta Tau International.
Spector, R. E. (2017). *Cultural diversity in health and illness* (9th ed.). New York, NY: Pearson.

- Ask how the client self-identifies his or her race/ethnicity. The client may have a preferred term, such as Latino rather than Hispanic. Make note of the client's preferences, and use the language preferred by the client.
- Find out what the client thinks about his or her health problems, illness, and treatments. Assess whether this information is congruent with the dominant healthcare culture. If the beliefs and practices are incongruent, determine the impact on the client's health.
- Always ask about anything you do not understand to avoid making assumptions about the client.
- Show respect for the client's values, beliefs, and practices, even if they differ from your own or from those of the dominant culture. If you do not agree with them, it is important to respect the client's right to hold these beliefs.
- Show respect for the client's support people. In some cultures, males in the family make decisions affecting the client, whereas in other cultures, females make the decisions.
- Make a concerted effort to obtain the client's trust, but do not be surprised if it develops slowly or not at all. A cultural assessment may take time and may need to extend over several meetings.
- Should you inadvertently do something to offend the client, be humble, admit that you made a mistake, and excuse yourself. Learn from experience.

Assessing

In creating a plan of care that is culturally responsive, many assessment tools are available. The tools are a way of interviewing and facilitating communication with clients and their families and may be used in any setting. The LEARN model and the 4 C's are quick assessment tools to better understand the client's perspective. LEARN is a commonly used tool (Berlin & Fowkes, 1983):

Listen actively with empathy to the client's perception of the problem.
Explain what you think you heard or ask for clarification.
Acknowledge the importance of what is said and what it means.
Recommend inclusive strategies.
Negotiate the plan of care by collaborating with the client and others.

The 4 C's of Culture were developed by Slavin, Galanti, and Kuo (Developed by Stuart Slavin, MD, Geri-Ann Galanti, PhD, and Alice Kuo, MD. www.ggalanti.org).

1. What do you *call* your problem? (Remember to ask "What do you think is wrong?" or "What is concerning or worrying you?" to get at the client's perception of the problem. You should not literally ask, "What do you call your problem?")
2. What do you think *caused* your problem? (This gets at the client's beliefs regarding the source of the problem.)
3. How do you *cope* with your condition? (You may want to phrase this as "What have you done to try to make it better? Who else have you been to for treatment?")
4. What are your *concerns* regarding the condition and/or recommended treatment? (This should address questions such as "How serious do you think this is?" "What potential complications do you fear?" "How does it interfere with your life, or your ability to function?" "Do you know anyone else who has tried the treatment I've recommended? What was their experience with it?")

The Heritage Assessment Interview (Spector, 2017) depicts the questions to ask when conducting a heritage assessment. It is designed to enhance the process in order to determine if clients are identifying with their traditional cultural heritage (**heritage consistent**) or if they have acculturated into the local culture in which they reside (**heritage inconsistent**). The tool may be used in any setting and is used to facilitate conversation and help in the planning of cultural care. When using the tool, the nurse may need to ask additional questions to allow the client to expand

EVIDENCE-BASED PRACTICE

Evidence-Based Practice

What Literature Is Available for Nurses About Older Amish Adults' Culture and Healthcare Experiences?

Older Amish adults are a growing population in the United States and have unique risks for healthcare disparities. Limited information is available about the caregiving needs of Amish older adults or their interactions with Western healthcare systems. This information is needed for nurses to develop interventions to reduce health disparity risks and promote culturally congruent care. Farrar, Kulig, and Sullivan-Wilson (2018) performed an integrative review of the literature between 1985 and 2016 about Amish older adult caregivers and their healthcare experiences. Twenty-seven publications were included in the final analysis, which addressed the characteristics of Amish caregivers of older adults, locations of caregiving, descriptive information about Amish older adult health and illness, and how decisions are made in Amish communities to access Western healthcare.

Implications

Nurses commonly care for clients whose culture and background are markedly different from their own. Research and descriptive publications, especially regarding smaller, unique groups of clients such as older Amish adults, can be essential to inform the nurse. This research provides specific material about the Amish but also highlights the importance of research and publications about underrepresented groups. In addition, the authors suggest that what is learned from studies of the Amish may have broader implications for other cultural groups in the United States.

on the yes or no answers. If appropriate, the nurse should modify the tool to add or eliminate items based on the nurse's cultural sensitivity. Once a conversation begins and the client describes aspects of cultural heritage, it becomes possible to develop an understanding of the client's unique health and illness beliefs, practices, and cultural needs. For example, you may discover that the individual participates in ethnic cultural events and social groups, such as religious festivals or national holidays, sometimes with singing, dancing, and costumes (Figure 21.4 ■).

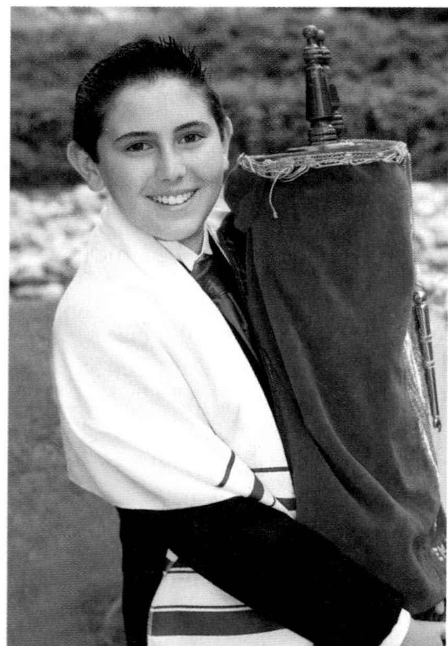

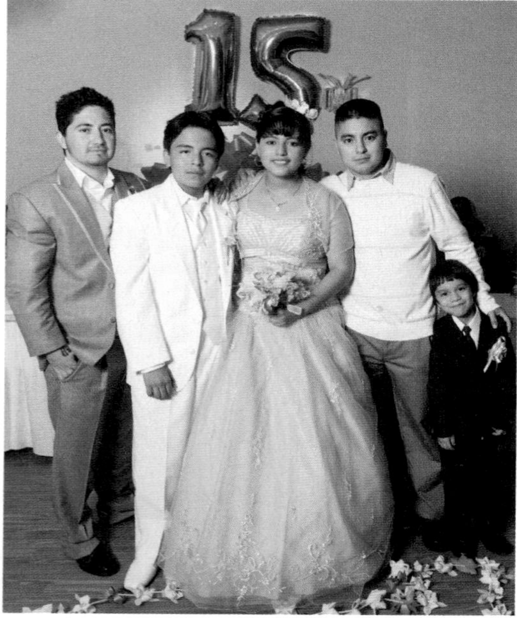

Figure 21.4 ■ Celebrations of the passage to adulthood are often based on culture or religion; for example, the Jewish bar mitzvah at age 13 and the Latin American quinceañera or fifteenth birthday celebration.
(Top) Gordon Swanson/Shutterstock; (Bottom) Erin Patrice O'Brien/Taxi/Getty Images.

Or you may learn that the client's childhood development occurred in the client's country of origin or in an immigrant community in the United States. For example, the client was raised in a specific ethnic neighborhood, such as an Italian, African American, Hispanic, or Jewish one, in a given part of a city and was exposed only to the culture, language, foods, and customs of that particular group. There are infinite examples of cultural influences on the client's health.

Diagnosing

The nursing diagnoses in the United States are focused on nursing care provided in that country and are based on European-centric cultural beliefs. It is essential to expand the understanding of nursing practice to include beliefs of other cultures when naming nursing diagnoses or problem statements. Nurses must provide appropriate care to clients of any culture. This is accomplished through developing cultural sensitivity and considering how a client's culture influences his or her responses to health conditions, much as the nurse considers how a client's age or gender influences a nursing diagnosis, the nursing plan, and the delivery of nursing care.

Planning

Providing culturally responsive care is an ongoing process that requires an individual or organization to develop along a continuum until diversity is accepted as a norm and the nurse has acquired greater understanding and capacity in a diverse environment. The knowledge and skills necessary to incorporate cultural care as a fundamental component of nursing require the acquisition of a broad base of knowledge about different cultures and social structures (Box 21.2). As one's knowledge and skills grow, the ability to convey cultural sensitivity also grows.

The following are examples of the necessary steps:

1. Become aware of one's own cultural heritage.
2. Become aware of the client's heritage and health traditions as described by the client.
3. Become aware of adaptations the client made to live in another culture. During this part of the interview, a nurse can also identify the client's preferences in health practices, diet, hygiene, and so on.
4. Form a nursing plan with the client that incorporates cultural beliefs regarding the maintenance, protection, and restoration of health. In this way, the client's cultural values, practices, and beliefs can be incorporated with the necessary nursing care.

Implementing

The implementation of culturally responsive nursing care includes (a) cultural preservation and maintenance and (b) cultural accommodation and negotiation. Cultural preservation may involve the use of cultural healthcare

ASSESSMENT INTERVIEW Heritage Assessment Tool

This set of questions is used to describe an individual's (or your own) ethnic, cultural, and religious background. The *heritage assessment* is helpful to determine how deeply a given individual identifies with his or her *traditional* heritage. This assessment is very useful in setting the stage for understanding an individual's traditional health and illness beliefs and practices and in helping to determine the family and community resources that will be appropriate for support when necessary. The greater the number of positive responses, the greater the degree to which the individual may identify with his or her traditional heritage. The one exception to positive answers is the question about whether an individual's name was changed.

1. Where was your mother born? ____
2. Where was your father born? ____
3. Where were your grandparents born?
  a. Your mother's mother? ____
  b. Your mother's father? ____
  c. Your father's mother? ____
  d. Your father's father? ____
4. How many brothers ____ and sisters ____ do you have?
5. What setting did you grow up in? Urban ____ Suburban ____ Rural ____
6. What country did your parents grow up in?
  Father ____
  Mother ____
7. How old were you when you came to the United States?
____
8. How old were your parents when they came to the United States?
  Mother ____
  Father ____
9. When you were growing up, who lived with you?
____
10. Have you maintained contact with
  1. Aunts, uncles, cousins? (1) Yes ____ (2) No ____
  2. Brothers and sisters? (1) Yes ____ (2) No ____
  3. Parents? (1) Yes ____ (2) No ____
  4. Your own children? (1) Yes ____ (2) No ____
11. Did most of your aunts, uncles, cousins live near your home?
  1. Yes ____
  2. No ____
12. Approximately how often did you visit family members who lived outside of your home?
  1. Daily ____
  2. Weekly ____
  3. Monthly ____
  4. Once a year or less ____
  5. Never ____
13. Was your original family name changed?
  1. Yes ____
  2. No ____
14. What is your religious preference?
  1. Catholic ____
  2. Jewish ____
  3. Protestant ______ Denomination ____
  4. Islam ____
  5. Buddhist ____
  6. Hindu ___
  7. Other ____
  8. None ____
15. Is your spouse/partner the same religion as you?
  1. Yes ____
  2. No ____
16. Is your spouse/partner from the same ethnic background as you?
  1. Yes ____
  2. No ____
17. What kind of school did you go to?
  1. Public ____
  2. Private ____
  3. Parochial ____
18. As an adult, do you live in a neighborhood where the neighbors are the same religion and ethnic background as you?
  1. Yes ____
  2. No ____
19. Do you belong to a religious institution?
  1. Yes ____
  2. No ____
20. Would you describe yourself as an active member?
  1. Yes ____
  2. No ____
21. How often do you attend your religious institution?
  1. More than once a week
  2. Weekly ____
  3. Monthly ____
  4. Special holidays only ____
  5. Never ____
22. Do you practice your religion in your home?
  1. Yes ____ (if yes, please specify by checking activities below)
    Praying ____
    Bible reading ____
    Diet ____
    Celebrating religious holidays ____
  2. No ____
23. Do you prepare foods special to your ethnic or religious background?
  1. Yes ____
  2. No ____
24. Do you participate in ethnic activities?
  1. Yes ____ (if yes, please specify) ____
    Singing ____
    Holiday celebrations ____
    Dancing ____
    Festivals ____
    Costumes ____
  2. No ____
25. Are your friends from the same religious background as you?
  1. Yes ____
  2. No ____
26. Are your friends from the same ethnic background as you?
  1. Yes ____
  2. No ____
27. What is your native language other than English? ____
28. Do you speak this language?
  1. Yes ____
  2. Occasionally ____
  3. No ____
29. Do you read your native (other than English) language?
  1. Yes
  2. No

From *Cultural Diversity in Health & Illness*, 9th ed. (pp. 276–278), by R. E. Spector, 2017, New York, NY: Pearson Education.

BOX 21.2 Selected Cultural Health-Related Practices

Note that these practices may or may not be applicable to the client you are caring for; they are generalizations of practices common among members of certain cultural groups. Caution must be exercised to not convert a generalization into a stereotype.

- Coining and cupping are traditional medical practices. They should not be misinterpreted as abuse.
- Fevers may be treated by wrapping the ill individual in warm blankets and having him or her drink warm liquids.
- Hot liquids, such as tea, may be preferred over ice water.
- Adherence to traditional treatment may be very different from the expected adherence to modern medicine. Care must be taken to fully explain instructions, such as taking antibiotics for the entire course, even after symptoms have disappeared.
- Menstruation may be viewed as the body's way of clearing dirty and excess blood. Too little flow may be viewed as "bad blood" staying in the body; too much flow may be viewed as weakening the body. May influence views of birth control.
- May avoid dairy products due to lactose intolerance. Check for family history.
- The focus on present time may interfere with the use of preventive medicine and follow-up care.
- Postpartum rest is valued.
- Sponge baths may be preferred to showers or tub baths after giving birth.
- Strong beliefs in fate and external control over events may lead to less adherence to medical regimens.

practices, such as giving herbal tea, chicken soup, or "hot" foods to the ill client. The tasks of accommodating a client's viewpoint and negotiating appropriate care require expert communication skills, such as responding empathetically, validating information, and effectively summarizing content. Negotiation is a collaborative process. It acknowledges that the nurse–client relationship is reciprocal and that different views exist of health, illness, and treatment. The nurse attempts to bridge the gap between the nurse's scientific and the client's cultural perspectives. During the negotiation process, the client's views are explored and acknowledged. Relevant scientific information is then provided. If the client's views reveal that certain behaviors would not affect the client's condition adversely, then they are incorporated into the care plan. If the client's views can lead to harmful behavior or outcomes, then an attempt is made to educate the client on the scientific view.

Nurses should determine precisely how a client is managing an illness, what practices could be harmful, and which practices can be safely combined. For example, reducing dosages of an antihypertensive medication or replacing insulin therapy with herbal measures may be detrimental. Some herbal remedies are synergistic with modern medicines, and others are antagonistic; therefore, it is necessary to fully inform the client about the possible outcomes. Consider these examples of potential conflicts between cultural beliefs or practices and the American healthcare system. The nurse does not assume that all members of a group make the same healthcare decisions and must always determine the particular client or family beliefs.

- Some women may value large body size and may be resistant to weight control.
- The decision to circumcise male infants, often made based on cultural and family beliefs, can occasionally conflict with medical advice.
- Some Hispanic/Latino or Asian clients may be unable to obtain hospice care if family members do not permit the client to be informed of the diagnosis or prognosis.
- Most members of the Jehovah's Witness faith do not accept blood transfusions even in life-threatening situations.
- Traditional Orthodox Sikhs do not cut their hair. This can conflict with the need to shave the hair for medical procedures.

When a client chooses to follow only cultural practices and declines all prescribed medical or nursing interventions, the nurse and client must adjust the client goals. Monitoring the client's condition to identify changes in health and to recognize impending crises before they become irreversible may be all that is realistically achievable. At a time of crisis, the opportunity may arise to renegotiate care.

Providing culturally responsive care can be challenging. It requires the discovery of the meaning of the client's behavior, flexibility, creativity, and knowledge to adapt nursing interventions. An effort must be made to learn from each experience. This knowledge will improve the delivery of culture-specific care to future clients.

Evaluating

In evaluating nursing care that incorporates the client's cultural perspectives, the actual client outcomes are compared with the goals and expected outcomes established following a comprehensive assessment that includes cultural sensitivity. However, if the outcomes are not achieved, the nurse should be especially careful to consider whether the client's belief system has been adequately included as an influencing factor.

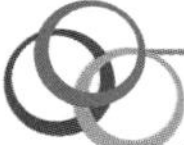

Critical Thinking Checkpoint

Rachel was born to a Jewish couple and lists her religion as Jewish. Her father died when she was 10 years old, and her mother remarried 3 years later. Rachel was legally adopted by her Italian stepfather, who was a devout Catholic. Although the family participated in Catholic and Italian traditions, Rachel's mother taught her many Jewish traditions as well so that her heritage would be preserved. Rachel is now 58 years old, practices traditions from both her Jewish and Italian upbringing, and is dying of cancer. You are the nurse caring for Rachel during her final days.

1. Differentiate between Rachel's culture and ethnicity.
2. How might Rachel's multicultural background affect you as her nurse or in working with her family?
3. How might Rachel's culture affect her approach to death and the care of her body following her death?
4. Of what benefit would a cultural assessment be to Rachel or her family given that she is dying?
5. How could nurses' culture or religion influence their care of clients who are racially or culturally different?

Answers to Critical Thinking Checkpoint questions are available on the faculty resources site. Please consult with your instructor.

Chapter 21 Review

CHAPTER HIGHLIGHTS

- Culturally responsive care requires the nurse to develop self-awareness and gain the attitudes, knowledge, and skills to incorporate each client's cultural perspectives into the plan of care.
- Individuals may live within their traditional heritage, or they may embrace both their original ethnocultural traditional heritage(s) and the culture of the country they are living in.
- Nurses should understand the *National Standards for Culturally and Linguistically Appropriate Services in Health Care* (CLAS) and apply them to their professional practice.
- *Healthy People 2020* calls for nursing to contribute to eliminating health disparities by gender, race or ethnicity, education, income, disability, geographic location, and sexual orientation.
- Racial and Ethnic Approaches to Community Health Across the United States (REACH U.S.) is an initiative that strives to eliminate racial and ethnic disparities in infant mortality, deficits in breast and cervical cancer screening/management, cardiovascular diseases, diabetes, HIV infections, AIDS, and child and adult immunizations.
- Acculturation is a two-way process. The minority groups accept the culture of their host country, and the host country is also influenced by the culture of the minority groups.
- Personal characteristics also modify an individual's cultural values, beliefs, and practices.
- Health beliefs and practices, family patterns, communication style, space and time orientation, and nutritional patterns may influence the relationship between the nurse and the client who have different cultural backgrounds.
- When assessing a client, the nurse considers the client's cultural values, beliefs, and practices related to health and healthcare.

TEST YOUR KNOWLEDGE

1. A community health nurse is learning about the REACH initiative and has decided to implement community education. Which of the following topics relate to this approach? Select those that apply.
   1. Child and adult immunizations
   2. Cardiovascular disease
   3. Chronic lower respiratory disease
   4. Stroke
   5. Infant mortality

2. A home health client participates in cultural health practices that the nurse feels may be detrimental to his health. In order to remain attentive to cultural sensitivity and provide appropriate cultural nursing care, what should the nurse do?
   1. Explain the right and wrong of the client's treatment and try to persuade him to follow the scientific perspective.
   2. Have the client's physician explain the care to the client in a firm but gentle manner.
   3. Validate the client's practices and understand that for this client it may be beneficial to continue with his preferences.
   4. Try to negotiate with the client by exploring his views and then provide relevant scientific information.

3. In initiating care for a client from a different culture than the nurse, which of the following would be an appropriate statement?
   1. "Because in your culture, individuals don't drink ice water, I will bring you hot tea."
   2. "Do you have any books I could read about individuals of your culture?"
   3. "Please let me know if I do anything that is not acceptable in your culture."
   4. "You will need to set aside your usual customs and practices while you are in the hospital."

4. Which of the following statements shows a nurse's understanding of the term *culture*? Select all that apply.
   1. "Culture involves groups who share biological markers."
   2. "Cultures seldom have diversity within them."
   3. "Male nurses are an example of a culture."
   4. "A culture is primarily exhibited through shared thoughts, actions, and beliefs."
   5. "A culture shapes its members' view of the world."

5. An outcome of achieving national cultural health goals would be which of the following?
1. All cultures receive the same healthcare.
2. All individuals have the same life expectancy.
3. All U.S. residents have access to the same quality of healthcare.
4. All cultures are fully assimilated into the dominant society.

6. Which nursing action primarily supports restoring HEALTH using traditional methods?
1. Herbal teas
2. Prayer
3. Wearing symbolic objects
4. Exercise

7. A client with strong preferences for folk healing methods would prefer which of the following to treat a sinus infection?
1. Hospitalization
2. Steam humidifier
3. Antibiotic therapy
4. "Watch and wait"

8. Which factors are most likely to be influenced by culture as opposed to personal characteristics? Select all that apply.
1. Value of older adults in society
2. Gender roles
3. Nonverbal gestures
4. Skill with technology
5. Intelligence
6. Diet

9. What does acculturation entail?
1. Changing careers.
2. Holidaying in a country whose culture differs from yours.
3. Changing one's lifestyle by picking up traits from another culture.
4. Being visited by friends from another country.

10. Which of the following actions would be the correct way for a nurse to provide culturally competent care to a client who has recently immigrated to Malta?
1. Explain to the client all about the culture of the host country.
2. Avoid making assumptions and clear doubts about client behavior that they do not understand.
3. Convince the client to conform and submit to the culture of the host country.

See Answers to Test Your Knowledge in Appendix A.

READINGS AND REFERENCES

Suggested Reading

Relf, M. V. (2016). Advancing diversity in academic nursing. *Journal of Professional Nursing*, *32*(5S), S42–S47. doi:10.1016/j.profnurs.2016.02.010

This article examines the role that accreditation agencies and innovative programs, such as pipeline programs and academic–service scholarship programs, could play in promoting diversity in the future nursing workforce.

Related Research

Hassankhani, H., Haririan, H., Porter, J. E., & Heaston, S. (2018). Cultural aspects of death notification following cardiopulmonary resuscitation. *Journal of Advanced Nursing, 74*(7), 1564–1572. doi:10.1111/jan.13558

Henderson, S., Horne, M., Hills, R., & Kendall, E. (2018). Cultural competence in healthcare in the community: A concept analysis. *Health & Social Care in the Community, 26*(4), 590–603. doi:10.1111/hsc.12556

References

Agency for Healthcare Research and Quality. (2018). *2017 national healthcare quality and disparities report* (AHRQ Publication No. 17-0001). Rockville, MD: Author. Retrieved from https://www.ahrq.gov/research/findings/nhqrdr/nhqdr17/index.html

Albougami, A.S., Pounds, K. G., & Alotaibi, J. S. (2016). Comparison of four cultural competence models in transcultural nursing: A discussion paper. *International Archives of Nursing and Health Care 2*. doi:10.23937/2469-5823/1510053

American Anthropological Association. (1998). *AAA statement on race*. Retrieved from http://www.aaanet.org/stmts/racepp.htm

American Association of Colleges of Nursing. (2008). *Cultural competency in baccalaureate nursing education*. Retrieved from https://www.aacnnursing.org/Portals/42/AcademicNursing/CurriculumGuidelines/Cultural-Competency-Bacc-Edu.pdf

American Nurses Association. (2015). *Nursing: Scope and standards of practice* (3rd ed.). Silver Spring, MD: Author.

Australian Bureau of Statistics. (2020). *3412.0 – Migration, Australia, 2018–19*. Retrieved from https://www.abs.gov.au/statistics/people/population/migration-australia/latest-release12018-19#:~:text=(c)%20Proportion%20of%20the%20total,cent%20who%20were%20international%20students

Australian Institute of Health and Welfare. (2019). *Australia's health 2018 – in brief*. Retrieved from: https://www.aihw.gov.au/getmedia/fe037cf1-0cd0-4663-a8c0-67cd09b1f30c/aihw-aus-222.pdf.aspx?inline=true

Baeten, R., Spasova, S., Vanherchke, B., & Coster, S. (2018). *Inequality in access to healthcare. A study of national policies 2018*. Brussels. European Commission.

Berlin, E. A., & Fowkes, W. C. (1983). A teaching framework for cross-cultural health care. *Western Journal of Medicine, 139*, 934–938.

Bhugun, D. (2017). Parenting advice for intercultural couples: a systematic perspective. *Journal of Family Therapy, (39)*3, 454–477. doi:10.1111/1467-6427.12156

Bornstein, M. H. (2015). Culture, Parenting, and Zero-to-Threes. *Zero Three, 35*(4), 2–9.

Brown, C., Harrison, D., Ziglio, E., & Burns, H. (2014). *Governance for Health Equity – taking forward equity values and goals of health 2020 in the WHO European Region*. Denmark. World Health Organization.

Campinha-Bacote, J. (2007). *The process of cultural competence in the delivery of healthcare services: The journey continues* (5th ed.). Cincinnati, OH: Transcultural C.A.R.E. Associates.

Centers for Disease Control and Prevention. (2018). *About CDC's Office of Minority Health & Health Equity: Mission*. Retrieved from https://www.cdc.gov/healthequity/about

Crippen, C. & Brew, L. (2007). Intercultural Parenting and the Transcultural Family: A Literature Review. *The Family Journal, (15)2*. doi:10.1177/1066480706297783.

Crippen, C. (2008). Cross-cultural parenting: experiences of intercultural parents and constructions of culturally diverse families (unpublished doctoral dissertation). University of New England, Australia.

Clarke, T. C., Barnes, P. M., Black, L. I., Stussman, B. J., & Nahin, R. L. (2018). *Use of yoga, meditation, and chiropractors among U.S. adults aged 18 and over* (National Center for Health Statistics Data Brief No. 325). Retrieved from https://www.cdc.gov/nchs/data/databriefs/db325-h.pdf

Eurostat. (2018). Database. Retrieved from https://ec.europa.eu/eurostat/data/database

Forster, T., Kentikelenis, A., & Bambra, C. (2018). *Health Inequalities in Europe: Setting the Stage for Progressive Policy Action*. Dublin, Ireland. TASC. Retrieved from https://www.researchgate.net/publication/328610704_Health_Inequalities_in_Europe_Setting_the_Stage_for_Progressive_Policy_Action

Farrar, H. M., Kulig, J. C., & Sullivan-Wilson, J. (2018). Older adult caregiving in the Amish: An integrative review. *Journal of Cultural Diversity, 25*(2), 54–65.

Ferro, M. A., Leis, A., Doll, R., Chiu, L., Chung, M., & Barroetavena, M.C. (2007). The impact of acculturation on the use of traditional Chinese medicine in newly diagnosed Chinese cancer patients. *Supportive Care in Cancer 15*(8), 985–992. doi:10.1007/s00520-007-0285-0

Giger, J. N. (2017). *Transcultural nursing: Assessment and intervention* (7th ed.). St. Louis. MO: Mosby.

Hu, P. (2018). Language barriers: How professional interpreters can enhance patient care. *Radiologic Technology, 89*(4), 409–412.

Humes, K. R., Jones, N. A., & Ramirez, R. R. (2011). *Overview of race and Hispanic origin: 2010*. Retrieved from http://www.census.gov/prod/cen2010/briefs/c2010br-02.pdf

International Monetary Fund. (2010). Republic of Tajikistan: Poverty Reduction Strategy Paper. Retrieved from https://www.imf.org/external/pubs/ft/scr/2010/cr10104.pdf

Jacobs, B., Ryan, A. M., Henrichs, K. S., & Weiss, B. D. (2018). Medical interpreters in outpatient practice. *Annals of Family Medicine, 16*(1), 70–76. doi:10.1370/afm.2154

Jeffreys, M. R. (2016). *Teaching cultural competence in nursing and health care: Inquiry, action, and innovation* (3rd ed.). New York, NY: Springer.

Karliner, L. S., Pérez-Stable, E. J., & Gregorich, S. E. (2017). Convenient access to professional interpreters in the hospital decreases readmission rates and estimated hospital expenditures for patients with limited English proficiency. *Medical Care, 55*(3), 199–206. doi:10.1097/MLR.0000000000000643

Mathews, K., Phelan, J., Jones, N. A., Konya, S., Marks, R., Pratt, B. M., . . . Bentley, M. (2017). *2015 National content test race and ethnicity analysis report*. U.S. Census Bureau. Retrieved from https://www2.census.gov/programs-surveys/decennial/2020/program-management/final-analysis-reports/2015nct-race-ethnicity-analysis.pdf

McFarland, M. R., & Wehbe-Alamah, H. B. (2018). *Leininger's culture care diversity and universality: A worldwide nursing theory* (4th ed.). New York, NY: McGraw-Hill.

Mladovski, P. (2007). *Migration and health in the EU*. European Commission. Retrieved from https://www.euro.who.int/__data/assets/pdf_file/0019/161560/e96458.pdf

National Center for Cultural Competence, Georgetown University Center for Child and Human Development, Georgetown University Medical Center. (2004). *Bridging the cultural divide in health care settings: The essential role of cultural broker programs*. Retrieved from https://nccc.georgetown.edu/culturalbroker//Cultural_Broker_EN.pdf

National Institutes of Health. (2015). *Racial and ethnic categories and definitions for NIH diversity programs and for other reporting purposes* (Notice Number: NOT-OD-15-089). Retrieved from http://grants.nih.gov/grants/guide/notice-files/NOT-OD-15-089.html

National Partnership for Action to End Health Disparities. (2011). *National stakeholder strategy for achieving health equity*. Retrieved from https://www.minorityhealth.hhs.gov/npa/files/Plans/NSS/CompleteNSS.pdf

Office of Management and Budget. (1997). Recommendations from the Interagency Committee for the review of the racial and ethnic standards to the Office of Management and Budget concerning changes to the standards for the classification of federal data on race and ethnicity. *Federal Register, 62*, 36874–36946.

Orgera, K., & Artiga, S. (2018). *Disparities in health and health care: Five key questions and answers*. Kaiser Family Foundation. Retrieved from http://files.kff.org/attachment/Issue-Brief-Disparities-in-Health-and-Health-Care-Five-Key-Questions-and-Answers

Owen, J. D. (2002). *Mixed matches: interracial marriage in Australia*. Sydney. University of New South Wales Press.

Parekh, N., & Rose, T. (2011). Health inequalities of the Roma in Europe: A literature review. *Central European Journal of Public Health, 19,* 139–142. doi:10.21101/cejph.a3661.

Public Health Scotland (2021). Improving Health. Retrieved from http://www.healthscotland.scot/reducing-health-inequalities/take-the-right-actions

Radford, J., & Budiman, A. (2018). *Facts on U.S. immigrants, 2016: Statistical portrait of the foreign-born population in the United States*. Pew Research Center. Retrieved from http://www.pewhispanic.org/2018/09/14/facts-on-u-s-immigrants-current-data

Russell, M., Pogemiller, H., & Barnett, E. D. (2018). *CDC health information for international travel: Newly arrived immigrants & refugees*. Retrieved from https://wwwnc.cdc.gov/travel/yellowbook/2018/advising-travelers-with-specific-needs/newly-arrived-immigrants-refugees

Schaefer, R. T. (2019). *Race and ethnicity in the United States* (9th ed.). New York, NY: Pearson.

Slavin, S., Galanti, G-A., & Kuo, A. (n. d.). *The 4 C's of culture: A mnemonic for healthcare professionals*. Retrieved from http://www.ggalanti.org/the-4cs-of-culture

Spector, R. E. (2004). *Cultural diversity in health and illness* (6th ed.). Upper Saddle River, NJ: Pearson Prentice Hall.

Spector, R. E. (2017). *Cultural diversity in health and illness* (9th ed.). New York, NY: Pearson.

Terry, D., Ali, M., & Lê, Q. (2011). Asian migrants' lived experience and acculturation to Western health care in rural Tasmania. *Australian Journal of Rural Health (19)*, 318–323. doi:10.1111/j.1440-1584.2011.01229.x

The Joint Commission. (2010). *Advancing effective communication, cultural competence, and patient- and family-centered care: A roadmap for hospitals*. Retrieved from https://www.jointcommission.org/assets/1/6/ARoadmapforHospitalsfinalversion727.pdf

Thresia, CU (2017). Health Inequalities in South Asia at the Launch of Sustainable Development Goals: Exclusions in Health in Kerala, India Need Political Interventions. *International Journal of Health Services*, doi:10.1177/0020731417738222

Tochluk, S. (2016). *Living in the tension: The quest for a spiritualized racial justice*. Roselle, NJ: Crandall, Dostie & Douglass.

UNDP (2015). Europe and the Commonwealth of Independent States PEI Regional Support Programme. Retrieved from https://www.unpei.org/europe-and-the-commonwealth-of-independent-states-pei-regional-support-programme/

U.S. Census Bureau. (2017). *2017 American Community Survey 1-year estimates*. Retrieved from https://www.census.gov/programs-surveys/acs/technical-documentation/table-and-geography-changes/2017/1-year.html

U.S. Census Bureau. (2018a). *2018 census test*. Retrieved from https://www.census.gov/newsroom/press-kits/2018/2018-census-test.html

U.S. Census Bureau. (2018b). *Population estimates by age, sex, race and Hispanic origin*. Retrieved from https://www.census.gov/newsroom/press-kits/2018/estimates-characteristics.html

U.S. Census Bureau. (2018c). *Projected race and Hispanic origin: Main projections series for the United States, 2017–2060*. Retrieved from https://www.census.gov/data/tables/2017/demo/popproj/2017-summary-tables.html

U.S. Department of Health and Human Services. (n.d.). *National standards for culturally and linguistically appropriate services in health care*. Retrieved from https://www.thinkculturalhealth.hhs.gov/clas/standards

U.S. Department of Health and Human Services. (2011). *HHS action plan to reduce racial and ethnic health disparities* Retrieved from http://minorityhealth.hhs.gov/npa/templates/content.aspx?lvl=1&lvlid=33&ID=285

U.S. Department of Health and Human Services, Office of Minority Health. (2018a). *National CLAS standards*. Retrieved from https://minorityhealth.hhs.gov/omh/browse.aspx?lvl=2&lvlid=53

U.S. Department of Health and Human Services, Office of Minority Health. (2018b). *What we do*. Retrieved from https://www.minorityhealth.hhs.gov/omh/browse.aspx?lvl=1&lvlid=2

U.S. Department of Labor, Bureau of Labor Statistics. (2019). *Labor force statistics from the current population survey: Employed persons by detailed occupation, sex, race, and Hispanic or Latino ethnicity*. Retrieved from http://www.bls.gov/cps/cpsaat11.htm

U.S. Department of State, Bureau of Consular Affairs. (2018). *Adoption statistics*. Retrieved from https://travel.state.gov/content/travel/en/Intercountry-Adoption/adopt_ref/adoption-statistics.html

World Health Organization – Europe (2008). The Tallinn Charter: Health Systems for Health and Wealth. Retrieved from https://www.euro.who.int/__data/assets/pdf_file/0008/88613/E91438.pdf

World Health Organization. How health systems can address health inequities linked to migration and ethnicity. Copenhagen, WHO Regional Office for Europe, 2010. Retrieved from https://www.euro.who.int/__data/assets/pdf_file/0005/127526/e94497.pdf

Zaharieva, R. (2020). Health inequalities: A persistent obstacle for Roma equality and inclusion. *European Public Health Alliance*. Retrieved from https://epha.org/health-inequalities-a-persistent-obstacle-for-roma-equality-and-inclusion/

Selected Bibliography

American Association of Colleges of Nursing. (2008). *Toolkit of resources for culturally competent education for baccalaureate nurses*. Washington, DC: Author.

CMS Office of Minority Health & RAND Corporation. (2017). *Racial and ethnic disparities by gender in health care in Medicare Advantage*. Retrieved from https://www.cms.gov/About-CMS/Agency-Information/OMH/Downloads/Health-Disparities-Racial-and-Ethnic-Disparities-by-Gender-National-Report.pdf

Expert Panel on Cultural Competence Education for Students in Medicine and Public Health (2012). *Cultural competence education for students in medicine and public health: Report of an expert panel*. Washington, DC: Association of American Medical Colleges and Association of Schools of Public Health.

Spector, R. E. (2016). Cultural Competence. *Cultura De Los Cuidados*, *20*(44), 9–14. doi:10.14198/cuid.2016.44.01

22 Complementary and Alternative Healing Modalities

LEARNING OUTCOMES

After completing this chapter, you will be able to:

1. Describe the basic concepts of alternative practices.
2. Give examples of healing environments.
3. Describe the basic principles of healthcare practices such as Ayurveda, traditional Chinese medicine, Native American healing, and curanderismo.
4. Explain how herbs are similar to many prescription drugs.
5. Discuss the principles of naturopathic medicine.
6. Identify the role of manual healing methods in health and illness.
7. Describe the goals that yoga, meditation, hypnotherapy, guided imagery, qi gong, and t'ai chi have in common.
8. Identify types of detoxification therapies.
9. Discuss uses of animals, prayer, and humor as treatment modalities.
10. Teach clients the uses of and safety precautions regarding complementary and alternative therapies.

KEY TERMS

acupressure, *425*
acupuncture, *425*
allopathic medicine, *418*
alternative medicine, *418*
animal-assisted therapy, *430*
aromatherapy, *423*
Ayurveda, *421*
balance, *420*
bioelectromagnetics, *430*
biofeedback, *428*
biomedicine, *418*
chiropractic, *425*
complementary medicine, *418*
conventional medicine, *418*
curanderismo, *422*
detoxification, *430*
Eastern medicine, *418*
energy, *420*
faith, *429*
guided imagery, *428*
hand-mediated biofield therapies, *426*
herbal medicine, *422*
holism, *419*
homeopathy, *423*
horticultural therapy, *431*
humanist, *420*
hypnotherapy, *427*
imagery, *427*
integrative medicine, *419*
massage therapy, *425*
meditation, *427*
music therapy, *429*
naturopathic medicine, *424*
Pilates, *428*
prayer, *429*
qi, *421*
qi gong, *428*
reflexology, *425*
spirituality, *420*
t'ai chi, *428*
traditional Chinese medicine (TCM), *421*
Western medicine, *418*
yoga, *426*

Introduction

Western medicine is an approach to health that focuses on the use of science in the diagnosis and treatment of health problems. This is in contrast to **Eastern medicine**, which places greater emphasis on prevention and natural healing. The differences between Western and Eastern medicine are not about geographic location because both Eastern and Western health practitioners exist in almost every part of the world. Nurses from the parts of the world where Western medicine is predominant are familiar and comfortable with biomedical beliefs, theories, practices, strengths, and limitations. In this chapter, the terms **conventional medicine**, **biomedicine**, and **allopathic medicine** are used to describe Western medical practices. Fewer nurses have studied Eastern medicine and as a result may lack information or even harbor misinformation about these healing practices.

The term *complementary and alternative medicine (CAM)* includes as many as 1800 other therapies practiced all over the world. Many of these have been handed down over thousands of years, both orally and as written records. They are based on the Eastern medical systems of ancient people, including Egyptians, Chinese, Asian Indians, Greeks, and Native Americans. Other therapies, such as bioelectromagnetics and chiropractic, evolved in the United States during the past two centuries. Still others, such as some of the mind–body approaches, are on the frontier of scientific knowledge and understanding. The CAM therapies described in this chapter are only some of the many used by clients. Nurses must learn about the ones being used by the clients in their specific practice settings.

Complementary medicine refers to the use of CAM *together with* conventional medicine. Most use of CAM by Americans is complementary. **Alternative medicine** refers to the use of CAM *in place of* conventional medicine. **Integrative medicine** combines treatments from conventional medicine and CAM for which there is some high-quality evidence of safety and effectiveness. It is also called *integrated medicine*.

The public interest in complementary and alternative therapies is extensive and growing, as evidenced by the proliferation of popular health books, health food stores, and clinics offering healing therapies. In 1998, the National Institutes of Health established the National Center for Complementary and Alternative Medicine to provide research, educational grants, and dissemination of information to the public. The final report of the White House Commission on Complementary and Alternative Medicine Policy (2002) identified several priorities, including the need for coordination of research to increase knowledge about CAM products, education and training of healthcare practitioners in CAM, reliable and useful information about CAM practices and products available to healthcare professionals, and guidance regarding appropriate access to and delivery of CAM. The National Health Interview Survey (NHIS) is an annual study, conducted by the National Center for Health Statistics (NCHS) of the Centers for Disease Control and Prevention (CDC), in which tens of thousands of Americans are interviewed about their health- and illness-related experiences. The complementary health approaches section of the NHIS, developed by the NCHS and National Center for Complementary and Integrative Health (NCCIH), was administered as a comprehensive survey in several years and as a focused survey on yoga, meditation, and chiropractic in 2017 (NCCIH, 2018b).

As with all interventions, the nurse must identify and comply with all legal issues related to the nurse's scope of practice in planning, implementing, evaluating, and documenting the use of CAM. In some cases, any nurse can perform a CAM intervention, whereas in other situations, the nurse must have special preparation, licensure, or certification to obtain a product or perform an intervention. In addition, the nurse must know whether CAM is included in the client's healthcare insurance coverage or if the fees will need to be paid directly by the client. In general, insurers will cover acupuncture and chiropractic. Other modalities may be covered and reimbursed through a health spending or flexible spending account. Encourage clients to investigate payment options according to their insurance plans.

Clinical Alert!

What constitutes traditional, alternative, complementary, or holistic to one individual may be considered mainstream to another. Do not assume anything about the client's belief system—be sure to assess and be open-minded.

Basic Concepts

Several concepts are common to most alternative practices. These are holism, humanism, balance, spirituality, energy, and healing environments.

Holism

Although they represent diverse approaches, alternative therapies share certain attributes. They are based on the paradigm of whole systems and the belief that individuals are more than physical bodies with fixable and replaceable parts. Combined mental, emotional, spiritual, relationship, and environmental components, referred to as **holism**, are considered to play crucial and equal roles in an individual's state of health. Interventions are individualized within the entire context of the individual's life.

Nurses have engaged in natural and traditional healing interactions since the finest traditions of Florence Nightingale. The modern nurse draws on biomedical and caring-healing models by utilizing technology and focusing on caring relationships and healing processes. "Nurses, by virtue of their education and relationships with clients, help clients assert their right to choose their own healing journey and the quality of their life and death experiences" (Fontaine, 2019, p. xiii).

The American Nurses Association (ANA) recognizes holistic nursing as a specialty practice and certifies nurses in the specialty at several different educational levels.

EVIDENCE-BASED PRACTICE

Evidence-Based Practice

What CAM Methods Do Individuals Use to Improve Athletic Performance?

In a secondary analysis of data from more than 30,000 respondents to the U.S. National Health Interview Study in 2012, the authors aimed to identify whether the CAM therapies reported as used by adults to improve athletic performance indicated that the therapies were helpful (Evans et al., 2018). The median age of the more than 10,000 respondents reporting specific use to improve athletic performance was slightly less than 38. Respondents were given 19 therapies to choose from, indicating their top three. The most used therapies were yoga, herbal supplements, manipulation, and massage. Females reported the therapies as helpful almost 3 times as often as males.

Implications

A number of conclusions were drawn from this analysis. Some therapies are self-administered and inexpensive, whereas others require significant training or specialized practitioners. Therapies are commonly used in combination. Some therapies have evidence-based effectiveness data, whereas others have not been well studied. Nurses can use the findings from this study in their work with clients aiming to improve athletic performance.

The mission statement of the American Holistic Nurses Association (AHNA, Reprinted with permission from the American Holistic Nurses Association, copyright 2019.) is "to illuminate holism in nursing practice, community, advocacy, research, and education."

Humanism

The **humanist** perspective includes propositions such as the following: The mind and body are indivisible, individuals have the power to solve their own problems and are responsible for the patterns of their lives, and well-being is a combination of personal satisfaction and contributions to the larger community. Nursing is in a unique position to take a leadership role in integrating alternative healing methods into Western healthcare systems. Nurses have historically used their hands, hearts, and heads in natural and traditional healing interactions.

Balance

In terms of optimal wellness, the concept of **balance** consists of finding a desirable point between opposite forces rather than being purely in one state or another. Balance has mental, physical, emotional, spiritual, and environmental components. Not only does each component have to be balanced; equilibrium is needed among the components. Physical aspects include optimal functioning of all body systems. Emotional aspects include the ability to feel and express the entire range of human emotions. Mental aspects include feelings of self-worth, a positive identity, a sense of accomplishment, and the ability to appreciate and create. Spiritual aspects involve moral values, a meaningful purpose in life, and a feeling of connectedness to others and a divine source. Environmental aspects include physical, biological, economic, social, and political conditions. Being in balance is a learned skill and one that must be practiced regularly to engage in the process of healthful living. This concept of balance appears throughout the various alternative therapies.

Spirituality

Spiritual healing techniques and spiritually based healthcare systems are among the most ancient healing practices. Spirit is the liveliness, richness, and beauty of one's life. It is who we are and how we are in the world. **Spirituality** includes the drive to become all that one can be and is bound to intuition, creativity, and motivation (see Chapter 41 ∞). It is the dimension that involves relationships with oneself, with others, and with a higher power. Spirituality is that which gives individuals meaning and purpose in their lives. It involves finding significance in the entirety of life, including illness and death.

Energy

The concept of energy has been recognized in most cultures for centuries. **Energy** is viewed as the force that integrates the body, mind, and spirit; it is that which connects everything.

Chinese Taoist scholars believed that energy was the basic building material of the universe. Albert Einstein and other physicists proved that matter and energy are the same and that energy is not only the raw material of the cosmos but the glue that holds it together. Modern scientists now look at the universe in terms of forces of tiny particles of matter. Their experimental findings are similar to the intuitive observation of China's ancient scholars. Everything in the world—animate and inanimate—is made of energy. Individuals are beings of energy, living in a universe composed of energy.

Two terms common in various healing practices and related to energy and balance are *grounding* and *centering*. *Grounding*, as its name suggests, relates to an individual's connection with the ground and, in a broader sense, to an individual's whole contact with reality. Being grounded suggests stability, security, independence, having a solid foundation, and living in the present rather than escaping into dreams. *Centering* refers to the process of bringing oneself to the center or middle. When individuals are centered, they are fully connected to the part of their bodies where all their energies meet. Centering is the process of focusing one's mind on the center of energy, allowing one to operate intuitively, with awareness, and to channel energy throughout the body.

Healing Environments

Nursing has always focused on creating healing environments for those who have been entrusted to their care. Healing environments are created when nurses empower clients by providing the knowledge, skills, and support that allow them to tap into their inner wisdom and make healthy decisions for themselves. Healing environments are a synthesis of the medical-curing approach and the nursing-healing approach. Nurses need a healthy balance between technology and compassion. Nurses create healing environments when they take the time to be with clients in deeply caring ways. It is when they become still and enter the other's subjective world that they are able to be wholly present for that client.

Nurses must also create their own healing environments. Working with clients can be draining work. Nurses need to learn how to restore their energy and replenish themselves. Nurses might compare their ability to care for others to a well of fresh, healing water. If the well is never dipped into, the water becomes stagnant and brackish. If the water is constantly drawn out and given away, with no source of replenishment, the well will soon run dry. What happens to nurses who do not sincerely care for others or take the time to replenish themselves? It soon becomes obvious by their behavior that they are stagnant or depleted; they are less patient, less tolerant, more irritable, and unhappy. Their state of "burnout" contaminates all aspects of their professional and personal lives.

Nurses can take a few simple steps to create a personal healing environment:

- Use good posture. You may spend many hours of your day walking incorrectly or slumped in a chair, which interrupts the flow of energy and oxygen through your body. Take a moment to sit up or stand straight. Imagine that a cord is attached to the top of your head, pulling it gently toward the sky. This image helps readjust your posture.
- Boost your energy. Take your shoes off; sit on the floor with your legs stretched out in front of you and your palms facing down at your sides. Point your toes as hard as you can and hold for 5 seconds, then dorsiflex your feet as hard as you can and hold for 5 seconds. Repeat 10 times.
- Sit comfortably and close your eyes. Simply notice your breathing without trying to change it. Pay attention to your inhale and your exhale. Now imagine that the breath is pouring into your heart with each inhalation and blowing out of your heart with each exhalation. Just feel the breath flowing in and out of your heart. Imagine the breath is pure love. Perform this breath awareness for 5 to 10 minutes. Now let your attention return to your environment, slowly open your eyes, get up, and move on. Think about the feeling throughout the day.

Healing Modalities

Ethnocentrism, the assumption that one's own cultural or ethnic group is superior to others, has often prevented Western healthcare practitioners from learning new ways to promote health and prevent chronic illness. With consumer demand for a broader range of options, we must open our minds to the idea that other cultures and countries have valid ways of preventing and curing diseases. Although the information may be new to us, many of these traditions are hundreds or even thousands of years old and have long been part of the medical mainstream in other cultures (see also Chapter 21 ∞). The nurse should inquire about healing modalities the client may have used previously (see Assessment Interview).

Systematized Healthcare Practices

A number of healthcare practices have been systematized throughout the centuries and throughout the world. These typically include an entire set of values, attitudes, and beliefs that generate a philosophy of life, not simply a group of remedies. Definitions and summaries of research in these practices can be found on the NCCIH website. The NCCIH, called the National Center for Complementary and Alternative Medicine prior to 2015, is a part of the U.S. Department of Health and Human Services' National Institutes of Health.

Ayurveda

The Indian system of medicine, **Ayurveda**, is at least 2500 years old. Illness is viewed as a state of imbalance among the body's systems. *Ayurveda* is from the Sanskrit words *ayur* life and *veda* science or knowledge. Ayurveda emphasizes the interdependence of the health of the individual and the quality of societal life. Mentally healthy individuals have good memory, comprehension, intelligence, and reasoning ability. Emotionally healthy individuals experience evenly balanced emotional states and a sense of well-being or happiness. Physically healthy individuals have abundant energy, with proper functioning of the senses, digestion, and elimination. From a spiritual perspective, healthy individuals have a sense of aliveness and richness of life; are developing in the direction of their full potential; and are in good relationships with themselves, other individuals, and the larger cosmos. Environmentally healthy individuals have minimal economic, social, and political stress.

Specific lifestyle interventions are a major preventive and therapeutic approach in Ayurveda. Each individual is prescribed an individualized diet and exercise program depending on *dosha* (body) type and the nature of the underlying *dosha* imbalance. Herbal preparations are added to the diet for preventive or regenerative purposes as well as for the treatment of specific disorders. Yoga, breathing exercises, and meditative techniques are also prescribed by the practitioner. This ancient system has adapted to modern science and technology, including biomedical science and quantum physics.

In the United States, most schools of Ayurveda award a certificate and only a few are accredited by the National Council on Ayurvedic Education. The first students in a state-approved Ayurvedic doctor program graduated in 2018 (Halpern, 2018).

Traditional Chinese Medicine

Traditional Chinese medicine (TCM) has developed over 3000 years and is based on the premise that the body's vital energy or **qi** (pronounced *chee*) circulates through pathways or meridians and can be accessed and manipulated

ASSESSMENT INTERVIEW Complementary and Alternative Therapies

- Tell me about your use of teas, herbs, vitamins, or other natural products to improve your health or treat diseases.
- What traditional or folk remedies do your family members use?
- Do you meditate, pray, or use relaxation techniques, music, or yoga for healing purposes?
- What alternative therapies have you used (e.g., acupuncture, touch therapies, magnets, hypnosis)?

through specific anatomic points along the surface of the body. Disease is described as an imbalance or interruption in the flow of qi. In TCM, the mind, body, spirit, and emotions are never separated. Thus, the heart is not just a blood pump; it also influences the individual's capacity for joy, sense of purpose in life, and connectedness with others. The kidneys filter fluids, but they also manage the individual's capacity for fear, will and motivation, and faith in life. The lungs breathe in air and breathe out waste products, but they also regulate an individual's capacity to grieve, as well as to acknowledge self and others. The liver cleanses the body, and it also influences an individual's feeling of anger as well as that of vision and creativity. The stomach has a part in digestion of food and influences the ability of an individual to be thoughtful, kind, and nurturing as well. These are just a few of the mind–body connections that TCM practitioners recognize.

Practitioners of TCM are trained to use a variety of ancient and modern therapeutic methods, including acupuncture, acupressure, herbal medicine, massage, heat therapy, qi gong, t'ai chi, and nutritional lifestyle counseling.

Native American Healing

There are more than 500 federally recognized Native American or American Indian tribes in the United States. Each tribe has its own origin stories, culture, customs, belief system, and language. Some tribes have adopted belief systems or religions from other cultures, such as Christianity, whereas others have not. Some Native Americans are traditional, meaning they adhere strictly to the old ways of life and avoid any form of biomedicine. Others have acculturated, or adapted to the mainstream culture, and use both native medicine and conventional medicine. A third group has become assimilated and has virtually abandoned all traditional ways in favor of the dominant culture and utilizes only biomedicine. Each of these groups will place different emphases on traditional health beliefs, practices, and use of healers.

Traditional Native American culture values the individual expression of each individual's uniqueness. Concepts common to many Native American tribes include connection to the land; balance or harmony between mind and body; the use of rituals as a part of the healing plan; cleansing such as through the traditional sweat lodge; use of music, drumming, chanting, and dancing as part of healing; and use of herbs and botanical treatments (Fontaine, 2019). Traditional Native American healers focus on the cause of an illness, which may require a ceremony to identify. The process of communication between the healer and the client may seem convoluted or indirect to outsiders (Spector, 2017).

Curanderismo

Curanderismo (pronounced *koo-rahn-dare-ees-mo*) is a cultural healing tradition found in Latin America and among many Latinos and Hispanics in the United States. Healers are called *curanderos* (men) and *curanderas* (women). They may specialize as herbalists, midwives, counselors, spine and joint workers, and massage therapists. They also utilize religious rituals, cleansing rites, and prayers in their healing practices. Healers work at one of three levels: the material level, the spiritual level, or the mental level (Fontaine, 2019).

Botanical Healing

Botanical (plant) healings are used by 80% of the world's population. These include herbs, aromatherapy, homeopathy, and naturopathy (Figure 22.1 ■).

Herbal Medicine

Before pharmaceutical companies existed, there was **herbal medicine**. In many parts of the world, treating illness with herbs is still the only medicine available. Even though only a tiny fraction of plants has been studied for medicinal benefits, conventional primary care providers use plant-derived products regularly. Many prescription drugs sold in the United States are derived from plants. Examples of herbal remedies that have been synthesized into modern drugs are reserpine from the Indian snakeroot plant, digoxin from foxglove, quinine from Peruvian bark, aspirin from willow tree bark, morphine from the opium poppy, cocaine from coca leaves, atropine from deadly nightshade, and paclitaxel (Taxol) found in Pacific yew bark.

Not all plant life is beneficial. Most plant-related poisonings are due to accidental consumption of toxic ornamental plants such as jade, holly, and poinsettia. The vast majority of herbal medicines present no danger if taken appropriately. Some can, however, cause serious adverse effects if taken in excess or, for some, if taken over a prolonged period of time. Herbs can also interact with drugs, and caution should be used when combining herbs with prescription and over-the-counter (OTC) medications. Pregnant and breastfeeding women should be cautioned not to take herbs internally except for mild herb teas.

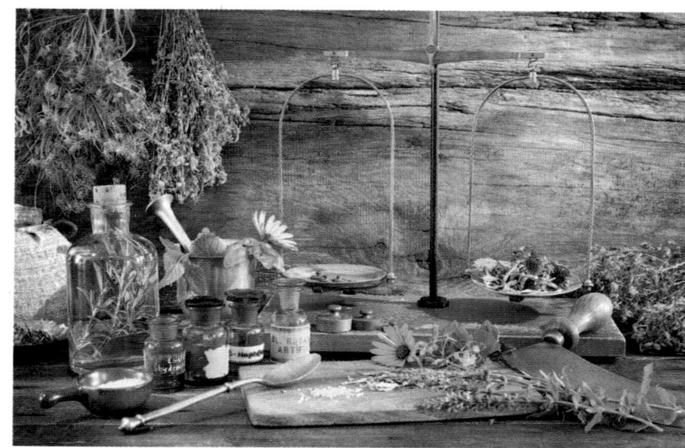

Figure 22.1 ■ Aromatherapy, homeopathy, and other botanical therapies may be used alone or in combination.
Alexander Raths/123RF.

Although herbs can be quite effective, it is important to caution individuals about becoming overdependent on them. If they have a life-threatening illness such as asthma, experience chest pain, or notice symptoms that persist for longer than a few days, they should seek medical attention. For example, although it may be healthy to take echinacea if an individual feels a cold coming on, any serious ailment should be diagnosed by a healthcare practitioner before undertaking an herbal cure. Conventional medicine is best used in crisis situations, and herbs are best used in noncrisis situations.

Nurses must be open to exploring and discussing their clients' uses of and questions regarding herbal medicine. This clinical screening allows for evaluation of herbal intake against known and potential adverse interactions with prescriptions and OTC medications. See the Practice Guidelines for some cautions and contraindications. In addition to the uses of herbs described in the Practice Guidelines, herbs may also be used in aromatherapy and homeopathy. These are only some of the examples of uses of medicinal herbs. When working with a client who is using herbal therapies, the nurse needs to learn as much as possible about the herbs so as to promote their positive effects and minimize any potential adverse effects.

Aromatherapy

Aromatherapy is the therapeutic use of essential oils of plants in which the odor or fragrance plays an important part. It is an offshoot of herbal medicine, with the basis of action being the same as that of modern pharmacology. The chemicals found in the essential oils are absorbed into the body, resulting in physiologic or psychologic benefit. Essential oils are extracted from plants and are massaged into the skin, inhaled, placed in baths, used as compresses, or mixed into ointments. Different oils may calm, stimulate, improve sleep, change eating habits, or boost the immune system.

Essential oils, other than lavender or tea tree oil, are quite potent and can irritate the skin, so they should be diluted with a carrier oil before being used on the skin. Carrier oils such as sunflower oil, grapeseed oil, and soy oil contain vitamins, proteins, and minerals that provide added nutrients to the body. Essential oils should not be ingested because even modest amounts can be fatal. Pregnant women and individuals with epilepsy should consult a knowledgeable healthcare practitioner or qualified aromatherapist prior to the use of essential oils. Some oils can trigger bronchial spasms, so individuals with asthma should consult their primary healthcare provider before using them. Table 22.1 describes oils that may be useful at home.

Homeopathy

Homeopathy is a self-healing system, assisted by small doses of remedies or medicines, which is useful in a variety of acute and chronic disorders. It was developed by Samuel Hahnemann, a German physician and chemist. He proposed the use of the *law of similars*, which claims that a natural substance that produces a given symptom in a healthy individual cures it in a sick individual. If taken

PRACTICE GUIDELINES Uses, Cautions, and Contraindications for Popular Herbal Preparations*

Herb	Traditional Uses	Selected Warnings
Echinacea	May boost immune system, enhance wound healing	May reduce the effectiveness of immunosuppressants
Feverfew	Prevents migraine headaches, arthritis; stimulates digestion	May increase the anticoagulant effects of aspirin and anticoagulant medications
Garlic	Reduces high blood pressure and cholesterol; antibiotic, antifungal; anticlotting agent	May increase the anticoagulant effects of aspirin and anticoagulant medications
Ginger	Aids digestion; relieves motion sickness, dizziness, and nausea	May increase the anticoagulant effects of aspirin and anticoagulant medications
Ginkgo	May improve memory function, relieve stress, treat dizziness	May increase the anticoagulant effects of aspirin and anticoagulant medications
Ginseng	Stimulates mental activity; enhances immune system, appetite	May interact with caffeine and cause irritability May decrease the effectiveness of glaucoma medications
Milk thistle	Enhances flow of bile, blood, and other substances in the gallbladder, liver, spleen, and stomach	Reduces the effectiveness of oral contraceptives
Saw palmetto	Treats prostate hyperplasia; anti-inflammatory	May give false low prostate-specific antigen (PSA) levels, thereby delaying diagnosis of prostate cancer
St. John's wort	Acts as antidepressant, anti-inflammatory; is antiviral	May potentiate antidepressant medications, causing severe agitation, nausea, confusion, and possible cardiac problems
Valerian	Sedative, tranquilizer; lowers blood pressure; helps menstrual cramps	May increase the sedative effects of antianxiety medication

*Some preparations may vary in efficacy and toxicity depending on the age of the client. Use extra caution with young children and older adults.

TABLE 22.1 Oils That May Be Useful to Have at Home

Oil	Use
Chamomile	Soothes muscle aches, sprains, swollen joints; gastrointestinal antispasmodic; rub on abdomen for colic, indigestion, gas; decreases anxiety, stress-related headaches; decreases insomnia.
Eucalyptus	Feels cool to skin and warm to muscles; decreases fever; relieves pain; anti-inflammatory; antiseptic, antiviral, and expectorant to respiratory system in steam inhalation; boosts immune system.
Ginger	Helps ward off colds; calms upset stomach, decreases nausea; soothes sprains, muscle spasms.
Jasmine	Uplifting and stimulating, antidepressant; massage abdomen and lower back for menstrual cramps.
Lavender	Calming, sedative for insomnia; massage around temples for headache; inhale to speed recovery from colds, flu; massage chest to decrease congestion; heals burns.
Tea tree	Antifungal, good for athlete's foot; soothes insect bites, stings, cuts, wounds; in bath for yeast infection; drops on handkerchief for coughs, congestion.

Note: Some oils are safe for children (e.g., chamomile, eucalyptus, orange), whereas others may be toxic (e.g., yellow camphor, horseradish, sassafras, tansy, wintergreen) and should only be used by qualified aromatherapists (Fontaine, 2019).

in large amounts, these natural compounds will produce symptoms of disease. In the doses used by homeopaths, however, these remedies stimulate an individual's self-healing capacity.

Natural healing compounds are prepared through a process of serial dilution and are taken orally. The compound is first dissolved in a water–alcohol mixture called the "mother tincture." One drop of the tincture is then mixed with 10 drops of water–alcohol, and this process is repeated hundreds or thousands of times depending on the potency being prepared. The remedies are diluted beyond the point at which any molecules of the substance can theoretically still be found in the solution. The homeopathic belief is that the more the substance is diluted, the more potent it becomes. No matter how many times a substance is diluted, a smaller but complete essence of the substance remains. Advances in quantum physics have led some scientists to suggest that electromagnetic energy in the remedies interacts with the body on some level. Researchers in physical chemistry have proposed the memory of water theory, in which the structure of the water–alcohol solutions is altered during the process of dilution and retains its new structure even after the substance is no longer present. It seems likely that remedies work through a bioenergetic or subatomic mechanism that we are not as yet capable of understanding. Homeopathic remedies are regulated by the U.S. Food and Drug Administration (FDA). However, the FDA does not evaluate the remedies for safety or effectiveness (NCCIH, 2018a).

Naturopathy

Naturopathic medicine is not only a system of medicine but also a way of life, with emphasis on client responsibility, education, health maintenance, and disease prevention. It may be the model health system of the future with the movement toward healthy lifestyles, healthy diets, and preventive healthcare.

The education of naturopathic practitioners is extensive and similar to that for conventional medical education. Four years of medical school follow a college degree in a biological science. Naturopathic medicine holds the same view of human physiology, body functions, and disease processes as conventional medicine. Naturopathic practitioners do not provide emergency care nor do they perform major surgery. They rarely prescribe drugs, and they treat clients in private practice and outpatient clinics, not in hospitals.

The goal of treatment is the restoration of health and normal body function, rather than the application of a particular therapy. Virtually every CAM therapy is utilized. Naturopaths mix and match different approaches, customizing treatment for each individual. The least invasive intervention to support the body's natural healing processes is a primary consideration. These interventions include dietetics, therapeutic nutrition, herbs, physical therapy, spinal manipulation, acupuncture, lifestyle counseling, stress management, exercise therapy, homeopathy, and aquatic (hydro-) therapy.

Nutritional Therapy

Nutritional therapy consists of the consumption of specific types of diets (see Chapter 46 ∞) or supplements, including vitamins, minerals, amino acids, herbs and other botanicals, and miscellaneous substances such as enzymes and fish oils, for the purpose of preventing or treating illness. Supplements are not considered medications. The Dietary Supplement Health and Education Act of 1994 requires that the companies selling these products determine their safety; however, the companies are not required to publicize this information or to inform the FDA of reports of adverse reactions.

Three major concerns are related to clients' use of nutritional supplements: efficacy, consistency, and safety. Often, research conducted to determine the effectiveness of supplements has been flawed in design or produced conflicting results. Nurses should assist clients in gathering reliable information about supplements, such as information available from the National Institutes of Health's Office of Dietary Supplements website. Supplements are manufactured by many different companies and often contain a variety of substances in varying amounts. The specific amount of a substance needed to produce the desired effect may not be known, and there is no guarantee that each dose (pill, capsule, tablet, or liquid) contains a consistent amount of the substance. There are no legal definitions of the words *standardized*, *certified*, or *verified* for supplements.

As mentioned in the discussion of herbs, not all supplements are harmless. Some supplements cause adverse effects such as diarrhea or high blood pressure, yet others become dangerous when taken in combination with certain medications (see earlier Practice Guidelines). Another safety concern with supplements is that they may be contaminated with dangerous substances such as mold, bacteria, pesticides, and metals (Rolfes, Pinna, & Whitney, 2018). Nurses must assess clients for the use of dietary supplements, and nurses' care planning should include teaching about the known benefits and risks of supplements.

Manual Healing Methods

Some manual healing methods come from ancient times; some were developed in the latter half of the 20th century. These healing practices include chiropractic, massage, acupuncture, acupressure, reflexology, and hand-mediated biofield therapies.

Chiropractic

Chiropractic focuses on the relationship between the body's structure—mainly the spine—and its functioning. Although practitioners may use a variety of treatment approaches, they primarily perform adjustments (manipulations) to the spine or other parts of the body, with the goal of correcting alignment problems, alleviating pain, improving function, and supporting the body's natural ability to heal itself.

Three primary clinical goals guide chiropractic intervention. The first clinical goal is to reduce or eliminate pain. The second goal is to correct the spinal dysfunction, thereby restoring biomechanical balance to reestablish shock absorption, leverage, and range of motion. In addition, muscles and ligaments are strengthened by spinal rehabilitative exercises to increase resistance to further injury. The third clinical goal is preventive maintenance to ensure the problem does not recur.

As holistic practitioners, chiropractors work with many facets of clients' lifestyles. They design exercise programs, plan rehabilitation measures, explain correct posture and lifting techniques, and assess activities of daily living (ADLs).

Massage

Massage therapy, the scientific manipulation of the soft tissues of the body, is a healing art, an act of physical caring, and a way of communicating without words. It is believed that massage aids the ability of the body to heal itself and is aimed at achieving or increasing health and well-being. In the United States, massage is considered an alternative or complementary treatment, whereas in many areas of the world, it is an integral part of health systems.

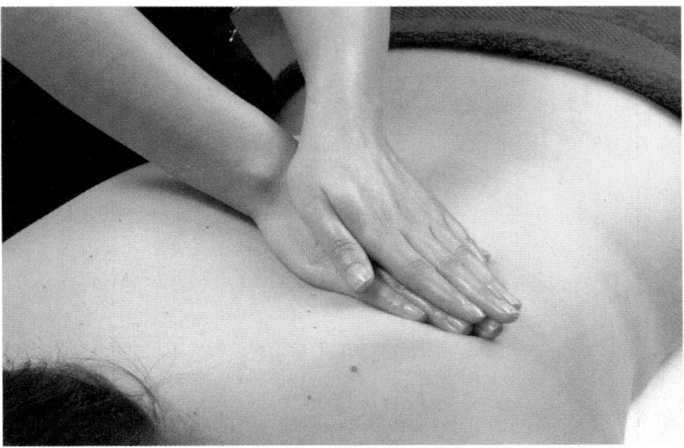

Figure 22.2 ■ Massaging the back.
Gareth Boden/Pearson Education Ltd.

Strong, sustained touch in massage can have an even greater effect than other forms of touch. A skilled massage therapist not only stretches and loosens muscle and connective tissue but also greatly improves blood flow and the movement of lymph fluid throughout the body (Figure 22.2 ■). Massage speeds the removal of metabolic waste products resulting from exercise or inactivity, allowing more oxygen and nutrients to reach the cells and tissues. The release of muscular tension also helps to unblock and balance the overall flow of life energy throughout the body.

On the physical level, massage relieves muscle tension, reduces muscle spasms, improves joint flexibility and range of motion, improves posture, lowers blood pressure, slows heart rate, promotes deeper and easier breathing, and improves the health of the skin. On the mental level, massage induces a relaxed state of alertness, reduces mental stress, and increases the capacity for clearer thinking. On the emotional level, massage satisfies the need for caring and nurturing touch, increases feelings of well-being, decreases mild depression, enhances self-image, reduces levels of anxiety, and increases awareness of the mind–body connection (Fontaine, 2019). For back massage techniques, see Skill 30.1 in Chapter 30 ∞.

Acupuncture, Acupressure, and Reflexology

Acupuncture and **acupressure** are techniques in which pressure or stimulation is applied to specific points on the body, known as acupuncture points, to relieve pain, cure certain illnesses, and promote wellness. Acupuncture uses needles (Figure 22.3 ■), whereas acupressure uses finger pressure. **Reflexology** is a form of acupressure most commonly performed on the feet, but the hands or ears may also be manipulated. Figure 22.4 ■ shows the foot reflex areas.

Acupuncture, acupressure, and reflexology are treatments rooted in the traditional Eastern philosophy that qi, or life energy, flows through the body along pathways known as *meridians*. As vital energy flows through the meridians, it forms tiny whirlpools close to the skin's surface at places called acupuncture points. These points function somewhat like gates to moderate the flow of qi.

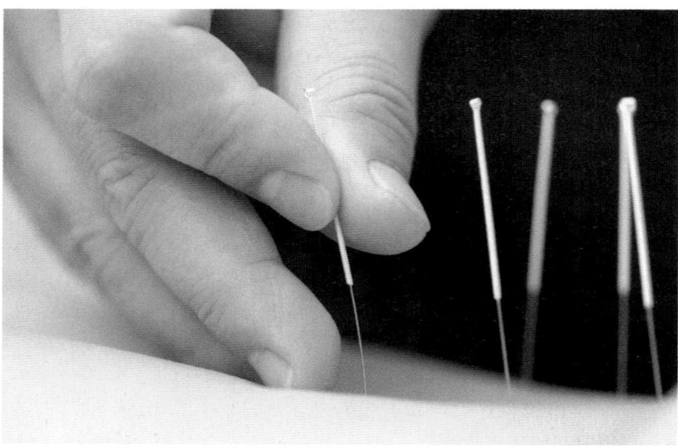

Figure 22.3 ■ Acupuncture involves the insertion of thin, sterile needles.
Bork/Shutterstock.

When the flow of energy becomes blocked or congested, individuals experience discomfort or pain on a physical level, may feel frustrated or irritable on an emotional level, and may experience a sense of vulnerability or lack of purpose in life on a spiritual level. The goal of care in wellness acupuncture is to recognize and manage the disruption before illness or disease occurs. Practitioners bring balance to the body's energies, which promotes optimal health and well-being and facilitates individuals' own healing capacity.

Examples of research on the effectiveness of acupuncture include the following:

- A study of acupuncture as a treatment for chronic pain with military veterans demonstrated positive effects (Plunkett et al., 2017).
- A study comparing medication with or without acupuncture or biofeedback as a treatment for insomnia found that sleep quality was statistically improved with acupuncture compared with the other treatment options (Huang, Lin, Lin, & Tzeng, 2017).

Hand-Mediated Biofield Therapies

The three most prominent **hand-mediated biofield therapies**, using the hands to alter the biofield, or energy field, are therapeutic touch (TT), healing touch, and Reiki. All three approaches could be defined as the use of the hands on or near the body with the intention to manipulate energy fields to help or to heal. The goals are to accelerate the individual's own healing process and to facilitate healing at all levels of body, mind, emotions, and spirit. All three are forms of treatment and are not designed to diagnose physical conditions, nor are they meant to replace conventional surgery, medicine, or drugs in treating organic disease.

Trained nurses can use TT, healing touch, and Reiki in almost any clinical setting, including hospitals, nursing homes, home healthcare, hospice, and private practice. These therapies are helpful for clients with a variety of medical and nursing diagnoses.

Mind–Body Therapies

In mind–body therapies, individuals focus on realigning or creating balance in mental processes to bring about healing. These therapies include yoga, meditation, hypnotherapy, guided imagery, biofeedback, qi gong, t'ai chi, and Pilates.

Yoga

Yoga has been practiced for thousands of years in India, where it is a way of life that includes ethical models for

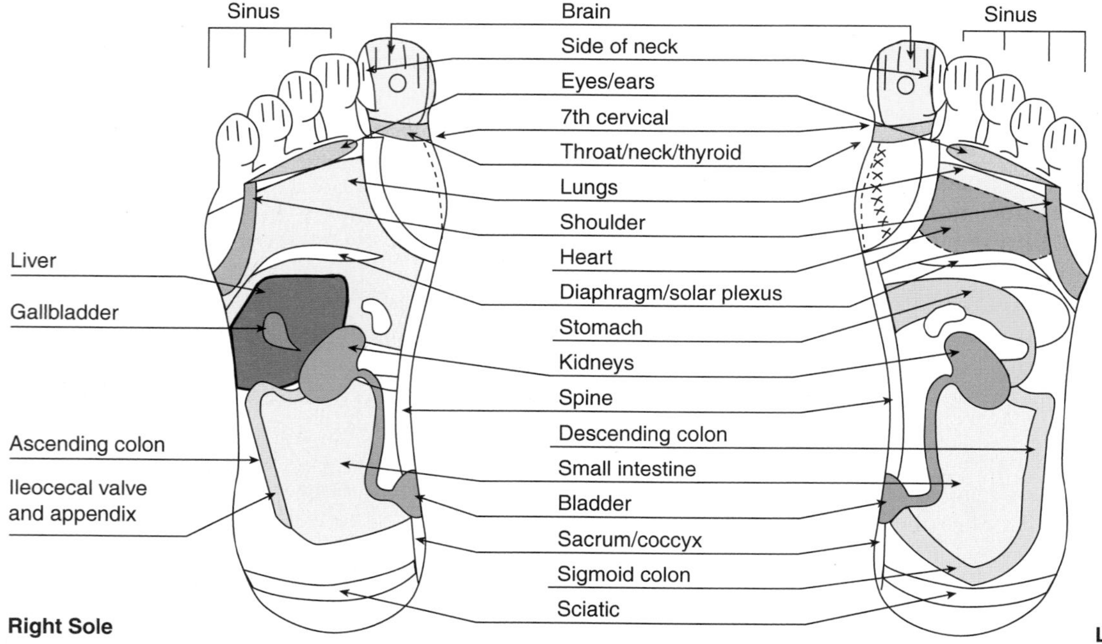

Figure 22.4 ■ Foot reflex areas.

behavior and mental and physical exercises aimed at producing spiritual enlightenment. It is a method for life that can complement and enhance any system of religion, or it can be practiced completely apart from religion. The Western approach to yoga tends to be more fitness oriented with the goal of managing stress, learning to relax, and increasing vitality and well-being. A typical yoga session lasts 20 minutes to an hour. Some individuals spend 30 minutes doing the poses and another 30 minutes doing breathing practices and meditations. Others spend the majority of the time doing poses and end with a short meditation or relaxation procedure. Even for those who are inactive and out of shape, sick, or weak, sets of easy exercises can help to loosen the joints and stimulate circulation. If practiced regularly, these simple exercises alone make a great difference in individuals' health and well-being.

The percentage of U.S. adults who used yoga increased from 9.5% to 14% between 2012 and 2017 and was the most common complementary health practice reported (Clarke, Barnes, Black, Stussman, & Nahin, 2018). In children aged 4–17, yoga practice more than doubled from 3.1% to 8.4% between 2012 and 2017 (Black, Barnes, Clarke, Stussman, & Nahin, 2018).

BOX 22.1 Guidelines for Meditation and Progressive Relaxation

1. Create a special time and place for meditation. Ideally, choose the early morning or evening, and wait at least 2 hours after eating so that complete energy is devoted to meditation rather than to digestive demands. A quiet, comfortable place, devoid of distractions, is helpful.
2. Sit either cross-legged on the floor or upright in a straight-backed chair, keeping the spine straight and the body relaxed. Avoid a lying position because it increases the tendency to fall asleep.
3. Support the palms on the thighs, and close the eyes.
4. Follow deep-breathing or progressive relaxation exercises.
    - Tense and tighten your right fist. Focus on the feeling of tension as you do so.
    - Allow the muscles in your right fist to relax. Contrast the difference in feeling from tension to relaxation.
    - Repeat the preceding two steps for the left fist.
    - Now tense and relax both your left and right fists.
    - Focus on and relish the feeling of relaxation.
    - Now tighten the muscles in both fists and both arms. Feel the tension, fully relax the muscles, and again focus on the sensation of relaxation.
    - Progressively tighten and relax each muscle group in the body: toes, ankles, knees, buttocks, and groin; stomach and lower back muscles; chest and upper back muscles; shoulders, forehead, and jaw muscles.
    - Couple deep breathing with progressive relaxation. While relaxing your muscles, inhale deeply, send the breath to the fist (or other muscle group), and exhale.
5. If using a mantra, repeat the word or phrase either aloud or silently while exhaling. When distracting thoughts arise, allow them to drift into and out of your mind without giving them undue attention; then refocus on your breathing or your mantra.
6. Practice this process daily for 10- to 20-minute periods.

Meditation

Meditation is a general term for a wide range of practices that involve relaxing the body and easing the mind. Meditation is a process that all individuals can use to calm themselves, cope with stress, and for those with spiritual inclinations, feel as one with God or the universe. It is one of the five most commonly used complementary treatments in the United States, used by almost as many adults as yoga and increasing numbers of children (Black et al., 2018; Clarke et al., 2018). Meditation can be practiced individually or in groups and is easy to learn. It requires no change in belief system and is compatible with most religious practices.

If practiced regularly, such as 20 minutes twice a day, meditation produces widespread positive effects on physical and psychologic functioning (Anselmo, 2016). The autonomic nervous system responds with a decrease in heart rate, lower blood pressure, decreased respiratory rate and oxygen consumption, and a lower arousal threshold. Individuals who meditate say that they have clearer minds and sharper thoughts. Meditation's residual effects—improved stress-coping abilities—are a protection against daily stress and anxiety. All other self-healing methods are improved with the practice of meditation. See Box 22.1 for guidelines for performing meditation.

Hypnotherapy

Hypnotherapy is the application of hypnosis in a wide variety of medical and psychologic disorders. Hypnosis is a trance state or an altered state of consciousness in which an individual's concentration is focused and distraction is minimized. Individuals in trances are aware of what is going on around them but choose not to focus on it and can return to normal awareness whenever they choose. Hypnosis is not a surrender of control; it is only an advanced form of relaxation. Hypnotherapy can be used to help individuals gain self-control, improve self-esteem, and become more autonomous. In some medical facilities, hypnosis is routinely used with a variety of conditions, usually in conjunction with other forms of medical, surgical, psychiatric, or psychologic treatment. It can be used with nonmedical clients as well, in working through problems of living or situations of performance anxiety and in changing bad habits. Depending on the complexity and seriousness of the complaint, treatment typically runs from 2 to 10 sessions. The American Society of Clinical Hypnosis and the American Council of Hypnotist Examiners share in the education and accreditation of individuals who meet professional requirements.

Guided Imagery

Imagery refers to a two-way communication between the conscious and unconscious mind and involves the whole body and all of its senses. Most of us imagine frequently throughout the day. Worry is the most common form of imagery that affects our health. In our imagination, we react to current stressors and anticipated dangers. Our bodies become aroused and tense, and we activate the fight-or-flight mechanism. **Guided imagery** is a state of focused attention, much like hypnosis, that encourages changes in attitudes, behavior, and physiologic reactions. Guided imagery can help us learn how to stop troublesome thoughts and focus on images that help us relax and decrease the negative impact of stressors.

In guided imagery, the images may be created by the therapist based on the needs and desires of the client. Clients can also create the images as a way to understand the meaning of symptoms or to access inner resources. Imagery stimulates changes in many body functions, such as heart rate, blood pressure, respiratory patterns, brain wave rhythms and patterns, electrical characteristics of the skin, local blood flow and temperature, gastrointestinal motility and secretions, sexual arousal, and levels of various hormones and neurotransmitters.

Imagery is used to promote healing; decrease pain and symptoms; minimize side effects; manage chronic illness; prepare for procedures, surgery, or childbirth; and access inner wisdom and resources. Table 22.2 describes several types of imagery.

Biofeedback

Biofeedback is a method by which an individual can learn to control certain physiologic responses of the body. The technique uses electronic equipment to provide clients with visible or audible evidence that they are controlling their bodies in the desired manner. For example, a sensor attached from an individual to a computer screen shows a wave pattern changing as the individual concentrates on processes such as increasing blood flow in the hands, decreasing sweat gland activity, lowering blood pressure, and controlling incontinence. The Biofeedback Certification International Alliance certifies practitioners in biofeedback, neurofeedback, and pelvic muscle dysfunction biofeedback.

Clinical Alert!

Although meditation, biofeedback, and imagery are different techniques, all three involve the process of physical resting and rhythmic breathing.

Qi Gong and T'ai Chi

A number of therapies focus on movement, body awareness, and breathing, and their purpose is to maintain health as well as to correct specific problems. **Qi gong** (pronounced *chee-goong*) is a Chinese discipline consisting of breathing and mental exercises combined with body movements. **T'ai chi** (pronounced *teye chee*) arose out of qi gong and is a discipline that combines physical fitness, meditation, and self-defense. Both disciplines consist of soft, slow, continuous movements that are circular in nature. The softness of movements develops energy without nervousness. The slowness of movements requires attentive control that quiets the mind and develops one's powers of awareness and concentration. The continuous circular nature of the movements develops strength and endurance.

Almost anyone can participate in movement-oriented therapies. They can be learned by the young and old, by individuals physically challenged or physically fit, and by those in good health and those recovering from long-term injury or illness. In China, 80-, 90-, and 100-year-old individuals get up every morning before dawn and go out to the parks to practice qi gong or t'ai chi, even in the middle of winter. These Eastern practices can be done alone, in pairs, or in large groups.

Pilates

Pilates (pronounced *pih-lah-tes*) is a method of physical movement and exercise designed to stretch, strengthen, and balance the body, in particular the core or center, including the abdominal region. It is based in principles of yoga, Zen meditation, and ancient Greek and Roman physical regimens. Pilates exercises were developed by Joseph Pilates, a German national in England at the outbreak of World War I, who was interned in a prison camp. While there, he devised his system of exercises to strengthen his frail asthmatic body, which he then taught to his fellow inmates. Exercises, coupled with focused breathing patterns, are done on the floor or with simple types of equipment. Benefits include increased lung capacity, improved flexibility and joint health, muscular coordination, increased bone density, and better posture and balance. Pilates can help rehabilitate back, knee, hip,

TABLE 22.2 Types of Imagery

Type	Description	Example
Cellular	Imagine events at cellular level.	Imagine natural killer cells surrounding and attacking cancer cells.
End state	Imagine self in the situation wished for.	See self as strong and healthy.
Energetic	Imagine free-flowing energy.	Feel self pulling up energy from the earth through the soles of the feet.
Feeling state	Move from a feeling state of tension to one of peace.	May imagine self at a beach or floating gently on the water.
Physiologic	Involves entire body.	Imagine all blood vessels relaxed and wider in order to lower blood pressure.
Psychologic	Involves perception of self.	Imagine a dialogue with an individual with whom one is in conflict in an effort to find a new solution to the problem.
Spiritual	Make contact with God or the Divine.	Imagine being held in the hands of God, where you are perfectly safe.

shoulder, and stress injuries; reduce risk for falls; and relieve muscle aches (Barker et al., 2016).

Spiritual Therapy

Healthcare sciences have begun to demonstrate that spirituality, faith, and religious commitment may play a role in promoting health and reducing illness. For more information about spirituality, see Chapter 41 ∞.

Faith and Prayer

Faith refers to our beliefs and expectations about life, ourselves, and others. In a religious context, faith refers to a belief in a Supreme Being who listens and responds to individuals and who cares about their well-being. In a spiritual context, faith is thought of as the power to accept the nature of life as it is and live in the present moment. It is a sense of letting go of the need to control while trusting and waiting for the moment when answers come.

Prayer is most often defined simply as a form of communication and fellowship with the Deity or Creator. The universality of prayer is evidenced by all cultures having some form of prayer. Prayer has been and continues to be used in times of difficulty and illness even in the most secular societies. In directed prayer, the praying individual asks for a specific outcome, such as for the cancer to go away or for the baby to be born healthy. In contrast, in nondirected prayer, no specific outcome is asked. The praying individual simply asks for the best thing to occur in a given situation.

Prayer can also be described according to form. *Colloquial* prayer is an informal talk with God, as if one were talking to a good friend. *Intercessory prayer* is asking God for things for oneself or others. The focus is on what God can provide. Intercessory prayer for others may be called "distant" prayer if the individual being prayed for is remote from the individual who is praying. This form of prayer is of interest to researchers. In one example, a prospective longitudinal design studied the feasibility and preliminary efficacy of 12 weeks of intercessory prayer by a group of nuns to reduce the disruptive behaviors of six late-stage dementia patients (Struve, Lu, Hart, & Keller, 2016). Although disruptive behavior decreased, it did not reach statistical significance.

Ritual prayer is the use of formal prayers or rituals, such as prayers from a prayer book or the Jewish siddur or the Catholic practice of saying the rosary. *Meditative* prayer, also known as contemplative prayer, is similar to meditation and is a process of focusing the mind on an aspect of spiritual belief for a period of time. Prayer is a self-care strategy that provides comfort, increases hope, and promotes healing and psychologic well-being.

Miscellaneous Therapies

Some therapies do not fit into any of the previously described categories. These include music therapy, humor and laughter, bioelectromagnetics, detoxifying therapies, animal-assisted therapy, and horticultural therapy.

Clinical Alert!

CAM modalities may be combined, for example, listening to music while being massaged with essential oils.

Music Therapy

Health is about balance or harmony of body, mind, and spirit. In a state of optimal health, all frequencies are in harmony, like a finely tuned piano. In fact, music is often used in healing, from the ancient sounds of the drum, rattle, bone flute, and other primitive instruments to the use of current music as a prescription for health.

Music therapy can be used in a variety of practice settings. Quiet, soothing music without words is often used to induce relaxation (Figure 22.5 ■). Music recordings are often used to relax and distract clients in operative settings, intensive care units, birthing rooms, rehabilitation and physical therapy units, and sleep induction units. In one research study, daily, long-term listening to classical music led to a positive relationship between mindfulness and spatial reasoning in a group of 76 African Americans (Bell, McIntyre, & Hadley, 2016). In another study, a 30-minute music therapy session consisting of either a relaxation intervention or a "song choice" intervention improved pain, anxiety, respiratory rate, and heart rate in patients in an intensive care unit (Golino et al., 2019). Music therapy can be performed independently or be combined with other therapies, such as dance and art.

Humor and Laughter

Healthcare professionals recently have focused on the positive effects of humor and laughter on health and disease, although Florence Nightingale wrote about the therapeutic effects of laughing in 1860. Humor involves the ability to discover, express, or appreciate the comical or bizarre; to be amused by one's own imperfections or the whimsical aspects of life; and to see the funny side of an otherwise serious situation. Humor in nursing can be a universal language among clients of all ages and cultures.

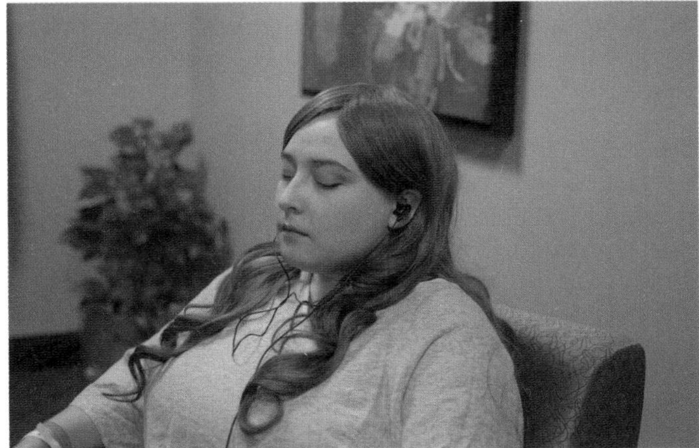

Figure 22.5 ■ Listening to music can provide a variety of therapeutic benefits.

Elaboration on these functions of humor in nursing situations follows:

- Establishing relationships. Humor decreases the social distance between individuals and assists in putting them at ease. When tension is decreased, individuals can focus on the message and on other individuals rather than on their own feelings. The use of humor helps the nurse establish rapport with clients, an important factor in achieving success in nursing interventions.
- Relieving tension and anxiety. The effective use of humor relieves the tension of emotionally charged events. The personal nature of humor, for example, helps clients deal with the impersonal nature of wearing a hospital gown and numbered ID band and with embarrassing questions and uncomfortable tests. Individuals can also use humor to decrease stress.
- Facilitating learning. Many lectures and presentations begin with a joke or cartoon. Humor not only reduces the presenter's anxiety but also gains the audience's attention. Individuals learn more when humor is used and anxiety levels are reduced. Individuals also recall more information when they associate information with a joke. Use of humor in instruction, however, needs to be carefully planned so that it will contribute to learning.

Humor also has physiologic benefits that involve alternating states of stimulation and relaxation. Laughter stimulates increases in respiratory rate, heart rate, muscular tension, and oxygen exchange. A state of relaxation follows laughter, during which heart rate, blood pressure, respiration, and muscle tension decrease. Humor stimulates the production of catecholamines and hormones. It also releases endorphins, thereby increasing pain tolerance.

Humor can bring out and integrate individuals' positive emotions: hope, faith, will to live, festivity, purpose, and determination. It therefore has healing properties. To use humor effectively, nurses need to be aware of their own feelings as well as the feelings of others and cultural variations in what individuals consider humorous. There may be a fine line between what is humorous to one individual and insulting to another. Resources for more information on humor in healthcare can be found on the Association for Applied and Therapeutic Humor website.

Bioelectromagnetics

Bioelectromagnetics is the emerging science that studies how living organisms interact with electromagnetic fields. It works on the principle that every animal, plant, and mineral has an electromagnetic field that enables organic beings and inorganic objects, such as crystals, to communicate and interact as part of a single, unified energy system. Magnetic fields are able to penetrate the body and affect the functioning of cells, tissues, organs, and systems. These therapies work best in combination with other healing modalities and are considered to be adjunct treatments to conventional medicine.

Magnet therapy is a common and controversial energy therapy. Contraindications for magnetic therapy include pregnancy, pacemakers, implanted defibrillators, aneurysm clips in the brain, cochlear implants, or other implanted electrical devices. It should not be used by individuals on anticoagulants, those with an actively bleeding or open wound, or those with a freshly torn muscle.

Detoxifying Therapies

Many cultures and religions, past and present, have rituals of purification. Some individuals adopt the concept of **detoxification**, the belief that physical impurities and toxins must be cleared from the body to achieve better health. These types of cleansing therapies may be included as a part of Ayurvedic practices.

Use of water as a healing treatment is known as hydrotherapy. The use of hot and cold moisture in the form of solid, liquid, or gas makes use of the body's response to heat and cold. Hydrotherapy is used to decrease pain, decrease fever, reduce swelling, reduce cramps, induce sleep, and improve physical and mental tone. It must be used with great care in the very young or old, who have poor heat regulation, and also with individuals experiencing a prolonged illness or fatigue.

Colonics, or colon therapy, is based on the idea that high-fat, Western diets lead to an accumulation of a substance in the colon, which in turn produces toxins that lead to disease. Colonics is the procedure for washing the inner wall of the colon by filling it with water or herbal solutions and then draining it. Colon cleansing is a controversial method of detoxification. Contraindications include individuals in a weakened state and those having ulcerative colitis, diverticulitis, Crohn's disease, severe hemorrhoids, or tumors of the large intestine or rectum.

Chelation therapy is the introduction of chemicals into the bloodstream that bind with heavy metals in the body. Ethylene diamine tetraacetic acid (EDTA) is a synthetic amino acid that readily binds to lead. The U.S. Food and Drug Administration has approved EDTA for the treatment of lead poisoning, hypercalcemia, and ventricular fibrillation secondary to digitalis toxicity, and initial studies suggest it may reduce the risk for repeated cardiac events in individuals who have had a heart attack (NCCIH, 2016).

Animal-Assisted Therapy

Animal-assisted therapy is the use of specifically selected animals as a treatment modality in health and human service settings. It has been shown to be a successful intervention for individuals with a variety of physical or psychologic conditions. Therapeutic horseback riding, or hippotherapy, is the use of the rhythmic movement of the horse to increase sensory processing and improve posture, balance, and mobility in individuals with movement dysfunctions.

Throwing an object for a dog to retrieve or brushing the animal increases upper extremity range of motion. Reaching for the object the dog has retrieved improves coordination. Ambulating with a dog improves mobility.

Recalling the animal's name helps with memory. Using simple commands to the animal increases language production. Attending to the animal and the situation increases attention and concentration.

Resident animals live at long-term healthcare facilities. Species include fish, birds, hamsters, gerbils, guinea pigs, rabbits, cats, and dogs. Some staff report that full-time pets become so perceptive that they actually gravitate to the rooms of clients who are the most isolated or depressed. The contributions companion animals (personal pets) make to the emotional well-being of clients include providing unconditional love and opportunities for affection; achievement of trust, responsibility, and empathy toward others; a reason to get up in the morning; and a source of reassurance.

Animal-assisted therapy is not the same thing as a service animal (dog or miniature horse). Service animals are trained to perform tasks for an individual with a physical or emotional disability. Because they are not considered a pet, they may legally go anywhere that an individual with disabilities goes. Some service animals are trained to "alert" the individual that a specific event is going to occur in the near future and are able to notify the human partner of this impending event. Other service animals are trained to act in a predetermined manner when a specific event occurs.

Horticultural Therapy

Horticultural therapy, also called gardening or a healing garden, is an adjunct therapy to occupational and physical therapy. Individuals may view nature, visit a healing garden or a wander garden, or actually participate in gardening. When it is a communal activity, gardening decreases social isolation by fostering interactions with others. Horticultural therapy stimulates the five senses, provides leisure activities, improves motor function, provides a sense of achievement, and improves self-esteem. Nurses must also be aware, however, that clients who are prone to infection should not come into contact with garden soil, perform activities that can cause skin punctures or scratches, or come in proximity to stagnant water that can contain insects or infectious organisms.

In summary, the CAM methods and modalities listed and described in this chapter are only a sample of those available. Others range from quite common and accepted oral supplements such as probiotics to ear candling, also called thermal-auricular therapy, which may be considered of no benefit or even to be dangerous. In every case, the nurse remains open-minded, reviews the literature for current evidence of therapeutic value, and advocates for the client in the use of the most beneficial approaches to healthcare.

LIFESPAN CONSIDERATIONS Examples of the Uses of Massage

Following are a few of the many examples illustrating the uses of massage in children and adults.

CHILDREN

Infant massage is gaining in popularity in the United States. Infant massage produces weight gain in premature infants, reduces complications in babies born to cocaine-addicted mothers, and helps depressed mothers soothe their babies. In healthy babies, it improves parent–infant bonding, eases painful procedures such as immunizations, reduces pain from teething and constipation, reduces colic, induces sleep, and makes parents feel they are doing something good for their baby.

ADULTS

- Massage is usually contraindicated until after the first trimester of pregnancy because of the danger of miscarriage during that time. During the second and third trimesters, massage can ease pain and provide comfort to the pregnant woman. Massage relaxes the woman and reduces the flow of stress hormones to the baby. It also nurtures the woman, which helps her nurture her baby after birth. Pregnancy massage is usually done in a side-lying position with plenty of pillows or cushions for support. The massage usually is done to the neck, arms, hands, back, pelvis, legs, and feet. Because not all massage therapists are trained in pregnancy massage, consumers must ask about the experience and credentials of a particular therapist.
- Massage is popular among athletes. Prior to the athletic event, massage loosens, warms, and readies the muscles for intensive use, especially when combined with stretching. Besides helping prevent injury, it can improve performance and endurance. Post-event massage relieves pain, prevents stiffness, and returns the muscles to their normal state more rapidly. The use of massage in sports healthcare is increasing rapidly in both training and competition. Recreational athletes have also discovered the benefits of sports massage as a regular part of their workouts.

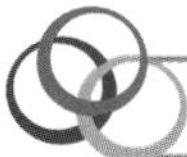

Critical Thinking Checkpoint

Tim Le is a 68-year-old accountant who has been diagnosed with gastric cancer. He lost a great deal of weight before the diagnosis and during treatment with chemotherapy and radiation. He is now admitted to the hospital with pain and weakness preventing him from working or performing many ADLs. His wife, Susan, stays with him the majority of the day. His elderly parents visit often and bring him homemade food and drink. They do not speak English. In the process of placing bathing items in Tim's bedside stand, the nurse notes several plastic bags of a tea-like product in the drawer.

1. What aspects of this case suggest that it would be appropriate for the nurse to discuss the use of alternative therapies with the client or family?
2. Which alternative therapies might be most useful for this client and are in keeping with the principle of "do no harm"?
3. How should the nurse respond to finding the bags in the client's drawer? What options should be considered, and what are the likely results of each?
4. How might the nurse's own belief system influence his or her interactions with the client and family regarding CAM?

Answers to Critical Thinking Checkpoint questions are available on the faculty resources site. Please consult with your instructor.

Chapter 22 Review

CHAPTER HIGHLIGHTS

- The concepts common to most alternative practices include holism, humanism, balance, spirituality, energy, and healing environments.
- We create healing environments when we provide holistic nursing care, take time to be with clients in deeply caring ways, and balance technology and compassion.
- If we do not create healing environments for ourselves, we are in danger of nursing "burnout."
- Ancient healthcare practices typically include an entire set of values, attitudes, and beliefs that generate a philosophy of life, not simply a group of remedies.
- Many prescription drugs sold in the United States are derived from plants.
- Although many botanical and nutritional supplements can be helpful in certain conditions, their effectiveness and safety are not all well studied.
- Manual healing methods include chiropractic, massage, acupuncture, acupressure, reflexology, and hand-mediated biofield therapies.
- Mind–body therapies such as yoga, meditation, hypnotherapy, guided imagery, biofeedback, qi gong, t'ai chi, and Pilates all focus on realigning or creating balance in mental and physical processes to bring about healing.
- Other CAM approaches include faith and prayer, music therapy, humor and laughter, bioelectromagnetics, detoxifying therapies, animal-assisted therapy, and horticultural therapy.

TEST YOUR KNOWLEDGE

1. A client asks the nurse the differences between traditional therapies and alternative therapies. What is the best response?
   1. Alternative therapies cost less than traditional therapies.
   2. Alternative therapies are used if traditional therapies are ineffective.
   3. Alternative therapies can be as effective as traditional therapies for some conditions.
   4. Alternative therapies utilize products from nature, but traditional therapies do not.

2. A client was in a motor vehicle crash where he sustained injury to his spinal cord that has resulted in difficulty with balance and holding his posture. Which of the following might the nurse working with the client suggest for consideration?
   1. Animal-assisted therapy
   2. Hypnotherapy
   3. Chelation therapy
   4. Detoxification

3. The nurse is working with a client who, during her interview, expresses feelings of groundedness. What does the nurse interpret this to mean about the client?
   1. The client is full of energy.
   2. The client feels connected to her reality.
   3. The client is focused on her center of energy.
   4. The client is "down in the dumps."

4. A client asks the nurse to state one of the primary principles associated with naturopathy. Which of the following is the best response?
   1. A higher being guides the learning needed to treat disease.
   2. It focuses on environmental causes when treating illnesses.
   3. It focuses on early detection and treatment of disease.
   4. It is a way of life to maintain health and prevent disease.

5. A client comes to the clinic with a chief complaint of feeling "dirty inside" and asks the nurse how colonics would work to improve the client's overall well-being. Which response is the most appropriate?
   1. "Colonics is a dangerous technique that no one should try."
   2. "There is much controversy about colonics. What do you know about it?"
   3. "This is a good way to get rid of toxins in your system."
   4. "You'd better ask your doctor about this."

6. A client asks how herbs are similar to prescribed medications. What is the nurse's best answer?
   1. "They are nothing alike. You should ask your doctor these types of questions."
   2. "Thirty percent of current prescription drugs are derived from plants."
   3. "Medications are much more effective than herbs."
   4. "Herbs are more dangerous than prescribed medications."

7. What is a rationale for the assessment of clients' use of herbs?
   1. There are potential adverse interactions between some herbs and some medications.
   2. Clients should not take anything that is not prescribed by the primary care provider.
   3. These data will contribute to the body of knowledge on the use of herbs.
   4. It is important to establish a pattern that clients tell nurses everything.

8. Which oils may be placed directly on the skin?
   1. Rose and orange
   2. Green apple and jasmine
   3. Clary sage and rosemary
   4. Lavender and tea tree

9. What are the effects of massage as a manual healing method? Select all that apply.
   1. Communication and caring
   2. Mental and physical relaxation
   3. Increased muscle strength
   4. Speeds the removal of waste products
   5. Lowers blood pressure and heart rate

10. Your friend is considering in vitro fertilization in hopes of becoming pregnant. Which one of the following is an accurate statement?
   1. "There is some evidence that acupuncture improves the chance of pregnancy in this situation."
   2. "Massage therapy may increase your sense of relaxation, which may help in getting pregnant."
   3. "Ask your doctor about which herbs will increase the likelihood of pregnancy."
   4. "Research suggests that yoga improves the chance of pregnancy in this situation."

See Answers to Test Your Knowledge in Appendix A.

READINGS AND REFERENCES

Suggested Readings

Dossey, B. M., & Keegan, L. (2016). *Holistic nursing: A handbook for practice* (7th ed.). Burlington, MA: Jones & Bartlett.

The 7th edition of this book received the AHNA Seal of Distinction. The authors state that it "continues the lifelong journey into understanding the wholeness of human existence." The book is organized around the five values stated in the holistic nursing scope and standards: philosophy, theories, and ethics; holistic caring process; communication, therapeutic healing environment, and cultural diversity; holistic education and research; and holistic nurse self-reflection and self-care.

Related Research

Field, T. (2016). Yoga research review. *Complementary Therapies in Clinical Practice*, *24*, 145–161. doi:10.1016/j.ctcp.2016.06.005

References

American Holistic Nurses Association. (n.d.). *Welcome*. Retrieved from http://www.ahna.org

Anselmo, J. (2016). Relaxation. In B. M. Dossey & L. Keegan (Eds.), *Holistic nursing: A handbook for practice* (7th ed., pp. 239–265). Burlington, MA: Jones & Bartlett.

Barker, A. L., Talevski, J., Bohensky, M. A., Brand, C. A., Cameron, P. A., & Morello, R. T. (2016). Feasibility of Pilates exercise to decrease falls risk: A pilot randomized controlled trial in community-dwelling older people. *Clinical Rehabilitation*, *30*, 984. doi:10.1177/0269215515606197

Bell, T. P., McIntyre, K. A., & Hadley, R. (2016). Listening to classical music results in a positive correlation between spatial reasoning and mindfulness. *Psychomusicology: Music, Mind, and Brain*, *26*, 226–235. doi:10.1037/pmu0000139

Black, L. I., Barnes, P. M., Clarke, C., Stussman, B. J., & Nahin, R. L. (2018). *Use of yoga, meditation, and chiropractors among U.S. children aged 4–17 years*. National Center for Health Statistics Data Brief No. 324. Retrieved from https://www.cdc.gov/nchs/data/databriefs/db324-h.pdf

Clarke, T. C., Barnes, P. M., Black, L. I., Stussman, B. J., & Nahin, R. L. (2018). *Use of yoga, meditation, and chiropractors among U.S. adults aged 18 and over*. National Center for Health Statistics Data Brief No. 325. Retrieved from https://www.cdc.gov/nchs/data/databriefs/db325-h.pdf

Evans Jr., M. W., Ndetan, H., Sekhon, V. K., Williams Jr., R., Oliver, B., Perko, M., . . . Singh, K. P. (2018). Adult use of complementary and integrative approaches to improve athletic performance. *Alternative Therapies in Health & Medicine*, *24*(1), 30–37.

Fontaine, K. L. (2019). *Complementary & alternative therapies for nursing practice* (5th ed.). New York, NY: Pearson.

Golino, A. J., Leone, R., Gollenberg, A., Christopher, C., Stanger, D., Davis, T. M., . . . Friesen, M. A. (2019). Impact of an active music therapy intervention on intensive care patients. *American Journal of Critical Care*, *28*(1), 48–55. doi:10.4037/ajcc2019792

Halpern, M. (2018). A review of the evolution of Ayurveda in the United States. *Alternative Therapies in Health & Medicine*, *24*(1), 12–14.

Huang, H-T., Lin, S-L, Lin, C-H, & Tzeng, D-S. (2017). Comparison between acupuncture and biofeedback as adjunctive treatments for primary insomnia disorder. *Alternative Therapies in Health & Medicine*, *23*(4), 8–15.

National Center for Complementary and Integrative Health. (2016). *Questions and answers: The NIH trials of EDTA chelation therapy for coronary heart disease*. Retrieved from https://nccih.nih.gov/health/chelation/TACT-questions

National Center for Complementary and Integrative Health. (2018a). *Homeopathy*. Retrieved from https://nccih.nih.gov/health/homeopathy

National Center for Complementary and Integrative Health. (2018b). *Use of complementary health approaches in the U.S. National Health Interview Survey (NHIS)*. Retrieved from https://nccih.nih.gov/research/statistics/NHIS/2012

Plunkett, A., Beltran, T., Haley, C., Kurihara, C., McCoart, A., Chen, L., . . . Cohen, S. P. (2017). Acupuncture for the treatment of chronic pain in the military population: Factors associated with treatment outcomes. *Clinical Journal of Pain*, *33*(10), 939–943. doi:10.1097/AJP.0000000000000518

Rolfes, S. R., Pinna, K., & Whitney, E. (2018). *Understanding normal and clinical nutrition* (11th ed.). Boston, CT: Cengage.

Spector, R. E. (2017). *Cultural diversity in health and illness* (9th ed.). New York, NY: Pearson.

Struve, A. R., Lu, D., Hart, L. K., & Keller, T. (2016). The use of intercessory prayer to reduce disruptive behaviors of patients with dementia. *Journal of Holistic Nursing*, *34*(2), 135–145. doi:10.1177/0898010115587400

White House Commission on Complementary and Alternative Medicine Policy. (2002). *Final report*. Retrieved from http://govinfo.library.unt.edu/whccamp/pdfs/fr2002_document.pdf

Selected Bibliography

Adekson, M. (2016). Similarities and differences between Yoruba traditional healers (YTH) and Native American and Canadian healers (NACH). *Journal of Religion and Health*, *55*, 1717–1728. doi:10.1007/s10943-016-0251-6

Beizaee, Y., Rejeh, N., Heravi-Karimooi, M., Tadrisi, S. D., Griffiths, P., & Vaismoradid, M. (2018). The effect of guided imagery on anxiety, depression and vital signs in patients on hemodialysis. *Complementary Therapies in Clinical Practice*, *33*, 184-190. doi:10.1016/j.ctcp.2018.10.008

Burns, D. S., Meadows, A. N., Althouse, S., Perkins, S. M., & Cripe, L. D. (2018). Differences between supportive music and imagery and music listening during outpatient chemotherapy and potential moderators of treatment effects. *Journal of Music Therapy*, *55*(1), 83–108. doi:10.1093/jmt/thy001

Clarke, T. C., Nahin, R. L., Barnes, P. M., & Stussman, B. J. (2016). *Use of complementary health approaches for musculoskeletal pain disorders among adults: United States, 2012*. National Center for Health Statistics Data Brief No. 98. Retrieved from https://www.cdc.gov/nchs/data/nhsr/nhsr098.pdf

Donaldson, J., Ingrao, C., Drake, D., & Ocampo, E. (2017). The effect of aromatherapy on anxiety experienced by hospital nurses. *MEDSURG Nursing*, *26*, 201–206.

Gamret, A. C., Price, A., Fertig, R. M., Lev-Tov, H., & Nichols, A. J. (2018). Complementary and alternative medicine therapies for psoriasis: A systematic review. *JAMA Dermatology*, *154*(11), 1330–1337. doi:10.1001/jamadermatol.2018.2972

Greenlee, H., DuPont-Reyes, M. J., Balneaves, L. G., Carlson, L. E., Cohen, M. R., Deng, G., . . . Tripathy, D. (2017). Clinical practice guidelines on the evidence-based use of integrative therapies during and after breast cancer treatment. *CA: A Cancer Journal for Clinicians*, *67*, 194–232. doi:10.3322/caac.21397

Medhurst, R. (2016). Further research in homeopathy. *Journal of the Australian Traditional-Medicine Society*, *22*(3), 146–147.

Micozzi, M. S. (2019). *Fundamentals of complementary, alternative, and integrative medicine* (6th ed.). St. Louis, MO: Saunders.

Müller, B. N., Gerasimova, A., & Ritter, S. M. (2016). Concentrative meditation influences creativity by increasing cognitive flexibility. *Psychology of Aesthetics, Creativity, and the Arts*, *10*, 278–286. doi:10.1037/a0040335

Nahin, R. L., Barnes, P. M., & Stussman, B. J. (2016). *Expenditures on complementary health approaches: United States, 2012*. National Center for Health Statistics Data Brief No. 95. Retrieved from https://www.cdc.gov/nchs/data/nhsr/nhsr095.pdf

Patricolo, G. E., LaVoie, A., Slavin, B., Richards, N. L., Jagow, D., & Armstrong, K. (2017). Beneficial effects of guided imagery or clinical massage on the status of patients in a progressive care unit. *Critical Care Nurse*, *37*, 62–69. doi:10.4037/ccn2017282

Sanchez, A. A. (2018). An examination of the folk healing practice of curanderismo in the Hispanic community. *Journal of Community Health Nursing*, *35*, 148–161. doi:10.1080/07370016.2018.1475801

Sheridan, C. B. (2016). *The mindful nurse: Using the power of mindfulness and compassion to help you thrive in your work*. Ireland: Rivertime.

Vashi, N. A., Patzelt, N., Wirya, S., Maymone, M. B. C., Zancanaro, P., & Kundu, R. V. (2018). Dermatoses caused by cultural practices: Therapeutic cultural practices. *Journal of the American Academy of Dermatology*, *79*(1), 1–16. doi:10.1016/j.jaad.2017.06.159

Wang, C., Preisser, J., Chung, Y., & Li, K. (2018). Complementary and alternative medicine use among children with mental health issues: Results from the National Health Interview Survey. *BMC Complementary and Alternative Medicine*, *18*, 241. doi:10.1186/s12906-018-2307-5

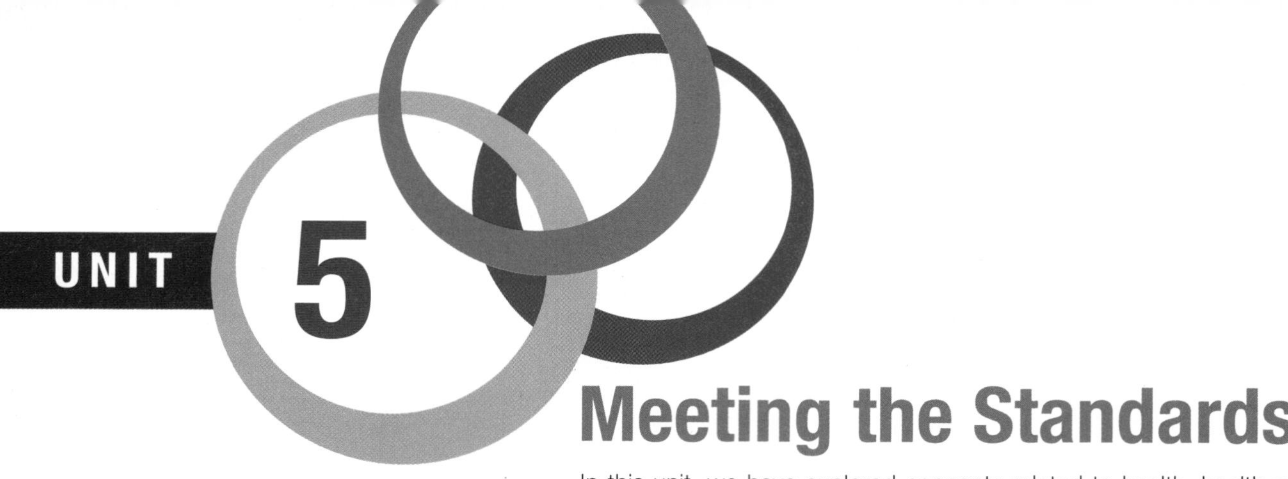

Meeting the Standards

In this unit, we have explored concepts related to health, health promotion, wellness, illness, culture and heritage, and complementary and alternative healing modalities. These topics heighten awareness of the individualistic nature of the relationship between the nurse and the client and the importance of assessing the breadth of factors that affect health decisions and behaviors. In the case described here, you will see how one client demonstrates complicated, interrelated, personal definitions of health and illness influenced by her medical condition, her heritage, and her demographic characteristics (e.g., age and family structure). These definitions and perspectives in turn influence her choices for care and support—including the role of her nurses.

CLIENT: Manuela AGE: 55
CURRENT MEDICAL DIAGNOSIS: Still's Disease

Medical History: Manuela has experienced some type of health challenge for most of her adult life. She was diagnosed with adult-onset Still's disease (AOSD) at about age 35 after several years of tests to try to determine exactly what syndrome her symptoms reflected. She complained of joint pain, rash, and fevers, which came and went, and she had an enlarged spleen and liver. This disease shares many similarities with rheumatoid and autoimmune diseases, but those conditions were all removed from consideration because the tests were negative. AOSD is a chronic condition for which there is no known cure. In addition to joint deterioration, it can progress to affect the lungs and heart. Initial treatment consists of steroids and nonsteroidal anti-inflammatory drugs (NSAIDs). If those are ineffective, other medications, such as gold and chemotherapeutics are used; however, they have severe side effects, such as kidney damage and bone marrow suppression. The condition worsens when the individual is under physical or emotional stress. Manuela underwent a hip replacement about 4 years ago and recently has had several hospitalizations for respiratory failure.

Personal and Social History: Manuela has never married and has lived near or with her parents or siblings for all her life. She has many friends, drives, and has an active social life when she is feeling well. She uses the computer extensively for communication, especially when having visitors or talking by phone is too exhausting. She must follow a strict diet of food and liquids that are easy to swallow and digest. She is a spiritual individual but not overly religious. She is quick to laugh and generally has an optimistic outlook, but she expresses awareness that her life could end at any time—certainly long before her full life expectancy.

Manuela is a college graduate but has been able to work only part time for most of her life. Recently, she was declared permanently disabled, which allows her access to financial and other support systems. She is creative in adapting her living situation to her disabilities and unwilling to give up her beloved pet dog.

Questions

American Nurses Association Standard of Practice #3 *is Outcomes Identification: The nurse collaborates with the healthcare consumer to define expected outcomes integrating the healthcare consumer's culture, values, and ethical considerations. As you learned in Chapter 19* ∞, Manuela's needs fall into the category of tertiary prevention in which rehabilitation and movement toward optimal levels of functionality within the individual's constraints are the focus.

1. What are some outcomes for Manuela that would reflect this focus?
2. Do you need to know her personal definitions of health and health beliefs (Chapter 20 ∞) before you can work with her to set expected outcomes?

American Nurses Association Standard of Practice #5b *is Health Teaching and Health Promotion: The nurse employs strategies to promote health and a safe environment.*

3. What are some aspects of Manuela's situation that you would consider incorporating into a teaching plan to maximize a safe environment for her?

American Nurses Association Standard of Professional Performance #10 *is Collaboration: Nurses partner with all stakeholders to create, implement, and evaluate a comprehensive plan.*

4. Which healthcare team members other than physicians and nurses would likely be important to include in Manuela's care plan?

American Nurses Association Standard of Professional Performance #13 *is Evidence-Based Practice and Research.*

5. What evidence might you have or seek to support the use of alternative or complementary treatment modalities in Manuela's care?

American Nurses Association. (2015). *Nursing: Scope and standards of practice* (3rd ed.). Silver Spring, MD: Author.

Answers to Meeting the Standards questions are available on the faculty resources site. Please consult with your instructor.

UNIT

6

Lifespan Development

23 Concepts of Growth and Development

LEARNING OUTCOMES

After completing this chapter, you will be able to:

1. Differentiate between the terms *growth* and *development*.
2. Describe essential principles related to growth and development.
3. List factors that influence growth and development.
4. Explain the concept of temperament.
5. Describe the stages of growth and development according to various theorists.
6. Describe characteristics and implications of Freud's five stages of development.
7. Identify Erikson's eight stages of development.
8. Identify developmental tasks associated with Havighurst's six age periods.
9. Compare Peck's and Gould's stages of adult development.
10. State the four characteristics of Bowlby's attachment theory.
11. Explain Piaget's theory of cognitive development.
12. Compare Kohlberg's and Gilligan's theories of moral development.
13. Compare Fowler's and Westerhoff's stages of spiritual development.

KEY TERMS

accommodation, *444*
adaptation, *444*
adaptive mechanisms, *439*
assimilation, *443*
attachment, *443*
cognitive development, *443*
defense mechanisms, *439*
development, *437*
developmental stages, *440*
developmental task, *441*
ego, *439*
fixation, *440*
growth, *436*
id, *439*
libido, *439*
maturation, *438*
moral, *446*
moral behavior, *446*
moral development, *446*
morality, *446*
personality, *438*
superego, *439*
temperament, *437*
unconscious mind, *439*

Introduction

Understanding the stages of growth and development is integral to the delivery of nursing care to the client and family. For example, recent literature has addressed the sandwich generation in the care of children and older adults in the family structure. Educating the caregivers of these clients on the developmental tasks inherent to both generations will enhance the totality of care delivered by the nurse and caregivers.

Abramson (2015) reported that the AARP (formerly the American Association of Retired Persons) in 2012 identified that 65.7 million individuals are functioning in the role of the caregiver for an aged parent or other relative or friend age 65 or older. It is important to educate these caregivers on how to deliver care. Further complicating nursing care, the terminology relating to the sandwich generation has expanded. The club sandwich generation identifies the adult aged 50–60 years who is caring for the aged parent, adult child, and grandchildren. An open-faced family is one in which an individual is caring for an older adult. The newest addition is the panini sandwich generation. These individuals are caring for an adult child, spouse, sibling, or grandchild while dealing with their own health-related needs due to aging (Abramson, 2015). Nurses who understand normal growth and development provide a framework for health assessment and health promotion throughout the lifespan. For example, teaching, a major nursing role, is more effective when the nurse incorporates growth and development needs and concepts. Furthermore, The Joint Commission, the accreditation body for hospitals and healthcare organizations, requires healthcare providers to be knowledgeable about the characteristics and needs of the age groups with which they come into contact. This ensures safe and effective age-specific client care.

The terms *growth* and *development* both refer to dynamic processes. Often used interchangeably, these terms have different meanings. **Growth** is physical change and an increase in size. It can be measured quantitatively. Indicators of growth include height, weight, bone size, and dentition. The pattern of physiologic growth is similar for all individuals. However, growth rates vary during different stages of growth and development. The growth rate is rapid during the prenatal, neonatal, infancy, and adolescent stages and slows during childhood. Physical growth is minimal during adulthood.

BOX 23.1 Principles of Growth and Development

- Growth and development are continuous, orderly, sequential processes influenced by maturational, environmental, and genetic factors.
- All humans follow the same pattern of growth and development.
- The sequence of each stage is predictable, although the time of onset, the length of the stage, and the effects of each stage vary with the individual.
- Learning can either help or hinder the maturational process, depending on what is learned.
- Each developmental stage has its own characteristics. For example, Piaget suggested that in the sensorimotor stage (birth to 2 years), children learn to coordinate simple motor tasks.
- Growth and development occur in a cephalocaudal direction, that is, starting at the head and moving to the trunk, the legs, and the feet (Figure 23.1 ■). This pattern is particularly obvious at birth, when the head of the infant is disproportionately large.
- Growth and development also occur in a proximodistal direction, that is, from the center of the body outward (see Figure 23.1). For example, infants can roll over before they can grasp an object with the thumb and second finger.
- Development proceeds from simple to complex, or from single acts to integrated acts. To accomplish the integrated act of drinking and swallowing from a cup, for example, the child must first learn a series of single acts: eye–hand coordination, grasping, hand–mouth coordination, controlled tipping of the cup, and then mouth, lip, and tongue movements to drink and swallow.
- Development becomes increasingly differentiated. Differentiated development begins with a generalized response and progresses to a skilled, specific response. For example, an infant's initial response to a stimulus involves the total body; a 5-year-old child can respond more specifically with laughter or fear.
- Certain stages of growth and development are more critical than others. It is known, for example, that the first 10 to 12 weeks after conception are critical. The incidence of congenital anomalies as a result of exposure to certain viruses, chemicals, or drugs is greater during this stage than others.
- The pace of growth and development is uneven. It is known that growth is greater during infancy than during childhood. Asynchronous development is demonstrated by the rapid growth of the head during infancy and the extremities at puberty.

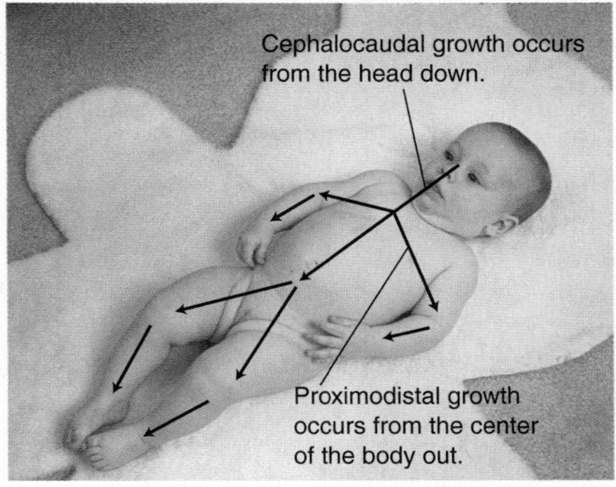

Figure 23.1 ■ Cephalocaudal and proximodistal growth.

Development is an increase in the complexity of function and skill progression. It is the capacity and skill of an individual to adapt to the environment. Development is the behavioral aspect of growth (e.g., an individual develops the ability to walk, talk, run, and think).

Growth and development are independent, interrelated processes. For example, an infant's muscles, bones, and nervous system must grow to a certain point before the infant is able to sit up, walk, or talk. Growth generally takes place during the first 20 years of life; development takes place during that time and also continues after that point. Principles of growth and development are shown in Box 23.1.

Factors Influencing Growth and Development

Many factors can influence growth and development. Knowledge of these factors helps the nurse to intervene to promote positive growth and development of the individual.

Genetics

The genetic inheritance of an individual is established at conception. It remains unchanged throughout life and determines such characteristics as gender, physical characteristics (e.g., eye color, potential height), and to some extent, temperament. Genetics plays a vital role in a client's growth and development. It is important that nurses understand the role genetics plays in the development of illness and disease. The client's genetic makeup influences weight, height, eye color, hair color, and skin pigmentation (Pierce, 2016). The client's genetic makeup influences the delivery of medical and nursing care. For example, the development of new chemotherapy agents is based on the genetic makeup of the tumor. The drugs developed in this process are referred to as targeted therapies. Targeted therapies use information from the tumor's DNA profile (Frandsen & Pennington, 2018).

Knowing a client's genetic inheritance provides awareness of the client's risk for developing disease. Many women develop breast cancer. Some forms of breast cancer are genetically transmitted, such as those resulting from the *BRCA* gene. Clients who know the risk of disease development based on their genetic profiles can receive genetic counseling to make an informed decision regarding health-related treatments.

Temperament

Temperament (i.e., the way individuals respond to their external and internal environment) sets the stage for the interactive dynamics of growth and development. Temperament may persist throughout the lifespan, although caution must be taken not to irrevocably label or categorize infants and children.

Family

The purpose of a family is to provide support and safety for the child. The family is the major constant in a child's life. Families are involved in their children's physical and psychologic well-being and development. Children are socialized through family dynamics. The parents set expected behaviors and model appropriate behavior.

Nutrition

Adequate nutrition is an essential component of growth and development. For example, poorly nourished children are more likely to have infections than are well-nourished children. In addition, poorly nourished children may not attain their full height potential.

Environment

A few environmental factors that can influence growth and development include the living conditions of the child (e.g., homelessness), socioeconomic status (e.g., impoverished versus financially stable), climate, and community (e.g., provides developmental support versus exposes the child to hazards).

Health

Illness, injury, or congenital conditions (e.g., congenital cardiac conditions) can affect growth and development. Being hospitalized is stressful for a child and can affect the coping mechanisms of the child and family. Prolonged or chronic illness may affect normal developmental processes.

Culture

Cultural customs can influence a child's growth and development. Nutritional practices may influence the rate of growth for infants. Childrearing practices may influence development.

Stages of Growth and Development

The rate of a person's growth and development is highly individual; however, the sequence of growth and development is predictable. Stages of growth usually correspond to certain developmental changes (Table 23.1).

Growth and development theories commonly include the following major components: biophysical, psychosocial, cognitive, moral, and spiritual. A discussion follows of some of the major theories relating to these components, as well as other well-known growth and development theories.

Growth and Development Theories

Researchers have advanced several theories about the various stages and aspects of growth and development, particularly with regard to infant and child development.

Biophysical Theory

Biophysical development theories describe the development of the physical body—how it grows and changes. These changes are compared against established norms. Arnold Gesell (1880–1961) is often identified as the "father of child development" in the United States. His theory states that development is directed by genetics. He conducted extensive research at Yale University in the 1920s and 1930s, asserting that child development is a process of **maturation**, or differentiation and refining of abilities and skills, based on an in-born "timetable." Although children benefit from experience, they will achieve maturational milestones such as rolling over, sitting, and walking at specific times. Gesell's (1934) most important work is found in *An Atlas of Infant Behavior*. His research documented a fixed sequence of developmental milestones of children from infancy through adolescence (Ball, 1977). Gesell observed children through a one-way mirror to determine their developmental milestones. As he collected data through observation, he also utilized photography to obtain an objective image of a child's developmental milestones. His goal was to produce a complete understanding of a child's development. The photographs were inspected, and 10 stages of development were identified. Each stage identified was assigned a percentage frequency for which the developmental milestone occurred (Varga, 2011).

Gesell's theory continues to play a significant role in determining causes and processes within neurologic developmental science and psychopathology, according to Green (2016). Gesell's information on embryology provides data for studies conducted today. In a study conducted in China by Liu et al. (2016), the adverse effects of prenatal and postnatal exposure to organophosphate pesticides were investigated. Gesell's theory was revised by the Beijing Mental Development Cooperative in 1985. The researchers utilized this information to assess neurologic development in children who had been exposed to organophosphate pesticides.

Psychosocial Theories

Psychosocial development refers to the development of personality. **Personality**, a complex concept that is difficult to define, can be considered as the outward (interpersonal)

TABLE 23.1 Stages of Growth and Development

Stage	Age	Significant Characteristics	Nursing Implications
Neonatal	Birth–28 days	Behavior is largely reflexive and develops toward more purposeful behavior.	Assist parents to identify and meet unmet needs.
Infancy	1 month–1 year	Physical growth is rapid.	Control the infant's environment so that physical and psychologic needs are met.
Toddlerhood	1–3 years	Motor development permits increased physical autonomy. Psychosocial skills increase.	Safety and risk-taking strategies must be balanced to permit growth.
Preschool	3–6 years	The preschooler's world is expanding. New experiences and the preschooler's social role are tried during play. Physical growth is slower.	Provide opportunities for play and social activity.
School age	6–12 years	Stage includes the preadolescent period (10–12 years). Peer group increasingly influences behavior. Physical, cognitive, and social development increase, and communication skills improve.	Allow time and energy for the school-age child to pursue hobbies and school activities. Recognize and support the child's achievements.
Adolescence	12–20 years	Self-concept changes with biological development. Values are tested. Physical growth accelerates. Stress increases, especially in the face of conflicts.	Assist adolescents to develop coping behaviors. Help adolescents develop strategies for resolving conflicts.
Young adulthood	20–40 years	A personal lifestyle develops. The individual establishes a relationship with a significant other and a commitment to something.	Accept the adult's chosen lifestyle and assist with necessary adjustments relating to health. Recognize the individual's commitments. Support change as necessary for health.
Middle adulthood	40–65 years	Lifestyle changes are due to other changes; for example, children leave home or occupational goals change.	Assist clients to plan for anticipated changes in life, to recognize the risk factors related to health, and to focus on strengths rather than weaknesses.
OLDER ADULTHOOD			
Young-old	65–74 years	Adaptation to retirement and changing physical abilities is often necessary. Chronic illness may develop.	Assist clients to keep physically and socially active and to maintain peer-group interactions.
Middle-old	75–84 years	Adaptation to decline in speed of movement, reaction time, and increasing dependence on others may be necessary.	Assist clients to cope with loss (e.g., hearing, sensory abilities and eyesight, death of loved one). Provide necessary safety measures.
Old-old	85 and over	Increasing physical problems may develop.	Assist clients with self-care as required, with maintenance of as much independence as possible.

expression of the inner (intrapersonal) self. It encompasses an individual's temperament, feelings, character traits, independence, self-esteem, self-concept, behavior, ability to interact with others, and ability to adapt to life changes.

Many theorists attempt to account for psychosocial development in humans, specifically the development of an individual's personality and the causes of behavior.

Freud (1856–1939)

Sigmund Freud introduced a number of concepts about development that are still used today. The concepts of the unconscious mind; defense mechanisms; and the id, ego, and superego are Freud's. The **unconscious mind** is the part of an individual's mental life of which the individual is unaware. This concept of the unconscious is one of Freud's major contributions to the field of psychiatry. The **id** resides in the unconscious and, operating on the pleasure principle, seeks immediate pleasure and gratification. The **ego**, the realistic part of the individual, balances the gratification demands of the id with the limitations of social and physical circumstances. The methods the ego uses to fulfill the needs of the id in a socially acceptable manner are called defense mechanisms. **Defense mechanisms**, or **adaptive mechanisms** as they are more commonly called today, are the result of conflicts between the id's impulses and the anxiety created by the conflicts due to social and environmental restrictions. The third aspect of the personality, according to Freud, is the superego. The **superego** contains the conscience and the ego ideal. The conscience consists of society's "do not's," usually as a result of parental and cultural expectations. The ego ideal comprises the standards of perfection toward which the individual strives. Freud proposed that the underlying motivation for human development is a dynamic, psychic energy, which he called **libido**.

According to Freud's theory of psychosexual development, the personality develops in five overlapping stages from birth to adulthood. The libido changes its location of

TABLE 23.2 Freud's Five Stages of Development

Stage	Age	Characteristics	Task to Be Attained
Oral	Birth–1½ years	Pleasure is accomplished by exploring the mouth and by sucking.	Weaning
Anal	1½–3 years	Pleasure is accomplished by exploring the organs of elimination.	Bowel and bladder control Toilet training
Phallic	4–6 years	Pleasure is accomplished by exploring the genitals. The child is attracted to the parent of the opposite sex.	Resolution of the Oedipus or Electra complex
Latency	6 years–puberty	Pleasure is directed by focusing on relationships with same-sex peers and the parent of the same sex.	Engagement in activities, such as sports, schoolwork, and socialization with same-sex peers
Genital	Puberty and after	Pleasure is directed in the development of sexual relationships.	Engagement in activities to promote independence

Adapted from *The Ego and the Mechanism of Defense*, by S. Freud, copyright 1946. New York, NY: International Universities Press.

emphasis within the individual from one stage to another. Therefore, a particular body area has special significance to a client at a particular stage. The first three stages (oral, anal, and phallic) are called *pregenital stages*. The culminating stage is the *genital stage*. Table 23.2 indicates characteristics for each stage. Freudian theory asserts that the individual must meet the needs of each stage in order to move successfully to the next developmental stage. For example, during an infant's oral stage, nurses can assist an infant's development by making feeding a pleasurable experience. This provides comfort and security for the infant. Freud also emphasized the importance of infant–parent interaction. Therefore, the nurse as a caregiver should provide a warm, caring atmosphere for an infant and assist parents to do so when the infant returns to their care.

If the individual does not achieve satisfactory progression at one stage, the personality becomes fixated at that stage. **Fixation** is immobilization or the inability of the personality to proceed to the next stage because of anxiety. For example, making toilet training a positive experience during the anal stage enhances the child's feeling of self-control. If, however, the toilet training was a negative experience, the resulting conflict or stress can delay or prolong progression through a stage or cause an individual to regress to a previous stage. Ideally, an individual progresses through each stage with a balance between the id, ego, and superego.

Erikson (1902–1994)

Erik H. Erikson (1963, 1964) adapted and expanded Freud's theory of development to include the entire lifespan, believing that individuals continue to develop throughout life. He described eight stages of development.

Erikson's theory proposes that life is a sequence of **developmental stages** or levels of achievement. Each stage signals a task that must be accomplished. The resolution of the task can be complete, partial, or unsuccessful. Erikson believed that the more success an individual has at each developmental stage, the healthier the personality of the individual. Failure to complete any developmental stage influences the individual's ability to progress to the next level. These developmental stages can be viewed as a series of crises or conflicts. Successful resolution of these crises supports healthy ego development. Failure to resolve the crises damages the ego.

Erikson's eight stages reflect both positive and negative aspects of the critical life periods. The resolution of the conflicts at each stage enables the individual to function effectively in society. Each phase has its own developmental task, and the individual must find a balance between, for example, trust versus mistrust (stage 1) or integrity versus despair (stage 8).

Stage 1 is trust versus mistrust, which is from birth to 18 months of age. The infant learns to trust the primary caregiver to meet the infant's needs for food, shelter, and personal care. In early childhood, age 18 months to 3 years, the development task is autonomy versus shame and doubt. The child begins to identify with the development of control of bodily functions (Erikson, 1963).

Initiative versus guilt is the developmental task of late childhood, between the ages of 3 and 5 years. At this stage, the child becomes assertive and is aware of her own behavior. If this task is not successfully achieved, the child will have decreased self-confidence, and feelings of fear will result (Erikson, 1963).

From age 6 to 12 years the developmental task is industry versus inferiority. Successful attainment indicates the child's ability to create. A negative response is withdrawal and a sense of hopelessness (Erikson, 1963).

The fifth stage of Erikson's theory is identity versus role confusion. This stage occurs from about 12 to 18 years. The individual searches for self and personal identity. A negative response would involve role confusion and inability to identify their place in society. From age 18 to 24 years, the central task is intimacy versus isolation. The individual is exploring relationships with other individuals while also exploring work experiences. A negative resolution would be the avoidance of a career or relationships.

The developmental task of adulthood is generativity versus stagnation. The adult age 25–65 years is creative and develops new interests. From age 65 years to death, the individual's central task is integrity versus despair.

The individual accepts his life and ultimate death (Erikson, 1963). See Figures 23.2 ■ and 23.3 ■.

When using Erikson's developmental framework, nurses should be aware of indicators of positive and negative resolution of each developmental stage. According to Erikson, the environment is highly influential in development. Nurses can enhance a client's development by being aware of the individual's developmental stage and assisting with the development of coping skills related to the stressors experienced at that specific level. Nurses can strengthen a client's positive resolution of a developmental task by providing appropriate opportunities and encouragement. For example, a 10-year-old child (industry versus inferiority) can be encouraged to be creative, to finish schoolwork, and to learn how to accomplish these tasks within the limitations imposed by health status.

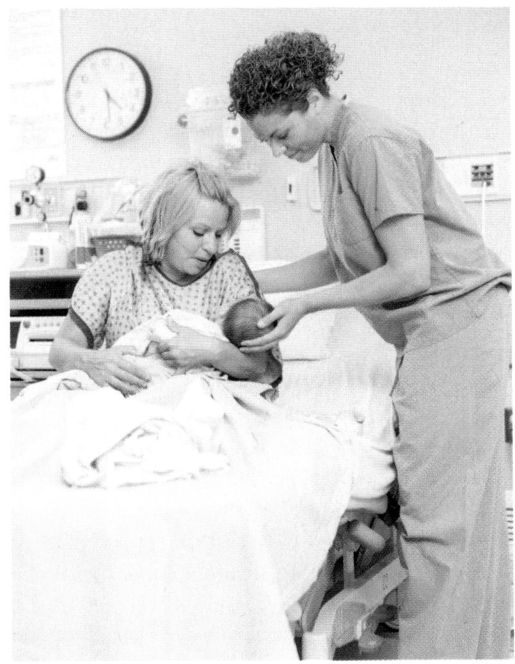

Figure 23.2 ■ Trust is established when the infant's basic needs are met.
Tyler Olson/123RF.

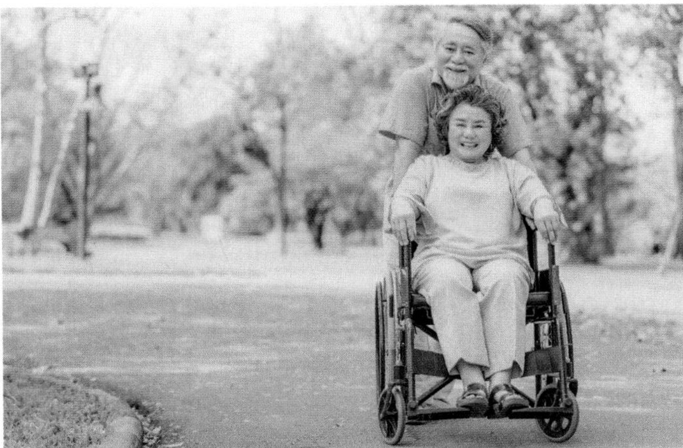

Figure 23.3 ■ Assistive devices help maintain independence and self-esteem, which also helps older adults maintain ego integrity and adapt to and cope with the realities of aging.
tidty/123RF.

Erikson emphasized that individuals must change and adapt their behavior to maintain control over their lives. In his view, no stage in personality development can be bypassed, but individuals can become fixated at one stage or regress to a previous stage under anxious or stressful conditions. For example, a middle-aged woman who has never satisfactorily accomplished the task of resolving identity versus role confusion might regress to an earlier stage when stressed by an illness with which she cannot cope.

Havighurst (1900–1991)

Robert Havighurst believed that learning is basic to life and that individuals continue to learn throughout life. He described growth and development as occurring during six stages, each associated with 6 to 10 tasks to be learned (Box 23.2).

Havighurst promoted the concept of developmental tasks in the 1950s. A **developmental task** is "a task which arises at or about a certain period in the life of an individual, successful achievement of which leads to his [*sic*] happiness and to success with later tasks, while failure leads to unhappiness in the individual, disapproval by society, and difficulty with later tasks" (Havighurst, 1972, p. 2).

Havighurst's developmental tasks provide a framework that the nurse can use to evaluate the client's general accomplishments. However, these tasks are presented as very broad categories and some nurses find them of limited use when assessing specific accomplishments, particularly those of infancy and childhood. Also, in a multicultural society, the definition of successful resolution of tasks may vary with values and belief systems (e.g., not all individuals may wish to marry or bear children), making these tasks less relevant for some.

Peck

Theories and models about adult development are relatively recent compared with theories of infant and child development. Research into adult development has been stimulated by a number of factors, including increased longevity and healthier old age. In the past, development was viewed as complete by the time of physical maturity, and aging was considered a decline following maturity. The emphasis was on the negative aspects rather than the positive aspects of aging. However, Robert Peck (1968) believes that although physical capabilities and functions decrease with old age, mental and social capacities tend to increase in the latter part of life.

Peck proposes three developmental tasks during old age, in contrast to Erikson's one (integrity versus despair):

1. ***Ego differentiation versus work-role preoccupation.*** Adults' identity and feelings of worth are highly dependent on their work roles. On retirement, individuals may experience feelings of worthlessness unless they derive their sense of identity from a number of roles so that one such role can replace the work role

BOX 23.2 Havighurst's Age Periods and Developmental Tasks

INFANCY AND EARLY CHILDHOOD

1. Learning to walk
2. Learning to take solid foods
3. Learning to talk
4. Learning to control the elimination of body wastes
5. Learning sex differences and sexual modesty
6. Achieving psychological stability
7. Forming simple concepts of social and physical reality
8. Learning to relate emotionally to parents, siblings, and other people
9. Learning to distinguish right from wrong and developing a conscience

MIDDLE CHILDHOOD

1. Learning the physical skills necessary for ordinary games
2. Building wholesome attitudes toward oneself as a growing organism
3. Learning to get along with age-mates
4. Learning an appropriate masculine or feminine social role
5. Developing fundamental skills in reading, writing, and calculating
6. Developing concepts necessary for everyday living
7. Developing conscience, morality, and a scale of values
8. Achieving personal independence
9. Developing attitudes toward social groups and institutions

ADOLESCENCE

1. Achieving new and more mature relations with age-mates of both sexes
2. Achieving a masculine or feminine social role
3. Accepting one's physique and using the body effectively
4. Achieving emotional independence from parents and other adults
5. Achieving assurance of economic independence
6. Selecting and preparing for an occupation
7. Preparing for marriage and family life
8. Developing intellectual skills and concepts necessary for civic competence
9. Desiring and achieving socially responsible behavior
10. Acquiring a set of values and an ethical system as a guide to behavior

EARLY ADULTHOOD

1. Selecting a mate
2. Learning to live with a partner
3. Starting a family
4. Rearing children
5. Managing a home
6. Getting started in an occupation
7. Taking on civic responsibility
8. Finding a congenial social group

MIDDLE AGE

1. Achieving adult civic and social responsibility
2. Establishing and maintaining an economic standard of living
3. Assisting teenage children to become responsible and happy adults
4. Developing adult leisure-time activities
5. Relating oneself to one's spouse as a person
6. Accepting and adjusting to the physiologic changes of middle age
7. Adjusting to aging parents

LATER MATURITY

1. Adjusting to decreasing physical strength and health
2. Adjusting to retirement and reduced income
3. Adjusting to death of a spouse
4. Establishing an explicit affiliation with one's age group
5. Meeting social and civil obligations
6. Establishing satisfactory physical living arrangements

or occupation as a source of self-esteem. For example, someone who likes to garden or golf can obtain ego rewards from those activities, replacing rewards formerly obtained from the individual's occupation.

2. ***Body transcendence versus body preoccupation.*** This task calls for the individual to adjust to decreasing physical capacities and at the same time maint ain feelings of well-being. Preoccupation with declining body functions reduces happiness and satisfaction with life.
3. ***Ego transcendence versus ego preoccupation.*** Ego transcendence is the acceptance, without fear, of one's death as inevitable. This acceptance includes being actively involved in one's own future beyond death. Ego preoccupation, by contrast, results in holding on to life and a preoccupation with self-gratification.

Gould

Roger Gould is another theorist who has studied adult development. He believes that transformation is a central theme during adulthood: "Adults continue to change over the period of time considered to be adulthood and developmental phases may be found during the adult span of life" (Gould, 1972, p. 33). According to Gould, the 20s is the time when an individual assumes new roles; in the 30s, role confusion often occurs; in the 40s, the individual becomes aware of time limitations in relation to accomplishing life's goals; and in the 50s, the acceptance of each stage as a natural progression of life marks the path to adult maturity. Gould's study of 524 men and women led him to describe seven stages of adult development:

- ***Stage 1 (ages 16–18).*** Individuals consider themselves part of the family rather than individuals and want to separate from their parents.
- ***Stage 2 (ages 18–22).*** Although individuals have established autonomy, they feel it is in jeopardy; they feel they could be pulled back into their families.
- ***Stage 3 (ages 22–28).*** Individuals feel established as adults and autonomous from their families. They see themselves as well defined but still feel the need to prove

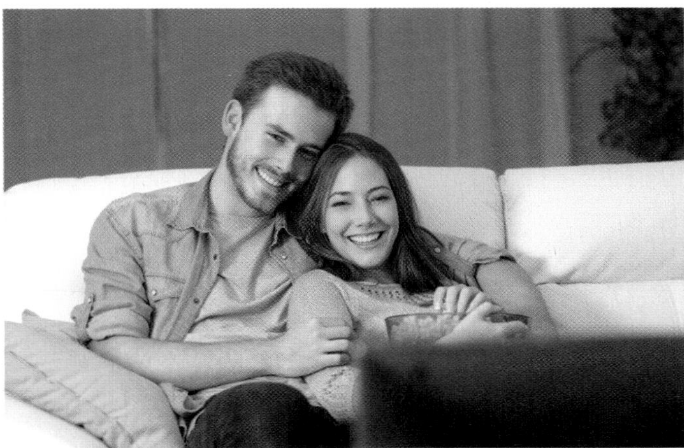

Figure 23.4 ■ Young adults develop meaningful relationships and begin considering a home and family for themselves.
Antonio Guillem/123RF.

themselves to their parents. They see this as the time for growing and building for the future (Figure 23.4 ■).

- *Stage 4 (ages 28–34).* Marriage and careers are well established. Individuals question what life is all about and wish to be accepted as they are, no longer finding it necessary to prove themselves.
- *Stage 5 (ages 34–43).* This is a period of self-reflection. Individuals question values and life itself. They see time as finite, with little time left to shape the lives of adolescent children.
- *Stage 6 (ages 43–50).* Personalities are seen as set. Time is accepted as finite. Individuals are interested in social activities with friends and spouse and desire both sympathy and affection from their spouses.
- *Stage 7 (ages 50–60).* This is a period of transformation, with a realization of mortality and a concern for health. There is an increase in warmth and a decrease in negativism. The spouse is seen as a valuable companion (Gould, 1972, pp. 525–527).

Temperament Theories

Early research on temperament, conducted in the 1950s by Stella Chess and Alexander Thomas, identified nine temperamental qualities seen in children's behavior (Table 23.3). Temperament is multidimensional, leading to the development of a child's personality traits. Temperament has a role in the development of anxiety, depression, attention-deficit/hyperactivity disorder (ADHD), and other types of behavior. When parents understand a child's temperament characteristics, they are better able to shape the environment to meet the child's needs. Rothbart and Bates (2006) developed Rothbart's Model of Temperament. There are three dimensions to the theory. The first is surgency (tendency toward positive affectation). Surgency in high levels in children will result in a high anxiety level. Negative affectivity, the second dimension, develops intense feelings of fear and anger. Effortful control (self-regulation), the third dimension, is a regulatory mechanism of temperament. A child with high effortful control is better able to regulate emotions. A study by Ullsperger, Nigg, and Nikolas (2016) investigated how a child's temperament and their parents' parenting practices relate to child ADHD symptoms. Inconsistent discipline by parents led to a lower level of conscientiousness and greater ADHD symptomatology. Thus, consistent parenting can have a positive impact on outcomes in a child's temperament and decrease ADHD symptomatology.

Attachment Theory

Attachment theory shares a common belief with Freud's psychoanalytic theory: that early childhood experiences have a strong influence on the child's development and later behavior. British psychologist and physician John Bowlby (1907–1990) worked extensively with children experiencing separation and loss during wartime, researching and explaining how they responded. He hypothesized that humans have an essential need for **attachment**, or lasting, strong emotional bonds, to others and that the infant–caregiver relationship is the first such attachment. Attachment, Bowlby believed, also serves as a protective or survival mechanism for the infant. Characteristics of Bowlby's attachment theory include the desire to be near the attachment figure, a return to the attachment figure when threatened or for comfort, the use of the attachment figure as a security base from which the child can explore the surrounding environment, and expression of anxiety (separation anxiety) when the attachment figure is absent (Bowlby, 1999).

Cognitive Theory

Cognitive development refers to the manner in which individuals learn to think, reason, and use language and other symbols. It involves an individual's intelligence, perceptual ability, and ability to process information. Cognitive development represents a progression of mental abilities from illogical to logical thinking, from simple to complex problem-solving, and from understanding concrete ideas to understanding abstract concepts.

The most widely known cognitive theorist is Jean Piaget (1896–1980). His theory of cognitive development has contributed to other theories, such as Kohlberg's theory of moral development and Fowler's theory of the development of faith, both discussed later in this chapter.

According to Piaget (1966), cognitive development is an orderly, sequential process in which a variety of new experiences (stimuli) must exist before intellectual abilities can develop. Piaget's cognitive developmental process is divided into five major phases: the sensorimotor phase, the preconceptual phase, the intuitive thought phase, the concrete operations phase (Figure 23.5 ■), and the formal operations phase.

An individual develops through each of these phases, each of which has its own unique characteristics (Table 23.4). In each phase, the individual uses three primary abilities: assimilation, accommodation, and adaptation. **Assimilation**

CONCEPT MAP

Overview of Growth and Development Psychosocial Theories and Theorists

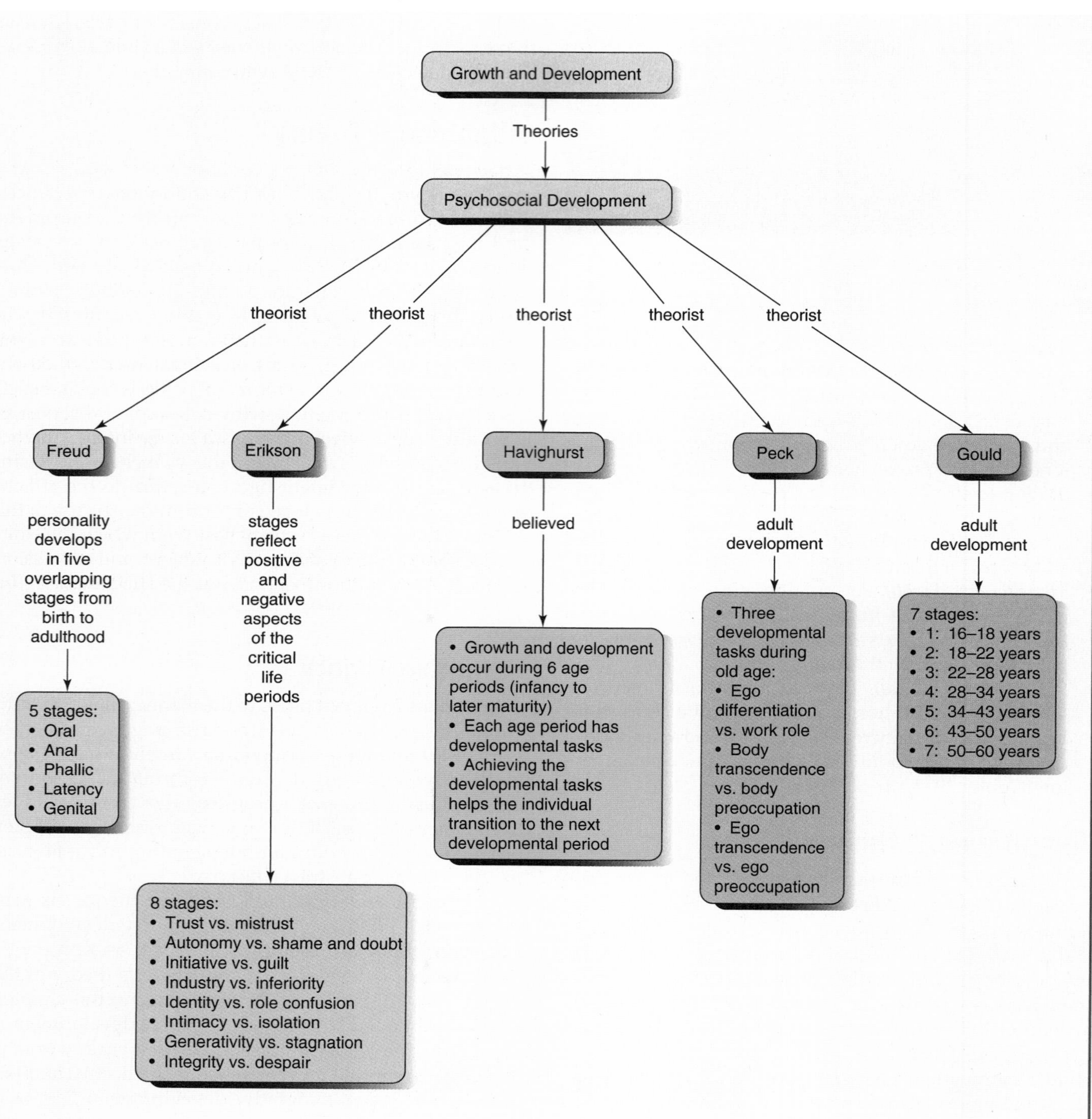

is the process by which humans encounter and react to new situations by using the mechanisms they already possess. In this way, individuals acquire knowledge and skills as well as insights into the world around them. **Accommodation** is a process of change whereby cognitive processes mature sufficiently to allow the individual to solve problems that were previously unsolvable. This adjustment is possible chiefly because new knowledge has been assimilated. **Adaptation**, or coping behavior, is the ability to handle the demands made by the environment.

Nurses can employ Piaget's theory of cognitive development when developing teaching strategies. For example,

TABLE 23.3 Characteristics of Temperament

Characteristic	Examples of Behavior Style
Activity level	Active, restless, always on the move versus quiet, inactive
Sensitivity	Apparently oblivious to stimuli versus reacts to minimal stimuli
Intensity	Minimal reaction to stimuli versus reacts strongly and intensely
Adaptability	Responds smoothly to unexpected events versus resists change
Distractibility	Focuses on tasks versus easily distracted by minimal stimuli
Approach or withdrawal	Jumps right into activities versus hesitant to engage, slow to warm up
Mood	Cheerful, happy versus serious, somber
Persistence	Sticks to tasks versus easily gives up
Regularity	Demonstrates patterns of behavior versus random activity

a nurse can expect a toddler to be egocentric and literal; therefore, explanations to the toddler should focus on the needs of the toddler rather than on the needs of others. A 13-year-old can be expected to use rational thinking and to reason; therefore, when explaining the need for a medication, the nurse can outline the consequences of taking and not taking the medication, enabling the adolescent to make a rational decision. Nurses must remember, however,

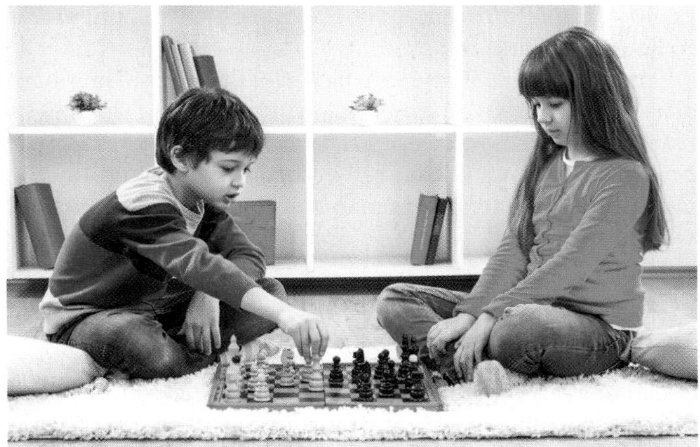

Figure 23.5 ■ School-age (7 to 11 years) children can understand cause-and-effect and concrete relationships or problems.
inesbazdar/123RF.

that the range of normal cognitive development is broad, despite the ages arbitrarily associated with each level. When teaching adults, nurses may become aware that some adults are more comfortable with concrete thought and slower to acquire and apply new information than are other adults.

Behaviorist Theory

Behaviorist theory states that learning takes place when an individual's response to a stimulus is either positively or negatively reinforced. The more rapid, consistent, and

TABLE 23.4 Piaget's Phases of Cognitive Development

Phases and Stages	Age	Significant Behavior
Sensorimotor phase	Birth–2 years	
Stage 1: Use of reflexes	Birth–1 month	The use of reflexes
Stage 2: Primary circular reaction	1–4 months	Sucking habits are developed, such as thumb sucking and the protrusion of the tongue when the infant is hungry. The infant acknowledges objects visually, grasps at objects, and is attracted by sounds.
Stage 3: Secondary circular reaction	4–8 months	The infant begins to discover and rediscover the external environment.
Stage 4: Coordination of secondary schemata	8–12 months	The first actual intellectual behavior patterns emerge. The infant begins to distinguish the ends and the means. The infant is utilizing cognitive development to attain a goal.
Stage 5: Tertiary circular reaction	12–18 months	The child discovers new ways of solving problems by utilizing experimentation.
Stage 6: Inventions of new means	18–24 months	The child possesses mental images of the environment and utilizes cognitive skills to solve problems. The child's playtime is an imitation of what has been seen, leading to pretend play.
Preconceptual phase	2–4 years	Uses an egocentric approach to accommodate the demands of an environment. Everything is significant and relates to "me." Explores the environment. Language development is rapid. Associates words with objects.
Intuitive thought phase	4–7 years	Egocentric thinking diminishes. Thinks of one idea at a time. Includes others in the environment. Words express thoughts.
Concrete operations phase	7–11 years	Solves concrete problems. Begins to understand relationships such as size. Understands right and left. Cognizant of viewpoints.
Formal operations phase	11–15 years	Uses rational thinking. Reasoning is deductive and futuristic.

Adapted from *The Origins of Intelligence in Children*, by J. Piaget, 1966, New York, NY: W. W. Norton and Company, Inc.; and *The Psychology of the Child*, by J. Piaget and B. Inhelder, 1969, New York, NY: Basic Books, HarperCollins.

positive the reinforcement is, the more likely a behavior is to be learned and retained.

B. F. Skinner (1904–1990) believed that organisms learn as they respond to or "operate on" their environment. His research led to the concept of *operant conditioning*, the basic premise of which is that rewarded or reinforced behavior will be repeated, whereas behavior that is punished will be suppressed. Most of his work was with laboratory animals.

Social Learning Theories

Social learning theory is based on the principle that individuals learn by observing and thinking about the behavior of the self and others and can be seen as spanning both behaviorist and cognitive learning theories.

Bandura

In contrast to Skinner's operant conditioning, Albert Bandura, a foremost social learning theorist, believes that learning occurs through imitation and practice and requires more awareness, self-motivation, and self-regulation of the individual. In Bandura's social learning theory, the individual actively interacts with the environment to learn new skills and behaviors. Social learning theorists contend that this process may not always lead to change in the individual's behavior; in contrast, behaviorist theory says that learning will result in a permanent change in behavior.

Vygotsky (1896–1934)

Lev Vygotsky, referred to as a social constructivist, explored the concept of cognitive development within a social, historical, and cultural context, arguing that adults guide children to learn and that development depends on the use of language, play, and extensive social interaction. These ideas also support the benefit of adult social learning opportunities via group interaction and observation. Vygotsky supported social learning and reinforcement through work, group discussion, and other means of interaction.

Ecologic Systems Theory

Urie Bronfenbrenner (1917–2005) expounded the ecologic systems theory of development. He viewed the child as interacting with the environment at different levels, or systems. Bronfenbrenner believed each child brings a unique set of genes—and specific attributes such as age, gender, health, and other characteristics—to his or her interactions with the environment.

The ecologic systems theory has five levels or systems. The microsystem includes close relationships the child has on a daily basis (e.g., home, school, friends). The mesosystem level includes relationships of microsystems with one another (e.g., the relationship between family and school). The exosystem includes those settings that may influence the child but with which the child does not have daily contact (e.g., parent's job, local school board). The macrosystem level includes the actions, attitudes, and beliefs of the child's culture and society. Finally, the chronosystem involves the time period in which the child is growing up and its influence on views of health and illness.

Theories of Moral Development

Moral development, a complex process that is not fully understood, involves learning what ought to be and what ought not to be done. It is more than imprinting parents' rules and virtues or values on children. The term **moral** means "relating to right and wrong." The terms *morality, moral behavior*, and *moral development* need to be distinguished from each other. **Morality** refers to the requirements necessary for individuals to live together in society; **moral behavior** is the way an individual perceives those requirements and responds to them; **moral development** is the pattern of change in moral behavior with age (see Chapter 4 ∞).

Kohlberg (1927–1987)

Lawrence Kohlberg's (1984) theory specifically addresses moral development in children and adults. The morality of an individual's decision was not Kohlberg's concern; rather, he focused on the reasons an individual makes a decision. According to Kohlberg, moral development progresses through three levels and six stages. Levels and stages are not always linked to a certain developmental stage or age because some individuals progress to a higher level of moral development than others.

At Kohlberg's first level, called the *premoral* or *preconventional level*, children are responsive to cultural rules and labels of good and bad, right and wrong. However, children interpret these in terms of the physical consequences of their actions, that is, punishment or reward. At the second level, the *conventional level*, the individual is concerned about maintaining the expectations of the family, group, or nation and sees this as right. The emphasis at this level is conformity and loyalty to one's own expectations as well as society's. Level three is called the *postconventional, autonomous*, or *principled level*. At this level, individuals make an effort to define valid values and principles without regard to outside authority or to the expectations of others (Table 23.5).

Gilligan (1936–Present)

After more than 10 years of research with female participants, Carol Gilligan reported that women often consider the dilemmas Kohlberg used in his research to be irrelevant. Women scored consistently lower on Kohlberg's scale of moral development despite the fact that they approached moral dilemmas with considerable sophistication. Gilligan believes that most frameworks for research in moral development do not include the concepts of caring and responsibility.

Gilligan (1982) contends that moral development proceeds through three levels and two transitions, with each level representing a more complex understanding of the relationship of self and others and each transition

CONCEPT MAP

Overview of Growth and Development Theories and Theorists

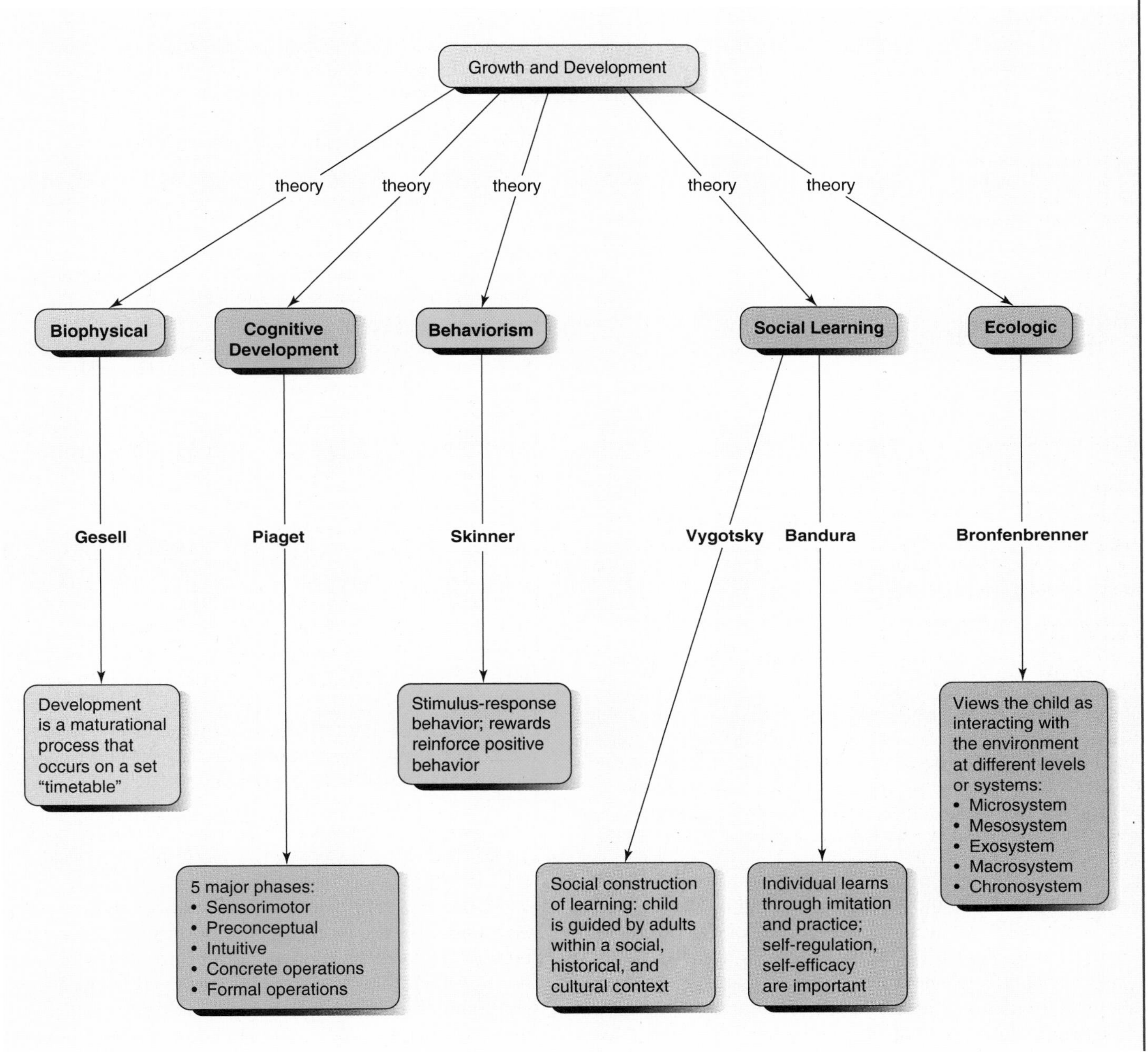

resulting in a crucial reevaluation of the conflict between selfishness and responsibility:

- ***Stage 1: caring for oneself.*** In this first stage of development, individuals are concerned only with caring for the self. They feel isolated, alone, and unconnected to others. There is no concern or conflict with the needs of others because the self is the most important. The focus of this stage is survival. The transition of this stage occurs when individuals begin to view this approach as selfish and move toward responsibility. Individuals begin to realize a need for relationships and connections with other people.
- ***Stage 2: caring for others.*** During this stage, individuals recognize the selfishness of earlier behavior and begin to understand the need for caring relationships with others. Caring relationships bring with them responsibility. The definition of responsibility includes self-sacrifice, where "good" is considered to be "caring for others." Individuals now approach relationships with a focus of not hurting others. This approach causes

TABLE 23.5 Kohlberg's Stages of Moral Development

Level	Stage
I. Preconventional **Egocentric Point of View** Individuals begin to understand the rules of right and wrong.	**1. Punishment and Obedience** Actions are judged in terms of physical consequences.
	2. Individual Instrumental Purpose and Exchange Individuals engage in actions that are right to meet their needs. Individuals separate their own interests from the interest of authorities.
II. Conventional Individuals are concerned about others and their feelings.	**3. Mutual Interpersonal Expectations, Relationships, and Conformity** Individuals are in relationships with others. Individuals pay attention to the feelings of others. Individuals put themselves in the other person's shoes.
Social Perspective Individuals are doing their duty to society.	**4. Social System and Conscience Maintenance** Individuals fulfill the duties assigned by authority figures, thus fulfilling obligations set forth by society's laws.
III. Postconventional Individuals uphold the basic rights, values, and legal contracts of the society.	**5. Prior Rights and Social Contract** Individuals have an obligation to obey the law. There is a commitment to family and work obligations. Individuals have a responsibility to consider the moral and legal point of view in ascertaining what will provide the greatest good for the greatest number.
Universal Focus	**6. Universal Ethical Principle** Individuals follow what is right in accordance with ethical principles.

Adapted from *Essays on Moral Development. Vol.1: The Philosophy of Moral Development*, 1981, by L. Kohlberg, San Francisco, CA: Harper & Row.

EVIDENCE-BASED PRACTICE

Evidence-Based Practice

How Does Socioeconomic Status Affect an Infant's Birth Outcomes?

Campbell and Seabrook (2016) reviewed health-related research to ascertain the effects of low socioeconomic status on adverse birth outcomes. The authors found that the most identified indicator of socioeconomic status was education. The lack of education resulted in adverse infant health outcomes. The infants of college educated women weighed 128 g more than those of women with a high school education. Low socioeconomic background also contributed to poor infant health outcomes. The overview of research collected concluded that decreased education, lower-socioeconomic neighborhood, and jobs requiring heavy lifting yielded adverse birth outcomes.

Implications

Public health and maternal child nurses must pay attention to the socioeconomic status of families under their care. The nurse must provide thorough client education, paying attention to primary prevention.

individuals to be more responsive and submissive to others' needs, excluding any thoughts of meeting their own needs. A transition from goodness to truth occurs when individuals recognize that this approach can cause difficulties with relationships because of the lack of balance between caring for the self and caring for others. Individuals make decisions based on personal intentions and the consequences of actions rather than on how they think others will react.

- *Stage 3: caring for self and others.* During this last stage, individuals see the need for a balance between caring for others and caring for the self. The concept of responsibility now includes responsibility for the self and for other people. Care remains the focus on which decisions are made. However, individuals recognize the interconnections between the self and others and realize that if their own needs are not met, other people may also suffer.

Gilligan (1982) believes that because women often see morality in the integrity of relationships and caring, the moral problems they encounter are different from those of men. Men tend to consider what is right to be what is just, whereas for women, taking responsibility for others as a self-chosen decision is what is right (p. 140). The ethic of justice, or fairness, is based on the idea of equality: Everyone should receive the same treatment. This is the development path usually followed by men and widely accepted by moral theorists. By contrast, the ethic of care is based on the premise of nonviolence: No one should be harmed. This is the path typically followed by women but given little attention in the literature of moral theory.

In the development of maturity, according to Gilligan (1982), both viewpoints blend "in the realization that just as inequality adversely affects both perspectives in an unequal relationship, so too violence is destructive for everyone involved" (p. 174). The blending of these two perspectives can give rise to a new view of human development and a better understanding of human relations.

Theories of Spiritual Development

The spiritual component of growth and development refers to individuals' understanding of their relationship with the universe and their perceptions about the direction and meaning of life. Spirituality and faith are distinctly different from religious beliefs, but religion may allow for their expression.

Fowler

James Fowler describes the development of faith as a force that gives meaning to an individual's life. He uses the term *faith* as a form of knowing, a way of being in relation to "an ultimate environment." To Fowler, "faith is a relational phenomenon; it is an active 'mode-of-being-in-relation' to another or others in which we invest commitment, belief, love, risk and hope" (Fowler & Keen, 1985, p. 18).

Fowler's theory and developmental stages were influenced by the work of Piaget, Kohlberg, and Erikson. Fowler believes that the development of faith is an interactive process between the individual and the environment (Fowler, Streib, & Keller, 2004). In each of Fowler's stages, new patterns of thought, values, and beliefs are added to those already held by the individual; therefore, the stages must follow in sequence. Faith stages, according to Fowler, are separate from the cognitive stages of Piaget: They evolve from a combination of knowledge and values. Stage 0 occurs from the age of 0 to 3. There is a formulation of concepts about self and the environment. The intuitive project stage occurs from the ages of 4 to 6. Children in this stage have a combination of images and beliefs. Children are introduced to images and beliefs from trusted individuals. They also utilize their own imagination and experiences in their spiritual development. The mythic-literal stage ranges from age 7 to 12 and encompasses symbols, stories, and myths that possess spiritual meaning. The synthetic-conventional stage begins with adolescence. The environment is structured by the expectations and judgment of others. After the age of 18, adults build their own spiritual systems. This is known as the individuating-reflexive stage. The paradoxical-consolidative phase occurs after 30 years of age with the awareness of truth from many different viewpoints. The last phase is universalizing. Individuals may not ever reach this stage In this stage, individuals express the principles of love and justice in their lives (Fowler & Keen, 1985).

Westerhoff

Westerhoff (2012) describes faith as a way of being and behaving that evolves from an experienced faith guided by parents and others during an individual's infancy and childhood to an owned faith that is internalized in adulthood and serves as a directive for personal action. The first stage is experienced faith. Infants through early adolescents interact with others in learning faith traditions. Affiliative faith occurs in late adolescence. At this stage, there is active participation in faith-based traditions. Teens feel a sense of belonging to their faith. In young adulthood, individuals begin the stage of searching faith. Young adults may doubt or question their faith. The stage of owned faith occurs in middle adulthood to old age. In this stage, faith becomes very personal, and individuals stand up for what they believe. For the client who is ill, faith—whether in a higher authority (e.g., God, Allah, Jehovah), in the client's own self, in the healthcare team, or in a combination of all—provides strength and trust.

Applying Growth and Development Concepts to Nursing Practice

Different theories explain one or more aspects of an individual's growth and development. Typically, theorists examine only one area of an individual's development, such as the cognitive, moral, or physical aspects. The area chosen for examination usually reflects the researcher's academic discipline and personal interest. Theorists may also limit the population that is studied to a particular part of the lifespan, such as infancy, childhood, or adulthood.

Although such theories can be useful, they have limitations. First, the theory chosen may explain only one aspect of the growth and development process. Yet an individual does not develop in fragmented sections but rather as a whole human being. Thus, the nurse may find it necessary to apply several theories for an adequate understanding of the growth and development of a client.

Another limitation of some theories is the suggestion that certain tasks are performed at a specific age. In most cases, the child or adult does accomplish the task at the time specified by the guidelines. In other cases, however, nurses may find that an individual does not accomplish the task or meet the milestone at the exact time suggested by the theory. Such individual differences are not easily defined or categorized by a single theory. Human development is a complex synthesis of biophysical, cognitive, psychologic, moral, and spiritual development. Nurses should expect individual variations and take these into consideration when applying theories about growth and development. In so doing, they will be better able to understand a client's development and plan effective nursing interventions.

In nursing, developmental theories can be useful in guiding assessment, explaining behavior, and providing a direction for nursing interventions. An understanding of a child's intellectual ability helps a nurse to anticipate and explain certain reactions, responses, and needs. Nurses can then encourage client behavior that is appropriate for that particular developmental stage.

CONCEPT MAP

Overview of Growth and Development Moral and Spiritual Theories and Theorists

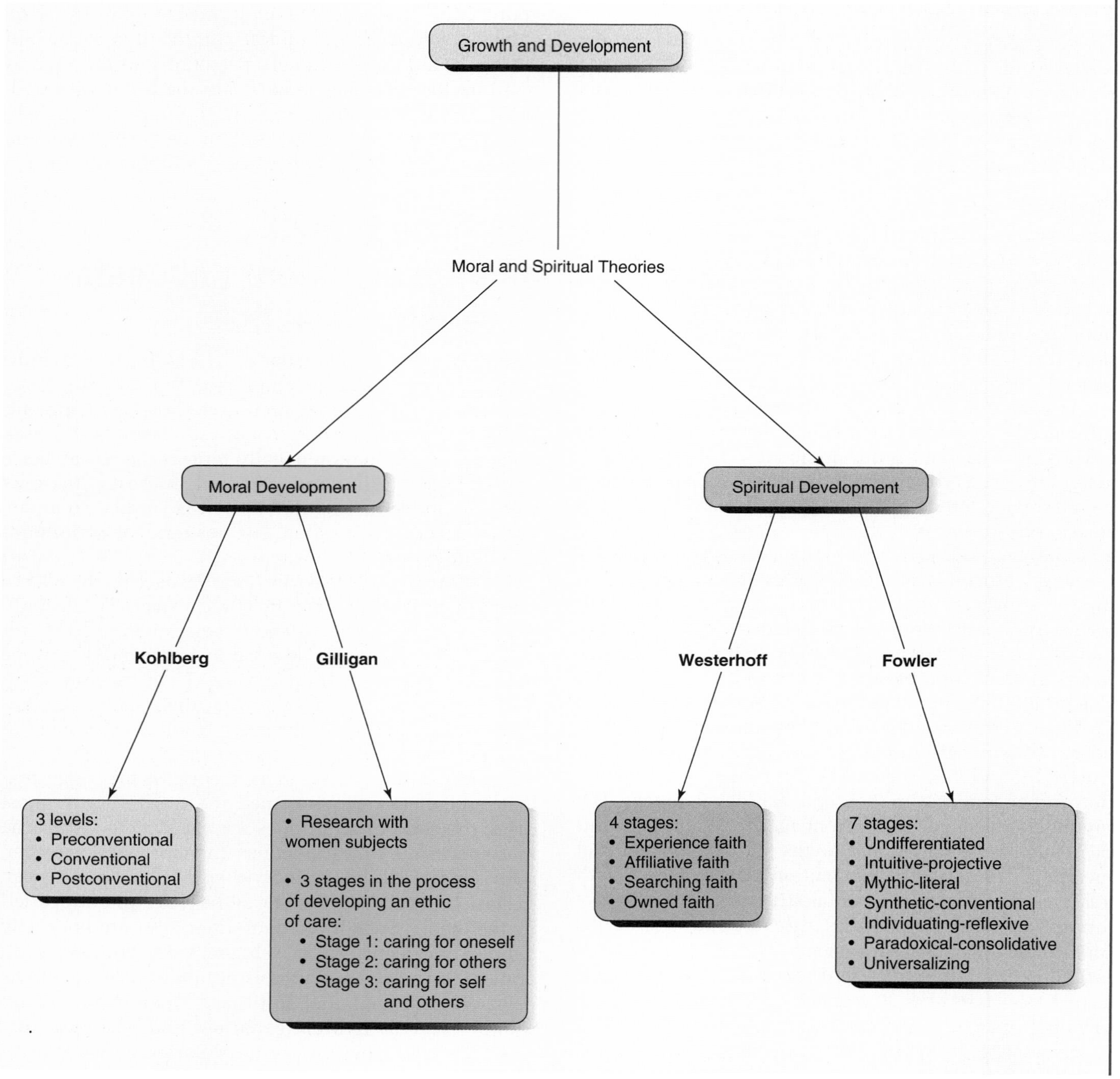

Growth and Development

Moral and Spiritual Theories

Moral Development

Kohlberg

3 levels:
- Preconventional
- Conventional
- Postconventional

Gilligan

- Research with women subjects
- 3 stages in the process of developing an ethic of care:
  - Stage 1: caring for oneself
  - Stage 2: caring for others
  - Stage 3: caring for self and others

Spiritual Development

Westerhoff

4 stages:
- Experience faith
- Affiliative faith
- Searching faith
- Owned faith

Fowler

7 stages:
- Undifferentiated
- Intuitive-projective
- Mythic-literal
- Synthetic-conventional
- Individuating-reflexive
- Paradoxical-consolidative
- Universalizing

Theories are also useful in planning a nursing intervention. For instance, choosing the appropriate toy for a 3-year-old child requires some knowledge of the physical and cognitive development of the child, as well as a sensitivity for individual preferences.

In adult care, knowledge about the physical, cognitive, and psychologic aspects of the aging process is a fundamental aspect of administering sensitive nursing care. For example, nurses can use their familiarity with the theories of development to help clients understand and anticipate the psychosocial changes that take place after retirement or the physical limitations that come with aging.

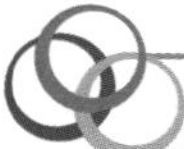

Critical Thinking Checkpoint

Finnegan, an inquisitive, energetic 2-year-old, is diagnosed with amblyopia (lazy eye) and far-sightedness in his stronger eye. Untreated, this condition will lead to blindness in the affected eye. Treatment includes wearing an eye patch over his stronger eye for 2 hours a day and wearing glasses with a corrective lens at all times when he is awake. Finnegan's mother says he resists actively when she or his father places the patch and that it is "almost impossible" to get him to leave his glasses on.

1. According to Erikson, at what stage of development is Finnegan?
2. What strategies could you suggest Finnegan's parents use to increase his cooperation with treatment?
3. Specifically describe strategies based on Piaget's theory of cognitive development and the theory of social learning.

Answers to Critical Thinking Checkpoint questions are available on the faculty resources site. Please consult with your instructor.

Chapter 23 Review

CHAPTER HIGHLIGHTS

- The terms *growth* and *development* represent independent, interrelated, and dynamic processes.
- Growth is physical change and an increase in size. The pattern of physiologic growth is similar for all individuals.
- Development is an increase in the complexity of function and skill progression. It is the capacity and skill of the individual to adapt to the environment.
- Temperament, the way in which individuals respond to their external and internal environments, influences the interactive dynamics of growth and development.
- The rate of an individual's growth and development is highly individual, but the sequence of growth and development is predictable.
- Components of growth and development are generally categorized as biophysical, psychosocial, cognitive, moral, and spiritual.
- Psychosocial development refers to the development of personality. Psychosocial theorists include Freud, Erickson, Havighurst, Peck, and Gould.
- Attachment theory states that humans have a need for a strong emotional bond to others. Bowlby lists four characteristics of attachment.
- Cognitive development refers to the manner in which individuals learn to think, reason, and use language. The most widely known cognitive theorist is Piaget.
- Behaviorist theory emphasizes stimulus–response patterns and either positive or negative reinforcement as the basis for learning and behavior change.
- Social learning theory states that learning can occur by observation. Role modeling and learning from watching role models are a part of social learning theory.
- Moral development, a complex process that is not fully understood, involves learning what ought to be and what ought not to be done. Kohlberg's theory focuses on the reasons an individual makes a decision. Gilligan posits that the moral development of women and men has a different focus, justice versus caring and responsibility.
- The spiritual component of growth and development refers to individuals' understanding of their relationship with the universe and their perceptions about the direction and meaning of life. Fowler and Westerhoff are two theorists who describe stages of spiritual development or faith.
- In nursing, developmental theories can be useful in guiding assessment, explaining behavior, and providing a direction for nursing interventions.

TEST YOUR KNOWLEDGE

1. When discussing human growth and development with the parents of a newborn, the nurse includes which of the following in her discussion? Select all that apply.
   1. Growth involves physical change and increase in size.
   2. Skills and function increase with growth.
   3. Most humans experience a similar pattern of growth.
   4. Being able to adapt to one's environment is an indicator of growth.
   5. Children's growth is monitored by height, weight, bone size, and dentition.
2. The nurse knows that the study of growth and development is an exploration of which of the following?
   1. Physical changes of the growing child
   2. Increasing complexity of function and skill progression of the growing child
   3. Environmental factors such as family, religion, and culture of the growing child
   4. Physical development and the increasing level and progression of function and skill of the growing child

3. The nurse examines a 2-year-old child recently hospitalized with pneumonia. Which pattern of behavior is most likely to be exhibited by the child?
1. Lies quietly while the nurse listens to the lungs
2. Asks many questions about what the nurse is doing and hearing
3. Fusses, cries, and pushes the nurse away during assessment of the breath sounds
4. Enjoys playing "nurse" with the stethoscope and listens to self and others' breath sounds

4. A 14-year-old is scheduled to have surgical repair of a spinal curvature (scoliosis). The adolescent will be hospitalized for about 2 weeks. Which nursing intervention will be most helpful during the hospital stay?
1. Have peers visit frequently during the day.
2. Instruct parents to room-in with her.
3. Encourage her to go to the recreation room.
4. Encourage her to arrange for her teachers to provide her with homework.

5. A 65-year-old man who recently retired from 40 years of work as an independent contractor is scheduled for a physical examination. The nurse should be concerned about which comment?
1. "My wife and I are planning to drive to Nebraska in June to visit our grandkids."
2. "Every day, when I wake up, it's hard to find a reason to get out of bed."
3. "I often take ibuprofen for the pain in my knees."
4. "People still call me for advice on building projects. I may never get to retire!"

6. A nurse is working with a school-age client who is learning how to use a peak flow meter to monitor his asthma. The child was frustrated at first, but now is able to give the reason to use the meter on a daily basis. Remembering the growth and development characteristics of the adolescent, which of the following is an appropriate response by the nurse?
1. "You should feel very proud for understanding and using your meter."
2. "Think of using the meter as one of your daily chores."
3. "Maybe you could make a game out of the daily use of your meter."
4. "It's too bad if you don't want to use the meter; it's just something you'll have to do."

7. A nurse decides that a review of which theorist would be helpful before teaching 4- and 5-year-olds in a preschool class how to brush their teeth?
1. Fowler
2. Erikson
3. Gould
4. Peck

8. A 5-year-old boy arrives for the preadmission workup for a surgical procedure. When the nurse brings in the intravenous (IV) control pump the child states: "It's going to bite me because I have been bad." Using knowledge of Piaget, Erikson, and Fowler, which is the best nursing action?
1. Reassure him by providing opportunities to touch and explore the machine, as well as explaining how it works.
2. Understand that his imagination is out of control. Tell him that his fears are unfounded and that he needs to be a "big boy."
3. Recognize that he is too young to understand and that he needs to be quickly distracted.
4. Acknowledge his need for fantasy by reassuring him that if he is a "good boy," the bad machine will not bite him.

9. A 15-month-old is admitted to the hospital for hernia surgery. When his mother leaves him, he cries inconsolably. Using knowledge of attachment theory and cognitive theory, which is the best nursing action?
1. Encourage his mother to stay with him as much as possible.
2. Put a picture of his mother in his crib to remind him that she will return soon.
3. Hold and cuddle him as much as possible.
4. Distract him with toys and music.

10. A community health nurse is planning adult health education classes. According to Erikson's stages of development, which task must the nurse address with this age group?
1. Industry versus inferiority
2. Identity versus role confusion
3. Intimacy versus isolation
4. Generativity versus stagnation

See Answers to Test Your Knowledge in Appendix A.

READINGS AND REFERENCES

Suggested Reading

Burrows, C. A., Usher, L. V., Schwartz, C. B., Mundy, P. C., & Henderson, H. A. (2016). Supporting the spectrum hypothesis: Self-reported treatment in children and adolescents with high functioning autism. *Journal of Autism and Developmental Disorders*, *46*, 1184–1195. doi:10.1007/s10803-015-2653-9

This study examined high-functioning children with autism. Children with high-functioning autism were able to report temperament and its association with parent-reported behavior problems.

Related Research

Kientrou, P. (2016). Influence of exercise and training on critical stages of bone growth and development. *Pediatric Exercise Science*, *28*(2), 178–186. doi:10.1123/pes.2015-0265

Wong, C. L., Ching, T. Y., Leigh, G., Cupples, G, Button, L., Marnane, V., . . . Martin, L. (2018). Psychosocial development of 5-year-old children with hearing loss: Risks and protective factors. *International Journal of Audiology*, *57*, S81–S92.

References

Abramson, T. A. (2015). Older adults: The "panini sandwich" generation. *Clinical Gerontologist*, *38*, 251–267. doi:10.1080/07317115.2015.1032466

Ball, R. S. (1977). The Gesell developmental schedules: Arnold Gesell (1880–1961). *Journal of Abnormal Child Psychology*, *5*, 233–239. doi:10.1007/BF00913694

Bowlby, J. (1999). *Attachment: Attachment and loss, Vol. 1* (2nd ed.). New York, NY: Basic.

Campbell, E. E., & Seabrook, J. A. (2016). The influence of socioeconomic status on adverse birth outcomes. *Canadian Journal of Midwifery Research and Practice*, *15*(2), 10–20.

Erikson, E. H. (1963). *Childhood and society* (2nd ed.). New York, NY: W. W. Norton. (Copyright renewed 1978 and 1991)

Erikson, E. H. (1964). *Insight and responsibility: Lectures on the ethical implications of psychoanalytic insight*. New York, NY: W. W. Norton.

Fowler, J., & Keen, S. (1985). *Life maps: Conversations in the journey of faith*. Waco, TX: Word.

Fowler, J. W., Streib, H., & Keller, B. (2004). *Manual for faith development research* (3rd ed.). Bielefeld, Germany: Research Center for Biographical Studies in Contemporary Religion, Bielefeld University; and Atlanta, GA: Center for Research in Faith and Moral Development, Emory University.

Frandsen, G., & Pennington, S. (2018). *Abrams' clinical drug therapy*. (11th ed). Philadelphia, PA: Lippincott, Williams, & Wilkins.

Freud, S. (1946). *The ego and the mechanism of defense*. New York, NY: International Universities.

Gesell, A. (1934). *An atlas of infant behavior: A systematic delineation of the forms and early growth of human behavior patterns*. New Haven, CT: Yale University.

Gilligan, C. (1982). *In a different voice: Psychological theory and women's development*. Cambridge, MA: Harvard University.

Gould, R. L. (1972). The phases of adult life: A study in developmental psychology. *American Journal of Psychiatry*, *129*, 33–43.

Green, J. (2016). Ingenious designs and causal inference in child psychology and psychiatry. [Editorial]. *Journal of Child*

Psychology and Psychiatry, *57*, 549–551. doi:10.1111/jcpp.12564

Havighurst, R. J. (1972). *Developmental tasks and education* (3rd ed.). New York, NY: Longman.

Kohlberg, L. (1981). *Essays on moral development. Vol. 1: The philosophy of moral development*. San Francisco, CA: Harper & Row.

Kohlberg, L. (1984). *Essays on moral development. Vol. 2: The psychology of moral development*. San Francisco, CA: Harper & Row.

Liu, P., Wu C., Chang, X., Qi, X., Zheng, M., & Zhou, Z. (2016). Adverse associations of both prenatal and postnatal exposure to organophosphate pesticides with infant neurodevelopment in an agricultural area of Jiangsu Province, China. *Environmental Health Perspectives*, *124*(10), 1637–1643. doi:10.1289/EHP196

Peck, R. (1968). Psychological developments in the second half of life. In B. L. Neugarten (Ed.), *Middle age and aging*. Chicago, IL: University of Chicago.

Piaget, J. (1966). *Origins of intelligence in children*. New York, NY: W. W. Norton.

Piaget, J., & Inhelder, B. (1969). *The psychology of the child*. New York, NY: Basic.

Pierce, B. A. (2016). *Genetics: A conceptual approach*. (6th ed). New York, NY: W. H. Freeman Macmillan Learning.

Rothbart, M. K., & Bates, J. E. (2006). Temperament. In N. Eisenberg, W. Damon, & R. M. Lerner (Eds.), *Handbook of child psychology. Volume 3: Social, emotional, and personality development* (6th ed., 99–166). Hoboken, NJ: John Wiley & Sons.

Ullsperger, J. M., Nigg, J. T., & Nikolas, M. A. (2016). Does child temperament play a role in the association between parenting practices and child attention/deficit hyperactivity disorder? *Journal of Abnormal Child Psychology*, *44*, 167–178. doi:10.1007/s10802-015-9982-1

Varga, D. (2011). Look—Normal: The colonized child of developmental science. *History of Psychology*, *14*(2), 137–157. doi:10.1037/a0021775

Westerhoff, J. (2012). *Will our children have faith?* (rev. ed.). New York, NY: Morehouse.

Selected Bibliography

De Pauw, S. W., & Mervielde, I. (2010). Temperament, personality, and developmental psychopathology: A review based on the conceptual dimensions underlying childhood traits. *Child Psychiatry and Human Development*, *41*, 313–329. doi:10.1007/s10578-009-0171-8

Fowler, J. W. (1995). *Stages of faith: The psychology of human development*. San Francisco, CA: HarperCollins.

Freud, S. (1923). *The ego and the id*. London, England: Hogarth.

Freud, S. (1961). *The ego and the id and other works* (Vol. 19) (J. Strachey, Trans.). London, England: Hogarth and the Institute of Psychoanalysis.

Havighurst, R. J. (1972). *Developmental tasks and education* (3rd ed.). New York, NY: Longman.

Hollander, A. (1980). *How to help your child have a spiritual life: A parent's guide to inner development*. New York, NY: A & W.

Keller-Dewild, A. (2017). The five temperaments: How the line of heredity is connected incarnation. *LILPOH*, *22*(87), 50–55.

Perkins, S. C., Finegood, E. D., & Swain, J. E. (2013). Poverty and language development: Roles of parenting and stress. *Innovations in Clinical Neuroscience*, *10*(4), 10–19.

24 Promoting Health from Conception Through Adolescence

LEARNING OUTCOMES

After completing this chapter, you will be able to:

1. Describe usual physical development from infancy through adolescence.
2. Identify tasks characteristic of different stages of development from infancy through adolescence.
3. Trace psychosocial development according to Erikson from infancy through adolescence.
4. Explain cognitive development according to Piaget from infancy through adolescence.
5. Describe moral development according to Kohlberg from childhood through adolescence.
6. Describe spiritual development according to Fowler throughout childhood and adolescence.
7. Identify assessment activities and expected characteristics from birth through late childhood.
8. Identify essential activities of health promotion and protection to meet the needs of infants, toddlers, preschoolers, school-age children, and adolescents.

KEY TERMS

abusive head trauma, *461*
adolescence, *473*
adolescent growth spurt, *473*
Ages & Stages Questionnaires (ASQ), *462*
amblyopia, *465*
Apgar scoring system, *461*
apocrine glands, *473*
Denver Developmental Screening Test (DDST-II), *462*
eccrine glands, *473*
ectoderm, *454*
ejaculation, *473*
embryonic phase, *454*
emmetropic, *466*
endoderm, *454*
entoderm, *454*
failure to thrive (FTT), *460*
fetal phase, *455*
fontanels, *457*
hyperopic, *466*
identification, *467*
imagination, *467*
inflicted traumatic brain injury, *461*
introjection, *467*
lanugo, *455*
menarche, *473*
mesoderm, *454*
myopic, *466*
normocephaly, *457*
peer groups, *474*
placenta, *455*
primary sexual characteristics, *473*
puberty, *473*
regression, *464*
repression, *467*
sebaceous glands, *473*
secondary sexual characteristics, *473*
self-concept, *464*
separation anxiety, *464*
shaken baby syndrome (SBS), *461*
stereognosis, *470*
strabismus, *465*
sudden infant death syndrome (SIDS), *461*
sutures, *457*
teratogen, *456*
trimesters, *454*
vernix caseosa, *455*

Introduction

Knowledge of growth and development is essential for nurses if they are to identify developmental needs and problems. This chapter applies the concepts of growth and development introduced in Chapter 23 ∞ to the prenatal period and to the neonate, infant, toddler, preschooler, school-age child, and adolescent. Each developmental stage includes physical, psychosocial, cognitive, moral, and spiritual aspects. Health assessment and promotion of health and wellness are emphasized.

Conception and Prenatal Development

Prenatal or intrauterine development lasts approximately 9 calendar months (10 lunar months) or 38 to 40 weeks, depending on the method of calculation. (A lunar month is 28 days.) If the time is calculated from the day of conception, this stage of life is about 38 weeks or $9\frac{1}{2}$ lunar months. If the time is calculated from the first day of the last menstrual period, it is 10 lunar months or 40 weeks.

Traditionally, pregnancy has been divided into three periods called **trimesters**, each of which lasts about 3 months. Each trimester includes certain landmarks for developmental changes in the mother and the fetus. There are two phases of intrauterine life, embryonic and fetal. The **embryonic phase**, occurring in the first trimester, is the period during which the fertilized ovum develops into an organism with most of the features of the human. This period is considered to encompass the first 8 weeks of pregnancy.

Within the first 3 weeks of life, the embryonic tissues differentiate into three layers—the **ectoderm** (outer layer), **mesoderm** (middle layer), and **endoderm** or **entoderm** (inner layer). The ectoderm and endoderm are formed by the second week; the mesoderm forms in the third week. The ectoderm forms a long tube for the development of the brain and spinal cord. The endoderm creates the gastrointestinal tract. A single tubular heart forms outside the body cavity of the embryo. Basic organ formation continues through the eighth week. By the eighth week, the umbilical cord and circulatory system are established (London et al., 2017). Three other events occur concurrently during the first 3 weeks:

1. The embryo is implanted in the endometrium of the uterus.
2. The fetal membranes differentiate into the chorion, precursor to the placenta, and the amnion, precursor to the amniotic sac.
3. Placental function starts. The **placenta** is a flat, disk-shaped organ that is highly vascular. It normally forms in the upper segment of the endometrium of the uterus. Its function is to facilitate the exchange of nutrients and gas between the embryo or fetus and the mother.

The **fetal phase** of development, occurring in the second and third trimester of pregnancy, is characterized by a period of rapid growth in the size of the fetus. Both genetic and environmental factors affect fetal growth.

At the end of the second trimester, or 6 lunar months, the fetus resembles a small baby. Because very little fat is present beneath the skin, the skin appears wrinkled, red, and transparent. Underlying vessels are visible. A protective covering called **vernix caseosa** begins to develop over the skin. This is a white, cheese-like substance that adheres to the skin and can become one-eighth inch thick by birth. **Lanugo**, a fine downy hair, also covers the body. At about 5 months, the mother can feel the movement of the fetus, and the first fetal heartbeat may be heard.

At the end of the third trimester ($9\frac{1}{2}$ lunar months), the fetus has developed to approximately 50 cm (20 in.) and 3.2 to 3.4 kg (7.0 to 7.5 lb). The lanugo has disappeared, and the skin is a more normal color and appears less wrinkled. A large amount of subcutaneous fat makes the baby look more rotund. The baby gains most of its weight during the last 2 months in utero. Box 24.1 lists maternal factors that can lead to impaired fetal development.

BOX 24.1 Maternal Factors That Contribute to Impaired Fetal Development

- Poor nutrition and inadequate weight gain
- Excessive nausea and vomiting (hyperemesis gravidarum)
- Low hemoglobin levels
- Gestational diabetes
- Positive protein in the urine
- Hypertension
- Maternal infection
- Smoking
- Drug use
- Teenage pregnancy
- Increased maternal age over 35 years
- Lack of adequate prenatal care
- Low socioeconomic status
- Previous pregnancy complications
- Genetic abnormalities

Health Promotion

During the intrauterine stage of development, the embryo or fetus relies on the maternal blood flow through the placenta to meet its basic survival needs. Good health of the mother is essential for proper growth and development.

Oxygen

To meet the fetal demands for oxygen, the pregnant mother gradually increases her normal blood flow by about one-third, peaking at about 8 months. Respiratory rate and cardiac output increase significantly during this period. Initially, the heart of the embryo lies outside its body. It is then repositioned in the chest early in the second trimester. Fetal circulation travels from the placenta through two umbilical arteries, which carry deoxygenated blood away from the fetus. By 20 weeks, the fetal heartbeat is audible through a fetoscope; the heartbeat is audible as early as the 10th week if a Doppler stethoscope with ultrasound is used.

Nutrition and Fluids

The fetus obtains nourishment from the placental circulation and by swallowing amniotic fluid. Nutritional needs are met when the mother eats a well-balanced diet containing sufficient calories and nutrients to meet both her needs and those of the fetus. Adequate folic acid, one of the B vitamins, is important in order to prevent neural tube defects (e.g., spina bifida) in the fetus. Two objectives of *Healthy People 2020* are to reduce the occurrence of neural tube defects and to increase the proportion of pregnancies begun with the recommended folic acid level (U.S. Department of Health and Human Services [USDHHS], n.d., 2010). Neural tube defects occur in the first few weeks of fetal development. As a result, it is recommended that all women capable of becoming pregnant consume 400 micrograms of folic acid daily. The nurse should teach the client about folic acid–rich foods (e.g., green leafy vegetables, oranges, dried beans, breakfast cereal) and suggest she take a vitamin supplement that contains folic acid.

Sleep and Activity

The fetus sleeps most of the time and develops a pattern of sleep and wakefulness that usually persists after birth. The mother can feel fetal activity at about the fifth lunar month of pregnancy.

Elimination

Throughout pregnancy, fetal feces are formed in the intestines from swallowed amniotic fluid but are normally not excreted until after birth. Inadequate oxygenation of the fetus during the third trimester can result in relaxation of the anal sphincter and passage of feces into the amniotic fluid. Urine normally is excreted into the amniotic fluid after the kidneys mature (16 to 20 weeks).

Temperature Maintenance

Amniotic fluid usually provides a safe and comfortable temperature for the fetus. Significant changes in maternal temperature can alter the temperature of the amniotic fluid and the fetus. Significant temperature increases due to illness, hot whirlpool baths, or saunas may result in birth defects. In the last weeks of gestation, the fetus develops subcutaneous fatty tissue stores that will help maintain body temperature at birth.

Safety

As stated earlier, the body systems form during the embryonic period. As a result, the embryo is particularly vulnerable to damage from a **teratogen**, which is anything that adversely affects normal cellular development in the embryo or fetus (Venes, 2017). It is important for the nurse to inquire about possible pregnancy when giving medications that are known teratogens and to ask when the woman is scheduled for tests that involve radiography (x-ray).

Smoking, alcohol, and drugs can affect the environment for the fetus. Exposure to environmental tobacco smoke has been associated with preterm births, stillbirth, miscarriage, and low-birth-weight infants. Witt et al. (2016) conducted a study to determine the relationships among stressful life events, a woman's alcohol consumption, and tobacco use in the preconception phase and during pregnancy. Women who experienced stress, consumed alcohol, and used tobacco were more likely to deliver very low-birth-weight babies. Women who smoked prior to conception and during the last trimester delivered low-birth-weight babies. Mothers who use drugs, alcohol, and tobacco have strong adverse birth consequences. Fetal alcohol spectrum disorders (FASDs) is a term that refers to specific diagnoses given to infants and children who have been exposed to alcohol prenatally. The adverse health effects of alcohol consumption during pregnancy include behavioral, emotional, cognitive, and adaptive functional deficits and congenital anomalies. In the general population, 8 of 1000 births have FASD (Lange et al., 2017).

Neonates and Infants (Birth to 1 Year)

Babies are considered neonates from birth to the end of the first month. Infants are babies from 1 month to 1 year of age.

Physical Development

A neonate's basic task is adjustment to the environment outside the uterus, which requires breathing, sleeping, sucking, eating, swallowing, digesting, and eliminating. Infants continue to grow and develop rapidly during the first year, learning more skills as they interact with their world. Infants undergo significant physiologic changes in weight, length, head growth, vision, hearing, smell, taste, touch, reflexes, and motor development. Some of these changes can be assessed using standardized growth charts based on the growth of groups of American children (Centers for Disease Control and Prevention [CDC], 2010). The *Child Growth Standards* from the World Health Organization (WHO, n.d.) provide documentation on physical growth curves and motor milestones to be achieved. Growth charts are available in a variety of languages. From 1997 to 2003, the WHO Multicentre Growth Reference Study was conducted to generate new growth curves for infants and children. A systematic review, meta-analysis, and meta-regression that evaluated the association between gestational weight gain above or below the Institute of Medicine's guidelines revealed that mothers from different ethnic groups who had insufficient gestational weight gain had a greater risk of premature birth and being small for gestational age (Goldstein et al., 2017).

EVIDENCE-BASED PRACTICE

Evidence-Based Practice

Does Project Step Up for Adolescents with Fetal Alcohol Spectrum Disorders Reduce Alcohol Use?

There is a wide range of disorders that can develop in a fetus exposed to alcohol. Fetal alcohol spectrum disorders (FASDs) and fetal alcohol syndrome lead to facial malformations, deficits in moral development, and deficiencies in growth patterns. O'Connor, Quattlebaum, Castañeda, and Dipple (2016) conducted a study on 54 adolescents who were diagnosed with FASDs. The adolescents participated in Project Step Up. Project Step Up was a 6-week 60-minute group intervention that educated the participants for the promotion of adapted responses to social pressures related to alcohol consumption. Following the education, participants reported a significant decrease in self-reported alcohol risk. Adolescents who did not consume alcohol reported no increase in alcohol use and resisted any social pressure to use alcohol.

Implications

Due to the positive results of Project Step Up, the program should be investigated further to increase the statistical evidence of its success.

Infants are at risk for the development of iron deficiency anemia. According to WHO (2016), supplemental iron is recommended for infants from 4 months to 23 months. Iron drops or syrup should be administered orally daily at a dosage of 10–12.5 mg elemental iron.

Weight

At birth, most babies weigh from 2.7 to 3.8 kg (6.0 to 8.5 lb). Just after birth, most infants lose 5% to 10% of their birth weight because of fluid loss. This weight loss is normal, and infants usually regain that weight in about 1 week. After several days, babies usually gain weight at the rate of 150 to 210 g (5 to 7 oz) weekly for 6 months. By 5 months of age, infants usually reach twice their birth weight, and by age 12 months, three times their birth weight. Studies have shown that increased weight gain in early infancy leads to an increased risk of obesity later in life (Savage, Birch, Marini, Anzman-Frasca, & Paul, 2016). Exclusive breastfeeding in the first 4 to 6 months may be helpful in preventing excessive weight gain.

Length

The average length of a European American newborn in the United States is about 50 cm (20 in.). Female babies are, on average, smaller than male babies. Babies from different ethnic groups may vary by height, weight, and head circumference, so ethnicity must be considered when determining what is "normal" for any particular infant. The WHO Multicentre Growth Reference Study, conducted from 1997 through 2003, demonstrates, however, that children worldwide who live in a healthy environment and are well fed (including exclusive breastfeeding for the first 4 to 6 months of life) will show similar patterns of growth (de Onis, 2011).

Two recumbent lengths are the crown-to-rump length (the sitting length) and the head-to-heel length (from the top of the head to the base of the heels) (Figure 24.1 ■). Normally, the crown-to-rump length is approximately the same as the head circumference. By 6 months, infants gain another 13.75 cm (5.5 in.) of height. By 12 months, they add another 7.5 cm (3 in.). The rate of increase in height is largely influenced by the baby's size at birth and by nutrition.

Head and Chest Circumference

Assessment of head circumference is particularly important in infants and children to determine the growth rate of the skull and the brain. An infant's head should be measured at every visit to the primary care provider or nurse until the child is 2 years old (Figure 24.2 ■). Normal head circumference (**normocephaly**) is often related to chest circumference. At birth, the average infant's head circumference is 35 cm (14 in.) and generally varies only 1 or 2 cm (0.5 in.). The chest circumference of the newborn is usually less than the head circumference by about 2.5 cm (1 in.). As the infant grows, the chest circumference becomes larger than the head circumference. At about 9 or 10 months, the head and chest circumferences are about the same, and after 1 year of age, the chest circumference is larger.

Head Molding

The heads of many newborn babies are misshapen because of the molding of the head that occurs during vaginal deliveries. Molding of the head is possible because of fontanels and sutures in the skull. **Fontanels** are unossified (i.e., without bone formation) membranous gaps in the bone structure of the skull. **Sutures** are junction lines of the skull bones that override to provide flexibility for molding of the head. Within a week, a newborn's head usually regains its symmetry, which is reassuring to the parents. The larger anterior fontanel (4 to 6 cm [1.6 to 2.4 in.] in diameter and diamond shaped) can increase in size for several months after birth. After 6 months, the size gradually decreases until closure occurs between 9 and 18 months. The posterior fontanel between the parietal bones and the occipital bone closes between 2 and 3 months after birth (Figure 24.3 ■).

Vision

The newborn can follow large moving objects and blinks in response to bright light and sound. The pupils of the newborn respond slowly, and the eyes cannot focus on

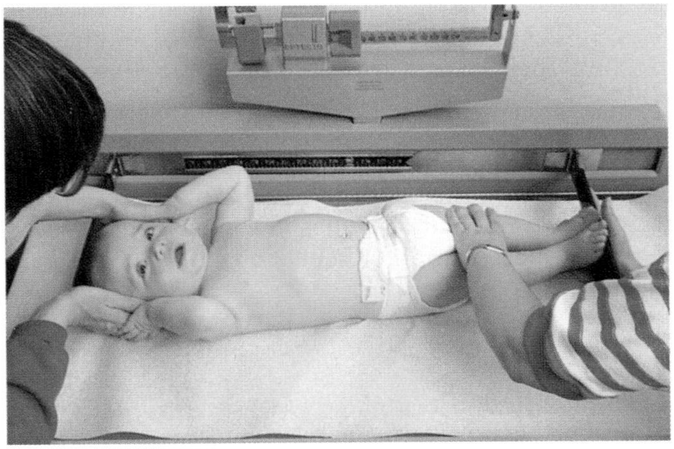

Figure 24.1 ■ Measuring an infant head to heel, from the top of the head to the base of the heels.

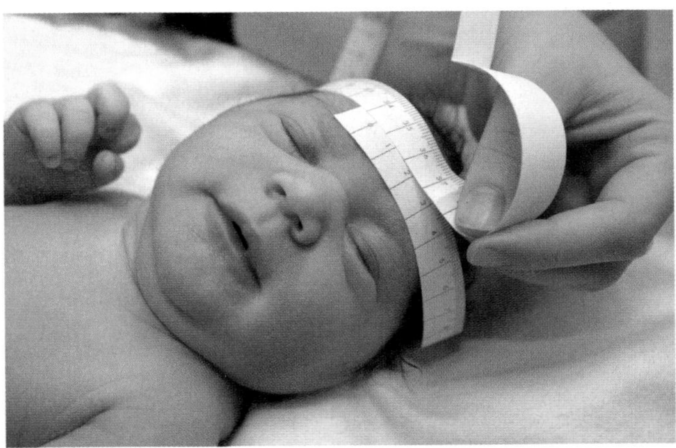

Figure 24.2 ■ An infant's head circumference is measured around the skull above the eyebrows, and around the occiput.
ChameleonsEye/Shutterstock.

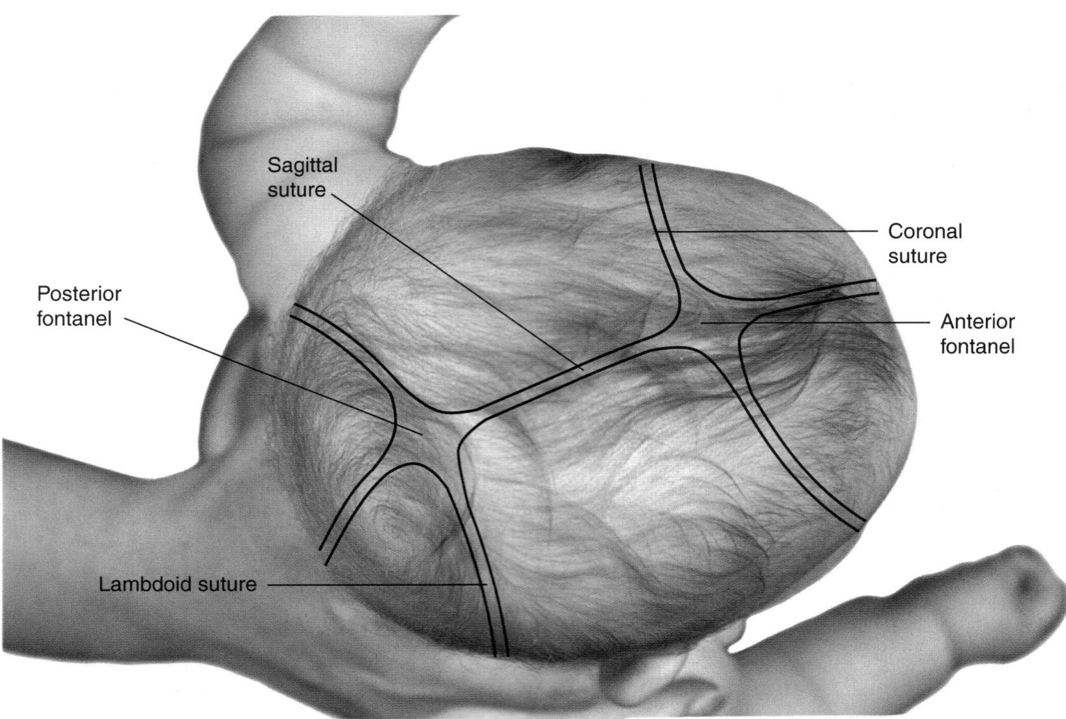

Figure 24.3 ■ The bones of the skull, showing the fontanelles and suture lines.

close objects. By 1 month, the infant can focus his or her gaze on objects and follow moving ones. At 4 months, the infant recognizes a parent's smile, although social smiles may appear as early as 2 months. The 4-month-old has almost complete color vision and follows objects through a 180-degree arc. A 5-month-old infant reaches for objects. Between 6 and 10 months, the infant can fix on an object and follow it in all directions. By 12 months, depth perception has fully developed, and the infant will consistently be able to recognize where a change in level occurs, such as at the edge of the bed.

Hearing

Newborns with intact hearing will react with a startle to a loud noise, a reaction called the *Moro reflex*. Within a few days, they are able to distinguish different sounds. For example, they can tell the difference between their mother's voice and that of another woman. By 2 to 3 months, they will actively coo, smile, or gurgle to sounds and voices. Between 3 and 6 months, the infant will look for sounds, pausing an activity to listen and responding with distress or pleasure to angry or happy voices. Between 6 and 9 months, individual words begin to take on meaning and the infant may look at named objects or individuals. The 9- to 12-month-old infant understands many words (e.g., "no," "hot," "dog"), uses gestures (e.g., waves "bye-bye"), may articulate one or two words with a specific reference (e.g., "mama," "dada"), and by 1 year of age, responds to simple commands.

Smell and Taste

The senses of smell and taste are functional shortly after birth. Newborns prefer sweet tastes and tend to decrease their sucking in response to liquids with a salty content. They are able to recognize the smell of their mother's milk and respond to this smell by turning toward the mother.

Touch

The sense of touch is well developed at birth. Skin-to-skin touching is important for an infant's development. The infant responds positively to the warmth, love, and security it perceives when touched, held, and cuddled. The newborn is sensitive to temperature extremes and has poor self-regulation of body temperature. In response to pain, young babies react diffusely, with a whole-body reaction, and cannot isolate the source of discomfort.

Reflexes

Reflexes of the newborn are unconscious, involuntary responses of the nervous system to external and internal stimuli. Reflexes normally present at birth are the sucking, rooting, Moro, palmar grasp, plantar, tonic neck, stepping, and Babinski reflexes (Box 24.2). Infant reflexes disappear during the first year of life in an ordered sequence, a process that allows the infant to develop voluntary movements. In addition, the abilities to yawn, stretch, sneeze, burp, and hiccup are all present at birth.

Motor Development

Motor development is the development of the baby's abilities to move and control the body. Initially, body movement is uncoordinated. At 1 month of age, the infant lifts the head momentarily when prone, turns the head when prone, and has a head lag when pulled to a sitting position. Head lag should be minimal by 4 months

BOX 24.2 Infant Reflexes

- *Sucking reflex:* A feeding reflex that occurs when the infant's lips are touched. The reflex persists throughout infancy.
- *Rooting reflex:* A feeding reflex elicited by touching the baby's cheek, causing the baby's head to turn to the side that was touched. The reflex usually disappears after 4 months.
- *Moro reflex:* Often assessed to estimate the maturity of the central nervous system. A loud noise, a sudden change in position, or an abrupt jarring of the crib elicits this reflex. The infant reacts by extending both arms and legs outward with the fingers spread, then suddenly retracting the limbs. Often the infant cries at the same time. This reflex disappears after 4 months.
- *Palmar grasp reflex:* Occurs when a small object is placed against the palm of the hand, causing the fingers to curl around it. This reflex disappears after 3 to 6 months.
- *Plantar reflex:* Similar to the palmar grasp reflex; an object placed just beneath the toes causes them to curl around it. This reflex disappears after 8 to 10 months.
- *Tonic neck reflex (TNR) or fencing reflex:* A postural reflex. When a baby who is lying on its back turns its head to, for example, the right side, the left side of the body shows a flexing of the left arm and the left leg. This reflex disappears after 4 to 6 months.
- *Stepping reflex (walking or dancing reflex):* Can be elicited by holding the baby upright so that the feet touch a flat surface. The legs then move up and down as if the baby were walking. This reflex usually disappears at about 2 months.
- *Babinski reflex:* When the sole of the foot is stroked, the big toe rises, and the other toes fan out. A newborn baby has a positive Babinski. After age 1, the infant exhibits a negative Babinski; that is, the toes curl downward. A positive Babinski after age 1 can indicate possible upper motor neuron damage.

of age. After 6 months, infants may sit without support (Figure 24.4 ■). At 9 months, they can reach, grasp a rattle, and transfer it from hand to hand. At 12 months, they can turn the pages of a book, put objects into a container, walk with some assistance, and help to dress themselves.

Psychosocial Development

According to Erikson (1963), the central crisis at this stage is trust versus mistrust. Resolution of this stage determines how the individual approaches subsequent developmental stages. During the first year of life, infants depend on the parents for all their physiologic and psychologic needs. Fulfillment of these needs is required for the infant to develop a basic sense of trust. Parents can enhance this sense of trust by (a) being sensitive to the infant's needs and meeting these needs promptly and skillfully, (b) responding consistently to an infant's needs, and (c) providing a predictable environment in which routines are established. Nurturing behavior, such as consistent care, handling, stroking, and cuddling, is essential for healthy psychosocial development. By 8 months, most infants exhibit attachment to their parents and may show displeasure when left with strangers.

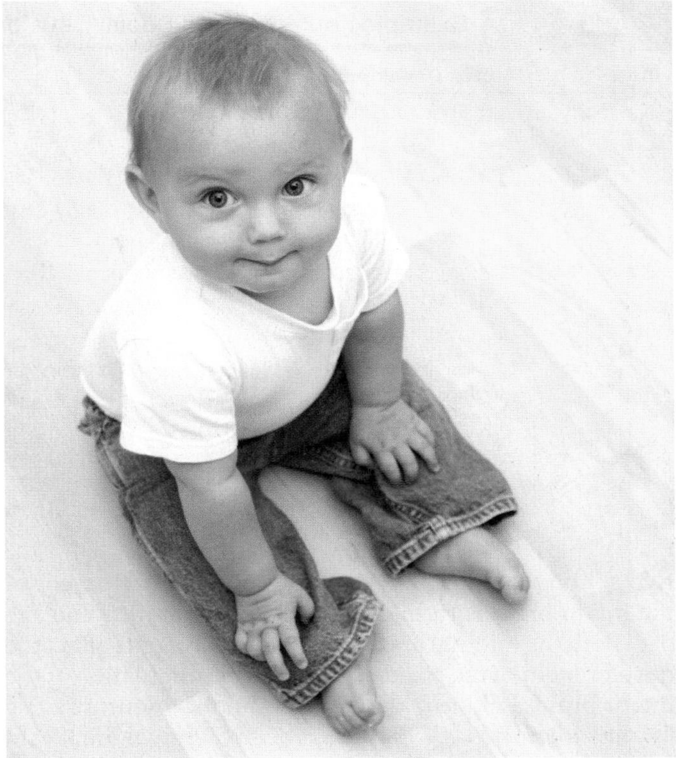

Figure 24.4 ■ An infant sits without support at 6 months of age.
D. Hurst/Alamy.

The newborn reacts socially to caregivers by paying attention to the face or voice and by cuddling when held. The baby is able to interact with the environment by responding to various stimuli such as touch and sound. Table 24.1 provides examples of motor and social development.

Infants have no understanding of waiting and no time frame by which to measure waiting. Crying is their initial reaction to stress and the major way they communicate stress. Infants learn gradually to tolerate stress. According to Freud, infants have an oral focus, many of their activities and pleasures are mouth centered, and they reduce tension by sucking and chewing on objects. Nurses and parents can reduce the stress of an infant by maintaining the infant's routine as much as possible and providing a consistent, predictable environment.

Cognitive Development

According to Piaget (1966), cognitive development is a result of interaction between an individual and the environment. Piaget referred to the initial period of cognitive development as the sensorimotor phase. This phase has six stages, three of which take place during the first year. From 4 to 8 months, infants begin to have perceptual recognition. By 6 months, they respond to new stimuli, and they remember certain objects and look for them for a short time. By 12 months, infants have a concept of both space and time. At 1 year of age, the infant has proceeded from the reflexive ability of the newborn to using one or

TABLE 24.1 Examples of Motor and Social Development in Infancy

Age	Motor Development	Social Development
Newborn	Turns head from side to side when in a prone position.	Displays displeasure by crying and satisfaction by soft vocalizations.
	Grasps by reflex when object is placed in palm of hand.	Attends to adult face and voice by eye contact and quieting.
4 months	Rolls over. Sits with support, holds head steady when sitting.	Babbles, laughs, and exhibits increased response to verbal play.
6 months	Lifts chest and shoulders off table when prone, bearing weight on hands.	Starts to imitate sounds. Vocalizes one-syllable sounds: "ma-ma," "da-da."
	Manipulates small objects.	
9 months	Creeps and crawls. Uses pincer grasp with thumb and forefinger.	Complies with simple verbal commands. Displays fear of being left alone (e.g., going to bed). Waves "bye-bye."
12 months	Walks alone with help.	Clings to mother in unfamiliar situations.
	Uses spoon to feed self.	Demonstrates emotions such as anger and affection.

two actions to attain a goal. The critical development of the infant brain is from 20 weeks' gestation until the age of 3. Both the internal and external environments affect the development of the mind and body. The stimulation of the infant brain enhances the development of neurons. The infant's interactions with the primary caregiver are key to enhancing infant brain development. Bernier, Calkins, and Bell (2016) conducted a longitudinal study that investigated the quality of mother–infant interactions and infant brain development. In this study, 352 mother–infant/toddler dyads came to the laboratory when the infants were 5, 10, and 24 months old. The infants were administered a resting-state encephalography (EEG). At the 5-month visit, the mother and infant were videotaped. The high-quality maternal and infant interactions predicted a higher frontal resting EEG activity, reflecting increased frontal brain activity. Thus, higher-quality maternal interaction resulted in an increase in brain development in the frontal lobe.

Moral Development

Infants are unable to understand right and wrong. When they receive abundant positive responses from the parent such as smiles, caresses, and voice tones of approval, in these early months, they learn that certain behaviors are "good" and that pleasure is the consequence. In later months and years, children can tell easily and quickly by changes in parental facial expressions and voice tones that their behavior is either approved or disapproved.

Health Risks

Neonates and infants are subject to a number of health problems that require interventions from healthcare personnel. Safety concerns are of particular importance.

Failure to Thrive

The term **failure to thrive (FTT)** is generally used to describe infants whose weight is less than normal for gestational age, gender, genetic potential, and medical condition. The CDC recommends the use of the WHO growth charts to assess the development of infants. Weight is altered initially, followed by length and head circumference. The child who falls below the fifth percentile for weight and height or whose growth declines across two percentiles on a standard growth chart over time should be considered for FTT. FTT may have organic causes (e.g., cardiac disease) or inorganic causes, which usually involve the parent–child relationship. Infants with inorganic FTT show delayed physical and emotional development without any physical cause. They are often malnourished and may be deprived of nurturing during infancy.

Infant Colic

Colic is acute abdominal pain caused by periodic contractions of the intestines. It occurs in infants as young as 2 weeks of age and, for most infants, disappears by 3 months of age. When an infant's crying lasts up to 10 to 12 hours a day, it is described as colicky. A crying or fussy period lasting 1 to 2 hours a day is usually considered normal. Although the direct cause is not known, colic tends to occur in babies with sensitive temperaments. Factors such as swallowing air, feeding too rapidly, allergies, taking excessive amounts of carbohydrates, infant emotional distress, and anxiety of the caregiver may be associated with colic.

To help relieve the colic, the nurse can assess the infant during feeding and suggest possible position changes. London et al. (2017) recommend the establishment of a warm and caring environment. An infant massage by a parent increases parent–newborn attachment and promotes relaxation to reduce the pain associated with infant colic. Cambron (2017) reviewed studies that utilized massage as an intervention to reduce colic. In one study, half of the mothers were taught to massage the baby, and the other half were instructed to rock their babies. The results of this study were statistically significant in the massage group. The number of hours the infant cried decreased, and the amount of sleep increased. In a second study, mothers were taught to use lavender and almond oil with the massage. The use of aromatherapy and massage on average decreased the episodes of crying by almost half.

Child Abuse

Reports of child abuse have increased in recent years, and the stress of having a baby with colic or excessive crying can put some parents at risk for child abuse. This abuse can take various forms, including physical abuse, physical neglect, sexual abuse, and emotional abuse and neglect. The term **shaken baby syndrome (SBS)** has been replaced by the term **abusive head trauma** or **inflicted traumatic brain injury**. Abusive head trauma is the most common cause of traumatic death in infants less than 1 year of age (Girard, Brunel, Dory-Lautrec, & Chabrol, 2016). This is classified as injuries caused by contact with rotational forces. The violent shaking of the infant causes whiplash and results in brain injury. The combined impact with a soft surface (e.g., mattress) can lead to retinal hemorrhages and subdural and subarachnoid hemorrhages. The infant may not display any external signs of trauma or may display the diagnostic signs of abusive brain injury. Cerebral damage, neurologic defects, blindness, and spinal cord damage can result. Nurses should teach parents about the dangers associated with shaking infants and the need to call their primary care provider if they feel they could harm their baby. Thomas (2016) states that it is essential that parents understand the reasons a baby cries and are knowledgeable about interventions to soothe the baby. Parents and caregivers must provide adequate nutrition, maintain a comfortable temperature, prevent overstimulation, and administer a soothing warm bath. These aspects of care can prevent crying and irritability and assist in preventing SBS or abusive head trauma.

Sudden Infant Death Syndrome

The sudden and unexpected death of an infant may be a case of **sudden infant death syndrome (SIDS)**. A postmortem examination usually fails to reveal a cause. The highest incidence of SIDS occurs in the second to fourth month of life, and boys are more susceptible than girls. Dr. Rachel Moon (2017) states that more than 3500 babies in the United States die suddenly due to SIDS each year. Research has shown that sleeping on the back (Figure 24.5 ■), not prone and not in a side-lying position, greatly decreases the risk of SIDS. Placing infants to sleep on their side is not recommended because they can easily roll onto the stomach. It is also recommended that infants be dressed in blanket sleepers and that no blankets, pillows, or stuffed animals be placed in the crib (American Academy of Pediatrics, 2017). The infant's mattress should be firm, and the use of wedges or positioners is not recommended. It is important for the infant to be in a smoke-free environment. The mother should also avoid smoking, consumption of alcohol, and the use of illicit drugs during pregnancy. All of these place the infant at risk for SIDS. It is important for the nurse to instruct the parents on the risk these activities have for an increased chance of SIDS. Lastly, nurses should encourage parents and caregivers to offer pacifiers to infants. The use of a pacifier during sleep reduces the risk of SIDS (Moon, 2017).

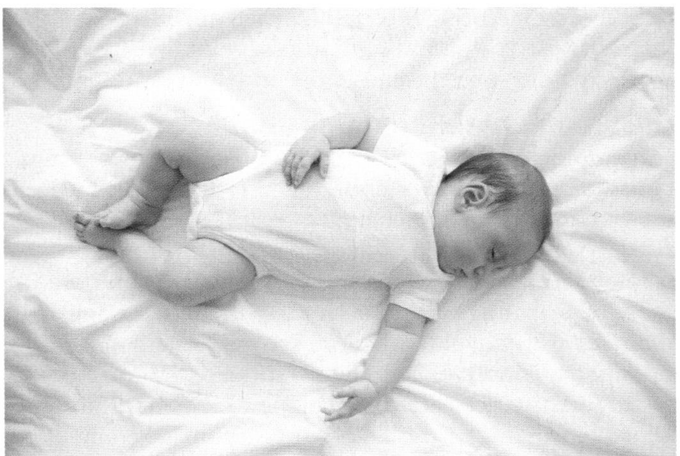

Figure 24.5 ■ Place infant on back for sleeping. Note the infant's tonic neck reflex.
Jamie Grill/Getty Images.

Health Assessment and Promotion

Physiologic health assessment occurs immediately at birth. Developmental assessment also begins at birth with the use of standardized tests. Ongoing nursing assessments continue for the promotion of wellness.

Apgar Scoring

Newborn babies can be assessed immediately by means of the **Apgar scoring system** (Table 24.2). This system provides a numeric indicator of the baby's physiologic capacities to adapt to extrauterine life. Each of five signs is assigned a maximum score of 2, so the maximum score achievable is 10. A score under 7 suggests that the baby is having difficulty, and a score under 4 indicates that the baby's condition is

TABLE 24.2 Apgar Scoring System to Assess the Newborn

	Score		
Sign	**0**	**1**	**2**
1. Heart rate	Absent	Slow (below 100 beats/ min)	Above 100 beats/min
2. Respirations	Absent	Slow, irregular	Regular rate, crying
3. Muscle tone	Flaccid	Some flexion of extremities	Active movements
4. Reflex irritability	None	Grimace	Cries
5. Color	Body pale, cyanotic	Body pink. For babies with dark skin (e.g., African American, some Latino, American Indian), check mucous membranes; extremities blue	Body completely pink, pink mucous membranes in babies with dark skin

critical. Apgar scoring is usually carried out 60 seconds after birth and is repeated in 5 minutes. Infants with very low scores require special resuscitative measures and care.

Developmental Screening Tests

Development can be assessed by observing the infant's behavior and by using standardized tests such as the **Denver Developmental Screening Test (DDST-II)**. The DDST-II is used to screen children from birth to 6 years of age. The test is intended to estimate the abilities of a child compared to those of an average group of children of the same age. Four main areas of development are screened: personal-social, fine motor adaptive, language, and gross motor. According to the American Academy of Neurology and the Child Neurology Society, the DDST-II is insensitive and lacks specificity. The **Ages & Stages Questionnaires (ASQ)** includes 19 age-specific surveys. Parents are asked about the developmental skills observed at ages 1 month to 5½ years. The ASQ assists healthcare professionals in identifying children who are at risk for social and emotional developmental delays (Hockenberry, Wilson, & Rodgers, 2019).

Ongoing Nursing Assessments

During ongoing assessments, the nurse examines and observes the infant, taking into account variations that occur with developmental age and activity. For example, the pulse of the baby at birth is affected by the child's activity, rising up to 170 when the infant is crying and falling to as low as 70 during sleep.

In addition, the nurse actively listens to the caregiver for possible problems or areas of concern and reviews with the parent the expected behavior or characteristics for the particular age group. It is important for the caregiver to know that certain behaviors, responses, and activities of the infant are normal and expected. It is also important to discuss the many individual differences that can, quite normally, occur.

The assessment interview is also a time to be supportive of the parent's role, to assess the attachment of the parent to the infant, and to observe the interactions between the infant and parent. Assessment guidelines for the infant are shown in the Developmental Assessment Guidelines.

The first month of life is critical for physical adjustments to extrauterine life and for the psychosocial adjustment of the parents. From 1 month to 1 year, infants experience rapid change, with advances in physical growth and psychosocial development. For a summary of health and wellness promotion, see Box 24.3.

Toddlers (1 to 3 Years)

Toddlers develop from having no voluntary control to being able to walk and speak. They also learn to control their bladder and bowels, and they acquire a wide variety of information about their environment.

Physical Development

Two-year-old children lose the baby look. Toddlers are usually chubby, with relatively short legs and a large head. The face appears small when compared to the skull, but as the toddler grows, the face seems to grow from under the skull and appears better proportioned. Toddlers have a pronounced lumbar lordosis and a protruding abdomen. The abdominal muscles develop gradually with growth, and the abdomen flattens.

Weight

Two-year-olds can be expected to weigh approximately 4 times their birth weight. The weight gain is about 2 kg (5 lb) between ages 1 and 2 years and about 1 to 2 kg (2 to 5 lb) between 2 and 3 years. The 3-year-old should weigh about 13.6 kg (30 lb).

Height

A toddler's height can be measured as height or length. Height is measured while the toddler stands, and length is measured while the toddler is in a recumbent position. Because the measurements differ slightly, nurses must specify which measurement is used. Between ages 1 and 2 years, the average growth in height is 10 to 12 cm (4 to 5 in.); between 2 and 3 years, it slows to 6 to 8 cm ($2\frac{1}{2}$ to $3\frac{1}{2}$ in.).

Head Circumference

The head circumference of the toddler increases about 2.5 cm (1 in.) each year. By 24 months, the head is 80% of the average adult size and the brain is 70% of its adult size.

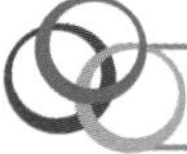

Developmental Assessment Guidelines — The Infant

In these five developmental areas, does the infant do the following?

PHYSICAL DEVELOPMENT

- Demonstrate physical growth (weight, length, head and chest circumference) within the normal range.
- Manifest appropriately sized fontanels for age.
- Exhibit vital signs within normal range for age.
- Display ability to habituate to stimuli and to calm self.

MOTOR DEVELOPMENT

- Perform gross and fine motor milestones within the normal range for age.
- Exhibit reflexes appropriate for age.
- Display symmetric movements.
- Exhibit no hyper- or hypotonia.

SENSORY DEVELOPMENT

- Follow a moving object within normal range for age.
- Respond to sounds, such as talking or clapping hands.
- Coo, babble, laugh, vocalize, and imitate sounds as expected for age.

PSYCHOSOCIAL DEVELOPMENT

- Interact appropriately with parent through body movements and vocalizations.

DEVELOPMENT IN ACTIVITIES OF DAILY LIVING

- Eat and drink appropriate amounts of breast milk, formula, and/or solid foods.
- Exhibit an elimination pattern within normal range for age.
- Exhibit a rest and sleep pattern appropriate for age.

BOX 24.3 Health Promotion Guidelines for Infants

HEALTH EXAMINATIONS
- Screening newborns for hearing loss at 1 month of age, diagnosis by 3 months of age, and intervention and treatment by 6 months of age, as recommended by the American Academy of Pediatrics and the Joint Committee on Infant Hearing (Krishnan & Van Hyfte, 2014)
- Physical exam at 2 weeks and at 2, 4, 6, 9, and 12 months

PROTECTIVE MEASURES
- Immunizations: diphtheria, tetanus, acellular pertussis (DTaP), inactivated poliovirus vaccine (IPV), pneumococcal (PVC), *Haemophilus influenzae* type B (HIB), hepatitis B (HepB), hepatitis A (HepA), rotavirus, and influenza vaccines as recommended. Varicella and measles-mumps-rubella (MMR) are not given before 12 months of age.
- Fluoride supplements for infants over 6 months of age if there is inadequate water fluoridation (less than 0.3 parts per million)
- Screening for tuberculosis
- Screening for metabolic conditions including phenylketonuria (PKU)
- Prompt attention for illnesses
- Appropriate skin hygiene and clothing

INFANT SAFETY
- Importance of supervision
- Car seat; crib with a firm mattress; playpen, bath, and home environment safety measures
- No stuffed animals, pillows, or blankets in the crib
- Positioning the infant on the back for sleep
- Feeding measures (e.g., avoid propping bottle)
- Providing toys with no small parts or sharp edges
- Elimination of toxins in the environment (e.g., tobacco, chemicals, radon, lead, mercury)
- Use of smoke and carbon monoxide (CO) detectors in the home

NUTRITION
- Exclusive breastfeeding for 4 to 6 months
- Solid foods between 4 and 6 months
- Need for iron supplements at 4 to 6 months
- Continued breastfeeding to age 12 months
- Breastfeeding and bottle-feeding techniques
- Formula preparation
- Feeding schedule

ELIMINATION
- Characteristics and frequency of stool and urine elimination
- Diarrhea and its effects

REST AND SLEEP
- Established routine for sleep and rest patterns
- Sensory stimulation
  - Touch: holding, cuddling, rocking
  - Vision: colorful, moving toys
  - Hearing: soothing voice tones, music, singing
  - Play: toys appropriate for development

Sensory Abilities

Visual acuity is fairly well established at 1 year; average estimates of acuity for the toddler are 20/70 at 18 months and 20/40 at 2 years of age. Accommodation to near and far objects is fairly well developed by 18 months and continues to mature with age. At 3 years of age, the toddler can look away from a toy prior to reaching out and picking it up. This ability requires the integration of visual and neuromuscular mechanisms.

The senses of hearing, taste, smell, and touch become increasingly developed and associated with each other. Hearing in the 3-year-old is at adult levels. The taste buds of the toddler are sensitive to the natural flavors of food, and the 3-year-old prefers familiar odors and tastes. Touch is a very important sense and a distressed toddler is often soothed by tactile sensations.

Motor Abilities

Fine muscle coordination and gross motor skills improve during the toddler years. At the age of 18 months, babies can pick up raisins or cereal pieces and place them in a receptacle. They can also hold a spoon and a cup and can walk upstairs with assistance. They will probably crawl down the stairs.

At 2 years, toddlers can hold a spoon and put it into the mouth correctly. They are able to run, their gait is steady, and they can balance on one foot and ride a tricycle (Figure 24.6 ■). In the third year, most children are toilet trained, although they still may have the occasional accident when playing or during the night.

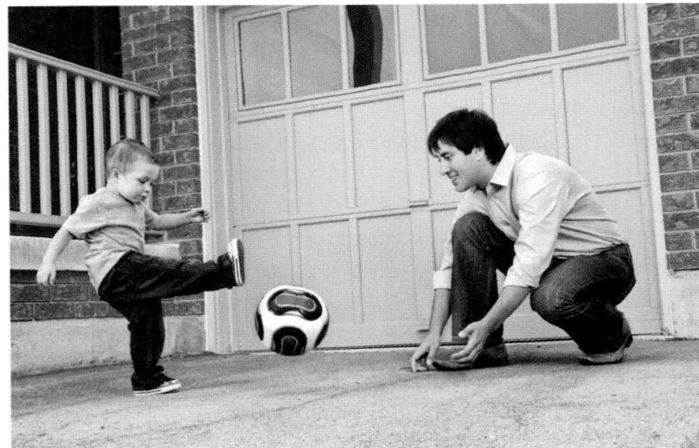

Figure 24.6 ■ A toddler has enough gross and fine motor ability to jump and kick a ball.
Elena Elisseeva/Shutterstock.

Psychosocial Development

According to Freud, the ages of 2 and 3 years represent the anal phase of development, when the rectum and anus are the especially significant areas of the body. Erikson viewed the period from 18 months to 3 years as the time when the central developmental task is autonomy versus shame and doubt.

Toddlers begin to develop their sense of autonomy by asserting themselves with frequent use of the word "no." They are often frustrated by restraints to their behavior and may have temper tantrums between ages 1 and 3. However, with the guidance of their caregivers, they slowly gain control over their emotions. Parents need to have a great deal of patience coupled with an understanding of the importance of this developmental milestone. To be effective, caregivers need to give the child some measure of control and at the same time be consistent in setting limits so that the child learns the results of misbehavior. The nurse can also assist the parents and caregivers in promoting the toddler's development by suggesting the activities summarized in Box 24.4.

BOX 24.4 Fostering the Toddler's Psychosocial Development

- Provide toys suitable for the toddler, including some toys challenging enough to motivate but not so difficult that the toddler will fail. (Failure can intensify feelings of self-doubt and shame.)
- Make positive suggestions rather than negative commands (e.g., "Don't get into that."). Avoid an emotional climate of negativism, blame, and punishment.
- Give the toddler choices, all of which are safe; however, limit the number to two or three.
- When the toddler has a temper tantrum, make sure the child is safe, and then leave.
- Help the toddler to develop inner control by setting and enforcing consistent, reasonable limits.
- Praise the toddler's accomplishments; give random and spontaneous feedback for positive behavior.

Self-concept refers to an individual's perception of his or her identity. A child's self-concept is formed by interpersonal experiences. It is formed in accordance with the child's ability to perform tasks, academic performance, social acceptance, and physical appearance. Children learn to develop a sense of self-concept through their immediate social environment, in which their parents play a significant role. If the children's social interactions with their parents are negative (e.g., constant disapproval regarding eating, toilet training, or other behavior), the children may begin to see themselves as bad. This perception is the basis of a negative self-concept. Parents need to give toddlers positive input so they can develop a positive and healthy self-concept. With a healthy self-concept, the toddler is better able to deal with periodic failures later in life.

Although toddlers like to explore the environment, they always need to have a significant individual nearby. Parents need to know that young children experience acute **separation anxiety**, the fear and frustration that come with parental absences. Abandonment is their greatest fear. At this age, the child may have difficulty accepting a babysitter or strongly resist being left by the parents at a daycare center. For example, toddlers may become highly anxious when separated from their parents and admitted to a hospital. **Regression**, or reverting to an earlier development stage, may be indicated by bed-wetting or using baby talk. Nurses can assist parents by helping them understand that this behavior is normal and indicates that these toddlers are trying to establish their position in the family.

Experience with separation helps the child cope with parental absences. Children need room for exploration and interaction with other children and adults. At the same time, they need to know that the parental bond of a loving and close relationship remains secure.

Toddlers assert their independence by saying "no" or by dawdling. During the toddler stage, receptive and expressive language skills develop quickly. Children can understand words and follow directions long before they can actually form sentences.

Cognitive Development

According to Piaget (1966), the toddler completes the fifth and sixth stages of the sensorimotor phase and starts the preconceptual phase at about 2 years of age. In the fifth stage, the toddler solves problems by a trial-and-error process. By stage 6, toddlers can solve problems mentally. For example, when given a new toy, the toddler will not immediately handle the toy to see how it works but will instead look at it carefully to think about how it works.

During Piaget's preconceptual phase, toddlers develop considerable cognitive and intellectual skills. They learn about the sequence of time. They have some symbolic thought; for example, a chair may represent a place of safety, and a blanket may symbolize comfort. Concepts start to form in late toddlerhood. A concept develops when the child learns words to represent classes of objects or thoughts. An example of a concrete concept is *table*, representing a number of articles of furniture that are all different but all tables.

Moral Development

According to Kohlberg (1981), the first level of moral development is the preconventional level, when children respond to punishment and reward. During the second year of life, children begin to know that some activities elicit affection and approval. They also recognize that certain rituals, such as repeating phrases from prayers, also elicit approval. This provides children with feelings of security. By 2 years of age, toddlers are learning what attitudes their parents hold about moral matters.

Spiritual Development

According to Fowler (1981), the toddler's stage of spiritual development is undifferentiated. Toddlers may be aware of some religious practices, but they are primarily involved in learning knowledge and emotional reactions rather than establishing spiritual beliefs. A toddler may repeat short prayers at bedtime, conforming to a ritual, because praise and affection result. This parental or caregiver response enhances the toddler's sense of security.

Health Risks

Toddlers experience significant health problems due to injuries, visual problems, dental caries, and respiratory and ear infections.

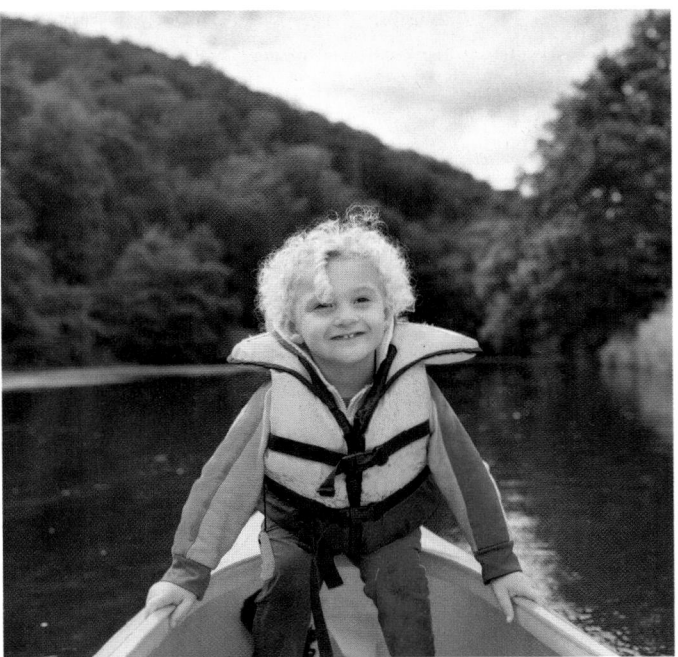

Figure 24.7 ■ Utilize safety equipment such as life jackets when near the water.
famveldman/123RF.

Injuries

Injuries are the leading cause of mortality of toddlers. Toddlers are curious and like to feel and taste everything. The most common causes of fatal injuries are automobile crashes, drowning, burns, poisoning, and falls. Parents or other caregivers need to take the appropriate preventive measures to guard against these health threats (Figure 24.7 ■).

Vision Problems

Early in the toddler years, the child should be screened for amblyopia. **Amblyopia** (a failure to establish normal neuropathways of vision that leads to reduced visual acuity in one eye) is usually the result of **strabismus** (cross-eye) but can be caused by refractive errors (e.g., myopia) or opacities in the lens. Initially, the child with amblyopia has straight eyes, but the condition can lead to deviation of the "lazy" eye and subsequent loss of vision.

Dental Caries

Dental caries occur frequently during the toddler period, resulting from the interaction between the tooth surface, the *Streptococcus mutans* bacterium, and carbohydrates, especially sugar, in the diet. Prolonged exposure of teeth to carbohydrates (e.g., use of the bottle during naps and at bedtime) can cause caries.

Respiratory Tract and Ear Infections

Respiratory and middle ear infections are common during the toddler years and contribute significantly to visits to the pediatric primary care provider; their incidence increases with exposure to other children (as in daycare centers or preschools), with use of a bottle during naps or at bedtime, or if bottles are propped for feedings.

Health Assessment and Promotion

Growth and development in the toddler and preschool years provide the basis for a child's future health and well-being. It is essential for nurses to perform accurate and timely assessments to promote health and detect problems early, thus allowing for early interventions. Providing health education, information about growth and development, and anticipatory guidance to parents is also an important nursing role. Assessment activities for the toddler are similar to those for the infant in terms of measuring weight, length (height), and vital signs (see the Developmental Assessment Guidelines).

Promoting health and wellness includes such areas as injury prevention, toilet training, and good dental hygiene. For a summary of health promotion for toddlers, see Box 24.5.

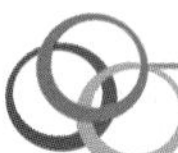

Developmental Assessment Guidelines — The Toddler

In these four developmental areas, does the toddler do the following?

PHYSICAL DEVELOPMENT

- Demonstrate physical growth (weight, height, and head circumference) within normal range.
- Manifest vital signs within normal range for age.
- Exhibit vision and hearing abilities within normal range.

MOTOR DEVELOPMENT

- Perform gross and fine motor milestones within the normal range for age. For example, by 3 years of age, is the toddler able to do the following?
  - Walk up steps without assistance.
  - Balance on one foot, jump, and walk on toes.
  - Copy a circle.
  - Build a bridge from blocks.
  - Ride a tricycle.

PSYCHOSOCIAL DEVELOPMENT

- Perform psychosocial developmental milestones for the child's age. For example, by 3 years of age, is the toddler able to do the following?
  - Express likes and dislikes.
  - Display curiosity and ask questions.
  - Accept separation from mother or primary caregiver for short periods of time.
  - Begin to play and communicate with children and others outside the immediate family.
  - Understand words such as *up*, *down*, *cold*, and *hungry.*
  - Speak in sentences of three to four words.
  - Imitate religious rituals of the family, if any.

DEVELOPMENT IN ACTIVITIES OF DAILY LIVING

- Feed self.
- Eat and drink a variety of foods.
- Begin to develop bowel and bladder control.
- Exhibit a sleep pattern appropriate for age.
- Dress self.

BOX 24.5 Health Promotion Guidelines for Toddlers

HEALTH EXAMINATIONS
- At 15 and 18 months and then as recommended by the primary care provider
- Dental visits starting at age 3 or earlier

PROTECTIVE MEASURES
- Immunizations: continuing acellular pertussis (DTaP), inactivated poliovirus vaccine (IPV), pneumococcal, measles-mumps-rubella (MMR), varicella, *Haemophilus influenzae* type B, hepatitis B, hepatitis A, influenza, and meningococcal vaccines as recommended
- Screenings for tuberculosis and lead poisoning
- Fluoride supplements if there is inadequate water fluoridation (less than 0.6 part per million)

TODDLER SAFETY
- Importance of constant supervision and teaching child to obey commands
- Home environment safety measures (e.g., lock medicine cabinet)
- Outdoor safety measures (e.g., close supervision near water and on sidewalks)
- Appropriate toys
- Elimination of toxins in environment (e.g., tobacco, pesticides, herbicides, mercury, lead, arsenic in playground materials)
- Use of smoke and carbon monoxide (CO) detectors in the home

NUTRITION
- Importance of nutritious meals and snacks
- Teaching simple mealtime manners
- Dental care
- Elimination
- Toilet-training techniques

REST AND SLEEP
- Dealing with sleep disturbances

PLAY
- Providing adequate space and a variety of activities
- Encouraging regular, vigorous physical activity
- Toys that allow "acting on" behaviors and provide motor and sensory stimulation

Preschoolers (4 and 5 Years)

During the preschool period, physical growth slows, but control of the body and coordination increase greatly. Preschoolers' worlds get larger as they meet relatives, friends, and neighbors.

Physical Development

Preschool-age children tend to grow more in height than in weight, so by the time children are 4 or 5 years old, they appear taller and thinner than toddlers. The posture of preschoolers gradually becomes more erect as the pelvis is straightened and the abdominal muscles become stronger. The extremities of the body grow more quickly than the body trunk, making the child's body appear somewhat out of proportion. The preschooler's brain almost reaches its adult size by 5 years.

Weight

Weight gain in preschool children is generally slow. By 5 years, they should have added only another 3 to 5 kg (7 to 12 lb) to their 3-year-old weight, increasing it to somewhere between 18 and 20 kg (40 and 45 lb).

Height

Preschool children grow about 5 to 6.25 cm (2.0 to 2.5 in.) each year. By 4 years of age, they have doubled their birth length and measure about 102 cm (41 in.).

Vision

Preschool children are generally **hyperopic** (farsighted), that is, unable to focus on near objects. As the eye grows in length, it becomes **emmetropic** (it refracts light normally). If the eyes become too long, the child becomes **myopic** (nearsighted), that is, unable to focus on objects that are far away. In severe cases of hyperopia or myopia, glasses may be prescribed. By the end of the preschool years, visual ability has improved; normal vision for the 5-year-old is approximately 20/30. The Snellen E chart can be used to assess the preschooler's vision.

Hearing and Taste

The hearing of the preschool child has reached optimal levels, and the ability to listen (attend to and comprehend what is said) has matured since the toddler age. As for the sense of taste, preschoolers show their preferences by asking for something "yummy" and may refuse something they consider "yucky." At about age 3, children may display food "jags," refusing to eat some foods or only eating a few particular foods. It is important that parents not engage the child in a "battle of wills" over food. If parents provide a variety of healthful foods in an environment that is pleasant and comfortable for eating, the child will eat what is needed.

Motor Abilities

By 5 years of age, children are able to wash their hands and face and brush their teeth (Figure 24.8 ■). They are self-conscious about exposing their bodies and go to the bathroom without telling others. Typically, preschool children run with increasing skill each year. By 5 years of age, they run skillfully and can jump three steps. Preschoolers can balance on their toes and dress themselves without assistance.

Psychosocial Development

For Erikson (1963), the major developmental crisis of the preschooler is initiative versus guilt. Preschoolers must solve problems in accordance with their consciences.

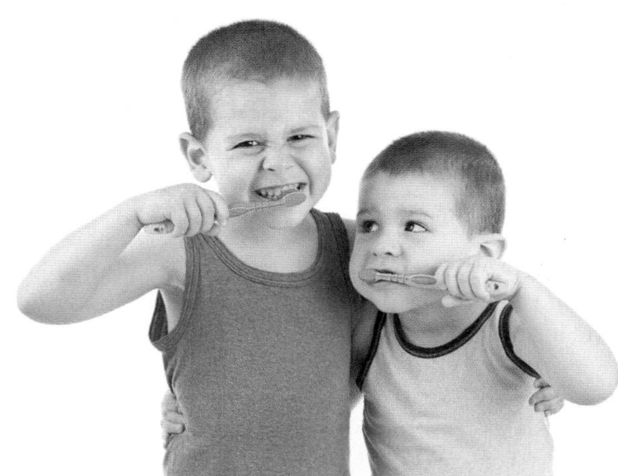

Figure 24.8 ■ Preschoolers brushing their teeth.
blendevo/123RF.

Their personalities continue to develop. Erikson viewed the success of this milestone as determining the individual's self-concept. According to Erikson, preschoolers must learn what they can do. As a result, preschoolers imitate behavior, and their imaginations and creativity become lively.

Parents can enhance the self-concept of the preschooler by providing opportunities for new achievements where the child can learn, repeat, and master. For example, a child obtains a two-wheel bike with safety wheels and quickly learns coordination, balance, use of the brakes, and bicycle safety. Mastery of these tasks provides the child with a sense of accomplishment. The child will soon be ready for the new challenge of mastering the two-wheeler without the safety wheels.

The self-concept of the preschooler is also based on gender identification. Preschoolers are aware of the two sexes and identify with their gender. They often imitate sexual stereotypes and usually begin by identifying with the parent of the same sex. They may mimic the parent's behavior, attitudes, and appearance (Figure 24.9 ■). Parents need to be aware that preschoolers are curious about their own bodies and sexual functions, as well as those of others, and will often ask questions. Parents should answer questions calmly and frankly, using words and concepts the child understands. Children do not have the social, emotional, or moral context that adults do, so a simple answer may be more than adequate. When parents overreact to a child's question, refuse to answer, or punish or shame the child, the child can become confused.

Freud theorized that the preschooler is in the phallic stage of development. The biological focus of the child during this stage is the genital area, and masturbation is common. The phase of close emotional relationships with both parents changes to the phase Freud referred to as the Electra or Oedipus complex. At this time, the child focuses feelings of love chiefly on the parent of the opposite sex, and the parent of the same sex may receive some hostile feelings. The child may express sexual curiosity, but it is without sexual connotations.

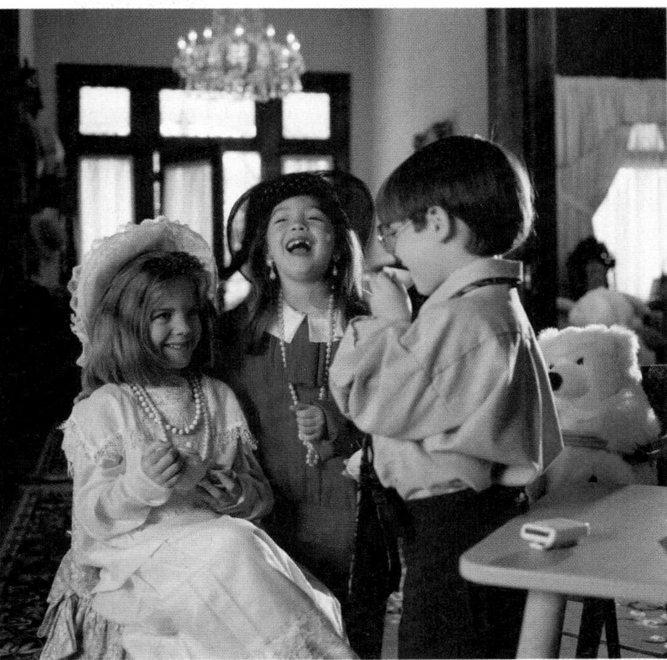

Figure 24.9 ■ Preschoolers often identify with the parent of the same sex and like to mimic behavior.
Stewart Cohen/Stockbyte/Getty Images.

During the preschool years, Freud asserted that four adaptive mechanisms are learned: identification, introjection, imagination, and repression. **Identification** occurs when the child perceives the self as similar to another individual and behaves like that individual. For example, a boy may internalize the attitudes and gender behavior of his father. **Introjection** is similar to identification. It is the assimilation of the attributes of others into oneself. When preschoolers observe their parents, they assimilate many of their values and attitudes, thus creating an ego and superego (conscience). **Imagination** is forming a mental image of something not present to the senses or never before experienced and is an important part of preschoolers' lives. Imagination helps children make sense of the world and gives them a sense of control and mastery. The preschooler has an active imagination and fantasizes in play; for example, a chair becomes a beautiful throne to a girl, and she is the ruler of all she sees. **Repression** is the removal of experiences, thoughts, and impulses from awareness. According to Freud, the preschooler generally represses thoughts related to the Oedipus or Electra complex.

Preschool children gradually emerge as social beings. At the age of 3 or 4, they learn to play with a small number of their peers. They gradually learn to play with more peers as they grow older. Preschoolers participate more in the family than they did previously. In associations with neighbors, family guests, and babysitters, too, they learn about social relationships.

In their speech, children of 4 years are often dogmatic; they tend to believe that what they know is right. Four-year-olds love nonsense words such as "jump-jump" and can string them together, much to an adult's exasperation. At age 4, children are aggressive in their speech and capable of long conversations, often mixing fact and fiction. By 5 years of age, speaking skills are well developed. Children use words purposefully and ask questions to acquire information. They do not merely practice speaking as 3- and 4-year-olds do but speak as a means of social interaction. Exaggeration is common among 4- and 5-year-olds.

Preschoolers become increasingly aware of themselves. They play with their bodies largely out of curiosity. They know where the body begins and ends as well as the correct names for the different parts. By 5 years of age, they are able to draw a person and include all the features. Preschoolers also learn about their feelings; they know the words *cry*, *sad*, and *laugh* and the feelings related to them. They begin to learn how to control their feelings and behavior. The preschooler uses the same types of coping mechanisms in response to stress as the toddler does, although protest behavior (kicking, screaming) is less likely to occur in the older preschooler. Preschoolers usually have greater ability to verbalize stress.

Preschoolers need to feel that they are loved and are an important part of the family. The child who has to compete with siblings for parental attention will often display jealousy. Parents and caregivers should be aware that preschoolers need time to adjust to a new baby and may need additional attention or special activities to help them through this adjustment period. Preschoolers with older siblings may also experience sibling rivalry. Siblings may fight and argue and become aggressive because of their daily proximity or competition for parental attention. Parents who can plan some special time or activity for each child will help that child to feel loved and may decrease the sibling rivalry.

Guidance and discipline are important parts of the parental role during the preschool years. As children seek independence from adults, they often test limits by refusing to cooperate and by repeatedly ignoring parental requests. Parents can help their children develop a sense of self-control and cooperative engagement in the family by setting reasonable expectations and consistent limits, reinforcing children's positive behaviors, and encouraging children to be responsible for their own behavior as much as possible. When conflict does occur, parents can employ mutual discussion and compromise.

Cognitive Development

The preschooler's cognitive development, according to Piaget, is the phase of intuitive thought. Children are still egocentric, but egocentrism gradually subsides as they experience their expanding world. Preschoolers learn through trial and error, observation, imitation, and practice in play and make-believe. They think of only one idea at a time. They do not fully understand relationships, such as those between mother and father or sister and brother. Preschoolers become concerned about death as something inevitable, but they do not explain it. They also associate death with others rather than themselves.

Reading and mathematical skills (e.g., recognizing and naming letters and numbers, counting, and "reading" age-appropriate books) begin to develop at this age. Young children like fairy tales and books about animals and other children, and they should be read to often.

Moral Development

Preschoolers are capable of prosocial behavior, that is, any action that an individual takes to benefit someone else. The term *prosocial* is synonymous with *kind* and connotes sharing, helping, protecting, giving aid, befriending, showing affection, and giving encouragement.

At this stage of development, preschoolers do not have a fully formed conscience; however, they do develop some internal controls. Moral behavior is largely learned by modeling, initially of parents and later significant others. The preschooler usually behaves well in social settings.

Children who perceive their parents as strict may become resentful or overly obedient. Preschoolers usually control their behavior because they want love and approval from their parents. Moral behavior to a preschooler may mean taking turns at play or sharing. Nurses can assist parents by discussing moral development and encouraging parents to give preschoolers recognition for actions such as sharing. It is also important for parents to answer preschoolers' "why" questions and discuss values with them.

Spiritual Development

Many preschoolers enroll in Sunday school or faith-oriented classes. The preschooler usually enjoys the social interaction of these classes. According to Fowler, children from the ages of 4 to 6 years are at the intuitive-projective stage of spiritual development. Faith at this stage is primarily a result of the teaching of significant others, such as parents and teachers. Children learn to imitate religious behavior, for example, bowing the head in prayer, although they don't understand the meaning of the behavior. Preschoolers require simple explanations, such as those in picture books, of spiritual matters. Children at this age use their imaginations to envision such ideas as angels or the devil.

Health Risks

Preschoolers often have health problems similar to those they had in the toddler years. Respiratory tract problems and communicable diseases frequently occur as the preschooler interacts with other children at nursery schools and daycare. Injuries and dental caries continue to be problems. Congenital abnormalities such as cardiac disorders and hernias are often corrected at this age.

Health Assessment and Promotion

During assessment, the preschooler can often participate in answering questions with assistance from parents or caregivers. For instance, children who attend preschool

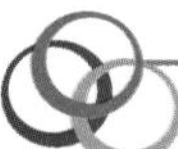

Developmental Assessment Guidelines — The Preschooler

In these four developmental areas, does the preschooler do the following?

PHYSICAL DEVELOPMENT
- Demonstrate physical growth (weight, height) within normal range.
- Manifest vital signs within normal range for age.
- Exhibit vision and hearing abilities within normal range.

MOTOR DEVELOPMENT
- Perform gross and fine motor milestones within the normal range for age. For example, by 5 years of age, is the preschooler able to do the following?
  - Jump rope and skip.
  - Climb playground equipment.
  - Ride a bicycle with training wheels.
  - Print letters and numbers.

PSYCHOSOCIAL DEVELOPMENT
- Perform psychosocial developmental milestones for age. For example, by 5 years of age, is the preschooler able to do the following?
  - Separate easily from parents.
  - Display imagination and creativity.
  - Enjoy playing with peers in cooperative activities.
  - Understand right from wrong and respond to others' expectations of behavior.
  - Identify four colors.
  - Exhibit increasing vocabulary using complete sentences and all parts of speech.
  - Cooperate in doing simple chores (e.g., putting away toys).
  - Demonstrate awareness of sexual differences.

DEVELOPMENT IN ACTIVITIES OF DAILY LIVING
- Demonstrate development of toilet training.
- Perform simple hygiene measures.
- Dress and undress self.
- Engage in bedtime rituals and demonstrate ability to put self to sleep.

can describe the typical lunch and how much of it they usually eat. Preschoolers can also describe the types of activities they enjoy. Guidelines for the preschooler are shown in the Developmental Assessment Guidelines.

Promoting health and wellness includes such areas as injury prevention, dental health, good nutrition, cognitive stimulation, and sufficient sleep. For a summary of health promotion, see Box 24.6.

BOX 24.6 Health Promotion Guidelines for Preschoolers

HEALTH EXAMINATIONS
- Every 1 to 2 years

PROTECTIVE MEASURES
- Immunizations: continuing acellular pertussis (DTaP), inactivated poliovirus vaccine (IPV), measles-mumps-rubella (MMR), hepatitis A and B, pneumococcal, influenza, varicella, and other immunizations as recommended
- Screenings for tuberculosis
- Vision and hearing screening
- Regular dental screenings and fluoride treatment if necessary

PRESCHOOLER SAFETY
- Educating child about simple safety rules (e.g., crossing the street)
- Teaching child to play safely (e.g., bicycle and playground safety)
- Educating to prevent poisoning; exposure to toxic materials

NUTRITION
- Importance of nutritious meals and snacks

ELIMINATION
- Teaching proper hygiene (e.g., washing hands after using bathroom)

REST AND SLEEP
- Dealing with sleep disturbances (e.g., night terrors, sleepwalking)

PLAY
- Encouraging regular, vigorous physical activity
- Providing times for group play activities
- Teaching child simple games that require cooperation and interaction
- Providing toys and dress-up clothing for role playing

School-Age Children (6 to 12 Years)

The school-age period starts when children are about 6 years of age and ends at about 12 years, with the onset of puberty. Because the average age of onset of puberty is 10 for girls and 12 for boys, some individuals define the school-age years as 6 to 10 for girls and 6 to 12 for boys. Skills learned during this stage are particularly important in relation to work later in life and willingness to try new tasks. In general, the period from 6 to 12 years is one of significant growth.

Physical Development

The school-age child gains weight rapidly and thus appears less thin than previously. Individual differences due to both genetic and environmental factors are obvious at this time.

Weight

At 6 years, boys tend to weigh about 21 kg (46 lb), about 1 kg (2 lb) more than girls. The weight gain of schoolchildren from 6 to 12 years of age averages about 3.2 kg (7 lb) per year, but the major weight gains occur from age 10 to 12 for boys and from 9 to 12 for girls. By 12 years of age, boys and girls weigh an average of 40 to 42 kg (88 to 95 lb); girls are usually heavier. Overweight and obesity are unlikely at this age if the child has demonstrated a pattern of good nutrition and regular, vigorous exercise in the infant, toddler, and preschool years.

Height

At 6 years, both boys and girls are about the same height, 115 cm (46 in.). They are about 150 cm (60 in.) by 12 years. Before puberty, children of both sexes have a growth spurt, girls between 10 and 12 years and boys between 12 and 14 years. Thus, girls may be taller than boys at 12 years.

The extremities tend to grow more quickly than the trunk; thus, school-age children's bodies appear somewhat ill-proportioned. By 6 years of age, the thoracic curvature starts to develop, and the lordosis disappears. Full adult posture is not assumed, however, until after the complete development of the skeletal musculature during adolescence.

Vision

The depth and distance perception of children 6 to 8 years of age is accurate. By age 6, children have full binocular vision. The eye muscles are well developed and coordinated, and both eyes can focus on one object at the same time. Because the shape of the eye changes during growth, the farsightedness of the preschool years gradually changes to 20/20 vision during the school-age years; 20/20 vision is usually well established between 9 and 11 years of age.

Hearing and Touch

Auditory perception is fully developed in school-age children, who are able to identify fine differences in voices, both in sound and in pitch. At this stage, children also have a well-developed sense of touch and are able to locate points of heat and cold on all body surfaces. They are able to identify an unseen object, such as a pencil or a book, simply by touch. This ability is called **stereognosis**.

Prepubertal Changes

Little change takes place in the reproductive and endocrine systems until the prepuberty period. During prepuberty, at about ages 9 to 13, endocrine functions slowly increase. This change in endocrine function can result in increased perspiration and more active sebaceous glands. Girls may have a sticky vaginal discharge (leukorrhea) prior to puberty.

Motor Abilities

During the middle years (ages 6 to 10), children perfect their muscular skills and coordination. By 9 years, many children are becoming skilled in games of interest, such as football, soccer, or baseball. These skills are often associated with school, and many of them are learned there. By 9 years, most children have sufficient fine motor control for such activities as drawing, building models, or playing musical instruments.

Psychosocial Development

According to Erikson, the central task of school-age children is industry versus inferiority. At this time, children begin to create and develop a sense of competence and perseverance. School-age children are motivated by activities that provide a sense of worth. They concentrate on mastering skills that will help them function in the adult world. Although children of this age work hard to succeed, they are always faced with the possibility of failure, which can lead to a sense of inferiority. If children have been successful in previous stages, they are motivated to be industrious and to cooperate with others toward a common goal.

Freud described the period from 6 through 12 years of age as the latency stage. During this time, the focus is on physical and intellectual activities, whereas sexual tendencies seem to be repressed. Curiosity about sexual matters is present, however, and children are aware of the messages related to sex in popular media, films, and on the Internet; parents need to set limits, answer questions, and provide guidance to help their children understand and cope with information and feelings.

In school, children have the restraints of the school system imposed on their behavior, and they learn to develop internal controls. Children tend to compare their skills with those of their peers in a number of areas, including motor development, social development, and language. This comparison assists in the development of self-concept.

As school-age children grow older, they learn to play in groups. The typical 6- and 7-year-old is a member of a peer group that is usually informal and transitory, with the leadership changing from time to time. During this period of socialization with others, children gradually become less self-centered and more cooperative within a group. Peers can have a greater influence than the family. During middle to late childhood, children may join a more formalized group of peers, which is often structured around common interests. These groups may consist of children of the same gender later in the school-age period.

Self-concept continues to mature during this period. Children recognize similarities and differences between themselves and others. School-age children compare themselves with others. Children who are successful and receive recognition for their efforts feel competent and in control of themselves and of their environment. Conversely, children who feel unaccepted by peers or constantly receive negative feedback and little recognition may experience feelings of inferiority and worthlessness. A major negative impact on psychosocial development is that of bullying. Bullying has become very common in all age groups, but it most commonly begins in the school years. Bullying is a complex social trend that needs to be addressed with strong school policies, parental awareness, and monitoring to combat the problem (Ali, Virani, & Alaman, 2017).

Although the focus of interest for this age group has moved to school, peers, and other activities, the home remains the crucial place for the child's development of high self-esteem.

Cognitive Development

According to Piaget, the ages 7 to 11 years mark the phase of concrete operations. During this stage, the child changes from egocentric interactions to cooperative interactions (Figure 24.10 ■). School-age children also develop an increased understanding of concepts that are associated with specific objects, for example, environmental conservation or wildlife preservation. Children at this time develop logical reasoning from intuitive reasoning. For example, they learn to add and subtract to obtain an answer to a problem. Children learn about cause-and-effect relationships at this age; for example, they know that a stone will not float because it is heavier than water.

Money is a concept that gains meaning for children when they start school. By the time they are 7 or 8 years old, children usually know the value of most coins. The concept of time is also learned at this age. Knowing the time of day and the day of the week are relatively easy for children because they relate time to routine activities. For example, a girl may go to school Monday through Friday, play on Saturday, go to Sunday school on Sunday morning, and go out with her father on Sunday afternoon. Children are beginning to read a clock by the time they are 6 years old; they can learn to read both digital and numerical clocks. However, it is not until 9 or 10 years of age that children are able to understand the long periods of time in the past.

Reading skills are usually well developed later in childhood, and what a child reads is largely influenced by the family. By 9 years of age, most children are self-motivated. They compete with themselves, and they like to plan in advance. By 12 years, they are motivated by inner drive rather than by competition with peers. They like to talk, discuss different subjects, and debate.

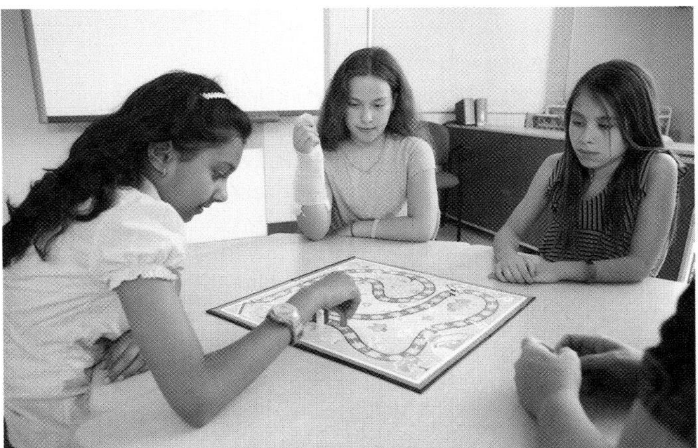

Figure 24.10 ■ Expanding cognitive skills enable school-age children to interact cooperatively in activities of an increasingly complex nature, as shown by the children playing an educational board game.
diane39/iStock/Getty Images.

Moral Development

Some school-age children are at Kohlberg's stage 1 of the preconventional level (punishment and obedience); that is, they act to avoid being punished. Some school-age children, however, are at stage 2 (instrumental-relativist orientation). These children do things to benefit themselves. Fairness, in which everyone gets a fair share or chance, becomes important. Later in childhood, most children progress to the conventional level. This level has two stages: Stage 3 is the "good boy–nice girl" stage, and stage 4 is the law-and-order orientation. Children usually reach the conventional level between the ages of 10 and 13. The child shifts from the concrete interests of individuals to the interests of groups. The motivation for moral action at this stage is to live up to what significant others think of the child.

Spiritual Development

According to Fowler, the school-age child is at stage 2 in spiritual development, the mythic-literal stage. Children learn to distinguish fantasy from fact. Spiritual facts are those beliefs that are accepted by a religious group, whereas fantasy is thoughts and images formed in the child's mind. Parents and the minister, rabbi, or priest help the child distinguish fact from fantasy. These individuals still influence the child more than peers in spiritual matters.

School-age children may ask many questions about God and religion in these years and will generally believe that God is good and always present to help. Just before puberty, children become aware that their prayers are not always answered and become disappointed. At this age, some children reject religion, whereas others continue to accept it. This decision is largely influenced by the parents. If a child continues religious training, the child is ready to apply reason rather than blind belief in most situations.

Health Risks

School-age children continue to have as many communicable diseases, dental caries, and unintentional injuries as preschoolers (Figure 24.11 ■). Another health concern in the United States is the increasing number of overweight children. Being overweight is a common nutritional problem among children and contributes to a wide range of health problems. School districts throughout the country are addressing the needs of students to decrease both fat and calories with healthier choices. The prevalence of childhood obesity from 2011–2014 remained stable at 17% of children and adolescents. The prevalence in Hispanic children is 21.9%, in Black non-Hispanic children is 19.5%, and in White non-Hispanic is 14.7% (CDC, 2018a).

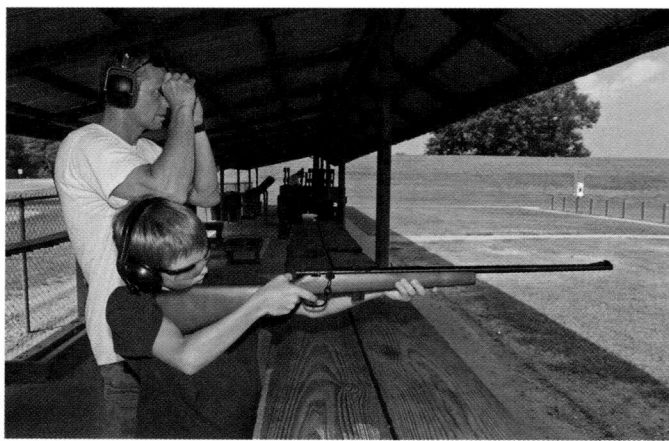

Figure 24.11 ■ Teach children never to touch guns without a parent present.
Dlewis33/E+/Getty Images.

Health Assessment and Promotion

During the assessment interview, the nurse responds to questions from the parent or other caregiver, gives appropriate feedback, and lends encouragement and support. The nurse also demonstrates an interest in the child and enthusiasm for the child's strengths and includes the child actively in the exam, explaining and encouraging the child to ask questions and participate. Guidelines for the school-age child are shown in the Developmental Assessment Guidelines.

Promoting health and wellness includes dental hygiene and regular dental examinations, safety measures to prevent injuries, promoting a healthy diet and physical fitness, supporting autonomy and self-esteem, and hygiene measures to prevent infections. Box 24.7 provides health promotion guidelines for this age group.

BOX 24.7 Health Promotion Guidelines for School-Age Children

HEALTH EXAMINATIONS
- Annual physical examination or as recommended

PROTECTIVE MEASURES
- Immunizations as recommended (e.g., human papillomavirus [HPV], measles-mumps-rubella [MMR], meningococcal, tetanus-diphtheria [Tdap], influenza)
- Screening for tuberculosis
- Periodic vision, speech, and hearing screenings
- Regular dental screenings and fluoride treatment
- Providing accurate information about sexual issues (e.g., reproduction, AIDS)

SCHOOL-AGE CHILD SAFETY
- Using proper equipment when participating in sports and other physical activities (e.g., helmets, pads)
- Encouraging child to take responsibility for own safety (e.g., participating in bicycle and water safety courses)

NUTRITION
- Importance of child not skipping meals and eating a balanced diet
- Experiences with food that may lead to obesity

ELIMINATION
- Utilizing positive approaches for elimination problems (e.g., enuresis)

PLAY AND SOCIAL INTERACTIONS
- Encouraging regular, vigorous physical activity
- Providing opportunities for a variety of organized group activities
- Accepting realistic expectations of child's abilities
- Acting as role models in acceptance of other individuals who may be different
- Providing a home environment that limits TV viewing and video games and encourages completion of homework and healthy exercise

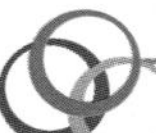

Developmental Assessment Guidelines — The School-Age Child

In these four developmental areas, does the school-age child do the following?

PHYSICAL DEVELOPMENT
- Demonstrate physical growth (weight, height) within normal range.
- Manifest vital signs within normal range for age.
- Exhibit vision and hearing abilities within normal range.
- Demonstrate male or female prepubertal changes within normal range.

MOTOR DEVELOPMENT
- Possess coordinated motor skills for age. For example, by 12 years of age, is the child able to do the following?
  - Do tricks on a bike or skateboard, climb a tree, and shimmy up a rope.
  - Throw and catch a small ball.
  - Play a musical instrument or do other activities requiring fine motor coordination.

PSYCHOSOCIAL DEVELOPMENT
- Perform psychosocial developmental milestones for age. For example, by 12 years of age, is the child able to do the following?
  - Make friends of the same sex and establish a peer group.
  - Become less dependent on family and venture away from them.
  - Interact well with parents.
  - Control strong and impulsive feelings.
  - Articulate an understanding of right and wrong.
  - Participate in organized competitions.
  - Read, print, and manipulate numbers and letters easily.
  - Express positive feelings about school and school activities.
  - Exhibit a concept of money and make change for small amounts of money.
  - Express self in a logical manner and talk through problems.
  - Enjoy riddles and read and understand comics.
  - Invest in a hobby or collection.
  - Like to help others.
  - Think of self as likable and healthy.

DEVELOPMENT IN ACTIVITIES OF DAILY LIVING
- Demonstrate concern for personal cleanliness and appearance.
- Express need for privacy.

Adolescents (12 to 18 Years)

Adolescence is the period during which an individual becomes physically and psychologically mature and acquires a personal identity. At the end of this critical period in development, the individual should be ready to enter adulthood and assume its responsibilities. The length of adolescence is culturally determined to some extent. In North America, adolescence is longer than in some cultures, extending to 18 or 20 years of age.

Puberty is the first stage of adolescence, in which sexual organs begin to grow and mature. **Menarche** (onset of menstruation) occurs in girls. **Ejaculation** (expulsion of semen) occurs in boys. For girls, puberty normally starts between 10 and 14 years; for boys, between 12 and 16 years. The adolescent period is often subdivided into three stages: early adolescence lasts from ages 12 to 13; middle adolescence extends from 14 to 16 years; and late adolescence extends from 17 to 18 or 20 years. Late adolescence is a more stable stage than the other two. In the late period, adolescents are involved mostly with planning their future and economic independence.

Physical Development

During puberty, growth is markedly accelerated compared to the slow, steady growth of the child. This period, marked by sudden and dramatic physical changes, is referred to as the **adolescent growth spurt**. In boys, the growth spurt usually begins between ages 12 and 16; in girls, it begins earlier, usually between ages 10 and 14. Because the growth spurt begins earlier in girls, many girls surpass boys in height at this time.

Physical Growth

Physical growth continues throughout adolescence. Growth is fastest for boys at about 14 years, and the maximum height is often reached at about 18 or 19 years. Some men add another 1 or 2 cm to their height during their 20s as the vertebral column gradually continues to grow. During the period from 10 to 18 years of age, the average American male doubles his weight, gaining about 32 kg (72 lb), and grows about 41 cm (16 in.). The fastest rate of growth in girls occurs at about age 12; they reach their maximum height at about 15 to 16 years. During ages 10 to 18, the average American female gains about 25 kg (55 lb) and grows about 24 cm (9 in.).

Physical growth during adolescence is greatly influenced by a number of factors, such as heredity, nutrition, medical care, illness, physical and emotional environment, family size, and culture. Generally, individuals in the United States have grown taller in recent years. This increase in average height is thought to be due to many of the preceding factors.

Growth is noted first in the musculoskeletal system. This growth follows a sequential pattern: The head, hands, and feet are the first to grow to adult status. Next, the extremities reach their adult size. Because the extremities grow before the trunk, the adolescent looks leggy, awkward, and uncoordinated. After the trunk grows to full size, the shoulders, chest, and hips grow. Skull and facial bones also change proportions: The forehead becomes more prominent, and the jawbones develop.

Glandular Changes

The eccrine and apocrine glands increase their secretions and become fully functional during puberty. The **eccrine glands**, found over most of the body, produce sweat. The **apocrine glands** develop in the axillae, in the anal and genital areas, in the external auditory canals, and around the umbilicus and the areola of the breasts. Apocrine sweat is released onto the skin in response to emotional stimuli only. **Sebaceous glands** also become active under the influence of androgens in both males and females. The sebaceous glands, which secrete sebum, become most active on the face, neck, shoulders, upper back, and chest and often contribute to an increased incidence of acne.

Sexual Characteristics

During puberty, both primary and secondary sexual characteristics develop. **Primary sexual characteristics** relate to the organs necessary for reproduction, such as the testes, penis, ovaries, vagina, and uterus. **Secondary sexual characteristics** differentiate the male from the female but do not relate directly to reproduction. Examples are pubic hair growth, breast development, and voice changes.

The first noticeable sign that puberty has begun in males is the appearance of pubic hair and the enlargement of the scrotum and testes. The milestone of male puberty is considered to be the first ejaculation, which commonly occurs at about 14 years of age. Fertility follows several months later. Sexual maturity is achieved by age 18.

Often the first noticeable sign of puberty in females is the appearance of breast buds (thelarche), although the appearance of hair along the labia may precede this. The milestone of female puberty is the menarche, which occurs about $1\frac{1}{2}$ to 2 years after breast buds appear. At first, menstrual periods are scanty and irregular and may occur without ovulation. Ovulation is usually established 1 to 2 years after menarche; ovulation and pregnancy, however, can occur early in menarche or as an immediate precursor to a girl's first menstruation. Female internal reproductive organs reach adult size by about age 18 to 20.

Psychosocial Development

According to Erikson, the psychosocial task of the adolescent is the establishment of identity. The danger of this stage is role confusion. The inability to settle on an occupational identity commonly disturbs the adolescent. Less commonly, doubts about sexual identity arise. Because of the adolescent's dramatic body changes, the development of a stable identity is difficult. Erikson says that adolescents help one another through this identity crisis by forming cliques and a separate youth culture. These cliques often exclude all those who are "different" in skin color, cultural background, aspects of dress, gestures, and tastes.

Adolescents are usually concerned about their bodies, their appearance, and their physical abilities. Hairstyling, skin care, and clothes become very important. In-groupers of an adolescent clique can be excessively clannish and cruel in excluding out-groupers; this intolerance is a temporary defense against identity confusion (Erikson, 1963, p. 236).

In their search for a new identity, adolescents have to reprocess many of the previous stages of development. The task of developing trust in self and others is again encountered when adolescents look for ideal individuals whom they can trust and with whom they can prove trustworthy. Development of autonomy is restaged in their search for ways to express the right to choose freely. The search for an occupational role that allows the expression of an autonomous, freely chosen direction is one example. Free choice and autonomy present conflicts to the adolescent. Conflict can arise between behaving well in the eyes of the parents and behaving in a manner that will lead to peer acceptance. The sense of initiative is also restaged. The adolescent has unlimited imagination and ambition and aspires to great accomplishments. The sense of industry is reenacted when the adolescent chooses a career. The extent to which the tasks of earlier stages have been successfully achieved influences the adolescent's ability to develop a healthy self-concept and self-identity.

The adolescent needs to establish a self-concept that accepts both personal strengths and weaknesses. Many adolescents experience temporary difficulty in developing a positive self-image. This is due to dramatic changes in body structure and function as well as greater expectations to assume responsibilities. Adolescents who are accepted, loved, and valued by family and peers generally tend to gain confidence and feel good about themselves. Teenagers with physical disabilities or illnesses are particularly vulnerable to peer rejection. Nurses and educators can promote peer understanding and acceptance by discussing within the peer group the problems an individual with a particular disability or condition might face. Establishing groups of peers who have similar problems can provide an opportunity for the individual to develop close relationships with others and feel valued and accepted.

Although sexual identification begins at about 3 or 4 years of age, it is a significant part of adolescence. Establishing a sense of sexual identity and clarifying one's sexual orientation occurs during late adolescence. Adolescents explore sexual images, fantasies, ideas, and roles. Experimenting with dress, language, and social interactions (e.g., dances, dating, youth activities, workplace) helps them define who they are. Adult role models (e.g., parents, movie stars, music idols) can influence greatly the way adolescents think and behave, helping teens to decide which aspects of masculinity or femininity to adopt or reject. Later, adolescents begin to establish intimacy with a partner or partners. This intimacy lays the groundwork for the commitments of adulthood. Sexual experimentation is not part of true intimacy, but once intimacy is achieved, sexual activity is often included. Homosexual youth may experience a great deal of confusion during this process because homosexuality is not openly accepted in all groups and their questions about self and identity may go unanswered.

Many adolescents are sexually active and may engage in masturbation as well as heterosexual and homosexual activity. The 2015 Youth Risk Behavior Surveillance survey was published in the *Morbidity Mortality Weekly Report* in 2016 (Kahn et al., 2016). It reported that 30.1% of high school students had had sexual intercourse during their lifetime. This is a significant decrease from 2011 and 2013. Nationwide, 30.1% of teens ages 15–19 were currently sexually active with at least one individual 3 months prior to the survey. Of these respondents, 56.9% reported they or their partner had used a condom during their last sexual intercourse. The CDC (2019) reported that the teenage pregnancy rate in 2017 was 18.8 births per 1000 women. The rate had declined by 7% since 2016. The rate of pregnancy for teens ages 15–19 is at a record low (CDC, 2019). It is unclear why the birth rate has declined, but it is hypothesized that fewer teens are sexually active and a greater number are using birth control.

Human papillomavirus (HPV) is the most commonly sexually transmitted infection in the United States. Since 2006 the prevalence of HPV has declined due to the administration of the HPV vaccine. HPV vaccine uptake is lower than the goal set for *Healthy People 2020.* The goal was set at 80%. The CDC (2018b) recommendations for the HPV vaccine are as follows; girls and boys age 11–12 should receive the first dose, and the second dose is recommended 6–12 months later. The vaccine can be administered as early as age 9. Two doses are recommended for ages 9–14. Teens and young adults age 15–26 years require three vaccines.

At about 15 years of age, many adolescents gradually draw away from the family and gain independence. This need for independence combined with the need for family support sometimes creates conflict within the adolescent and between the adolescent and the family. The young individual may appear hostile or depressed at times. At this age, adolescents prefer to be with their peers rather than their parents and may seek advice from adults other than their parents. Parents sometimes are bewildered by this stage of development; instead of reducing controls, they increase them, causing the adolescent to rebel.

Adolescents also have to resolve their ambivalent feelings toward the parent of the opposite gender. As part of the resolution, adolescents may develop brief crushes on adults outside the family—teachers or neighbors, for example. Adolescents sometimes adopt some of the attributes of the adults with whom they are infatuated. This modeling can be helpful in the maturing process.

Some of the discord in the family at this time is due to the generation gap. The values of the adolescent may differ from those of the parents. This difference may be difficult for the parents to understand and to accept. Adolescents still need guidance from their parents, although they appear to neither want it nor need it. However, adolescents need to know that their parents care about them and that their parents still want to help them. Discipline and guidance need to be presented in a manner that makes adolescents feel loved. They need consistency in guidance and fewer restrictions than previously. They should have the independence they can handle yet know that their parents will assist them when they need help.

During adolescence, **peer groups** assume great importance (Figure 24.12 ■). The peer group has a number of

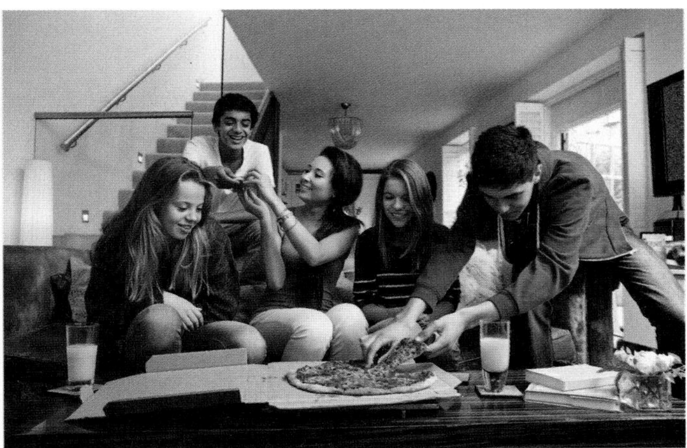

Figure 24.12 ■ Adolescent peer-group relationships enhance a sense of belonging, self-esteem, and self-identity.
Source: Image Source/Getty Images.

functions. It provides a sense of belonging, pride, social learning, and sexual roles. Most peer groups have well-defined, sex-specific modes of acceptable behavior. In adolescence, the peer groups change with age. They start as single-sex groups, evolve to mixed groups, and finally narrow to couples whose members share activities.

Not all adolescents are heterosexual. For homosexuals, adolescence is a difficult time. Because peer acceptance is crucial to self-acceptance, lesbian and gay adolescents usually conform to the heterosexual codes and behaviors of their peer groups even though these do not feel natural or correct and conforming may exact a great personal cost. Adolescents who choose to be openly gay or lesbian face not only the ostracism of their peers but also the misunderstanding and hostility of parents, teachers, and other important adults.

Cognitive Development

Cognitive abilities mature during adolescence. Between the ages of 11 and 15, the adolescent begins Piaget's formal operations stage of cognitive development. The main feature of this stage is that individuals can think beyond the present and beyond the world of reality. Adolescents are highly imaginative and idealistic. They consider things that do not exist but that might be and consider ways things could be or ought to be. This type of thinking requires logic, organization, and consistency. In social interactions, adolescents often practice this increasing ability to think abstractly, and parents may misunderstand their child's intent, seeing the teen as arguing or being contrary, which can lead to unnecessary confusion and conflict.

The adolescent becomes more informed about the world and environment. Adolescents use new information to solve everyday problems and can communicate with adults on most subjects. The adolescent's capacity to absorb and use knowledge is great. Adolescents usually select their own areas for learning; they explore interests from which they may evolve a career plan. Study habits and learning skills developed in adolescence are used throughout life.

Moral Development

According to Kohlberg, the young adolescent is usually at the conventional level of moral development. Most still accept the Golden Rule and want to abide by social order and existing laws. Adolescents examine their values, standards, and morals. They may discard some of the values they have adopted from parents in favor of values they consider more suitable.

When adolescents move into the postconventional or principled level, they start to question the rules and laws of society. Right thinking and right action become a matter of personal values and opinions, which may conflict with societal laws. Adolescents consider the possibility of rationally changing the law and emphasize individual rights. Not all adolescents or even adults proceed to this postconventional level. See the discussion about Kohlberg's stages of moral development in Chapter 23 ∞.

Spiritual Development

According to Fowler, the adolescent or young adult reaches the synthetic-conventional stage of spiritual development. As adolescents encounter different groups in society, they are exposed to a wide variety of opinions, beliefs, and behaviors regarding religious matters. The adolescent may reconcile the differences in one of the following ways:

- Deciding any differences are wrong
- Compartmentalizing the differences (For example, a friend may not be able to go to dances on Friday evenings because of religious observances, but the friend can share activities on other days.)
- Obtaining advice from a significant other, such as a parent or a minister.

Often, the adolescent believes that various religious beliefs and practices have more similarities than differences. At this stage, the adolescent's focus is often on interpersonal rather than conceptual matters.

Nursing activities relative to this stage of spiritual development include:

- Presenting an open, accepting attitude to adolescents' questions and statements regarding spiritual matters and their implications for health
- Arranging for adolescents to see a member of their religious faith if so desired or to talk with members of their church peer group for support
- Providing a comfortable environment in which adolescents can practice the rituals of their faith.

Health Risks

Adolescents face many health risks as they negotiate the intricate process of becoming young adults. Principal among these are consequences of risky behavior. The psychologic and emotional challenges of adolescence may lead to psychologic problems. Also, the developing brain is susceptible to addiction. The first manifestation of schizophrenia may appear as early as 13 years of age and reaches a peak incidence of onset at age 15–25 years (Videbeck, 2017). With communal living (e.g., in college dormitories), late adolescents are also at increased risk for infectious diseases, such as measles and pneumococcal meningitis. A booster dose of meningococcal conjugate vaccine is recommended for adolescents and young adults age 16–23 (CDC, 2017). They should also be vaccinated with the serogroup B meningococcal vaccine.

High-Risk Behaviors

The 2017 Youth Risk Behavior Surveillance survey identified six high-priority risks:

- Behaviors contributing to unintentional injury or violence
- Tobacco use
- Alcohol or other drug use
- Sexual activity that contributes to pregnancy and sexually transmitted infections, including HIV
- Unhealthy diet
- Physical inactivity.

The consequences of high-risk behavior can be severe. Seventy-four percent of all deaths in the 10- to 24-year-old age group resulted from four causes:

- Motor vehicle crashes (Figure 24.13 ■)
- Other unintentional injuries (e.g., falls, drowning, poisoning)
- Homicides
- Suicide.

During the 30 days prior to the Youth Risk Behavior Surveillance survey, high school students engaged in the following risky behaviors:

- 5.5% drove a car or other vehicle after drinking alcohol
- 39.2% drove a car while texting or emailing
- 13.0% drove a car after having used marijuana
- 15.7% had carried a weapon
- 4.8% had carried a gun
- 6.7% had not gone to school because they feared violence at or on the way to or from school
- 28.9% had smoked cigarettes.

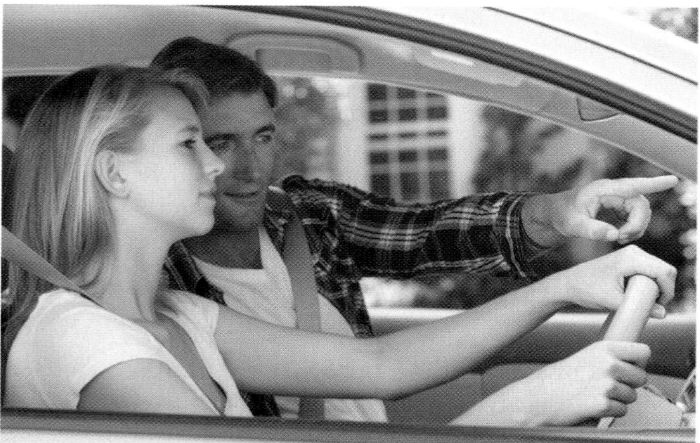

Figure 24.13 ■ To prevent motor vehicle crashes, insist on driver's education classes, and enforce rules about safe driving.
Source: Cathy Yeulet/123RF.

In the 12 months prior to the survey, high school students nationwide indicated the following:

- 7.4% of students had been forced to do sexual things they did not want to
- 6.0% had been threatened or injured one or more times on school property
- 19% had been bullied on school property
- 14.9% had been electronically bullied
- 7.4% had attempted suicide one or more times (CDC, 2018c).

The rate of attempted suicide in female adolescents is higher than for males. There has been a linear decline in the prevalence of adolescents who have seriously considered suicide. This decline has been documented from 1991 through 2017. The prevalence in 38 states ranged from 5.4% to 16.3%. In 21 large urban school districts, the prevalence of attempted suicides ranged from 5.6% to 19.5% (CDC, 2018c). Suicide by an adolescent may be reported as an accidental death. Motor vehicle crashes, drug and alcohol overdoses, firearm injuries, and even homicides can be disguised suicides. Psychologic, social, and physiologic stressors are apparent causes for many suicides. Other adolescent health problems are cardiovascular disease, depression, tooth decay, gingivitis, malalignment of teeth, neglect, and abuse.

Violence

School bullying among adolescents affects school achievement and psychologic well-being for both victims and perpetrators. Bullying is a documented problem in adolescence throughout the world. Bullying is a form of aggression in which an individual is victimized by one or more students. Adolescent bullying can take different forms: physical (e.g., hitting, pushing, and kicking), verbal (e.g., name-calling), relational or social (e.g., social exclusion, spreading rumors), and the emerging new form of cyber- or electronic bullying. Salmeron and Christian (2016) conducted a study in the Pinellas, Florida school district and provided education to school nurses and unlicensed healthcare professionals to assist them in identifying bullied children and bullies.

School shootings have occurred during the past decade, resulting in increased fear among educators, parents, and students. Investigations have been conducted to try to determine factors contributing to violence in and around schools.

Eating Disorders

Eating disorders are complex conditions that result in negative effects on memory, attention, and concentration. These disorders lead to personal, family, and social difficulties for the adolescent. The highest nutrient and energy demands occur during the growth spurt in adolescence. The addition of sports and other physical activities increases these demands. Obesity among adolescents has increased significantly over the years. Increasing obesity rates are making type 2 diabetes more common among teens. There is also an inherited form of diabetes, maturity-onset diabetes of the young (MODY), that can cause diabetic complications as early as the teens. MODY3 is a subtype of MODY. According to Wedrychowicz et al. (2017), there are 800 mutations of

MODY. Glucokinase-maturity-onset diabetes is most common in nonobese young clients. The adolescent may need genetic counseling and genetic testing. As discussed in Chapter 46 ∞, common problems related to nutrition and self-esteem among adolescents include obesity, anorexia nervosa, and bulimia. Nurses need to help adolescents create a wellness plan that addresses body image, diet, weight concerns, and exercise.

Nonsuicidal Self-Injury

The number of adolescents who engage in nonsuicidal self-injury (NSSI) appears to be increasing internationally, with self-injury involving intentional cutting as a primary form of self-harm (Videbeck, 2017). NSSI is the result of negative thoughts and feelings that create emotional, physical, and social consequences. It can occur with or without other specific psychiatric syndromes. Eating disorders and self-injury are often related. Alasaarela, Hakko, Riala, and Riipinen (2017) conducted a study on impulsivity and its association with nonsuicidal self-injury. The study revealed that among psychiatric inpatients, self-reported impulsivity increases the likelihood of girls experiencing suicidal ideations.

Health Assessment and Promotion

Guidelines for growth and development of the adolescent are shown in the Developmental Assessment Guidelines.

Adolescents are usually self-directed in meeting their health needs. Because of maturation changes, however, they need teaching and guidance in a number of healthcare areas.

Promoting health and wellness includes screening for tobacco, alcohol, and drug use; screening for sexual practices; screening for mental health status; checking blood pressure, height, and weight; and ensuring that immunizations are current. For a summary of health promotion, see Box 24.8.

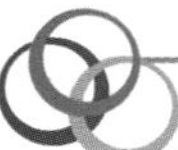

Developmental Assessment Guidelines — The Adolescent

In these three developmental areas, does the adolescent do the following?

PHYSICAL DEVELOPMENT

- Exhibit physical growth (weight, height) within normal range for age and sex.
- Demonstrate male or female sexual development consistent with standards.
- Manifest vital signs within normal range for age and sex.
- Exhibit vision and hearing abilities within normal range.

PSYCHOSOCIAL DEVELOPMENT

- Interact well with parents, teachers, peers, siblings, and individuals in authority.
- Like self.
- Think and plan for the future, such as college or a career.
- Choose a lifestyle and interests that fit own identity.
- Determine own beliefs and values.
- Begin to establish a sense of identity in the family.
- Seek help from appropriate individuals about problems.

DEVELOPMENT IN ACTIVITIES OF DAILY LIVING

- Demonstrate knowledge of physical development, menstruation, reproduction, and birth control.
- Exhibit healthy lifestyle practices in nutrition, exercise, recreation, sleep patterns, and personal habits.
- Demonstrate concern for personal cleanliness and appearance.

BOX 24.8 Health Promotion Guidelines for Adolescents

HEALTH EXAMINATIONS

- As recommended by the primary care provider

PROTECTIVE MEASURES

- Immunizations as recommended, such as adult tetanus-diphtheria vaccine, measles-mumps-rubella (MMR), pneumococcal, human papillomavirus (HPV), and hepatitis B vaccine
- Screening for tuberculosis
- Periodic vision and hearing screenings
- Regular dental assessments
- Obtaining and providing accurate information about sexual issues
- Assessing for mental health status

ADOLESCENT SAFETY

- Adolescents taking responsibility for using motor vehicles safely (e.g., completing a driver's education course, wearing seat belt and helmet)
- Making certain that proper precautions are taken during all athletic activities (e.g., medical supervision, proper equipment)
- Parents keeping lines of communication open and being alert to signs of substance abuse and emotional disturbances in the adolescent

NUTRITION AND EXERCISE

- Importance of healthy snacks and appropriate patterns of food intake and exercise
- Factors that may lead to nutritional problems (e.g., obesity, anorexia nervosa, bulimia)
- Engaging in regular vigorous exercise, at least three times a week for 1 hour each time

SOCIAL INTERACTIONS

- Encouraging and facilitating adolescent success in school
- Encouraging adolescents to establish relationships that promote discussion of feelings, concerns, and fears
- Parents encouraging adolescent peer-group activities that promote appropriate moral and spiritual values
- Parents acting as role models for appropriate social interactions
- Parents providing a comfortable home environment for appropriate adolescent peer group activities
- Expecting adolescents to participate in and contribute to family activities

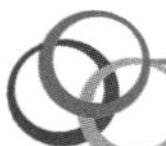

Critical Thinking Checkpoint

Shireena, an 8-year-old, comes to your clinic with her mother, complaining of pain in both ears for about 4 days. Although she has a history of recurrent ear infections as a child and had tympanostomy tubes placed 3 years ago, her mother says she has not had an ear infection for at least 2 years. Shireena participated in summer day camp last week, which involved swimming in a local lake. She says, "I didn't put my head under water. I know better than that!" The nurse practitioner diagnoses Shireena with acute external otitis media with swelling and exudate; she prescribes a topical antibiotic with corticosteroid (otic drops) three times a day for 10 days. As the clinic nurse, you provide Shireena and her mother with health education.

1. According to Piaget, at what stage of cognitive development is Shireena?
2. Based on knowledge of Shireena's cognitive development, how would you approach her to discuss her condition? Describe how you will include both Shireena and her mother in the discussion.
3. What strategies will you suggest to ensure compliance with the nurse practitioner's orders? Discuss how Shireena can be actively involved in her medical treatment.

Answers to Critical Thinking Checkpoint questions are available on the faculty resources website. Please consult with your instructor.

Chapter 24 Review

CHAPTER HIGHLIGHTS

- Prenatal or intrauterine development lasts approximately 9 calendar months.
- The embryonic phase is the 8-week period during which the fertilized ovum develops into an organism with most of the features of a human.
- The infant's weight, length, head and chest circumferences, fontanel size and status, vision, hearing, smell and taste, touch, reflexes, and motor development are important indicators of the newborn's growth and health.
- Infants from birth to 12 months reveal marked growth in size and stature with appropriate nutrition and care: Birth weight doubles by about 5 months and triples by 12 months.
- Rapid weight gain in the first 5 to 6 months of life appears to be related to overweight and obesity in childhood and as an adult.
- During infancy, motor development is notable: At 1 month, infants can lift their heads momentarily when prone; at 6 months, they can sit unsupported; and at 12 months, they can walk with help.
- Fulfillment of the infant's physiologic and psychologic needs is required to develop a basic sense of trust. Parents can enhance this sense of trust by being sensitive to the infant's needs and meeting those needs skillfully, promptly, and consistently and providing a predictable environment in which routines are established.
- For the infant, cognitive development is a result of interaction between an individual and the environment. The infant needs a variety of sensory and motor stimuli.
- Those in the toddler group, ages 12 months to 3 years, are, according to Erikson, developing a sense of autonomy. Voluntary control increases and these children learn to walk and speak. They also learn to control their bladders and bowels, and they acquire all kinds of information about their environment.
- During the preschool years, ages 4 to 5, physical growth slows, but control of the body and coordination increase greatly. Preschoolers' worlds get larger as they meet relatives, friends, and neighbors. They are engaged in Erikson's task of initiative versus guilt.
- The school-age period starts when children are about 6 years of age. In general, this period from 6 to 12 years is one of significant change. Skills learned during this stage are particularly important in relation to work later in life and the willingness to try new tasks.
- During psychosocial development, school-age children face Erikson's conflict of industry versus inferiority.
- School-age children change from being egocentric to having cooperative interactions, and they begin to understand cause-and-effect relationships. According to Piaget, they are in the concrete operations phase of cognitive development.
- Most school-age children progress to the conventional level of moral development and to the mythic-literal stage of spiritual development.
- Rapid growth in height, development of secondary sexual characteristics, sexual maturity, and increasing independence from the family are major landmarks of adolescence.
- Peer groups assume great importance during adolescence; they provide a sense of belonging, pride, social learning, and sexual roles.
- Adolescents between the ages of 11 and 15 begin the formal operations stage of cognitive development; they are able to think logically, rationally, and futuristically and can conceptualize things as they could be rather than as they are.
- The adolescent is at Kohlberg's conventional level of moral development, and some proceed to the postconventional or principled level.
- Adolescents are at Fowler's synthetic-conventional stage of spiritual development.
- The four leading causes of adolescent death are motor vehicle crashes, other unintentional injuries, homicide, and suicide.

TEST YOUR KNOWLEDGE

1. The parent of an 8-month-old girl who has been admitted to the hospital with pneumonia is worried about the infant having sudden infant death syndrome (SIDS). The parent stated, "My sister's baby died at the age of 2 months, and all he had was a little cold." Which is the nurse's best response?
   1. "You don't need to worry. Your daughter is too old for SIDS."
   2. "Girls are less likely to have SIDS than boys are."
   3. "We don't know what causes SIDS, so I would try not to worry about it."
   4. "You must be very anxious; let's talk about SIDS and what you are thinking."

2. Four-year-old Angie, whose grandmother recently died, tells the nurse, "My grandma has wings just like angels. She flew to heaven yesterday, and tomorrow she'll be back." Which is the nurse's best response?
   1. "She's not coming back, honey."
   2. "It is normal for a little one to make-believe."
   3. "You must miss your grandma a lot."
   4. "When people get old, they die."

3. Because near-drowning is one of the leading causes of vegetative state in young children, which is the best instruction for the nurse to teach parents?
   1. Supervise children at all times when near any source of water.
   2. Enroll children in swimming classes at an early age to ensure water safety.
   3. Make bathroom doors and toilets easily accessible and appropriate for a toddler's size.
   4. Allow unsupervised play only in "kiddy pools" designated for young children.

4. Which statement most accurately describes physical development during the school-age years?
   1. Child's weight almost triples.
   2. Child acquires stereognosis.
   3. Few physical changes occur during middle childhood.
   4. Fat gradually increases, which contributes to the child's heavier appearance.

5. An adolescent comes to the school nurse's office seeking advice about his friends and feeling pressure to participate in activities he isn't comfortable with (i.e., drinking parties and sexual explorations). What should the nurse's response be?
   1. Tell the adolescent to stay away from "friends like that."
   2. Be open to the concerns and provide accurate information about any questions.
   3. Encourage the adolescent to accept psychosocial counseling.
   4. Give the adolescent pamphlets on sexually transmitted diseases.

6. Parents of a newborn ask the nurse why their newborn's head seems lopsided and not round, as they thought it should be. Which is the nurse's best response?
   1. "I don't think it looks unusual; actually, the head is beautifully shaped."
   2. "Your baby's head had to shape itself to the birth canal. It will look round in a few days."
   3. "You're right. We'll make sure your doctor checks this out."
   4. "Babies' heads always look funny. Once his hair grows out, you'll hardly notice it."

7. During a physical examination, a 24-month-old child clings to the parent and cries every time the nurse attempts to touch her. From knowledge of psychosocial development, the nurse makes which conclusion about the child?
   1. The child is displaying normal toddler development.
   2. The child needs further psychologic evaluation.
   3. The child is manipulative and should be taken from the parent to be examined.
   4. The child is showing signs of regression.

8. A toilet-trained 4-year-old hospitalized for several days with an acute illness has been wetting the bed at night and is having incontinence accidents during the day. The nurse addresses the parents' concerns with the following statement:
   1. "Maybe your child should be seen by a specialist, just to make sure there are no physical problems."
   2. "It is normal for some children to go through a stage of regression after separation from their family or after an acute illness. Try not to be too discouraged."
   3. "You'll have to be very strict with discipline, so your child knows this behavior is not acceptable."
   4. "I'd be upset too. It must be hard to go back to using diapers."

9. According to Piaget's theory of cognitive development, the movement from intuitive reasoning to logical reasoning in school-age children is called the concrete operations phase. Which is an example of this phase?
   1. A science-fair project comparing how fast different objects fall from a set height
   2. Feeling responsible for wishing that a sibling would go away, and now that sibling is ill and hospitalized
   3. Understanding how geometric figures might fit into a futuristic and idealistic world
   4. Learning to ride a bike

10. Parents ask the nurse how they will know that their daughter has reached puberty. Which is the best response by the nurse?
   1. "The first noticeable sign of puberty in females is the appearance of the breast bud."
   2. "The growth spurt usually begins between ages 10 and 14."
   3. "The apocrine glands, found over most of the body, begin to produce sweat."
   4. "The adolescent will display significant mood swings."

See Answers to Test Your Knowledge in Appendix A.

READINGS AND REFERENCES

Suggested Reading

Sills, J., Rowse, G., & Emerson, L. M., (2016). The role of collaboration in cognitive development of young children: A systemic review. *Child: Care, Health, and Development*, *42*, 313–324. doi:10.1111/cch.12330

Collaboration is a coordinated synchronous activity to promote the development of verbal, cognitive, and social skills. The study revealed that collaboration is beneficial and enhances problem-solving abilities.

Related Research

Alasaarela, L., Hakko, H., Kaisa, R., & Riipinen, P. (2017). Association of self-reported impulsivity to nonsuicidal self injury, suicidality, and mortality in adolescent psychiatric inpatients. *Journal of Nervous & Mental Disorders*, *205*(3), 340–345.

Brabcova, D., Zarubova, J., Kohout, J., Jost J., & Krsek, P. (2015). Effect of learning disabilities on academic self-concept in children with epilepsy and on their quality of life. *Research in Developmental Disabilities*, *45*(46), 120–128. doi:10.1016/j.ridd.2015.07.018

Bullock, A., Sheff, K., Moore, K., & Manson, S. (2017). Obesity and overweight in American Indian and Alaska Native children, 2006–2015. *American Journal of Public Health*, *107*, 1502–1507. doi:10.2105/AJPH.2017.303904

References

Ali, M. M., Virani, S. F., & Alaman, A. (2017). Bullying: Its impact on child's personality. *I-Manager's Journal on Nursing*, *6*(4), 1–5. doi:10.26634/jnur.6.4.10338

American Academy of Pediatrics. (2017). *Back to sleep, tummy to play*. Retrieved from https://www.healthychildren.org/English/ages-stages/baby/sleep/Pages/Back-to-Sleep-Tummy-to-Play.aspx

Bernier, A., Calkins, S. D., & Bell, M. A. (2016). Longitudinal associations between the quality of mother-infant interactions and brain development across infancy. *Child Development*, *87*, 1159–1174. doi:10.1111/cdev.12518

Cambron, J. (2017). Massage for infantile colic. *Massage & Bodywork*, *2*, 48–49.

Centers for Disease Control and Prevention. (2010). *2000 CDC growth charts for the United States*. Retrieved from https://www.cdc.gov/nchs/data/series/sr_11/sr11_246.pdf

Centers for Disease Control and Prevention. (2017). *Vaccines and preventable diseases*. Retrieved from https://www.cdc.gov/vaccines/vpd/mening/public/index.html

Centers for Disease Control and Prevention. (2018a). *Childhood obesity facts*. Retrieved from https://www.cdc.gov/obesity/data/childhood.html

Centers for Disease Control and Prevention. (2018b). *HPV vaccines: vaccinating your preteen or teen*. Retrieved from https://www.cdc.gov/hpv/parents/vaccine.html

Centers for Disease Control and Prevention. (2018c). Youth risk behavior surveillance-United states, 2017. *Morbidity and Mortality Weekly Report Surveillance Summaries*. *67*(8), 1–479

Centers for Disease Control and Prevention. (2019). *About teen pregnancy*. Retrieved from https://www.cdc.gov/teen-pregnancy/about/index.htm

de Onis, M. (2011) New WHO child growth standards catch on. *Bulletin of the World Health Organization*, *89*, 250–251. doi:10.2471/BLT.11.040411

Erikson, E. H. (1963). *Childhood and society* (2nd ed.). New York, NY: W. W. Norton.

Fowler, J. W. (1981). *Stages of faith: The psychology of human development and the quest for meaning*. New York, NY: Harper & Row.

Girard, N., Brunel, H., Dory-Lautrec, P., & Chabrol, B. (2016). Neuroimaging differential diagnosis to abusive head trauma. *Pediatric Radiology*, *46*, 603–614. doi:10.1007/s00247-015-3509-3

Goldstein, R. F., Abel, S. K., Ranisinha, S., Misso, M., Boyle, J. A., Black, M. H., . . . Teede, H. J. (2017). Association of gestational weight gain with maternal and infant outcomes: A systematic review and meta-analysis. *JAMA*, *317*, 2207–2225. doi:10.1001/jama.2017.3635

Hockenberry, M., Wilson, D., & Rodgers, C. C. (2019). *Wong's nursing care of infants and children* (11th edition). St. Louis, MO: Mosby.

Kann, L., McManus, T., Harris, W. A., Shanklin, S. L., Flint, K. H., Hawkins, J., . . . Zaza, S. (2016). Youth risk behavior surveillance—United States, 2015. *Morbidity and Mortality Weekly Report, 65*(6), 1–174. doi:10.15585/mmwr.ss6506a1

Kohlberg, L. (1981). *Essays on moral development. Vol. 1: The philosophy of moral development*. San Francisco, CA: Harper & Row.

Krishnan, L. A., & Van Hyfte, S. (2014). Effects of policy changes to universal newborn hearing screening follow-up in a university clinic. *American Journal of Audiology*, *23*, 282–292. doi:10.1044/2014_AJA-14-0008

Lange, S., Probst, C., Gmel, G., Rehm, J., Burd, L., & Popova, S. (2017). Global prevalence of fetal alcohol spectrum disorder among children and youth: A systematic and meta-analysis. *JAMA Pediatrics, 171*(10), 948–956. doi:10.1001/jamapediatrics.2017.1919

London, M. L., Ladewig, P. A., Davidson, M., Ball, J. W., Bindler, R. C., & Cowen, K. J. (2017). *Maternal and child nursing care* (5th ed.). Hoboken, NJ: Pearson.

Lumeng, J. C. (2016). Infant eating behaviors and risk for overweight. *JAMA*, *316*, 2036–2037. doi:10.1001/jama.2016.16899

Moon, R. Y. (2017). *How to keep your sleeping baby safe: AAP policy explained*. Retrieved from https://www.healthychildren.org/English/ages-stages/baby/sleep/Pages/A-Parents-Guide-to-Safe-Sleep.aspx

O'Connor, M. J., Quattlebaum, J., Castañeda, M., & Dipple, K. M. (2016). Alcohol intervention for adolescents with fetal alcohol spectrum disorders: Project Step Up, a treatment development study. *Alcoholism: Clinical and Experimental Research, 40*(8), 1744–1751. doi:10.1111/acer.13111

Piaget, J. (1966). *Origins of intelligence in children*. New York, NY: W. W. Norton.

Salmeron, P. A., & Christian, B. J. (2016). Evaluation of an educational program to improve school nursing staff perceptions of bullying in Pinellas County, Florida. *Pediatric Nursing, 42*(6), 283–292.

Savage, J. S., Birch, L. L., Marini, M., Anzman-Frasca, S., & Paul, I. M. (2016). Effects of the INSIGHT responsive parenting intervention on rapid infant weight gain and overweight status at age 1 year: A randomized clinical trial. *JAMA, 170*(8), 742–749. doi:10.1001/jamapediatrics.2016.0445

Thomas, S. (2016). Soothing crying babies and preventing shaken baby syndrome. *International Journal of Nursing Education, 8*(2), 34–36. doi:10.5958/0974-9357.2016.00043.X

U.S. Department of Health and Human Services. (n.d.). *MICH-14 increase the proportion of women of child-bearing potential with intake of at least 400 micrograms of folic acid from fortified foods or dietary supplements*. Retrieved from https://www.healthypeople.gov/node/4842/data_details

U.S. Department of Health and Human Services. (2010). *Healthy people 2020: Topics and objectives: Maternal, infant, and child health*. Retrieved from http://www.healthypeople.gov/2020/topicsobjectives2020/default.aspx

Venes, D. (Ed.). (2017). *Taber's cyclopedic medical dictionary* (26nd ed.). Philadelphia, PA: F. A. Davis.

Videbeck, S. L. (2017). *Psychiatric mental health nursing* (7th ed.). Philadelphia, PA: Lippincott, Williams, & Wilkins.

Wedrychowicz, A., Tobor, E., Wilk, M., Ziolkowska-Ledwith, E., Rams, A., Wzorek, . . . Starzyk, J. B. (2017). Phenotype heterogeneity in glucokinase-maturity onset diabetes of the young (GCK-MODY) patients. *Journal of Clinical Research in Pediatric Endocrinology, 9*(3), 246–252. doi:10.4274/jcrpe.4461

Witt, W. P., Mandell, K. C., Wisk, L. E., Cheng, E., Chatterjee, D., Wakeel, F., . . . Zarak, D. (2016). Infant birthweight in the U.S.: The role of preconception stressful life events and substance use. *Archives of Women's Mental Health, 19*, 529–542. doi:1007/s00737-015-0595-z

World Health Organization. (n.d.). The *WHO child growth standards*. Retrieved from http://www.who.int/childgrowth/en

World Health Organization. (2016). *Guideline: Daily iron supplementation in infants and children*. Retrieved from http://apps.who.int/iris/bitstream/10665/204712/1/9789241549523_eng.pdf?ua=1&ua=1

Selected Bibliography

American Academy of Pediatrics Committee on Nutrition. (2013). *Pediatric nutrition*. (7th ed.). Elk Grove Village, IL: American Academy of Pediatrics.

Edelman, C. L., & Kudzma, E. (2018). *Health promotion throughout the life span* (9th ed.). St. Louis, MO: Mosby.

Leifer, G. (2019). *Introduction to maternity and pediatric nursing* (8th ed.). St Louis, MO: Saunders.

McKinney, E. S. (2018). *Maternal–child nursing* (5th ed.). St. Louis, MO: W. B. Saunders.

Murdaugh, C. L., Parsons, M. A., & Pender, N. J. (2019). *Health promotion in nursing practice* (8th ed.). New York, NY: Pearson.

Rudd, K., & Kocisko, D. (2019). *Pediatric nursing: The critical components of nursing care*. (2nd ed.). Philadelphia, PA: F. A. Davis.

Ward, S. L., Hisley, S. M., & Kennedy, A. M. (2016). *Maternal–child nursing care*. (2nd edition). Philadelphia, PA: F. A. Davis.

Promoting Health in Young and Middle-Aged Adults

25

LEARNING OUTCOMES

After completing this chapter, you will be able to:

1. Compare and contrast the following generational groups: baby boomers, Generation X, Generation Y, and the iGeneration.
2. Describe the usual physical development occurring during young and middle adulthood.
3. Identify characteristic tasks of psychosocial development during young and middle adulthood.
4. Explain changes in cognitive development throughout adulthood.
5. Describe moral development according to Kohlberg throughout adulthood.
6. Describe spiritual development according to Fowler throughout adulthood.
7. Identify selected health risks associated with young and middle-aged adults.
8. Identify developmental assessment guidelines for young and middle-aged adults.
9. List examples of health promotion topics for young and middle adulthood.

KEY TERMS

baby boomers, *481*
boomerang kids, *482*
climacteric, *488*
Generation X, *481*
Generation Y, *481*
generativity, *488*
iGeneration, *481*
intimacy, *482*
maturity, *487*
menopause, *487*
Papanicolaou (Pap) test, *486*

Introduction

The adult phase of development encompasses the years from the end of adolescence to death. Because the developmental tasks of young adults differ from those of older adults, adulthood is often divided into three phases: young adulthood, middle adulthood, and late adulthood. In this text, young adults are defined as individuals 20 to 40 years old, and middle-aged adults are those aged 40 to 65.

Today's adult age span includes three very different generations: the **baby boomers** (born in years 1945–1964), **Generation X** (birth years 1965–1980), and **Generation Y** or the Millennials (birth years 1981–1994). The newest cohort is known as the **iGeneration** or iGens. This cohort has been identified by Twenge (2017) as those born between 1995 and 2012. Each cohort has shared specific life events and has its own worldview, making them quite diverse in some ways. It is unclear if these generational differences will prompt new developmental theories or if the differences are in "generational personalities" and values. At this time, younger baby boomers are in the middle-adult stage of development, and older baby boomers are in the late-adult stage of development. Given this age span, they will be discussed in this chapter and in Chapter 26 ∞. Baby boomers are usually well educated, and many have chosen to continue working beyond the normal retirement age. They lead a healthier lifestyle, incorporating exercise and good nutrition, than members of past generations. They also find or continue employment past the usual retirement age to increase companionship and self-esteem (Badley, Canizares, Perruccio, Hogg-Johnson, & Gignac, 2015; Paul & Mayho, 2017). Baby boomers have a strong work ethic. Those in retirement are motivated to find opportunities that enhance their older years and provide meaningful experiences (Clark, 2017). Generation Xers were frequently raised in two-worker households where long hours at work were common. They may now be less impressed with corporate values, be more skeptical, resist authority, and enjoy challenges and opportunities to creatively problem solve. Generation Ys (or Millennials) have come of age in an increasingly multicultural America, are technologically sophisticated (and dependent), and enjoy public affirmation of their efforts. The iGens are also known as Generation Z. This group of individuals has never been without the internet. They are multitaskers. According to Twenge (2017), the iGens are obsessed with safety. They are fearful about the economy and have no tolerance for inequality of gender, race, or sexual orientation. Twenge goes further to state that they are on the front lines of a mental health crisis. The rate of teen depression and suicide has increased since 2011. In regard to their nursing careers, they prefer to have face-to-face communication with their nurse managers. Over half are opposed to emails. They seek to balance work and social obligations (Smith-Trudeau, 2016).

This chapter applies the concepts of growth and development introduced in Chapter 24 ∞ to the young adult and the middle-aged adult. Each developmental stage includes physical, psychosocial, cognitive, moral, and spiritual aspects. Also discussed are health problems and health assessment and promotion guidelines.

Young Adults (20 to 40 Years)

The age at which an individual is considered an adult depends on how adulthood is described in the social context of the individual, and this defining age is changing. Legally, an individual in the United States can vote at 18 years. Since the passage of the National Minimum Drinking Age Act in 1984, the legal age for alcohol consumption outside the home is 21 years, making the 21st birthday an important developmental milestone in the United States. A study conducted by Geisner et al. (2017) determined that positive social expectancies, such as socialization, are greater for the 21st birthday compared with other occasions. Another criterion of adulthood is financial independence, which is also highly variable. Some adolescents support themselves as early as 16 years of age, usually because of family circumstances. By contrast, some adults are financially dependent on their families for many years, for example, during prolonged periods of education.

Adulthood may also be indicated by moving away from home and establishing one's own living arrangements. Yet this independence also varies greatly. Some adolescents leave home because of family problems. In recent years, however, **boomerang kids** have evolved as young adults have moved back into their parents' homes after an initial period of independent living. The factors contributing to this trend include high housing costs, high divorce rates, high unemployment rates, and the problems resulting from substance abuse and maladaptive behaviors. Some young individuals who are employed full time receive only minimum wage and are unable to earn enough money to be self-supporting.

Young adults are typically busy and face many challenges. They are expected to assume new roles at work, in the home, and in the community and to develop interests, values, and attitudes related to these roles.

Physical Development

Individuals in their early 20s are in their prime physical years. The human body is at its most efficient functioning at about age 25 years. The musculoskeletal system is well developed and coordinated. This is the period when athletic endeavors reach their peak. All other systems of the body (e.g., cardiovascular, visual, auditory, and reproductive) are also functioning at peak efficiency. Emerging or young adults, however, tend to be risk takers, placing their high-functioning bodies at substantial risk of serious injury.

Although physical changes are minimal during this stage, weight and muscle mass may change as a result of diet and exercise. Health outcomes in middle age and older adulthood may have their beginnings in younger-adult behaviors. In addition, extensive physical and psychosocial changes occur in pregnant and lactating women. These changes are discussed in maternal and pediatric textbooks.

Psychosocial Development

In contrast to the minimal physical changes, the psychosocial development of the young adult is great. Box 25.1 reviews this psychosocial development according to the theories of Freud, Erikson, Havighurst, and Newman and Newman. The basic developmental task is establishing **intimacy** or very close friendships. Establishing a firm sense of self, then reaching out to others to develop loving, intimate relationships is key. The choice of a lifelong partner and considerations of childbearing depend on successful negotiation of intimacy.

BOX 25.1 Psychosocial Development: Young Adult

The young adult:

- Is in the genital stage, in which energy is directed toward attaining a mature sexual relationship, according to Freud's theory
- Is in the intimacy versus isolation phase of Erikson's stages of development
- Has the following developmental tasks, according to Havighurst:
  - Selecting a mate
  - Learning to live with a partner
  - Starting a family
  - Rearing children
  - Managing a home
  - Getting started in an occupation
  - Taking on civic responsibility
  - Finding a congenial social group.
- Has the following characteristics, according to Newman and Newman (2015):
  - Identifies social and occupational roles
  - Experiences stress related to changing roles
  - Experiences conflict related to the demands of roles
  - Is interested in personal discovery and self-discovery.

Young adults face a number of new experiences and changes in lifestyle as they progress toward maturity. They make choices about education and employment, about whether to marry or remain single, about starting a home, and about rearing children. Social responsibilities include forming new friendships and assuming some community activities.

Many young adults have experienced the stressors of the divorce of their parents and being raised in stepfamilies. As children of divorce, feelings of being "caught" between two divorced parents may be heavy burdens as they move into young adulthood. These added concerns may have implications for the development of intimate relationships.

Occupational choice and education are largely inseparable. Education influences occupational opportunities; conversely, an occupation, once chosen, can determine the education needed and sought. Education enhances employment opportunities and usually ensures economic survival. As the role of women has changed, many women now choose to assume active careers and civic roles in society in addition to their roles as mother and wife or partner (Figure 25.1 ■).

Remaining single is becoming the lifestyle of more and more young adults. Many individuals choose to remain single, perhaps to pursue an education and then to have the freedom to pursue their chosen vocation. Some unmarried individuals choose to live with another individual of the opposite or same gender and share living arrangements and certain expenses. Some individuals who are gay or lesbian commit themselves legally to a partner through marriage, whereas others who are not legally married have made a lifelong commitment and do not consider themselves to be single.

Although nontraditional lifestyles are becoming more acceptable in society, attitudes toward these various lifestyles can contribute social pressures that lead to stress responses. The multiple roles of adulthood (citizen, worker, taxpayer, homeowner, wife or husband, daughter or son, brother or sister, parent, friend, and so on) may also create role conflict, which can result in stress.

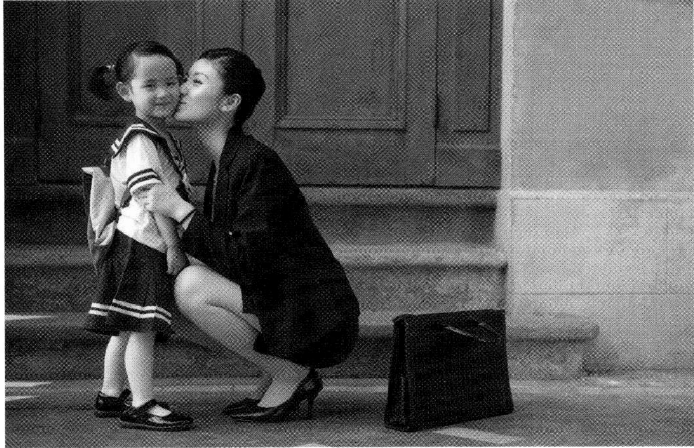

Figure 25.1 ■ Many young women combine active careers with motherhood.
blue jean images/Getty Images.

Cognitive Development

Young adults are able to use formal operations, characterized by the ability to think abstractly and employ logic. For example, young adults are able to generate hypotheses about what will happen, given a set of circumstances, and do not have to engage in trial-and-error behavior.

Recently, researchers in the field of psychology have suggested that Piaget's (1966) formal operational stage is not the last stage of human development. Some have proposed a concept of postformal thought, which is thinking that goes beyond Piaget's formal operations. *Postformal thought* includes creativity, intuition, and the ability to consider information in relation to other ideas. Postformal thinkers possess an understanding of the temporary or relative nature of knowledge. They can proceed from abstract reasoning to practical considerations. They are aware that most problems have more than one cause and more than one answer and that some solutions will work better than others. They are able to comprehend and become more specialized and focused in particular areas of interest (Beckett & Taylor, 2016). Meditation and other insight-oriented practices facilitate becoming a postformal thinker.

Moral Development

Young adults who have mastered the previous stages of Kohlberg's theory of moral development enter the postconventional level. At this time, the individual is able to separate self from the expectations and rules of others and to define morality in terms of personal principles. When individuals perceive a conflict with society's rules or laws, they judge according to their own principles. For example, an individual may intentionally break the law and join a protest group to stop hunters from killing wild animals, believing that the principle of wildlife conservation justifies the protest action. This type of reasoning is called *principled reasoning*. See also Gilligan's ethic of care in Chapter 23 ∞. Gilligan argues that as individuals approach young adulthood, men and women tend to define moral problems somewhat differently. Men often use an "ethic of justice" and define moral problems in terms of rules and rights. Women, by contrast, often define moral problems in terms of the obligation to care and to avoid harm.

Spiritual Development

According to Fowler (1981), the individual enters the individuating-reflective period sometime after 18 years of age. During this period, the individual focuses on reality. The religious teaching that the young adult had as a child may now be accepted or redefined. Paterson and Francis (2017) report a lack of research exploring the influence of religious or spiritual beliefs on response to psychologic therapies. Their results also revealed a positive relationship between the levels of religiosity and the response to the implementation of psychologic therapy. Young adults are noted as spiritual but not necessarily religious.

Health Risks

Young adulthood is generally a healthy time of life. Health risks that do occur and are common in this age group include injury and violence, suicide, hypertension, substance abuse, sexually transmitted infections (STIs), eating disorders, and certain malignancies. Some of the problems, such as injuries, substance abuse, and STIs, are related to behaviors that could possibly be prevented through appropriate education and other primary prevention strategies.

Injury and Violence

Healthy People 2020 (U.S. Department of Health and Human Services [USDHHS], n.d.) established the goal of preventing unintentional injuries and violence and reducing both fatal and nonfatal injuries. The leading causes of death differ among the various population groups. For example, unintentional injuries (primarily motor vehicle crashes) are the fifth leading cause of death for the total population but the leading cause of death for individuals 1 to 44 years of age. Education about safety precautions and injury prevention is a major role of the nurse in promoting the health of young adults. For a further discussion of safety education for young adults, see Chapter 32 ∞.

Violence has spread throughout the United States and claims lives or threatens the well-being of individuals of all ages. Homicide is one of the leading causes of death in adult women under the age of 44. Approximately half of those deaths are due to current or former male intimate partners. The actual or threatened abuse of a current or former partner, whether male or female, is called intimate partner violence (IPV). The abuse can be physical, sexual, or psychologic. It is estimated that 42% of women and 14% of men experience intimate partner violence (McKay et al., 2016). Some risk factors identified include being young, having a low income, being an immigrant, being unmarried, and having a mental illness. The victims of IPV may engage in risk-taking behaviors such as substance abuse. In a study by Stover and Coates (2016), the children of fathers with a concurrent history of IPV and substance abuse avoided their fathers and experienced dyadic tension. Nurses have a responsibility to address IPV and can play an important part in screening, assistance, and support. Screening tools are often very effective in assessing IPV. During the screening process, the nurse must calmly assure the client that confidentiality will be maintained. All screening should take place in a quiet environment without children, spouses, friends, or family. The nurse should ask if the client feels safe at home instead of asking if the client is being abused. Efforts to prevent violence can occur at the primary, secondary, or tertiary level of prevention. Thus, the nurse needs to become familiar with community resources, such as adult protective services, shelters, Partners Anonymous, advocacy programs, victim assistance programs, and hotlines. The Centers for Disease Control and Prevention (CDC) has recommended that young women and men be educated on safe and healthy relationship skills as well as the ability to recognize situations or behaviors that result in violence (Petrosky et al., 2017).

Mass shootings in workplaces, schools, grocery store parking lots, movie theaters, and other public areas have become all too commonplace. According to Metzl and MacLeish (2015), four central assumptions arise after a mass shooting. The first is that mental illness is a cause of gun violence. Second, a psychiatric diagnosis can predict a gun crime prior to the crime event. Third, U.S. mass shootings teach citizens to fear loners with mental illness. Lastly, the complex psychiatric histories of mass shooters cannot be prevented by gun control. Based on these assumptions, Metzl and MacLeish believe that care of the mentally ill can assist in the prevention of mass-shooting events.

Suicide

The suicide rate for young adults ages 15–24 is 14.46 per 100,000. Adults age 45–54 years have the highest rate of suicide at 20.02 per 100,000 (American Foundation for Suicide Prevention, 2017). The rate of suicide is increasing in this group of individuals. In 2017, 47,173 Americans died by suicide. On average in the United States, 123 suicides are committed per day. Many suicides may actually be mistaken for unintentional death (motor vehicle crashes, combining alcohol and barbiturates, or discharging a gun while cleaning it). Suicide may result from problems with close relationships, such as those

EVIDENCE-BASED PRACTICE

Evidence-Based Practice

What Is the Prevalence of Ophthalmologic Injury Related to Intimate Partner Violence?

Cohen, Renner, and Shriver (2017) conducted a literature review of population-based studies on intimate partner violence. The study examined the prevalence, the associated injury patterns, and the impact intimate partner violence has in causing ocular and orbital trauma. The authors summarized the literature regarding the impact of intimate partner violence on ophthalmologic injuries. Based on 48 population-based studies, the lifetime prevalence of head and neck trauma was found to be 7.5 times more likely in female clients presenting to the emergency department (ED) than other clients who have from injuries with other etiologies.

Implications

With the high prevalence of intimate partner violence resulting in orbital and ocular injuries, all members of the ED must be trained in identifying intimate partner violence and screening for ophthalmologic injuries.

with marriage partners or parents, or from depression related to perceived occupational, academic, or financial failure. In general, suicide results from the young adult's inability to cope with the pressures, responsibilities, and expectations of adulthood.

The nurse's role in the prevention of suicide includes identifying behaviors that may indicate potential problems: depression; a variety of physical complaints, including weight loss, sleep disturbances, and digestive disorders; and decreased interest in social and work roles along with an increase in isolation. A young adult identified as at risk for suicide must be referred to a mental health specialist or a crisis center. A suicide threat should never be ignored. Nurses can also reduce the incidence of suicide by participating in educational programs that provide information about the early signs of suicide.

Hypertension

Hypertension is a major problem for young African American adults, particularly men. Many of the causes for this higher incidence of hypertension are unknown. In addition to biological inheritance, contributing factors may include smoking, obesity, a high-sodium diet, and high stress levels. Hypertension is a major risk factor in the development of chronic heart disease and stroke (cerebrovascular accidents). Blood pressure measurements are usually advised at least every 2 years for young adults to screen for hypertension.

Substance Abuse

Substance abuse is a major threat to the health of young adults. Alcohol, marijuana, amphetamines, and cocaine, for example, can bring about feelings of well-being that may be highly valued by individuals with adjustment problems. Prolonged use can lead to physical and psychologic dependency and subsequent health problems. Addiction, or physical and psychologic dependence on a substance, is related to the properties of the substance, the individual user, and the social network of the individual. For example, drug abuse during pregnancy can lead to fetal damage. Prolonged use of alcohol can lead to such diseases as cirrhosis of the liver and cancer of the esophagus.

Nursing strategies related to drug abuse include teaching about the complications of their use, changing individual attitudes toward drug abuse, and counseling regarding problems that lead to drug abuse. In addition, assessment of the young adult for substance abuse may help the nurse identify a problem early on and assist the young adult client in accessing intervention services.

Smoking is another type of substance abuse, and it can lead to lung cancer and cardiovascular disease. According to the level of education, the highest rate of smoking is among individuals 25 years and older who have attained a General Education Diploma (GED), at 34.1%, followed by those with less than a high school diploma at 24.1%. Those with graduate degrees have the lowest rate at 4.5% (CDC, 2019a).

The most common reasons for smoking in the young adult population are independence from parents, reaching the legal age to purchase tobacco, and the use of substances such as alcohol. The nurse's role regarding smoking is to (a) serve as a role model by not smoking; (b) provide educational information regarding the dangers of smoking; (c) help make smoking socially unacceptable, for example, by posting No Smoking signs in client lounges and offices; and (d) suggest resources such as hypnosis, lifestyle training, and behavior modification to clients who desire to stop smoking. Nurses can also promote health related to tobacco by being aware of marketing efforts that target young adults.

Sexually Transmitted Infections

STIs such as genital herpes, AIDS, syphilis, and gonorrhea are common infections in young adults. Chlamydia is the most prevalent STI, and in fact, it is the most prevalent infectious disease in the United States. The rate of chlamydia cases increased by 6.9% during 2016–2017 (CDC, 2018). Other STIs, such as gonorrhea, are becoming resistant to multiple antibiotics and therefore cause an increased risk for future health problems. Nursing functions are largely educational. The use of condoms greatly reduces the transfer of infectious microorganisms from one partner to another. Knowledge about the symptoms of these diseases can help the client obtain early treatment. In dealing with clients with an STI, the nurse must be nonjudgmental and accepting of the client's lifestyle and treat any information obtained as confidential (see Chapter 40 ∞).

Eating Disorders

Many young adults battle with obesity. According to *Healthy People 2020* goals and objectives for nutrition and weight status, all Americans will avoid unhealthy weight gain (USDHHS, n.d.). The nurse needs to assess nutritional concerns, discuss diet and exercise patterns with the client, and assist in the development of an individualized wellness plan. Other areas of nutritional needs for young women include meeting calcium requirements and ensuring proper nutrition during the childbearing years (see Chapter 46 ∞).

Malignancies

Testicular cancer is the most common neoplasm in young men. Seminoma testicular cancer most commonly affects men ages 30 to 45. The yolk sac tumor is most common in 20- to 35-year-olds. More recent recommendations from the American Cancer Society (ACS) are that men should have a testicular exam as part of a yearly physical exam. Men who have risk factors for testicular cancer should discuss monthly testicular self-examination with their primary care provider. According to the ACS (2018), the risk factors for testicular cancer include the following:

- An undescended testicle
- Family history of testicular cancer
- HIV infection

- Carcinoma in situ of the testicle
- Body size
- Race or ethnicity (White men are 4 to 5 times more likely to get testicular cancer than Black men, American Indians, or Asians. According to a research study conducted in Seattle, Washington, in 2014, researchers found that testicular cancer was on the rise in the U.S. Latino population. From 1992–2010, the rate of testicular cancer increased by 58% [ACS, 2014]).

Breast cancer is the most common cause of cancer in American women (ACS, 2019). Approximately one in eight women is diagnosed each year. It is the second leading cause of cancer death in women; the first leading cause of death is lung cancer (ACS, 2017b). Death rates from breast cancer have been declining, with the greatest decline in women younger than age 50. This is thought to be because of earlier detection, increased awareness, and improved treatment. The ACS (2017a) recommends the following guidelines for women at average risk of developing breast cancer:

- Breast self-exam (BSE) is an *option* for women starting in their 20s.
- Women between 40 and 44 years should begin yearly screening.
- Women ages 45 to 54 should get mammograms every year.
- Women ages 55 and older can switch to a mammogram every other year, or they can choose to continue yearly mammograms. Screening should continue as long as a woman is in good health and is expected to live 10 more years or longer.

For detailed information, see Chapter 29 ∞. The earlier a breast lump is discovered, the greater the effectiveness of treatment.

It is important that young women and men become vaccinated against human papillomavirus (HPV). Women who become infected are at risk of developing cervical cancer. The Advisory Committee on Immunization Practices (ACIP) is a chartered federal advisory committee that provides guidance to the director of the CDC on the use of vaccines (Meites, Kempe, & Markowitz, 2016). Routine HPV vaccination should begin at age 11 to 12 years. Three doses are recommended for women aged 15 to 26 years. The ACIP recommends the following catch-up schedule: females through the age of 26 years and males through 21 years who have not been vaccinated should be vaccinated. All women should be screened for cervical cancer by age 21. Women ages 21 to 29 should be screened every 3 years. At age 30, screening should be combined with an HPV test every 5 years. Screening for cervical cancer is done by having a routine **Papanicolaou (Pap) test**. A Pap test is done by obtaining and examining cells from the uterine cervical os. The cells are obtained during a pelvic examination. For more information on the vaginal exam, see Chapter 29 ∞. The nurse should also screen for high-risk factors for cervical cancer: sexual activity at an early age; multiple sexual partners; or a history of syphilis, herpes genitalis, or *Trichomonas vaginalis*. Many young adults are reluctant to have these examinations and screenings. Therefore, it is important for nurses to explain the purpose of the test and to encourage all young women to begin this preventive measure. See the cancer screening guidelines in Chapter 29 ∞.

Health Assessment and Promotion

Assessment guidelines for the growth and development of the young adult are shown in the accompanying Developmental Assessment Guidelines.

Young adults are usually interested in meeting their health needs. However, because of the many stresses and changes that occur throughout the 20-year period from ages 20 to 40, the nurse needs to offer teaching and guidance in several healthcare areas. The nurse may wish to discuss some or all of the health promotion topics outlined in Box 25.2. These topics are discussed in detail in subsequent chapters throughout the text.

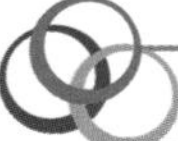

Developmental Assessment Guidelines — The Young Adult

In these three developmental areas, does the young adult do the following?

PHYSICAL DEVELOPMENT

- Exhibit weight within normal range for age and sex.
- Manifest vital signs (e.g., blood pressure) within normal range for age and sex.
- Demonstrate visual and hearing abilities within normal range.
- Exhibit appropriate knowledge (e.g., about STIs) and attitudes about sexuality.

PSYCHOSOCIAL DEVELOPMENT

- Feel independent from parents.
- Have a realistic self-concept.
- Like self and direction life is going.
- Interact well with family.
- Cope with the stresses of change and growth.
- Have well-established bonds with significant others, such as marriage partner or close friends.
- Have a meaningful social life.
- Demonstrate emotional, social, and economic responsibility for own life.
- Have a set of values that guide behavior.

DEVELOPMENT IN ACTIVITIES OF DAILY LIVING

- Have a healthy lifestyle.

BOX 25.2 Health Promotion Guidelines for Young Adults

HEALTH TESTS AND SCREENINGS
- Routine physical examination (every 1 to 3 years for females; every 5 years for males)
- Immunizations as recommended, such as tetanus-diphtheria boosters every 10 years, meningococcal vaccine if not given in early adolescence, hepatitis B vaccine
- Human papillomavirus (HPV) vaccination is recommended at age 11–12 years for females and males. There is a 2-dose schedule for females and males age 9–14 years. Three doses are recommended for individuals who initiate the vaccination series at ages 15–26 years (CDC, 2019d).
- Regular dental assessments (every 6 months)
- Periodic vision and hearing screenings
- Professional breast examination every 1 to 3 years
- Papanicolaou smear annually within 3 years of onset of sexual activity
- Testicular examination every year
- Screening for cardiovascular disease (e.g., cholesterol test every 5 years if results are normal; blood pressure to detect hypertension; baseline electrocardiogram at age 35)
- Tuberculosis skin test every 2 years
- Smoking: history and counseling, if needed

SAFETY
- Motor vehicle safety reinforcement (e.g., using designated drivers when drinking, maintaining brakes and tires)
- Sun protection measures
- Workplace safety measures
- Water safety reinforcement (e.g., no diving in shallow water)

NUTRITION AND EXERCISE
- Importance of adequate iron intake in diet
- Nutritional and exercise factors that may lead to cardiovascular disease (e.g., obesity, cholesterol and fat intake, lack of vigorous exercise)

SOCIAL INTERACTIONS
- Encouraging personal relationships that promote discussion of feelings, concerns, and fears
- Setting short- and long-term goals for work and career choices

Middle-Aged Adults (40 to 65 Years)

The middle years, from 40 to 65, have been called the years of stability and consolidation. For most individuals, it is a time when children have grown and moved away or are moving away from home. Thus, partners generally have more time for and with each other and time to pursue interests they may have deferred for years (Figure 25.2 ■).

Maturity is the state of maximal function and integration, or the state of being fully developed. Many other characteristics are generally recognized as representative of maturity. Mature individuals are guided by an underlying philosophy of life. They take many perspectives into account and are tolerant of the views of others. A comprehensive philosophy allows an individual to make sense out of life and thus helps that individual maintain a sense of purpose and hope in the face of human tragedies. Mature individuals are open to new experiences and continued growth; they can tolerate ambiguity, are flexible, and can adapt to change. In addition, mature individuals have the quality of self-acceptance; they are able to be reflective and insightful about life and to see themselves as others see them. Mature individuals also assume responsibility for themselves and expect others to do the same. They confront the tasks of life in a realistic and mature manner, make decisions, and accept responsibility for those decisions.

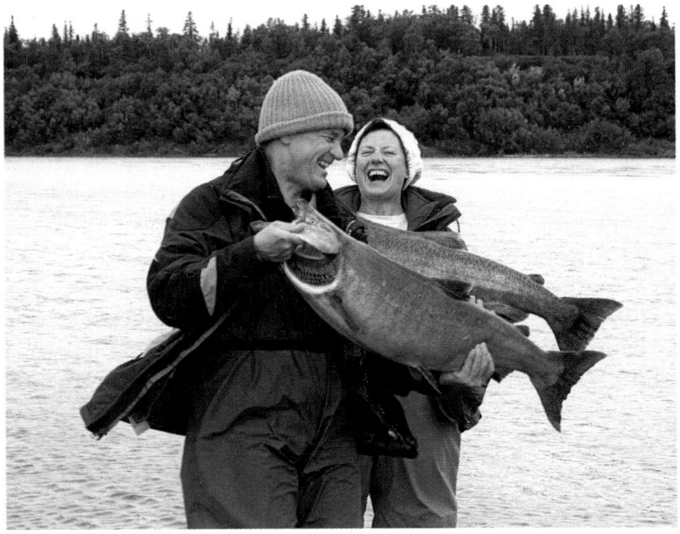

Figure 25.2 ■ Middle-aged adults have time to pursue interests that may have been put aside for child care.
Jessica Lynn Culver/Moment Select/Getty Images.

Physical Development

A number of changes that start when young adults are in their mid-20s become noticeable as the fifth decade approaches. At 40, most adults can function as effectively as they did in their 20s. However, during ages 40 to 65, many physical changes take place. These are summarized in Table 25.1.

Both men and women experience decreasing hormonal production during the middle years. The term **menopause** refers to the so-called "change of life" in women, when menstruation ceases. It is said to occur when a woman has not had a menstrual period for 12 months. The menopause usually occurs sometime between ages 40 and 55. The average is about 47 years. At this time, ovarian activity declines until ovulation ceases. Common symptoms, related to a decline in estrogen, are hot flashes, chilliness,

TABLE 25.1 Physical Changes of the Middle-Aged Adult

Category	Description
Appearance	Hair begins to thin, and gray hair appears. Skin turgor and moisture decrease, subcutaneous fat decreases, and wrinkling occurs. Fatty tissue is redistributed, resulting in fat deposits in the abdominal area.
Musculoskeletal system	Skeletal muscle bulk decreases at about age 60. Thinning of the intervertebral disks causes a decrease in height of about 1 inch. Calcium loss from bone tissue is more common among postmenopausal women. Muscle growth continues in proportion to use.
Cardiovascular system	Blood vessels lose elasticity and become thicker.
Sensory perception	Visual acuity declines, often by the late 40s, especially for near vision (presbyopia). Auditory acuity for high-frequency sounds also decreases (presbycusis), particularly in men. Taste sensations also diminish.
Metabolism	Metabolism slows, which may result in weight gain.
Gastrointestinal system	Gradual decrease in tone of large intestine may predispose the individual to constipation.
Urinary system	Nephron units are lost during this time, and the glomerular filtration rate decreases.
Sexuality	Hormonal changes take place in both men and women.

a tendency of the breasts to become smaller and less dense, and a decrease in metabolic rate that may lead to weight gain. Insomnia and headaches may also occur. Psychologically, the menopause can be an anxiety-producing time, especially if the ability to bear children is an integral part of the woman's self-concept. For other women, menopause may produce few symptoms, physically or psychologically.

Sexual arousal in both men and women takes longer after midlife than in younger adulthood. In men, there is no change comparable to the menopause in women, although the term **climacteric** (andropause) has been used to denote the change in sexual response in men. Androgen levels decrease very slowly; however, men can father children even in late life. Some men may have difficulties achieving sexual arousal for psychologic reasons, such as anxiety. See Chapter 40 ∞ for further details about sexual health.

Psychosocial Development

Before the mid-1990s, the developmental tasks of middle-aged adults received little attention. Havighurst (1972) outlined nine tasks for this age group (Box 25.3). Erikson (1963, p. 266) viewed the developmental choice of the middle-aged adult as generativity versus stagnation. **Generativity** is defined as the concern for establishing and guiding the next generation. In other words, the concern about providing for the welfare of mankind is equal to the concern of providing for self. Individuals in their 20s and 30s tend to be self- and family-centered. In middle age, the individual collaborates with others to guide the next generation. Marriage partners refocus the marriage relationship (Kaakinen, Coehlo, Steele, Tabacco, & Hanson, 2015). They have more time for companionship and recreation; thus, marriage may be more satisfying in the middle years of life. Partners have time to work together in volunteer activities and time to enjoy separate activities, such as one partner going out for lunch while the other goes fishing. Generative middle-aged individuals are able to feel a sense of comfort in their lifestyle and receive gratification from charitable endeavors.

BOX 25.3 Psychosocial Development: Middle-Aged Adult

The middle-aged adult:

- Is in the generativity versus stagnation phase of Erikson's stages of development
- According to Havighurst, has the following developmental tasks:
  - Achieving adult civic and social responsibility
  - Establishing and maintaining an economic standard of living
  - Assisting teenage children to become responsible and happy adults
  - Developing adult leisure-time activities
  - Relating oneself to one's spouse as an individual
  - Accepting and adjusting to the physiologic changes of middle age
  - Adjusting to aging parents
  - Balancing the needs of multiple constituencies (children, parents, work, etc.)
  - Having work as a central theme.

Erikson (1963) wrote that individuals who are unable to expand their interests at this time and who do not assume the responsibilities of middle age experience a sense of boredom and impoverishment, that is, stagnation. These individuals have difficulty accepting their aging bodies and become withdrawn and isolated. They are preoccupied with self and unable to give to others. Some may regress to younger patterns of behavior, for example, adolescent behavior.

Middle adulthood is the time when most individuals become increasingly aware of the gradual changes in their bodies that mark the aging process. Individuals usually accept the fact that they are aging; however, some try to defy the years by changing their dress and even their actions. A new freedom to be independent and follow one's individual interests arises. Prior to this period, the marriage partner or lover and other individuals were crucial to a definition of self. Now the middle-aged individual does not make comparisons with others, often no longer fears aging or death, relaxes the sense of competitiveness, and enjoys the independence and freedom of middle age. Other individuals' opinions become less important, and the earlier habit of trying to please everyone is overcome. The individual establishes ethical and moral standards that are independent of the standards of others. The focus shifts from inner self and being to others and doing. Religious and philosophical concerns become important.

The "midlife crisis" is a popular idea and one that is the source of many jokes and humorous anecdotes. This crisis occurs when individuals recognize that they have reached the halfway mark of life. The midlife crisis is *not* universal and is more common in the male. The midlifer begins to recognize that time is at a premium and that life is finite. Youthfulness and physical strength can no longer be taken for granted.

Cognitive Development

The middle-aged adult's cognitive and intellectual abilities change very little. Cognitive processes include reaction time, memory, perception, learning, problem-solving, and creativity. Reaction time during the middle years stays much the same or diminishes during the latter part of the middle years. Memory and problem-solving are maintained throughout middle adulthood. Learning continues and can be enhanced by increased motivation at this time in life.

Adults in their middle years may have difficulties dealing with the new challenges in this stage of life. The difficulties in the challenges may be related to a lack of development in earlier stages (Beckett & Taylor, 2016). The professional, social, and personal life experiences of middle-aged individuals will be reflected in their cognitive performance. Thus, approaches to problem-solving and task completion will vary considerably in a middle-aged group.

Moral Development

According to Kohlberg, the adult can move beyond the conventional level to the postconventional level (see Chapter 23 ∞). Kohlberg believed that extensive experience of personal moral choice and responsibility is required before individuals can reach the postconventional level. Kohlberg found that few of his subjects achieved the highest level of moral reasoning. To move from stage 4, a law and order orientation, to stage 5, a social contract orientation, requires that the individual move to a stage in which rights of others take precedence.

Spiritual Development

Not all adults progress through Fowler's stages to the fifth, called the paradoxical-consolidative stage. At this stage, the individual can view "truth" from a number of viewpoints. Fowler's fifth stage corresponds to Kohlberg's fifth stage of moral development. Fowler believes that only some individuals reach this stage after the age of 30 years.

In middle age, individuals tend to be less dogmatic about religious beliefs, and religion often offers more comfort to the middle-aged individual than it did previously. Individuals in this age group often rely on spiritual beliefs to help them deal with illness, death, and tragedy.

Health Risks

Many middle-aged adults remain healthy; however, the risk of developing a health problem is greater than that of the young adult. Leading causes of death in this age group include motor vehicle and occupational injuries, chronic disease such as cancer, and cardiovascular disease. Lifestyle patterns in combination with aging, family history, and developmental stressors (e.g., menopause, climacteric) and situational stressors (e.g., divorce) are often related to health problems that do arise. For example, smoking and excessive alcohol consumption place an individual at greater risk of developing chronic respiratory problems, lung cancer, and liver disease. Overeating can result in obesity, diabetes mellitus, and atherosclerosis and their associated risks for hypertension and coronary artery disease. Many diseases of older age may be decreased by health-conscious and lifestyle decisions made, and acted on, in midlife. The nurse can play an important role in teaching middle-aged clients about preventive healthcare to avoid or minimize the risk of such health problems.

Injuries

Changing physiologic factors, as well as concern over personal and work-related responsibilities, may contribute to the injury rate of middle-aged individuals. Motor vehicle crashes are the most common cause of unintentional death in this age group. Decreased reaction times and visual acuity may make the middle-aged adult prone to injury. Other unintentional causes of death for middle-aged adults include falls, fires, burns, poisonings, and drownings. Work-related injuries continue to be a significant safety hazard during the middle years.

Cancer

Cancer is the fourth leading cause of death for males in middle adulthood years (CDC, 2019c). For women, cancer is the leading cause of death as reported by the

CDC (2019b). The patterns of cancer types and incidences for men and women have changed during the past several decades. The ACS (2016) states that men have a high incidence of cancer of the lung, prostate, and colon. In women, lung cancer is highest in incidence, followed by breast cancer and colon cancer. Screening guidelines for the early detection of cancer are constantly evolving as new data are analyzed.

Cardiovascular Disease

Heart disease and cancer are the leading causes of death during middle adulthood (CDC, 2019c, 2019d). Risk factors for heart disease include smoking, obesity, hypertension, hyperlipidemia, diabetes mellitus, sedentary lifestyle, a family history of myocardial infarction or sudden death in a father less than 55 years old or in a mother less than 65 years old, and the individual's age. A newly recognized cluster of risk factors that often occur together, termed *metabolic syndrome*, increases the risk for heart disease. This syndrome includes the following risk factors: obesity with excessive abdominal fat, hypertension, high lipid levels, and insulin resistance (Huether, McCance, Brashers & Rote, 2017). Lifestyle activities and behaviors, such as diet modifications and increasing physical activity, play an important role in preventing the development of metabolic syndrome risk factors.

Obesity

Middle-aged adults who gain weight may not be aware of some common facts about this age period. Decreased metabolic activity and decreased physical activity mean a decrease in caloric need. The nurse's role in nutritional health promotion is to counsel clients to prevent obesity by reducing caloric intake and participating in regular exercise. Clients should also be educated that being overweight is a risk factor for many chronic diseases, such as diabetes and hypertension, and for problems of mobility, such as arthritis. Recent changes in the Food Guide Pyramid propagated by the U.S. Department of Agriculture now encourage nutrient intake based on physical activity, age, and gender. Clients may be directed to the new MyPlate website to design a customized, healthy diet plan for themselves. Clients should seek medical advice before considering any major changes in their diets.

Alcoholism

The excessive use of alcohol can result in unemployment, disrupted homes, injuries, and diseases. It is estimated that 4 million individuals in the United States are dependent on alcohol and can be considered alcoholics. Alcohol use may exacerbate other health problems. Nurses can help clients by providing information about the dangers of excessive alcohol use, by helping the individual clarify values about health, and by referring the client who abuses alcohol to special groups such as Alcoholics Anonymous.

Mental Health Alterations

Developmental stressors, such as menopause, the climacteric, aging, and impending retirement, and situational stressors, such as divorce, unemployment, and the death of a spouse, can precipitate increased anxiety and depression in middle-aged adults. Clients may benefit from support groups or individual therapy to help them cope with specific crises.

Health Assessment and Promotion

Assessment guidelines for the growth and development of the middle-aged adult are shown in the accompanying Developmental Assessment Guidelines. Middle-aged adults usually take care of their health needs and are interested in maintaining health and preventing the acceleration of the aging process.

The nurse may choose to discuss some or all of the health promotion topics listed in Box 25.4 with the middle-aged adult client. These topics are discussed in detail in subsequent chapters throughout the text.

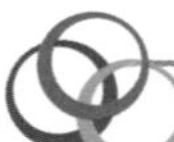

Developmental Assessment Guidelines — The Middle-Aged Adult

In these three developmental areas, does the middle-aged adult do the following?

PHYSICAL DEVELOPMENT

- Exhibit weight within normal range for age and sex.
- Manifest vital signs (e.g., blood pressure) within normal range for age and sex.
- Manifest visual and hearing abilities within normal range.
- Exhibit appropriate knowledge and attitudes about sexuality (e.g., about menopause).
- Verbalize any changes in eating, elimination, or exercise.

PSYCHOSOCIAL DEVELOPMENT

- Accept aging body.
- Feel comfortable and respect self.
- Enjoy new freedom to be independent.
- Accept changes in family roles (e.g., having teenage children and aging parents).
- Interact effectively and share companionable activities with life partner.
- Expand and renew previous interests.
- Pursue charitable and altruistic activities.
- Have a meaningful philosophy of life.

DEVELOPMENT IN ACTIVITIES OF DAILY LIVING

- Follow preventive health practice.

BOX 25.4 Health Promotion Guidelines for Middle-Aged Adults

HEALTH TESTS AND SCREENING
- Annual physical examination
- Immunizations as recommended, such as a tetanus booster every 10 years and current recommendations for influenza vaccine
- Regular dental assessments (e.g., every 6 months)
- Tonometry for signs of glaucoma and other eye diseases every 2 to 3 years or annually if indicated
- Breast examination annually by primary care provider
- Testicular examination annually by primary care provider
- Screenings for cardiovascular disease (e.g., blood pressure measurement; electrocardiogram and cholesterol test as directed by the primary care provider)
- Screenings for colorectal, breast, cervical, uterine, and prostate cancer (see cancer screening guidelines in Chapter 29)
- Screening for tuberculosis every 2 years
- Smoking: history and counseling, if needed

SAFETY
- Motor vehicle safety reinforcement, especially when driving at night
- Workplace safety measures
- Home safety measures: keeping hallways and stairways lighted and uncluttered, using smoke detectors, using nonskid mats and handrails in the bathrooms

NUTRITION AND EXERCISE
- Importance of adequate protein, calcium, and vitamin D in diet
- Nutritional and exercise factors that may lead to cardiovascular disease (e.g., obesity, cholesterol and fat intake, lack of vigorous exercise)
- An exercise program that emphasizes skill and coordination

SOCIAL INTERACTIONS
- The possibility of a midlife crisis: encourage discussion of feelings, concerns, and fears
- Providing time to expand and review previous interests
- Retirement planning (financial and possible diversional activities), with partner if appropriate

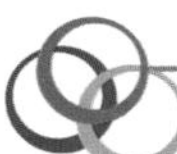

Critical Thinking Checkpoint

Mark Jones, a 22-year-old construction worker, comes into the health center for a "physical." He states that the last time he saw a healthcare provider was during high school, and he is only here today because his employer required that he be examined prior to returning to work. Mr. Jones has been off the job for 2 weeks following an injury in which he fell off a ladder, sustaining multiple contusions and a concussion. He mentions that he and "his buddies" have enjoyed his 2 weeks off from work and have used the time to "drink beer and chase women."

1. What questions would you ask Mr. Jones about his usual health promotion activities?
2. How would you ask Mr. Jones about his risk for sexually transmitted infections?
3. What health conditions are young adults at risk for, and how would you explain these to Mr. Jones?
4. What health screening activities would you suggest to Mr. Jones? How would you explain the rationale to him?
5. How would you assess Mr. Jones's psychosocial development?

Answers to Critical Thinking Checkpoint questions are available on the faculty resources site. Please consult with your instructor.

Chapter 25 Review

CHAPTER HIGHLIGHTS

- Three distinct generations are included in adulthood: baby boomers, Generation Xers, and Generation Ys. Each group has its own worldview.
- Emerging and young adults develop self-identity and prepare for intimate relationships with others.
- Moral development continues throughout adulthood.
- Health risks for young adults are primarily related to lifestyle and behavior.
- Midlife adults begin to notice physical changes associated with aging.
- The developmental issue for midlife adults is generativity.
- Adults in midlife must balance the needs of many, including their own parents and children.
- Health decisions made by midlife adults may affect their health in later life.
- A variety of health threats, including cancer and heart disease, begin to affect individuals in their middle age.
- Physical activity, healthy nutrition choices, and routine care by a health provider are important throughout the adult years.

TEST YOUR KNOWLEDGE

1. Because a 45-year-old woman is worried that she still has regular menstrual periods, she asks about menopause. Which answer by the nurse is most appropriate?
   1. "Regular menses in a 45-year-old woman should be promptly evaluated by a gynecologist."
   2. "Although you continue to have menstrual periods, you are unlikely to become pregnant."
   3. "It is common for women to experience menopause in their late 40s."
   4. "Many women dread menopause because it is an unpleasant experience."

2. The nurse is providing pre-employment physicals to a group of adults, aged 30 to 40. This age group is representative of:
   1. Baby Boomers
   2. Generation X
   3. Generation Y
   4. Millennials

3. A woman is seen at her primary care provider's office. She has been losing weight and not feeling well. She is 44 years old. What is the leading cause of cancer death in female clients between the ages of 25 and 64?
   1. Breast cancer
   2. Lymphoma
   3. Lung cancer
   4. Colon cancer

4. A nurse is working in a community health office that is often frequented by young adults. In assessing for potential problems, the nurse realizes that a leading cause of death in this age group is suicide. Which of the following factors may indicate a problem in this area?
   1. Decreased interest in work
   2. Weight loss
   3. Depression
   4. Brain dysfunction, including tumors
   5. Sleep disturbances

5. Which statement about moral development in adults is the most correct?
   1. Moral development is completed during adolescence.
   2. Moral development continues throughout adulthood.
   3. Moral development is highly individualized.
   4. Moral development correlates with spiritual development.

6. If the nurse is assessing the status of a middle-aged client's psychosocial development, which activity should be the focus?
   1. Selecting a life partner
   2. Balancing the needs of others
   3. Reviewing one's life course
   4. Establishing a sense of self

7. An occupational health nurse is providing a hypertension screening at a local manufacturing plant. What is the primary focus group of the intervention among the employees?
   1. Male and female, equally
   2. African American males
   3. Asian American females
   4. White females

8. When planning a screening program for cardiovascular disease in the middle-aged adult, the nurse has limited funds and decides to address which significant elements? Select all that apply.
   1. Blood pressure measurement
   2. Electrocardiogram
   3. Cholesterol measurement
   4. Sexual performance
   5. Activity level

9. A woman comes into the emergency department with multiple bruises on her face and head. The nurse suspects that intimate partner violence (IPV) may be related to the injuries. What is the most appropriate action for the nurse to take at this time?
   1. Ask the woman if she is afraid of someone at home who is hurting her.
   2. Refer the woman to a shelter for battered women.
   3. Call a social worker to assess the woman for IPV.
   4. Document the concern in the chart, but do nothing else.

10. The nurse is completing a health history on a 24-year-old male. Which activity is the best indicator of appropriate psychosocial development?
   1. Creating a scrapbook of his life experiences
   2. Joining the board of directors for three charities
   3. Decorating his new apartment
   4. Attending seminars on choosing a career

See Test Your Knowledge Answers in Appendix A.

READINGS AND REFERENCES

Suggested Readings

Song, S., Kim, J., & Kim, J. (2018). Gender differences in the association between dietary pattern and the incidence of hypertension in middle aged and older adults. *Nutrients, 10*(2), 252. doi:10.3390/nu10020252

The purpose of this study was to determine the association of dietary patterns and the risk of hypertension. A diet that includes whole grains and legumes is not associated with an increased risk of hypertension.

Towne, S. D., Won, J., Lee, S., Ory, M. G., Forjuoh, S. N., Wang, S., & Lee, C. (2016). Using Walk Score™ and neighborhood perceptions to assess walking among middle-aged and older adults. *Journal of Community Health, 41*, 977–988. doi:10.1007/s10900-016-0180-z

The aim of the study was to determine the relationship between neighborhood characteristics such as, walkability and safety. The outcome of the study revealed that the identification of factors to promote safety in walking will allow the community's stakeholders to build an environment that promotes walking.

Related Research

Arbour, C., Gosselin, N., Levert, M., Gauvin-Lepage, J., Michallet, B., & Lefebvre, H. (2017). Does age matter? A mixed methods study examining determinants of good recovery and resilience in young and middle-aged adults following moderate to severe traumatic brain injury. *Journal of Advanced Nursing, 73*(12), 3133–3143. doi:10.1111/jan.13376

Xiang, S., & An, R. (2015). Depression and onset of cardiovascular disease in the US middle-aged and older adults. *Aging and Mental Health, 19*, 1084–1092. doi:10.1080/13607863.2014.1003281

References

American Cancer Society. (2014). *Rates of testicular cancer increasing in young Hispanic men*. Retrieved from https://www.cancer.org/latest-news/rates-of-testicular-cancer-increasing-in-young-hispanic-men.html

American Cancer Society. (2016). *Cancer facts & figures 2016*. Retrieved from https://www.cancer.org/content/dam/cancer-org/research/cancer-facts-and-statistics/annual-cancer-facts-and-figures/2016/cancer-facts-and-figures-2016.pdf

American Cancer Society. (2017a). *American Cancer Society recommendations for the early detection of breast cancer*. Retrieved from https://www.cancer.org/cancer/breast-cancer/screening-tests-and-early-detection/american-cancer-society-recommendations-for-the-early-detection-of-breast-cancer.html

American Cancer Society. (2017b). *Cancer facts and figures 2017*. Retrieved from https://www.cancer.org/content/dam/cancer-org/research/cancer-facts-and-statistics/annual-cancer-facts-and-figures/2017/cancer-facts-and-figures-2017.pdf

American Cancer Society. (2018). *What are the risk factors for testicular cancer?* Retrieved from https://www.cancer.org/cancer/testicular-cancer/causes-risks-prevention/risk-factors.html

American Cancer Society. (2019). *How common is breast cancer?* Retrieved from https://www.cancer.org/cancer/breast-cancer/about/how-common-is-breast-cancer.html

American Foundation for Suicide Prevention. (2017). *Suicide statistics*. Retrieved from https://afsp.org/about-suicide/suicide-statistics

Badley, E., Canizares, M. Peruccio, A., Hogg-Johnson, S., & Gignac, M. (2015). Benefits gained, benefits lost: Comparing baby boomers to other generations in a longitudinal cohort study of self-rated health. *Milbank Quarterly*, *93*, 40–72. doi:10.1111/1468-0009.12105

Beckett, C., & Taylor, H. (2016). *Human growth and development* (3rd ed.). Thousand Oaks, CA: Sage.

Centers for Disease Control and Prevention. (2018). *Sexually transmitted disease surveillance 2017*. Retrieved from https://www.cdc.gov/std/stats17/chlamydia.htm

Centers for Disease Control and Prevention. (2019a). *Current cigarette smoking among adults in the United States*. Retrieved from https://www.cdc.gov/tobacco/data_statistics/fact_sheets/adult_data/cig_smoking/index.htm

Centers for Disease Control and Prevention. (2019b). *Preventing cancer just got easier*. Retrieved from https://www.cdc.gov/hpv/downloads/hpv-2-dose-decision-tree.pdf

Centers for Disease Control and Prevention. (2019c). *Leading causes of death in males (LCOD), by age group, all males—United States, 2015*. Retrieved from https://www.cdc.gov/healthequity/lcod/men/2015/all-males/index.htm

Centers for Disease Control and Prevention. (2019d). *Leading causes of death (LCOD), by age group, all females—United States, 2015 (current listing)*. Retrieved from https://www.cdc.gov/women/lcod/2015/all-females/index.htm

Clark, K. R. (2017). Managing multiple generations in the workplace. *Radiologic Technology*, *88*, 379–398.

Cohen, A. R., Renner, L. M., & Shriver, E. M. (2017). Intimate partner violence in ophthalmology: A global call to action. *Current Opinion in Ophthalmology*, *28*(5), 534–538. doi:10.1097/ICU.0000000000000397

Erikson, E. H. (1963). *Childhood and society* (2nd ed.). New York, NY: W. W. Norton.

Fowler, J. W. (1981). *Stages of faith: The psychology of human development and the quest for meaning*. New York, NY: Harper & Row.

Geisner, I. M., Rhew, I. C., Ramirez, J. J., Lewis, M. E., Larimer, M. E., & Lee, C. M. (2017). Not all drinking events are the same: Exploring 21st birthday and typical alcohol expectancies as a risk factor for high-risk drinking and alcohol problems. *Addictive Behaviors*, *70*, 97–101. doi:10.1016/j.addbeh.2017.02.021

Havighurst, R. J. (1972). *Developmental tasks and education* (3rd ed.). New York, NY: Longman.

Huether, S. E., McCance, K. L., Brashers, V. L., & Rote, N. S. (2017). *Understanding pathophysiology* (6th ed.). St. Louis, MO: Elsevier.

Kaakinen, J. R., Coehlo, D. P., Steele, R., Tabacco, A., & Hanson, S. M. H. (2015). *Family and health care nursing: Theory, practice, and research* (5th ed.). Philadelphia, PA: F. A. Davis.

McKay, T., Cohen, J., Kan, M., Bir, A., Grove, L., & Cutbush, S. (2016). Intimate partner violence prevalence and experiences among healthy relationship program target populations. Office of Planning, Research, & Evaluation (OPRE) Report 2016-40. Retrieved from https://www.acf.hhs.gov/sites/default/files/opre/rivir_paper_1_prevalence_3_29_16_complete_b508.pdf

Meites, E., Kempe, A., & Markowitz, L. E. (2016). Use of a 2-dose schedule for human papillomavirus vaccination—Updated recommendations of the Advisory Committee on Immunization Practices. *Morbidity and Mortality Weekly Report*, *65*, 1405–1408. doi:10.15585/mmwr.mm6549a5

Metzl, J. M., & MacLeish, K. T. (2015). Mental illness, mass shootings, and the politics of American firearms. *American Journal of Public Health*, *105*(2), 240–249. doi:10.2105/AJPH.2014.302242

Newman, B. M., & Newman, P. R. (2015). *Development through life: A psychosocial approach*. (12th ed.). Stamford, CT: Cengage.

Paterson, J. & Francis, A. J. P. (2017). Influence of religiosity on self-reported response to psychological therapies. *Mental Health, Religion, & Culture*, *25*(5), 428–448. https://doi.org/10.1080/13674676.2017.1355898

Paul, J., & Mayho, G. V. (2017). Aging and employment: Are patients too old to work? *British Journal of General Practice*, *67*(654), 6–7. doi:10.3399/bjgp17X688441

Petrosky, E., Blair, J. M., Betz, C. J., Fowler, K. A., Jack, S., & Lyons, B. H. (2017). Racial and ethnic differences in homicides of adult women and the role of intimate partner violence—United States, 2003–2014. *Morbidity and Mortality Weekly Report*, *66*(28), 741–768. doi:10.15585/mmwr.mm6628a1

Piaget, J. (1966). *Origins of intelligence in children*. New York, NY: W. W. Norton.

Smith-Trudeau, P. (2016, April–June). Generation Z nurses have arrived, Are you ready? *New Hampshire Nursing News*, 13–14.

Stover, C. S., & Coates, E. E. (2016). The relationship of reflective functioning to parent child interactions in a sample of fathers with concurrent intimate partner violence perpetration and substance abuse problems. *Journal of Family Violence*, *31*, 433–442. doi:10.1007/s10896-015-9775-x

Twenge, J. M. (2017). *iGen: Why today's super-connected kids are growing up less rebellious, more tolerant, less happy and completely unprepared for adulthood*. New York, NY: Atria.

U.S. Department of Health and Human Services. (n.d.). *NWS-11.5 (developmental): Prevent inappropriate weight gain in adults aged 20 years and older*. Retrieved from https://www.healthypeople.gov/2020/topics-objectives/objective/nws-115

Selected Bibliography

Edelman, C., & Kudzman, E. (2018). *Health promotion throughout the lifespan* (9th ed.). St. Louis, MO: Elsevier.

Erikson, E. H. (1982). *The life cycle completed: A review*. New York, NY: W. W. Norton.

Freud, S. (1922). *The ego and the id*. London, UK: Hogarth.

Gilligan, C. (1982). *In a different voice: Psychological theory and women's development*. Cambridge, MA: Harvard University.

Kohlberg, L. (1971). *Recent research in moral development*. New York, NY: Holt, Rinehart & Winston.

Kohlberg, L. (1981). *The psychology of moral development: Moral stages and the idea of justice*. San Francisco, CA: Harper & Row.

Kohlberg, L. (1984). *The psychology of moral development: The nature and validity of moral stages*. San Francisco, CA: Harper & Row.

Maslow, A. H. (1970). *Motivation and personality*. New York, NY: Harper & Row.

Ng Fat, L., & Shelton, N. (2012). Associations between self-reported illness and non-drinking in young adults. *Addiction*, *107*, 1612–1620. doi:10.1111/j.1360-0443.2012.03878.x

Peters, B. S., Verly, E., Marchioni, D. M., Fisberg, M., & Martinin, L. A. (2011). The influence of breakfast and dairy products on dietary calcium and vitamin D intake in postpubertal adolescents and young adults. *Journal of Human Nutrition and Dietetics*, *25*, 69–74. doi:10.1111/j.1365-277X.2011.01166.x

Shay, C. M., Ning, H., Allen, N. B., Carnethon, M. R., Chiuve, S. E., Greenlund, K. J., . . . Lloyd-Jones, D. M. (2012). Status of cardiovascular health in U.S. adults: Prevalence estimates from the national health and nutrition examination surveys 2003–2008. *Circulation*, *125*, 45–56. doi:10.1161/CIRCULATIONAHA.111.035733

Sheehy, G. (1995). *New passages. Mapping your life across time*. New York, NY: Ballantine.

Stevenson, J. S. (1977). *Issues and crises during middlescence*. New York, NY: Appleton-Century-Crofts.

Touhy, T. A., & Jett, K. F. (2013). *Ebersole and Hess' gerontological nursing & healthy aging* (4th ed.). St. Louis, MO: Mosby Elsevier.

26 Promoting Health in Older Adults

LEARNING OUTCOMES

After completing this chapter, you will be able to:

1. Describe the demographic, socioeconomic, ethnicity, and health characteristics of older adults in the United States.
2. Identify the different categories of older adults as they range from 65 to 100 years of age.
3. Describe ageism and its contribution to the development of negative stereotypes about older adults.
4. Compare and contrast gerontology and geriatrics.
5. Describe the development of gerontological nursing and the roles of the gerontological nurse.
6. Describe the different care settings for older adults.
7. List the common biological theories of aging.
8. Describe the usual physical changes that occur during older adulthood.
9. List the common psychosocial theories about aging.
10. Describe developmental tasks of the older adult.
11. Describe psychosocial changes to which the older adult adjusts during the aging process.
12. Explain changes in cognitive abilities that occur during the aging process.
13. Compare and contrast Kohlberg's and Gilligan's theories of moral reasoning in older adults.
14. Describe how spirituality and aging interact.
15. Describe selected health problems associated with older adults.
16. List examples of health promotion topics for older adulthood.

KEY TERMS

activity theory, *507*
adult daycare, *498*
ageism, *496*
Alzheimer's disease (AD), *498*
assisted living, *498*
cataracts, *504*
continuity theory, *507*
dementia, *513*
disengagement theory, *507*
dyspnea, *504*
e-health, *508*
geriatrics, *497*
gerontology, *497*
hypothermia, *512*
kyphosis, *502*
long-term memory, *510*
osteoporosis, *502*
pathologic fractures, *502*
perception, *510*
presbycusis, *504*
presbyopia, *504*
recent memory, *510*
sarcopenia, *500*
sensory memory, *510*
short-term memory, *510*

Introduction

The birth of baby boomers began in the mid-1940s. According to the Joint Center for Housing Studies of Harvard University (2016), this population of baby boomers is over the age of 70. In the next 20 years, we will see a growth in the population aged 70 or older by 28 million. In the same period, the population aged 80 and older will more than double. By 2035, one in five individuals will be over the age of 65 years. This increase has been termed the "graying of America." By 2035, one out of every three households will be headed by an individual 65 years or older. Low income older adults will experience difficulties paying for housing, forcing them to reduce the resources needed for food and healthcare. Because the population will be older and greater in number in the coming years, overall U.S. healthcare costs are projected to increase 25% by 2030 (Tabloski, 2019, p. 11). The states with the greatest population of older Americans are Florida, West Virginia, Maine, Pennsylvania, and Iowa.

Characteristics of Older Adults in the United States

Older adults represent an increasingly diverse population in the United States. A review of the major characteristics of the older population includes demographic, socioeconomic, ethnicity, and health characteristics.

Demographics

At one time, all individuals over the age of 65 were considered old. With advancements in disease control, living conditions, and health technology, individuals are living longer. The number of individuals over the age of 65 in the United States is 47.8 million (U.S. Census Bureau, 2017b). This represents a growth of 1.6 million since 2014 (U.S. Census Bureau, n.d.). As of 2017, there were 44,389,997 individuals over the age of 65 years, with 6,468,682 over 85 (U.S. Census Bureau, 2017a). Older adults are as

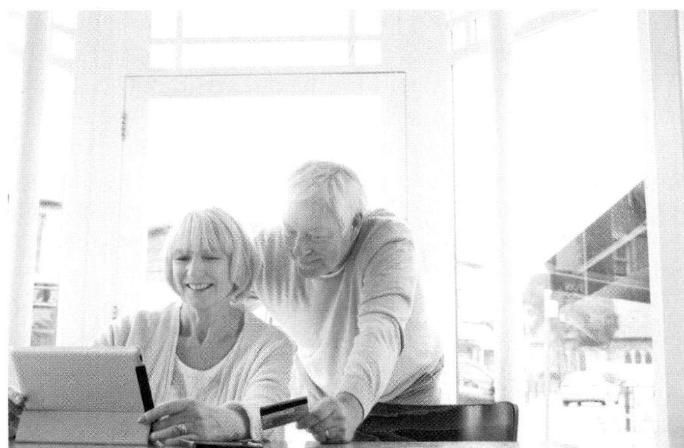

Figure 26.1 ■ Older adults are the fastest-growing group of computer users.
Bloom Productions/Taxi/Getty Images.

heterogeneous as any other age group that spans 40 years or more. The categories of older adults established by Eliopoulos (2018) include the young-old, ages 65–74 years; the old adult, age 75–84 years; and the oldest-old, ages 85 and above. Each of these groups has a distinct set of interests and healthcare needs.

Baby boomers is a term used to describe those born from 1946 to 1964, reflecting a large increase in the U.S. birthrate. Starting in 2011 (and expected to continue through 2030), they began to enter their senior years with better education, higher household incomes, and very active lifestyles compared with previous generations of seniors. They tend to be informed consumers of healthcare and may research information on the internet prior to seeing a healthcare provider (Eliopoulos, 2018; Miller, 2019) (Figure 26.1 ■).

Socioeconomic

Socioeconomic characteristics, such as gender, marital status, education, income, and living arrangements, vary among the young-old and old-old groups (Miller, 2019). Women outnumber men because they have a longer life expectancy than men. In addition, women are more likely than men to be widowed, and older men have higher remarriage rates.

The level of education can affect the socioeconomic status of the older adult. Higher education is usually associated with higher incomes. According to Miller (2019), educational levels for older adults are gradually increasing, as indicated by the increasing percentages of individuals 65 years and older who have completed high school. However, there is significant variation among racial and ethnic groups. In previous decades, older adults were the most economically disadvantaged group. However, the current trend is that older adults are doing better economically. Women over the age of 75 years are more economically disadvantaged than men of the same age. Widowed women and those living alone are the largest group of older adults living in poverty (Miller, 2019, p. 106).

The living arrangements of older adults are linked not only to income but also to health status. Most live in a variety of community settings, with only 4% living in nursing homes. Older men are more likely to live with a spouse as compared with older women, who are more likely to live alone. Women are more likely to live with their children than are men.

Ethnicity

The older population will become more racially and ethnically diverse, although significant shifts will not happen until today's more diverse Generation X and millennials reach retirement age. Still, by 2035, the non-Hispanic White share of the older population will fall from 78% to 69%, with rising shares of non-Hispanic Black, Hispanic, Asian, and other races filling out the remaining 31% share. The share of foreign-born older adults is expected to increase from 13% to 19% over the next 2 decades (Joint Center for Housing Studies of Harvard University, 2016).

According to the 2016 *Older Americans Key Indicators of Well-Being*, life expectancy varies by race. However, the variations decrease with decreases in the client's age. As of 2014, at age 65, White Americans were expected to live 1.1 years longer than Black Americans (Federal Interagency Forum on Aging-Related Statistics [FIFAS], 2016).

From 2014 through 2060, the entire population aged 65 and over is expected to increase from 15% to 24% of the total population. According to the U.S. Census Bureau (Colby & Ortman, 2015), the native and foreign-born populations over age 65 are expected to increase; the foreign-born increase will be greater. The native-born population 65 years and older will increase by 7% to constitute 22% of the total population. The foreign-born population is expected to increase by 18% to constitute 32% of the total population. The growing population of older adults consists primarily of increasing numbers of individuals of color. Between 2030 and 2060, the older White, non-Hispanic population will drop by 17%, whereas the Hispanic population will double (Mather, Jacobsen, & Pollard, 2016). These numbers emphasize the importance of nurses being culturally sensitive and competent. See Table 26.1 for a comparison of the older adult population growth.

TABLE 26.1 Comparison of Older Population for 2014 Census and Projected Older Population for 2060 Census by Ethnicity

Ethnicity	2014	2060 Projection
White	254,009,000	55,558,000
Black	45,562,000	28,968,000
Asian	19,983,000	28,592,000
Hispanic	55,410,000	63,635,000
American Indian/ Alaskan Natives	6,528,000	3,640,000
Hawaiian/Pacific Islander	1,458,000	1,470,000

From "Projections of the Size and Composition of the U.S. Population: 2014 to 2060," by S. Colby and J. M. Ortman, 2015. Retrieved from https://www.census.gov/content/dam/Census/library/publications/2015/demo/p25-1143.pdf

Health

Chronic health problems and disabilities increase as individuals age. However, disease is *not* a normal outcome of aging. Older adults in the United States are living longer with less disability than previous generations (Mather et al., 2016). In 2015, 39% of noninstitutionalized older Americans 75 years and older rated their health as excellent or very good. Most older individuals have at least one chronic condition, and many have multiple chronic conditions. *Healthy People 2030* continues the tradition of improving health, equity, and well-being in America. This decade will focus on building a culture of health. The desired outcome is that every American lives a healthier life. A major focus is to address the health of populations. Given the fact that chronic conditions are of primary concern in the older adult population, the highest goal established for 2030 is the response to the rise in noncommunicable diseases. The new director of the World Health Organization (WHO) asserts that everyone must have the highest attainable standards of health (Gostin et al., 2016).

Attitudes Toward Aging

The graying of America impacts the nursing profession. With the increase in numbers, many nurses will be caring for older adults at some point. It is important for nurses to be aware of their own values and attitudes toward aging and examine whether myths or stereotypes influence those attitudes.

Ageism

American society values youth. The term **ageism** is used to describe negative attitudes toward aging or older adults. It is defined as stereotyping, prejudice, or discrimination against individuals because of their chronological age (Ayalon & Tesch-Romer, 2017). These attitudes often arise from negative past experiences (Mauk, 2018, p. 9). Raposo and Carstensen (2015) identify an important change. The United States is undergoing a transformation to an old-age society. The population of older adults is greater than any other age group. These authors state that pessimism about the age-related decline in society reduces the likelihood that problems will be solved to improve the quality of life. In a review of the ageism literature, Ayalon and Tesch-Romer (2017) found ageism to be prevalent in the healthcare sector. One phenomenon researchers identified is that older adults impose a great burden on the healthcare system. In addition, some healthcare professionals communicate in a disrespectful manner and do not include older adults in treatment decisions.

It is important to identify strategies to prevent the development of negative attitudes toward aging. Raposo and Carstensen (2015) found that ageism impedes the engagement of the older individuals in our society. Baby boomers are working longer than the members of the old-old group did. It is recommended that research be conducted to identify working conditions and roles that enhance the performance of all ages. Technologic advances can assist in reducing injury and improving the safety of older workers. In addition, Raposo and Carstensen recommend that pharmaceutical research should focus on the older adult to enhance outcomes of care.

Myths and Stereotypes

Ageism contributes to the development of negative stereotypes about older adults. Stereotypes occur when younger individuals do not understand or identify with older adults as unique human beings. Instead, they generalize undesirable characteristics (e.g., senile, old-fashioned, unproductive, inflexible) to all older adults. Many negative attitudes about aging are based on myths and incorrect information regarding growing old. For example, an older client only experiences loss of memory related to the onset of a neurologic disease. Most causes of disability are related to the adverse effects of many drugs, such as pain medications. Disease processes also increase the client's risk of developing disabling conditions. For example, diabetes mellitus can result in loss of feeling in the extremities, diminished kidney function, and loss of vision. As a result, it is important for nurses to provide accurate information about aging. This has been found to be an effective intervention for reducing negative stereotypes and improving attitudes about aging (Miller, 2019, p. 7).

EVIDENCE-BASED PRACTICE

Evidence-Based Practice

Do Nurses Support Fewer Treatment Modalities in an Older Adult Compared with a Younger Adult?

Schroyen, Missotten, Jerusalem, Gilles, and Adam (2016) conducted a study on ageism in nursing. In this study, they distributed vignettes about immunotherapy, adjuvant chemotherapy, and breast reconstruction to 76 nurses. The outcome of the care provided by the nurses for clients aged 35, 55, and 75 years revealed that the support for immunotherapy, breast reconstruction, and chemotherapy was lower for the patient aged 75 years versus the 35-year-old and 55-year-old, respectively. Based on the results, the authors concluded that nurses and other healthcare providers should receive specialized training about ageism and its consequences related to adequate client care.

Implications

It is important that clients be provided all options in medical and nursing care regardless of age and cost. Clients should be afforded every option in their care.

Gerontological Nursing

The older adult population is characterized by unique and diverse individuals who may require a variety of professionals to meet their healthcare needs. **Gerontology** is the term used to define the study of aging and older adults. Gerontology is multidisciplinary and is a specialized area within various disciplines, such as nursing, psychology, and social work. **Geriatrics** is associated with the medical care (e.g., diseases and disabilities) of older adults.

Development

Gerontological nursing involves advocating for the health of older adults at all levels of prevention (Mauk, 2018). In the 1960s, gerontological nursing became a subspecialty of nursing. In the 1980s, gerontological nursing leaders stated that most practicing nurses did not have sufficient knowledge about gerontology. This prompted discussion of how to prepare nurses for gerontological nursing. Since the late 1990s, the nursing profession has recognized the importance of preparing all practicing nurses with basic gerontological knowledge. As a result, schools of nursing provide classes or courses about the nursing care of older clients. Practicing gerontological nurses can obtain gerontological nursing certification through the American Nurses Association. Advanced practice in gerontological nursing requires a master's degree in nursing, for which there are two options: the gerontological clinical nurse specialist and the gerontological nurse practitioner.

Roles

The gerontological nurse has many roles: provider of care, teacher, manager, advocate, and research consumer. As a provider of care, the nurse gives direct care to older adults in a variety of settings. The teaching of gerontological nurses often focuses on modifiable risk factors (e.g., healthy diet, physical activity, stress management). Gerontological nurse managers balance the concerns of the older client and family, as well as the concerns of nurses and other interdisciplinary team members. As an advocate, the gerontological nurse empowers older adults by helping them remain independent and strengthen their autonomy and decision-making ability. Being a research consumer requires nurses to read the latest professional literature for evidence-based practice to improve the quality of nursing care for older clients.

Care Settings for Older Adults

Gerontological nurses practice in many settings. Older adults are the primary users of healthcare services that range from acute care facilities to rehabilitation, long-term care, and the community (Eliopoulos, 2018). Regardless of the setting, older adults require health assessment and promotion.

Acute Care Facilities

Older adults are the majority of clients cared for in acute care. In 2013 Medicare adopted a transitional care management services system. This system was designed to furnish transitional care management services for Medicare beneficiaries. The goal of these services was to improve discharge outcomes and reduce readmission to acute care facilities. Bindman and Cox (2018) conducted a retrospective cohort analysis of all Medicare fee-for-service claims from January 1, 2013, to December 31, 2015. Discharges from hospitals, inpatient psychiatric facilities, long-term hospitals, skilled nursing, inpatient rehabilitation, and observational stay were examined. The authors stated that despite the apparent benefits of transition-of-care-management services, the use of the services is low. It is important that an assessment of the interventions be made to increase the use of these services. Transition-of-care services may reduce readmission and enhance the outcomes of care.

Nurses in an acute care setting focus on protecting the health of the older adult, with the goal of the older adult returning to his or her prior level of independence. Examples include the following:

- Preventing healthcare-associated infections (e.g., urinary tract infections, pneumonia)
- Preventing therapy-related problems (e.g., confusion, sleeplessness, dehydration, decreased nutrition)
- Treating the health problem that resulted in the older adult's admission and assessing for potential undiagnosed health problems (e.g., depression, drug or alcohol abuse)
- Preventing complications (e.g., pressure injury).

Older adults often perceive that hospitalization could change their ability to be autonomous and independent. As a result, nurses need to assess the older adult's stage or perception of the need for control and autonomy during hospitalization and his or her fears and hopes about being discharged from the hospital setting.

Long-Term Care Facilities

Long-term care is the provision of healthcare and personal care assistance to clients who have a chronic disease or disability. Long-term care facilities are also known as nursing facilities. *Nursing facility* is a new term that includes providers of care who are certified by Medicare and institutions previously referred to as *intermediate care*. The primary difference between institutions is the care offered and the level of care provided to the client (Pratt, 2018, p. 17). In the long-term care setting or nursing facilities, the individual is referred to as a resident. Care includes many different levels of care. These may include assisted living, intermediate care, skilled care, and Alzheimer's units. Older adults who do not feel safe living alone or require additional help with activities of daily living (ADLs) may desire **assisted living**. Individuals in assisted living facilities usually have their own apartment. The assisted living facility provides meals, weekly activities, and a pleasant environment for socializing with other residents. Some assisted living units are part of a larger facility. When residents require additional assistance, they may enter intermediate care. The term *intermediate care* was formerly used to describe a nursing facility that provided less advanced services than a skilled nursing facility (Pratt, 2018, p. 545).

Skilled care units or skilled nursing facilities (SNFs) are designed to provide for the needs of clients whose acuity levels require a higher level of nursing care. Gerontological nurses working in SNFs often care for clients who require tube feedings, intravenous therapy, chronic wound therapy, and mechanical ventilators.

Many long-term care facilities offer specialized units for clients with **Alzheimer's disease (AD)**. AD is characterized by progressive dementia, memory loss, and the inability to care for oneself. Gerontological nurses working in AD units have specialized knowledge and help family members understand and cope with the disease process affecting their loved one.

Hospice

Gerontological nurses may also work in hospice and care for dying clients and their families. The majority of hospice clients are older adults. Hospice requires a great deal of patience, expertise, understanding, interdisciplinary communication, and compassion on the part of gerontological nurses. The goal of hospice care is to provide the client with a comprehensive set of services to be identified and coordinated by an interdisciplinary group for the provision of physical, psychosocial, spiritual, and emotional care to meet the needs of the individual client and family members (American Association of Colleges of Nursing, 2016).

Rehabilitation

Gerontological rehabilitation nursing combines expertise in gerontological nursing with rehabilitation concepts and practice. Nurses working in gerontological rehabilitation often care for older adults with chronic illnesses and long-term functional limitations (e.g., orthopedic surgery, stroke, or amputation). This rehabilitative care may be found in several settings: acute care hospitals, subacute or transitional care centers, and long-term care facilities. The nurse is an important member of the interdisciplinary rehabilitation team. The role of the nurse is often as a healthcare coordinator, manager, and counselor for older adults and their families. For example, nurses monitor the client's healthcare, assist with ADLs, and assist older adults in regaining and maintaining the highest level of function and independence possible while preventing complications and enhancing quality of life (Mauk, 2018, p. 10).

Community

Gerontological nurses provide nursing care in many types of community settings. Nurses often assess the older client's needs and then try to match the need with a community resource. Examples of the different community areas in which gerontological nurses practice include the following:

- ***Home healthcare.*** Home care is designed for those who are homebound due to the severity of illness or disability. The Medicare guidelines describe these clients as homebound and unable to leave the home without a considerable amount of effort. Services are provided by a primary care provider and require skilled or rehabilitation nursing. The provision of nursing care and monitoring of the client's health status are integral in preventing hospital readmissions.
- ***Nurse-run clinics.*** These clinics focus on managing chronic illness. Nurses follow up with either telephone contacts or home visits within a week after discharge from a hospital. Again, this often helps decrease hospital readmissions.
- ***Adult daycare.*** The older adult may receive **adult daycare**, where the focus is on social activities and healthcare (Figure 26.2 ■). The level of nursing care can vary (e.g., bathing, medication administration, wound dressing). Family caregivers who may need to work during the day or need some respite from the continual care often use these services. This is an alternative to institutionalizing an older adult.

Physiologic Aging

In the past half century, scientists have proposed numerous theories of why individuals age. More recently, as both the absolute number and the population percentage of older adults increase, there is renewed interest in why and how individuals age and what factors affect the physical, psychologic, and functional status of older individuals. This interest has resulted in the development of additional theories about the aging process. There are many different theories of aging in the biological, psychologic, and social sciences. Three nursing theories of aging have been developed in the past 20 years. Miller (2019) developed the functional consequences theory in 1990. Functional consequences are age-related changes, actions that have placed the client at risk for illness or injury, and risk factors for disease. The nurse should design interventions that promote safety and improve the client's quality of life. Haight, Barba, Courts, and Tesh's (2002) theory of thriving asserts that nurses must intervene to promote the older adult's growth and development. The third theory is a middle-range theory. It is the nursing theory of successful

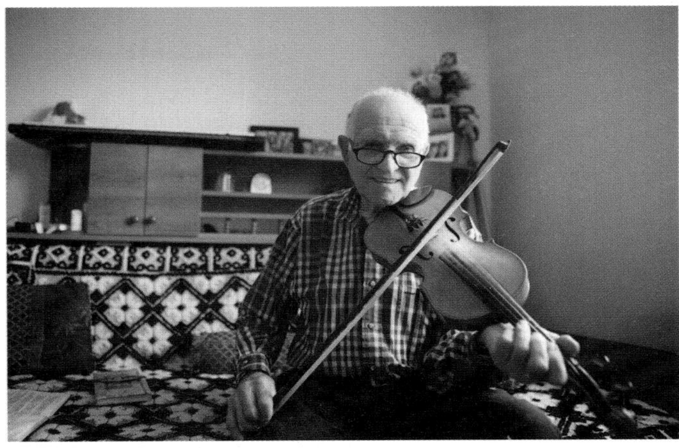
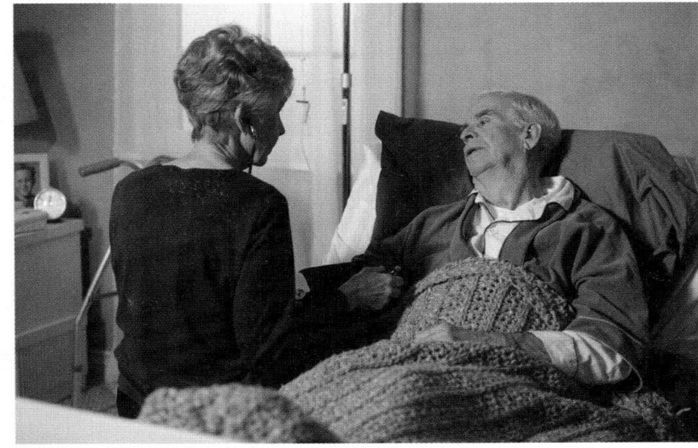
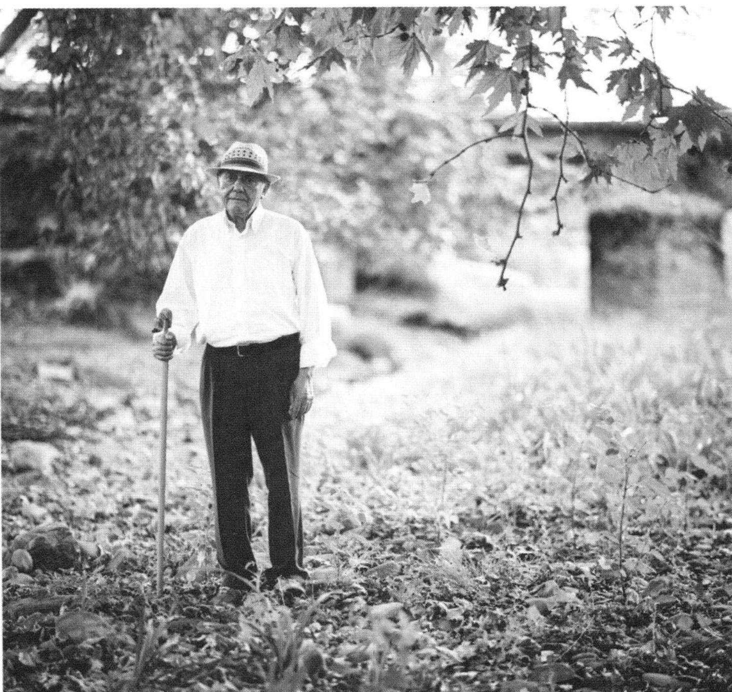
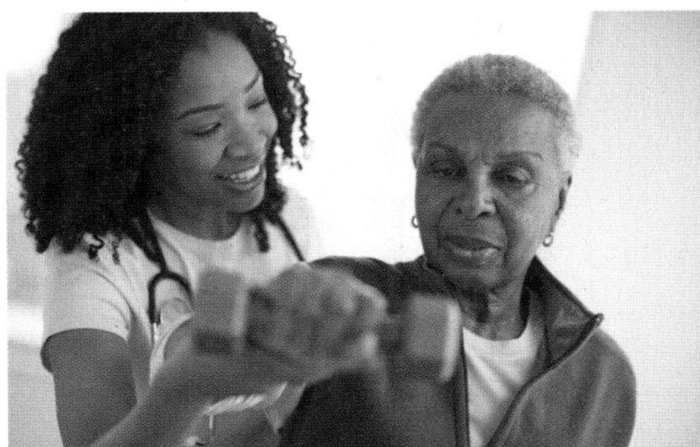
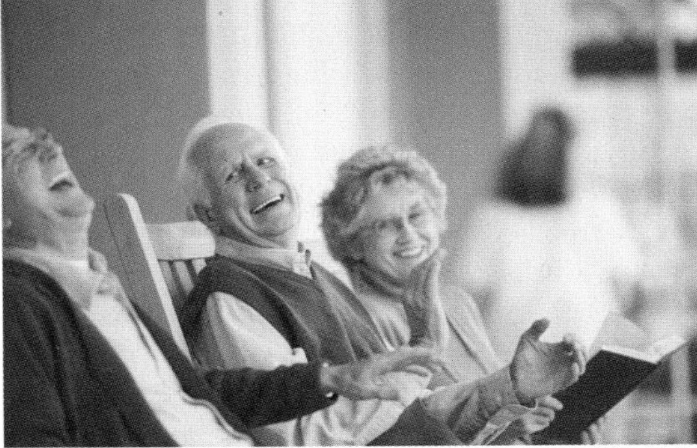

Figure 26.2 ■ Adult daycare centers focus on social activities and healthcare.
Cavan Images/Getty Images, Thanasis Zovoilis/Moment/Getty Images, Photodisc/Getty Images, Blend Images - JGI/Tom Grill/Getty Images, Comstock/Stockbyte/Getty Images.

aging developed by Flood. Flood (2005) defines successful aging as the "cumulative physiologic and functional alterations associated with the passage of time" (p. 36). The client experiences spiritual connections and a sense of meaning and worth. Nurses must target interventions for the older adult in the promotion of mental, physical, and spiritual health throughout the aging process. Mauk (2018) asserted that nursing theories on aging lack all holistic elements that influence aging. Nurses must be aware of a client's socioeconomic resources. It is important for future theoretical development to address the client's cultural, spiritual, geographic, psychosocial, physiologic, and environmental elements that are influential in the aging process (Mauk, 2018, p. 88). Examples of theories for explaining physical aging include wear-and-tear, endocrine, free-radical, genetic, cross-linking, and immunologic theories. Table 26.2 describes the various biological theories of aging.

At this point, it is helpful to distinguish between normal or usual aging (the typical aging course with concomitant diseases and disabilities) and successful aging (the aging course without disease). Arthritis, heart disease, cancer, and diabetes are the leading causes of disability or death in the United States. Adams (2017) reported for the Centers for Disease Control and Prevention (CDC) that the healthcare costs to treat chronic diseases in adults and adults over the age of 65 years is similar. The expenditure for the entire adult population with two or three chronic conditions is approximately $3700 annually. Individuals with four or more chronic conditions

TABLE 26.2 Common Biological Theories of Aging

Theory Type	Hypotheses
Wear-and-tear theory	Proposes that humans, like automobiles, have vital parts that run down with time, leading to aging and death. Proposes that the faster an organism lives, the quicker it dies. Proposes that cells wear out through exposure to internal and external stressors, including trauma, chemicals, and buildup of natural wastes.
Endocrine theory	Proposes that events occurring in the hypothalamus and pituitary are responsible for changes in hormone production and response that result in the organism's decline.
Free-radical theory	Proposes that unstable free radicals (groups of atoms) result from the oxidation of organic materials, such as carbohydrates and proteins. These radicals cause biochemical changes in the cells, and the cells cannot regenerate themselves.
Genetic theory	Proposes that the organism is genetically programmed for a predetermined number of cell divisions, after which the cell or organism dies. Proposes that when damage to protein synthesis occurs, faulty proteins will be synthesized and will gradually accumulate, causing a progressive decline in the organism.
Cross-linking theory	Proposes that the irreversible aging of proteins such as collagen is responsible for the ultimate failure of tissues and organs. Proposes that as cells age, chemical reactions create strong bonds, or cross-linkages, between proteins. These bonds cause loss of elasticity, stiffness, and eventual loss of function.
Immunologic theory	Proposes that the immune system becomes less effective with age, resulting in reduced resistance to infectious disease and viruses. Proposes that a decrease in immune function may result in an increase in autoimmune responses, causing the body to produce antibodies that attack itself.

will note expenditures of $8900 annually. As an individual ages, many physical changes occur; some are visible, whereas others are not. In general, lean body mass is reduced, fat tissue increases, and bone mass decreases. Extracellular fluid remains constant; however, intracellular fluid decreases and leads to reduced total body fluid. Thus, older adults are at risk of developing dehydration. Table 26.3 provides a summary of the normal physical changes associated with aging.

Integumentary

Obvious changes occur in the integumentary system (skin, hair, nails) with age. The skin becomes drier, less elastic, and more fragile, making the older individual more susceptible to skin tears and shearing injuries. The hair loses color, the fingernails and toenails become thickened and brittle, and in women over age 60, facial hair increases.

Responses to these changes vary among individuals and cultures. For example, one individual may feel distinguished with gray hair, whereas another may feel embarrassed or depressed, interpreting gray hair as a sign of losing one's youth.

These integumentary changes accompany progressive losses of subcutaneous fat and muscle tissue, muscle atrophy, and loss of elastic fiber, resulting in a "double" chin, sagging of eyelids and earlobes, and wrinkling of the skin, especially in areas exposed to the sun. Bony prominences may become visible. In older women, the breasts become less firm and may sag. Loss of subcutaneous fat also decreases older adults' tolerance of cold.

Health promotion teaching about skin care for older adults can include the following:

- Maintaining healthy skin:
  - Ensure optimal nutrition.
  - Maintain adequate hydration.
  - Prevent skin dryness by using emollient lotions after bathing or showering, when the skin is still moist.
  - Avoid skin products that contain perfume or alcohol.
  - Assess the frequency of bathing and showering.
- Avoiding sun damage:
  - Use sun-screening lotions with a sun protection factor (SPF) of 15 or higher.
  - Wear wide-brimmed hats, sun visors, and sunglasses when exposed to the sun.
  - Observe for any skin changes (e.g., new lesions, change in mole size or color) and seek medical evaluation.
- Preventing skin injury:
  - Do not use strong detergent to launder clothes.
  - Avoid rough texture in clothing.
  - Avoid highly starched linens.
  - Use soft washcloths, towels, and bed linens.

Neuromuscular

With aging comes a gradual reduction in the speed and power of skeletal or voluntary muscle contractions and sustained muscular effort. Exercise can strengthen weakened muscles, and up to about age 50, the skeletal muscles can increase in bulk and density. **Sarcopenia** is a syndrome that

TABLE 26.3 Normal Physical Changes Associated with Aging

Physical Changes	Rationale
INTEGUMENTARY	
Increased skin dryness	Decrease in sebaceous gland activity and tissue fluid
Increased skin pallor	Decreased vascularity
Increased skin fragility	Reduced thickness and vascularity of the dermis; loss of subcutaneous fat
Progressive wrinkling and sagging of the skin	Loss of skin elasticity, increased dryness, and decreased subcutaneous fat
Brown "age spots" (lentigo senilis) on exposed body parts (e.g., face, hands, arms)	Clustering of melanocytes (pigment-producing cells)
Decreased perspiration	Reduced number and function of sweat glands
Thinning and graying of scalp, pubic, and axillary hair	Progressive loss of pigment cells from the hair bulbs
Slower nail growth and increased thickening with ridges	Increased calcium deposition
NEUROMUSCULAR	
Decreased speed and power of skeletal muscle contractions	Decrease in muscle fibers
Slowed reaction time	Diminished conduction speed of nerve fibers and decreased muscle tone
Loss of height (stature)	Atrophy of intervertebral disks, increased flexion at hips and knees
Loss of bone mass	Bone reabsorption outpaces bone reformation
Joint stiffness	Drying and loss of elasticity in joint cartilage
Impaired balance	Decreased muscle strength, reaction time, and coordination; change in center of gravity
Greater difficulty in complex learning and abstraction	Fewer cells in cerebral cortex
SENSORY/PERCEPTUAL	
Loss of visual acuity	Degeneration leading to lens opacity (cataracts), thickening, and inelasticity (presbyopia)
Increased sensitivity to glare and decreased ability to adjust to darkness	Changes in the ciliary muscles; rigid pupil sphincter; decrease in pupil size
Partial or complete glossy white circle around the periphery of the cornea (arcus senilis)	Fatty deposits
Progressive loss of hearing (presbycusis)	Changes in the structures and nerve tissues in the inner ear; thickening of the eardrum
Decreased sense of taste, especially the sweet sensations at the tip of the tongue	Decreased number of taste buds in the tongue because of tongue atrophy
Decreased sense of smell	Atrophy of the olfactory bulb at the base of the brain (responsible for smell perception)
Increased threshold for sensations of pain, touch, and temperature	Possible nerve conduction and neuron changes
PULMONARY	
Decreased ability to expel foreign or accumulated matter	Decreased elasticity and ciliary activity
Decreased lung expansion, less effective exhalation, reduced vital capacity, and increased residual volume	Weakened thoracic muscles; calcification of costal cartilage, making the rib cage more rigid with increased anterior-posterior diameter; dilation from inelasticity of alveoli
Difficult, short, heavy, rapid breathing (dyspnea) following intense exercise	Diminished delivery and diffusion of oxygen to the tissues to repay the normal oxygen debt because of exertion or changes in both respiratory and vascular tissues
CARDIOVASCULAR	
Reduced cardiac output and stroke volume, particularly during increased activity or unusual demands; may result in shortness of breath on exertion and pooling of blood in the extremities	Increased rigidity and thickness of heart valves (hence, decreased filling and emptying abilities); decreased contractile strength
Reduced elasticity and increased rigidity of arteries	Increased calcium deposits in the muscular layer
Increase in diastolic and systolic blood pressure	Inelasticity of systemic arteries and increased peripheral resistance
Orthostatic hypertension	Reduced sensitivity of the blood pressure–regulating baroreceptors

Continued on page 502

TABLE 26.3 Normal Physical Changes Associated with Aging—*continued*

Physical Changes	Rationale
GASTROINTESTINAL	
Delayed swallowing time	Alterations in the swallowing mechanism
Increased tendency for indigestion	Gradual decrease in digestive enzymes, reduction in gastric acid production, and slower absorption rate
Increased tendency for constipation	Decreased muscle tone of the intestines; decreased peristalsis; decreased free body fluid
URINARY	
Reduced filtering ability of the kidney and impaired renal function	Decreased number of functioning nephrons (basic functional units of the kidney) and arteriosclerotic changes in blood flow
Less effective concentration of urine	Decreased tubular function
Urinary urgency and urinary frequency	Enlarged prostate gland in men; weakened muscles supporting the bladder or weakness of the urinary sphincter in women
Tendency for nocturnal frequency and retention of residual urine	Decreased bladder capacity and tone
GENITALS	
Prostate enlargement (benign) in men	Exact mechanism is unclear; possible endocrine changes
Multiple changes in women (shrinkage and atrophy of the vulva, cervix, uterus, fallopian tubes, and ovaries; reduction in secretions; and changes in vaginal flora)	Diminished secretion of female hormones and more alkaline vaginal pH
Increased time to sexual arousal	Changes in blood supply to penis, clitoris
Decreased firmness of erection, increased refractory period (men)	Changes in blood supply
Decreased vaginal lubrication and elasticity (women)	Loss of estrogen effects
IMMUNOLOGIC	
Decreased immune response; lowered resistance to infections	T cells less responsive to antigens; B cells produce fewer antibodies
Poor response to immunization	
Decreased stress response	
ENDOCRINE	
Increased insulin resistance	Immune system changes may precipitate insulin resistance
Decreased thyroid function	Unclear mechanism

results in muscle weakness leading to diminished independence and contributes to the client's decreased ability to perform ADLs. This condition leads to alterations in balance and gait, leading to falls and, ultimately, fractures (Taani, Siglinksy, Kovach, & Buehring, 2018). The authors studied the relationship of muscle strength and function with the psychosocial factors among older residents of a residential care apartment complex. Their findings showed a trend that older individuals who were active and exercised exhibited a higher self-efficacy with a strong social network. They also possessed greater muscle strength and function.

The reduction of skeletal muscle strength and diminished muscular contraction increase the risk of falls in the older adult. Falls contribute to the development of fractures in older adults. Maritz and Silbernagel (2016) conducted a study that identified the importance of unilateral calf muscle strength and its association with fall risk in older adults. Older adults in a community living setting had improved balance, increased calf muscle strength, and greater balance confidence. Thus, exercise that improves muscle strength can lead to fall prevention in the older adult population. Each of these studies provides evidence that older adults need to maintain or increase activity in the prevention of falls and related musculoskeletal disability.

The individual's reaction time slows with age. Reaction time can be delayed further by decreased muscle tone as a result of diminished physical activity. Older adults compensate for this reaction difference by being exceptionally cautious, for instance, in their driving habits, which exasperates some impatient younger drivers.

A loss in overall stature occurs with age. This can be exaggerated by muscular weakness, resulting in a stooping posture and **kyphosis** (humpback of the upper spine). Imbalance in the rates of absorption and formation of bone tissue occurs with aging, so older adults have more porous and fragile bones than do younger adults, making older adults prone to serious fractures. **Osteoporosis**, a pathologic decrease in bone density that is more common in older than younger adults, may lead to spontaneous (i.e., without a fall or other trauma to the bone) fractures that are called **pathologic fractures**. Osteoporosis occurs more frequently in individuals with insufficient intake of dietary calcium, in women after menopause, in Caucasians and Asians, and in individuals who are immobilized or physically inactive. Often considered a disease of women, it is important to remember that osteoporosis also affects men (Eliopoulos, 2018). Osteoporosis occurs in both women and men with fractures of the proximal femur, proximal humerus, or forearm. The client may have low bone mineral density in the lumbar spine and hip. Testosterone increases longitudinal and appositional bone growth in children. Estrogen produces epiphyseal closure. As the male ages, testosterone and estradiol levels decrease. The risk of fracture in male clients is associated with a decline in estradiol levels.

In 2018 the American College of Physicians (ACP) updated the 2008 ACP recommendations on the treatment of low bone density and osteoporosis for the prevention of fractures in men and women (Qaseen, Forciea, McLean, & Denberg, 2017). The ACP Clinical Guidelines Committee performed a systematic review of studies conducted from January 2, 2005 through June 3, 2011. Two additional updates were conducted in July and October of 2016. These updates examined the risks and benefits of short- and long-term pharmacologic treatments for low bone density. The 2018 clinical guidelines are listed in Table 26.4.

Joints and their supporting structures change with age. Decreased elasticity, strength, and hydration of the tendons and ligaments make movement stiffer and more restricted. Stiffness is aggravated by inactivity; for example, if an individual sits too long, the joints become stiff, and the individual has difficulty standing and walking. These changes may be compounded by osteoarthritis. A continual program of physical activity and proper nutrition will slow bone density loss and decrease muscle atrophy and stiffness (Figure 26.3 ■).

These age-related changes may affect the mobility and safety of the older adult. For example, decreased muscle strength, decreased balance, and osteoporosis put the older adult at risk for falls and fractures. For health promotion, the nurse assesses the musculoskeletal functioning of the older adult and identifies any risk factors that may contribute to falls or the ability of the older adult to perform ADLs. Health promotion interventions often include providing information about the risk factors for osteoporosis and the importance of adequate intake of calcium and vitamin D.

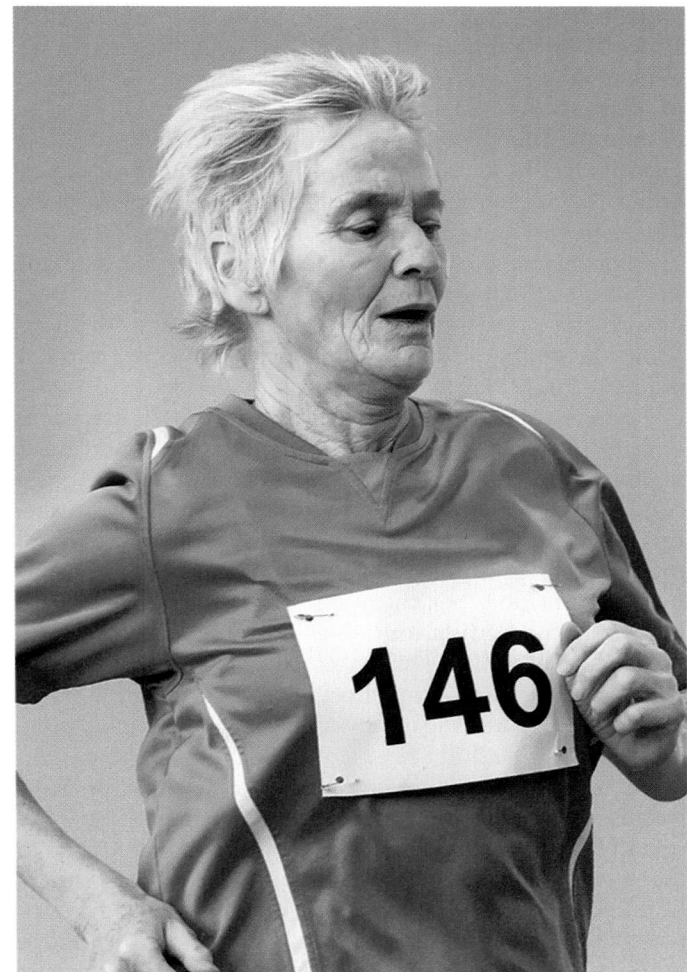

Figure 26.3 ■ A regular program of exercise is important for maintaining joint mobility and muscle tone.
mezzotint/Shutterstock.

Sensory-Perceptual

Each of the five senses becomes less efficient in older adulthood. Changes in vision associated with aging include the obvious changes around the eye, such as the shrunken

TABLE 26.4 American College of Physicians Recommendations on Low Bone Density and Osteoporosis to Prevent Fractures in Men and Women

Recommendation	Guideline
Recommendation 1	Clinicians offer pharmacologic treatment with alendronate, risedronate, zoledronic acid, or denosumab to reduce the risk of hip and vertebral fractures in women who have osteoporosis.
Recommendation 2	Clinicians treat women with osteoporosis with pharmacologic therapy for 5 years.
Recommendation 3	Clinicians offer pharmacologic treatment with bisphosphonates to reduce the risk of vertebral fracture in men who have clinically recognized osteoporosis.
Recommendation 4	No bone density monitoring during the 5-year pharmacologic treatment period for women with osteoporosis.
Recommendation 5	No use of menopausal estrogen therapy or menopausal estrogen plus progesterone therapy or raloxifene for the treatment of osteoporosis in women.
Recommendation 6	Clinicians should make the decision whether to treat osteopenic women 65 years and older who are at high risk for fracture based on a discussion of patient preferences; fracture risk profile; and benefits, harms, and cost of medications.

From "Clinical Guideline Treatment of Low Bone Density or Osteoporosis to Prevent Fractures in Men and Women: A Clinical Practice Guideline Update from the American College of Physicians," by A. Qaseen, M. A., Forciea, R. M. McLean, and T. D. Denberg, 2017, *Annals of Internal Medicine*, *166*, 818–839.

appearance of the eyes due to the loss of orbital fat, the slowed blink reflex, and diminished eyelid muscle tone. Other changes result in decreased visual acuity, less power of adaptation to darkness and dim light, and decreased accommodation to near and far objects. Loss of peripheral vision; atrophy of lacrimal glands resulting in dry eyes; and difficulty in discriminating similar colors, especially blues, greens, and purples, also occur.

Presbyopia, the inability to focus or accommodate due to a loss of flexibility of the lens, causes decreased near vision. This process generally starts around age 40. Visual acuity lessens gradually after age 50 and more rapidly after age 70 (Miller, 2019).

By the age of 80, nearly all older adults have some lens opacity (**cataracts**) that reduces visual acuity and causes glare to be a problem. In addition to cataracts, three other conditions result in visual impairment and blindness: age-related macular degeneration (ARMD), glaucoma, and diabetic retinopathy (Miller, 2019). It is important for the nurse to promote health by informing older clients that they should schedule routine eye examinations to maintain and protect their vision. Also, wearing sunglasses will help avoid the damaging effect of ultraviolet light.

The loss of hearing ability related to aging, called **presbycusis**, affects adults over age 65. Gradual loss of hearing is more common among men than women, perhaps because men work in noisy work environments more frequently. Hearing loss is greater in the higher frequencies than the lower. Thus, older adults with hearing loss usually hear speakers with low, distinct voices best. Hard consonants (e.g., *k, d, t*) and long vowel sounds (e.g., *ay, ee*) are more easily recognized, and sibilant sounds (e.g., *s, th, f*) are the most difficult to hear. Older adults may have more difficulty compensating for hearing loss than the young, who pay closer attention to the lip movements of the speaker.

If family members notice communication problems or social withdrawal, the nurse should provide health promotion teaching by suggesting a referral for hearing screening. Also, the older adult's ears should be checked for impacted earwax. If hearing has diminished, assistive listening devices are available, and the nurse can provide information to the older adult and family. To help avoid increased hearing loss, inform the older adult to use ear protection devices when working in or around activities that produce loud noises.

Older adults have a poorer sense of taste and smell and are less stimulated by food than the young. It is common for the sense of smell to decline more than the sense of taste. These changes significantly affect appetite in the older adult, contributing to poor nutrition. Decreased or absent sense of smell and taste also add to the health hazard of increased salt usage and safety issues (e.g., being unable to smell a gas leak). It is important for the nurse to teach the older client and family about the safety issues involved with a decreased sense of taste and smell and what strategies can be implemented to promote the older adult's safety (e.g., dating and labeling foods, using smoke alarms).

Loss of skin receptors takes place gradually, producing an increased threshold for sensations of pain, touch, and temperature. The older adult may not be able to distinguish hot from cold or the intensity of heat. Stimuli causing severe pain in a younger individual may cause only minor sensation or pressure in older adults. This places the older adult at higher risk for burns and other injuries. Again, it is important for the nurse to teach about the involved safety risks and subsequent interventions (e.g., setting the temperature of the water heater to 110°F to prevent scalding).

Pulmonary

Respiratory efficiency declines with age. Tidal volume (the measurement of air moved in and out during normal respiration) remains the same. However, the older adult has a decreased vital capacity. This means the older adult is unable to compensate for increased oxygen need by significantly increasing the amount of air inspired. **Dyspnea** (difficult breathing) often occurs with physically

EVIDENCE-BASED PRACTICE

Evidence-Based Practice

What Is the Result of Social Support and Coping on the Quality of Life Among Older Clients with Age-Related Hearing Loss?

Moser, Luxenberger, and Freidl (2017) conducted a study on 65 older adults with age-related hearing loss. Each participant completed the Hearing Handicap Inventory for the Elderly, Assessment for Coping and Stress, the short form of the Social Support Questionnaire, and the World Health Organization Quality of Life Scale—Brief Version. The purpose of the study was to determine the set of psychosocial factors that influence the quality of life in older adults who have age-related hearing loss. The study participants had mild to moderate hearing loss. The participants with hearing loss who consistently received social support from significant others and family had an increased quality of life. It is a recommendation of the study that counseling of the hearing impaired can contribute to an increased quality of life.

Implications

It is important for nurses to encourage older adults with impaired hearing to seek counseling to assist in developing coping strategies to enhance their quality of life. In addition, family and individuals close to the older client should be educated on strategies to provide social support to the client with hearing loss. It is also important to provide listening devices and hearing aids to compensate for hearing loss.

demanding activities, such as running for a bus or carrying heavy parcels upstairs. A greater volume of residual air is left in the lungs after expiration, and the capacity to cough efficiently decreases because of weaker expiratory muscles. Mucous secretions tend to collect more readily in the respiratory tree. Thus, susceptibility to respiratory infections increases in older adults.

Health promotion teaching includes information about the following:

- Cessation of smoking, if appropriate
- Preventing respiratory infections by washing hands
- Ensuring that influenza and pneumonia vaccinations are up to date.

Cardiovascular

The working capacity of the heart diminishes with age. This is particularly evident when increased demands are made on the heart, such as during periods of exercise or emotional stress. The heart rate at normal rest may decrease with age. However, the heart rate of the older adult is slower to respond to stress and slower to return to normal after periods of physical activity.

Changes in the arteries occur concurrently. Reduced arterial elasticity may result in diminished blood supply to, for instance, the legs and the brain, resulting in pain on exertion in the calf muscles and dizziness, respectively. In addition, there may be a delay in the circulatory adjustments required when an individual quickly stands up from a lying or sitting position. The delay results in an abrupt drop in systolic blood pressure known as *orthostatic hypotension*.

For blood pressure measurements, it is not unusual to have a slight increase in the systolic pressure while the diastolic pressure remains the same. For many years, isolated systolic hypertension was considered to be "normal" in older adults and was frequently not treated. Newer evidence indicates that a systolic pressure at or greater than 140 mmHg is as problematic in older adults as in younger ones and should be as aggressively treated with antihypertensive agents, diet, and exercise. Obese older adults with hypertension will have pathophysiologic changes affecting the heart, blood vessels, and kidneys. Damage to the renal system with comorbid cardiovascular disease increases the client's risk of death (Porth, 2015). The reduction in blood pressure will preserve kidney function and reduce heart disease and stroke risk.

Health promotion activities are aimed at detecting and reducing risks for cardiovascular disease. To detect risks, blood pressure and cholesterol levels should be checked annually and more frequently with abnormal results. To reduce the risk of cardiovascular disease, the nurse should inform the older adult about the importance of the following: smoking cessation (if applicable), maintaining ideal body weight, exercising daily, avoiding foods high in sodium and fat and eating fruits and vegetables, and discussing the use of low-dose aspirin therapy with the primary care provider (Miller, 2019).

DRUG CAPSULE

Angiotensin-Converting Enzyme Inhibitor: enalapril and thiazide diuretic hydrochlorothiazide

A 65-year-old male client has been experiencing headaches and edema in his lower extremities. On three occasions, his systolic blood pressure has been greater than 150 and his diastolic greater than 100. The primary care provider prescribes enalapril (Vasotec) 10 mg orally every day and hydrochlorothiazide (Microzide) 25 mg orally every morning.

THE CLIENT TAKING MEDICATIONS FOR HYPERTENSION

Thiazide diuretics are used as monotherapy or in combination with angiotensin-converting enzyme (ACE) inhibitors, angiotensin-receptor blockers (ARBs) or calcium-channel blockers (CCBs).

Due to the narrowing of the arterial walls by sclerosis, the workload on the heart increases. This activity can lead to hypertrophy of the myocardial tissue, leading to heart failure. Necrosis may develop in arteries, and the arteries may rupture if high blood pressure is sustained.

Enalapril is an ACE inhibitor that blocks the conversion of angiotensin I to the potent constrictor angiotensin II. Blocking the production of angiotensin II results in a decrease of vascular constriction and a decrease in the production of aldosterone, reducing the retention of sodium and water. The ACE inhibitor will also inhibit the breakdown of bradykinin, prolonging vasodilating effects.

Hydrochlorothiazide decreases the reabsorption of sodium, water, chloride, and bicarbonate in the distal convoluted tubule. It is used to treat hypertension with edema. The following information is applicable to all medications administered to lower blood pressure unless a specific medication is identified.

NURSING RESPONSIBILITIES

- Assess the client's response to medication and the blood pressure, which should be less than 120 systolic and less than 80 diastolic (American Heart Association, 2017).
- Assess for hypotension with the initial dose of enalapril.
- Assess for acute hypotension.
- Monitor serum potassium level for hyperkalemia.
- Assess for decrease in lower extremity edema.
- Assess for persistent cough.

CLIENT AND FAMILY TEACHING

- Explain the drug regimen and the action of the medications to reduce blood pressure.
- Teach the client to avoid using salt substitutes due to the risk of hyperkalemia.
- Instruct to control weight, salt, and fat intake.
- Instruct to notify primary care provider with symptoms of dizziness or feeling faint, indicative of hypotension.
- Instruct that treatment of hypertension is long term (Frandsen & Pennington, 2018).

Gastrointestinal

Age-related changes in the gastrointestinal system include the following:

- Periodontal disease can lead to tooth loss. With age, tooth enamel becomes harder and more brittle, making teeth more susceptible to fractures. The root of the tooth shrinks, and the gingiva retracts. The bones that support the teeth decrease in density and height, all leading to tooth loss.
- Reduced production of saliva may lead to xerostomia (dry mouth) and make the oral mucosa more susceptible to infection.
- Decreased esophageal motility can slow the esophageal emptying process.
- Stomach motility and emptying time are decreased. Also, a higher pH of the stomach contributes to increased incidence of gastric irritation in the older adult.
- The production of intrinsic factor (protein needed to make vitamin B_{12}) is decreased, leading to pernicious anemia.
- Intestinal absorption, motility, and blood flow are decreased.

Health promotion teaching for older adults includes effective oral hygiene and preventive dental care (e.g., semiannual teeth cleaning). Nutrition is important, including appropriate diet and sufficient fluid intake. Maintenance of a regular bowel routine is helpful, and screening for colorectal cancer is important (e.g., annual fecal occult blood test, sigmoidoscopy every 5 years, and colonoscopy every 10 years) (Miller, 2019).

Urinary

The excretory function of the kidney diminishes with age but usually not significantly below normal levels unless a disease process intervenes. The kidney's filtering abilities may also be impaired; thus, waste products may be filtered and excreted more slowly. For this reason, the nurse should be aware of whether medications that are administered are excreted via the kidney or liver. Drugs that are metabolized predominantly in the kidney may accumulate in the older adult, and the nurse should watch for signs of toxicity.

More noticeable changes are those related to the bladder. Complaints of urinary urgency and urinary frequency are common. The capacity of the bladder and its ability to completely empty diminish with age. Many older adults need to void during the night (nocturia) and may experience retention of residual urine, predisposing them to bladder infections.

Although older adults are susceptible to urinary incontinence (UI) because of changes in the kidney and bladder, UI is *never* normal. The nurse must promptly investigate UI, particularly when of new onset. Urinary incontinence has many ill effects on older adults, including social isolation, falls, and skin breakdown.

The nurse can teach the following health promotion activities for good urinary function:

- Drink sufficient fluids daily (e.g., 8 to 10 glasses of noncaffeinated liquid).
- Drink fluids even if not thirsty. (The thirst mechanism in older adults is diminished.)
- Avoid foods that can irritate the bladder (e.g., sugar, caffeine, alcohol, chocolate, artificial sweeteners, and spicy and acidic foods).
- Practice pelvic muscle exercises to stop or control stress incontinence.
- The nurse should explain that incontinence is not a normal change related to aging.

Genitals

Degenerative changes in the gonads are gradual in men. Production of testosterone continues, and the testes can produce sperm well into old age although there is a gradual decrease in the number of sperm produced. In women, the degenerative changes in the ovaries are noted by the cessation of menses in middle age during the menopause.

Changes in the gonads of older women result from diminished secretion of the ovarian hormones. Some changes, such as the shrinking of the uterus and ovaries, go unnoticed. Other changes are obvious. The breasts atrophy, and lubricating vaginal secretions are reduced. Reduced natural lubrication may be the cause of painful intercourse, which may be addressed through the use of water-soluble lubricants.

The older man will notice several age-related changes in his sexual response and performance, but it is important for both the client and nurse to know that sexual response and performance should be present in the older adult. There is a decline in sex hormones, with a more gradual decline in the male than the female (Miller, 2019). For both men and women, the major age-related change in sexual response is timing. It takes longer to become sexually aroused, longer to complete intercourse, and longer before sexual arousal can occur again. In general, the older man's libido may decrease, but it does not disappear. If an older man reports a loss in sexual interest, the nurse should be as concerned as when a younger man reports a loss of interest in sexual activity. Older men achieve an erection that is less firm than in younger men but still capable of penetration. Ejaculation may take longer to occur, and the older man may have difficulty anticipating or delaying ejaculation. During orgasm, the urethral contractions are decreased, and there is a decrease in seminal fluid and lessened force of ejaculation (Tabloski, 2019).

The risk of erectile dysfunction (ED) increases with each decade of age (Tabloski, 2019). The many possible causes of ED include atherosclerosis, diabetes, hypertension, medications, and psychologic factors. Various treatment options are available, such as oral medication, vacuum pump devices, penile implants, and drugs injected into the penis. Oral medication is the first line of therapy used if there are no contraindications to the drug. Sildenafil (Viagra), vardenafil (Levitra), and tadalafil (Cialis) are the three oral medications used for ED.

Older women also experience changes in their sexual responses. Sexual dysfunction in older women may be related to an imbalance in the neurotransmitters that increase sexual desire, lowered estrogen levels, cardiovascular disease that decreases normal blood flow, joint pain, pharmacologic adverse effects, or psychosocial or sociocultural issues. Women may experience vaginal dryness, vaginal bleeding with intercourse, reduced sexual response, and inability to experience sexual arousal (Mayo Clinic, 2018). The clitoris remains an important part of orgasm, but it may become irritated more easily because the clitoral hood is less protective than in younger women. During orgasm, the uterus will contract less frequently, but the contractions remain vigorous, and orgasm is as intense as in younger women.

The nurse needs excellent communication skills when providing health education about sexual function to the older adult. It is important to avoid the use of medical terminology. A quiet, private room to discuss sensitive issues related to sexuality is essential. Older adults are fully capable of enjoying sexual activity. If they experience problems with sexual function, they are encouraged to seek professional advice from their primary care provider or other appropriate healthcare professional (Miller, 2019).

Psychosocial Aging

A number of theories have attempted to explain psychosocial aging. These theories focus on behavior and attitude changes during the aging process. One of the earliest, **disengagement theory**, developed in the early 1960s, proposed that aging involves mutual withdrawal (disengagement) between the older adult and others in the older adult's environment (Tabloski, 2019). It has been widely criticized for the assumption that disengagement is appropriate for the older adult. According to Havighurst's (1972) **activity theory**, the best way to age is to stay active physically and mentally. The **continuity theory** proposes that individuals maintain their values, habits, and behavior in old age. An individual who is accustomed to having others around will continue to do so, and the individual who prefers not to be involved with others is more likely to disengage (Tabloski, 2019). This theory accounts for the great variety of behavior seen in older adults.

According to Erikson, the developmental task at this time is ego integrity versus despair. Individuals who attain ego integrity view life with a sense of wholeness and derive satisfaction from past accomplishments. They view death as an acceptable completion of life. Individuals who develop integrity accept "one's one and only life cycle" (Erikson, 1963, p. 263). By contrast, individuals who despair often believe they have made poor choices during life and wish they could live life over.

Acknowledging that the young-old and old-old differ not only in physical characteristics but also in psychosocial responses, many individuals have difficulty with Erikson's singular developmental task. Peck (1968) proposed the following three developmental tasks of the older adult in contrast to Erikson's task of ego integrity versus despair:

1. Ego differentiation versus work-role preoccupation
2. Body transcendence versus body preoccupation
3. Ego transcendence versus ego preoccupation.

For details about these tasks, see Chapter 23 ∞.

Retirement

The ability to retire at the age of 65 is becoming increasingly more challenging for older adults based on the changes within the U.S. labor force. Economic risk has risen in the past several years. Today's seniors may lack the assets needed to retire. Complicating this situation are rising healthcare costs and inadequate monthly income to meet the needs of seniors. According to Morley (2017), with the rate of inflation at 3% per year and the longevity of life in retirement, the money baby boomers retire with will be worth at least one-half of what it is worth today. Older adults may find that their retirement income has not kept up with inflation. They may need to continue working to meet medical, insurance, and housing costs. These older adults must also adopt a healthy lifestyle (Morley, 2017).

Retirement can be a time when projects or recreational activities deferred for a long time can be pursued, or it can be a difficult time of adjustment. Either way, retirement requires a process of adaptation (Figure 26.4 ■). Retired individuals are no longer governed by an alarm clock and can get up and go to bed when they please. Physical

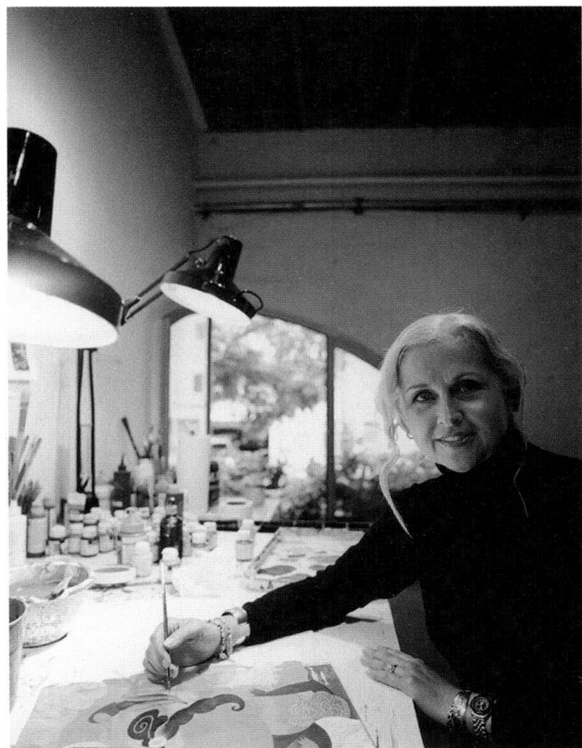

Figure 26.4 ■ Many older adults find creative outlets during retirement.
Zia Soleil/Getty Images.

activity is often a measure of how an individual's health and wellness are judged. Those who are accustomed to activity find many outlets, including jobs, community projects, travel, volunteer services, intellectual or recreational pursuits, or hobbies (Figure 26.5 ■). Research in gerontological exercise physiology indicates that the maintenance of a physically active lifestyle delays or improves age changes associated with cardiovascular, respiratory, and musculoskeletal function. Physical inactivity, on the other hand, is a risk factor for many chronic diseases experienced by older adults, including obesity, diabetes, cardiovascular disease, and respiratory diseases (Touhy & Jett, 2016).

The lifestyle of later years is to a large degree formulated in youth. Individuals who attempt suddenly to refocus and enrich their lives at retirement usually have difficulty. Those who learned early in life to live well-balanced and fulfilling lives are generally more successful in retirement. The woman who has been concerned only with the accomplishments of her children or the man who has been concerned only with his salary and job status can be left with a feeling of emptiness when children leave and the job no longer exists. The later years can foster a sense of integrity and continuity, or they can be years of despair.

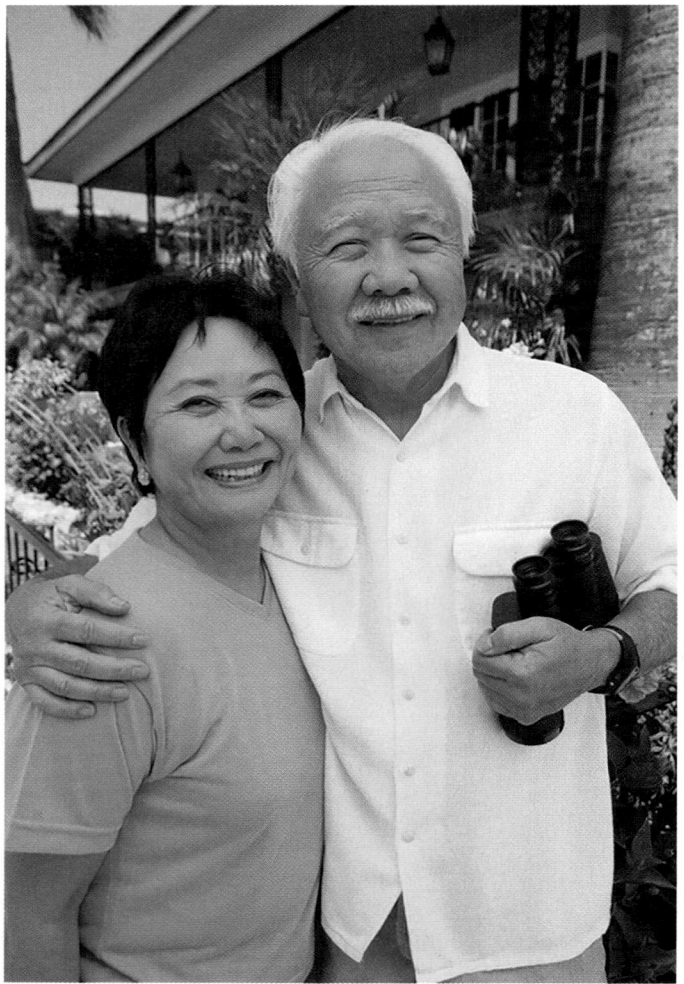

Figure 26.5 ■ Retirement provides time for enjoying hobbies.
sirtravelalot/Shutterstock.

E-Health

In retirement, seniors may take a class to learn to use a computer, or they may retire having already learned computer skills. The term **e-health** is used to describe the use of technology in the delivery of healthcare and health information. Seniors have been the fastest-growing age group using the internet. They are now ranked as the fastest-growing users of social media. The use of social networking sites by seniors increases so that seniors can stay connected with kin and non-kin relations (Yu, McCammon, Ellison, & Langa, 2016). Searches on the internet often include healthcare or disease information. Blogs and online discussions are utilized by seniors to search for information related to living with chronic disease and answers to health-related questions (Mauk, 2018).

Economic Change

The financial needs of older adults vary considerably. Although most need less money for clothing, entertainment, and work, and although some own their homes outright, costs continue to rise, making it difficult for some to manage. Food and medical costs alone are often a financial burden. Adequate financial resources enable the older adult to remain independent.

Problems with income are often related to low retirement benefits, lack of pension plans for many workers, and the increased length of the retirement years. Older individuals of color and women often have greater financial problems than older White men (Eliopoulos, 2018). Older women of all ages usually have lower incomes than men, and the oldest women may be the poorest.

Nurses should be aware of the costs of healthcare. For example, while assisting a client in planning a diet, the nurse must consider which foods the client can afford to buy. The nurse or the client can request the primary care provider to order lower-priced medications or assist the older client in applying for medication assistance programs operated by pharmaceutical companies. In addition, the supplies used in a client's care should be as economical as possible.

Grandparenting

Grandparents traditionally provide gifts, money, and other forms of support (e.g., babysitting) for younger family members. They also provide a sense of continuity, family heritage, rituals, and folklore (Giger, 2017). However, the rate of grandparents being the primary caregiver for their grandchildren is increasing. The major reasons for grandparents raising grandchildren include substance abuse, incarceration, teen pregnancy, emotional problems, and parental death. The terms used to describe families in which grandparents serve as the parents are kinship families, grandfamilies, or skipped-generation families. These families provide the primary care of the child or children. Lee and Blitz (2016) conducted a qualitative study in which they interviewed grandparents who are raising their grandchildren. The study identified how the grandparents were engaged in their grandchildren's upbringing from school age to the high school years. Five major themes emerged during these interviews. Grandparents stated they often deal with role conflict due to the fact they are grandparents and not parents when engaged in the child's school environment. They were challenged when communicating with their grandchildren's teachers and with any bullying issues. They identified poor relationships and difficulty in communicating with teachers due to the teachers' lack of understanding of multigenerational caregiving. They also identified that they were dealing with their own aging issues. Grandparents caring for grandchildren often experience stress, anxiety, financial hardship, and deteriorating health. For example, they must cope with their own chronic health problems while caring for their grandchildren.

It is important for nurses to assess and help maintain the health of the grandparents.

Relocation

During late adulthood, many individuals experience relocation. A variety of factors may lead to this decision. The house or apartment may be too large or too expensive. The work involved in maintaining the house may become burdensome or impossible for an older individual or couple. Some older adults with decreased mobility desire living arrangements that are all on one floor or need more accessible bathroom facilities.

Making the decision to move is stressful. Moving to an apartment may mean leaving the comfort of the family home and the neighbors and friends of several decades. Some older adults need to move nearer to their children for general support and supervision. For many, this decision is difficult and stressful. For others, relocation is voluntary. The individual may be seeking a more moderate climate with better recreational facilities geared to a more leisurely lifestyle. The adjustment will be much easier for the older adult making a voluntary move.

More living choices and options are available for older adults today. Depending on their needs, examples include the following:

- ***Assisted living.*** This is a facility that meets the needs of the older adult (e.g., wide doorways, grab bars in the bathroom, a call light). Various degrees of personal care assistance may be provided.
- ***Adult daycare.*** The older adult who lives at home can attend a daycare center that provides health and social services to older individuals. While the older adult is at daycare, the caregiver has a respite from the daily care tasks.
- ***Adult foster care and group homes.*** These programs offer services to individuals who can care for themselves but require some form of supervision for safety purposes.

Some older adults, however, must relocate to long-term care facilities or nursing homes. The decision to enter a nursing home is frequently made when older adults can no longer care for themselves, often because of problems with mobility and memory impairment. The facilities in nursing homes differ in many ways and offer varying degrees of independence to the residents. All provide meals but vary in providing other services, such as assistance with hygiene and dressing, physical therapy or exercise, recreational activities, transportation services, and medical and nursing supervision.

Nurses in hospitals should find out whether a client is being discharged to a nursing home or to a private home. Nursing homes require appropriate information to provide for continuity of care. Clients returning home, however, may require the assistance of a home care nurse.

Maintaining Independence and Self-Esteem

Most older Americans thrive on independence. It is important to them to be able to look after themselves even if they have to struggle to do so. Although it may be difficult for younger family members to watch an older individual completing tasks in a slow, determined way, older adults need this sense of accomplishment. Children might notice that the aging father or mother with failing vision cannot keep the kitchen as clean as before. The aging parent may be slower and less meticulous in carpentry tasks or gardening. To maintain the older adult's sense of self-respect, nurses and family members need to encourage them to do as much as possible for themselves, provided that safety is maintained. Many young individuals, including nurses, mistakenly think that they are being helpful to older adults when they take over for them and do the job much faster and more efficiently.

Nurses need to acknowledge the older adult's ability to think, reason, and make decisions. Most older adults are willing to listen to suggestions and advice, but they do not want to be ordered around. The nurse can support a decision by an older adult even if eventually the decision is reversed because of failing health.

Older adults appreciate the same thoughtfulness, consideration, and acceptance of their abilities as younger adults do. There is as much diversity among older adults as there is in any other population group, and the nurse should be just as wary of stereotyping older adults as with stereotyping any other group. The values and standards held by older adults need to be accepted, whether they are related to ethical, religious, or household matters. For example, the nurse should respect an older individual's decision to hang the laundry outside rather than to use a dryer or to cook on a conventional stove rather than in a microwave oven.

Facing Death and Grieving

Well-adjusted aging couples usually thrive on companionship. Many couples rely increasingly on their partners for this company and may have few outside friends. Great bonds of affection and closeness can develop during this period of aging together and nurturing each other. When a mate dies, the remaining partner inevitably experiences feelings of loss, emptiness, and loneliness. Many are capable of living alone and can manage to do so; however, reliance on younger family members may increase as age advances and ill health occurs. Some widows and widowers remarry, particularly the latter because most widowers are less inclined than widows to maintain a household. More women than men face bereavement and solitude because women usually live longer. Following the death of a spouse, women experience burdens due to the complexities related to financial and administrative obligations that follow the death. Both women and men may also experience alterations in health due to the stress of caring for the spouse (Matzo, 2019). Older adults are often reminded of the brevity of life by the death of friends. It is a time when they review their lives with happiness or regret. Feelings of serenity or guilt and inadequacy can arise. Survivor coping ability improves when the individual is aware that death and bereavement can lead to growth (Touhy & Jett, 2016). This coping can result from the anticipatory grief related to the premature detachment from the individual who is dying. It is the goal of the gerontological nurse to support those who are grieving. See Chapter 43 ∞ for a discussion about facing death.

Nurses help clients who are alone a great deal to adjust their living arrangements or lifestyle so that they have more companionship. Moving to a retirement home that has other individuals in similar circumstances and organized social activities is one example. Many communities provide social centers for older adults, for example, drop-in centers or community centers that offer day trips for seniors. Nurses refer clients to services and encourage them to obtain companionship.

Cognitive Abilities and Aging

Piaget's phases of cognitive development end with the formal operations phase. However, considerable research on cognitive abilities and aging is currently being conducted. Intellectual capacity includes perception, cognitive agility, memory, and learning.

Perception

Perception, or the ability to interpret the environment, depends on the acuteness of the senses. If the aging adult's senses are impaired, the ability to perceive the environment and react appropriately is diminished. Changes in the nervous system may also affect perceptual capacity.

Changes in cognitive structures occur as an individual ages. The brain loses mass with aging. In addition, blood flow to the brain decreases, the meninges thicken, and brain metabolism slows. As yet, little is known about the effect of these physical changes on the cognitive functioning of the older adult. Lifelong mental activity, particularly verbal activity, helps the older adult retain a high level of cognitive function and helps maintain long-term memory.

Cognitive Agility

In older adults, changes in cognitive abilities are more often a difference in speed than in ability. Overall, the older adult maintains intelligence, problem-solving, judgment, creativity, and other well-practiced cognitive skills. Intellectual loss generally reflects a disease process such as atherosclerosis, which causes the blood vessels to narrow and diminishes perfusion of nutrients to the brain. Most older adults do not experience cognitive impairments. Dementia affects 2.4 to 5.5 million Americans. Mild cognitive impairment is different from dementia because the client is able to perform ADLs independently. Touhy and Jett (2016) conducted a qualitative research study on clients with mild cognitive impairment. At the start of every session, the older client was read a story and then engaged in activities to test memory. This activity advanced verbal skills and allowed for creative memories. It is important to note that memory impairment is more prevalent in individuals over age 85 than individuals between the ages of 65 and 69. Cognitive impairment that interferes with normal life is not considered part of normal aging. A decline in intellectual abilities that interferes with social or occupational functions should always be regarded as abnormal. Family members should be advised to seek prompt medical evaluation.

Memory

Memory is also a component of intellectual capacity that involves the following steps:

1. Momentary perception of stimuli from the environment, referred to as **sensory memory**.
2. Storage in **short-term memory** (information held in the brain for immediate use or what one has in mind at a given moment). An example of this type of memory is when you call information for a telephone number and remember the number only for the brief time needed to dial the number. Short-term memory also deals with activities of the recent past of minutes to a few hours, often referred to as **recent memory**.
3. Encoding, during which the information leaves short-term memory and enters **long-term memory**, the repository for information stored for periods longer than 72 hours and usually weeks and years. Memories of childhood friends, teachers, and events are stored in long-term memory. Older individuals who remember the flowers in their wedding bouquet or the names of the boys on their dance card are drawing from long-term memory.

In older adults, retrieval of information from long-term memory can be slower, especially if the information is not frequently used. Most age-related differences, however, occur in short-term memory. Older adults tend to forget the recent past. This forgetfulness can be improved with the use of memory aids, by making notes or lists, and by placing objects in consistent locations.

Learning

Older clients need additional time for learning, largely because of the problem of retrieving information. Motivation is also important. Older clients have more difficulty than younger ones in learning information they do not consider meaningful; therefore, the nurse should be particularly careful to discover what is meaningful to the older client before attempting client education. See Chapter 17 ∞.

Moral Reasoning

Much of the theoretical and empirical work related to moral development in older adults was conducted in the 1980s, and few current studies can be found. According to Kohlberg (1984), moral development is completed in the early adult years. Kohlberg hypothesized that an older adult at the preconventional level obeys rules to avoid pain and the displeasure of others. At stage 1, an individual defines good and bad in relation to self, whereas older individuals at stage 2 may act to meet another's needs as well as their own. Older adults at the conventional level follow society's rules of conduct in response to the expectations of others. Pratt, Diessner, Pratt, Hunsberger, and Pancer (1996) found that moral reasoning does not decline in old age.

Gilligan (1982), however, challenged Kohlberg's stages as not being applicable to women. She developed a theory of moral reasoning based on the concept of caring. She believed that women base moral judgments on connectedness to others and the value of relationships, whereas Kohlberg based his stages on the concepts of justice, objectivity, and preservation of rights. Subsequent research has demonstrated that men and women make moral decisions differently, representing the theories of Kohlberg (men) and Gilligan (women) along gender lines. Older adults, however, begin to make moral decisions that are consistent with *both* Kohlberg and Gilligan. Older men consider relationships, as well as justice, in moral decisions, and older women add justice to the factors they consider in moral situations.

The value and belief patterns that are important to older adults may be different from those held by younger adults because they developed during a time that was very different from today. Cultural background, life experiences, gender, religion, and socioeconomic status all influence an individual's values. The nurse must identify and consider the specific values of the older client when planning nursing care.

Spirituality and Aging

Older adults can contemplate new religious and philosophic views and try to understand ideas missed previously or interpreted differently. The older adult may derive a sense of worth by sharing experiences or views. In contrast, the older adult who has not matured spiritually may feel impoverishment or despair as the drive for economic and professional success lessens.

Many older adults take their faith and religious practice very seriously and display a high level of spirituality. It would be a mistake, however, to assume that religiosity increases with age. Today's older adults grew up in a time when religion was much more important than it is for younger adults today. The continuing participation in religious practices provides an inner strength that enhances coping. In the event the client wishes to engage in prayer or attend religious services, it is the nurse's role to support the practice of religion. If the nurse is unfamiliar with the client's religious practices, referrals should be made to other members of the healthcare team with skills and knowledge in that area (Eliopoulos, 2018). Many older adults have strong religious convictions and continue to attend religious meetings or services. Involvement in religion often helps the older adult to resolve issues related to the meaning of life, adversity, or good fortune. Religion may also be an important coping resource, leading to enhanced well-being. The "old-old" individual who cannot attend formal services often continues religious participation in a more private manner. Assisting the older adult to participate in religious and spiritual practices is an important nursing responsibility.

Health Problems

Health problems that older adults may experience include injuries, chronic disabling disease such as hypertension and arthritis, drug abuse and misuse, alcoholism, dementia, and mistreatment. The leading causes of death in individuals ages 65 and over are heart disease, cancer, cerebrovascular disease (stroke), lower respiratory disease, pneumonia or influenza, and diabetes mellitus (FIFAS, 2016).

Injuries

Injury prevention is a major concern for older adults. Falls are a leading cause of morbidity and mortality among older adults (Edelman & Kudzma, 2018). Because vision is limited, reflexes are slowed, and bones are brittle, caution is required in climbing stairs, driving a car, and even walking. Driving, particularly night driving, requires caution because the accommodation of the eye to light is impaired and peripheral vision is diminished. Older adults need to learn to turn the head before changing lanes and should not rely on side vision, for example, when crossing a street. Driving in fog or other hazardous conditions should be avoided.

Fires are a hazard for the older adult with a failing memory. Older adults may forget that the iron or stove is left on or may not extinguish a cigarette completely. Because of reduced sensitivity to pain and heat, care must be taken to prevent burns when the individual bathes or uses heating devices.

Many older adults experience hypothermia each year, with some of these cases leading to death. **Hypothermia** is a body temperature below normal. A lowered metabolism and loss of normal insulation from thinning subcutaneous tissue decrease the older client's ability to retain heat. The older adult who spends time outdoors in cold weather or who does not turn on the heat in the home is at significant risk for hypothermia.

Nurses can help older adults make the home environment safe by identifying and correcting specific hazards, for example, installing handrails on staircases. The nurse teaches the importance of taking only prescribed medications and contacting a health professional at the first indication of intolerance to them.

Individuals with AD or other types of dementia experience increasing safety needs as their condition deteriorates. Judgment becomes impaired as the disease progresses, and some environmental modification is needed to help the older adult remain safe. Some of these are keeping poisons and medications out of reach (preferably locked up), taking knobs off kitchen stoves to prevent burns and fires, and putting special locks on doors for individuals who tend to wander. Attention should be given to these potential problems whether the client lives at home or is in a healthcare facility.

Guidelines for injury prevention for the older adult are detailed in Chapter 32 ∞.

Chronic Disabling Illness

Many older adults function well within the community without impairments; others are afflicted with one or more chronic illnesses that may seriously impair their functioning. Examples of these are arthritis, osteoporosis, heart disease, stroke, obstructive lung disease, hearing and visual alterations, and cognitive dysfunctions. In addition, acute illnesses such as pneumonia and fractures and trauma from falls, motor vehicle crashes, or other incidents may create chronic health problems. Chronic illness brings many changes to the client and the family members. The client, for example, may need increasing help with the ADLs of ambulation, feeding, hygiene, and so on; healthcare expenses often escalate and may become an economic concern; family roles may need to be altered; and family members may need to change their lifestyle to meet caregiving needs.

Drug Abuse and Misuse

The use of prescription drugs has increased over the past 40 years due to increased medical need, prescription drug development, drug advertising, and the expansion of prescription drug insurance coverage. The CDC (2017) reports that prescription drug utilization increased by 17.2% in those 65 and older. The increased use of prescriptions leads to concerns related to polypharmacy. The definition of *polypharmacy* is taking five or more medications. Added to this, older adults may purchase over-the-counter (OTC) drugs to remedy common discomforts related to aging, such as constipation, sleep disturbance, and joint pain. The ingestion of numerous medications increases the client's risk for drug interactions, adverse drug events, and nonadherence (CDC, 2017). During the past few years, the use of vitamins, food supplements, and herbal remedies has increased. These agents fall under the category of OTC drugs and are often not reported by clients as part of their medication regimen. An accurate assessment should include a listing of all these agents. Many of these agents have not had adequate testing for effectiveness, side effects, or interactions with other medications.

The complexities involved in the self-administration of medication may lead to a variety of misuse situations, including taking too much or too little medication, combining alcohol and medication, combining prescribed medications with OTC drugs causing increased risk for drug interactions and adverse events, taking medications at the wrong time, or taking someone else's medication. Other potential misuse situations occur when more than one primary care provider prescribes medications and the client fails to tell each primary care provider what has been previously prescribed.

Additionally, the pharmacodynamics of drugs are altered in older adults. The variations in absorption, distribution, metabolism, and excretion of drugs are related to physiologic changes associated with aging. These variations are discussed in Chapter 35 ∞.

Most older adults living independently in the community take their medications with no supervision. Therefore, education about medications is important for safe medication-taking behaviors. The following strategies, taught by the nurse, can promote safe medication use by the older adult:

- Write a list of all the medications you are taking, including OTC drugs and herbal supplements. Include any medication allergies on the list. Keep the list current and carry it in your purse or billfold.
- Know the reason you are taking each medication. Ask your primary care practitioner the reason for any new medication.
- Consider using a "pill organizer" system to help you remember to take your medications. This is helpful if you have many medications to take each day.
- Ask your pharmacist for easy-to-open containers if you have difficulty opening the medications.
- If possible, obtain all medications from the same pharmacy. This allows the pharmacist to monitor for drug duplications and interactions.

Alcoholism

There are two types of older alcoholics: those who began drinking alcohol in their youth and those who began excessive alcohol use later in life to help them cope with the changes and problems of their older years. Approximately one-third of older alcoholics are late-onset drinkers (after age 60), and that number includes a higher number of women (Touhy & Jett, 2016, p. 339).

Chronic drinking has major effects on all body systems, causes progressive liver and kidney damage, damages the stomach and related organs, and slows mental response, frequently leading to injuries and death. Alcohol interacts with various drugs, altering the normal effect of the medication on the body. Some medications have an increased effect when taken with alcohol (e.g., anticoagulants and narcotics), whereas the action of other medications (e.g., antibiotics) is inhibited. For the older adult who has a chronic illness and takes many medications, the combination of drugs and alcohol can lead to a serious drug overdose.

Clients with alcoholism should not be stereotyped or prejudged by the nurse. Rather, they should be accepted, listened to, and offered help. The nurse should assess the number and type of alcoholic beverages consumed as well as the pattern and frequency of consumption. It is important for the nurse to discuss any medications the client is taking and review the side effects and interaction effects of alcohol and medication. The role of the nurse is to act as a client advocate and facilitate the treatment of the drinking problem in addition to the prevention of possible complications.

Dementia

Dementia is a progressive loss of cognitive function. It is critical that dementia be differentiated from delirium, which is an acute and reversible syndrome. Both may be characterized by changes in memory, judgment, language, mathematical calculation, abstract reasoning, and problem-solving ability. The most common causes of *delirium* are infection, medications, and dehydration. The most common type of *dementia* is AD, of which the cause is unknown. The course of this disease is slow and insidious, affecting about 5.8 million individuals in the United States. Of this number, in those 65 and older, it affects 5.6 million individuals. One in 10 individuals over the age of 65 is affected, and 17% of individuals age 75–84 have AD. In addition, more women than men are affected. Unless a prevention or cure is found, it is estimated that 13.8 million Americans 65 and older will have AD by the year 2050 (Alzheimer's Association, 2019).

The symptoms of AD vary from client to client. The most prominent symptoms are cognitive dysfunctions, including a decline in memory, learning, attention, judgment, orientation, and language skills. The symptoms are progressive, leading to a steady decline in cognitive and physical abilities, lasting between 7 and 15 years, and ending in death. In the last stage, the client requires total assistance, is unable to communicate, is incontinent, and is often unable to walk. There is no cure or specific treatment for AD. Several drugs have been developed, but none has been shown consistently to reverse the progression of the disease.

The Alzheimer's Association (2019) reported that an estimated 18.5 billion hours of unpaid assistance were provided to AD clients. There are three primary reasons why care is provided in the home environment: the need to keep the client at home, the proximity of the caregiver to the client with dementia, and the caregiver's obligation as a spouse or partner. The burden of care is frequently on women—wives and daughters—who are themselves aging. AD is devastating for the families and caregivers of its victims. Caregivers may experience physical and emotional exhaustion while rendering continuous care to their loved one. Caregiving is complicated when the client no longer recognizes family members or close friends. The nurse's responsibility is to provide supportive nursing care, accurate information, and referral assistance when placement in a nursing care facility is deemed necessary. Help by the nurse in facilitating the provision of respite services may also be helpful to the caregiver. Ongoing nursing assessment of both the client and the caregiver is important, especially as the client's condition deteriorates.

Mistreatment of Older Adults

Approximately 1.6 to 2 million Americans over the age of 65 have been abused, neglected, or exploited by someone on whom they depend for protection and care (National Council on Child Abuse & Family Violence, n.d.). Mistreatment of older adults may affect either gender. However, the victims most often are women over 75 years of

DRUG CAPSULE

Parasympathomimetic or Cholinesterase Inhibitor: donepezil (Aricept)

THE CLIENT WITH ALZHEIMER'S DISEASE

Cholinesterase inhibitors improve cholinergic function by inhibiting acetylcholinesterase, thus increasing the amount of acetylcholine in the brain.

In normal brain function, acetylcholine is an essential neurotransmitter and plays an important role in cognitive function, including memory storage and retrieval (Frandsen & Pennington, 2018).

Cholinesterase inhibitors do not alter AD but may stabilize the older client at the current level of dementia or lessen symptoms for a short period of time (e.g., average of 6 months).

NURSING RESPONSIBILITIES

- Assess the cognitive ability of the client.
- Monitor heart rate because bradycardia may occur.

CLIENT AND FAMILY TEACHING

- Explain that donepezil may cause dizziness and that the client may want to take the medication in the evening before going to bed.
- Teach that the medication can be taken with or without food.
- Emphasize the importance of taking the medication every day. A missed dose should be skipped, and the client should return to the regular schedule the next day.
- Explain that the medication is started at a lower dose, with a gradual increase in dosage. Higher doses may not increase the effects but may increase the side effects (gastrointestinal disturbance, sleep disturbance, and sedation).

Note: Prior to administering any medication, review all aspects in a current drug handbook or other reliable source.

age who are physically or mentally impaired and dependent for care on the abuser. The abuse may be physical, psychologic, or emotional in nature. Sexual abuse, financial abuse, violation of human or civil rights, and active or passive neglect have also been documented.

When mistreatment involves physical neglect, victims may experience dehydration, malnutrition, and oversedation. The victim may be deprived of necessary articles, such as glasses, hearing aids, or walkers. Psychologically, the individual may experience verbal assaults, threats, humiliation, or harassment. Abuse may also include the failure to provide appropriate medications or medical treatment, isolation, unreasonable confinement, lack of privacy, an unsafe environment, and involuntary servitude. Some are financially exploited by relatives who steal from them or misuse their property or funds. Others are beaten and even raped by family members. Most victims experience two or more forms of abuse.

Abuse or neglect of older adults may occur in private homes, senior citizens' homes, nursing homes, hospitals, and long-term care facilities. Many of the abusers are either sons or daughters; others include spouses, relatives (grandchildren, siblings, nieces, and nephews), and in some instances, healthcare providers.

Older adults at home may fail to report abuse or neglect for many reasons. They may be ashamed to admit that their children have mistreated them or fear retaliation if they seek help. They may fear being sent to an institution. They frequently lack financial resources or lack the mental capacity to be aware of abuse or neglect and report the situation. Examples of crimes are assault and financial abuse of an older adult who is physically or mentally incompetent and has no trustworthy friend or relative to help. In some instances, nurses can intervene by educating caregivers about the needs of older adults and available resources to provide increased home support. They should also report the situation to the appropriate individual in the healthcare agency.

Nurses should be familiar with the laws of their particular state regarding the reporting of suspected or known abuse. The legally competent adult cannot be forced, however, to leave the abusive situation and, in many cases, may decide to stay. If the client is not legally competent, court proceedings to attain guardianship can be initiated.

Health Assessment and Promotion

Assessment guidelines for the development of the older adult are shown in the accompanying Developmental Assessment Guidelines. Assessment activities include measurement of weight, height, and vital signs; observation of the skin for hydration status or presence of lesions; examination of visual acuity using the Snellen chart; examination of hearing acuity using the Weber and Rinne tests (see Chapter 29 ∞); and questions about the following:

- Usual dietary pattern
- Bowel or urinary elimination problems
- Activity, exercise, and sleep patterns
- Family and social activities and interests
- Reading, writing, or problem-solving difficulties
- Adjustment to retirement or the loss of a partner.

Healthcare professionals should also be alert for these signs:

- Symptoms of depression
- Risk factors for suicide
- Signs of abnormal bereavement
- Changes in cognitive function
- Medications that increase the risk of falls
- Signs of physical abuse or neglect
- Skin lesions (malignant and peripheral)
- Tooth decay, gingivitis, and loose teeth
- Peripheral arterial disease.

Older adults are usually concerned about their health and interested in information and behavioral strategies directed toward improving it. The nurse may wish to discuss some or all of the health promotion topics outlined in Box 26.1. These topics are discussed in detail in subsequent chapters throughout this text.

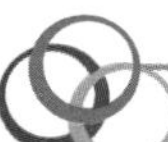

Developmental Assessment Guidelines — The Older Adult

In these three developmental areas, does the older adult do the following?

PHYSICAL DEVELOPMENT

- Adjust to physiologic changes (e.g., appearance, sensory-perceptual, musculoskeletal, neurologic, cardiovascular).
- Adapt lifestyle to diminishing energy and ability.
- Maintain vital signs (especially blood pressure) within normal range for age and gender.

PSYCHOSOCIAL DEVELOPMENT

- Manage retirement years in a satisfying manner.
- Participate in social and leisure activities.
- Have a social network of friends and support people.
- View life as worthwhile.
- Have high self-esteem.
- Gain support from value system and/or spiritual philosophy.
- Accept and adjust to the death of significant others.

DEVELOPMENT IN ACTIVITIES OF DAILY LIVING

- Exhibit healthy practices in nutrition, exercise, recreation, sleep patterns, and personal habits.
- Have the ability to care for self or to secure appropriate help with ADLs.
- Have satisfactory living arrangements and income to meet changing needs.

BOX 26.1 Health Promotion Guidelines for Older Adults

HEALTH TESTS AND SCREENING

- Total cholesterol and high-density lipoprotein measurement every 3 to 5 years until age 75
- Aspirin, 81 mg, daily, if in high-risk group
- Diabetes mellitus screen every 3 years, if in high-risk group
- Smoking cessation
- Screening mammogram every 1 to 2 years (women)
- Clinical breast exam annually (women)
- Women 30–65 years should have both a Pap test and an HPV test every 5 years. This is the preferred approach, but it is also OK to have a Pap test alone every 3 years (American Cancer Society, 2016).
- Annual digital rectal exam
- Annual prostate-specific antigen (PSA)
- Annual fecal occult blood test (FOBT)
- Sigmoidoscopy every 5 years; colonoscopy every 10 years
- Visual acuity screen annually
- Hearing screen annually
- Depression screen periodically
- Family violence screen periodically
- Height and weight measurements annually
- Sexually transmitted infection testing, if in high-risk group
- Annual flu vaccine if over age 65 or in high-risk group
- Pneumococcal vaccine at age 65 and every 10 years thereafter
- Single dose of shingles vaccine for adults 60 years of age or older
- Tetanus booster every 10 years

SAFETY

- Home safety measures to prevent falls, fire, burns, scalds, and electrocution
- Working smoke detectors and carbon monoxide detectors in the home
- Motor vehicle safety reinforcement, especially when driving at night
- Older driver skills evaluation (some states require for license renewal)
- Precautions to prevent pedestrian accidents

NUTRITION AND EXERCISE

- Importance of a well-balanced diet with fewer calories to accommodate lower metabolic rate and decreased physical activity
- Importance of sufficient amounts of vitamin D and calcium to prevent osteoporosis
- Nutritional and exercise factors that may lead to cardiovascular disease (e.g., obesity, cholesterol and fat intake, lack of exercise)
- Importance of 30 minutes of moderate physical activity daily; 20 minutes of vigorous physical activity 3 times per week

ELIMINATION

- Importance of adequate roughage in the diet, adequate exercise, and at least six 8-ounce glasses of fluid daily to prevent constipation

SOCIAL INTERACTIONS

- Encouraging intellectual and recreational pursuits
- Encouraging personal relationships that promote discussion of feelings, concerns, and fears
- Assessment of risk factors for maltreatment
- Availability of social community centers and programs for seniors

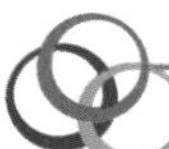

Critical Thinking Checkpoint

Alice Green, a 78-year-old female, has had a bone density scan as part of a regular physical exam and has been told that she has severe osteoporosis. Her primary care provider has ordered alendronate, which is supposed to maintain bone mass in clients with osteoporosis. She lives alone in her own home and is able to perform ADLs independently.

1. How would you define osteoporosis to Mrs. Green?
2. What risk factors related to osteoporosis should be included in an assessment of Mrs. Green?
3. Which of the risk factors are modifiable or can be altered by a change in lifestyle?
4. What medication teaching is essential when a client is taking medications to increase or maintain bone mass in osteoporosis?
5. What preventive measures should be taught to decrease the risk of fractures and to maintain bone mass?

Answers to Critical Thinking Checkpoint questions are available on the faculty resources website. Please consult with your instructor.

Chapter 26 Review

CHAPTER HIGHLIGHTS

- The older adult population is steadily growing and projected to outnumber the young population by the middle of the 21st century.
- Older adults are categorized into young-old (60–74 years), old (75–84) and oldest-old (85 and older).
- Older adults represent a diverse population in the United States. For example, women outnumber men, older Hispanics are the fastest-growing subpopulation group, and the majority of older adults rate their health as good.
- It is important for nurses to be aware of their own values and attitudes toward aging to avoid ageism and to examine whether myths or stereotypes influence their personal attitudes and beliefs.

- The gerontological nurse has many roles: care provider, teacher, manager, advocate, and research consumer.
- Older adults are primary users of healthcare services in different types of care settings, including acute care, rehabilitation, long-term care, and the community. Regardless of the setting, the older adult requires health assessment and health promotion.
- Several theories have been proposed to account for the biological aging process: wear-and-tear, endocrine, free-radical, genetic, cross-linking, and immunologic theories.
- Older adults experience many physical changes associated with aging. All body systems undergo change: integumentary, neuromuscular, sensory-perceptual, pulmonary, cardiovascular, gastrointestinal, and genitourinary.
- Psychosocial theories about aging include the disengagement, activity, and continuity theories.
- The older adult has to adjust to possible psychosocial changes, including retirement (which necessitates financial and social adjustments), grandparenting, relocation, increasing dependence on others, and coping with losses and death.
- The cognitive abilities of the healthy older adult undergo some changes in perception, cognitive agility, memory, and learning.
- In the realm of moral reasoning, most older adults begin to blend concepts of justice and caring relationships into their moral decision making.
- Many older adults take their faith and religious practice seriously and display a high level of spirituality.
- Health problems of older adults include injuries, chronic disabling illness, drug abuse and misuse, alcoholism, dementia, and mistreatment.
- Health promotion information for all adults needs to include positive health practices that can promote health and wellness. These include (a) recommended physical, visual, hearing, and dental assessments; (b) screenings for cardiovascular disease and tuberculosis; (c) breast and testicular self-examinations; (d) immunizations; (e) Papanicolaou smears for some older women; (f) safety precautions to prevent injuries; (g) the importance of appropriate nutrition and exercise; and (h) the importance of measures to prevent constipation.

TEST YOUR KNOWLEDGE

1. A nurse is working with clients in an assisted living facility. In the past month, there have been several deaths among the residents and their spouses. In helping the remaining residents deal with these deaths, the nurse understands that adjustment may be easier for which of the following residents?
   1. A resident who spent most of her days attending to her partner who is now deceased
   2. A resident who had a wide circle of friends, besides her spouse
   3. A resident who was not inclined to participate in any activities offered at the facility
   4. A resident who started to become more dependent on the nursing staff at the facility

2. A nurse in a long-term care facility is caring for several older adults with noticeable hearing loss. Which is the best way for the nurse to communicate with these clients?
   1. Speak slowly using the proper volume and as few words as possible.
   2. Write the information using large lettering.
   3. Speak in a low and distinct voice tone.
   4. Have the clients increase the volume on their hearing aids.

3. During care activities, an 80-year-old client talks about "the good old days" and often repeats the same stories. What action should the nurse plan?
   1. Request a psychological consult for the client.
   2. Support this as reminiscence therapy.
   3. Redirect the client to other topics of conversation.
   4. Vary caregivers assigned to the client.

4. The home health nurse evaluates an older adult for depression. The client's daughter is present and comments, "I don't see the need for this evaluation. Aren't all older adults depressed?" Which is the nurse's best initial response?
   1. "How many losses has your mother had?"
   2. "Your mother looks so depressed."
   3. "How long has she been depressed?"
   4. "Depression is not a normal part of aging."

5. An elderly client comes to the clinic reporting gastrointestinal problems, including frequent constipation and indigestion but denies any recent weight loss. What does the nurse initially recognize about these symptoms?
   1. They indicate a concern and could be caused by cancer.
   2. They indicate the need for an upper and lower GI X-ray series.
   3. They could be related to normal changes in muscle tone and activity.
   4. They are probably indicative of a gastric ulcer or colitis.

6. The nurse notices that when an 80-year-old man rises from a seated position, he uses both arms to push himself up, and he also "rocks" back and forth before finally standing. What is the most appropriate nursing intervention for this client?
   1. Suggest a referral to physical therapy for strengthening exercises.
   2. Request a waist restraint to remind the client not to stand by himself.
   3. Praise the client for his attempts to remain independent.
   4. Assist the client to rise by grasping both his shoulders and pulling forward.

7. A healthy 78-year-old woman who is considering marriage to a healthy 79-year-old neighbor tells the nurse that she wonders if they will be able to have sexual intercourse. Which is the nurse's most appropriate response?
   1. "Sexual activity may be too demanding for your heart."
   2. "Older women maintain sexual function, but most older men are impotent."
   3. "Most older adults are not interested in sexual activity."
   4. "Both of you may have slower responses to sexual stimulation."

8. The client complains of having difficulty clearly seeing the words in the newspaper unless he holds the newspaper an arm's length away. The nurse uses which terminology to document this assessment?
1. Presbycusis
2. Xerostomia
3. Presbyopia
4. Presbyesophagus

9. The nursing student is planning care for an older adult who had a total knee replacement yesterday evening. Which nursing intervention would be *most* appropriate?
1. Ask the client how much of his bath he can independently perform.
2. Ask the client if he has any questions regarding discharge from the hospital.
3. Tell the client that he needs to decide when he wants his medications.
4. Tell the client that he needs to rest and will be given a complete bed bath.

10. A 76-year-old woman with dementia lives in an assisted living facility and often asks, "When will my sister come to visit me this afternoon?" The sister passed away last year. Which is the best response from the nurse?
1. "This is so sad. I'm sorry to tell you, but your sister died last year."
2. "She won't be coming to visit today."
3. "I understand you want her to visit you. Where did you and your sister grow up?"
4. "Wait and see if she comes to visit today."

See Answers to Test Your Knowledge in Appendix A.

READINGS AND REFERENCES

Suggested Readings

Buurman, B. M., Parlevliet, J. L., Allore, H. G., Blok, W., vanDeelen, B. A. J., Moll van Charante, E. P., . . . Rooij, S. E. (2016). Comprehensive geriatric assessment and transitional care in acutely hospitalized patients: The transitional care bridge randomized clinical trial. *JAMA Internal Medicine*, *176*, 302–309. doi:10.1001/jamainternmed.2015.8042

The objective of this study was to determine whether an intervention using a systemic comprehensive geriatric assessment would improve the ADLs. The intervention was implemented by a community care registered nurse and continued after discharge. The intervention resulted in a lower risk for death within 6 months of admission.

Todde, F., Melis, F., Mura, R., Pau, M., Fois, F., Magnani, S., . . . Tocco, F. (2016). A 12 week vigorous exercise protocol in a health group of persons over 65: Study of physical function by means of the senior fitness test. *BioMed Research International, 2016*, Article ID 7639842. doi:10.1155/2016/7639842

This study assessed the effects of vigorous exercise on functional abilities with the implementation of a senior fitness test. The results noted an improvement in functional mobility in clients over 65 years.

Related Research

Lund, J. L., Meyer, A. M., Deal, A. M., Choi, B. J., Chang, Y., Williams, G. R., . . . Sanoff, H. K. (2017). Data linkage to improve geriatric oncology research: A feasibility study. *The Oncologist*, *22*, 1002–1005. doi:10.1634/theoncologist.2016-0418

Theou, O., Blodgett, J. M., Godin, J., & Rockwood, K. (2017). Association between sedentary time and mortality across levels of frailty. *Canadian Medical Association Journal*, *189*, E1056–E1064. doi:10.1503/cmaj.161034

References

Adams, M. L. (2017). Differences between younger and older U.S. adults with multiple chronic conditions. *Preventing Chronic Disease*, *14*, 160613. doi:10.5888/pcd14.160613

Alzheimer's Association. (2019). *2019 Alzheimer's disease facts and figures*. Retrieved from https://www.alz.org/alzheimers-dementia/facts-figures

American Association of Colleges of Nursing. (2016). *CARES: Competencies and recommendations for educating undergraduate nursing students: Preparing nurses to care for the seriously ill and their families*. Retrieved from https://www.aacnnursing.org/Portals/42/ELNEC/PDF/New-Palliative-Care-Competencies.pdf

American Heart Association. (2017). *Understanding blood pressure readings*. Retrieved from http://www.heart.org/HEARTORG/Conditions/HighBloodPressure/KnowYourNumbers/Understanding-Blood-Pressure-Readings_UCM_301764_Article.jsp#.Wka4BjdMG70

Ayalon, L., & Tesch-Romer, C. (2017). Taking a closer look at ageism: Self and other self-directed ageist attitudes and discrimination. *European Journal of Aging*, *14*, 1–4. doi:10.1007/s10433-016-0409-9

Bindman, A. B., & Cox, D. F. (2018). Changes in health care costs and mortality associated with transitional care management services after a discharge among Medicare beneficiaries. *JAMA Internal Medicine*, *178*(9), 1165–1171. doi:10.1001/jamainternmed.2018.2572

Centers for Disease Control and Prevention. (2017). *Health, United States, 2016 with chartbook on long-term trends in health*. Retrieved from https://www.cdc.gov/nchs/data/hus/hus16.pdf#079

Colby, S. L., & Ortman, J. M. (2015). *Projections of the size and composition of the U. S. population: 2014 to 2060*. Retrieved from https://census.gov/content/dam/Census/library/publications/2015/demo/p25-1143.pdf

Edelman, C. L., & Kudzma, E. C. (2018). *Health promotion throughout the lifespan* (9th ed.). St. Louis, MO: Mosby Elsevier.

Eliopoulos, C. (2018). *Gerontological nursing* (9th ed.). Philadelphia, PA: Lippincott Williams & Wilkins.

Erikson, E. H. (1963). *Childhood and society* (2nd edition). New York, NY: W. W. Norton.

Federal Interagency Forum on Aging-Related Statistics. (2016). *2016 older Americans key indicators of well-being*. Retrieved from https://agingstats.gov/docs/LatestReport/Older-Americans-2016-Key-Indicators-of-WellBeing.pdf

Flood, M. (2005). A mid-range nursing theory of successful aging. *Journal of Theory Construction & Testing*, *9*(2), 35–39.

Frandsen, G., & Pennington, S. (2018). *Abrams' clinical drug therapy rationales for nursing practice* (11th ed.). Philadelphia, PA: Lippincott Williams & Wilkins.

Giger, J. N. (2017). *Transcultural nursing: Assessment and intervention* (7th ed.). St. Louis, MO: Mosby.

Gilligan, C. (1982). *In a different voice: Psychological theory and women's development*. Cambridge, MA: Harvard University.

Gostin, L. O., Friedman, E. A., Buss, P., Chowdhury, M., Grover, A., Heywood, M., . . . Zewdie, D. (2016). The next WHO director general's highest priority: A global treaty on the human right to health. *The Lancet Global Health*, *4*(12), e890–e892. doi:10.1016/S2214-109X(16)30219-4

Haight, B. K., Barba, B. E., Courts, N. F., & Tesh, A. S. (2002). Thriving: A life span theory. *Journal of Gerontological Nursing*, *29*(3), 14–22.

Havighurst, R. J. (1972). *Developmental tasks and education* (3rd ed.). New York, NY: Longman.

Joint Center for Housing Studies of Harvard University. (2016). *Projections & implications for housing a growing population: Older households 2015–2035*. Retrieved from http://www.jchs.harvard.edu/sites/jchs.harvard.edu/files/harvard_jchs_housing_growing_population_2016.pdf

Kohlberg, L. (1984). *The psychology of moral development: The nature and validity of moral stages*. San Francisco, CA: Harper & Row.

Lee, Y., & Blitz, L. V. (2016). We're grand: A qualitative design and development pilot project addressing the needs and strengths of grandparents raising grandchildren. *Child and Family Social Work*, *21*, 381–390. doi:10.1111/cfs.12153

Maritz, C. A., & Silbernagel, K. G. (2016). A prospective cohort study on the effect of a balance training program, including calf muscle strengthening in community-dwelling older adults. *Journal of Geriatric Physical Therapy*, *39*(3), 125–131. doi:10.1519/JPT.0000000000000059

Mather, M., Jacobsen, L. A., & Pollard, K. M. (2016). Aging in the United States. *Population Bulletin*, *70*(2), 1–23. Retrieved from http://www.prb.org/pdf16/aging-us-population-bulletin.pdf

Matzo, M. (2019). *Palliative care nursing*. (5th edition). NY: Springer.

Mauk, K. L. (2018). *Gerontological nursing: Competencies for care* (4th ed.). Sudbury, MA: Jones & Bartlett.

Mayo Clinic. (2018). Low sex drive in women—Feature on rediscovering lost libido. *Mayo Clinic Health Letter*, *36*(1), 4–5.

Miller, C. A. (2019). *Nursing for wellness in older adults: Theory and practice* (8th ed.). Philadelphia, PA: Lippincott Williams & Wilkins.

Morley, J. E. (2017). Vicissitudes: Retirement with a long post-retirement future. *Generations: Journal of the American Society on Aging*, *41*(2), 101–109.

Moser, S., Luxenberger, W., & Freidl, W. (2017). The influence of social support and coping on quality of life among elderly with age-related hearing loss. *American Journal of Audiology*, *26*, 170–179. doi:10.1044/2017_AJA-16-0083

National Council on Child Abuse & Family Violence. (n.d). *Elder abuse information*. Retrieved from https://www.nccafv.org/elder-abuse

Peck, R. (1968). Psychological development in the second half of life. In B. L. Neugarten (Ed.), *Middle age and aging* (pp. 88–92). Chicago, IL: University of Chicago Press.

Porth, C. M. (2015). *Essentials of pathophysiology* (4th ed.) Philadelphia, PA: Lippincott Williams & Wilkins.

Pratt, J. R. (2018). *Long-term care managing across the continuum* (4th ed.). Boston, MA: Jones & Bartlett.

Pratt, M. W., Diessner, R., Pratt, A., Hunsberger, B., & Pancer, S. M. (1996). Moral and social reasoning and perspective taking in later life: A longitudinal study. *Psychology and Aging*, *11*, 66–73. doi:10.1037/0882-7974.11.1.66

Qaseen, A., M. A., Forciea, M. A., McLean, R. M., and Denberg, T. D. (2017). Clinical guideline treatment of low bone density or osteoporosis to prevent fractures in men and women: A clinical practice guideline update from the American College of Physicians. *Annals of Internal Medicine*, *166*, 818–839. doi:10.7326/M15-1361

Raposo, S., & Carstensen, L. L. (2015). Developing a research agenda to combat ageism. *Generations: Journal of the American Society on Aging*, *39*(3), 79–85.

Schroyen, S., Missotten, P., Jerusalem, G., Gilles, C., & Adam, S. (2016). Ageism and caring attitudes among nurses in oncology. *International Psychogeriatric*, *28*, 749–757. doi:10.1017/S1041610215001970

Taani, M. H., Siglinsky, E., Kovach, C. R., & Buehring, B. (2018). Psychosocial factors associated with reduced muscle mass, strength, and function in residential care apartment complex residents. *Researching Gerontological Nursing*, *11*, 238–248. doi:10.3928/19404921-20180810-02

Tabloski, P. A. (2019). *Gerontological nursing* (4th ed.). New York, NY: Pearson.

Touhy, T. A., & Jett, K. F. (2016). *Ebersole & Hess' toward healthy aging: Human needs and nursing responses* (9th ed.). St. Louis, MO: Elsevier.

U.S. Census Bureau. (n.d.). *An aging nation*. Retrieved from https://www.census.gov/content/dam/Census/newsroom/facts-for-features/2017/cb17-ff08_graphic_olderamericans.pdf

U.S. Census Bureau. (2017a). *American fact finder*. Retrieved from https://factfinder.census.gov/faces/tableservices/jsf/pages/productview.xhtml?pid=PEP_2017_PEPAGESEX&prodType=table

U.S. Census Bureau. (2017b). *Older Americans month: May 2017*. Retrieved from https://www.census.gov/content/dam/Census/newsroom/facts-for-features/2017/cb17-ff08.pdf

Yu, R. P., McCammon, R. J., Ellison, N. B., & Langa, K. M. (2016). The relationships that matter: Social network site use and social wellbeing among older adults in the United States of America. *Aging and Society*, *36*, 1826–1852. doi:10.1017/S0144686X15000677

Selected Bibliography

American Geriatrics Society 2015 Beers Criteria Update Expert Panel. (2015). American Geriatric Society 2015 updated Beers criteria for potentially inappropriate medication use in older adults. *Journal of the American Geriatric Society*, *63*(11), 2227–2246. doi:10.1111/jgs.13702

Capezuti, E. A., Malone, M. L., Gardener, D. S., Khan, A., Baumann, S. (2018). *The encyclopedia of elder care*. (4th ed.). New York, NY: Springer.

Erikson, E. H. (1982). *The life cycle completed: A review*. New York, NY: W. W. Norton.

Frankl, V. (2006). *Man's search for meaning*. Boston, MA: Beacon.

Freud, S. (1923). *The ego and the id*. London, England: Hogarth.

Kohlberg, L. (1971). *Recent research in moral development*. New York, NY: Holt, Rinehart & Winston.

Kohlberg, L. (1981). *The psychology of moral development: Moral stages and the idea of justice*. San Francisco, CA: Harper & Row.

Piaget, J. (1966). *Origins of intelligence in children*. New York, NY: W. W. Norton.

Raeifar, E., Halkett, A., Lohman, M. C., & Sirey, J. A. (2017). The relation between mastery, anticipated stigma, and depression among older adults in a primary care setting. *Journal of Nervous and Mental Disease*, *205*, 801–804. doi:10.1097/NMD.0000000000000686

Smith, A. K., Ritchie, C. S., & Wallhagen, M. L. (2016). Hearing loss in hospice and palliative care: A national survey of providers. *Journal of Pain and Symptom Management*, *52*(2), 254–258. doi:10.1016/j.jpainsymman.2016.02.007

Yuan, S., Hussain, S. A., Hales, K. D., & Cotton, S. (2016). What do they like? Communication preferences and patterns of older adults in the United States: The role of technology. *Educational Gerontology*, *42*(3), 163–174. doi:10.1080/03601277.2015.1083392

Promoting Family Health 27

LEARNING OUTCOMES

After completing this chapter, you will be able to:

1. Describe the functions of the family.
2. Describe different types of families.
3. Identify theoretical frameworks used in family health promotion.
4. Identify the components of a family health assessment.
5. Identify common risk factors for family health problems.
6. Develop nursing diagnoses, outcomes, and interventions pertaining to family functioning.

KEY TERMS

ecomap, *523*
extended family, *520*
family, *519*
family-centered nursing, *519*
genogram, *523*
nuclear family, *520*

Introduction

Nurses assess and plan healthcare for three types of clients: the individual, the family, and the community. The beliefs and values of each individual and the support he or she receives come in large part from the family and are reinforced by the community. Thus, an understanding of family dynamics and the context of the community assists the nurse in planning care. When a family is the client, the nurse determines the health status of the family and its individual members, the level of family functioning, family interaction patterns, and family strengths and weaknesses.

Family Health

The **family** is a basic unit of society. It consists of those individuals, male or female, youth or adult, legally or not legally related, genetically or not genetically related, who are considered by the others to represent significant individuals. In the nursing profession, interest in the family unit and its impact on the health, values, and productivity of individual family members is expressed by **family-centered nursing**: nursing that considers the health of the family as a unit in addition to the health of individual family members.

Functions of the Family

The economic resources needed by the family are secured by adult members. The family protects the physical health of its members by providing adequate nutrition and healthcare services. The nutritional and lifestyle practices of the family also directly affect the developing health attitudes and lifestyle practices of the children.

In addition to providing an environment conducive to physical growth and health, the family creates an atmosphere that influences the cognitive and the psychosocial growth of its members. Children and adults in healthy, functional families receive support, understanding, and encouragement as they progress through predictable developmental stages, as they move in or out of the family unit, and as they establish new family units. In families where members are physically and emotionally nurtured, individuals are challenged to achieve their potential in the family unit. As individual needs are met, family members are able to reach out to others in the family and the community and to society.

Families from different cultures are an integral part of North America's rich heritage. Each family has values and beliefs that are unique to their culture of origin and that shape the family's structure, methods of interaction, healthcare practices, and coping mechanisms. These factors interact to influence the health of families. Families of a particular culture may cluster to form mutual support systems and to preserve their heritage; however, this practice may isolate them from the larger society (Figure 27.1 ■).

Becoming acculturated is a slow, stressful process of learning the language and customs of a new country. Children in cultural clusters often have greater contact with the world around them than do adults; through school, children become more proficient in a new language and more comfortable with new customs and behaviors. Sometimes children create conflict in the family when they bring home new ideas and values. For more information about the cultural aspects of the health of individuals and families, see Chapter 21 ∞.

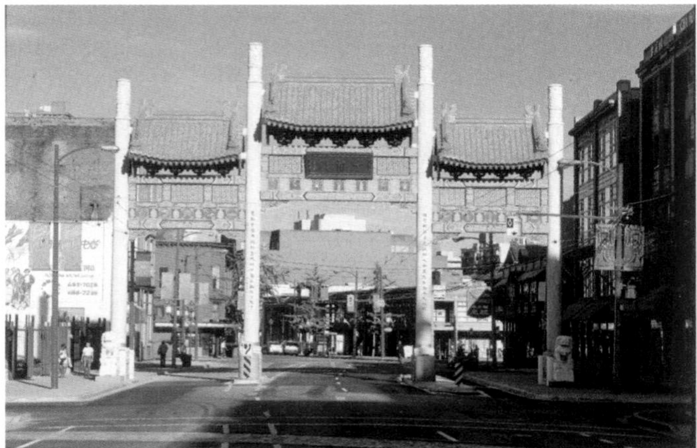

Figure 27.1 ■ Cultural separation.
Dorling Kindersley ltd/Alamy Stock Photo.

Types of Families in Today's Society

Families consist of individuals (structure) and their responsibilities within the family (roles). Government data are grouped by types of *households*: married couples with children, married couples without children, other family households (single-parent families), men living alone, women living alone, and other nonfamily households. A family structure of parents and their offspring is known as the **nuclear family**. The relatives of nuclear families, such as grandparents or aunts and uncles, compose the **extended family**. In some families, members of the extended family live with the nuclear family. Although members of the extended family may live in different areas, they may be a source of emotional or financial support for the family.

Some families live in houses, some in apartments; some live in urban areas, some in rural towns; and some are homeless. Annually, the U.S. Conference of Mayors publishes a Hunger and Homelessness Survey. In the 2016 report, the mayors joined with the National Alliance to End Homelessness to assist in solving the problem of homelessness in the U.S. cities represented at the conference. The report contains the results of surveys from 38 cities across the country. In 2016, it reported that on a single night, 544,084 individuals experience homeless in the United States. The homelessness rate in the cities studied was 51 individuals per 10,000. This rate is higher than the reported national average of 17 individuals per 10,000. The cities studied identified that if every shelter bed or traditional housing bed was filled, over 34,000 individuals would remain unsheltered nationwide. The lack of affordable housing for families has been established as the key reason for this increase (U.S. Conference of Mayors, 2016).

Traditional Family

The traditional family is viewed as an independent unit in which both parents reside in the home with their children, with the mother often assuming the nurturing role and the father providing the necessary economic resources. In today's society, both males and females are less bound to traditional role patterns. For example, fathers are more likely to be involved with the household chores, their children, and family life (Figure 27.2 ■). The U.S. Census Bureau (2018a) reported 37.4 million fathers in married-couple families, 190,000 of whom were stay-at-home fathers, in 2018 (U.S. Census Bureau, 2018f). In 2018, 54% of young adults aged 18–24 lived with their parents, and 16% of young adults aged 25–34 years lived in the parental home (U.S. Census Bureau, 2018g).

Two-Career Family

In two-career (or dual-career) families, both partners are employed. They may or may not have children. As of 2018, there were 24,555,000 married couples with both spouses employed outside of the home (U.S. Census Bureau, 2018e). Two-career families have steadily increased since the 1960s because of increased career opportunities for women, a desire to increase the family's standard of living, and economic necessity. Finding good-quality, affordable child care is one of the greatest stresses faced by working parents.

Single-Parent Family

Since 1970, the number of single-parent households has been increasing. In 2018, 12,805,000 children lived with a single mother, and 3,881,000 lived with a single father

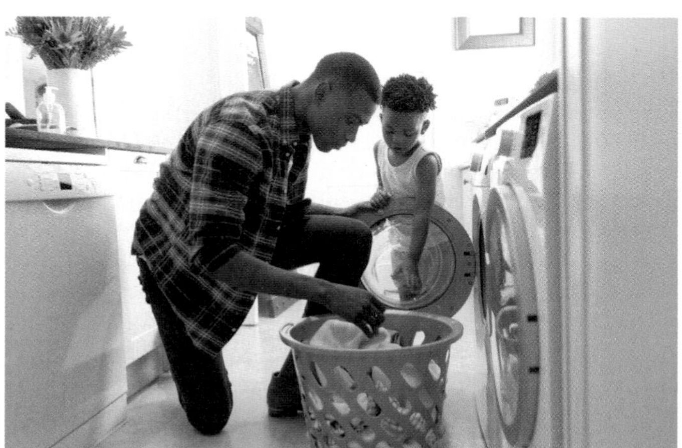

Figure 27.2 ■ Role patterns within traditional families are changing.
wavebreakmedia/Shutterstock.

(U.S. Census Bureau, 2018b). The U.S. Census Bureau (2018c) has compiled a snapshot of fathers in the United States. Approximately 6 in 10 males are fathers. Of these fathers, 54% have adult children aged 18 years or older. They have at least one minor child less than 18 years of age. Of the 35 million fathers of minor children, 2% are single fathers living with at least one child under the age of 18 years. The stresses of single parenthood are many: child-care concerns, financial concerns, role overload, fatigue in managing daily tasks, and social isolation.

Adolescent Family

Birthrates among teenagers have declined since the early 1990s. A 9% drop in teen pregnancy was noted in 2015–2016. The teen birthrate was 61.8 per 1000 teens in 1991. By 2015, that birth rate had dropped to 22.3 per 1000 births (U.S. Department of Health and Human Services [USDHHS], 2018a). The Teen Pregnancy Prevention Program is a national program that funds diverse organizations that assist in teenage pregnancy prevention initiatives (USDHHS, 2018b). Teen births declined in all ethnicities from 2015 to 2016. The birth rate for women aged 15–19 years was 20.3 births per 1000 women. The birth rate for non-Hispanic Asian teens aged 15–19 was 3.9. For non-Hispanic White teens of this age group, the birth rate was 14.3, and for non-Hispanic Black teens, the rate was 28.6. The non-Hispanic American Indian and Alaskan Native birth rate for those aged 15–19 was 35.1 (Martin, Hamilton, Osterman, Driscoll, & Drake, 2018). These young parents are often developmentally, physically, emotionally, and financially ill prepared to undertake the responsibility of parenthood. Adolescent pregnancies frequently interrupt or stop formal education. Children born to an adolescent are often at greater risk for health and social problems, and they have few role models to assist in breaking out of the cycle of poverty.

Foster Family

Children who can no longer live with their birth parents may require placement with a family that has agreed to include them temporarily. The legal agreement between the foster family and the court to care for the child includes the expectations of the foster parents and the financial compensation they will receive. A family (with or without their own children) may house more than one foster child at a time or different children over many years. Hopefully, at some time, the fostered child can return to the birth parent(s) or be legally and permanently adopted by other parents.

Blended Family

Existing family units that join together to form new families are known as *blended* or *stepfamilies*. There are no official statistics on the number of blended families, but a commonly accepted view is that about one of every three Americans is a member of a stepfamily. Family integration requires time and effort. Stresses occur as blended families become acquainted with each other, respect differences, and establish new patterns of behavior. When blended families with children form following the divorce or death of a parent, adjustment can be particularly challenged by the normal processes of grief and loss (see Chapter 43 ∞).

Intragenerational Family

In some cultures, and as individuals live longer, more than two generations may live together. Children may continue to live with their parents even after having their own children, or the grandparents may move in with their grown children's families after some years of living apart. The U.S. Census Bureau reported the number of children living with their grandparents from 1970 to 2014. In 1970, a total of 69,276,000 children under the age of 18 lived in the United States. Of this population, 2,214,000 were living with their grandparents. In 2014, the total number of children under the age of 18 in the United States had risen to 73,692,000, with 4,834,000 living with their grandparents. The total population of children under 18 increased by 106% from 1970 to 2014. However, the number of children under the age of 18 years living with their grandparents increased by 199% (U.S. Census Bureau, 2018d). It is imperative that nurses understand the implications this information may have on the care of these children. Most grandparents are on a fixed income and may be dealing with their own health issues. These factors can impede the healthcare needs of the child.

Cohabiting Family

Cohabiting (or communal) families consist of unrelated individuals or families living under one roof. Reasons for cohabiting may be a need for companionship, a desire to achieve a sense of family, testing a relationship or commitment, or sharing expenses and household management. Cohabiting families illustrate the flexibility and creativity of the family unit in adapting to individual challenges and changing societal needs. There is a lack of data collected on households with communal families.

Gay and Lesbian Family

On June 26, 2015, the U.S. Supreme Court ruled to legalize same-sex marriage. In this ruling, the Supreme Court justices stated that states cannot ban same-sex marriage. De Vogue and Diamond (2015) reported what Justice Kennedy wrote: "No union is more profound than marriage, for it embodies the highest ideals of love, fidelity, devotion, sacrifice, and family. In forming a marital union, two individuals become something greater than they once were. Their hope is not to be condemned to live in loneliness, excluded from one of civilizations oldest institutions. They ask for dignity in the eyes of the law. The Constitution grants them this right."

Gay and lesbian adults form families based on the same goals of caring and commitment seen in heterosexual relationships. In addition, the structure of gay and lesbian families is as diverse as that of heterosexual families, including stepfamilies and single-parent families. Children raised in these family units develop sex-role orientations and behaviors similar to those of children in the general population.

Single Adults Living Alone

Individuals who live by themselves represent a significant portion of today's society—about 45%. Unmarried individuals in America aged 18 or older total 109 million, with 53% representing women and 47% representing men in 2015 (U.S. Census Bureau, 2016). It is noted that 63% of these individuals were never married, 24% were divorced, and 13% were widowed.

In younger single adults 18 to 34 years of age, there is little variation in the percentages between males and females who are living alone. Singles include young self-supporting adults who have recently left the nuclear family as well as older adults living alone. Young adults typically move in and out of living situations and may have membership in the categories of family households, nonfamily households, and living alone at several different times. Older adults may find themselves single through divorce, separation, or the death of a spouse or significant other but generally remain living alone for the remainder of their lives.

Applying Theoretical Frameworks to Families

Theoretical frameworks provide the nurse with a context or structure from which to view health and health promotion for families across the lifespan. Nurses generally use a combination of theoretical frameworks in promoting the health of individuals and families. Two major theoretical frameworks that nurses use in promoting the health of families are systems theory and structural–functional theory.

Systems Theory

Systems theory was introduced in Chapter 19 ∞. Nurses are increasingly using systems theory to understand not only biological systems but also systems in families, communities, and nursing and healthcare. Family system members are interdependent, working toward specific purposes and goals. Families, as open systems, are continually interacting with and influenced by other systems in the community. Boundaries regulate the input from other systems that interact with the family system; they also regulate output from the family system to the community or to society. Boundaries protect the family from the demands and influences of other systems. Healthy families are likely to welcome input from the outside, encourage individual members to adapt beliefs and practices to meet the changing demands of society, seek out healthcare information, and use community resources.

When using systems theory for health promotion of the family, the nurse considers how each element of the system affects the others. For example, if a child is seriously injured in a home incident, other siblings may feel left out of the considerable attention devoted to the child, a parent may withdraw if there are feelings of guilt for not preventing the injury, and other family members may be recruited to assist with finances or chores while the nuclear family focuses on the injured child. The nurse will facilitate a care plan that includes diagnoses and problems affecting the different components of the family system.

Structural–Functional Theory

The structural–functional theory, as the name implies, focuses on family structure and function. The structural component of the theory addresses the membership of the family and the relationships among family members. Intrafamily relationships are complex because of the numerous relationships that exist within the family structure—mother–daughter, brother–sister, spouse–partner, and so on. These relationships are constantly evolving as children mature and leave the family nest and adults age and become more dependent on others to meet their daily needs.

The functional aspect of the theory examines the effects of intrafamily relationships on the family system, as well as their effects on other systems. Some of the main functions of the family include developing a sense of family purpose and affiliation, adding and socializing new members, and providing and distributing care and services to members. A healthy family organizes its members and resources in meeting family goals; it functions in harmony, working toward shared goals.

Using this theory to examine the case described earlier in which one child in a family is seriously injured, the nurse considers how the family is structured. The members of the family are parents and more than one child plus extended family, but we do not know exactly how they communicate. Who is the decision maker and in which directions do communication occur? Then, how is the family functioning? In this case, the most important functional aspects are likely to be the economic and emotional stability of the family members. The nurse will facilitate a care plan that includes diagnoses and problems from the perspective of stabilizing or enhancing the family structure and function during this episode of disruption.

●○● NURSING MANAGEMENT

Assessing

The purpose of family assessment is to determine the level of family functioning, clarify family interaction patterns, identify family strengths and weaknesses, and describe the health status of the family and its individual members. Also important are family living patterns, including communication, childrearing, coping strategies, and health practices. The family assessment gives an overview of the family process and helps the nurse identify areas that need further investigation (Box 27.1). Nurses carry out a detailed assessment in specific target areas as they become

BOX 27.1 Family Assessment Guide

FAMILY STRUCTURE
- Size and type: nuclear, extended, or other type of family
- Age and gender of family members

FAMILY ROLES AND FUNCTIONS
- Family members working outside the home; type of work and satisfaction with it
- Household roles and responsibilities and how tasks are distributed
- Ways childrearing responsibilities are shared
- Major decision maker and methods of decision-making
- Family members' satisfaction with roles, the way tasks are divided, and the way decisions are made

PHYSICAL HEALTH STATUS
- Current physical health status of each member
- Perceptions of own and other family members' health
- Preventive health practices (e.g., status of immunizations, oral hygiene practices, regularity of visual examinations)
- Previous acute illnesses and presence of chronic conditions of any member
- Screening for and knowledge of any genetic disorders
- Routine healthcare, when and why primary care provider last seen

INTERACTION PATTERNS
- Ways of expressing emotions (e.g., affection, love, sorrow, anger)
- Most significant family member in the individual's life
- Openness of communication with all family members

FAMILY VALUES
- Cultural and religious orientations; degree to which cultural and religious practices are followed
- Use of leisure time and whether leisure time is shared with total family unit
- Family's view of education, teachers, and the school system
- Health values: how much emphasis is put on exercise, diet, and preventive healthcare

COPING RESOURCES
- Degree of emotional support offered to one another
- Availability of support people and affiliations outside the family (e.g., friends, co-workers, church memberships)
- Sources of stress
- Methods of handling stressful situations and conflicting goals of family members
- Financial ability to meet current and future needs

more acquainted with the family and begin to understand family needs and strengths more fully. In planning interventions, nurses need to focus not only on problems but also on family strengths and resources as part of the nursing care plan.

The assessment begins with a complete health history. The nurse focuses first on the family unit and then on the individuals in that family. The health history is one of the most effective ways of identifying existing or potential health problems. The history is followed by a physical assessment of family members.

Employment of a genogram will help the nurse visualize how all family members are genetically related to each other and to grasp how patterns of chronic conditions are present within the family unit. A **genogram** is composed of visual representations of gender and lines of birth descent through the generations (Figure 27.3 ■). If further evaluation is indicated, a referral is made to the appropriate healthcare professional.

The nurse should also develop an ecomap for family members individually and as a group to document the family unit's energy expenditures within the community setting. An **ecomap** provides a visualization of how the family unit interacts with the external community environment, such as schools, religious commitments, occupational duties, and recreational pursuits (Figure 27.4 ■). When the focus is on health, the appraisal includes information on lifestyle behaviors and health beliefs. The nurse uses data from the health appraisal to formulate a health profile. The health profile provides the data necessary to determine wellness or to establish a nursing diagnosis and to plan appropriate nursing interventions to promote optimal health through lifestyle modification.

Health Beliefs

To promote health, the nurse must understand the health beliefs of individuals and families. Health beliefs may reflect a lack of information or misinformation about health or disease. They may also include folklore and practices from different cultures. Because of the many advances in medicine and healthcare during the past few decades, clients may have outdated information about health, illness, treatment, and prevention. The nurse is frequently in a position to give information or correct misconceptions. This function is an important component of the nursing care plan. For additional information on health beliefs, see Chapter 20 ∞.

Family Communication Patterns

The effectiveness of family communication determines the family's ability to function as a cooperative, growth-producing unit. Messages are constantly being communicated among family members, both verbally and nonverbally. The information transmitted influences how members work together, fulfill their assigned roles in the family, incorporate family values, and develop skills to function in society. Intrafamily communication plays a significant role in the development of self-esteem, which is necessary for the growth of personality.

Families that communicate effectively transmit messages clearly. Members are free to express their feelings without fear of jeopardizing their standing in the family. Family members support one another and have the ability to listen, empathize, and reach out to one another in times of crisis. When the needs of family members are met, they are more able to reach out to meet the needs of others in society.

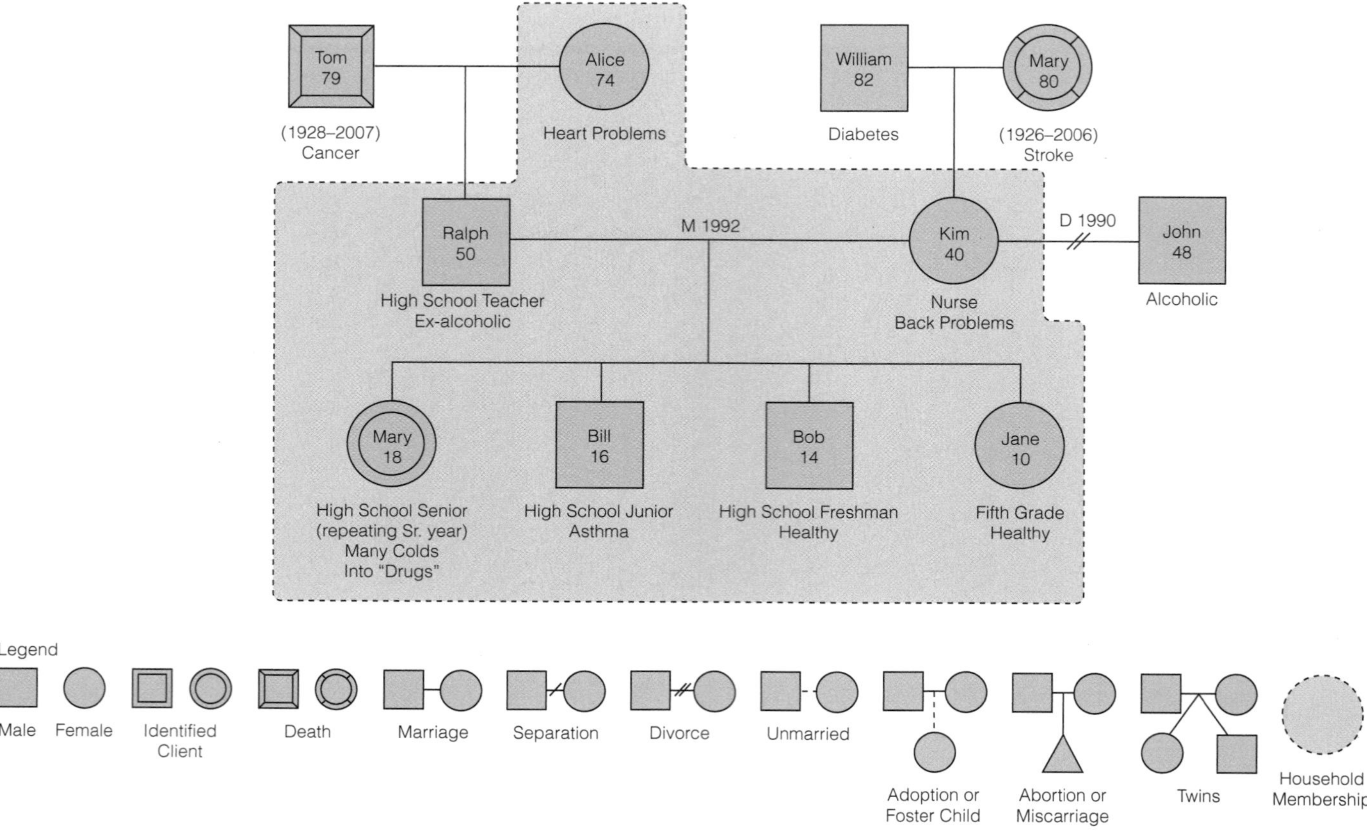

Figure 27.3 ■ Example of a family genogram with accompanying legend (symbols used in genograms).

When patterns of communication among family members are dysfunctional, messages are often communicated unclearly. Verbal communication may be incongruent with nonverbal messages. Power struggles may be evidenced by hostility, anger, or silence. Members may be cautious in expressing their feelings because they cannot predict how others in the family will respond. When family communication is impaired, the growth of individual members is stunted. Members often turn to other systems to seek personal validation and gratification.

The nurse needs to observe intrafamily communication patterns closely. Nurses should pay special attention to who does the talking for the family, which members are silent, how disagreements are handled, and how well the members listen to one another and encourage the participation of others. Nonverbal communication is important because it gives valuable clues about what individuals are feeling.

Family Coping Mechanisms

Family coping mechanisms are the behaviors families use to deal with stress or changes imposed from either within or without. The use of coping mechanisms can be viewed as an active method of problem-solving developed to meet life's challenges. The coping mechanisms families and individuals develop reflect their individual resourcefulness. Families may use coping patterns rather consistently over time or may change their coping strategies when new demands are made on the family. The success of a family largely depends on how well it copes with the stresses it experiences.

Nurses working with families realize the importance of assessing coping mechanisms as a way of determining how families relate to stress. Also important are the resources available to the family. Internal resources, such as knowledge, skills, effective communication patterns, and a sense of mutuality and purpose within the family, assist in the problem-solving process. In addition, external support systems promote coping and adaptation. These external systems may be extended family, friends, religious affiliations, healthcare professionals, or social services. The development of social support systems is particularly valuable today because many families, due to stress, mobility, or poverty, are isolated from the resources that would traditionally have helped them cope.

Family Violence

The incidence of family violence has increased in recent years. Statistics are not accurate because many cases remain unreported. Family violence includes abuse between intimate partners, child abuse, and elder abuse and may include physical, mental, and verbal abuse, as well as neglect. Early symptoms are evident in burns, cuts, fractures, and even death. Other manifestations often seen are depression, alcohol and substance abuse, and suicide attempts. Nurses should be alert to the symptoms of family violence and act appropriately to report it and obtain

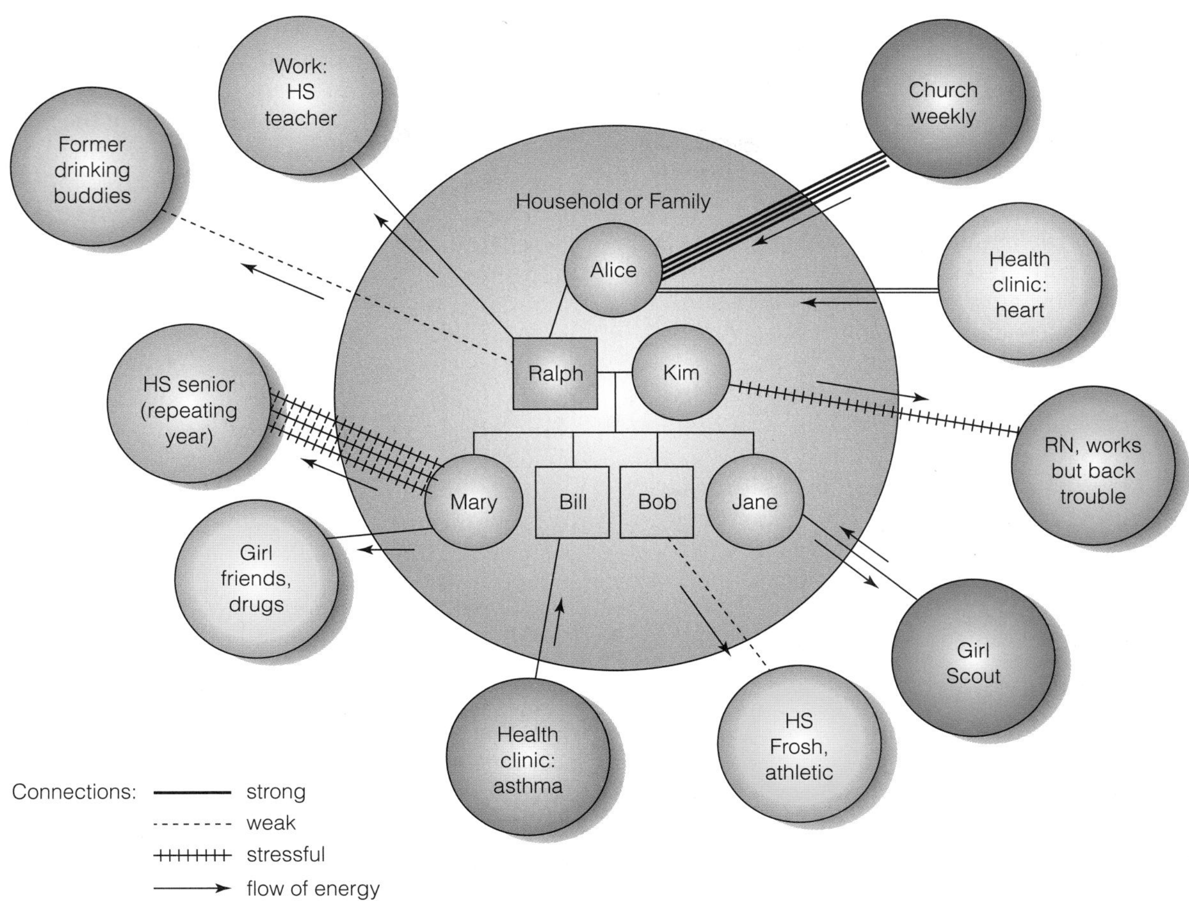

Figure 27.4 ■ Example of a family ecomap. Many more components may be added to the map.

resources for the family. In most circumstances, laws require that the nurse report suspected abuse.

Risk for Health Problems

Risk assessment helps the nurse identify individuals and groups at higher risk than the general population of developing specific health problems, such as stroke, diabetes, and lung cancer. The vulnerability of family units to health problems may be based on the maturity level of individual family members, hereditary or genetic factors, sex or ethnicity, sociologic factors, and lifestyle practices.

Maturity Factors

Families with members at both ends of the age continuum are at risk of developing health problems. Families entering childbearing and childrearing phases experience many changes in roles, responsibilities, and expectations. The many, often conflicting, demands on the family cause stress and fatigue, which may impede the growth of individual family members and the functioning of the group as a unit. Adolescent mothers, because of their developmental level and lack of knowledge about parenthood, and single-parent families, because of role overload experienced by the head of the household, are more likely to develop health problems. Older adults may feel a lack of purpose and decreased self-esteem. These feelings, in turn, reduce their motivation to engage in health-promoting behaviors, such as exercise or community and family involvement. Adults who simultaneously help care for their own parents and their children may have particular challenges.

Hereditary Factors

Individuals born into families with a history of certain diseases, such as diabetes or cardiovascular disease, are at greater risk of developing these conditions. A detailed family health history, including genetically transmitted disorders, is crucial to the identification of individuals and families at risk. These data are used to monitor the health of individual family members and to recommend health practices that reduce risk, minimize consequences, or postpone the development of genetically related conditions.

Sex or Ethnicity

Some family units or family members may be at risk of developing a disease because of sex or ethnicity. Males, for example, are at greater risk of having cardiovascular disease at an earlier age than females, and females are at greater risk of developing osteoporosis, particularly after menopause. Although it is sometimes difficult to separate genetic factors from cultural factors, certain risk factors seem to be related to ethnicity. Sickle cell disease, for example, is a hereditary disease that occurs primarily in individuals of African descent, and Tay–Sachs is a neurodegenerative disease that occurs primarily in descendants of Eastern European Jews.

Sociologic Factors

Poverty is a major problem that affects not only the family but also the community and society. Poverty is a real concern among the rising number of single-parent families. As the number of these families increases, poverty will affect a large number of growing children.

When ill, the poor are likely to put off seeking services until the illness reaches an advanced state and requires longer or more complex treatment. Although the health of the individuals of industrialized nations has improved significantly during the past century, this progress has not benefited all segments of society, particularly the poor. Those affected by homelessness and violence experience similar challenges.

Lifestyle Practices

Many diseases are preventable, the effects of some diseases can be minimized, or the onset of disease can be delayed through lifestyle modifications. Certain cancers, cardiovascular disease, adult-onset diabetes, and tooth decay are among the lifestyle diseases. The incidence of lung cancer, for example, would be greatly reduced if individuals stopped smoking. Good nutrition, dental hygiene, and the use of fluoride—in the water supply, in toothpaste, as a topical application, or as a supplement—have been shown to reduce dental decay or caries, one of America's most prevalent health problems. Many diseases can be prevented through immunizations such as rubella, pertussis, and hepatitis B. Most of these immunizations are given in childhood but they can be given to adults who have not developed immunity. Other important lifestyle considerations are exercise, stress management, and sleep.

Today, health professionals have the knowledge to prevent or minimize the effects of some of the main causes of disease, disability, and death. The challenge is to disseminate information about prevention and to motivate families to make lifestyle changes prior to the onset of illness.

Diagnosing and Planning

Data gathered during a family assessment may lead to the following nursing diagnoses: impairment in caregiver role, impaired family coping, interrupted family dynamics, ineffective home maintenance, alteration in parenting, alteration in family relations, and willingness to improve family coping.

Being sensitive to cultural differences is important during assessment and when planning care. Knowing who makes most of the decisions in the family, especially healthcare decisions, helps the nurse know to whom to direct questions in order to obtain information and to whom to give instructions. The extended family unit is found in many cultures, and there may be a difference in health beliefs and health practices within the family. Older members of the family may use their traditional practices, whereas younger members may have had more exposure to modern practices. Building a trusting relationship with these families is the first step toward planning care that is more effective by being able to talk to the family members about their beliefs and practices.

Nurses need to focus on assisting the family to plan realistic goals or outcomes and strategies that enhance family functioning, such as improving communication skills, identifying and utilizing support systems, and developing and rehearsing parenting skills. Anticipatory guidance may assist well-functioning families in preparing for the predictable developmental transitions that occur in the life of families.

The Family Experiencing a Health Crisis

The illness of a family member is a crisis that affects the entire family system. The family is disrupted as members abandon their usual activities and focus their energy on restoring family equilibrium. Roles and responsibilities previously assumed by the ill family member are delegated to other family members, or those functions may remain undone for the duration of the illness. The family experiences anxiety because members are concerned about the sick individual and the resolution of the illness. This anxiety is compounded by additional responsibilities when there is less time or motivation to complete the normal tasks of daily living. See Box 27.2 for some factors that determine the impact of illness on the family unit.

BOX 27.2 Factors That Determine the Impact of Illness on the Family

- The nature of the illness, which can range from minor to life threatening
- The duration of the illness, which ranges from short term to long term
- The residual effects of the illness, including none to permanent disability
- The meaning of the illness to the family and its significance to family systems
- The financial impact of the illness, which is influenced by factors such as insurance and ability of the ill member to return to work
- The effect of the illness on future family functioning (e.g., previous patterns may be restored, or new patterns may be established)

The family's ability to deal with the stress of illness depends on the members' coping skills. Families with good communication skills are better able to discuss how they feel about the illness and how it affects family functioning. They can plan for the future and are flexible in adapting these plans as the situation changes. An established social support network provides strength, encouragement, and services to the family during the illness. During health crises, families need to realize that it is a strength, not a sign of weakness, to turn to others for support. Nurses can be part of the support system for families, or they can identify other sources of support in the community.

During a crisis, families are often drawn together by a common purpose. In this time of closeness, family members have the opportunity to reaffirm personal and family values and their commitment to one another. Indeed, illness may provide a unique opportunity for family growth.

The Nurse's Role with Families Experiencing Illness

Nurses committed to family-centered care involve both the ill individual and the family in the nursing process. Through their interaction with families, nurses can give support and information. Nurses make sure that not only the individual but also each family member understands the health condition, its management, and the effect of these two factors on family functioning. The nurse also assesses the family's readiness and ability to provide continued care and supervision at home when warranted. After carefully planned instruction and practice, families are given an opportunity to demonstrate their ability to provide care under the supportive guidance of the nurse. When the care indicated is beyond the capability of the family, nurses work with families to identify available resources that are socially and financially acceptable.

In helping families reintegrate the ill individual into the home, nurses use data gathered during the family assessment to identify family resources and deficits. By formulating mutually acceptable goals for reintegration, nurses help families cope with the realities of the illness and the changes it may have brought about, which may include new roles and functions of family members or the need to provide continued medical care to the ill or recovering individual. Working together, nurses and families can create environments that restore or reorganize family functioning during illness and throughout the recovery process.

Death of a Family Member

The death of a family member often has a profound effect on the family. After the death, families may need counseling to deal with their feelings and to talk about the individual who died. Individual members experience a sense of loss. They grieve for the lost individual, and they grieve for the family the way that it once was. Family disorganization may occur. The structure of the family is altered, and this change may, in turn, affect how it functions as a unit. Members may also want to talk about their fears and hopes for the future. At this time, families often derive comfort from their religious beliefs and their spiritual advisers. Support groups are also available for families experiencing the pain of death. This painful blow takes time to heal. However, as the family begins to recover, a new sense of normalcy develops, the family reintegrates its roles and functions, and it comes to grips with the reality of the situation.

It is often difficult for nurses to deal with grieving families because the nurses also feel the loss and may feel inadequate in knowing what to say or do. By understanding the effect death has on families, nurses can help families resolve their grief and move ahead with life. (See Chapter 43 ∞ for a discussion of loss and grieving.)

Implementing and Evaluating

Nursing interventions are based on the medical diagnoses, nursing diagnoses, and selected goals or outcomes. In evaluating the success of the family care plan, the nurse assesses for the presence of the indicators identified for the chosen outcomes. If the indicators are present, it is likely that the outcome has been achieved. If the indicators or outcomes are partially or not met, all aspects of the family situation must be reexamined: Have the intervention activities been carried out? Are the indicators and outcomes appropriate? Is the nursing diagnosis proper? Has the medical condition or diagnosis changed?

Recognition of individual and family strengths helps to maintain wellness and directs behavior in crisis situations. If a plan of care has to be modified to be more effective, these strengths should be identified and utilized.

EVIDENCE-BASED PRACTICE

Evidence-Based Practice

Do Child Health Outcomes Differ for Same-Sex and Different-Sex Parenting Households?

In this national survey of children's health, Bos, Knox, Rijn-van Gelderen, and Gartrell (2016) utilized the 2011–2012 National Survey of Children's Health data set. In their research, they compared the spousal and parent relationship as well as the parent and child relationship regarding parenting stress and each child's general health and ability to cope and learn. The study participants included 95 same-sex and 95 different-sex couples with children age 6–17 years. The researchers found that no differences were observed between the household types. The only difference that was reported in the study involved parental stress. The same-sex parents revealed increases in parental stress.

Implications

When caring for parents and children, it is important to assess all physiologic and psychosocial stressors experienced by the individuals and the family unit.

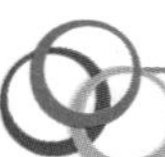

Critical Thinking Checkpoint

Linda is a young mother of three children who has developed a severe arthritic condition that has affected her ability to work and adequately care for her family. Her illness has created a financial hardship for the family and has strained their roles. Linda and her husband have custody of their children from previous marriages as well as a daughter of their own. They are reluctant to seek assistance from outside sources because they fear interference from their ex-spouses with regard to their children.

1. What aspects of Linda's physical problem must the nurse be concerned about as they relate to the other issues occurring in Linda's life?
2. Explain why Linda's family is considered to be in a health crisis when only Linda is experiencing an illness.
3. What are the advantages or disadvantages of facing illness as a member of a family as opposed to individually?
4. Describe Linda's family from the perspective of general systems theory.

Answers to Critical Thinking Checkpoint questions are available on the faculty resources site. Please consult with your instructor.

Chapter 27 Review

CHAPTER HIGHLIGHTS

- The family is the basic unit of society.
- Family-centered nursing addresses the health of the family as a unit, as well as the health of individual family members.
- In today's society, many types of families exist: traditional, two-career, single-parent, those headed by one or more adolescent parents, foster, blended, intragenerational, cohabiting, and gay and lesbian families. In addition, many single adults live alone.
- Theoretical frameworks provide the nurse with a structure for viewing the health promotion of families across the lifespan.
- The purpose of family assessment is to determine the level of family functioning, clarify family interaction patterns, identify family strengths and weaknesses, and describe the health status of the family and its individual members.
- Information on how family members are genetically related is gathered via a genogram. An ecomap allows the nurse to see where the family's energy is being expended.
- Families may be considered as being at risk for health problems based on individual family members' maturity levels, the presence of hereditary factors, sex or ethnicity, sociologic factors, and lifestyle practices.
- Nursing diagnoses that relate to family health needs and problems include impairment in caregiver role, impaired family coping, interrupted family dynamics, ineffective home maintenance, alteration in parenting, alteration in family relations, and willingness to improve family copings.

TEST YOUR KNOWLEDGE

1. Because a severely injured middle-aged client informed the nurse that he did not have any immediate family members, the nurse contacted extended family members. Which of the following is most representative of extended family members?
   1. Grandparents, aunts, and uncles
   2. Parents and spouse
   3. Children who no longer live at home
   4. Roommates and close family friends

2. A nurse is performing a family risk assessment. Which of the following factors would indicate that this family is at risk of developing health problems?
   1. The family is an elderly couple who are active in their retirement community.
   2. The family is a teenage mother and child. The mother is enrolled in parenting classes at the high school.
   3. The family belongs to the local synagogue and has family members still living in Germany.
   4. The family depends on two incomes with a limit on their health insurance spending.

3. What should a nurse instruct a client who identifies the "family" as two college roommates, a dog, and a cat when completing a family health history form?
   1. Include all information about blood relatives and the animals and roommates that might influence his health.
   2. Include only information about genetic, hereditary, and environmental illnesses of blood relatives.
   3. Leave the area blank because the client does not live with blood relatives.
   4. Use the client's own judgment in completing the area because the physical exam is more important than the history.

4. A visual representation of family members by sex, age, health status, and lines of relationships through the generations is referred to as a(n) __________.

5. To assess the impact of illness on the family as a unit, it is essential for the nurse to assess which factors? Select all that apply.
1. The duration of the illness
2. The meaning of the illness to the family and its significance to family systems
3. The coping mechanisms used by other families with similar illnesses
4. The financial impact of the illness (including factors such as insurance and the ability of the ill member to work)
5. The incidence of the illness in the community at large

6. An adult child brings a parent to an agency with signs and symptoms of potential fluid retention (e.g., high blood pressure, swollen feet), possibly related to excessive sodium intake. Further nursing assessment indicates inadequate food storage and preparation techniques in the home. Which would be the most appropriate nursing diagnosis?
1. Willingness to improve family coping
2. Impaired family coping
3. Alteration in parenting
4. Impairment in caregiver role

7. A family struggles with clear communication, and members of the family often seek the help of other systems for personal validation and gratification. What would be an appropriate nursing diagnosis for this family?
1. Altered family processes related to communication patterns
2. Impaired verbal communication related to inability to communicate
3. Ineffective family coping evidenced by assistance from outside sources
4. Knowledge deficiency (communication patterns) related to dysfunctional patterns of communication

8. Nurses often utilize systems theory to assess family units. Which example illustrates a family unit that does NOT meet the criteria of a well-functioning system?
1. The family members allow input from outside the family unit.
2. The family members are interdependent.
3. Each member's personal boundaries are well defined.
4. The primary activities of each member focus on personal purposes.

9. What is a primary function of a family?
1. Provide everything each member wants.
2. Provide an environment that supports the growth of individuals
3. Ensure that the members are accepted into society.
4. Ensure that family resources are not shared with the broader community

10. A nurse has been working with a family at the community health office and is alert to signs of family violence. Which of the following would the nurse find most concerning?
1. The baby always seems to have a cold.
2. One of the children never speaks and seems "on guard" when in the presence of a parent.
3. The family's clothes are relatively clean, but the children usually have some kind of dirt stain on their shirt or pants.
4. The family does not have a regular physician.

See Answers to Test Your Knowledge in Appendix A.

READINGS AND REFERENCES

Suggested Reading

Farr, R. H. (2017). Does parental sexual orientation matter? A longitudinal follow-up of adoptive families with school-age children. *Developmental Psychology*, *53*(2), 252–264. doi:10.1037/dev0000228

This study found that school-age children in same-sex parenting families experienced behavior problems if they experienced poor family functioning and high levels of stress. The adjustment among children, parents, and couples and the family's functioning were not different based on the parenting structure. It was positive parenting that resulted in the children's positive behaviors.

Related Research

Von Doussa, H., Power, J., McNair, R., Brown, R., Schofield, M., Perlesz, A., . . . Bickerdike, A. (2016). Building health-care workers' confidence to work with same-sex parented families. *Health Promotion International*, *31*, 459–469. doi:10.1093/heapro/dav010

References

Bos, H. M. W., Knox, J. R., van Rijn-van Gelderen, L., & Gartrell, N. K. (2016). Same-sex and different-sex parent households and child health outcomes: Findings from the National Survey of Children's Health. *Journal of Developmental & Behavioral Pediatrics*, *37*, 179–187. doi:10.1097/DBP.0000000000000288

de Vogue, A., & Diamond, J. (2015). *Supreme Court rules in favor of same-sex marriage nationwide*. Retrieved from https://www.cnn.com/2015/06/26/politics/supreme-court-same-sex-marriage-ruling/index.html

Martin, J. A., Hamilton, B. E., Osterman, M. J. K., Driscoll, A. K., & Drake, P. (2018). Births: Final data for 2016. *National Vital Statistics*, *67*(1), 1–12. Retrieved from https://www.cdc.gov/nchs/data/nvsr/nvsr67/nvsr67_01.pdf

U.S. Census Bureau (2016). *Ummarried and single Americans week: Sept. 18–24, 2016*. Retrieved from https://www.census.gov/newsroom/facts-for-features/2016/cb16-ff18.html

U.S. Census Bureau. (2018a). Table FG.7 *Family groups by family type and sex of reference persons: 2018*. Retrieved from https://www.census.gov/data/tables/2018/demo/families/cps-2018.html

U.S. Census Bureau. (2018b). *Family households by type, age of own children, age of family members, and age of householder*. Retrieved from https://www.census.gov/data/tables/2018/demo/families/cps-2018.html

U.S. Census Bureau. (2018c). *Fatherly figures: A snapshot of dads today*. Retrieved from https://www.census.gov/content/dam/Census/library/visualizations/2018/comm/fathers-day.jpg

U.S. Census Bureau. (2018d). *Grandchildren under age 18 living in the home of the grandparents 1970–2014*. Retrieved from https://www.census.gov/data/tables/time-series/demo/families/children.html

U.S. Census Bureau. (2018e). *Married couple family groups by labor force status of both spouses 2018*. Retrieved from https://www.census.gov/data/tables/2018/demo/families/cps-2018.html

U.S. Census Bureau. (2018f). *Patients and children in stay-at-home parent family groups: 1994–present. Table SHP-1* Retrieved from https://www.census.gov/newsroom/stories/2018/fathers-day.html

U.S. Census Bureau. (2018g). *U.S. Census Bureau releases 2018 families and living arrangements tables*. Retrieved from https://www.census.gov/newsroom/press-releases/2018/families.html

U.S. Conference of Mayors. (2016). *The U.S. conference of mayor's report on hunger and homelessness: A status report on homelessness and hunger in America's cities, December 2016*. Retrieved from https://endhomelessness.atavist.com/mayorsreport2016

U.S. Department of Health and Human Services. (2018a). *Teen pregnancy and childbearing*. Retrieved from https://www.hhs.gov/ash/oah/adolescent-development/reproductive-health-and-teen-pregnancy/teen-pregnancy-and-childbearing

U.S. Department of Health and Human Services. (2018b). *Teen pregnancy prevention program*. Retrieved from https://www.hhs.gov/ash/oah/grant-programs/teen-pregnancy-prevention-program-tpp/index.html

Selected Bibliography

Edelman, C. L, & Kudzma, E. (2018). *Health promotion throughout the life span* (9th ed.). St. Louis, MO: Mosby Elsevier.

Giger, J. (2017). *Transcultural nursing: Assessment and intervention* (7th ed.). St. Louis, MO: Elsevier.

Kaakinin, J., Coehlo, D. P., Steele, R., & Robinson, M. (2018). *Family health care nursing: Theory, practice & research* (6th ed.). Philadelphia, PA: F. A. Davis.

Kenner, C., & Lewis, J. A. (2013). *Genetics and genomics for nursing*. Upper Saddle River, NJ: Pearson.

McGoldrick, M., Gerson, R., & Petry, S. S. (2008). *Genograms: Assessment and intervention* (3rd ed.). New York, NY: W. W. Norton.

McGoldrick, M., Preto, N. G., & Carter, B. (2016). *The expanding family life cycle: Individual, family, and social perspectives* (5th ed.). Boston, MA: Allyn & Bacon.

Shajani, Z., & Snell, D. (2019). *Wright & Leahey's nurses and families: A guide to family assessment and intervention* (7th ed.). Philadelphia, PA: F. A. Davis.

Thomlinson, B. (2016). *Family assessment handbook: An introductory practical guide to family assessment* (4th ed.). Boston, MA: Cengage.

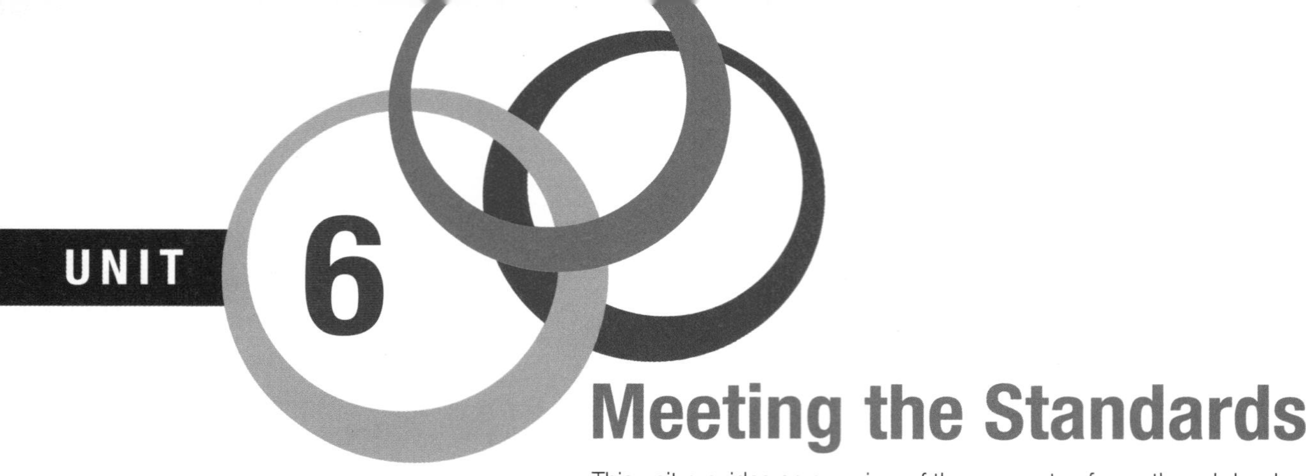

Meeting the Standards

This unit provides an overview of the concepts of growth and development, focusing on health promotion across the lifespan and within the family. In order for nurses to deliver developmentally appropriate care, nurses must be knowledgeable about normal growth and development and the age-specific risks faced by individuals in each stage of development. Knowledge of growth and development provides a framework for health assessment and health promotion across the lifespan. An understanding of the role of the family in the client's life, as well as how the family impacts health beliefs, will improve the nurse's care of the individual.

In the case described here, the family is coping with an illness of one member that impacts all members in unique ways based on their developmental stages and tasks. The nurse acts to provide support, resources, and coping strategies to help each member meet his or her developmental needs.

CLIENT: Carmelita AGE: 76
CURRENT MEDICAL DIAGNOSIS: Alzheimer's Disease

Medical History: Carmelita is a healthy Latino woman of Colombian descent. She was diagnosed with Alzheimer's disease 5 years ago and is now in stage II. She is usually unable to identify her daughter and son-in-law, and she wanders frequently, requiring constant watching. She is unable to sleep most nights and takes naps periodically throughout the day. Her daughter reports that she is easily upset and will scream and strike out when frustrated. She has no other health problems and is very active, enjoying walking with her daughter or grandchildren around the neighborhood or to the local park. Lately however, her grandchildren have found it difficult to control her behavior during walks and are reluctant to be alone with her.

Personal and Social History: Carmelita lives with her daughter and son-in-law and their five children ages 19, 15, 10, 5, and 2 years of age. Her husband of 43 years died 4 years ago, and Carmelita was unable to live independently. She used to speak some English but is increasingly only able to communicate in Spanish. The family lives in a single-family home with three bedrooms. Four children have to share a room, while the oldest child, a boy, sleeps on a couch in the basement in order to provide the client with her own room. They tried having one of the girls share Carmelita's room, but her late-night sleeplessness and wandering interfered with the girl's sleep. Carmelita's daughter admits to feeling tired all of the time as well as often feeling pulled in many different directions when her children and her mother need her attention or help at the same time. Carmelita often calls her son-in-law by her husband's name, making him uncomfortable in caring for her. The family has considered moving Carmelita into a long-term care facility, but her daughter promised her shortly after the diagnosis that she would take care of her mother for as long as necessary. Now she cannot bring herself to break her promise.

Questions

American Nurses Association Standard of Practice #5B is Health Teaching and Health Promotion: *The nurse employs strategies to promote health and a safe environment by using health promotion and health teaching methods appropriate to the situation and the healthcare consumer's values, beliefs, health practices, developmental level, learning needs, readiness and ability to learn, language preference, spirituality, culture, and socioeconomic status.*

1. What health promotion teaching would you provide this family?
2. What recommendations would you make to each family member to promote health based on each member's current developmental level?
3. How will Carmelita's condition impact her own development and health promotion needs?

American Nurses Association Standard of Practice #15 is Professional Practice Evaluation: *The nurse engages in self-reflection and self-evaluation to provide age-appropriate and developmentally appropriate care in a culturally and ethnically sensitive manner.*

4. The nurse assesses that Carmelita's condition is likely to have what impact on the developmental tasks of the other members of her family?
5. The nurse anticipates that Carmelita's condition is likely to have what impact on the health of the family, both physically and psychologically?

American Nurses Association. (2016). *Nursing: Scope and standards of practice* (3rd ed.). Silver Spring, MD: Author.

Answers to Meeting the Standards questions are available on the faculty resources site. Please consult with your instructor.

UNIT 7

Assessing Health

28 Vital Signs

LEARNING OUTCOMES

After completing this chapter, you will be able to:

1. Describe factors that affect the vital signs and accurate measurement of them.
2. Identify the variations in normal body temperature, pulse, respirations, and blood pressure that occur from infancy to old age.
3. Verbalize the steps used in:
   a. Assessing body temperature.
   b. Assessing a peripheral pulse.
   c. Assessing the apical pulse and the apical-radial pulse.
   d. Assessing respirations.
   e. Assessing blood pressure.
   f. Assessing blood oxygenation using pulse oximetry.
4. Describe appropriate nursing care for alterations in vital signs.
5. Identify nine sites used to assess the pulse and state the reasons for their use.
6. List the characteristics that should be included when assessing pulses.
7. Describe the mechanics of breathing and the mechanisms that control respirations.
8. Recognize when it is appropriate to assign or delegate measurement of vital signs to assistive personnel.
9. Demonstrate appropriate documentation and reporting of vital signs.

KEY TERMS

afebrile, *535*
apical pulse, *543*
apical-radial pulse, *551*
apnea, *553*
arrhythmia, *545*
arterial blood pressure, *556*
arteriosclerosis, *556*
auscultatory gap, *560*
basal metabolic rate (BMR), *533*
body temperature, *533*
bradycardia, *545*
bradypnea, *553*
cardiac output, *542*
compliance, *542*
conduction, *534*
constant fever, *535*
convection, *534*
core temperature, *533*
costal (thoracic) breathing, *552*
diaphragmatic (abdominal) breathing, *552*
diastolic pressure, *556*
dysrhythmia, *545*
evaporation, *534*
exhalation, *552*
expiration, *552*
febrile, *535*
fever, *535*
fever spike, *535*
heat balance, *533*
heat exhaustion, *535*
heat stroke, *535*
hematocrit, *556*
hyperpyrexia, *535*
hypertension, *557*
hyperthermia, *535*
hyperventilation, *554*
hypotension, *557*
hypothermia, *536*
hypoventilation, *554*
inhalation, *552*
insensible heat loss, *534*
insensible water loss, *534*
inspiration, *552*
intermittent fever, *535*
Korotkoff sounds, *560*
mean arterial pressure (MAP), *556*
orthostatic hypotension, *557*
oxygen saturation (SpO_2), *564*
peripheral pulse, *543*
point of maximal impulse (PMI), *543*
pulse, *542*
pulse deficit, *551*
pulse oximeter, *564*
pulse pressure, *556*
pulse rhythm, *545*
pulse volume, *545*
pyrexia, *535*
radiation, *534*
relapsing fever, *535*
remittent fever, *535*
respiration, *552*
respiratory character, *554*
respiratory quality, *554*
respiratory rhythm, *554*
sphygmomanometer, *558*
surface temperature, *533*
systolic pressure, *556*
tachycardia, *545*
tachypnea, *553*
tidal volume, *554*
ventilation, *552*
vital signs, *532*

Introduction

The traditional **vital signs** are body temperature, pulse, respirations, and blood pressure. Many agencies such as the Veterans Administration, American Pain Society, and The Joint Commission have designated pain as a fifth vital sign, to be assessed at the same time as each of the other four. Pain assessment is covered in Chapter 30 ∞. Oxygen saturation is also commonly measured at the same time as the traditional vital signs and could be considered the sixth vital sign. Vital signs, which should be looked at in total, are checked to monitor the functions of the body. The signs reflect changes in function that otherwise might not be observed. Monitoring a client's vital signs should not be an automatic or routine procedure; it should be a thoughtful, scientific assessment. Vital signs should be evaluated with reference to clients' present and prior health status, their usual vital sign results (if known), and accepted standards.

When and how often to assess a specific client's vital signs are chiefly nursing judgments, depending on the client's health status. Some agencies have policies about when to take clients' vital signs. The primary care provider may specifically order a vital sign (e.g., "Blood pressure q2h"). Ordered vital sign measurements, however, should be considered the minimum; a nurse should assess vital signs more often if the client's health status requires it. Examples of times to assess vital signs are listed in Box 28.1.

BOX 28.1 Times to Assess Vital Signs

- On admission to a healthcare agency to obtain baseline data
- When a client has a change in health status or reports symptoms such as chest pain or feeling hot or faint
- Before and after surgery or an invasive procedure
- Before and after the administration of a medication that could affect the respiratory or cardiovascular systems; for example, before giving a digitalis preparation
- Before and after any nursing intervention that could affect the vital signs (e.g., ambulating a client who has been on bedrest)

Often, someone other than the nurse measures the client's vital signs. Prior to assigning this task to assistive personnel (AP), however, the nurse must have assessed the client and determined that the client is medically stable or in a chronic condition and not fragile and that the vital sign measurement is considered routine for this client. Under those circumstances, the AP may measure, record, and report vital signs; however, real assessment, or interpretation of the measurements, rests with the registered nurse.

Body Temperature

Body temperature reflects the balance between the heat produced and the heat lost from the body, and is measured in heat units called degrees. There are two kinds of body temperature: core temperature and surface temperature. **Core temperature** is the temperature of the deep tissues of the body, such as the abdominal cavity and pelvic cavity. It remains relatively constant. The normal core body temperature is a range of temperatures (Figure 28.1 ■). The **surface temperature** is the temperature of the skin, the subcutaneous tissue, and fat. It, by contrast, rises and falls in response to the environment.

The body continually produces heat as a by-product of metabolism. When the amount of heat produced by the body equals the amount of heat lost, the client is in **heat balance** (Figure 28.2 ■).

A number of factors affect the body's heat production. The most important are these five:

1. ***Basal metabolic rate.*** The **basal metabolic rate (BMR)** is the rate of energy utilization in the body required to maintain essential activities such as breathing. Metabolic rates decrease with age. In general, the younger the client, the higher the BMR.
2. ***Muscle activity.*** Muscle activity, including shivering, increases the metabolic rate.
3. ***Thyroxine output.*** Increased thyroxine output increases the rate of cellular metabolism throughout the body.
4. ***Epinephrine and norepinephrine and sympathetic nervous system stimulation (such as with stress).*** Epinephrine and norepinephrine immediately increase the rate of cellular metabolism in many body tissues.
5. ***Fever.*** Fever increases the cellular metabolic rate and thus increases the body's temperature further.

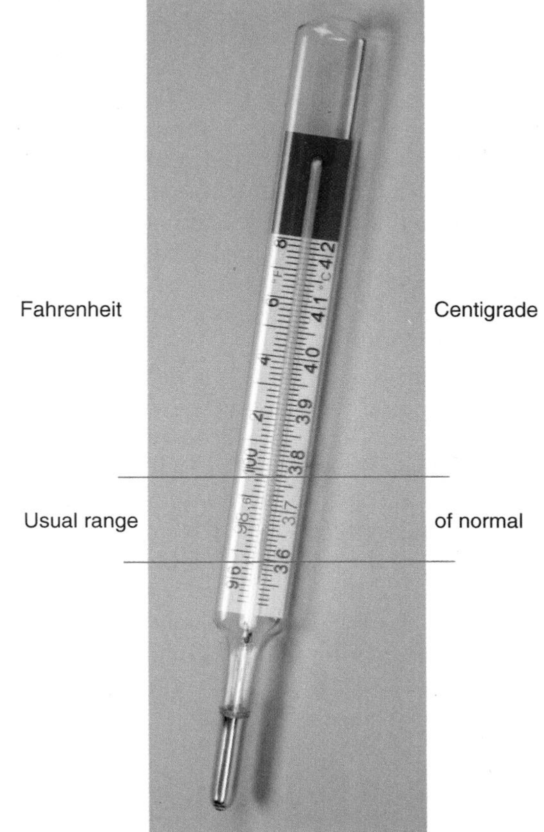

Figure 28.1 ■ Estimated ranges of body temperatures in healthy adults.

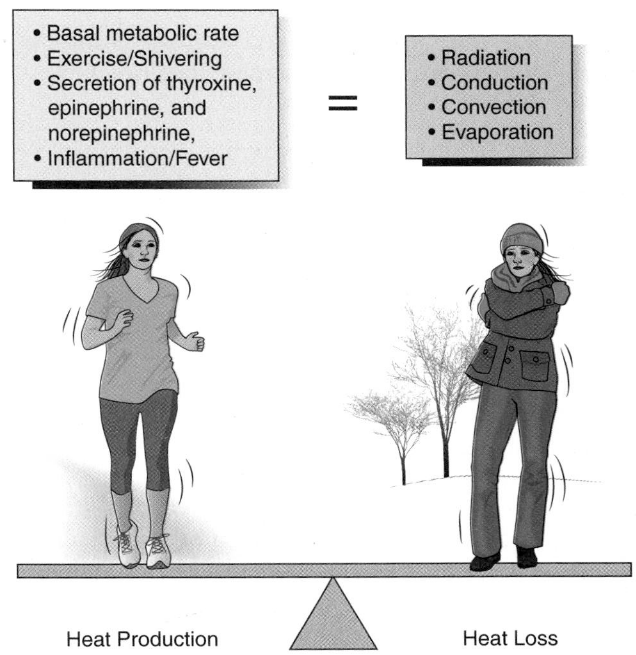

Figure 28.2 ■ As long as heat production and heat loss are properly balanced, body temperature remains constant. Factors contributing to heat production (and temperature rise) are shown on the left; those contributing to heat loss (and temperature fall) are shown on the right.

Heat is lost from the body through radiation, conduction, convection, and evaporation. **Radiation** is the transfer of heat from the surface of one object to the surface of another without contact between the two objects, mostly in the form of infrared rays. **Conduction** is the transfer of heat from one molecule to a molecule of lower temperature. Conductive transfer cannot take place without contact between the molecules and normally accounts for minimal heat loss except, for example, when a body is immersed in cold water. The amount of heat transferred depends on the temperature difference and the amount and duration of the contact.

Convection is the dispersion of heat by air currents. The body usually has a small amount of warm air adjacent to it. This warm air rises and is replaced by cooler air, so people always lose a small amount of heat through convection.

Evaporation is continuous vaporization of moisture from the respiratory tract and from the mucosa of the mouth and from the skin. This continuous and unnoticed water loss is called **insensible water loss**, and the accompanying heat loss is called **insensible heat loss**. Insensible heat loss accounts for about 10% of basal heat loss. When the body temperature increases, vaporization accounts for greater heat loss.

Regulation of Body Temperature

The system that regulates body temperature has three main parts: sensors in the periphery and in the core, an integrator in the hypothalamus, and an effector system that adjusts the production and loss of heat. Most sensors or sensory receptors are in the skin. The skin has more receptors for cold than warmth. Therefore, skin sensors detect cold more efficiently than warmth.

When the skin becomes chilled over the entire body, three physiologic processes to increase the body temperature take place:

1. Shivering increases heat production.
2. Sweating is inhibited to decrease heat loss.
3. Vasoconstriction decreases heat loss.

The hypothalamic integrator is the center that controls the core temperature. When the integrator detects heat, it sends out signals intended to reduce the temperature, that is, to decrease heat production and increase heat loss. In contrast, when the cold sensors are stimulated, the integrator sends out signals to increase heat production and decrease heat loss.

The signals from the cold-sensitive receptors of the hypothalamus initiate effectors, such as vasoconstriction, shivering, and the release of epinephrine, which increases cellular metabolism and hence heat production. When the warmth-sensitive receptors in the hypothalamus are stimulated, the effector system sends out signals that initiate sweating and peripheral vasodilation. Also, when this system is stimulated, the individual consciously makes appropriate adjustments, such as putting on additional clothing in response to cold or turning on a fan in response to heat.

Factors Affecting Body Temperature

Nurses should be aware of the factors that can affect a client's body temperature so that they can recognize normal temperature variations and understand the significance of body temperature measurements that deviate from normal. Among the factors that affect body temperature are the following:

1. ***Age.*** Infants are greatly influenced by the temperature of the environment and must be protected from extreme changes. Children's temperatures vary more than those of adults do until puberty. Many older people, particularly those over 75 years, are at risk of hypothermia (temperatures below 36°C, or 96.8°F) for a variety of reasons, such as inadequate diet, loss of subcutaneous fat, lack of activity, and reduced thermoregulatory efficiency. Older adults are also particularly sensitive to extremes in the environmental temperature due to decreased thermoregulatory controls.
2. ***Diurnal variations (circadian rhythms).*** Body temperatures normally change throughout the day, varying as much as 1.0°C (1.8°F) between the early morning and the late afternoon. The point of highest body temperature is usually reached between 1600 and 1800 hours (4:00 p.m. and 6:00 p.m.), and the lowest point is reached during sleep between 0400 and 0600 hours (4:00 a.m. and 6:00 a.m.) (Figure 28.3 ■). Older adults' temperatures may vary less than those of younger individuals due to the changes in autonomic functioning common in aging (Parashar, Amir, Pakhare, Rathi, & Chaudhary, 2016).
3. ***Exercise.*** Hard work or strenuous exercise can increase body temperature to as high as 38.3°C to 40°C (101°F to 104°F) measured rectally.
4. ***Hormones.*** Women usually experience more hormone fluctuations than men. In women, progesterone secretion at the time of ovulation raises body temperature by about 0.3°C to 0.6°C (0.5°F to 1.0°F) above basal temperature.
5. ***Stress.*** Stimulation of the sympathetic nervous system can increase metabolic activity and heat production. Nurses should anticipate that a highly stressed or anxious client could have an elevated body temperature for that reason.

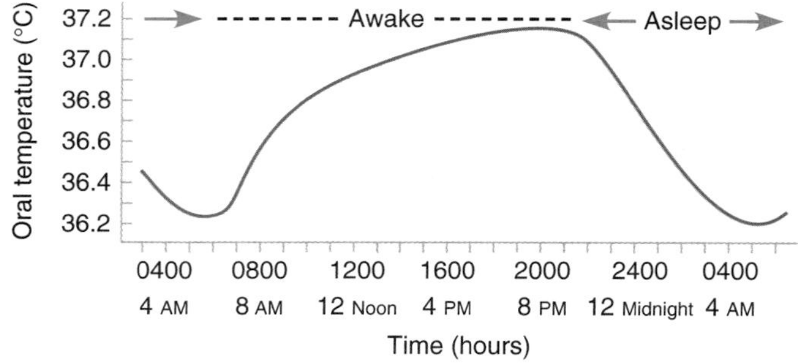

Figure 28.3 ■ Range of oral temperatures during 24 hours for a healthy young adult.

6. ***Environment.*** Extremes in environmental temperatures can affect a client's temperature regulatory systems. If the body temperature is assessed in a very warm room and cannot be modified by convection, conduction, or radiation, the temperature will be elevated. Similarly, if the client has been outside in cold weather without suitable clothing, or if a medical condition prevents the client from controlling the temperature in the environment (e.g., the client has altered mental status or cannot dress self), the body temperature may be low.

Alterations in Body Temperature

The normal range for adults is considered to be between 36°C and 37.5°C (96.8°F to 99.5°F). There are two primary alterations in body temperature: pyrexia and hypothermia.

Pyrexia

A body temperature above the usual range is called **pyrexia**, **hyperthermia**, or (in lay terms) **fever**. A very high fever, such as 41°C (105.8°F), is called **hyperpyrexia** (Figure 28.4 ■). The client who has a fever is referred to as **febrile**; the one who does not is **afebrile**.

Four common types of fevers are intermittent, remittent, relapsing, and constant. During an **intermittent fever**, the body temperature alternates at regular intervals between periods of fever and periods of normal or subnormal temperatures. An example is with the disease malaria. During a **remittent fever**, such as with a cold or influenza, a wide range of temperature fluctuations (more than 2°C [3.6°F]) occurs over a 24-hour period, all of which are above normal. In a **relapsing fever**, short febrile periods of a few days are interspersed with periods of 1 or 2 days of normal temperature. During a **constant fever**, the body temperature fluctuates minimally but always remains above normal. This can occur with typhoid fever. A temperature that rises to fever level rapidly following a normal temperature and then returns to normal within a few hours is called a **fever spike**. Bacterial blood infections often cause fever spikes.

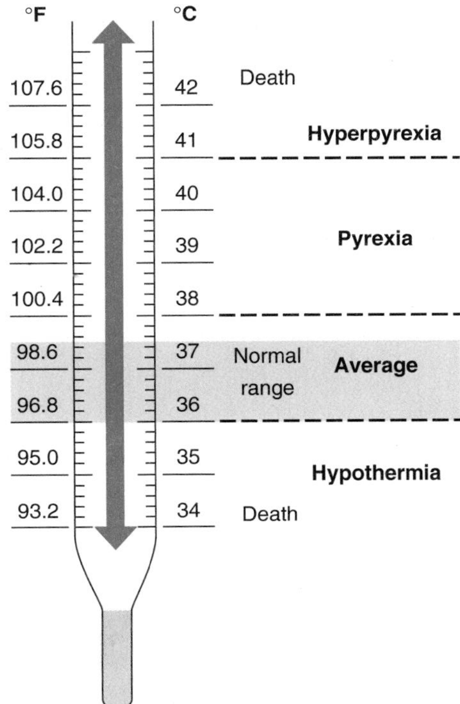

Figure 28.4 ■ Terms used to describe alterations in body temperature (oral measurements) and ranges in Fahrenheit and Celsius (centigrade) scales.

In some conditions, an elevated temperature is not a true fever. Two examples are heat exhaustion and heat stroke. **Heat exhaustion** is a result of excessive heat and dehydration. Signs of heat exhaustion include paleness, dizziness, nausea, vomiting, fainting, and a moderately increased temperature (38.3°C to 38.9°C [101°F to 102°F]). Individuals experiencing **heat stroke** generally have been exercising in hot weather, have warm, flushed skin, and often do not sweat. They usually have a temperature of 41.1°C (106°F) or higher, and may be delirious, unconscious, or having seizures.

The clinical signs of fever vary with the onset, course, and abatement stages of the fever (Box 28.2). These signs occur as a result of changes in the set point of the temperature control mechanism regulated by the hypothalamus. Under normal conditions, whenever the core temperature rises, the rate of heat loss is increased, resulting in a fall in

BOX 28.2 Fever

ONSET (COLD OR CHILL PHASE)

- Increased heart rate
- Increased respiratory rate and depth
- Shivering
- Pallid, cold skin
- Complaints of feeling cold
- Cyanotic nail beds
- "Gooseflesh" appearance of the skin
- Cessation of sweating

COURSE (PLATEAU PHASE)

- Absence of chills
- Skin that feels warm
- Photosensitivity
- Glassy-eyed appearance
- Increased pulse and respiratory rates
- Increased thirst
- Mild to severe dehydration
- Drowsiness, restlessness, delirium, or convulsions
- Herpetic lesions of the mouth
- Loss of appetite (if the fever is prolonged)
- Malaise, weakness, and aching muscles

DEFERVESCENCE (FEVER ABATEMENT AND FLUSH PHASE)

- Skin that appears flushed and feels warm
- Sweating
- Decreased shivering
- Possible dehydration

temperature toward the set-point level. Conversely, when the core temperature falls, the rate of heat production is increased, resulting in a rise in temperature toward the set point.

In a fever, however, the set point of the hypothalamic thermostat changes suddenly from the normal level to a higher than normal value (e.g., 39.5°C [103.1°F]) as a result of the effects of tissue destruction, pyrogenic substances, or dehydration on the hypothalamus. Although the set point changes rapidly, the core body temperature (i.e., the blood temperature) reaches this new set point only after several hours. During this interval, the usual heat production responses that cause elevation of the body temperature occur: chills, feeling of coldness, cold skin due to vasoconstriction, and shivering. This is referred to as the chill phase.

When the core temperature reaches the new set point, the individual feels neither cold nor hot and no longer experiences chills (the plateau phase). Depending on the degree of temperature elevation, other signs may occur during the course of the fever. Very high temperatures, such as 41°C to 42°C (106°F to 108°F), damage the parenchyma of cells throughout the body, particularly in the brain, where destruction of neuronal cells is irreversible. Damage to the liver, kidneys, and other body organs can also be great enough to disrupt functioning and eventually cause death.

When the cause of the high temperature is suddenly removed, the set point of the hypothalamic thermostat is suddenly reduced to a lower value, perhaps even back to the original normal level. In this instance, the hypothalamus now attempts to lower the temperature, and the usual heat loss responses that cause a reduction of the body temperature occur: excessive sweating and hot, flushed skin due to sudden vasodilation. This is referred to as the flush phase. Nursing interventions for a client who has a fever are designed to support the body's normal physiologic processes, provide comfort, and prevent complications. During the course of a fever, the nurse needs to monitor the client's vital signs closely.

Nursing interventions during the chill phase are designed to help the client decrease heat loss. At this time, the body's physiologic processes are attempting to raise the core temperature to the new set-point temperature. During the flush or crisis phase, the body processes are attempting to lower the core temperature to the reduced or normal set-point temperature. At this time, the nurse takes measures to increase heat loss and decrease heat production. Nursing interventions for a client with fever are shown in Box 28.3.

Hypothermia

Hypothermia is a core body temperature below the lower limit of normal. The three physiologic mechanisms of hypothermia are (a) excessive heat loss, (b) inadequate heat production to counteract heat loss, and (c) impaired hypothalamic thermoregulation. The clinical signs of hypothermia are listed in Box 28.4.

BOX 28.3 Nursing Interventions for Clients with Fever

- Monitor vital signs.
- Assess skin color and temperature.
- Monitor white blood cell count, hematocrit value, and other pertinent laboratory reports for indications of infection or dehydration.
- Remove excess blankets when the client feels warm, and provide extra warmth when the client feels chilled.
- Provide adequate nutrition and fluids (e.g., 2500–3000 mL/day) to meet the increased metabolic demands and prevent dehydration.
- Measure intake and output.
- Reduce physical activity to limit heat production, especially during the flush stage.
- Administer antipyretics (drugs that reduce the level of fever) as ordered.
- Provide oral hygiene to keep the mucous membranes moist.
- Provide a tepid sponge bath to increase heat loss through conduction.
- Provide dry clothing and bed linens.

Hypothermia may be induced or accidental. Induced hypothermia is the deliberate lowering of the body temperature to decrease the need for oxygen by the body tissues such as during certain surgeries. Accidental hypothermia can occur as a result of (a) exposure to a cold environment, (b) immersion in cold water, and (c) lack of adequate clothing, shelter, or heat. In older adults, the problem can be compounded by a decreased metabolic rate and the use of sedative medications. If skin and underlying tissues are damaged by freezing cold, this results in frostbite. Frostbite most commonly occurs in hands, feet, nose, and ears.

Managing hypothermia involves removing the client from the cold and rewarming the client's body. For the client with mild hypothermia, the body is rewarmed by applying blankets; for the client with severe hypothermia, a hyperthermia blanket (an electronically controlled blanket that provides a specified temperature) is applied, and warm IV fluids are given. Wet clothing, which increases heat loss because of the high conductivity of water, should be replaced with dry clothing. See Box 28.5 for nursing interventions for clients who have hypothermia.

BOX 28.4 Hypothermia

- Decreased body temperature, pulse, and respirations
- Severe shivering (initially)
- Feelings of cold and chills
- Pale, cool, waxy skin
- Frostbite (discolored, blistered nose, fingers, toes)
- Hypotension
- Decreased urinary output
- Lack of muscle coordination
- Disorientation
- Drowsiness progressing to coma

BOX 28.5 Nursing Interventions for Clients with Hypothermia

- Provide a warm environment.
- Provide dry clothing.
- Apply warm blankets.
- Keep limbs close to the body.
- Cover the client's scalp with a cap or turban.
- Supply warm oral or IV fluids.
- Apply warming pads.

Assessing Body Temperature

The most common sites for measuring body temperature are oral, rectal, axillary, tympanic membrane, and temporal artery. Each of the sites has advantages and disadvantages (Table 28.1).

The body temperature may be measured *orally*. If a client has been taking cold or hot food or fluids or smoking, the nurse should wait 30 minutes before taking the temperature orally to ensure that the temperature of the mouth is not affected by the temperature of the food, fluid, or warm smoke.

Rectal temperature readings are considered to be very accurate. Rectal temperatures are contraindicated for clients who are undergoing rectal surgery, have diarrhea or diseases of the rectum, are immunosuppressed, have a clotting disorder, or have significant hemorrhoids.

The *axilla* is often the preferred site for measuring temperature in newborns because it is accessible and safe. Axillary temperatures are lower than rectal temperatures. Some clinicians recommend rechecking an elevated axillary temperature with one taken from another site to confirm the degree of elevation. Nurses should check agency protocol when taking the temperature of newborns, infants, toddlers, and children. Adult clients for whom the axillary method of temperature assessment is appropriate include those for whom other temperature sites are contraindicated.

The *tympanic membrane*, or nearby tissue in the ear canal, is a frequent site for estimating core body temperature. However, proper technique must be used. If the probe fits too loosely in the ear canal, the reading can be lower than the true value. If too tight, the probe can be uncomfortable. Research has shown no significant difference in tympanic temperature readings between normal left and right ears (Salota, Slovakova, Panes, Nundlall, & Goonasekera, 2016). Electronic tympanic thermometers are found extensively in both inpatient and ambulatory care settings.

The temperature may also be measured on the forehead using a chemical thermometer or a *temporal artery* thermometer. Forehead temperature measurements are useful for infants and children when a more invasive measurement is not necessary. Temporal artery thermometry is also beneficial for adults when any invasive or uncomfortable measure should be avoided, such as with cancer patients (Mason et al., 2017).

Types of Thermometers

Traditionally, body temperatures were measured using mercury-in-glass thermometers. Such thermometers, however, can be hazardous due to exposure to mercury, which is toxic to humans, and broken glass should the thermometer crack or break. In 1998, the U.S. Environmental Protection Agency and the American Hospital Association agreed to the goal of eliminating mercury from healthcare environments. Hospitals no longer use mercury-in-glass thermometers, and several cities have banned the sale and manufacture of them. However, the nurse may still encounter this type of thermometer, especially in the home. In some cases, plastics have replaced glass and safer chemicals (e.g., gallium) have replaced mercury in modern versions of the thermometer.

TABLE 28.1 Advantages and Disadvantages of Sites Used for Body Temperature Measurements

Site	Advantages	Disadvantages
Oral	Accessible and convenient	Thermometers can break if bitten. Inaccurate if client has just ingested hot or cold food or fluid or smoked. Could injure the mouth following oral surgery.
Rectal	Reliable measurement	Inconvenient and more unpleasant for clients; difficult for client who cannot turn to the side. Could injure the rectum. Presence of stool may interfere with thermometer placement.
Axillary	Safe and noninvasive	The thermometer may need to be left in place a long time to obtain an accurate measurement.
Tympanic membrane	Readily accessible; reflects the core temperature; very fast	Can be uncomfortable and involves risk of injuring the membrane if the probe is inserted too far. Repeated measurements may vary. Right and left measurements can differ if there are anatomic or pathologic differences (e.g., infection). Presence of cerumen can affect the reading.
Temporal artery	Safe and noninvasive; very fast	Requires electronic equipment that may be expensive or unavailable. Variation in technique needed if the client has perspiration on the forehead.

Safety Alert! SAFETY

Whenever mercury-in-glass thermometers are encountered, the nurse should recommend their immediate replacement with less hazardous thermometers and their safe disposal.

Electronic thermometers can provide a reading in only 2 to 60 seconds, depending on the model. The equipment consists of an electronic base, a probe, and a probe cover, which is usually disposable (Figure 28.5 ■). Some institutional models have a different circuit and probe for oral and rectal measurement.

Chemical disposable thermometers have liquid crystal dots or bars that change color to indicate temperature. Some of these are single use and others may be reused several times. One type that has small chemical dots at one end is shown in Figure 28.6 ■. To read the temperature, the nurse notes the highest reading among the dots that have changed color. These thermometers can be used orally, rectally, or in the axilla.

Temperature-sensitive tape does not indicate the core temperature. The tape contains liquid crystals that change color according to temperature. When applied to the skin, usually of the forehead or abdomen, the temperature digits on the tape respond by changing color (Figure 28.7 ■). The skin area should be dry. After the length of time specified by the manufacturer (e.g., 15 seconds), a color appears on the tape. This method is particularly useful at home and for infants whose temperatures are to be monitored.

Infrared thermometers sense body heat in the form of infrared energy given off by a heat source, which, in the ear canal, is primarily the tympanic membrane (Figure 28.8 ■). The infrared thermometer makes no contact with the tympanic membrane.

Temporal artery thermometers determine temperature using a scanning infrared thermometer that compares the arterial temperature in the temporal artery of the forehead to the temperature in the room and calculates the heat balance to approximate the core temperature of the blood in the pulmonary artery. The probe is placed in the middle of the forehead and then drawn laterally to the hairline. If the client has perspiration on the forehead, the probe is also touched behind the earlobe so the thermometer can compensate for evaporative cooling (Figure 28.9 ■).

The latest innovation in thermometers is *noncontact thermometers*. These are held about 1 inch from the forehead and use infrared light to estimate temperature in a few seconds. The accuracy of these thermometers is similar to temporal artery or axillary thermometer measurements, and they are particularly useful in conditions where reusable thermometer contact with the client should be minimized, such as communicable diseases or infants in incubators (Schuman, 2016).

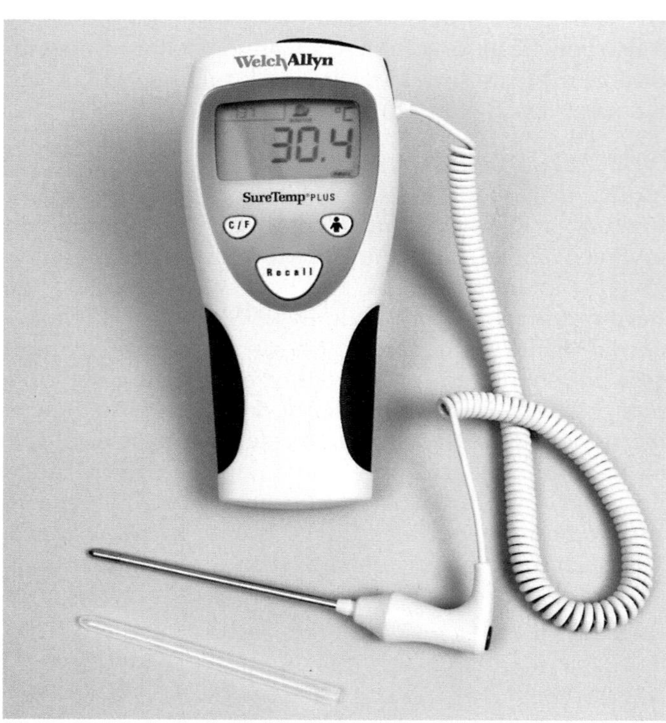

A

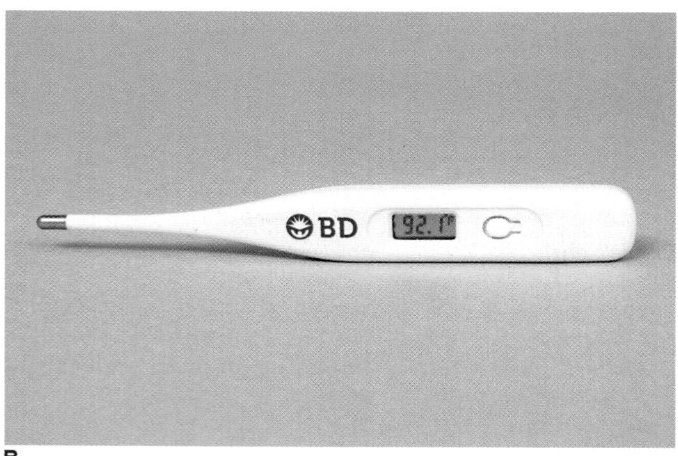

B

Figure 28.5 ■ Electronic thermometers: *A*, institutional model (note the probe and probe cover); *B*, one-piece home electronic thermometer.

Temperature Scales

Sometimes a nurse needs to convert a body temperature reading in Celsius (centigrade) to Fahrenheit, or vice versa. Although the conversion can be accomplished using several different formulas, the most common is described here. To convert from Fahrenheit to Celsius, deduct 32 from the Fahrenheit reading and then multiply by the fraction 5/9; that is:

$$C = (\text{Fahrenheit temperature} - 32) \times 5/9$$

For example, when the Fahrenheit reading is 100:

$$C = (100 - 32) \times 5/9 = (68) \times 5/9 = 37.8$$

To convert from Celsius to Fahrenheit, multiply the Celsius reading by the fraction 9/5 and then add 32; that is:

$$F = (\text{Celsius temperature} \times 9/5) + 32$$

For example, when the Celsius reading is 40:

$$F = (40 \times 9/5) + 32 = (72 + 32) = 104$$

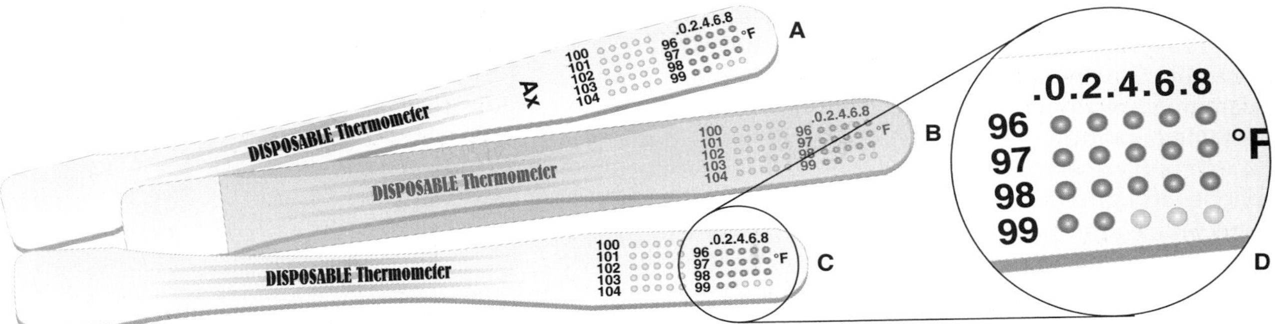

Figure 28.6 ■ Chemical dot thermometers: *A*, axillary (note the “Ax” on the stem); *B*, rectal (note the plastic cover); *C*, oral; *D*, an enlargement showing a reading of 99.2°F.

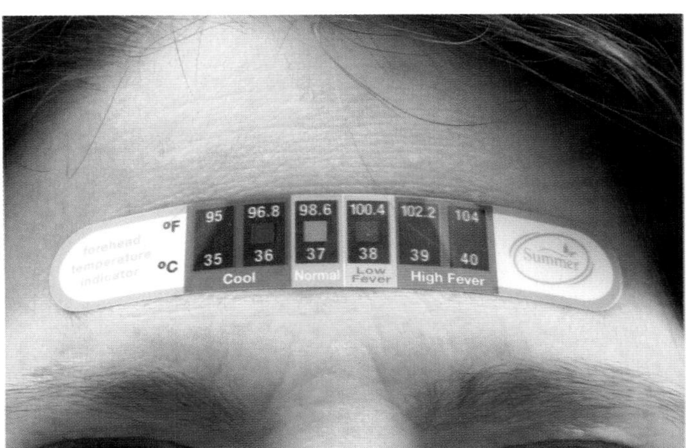

Figure 28.7 ■ A temperature-sensitive skin tape.

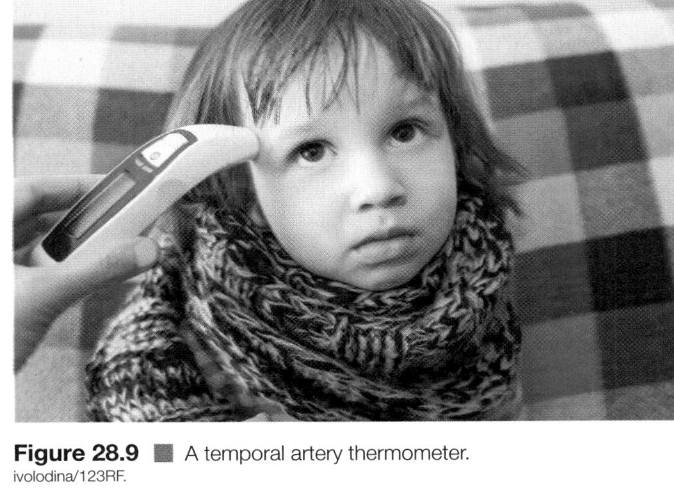

Figure 28.9 ■ A temporal artery thermometer.
ivolodina/123RF.

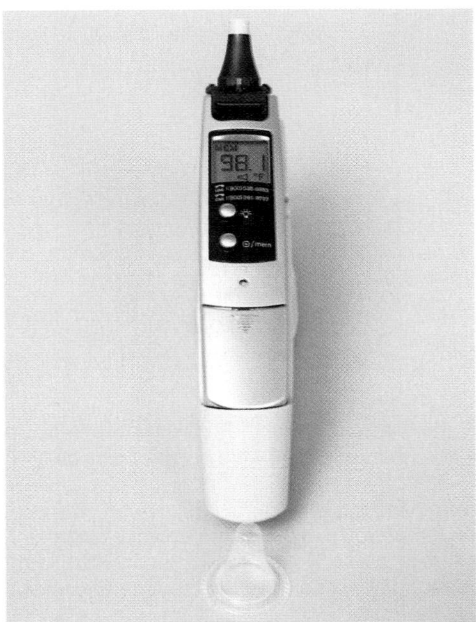

Figure 28.8 ■ An infrared (tympanic) thermometer used to measure the tympanic membrane temperature.

QSEN Patient-Centered Care: Temperature

In addition to measuring the temperature while the client is at a healthcare facility, the nurse provides guidance for clients at home. When making a home visit, take a thermometer with you in case the client does not own a functional thermometer.

Observe the client or caregiver taking and reading a temperature. Examine the home thermometer for safety and proper functioning. Facilitate the replacement of mercury thermometers with nonmercury ones. Ensure that the client has water-soluble lubricant if using a rectal thermometer. Reinforce the importance of reporting the site and type of thermometer used and using the same site and thermometer consistently. Check that the client knows how to record the temperature and provide a recording chart if indicated. Discuss means of cleaning the thermometer, such as warm water and soap, and avoiding cross contamination.

Instruct the client or family member to notify the healthcare provider if the temperature is 38.5°C (101.3°F) or higher. Discuss environmental control modifications that should be made during illness or extreme climate conditions (e.g., heating, air conditioning, appropriate clothing and bedding).

Pacifier thermometers (Figure 28.10 ■) may be used in the home setting for children under 2 years old. The manufacturer's instructions must be followed carefully since many require adding 0.28°C (0.5°F) in order to estimate rectal temperature.

"Smart thermometers" are available that connect to smartphones and can communicate with electronic health records. A phone application calibrates the thermometer, records the time of the temperature, and enables the client to record symptoms and document the time that a medication such as an antipyretic was administered (Miller, Singh, Koehler, & Polgreen, 2018).

Skill 28.1 explains how to assess body temperature.

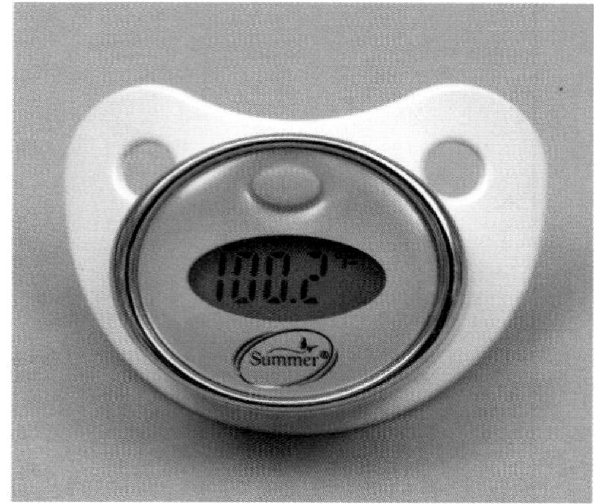

Figure 28.10 ■ A pacifier thermometer.

SKILL 28.1

Assessing Body Temperature

PURPOSES

- To establish baseline data for subsequent evaluation
- To identify whether the core temperature is within normal range
- To determine changes in the core temperature in response to specific therapies (e.g., antipyretic medication, immunosuppressive therapy, invasive procedure)
- To monitor clients at risk for imbalanced body temperature (e.g., clients at risk for infection or diagnosis of infection; those who have been exposed to temperature extremes)

ASSESSMENT

Assess

- Clinical signs of fever
- Clinical signs of hypothermia
- Site and method most appropriate for measurement
- Factors that may alter core body temperature

PLANNING

Assignment

Routine measurement of the client's temperature can be assigned to AP or be performed by family members or caregivers in nonhospital settings. The nurse must explain the appropriate type of thermometer and site to be used and ensure that the individual knows when to report an abnormal temperature and how to record the finding. The nurse interprets an abnormal temperature and determines appropriate responses.

Equipment

- Thermometer
- Thermometer sheath or cover
- Water-soluble lubricant for a rectal temperature
- Clean gloves for a rectal temperature
- Towel for axillary temperature
- Tissues or wipes

IMPLEMENTATION

Preparation

Check that all equipment is functioning normally.

Performance

1. Prior to performing the procedure, introduce self and verify the client's identity using agency protocol. Explain to the client what you are going to do, why it is necessary, and how to participate. Discuss how the results will be used in planning further care or treatments.
2. Perform hand hygiene and observe appropriate infection prevention procedures. Apply gloves if performing a rectal temperature.
3. Provide for client privacy.
4. Position the client appropriately (e.g., lateral or Sims' position for inserting a rectal thermometer).
5. Place the thermometer (Box 28.6).
   - Apply a protective sheath or probe cover if appropriate.
   - Lubricate a rectal thermometer.
6. Wait the appropriate amount of time. Electronic and tympanic thermometers will indicate that the reading is complete through a light or tone. Check package instructions for length of time to wait prior to reading chemical dot or tape thermometers.

Clinical Alert!

Be sure to record the temperature from an electronic thermometer before replacing the probe into the charging unit. With many models, replacing the probe erases the temperature from the display.

7. Remove the thermometer and discard the cover or wipe with a tissue if necessary. If gloves were applied, remove and discard them.
   - Perform hand hygiene.
8. Read the temperature and record it on your worksheet. If the temperature is markedly high, low, or inconsistent with the client's condition, recheck it with a thermometer known to be functioning properly.
9. Wash the thermometer if necessary and return it to the storage location.

Assessing Body Temperature—*continued*

10. Document the temperature in the client record. ❶ A rectal temperature may be recorded with an "R" next to the value or with the mark on a graphic sheet circled. An axillary temperature may be recorded with "AX" or marked on a graphic sheet with an "X."

EVALUATION

- Compare the temperature measurement to baseline data, normal range for age of client, and client's previous temperatures. Analyze considering time of day and any additional influencing factors and other vital signs.
- Conduct appropriate follow-up such as notifying the primary care provider if a temperature is outside of a specific range or is not responding to interventions, giving a medication, or altering the client's environment. This includes teaching the client how to lower an elevated temperature through actions such as increasing fluid intake, coughing and deep breathing, cool compresses, or removing heavy coverings. Interventions for hypothermia include intake of warm fluids and use of warm or electric blankets.

SKILL 28.1

Pulse ▾ | Entered in Error | Enter Vitals

Vitals	04-23-20 14:00:00	04-23-20 12:00:00	04-23-20 10:00:00
Temp.	97.6	98	100
Pulse	76	86	88
Resp.	22*	20*	22*
B/P	120/80	130/80	110/60*
P Ox%	98	99	98
Pain	0	0	0
Ht (in)	68.8980	68.8980	68.8980
Wt (lbs.)	171.96	171.96	154.32
BMI	25.52	25.52	22.90
C/G	68	68	60
CVP (cmH20)			
Location	CARDIOLOGY	CARDIOLOGY	CARDIOLOGY
Entered By	GEORGE,ROSILY	GEORGE,ROSILY	GEORGE,ROSILY
Data Source	Vitals	Vitals	Vitals

❶ Vital signs record.
iCare.

BOX 28.6 Thermometer Placement

Oral

- Place the tip on either side of the frenulum. ❶

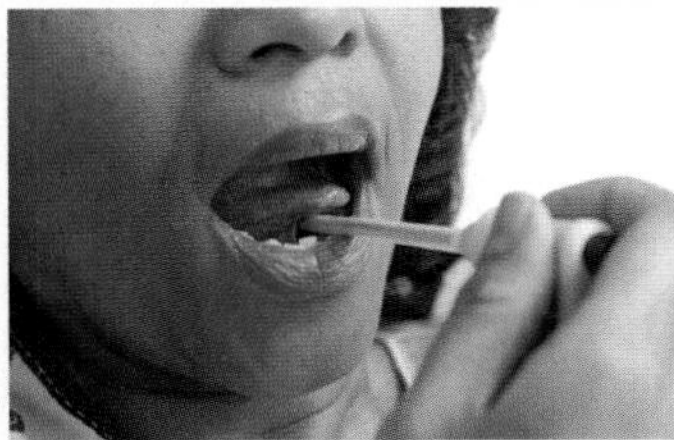

❶ Oral thermometer placement

Rectal

- Apply clean gloves.
- Instruct the client to take a slow deep breath during insertion. ❷
- Never force the thermometer if resistance is felt.
- Insert 3.5 cm (1.5 in.) in adults.

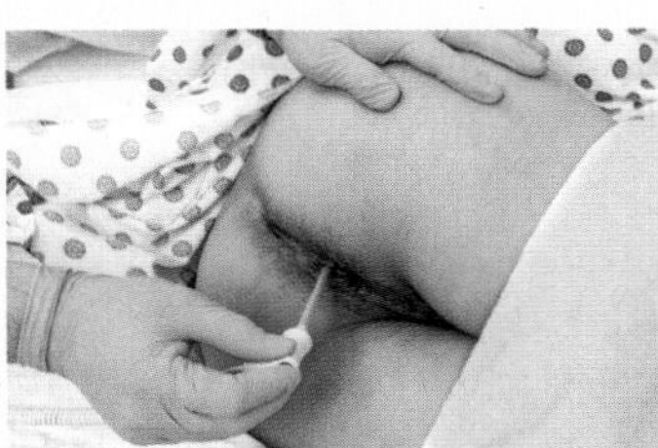

❷ Inserting a rectal thermometer.

Axillary

- Pat the axilla dry if very moist.
- Place the tip in the center of the axilla. ❸

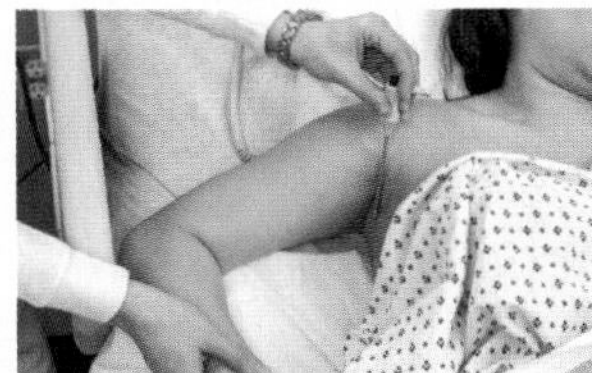

❸ Placing the tip of the thermometer in the center of the axilla.

Tympanic

- Pull the pinna slightly upward and backward for an adult. ❹
- Point the probe slightly anteriorly, toward the eardrum.
- Insert the probe slowly using a rotating motion until snug.

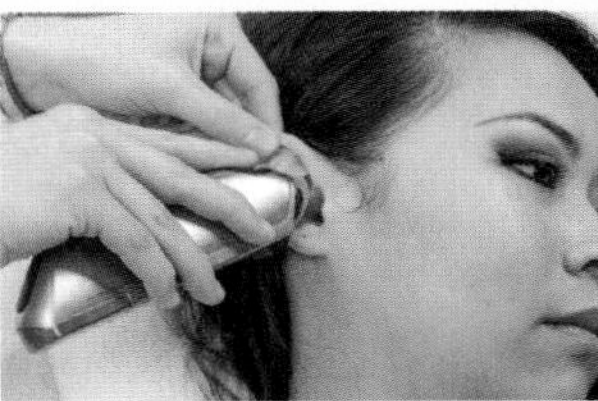

❹ Pull the pinna of the ear up and back for an adult while inserting the tympanic thermometer.

Continued on page 542

BOX 28.6 Thermometer Placement—*continued*

Temporal Artery

- Brush hair aside if covering the temporal artery area. With the probe flush on the center of the forehead, depress the red button; keep depressed. Slowly slide the probe midline across the forehead to the hairline, not down the side of the face. Lift the probe from the forehead and touch on the neck just behind the earlobe. Release the button. ⑤

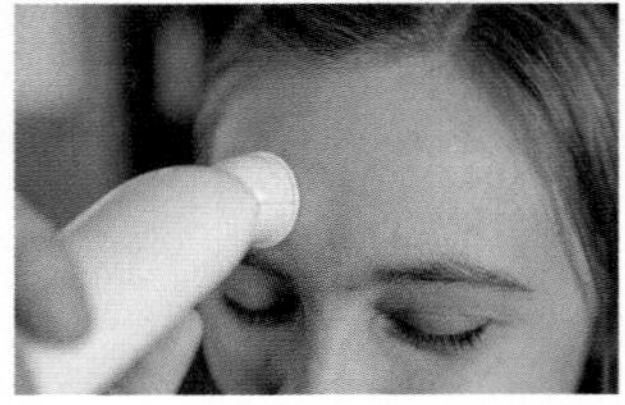

⑤ Positioning a temporal artery thermometer.

LIFESPAN CONSIDERATIONS Temperature

INFANTS

- The body temperature of newborns is extremely labile, and newborns must be kept warm and dry to prevent hypothermia.
- Using the axillary site, you need to hold the infant's arm against the chest (Figure 28.11 ■).
- The axillary route may not be as accurate as other routes for detecting fevers in children.
- The tympanic route is fast and convenient. Place the infant supine and stabilize the head. Pull the pinna straight back and slightly downward. Remember that the pinna is pulled upward for children over 3 years of age and adults, but downward for children younger than age 3. Direct the probe tip anteriorly and insert far enough to seal the canal. The tip will not touch the tympanic membrane.
- Avoid the tympanic route in a child with active ear infections or tympanic membrane drainage tubes.
- The tympanic membrane route may be more accurate in determining temperature in febrile infants.
- The rectal route is least desirable in infants.

CHILDREN

- Tympanic or temporal artery sites are preferred.
- For the tympanic route, have the child held on an adult's lap with the child's head held gently against the adult for support. Pull the pinna straight back and upward for children over age 3 (Figure 28.12 ■).
- Avoid the tympanic route in a child with active ear infections or tympanic membrane drainage tubes.
- The oral route may be used for children over age 3, but nonbreakable, electronic thermometers are recommended.
- For a rectal temperature, place the child prone across your lap or in a side-lying position with the knees flexed. Insert the thermometer 2.5 cm (1 in.) into the rectum.

OLDER ADULTS

- Older adults' temperatures tend to be lower than those of middle-aged adults.
- Older adults' temperatures are strongly influenced by both environmental and internal temperature changes. Their thermoregulation control processes are not as efficient as when they were younger, and they are at higher risk for both hypothermia and hyperthermia.
- Older adults can develop significant buildup of ear cerumen (earwax) that may interfere with tympanic thermometer readings.
- Older adults are more likely to have hemorrhoids. Inspect the anus before taking a rectal temperature.
- Older adults' temperatures may not be a valid indication of the seriousness of the pathology of a disease. They may have pneumonia or a urinary tract infection and have only a slight temperature elevation. Other symptoms, such as confusion and restlessness, may be displayed and need follow-up to determine if there is an underlying process.

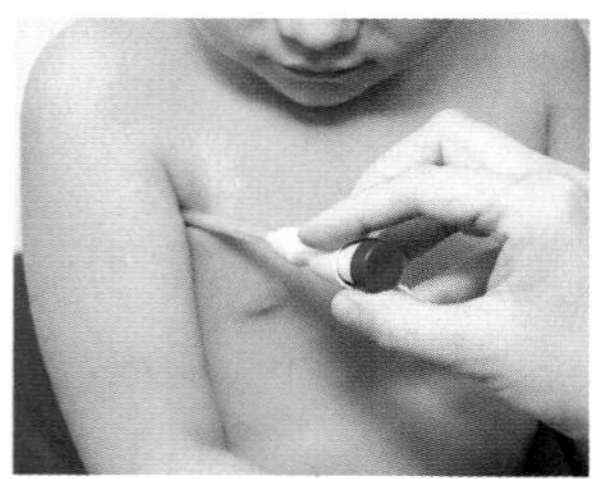

Figure 28.11 ■ Axillary thermometer placement for a child.

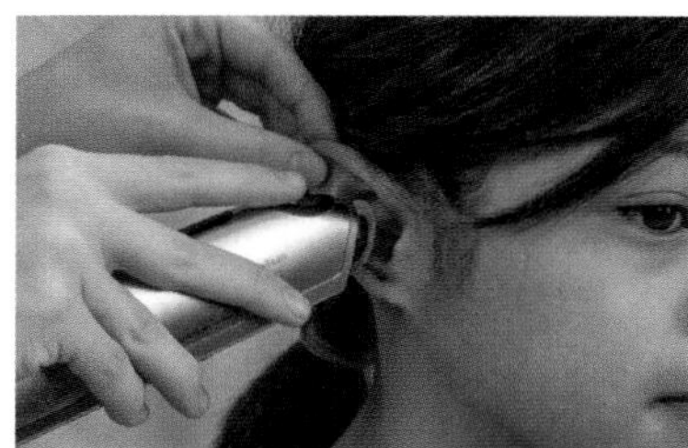

Figure 28.12 ■ Pull the pinna of the ear back and up for placement of a tympanic thermometer in a child over 3 years of age; back and down for children under age 3.

Pulse

The **pulse** is a wave of blood created by contraction of the left ventricle of the heart. Generally, the pulse wave represents the stroke volume output or the amount of blood that enters the arteries with each ventricular contraction. **Compliance** of the arteries is their ability to contract and expand. When an individual's arteries lose their distensibility, as can happen with age, greater pressure is required to pump the blood into the arteries.

Cardiac output is the volume of blood pumped into the arteries by the heart and equals the result of the stroke volume (SV) times the heart rate (HR) per minute. For example, 65 mL × 70 beats per minute = 4.55 L per minute. When an adult is resting, the heart pumps about 5 liters of blood each minute.

In a healthy individual, the pulse reflects the heartbeat; that is, the pulse rate is the same as the rate of the ventricular contractions of the heart. However, in some conditions, the heartbeat and pulse rates can differ. For example, a client's heart may produce very weak pulse waves that are not detectable in a pulse far from the heart. In these instances, the nurse should assess both the heartbeat (apical pulse) and the peripheral pulse. A **peripheral pulse** is a pulse located away from the heart, for example, in the foot or wrist. The **apical pulse**, in contrast, is a central pulse; that is, it is located at the apex of the heart. It is also referred to as the **point of maximal impulse (PMI)**.

Factors Affecting the Pulse

The rate of the pulse is expressed in beats per minute (beats/min). Consider each of the following factors when assessing a client's pulse:

- *Age.* As age increases, the average pulse rate gradually decreases. See Table 28.2 for specific variations in pulse rates from birth to adulthood.
- *Sex.* After puberty, the average male's pulse rate is slightly lower than the female's.
- *Exercise.* The pulse rate normally increases with activity. The rate of increase in the professional athlete is often less than in the average individual because of greater cardiac size, strength, and efficiency.
- *Fever.* The pulse rate increases (a) in response to the lowered blood pressure that results from peripheral vasodilation associated with elevated body temperature and (b) because of the increased metabolic rate.
- *Medications.* Some medications decrease the pulse rate, and others increase it. For example, cardiotonics (e.g., digitalis preparations) decrease the heart rate, whereas epinephrine increases it.
- *Hypovolemia or dehydration.* Loss of fluid from the vascular system increases the pulse rate. The loss of circulating volume results in an adjustment of the heart rate to increase blood pressure as the body compensates for the lost blood volume.

TABLE 28.2 Variations in Pulse and Respirations by Age

Age	Pulse Average (and Ranges)	Respirations Average (and Ranges)
Newborn	130 (80–180)	35 (30–60)
1 year	120 (80–140)	30 (20–40)
5–8 years	100 (75–120)	20 (15–25)
10 years	70 (50–90)	19 (15–25)
Teen	75 (50–90)	18 (15–20)
Adult	80 (60–100)	16 (12–20)
Older adult	70 (60–100)	16 (15–20)

- *Stress.* In response to stress, sympathetic nervous stimulation increases the overall activity of the heart. Stress increases the rate as well as the force of the heartbeat. Fear and anxiety as well as acute pain stimulate the sympathetic system.
- *Position.* When a client is sitting or standing, blood usually pools in dependent vessels of the venous system. Pooling results in a transient decrease in the venous blood return to the heart and a subsequent reduction in blood pressure and increase in heart rate.
- *Pathology.* Certain diseases such as some heart conditions or those that impair oxygenation can alter the resting pulse rate.

Pulse Sites

A pulse is commonly measured in nine sites (Figure 28.13 ■):

1. Temporal, where the temporal artery passes over the temporal bone of the head. The site is superior (above) and lateral to (away from the midline of) the eye.

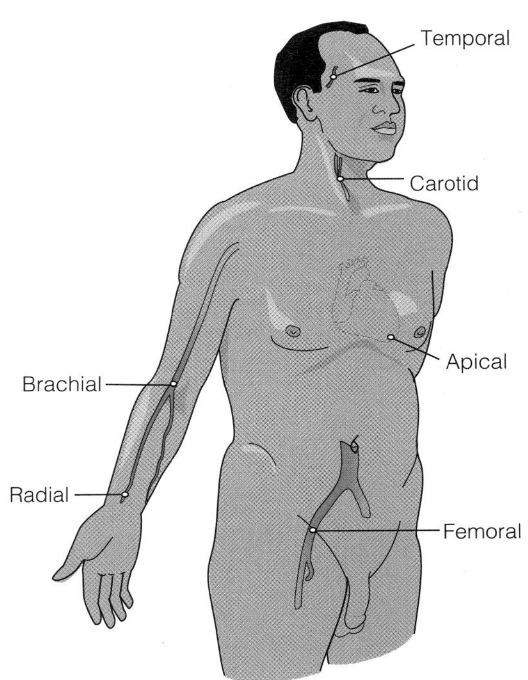

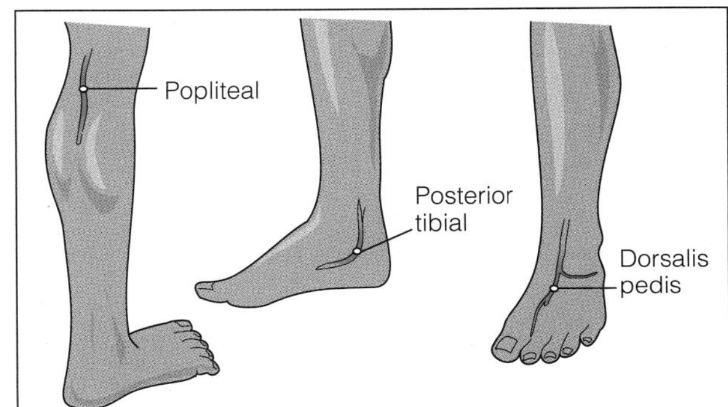

Figure 28.13 ■ Nine sites for assessing pulse.

2. Carotid, at the side of the neck where the carotid artery runs between the trachea and the sternocleidomastoid muscle.

Clinical Alert!

Never press both carotids at the same time because this can cause a reflex drop in blood pressure or pulse rate.

3. Apical, at the apex of the heart. In an adult, this is located on the left side of the chest, about 8 cm (3 in.) to the left of the sternum (breastbone) at the fifth intercostal space (area between the ribs). In older adults, the apex may be further left if conditions are present that have led to an enlarged heart. Before 4 years of age, the apex is left of the midclavicular line (MCL); between 4 and 6 years, it is at the MCL (Figure 28.14 ■). For a child 7 to 9 years of age, the apical pulse is located at the fourth or fifth intercostal space.
4. Brachial, at the inner aspect of the biceps muscle of the arm or medially in the antecubital space.
5. Radial, where the radial artery runs along the radial bone, on the thumb side of the inner aspect of the wrist.
6. Femoral, where the femoral artery passes alongside the inguinal ligament.
7. Popliteal, where the popliteal artery passes behind the knee.
8. Posterior tibial, on the medial surface of the ankle where the posterior tibial artery passes behind the medial malleolus.
9. Dorsalis pedis, where the dorsalis pedis artery passes over the bones of the foot, on an imaginary line drawn from the middle of the ankle to the space between the big and second toes.

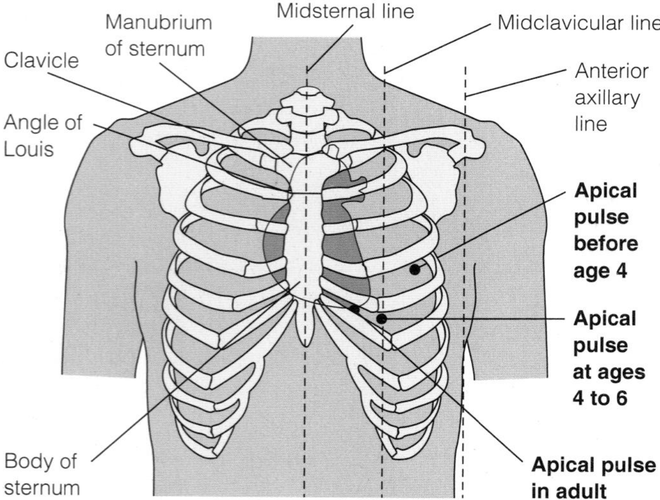

Figure 28.14 ■ Location of the apical pulse for a child under 4 years, a child 4 to 6 years, and an adult.

TABLE 28.3 Reasons for Using Specific Pulse Site

Pulse Site	Reasons for Use
Radial	Readily accessible
Temporal	Used when radial pulse is not accessible
Carotid	Used during cardiac arrest or shock in adults
	Used to determine circulation to the brain
Apical	Routinely used for infants and children up to 3 years of age
	Used to determine discrepancies with radial pulse
	Used in conjunction with some medications
Brachial	Used to measure blood pressure
	Used during cardiac arrest for infants
Femoral	Used in cases of cardiac arrest or shock
	Used to determine circulation to a leg
Popliteal	Used to determine circulation to the lower leg
Posterior tibial	Used to determine circulation to the foot
Dorsalis pedis	Used to determine circulation to the foot

The radial site is most commonly used in adults. It is easily found in most people and readily accessible. Some reasons for use of each site are given in Table 28.3.

Assessing the Pulse

A pulse is commonly assessed by palpation (feeling) or auscultation (hearing). The middle three fingertips are used for palpating all pulse sites except the apex of the heart. A stethoscope is used for assessing apical pulses. A Doppler ultrasound stethoscope (DUS; Figure 28.15 ■)

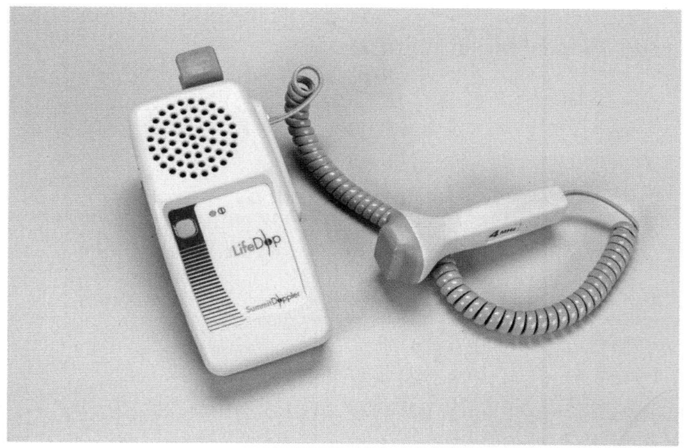

Figure 28.15 ■ A Doppler ultrasound stethoscope (DUS).

is used for pulses that are difficult to assess. The DUS has a headset with earpieces similar to standard stethoscope earpieces or a speaker, and an ultrasound transducer. The DUS detects movement of red blood cells through a blood vessel. In contrast to the conventional stethoscope, it eliminates environmental sounds and, thus, is useful in noisy settings.

A pulse is normally palpated by applying moderate pressure with the three middle fingers of the hand. The pads on the most distal aspects of the finger are the most sensitive areas for detecting a pulse. With excessive pressure, one can obliterate a pulse, whereas with too little pressure one may not be able to detect it. Before the nurse assesses the resting pulse, the client should assume a comfortable position. The nurse should also be aware of the following:

- Any medication that could affect the heart rate.
- Whether the client has been physically active. If so, wait 10 to 15 minutes until the client has rested and the pulse has slowed to its usual rate.
- Any baseline data about the normal heart rate for the client. For example, a physically fit athlete may have a resting heart rate below 60 beats/min.
- Whether the client should assume a particular position (e.g., sitting). In some clients, the rate changes with the position because of changes in blood flow volume and autonomic nervous system activity.

When assessing the pulse, the nurse collects the following data: the rate, rhythm, volume, arterial wall elasticity, and presence or absence of bilateral equality. An excessively fast heart rate (e.g., over 100 beats/min in an adult) is referred to as **tachycardia**. A heart rate in an adult of less than 60 beats/min is called **bradycardia**. If a client has either tachycardia or bradycardia, the apical pulse should be assessed.

The **pulse rhythm** is the pattern of the beats and the intervals between the beats. Equal time elapses between beats of a normal pulse. A pulse with an irregular rhythm is referred to as a **dysrhythmia** or **arrhythmia**. It may consist of random, irregular beats or a predictable pattern of irregular beats (documented as "regularly irregular"). When a dysrhythmia is detected, the apical pulse should be assessed. An electrocardiogram (ECG or EKG) is necessary to define the dysrhythmia further.

Pulse volume, also called the pulse strength or amplitude, refers to the force of blood with each beat. Usually, the pulse volume is the same with each beat. It can range from absent to bounding. A normal pulse can be felt with moderate pressure of the fingers and can be obliterated with greater pressure. A forceful or full blood volume that is obliterated only with difficulty is called a full or bounding pulse. A pulse that is readily obliterated with pressure from the fingers is referred to as weak, feeble, or thready.

The elasticity of the arterial wall reflects its expansibility or its deformities. A healthy, normal artery feels straight, smooth, soft, and pliable. Older adults often have inelastic arteries that feel twisted (tortuous) and irregular on palpation.

When assessing a peripheral pulse to determine the adequacy of blood flow to a particular area of the body (perfusion), the nurse should also assess the corresponding pulse on the other side of the body. The second assessment gives the nurse data with which to compare the pulses. For example, when assessing the blood flow to the right foot, the nurse assesses the right dorsalis pedis pulse and then the left dorsalis pedis pulse. If the client's right and left pulses are the same volume and elasticity, the client's dorsalis pedis pulses are bilaterally equal. The pulse rate does not need to be counted when assessing for perfusion and equality.

When a peripheral pulse is located, it indicates that pulses more proximal to that location will also be present. For example, if the dorsalis pedis, the most distal pulse of the lower extremity, cannot be felt, the nurse next palpates for the posterior tibial pulse. If it is not felt, the popliteal pulse must be assessed. If the popliteal pulse is found, it is not necessary to assess the femoral pulse since it must also be present in order for the more distal pulse to exist.

QSEN Patient-Centered Care: Pulse

In addition to measuring the pulse while the client is at a healthcare facility, the nurse provides guidance for clients at home.

- Teach the client to monitor the pulse prior to taking medications that affect the heart rate. Tell the client to report any notable changes in heart rate or rhythm (regularity) to the healthcare provider.
- Inform the client or family of activities known to significantly affect pulse rate such as emotional stress, exercise, ingesting caffeine, and sleep. Clients sensitive to pulse rate changes should consider whether any of these activities should be modified in order to stabilize the pulse.
- Some clients require lengthy monitoring of the pulse and ECG. A special device, often referred to as a Holter monitor, is used for this type of monitoring. It is usually applied in an office or clinic setting, and the client wears the portable recorder for 24 hours or longer. Other portable devices used for recording episodic arrhythmias include cardiac event monitors. The client activates the device during times when symptoms appear and then the recorded data can be transmitted to a central location through a telephone.

Skill 28.2 provides guidelines for assessing a peripheral pulse.

Assessing a Peripheral Pulse

PURPOSES

- To establish baseline data for subsequent evaluation
- To identify whether the pulse rate is within normal range
- To determine the pulse volume and whether the pulse rhythm is regular
- To determine the equality of corresponding peripheral pulses on each side of the body
- To monitor and assess changes in the client's health status
- To monitor clients at risk for pulse alterations (e.g., those with a history of heart disease or experiencing cardiac arrhythmias, hemorrhage, acute pain, infusion of large volumes of fluids, or fever)
- To evaluate blood perfusion to the extremities

ASSESSMENT

Assess

- Clinical signs of cardiovascular alterations such as dyspnea (difficult respirations), fatigue, pallor, cyanosis (bluish discoloration of skin and mucous membranes), palpitations, syncope (dizziness or fainting), or impaired peripheral tissue perfusion (as evidenced by skin discoloration and cool temperature)
- Factors that may alter pulse rate (e.g., emotional status and activity level)
- Which site is most appropriate for assessment based on the purpose

PLANNING

Assignment

Measurement of the client's radial or brachial pulse can be assigned to AP, or be performed by family members or caregivers in nonhospital settings. Reports of abnormal pulse rates or rhythms require reassessment by the nurse, who also determines appropriate action if the abnormality is confirmed. AP are generally not delegated these techniques due to the skill required in locating and interpreting peripheral pulses other than the radial or brachial artery and in using Doppler ultrasound devices.

Equipment

- Clock, timer, or watch with a sweep second hand or digital seconds indicator
- If using a DUS: transducer probe, stethoscope headset (some models), transmission gel, and tissues or wipes

IMPLEMENTATION

Preparation

If using a DUS, check that the equipment is functioning normally.

Performance

1. Prior to performing the procedure, introduce self and verify the client's identity using agency protocol. Explain to the client what you are going to do, why it is necessary, and how to participate. Discuss how the results will be used in planning further care or treatments.
2. Perform hand hygiene and observe appropriate infection prevention procedures.
3. Provide for client privacy.
4. Select the pulse point. Normally, the radial pulse is taken, unless it cannot be reached or circulation to another body area is to be assessed.
5. Assist the client to a comfortable resting position. When the radial pulse is assessed, with the palm facing downward, the client's arm can rest alongside the body or the forearm can rest at a 90-degree angle across the chest. For the client who can sit, the forearm can rest across the thigh, with the palm of the hand facing downward or inward.
6. Palpate and count the pulse. Place two or three middle fingertips lightly and squarely over the pulse point. ❶ **Rationale:** *Using the thumb is contraindicated because the nurse's thumb has a pulse that could be mistaken for the client's pulse.*
   - Count for 15 seconds and multiply by 4. Record the pulse in beats per minute on your worksheet. If taking a client's pulse for the first time, when obtaining baseline data, or if the pulse is irregular, count for a full minute. If an irregular pulse is found, also take the apical pulse.
7. Assess the pulse rhythm and volume.
   - Assess the pulse rhythm by noting the pattern of the intervals between the beats. A normal pulse has equal time periods between beats. If this is an initial assessment, assess for 1 minute.
   - Assess the pulse volume. A normal pulse can be felt with moderate pressure, and the pressure is equal with each beat. A forceful pulse volume is full; an easily obliterated pulse is weak. Record the rhythm and volume on your worksheet.
8. Document the pulse rate, rhythm, and volume and your actions in the client record (see Figure ❶ in Skill 28.1). Also record in the nurse's notes pertinent related data such as variation in pulse rate compared to normal for the client and abnormal skin color and skin temperature.

❶ Assessing pulses: *A*, Radial

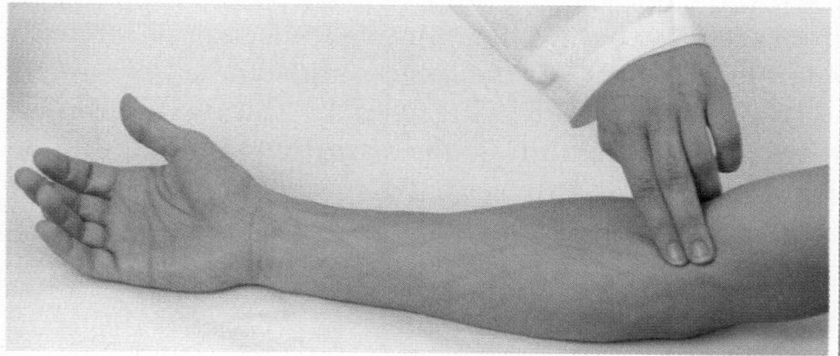

❶ *B*, Brachial

Assessing a Peripheral Pulse—*continued*

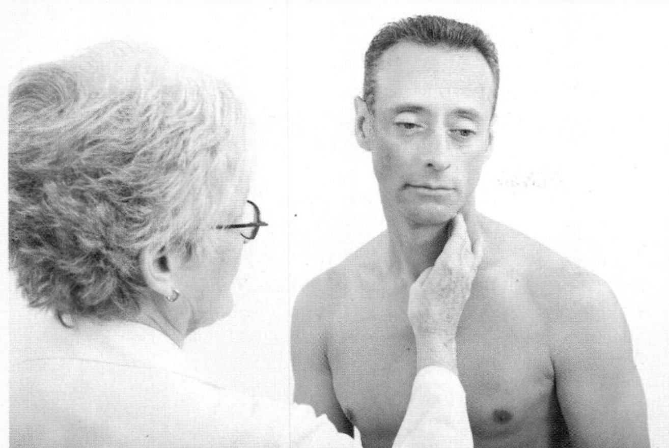

❶ *C,* Carotid

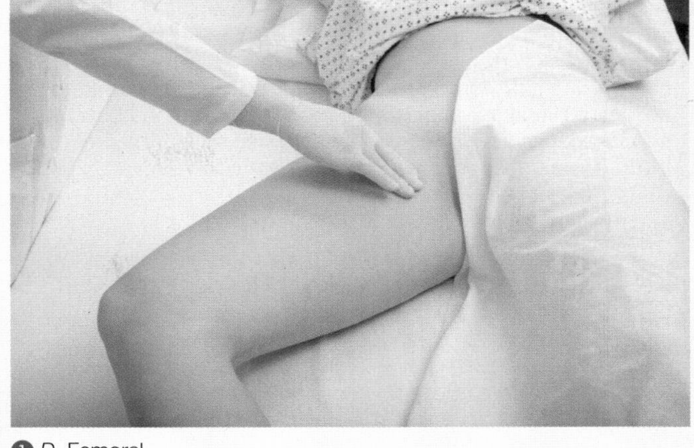

❶ *D,* Femoral

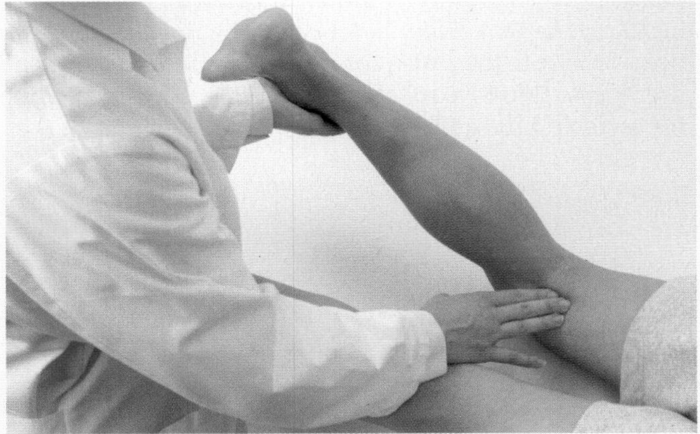

❶ *E,* Popliteal

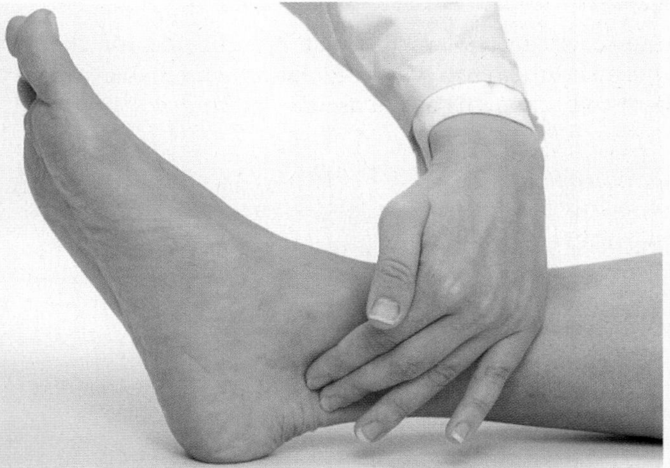

❶ *F,* Posterior tibial

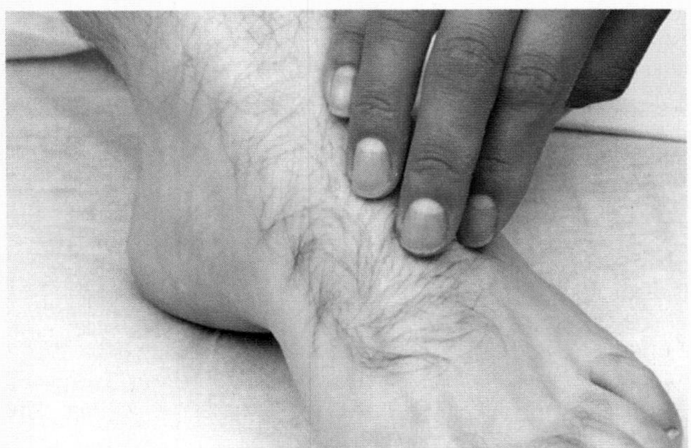

❶ *G,* Dorsalis pedis

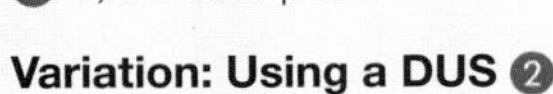

Variation: Using a DUS ❷

- If used, plug the stethoscope headset into one of the two output jacks located next to the volume control. DUS units may have two jacks so that a second individual can listen to the signals.
- Apply transmission gel either to the probe at the narrow end of the plastic case housing the transducer, or to the client's skin. **Rationale:** *Ultrasound beams do not travel well through air. The gel makes an airtight seal, which then promotes optimal ultrasound wave transmission.*
- Press the "on" button.

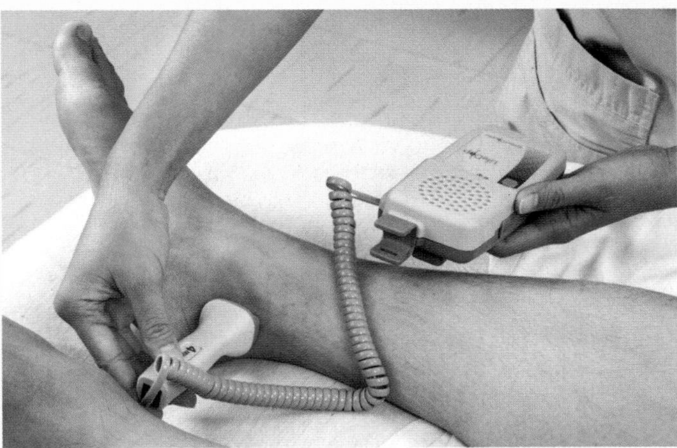

❷ Using a DUS to assess the posterior tibial pulse.

- Hold the probe against the skin over the pulse site. Use light pressure, and keep the probe in contact with the skin. **Rationale:** *Too much pressure can stop the blood flow and obliterate the signal.*

Continued on page 548

SKILL 28.2

Assessing a Peripheral Pulse—*continued*

- Adjust the volume if necessary. Distinguish artery sounds from vein sounds. The artery sound (signal) is distinctively pulsating and has a pumping quality. The venous sound is intermittent and varies with respirations. Both artery and vein sounds are heard simultaneously through the DUS because major arteries and veins are situated close together throughout the body. If arterial sounds cannot be easily heard, reposition the probe. If you cannot hear any pulse, move the probe to several different locations in the same area before determining that no pulse is present.
- After assessing the pulse, use a tissue or wipe to remove all gel from the probe to prevent damage to the surface. Clean the transducer with water-based solution. **Rationale:** *Alcohol or other disinfectants may damage the face of the transducer.*
- Remove all gel from the client, using a tissue or wipe.

EVALUATION

- Compare the pulse rate to recent, baseline, or usual range for the age of the client. If other members of the healthcare team have also assessed the pulse, such as during activity with a physical therapist, also compare your findings to theirs.
- Relate pulse rate and volume to other vital signs; relate pulse rhythm and volume to baseline data and health status.
- If assessing peripheral pulses, evaluate equality, rate, and volume in corresponding extremities.
- Conduct appropriate follow-up such as notifying the primary care provider or giving medication.

Apical Pulse Assessment

Assessment of the apical pulse is indicated for clients whose peripheral pulse is irregular or unavailable and for clients with known cardiovascular, pulmonary, and renal diseases. It is commonly assessed prior to administering medications that affect heart rate. The apical site is also used to assess the pulse for newborns, infants, and children up to 2 to 3 years old. Skill 28.3 presents guidelines for assessing the apical pulse.

SKILL 28.3

Assessing an Apical Pulse

PURPOSES

- To obtain the heart rate of an adult with an irregular peripheral pulse
- To establish baseline data for subsequent evaluation
- To determine whether the cardiac rate is within normal range and the rhythm is regular
- To monitor clients with cardiac, pulmonary, or renal disease and those receiving medications to improve heart action

ASSESSMENT

Assess

- Clinical signs of cardiovascular alterations such as dyspnea (difficult respirations), fatigue, weakness, pallor, cyanosis (bluish discoloration of skin and mucous membranes), palpitations, syncope (dizziness or fainting), or impaired peripheral tissue perfusion as evidenced by skin discoloration and cool temperature
- Factors that may alter pulse rate (e.g., emotional status, activity level, and medications that affect heart rate such as digoxin, beta-blockers, or calcium channel blockers)

PLANNING

Assignment

Due to the degree of skill and knowledge required, AP are generally not responsible for assessing apical pulses.

Equipment

- Clock, timer, or watch with a sweep second hand or digital seconds indicator
- Stethoscope
- Antiseptic wipes
- If using a DUS: the transducer probe, the stethoscope headset, transmission gel, and tissues or wipes

IMPLEMENTATION

Preparation

If using a DUS, check that the equipment is functioning normally.

Performance

1. Prior to performing the procedure, introduce self and verify the client's identity using agency protocol. Explain to the client what you are going to do, why it is necessary, and how to participate. Discuss how the results will be used in planning further care or treatments.
2. Perform hand hygiene and observe appropriate infection prevention procedures.
3. Provide for client privacy.
4. Position the client appropriately in a comfortable supine position or in a sitting position. Expose the area of the chest over the apex of the heart.
5. Locate the apical impulse. This is the point over the apex of the heart where the apical pulse can be most clearly heard.
   - Palpate the angle of Louis (the angle between the manubrium, the top of the sternum, and the body of the sternum). It is palpated just below the suprasternal notch and is felt as a prominence (see Figure 28.14).
   - Slide your index finger just to the left of the sternum, and palpate the second intercostal space. ❶

Assessing an Apical Pulse—*continued*

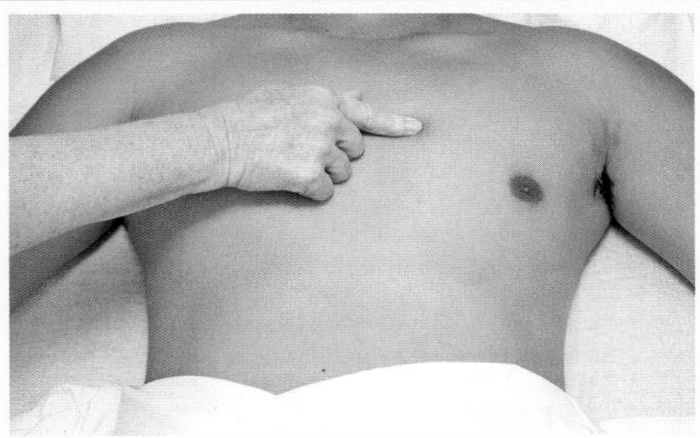

❶ Second intercostal space.
Shirlee Snyder.

Clinical Alert!

When "left" and "right" are used to describe the nurse's hand placement on the client, the terms refer to the client's right or left side, not the nurse's.

- Place your middle or next finger in the third intercostal space, and continue palpating downward until you locate the fifth intercostal space. ❷
- Move your index finger laterally along the fifth intercostal space toward the MCL. ❸
- Normally, the apical impulse is palpable at or just medial to the MCL (see Figure 28.14).

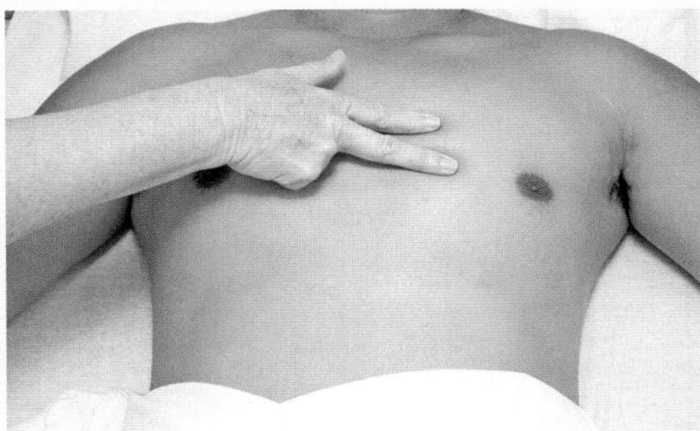

❷ Third intercostal space.
Shirlee Snyder.

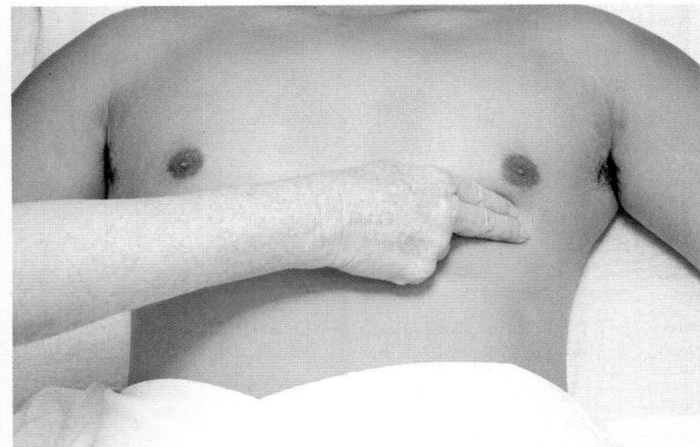

❸ Fifth intercostal space, MCL.
Shirlee Snyder.

6. Auscultate and count heartbeats.
- Use antiseptic wipes to clean the earpieces and diaphragm of the stethoscope. **Rationale:** *The diaphragm needs to be cleaned and disinfected on a regular basis. Both earpieces and diaphragms have been shown to harbor pathogenic bacteria (Bansal, Sarath, Bhan, Gupta, & Purwar, 2019).*
- Warm the diaphragm of the stethoscope by holding it in the palm of the hand for a moment. **Rationale:** *The metal of the diaphragm is usually cold and can startle the client when placed immediately on the chest.*
- Insert the earpieces of the stethoscope into your ears in the direction of the ear canals, or slightly forward. **Rationale:** *This position facilitates hearing.*
- Tap your finger lightly on the diaphragm. **Rationale:** *This ensures it is the active side of the head. If necessary, rotate the head to select the diaphragm side.* ❹
- Place the diaphragm of the stethoscope over the apical impulse and listen for the normal S_1 and S_2 heart sounds, which are heard as "lub-dub." ❺ **Rationale:** *The heartbeat is normally loudest over the apex of the heart.* Each lub-dub is counted as one heartbeat. **Rationale:** *The two heart sounds are produced by closure of the heart valves. The S_1 heart sound (lub) occurs when the atrioventricular valves close after the ventricles have been sufficiently filled. The S_2 heart sound (dub) occurs when the semilunar valves close after the ventricles empty.*

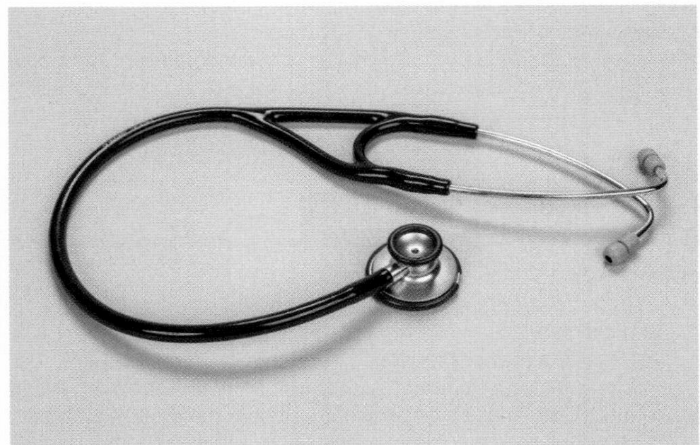

A

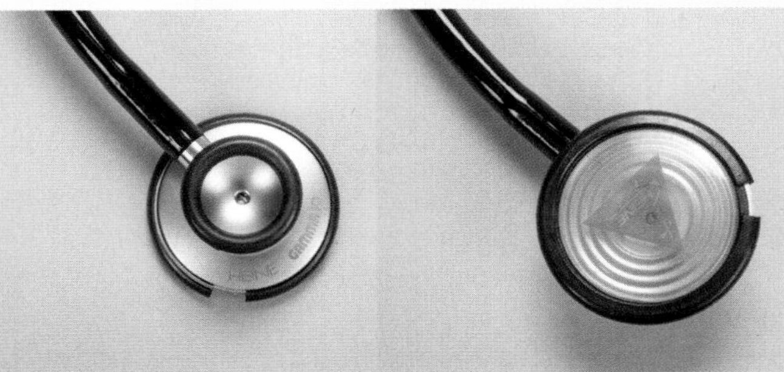

B

❹ *A*, Stethoscope with both a bell and a diaphragm. *B*, Close-up of a bell (left) and a diaphragm (right).

Continued on page 550

SKILL 28.3

Assessing an Apical Pulse—*continued*

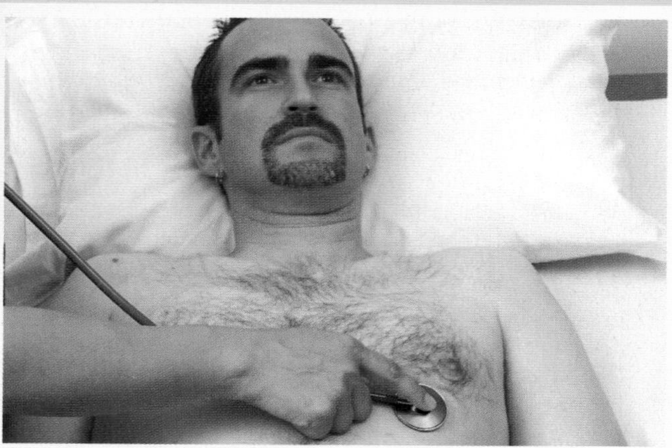

5 Taking an apical pulse using the flat-disc stethoscope. Note how the diaphragm is held against the chest.

- If you have difficulty hearing the apical pulse, ask the supine client to roll onto his or her left side or the sitting client to lean slightly forward. **Rationale:** *This positioning moves the apex of the heart closer to the chest wall.*
- If the rhythm is regular, count the heartbeats for 30 seconds and multiply by 2. If the rhythm is irregular or for giving certain medications such as digoxin, count the beats for 60 seconds. **Rationale:** *A 60-second count provides a more accurate assessment of an irregular pulse than a 30-second count.*

7. Assess the rhythm and the strength of the heartbeat.
- Assess the rhythm of the heartbeat by noting the pattern of intervals between the beats. A normal pulse has equal time periods between beats.
- Assess the strength (volume) of the heartbeat. Normally, the heartbeats are equal in strength and can be described as strong or weak.

8. Document the pulse rate and rhythm, and nursing actions in the client record. Also record pertinent related data such as variation in pulse rate compared to normal for the client and abnormal skin color and skin temperature.

SAMPLE DOCUMENTATION

2/24/2020 1000 Radial pulse 116 & irregular. Had been 82 & regular at 0600. T, R, & BP within client's usual range. C/o being a "little dizzy." Skin warm & dry. Apical pulse 120, irregular, with brief pause after q 3rd beat. MD notified & ECG ordered. G. Chapman, RN

EVALUATION

- Relate the pulse rate to other vital signs. Relate the pulse rhythm to baseline data and health status.
- Report to the primary care provider and other relevant members of the healthcare team any abnormal findings such as irregular rhythm, reduced ability to hear the heartbeat, pallor, cyanosis, dyspnea, tachycardia, or bradycardia.
- Conduct appropriate follow-up such as administering medication ordered based on apical heart rate.

LIFESPAN CONSIDERATIONS Pulse

INFANTS

- Use the apical pulse for the heart rate of newborns, infants, and children 2 to 3 years old to establish baseline data for subsequent evaluation, to determine whether the cardiac rate is within normal range, and to determine if the rhythm is regular.
- Place a baby in a supine position, and offer a pacifier if the baby is crying or restless. Crying and physical activity will increase the pulse rate. For this reason, take the resting apical pulse rate of infants and small children prior to other uncomfortable procedures so that the rate is not artificially elevated by the discomfort.
- Locate the apical pulse in the left fourth intercostal space, lateral to the midclavicular line during infancy.
- Brachial, popliteal, and femoral pulses may be palpated. Due to a normally low blood pressure and rapid heart rate, infants' other distal pulses may be hard to feel.
- Newborn infants may have heart murmurs that are not pathologic, but reflect functional incomplete closure of fetal heart structures (ductus arteriosus or foramen ovale).

CHILDREN

- To take a peripheral pulse, position the child comfortably in the adult's arms or have the adult remain close by. This may decrease anxiety and yield more accurate results.
- To assess the apical pulse, assist a young child to a comfortable supine or sitting position.
- Demonstrate the procedure to the child using a stuffed animal or doll, and allow the child to handle the stethoscope before beginning the procedure. This will decrease anxiety and promote cooperation.
- The apex of the heart is normally located in the left fourth intercostal space in young children and in the fifth intercostal space in children 7 years of age and over, between the MCL and the anterior axillary line (see Figure 28.14).
- Count the pulse prior to other uncomfortable procedures so that the rate is not artificially elevated by the discomfort.

OLDER ADULTS

- If the client has severe hand or arm tremors, the radial pulse may be difficult to count.
- Cardiac changes in older adults, such as decrease in cardiac output, sclerotic changes to heart valves, and dysrhythmias, may suggest that obtaining an apical pulse will be more accurate than a peripheral pulse.
- Older adults often have decreased peripheral circulation. To detect these, pedal pulses should also be checked for regularity, volume, and symmetry.
- The pulse returns to baseline after exercise more slowly than with other age groups.

Apical-Radial Pulse Assessment

An **apical-radial pulse** may need to be assessed for clients with certain cardiovascular disorders. Normally, the apical and radial rates are identical. An apical pulse rate greater than a radial pulse rate can indicate that the thrust of the blood from the heart is too weak for the wave to be felt at the peripheral pulse site, or it can indicate that vascular disease is preventing impulses from being transmitted. Any discrepancy between the two pulse rates is called a **pulse deficit** and needs to be reported promptly. In no instance is the radial pulse greater than the apical pulse.

An apical-radial pulse can be taken by two nurses or one nurse, although the two-nurse technique may be more accurate. Skill 28.4 outlines the steps for assessing an apical-radial pulse.

Assessing an Apical-Radial Pulse

SKILL 28.4

PURPOSE

- To determine adequacy of peripheral circulation or presence of pulse deficit

ASSESSMENT

Assess

- Clinical signs of hypovolemic shock (hypotension, pallor, cyanosis, and cold, clammy skin)

PLANNING

Assignment

AP are generally not responsible for assessing apical-radial pulses using the one-nurse technique. AP or any healthcare provider who is trained to assess a radial pulse may perform the radial pulse count using the two-nurse technique.

Equipment

- Clock, timer, or watch with a sweep second hand or digital seconds indicator
- Stethoscope
- Antiseptic wipes

IMPLEMENTATION

Preparation

If using the two-nurse technique, ensure that the other nurse is available at this time.

Performance

1. Prior to performing the procedure, introduce self and verify the client's identity using agency protocol. Explain to the client what you are going to do, why it is necessary, and how to participate. Discuss how the results will be used in planning further care or treatments.
2. Perform hand hygiene and observe appropriate infection prevention procedures.
3. Provide for client privacy.
4. Position the client appropriately. Assist the client to a comfortable supine or sitting position. Expose the area of the chest over the apex of the heart. If previous measurements were taken, use the same position. **Rationale:** *This ensures an accurate comparative measurement*.
5. Locate the apical and radial pulse sites. In the two-nurse technique, one nurse locates the apical impulse by palpation or with the stethoscope while the other nurse palpates the radial pulse site (see Skills 28.2 and 28.3).
6. Count the apical and radial pulse rates.

   Two-Nurse Technique ❶
   - If a clock or timer is not visible, the nurse who is taking the radial pulse needs to have a watch. The nurse taking the radial pulse decides on when to begin and says, "Start." **Rationale:** *This ensures that simultaneous counts are begun*.
   - Each nurse counts the pulse rate for 60 seconds. Both nurses end the count when the nurse taking the radial pulse says, "Stop." **Rationale:** *A full 60-second count is necessary for accurate assessment of any discrepancies between the two pulse sites*.
   - The nurse who assesses the apical rate also assesses the apical pulse rhythm and volume (i.e., whether the heartbeat is strong or weak). If the pulse is irregular, note whether the irregular beats come at random or at predictable times.
   - The nurse assessing the radial pulse rate also assesses the radial pulse rhythm and volume.

   One-Nurse Technique
   - Feel the radial pulse at the same time as listening to the apical pulse. ❷ You will be able to detect if they are not synchronized.
   - If the two pulses are not the same, to determine the pulse deficit assess the apical pulse for 60 seconds, and then immediately assess the radial pulse for 60 seconds.
7. Document the apical and radial (AR) pulse rates, rhythm, volume, and any pulse deficit in the client record. Also record related data such as variation in pulse rate compared to normal for the client and other pertinent observations, such as pallor, cyanosis, or dyspnea.

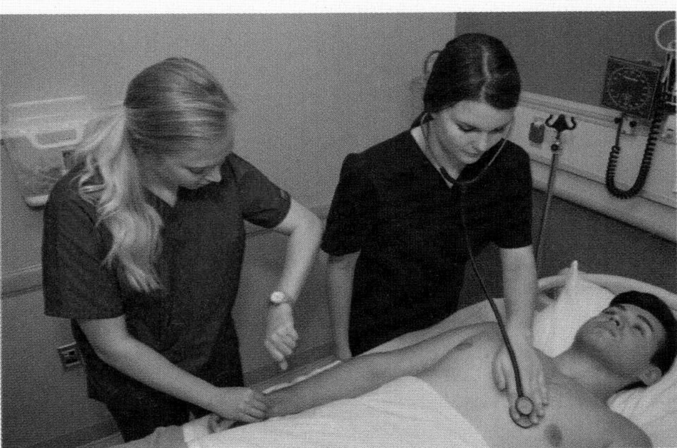

❶ Apical-radial pulse check with two nurses.

Continued on page 552

SKILL 28.4

Assessing an Apical-Radial Pulse—*continued*

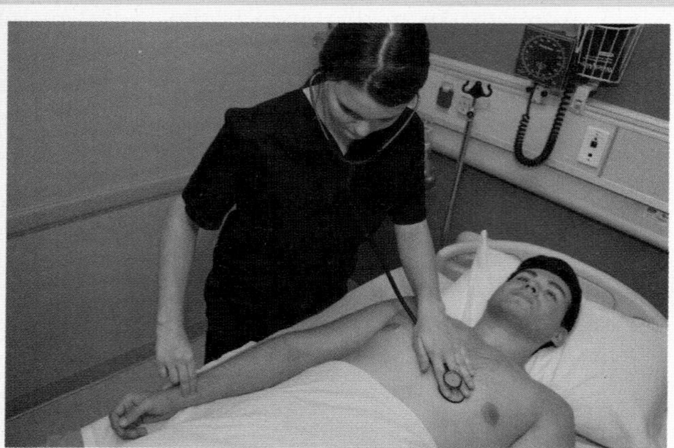

2 Apical-radial pulse check with one nurse.

EVALUATION

- Relate pulse rate and rhythm to other vital signs, to baseline data, and to general health status.
- Report to the primary care provider any changes from previous measurements or any discrepancy between the two pulse rates.

DRUG CAPSULE

Cardiac Glycoside or Digitalis Glycoside: digoxin (Lanoxin)

CLIENT WITH CARDIAC MEDICATIONS THAT AFFECT HEART RATE

Cardiac glycosides increase cardiac contractility, which increases cardiac output. As a result, perfusion to the kidneys is increased, which increases the production of urine. Cardiac glycosides also decrease heart rate by prolonging cardiac conduction.

Digoxin is commonly used for the clinical management of heart failure, atrial fibrillation, atrial flutter, and paroxysmal atrial tachycardia.

NURSING RESPONSIBILITIES

- Take the apical pulse for 1 minute before administering the dose. If the apical pulse is less than 60 beats/min or another specific parameter set by the healthcare provider, do not administer the dose and retake the pulse in 1 hour. If pulse remains less than 60, call the prescriber. *Note*: If the initial resting pulse is significantly less than 60 or the client has symptoms of bradycardia such as dizziness, notify the primary care provider without waiting to retake.
- Monitor electrolyte levels: Low potassium and low magnesium and high levels of calcium place the client at risk for digitalis toxicity. Check the client's most recent electrolyte laboratory work for safe levels before administering the dose.
- Avoid giving with meals because this will delay absorption.
- Monitor for therapeutic drug levels: 0.5–2 ng/mL. Digoxin has a narrow therapeutic index, which means that there is not much difference between a therapeutic effect and a toxic effect.
- Assess for signs of digoxin toxicity: anorexia, nausea, vomiting, diarrhea, blurred or "yellow" vision, unusual fatigue and weakness.

CLIENT AND FAMILY TEACHING

- Explain the reason for taking digoxin and the importance of medical checkups that may include laboratory work to evaluate the effects and dosage of the drug.
- Teach the client and family how to check the radial or carotid pulse for a full minute. Inform them to take the pulse at the same time each day and to write it on the calendar. Provide pulse parameters and tell them when it is appropriate to call the healthcare provider.
- Caution the client not to stop taking the digoxin without approval of the healthcare provider.
- Caution the client to avoid over-the-counter drugs, except on the advice of the healthcare provider, because many can interact with digoxin.
- Explain the signs and symptoms of digoxin toxicity and the importance of calling the healthcare provider.

Note: Prior to administering any medication, review all aspects with a current drug handbook or other reliable source.

Respirations

Respiration is the act of breathing. **Inhalation** or **inspiration** refers to the intake of air into the lungs. **Exhalation** or **expiration** refers to breathing out or the movement of gases from the lungs to the atmosphere. **Ventilation** is also used to refer to the movement of air into and out of the lungs.

There are basically two types of breathing: **costal (thoracic) breathing** and **diaphragmatic (abdominal) breathing**. Costal breathing involves the external intercostal muscles and other accessory muscles, such as the sternocleidomastoid muscles. It can be observed by the movement of the chest upward and outward. By contrast, diaphragmatic breathing involves the contraction and relaxation of the diaphragm, and it is observed by the movement of the abdomen, which occurs as a result of the diaphragm's contraction and downward movement.

Mechanics and Regulation of Breathing

During inhalation, the following processes normally occur (Figure 28.16 ■): The diaphragm contracts (flattens), the

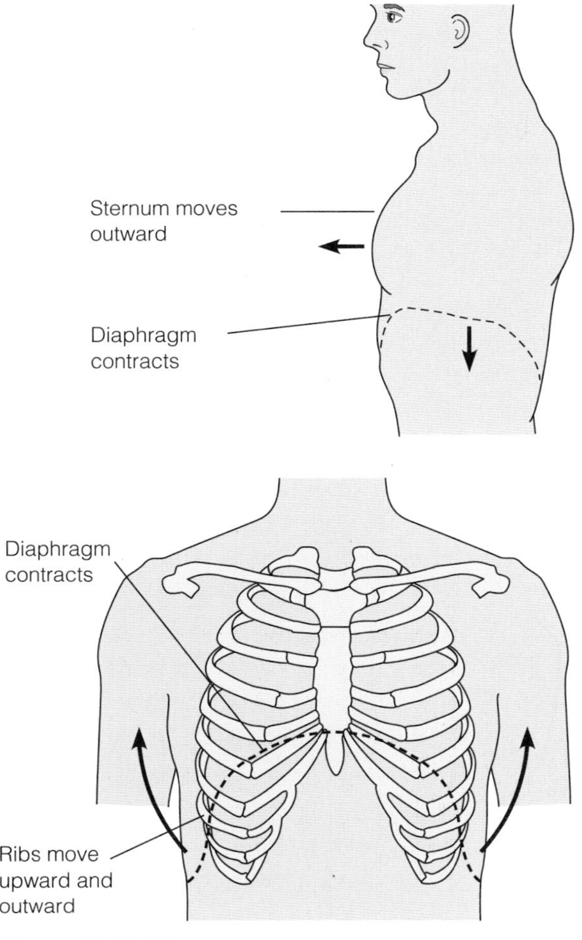

Figure 28.16 ■ Respiratory inhalation: *top*: lateral view; *bottom*: anterior view.

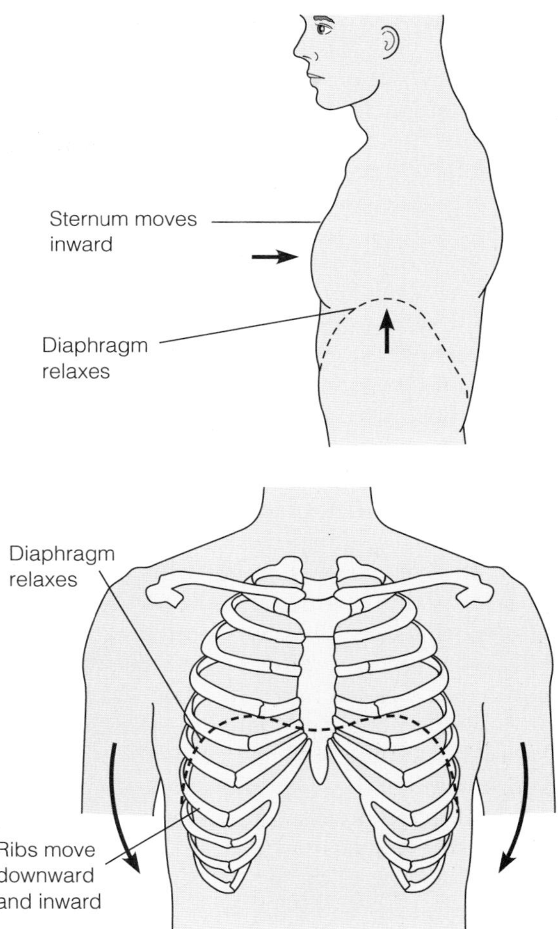

Figure 28.17 ■ Respiratory exhalation: *top*: lateral view; *bottom*: anterior view.

ribs move upward and outward, and the sternum moves outward, thus enlarging the thorax and permitting the lungs to expand. During exhalation (Figure 28.17 ■), the diaphragm relaxes, the ribs move downward and inward, and the sternum moves inward, thus decreasing the size of the thorax as the lungs are compressed. Normal breathing is automatic and effortless. A normal adult inspiration lasts 1 to 1.5 seconds, and an expiration lasts 2 to 3 seconds.

Respiration is controlled by (a) respiratory centers in the medulla oblongata and the pons of the brain and (b) chemoreceptors located centrally in the medulla and peripherally in the carotid and aortic bodies. These centers and receptors respond to changes in the concentrations of oxygen (O_2), carbon dioxide (CO_2), and hydrogen (H^+) in the arterial blood. See Chapter 49 ∞ for details.

Assessing Respirations

Resting respirations should be assessed when the client is relaxed because exercise affects respirations, increasing their rate and depth. Anxiety is likely to affect respiratory rate and depth as well. Respirations may also need to be assessed after exercise to identify the client's tolerance to activity. Before assessing a client's respirations, a nurse should be aware of the following:

- The client's normal breathing pattern
- The influence of the client's health problems on respirations
- Any medications or therapies that might affect respirations
- The relationship of the client's respirations to cardiovascular function.

The rate, depth, rhythm, quality, and effectiveness of respirations should be assessed. The respiratory rate is normally described in breaths per minute. Breathing that is normal in rate and depth is called *eupnea*. Abnormally slow respirations are referred to as **bradypnea**, and abnormally fast respirations are called **tachypnea** or *polypnea*. **Apnea** is the absence of breathing. For the respiratory rates for different age groups, see Table 28.2 on page 543.

Clinical Alert!

An adult sleeping client's respirations can fall to fewer than 10 shallow breaths per minute. Use other vital signs to validate the client's condition.

Factors Affecting Respirations

Several factors influence respiratory rate. Those that increase the rate include exercise (increases metabolism), stress (readies the body for "fight or flight"), increased environmental temperature, and lowered oxygen concentration at increased altitudes. Factors that may decrease the respiratory rate include decreased environmental temperature, certain medications (e.g., narcotics), and increased intracranial pressure.

The depth of an individual's respirations can be established by watching the movement of the chest. Respiratory depth is generally described as normal, deep, or shallow. Deep respirations are those in which a large volume of air is inhaled and exhaled, inflating most of the lungs. Shallow respirations involve the exchange of a small volume of air and often the minimal use of lung tissue. During a normal inspiration and expiration, an adult takes in about 500 mL of air. This volume is called the **tidal volume**. For further information about pulmonary volumes and pulmonary capacities, see Chapter 49 ∞.

Body position also affects the amount of air that can be inhaled. People in a supine position experience two physiologic processes that suppress respiration: an increase in the volume of blood inside the thoracic cavity and compression of the chest. Consequently, clients lying on their back have poorer lung aeration, which predisposes them to the stasis of fluids and subsequent infection. Certain medications also affect the respiratory depth. For example, narcotics such as morphine and large doses of barbiturates such as pentobarbital depress the respiratory centers in the brain, thereby depressing the respiratory rate and depth. **Hyperventilation** refers to very deep, rapid respirations; **hypoventilation** refers to very shallow respirations.

Respiratory rhythm refers to the regularity of the expirations and the inspirations. Normally, respirations are evenly spaced. Respiratory rhythm can be described as regular or irregular. An infant's respiratory rhythm may be less regular than an adult's. See Chapter 49 ∞ for details about abnormal respiratory rhythms.

Respiratory quality or **character** refers to those aspects of breathing that are different from normal, effortless breathing. Two of these aspects are the amount of effort a client must exert to breathe and the sound of breathing. Usually, breathing does not require noticeable effort. Sometimes, however, clients can breathe only with substantial effort—this is referred to as labored breathing.

The sound of breathing is also significant. Normal breathing is silent, but a number of abnormal sounds such as a wheeze are obvious to the nurse's ear. Many sounds occur as a result of the presence of fluid in the lungs and are most clearly heard with a stethoscope. See Chapter 29 ∞ for methods used to assess lung sounds. For details about altered breathing patterns and terms used to describe various patterns and sounds, see Box 28.7.

BOX 28.7 Altered Breathing Patterns and Sounds

BREATHING PATTERNS

Rate
- Tachypnea—quick, shallow breaths
- Bradypnea—abnormally slow breathing
- Apnea—cessation of breathing

Volume
- Hyperventilation—overexpansion of the lungs characterized by rapid and deep breaths
- Hypoventilation—underexpansion of the lungs, characterized by shallow respirations

Rhythm
- Biot breathing—several short breaths followed by long irregular periods of apnea
- Cheyne-Stokes breathing—rhythmic waxing and waning of respirations, from very deep to very shallow breathing and temporary apnea

Ease or Effort
- Dyspnea—difficult and labored breathing during which the individual has a persistent, unsatisfied need for air and feels distressed
- Orthopnea—ability to breathe only in upright sitting or standing positions

BREATH SOUNDS

Audible Without Amplification
- Stridor—a shrill, harsh sound heard during inspiration with laryngeal obstruction
- Stertor—snoring or sonorous respiration, usually due to a partial obstruction of the upper airway
- Wheeze—continuous, high-pitched musical squeak or whistling sound occurring on expiration and sometimes on inspiration when air moves through a narrowed or partially obstructed airway
- Bubbling—gurgling sounds heard as air passes through moist secretions in the respiratory tract

CHEST MOVEMENTS
- Intercostal retraction—indrawing between the ribs
- Substernal retraction—indrawing beneath the breastbone
- Suprasternal retraction—indrawing above the clavicles

SECRETIONS AND COUGHING
- Hemoptysis—the presence of blood in the sputum
- Productive cough—a cough accompanied by secretions
- Nonproductive cough—a dry, harsh cough without secretions

The effectiveness of respirations is measured in part by the uptake of oxygen from the air into the blood and the release of carbon dioxide from the blood into expired air. The amount of hemoglobin in arterial blood that is saturated with oxygen can be measured indirectly through pulse oximetry. A pulse oximeter provides a digital readout of both the client's pulse rate and the oxygen saturation (see Skill 28.7 later in this chapter).

Skill 28.5 outlines the steps for assessing respirations.

Assessing Respirations

PURPOSES

- To acquire baseline data against which future measurements can be compared
- To monitor abnormal respirations and respiratory patterns and identify changes
- To monitor respirations before or after the administration of a general anesthetic or any medication that influences respirations
- To monitor clients at risk for respiratory alterations (e.g., those with fever, pain, acute anxiety, chronic obstructive pulmonary disease, asthma, respiratory infection, pulmonary edema or emboli, chest trauma or constriction, brainstem injury)

ASSESSMENT

Assess

- Skin and mucous membrane color (e.g., cyanosis or pallor)
- Position assumed for breathing (e.g., use of orthopneic position)
- Signs of lack of oxygen to the brain (e.g., irritability, restlessness, drowsiness, or loss of consciousness)
- Chest movements (e.g., retractions between the ribs or above or below the sternum)
- Activity tolerance
- Chest pain
- Dyspnea
- Medications affecting respiratory rate
- History of pulmonary conditions, smoking, exposure to toxic fumes, and living with others who smoke

PLANNING

Assignment

Counting and observing respirations may be assigned to AP. The nurse does the follow-up assessment, interprets abnormal respirations, and determines appropriate interventions.

Equipment

- Clock, timer, or watch with a sweep second hand or digital seconds indicator

IMPLEMENTATION

Preparation

For a routine assessment of respirations, determine the client's activity schedule and choose a suitable time to monitor the respirations. A client who has been exercising will need to rest for a few minutes to permit the accelerated respiratory rate to return to normal.

Performance

1. Prior to performing the procedure, introduce self and verify the client's identity using agency protocol. Explain to the client what you are going to do, why it is necessary, and how to participate. Discuss how the results will be used in planning further care or treatments.
2. Perform hand hygiene and observe appropriate infection prevention procedures.
3. Provide for client privacy.
4. Observe or palpate and count the respiratory rate.
   - The client's awareness that the nurse is counting the respiratory rate could cause the client to purposefully alter the respiratory pattern. If you anticipate this, place a hand against the client's chest to feel the chest movements with breathing, or place the client's arm across the chest and observe the chest movements while supposedly taking the radial pulse.
   - Count the respiratory rate for 30 seconds if the respirations are regular. Count for 60 seconds if they are irregular. An inhalation and an exhalation count as one respiration.
5. Observe the depth, rhythm, and character of respirations.
   - Observe the respirations for depth by watching the movement of the chest. **Rationale:** *During deep respirations, a large volume of air is exchanged; during shallow respirations, a small volume is exchanged.*
   - Observe the respirations for regular or irregular rhythm. **Rationale:** *Normally, respirations are evenly spaced.*
   - Observe the character of respirations—the sound they produce and the effort they require. **Rationale:** *Normally, respirations are silent and effortless.*
6. Document the respiratory rate, depth, rhythm, and character on the appropriate record (see ❶ in Skill 28.1).

SAMPLE DOCUMENTATION

5/17/2020 1320 Respirations irregular, from 18–34/min in past hour. Shallower respirations during tachypnea. Inspiratory wheeze noted. Respiratory therapist called to provide treatment. D. Katano, RN

EVALUATION

- Relate respiratory rate to other vital signs, in particular pulse rate; relate respiratory rhythm and depth to baseline data and health status.
- Report to the primary care provider a respiratory rate significantly above or below the normal range and any notable change in respirations from previous assessments; irregular respiratory rhythm; inadequate respiratory depth; abnormal character of breathing (e.g., orthopnea, wheezing, stridor, or bubbling); and any complaints of dyspnea.
- Collaborate with other healthcare team members, such as the respiratory therapist, regarding the care plan to address any respiratory issues.

LIFESPAN CONSIDERATIONS Respirations

INFANTS AND CHILDREN

- An infant or child who is crying will have an abnormal respiratory rate and rhythm and needs to be quieted before respirations can be accurately assessed.
- Have an adult hold a child gently to reduce movement while counting respirations.
- Infants and young children use their diaphragms for inhalation and exhalation. If necessary, place your hand gently on the infant's abdomen to feel the rapid rise and fall during respirations.
- Most newborns are complete nose breathers, so nasal obstruction can be life-threatening.
- Some newborns display "periodic breathing" in which they pause for a few seconds between respirations. This condition can be normal, but parents should be alert to prolonged or frequent pauses (apnea) that require medical attention.
- Compared to adults, infants have fewer alveoli and their airways have a smaller diameter. As a result, infants' respiratory rate and effort of breathing will increase with respiratory infections.
- Count respirations prior to uncomfortable procedures so that the respiratory rate is not artificially elevated by the discomfort.

OLDER ADULTS

- Ask the client to remain quiet, or count respirations after taking the pulse.
- Older adults experience anatomic and physiologic changes that cause the respiratory system to be less efficient. Any changes in rate or type of breathing should be reported immediately.

Blood Pressure

Arterial blood pressure is a measure of the pressure exerted by the blood as it flows through the arteries. Because the blood moves in waves, there are two blood pressure measurements. The **systolic pressure** is the pressure of the blood as a result of contraction of the ventricles, that is, the pressure of the height of the blood wave. The **diastolic pressure** is the pressure when the ventricles are at rest. Diastolic pressure, then, is the lower pressure, present at all times within the arteries. The difference between the diastolic and the systolic pressures is called the **pulse pressure**. A normal pulse pressure is about 40 mmHg but can be as high as 100 mmHg during exercise.

Blood pressure is measured in millimeters of mercury (mmHg) and recorded as a fraction: systolic pressure over the diastolic pressure. A typical blood pressure for a healthy adult is 120/80 mmHg (pulse pressure of 40). Because blood pressure can vary considerably among individuals, it is important for the nurse to know a specific client's baseline blood pressure. For example, if a client's usual blood pressure is 180/100 mmHg, and it is assessed following surgery to be 120/80 mmHg, this significant drop in pressure may indicate complications and must be reported to the primary care provider.

A consistently elevated pulse pressure occurs in arteriosclerosis. A low pulse pressure (e.g., less than 25 mmHg) occurs in conditions such as severe heart failure. Sometimes, it is useful to also determine the **mean arterial pressure (MAP)** because this represents the pressure actually delivered to the body's organs. The MAP can be calculated in several different ways, one of which is to add two-thirds of the diastolic pressure to one-third of the systolic pressure. A normal MAP is 70 to 110 mmHg.

Determinants of Blood Pressure

Arterial blood pressure is the result of several factors: the pumping action of the heart, the peripheral vascular resistance (the resistance supplied by the blood vessels through which the blood flows), and the blood volume and viscosity.

Pumping Action of the Heart

When the pumping action of the heart is weak, less blood is pumped into arteries (lower cardiac output), and the blood pressure decreases. When the heart's pumping action is strong and the volume of blood pumped into the circulation increases (higher cardiac output), the blood pressure increases.

Peripheral Vascular Resistance

Peripheral resistance can increase blood pressure. The diastolic pressure especially is affected. Some factors that create resistance in the arterial system are the capacity of the arterioles and capillaries, the compliance of the arteries, and the viscosity of the blood.

The internal diameter or capacity of the arterioles and the capillaries determines in great part the peripheral resistance to the blood in the body. The smaller the space within a vessel, the greater the resistance. Normally, the arterioles are in a state of partial constriction. Increased vasoconstriction, such as occurs with smoking, raises the blood pressure, whereas decreased vasoconstriction lowers the blood pressure.

If the elastic and muscular tissues of the arteries are replaced with fibrous tissue, the arteries lose much of their ability to constrict and dilate. This condition, most common in middle-aged and older adults, is known as **arteriosclerosis**.

Blood Volume

When the blood volume decreases (for example, as a result of a hemorrhage or dehydration), the blood pressure decreases because of decreased fluid in the arteries. Conversely, when the volume increases (for example, as a result of a rapid IV infusion), the blood pressure increases because of the greater fluid volume within the circulatory system.

Blood Viscosity

Blood pressure is higher when the blood is highly viscous (thick), that is, when the proportion of red blood cells to the blood plasma is high. This proportion is referred to as the **hematocrit**. The viscosity increases markedly when the hematocrit is more than 60% to 65%.

Factors Affecting Blood Pressure

Among the factors influencing blood pressure are age, exercise, stress, race, sex, medications, obesity, diurnal variations, medical conditions, and temperature.

- *Age.* Newborns have a systolic pressure of about 75 mmHg. The pressure rises with age, reaching a peak at the onset of puberty, and then tends to decline somewhat. In older adults, elasticity of the arteries is decreased—the arteries are more rigid and less yielding to the pressure of the blood. This produces an elevated systolic pressure. Because the walls no longer retract as flexibly with decreased pressure, the diastolic pressure may also be high.
- *Exercise.* Physical activity increases the cardiac output and hence the blood pressure. For reliable assessment of resting blood pressure, wait 20 to 30 minutes following exercise.
- *Stress.* Stimulation of the sympathetic nervous system increases cardiac output and vasoconstriction of the arterioles, thus increasing the blood pressure reading; however, severe pain can decrease blood pressure greatly by inhibiting the vasomotor center and producing vasodilation.
- *Race.* African American individuals older than 35 years tend to have higher blood pressures than other races of the same age, and African American women have higher rates of high blood pressure than African American men (Mozzafarian et al., 2016).
- *Sex.* After puberty, females usually have lower blood pressures than males of the same age; this difference is thought to be due to hormonal variations. After menopause, women generally have higher blood pressures than before. After age 65, the rate of high blood pressure is higher in women than it is in men of the same age (Mozzafarian et al., 2016).
- *Medications.* Many medications, including caffeine, may increase or decrease the blood pressure.
- *Obesity.* Both childhood and adult obesity predispose to hypertension.
- *Diurnal variations.* Pressure is usually lowest early in the morning, when the metabolic rate is lowest, then rises throughout the day and peaks in the late afternoon or early evening.
- *Medical conditions.* Any condition affecting the cardiac output, blood volume, blood viscosity, or compliance of the arteries has a direct effect on the blood pressure.
- *Temperature.* Because of increased metabolic rate, fever can increase blood pressure. However, external heat causes vasodilation and decreased blood pressure. Cold causes vasoconstriction and elevates blood pressure.

Hypertension

A blood pressure that is persistently above normal is called **hypertension**. A single elevated blood pressure reading indicates the need for reassessment. Hypertension cannot be diagnosed unless an elevated blood pressure is found when measured twice at different times. It is usually asymptomatic and is often a contributing factor to myocardial infarctions (heart attacks). An elevated blood pressure of unknown cause is called *primary hypertension*. An elevated blood pressure of known cause is called *secondary hypertension*. Hypertension is a widespread health problem. Exact definitions of hypertension vary somewhat according to the agency. The American College of Cardiology and the American Heart Association (Cifu & Davis, 2017) define normal blood pressure as systolic less than 120 mmHg and diastolic less than 80 mmHg (see Table 28.4). Above those values, intervention is recommended. The stage of hypertension is determined by the higher of the two values. For example, if either of the systolic or diastolic values falls in the stage 2 range, stage 2 hypertension is assigned. By contrast, the European Society of Cardiology and the European Society of Hypertension recommend treatment only when the blood pressure is greater than 140/90 (Whelton & Williams, 2018).

Factors associated with hypertension include thickening of the arterial walls, which reduces the size of the arterial lumen, and inelasticity of the arteries, as well as such lifestyle factors as cigarette smoking, obesity, heavy alcohol consumption, lack of physical exercise, high blood cholesterol levels, and continued exposure to stress.

Hypotension

Hypotension is a blood pressure that is below normal, that is, a systolic reading consistently between 85 and 110 mmHg in an adult whose normal pressure is higher than this. **Orthostatic hypotension** (or postural hypotension) is a blood pressure that decreases when the client changes from a supine to a sitting or standing position. It is usually the result of peripheral vasodilation in which blood leaves the central body organs, especially the brain, and moves to the periphery, often causing the client to feel faint. Hypotension can also be caused by analgesics such as meperidine hydrochloride (Demerol), bleeding, severe burns, and dehydration. It is important to monitor hypotensive clients carefully to prevent falls. When assessing for orthostatic hypotension:

- Place the client in a supine position for at least 5 minutes.
- Record the client's pulse and blood pressure.

TABLE 28.4 Classification of Blood Pressure

Category	Systolic BP (mmHg)		Diastolic BP (mmHg)
Normal	<120	and	<80
Elevated	120–129	or	<80
Hypertension, stage 1	130–139	or	80–89
Hypertension, stage 2	>140	or	>90

Source: From "Prevention, Detection, Evaluation, and Management of High Blood Pressure in Adults," by A. S. Cifu and A. M. Davis, 2017, *Journal of the American Medical Association*, *318*(21), pp. 2132–2134.

- Assist the client to slowly sit or stand. Support the client in case of faintness.
- Immediately recheck the pulse and blood pressure in the same sites as previously.
- Measure the pulse and blood pressure again after 3 minutes. Some research indicates that BP and pulse should be measured at 30, 60, 120, and 180 seconds after standing, although the 1- and 3-minute measurements are the most valuable (Jones & Kuritzky, 2018).
- Record the results. A drop in blood pressure of 20 mmHg systolic or 10 mmHg diastolic or an increase in pulse of 20 beats/min indicates orthostatic hypotension (Jones & Kuritzky, 2018).

Assessing Blood Pressure

Manual blood pressure measurement is performed with a blood pressure cuff, a sphygmomanometer, and a stethoscope. The blood pressure cuff consists of a bag, called a bladder, that can be inflated with air (Figure 28.18 ■). It has two tubes attached to it. One tube connects to a bulb that inflates the bladder. A small valve on the side of this bulb traps and releases the air in the bladder.

The other tube is attached to a sphygmomanometer. The **sphygmomanometer** indicates the pressure of the air within the bladder. There are two types of sphygmomanometers: aneroid and digital. The aneroid sphygmomanometer has a calibrated dial with a needle that points to the calibrations (Figure 28.19 ■).

Many agencies use digital (electronic) sphygmomanometers (Figure 28.20 ■), which eliminate the need to listen for the sounds of the client's systolic and diastolic blood pressures through a stethoscope. Electronic blood pressure devices should be calibrated periodically to check accuracy. All healthcare facilities should have manual blood pressure equipment available as backup.

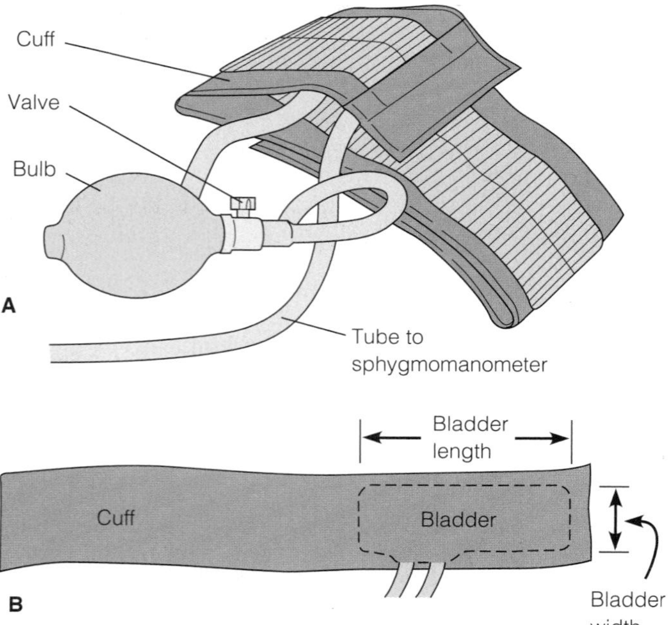

Figure 28.18 ■ *A*, Blood pressure cuff and bulb; *B*, bladder inside the cuff.

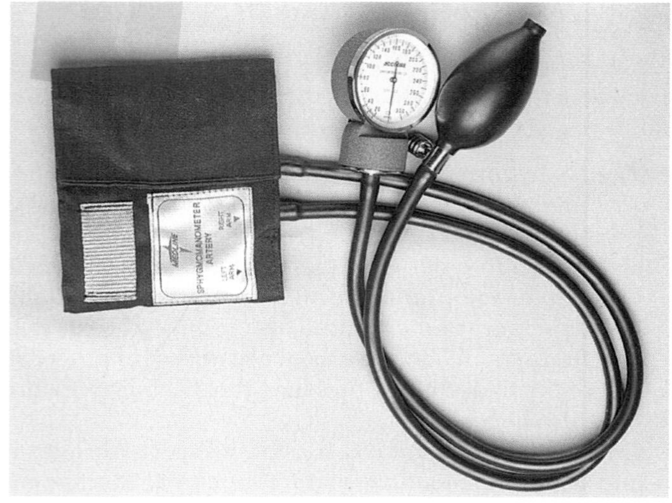

Figure 28.19 ■ Blood pressure equipment: an aneroid manometer and cuff.

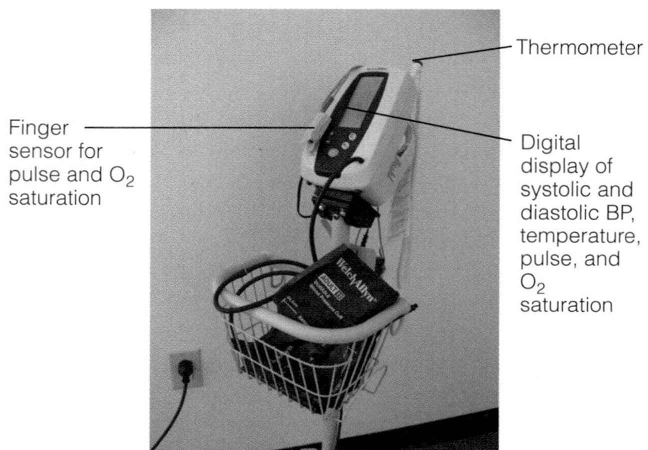

Figure 28.20 ■ Electronic blood pressure monitors register blood pressures.

Doppler ultrasound stethoscopes are also used to assess blood pressure (see Figure 28.15). These are of particular value when blood pressure sounds are difficult to hear, such as in infants, obese clients, and clients in shock. Systolic pressure may be the only blood pressure obtainable with some ultrasound models.

Blood pressure cuffs come in various sizes because the bladder must be the correct width and length for the client's arm (Figure 28.21 ■). If the bladder is too narrow, the blood pressure reading will be erroneously elevated; if it is too wide, the reading will be

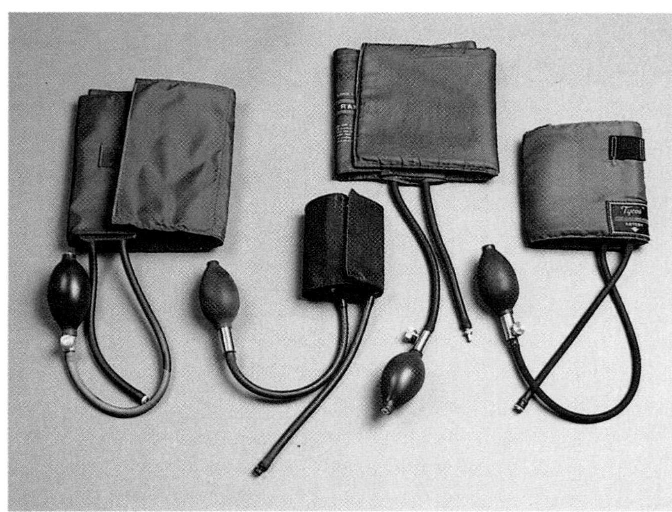

Figure 28.21 ■ Standard cuff sizes: smaller cuffs are used for infants, small children, or frail adults; midsize cuffs are used for most adults; and larger cuffs are used for measuring the blood pressure on the leg or arm of an adult with obesity.

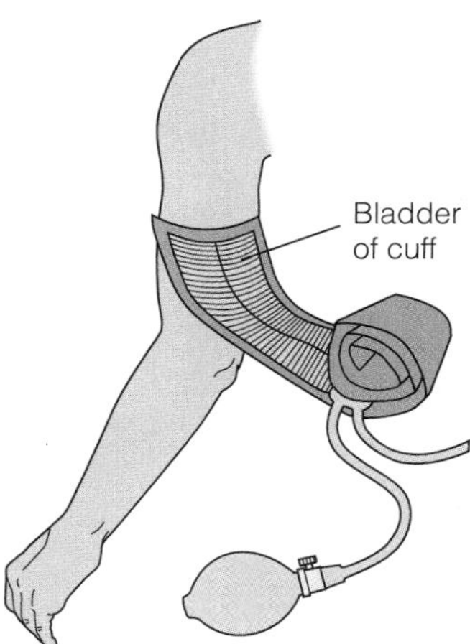

Figure 28.22 ■ Determining that the bladder width of a blood pressure cuff is 40% of the arm circumference or 20% wider than the diameter of the midpoint of the limb.

erroneously low. The width should be 40% of the circumference, or 20% wider than the diameter of the midpoint, of the limb on which it is used. Sometimes, the cuff is referred to as an *adult*, *child*, or *pediatric* cuff. However, the arm circumference, not the age of the client, should always be used to determine bladder size. The nurse can determine whether the width of a blood pressure cuff is appropriate: Lay the cuff lengthwise at the midpoint of the upper arm, and hold the outermost side of the bladder edge laterally on the arm. With the other hand, wrap the width of the cuff around the arm, and ensure that the width is 40% of the arm circumference (Figure 28.22 ■).

The length of the bladder also affects the accuracy of measurement. The bladder should be sufficiently long to cover at least two-thirds of the limb's circumference.

Blood pressure cuffs are made of nondistensible material so that an even pressure is exerted around the limb. Most cuffs are held in place by hooks, snaps, or hook-and-loop fabric. Others have a cloth bandage that is long enough to encircle the limb several times; this type is closed by tucking the end of the bandage into one of the bandage folds.

QSEN Patient-Centered Care: Blood Pressure

- If the client takes blood pressure readings at home, during a home visit the nurse should use the same equipment or calibrate it against a system known to be accurate.
- Observe the client or family member taking the blood pressure and provide feedback if further instruction is needed.
- Home blood pressure measurement done by the client or family can be compared to pressures found when the client is seen in a clinic or office setting. The 2017 hypertension guidelines make a strong recommendation for individuals to do out-of-office (home) BP monitoring (Cifu & Davis, 2017). If there are differences in the readings, they may be because of so-called white coat elevation, which is an increase in blood pressure due to mild anxiety associated with the healthcare provider's presence—who historically wore a white laboratory coat. Some estimates are that white coat hypertension occurs in more than 20% of the U.S. population (Headley, Wall, & Cushman, 2017). If the differences between office and home measurements are large, the client should take the home equipment to the medical office, where simultaneous readings using both the home and office equipment can be done to determine the accuracy of the home device.

Blood Pressure Assessment Sites

The blood pressure is commonly assessed in the client's upper arm. In some settings, blood pressure may be routinely measured on the forearm or wrist, usually using an electronic blood pressure monitor (Figure 28.23 ■).

Assessing the blood pressure on a client's thigh is indicated in these situations:

- The blood pressure cannot be measured on either arm (e.g., because of burns or other trauma).
- The blood pressure in one thigh is to be compared with the blood pressure in the other thigh.

Blood pressure is not measured on a particular client's limb in the following situations:

- The shoulder, arm, or hand (or the hip, knee, or ankle) is injured or diseased.
- A cast or bulky bandage is on any part of the limb.
- The client has had surgical removal of breast or axillary (or inguinal) lymph nodes on that side.

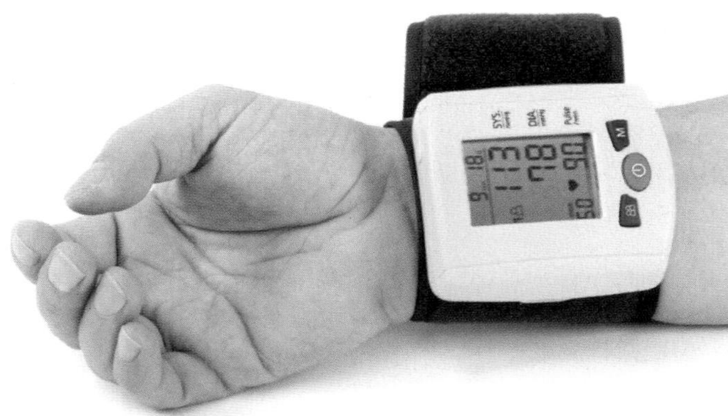

Figure 28.23 ■ In many outpatient settings, the electronic blood pressure monitor is used on the wrist instead of the upper arm.
Werner Muenzker/123RF.

- The client has an IV infusion or blood transfusion in that limb.
- The client has an arteriovenous fistula (e.g., for renal dialysis) in that limb.

Methods

Blood pressure can be assessed directly or indirectly. Direct (invasive monitoring) measurement involves the insertion of a catheter into the brachial, radial, or femoral artery. Arterial pressure is represented as wavelike forms displayed on a monitor. With correct placement, this pressure reading is highly accurate.

Two noninvasive indirect methods of measuring blood pressure are the auscultatory and palpatory methods. The auscultatory method is most commonly used in hospitals, clinics, and homes. When taking a blood pressure using a stethoscope, the nurse identifies phases in the series of sounds called **Korotkoff sounds** (Figure 28.24 ■). Five phases occur but may not always be audible (Box 28.8).The systolic pressure is the point where the first tapping sound is heard (phase 1). In adults, the diastolic pressure is the point where the sounds become inaudible (phase 5). The phase 5 reading may be zero; that is, the muffled sounds are heard even when there is no air pressure in the blood pressure cuff. For complete accuracy, the phase 4 and 5 readings should be recorded.

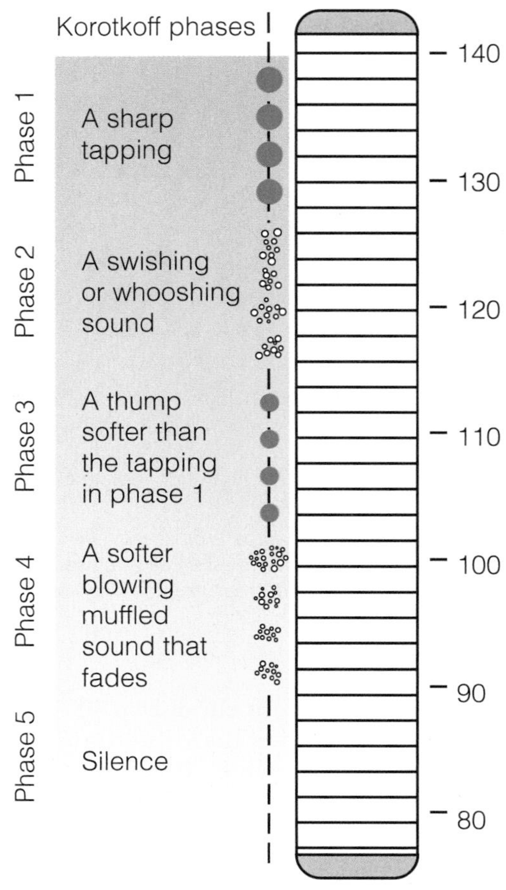

Figure 28.24 ■ Korotkoff sounds can be differentiated into five phases. In the illustration the blood pressure is 138/90 or 138/102/90 mmHg.

The palpatory method is sometimes used when Korotkoff sounds cannot be heard and electronic equipment to amplify the sounds is not available, or to prevent misdirection from the presence of an auscultatory gap. An **auscultatory gap**, which occurs particularly in hypertensive clients, is the temporary disappearance of sounds normally heard over the brachial artery when the

BOX 28.8 Korotkoff Sounds

- *Phase 1*: The pressure level at which the first faint, clear tapping or thumping sounds are heard. These sounds gradually become more intense. To ensure that they are not extraneous sounds, the nurse should identify at least two consecutive tapping sounds. The first tapping sound heard during deflation of the cuff is the systolic blood pressure.
- *Phase 2*: The period during deflation when the sounds have a muffled, whooshing, or swishing quality.
- *Phase 3*: The period during which the blood flows freely through an increasingly open artery and the sounds become crisper and more intense and again assume a thumping quality but softer than in phase 1.
- *Phase 4*: The time when the sounds become muffled and have a soft, blowing quality.
- *Phase 5*: The pressure level when the last sound is heard. This is followed by a period of silence. The pressure at which the last sound is heard is the diastolic blood pressure in adults.*

*In agencies where the fourth phase is considered the diastolic pressure, three measures are recommended (systolic pressure, diastolic pressure, and phase 5). These may be referred to as systolic, first diastolic, and second diastolic pressures. The phase 5 (second diastolic pressure) reading may be zero; that is, the muffled sounds are heard even when there is no air pressure in the blood pressure cuff. In some instances, muffled sounds are never heard, in which case a dash is inserted where the reading would normally be recorded (e.g., /–/110).

TABLE 28.5 Selected Sources of Error in Blood Pressure Assessment

Error	Effect
Bladder cuff too narrow	Erroneously high
Bladder cuff too wide	Erroneously low
Arm unsupported	Erroneously high
Insufficient rest before the assessment	Erroneously high
Repeating assessment too quickly	Erroneously high systolic or low diastolic readings
Cuff wrapped too loosely or unevenly	Erroneously high
Deflating cuff too quickly	Erroneously low systolic and high diastolic readings
Deflating cuff too slowly	Erroneously high diastolic reading
Failure to use the same arm consistently	Inconsistent measurements
Arm above level of the heart	Erroneously low
Assessing immediately after a meal or while client smokes or has pain	Erroneously high
Failure to identify auscultatory gap	Erroneously low systolic pressure and erroneously low diastolic pressure

cuff pressure is high followed by the reappearance of the sounds at a lower level. This temporary disappearance of sounds occurs in the latter part of phase 1 and phase 2 and may cover a range of 40 mmHg. If a palpated estimation of the systolic pressure is not made prior to auscultation, the nurse may begin listening in the middle of this range and underestimate the systolic pressure. In the palpatory method of blood pressure determination, instead of listening for the blood flow sounds, the nurse uses light to moderate pressure to palpate the pulsations of the artery as the pressure in the cuff is released. The pressure is read from the sphygmomanometer when the first pulsation is felt. A single whiplike vibration, felt in addition to the pulsations, identifies the point at which the pressure in the cuff nears the diastolic pressure. This vibration is no longer felt when the cuff pressure is below the diastolic pressure.

Common Errors in Assessing Blood Pressure

The importance of the accuracy of blood pressure assessments cannot be overemphasized. Many judgments about a client's health are made based on blood pressure. It is an important indicator of the client's condition and is used extensively as a basis for nursing interventions. Two possible reasons for blood pressure errors are hurrying on the part of the nurse and subconscious bias in which a nurse may be influenced by the client's previous blood pressure measurements or diagnosis and "hear" a value consistent with the nurse's expectations. Some reasons for erroneous blood pressure readings are given in Table 28.5.

Skill 28.6 provides guidelines for assessing blood pressure.

Assessing Blood Pressure

SKILL 28.6

PURPOSE

- To obtain a baseline measurement of arterial blood pressure for subsequent evaluation
- To determine the client's hemodynamic status (e.g., cardiac output: stroke volume of the heart and blood vessel resistance)
- To identify and monitor changes in blood pressure resulting from a disease process or medical therapy (e.g., presence or history of cardiovascular disease, renal disease, circulatory shock, or acute pain; rapid infusion of fluids or blood products)

ASSESSMENT

Assess

- Signs and symptoms of hypertension (e.g., headache, ringing in the ears, flushing of face, nosebleeds, fatigue)
- Signs and symptoms of hypotension (e.g., tachycardia, dizziness, mental confusion, restlessness, cool and clammy skin, pale or cyanotic skin)
- Factors affecting blood pressure (e.g., activity, emotional stress, pain, and time the client last smoked or ingested caffeine)
- Some blood pressure cuffs contain latex. Assess the client for latex allergy and obtain a latex-free cuff if indicated.

PLANNING

Assignment

Blood pressure measurement may be assigned to AP. The nurse interprets abnormal blood pressure readings and determines appropriate responses.

Equipment

- Stethoscope or DUS
- Blood pressure cuff of the appropriate size
- Sphygmomanometer

Continued on page 562

Assessing Blood Pressure—*continued*

IMPLEMENTATION

Preparation

1. Ensure that the equipment is intact and functioning properly. Check for leaks in the tubing between the cuff and the sphygmomanometer.
2. Make sure that the client has not smoked or ingested caffeine within 30 minutes prior to measurement. **Rationale:** *Smoking constricts blood vessels, and caffeine increases the pulse rate. Both of these cause a temporary increase in blood pressure.*

Performance

1. Prior to performing the procedure, introduce self and verify the client's identity using agency protocol. Explain to the client what you are going to do, why it is necessary, and how to participate. Discuss how the results will be used in planning further care or treatments.
2. Perform hand hygiene and observe appropriate infection prevention procedures.
3. Provide for client privacy.
4. Position the client appropriately.
   - The adult client should be sitting unless otherwise specified. Both feet should be flat on the floor. **Rationale:** *Legs crossed at the knee results in elevated systolic and diastolic blood pressures (Wilson & Giddens, 2017).*
   - The elbow should be slightly flexed with the palm of the hand facing up and the arm supported at heart level. Readings in any other position should be specified. The blood pressure is normally similar in sitting, standing, and lying positions, but it can vary significantly by position in certain clients. **Rationale:** *The blood pressure increases when the arm is below heart level and decreases when the arm is above heart level.*
   - Expose the upper arm.
5. Wrap the deflated cuff evenly around the upper arm. Locate the brachial artery (see Figure 28.13, page 543). Apply the center of the bladder directly over the artery. **Rationale:** *The bladder inside the cuff must be directly over the artery to be compressed if the reading is to be accurate.*
   - For an adult, place the lower border of the cuff approximately 2.5 cm (1 in.) above the antecubital space.
6. If this is the client's initial examination, perform a preliminary palpatory determination of systolic pressure. **Rationale:** *The initial estimate tells the nurse the maximal pressure to which the sphygmomanometer needs to be elevated in subsequent determinations. It also prevents underestimation of the systolic pressure or overestimation of the diastolic pressure should an auscultatory gap occur.*
   - Palpate the brachial artery with the fingertips ❶.
   - Close the valve on the bulb.
   - Pump up the cuff until you no longer feel the brachial pulse. At that pressure the blood cannot flow through the artery. Note the pressure on the sphygmomanometer at which pulse is no longer felt. **Rationale:** *This gives an estimate of the systolic pressure.*
   - Release the pressure completely in the cuff, and wait 1 to 2 minutes before making further measurements. **Rationale:** *A waiting period gives the blood trapped in the veins time to be released. Otherwise, false readings will occur.*
7. Position the stethoscope appropriately.
   - Cleanse the earpieces with antiseptic wipe.
   - Insert the ear attachments of the stethoscope in your ears so that they tilt slightly forward. **Rationale:** *Sounds are heard more clearly when the ear attachments follow the direction of the ear canal.*

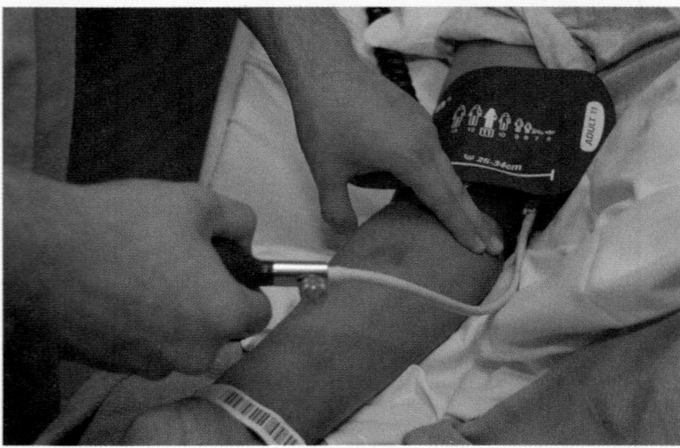

❶ Locate the brachial artery to perform a palpatory blood pressure.

   - Ensure that the stethoscope hangs freely from the ears to the amplifier. **Rationale:** *If the stethoscope tubing rubs against an object, the noise can interfere with the sounds of the blood within the artery.*
   - Place the amplifier of the stethoscope over the brachial pulse site. Because the blood pressure is a low-frequency sound, it may be best heard with the bell-shaped diaphragm. The American Heart Association states that either the bell or diaphragm can be used to auscultate blood pressure, but some research has shown that the diastolic pressure reads slightly lower when using the diaphragm (Liu, Griffiths, Murray, & Zheng, 2016).
   - Place the stethoscope directly on the skin, not on clothing over the site. **Rationale:** *This is to avoid noise made from rubbing the amplifier against cloth.*
   - Hold the amplifier with the thumb and index finger.
8. Auscultate the client's blood pressure.
   - Pump up the cuff until the sphygmomanometer reads 30 mmHg above the point where the brachial pulse disappeared.
   - Release the valve on the cuff carefully so that the pressure decreases at the rate of 2 to 3 mmHg per second. **Rationale:** *If the rate is faster or slower, an error in measurement may occur.*
   - As the pressure falls, identify the manometer reading at Korotkoff phases 1, 4, and 5. **Rationale:** *There is no clinical significance to phases 2 and 3.*
   - After hearing phase 5, deflate the cuff rapidly and completely.
   - Wait 1 to 2 minutes before making further determinations. **Rationale:** *This permits blood trapped in the veins to be released.*
   - Repeat the above steps to confirm the accuracy of the reading—especially if it falls outside the normal range (although this may not be routine procedure for hospitalized or well clients). If there is greater than 5 mmHg difference between the two readings, additional measurements may be taken and the results averaged.
9. If this is the client's initial examination, repeat the procedure on the client's other arm. There should be a difference of no more than 10 mmHg between the arms. Inter-arm differences greater than 10 mmHg occur more commonly in hypertensive and diabetic clients and should be evaluated further (Clark, 2017).

Variation: Obtaining a Blood Pressure by the Palpation Method

If it is not possible to use a stethoscope to obtain the blood pressure or if the Korotkoff sounds cannot be heard, palpate the radial or brachial pulse site as the cuff pressure is released. The manometer reading at the point where the pulse reappears is an estimate of systolic value.

Assessing Blood Pressure—*continued*

Variation: Taking a Thigh Blood Pressure

- Help the client to assume a prone position. If the client cannot assume this position, measure the blood pressure while the client is in a supine position with the knee slightly flexed. Slight flexing of the knee will facilitate placing the stethoscope on the popliteal space.
- Expose the thigh, taking care not to expose the client unduly.
- Locate the popliteal artery (see Figure 28.13).
- Wrap the cuff evenly around the midthigh with the compression bladder over the posterior aspect of the thigh and the bottom edge above the knee. ❷ **Rationale:** *The bladder must be directly over the posterior popliteal artery if the reading is to be accurate.*
- If this is the client's initial examination, perform a preliminary palpatory determination of systolic pressure by palpating the popliteal artery.
- In adults, the systolic pressure in the popliteal artery is usually 20 to 30 mmHg higher than that in the brachial artery; the diastolic pressure is usually the same.

Variation: Using an Electronic Indirect Blood Pressure Monitoring Device (see Figure 28.20, page 558)

The results of a large research study have led to recommendations including presetting the automated machine to wait five minutes before taking the first measurement, taking multiple blood pressure readings, and averaging them while the client is resting quietly, seated in a chair (with back support—not on an examination table) and alone in the room (Headley, 2017).

- Place the blood pressure cuff on the extremity according to the manufacturer's guidelines.
- Turn on the power switch.
- If appropriate, set the device for the desired number of minutes between automatic blood pressure determinations.
- When the device has determined the blood pressure reading, note the digital results.

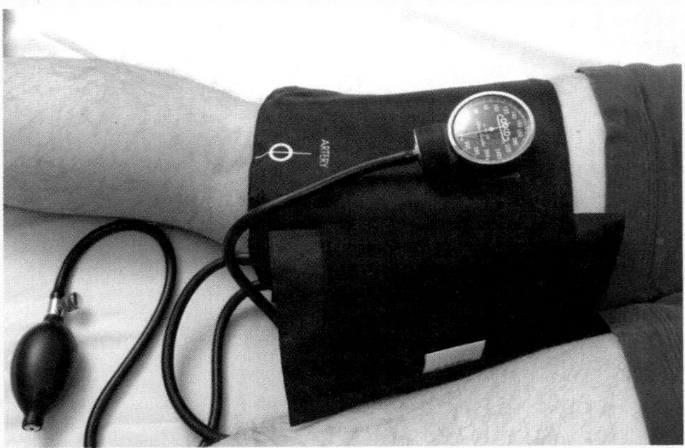

❷ Measuring blood pressure in a client's thigh.

10. Remove the cuff from the client's arm.

Safety Alert! SAFETY

Electronic or automatic blood pressure cuffs can be left in place for many hours. Remove the cuff and check skin condition periodically.

11. Wipe the cuff with an approved disinfectant. **Rationale:** *Cuffs can become significantly contaminated.*
- Many institutions use disposable blood pressure cuffs. The client uses it for the length of stay and then it is discarded. **Rationale:** *This decreases the risk of spreading infection by sharing cuffs.*

12. Document and report pertinent assessment data according to agency policy. Record two pressures in the form "130/80" where "130" is the systolic (phase 1) and "80" is the diastolic (phase 5) pressure. Record three pressures in the form "130/90/0," where "130" is the systolic, "90" is the first diastolic (phase 4), and sounds are audible even after the cuff is completely deflated. Use the abbreviations RA or RL for right arm or right leg and LA or LL for left arm or left leg.

EVALUATION

- Relate blood pressure to other vital signs, to baseline data, and to health status. If the findings are significantly different from previous values without obvious reasons, consider possible causes (see Table 28.5).
- Report any significant change in the client's blood pressure. Also report these findings for an adult if they are consistent over time:
  - Systolic blood pressure above 140 mmHg
  - Diastolic blood pressure above 90 mmHg
  - Systolic blood pressure below 100 mmHg
  - Inter-arm differences of greater than 10 mmHg.

LIFESPAN CONSIDERATIONS Blood Pressure

INFANTS

- Use a pediatric stethoscope.
- The lower edge of the blood pressure cuff can be closer to the antecubital space of an infant.
- Use the palpation method if auscultation with a stethoscope or DUS is unsuccessful.
- Arm and thigh pressures are equivalent in children under 1 year of age.
- The systolic blood pressure of a newborn averages about 70 mmHg but, because of the technical difficulty, is not commonly measured unless a problem is suspected (D'Amico & Barbarito, 2016).

CHILDREN

- Blood pressure should be measured in all children over 3 years of age and in children less than 3 years of age with certain medical conditions (e.g., congenital heart disease, renal malformation, medications that affect blood pressure).
- Explain each step of the process and what it will feel like. Demonstrate on a doll.
- Use the palpation technique for children under 3 years old.
- Cuff bladder width should be 40% and length should be 80% to 100% of the arm circumference (Figure 28.25 ■).

Continued on page 564

LIFESPAN CONSIDERATIONS **Blood Pressure—*continued***

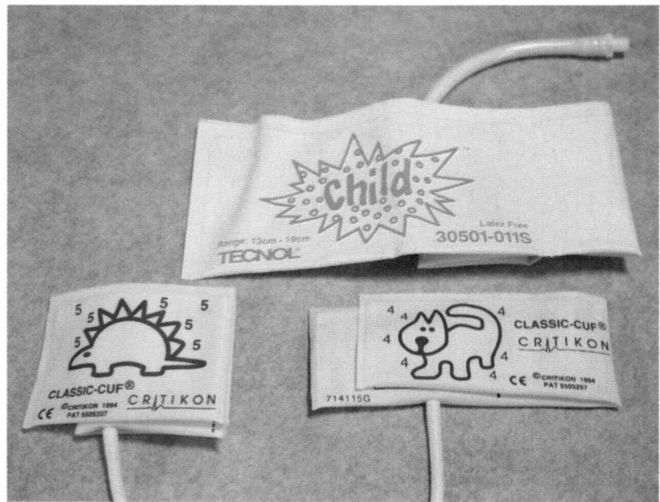

Figure 28.25 ■ Pediatric blood pressure cuffs.

- Take the blood pressure prior to other uncomfortable procedures so that the blood pressure is not artificially elevated by the discomfort.
- In children, the diastolic pressure is considered to be the onset of phase 4, where the sounds become muffled.
- In children, the thigh pressure is about 10 mmHg higher than the arm pressure.
- One quick way to determine the normal systolic blood pressure of a child is to use the following formula:

$$\text{Normal systolic BP} = 80 + (2 \times \text{child's age in years})$$

OLDER ADULTS

- Skin may be very fragile. Do not allow cuff pressure to remain high any longer than necessary.
- Determine if the client is taking antihypertensives and, if so, when the last dose was taken.
- Medications that cause vasodilation (antihypertensive medications) and also the loss of baroreceptor efficiency in older clients place them at increased risk for having orthostatic hypotension. Measuring blood pressure while the client is in the lying, sitting, and standing positions—and noting any changes—can determine this.
- If the client has arm contractures, assess the blood pressure by palpation, with the arm in a relaxed position. If this is not possible, take a thigh or wrist blood pressure.

Oxygen Saturation

A **pulse oximeter** is a noninvasive device that estimates a client's blood **oxygen saturation** (SpO_2) by means of a sensor attached to the client's finger (Figure 28.26 ■), toe, nose, earlobe, or forehead (or around the hand or foot of a neonate). The oxygen saturation value is the percent of all hemoglobin binding sites that are occupied by oxygen. The pulse oximeter can detect hypoxemia (low oxygen saturation) before clinical signs and symptoms, such as a dusky color to skin and nail beds, develop.

The pulse oximeter's sensor has two parts: (a) two light-emitting diodes (LEDs)—one red, the other infrared—that transmit light through nails, tissue, venous blood, and arterial blood; and (b) a photodetector placed directly opposite the LEDs (e.g., the other side of the finger, toe, or nose). Because the photodetector measures the amount of red and infrared light absorbed by oxygenated and deoxygenated hemoglobin in *peripheral* arterial blood, it is reported as *SpO_2*. Normal oxygen saturation is 95% to 100%; below 90% should be evaluated and treated, and below 70% is life-threatening.

Pulse oximeters with various types of sensors are available from many manufacturers and the specific components vary accordingly. Generally, the oximeter unit consists of an inlet connection for the sensor cable, and a faceplate that indicates (a) the oxygen saturation measurement and (b) the pulse rate. Cordless units are also available (Figure 28.27 ■). A preset alarm system signals high and low SpO_2 measurements and a high

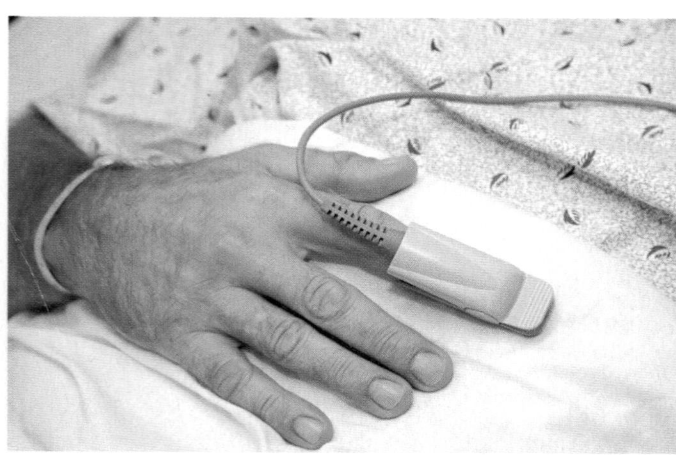

Figure 28.26 ■ Fingertip oximeter sensor (adult).

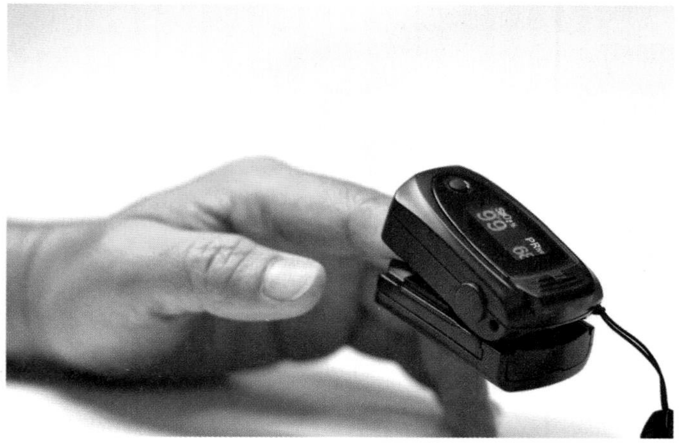

Figure 28.27 ■ Fingertip oximeter sensor (cordless).
toysf400/Shutterstock.

and low pulse rate. The high and low SpO_2 levels are generally preset at 100% and 85%, respectively, for adults. The high and low pulse rate alarms are usually preset at 140 and 50 beats/min for adults. These alarm limits can, however, be changed using the manufacturer's directions.

Factors Affecting Oxygen Saturation Readings

Among the factors influencing oxygen saturation readings are hemoglobin levels, circulation, activity, and exposure to carbon monoxide.

- ***Hemoglobin.*** If the hemoglobin is fully saturated with oxygen, the SpO_2 will appear normal even if the total hemoglobin level is low. Thus, the client could be severely anemic and have inadequate oxygen to supply the tissues but the pulse oximeter would return a normal value.
- ***Circulation.*** The oximeter will not return an accurate reading if the area under the sensor has impaired circulation.
- ***Activity.*** Shivering or excessive movement of the sensor site may interfere with accurate readings.
- ***Carbon monoxide poisoning.*** Pulse oximeters cannot discriminate between hemoglobin saturated with carbon monoxide versus oxygen. In this case, other measures of oxygenation are needed.

Skill 28.7 outlines the steps in measuring oxygen saturation.

EVIDENCE-BASED PRACTICE

Evidence-Based Practice

Is a Pocket Pulse Oximeter as Accurate as a Standard One?

With the increasing use and decreasing cost of pulse oximeters in the outpatient setting, da Costa, Faustino, Lima, Ladeira, and Guimarães (2016) aimed to determine if more inexpensive, portable devices were as accurate as more traditional devices and arterial blood gases. Ninety-five clients participated in the study, excluding any with acute disease or receiving oxygen therapy. The mean difference between the readings on the two oximeters was 0.01%, and the difference between each of the oximeters and the arterial blood sample was the same.

Implications

Although this study was performed using only one brand of each of the oximeters, and the participants' activity during measurement was controlled, the results support the self-monitoring of SpO_2 using the pocket pulse oximeter. The study reflects an issue of importance to nurses: The least expensive but still accurate and easy-to-use method should be implemented. Further research should be conducted on additional devices and under more variable circumstances.

Assessing Oxygen Saturation

SKILL 28.7

PURPOSES

- To estimate the arterial blood oxygen saturation
- To detect the presence of hypoxemia before visible signs develop

ASSESSMENT

Assess

- The best location for a pulse oximeter sensor based on the client's age and physical condition. Unless contraindicated, the finger is usually selected for adults.
- The client's overall condition including risk factors for development of hypoxemia (e.g., respiratory or cardiac disease) and hemoglobin level
- Vital signs, skin color and temperature, nail bed color, and tissue perfusion of extremities as baseline data
- Adhesive allergy

PLANNING

Most hospitals and clinics have pulse oximeters readily available for use with other vital signs equipment (or even as an integrated part of the electronic blood pressure device). Other facilities may have a limited supply of oximeters.

Assignment

Application of the pulse oximeter sensor and recording of the SpO_2 value may be assigned to AP. The nurse interprets the oxygen saturation value and determines appropriate responses.

Equipment

- Nail polish remover as needed
- Pulse oximeter

Continued on page 566

SKILL 28.7

Assessing Oxygen Saturation—*continued*

IMPLEMENTATION

Preparation

Check that the oximeter equipment is functioning normally.

Performance

1. Prior to performing the procedure, introduce self and verify the client's identity using agency protocol. Explain to the client what you are going to do, why it is necessary, and how to participate. Discuss how the results will be used in planning further care or treatments.
2. Perform hand hygiene and observe appropriate infection prevention procedures.
3. Provide for client privacy.
4. Choose a sensor appropriate for the client's size and desired location. A pediatric sensor could be used for a small adult.
   - If the client is allergic to adhesive, use a clip or sensor without adhesive.
   - If using an extremity, apply the sensor only if the proximal pulse and capillary refill at the point closest to the site are present. If the client has low tissue perfusion due to peripheral vascular disease or therapy using vasoconstrictive medications, use a nasal sensor or a reflectance sensor on the forehead. Avoid using lower extremities that have a compromised circulation and extremities that are used for infusions or other invasive monitoring.
5. Prepare the site.
   - If visibly soiled, clean the site before applying the sensor.
   - It may be necessary to remove a female client's dark nail polish. **Rationale:** *Nail polish may interfere with accurate measurements, although the data about this are inconsistent*.
   - Alternatively, position the sensor on the side of the finger rather than perpendicular to the nail bed.
6. Apply the sensor, and connect it to the pulse oximeter.
   - Make sure the LED and photodetector are accurately aligned, that is, opposite each other on either side of the finger, toe, nose, or earlobe. Many sensors have markings to facilitate correct alignment of the LEDs and photodetector.
   - Attach the sensor cable to the connection outlet on the oximeter. Turn on the machine according to the manufacturer's directions. Appropriate connection will be confirmed by an audible beep indicating each arterial pulsation.
   - Ensure that the light or waveform on the face of the oximeter fluctuates with each pulsation.
7. Set and turn on the alarm when using continuous monitoring.
   - Check the preset alarm limits for high and low oxygen saturation and high and low pulse rates. Change these alarm limits according to the agency policy. Ensure that the audio and visual alarms are on before you leave the client.
8. Ensure client safety.
   - Inspect and change the location of an adhesive toe or finger sensor every 4 hours and a spring-tension sensor every 2 hours.
   - Inspect the sensor site tissues for irritation from adhesive sensors.
9. Ensure the accuracy of measurement.
   - Minimize motion artifacts by using an adhesive sensor, changing the sensor location, or immobilizing the client's monitoring site if absolutely necessary. **Rationale:** *Movement of the client's finger or toe may be misinterpreted by the oximeter*.
   - If indicated, cover the sensor with a sheet or towel to block large amounts of light from external sources (e.g., sunlight, procedure lamps, or bilirubin lights in the nursery). **Rationale:** *Bright room light may be sensed by the photodetector and alter the* SpO_2 *value*.
   - Compare the pulse rate indicated by the oximeter to the radial pulse periodically. **Rationale:** *A large discrepancy between the two values may indicate oximeter malfunction*.
10. Document the oxygen saturation on the appropriate record at designated intervals.

EVALUATION

- Compare the oxygen saturation to the client's previous oxygen saturation level. Relate to pulse rate and other vital signs.
- Conduct appropriate follow-up such as notifying the primary care provider, adjusting oxygen therapy, or providing breathing treatments.

LIFESPAN CONSIDERATIONS Pulse Oximetry

INFANTS

- If an appropriate-sized finger, foot, or toe sensor is not available, consider using an earlobe or forehead sensor.
- The high and low SpO_2 levels are generally preset at 100% and 90%, respectively, for neonates.
- The high and low pulse rate alarms are usually preset at 200 and 100, respectively, for neonates.
- The oximeter may need to be taped, wrapped with an elastic bandage, or covered by a stocking to keep it in place.

CHILDREN

- Instruct the child that the sensor does not hurt. Disconnect the probe whenever possible to allow for movement of the child.

OLDER ADULTS

- Use of vasoconstrictive medications, poor circulation, or thickened nails may make finger or toe sensors inaccurate.
- Use a forehead or earlobe sensor if indicated (Figure 28.28 ■).

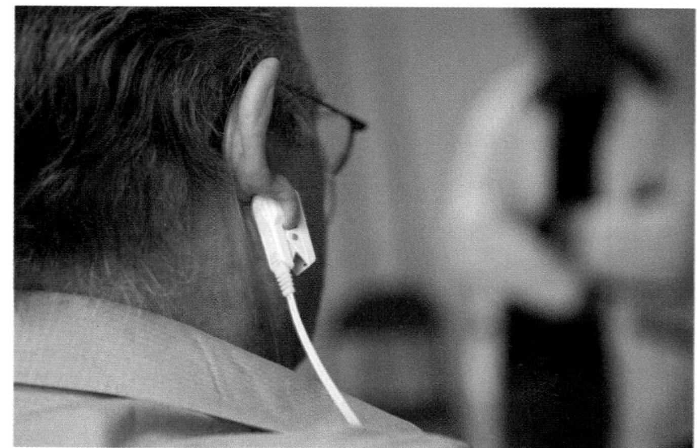

Figure 28.28 ■ Earlobe oximeter sensor.
Bruno Boissonnet/Science Source.

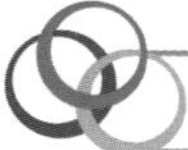

Critical Thinking Checkpoint

1. When you approach your older client to take her blood pressure, she tells you she doesn't want you to take it. What questions will you ask the client at this time?
2. After much exploration, the client agrees to let you take the blood pressure. After pumping up the cuff, you are unable to hear any sounds during release of the valve. What would you say to her?
3. Once you are able to measure the blood pressure, your reading is 180/110 mmHg. Before taking any action on this blood pressure, what do you need to know?
4. The pulse oximeter on the client's finger reads 85%. Her skin is warm and its color is normal, she is awake and oriented, temperature is 37.1°C (98.8°F), and apical pulse is 78. What would be your next actions and why?

Answers to Critical Thinking Checkpoint questions are available on the faculty resources site. Please consult with your instructor.

Chapter 28 Review

CHAPTER HIGHLIGHTS

- Vital signs reflect changes in body function that otherwise might not be observed.
- Body temperature is the balance between heat produced by and heat lost from the body.
- Factors affecting body temperature include age, diurnal variations, exercise, hormones, stress, and environmental temperatures.
- Four common types of fever are intermittent, remittent, relapsing, and constant.
- During a fever, the set point of the hypothalamic thermostat changes suddenly from the normal level to a higher than normal level, but several hours elapse before the core temperature reaches the new set point.
- Hypothermia involves three mechanisms: excessive heat loss, inadequate heat production by body cells, and increasing impairment of hypothalamic thermoregulation.
- The nurse selects the most appropriate site to measure temperature according to the client's age and condition.
- Pulse rate and volume reflect the stroke volume output, the compliance of the client's arteries, and the adequacy of blood flow.
- Normally a peripheral pulse reflects the client's heartbeat, but it may differ from the heartbeat in clients with certain cardiovascular diseases; in these instances, the nurse takes an apical pulse and compares it to the peripheral pulse.
- Many factors may affect an individual's pulse rate: age, sex, exercise, presence of fever, certain medications, hypovolemia, dehydration, stress (in some situations), position changes, and pathology.
- Although the radial pulse is the site most commonly used, eight other sites may be used in certain situations.
- The difference between the apical and radial pulses is called the pulse deficit.
- Respirations are assessed by observing respiratory rate, depth, rhythm, quality, and effectiveness.
- Blood pressure reflects the pumping action of the heart, peripheral vascular resistance, blood volume, and blood viscosity.
- Among the factors influencing blood pressure are age, exercise, stress, race, sex, medications, obesity, diurnal variations, medical conditions, and temperature.
- Orthostatic hypotension occurs when the blood pressure falls as the client assumes an upright position.
- A blood pressure cuff that is too narrow or too wide will give false readings.
- During blood pressure measurement, the artery must be held at heart level.
- A pulse oximeter measures the percent of hemoglobin saturated with oxygen. A normal result is 95% to 100%.
- Pulse oximeter sensors may be placed on the finger, toes, nose, earlobe, or forehead, or around the hand or foot of the neonate.

TEST YOUR KNOWLEDGE

1. Which of the following sites would be the most appropriate choice to use to measure the temperature of a client who has a history of heart disease and has eaten a bowl of vegetable soup 45 minutes ago?
   1. Axilla
   2. Oral
   3. Popliteal
   4. Rectal
2. Which client meets the criteria for selection of the apical site for assessment of the pulse rather than a radial pulse?
   1. A client who is in shock
   2. A client whose pulse changes with body position changes
   3. A client with an arrhythmia
   4. A client who had surgery less than 24 hours ago

3. Which of the following positions should an RN assist the client in to *best* assess respiratory status?
   1. Prone
   2. Semi-Fowler's
   3. Side-lying
   4. Supine
4. For a client with a previous blood pressure of 138/74 mmHg and pulse of 64 beats/min, approximately how long should the nurse take to release the blood pressure cuff in order to obtain an accurate reading?
   1. 10–20 seconds
   2. 30–45 seconds
   3. 1–1.5 minutes
   4. 3–3.5 minutes
5. An RN needs vital signs assessed for four clients. Which client should the nurse address and not assign to a UAP?
   1. Cardiac catheterization client returning to the nursing unit
   2. COPD client on 2 Lpm oxygen via nasal cannula
   3. Pneumonia client nearing discharge
   4. Post-op client of two days from gallbladder surgery
6. An 85-year-old client has had a stroke resulting in right-sided facial drooping, difficulty swallowing, and the inability to move self or maintain position unaided. The nurse determines that which sites are most appropriate for taking the temperature? Select all that apply.
   1. Oral
   2. Rectal
   3. Axillary
   4. Tympanic
   5. Temporal artery
7. A nursing diagnosis of impaired perfusion of peripheral tissue would be validated by which one of the following?
   1. Bounding radial pulse
   2. Irregular apical pulse
   3. Carotid pulse stronger on the left side than the right
   4. Absent posterior tibial and pedal pulses
8. The nurse reports that the client has dyspnea when ambulating. The nurse is most likely to have assessed which of the following?
   1. Shallow respirations
   2. Wheezing
   3. Shortness of breath
   4. Coughing up blood
9. When auscultating the blood pressure, the nurse hears:
   From 200 to 180 mmHg: silence; then:
   a thumping sound continuing down to 150 mmHg:
   muffled sounds continuing down to 130 mmHg;
   soft thumping sounds continuing down to 105 mmHg;
   muffled sounds continuing down to 95 mmHg;
   then silence.
   The nurse records the blood pressure as _______.
10. In Figure 28.29 ■, which number indicates the client's oxygen saturation as measured by pulse oximetry? _______

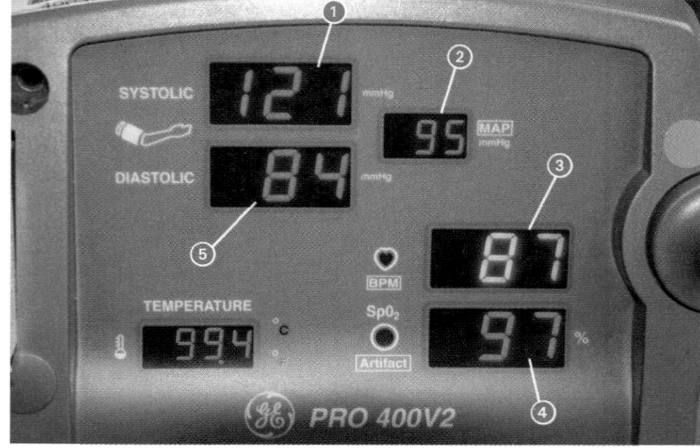

Figure 28.29 ■ Vital signs monitor.

See Answers to Test Your Knowledge in Appendix A.

READINGS AND REFERENCES

Suggested Reading

Breen, A. E., & Hessels, A. J. (2017). Stethoscopes: Friend or fomite? *Nursing Management*, *48*(12), 9–11. doi:10.1097/01.NUMA.0000526917.85088.eb

The article discusses some studies claiming that many stethoscopes when tested were found to harbor disease-causing bacteria, including methicillin-resistant strains. Topics mentioned include meticulous hand hygiene as the best defense against bacteria transmission, link of stethoscope ear pieces to infections in a neonatal intensive care unit, and use of ethanol-based cleaners during hand cleaning by healthcare professionals.

Related Research

Juraschek, S. P., Appel, L. J., Miller, E. R., Mukamal, K. J., & Lipsitz, L. A. (2018). Hypertension treatment effects on orthostatic hypotension and its relationship with cardiovascular disease. *Hypertension*, *72*, 986–993. doi:10.1161/HYPERTENSIONAHA.118.11337

Mickley, J. P., Evans, K. D., Tatarski, R. L., & Sommerich, C. M. (2018). Pilot application of varied equipment and procedural techniques to determine clinical blood pressure measurements. *Journal of Diagnostic Medical Sonography*, *34*, 446–457. doi:10.1177/8756479318800303

References

Bansal, A., Sarath, R. S., Bhan, B. D., Gupta, K., & Purwar, S. (2019). To assess the stethoscope cleaning practices, microbial load and efficacy of cleaning stethoscopes with alcohol-based disinfectant in a tertiary care hospital. *Journal of Infection Prevention*, *20*(1), 46–50. doi:10.1177/1757177418802353

Cifu, A. S., & Davis, A. M. (2017). Prevention, detection, evaluation, and management of high blood pressure in adults, *JAMA*, *318*(21), 2132–2134. doi:10.1001/jama.2017.18706

Clark, C. E. (2017). The interarm blood pressure difference: Do we know enough yet? *Journal of Clinical Hypertension*, *19*, 462–465. doi:10.1111/jch.12982

da Costa, J. C., Faustino, P., Lima, R., Ladeira, I., & Guimarães, M. (2016). Comparison of the accuracy of a pocket versus standard pulse oximeter. *Biomedical Instrumentation & Technology*, *50*, 190–193. doi:10.2345/0899-8205-50.3.190

D'Amico, D., & Barbarito, C. (2016). *Health and physical assessment in nursing* (3rd ed.). Boston, MA: Pearson.

Headley, C. (2017). A roundtable discussion with the experts. *Nephrology Nursing Journal*, *44*, 69–71.

Headley, C. M., Wall, B. M., & Cushman, W. C. (2017). Nephrology nursing roundtable: A blood pressure you can believe in. *Nephrology Nursing Journal*, *44*(1), 57–72.

Jones, J., & Kuritzky, L. (2018). Recognition and management of orthostatic hypotension in primary care. *Journal of Family Practice*, *67*(8 Suppl.), S25–S30.

Liu, C. C., Griffiths, C., Murray, A., & Zheng, D. (2016). Comparison of stethoscope bell and diaphragm, and of stethoscope tube length, for clinical blood pressure measurement. *Blood Pressure Monitoring*, *21*, 178–183. doi:10.1097/MBP.0000000000000175

Mason, T. M., Boubekri, A., Lalau, J., Patterson, A., Hartranft, S. R., & Sutton, S. K. (2017). Equivalence study of two temperature-measurement methods in febrile adult patients with cancer. *Oncology Nursing Forum*, *44*, E82–E87. doi:10.1188/17.ONF.E82-E87

Miller, A. C., Singh, I., Koehler, E., & Polgreen, P. M. (2018). A smartphone-driven thermometer application for real-time population- and individual-level influenza surveillance.

Clinical Infectious Diseases, *67*, 388–397. doi:10.1093/cid/ciy073

Mozzafarian, D., Benjamin, E. J., Go, A. S., Arnett, D. K., Blaha, M. J., Cushman, M., . . . Turner, M. B. (2016). Heart disease and stroke statistics—2016 update: A report from the American Heart Association. *Circulation*, *133*, e38–e360. doi:10.1161/CIR.0000000000000350

Parashar, R., Amir, M., Pakhare, A., Rathi, P., & Chaudhary, L. (2016). Age related changes in autonomic functions. *Journal of Clinical and Diagnostic Research*, *10*(3), CC11–CC15. doi:10.7860/JCDR/2016/16889.7497

Salota, V., Slovakova, Z., Panes, C., Nundlall, A., & Goonasekera, C. (2016). Is postoperative tympanic membrane temperature measurement effective? *British Journal of Nursing*, *25*(9), 490–493. doi:10.12968/bjon.2016.25.9.490

Schuman, A. J. (2016). Clinical thermometry. *Contemporary Pediatrics*, *33*(3), 37–40.

Whelton, P. K., & Williams, B. (2018). The 2018 European Society of Cardiology/European Society of Hypertension and 2017 American College of Cardiology/American Heart Association blood pressure guidelines: More similar than different. *JAMA*, *320*(17), 1749–1750. doi:10.1001/jama.2018.16755

Wilson, S. F., & Giddens, J. F. (2017). *Health assessment for nursing practice* (6th ed.). St. Louis, MO: Elsevier.

Selected Bibliography

Álvarez, J. A., Ruíz, S. R., Mosqueda, J. L., León, X., Arreguín, V., Macías, A. E., & Macias, J. H. (2016). Decontamination of stethoscope membranes with chlorhexidine: Should it be recommended? *American Journal of Infection Control*, *44*(11), e205–e209. doi:10.1016/j.ajic.2016.07.012

Anast, N., Olejniczak, M., Ingrande, J., & Brock-Utne, J. (2016). The impact of blood pressure cuff location on the accuracy of noninvasive blood pressure measurements in obese patients: An observational study. *Canadian Journal of Anaesthesia*, *63*(3), 298–306. doi:10.1007/s12630-015-0509-6

Banker, A., Bell, C., Gupta-Malhotra, M., & Samuels, J. (2016). Blood pressure percentile charts to identify high or low blood pressure in children. *BMC Pediatrics*, *16*, 1–7. doi:10.1186/s12887-016-0633-7

Chen, D., Chen, F., & Zheng, D. (2016). Respiratory modulation of oscillometric cuff pressure pulses and Korotkoff sounds during clinical blood pressure measurement in healthy adults. *Biomedical Engineering Online*, *15*, 53. doi:10.1186/s12938-016-0169-y

Clark, C. E., Taylor, R. S., Shore, A. C., & Campbell, J. L. (2016). Prevalence of systolic inter-arm differences in blood pressure for different primary care populations: Systematic review and meta-analysis. *British Journal of General Practice*, *66*, e838–e847. doi:10.3399/bjgp16X687553

DuBois, E. F. (1948). *Fever and the regulation of body temperature*. Springfield, IL: Charles C. Thomas.

Feenstra, R. K., Allaarta, C. P., Berkelmans, G. F. N., Westerhof, B. E., Smulders, Y. M., & Allaart, C. P. (2018). Accuracy of oscillometric blood pressure measurement in atrial fibrillation. *Blood Pressure Monitoring*, *23*(2), 59–63. doi:10.1097/MBP.0000000000000305

Fletcher, B. R., Hinton, L., Hartmann-Boyce, J., Roberts, N. W., Bobrovitz, N., & McManus, R. J. (2016). Self-monitoring blood pressure in hypertension, patient and provider perspectives: A systematic review and thematic synthesis. *Patient Education & Counseling*, *99*(2), 210–219. doi:10.1016/j.pec.2015.08.026

Get the alcohol out: Your stethoscopes are dirtier than you think they are. (2019). *Medical Environment Update*, *29*(2), 7–9.

Haun, N., Hooper-Lane, C., & Safdar, N. (2016). Healthcare personnel attire and devices as fomites: A systematic review. *Infection Control & Hospital Epidemiology*, *37*(11), 1367–1373.

How dirty is your stethoscope? (2016). *Imprint (00193062)*, *63*(4), 54–55.

Jarvis, C. (2016). *Physical examination and health assessment* (7th ed.). St. Louis, MO: Elsevier.

Kelly, C. (2018). Respiratory rate 1: Why measurement and recording are crucial. *Nursing Times*, *114*(4), 151.

Lakhal, K., Martin, M., Ehrmann, S., Faiz, S., Rozec, B., & Boulain, T. (2018). Non-invasive blood pressure monitoring with an oscillometric brachial cuff: Impact of arrhythmia. *Journal of Clinical Monitoring & Computing*, *32*, 707–715. doi:10.1007/s10877-017-0067-2

Mol, A., Reijnierse, E. M., Trappenburg, M. C., van Wezel, R. J. A., Maier, A. B., & Meskers, C. G. M. (2018). Rapid systolic blood pressure changes after standing up associate with impaired physical performance in geriatric outpatients. *Journal of the American Heart Association*, *7*(21), 1–10. doi:10.1161/JAHA.118.010060

O'Brien, E., Dolan, E., & Stergiou, G. S. (2018). Achieving reliable blood pressure measurements in clinical practice: It's time to meet the challenge. *Journal of Clinical Hypertension*, *20*, 1084–1088. doi:10.1111/jch.13323

Rushton, M., & Smith, J. (2016). How to measure blood pressure manually. *Nursing Standard*, *30*(21), 36–39.

Sarafis, Z. K., Monga, A. K., Phillips, A. A., & Krassioukov, A. V. (2018). Is technology for orthostatic hypotension ready for primetime? *PM & R: Journal of Injury, Function & Rehabilitation*, *10*(9, Suppl. 2), S249–S263. doi:10.1016/j.pmrj.2018.04.011

Schaffer, J. T., Keim, S. M., Hunter, B. R., Kirschner, J. M., & De Lorenzo, R. A. (2018). Do orthostatic vital signs have utility in the evaluation of syncope? *Journal of Emergency Medicine (0736-4679)*, *55*, 780–787. doi:10.1016/j.jemermed.2018.09.011

Scott-Rimington, R. B., Klim, S., & Kelly, A. (2017). How clean is your stethoscope? *Emergency Medicine Australasia*, *29*, 122–123. doi:10.1111/1742-6723.12729

Sharman, J. E., Howes, F. S., Head, G. A., McGrath, B. P., Stowasser, M., Schlaich, M., . . . Nelson, M. (2016). How to measure home blood pressure: Recommendations for healthcare professionals and patients. *Australian Family Physician*, *45*, 31–34.

Tompson, A. C., Schwartz, C. L., Fleming, S., Ward, A. M., Greenfield, S. M., Grant, S., . . . McManus, R. J. (2018). Patient experience of home and waiting room blood pressure measurement: A qualitative study of patients with recently diagnosed hypertension. *British Journal of General Practice*, *68*(677), e835–e843. doi:10.3399/bjgp18X699761

Viera, A. J., Tuttle, L., & Zeng, J. (2016). Dollars and discomfort: What will people be willing to give for better blood pressure assessment? *Journal of Clinical Hypertension*, *18*, 422–423. doi:10.1111/jch.12680

Vongpatanasin, W. (2018). Accurate blood pressure in the office. *Circulation*, *138*, 1771–1773. doi:10.1161/CIRCULATIONAHA.118.036209

Whelton, P. K., Carey, R. M., Aronow, W. S., Casey, D. E., Collins, K. J., Dennison, C., . . . Wright, J. T. (2017). 2017 guideline for the prevention, detection, evaluation, and management of high blood pressure in adults. *Journal of the American College of Cardiology*, *70*(19), e127–e248. doi:10.1016/j.jacc.2017.11.006

29 Health Assessment

LEARNING OUTCOMES

After completing this chapter, you will be able to:

1. Identify the purposes of the physical examination.
2. Explain the four techniques used in physical examination: inspection, palpation, percussion, and auscultation.
3. Identify expected findings during health assessment.
4. Verbalize the steps used in performing selected examination procedures:
   a. Assessing appearance and mental status.
   b. Assessing the skin.
   c. Assessing the hair.
   d. Assessing the nails.
   e. Assessing the skull and face.
   f. Assessing the eye structures and visual acuity.
   g. Assessing the ears and hearing.
   h. Assessing the nose and sinuses.
   i. Assessing the mouth and oropharynx.
   j. Assessing the neck.
   k. Assessing the thorax and lungs.
   l. Assessing the heart and central vessels.
   m. Assessing the peripheral vascular system.
   n. Assessing the breasts and axillae.
   o. Assessing the abdomen.
   p. Assessing the musculoskeletal system.
   q. Assessing the neurologic system.
   r. Assessing the female genitals and inguinal area.
   s. Assessing the male genitals and inguinal area.
   t. Assessing the anus.
5. Describe suggested sequencing to conduct a physical health examination in an orderly fashion.
6. Discuss variations in examination techniques appropriate for clients of different ages.
7. Recognize when it is appropriate to assign data collection skills to assistive personnel.
8. Demonstrate appropriate documentation and reporting of health assessment.

KEY TERMS

adventitious breath sounds, *610*
alopecia, *585*
angle of Louis, *608*
antihelix, *595*
aphasia, *633*
astigmatism, *589*
auricle, *595*
auscultation, *576*
blanch test, *587*
bruit, *616*
caries, *600*
cataracts, *590*
cerumen, *595*
clubbing, *586*
cochlea, *595*
conductive hearing loss, *596*
conjunctivitis, *590*
cyanosis, *580*
dacryocystitis, *590*
diastole, *615*
dullness, *576*
duration, *577*
edema, *580*
erythema, *580*
eustachian tube, *595*
exophthalmos, *588*
external auditory meatus, *595*
extinction, *635*
fasciculation, *631*
flatness, *576*
fremitus, *612*
gingivitis, *600*
glaucoma, *590*
glossitis, *600*
helix, *595*
hernia, *646*
hordeolum (sty), *590*
hyperopia, *589*
hyperresonance, *576*
incus, *595*
inspection, *574*
intensity, *577*
intention tremor, *631*
jaundice, *580*
lift, *615*
lobule, *595*
malleus, *595*
manubrium, *608*
mastoid, *595*
miosis, *591*
mixed hearing loss, *596*
mydriasis, *591*
myopia, *589*
normocephalic, *588*
nystagmus, *593*
one-point discrimination, *635*
ossicles, *595*
otoscope, *595*
pallor, *580*
palpation, *575*
parotitis, *600*
percussion, *575*
perfusion, *620*
periodontal disease, *600*
PERRLA, *592*
pinna, *595*
pitch, *577*
plaque, *600*
pleximeter, *576*
plexor, *576*
precordium, *615*
presbyopia, *589*
proprioceptors, *634*
pyorrhea, *600*
quality, *577*
reflex, *634*
resonance, *576*
resting tremor, *631*
S_1, *615*
S_2, *615*
semicircular canals, *595*
sensorineural hearing loss, *596*
sordes, *600*
stapes, *595*
stereognosis, *635*
sternum, *608*
strabismus, *593*
systole, *615*
tartar, *600*
thrill, *616*
tragus, *595*
tremor, *631*
triangular fossa, *595*
two-point discrimination, *635*
tympanic membrane, *595*
tympany, *576*
vestibule, *595*
visual acuity, *589*
visual fields, *589*
vitiligo, *580*

Introduction

Assessing a client's health status is a major component of nursing care and has two aspects: (1) the nursing health history discussed in Chapter 10 ∞ and (2) the physical examination discussed in this chapter. A physical examination can be any of several types: (1) a comprehensive initial assessment (e.g., when a client is admitted to a healthcare agency), (2) a focused examination of a body system (e.g., the cardiovascular system) or body area (e.g., the lungs, when difficulty with breathing is observed), or (3) a functional assessment that examines one or more aspects of the client's abilities (e.g., nutrition and metabolism, elimination, or sleep and rest). *Note:* Some nurses consider *assessment* to be the broad term used in applying the nursing process to health data and *examination* to be the physical process used to gather the data. In this text, the terms *assessment* and *examination* are sometimes used interchangeably—both referring to a critical investigation and evaluation of client status.

As described in Chapter 10 ∞, assessing is considered the first phase or step of the nursing process. Performing the health history and physical examination is part of assessing, which includes data collection, organization, validation, and documentation. The new nurse learns the detailed steps of assessment for each system and then can select only those aspects of the assessment needed in a particular practice situation.

Physical Health Assessment

These are some purposes of the physical examination:

- To obtain baseline data about the client's functional abilities
- To supplement, confirm, or refute data obtained in the nursing history
- To obtain data that will help establish nursing diagnoses and plans of care
- To evaluate the physiologic outcomes of healthcare and thus the progress of a client's health problem
- To make clinical judgments about a client's health status
- To identify areas for health promotion and disease prevention.

Assessments are conducted using a framework or approach to gathering the data. The most common framework for a comprehensive assessment is the head-to-toe assessment. However, the procedure can vary according to the age of the individual, the health status of the individual, the preferences of the nurse, the location of the examination, and the agency's priorities and procedures. The order of head-to-toe assessment is given in Box 29.1. Regardless of the procedure used, the client's energy and time need to be considered. The health assessment is therefore conducted in a systematic and efficient manner that results in the fewest position changes for the client.

With hospitalized clients, a quick assessment is done at the beginning of the shift to use as a baseline for comparing with later data. This shift assessment is focused on immediate needs and problems and includes evaluating the status of environmental factors such as tubes, devices, and dressings. One possible structure for this shift assessment is the following:

1. Observe
   a. Level of consciousness
   b. Skin color
   c. Respiratory effort

BOX 29.1 Head-to-Toe Framework

- General survey
- Vital signs
- Head
  - Hair, scalp, face
  - Eyes and vision
  - Ears and hearing
  - Nose
  - Mouth and oropharynx
- Neck
  - Muscles
  - Lymph nodes
  - Trachea
  - Thyroid gland
  - Carotid arteries
  - Neck veins
- Upper extremities
  - Skin and nails
  - Muscle strength and tone
  - Joint range of motion
  - Brachial and radial pulses
  - Sensation
- Chest and back
  - Skin
  - Thorax shape and size
  - Lungs
  - Heart
  - Spinal column
  - Breasts and axillae
- Abdomen
  - Skin
  - Abdominal sounds
  - Femoral pulses
- External genitals
- Anus
- Lower extremities
  - Skin and toenails
  - Gait and balance
  - Joint range of motion
  - Popliteal, posterior tibial, and dorsalis pedis pulses

   d. Nutritional status
   e. Body position (e.g., does the client appear in pain?)
   f. Speech
   g. Hygiene and grooming
2. Check vital signs including pain. Include pedal pulses.
3. Auscultate lungs and apical pulse
4. Check capillary refill and peripheral edema
5. Auscultate bowel sounds
6. Observe skin turgor and surfaces for lesions (anterior and posterior, especially bony prominences)
7. Observe mobility (all four extremities, weight bearing)
8. Examine drains, catheters, wound dressings or tubes: location, patency, and description of drainage, if any.

Frequently, nurses assess a specific body area instead of the entire body. These specific assessments are made in relation to client complaints, the nurse's own observation of problems, the client's presenting problem, nursing interventions provided, and medical therapies. Examples of these situations and assessments are provided in Table 29.1.

Nurses use national guidelines and evidence-based practice to focus health assessment on specific conditions. The nurse's judgment is key when the evidence is inconclusive or conflicting. For example, when screening for cancer, nurses should remember the American Cancer Society's guidelines for early detection (Box 29.2). However, whereas those guidelines call for mammography every year between ages 45 to 54, the U.S. Preventive Services Task Force (2016) recommends breast mammography only every 2 years for females ages 50 to 74 and none thereafter.

Preparing the Client

Most people need an explanation of the physical examination. Often clients are anxious about what the nurse will find. They can be reassured during the examination by explanations at each step. The nurse should explain when and where the examination will take place, why it is important, and what will happen. Instruct the client that all information gathered and documented during the assessment is kept confidential under the Health Insurance Portability and Accountability Act (HIPAA). This means that only those who legitimately need to know the client's information will have access to it.

Health examinations are usually painless. Determine in advance any positions that are contraindicated for a particular

TABLE 29.1 Nursing Assessments Addressing Selected Client Situations

Situation	Physical Assessment
Client complains of abdominal pain.	Inspect, auscultate, percuss, and palpate the abdomen; assess vital signs.
Client is admitted with a head injury.	Assess level of consciousness using Glasgow Coma Scale (see Table 29.10 later in this chapter); assess pupils for reaction to light and accommodation; assess vital signs.
The client has just had a cast applied to the lower leg.	Assess peripheral perfusion of toes, capillary blanch test, pedal pulse if able, and vital signs.
The client's fluid intake is minimal.	Assess tissue turgor, fluid intake and output, and vital signs.

BOX 29.2 Cancer Screening Guidelines for Average-Risk, Asymptomatic People

COLORECTAL CANCER (MALES AND FEMALES)
Beginning at age 45 and until age 75, one of the following:
- Fecal occult blood test or
- Fecal immunochemical test annually or
- Stool DNA test every 3 years or
- Flexible sigmoidoscopy every 5 years or
- Colonoscopy every 10 years or
- Computerized tomography colonography every 5 years.

At age 76 to 85, screening should be individualized based on patient preference, health status, and prior screenings. Screening after age 85 is discouraged.

BREAST CANCER (FEMALES)
- Beginning in their early 20s, females should be told about the benefits and limitations of breast self-examination (BSE) and the importance of reporting breast symptoms to a health professional. Those who choose to perform BSE should receive instruction and have their technique reviewed regularly. Females may perform BSE regularly, occasionally, or not at all.
- Females should have the opportunity to begin annual screening between ages 40 and 44.
- Females with an average risk of breast cancer should undergo regular screening mammography starting at age 45.
- Females ages 45 to 54 should be screened annually.
- Females aged 55 or older should transition to biennial screening or can continue screening annually.
- Females should continue screening mammography as long as their overall health is good and they have a life expectancy of 10 or more years.

CERVICAL AND UTERINE CANCER (FEMALES)
- For females ages 21 to 29, screening every 3 years with Pap tests.
- For females ages 30–65, screening every 5 years with both HPV test and the Pap test, or every 3 years with the Pap test alone.
- Females ages 65 and older who have had 3 or more consecutive negative Pap tests or 2 or more consecutive negative HPV and Pap tests in the last 10 years, the most recent test in the last 5 years, and females who have had a total hysterectomy should stop cervical cancer screening.

PROSTATE CANCER (MALES)
- For men aged 50 and older who have at least a 10-year life expectancy, discussion with the primary care provider about the benefits, risks, and uncertainties associated with prostate cancer screening.

From "A Blueprint for Cancer Screening and Early Detection: Advancing Screening's Contribution to Cancer Control" by R. C. Wender, O. W. Brawley, S. A. Fedewa, T. Gansler, & R. A. Smith, 2019, *CA: A Cancer Journal for Clinicians*, *69*, pp. 50–79. doi:10.3322/caac.21550

client. The nurse assists the client as needed to undress and put on a gown. Clients should empty their bladders before the examination. Doing so helps them feel more relaxed and facilitates palpation of the abdomen and pubic area.

When assessing adults it is important to recognize that people of the same age differ markedly. Box 29.3 provides special considerations for assessing adults, especially older adults.

The sequence of the assessment differs with children and adults. With children, always proceed from the least invasive or uncomfortable aspect of the exam to the more invasive. Examination of the head and neck, heart and lungs, and range of motion can be done early in the process, with the ears, mouth, abdomen, and genitals being left for the end of the exam.

Preparing the Environment

Prepare the environment before starting the assessment. The time should be convenient to both the client and the nurse. The environment needs to be well lighted and the equipment should be organized for efficient use. The room should be warm enough to be comfortable for the client. Providing privacy is important. Most people are embarrassed if their bodies are exposed or if others can overhear or view them during the assessment. Culture, age, and gender of both the client and the nurse influence how comfortable the client will be and what special arrangements might be needed. Family and friends should not be present unless the client asks for someone.

BOX 29.3 Health Assessment of the Adult

- Be aware of normal physiologic changes that occur with aging (see the Lifespan Considerations later in this chapter).
- Be aware of stiffness of muscles and joints from aging or history of orthopedic surgery. The client may need modification of the usual positioning.
- Permit ample time for the client to answer your questions and assume the required positions.
- Be aware of cultural differences. The client may want a family member present during undressing.
- Arrange for an interpreter if the client's language differs from that of the nurse.
- Ask clients how they wish to be addressed, such as "Mrs." or "Miss."
- Adapt assessment techniques to any sensory impairment; for example, have clients use their eyeglasses or hearing aids.
- If clients are frail, it is wise to conduct the assessment in several segments in order to avoid overtiring them.

Positioning

Several positions are required during the physical assessment. The client's physical condition, energy level, and age should be considered. Some positions are embarrassing and uncomfortable and therefore should not be maintained for long. The assessment is organized so several body areas can be assessed in one position, thus minimizing the number of position changes needed (Table 29.2).

Draping

Drapes should be arranged so that the area to be assessed is exposed and other body areas are covered. Exposure of the body is frequently embarrassing to clients. Drapes provide not only a degree of privacy but also warmth. Drapes are made of paper, cloth, or bed linen.

Instrumentation

All equipment required for the health assessment should be clean, in good working order, and readily accessible. Equipment is frequently set up on trays, ready for use. Various instruments are shown in Table 29.3. If the assessment is being conducted outside of a healthcare setting, be sure you obtain all the needed equipment, including adequate lighting.

TABLE 29.2 Client Positions and Body Areas Assessed

Position	Description	Areas Assessed	Cautions
Sitting	A seated position, back unsupported and legs hanging freely	Head, neck, posterior and anterior thorax, lungs, breasts, axillae, heart, vital signs, upper and lower extremities, reflexes	Older adults and weak clients may require support.
Supine (horizontal recumbent)	Back-lying position with legs extended; with or without pillow under the head	Head, neck, axillae, anterior thorax, lungs, breasts, heart, vital signs, abdomen, extremities, peripheral pulses	Tolerated poorly by clients with cardiovascular and respiratory problems.

Continued on page 574

TABLE 29.2 Client Positions and Body Areas Assessed—*continued*

Position	Description	Areas Assessed	Cautions
Semi-Fowler's (30° – 45°)	Back-lying with head of the bed elevated approximately 30° – 45°	Jugular vein distension	May be uncomfortable unless the foot or knee is elevated slightly.
Sims'	Side-lying position with lowermost arm behind the body, uppermost leg flexed at hip and knee, upper arm flexed at shoulder and elbow	Rectum, vagina	Difficult for older adults and people with limited joint movement.
Dorsal recumbent	Back-lying position with knees flexed and hips externally rotated; small pillow under the head; soles of feet on the surface	Female genitals, rectum, and female reproductive tract	May be contraindicated for clients with cardiopulmonary problems.

TABLE 29.3 Equipment and Supplies Used for a Health Examination

Supplies		Purpose
Flashlight or penlight		To assist viewing of the pharynx or to determine the reactions of the pupils of the eye
Ophthalmoscope		A lighted instrument to visualize the interior of the eye
Otoscope		A lighted instrument to visualize the eardrum and external auditory canal (a nasal speculum may be attached to the otoscope to inspect the nasal cavities)
Percussion (reflex) hammer		An instrument with a rubber head to test reflexes
Tuning fork		A two-pronged metal instrument used to test hearing acuity and vibratory sense
Gloves		To protect the nurse
Tongue blades (depressors)		To depress the tongue during assessment of the mouth and pharynx

Methods of Examining

Four primary techniques are used in the physical examination: inspection, palpation, percussion, and auscultation. These techniques are discussed throughout this chapter as they apply to each body system.

Inspection

Inspection is the visual examination, which is assessing by using the sense of sight. It should be deliberate, purposeful, and systematic. The nurse inspects with the naked eye and with a lighted instrument such as an otoscope (used to view the ear). In addition to visual observations, olfactory (smell) and auditory (hearing) cues are noted. Nurses frequently use visual inspection to assess moisture, color, and texture of body surfaces, as well as shape, position, size, color, and symmetry of the body. Lighting must be sufficient for the nurse to see clearly; either natural or artificial light can be used. When using the auditory senses, it is important to have a quiet environment for accurate hearing. Inspection can be combined with the other assessment techniques.

Palpation

Palpation is the examination of the body using the sense of touch. The pads of the fingers are used because their concentration of nerve endings makes them highly sensitive to tactile discrimination. Palpation is used to determine (a) texture (e.g., of the hair); (b) temperature (e.g., of a skin area); (c) vibration (e.g., of a joint); (d) position, size, consistency, and mobility of organs or masses; (e) distention (e.g., of the urinary bladder); (f) pulsation; and (g) tenderness or pain.

There are two types of palpation: light and deep. *Light* (superficial) *palpation* should always precede *deep palpation* because heavy pressure on the fingertips can dull the sense of touch. For light palpation, the nurse extends the dominant hand's fingers parallel to the skin surface and presses gently while moving the hand in a circle (Figure 29.1 ■). With light palpation, the skin is slightly depressed. If it is necessary to determine the details of a mass, the nurse presses lightly several times rather than holding the pressure. See Box 29.4 for the characteristics of masses.

Deep palpation is usually not done during a routine examination and requires significant practitioner skill. It is performed with extreme caution because pressure can damage internal organs. It is usually not indicated in clients who have acute abdominal pain or pain that is not yet diagnosed.

Deep palpation is done with two hands (bimanually) or one hand. In deep bimanual palpation, the nurse extends the dominant hand as for light palpation, then places the finger pads of the nondominant hand on the dorsal surface of the distal interphalangeal joint of the middle three fingers of the dominant hand (Figure 29.2 ■). The top hand applies pressure while the lower hand remains relaxed to perceive the tactile sensations. For deep palpation using one hand, the finger pads of the dominant hand press over the area to be palpated. Often the other hand is used to support from below (Figure 29.3 ■).

To test skin temperature, it is best to use the dorsum (back) of the hand and fingers, where the examiner's skin is thinnest. To test for vibration, the nurse should use the palmar surface of the hand. General guidelines for palpation include the following:

- The nurse's hands should be clean and warm, and the fingernails short.
- Areas of tenderness should be palpated last.
- Deep palpation should be done after superficial palpation.

The effectiveness of palpation depends largely on the client's relaxation. Nurses can assist a client to relax by (a) gowning and draping the client appropriately, (b) positioning the client comfortably, and (c) ensuring that their own hands are warm before beginning. During palpation, the nurse should be sensitive to the client's verbal and facial expressions indicating discomfort.

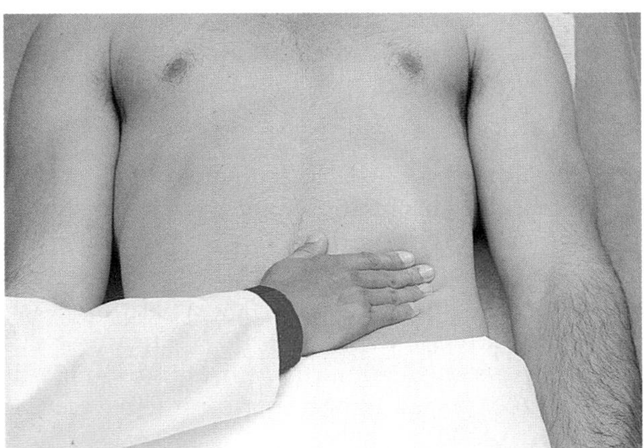

Figure 29.1 ■ The position of the hand for light palpation.

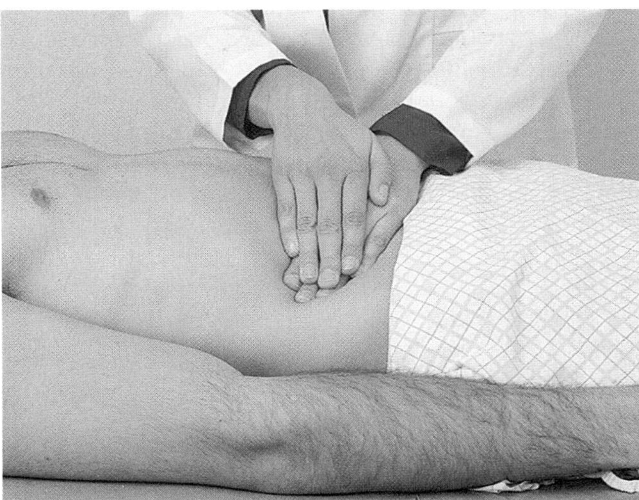

Figure 29.2 ■ The position of the hands for deep bimanual palpation.

BOX 29.4 Characteristics of Masses

Location—site on the body, dorsal or ventral surface
Size—length and width in centimeters
Shape—oval, round, elongated, irregular
Consistency—soft, firm, hard
Surface—smooth, nodular
Mobility—fixed, mobile
Pulsatility—present or absent
Tenderness—degree of tenderness to palpation

Percussion

Percussion is the act of striking the body surface to elicit sounds that can be heard or vibrations that can be felt. There are two types of percussion: direct and indirect.

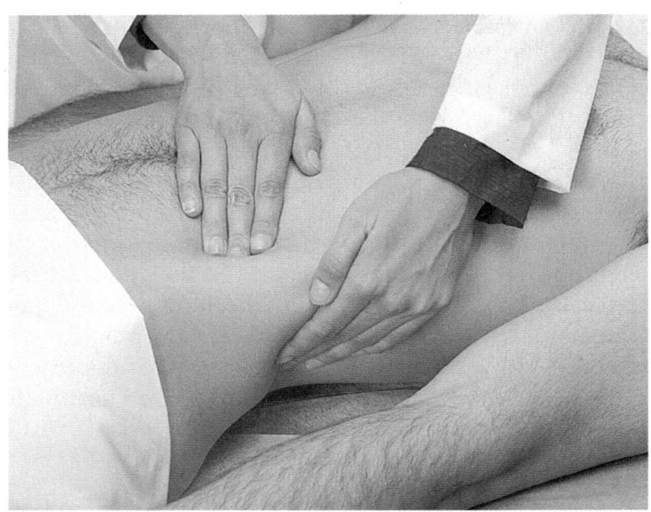

Figure 29.3 ■ Deep palpation using the lower hand to support the body while the upper hand palpates the organ.

In *direct percussion*, the nurse strikes the area to be percussed directly with the pads of two, three, or four fingers or with the pad of the middle finger. The strikes are rapid, and the movement is from the wrist. This technique is useful in percussing an adult's sinuses (Figure 29.4 ■).

Indirect percussion is the striking of an object (e.g., a finger) held against the body area to be examined. In this technique, the middle finger of the nondominant hand, referred to as the **pleximeter**, is placed firmly on the client's skin. Only the distal phalanx and joint of this finger should be in contact with the skin. Using the tip of the flexed middle finger of the other hand, called the **plexor**, the nurse strikes the pleximeter, usually at the distal interphalangeal joint or a point between the distal and proximal joints (Figure 29.5 ■). The striking motion comes from the wrist; the forearm remains stationary. The angle between the plexor and the pleximeter should be 90°, and the blows must be firm, rapid, and short to obtain a clear sound.

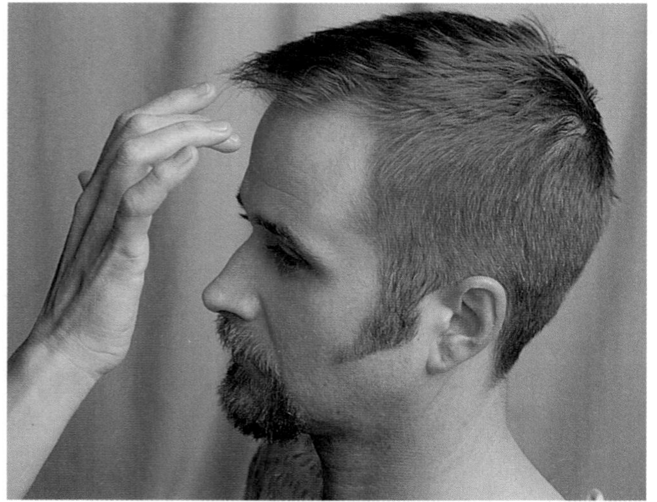

Figure 29.4 ■ Direct percussion using one hand to strike the surface of the body.

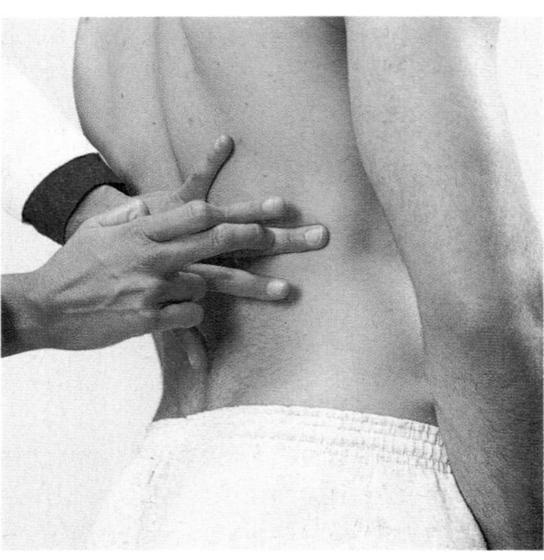

Figure 29.5 ■ Indirect percussion using the finger of one hand to tap the finger of the other hand.

Percussion is used to determine the size and shape of internal organs by establishing their borders. It indicates whether tissue is fluid filled, air filled, or solid. Percussion elicits five types of sound: flatness, dullness, resonance, hyperresonance, and tympany. **Flatness** is an extremely dull sound produced by very dense tissue, such as muscle or bone. **Dullness** is a thudlike sound produced by dense tissue such as the liver, spleen, or heart. **Resonance** is a hollow sound such as that produced by lungs filled with air. **Hyperresonance** is not produced in the normal body. It is described as booming and can be heard over an emphysematous lung. **Tympany** is a musical or drumlike sound produced from an air-filled stomach. On a continuum, flatness reflects the most dense tissue (the least amount of air) and tympany the least dense tissue (the greatest amount of air). A percussion sound is described according to its intensity, pitch, duration, and quality (Table 29.4).

Auscultation

Auscultation is the process of listening to sounds produced within the body. Auscultation may be direct or indirect. *Direct auscultation* is performed using the unaided ear, for example, to listen to a respiratory wheeze or the grating of a moving joint. *Indirect auscultation* is performed using a stethoscope, which transmits sounds to the nurse's ears. A stethoscope is used primarily to listen to sounds from within the body, such as bowel sounds or valve sounds of the heart and blood pressure.

The stethoscope tubing should be 30 to 35 cm (12 to 14 in.) long, with an internal diameter of about 0.3 cm (1/8 in.). It should have both a flat-disk diaphragm and a bell-shaped amplifier (see Figure 4 in Skill 28.3 on page 549). The diaphragm best transmits high-pitched sounds (e.g., bronchial sounds), and the bell best transmits low-pitched sounds such as some heart sounds. The earpieces of the stethoscope should fit comfortably into the nurse's ears, facing forward. The amplifier of the stethoscope is placed firmly but lightly against the client's skin. If the client has excessive hair, it may be necessary to dampen the hairs with a moist cloth so that they will lie flat against the skin and not interfere with clear sound transmission.

TABLE 29.4 Percussion Sounds and Tones

Sound	Intensity	Pitch	Duration	Quality	Example of Location
Flatness	Soft	High	Short	Extremely dull	Muscle, bone
Dullness	Medium	Medium	Moderate	Thudlike	Liver, heart
Resonance	Loud	Low	Long	Hollow	Normal lung
Hyperresonance	Very loud	Very low	Very long	Booming	Emphysematous lung
Tympany	Loud	High (distinguished mainly by musical timbre)	Moderate	Musical	Stomach filled with gas (air)

Auscultated sounds are described according to their pitch, intensity, duration, and quality. The **pitch** is the frequency of the vibrations (the number of vibrations per second). Low-pitched sounds, such as some heart sounds, have fewer vibrations per second than high-pitched sounds, such as bronchial sounds. The **intensity** (amplitude) refers to the loudness or softness of a sound. Some body sounds are loud, for example, bronchial sounds heard from the trachea; others are soft, for example, normal breath sounds heard in the lungs. The **duration** of a sound is its length (long or short). The **quality** of sound is a subjective description of a sound, for example, whistling, gurgling, or snapping.

QSEN Teamwork and Collaboration: Interprofessional Practice

Obtaining a health history and performing physical assessment of various aspects of the client are within the scope of practice of many healthcare providers other than nurses before, during, and after their treatments of clients. Although these providers may verbally communicate their findings and plan to other healthcare team members, the nurse must also know where to locate their documentation in the client's medical record. The nursing care plan should incorporate interprofessional considerations when appropriate.

General Survey

Health assessment begins with a general survey that involves observation of the client's general appearance, level of comfort, and mental status, and measurement of vital signs, height, and weight. Many components of the general survey are assessed while taking the client's health history, such as the client's body build, posture, hygiene, and mental status (see Chapter 10 ∞).

Appearance and Mental Status

The general appearance and behavior of an individual must be assessed in relationship to culture, educational level, socioeconomic status, and current circumstances. For example, an individual who has recently experienced a personal loss may appropriately appear depressed (sad expression, slumped posture). The client's age, sex, and race are also useful factors in interpreting findings that suggest increased risk for known conditions. Skill 29.1 describes how to assess general appearance and mental status. Skill 29.17 later in this chapter describes a mental status examination in detail.

Assessing Appearance and Mental Status

SKILL 29.1

PLANNING

Assignment

Due to the substantial knowledge and skill required, assessment of general appearance and mental status is not assigned to assistive personnel (AP). However, many aspects are observed during usual care and may be recorded by individuals other than the nurse. Abnormal findings must be validated and interpreted by the nurse.

Equipment

None

IMPLEMENTATION

Performance

1. Prior to performing the assessment, introduce self and verify the client's identity using agency protocol. Explain to the client what you are going to do, why it is necessary, and how to participate. Discuss how the results will be used in planning further care or treatments.
2. Perform hand hygiene and observe other appropriate infection prevention procedures.
3. Provide for client privacy.

Assessment	Normal Findings	Deviations from Normal
4. Observe for signs of distress in posture or facial expression.	No distress noted	Bending over because of abdominal pain, wincing, frowning, or labored breathing
5. Observe general body build, height, and weight.	Proportionate, varies with lifestyle	Excessively thin or obese

Continued on page 578

SKILL 29.1

Assessing Appearance and Mental Status—*continued*

Assessment	Normal Findings	Deviations from Normal
6. Observe client's posture and gait, standing, sitting, and walking.	Relaxed, erect posture; coordinated movement	Tense, slouched, bent posture; uncoordinated movement, tremors, unbalanced gait
7. Observe client's overall hygiene and grooming.	Clean, neat	Dirty, unkempt
8. Note body and breath odor.	No body odor or minor body odor relative to work or exercise; no breath odor	Foul body odor; ammonia odor; acetone breath odor; foul breath
9. Note obvious signs of health or illness (e.g., in skin color or breathing).	Well developed, well nourished, intact skin, easy breathing	Pallor (paleness); weakness; lesions, cough
10. Assess the client's attitude (frame of mind).	Cooperative, able to follow instructions	Negative, hostile, withdrawn, anxious
11. Note the client's affect and mood; assess the appropriateness of the client's responses.	Appropriate to situation	Inappropriate to situation, sudden mood change, paranoia
12. Listen for quantity of speech (amount and pace), quality (loudness, clarity, inflection).	Understandable, moderate pace; clear tone and inflection	Rapid or slow pace; overly loud or soft
13. Listen for relevance and organization of thoughts.	Logical sequence; makes sense; has sense of reality	Illogical sequence; flight of ideas; confusion; generalizations; vague

14. Document findings in the client record using printed or electronic forms and checklists supplemented by narrative notes when appropriate. ❶

EVALUATION

- Perform a detailed follow-up examination of specific systems based on findings that deviated from expected or normal for the client. Relate findings to previous assessment data if available.
- Report significant deviations from expected or normal findings to the primary care provider.

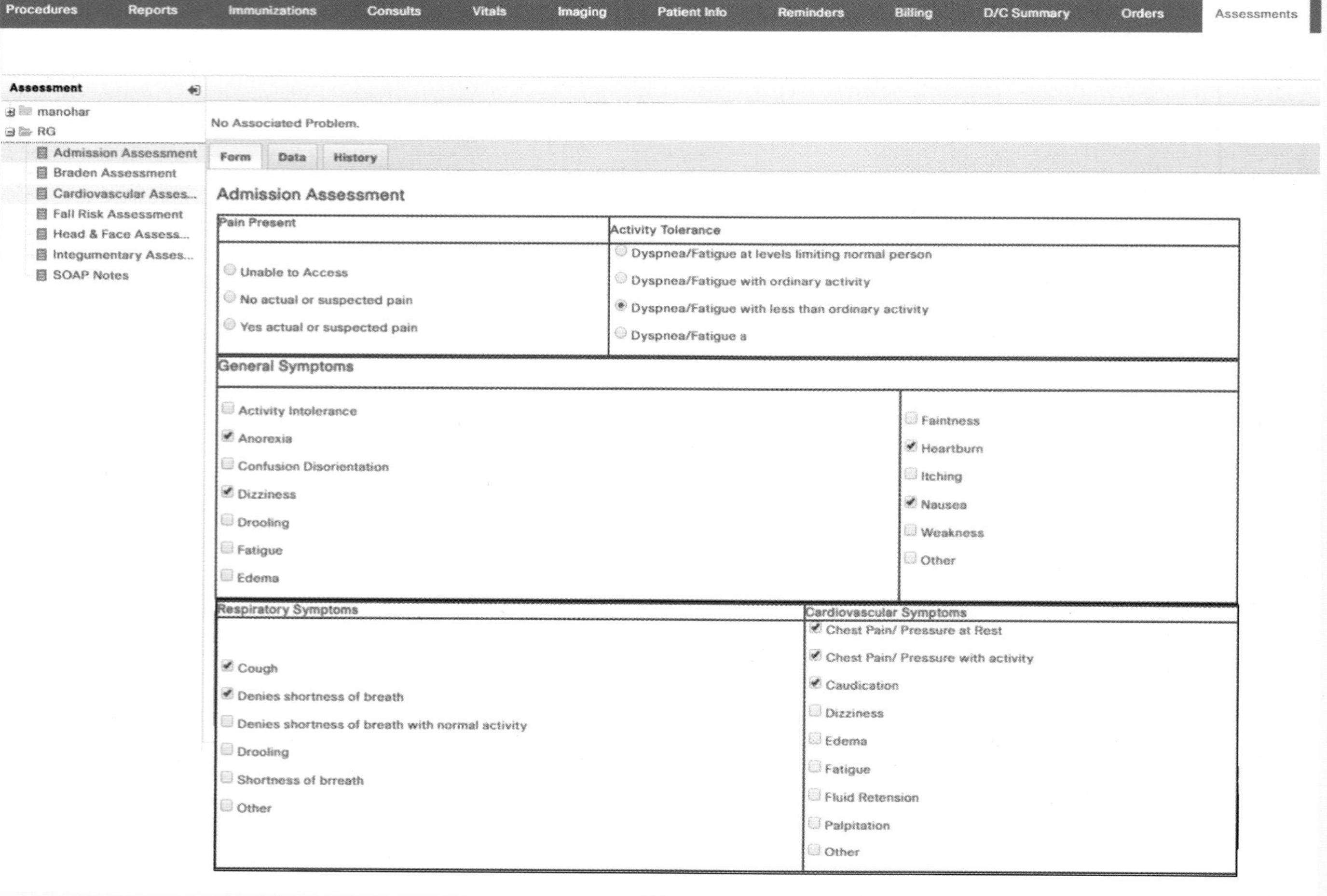

Procedures | Reports | Immunizations | Consults | Vitals | Imaging | Patient Info | Reminders | Billing | D/C Summary | Orders | Assessments

Assessment
- manohar
- RG
  - Admission Assessment
  - Braden Assessment
  - Cardiovascular Asses...
  - Fall Risk Assessment
  - Head & Face Assess...
  - Integumentary Asses...
  - SOAP Notes

No Associated Problem.

Form | Data | History

Admission Assessment

Pain Present
- ☐ Unable to Access
- ☐ No actual or suspected pain
- ☐ Yes actual or suspected pain

Activity Tolerance
- ○ Dyspnea/Fatigue at levels limiting normal person
- ○ Dyspnea/Fatigue with ordinary activity
- ◉ Dyspnea/Fatigue with less than ordinary activity
- ○ Dyspnea/Fatigue a

General Symptoms
- ☐ Activity Intolerance
- ☑ Anorexia
- ☐ Confusion Disorientation
- ☑ Dizziness
- ☐ Drooling
- ☐ Fatigue
- ☐ Edema
- ☐ Faintness
- ☑ Heartburn
- ☐ Itching
- ☑ Nausea
- ☐ Weakness
- ☐ Other

Respiratory Symptoms
- ☑ Cough
- ☑ Denies shortness of breath
- ☐ Denies shortness of breath with normal activity
- ☐ Drooling
- ☐ Shortness of brreath
- ☐ Other

Cardiovascular Symptoms
- ☑ Chest Pain/ Pressure at Rest
- ☑ Chest Pain/ Pressure with activity
- ☑ Caudication
- ☐ Dizziness
- ☐ Edema
- ☐ Fatigue
- ☐ Fluid Retension
- ☐ Palpitation
- ☐ Other

❶ Nursing assessment form.
iCare.

Clinical Alert!

Review the agency charting form before beginning your assessment to ensure that you know which data you will need to collect, have all the equipment you require, and know how to perform the assessment in a systematic manner.

Vital Signs

Vital signs are measured (a) to establish baseline data against which to compare future measurements and (b) to detect actual and potential health problems. See Chapter 28 ∞ for measurements of temperature, pulse, respirations, blood pressure, and oxygen saturation. See Chapter 30 ∞ for pain assessment.

Height and Weight

In adults, the ratio of weight to height provides a general measure of health. By asking clients about their height and weight before actually measuring them, the nurse obtains some idea of the client's self-image. Excessive discrepancies between the client's responses and the measurements may provide clues to actual or potential problems in self-concept. Take note of any unintentional weight gain or loss lasting or progressing over several weeks.

The nurse measures height with a measuring stick attached to weight scales or to a wall. The client should remove the shoes and stand erect, with heels together, and the heels, buttocks, and back of the head against the measuring stick; eyes should be looking straight ahead. The nurse raises the L-shaped sliding arm until it rests on top of the client's head, or places a small flat object such as a ruler or book on the client's head. The edge of the flat object should abut the measuring guide.

Weight is usually measured when a client is admitted to a healthcare agency and then often regularly thereafter, for example, each morning before breakfast and after emptying the bladder. Scales measure in pounds (lb) or kilograms (kg), and the nurse may need to convert between the two systems. One kilogram is equal to 2.2 pounds. When accuracy is essential, the nurse should use the same scale each time (because every scale weighs slightly differently), take the measurements at the same time each day, and make sure the client has on a similar kind of clothing and no footwear. The weight is read from a digital display panel or a balancing arm. Clients who cannot stand are weighed on chair (Figure 29.6 ■) or bed scales. The bed scales (Figure 29.7 ■) have canvas straps or a stretcher-like apparatus to support the client. A machine lifts the client above the bed, and the weight is reflected either on a digital display panel or on a balance arm like that of a standing scale. Newer hospital beds have built-in scales.

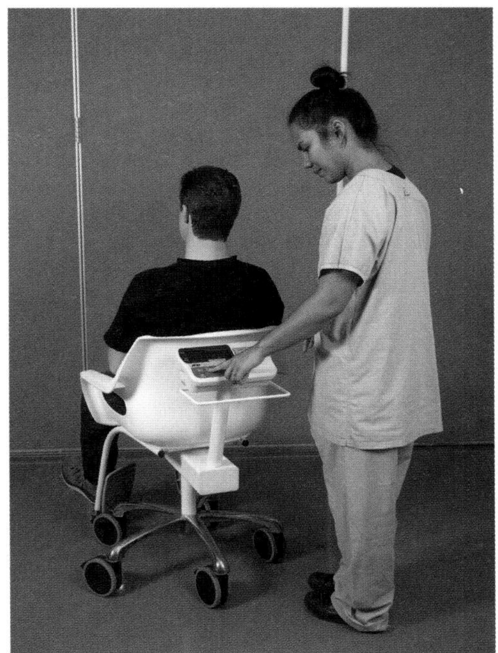

Figure 29.6 ■ Chair scale.
Sian Bradfield/Pearson Education Australia Pty Ltd.

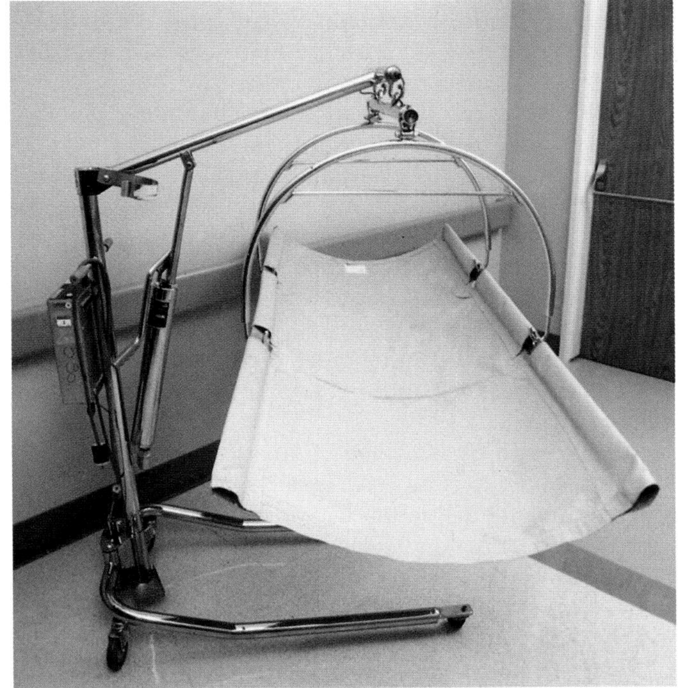

Figure 29.7 ■ Bed scale.

Integument

The integument includes the skin, hair, and nails. The examination begins with a generalized inspection using a good source of lighting, preferably indirect natural daylight.

LIFESPAN CONSIDERATIONS General Survey

INFANTS

- Observation of children's behavior can provide important data for the general survey, including physical development, neuromuscular function, and social and interactional skills.
- It may be helpful to have parents hold older infants and very young children for part of the assessment.
- Measure height of children under age 2 in the supine position with knees fully extended.
- Weigh without clothing.
- Include measurement of head circumference until age 2. Standardized growth charts include head circumference up to age 3.

CHILDREN

- Anxiety in preschool-age children can be decreased by letting them handle and become familiar with examination equipment.
- School-age children may be very modest and shy about exposing parts of the body.
- Adolescents should be examined without parents present.
- Weigh children without shoes and with as little clothing as possible.

OLDER ADULTS

- Allow extra time for clients to answer questions.
- Adapt questioning techniques as appropriate for clients with hearing or visual limitations.
- Older adults can lose several inches in height. Be sure to document height and ask if they are aware of becoming shorter in height.
- When asking about weight loss, be specific about amount and time frame, for example, "Have you lost more than five pounds in the last two months?" "How much did you weigh one year ago?"

Skin

Assessment of the skin involves inspection and palpation. The entire skin surface may be assessed at one time or as each aspect of the body is assessed. The nurse may also use the olfactory sense to detect unusual skin odors; these are usually most evident in the skinfolds or in the axillae. Pungent body odor is frequently related to poor hygiene, hyperhidrosis (excessive perspiration), or bromhidrosis (foul-smelling perspiration).

Pallor is the result of inadequate circulating blood or hemoglobin and subsequent reduction in tissue oxygenation. In clients with dark skin, it is usually characterized by the absence of underlying red tones in the skin and may be most readily seen in the buccal mucosa. In brown-skinned clients, pallor may appear as a yellowish brown tinge; in black-skinned clients, the skin may appear ashen gray. Pallor in all people is usually most evident in areas with the least pigmentation such as the conjunctiva, oral mucous membranes, nail beds, palms of the hand, and soles of the feet.

Cyanosis (a bluish tinge) is most evident in the nail beds, lips, and buccal mucosa. In dark-skinned clients, close inspection of the palpebral conjunctiva (the lining of the eyelids) and palms and soles may also show evidence of cyanosis. **Jaundice** (a yellowish tinge) may first be evident in the sclera of the eyes and then in the mucous membranes and the skin. Nurses should take care not to confuse jaundice with the normal yellow pigmentation in the sclera of a dark-skinned client. If jaundice is suspected, the posterior part of the hard palate should also be inspected for a yellowish color tone. **Erythema** is skin redness associated with a variety of rashes and other conditions.

Localized areas of hyperpigmentation (increased pigmentation) and hypopigmentation (decreased pigmentation) may occur as a result of changes in the distribution of melanin (the dark pigment) or in the function of the melanocytes in the epidermis. An example of hyperpigmentation in a defined area is a birthmark; an example of hypopigmentation is vitiligo. **Vitiligo**, seen as patches of hypopigmented skin, is caused by the destruction of melanocytes in the area. Albinism is the complete or partial lack of melanin in the skin, hair, and eyes. Other localized color changes may indicate a problem such as edema or a localized infection. Dark-skinned clients normally have areas of lighter pigmentation, such as the palms, lips, and nail beds.

Edema is the presence of excess interstitial fluid. An area of edema appears swollen, shiny, and taut and tends to blanch the skin color or, if accompanied by inflammation, may redden the skin. Generalized edema is most often an indication of impaired venous circulation and in some cases reflects cardiac dysfunction or venous abnormalities.

A skin lesion is an alteration in a client's normal skin appearance. Primary skin lesions are those that appear initially in response to some change in the external or internal environment of the skin (Figure 29.8 ■, ❶–❽). Secondary skin lesions are those that do not appear initially but result from modifications such as chronicity, trauma, or infection of the primary lesion. For example, a vesicle or blister (primary lesion) may rupture and cause an erosion (secondary lesion). Table 29.5 illustrates secondary lesions. Nurses are responsible for describing skin lesions accurately in terms of location (e.g., face), distribution (i.e., body regions involved), and configuration (the arrangement or position of several lesions) as well as color, shape, size, firmness, texture, and characteristics of individual lesions. Skill 29.2 describes how to assess the skin.

Clinical Alert!

If you have not already gathered relevant information about the client's history as it relates to the specific area being assessed, do so before beginning the physical examination. This allows you to focus the examination, customizing it to the individual client history and current status.

Macule, Patch Flat, unelevated change in color. Macules are 1 mm to 1 cm (0.04 to 0.4 in.) in size and circumscribed. Examples: freckles, measles, petechiae, flat moles. Patches are larger than 1 cm (0.4 in.) and may have an irregular shape. Examples: port wine birthmark, vitiligo (white patches), rubella. 1

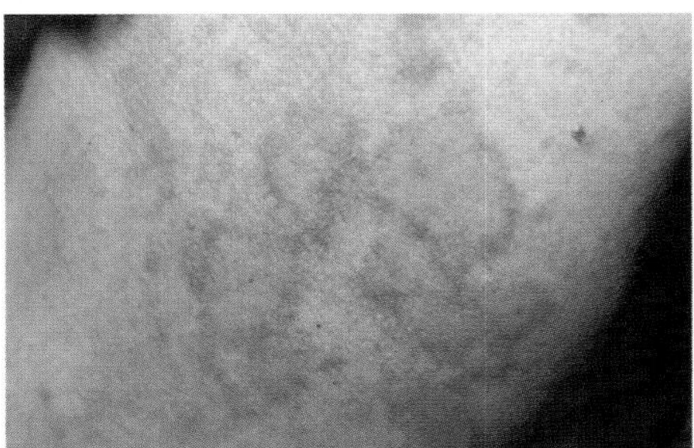

1 **A café-au-lait macule**

Papule Circumscribed, solid elevation of skin. Papules are less than 1 cm (0.4 in.). Examples: warts, acne, pimples, elevated moles. 2

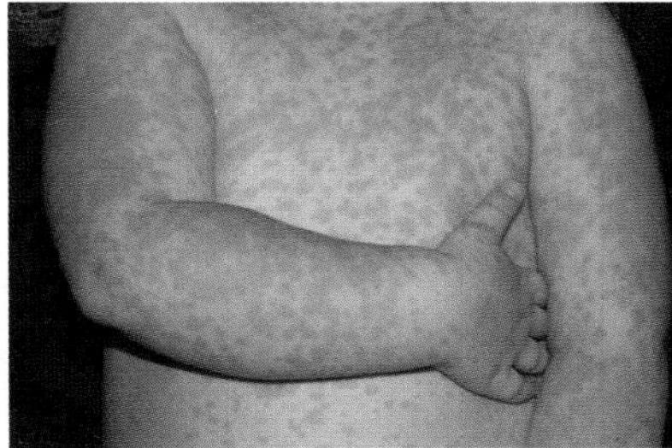

2 **Papular drug eruption**

Plaque Plaques are larger than 1 cm (0.4 in.). Examples: psoriasis, rubeola. 3

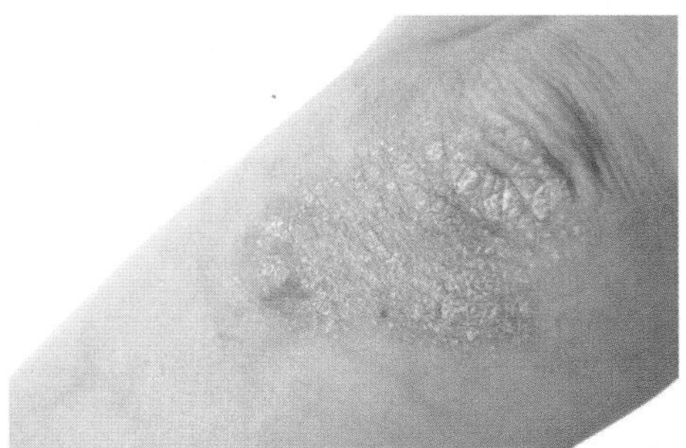

3 **Psoriasis**

Nodule, Tumor Elevated, solid, hard mass that extends deeper into the dermis than a papule. Nodules have a circumscribed border and are 0.5 to 2 cm (0.2 to 0.8 in.). Examples: squamous cell carcinoma, fibroma. Tumors are larger than 2 cm (0.8 in.) and may have an irregular border. Examples: malignant melanoma, hemangioma. 4

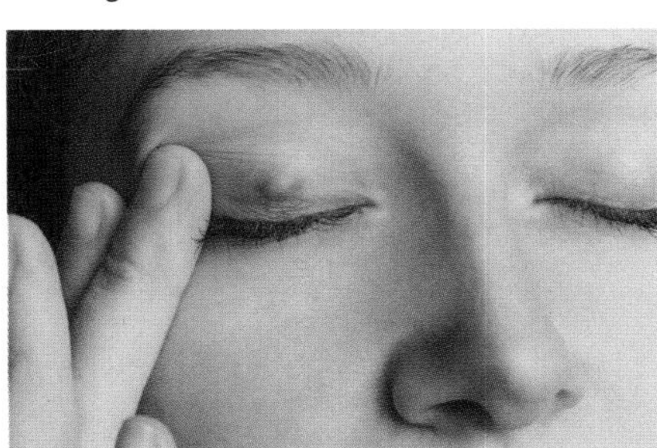

4 Chalazion

Pustule Vesicle or bulla filled with pus. Examples: acne vulgaris, impetigo. 5

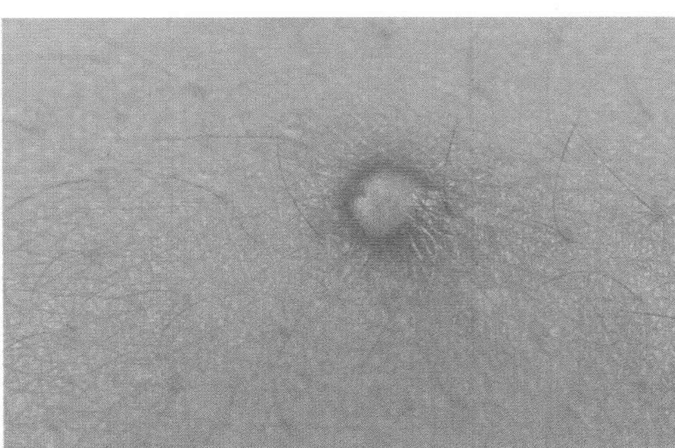

5 Acne pimple

Vesicle, Bulla A circumscribed, round or oval, thin translucent mass filled with serous fluid or blood. Vesicles are less than 0.5 cm (0.2 in.). Examples: herpes simplex, early chicken pox, small burn blister. Bullae are larger than 0.5 cm (0.2 in.). Examples: large blister, second-degree burn, herpes simplex. 6

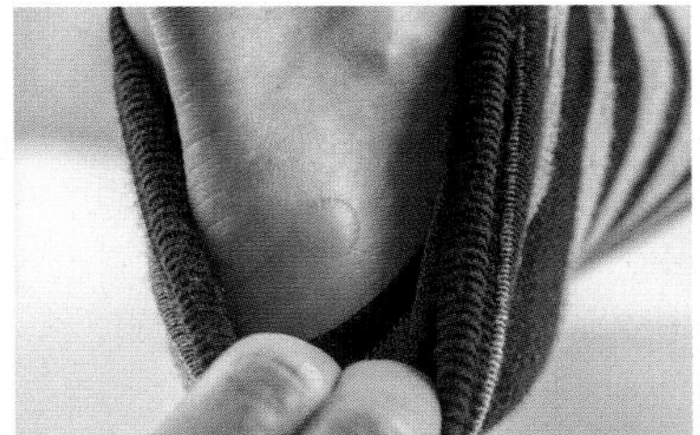

6 Blister

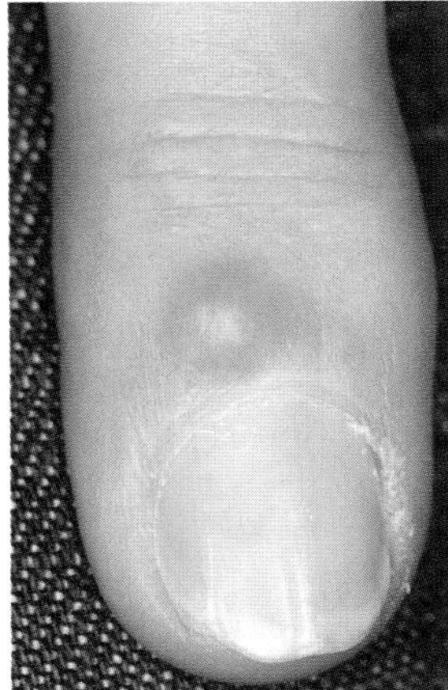

Cyst A 1-cm (0.4 in.) or larger, elevated, encapsulated, fluid-filled or semisolid mass arising from the subcutaneous tissue or dermis. Examples: sebaceous and epidermoid cysts. 7

7 **Digital mucous cyst**

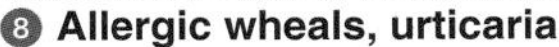

Wheal A reddened, localized collection of edema fluid; irregular in shape. Size varies. Examples: hives, mosquito bites. 8

8 **Allergic wheals, urticaria**

Figure 29.8 ■ Primary skin lesions.

Figures 1 Dr. Marazzi/Science Source; 2 Scott Camazine/Alamy; 3 hriana/123RF; 4 Elena Shishkina/123RF; 5 Faiz Zaki/Shutterstock; 6 gajus/123RF; 7 Hercules Robinson/Alamy; 8 ipen/Shutterstock.

TABLE 29.5 **Secondary Skin Lesions**

Lesion	Description	Lesion	Description
Atrophy 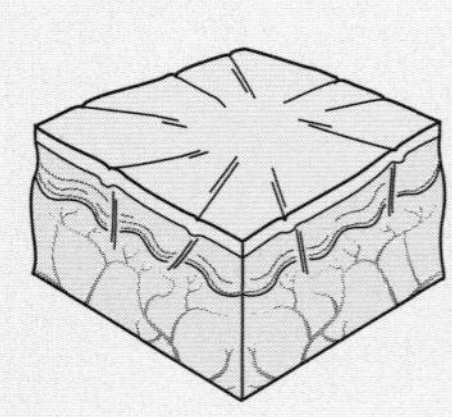	A translucent, dry, paper-like, sometimes wrinkled skin surface resulting from thinning or wasting of the skin due to loss of collagen and elastin. **Examples:** striae, aged skin	Ulcer 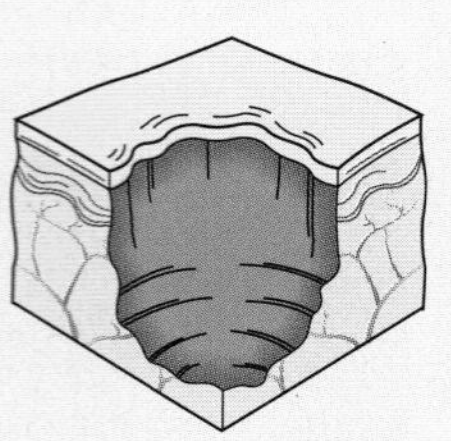	Deep, irregularly shaped area of skin loss extending into the dermis or subcutaneous tissue. May bleed. May leave scar. **Examples:** pressure injuries, stasis ulcers, chancres
Erosion 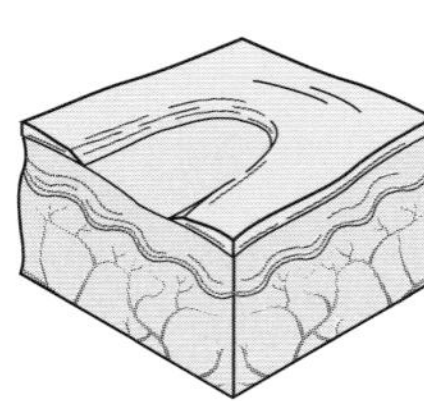	Wearing away of the superficial epidermis causing a moist, shallow depression. Because erosions do not extend into the dermis, they heal without scarring. **Examples:** scratch marks, ruptured vesicles	Fissure 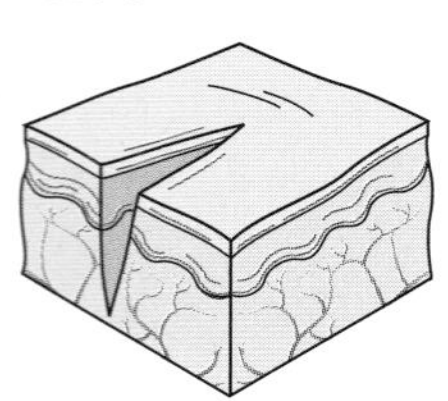	Linear crack with sharp edges, extending into the dermis. **Examples:** cracks at the corners of the mouth or in the hands, athlete's foot
Lichenification 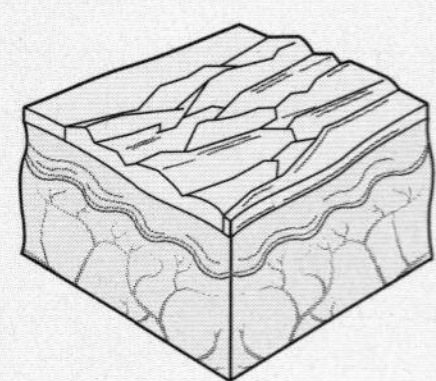	Rough, thickened, hardened area of epidermis resulting from chronic irritation such as scratching or rubbing. **Examples:** chronic dermatitis	Scar 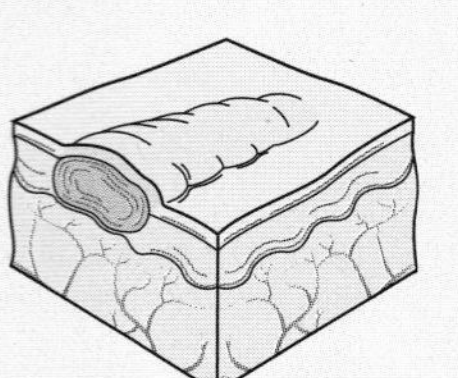	Flat, irregular area of connective tissue left after a lesion or wound has healed. New scars may be red or purple; older scars may be silvery or white. **Examples:** healed surgical wound or injury, healed acne
Scales 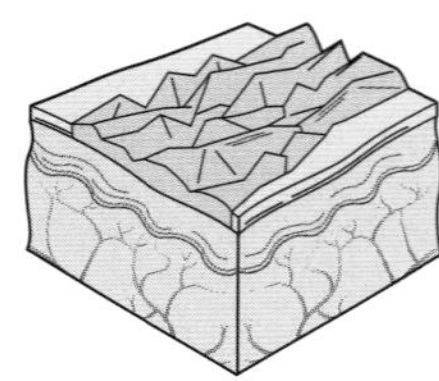	Shedding flakes of greasy, keratinized skin tissue. Color may be white, gray, or silver. Texture may vary from fine to thick. **Examples:** dry skin, dandruff, psoriasis, and eczema	Keloid 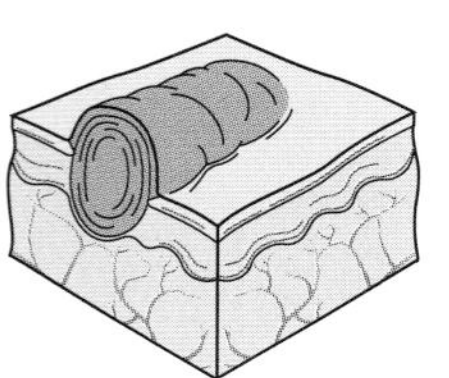	Elevated, irregular, darkened area of excess scar tissue caused by excessive collagen formation during healing. Extends beyond the site of the original injury. Higher incidence in people of African descent. **Examples:** keloid from ear piercing or surgery
Crust 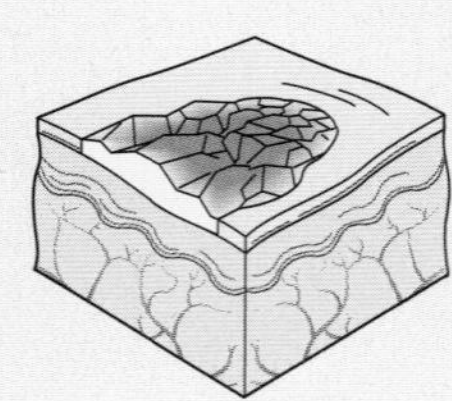	Dry blood, serum, or pus left on the skin surface when vesicles or pustules burst. Can be red-brown, orange, or yellow. Large crusts that adhere to the skin surface are called scabs. **Examples:** eczema, impetigo, herpes, or scabs following abrasion	Excoriation 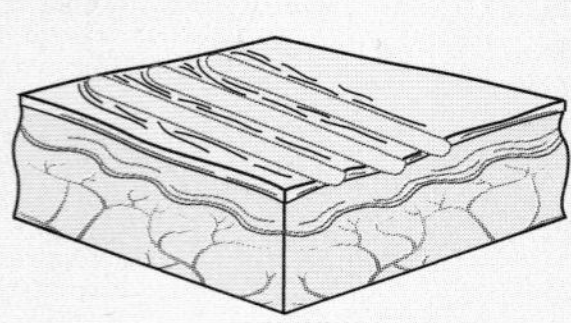	Linear erosion. **Examples**: scratches, some chemical burns

Assessing the Skin

SKILL 29.2

PLANNING

- Review characteristics of primary and secondary skin lesions if necessary (see Figure 29.8 and Table 29.5).
- Ensure that adequate lighting is available.

Assignment

Due to the substantial knowledge and skill required, assessment of the skin is not assigned to AP. However, the skin is observed during usual care and AP should record their findings. Abnormal findings must be validated and interpreted by the nurse.

Equipment

- Millimeter ruler
- Clean gloves
- Magnifying glass

Assessing the Skin—*continued*

IMPLEMENTATION

Performance

1. Prior to performing the assessment, introduce self and verify the client's identity using agency protocol. Explain to the client what you are going to do, why it is necessary, and how to participate. Discuss how the results will be used in planning further care or treatments.
2. Perform hand hygiene and observe other appropriate infection prevention procedures.
3. Provide for client privacy.
4. Inquire if the client has any history of the following: pain or itching; presence and spread of lesions, bruises, abrasions, pigmented spots; previous experience with skin problems; associated clinical signs; family history; presence of problems in other family members; related systemic conditions; use of medications, lotions, home remedies; excessively dry or moist feel to the skin; tendency to bruise easily; association of the problem to season of year, stress, occupation, medications, recent travel, housing, and so on; recent contact with allergens (e.g., metal paint).

Assessment	Normal Findings	Deviations from Normal
5. Inspect skin color (best assessed under natural light and on areas not exposed to the sun).	Varies from light to deep brown; from ruddy pink to light pink; from yellow overtones to olive	Pallor, cyanosis, jaundice, erythema
6. Inspect uniformity of skin color.	Generally uniform except in areas exposed to the sun; areas of lighter pigmentation (palms, lips, nail beds) in dark-skinned people	Areas of either hyperpigmentation or hypopigmentation
7. Assess edema, if present (i.e., location, color, temperature, shape, and the degree to which the skin remains indented or pitted when pressed by a finger). Measuring the circumference of the extremity with a millimeter tape may be useful for future comparison.	No edema	See the scale for describing edema. ❶
8. Inspect, palpate, and describe skin lesions. Apply gloves if lesions are open or draining. Palpate lesions to determine shape and texture. Describe lesions according to location, distribution, color, configuration, size, shape, type, or structure (Box 29.5 on page 584). Use the millimeter ruler to measure lesions. • Another method that can be used to record lesion size and shape is to lay clean double-thick clear plastic over the lesion or wound and trace the shape with a permanent marker. Dispose of the bottom layer that came in contact with the client and place the top layer in the client record. Use this method only if contact with the plastic does not contaminate the wound. • If gloves were applied, remove and discard gloves. • Perform hand hygiene.	Freckles, some birthmarks that have not changed since childhood, and some long-standing vascular birthmarks such as strawberry or port-wine hemangiomas, some flat and raised nevi; no abrasions or other lesions	Various interruptions in skin integrity; irregular, multicolored, or raised nevi, some pigmented birthmarks such as melanocystic nevi, and some vascular birthmarks such as cavernous hemangiomas. Even these deviations from normal may not be dangerous or require treatment. Assessment by an advanced-level practitioner is required. If skin lesions are suggestive of physical abuse, follow state regulations for follow-up and reporting. Signs of abuse may include bruises, unusual location of burns, or lesions that are not easily explainable. If lesions are present in adults or verbal-age children, conduct the interview and assessment in private.

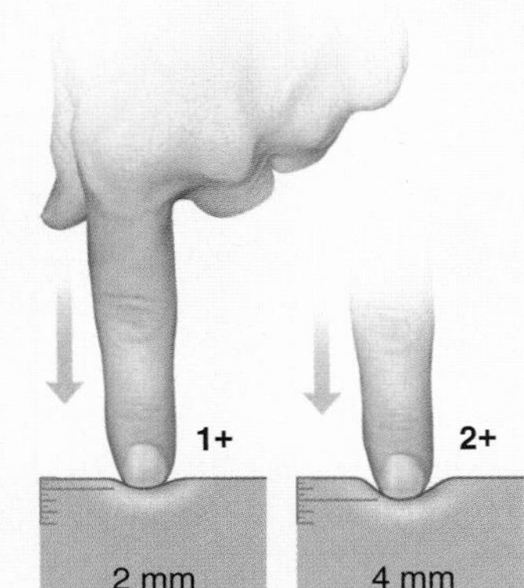

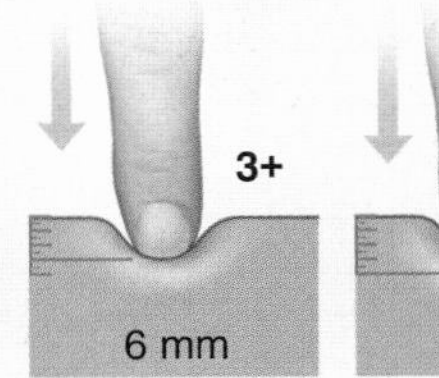

❶ Scale for grading edema.

Assessment	Normal Findings	Deviations from Normal
9. Observe and palpate skin moisture.	Moisture in skinfolds and the axillae (varies with environmental temperature and humidity, body temperature, and activity)	Excessive moisture (e.g., in hyperthermia); excessive dryness (e.g., in dehydration)
10. Palpate skin temperature. Compare the two feet and the two hands, using the backs of your fingers.	Uniform; within normal range	Generalized hyperthermia (e.g., in fever); generalized hypothermia (e.g., in shock); localized hyperthermia (e.g., in infection); localized hypothermia (e.g., in arteriosclerosis)
11. Note skin turgor (fullness or elasticity) by lifting and pinching the skin on an extremity or on the sternum.	When pinched, skin springs back to previous state (is elastic); may be slower in older adults.	Skin stays pinched or tented or moves back slowly (e.g., in dehydration). Count in seconds how long the skin remains tented.

Continued on page 584

SKILL 29.2

Assessing the Skin—*continued*

Assessment	Normal Findings	Deviations from Normal
12. Document findings in the client record using printed or electronic forms or checklists supplemented by narrative notes when appropriate. Draw location of skin lesions on body surface diagrams. ❷		

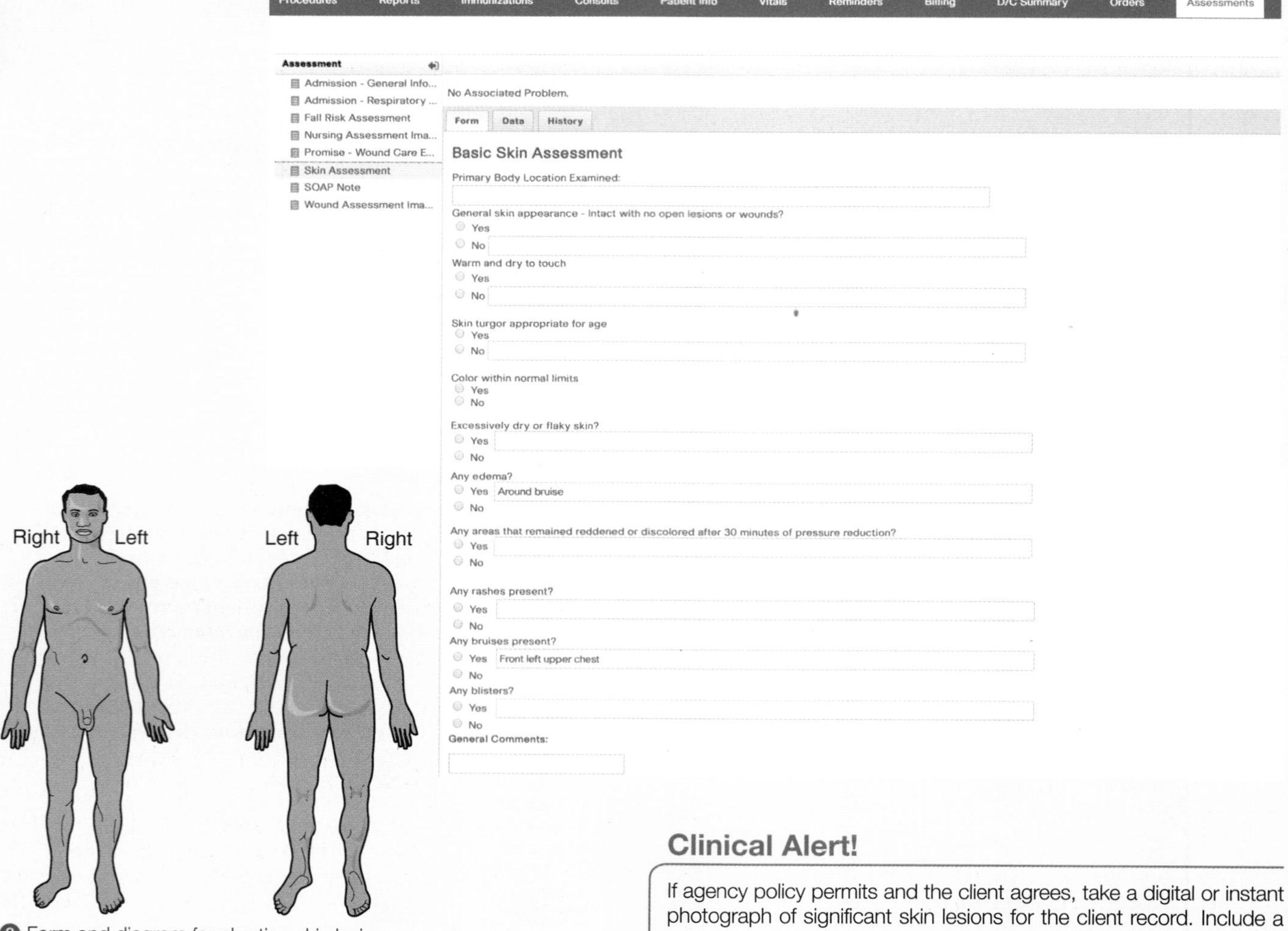

Procedures | Reports | Immunizations | Consults | Patient Info | Vitals | Reminders | Billing | D/C Summary | Orders | Assessments

Assessment
- Admission - General Info...
- Admission - Respiratory ...
- Fall Risk Assessment
- Nursing Assessment Ima...
- Promise - Wound Care E...
- Skin Assessment
- SOAP Note
- Wound Assessment Ima...

No Associated Problem.

Form | Data | History

Basic Skin Assessment

Primary Body Location Examined:

General skin appearance - Intact with no open lesions or wounds?
○ Yes
○ No

Warm and dry to touch
○ Yes
○ No

Skin turgor appropriate for age
○ Yes
○ No

Color within normal limits
○ Yes
○ No

Excessively dry or flaky skin?
○ Yes
○ No

Any edema?
○ Yes Around bruise
○ No

Any areas that remained reddened or discolored after 30 minutes of pressure reduction?
○ Yes
○ No

Any rashes present?
○ Yes
○ No

Any bruises present?
○ Yes Front left upper chest
○ No

Any blisters?
○ Yes
○ No

General Comments:

❷ Form and diagram for charting skin lesions.
iCare.

Clinical Alert!

If agency policy permits and the client agrees, take a digital or instant photograph of significant skin lesions for the client record. Include a measuring guide (ruler or tape) in the picture to demonstrate lesion size.

EVALUATION

- Compare findings to previous skin assessment data if available to determine if lesions or abnormalities are changing.
- Report significant deviations from expected or normal findings to the primary care provider.

BOX 29.5 Describing Skin Lesions

- *Type or structure.* Skin lesions are classified as primary (those that appear initially in response to some change in the external or internal environment of the skin) and secondary (those that do not appear initially but result from modifications such as chronicity, trauma, or infection of the primary lesion). For example, a vesicle (primary lesion) may rupture and cause an erosion (secondary lesion).
- *Size, shape, and texture.* Note size in millimeters and whether the lesion is circumscribed or irregular; round or oval shaped; flat, elevated, or depressed; solid, soft, or hard; rough or thickened; fluid filled or has flakes.
- *Color.* There may be no discoloration; one discrete color (e.g., red, brown, or black); or several colors, as with ecchymosis (a bruise), in which an initial dark red or blue color fades to a yellow color. When color changes are limited to the edges of a lesion, they are described as *circumscribed*; when spread over a large area, they are described as *diffuse*.
- *Distribution.* Distribution is described according to the location of the lesions on the body and symmetry or asymmetry of findings in comparable body areas.
- *Configuration.* Configuration refers to the arrangement of lesions in relation to each other. Configurations of lesions may be annular (arranged in a circle), clustered together (grouped), linear (arranged in a line), arc or bow shaped, or merged (indiscrete); may follow the course of cutaneous nerves; or may be meshed in the form of a network.

LIFESPAN CONSIDERATIONS Assessing the Skin

INFANTS

- Physiologic jaundice may appear in newborns 2 to 3 days after birth and usually lasts about 1 week. Pathologic jaundice, or that which indicates a disease, appears within 24 hours of birth and may last more than 8 days.
- Newborns may have milia (whiteheads), small white nodules over the nose and face, and vernix caseosa (white cheesy, greasy material on the skin).
- Premature infants may have lanugo, a fine downy hair covering their shoulders and back.
- In dark-skinned infants, areas of hyperpigmentation may be found on the back, especially in the sacral area.
- Diaper dermatitis may be seen in infants.
- If a rash is present, inquire in detail about immunization history.
- Assess skin turgor by pinching the skin on the abdomen.

CHILDREN

- Children normally have minor skin lesions (e.g., bruising or abrasions) on arms and legs due to their high activity level. Lesions on other parts of the body may be signs of disease or abuse, and a thorough history should be taken.
- Secondary skin lesions may occur frequently as children scratch or expose a primary lesion to microbes.
- With puberty, oil glands become more productive, and children may develop acne. Most individuals ages 12 to 24 have some acne.
- In dark-skinned children, areas of hyperpigmentation may be found on the back, especially in the sacral area.
- If a rash is present, inquire in detail about immunization history.

OLDER ADULTS

- Changes in lighter colored skin occur at an earlier age than in darker skin.
- The skin loses its elasticity, resulting in wrinkles. Wrinkles first appear on the skin of the face and neck, which are abundant in collagen and elastic fibers.
- The skin appears thin and translucent because of loss of dermis and subcutaneous fat.
- The skin is increasingly dry and flaky because sebaceous and sweat glands are less active. Dry skin is more prominent on the extremities.
- The skin takes longer to return to its natural shape after being tented between the thumb and finger.
- Due to the normal loss of peripheral skin turgor in older adults, assess for hydration by checking skin turgor over the sternum or clavicle.
- Flat tan to brown-colored macules, referred to as *senile lentigines* or *melanotic freckles*, are normally apparent on the back of the hand and other skin areas that are exposed to the sun. These macules may be as large as 1 to 2 cm (0.4 to 0.8 in.).
- Warty lesions (*seborrheic keratosis*) with irregularly shaped borders and a scaly surface often occur on the face, shoulders, and trunk. These benign lesions begin as yellowish to tan and progress to a dark brown or black.
- Vitiligo tends to increase with age and is thought to result from an autoimmune response.
- Cutaneous tags (*acrochordons*) are most commonly seen in the neck and axillary regions. These skin lesions vary in size and are soft, often flesh colored, and pedicled.
- Visible, bright red, fine dilated blood vessels (*telangiectasias*) commonly occur as a result of the thinning of the dermis and the loss of support for the blood vessel walls.
- Pink to slightly red lesions with indistinct borders (*actinic keratoses*) may appear at about age 50, often on the face, ears, backs of the hands, and arms. They may become malignant if untreated.

Hair

Assessing a client's hair includes inspecting the hair, considering developmental changes and ethnic differences, and determining the individual's hair care practices and factors influencing them. Much of the information about hair can be obtained by questioning the client.

Normal hair is resilient and evenly distributed. In people with severe protein deficiency (kwashiorkor), the hair color is faded and appears reddish or bleached, and the texture is coarse and dry. Some therapies cause **alopecia** (hair loss), and some disease conditions and medications affect the coarseness of hair. For example, hypothyroidism can cause very thin and brittle hair. Skill 29.3 describes how to assess the hair.

Assessing the Hair

SKILL 29.3

PLANNING

Assignment

Due to the substantial knowledge and skill required, assessment of the hair is not assigned to AP. However, many aspects are observed during usual care and may be recorded by individuals other than the nurse. Abnormal findings must be validated and interpreted by the nurse.

Equipment

- Clean gloves

IMPLEMENTATION

Performance

1. Prior to performing the assessment, introduce self and verify the client's identity using agency protocol. Explain to the client what you are going to do, why it is necessary, and how to participate. Discuss how the results will be used in planning further care or treatments.
2. Perform hand hygiene, apply gloves, and observe other appropriate infection prevention procedures.
3. Provide for client privacy.
4. Inquire if the client has any history of the following: recent use of hair dyes, rinses, or curling or straightening preparations; recent chemotherapy (if alopecia is present); presence of disease, such as hypothyroidism, which can be associated with dry, brittle hair.
5. Ask about the products and equipment (e.g., combs, brushes, dryers, irons) the client usually uses on the hair. Assist the client to determine if the products are appropriate for the client's type of hair and scalp (e.g., for dry or oily hair). Provide education regarding hygiene of the hair and scalp.

Continued on page 586

SKILL 29.3

Assessing the Hair—*continued*

Assessment	Normal Findings	Deviations from Normal
6. Inspect the evenness of growth over the scalp.	Evenly distributed hair	Patches of hair loss (i.e., alopecia)
7. Inspect hair thickness or thinness.	Thick hair	Very thin hair (e.g., in hypothyroidism)
8. Inspect hair texture and oiliness.	Silky, resilient hair	Brittle hair (e.g., hypothyroidism); excessively oily or dry hair
9. Note presence of infections or infestations by parting the hair in several areas, checking behind the ears and along the hairline at the neck.	No infection or infestation	Flaking, sores, lice, nits (lice eggs), and ringworm
10. Inspect amount of body hair.	Variable	Hirsutism (excessive hairiness); naturally absent or sparse leg hair (poor circulation)

11. Remove and discard gloves.
- Perform hand hygiene.

12. Document findings in the client record using printed or electronic forms or checklists supplemented by narrative notes when appropriate.

EVALUATION

- Perform a detailed follow-up examination based on findings that deviated from expected or normal for the client. Relate findings to previous assessment data if available.
- Report significant deviations from expected or normal findings to the primary care provider.

LIFESPAN CONSIDERATIONS Assessing the Hair

INFANTS

- It is normal for infants to have either very little or a great deal of body and scalp hair.

CHILDREN

- As puberty approaches, axillary and pubic hair will appear (see Box 29.9 later in this chapter).

OLDER ADULTS

- Older adults may experience a loss of scalp, pubic, and axillary hair.
- Hairs of the eyebrows, ears, and nostrils become coarse.

Nails

Nails are inspected for nail plate shape, angle between the fingernail and the nail bed, nail texture, nail bed color, and the intactness of the tissues around the nails. The parts of the nail are shown in Figure 29.9 ■.

The nail plate is normally colorless and has a convex curve. The angle between the fingernail and the nail bed is normally 160 degrees (Figure 29.10*A* ■). One nail abnormality is the spoon shape, in which the nail curves upward from the nail bed (Figure 29.10*B*). This condition, called koilonychia, may be seen in clients with iron deficiency anemia. **Clubbing** is a condition in which the angle between the nail and the nail bed is 180 degrees, or greater (Figures 29.10*C* and *D*). Clubbing may be caused by a long-term lack of oxygen.

Nail texture is normally smooth. Excessively thick nails can appear in older adults, in the presence of poor circulation, or in relation to a chronic fungal infection. Excessively thin nails or the presence of grooves or furrows can reflect prolonged iron deficiency anemia. Beau's lines are horizontal depressions in the nail that can result from injury or severe illness (Figure 29.10*E*). The nail bed is highly vascular, a characteristic that accounts for its color. A bluish or purplish tint to the nail bed may reflect cyanosis, and pallor may reflect poor arterial circulation. Should the client report a history of nail fungus (onychomycosis), a referral to a podiatrist or dermatologist for treatment of nail fungus may be appropriate. Symptoms of nail fungus include brittleness, discoloration, thickening, distortion of nail shape, crumbling of the nail, and loosening (detaching) of the nail.

Nail root
Nail body
Nail bed

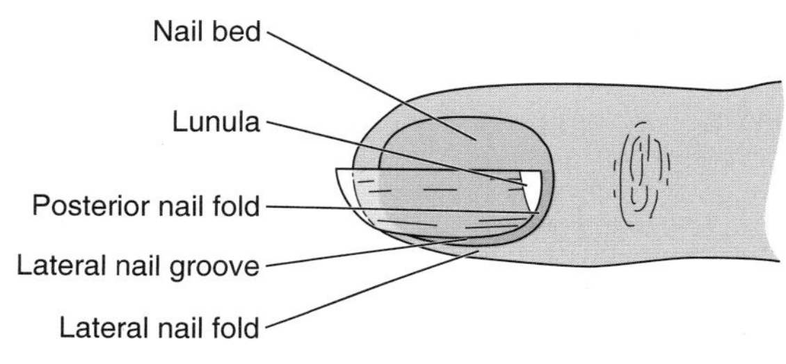

Figure 29.9 ■ The parts of a nail.

About 160° Normal

A

Koilonychia

B

Flattened angle (180°)

C

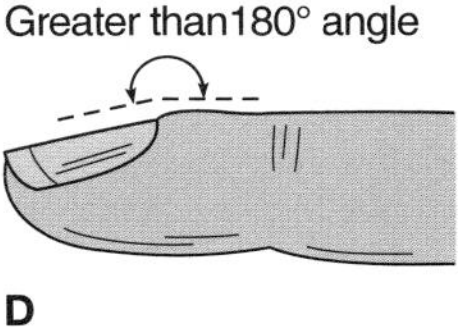

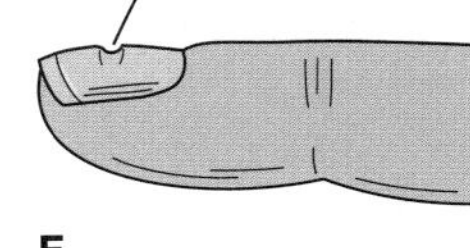

Figure 29.10 ■ *A*, A normal nail; *B*, a spoon-shaped nail; *C*, early clubbing; *D*, late clubbing; *E*, Beau's lines.

The tissue surrounding the nails is normally intact epidermis. Paronychia is an inflammation of the tissues surrounding a nail. The tissues appear inflamed and swollen, and tenderness is usually present.

A **blanch test** can be carried out to test the capillary refill, that is, peripheral circulation. Normal nail bed capillaries blanch when pressed, but quickly turn pink or their usual color when pressure is released. A slow rate of capillary refill may indicate circulatory problems. Skill 29.4 describes how to assess the nails.

Assessing the Nails

SKILL 29.4

PLANNING

Assignment

Due to the substantial knowledge and skill required, assessment of the nails is not assigned to AP. However, many aspects are observed during usual care and may be recorded by individuals other than the nurse. Abnormal findings must be validated and interpreted by the nurse.

Equipment

None

IMPLEMENTATION

Performance

1. Prior to performing the assessment, introduce self and verify the client's identity using agency protocol. Explain to the client what you are going to do, why it is necessary, and how to participate. Discuss how the results will be used in planning further care or treatments. In most situations, clients with artificial nails or polish on fingernails or toenails are not required to remove these for assessment; however, if the assessment cannot be conducted due to the presence of polish or artificial nails, document this in the record.
2. Perform hand hygiene and observe other appropriate infection prevention procedures.
3. Provide for client privacy.
4. Inquire if the client has any history of the following: presence of diabetes mellitus, peripheral circulatory disease, previous injury, or severe illness.

Assessment	Normal Findings	Deviations from Normal
5. Inspect fingernail plate shape to determine its curvature and angle.	Convex curvature; angle of nail plate about 160° (Figure 29.10*A*)	Spoon nail (Figure 29.10*B*); clubbing (180° or greater) (Figures 29.10*C* and *D*)
6. Inspect fingernail and toenail texture.	Smooth texture	Excessive thickness or thinness or presence of grooves or furrows; Beau's lines (Figure 29.10*E*); discolored or detached nail
7. Inspect fingernail and toenail bed color.	Highly vascular and pink in light-skinned clients; dark-skinned clients may have brown or black pigmentation in longitudinal streaks	Bluish or purplish tint (may reflect cyanosis); pallor (may reflect poor arterial circulation)
8. Inspect tissues surrounding nails.	Intact epidermis	Hangnails; paronychia (inflammation). If indicated, teach the client or family member about proper nail care including how to trim and shape the nails to avoid paronychia.
9. Perform blanch test of capillary refill. Press the nail bed between your thumb and index finger; look for blanching and return of pink color to nail bed. Perform on at least one nail on each hand and foot.	Prompt return of pink or usual color (generally less than 2 seconds)	Delayed return of pink or usual color (may indicate circulatory impairment)

10. Document findings in the client record using printed or electronic forms or checklists supplemented by narrative notes when appropriate.

EVALUATION

- Perform a detailed follow-up examination of other systems based on findings that deviated from expected or normal for the client. Relate findings to previous assessment data if available.
- Report significant deviations from expected or normal to the primary care provider.

LIFESPAN CONSIDERATIONS **Assessing the Nails**

INFANTS

- Newborns' nails grow very quickly, are extremely thin, and tear easily.

CHILDREN

- Bent, bruised, or ingrown toenails may indicate shoes that are too tight.
- Nail biting should be discussed with an adult family member because it may be a symptom of stress.

OLDER ADULTS

- The nails grow more slowly and thicken.
- Longitudinal bands commonly develop, and the nails tend to split.
- Bands across the nails may indicate protein deficiency; white spots, zinc deficiency; spoon-shaped nails may indicate iron deficiency.
- Toenail fungus is more common and difficult to eliminate (although not dangerous to health).

Head

During assessment of the head, the nurse inspects and palpates simultaneously and also auscultates. The nurse examines the skull, face, eyes, ears, nose, sinuses, mouth, and pharynx.

Skull and Face

There is a large range of normal shapes of skulls. A normal head size is referred to as **normocephalic**. If head size appears to be outside of the normal range, the circumference can be compared to standard size tables. Measurements more than two standard deviations from the norm for the age, sex, and race of the client are abnormal and should be reported to the primary care provider. Names of areas of the head are derived from names of the underlying bones: frontal, parietal, occipital, mastoid process, mandible, maxilla, and zygomatic (Figure 29.11 ■).

Many disorders cause a change in facial shape or condition. Kidney or cardiac disease can cause edema of the eyelids. Hyperthyroidism can cause **exophthalmos**, a protrusion of the eyeballs with elevation of the upper eyelids, resulting in a startled or staring expression. Hypothyroidism, or myxedema, can cause a dry, puffy face with dry skin and coarse features and thinning of scalp hair and eyebrows. Increased adrenal hormone production or administration of steroids can cause a round face with reddened cheeks, referred to as *moon face*, and excessive hair growth on the upper lips, chin, and sideburn areas. Prolonged illness, starvation, and dehydration can result in sunken eyes, cheeks, and temples. Skill 29.5 describes how to assess the skull and face.

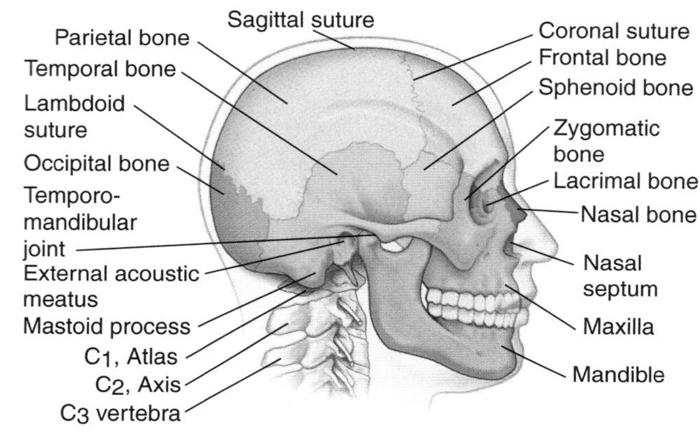

Figure 29.11 ■ Bones of the head.

SKILL 29.5

Assessing the Skull and Face

PLANNING

Assignment

Due to the substantial knowledge and skill required, assessment of the skull and face is not assigned to AP. However, many aspects are observed during usual care and may be recorded by individuals other than the nurse. Abnormal findings must be validated and interpreted by the nurse.

Equipment

None

IMPLEMENTATION

Performance

1. Prior to performing the assessment, introduce self and verify the client's identity using agency protocol. Explain to the client what you are going to do, why it is necessary, and how to participate. Discuss how the results will be used in planning further care or treatments.
2. Perform hand hygiene and observe other appropriate infection prevention procedures.
3. Provide for client privacy.
4. Inquire if the client has any history of the following: past problems with lumps or bumps, itching, scaling, or dandruff; history of loss of consciousness, dizziness, seizures, headache, facial pain, or injury; when and how any lumps occurred; length of time any other problem existed; any known cause of problem; associated symptoms, treatment, and recurrences.

Assessing the Skull and Face—*continued*

Assessment	Normal Findings	Deviations from Normal
5. Inspect the skull for size, shape, and symmetry.	Rounded (normocephalic and symmetric, with frontal, parietal, and occipital prominences); smooth skull contour	Lack of symmetry; increased skull size with more prominent nose and forehead; longer mandible (may indicate excessive growth hormone or increased bone thickness)
6. Inspect the facial features (e.g., symmetry of structures and of the distribution of hair).	Symmetric or slightly asymmetric facial features; palpebral fissures equal in size; symmetric nasolabial folds	Increased facial hair; low hair line; thinning of eyebrows; asymmetric features; exophthalmos; myxedema facies; moon face
7. Inspect the eyes for edema or hollowness.	No edema	Periorbital edema; sunken eyes
8. Note symmetry of facial movements. Ask the client to elevate the eyebrows, frown, or lower the eyebrows, close the eyes tightly, puff the cheeks, and smile and show the teeth.	Symmetric facial movements	Asymmetric facial movements (e.g., eye cannot close completely); drooping of lower eyelid and mouth; involuntary facial movements (i.e., tics or tremors)
9. Document findings in the client record using printed or electronic forms or checklists supplemented by narrative notes when appropriate.		

EVALUATION

- Perform a detailed follow-up examination of other systems based on findings that deviated from expected or normal for the client. Relate findings to previous assessment data if available.
- Report deviations from expected or normal findings to the primary care provider.

LIFESPAN CONSIDERATIONS Assessing the Skull and Face

INFANTS

- Newborns delivered vaginally can have elongated, molded heads, which take on more rounded shapes after a week or two. Infants born by cesarean birth tend to have smooth, rounded heads.
- The posterior fontanel (soft spot) is about 1 cm (0.4 in.) in size and usually closes by 8 weeks. The anterior fontanel is larger, about 2 to 3 cm (0.8 to 1.2 in.) in size. It closes by 18 months.
- Newborns can lift their heads slightly and turn them from side to side. Voluntary head control is well established by 4 to 6 months.

Eyes and Vision

To maintain optimum vision, people need to have their eyes examined regularly throughout life. It is recommended that people under age 40 have their eyes tested every 3 to 5 years, or more frequently if there is a family history of diabetes, hypertension, blood dyscrasia, or eye disease (e.g., glaucoma). After age 40, an eye examination is recommended every 2 years.

Examination of the eyes includes assessment of the external structures, **visual acuity** (the degree of detail the eye can discern in an image), ocular movement, and **visual fields** (the area an individual can see when looking straight ahead). Most eye assessment procedures involve inspection. Consideration is also given to developmental changes and to individual hygienic practices, if the client wears contact lenses or has an artificial eye. For the anatomic structures of the eye, see Figure 29.12 ■ and Figure 29.13 ■.

Many people wear eyeglasses or contact lenses to correct common refractive errors of the lens of the eye. These errors include **myopia** (nearsightedness), **hyperopia** (farsightedness), and **presbyopia** (loss of elasticity of the lens and thus loss of ability to see close objects). Presbyopia begins at about 45 years of age. People notice that they have difficulty reading newsprint. When both far and near vision require correction, two lenses (bifocals) are required. **Astigmatism**, an uneven curvature of the cornea that prevents horizontal and vertical rays from focusing on the retina, is a common problem that may occur in conjunction with myopia and hyperopia. Astigmatism may be corrected with glasses or surgery.

Three types of eye charts are available to test visual acuity (Figure 29.14 ■). People with denominators of 40 or more on the Snellen chart with or without corrective lenses need to be referred to an optometrist or ophthalmologist.

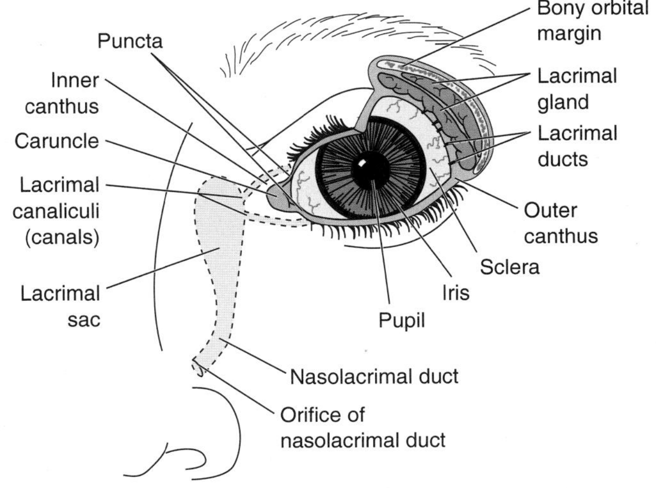

Figure 29.12 ■ The external structures and lacrimal apparatus of the left eye.

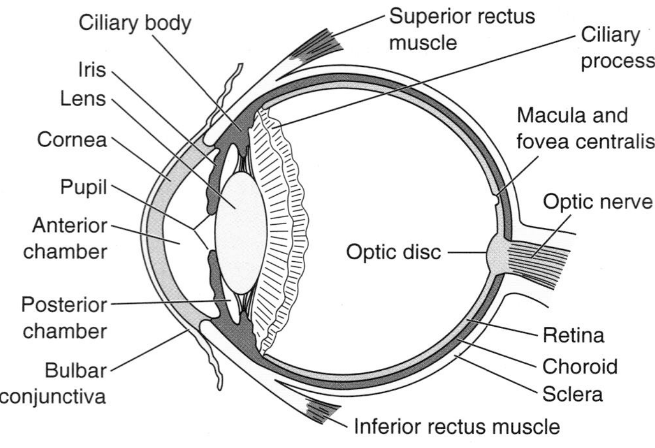

Figure 29.13 ■ Anatomic structures of the right eye, lateral view.

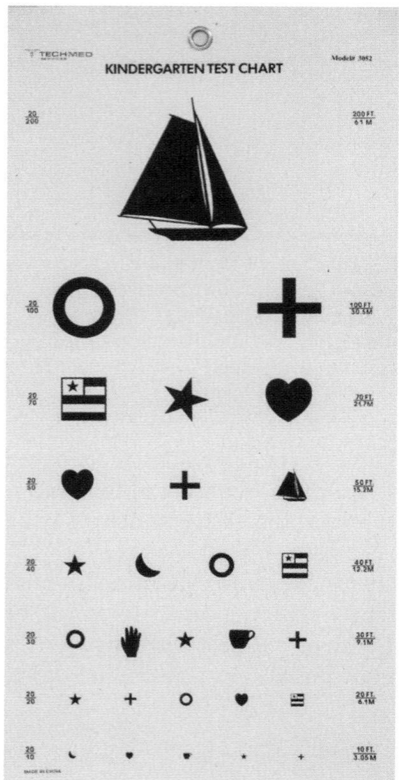

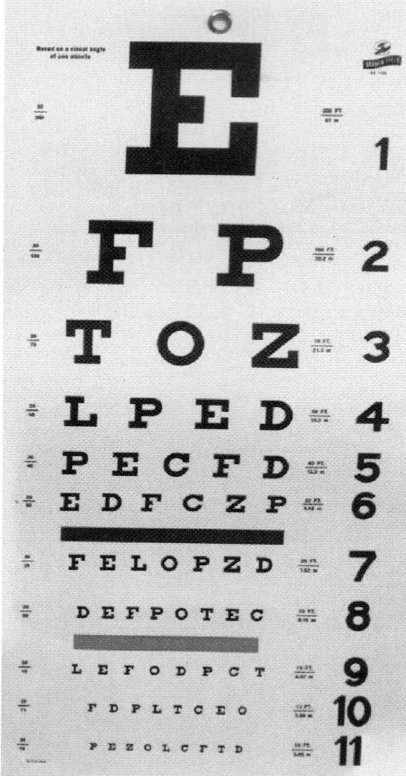

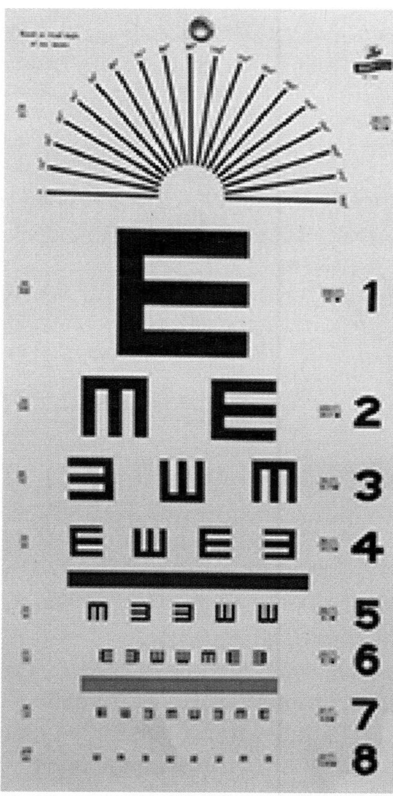

Figure 29.14 ■ Three types of eye charts: *left*, the preschool children's chart; *center*, the Snellen standard chart; *right*, Snellen E chart for clients unable to read the Roman alphabet.

Common inflammatory visual problems that nurses may encounter in clients include conjunctivitis, dacryocystitis, hordeolum, iritis, and contusions or hematomas of the eyelids and surrounding structures. **Conjunctivitis** (inflammation of the bulbar and palpebral conjunctiva) may result from foreign bodies, chemicals, allergenic agents, bacteria, or viruses. Redness, itching, tearing, and mucopurulent discharge occur. During sleep, the eyelids may become encrusted and matted together. **Dacryocystitis** (inflammation of the lacrimal sac) is manifested by tearing and a discharge from the nasolacrimal duct. **Hordeolum (sty)** is a redness, swelling, and tenderness of the hair follicle and glands that empty at the edge of the eyelids. *Iritis* (inflammation of the iris) may be caused by local or systemic infections and results in pain, tearing, and photophobia (sensitivity to light). Contusions or hematomas are "black eyes" resulting from injury.

Cataracts tend to occur in individuals over 65 years old although they may be present at any age. This opacity of the lens or its capsule, which blocks light rays, is frequently removed and replaced by a lens implant. Cataracts may also occur in infants due to a malformation of the lens if the mother contracted rubella in the first trimester of pregnancy. **Glaucoma** (a disturbance in the circulation of aqueous fluid, which causes an increase in intraocular pressure) is the most frequent cause of blindness in people over age 40 although it can occur at younger ages. It can be controlled if diagnosed early. Danger signs of glaucoma include blurred or foggy vision, loss of peripheral vision, difficulty focusing on close objects, difficulty adjusting to dark rooms, and seeing rainbow-colored rings around lights.

Upper eyelids that lie at or below the pupil margin are referred to as ptosis and are usually associated with aging, edema from drug allergy or systemic disease (e.g., kidney disease), congenital lid muscle dysfunction, neuromuscular disease (e.g., myasthenia gravis), and third cranial nerve impairment. Eversion, an outturning of the eyelid, is called ectropion; inversion, an inturning of the lid, is called entropion. These abnormalities are often associated with scarring injuries or the aging process.

Pupils are normally black, are equal in size (about 3 to 7 mm in diameter), and have round, smooth borders. Cloudy pupils are often indicative of cataracts. **Mydriasis** (enlarged pupils) may indicate injury or glaucoma, or result from certain drugs (e.g., atropine, cocaine, amphetamines). **Miosis** (constricted pupils) may indicate an inflammation of the iris or result from such drugs as morphine or heroin and other narcotics, barbiturates, or pilocarpine. It is also an age-related change in older adults. *Anisocoria* (unequal pupils) may result from a central nervous system disorder; however, slight variations may be normal. The iris is normally flat and round. A bulging toward the cornea can indicate increased intraocular pressure. Skill 29.6 describes how to assess a client's eye structures and visual acuity.

Assessing the Eye Structures and Visual Acuity

SKILL 29.6

PLANNING

Place the client in an appropriate room for assessing the eyes and vision. The nurse must be able to control natural and overhead lighting during some portions of the examination.

Equipment

- Millimeter ruler
- Penlight
- Eye chart
- Opaque card

Assignment

Due to the substantial knowledge and skill required, assessment of the eyes and vision is not assigned to AP. However, many aspects are observed during usual care and may be recorded by individuals other than the nurse. Abnormal findings must be validated and interpreted by the nurse.

IMPLEMENTATION

Performance

1. Prior to performing the assessment, introduce self and verify the client's identitwy using agency protocol. Explain to the client what you are going to do, why it is necessary, and how to participate. Discuss how the results will be used in planning further care or treatments.
2. Perform hand hygiene and observe other appropriate infection prevention procedures.
3. Provide for client privacy.
4. Inquire if the client has any history of the following: family history of diabetes, hypertension, blood dyscrasia, or eye disease, injury, or surgery; client's last visit to a provider who specifically assessed the eyes (e.g., ophthalmologist or optometrist); current use of eye medications; use of contact lenses or eyeglasses; hygienic practices for corrective lenses; current symptoms of eye problems (e.g., changes in visual acuity, blurring of vision, tearing, spots, photophobia, itching, or pain). Use this opportunity to reinforce proper eye care and need for regular vision testing.

Assessment	Normal Findings	Deviations from Normal
EYE STRUCTURES		
5. Inspect the eyebrows for hair distribution and alignment and skin quality and movement (ask client to raise and lower the eyebrows).	Hair evenly distributed; skin intact Eyebrows symmetrically aligned; equal movement	Loss of hair; scaling and flakiness of skin Unequal alignment and movement of eyebrows
6. Inspect the eyelashes for evenness of distribution and direction of curl.	Equally distributed; curled slightly outward	Turned inward
7. Inspect the eyelids for surface characteristics (e.g., skin quality and texture), position in relation to the cornea, ability to blink, and frequency of blinking.	Skin intact; no discharge; no discoloration Lids close symmetrically Approximately 15 to 20 involuntary blinks per minute; bilateral blinking When lids open, no visible sclera above corneas, and upper and lower borders of cornea are slightly covered	Redness, swelling, flaking, crusting, plaques, discharge, nodules, lesions Lids close asymmetrically, incompletely, or painfully Rapid, monocular, absent, or infrequent blinking Ptosis, ectropion, or entropion; rim of sclera visible between lid and iris
8. Inspect the bulbar conjunctiva (that lying over the sclera) for color, texture, and the presence of lesions.	Transparent; capillaries sometimes evident; sclera appears white (darker or yellowish and with small brown macules in dark-skinned clients)	Jaundiced sclera (e.g., in liver disease); excessively pale sclera (e.g., in anemia); reddened sclera (marijuana use, rheumatoid disease); lesions or nodules (may indicate damage by mechanical, chemical, allergenic, or bacterial agents)

Continued on page 592

SKILL 29.6

Assessing the Eye Structures and Visual Acuity—*continued*

Assessment	Normal Findings	Deviations from Normal
9. Inspect the cornea for clarity and texture. Ask the client to look straight ahead. Hold a penlight at an oblique angle to the eye, and move the light slowly across the corneal surface.	Transparent, shiny, and smooth; details of the iris are visible In older people, a thin, grayish white ring around the margin, called arcus senilis, may be evident	Opaque; surface not smooth (may be the result of trauma or abrasion) Arcus senilis in clients under age 40
10. Inspect the pupils for color, shape, and symmetry of size. Pupil charts are available in some agencies. See ❶ for variations in pupil diameters.	Black in color; equal in size; normally 3 to 7 mm in diameter; round, smooth border, iris flat and round	Cloudiness, mydriasis, miosis, anisocoria; bulging of iris toward cornea

1 2 3 4 5 6 7 8 9 10

❶ Variations in pupil diameters in millimeters.

Assessment	Normal Findings	Deviations from Normal
11. Assess each pupil's direct and consensual reaction to light to determine the function of the third (oculomotor) and fourth (trochlear) cranial nerves.	Illuminated pupil constricts (direct response) Nonilluminated pupil constricts (consensual response)	Neither pupil constricts Unequal responses
• Partially darken the room. • Ask the client to look straight ahead. • Using a penlight and approaching from the side, shine a light on the pupil. • Observe the response of the illuminated pupil. It should constrict (direct response). • Shine the light on the pupil again, and observe the response of the other pupil. It should also constrict (consensual response).	Response is brisk	Response is sluggish Absent responses
12. Assess each pupil's reaction to accommodation. • Hold an object (a penlight or pencil) about 10 cm (4 in.) from the bridge of the client's nose. • Ask the client to look first at the top of the object and then at a distant object (e.g., the far wall) behind the penlight. Alternate the gaze from the near to the far object. Observe the pupil response.	Pupils constrict when looking at near object; pupils dilate when looking at far object	One or both pupils fail to constrict, dilate, or converge
• Next, ask the client to look at the near object and then move the penlight or pencil toward the client's nose.	Pupils converge when near object is moved toward nose. To record normal assessment of the pupils, use the abbreviation **PERRLA** (pupils equally round and react to light and accommodation).	
VISUAL FIELDS		
13. Assess peripheral visual fields to determine function of the retina and neuronal visual pathways to the brain and second (optic) cranial nerve. • Have the client sit directly facing you at a distance of 60 to 90 cm (2 to 3 ft). • Ask the client to cover the right eye with a card and look directly at your nose.	When looking straight ahead, client can see objects in the periphery	Visual field smaller than normal (possible glaucoma); one-half vision in one or both eyes (possible nerve damage)
• Cover or close your eye directly opposite the client's covered eye (i.e., your left eye), and look directly at the client's nose.	Temporally, peripheral objects can be seen at right angles (90°) to the central point of vision. The upward field of vision is normally 50°, because the orbital ridge is in the way. The downward field of vision is normally 70°, because the cheekbone is in the way.	

Assessing the Eye Structures and Visual Acuity—*continued*

Assessment	Normal Findings	Deviations from Normal
• Hold an object (e.g., a penlight or pencil) in your fingers, extend your arm, and move the object into the visual field from various points in the periphery. The object should be at an equal distance from the client and yourself. Ask the client to tell you when the moving object is first spotted. a. To test the temporal field of the left eye, extend and move your right arm in from the client's right periphery. b. To test the upward field of the left eye, extend and move the right arm down from the upward periphery. c. To test the downward field of the left eye, extend and move the right arm up from the lower periphery. d. To test the nasal field of the left eye, extend and move your left arm in from the periphery. ❷ • Repeat the above steps for the right eye, reversing the process.	The nasal field of vision is normally 50° away from the central point of vision because the nose is in the way. 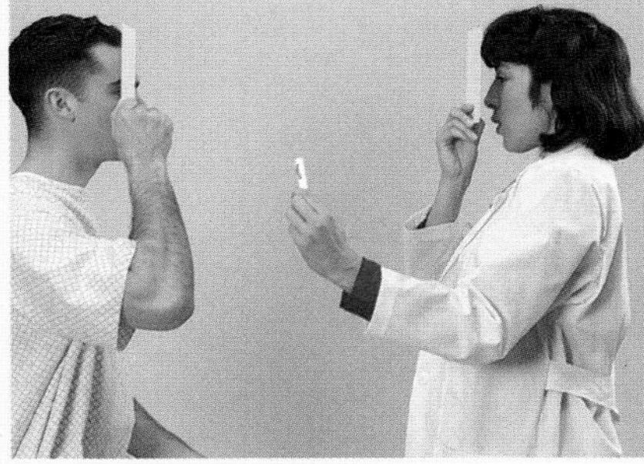 ❷ Assessing the client's left peripheral visual field.	
EXTRAOCULAR MUSCLE TESTS		
14. Assess six ocular movements to determine eye alignment and coordination. • Stand directly in front of the client and hold the penlight at a comfortable distance, such as 30 cm (1 ft) in front of the client's eyes. • Ask the client to hold the head in a fixed position facing you and to follow the movements of the penlight with the eyes only. • Move the penlight in a slow, orderly manner through the six cardinal fields of gaze, that is, from the center of the eye along the lines of the arrows in ❸ and back to the center. • Stop the movement of the penlight periodically so that nystagmus can be detected.	Both eyes coordinated, move in unison, with parallel alignment 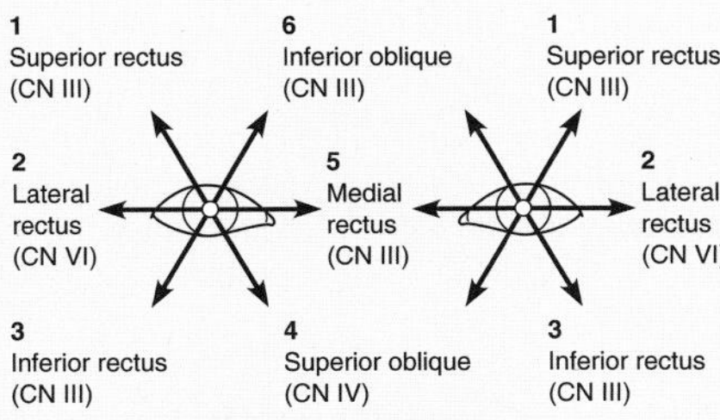 ❸ The six muscles that govern eye movement and their cranial nerves (CNs).	Eye movements not coordinated or parallel; one or both eyes fail to follow a penlight in specific directions, e.g., **strabismus** (cross-eye) **Nystagmus** (rapid involuntary rhythmic eye movement) other than at end point may indicate neurologic impairment 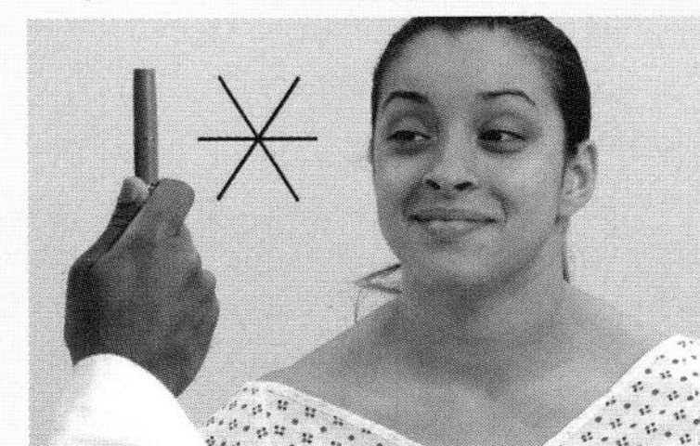
15. Assess for location of light reflex by shining penlight on the corneal surface (Hirschberg test).	Light falls symmetrically (e.g., at "6 o'clock" on both pupils)	Light falls off center on one eye
16. Have client fixate on a near or far object. Cover one eye and observe for movement in the uncovered eye (cover test).	Uncovered eye does not move	If misalignment is present, when dominant eye is covered, the uncovered eye will move to focus on object
VISUAL ACUITY		
17. If the client can read, assess near vision by providing adequate lighting and asking the client to read from a magazine or newspaper held at a distance of 36 cm (14 in.). If the client normally wears corrective lenses, the glasses or lenses should be worn during the test. The document must be in a language the client can read.	Able to read newsprint	Difficulty reading newsprint unless due to aging process

Clinical Alert!

A Rosenbaum eye chart may be used to test near vision. It consists of paragraphs of text or characters in different sizes. Be sure the client has a literacy level appropriate for the text used.

Continued on page 594

SKILL 29.6

Assessing the Eye Structures and Visual Acuity—*continued*

Assessment	Normal Findings	Deviations from Normal
18. Assess distance vision by asking the client to wear corrective lenses, unless they are used for reading only (i.e., for distances of only 36 cm [14 in.]). • Ask the client to stand or sit 6 m (20 ft) from an eye chart, ❹ cover the eye not being tested, and identify the letters or characters on the chart. • Take three readings: right eye, left eye, both eyes. • Record the readings of each eye and both eyes (i.e., the smallest line from which the client is able to read one-half or more of the letters). At the end of each line of the chart are standardized numbers (fractions). The top line is 20/200. The numerator (top number) is always 20, the distance the client stands from the chart. The denominator (bottom number) is the distance from which the normal eye can read the chart. Therefore, a client who has 20/40 vision can see at 20 feet from the chart what a normal-sighted client can see at 40 feet from the chart. Visual acuity is recorded as "sc" (without correction), or "cc" (with correction). You can also indicate how many letters were misread in the line, e.g., "visual acuity 20/40 – 2 cc" indicates that two letters were misread in the 20/40 line by a client wearing corrective lenses.	20/20 vision on Snellen-type chart 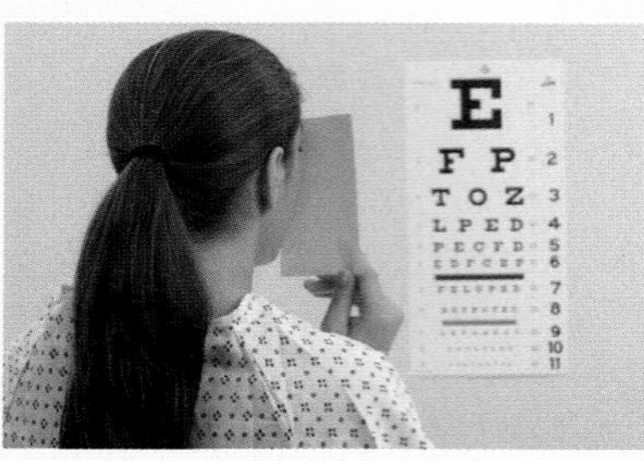 ❹ Testing distance vision.	Denominator of 40 or more on Snellen-type chart with corrective lenses
19. If the client is unable to see even the top line (20/200) of the chart, perform selected vision tests (Box 29.6).		Limited vision only (e.g., light perception, hand movements, counting fingers at 30 cm (1 ft)
20. Document findings in the client record using printed or electronic forms or checklists supplemented by narrative notes when appropriate.		

EVALUATION

- Perform a detailed follow-up examination of other systems based on findings that deviated from expected or normal for the client. Relate findings to previous assessment data if available.
- Report deviations from expected or normal findings to the primary care provider. Individuals with denominators of 40 or more on the Snellen or character chart, with or without corrective lenses, may need to be referred to an optometrist or ophthalmologist.

LIFESPAN CONSIDERATIONS Assessing the Eyes and Vision

INFANTS

- Infants 4 weeks of age should gaze at and follow objects.
- Ability to focus with both eyes should be present by 6 months of age.
- Infants do not have tears until about 3 months of age.
- Visual acuity is about 20/300 at 4 months and progressively improves.

CHILDREN

- Epicanthal folds, common in individuals of Asian cultures, may cover the medial canthus and cause eyes to appear misaligned. Epicanthal folds may also be seen in young children of any race before the bridge of the nose begins to elevate.
- Preschool children's acuity can be checked with picture cards or the Snellen E chart. Acuity should approach 20/20 by 6 years of age.
- A cover test and the corneal light reflex (Hirschberg) test should be conducted on young children to detect misalignment early and prevent amblyopia.
- Always perform the acuity test with glasses on if a child has prescription lenses.
- Children should be tested for color vision deficit. About 8% of males and 0.4% of females have this deficit (Barry, Mollan, Burdon, Jenkins, & Denniston, 2017). The Ishihara or Hardy-Rand-Rittler test can be used.

OLDER ADULTS

Visual Acuity

- Visual acuity decreases as the lens of the eye ages and becomes more opaque and loses elasticity.
- The ability of the iris to accommodate to darkness and dim light diminishes.

LIFESPAN CONSIDERATIONS **Assessing the Eyes and Vision—*continued***

- Peripheral vision diminishes.
- The adaptation to light (glare) and dark decreases.
- Accommodation to far objects often improves, but accommodation to near objects decreases.
- Color vision declines; older people are less able to perceive purple colors and to discriminate pastel colors.
- Many older adults wear corrective lenses; they are most likely to have hyperopia. Visual changes are due to loss of elasticity (presbyopia) and transparency of the lens.

External Eye Structures
- The skin around the orbit of the eye may darken.
- The eyeball may appear sunken because of the decrease in orbital fat.
- Skinfolds of the upper lids may seem more prominent, and the lower lids may sag.
- The eyes may appear dry and dull because of the decrease in tear production from the lacrimal glands.
- A thin, grayish white arc or ring (*arcus senilis*) appears around part or all of the cornea. It results from an accumulation of a lipid substance on the cornea. The cornea tends to cloud with age.
- The iris may appear pale with brown discolorations as a result of pigment degeneration.
- The conjunctiva of the eye may appear paler than that of younger adults and may take on a slightly yellow appearance because of the deposition of fat.
- Pupil reaction to light and accommodation is normally symmetrically equal but may be less brisk.
- The pupils can appear smaller in size, unequal, and irregular in shape because of sclerotic changes in the iris.

BOX 29.6 **Performing Selected Vision Tests**

LIGHT PERCEPTION (LP)
Shine a penlight into the client's eye from a lateral position, and then turn the light off. Ask the client to tell you when the light is on or off. If the client knows when the light is on or off, the client has light perception, and the vision is recorded as "LP."

HAND MOVEMENTS (H/M)
Hold your hand 30 cm (1 ft) from the client's face and move it slowly back and forth, stopping it periodically. Ask the client to tell you when your hand stops moving. If the client knows when your hand stops moving, record the vision as "H/M 1 ft."

COUNTING FINGERS (C/F)
Hold up some of your fingers 30 cm (1 ft) from the client's face, and ask the client to count your fingers. If the client can do so, note on the vision record "C/F 1 ft."

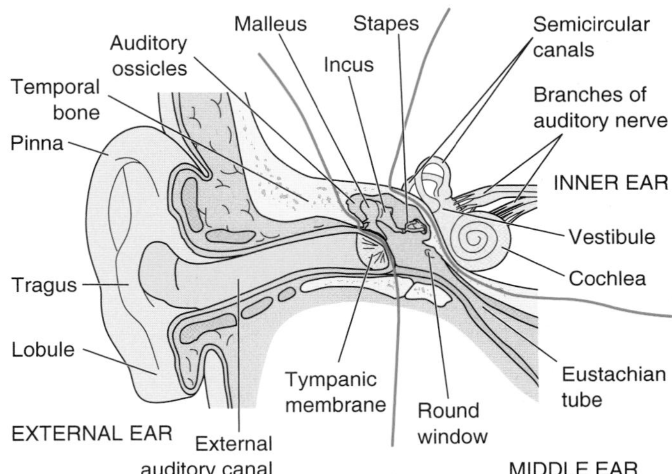

Figure 29.15 ■ Anatomic structures of the external, middle, and inner ear.

Ears and Hearing

Assessment of the ear includes direct inspection and palpation of the external ear, inspection of the internal parts of the ear by an **otoscope** (instrument for examining the interior of the ear, especially the eardrum, consisting essentially of a magnifying lens and a light), and determination of auditory acuity. The ear is usually assessed during an initial physical examination; periodic reassessments may be necessary for long-term clients or those with hearing problems. In some practice settings, only advanced practice nurses perform otoscopic examinations.

The ear is divided into three parts: external ear, middle ear, and inner ear. Many of the structures discussed next are illustrated in Figure 29.15 ■. The external ear includes the **auricle** or **pinna**, the external auditory canal, and the **tympanic membrane**, or eardrum. Landmarks of the auricle include the **lobule** (earlobe), **helix** (the posterior curve of the auricle's upper aspect), **antihelix** (the anterior curve of the auricle's upper aspect), **tragus** (the cartilaginous protrusion at the entrance to the ear canal), **triangular fossa** (a depression of the antihelix), and **external auditory meatus** (the entrance to the ear canal). Although not part of the ear, the **mastoid**, a bony prominence behind the ear, is another important landmark. The external ear canal is curved, is about 2.5 cm (1 in.) long in the adult, and ends at the tympanic membrane. It is covered with skin that has many fine hairs, glands, and nerve endings. The glands secrete **cerumen** (earwax), which lubricates and protects the canal.

The curvature of the external ear canal differs with age. In the infant and toddler, the canal has an upward curvature. By age 3, the ear canal assumes the more downward curvature of adulthood.

The middle ear is an air-filled cavity that starts at the tympanic membrane and contains three **ossicles** (bones of sound transmission): the **malleus** (hammer), the **incus** (anvil), and the **stapes** (stirrups). The **eustachian tube**, another part of the middle ear, connects the middle ear to the nasopharynx. The tube stabilizes the air pressure between the external atmosphere and the middle ear, thus preventing rupture of the tympanic membrane and discomfort produced by marked pressure differences.

The inner ear contains the **cochlea**, a seashell-shaped structure essential for sound transmission and hearing, and the **vestibule** and **semicircular canals**, which contain the organs of equilibrium.

Sound transmission and hearing are complex processes. In brief, sound can be transmitted by air conduction or bone conduction. Air-conducted transmission occurs by this process:

1. A sound stimulus enters the external canal and reaches the tympanic membrane.
2. The sound waves vibrate the tympanic membrane and reach the ossicles.
3. The sound waves travel from the ossicles to the opening in the inner ear (oval window).
4. The cochlea receives the sound vibrations.
5. The stimulus travels to the auditory nerve (the eighth cranial nerve) and the cerebral cortex.

Bone-conducted sound transmission occurs when skull bones transport the sound directly to the auditory nerve.

Audiometric evaluations, which measure hearing at various decibels, are recommended for children and older adults. A common hearing deficit with age is loss of ability to hear high-frequency sounds, such as *f*, *s*, *sh*, and *ph*. This neurosensory hearing deficit does not respond well to use of a hearing aid.

Conductive hearing loss is the result of interrupted transmission of sound waves through the outer and middle ear structures. Possible causes are a tear in the tympanic membrane or an obstruction, due to swelling or other causes, in the auditory canal. **Sensorineural hearing loss** is the result of damage to the inner ear, the auditory nerve, or the hearing center in the brain. **Mixed hearing loss** is a combination of conduction and sensorineural loss. Skill 29.7 describes how to assess the ears and hearing.

Hearing loss is the third most common chronic health condition in the United States, and about 40 million adults

SKILL 29.7

Assessing the Ears and Hearing

PLANNING

It is important to conduct the ear and hearing examination in an area that is quiet. In addition, the location should allow the client to be positioned sitting or standing at the same level as the nurse.

Equipment

- Tuning fork

Assignment

Due to the substantial knowledge and skill required, assessment of the ears and hearing is not assigned to AP. However, many aspects are observed during usual care and may be recorded by individuals other than the nurse. Abnormal findings must be validated and interpreted by the nurse.

IMPLEMENTATION

Performance

1. Prior to performing the assessment, introduce self and verify the client's identity using agency protocol. Explain to the client what you are going to do, why it is necessary, and how to participate. Discuss how the results will be used in planning further care or treatments.
2. Perform hand hygiene and observe other appropriate infection prevention procedures.
3. Provide for client privacy.
4. Inquire if the client has any history of the following: family history of hearing problems or loss; exposure to loud noises at home or work; presence of ear problems or pain; medication history, especially if there are complaints of ringing in the ears (tinnitus); hearing difficulty: its onset, factors contributing to it, and how it interferes with activities of daily living; use of a corrective hearing device: when and from whom it was obtained.
5. Position the client comfortably, seated if possible.

Assessment	Normal Findings	Deviations from Normal
AURICLES		
6. Inspect the auricles for color, symmetry of size, and position. To inspect position, note the level at which the superior aspect of the auricle attaches to the head in relation to the eye.	Color same as facial skin Symmetrical Auricle aligned with outer canthus of eye, about 10°, from vertical ❶	Bluish color of earlobes (e.g., cyanosis); pallor (e.g., frostbite); excessive redness (inflammation or fever) Asymmetry Low-set ears (associated with a congenital abnormality, such as Down syndrome)

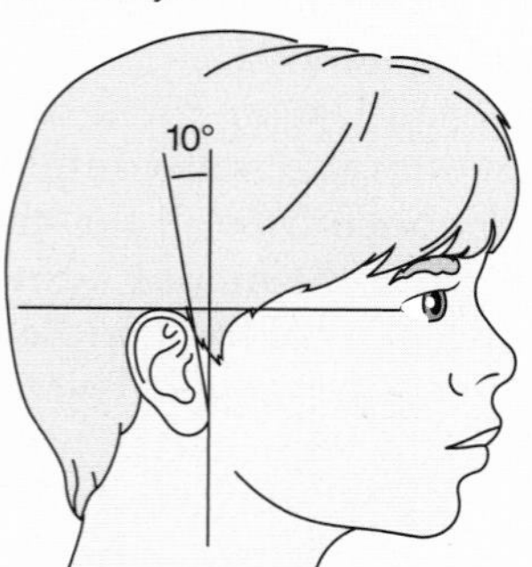

Normal alignment

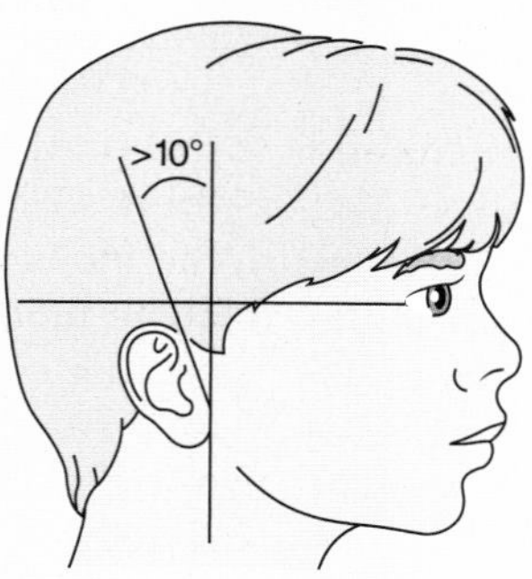

Low-set ears and deviation in alignment

❶ Alignment of the ears.

Assessing the Ears and Hearing—*continued*

Assessment	Normal Findings	Deviations from Normal
7. Palpate the auricles for texture, elasticity, and areas of tenderness. • Gently pull the auricle upward, downward, and backward. • Fold the pinna forward (it should recoil). • Push in on the tragus. • Apply pressure to the mastoid process.	Mobile, firm, and not tender; pinna recoils after it is folded	Lesions (e.g., cysts); flaky, scaly skin (e.g., seborrhea); tenderness when moved or pressed (may indicate inflammation or infection of external ear)
EXTERNAL EAR CANAL		
8. Inspect the external ear canal for cerumen, skin lesions, pus, and blood.	Distal third contains hair follicles and glands Dry cerumen, grayish-tan color; or sticky, wet cerumen in various shades of brown	Redness and discharge Scaling Excessive cerumen obstructing canal
GROSS HEARING ACUITY TESTS		
9. Assess client's response to normal voice tones. If client has difficulty hearing the normal voice, proceed with the following tests.	Normal voice tones audible	Normal voice tones not audible (e.g., requests nurse to repeat words or statements, leans toward the speaker, turns the head, cups the ears, or speaks in loud tone of voice)
10A. Perform the whisper test to assess high-frequency hearing. • Have the client occlude one ear. Out of the client's sight, at a distance of 0.3 to 0.6 m (1 to 2 ft), whisper a simple phrase such as "The weather is hot today." • Ask the client to repeat the phrase. • Repeat with the other ear using a different phrase.	Able to repeat the phrases correctly in both ears	Unable to repeat the phrases in one or both ears
10B. *Tuning Fork Tests*. Perform Weber test to assess bone conduction by examining the lateralization (sideward transmission) of sounds. • Hold the tuning fork at its base. Activate it by tapping the fork gently against the back of your hand near the knuckles or by stroking the fork between your thumb and index fingers. It should be made to ring softly. • Place the base of the vibrating fork on top of the client's head ❷ and ask where the client hears the noise. Conduct the Rinne test to compare air conduction to bone conduction.	Sound is heard in both ears or is localized at the center of the head (Weber negative) ❷ Placing the base of the activated tuning fork on the client's skull (Weber test).	Sound is heard better in impaired ear, indicating a bone-conductive hearing loss; or sound is heard better in ear without a problem, indicating a sensorineural disturbance (Weber positive)

Continued on page 598

SKILL 29.7

Assessing the Ears and Hearing—*continued*

Assessment	Normal Findings	Deviations from Normal
• Hold the handle of the activated tuning fork on the mastoid process of one ear ③ *A* until the client states that the vibration can no longer be heard. • Immediately hold the still vibrating fork prongs in front of the client's ear canal. ③ *B* Push aside the client's hair if necessary. Ask whether the client now hears the sound. Sound conducted by air is heard more readily than sound conducted by bone. The tuning fork vibrations conducted by air are normally heard longer.	Air-conducted (AC) hearing is greater than bone-conducted (BC) hearing, i.e., AC > BC (positive Rinne)	Bone conduction time is equal to or longer than the air conduction time, i.e., BC > AC or BC = AC (negative Rinne; indicates a conductive hearing loss)

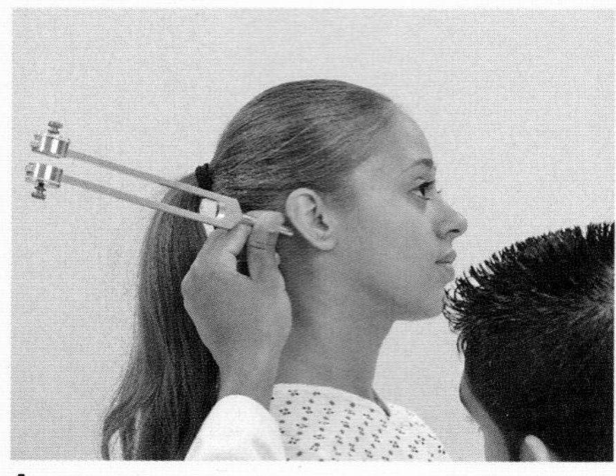

A

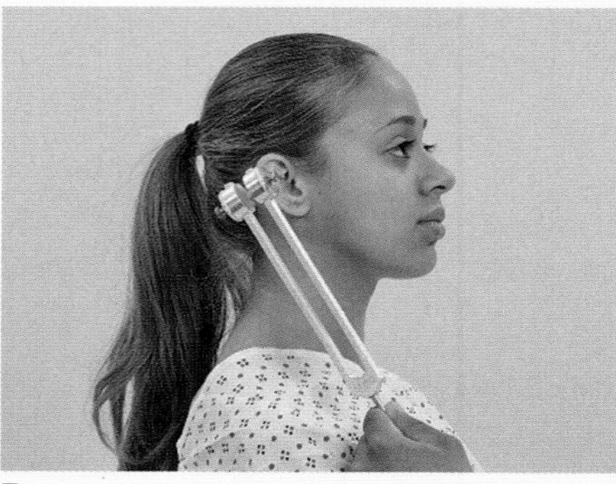

B

③ Rinne test activated tuning fork placement: *A*, base of the tuning fork on the mastoid process; *B*, tuning fork prongs placed in front of the client's ear.

11. Document findings in the client record using printed or electronic forms or checklists supplemented by narrative notes when appropriate.

EVALUATION

- Perform a detailed follow-up examination of other systems based on findings that deviated from expected or normal for the client. Relate findings to previous assessment data if available.
- Report deviations from expected or normal findings to the primary care provider.

LIFESPAN CONSIDERATIONS Assessing the Ears and Hearing

INFANTS

- To assess gross hearing, ring a bell from behind the infant or have the parent call the child's name to check for a response. Newborns will quiet to the sound and may open their eyes wider. By 3 to 4 months of age, the child will turn head and eyes toward the sound.
- All newborns should be assessed for hearing prior to discharge from the hospital. Most states and many countries have a law or regulation requiring universal newborn hearing screening.

CHILDREN

- To inspect the external canal in children less than 3 years old, pull the pinna down and back. If necessary, ask an adult present to assist in holding the child during the examination.
- Perform routine hearing checks and follow up on abnormal results. In addition to congenital or infection-related causes of hearing loss, noise-induced hearing loss is becoming more common in adolescents and young adults as a result of exposure to loud music and prolonged use of headsets at extremely loud volumes plus environmental noise (Neitzel, Swinburn, Hammer, & Eisenberg, 2017). Teach that music loud enough to prevent hearing a normal conversation can damage hearing.

OLDER ADULTS

- The skin of the ear may appear dry and be less resilient because of the loss of connective tissue.
- Increased coarse hair growth occurs along the helix, antihelix, and tragus.
- The pinna increases in both width and length, and the earlobe elongates.
- Earwax is drier.
- Sensorineural hearing loss occurs. Ensure that the examination is conducted in a quiet place. In particular, older adults will have difficulty accurately reporting results of hearing tests if excessive noise is present.
- Generalized hearing loss (presbycusis) occurs in all frequencies, although the first symptom is the loss of high-frequency sounds: the *f*, *s*, *sh*, and *ph* sounds. To such individuals, conversation can be distorted and result in what appears to be inappropriate or confused behavior.

have hearing loss resulting from nonoccupational exposure to loud noises (Centers for Disease Control and Prevention [CDC], 2017). The CDC reports that exposure as little as 2 minutes at a rock concert can cause hearing damage. Many adults are unaware that they have hearing loss.

Nose and Sinuses

A nurse can inspect the nasal passages very simply with a flashlight or penlight. Assessment of the nose includes inspection and palpation of the external nose (the upper third of the nose is bone; the remainder is cartilage) and patency of the nasal cavities.

If the client reports difficulty or abnormality in smell, the nurse may test the client's olfactory sense by asking the client to identify common odors such as coffee or mint. This is done by asking the client to close the eyes and placing vials containing the scent under the client's nose.

The nurse also inspects and palpates the facial sinuses (Figure 29.16 ■). Skill 29.8 describes how to assess the nose and sinuses.

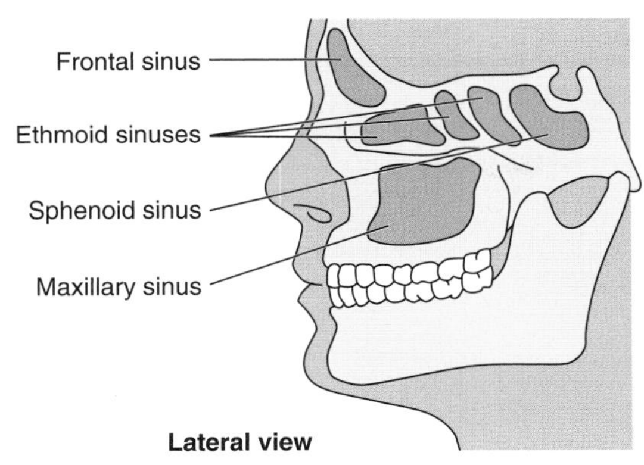

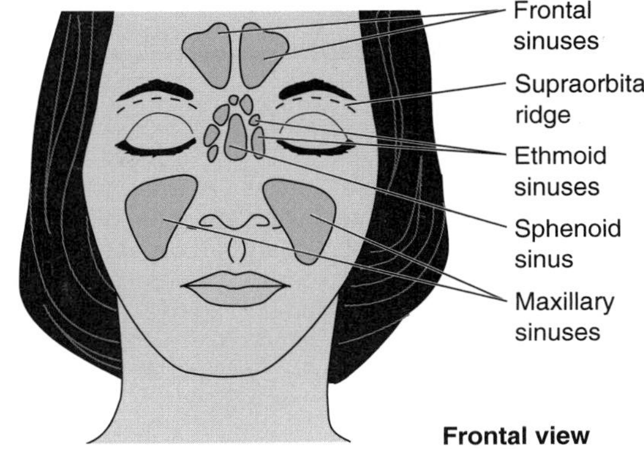

Figure 29.16 ■ The facial sinuses.

Assessing the Nose and Sinuses

SKILL 29.8

PLANNING

Assignment

Due to the substantial knowledge and skill required, assessment of the nose and sinuses is not assigned to AP. However, many aspects are observed during usual care and may be recorded by individuals other than the nurse. Abnormal findings must be validated and interpreted by the nurse.

Equipment

- Flashlight or penlight

IMPLEMENTATION

Performance

1. Prior to performing the assessment, introduce self and verify the client's identity using agency protocol. Explain to the client what you are going to do, why it is necessary, and how to participate. Discuss how the results will be used in planning further care or treatments.
2. Perform hand hygiene and observe other appropriate infection prevention procedures.
3. Provide for client privacy.
4. Inquire if the client has any history of the following: allergies, difficulty breathing through the nose, sinus infections, injuries to nose or face, nosebleeds; medications taken; changes in sense of smell.
5. Position the client comfortably, seated if possible.

Assessment	Normal Findings	Deviations from Normal
NOSE		
6. Inspect the external nose for any deviations in shape, size, or color and flaring or discharge from the nares.	Symmetric and straight No discharge or flaring Uniform color	Asymmetric Discharge from nares Localized areas of redness or presence of skin lesions
7. Lightly palpate the external nose to determine any areas of tenderness, masses, and displacements of bone and cartilage.	Not tender; no lesions	Tenderness on palpation; presence of lesions
8. Determine patency of both nasal cavities. Ask the client to close the mouth, exert pressure on one naris, and breathe through the opposite naris. Repeat the procedure to assess patency of the opposite naris.	Air moves freely as the client breathes through the nares	Air movement is restricted in one or both nares
9. Observe for the presence of redness, swelling, growths, and discharge.	Mucosa pink Clear, watery discharge No lesions	Mucosa red, edematous Abnormal discharge (e.g., pus) Presence of lesions (e.g., polyps)
10. Inspect the nasal septum between the nasal chambers.	Nasal septum intact and in midline	Septum deviated to the right or to the left
SINUSES		
11. Palpate the maxillary and frontal sinuses for tenderness.	Not tender	Tenderness in one or more sinuses

12. Document findings in the client record using printed or electronic forms or checklists supplemented by narrative notes when appropriate.

EVALUATION

- Perform a detailed follow-up examination of other systems based on findings that deviated from expected or normal for the client. Relate findings to previous assessment data if available.
- Report deviations from expected or normal findings to the primary care provider.

LIFESPAN CONSIDERATIONS **Assessing the Nose and Sinuses**

INFANTS AND CHILDREN

- Push the tip of the nose gently upward with the thumb and shine a light into the nares.
- Ethmoid and maxillary sinuses are present at birth; frontal sinuses begin to develop by 1 to 2 years of age; and sphenoid sinuses develop later in childhood. Infants and young children have fewer sinus problems than older children and adolescents.
- Ethmoid sinuses continue to develop until age 12.
- Cough and runny nose are the most common signs of sinusitis in preadolescent children. Adolescents with sinusitis may have headaches, facial tenderness, and swelling.

OLDER ADULTS

- The sense of smell markedly diminishes because of a decrease in the number of olfactory nerve fibers and atrophy of the remaining fibers. Older adults are less able to identify and discriminate odors.
- Nosebleeds may result from hypertensive disease or other arterial vessel changes.

Mouth and Oropharynx

The mouth and oropharynx are composed of a number of structures: lips, oral mucosa, the tongue and floor of the mouth, teeth and gums, hard and soft palate, uvula, salivary glands, tonsillar pillars, and tonsils. Anatomic structures of the mouth are shown in Figure 29.17 ■. By age 25, most people have all their permanent teeth. For information about structures of the teeth, see Chapter 33 ∞.

Normally, three pairs of salivary glands empty into the oral cavity: the parotid, submandibular, and sublingual glands. The *parotid gland* is the largest and empties through the Stensen duct opposite the second molar. The *submandibular gland* empties through the Wharton duct, which is situated on either side of the frenulum on the floor of the mouth. The *sublingual salivary gland* lies in the floor of the mouth and has numerous openings.

Dental **caries** (cavities) and **periodontal disease** (or **pyorrhea**) are the two problems that most frequently affect the teeth. Both problems are commonly associated with plaque and tartar deposits. **Plaque** is an invisible soft film that adheres to the enamel surface of teeth; it consists of bacteria, molecules of saliva, and remnants of epithelial cells and leukocytes. When plaque is unchecked, tartar (dental calculus) forms. **Tartar** is a visible, hard deposit of plaque and dead bacteria that forms at the gum lines. Tartar buildup can alter the fibers that attach the teeth to the gum and eventually disrupt bone tissue. Periodontal disease is characterized by **gingivitis** (red, swollen gingiva [gum]), bleeding, receding gum lines, and the formation of pockets between the teeth and gums.

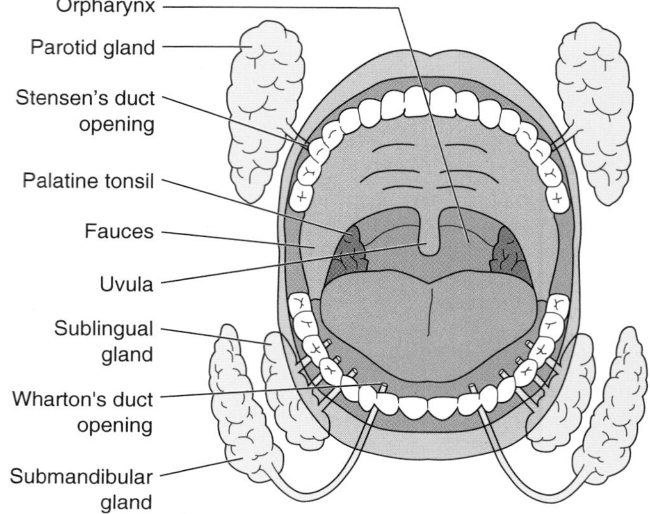

Figure 29.17 ■ Anatomic structures of the mouth.

Other problems nurses may see are **glossitis** (inflammation of the tongue), *stomatitis* (inflammation of the oral mucosa), and **parotitis** (inflammation of the parotid salivary gland). A variety of mouth sores also may occur including those referred to as canker sores, cold sores, or fever blisters. Some of those may be minor and self-limiting while others may be caused by the highly contagious herpes simplex virus. The accumulation of foul matter (food, microorganisms, and epithelial elements) on the teeth and gums is referred to as **sordes**. Skill 29.9 describes assessment of the mouth and oropharynx.

SKILL 29.9

Assessing the Mouth and Oropharynx

PLANNING

If possible, arrange for the client to sit with the head against a firm surface such as a headrest or examination table. This makes it easier for the client to hold the head still during the examination.

Equipment

- Clean gloves
- Tongue depressor
- 2×2 gauze pads
- Penlight

Assignment

Due to the substantial knowledge and skill required, assessment of the mouth and oropharynx is not assigned to AP. However, many aspects are observed during usual care and may be recorded by individuals other than the nurse. Abnormal findings must be validated and interpreted by the nurse.

Assessing the Mouth and Oropharynx—*continued*

IMPLEMENTATION

Performance

1. Prior to performing the assessment, introduce self and verify the client's identity using agency protocol. Explain to the client what you are going to do, why it is necessary, and how to participate. Discuss how the results will be used in planning further care or treatments.
2. Perform hand hygiene and observe other appropriate infection prevention procedures.
3. Provide for client privacy.
4. Inquire if the client has any history of the following: routine pattern of dental care, last visit to dentist; length of time ulcers or other lesions have been present; denture discomfort; medications client is receiving.
5. Position the client comfortably, seated if possible.

Assessment	Normal Findings	Deviations from Normal
LIPS AND BUCCAL MUCOSA		
6. Inspect the outer lips for symmetry of contour, color, and texture. Ask the client to purse the lips as if to whistle.	Uniform pink color (darker, e.g., bluish hue, in Mediterranean groups and dark-skinned clients) Soft, moist, smooth texture Symmetry of contour Ability to purse lips	Pallor; cyanosis Blisters; generalized or localized swelling; fissures, crusts, or scales (may result from excessive moisture, nutritional deficiency, or fluid deficit) Inability to purse lips (may indicate facial nerve damage)
7. Inspect and palpate the inner lips and buccal mucosa for color, moisture, texture, and the presence of lesions.	Uniform pink color (freckled brown pigmentation in dark-skinned clients)	Pallor; leukoplakia (white patches), red, bleeding
• Apply clean gloves. • Ask the client to relax the mouth for better visualization. • Grasp the lip on each side between the thumb and index finger. ❶ • Pull the lip outward and away from the teeth.	Moist, smooth, soft, glistening, and elastic texture (drier oral mucosa in older clients due to decreased salivation)	Excessive dryness Mucosal cysts; irritations from dentures; abrasions, ulcerations; nodules

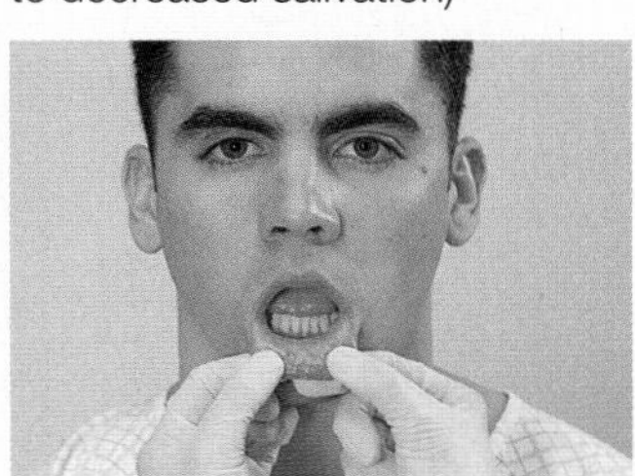

❶ Inspecting the mucosa of the lower lip.

Assessment	Normal Findings	Deviations from Normal
TEETH AND GUMS		
8. Inspect the teeth and gums while examining the inner lips and buccal mucosa.	32 adult teeth Smooth, white, shiny tooth enamel	Missing teeth; ill-fitting dentures Brown or black discoloration of the enamel (may indicate staining or the presence of caries)
• Ask the client to open the mouth. Using a tongue depressor, retract the cheek. ❷ View the surface buccal mucosa from top to bottom and back to front. Repeat the procedure for the other side.	Pink gums (bluish or brown patches in dark-skinned clients) Moist, firm texture to gums No retraction of gums	Excessively red gums Spongy texture; bleeding; tenderness (may indicate periodontal disease) Receding, atrophied gums; swelling that partially covers the teeth
• Examine the back teeth. For proper vision of the molars, use the index fingers of both hands to retract the cheek. ❸ Ask the client to relax the lips and first close, then open, the jaw. **Rationale:** *Closing the jaw assists in observation of tooth alignment and loss of teeth; opening the jaw assists in observation of dental fillings and caries.* • Observe the number of teeth, tooth color, the state of fillings, dental caries, and tartar along the base of the teeth. Note the presence and fit of partial or complete dentures. • Inspect the gums. Observe for bleeding, color, retraction (pulling away from the teeth), edema, and lesions.		

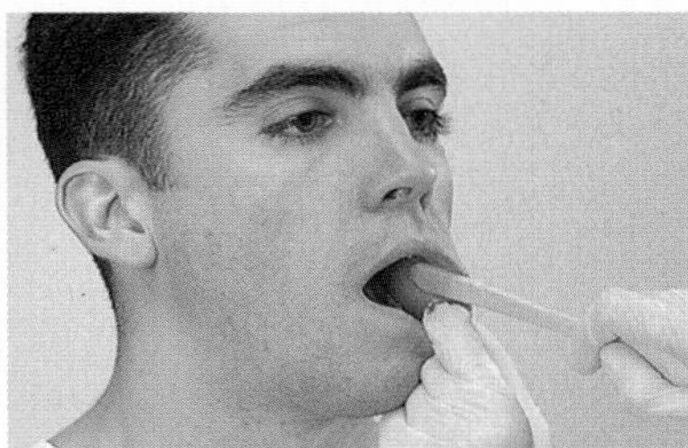

❷ Inspecting the buccal mucosa using a tongue depressor.

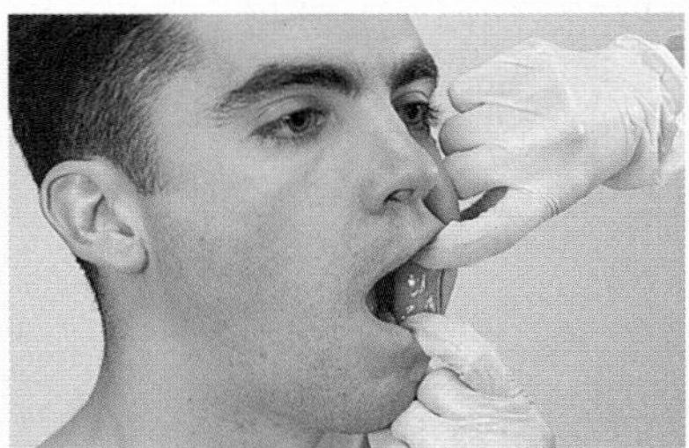

❸ Inspecting the back teeth.

Continued on page 602

SKILL 29.9

Assessing the Mouth and Oropharynx—*continued*

Assessment	Normal Findings	Deviations from Normal
9. Inspect the dentures. Ask the client to remove complete or partial dentures. Inspect their condition, noting in particular broken or worn areas. Examine the gums beneath the dentures for sore areas.	Smooth, intact dentures	Ill-fitting dentures; irritated and excoriated area under dentures
TONGUE AND FLOOR OF THE MOUTH		
10. Inspect the surface of the tongue for position, color, and texture. Ask the client to extend the tongue.	Central position Pink color (some brown pigmentation on tongue borders in dark-skinned clients); moist; slightly rough; thin whitish coating Smooth, lateral margins; no lesions Raised papillae (taste buds)	Deviated from center (may indicate damage to hypoglossal [12th cranial] nerve); excessive trembling Smooth red tongue (may indicate iron, vitamin B_{12}, or vitamin B_3 deficiency) Dry, furry tongue (associated with fluid deficit), white coating (may be oral yeast infection) Nodes, ulcerations, discolorations (white or red areas); areas of tenderness
11. Inspect tongue movement. Ask the client to roll the tongue upward and move it from side to side.	Moves freely; no tenderness	Restricted mobility
12. Inspect the base of the tongue, the mouth floor, and the frenulum. Ask the client to place the tip of the tongue against the roof of the mouth.	Smooth tongue base with prominent veins	Swelling, ulceration
PALATES AND UVULA		
13. Inspect the hard and soft palate for color, shape, texture, and the presence of bony prominences. Ask the client to open the mouth wide and tilt the head backward. Then, depress tongue with a tongue depressor as necessary, and use a penlight for appropriate visualization.	Light pink, smooth, soft palate Lighter pink hard palate, more irregular texture	Discoloration (e.g., jaundice or pallor) Palates the same color Irritations Exostoses (bony growths) growing from the hard palate
14. Inspect the uvula for position and mobility while examining the palates. To observe the uvula, ask the client to say "ah" so that the soft palate rises.	Positioned in midline of soft palate, rises during vocalization	Deviation to one side from tumor or trauma; immobility (may indicate damage to trigeminal [5th cranial] nerve or vagus [10th cranial] nerve)
OROPHARYNX AND TONSILS		
15. Inspect the oropharynx for color and texture. Inspect one side at a time to avoid eliciting the gag response. To expose one side of the oropharynx, press a tongue depressor against the tongue on the same side about halfway back while the client tilts the head back and opens the mouth wide. Use a penlight for illumination, if needed.	Pink and smooth posterior wall	Reddened or edematous; presence of lesions, plaques, or drainage
16. Inspect the tonsils (behind the fauces) for color, discharge, and size.	Pink and smooth No discharge Of normal size or not visible • Grade 1 (normal): The tonsils are behind the tonsillar pillars (the soft structures supporting the soft palate).	Inflamed Presence of discharge Swollen • Grade 2: The tonsils are between the pillars and the uvula. • Grade 3: The tonsils touch the uvula. • Grade 4: One or both tonsils extend to the midline of the oropharynx.

17. Remove and discard gloves.
- Perform hand hygiene.

18. Document findings in the client record using printed or electronic forms or checklists supplemented by narrative notes when appropriate.

EVALUATION

- Perform a detailed follow-up examination of other systems based on findings that deviated from expected or normal for the client. Relate findings to previous assessment data if available.
- Report deviations from expected or normal findings to the primary care provider.

LIFESPAN CONSIDERATIONS Assessing the Mouth and Oropharynx

INFANTS

- Inspect the palate and uvula for a cleft. A bifid (forked) uvula may indicate an unsuspected cleft palate (i.e., a cleft in the cartilage that is covered by skin).
- Newborns may have pearly white nodules on their gums, which resolve without treatment.
- The first teeth erupt at about 6 to 7 months of age. Assess for dental hygiene; parents should cleanse the infant's teeth daily with a soft cloth or soft toothbrush.
- Fluoride supplements should be given by 6 months if the child's drinking water contains less than 0.3 parts per million (ppm) fluoride.
- Children should see a dentist by 1 year of age.

CHILDREN

- Tooth development should be appropriate for age.
- White spots on the teeth may indicate excessive fluoride ingestion.
- Drooling is common up to 2 years of age.
- The tonsils are normally larger in children than in adults and commonly extend beyond the palatine arch until the age of 11 or 12 years.

OLDER ADULTS

- The oral mucosa may be drier than that of younger people because of decreased salivary gland activity. Decreased salivation occurs in older people taking medications such as antidepressants, antihistamines, decongestants, diuretics, antihypertensives, tranquilizers, antispasmodics, and antineoplastics. Extreme dryness is associated with dehydration.
- Some receding of the gums occurs, giving an appearance of increased toothiness.
- Taste sensations diminish. Sweet and salty tastes are lost first. Older people may add more salt and sugar to food than they did when they were younger. Diminished taste sensation is due to atrophy of the taste buds and a decreased sense of smell. It indicates diminished function of the fifth and seventh cranial nerves.
- Tiny purple or bluish black swollen areas (varicosities) under the tongue, known as *caviar spots*, are not uncommon.
- The teeth may show signs of staining, erosion, chipping, and abrasions due to loss of dentin. Older adults with limited incomes may delay or avoid professional dental care.
- Tooth loss occurs as a result of dental disease but is preventable with good dental hygiene.
- Check that full or removable partial dentures fit properly. Bone loss and weight loss or gain can change the way these prosthetics fit.
- The gag response may be slightly sluggish.
- Older adults who are homebound or are in long-term care facilities often have teeth or dentures in need of repair, due to the difficulty of obtaining dental care in these situations. Do a thorough assessment of missing teeth and those in need of repair, whether they are natural teeth or dentures.

Neck

Examination of the neck includes the muscles, lymph nodes, trachea, thyroid gland, carotid arteries, and jugular veins. Areas of the neck are defined by the sternocleidomastoid muscles, which divide each side of the neck into two triangles: the anterior and posterior (Figure 29.18 ■). The trachea, thyroid gland, anterior cervical nodes, and carotid artery lie within the anterior triangle (Figure 29.19 ■); the carotid artery runs parallel and anterior to the sternocleidomastoid muscle. The posterior lymph nodes lie within the posterior triangle (Figure 29.20 ■).

Each sternocleidomastoid muscle extends from the upper sternum and the medial third of the clavicle to the mastoid process of the temporal bone behind the ear. These muscles turn and laterally flex the head. Each trapezius muscle extends from the occipital bone of the skull to the lateral third of the clavicle. These muscles draw the head to the side and back, elevate the chin, and elevate the shoulders to shrug them.

Lymph nodes in the neck that collect lymph from the head and neck structures are grouped serially and referred to as *chains*. See Figure 29.20 and Table 29.6. The deep cervical chain is not shown in Figure 29.20 because it lies beneath the sternocleidomastoid muscle. Skill 29.10 describes how to assess the neck.

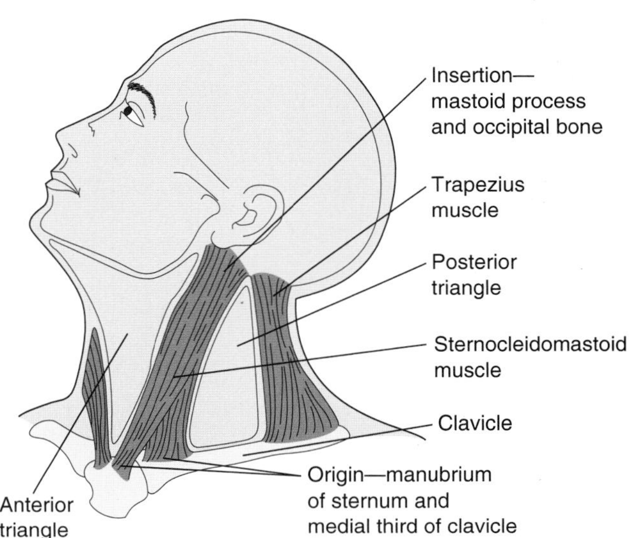

Figure 29.18 ■ Major muscles of the neck.

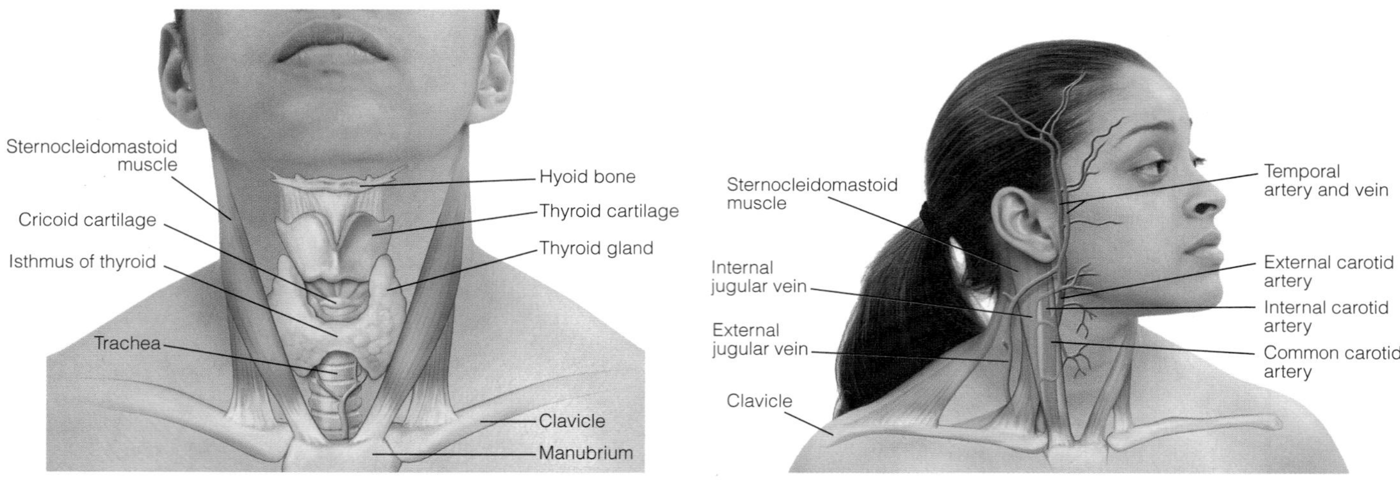

Figure 29.19 ■ Structures and vessels of the neck.
From *Health Assessment and Physical Assessment* (3rd ed., p. 263), by D. D'Amico and C. Barbarito, 2016. Boston, MA: Pearson.

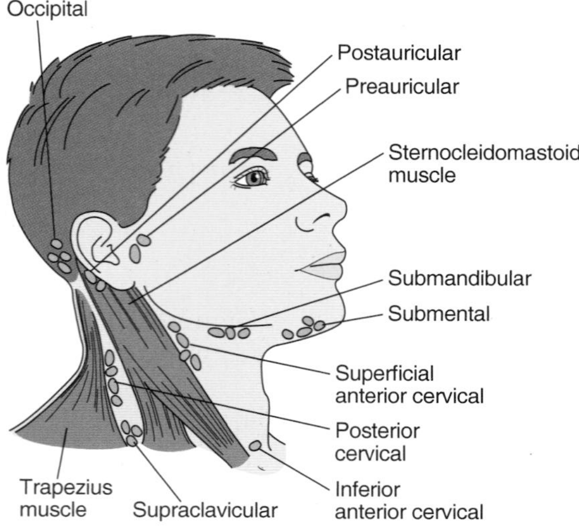

Figure 29.20 ■ Lymph nodes of the neck.

Thorax and Lungs

Assessing the thorax and lungs is frequently critical to assessing the client's oxygenation status (also see Chapter 49 ∞). Changes in the respiratory system can occur slowly or quickly. In clients with chronic obstructive pulmonary disease (COPD), such as chronic bronchitis, emphysema, and asthma, changes are frequently gradual. The onset of conditions such as pneumonia or pulmonary embolus is generally more acute or sudden.

Chest Landmarks

Before beginning the assessment, the nurse must be familiar with a series of imaginary lines on the chest wall and be able to locate the position of each rib and some spinous processes. These landmarks help the nurse to identify the position of

TABLE 29.6 Lymph Nodes of the Head and Neck

Node Center	Location	Area Drained
HEAD		
Occipital	At the posterior base of the skull	The occipital region of the scalp and the deep structures of the back of the neck
Postauricular (mastoid)	Behind the auricle of the ear or in front of the mastoid process	The parietal region of the head and part of the ear
Preauricular	In front of the tragus of the ear	The forehead and upper face
FLOOR OF MOUTH		
Submandibular (submaxillary)	Along the medial border of the mandible, halfway between the angle of the jaw and the chin	The chin, upper lip, cheek, nose, teeth, eyelids, part of the tongue and floor of the mouth
Submental	Behind the tip of the mandible in the midline, under the chin	The anterior third of the tongue, gums, and floor of the mouth

TABLE 29.6 Lymph Nodes of the Head and Neck—*continued*

Node Center	Location	Area Drained
NECK		
Superficial anterior cervical (tonsillar)	Along the mandible, anterior to the sternocleidomastoid muscle	The skin and neck
Posterior cervical	Along the anterior aspect of the trapezius muscle	The posterior and lateral regions of the neck, occiput, and mastoid
Deep cervical	Under the sternocleidomastoid muscle	The larynx, thyroid gland, trachea, and upper part of the esophagus
Supraclavicular	Above the clavicle, in the angle between the clavicle and the sternocleidomastoid muscle	The lateral regions of the neck and lungs

Assessing the Neck

SKILL 29.10

PLANNING

Assignment

Due to the substantial knowledge and skill required, assessment of the neck is not assigned to AP. However, many aspects are observed during usual care and may be recorded by individuals other than the nurse. Abnormal findings must be validated and interpreted by the nurse.

Equipment

None

IMPLEMENTATION

Performance

1. Prior to performing the assessment, introduce self and verify the client's identity using agency protocol. Explain to the client what you are going to do, why it is necessary, and how to participate. Discuss how the results will be used in planning further care or treatments.
2. Perform hand hygiene and observe other appropriate infection prevention procedures.
3. Provide for client privacy.
4. Inquire if the client has any history of the following: problems with neck lumps; neck pain or stiffness; when and how any lumps occurred; previous diagnoses of thyroid problems; and other treatments provided (e.g., surgery, radiation).

Assessment	Normal Findings	Deviations from Normal
NECK MUSCLES		
5. Inspect the neck muscles (sternocleidomastoid and trapezius) for abnormal swellings or masses. Ask the client to hold the head erect.	Muscles equal in size; head centered	Unilateral neck swelling; head tilted to one side (indicates presence of masses, injury, muscle weakness, shortening of sternocleidomastoid muscle, scars)
6. Observe head movement. Ask client to:	Coordinated, smooth movements with no discomfort	Muscle tremor, spasm, or stiffness
• Bend the chin to the chest. **Rationale:** *This determines function of the sternocleidomastoid muscle.*	Head flexes 45°	Limited range of motion; painful movements; involuntary movements (e.g., up-and-down nodding movements associated with Parkinson's disease)
• Bend the head back so that the chin points upward. **Rationale:** *This determines function of the trapezius muscle.*	Head hyperextends 60°	Head hyperextends less than 60°
• Tilt the head so that the ear is moved toward the shoulder on each side. **Rationale:** *This determines function of the sternocleidomastoid muscle.*	Head laterally flexes 40°	Head laterally flexes less than 40°
• Turn the head to the right and to the left. **Rationale:** *This determines function of the sternocleidomastoid muscle.*	Head laterally rotates 70°	Head laterally rotates less than 70°

Continued on page 606

Assessing the Neck—*continued*

Assessment	Normal Findings	Deviations from Normal
7. Assess muscle strength. • Ask the client to turn the head to one side against the resistance of your hand. Repeat with the other side. **Rationale:** *This determines the strength of the sternocleidomastoid muscle.*	Equal strength	Unequal strength
• Ask the client to shrug the shoulders against the resistance of your hands. **Rationale:** *This determines the strength of the trapezius muscles.*	Equal strength	Unequal strength
LYMPH NODES		
8. Palpate the entire neck for enlarged lymph nodes. • Face the client, and bend the client's head forward slightly or toward the side being examined. **Rationale:** *This relaxes the soft tissue and muscles.* • Palpate the nodes using the pads of the fingers. Move the fingertips in a gentle rotating motion. • When examining the submental and submandibular nodes, place the fingertips under the mandible on the side nearest the palpating hand, and pull the skin and subcutaneous tissue laterally over the mandibular surface so that the tissue rolls over the nodes. • When palpating the supraclavicular nodes, have the client bend the head forward to relax the tissues of the anterior neck and to relax the shoulders so that the clavicles drop. Use your hand nearest the side to be examined when facing the client (i.e., your left hand for the client's right nodes). Use your free hand to flex the client's head forward if necessary. Hook your index and third fingers over the clavicle lateral to the sternocleidomastoid muscle. ❶ • When palpating the anterior cervical nodes and posterior cervical nodes, move your fingertips slowly in a forward circular motion against the sternocleidomastoid and trapezius muscles, respectively. • To palpate the deep cervical nodes, bend or hook your fingers around the sternocleidomastoid muscle.	Not palpable	Enlarged, palpable, possibly tender (associated with infection and tumors)
TRACHEA		
9. Palpate the trachea for lateral deviation. Place your fingertip or thumb on the trachea in the suprasternal notch (see Figure 29.19, earlier), and then move your finger laterally to the left and the right in spaces bordered by the clavicle, the anterior aspect of the sternocleidomastoid muscle, and the trachea.	Central placement in midline of neck; spaces are equal on both sides	Deviation to one side, indicating possible neck tumor; thyroid enlargement; enlarged lymph nodes

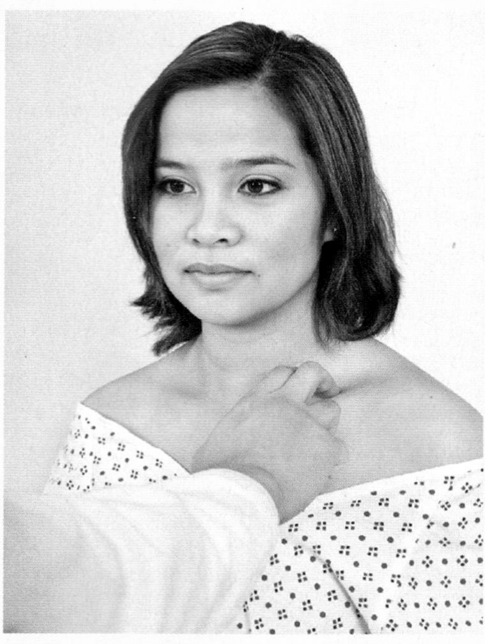

❶ Palpating the supraclavicular lymph nodes.
From *Health and Physical Assessment* (3rd ed. p. 275), by D. D'Amico and C. Barbarito, 2016. Boston, MA: Pearson.

Assessing the Neck—*continued*

Assessment	Normal Findings	Deviations from Normal
THYROID GLAND		
10. Inspect the thyroid gland. • Stand in front of the client. • Observe the lower half of the neck overlying the thyroid gland for symmetry and visible masses.	Not visible on inspection	Visible diffuseness or local enlargement
• Ask the client to extend the head and swallow. If necessary, offer a glass of water to make it easier for the client to swallow. **Rationale:** *This action determines how the thyroid and cricoid cartilages move and whether swallowing causes a bulging of the gland.*	Gland ascends during swallowing but is not visible	Gland is not fully movable with swallowing

11. Document findings in the client record using printed or electronic forms or checklists supplemented by narrative notes when appropriate.

EVALUATION

- Perform a detailed follow-up examination of other systems based on findings that deviated from expected or normal for the client. Relate findings to previous assessment data if available.
- Report deviations from expected or normal findings to the primary care provider.

LIFESPAN CONSIDERATIONS Assessing the Neck

INFANTS AND CHILDREN

- Examine the neck while the infant or child is lying supine. Lift the head and turn it gently from side to side to determine neck mobility.
- An infant's neck is normally short, lengthening by about age 3 years. This makes palpation of the trachea difficult.

underlying organs (e.g., lobes of the lung) and to record abnormal assessment findings. Figure 29.21 ■ shows the anterior, lateral, and posterior series of lines. The midsternal line is a vertical line running through the center of the sternum. The midclavicular lines (right and left) are vertical lines from the midpoints of the clavicles. The anterior axillary lines (right and left) are vertical lines from the anterior axillary folds (Figure 29.21*A*). Figure 29.21*B* shows the three imaginary lines of the lateral chest. The posterior axillary line is a vertical line from the posterior axillary fold. The midaxillary line is a vertical line from the apex of the axilla. Figure 29.21*C* shows the posterior chest landmarks. The vertebral line is a vertical line along the spinous processes. The scapular lines (right and left) are vertical lines from the inferior angles of the scapulae.

Locating the position of each rib and certain spinous processes is essential for identifying underlying lobes of the lung. Figure 29.22*A* ■ shows an anterior view of the chest and underlying lungs; Figure 29.22*B*, a posterior view; and Figure 29.22*C*, right and left lateral views.

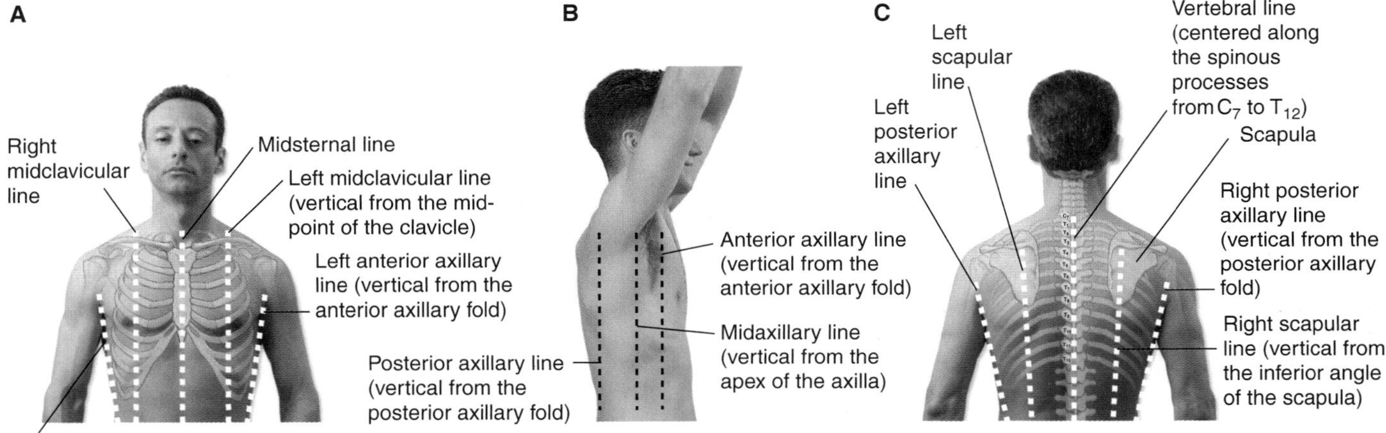

Figure 29.21 ■ Chest wall landmarks: *A*, anterior chest; *B*, lateral chest; *C*, posterior chest.

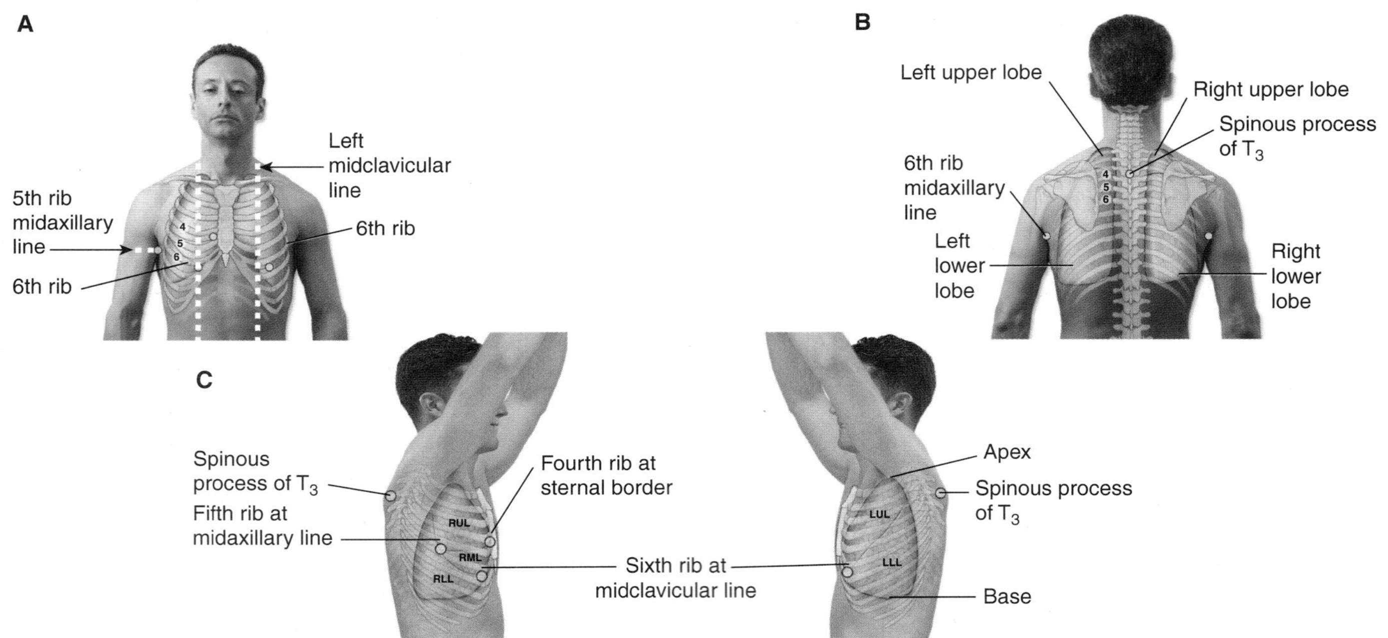

Figure 29.22 ■ Chest landmarks: *A*, anterior chest landmarks and underlying lungs; *B*, posterior chest landmarks and underlying lungs; *C*, lateral chest landmarks and underlying lungs.

Each lung is first divided into the upper and lower lobes by an oblique fissure that runs from the level of the spinous process of the third thoracic vertebra (T_3) to the level of the sixth rib at the midclavicular line. The right upper lobe is abbreviated RUL; the right lower lobe, RLL. Similarly, the left upper lobe is abbreviated LUL; the left lower lobe, LLL. The right lung is further divided by a minor fissure into the right upper lobe and right middle lobe (RML).

These specific landmarks (i.e., T_3 and the fourth, fifth, and sixth ribs) are located as follows. The starting point for locating the ribs anteriorly is the **angle of Louis**, the junction between the body of the **sternum** (breastbone) and the **manubrium** (the handle-like superior part of the sternum that joins with the clavicles). The superior border of the second rib attaches to the sternum at this manubrio-sternal junction (Figure 29.23 ■). The nurse can identify the manubrium by first palpating the clavicle and following its course to its attachment at the manubrium. The nurse then palpates and counts distal ribs and intercostal spaces (ICSs) from the second rib. It is important to note that an ICS is numbered according to the number of the rib immediately *above* the space. When palpating for rib identification, the nurse should palpate along the midclavicular line rather than the sternal border because the rib cartilages are very close at the sternum. Only the first seven ribs attach directly to the sternum.

The counting of ribs is more difficult on the posterior than on the anterior thorax. For identifying underlying lung lobes, the pertinent landmark is T_3. The starting point for locating T_3 is the spinous process of the seventh cervical vertebra (C_7) (Figure 29.24 ■). When the client flexes the neck anteriorly, a prominent process can be observed and palpated. This is the spinous process of the seventh cervical vertebra. If two spinous processes are observed, the superior one is C_7, and the inferior one is the spinous process of the first thoracic vertebra (T_1). The nurse then palpates and counts the

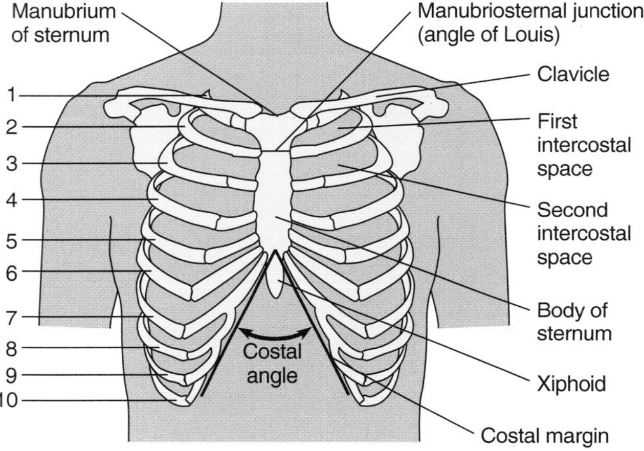

Figure 29.23 ■ Location of the anterior ribs, the angle of Louis, and the sternum.

spinous processes from C_7 to T_3. Each spinous process up to T_4 is adjacent to the corresponding rib number; for example, T_3 is adjacent to the third rib. After T_4, however, the spinous processes project obliquely, causing the spinous process of the vertebra to lie, not over its correspondingly numbered rib, but over the rib below. Thus, the spinous process of T_5 lies over the body of T_6 and is adjacent to the sixth rib.

Chest Shape and Size

In healthy adults, the thorax is oval. Its anteroposterior diameter is half its transverse diameter (Figure 29.25 ■). The overall shape of the thorax is elliptical; that is, its transverse diameter is smaller at the top than at the base. In older adults, kyphosis and osteoporosis alter the size of the chest cavity as the ribs move downward and forward.

There are several deformities of the chest (Figure 29.26 ■). Pigeon chest (*pectus carinatum*), a permanent

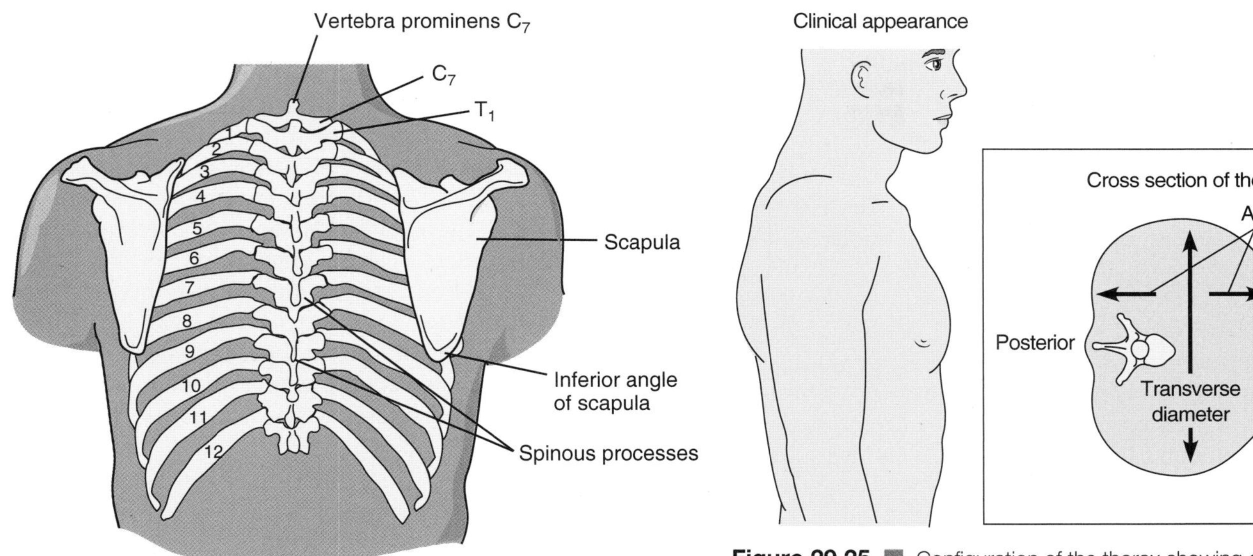

Figure 29.24 ■ Location of the posterior ribs in relation to the spinous processes.

Figure 29.25 ■ Configuration of the thorax showing oval shape, anteroposterior diameter, and transverse diameter.

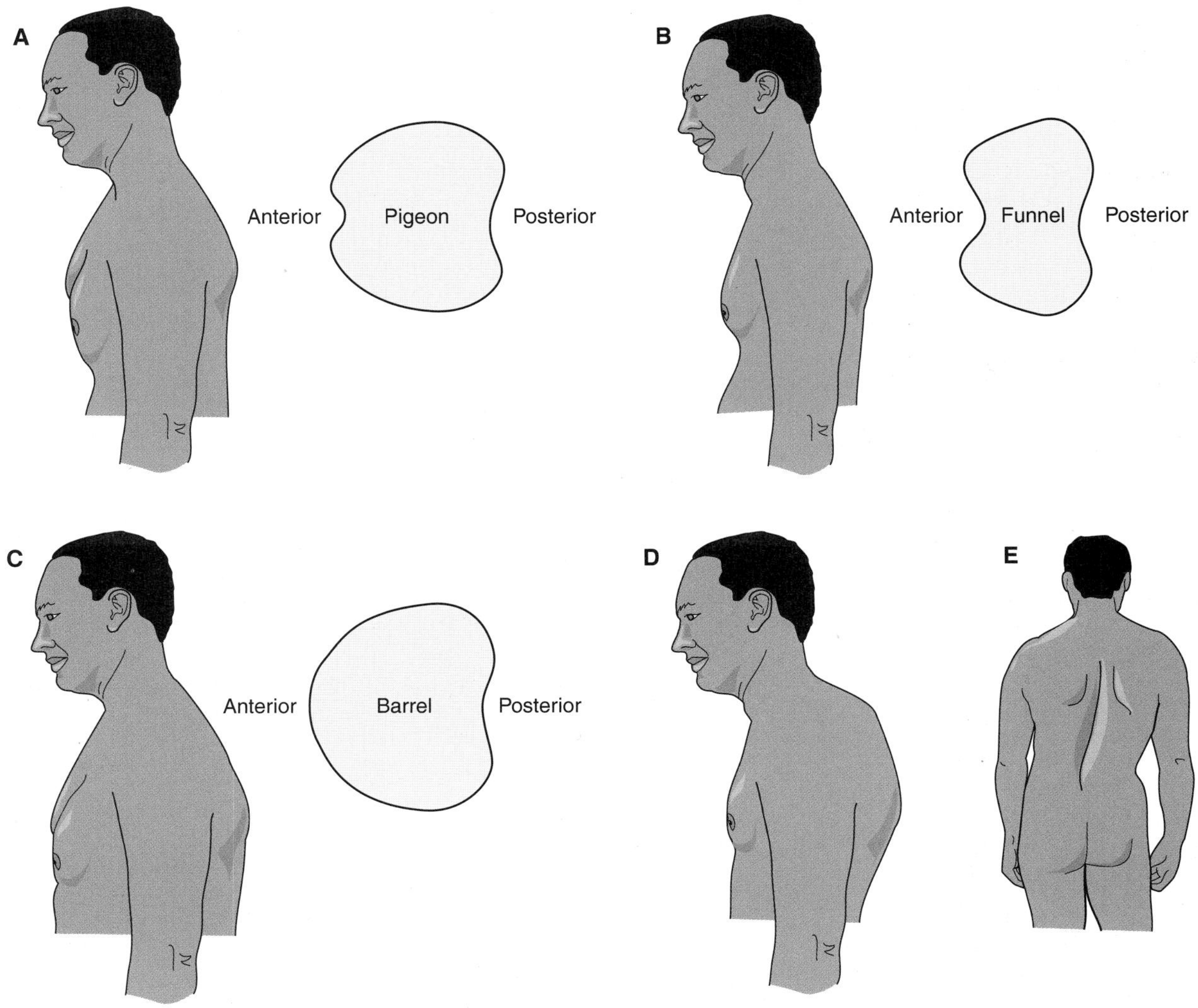

A

Anterior Pigeon Posterior

B

Anterior Funnel Posterior

C

Anterior Barrel Posterior

D

E

Figure 29.26 ■ Chest deformities: *A*, pigeon chest; *B*, funnel chest; *C*, barrel chest; *D*, kyphosis; *E*, scoliosis.

deformity, may be caused by rickets (abnormal bone formation due to lack of dietary calcium). A narrow transverse diameter, an increased anteroposterior diameter, and a protruding sternum characterize pigeon chest. A funnel chest (*pectus excavatum*), a congenital defect, is the opposite of pigeon chest in that the sternum is depressed, narrowing the anteroposterior diameter. Because the sternum points posteriorly in clients with a funnel chest, abnormal pressure on the heart may result in altered function. A barrel chest, in which the ratio of the anteroposterior to transverse diameter is 1 to 1, is seen in clients with thoracic kyphosis (excessive convex curvature of the thoracic spine) and emphysema (chronic pulmonary condition in which the air sacs, or alveoli, are dilated and distended). Scoliosis is a lateral deviation of the spine.

Breath Sounds

Abnormal breath sounds, called **adventitious breath sounds**, occur when air passes through narrowed airways or airways filled with fluid or mucus, or when pleural linings are inflamed. Table 29.7 describes normal breath sounds. Adventitious sounds are often superimposed over normal sounds (Table 29.8). Absence of breath sounds over some lung areas is also a significant finding that is associated with collapsed and surgically removed lobes or severe pneumonia.

Assessment of the lungs and thorax includes all methods of examination: inspection, palpation, percussion, and auscultation. Skill 29.11 describes how to assess the thorax and lungs.

TABLE 29.7 Normal Breath Sounds

Type	Description	Location	Characteristics
Vesicular	Soft-intensity, low-pitched, "gentle sighing" sounds created by air moving through smaller airways (bronchioles and alveoli)	Over peripheral lung; best heard at base of lungs	Best heard on inspiration, which is about 2.5 times longer than the expiratory phase (5:2 ratio)
Bronchovesicular	Moderate-intensity and moderate-pitched "blowing" sounds created by air moving through larger airway (bronchi)	Between the scapulae and lateral to the sternum at the first and second intercostal spaces	Equal inspiratory and expiratory phases (1:1 ratio)
Bronchial (tubular)	High-pitched, loud, "harsh" sounds created by air moving through the trachea	Anteriorly over the trachea; not normally heard over lung tissue	Louder than vesicular sounds; have a short inspiratory phase and long expiratory phase (1:2 ratio)

TABLE 29.8 Adventitious Breath Sounds

Name	Description	Cause	Location
Crackles (rales)	Fine, short, interrupted crackling sounds; alveolar rales are high pitched. Sound can be simulated by rolling a lock of hair near the ear. Best heard on inspiration but can be heard on both inspiration and expiration. May not be cleared by coughing.	Air passing through fluid or mucus in any air passage	Most commonly heard in the bases of the lower lung lobes
Gurgles (rhonchi)	Continuous, low-pitched, coarse, gurgling, harsh, louder sounds with a moaning or snoring quality. Best heard on expiration but can be heard on both inspiration and expiration. May be altered by coughing.	Air passing through narrowed air passages as a result of secretions, swelling, tumors	Loud sounds can be heard over most lung areas but predominate over the trachea and bronchi
Friction rub	Superficial grating or creaking sounds heard during inspiration and expiration. Not relieved by coughing.	Rubbing together of inflamed pleural surfaces	Heard most often in areas of greatest thoracic expansion (e.g., lower anterior and lateral chest)
Wheeze	Continuous, high-pitched, squeaky musical sounds. Best heard on expiration. Not usually altered by coughing.	Air passing through a constricted bronchus as a result of secretions, swelling, tumors	Heard over all lung fields

Assessing the Thorax and Lungs

PLANNING

For efficiency, the nurse usually examines the posterior thorax first, then the anterior thorax. For posterior and lateral thorax examinations, the client is uncovered to the waist and in a sitting position. A sitting or lying position may be used for anterior thorax examination. The sitting position is preferred because it maximizes thorax expansion. Good lighting is essential, especially for thorax inspection.

Equipment

- Stethoscope

Assignment

Due to the substantial knowledge and skill required, assessment of the thorax and lungs is not assigned to AP. However, many aspects of breathing are observed during usual care and may be recorded by individuals other than the nurse. Abnormal findings must be validated and interpreted by the nurse.

IMPLEMENTATION

Performance

1. Prior to performing the assessment, introduce self and verify the client's identity using agency protocol. Explain to the client what you are going to do, why it is necessary, and how to participate. Discuss how the results will be used in planning further care or treatments.
2. Perform hand hygiene and observe other appropriate infection prevention procedures.
3. Provide for client privacy. For females, drape the anterior thorax when it is not being examined.
4. Inquire if the client has any history of the following: family history of illness, including cancer, allergies, tuberculosis; lifestyle habits such as smoking and occupational hazards (e.g., inhaling fumes); medications being taken; current problems (e.g., swellings, coughs, wheezing, pain).

Assessment	Normal Findings	Deviations from Normal
POSTERIOR THORAX		
5. Inspect the shape and symmetry of the thorax from posterior and lateral views. Compare the anteroposterior diameter to the transverse diameter.	Anteroposterior to transverse diameter in ratio of 1:2 Thorax symmetric	Barrel chest; increased anteroposterior to transverse diameter Thorax asymmetric
6. Inspect the spinal alignment for deformities if the client can stand. From a lateral position, observe the three normal curvatures: cervical, thoracic, and lumbar.	Spine vertically aligned	Exaggerated spinal curvatures (kyphosis, lordosis)
• To assess for lateral deviation of spine (scoliosis), observe the standing client from the rear. Have the client bend forward at the waist and observe from behind.	Spinal column is straight, right and left shoulders and hips are at same height.	Spinal column deviates to one side, often accentuated when bending over. Shoulders or hips not even.
7. Palpate the posterior thorax.		
• Assess the temperature and integrity of all chest skin.	Skin intact; uniform temperature	Skin lesions; areas of hyperthermia
• For clients who have respiratory complaints, palpate all thorax areas for bulges, tenderness, or abnormal movements. Avoid deep palpation for painful areas, especially if a fractured rib is suspected. In such a case, deep palpation could lead to displacement of the bone fragment against the lungs.	Chest wall intact; no tenderness; no masses	Lumps, bulges; depressions; areas of tenderness; movable structures (e.g., rib)
8. Palpate the posterior thorax for thoracic expansion. Place the palms of both your hands over the lower thorax with your thumbs adjacent to the spine and your fingers stretched laterally. ❶ Ask the client to take a deep breath while you observe the movement of your hands and any lag in movement.	Full and symmetric thorax expansion (i.e., when the client takes a deep breath, your thumbs should move apart an equal distance and at the same time; normally the thumbs separate 3 to 5 cm [1.2 to 2 in.] during deep inspiration)	Asymmetric or decreased thorax expansion

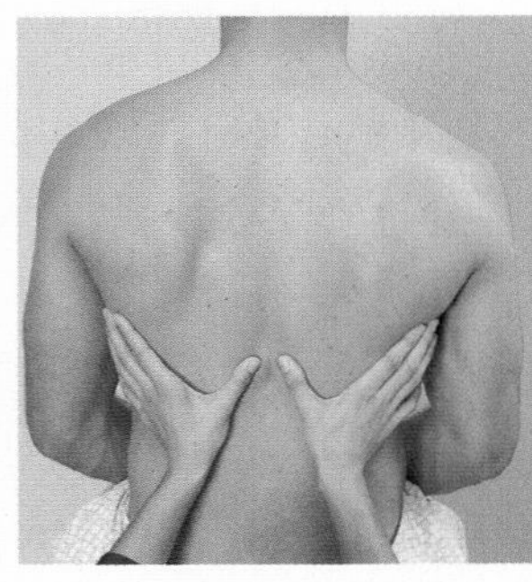

❶ Position of the nurse's hands when assessing respiratory expansion on the posterior thorax.

Continued on page 612

SKILL 29.11

Assessing the Thorax and Lungs—*continued*

Assessment	Normal Findings	Deviations from Normal
9. Palpate the thorax for **fremitus**, the faintly perceptible vibration felt through the chest wall when the client speaks (tactile fremitus). • Place the palmar surfaces of your fingertips or the ulnar aspect of your hand or closed fist on the posterior thorax, starting near the apex of the lungs (see ❷, position A). • Ask the client to repeat such phrases as "blue moon" or "one, two, three." • Repeat the two steps, moving your hands sequentially to the base of the lungs, through positions B–E in ❷. • Compare the fremitus on both lungs and between the apex and the base of each lung, using either one hand and moving it from one side of the client to the corresponding area on the other side *or* using two hands that are placed simultaneously on the corresponding areas of each side of the thorax.	Bilateral symmetry of fremitus Fremitus is felt most clearly at the apex of the lungs Low-pitched voices of males are more readily palpated than higher pitched voices of females	Decreased or absent fremitus (associated with pneumothorax) Increased fremitus (associated with consolidated lung tissue, as in pneumonia)

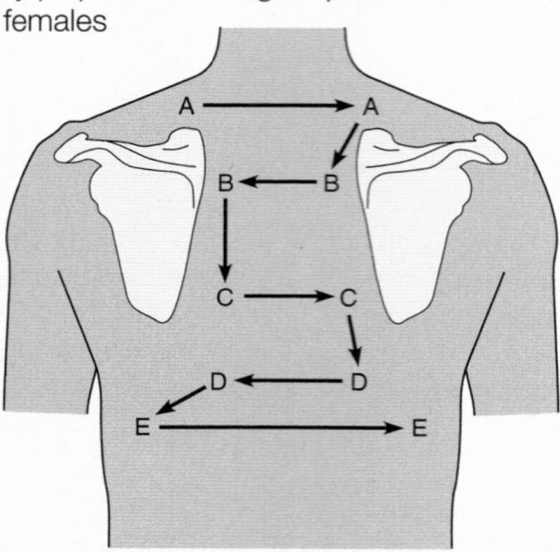

❷ Areas and sequence in palpating for tactile fremitus on the posterior thorax.

Assessment	Normal Findings	Deviations from Normal
10. Percuss the thorax. Percussion of the thorax is performed to determine whether underlying lung tissue is filled with air, liquid, or solid material and to determine the positions and boundaries of certain organs. Because percussion penetrates to a depth of 5 to 7 cm (2 to 3 in.), it detects superficial rather than deep lesions (see ❸ and Table 29.4, earlier). • Ask the client to bend the head and fold the arms forward across the chest. **Rationale:** *This separates the scapula and exposes more lung tissue to percussion*. • Percuss in the intercostal spaces at about 5-cm (2-in.) intervals in a systematic sequence. ❹ • Compare one side of the lung with the other. • Percuss the lateral thorax every few inches, starting at the axilla and working down to the eighth rib.	Percussion notes resonate, except over scapula Lowest point of resonance is at the diaphragm (i.e., at the level of the 8th to 10th rib posteriorly) *Note:* Percussion on a rib normally elicits dullness.	Asymmetry in percussion notes Areas of dullness or flatness over lung tissue (associated with consolidation of lung tissue or a mass)
11. Auscultate the thorax using the flat-disk diaphragm of the stethoscope. **Rationale:** *The diaphragm of the stethoscope is best for transmitting the high-pitched breath sounds*. • Use the systematic zigzag procedure used in percussion. • Ask the client to take slow, deep breaths through the mouth. Listen at each point to the breath sounds during a complete inspiration and expiration. • Compare findings at each point with the corresponding point on the opposite side of the thorax.	Vesicular and bronchovesicular breath sounds (see Table 29.7)	Adventitious breath sounds (e.g., crackles, gurgles, wheeze, friction rub; see Table 29.8) Absence of breath sounds

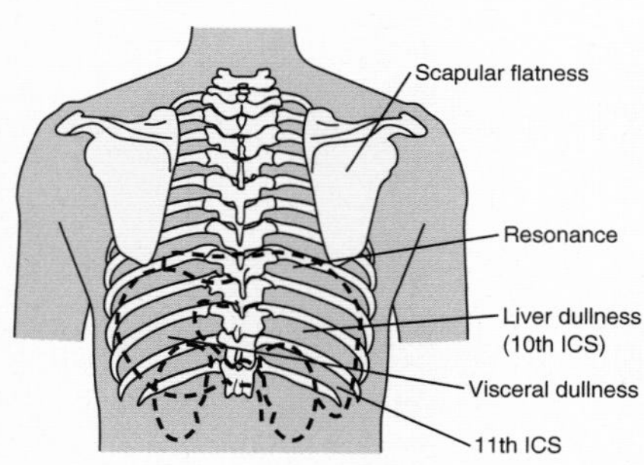

❸ Normal percussion sounds on the posterior thorax.

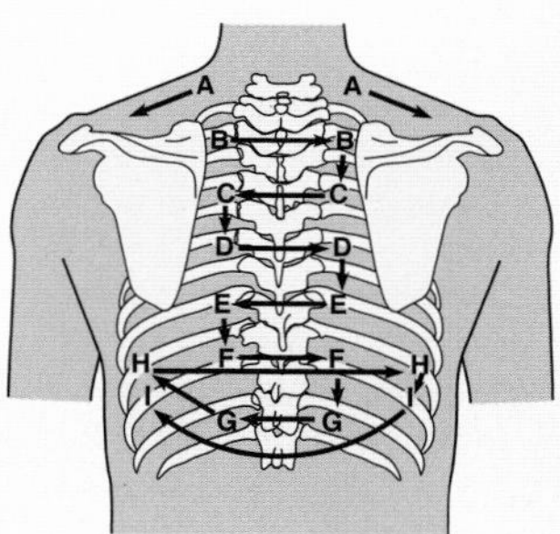

❹ Sequence for posterior thorax percussion.

Assessing the Thorax and Lungs—*continued*

Assessment	Normal Findings	Deviations from Normal
ANTERIOR THORAX		
12. Inspect breathing patterns (e.g., respiratory rate and rhythm).	Quiet, rhythmic, and effortless respirations (see Chapter 28 ∞, page 532)	See Chapter 28 ∞, Box 28.7 on page 554, for abnormal breathing patterns and sounds.
13. Inspect the costal angle (angle formed by the intersection of the costal margins) and the angle at which the ribs enter the spine.	Costal angle is less than 90°, and the ribs insert into the spine at approximately a 45° angle (see Figure 29.23, earlier)	Costal angle is widened (associated with chronic obstructive pulmonary disease)
14. Palpate the anterior thorax (see posterior thorax palpation).		
15. Palpate the anterior thorax for respiratory expansion. • Place the palms of both your hands on the lower thorax, with your fingers laterally along the lower rib cage and your thumbs along the costal margins. ❺ • Ask the client to take a deep breath while you observe the movement of your hands.	Full symmetric expansion; thumbs normally separate 3 to 5 cm (1.2 to 2 in.) 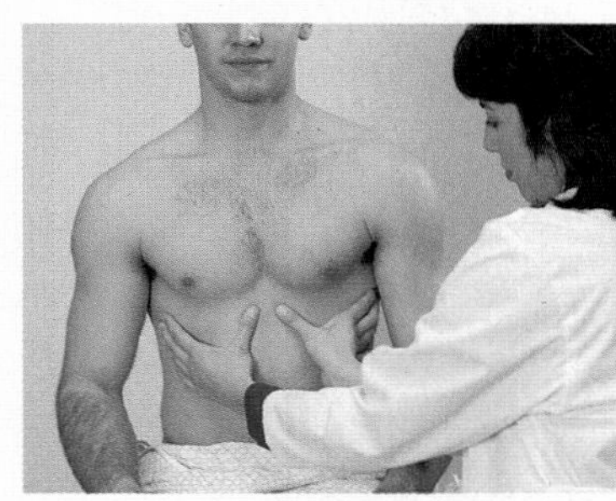 ❺ Position of the nurse's hands when assessing respiratory expansion on the anterior thorax.	Asymmetric or decreased respiratory expansion
16. Palpate for tactile fremitus in the same manner as for the posterior thorax and using the sequence shown in ❻. If the breasts are large and cannot be retracted adequately for palpation, this part of the examination is usually omitted.	Same as posterior fremitus; fremitus is normally decreased over heart and breast tissue 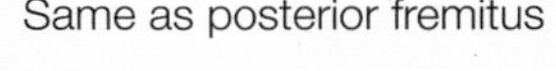 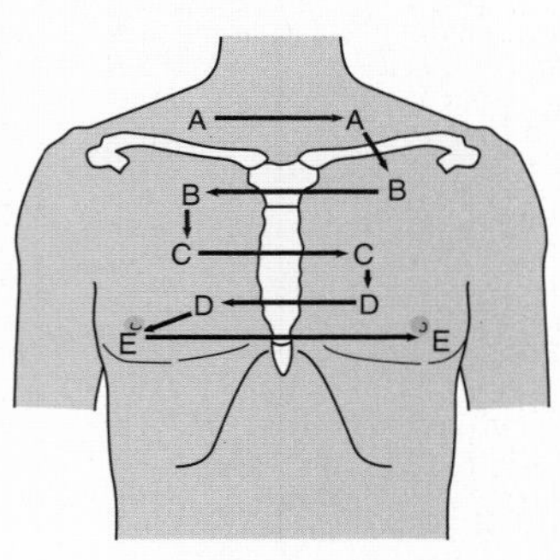 ❻ Areas and sequence in palpating for tactile fremitus on the anterior thorax.	Same as posterior fremitus
17. Percuss the anterior thorax systematically. • Begin above the clavicles in the supraclavicular space, and proceed downward to the diaphragm. ❼ • Compare the lung on one side to the lung on the other side. • Displace female breasts to facilitate percussion of the lungs.	Percussion notes resonate down to the sixth rib at the level of the diaphragm but are flat over areas of heavy muscle and bone, dull on areas over the heart and the liver, and tympanic over the underlying stomach. ❽ 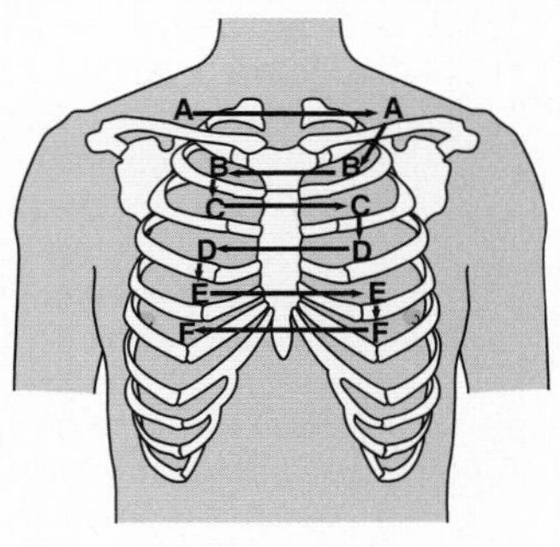 ❼ Sequence for anterior thorax percussion. 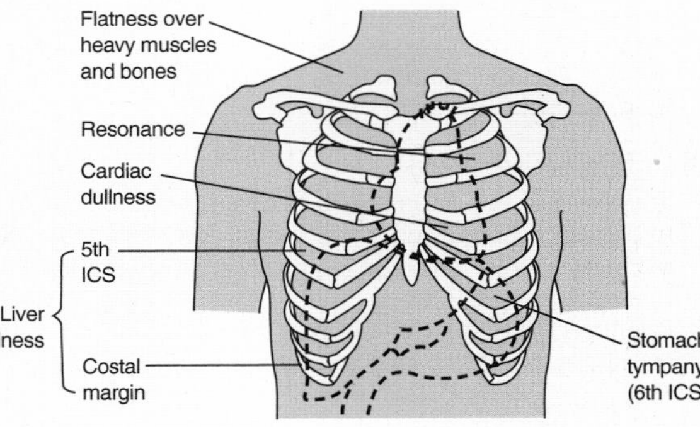 ❽ Normal percussion sounds on the anterior thorax.	Asymmetry in percussion notes Areas of dullness or flatness over lung tissue

Continued on page 614

SKILL 29.11

Assessing the Thorax and Lungs—*continued*

Assessment	Normal Findings	Deviations from Normal
18. Auscultate the trachea	Bronchial and tubular breath sounds (see Table 29.7 on page 610)	Adventitious breath sounds (see Table 29.8 on page 610)
19. Auscultate the anterior thorax. Use the sequence used in percussion 7, beginning over the bronchi between the sternum and the clavicles.	Bronchovesicular and vesicular breath sounds (see Table 29.7)	Adventitious breath sounds (see Table 29.8)

20. Document findings in the client record using printed or electronic forms or checklists supplemented by narrative notes when appropriate.

SAMPLE DOCUMENTATION

5/28/2020 0830 Lungs clear to auscultation except for fine crackles over both posterior lower lobes, partially cleared after coughing. Rarely moves in bed. Assisted to a chair and reviewed deep-breathing exercises. Effective return demonstration. N. Schmidt, RN

EVALUATION

- Perform a detailed follow-up examination based on findings that deviated from expected or normal for the client. Relate findings to previous assessment data if available.
- Report deviations from expected or normal findings to the primary care provider.

LIFESPAN CONSIDERATIONS Assessing the Thorax and Lungs

INFANTS

The thorax is rounded; that is, the diameter from the front to the back (anteroposterior) is equal to the transverse diameter (Figure 29.27 ■). It is also cylindrical, having a nearly equal diameter at the top and the base. This makes it harder for infants to expand their thoracic space.

- To assess tactile fremitus, place the hand over the crying infant's thorax.
- Infants tend to breathe using their diaphragm; assess rate and rhythm by watching the abdomen, rather than the thorax, rise and fall.
- The right bronchial branch is short and angles down as it leaves the trachea, making it easy for small objects to be inhaled. Sudden onset of cough or other signs of respiratory distress may indicate the infant has inhaled a foreign object.

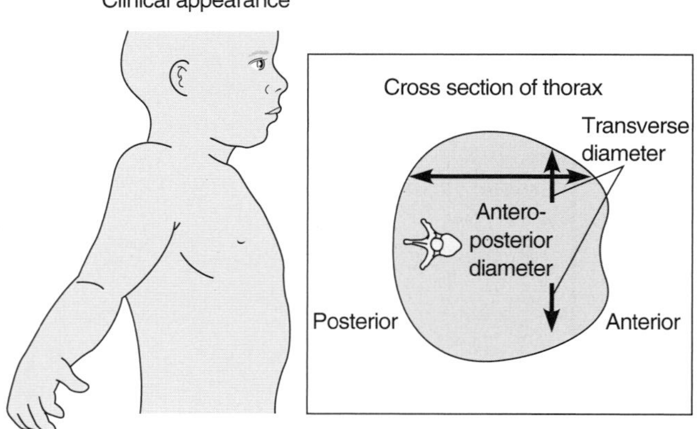

Figure 29.27 ■ Configuration of the infant's thorax showing round shape, anteroposterior diameter, and transverse diameter.

CHILDREN

- By about 6 years of age, the anteroposterior diameter has decreased in proportion to the transverse diameter, with a 1:2 ratio present.
- Children tend to breathe more abdominally than thoracically up to age 6.
- During the rapid growth spurts of adolescence, spinal curvature and rotation (scoliosis) may appear. Children should be assessed for scoliosis by age 12 and annually until their growth slows. Curvature greater than 10% should be referred for further medical evaluation.

OLDER ADULTS

- The thoracic curvature may be accentuated (kyphosis) because of osteoporosis and changes in cartilage, resulting in collapse of the vertebrae. This can also compromise and decrease normal respiratory effort.
- Kyphosis and osteoporosis alter the size of the thorax cavity as the ribs move downward and forward.
- The anteroposterior diameter of the thorax widens, giving the individual a barrel-chested appearance. This is due to loss of skeletal muscle strength in the thorax and diaphragm and constant lung inflation from excessive expiratory pressure on the alveoli.
- Breathing rate and rhythm are unchanged at rest; the rate normally increases with exercise but may take longer to return to the pre-exercise rate.
- Inspiratory muscles become less powerful, and the inspiration reserve volume decreases. A decrease in depth of respiration is therefore apparent.
- Expiration may require the use of accessory muscles. The expiratory reserve volume significantly increases because of the increased amount of air remaining in the lungs at the end of a normal breath.
- Deflation of the lung is incomplete.
- Small airways lose their cartilaginous support and elastic recoil; as a result, they tend to close, particularly in basal or dependent portions of the lung.
- Elastic tissue of the alveoli loses its stretchability and changes to fibrous tissue. Exertional capacity decreases.
- Cilia in the airways decrease in number and are less effective in removing mucus; older clients are therefore at greater risk for pulmonary infections.

Cardiovascular and Peripheral Vascular Systems

The cardiovascular system consists of the heart and the central blood vessels (primarily the pulmonary, coronary, and neck arteries and veins). The peripheral vascular system includes those arteries and veins distal to the central vessels, extending all the way to the brain and to the extremities.

Heart

Nurses assess the heart through inspection, palpation, and auscultation, in that sequence. Auscultation is more meaningful when other data are obtained first. The heart is usually assessed during an initial physical assessment; periodic reassessments may be necessary for long-term or at-risk clients or those with cardiac problems. Also see Chapter 50 ∞.

In the average adult, most of the heart lies behind and to the left of the sternum. A small portion (the right atrium) extends to the right of the sternum. The upper portion of the heart (both atria), referred to as its *base*, lies toward the back. The lower portion (the ventricles), referred to as its *apex*, points anteriorly. The apex of the left ventricle actually touches the chest wall at or medial to the left midclavicular line (MCL) and at or near the fifth left intercostal space (LICS), which is slightly below the left nipple (see Figure 2 in Skill 29.12 on page 617). The point where the apex touches the anterior chest wall and heart movements are most easily observed and palpated is known as the point of maximal impulse (PMI).

Clinical Alert!

Remember that the base of the lungs is the lower (inferior) portion, and the base of the heart is the upper (superior) portion.

The **precordium**, the area of the chest overlying the heart, is inspected and palpated for the presence of abnormal pulsations or lifts or heaves. The terms **lift** and *heave*, often used interchangeably, refer to a rising along the sternal border with each heartbeat. A lift occurs when cardiac action is very forceful. It should be confirmed by palpation with the palm of the hand. Enlargement or overactivity of the left ventricle produces a heave lateral to the apex, whereas enlargement of the right ventricle produces a heave at or near the sternum.

Heart sounds can be heard by auscultation. The normal first two heart sounds are produced by closure of the valves of the heart. The first heart sound, **S_1**, occurs when the atrioventricular (AV) valves close. These valves close when the ventricles have been sufficiently filled. Although the AV valves do not close simultaneously, the closure occurs closely enough to be heard as one sound. S_1 is a dull, low-pitched sound described as "lub." After the ventricles empty the blood into the aorta and pulmonary arteries, the semilunar valves close, producing the second heart sound, **S_2**, described as "dub." S_2 has a higher pitch than S_1 and is shorter in duration. These two sounds, S_1 and S_2 ("lub-dub"), occur within 1 second or less, depending on the heart rate.

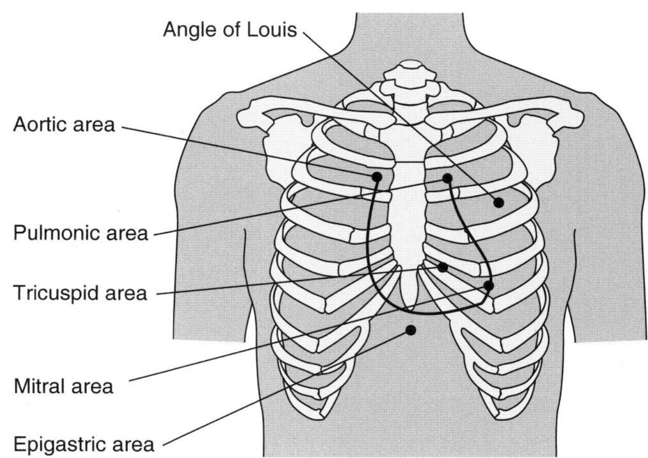

Figure 29.28 ■ Anatomic sites of the precordium.

The two heart sounds are audible anywhere on the precordial area, but they are best heard over the aortic, pulmonic, tricuspid, and mitral areas (Figure 29.28 ■). Each area is associated with the closure of heart valves: the aortic area with the aortic valve (inside the aorta as it arises from the left ventricle); the pulmonic area with the pulmonic valve (inside the pulmonary artery as it arises from the right ventricle); the tricuspid area with the tricuspid valve (between the right atrium and ventricle); and the mitral area (sometimes referred to as the apical area) with the mitral valve (between the left atrium and ventricle).

Associated with these sounds are systole and diastole. **Systole** is the period in which the ventricles contract. It begins with S_1 and ends at S_2. Systole is normally shorter than diastole. **Diastole** is the period in which the ventricles relax. It starts with S_2 and ends at the subsequent S_1. Normally no sounds are audible during these periods (Figure 29.29 ■). The experienced nurse, however, may perceive extra heart sounds (S_3 and S_4) during diastole. Both sounds are low in pitch and heard best at the apex, with the bell of the stethoscope, and with the client lying on the left side. S_3 occurs early in diastole right after S_2 and sounds like "lub-dub-*ee*" (S_1, S_2, S_3) or "Kentuc-*ky*." It often disappears when the client sits up. S_3 is normal in children and young adults. In older adults, it may indicate heart failure. The S_4 sound (ventricular gallop) occurs near the very end of diastole just before S_1 and creates the sound of "*dee*-lub-dub" (S_4, S_1, S_2) or "*Ten*-nessee." S_4 may be heard in older clients and can be a sign of hypertension.

Normal heart sounds are summarized in Table 29.9. The nurse may also hear abnormal heart sounds, such as clicks, rubs, and murmurs. These are caused by valve disorders or impaired blood flow within the heart and require advanced training to diagnose.

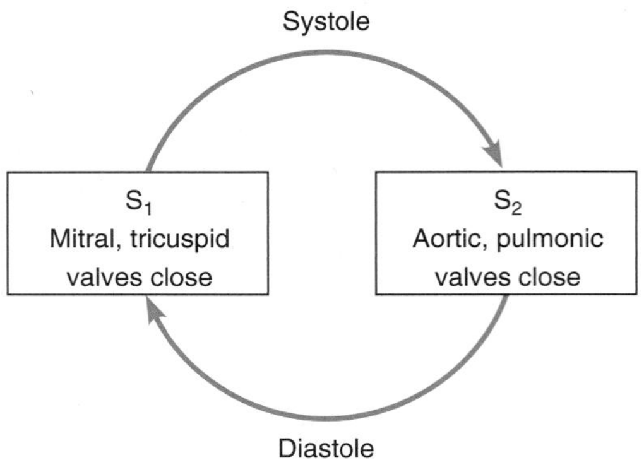

Figure 29.29 ■ Relationship of heart sounds to systole and diastole.

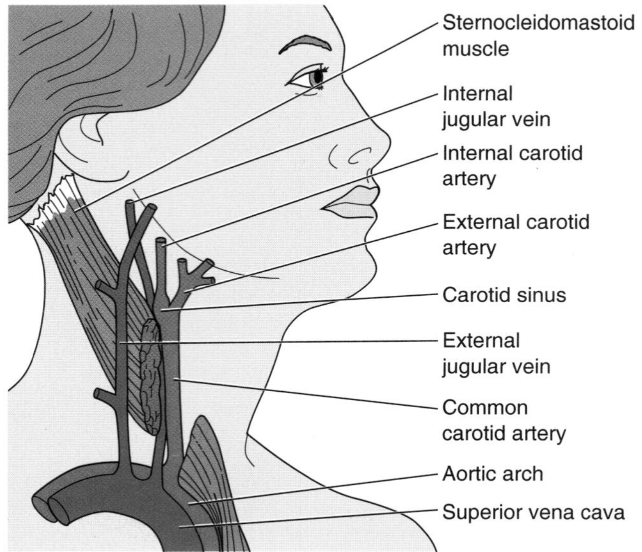

Figure 29.30 ■ Arteries and veins of the right side of the neck.

Central Vessels

The carotid arteries supply oxygenated blood to the head and neck (Figure 29.30 ■). Because they are the only source of blood to the brain, prolonged occlusion of these arteries can result in serious brain damage. The carotid pulses correlate with central aortic pressure, thus reflecting cardiac function better than the peripheral pulses. When cardiac output is diminished, the peripheral pulses may be difficult or impossible to feel, but the carotid pulse should be felt easily.

The carotid is also auscultated for a bruit. A **bruit** (a blowing or swishing sound) is created by turbulence of blood flow due either to a narrowed arterial lumen (a common development in older people) or to a condition, such as anemia or hyperthyroidism, that elevates cardiac output. If a bruit is found, the carotid artery is then palpated for a thrill. A **thrill**, which frequently accompanies a bruit, is a vibrating sensation like the purring of a cat or water running through a hose. It, too, indicates turbulent blood flow due to arterial obstruction.

The jugular veins drain blood from the head and neck directly into the superior vena cava and right side of the heart. The external jugular veins are superficial and may be visible above the clavicle. The internal jugular veins lie deeper along the carotid artery and may transmit pulsations onto the skin of the neck. Normally, external neck veins are distended and visible when a client lies down; they are flat and not as visible when a client stands up, because gravity promotes venous drainage. By inspecting the jugular veins for pulsations and distention, the nurse can assess the adequacy of function of the right side of the heart and venous pressure. Bilateral jugular venous distention (JVD) may indicate right-sided heart failure. Skill 29.12 describes how to assess the heart and central vessels.

TABLE 29.9 Normal Heart Sounds

			Area		
Sound or Phase	**Description**	**Aortic**	**Pulmonic**	**Tricuspid**	**Mitral**
S_1	Dull, low pitched, and longer than S_2; sounds like "lub"	Less intensity than S_2	Less intensity than S_2	Louder than or equal to S_2	Louder than or equal to S_2
Systole	Normally silent interval between S_1 and S_2				
S_2	Higher pitch than S_1; sounds like "dub"	Louder than S_1	Louder than S_1; abnormal if louder than the aortic S_2 in adults over 40 years of age	Less intensity than or equal to S_1	Less intensity than or equal to S_1
Diastole	Normally silent interval between S_2 and next S_1				

Assessing the Heart and Central Vessels

SKILL 29.12

PLANNING

Heart examination is usually performed while the client is in a semi-Fowler's position. The practitioner usually stands at the client's right side and auscultates and palpates with the right hand, but this may be reversed if the nurse is left-handed.

Assignment

Due to the substantial knowledge and skill required, assessment of the heart and central vessels is not assigned to AP. However, many aspects of cardiac function are observed during usual care and may be recorded by individuals other than the nurse. Abnormal findings must be validated and interpreted by the nurse.

Equipment

- Stethoscope
- Centimeter ruler

IMPLEMENTATION

Performance

1. Prior to performing the assessment, introduce self and verify the client's identity using agency protocol. Explain to the client what you are going to do, why it is necessary, and how to participate. Discuss how the results will be used in planning further care or treatments.
2. Perform hand hygiene and observe other appropriate infection prevention procedures.
3. Provide for client privacy.
4. Inquire if the client has any of the following: family history of incidence and age of heart disease, high cholesterol levels, high blood pressure, stroke, obesity, congenital heart disease, arterial disease, hypertension, and rheumatic fever; client's past history of rheumatic fever, heart murmur, heart attack, varicosities, or heart failure; present symptoms indicative of heart disease (e.g., fatigue, dyspnea, orthopnea, edema, cough, chest pain, palpitations, syncope, hypertension, wheezing, hemoptysis); presence of diseases that affect the heart (e.g., obesity, diabetes, lung disease, endocrine disorders); treatments that affect the heart (e.g., radiation therapy to the chest, cardiotoxic medications); lifestyle habits that are risk factors for cardiac disease (e.g., smoking, alcohol intake, eating and exercise patterns, areas and degree of stress perceived).

Assessment	Normal Findings	Deviations from Normal

5. Simultaneously inspect and palpate the precordium for the presence of abnormal pulsations, lifts, or heaves. Locate the valve areas of the heart:
   - Locate the angle of Louis. It is felt as a prominence on the sternum.
   - Move your fingertips laterally from each side of the angle until you feel the second intercostal spaces. At the edge of the sternum, the client's right second intercostal space is the aortic area, and the left second intercostal space is the pulmonic area. ❶ From the pulmonic area, move your fingertips down three left intercostal spaces along the edge of the sternum. The left fifth intercostal space close to the sternum is the tricuspid or right ventricular area.
   - From the tricuspid area, move your fingertips laterally 5 to 7 cm (2 to 3 in.) to the left midclavicular line. ❷ This is the apical or mitral area, or point of maximal impulse (PMI). If you have difficulty locating the PMI, have the client roll onto the left side to move the apex closer to the chest wall.

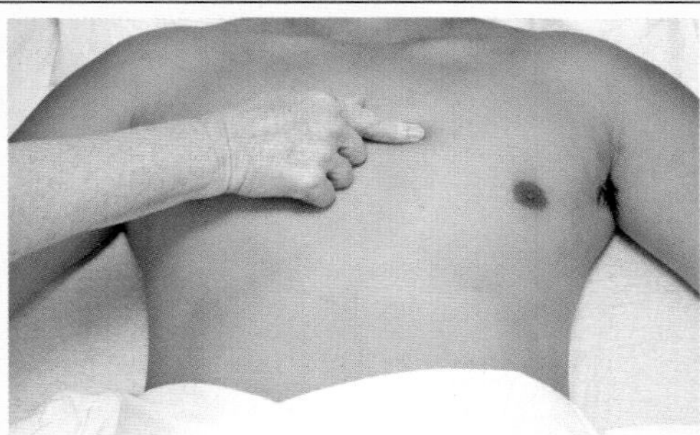

❶ Left second intercostal space.
Shirlee Snyder.

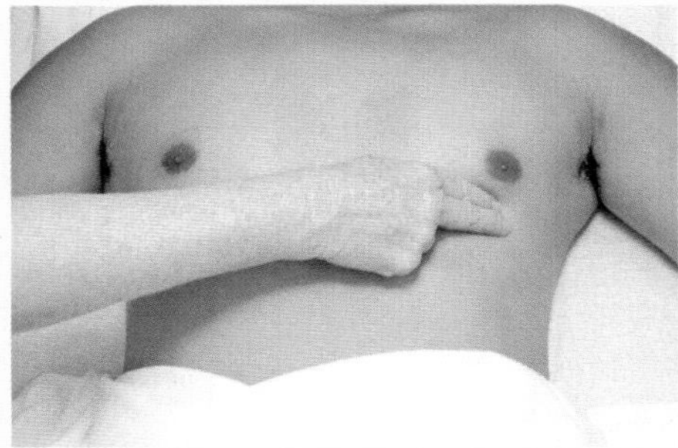

❷ Left fifth intercostal space, MCL.
Shirlee Snyder.

Continued on page 618

Assessing the Heart and Central Vessels—*continued*

Assessment	Normal Findings	Deviations from Normal
• Inspect and palpate the aortic and pulmonic areas, observing them at an angle to note the presence or absence of pulsations. Observing these areas at an angle increases the likelihood of seeing pulsations.	No pulsations	Pulsations
• Inspect and palpate the tricuspid area for pulsations and heaves or lifts.	No pulsations No lift or heave	Pulsations Diffuse lift or heave, indicating enlarged or overactive right ventricle
• Inspect and palpate the apical area for the strongest pulsation, noting its location (it may be displaced laterally or lower). If displaced laterally, record the distance between the apex and the MCL in centimeters.	Pulsations visible in 50% of adults and palpable in most PMI in fifth LICS at or medial to MCL No lift or heave	 PMI displaced laterally or lower indicates enlarged heart Diffuse lift or heave lateral to apex indicates enlargement or overactivity of left ventricle
• Inspect and palpate the epigastric area at the base of the sternum for abdominal aortic pulsations.	Aortic pulsations	Bounding abdominal pulsations (e.g., aortic aneurysm)
6. Auscultate the heart in all four anatomic sites: aortic, pulmonic, tricuspid, and apical (mitral). Auscultation need not be limited to these areas; the nurse may need to move the stethoscope to find the most audible sounds for each client. • Eliminate all sources of room noise. **Rationale:** *Heart sounds are of low intensity, and other noise hinders the nurse's ability to hear them*.	S_1: usually heard at all sites Usually louder at apical area S_2: usually heard at all sites Usually louder at base of heart Systole: silent interval; slightly shorter duration than diastole at normal heart rate (60 to 90 beats/min) Diastole: silent interval; slightly longer duration than systole at normal heart rates	Increased or decreased intensity Varying intensity with different beats Increased intensity at aortic area Increased intensity at pulmonic area Sharp-sounding ejection clicks
• Keep the client in a supine position with head elevated 15° to 45°. • Use both the diaphragm and the bell to listen to all areas. • In every area of auscultation, distinguish both S_1 and S_2 sounds. • When auscultating, concentrate on one particular sound at a time in each area: the first heart sound, followed by systole, then the second heart sound, then diastole. Systole and diastole are normally silent intervals. • Later, re-examine the heart while the client is in the upright sitting position. **Rationale:** *Certain sounds are more audible in certain positions*.	S_3 in children and young adults S_4 in many older adults	S_3 in older adults S_4 may be a sign of hypertension
CAROTID ARTERIES		
7. Palpate the carotid artery, using extreme caution.	Symmetric pulse volumes	Asymmetric volumes (possible stenosis or thrombosis)
• Palpate only one carotid artery at a time. **Rationale:** *This ensures adequate blood flow to the brain through the other artery.* • Avoid exerting too much pressure or massaging the area. **Rationale:** *Pressure can occlude the artery, and carotid sinus massage can precipitate bradycardia*. The carotid sinus is a small dilation at the beginning of the internal carotid artery just above the bifurcation of the common carotid artery, in the upper third of the neck. • Ask the client to turn the head slightly toward the side being examined. This makes the carotid artery more accessible.	Full pulsations, thrusting quality Quality remains same when client breathes, turns head, and changes from sitting to supine position Elastic arterial wall	Decreased pulsations (may indicate impaired left cardiac output) Increased pulsations Thickening, hard, rigid, beaded, inelastic walls (indicate arteriosclerosis)

Assessing the Heart and Central Vessels—*continued*

Assessment	Normal Findings	Deviations from Normal
8. Auscultate the carotid artery. • Turn the client's head slightly away from the side being examined. **Rationale:** *This facilitates placement of the stethoscope.* • Auscultate the carotid artery on one side and then the other. • Listen for the presence of a bruit. If you hear a bruit, gently palpate the artery to determine the presence of a thrill.	No sound heard on auscultation	Presence of bruit in one or both arteries (suggests occlusive artery disease)
JUGULAR VEINS		
9. Inspect the jugular veins for distention while the client is placed in the semi-Fowler's position (30° to 45° angle), with the head supported on a small pillow.	Veins not visible (indicating right side of heart is functioning normally)	Veins visibly distended (indicating advanced cardiopulmonary disease)
10. If jugular distention is present, assess the jugular venous pressure (JVP). • Locate the highest visible point of distention of the internal jugular vein. Although either the internal or the external jugular vein can be used, the internal jugular vein is more reliable. **Rationale:** *The external jugular vein is more easily affected by obstruction or kinking at the base of the neck.* • Measure the vertical height of this point in centimeters from the sternal angle, the point at which the clavicles meet. ❸ Repeat the preceding steps on the other side.	Distension less than 3 cm (1.2 in.)	Bilateral measurements above 3 to 4 cm (1.2 to 1.6 in.) are considered elevated (may indicate right-sided heart failure) Unilateral distention (may be caused by local obstruction)
11. Document findings in the client record using printed or electronic forms or checklists supplemented by narrative notes when appropriate.		

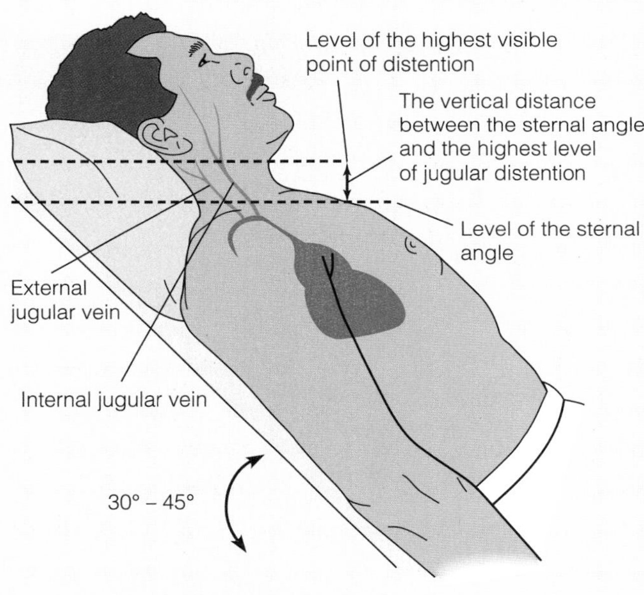

❸ Assessing the highest point of distention of the jugular vein.

EVALUATION

- Perform a detailed follow-up examination of other systems based on findings that deviated from expected or normal for the client. Relate findings to previous assessment data if available.
- Report deviations from expected or normal findings to the primary care provider.

LIFESPAN CONSIDERATIONS Assessing the Heart and Central Vessels

INFANTS

- Physiologic splitting of the second heart sound (S_2) may be heard when the child takes a deep breath and the aortic valve closes a split second before the pulmonic valve. If splitting of S_2 is heard during normal respirations, it is abnormal and may indicate an atrial-septal defect, pulmonary stenosis, or another heart problem.
- Infants may normally have sinus arrhythmia that is related to respiration. The heart rate slows during expiration and increases when the child breathes in.
- Murmurs may be heard in newborns as the structures of fetal circulation, especially the ductus arteriosus, close.

Continued on page 620

LIFESPAN CONSIDERATIONS Assessing the Heart and Central Vessels—*continued*

CHILDREN

- Heart sounds may be louder because of the thinner chest wall.
- A third heart sound (S_3), caused as the ventricles fill, is best heard at the apex, and is present in about one third of all children.
- The PMI is higher and more medial in children under 8 years old.

OLDER ADULTS

- If no disease is present, heart size remains the same size throughout life.
- Cardiac output and strength of contraction decrease, thus lessening the older individual's activity tolerance.
- The heart rate returns to its resting rate more slowly after exertion than it did when the individual was younger.
- S_4 heart sound is considered normal in older adults.
- Extra systoles commonly occur. Ten or more systoles per minute are considered abnormal.
- Sudden emotional and physical stresses may result in cardiac arrhythmias and heart failure.

Peripheral Vascular System

Assessing the peripheral vascular system includes measuring the blood pressure, palpating peripheral pulses, and inspecting the skin and tissues to determine **perfusion** (blood supply to an area) to the extremities. Certain aspects of peripheral vascular assessment are often incorporated into other parts of the assessment procedure. For example, blood pressure is usually measured at the beginning of the physical examination (see the section on assessing blood pressure in Chapter 28 ∞). Pulse sites and pulse assessments are described in Chapter 28 ∞. Skill 29.13 describes how to assess the peripheral vascular system.

SKILL 29.13

Assessing the Peripheral Vascular System

PLANNING

Assignment

Due to the substantial knowledge and skill required, assessment of the peripheral vascular system is not assigned to AP. However, many aspects of the vascular system are observed during usual care and may be recorded by individuals other than the nurse. Abnormal findings must be validated and interpreted by the nurse.

Equipment

- None

IMPLEMENTATION

Performance

1. Prior to performing the assessment, introduce self and verify the client's identity using agency protocol. Explain to the client what you are going to do, why it is necessary, and how to participate. Discuss how the results will be used in planning further care or treatments.
2. Perform hand hygiene and observe other appropriate infection prevention procedures.
3. Provide for client privacy.
4. Inquire if the client has any of the following: past history of heart disorders, varicosities, arterial disease, and hypertension; lifestyle habits such as exercise patterns, activity patterns and tolerance, smoking, and use of alcohol.

Assessment	Normal Findings	Deviations from Normal
PERIPHERAL PULSES		
5. Palpate the peripheral pulses on both sides of the client's body individually, simultaneously (except the carotid pulse), and systematically to determine the symmetry of pulse volume. If you have difficulty palpating some of the peripheral pulses, use a Doppler ultrasound stethoscope.	Symmetric pulse volumes	Asymmetric volumes (indicate impaired circulation) Absence of pulsation (indicates arterial spasm or occlusion) Decreased, weak, thready pulsations (indicate impaired cardiac output) Full or bounding pulse volume (may indicate hypertension, high cardiac output, or circulatory overload)
PERIPHERAL VEINS		
6. Inspect the peripheral veins in the arms and legs for the presence or appearance of superficial veins when limbs are dependent and when limbs are elevated.	In dependent position, presence of distention and nodular bulges at calves When limbs are elevated, veins collapse (veins may appear tortuous or distended in older people)	Distended veins in the thigh or lower leg or on posterolateral part of calf from knee to ankle

Assessing the Peripheral Vascular System—*continued*

Assessment	Normal Findings	Deviations from Normal
7. Assess the peripheral leg veins for signs of phlebitis. • Inspect the calves for redness and swelling over vein sites. • Palpate the calves for firmness or tension of the muscles, the presence of edema over the dorsum of the foot, and areas of localized warmth. **Rationale:** *Palpation augments inspection findings, particularly in darker pigmented people in whom redness may not be visible.* • Push the calves from side to side to test for tenderness. • Firmly dorsiflex the client's foot while supporting the entire leg in extension (Homans test), or have the client stand or walk.	Symmetric in size Limbs not tender	Swelling of one calf or leg Tenderness on palpation Pain in calf muscles with forceful dorsiflexion of the foot (positive Homans test) Warmth and redness over vein No one sign or symptom consistently confirms or excludes the presence of phlebitis or a deep vein thrombosis. Homans test has been found to give inconsistent results (D'Amico & Barbarito, 2016).
PERIPHERAL PERFUSION		
8. Inspect the skin of the hands and feet for color, temperature, edema, and skin changes.	Skin color pink	Cyanotic (venous insufficiency) Pallor that increases with limb elevation Dependent rubor, a dusky red color when limb is lowered (arterial insufficiency) Brown pigmentation around ankles (arterial or chronic venous insufficiency)
	Skin temperature not excessively warm or cold	Skin cool (arterial insufficiency)
	No edema	Mild edema (arterial insufficiency) Marked edema (venous insufficiency)
	Skin texture resilient and moist	Skin thin and shiny or thick, waxy, shiny, and fragile, with reduced hair and ulceration (venous or arterial insufficiency)
9. Assess the adequacy of arterial flow if arterial insufficiency is suspected.		
CAPILLARY REFILL TEST • Press at least one nail and pad on each hand and foot between your thumb and index finger sufficiently to cause blanching (about 5 seconds). ❶ • Release the pressure, and observe how quickly normal color returns (less than 2 seconds).	Immediate return of color	Delayed return of color (arterial insufficiency)
OTHER ASSESSMENTS • Inspect the fingernails for changes indicative of circulatory impairment. See the section on assessment of nails earlier in this chapter. • See also peripheral pulse assessment earlier.		
10. Document findings in the client record using printed or electronic forms or checklists supplemented by narrative notes when appropriate.		

❶ Apply pressure to the nailbed until it turns white.

SAMPLE DOCUMENTATION

5/28/2020 0830 Legs mottled red bilaterally toes to mid-calf. States "actually looks a bit better." Capillary refill 4–5 seconds in toes on both feet. Pedal pulses present but weak. Homans test negative. c/o pain in calves after walking 100 feet. N. Schmidt, RN

EVALUATION

- Perform a detailed follow-up examination of other systems based on findings that deviated from expected or normal for the client. Relate findings to previous assessment data if available.
- Report deviations from expected or normal findings to the primary care provider.

LIFESPAN CONSIDERATIONS **Assessing the Peripheral Vascular System**

INFANTS

- Screen for coarctation of the aorta by palpating the peripheral pulses and comparing the strength of the femoral pulses with the radial pulses and apical pulse. If coarctation is present, femoral pulses will be diminished and radial pulses will be stronger.

CHILDREN

- Changes in the peripheral vasculature, such as bruising, petechiae, and purpura, can indicate serious systemic diseases in children (e.g., leukemia, meningococcemia).

OLDER ADULTS

- The overall efficiency of blood vessels decreases as smooth muscle cells are replaced by connective tissue. The lower extremities are more likely to show signs of arterial and venous impairment because of the more distal and dependent position.
- Peripheral vascular assessment should always include upper and lower extremities' temperature, color, pulses, edema, skin integrity, and sensation. Any differences in symmetry of these findings should be noted.
- Proximal arteries become thinner and dilate.
- Peripheral arteries become thicker and dilate less effectively because of arteriosclerotic changes in the vessel walls.
- Blood vessels lengthen and become more tortuous and prominent. Varicosities occur more frequently.
- In some instances, arteries may be palpated more easily because of the loss of supportive surrounding tissues. Often, however, the most distal pulses of the lower extremities are more difficult to palpate because of decreased arterial perfusion.
- Systolic and diastolic blood pressures increase, but the increase in the systolic pressure is greater. As a result, the pulse pressure widens. Any client with a blood pressure reading above 140/90 mmHg should be referred for follow-up assessments.
- Peripheral edema is frequently observed and is most commonly the result of chronic venous insufficiency or low protein levels in the blood (hypoproteinemia).
- Use the assessment as an opportunity to provide teaching regarding appropriate care of the extremities in those at high risk for or with actual vascular impairment. Educate clients and families regarding skin and nail care, exercise, and positioning to promote circulation.

Breasts and Axillae

The breasts of males and females need to be inspected and palpated. Males have some glandular tissue beneath each nipple, a potential site for malignancy, whereas mature females have glandular tissue throughout the breast. In females, the largest portion of glandular breast tissue is located in the upper outer quadrant of each breast. A projection of breast tissue from this quadrant extends into the *axilla*, called the *axillary tail of Spence* (Figure 29.31 ■). The majority of breast tumors are located in this upper outer breast quadrant including the tail of Spence. During assessment, the nurse can localize specific findings by dividing the breast into quadrants and the axillary tail. Skill 29.14 describes how to assess the breasts and axillae.

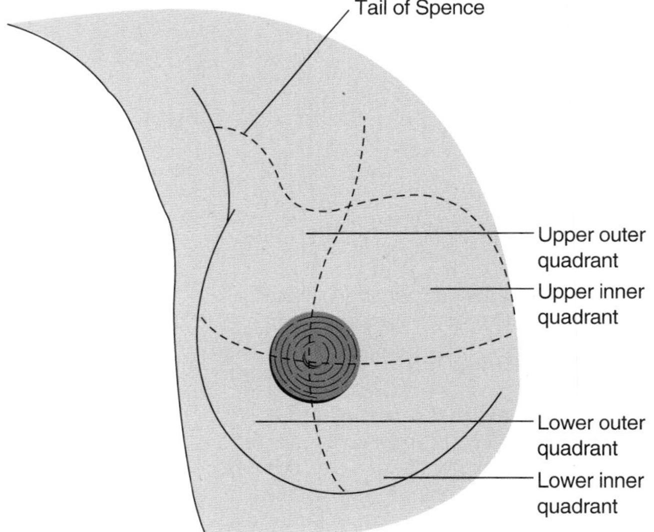

Figure 29.31 ■ The four breast quadrants and the axillary tail of Spence.

SKILL 29.14 Assessing the Breasts and Axillae

PLANNING

Assignment

Due to the substantial knowledge and skill required, assessment of the breasts and axillae is not assigned to AP. However, individuals other than the nurse may record aspects observed during usual care. Abnormal findings must be validated and interpreted by the nurse.

Equipment

- Centimeter ruler

IMPLEMENTATION

Performance

1. Prior to performing the assessment, introduce self and verify the client's identity using agency protocol. Explain to the client what you are going to do, why it is necessary, and how to participate. Inquire whether the client has ever had a clinical breast exam previously. Discuss how the results will be used in planning further care or treatments.
2. Perform hand hygiene and observe other appropriate infection prevention procedures.
3. Provide for client privacy.

Assessing the Breasts and Axillae—*continued*

4. Inquire if the client has any history of the following: breast masses and what was done about them; pain or tenderness in the breasts and relation to the female's menstrual cycle; discharge from the nipple; medication history (some medications, e.g., oral contraceptives, steroids, digitalis, and diuretics, may cause nipple discharge; estrogen replacement therapy may be associated with the development of cysts or cancer); risk factors that may be associated with development of breast cancer (e.g., mother, sister, aunt with breast cancer; alcohol consumption, high-fat diet, obesity, use of oral contraceptives, menarche before age 12, menopause after age 55, age 30 or more at first pregnancy). Inquire if the client performs breast self-examination; technique used and when performed in relation to the menstrual cycle.

Assessment	Normal Findings	Deviations from Normal
5. Inspect the breasts for size, symmetry, and contour or shape while the client is in a sitting position.	*Females*: rounded shape; slightly unequal in size; generally symmetric *Males*: breasts even with the chest wall; if obese, may be similar in shape to female breasts	Recent change in breast size; swellings; marked asymmetry
6. Inspect the skin of the breast for localized discolorations or hyperpigmentation, retraction or dimpling, localized hypervascular areas, swelling or edema. ❶	Skin uniform in color (similar to skin of abdomen if not tanned) Skin smooth and intact Diffuse symmetric horizontal or vertical vascular pattern in light-skinned people Striae (stretch marks); moles and nevi	Localized discolorations or hyperpigmentation Retraction or dimpling (result of scar tissue or an invasive tumor) Unilateral, localized hypervascular areas (associated with increased blood flow) Swelling or edema appearing as pig skin or orange peel due to exaggeration of the pores

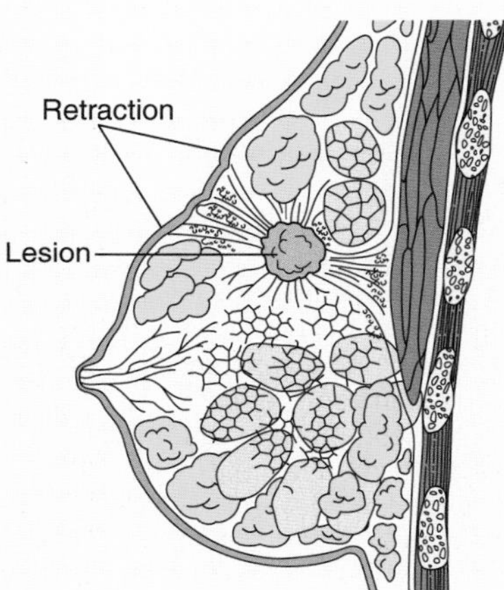

❶ A lesion causing retraction of the skin.

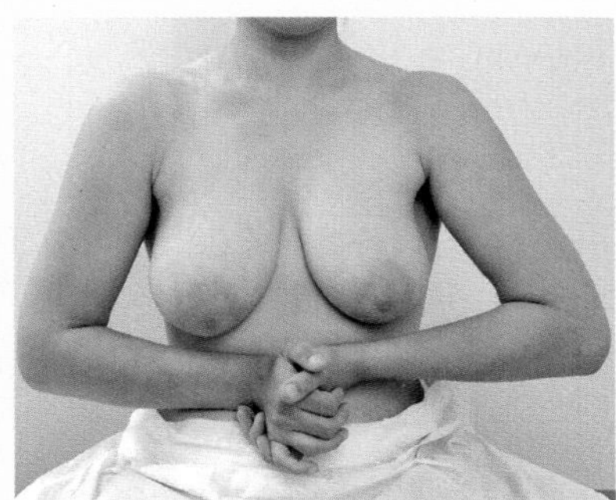

❷ Pushing the hands together to accentuate retraction of breast tissue.

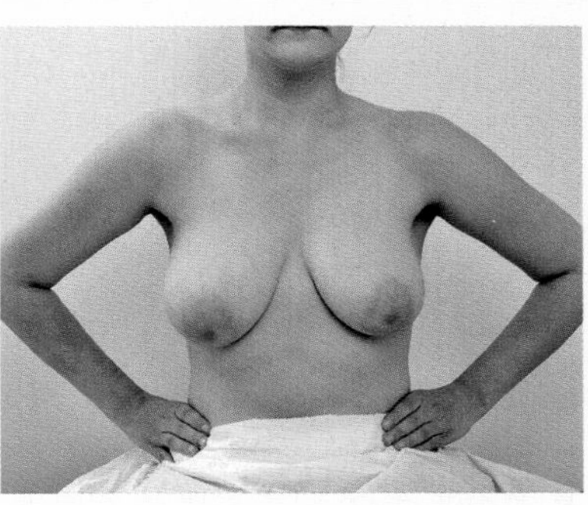

❸ Pressing the hands down on the hips to accentuate retraction of breast tissue.

Assessment	Normal Findings	Deviations from Normal
7. Emphasize any retraction by having the client: • Raise the arms above the head. • Push the hands together, with elbows flexed. ❷ • Press the hands down on the hips. ❸		
8. Inspect the areola area for size, shape, symmetry, color, surface characteristics, and any masses or lesions.	Round or oval and bilaterally the same Color varies widely, from light pink to dark brown Irregular placement of sebaceous glands on the surface of the areola (Montgomery's tubercles)	Any asymmetry, mass, or lesion
9. Inspect the nipples for size, shape, position, color, discharge, and lesions.	Round, everted, and equal in size; similar in color; soft and smooth; both nipples point in same direction (out in young females and males, downward in older females) No discharge, except from pregnant or breastfeeding females Inversion of one or both nipples that is present from puberty	Asymmetrical size and color Presence of discharge, crusts, or cracks Recent inversion of one or both nipples

Continued on page 624

Assessing the Breasts and Axillae—*continued*

Assessment	Normal Findings	Deviations from Normal
10. Palpate the axillary, subclavicular, and supraclavicular lymph nodes ❹ while the client sits with the arms abducted and supported on the nurse's forearm. See discussion on palpation of clavicular lymph nodes in Skill 29.10. Use the flat surfaces of all fingertips to palpate the four areas of the axilla: • The edge of the greater pectoral muscle (musculus pectoralis major) along the anterior axillary line • The thoracic wall in the midaxillary area • The upper part of the humerus • The anterior edge of the latissimus dorsi muscle along the posterior axillary line.	No tenderness, masses, or nodules	Tenderness, masses, or nodules

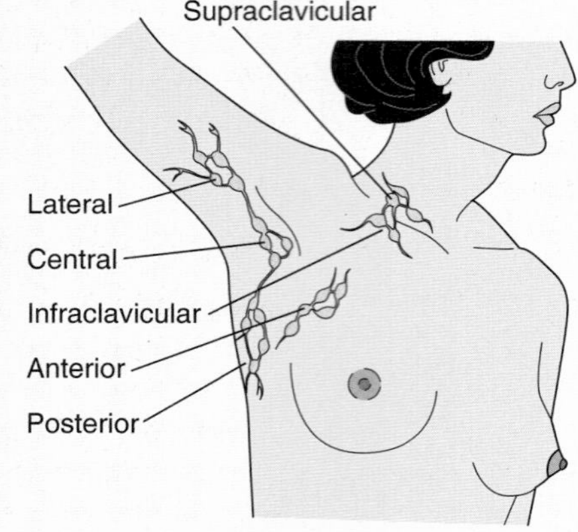

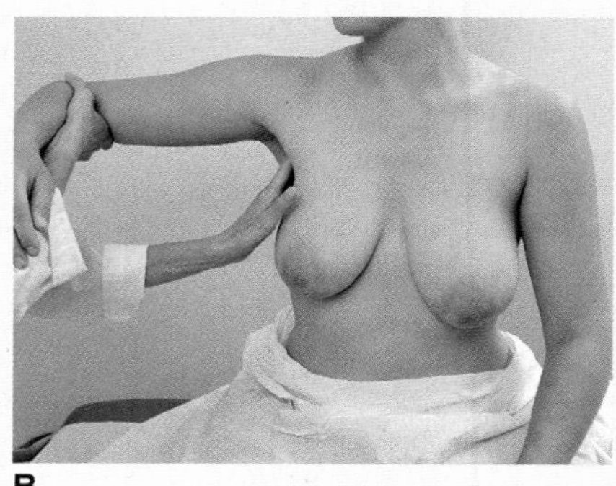

❹ Location and palpation of the lymph nodes that drain the lateral breast: *A*, lymph nodes; *B*, palpating the axilla.

Assessment	Normal Findings	Deviations from Normal
11. Palpate the breast for masses, tenderness, and any discharge from the nipples. Palpation of the breast is generally performed while the client is supine. **Rationale:** *In the supine position, the breasts flatten evenly against the chest wall, facilitating palpation*. For clients who have a past history of breast masses, who are at high risk for breast cancer, or who have pendulous breasts, examination in both a supine and a sitting position is recommended. • If the client reports a breast lump, start with the "normal" breast to obtain baseline data that will serve as a comparison to the reportedly involved breast. • To enhance flattening of the breast, instruct the client to abduct the arm and place her hand behind the head. Then place a small pillow or rolled towel under the client's shoulder. • For palpation, use the palmar surface of the middle three fingertips (held together) and make a gentle rotary motion on the breast. • Choose one of three patterns for palpation: a. Hands-of-the-clock or spokes-on-a-wheel ❺ b. Concentric circles ❻ c. Vertical strips pattern. ❼ • Start at one point for palpation, and move systematically to the end point to ensure that all breast surfaces are assessed. • Pay particular attention to the upper outer quadrant area and the tail of Spence.	No tenderness, masses, nodules, or nipple discharge	Tenderness, masses, nodules, or nipple discharge • If you detect a mass, record the following data: a. Location: the exact location relative to the quadrants and axillary tail, or the clock 5 and the distance from the nipple in centimeters. b. Size: the length, width, and thickness of the mass in centimeters. If you are able to determine the discrete edges, record this fact. c. Shape: whether the mass is round, oval, lobulated, indistinct, or irregular. d. Consistency: whether the mass is hard or soft. e. Mobility: whether the mass is movable or fixed. f. Skin over the lump: whether it is reddened, dimpled, or retracted. g. Nipple: whether it is displaced or retracted. h. Tenderness: whether palpation is painful.

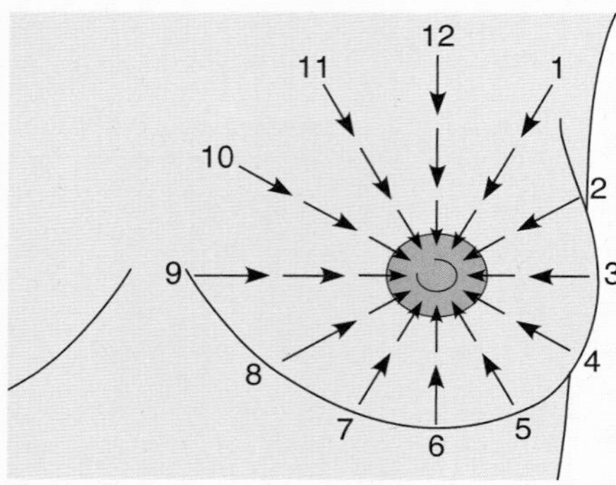

❺ Hands-of-the-clock or spokes-on-a-wheel pattern of breast palpation.

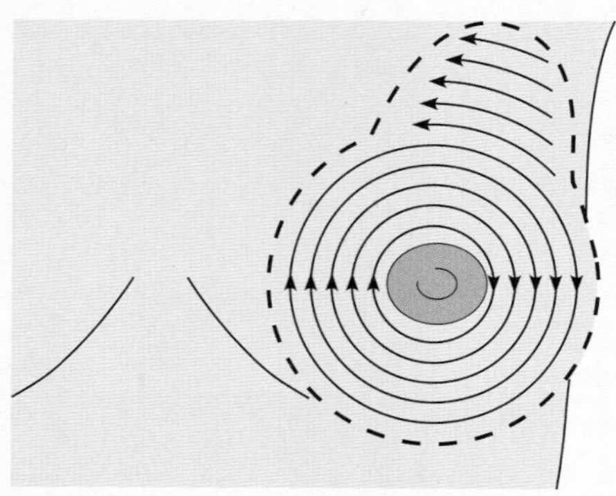

❻ Concentric circles pattern of breast palpation.

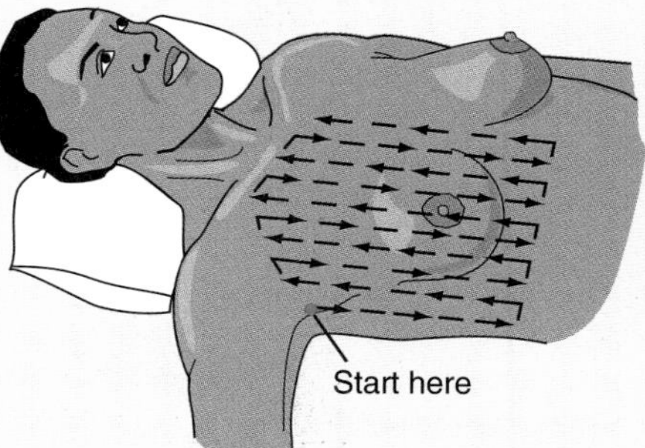

❼ Vertical strips pattern of breast palpation.

Assessing the Breasts and Axillae—*continued*

Assessment	Normal Findings	Deviations from Normal
12. Palpate the areolae and the nipples for masses. Compress each nipple to determine the presence of any discharge. If discharge is present, milk the breast along its radius to identify the discharge-producing lobe. Assess any discharge for amount, color, consistency, and odor. Note also any tenderness on palpation.	No tenderness, masses, nodules, or nipple discharge	Tenderness, masses, nodules, or nipple discharge
13. If the client wishes, teach the technique of breast self-examination (see Chapter 40 ∞).		

14. Document findings in the client record using printed or electronic forms or checklists supplemented by narrative notes when appropriate.

EVALUATION

- Perform a detailed follow-up examination of other systems based on findings that deviated from expected or normal for the client. Relate findings to previous assessment data if available.
- Report deviations from expected or normal findings to the primary care provider.

LIFESPAN CONSIDERATIONS Assessing the Breasts and Axillae

INFANTS

- Newborns up to 2 weeks of age, both males and females, may have breast enlargement and white discharge from the nipples (witch's milk).
- Supernumerary ("extra") nipples infrequently are present as small dimples along the mammary chain; these may be associated with renal anomalies.

CHILDREN

- Female breast development begins between 9 and 13 years of age and occurs in five stages (Tanner stages). One breast may develop more rapidly than the other, but at the end of development, they are more or less the same size.
  Stage 1: prepubertal with no noticeable change
  Stage 2: breast bud with elevation of nipple and enlargement of the areola
  Stage 3: enlargement of the breast and areola with no separation of contour
  Stage 4: projection of the areola and nipple
  Stage 5: recession of the areola by about age 14 or 15, leaving only the nipple projecting.
- Males may develop breast buds and have slight enlargement of the areola in early adolescence. Further enlargement of breast tissue (gynecomastia) can occur. This growth is transient, usually lasting about 2 years, resolving completely by late puberty.
- Axillary hair usually appears in Tanner stages 3 or 4 and is related to adrenal rather than gonadal changes.

PREGNANT FEMALES

- Breast, areola, and nipple size increase.
- The areolae and nipples darken; nipples may become more erect; areolae contain small, scattered, elevated Montgomery's glands.
- Superficial veins become more prominent, and jagged linear stretch marks may develop.
- A thick yellow fluid (colostrum) may be expressed from the nipples after the first trimester.

OLDER ADULTS

- In the postmenopausal female, breasts change in shape and often appear pendulous or flaccid; they lack the firmness they had in younger years.
- The presence of breast lesions may be detected more readily because of the decrease in connective tissue.
- General breast size remains the same. Although glandular tissue atrophies, the amount of fat in breasts (predominantly in the lower quadrants) increases in most females.

Abdomen

The nurse locates and describes abdominal findings using two common methods of subdividing the abdomen: quadrants and regions. To divide the abdomen into quadrants, the nurse imagines two lines: a vertical line from the xiphoid process to the pubic symphysis, and a horizontal line across the umbilicus (Figure 29.32 ■). These quadrants are labeled right upper quadrant, left upper quadrant, right lower quadrant, and left lower quadrant. Using the second method, division into nine regions, the nurse imagines two vertical lines that extend superiorly from the midpoints of the inguinal ligaments, and two horizontal lines, one at the level of the edge of the lower ribs and the

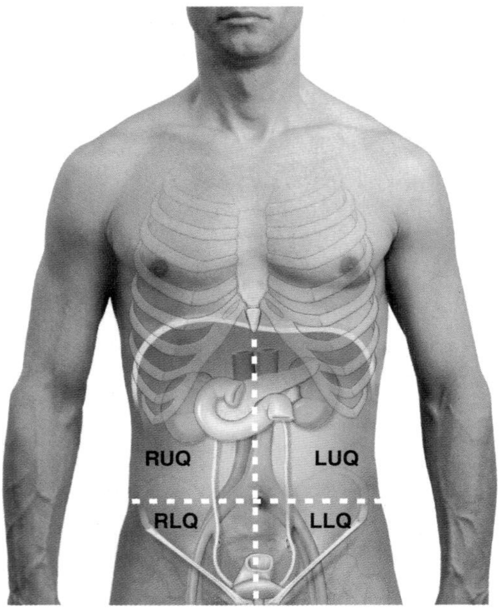

Figure 29.32 ■ The four abdominal quadrants and the underlying organs: RUQ, right upper quadrant; LUQ, left upper quadrant; RLQ, right lower quadrant; LLQ, left lower quadrant.

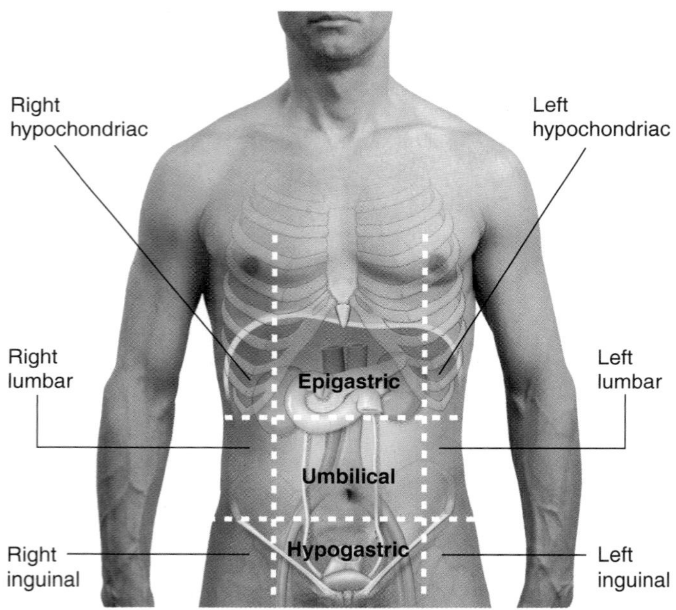

Figure 29.33 ■ The nine abdominal regions: epigastric; left and right hypochondriac; umbilical; left and right lumbar; hypogastric; left and right inguinal or iliac.

other at the level of the iliac crests (Figure 29.33 ■). Specific organs or parts of organs lie in each abdominal region (Boxes 29.7 and 29.8).

In addition, practitioners often use certain landmarks to locate abdominal signs and symptoms. These are the xiphoid process of the sternum, the costal margins, the anterosuperior iliac spine, the umbilicus, the inguinal ligaments, and the superior margin of the pubic symphysis (Figure 29.34 ■).

BOX 29.7 Organs in the Four Abdominal Quadrants

RIGHT UPPER QUADRANT
Liver
Gallbladder
Duodenum
Head of pancreas
Right adrenal gland
Upper lobe of right kidney
Hepatic flexure of colon
Section of ascending colon
Section of transverse colon

LEFT UPPER QUADRANT
Left lobe of liver
Stomach
Spleen
Upper lobe of left kidney
Pancreas
Left adrenal gland
Splenic flexure of colon
Section of transverse colon
Section of descending colon

RIGHT LOWER QUADRANT
Lower lobe of right kidney
Cecum
Appendix
Section of ascending colon
Right ovary
Right fallopian tube
Right ureter
Right spermatic cord
Part of uterus

LEFT LOWER QUADRANT
Lower lobe of left kidney
Sigmoid colon
Section of descending colon
Left ovary
Left fallopian tube
Left ureter
Left spermatic cord
Part of uterus

BOX 29.8 Organs in the Nine Abdominal Regions

RIGHT HYPOCHONDRIAC
Right lobe of liver
Gallbladder
Part of duodenum
Hepatic flexure of colon
Upper half of right kidney
Suprarenal gland

RIGHT LUMBAR
Ascending colon
Lower half of right kidney
Part of duodenum and jejunum

RIGHT INGUINAL
Cecum
Appendix
Lower end of ileum
Right ureter
Right spermatic cord
Right ovary

EPIGASTRIC
Aorta
Pyloric end of stomach
Part of duodenum
Pancreas
Part of liver

UMBILICAL
Omentum
Mesentery
Lower part of duodenum
Part of jejunum and ileum

HYPOGASTRIC (PUBIC)
Ileum
Bladder
Uterus

LEFT HYPOCHONDRIAC
Stomach
Spleen
Tail of pancreas
Splenic flexure of colon
Upper half of left kidney
Suprarenal gland

LEFT LUMBAR
Descending colon
Lower half of left kidney
Part of jejunum and ileum

LEFT INGUINAL
Sigmoid colon
Left ureter
Left spermatic cord
Left ovary

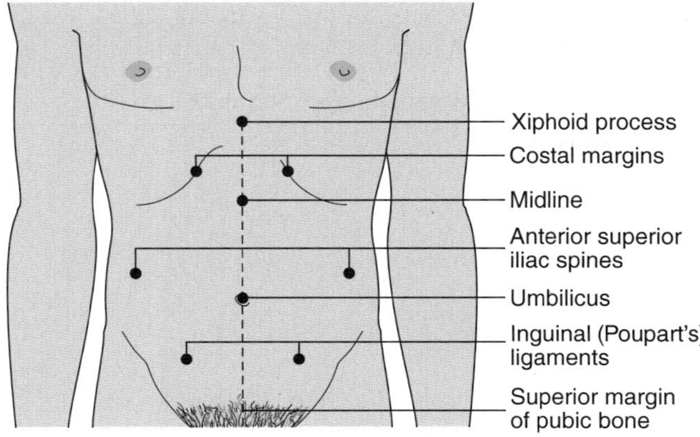

Figure 29.34 ■ Landmarks commonly used to identify abdominal areas.

Assessment of the abdomen involves all four methods of examination (inspection, auscultation, palpation, and percussion). When assessing the abdomen, the nurse performs inspection first, followed by auscultation, percussion, and/or palpation. Auscultation is done before palpation and percussion because palpation and percussion cause movement or stimulation of the bowel, which can increase bowel motility and thus heighten bowel sounds, creating false results. Skill 29.15 describes how to assess the abdomen.

Assessing the Abdomen

SKILL 29.15

PLANNING

- Ask the client to urinate since an empty bladder makes the assessment more comfortable.
- Ensure that the room is warm since the client will be exposed.

Assignment

Due to the substantial knowledge and skill required, assessment of the abdomen is not assigned to AP. However, signs and symptoms of problems may be observed during usual care and should be recorded by those individuals. Abnormal findings must be validated and interpreted by the nurse.

Equipment

- Tape measure (metal or unstretchable material)
- Skin-marking pen
- Stethoscope

IMPLEMENTATION

Performance

1. Prior to performing the assessment, introduce self and verify the client's identity using agency protocol. Explain to the client what you are going to do, why it is necessary, and how to participate. Discuss how the results will be used in planning further care or treatments.
2. Perform hand hygiene and observe other appropriate infection prevention procedures.
3. Provide for client privacy.
4. Inquire if the client has any history of the following: incidence of abdominal pain; its location, onset, sequence, and chronology; its quality (description); its frequency; associated symptoms (e.g., nausea, vomiting, diarrhea); incidence of constipation or diarrhea (have client describe what client means by these terms); change in appetite, food intolerances, and foods ingested in past 24 hours; specific signs and symptoms (e.g., heartburn, flatulence and/or belching, difficulty swallowing, hematemesis [vomiting blood], blood or mucus in stools, and aggravating and alleviating factors); previous problems and treatment (e.g., stomach ulcer, gallbladder surgery, history of jaundice).
5. Assist the client to a supine position, with the arms placed comfortably at the sides. Place small pillows beneath the knees and the head to reduce tension in the abdominal muscles. Expose the client's abdomen only from the chest line to the pubic area to avoid chilling and shivering, which can tense the abdominal muscles.

Assessment	Normal Findings	Deviations from Normal
INSPECTION OF THE ABDOMEN		
6. Inspect the abdomen for skin integrity (refer to the discussion of skin assessment earlier in this chapter).	Unblemished skin Uniform color Silver-white striae (stretch marks) or surgical scars	Presence of rash or other lesions Tense, glistening skin (may indicate ascites, edema) Purple striae (associated with Cushing's disease or rapid weight gain and loss)
7. Inspect the abdomen for contour and symmetry:		
• Observe the abdominal contour (profile line from the rib margin to the pubic bone) while standing at the client's side when the client is supine.	Flat, rounded (convex), or scaphoid (concave)	Distended
• Ask the client to take a deep breath and to hold it. **Rationale:** *This makes an enlarged liver or spleen more obvious.*	No evidence of enlargement of liver or spleen	Evidence of enlargement of liver or spleen
• Assess the symmetry of contour while standing at the foot of the bed.	Symmetric contour	Asymmetric contour, e.g., localized protrusions around umbilicus, inguinal ligaments, or scars (possible hernia or tumor)

Continued on page 628

SKILL 29.15

Assessing the Abdomen—*continued*

Assessment	Normal Findings	Deviations from Normal
• If distention is present, measure the abdominal girth by placing a tape around the abdomen at the level of the umbilicus. ❶ If girth will be measured repeatedly, use a skin-marking pen to outline the upper and lower margins of the tape placement for consistency of future measurements.	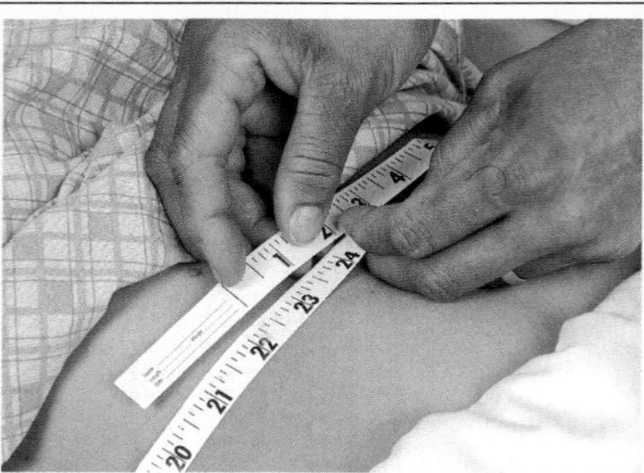 ❶ Measuring abdominal girth.	
8. Observe abdominal movements associated with respiration, peristalsis, or aortic pulsations.	Symmetric movements caused by respiration Visible peristalsis in very lean people Aortic pulsations in thin people at epigastric area	Limited movement due to pain or disease process Visible peristalsis in nonlean clients (possible bowel obstruction) Marked aortic pulsations
9. Observe the vascular pattern.	No visible vascular pattern	Visible venous pattern (dilated veins) is associated with liver disease, ascites, and venocaval obstruction
AUSCULTATION OF THE ABDOMEN **10.** Auscultate the abdomen for bowel sounds, vascular sounds, and peritoneal friction rubs. Warm the hands and the stethoscope diaphragms. **Rationale:** *Cold hands and a cold stethoscope may cause the client to contract the abdominal muscles, and these contractions may be heard during auscultation.* **FOR BOWEL SOUNDS** • Use the flat-disk diaphragm. ❷ **Rationale:** *Intestinal sounds are relatively high pitched and best accentuated by the diaphragm.* Light pressure with the stethoscope is adequate. • Ask when the client last ate. **Rationale:** *Shortly after or long after eating, bowel sounds may normally increase. They are loudest when a meal is long overdue.* Four to 7 hours after a meal, bowel sounds may be heard continuously over the ileocecal valve area (right lower quadrant) while the digestive contents from the small intestine empty through the valve into the large intestine. • Place diaphragm of the stethoscope in each of the four quadrants of the abdomen. • Listen for active bowel sounds—irregular gurgling noises occurring about every 5 to 20 seconds. The duration of a single sound may range from less than a second to more than several seconds.	Audible bowel sounds 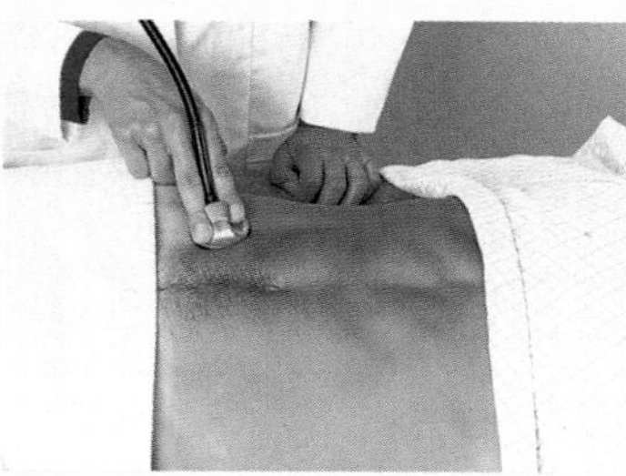 ❷ Auscultating the abdomen for bowel sounds.	Hypoactive, i.e., extremely soft and infrequent (e.g., one per minute). Hypoactive sounds indicate decreased motility and are usually associated with manipulation of the bowel during surgery, inflammation, paralytic ileus, or late bowel obstruction. True absence of sounds (none heard in 3 to 5 minutes) indicates a cessation of intestinal motility. Hyperactive or increased, i.e., high-pitched, loud, rushing sounds that occur frequently (e.g., every 3 seconds) also known as borborygmi. Hyperactive sounds indicate increased intestinal motility and are usually associated with diarrhea, an early bowel obstruction, or the use of laxatives.

Assessing the Abdomen—*continued*

SKILL 29.15

Assessment	Normal Findings	Deviations from Normal
FOR VASCULAR SOUNDS • Use the bell of the stethoscope over the aorta, renal arteries, iliac arteries, and femoral arteries. ❸ • Listen for bruits.	Absence of arterial bruits	Loud bruit over aortic area (possible aneurysm) Bruit over renal or iliac arteries

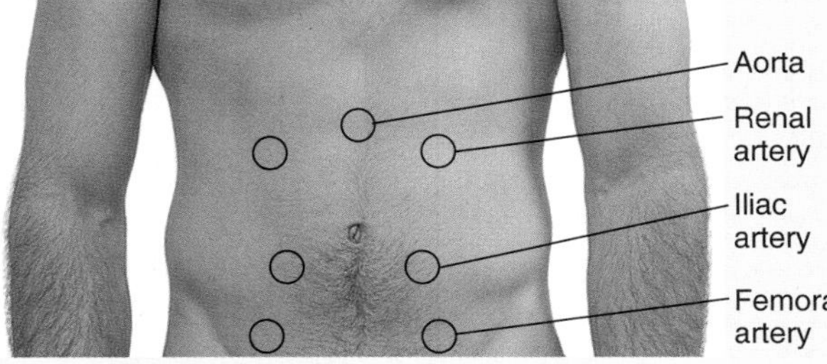

❸ Sites for auscultating the vascular sounds.

Assessment	Normal Findings	Deviations from Normal
PERITONEAL FRICTION RUBS • Peritoneal friction rubs are rough, grating sounds like two pieces of leather rubbing together. Friction rubs may be caused by inflammation, infection, or abnormal growths.	Absence of friction rub	Friction rub
PERCUSSION OF THE ABDOMEN **11.** Percuss several areas in each of the four quadrants to determine presence of tympany (sound indicating gas in stomach and intestines) and dullness (decrease, absence, or flatness of resonance over solid masses or fluid). Use a systematic pattern: Begin in the lower right quadrant, proceed to the upper right quadrant, the upper left quadrant, and the lower left quadrant. ❹	Tympany over the stomach and gas-filled bowels; dullness, especially over the liver and spleen, or a full bladder	Large dull areas (associated with presence of fluid or a tumor)

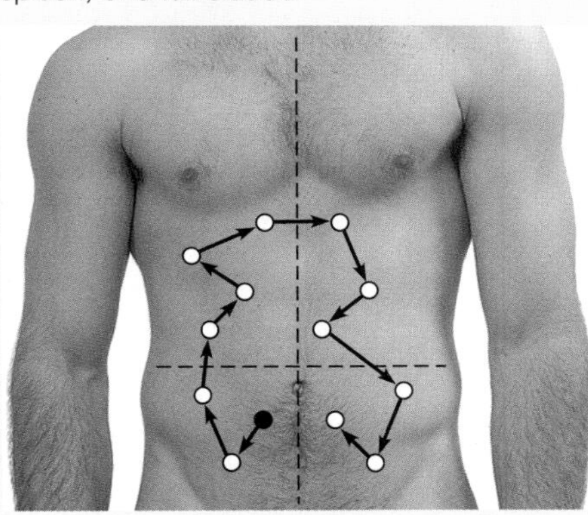

❹ Systematic percussion sites for all four quadrants.

Assessment	Normal Findings	Deviations from Normal
PALPATION OF THE ABDOMEN **12.** Perform light palpation to detect areas of tenderness and/or muscle guarding. Systematically explore all four quadrants. Ensure that the client's position is appropriate for relaxation of the abdominal muscles, and warm the hands. **Rationale:** *Cold hands can elicit muscle tension and thus impede palpatory evaluation*. • Hold the palm of your hand slightly above the client's abdomen, with your fingers parallel to the abdomen. • Depress the abdominal wall lightly, about 1 cm or to the depth of the subcutaneous tissue, with the pads of your fingers. ❺ • Move the finger pads in a slight circular motion.	No tenderness; relaxed abdomen with smooth, consistent tension	Tenderness and hypersensitivity Superficial masses Localized areas of increased tension

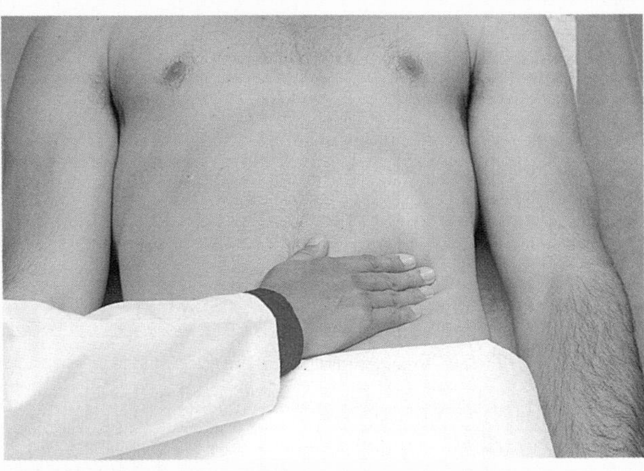

❺ Light palpation of the abdomen.

Continued on page 630

SKILL 29.15

Assessing the Abdomen—*continued*

Assessment	Normal Findings	Deviations from Normal
• Note areas of tenderness or superficial pain, masses, and muscle guarding. To determine areas of tenderness, ask the client to tell you about them and watch for changes in the client's facial expressions. • If the client is excessively ticklish, begin by pressing your hand on top of the client's hand while pressing lightly. Then slide your hand off the client's and onto the abdomen to continue the examination.		
PALPATION OF THE BLADDER		
13. Palpate the area above the pubic symphysis if the client's history indicates possible urinary retention. ❻	Not palpable	Distended and palpable as smooth, round, tense mass (indicates urinary retention)

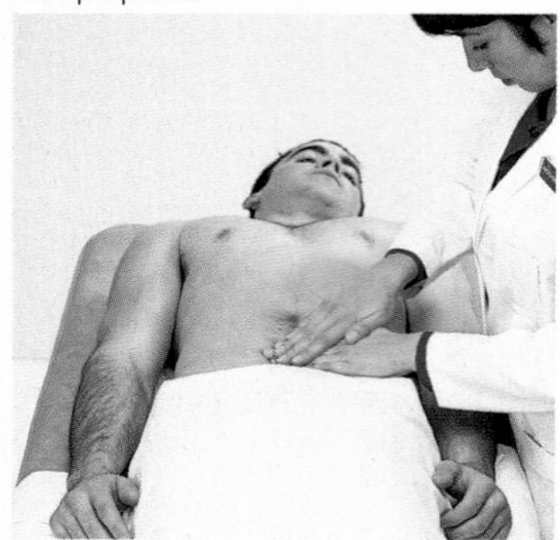

❻ Palpating the bladder.

14. Document findings in the client record using printed or electronic forms or checklists supplemented by narrative notes when appropriate.

SAMPLE DOCUMENTATION

5/28/2020 0945 c/o "gassy" pain LRQ. No BM x 48 hrs. Ate 75% regular diet yesterday. Abdomen flat. Active bowels sounds all 4 quadrants. Tympany above umbilicus, dull below. No masses palpated. 30 mL milk of magnesia given. N. Schmidt, RN

EVALUATION

- Perform a detailed follow-up examination of other systems based on findings that deviated from expected or normal for the client. Relate findings to previous assessment data if available.
- Report deviations from expected or normal findings to the primary care provider.

LIFESPAN CONSIDERATIONS Assessing the Abdomen

INFANTS

- Internal organs of newborns and infants are proportionately larger than those of older children and adults, so their abdomens are rounded and tend to protrude.
- The infant's liver may be palpable 1 to 2 cm (0.4 to 0.8 in.) below the right costal margin.
- Umbilical hernias may be present at birth.

CHILDREN

- Toddlers have a characteristic "potbelly" appearance, which can persist until age 3 to 4 years.
- Late preschool and school-age children are leaner and have a flat abdomen.
- Peristaltic waves may be more visible than in adults.
- Children may not be able to pinpoint areas of tenderness; by observing facial expressions the examiner can determine areas of maximum tenderness.
- The liver is relatively larger than in adults. It can be palpated 1 to 2 cm (0.4 to 0.8 in.) below the right costal margin.
- If the child is ticklish, guarding, or fearful, use a task that requires concentration (such as squeezing the hands together) to distract the child, or have the child place his or her hands on yours as you palpate the abdomen, "helping" you to do the exam.

OLDER ADULTS

- The rounded abdomens of older adults are due to an increase in adipose tissue and a decrease in muscle tone.

LIFESPAN CONSIDERATIONS **Assessing the Abdomen—*continued***

- The abdominal wall is slacker and thinner, making palpation easier and more accurate than in younger clients. Muscle wasting and loss of fibroconnective tissue occur.
- The pain threshold in older adults is often higher; major abdominal problems such as appendicitis or other acute emergencies may therefore go undetected.
- Gastrointestinal pain needs to be differentiated from cardiac pain. Gastrointestinal pain may be located in the chest or abdomen, whereas cardiac pain is usually located in the chest. Factors aggravating gastrointestinal pain are usually related to either ingestion or lack of food intake; gastrointestinal pain is usually relieved by antacids, food, or assuming an upright position. Common factors that can aggravate cardiac pain are activity or anxiety; rest or nitroglycerin relieves cardiac pain.
- Stool passes through the intestines at a slower rate in older adults, and the perception of stimuli that produce the urge to defecate often diminishes.
- Fecal incontinence may occur in adults who are confused or have a neurologic impairment.
- Many older adults believe that the absence of a daily bowel movement signifies constipation. When assessing for constipation, the nurse must consider the client's diet, activity, medications, and characteristics and ease of passage of feces as well as the frequency of bowel movements.
- The incidence of colon cancer is higher among older adults than younger adults. Symptoms include a change in bowel function, rectal bleeding, and weight loss. Changes in bowel function, however, are associated with many factors, such as diet, exercise, and medications.
- Decreased absorption of oral medications often occurs with aging.
- In the liver, impaired metabolism of some drugs may occur with aging.

Musculoskeletal System

The musculoskeletal system encompasses the muscles, bones, and joints. The completeness of an assessment of this system depends largely on the needs and problems of the individual client. The nurse usually assesses the musculoskeletal system for muscle strength, tone, size, and symmetry of muscle development, and for tremors. A **tremor** is an involuntary trembling of a limb or body part. Tremors may involve large groups of muscle fibers or small bundles of muscle fibers. An **intention tremor** becomes more apparent when an individual attempts a voluntary movement, such as holding a cup of coffee. A **resting tremor** is more apparent when the client is relaxed and diminishes with activity. A **fasciculation** is an abnormal contraction of a bundle of muscle fibers that appears as a twitch.

Bones are assessed for normal form. Joints are assessed for tenderness, swelling, thickening, crepitation (a crackling, grating sound), and range of motion. Body posture is assessed for normal standing and sitting positions. For information about body posture, see Chapter 44 ∞. Skill 29.16 describes how to assess the musculoskeletal system.

Assessing the Musculoskeletal System

SKILL 29.16

PLANNING

Assignment

Due to the substantial knowledge and skill required, assessment of the musculoskeletal system is not assigned to AP. However, many aspects of its functioning are observed during usual care and may be recorded by individuals other than the nurse. Abnormal findings must be validated and interpreted by the nurse.

Equipment

- Tape measure

IMPLEMENTATION

Performance

1. Prior to performing the assessment, introduce self and verify the client's identity using agency protocol. Explain to the client what you are going to do, why it is necessary, and how to participate. Discuss how the results will be used in planning further care or treatments.
2. Perform hand hygiene and observe other appropriate infection prevention procedures.
3. Provide for client privacy.
4. Inquire if the client has any history of the following: muscle pain: onset, location, character, associated phenomena (e.g., redness and swelling of joints), and aggravating and alleviating factors; limitations to movement or inability to perform activities of daily living; previous sports injuries; loss of function without pain.

Assessment	Normal Findings	Deviations from Normal
MUSCLES		
5. Inspect the muscles for size. Compare the muscles on one side of the body (e.g., of the arm, thigh, and calf) to the same muscle on the other side. For any discrepancies, measure the muscles with a tape.	Equal size on both sides of body	Atrophy (a decrease in size) or hypertrophy (an increase in size), asymmetry
6. Inspect the muscles and tendons for contractures (shortening).	No contractures	Malposition of body part, e.g., foot drop (foot flexed downward)

Continued on page 632

SKILL 29.16

Assessing the Musculoskeletal System—*continued*

Assessment	Normal Findings	Deviations from Normal
7. Inspect the muscles for tremors, for example by having the client hold the arms out in front of the body.	No tremors	Presence of tremor
8. Test muscle strength. Compare the right side with the left side. *Sternocleidomastoid:* Client turns the head to one side against the resistance of your hand. Repeat with the other side. *Trapezius:* Client shrugs the shoulders against the resistance of your hands. *Deltoid:* Client holds arm up and resists while you try to push it down. *Biceps:* Client fully extends each arm and tries to flex it while you attempt to hold arm in extension. *Triceps:* Client flexes each arm and then tries to extend it against your attempt to keep arm in flexion. *Wrist and finger muscles:* Client spreads the fingers and resists as you attempt to push the fingers together. *Grip strength:* Client grasps your index and middle fingers while you try to pull the fingers out. *Hip muscles:* Client is supine, both legs extended; client raises one leg at a time while you attempt to hold it down. *Hip abduction:* Client is supine, both legs extended. Place your hands on the lateral surface of each knee; client spreads the legs apart against your resistance. *Hip adduction:* Client is in same position as for hip abduction. Place your hands between the knees; client brings the legs together against your resistance. *Hamstrings:* Client is supine, both knees bent. Client resists while you attempt to straighten the legs. *Quadriceps:* Client is supine, knee partially extended; client resists while you attempt to flex the knee. *Muscles of the ankles and feet:* Client resists while you attempt to dorsiflex the foot and again resists while you attempt to flex the foot.	Equal strength on each body side	**Grading Muscle Strength** 0: 0% of normal strength; complete paralysis 1: 10% of normal strength; no movement, contraction of muscle is palpable or visible 2: 25% of normal strength; full muscle movement against gravity, with support 3: 50% of normal strength; normal movement against gravity 4: 75% of normal strength; normal full movement against gravity and against minimal resistance 5: 100% of normal strength; normal full movement against gravity and against full resistance
BONES		
9. Inspect the skeleton for structure.	No deformities	Bones misaligned
10. Palpate the bones to locate any areas of edema or tenderness.	No tenderness or swelling	Presence of tenderness or swelling (may indicate fracture, neoplasms, or osteoporosis)
JOINTS		
11. Inspect the joint for swelling. Palpate each joint for tenderness, smoothness of movement, swelling, crepitation, and presence of nodules.	No swelling No tenderness, swelling, crepitation, or nodules Joints move smoothly	One or more swollen joints Presence of tenderness, swelling, crepitation, or nodules
12. Assess joint range of motion. See Chapter 44 ∞ for the types of joint movements.	Varies to some degree in accordance with a client's genetic makeup and degree of physical activity	Limited range of motion in one or more joints
13. Document findings in the client record using printed or electronic forms or checklists supplemented by narrative notes when appropriate.		

EVALUATION

- Perform a detailed follow-up examination of other systems based on findings that deviated from expected or normal for the client. Relate findings to previous assessment data if available.
- Report deviations from expected or normal findings to the primary care provider.

LIFESPAN CONSIDERATIONS Assessing the Musculoskeletal System

INFANTS

- Palpate the clavicles of newborns. A mass and crepitus may indicate a fracture experienced during vaginal delivery. The newborn may also have limited movement of the arm and shoulder on the affected side.
- When the arms and legs of newborns are pulled to extension and released, newborns naturally return to the flexed fetal position.
- Check muscle strength by holding the infant lightly under the arms with feet placed lightly on a table. Infants should not fall through the hands and should be able to bear body weight on their legs if normal muscle strength is present.
- Check infants for developmental dysplasia of the hip (congenital dislocation) by examining for asymmetric gluteal folds, asymmetric abduction of the legs (Ortolani and Barlow tests), or apparent shortening of the femur.
- Infants should be able to sit without support by 8 months of age, crawl by 7 to 10 months, and walk by 12 to 15 months.
- Observe for symmetry of muscle mass, strength, and function.

CHILDREN

- Pronation and "toeing in" of the feet are common in children between 12 and 30 months of age.
- Genu varum (bowleg) is normal in children for about 1 year after beginning to walk.
- Genu valgus (knock-knee) is normal in preschool and early school-age children.
- Lordosis (swayback) is common in children before age 5.
- Observe the child in normal activities to determine motor function.
- During the rapid growth spurts of adolescence, spinal curvature and rotation (scoliosis) may appear. Children should be assessed for scoliosis by age 12 and annually until their growth slows. Curvature greater than 10% should be referred for further medical evaluation.
- Muscle mass increases in adolescence, especially as children engage in strenuous physical activity, and requires increased nutritional intake.
- Children are at risk for injury related to physical activity and should be assessed for nutritional status, physical conditioning, and safety precautions in order to prevent injury.
- Adolescent females who participate extensively in strenuous athletic activities are at risk for delayed menses, osteoporosis, and eating disorders; assessment should include a history of these factors (Prather et al., 2016).

OLDER ADULTS

- Muscle mass decreases progressively with age, but wide variations are seen among different individuals.
- The decrease in speed, strength, resistance to fatigue, reaction time, and coordination in the older adult is due to a decrease in nerve conduction and muscle tone.
- The bones become more fragile and osteoporosis leads to a loss of total bone mass. As a result, older adults are predisposed to fractures and compressed vertebrae.
- In most older adults, osteoarthritic changes in the joints can be observed.
- Note any surgical scars from joint replacement surgeries.

Neurologic System

A thorough neurologic examination may take 1 to 3 hours; however, routine screening tests are usually done first. If the results of these tests raise questions, more extensive evaluations are made. Three major considerations determine the extent of a neurologic exam: (1) the client's chief complaints, (2) the client's physical condition (i.e., level of consciousness and ability to ambulate) because many parts of the examination require movement and coordination of the extremities, and (3) the client's willingness to participate and cooperate.

Examination of the neurologic system includes assessment of (a) mental status including level of consciousness, (b) the cranial nerves, (c) reflexes, (d) motor function, and (e) sensory function. Parts of the neurologic assessment are performed throughout the health examination. For example, the nurse performs a large part of the mental status assessment during the taking of the history and when observing the client's general appearance. Also, the nurse assesses the function of cranial nerves II, III, IV, V, and VI (ophthalmic branch) with the eyes and vision, and cranial nerve VIII (cochlear branch) with the ears and hearing.

Mental Status

Assessment of mental status reveals the client's general cerebral function. These functions include intellectual (cognitive) as well as emotional (affective) functions.

If problems with use of language, memory, concentration, or thought processes are noted during the nursing history, a more extensive examination is required during neurologic assessment. Major areas of mental status assessment include language, orientation, memory, and attention span and calculation.

Language

Any defects in or loss of the power to express oneself by speech, writing, or signs, or to comprehend spoken or written language due to disease or injury of the cerebral cortex, is called **aphasia**. Aphasias can be categorized as sensory or receptive aphasia, and motor or expressive aphasia.

Sensory or receptive aphasia is the loss of the ability to comprehend written or spoken words. Two types of sensory aphasia are auditory (or acoustic) aphasia and visual aphasia. Clients with auditory aphasia have lost the ability to understand the symbolic content associated with sounds. Clients with visual aphasia have lost the ability to understand printed or written figures. Motor or expressive aphasia involves loss of the power to express oneself by writing, making signs, or speaking.

Orientation

This aspect of the assessment determines the client's ability to recognize other people (*person*), awareness of when and where they presently are (*time* and *place*), and who they, themselves, are (*self*). The terms *disorientation* and *confusion* are often used synonymously although there are differences. It is always preferable to describe the client's actions or statements rather than to label them.

Clinical Alert!

Nurses often chart that the client is "awake, alert, & oriented ×3" (or "times three"). This refers to accurate awareness of persons, time, and place. Remember, "person" indicates that the client recognizes others, not that the client can state what his or her own name is.

Memory

The nurse assesses the client's recall of information presented seconds previously (immediate recall), events or information from earlier in the day or examination (recent memory), and knowledge recalled from months or years ago (remote or long-term memory).

Attention Span and Calculation

This component determines the client's ability to focus on a mental task that is expected to be able to be performed by individuals of normal intelligence.

Level of Consciousness

Level of consciousness (LOC) can lie anywhere along a continuum from a state of alertness to coma. A fully alert client responds to questions spontaneously; a comatose client may not respond to verbal stimuli. The Glasgow Coma Scale was originally developed to predict recovery from a head injury; however, it is used by many professionals to assess LOC. It tests in three major areas: eye response, motor response, and verbal response. An assessment totaling 15 points indicates the client is alert and completely oriented. A comatose client scores 7 or less (see Table 29.10).

TABLE 29.10 Levels of Consciousness: Glasgow Coma Scale

Faculty Measured	Response	Score
Eye opening	Spontaneous	4
	To verbal command	3
	To pain	2
	No response	1
Motor response	To verbal command	6
	To localized pain	5
	Flexes and withdraws	4
	Flexes abnormally	3
	Extends abnormally	2
	No response	1
Verbal response	Oriented, converses	5
	Disoriented, converses	4
	Uses inappropriate words	3
	Makes incomprehensible sounds	2
	No response	1

Cranial Nerves

The nurse needs to be aware of specific nerve functions and assessment methods for each cranial nerve to detect abnormalities. In some cases, each nerve is assessed; in other cases only selected nerve functions are evaluated.

Reflexes

A **reflex** is an automatic response of the body to a stimulus. It is not voluntarily learned or conscious. The deep tendon reflex (DTR) is activated when a tendon is stimulated (tapped) and its associated muscle contracts. The quality of a reflex response varies among individuals and by age. As a client ages, reflex responses may become less intense.

Reflexes are tested using a percussion hammer. The response is described on a scale of 0 to 4. Experience is necessary to determine appropriate scoring for an individual. Generalist nurses do not commonly assess each of the deep tendon reflexes except for possibly the plantar (Babinski) reflex, indicative of possible spinal cord injury.

Motor Function

Neurologic assessment of the motor system evaluates proprioception and cerebellar function. Structures involved in proprioception are the proprioceptors, the posterior columns of the spinal cord, the cerebellum, and the vestibular apparatus (which is innervated by cranial nerve VIII) in the labyrinth of the internal ear.

Proprioceptors are sensory nerve terminals that occur chiefly in the muscles, tendons, joints, and internal ear. They give information about movements and the position of the body. Stimuli from the proprioceptors travel through the posterior columns of the spinal cord. Deficits of function of the posterior columns of the spinal cord result in impairment of muscle and position sense. Clients with such impairment often must watch their own arm and leg movements to ascertain the position of the limbs.

The cerebellum (a) helps to control posture, (b) acts with the cerebral cortex to make body movements smooth and coordinated, and (c) controls skeletal muscles to maintain equilibrium.

Sensory Function

Sensory functions include touch, pain, temperature, position, and tactile discrimination. The first three are routinely tested. Generally, the face, arms, legs, hands, and feet are tested for touch and pain, although all parts of the body can be tested. If the client complains of numbness, peculiar sensations, or paralysis, the practitioner should check sensation more carefully over flexor and extensor surfaces of limbs, mapping out clearly any abnormality of touch or pain by examining responses in the area about every 2 cm (1 in.). This is a lengthy procedure and may be performed by a specialist. Abnormal responses to touch stimuli include loss of sensation (anesthesia); more than normal sensation (hyperesthesia); less than normal sensation (hypoesthesia); or an abnormal sensation such as burning, pain, or an electric shock (paresthesia).

A variety of common health conditions, including diabetes and arteriosclerotic heart disease, result in loss of the protective sensation in the lower extremities. This loss can lead to severe tissue damage. In efforts to identify clients at increased risk for damage to the feet, the Bureau of Primary Health Care of the U.S. government has established the Lower Extremity Amputation Prevention (LEAP) program. The most important aspect of LEAP is assessment of sensation using a special monofilament that delivers 10 grams of force. Healthcare providers should perform an initial foot screen on all clients with diabetes and at least annually thereafter. Clients who are at risk should have their feet and shoes evaluated at least 4 times a year to help prevent foot problems from occurring.

A detailed neurologic examination includes position sense, temperature sense, and tactile discrimination. Three types of tactile discrimination are generally tested: **one- and two-point discrimination**, the ability to sense whether one or two areas of the skin are being stimulated by pressure; **stereognosis**, the act of recognizing objects by touching and manipulating them; and **extinction**, the failure to perceive touch on one side of the body when two symmetric areas of the body are touched simultaneously. Skill 29.17 describes how to assess the neurologic system.

Assessing the Neurologic System

SKILL 29.17

PLANNING

If possible, determine whether a screening or full neurologic examination is indicated. This impacts preparation of the client, equipment, and timing.

Assignment

Due to the substantial knowledge and skill required, assessment of the neurologic system is not assigned to AP. However, many aspects of neurologic behavior are observed during usual care and may be recorded by individuals other than the nurse. Abnormal findings must be validated and interpreted by the nurse.

Equipment (Depending on Components of Examination)

- Percussion hammer
- Wisps of cotton to assess light-touch sensation
- Sterile safety pin for tactile discrimination

IMPLEMENTATION

Performance

1. Prior to performing the assessment, introduce self and verify the client's identity using agency protocol. Explain to the client what you are going to do, why it is necessary, and how to participate. Discuss how the results will be used in planning further care or treatments.
2. Perform hand hygiene and observe other appropriate infection prevention procedures.
3. Provide for client privacy.
4. Inquire if the client has any history of the following: presence of pain in the head, back, or extremities, as well as onset and aggravating and alleviating factors; disorientation to time, place, or person; speech disorder; loss of consciousness, fainting, convulsions, trauma, tingling or numbness, tremors or tics, limping, paralysis, uncontrolled muscle movements, loss of memory, mood swings; or problems with smell, vision, taste, touch, or hearing.

Clinical Alert!

All questions and tests used in a neurologic examination must be age, language, education level, and culturally appropriate. Individualize questions and tests before using them.

Language

5. If the client displays difficulty speaking:
   - Point to common objects, and ask the client to name them.
   - Ask the client to read some words and to match the printed and written words with pictures.
   - Ask the client to respond to simple verbal and written commands (e.g., "point to your toes" or "raise your left arm").

Orientation

6. Determine the client's orientation to *time*, *place*, and *person* by tactful questioning. Ask the client the time of day, date, day of the week, duration of illness, city and state of residence, and names of family members.

   Ask the client why he or she is seeing a healthcare provider. Orientation is lost gradually, and early disorientation may be very subtle. "Why" questions may elicit a more accurate clinical picture of the client's orientation status than questions directed to time, place, and person. To evaluate the response, you must know the correct answer.

   More direct questioning may be necessary for some people (e.g., "Where are you now?" "What day is it today?"). Most people readily accept these questions if initially the nurse asks, "Do you get confused at times?" If the client cannot answer these questions accurately, also include assessment of the *self* by asking the client to state his or her full name.

Memory

7. Listen for lapses in memory. Ask the client about difficulty with memory. If problems are apparent, three categories of memory are tested: immediate recall, recent memory, and remote memory.

To Assess Immediate Recall

- Ask the client to repeat a series of three digits (e.g., 7–4–3), spoken slowly.
- Gradually increase the number of digits (e.g., 7–4–3–5, 7–4–3–5–6, and 7–4–3–5–6–7–2) until the client fails to repeat the series correctly.
- Start again with a series of three digits, but this time ask the client to repeat them backward. The average individual can repeat a series of five to eight digits in sequence and four to six digits in reverse order.

To Assess Recent Memory

- Ask the client to recall the recent events of the day, such as how the client got to the clinic. This information must be validated, however.
- Ask the client to recall information given early in the interview (e.g., the name of a doctor).
- Provide the client with three facts to recall (e.g., a color, an object, and an address) or a three-digit number, and ask the client to repeat all three. Later in the interview, ask the client to recall all three items.

Continued on page 636

SKILL 29.17

Assessing the Neurologic System—*continued*

To Assess Remote Memory

- Ask the client to describe a previous illness or surgery (e.g., 5 years ago) or a birthday or anniversary. Generally remote memory will be intact until late in neurologic pathology. It is least useful in assessing acute neurologic problems.

Attention Span and Calculation

8. Test the ability to concentrate or maintain *attention span* by asking the client to recite the alphabet or to count backward from 100. Test the ability to calculate by asking the client to subtract 7 or 3 progressively from 100 (i.e., 100, 93, 86, 79, or 100, 97, 94, 91), a task that is referred to as *serial sevens* or *serial threes*. Normally, an adult can complete the serial sevens test in about 90 seconds with three or fewer errors. Because educational level, language, or cultural differences affect calculating ability, this test may be inappropriate for some people.

Level of Consciousness

9. Apply the Glasgow Coma Scale (see Table 29.10 on page 634): eye response, motor response, and verbal response. An assessment totaling 15 points indicates the client is alert and completely oriented. A comatose client scores 7 or less.

Cranial Nerves

10. For the specific functions and assessment methods of each cranial nerve, see Table 29.11 on page 641. Test each nerve not already evaluated in another component of the health assessment. A quick way to remember which cranial nerves are assessed in the face is shown in ❶.

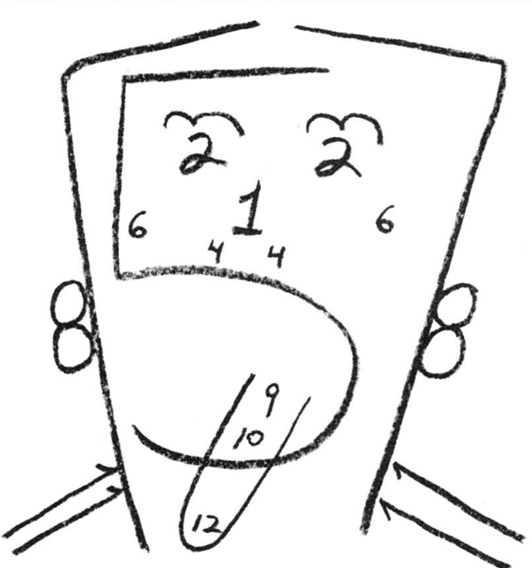

❶ Cranial nerves by the numbers. The next time you're trying to remember the locations and functions of the cranial nerves, picture this drawing. All the cranial nerves are represented, though some may be a little harder to spot than others. For example, the shoulders are formed by the number "11" because cranial nerve XI controls neck and shoulder movement. If you immediately recognize that the sides of the face and the top of the head are formed by the number "7" you're well on your way to using this memory device.

Clinical Alert!

The names and order of the cranial nerves can be recalled by a mnemonic device such as "On old Olympus' treeless top, a Finn and German viewed a hop." The first letter of each word in the sentence is the same as the first letter of the name of the cranial nerve, in order.

Assessment	Normal Findings	Deviations from Normal
Reflexes **11.** Test reflexes using a percussion hammer, comparing one side of the body with the other to evaluate the symmetry of response. 0 No reflex response +1 Minimal activity (hypoactive) +2 Normal response +3 More active than normal +4 Maximal activity (hyperactive) *Plantar (Babinski) Reflex* The plantar, or Babinski, reflex is superficial. It may be absent in adults without pathology or overridden by voluntary control. • Use a moderately sharp object, such as the handle of the percussion hammer, a key, or an applicator stick. • Stroke the lateral border of the sole of the client's foot, starting at the heel, continuing to the ball of the foot, and then proceeding across the ball of the foot toward the big toe. ❷ • Observe the response.	Normally, all five toes bend downward; this reaction is negative Babinski. 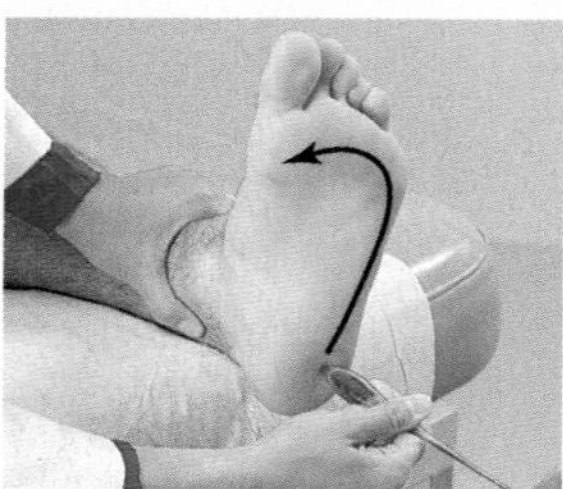 ❷ Testing the plantar (Babinski) reflex.	In an abnormal (positive) Babinski response, the toes spread outward and the big toe moves upward.

Assessing the Neurologic System—*continued*

Assessment	Normal Findings	Deviations from Normal
MOTOR FUNCTION **12.** *Gross Motor and Balance Tests* Generally, the Romberg test and one other gross motor function and balance test are used.		
WALKING GAIT Ask the client to walk across the room and back, and assess the client's gait.	Has upright posture and steady gait with opposing arm swing; walks unaided, maintaining balance	Has poor posture and unsteady, irregular, staggering gait with wide stance; bends legs only from hips; has rigid or no arm movements
ROMBERG TEST Ask the client to stand with feet together and arms resting at the sides, first with eyes open, then closed. Stand close during this test. **Rationale:** *This prevents the client from falling.*	Negative Romberg: may sway slightly but is able to maintain upright posture and foot stance	Positive Romberg: cannot maintain foot stance; moves the feet apart to maintain stance If client cannot maintain balance with the eyes shut, client may have sensory ataxia (lack of coordination of the voluntary muscles) If balance cannot be maintained whether the eyes are open or shut, client may have cerebellar ataxia
STANDING ON ONE FOOT WITH EYES CLOSED Ask the client to close the eyes and stand on one foot. Repeat on the other foot. Stand close to the client during this test.	Maintains stance for at least 5 seconds	Cannot maintain stance for 5 seconds
HEEL-TOE WALKING Ask the client to walk a straight line, placing the heel of one foot directly in front of the toes of the other foot. ❸	Maintains heel-toe walking along a straight line 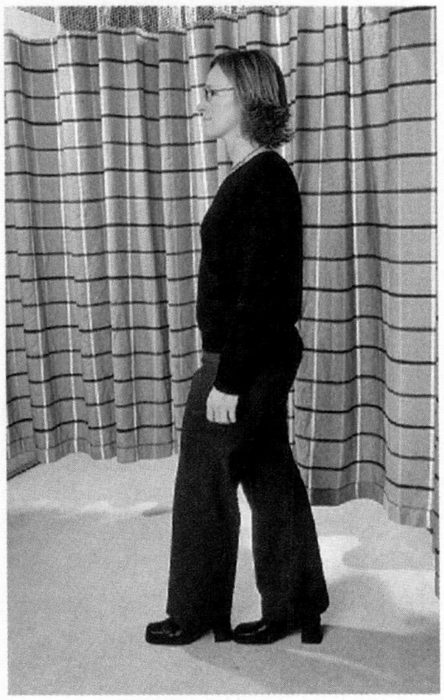 ❸ Heel-toe walking test.	Assumes a wider foot gait to stay upright
TOE OR HEEL WALKING Ask the client to walk several steps on the toes and then on the heels.	Able to walk several steps on toes or heels	Cannot maintain balance on toes and heels

Continued on page 638

Assessing the Neurologic System—*continued*

Assessment	Normal Findings	Deviations from Normal
13. Fine Motor Tests for the Upper Extremities		
FINGER-TO-NOSE TEST Ask the client to abduct and extend the arms at shoulder height and then rapidly touch the nose alternately with one index finger and then the other. The client repeats the test with the eyes closed if the test is performed easily. ❹	Repeatedly and rhythmically touches the nose 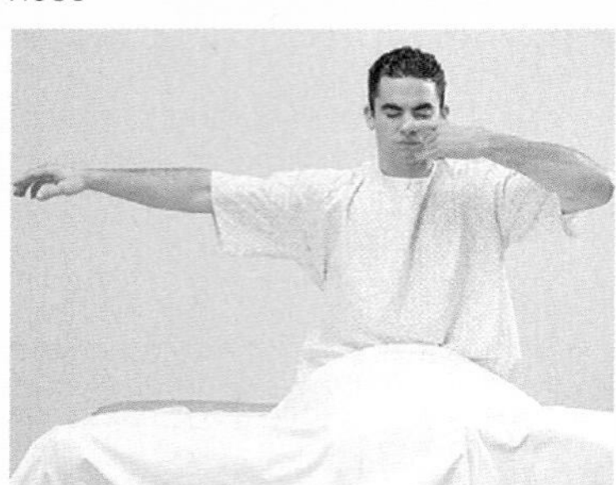 ❹ Finger-to-nose test.	Misses the nose or gives slow response
ALTERNATING SUPINATION AND PRONATION OF HANDS ON KNEES Ask the client to pat both knees with the palms of both hands and then with the backs of the hands alternately at an ever-increasing rate. ❺	Can alternately supinate and pronate hands at rapid pace 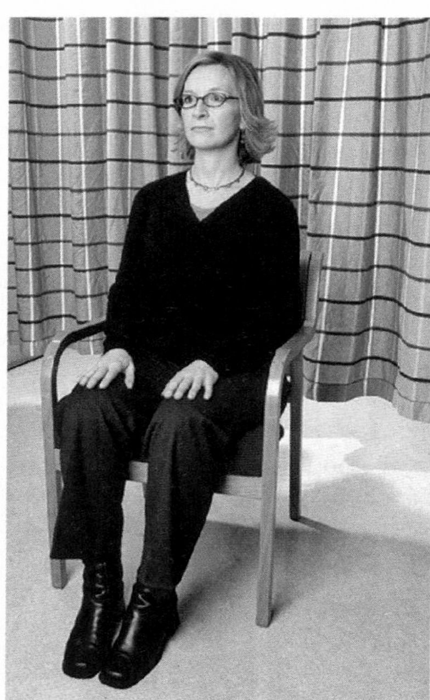	Performs with slow, clumsy movements and irregular timing; has difficulty alternating between supination and pronation 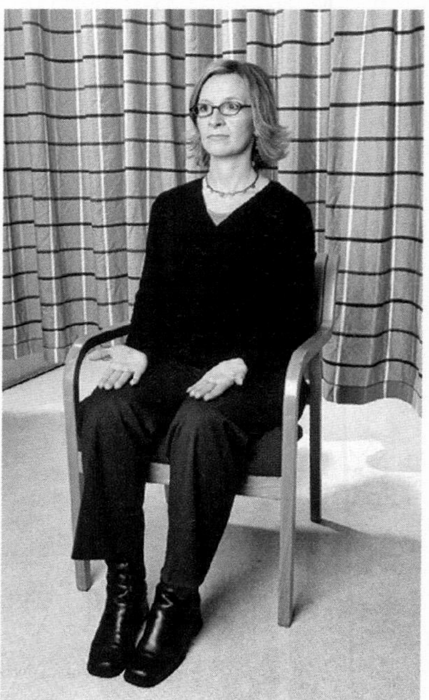
	❺ Alternating supination and pronation of hands on knees test.	
FINGER-TO-NOSE AND TO THE NURSE'S FINGER Ask the client to touch the nose and then your index finger, held at a distance of about 45 cm (18 in.), at a rapid and increasing rate. ❻	Performs with coordination and rapidity 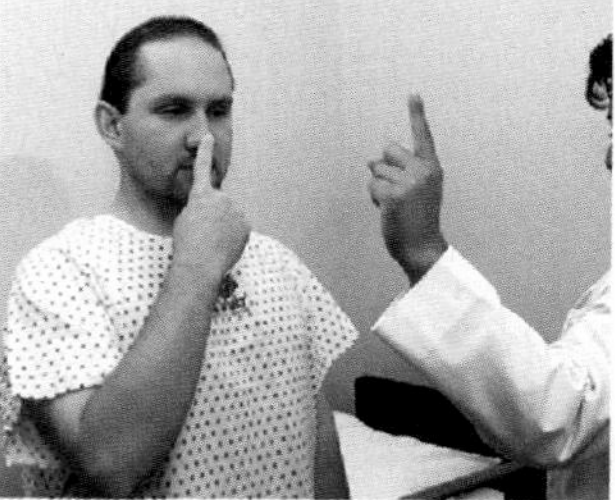 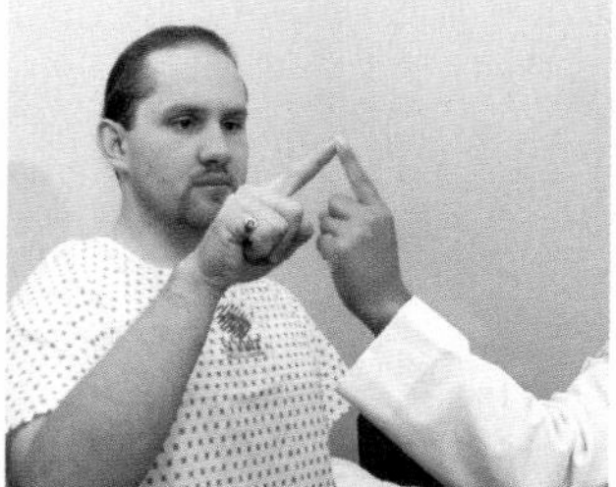 ❻ Finger-to-nose and to the nurse's finger test.	Misses the finger and moves slowly

Assessing the Neurologic System—*continued*

Assessment	Normal Findings	Deviations from Normal
FINGERS-TO-FINGERS Ask the client to spread the arms broadly at shoulder height and then bring the fingers together at the midline, first with the eyes open and then closed, first slowly and then rapidly. ❼	Performs with accuracy and rapidity	Moves slowly and is unable to touch fingers consistently

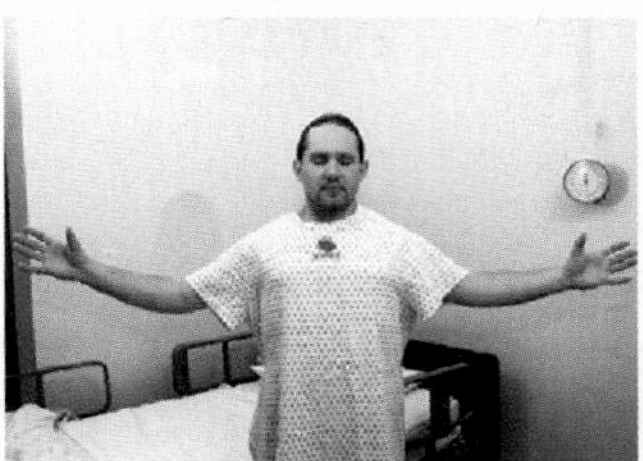

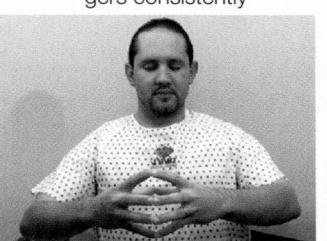

❼ Fingers-to-fingers test.

Assessment	Normal Findings	Deviations from Normal
FINGERS-TO-THUMB (SAME HAND) Ask the client to touch each finger of one hand to the thumb of the same hand as rapidly as possible. ❽	Rapidly touches each finger to thumb with each hand	Cannot coordinate this fine discrete movement with either one or both hands

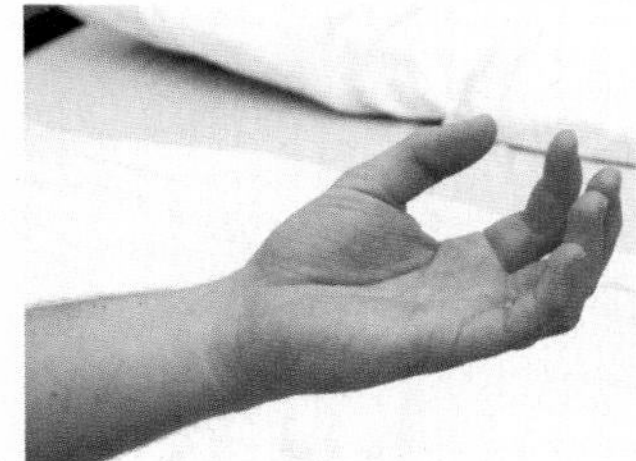

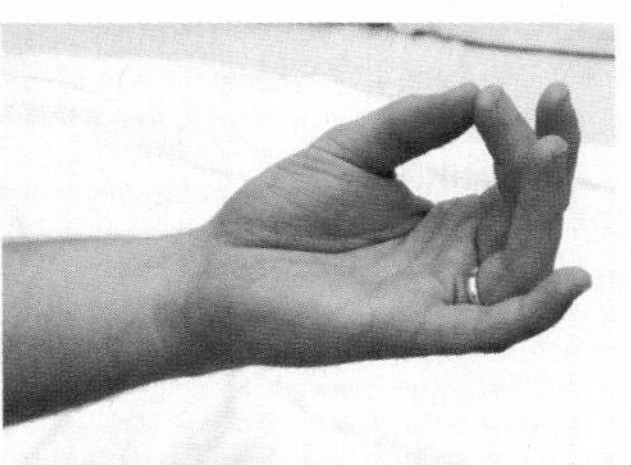

❽ Fingers-to-thumb (same hand) test.

14. Fine Motor Tests for the Lower Extremities
Ask the client to lie supine and to perform these tests.

Assessment	Normal Findings	Deviations from Normal
HEEL DOWN OPPOSITE SHIN Ask the client to place the heel of one foot just below the opposite knee and run the heel down the shin to the foot. Repeat with the other foot. The client may also use a sitting position for this test. ❾	Demonstrates bilateral equal coordination	Has tremors or is awkward; heel moves off shin

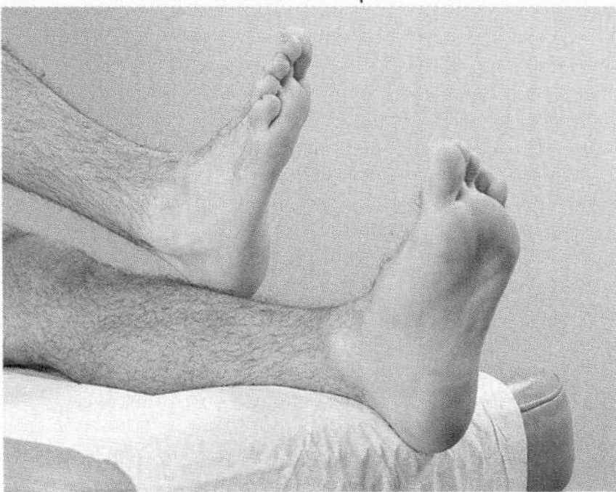

❾ Heel down opposite shin test.

Assessment	Normal Findings	Deviations from Normal
TOE OR BALL OF FOOT TO THE NURSE'S FINGER Ask the client to touch your finger with the large toe of each foot. ❿	Moves smoothly, with coordination	Misses your finger; cannot coordinate movement

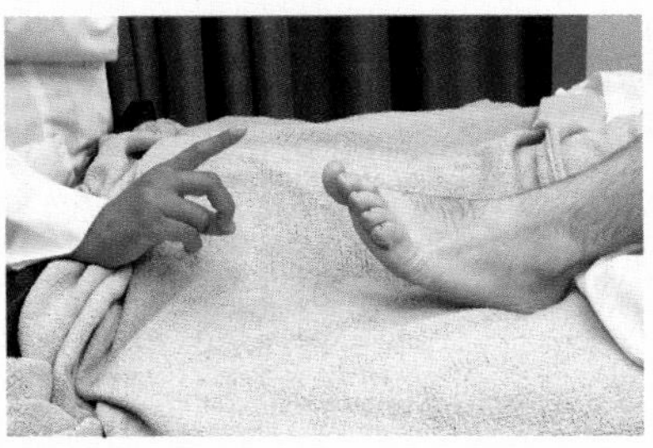

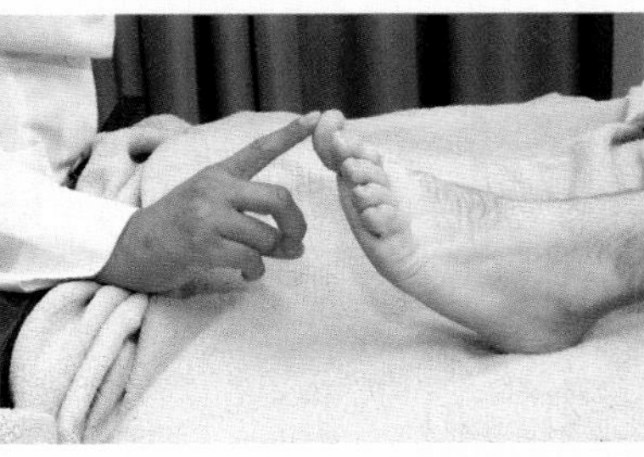

❿ Toe or ball of foot to nurse's finger test.

Continued on page 640

Assessing the Neurologic System—*continued*

Assessment	Normal Findings	Deviations from Normal
15. Light-Touch Sensation Compare the light-touch sensation of symmetric areas of the body. **Rationale:** *Sensitivity to touch varies among different skin areas.* • Ask the client to close the eyes and to respond by saying "yes" or "now" whenever the client feels the cotton wisp touching the skin. • With a wisp of cotton, lightly touch one specific spot and then the same spot on the other side of the body. ⓫ • Test areas on the forehead, cheek, hand, lower arm, abdomen, foot, and lower leg. Check a distal area of the limb first (i.e., the hand before the arm and the foot before the leg). **Rationale:** *The sensory nerve may be assumed to be intact if sensation is felt at its most distal part.* • If areas of sensory dysfunction are found, determine the boundaries of sensation by testing responses about every 2.5 cm (1 in.) in the area. Make a sketch of the sensory loss area for recording purposes.	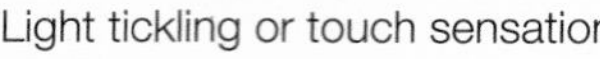Light tickling or touch sensation 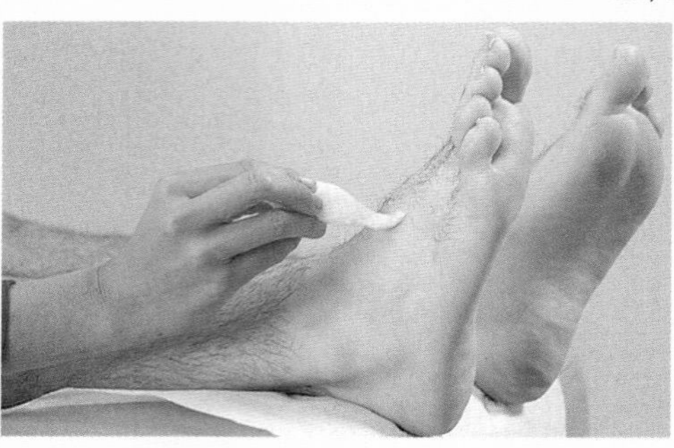 ⓫ Assessing light-touch sensation.	Anesthesia, hyperesthesia, hypoesthesia, or paresthesia
16. Pain Sensation Assess pain sensation as follows: • Ask the client to close the eyes and to say "sharp," "dull," or "don't know" when the sharp or dull end of a safety pin is felt. • Alternately, use the sharp and dull end to lightly prick designated anatomic areas at random (e.g., hand, forearm, foot, lower leg, abdomen). *Note*: The face is not tested in this manner. • Allow at least 2 seconds between each test to prevent summation effects of stimuli (i.e., several successive stimuli perceived as one stimulus).	Able to discriminate "sharp" and "dull" sensations	Areas of reduced, heightened, or absent sensation (map them out for recording purposes)
17. Position or Kinesthetic Sensation Commonly, the middle fingers and the large toes are tested for the kinesthetic sensation (sense of position). • To test the fingers, support the client's arm and hand with one hand. To test the toes, place the client's heels on the examining table. • Ask the client to close the eyes. • Grasp a middle finger or a big toe firmly between your thumb and index finger, and exert the same pressure on both sides of the finger or toe while moving it. ⓬ • Move the finger or toe until it is up, down, or straight out, and ask the client to identify the position. • Use a series of brisk, gentle up-and-down movements before bringing the finger or toe suddenly to rest in one of the three positions.	Can readily determine the position of fingers and toes 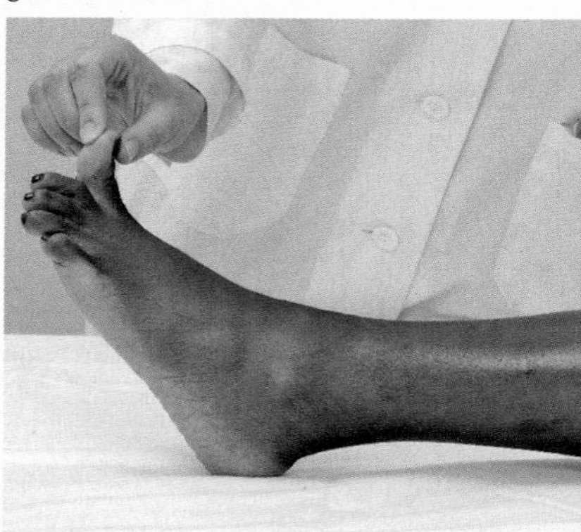 ⓬ Position or kinesthetic sensation.	Unable to determine the position of one or more fingers or toes

18. Document findings in the client record using printed or electronic forms or checklists supplemented by narrative notes when appropriate. Describe any abnormal findings in objective terms, for example, "When asked to count backwards by threes, client made seven errors and completed the task in 4 minutes."

EVALUATION

- Perform a detailed follow-up examination of specific systems based on findings that deviated from expected or normal for the client. Relate findings to previous assessment data if available.
- Report significant deviations from expected or normal findings to the primary care provider.

LIFESPAN CONSIDERATIONS Assessing the Neurologic System

INFANTS

- Reflexes commonly tested in newborns include:
  - *Rooting:* Stroke the side of the face near mouth; infant opens mouth and turns to the side that is stroked.
  - *Sucking:* Place nipple or finger 3 to 4 cm (1.2 to 1.6 in.) into mouth; infant sucks vigorously.
  - *Tonic neck:* Place infant supine, turn head to one side; arm on side to which head is turned extends; on opposite side, arm curls up (fencer's pose).
  - *Palmar grasp:* Place finger in infant's palm and press; infant curls fingers around.
  - *Stepping:* Hold infant as if weight bearing on surface; infant steps along, one foot at a time.
  - *Moro:* Present loud noise or unexpected movement; infant spreads arms and legs, extends fingers, then flexes and brings hands together; may cry.
- Most of these reflexes disappear between 4 and 6 months of age.

CHILDREN

- Present the procedures as games whenever possible.
- Positive Babinski reflex is abnormal after the child ambulates or at age 2.
- For children under age 5, the Denver Developmental Screening Test II provides a comprehensive neurologic evaluation, particularly for motor function.
- Note the child's ability to understand and follow directions.
- Assess immediate recall or recent memory by using names of movie or cartoon characters who would be known to that child. Normal recall in children is one less than age in years.
- Assess for signs of hyperactivity or abnormally short attention span.
- Children should be able to walk backward by age 2, balance on one foot for 5 seconds by age 4, heel-toe walk by age 5, and heel-toe walk backward by age 6.
- Use of the Romberg test is appropriate for children ages 3 and older.

OLDER ADULTS

- Because older adults tire more easily than younger clients, a total neurologic assessment is often done at a different time than the other parts of the physical assessment.
- A full neurologic assessment can be lengthy. Conduct in several sessions if indicated, and cease the tests if the client is noticeably fatigued.
- A decline in mental status is not a normal result of aging. Changes are more the result of physical or psychologic disorders (e.g., fever, fluid and electrolyte imbalances, medications). Acute, abrupt-onset mental status changes are usually caused by delirium. These changes are often reversible with treatment. Chronic subtle mental health changes are usually caused by dementia and are usually irreversible.
- Intelligence and learning ability are unaltered with age. Many factors, however, inhibit learning (e.g., anxiety, illness, pain, cultural barrier).
- Short-term memory is often less efficient. Long-term memory is usually unaltered.
- Because old age is often associated with loss of support persons, depression can occur. Mood changes, weight loss, anorexia, constipation, and early morning awakening may be symptoms of depression.
- The stress of being in unfamiliar situations can cause confusion in older adults.
- As an individual ages, reflex responses may become less intense.
- Although there is a progressive decrease in the number of functioning neurons in the central nervous system and in the sense organs, older adults usually function well because of the abundant reserves in the number of brain cells.
- Impulse transmission and reaction to stimuli are slower.
- Many older adults have some impairment of hearing, vision, smell, temperature and pain sensation, memory, or mental endurance.
- Coordination changes and includes slower fine finger movements. Standing balance remains intact, and Romberg's test remains negative.
- Reflex responses may slightly increase or decrease. Many show loss of Achilles reflex, and the plantar reflex may be difficult to elicit.
- When testing sensory function, the nurse needs to give older adults time to respond. Normally, older adults have unaltered perception of light touch and superficial pain, decreased perception of deep pain, and decreased perception of temperature stimuli. Many also reveal a decrease or absence of position sense in the large toes.

TABLE 29.11 Cranial Nerve Functions and Assessment Methods

Cranial Nerve	Name	Type	Function	Assessment Method
I	Olfactory	Sensory	Smell	Ask client to close eyes and identify different mild aromas, such as coffee, vanilla, peanut butter, orange, lemon, chocolate.
II	Optic	Sensory	Vision and visual fields	Ask client to read Snellen-type chart; check visual fields by confrontation; and conduct an ophthalmoscopic examination (see Skill 29.6).
III	Oculomotor	Motor	Extraocular eye movement (EOM); movement of sphincter of pupil; movement of ciliary muscles of lens	Assess six ocular movements and pupil reaction (see Skill 29.6).
IV	Trochlear	Motor	EOM; specifically, moves eyeball downward and laterally	Assess six ocular movements (see Skill 29.6).

Continued on page 642

TABLE 29.11 Cranial Nerve Functions and Assessment Methods—*continued*

Cranial Nerve	Name	Type	Function	Assessment Method
V	Trigeminal Ophthalmic branch	Sensory	Sensation of cornea, skin of face, and nasal mucosa	While client looks upward, lightly touch the lateral sclera of the eye with sterile gauze to elicit blink reflex. To test light sensation, have client close eyes, wipe a wisp of cotton over client's forehead and paranasal sinuses. To test deep sensation, use alternating blunt and sharp ends of a safety pin over same areas.
	Maxillary branch	Sensory	Sensation of skin of face and anterior oral cavity (tongue and teeth)	Assess skin sensation as for ophthalmic branch above.
	Mandibular branch	Motor and sensory	Muscles of mastication; sensation of skin of face	Ask client to clench teeth.
VI	Abducens	Motor	EOM; moves eyeball laterally	Assess directions of gaze.
VII	Facial	Motor and sensory	Facial expression; taste (anterior two thirds of tongue)	Ask client to smile, raise the eyebrows, frown, puff out cheeks, close eyes tightly. Ask client to identify various tastes placed on tip and sides of tongue: sugar (sweet), salt, lemon juice (sour), and quinine (bitter); identify areas of taste.
VIII	Auditory			
	Vestibular branch	Sensory	Equilibrium	Perform Romberg test (see page 637).
	Cochlear branch	Sensory	Hearing	Assess client's ability to hear spoken word and vibrations of tuning fork.
IX	Glossopharyngeal	Motor and sensory	Swallowing ability, tongue movement, taste (posterior tongue)	Apply tastes on posterior tongue for identification. Ask client to move tongue from side to side and up and down.
X	Vagus	Motor and sensory	Sensation of pharynx and larynx; swallowing; vocal cord movement	Assessed with cranial nerve IX; assess client's speech for hoarseness.
XI	Accessory	Motor	Head movement; shrugging of shoulders	Ask client to shrug shoulders against resistance from your hands and turn head to side against resistance from your hand (repeat for other side).
XII	Hypoglossal	Motor	Protrusion of tongue; moves tongue up and down and side to side	Ask client to protrude tongue at midline, then move it side to side.

Female Genitals and Inguinal Area

The examination of the genitals and reproductive tract of females includes assessment of the inguinal lymph nodes and inspection and palpation of the external genitals. Completeness of the assessment of the genitals and reproductive tract depends on the needs and problems of the individual client. In most practice settings, generalist nurses perform only inspection of the external genitals and palpation of the inguinal lymph nodes.

For sexually active adolescent and adult females, a Papanicolaou test (Pap test) is used to detect cancer of the cervix. If there is an increased or abnormal vaginal discharge, specimens should be taken to check for a sexually transmitted infection.

Examination of the genitals usually creates uncertainty and apprehension, and the lithotomy position required for an internal examination can cause embarrassment. The nurse must explain each part of the examination in advance and perform the examination in an objective, supportive, and efficient manner. Not all agencies permit male practitioners to examine the female genitals. Some agencies may require the presence of another female during the examination so that there is no question of unprofessional behavior. Most female clients accept examination by a male, especially if he is emotionally comfortable about performing it and does so in a matter-of-fact and competent manner. If the male nurse does not feel comfortable about this part of the examination or if the client is reluctant to be examined by a man, the nurse should refer this part of the examination to a female practitioner. Skill 29.18 describes how to assess the female genitals and inguinal area.

Assessing the Female Genitals and Inguinal Area

SKILL 29.18

PLANNING

Assignment

Due to the substantial knowledge and skill required, assessment of the female genitals and inguinal lymph nodes is not assigned to AP. However, individuals other than the nurse may record any aspect that is observed during usual care. Abnormal findings must be validated and interpreted by the nurse.

Equipment

- Clean gloves
- Drape
- Supplemental lighting, if needed

IMPLEMENTATION

Performance

1. Prior to performing the assessment, introduce self and verify the client's identity using agency protocol. Explain to the client what you are going to do, why it is necessary, and how to participate. Discuss how the results will be used in planning further care or treatments.
2. Perform hand hygiene, apply gloves, and observe other appropriate infection prevention procedures.
3. Provide for client privacy. Request the presence of another healthcare provider if desired, required by agency policy, or requested by the client.
4. Inquire about the following: age of onset of menstruation, last menstrual period (LMP), regularity of cycle, duration, amount of daily flow, and whether menstruation is painful; incidence of pain during intercourse; vaginal discharge; number of pregnancies, number of live births, labor or delivery complications; urgency and frequency of urination at night; blood in urine, painful urination, incontinence; history of sexually transmitted infection, past and present.
5. Cover the pelvic area with a sheet or drape at all times when the client is not actually being examined. Position the client supine.

Assessment	Normal Findings	Deviations from Normal
6. Inspect the distribution, amount, and characteristics of pubic hair.	There are wide variations; generally kinky in the menstruating adult, thinner and straighter after menopause	Scant pubic hair (may indicate hormonal problem)
	Distributed in the shape of an inverse triangle	Hair growth should not extend over the abdomen
7. Inspect the skin of the pubic area for parasites, inflammation, swelling, and lesions. To assess pubic skin adequately, separate the labia majora and labia minora.	Pubic skin intact, no lesions Skin of vulva area slightly darker than the rest of the body Labia round, full, and relatively symmetric in adult females	Lice, lesions, scars, fissures, swelling, erythema, excoriations, varicosities, or leukoplakia
8. Inspect the clitoris, urethral orifice, and vaginal orifice when separating the labia minora.	Clitoris does not exceed 1 cm (0.4 in.) in width and 2 cm (0.8 in.) in length Urethral orifice appears as a small slit and is the same color as surrounding tissues	Presence of lesions
	No inflammation, swelling, or discharge	Presence of inflammation, swelling, or discharge
9. Palpate the inguinal lymph nodes. ❶ Use the pads of the fingers in a rotary motion, noting any enlargement or tenderness.	No enlargement or tenderness	Enlargement and tenderness

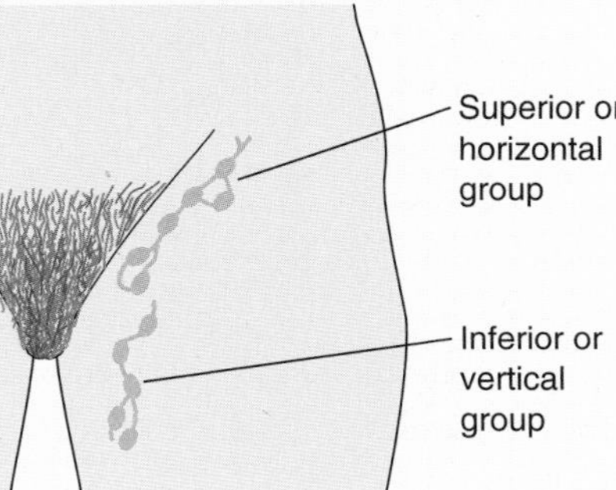

❶ Lymph nodes of the groin area.

10. Remove and discard gloves. Perform hand hygiene.
11. Document findings in the client record using printed or electronic forms or checklists supplemented by narrative notes when appropriate.

EVALUATION

- Perform a detailed follow-up examination of other systems based on findings that deviated from expected or normal for the client. Relate findings to previous assessment data if available.
- Significant deviations from normal indicate the need for an internal vaginal examination.

LIFESPAN CONSIDERATIONS Assessing the Female Genitals and Inguinal Area

INFANTS

- Infants can be held in a supine position on the parent's lap with the knees supported in a flexed position and separated.
- In newborns, because of maternal estrogen, the labia and clitoris may be edematous and enlarged, and there may be a small amount of white or bloody vaginal discharge.
- Assess the mons and inguinal area for swelling or tenderness that may indicate presence of an inguinal hernia.

CHILDREN

- Ensure that you have the parent or guardian's approval to perform the examination and then tell the child what you are going to do. Preschool children are taught not to allow others to touch their "private parts."
- Females should be assessed for Tanner staging of pubertal development (Box 29.9).
- Females should have a Papanicolaou (Pap) test done if sexually active, or by age 18 years.
- The clitoris is a common site for syphilitic chancres in younger females.

OLDER ADULTS

- Labia are atrophied and flattened.
- The clitoris is a potential site for cancerous lesions.
- The vulva atrophies as a result of a reduction in vascularity, elasticity, adipose tissue, and estrogen levels. Because the vulva is more fragile, it is more easily irritated.
- The vaginal environment becomes drier and more alkaline, resulting in an alteration of the type of flora present and a predisposition to vaginitis. Dyspareunia (difficult or painful intercourse) is also a common occurrence.
- The cervix and uterus decrease in size.
- The fallopian tubes and ovaries atrophy.
- Ovulation and estrogen production cease.
- Vaginal bleeding unrelated to estrogen therapy is abnormal in older females.
- Prolapse of the uterus can occur in older females, especially those who have had multiple pregnancies.

BOX 29.9 Five Stages of Pubic Hair Development in Females

Stage 1: Preadolescence. No pubic hair except for fine body hair.
Stage 2: Usually occurs at ages 11 and 12. Sparse, long, slightly pigmented curly hair develops along the labia.
Stage 3: Usually occurs at ages 12 and 13. Hair becomes darker in color and curlier and develops over the pubic symphysis.
Stage 4: Usually occurs between ages 13 and 14. Hair assumes the texture and curl of the adult but is not as thick and does not appear on the thighs.
Stage 5: Sexual maturity. Hair assumes adult appearance and appears on the inner aspect of the upper thighs (Figure 29.35 ■).

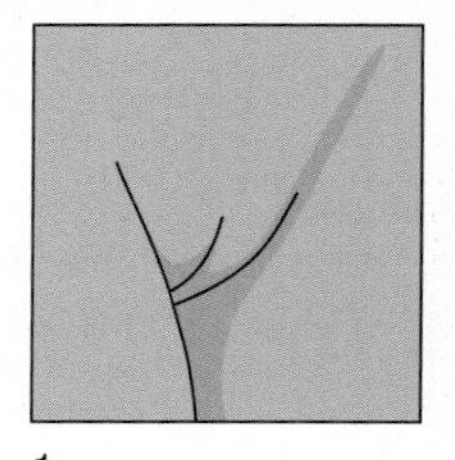
1

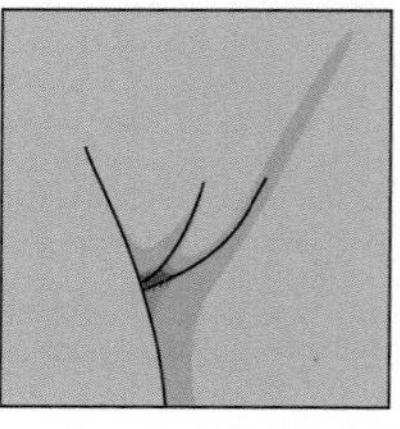
2

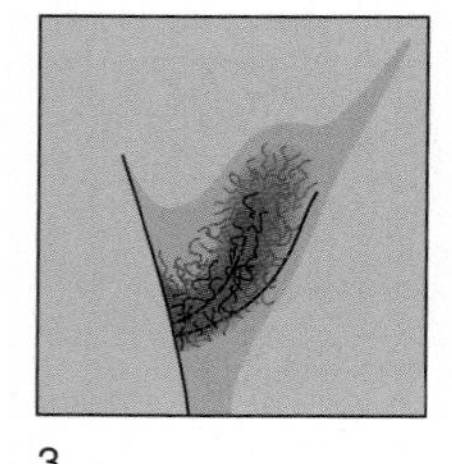
3

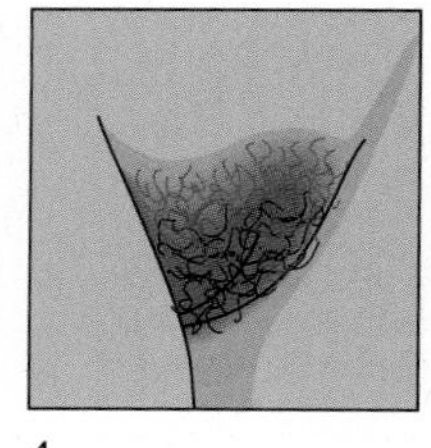
4

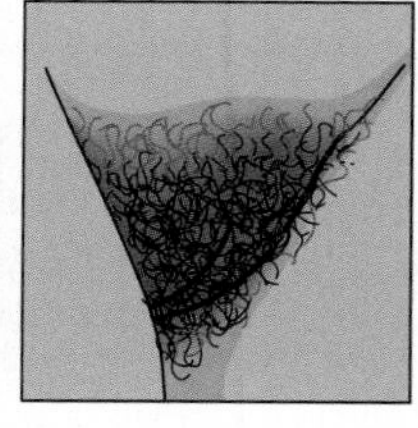
5

Figure 29.35 ■ Stages of female pubic hair development.

In many agencies only nurse practitioners examine the internal genitals. However, generalist nurses often assist with this examination and need to be familiar with the procedure. Examination of the internal genitals involves (a) palpating Skene's and Bartholin's glands, (b) assessing the pelvic musculature, (c) inserting a vaginal speculum to inspect the cervix and vagina, and (d) obtaining a Papanicolaou smear.

The speculum examination of the vagina involves the insertion of a plastic or metal speculum that consists of two blades and an adjustable thumb screw. Various sizes are available (small, medium, and large); the appropriate size needs to be selected for each client (Figure 29.36 ■). The speculum may be lubricated with water-soluble lubricant if specimens are not being collected. Most examiners lubricate the speculum with warm water. After visualizing the cervix, the examiner takes smear specimens from one or more of the sites.

The nurse's responsibilities when assisting with an examination of the internal female genitals include the following:

1. ***Assembling equipment.*** These include drapes, gloves, vaginal speculum, warm water or lubricant, and supplies for cytology and culture studies.
2. ***Preparing the client.*** Explain the procedure. It should take only 5 minutes and is normally not painful. Position the client as needed, and drape her appropriately.

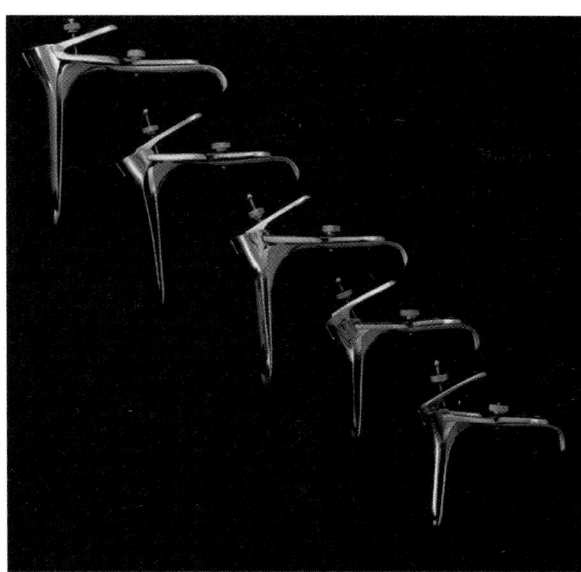

Figure 29.36 ■ Different sizes of metal vaginal specula.

3. *Supporting the client during the procedure.* This involves explaining the procedure as needed, and encouraging the client to take deep breaths that will help the pelvic muscles relax.
4. *Monitoring and assisting the client after the procedure.* Assist the client to a comfortable position and with perineal care as needed.
5. *Documenting the procedure.* Include the date and time it was performed, the name of the examiner, and any nursing assessments and interventions.

Male Genitals and Inguinal Area

In adult males, a complete examination includes assessment of the external genitals and prostate gland, and for the presence of any hernias. Nurses in some practice settings performing routine assessment of clients may assess only the external genitals. The male reproductive and urinary systems (Figure 29.37 ■) share the urethra, which is the passageway for both urine and semen. Therefore, in physical assessment of the male these two systems are frequently assessed together.

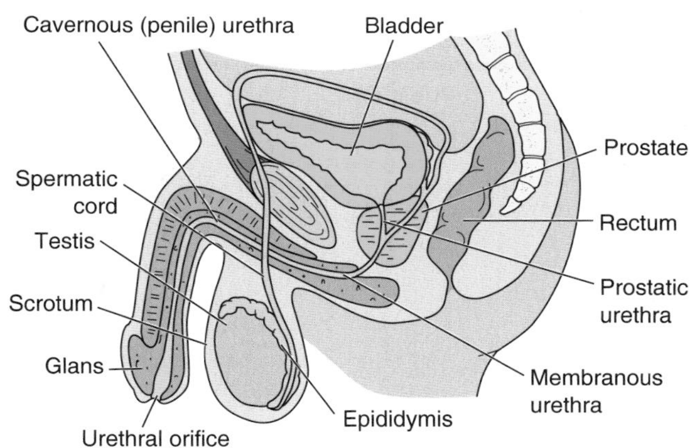

Figure 29.37 ■ The male urogenital tract.

Examination of the male genitals by a female practitioner is becoming increasingly common, although not all agencies permit a female practitioner to examine the male genitals. Some agencies may require the presence of another individual during the examination so that there is no question of unprofessional behavior. Most male clients accept examination by a female, especially if she is emotionally comfortable about performing it and does so in a matter-of-fact and competent manner. If the female nurse does not feel comfortable about this part of the examination or if the client is reluctant to be examined by a female, the nurse should refer this part of the examination to a male practitioner.

Development of secondary sex characteristics is assessed in relationship to the client's age. See Table 29.12 for the five Tanner stages of the development of pubic hair, the penis, and the testes and scrotum during puberty.

TABLE 29.12 Tanner Stages of Male Pubic Hair and External Genital Development (12 to 16 Years)

Stage	Pubic Hair	Penis	Testes, Scrotum
1	None, except for body hair like that on the abdomen	Size is relative to body size, as in childhood	Size is relative to body size, as in childhood
2	Scant, long, slightly pigmented at base of penis	Slight enlargement occurs	Becomes reddened in color and enlarged

Continued on page 646

TABLE 29.12 Tanner Stages of Male Pubic Hair and External Genital Development (12 to 16 Years)—*continued*

Stage	Pubic Hair	Penis	Testes, Scrotum
3	Darker, begins to curl and becomes more coarse; extends over pubic symphysis	Elongation occurs	Continuing enlargement
4	Continues to darken and thicken; extends on the sides, above and below	Increase in both breadth and length; glans develops	Continuing enlargement; color darkens
5	Adult distribution that extends to inner thighs, umbilicus, and anus	Adult appearance	Adult appearance

All male clients should be screened for the presence of inguinal or femoral hernias. A **hernia** is a protrusion of the intestine through the inguinal wall or canal. Cancer of the prostate gland is the most common cancer in adult males and occurs primarily in males over age 50. Examination of the prostate gland is performed with the examination of the rectum and anus (see Skill 29.20).

Testicular cancer is much rarer than prostate cancer and occurs primarily in young males ages 15 to 35. Testicular cancer is most commonly found on the anterior and lateral surfaces of the testes. Testicular self-examination should be conducted monthly (see Chapter 40 ∞).

The techniques of inspection and palpation are used to examine the male genitals. Skill 29.19 describes how the nurse can conduct an assessment of the male genitals and inguinal area.

SKILL 29.19 Assessing the Male Genitals and Inguinal Area

PLANNING

Assignment

Due to the substantial knowledge and skill required, assessment of the male genitals and inguinal area is not assigned to AP. However, individuals other than the nurse may record any aspect that is observed during usual care. Abnormal findings must be validated and interpreted by the nurse.

Equipment

- Clean gloves

IMPLEMENTATION

Performance

1. Prior to performing the assessment, introduce self and verify the client's identity using agency protocol. Explain to the client what you are going to do, why it is necessary, and how to participate. Discuss how the results will be used in planning further care or treatments.
2. Perform hand hygiene, apply gloves, and observe other appropriate infection prevention procedures.
3. Provide for client privacy. Request the presence of another healthcare provider if desired, required by agency policy, or requested by the client.
4. Inquire about the following: usual voiding patterns and changes, bladder control, urinary incontinence, frequency, urgency, abdominal pain; symptoms of sexually transmitted infection; swellings that could indicate presence of hernia; family history of nephritis, malignancy of the prostate, or malignancy of the kidney.
5. Cover the pelvic area with a sheet or drape at all times when not actually being examined.

Assessing the Male Genitals and Inguinal Area—*continued*

Assessment	Normal Findings	Deviations from Normal
PUBIC HAIR		
6. Inspect the distribution, amount, and characteristics of pubic hair.	Triangular distribution, often spreading up the abdomen	Scant amount or absence of hair
PENIS		
7. Inspect the penile shaft and glans penis for lesions, nodules, swellings, and inflammation.	Penile skin intact Appears slightly wrinkled and varies in color as widely as other body skin Foreskin easily retractable from the glans penis Small amount of thick white smegma between the glans and foreskin	Presence of lesions, nodules, swellings, or inflammation Foreskin not retractable Large amount, discolored, or malodorous substance
8. Inspect the urethral meatus for swelling, inflammation, and discharge.	Pink and slitlike appearance Positioned at the tip of the penis	Inflammation; discharge Variation in meatal locations (e.g., hypospadias, on the underside of the penile shaft, and epispadias, on the upper side of the penile shaft)
SCROTUM		
9. Inspect the scrotum for appearance, general size, and symmetry. • Inspect all skin surfaces by spreading the rugated surface skin and lifting the scrotum as needed to observe posterior surfaces.	Scrotal skin is darker in color than that of the rest of the body and is loose Size varies with temperature changes (the dartos muscles contract when the area is cold and relax when the area is warm) Scrotum appears asymmetric (left testis is usually lower than right testis)	Discolorations; any tightening of skin (may indicate edema or mass) Marked asymmetry in size
INGUINAL AREA		
10. Inspect both inguinal areas for bulges while the client is standing, if possible. • First, have the client remain at rest. • Next, have the client hold his breath and strain or bear down as though having a bowel movement. Bearing down may make the hernia more visible.	No swelling or bulges	Swelling or bulge (possible inguinal or femoral hernia)

11. Remove and discard gloves. Perform hand hygiene.

12. Document findings in the client record using printed or electronic forms or checklists supplemented by narrative notes when appropriate.

EVALUATION

- Perform a detailed follow-up examination of other systems based on findings that deviated from expected or normal for the client. Relate findings to previous assessment data if available.
- Report deviations from expected or normal findings to the primary care provider.

LIFESPAN CONSIDERATIONS Assessing the Male Genitals and Inguinal Area

INFANTS

- The foreskin of the uncircumcised infant is normally tight at birth and should not be retracted. It will gradually loosen as the baby grows and is usually fully retractable by 2 to 3 years of age. Assess for cleanliness, redness, or irritation.
- Assess for placement of the urethral meatus.
- Palpate the scrotum to determine if the testes are descended; in the newborn and infant, the testes may retract into the inguinal canal, especially with stimulation of the cremasteric reflex.
- Assess the inguinal area for swelling or tenderness that may indicate the presence of an inguinal hernia.

CHILDREN

- Ensure that you have the parent or guardian's approval to perform the examination and then tell the child what you are going to do. Preschool children are taught to not allow others to touch their "private parts."
- In young males, the cremasteric reflex can cause the testes to ascend into the inguinal canal. If possible have the child sit cross-legged, which stretches the muscle and decreases the reflex.
- Table 29.12 on page 645 shows the five Tanner stages of development of pubic hair, penis, testes, and scrotum.

OLDER ADULTS

- The penis decreases in size with age; the size and firmness of the testes decrease.
- Testosterone is produced in smaller amounts.
- More time and direct physical stimulation are required for an older man to achieve an erection, but he may have less premature ejaculation than he did at a younger age.
- Seminal fluid is reduced in amount and viscosity.
- Urinary frequency, nocturia, dribbling, and problems with beginning and ending the stream are usually the result of prostatic enlargement.

Anus

For the generalist nurse, anal examination, an essential part of every comprehensive physical examination, involves only inspection. Skill 29.20 describes how to assess the rectum and anus.

SKILL 29.20

Assessing the Anus

PLANNING

Assignment

Due to the substantial knowledge and skill required, assessment of the anus is not assigned to AP. However, many aspects are observed during usual care and may be recorded by individuals other than the nurse. Abnormal findings must be validated and interpreted by the nurse.

Equipment

- Clean gloves

IMPLEMENTATION

Performance

1. Prior to performing the assessment, introduce self and verify the client's identity using agency protocol. Explain to the client what you are going to do, why it is necessary, and how to participate. Discuss how the results will be used in planning further care or treatments.
2. Perform hand hygiene, apply gloves, and observe other appropriate infection prevention procedures for all rectal examinations.
3. Provide for client privacy. Drape the client appropriately to prevent undue exposure of body parts.
4. Inquire if the client has any history of the following: bright blood in stools, tarry black stools, diarrhea, constipation, abdominal pain, excessive gas, hemorrhoids, or rectal pain; family history of colorectal cancer; when last stool specimen for occult blood was performed and the results; and for males, if not obtained during the genitourinary examination, signs or symptoms of prostate enlargement (e.g., slow urinary stream, hesitance, frequency, dribbling, and nocturia).
5. Position the client. In adults, a left lateral or Sims' position with the upper leg acutely flexed is required for the examination. A dorsal recumbent position with hips externally rotated and knees flexed or a lithotomy position may be used. For males, a standing position while the client bends over the examining table may also be used.

Assessment	Normal Findings	Deviations from Normal
6. Inspect the anus and surrounding tissue for color, integrity, and skin lesions. Then, ask the client to bear down as though defecating. Bearing down creates slight pressure on the skin that may accentuate rectal fissures, rectal prolapse, polyps, or internal hemorrhoids. Describe the location of all abnormal findings in terms of a clock, with the 12 o'clock position toward the pubic symphysis.	Intact perianal skin; usually slightly more pigmented than the skin of the buttocks Anal skin is normally more pigmented, coarser, and moister than perianal skin and is usually hairless	Presence of fissures (cracks), ulcers, excoriations, inflammations, abscesses, protruding hemorrhoids (dilated veins seen as reddened protrusions of the skin), lumps or tumors, fistula openings, or rectal prolapse (varying degrees of protrusion of the rectal mucous membrane through the anus)

7. Remove and discard gloves. Perform hand hygiene.
8. Document findings in the client record using printed or electronic forms or checklists supplemented by narrative notes when appropriate.

EVALUATION

- Perform a detailed follow-up examination based on findings that deviated from expected or normal for the client. Relate findings to previous assessment data if available.
- Report deviations from expected or normal findings to the primary care provider.

LIFESPAN CONSIDERATIONS Assessing the Anus

INFANTS

- Lightly touching the anus should result in a brief anal contraction ("wink" reflex).

CHILDREN

- Erythema and scratch marks around the anus may indicate a pinworm parasite. Children with this condition may be disturbed by itching during sleep.

OLDER ADULTS

- Chronic constipation and straining at stool cause an increase in the frequency of hemorrhoids and rectal prolapse.

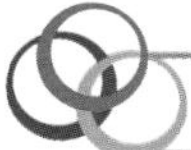

Critical Thinking Checkpoint

A 75-year-old female is admitted to your unit for evaluation after being found unconscious on the floor of her apartment. She is now awake but moving slowly. Her vital signs are within normal limits.

1. In the hospital, it is unrealistic to expect to be able to spend an uninterrupted 30 to 60 minutes with a single client performing an admission assessment. Which three systems would have top priority for her initial assessment and why?
2. While gathering relevant history data, what should you do if the client answers with simple one-word answers or gestures?
3. Because the client may be in significant discomfort from her fall, it is not easy for her to move about for the examination. How might you organize your assessment to minimize her need to change positions frequently?
4. If the client is unable to provide a detailed recent history, what other sources of these data could you consider?

Answers to Critical Thinking Checkpoint questions are available on the faculty resources site. Please consult with your instructor.

Chapter 29 Review

CHAPTER HIGHLIGHTS

- The health examination is conducted to assess the function and integrity of the client's body parts. Initial findings provide baseline data against which subsequent assessment findings are compared.
- The health examination may entail a complete head-to-toe assessment or individual assessment of a body system or body part.
- The health assessment is conducted in a systematic manner that requires the fewest position changes for the client.
- Data obtained in the physical health examination supplement, confirm, or refute data obtained during the nursing history.
- Aspects of the physical assessment procedures should be incorporated in the assessment, intervention, and evaluation phases of the nursing process.
- Nursing history data help the nurse focus on specific aspects of the physical health examination.
- Data obtained in the physical health examination help the nurse establish nursing diagnoses, plan the client's care, and evaluate the outcomes of nursing care.
- Skills in inspection, palpation, percussion, and auscultation are required for the physical health examination; these skills are used in that order throughout the examination except during abdominal assessment, when auscultation follows inspection and precedes percussion and palpation.
- Knowledge of the normal structure and function of body parts and systems is an essential requisite to conducting physical assessment.

TEST YOUR KNOWLEDGE

1. Which is a normal finding on auscultation of the lungs?
   1. Tympany over the right upper lobe
   2. Resonance over the left upper lobe
   3. Hyperresonance over the left lower lobe
   4. Dullness above the left 10th intercostal space

2. A nurse is utilizing the technique of inspection during a client's physical examination. When using this technique, what will the nurse do? Select all that apply.
   1. Visually observe a body area
   2. Obtain information through the sense of smell
   3. Obtain information through the sense of hearing
   4. Examine the body through the use of touch
   5. Strike the body to elicit a sound from a body part

3. After auscultating the abdomen, the nurse should report which finding to the primary care provider?
   1. Bruit over the aorta
   2. Absence of bowel sounds for 60 seconds
   3. Continuous bowel sounds over the ileocecal valve
   4. A completely irregular pattern of bowel sounds

4. If unable to locate the client's popliteal pulse during a routine examination, what should the nurse do next?
   1. Check for a pedal pulse.
   2. Check for a femoral pulse.
   3. Take the client's blood pressure on that thigh.
   4. Ask another nurse to try to locate the pulse.

5. Which of the following is an expected finding during assessment of the older adult?
   1. Facial hair that becomes finer and softer
   2. Decreased peripheral, color, and night vision
   3. Increased sensitivity to odors
   4. An irregular respiratory rate and rhythm at rest

6. List five aspects of the skin that the nurse assesses during a routine examination.
   1.
   2.
   3.
   4.
   5.

7. If the client reports loss of short-term memory, the nurse would assess this using which one of the following?
   1. Have the client repeat a series of three numbers, increasing to eight if possible.
   2. Have the client describe his or her childhood illnesses.
   3. Ask the client to describe what was eaten for breakfast.
   4. Ask the client to count backward from 100 subtracting seven each time.
8. Refer back to Figure 29.14. If the client can accurately read only the top three lines, what would be an appropriate nursing diagnosis?
   1. Inability to read
   2. Altered memory
   3. Myopia
   4. Potential for injury
9. What will a nurse do when performing indirect percussion of an area of a client's body during a physical examination? Select all that apply.
   1. Place the middle finger of the non-dominant hand on the client's skin.
   2. Use the tip of the flexed middle finger of the other hand to strike the middle finger of the non-dominant hand.
   3. Perform a striking motion by moving the wrist.
   4. Perform short, rapid, firm blows.
   5. Use a stethoscope to transmit sounds to the ears.
10. For a client whose assessment of the musculoskeletal system is normal, which does the nurse check on the medical record? (Select all that apply.)
    1. ____ Atrophied
    2. ____ Contractured
    3. ____ Crepitation
    4. ____ Equal
    5. ____ Firm
    6. ____ Flaccid
    7. ____ Hypertrophied
    8. ____ Spastic
    9. ____ Symmetrical
    10. ____ Tremor

See Answers to Test Your Knowledge in Appendix A.

READINGS AND REFERENCES

Suggested Reading

Fennessey, A. G. (2016). The relationship of burnout, work environment, and knowledge to self-reported performance of physical assessment by registered nurses. *MEDSURG Nursing, 25*, 346–350.

The author of this descriptive study noted in clinical practice that nurses often rushed through their assessments. The research aimed to determine if there was a correlation between burnout and nurses' self-reports of aspects of physical assessment, including how knowledgeable they were, how important they thought the assessment was, and how frequently the assessment was performed. No correlations were found. However, the study did show that those assessments the participants viewed as important did not match those identified by expert panels. Several areas for further research and consideration are identified.

Related Research

Celik, G. G., & Eser, I. (2017). Examination of intensive care unit patients' oral health. *International Journal of Nursing Practice, 23*(6), 12592. doi:10.1111/ijn.12592

Kohtz, C., Brown, S. C., Williams, R., & O'Connor, P. A. (2017). Physical assessment techniques in nursing education: A replicated study. *Journal of Nursing Education, 56*, 287–291. doi:10.3928/01484834-20170421-06

References

Barry, J. A., Mollan, S., Burdon, M. A., Jenkins, M., & Denniston, A. K. (2017). Development and validation of a questionnaire assessing the quality of life impact of colour blindness (CBQoL). *BMC Ophthalmology, 17*, 171–177. doi:10.1186/s12886-017-0579-z

Centers for Disease Control and Prevention. (2017). *Too loud! For too long! Loud noises damage hearing*. Retrieved from https://www.cdc.gov/vitalsigns/hearingloss

D'Amico, D., & Barbarito, C. (2016). *Health and physical assessment in nursing* (3rd ed.). Boston, MA: Pearson.

Neitzel, R. L., Swinburn, T. K., Hammer, M. S., & Eisenberg, D. (2017). Economic impact of hearing loss and reduction of noise-induced hearing loss in the United States. *Journal of Speech, Language and Hearing Research, 60*, 182–189. doi:10.1044/2016_JSLHR-H-15-0365

Prather, H., Hunt, D., McKeon, K., Simpson, S., Meyer, E. B., Yemm, T., & Brophy, R. (2016). Are elite female soccer athletes at risk for disordered eating attitudes, menstrual dysfunction, and stress fractures? *PM&R, 8*, 208–213. doi:10.1016/j.pmrj.2015.07.003

U.S. Preventive Services Task Force. (2016). *Breast cancer: Screening*. Retrieved from https://www.uspreventiveservicestaskforce.org/Page/Document/UpdateSummaryFinal/breast-cancer-screening1

Wender, R. C., Brawley, O. W., Fedewa, S. A., Gansler, T., & Smith, R. A. (2019). A blueprint for cancer screening and early detection: Advancing screening's contribution to cancer control. *CA: A Cancer Journal for Clinicians, 69*, 50–79. doi:10.3322/caac.21550

Selected Bibliography

Bickley, L. S. (2017). *Bates' guide to physical examination and history taking* (12th ed.). Philadelphia, PA: Lippincott Williams & Wilkins.

Donnelly, M., & Martin, D. (2016). History taking and physical assessment in holistic palliative care. *British Journal of Nursing, 25*, 1250–1255. doi.10.12968/bjon.2016.25.22.1250

Jarvis, C. (2020). *Physical examination & health assessment* (8th ed.). St. Louis, MO: Elsevier.

Wilson, S. F., & Giddens, J. F. (2017). *Health assessment for nursing practice* (6th ed.). St. Louis, MO: Elsevier.

Pain Assessment and Management 30

LEARNING OUTCOMES

After completing this chapter, you will be able to:

1. Discriminate between nociceptive and neuropathic pain categories.
2. Describe the four processes involved in nociception and how pain interventions can work during each process.
3. Describe factors that can affect a client's perception of and reaction to pain.
4. Identify subjective and objective data to collect and analyze when assessing pain.
5. Identify examples of nursing diagnoses for clients with pain.
6. Individualize a pain treatment plan based on clinical and personal goals, while setting objective outcome criteria by which to evaluate a client's response to interventions for pain.
7. Compare barriers to effective pain management affecting nurses and clients.
8. Differentiate tolerance, physical dependence, and addiction.
9. Describe the benefits of multimodal pain management.
10. Describe pharmacologic interventions for pain.
11. Describe the World Health Organization's three-step analgesic ladder approach developed for cancer pain control.
12. Identify risks and benefits of patient-controlled analgesia.
13. Describe nonpharmacologic pain control interventions.
14. Verbalize the steps used in performing a back massage.
15. Recognize when it is appropriate to assign aspects of back massage to assistive personnel.
16. Demonstrate appropriate documentation and reporting of back massage.
17. List three nonpharmacologic interventions directed at each of the following: the body, the mind, the spirit, and social interactions.

KEY TERMS

acute pain, *653*
addiction, *670*
adjuvant, *675*
cancer-related pain, *653*
chronic pain, *653*
effleurage, *680*
equianalgesia, *675*
mild pain, *653*
moderate pain, *653*
multimodal pain management, *671*
neuropathic pain, *653*
nociception, *654*
nociceptive pain, *653*
nociceptors, *654*
nonsteroidal anti-inflammatory drugs (NSAIDs), *672*
pain, *651*
pain management, *651*
pain threshold, *653*
pain tolerance, *653*
patient-controlled analgesia (PCA), *677*
physical dependence, *670*
placebo, *677*
preemptive analgesia, *671*
range orders, *675*
referred pain, *652*
severe pain, *653*
somatic pain, *653*
tolerance, *670*
transcutaneous electrical nerve stimulation (TENS), *682*
visceral pain, *652*

Introduction

Pain is an unpleasant and highly personal experience that may be imperceptible to others, while consuming all parts of an individual's life. The best definition of pain comes from Margo McCaffery, an internationally known nurse expert on pain. Her often-quoted definition of pain states, "pain is whatever the person says it is, and exists whenever he says it does" (Pasero & McCaffery, 2011, p. 21). This definition certainly portrays how subjective pain is. Another widely agreed-on definition of **pain** is "an unpleasant sensory and emotional experience associated with actual or potential tissue damage, or described in terms of such damage" (American Pain Society, 2016, p. 2). Three aspects of these definitions have important implications for nurses. First, pain is a physical *and* emotional experience, not all in the body or all in the mind. Second, it is in response to actual *or* potential tissue damage, so laboratory or radiographic reports may not be abnormal despite the real pain. Finally, pain is described in terms of such damage (e.g., neuropathic pain). Given that some clients are reluctant to disclose the presence of pain unless asked, nurses will be unaware of a client's pain until they assess for it. Additionally, clients who are nonverbal (e.g., preverbal children, intubated clients, people with cognitive impairments or those who are unconscious) are at risk for undertreatment of pain. They often experience pain that demands nursing assessment and treatment even though the clients are unable to describe their discomfort. Pain interferes with functional abilities and quality of life. Severe or persistent pain affects all body systems, causing potentially serious health problems while increasing the risk of complications and delays in healing (Polomano & Jungquist, 2017).

Pain management is the alleviation of pain or a reduction in pain to a level of comfort that is acceptable to the client. Even if the original cause of the pain heals, the changes in the nervous system resulting from suboptimal pain management may increase the risk of the development of persistent or chronic pain. Persistent pain also contributes to insomnia, weight gain or loss, constipation, hypertension, deconditioning, chronic stress, and depression. These effects can interfere with work, recreation, domestic activities, and personal care activities to the point at which many sufferers question whether life is worth living. Effective pain management is an important aspect of nursing care to promote healing, prevent complications, reduce suffering, and prevent the development of incurable pain states. To be a true client advocate, nurses must realize their role as advocates for pain relief.

Pain is more than a symptom of a problem; it can be a high-priority problem. Pain presents both physiologic and psychologic dangers to health and recovery. Severe pain requires prompt professional attention and treatment.

The Nature of Pain

Although pain is a universal experience, the nature of the experience is unique to the individual based, in part, on the type of pain experienced, the psychosocial meaning, and the response. Adding to the complexity, pain may be a physiologic warning system alerting the nurse to a problem or unmet need demanding attention; or it may be a diseased, malfunctioning segment of the nervous system. Advances in the understanding of physiologic mechanisms may someday help to create a warning system that will replace the currently used categories of acute pain or chronic (persistent) pain. In addition to the underlying mechanisms, nurses need to consider a holistic view of care and how these physiologic signals affect the mind, body, spirit, and social interactions. This section includes the scientific, theoretical, and clinical concepts that form the foundation of knowledge needed by nurses to assess and treat clients with pain in a holistic, comprehensive manner.

Types of Pain

Pain may be described in terms of location, duration, intensity, and etiology.

Location

Classifications of pain based on location (e.g., head, back, chest) may be problematic. For example, the International Headache Society (n.d.) recognizes numerous different types of headaches. Many have similar clinical presentations but different clinical needs. Nevertheless, location of pain is an important consideration. For example, if after knee surgery, a client reports moderately severe chest pain, the nurse must act immediately to further evaluate and treat this discomfort. The ability to discriminate between cardiac and noncardiac chest pain challenges even expert clinicians, but the fact that chest pain is evaluated and treated differently than knee pain in this client is understandable. Complicating the categorization of pain by location is the fact that some pains radiate (spread or extend) to other areas (e.g., low back to legs). Pain may also be **referred** (appear to arise in different areas) to other parts of the body. For example, cardiac pain may be felt in the shoulder or left arm, with or without chest pain (Figure 30.1 ■). **Visceral pain** (pain arising from organs or

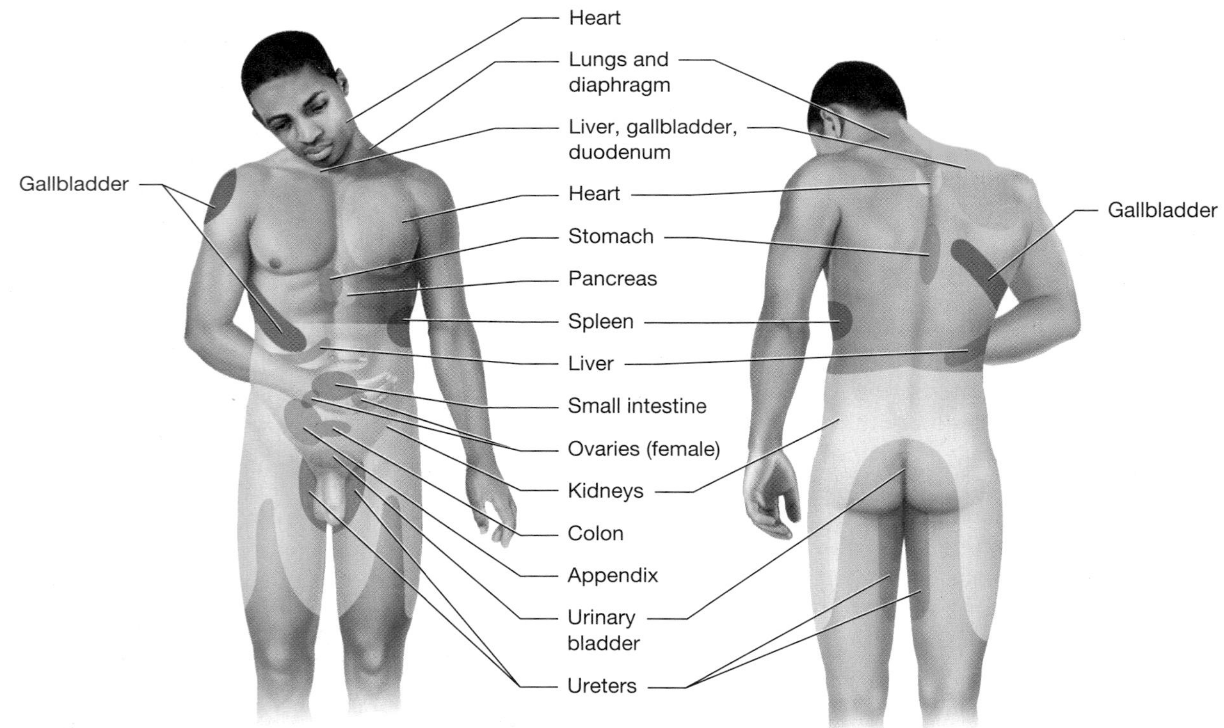

Figure 30.1 ■ Common sites of referred pain from various body organs.

hollow viscera) is often perceived in an area remote from the organ causing the pain.

Duration

When pain lasts only through the expected recovery period of less than 3 months, it is described as **acute pain**, whether it has a sudden or slow onset, regardless of its intensity. **Chronic pain**, also known as persistent pain, is caused by pain signals firing in the nervous system beyond 3 months to even years. The pain may have been initiated by an injury (e.g., sprained back) or may exist because of an ongoing cause of pain, such as arthritis (Cox, 2018; National Institute of Neurological Disorders and Stroke [NINDS], 2019). **Cancer-related pain** may result from the direct effects of the disease and its treatment, such as radiation or chemotherapy. Acute pain and chronic pain produce different physiologic and behavioral responses, as shown in Table 30.1.

Intensity

Most practitioners classify intensity of pain by using a numeric scale: 0 (no pain) to 10 (worst pain imaginable). Linking the rating to health and functioning scores, pain in the 1 to 3 range is considered **mild pain**, a rating of 4 to 6 is **moderate pain**, and pain reaching 7 to 10 is viewed as **severe pain** and is associated with the worst outcomes.

Etiology

Designating types of pain by etiology can be done under the broad categories of nociceptive pain and neuropathic pain. The process of pain awareness is nociception. **Nociceptive pain** is experienced when an intact, properly functioning nervous system sends signals that tissues are damaged, requiring attention and proper care. For example, the pain experienced following a cut or broken bone alerts the individual to avoid further damage until it is properly healed. Once stabilized or healed, the pain goes away; thus, this pain is temporary. There may also be persistent forms of nociceptive pain. An example is an individual who has lost the protective cartilage in joints. Pain will occur when the joints are stressed because the bone-to-bone contact damages tissues. This common form of osteoarthritis produces pain in millions of individuals, some of whom have intermittent pain whereas others have constant pain for years.

Subcategories of nociceptive pain include somatic and visceral. **Somatic pain** originates in the skin, muscles, bone, or connective tissue. The sharp sensation of a paper cut or aching of a sprained ankle are common examples of somatic pain. Visceral pain results from activation of pain receptors in the organs or hollow viscera and tends to be characterized by cramping, throbbing, pressing, or aching qualities. Often visceral pain is associated with feeling sick (e.g., sweating, nausea, or vomiting) as in the examples of labor pain, angina pectoris, or irritable bowel.

Neuropathic pain is associated with damaged or malfunctioning nerves due to illness (e.g., post-herpetic neuralgia, diabetic peripheral neuropathy), injury (e.g., phantom limb pain, spinal cord injury pain), or undetermined reasons. Neuropathic pain is typically chronic; it is often described as burning, "electric-shock," or tingling, painful numbness, dull, and aching. Episodes of sharp, shooting pain can also be experienced. Neuropathic pain tends to be difficult to treat.

Common chronic pain syndromes are briefly described in Box 30.1.

TABLE 30.1 Comparison of Acute and Chronic Pain

Acute Pain	Chronic Pain
Mild to severe	Mild to severe
Sympathetic nervous system responses: • Increased pulse rate • Increased respiratory rate • Elevated blood pressure • Diaphoresis • Dilated pupils	Parasympathetic nervous system responses: • Vital signs normal • Dry, warm skin • Pupils normal or dilated
Related to tissue injury; resolves with healing	Continues beyond healing
Client may be restless and anxious	Client is usually depressed and withdrawn
Client reports pain	Client often does not mention pain unless asked
Client may exhibit behavior indicative of pain: crying, rubbing area, holding area	Pain behavior often absent

Concepts Associated with Pain

It is useful for nurses to differentiate pain threshold from pain tolerance. **Pain threshold** is the least amount of stimuli that is needed for someone to label a sensation as pain. It may vary slightly from individual to individual, and may be related to age, gender, or race, but it changes little in the same individual over time. **Pain tolerance** is the maximum amount of painful stimuli that an individual is willing to withstand without seeking avoidance of the pain or relief. Pain tolerance varies significantly among individuals, even within the same individual at different times and in different circumstances. For example, a woman may tolerate a considerable amount of labor pain because she does not want to alter her level of alertness or the health of her baby. She likely would not tolerate a fraction of that pain during a routine dental procedure before requesting appropriate pain relief medicine. See Box 30.2 for a review of concepts associated with pain.

Physiology of Pain

The transmission and perception of pain are complex processes. The central nervous system's structure constantly changes, and the constituency and function of its chemical mediators are not well understood. The extent to which pain is perceived depends on the interaction between the body's analgesia system, the nervous system's transmission, and the mind's interpretation of stimuli and its meaning.

BOX 30.1 Common Chronic Pain Syndromes

- *Post-herpetic neuralgia.* This pain occurs when a case of herpes zoster (shingles) typically erupts decades after a primary infection (chickenpox) during a period of stress or compromised immune functioning. After the painful unilateral vesicular rash fades, burning or electric-shock pain in the area may persist for months or years. Advancing age is a risk factor for persistent post-herpetic neuralgia. A vaccine has been approved and is recommended for all people over the age of 60 to prevent shingles and the possibility of post-herpetic neuralgia.
- *Phantom pain.* Phantom sensations, the feeling that a lost body part is present, occur in most people after amputation. For many, this sensation is painful and it may occur spontaneously or be evoked (e.g., by a poor-fitting prosthesis). When the amputation involves a limb, it is termed *phantom limb pain*, whereas following breast surgery, it is called *postmastectomy pain*. If the limb was painful or mangled before the amputation, that is commonly the sensation that is experienced (unless the discomfort is completely relieved prior to surgery). It is important for the nurse to remember to explain the reasons for phantom limb pain, as clients may have difficulty understanding why they have pain when the limb is gone. They may start to question their sanity.
- *Trigeminal neuralgia.* This is an intense stablike pain that is distributed by one or more branches of the trigeminal nerve (fifth cranial). The pain is usually experienced on parts of the face and head. It is so severe that it produces facial muscle spasms.
- *Headache.* This commonly occurring painful condition can be caused by either intracranial or extracranial problems, or serious or benign conditions. To establish a plan to prevent or treat headache, the nurse needs to assess the quality, location, onset, duration, and frequency of the pain, as well as any signs and symptoms that precede the headache. There are many types of headaches, but the three most common include migraine, tension, and cluster. Migraine and tension headaches are 3 times more common in women than in men, while cluster headaches occur primarily in men.
- *Low back pain.* Nearly everyone suffers from low back pain at some time during their lives. Most occurrences of low back pain go away within a few days. Chronic back pain (CBP) is often progressive and the cause can be difficult to determine. *Healthy People 2020* includes objectives about CBP because it is common, costly, and potentially disabling (Office of Disease Prevention and Health Promotion, n.d.).
- *Fibromyalgia.* This chronic disorder is characterized by widespread musculoskeletal pain, fatigue, and multiple tender points. This disease is poorly understood and primarily occurs in women. "Tender points" refers to tenderness that occurs in precise, localized areas, particularly in the neck, spine, shoulders, and hips. People with this syndrome may also experience sleep disturbances, morning stiffness, irritable bowel syndrome, anxiety, and other symptoms. Although the symptoms present as muscle pain, stiffness, and weakness, it is considered by many to be a problem of abnormal central nervous system (CNS) functioning, particularly as it relates to the way nerves process pain.

BOX 30.2 Concepts Associated with Pain

Acute pain: Pain that is directly related to tissue injury and resolves when tissue heals. Usually lasts less than 3 months.

Cancer-related pain: Pain associated with the disease, treatment, or some other factor in individuals with cancer. Can be acute, recurrent, or chronic.

Chronic or persistent pain: Pain that persists beyond 3 to 6 months secondary to chronic disorders or nerve malfunctions that produce ongoing pain after healing is complete.

Intractable pain: A pain state (generally severe) for which no cure is possible even after accepted medical evaluation and treatments have been implemented. The focus of treatment turns from cure to pain reduction, functional improvement, and the enhancement of quality of life.

Neuropathic pain: Pain that is related to damaged or malfunctioning nervous tissue in the peripheral or CNS.

Nociceptive pain: Pain that is directly related to tissue damage. May be somatic (e.g., damage to skin, muscle, bone) or visceral (e.g., damage to organs).

Pain threshold: The least amount of stimuli necessary for an individual to label a sensation as pain.

Pain tolerance: The most pain an individual is willing or able to tolerate before taking evasive actions.

Procedural pain: Pain associated with any medical intervention. Nurses need to anticipate type of expected pain and provide appropriate interventions.

The following states indicate abnormal nerve functioning, and the associated cause needs to be identified and treated (as soon as possible) before irreversible damage occurs:

Allodynia: Sensation of pain from a stimulus that normally does not produce pain (e.g., light touch).

Dysesthesia: An unpleasant abnormal sensation that can be either spontaneous or evoked.

Hyperalgesia: Increased sensation of pain in response to a normally painful stimulus.

The following concepts are important reasons to prevent pain or treat it as soon as possible to prevent the amplification, spread, and persistence of pain:

Sensitization: An increased sensitivity of a receptor after repeated activation by noxious stimuli.

Windup: Progressive increase in excitability and sensitivity of spinal cord neurons, leading to persistent, increased pain.

Nociception

The peripheral nervous system includes specialized primary sensory neurons that detect mechanical, thermal, or chemical conditions associated with potential tissue damage. When these nociceptors are activated, signals are transduced and transmitted to the spine and brain where the signals are modified before they are ultimately understood and then "felt." The physiologic processes related to pain perception are described as **nociception**. Four physiologic processes are involved in nociception: transduction, transmission, perception, and modulation.

Transduction

Specialized pain receptors or **nociceptors** can be excited by mechanical, thermal, or chemical stimuli (Table 30.2).

TABLE 30.2 Types of Pain Stimuli

Stimulus Type	Physiologic Basis of Pain
MECHANICAL	
1. Trauma to body tissues (e.g., surgery)	Tissue damage; direct irritation of the pain receptors; inflammation
2. Alterations in body tissues (e.g., edema)	Pressure on pain receptors
3. Blockage of a body duct	Distention of the lumen of the duct
4. Tumor	Pressure on pain receptors; irritation of nerve endings
5. Muscle spasm	Stimulation of pain receptors (also see chemical stimuli)
THERMAL	
Extreme heat or cold (e.g., burns)	Tissue destruction; stimulation of thermosensitive pain receptors
CHEMICAL	
1. Tissue ischemia (e.g., blocked coronary artery)	Stimulation of pain receptors because of accumulated lactic acid (and other chemicals, such as bradykinin and enzymes) in tissues
2. Muscle spasm	Tissue ischemia secondary to mechanical stimulation (see above)

During the transduction phase, harmful stimuli trigger the release of biochemical mediators, such as prostaglandins, bradykinin, serotonin, histamine, and substance P, which sensitize nociceptors. Painful stimulation also causes movement of ions across cell membranes, which excites nociceptors. Pain medications can work during this phase by blocking the production of prostaglandin (e.g., nonsteroidal anti-inflammatory drugs [NSAIDs]) or by decreasing the movement of ions across the cell membrane (e.g., topical local anesthetic). Another example is the topical analgesic capsaicin, which depletes the accumulation of substance P and blocks transduction.

Transmission

The second process of nociception, transmission of pain, includes three segments. During the first segment of transmission, the pain impulses travel from the peripheral nerve fibers to the spinal cord. Substance P serves as a neurotransmitter, enhancing the movement of impulses across the nerve synapse from the primary afferent neuron to the second-order neuron in the dorsal horn of the spinal cord (Figure 30.2 ■). Two types of nociceptor fibers cause this transmission to the dorsal horn of the spinal cord: unmyelinated C fibers, which transmit dull, aching pain, and thin A-delta fibers, which transmit sharp, localized pain. The second segment is transmission of the pain signal through an ascending pathway in the spinal cord to the brain (Figure 30.3 ■). The third segment involves transmission of information to the brain where pain perception occurs. Only microseconds are required for the signal to be conducted from the site of injury (transduction process) to the brain, where pain is perceived (perception process).

Pain control can take place during this second process of transmission. For example, opioids block the release of neurotransmitters, particularly substance P, which stops the pain at the spinal level. The gabapentinoids (i.e., gabapentin and pregabalin) treat neuropathic pain by inhibiting the transmission of painful stimuli in the dorsal horn (Polomano et al., 2017).

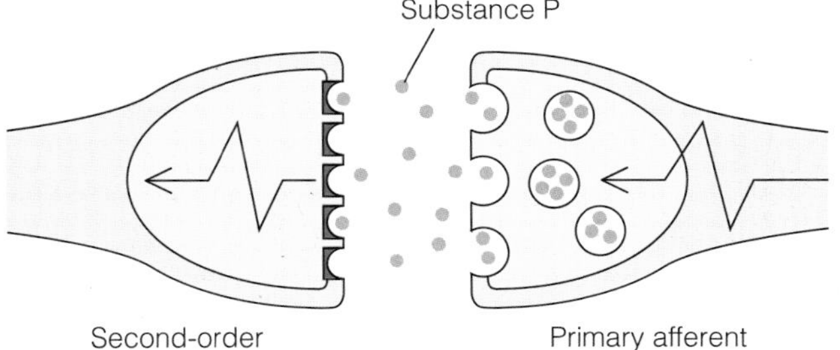

Figure 30.2 ■ Substance P assists the transmission of impulses across the synapse from the primary afferent neuron to a second-order neuron in the spinothalamic tract.

Perception

The third process, perception, is when the client becomes conscious of the pain. Pain perception is the sum of complex activities in the central nervous system (CNS) that may shape the character and intensity of pain perceived (e.g., sharp, burning, pressure) and give meaning to the pain. The psychosocial context of the situation and the meaning of the pain based on past experiences and future hopes and dreams help to shape the behavioral response that follows. Nonpharmacologic interventions such as distraction, imagery, massage, and acupuncture have been used to influence pain perception.

Modulation

Often described as the "descending system," this final process occurs when neurons in the brain send signals back down to the dorsal horn of the spinal cord. These descending fibers release substances such as endogenous opioids, serotonin, and norepinephrine, which can inhibit or reduce the ascending painful impulses in the dorsal horn. In contrast, excitatory amino acids (e.g., glutamate, N-methyl-d-aspartate [NMDA]) can increase these pain signals. The effects of excitatory amino acids tend to continue, while the effects of the inhibitory neurotransmitters (endogenous opioids, serotonin, and norepinephrine)

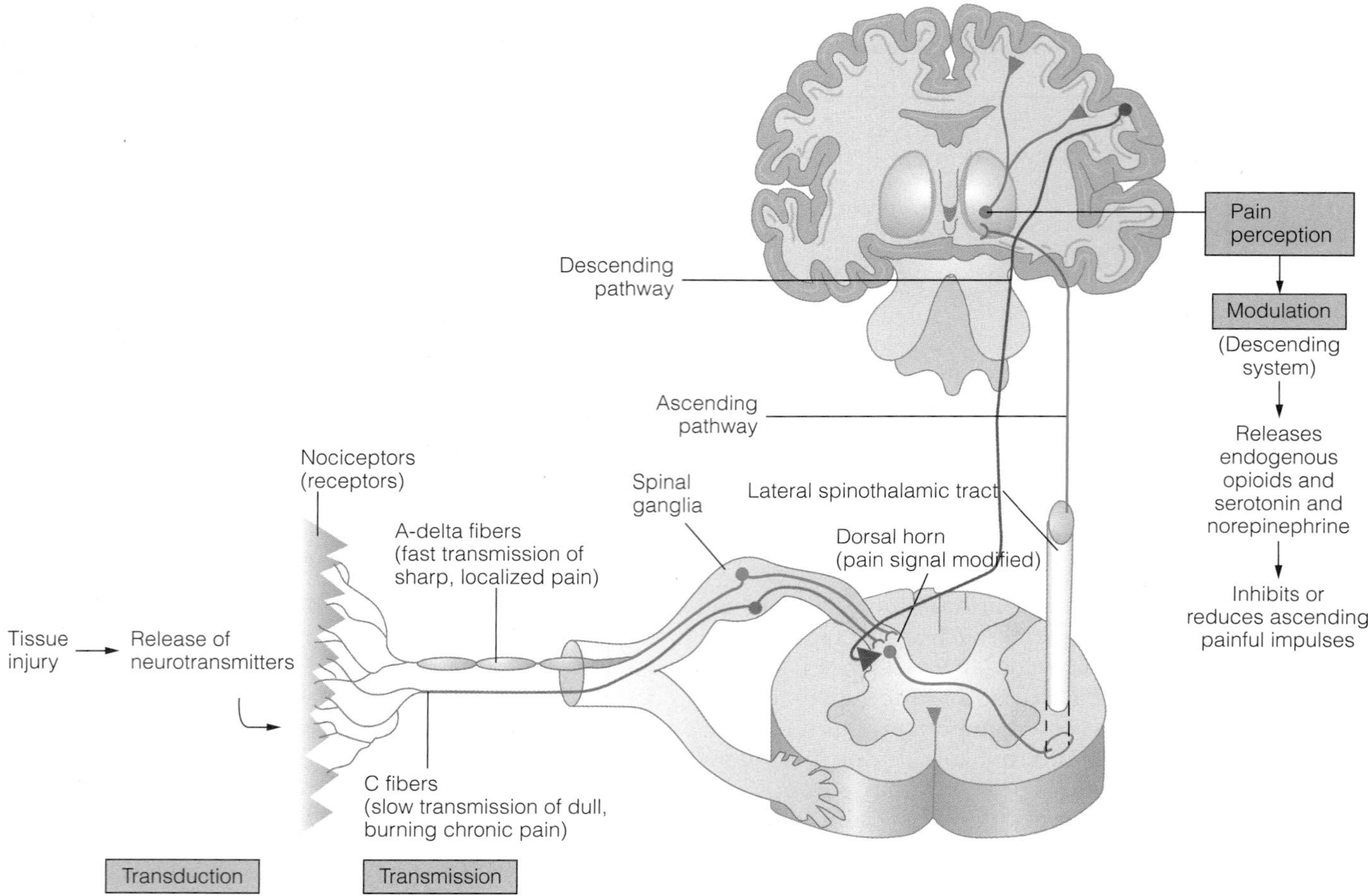

Figure 30.3 ■ Physiology of pain perception. Pain processing involves the ascending (in red) and descending (in blue) pathways.

tend to be short lived because they are reabsorbed into the nerves. Tricyclic antidepressants can relieve pain by blocking the resorption of norepinephrine and serotonin, making them more available to fight pain; or NMDA-receptor antagonists (e.g., ketamine, dextromethorphan) or opioids may be used to help diminish the pain signals.

Pain Management Models and Theories

The foundation for pain management is built on multiple theories and models. For example, theories in the 17th and 18th century suggested the existence of specific pain pathways. In the 19th century, theories specifically outlined the anatomy and physiology of pain, including receptors sensitive to pain. In 1965, Melzack and Wall developed the Gate Control Theory, which expanded the physiologic models of pain and led to the development of the psychosocial and behavioral theories that are part of current pain management strategies. Nursing models for the delivery of pain management continue to evolve (American Nurses Association [ANA], 2016, pp. 14–15).

Responses to Pain

The body's response to pain is a complex process. It has both physiologic and psychosocial aspects. Initially, with acute pain, the sympathetic nervous system responds, resulting in the fight-or-flight response, with a noticeable increase in pulse and blood pressure. The client may hold his or her breath, or have short, shallow breathing. There may also be some reflexive movements as the client withdraws from the painful stimuli (Figure 30.4 ■). Over a matter of minutes, or hours, the pulse and blood pressure return to baseline despite the persistence of pain. Contrary to the adaptation noted in vital signs, the pain fibers themselves adapt very little and become sensitized in a way that intensifies, prolongs, or spreads the pain.

Unrelieved pain has a potentially harmful effect on an individual's well-being. For example, pain interferes with sleep, affects appetite, and lowers the quality of life for clients and their family members. A natural response to pain is to stop activity, tense muscles, and withdraw from the pain-provoking activities. This reduced mobility may produce muscle atrophy and painful spasm, putting the client at risk of complications related to immobility or cardiopulmonary deconditioning. Uncontrolled pain impairs immune function, which slows healing and increases susceptibility to infections and pressure injuries. The short, shallow breathing that accompanies pain produces atelectasis, lowers circulating oxygen levels, and increases cardiac workload. The physical stress and emotional distress of severe or prolonged pain can contribute to the

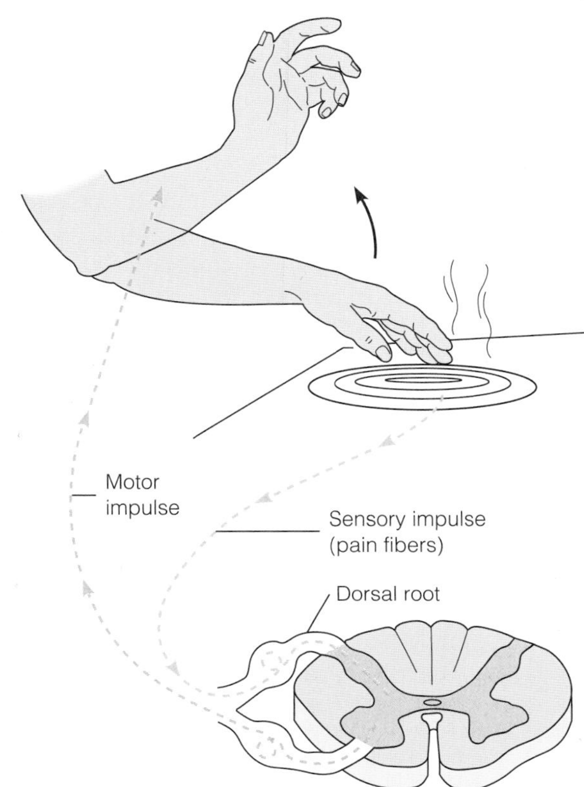

Figure 30.4 ■ Proprioceptive reflex to a pain stimulus.

development of a wide variety of physical and emotional disorders.

Persistent, severe pain changes the nervous system in a way that intensifies, spreads, and prolongs the pain, risking the development of incurable chronic pain syndromes. Beginning at 24 hours, persistent, unrelieved, severe acute pain changes the structure and function of the nervous system in a way that prolongs and intensifies the pain experience. This complex process contributes to the pathogenesis of chronic pain (Jungquist, Vallerand, Sicoutris, Kwon, & Polomano, 2017). Thus, to prevent the development of persistent pain and promote overall health and well-being, the nurse must act to promote optimal and appropriate pain control.

Factors Affecting the Pain Experience

Numerous factors can affect an individual's perception of and reaction to pain. These include the individual's ethnic and cultural values, developmental stage, environment and support people, previous pain experiences, the meaning of the current pain, and emotional responses to pain.

Ethnic and Cultural Values

Ethnic background and cultural heritage are factors that can influence both an individual's reaction to pain and the expression of that pain. Behavior related to pain is a part of the socialization process. For example, individuals in one culture may learn to be expressive about pain, whereas individuals from another culture may have learned to keep those feelings to themselves.

Nurses must recognize their own attitudes and expectations about pain. To provide culturally sensitive pain management, nurses must first be aware of their own personal beliefs, values, and behaviors about pain, and subsequently, be open to the cultural effects of how clients perceive and react to pain. For example, a growing body of research indicates that members of some racial and ethnic groups are less likely to receive adequate pain management (Hoffman, Trawalter, Axt, & Oliver, 2016; Jungquist, Vallerand, et al., 2017). This may be because of a hidden bias that nurses are not aware of at a conscious level. Nurses who deny, refute, or downplay the pain they observe in others may be culturally incompetent (unaware and emotionally apathetic toward others' viewpoints). To become culturally competent, nurses must become knowledgeable about differences in the meaning of and responses to pain. They must be sympathetic to concerns and develop the skills needed to address pain in a culturally sensitive way. It is important, therefore, to develop an effective and caring relationship with the client. This relationship is based on respect, that is, respecting the client's statement of pain and asking about the client's beliefs and how the client copes with pain. This means respecting the client's response to pain by recognizing that expressions of pain vary widely and no expression is good or bad, just different.

QSEN Patient-Centered Care: Responses to Pain

Expressions of pain vary from culture to culture and may vary from individual to individual *within* a culture. It is important to avoid stereotyping. Treat each client as an individual and provide the type of pain relief that is the best fit for the client. There are variations in how clients may respond to pain, including the following:

- Believe pain and suffering is a part of life and is to be endured.
- Deny or avoid dealing with pain until it becomes unbearable.
- View pain as a part of life and as an indicator of the seriousness of an illness.
- Believe that enduring pain is a sign of strength.
- May be loud and outspoken in their expressions of pain. This may be a socially learned way to cope, and it is important for the nurse to not judge or disapprove.
- May be quiet when in pain because they do not want to cause dishonor to themselves and their family. The nurse can offer pain medications to determine if the individual will agree to the use of pain medications.
- May believe that pain is "God's will" and therefore to be endured, not expressed, and refuse pain medication.
- Remain calm when in pain because pain is viewed as bringing the individual to a higher state of being.
- Regard pain as unpleasant and anticipate immediate relief from their symptoms. Expressive emotional and

vocal responses to pain may be reserved only for immediate family, not for health professionals. As a result, this may lead to conflicting perceptions among the family members and the nurse regarding the effectiveness of the client's pain relief. For example, the nurse may believe the client has adequate pain management, whereas the family is requesting additional pain medication for their family member.

The above list of examples reflects the uniqueness of clients and, thus, the importance for the nurse to partner with clients and support people to implement a culturally responsive and client-centered pain management plan.

Developmental Stage

The age and developmental stage of a client is an important variable that will influence both the reaction to and the expression of pain. Age variations and related nursing interventions are presented in Table 30.3.

The field of pain management for infants and children has grown significantly. It is now accepted that anatomic, physiologic, and biochemical elements necessary for pain transmission are present in newborns, regardless of their gestational age. For many years, people believed the myth that infants and children do not feel pain. Now, it is universally accepted that environmental, nonpharmacologic,

TABLE 30.3 Age Variations in the Pain Experience

Age Group	Pain Perception and Behavior	Selected Nursing Interventions
Infant	Perceives pain. Responds to pain with increased sensitivity. Older infant tries to avoid pain; for example, turns away and physically resists.	Give a glucose pacifier. Use tactile stimulation. Play music or tapes of a heartbeat.
Toddler and preschooler	Develops the ability to describe pain and its intensity and location. Often responds with crying and anger because child perceives pain as a threat to security. Reasoning with child at this stage is not always successful. May consider pain a punishment. Feels sad. May learn there are gender differences in pain expression. Tends to hold someone accountable for the pain.	Distract the child with toys, books, pictures. Involve the child in blowing bubbles as a way of "blowing away the pain." Appeal to the child's belief in magic by using a "magic" blanket or glove to take away pain. Hold the child to provide comfort. Explore misconceptions about pain.
School-age child	Tries to be brave when facing pain. Rationalizes in an attempt to explain the pain. Responsive to explanations. Can usually identify the location and describe the pain. With persistent pain, may regress to an earlier stage of development.	Use imagery to turn off "pain switches." Provide a behavioral rehearsal of what to expect and how it will look and feel. Provide support and nurturing.
Adolescent	May be slow to acknowledge pain. Recognizing pain or "giving in" may be considered weakness. Wants to appear brave in front of peers and not report pain.	Provide opportunities to discuss pain. Provide privacy. Present choices for dealing with pain. Encourage music or TV for distraction.
Adult	Behaviors exhibited when experiencing pain may be gender-based behaviors learned as a child. May ignore pain because to admit it is perceived as a sign of weakness or failure. Fear of what pain means may prevent some adults from taking action.	Deal with any misconceptions about pain. Focus on the client's control in dealing with the pain. Alleviate fears and anxiety when possible.
Older Adult	May have multiple conditions presenting with vague symptoms. May perceive pain as part of the aging process. May have decreased sensations or perceptions of the pain. Lethargy, anorexia, and fatigue may be indicators of pain. May withhold statements of pain because of fear of the treatment, of any lifestyle changes that may be involved, or of becoming dependent. May describe pain differently, that is, as "ache," "hurt," or "discomfort." May consider it unacceptable to admit or show pain.	Take a thorough history and assessment. Spend time with the client and listen carefully. Clarify misconceptions. Encourage independence whenever possible.

and pharmacologic interventions are to be used to prevent, reduce, or eliminate pain in neonates. Physiologic indicators may vary in infants, so behavioral observation is recommended for pain assessment. Children may be less able than an adult to articulate their experience or needs related to pain, which may result in their pain being undertreated. However, children as young as 3 years, if evaluated properly, can accurately report the location and intensity of their pain.

With puberty comes the emergence of some pain syndromes, particularly in young women. Women are overrepresented in many painful disorders, including headaches, fibromyalgia, lupus, and menstrual-related disorders. Men are more vulnerable to pain related to their occupational or risk-taking patterns, including burn pain and post-trauma pain. Also, as stated earlier, studies report that racial disparities in pain and health exist.

About 30% of adults over age 60 have persistent pain resulting in pain emerging as a geriatric syndrome. This health condition has unique implications for function and quality of life. Studies show that pain is underassessed in this population (Booker & Haedtke, 2016, p. 65). With the number of older individuals in our society increasing dramatically, nurses will be caring for older adults in all settings of care in greater numbers.

Older adults constitute the largest group of clients seeking healthcare services. The prevalence of pain in the older population is generally higher due to both acute and chronic disease conditions. Pain threshold does not appear to change with aging, although the effect of analgesics may increase due to physiologic changes related to drug metabolism and excretion.

Environment and Support People

A strange environment such as a hospital, with its noises, lights, and activity, can compound pain. In addition, the lonely client who is without a support network may perceive pain as severe, whereas the client who has supportive people around may perceive less pain. Some clients prefer to withdraw when they are in pain, whereas others prefer the distraction of people and activity around them. Family caregivers can provide significant support to a client in pain. With the increase in outpatient and home care, families are assuming an increased responsibility for the management of pain. Education related to the assessment and management of pain can positively affect the perceived quality of life for both clients and their caregivers.

Expectations of significant others can affect an individual's perceptions of and responses to pain. In some situations, girls may be permitted to express pain more openly than boys. Family role can also affect how a client perceives or responds to pain. For instance, a single mother supporting three children may ignore pain because of her need to stay on the job. The presence of support people often modifies a client's reaction to pain. For example, toddlers often tolerate pain more readily when supportive parents or nurses are nearby.

Previous Pain Experiences

Previous pain experiences alter a client's sensitivity to pain. Clients who have personally experienced pain or who have been exposed to the suffering of someone close

LIFESPAN CONSIDERATIONS Pain

CHILDREN

Children often receive inadequate medication to treat their pain. This may be due to nurses' lack of knowledge about how to evaluate pain in children. The pain of infants and young children who cannot verbalize well is particularly difficult to assess. Nurses will benefit from learning how to use pain assessment tools and by being alert to the possibility that children may be experiencing significant levels of pain, even if they do not appear to be in pain.

OLDER ADULTS

The presentation of pain may vary in older adults for a variety of reasons. Changes in nerve structure and functioning or vascular changes with aging may cause a variation in the pain sensation. Sometimes the pain is heightened in those whose nervous systems have been sensitized from previous unresolved pain, whereas at other times significant tissue damage (e.g., silent heart attack) may occur without pain being experienced. In some situations, pain presents itself with atypical symptoms, such as confusion, restlessness, aggression, and change in mood, activity patterns, or function. This is especially true in clients with dementia who have a difficult time understanding and verbalizing what they are feeling.

Maintaining optimal function is especially crucial for a high quality of life in older clients. If pain is not effectively controlled, the following areas are often affected in their daily lives:

- Activity tolerance
- Mobility
- Ability to socialize
- Sleep disturbance
- Ability to perform ADLs
- Ability to remain as independent as possible.

All efforts, pharmacologic and nonpharmacologic, should be used to help provide pain reduction, while maintaining or enhancing functional ability. Involvement of the client and family is important when working with the primary care provider, pharmacist, and nurse to plan which treatment is most appropriate and most acceptable to the client.

The principle "start low and go slow" is especially important when ordering dosages and pain medications for older adults. Typically, the starting dose of medicines for older adults is reduced by 25% to 50%, and then titrated for effect. Decreased renal and liver function may prolong the duration of action, but it also increases the risk of toxicity from pain medications in older clients. For example, risk of silent gastrointestinal bleeding and renal damage from NSAIDs increases, so dosages and laboratory work need to be carefully monitored related to hematocrit and renal function (liver function is monitored with acetaminophen). Comorbid conditions may also affect medication selection in older adults; for example, clients with gastric ulcers, hypertension, or the combination of asthma and nasal polyps should not receive NSAIDs. Older adults with chronic obstructive pulmonary disease (COPD) must have their respiratory rate carefully monitored when placed on an opioid pain reliever, especially at night when respirations slow and the risk of oxygen desaturation is high.

to them are often more threatened by anticipated pain than those without a pain experience. In addition, the success or lack of success of pain relief measures influences a client's expectations for relief and future response to interventions. For example, a client who has tried several nondrug pain relief measures without success may have little hope about the helpfulness of nursing interventions and may demand medication as the only thing that helps the pain.

Meaning of Pain

Some clients may accept pain more readily than others, depending on the circumstances and the client's interpretation of its significance. A client who associates the pain with a positive outcome may withstand the pain amazingly well. For example, a woman giving birth to a child or an athlete undergoing knee surgery to prolong her career may tolerate pain better because of the benefit associated with it. These clients may view the pain as a temporary inconvenience rather than a potential threat or disruption to daily life.

By contrast, clients with unrelenting chronic, persistent pain may suffer more intensely. Persistent pain affects the body, mind, spirit, and social relationships in an undesirable way. Physically, the pain limits functioning and contributes to the disuse or deconditioning alluded to previously. For many, the change in activities of daily living (ADLs), such as eating, sleeping, and toileting, also takes a toll. The side effects of the many medications used to try to control the pain also place a heavy burden on the body.

Mentally, clients with chronic pain change their outlook, becoming more pessimistic, often to the point of helplessness and hopelessness. Mood often becomes impaired when pain persists, because the sadness of being unable to do important or enjoyable activities combines with self-doubts and learned helplessness to produce depression. Anxiety, worry, and uncertainty about coping with the pain may escalate emotionally, to the point of panic. Spiritually, pain may be viewed in a variety of ways. It may be perceived as a punishment for wrongdoing, a betrayal by a higher power, a test of fortitude, or a threat to the essence of who the client is. Pain may be a source of spiritual distress, or it may be a source of strength and enlightenment. Socially, pain often strains valued relationships, in part because of the impaired ability to fulfill role expectations.

Emotional Responses to Pain

Anxiety often accompanies pain. Prolonged anxiety associated with pain can lead to other emotional disturbances, such as depression or difficulty coping. Fear of the unknown and the inability to control the pain or the events surrounding it often raises pain perception. When clients are experiencing pain, they often become fatigued. Fatigue reduces a client's ability to cope, thereby increasing pain perception. With anxiety, depression, and fatigue, sleep disturbances can occur. When pain interferes with sleep, fatigue and muscle tension often result and increase the pain; thus, a cycle of pain, fatigue, and increased pain develops. Assessing clients with chronic pain for the presence of insomnia, major depression, and suicide potential is vitally important.

Some anxious clients in pain think about the worst consequence they can imagine happening, which leads them to perceive that their pain is extremely life-threatening. This process, called *catastrophizing*, has been associated with pain disability, avoiding activity, and higher levels of pain intensity. Cognitive–behavioral interventions may help avoid this process (ANA, 2016).

Clients in pain who believe that they have control of their pain have less fear and anxiety, which decreases their pain perception. A perception of lacking control or a sense of helplessness tends to increase pain perception.

●○● NURSING MANAGEMENT

The ANA's *Pain Management Nursing: Scope and Standards of Practice* states that "the foundation of pain management nursing applies the nursing process through prevention, assessment, treatment, evaluation, and rehabilitation with a readiness to consider the individualized, multidimensional aspects of client care" (ANA, 2016, p. 14).

Assessing

Accurate pain assessment is essential for effective pain management. Given the highly subjective and individually unique nature of pain, a comprehensive assessment of the pain experience (physiologic, psychologic, behavioral, emotional, spiritual, and sociocultural) provides the necessary foundation for optimal pain control. It is important to base clinical decision making on client assessment versus relying only on a severity rating score.

The extent and frequency of the pain assessment varies according to the situation and the organizational policy. For clients experiencing severe acute pain, the nurse may focus only on location, quality, and severity, and provide interventions to control the pain before conducting a more detailed evaluation. Clients with mild or moderate acute pain or chronic pain can usually provide a more detailed description of the experience. A simple screening question such as "Are you experiencing any discomfort right now?" will usually be adequate. Frequency of pain assessment may vary depending on the pain control measures being used and the clinical circumstances. For example, in the initial postoperative period, vital signs are taken as frequently as every 15 minutes. Assessing for pain this frequently is justifiable because there is a high incidence of pain during this period as local, regional, or general anesthesia may be wearing off.

BOX 30.3 Why Clients May Be Reluctant to Report Pain

- Unwillingness to trouble staff who are perceived as busy
- Do not want to be labeled as a "complainer" or "bad"
- Fear of the injectable route of analgesic administration—especially children
- Belief that unrelieved pain is an expected, normal part of recovery or aging
- Belief that others will think they are weak if they express pain
- Difficulty or inability to communicate their discomfort
- Concern about risks associated with opioid drugs (e.g., addiction)
- Concern about unwanted side effects, especially of opioid drugs
- Concern that use of drugs now will make the drug inefficient later in life
- Fear that reporting pain will lead to further tests and expenses
- Belief that nothing can be done to control pain
- Belief that enduring pain and suffering may lead to spiritual enlightenment
- Differences in behavioral responses to pain and treatment preferences (e.g., some individuals are comfortable expressing pain while others are stoic and are not comfortable expressing or reporting pain)

Major barriers to better pain control for both nurses and clients relate to failure to assess pain, underestimation of pain, failure to accept the client's report of pain, failure to act on the client's report of pain, and concerns about addiction (Pasero & McCaffery, 2011). Given that many clients will not voice their pain unless asked about it, the nurse *must* initiate pain assessments. Some of the many reasons clients may be reluctant to report pain are listed in Box 30.3. Because the words *pain* or *complain* may have emotional or sociocultural meaning attached, it is better to ask, "Do you have any discomfort to report?" rather than "Do you have any complaints of pain?" It is also essential that nurses listen to and believe the client's statements of pain. Believing the client's statement is crucial in establishing the sense of trust needed to develop a therapeutic relationship.

Pain assessments consist of two major components: (a) a pain history to obtain facts from the client and (b) direct observation of behaviors, physical signs of tissue damage, and secondary physiologic responses of the client. It is important to remember that behaviors can vary greatly among clients; thus, behavior is only one aspect of a comprehensive pain assessment. The goal of assessment is to gain an objective understanding of a subjective experience.

Pain History

While taking a pain history, the nurse must provide an opportunity for clients to express in their own words how they view the pain. This will help the nurse understand what the pain means to the client and how the client is coping with it. Remember that each individual's pain experience is unique and that the client is the best interpreter of the experience. This history should be geared to the specific client. For example, questions asked of a car crash victim would be different from those asked of a postoperative client or someone suffering from chronic pain. The initial pain assessment for someone in severe acute pain may consist of only a few questions before intervention occurs. In contrast, for the client with chronic pain, the nurse may focus on the client's coping mechanisms, effectiveness of current pain management, and ways in which the pain has affected the client's body, thoughts and feelings, activities, and relationships.

ASSESSMENT INTERVIEW Pain History

- *Precipitating factors:* What triggers the pain or makes it worse? What measures or methods have you found helpful in reducing or relieving the pain? What pain medications do you use?
- *Quality:* Tell me what your discomfort feels like.
- *Region/Radiation:* Where is your discomfort? Ask client to point to the location and document the exact location (e.g., left lower abdomen instead of abdominal pain).

  Do you feel the pain moving to other parts of the body? If yes, where?
- *Severity:* On a scale of 0 to 10, with '0' representing no pain (substitute the term client uses e.g., 'no burning') and '10' representing the worst pain imaginable (e.g., 'burning sensation'), how would you rate the degree of discomfort you are in right now?
- *Timing:*
  a. Time of onset: When did or does the pain start?
  b. Duration: How long have you had it, or how long does it usually last?
  c. Constancy: Do you have pain-free periods? And for how long?
- *Understanding:* What does experiencing this pain mean to you? Does it signal something about the future or the past? What worries or scares you the most about your pain?
- *Associated symptoms:* Do you have any other symptoms (e.g., nausea, dizziness, shortness of breath) before, during, or after your pain?
- *Coping resources:* What do you usually do to deal with pain?
- *Affective response:* How does the pain make you feel? Anxious? Depressed? Frightened? Tired? Burdensome?
- *Past pain experience:* Tell me about past pain experiences you have had and what was done to relieve the pain.
- *Effects on ADLs:* How does the pain affect your daily life? (e.g., eating, working, sleeping, and social and recreational activities)?

Data that should be obtained in a comprehensive pain history include pain location, intensity, quality, pattern, precipitating factors, alleviating factors, associated symptoms, effect on ADLs, coping resources, and affective responses. Other data include past pain experiences and the meaning of pain to the client, as previously discussed. Questions to elicit these data are shown in the Assessment Interview.

Location

To ascertain the specific location of the pain, ask the client to point to the site of the discomfort. A chart consisting of drawings of the body can assist in identifying pain locations. The client marks the location of pain on the chart. This tool can be especially effective with clients who have more than one source of pain. A client who has multiple pain sites of different character can use symbols to draw the distribution of different pain types (e.g., circle aching areas, mark areas where shock-like pain is felt with an *X*).

When assessing the location of a child's pain, the nurse needs to understand the child's vocabulary. For example, "tummy" might refer either to the abdomen or to part of the chest. Asking the child to point to the pain helps clarify the child's word usage to identify location. The use of figure drawings can assist in identifying pain locations. Parents can also be helpful in interpreting the meaning of a child's words.

When documenting pain location the nurse may use various body landmarks. Further clarification is possible with the use of terms such as *proximal*, *distal*, *medial*, *lateral*, and *diffuse*.

Pain Intensity or Rating Scales

The single most important indicator of the existence and intensity of pain is the client's report of pain. Pain assessment that is inaccurate or incomplete leads to undertreatment of pain. Appropriate pain assessment tools based on age, developmental level, and cognitive function should be used. The use of pain intensity scales is an easy method of determining the client's pain intensity. Such scales provide consistency for nurses to communicate with the client (adults and children) and other health-care providers.

To avoid confusion, numeric rating scales (NRS) should use a 0-to-10 range with 0 indicating "no pain" and 10 indicating the "worst pain imaginable" for that individual. An 11-point (0–10) rating scale is shown in Figure 30.5 ■. The inclusion of word modifiers on the scale can assist some clients who find it difficult to apply a number level to their pain. For example, after ruling out "0" and "10" (neither no pain nor the worst imaginable pain), a nurse can ask the client if it is mild (ratings in the 1–3 range), moderate (ratings in the 4–6 range), or severe (ratings in the 7–10 range).

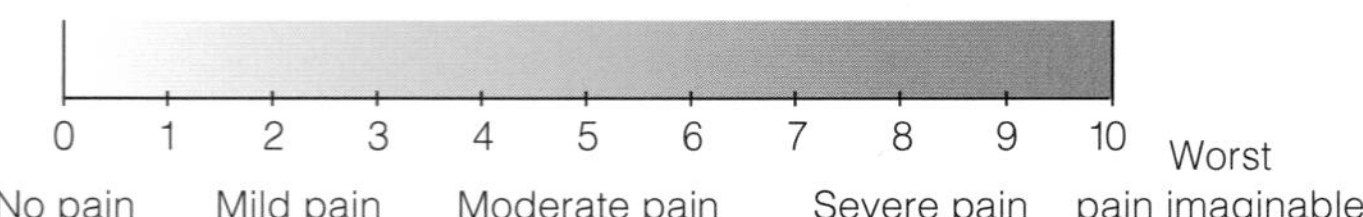

Figure 30.5 ■ An 11-point numeric pain intensity rating scale with word modifiers.

Another way to evaluate the intensity of pain for clients who are unable to use the numeric rating scales is to determine the extent of pain awareness and degree of interference with functioning. For example, 0 = no pain; 2 = awareness of pain only when paying attention to it; 4 = can ignore pain and do things; 6 = cannot ignore pain, interferes with functioning; 8 = impairs ability to function or concentrate; and 10 = intense incapacitating pain. It is believed that the degree to which pain interferes with functioning is a good marker for the severity of pain, especially for those with chronic pain.

Clinical Alert!

Perception is reality. The client's self-report of pain is what must be used to determine pain intensity. The nurse is obligated to record the pain intensity as reported by the client. By challenging the believability of the client's report, the nurse is undermining the therapeutic relationship and preventing the fulfillment of advocacy and helping clients with pain.

Nursing literature has noted that although pain screening using the NRS has existed for many years, there is little research evaluating its accuracy and effectiveness. The American Society for Pain Management Nursing (ASPMN) holds the position that the practice of prescribing opioid analgesics based *only* on a client's pain intensity or a score from a behavioral (observational) pain assessment tool should be avoided because they are subjective and ignore other important assessment elements (Pasero, Quinlan-Colwell, Rae, Broglio, & Drew, 2016). ASPMN advocates that safe and effective opioid doses should be dependent on careful assessment of objective measures such as age, other diseases or conditions, client's response to previous opioids, sedation level, concurrent medications, respiratory status, and functional status, in addition to the subjective measure of pain intensity.

Not all clients understand or relate to numeric rating scales. These include preverbal children, older adults with impairments in cognition or communication, and people who do not speak English. Given the diversity of pain and behaviors among clients spanning a broad range of age and physical and mental capabilities, it is unrealistic to believe a single pain assessment tool can be applied across all populations. The pain scale needs to fit the client being assessed.

When clients are unable to verbalize their pain due to age, being nonverbal or cognitively impaired, medical interventions, or other reasons, nurses need to accurately assess the intensity of their pain and the effectiveness of the pain management interventions. For these clients, the nurse must rely on observation of behavior. For example, the Neonatal Infant Pain Scale (NIPS) can be used for premature infants to 3 months of age. The FLACC scale has been validated in children 2 months up to adolescence and rates pain behaviors as manifested by **F**acial expressions, **L**eg movement, **A**ctivity, **C**ry, and **C**onsolability measures that yield a score of 0 to 10. The Wong-Baker FACES scale can also be used for clients ranging in age from 3 months to adults. It includes a number scale along with an illustrated facial expression so that the pain intensity can be documented. When using the FACES rating scale, it is important to remember that the client's facial expression does not need to match the picture. The client points to the picture that represents how much pain the client is experiencing. The Faces Pain Scale—Revised is another scale that uses illustrations of facial expressions. It can be used with clients ranging from 3 years to adults. It is recommended over the Wong-Baker FACES scale for older adults because the illustrations look less cartoonish and uses impersonal, more realistic expressions, and the absence of smiles and tears seems more appropriate to older or stoic clients (Booker & Haedtke, 2016). A scale specifically designed for older adults with advanced dementia is PAINAD. This scale looks at five specific indicators: breathing, vocalization, facial expression, body language, and consolability (ANA, 2016; Pasero & McCaffery, 2011).

When noting pain intensity, it is important to determine any related factors that may be affecting the pain. When the intensity changes the nurse needs to consider the possible cause. For example, the abrupt cessation of acute abdominal pain may indicate a ruptured appendix. Several factors affect the perception of intensity: (a) the amount of distraction, or the client's concentration on another event; (b) the client's state of consciousness; (c) the level of activity; and (d) the client's expectations.

For effective use of pain rating scales, clients need to understand the use of the scale and how the information will be used to determine changes in their condition and the effectiveness of pain management interventions. Clients should also be asked to indicate what level of comfort is acceptable so that they can perform specific activities. To support the client's goals and expectations with reality, it is important to note that acute pain can typically be decreased by 50% and chronic pain can be decreased by 25%. To ensure that optimal pain management is achieved, the client works together with professionals toward established goals of pain reduction and functional improvement. A rating scale can be used in acute, outpatient, and home care settings. See Figure 30.6 ■ for an example of a pain documentation form in an electronic health record (EHR).

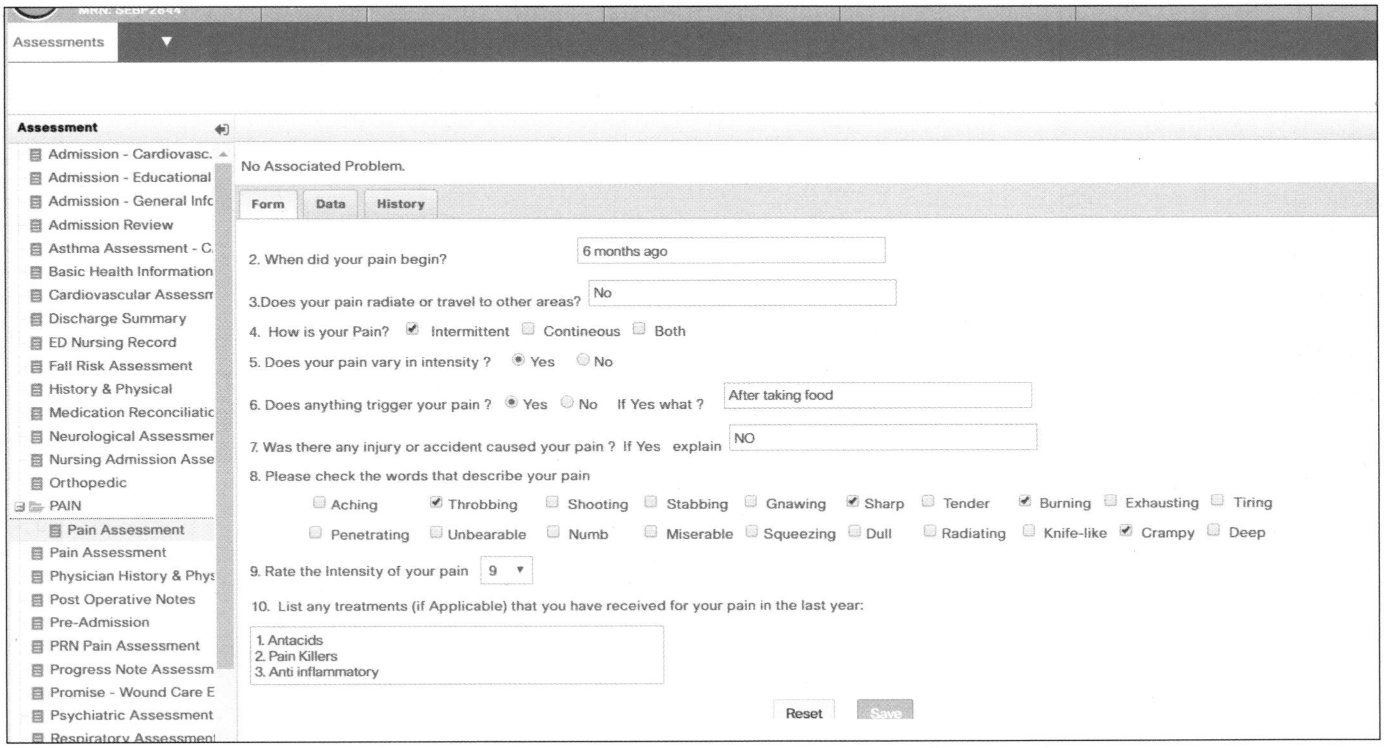

Assessments

Assessment

Admission - Cardiovasc.
Admission - Educational
Admission - General Infc
Admission Review
Asthma Assessment - C.
Basic Health Information
Cardiovascular Assessm
Discharge Summary
ED Nursing Record
Fall Risk Assessment
History & Physical
Medication Reconciliatic
Neurological Assessmer
Nursing Admission Asse
Orthopedic
PAIN
Pain Assessment
Pain Assessment
Physician History & Phys
Post Operative Notes
Pre-Admission
PRN Pain Assessment
Progress Note Assessm
Promise - Wound Care E
Psychiatric Assessment
Respiratory Assessment

No Associated Problem.

Form | Data | History

2. When did your pain begin? 6 months ago
3.Does your pain radiate or travel to other areas? No
4. How is your Pain? ☑ Intermittent ☐ Contineous ☐ Both
5. Does your pain vary in intensity ? ◉ Yes ○ No
6. Does anything trigger your pain ? ◉ Yes ○ No If Yes what ? After taking food
7. Was there any injury or accident caused your pain ? If Yes explain NO
8. Please check the words that describe your pain
☐ Aching ☑ Throbbing ☐ Shooting ☐ Stabbing ☐ Gnawing ☑ Sharp ☐ Tender ☑ Burning ☐ Exhausting ☐ Tiring
☐ Penetrating ☐ Unbearable ☐ Numb ☐ Miserable ☐ Squeezing ☐ Dull ☐ Radiating ☐ Knife-like ☑ Crampy ☐ Deep
9. Rate the Intensity of your pain 9
10. List any treatments (if Applicable) that you have received for your pain in the last year:
1. Antacids
2. Pain Killers
3. Anti inflammatory

Reset Save

Figure 30.6 ■ Pain management flow sheet in an electronic health record.
iCare.

Pain Quality

Descriptive adjectives help people communicate the quality of pain. A headache may be described as "unbearable" or an abdominal pain as "piercing like a knife." The smart clinician can collect subtle clinical clues from the quality of the pain described; thus, it is important to record the description exactly as described by the client. Some of the commonly used pain descriptors are listed in Table 30.4. Note that the term "unbearable" is listed as an affective term and "piercing" is a sensory term. Both pains are real physical conditions signaling an underlying condition, but the affective description "unbearable" suggests that there is a coexisting emotional distress that needs to be addressed as well. Pain described as burning or shock-like tends to be neuropathic in origin and may be responsive to anticonvulsants (e.g., gabapentin or pregabalin).

Pattern

The pattern of pain includes time of onset, duration, and recurrence or intervals without pain. The nurse therefore determines when the pain began; how long it lasts; whether it recurs and, if so, the length of the interval without pain; and when the pain last occurred. Attention to the pattern of pain helps the nurse anticipate and meet the needs of the client, as well as recognize patterns of serious concern (e.g., chest pain only on exertion).

Precipitating Factors

Certain activities sometimes precede pain. For example, physical exertion may precede chest pain, or abdominal pain may occur after eating. These observations can help prevent pain and determine its cause. Environmental factors such as extreme cold or heat and extremes of humidity can affect some types of pain. For example, clients with rheumatic conditions have worse pain on cold, damp days or just before a storm. Physical and emotional stressors can also precipitate pain. Strong emotions can trigger a migraine headache or an episode of chest pain. Extreme physical exertion can trigger muscle spasms in the neck, shoulders, or back.

TABLE 30.4 Commonly Used Pain Descriptors

Term	Sensory Words	Affective Words
Pain	Searing Scalding Sharp Piercing Drilling Wrenching Shooting Burning Crushing Penetrating	Unbearable Killing Intense Torturing Agonizing Terrifying Exhausting Suffocating Frightful Punishing Miserable
Hurt	Hurting Pricking Pressing Tender	Heavy Throbbing
Ache	Numb Cold Flickering Radiating Dull Sore Aching Cramping	Annoying Nagging Tiring Troublesome Gnawing Uncomfortable Sickening Tender

Alleviating Factors

Nurses must ask clients to describe anything that they have done to alleviate the pain (e.g., home remedies such as herbal teas, medications, rest, applications of heat or cold, prayer, or distractions like TV). It is important to explore the effect any of these measures had on the pain, if relief was obtained, or whether the pain became worse. It is helpful to recommend a diary be kept for gathering this information.

Associated Symptoms

Also included in the clinical appraisal of pain are associated symptoms such as nausea, vomiting, dizziness, and diarrhea. These symptoms may relate to the onset of the pain or they may result from the presence of the pain.

Effect on Activities of Daily Living

Knowing how ADLs are affected by pain helps the nurse understand the client's perspective on the pain's severity. The nurse should ask the client to describe how the pain has affected the following aspects of life:

- Sleep
- Appetite
- Concentration
- Work or school
- Interpersonal relationships
- Marital relations or sex
- Home activities
- Driving and walking
- Leisure activities
- Emotional status (mood, irritability, depression, anxiety).

A rating scale of none, a little, or a great deal, or another range can be used to determine the degree of alteration in ADLs.

Coping Resources

Everyone exhibits personal ways of coping with pain. Strategies may relate to earlier pain experiences or the specific meaning of the pain; some may reflect religious or cultural influences. Nurses can encourage and support the client's use of methods known to have helped in modifying pain, unless they are specifically contraindicated. Strategies may include seeking quiet and solitude, learning about their condition, pursuing interesting or exciting activities (for distraction), saying prayers (or engaging in other meaningful rituals), or socializing (with family, friends, support groups, etc.).

Affective Responses

Affective responses vary according to the situation, the degree and duration of pain, the interpretation of it, and many other factors. The nurse needs to explore the client's feelings of anxiety, fear, exhaustion, level of function, depression, or a sense of failure. Because many people with chronic pain become depressed and potentially suicidal, it may also be necessary to assess the client's suicide risk. In such situations, the nurse needs to ask the client, "Do you ever feel so bad that you want to die? Have you considered harming yourself or others recently?" Most chronic pain sufferers, however, are not actively suicidal and do not have a specific, lethal plan. For those who express suicidal intent, nurses need to be familiar with state regulations, organizational policies, and resources available to guide practice in this area.

Observation of Behavioral and Physiologic Responses

A client's self-report is an important component for pain assessment. Not all clients, however, are able to self-report. This group, referred to as "nonverbal" clients, includes the very young; individuals who are cognitively impaired, critically ill, or comatose; and some individuals at end of life. These clients are a challenge as the nurse provides effective pain management.

There are wide variations in nonverbal responses to pain. Facial expression is often the first indication of pain, and it may be the only one. Clenched teeth, tightly closed eyes, rapid blinking, biting of the lower lip, and other facial grimaces may indicate pain. Vocalizations such as sighing, moaning and groaning, crying, and screaming are sometimes associated with pain.

Immobilization of the body or a part of the body may also indicate pain. The client with chest pain often holds the left arm across the chest. A client with abdominal pain may assume the position of greatest comfort, often with the knees and hips flexed, and move reluctantly.

Purposeless body movements can also indicate pain—for example, tossing and turning in bed or flinging the arms about. Involuntary movements such as a reflexive jerking away from a needle inserted through the skin indicate pain. An adult may be able to control this reflex; however, a child may be unable or unwilling to do so.

Behavioral changes such as irritability, confusion, and restlessness may be indicators of pain in both cognitively intact and cognitively impaired clients. Older adults with chronic pain may become agitated or aggressive.

Rhythmic body movements or rubbing may indicate pain. An adult or child may assume a fetal position and rock back and forth when experiencing abdominal pain. During labor a woman may massage her abdomen rhythmically with her hands.

It is important to note that because behavioral responses are controllable, they may not be very revealing. When pain is chronic, behavioral responses are rarely apparent because the individual develops personal coping styles for dealing with pain, discomfort, or suffering.

Physiologic responses vary with the origin and duration of the pain. Early in the onset of acute pain, the sympathetic nervous system is stimulated, resulting in increased blood pressure, pulse rate, respiratory rate, pallor, diaphoresis, and pupil dilation. The body does not sustain the increased sympathetic function over a prolonged period and, therefore, the sympathetic nervous system adapts, causing the responses to be less evident or even absent. Physiologic responses are likely to be absent in clients with chronic pain because of autonomic nervous system adaptation. Thus, measures of physiologic responses (e.g., pulse, blood pressure) are poor indicators of the presence, absence, or severity of pain.

Daily Pain Diary

For clients who experience chronic pain, a daily diary may help the client and healthcare provider identify pain patterns and factors that worsen or resolve the pain experience. In home care, the family or other caregiver can be taught to complete the diary with the family member who is unable to do so alone. The record could include the following:

- Time of onset of pain
- Activity or situation
- Physical pain character (quality) and intensity level (0–10)
- Emotions experienced and intensity level (0–10)
- Use of analgesics or other relief measures (intervention)
- Pain rating after intervention taken
- Comments.

Pain diaries have been shown to improve pain management. They avoid "recall bias" and allow clients to understand and express their pain experience and possibly determine patterns that can help providers suggest better interventions. The diary may also increase clients' sense of control by helping them use medication more effectively. For example, a pain diary may show the client that waiting too long to take an analgesic means that it takes longer to control the pain.

The recorded data in the diary provide the basis for developing or modifying the plan for care. For this tool to be effective, it is important for the nurse to educate the client and family about the value and use of the diary in achieving effective pain control. Review the diary each visit, asking questions, sharing observations, and providing hints. Determining the client's ability to use the diary is essential.

Diagnosing

Examples of nursing diagnoses for clients experiencing pain or discomfort can include mild acute pain, moderate acute pain, severe acute pain, and chronic pain. When writing the diagnostic statement, the nurse should specify the location (e.g., right ankle pain or left frontal headache).

CLIENT TEACHING Monitoring Pain in the Home Setting

- Teach the client to keep a pain diary to monitor pain onset, activity before pain, pain intensity, use of analgesics or other relief measures, and so on.
- Instruct the client to contact a healthcare professional if planned control measures are ineffective.

PAIN CONTROL

- Teach the use of preferred and selected nonpharmacologic techniques such as relaxation, guided imagery, distraction, music therapy, massage, heat, and cold.
- Discuss the actions, side effects, dosages, and frequency of administration of prescribed analgesics.
- Suggest ways to handle side effects of medications.
- Provide accurate information about tolerance, physical dependence, and addiction if opioid analgesics are prescribed.
- Instruct the client to use pain control measures before the pain becomes severe.
- Inform the client of the effects of untreated pain.
- Demonstrate and have the client or caregiver in return demonstrate appropriate skills to administer analgesics (e.g., skin patches, injections, infusion pumps, or patient-controlled analgesia). If a home infusion pump is to be used, caregivers need to be able to:
  a. Demonstrate stopping and starting the pump.
  b. Change the medication cartridge and tubing.
  c. Adjust the delivery dose.
  d. Demonstrate site care.
  e. Identify signs indicating the need to change an injection site.
  f. Describe care of the pump and insertion site when the client is ambulatory, bathing, sleeping, or traveling.
  g. Perform problem solving for pumps when alarms are activated.
  h. Change the battery.

RESOURCES

- Provide appropriate information about how to access community resources, home care agencies, and associations that offer self-help groups and educational materials.

Related factors, when known, should also be part of the diagnostic statement. These may include both physiologic and psychologic factors. For example, in addition to the injurious agent, related factors may include lack of knowledge of pain management techniques or fear of drug addiction.

Because the presence of pain can affect so many aspects of a client's functioning, pain may be the etiology of other nursing diagnoses. Examples of such nursing diagnoses follow:

- Impaired coping related to prolonged continuous back pain, ineffective pain management, and inadequate support systems
- Altered physical mobility related to pain and inflammation secondary to arthritic pain in knee and ankle joints
- Impaired sleep related to increased pain perception at night.

Planning

The established goals for the client will vary according to the diagnosis and its signs and symptoms. Specific nursing interventions can be selected to meet the individual needs of the client.

Planning Independent of Setting

When planning, nurses need to choose pain relief measures appropriate for the client, based on the assessment data and input from the client or support people. Nursing interventions may include a variety of pharmacologic and nonpharmacologic strategies. Developing a plan that incorporates a wide range of approaches is usually most effective. Whether in acute care, home care, or long-term care settings, it is important for everyone involved in pain management to understand the plan of care. The plan should be documented in the client's record; in home care, a copy needs to be made available to the client, support people, and caregivers.

When the client's pattern and level of pain can be anticipated or is already known, regular or scheduled administration of analgesics can provide a steady serum level. Frequency of administration can be adjusted to prevent pain from recurring. Nonpharmacologic interventions should also be regularly scheduled. An additional advantage of scheduling is that the client spends less time in pain and therefore does not experience as much anxiety or fear of the recurrence of pain or the helplessness of not knowing what to do when it flares.

Planning for Home Care

In preparation for discharge, the nurse should determine the client's and family's needs, strengths, and resources.

QSEN Patient-Centered Care: Pain Assessment

The following home care assessments describe the specific assessment data required for the client, family, and available resources when establishing a discharge plan. Using the assessment data, the nurse creates a personalized teaching plan for the client and family. The nurse needs to assess the *client* for the following:

- *Level of knowledge:* pharmacologic and nonpharmacologic pain relief measures selected; adverse effects and measures to counteract these effects; warning signs to report to primary care provider
- *Self-care abilities for analgesic administration:* ability to use analgesics appropriately (e.g., to prepare correct dosages of analgesics and adhere to scheduled administration); physical dexterity to take pills or to administer IV

PRACTICE GUIDELINES **Individualizing Care For Clients with Pain**

- *Establish a trusting relationship.* Convey your concern, and acknowledge that you believe that the client is experiencing pain. Saying "I believe you are in pain, and I am going to do whatever I can to help you" will promote this trusting relationship.
- *Consider the client's ability and willingness to participate actively in pain relief measures.* Clients who are excessively fatigued, are sedated, or have altered levels of consciousness are less able to participate actively. For example, a client with an altered level of consciousness or altered thought processes cannot safely or effectively use patient-controlled analgesia. In contrast, a fatigued client may express a willingness to use pain relief measures that require little effort, such as listening to music or performing relaxation techniques.
- *Use a variety of pain relief measures.* It is thought that using more than one measure has an additive, if not synergistic, effect in relieving pain. Two types of relief measures that should be part of any pain treatment plan are active (relief strategies that are self-initiated) and passive (relief strategies that require the assistance of others). Establishing rapport and client teaching are necessary components of all therapeutic encounters. Because a client's pain may vary throughout a 24-hour period, different types of pain relief or preemptive interventions may be scheduled (e.g., medication 1 hour before dressing change, relaxation techniques with pleasant imagery after bedtime medication).
- *Provide measures to relieve pain before it becomes severe.* For example, providing an analgesic before the onset of pain is preferable to waiting for the client to report pain, when a larger dose may be required.
- *Use pain-relieving measures that the client believes are effective.* It has been recognized that clients are the authorities about their own pain. Thus, incorporating the client's preferred methods of relieving their pain into the treatment plan should be seriously considered.
- *The selection of pain relief measures should be aligned with the client's report of the severity of the pain.* If a client reports mild pain, an analgesic such as acetaminophen may be indicated, whereas a client who reports severe pain often requires a more potent relief measure. Telling a client to ignore the pain (e.g., through distraction techniques) when he or she is reporting severe pain is an example of a misalignment (no correlation) between the pain severity and intervention selected.
- *Maintain an unbiased attitude (open mind) about what may relieve pain.* New ways to relieve pain are continually being developed. It is not always possible to explain the effectiveness of particular pain relief measures; however, using approaches the client believes will work should be considered.
- *Keep trying.* Do not ignore a client because pain persists despite failed attempts to alleviate the discomfort. In these circumstances, reassess the pain and consider other relief measures.
- *Prevent harm to the client.* Pain therapy should not increase discomfort or harm the client. Some pain relief measures may have adverse effects, such as fatigue, but they should not disable the client.
- *Educate the client and caregivers about pain.* Clients and support people need to be informed about possible causes of pain, precipitating and alleviating factors, and alternatives to drug therapy. Misconceptions also need to be corrected.

medications and to store medications safely; and ability to obtain prescriptions or over-the-counter (OTC) medications at the pharmacy

The nurse assesses the *family* for the following:

- *Caregiver availability, skills, and willingness:* ability and willingness to assist with pain management; ability to do shopping if the client has a restricted activity level; ability to comprehend selected therapies (e.g., infusion pumps, imagery, massage, positioning, and relaxation techniques) and perform them or assist the client with them as needed
- *Family role changes and coping:* effect on financial status, parenting and spousal roles, sexuality, and social roles
- *Community resources:* availability of and familiarity with resources such as supplies, home health aide, or financial assistance.

Implementing

Nursing management of pain consists of both independent and collaborative nursing actions. In general, noninvasive measures may be performed as an independent nursing function, whereas administration of analgesic medication generally requires a medical order from a primary care provider.

Generally, a combination of strategies works best for the client in pain, especially chronic pain. Some strategies need to be modified until the client obtains effective pain relief. See the Practice Guidelines for individualizing care for clients with pain.

Barriers to Pain Management

Misconceptions and biases about pain involve attitudes of the nurse or the client as well as knowledge deficiencies. Clients can respond to pain experiences based on their culture, personal experiences, and the meaning the pain has for them. For many clients, pain is expected and accepted as a normal part of illness. Clients and families may lack knowledge of the adverse effects of pain and may have been provided incorrect information regarding the use of analgesics. Clients may not report pain because they expect that nothing can be done, or think the pain is not severe enough, or feel it would distract or prejudice the healthcare provider. Other common misconceptions are shown in Table 30.5.

Over the last 20 years, opioid misuse and abuse has become an increasing problem in our society (Assil, 2016). The Centers for Disease Control and Prevention (CDC, 2018) provided data that showed the rise in opioid overdose deaths occurred in three distinct waves. The first wave began with increased prescribing of

TABLE 30.5 Misconceptions About Pain

Misconception	Correction
Clients experience severe pain only when they have had major surgery.	Even after minor surgery, clients can experience intense pain.
The nurse or other healthcare professionals are the authorities about a client's pain.	The individual who experiences the pain is the only authority about its existence and nature.
The amount of tissue damage is directly related to the amount of pain.	Pain is a subjective experience, and the intensity and duration of pain vary considerably among individuals.
Visible physiologic or behavioral signs accompany pain and can be used to verify its existence.	Even with severe pain, periods of physiologic and behavioral adaptation can occur.

opioids in the 1990s, with overdose deaths involving prescription opioids. Prescribers started using opioids to treat chronic noncancer pain. This prevalence of opioid misuse and dependence increased the availability of opioids, allowing diversion of prescription opioids to recreational users. For example, many of those who use prescription opioids for nonmedical reasons obtained them from a friend or relative. The second wave began in 2010, with rapid increases in overdose deaths involving heroin (CDC, 2018). Individuals, cut off from prescription analgesics, turned to heroin on the street, which was purer and cheaper than pills (Stempniak, 2016, pp. 25–26). The third wave began in 2013, with significant increases in overdose deaths involving synthetic opioids, particularly those involving illicitly manufactured fentanyl (CDC, 2018).

As a result, drug overdose became the leading cause of unintentional injury deaths in the United States, and most of those deaths involved an opioid (National Academies of Sciences, Engineering, and Medicine, 2017, p. 2). The CDC determined that there had been a 200% increase in the rate of overdose deaths involving opioid pain relievers and heroin (Windle, 2016, p. 11). These increasing numbers caused the phrase "the opioid addiction epidemic." This epidemic resulted in the declaration of a public health emergency in October 2017 (ANA, 2018). In 2018, the CDC stated that on average, 130 Americans died every day from an opioid overdose (para. 1).

The Comprehensive Addiction and Recovery Act of 2016 allocated $181 million with the expectations that lawmakers approve $500 million more for grants to address prescription opioid use in communities and review best practices for pain management ("Tackling Nation's," 2016, p. 15). Federal agencies were directed by the White House to ensure that those involved in prescribing controlled substances complete training regarding the appropriate use of opioid drugs (Traynor, 2016). Furthermore, to solve the physician-driven epidemic (Windle, 2016), the CDC issued guidelines for prescribing opioids for chronic pain. In 2018, Congress passed a federal spending bill that included a $3.3 billion increase in funding to go toward prevention, treatment, and law enforcement activities to help state and local governments. Many health policy experts, however, argued that it was not enough to make a meaningful impact (Quinn, 2018).

Evidence supports *short-term* effectiveness of opioids for reducing pain and improving function in noncancer nociceptive and neuropathic pain (ANA, n.d.). Few studies have assessed the long-term benefits of opioids for chronic pain, while several studies have shown nonopioid pharmacologic and nonpharmacologic treatments to be effective and preferred in managing chronic pain (Dowell, Haegerich, & Chou, 2016, p. 12). The CDC's *Guideline for Prescribing Opioids for Chronic Pain* (2017; CDC, n.d.) provides 12 recommendations grouped into three areas: (1) determining when to initiate or continue opioids for chronic pain; (2) opioid selection, dosage, duration, follow-up, and discontinuation; and (3) assessing risk and addressing harms of opioid use. An important focus of the *Guideline* is to start with nonpharmacologic therapy and nonopioid pharmacologic therapy.

The National Academies of Sciences, Engineering, and Medicine (2017) reports four strategies, each with a variety of approaches, to address the opioid epidemic while meeting the needs of clients. These strategies include the following:

- ***Restricting the supply of opioids.*** One example is to limit the number of days' supply of opioid medications for a client. Another approach is to increase the number of drug take-back programs, thereby increasing the safe disposal or return of unused drugs. Currently many drug take-back programs are once-a-year events. This approach would allow individuals to return drugs to any pharmacy on any day of the year. The U.S. Food and Drug Administration (FDA, 2018) now provides a list of medicines that can be flushed when they are no longer needed. The FDA believes that "the known risk of harm, including death, to humans from accidental exposure to certain medicines, especially potent opioid medicines, far outweighs any potential risk to humans or the environment from flushing these medicines when a take-back option is not readily available" (p. 2).

- ***Influencing prescribing practices.*** This strategy recommends establishing comprehensive pain education materials and curricula for healthcare providers. Another approach is to improve the use of prescription drug monitoring programs (PDMPs), which are electronic databases that can provide a prescriber or pharmacist information about a client's prescription history. This information may identify clients who knowingly or unknowingly misuse medications.
- ***Reducing demand.*** This strategy includes changing the client's expectations for the treatment and management of chronic pain, specifically, educating the public about the risks and benefits of opioid therapy and the effectiveness of nonopioid analgesics and nonpharmacologic interventions.
- ***Reducing harm.*** One of the approaches for this strategy is to expand access to naloxone, an opioid antagonist, to reverse overdose. This life-saving medication is currently available to health professionals in the prehospital and hospital settings. Most states now have legislation allowing the layperson to access naloxone, generally in intranasal form. Naloxone overdose prevention laws generally protect professional and lay responders from civil or criminal liability related to opioid antagonist administration (Strickler, James, O'Leary, & Dube-Clark, 2018, p. 43).

Another barrier to effective pain management is the fear of becoming addicted. Both nurses and clients often hold this fear. It is important that all individuals know the difference between tolerance, physical dependence, and addiction.

EVIDENCE-BASED PRACTICE

Evidence-Based Practice

Is There a Relationship Between Nurses' Knowledge and Clients' Knowledge About Their Opioid Prescriptions?

Many clients receive a prescription for opioid analgesia after a surgical procedure or a visit to the emergency department. The literature reports that the increase in the number of opioid prescriptions has also been associated with an increase in nonmedical use of opioids. This nonmedical use of opioids has led to adverse outcomes, such as substance abuse, falls and fractures in older adults, overdose, and death. Clients may begin nonmedical use of opioids due to a lack of education at the time they receive their prescriptions at discharge. It is important for clients to know that an opioid prescription is intended to manage pain at an acceptable level to allow activities of daily living, not to provide complete freedom from pain. They should take the smallest amount needed to achieve an acceptable pain intensity. Clients should also receive information on side effects of opioids, including psychomotor and cognitive effects, and potential risks of tolerance, addiction, physical dependence, and withdrawal. Recently the FDA recommended that all clients have information on safe use, storage, and disposal of opioids. However, evidence suggests that nurses may lack knowledge of these important concepts. Costello, Thompson, Aurelien, and Luc (2016) conducted a study to determine if an educational intervention improved nurses' and subsequently clients' knowledge of the safe use of opioids. Their review of the literature revealed the following concerns regarding opioid prescriptions: Clients often did not use all the pills and kept the medications at home long after they were needed; clients often stored unused opioids unsecured in their homes; parents with children in their households did not store their medications out of reach; and clients never received instructions on disposal of unused opioids. One study found that less than 75% of nurses answered only 24 of 50 questions correctly on a test of opioid knowledge. No literature was found that addressed the role of nurses in educating clients on safe use of prescription opioids.

The researchers conducted a quasi-experimental pretest–posttest design to evaluate nurses' knowledge of opioids on a gastrointestinal (GI) surgical unit at an academic medical center in the northeastern United States. All 83 nurses who worked on the nursing unit were invited to participate, with 64% taking a pretest of 11 demographic questions and 10 questions about knowledge of safe use of opioids. The nurses received a 40-minute presentation and the posttest was administered immediately after the education. Before the educational presentation, nurses were given the option of using computer-generated instructions that included a list of medications, routes of administration, and schedule. After the educational intervention for the nurses, the researchers developed an instructional sheet for nurses to use with clients during opioid education.

Before the nurses received their educational presentation, a research assistant, through a telephone survey, contacted clients who had undergone a surgical procedure and were discharged with an oral opioid prescription. Data were collected for 93 clients. The same research assistant contacted an additional 100 clients one week after the nurses received education.

The findings indicated a significant difference in the nurses' knowledge before and after the educational intervention. In addition, there was a significant difference in knowledge between the clients who were educated before and after the nurses' educational intervention. The percentage of clients who received education from nurses increased after intervention on the following topics regarding opioids: safe storage, disposal, decreased use with decreased pain, avoidance of use other than for pain, and not sharing.

Implications

The authors address the limitations of the study: Bias may be a concern due to the self-reported nature of the surveys and the narrow scope of the sample. The study found that clients have a clearer understanding of safe opioid use when nurses also have a better understanding of safe practices around prescription opioids. The results support the use of a short educational activity to increase nurses' knowledge of clients' safe use of opioids. More effective education for clients about their opioid prescriptions may contribute to decreased nonmedical use of opioids.

Tolerance occurs when the client's opioid dose, over time, leads to a decreased sensitivity to the drug's analgesic effect. In other words, increasing doses of the opioid are needed to provide the same level of pain relief. **Physical dependence** is an expected physical response when a client who is on long-term opioid therapy has the opioid significantly reduced or withdrawn. The client experiences withdrawal symptoms consistent with the substance. Physical dependence is associated with *physiologic* dependence (potential ability for withdrawal), whereas addiction is associated with a *psychologic* dependence on the drug. **Addiction** is a chronic, relapsing, treatable disease influenced by genetic, developmental, and environmental factors. Research has shown that prevention programs involving families, schools, communities, and the media are effective for preventing or reducing drug use and addiction (National Institute on Drug Abuse, 2018). Pasero and McCaffery (2011) remind us that it is important for the nurse to remember that tolerance, physical dependence, and addiction are separate conditions, with each requiring different treatment (p. 33).

Nurses will provide care for clients who have substance use disorders (SUD). For example, a client who has a SUD could come to the acute care setting for an elective surgery, come to the emergency department, or have cancer. Thus, the nurse will be caring for a client who has two separate problems: pain and SUD. Unfortunately, clients with a present or past history of SUD may suffer a great deal of pain needlessly. This is likely due to nurses' fear of addiction when administering opioid medications. It is important to treat the pain. A myth held by some nurses is that if they treat the pain, they are contributing to the SUD, but this is not true. In fact, undertreating the pain may cause clients with SUDs to increase their drug use. Often, clients who have SUDs require more pain medication than usual, often more than the nurse is comfortable giving. To best help the client, if possible, nurses should consult with a pain management expert and a substance abuse specialist.

Nurses may also care for clients who are receiving medication-assisted treatment for opioid use disorder (OUD). Such medication-assisted treatment incorporates methadone, buprenorphine, or naltrexone (do not confuse with naloxone). Many nurses may be unaware of how to manage acute pain in such clients. For example, acute pain management may be insufficient with the once-daily dose of methadone typically used in OUD treatment. If buprenorphine is discontinued during hospitalization, the client may require higher doses of other opioids to achieve pain relief. Naltrexone must be discontinued if the client needs pain management with opioids. If clients require opioids for pain management and have naltrexone in their system, they may require 10 to 20 times the usual opioid dose (Broglio & Matzo, 2018, pp. 30–37). Clients with OUD and a serious illness worry about receiving effective pain management. By learning about OUD and its treatment, nurses can provide the most effective nursing care.

Because addiction is a disease, clients must be cared for appropriately. The ANA's *Pain Management Nursing: Scope and Standards of Practice* (2nd ed.) states that "the registered nurse practices ethically in the delivery of care, including pain management. The registered nurse provides care without prejudice and with compassion and respect; honoring the rights, lifestyle, values, beliefs, dignity, worth, and uniqueness of each individual regardless of race, ethnicity, gender, literacy, social or economic status, or coexisting diseases such as substance use disorder" (ANA, 2016, p. 57).

Key Strategies in Pain Management

Key strategies to reduce pain include acknowledging and accepting the client's pain, assisting support people, reducing misconceptions about pain, reducing fear and anxiety, and preventing pain.

Acknowledging and Accepting Clients' Pain

According to the professional standards of conduct, nurses have a duty to ask clients about their pain and to believe their reports of discomfort. Challenging the client's report of discomfort undermines the environment of trust that is an essential component in the therapeutic relationship. See the Practice Guidelines for strategies for colleague accountability in pain management. Consider these four ways of communicating this belief:

1. Acknowledge the possibility of the pain. "Many people with your condition are bothered by leg pain. Are you experiencing any leg discomfort? What does it feel like? How concerned or upset are you about it?"
2. Listen attentively to what the client says about the pain, restating your understanding of the reported discomfort. Adding an empathetic statement like "I'm sorry you are hurting, it must be very upsetting. I want to help you feel better" lets the client know you believe the pain is real and intend to help.
3. Convey that you need to ask about the pain because, despite some similarities, everybody's experience is unique, for example, "Many people with your condition report having some discomforts. Do you have any discomfort or pain?"
4. Attend to the client's needs promptly. It is unacceptable to believe the client's report of pain and then do nothing. After determining the client has pain, discuss options and plan actions for providing relief.

Clinical Alert!

So what if you are fooled by a client's self-report of pain? Evidence suggests 5% of people reporting pain are dishonest and seeking some secondary gain. By believing everyone, you will not short change the 95% of people who so desperately need to have help controlling their pain, providing them with competent, compassionate, and appropriate nursing care based on the best available information.

Assisting Support People

Support people (e.g., family, significant others, caregivers) often need assistance to respond in a helpful manner to the client experiencing pain. Nurses can help by giving them accurate information about the pain and providing

PRACTICE GUIDELINES Strategies for Colleague Accountability in Pain Management

What do we do if the healthcare team does not respond positively to the client's report of pain?

- Speak up! Inappropriate professional behavior will persist if not challenged. If necessary, file an "incident" or "variance" report for persistent patterns or unacceptable violations of standards of care. These types of behaviors (ignoring reports of pain, failing to treat or mistreating people with pain) are not only unethical, but legally indefensible because a standard of care is not being met.
- Clarify that the sensation of pain is subjective and that professionals have a duty to believe clients' reports of their symptoms.
- Cite recommendations from evidence-based clinical practice guidelines (e.g., American Pain Society, Agency for Health Care Policy and Research), The Joint Commission standards, organization-specific documents (e.g., mission statement, patient bill of rights, practice standards), or relevant research and quality reports. As necessary, distribute or post with key passages highlighted.
- Involve key committees, managers, and administrators in studying and addressing the problem from a cost, quality, competency, and credentialing perspective.

opportunities for them to discuss their emotional reactions, which may include anger, fear, frustration, and feelings of inadequacy. Teaching the support people about the disease and medications (including warning signs to report) and nondrug pain-relieving techniques they can help with (e.g., massage, application of ice, coached relaxation techniques) may diminish their feelings of helplessness and strengthen their relationship. Support people also may need the nurse's understanding and reassurance and perhaps access to resources that will help them cope as they add the caregiver role to an already stressful life circumstance.

Reducing Misconceptions About Pain

Reducing a client's misconceptions about pain and its treatment will remove one of the barriers to optimal pain relief. The nurse should explain to the client that pain is a highly individual experience and that it is only the client who really experiences the pain, although others can understand and empathize. Misconceptions are also dealt with when the nurse and client discuss the context of pain control as part of the healing process. For example, a client may refuse pain medicine out of concern for addiction, explaining that the pain is more tolerable as long as he or she remains totally still. This misconception overstates the risk of addiction (estimated at less than 5% of clients without a history of substance abuse when treated for acute pain) while underestimating the risks associated with immobility (e.g., atelectasis, muscle atrophy, pressure injuries, infections).

Clinical Alert!

Emphasize to the client that at times, treatment may need to balance the demands of providing pain reduction with functional improvement. Too much pain medicine might impair alertness or gait; too much pain impairs alertness and ability to move. Thus, nurses may have to explain to clients that the aim is to prevent and control pain in order to maximize functioning and recovery (e.g., cough, deep breathe, and walk).

Reducing Fear and Anxiety

It is important to help relieve strong emotions capable of amplifying pain (e.g., anxiety, anger, and fear). When clients have no opportunity to talk about their pain and associated fears, their perceptions and reactions to the pain can be intensified. Often, these emotions are related to uncertainty about the future, feeling mistreated in the past, or having unmet expectations. By providing accurate information, the nurse can reduce many of the client's fears or anxiety, while clarifying expectations can minimize frustration and anger. Specifically, client education about the range of pain that is considered normal for the condition as well as the types of discomforts that signal a potential for problems will help lessen this fear and anxiety.

Preventing Pain

A preventive approach to pain management involves the provision of measures to treat the pain before it occurs or before it becomes severe. **Preemptive analgesia** is the administration of analgesics *before* surgery to decrease or relieve pain *after* surgery and reduce the need for opioid pain control. Some authors, however, believe the term "preventive" analgesia better explains the assumption of the practice—that the only way to prevent central sensitization might be to block any pain and afferent signals from the surgical wound from the time of incision until final wound healing (Polomano et al., 2017, p. S13).

Nurses can use a preemptive approach by providing an analgesic around the clock (ATC), and supplementing with as-needed (prn) doses after surgery or prior to painful procedures (e.g., dressing changes, physical therapy). This strategy prevents the windup and sensitization (described earlier in Box 30.2) that spreads, intensifies, and prolongs pain.

Multimodal Pain Management

Multimodal pain management incorporates both pharmacologic and nonpharmacologic approaches to achieve the best possible outcomes for the client. Multimodal analgesia combines analgesics from two or more drug classes and a variety of delivery approaches for the analgesics that result in reducing, and often eliminating, the need for opioids. This is also referred to as *opioid-sparing therapy*. Multimodal pain therapies include therapies that are independent of or in addition to pharmacologic therapy and include nonpharmacologic therapies such as yoga, massage, biofeedback, acupuncture, mind–body therapies, and physical therapies. The literature reflects that multimodal pain management is effective for both acute and chronic pain (ANA, 2016, pp. 29–30; Chou et al., 2016; Polomano et al., 2017).

Pharmacologic Approaches

Pharmacologic approaches can involve the use of nonopioids such as NSAIDs, opioids, and adjuvant drugs (Box 30.4). Because many analgesics are ordered to be administered on a prn basis, the decision to administer the prescribed medication is frequently the nurse's, requiring judgment as to the dose and the time of administration.

Nonopioids

Nonopioids include acetaminophen, aspirin and **nonsteroidal anti-inflammatory drugs (NSAIDs)** such as ibuprofen. All are useful for the management of acute and chronic pain.

Acetaminophen (Tylenol) does not affect platelet function and rarely causes GI distress. It does, however, have serious side effects such as hepatotoxicity and possible renal toxicity, especially with high doses or with long-term use. Even at recommended doses up to 4 grams per day, some individuals taking acetaminophen on a regular basis or who have pre-existing liver disease or regular alcohol intake may be at an increased risk for liver toxicity. FDA currently requires warnings on acetaminophen labels against taking alcohol with acetaminophen. Because acetaminophen is so well tolerated, it is often an ingredient in OTC remedies (e.g., pain, fever, allergy, cough and cold preparations), so clients must be instructed to read the ingredient list of all OTC medicines they take. Box 30.5 lists common prescription medications that contain acetaminophen.

Aspirin is the oldest nonopioid analgesic and is available OTC. Because it can prolong bleeding time, clients should stop taking it 1 week prior to any surgical procedure. Aspirin should never be given to children under 12 years of age due to the possibility of Reye's syndrome. The nurse must also be aware that aspirin can cause excessive anticoagulation if a client is taking the anticoagulant warfarin.

Clinical Alert!

Many healthcare professionals underestimate the effectiveness of ordinary aspirin and acetaminophen. The ordinary dose of aspirin or acetaminophen relieves as much pain as 1.5 mg of parenteral morphine, whereas standard doses of mixed analgesics (e.g., Tylenol No. 3 or Percocet) are approximately equivalent to 2.5 to 5 mg of morphine.

NSAIDs have anti-inflammatory, analgesic, and antipyretic effects. All NSAIDs relieve pain by inhibiting the enzyme cyclooxygenase (COX), a chemical that is activated by damaged tissue, resulting in decreased synthesis of prostaglandins. The COX-1 specific isoforms (proteins) are found in platelets, the GI tract, kidneys, and most other tissue, and are believed to be the cause of the well-known adverse effects of NSAIDs (e.g., GI bleed, diminished renal blood flow, and inhibited clotting).

In the 1990s a second isoform (COX-2) was found and believed to be specific only for pain and inflammation. The resulting new "safer" (COX-2 selective) NSAIDs were tested, approved, and widely used. These drugs demonstrated significantly less GI bleeding, but uncommon cardiovascular events and rare skin problems occurred in susceptible individuals. The only COX-2 currently available in the United States is celecoxib (Celebrex). Although the COX-2 NSAIDs have fewer GI side effects, they are no safer on renal function than the COX-1 NSAIDs. All prescription NSAIDs now must carry the strong "black box" warning of the risks of using these drugs. Even nonprescription NSAIDs (e.g., aspirin, ibuprofen, naproxen) must be relabeled to warn consumers of their potential dangers.

Individual drugs in this category vary little in their analgesic potency, but do vary in their anti-inflammatory properties, metabolism, excretion, and side effects. These drugs have a ceiling effect and a narrow therapeutic index. The *ceiling effect* means that once the maximum analgesic benefit is achieved, additional amounts of the drug will *not* produce more analgesia; however, more toxicity may

BOX 30.4 Categories and Examples of Analgesics

NONOPIOID ANALGESICS FOR MILD PAIN
- Acetaminophen
- Acetylsalicylic acid
- Celecoxib
- Ibuprofen
- Ketorolac
- Meloxicam
- Naproxen
- Piroxicam

OPIOID ANALGESICS FOR MODERATE PAIN
- Hydrocodone
- Codeine
- Tramadol
- Pentazocine
- Buprenorphine

OPIOID ANALGESICS FOR SEVERE PAIN
- Fentanyl
- Hydromorphone
- Methadone
- Morphine sulfate
- Oxycodone
- Oxymorphone

ADJUVANTS
- Anticonvulsants
- Topical local anesthetic
- Tricyclic antidepressants
- Duloxetine
- Amitriptyline
- Gabapentin
- Pregabalin

BOX 30.5 Common Prescription Pain Medications Containing Acetaminophen

MEDICATION
- Lortab (500 mg acetaminophen/5, 7.5, or 10 mg hydrocodone)
- Percocet (325 mg acetaminophen/5 mg oxycodone)
- Tylenol with codeine (325 mg acetaminophen/30 mg codeine)
- Tylox (500 mg acetaminophen/5 mg oxycodone)
- Vicodin (500 mg acetaminophen/5 mg hydrocodone)
- Vicodin ES (750 mg acetaminophen/7.5 mg hydrocodone)

occur. The *narrow therapeutic index* indicates that there is not much margin for safety between the dose that produces a desired effect and the dose that may produce a toxic, even lethal effect. The most common adverse effect of NSAIDs is GI, such as heartburn or indigestion. These effects can become toxic or lethal if silent GI bleeding occurs. Given the interference with platelet aggregation, a small stomach ulcer can bleed a great deal, making it a potentially life-threatening condition. Clients should be taught to take NSAIDs with food and a full glass of water. Routine monitoring by a health professional is indicated if these preparations are taken daily for more than 2 weeks.

Opioids

An opioid analgesic is a natural or synthetic morphine-like substance responsible for reducing moderate to severe pain (Adams, Holland, & Urban, 2020, p. 227). In addition to knowing the pharmacodynamics (how the medication affects the body) of the various opioid analgesics, it is important for the nurse to be aware of the potential side effects.

Opioid Analgesics for Moderate Pain These include drugs such as codeine, hydrocodone, and tramadol. Most of these drugs are combinations of a nonopioid with an opioid. These medicines are generally 2 to 4 times more potent than nonopioids alone, and share some of the risks of both drug classes. They are controlled substances and must be ordered by a physician or nurse practitioner, adhering to applicable federal and state laws. They also have a ceiling effect due to the nonopioid and a maximum daily dose limit. There are advantages to giving combination drugs, such as lowering the amount of any one medicine needed in a 24-hour period, thus reducing the potential for adverse effects or toxicity; however, nurses need to be familiar with each medication and be aware of daily dose limits of the ingredients as well as the potential to receive duplicate medications for different clinical indications (e.g., acetaminophen for fever and acetaminophen in a headache preparation).

These opioids have a narrow therapeutic index. Codeine at doses of 30 to 60 mg produces dose-limiting GI distress in many people. A specific enzyme in the body (CYP2D6) is required to make codeine active in order for analgesia to be achieved. This enzyme and others can affect how an opioid is metabolized. For example, codeine and tramadol require conversion to an active metabolite to have an analgesic effect, and the CYP2D6 enzyme is responsible for their metabolism. Some people may have poor metabolism of this enzyme resulting in little or no analgesic effect. Others may have ultra-rapid metabolism resulting in increased side effects and a decrease in duration of analgesia. Pharmacogenomic data support that individuals vary in their metabolism of codeine and tramadol (American Pain Society, 2016). Thus, it is important for nurses to understand that clients can respond differently and that it is critical to observe for toxicity even with normal dosages and to assess if the codeine or tramadol is providing pain relief.

Opioid Analgesics for Severe Pain Pure agonist opioid analgesics bind tightly to mu receptor sites in the peripheral and central nervous systems, producing maximum pain inhibition, an agonist effect. These analgesics include opium derivatives, such as morphine (the gold standard opioid), hydromorphone, oxycodone, fentanyl, and methadone. There is no ceiling on the level of analgesia from these drugs; their dose can be steadily increased to relieve pain. There is also no maximum daily dose limit unless they are in combination with a nonopioid analgesic drug.

Opioid is the pharmacologic class of pain relievers and is the correct medical term. Many opioids are "scheduled" as a controlled substance due to the potential for misuse. In addition to pain reduction, changes in mood may make the client feel more comfortable even though the pain persists. As the most potent class of pain relievers, these drugs are indicated for severe pain, or when other medications have failed to control moderately severe or worse pain.

Methadone is a synthetic opioid used for severe pain. The nurse needs to be aware of the potential for serious problems when a client is on methadone. Due to its long half-life (15 to 60 hours), there is an increased risk of sedation and respiratory depression, especially in older adults.

Clinical Alert!

Combining opioid and nonopioid analgesics is a useful way to manage pain, and is frequently overlooked. Each has different mechanisms of action, side effects, and toxicity profiles. Alternating the two or giving them at the same time creates no danger and often produces a synergistic rather than merely additive effect. By combining nonopioids and opioids, pain management can be enhanced, reducing doses of analgesics and decreasing the risks of side effects for both.

Opioid Side Effects When administering any analgesic, the nurse must review adverse effects. Adverse effects of the opioids typically include sedation, respiratory depression, nausea, vomiting, constipation, urinary retention, blurred vision, and sexual dysfunction.

The most concerning adverse effect of opioids is respiratory depression (e.g., 8 breaths per minute or less), which usually occurs early in therapy among opioid-naïve clients (individuals who have not taken opioids for 1 week or longer), with dose escalation, or in clients with drug–drug or drug–disease interactions. Clinically, the client will appear overly sedated, and respirations will be slow and deep with periods of apnea. The nurse should assess a client's level of alertness and respiratory rate for baseline data before administering opioids.

A variety of mechanisms are available to assess respiratory status of a client receiving opioids. Intermittent pulse oximetry is the minimum standard of care. Continuous pulse oximetry monitoring is more accurate and allows for trending of the readings. Capnography, which measures end-tidal carbon dioxide level, is more sensitive than pulse oximetry. Another mechanism to measure respiratory status is minute ventilation technology, which uses two chest leads to assess tidal volume and respiratory rate (Jungquist, Smith, Nicely, & Polomano, 2017, p. S31).

Clients will often exhibit an increase in sedation *before* the result of opioid-induced respiratory depression (OIRD).

Risk factors for OIRD can include age greater than 55 years, obesity, untreated obstructive sleep apnea, smoker, pulmonary or cardiac disease or dysfunction, and first 24 hours after surgery (Jungquist, Smith, et al., 2017, p. S29).

The use of a sedation scale during opioid pain management is common in hospitals in the United States. A number of sedation scales are available; thus, it is important for nurses to know how to use their facility's choice of sedation scale. A commonly used scale is the Pasero Opioid-Induced Sedation Scale (POSS), which uses a scale ranging from S (sleep, easy to arouse) to 1 (alert and awake) to 2 (slightly drowsy, easily aroused) to 3 (frequently drowsy, arousable, drifts off to sleep during conversation) to 4 (minimal or no response to verbal and physical stimulation) (Pasero & McCaffery, 2011, p. 510). Pasero and McCaffery (2011) suggest that an easy way for the nurse to assess sedation is to ask the client a simple question, such as "What did you have for breakfast today?" and observe the client's ability to stay awake and answer the question (p. 509). The client who is excessively sedated, will fall asleep in the middle of answering the question. This behavior is unacceptable and requires close monitoring of respiratory rate and sedation level. Early recognition of an increasing level of sedation or respiratory depression will enable the nurse to implement appropriate measures promptly.

Box 30.6 provides suggested measures to prevent and treat side effects of opioid analgesics. Tolerance to

Clinical Alert!

Constipation is an almost universal adverse effect of opioid use. All clients should receive prophylactic stimulant laxative therapy, unless contraindicated. Stool softeners are not useful alone, but are a good choice when combined with a stimulant laxative (e.g., Senokot-S). If those products are ineffective, a regimen of cathartic laxatives (e.g., bisacodyl), followed by more aggressive forms of treatment (e.g., osmotic laxatives, enema, manual disimpaction) may be necessary. There are also prescription medications (naloxegol, methylnaltrexone, lubiprostone) for opioid-induced constipation (OIC) that stop opioids from attaching to receptors in the intestine.

Safety Alert! SAFETY

Assessing for sedation and respiratory status is critical during the first 12 to 24 hours after starting opioid therapy. The most critical period is during the peak effect of the first dose (15 minutes if administered IV; first hour after IM, oral, or rectal route). An exception is with opioids administered via the spinal route. Respiratory depression may increase over time with epidural infusions and with intrathecal analgesia; respiratory depression may manifest 24 hours after the spinal injection even after the analgesic effect has worn off. In general, the longer the client receives opioids, the wider the safety margin as the client develops a tolerance to the sedative and respiratory depressive effects of the drug.

BOX 30.6 Common Opioid Side Effects with Preventive and Treatment Measures

SEDATION

- Inform client that tolerance usually develops over 3 to 5 days.
- Consider the administration of a stimulant in the morning (e.g., caffeine, Dexedrine, or Ritalin for adult clients) or an alternative route of administration (e.g., epidural) to counteract sedation.
- Observe client for evidence of respiratory depression that may occur with sedation.

RESPIRATORY DEPRESSION

- Administer an opioid antagonist, such as naloxone hydrochloride (Narcan), cautiously by diluting 1 ampule in 10 mL of saline and then administering 1 mL/min until the respirations are equal to or more than 10/min. Make provisions for repeat administration, continuous infusion, or a longer acting version of a reversal agent because the half-life of naloxone is considerably shorter than that of most opioids being reversed.
- Remember to titrate naloxone to prevent seizures, arrhythmias, and returning pain.
- Attempt to stimulate the client to take deep breaths every 15 to 30 minutes. Stop, change, or slow the administration of opioids until respirations are restored.
- Be aware of the CNS depression risks of other medications such as hypnotics, benzodiazepines, and sedatives, especially in the opioid-naïve client.

NAUSEA AND VOMITING

- Inform the client that tolerance to this emetic effect generally develops after several days of opioid therapy.
- Provide an antiemetic: the 5HT antagonist ondansetron (Zofran), phenothiazines (Phenergan), or the GI stimulant metoclopramide (Reglan).
- Change the dose or analgesic agent as indicated.

CONSTIPATION

- Increase fluid intake (e.g., 6 to 8 glasses daily).
- Increase fiber and bulk-forming agents to the diet (e.g., fresh fruits and vegetables). Increasing exercise is often ineffective in controlling this type of constipation.
- Administer daily stool softeners combined with a mild laxative (e.g., Senokot-S) as prevention against constipation for clients on opioid maintenance therapy.
- Stimulants (bisacodyl), osmotic laxatives (lactulose, sorbitol, and polyethylene glycol), enemas (tap water and sodium phosphate), and even prokinetic agents (metoclopramide) may be needed for refractory cases of constipation.
- Two medications, methylnaltrexone (Relistor) and naloxegol (Movantik) are specifically used to treat opioid-induced constipation in clients with advanced illness who are receiving opioids. When opioids occupy the mu receptors in the GI tract, they slow the transit of intestinal contents, causing constipation. These drugs act by blocking opioid mu receptors in the GI tract. Blocking the mu receptor occurs without affecting opioid-induced analgesia.

PRURITUS

- Apply cool packs, lotion, and diversional activity.
- Administer antihistamines, for example, diphenhydramine hydrochloride (Benadryl) or chlorphenamine (Piriton). Instruct client about sedation effects. In some instances, Naloxone can also be administered, but the client needs to be cautioned about possible withdrawal.
- Inform the client that tolerance also develops to pruritus within a few days; otherwise, as with other unresolved side effects, switching to another opioid may prove beneficial.

URINARY RETENTION

- May need to catheterize client, or change or lower the analgesic dose.

all opioid side effects usually occurs within a few days, except for constipation. Because of this, the nurse must initiate and continue measures to prevent constipation during the entire time the client receives opioids.

Range Orders

Range orders are medication orders in which the selected dose varies over a prescribed range according to the client's situation and status. For example, a prn range order for morphine 2 to 6 mg IV every 2 h for pain or for oxycodone 5 to 10 mg PO every 4 h prn for pain provides flexibility in dosing to meet individual client analgesic needs. In the past, there was an inconsistent understanding of how to interpret and carry out prn range orders. As a result, the American Society of Pain Management Nurses and the American Pain Society published a position statement on the use of "as-needed" range orders for opioid analgesics (Drew, Gordon, Morgan, & Manworren, 2018). It is important to check the agency policy as it may be more specific on how to interpret the dose range order. These changes to the way prn range orders are written provide more structure than in the past; however, clients' responses to analgesics can vary greatly. Professional nursing judgment remains a key factor in relieving pain by determining which medication in what dosage would best meet the client's comfort needs. As a result, professional nursing judgment needs to include those factors that influence this variability, such as pain severity, prior opioid exposure (opioid naïveté or tolerance), age, kidney function, and other health disorders affecting the client. Other influencing factors include drug pharmacokinetics and other medications the client is receiving, such as sedatives (Drew et al., 2018, p. 208).

Range orders enable safe adjustments in doses based on individual responses to treatment. However, to do so, it is important that primary care providers, nurses, and pharmacists share a common understanding of how to properly prescribe, interpret, and carry out prn range orders (Drew et al., 2018, p. 208).

Recommendations from the position statement on prn range orders that relate to the prescriber include: The order should provide a dosage range with a fixed time interval. Avoid duplication of different opioids by the same route (e.g., IV morphine and IV hydromorphone). Limit opioid dose ranges to 2 to 3 times the lower dose. It is unsafe to order more than one analgesic by different routes *unless* the orders provide clear guidelines for use. For example, an order might state: prn IV hydromorphone for severe pain, PO hydrocodone for moderate pain, and PO ibuprofen for mild pain. Written orders for the same opioid but different routes should provide clear direction for use (e.g., use oral route unless client is NPO, nauseous, or vomiting).

Recommendations that relate to nurses include: Make decisions about the range order based on a thorough pain assessment and knowledge of the pharmacokinetics of the analgesic. Avoid administering small, frequent partial doses (e.g., giving oxycodone 10 mg every 2 hours when the order reads oxycodone 10 to 20 mg every 3 hours prn). If the half-life of the drug is longer than the dosing frequency, the drug may accumulate and lead to overdosing. If a partial dose is administered first, wait until the peak effect has been reached before giving a subsequent dose. Avoid making a client wait the full time interval after giving an additional partial dose within the allowed range (p. 209).

In addition, the *Guidelines for Safe Electronic Communication of Medication Information* (Institute for Safe Medication Practices, 2019) states the following: Do not allow single orders for medications with range doses, various frequencies, or more than one route of administration. If orders for the same drug are prescribed at different doses, frequencies, or routes, require separate orders for each that specify objective measures to guide determination of which dose to administer at which frequency and by which route. Examples of pain assessment measures that may be used to guide determination of the dose, route, or frequency of medication include severity, chronicity, quality of pain, and prior response to analgesics) (p. 7).

Equianalgesic Dosing

The term **equianalgesia** refers to the relative potency of various opioid analgesics compared to a standard dose of parenteral morphine. This tool helps professionals individualize the analgesic regimen by guiding the adjustment of medication, dose, time interval, and route of administration. An equianalgesic table can be used to help provide doses of approximately equal ability to relieve pain.

Adjuvants

An **adjuvant** is a medication that is not classified as a pain medication. However, adjuvants have properties that may reduce pain alone or in combination with other analgesics, relieve other discomforts, potentiate the effect of pain medications, or reduce the pain medication's side effects. Examples of adjuvants that relieve pain are antidepressants (increase pain relief, improve mood, and improve sleep), anticonvulsants (stabilize nerve membranes, reducing excitability and spontaneous firing), and local anesthetics (block the transmission of pain signals). Anxiolytics, sedatives, and antispasmodics are examples of medicines that relieve other discomforts; however, they do not alleviate pain and thus should be used in addition to rather than instead of analgesics. Examples of medications used to reduce the adverse effects of analgesics include stimulants, laxatives, and antiemetics.

Adjuvants appear to be particularly beneficial for the management of neuropathic pain. Tricyclic antidepressant drugs are prescribed for central neuropathic pain, which often manifests as pain with a burning, unusual, or stinging quality. Anticonvulsant drugs, such as gabapentin (Neurontin) or pregabalin (Lyrica), are used for peripheral neuropathic conditions that often present with a stabbing, shooting, or electrical-shock quality. Local anesthetics such as the Lidoderm patch also alleviate neuropathic as well as other types of pain, and are particularly useful for clients with the skin sensitivity known as allodynia. There is a growing scientific and clinical basis for the use of these medications in relieving pain, especially for persistent pain.

World Health Organization Three-Step Analgesic Ladder
According to the World Health Organization (WHO, n.d.) guideline *Cancer Pain Relief* (2nd ed.), pain treatment for cancer and noncancer chronic pain should be prescribed in three steps (see Figure 30.7 ■). For clients with mild pain (1 to 3 on a 0-to-10 scale), step 1 of the analgesic ladder, nonopioid analgesics (with or without an adjuvant) is the appropriate starting point. If the client has mild pain that persists or increases despite using full doses of step 1 medications, or if the pain is moderate (4 to 6 on a 0-to-10 scale), then a step 2 routine is appropriate. At the second step, a weak-acting opioid for moderate pain (e.g., codeine, tramadol) or a combination of opioid and nonopioid medicine (e.g., oxycodone with acetaminophen, hydrocodone with ibuprofen) is provided with or without adjuvant medications. If the client has moderate pain that persists or increases despite using full doses of step 2 medications, or if the pain is severe (7 to 10 on a 0-to-10 scale), then at the third step, a strong-acting opioid for severe pain (e.g., morphine, hydromorphone, fentanyl) is administered. Nonopioid analgesics and adjuvants can be added.

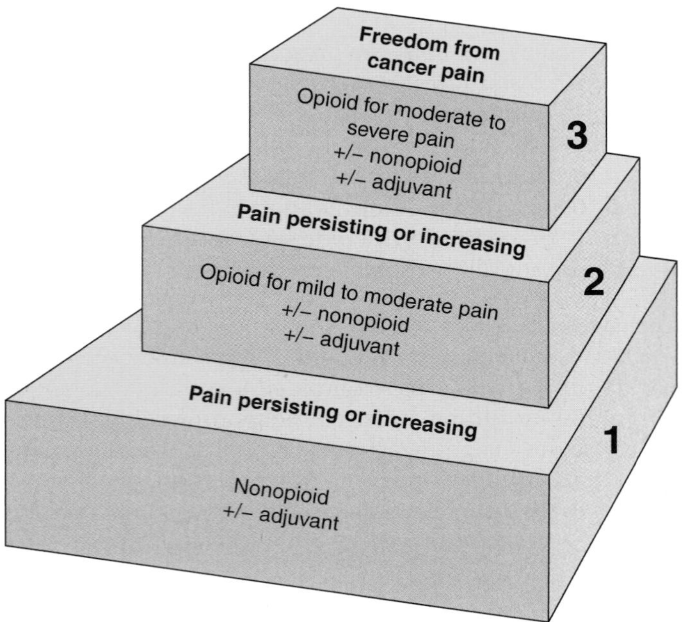

Figure 30.7 ■ The World Health Organization (WHO) three-step analgesic ladder.
Reprinted from 'WHO's cancer pain ladder for adults', World Health Organization.

The WHO first developed the pain ladder in 1986 and updated it in 1996 as a framework for the management of cancer-related pain. It is not an evidence-based guideline (WHO, 2012). It has been unofficially adopted for use in other pain syndromes. Over the years, there have been major developments in the understanding of pain, pain control, and new methods for treating pain. As a result, in the professional literature, clinicians have proposed that the WHO ladder continue to be used but that clinicians should feel free to modify it as needed for individual clients, reflecting modern pain practice (Pergolizzi & Raffa, 2015, p. 1). Candido, Kusper, and Knezevic (2017) also recommend, in keeping with the current multimodal pain treatment approach, the addition of a step 4 for severe to very severe pain. This step would include interventional treatments (e.g., intrathecal drug administration and nerve blocks) with or without the use of nonopioids and adjuvant therapy. They also recommend that the prescriber does not need to "climb"

DRUG CAPSULE

Opioid Analgesic: oxycodone (OxyContin), oxycodone/acetaminophen (Percocet), oxycodone/aspirin (Percodan)

CLIENT WITH PAIN

Opioids relieve moderate to severe pain by inhibiting the release of substance P in both central and peripheral nerves, reducing the perception of pain, producing sedation, and decreasing the emotional stress of pain.

Oxycodone is a semisynthetic derivative of codeine and a Schedule II controlled substance. It is often administered as a combination drug with acetaminophen (Percocet, Tylox) or aspirin (Percodan). It is also available as a single-agent, controlled-release medication (OxyContin).

NURSING RESPONSIBILITIES

- Assess pain prior to and 60 minutes after administration.
- Assess bowel function to prevent constipation.
- Keep track of the total amount of acetaminophen or aspirin the client is receiving when taking a combination drug. The maximum daily dose of acetaminophen is 4000 mg unless the client is at risk for liver problems (e.g., older adult, malnourished, or hepatic problems). For these clients, the maximum amount is lowered.

CLIENT AND FAMILY TEACHING

- Take with food to decrease GI upset.
- Avoid crushing or chewing long-acting tablets (e.g., OxyContin).
- Avoid alcohol or other CNS depressants.
- Explain that the medication may cause dizziness, and instruct to make position changes slowly.
- Instruct that constipation is a common side effect. Discuss preventive measures.
- Take only as prescribed.

Note: Prior to administering any medication, review all aspects with a current drug handbook or other reliable source.

the ladder rung by rung, but that it is acceptable to skip steps when going upward or to start high and move back down the ladder. The starting point should be controlled by the needs of the client and his or her response to the prescribed treatment (p. 2).

Routes for Opioid Delivery

Opioids can be given in the following routes: oral, transnasal, transdermal, transmucosal, rectal, topical, subcutaneous, intramuscular, IV (bolus and continuous), and intraspinal (epidural and intrathecal) and as continuous local anesthetics. For further details of these various methods of opioid administration, see Chapter 35 ∞.

Administration of Placebos

A **placebo** is "any sham medication or procedure designed to be void of any known therapeutic value" (Arnstein, Broglio, Wuhrman, & Kean, 2011, p. 226). An example would be a sugar pill or an injection of saline. In contrast, the *placebo effect* is "the positive response some patients/participants experience after receiving a placebo" (Arnstein et al., 2011, p. 226). Some professionals try to justify the use of placebos to elicit the desirable placebo effect or in a misguided attempt to determine if the client's pain is "real." The use of placebos, outside the context of an approved research study, is deceptive and represents fraudulent and unethical treatment. Many professional and pain management organizations (e.g., American Society for Pain Management Nursing) have published position papers that adamantly oppose the use of placebos without consent.

Patient-Controlled Analgesia

Patient-controlled analgesia (PCA) is an interactive method of pain management that permits clients to treat their pain by self-administering doses of analgesics. The IV route is the most common in an acute care setting. Its use for postoperative pain has been well documented. It is also helpful when oral pain management is not possible. The PCA mode of therapy minimizes the roller-coaster effect of peaks of sedation and valleys of pain that occur with the traditional method of prn dosing. With the parenteral routes, the client administers a predetermined dose of an opioid by an electronic infusion pump. This allows the client to maintain a more constant level of relief yet requires less medication for pain relief. PCA can be effectively used for clients with acute pain related to a surgical incision, traumatic injury, or labor and delivery, and for chronic pain as with cancer.

The prescriber orders the analgesic, dose, demand (bolus) dose interval, and lockout interval. Standardized medications and order sets are recommended. The most commonly used opioids for PCA are morphine, hydromorphone (Dilaudid), and fentanyl. Whether in an acute hospital setting, in an ambulatory clinic, or with home care, the nurse is responsible for the initial instruction regarding use of the PCA. To avoid incorrect pump programming, two registered nurses should double-check the pump settings at the start of the PCA therapy, the beginning of each shift, change of infusion container, or change in PCA order (Infusion Nurses Society, 2016, p. 247). The nurse also is responsible for ongoing monitoring of the therapy (e.g., checking every 2 to 4 hours). The client's pain level, respiratory rate, sedation level, ability to understand, and use of the device must be assessed at regular intervals. Postoperative clients may also have oxygen levels or carbon dioxide levels monitored. Some PCA pumps have an in-line capnography system that monitors carbon dioxide levels while the PCA is being used. Analgesic use is documented in the client's record. The most significant adverse effects are respiratory depression and hypotension.

Safety Alert! **SAFETY**

As a precaution, have naloxone (Narcan), sodium chloride 0.9% diluent, and injection equipment on hand for each client receiving an opioid-containing epidural infusion.

Although PCA pumps vary in design, they all have similar protective features. The line of the PCA pump, a syringe-type pump, is usually introduced into the injection port of a primary IV fluid line (Figure 30.8 ■). The primary care provider determines the drug concentration (amount of drug per milliliter of solution), the PCA bolus dose (amount of medication the client will receive when a bolus is self-administered), and the lockout, which is also called the delay interval (the amount of time that must pass between PCA doses). When clients need a dose of analgesic, they push a button attached to the infusion pump and a preset dose (bolus) is delivered. The lockout interval is usually set at 6 or 8 minutes for postoperative clients. This means that the client can give him- or herself a dose of medication every 6 or 8 minutes. Even

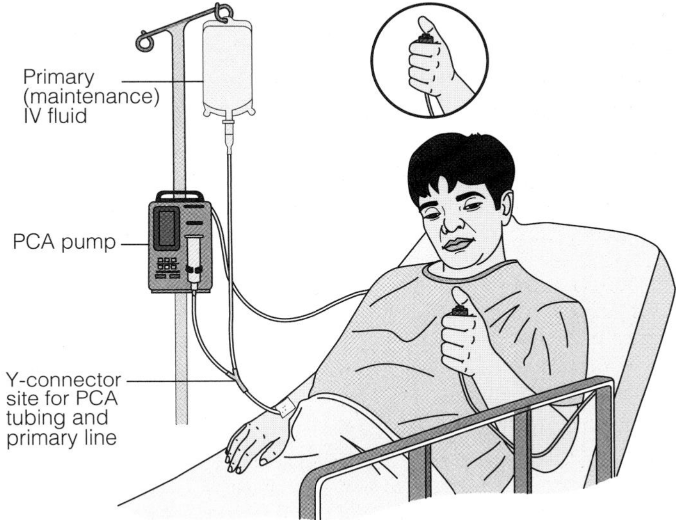

Figure 30.8 ■ PCA line introduced into the injection port of a primary IV line.

if the client pushes the button more frequently, the client will receive only one bolus dose during the lockout interval. The primary care provider can also prescribe an hour interval, which determines the maximum amount of opioid a client can receive in an hour-limit time period. Most PCA pumps can be programmed for a 1-hour or a 4-hour limit. The 1-hour limit is preferable because it allows for closer PCA monitoring by the nurse; that is, the nurse is alerted earlier if the client is not receiving adequate analgesia and requires an increase in opioid dose. Many pumps are capable of delivering a basal rate (continuous infusion), with or without additional PCA doses administered by the client. This practice is no longer recommended for opioid-naïve clients due to the risk of oversedation. It is more appropriate, if not necessary, for the client who is opioid tolerant and experiencing chronic pain.

As PCA has increased in use, so have errors and other problems, such as adverse (untoward, undesirable, and usually unanticipated) events. Problems that reduce PCA safety include improper client selection, programming errors, and PCA by proxy.

Clients who use PCA must be able to understand how to use PCA and be able to physically push the button independently. Clients who are not good candidates for PCA include infants and young children who do not understand how to safely use PCA, confused older clients, individuals who are obese or have asthma or sleep apnea, and clients taking other drugs that potentiate opioids, such as muscle relaxants.

Improperly programming the PCA pump is the most common human error (Pasero & McCaffery, 2011). Examples of errors include confusing milliliters and milligrams, decimal point errors (i.e., order is for 0.5 mg and the pump is programmed for 5 mg), using the loading dose for the bolus dose, and wrong lockout settings. To increase safety upon PCA initiation, many institutions now require that two nurses independently check client identity, drug and concentration, and PCA pump settings.

PCA by proxy is a term that describes activation of the PCA pump by *anyone other than the client*. For example, a well-intentioned family member may push the button when the client is sleeping or already sedated, leading to oversedation. A natural safety feature of PCA is that a client who is sleeping or sedated will not push the button and overmedicate him- or herself. That is why it is important that the client be the only one to push the button. To counteract this, some institutions put signs on the PCA pump stating "only the client is to push the PCA button."

The ASPMN differentiates between PCA by proxy (unauthorized activation of the pump) and authorized agent–controlled analgesia (AACA). AACA is a method of pain control in which a consistently available and competent individual is authorized by a prescriber and properly educated to push the PCA button when the client is unable to and in response to the client's pain (Infusion Nurses Society, 2016, p. 247). AACA is not appropriate if the client is determined to be able to use PCA. Parent/nurse-controlled analgesia (PNCA) is the term used when the authorized individual is the parent or nurse responsible for an infant client.

QSEN Safety: PCA Pump

In the home setting, the nurse needs to inform the client's support people to monitor for signs and symptoms of oversedation such as excessive drowsiness, slowed respiratory rate, or change in mental state. No one should adjust settings without consulting the appropriate primary care provider. The caregiver should tape the following emergency contact numbers to the back of the pump: emergency medical services, primary care provider, home care agency, and pump manufacturer.

Oral medication on demand (MOD) is another electronic delivery device that permits client-controlled access to oral medications prescribed on a prn basis, within preset time intervals (Avancen, n.d.). The patient-controlled oral analgesia device is placed on an IV pole within easy reach of the client. It has functions such as keypads allowing clients to input their pain intensity rating before swiping a radio frequency identification (RFID) wristband individual to each client. After waving the RFID wristband in front of the locked, preprogrammed device, the client removes the oral prn medication. A green light signals the client when the next dose is available (see Figure 30.9 ■). In addition, the device has the potential to interface with network, inventory, and billing systems.

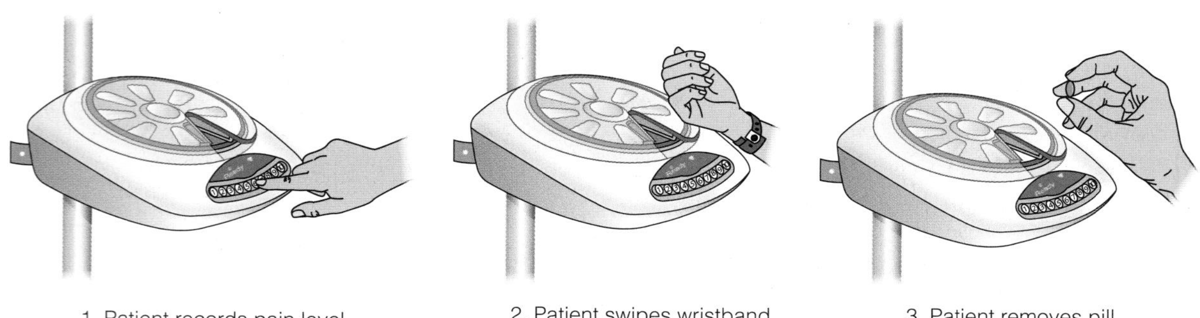

1. Patient records pain level
2. Patient swipes wristband
3. Patient removes pill

Figure 30.9 ■ Patient-controlled oral analgesia delivery device (MOD®).

CLIENT TEACHING **Client Self-Management of Pain Using IV PCA**

Choose a time to teach the client about pain management when the pain is controlled so that the client is able to focus on the teaching. Teaching about self-management of pain may include the following:

- Demonstrate the operation of the PCA pump and explain that the client can safely push the button without fear of overmedicating. Sometimes it helps clients who are reluctant to repeatedly push the button to know that they must dose themselves (i.e., push the button) 5 to 10 times to receive the same amount of medication (10 mg morphine equivalent) they would receive in a standard dose.
- Describe the use of the pain scale and encourage the client to respond in order to demonstrate understanding.
- Explore a variety of nonpharmacologic pain relief techniques that the client is willing to learn and use to promote pain relief and optimize functioning.
- Explain to the client the need to notify staff when ambulation is desired (e.g., for bathroom use) if applicable.

LIFESPAN CONSIDERATIONS **PCA Pump**

CHILDREN

- Include the parents in teaching.
- Assess the child's ability to understand and use the client control button. Pasero and McCaffery (2011) report that "PCA has been used effectively and safely in developmentally normal children as young as 4 years old" (p. 314).
- Use distraction techniques to avoid dislodgement or disconnection by the child.
- Use pediatric elbow immobilizers (no-nos, Snuggle Wraps) if distraction is not effective in keeping the child from playing with tubing and ports.

OLDER ADULTS

- Carefully monitor for drug side effects.
- Use cautiously for individuals with impaired pulmonary or renal function.
- Assess the client's cognitive and physical ability to use the client control button.

The traditional method of administering prn oral pain medications can mean delays in delivery to the client, especially if a busy nurse caring for six to eight clients has three requests for prn medications at the same time. This device allows clients autonomy with their pain management and frees up time for the nurse to deliver other important client care. The device should be made available only to clients who are awake, alert, able to accept device responsibilities and remember instruction on how to use the device, and with no swallowing difficulties and no drug-seeking behavior.

Nonpharmacologic Approaches

Nonpharmacologic pain management consists of a variety of physical, cognitive–behavioral, and lifestyle pain management strategies that target the body, mind, spirit, and social interactions (Table 30.6). Physical modalities include cutaneous stimulation, ice or heat, immobilization or therapeutic exercises, transcutaneous electrical nerve stimulation (TENS), and acupuncture. Mind–body (cognitive–behavioral) interventions include distracting activities, relaxation techniques, imagery, meditation, biofeedback, hypnosis, cognitive reframing, emotional counseling, and spiritually directed approaches such as therapeutic touch or Reiki. Lifestyle management approaches include symptom monitoring, stress management, exercise, nutrition, disability management, and other approaches needed by many clients with persistent pain that has drastically changed their life. For further information on selected mind–body interventions and acupuncture, see Chapter 22 ∞. This discussion is limited to selected physical and cognitive–behavioral interventions.

TABLE 30.6 Nonpharmacologic Interventions for Pain Control

Target Domain of Pain Control	Intervention
Body	Reducing pain triggers, promoting comfort Deep, slow breathing Massage Applying heat or ice Electrical stimulation (TENS) Positioning, bracing (selective immobilization) Acupressure, acupuncture Diet, nutritional supplements Exercise, pacing activities Invasive interventions (e.g., nerve blocks) Sleep hygiene
Mind	Relaxation, imagery Self-hypnosis Pain diary, journal writing Distracting attention Repatterning thinking Attitude adjustment Reducing fear, anxiety, stress Reducing sadness, helplessness Information about pain
Spirit	Music therapy Prayer, meditation Self-reflection regarding life and pain Meaningful rituals Energy work (e.g., therapeutic touch, Reiki) Spiritual healing
Social interactions	Functional restoration Improved communication Pet therapy Family therapy Problem solving Vocational training Volunteering Support groups

Physical Interventions: Cutaneous Stimulation

The goals of physical intervention include providing comfort, altering physiologic responses to reduce pain perception, and optimizing functioning. Cutaneous stimulation can provide effective temporary pain relief. It distracts the client and focuses attention on the tactile stimuli, away from the painful sensations, thus reducing pain perception. Cutaneous stimulation is also believed to interrupt the pain pathway. Selected cutaneous stimulation techniques include the following:

- Massage
- Application of heat or cold
- Acupressure
- Contralateral stimulation.

Cutaneous stimulation can be applied directly to the painful area, proximal to the pain or distal to the pain (along the nerve path or dermatome), and contralateral (exact location, opposite side of the body) to the pain. Cutaneous stimulation is contraindicated in areas of skin breakdown or impaired neurologic functioning.

Massage Massage affects both body and mind. Research provides evidence of the benefits of massage such as lowering stress levels, improving pain management, triggering the body's relaxation response, reducing signs of inflammation, and promoting healing after burns (Westman & Blaisdell, 2016). The human touch in massage communicates caring and strengthens the relationship between client and nurse. Massage can involve the back and neck, hands and arms, or feet. The use of ointments or liniments may provide localized pain relief with joint or muscle pain. Massage is contraindicated in areas of skin breakdown, suspected clots, or infections.

Ironically, nurses in acute care settings seldom use this basic nursing skill. The intensity of the acute care environment and the time demands of high-technology nursing may be contributing factors leading to the disappearance of the back massage. Nurses, however, need to reconsider this simple, effective, traditional skill because research supports the many positive client outcomes and few adverse effects. Skill 30.1 provides guidelines for giving a back massage.

SKILL 30.1

Providing a Back Massage

Effleurage is a type of massage consisting of long, slow, gliding strokes. Research demonstrates that back massage can enhance client comfort, relaxation, and sleep.

PURPOSES

- To relieve muscle tension
- To decrease pain intensity
- To promote physical and mental relaxation

ASSESSMENT

Assess

- Behaviors indicating potential need for a back massage, such as a complaint of stiffness, muscle tension in the back or shoulders, or difficulty sleeping related to tenseness or anxiety
- Whether the client is willing to have a massage, because some individuals may not enjoy a massage
- Contraindications for back massage (e.g., coagulation issues, clots, impaired skin integrity, back surgery, vertebral issues, or risk of fracture)

PLANNING

Ensure that you have adequate time available for the massage. Although the actual skill may require only about 5 minutes, the entire process should be conducted in a calm and unhurried manner.

Assignment

The nurse can assign this skill to assistive personnel (AP); however, the nurse should first assess for the AP's comfort and ability, any contraindications, and client willingness to participate.

Equipment

- Lotion
- Towel for excess lotion

IMPLEMENTATION

Preparation

Determine (a) previous assessments of the skin, (b) special lotions to be used, and (c) positions contraindicated for the client. Create a quiet, calming environment with no interruptions to promote maximum effect of the back massage.

Performance

1. Prior to performing the procedure, introduce self and verify the client's identity using agency protocol. Explain to the client what you are going to do, why it is necessary, and how to participate. Invite feedback as to the amount of pressure, position, and length of time during the back massage.
2. Perform hand hygiene and observe other appropriate infection prevention procedures.
3. Provide for client privacy.
4. Prepare the client.
   - Assist the client to move to the near side of the bed within your reach and adjust the bed to a comfortable working height. **Rationale:** *This prevents back strain.*

Providing a Back Massage—*continued*

- Establish which position the client prefers. The prone position is recommended for a back massage. The side-lying position can be used if a client cannot assume the prone position.
- Expose the back from the shoulders to the sacral area. Cover the remainder of the body. **Rationale:** *This is to prevent chilling and minimize exposure.*

5. Massage the back.
   - Warm the lotion or oil in your hands before touching the client. The lotion bottle can also be placed in a bath basin filled with warm water. **Rationale:** *Back massage preparations tend to feel uncomfortably cold to people. Warming the solution facilitates client comfort.*
   - Using your palm, begin in the sacral area using smooth, circular strokes.
   - Move your hands up the center of the back and then over both scapulae.
   - Massage in a circular motion over the scapulae.
   - Move your hands down the sides of the back.
   - Massage the areas over the right and left iliac crests. Massage the back in an orderly pattern using a variety of strokes and appropriate pressure.❶
   - Apply firm, continuous pressure without breaking contact with the client's skin.
   - Repeat above for 3 to 5 minutes, obtaining more lotion as necessary.
   - While massaging the back, assess for skin redness and areas of decreased circulation.
   - Pat dry any excess lotion with a towel.
6. Document that a back massage was performed and the client's response. Record any unusual findings.

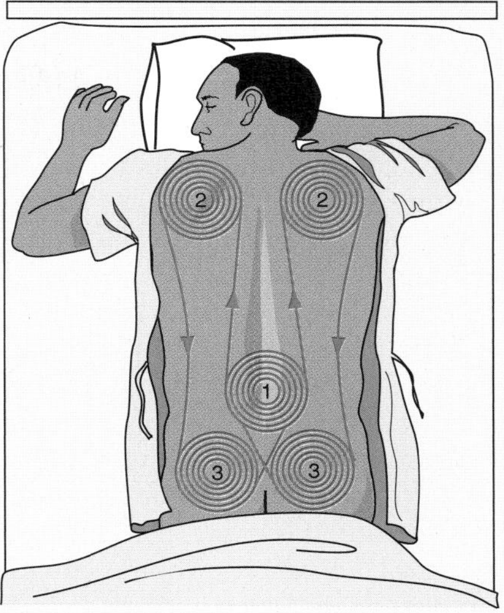

❶ One suggested pattern for a back massage.

SAMPLE DOCUMENTATION

6/22/2020 1400 Reports aching, intermittent back pain. Wincing and grimacing when attempting to move in bed. Rates pain at 4–5 on 0–10 scale. States uses massage to help relieve pain when at home. Back massaged. Stated the massage helped him "to relax." Lights dimmed and door to room closed. D. Aubrey, RN

1430 Reports pain at 1–2/10. States feels "much more comfortable." Moving in bed with ease. D. Aubrey, RN

EVALUATION

Compare the client's current response to his or her previous response. Is there a positive client outcome such as increased relaxation and decrease in pain and anxiety because of the back massage?

Heat and Cold Applications A warm bath, heating pads, ice bags, ice massage, hot or cold compresses, and warm or cold sitz baths in general relieve pain and promote healing of injured tissues (see Chapter 36 ∞). Cold works best when applied within the first 24 hours of injury or condition, while heat is primarily used to treat the chronic phase of an injury or condition, usually 48 hours after an acute injury.

Acupressure Acupressure developed from the ancient Chinese healing system of acupuncture. The therapist applies finger pressure to points that correspond to many of the points used in acupuncture (see Chapter 22 ∞).

Contralateral Stimulation Contralateral stimulation can be accomplished by stimulating the skin in an area opposite to the painful area (e.g., stimulating the left knee if the pain is in the right knee). The contralateral area may be scratched for itching, massaged for cramps, or treated with cold packs, heat application, or analgesic ointments. This method is particularly useful when the painful area cannot be touched because it is hypersensitive, when it is inaccessible by a cast or bandages, or when the pain is felt in a missing part (phantom pain). The nurse should explain the rationale to the client in that nerves are crossed in the spinal cord, and that is why these techniques may work contralaterally.

Immobilization and Bracing

Immobilizing or restricting the movement of a painful body part (e.g., arthritic joint, traumatized limb) may help to manage episodes of acute pain. Splints or supportive devices should hold joints in the position of optimal function and should be removed regularly in accordance with agency protocol to provide range-of-motion (ROM) exercises. Prolonged immobilization can result in joint contracture, muscle atrophy, and cardiovascular problems. Therefore, clients should be encouraged to participate in self-care activities and remain as active as possible, with frequent ROM exercises.

Transcutaneous Electrical Nerve Stimulation

Transcutaneous electrical nerve stimulation (TENS) is a method of applying low-voltage electrical stimulation directly over identified pain areas, at an acupressure point, along peripheral nerve areas that innervate the pain area, or along the spinal column. The TENS unit consists of a portable, battery-operated device with lead wires and electrode pads that are applied to the chosen area of skin (Figure 30.10 ■). Cutaneous stimulation from the TENS unit is thought to activate large-diameter fibers that modulate the transmission of the nociceptive impulse in the peripheral and central nervous systems, resulting in pain relief. This stimulation may also cause a release of endorphins from the CNS centers. The use of TENS is contraindicated for clients with pacemakers or arrhythmias, or in areas of skin breakdown. It is generally not used on the head or over the chest.

Cognitive–Behavioral Interventions

The goals of cognitive–behavioral interventions include providing comfort, altering psychologic responses to reduce pain perception, and optimizing functioning. Selected cognitive–behavioral interventions include distraction, producing the relaxation response, repatterning unhelpful thinking, and facilitating coping with emotions.

Distraction Distraction draws the client's attention away from the pain and lessens the perception of pain. In some instances, it can make a client completely unaware of pain. Distraction makes the client unaware of the pain only for the amount of time and to the extent that the distracting activity holds his or her "undivided" attention. For example, a client recovering from surgery may feel no pain while watching a football game on television, yet feel pain again during commercials or when the game is over. Nurses and caregivers need to be aware of the use of distraction and avoid labeling individuals as not "looking like" they are in pain (Ward, 2016).

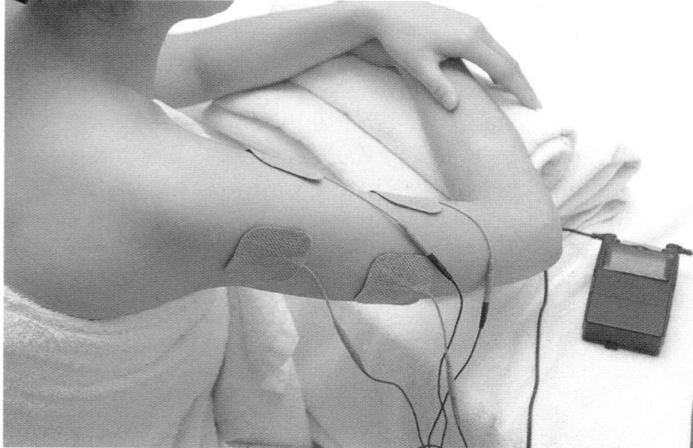

Figure 30.10 ■ A transcutaneous electrical nerve stimulator (TENS).
plepraisaeng/123RF.

Different types of distractions are shown in Box 30.7. Using multiple forms of distraction simultaneously adds value to the activity. For example, listening to music can be distracting; however, value can be added by tapping to the music, singing along, or playing along on a musical instrument. Play therapy can be a distraction for children.

The Relaxation Response Stress increases pain, in part by increasing muscle tension, activating the sympathetic nervous system, and putting the client at risk for stress-related types of pain (e.g., tension headaches). The relaxation response decreases and counteracts the harmful effects of stress, including the effect it has on physical, cognitive, and emotional functioning. Producing this response requires more than simply helping someone to relax; rather, it involves a structured technique designed to focus the mind and relax muscle groups. Basic techniques with helpful scripts are available for common techniques including progressive relaxation, breath-focus relaxation, and meditation. The nurse can coach the client, urge self-directed meditation, or provide an electronic guide to help elicit the relaxation response. Many clients can achieve the desired state after a few attempts, but mastery of this skill requires daily practice over a few weeks. In general, relaxation techniques by themselves do not have remarkable pain-relieving properties; however, they can

BOX 30.7 Types of Distraction

VISUAL DISTRACTION
- Reading or watching television
- Video and computer games (also tactile)
- Watching a baseball game
- Guided imagery

AUDITORY DISTRACTION
- Humor
- Music

TACTILE DISTRACTION
- Slow, rhythmic breathing
- Massage
- Needlework such as knitting, embroidery, cross-stitch (also intellectual)
- Holding or stroking a pet or toy

INTELLECTUAL DISTRACTION
- Crossword puzzles, Sudoku number puzzles
- Card games
- Hobbies

reduce pain that may have been exacerbated by stress. Some clients may become more consciously aware of their pain while practicing relaxation techniques before they have learned mastery of controlling "mind chatter" and remaining mentally focused.

Once the client has mastered the basic skills for producing the relaxation response, techniques of imagery or self-hypnosis can be used. Both imagery and hypnosis begin with attaining a deep state of relaxation and are capable of altering the experience of pain, for example, having the client replace the pain with a feeling of pleasant numbness. Additional post-hypnotic suggestions can then be made, linking these pleasant numb sensations to coping efforts used during the day (e.g., "Every time you stop to take a slow, deep, diaphragmatic breath, you will feel this pleasant numbness instead of pain").

Music therapy can also be useful for providing relaxation and distraction from pain. With iPods and smartphones, clients can listen to their favorite tunes as a helpful distraction from pain.

Repatterning Unhelpful Thinking Some clients harbor strong self-doubts, unrealistic expectations (e.g., "I just want someone to make the pain go away"), rumination (e.g., "I keep thinking about my pain and the person who did this to me"), helplessness (e.g., "I can't do anything"), and magnification (e.g., "My life is ruined, I'll never be a good parent because of my pain"). These cognitive patterns have been identified as important contributors to treatment failures and the intensification of pain, disability, and depression. Nurses can help by challenging the truthfulness and helpfulness of these thoughts and replacing them with realistic and confidence-building ones that are particularly powerful predictors of more effective coping, better clinical outcomes, and improved quality of life.

Facilitating Coping Nurses can help by intervening with clients who are anxious, are sad, or express overly pessimistic or helpless points of view. Awareness of the client's misperceptions or unrealistic expectations also helps the professional avoid a common cause of therapeutic failure. Therapeutic communication with an emphasis on listening, providing encouragement, teaching self-management skills, and persuading clients to act on their own behalf are strategies that enhance coping. Helping clients to better communicate with the professional staff, family members, and friends can also promote coping. Counseling from trained professionals may be indicated for those clients with severe emotional distress, but must be offered to them in a sensitive way that does not convey the notion that pain is "in their head." Chronic pain support groups have been effective for many clients.

Selected Spiritual Interventions

The spiritual dimension encompasses a client's innermost concerns and values, including the purpose, meaning, and driving force in his or her life. It may include rituals that help the individual become part of a community or feel a bond with the universe that is not necessarily religious in nature. For those who express their spirituality in a religious context, it is appropriate to offer prayer, intercessory prayer (being prayed for by others), or access to meaningful rituals. For some clients, a caring presence, attentive listening, and facilitating the process of acceptance can help reduce spiritual distress, whereas other clients benefit from manipulation of energy patterns (e.g., therapeutic touch).

Some clients may view pain as a punishment from God. For them, it could be helpful to provide opportunities to discuss their situation with a resource person well versed in theology (e.g., a clergyperson). To hold such beliefs inside without attempting to increase understanding can contribute to pain and suffering.

When using imagery techniques with clients, multisensory input relating to spiritual and religious experience can be powerfully healing. Seek understanding of the client's needs, preferences, and fears in this area. For some, imagining themselves being held in the loving arms or presence of healing light, God, the mother Mary, Buddha, or some other figure can be very comforting.

When using relaxation breathing techniques with clients, the breath can be viewed as a direct connection with God and life energy. The word *inspiration* means "to take in the spirit." The image of breathing in the healing spirit, and breathing out the pain, can be calming and empowering. To say to oneself while breathing in, "I am breathing in the healing power of God," and out, "I am releasing my pain as I breathe out," can serve as powerful, faith-based affirmations for cognitive restructuring.

QSEN Patient-Centered Care: Pain Management

At discharge or in the home setting, the nurse can provide helpful information to the client and the caregiver about pain management. Examples include teaching the client:

- To keep a pain diary to monitor pain onset, activity before pain, pain intensity, use of analgesics, or other relief measures and effectiveness of each measure.
- To contact a healthcare professional if planned pain control measures are ineffective.
- To use preferred and selected nonpharmacologic techniques such as relaxation, guided imagery, distraction, music therapy, and massage.
- To use pain control measures before the pain becomes severe.
- The effects of untreated pain.
- Appropriate information about how to access community resources, home care agencies, and associations that offer self-help groups and educational materials.

LIFESPAN CONSIDERATIONS **Pain Management**

INFANTS

- Giving an infant, particularly a very-low-birth-weight infant, a water and sucrose solution administered through a pacifier provides some pain reduction during procedures that may be painful, but should not be a substitute for anesthetic or analgesic medications.

CHILDREN

- Distract the child with toys, books, or pictures.
- Hold the child (or ask the parent to hold) to console and promote comfort.
- Explore misconceptions about pain and correct in understandable terms. Be aware of how your explanations may be misunderstood. For example, telling a child he won't hurt during surgery because he will be "put to sleep" will be very upsetting to a child who knows of an animal that was "put to sleep."
- Children can use their imagination during guided imagery. Ask the child to imagine a "pain switch" (even give it a color) and to visualize turning the switch off in the area where there is pain. A "magic glove" or "magic blanket" is an imaginary object that the child applies on areas of the body (e.g., hand, thigh, back, hip) to lessen discomfort.

OLDER ADULTS

- Promote clients' use of pain control measures that have worked for them in the past.
- Spend time with clients and listen carefully.
- Clarify misconceptions. Encourage independence whenever possible.
- Carefully review the treatment plan to avoid drug–drug, food–drug, or disease–drug interactions.
- Physicians and nurse practitioners with advanced certification in hospice and palliative medicine (HPM) are often members of the intraprofessional team that works with the client and family to provide the best possible hospice care.

Clinical Alert!

The statement "Please tell me how I can best help you control your pain" sends a couple of subtle messages that are an important part of treatment planning and evaluation of care. First, it places the ownership and responsibility for controlling pain on the client. Second, it acknowledges that the client may be the best judge of what is needed, respecting the cultural meaning of pain and acceptable ways of expressing and controlling pain. Third, it establishes the nurse's role in helping the client be more comfortable and in control of his or her condition.

Evaluating

The goals established in the planning phase are evaluated according to specific desired outcomes, also established in that phase. To assist in the evaluation process, flow sheet records in the client's EHR or a client diary may be helpful. A weekly log can also be developed for the individual client. For example, columns including day, time, onset of pain, activity before pain, pain relief measure, and duration of pain can help the client and nurse determine the effectiveness of pain relief strategies.

If outcomes are not achieved, the nurse and client need to explore the reasons before modifying the care plan. The nurse might consider the following questions:

- Is adequate analgesia being given? Would the client benefit from a change in dose or in the time interval between doses or in the type of analgesic?
- Were the client's beliefs, expectations, and values about pain therapy considered?
- Did the client understate the pain experience for some reason?
- Were appropriate instructions provided to prevent misconceptions about pain management?
- Did the client and support people understand the instructions about pain management techniques?
- Is the client receiving adequate support for both physical pain and emotional distress?
- Has the client's physical condition changed, necessitating modifications in interventions?
- Should selected intervention strategies be re-evaluated?

See the Nursing Care Plan and the Concept Map.

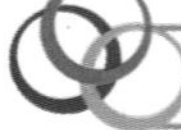

Critical Thinking Checkpoint

Mrs. Lundahl underwent abdominal surgery approximately 6 hours ago. She has a 15-cm midline incision that is covered with a dry, intact surgical dressing. On assessment, you note that Mrs. Lundahl is perspiring, lying in a rigid position, holding her abdomen, and grimacing. Her blood pressure is 150/90 mmHg, heart rate 100 beats/min, and respiratory rate 32/min. When asked to rate her pain on a scale of 0 to 10, Mrs. Lundahl rates her pain as 5 as long as she remains perfectly still. There is a sharp area of pain at her incision; however, the most bothersome pain is crampy and dull, as if she was "kicked in the stomach" with severe exacerbations that come in unpredictable waves.

1. What conclusions, if any, can be drawn about Mrs. Lundahl's pain status?
2. Does Mrs. Lundahl's rating her pain as 5 mean that she is not experiencing pain severe enough to warrant intervention?
3. What type of pain is Mrs. Lundahl experiencing?
4. What interventions, in addition to pain medication, may be useful in reducing Mrs. Lundahl's pain?
5. How will you know if your interventions have been effective in reducing Mrs. Lundahl's pain?

Answers to Critical Thinking Checkpoint questions are available on the faculty resources site. Please consult with your instructor.

NURSING CARE PLAN Acute Pain

ASSESSMENT DATA	NURSING DIAGNOSIS	DESIRED OUTCOMES*
NURSING ASSESSMENT Mr. C. is a 57-year-old businessman who was admitted to the surgical unit for treatment of a possible strangulated inguinal hernia. Two days ago he had a partial bowel resection. Postoperative orders include NPO, IV infusion of D_5 1/2 NS at 125 mL/h left forearm, nasogastric tube to low intermittent suction. Mr. C. is in a dorsal recumbent (supine) position and is attempting to draw up his legs. He appears restless and is complaining of abdominal pain (7 on a scale of 0–10). **Physical Examination** Height: 188 cm (6′ 3″) Weight: 90.0 kg (200 lb) Temperature: 37°C (98.6°F) Pulse: 90 beats/min Respirations: 24/min Blood pressure: 158/82 mmHg Skin pale and moist, pupils dilated. Midline abdominal incision, sutures dry and intact. **Diagnostic Data** Chest x-ray and urinalysis negative, WBC 12,000	Severe acute pain related to tissue injury secondary to surgical intervention (as evidenced by restlessness; pallor; elevated pulse, respirations, and systolic blood pressure; dilated pupils; and report of 7/10 abdominal pain)	Pain Control [1605] as evidenced by often demonstrating ability to: • Use analgesics as recommended. • Use nonanalgesic relief measures. • Report uncontrolled symptoms to healthcare professional. Pain Level [2102] as evidenced by mild to no: • Reported pain • Restlessness • Diaphoresis • Change in BP, HR, R from normal baseline data.

NURSING INTERVENTIONS*/SELECTED ACTIVITIES	RATIONALE
PAIN MANAGEMENT: ACUTE [1410]	
Perform a comprehensive assessment of pain to include location, characteristics, onset, duration, frequency, quality, intensity or severity, and precipitating factors of pain.	*Pain is a subjective experience and must be described by the client in order to plan effective treatment.*
Explore Mr. C.'s knowledge and beliefs about pain, including cultural influences.	*Each client experiences and expresses pain in an individual manner using a variety of sociocultural adaptation techniques.*
Question Mr. C. regarding the level of pain that allows a state of comfort and appropriate function and attempt to keep pain at or lower than identified level.	*Factors that may be precipitating or augmenting pain should be reduced or eliminated to enhance the overall pain management program.*
Ensure that Mr. C. receives prompt analgesic care before the pain becomes severe or before pain-inducing activities.	*Each client has a right to expect maximum pain relief. Turning and ambulation activities will be enhanced if pain is controlled or tolerable.*
Incorporate nonpharmacologic interventions to the pain etiology and client preference, as appropriate.	*The use of noninvasive pain relief measures can increase the release of endorphins and enhance the therapeutic effects of pain relief medications.*
ANALGESIC ADMINISTRATION [2210]	
Check medical order for drug, dose, and frequency of analgesic prescribed.	*Ensures that the nurse has the right drug, right route, right dosage, right client, right frequency.*
Determine analgesic selections (opioid or nonopioid, or NSAIDs) based on type and severity of pain.	*Various types of pain (e.g., acute, chronic, nociceptive, neuropathic) require different analgesic approaches. Some types of pain respond to nonopioid drugs alone, while others can be relieved by combining a low-dose opioid with a nonopioid.*
Institute safety precautions as appropriate if Mr. C. receives opioid analgesics.	*Side effects of opioids include drowsiness and sedation.*
Instruct Mr. C. to request prn pain medication *before* the pain is severe.	*Severe pain is more difficult to control and increases the client's anxiety and fatigue. The preventive approach to pain management can reduce the total 24-hour analgesic dose.*
Evaluate the effectiveness of analgesic at regular, frequent intervals after each administration and especially after the initial doses.	*The analgesic dose may not be adequate to raise the client's pain threshold or may be causing intolerable or dangerous side effects or both. Ongoing evaluation will assist in making necessary adjustments for effective pain management.*

Continued on page 686

NURSING CARE PLAN Acute Pain—*continued*

ASSESSMENT DATA	NURSING DIAGNOSIS / DESIRED OUTCOMES*
Document Mr. C.'s response to analgesics and any untoward effects.	*Documentation facilitates pain management by communicating effective and noneffective pain management strategies to the entire healthcare team.*
Implement actions to decrease untoward effects of analgesics (e.g., sedation, respiratory depression, nausea and vomiting, dry mouth, constipation, gastric irritation).	*Constipation is the most common side effect of opioids, and a treatment plan to prevent occurrence should be instituted at the beginning of analgesic therapy. For Mr. C., constipation could result from his primary condition or his analgesia. Assess for overall GI functioning, possible complications of surgery (e.g., ileus), as well as opioid-induced constipation or NSAID-induced gastritis.*

NURSING INTERVENTIONS*/SELECTED ACTIVITIES	RATIONALE
RELAXATION THERAPY [6040]	
Consider Mr. C.'s willingness and ability to participate, preference, past experiences, and contraindications before selecting a specific relaxation strategy.	*The client must feel comfortable trying a different approach to pain management. To avoid ineffective strategies, the client should be involved in the planning process.*
Elicit behaviors that are conditioned to produce relaxation, such as deep breathing, yawning, abdominal breathing, or peaceful imaging.	*Relaxation techniques help reduce skeletal muscle tension, which will reduce the intensity of the pain.*
Create a quiet, nondisruptive environment with dim lights and comfortable temperature when possible.	*Comfort and a quiet atmosphere promote a relaxed feeling and permit the client to focus on the relaxation technique rather than external distraction.*
Individualize the content of the relaxation intervention (e.g., by asking for suggestions about what Mr. C. enjoys or finds relaxing).	*Each client may find different images or approaches to relaxation more helpful than others. The nurse should have a variety of relaxation scripts or audiovisual aids to help clients find the best one for them.*
Demonstrate and practice the relaxation technique with Mr. C.	*Return demonstrations by the participant provide an opportunity for the nurse to evaluate the effectiveness of teaching sessions.*
Evaluate and document his response to relaxation therapy.	*Conveys to the healthcare team effective strategies in reducing or eliminating pain.*

EVALUATION

Outcomes partially met. The client verbalizes pain and discomfort, requesting analgesics at onset of pain. States "the pain is a 2" (on a scale of 0–10) 30 minutes after an IV analgesic administration. Requests analgesic 30 minutes before ambulation. States willingness to try relaxation techniques; however, has not attempted to do so.

*The NOC # for desired outcomes and the NIC # for nursing interventions are listed in brackets following the appropriate outcome or intervention. Outcomes, indicators, interventions, and activities selected are only a sample of those suggested by NOC and NIC and should be further individualized for each client.

APPLYING CRITICAL THINKING

1. Is there any other assessment data you would want to gather to help plan Mr. C.'s pain management?
2. Mr. C. does not have a PCA. What nursing interventions are important?
3. What kind of data would you gather prior to having a discussion with the primary care provider about options for improving pain control in this client?

Answers to Applying Critical Thinking questions are available on the faculty resources site. Please consult with your instructor.

CONCEPT MAP

Severe Acute Pain

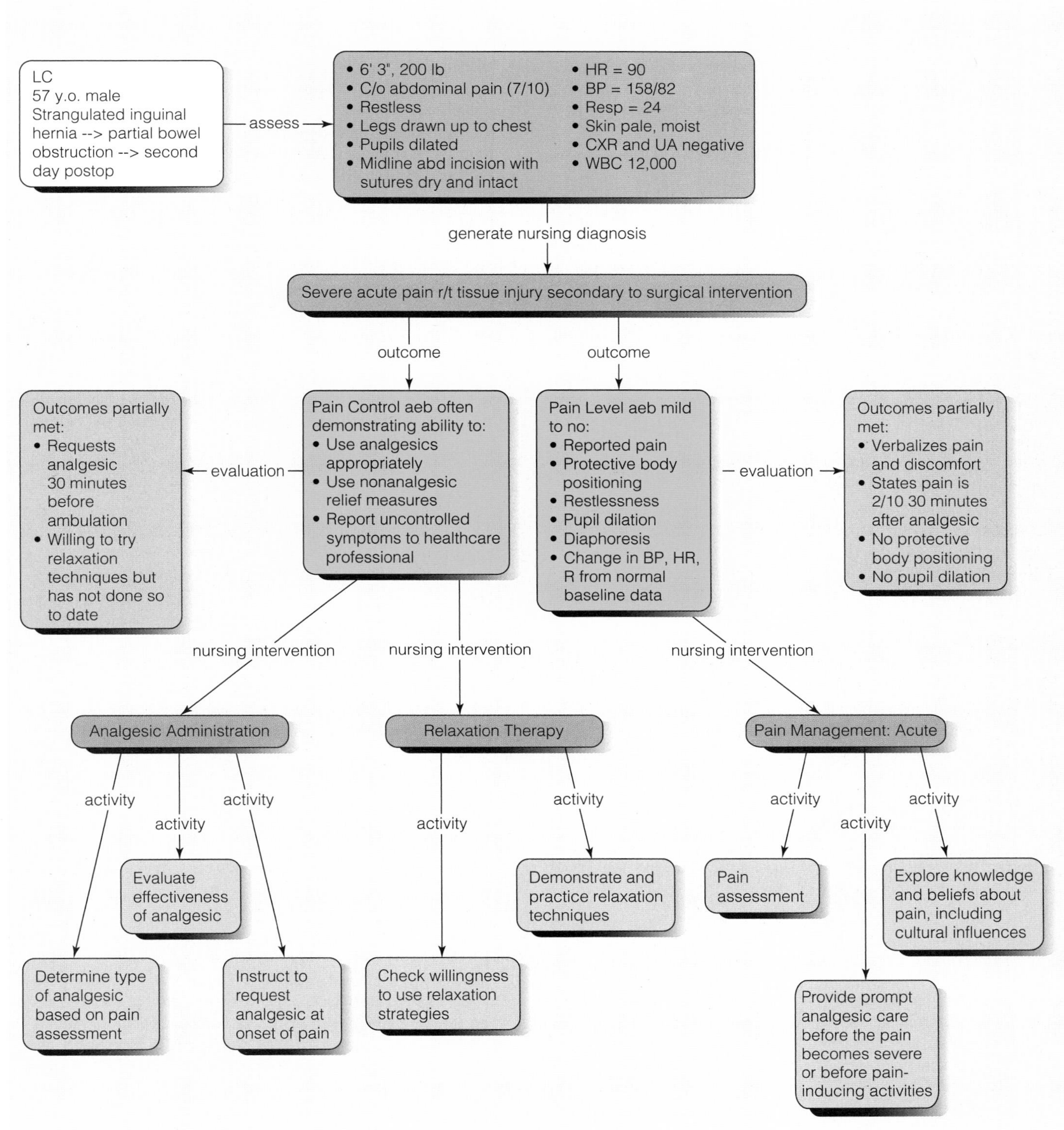

Chapter 30 Review

CHAPTER HIGHLIGHTS

- Pain is "whatever the person says it is, and exists whenever he says it does." It is a subjective sensation to which no two people respond in the same way. It can directly impair health and prolong recovery from surgery, disease, and trauma.
- Types of pain may be described in terms of location, duration, intensity, and etiology.
- Pain threshold is generally similar in all people, but pain tolerance and response vary considerably among individuals.
- The physiologic processes related to pain perception are described as nociception. Four processes are involved in nociception: transduction, transmission, perception, and modulation.
- For nociceptive pain to be perceived, nociceptors must be stimulated. Three types of pain stimuli are mechanical, thermal, and chemical.
- Numerous factors influence a client's perception and reaction to pain: ethnic and cultural values, developmental stage, environment and support people, previous pain experiences, and meaning of pain.
- Pain is subjective, and the most reliable indicator of the presence or intensity of pain is the client's self-report. Assessment of a client who is experiencing pain, however, should also include subjective and objective data.
- Although the nursing diagnosis given to clients experiencing pain can be mild acute pain, moderate acute pain, severe acute pain, or chronic pain, the pain itself may also be the etiology of other nursing diagnoses.
- Overall client goals include preventing, modifying, or eliminating pain so that the client is able to partly or completely resume usual daily activities and to cope more effectively with the pain experience.
- When planning, nurses need to choose pain relief measures appropriate for the client, based on assessment data.
- Multimodal pain management incorporates both pharmacologic and nonpharmacologic approaches to achieve the best possible outcomes for the client.
- Key strategies to reduce pain include acknowledging and accepting the client's pain, assisting support people, reducing misconceptions about pain, reducing fear and anxiety, and preventing pain.
- Pharmacologic interventions, ordered by the physician (or nurse practitioner), include the use of opioids, nonopioids, and adjuvant drugs.
- The World Health Organization recommends a three-step analgesic ladder approach to manage chronic cancer pain. This model establishes the pharmacologic foundation on which other types of pain are managed.
- Placebos should never be used to determine whether or not someone is in pain. Deceptive use of placebos is unethical.
- Analgesic medication can be delivered through a variety of routes and methods to meet the specific needs of the client. Additional information is found in Chapter 35 ∞.
- Patient-controlled analgesia enables the client to exercise control and treat the pain by self-administering doses of analgesics.
- Physical modalities of nonpharmacologic pain interventions include cutaneous stimulation such as massage, hot and cold applications, acupressure, and contralateral stimulation; immobilization and bracing; and transcutaneous electrical nerve stimulation (TENS).
- Cognitive–behavioral interventions include distraction techniques, eliciting the relaxation response, repatterning thinking, facilitating coping, and selected spiritual interventions.
- Evaluation of the client's pain therapy includes the response of the client, the changes in the pain, and the client's perceptions of the effectiveness of the therapy. Ongoing verbal or written feedback from the client and family is integral to this process.

TEST YOUR KNOWLEDGE

1. A client experiencing pain has been prescribed aspirin. Which pain process will this medication affect?
   1. Transduction
   2. Transmission
   3. Perception
   4. Modulation

2. When a client has arrived at the nursing unit from surgery, the nurse is most likely to give priority to which of the following assessments?
   1. Pain tolerance
   2. Pain intensity
   3. Location of pain
   4. Pain history

3. Which pain assessment tool would a nurse use to assess pain in an older adult with cognitive impairment?
   1. The NRS
   2. The FLACC scale
   3. The Faces Pain Scale—Revised
   4. PAINAD

4. A 60-year-old client with a history of untreated obstructive sleep apnea has been given a PRN IV dose of morphine following an ankle fracture. As he falls asleep, he has difficulty engaging in a conversation. Which of the following checks should a nurse perform immediately?
   1. Respiratory rate
   2. Level of alertness
   3. Blood pressure
   4. Pain intensity score

5. Which of the following objective assessment data will the nurse obtain before administering a prescribed opioid medication to a client?
1. Pain level as stated by client
2. Any nausea the client may be feeling
3. Respiratory rate
4. Color of skin

6. While discussing pain history, a client with a below-the-knee amputation of the right leg reveals to the nurse that he experiences sudden "electric shock-like" pain attacks in his stump. He has been prescribed Gabapentin to further manage his pain. What type of pain does the client have?
1. Visceral
2. Somatic
3. Neuropathic
4. Procedural pain

7. A client with arthritis has been taking over-the-counter NSAIDs for the past year. Which questions would the nurse ask during a health history? Select all that apply.
1. "How often do you take this drug?"
2. "How often do you get your blood pressure checked?"
3. "Have you noticed any problems with your breathing?"
4. "Do you take the drug with food?"
5. "Have you ever vomited blood or had very dark stools?"

8. Which statement best reflects a nurse's assessment of pain?
1. "Do you have any complaints?"
2. "Are you experiencing any discomfort?"
3. "Is there anything I can do for you now?"
4. "Do you have any complaints of pain?"

9. When planning care for pain control of older clients, which principles should the nurse apply? Select all that apply.
1. Pain is a natural outcome of the aging process.
2. Pain perception increases with age.
3. The client may deny pain.
4. The nurse should avoid use of opioids.
5. The client may describe pain as an "ache" or "discomfort."

10. A client recovering from abdominal surgery refuses analgesia, saying that he is "fine, as long as he doesn't move." Which nursing diagnosis should be a priority?
1. Lack of knowlege (pain control measures)
2. Fear of drug addiction
3. Difficulty maintaining a clear airway
4. Altered physical mobility

See Answers to Test Your Knowledge in Appendix A.

READINGS AND REFERENCES

Suggested Readings

American Nurses Association. (2018). *Position statement: The ethical responsibility to manage pain and the suffering it causes.* Retrieved from https://www.nursingworld.org/~495e9b/globalassets/docs/ana/ethics/theethicalresponsibilitytomanagepainandthesufferingitcauses2018.pdf
The purpose of this position statement is to provide ethical guidance and support to nurses as they fulfill their responsibility to provide optimal care to clients experiencing pain.

Jungquist, C. R., Smith, K., Nicely, K. L. W., & Polomano, R. C. (2017). Monitoring hospitalized adult patients for opioid-induced sedation and respiratory depression. *American Journal of Nursing*, *117*(3 Suppl. 1), S27–S35. doi:10.1097/01.NAJ.0000513528.79557.33
The authors review the literature on opioid-induced sedation and respiratory depression and present evidence-based recommendations for clinical decision making.

Related Research

Moreland Lewis, M. J., Kohtz, C., Emmerling, S., Fisher, M., & McGarvey, J. (2018). Pain control and nonpharmacologic interventions. *Nursing*, *48*(9), 65–68.doi:10.1097/01.NURSE.0000544231.59222.ab

Notte, B. B., Fazzini, C., & Mooney, R. A. (2016). Reiki's effect on patients with total knee arthroplasty: A pilot study. *Nursing*, *46*(2), 17–23. doi:10.1097/01.NURSE.0000476246.16717.65

Quinn, B. L., Solodiuk, J. C., Morrill, D., & Mauskar, S. (2018). Pain in nonverbal children with medical complexity: A two-year retrospective study. *American Journal of Nursing*, *118*(8), 28–37. doi:10.1097/01.NAJ.0000544137.55887.5a

Ramira, M. L., Instone, S., & Clark, M. J. (2016). Pain management: An evidence-based approach. *Pediatric Nursing*, *42*(1), 39–49.

Waszak, D. L., Mitchell, A. M., Ren, D., & Fennimore, L. A. (2018). A quality improvement project to improve education provided by nurses to ED patients prescribed opioid analgesics at discharge. *Journal of Emergency Nursing*, *44*(4), 336–344. doi:10.1016/j.jen.2017.09.010

References

Adams, M. P., Holland, N., & Urban, C. (2020). *Pharmacology for nurses: A pathophysiologic approach* (6th ed.). New York, NY: Pearson.

American Nurses Association. (n.d.). *Opioid epidemic: Pain management*. Retrieved from https://www.nursingworld.org/practice-policy/work-environment/health-safety/opioid-epidemic

American Nurses Association. (2016). *Pain management nursing: Scope and standards of practice* (2nd ed.). Silver Spring, MD: Author.

American Nurses Association. (2018). *The opioid epidemic: The evolving role of nursing*. Retrieved from https://www.nursingworld.org/~4a4da5/globalassets/practiceandpolicy/work-environment/health--safety/opioid-epidemic/2018-ana-opioid-issue-brief-vfinal-pdf-2018-08-29.pdf

American Pain Society. (2016). *Principles of analgesic ese* (7th ed.). Chicago, IL: Author.

Arnstein, P., Broglio, K., Wuhrman, E., & Kean, M. B. (2011). Use of placebos in pain management. *Pain Management Nursing*, *12*(4), 225–229. doi:10.1016/j.pmn.2010.10.033

Assil, K. (2016). *Opioids: Prescribe with care*. Retrieved from https://www.painedu.org/opioids-prescribe-care

Avancen. (n.d.). *The Avancen MOD® 2.0 system*. Retrieved from https://www.avancen.com/the-avancen-mod-oral-pca-system

Booker, S. Q., & Haedtke, C. (2016). Assessing pain in verbal older adults. *Nursing*, *46*(2), 65–68. doi:10.1097/01.NURSE.0000473408.89671.52

Broglio, K., & Matzo, M. (2018). Acute pain management for people with opioid use disorder. *American Journal of Nursing*, *118*(10), 39–38. doi:10.1097/01.NAJ.0000546378.81550.84

Butcher, H. K., Bulechek, G. M., Dochterman, J. M., & Wagner, C. M. (Eds.). (2018. *Nursing interventions classification (NIC)* (7th ed.). St. Louis, MO: Elsevier.

Candido, K. D., Kusper, T. M., & Knezevic, N. N. (2017). New cancer pain treatment options. *Current Pain and Headache Reports*, *21*(2), 1–12. doi:10.1007/s11916-017-0613-0

Centers for Disease Control and Prevention. (n.d.). *Guideline for prescribing opioids for chronic pain: Improving practice through recommendations*. Retrieved from https://www.cdc.gov/drugoverdose/pdf/Guidelines_Factsheet-a.pdf

Centers for Disease Control and Prevention. (2017). *CDC guideline for prescribing opioids for chronic pain*. Retrieved from https://www.cdc.gov/drugoverdose/prescribing/guideline.html

Centers for Disease Control and Prevention. (2018). *Understanding the epidemic*. Retrieved from https://www.cdc.gov/drugoverdose/epidemic/index.html

Chou, R., Gordon, D. B., deLeon-Casasola, O. A., Rosenberg, J. M., Bickler, S., Brennan, T., . . . Wu, C. L. (2016). Management of postoperative pain. *The Journal of Pain*, *17*, 131–157. doi:10.1016/j.jpain.2015.12.008

Costello, M., Thompson, S., Aurelien, J., & Luc, T. (2016). Patient opioid education: Research shows nurses' knowledge of opioids makes a difference. *MEDSURG Nursing*, *25*(5), 307–311, 333.

Cox, F. (2018). Advances in the pharmacological management of acute and chronic pain. *Nursing Standard*, *33*(3), 37–42.

Dowell, D., Haegerich, T. M., & Chou, R. (2016). CDC guideline for prescribing opioids for chronic pain—United States, 2016. *MMWR Recommendations and Reports*, *65*(1), 1–49.

Drew, D. J., Gordon, D. B., Morgan, B., & Manworren, R. C. B. (2018). "As-needed" range orders for opioid analgesics in the management of pain: A consensus statement of the American Society for Pain Management Nursing and the American Pain Society. *Pain Management Nursing*, *19*(3), 207–210. doi:10.1016/j.pmn.2018.03.003

Hoffman, K. M., Trawalter, S., Axt, J. R., & Oliver, M. N. (2016). Racial bias in pain assessment and treatment recommendations, and false beliefs about biological differences between blacks and whites. *Proceedings of the National Academy of Sciences of the United States of America*, *113*(16), 4296–4301. doi:10.1073/pnas.1516047113

Infusion Nurses Society. (2016). *Policies and procedures for infusion therapy* (5th ed.). Norwood, MA: Author.

Institute for Safe Medication Practices. (2019). *Guidelines for safe electronic communication of medication information*. Retrieved from https://www.ismp.org/resources/guidelines-safe-electronic-communication-medication-information

International Association for the Study of Pain. (2001). *Faces pain scale–revised home*. Retrieved from https://www.iasp-pain.org/Education/Content.aspx?ItemNumber=1519

International Headache Society. (n.d.). *IHS Classification ICHD-3 Beta: Classification outline*. Retrieved from https://www.ichd-3.org/classification-outline

Jungquist, C. R., Smith, K., Nicely, K. L. W., & Polomano, R. C. (2017). Monitoring hospitalized adult patients for opioid-induced sedation and respiratory depression.

American Journal of Nursing, 117(3 Suppl. 1), S27–S35. doi:10.1097/01.NAJ.0000513528.79557.33

Jungquist, C. R., Vallerand, A. H., Sicoutris, C., Kwon, K. N., & Polomano, R. C. (2017). Assessing and managing acute pain: A call to action. *American Journal of Nursing*, *117*(3 Suppl. 1), S4–S11. doi:10.1097/01.NAJ.0000513526.33816.0e

Moorhead, S., Swanson, E., Johnson, M., & Maas, M. L. (Eds.). (2018). *Nursing outcomes classification (NOC)* (6th ed.). St. Louis, MO: Elsevier.

Office of Disease Prevention and Health Promotion. (n.d.). *Arthritis, osteoporosis, and chronic back conditions*. Retrieved from https://www.healthypeople.gov/2020/topics-objectives/topic/Arthritis-Osteoporosis-and-Chronic-Back-Conditions/objectives

National Academies of Sciences, Engineering, and Medicine. (2017). *Pain management and the opioid epidemic: Balancing societal and individual benefits and risks of prescription opioid use*. Washington, DC: The National Academies Press.

National Institute on Drug Abuse. (2018). *Understanding drug use and addiction*. Retrieved from https://www.drugabuse.gov/publications/drugfacts/understanding-drug-use-addiction

National Institute of Neurological Disorders and Stroke. (2019). *Chronic pain information page*. Retrieved from https://www.ninds.nih.gov/Disorders/All-Disorders/Chronic-pain-Information-Page

Pasero, C., & McCaffery, M. (2011). *Pain assessment and pharmacologic management*. St. Louis, MO: Mosby.

Pasero, C., Quinlan-Colwell, A., Rae, D., Broglio, K., & Drew, D. (2016). Prescribing and administering opioid doses based solely on pain intensity. *Pain Management Nursing*, *17*, 170–180. doi:10.1016/j.pmn.2016.03.001

Pergolizzi, J. V., & Raffa, R. B. (2015). *The WHO pain ladder: Do we need another step?* Retrieved from https://www.practicalpainmanagement.com/resources/who-pain-ladder-do-we-need-another-step?page=0,3

Polomano, R. C., Fillman, M., Giordano, N. A., Vallerand, A. H., Nicely, K. L. W., & Jungquist, C. R. (2017). Multimodal analgesia for acute postoperative and trauma-related pain. *American Journal of Nursing*, *117*(3 Suppl. 1), S12–S26. doi:10.1097/01.NAJ.0000513527.71934.73

Polomano, R. C., & Jungquist, C. R. (2017). Foreword. *American Journal of Nursing*, *117*(3), S3. doi:10.1097/01.NAJ.0000513525.26192.18

Quinn, M. (2018). *6 months since Trump declared an opioid emergency, what's changed?* Retrieved from http://www.governing.com/topics/health-human-services/gov-opioid-emergency-declaration-trump.html

Stempniak, M. (2016). How hospitals are fighting on the frontlines of the opioid crisis. *H&HN: Hospitals & Health Networks*, *90*(3), 22–28.

Strickler, J., James, A., O'Leary, S., & Dube-Clark, G. (2018). Portrait of an epidemic: Acute opioid intoxication in adults. *Nursing*, *48*(9), 41–43. doi:10.1097/01.NURSE.0000541389.52104.65

Tackling nation's opioid epidemic. (2016). *The American Nurse*, *48*(4), 15.

Traynor, K. (2016). White House expands opioid addiction response. *American Journal of Health-System Pharmacy*, *73*(1), e1–e2. doi:10.2146/news160001

U.S. Food and Drug Administration. (2018). *Disposal of unused medicines: What you should know*. Retrieved from https://www.fda.gov/Drugs/ResourcesForYou/Consumers/BuyingUsingMedicineSafely/EnsuringSafeUseofMedicine/SafeDisposalofMedicines/ucm186187.htm#Medicines_recommended

Ward, C. W. (2016). Non-pharmacologic methods of postoperative pain management. *MedSurg Matters*, *25*(1), 9–10.

Westman, K. F., & Blaisdell, C. (2016). Many benefits, little risk: The use of massage in nursing practice. *American Journal of Nursing*, *116*(1), 34–39. doi:10.1097/01.NAJ.0000476164.97929.f2

Windle, M. (2016). Has the federal government declared war on chronic pain patients? *MedSurg Matters*, *25*(3), 11–15.

World Health Organization. (n.d.). *Impact of impaired access to controlled medications*. Retrieved from http://www.who.int/medicines/areas/quality_safety/Impaired_Access/en

World Health Organization. (2012). *Scoping document for WHO guidelines for the pharmacological treatment of persisting pain in adults with medical illnesses*. Retrieved from http://www.who.int/medicines/areas/quality_safety/Scoping_WHO_GLs_PersistPainAdults_webversion.pdf?ua=1

Selected Bibliography

Adams, J., Bledsoe, G. H., & Armstrong, J. H. (2016). Are pain management questions in patient satisfaction surveys driving the opioid epidemic? *American Journal of Public Health*, *106*(6), 985–986. doi:10.2105/AJPH.2016.303228

Booker, S. Q., & Haedtke, C. (2016). Assessing pain in nonverbal older adults. *Nursing*, *46*(5), 66–69. doi:10.1097/01.NURSE.0000480619.08039.50

Booker, S. Q., & Haedtke, C. (2016). Evaluating pain management in older adults. *Nursing*, *46*(6), 66–69. doi:10.1097/01.NURSE.0000482868.40461.06

Contreras, G. W., Bellomo, T. L., & Cichminski, L. (2017). Epidemic! Opioid overdose in America. *Nursing Made Incredibly Easy!*, *15*(2), 27–31. doi:10.1097/01.NME.0000511843.62892.6c

Cornelius, R., Herr, K. A., Gordon, D. B., Kretzer, K., & Butcher, H. K. (2017). Evidence-based guideline: Acute pain management in older adults. *Journal of Gerontological Nursing*, *43*(2), 18–27. doi:10.3928/00989134-20170111-08

Dever, C. (2017). Treating acute pain in the opiate-dependent patient. *Journal of Trauma Nursing*, *24*(5), 292–299. doi:10.1097/JTN.0000000000000309

Johnson, S. R. (2016). The racial divide in the opioid epidemic. *Modern Healthcare*, *46*(9), 12.

Mallick-Searle, T. (2018). Commonly used nonopioid analgesics in adults. *Nursing*, *48*(5), 61–63. doi:10.1097/01.NURSE.0000530985.53988.37

Manworren, R. C. B., Gordon, D. B., & Montgomery, R. (2018). Managing postoperative pain. *American Journal of Nursing*, *118*(1), 36–43. doi:10.1097/01.NAJ.0000529695.38192.67

National Consensus Project for Quality Palliative Care. (2018). *Clinical practice guidelines for quality palliative care* (4th ed.). Richmond, VA: Author.

Pich, J. (2018). The analgesic efficacy of opioids in cancer pain. *American Journal of Nursing*, *118*(12), 22. doi:10.1097/01.NAJ.0000549686.66629.f6

Robinson-Lane, S. G., & Booker, S. Q. (2017). Culturally responsive pain management for black older adults. *Journal of Gerontological Nursing*, *43*(8), 33–41. doi:10.3928/00989134-20170224-03

Rosa, W. E. (2018). Transcultural pain management: Theory, practice, and nurse-client partnerships. *Pain Management Nursing*, *19*(1), 23–33. doi:10.1016/j.pmn.2017.10.007

Sampson, J., & Allbright, R. (2018). Distracting pediatric patients during painful procedures. *Nursing*, *48*(7), 56–57. doi:10.1097/01.NURSE.0000534109.96519.25

Stempniak. M. (2016). 12 steps providers can take to fight the opioid epidemic. *H&HN: Hospitals & Health Networks*, *90*(3), 29.

Sullivan, D., Lyons, M., Montgomery, R., & Quinlan-Colwell, A. (2016). Exploring opioid-sparing multimodal analgesia options in trauma: A nursing perspective. *Journal of Trauma Nursing*, *23*, 361–375. doi:10.1097/JTN.0000000000000250

Tierney, M. (2016). Improving nurses' attitudes toward patients with substance use disorders. *American Nurse Today*, *11*(11), 6–9.

Valdez, A. M. (2019). Will you save me? Injury prevention strategies to prevent opioid overdose. *Journal of Emergency Nursing*, *45*(1), 90–93. doi:10.1016/j.jen.2018.11.005

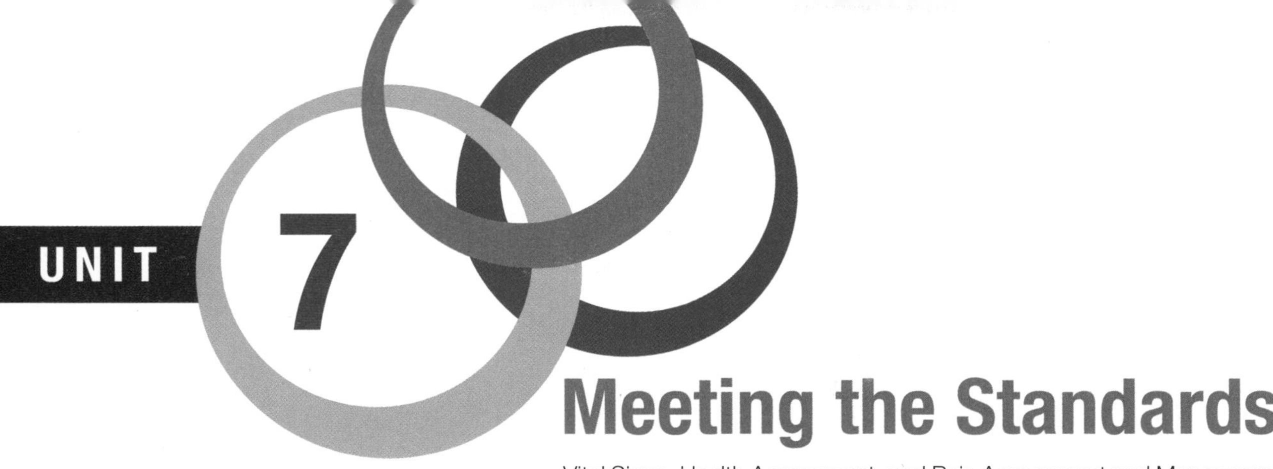

Meeting the Standards

Vital Signs, Health Assessment, and Pain Assessment and Management, the chapters in Unit 7 of *Fundamentals of Nursing: Concepts, Process, and Practice*, cover the most common knowledge, skills, and attitudes required of every registered nurse. Although the nurse does not perform the full spectrum of these activities during each encounter, at least some of the assessments are always essential in providing professional nursing care. Many other practitioners also perform the techniques of gathering the available data regarding clients' temperature, pulses, respirations, blood pressure, oxygen saturation, pain status, and systems functioning. However, it is the nurse's interpretation and responses to the data that have an impact on the client's health.

Scenario: Imagine that you are working the evening shift in a hospital on a general medical unit. As the registered nurse, you share an assignment of clients with assistive personnel (AP). You have worked with this certified nursing assistant (CNA) previously and know that she does her work in an efficient and accurate manner. You are able to communicate effectively with her because she asks questions when she needs clarification and she reports relevant client data as indicated.

Among the clients you and the CNA are caring for are a female adult receiving IV chemotherapy for lung cancer, a female adult with a possible deep vein thrombosis (DVT), a male adult who has chronic obstructive lung disease (COPD), and a male adult admitted for acute appendicitis who also has a substance use disorder (SUD).

Questions

American Nurses Association Standard of Professional Performance #14 is Quality of Practice: *The registered nurse contributes to quality nursing practice.* This involves ensuring that nursing practice is safe, effective, and client-centered, identifying barriers and opportunities to improve healthcare safety and client-centeredness, and using creativity and quality improvement strategies to enhance client care.

When you auscultate the lungs of the client with lung disease, you hear bronchovesicular sounds in the upper and middle lobes and adventitious sounds in both left and right lower lobes. The client reports no significant changes in the previous 24 hours and vital signs are substantially the same as previously. The day shift nurse had reported that the client's lungs were clear throughout, and the previous night shift nurse did not record the results of auscultated lung sounds in the client record.

1. How does this situation relate to Standard #14? Do you see opportunities to improve the quality of practice? Beyond the care of this individual client, what might you do to ensure that the nurses on this unit meet the competencies of the standard?
2. When you perform a pain assessment for the client admitted for appendicitis, he rates his pain level at a 9 to 10. He is loudly demanding more of the IV opioid that is prescribed for him. You remember from report that his pain ratings have been consistently in the severe pain range (7 to 10) and that he watches the clock and knows when he can receive the next dose. Considering the standard, what actions would be consistent with client-centered, safe, and effective nursing practice for this client?

American Nurses Association Standard of Professional Performance #15 is Professional Practice Evaluation: *The registered nurse evaluates one's own and others' nursing practice.* This evaluation includes engaging in self-evaluation of nursing practice; following guidelines for professional practice; uses peer feedback; and incorporates evidence-based actions as part of the evaluation process.

3. Imagine that when you assess the peripheral pulses of the client with a suspected thrombus, you have difficulty feeling the dorsalis pedis or posterior tibial pulses on either leg. Considering the standard, what actions would be consistent with professional practice evaluation? Would your actions differ if this was the first time you had such difficulty or if you frequently find you are unable to palpate pedal pulses?

American Nurses Association Standard of Professional Performance #16 is Resource Utilization: *The registered nurse utilizes appropriate resources to plan, provide, and sustain evidence-based nursing services that are safe, effective, and fiscally responsible.* This standard holds the registered nurse accountable for assessing client needs, allocating resources based on client needs, delegating care to others, and advocating for resources as needed.

In the scenario described, you will likely do all of those things. You have assigned the measurement of vital signs for all three clients to the AP.

4. The AP measures vital signs at 1600 and reports to you immediately that the client receiving chemotherapy has an oral temperature of 40°C (104°F). Describe your thinking in interpreting this data. What would be your response and next steps? List at least four things you would do and explain why they are necessary and appropriate.
5. In retrospect, do you think you should not have assigned measuring the vital signs on this client to the AP? Why or why not?

American Nurses Association. (2015). *Nursing: Scope and standards of practice* (3rd ed.). Silver Spring, MD: Author.

Answers to Meeting the Standards questions are available on the faculty resource site. Please consult with your instructor.

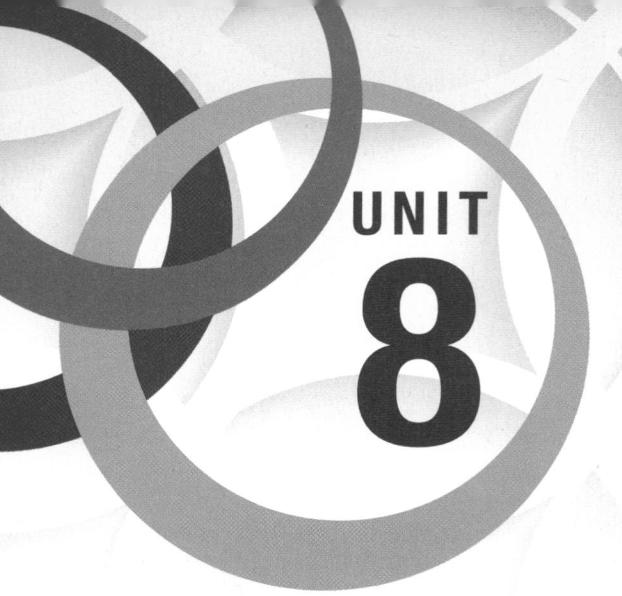

Integral Components of Client Care

Asepsis and Infection Prevention 31

LEARNING OUTCOMES

After completing this chapter, you will be able to:

1. Explain the concepts of medical and surgical asepsis.
2. Identify signs of localized and systemic infections and inflammation.
3. Identify risks for nosocomial and healthcare-associated infections.
4. Identify factors influencing a microorganism's ability to produce an infectious process.
5. Identify anatomic and physiologic barriers that defend the body against microorganisms.
6. Differentiate active from passive immunity.
7. Identify relevant nursing diagnoses and contributing factors for clients at risk for infection and who have an infection.
8. Identify interventions to reduce risks for infections.
9. Identify measures that break each link in the chain of infection.
10. Compare and contrast category-specific, disease-specific, standard, and transmission-based isolation precaution systems.
11. Verbalize the steps used in:
    a. Performing hand hygiene.
    b. Applying and removing a gown, face mask, eyewear, and clean gloves.
    c. Establishing and maintaining a sterile field.
    d. Applying and removing sterile gloves by the open method.
12. Recognize when it is appropriate to assign infection prevention skills to assistive personnel.
13. Describe the steps to take in the event of a bloodborne pathogen exposure.

KEY TERMS

acquired immunity, *700*
active immunity, *700*
acute infections, *695*
airborne precautions, *711*
antibodies, *700*
antigen, *699*
antiseptics, *708*
asepsis, *694*
autoantigen, *699*
bacteremia, *695*
bacteria, *694*
bloodborne pathogens, *708*
carrier, *696*
cell-mediated defenses, *700*
cellular immunity, *700*
chronic infections, *695*
circulating immunity, *700*
clean, *694*
colonization, *694*
communicable disease, *694*
compromised host, *698*
contact precautions, *711*
cultures, *702*
dirty, *694*
disease, *694*
disinfectants, *708*
droplet nuclei, *697*
droplet precautions, *711*
endogenous, *695*
exogenous, *695*
exudate, *699*
fungi, *694*
granulation tissue, *699*
healthcare-associated infection (HAI), *695*
humoral immunity, *700*
iatrogenic infections, *696*
immune defenses, *698*
immunity, *699*
immunoglobulins, *700*
infection, *694*
inflammation, *699*
isolation, *709*
leukocytes, *699*
leukocytosis, *699*
local infection, *695*
medical asepsis, *694*
nonspecific defenses, *698*
nosocomial infections, *695*
occupational exposure, *723*
opportunistic pathogen, *694*
parasites, *694*
passive immunity, *700*
pathogenicity, *694*
personal protective equipment (PPE), *709*
regeneration, *699*
reservoirs, *696*
resident flora, *693*
respiratory hygiene or cough etiquette, *709*
sepsis, *694*
septicemia, *695*
specific defenses, *698*
standard precautions (SP), *709*
sterile field, *717*
sterile technique, *694*
sterilization, *708*
surgical asepsis, *694*
systemic infection, *695*
universal precautions (UP), *709*
vector-borne transmission, *696*
vehicle-borne transmission, *696*
virulence, *694*
viruses, *694*

Introduction

Nurses are directly involved in providing a biologically safe environment. Microorganisms exist everywhere: in water, in soil, and on body surfaces such as the skin, intestinal tract, and other areas open to the outside (e.g., mouth, upper respiratory tract, vagina, and lower urinary tract). Most microorganisms are harmless and some are even beneficial in that they perform essential functions in the body. Some microorganisms found in the intestines (e.g., enterobacteria) produce substances called *bacteriocins*, which are lethal to related strains of bacteria. Others produce substances that repress the growth of other microorganisms. Some microorganisms are normal **resident flora** (the collective vegetation in a given area) in one part of the body, yet produce infection in another. For example, *Escherichia coli*, commonly referred to as *E. coli*, is a normal inhabitant of the large intestine but a common cause of infection of the urinary tract. Table 31.1 provides a list of common resident microorganisms.

TABLE 31.1 Examples of Common Resident Microorganisms

Body Area	Microorganisms
Skin	*Staphylococcus epidermidis*
	Propionibacterium acnes
	Staphylococcus aureus
	Corynebacterium xerosis
	Pityrosporum ovale (yeast)
Nasal passages	*Staphylococcus aureus*
	Staphylococcus epidermidis
Oropharynx	*Streptococcus pneumoniae*
Mouth	*Streptococcus mutans*
	Lactobacillus
	Bacteroides
	Actinomyces
Intestine	*Bacteroides*
	Fusobacterium
	Eubacterium
	Lactobacillus
	Streptococcus
	Enterobacteriaceae
	Shigella
	Escherichia coli
Urethral orifice	*Staphylococcus epidermidis*
Urethra (lower)	*Proteus*
Vagina	*Lactobacillus*
	Bacteroides
	Clostridium
	Candida albicans

An **infection** is the growth of microorganisms in body tissue where they are not usually found. Such a microorganism is called an *infectious agent*. If the microorganism produces no clinical evidence of disease, the infection is called *asymptomatic* or *subclinical*. Some subclinical infections can cause considerable damage. For example, cytomegalovirus (CMV) infection in a pregnant woman can lead to significant disease in the unborn child. A detectable alteration in normal tissue function, however, is called **disease**.

Microorganisms vary in their **virulence** (i.e., their ability to produce disease). Microorganisms also vary in the severity of the diseases they produce and their degree of communicability. For example, the common cold virus is less severe but more readily transmitted than the bacillus that causes leprosy (*Mycobacterium leprae*). If the infectious agent can be transmitted to an individual by direct or indirect contact or as an airborne infection, the resulting condition is called a **communicable disease**.

Pathogenicity is the ability to produce disease; thus, a pathogen is a microorganism that causes disease. Many microorganisms that are normally harmless can cause disease under certain circumstances. A "true" pathogen causes disease or infection in a healthy individual. An **opportunistic pathogen** causes disease only in a susceptible individual.

Infectious diseases are a major cause of death worldwide. The control of the spread of microorganisms and the protection of people from communicable diseases and infections are carried out on international, national, state, community, and individual levels. The World Health Organization (WHO) is the major regulatory agency at the international level. In the United States, the Centers for Disease Control and Prevention (CDC) is the principal national public health agency concerned with disease prevention and control. At the state and county level, health departments track and respond to epidemics and illnesses.

Asepsis is the freedom from disease-causing microorganisms. To decrease the possibility of transferring microorganisms from one place to another, aseptic technique is used. The two basic types of asepsis are medical and surgical. **Medical asepsis** includes all practices intended to confine a specific microorganism to a specific area, limiting the number, growth, and transmission of microorganisms. In medical asepsis, objects are referred to as **clean**, which means the absence of almost all microorganisms, or **dirty** (soiled, contaminated), which means likely to have microorganisms, some of which may be capable of causing infection.

Surgical asepsis, or **sterile technique**, refers to those practices that keep an area or object free of all microorganisms; it includes practices that destroy all microorganisms and spores (microscopic dormant structures formed by some pathogens that are very hardy and often survive common cleaning techniques). Surgical asepsis is used for all procedures involving the sterile areas of the body. **Sepsis** is the condition in which acute organ dysfunction occurs secondary to infection.

Four major categories of microorganisms cause infection in humans: bacteria, viruses, fungi, and parasites. **Bacteria** are by far the most common infection-causing microorganisms. Several hundred species can cause disease in humans and can live and be transported through air, water, food, soil, body tissues and fluids, and inanimate objects. Most of the microorganisms in Table 31.1 are bacteria. **Viruses** consist primarily of nucleic acid and therefore must enter living cells in order to reproduce. Common virus families include the rhinovirus (causes the common cold), hepatitis, herpes, and HIV. **Fungi** include yeasts and molds. *Candida albicans* is a yeast considered to be normal flora in the human vagina. **Parasites** live on other living organisms. They include protozoa such as the one that causes malaria, helminths (worms), and arthropods (mites, fleas, ticks).

Types of Infections

Colonization is the process by which strains of microorganisms become resident flora. In this state, the microorganisms may grow and multiply but do not cause disease. Infection occurs when newly introduced or resident microorganisms succeed in invading a part of the body where the host's defense mechanisms are ineffective and the pathogen causes tissue damage. The infection becomes a disease when the signs and symptoms of the infection are unique and can be differentiated from other conditions.

Infections can be local or systemic. A **local infection** is limited to the specific part of the body where the microorganisms remain. If the microorganisms spread and damage different parts of the body, the infection is a **systemic infection**. When a culture of the individual's blood reveals microorganisms, the condition is called **bacteremia**. When bacteremia results in systemic infection, it is referred to as **septicemia**. Unfortunately, septicemia has become more common over time.

There are also **acute** and **chronic infections**. Acute infections generally appear suddenly or last a short time. A chronic infection may occur slowly, over a very long period, and may last months or years.

Nosocomial and Healthcare-Associated Infections

Nosocomial infections are classified as infections that originate in the hospital. Nosocomial infections can either develop during a client's stay in a facility or manifest after discharge. Nosocomial microorganisms may also be acquired by personnel working in the facility and can cause significant illness and time lost from work. Nosocomial infections are a subgroup of **healthcare-associated infections (HAIs)**—those that originate in any healthcare setting—and of hospital-acquired conditions (HACs), which include other types of conditions besides infections.

HAIs have received increasing attention in recent years and are believed to involve about 1 million clients per year. The Joint Commission (2019) includes reducing the risk of HAIs as one of the National Patient Safety Goals. The CDC (2016) reports that central intravenous line–associated bloodstream infections, catheter-associated urinary tract infections, surgical site infections, and ventilator-associated pneumonia account for the majority of HAIs. The microorganisms that cause nosocomial infections can originate from the clients themselves (an **endogenous** source) or from the hospital environment and hospital personnel (**exogenous** sources). See Table 31.2 for a list of microorganisms and the conditions they cause. Most nosocomial infections appear to have endogenous sources. *E. coli*, *Staphylococcus aureus*, and enterococci are common infecting microorganisms. *Clostridium difficile (C. difficile)*, a spore-forming bacillus that infects the gastrointestinal (GI) tract following treatment of other infections with antibiotics, is one of the HAIs increasing in frequency. *C. difficile* spores are transferred to clients mainly via the hands of healthcare personnel who have touched a contaminated surface or item.

TABLE 31.2 Nosocomial Infections

Most Common Microorganisms	Causes
URINARY TRACT	
Escherichia coli	Improper catheterization technique
Enterococcus species	Contamination of closed drainage system
Pseudomonas aeruginosa	Inadequate hand hygiene
SURGICAL SITES	
Staphylococcus aureus (including methicillin-resistant strains—MRSA)	Inadequate hand hygiene
Enterococcus species (including vancomycin-resistant strains—VRE)	Improper dressing change technique
Pseudomonas aeruginosa	
BLOODSTREAM	
Coagulase-negative staphylococci	Inadequate hand hygiene
Staphylococcus aureus *Enterococcus* species	Improper intravenous fluid, tubing, and site care technique
PNEUMONIA	
Staphylococcus aureus	Inadequate hand hygiene
Pseudomonas aeruginosa *Enterobacter* species	Improper suctioning technique

Safety Alert! SAFETY

2019 The Joint Commission National Patient Safety Goals

Goal 7: Reduce the Risk of Healthcare-Associated Iinfections.

- Comply with either the current CDC hand hygiene guidelines or the current WHO hand hygiene guidelines. **Rationale:** *Following the best practices identified in these guidelines helps ensure standardized, proven approaches to hand hygiene.*
- Implement evidence-based practices to prevent HAIs due to multidrug-resistant organisms (MDROs) in acute care hospitals. **Rationale:** *Each healthcare agency needs to determine which practices are most appropriate for its unique client population and circumstances that lead to prevalence of particular MDROs.*
- Implement evidence-based practices to prevent central line–associated bloodstream infections (CLABSIs). *Note:* This requirement covers short- and long-term central venous catheters and peripherally inserted central catheter (PICC) lines.
- Implement evidence-based practices for preventing surgical site infections (SSIs).
- Implement evidence-based practices to prevent indwelling catheter-associated urinary tract infections (CAUTIs).

A number of factors contribute to nosocomial infections. **Iatrogenic infections** are the direct result of diagnostic or therapeutic procedures. One example of an iatrogenic infection is bacteremia that results from an intravascular infusion line. Not all nosocomial infections are iatrogenic, nor are all nosocomial infections preventable. Another factor contributing to the development of nosocomial infections is the compromised host, that is, a client whose normal defenses have been lowered by treatments or illness.

The hands of healthcare personnel are a common vehicle for the spread of microorganisms. Insufficient hand hygiene is thus an important factor contributing to the spread of nosocomial microorganisms.

Safety Alert! SAFETY

An individual does not need to have an identified infection in order to pass potentially infective microorganisms to another individual. Even normal microorganisms for one individual can infect another individual.

The cost of nosocomial infections to the client, the facility, and funding sources (e.g., insurance companies and federal, state, or local governments) is great. Nosocomial infections extend hospitalization time, increase clients' time away from work, cause disability and discomfort, and even result in loss of life.

Chain of Infection

Six links make up the chain of infection (Figure 31.1 ■): the etiologic agent, or microorganism; the place where the organism naturally resides (reservoir); a portal of exit from the reservoir; a method (mode) of transmission; a portal of entry into a host; and the susceptibility of the host.

Etiologic Agent

The extent to which any microorganism is capable of producing an infectious process depends on the number of microorganisms present, the virulence and potency of the microorganisms (pathogenicity), the ability of the microorganisms to enter the body, the susceptibility of the host, and the ability of the microorganisms to live in the host's body.

Some microorganisms, such as the smallpox virus, have the ability to infect almost all susceptible people after exposure. By contrast, microorganisms such as the tuberculosis bacillus infect a relatively small number of the population who are susceptible and exposed, usually people who are poorly nourished, who are living in crowded conditions, or whose immune systems are less competent (such as older adults or those with HIV or cancer).

Reservoir

There are many **reservoirs**, or sources of microorganisms. Common sources are other humans, the client's own microorganisms, plants, animals, medical equipment, or the general environment (e.g., soil and water). People are the most common source of infection for others and for themselves. For example, the individual with an influenza virus frequently spreads it to others. A **carrier** is a human or animal reservoir of a specific infectious agent that usually does not manifest any clinical signs of disease. The *Anopheles* mosquito reservoir carries the malaria parasite but is unaffected by it. The carrier state may also exist in individuals with a clinically recognizable disease such as the dog with rabies. Under either circumstance, the carrier state may be of short duration (temporary or transient carrier) or long duration (chronic carrier). Food, water, and feces also can be reservoirs.

Portal of Exit from Reservoir

Before an infection can establish itself in a host, the microorganisms must leave the reservoir. Common human reservoirs and their associated portals of exit are summarized in Table 31.3.

Method of Transmission

After a microorganism leaves its source or reservoir, it requires a means of transmission to reach another individual or host through a receptive portal of entry. There are three mechanisms:

1. ***Direct transmission.*** Direct transmission involves immediate and direct transfer of microorganisms from individual to individual through touching, biting, kissing, or sexual intercourse. Droplet spread is also a form of direct transmission but can occur only if the source and the host are within 1 m (3 ft) of each other. Sneezing, coughing, spitting, singing, or talking can project droplet spray into the conjunctiva or onto the mucous membranes of the eye, nose, or mouth of another individual.
2. ***Indirect transmission.*** Indirect transmission may be either vehicle borne or vector borne:
   a. **Vehicle-borne transmission**. A *vehicle* is any substance that serves as an intermediate means to transport and introduce an infectious agent into a susceptible host through a suitable portal of entry. Fomites (inanimate materials or objects), such as handkerchiefs, toys, soiled clothes, cooking or eating utensils, and surgical instruments or dressings, can act as vehicles. Water, food, blood, serum, and plasma are other vehicles. For example, food or water may become contaminated by a food handler who carries the hepatitis A virus. The food is then ingested by a susceptible host.
   b. **Vector-borne transmission**. A *vector* is an animal or flying or crawling insect that serves as an intermediate means of transporting the infectious agent. Transmission may occur by injecting salivary fluid during biting or by depositing feces or other materials on the skin through the bite wound or a traumatized skin area.

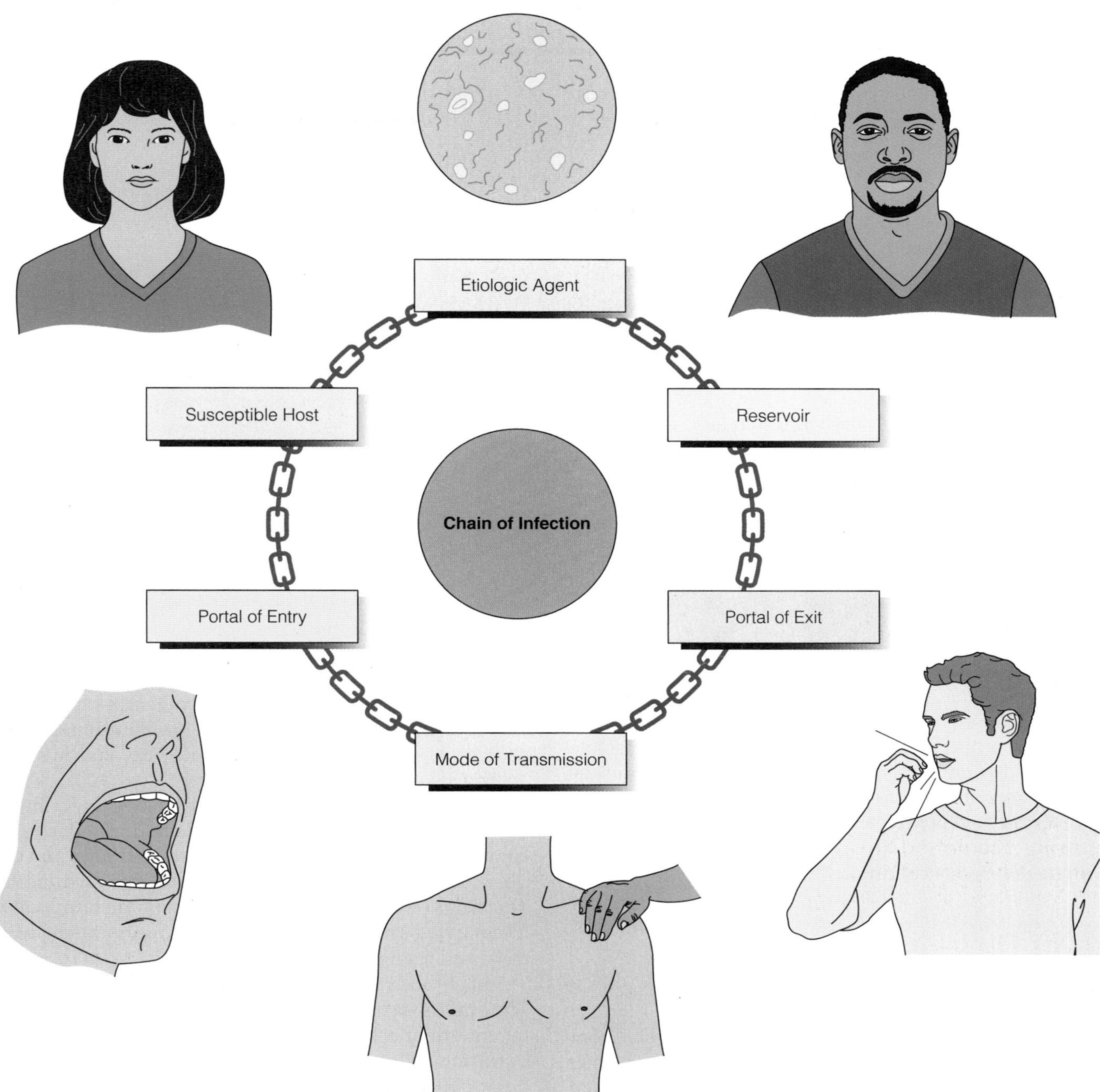

Figure 31.1 ■ The chain of infection.

3. ***Airborne transmission.*** Airborne transmission may involve droplets or dust. **Droplet nuclei**, the residue of evaporated droplets emitted by an infected host such as someone with tuberculosis, can remain in the air for long periods. Dust particles containing the infectious agent (e.g., *C. difficile,* spores from the soil) can also become airborne. The material is transmitted by air currents to a suitable portal of entry, usually the respiratory tract, of another individual.

Portal of Entry to the Susceptible Host

Before an individual can become infected, microorganisms must enter the body. The skin is a barrier to infectious agents; however, any break in the skin can readily serve as a portal of entry. Medical interventions such as tubes, catheters, and surgical wounds are common portals of entry. Often, microorganisms enter the body of the host by the same route they used to leave the source.

TABLE 31.3 Human Body Area Reservoirs, Common Infectious Microorganisms, and Portals of Exit

Body Area Reservoir	Common Infectious Microorganisms	Portals of Exit
Respiratory tract	Parainfluenza virus *Mycobacterium tuberculosis* *Staphylococcus aureus*	Nose or mouth through sneezing, coughing, breathing, or talking
Gastrointestinal tract	Hepatitis A virus *Salmonella* species *C. difficile*	Mouth: saliva, vomitus Anus: feces Ostomies: feces
Urinary tract	*Escherichia coli* enterococci *Pseudomonas aeruginosa*	Urethral meatus and urinary diversion
Reproductive tract	*Neisseria gonorrhoeae Treponema pallidum* Herpes simplex virus type 2 Hepatitis B virus (HBV)	Vagina: vaginal discharge Urinary meatus: semen, urine
Blood	HBV HIV *Staphylococcus aureus* *Staphylococcus epidermidis*	Open wound, needle puncture site, any disruption of intact skin or mucous membrane surfaces
Tissue	*Staphylococcus aureus* *Escherichia coli* *Proteus* species *Streptococcus* beta-hemolytic A or B	Drainage from a cut or wound

Susceptible Host

A susceptible host is any individual who is at risk for infection. A **compromised host** is someone at increased risk, an individual who for one or more reasons is more likely than others to acquire an infection. Impairment of the body's natural defenses and a number of other factors can affect susceptibility to infection. Examples include age (the very young or the very old); clients receiving immune suppression treatment for cancer, for chronic illness, or following a successful organ transplant; and those with immune deficiency conditions.

Body Defenses Against Infection

Individuals have defenses that protect the body from infection. These defenses can be categorized as nonspecific and specific. **Nonspecific defenses** protect the individual against all microorganisms, regardless of prior exposure. **Specific (immune) defenses**, by contrast, are directed against identifiable bacteria, viruses, fungi, or other infectious agents.

Nonspecific Defenses

Nonspecific body defenses include anatomic and physiologic barriers and the inflammatory response.

Anatomic and Physiologic Barriers

Intact skin and mucous membranes are the body's first line of defense against microorganisms. Unless the skin and mucosa become broken, they are an effective barrier against bacteria. Fungi can live on the skin, but they cannot penetrate it. The dryness of the skin also is a deterrent to bacteria. Bacteria are most plentiful in moist areas of the body, such as the perineum and axillae. Resident bacteria of the skin also prevent other bacteria from multiplying. They use up the available nourishment, and the end products of their metabolism inhibit other bacterial growth. Normal secretions make the skin slightly acidic; acidity also inhibits bacterial growth.

The nasal passages have a defensive function. As entering air follows the tortuous route of the passage, it comes in contact with moist mucous membranes and cilia. These trap microorganisms, dust, and foreign materials. The lungs have alveolar macrophages (large phagocytes). Phagocytes are cells that ingest microorganisms, dead cells, and foreign particles.

Each body orifice also has protective mechanisms. The oral cavity regularly sheds mucosal epithelium to rid the mouth of colonizers. The flow of saliva and its partial buffering action help prevent infections. Saliva contains microbial inhibitors, such as lactoferrin, lysozyme, and secretory IgA.

The eye is protected from infection by tears, which continually wash microorganisms away and contain inhibiting lysozyme. The GI tract also has defenses against infection. The high acidity of the stomach normally prevents microbial growth. The resident flora of the large intestine help prevent the establishment of disease-producing microorganisms. Peristalsis also tends to move microbes out of the body.

The vagina also has natural defenses against infection. When a girl reaches puberty, lactobacilli ferment sugars in the vaginal secretions, creating a vaginal pH of 3.5 to 4.5. This low pH inhibits the growth of many disease-producing microorganisms. The entrance to the urethra normally harbors many microorganisms. These include

Staphylococcus epidermidis coagulase (from the skin) and *E. coli* (from feces). Urine flow has a flushing and bacteriostatic action that keeps the bacteria from ascending the urethra. An intact mucosal surface also acts as a barrier.

Inflammatory Response

Inflammation is a local and nonspecific defensive response of the tissues to an injurious or infectious agent. It is an adaptive mechanism that destroys or dilutes the injurious agent, prevents further spread of the injury, and promotes the repair of damaged tissue. It is characterized by five signs: (1) pain, (2) swelling, (3) redness, (4) heat, and (5) impaired function of the part, if the injury is severe. Commonly, words with the suffix *itis* describe an inflammatory process. For example, *appendicitis* means inflammation of the appendix; *gastritis* means inflammation of the stomach.

Clinical Alert!

An easy way to remember the signs of inflammation are the rhyming Latin words *rubor* (redness), *tumor* (swelling), *color/calor* (heat), and *dolor* (pain).

Injurious agents can be categorized as physical agents, chemical agents, and microorganisms. *Physical agents* include mechanical objects causing trauma to tissues, excessive heat or cold, and radiation. *Chemical agents* include external irritants (e.g., strong acids, alkalis, poisons, and irritating gases) and internal irritants (substances manufactured within the body such as excessive hydrochloric acid in the stomach). *Microorganisms* include the broad groups of bacteria, viruses, fungi, and parasites.

A series of dynamic events is commonly referred to as the three stages of the inflammatory response:

First stage: vascular and cellular responses
Second stage: exudate production
Third stage: reparative phase.

VASCULAR AND CELLULAR RESPONSES

At the start of the first stage of inflammation, blood vessels at the site of injury constrict. This is rapidly followed by dilation of small blood vessels (occurring as a result of histamine released by the injured tissues). Thus, more blood flows to the injured area. This marked increase in blood supply is referred to as hyperemia and is responsible for the characteristic signs of redness and heat.

Vascular permeability increases at the site with dilation of the vessels in response to cell death, the release of chemical mediators (e.g., bradykinin, serotonin, and prostaglandin), and the release of histamine. Fluid, proteins, and **leukocytes** (white blood cells) leak into the interstitial spaces, and the signs of inflammation—swelling (edema) and pain—appear. Pain is caused by the pressure of accumulating fluid on nerve endings and the irritating chemical mediators. Fluid pouring into areas such as joints impairs function.

In response to the exit of leukocytes from the blood, the bone marrow produces large numbers of leukocytes and releases them into the bloodstream. This is called **leukocytosis**. A normal leukocyte count of 4500 to 11,000 per cubic millimeter of blood can rise to 20,000 or more when inflammation occurs.

EXUDATE PRODUCTION

In the second stage of inflammation, **exudate** is produced, consisting of fluid that escaped from the blood vessels, dead phagocytic cells, and dead tissue cells and products that they release. The plasma protein fibrinogen (which is converted to fibrin when it is released into the tissues), thromboplastin (released by injured tissue cells), and platelets together form an interlacing network to wall off the area and prevent spread of the injurious agent. During this stage, the injurious agent is overcome, and the exudate is cleared away by lymphatic drainage.

The nature and amount of exudate vary according to the tissue involved and the intensity and duration of the inflammation. The major types of exudate are serous, purulent, and hemorrhagic (sanguineous). Descriptions of these exudates are provided in Chapter 36 ∞.

REPARATIVE PHASE

The third stage of the inflammatory response involves the repair of injured tissues by regeneration or replacement with fibrous tissue (scar) formation. **Regeneration** is the replacement of destroyed tissue cells by cells that are identical or similar in structure and function. Damaged cells are replaced one by one, but the cells are also organized so that the architectural pattern and function of the tissue are restored. The ability to regenerate cells varies considerably from one type of tissue to another. Epithelial tissues of the skin and of the digestive and respiratory tracts have a good regenerative capacity if their underlying support structures are intact. The same holds true for osseous, lymphoid, and bone marrow tissues. Tissues that have little regenerative capacity include nervous, muscular, and elastic tissues.

When regeneration is not possible, repair occurs by scar formation. The inflammatory exudate with its interlacing fibrin network provides the framework for this tissue to develop. Damaged tissues are replaced with the connective tissue elements of collagen, blood capillaries, lymphatics, and other tissue-bound substances. In the early stages of this process, the tissue is called **granulation tissue**. It is a fragile, gelatinous tissue, appearing pink or red because of the many newly formed capillaries. Later in the process, the tissue shrinks (the capillaries are constricted, even obliterated) and the collagen fibers contract, so that a firmer fibrous tissue remains. This is called cicatrix, or scar.

Specific Defenses

Specific defenses of the body involve the immune system. An **antigen** is a substance that induces a state of sensitivity or immune responsiveness (**immunity**). If the proteins originate in an individual's own body, the antigen is called an **autoantigen**.

The immune response has two components: antibody-mediated defenses and cell-mediated defenses. These two systems provide distinct but overlapping protection.

Antibody-Mediated Defenses

Another name for the *antibody-mediated defenses* is **humoral** (or **circulating**) **immunity** because these defenses reside ultimately in the B lymphocytes and are mediated by antibodies produced by B cells. **Antibodies**, also called **immunoglobulins**, are part of the body's plasma proteins. The antibody-mediated responses defend primarily against the extracellular phases of bacterial and viral infections.

The two major types of immunity are active and passive (Table 31.4). In **active immunity**, the host produces antibodies in response to natural antigens (e.g., infectious microorganisms) or artificial antigens (e.g., vaccines). B cells are activated when they recognize the antigen. They then differentiate into plasma cells, which secrete the antibodies and serum proteins that bind specifically to the foreign substance and initiate a variety of elimination responses. The B cell may produce antibody molecules of five classes of immunoglobulins designated by letters and usually written as IgM, IgG, IgA, IgD, and IgE. The presence of IgM in a laboratory analysis shows current infection. Before the antibody response can become effective, the phagocytic cells of the blood bind and ingest foreign substances. The rate of binding and phagocytosis increases if IgG antibodies (which indicate past infection and subsequent immunity) are present. With **passive** (or **acquired**) **immunity**, the host receives natural (e.g., from a nursing mother) or artificial (e.g., from an injection of immune serum) antibodies produced by another source.

Cell-Mediated Defenses

The **cell-mediated defenses**, or **cellular immunity**, occur through the T-cell system. On exposure to an antigen, the lymphoid tissues release large numbers of activated T cells into the lymph system. These T cells pass into the general circulation. There are three main groups of T cells: (1) helper T cells, which help in the functions of the immune system; (2) cytotoxic T cells, which attack and kill microorganisms and sometimes the body's own cells; and (3) suppressor T cells, which can suppress the functions of the helper T cells and the cytotoxic T cells. When cell-mediated immunity is lost, as occurs with HIV infection, an individual is "defenseless" against most viral, bacterial, and fungal infections.

Factors Increasing Susceptibility to Infection

Whether a microorganism causes an infection or not depends on a number of factors already mentioned. One of the most important factors is host susceptibility, which is affected by age, heredity, level of stress, nutritional status, current medical therapy, and pre-existing disease processes.

Newborns and older adults have reduced defenses against infection. Newborns have immature immune systems and are protected only for the first 2 or 3 months by immunoglobulins passively received from the mother. Between 1 and 3 months of age, infants begin to synthesize their own immunoglobulins. Immunizations against hepatitis B can begin at birth, while diphtheria, tetanus, and pertussis are usually started at 2 months, when the infant's immune system can respond. Children who missed immunizations at earlier ages can receive them later. Each year, the CDC's Advisory Committee on Immunization Practices (ACIP) approves immunization schedules for people living in the United States. The immunization schedule for children and adolescents aged 18 years or younger provides a summary of ACIP recommendations on the use of routinely recommended vaccines.

Immunity to infection decreases with advancing age. Because of the prevalence of influenza and its potential for causing death, the CDC recommends annual immunization against influenza for older adults and for individuals with chronic cardiac, respiratory, metabolic, and renal disease. Pneumococcal vaccine is recommended for older adults last vaccinated more than 5 years previously.

Vaccine-preventable diseases continue to cause significant morbidity and mortality in the United States despite the availability of safe and effective vaccines. Adult immunization rates in the United States are well below *Healthy People 2020* targets. Vaccines have been studied repeatedly and are a safe and effective intervention for protecting the public's health and should be advocated at every healthcare encounter (Hogue & Meador, 2016).

Heredity influences the development of infection in that some individuals have a genetic susceptibility to certain infections. For example, some may be deficient in serum immunoglobulins, which play a significant role in the internal defense mechanism of the body.

TABLE 31.4 Types of Immunity

Type	Antigen or Antibody Source	Duration
1. Active	Antibodies are produced by the body in response to an antigen.	Long
a. Natural	Antibodies are formed in the presence of active infection in the body.	Lifelong
b. Artificial	Antigens (vaccines or toxoids) are administered to stimulate antibody production.	Many years; the immunity must be reinforced by booster
2. Passive (acquired)	Antibodies are produced by another source, animal or human.	Short
a. Natural	Antibodies are transferred naturally from an immune mother to her baby through the placenta or in colostrum.	6 months to 1 year
b. Artificial	Immune serum (antibody) from an animal or another human is injected.	2–3 weeks

The nature, number, and duration of physical and emotional stressors can influence susceptibility to infection. Stressors elevate blood cortisol. Prolonged elevation of blood cortisol decreases anti-inflammatory responses, depletes energy stores, leads to a state of exhaustion, and decreases resistance to infection. For example, an individual recovering from a major operation or injury is more likely to develop an infection than a healthy individual.

Resistance to infection depends on adequate nutritional status. Because antibodies are proteins, the ability to synthesize antibodies may be impaired by inadequate nutrition, especially when protein reserves are depleted (e.g., as a result of injury, surgery, or a debilitating disease).

Some medical therapies predispose a client to infection. For example, radiation treatments for cancer destroy not only cancerous cells but also some normal cells, thereby rendering them more vulnerable to infection. Some diagnostic procedures may also predispose the client to an infection, especially when the skin is broken or sterile body cavities are penetrated during the procedure.

Certain medications also increase susceptibility to infection. Antineoplastic (anticancer) medications may depress bone marrow function, resulting in inadequate production of white blood cells necessary to combat infections. Anti-inflammatory medications, such as adrenal corticosteroids, inhibit the inflammatory response, an essential defense against infection. Even some antibiotics used to treat infections can have adverse effects. Antibiotics may kill resident flora, allowing the proliferation of strains that would not grow and multiply in the body under normal conditions.

Clinical Alert!

Some common medications such as aspirin and ibuprofen are analgesic (pain relieving), antipyretic (fever reducing), and anti-inflammatory. Acetaminophen, however, is analgesic and antipyretic, but not anti-inflammatory.

Studies indicate that many antibiotics prescribed in hospitals are unnecessary or inappropriate. These practices increase rates of *C. difficile* and antibiotic-resistant bacteria. This resistance has become so widespread that the CDC has created a 12-step campaign to prevent antimicrobial resistance in healthcare settings called "Get Smart for Healthcare," consisting of four strategies: preventing infection, diagnosing and treating infection effectively, using antimicrobials wisely, and preventing transmission. Studies demonstrate that improving prescribing practices in hospitals can reduce rates of *C. difficile* infection and antibiotic resistance, improve patient outcomes, and reduce healthcare costs.

Any disease that lessens the body's defenses against infection places the client at risk. Examples are chronic pulmonary disease, which impairs ciliary action and weakens

LIFESPAN CONSIDERATIONS Infections

CHILDREN

Infections are an expected part of childhood, with most children experiencing some kind of infection from time to time. The majority of these infections are caused by viruses, and for the most part are transient, relatively benign, and able to be overcome by the body's natural defenses and supportive care. In some cases, severe, even life-threatening infections occur. Considerations related to children include the following:

- Newborns may not be able to respond to infections due to an underdeveloped immune system. As a result, in the first few months of life, infections may not be associated with typical signs and symptoms (e.g., an infant with an infection may not have a fever).
- Newborns are born with some naturally acquired immunity transferred from the mother across the placenta.
- Breastfed infants experience higher levels of immunity against infections than formula-fed infants.
- Children between 6 months and 5 years are at higher risk for fever-induced (febrile) seizures. Febrile seizures are not associated with neurologic seizure disorders (e.g., epilepsy).
- Children who are immune compromised (e.g., leukemia, HIV) or have a chronic health condition (e.g., cystic fibrosis, sickle cell disease, congenital heart disease) need extra precautions to prevent exposure to infectious agents.
- Hand hygiene, comprehensive immunizations, good nutrition, adequate hydration, and appropriate rest are essential to preventing and treating infections in children.
- Hand washing and good hygiene in daycare facilities and schools are important to prevent the spread of infections.
- Adolescents are at high risk for sexually transmitted infections and should be well educated about how to prevent them.

OLDER ADULTS

Changes take place in the skin, respiratory tract, GI system, kidneys, and immune system. If unchallenged, these systems work well to maintain homeostasis for the individual, but if compromised by stress, illness, infections, treatments, or surgeries, they find it difficult to keep up and therefore are not able to provide adequate protection. Considerations for older adults include the following:

- Certain nutritional components, especially adequate protein, are necessary to build up and maintain the immune system.
- Diabetes mellitus, which occurs more frequently in older adults, increases the risk of infection and delayed healing by causing an alteration in nutrition and impaired peripheral circulation, which decrease oxygen transport to the tissues.
- The immune system reacts slowly to the introduction of antigens, allowing the antigen to reproduce itself several times before it is recognized by the immune system.
- The normal inflammatory response is delayed. This often causes atypical responses to infections. Instead of displaying the redness, swelling, and fever usually associated with infections, atypical symptoms such as confusion and disorientation, agitation, incontinence, falls, lethargy, and general fatigue are often seen first.

Recognizing these changes in older adults is important in early detection and treatment of related potential for infections and delayed healing. Nursing interventions to promote prevention include the following:

- Provide and teach ways to improve nutritional status.
- Use strict aseptic technique to decrease chance of infections (especially HAIs).
- Encourage older adults to have regular immunizations for flu and pneumonia.
- Be alert to subtle atypical signs of infection and act quickly to diagnose and treat.

the mucous barrier; peripheral vascular disease, which restricts blood flow; burns, which impair skin integrity; chronic or debilitating diseases, which deplete protein reserves; and immune system diseases such as leukemia and aplastic anemia, which alter the production of white blood cells. Diabetes mellitus is a major underlying disease predisposing clients to infection because compromised peripheral vascular status and increased serum glucose levels increase susceptibility.

●○● NURSING MANAGEMENT

Assessing

During the assessing phase of the nursing process, the nurse obtains the client's history, conducts the physical assessment, and gathers laboratory data.

Nursing History

During the nursing history, the nurse assesses (a) the degree to which a client is at risk of developing an infection and (b) any client complaints suggesting the presence of an infection. To identify clients at risk, the nurse reviews the client's chart and structures the nursing interview to collect data regarding the factors influencing the development of infection, especially existing disease process, history of recurrent infections, current medications and therapeutic measures, current emotional stressors, nutritional status, and history of immunizations (see the Assessment Interview).

Physical Assessment

Signs and symptoms of an infection vary according to the body area involved. For example, sneezing, watery or mucoid discharge from the nose, and nasal stuffiness commonly occur with an infection of the nose and sinuses; urinary frequency and cloudy or discolored urine often occur with a urinary infection. Commonly, the skin and mucous membranes are involved in a local infectious process, resulting in the following:

- Localized swelling
- Localized redness
- Pain or tenderness with palpation or movement
- Palpable heat at the infected area
- Loss of function of the body part affected, depending on the site and extent of involvement.

In addition, open wounds may exude drainage of various colors.

Signs of systemic infection include the following:

- Fever
- Increased pulse and respiratory rate if the fever is high
- Malaise and loss of energy
- Anorexia and, in some situations, nausea and vomiting
- Enlargement and tenderness of lymph nodes that drain the area of infection.

Laboratory Data

Laboratory data that may indicate the presence of an infection include the following:

- Elevated leukocyte (white blood cell [WBC]) count (4500 to 11,000/mL^3 is normal).
- Increases in specific types of leukocytes as revealed in the differential WBC count. Specific types of WBCs are increased or decreased in certain infections. See Chapter 34 ∞ for normal values for the adult.
- Elevated erythrocyte sedimentation rate (ESR) and C-reactive protein blood tests. Both test values increase in the presence of an inflammatory process.
- Urine, blood, sputum, or other drainage **cultures** (laboratory cultivations of microorganisms in a special growth medium) that indicate the presence of pathogenic microorganisms.
- Elevated serum lactate. Lactate may be elevated in conditions of infection that are worsening and approaching sepsis.

Diagnosing

Nursing diagnostic terms for problems associated with the transmission of microorganisms include phrases relating to actual or potential infections. Supporting assessment data for these nursing diagnoses or problem statements include broken skin (unintentional or surgical), trauma, impaired ciliary action, stasis of body fluids, change in pH of secretions, or altered peristalsis. Conditions such as

ASSESSMENT INTERVIEW Client at Risk for Infections

- When were you last immunized for diphtheria, tetanus, poliomyelitis, rubella, measles, influenza, hepatitis, and pneumococcal pneumonia?
- When did you last have a tuberculin skin test?
- What infections have you had in the past, and how were these treated? Have any of these infections recurred?
- Are you taking any antibiotics, anti-inflammatory medications such as aspirin or ibuprofen, or medications for cancer?
- Have you had any recent diagnostic procedure or therapy that penetrated through your skin or a body cavity?
- What past surgeries have you had?
- How would you describe your eating habits? Do you eat a variety of types of foods?
- Do you take vitamins?
- On a scale of 1 to 10, how would you rate the stress you have experienced in the last 6 months?
- Have you experienced any loss of energy, loss of appetite, nausea, headache, or other signs associated with specific body systems (e.g., difficulty urinating, urinary frequency, or a sore throat)?

Note: As with all history taking, the nurse must individualize the specific terms used, examples given to the client, and teaching techniques used to validate agreement on the meaning of words according to the client's culture, language spoken, and education or intellectual abilities.

leukopenia, immunosuppression, anemia, or suppressed inflammatory response contribute to the potential for developing an infection.

Clients who have or have potential for an existing infection are prime candidates for other physical and psychologic problems. Examples of nursing diagnoses or collaborative problems that may arise from the actual presence of an infection include nutritional deficiencies if the client is too ill to eat adequately, pain if the client is experiencing tissue damage and discomfort, changes in social life if the client is required to be separated from others during a contagious episode, and anxiety if the client is apprehensive regarding changes in life activities resulting from the infection or its treatment such as absence from work or inability to perform usual functions.

Planning

The major goals for clients susceptible to infection are to:

- Maintain or restore defenses.
- Avoid the spread of infectious organisms.
- Reduce or alleviate problems associated with the infection.

Desired outcomes depend on the individual client's condition. Nursing strategies to meet the three broad goals generally include using meticulous aseptic techniques to prevent the spread of potentially infectious microorganisms, implementing measures to support the defenses of a susceptible host, and teaching clients about protective measures to prevent infections and the spread of infectious agents when an infection is present.

Planning for Home Care

Clients being discharged following hospital care for an infection often require continued care to completely eliminate the infection or to adapt to a chronic state. In addition, such clients may be at increased risk for reinfection or development of an opportunistic infection following therapy for existing pathogens.

In preparation for discharge, the nurse needs to know the client's and family's risks, needs, strengths, and resources. Using data gathered about the home situation, the nurse tailors the teaching plan for the client and family (see Client Teaching: Infection Prevention and Control).

CLIENT TEACHING Infection Prevention and Control

ENVIRONMENTAL MANAGEMENT

- Discuss injury-proofing the home to prevent the possibility of further tissue injury (e.g., use of padding, handrails, removal of hazards).
- Explore ways to control the environmental temperature and airflow (especially if the client has an airborne pathogen).
- Determine the advisability of visitors and family members being in proximity to the client.
- Describe ways to manipulate the bed, the room, and other household facilities to prevent additional injury or to contain possible cross-contamination.
- Instruct to clean obviously soiled linen separately from other laundry. Rinse in cold water, wash in hot water if possible, and add a cup of bleach or phenol-based disinfectant such as Lysol concentrate to the wash.

INFECTION CONTROL

- Based on assessment of client and family knowledge, teach proper hand hygiene (e.g., before handling foods, before eating, after toileting, before and after any required home care treatment, and after touching any body substances such as wound drainage) and related hygienic measures to all family members.
- Discuss hand soaps and effective disinfectants.
- Promote nail care: keep fingernails short, clean, and manicured to eliminate rough edges or hangnails, which can harbor microorganisms.
- Instruct not to share personal care items such as toothbrushes, washcloths, and towels. Describe the rationale of how infections can be transmitted from shared personal items.
- Ensure access to and proper use of gloves and other barriers as indicated by the type of infection or risk.
- Discuss the relationship between hygiene, rest, activity, and nutrition in the chain of infection.
- Instruct about proper administration of medication.
- Instruct about cleaning reusable equipment and supplies using soap and water or appropriate disinfectants.

INFECTION PREVENTION

- Teach the client and family members the signs and symptoms of infection, and when to contact a healthcare provider. After each teaching session, determine the level of understanding on the topic by verbal questioning.
- Teach the client and family members how to avoid infections. Include information on the importance of adequate nutrition in supporting the body's ability to resist infection (see Chapter 46 ∞).
- Suggest techniques for safe food preservation and preparation (e.g., wash raw fruits and vegetables before eating them, refrigerate all opened and unpackaged foods).
- Remind to avoid coughing, sneezing, or breathing directly on others. Cover the mouth and nose to prevent the transmission of airborne microorganisms.
- Inform of the importance of maintaining sufficient fluid intake to promote urine production and output. This helps flush the bladder and urethra of microorganisms.
- Emphasize the need for proper immunizations of all family members.

WOUND CARE

- Teach the client and family the signs of wound healing and wound infection and why monitoring of the wound is important.
- Delineate factors that promote wound healing.
- Explain the proper technique for changing the dressing and disposing of the soiled one. Reinforce the need to place contaminated dressings and other disposable items containing body fluids in moisture-proof plastic bags.
- Advise to put used needles in a puncture-resistant container. Label so as not to discard in the garbage.
- Have client or family repeat instructions and demonstrate skills.

REFERRALS

- Provide appropriate information regarding how to access community resources, home care agencies, sources of supplies, and community or public health departments for immunizations.

Implementing

The nurse implements strategies to prevent infection. If infection cannot be prevented, the nurse's goal is to prevent the spread of the infection within and between individuals, and to treat the existing infection. In the sections that follow, nursing activities are described that interfere with the chain of infection to prevent and control transmission of infectious organisms, and that promote care of the infected client. These activities are summarized in Table 31.5.

Preventing Healthcare-Associated Infections

Meticulous use of medical and surgical asepsis is necessary to prevent transport of potentially infectious microorganisms. Many HAIs can be prevented by using proper hand hygiene techniques, environmental controls, sterile technique when warranted, and identification and management of clients at risk for infections.

Hand Hygiene

Hand hygiene is important in every setting, including hospitals. It is considered one of the most effective infection prevention measures. Any client may harbor microorganisms that are currently harmless to the client yet potentially harmful to another individual or to the same client if they find a portal of entry. It is important for both the nurses' and the clients' hands to be cleansed at the following times to prevent the spread of microorganisms: before eating, after using the bedpan or toilet, and after the hands have come in contact with any body substances, such as sputum or drainage from a wound. In addition, healthcare workers should cleanse their hands before and after giving care of any kind.

Because hand hygiene is performed so frequently, it provides a good opportunity for the nurse to take a moment to breathe and prepare for the next client encounter. By allowing a full, quiet breath in and a slow, complete exhalation, the nurse can focus attention and intention to remain mindful. This mindful attitude enhances the nurse's therapeutic presence and increases the effectiveness and safety of care.

For routine client care, vigorous hand washing under a stream of water for 15 to 20 seconds using soap at the beginning of the nurse's shift, when hands are visibly soiled, and after using the toilet is recommended (WHO, 2009). Note that in late 2016, the U.S. Food and Drug Administration (FDA) issued a final rule establishing that over-the-counter consumer antiseptic wash products (sometimes labeled as antimicrobial soap) containing certain active ingredients such as triclosan can no longer be marketed to the public because they have not been shown to be effective and may be unsafe (FDA, 2016b). *Note:* The chemical triclosan, itself, is not banned and may be found in products such as toothpaste and cosmetics.

Hand washing with soap and water may be inadequate to sufficiently remove pathogens, particularly because healthcare personnel tend to not wash thoroughly. After the initial soap and water hand washing, the CDC recommends the use of alcohol-based antiseptic hand rubs (rinses, gels, or foams) before and after each direct client contact. If there is visible dirt or matter, or if *C. difficile* may be present, alcohol-based rubs will not be sufficient, and soap and water washing is necessary for each hand cleansing (WHO, 2009). Even if soap and water or alcohol-based rubs are used appropriately, gloves are still required in some situations such as when caring for clients with *C. difficile*.

Alcohol-based hand rubs (foam or gel):

- Kill bacteria more effectively and more quickly than hand washing with soap and water.
- Are less damaging to skin than repeated soap and water, resulting in less dryness and irritation.
- Require less time than hand washing with soap and water.
- Can be placed at the point of care in bottles or dispensers so they are more accessible.
- Proper use of alcohol-based products includes these steps:
  - Apply a palmful of product into cupped hand—enough to cover all surfaces of both hands.
  - Rub palm against palm.
  - Interlace fingers palm to palm.
  - Rub palms to back of hands.
  - Rub all surfaces of each finger with opposite hand.
  - Continue until product is dry—about 20 to 30 seconds.

Clinical Alert!

Although some religions prohibit drinking alcohol, most accept the value of using alcohol-based hand rubs in healthcare settings. Nurses must use cultural sensitivity with both colleagues and clients regarding acceptance of using alcohol-based products.

In the following situations, the CDC recommends hospital-grade antimicrobial hand hygiene agents such as chlorhexidine :

- When there are known multiple resistant bacteria
- Before invasive procedures
- In special care units, such as nurseries and intensive care units (ICUs)
- Before caring for severely immunocompromised clients.

It is important to recognize that performing frequent hand hygiene with either soap or alcohol-based cleansers can damage the skin through the drying effect of the detergents or chemicals. If the nurse develops dermatitis, the client may be at higher risk because hand washing does not decrease bacterial counts on skin with dermatitis. The nurse is also at higher risk because the normal skin barrier has been broken. Although lotions, moisturizers, and emollients have been tried, no research has yet confirmed their effectiveness in decreasing the damage.

Skill 31.1 describes proper hand hygiene techniques using soap and water.

TABLE 31.5 Nursing Interventions That Break the Chain of Infection

Link	Interventions	Rationales
Etiologic agent (microorganism)	Ensure that articles are correctly cleaned and disinfected or sterilized before use.	Correct cleaning, disinfecting, and sterilizing reduce or eliminate microorganisms.
	Educate clients and support people about appropriate methods for cleaning, disinfecting, and sterilizing articles.	Knowledge of ways to reduce or eliminate microorganisms reduces the likelihood of transmission.
Reservoir (source)	Change dressings and bandages when they are soiled or wet.	Moist dressings are ideal environments for microorganisms to grow and multiply.
	Assist clients to carry out appropriate skin and oral hygiene.	Hygienic measures reduce the numbers of resident and transient microorganisms and the likelihood of infection.
	Dispose of damp, soiled linens appropriately.	Damp, soiled linens harbor more microorganisms than dry linens.
	Dispose of feces and urine in appropriate receptacles.	Urine and feces may contain many microorganisms.
	Ensure that all fluid containers, such as bedside water jugs and suction and drainage bottles, are covered or capped.	Prolonged exposure to room air increases the risk of contamination and promotes microbial growth.
	Empty suction and drainage bottles at the end of each shift or before they become full, or according to agency policy.	Drainage harbors microorganisms that, if left for long periods, proliferate and can be transmitted to others.
Portal of exit from the reservoir	Avoid talking, coughing, or sneezing over open wounds or sterile fields, and cover the mouth and nose when coughing and sneezing.	These measures limit the number of microorganisms that escape from the respiratory tract.
Method of transmission	Cleanse hands between client contacts, after touching body substances, and before performing invasive procedures or touching open wounds.	Hand hygiene is an important means of controlling and preventing the transmission of microorganisms.
	Instruct clients and support people to cleanse hands before handling food or eating, after eliminating, and after touching infectious material.	Hand hygiene helps prevent transfer of microorganisms from one individual or body area to another.
	Wear gloves when handling secretions and excretions.	Gloves prevent soiling of the hands.
	Wear gowns if there is danger of soiling clothing with body substances.	Gowns prevent soiling of the clothing.
	Place discarded soiled materials in moisture-proof refuse bags.	Moisture-proof bags prevent the spread of microorganisms to others.
	Hold used bedpans steadily to prevent spillage, and dispose of urine and feces in appropriate receptacles.	Urine and feces contain many microorganisms.
	Initiate and implement infection prevention strategies for all clients.	All clients may harbor potentially infectious microorganisms that can be transmitted to others.
	Wear mask and eye protection when in close contact with clients who have infections transmitted by droplets from the respiratory tract.	Masks and eyewear reduce the spread of droplet-transmitted microorganisms.
	Wear mask and eye protection when sprays of body fluid are possible (e.g., during irrigation procedures).	Masks and eye protection provide protection from microorganisms in clients' body substances.
Portal of entry to the susceptible host	Use aseptic technique for invasive procedures (e.g., injections, catheterizations).	Invasive procedures penetrate the body's natural protective barriers to microorganisms.
	Use aseptic technique when exposing open wounds or handling dressings.	Open wounds are vulnerable to microbial infection.
	Place used disposable needles and syringes in puncture-resistant containers for disposal.	Injuries from needles contaminated by blood or body fluids from an infected client or carrier are a primary cause of HBV and HIV transmission to healthcare workers.
	Provide all clients with their own personal care items.	Individuals have less resistance to another individual's microorganisms than to their own.
Susceptible host	Maintain the integrity of the client's skin and mucous membranes.	Intact skin and mucous membranes protect against invasion by microorganisms.
	Ensure that the client receives a balanced diet.	A balanced diet supplies proteins and vitamins necessary to build or maintain body tissues.
	Educate the public about the importance of immunizations.	Certain immunizations may protect individuals against virulent infectious diseases.
	Encourage deep, slow, full breathing, ambulation, and movement.	These actions enhance ventilation and circulation throughout the body.
	Offer stress management strategies and encourage healthy relationships.	Tap into the mind–body connection to enhance healing.

SKILL 31.1

Performing Hand Washing

PURPOSES

- To reduce the risk of transmission of microorganisms to clients
- To reduce the risk of cross-contamination among clients
- To reduce the risk of transmission of infectious organisms to oneself

ASSESSMENT

Determine the client's:

- Presence of factors increasing susceptibility to infection and possibility of undiagnosed infection (e.g., HIV)
- Use of immunosuppressive medications
- Recent diagnostic procedures or treatments that penetrated the skin or a body cavity
- Current nutritional status
- Signs and symptoms indicating the presence of an infection:
  - Localized signs: swelling, redness, pain or tenderness with palpation or movement, palpable heat at site, loss of function of affected body part, presence of exudate
  - Systemic indications: fever, increased pulse and respiratory rates, lack of energy, anorexia, enlarged lymph nodes

PLANNING

Determine the location of running water and soap.

Assignment

The skill of hand hygiene is identical for all healthcare providers, including assistive personnel (AP). Healthcare team members are accountable for themselves and others to implement appropriate hand washing procedures.

Equipment

- Soap
- Warm running water
- Paper towels

IMPLEMENTATION

Preparation

Assess your hands:

- Nails should be kept short. Most agencies do not permit healthcare workers in direct contact with clients to have any form of artificial nails. The CDC guidelines prohibit artificial nails in caring for high-risk clients, and the WHO guidelines prohibit artificial nails in all settings. **Rationale:** *Short, natural nails are less likely to harbor microorganisms, scratch a client, or puncture gloves*.
- Removal of all jewelry is recommended. **Rationale:** *Although the research is controversial, microorganisms can lodge in the settings of jewelry and under rings. Removal facilitates proper cleaning of the hands and forearms*.
- Check hands for breaks in the skin, such as hangnails or cuts. **Rationale:** *A nurse who has open sores may require a work assignment with decreased risk for transmission of infectious organisms due to the chance of acquiring or passing on an infection*.

Performance

1. If you are washing your hands where the client can observe you, introduce self and explain to the client what you are going to do and why it is necessary.
2. Turn on the water and adjust the flow.
   - There are five common types of faucet controls:
     a. Hand-operated handles.
     b. Knee levers.
     c. Foot pedals.
     d. Elbow controls. Move these with the elbows instead of the hands.
     e. Infrared control. Motion in front of the sensor causes water to start and stop flowing automatically.
   - If possible, adjust the flow so that the water is warm. **Rationale:** *Warm water removes less of the protective oil of the skin than hot water*.
3. Wet the hands thoroughly by holding them under the running water and apply soap to the hands.
   - Hold the hands lower than the elbows so that the water flows from the arms to the fingertips. **Rationale:** *The water should flow from the least contaminated to the most contaminated area; the hands are generally considered more contaminated than the lower arms.* Note that this is a different technique than is used when performing surgical hand washing. Nurses will learn to perform that level of hand washing if they are working in the operating room.
   - If the soap is liquid, apply 4 to 5 mL (1 tsp). If it is bar soap, granules, or sheets, rub them firmly between the hands.
4. Thoroughly wash and rinse the hands.
   - Use firm, rubbing, and circular movements to wash the palm, back, and wrist of each hand. Be sure to include the heel of the hand. Interlace the fingers and thumbs, and move the hands back and forth. ❶ The WHO (2009) recommends these steps:
     a. Right palm over left dorsum with interlaced fingers and vice versa
     b. Palm to palm with fingers interlaced
     c. Backs of fingers to opposing palms with fingers interlocked
     d. Rotational rubbing of left thumb clasped in right palm and vice versa.

     Continue these motions for about 20 seconds. **Rationale:** *The circular action creates friction that helps remove microorganisms mechanically. Interlacing the fingers and thumbs cleans the interdigital spaces*.
   - Rub the fingertips against the palm of the opposite hand. **Rationale:** *The nails and fingertips are commonly missed during hand hygiene*.
   - Rinse the hands.
5. Thoroughly pat dry the hands and arms.
   - Dry hands and arms thoroughly with a paper towel without scrubbing. **Rationale:** *Moist skin becomes chapped readily as does dry skin that is rubbed vigorously; chapping produces lesions*.
   - Discard the paper towel in the appropriate container.
6. Turn off the water.
   - Use a new paper towel to grasp a hand-operated control. ❷ **Rationale:** *This prevents the nurse from picking up microorganisms from the faucet handles*. Apply hand lotion if desired. Use only agency-approved hand lotions and dispensers. Other lotions may make hand hygiene less effective, cause the breakdown of latex gloves, and become contaminated with bacteria if dispensers are refilled.

Performing Hand Washing—*continued*

A

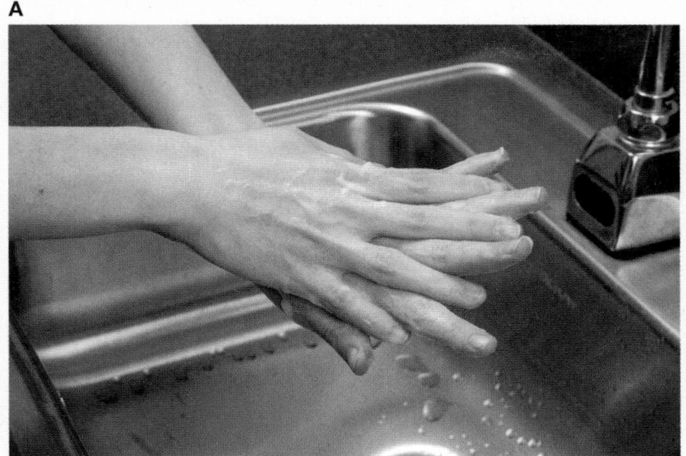

D

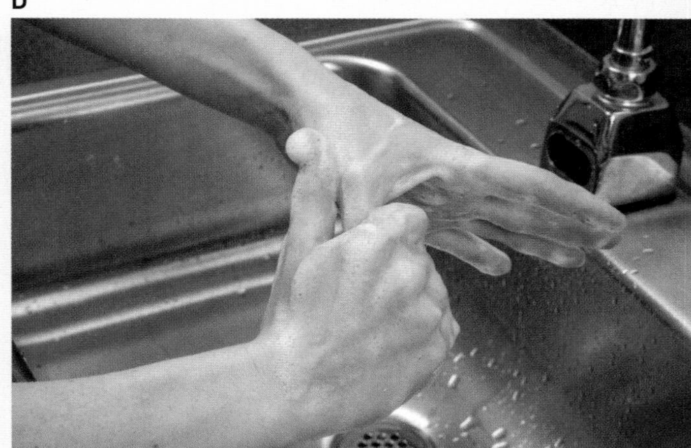

❶ Hand washing steps.

B

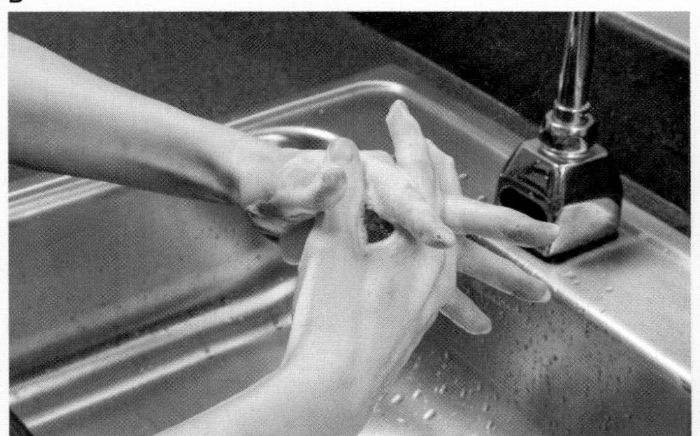

C

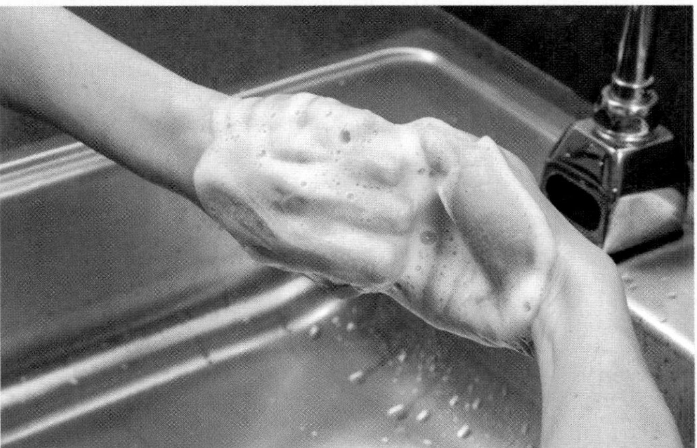

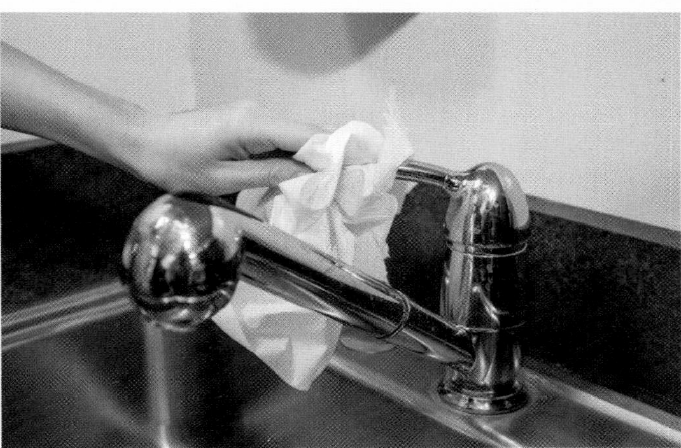

❷ Using a paper towel to grasp the handle of a hand-operated faucet.

Variation: Hand Washing Before Performing Sterile Skills

- Apply the soap and wash as described in step 4, but hold the hands higher than the elbows during this hand wash. Wet the hands and forearms under the running water, letting it run from the fingertips to the elbows so that the hands become cleaner than the elbows. **Rationale:** *In this way, the water runs from the area that now has the fewest microorganisms to areas with a relatively greater number of pathogens.*
- After washing and rinsing, use a towel to dry one hand thoroughly in a rotating motion from the fingers to the elbow. Use a new towel to dry the other hand and arm. **Rationale:** *A clean towel prevents the transfer of microorganisms from one elbow (least clean area) to the other hand (cleanest area).*
- Apply sterile gloves before touching any unsterile items (see Skill 31.4).

EVALUATION

- There is no traditional evaluation of the effectiveness of the individual nurse's hand washing practices. Institutional quality control departments monitor the occurrence of client infections and investigate those situations in which healthcare providers are implicated in the transmission of infectious organisms. Research has repeatedly shown the positive impact of careful hand hygiene on client health associated with prevention of infection. More researchers are focusing on the relationship between quality of hand hygiene products (gentle, nondrying, aromatic) and adherence to recommended protocols.

Note: In some agencies, clients are encouraged to ask the provider if they have cleansed their hands before allowing them to perform procedures, although not all clients are comfortable asking (AHC Media, 2018).

Disinfecting and Sterilizing

The first links in the chain of infection, the etiologic agent and the reservoir, are interrupted by the use of **antiseptics** (agents that inhibit the growth of some microorganisms) and **disinfectants** (agents that destroy pathogens other than spores) and by sterilization.

Disinfecting

An antiseptic is a chemical preparation used on skin or tissue. A disinfectant is a chemical preparation, such as phenol or iodine compounds, used on inanimate objects. Disinfectants are frequently caustic and toxic to tissues. Antiseptics and disinfectants often have similar chemical components, but the disinfectant is a more concentrated solution.

Both antiseptics and disinfectants are said to have bactericidal or bacteriostatic properties. A *bactericidal* preparation destroys bacteria, whereas a *bacteriostatic* preparation prevents the growth and reproduction of some bacteria. An agent known to be effective against a particular type of bacteria should be selected. Spore-forming bacteria such as *C. difficile*, which is a frequent cause of nosocomial diarrhea, and *Bacillus anthracis* (anthrax) may be inhibited by only a few of the agents normally effective against other forms of bacteria. Table 31.6 lists commonly used antiseptics and disinfectants.

When disinfecting, nurses need to follow agency protocol and consider the following:

1. The type and number of infectious organisms. Some microorganisms are readily destroyed, whereas others require longer contact with the disinfectant.
2. The recommended concentration of the disinfectant and the duration of contact.
3. The presence of soap. Some disinfectants are ineffective in the presence of soap or detergent.
4. The presence of organic materials. The presence of saliva, blood, pus, or excretions can readily inactivate many disinfectants.
5. The surface areas to be treated. The disinfecting agent must come into contact with all surfaces and areas.

Sterilizing

Sterilization is a process that destroys all microorganisms, including spores and viruses. Four commonly used methods of sterilization are moist heat, gas, boiling water, and radiation.

Moist Heat

To sterilize with moist heat (such as with an autoclave), steam under pressure is used because it attains temperatures higher than the boiling point.

Gas

Ethylene oxide destroys microorganisms by interfering with their metabolic processes. It is also effective against spores. Its advantages are good penetration and effectiveness for heat-sensitive items. Its major disadvantage is its toxicity to humans.

Boiling Water

This is the most practical and inexpensive method for sterilizing in the home. The main disadvantage is that spores and some viruses are not killed by this method. Boiling a minimum of 15 minutes is advised for disinfection of articles in the home.

Radiation

Both ionizing (such as alpha, beta, and x-rays) and nonionizing (ultraviolet light) radiation are used for disinfection and sterilization. The main drawback to ultraviolet light is that the rays do not penetrate deeply. Ionizing radiation is used effectively in industry to sterilize foods, drugs, and other items that are sensitive to heat. Its main advantage is that it is effective for items difficult to sterilize; its chief disadvantage is that the equipment is very expensive.

Infection Prevention and Control

Because it is not always possible to know which clients may have infectious organisms, guidelines are established by the CDC and other organizations outlining steps all healthcare workers must follow to reduce the chances that organisms in blood (**bloodborne pathogens**) and potentially infectious organisms from other body tissues will

TABLE 31.6 Commonly Used Antiseptics and Disinfectants and Their Effectiveness and Use

	Effective Against					
Agent	**Bacteria**	**Tuberculosis**	**Spores**	**Fungi**	**Viruses**	**Use on**
Isopropyl and ethyl alcohol	X	X		X	X	Hands, vial stoppers
Chlorine (bleach)	X	X	X	X	X	Blood spills
Hydrogen peroxide	X	X	X	X	X	Surfaces
Iodophors	X	X	X	X	X	Equipment; intact skin and tissues if diluted
Phenol	X	X		X	X	Surfaces
Chlorhexidine gluconate (Hibiclens)	X				X	Hands

DRUG CAPSULE

Macrolide Antibiotic: azithromycin (Zithromax)

Macrolide antibiotics prevent bacteria from growing by interfering with their ability to make proteins. Due to the differences in the way proteins are made in bacteria and humans, the macrolide antibiotics do not interfere with humans' ability to make proteins. They are effective against a wide variety of bacterial organisms, including *Haemophilus influenzae*, *Streptococcus pneumoniae*, *Mycoplasma pneumoniae*, *S. aureus*, and *Mycobacterium avium*. Azithromycin is unusual in that it stays in the body for quite a while, allowing for once-a-day dosing and for shorter treatment courses for most infections. It may be prescribed for infections from susceptible microorganisms such as those that occur in the lungs (bronchitis), ears, skin, and throat. A common oral azithromycin treatment consists of a double dose of medication on the first day of treatment and then a single dose for an additional 4 or 5 days. This is often dispensed and referred to as a "Z-Pak" that contains all the pills needed for the full course: two tablets on the first day and one tablet once daily for the next 4 or 5 days.

NURSING RESPONSIBILITIES

- Assess the client for any drug allergies—especially to other antibiotics and particularly those from the erythromycin family. Do not administer azithromycin to clients with stated allergies unless the primary care provider has given approval.
- Assess for signs of possible allergic reaction: rash, hives, itching, swelling of the face or mouth, and difficulty breathing or swallowing. If any are detected, contact the primary care provider immediately—this is an emergency.
- Azithromycin may be given with meals or on an empty stomach.
- It is available in capsule form or as an oral liquid suspension.
- Drug interactions can occur with anticoagulants, digoxin, and several other medications. Always check the list of client medications for possible interactions.
- Adverse effects are generally limited to GI upset.

CLIENT AND FAMILY TEACHING

- Assess and document client's level of understanding related to medication therapy. Develop a teaching plan to augment any lack of knowledge on the part of the client or family caregiver.
- Teach the client to take azithromycin with a full glass of water, with or without food, but at least 2 hours after antacids.
- Teach the client to complete the entire course of therapy. Stress that the client should not stop taking the medication even if he or she feels better before finishing the course of therapy.
- Instruct to store the medication away from heat and moisture—not in the bathroom.
- Be sure the client understands not to keep leftover medication or share it with other individuals.

Note: Prior to administering any medication, review all aspects with a current drug handbook or other reliable source.

be transmitted from the client to other individuals. The guidelines contain a two-tiered approach. The first tier is **standard precautions (SP)**. Some agencies may use an earlier term—**universal precautions (UP)**—reflecting their applicability in all client care situations.

The recommendations reinforce the need for effective hand hygiene, use of personal protective equipment, and environmental controls. They also include respiratory hygiene or cough etiquette. Healthcare professionals use SP when providing care to all clients. That is, the risk of caregiver exposure to client body tissues and fluids rather than the suspected presence or absence of infectious organisms determines the use of clean gloves, gowns, masks, and eye protection.

If the client is known to have an infection, the CDC's second tier, transmission-based precautions, are used to protect the nurse and others from acquiring the infectious organism. These precautions are used in addition to SP when those precautions do not completely block the chain of infection and the infections are spread in one of three ways: by airborne or droplet transmission or by contact. Transmission-based precautions may be used singly or in combination.

Isolation refers to measures designed to prevent the spread of infections or potentially infectious microorganisms to health personnel, clients, and visitors. Several sets of guidelines have been used in hospitals and other healthcare settings.

Category-specific isolation precautions use seven categories: strict isolation, contact isolation, respiratory isolation, tuberculosis isolation, enteric precautions, drainage and secretions precautions, and blood and body fluid precautions.

Disease-specific isolation precautions provide precautions for specific diseases. These precautions delineate use of private rooms with special ventilation, having the client share a room with other clients infected with the same organism, and gowning to prevent gross soilage of clothes for specific infectious diseases.

Standard Precautions

Standard precautions are used in any situations involving blood; all body fluids, excretions, and secretions except sweat; nonintact skin; and mucous membranes (whether or not blood is present or visible). SP include (a) hand hygiene; (b) use of **personal protective equipment (PPE)**, which includes gloves, gowns, eyewear, and masks; (c) safe injection practices; (d) safe handling of potentially contaminated equipment or surfaces in the client environment; and (e) **respiratory hygiene or cough etiquette** that calls for covering the mouth and nose when sneezing or coughing, proper disposal of tissues, and separating potentially infected individuals from others by at least 1 m (3 ft) or having them wear a surgical mask.

Transmission-Based Precautions

Transmission-based precautions are used in addition to standard precautions for clients with known or suspected infections that are spread in one of three ways: by airborne or droplet transmission, or by contact. The three types of transmission-based precautions may be used alone or in combination but always in addition to SP. Recommended practices for standard and transmission-based precautions are shown in Box 31.1.

BOX 31.1 Recommended Infection Precautions in Hospitals

STANDARD PRECAUTIONS

- Designed for all clients in hospital.
- These precautions apply to (a) blood; (b) all body fluids, excretions, and secretions except sweat; (c) nonintact (broken) skin; and (d) mucous membranes.
- Designed to reduce risk of transmission of microorganisms from recognized and unrecognized sources.

1. Perform proper hand hygiene after contact with blood, body fluids, secretions, excretions, and contaminated objects whether or not gloves are worn.
   a. Perform proper hand hygiene immediately after removing gloves.
   b. Use a nonantimicrobial product for routine hand hygiene.
   c. Use an antimicrobial agent or an antiseptic agent for the control of specific outbreaks of infection.
2. Wear clean gloves when touching blood, body fluids, secretions, excretions, and contaminated items (i.e., soiled gowns).
   a. Clean gloves can be unsterile unless their use is intended to prevent the entrance of microorganisms into the body. See the discussion of sterile gloves in this chapter.
   b. Remove gloves before touching noncontaminated items and surfaces.
   c. Perform proper hand hygiene immediately after removing gloves.
3. Wear a mask, eye protection, or a face shield if splashes or sprays of blood, body fluids, secretions, or excretions can be expected.
4. Wear a clean, nonsterile, water-resistant gown if client care is likely to result in splashes or sprays of blood, body fluids, secretions, or excretions. The gown is intended to protect clothing.
   a. Remove a soiled gown carefully to avoid the transfer of microorganisms to others (i.e., clients or other healthcare workers).
   b. Cleanse hands after removing gown.
5. Handle client care equipment that is soiled with blood, body fluids, secretions, or excretions carefully to prevent the transfer of microorganisms to others and to the environment.
   a. Make sure reusable equipment is cleaned and reprocessed correctly.
   b. Dispose of single-use equipment correctly.
6. Handle all soiled linen as little as possible. Do not shake it. Bundle it up with the clean side out and dirty side in, and hold away from self so that the nurse's uniform or clothing is not contaminated.
7. Place used needles and other "sharps" directly into puncture-resistant containers as soon as their use is completed. Do not attempt to recap needles or place sharps back in their sheaths. This can result in a needlestick puncture injury if the nurse accidentally misses the cover.

TRANSMISSION-BASED PRECAUTIONS

Airborne Precautions

Use standard precautions as well as the following:

1. Place client in an airborne infection isolation room (AIIR). An AIIR is a private room that has negative air pressure, 6 to 12 air changes per hour, and either discharge of air to the outside or a filtration system for the room air.
2. If a private room is not available, place client with another client who is infected with the same microorganism.
3. Wear an N95 respirator mask when entering the room of a client who is known to have or suspected of having primary tuberculosis. See the Practice Guidelines on using a respirator mask.
4. Susceptible individuals should not enter the room of a client who has rubeola (measles) or varicella (chickenpox). If they must enter, they should wear a respirator mask.
5. Limit movement of the client outside the room to essential purposes. Place a surgical mask on the client during transport.

Droplet Precautions

Use standard precautions as well as the following:

1. Place client in private room.
2. If a private room is not available, place client with another client who is infected with the same microorganism.
3. Wear a mask if working within 1 m (3 ft) of the client.
4. Limit movement of client outside the room to essential purposes. Place a surgical mask on the client while outside the room.

Contact Precautions

Use standard precautions as well as the following:

1. Place client in private room.
2. If a private room is not available, place client with another client who is infected with the same microorganism.
3. Wear gloves as described in standard precautions.
   a. Change gloves after contact with infectious material.
   b. Remove gloves before leaving client's room.
   c. Cleanse hands immediately after removing gloves. Use an antimicrobial agent. *Note:* If the client is infected with *C. difficile*, do not use an alcohol-based hand rub because it is not effective on these spores. Use soap and water (Sanyal & Strelczyk, 2018).
   d. After hand hygiene, do not touch possibly contaminated surfaces or items in the room.
4. Wear a gown (see standard precautions) when entering a room if there is a possibility of contact with infected surfaces or items, or if the client is incontinent or has diarrhea, a colostomy, or wound drainage not contained by a dressing.
   a. Remove gown in the client's room.
   b. Make sure uniform does not contact possible contaminated surfaces.
5. Limit movement of client outside the room.
6. Dedicate the use of noncritical client care equipment to a single client or to clients with the same infecting microorganisms.

Adapted from "2007 Guidelines for Isolation Precautions Preventing Transmission of Infectious Agents in Healthcare Settings," by J. D. Siegel, E. Rhinehart, M. Jackson, L. Chiarello, and the Healthcare Infection Control Practices Advisory Committee, 2007. Retrieved from https://www.cdc.gov/infectioncontrol/guidelines/isolation/index.html

Airborne precautions are used for clients known to have or suspected of having serious illnesses transmitted by airborne droplet nuclei smaller than 5 microns. Examples of such illnesses include measles (rubeola), varicella (including disseminated zoster), and tuberculosis. The CDC has prepared special guidelines for preventing the transmission of tuberculosis. The most current information may be found on the CDC Division of Tuberculosis Elimination website.

Droplet precautions are used for clients known to have or suspected of having serious illnesses transmitted by particle droplets larger than 5 microns. Examples of such illnesses are diphtheria (pharyngeal); mycoplasma pneumonia; pertussis; mumps; rubella; streptococcal pharyngitis, pneumonia, or scarlet fever in infants and young children; and pneumonic plague.

Contact precautions are used for clients known to have or suspected of having serious illnesses easily transmitted by direct client contact or by contact with items in the client's environment. According to the CDC, such illnesses include GI, respiratory, skin, or wound infections or colonization with multidrug-resistant bacteria; specific enteric infections such as *C. difficile* and enterohemorrhagic *E. coli O157:H7*, *Shigella*, and hepatitis A, for diapered or incontinent clients; respiratory syncytial virus, parainfluenza virus, or enteroviral infections in infants and young children; and highly contagious skin infections such as herpes simplex virus, impetigo, pediculosis, and scabies.

Another organism requiring contact precautions is methicillin-resistant *S. aureus* (MRSA). Approximately half of all MRSA infections are acquired in the hospital, one-fourth are associated with having received healthcare but onset is in the community, and the remainder are considered community acquired. Due to aggressive healthcare emphasis on prevention of MRSA transmission using standard and contact precautions, rates have decreased but are still unacceptably high. More Americans die each year from MRSA than from AIDS (MRSA Research Center, 2017).

Some diseases require a combination of transmission-based precautions. For clients infected with the coronavirus that causes severe acute respiratory syndrome (SARS-CoV), standard (including eye protection), contact, and airborne precautions are indicated (Siegel, Rhinehart, Jackson, Chiarello, & the Healthcare Infection Control Practices Advisory Committee, 2007).

When certain conditions exist, transmission-based precautions are indicated until the presence or absence of the suspected agent has been confirmed. For example, for a generalized petechial rash with fever and a history of travel in an area known to have viral hemorrhagic fever, droplet and contact precautions are used until viruses such as Ebola or Lassa have been ruled out. In contrast, airborne precautions should be initiated if a maculopapular rash with fever, cough, and nasal congestion is present and rubeola has not been eliminated as a possible cause.

Compromised Clients

Compromised clients (those highly susceptible to infection) are often infected by their own microorganisms, by microorganisms on the inadequately cleansed hands of healthcare personnel, and by nonsterile items (food, water, air, and client-care equipment). Clients who are severely compromised include those who:

- Have diseases, such as leukemia, or treatments such as chemotherapy, that depress the client's resistance to infectious organisms.
- Have extensive skin impairments, such as severe dermatitis or major burns, which cannot be effectively covered with dressings.

The 2007 CDC guidelines (Siegel et al., 2007) for care of severely compromised (immunocompromised) clients include the use of SP as described earlier.

Isolation Practices

Initiation of practices to prevent the transmission of microorganisms is generally a nursing responsibility and is based on a comprehensive assessment of the client. This assessment takes into account the status of the client's normal defense mechanisms, the client's ability to implement necessary precautions, and the source and mode of transmission of the infectious agent. The nurse then decides whether to wear gloves, gowns, masks, and protective eyewear. In all client situations, *nurses must cleanse their hands before and after giving care.*

Personal Protective Equipment

All healthcare providers must apply PPE (clean or sterile gloves, gowns, masks, and protective eyewear) according to the risk of exposure to potentially infective materials.

Gloves

Gloves are worn for three reasons: First, they protect the hands when the nurse is likely to handle any body substances, for example, blood, urine, feces, sputum, and nonintact skin. Second, gloves reduce the likelihood of nurses transmitting their own endogenous microorganisms to individuals receiving care. Nurses who have open sores or cuts on the hands must wear gloves for protection. Third, gloves reduce the chance that the nurse's hands will transmit microorganisms from one client or an object to another client. In all situations, gloves are changed between client contacts. The hands are cleansed each time gloves are removed for two primary reasons: (1) The gloves may have imperfections or be damaged during wearing so that they could allow microorganism entry and (2) the hands may become contaminated during glove removal.

Skill 31.2 describes application and removal of gloves.

SKILL 31.2

Applying and Removing Personal Protective Equipment (Gloves, Gown, Mask, Eyewear)

PURPOSE

- To protect healthcare workers and clients from transmission of potentially infective materials

ASSESSMENT

Consider which activities will be required while the nurse is in the client's room at this time. **Rationale:** *This will determine which equipment is required.*

PLANNING

- Application and removal of PPE can be time consuming. Prioritize care and arrange for personnel to care for your other clients if indicated.
- Determine which supplies are present within the client's room and which must be brought to the room.
- Consider if special handling is indicated for removal of any specimens or other materials from the room.

Assignment

Use of PPE is identical for all healthcare providers. Clients whose care requires use of PPE may be assigned to AP. Healthcare team members are accountable for proper implementation of these procedures by themselves and others.

Equipment

As indicated according to which activities will be performed, ensure that extra supplies are easily available.

- Gown
- Mask
- Eyewear
- Clean gloves

IMPLEMENTATION

Preparation

Remove or secure all loose items such as name tags or jewelry.

Performance

1. Prior to performing the procedure, introduce self and verify the client's identity using agency protocol. Explain to the client what you are going to do, why it is necessary, and how to participate.
2. Perform hand hygiene.
3. Apply a clean gown.
   - Pick up a clean gown, and allow it to unfold in front of you without allowing it to touch any area soiled with body substances.
   - Slide the arms and the hands through the sleeves.
   - Fasten the ties at the neck to keep the gown in place.
   - Overlap the gown at the back as much as possible, and fasten the waist ties or belt. ❶ **Rationale:** *Overlapping securely covers the uniform at the back. Waist ties keep the gown from falling away from the body, which can cause inadvertent soiling of the uniform.*
4. Apply the face mask.
   - Locate the top edge of the mask. The mask usually has a narrow metal strip along the edge.
   - Hold the mask by the top two strings or loops.
   - Place the upper edge of the mask over the bridge of the nose, and tie the upper ties at the back of the head or secure the loops around the ears. If glasses are worn, fit the upper edge of the mask under the glasses. ❷ **Rationale:** *With the edge of the mask under the glasses, clouding of the glasses is less likely to occur.*
   - Secure the lower edge of the mask under the chin, and tie the lower ties at the nape of the neck. **Rationale:** *To be effective, a mask must cover both the nose and the mouth, because air moves in and out of both.*
   - If the mask has a metal strip, adjust this firmly over the bridge of the nose. **Rationale:** *A secure fit prevents both the escape and the inhalation of microorganisms around the edges of the mask and the fogging of eyeglasses.*

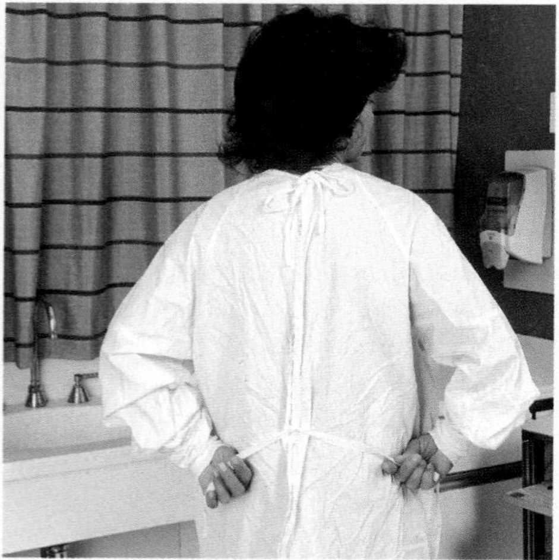

❶ Overlapping the gown at the back to cover the nurse's uniform.

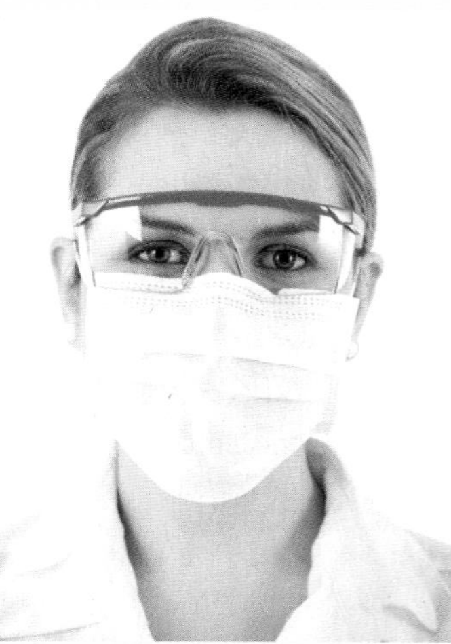

❷ A face mask tucked under eye protection.
ESB Basic/Shutterstock.

Applying and Removing Personal Protective Equipment—*continued*

- Wear the mask only once, and do not wear any mask longer than the manufacturer recommends or once it becomes wet. **Rationale:** *A mask should be used only once because it becomes ineffective when moist from exhaled breath.*
- Do not leave a used face mask hanging around the neck.
- The Practice Guidelines provide further instructions on using a face mask.

5. Apply protective eyewear if it is not combined with the face mask.

6. Apply clean gloves.
- No special technique is required.
- If wearing a gown, pull the gloves up to cover the cuffs of the gown. If not wearing a gown, pull the gloves up to cover the wrists.

7. To remove soiled PPE, remove the gloves first since they are the most soiled.
- If wearing a gown that is tied at the waist in front, undo the ties before removing gloves.
- Remove the first glove by grasping it on its palmar surface, taking care to touch only glove to glove. ❸ **Rationale:** *This keeps the soiled parts of the used gloves from touching the skin of the wrist or hand.*

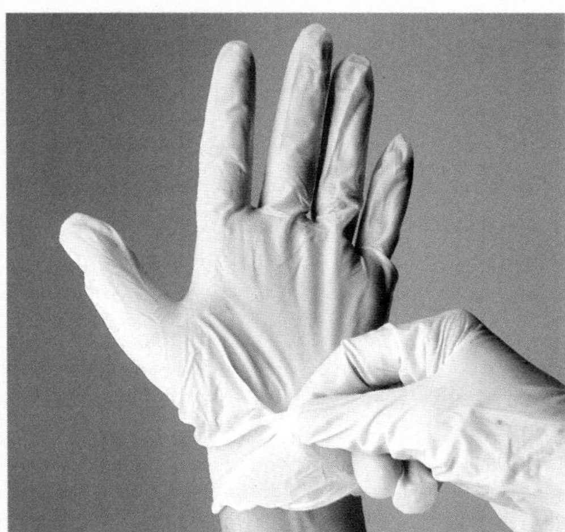

❸ Plucking the palmar surface of a contaminated glove.

- Pull the first glove completely off by inverting or rolling the glove inside out.
- Continue to hold the inverted removed glove by the fingers of the remaining gloved hand. Place the first two fingers of the bare hand inside the cuff of the second glove. ❹ **Rationale:** *Touching the outside of the second soiled glove with the bare hand is avoided.*
- Pull the second glove off to the fingers by turning it inside out. This pulls the first glove inside the second glove. **Rationale:** *The soiled part of the glove is folded to the inside to reduce the chance of transferring any microorganisms by direct contact.*
- Using the bare hand, continue to remove the gloves, which are now inside out, and dispose of them in the refuse container. ❺

8. Perform hand hygiene. **Rationale:** *Contact with microorganisms may occur while removing PPE.*

9. Remove protective eyewear and dispose of properly or place in the appropriate receptacle for cleaning.

10. Remove the gown when preparing to leave the room.
- Avoid touching soiled parts on the outside of the gown, if possible. **Rationale:** *The top part of the gown may be soiled, for example, if you have been holding an infant with a respiratory infection.*
- Grasp the gown along the inside of the neck and pull down over the shoulders. Do not shake the gown.
- Roll up the gown with the soiled part inside, and discard it in the appropriate container.

11. Remove the mask.
- Remove the mask at the doorway to the client's room. If using a respirator mask, remove it after leaving the room and closing the door.
- If using a mask with strings, first untie the lower strings of the mask. **Rationale:** *This prevents the top part of the mask from falling onto the chest.*
- Untie the top strings and, while holding the ties securely, remove the mask from the face. If side loops are present, lift the side loops up and away from the ears and face. Do not touch the front of the mask. **Rationale:** *The front of the mask through which the nurse has been breathing is contaminated.*
- Discard a disposable mask in the waste container.
- Perform proper hand hygiene again.

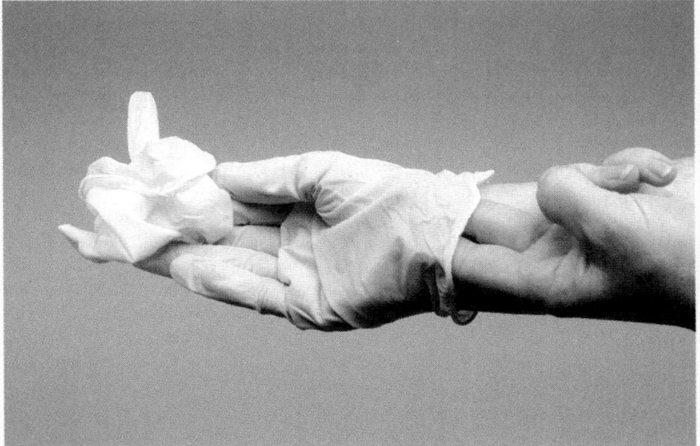

❹ Inserting fingers to remove the second contaminated glove.

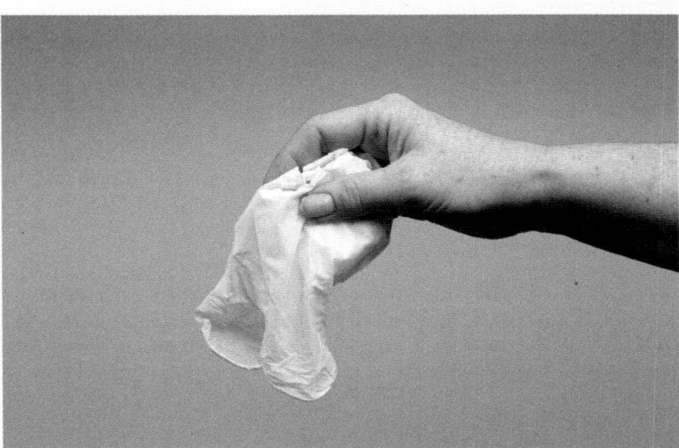

❺ Holding contaminated gloves that are inside out.

EVALUATION

- Conduct any follow-up indicated during your care of the client. If there has been any failure of the equipment and exposure to potentially infective materials is suspected, follow the procedure in the Practice Guidelines: Steps to Follow After Occupational Exposure to Bloodborne Pathogens later in this chapter.
- Ensure that an adequate supply of equipment is available for the next healthcare provider.

Gowns

Clean or disposable impervious (water-resistant) gowns or plastic aprons are worn during procedures when the nurse's uniform is likely to become soiled. Sterile gowns may be indicated when the nurse changes the dressings of a client with extensive wounds (e.g., burns). *Single-use gown technique* (using a gown only once before it is discarded or laundered) is the usual practice in hospitals. After the gown is worn, the nurse discards it (if it is paper) or places it in a laundry hamper. Plastic aprons should be discarded after use. Skill 31.2 describes the steps for applying and removing a gown. Before leaving the client's room, the nurse cleanses his or her hands.

Clinical Alert!

Wearing a client hospital gown over your uniform serves no infection prevention purpose.

Face Masks

Masks are worn to reduce the risk for transmission of organisms by the droplet contact and airborne routes and by splatters of body substances. The CDC recommends that masks be worn:

- By those close to the client if the infection (e.g., measles, mumps, or acute respiratory diseases in children) is transmitted by large-particle aerosols (droplets). Large-particle aerosols are transmitted by close contact and generally travel short distances (about 1 m, or 3 ft).
- By all individuals entering the room if the infection (e.g., pulmonary tuberculosis and SARS-CoV) is transmitted by small-particle aerosols (droplet nuclei). Small-particle aerosols remain suspended in the air and thus travel greater distances by air. Special masks that provide a tighter face seal and better filtration may be used for these infections.

Various types of masks differ in their filtration effectiveness and fit. Single-use disposable surgical masks are effective for use while the nurse provides care to most clients but should be changed if they become wet or soiled. These masks are discarded in the waste container after use. Disposable particulate respirators of different types may be effective for droplet transmission, splatters, and airborne microorganisms. Some respirators now available are effective in preventing inhalation of tuberculin organisms. The National Institute for Occupational Safety and Health (NIOSH), part of the CDC and a research agency of the U.S. Department of Health and Human Services, tests and certifies such respirators. Currently, the category "N" respirator at 95% efficiency (referred to as an N95 respirator) meets tuberculosis, SARS, and influenza control criteria.

During certain techniques requiring surgical asepsis (sterile technique), masks are worn (a) to prevent droplet contact transmission of exhaled microorganisms to the sterile field or to a client's open wound and (b) to protect the nurse from splashes of body substances from the client.

Guidelines for applying and removing face masks are shown in Skill 31.2 and in the Practice Guidelines.

Eyewear

Protective eyewear (goggles, glasses, or face shields) and masks are indicated in situations where body substances may splatter the face (see Skill 31.2). If the nurse wears prescription eyeglasses, goggles must still be worn over the glasses because the protection must extend around the sides of the glasses.

Disposal of Soiled Equipment and Supplies

Many pieces of equipment are supplied for single use only and are disposed of after use. Some items, however, are reusable. Agencies have specific policies and procedures for handling soiled equipment (e.g., disposal, cleaning, disinfecting, and sterilizing); the nurse needs to become familiar with these practices in the employing agency. Appropriate handling of soiled equipment and supplies is essential for these reasons:

- To prevent inadvertent exposure of healthcare workers to articles contaminated with body substances
- To prevent contamination of the environment.

Articles contaminated, or likely to have been contaminated, with infective material such as pus, blood, body fluids, feces, or respiratory secretions (biohazard waste) need to be enclosed in a sturdy container impervious to microorganisms before they are removed from the room

PRACTICE GUIDELINES Using an N95 Respirator Mask

If respirators are used for people performing work-related duties, employers must comply with the Occupational Safety and Health Administration's (OSHA) Respiratory Protection Standard, 29 CFR 1910.134.

- A respirator fit test is required to confirm the fit of any respirator that forms a tight seal on the wearer's face before it is to be used in the workplace.
- Because each brand, model, and size fits slightly differently, you should have a fit test every time a new model, manufacture type or brand, or size is worn. Also, if your weight fluctuates or facial or dental alterations occur, a fit test should be done again to ensure the respirator remains effective. Otherwise, fit testing should be completed at least annually to ensure continued adequate fit (Zhuang et al., 2016).
- Before handling the respirator, wash hands thoroughly with soap and water.
- Inspect the respirator for damages. If your respirator has been damaged, DO NOT USE IT. Get a new one.
- Anything that comes between the respirator and your face will make the respirator less effective. Do not allow facial hair, hair, jewelry, glasses, or clothing to come between your face and the respirator or interfere with the placement of the respirator on the face.

EVIDENCE-BASED PRACTICE

Evidence-Based Practice

How Effectively Do Providers Use PPE?

Events such as the 2014 Ebola outbreak demonstrate that there is lack of consensus regarding the proper use of PPE in some situations and that healthcare workers may be vulnerable to infection even when they believe they are using PPE correctly. Kang et al. (2017) conducted 130 simulated situations in which providers (80% were nurses) applied and removed both routine and full-body PPE. The sessions were recorded and contamination was determined using fluorescent powder. Even though they knew they were being taped, and even after receiving individual feedback prior to being rerecorded, the contamination rate was 80%. When surveyed, participants stated that barriers to effective use of PPE included the time required, that functioning with PPE in place was awkward, and that PPE might not even be effective.

Implications

The study authors concluded that better standardized PPE protocols and implementing innovative PPE education were necessary. It is evident that existing education of students does not translate into effective practice. Although time consuming and expensive, it may be that stricter regulations on training, feedback, demonstrated competence, and peer support may be necessary on an annual basis for all providers.

of any client. Some agencies use labels or containers of a particular color (usually red) that designates them as infective wastes.

CDC guidelines recommend the following methods:

- A single bag or container, if it is sturdy and impervious to microorganisms, and if the contaminated articles can be placed without soiling or contaminating its outside.
- Double-bagging if the above conditions are not met.
- Follow agency protocol, or use the following CDC guidelines to handle and bag soiled items:
  - Place garbage and soiled *disposable* equipment, including dressings and tissues but not sharps, in the appropriate and labeled bag or container and immediately close it. If the bag is sturdy and impermeable to microorganisms (waterproof or solid enough to prevent organisms from moving through it even when wet), a single bag is adequate. If not, place the first bag inside another impermeable bag. Some agencies have a particular location where such garbage is to be placed. Some also separate dry and wet waste material and incinerate dry items, such as paper towels and disposable items. No special precautions are required for disposable equipment that is not contaminated.
  - Place *nondisposable* or *reusable* equipment that is visibly soiled in a labeled container before removing it from the client's room or cubicle, and send it to a central processing area for decontamination. Some agencies may require that glass bottles or jars and metal items be placed in separate bags from plastic items.
  - Disassemble special procedure trays into component parts. Some components are disposable; others need to be sent to the laundry or central services for cleaning and decontaminating.
- Bag soiled client clothing before sending it home or to the agency laundry.

Linens

Handle soiled linen as little as possible and with the least agitation possible. Roll the linen with the soiled side in before placing it in the laundry hamper. This prevents gross microbial contamination of the air and individuals handling the linen. Close the bag before sending it to the laundry in accordance with agency practice.

Laboratory Specimens

Laboratory specimens, if placed in a leakproof container with a secure lid with a biohazard label, need no special precautions. Use care when collecting specimens to avoid contaminating the outside of the container. Containers that are visibly contaminated on the outside should be placed inside a sealable plastic bag before sending them to the laboratory. This prevents personnel from having hand contact with potentially infective material.

Dishes and Utensils

Dishes and utensils require no special precautions. Soiling can largely be prevented by encouraging clients to cleanse their hands before eating. Some agencies use disposable dishes for convenience.

Blood Pressure Equipment

Blood pressure equipment needs no special precautions unless it becomes contaminated with infective material. If it does become contaminated, follow agency policy to decontaminate it. Cleaning procedures vary according to whether it is a wall or portable unit. In some agencies, a disposable cuff is used. Stethoscopes should be cleaned frequently and between clients to remove gross contamination. Dedicated stethoscopes are used when a client is in isolation.

Disposable Needles, Syringes, and Sharps

Place all needles, syringes, and "sharps" (e.g., lancets, scalpels, and broken glass) into a labeled, puncture-resistant container approved only for this use. To avoid puncture wounds, use safety or needleless systems and do not detach needles from the syringe or recap the needle before disposal. See Chapter 35 ∞ for how to prevent needlestick injuries.

Clinical Alert!

Federal rules protecting the privacy of personal health information (PHI) may extend to the client labels placed on disposable supplies such as intravenous fluid containers. Agencies may require the nurse to remove the label or return the supplies to the pharmacy so that personal information may be removed before disposal. Never place items with PHI in the regular trash. Check agency policy.

Transporting Clients with Infections

Avoid transporting clients with infections outside their own rooms unless absolutely necessary. If a client must be moved, the nurse implements appropriate precautions and measures to prevent contamination of the environment. For example, the nurse ensures that any draining wound is securely covered or places a surgical mask on the client who has an airborne infection. In addition, the nurse notifies personnel at the receiving area of any infection risk so that they can maintain necessary precautions. Follow agency protocol.

Psychosocial Needs of Isolation Clients

Clients requiring isolation precautions can develop several problems as a result of the separation from others and of the special precautions taken in their care. Two of the most common are sensory deprivation and decreased self-esteem related to feelings of inferiority. *Sensory deprivation* occurs when the environment lacks normal stimuli for the client, for example, communication with others. Nurses should therefore be alert to common clinical signs of sensory deprivation: boredom, inactivity, slowness of thought, daydreaming, increased sleeping, thought disorganization, anxiety, hallucinations, and panic.

Chapter 39 ∞ provides information on the development of self-esteem and self-esteem disturbances. A client's *feeling of inferiority* can be due to the perception of the infection itself or to the required precautions. In North America, many people place a high value on cleanliness, and the idea of being "soiled," "contaminated," or "dirty" can give clients the feeling that they have done something bad. The infected clients may feel "not as good" as others and blame themselves. An appropriate nursing diagnosis may be potential alteration in self-esteem.

Nurses need to provide care that prevents these two problems or that deals with them positively. Nursing interventions include the following:

1. Assess the client's need for stimulation.
2. Initiate measures to help meet the need, including regular communication with the client and diversionary activities, such as toys for a child, and telephone, books, television, computer, or radio for an adult; provide a variety of foods to stimulate the client's sense of taste; stimulate the client's visual sense by providing a view or an activity to watch.
3. Explain the infection and the associated procedures to help clients and their support persons understand and accept the situation.
4. Demonstrate warm, accepting behavior. Avoid conveying to the client any sense of annoyance about the precautions or any feelings of revulsion about the infection.
5. Use the least strict precautions indicated by the diagnosis or the client's condition.

Sterile Technique

An object is sterile only when it is free of all microorganisms. It is well known that sterile technique is practiced in operating rooms and special diagnostic areas. Less known perhaps is that sterile technique is also employed for many procedures in general care areas (such as when administering injections, changing wound dressings, performing urinary catheterizations, and administering intravenous therapy). The basic principles of surgical asepsis, and practices that relate to each principle, appear in Table 31.7.

TABLE 31.7 Principles and Practices of Surgical Asepsis

Principles	Practices
All objects used in a sterile field must be sterile.	Always check a package containing a sterile object for intactness, dryness, and expiration date. Sterile articles can be stored for only a prescribed time; after that, they are considered unsterile. Any package that appears already open, torn, punctured, or wet is considered unsterile.
	Storage areas should be clean, dry, off the floor, and away from sinks.
	Always check indicators of sterilization before using a package. The indicator is often a tape used to fasten the package or contained inside the package. The indicator changes color during sterilization, indicating that the contents have undergone a sterilization procedure. If the color change is not evident, the package is considered unsterile. Commercially prepared sterile packages may not have indicators but are marked with the word *sterile*.
Sterile objects become unsterile when touched by unsterile objects.	Handle sterile objects that will touch open wounds or enter body cavities only with sterile forceps or sterile gloved hands.
	Discard or resterilize objects that come into contact with unsterile objects.
	Whenever the sterility of an object is questionable, assume the article is unsterile.

TABLE 31.7 Principles and Practices of Surgical Asepsis—*continued*

Principles	Practices
Sterile objects that are out of sight or below the waist or table level are considered unsterile.	Once left unattended, a sterile field is considered unsterile. Sterile objects are always kept in view. Nurses do not turn their backs on a sterile field. Only the front part of a sterile gown, from shoulder to waist (or table height, whichever is higher), and the cuff of the sleeves to 5 cm (2 in.) above the elbows are considered sterile. Always keep sterile gloved hands in sight and above waist or table level; touch only objects that are sterile. Sterile draped tables in the operating room or elsewhere are considered sterile only at surface level.
Sterile objects can become unsterile by exposure to airborne microorganisms.	Keep doors closed and traffic to a minimum in areas where a sterile procedure is being performed, because moving air can carry dust and microorganisms. Keep areas in which sterile procedures are carried out as clean as possible by frequent damp cleaning with detergent germicides to minimize contaminants in the area. Prevent hair from falling on sterile objects. Microorganisms on the hair can make a sterile field unsterile. Refrain from sneezing or coughing over a sterile field. Droplets from sneezing or coughing contain microorganisms from the respiratory tract that can travel 1 m (3 ft). Some agencies recommend that masks covering the mouth and the nose be worn by anyone working over a sterile field or an open wound. When working over a sterile field, keep talking to a minimum. To prevent microorganisms from falling over a sterile field, refrain from reaching over a sterile field unless sterile gloves are worn and refrain from moving unsterile objects over a sterile field.
Fluids flow in the direction of gravity.	Unless gloves are worn, always hold wet forceps with the tips below the handles. When the tips are held higher than the handles, fluid can flow onto the handle and become contaminated by the hands. When the forceps are again pointed downward, the contaminated fluid flows back down and contaminates the tips. During a surgical hand wash, hold the hands higher than the elbows to prevent contaminants from the forearms from reaching the hands.
Moisture that passes through a sterile object draws microorganisms from unsterile surfaces above or below to the sterile surface by capillary action.	Sterile moisture-proof barriers are used beneath sterile objects. Liquids are frequently poured into containers on a sterile field. If they are spilled onto the sterile field, the barrier keeps the liquid from seeping beneath it. Keep the sterile covers on sterile equipment dry. Damp surfaces can attract microorganisms in the air. Replace sterile drapes that do not have a sterile barrier underneath when they become moist.
The edges of a sterile field are considered unsterile.	A 2.5-cm (1-in.) margin at each edge of an opened drape is considered unsterile because the edges are in contact with unsterile surfaces. Place all sterile objects more than 2.5 cm (1 in.) inside the edges of a sterile field. Any article that falls outside the edges of a sterile field is considered unsterile.
The skin cannot be sterilized and is unsterile.	Use sterile gloves or sterile forceps to handle sterile items. Prior to a surgical aseptic procedure, cleanse the hands to reduce the number of microorganisms on them.
Conscientiousness, alertness, and honesty are essential qualities in maintaining surgical asepsis.	When a sterile object becomes unsterile, it does not necessarily change in appearance. The staff member who sees a sterile object become contaminated must correct or report the situation. Do not set up a sterile field ahead of time for future use.

Sterile Field

A **sterile field** is a microorganism-free area. Nurses often establish a sterile field by using the innermost side of a sterile wrapper or by using a sterile drape. When the field is established, sterile supplies can be placed on it. Sterile forceps are used in many instances to handle and transfer sterile supplies.

So that sterility can be maintained, supplies may be wrapped in a variety of materials. Commercially prepared items are frequently wrapped in plastic, paper, or glass. Sterile liquids (e.g., sterile water for irrigations) are preferably packaged in amounts adequate for one use only because once a container has been opened, there is no assurance that it will remain sterile. Any leftover liquid is discarded.

Skill 31.3 describes how to establish and maintain a sterile field.

SKILL 31.3

Establishing and Maintaining a Sterile Field

PURPOSE

- To ensure that sterile items remain sterile

ASSESSMENT

Review the client's record or discuss with the client exactly what procedure will be performed that requires a sterile field. Assess the client for the presence of or risk for infection and ability to participate with the procedure.

PLANNING

Determine, if possible, what supplies and techniques have been used in the past to perform the sterile procedure for this client. Also, attempt to determine if the procedure will be performed again in the future, so you can conduct appropriate client teaching and ensure that adequate supplies will be available.

Schedule the procedure at a time consistent with the primary care provider's order, the need for the procedure, and the client's other activities.

Assignment

Sterile procedures are not assigned to AP.

Equipment

- Package containing a sterile drape
- Sterile equipment as needed (e.g., wrapped sterile gauze, wrapped sterile bowl, antiseptic solution, sterile forceps)

IMPLEMENTATION

Preparation

- Ensure that the package is clean and dry; if moisture is noted on the inside of a plastic-wrapped package or the outside of a cloth-wrapped package, it is considered contaminated and must be discarded.
- Check the sterilization expiration dates on the package, and look for any indications that it has been previously opened. Spots or stains on cloth or paper-wrapped objects may indicate contamination, and the objects should not be used.
- Follow agency practice for disposal of possibly contaminated packages.

Performance

1. Prior to performing the procedure, introduce self and verify the client's identity using agency protocol. Explain to the client what you are going to do, why it is necessary, and how to participate. Discuss how the results will be used in planning further care or treatments.
2. Perform hand hygiene and observe other appropriate infection prevention procedures (see Skills 31.1 and 31.2).
3. Provide for client privacy.
4. Open the package. If the package is inside a plastic cover, remove the cover.

To Open a Wrapped Package on a Surface

- Cleanse the work surface with soap and water or agency-approved disinfectant and dry it.
- Place the package in the work area so that the top flap of the wrapper opens away from you.
- Reaching around the package (not over it), pinch the first flap on the outside of the wrapper between the thumb and index finger. ❶ **Rationale:** *Touching only the outside of the wrapper maintains the sterility of the inside of the wrapper.* Pull the flap open, laying it flat on the far surface.
- Repeat for the side flaps, opening the topmost one first. Use the right hand for the right flap, and the left hand for the left flap. ❷ **Rationale:** *By using both hands, you avoid reaching over the sterile contents.*
- Pull the fourth flap toward you by grasping the corner that is turned down. ❸

Variation: Opening a Wrapped Package While Holding It

- Hold the package in one hand with the top flap opening away from you.
- Using the other hand, open the package as described above, pulling the corners of the flaps well back. ❹ Tuck each of the corners into the hand holding the package so that they do not flutter and contaminate sterile objects. The hands are considered contaminated, and at no time should they touch the contents of the package.

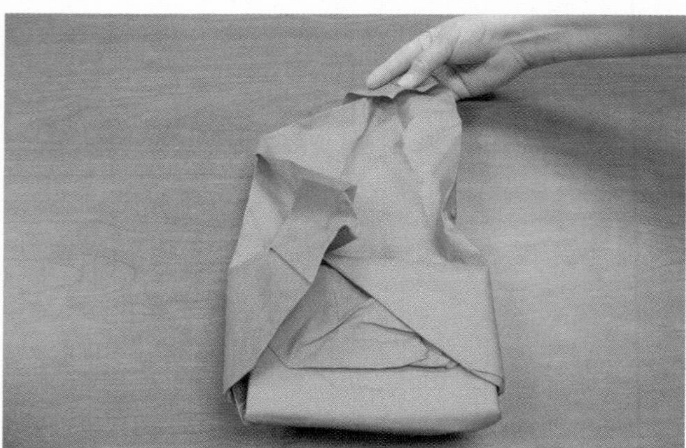

❶ Opening the first flap of a sterile wrapped package.

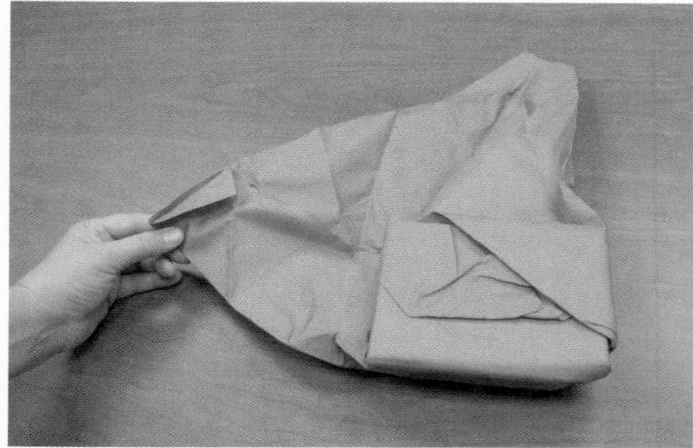

❷ Opening the second flap to the side.

Establishing and Maintaining a Sterile Field—*continued*

SKILL 31.3

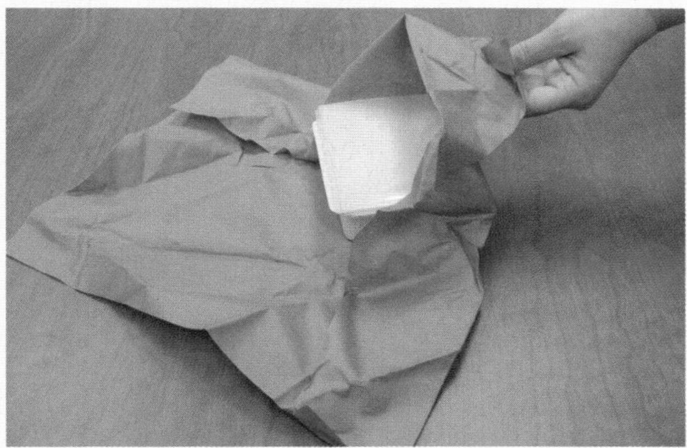
3 Pulling the last flap toward oneself by grasping the corner.

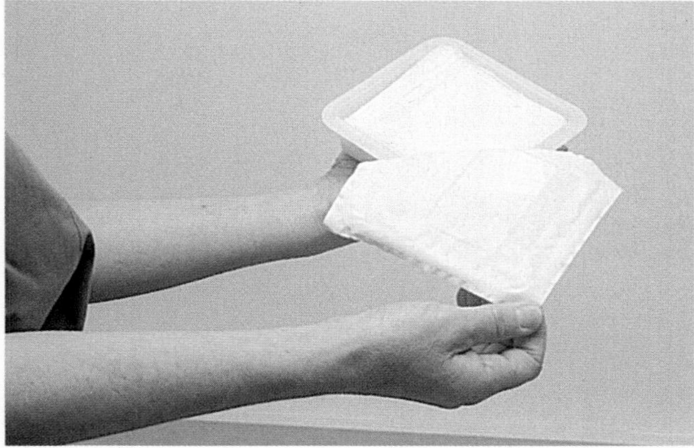
5 Opening a sterile package that has an unsealed corner.

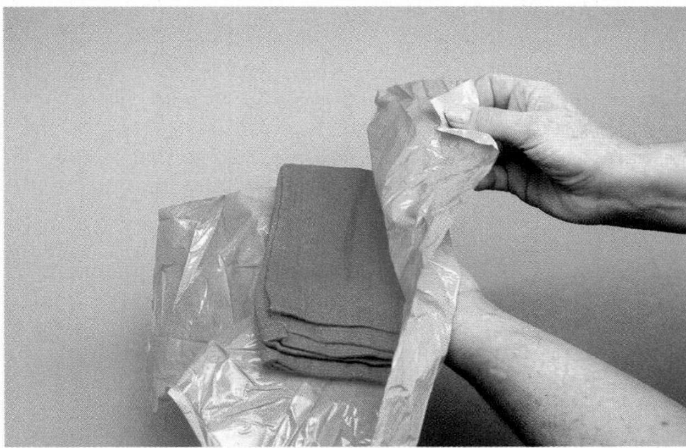
4 Opening a wrapped package while holding it.

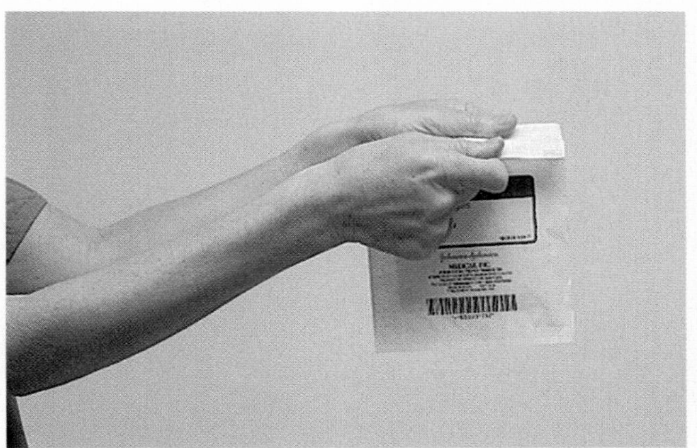
6 Opening a sterile package that has a partially sealed edge.

Variation: Opening Commercially Prepared Packages

- If the flap of the package has an unsealed corner, hold the package in one hand, and pull back on the flap with the other hand. 5
- If the package has a partially sealed edge, grasp both sides of the edge, one with each hand, and pull apart gently. 6

5. Establish a sterile field by using a drape.
   - Open the package containing the drape as described above.
   - With one hand, pluck the corner of the drape that is folded back on the top touching only one side of the drape.
   - Lift the drape out of the cover, and allow it to open freely without touching any objects. 7 **Rationale:** *If the drape touches the outside of the package or any unsterile surface, it is considered contaminated*.
   - With the other hand, carefully pick up another corner of the drape, holding it well away from you and, again, touching only the same side of the drape as the first hand.
   - Lay the drape on a clean and dry surface, placing the bottom (i.e., the freely hanging side) farthest from you. 8 **Rationale:** *By placing the lowermost side farthest away, you avoid leaning over the sterile field and contaminating it*.
6. Add necessary sterile supplies, being careful not to touch the drape with the hands.

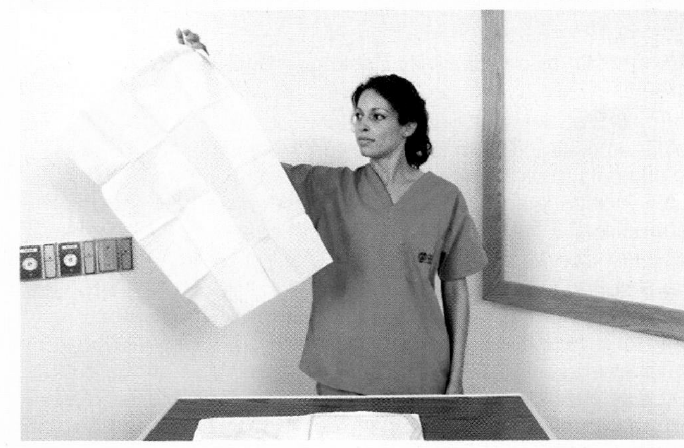
7 Allowing a drape to open freely without touching any objects.

To Add Wrapped Supplies to a Sterile Field

- Open each wrapped package as described in the preceding steps.
- With the free hand, grasp the corners of the wrapper, and hold them against the wrist of the other hand. 9 **Rationale:** *The sterile wrapper now covers the unsterile hand*.
- Place the sterile bowl, drape, or other supply on the sterile field by approaching from an angle rather than holding the arm over the field. Discard the wrapper.

Continued on page 720

SKILL 31.3

Establishing and Maintaining a Sterile Field—*continued*

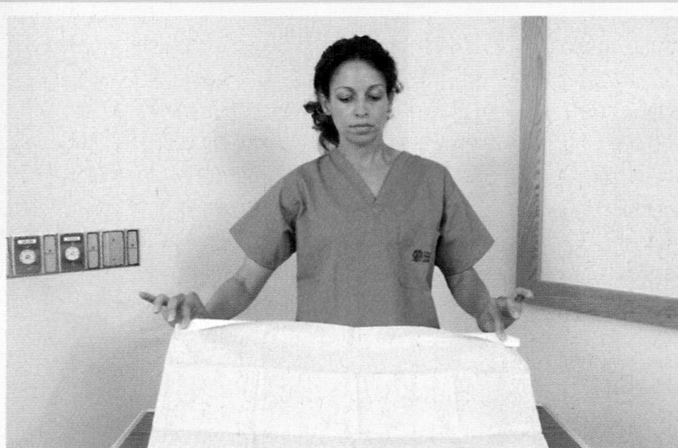

8 Placing a drape on a surface.

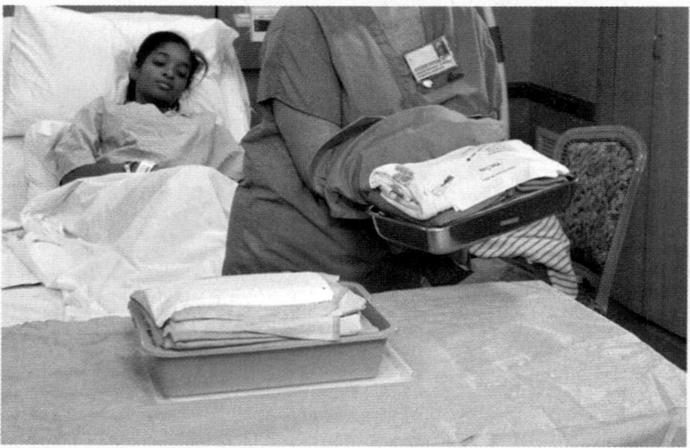

9 Adding wrapped sterile supplies to a sterile field.

Variation: Adding Commercially Packaged Supplies to a Sterile Field

- Open each package as previously described.
- Hold the package 15 cm (6 in.) above the field, and allow the contents to drop on the field. 10 Keep in mind that 2.5 cm (1 in.) around the edge of the field is considered contaminated. **Rationale:** *At a height of 15 cm (6 in.), the outside of the package is not likely to touch and contaminate the sterile field.*

Adding Solution to a Sterile Bowl

Liquids (e.g., normal saline) may need to be poured into containers within a sterile field. Unwrapped bottles that contain sterile solution are considered sterile on the inside and contaminated on the outside because the bottle may have been handled. Bottles used in an operating room may be sterilized on the outside as well as the inside, however, and these are handled with sterile gloves.

- Obtain the exact amount of solution, if possible. **Rationale:** *Once a sterile bottle has been opened, its sterility cannot be ensured for future use. Follow agency policy for reuse of opened sterile solution bottles.*
- Before pouring any liquid, read the label 3 times to make sure you have the correct solution and concentration (strength). Wipe the outside of the bottle with a damp towel to remove any large particles that could fall into the bowl or field.
- Remove the lid or cap from the bottle and invert the lid before placing it on a surface that is not sterile. **Rationale:** *Inverting the lid maintains the sterility of the inside surface because it is not allowed to touch an unsterile surface.*

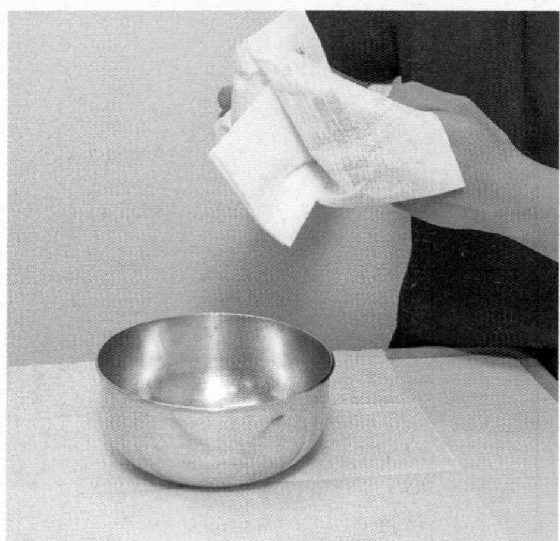

10 Adding commercially packaged gauze to a sterile field.

- Hold the bottle so that the label is against the palm of the hand. **Rationale:** *Any solution that flows down the outside of the bottle during pouring will not damage or obliterate the label.*
- Hold the bottle of fluid at a height of 10 to 15 cm (4 to 6 in.) over the bowl and to the side of the sterile field so that as little of the bottle as possible is over the field. 11 **Rationale:** *At this height, there is less likelihood of contaminating the sterile field by touching the field or by reaching an arm over it.*
- Pour the solution gently to avoid splashing the liquid. **Rationale:** *If a barrier drape (one that has a water-resistant layer) is not used and the drape is on an unsterile surface, moisture will contaminate the field by wicking microorganisms through the drape.*
- Tilt the neck of the bottle back to vertical quickly when done pouring so that none of the liquid flows down the outside of the bottle. **Rationale:** *Such drips would contaminate the sterile field if the outside of the bottle is not sterile.*
- If the bottle will be used again, replace the lid securely and write on the label the date and time of opening. **Rationale:** *Replacing the lid immediately maintains the sterility of the inner aspect of the lid and the solution.* Depending on agency policy, a sterile container of solution that is opened may be used only once and is then discarded (such as in the operating room). In other settings, policy may permit recapped bottles to be reused within 24 hours.

7. Use sterile forceps to handle sterile supplies. Forceps are used to move a sterile article from one place to another, for example, transferring sterile gauze from its package to a sterile dressing tray. Forceps may be disposable or resterilized after use. Commonly used forceps include hemostats 12 and tissue forceps. 13

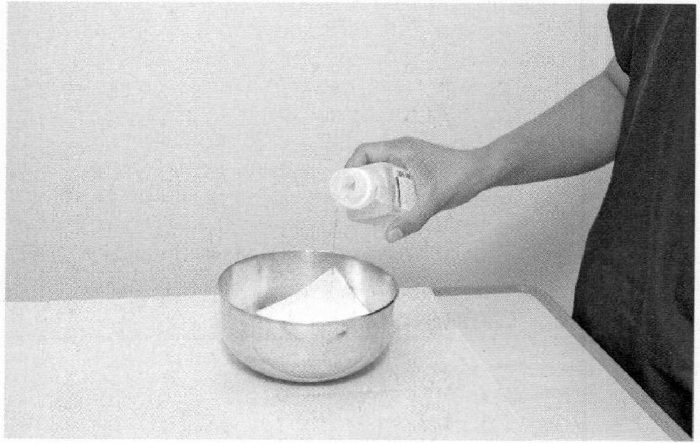

11 Adding a liquid to a sterile bowl.

Establishing and Maintaining a Sterile Field—*continued*

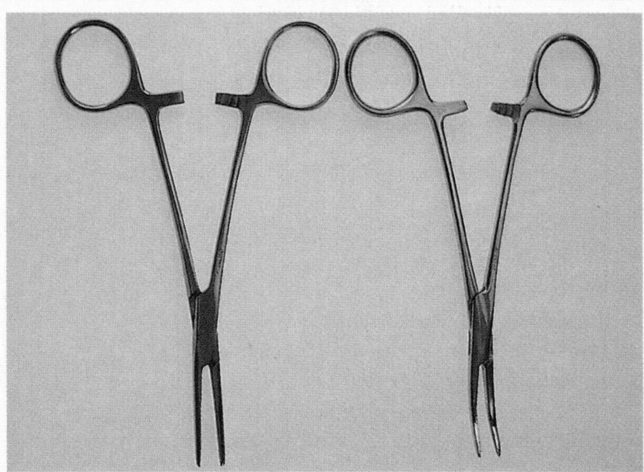

⓬ Hemostats: *Left*, straight; *Right*, curved.

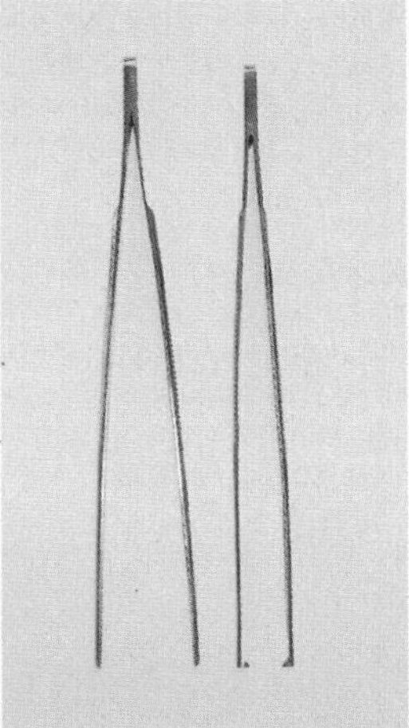

⓭ Tissue forceps: *Left*, plain; *Right*, toothed.

- If forceps tips are wet, keep the tips lower than the wrist at all times, unless you are wearing sterile gloves. ⓮ **Rationale:** *Gravity prevents liquids on the tips of the forceps from flowing to the unsterile handles and later back to the tips.*

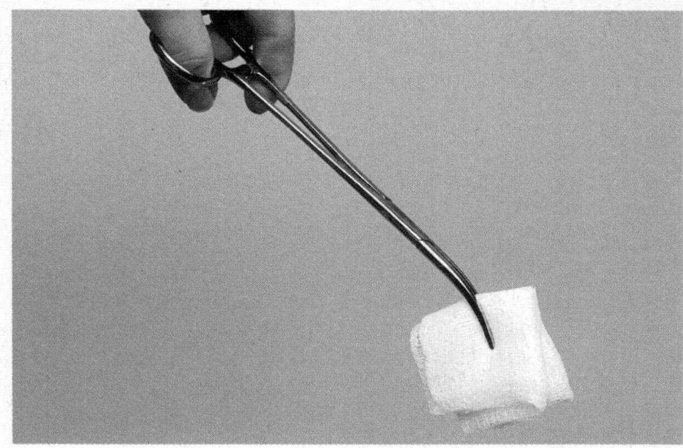

⓮ Holding forceps with an ungloved hand, keeping the tips lower than the wrist.

- Hold sterile forceps above waist or table level, whichever is higher. **Rationale:** *Items held below waist or table level are considered contaminated.*
- Hold sterile forceps within sight. **Rationale:** *While out of sight, forceps may, unknown to the user, become unsterile. Any forceps that go out of sight should be considered unsterile.*
- When using forceps to lift sterile supplies, be sure that the forceps do not touch the edges or outside of the wrapper. **Rationale:** *The edges and outside of the sterile field are considered unsterile.*
- When placing forceps whose handles were in contact with the bare hand, position the handles outside the sterile area. **Rationale:** *The handles of these forceps harbor microorganisms from the bare hand.*
- Deposit a sterile item on a sterile field without permitting moist forceps to touch the sterile field when the surface under the absorbent sterile field is unsterile and a barrier drape is not used.

8. Document that sterile technique was used in the performance of the procedure.

EVALUATION

- Conduct any follow-up indicated during your care of the client. Ensure that adequate numbers and types of sterile supplies are available for the next healthcare provider.

Sterile Gloves

Sterile gloves may be applied by the open method or the closed method. The open method is most frequently used outside the operating room because the closed method requires that the nurse wear a sterile gown. Gloves are worn during many procedures to enable the nurse to handle sterile items freely and to prevent clients at risk (e.g., those with open wounds) from becoming infected by microorganisms on unsterile gloves or the nurse's hands.

Sterile gloves are packaged with a cuff of about 5 cm (2 in.) and with the palms facing upward when the package is opened. The package usually indicates the size of the glove (e.g., size 6 or 7 1/2 or small, medium, large).

Sterile gloves protect the nurse from contact with blood and body fluids. Nitrile gloves are more flexible than vinyl, mold to the wearer's hands, and allow freedom of movement. Wear nitrile gloves when performing tasks (a) that demand flexibility, (b) that place stress on the material (e.g., turning stopcocks, handling sharp instruments or tape), and (c) that involve a high risk of exposure to pathogens. Vinyl gloves should be chosen for tasks unlikely to stress the glove material, requiring minimal precision, and with minimal risk of exposure to pathogens. As of January 2017, the FDA has banned the use of powder in surgical and examination gloves (FDA, 2016a).

Skill 31.4 describes how to apply and remove sterile gloves by the open method.

SKILL 31.4

Applying and Removing Sterile Gloves (Open Method)

PURPOSES

- To enable the nurse to handle or touch sterile objects freely without contaminating them
- To prevent transmission of potentially infective organisms from the nurse's hands to clients at high risk for infection

ASSESSMENT

Review the client's record and orders to determine exactly what procedure will be performed that requires sterile gloves. Use nonlatex gloves whenever possible.

PLANNING

Think through the procedure, planning which steps need to be completed before the gloves can be applied. Determine what additional supplies are needed to perform the procedure for this client. Always have an extra pair of sterile gloves available.

Assignment

Sterile procedures are not assigned to AP.

Equipment

- Packages of sterile gloves

IMPLEMENTATION

Preparation

Ensure the sterility of the package of gloves.

Performance

1. Prior to performing the procedure, introduce self and verify the client's identity using agency protocol. Explain to the client what you are going to do, why it is necessary.
2. Perform hand hygiene and observe other appropriate infection prevention procedures (see Skills 31.1, 31.2, and 31.3).
3. Provide for client privacy.
4. Open the package of sterile gloves.
   - Place the package of gloves on a clean, dry surface. **Rationale:** *Any moisture on the surface could contaminate the gloves.*
   - Some gloves are packed in an inner as well as an outer package. Open the outer package without contaminating the gloves or the inner package. See Skill 31.3.
   - Remove the inner package from the outer package.
   - Open the inner package as in step 4 of Skill 31.3 or according to the manufacturer's directions. Some manufacturers provide a numbered sequence for opening the flaps and folded tabs to grasp for opening the flaps. If no tabs are provided, pluck the flap so that the fingers do not touch the inner surfaces. **Rationale:** *The inner surfaces, which are next to the sterile gloves, will remain sterile.*
5. Put the first glove on the dominant hand.
   - If the gloves are packaged so that they lie side by side, grasp the glove for the dominant hand by its folded cuff edge (on the palmar side) with the thumb and first finger of the nondominant hand. Touch only the inside of the cuff. ❶ **Rationale:** *The hands are not sterile. By touching only the inside of the glove, the nurse avoids contaminating the outside.*
   - If the gloves are packaged one on top of the other, grasp the cuff of the top glove as above, using the opposite hand.
   - Insert the dominant hand into the glove and pull the glove on. Keep the thumb of the inserted hand against the palm of the hand during insertion. ❷ **Rationale:** *If the thumb is kept against the palm, it is less likely to contaminate the outside of the glove.*
   - Leave the cuff in place once the unsterile hand releases the glove. **Rationale:** *Attempting to further unfold the cuff is likely to contaminate the glove.*
6. Put the second glove on the nondominant hand.
   - Pick up the other glove with the sterile gloved hand, inserting the gloved fingers under the cuff and holding the gloved thumb close to the gloved palm. ❸

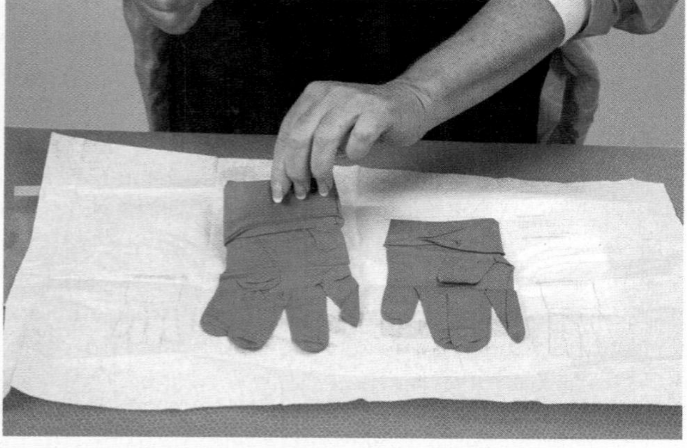

❶ Picking up the first sterile glove.

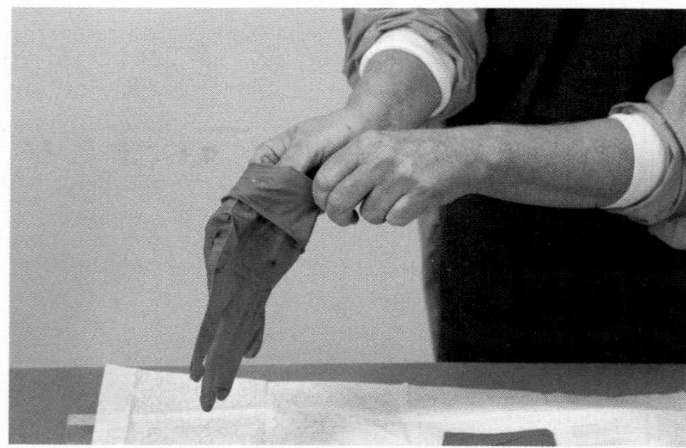

❷ Putting on the first sterile glove.

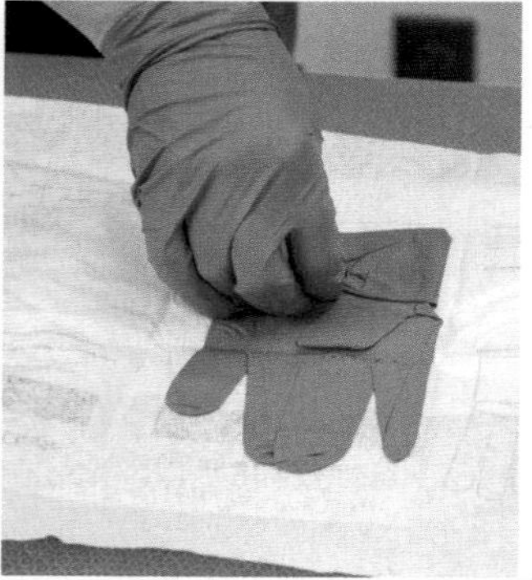

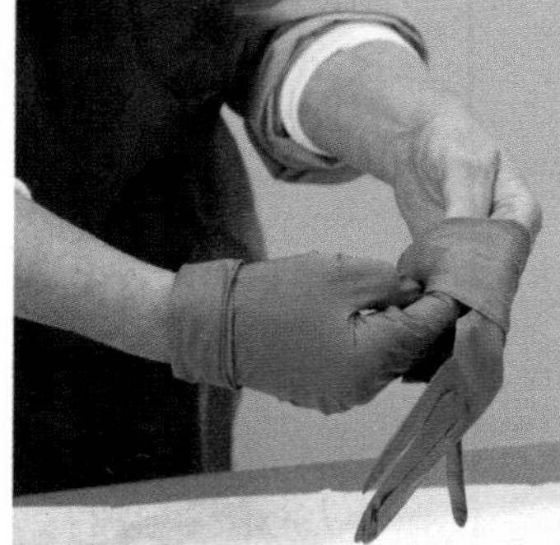

❸ Picking up the second sterile glove.

Applying and Removing Sterile Gloves (Open Method)—*continued*

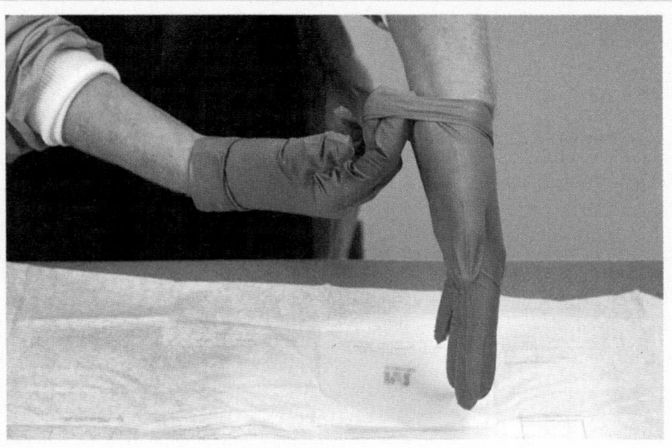

4 Putting on the second sterile glove.

- Pull on the second glove carefully. Hold the thumb of the gloved first hand as far as possible from the palm. 4 **Rationale:** *In this position, the thumb is less likely to touch the arm and become contaminated.*
- Adjust each glove so that it fits smoothly, and carefully pull the cuffs up by sliding the fingers under the cuffs.

7. Remove and dispose of used gloves.
   - There is no technique for removing sterile gloves that is different from removing unsterile gloves. If they are soiled with secretions, remove them by turning them inside out. See removal of gloves in Skill 31.2.
   - Perform hand hygiene.
8. Document that sterile technique was used in the performance of the procedure.

EVALUATION

- Conduct any follow-up indicated during your care of the client. Ensure that adequate numbers and types of sterile supplies are available for the next healthcare provider.

Infection Prevention for Healthcare Workers

NIOSH investigates potentially hazardous working conditions and publishes recommendations for preventing workplace illnesses and injuries.

OSHA, an agency of the U.S. Department of Labor, publishes and enforces regulations to protect healthcare workers from occupational injuries, including exposure to bloodborne pathogens in the workplace. **Occupational exposure** is defined as skin, eye, mucous membrane, or parenteral contact with blood or other potentially infectious materials that may result from the performance of an employee's duties.

There are three major modes of transmission of infectious materials in the clinical setting:

- Puncture wounds from contaminated needles or other sharps
- Skin contact, which allows infectious fluids to enter through wounds and broken or damaged skin
- Mucous membrane contact, which allows infectious fluids to enter through mucous membranes of the eyes, mouth, or nose.

Using proper precautions with general medical asepsis, appropriately using PPE (gloves, masks, gowns, goggles, special resuscitative equipment), and avoiding carelessness in the clinical area will place the caregiver at significantly less risk for injury. The chance of a healthcare worker becoming infected following exposure to pathogens varies widely; estimates range from 6% to 30% for HBV nonimmune workers (depending on the antigen status of the source individual), to 1.8% for hepatitis C (HCV), to 0.3% for an HIV needlestick or cut exposure—and even less for a skin or mucous membrane exposure (Kuhar et al., 2013). HCV, a worldwide epidemic greater than HIV, has become a significant concern to all healthcare workers because no vaccine against the virus or postexposure prophylaxis currently exists. Prevention remains the primary goal. Measures to be taken in case of possible exposure to these viruses are delineated by the U.S. Public Health Service (Kerns & Sheridan, 2019) and outlined in the accompanying Practice Guidelines. You should consider in advance whether you would want prophylaxis for HIV exposure since this is optimally begun within hours of exposure.

OSHA requires that healthcare employers make the HBV vaccine and vaccination series available to all employees. Other vaccinations may also be made available (e.g., nurses working in an obstetric area should be vaccinated against rubella to protect pregnant clients and their fetuses).

Role of the Infection Prevention Nurse

All healthcare organizations must have interdisciplinary infection prevention committees. Representatives from the clinical laboratory, housekeeping, maintenance, dietary, and client care areas are included. An important member of this committee is the infection prevention nurse. This nurse is specially trained to be knowledgeable about the latest research and practices in preventing, detecting, and treating infections. All infections are reported to the nurse in a manner that allows for recording and analyzing statistics that can assist in improving infection prevention practices. In addition, the infection prevention nurse may be involved in employee education and implementation of the bloodborne pathogen exposure plan mandated by OSHA.

PRACTICE GUIDELINES **Steps to Follow After Occupational Exposure to Bloodborne Pathogens**

- Report the incident immediately to appropriate personnel within the agency.
- Complete an injury or accident report and an incident report if required by the agency.
- Seek appropriate evaluation and follow-up. This includes:
  - Identification and documentation of the source individual when feasible and legal. Sometimes the source individual is unknown or the individual's identity is protected by law.
  - Testing of the source for HBV, HCV, and HIV when feasible and consent is given.
  - Making results of the test available to the source individual's healthcare provider.
  - Testing of blood of exposed nurse (with consent) for HBV, HCV, and HIV antibodies.
  - Postexposure prophylaxis if medically indicated.
  - Medical and psychologic counseling regarding personal risk of infection or risk of infecting others.
  - Counseling to use precautions (e.g., use of barrier contraception and avoidance of blood or tissue donations, pregnancy, and, if possible, breastfeeding) to prevent secondary transmission, especially during the first 6 to 12 weeks after exposure.
- For a puncture or laceration:
  - Allow some bleeding to drain the site but do not squeeze the tissues.
  - Clean the area with soap and water.
  - Initiate first aid and seek treatment if indicated.
- For a mucous membrane exposure (eyes, nose, mouth), saline or water flush for 5 to 10 minutes.

POSTEXPOSURE PROTOCOL (PEP)

HIV

- Treatment should be started as soon as possible, preferably within hours after exposure. Treatment may be less effective when started more than 24 hours after exposure. Starting treatment after a longer period (e.g., 1 week) should be considered for high-risk exposures previously untreated.
- Treatment with three or more antiviral drugs is recommended.
- Drug prophylaxis continues for 4 weeks. If the source is determined to be HIV negative, PEP should be discontinued.
- Drug regimens vary and new drugs and regimens are continuously being developed.
- HIV antibody tests should be done shortly after exposure (baseline), and 6 weeks, 3 months, and 6 months afterward. If a fourth-generation combination HIV p24 antigen–HIV antibody test is being utilized, then testing can be performed at baseline, 6 weeks, and ended at 4 months.

Hepatitis B

- Anti-HBs testing after last vaccine dose.
- Hepatitis B immune globulin and/or hepatitis B vaccine within 1 to 7 days following exposure for nonimmune workers.

Hepatitis C

- Anti-HCV and liver enzymes (e.g., alanine transaminase) at baseline and 4 to 6 months after exposure.

Evaluating

Using data collected during care—vital signs, lung sounds, skin status, characteristics of urine or other drainage, laboratory blood values, and so on—the nurse judges whether client outcomes have been achieved.

If outcomes have not been achieved, the nurse may need to consider questions such as the following:

- Were appropriate measures implemented to prevent skin breakdown and lung infection?
- Was strict aseptic technique implemented for invasive procedures?
- Are prescribed medications affecting the immune system?
- Is client placement appropriate to reduce the risk of transmission of microorganisms?
- Did the client and family misunderstand or fail to comply with necessary instructions?

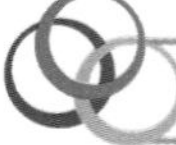

Critical Thinking Checkpoint

Mrs. Cortez is a 76-year-old woman who is independent, lives alone, and prefers not to rely on others unless absolutely necessary. She was active and healthy until about 6 months ago, at which time she developed a persistent upper respiratory infection. Because she was unable to obtain or prepare foods, she lost weight and became very weak. She finally sought medical attention, but she has not yet fully recovered. Her primary care provider has admitted Mrs. Cortez to the hospital for shortness of breath, productive cough, dehydration, and nutritional deficiency.

1. Mrs. Cortez's primary care provider suspects that Mrs. Cortez has pneumonia. What data support Mrs. Cortez's increased risk for such an infection?
2. What other information or assessment data would be helpful to you when planning care for Mrs. Cortez?
3. You recognize that SP are instituted for all hospitalized clients. Explain why the use of such precautions may not prevent the spread of Mrs. Cortez's respiratory infection to other susceptible clients.
4. What can you do to prevent the spread of Mrs. Cortez's infection to other hospitalized clients and at the same time prevent Mrs. Cortez from getting infections from other clients?
5. You see the nursing assistant leaving Mrs. Cortez's room. She stops to wash her hands. She turns on the water handles and soaps and rubs her hands together under running water for about 5 seconds. She then turns off the faucets with her bare hands and proceeds with drying her hands. Should you intervene and, if so, what should you do?

Answers to Critical Thinking Checkpoint questions are available on the faculty resources site. Please consult with your instructor.

Chapter 31 Review

CHAPTER HIGHLIGHTS

- Microorganisms are everywhere. Most are harmless and some are beneficial; however, many can cause infection in susceptible individuals.
- Effective prevention and control of infectious disease is an international, national, community, and individual responsibility.
- Asepsis is the freedom from disease-causing microorganisms.
- Medical aseptic practices limit the number, growth, and transmission of microorganisms.
- Surgical aseptic practices keep an area or objects free of all microorganisms.
- The incidence of healthcare-associated infections is significant. Major sites for these infections are the respiratory and urinary tracts, the bloodstream, and wounds.
- Factors that contribute to nosocomial and healthcare-associated infection risks are invasive procedures, medical therapies, the existence of a large number of susceptible individuals, inappropriate use of antibiotics, and insufficient hand hygiene after client contact and after contact with body substances.
- An infection can develop if the links in the chain of infection—etiologic agent, reservoir, portal of exit, mode of transmission, portal of entry, and susceptible host—are not interrupted.
- Intact skin and mucous membranes are the body's first line of defense against microorganisms.
- Some body secretions (e.g., saliva and tears) contain enzymes that act as antibacterial agents.
- The inflammatory response limits physical, chemical, and microbial injury and promotes repair of injured tissue.
- Immunity is the specific resistance of the body to infectious agents.
- Immunity is active or passive and in either case may be naturally or artificially induced.
- Individuals especially at risk of acquiring an infection are the very young or old; those with a deficiency of serum immunoglobulins, multiple stressors, poor nutritional status, or insufficient immunizations; those receiving certain medical therapies; and those who have an existing disease process.
- Preventing infections in healthy or ill individuals and preventing the transmission of microorganisms from infected clients to others are major nursing functions.
- All healthcare providers must apply clean or sterile gloves, gowns, masks, and protective eyewear according to the risk of exposure to potentially infective materials.
- Should a healthcare worker be exposed to substances with a high risk of transmitting bloodborne pathogens, postexposure practices and consideration of prophylactic treatment must be followed immediately.

TEST YOUR KNOWLEDGE

1. A client diagnosed with tuberculosis is being admitted to a care area. Which nursing action prevents the transmission of the disease?
   1. Have the client wear a mask when coming from admission.
   2. Stock the supply cart at the beginning of each shift.
   3. Wash the hands only after leaving the room.
   4. Wear a mask when exiting the room.

2. A client is being discharged after a surgical procedure. Regarding what should the nurse instruct the client to reduce the risk of infection? Select all that apply.
   1. Handwashing technique
   2. The importance of adequate nutrition
   3. Covering the mouth and nose when coughing or sneezing
   4. Increasing contact with others
   5. Restricting rest period

3. Which items should a nurse ensure are included in the room of a client who is on contact isolation?
   1. Cabinet stocked with gloves and gowns
   2. Cards and records
   3. Paper towels, sink, and blood pressure cuff
   4. Sign on the door

4. When caring for a single client during one shift, it is appropriate for the nurse to reuse only which of the following personal protective equipment?
   1. Goggles
   2. Gown
   3. Surgical mask
   4. Clean gloves

5. While applying sterile gloves, the cuff of the first glove rolls under itself about 0.5 cm (1/4 in.). What is the best action for the nurse to take?
   1. Remove the glove and start over with a new pair.
   2. Wait until the second glove is in place and then unroll the cuff with the other sterile hand.
   3. Ask a colleague to assist by unrolling the cuff.
   4. Leave the cuff rolled under.

6. Which steps are appropriate when utilizing an alcohol-based hand hygiene product? Select all that apply.
   1. Apply a palmful of product into a cupped hand—enough to cover all surfaces of both hands.
   2. Rub palm against palm.
   3. Interlace fingers palm to palm.
   4. Rub palms to back of hands.
   5. Rub all surfaces of each finger with the opposite hand.
   6. Continue for about 10 to 15 seconds.

7. A client with poor nutrition enters the hospital for treatment of a puncture wound. An appropriate nursing diagnosis would be ____________.

8. After teaching a client and family strategies to prevent infection, which statement by the client would indicate effective learning has occurred?
   1. "We will use antimicrobial soap and hot water to wash our hands at least 3 times per day."
   2. "We must wash or peel all raw fruits and vegetables before eating."
   3. "A wound or sore is not infected unless we see it draining pus."
   4. "We should not share toothbrushes but it is OK to share towels and washcloths."

9. Which of the numbered areas is considered sterile on a healthcare provider in the operating room? You may assume that all articles were sterile when applied.

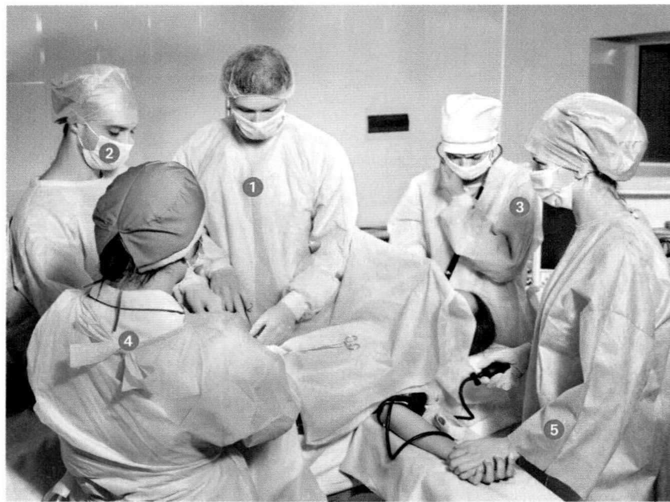

Poznyakov/Shutterstock.

10. The nurse determines that a field remains sterile if which of the following conditions exist?

1. Tips of wet forceps are held upward when held in ungloved hands.
2. The field was set up 1 hour before the procedure.
3. Sterile items are 2 inches from the edge of the field.
4. The nurse reaches over the field rather than around the edges.

See Answers to Test Your Knowledge in Appendix A.

READINGS AND REFERENCES

Suggested Reading

Hogue, M. D., & Meador, A. E. (2016). Vaccines and immunization practice. *Nursing Clinics*, *51*, 121–136. doi:10.1016/j.cnur.2015.10.005

Key points made in this article are that vaccine-preventable diseases continue to cause significant morbidity and mortality in the United States despite the availability of safe and effective vaccines; adult immunization rates are well below Healthy People 2020 *targets for all vaccine-preventable diseases and require nurses and other healthcare professionals to take more proactive, intentional approaches to immunizing patients; and vaccines are a safe and effective intervention for protecting the public's health and should be advocated at every healthcare encounter.*

Related Research

Rhodes, A., Evans, L. E., Alhazzani, W., Levy, M. M., Antonelli, M., Ferrer, R., . . . Dellinger, R. P. (2017). Surviving sepsis campaign: International guidelines for management of sepsis and septic shock: 2016. *Critical Care Medicine*, *45*, 486–552. doi:10.1097/CCM.0000000000002255

References

AHC Media. (2018). Empowering patients to prompt hand hygiene. *Hospital Infection Control & Prevention*, *45*(9).

Centers for Disease Control and Prevention. (2016). *HAI data and statistics*. Retrieved from https://www.cdc.gov/HAI/surveillance/index.html

The Joint Commission. (2019). *2019 National Patient Safety Goals*. Retrieved from https://www.jointcommission.org/assets/1/6/NPSG_Chapter_HAP_Jan2019.pdf

Kang, J., O'Donnell, J. M., Colaianne, B., Bircher, N., Ren, D., & Smith, K. J. (2017). Use of personal protective equipment among health care personnel: Results of clinical observations and simulations. *American Journal of Infection Control*, *45*, 17–23. doi:10.1016/j.ajic.2016.08.011

Kerns, R., & Sheridan, D. (2019). HIV postexposure prophylaxis for healthcare professionals. *Nursing*, *49*(1), 67–68. doi:10.1097/01.NURSE.0000547727.22976.53

Kuhar, D. T., Henderson, D. K., Struble, K. A., Heneine, W., Thomas, V., Cheever, L. W., . . . U.S. Public Health Service Working Group. (2013). Updated US Public Health Service guidelines for the management of occupational exposures to human immunodeficiency virus and recommendations for postexposure prophylaxis. *Infection Control and Hospital Epidemiology*, *34*, 875–892. doi:10.1086/672271

MRSA Research Center. (2017). *What disease kills more Americans a year than AIDS? If you don't know about MRSA, you're not alone*. Retrieved from http://mrsa-research-center.bsd.uchicago.edu/index.html

Sanyal, K., & Strelczyk, K. (2018). Preventing the spread of *Clostridium difficile* infection. *American Nurse Today*, *13*(6), 8–11.

Siegel, J. D., Rhinehart, E., Jackson, M., Chiarello, L., & the Healthcare Infection Control Practices Advisory Committee. (2007). *Guidelines for isolation precautions: Preventing transmission of infectious agents in healthcare settings (2007)*. Retrieved from https://www.cdc.gov/infectioncontrol/guidelines/isolation/index.html

U.S. Food and Drug Administration. (2016a). Banned devices; powdered surgeon's gloves, powdered patient examination gloves, and absorbable powder for lubricating a surgeon's glove. *Federal Register*, *81*(243), 91722–91731.

U.S. Food and Drug Administration. (2016b). Safety and effectiveness of consumer antiseptics: Topical antimicrobial drug products for over-the-counter human use. *Federal Register*, *81*(172), 61106–611030.

World Health Organization. (2009). *WHO guidelines on hand hygiene in health care*. Geneva, Switzerland: Author.

Zhuang, Z., Bergman, M., Brochu, E., Palmiero, A., Niezgoda, G., He, X., . . . Shaffer, R. (2016). Temporal changes in filtering facepiece respirator fit. *Journal of Occupational and Environmental Hygiene*, *13*, 265–274. doi:10.1080/15459624.2015.1116692

Selected Bibliography

Albright, J., White, B., Pedersen, D., Carlson, P., Yost, L., & Littau, C. (2018). Use patterns and frequency of hand hygiene in healthcare facilities: Analysis of electronic surveillance data. *American Journal of Infection Control*, *46*(10), 1104–1109. doi:10.1016/j.ajic.2018.04.205

Almyroudis, N. G., Osawa, R., Samonis, G., Wetzler, M., Wang, E. S., McCarthy, P. L., & Segal, B. H. (2016). Discontinuation of systematic surveillance and contact precautions for vancomycin-resistant Enterococcus (VRE) and its impact on the incidence of VRE faecium bacteremia in patients with hematologic malignancies. *Infection Control & Hospital Epidemiology*, *37*, 398–403. doi:10.1017/ice.2015.310

Boyce, J. M. (2016). Modern technologies for improving cleaning and disinfection of environmental surfaces in hospitals. *Antimicrobial Resistance and Infection Control*, *5*, 10. doi:10.1186/s13756-016-0111-x

Centers for Disease Control and Prevention. (2018). *2016 national and state healthcare-associated infections progress report*. Retrieved from https://www.cdc.gov/hai/progress-report/index.html

Deresinski, S. (2017). VRE and MRSA: Should we stop routine contact precautions? *Hospital Infection Control & Prevention*, *44*(1), 1–2.

Deshpande, A., Fox, J., Wong, K. K., Cadnum, J. L., Sankar, T., Jencson, A., . . . Gordon, S. (2018). Comparative antimicrobial efficacy of two hand sanitizers in intensive care units common areas: A randomized, controlled trial. *Infection Control & Hospital Epidemiology*, *39*(3), 267–271. doi:10.1017/ice.2017.293

Evans, M. E., Kralovic, S. M., Simbarti, L. A., Jain, R., & Roselle, G. A. (2017). Eight years of decreased methicillin-resistant *Staphylococcus aureus* health care-associated infections associated with a Veterans Affairs prevention initiative. *American Journal of Infection Control*, *45*(1), 13–16. doi:10.1016/j.ajic.2016.08.010

Gellin, B. G., Shen, A. K., Fish, R., Zettle, M. A., Uscher-Pines, L., & Ringel, J. S. (2016). The national adult immunization plan: Strengthening adult immunization through coordinated action. *American Journal of Preventive Medicine*, *51*, 1079–1083. doi:10.1016/j.amepre.2016.04.014

Hospitals explore a new approach to MRSA and VRE: Eliminating contact precautions. (2016). *Patient Safety Monitor Journal*, *17*(10), 5–7.

Isenman, H., & Fisher, D. (2016). Advances in prevention and treatment of vancomycin-resistant Enterococcus infection. *Current Opinion in Infectious Diseases*, *29*, 577–582. doi:10.1097/QCO.0000000000000311

Jarrett, N. M., & Callaham, M. (2016). *Evidence-based guidelines for selected hospital-acquired conditions: Final report*. Retrieved from https://www.cms.gov/Medicare/Medicare-Fee-for-Service-Payment/HospitalAcqCond/Downloads/2016-HAC-Report.pdf

Jo, K. W. (2017). Preventing the transmission of tuberculosis in health care settings: Administrative control. *Tuberculosis and Respiratory Diseases*, *80*, 21–26. doi:10.4046/trd.2017.80.1.21

Lee, S. M., & An, W. S. (2016). New clinical criteria for septic shock: Serum lactate level as new emerging vital sign. *Journal of Thoracic Disease*, *8*, 1388–1390. doi:10.21037/jtd.2016.05.55

Paiva, J., & Eggimann, P. (2017). Treatment of severe MRSA infections: Current practice and further development. *Intensive Care Medicine*, *43*, 233–236. doi:10.1007/s00134-016-4572-4

Warren, C., Medei, M. K., Wood, B., & Schutte, D. (2019). A nurse-driven oral care protocol to reduce hospital-acquired pneumonia. *American Journal of Nursing*, *119*(2), 44–51. doi:10.1097/01.NAJ.0000553204.21342.01

Whelan, A. M. (2016). Lowering the age of consent: Pushing back against the anti-vaccine movement. *The Journal of Law, Medicine & Ethics*, *44*, 462–473. doi:10.1177/1073110516667942

Safety 32

LEARNING OUTCOMES

After completing this chapter, you will be able to:

1. Discuss factors that affect individuals' ability to protect themselves from injury.
2. Describe methods to assess a client's risk for injury.
3. Discuss the National Patient Safety Goals.
4. Identify common potential hazards throughout the lifespan.
5. Plan strategies to maintain safety in the healthcare setting, home, and community, including prevention strategies across the lifespan for falls, seizures, thermal injury, fires, carbon monoxide and other types of poisoning, suffocation or choking, excessive noise, electrical hazards, firearms, radiation, and disasters.
6. Explain interventions to prevent falls.
7. Discuss implementation of seizure precautions.
8. Discuss the use and legal implications of restraints.
9. Describe alternatives to restraints.
10. List desired outcomes to use in evaluating the selected strategies for injury prevention.
11. Verbalize the steps for:
    a. Using a bed or chair exit safety monitoring device.
    b. Implementing seizure precautions.
    c. Applying restraints.
12. Recognize when it is appropriate to assign using a bed or chair exit safety monitoring device, implementing seizure precautions, and applying restraints of clients to assistive personnel.
13. Demonstrate appropriate documentation and reporting of using a bed or chair exit safety monitoring device, implementing seizure precautions, and applying restraints.

KEY TERMS

asphyxiation, *743*
burn, *742*
carbon monoxide, *743*
chemical restraints, *746*
electric shock, *745*
Heimlich maneuver, *743*
physical restraints, *746*
restraints, *746*
safety monitoring devices, *738*
scald, *742*
seclusion, *746*
seizure, *740*
seizure precautions, *740*

Introduction

A fundamental concern of nurses, which extends from the bedside to the home to the community, is preventing injuries and assisting the injured. Motor vehicle crashes, falls, drowning, fire and burns, poisoning, inhalation and ingestion of foreign objects, and firearm use are major causes of injury and death.

Nurses need to be aware of what constitutes a safe environment for a particular individual or for a group of individuals in home and community settings. Injuries are often caused by human conduct and can be prevented.

Factors Affecting Safety

The ability of individuals to protect themselves from injury is affected by such factors as age and development, lifestyle, mobility and health status, sensory–perceptual alterations, cognitive awareness, emotional state, ability to communicate, safety awareness, and environmental factors. Nurses need to assess each of these factors when they plan care or teach clients to protect themselves.

Age and Development

Through knowledge and accurate assessment of the environment, individuals learn to protect themselves from many injuries. Children walking to school learn to stop before crossing the street and wait for oncoming traffic. They also learn not to touch a hot stove. For the very young, learning about the environment is essential. Only through knowledge and experience do children learn what is potentially harmful.

Older adults can have difficulty with movement and diminished sensory–neurologic acuity, which can contribute to the likelihood of injury. Specific age-related potential hazards and preventive measures are discussed later in this chapter. Box 32.1 summarizes selected hazards for each age group.

Lifestyle

Lifestyle factors that place individuals at risk for injury include unsafe work environments; residence in neighborhoods with high crime rates; access to firearms; insufficient income to purchase safety equipment or make necessary repairs; and access to illicit drugs, which may also be contaminated by harmful additives. Risk-taking behaviors are contributing factors in some unintentional injuries.

BOX 32.1 Selected Safety Hazards Throughout the Lifespan*

- *Developing fetus:* exposure to maternal smoking, alcohol consumption, addictive drugs, x-rays (first trimester), certain pesticides
- *Newborns and infants:* falling, suffocation in crib, placement in the prone position, suffocation when entangled in cords, choking from aspirated milk or ingested objects, burns from hot water or other spilled hot liquids, automobile crashes, crib or playpen injuries, electric shock, poisoning
- *Toddlers:* physical trauma from falling, running into objects, aspiration of small toys, getting cut by sharp objects; automobile crashes; burns; poisoning; drowning; electric shock
- *Preschoolers:* injury from traffic, playground equipment, and other objects; choking, suffocation, and obstruction of airway or ear canal by foreign objects; poisoning; drowning; fire and burns; harm from other people or animals
- *Adolescents:* vehicular (automobile, bicycle) crashes, recreational injuries, firearms, substance abuse
- *Older adults:* falling, burns, pedestrian and automobile crashes

*Preventive measures are discussed later in this chapter.

Mobility and Health Status

Alterations in mobility related to paralysis, muscle weakness, diminished balance, and lack of coordination place clients at risk for injury. Spinal cord injuries or paralysis impair the client's ability to perceive discomfort, increasing the risk for injury or skin breakdown. Clients who have impaired mobility such as hemiplegia or leg casts are prone to falls related to poor balance. Clients weakened by illness or surgery may have impaired levels of alertness, placing them at risk for falls or injury.

Sensory–Perceptual Alterations

Accurate sensory perception of environmental stimuli is vital to safety. People with impaired touch perception, hearing, taste, smell, and vision are highly susceptible to injury. A client with impaired vision may trip over a toy or not see an electric cord. A client with impaired hearing may not hear a siren in traffic. A client with impaired olfactory sense may not smell burning food or the sulfur aroma of escaping gas.

Cognitive Awareness

Awareness is the ability to perceive environmental stimuli and body reactions and to respond appropriately through thought and action. Clients with impaired awareness include individuals who lack sleep; are unconscious or semiconscious; are disoriented and may not understand where they are or what to do to help themselves; perceive stimuli that do not exist; and whose judgment is altered by disease or medications, such as opioids, tranquilizers, hypnotics, and sedatives. Mildly confused clients may momentarily forget where they are, wander from their rooms, misplace personal belongings, and so forth.

Emotional State

Extreme emotional states can alter the ability to perceive environmental hazards. Stressful situations can reduce a client's level of concentration, cause errors of judgment, and decrease awareness of external stimuli. Clients with depression may think and react to environmental stimuli more slowly than usual.

Ability to Communicate

Individuals with diminished ability to receive and convey information are at risk for injury. They include clients with aphasia, language barriers, or the inability to read. For example, the client unable to interpret the sign "No smoking—oxygen in use" could cause a fire.

Safety Awareness

Information is crucial to safety. Clients in unfamiliar environments frequently need specific safety information. Lack of knowledge about unfamiliar equipment, such as oxygen tanks, IV tubing, and hot packs, is a potential hazard. Healthy clients need information about water safety, car safety, fire prevention, ways to prevent the ingestion of harmful substances, and many preventive measures related to specific age-related hazards.

Environmental Factors

Client safety is affected by the healthcare setting. Depending on the client situation, the nurse may need to assess

LIFESPAN CONSIDERATIONS Preventing Falls

OLDER ADULTS

- Assess for potential personal causes of falls: hypotension, unsteady gait, altered mental status (such as from medications), poor vision, foot pathology, cognitive changes, and fear.
- In the home or community setting, assess for potential environmental causes of falls:
  - *Lighting:* inadequate amount, inaccessible or inconvenient switches
  - *Floors:* presence of electrical cords, loose rugs, clutter, slippery surfaces
  - *Stairs:* absent or unsteady railings, uneven step height or surfaces
  - *Furniture:* unsteady base, lack of armrests, cabinets too high or too low, chairs with wheels
  - *Bathroom:* inappropriate toilet height, slippery floors or tub, absence of grab bars.
- In the home, consider alternatives to hospital or regular bed if client is extremely prone to fall out of bed:
  - Place the mattress directly onto the floor.
  - Place padding on floor next to bed or between client and side rails.

the environment of the workplace, home, or community. Natural disasters are national safety concerns.

Healthcare Setting

It has been 20 years since the Institute of Medicine (IOM) released its reports on client safety and medical errors: *To Err Is Human: Building a Safer Health System* and *Crossing the Quality Chasm: A New Health System for the 21st Century* (American Nurses Association, n.d.). These landmark reports attracted a great deal of attention when they reported the numbers of individuals who died in hospitals each year because of medical errors, and that many more were seriously harmed. As a result, organizations such as The Joint Commission and the Agency for Healthcare Research and Quality (AHRQ) developed or continued to accelerate work around client safety. In addition, the Quality and Safety Education for Nurses (QSEN) project developed guidelines that would enable future nurses to have the knowledge, skills, and attitudes necessary to improve the quality and safety of the healthcare systems within which they work.

Historically, medical professionals were blamed and punished for errors, which were often unintended. This punitive approach discouraged individuals from reporting errors, which blocked responsibility for client safety. The clear message of the IOM reports was that errors were not usually the result of one individual but of a complex system-related problem. IOM recommended that healthcare organizations create safety systems. As a result, The Joint Commission created the National Patient Safety Goals (NPSGs) program to help organizations target areas most in need of improvement.

It is important for health organizations to create an environment in which safety is a top priority; this is also known as providing a "culture of safety." The foundation for a culture of safety is a blame-free work environment, transparency, and a process designed to prevent errors. An example is a willingness to share information and learn from errors.

The AHRQ conducts an annual hospital survey on client safety culture. The 2018 database report (Famolaro et al., 2018) from 630 hospitals and over 382,000 hospital provider and staff respondents revealed the three areas with the highest percentage of positive responses and the three areas with the lowest percentage of positive responses. The highest percentage of positive responses included *Teamwork Within Units*, where staff supported each other, treated each other with respect, and worked as a team; *Management Support for Patient Safety*, where hospital management provided a work climate that promoted client safety and showed that client safety was a top priority; and *Organizational Learning–Continuous Improvement*, where mistakes led to positive changes and those changes were evaluated for effectiveness. The three areas that indicated potential for improvement included *Nonpunitive Response to Error*, where some staff felt that their mistakes were held against them; *Handoffs and Transitions*, where client care information during shift change or across hospital units could still be improved; and *Staffing*, where more staff were needed for the workload and work hours to improve (p. 4). Nurses have been active participants in improving client safety; however, client safety requires *everyone* to be continuously involved in identifying opportunities where client safety can be improved.

Workplace

In the workplace, machinery, industrial belts and pulleys, and chemicals may create danger. Worker fatigue, noise, and air pollution, or working at great heights or in subterranean areas may also create occupational hazards. The work environment of the nurse may also be unsafe. The Bureau of Labor Statistics (2018) reports that nursing has many hazards. Some of the hazards identified are exposure to infectious diseases; activities in client care that require lifting, bending, and walking; exposure to hazardous compounds; and unintentional needlesticks. Nurses must follow standardized guidelines to prevent injury or disease.

Home

A safe home requires well-maintained flooring and carpets, a nonskid bathtub or shower surface, handrails, functioning smoke alarms that are strategically placed, and knowledge of fire escape routes. Outdoor areas, where steps or stairs increase the risk for falls, may need ramps instead. Swimming pools need to be safely secured and maintained. Adequate lighting, both inside and out, will minimize the potential for unintentional injuries.

Community

Adequate street lighting, safe water and sewage treatment, and regulation of sanitation in food buying and handling all contribute to a healthy, hazard-free community. A safe and secure community strives to be free of excess noise, crime, traffic congestion, rundown housing, or unprotected creeks and landfills.

Disaster Planning

Nursing personnel play a key role in disaster management and client care throughout all aspects of the healthcare industry. Nurses are employed in acute care facilities, ambulatory care facilities, long-term care facilities, and within community agencies, including home care and public health. The terrorist events of September 11, 2001; natural disasters such as hurricanes, floods, earthquakes, and wild fires; mass casualty events; bioterrorism; and international health situations such as the Ebola outbreak and the Zika virus provide evidence that nursing and healthcare organizations must plan for emergency management during a disaster.

All institutions are either required or encouraged to have emergency operations plans, and personnel with a direct role in emergency preparedness are required by the Homeland Security Presidential Directive to have National Incident Management Systems (NIMS) training (Nielson, 2017, p. 54). NIMS is a proactive, organized approach to provide a nationwide guide to enable the whole community to work together in managing all threats and hazards (Federal Emergency Management Agency, 2019; Nielson, 2017). Training is designed to provide basic information for first responders (emergency management technicians, firefighters, and RNs) and additional information for emergency management personnel.

●○● NURSING MANAGEMENT

Assessing

Assessing clients at risk for injury involves (a) noting pertinent indicators in the nursing history and physical examination, (b) using specifically developed risk assessment tools, and (c) evaluating the client's home environment.

Nursing History and Physical Examination

The nursing history and physical examination can reveal considerable data about the client's safety practices and risks for injury. Data include age and developmental level; general health status; mobility status; presence or absence of physiologic or perceptual deficits such as olfactory, visual, tactile, taste, or other sensory impairments; altered thought processes or other impaired cognitive or emotional capabilities; substance abuse; any indications of abuse or neglect; and an accident and injury history. A safety history also needs to include the client's awareness of hazards, knowledge of safety precautions both at home and at work, and any perceived threats to safety (Figure 32.1 ■).

Risk Assessment Tools

Risk assessment tools are available to determine clients at risk both for specific types of injury, such as falls, or for the general safety of the home and healthcare setting. In general, these tools direct the nurse to evaluate the factors affecting safety as previously discussed. The tools summarize specific data contained in the client's nursing history and physical examination. Client risk factors and environmental hazards for falls are discussed later in this chapter (see the Falls section).

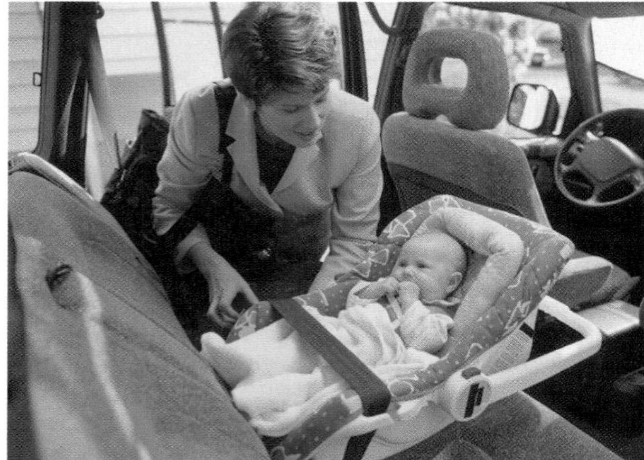

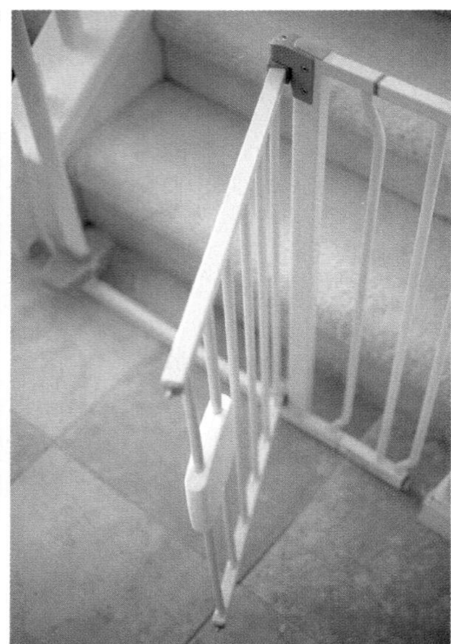

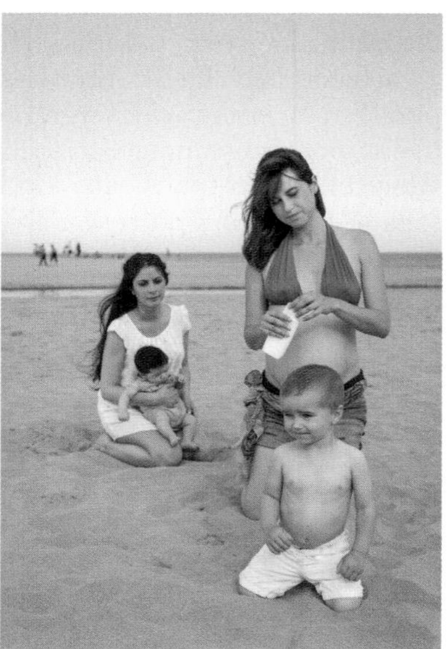

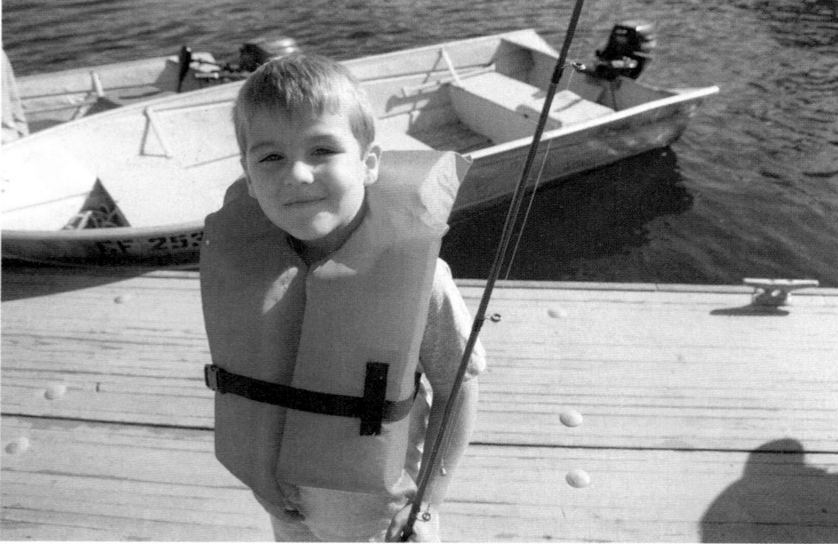

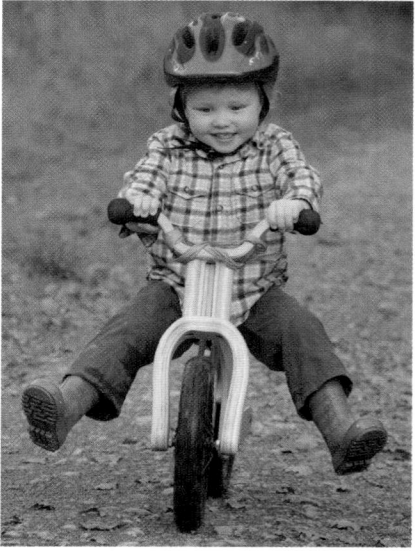

Figure 32.1 ■ Nurses need to teach clients about safety and how to prevent unintentional injuries by using infant car seats, guard gates on stairs, and sunburn protection, life jackets, and helmets.

Home Hazard Appraisal

Hazards in the home are major causes of falls, fire, poisoning, suffocation, and other unintentional injuries, such as those caused by improper use of household equipment, tools, and cooking utensils. See Chapter 7 ∞ for a summary of specific data necessary for a home hazard appraisal.

National Patient Safety Goals

Because of IOM's report *To Err Is Human* (2000), the healthcare industry and national organizations (e.g., National Patient Safety Foundation) increased their awareness of the need to improve client safety. For example, since 2002, The Joint Commission has required its accredited agencies to meet specific NPSGs. See Box 32.2 for The Joint Commission's 2019 National Patient Safety Goals. It is important to remember that the focus of the NPSGs is on system-wide solutions. This is an important change from the traditional method of finding out who made the error (i.e., creating an environment of fear and scapegoating) to analyzing the system to find out why the error was made (i.e., creating an environment of learning and improvement).

Disasters

Nurses need to be able to respond to disasters in the community as well as keep clients who are already in the healthcare setting safe. The Joint Commission has standards requiring healthcare organizations to develop disaster plans. The role that nurses play in disaster planning is to know and understand the chain of command. The line of authority during a disaster is different from that of day-to-day operations. For example, the chain of command may be under the control of an outside agency instead of the nurse's healthcare institution. For the bedside nurse, the client's safety is top priority, and it is essential for the nurse to know the organization's disaster response plan. Many organizations conduct disaster drills for this reason.

BOX 32.2 The Joint Commission's 2019 National Patient Safety Goals for Hospitals and Nursing Care Centers (i.e., nursing homes, long-term care, Medicare and Medicaid skilled nursing facilities)

GOAL: IMPROVE THE ACCURACY OF PATIENT IDENTIFICATION.

- Use at least two patient identifiers when providing care, treatment, and services. [Hospital and Nursing Care Center]
    - Note: In the Nursing Care Center, at the first encounter, the requirement for two identifiers is appropriate; thereafter, and in any situation of continuing one-on-one care in which the clinician knows the patient or resident, one identifier can be facial recognition.
- Eliminate transfusion errors related to patient misidentification. [Hospital]

GOAL: IMPROVE THE EFFECTIVENESS OF COMMUNICATION AMONG CAREGIVERS.

- Report critical results of tests and diagnostic procedures on a timely basis. [Hospital]

GOAL: IMPROVE THE SAFETY OF USING MEDICATIONS.

- Label all medications, medication containers, and other solutions on and off the sterile field in perioperative and other procedural settings. [Hospital]
- Reduce the likelihood of patient harm associated with the use of anticoagulant therapy. [Hospital and Nursing Care Center]
- Maintain and communicate accurate patient medication information. [Hospital and Nursing Care Center]

GOAL: REDUCE THE HARM ASSOCIATED WITH CLINICAL ALARM SYSTEMS.

- Improve the safety of clinical alarm systems. [Hospital]

GOAL: REDUCE THE RISK OF HEALTHCARE-ASSOCIATED INFECTIONS.

- Comply with either the current Centers for Disease Control and Prevention (CDC) hand hygiene guidelines or the current World Health Organization (WHO) hand hygiene guidelines. [Hospital and Nursing Care Center]
- Implement evidence-based practices to prevent healthcare–associated infections due to multidrug-resistant organisms in acute care hospitals and in nursing care centers. [Hospital and Nursing Care Center]
- Implement evidence-based practices to prevent central line–associated bloodstream infections. [Hospital and Nursing Care Center]
- Implement evidence-based practices for preventing surgical site infections. [Hospital]
- Implement evidence-based practices to prevent indwelling catheter-associated urinary tract infections (CAUTI). [Hospital and Nursing Care Center]

GOAL: REDUCE THE RISK OF PATIENT AND RESIDENT HARM RESULTING FROM FALLS.

- Reduce the risk of falls. [Nursing Care Center]

GOAL: PREVENT HEALTHCARE–ASSOCIATED PRESSURE ULCERS (DECUBITUS ULCERS).

- Assess and periodically reassess each patient's and resident's risk for developing a pressure ulcer and take action to address any identified risks. [Nursing Care Center]

GOAL: THE HOSPITAL IDENTIFIES SAFETY RISKS INHERENT IN ITS PATIENT POPULATION.

- Identify patients at risk for suicide. [Hospital]
    - Note: This requirement applies only to psychiatric hospitals and patients being treated for emotional or behavioral disorders in general hospitals.

UNIVERSAL PROTOCOL FOR PREVENTING WRONG SITE, WRONG PROCEDURE, AND WRONG PERSON SURGERY [HOSPITALS]

The Universal Protocol applies to all surgical and nonsurgical invasive procedures. Hospitals can enhance safety by correctly identifying the patient, the appropriate procedure, and the correct site of the procedure.

- Conduct a preprocedure verification process.
- Mark the procedure site.
- A time-out is performed before the procedure.

Diagnosing

Examples of nursing diagnoses for clients with potential for injury are most helpful when specific labels are used to provide clear direction for nursing care. Nursing diagnoses that describe potential for injury more specifically can include but are not limited to potential for: falls, infection, suffocation, poisoning, and suicide. Other diagnoses the nurse may choose to use are lack of knowledge (unintentional injury prevention) or the wellness diagnosis of willingness for knowledge enhancement (unintentional injury prevention).

Planning

When planning care to prevent unintentional injury, the nurse considers all factors affecting the client's safety, specifies desired outcomes, and selects nursing activities to meet these outcomes. The major goal for clients with safety risks is to prevent unintentional injury. To meet this goal, clients often need to change their health behaviors and may need to modify the environment.

Desired outcomes associated with preventing injury depend on the individual client. Examples of desired outcomes, although established in the planning phase, are provided in the Evaluating section on page 749.

Nursing interventions to meet desired outcomes are largely directed toward helping the client and family to accomplish the following:

- Identify environmental hazards in the home and community.
- Demonstrate safety practices appropriate to the home healthcare agency, community, and workplace.
- Experience a decrease in the frequency or severity of injury.
- Demonstrate safe childrearing practices or lifestyle practices.

Implementing

Hazards to safety occur at all ages and vary according to the age and developmental level of the individual.

Promoting Safety Across the Lifespan

Measures to ensure the safety of clients of all ages focus on (a) observation or prediction of potentially harmful situations so that harm can be avoided and (b) client education that empowers clients to protect themselves and their families from injury. Safety measures covering the lifespan from infancy to older adults are listed in the accompanying Client Teaching.

CLIENT TEACHING Safety Measures Throughout the Lifespan

NEWBORNS AND INFANTS

- Use a federally approved car seat at all times (including coming home from hospital). It should be in the back seat, facing backward.
- Never leave the infant unattended on a raised surface.
- Check the temperature of the infant's bath water and formula prior to using.
- Hold the infant upright during feeding. Do not prop the bottle. Cut food in small pieces, and do not feed the infant peanuts or popcorn. Slice hot dogs lengthwise in two pieces then into small pieces.
- Investigate the infant's crib for compliance with federal safety regulations: slats no more than 6 cm (2.4 in.) apart, lead-free paint, height of crib sides, tight fit of mattress to crib.
- Use a playpen with sides made of small-size netting. Never leave playpen sides down.
- Provide large soft toys with no small detachable or sharp-edged parts.
- Use guard gates on stairs and screens on windows. Supervise the infant in swings and highchairs.
- Cover electric outlets. Coil cords out of reach.
- Place plants, household cleaners, and wastebaskets out of reach. Lock away potential poisons, such as medicines, paint, and gasoline.

TODDLERS

- Continue to use federally approved car seats at all times. Place children in back seat when traveling in a car.
- Teach children not to put objects in the mouth, including pills (unless given by parent).
- Keep objects with sharp edges (such as furniture and knives) out of children's reach. Keep plastic bags out of reach.
- Place hot pots on back burners with handles turned inward.
- Keep cleaning solutions, insecticides, and medicines in locked cupboards.
- Keep windows and balconies screened.
- Supervise toddlers in the tub.
- Fence in pools, and supervise toddlers at all times when in or near pools. Do not overfill bathtub. Do not let toddlers play near ditches or wells.
- Teach children not to run or ride a tricycle into the street.
- Obtain a low bed when the child begins to climb.
- Cover outlets with safety covers or plugs.

PRESCHOOLERS

- Do not allow children to run with candy or other objects in the mouth.
- Teach children not to put small objects in the mouth, nose, and ears.
- Remove doors from unused equipment such as refrigerators.
- Always supervise preschoolers crossing streets and begin safety teaching about obeying traffic signals and looking both ways.
- Check Halloween treats before allowing children to eat them. Discard loose or open candy.
- Teach children to play in "safe" areas, not on streets and railroad tracks.
- Teach preschoolers the dangers of playing with matches and playing near charcoal, fire, and heating appliances.
- Teach children to avoid strangers and keep parents informed of their whereabouts.
- Teach preschoolers not to walk in front of swings and not to push others off playground equipment.

SCHOOL-AGE CHILDREN

- Teach children safety rules for recreational and sports activities: Never swim alone, always wear a life jacket when in a boat, and wear a protective helmet and knee and elbow pads when needed.
- Supervise contact sports and activities in which children aim at a target.

CLIENT TEACHING **Safety Measures Throughout the Lifespan**—*continued*

- Teach children to obey all traffic and safety rules for bicycling, skateboarding, and roller skating.
- Teach children to use light or reflective clothing when walking or cycling at night.
- Teach children safe ways to use the stove, garden tools, and other equipment.
- Supervise children when they use saws, electric appliances, tools, and other potentially dangerous equipment.
- Teach children not to play with fireworks, gunpowder, or firearms. Keep firearms unloaded, locked up, and out of reach.
- Teach children to avoid excavations, quarries, vacant buildings, and playing around heavy machinery.
- Teach children the health hazards of smoking. If you smoke, stop.
- Teach children the effects of drugs and alcohol on judgment and coordination.

ADOLESCENTS

- Have adolescents complete a driver's education course, and take practice drives with them in various types of weather.
- Set firm limits on automobile use, namely, never to drive after drinking or using drugs, and never to ride with a driver who has done so. Encourage adolescents to call home for a ride if they have been drinking, assuring them they can do so without a reprimand.
- Restrict number of passengers in car during the first year of driving.
- Teach adolescents to wear a safety helmet when riding motorcycles, scooters, and other sports vehicles. Teach safety rules for water sports.
- Encourage adolescents to use proper equipment when participating in sports. Schedule a physical examination before participation, and be certain there is medical supervision for all athletic activities.
- Encourage adolescents to swim, jog, and go boating in groups so they can obtain help in case of an unintentional injury.
- Teach safety measures for use of power tools.
- Teach rules for hunting and the proper care and use of firearms.
- Inform the adolescent of the dangers of drugs, alcohol, and unprotected sex. Include teaching about date rape prevention and defense.
- Teach dangers of sunbathing and tanning beds, as well as the proper use of sun block and protective clothing when doing outdoor activities.
- Be alert to changes in the adolescent's mood and behavior. Listen to and maintain open communication with the adolescent. Open communication is a powerful preventive measure.
- Set a good example of behavior that the adolescent can follow.

YOUNG ADULTS

- Reinforce motor vehicle safety: Drive defensively, use "designated drivers" if alcohol is consumed, routinely check brakes and tires, and use seat and shoulder belts or car seats for all passengers.
- Remind the young adult to repair potential fire hazards, such as electric wiring.
- Reinforce water safety: Know the depth of a pool or lake before diving; supervise backyard pools and other water activities.
- Discuss evaluating the potential for workplace injuries or death when making decisions about a career or occupation. Encourage the young adult to participate actively in programs that reduce occupational hazards.
- Discuss avoiding excessive sun radiation by limiting exposure, using sun-blocking agents, and wearing protective clothing. Explain the skin changes that may indicate a cancerous condition.
- Encourage young adults who are unable to cope with the pressures, responsibilities, and expectations of adulthood to seek counseling.
- Discuss the dangers associated with the internet and social networking.

MIDDLE-AGED ADULTS

- Reinforce motor vehicle safety: Use seat belts and drive within the speed limit, especially at night. Test visual acuity periodically.
- Make certain stairways are well lighted and uncluttered.
- Equip bathrooms with hand grasps and nonskid bath mats.
- Test carbon monoxide detectors, smoke detectors, and fire alarms regularly.
- Keep all machines and tools in good working condition at work and at home. Follow safety precautions when using machinery.
- Reinforce safety measures taught earlier in life, such as the hazards of excessive sun exposure.

OLDER ADULTS

- Encourage the client to have regular vision and hearing tests.
- Assist the client to have a home hazard appraisal.
- Encourage the client to keep as active as possible.
- Ensure eyeglasses are functional.
- Ensure appropriate lighting.
- Mark doorways and edges of steps as needed.
- Keep the environment tidy and uncluttered.
- Set safe limits to activities.
- Remove unsafe objects.
- Wear shoes or well-fitted slippers with nonskid soles.
- Use ambulatory devices as necessary (cane, crutches, walker, braces, wheelchair).
- Provide assistance with ambulation as needed.
- Monitor gait and balance.
- Adapt living arrangements to one floor if necessary.
- Encourage exercise and activity as tolerated to maintain muscle strength, joint flexibility, and balance.
- Ensure uncluttered environment with securely fastened rugs.
- Encourage the client to request assistance.
- Keep the bed in the low position.
- Install grab bars in the bathroom.
- Provide a raised toilet seat.
- Instruct the client to rise slowly from a lying to sitting to standing position, and to stand in place for several seconds before walking.
- Provide a bedside commode as needed.
- Assist with voiding on a frequent and scheduled basis.
- Encourage the client to summon help.
- Monitor activity tolerance.
- Attach side rails to the bed.
- Keep rails in place when the bed is in the lowest position.
- Monitor orientation and alertness status.
- Encourage annual or more frequent review of all prescribed medications.

Newborns and Infants

Unintentional injuries are a leading cause of death during the first year of life. Infants are completely dependent on others for care; they are oblivious to such dangers as falling or ingesting harmful substances. Parents need to learn the amount of observation necessary to maintain infant safety. They also need help to identify and remove common hazards in and around the home, and first aid information that includes cardiopulmonary resuscitation and interventions for airway obstruction. Common injuries during infancy include burns, suffocation or choking, automobile crashes, falls, and poisoning. Education and support of parents can make them more knowledgeable and better prepared to protect their children from injuries.

Toddlers

Toddlers are curious and like to feel and taste everything. They are fascinated by potential dangers, such as pools and busy streets, so they need constant supervision and protection. Parents prevent many injuries by "toddler-proofing" the home or other setting where the child will be (Figure 32.2 ■). This practice extends to the use of federally approved car restraints and removing or securing all items that can pose a safety hazard to the child in any setting. It may be necessary to inspect for and remove sources of lead from the environment. Lead poisoning (plumbism) is a risk for children exposed to lead paint chips, imported toys, pottery with leaded glaze, imported candy, drinking water, and secondhand smoke (Winslow, 2016, p. 36).

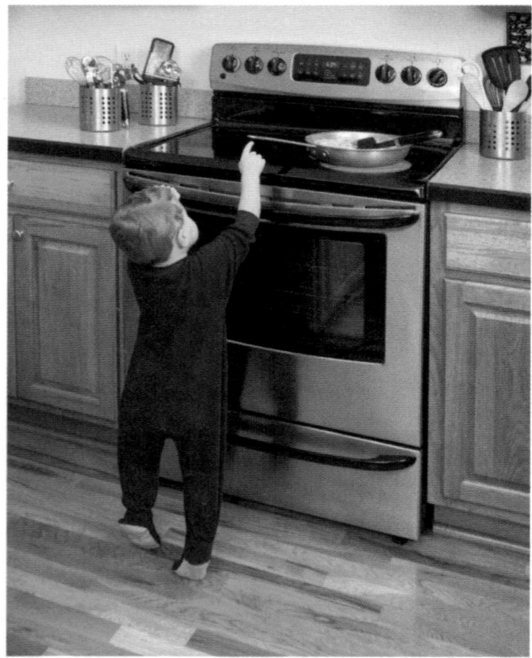

Figure 32.2 ■ Promoting safety (e.g., by placing hot pots on back burners with handles turned inward) is required to keep children from injury.
HKPNC/E+/Getty Images.

Clinical Alert!

The remodeling and renovation of older homes (e.g., those built before 1978) accounts for some of the lead poisoning seen today. Nurses need to educate families living in older homes about their children's risk for lead poisoning and provide lead poisoning prevention advice.

Preschoolers

Children of preschool age are active and often very clumsy, making them susceptible to injury. Control of the environment must continue, keeping hazards such as matches, medicines, and other potential poisons out of reach. Safety education for the child must begin early. Education of the preschooler involves learning how to cross streets, what traffic signals mean, and how to ride bicycles and other wheeled toys safely. It is important to warn children to avoid hazards, such as busy streets, swimming pools, and other potentially dangerous areas. Parents must maintain careful surveillance; the developmental level of the preschooler does not allow for self-reliance in matters of safety. Parents must also keep in mind that their child's cognitive and motor skills increase quickly; thus, safety measures must keep up with the acquisition of new skills.

School-Age Children

By the time children attend school, they are learning to think before they act. They often prefer adult equipment to toys. They want to play with other children in such activities as bicycling, hiking, swimming, and boating. Although sensitive to peer pressure, the school-age child will respond to rules. Children of this age engage in fantasy and magical thinking. They often imitate the actions of parents and superheroes with whom they identify.

Unintentional injuries are the leading cause of death in school-age children. The most frequent causes of fatalities, in descending order, are motor vehicle crashes, drownings, fires, and firearms. School-age children are also involved in many minor injuries, frequently resulting from outdoor activities and recreational equipment such as swings, bicycles, skateboards, and swimming pools.

Adolescents

Obtaining a driver's license is an important event in the life of an adolescent in the United States, but the privilege is not always wisely handled. Teenagers may use driving as an outlet for stress, as a way to assert independence, or as a way to impress peers. When setting limits on automobile use, parents need to assess the teenager's level of responsibility, common sense, and ability to resist peer pressure. The age of the teenager alone does not determine readiness to handle this responsibility.

Adolescents are at risk for sports injuries because their coordination skills are not fully developed. However, sports activities are important to the adolescent's self-esteem and overall development. In addition to providing beneficial exercise, sports activities enhance social and personal development. They help the adolescent experience competition, teamwork, and conflict resolution.

Lee and Mannix (2018) report recent trends that show that unintentional injuries (including motor vehicle crashes, poisoning, and drowning), suicide, and homicide are the three leading causes of death in teenagers and young adults 15 to 34 years old (p. 543). Unintentional deaths from poisoning are related to narcotics and hallucinogens, including heroin, fentanyl, and oxycodone. Deaths from these legal and illicit substances are classified as poisonings in the Centers for Disease Control and Prevention (CDC) database. In the 15- to 24-year-old age group, narcotic and hallucinogen overdoses resulted in 50% of the poisoning-related deaths in 2016. The effects of the opioid epidemic on this younger age group have been less publicized, although increased hospitalizations have been reported (p. 543). Another concern is the increasing fatalities from firearms. For example, firearm suicides and firearm homicides have increased more than 20% among the 15- to 24-year-old group (Lee & Mannix, 2018, p. 544).

Young Adults

Motor vehicle fatalities have increased for this group. Reasons for this increase include distracted driving. For example, these drivers are more likely to send text messages or emails while driving (Lee & Mannix, 2018, p. 543). The trends reported by Lee and Mannix (2018) also reflect increasing firearm suicides and homicides among young adults aged 25 to 34 years (p. 544).

The nurse's role in the prevention of suicide includes identifying behaviors that may indicate potential problems: depression; a variety of physical complaints including weight loss, sleep disturbances, and digestive disorders; and decreased interest in social and work roles along with an increase in isolation. A young adult identified as at risk for suicide should be referred to a mental health professional or a crisis center. Nurses can also reduce the incidence of suicide by participating in educational programs that provide information about the early signs of suicide.

Middle-Aged Adults

Changing physiologic factors, as well as concern over personal and work-related responsibilities, may contribute to the injury rate of middle-aged adults. Motor vehicle crashes are the most common cause of unintentional death in this age group. Decreased reaction times and visual acuity may make the middle-aged adult prone to unintentional injuries. Other unintentional causes of death for middle-aged adults include falls, fires, burns, poisonings, and drownings. Occupational injuries continue to be a significant safety hazard during the middle years.

Older Adults

Unintentional injury prevention is a major concern for older adults. Because vision is limited, reflexes are slower, and bones are brittle, activities such as climbing stairs, driving a car, and even walking require caution. Driving, particularly at night, requires caution because accommodation of the eye to light is impaired and peripheral vision is diminished. Driving in fog or other hazardous conditions should be avoided. The CDC (2017b) offers actions that older adults can take to stay safe on the road: exercising regularly to increase strength and flexibility, having eyes checked annually, driving during daylight and in good weather, planning the route before driving, keeping a safe distance behind the car in front of them, avoiding distractions while driving, and considering alternatives to driving (e.g., riding with a friend, public transportation).

Fires are a hazard for the older adult with a failing memory. The older adult may forget that the iron or stove has been left on or may not extinguish a cigarette completely. Because of reduced sensitivity to pain and heat, care must be taken to prevent burns when the individual bathes or uses heating devices.

Older adults at risk for wandering due to organic brain syndromes need to wear identification devices. They can also be registered with the local Alzheimer Association Safe Return program.

Because older adults who take analgesics or sedatives may become lethargic or confused, they should be monitored regularly and closely. Other measures to induce sleep should be used whenever possible. Nurses can help older clients make the home environment safe. Specific hazards should be identified and corrected; for example, handrails can be installed on staircases. The nurse teaches the importance of taking only prescribed medications and contacting a health professional at the first indication of medication intolerance.

Safety Alert! SAFETY

Older adults have trouble seeing the edges of stairs. Painting white stripes on the edges of the steps will help increase contrast and may prevent falls.

Safety Problems Across the Lifespan

Domestic violence involves individuals of all ages. It includes child abuse, intimate partner abuse, and older adult abuse and affects the health and safety of families and the community. Statistics are inaccurate due to the underreporting of incidents. Nurses are involved in working with all phases of domestic violence: prevention, screening, referrals for treatment, and follow-up care. This usually necessitates collaborative planning with primary care providers, law enforcement agencies, social services, and other community agencies. Nurses also have the opportunity to become advocates for community support programs for domestic violence and can become involved in educating other professionals regarding prevention, screening, and treatment. Domestic violence takes on extra importance because it is known that people who were abused as children often display abusive behavior as an adult. This fact points to the need for prevention and early intervention to prevent the cycle from continuing. Nurses can be of assistance in restoring dignity, health, and safety to vulnerable individuals.

Nurses are on the frontline of client care and need to be aware of disease trends not only in the United States but worldwide, given the frequency of international travel (Lamprecht, 2016). Travel health can be complicated and advice for health professionals is ever-changing (Chiodini, 2016). The CDC (2019) provides three types of travel health notices: Watch Level 1—Practice usual precautions, Alert Level 2—Practice enhanced precautions, and Warning Level 3—Avoid nonessential travel. Each notice level includes information for traveler action and risk to traveler. Examples of travel-related disease notices include outbreaks of Ebola, the Zika virus, measles, and polio (CDC, 2019). The CDC provides helpful information for the traveler and the clinician about vaccines and medicines, non–vaccine-preventable diseases, client counseling, and travel health notices depending upon the specific country. The World Health Organization (WHO) also provides information. For example, WHO advises individuals traveling to areas with Zika virus outbreaks to seek up-to-date advice on potential risks and appropriate measures to reduce the possibility of exposure to mosquito bites and sexual transmission of Zika. With this in mind, nurses should take the opportunity to discuss the Zika virus with their clients and repeat the travel health information that is available.

Promoting Safety in the Healthcare Setting

Client safety in the healthcare setting is of primary importance. One of the primary interventions healthcare institutions must enact is a climate of change and trust. There is a need to change the culture in healthcare from placing blame to examining how to improve care. Trust needs to be developed and sustained for people to feel open to discuss and share experiences about their safety. Communication is of utmost importance to protect clients from errors and maintain continuity of care. Nurses are the frontline managers of client care and must be actively involved in the priority of client safety and the prevention of medical errors.

Preventing Specific Hazards

Implementing measures to prevent specific hazards or injuries such as burns, fires, falls, seizures, poisoning, suffocation, and so on are critical aspects of nursing care. Teaching clients about safety is another important aspect. Nurses usually have opportunities to teach while providing care.

Falls

People of any age can fall, but infants and older adults are particularly prone to falling and causing serious injury. Older adults experience a decrease in muscle strength as they age that affects their balance and increases their risk of falling. More than one out of four older people fall each year, with less than half telling their doctor. Moreover, more than 95% of hip fractures are caused by falls, and they are the most common reason for hospital admission (CDC, 2017a; Falls Prevention, 2016). Most falls occur in the home and are a major threat to the independence of older adults. Fear of falling is common in older adults, even in those who have not experienced a fall. This fear is of particular concern for those who live alone and who anticipate being helpless and unable to summon help after a fall. For these individuals the nurse should encourage daily or more frequent contact with a friend or family member, installation of a personal emergency response system, and measures to maintain a physical environment that prevents falls. Risk factors and associated preventive measures are shown in Table 32.1.

Clinical Alert!

Falls can break bones and self-confidence, leading to fear of falling, which can cause a decreased activity level and decreased muscle strength. All increase the risk of falling.

Healthcare facilities have strong incentives to reduce the number of client falls. The Centers for Medicare and Medicaid Services (CMS) include falls in their list of hospital-acquired conditions for which hospitals are not reimbursed (Chu, 2017). Fall-related injuries lead to longer times spent in the hospital, with an average of 6–12 additional days (Dykes et al., 2018).

It is important to assess clients for fall risk on admission, whenever a change in physical or mental status occurs, on transfer, and before discharge. Many assessment tools to determine a client's risk of falling are available. Most assess for age, number of diseases, medications, environment, physical ability, vision, and history of falls. Assessing the client for fall risks gives the nurse information needed to develop an individualized care plan. Assessing a client's risk for falls is within the scope of practice of several healthcare providers. For example, in addition to nurses, both physical therapists and occupational therapists assess for fall risk.

Most falls in the acute hospital setting occur in the client's room, generally around the bed and in the bathroom, with many of the falls not being observed. The major reason for these falls relates to toileting and a client's fear of having "an accident." Evidence reveals an association between being in a hurry to get to the bathroom and falls. As a result, one proactive intervention is to schedule regular client rounds to provide for client needs. This is where the nurse conducts hourly visits between 6 a.m. and 10 p.m. and visits every 2 hours between 10 p.m. and 6 a.m. The hourly rounding can be alternated between the nurse and assistive personnel (AP). The rounding usually includes pain assessment, offering help with toileting, offering hydration or nutrition, positioning the client if needed, making sure client's call light and personal items are within safe reach, and asking the client and family to use the call light if the client needs to get out of bed. For information on preventing falls and subsequent injury of clients, see the Practice Guidelines.

TABLE 32.1 Risk Factors and Preventive Measures for Falls

Risk Factor	Preventive Measures
Poor vision	Ensure eyeglasses are functional. Ensure appropriate lighting. Mark doorways and edges of steps as needed. Keep the environment tidy.
Cognitive dysfunction (confusion, disorientation, impaired memory or judgment)	Set safe limits to activities. Remove unsafe objects.
Impaired gait or balance and difficulty walking because of lower extremity dysfunction (e.g., arthritis)	Wear shoes or well-fitted slippers with nonskid soles. Use ambulatory devices as necessary (cane, crutches, walker, braces, wheelchair). Provide assistance with ambulation as needed. Monitor gait and balance. Adapt living arrangements to one floor if necessary. Encourage exercise and activity as tolerated to maintain muscle strength, joint flexibility, and balance. Ensure uncluttered environment with securely fastened rugs.
Difficulty getting in and out of a chair or in and out of bed	Encourage client to request assistance. Keep the bed in the low position. Install grab bars in bathroom. Provide a raised toilet seat.
Orthostatic hypotension	Instruct client to rise slowly from a lying to sitting to standing position, and to stand in place for several seconds before walking.
Urinary frequency or receiving diuretics	Provide a bedside commode. Assist with voiding on a frequent and scheduled basis.
Weakness from disease process or therapy	Encourage client to summon help. Monitor activity tolerance.
Current medication regimen that includes sedatives, hypnotics, tranquilizers, narcotic analgesics, diuretics	Attach one-quarter to one-half length side rails to the bed if appropriate. Keep the rails in place when the bed is in the lowest position. Monitor orientation and alertness status. Discuss how alcohol contributes to fall-related injuries. Encourage client not to mix alcohol and medications and to avoid alcohol when necessary. Encourage annual or more frequent review of all medications prescribed.

PRACTICE GUIDELINES Preventing Falls in Healthcare Agencies

- On admission, orient clients to their surroundings and explain the call system.
- Carefully assess the client's ability to ambulate and transfer. Provide nonskid footwear, walking aids, and assistance as required.
- Closely supervise the clients at risk for falls, especially at night. Implement hourly rounding and toileting schedule, as needed.
- Encourage the client to use the call light to request assistance. Ensure that the light is within easy reach.
- Place bedside tables and overbed tables near the bed or chair so that clients do not overreach and consequently lose their balance.
- Always keep hospital beds in the low position and wheels locked when not providing care so that clients can move in or out of bed easily.
- Encourage clients to use grab bars mounted in toilet and bathing areas and railings along corridors.
- Make sure nonskid bath mats are available in tubs and showers.
- Keep the environment tidy; keep light cords from underfoot and furniture out of the way.
- Use individualized interventions (e.g., alarm sensitive to client position) rather than side rails for confused clients.
- Use mechanical or electronic ceiling lifts to transfer dependent clients.
- Assess for medication side effects (e.g., sedation, dizziness, lightheadedness, unsteadiness) and develop appropriate management plan.

Clinical Alert!

When a client falls, the nurse's first duty is to the client. First, assess for injuries. Then, notify the primary care provider.

Although it may seem that raising the side rails on a bed is an effective method of preventing falls, do not routinely raise rails for this purpose. Research has shown that individuals with memory impairment, altered mobility, nocturia, and other sleep disorders are prone

EVIDENCE-BASED PRACTICE

Evidence-Based Practice

What Client Behaviors Predict or Precede a Fall?

Klymko, Etcher, Munchiando, and Royse (2016) relate that almost one million falls occur annually in acute care settings in the United States. Thus, ongoing research aimed at advancing methods to detect and prevent falls is important. They believe that understanding behaviors leading to client falls may facilitate the design of reliable, valid tools for concurrent use with video monitoring (VM) intervention in hospital settings. From a review of the literature, they found that interventions using technology for fall prevention (e.g., electronic sensors, bed alerts, pressure sensors, cameras, and VM) are gaining attention because they provide a means of examining falls in a new way. VM uses in-room cameras to provide real-time viewing of client activity via a computer. VM staff members are trained to view the screen, detect an impending fall, and intervene. The purpose of their qualitative study was to explore behaviors leading to falls in the acute care setting from the experiences of a diverse sample of expert health professionals, client care assistants (1:1 safety sitters), VM technicians, nurses, and fall prevention experts (p. 329).

The setting of the study was an academic medical center where VM had been implemented in five rooms to allow for concurrent viewing of eight clients. The clients had to meet criteria to be placed in a VM monitored bed: 65 years or older with an acute illness at risk for or displaying delirium or at high risk for a fall. The participants in the study were recruited from the hospital, and the sample consisted of 34 participants in four similar groups: fall prevention experts (expert nurses, geriatricians [$n = 9$]), RNs from the VM unit ($n = 10$), VM technicians ($n = 6$), and client care assistants ($n = 9$). The researchers conducted focus groups with the participants with each focus group lasting 60 to 90 minutes. The questions asked at the focus groups related to the study's purpose (e.g., what behaviors predicted or preceded a fall, how would those behaviors appear, and what specific behaviors would alert you to take action to prevent a fall?).

The findings included the major themes of environmental factors and behavioral representations. Challenging hazards within the rooms included overcrowding, extreme room temperatures, and lines attached to or close to the client (e.g., feeding tube, IV line, urinary catheter bag, monitoring lines) that could cause the client to become entangled or trip when getting out of bed or ambulating. Also, soiled bedding or clothing often caused the client to try to get out of bed. Bedside tables containing personal items that were too far away to reach caused clients to reach unsafely. Vulnerable times for a fall to occur included the day of admission or discharge, waking up in the morning, meal times, shift changes, staff breaks, and when people entered or left a client's room.

Behavioral conduct consisted of two subthemes: physical and psychologic or emotional. Frequent physical behaviors were restlessness and picking at or touching whatever was around before trying to climb out of bed. A pattern and order of movements was reported. For example, the client would initially be restless and picking around, followed by more gross movement such as sitting up suddenly or scooting to the side of the bed. Issues that were associated with ambulation that preceded a fall included improper use of unfamiliar assistive devices, excessive speed in walking, foot dragging, unsteadiness, and verbalizations of dizziness. The psychologic and emotional behaviors described were observed when cognitive changes occurred suddenly, such as in a client who had a urinary tract infection.

Implications

The researchers described the limitations to the study: self-selected groups, one hospital setting, and lack of a focus group of clients who had experienced a hospital fall. The preceding behaviors to hospital falls, as described by the study participants, were consistent with client-specific factors and environmental risk factors already described in the literature and added to the existing knowledge. The findings may assist nurses who are planning to implement a VM intervention in their hospitals. Further investigations are needed on the characteristics of clients who may be best served by VM.

to becoming entrapped in side rails and may, in fact, be more likely to fall trying to get out around raised rails. Clients may even become entrapped between the mattress and side rails, leading to asphyxiation deaths. In some settings, side rails are not used at all. Instead, beds are lowered fully, and long pads are placed on each side of the bed.

Healthcare environments should be safety oriented with systems in place to allow objective evaluation of outcomes. Environments should be designed with many safety features to reduce the risk of falls, such as regular toileting and orientation of clients who are confused or impaired; the use of fall risk alerts such as client ID wrist bands or client gown of a specific color and fall precaution signs on the door and in the room; railings along corridors; call lights at each bedside; safety bars in toilet areas; locks on beds, wheelchairs, and stretchers; well-maintained and appropriately sized wheelchairs; one-quarter to one-half length side rails on beds or pads beside beds; night lights; freedom from clutter; and so on.

Electronic **safety monitoring devices** are available to detect when clients are attempting to move or get out of bed. For example, a bed or chair safety monitor has a position-sensitive switch that triggers an audio alarm when the client attempts to get out of the bed or chair. A magnetic box mobility monitor mounted on a bed or chair connects with a clip to clothing. It will pull apart should the client try to move away from the chair or bed, triggering an alarm. There are also dual-sensor systems that have a pressure-sensitive sensor combined with an infrared beam detector. These monitors, however, can alarm with normal position changes, so nurses must be careful to assess whether or not the client is actually trying to exit the bed or chair. Some hospital beds have a built-in alarm to alert staff when a client tries to get out of bed. Bed and chair alarms should be used only for clients who are confused or will not reliably call for help. Dykes et al. (2018) point out that research has shown that alarms are ineffective for clients who are mentally alert and only contribute noise to the environment (p. 11). Skill 32.1 describes how to use these devices.

Using a Bed or Chair Exit Safety Monitoring Device

PURPOSES

- To alert the nurse that the client is attempting to get out of bed
- To help decrease the risk of client falls

ASSESSMENT

Assess

- Fall risk
- Mobility status
- Judgment about the ability to get out of bed safely
- Client's pattern of exiting the bed (e.g., using upper extremities to pull the body up before lowering the feet to the floor or leaning toward the edge of the bed prior to dropping the legs over the side)
- Proximity of client's room to nurses' station
- Position of side rails
- Functioning status of call light

PLANNING

Determine the best type of device and appropriate location for the device. No matter where the device is applied, choose a location where skin is intact.

Assignment

Risk factors for falls may be observed and recorded by individuals other than the nurse. The nurse is responsible for assessing the client and confirming that there is a risk of the client falling when getting out of a chair or bed unassisted. The nurse develops a plan of care that includes a variety of interventions that will protect the client. If indicated, use of a safety monitoring device may be assigned to AP who have been trained in their application and monitoring.

Equipment

- Alarm and control device
- Sensor
- Connection to nurse call system

IMPLEMENTATION

Performance

1. Prior to performing the procedure, introduce self and verify the client's identity using agency protocol. Explain to client and family the purpose and procedure of using a safety monitoring device. Explain that the device does not limit mobility in any manner; rather, it alerts the staff when the client is about to get out of bed or a chair. Explain that the nurse must be called when the client needs to get out of bed or a chair.
2. Perform hand hygiene and observe other appropriate infection prevention procedures.
3. Provide for client privacy.
4. Test the battery device and alarm sound. **Rationale:** *Testing ensures that the device is functioning properly prior to use.*
5. Apply the leg band or sensor pad.
   - Place the leg band according to the manufacturer's recommendation. Place the client's leg in a straight horizontal position. **Rationale:** *The alarm device is position sensitive; that is, when it approaches a near-vertical position (such as in walking, crawling, or kneeling as the client attempts to get out of bed), the audio alarm will be triggered.*
   - For the bed or chair device, the sensor is usually placed under the buttocks area. ❶
   - For a bed or chair device, set the time delay from 1 to 12 seconds for determining the client's movement patterns.
   - Connect the sensor pad to the control unit and the nurse call system.
6. Instruct the client to call the nurse when the client wants or needs to get up, and assist as required.
   - When assisting the client up, deactivate the alarm.
   - Assist the client back to the bed or chair, and reattach the alarm device.
7. Ensure client safety with additional safety precautions.
   - Place call light within client reach, lift side rails per agency policy, and lower the bed to its lowest position. **Rationale:** *The alarm device is not a substitute for other precautionary measures.*
   - Place fall precaution signs on the client's door, chart, and other relevant locations per facility policy.
8. Document the type of alarm used, where it was placed, and its effectiveness in the client record using forms or checklists supplemented by narrative notes when appropriate. Record all additional safety precautions and interventions discussed and employed.

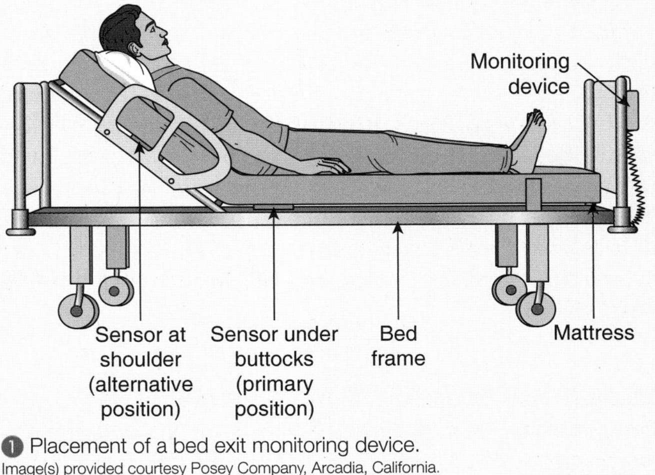

❶ Placement of a bed exit monitoring device.
Image(s) provided courtesy Posey Company, Arcadia, California.

Continued on page 740

SKILL 32.1

Using a Bed or Chair Exit Safety Monitoring Device—*continued*

9. If the device is used in the home, instruct caregivers to do the following:
   - Test the monitoring device every 12 to 24 hours to ensure that it is working.
   - Check the volume of the alarm to ascertain that they can hear it.
   - Investigate all alarms and do not assume a false alarm. They may, however, adjust the alarm controls.

SAMPLE DOCUMENTATION

7/2/2020 1130 Found out of bed. Frequent reminders previously given to use the call light for assistance. Explained about the use of a magnetic box mobility alarm to ensure own safety from possible fall. Verbalized agreement. Alarm device applied. Reminded again of importance to call the nurse for assistance. Call light placed within client's reach. T. Kyle, RN

EVALUATION

- If the alarm is too sensitive to client movement that is not an attempt to move from bed or chair, reassess and modify alarm controls accordingly.
- Conduct appropriate follow-up relating to effectiveness of safety precautions.
- Report any difficulties using the device or any falls to the primary care provider.

Seizures

A **seizure** is a single temporary event that consists of uncontrolled electrical neuronal discharge of the brain that interrupts normal brain function. The etiology or cause of the seizure can be different based on the age of the client. Trauma during birth is the leading cause of seizures in newborns. Infants and children develop seizures as a result of fever, trauma, and infections of the central nervous system. The development of seizures in the adult population is most commonly related to structural abnormalities of the brain such as tumors, strokes, and trauma.

Seizures are classified into two categories: partial and generalized. Partial seizures (also called focal) involve electrical discharges from one area of the brain. In contrast, generalized seizures affect the whole brain. Each of these seizure categories includes different types of seizures, depending on the characteristics of the seizure activity (e.g., loss of consciousness versus no impairment to consciousness). Thus, it is important for nurses to thoroughly describe their observations before, during, and after a client's seizure episode. Clients are at risk for injury if they experience seizures that involve the entire body such as *grand mal* (tonic–clonic) seizures or any seizure that includes loss of consciousness. **Seizure precautions** are safety measures taken by the nurse to protect clients from injury should they have a seizure. Skill 32.2 describes how to implement seizure precautions in the acute care setting.

Seizure precautions in the home care setting include the following considerations:

- If clients have frequent or recurrent seizures or take anticonvulsant medications, they should wear a medical identification tag (bracelet or necklace) and carry a card listing any medications they take.
- When making home visits, inspect antiepileptic medications and confirm that clients are taking them correctly. Blood samples may be required periodically to measure the level of medication in the blood.
- Discuss safety precautions for inside and outside of the home. If seizures are not well controlled, activities that may require restriction or direct supervision by others include bathing (i.e., tub and showering), swimming, cooking, using electric equipment or machinery, and driving.
- Discuss with the client and family factors that may precipitate a seizure.
- Assist clients in determining who in the community should or must be informed of their seizure disorder (e.g., employers, healthcare providers such as dentists, motor vehicle department if driving, and companions).

SKILL 32.2

Implementing Seizure Precautions

PURPOSE

- To protect the client from injury

ASSESSMENT

Assess the history of seizures during the admission assessment. If the client has experienced a seizure previously, ask for detailed information, including characteristics of an aura or warning symptoms that indicate the seizure is beginning, duration and frequency of the seizures, consequences of the seizures (e.g., incontinence or difficulty breathing), and actions that should be taken to prevent or reduce seizure activity.

Implementing Seizure Precautions—*continued*

PLANNING

Review emergency procedures because respiratory arrest or other injury can result from a seizure.

Assignment

AP should be familiar with establishing and implementing seizure precautions and methods of obtaining assistance during a client's seizure. Care of the client during a seizure, however, is the responsibility of the nurse due to the importance of careful assessment of respiratory status and the potential need for intervention.

Equipment

- Blankets or other linens to pad side rails
- Oral suction equipment
- Oxygen equipment
- Clean gloves

IMPLEMENTATION

Performance

1. Prior to performing the procedure, introduce self and verify the client's identity using agency protocol. Explain to the client what you are going to do, why it is necessary, and how to participate.
2. Perform hand hygiene and observe other appropriate infection prevention procedures. If the client is actively seizing, apply clean gloves in preparation for performing respiratory care measures.
3. Provide for client privacy.
4. Pad the bed of any client who might have a seizure. Secure blankets or other linens around the head, foot, and side rails of the bed. ❶
5. Put oral suction equipment in place and test to ensure that it is functional. **Rationale:** *Suctioning may be needed to prevent aspiration of oral secretions*.
6. If a seizure occurs:
   - Remain with the client and call for assistance. Do not restrain the client.
   - If the client is not in bed, assist the client to the floor and protect the client's head by holding it in your lap or on a pillow. Loosen any clothing around the neck and chest.
   - Turn the client to a lateral position if possible. This may not be possible during the seizure but is required after the seizure. **Rationale:** *Turning to the side allows secretions to drain out of the mouth, decreasing the risk of aspiration, and helps keep the tongue from occluding the airway*.
   - Move items in the environment to ensure the client does not experience an injury.
   - Do not insert anything into the client's mouth.
   - Time the seizure duration.
   - Observe the progression of the seizure, noting the sequence and type of limb involvement. Observe skin color. When the seizure allows, assess pulse, respirations, and oxygen saturation.
   - Apply gloves and use equipment to suction the oral airway if the client vomits or has excessive oral secretions.
   - Apply oxygen to the client via mask or nasal cannula.
   - Administer anticonvulsant medications, as ordered.
   - When the seizure has subsided, assist client to a comfortable position. Reorient. Explain what happened. Reassure the client. Provide hygiene as necessary. Allow the client to verbalize feelings about the seizure.
   - Status epilepticus clients may stop breathing after the seizure. Begin CPR immediately. Bring the emergency cart to the bedside. Apply oxygen per nasal cannula or mask when breathing resumes.
   - If applied, remove and discard gloves.
   - Perform hand hygiene.
7. Document the event in the client record using forms or checklists supplemented by narrative notes when appropriate.

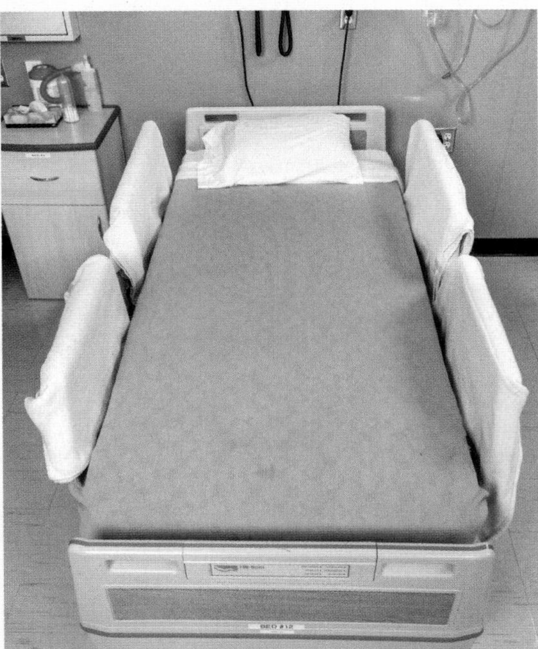

❶ Padding a bed for seizure precautions.

SAMPLE DOCUMENTATION

7/8/2020 1815 Upon entering room, observed generalized muscle spasms/contractions of arms and legs lasting 25 seconds. Seizure padding previously placed on bed. Incontinent of urine. Cyanotic. Placed on left side. Suctioned. Airway clear. Respirations 14/min with irregular pattern. Oxygen applied at 4 L/min via mask. Oxygen sat 90% on O_2. Not currently responding to verbal stimuli. Dr. Smith notified. Diazepam 10 mg given IV per order. VS taken every 15 min. See neuro flow sheet. T B. Gill, RN

1835 Respirations 15/min regular. Responding to verbal stimuli. Oriented to person, place, and time. Oxygen saturation 95% on O_2. Oxygen discontinued per doctor's order. VS continue every 15 min. See neuro flow sheet. T B. Gill, RN

EVALUATION

- Perform a detailed follow-up examination of the client. Assess the client for any signs of injury that may have occurred during the seizure. Administer medications if indicated and ordered.
- Report significant deviations from normal to the primary care provider.

LIFESPAN CONSIDERATIONS **Implementing Seizure Precautions**

CHILDREN

- Febrile seizures occur more commonly in children than in adults and are usually preventable through the use of antipyretics and tepid baths.
- Determine oxygenation. Apply oxygen if pulse oximetry reading is less than 95% (see Chapter 49). Oxygen can be applied via head hood, tent, nasal cannula, or mask, depending on the age and response of the child. Oxygen is drying and must be humidified. Tents are cooling, and the child's thermal balance must be monitored. The concentration of oxygen in tents is more difficult to regulate.
- Children who have frequent seizures may need to wear helmets for protection.
- Children on antiepileptic medications should wear a medical identification tag (bracelet or necklace).

Scalds and Burns

A **scald** is a burn from a hot liquid or vapor, such as steam. A **burn** results from excessive exposure to thermal, chemical, electric, or radioactive agents.

Common home hazards causing scalds include the following:

- Pot handles that protrude over the edge of a stove
- Electric appliances used to heat liquids or oils, especially those with dangling cords that are within reach of crawling infants and young children
- Excessively hot bath water.

In healthcare agencies, the risk of scalds and burns is greater for clients whose skin sensitivity to temperature is impaired. Scalds can occur from overly hot bath water, and burns can occur from therapeutic applications of heat (see Chapter 36). It is important for the nurse to assess how well clients can protect themselves and what special precautions, if any, need to be taken.

Fires

Fires continue to be a constant risk in both healthcare settings and homes. Agency fires usually result from malfunctioning electric equipment or combustion of anesthetic gas. Home fires most frequently result from careless disposal of burning cigarettes or matches, from grease, or from faulty electric wiring.

Agency Fires

In healthcare agencies, fire is particularly hazardous when individuals are incapacitated and unable to leave the building without assistance. This incapacity makes it extremely important for nurses to be aware of the fire safety regulations and fire prevention practices of the agencies in which they work. When smoke or fire is detected, two mnemonics can help the nurse remember the steps to follow. First is the RACE protocol:

1. **R**escue: If the area is safe to enter, protect and evacuate clients who are in immediate danger.
2. **A**larm: Pull the fire alarm and report the fire details and location to the hospital's fire emergency extension.
3. **C**onfine: Contain the fire by closing the doors to all rooms and the fire doors at each entrance to the unit.
4. **E**xtinguish: Extinguish the fire. Use the appropriate type of fire extinguisher (see the PASS mnemonic) OR **E**vacuate the area if the fire is too large for a fire extinguisher.

Extinguishing the fire requires knowledge of three categories of fire, classified according to the type of material that is burning:

Class A: paper, wood, upholstery, rags, ordinary rubbish
Class B: flammable liquids and gases
Class C: electrical.

The right type of extinguisher must be used to fight the fire. Extinguishers have picture symbols showing the type of fire for which they are to be used. Directions for use are also attached. See Figure 32.3 ■. The nurse follows the mnemonic PASS when using a fire extinguisher:

Pull out the extinguisher's safety pin.
Aim the hose at the base of the fire.
Squeeze or press the handle to discharge the material onto the fire.
Sweep the hose from side to side across the base of the fire until the fire appears to be out.

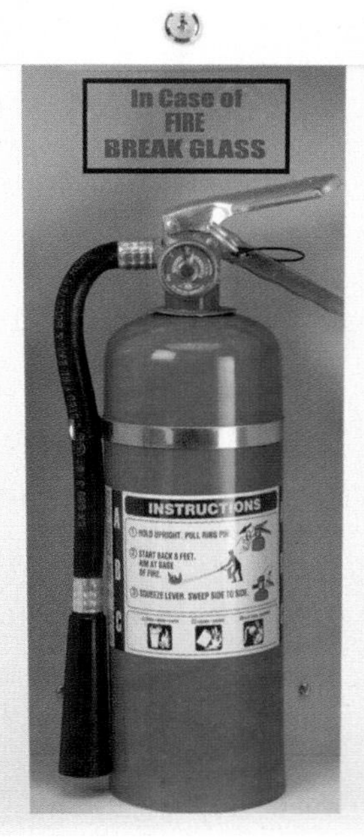

Figure 32.3 ■ Fire extinguisher.
C Squared Studios/Getty Images.

Home Fires

Nursing interventions for home fires focus on teaching fire safety. Preventive measures include the following:

- Keep emergency numbers near the telephone, or stored for speed dialing.
- Be sure the smoke alarms are operable and appropriately located.
- Teach clients to change the batteries in their smoke alarms annually on a special day such as a birthday or January 1.
- Have a family fire drill plan. Every member needs to know the plan for the nearest exit from different locations of the home.
- Keep fire extinguishers available and in working order.
- Close windows and doors if possible, cover the mouth and nose with a damp cloth when exiting through a smoke-filled area, and avoid heavy smoke by assuming a bent position with the head as close to the floor as possible.

Carbon Monoxide Poisoning

Carbon monoxide (CO) is an odorless, colorless, tasteless gas that is very toxic. Exposure to CO can cause symptoms that include headaches, dizziness, weakness, nausea, vomiting, or loss of muscle control. Prolonged exposure to CO can lead to unconsciousness, brain damage, or death. Learning the steps to prevent CO exposure is particularly important because all gasoline-powered vehicles, lawn mowers, kerosene stoves, barbecues, and burning wood emit CO. Incomplete or faulty combustion of any fuel, including natural gas used in furnaces, also produces CO. Carbon monoxide detectors are available for the home (Figure 32.4 ■).

Poisoning

Inadequate supervision and improper storage of many household toxic substances are the major reasons for poisoning in children. Implementing poison prevention for children is focused on teaching parents to "childproof" the environment, including disposing of unused medications properly (see Chapter 35 ∞). Adolescent and adult poisonings are usually caused by insect or snake bites and drugs used for recreation or in suicide attempts. Implementing poison prevention in these age groups focuses on providing information and counseling. Poisoning in older adults usually results from unintentional ingestion of a toxic substance (e.g., due to failing eyesight) or an overdose of a prescribed medication (e.g., due to impaired memory). Implementing poison prevention with older adults focuses on protecting the environment and monitoring the main problems.

In older adults who have dementia, poisoning is often a safety problem. As cognitive abilities deteriorate, the same precautions need to be taken as with children. Older adults who have dementia have the need to feel everything and will put anything in their mouths, including plants, flowers, candles, small objects, and medications. These and other potentially dangerous items need to be locked up or kept out of reach. A telephone number for the nearest poison control center should be readily available. These precautions are important whether the individual with dementia is being cared for at home or in a healthcare setting.

In response to the ever-increasing number of poison hazards, many countries have established poison control centers that provide accurate, up-to-date information about potential hazards and recommend treatment as needed. For certain poisons, specific antidotes or treatments are available; for many, there is no specific therapy.

Nurses intervene in community settings by educating the public about what to do in the event of poisoning: Identify the specific poison by searching for an opened container, empty bottle, or other evidence. Contact the poison control center, indicate the exact quantity of poison ingested and state the individual's age and apparent symptoms. Keep the individual as quiet as possible and lying on the side or sitting with head placed between the legs to prevent aspiration of vomitus. The Client Teaching feature provides additional guidelines for teaching clients to prevent poisoning.

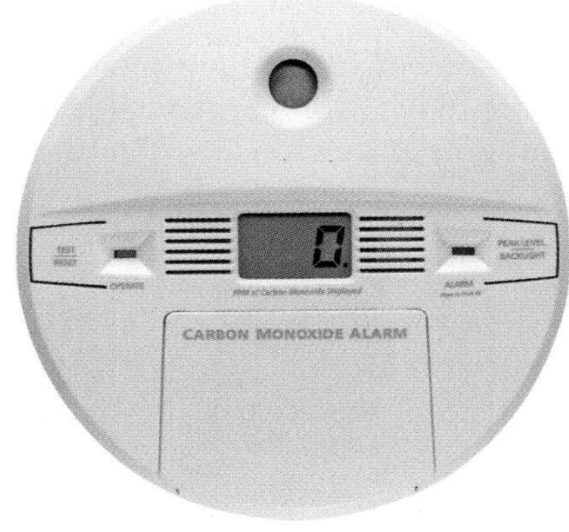

Figure 32.4 ■ Carbon monoxide detector.
dehooks/iStock/Getty Images.

Suffocation or Choking

Suffocation, or **asphyxiation**, is lack of oxygen due to interrupted breathing. Suffocation occurs when the air source is cut off for any reason. One common reason for choking is that food or a foreign object has become lodged in the throat. The universal sign of distress is the victim's grasping the anterior neck and being unable to speak or cough. The emergency response is the **Heimlich maneuver** or abdominal thrust, which can dislodge the foreign object and reestablish an airway. See Figure 32.5 ■.

Other causes of suffocation are drowning, gas or smoke inhalation, unintentional coverage of the nose and mouth by a piece of plastic, unintentional strangulation by the shoulder harness of a seat belt, and being trapped in a confined space (e.g., a discarded refrigerator). If an individual does not receive immediate relief from suffocation, the interrupted breathing leads to respiratory and cardiac

CLIENT TEACHING Preventing Poisoning

- Lock potentially toxic agents, including drugs and cleaning agents, in a cupboard, or attach special plastic hooks to the insides of cabinet doors to keep them securely closed. Unlatching these hooks requires firmer thumb pressure than small children can usually exert. Do not let children watch you open the latches. Kids learn fast!
- Avoid storing toxic liquids or solids in food containers, such as soft drink bottles, peanut butter jars, or milk cartons.
- Do not remove container labels or reuse empty containers to store different substances. Laws mandate that the labels of all poisons specify antidotes.
- Do not rely on cooking to destroy toxic chemicals in plants. Never use anything prepared from nature as a medicine or "tea."
- Teach children never to eat any part of an unknown plant or mushroom and not to put leaves, stems, bark, seeds, nuts, or berries from any plant into their mouths.
- Place poison warning stickers designed for children on containers of bleach, lye, kerosene, solvent, and other toxic substances.
- Do not refer to medicine as candy or pretend false enjoyment when taking medications in front of children; allow them to see the necessity of the medicine without glamorizing it.
- Read and follow label directions on all products before using them.
- Keep syrup of ipecac on hand at all times. Syrup of ipecac is a nonprescription emetic available in single-dose 15-mL vials in all drugstores. Use it only after getting advice from the local poison control center or the family primary care provider.
- Do not keep poisonous plants in the home, and avoid planting poisonous plants in the yard. The cooperative extension agency in your county can provide a list of poisonous plants.
- Display the phone number of the poison control center near or on all telephones in the home so that it is available to babysitters, family, and friends.

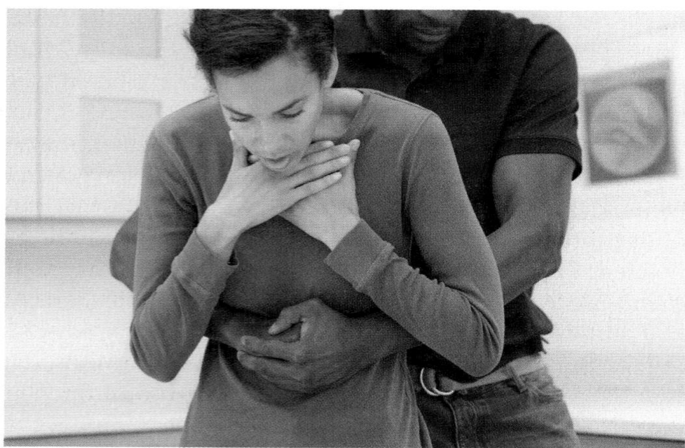

Figure 32.5 ■ Performing the Heimlich maneuver.
Science Photo Library/Getty Images.

arrest and death. Any obstruction to the air passages must be immediately removed and life support measures instituted when an arrest occurs.

Excessive Noise

Excessive noise is a health hazard that can cause hearing loss, depending on (a) the overall level of noise, (b) the frequency range of the noise, and (c) the duration of exposure and individual susceptibility. Sound levels above 120 decibels (dB; units of loudness) are painful and may cause hearing damage even if an individual is exposed for only a short period. Exposure to 85 to 95 dB for several hours a day can lead to progressive or permanent hearing loss. Noise levels below 85 dB usually do not affect hearing.

Tolerance of noise is largely individual. The rural dweller may find the city noisy, whereas the city dweller may be oblivious to urban sounds.

When ill or injured, people are frequently sensitive to noises that normally would not disturb them. Loud voices, the clatter of dishes, and even a nearby television can disturb clients, some of whom react angrily. Physiologic effects of noise include (a) increased heart and respiratory rates, (b) increased muscular activity, (c) nausea, and (d) hearing loss, if the noise is sufficiently loud.

Noise can be minimized in several ways. Acoustic tiles on ceilings, walls, and floors as well as drapes and carpeting absorb sound. Background music can mask noise and have a calming effect on some people. It is important for nurses to minimize noise in the hospital setting and to encourage clients to protect their hearing as much as possible.

Electrical Hazards

All electric equipment must be properly grounded. The electric plug of grounded equipment has three prongs. The two short prongs transmit the power to the equipment. The third, longer prong is the grounding device, which carries short circuits or stray electric current to the ground (Figure 32.6 ■). Grounding prongs offer a path of least resistance to stray electric currents.

Faulty equipment such as equipment with a frayed cord presents a danger of electric shock or may start a fire. For example, an electric spark near certain anesthetic gases or a high concentration of oxygen can cause a serious fire. Actions to reduce electrical hazards are described in Client Teaching.

When major electrical injury (macroshock) does occur, the victim may sustain both superficial and deep burns, muscle contractions, and cardiac and respiratory

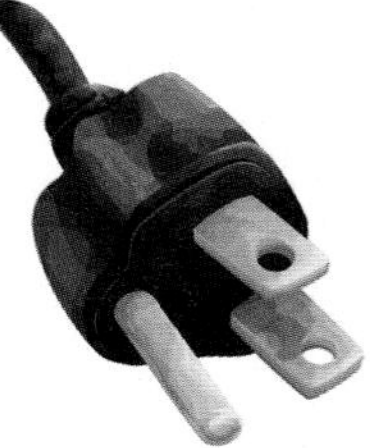

Figure 32.6 ■ Three-pronged grounded plug.
Scott Weichert/Imagezoo/Getty Images.

arrest, necessitating cardiopulmonary resuscitation and life support. **Electric shock** occurs when a current travels through the body to the ground rather than through electric wiring, or from static electricity that builds up on the body. Using machines in good repair, wearing shoes with rubber soles, standing on a nonconductive floor, and using nonconductive gloves can prevent macroshock. However, even with such precautions the rescuer must know that the victim is not to be touched until the electricity is shut off or the victim has been removed from contact with the electric current; otherwise the rescuer may also receive electrical injury.

Firearms

Parents who bring a firearm into the home must accept full responsibility for teaching safety rules to any children who have knowledge of the presence of firearms. The following basic firearm safety rules must be implemented for any gun:

- Store all firearms in sturdy locked cabinets without glass and make sure the keys are inaccessible to children.
- Store the bullets in a different location from the guns.
- Tell children never to touch a firearm or stay in a friend's house where a firearm is nearby.
- Teach children never to point the barrel of a firearm at anyone.
- Ensure the firearm is unloaded and the action is open when handing it to someone else.
- Do not handle firearms while affected by alcohol or drugs of any kind, including pharmaceuticals.
- When cleaning or dry firing a firearm, remove all ammunition to another room, and double-check the firearm when you enter the room you will be using to clean the firearm.
- Have firearms that are regularly used inspected by a qualified gunsmith at least every 2 years.

Radiation

Radiation injury can occur from overexposure to radioactive materials used in diagnostic and therapeutic procedures. Clients being examined using radiography or fluoroscopy generally receive minimal exposure and few precautions are necessary. Nurses need to protect themselves, however, from radiation when some clients are receiving radiation therapy. Exposure to radiation can be minimized by (a) limiting the time near the source, (b) providing as much distance as possible from the source, and (c) using shielding devices such as lead aprons when near the source. Nurses need to become familiar with agency protocols related to radiation therapy.

Disasters

No one knows when a disaster will occur. Thus, it is important that healthcare personnel and facilities plan and prepare for the unknown. The Joint Commission requires its accredited healthcare organizations to meet established disaster preparedness standards. In 2001, these standards were expanded to introduce the concepts of emergency management and community involvement in the preparedness process. Healthcare organizations are now expected to address four specific phases of disaster planning—mitigation, preparedness, response, and recovery—as well as to participate annually in at least one community-wide practice drill.

Nurses must also care for themselves in the event of a disaster. For example, they must be prepared to deal with the stress associated with the disaster, and to be separated from their families for extended periods of time. It is imperative that nurses set up their own emergency action plans with their families.

It is important for the nurse to understand work-related expectations during times of disaster, including termination if employer obligations cannot be met. Nurse attorney Stokes (2018) points out that when searching for a new employer, the nurse should know

CLIENT TEACHING **REDUCING ELECTRICAL HAZARDS**

- Check cords for fraying or other signs of damage before using an appliance. Do not use if damage is apparent.
- Avoid overloading outlets and fuse boxes with too many appliances.
- Use only grounded outlets and plugs.
- Always pull a plug from the wall outlet by firmly grasping the plug and pulling it straight out. Pulling a plug by its cord can damage the cord and plug unit.
- Never use electric appliances near sinks, bathtubs, showers, or other wet areas, because water readily conducts electricity.
- Keep electric cords and appliances out of the reach of young children.
- Place protective covers over wall outlets to protect young children.
- Have all noninsulated wiring in the home altered to meet safety standards.
- Carefully read instructions before operating electric equipment. Clients who do not understand how to operate the equipment should seek advice.
- Always disconnect appliances before cleaning or repairing them.
- Unplug any appliance that has given a tingling sensation or shock and have an electrician evaluate it for stray current.
- Keep electric cords coiled or taped to the ground away from areas of traffic to prevent others from damaging the cords or tripping over them.

the emergency response plans and state and local disaster preparedness expectations. Also, nurses need to know the legal obligations in their state of practice because some states have laws requiring healthcare providers to respond, and refusal to comply can be punishable. Nielson (2017) states that hospitals should have policies that inform nurses of their responsibilities during a disaster and protect nurses acting in good faith from charges of negligence or malpractice (p. 56). After the disaster, organizations need to provide stress management opportunities to minimize the impact of the stress incurred during the disaster.

Some nurses would like to help out and volunteer their services during a disaster. Organized response registries for healthcare professionals exist at both state and federal levels. The interested nurse should determine which organization best suits his or her needs and should register with only one system. Then the nurse needs to register in advance with one of these response systems to receive appropriate training.

Procedure- and Equipment-Related Unintentional Injuries

Risk assessment in the healthcare setting must include risks related to procedures and equipment. Nurses need to follow safeguards to prevent errors or unintentional injuries whether giving a medication or assisting a client out of bed. Most healthcare agencies establish protocols that are designed to prevent unintentional injuries. When in doubt about a course of action, the nurse should consult the appropriate written guidelines before proceeding.

When an unintentional injury or error does occur, most agencies require that the incident be reported. The nurse completes the report immediately after taking whatever action is required to safeguard the client and notifying the charge nurse. For additional information about incident reports, see Chapter 3 ∞.

Restraining Clients

Restraints are devices used to reduce or prevent physical activity of a client or a part of the body when the client is unable to remove the device. The CMS states that "all patients have the right to be free from physical or mental abuse, and corporal punishment. All patients have the right to be free from restraint or seclusion, of any form, imposed as a means of coercion, discipline, convenience, or retaliation by staff. Restraint or seclusion may only be imposed to ensure the immediate physical safety of the patient, a staff member, or others and must be discontinued at the earliest possible time" (2008, p. 83). Physical restraints have been shown to *not* prevent the safety problems that they are used to prevent, such as avoiding falls and pulling out medical devices (e.g., IV, Foley catheter, endotracheal tube). In fact, evidence has shown that the use of physical restraint can result in a variety of injuries including death. Research has also shown that progress in reducing physical restraint has been made in long-term care settings; however, restraint use continues to be a routine practice in hospitals with wide variability within hospitals and across hospitals (Lach, Leach, & Butcher, 2016). The desired outcome is to use other means for controlling behaviors that may pose a threat to self or others, referred to as a *restraint-free environment*. Unfortunately, Lach and colleagues (2016) found that "nurses continue to have misconceptions of restraint use, and believe they do not have satisfactory alternative options" (p. 19).

The decision to use a restraint is usually initiated by nurses, despite needing a healthcare provider's order. It is important that the nurse base the decision on a comprehensive, individualized client assessment. Client safety is a primary concern of nurses. Identifying clients who are at risk for unsafe behaviors is part of the assessment. Examples include clients who are incontinent, restless, or cognitively impaired; who get up without asking for assistance; and who have medical devices as part of their care. The goal is to provide interventions that will be successful in preventing the problem behaviors. For example, conduct frequent toileting rounds, secure anchoring of tubes, keep tubing out of client's vision, and reorient the confused client. The assessment needs to determine whether the use of alternative measures is a greater risk than the risk of using a restraint (CMS, 2008, p. 83). Restraints should not be considered a part of routine client care and should not be included in a fall prevention program. A request from a family member to apply a restraint is not sufficient cause to apply a restraint. It should, however, encourage the nurse to assess the client and current situation to determine if a restraint intervention is needed. The assessment and determination that a restraint is needed must be documented and reflect that an alternative intervention was attempted.

There are three types of restraints: physical, chemical, and seclusion. **Physical restraints**, which are used most commonly, involve "use of an intervention or device that hinders the client from moving or restricts the individual from contact with his or her body" (Bauer & Weust, 2017, p. 352). Examples can include leather or cloth wrist and ankle restraints, soft belts or vests, hand mitts, enclosure beds, gerichairs, and overchair tables. They cannot be removed easily and they restrict the client's movement. Generally, if a client can easily remove a device, the device would not be considered a restraint. **Chemical restraints** involve using a medication to control behavior or to restrict the client's freedom of movement and is *not* a standard treatment for the client's medical or psychologic condition (CMS, 2008). **Seclusion** is the involuntary confinement of a client alone in a room or area from which the client is physically prevented from leaving (CMS, 2008).

Improper use of restraints and lack of monitoring can lead to injury and death and to psychologic harm. Restraints can cause injury to clients through the hazards of immobility, confusion, boredom and loneliness, depression, and loss of dignity. Death can result due to strangulation, suffocation, broken necks, burns, pneumonia, and sepsis. Cases have been documented in which restrained individuals have not received proper care related to hygiene, skin assessments, hydration, nutritional requirements, elimination, pain assessment, and appropriate assessments and monitoring of vital signs. The recent focus in healthcare safety is to explore ways to prevent, reduce, and hopefully eliminate the use of restraints while still protecting a client's safety, rights, and dignity. Attention to the legal and ethical rights of clients has increased movement toward restraint-free environments.

Restrained clients must be monitored regularly, and the new standards allow hospital policies to guide staff in determining appropriate intervals for assessment and monitoring. However, in the case of clients in seclusion, continual, ongoing monitoring is required.

Standards require that a primary care provider's order for restraints include explanation of the reason for, specific time frame (only for violent or self-destructive behavior), and type of restraint necessary. Restraint or seclusion must be discontinued at the earliest possible time, regardless of the length of time identified in the order. "As-needed" (prn) orders for restraints are forbidden. *In all cases, restraints should be used only after every other possible means of ensuring safety has been unsuccessful and documented.* See alternatives to the use of restraints in Box 32.3. Restrained clients often become more restless and anxious because of the loss of self-control. Nurses must document that the need for the restraint was made clear both to the client and to support people such as family members.

Clients have the right to be free from restraints that are not medically necessary. As a result, there must be justification that the use of restraints will protect the client and that less restrictive alternative measures were attempted and found ineffective. Restraints *cannot* be used for staff convenience or client punishment. Given that the above conditions are met and restraints are needed, it is important for the nurse to be able to correctly apply restraints without endangering client safety.

Selecting a Restraint

Before selecting a restraint, nurses need to understand its purpose clearly and measure it against the following five criteria:

BOX 32.3 Alternative Interventions to the Use of Restraints

TO PREVENT:

Physiologic Causes of Unsafe Behavior:

- Assess for pain and treat appropriately before potentially painful procedures to avoid agitation.
- Stay with a client using a bedside commode or bathroom if the client is confused or sedated or has a gait disturbance or a high-risk score for falling.
- Provide frequent toileting, if needed; provide a bedside commode.
- Guide the client to feel and become familiar with tubes or other equipment.
- Overdress wounds; use abdominal binders to cover wound dressings.

Psychologic Causes of Unsafe Behavior:

- Increase communication by explaining devices and active listening; use translators as needed.
- Ask family members or significant others to stay with the client; ask family to bring photographs or familiar objects.
- Place a photograph or other personal item on the door to clients' rooms to help them identify their room.
- Prepare clients before a move to limit relocation shock and resultant confusion.
- Use rocking chairs to help confused clients expend some of their energy so that they will be less inclined to wander.
- To quiet agitated clients, try a warm beverage, soft lights, a back massage, or a walk.
- Reorient the confused client; provide reality links (e.g., calendar, clock); introduce self each time you enter the room.

Environmental Causes of Unsafe Behavior:

- Remove hazards and clutter that could cause injury.
- Support sensory input by ensuring the client has eyeglasses or hearing aids to interpret the environment.
- Provide adequate lighting.
- Conduct frequent nursing rounds.
- Place unstable clients in an area that is constantly and closely supervised.
- Reduce excessive or annoying stimulation (e.g., noise, lights); play soothing music.
- Position beds at their lowest level to facilitate getting in and out of bed.
- Use alternative seating such as an Adirondack chair or bean bag chair, which uses gravity to secure the client.
- Replace full-length side rails with half- or three-quarter-length rails to prevent confused clients from climbing over rails or falling from the end of the bed.
- Wedge pillows or pads against the sides of wheelchairs to keep clients safely positioned.
- Place a removable lap tray on a wheelchair to provide support and help keep the client in place.
- Use "environmental restraints," such as pieces of furniture or large plants as barriers, to keep clients from wandering beyond appropriate areas.

Other Causes of Unsafe Behavior:

- Assign nurses in pairs to act as "buddies" so that one nurse can observe the client when the other leaves the unit.
- Monitor all the client's medications and, if possible, attempt to lower or eliminate dosages of sedatives or psychotropics.
- Establish ongoing assessment to monitor changes in physical and cognitive functional abilities and risk factors.

1. It restricts the client's movement as little as possible. If a client needs to have one arm restrained, do not restrain the entire body.
2. It is safe for the client. Choose a restraint with which the client cannot self-inflict injury. For example, a physically restrained client could suffer injury trying to climb out of bed if one wrist is tied to the bed frame. A jacket restraint would restrain the client more safely.
3. It does not interfere with the client's treatment or health problem. If a client has poor blood circulation to the hands, apply a restraint that will not aggravate that circulatory problem.
4. It is readily changeable. Restraints need to be changed frequently, especially if they become soiled. Keeping other guidelines in mind, choose a restraint that can be changed with minimal disturbance to the client.
5. It is as discreet as possible. Both clients and visitors are often embarrassed by a restraint, even though they understand why it is being used. The less obvious the restraint, the more comfortable people feel.

Types of Restraints

Several types of restraints are available. Among the most common for adults are jacket or vest restraints, roll belts, belt restraints, mitt or hand restraints, and limb restraints. Geri-chairs, wheelchairs with lap trays, and bedrails can also be considered restraints. When using restraints, the nurse may find the accompanying Practice Guidelines helpful.

When evaluating if a device is a restraint or not, determine the intended use (e.g., physical restriction), its involuntary application, or the client need for the restraint. For example, if all of the bed's side rails are up and restrict the client's freedom to leave the bed, and the client did not voluntarily request all rails to be up, they are a restraint. If, however, one side rail is up to assist the client to get in and out of the bed, it is not a restraint because it is helping the client to exit the bed. Also, if the client can release or remove a device, it would not be considered a restraint.

There are several types of vest restraints, but all are essentially sleeveless jackets or vests with straps (tails) that can be tied to the bed frame under the mattress or wheelchair frame. These body restraints are used to ensure the safety of confused or sedated clients in beds or wheelchairs. The U.S. Food and Drug Administration (FDA) advises that manufacturers place "front" and "back" labels on vest restraints.

Roll belts allow clients to roll from side to side in bed or to sit up in bed (Figure 32.7 ■). This less-restrictive belt is often used in the home setting with home hospital beds.

Belt or safety strap body restraints are used to ensure the safety of all clients who are being moved on stretchers or in wheelchairs. Some wheelchairs have a soft, padded safety bar that attaches to side brackets that are installed under the armrests. To prevent the client from slumping forward, the nurse then attaches a shoulder "Y" strap to the bar and over the client's shoulders to the rear handles. Other safety belt models have a three-loop design. One loop surrounds the client's waist and attaches to the rear handles.

A mitt or hand restraint (Figure 32.8 ■) is used to prevent clients of any age from using their hands or fingers to scratch and injure themselves. For example, a confused client may need to be prevented from pulling at IV tubing or a head bandage following brain surgery. Hand or mitt restraints allow the client to be ambulatory

PRACTICE GUIDELINES Applying Restraints

- Obtain consent from the client or guardian.
- Ensure that a primary care provider's order has been provided or, in an emergency, obtain one within the time frame specified in agency policy.
- Assure the client and the client's support people that the restraint is temporary and protective. A restraint must never be applied as punishment for any behavior or merely for the nurse's convenience.
- Apply the restraint in such a way that the client can move as freely as possible while remaining safe.
- Ensure that limb restraints are applied securely but not so tightly that they impede blood circulation to any body area or extremity.
- Pad bony prominences (e.g., wrists and ankles) before applying a restraint over them. The movement of a restraint without padding over such prominences can quickly abrade the skin.
- Always tie a limb restraint with a knot (e.g., a clove hitch) that will not tighten when pulled.
- Tie the ends of a body restraint to the part of the bed that moves to elevate the head. Never tie the ends to a side rail or to the fixed frame of the bed if the bed position is to be changed.
- Assess the restraint per agency protocol time frame. Some facilities have specific forms to be used to record ongoing assessment. This may be a visual check to ensure client safety and no signs of injury.
- Assess skin integrity per agency protocol (e.g., every 2 hours), and provide range-of-motion (ROM) exercises (see Chapter 44 ∞) and skin care when restraints are removed (see Chapter 36 ∞).
- Assess and assist with basic needs: nutrition, hydration, hygiene, elimination.
- Reassess the continued need for the restraint. Include an assessment of the underlying cause of the behavior necessitating use of the restraints.
- When a restraint is temporarily removed, do not leave the client unattended.
- Immediately report to the nurse in charge and record on the client's chart any persistent reddened or broken skin areas under the restraint.
- At the first indication of cyanosis or pallor, coldness of a skin area, or a client's complaint of a tingling sensation, pain, or numbness, loosen the restraint and exercise the limb.
- Apply a restraint so that it can be released quickly in case of an emergency and with the body part in a normal anatomic position.
- Provide emotional support verbally and through touch.

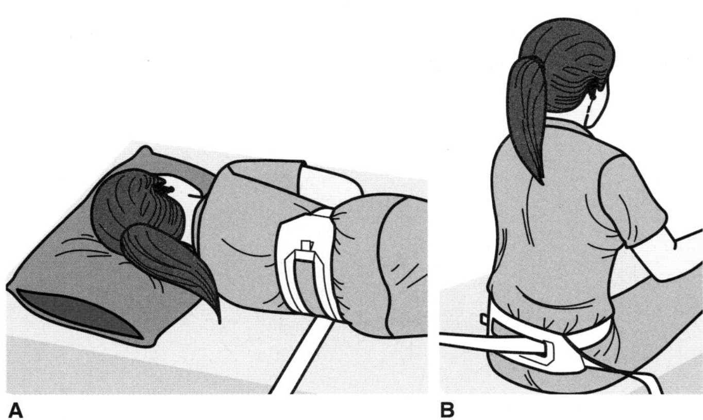

Figure 32.7 ■ A roll belt allows the client to (*A*) roll from side to side in bed or (*B*) to sit up in bed.

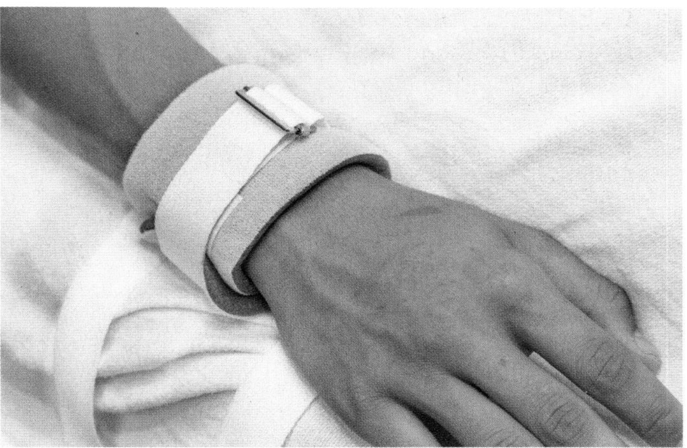

Figure 32.9 ■ A limb restraint.

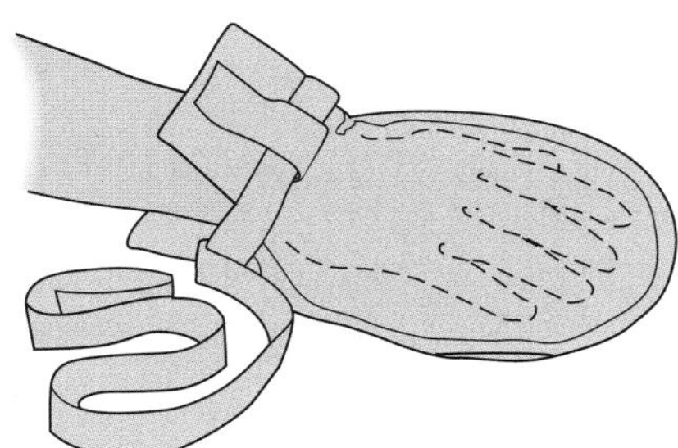

Figure 32.8 ■ A mitt restraint.

and to move the arm freely rather than be confined to a bed or a chair. Mitts need to be removed on a regular basis to permit the client to wash and exercise the hands. The nurse also needs to take off the mitt to check the circulation to the hand. A mitt is considered an alternative if it is not attached to the bed and a client could easily remove them.

Limb restraints (Figure 32.9 ■), which are generally made of cloth, may be used to immobilize a limb, primarily for therapeutic reasons (e.g., to maintain an IV infusion). Commonly used with children, elbow restraints (e.g., no-no's) prevent flexion of the joint so that tubing, connections, catheters, and bandages cannot be reached. Restraints for infants and children include mummy restraints, elbow restraints, and crib nets (see Lifespan Considerations later in chapter).

The enclosure bed is a restraint that allows confused or agitated clients, who try to leave the bed when it is unsafe to do so, to enjoy freedom of body movement while reducing risk of falls and entrapment in the side rails. This device is used most often as an alternative to vest or wrist restraints (Bauer & Weust, 2017; Kim, Hughes, & Fields, 2018). An enclosure bed (Figure 32.10 ■) is a hospital bed that has a soft mesh canopy with zippered panels to allow access to the client on all four sides. Four slots also allow access for tube and equipment management. It is considered a physical restraint and therefore, a provider's order is required. A study explored nurses' perceptions of enclosure beds and found that nurses valued knowing that the client was not tied down, could move around, and could not fall out of bed. Staff initially thought that the client would feel trapped but reported that the enclosure bed actually calmed agitated clients. The nurses did find that providing nursing care (e.g., assessments and interventions) was more difficult (e.g., having to unzip the bed). However, the nurses accepted these challenges knowing that the enclosed bed protected the client (Kim, Hughes, & Fields, 2018). See Skill 32.3 for applying restraints.

Evaluating

To prevent client injury, the nurse's role is largely educative, and desired outcomes reflect the client's acquisition of knowledge of hazards, behaviors that incorporate safety practices, and skills to perform in the event of certain emergencies. The nurse needs to individualize these

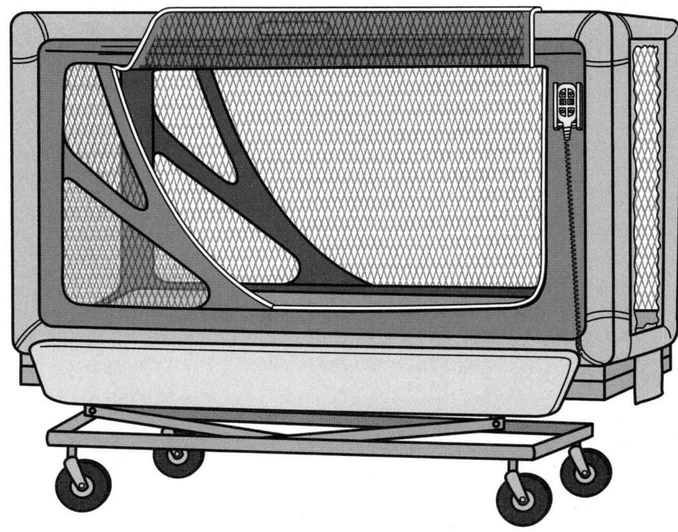

Figure 32.10 ■ An enclosure bed can help calm agitated clients who may injure themselves.

SKILL 32.3

Applying Restraints

PURPOSES

- To promote safety and prevent injury
- To allow a medical or surgical treatment to proceed without client interference (e.g., to prevent movements that would disrupt therapy to a limb connected to tubes or appliance)

ASSESSMENT

Assess

- The behavior indicating the possible need for a restraint
- Underlying cause for assessed behavior
- What other protective measures may be implemented before applying a restraint
- Status of skin to which restraint is to be applied
- Circulatory status distal to restraints and of extremities
- Effectiveness of available alternative safety precautions

PLANNING

Review institutional policy for restraints and seek consultation as appropriate before independently deciding to apply a restraint. All other possible interventions that are less restrictive *must* have been tried and their failure documented. The primary care provider must be notified prior to using a restraint, unless there is a danger to self or others. In that case the primary care provider must be notified within the prescribed time frame per the agency protocol.

Assignment

The nurse must make the determination that restraints are appropriate in specific situations, select the proper type of restraints, evaluate the effectiveness of the restraints, and assess for potential complications from their use. Application of ordered restraints and their temporary removal for skin monitoring and care may be assigned to AP who have been trained in their use.

Equipment

- Appropriate type and size of restraint

IMPLEMENTATION

Performance

1. Prior to performing the procedure, introduce self and verify the client's identity using agency protocol. Explain to the client and family what you are going to do, why it is necessary, and how to participate. Allow time for the client to express feelings about being restrained. Provide needed emotional reassurance that the restraints will be used only when absolutely necessary and that there will be close contact with the client in case assistance is required.
2. Perform hand hygiene and observe other appropriate infection prevention procedures.
3. Provide for client privacy if indicated.
4. Apply the selected restraint.

Belt Restraint (Safety Belt)

- Determine that the safety belt is in good order. If a Velcro safety belt is to be used, make sure that both pieces of Velcro are intact.
- If the belt has a long portion and a shorter portion, place the long portion of the belt behind (under) the bedridden client and secure it to the movable part of the bed frame. **Rationale:** *The long attached portion will then move up when the head of the bed is elevated and will not tighten around the client.*
  Place the shorter portion of the belt around the client's waist, over the gown. There should be a finger's width between the belt and the client.
  or
- Attach the belt around the client's waist, and fasten it at the back of the chair.
  or
- If the belt is attached to a stretcher, secure the belt firmly over the client's hips or abdomen. **Rationale:** *Belt restraints must be applied to all clients on stretchers even when the side rails are up.*

Roll Belt

- Position the client in a sitting position while in bed.
- Place the belt on the center of the bed at the client's waistline with the soft flannel side up.
- Secure the short strap to the bed with a quick-release tie. **Rationale:** *A quick-release knot does not tighten or slip when the attached end is pulled, but unties easily when the loose end is pulled.*
- Bring the long strap over and around the client's waist. Continue bringing the long strap behind the client's back and thread the strap through the slot in the back pad.
- Once the belt is secured around the client's waist, position the client on his or her back.
- Secure the long strap to the bed with a quick-release tie. Secure it to a movable part of the bed frame. **Rationale:** *The long attached portion will then move up when the head of the bed is elevated and will not tighten around the client.*
- Confirm that two fingers can fit between the belt and the client. **Rationale:** *This avoids impaired circulation.*

Vest Restraint

- Place vest on the client, with opening at the front or the back, depending on the type.
- Pull the tie on the end of the vest flap across the chest, and place it through the slit in the opposite side of the chest.
- Repeat for the other tie.
- Use a half-bow knot (a type of quick-release knot) to secure each tie around the movable bed frame or behind the chair to a chair leg. ❶ **Rationale:** *A half-bow (quick-release) knot does not tighten or slip when the attached end is pulled but unties easily when the loose end is pulled.*
  or
- Fasten the ties together behind the chair using a slip or quick-release knot.
- Ensure that the client is positioned appropriately to enable maximum chest expansion for breathing.

Mitt Restraint

- Apply the commercial thumbless mitt (see Figure 32.8) to the hand to be restrained. Make sure the fingers can be slightly flexed and are not caught under the hand. Ensure that the restraint is not too tight by checking that one to two fingers can fit under the strap before securing around the client's wrist. **Rationale:** *This avoids impaired blood circulation.*
- Follow the manufacturer's directions for securing the mitt.
- Assess the client's circulation to the hands shortly after the mitt is applied and at regular intervals. **Rationale:** *Client complaints*

Applying Restraints—*continued*

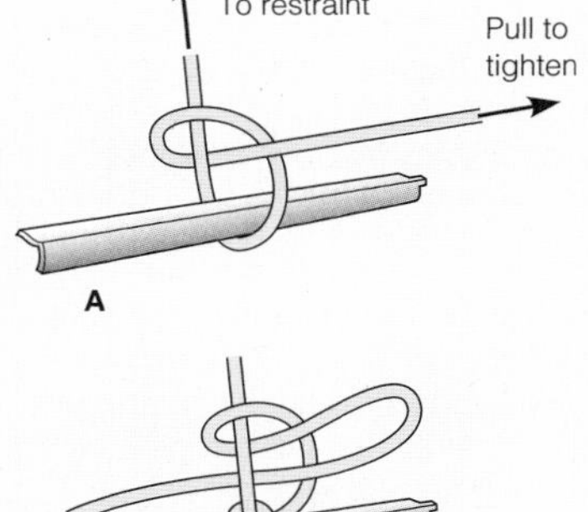

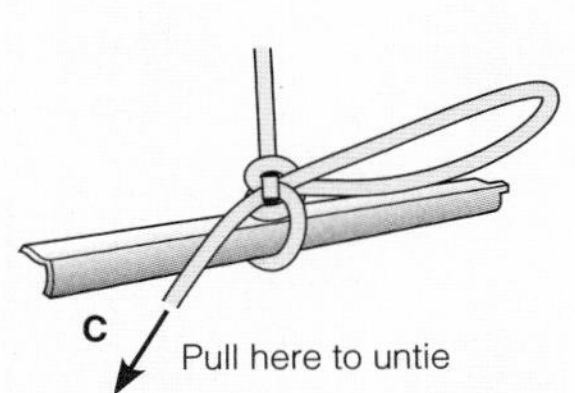

❶ To make a half-bow (quick-release) knot, first place the restraint tie under the side frame of the bed (or around a chair leg). *A*, Bring the free end up, around, under, and over the attached end of the tie and pull it tight. *B*, Again, take the free end over and under the attached end of the tie, but this time make a half-bow loop. *C*, Tighten the free end of the tie and the bow until the knot is secure. To untie the knot, pull the end of the tie and then loosen the first cross over the tie.

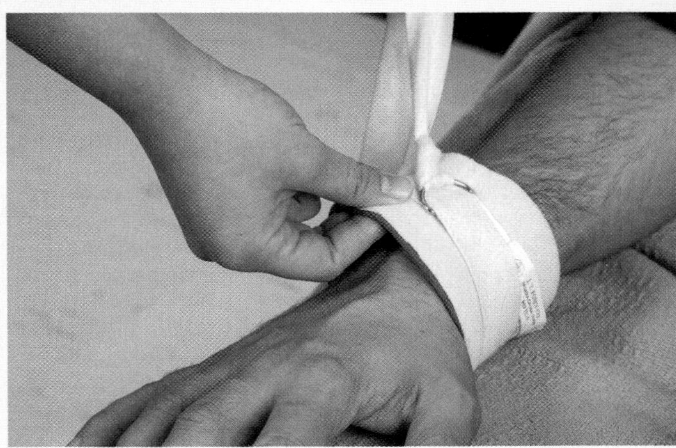

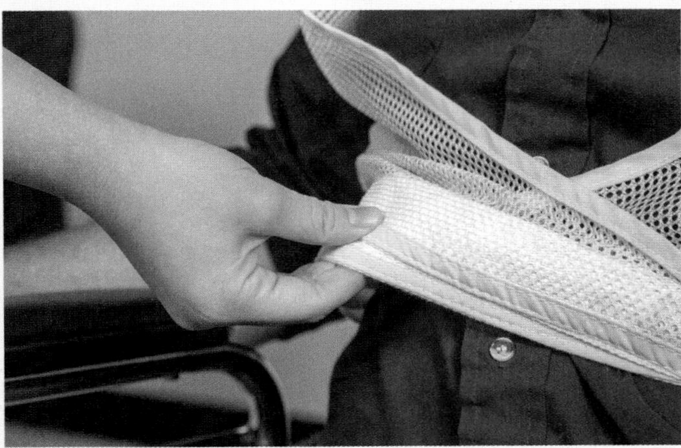

❷ Ensure that two fingers can be inserted between the restraint and *A*, the wrist, and *B*, the chest.

of numbness, discomfort, or inability to move the fingers could indicate impaired blood circulation to the hand.
- If a mitt is to be worn for several days, remove it at regular intervals per agency protocol. Wash and exercise the client's hand, then reapply the mitt. Check agency policies about recommended intervals for removal.

Wrist or Ankle Restraint
- Pad bony prominences on the wrist or ankle if needed to prevent skin breakdown.
- Apply the padded portion of the restraint around the ankle or wrist.
- Pull the tie of the restraint through the slit in the wrist portion or through the buckle and ensure that the restraint is not too tight. ❷
- Using a half-bow quick-release knot, attach the other end of the restraint to the movable portion of the bed frame. **Rationale:** *If the ties are attached to the movable portion, the wrist or ankle will not be pulled when the bed position is changed.*

5. Adjust the plan of care as required, for example, to include releasing the restraint (always stay with a client whose restraint is temporarily removed), providing skin care, range-of-motion exercises, and attending to the client's physical needs by providing fluids, nutrition, and toileting.
6. Document on the client's chart the behavior(s) indicating the need for the restraint, all other interventions implemented to avoid the use of restraints and their outcomes, and the time the primary care provider was notified of the need for restraint. Also record:
   - The type of restraint applied, the time it was applied, and the goal for its application
   - The client's response to the restraint, including a rationale for its continued use
   - The times that the restraints were removed and skin care given
   - Any other assessments and interventions
   - Explanations given to the client and significant others.
7. Restraints may be necessary for clients in the home. The above safety guidelines apply. Assess the knowledge and skill of all caregivers in the use of restraints and educate as indicated.

SAMPLE DOCUMENTATION

7/10/2020 2300 Confused. Disoriented to time and place. Reoriented frequently. Pulling at central IV line, NG tube, and chest tube. Medicated for pain relief. Lights dimmed. C. Murphy, RN

0100 Continues to pull at IV and tubes. Dr. Jones called. Received an order to apply mitt restraints. Family notified and situation explained. Stated that a family member will come and sit with client. Mitt restraints applied, relaxation music initiated. C. Murphy, RN

0130 Son arrived and sitting with client. Calm though remains disoriented to time and place. Mitts removed, skin intact, hands warm and pink. Vital signs stable. C. Murphy, RN

EVALUATION

- Perform a detailed follow-up of the need for the restraints and the client's response. Relate these findings to previous data if available.
- Evaluate circulatory status of restrained limbs.
- Evaluate skin status beneath restraints.
- Remove the restraints as soon as they are no longer needed and document.
- Report significant deviations from normal to the primary care provider.

LIFESPAN CONSIDERATIONS Restraints

INFANTS

Elbow restraints (Figure 32.11 ■) are used to prevent infants or small children from flexing their elbows to touch or reach their face or head, especially after surgery. Ready-made elbow restraints are available commercially.

A mummy restraint (Figure 32.12 ■) is a special folding of a blanket or sheet around an infant to prevent movement during a procedure such as gastric washing, eye irrigation, or collection of a blood specimen. This procedural restraint is temporary and does not require the documentation and orders as the restraints previously discussed.

- Obtain a blanket or sheet large enough so that the distance between opposite corners is about twice the length of the infant's body. Lay the blanket or sheet on a flat, dry surface.
- Fold down one corner, and place the baby on it in the supine position.
- Fold the right side of the blanket over the infant's body, leaving the left arm free (Figure 32.12*A*). The right arm is in a natural position at the side.
- Fold the excess blanket at the bottom up under the infant (Figure 32.12*B*, 2).
- With the left arm in a natural position at the baby's side, fold the left side of the blanket over the infant, including the arm, and tuck the blanket under the body (Figure 32.12*B*, 3).
- Remain with the infant who is in a mummy restraint until the specific procedure is completed.

CHILDREN

A crib net is simply a device placed over the top of a crib to prevent active young children from climbing out of the crib. At the same time, it allows them freedom to move about in the crib. The crib net or dome is not attached to the movable parts of the crib so that the caregiver can have access to the child without removing the dome or net.

- Place the net over the sides and ends of the crib.
- Secure the ties to the springs or frame of the crib. The crib sides can then be freely lowered without removing the net.
- Test with your hand that the net will stretch if the child stands against it in the crib.

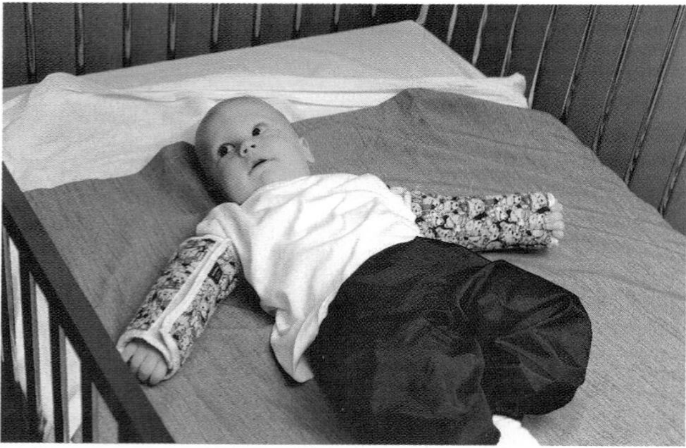

Figure 32.11 ■ Infant with elbow restraints.

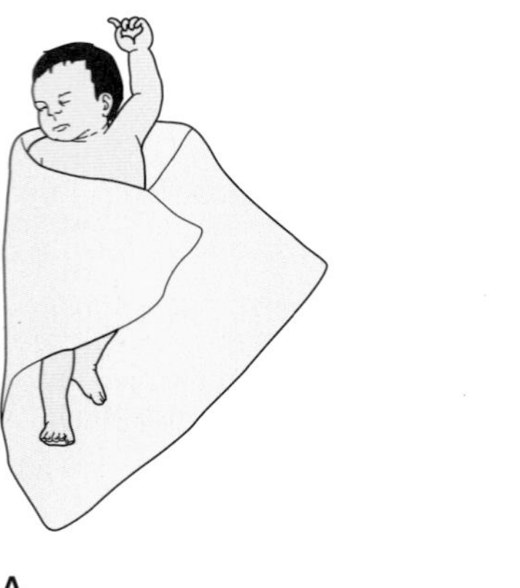

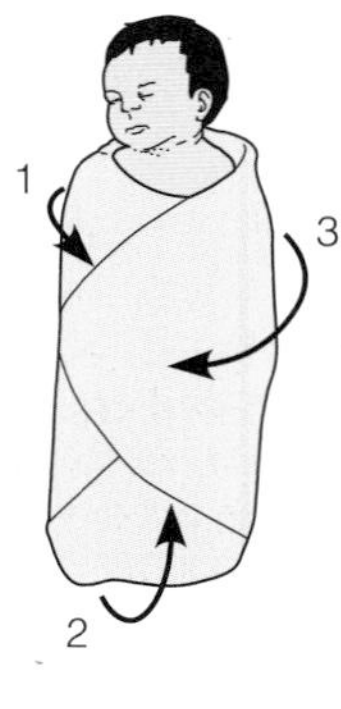

Figure 32.12 ■ Making a mummy restraint.

LIFESPAN CONSIDERATIONS Safety

OLDER ADULTS

Some of the changes due to aging that place the older adult at higher risk for safety concerns are:

- Decrease in visual and hearing acuity
- Decrease in response of reflexes
- Fragility of bones and decrease in flexibility of joints and muscles
- Decrease in temperature regulation, increasing the risk of hypothermia and hyperthermia
- Decrease in kidney function, which increases risk of toxicity from medications.

A home environment that was safe when they were younger may need modifications for older adults to decrease the risk of injury. A plan and telephone numbers of those to call in an emergency situation should be available.

for clients. Examples of desired outcomes include the client being able to do the following:

- Describe methods to prevent specific hazards (e.g., falls, suffocation, choking, fires, drowning, electric shock).
- Report use of home safety measures (e.g., fire safety measures, smoke detector maintenance, fall prevention strategies, burn prevention measures, poison prevention measures, safe storage of hazardous materials, firearm safety precautions, electrocution prevention, water safety precautions, bicycle safety, motor vehicle safety).
- Alter home physical environment to reduce the risk of injury.
- Describe emergency procedures for poisoning and fire.
- Describe age-specific risks, work safety risks, or community safety risks.
- Demonstrate correct use of child safety seats.
- Demonstrate correct administration of cardiopulmonary resuscitation.

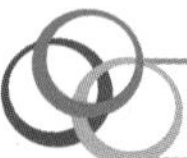

Critical Thinking Checkpoint

Mr. Moore is a 72-year-old widower who is recovering from a fall in which he fractured his hip and underwent surgical repair 1 week ago. He will be staying with his son for 2 weeks after he is discharged from the hospital, but he is eager to return to his own home. Once he is home, his son will visit nightly after work, he will receive Meals-on-Wheels once a day, and a home healthcare attendant will visit weekly to assist him with hygienic care until he is more independent. Mr. Moore's wife died 3 years ago, but he has remained independent and continued his social functions. He lives in a small single-level house with his dog and cat, and he enjoys gardening. Prior to fracturing his hip he walked his dog daily. You will be his home healthcare nurse.

1. While hospitalized, Mr. Moore experienced some mild confusion during the night, but his nurses decided not to restrain him. What are the best reasons for avoiding the use of restraints for clients such as Mr. Moore?
2. What are some of the more obvious factors that may affect Mr. Moore's safety as he returns home?
3. What do you need to assess with regard to Mr. Moore's safety and what suggestions can you make for enhancing his safety?
4. What strengths do you note about Mr. Moore that may protect him from injury when he returns home?

Answers to Critical Thinking Checkpoint questions are available on the faculty resources site. Please consult with your instructor.

Chapter 32 Review

CHAPTER HIGHLIGHTS

- Injuries are a major cause of death among individuals of all ages in the United States.
- Nurses need awareness of what constitutes a safe environment for specific individuals and for groups of people in the home, community, and workplace.
- Hazards to safety occur at all ages and vary according to the age and development of the individual.
- Nursing assessment of safety includes assessing factors that can affect safety, for example, age and developmental level, lifestyle, mobility and health status, sensory–perceptual alterations, cognitive awareness, ability to communicate, safety awareness, and environmental factors.
- Nurses assess clients at risk for injury through methods such as nursing history and physical examination, risk assessment tools, and home hazard appraisal.
- The landmark report *To Err Is Human* increased the awareness in the healthcare industry of the need to improve client safety. As a result, National Patient Safety Goals (NPSGs) were initiated and are required to be implemented by The Joint Commission. The QSEN project developed guidelines to help future nurses develop the knowledge, skills, and attitudes required to improve client safety. The foundation for a culture of safety is a blame-free environment, transparency, and a process designed to prevent error.
- Nurses need to be able to respond to disasters in the community as well as keep safe clients who are already in the healthcare setting. The Joint Commission has standards requiring healthcare organizations to develop disaster plans. The role that nurses play in disaster planning is to know and understand the chain of command. The line of authority during a disaster is different from that of day-to-day operations.
- Examples of nursing diagnoses for clients with potential for injury are most helpful when specific labels are used to provide clear direction for nursing care (e.g., potential for: falls, infection, suffocation, poisoning, and suicide). Other diagnoses the nurse may choose to use are lack of knowledge (unintentional injury prevention) or the wellness diagnosis of willingness for knowledge enhancement (unintentional injury prevention).
- Measures to ensure the safety of clients of all ages focus on (a) observation or prediction of situations that are potentially harmful and (b) client education that empowers clients to safeguard themselves and their families from injury.
- Falls are a common cause of injury among older adults.
- Side rails do not protect hospitalized clients from falls. It is more likely the client will fall trying to get out around raised rails.
- Prevention of falls in healthcare agencies is an ongoing concern.
- Seizure precautions are safety measures taken by the nurse to protect clients from injury should they have a seizure.
- Nurses must be familiar with the fire procedures in the healthcare agencies where they practice. In the event of a fire, the nurse can use two mnemonics to remember the steps to follow: RACE and PASS.
- Major reasons for poisoning in children are inadequate supervision and improper storage of household toxic substances.
- Suffocation can occur when foreign objects become lodged in the throat, cutting off an individual's oxygen supply.
- Prolonged exposure to excessive noise can cause hearing loss.
- Improper grounding and faulty electric equipment pose health hazards in the hospital and the home. Injuries can be prevented by using grounded outlets and plugs, putting protective covers over outlets, keeping appliances in good repair, and making sure that electric wiring and circuits meet safety standards.
- Firearms pose a risk to individuals of all ages. Adults must take full responsibility for following safety procedures when keeping firearms in the home, including storage of ammunition in a separate location.
- In hospitals, radioactive substances are used for both diagnostic and treatment purposes; agency policy must be followed to safeguard clients and staff from unsafe exposure.
- Various alternatives to restraints must be considered before a restraint is applied.
- Because restraints restrict a client's basic freedom to move, careful assessment and accurate, complete documentation are important when restraints are used.

TEST YOUR KNOWLEDGE

1. A nurse sees smoke emerging from the suction equipment being used. Which is the greatest priority in the event of a fire?
   1. Report the fire.
   2. Extinguish the fire.
   3. Protect the clients.
   4. Contain the fire.

2. What should the nurse point out as a safety hazard for the developing fetus when instructing a pregnant client?
   1. Banging into objects
   2. Bicycle rides
   3. Recreational activities
   4. X-rays

3. An older client is observed having difficulty moving from a sitting to a standing position and has an unsteady gait. What should the nurse assess in this client to promote home safety? Select all that apply.
   1. Presence of grab bars in the bathroom
   2. Absence of scatter rugs on the floors
   3. Correct use of cane to ambulate
   4. Ability to stand in place for a minute before ambulating
   5. Alcohol use with prescribed medications

4. A mother and her 3-year-old live in a home built in 1972. Which nursing diagnosis is most applicable for this child?
   1. Potential for suffocation
   2. Potential for injury
   3. Potential for poisoning
   4. Potential for decline in health

5. A 75-year-old client, hospitalized with a stroke, becomes disoriented at times and tries to get out of bed, but is unable to ambulate without help. What is the most appropriate safety measure?
   1. Restrain the client in bed.
   2. Ask a family member to stay with the client.
   3. Check the client every 15 minutes.
   4. Use a bed exit safety monitoring device.

6. A client is being admitted to the hospital because of a seizure that occurred at his home. The client has no previous history of seizures. In planning the client's nursing care, which of the following measures is most essential at this time of admission? Select all that apply.
   1. Place a padded tongue depressor at the head of the bed.
   2. Pad the bed with blankets.
   3. Inform the client about the importance of wearing a medical identification tag.
   4. Teach the client about epilepsy.
   5. Test oral suction equipment.

7. What can a nurse do to promote a safe environment for a client?
   1. Keep clutter to a minimum in the client's room.
   2. Have the client wear terry cloth slippers.
   3. Provide adequate lighting.
   4. Turn off alarms to reduce noise.

8. A confused client is touching his IV line and the nurse is concerned for his safety. The nurse wants to consider options for keeping the IV line from being pulled out. Which of the following options would best meet the needs of the client and nurse? Select all that apply.
   1. Explain the purpose of the IV line.
   2. Reorient the client by telling him the day and time.
   3. Cover up the IV site with a long-sleeved gown.
   4. Apply wrist restraints to both wrists.
   5. Apply a mitt to both hands without attaching straps to the bed.

9. When planning to teach healthcare topics to a group of male adolescents, which topic should the nurse consider a priority?
   1. Sports contribute to an adolescent's self-esteem.
   2. Sunbathing and tanning beds can be dangerous.
   3. Guns are the most frequently used weapon for adolescent suicide.
   4. A driver's education course is mandatory for safety.

10. The nurse, at change-of-shift report, learns that one of the clients in his care has bilateral soft wrist restraints. The client is confused, is trying to get out of bed, and had pulled out the IV line, which was subsequently reinserted. Which action(s) by the nurse is appropriate? Select all that apply.
   1. Document the behavior(s) that require continued use of the restraints.
   2. Ensure that the restraints are tied to the side rails.
   3. Provide range-of-motion exercises when the restraints are removed.
   4. Orient the client.
   5. Assess the tightness of the restraints.

See Answers to Test Your Knowledge in Appendix A.

READINGS AND REFERENCES

Suggested Readings

American Nurses Association. (2017). *Who will be there? Ethics, the law, and a nurse's duty to respond in a disaster.* Retrieved from https://www.nursingworld.org/~4ad845/globalassets/docs/ana/who-will-be-there_disaster-preparedness_2017.pdf
A thought provoking article that brings up relevant questions that nurses may ask when a disaster strikes.

Campbell, B. (2016). Patient falls: Preventable, not inevitable. *Nursing made Incredibly Easy!, 14*(1), 14–18. doi:10.1097/01.NME.0000475168.08103.37
The author provides helpful information about the numerous tools to screen clients for the risk of falling.

Heavey, E. (2016). Lead poisoning. When an entire community is exposed. *Nursing, 46*(9), 29–33. doi:10.1097/01.NURSE.0000490212.15944.5e
This article discusses how to identify and control exposure to lead, how to implement appropriate screening and intervention for children and others at risk, and racial and economic disparities associated with lead poisoning.

Williams, A. P., & Estrada, R. D. (2016). Carbon monoxide poisoning: The silent killer. *American Nurse Today, 11*(9), 7–9
This article describes how to identify and manage victims of carbon monoxide (CO) and prevent CO exposures.

Related Research

Gaffney, T. A., Hatcher, B. J., Milligan, R., & Trickey, A. (2016). Enhancing patient safety: Factors influencing medical error recovery among medical-surgical nurses. *The Online Journal of Issues in Nursing, 21*(3), 1. doi:10.3912/OJIN.Vol21No03Man06

Hester, A. L., Tsai, P. F., Rettiganti, M., & Mitchell, A. (2016). Original research. Predicting injurious falls in the hospital setting: Implications for practice. *American Journal of Nursing, 116*(9), 24–32. doi:10.1097/01.NAJ.0000494688.10004.85

Hevener, S., Rickabaugh, B., & Marsh, T. (2016). Using a decision wheel to reduce use of restraints in a medical-surgical intensive care unit. *American Journal of Critical Care, 25*, 479–486. doi:10.4037/ajcc2016929

Johnston, Y. A., Bergen, G., Bauer, M., Parker, E. M., Wentworth, L., McFadden, M., . . . Garnett, M. (2018). Implementation of the stopping elderly accidents, deaths, and injuries initiative in primary care: An outcome evaluation. *The Gerontologist, XX*(XX), 1–10. doi:10.1093/geront/gny101

Stinson, K. J. (2016). Nurses' attitudes, clinical experience, and practice issues with use of physical restraints in critical care units. *American Journal of Critical Care*, *25*, 21–26. doi:10.4037/ajcc2016428

References

American Nurses Association. (n.d.). *Culture of safety*. Retrieved from https://www.nursingworld.org/practice-policy/work-environment/health-safety/culture-of-safety

Bauer, R. N., & Weust, J. (2017). Safety regarding restraints. *MEDSURG Nursing*, *26*(5), 352–355.

Bureau of Labor Statistics. (2018). *Occupational outlook handbook, registered nurses: Work environment*. Retrieved from https://www.bls.gov/ooh/healthcare/registered-nurses.htm#tab-3

Centers for Disease Control and Prevention. (2017a). *Important facts about falls*. Retrieved from http://www.cdc.gov/homeandrecreationalsafety/falls/adultfalls.html

Centers for Disease Control and Prevention. (2017b). *Older adult drivers*. Retrieved from https://www.cdc.gov/motor-vehiclesafety/older_adult_drivers/index.html

Centers for Disease Control and Prevention. (2019). *Travel health notices*. Retrieved from https://wwwnc.cdc.gov/travel/notices

Centers for Medicare and Medicaid Services. (2008). *Hospitals—restraint/seclusion interpretive guidelines & updated state operations manual (SOM) Appendix A*. Retrieved from https://www.cms.gov/Medicare/Provider-Enrollment-and-Certification/SurveyCertificationGenInfo/downloads/SCLetter08-18.pdf

Chiodini, J. (2016). Travel health update. *Practice Nurse*, *46*(5), 42.

Chu, R. Z. (2017). Preventing in-patient falls: The nurse's pivotal role. *Nursing*, *47*(3), 24–30. doi:10.1097/01.NURSE.0000512872.83762.69

Dykes, P. C., Adelman, J., Adkison, L., Bogaisky, M., Carroll, D. L., Carter, E., . . . Yu, S. P. (2018). Preventing falls in hospitalized patients. Engage patients and families in a three-step prevention process to reduce the risk of falls. *American Nurse Today*, *13*(9), 3–13.

Falls Prevention. (2016). *Australian Nursing & Midwifery Journal*, *24*(1), 32–33.

Famolaro, T., Yount, N., Hare, R., Thornton, S., Meadows, K., Fan, L., . . . Sorra, J. (2018). Hospital survey on patient safety culture 2018 user database report. Retrieved from https://www.ahrq.gov/sites/default/files/wysiwyg/sops/quality-patient-safety/patientsafetyculture/2018hospitalsopsreport.pdf

Federal Emergency Management Agency. (2019). *National Incident Management System*. Retrieved from https://www.fema.gov/national-incident-management-system

Institute of Medicine. (2000). *To err is human: Building a safer health system*. Washington, DC: National Academy of Sciences.

The Joint Commission. (2019a). *National patient safety goals effective January 2019: Hospital accreditation program*. Retrieved from https://www.jointcommission.org/assets/1/6/NPSG_Chapter_HAP_Jan2019.pdf

The Joint Commission. (2019b). *National patient safety goals effective January 2019: Nursing care center accreditation program*. Retrieved from https://www.jointcommission.org/assets/1/6/NPSG_Chapter_NCC_Jan2019.pdf

Kim, C., Hughes, M., & Fields, W. (2018). Nurses' reactions to enclosure beds. *MEDSURG Nursing*, *27*(2), 87–91, 107.

Klymko, K., Etcher, L., Munchiando, J., & Royse, M. (2016). Video monitoring: A room with a view, or a window to challenges in falls prevention research? *MEDSURG Nursing*, *25*(5), 329–333.

Lach, H. W., Leach, K. M., & Butcher, H. K. (2016). Evidence-based practice guideline: Changing the practice of physical restraint use in acute care. *Journal of Gerontological Nursing*, *42*(2), 17–25. doi:10.3928/00989134-20160113-04

Lamprecht, S. (2016). Infection control and international travel. *Nevada RNformation*, *25*(4), 3.

Lee, L. K., & Mannix, R. (2018). Increasing fatality rates from preventable deaths in teenagers and young adults. *JAMA*, *320*(6), 543–544. doi:10.1001/jama.2018.6566

Nielson, M. H. (2017). When disaster strikes, will you be ready? *Nursing*, *47*(12), 52–56. doi:10.1097/01.NURSE.0000526891.17929.d4

Stokes, L. (2018). Conflict in duty to provide care when disaster strikes. *American Nurse Today*, *13*(8), 29.

Winslow, A. (2016). Testing those most at risk for blood lead exposure. *MLO: Medical Laboratory Observer*, *48*(11), 34–36.

Selected Bibliography

Agency for Healthcare Research and Quality. (2018). *Six domains of health care quality*. Retrieved from http://www.ahrq.gov/professionals/quality-patient-safety/talkingquality/create/sixdomains.html

Benton, D. (2018). Disasters, regulation, and proactive response. *American Nurse Today*, *13*(1), 32–33.

Centers for Disease Control and Prevention. (2019). *STEADI—older adult fall prevention*. Retrieved from https://www.cdc.gov/steadi

Glasofer, A., & Laskowski-Jones, L. (2018). Mass shootings. *Nursing*, *48*(12), 50–55. doi:10.1097/01.NURSE.0000549496.58492.26

Grimley-Baker, K. (2018). Preventing suicide beyond psychiatric units. *Nursing*, *48*(3), 59–61. doi:10.1097/01.NURSE.0000529816.67148.e9

Haddad, Y. K., Bergen, G., & Luo, F. (2018). Reducing fall risk in older adults. *American Journal of Nursing*, *118*(7), 21–22. doi:10.1097/01.NAJ.0000541429.36218.2d

Hodges, K. T., & Gilbert, J. H. (2016). Eliminating infant falls. *Nursing Made Incredibly Easy!*, *14*(1), 20–25. doi:10.1097/01.NME.0000475169.08103.7e

Hollenback, R., Simpson, A., & Mueller, L. (2017). Falls simulation room: Do you see what your patient sees? *Nursing*, *47*(9), 65–67. doi:10.1097/01.NURSE.0000522020.45924.3a

Li, F., Harmer, P., & Fitzgerald, K. (2016). Implementing an evidence-based fall prevention intervention in community senior centers. *American Journal of Public Health*, *106*, 2026–2031. doi:10.2105/AJPH.2016.303386

Lupton, K. (2016). Zika virus disease: A public health emergency of international concern. *British Journal of Nursing*, *25*(4), 198–202. doi:10.12968/bjon.2016.25.4.198

NewsCAP. (2018). Each year an estimated 600 to 1,600 newborns fall or are dropped while in the hospital. *American Journal of Nursing*, *118*(7), 16. doi:10.1097/01.NAJ.0000541422.98099.bf

Reducing "never events," measuring progress in patient safety. (2016). *AACN Bold Voices*, *8*(2), 10.

Simon, R. B., & Carpenetti, T. L. (2016). Zika virus: Facing a new threat. *Nursing*, *46*(8), 24–31. doi:10.1097/01.NURSE.0000484957.70486.d0

Sofer, D. (2018). Responding to mass shootings: Are hospitals and nurses fully prepared? *American Journal of Nursing*, *118*(9), 18–19. doi:0.1097/01.NAJ.0000544970.28486.90

Trossman, S. (2015). A matter of life or death. *American Nurse*, *47*(6), 1–8.

Trossman, S. (2016). Creating a culture of safety. *American Nurse*, *48*(1), 9.

Walters, D. (2017). Enclosure bed: A tool for calming agitated patients. *American Nurse Today*, *12*(9), 25–26.

West, G. F., Rose, T., & Throop, M. D. (2018). Assessing nursing interventions to reduce patient falls. *Nursing*, *48*(8), 59–60. doi:10.1097/01.NURSE.0000541404.79920.4e

33 Hygiene

LEARNING OUTCOMES

After completing this chapter, you will be able to:

1. Describe hygienic care that nurses provide to clients.
2. Identify factors influencing personal hygiene.
3. Identify normal and abnormal assessment findings while providing hygiene care.
4. Apply the nursing process to common problems related to hygienic care of the:
   - Skin
   - Feet
   - Nails
   - Mouth
   - Hair
   - Eyes
   - Ears.
5. Identify the purposes of bathing.
6. Describe various types of baths.
7. Compare and contrast the task-centered approach and the client-centered approach to bathing.
8. Describe guidelines for bathing individuals with dementia.
9. Discuss the different types of contact lenses.
10. Discuss the different types of hearing aids.
11. Discuss factors that support a positive and safe environment for the client.
12. Identify safety and comfort measures underlying bedmaking procedures.
13. Verbalize the steps used in:
    a. Bathing an adult client
    b. Providing perineal-genital care
    c. Providing foot care
    d. Brushing and flossing the teeth
    e. Providing special oral care
    f. Providing hair care
    g. Removing, cleaning, and inserting a hearing aid
    h. Changing an unoccupied bed
    i. Changing an occupied bed.
14. Recognize when it is appropriate to assign hygiene skills for clients to assistive personnel.
15. Demonstrate appropriate documentation and reporting of hygiene skills.

KEY TERMS

alopecia, *785*
callus, *771*
caries, *776*
cerumen, *791*
cleansing baths, *762*
corn, *772*
cross-contamination, *769*
dandruff, *785*
fissures, *772*
gingiva, *776*
gingivitis, *777*
hirsutism, *786*
hygiene, *756*
ingrown toenail, *772*
lanugo, *785*
pediculosis, *786*
periodontal disease, *776*
plantar warts, *772*
plaque, *776*
pyorrhea, *777*
scabies, *786*
tartar, *777*
therapeutic baths, *763*
ticks, *785*
tinea pedis, *772*
xerostomia, *778*

Introduction

Hygiene is the science of health and its maintenance. Personal hygiene is the self-care by which individuals attend to such functions as bathing, toileting, general body hygiene, and grooming. Hygiene is a highly personal matter determined by individual and cultural values and practices. It involves care of the skin, feet, nails, oral and nasal cavities, teeth, hair, eyes, ears, and perineal-genital areas.

It is important for nurses to know exactly how much assistance a client needs for hygienic care. Clients may require help after urinating or defecating, after vomiting, and whenever they become soiled, for example, from wound drainage or from profuse perspiration. In addition, culture-specific beliefs and practices influence hygienic care. Table 33.1 lists factors that influence hygienic practices.

Hygienic Care

The types of hygienic care are often described by when they occur. For example, *early morning care* is provided to clients as they awaken in the morning. This care consists of providing a urinal or bedpan to the client confined to bed, washing the face and hands, and giving oral care. *Morning care* is often provided after clients have breakfast, although it may be provided before breakfast. It usually includes providing for elimination needs, a bath or shower, perineal care, back massages, and oral, nail, and hair care. Making the client's bed is part of morning care. *Hour of sleep* or *PM care* is provided to clients before they retire for the night. It usually involves providing for elimination needs, washing face and hands, giving oral care, and giving a back massage. *As-needed (prn) care* is

TABLE 33.1 Factors Influencing Individual Hygienic Practices

Factor	Variables
Culture	Some cultures place a high value on cleanliness. For example, some individuals may bathe or shower once or twice a day, whereas people from other cultures may bathe once a week. Some cultures consider privacy essential for bathing, whereas others practice communal bathing. Body odor is offensive in some cultures and accepted as normal in others.
Religion	Ceremonial washings are practiced by some religions.
Environment	Finances may affect the availability of facilities for bathing. For example, individuals who are homeless may not have warm water available; soap, shampoo, shaving lotion, and deodorants may be too expensive for individuals who have limited resources.
Developmental level	Children learn hygiene in the home. Practices vary according to the individual's age; for example, preschoolers can carry out most tasks independently with encouragement.
Health and energy	Individuals who are ill may not have the motivation or energy to attend to hygiene. Some clients who have neuromuscular impairments may be unable to perform hygienic care.
Personal preferences	Some clients prefer a shower to a tub bath. The time of bathing varies (e.g., morning versus evening).

provided as required by the client. For example, a client who is diaphoretic (sweating profusely) may need more frequent bathing and a change of clothes and linen.

Skin

The skin is the largest organ of the body. It serves five major functions:

1. It protects underlying tissues from injury by preventing the passage of microorganisms. The skin and mucous membranes are considered the body's first line of defense.
2. It regulates the body temperature.
3. It secretes sebum, an oily substance that (a) softens and lubricates the hair and skin, (b) prevents the hair from becoming brittle, and (c) decreases water loss from the skin when the external humidity is low.
4. It transmits sensations through nerve receptors, which are sensitive to pain, temperature, touch, and pressure.
5. It produces and absorbs vitamin D in conjunction with ultraviolet rays from the sun, which activate a vitamin D precursor present in the skin.

The normal skin of a healthy individual has transient and resident microorganisms that are not usually harmful. See Chapter 36 ∞.

●○● NURSING MANAGEMENT

Assessing

Assessment of the client's skin and hygienic practices includes (a) a nursing health history to determine the client's skin care practices, self-care abilities, and past or current skin problems; and (b) physical assessment of the skin.

Nursing History

Data about the client's skin care practices enable the nurse to incorporate the client's needs and preferences as much as possible in the plan of care. Some individuals try to disguise natural body odors by bathing frequently and using deodorant, cologne, or perfumes. Individuals in countries where water is scarce may bathe less often than those in countries where water is more accessible.

Assessment of the client's self-care abilities determines the amount of nursing assistance and the type of bath (e.g., bed, tub, or shower) best suited for the client. Important considerations include the client's balance (for tub and shower), ability to sit unsupported (in the tub or bed), activity tolerance, coordination, adequate muscle strength, appropriate joint range of motion, vision, and preferences. Cognition and motivation are also essential. Clients whose cognitive function is impaired or whose illness alters energy levels and motivation will usually need more assistance. It is important for the nurse to determine each client's functional level and to maintain and promote as much client independence as possible. This also enables the nurse to identify a client's potential for growth and rehabilitation. There are several models of functional levels of self-care. One example is shown in Table 33.2.

The presence of past or current skin problems alerts the nurse to specific nursing interventions or referrals the client may require. Many skin care conditions have implications for hygienic care. The client may provide descriptions of these problems during the nursing health history, or the nurse may observe some during the physical examination that follows. Common skin problems and implications for nursing interventions are shown in Table 33.3. Questions to elicit data about the client's skin care practices, self-care abilities, and skin problems are shown in the accompanying Assessment Interview.

Physical Assessment

Physical assessment of the skin, which involves inspection and palpation, is described in Chapter 29 ∞. When assisting with bathing and other hygienic care, the nurse often has the opportunity to collect data about skin color, uniformity of color, texture, turgor, temperature, intactness, and lesions.

TABLE 33.2 Definitions and Descriptors for Functional Level

	(0) Completely Independent	(+1) Requires Use of Equipment or Device	Semidependent (+2) Requires Help from Another Person for Assistance, Supervision, or Teaching	Moderately Dependent (+3) Requires Help from Another Person and Equipment or Device	Totally Dependent (+4) Does Not Participate in Activity
Bathing			Nurse provides all equipment; positions client in bed or bathroom. Client completes bath, except for back and feet.	Nurse supplies all equipment; positions client; washes back, legs, perineum, and all other parts, as needed. Client can assist.	Client needs complete bath; cannot assist at all.
Oral hygiene			Nurse provides equipment; client does task.	Nurse prepares brush, rinses mouth, positions client.	Nurse completes entire procedure.
Dressing/grooming			Nurse gathers items for client; may button, zip, or tie clothing. Client dresses self.	Nurse combs client's hair, assists with dressing, buttons and zips clothing, ties shoes.	Client needs to be dressed and cannot assist the nurse; nurse combs client's hair.
Toileting			Client can walk to bathroom or commode with assistance; nurse helps with clothing.	Nurse provides bedpan, positions client on or off bedpan, places client on commode.	Client is incontinent; nurse places client on bedpan or commode.

From *Pearson Nursing Diagnosis Handbook*, 11th ed. (pp. 725, 730, 739), by J. M. Wilkinson and L. Barcas, 2017. Reprinted and electronically reproduced by permission of Pearson Education, Inc., New York, NY.

TABLE 33.3 Common Skin Problems

Problem and Appearance	Nursing Implications
ABRASION Superficial layers of the skin are scraped or rubbed away. Area is reddened and may have localized bleeding or serous weeping.	1. Prone to infection; therefore, wound should be kept clean and dry. 2. Do not wear rings or jewelry when providing care to avoid causing abrasions to clients. 3. Lift, do not pull, a client across a bed. 4. Use two or more people for assistance.
EXCESSIVE DRYNESS Skin can appear flaky and rough.	1. Prone to infection if the skin cracks; therefore, provide alcohol-free lotions to moisturize the skin and prevent cracking. 2. Bathe client less frequently; use no soap, or use nonirritating soap and limit its use. Rinse skin thoroughly because soap can be irritating and drying. 3. Encourage increased fluid intake if health permits to prevent dehydration.
AMMONIA DERMATITIS (DIAPER RASH) Caused by skin bacteria reacting with urea in the urine. The skin becomes reddened and is sore.	1. Keep skin dry and clean by applying protective ointments containing zinc oxide to areas at risk (e.g., buttocks and perineum). 2. Boil an infant's diapers or wash them with an antibacterial detergent to prevent infection. Rinse diapers well because detergent is irritating to an infant's skin.
ACNE Inflammatory condition with papules and pustules.	1. Keep the skin clean to prevent secondary infection. 2. Treatment varies widely.
ERYTHEMA Redness associated with a variety of conditions, such as rashes, exposure to sun, elevated body temperature.	1. Wash area carefully to remove excess microorganisms. 2. Apply antiseptic spray or lotion to prevent itching, promote healing, and prevent skin breakdown.
HIRSUTISM Excessive hair on the body and face, particularly in women.	1. Remove unwanted hair by using depilatories, shaving, electrolysis, or tweezing. 2. Enhance client's self-concept.

ASSESSMENT INTERVIEW Skin Hygiene

SKIN CARE PRACTICES

- What are your usual showering or bathing times?
- What hygienic products do you routinely use (e.g., bath oils, powder, facial cleansing creams, body lotions or creams, deodorants, antiperspirants)?
- What facial cosmetic products do you use?
- How and when do you clean makeup applicators and puffs? (Applicators should be kept clean, and products used around the eyes in particular should be discarded after 4 months to prevent bacterial and fungal infections.)
- What hygienic or cosmetic products do you not use because of the skin problems they create (e.g., skin dryness or allergic reactions)?

SELF-CARE ABILITIES

- Do you have any problems managing your hygienic practices (e.g., baths and facial care)? If so, what are these?
- How can the nurses best help you?

SKIN PROBLEMS

- Do you have any tendency toward skin dryness, itchiness, rashes, bruising, excessive perspiration, or lack of perspiration? Have you had skin or scalp lesions in the past?
- Do you have any allergic tendencies? If so, what?

Positive responses to any of these require further exploration in terms of duration (When did it start?); frequency (How often have you had this?); description of lesion or rash; any associated signs, such as fever or nausea; aggravating factors (e.g., season of the year, stress, occupation, medication, recent travel, housing, personal contact); alleviating factors (e.g., medications, lotions, home remedies); and any family history of the problem.

Diagnosing

Examples of nursing diagnoses for clients with self-care problems need to specify the problem, such as bathing, feeding, toileting, or dressing. The nursing diagnoses, specified as altered self-care (bathing), altered self-care (dressing), and altered self-care (toileting), are discussed in this chapter. Another altered self-care nursing diagnosis, altered self-care (feeding), is discussed in Chapter 46 ∞.

Difficulties encountered by the client in performing bathing activities include the inability to wash the body or body parts, to obtain or get to a water source, and to regulate water temperature or flow. Difficulties in dressing and grooming include inability to obtain, put on, take off, fasten, or replace articles of clothing and to maintain appearance at a satisfactory level. Toileting problems may involve difficulties getting to the toilet or commode or sitting on and rising from it. In addition, the client may experience problems manipulating clothing for toileting, carrying out proper toilet hygiene, or flushing the toilet or emptying the commode. The reasons (etiologies or related factors) for these problems are varied (e.g., weakness, fatigue, pain, altered physical mobility).

The nursing diagnoses, potential for developing altered skin integrity, and altered skin integrity are discussed in Chapter 36 ∞.

Planning

In planning care, the nurse and, if appropriate, the client and family set outcomes for each nursing diagnosis. The nurse then performs nursing interventions and activities to achieve the client outcomes.

The specific, detailed nursing activities provided by the nurse may include assisting dependent clients with bathing, skin care, and perineal care; providing back massages to promote circulation; instructing clients and families about appropriate hygienic practices and alternative methods for dressing; and demonstrating use of assistive equipment and adaptive activities. Although the nursing interventions discussed in this chapter focus on hygienic measures, the etiology of the nursing diagnoses established may point to other interventions that promote circulation, promote self-esteem, restore nutritional status, correct fluid deficits or excesses, or prevent problems associated with immobility. Nursing strategies to deal with these etiologies are provided in other chapters.

Planning to assist a client with personal hygiene includes consideration of the client's personal preferences, health, and limitations; the best time to give the care; and the equipment, facilities, and personnel available. A client's personal preferences—about when and how to bathe, for example—should be followed as long as they are compatible with the client's health and the equipment available. Another consideration for the nurse is to assess the client's comfort level with the gender of the caregiver. Hygienic care, particularly bathing, can be embarrassing and stressful to modest individuals. Nurses must respect a client's modesty, whether male or female, and provide adequate privacy and sensitivity. If possible, try to provide a caregiver of the same gender. Nurses need to provide whatever assistance the client requires, either directly or by assigning this task to other assistive personnel, or including a family caregiver in the task if the client prefers.

Planning for Home Care

To provide for continuity of care, the nurse should assess the client's and family's abilities to provide self-care and the need for referrals and home health services. In addition, the nurse needs to determine the client's learning needs.

QSEN Patient-Centered Care: Assessing the Client and the Home Environment

Assessments of the client and environment should include:

- *Self-care abilities for hygiene:* Assess the client's ability to bathe, to regulate water faucets, to dress and undress, to groom, and to use the toilet.
- *Self-care aids required:* Determine if there is a need for a tub or shower seat (Figure 33.1 ■), a hand shower, a nonskid surface or mat in the tub or shower, hand bars on the sides of the tub (Figure 33.2 ■), or a raised toilet seat.
- *Facilities:* Check for the presence of laundry facilities and running water.
- *Mechanical barriers:* Note furniture obstructing access to the bathroom and toilet, or a doorway too narrow for a wheelchair.

Assessments of the family should include:

- *Caregiver availability, skills, and responses:* Determine whether individuals are available and able to assist with bathing, dressing, toileting, nail care, hair shampooing, or shopping for hygienic or grooming aids.
- *Education needs:* Assess whether the caregiver needs instruction in how to assist the client in and out of the tub, on and off the toilet, and so on.
- *Family role changes and coping:* Assess the effects of client's illness on financial status, parenting, spousal roles, sexuality, and social roles.

Assessments of the community should include:

- Explore resources that will provide assistance with bathing, laundry, and foot care (e.g., home health aide, podiatrist).
- Consult a social worker as needed to coordinate placement of a client unable to remain in the home or to identify community resources that will help the client stay in the home.
- Consider a consult with (a) a physical therapist to assess, develop, and improve the client's motor function; (b) a home health nurse to provide follow-up for care, teaching, and support; and (c) an occupational therapist to assess and develop abilities to perform activities of daily living.

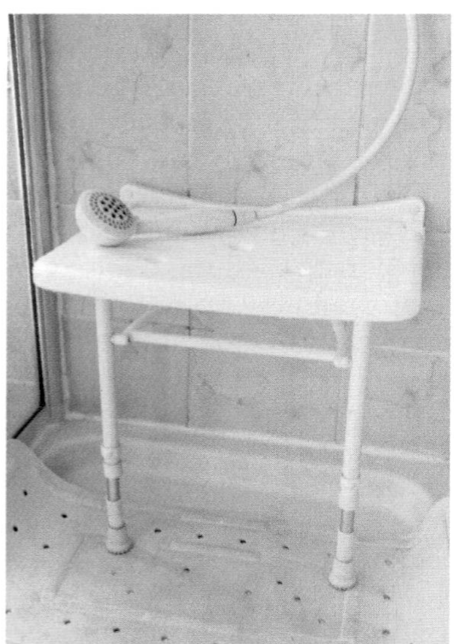

Figure 33.1 ■ A shower seat.
stocksolutions/123RF.

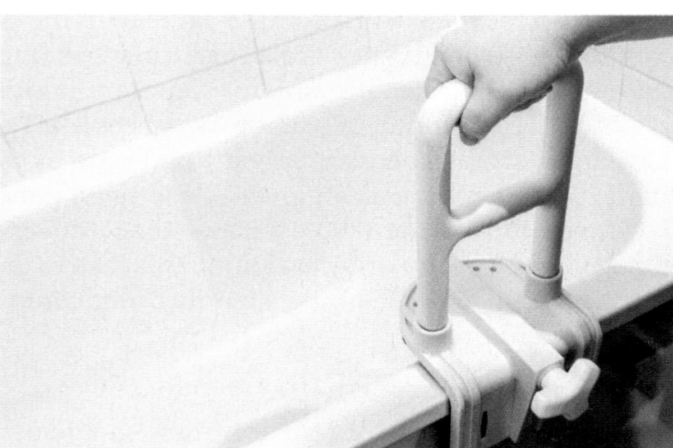

Figure 33.2 ■ A hand bar on the side of the bathtub.
Oleg Doroshin/123RF.

Implementing

The nurse applies the general guidelines for skin care while providing one of the various types of baths available to clients. Skill 33.1 describes how to bathe an adult client.

General Guidelines for Skin Care

1. ***Intact, healthy skin is the body's first line of defense.*** Nurses need to ensure that all skin care measures prevent injury and irritation. Scratching the skin with jewelry or long, sharp fingernails must be avoided. Harsh rubbing or use of rough towels and washcloths can cause tissue damage, particularly when the skin is irritated or when circulation or sensation is diminished. Bottom bed sheets are kept taut and free from wrinkles to reduce friction and abrasion to the skin. Top bed linens are arranged to prevent undue pressure on the toes. When necessary, footboards are used to keep bedclothes off the feet.
2. ***The degree to which the skin protects the underlying tissues from injury depends on the general health of the cells, the amount of subcutaneous tissue, and the dryness of the skin.*** Skin that is poorly nourished and dry is less easily protected and more vulnerable to injury. When the skin is dry, lotions or creams with lanolin can be applied, and bathing is limited to once or twice a week because frequent bathing removes the natural oils of the skin and causes dryness.

3. ***Moisture in contact with the skin for more than a short time can result in increased bacterial growth and irritation.*** After a bath, the client's skin is dried carefully. Particular attention is paid to areas such as the axillae, the groin, beneath the breasts, and between the toes, where the potential for irritation and fungal infection is greatest. A nonirritating dusting powder tends to reduce moisture and can be applied to these areas after they are dried. Clients who are incontinent of urine or feces or who perspire excessively are provided with immediate skin care to prevent skin irritation.
4. ***Body odors are caused by resident skin bacteria acting on body secretions.*** Cleanliness is the best deodorant. Commercial deodorants and antiperspirants can be applied only after the skin is cleaned. Deodorants diminish odors, whereas antiperspirants reduce the amount of perspiration. Neither is applied immediately after shaving because of the possibility of skin irritation, nor are they used on skin that is already irritated.
5. ***Skin sensitivity to irritation and injury varies among individuals and in accordance with their health.*** Generally speaking, skin sensitivity is greater in infants, very young children, and older adults. A client's nutritional status also affects sensitivity. Individuals who are emaciated or obese tend to experience more skin irritation and injury. The same tendency is seen in individuals with poor dietary habits and insufficient fluid intake. Even in healthy individuals, skin sensitivity is highly variable. Some individuals' skin is sensitive to the chemicals used in skin care agents and cosmetics. Hypoallergenic cosmetics and soaps or soap substitutes are now available for them. The nurse needs to ascertain whether the client has any sensitivities and what agents are appropriate to use.
6. ***Agents used for skin care have selective actions and purposes.*** Commonly used agents are described in Table 33.4.

TABLE 33.4 Agents Commonly Used on the Skin

Soap	Lowers surface tension and thus helps in cleaning. Some soaps contain antibacterial agents, which can change the natural flora of the skin.
Chlorhexidine gluconate (CHG)	A disposable cloth saturated with 2% CHG and skin-moisturizing substances. An advantage is continued antimicrobial activity after application. These cloths are often used in critical-care settings.
Bath oil	Used in bathwater; provides an oily film on the skin that softens and prevents chapping. Oils can make the tub surface slippery, and clients should be instructed about safety measures (e.g., using nonskid tub surface or mat).
Skin cream, lotion	Provides a film on the skin that prevents evaporation and therefore chapping.
Powder	Can be used to absorb water and prevent friction. For example, powder under the breasts can prevent skin irritation. Some powders are antibacterial.
Deodorant	Masks or diminishes body odors.
Antiperspirant	Reduces the amount of perspiration.

CLIENT TEACHING Skin Problems and Care

DRY SKIN

- Use cleansing creams to clean the skin rather than soap or detergent, which cause drying and, in some cases, allergic reactions.
- Use bath oils, but take precautions to prevent falls caused by slippery tub surfaces.
- Thoroughly rinse soap or detergent, if used, from the skin.
- Bathe less frequently when environmental temperature and humidity are low.
- Increase fluid intake.
- Humidify the air with a humidifier or by keeping a tub or sink full of water.
- Use moisturizing or emollient creams that contain lanolin, petroleum jelly, or cocoa butter to retain skin moisture.

SKIN RASHES

- Keep the area clean by washing it with a mild soap. Rinse the skin well, and pat it dry.
- To relieve itching, try a tepid bath or soak. Some over-the-counter preparations, such as Caladryl lotion, may help but should be used with full knowledge of the product.
- Avoid scratching the rash to prevent inflammation, infection, and further skin lesions.
- Choose clothing carefully. Too much can cause perspiration and aggravate a rash.

ACNE

- Wash the face frequently with soap or detergent and hot water to remove oil and dirt.
- Avoid using oily creams, which aggravate the condition.
- Avoid using cosmetics that block the ducts of the sebaceous glands and the hair follicles.
- Never squeeze or pick at the lesions. This increases the potential for infection and scarring.

Bathing

Bathing removes accumulated oil, perspiration, dead skin cells, and some bacteria. The nurse can appreciate the quantity of oil and dead skin cells produced when observing a client after the removal of a cast that has been on for several weeks. The skin is crusty, flaky, and dry underneath the cast. Applications of oil over several days are usually necessary to remove the debris.

Excessive bathing, however, can interfere with the intended lubricating effect of the sebum, causing dryness of the skin. This is an important consideration, especially for older adults, who produce less sebum.

In addition to cleaning the skin, bathing also stimulates circulation. A warm or hot bath dilates superficial arterioles, bringing more blood and nourishment to the skin. Vigorous rubbing has the same effect. Rubbing with long, smooth strokes from the distal to proximal parts of extremities (from the point farthest from the body to the point closest) is particularly effective in facilitating venous blood flow return unless there is some underlying condition (e.g., thrombosis) that would contraindicate this action. Vigorous rubbing is avoided in older clients with little subcutaneous tissue and those on medications that thin skin or cause easy bruising such as steroids or anticoagulants.

Bathing also produces a sense of well-being. It is refreshing and relaxing and frequently improves morale, appearance, and self-concept. Some people take a morning shower for its refreshing, stimulating effect. Others prefer an evening bath because it is relaxing. These effects are more evident when an individual is ill. For example, it is not uncommon for clients who have had a restless or sleepless night to feel relaxed, comfortable, and sleepy after a morning bath.

Bathing offers an excellent opportunity for the nurse to assess clients and provides an opportunity for establishing trust. The nurse can observe the client's skin for conditions such as sacral edema or rashes. While assisting a client with a bath, the nurse can also assess the client's psychosocial needs, such as orientation to time, ability to cope with the illness, and physical ability to implement self-care. Learning needs, such as the need for a client who has diabetes to learn foot care, can also be assessed.

Categories

Two categories of baths are given to clients: cleansing and therapeutic. **Cleansing baths** are given chiefly for hygiene purposes and include these types:

- ***Complete bed bath.*** The nurse washes the entire body of a dependent client in bed.
- ***Self-help (assisted) bed bath.*** Clients confined to bed are able to bathe themselves with help from the nurse for washing the back and perhaps the feet.
- ***Partial bath.*** Only the parts of the client's body that might cause discomfort or odor, if neglected, are washed: the face, hands, axillae, perineal area, and back. Omitted are the arms, chest, abdomen, legs, and feet. The nurse provides this care for dependent clients and assists self-sufficient clients confined to bed by washing their backs. Some ambulatory clients prefer to take a partial bath at the sink. The nurse can assist them by washing their backs.
- ***Bag bath.*** This bath is a commercially prepared product that contains 10 to 12 presoaked disposable washcloths that contain no-rinse cleanser solution. The package is warmed in a microwave. The warming time is about 1 minute, but the nurse needs to determine how long it takes to attain a desirable temperature. Each area of the body is cleaned with a different cloth and then air dried. Because the body is not rubbed dry, the emollient in the solution remains on the skin. The disposable bag bath is often a desirable form for bathing clients in critical care and in some long-term care settings.
- ***Towel bath.*** This bath is similar to a bag bath but uses regular towels. It is useful for clients who are bedridden and clients with dementia. The client is covered and kept warm throughout the bathing process by a bath blanket. The nurse gradually replaces the bath blanket with a large towel that has been soaked with warm water and no-rinse soap. The client is then gently massaged with the warm, wet, soapy towel. The wet towel is replaced with a large dry towel for drying the client's skin.
- ***Tub bath.*** Tub baths are often preferred to bed baths because it is easier to wash and rinse in a tub. Tubs are also used for therapeutic baths. The amount of assistance the nurse offers depends on the abilities of the client. There are specially designed tubs for dependent clients. These tubs greatly reduce the work of the nurse in lifting clients in and out of the tub and offer greater benefits than a sponge bath in bed.

  Sponge baths are suggested for the newborn because daily tub baths are not considered necessary. After the bath, the infant should be immediately dried and wrapped to prevent heat loss. Parents need to be advised that the infant's ability to regulate body temperature has not yet fully developed. Infants perspire minimally, and shivering starts at a lower temperature than it does in adults; therefore, infants lose more heat before shivering begins. In addition, because the infant's body surface area is very large in relation to body mass, the body loses heat readily.
- ***Shower.*** Many ambulatory clients are able to use shower facilities and require only minimal assistance from the nurse. Clients in long-term care settings are often given showers with the aid of a shower chair. The shower chair also has a commode seat to facilitate cleansing of the client's perineal area during the shower process (Figure 33.3 ■).

The water for a bath should feel comfortably warm to the client. People vary in their sensitivity to heat; generally, the temperature should be 43°C to 46°C (110°F to 115°F). Most clients will verify a suitable temperature. Clients with

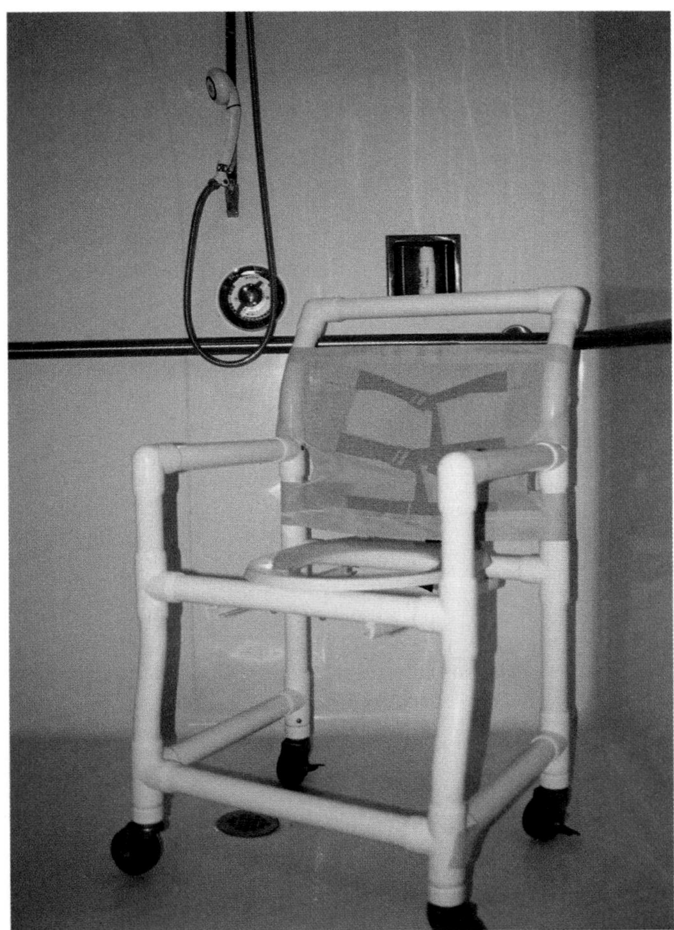

Figure 33.3 ■ A shower chair.
Shirlee Snyder.

decreased circulation or cognitive problems, however, will not be able to verify the temperature. Therefore, the nurse must check the water temperature to avoid burning the client with water that is too hot. The water for a bed bath should be changed when it becomes dirty or cold.

Therapeutic baths are given for physical effects, such as to soothe irritated skin or to treat an area (e.g., the perineum). Two common types are the sitz bath and the medicated bath. For the sitz bath, the client sits in warm water to help soothe and heal the perineum. For example, mothers after childbirth or clients who have had rectal surgery may find a sitz bath soothing. Some clients may also use a sitz bath to help alleviate discomfort from hemorrhoids. A bathtub can be used for a sitz bath, or a disposable plastic sitz bath unit that sits over a toilet bowl can be used.

The medicated therapeutic bath is generally taken in a tub one-third or one-half full with water at a comfortable temperature. Medications may be placed in the water (e.g., sodium bicarbonate, Aveeno oatmeal products, bath oils). The baths are useful for soothing irritated or itchy skin (e.g., from sunburn, hives, skin diseases). The client usually remains in the bath for no longer than 20 to 30 minutes. If the client's back, chest, and arms are to be treated, these areas need to be immersed in the solution. For safety reasons, advise the client to use a bath mat, especially if the product added to the water will make the surface of the tub slippery. Skill 33.1 provides guidelines for bathing clients.

QSEN Safety: Bathing at Home

For bathing and hygiene in the home setting, the nurse can suggest that the client or caregiver do the following:

- Consider purchasing a bath seat that fits in the bathtub or shower.
- Install a hand shower for use with a bath seat and shampooing.
- Use a nonskid surface on the tub or shower.
- Install hand bars on both sides of the tub or shower to facilitate transfers in and out of the tub or shower.
- Carefully monitor the temperature of the bathwater.
- Apply lotion and oil after a bath, not during, because these solutions can make a tub surface slippery.

Bathing an Adult Client

SKILL 33.1

PURPOSES

- To remove transient microorganisms, body secretions and excretions, and dead skin cells
- To stimulate circulation to the skin
- To promote a sense of well-being
- To produce relaxation and comfort
- To prevent and eliminate unpleasant body odors

ASSESSMENT

Assess

- Physical or emotional factors (e.g., fatigue, sensitivity to cold, need for control, anxiety or fear)
- Condition of the skin (color, texture and turgor, presence of pigmented spots, temperature, lesions, excoriations, abrasions, and bruises). Areas of erythema (redness) on the sacrum, bony prominences, and heels should be assessed for possible pressure sores.
- Presence of pain and need for additional measures (e.g., an analgesic) before the bath
- Range of motion of the joints
- Any other aspect of health that may affect the client's bathing process (e.g., mobility, strength, cognition)
- Need for use of clean gloves during the bath
- Fall risk of clients who wish to shower
- Some clients may have body piercings. Ask the client what hygienic measures are needed for the care of the piercings.

Continued on page 764

SKILL 33.1

Bathing an Adult Client—*continued*

PLANNING

Assignment

The nurse often assigns the skill of bathing to assistive personnel (AP). The nurse, however, remains responsible for assessment and client care. The nurse needs to do the following:

- Inform the AP of the type of bath appropriate for the client and precautions, if any, specific to the needs of the client.
- Remind the AP to notify the nurse of any concerns or changes (e.g., redness, skin breakdown, rash) so the nurse can assess, intervene if needed, and document.
- Instruct the AP to encourage the client to perform as much self-care as appropriate in order to promote independence and self-esteem.
- Obtain a complete report about the bathing experience from the AP.

Equipment

- Basin or sink with warm water (between 43°C and 46°C [110°F and 115°F])
- Soap and soap dish
- Linens: bath blanket, bath towels, and washcloths as determined by client need; clean gown or pajamas or clothes as needed; additional bed linen and towels, if required
- Clean gloves, if appropriate (e.g., presence of body fluids or open lesions)
- Personal hygiene articles (e.g., deodorant, lotions)
- Shaving equipment
- Table for bathing equipment
- Bag for soiled linens

IMPLEMENTATION

Preparation

Before bathing a client, determine (a) the purpose and type of bath the client needs; (b) self-care ability of the client; (c) any movement or positioning precautions specific to the client; (d) other care the client may be receiving, such as physical therapy or x-rays, in order to coordinate all aspects of healthcare and prevent unnecessary fatigue; (e) client's comfort level with being bathed by someone else; and (f) necessary bath equipment and linens.

Caution is needed when bathing clients who are receiving IV therapy. Easy-to-remove gowns that have Velcro or snap fasteners along the sleeves may be used. If a special gown is not available, the nurse needs to pay special attention when changing the client's gown after the bath (or whenever the gown becomes soiled). In addition, special attention is needed to reassess the IV site for security of IV connections and appropriate taping around the IV site.

The nurse should use standard precautions when bathing a client, particularly when performing perineal care. It is not necessary, however, to wear gloves while providing a bath, and the nurse should use clinical judgment when deciding to wear gloves and offer an explanation to the client.

Performance

1. Prior to performing the procedure, introduce self and verify the client's identity using agency protocol. Explain to the client what you are going to do, why it is necessary, and how to participate. Discuss with the client his or her preferences for bathing and explain any unfamiliar procedures.
2. Perform hand hygiene and observe other appropriate infection prevention procedures.
3. Provide for client privacy by drawing the curtains around the bed or closing the door to the room. Some agencies provide signs indicating the need for privacy. **Rationale:** *Hygiene is a personal matter*.
4. Prepare the client and the environment.
   - Invite a family member or significant other to participate if desired or requested by the client.
   - Close windows and doors to ensure the room is a comfortable temperature. **Rationale:** *Air currents increase loss of heat from the body by convection*.
   - Offer the client a bedpan or urinal or ask whether the client wishes to use the toilet or commode. **Rationale:** *Warm water and activity can stimulate the need to void. The client will be more comfortable after voiding, and voiding before cleaning the perineum is advisable*.
   - Encourage the client to perform as much personal self-care as possible. **Rationale:** *This promotes independence, exercise, and self-esteem*.
   - During the bath, assess each area of the skin carefully.

For a Bed Bath

5. Prepare the bed and position the client appropriately.
   - Position the bed at a comfortable working height. Lower the side rail on the side close to you. Keep the other side rail up. Assist the client to move near you. **Rationale:** *This avoids undue reaching and straining and promotes good body mechanics. It also ensures client safety*.
   - Place the bath blanket over top sheet. Remove the top sheet from under the bath blanket by starting at client's shoulders and moving linen down toward client's feet. ❶ Ask the client to grasp and hold the top of the bath blanket while pulling linen to the foot of the bed. **Rationale:** *The bath blanket provides comfort, warmth, and privacy*.

   Note: If the bed linen is to be reused, place it over the bedside chair. If it is to be changed, place it in the linen hamper, not on the floor.
   - Remove the client's gown while keeping the client covered with the bath blanket. Place gown in linen hamper.
6. Make a bath mitt with the washcloth. **Rationale:** *A bath mitt retains water and heat better than a cloth loosely held and prevents ends of washcloth from dragging across the skin*.
7. Wash the face. **Rationale:** *Begin the bath at the cleanest area and work downward toward the feet*.
   - Place towel under the client's head.
   - Wash the client's eyes with water only and dry them well. Use a separate corner of the washcloth for each eye. **Rationale:** *Using separate corners prevents transmitting microorganisms from one eye to the other*. Wipe from the

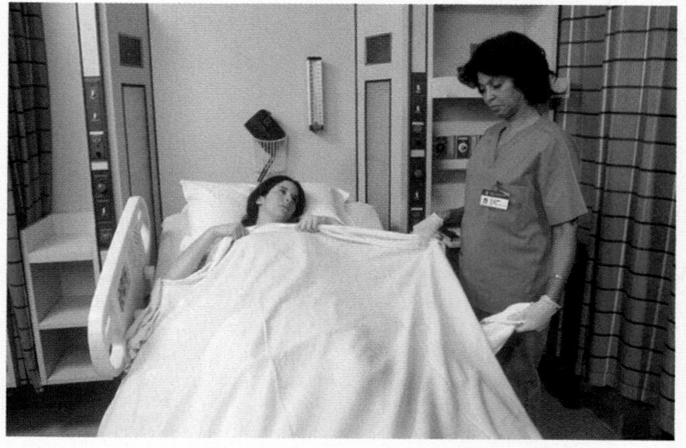

❶ Remove the top sheet from under the bath blanket.

Bathing an Adult Client—*continued*

inner to the outer canthus. ❷ **Rationale:** *This prevents secretions from entering the nasolacrimal ducts*.
- Ask whether the client wants soap used on the face. **Rationale:** *Soap has a drying effect, and the face, which is exposed to the air more than other body parts, tends to be drier*.
- Wash, rinse, and dry the client's face, ears, and neck.
- Remove the towel from under the client's head.

8. Wash the arms and hands. (Omit the arms for a partial bath.)
- Place a towel lengthwise under the arm away from you. **Rationale:** *It protects the bed from becoming wet*.
- Wash, rinse, and dry the arm by elevating the client's arm and supporting the client's wrist and elbow. ❸ Use long, firm strokes from wrist to shoulder, including the axillary area. **Rationale:** *Firm strokes from distal to proximal areas promote circulation by increasing venous blood return*.
- Apply deodorant or powder if desired. Special caution is needed for clients with respiratory alterations. **Rationale:** *Powder is not recommended for these clients due to the potential respiratory adverse effects*.
- Optional: Place a towel on the bed and put a washbasin on it. Place the client's hands in the basin. **Rationale:** *Many clients enjoy immersing their hands in the basin and washing themselves*. Soaking loosens dirt under the nails. Assist the client as needed to wash, rinse, and dry the hands, paying particular attention to the spaces between the fingers.

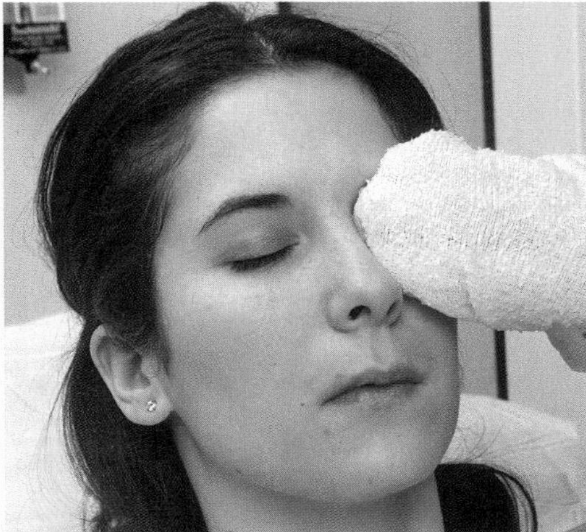

❷ Using a separate corner of the washcloth for each eye, wipe from the inner to the outer canthus.

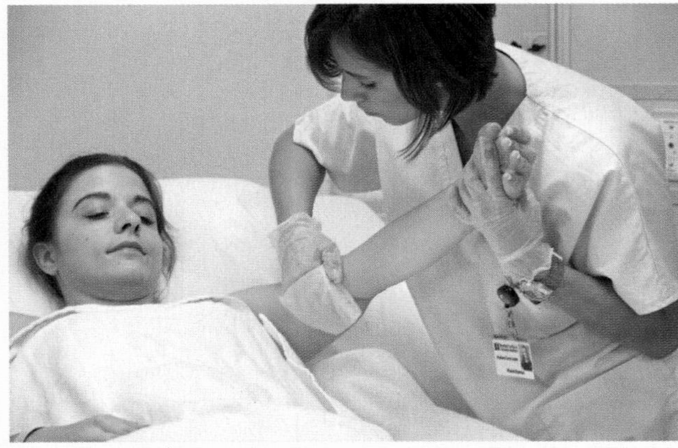

❸ Washing the arm using long, firm strokes from wrist to shoulder area.

- Repeat for hand and arm nearest you. Exercise caution if an IV infusion is present, and check its flow after moving the arm. Avoid submersing the IV site if the dressing site is not a clear, transparent dressing. **Rationale:** *A clear, transparent dressing will keep water from an IV site; however, a gauze dressing becomes contaminated when it becomes wet with the water*.

9. Wash the chest and abdomen. (Omit the chest and abdomen for a partial bath. However, the areas under a woman's breasts may require bathing if this area is irritated or if the client has significant perspiration under the breast.)
- Place bath towel lengthwise over chest. Fold bath blanket down to the client's pubic area. **Rationale:** *Keeps the client warm while preventing unnecessary exposure of the chest*.
- Lift the bath towel off the chest, and bathe the chest and abdomen with your mitted hand using long, firm strokes. ❹ Give special attention to the skin under the breasts and any other skinfolds, particularly if the client is overweight. Rinse and dry well.
- Replace the bath blanket when the areas have been dried.

10. Wash the legs and feet. (Omit legs and feet for a partial bath.)
- Expose the leg farthest from you by folding the bath blanket toward the other leg, being careful to keep the perineum covered. **Rationale:** *Covering the perineum promotes privacy and maintains the client's dignity*.
- Lift leg and place the bath towel lengthwise under the leg. Wash, rinse, and dry the leg using long, smooth, firm strokes from the ankle to the knee to the thigh. ❺ **Rationale:** *Washing from the distal to proximal areas promotes circulation by stimulating venous blood flow*.
- Reverse the coverings and repeat for the other leg.
- Wash the feet by placing them in the basin of water.
- Dry each foot. Pay particular attention to the spaces between the toes. If preferred, wash one foot after that leg before washing the other leg.

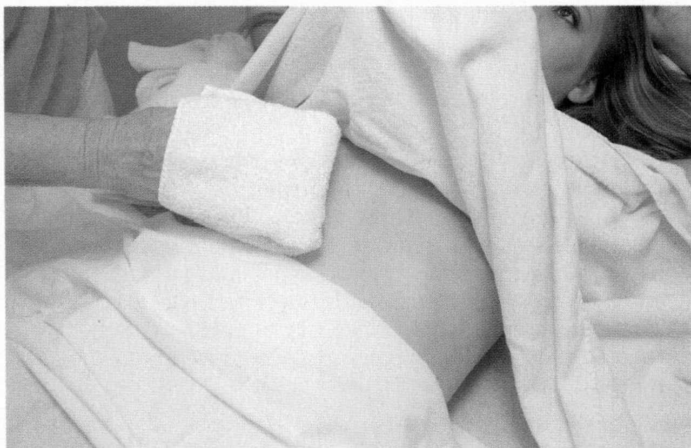

❹ Washing the chest and abdomen.

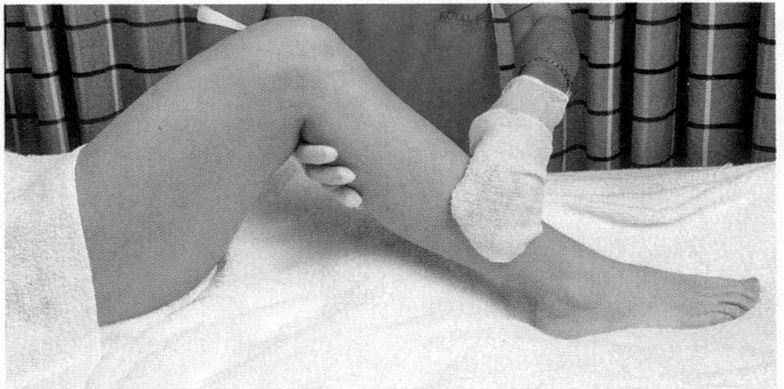

❺ Washing the far leg.

SKILL 33.1

Continued on page 766

SKILL 33.1

Bathing an Adult Client—*continued*

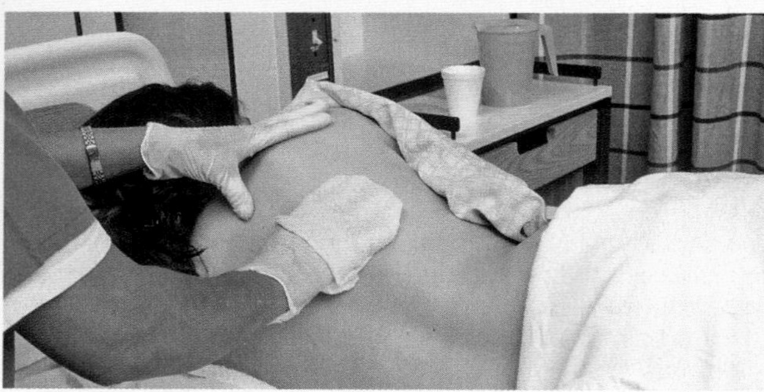

6 Washing the back.

- Obtain fresh, warm bathwater now or when necessary. **Rationale:** *Water may become dirty or cold.* Because surface skin cells are removed with washing, the bathwater from dark-skinned clients may be dark, however, this does not mean the client is dirty. Lower the bed and raise the side rails when refilling the basin. **Rationale:** *This ensures the safety of the client.*

11. Wash the back and then the perineum.
- Assist the client into a prone or side-lying position facing away from you. Place the bath towel lengthwise alongside the back and buttocks while keeping the client covered with the bath blanket as much as possible. **Rationale:** *This provides warmth and prevents undue exposure.*
- Wash and dry the client's back, moving from the shoulders to the buttocks, and upper thighs, paying attention to the gluteal folds. 6
- Remove and discard gloves if used.
- Perform a back massage now or after completion of the bath. (See Skill 30.1, page 680.)
- Assist the client to the supine position and determine whether the client can wash the perineal area independently. If the client cannot do so, drape the client as shown in Skill 33.2 and wash the area.

12. Assist the client with grooming aids such as powder, lotion, or deodorant.
- Use powder sparingly. Do not shake directly onto the client; put in hands and lightly dust skin. Release as little as possible into the atmosphere. **Rationale:** *This will avoid irritation of the respiratory tract by powder inhalation. Excessive powder can cause caking, which leads to skin irritation.*
- Help the client put on a clean gown or pajamas.
- Assist the client to care for hair, mouth, and nails. Some people prefer or need mouth care prior to their bath.

For a Tub Bath or Shower

13. Prepare the client and the tub.
- Fill the tub about one-third to one-half full of water at 43°C to 46°C (110°F to 115°F). **Rationale:** *Sufficient water is needed to cover the perineal area.*
- Cover all IV catheters or wound dressings with plastic coverings, and instruct the client to prevent wetting these areas if possible.
- Put a rubber bath mat or towel on the floor of the tub if safety strips are not on the tub floor. **Rationale:** *These prevent slippage of the client during the bath or shower.*

14. Assist the client into the shower or tub.
- Assist the client taking a standing shower with the initial adjustment of the water temperature and water flow pressure, as needed. Some clients need a chair to sit on in the shower because of weakness. Hot water can cause older clients to feel faint due to vasodilation and decreased blood pressure from positional changes.
- If the client requires considerable assistance with a tub bath, a hydraulic bathtub chair may be required (see Variation).
- Explain how the client can signal for help, leave the client for 2 to 5 minutes, and place an "occupied" sign on the door. For safety reasons, do not leave a client with decreased cognition or clients who may be at risk (e.g., history of seizures, syncope).

15. Assist the client with washing and getting out of the tub.
- Wash the client's back, lower legs, and feet, if necessary.
- Assist the client out of the tub. If the client is unsteady, place a bath towel over the client's shoulders and drain the tub of water before the client attempts to get out of it. **Rationale:** *Draining the water first lessens the likelihood of a fall. The towel prevents chilling.*

16. Dry the client, and assist with follow-up care.
- Follow step 12.
- Assist the client back to his or her bed.
- Clean the tub or shower in accordance with agency practice, discard the used linen in the laundry hamper, and place the "unoccupied" sign on the door.

17. Document the following:
- Type of bath given (e.g., complete, partial, or self-help with assistance). This is usually recorded on a flow sheet.
- Skin assessment, such as excoriation, erythema, exudates, rashes, drainage, or skin breakdown.
- Nursing interventions related to skin integrity.
- Ability of the client to assist or participate with bathing.
- Client response to bathing. Also, document the need for reassessment of vital signs if appropriate.
- Educational needs regarding hygiene.
- Information or teaching shared with the client or family.

Variation: Bathing Using a Hydraulic Bathtub Chair

A hydraulic chair lift, often used in long-term care or rehabilitation settings, can facilitate the transfer of a client who is unable to ambulate to a tub. The lift also helps eliminate strain on the nurse's back.

- Bring the client to the tub room in a wheelchair or shower chair.
- Fill the tub and check the water temperature according to agency protocol. **Rationale:** *This avoids thermal injury to the client.*
- Lower the hydraulic chair lift to its lowest point, outside the tub.
- Transfer the client to the chair lift and secure the seat belt.
- Raise the chair lift above the tub.
- Support the client's legs as the chair is moved over the tub. **Rationale:** *This avoids injury to the legs.*
- Position the client's legs down into the water and slowly lower the chair lift into the tub.
- Assist in bathing the client, if appropriate.
- Reverse the procedure when taking the client out of the tub.
- Dry the client and transport him or her to the room.

EVALUATION

- Note the client's tolerance of the procedure (e.g., respiratory rate and effort, pulse rate, behaviors of acceptance or resistance, statements regarding comfort).
- Conduct appropriate follow-up, such as determining:
  - Condition and integrity of skin (dryness, turgor, redness, lesions, and so on).
  - Client strength. Note range of motion and circulation, movement, and sensation for all extremities.
  - Percentage of bath done without assistance.
- Compare to prior assessment data, if available.

LIFESPAN CONSIDERATIONS Bathing

INFANTS

- Sponge baths are suggested for the newborn because daily tub baths are not considered necessary. After the bath, the infant should be immediately dried and wrapped. Parents need to be advised that the infant's ability to regulate body temperature has not yet fully developed and newborns' bodies lose heat readily.

CHILDREN

- Encourage a child's participation as appropriate for developmental level.
- Closely supervise children in the bathtub. Do not leave them unattended.

ADOLESCENTS

- Assist adolescents as needed to choose deodorants and antiperspirants. Secretions from newly active sweat glands react with bacteria on the skin, causing a pungent odor.

OLDER ADULTS

- Changes of aging can decrease the protective function of the skin in older adults. These changes include fragile skin, less oil and moisture, and a decrease in elasticity.
- To minimize skin dryness in older adults, avoid excessive use of soap. The ideal time to moisturize the skin is immediately after bathing.
- Avoid excessive powder because it causes moisture loss and is a hazardous inhalant. Cornstarch should also be avoided because in the presence of moisture it breaks down into glucose and can facilitate the growth of organisms.
- Protect older adults and children from injury related to hot water burns.

EVIDENCE-BASED PRACTICE

Evidence-Based Practice

What Is the Impact of Chlorhexidine Bathing on Healthcare-Associated Infections?

According to Denny and Munro (2017), approximately 4% of hospitalized clients contract a healthcare-associated infection (HAI) during their hospitalizations. These infections frequently result in increased morbidity, mortality, and length of hospital stay. Skin bacterial colonization aids in the transmission and development of HAIs. Nurses frequently use bathing with chlorhexidine gluconate (CHG) to reduce bacterial colonization on the client's skin. Studies have shown that bathing with CHG products has had mixed results in the prevention of HAIs. As a result, the authors performed a literature review to examine the current evidence on the impact of CHG bathing on HAIs. The literature search identified peer-reviewed studies and meta-analyses that examined the impact of CHG bathing in preventing HAIs, specifically surgical site infections (SSIs), central line–associated bloodstream infections (CLABSIs), ventilator-associated pneumonias (VAP), catheter-associated urinary-tract infections (CAUTIs), and *Clostridium difficile*–associated disease. The search resulted in 23 articles for review.

The findings concluded that there was good evidence to support using a CHG bathing regimen to reduce the incidence of CLABSIs, SSIs, vancomycin-resistant enterococci (VRE), and methicillin-resistant *Staphylococcus aureus* (MRSA) HAIs.

The authors, based on the literature search, raised questions for further research, including the value of using CHG liquid soap versus CHG-impregnated washcloths. Research has shown that application of CHG on the client's body without rinsing has greater impact than applying CHG followed by rinsing the body. Do CHG-impregnated washcloths have an advantage because the CHG in the wipes is not rinsed from the skin? Another issue raised by the authors was that most studies were conducted in targeted populations (e.g., intensive care units). They suggest that more research is needed on the benefits of bathing all clients versus a targeted (bathing only at-risk clients) approach.

IMPLICATIONS

Hospitals are beginning to replace the traditional soap and water bathing with CHG bathing in order to prevent HAIs. As the authors suggested, nurses need to assess for adverse reactions to the use of CHG and increase their awareness that, with the increasing use of CHG, organisms may develop resistance to the antiseptic.

Long-Term Care Setting

From a historical perspective, the bath has always been a part of the art of nursing care and considered a component of nursing. In today's nursing world, however, the bath is seen as a necessary, routine task and is often assigned to AP.

In spite of the previously listed beneficial values associated with bathing, the choice of bathing procedure often depends on the amount of time available to the nurses or AP and the client's self-care ability. The bath routine (e.g., day, time, and number per week) for clients in healthcare settings is often determined by agency policy, which often results in the bath becoming routine and depersonalized versus therapeutic, satisfying, and client focused. New models and a culture change process are occurring in long-term care and residential care settings. That is, these settings are trying to become less about tasks and more about individuals and the relationships between individuals. This client-focused approach to bathing is especially important for the older client in a long-term care setting. Bathing needs to focus on the experience for the client rather than the outcome (i.e., getting a bath or shower).

A nurse who provides client-focused care asks such questions as: What is the client's usual method of maintaining cleanliness? Are there any past negative experiences related to bathing? Are factors such as pain or fatigue increasing the client's difficulty with the demands and stimuli associated with bathing or showering? A client's resistance to the bathing experience can be a cue to the nurse to consider other methods of maintaining cleanliness. For example, if the shower causes distress, is there another form of bathing (such as the bag or towel bath) that may be more therapeutic and comforting?

An individualized approach focusing on therapeutic and comforting outcomes of bathing is especially important for clients with dementia. Alzheimer's disease is the most common cause of dementia among people ages 65 and older. As the incidence of dementia increases, so does the need to preserve the dignity of clients with dementia.

Providing personal hygiene to a client with dementia is often an ongoing challenge. Being sensitive to the rhythm of the client's behavior and looking for cues can often offset problems related to this. Clients with dementia, whether they are at home or in a healthcare facility, often have certain times of the day when they are more agitated—these are times to avoid doing things that will increase their fear and agitation. When increased agitation occurs, the nurse should stop and change the approach. It is also sometimes helpful to wait (e.g., half an hour or so) and then try giving the bath because the client may forget protesting and be willing to participate.

Interventions that use the client-focused approach can include the following: preparing the environment for bathing by gathering everything before approaching the client, ensuring privacy, allowing sufficient time, speaking with a pleasant voice, giving the client choices, describing bathing activities before performing them, and keeping parts of the body covered while washing one section at a time (Alzheimer's Association, n.d.). Playing music, based on the client's preference or a family member's suggestion, may reduce resistance to care during personal care activities.

In addition, collaboration between the nurse and AP is a critical element to implementing the individualized client-focused approach for those with cognitive impairments who show aggressive behavior during bathing. The nurse, after observing a difficult bathing situation, should discuss with the AP possible alternative strategies or methods they might implement for the client. More than one intervention may be required (e.g., reassurance, simple explanations, moving slowly). It is important for the nurse to subsequently evaluate the client's response to the new intervention(s). The nurse has a role in educating AP about dementia and collaboratively problem-solving bathing challenges.

Perineal-Genital Care

Perineal-genital care is also referred to as perineal care or pericare. Perineal care as part of the bed bath is embarrassing for many clients. Nurses also may find it embarrassing initially, particularly with clients of the opposite sex. Most clients who require a bed bath from the nurse are able to clean their own genital areas with minimal assistance. The nurse may need to hand a moistened washcloth and soap to the client, rinse the washcloth, and provide a towel.

Because some clients are unfamiliar with terminology for the genitals and perineum, it may be difficult for nurses to explain what is expected. Most clients, however, understand what is meant if the nurse simply says, "I'll give you a washcloth to finish your bath in privacy." Some older clients may be familiar with the term *private parts*. Whatever expression the nurse uses, it needs to be one that the client understands and one that is comfortable for the nurse to use.

The nurse needs to provide perineal care efficiently and in a matter-of-fact manner. Nurses should wear gloves while providing this care for the comfort of the client and to protect themselves from infection. Skill 33.2 explains how to provide perineal-genital care.

Client Teaching

Clients often need information about dry skin, skin rashes, and acne.

Clinical Alert!

Always wash or wipe from "clean to dirty." For a female, cleanse the perineal area from front to back. For a male, cleanse the urinary meatus by moving in a circular motion from the center of the urethral opening around the glans.

SKILL 33.2 Providing Perineal-Genital Care

PURPOSES

- To remove normal perineal secretions and odors
- To promote client comfort

ASSESSMENT

Assess for the presence of

- Irritation, excoriation, inflammation, swelling
- Excessive discharge
- Odor; pain or discomfort
- Urinary or fecal incontinence
- Recent rectal or perineal surgery
- Indwelling catheter

Determine

- Perineal-genital hygiene practices
- Self-care abilities

PLANNING

Assignment

Perineal-genital care can be assigned to AP; however, if the client has recently had perineal, rectal, or genital surgery, the nurse needs to assess if it is appropriate for the AP to perform the care.

Equipment

- Perineal-genital care provided in conjunction with the bed bath:
  - Bath towel
  - Bath blanket
  - Clean gloves

Providing Perineal-Genital Care—*continued*

- Bath basin with warm water at 43°C to 46°C (110°F to 115°F)
- Soap
- Washcloth

Special perineal-genital care:

- Bath towel
- Bath blanket
- Clean gloves
- Solution bottle, pitcher, or container filled with warm water or a prescribed solution
- Bedpan to receive rinse water
- Perineal pad

SKILL 33.2

IMPLEMENTATION

Preparation

- Determine whether the client is experiencing any discomfort in the perineal-genital area.
- Obtain and prepare the necessary equipment and supplies.

Performance

1. Prior to performing the procedure, introduce self and verify the client's identity using agency protocol. Explain to the client what you are going to do, why it is necessary, and how to participate, being particularly sensitive to any embarrassment displayed by the client.
2. Perform hand hygiene and observe other appropriate infection prevention procedures.
3. Provide for client privacy by drawing the curtains around the bed or closing the door to the room. Some agencies provide signs indicating the need for privacy. **Rationale:** *Hygiene is a personal matter*.
4. Prepare the client:
    - Fold the top bed linen to the foot of the bed and fold the gown up to expose the genital area.
    - Place a bath towel under the client's hips. **Rationale:** *The bath towel prevents the bed from becoming soiled*.
5. Position and drape the client and clean the upper inner thighs and inguinal areas.

For Female Clients

- Position the female in a back-lying (lithotomy) position with the knees flexed and spread well apart.
- Cover her body and legs with the bath blanket positioned so a corner is at her head, the opposite corner at her feet, and the other two on the sides. Drape the legs by tucking the bottom corners of the bath blanket under the inner sides of the legs. ❶ **Rationale:** *Minimum exposure lessens embarrassment and helps to provide warmth*. Bring the middle portion of the base of the blanket up and then over the pubic area.
- Apply gloves. Wash and dry the upper inner thighs and inguinal areas.

For Male Clients

- Position the male client in a supine position with knees slightly flexed and hips slightly externally rotated.
- Drape him by placing a towel or bath blanket over his abdomen and covering his legs with a sheet or towel. **Rationale:** *Minimum exposure lessens embarrassment and helps to provide warmth. When ready to begin care, fold the sheet or towel back to expose the penis and perineal area*.
- Apply gloves and wash and dry the upper inner thighs and inguinal areas.

6. Inspect the perineal area.
    - Note particular areas of inflammation, excoriation, or swelling, especially between the labia in females and the scrotal folds in males.
    - Also note excessive discharge or secretions from the orifices and the presence of odors.
7. Wash and dry the perineal-genital area.

For Female Clients

- Clean the labia majora and perineum from front to back, from pubis to the rectum. ❷ Use a separate clean area of the washcloth for each area or a new washcloth for each stroke. **Rationale:** *Using separate quarters of the washcloth or new wipes prevents the transmission of microorganisms from one area to the other. Wipe from the area of least contamination (the pubis) to that of greatest (the rectum)*. Do not place the washcloth in the basin. **Rationale:** *This prevents* ***cross-contamination*** *(the movement of microorganisms from one client to another)*.
- Separate the labia with one hand to expose the urethra and vaginal opening. Using a different washcloth, wash the labia minora from front to back on one side. Take a separate clean area of the washcloth or a new cloth and wash the other side from top to bottom. **Rationale:** *Secretions that tend to collect around the labia minora facilitate bacterial growth*.

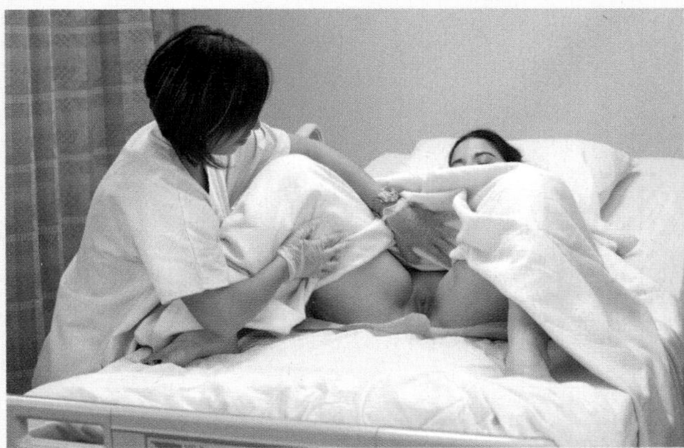

❶ Draping the female client for perineal-genital care.

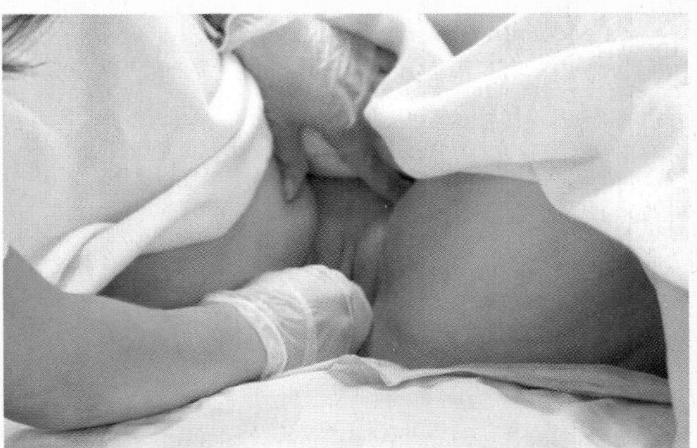

❷ Cleaning the labia.

Continued on page 770

Providing Perineal-Genital Care—*continued*

- Using a separate clean area of the washcloth or a new washcloth, wash the urethra from front to back, in a downward motion. **Rationale:** *This action uses the principle of washing from a clean to dirty area to prevent a urinary tract infection.*
- For menstruating women and clients with indwelling catheters, use clean wipes instead of washcloths. Use a clean wipe for each stroke.
- Rinse the area well. You may place the client on a bedpan and use Peri-Wash or a solution bottle to pour warm water over the area. Dry the perineum thoroughly, paying particular attention to the folds between the labia. **Rationale:** *Moisture supports the growth of many microorganisms.*

For Male Clients

- If the client is uncircumcised, retract the prepuce (foreskin) to expose the glans penis (the tip of the penis) for cleaning. Replace the foreskin after cleaning and drying the glans penis. ❸ **Rationale:** *Retracting the foreskin is necessary to remove the smegma (thick, cheesy secretion) that collects under the foreskin and facilitates bacterial growth. Replacing the foreskin prevents constriction of the penis, which may cause edema.*
- Hold the shaft of the penis gently and securely in one hand. ❹
- Clean the tip of the penis at the urethral meatus in a circular motion from the center outward and wash down the shaft with soap and water. ❺ Use a clean area of the washcloth or a new washcloth when washing a new area. **Rationale:** *This prevents cross-contamination.*
- Rinse and dry with new washcloth.
- Wash and dry the scrotum. The posterior folds of the scrotum may need to be cleaned when the buttocks are cleaned (see step 9). **Rationale:** *The scrotum tends to be more soiled than the penis because of its proximity to the rectum; thus it is usually cleaned after the penis. This follows the principle of cleaning from the least contamination to that of the greatest.*

8. Inspect perineal orifices for intactness.
   - Inspect particularly around the urethra in clients with indwelling catheters. **Rationale:** *A catheter may cause excoriation around the urethra.*
9. Clean between the gluteal folds and the entire buttocks.
   - Assist the client to turn onto the side facing away from you.
   - Pay particular attention to the anal area and posterior folds of the scrotum in males. Clean the anus with a wipe or toilet tissue before washing it, if necessary.
   - Dry the area well.
   - For postdelivery or menstruating women, apply a perineal pad as needed from front to back. **Rationale:** *This prevents contamination of the vagina and urethra from the anal area.*
10. Remove and discard gloves.
11. Perform hand hygiene.
12. Document any unusual findings such as redness, excoriation, skin breakdown, discharge or drainage, and any localized areas of tenderness.

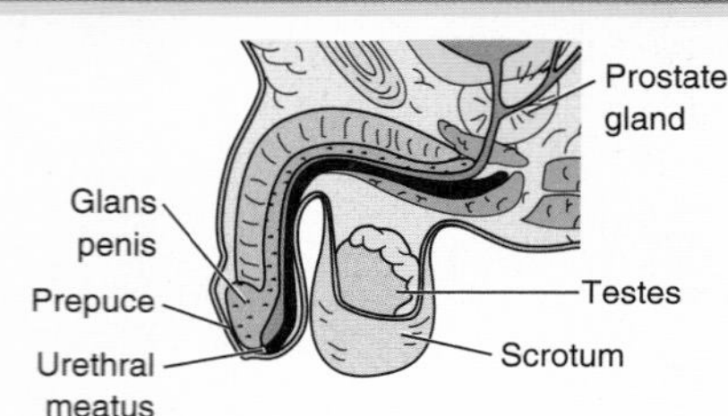

❸ Male genitals.

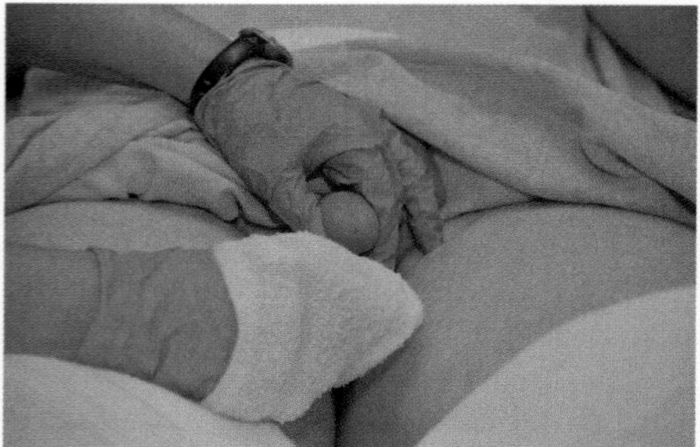

❹ Hold shaft of penis in one hand.

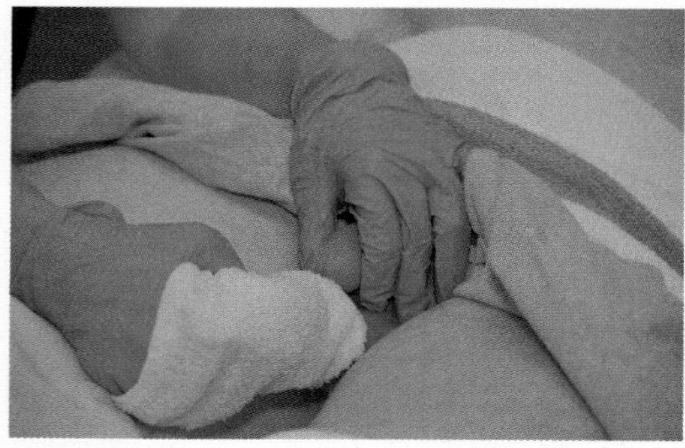

❺ Use circular motion, starting at tip of penis and wash toward shaft.

EVALUATION

- Compare current assessments to previous assessments.
- Conduct appropriate follow-up such as prescribed ointment for excoriation.
- Report any deviation from normal to the primary care provider.

Evaluating

Using data collected during care, the nurse judges whether desired outcomes have been achieved. If the outcomes have not been achieved, the nurse explores reasons why. For example:

- Did the nurse overestimate the client's functional abilities (physical, mental, emotional) for self-care?
- Were provided instructions clear?
- Were appropriate assistive devices or supplies available to the client?
- Did the client's condition change?
- Were required analgesics provided before hygienic care?
- What currently prescribed medications and therapies could affect the client's abilities or tissue integrity?
- Is the client's fluid and food intake adequate or appropriate to maintain skin and mucous membrane moisture and integrity?

Feet

The feet are essential for ambulation and merit attention even when people are confined to bed. Each foot contains 26 bones, 107 ligaments, and 19 muscles. These structures function together for both standing and walking.

Developmental Variations

At birth, a baby's foot is relatively unformed. The arches, supported by fatty pads, do not take their full shape until 5 to 6 years of age. During childhood, tight, binding stockings and ill-fitting shoes easily damage the bones and small muscles of the feet. For normal development, it is important that the arches be supported and that the bony structure and the feet grow with no external restrictions. Feet are not fully grown until about age 20. The average individual takes 10,000 steps per day. Each step places 2 to 3 times the force of the body weight on the feet. This repetitive use leads to normal changes associated with aging. Changes include wider and longer feet, mild settling of the arches, and loss of natural padding on the bottom of the heels. The cartilage around the joints also deteriorates, producing loss of normal range of motion of the foot and ankle. All older clients should know about foot care. Some older clients, however, require special attention for their feet. For example, reduced blood supply and accompanying arteriosclerosis can make a foot prone to ulcers and infection following trauma. Decreased flexibility or poor eyesight can make self-care of the feet impossible for the older client.

Safety Alert! SAFETY

Clients with diabetes are at high risk for lower extremity amputations (LEAs). Routine foot assessment and client education in proper foot care can significantly reduce the risk for LEAs.

●○● NURSING MANAGEMENT

Assessing

Assessment of the client's feet includes a nursing health history, physical assessment of the feet, and identifying clients at risk for foot problems.

Nursing History

The nurse determines the client's history of (a) normal nail and foot care practices, (b) type of footwear worn, (c) self-care abilities, (d) presence of risk factors for foot problems, (e) any foot discomfort, and (f) any perceived problems with foot mobility. To obtain such data, the nurse asks the client the questions provided in the accompanying Assessment Interview.

Physical Assessment

Inspect each foot and toe for shape, size, and presence of lesions and palpate to assess areas of tenderness, edema, and circulatory status. Normally, the toes are straight and flat. Table 33.5 lists physical assessment methods for the feet. Common foot problems include calluses, corns, unpleasant odors, plantar warts, fissures between the toes, fungal infections such as athlete's foot, and ingrown toenails.

A **callus** is a thickened portion of epidermis, a mass of keratotic material. Most calluses are painless and flat and are found on the bottom or side of the foot over a bony

TABLE 33.5 Assessment of the Feet

Method	Normal Findings	Deviations from Normal
Inspect all skin surfaces, particularly between the toes, for cleanliness, odor, dryness, inflammation, swelling, abrasions, or other lesions.	Intact skin Absence of swelling or inflammation	Excessive dryness Areas of inflammation or swelling (e.g., corns, calluses) Fissures Scaling and cracking of skin (e.g., athlete's foot) Plantar warts
Palpate anterior and posterior surfaces of ankles and feet for edema.	No swelling	Swelling or pitting edema
Palpate dorsalis pedis pulse on dorsal surface of foot.	Strong, regular pulses in both feet	Weak or absent pulses
Compare skin temperature of both feet.	Warm skin temperature	Cool skin temperature in one or both feet

ASSESSMENT INTERVIEW Foot Hygiene

FOOT CARE PRACTICES
- How often do you wash your feet and cut your toenails?
- What hygiene products do you usually use on your feet (e.g., soap, foot powder or deodorant, lotion, or cream)?
- What type of shoes and socks do you wear?
- How often do you put on clean socks?
- Do you ever go barefoot? If so, when, where, and how often?

SELF-CARE ABILITIES
- Do you have any problems managing your foot care? If so, what are these?
- How can the nurses best help you?

FOOT PROBLEMS AND RISK FACTORS
- Do you have any problems with foot odor?
- Do you have any foot discomfort? If so, where? When does this occur? What do you do to relieve the discomfort? Does this discomfort affect how you walk?
- Have you noticed any problems with foot mobility (e.g., joint stiffness)?
- Do you have diabetes, any circulatory problems with feet (e.g., swelling, changes in skin color, arthritis), or any instances of prolonged exposure to chemicals or water?

prominence. Calluses are usually caused by pressure from shoes. They can be softened by soaking the foot in warm water with Epsom salts, and abraded with pumice stones or similar abrasives. Creams with lanolin help to keep the skin soft and prevent the formation of calluses.

A **corn** is a keratosis caused by friction and pressure from a shoe. It commonly occurs on the fourth or fifth toe, usually on a bony prominence such as a joint. Corns are usually circular and raised. The base is the surface of the corn and the apex is in deeper tissues, sometimes even attached to bone. Corns are generally removed surgically. They are prevented from re-forming by relieving the pressure on the area (i.e., wearing comfortable shoes) and by massaging the tissue to promote circulation. The use of oval corn pads should be avoided because they increase pressure and decrease circulation.

Unpleasant odors occur as a result of perspiration and its interaction with microorganisms. Regular and frequent washing of the feet and wearing clean hosiery help to minimize odor. Foot powders and deodorants also help to prevent this problem.

Plantar warts appear on the sole of the foot. These warts are caused by the papovavirus hominis virus. They are moderately contagious. The warts are frequently painful and often make walking difficult. The primary care provider may curettage the warts, freeze them with solid carbon dioxide several times, or apply salicylic acid.

Fissures, or deep grooves, frequently occur between the toes as a result of dryness and cracking of the skin. The treatment of choice is good foot hygiene and application of an antiseptic to prevent infection. Often a small piece of gauze is inserted between the toes in applying the antiseptic and left in place to assist healing by allowing air to reach the area.

Clinical Alert!

Clients with diabetes often have extremely dry skin. Tell them to use a nonperfumed lotion and to avoid putting lotion between the toes. Advise to not soak their feet in water because it is drying to the skin.

Athlete's foot, or **tinea pedis** (ringworm of the foot), is caused by a fungus. The symptoms are scaling and cracking of the skin, particularly between the toes. Sometimes small blisters form, containing a thin fluid. In severe cases, the lesions may also appear on other parts of the body, particularly the hands. Treatments usually involve the application of commercial antifungal ointments or powders. Prevention is important. Common preventive measures are keeping the feet well ventilated, drying the feet well after bathing, wearing clean socks or stockings, and not going barefoot in public showers.

An **ingrown toenail**, the growing inward of the nail into the soft tissues around it, most often results from improper nail trimming. Pressure applied to the area causes localized pain. Treatment involves frequent, hot antiseptic soaks and surgical removal of the portion of nail embedded in the skin. Preventing recurrence involves appropriate instruction and adherence to proper nail-trimming techniques.

Identifying Clients at Risk

Because of reduced peripheral circulation to the feet, clients with diabetes or peripheral vascular disease or on long-term steroid therapy are particularly prone to infection if skin breakage occurs. Many foot problems can be prevented by teaching the client simple foot care guidelines (see Client Teaching).

Diagnosing

A number of nursing diagnoses may apply to clients with foot or foot care problems. Following are examples of common nursing diagnoses, along with possible related or contributing factors:

- Altered self-care (foot care) related to:
  a. Visual impairment
  b. Impaired hand coordination.
- Potential for infection related to:
  a. Altered skin integrity (ingrown toenail, corn, trauma)
  b. Insufficient nail or foot care.

CLIENT TEACHING **Foot Care**

- Wash the feet daily, and dry them well, especially between the toes.
- When washing, inspect the skin of the feet for breaks or red or swollen areas. Use a mirror if needed to visualize all areas.
- To prevent burns, check the water temperature before immersing the feet.
- Cover the feet, except between the toes, with creams or lotions to moisten the skin. Lotion will also soften calluses. A lotion that reduces dryness effectively is a mixture of lanolin and mineral oil.
- To prevent or control an unpleasant odor due to excessive foot perspiration, wash the feet frequently and change socks and shoes at least daily. Special deodorant sprays or absorbent foot powders are also helpful.
- File the toenails rather than cutting them to avoid skin injury. File the nails straight across the ends of the toes. If the nails are too thick or misshapen to file, consult a podiatrist.
- Wear clean stockings or socks daily. Avoid socks with holes that can cause pressure areas.
- Wear comfortable, well-fitting shoes that neither restrict the foot nor rub on any area; rubbing can cause corns and calluses. Check worn shoes for rough spots in the lining. Break in new shoes gradually by increasing the wearing time 30 to 60 minutes each day.
- Avoid walking barefoot, because injury and infection may result. Wear slippers in public showers and in change areas to avoid contracting athlete's foot or other infections.
- Several times each day exercise the feet to promote circulation. Point the feet upward, point them downward, and move them in circles.
- Avoid wearing constricting garments such as knee-high elastic stockings and avoid sitting with the legs crossed at the knees, which may decrease circulation.
- When the feet are cold, use extra blankets and wear warm socks rather than using heating pads or hot water bottles, which may cause burns. Test bathwater before stepping into it.
- Wash any cut on the foot thoroughly, apply a mild antiseptic, and notify the primary care provider.
- Avoid self-treatment for corns or calluses. Pumice stones and some callus and corn applications are injurious to the skin. Do not cut calluses or corns. Consult a podiatrist or the primary care provider first.
- Notify the primary care provider if you notice abnormal sores or drainage, pain, or changes in temperature, color, and sensation of the foot.

Planning

Planning involves (a) identifying nursing interventions that will help the client maintain or restore healthy foot care practices and (b) establishing desired outcomes for each client. Interventions may include teaching the client about correct nail and foot care, proper footwear, wearing the correct size, and ways to prevent potential foot problems (e.g., infection, injury, and decreased circulation). For clients with self-care difficulties, the nurse plans a schedule for soaking the client's feet and assisting with regular cleaning and trimming of nails (if not contraindicated). Foot and nail care are often provided during the client's bath but may be provided at any time of the day to accommodate the client's preference or schedule. The frequency of foot care is determined by the nurse and client and is based on objective assessment data and the client's specific problems. For some clients, the feet need to be bathed daily; for those whose feet perspire excessively, bathing more than once a day may be necessary.

Implementing

Skill 33.3 describes how to provide foot care. See also the next section's discussion of nails. During these procedures, the nurse has the opportunity to teach the client appropriate methods for foot care, including those designed to prevent tissue injury and infection (see Client Teaching feature on foot care).

Providing Foot Care

SKILL 33.3

PURPOSES

- To maintain the skin integrity of the feet
- To prevent foot infections
- To prevent foot odors
- To assess or monitor foot problems

ASSESSMENT

Determine

- History of any problems with foot discomfort, foot odor, foot mobility, circulatory problems (e.g., swelling, changes in skin color or temperature, and pain), structural problems (e.g., bunion, hammer toe, or overlapping digits)
- Usual foot care practices (e.g., frequency of washing feet and cutting nails, foot hygiene products used, how often socks are changed, whether the client ever goes barefoot, whether the client sees a podiatrist)

Assess

- Skin surfaces for cleanliness, odor, dryness, and intactness
- Each foot and toe for shape, size, presence of lesions (e.g., corn, callus, wart, or rash), and areas of tenderness; ankle edema
- Heels for erythema, blisters, or breaks in skin integrity
- Skin temperatures of both feet to assess circulatory status:
  - Pedal pulses: dorsalis pedis and posterior tibialis
  - Feet of bedbound clients for foot drop
- Self-care abilities (e.g., any problems managing foot care)

Continued on page 774

SKILL 33.3

Providing Foot Care—*continued*

PLANNING

Assignment

Foot care for the nondiabetic client can be assigned to AP. Remind the AP to notify the nurse of anything that looks out of the ordinary. Review with the AP the agency policy about cutting or trimming nails.

Equipment

- Washbasin containing warm water
- Pillow
- Moisture-resistant disposable pad
- Towels
- Soap
- Washcloth
- Toenail cleaning and trimming equipment, if agency policy permits
- Lotion or foot powder

IMPLEMENTATION

Preparation

Assemble all the necessary equipment and supplies if nails need trimming and agency policy permits.

Performance

1. Prior to performing the procedure, introduce self and verify the client's identity using agency protocol. Explain to the client what you are going to do, why it is necessary, and how to participate.
2. Perform hand hygiene and observe other appropriate infection prevention procedures.
3. Provide for client privacy by drawing the curtains around the bed or closing the door to the room. Some agencies provide signs indicating the need for privacy. **Rationale:** *Hygiene is a personal matter*.
4. Prepare the equipment and the client.
   - Fill the washbasin with warm water at about 40°C to 43°C (105°F to 110°F). **Rationale:** *Warm water promotes circulation, provides comfort, and refreshes*.
   - Assist the ambulatory client to a sitting position in a chair, or the bed client to a supine or semi-Fowler's position.
   - Place a pillow under the bed client's knees. **Rationale:** *This provides support and prevents muscle fatigue*.
   - Place the washbasin on the moisture-resistant pad at the foot of the bed for a bed client or on the floor in front of the chair for an ambulatory client. For a bed client, pad the rim of the washbasin with a towel. **Rationale:** *The towel prevents undue pressure on the skin*.
5. Wash the foot and soak it.
   - Place one of the client's feet in the basin and wash it with soap, paying particular attention to the interdigital areas. Prolonged soaking is generally not recommended for clients with diabetes or individuals with peripheral vascular disease. **Rationale:** *Prolonged soaking may remove natural skin oils, thus drying the skin and making it more susceptible to cracking and injury*.
   - Rinse the foot well to remove soap. **Rationale:** *Soap irritates the skin if not completely removed*.
   - Rub callused areas of the foot with the washcloth. **Rationale:** *This helps remove dead skin layers*.
   - If the nails are brittle or thick and require trimming, replace the water and allow the foot to soak for 10 to 20 minutes. **Rationale:** *Soaking softens the nails and loosens debris under them*.
   - Clean the nails as required with an orange stick, if agency policy permits. **Rationale:** *This removes excess debris that harbors microorganisms*. Use gently, especially with clients who are at risk for injury (e.g., clients with diabetes or peripheral vascular disease).
   - Remove the foot from the basin and place it on the towel.
6. Dry the foot thoroughly and apply lotion or foot powder.
   - Blot the foot gently with the towel to dry it thoroughly, particularly between the toes. **Rationale:** *Harsh rubbing can damage the skin. Thorough drying reduces the risk of infection*.
   - Apply lotion or lanolin cream to the foot but not between the toes. **Rationale:** *This lubricates dry skin and keeps the area between the toes dry*.

     or
   - Apply a foot powder containing a nonirritating deodorant if the feet tend to perspire excessively. **Rationale:** *Foot powders have greater absorbent properties than regular bath powders; some also contain menthol, which makes the feet feel cool*.
7. If agency policy permits, trim the nails of the first foot while the second foot is soaking.
   - See the discussion on nails for the appropriate method to trim nails. Note that in many agencies toenail trimming requires a primary care provider's order or is contraindicated for clients with diabetes mellitus, toe infections, and peripheral vascular disease, unless performed by a podiatrist, general practice physician, or advanced practice provider such as a nurse practitioner.
8. Document any foot problems observed.
   - Foot care is not generally recorded unless problems are noted.
   - Record any signs of inflammation, infection, breaks in the skin, corns, troublesome calluses, bunions, and pressure areas. This is of particular importance for clients with peripheral vascular disease and diabetes.

EVALUATION

- Inspect nails and skin after the soak.
- Compare to prior assessment data.
- Report any abnormalities to the primary care provider.

Evaluating

Examples of desired outcomes for foot hygiene include the client being able to:

- Participate in self-care (foot hygiene) to optimal level of capacity (specify).
- Describe hygienic and other interventions (e.g., proper footwear) to maintain skin integrity, prevent infection, and maintain peripheral tissue perfusion.
- Demonstrate optimal foot hygiene, as evidenced by:
  a. Intact, pink, smooth, soft, hydrated, and warm skin
  b. Intact cuticles and skin surrounding nails
  c. Correct foot care and nail care practices.

Nails

Nails are normally present at birth. They continue to grow throughout life and change very little until people are older. At that time, the nails tend to be tougher, more brittle, and in some cases thicker. The nails of an older adult normally grow less quickly than those of a younger individual and may be ridged and grooved.

●○● NURSING MANAGEMENT

Assessing

During the nursing health history, the nurse explores the client's usual nail care practices, self-care abilities, and any problems associated with them (see accompanying Assessment Interview). Physical assessment involves inspection of the nails (e.g., nail shape and texture, nail bed color, and tissues surrounding the nails). See Chapter 29 ∞.

Diagnosing

Nursing diagnoses related to nail care and nail problems include altered self-care and potential for infection. Examples of these nursing diagnoses and contributing factors follow:

- Altered self-care (nail care) related to:
  a. Impaired vision
  b. Cognitive impairment.
- Potential for infection around the nail bed related to:
  a. Impaired skin integrity of cuticles
  b. Altered peripheral circulation.

Planning

The nurse identifies measures that will assist the client to develop or maintain healthy nail care practices. A schedule of nail care needs to be established.

Implementing

To provide nail care, the nurse needs a nail clipper, a nail file, an orange stick to push back the cuticle, hand lotion or mineral oil to lubricate any dry tissue around the nails, and a basin of water to soak the nails if they are particularly thick or hard. Check the agency's policy regarding nail care. Often, podiatrists must be consulted for clients with diabetes, peripheral vascular disease, long-term steroid therapy, and anticoagulant therapy.

One hand or foot is soaked, if needed, and dried; then the nail is cut or filed straight across beyond the end of the finger or toe (Figure 33.4 ■). Avoid trimming or digging into nails at the lateral corners. This predisposes the client to ingrown toenails. Clients who have diabetes or circulatory problems should have their nails filed rather than cut; inadvertent injury to tissues can occur if scissors are used. After the initial cut or filing, the nail is filed to round the corners, and the nurse cleans under the nail. The nurse then gently pushes back the cuticle, taking care not to injure it. The next finger or toe is cared for in the same manner. Any abnormalities, such as an infected cuticle or inflammation of the tissue around the nail, are recorded and reported.

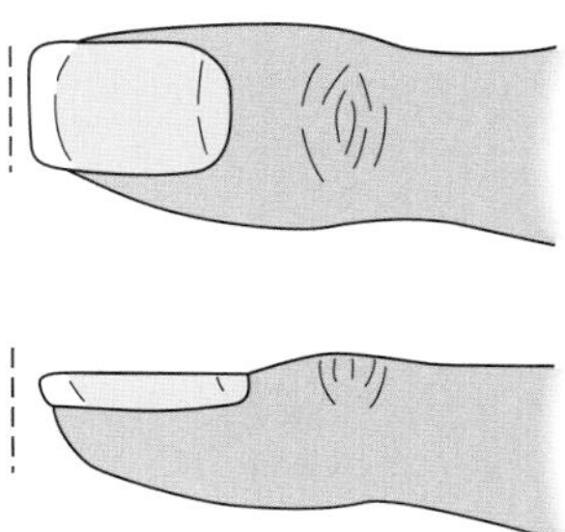

Figure 33.4 ■ Fingernails are trimmed straight across.

Evaluating

Examples of desired outcomes for nail hygiene include the client being able to:

- Demonstrate healthy nail care practices, as shown by:
  a. Clean, short nails with smooth edges
  b. Intact cuticles and hydrated surrounding skin.
- Describe factors contributing to the nail problem.
- Describe preventive interventions for the specific nail problem.
- Demonstrate nail care as instructed.

In addition, the client should have pink nail beds and quick return of nail bed color after the blanch test.

Mouth

Each tooth has three parts: the crown, the root, and the pulp cavity (Figure 33.5 ■). The crown is the exposed part of the tooth, which is outside the gum. It is covered with a hard substance called enamel. The ivory-colored internal part of the crown below the enamel is the dentin. The root of a tooth is embedded in the jaw and covered by a bony tissue called cementum. The pulp cavity in the center of the tooth contains the blood vessels and nerves.

ASSESSMENT INTERVIEW Nail Hygiene

- What are your usual nail care practices?
- Do you have any problems managing your nail care? If so, what are they?
- Have you had any problems associated with your nails (e.g., inflammation of the tissue surrounding the nail, injury, prolonged exposure to water or chemicals, circulatory problems)?

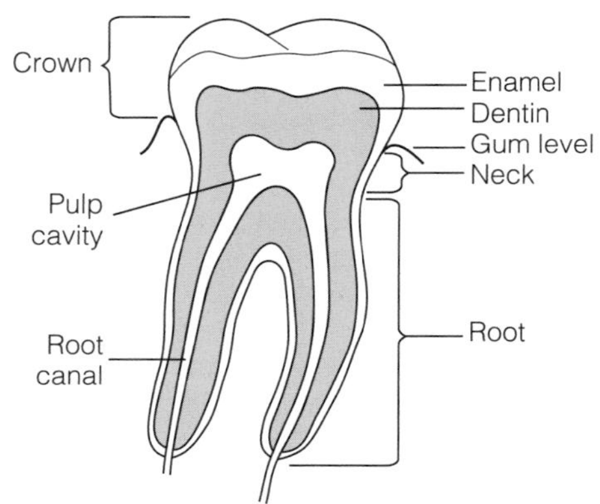

Figure 33.5 ■ The anatomic parts of a tooth.

Developmental Variations

Teeth usually appear 5 to 8 months after birth. Early childhood **caries** (cavities) occur when an infant or toddler is allowed to drink formula, milk, or fruit juice from a bottle for long periods, especially when sleeping (Ball, Bindler, Cowen, & Shaw, 2017). The carbohydrates in the solution cause demineralization of the tooth enamel, which leads to tooth decay. If the child wants a bottle at bedtime, it should contain only water.

By the time children are 2 years old, they usually have all 20 of their temporary teeth. At about age 6 or 7, children start losing their deciduous teeth, and these are gradually replaced by the 33 permanent teeth. By age 25, most people have all of their permanent teeth.

The incidence of periodontal disease increases during pregnancy because the rise in female hormones affects gingival tissue and increases its reaction to bacterial plaque. Many pregnant women experience more bleeding from the gingival sulcus during brushing and increased redness and swelling of the **gingiva** (the gum).

Teeth turn yellowish in color as a part of the aging process. Teeth are normally off-white and with age, the enamel thins and the yellow-gray color of the inner portion of the teeth begins to show. In addition, coffee drinking and cigarette smoking can stain the teeth. Commercial teeth-whitening products and treatments offered at dental offices are available to consumers who desire whiter teeth for cosmetic reasons.

Lack of fluoridated water and preventive dentistry during their developmental years have caused tooth and gum problems in older adults. As a result, some older adults may have few permanent teeth left, and some have dentures. Loss of teeth occurs mainly because of **periodontal disease** (gum disease) rather than dental caries; however, caries are also common in middle-aged adults.

Some receding of the gums and a brownish pigmentation of the gums occur with age. Because saliva production decreases with age, dryness of the oral mucosa is a common finding in older people.

●○● NURSING MANAGEMENT

Assessing

Assessment of the client's mouth and hygiene practices includes (a) a nursing health history, (b) physical assessment of the mouth, and (c) identification of clients at risk for developing oral problems.

Nursing History

During the nursing health history, the nurse obtains data about the client's oral hygiene practices, including dental visits, self-care abilities, and past or current mouth problems. Data about the client's oral hygiene help the nurse determine learning needs and incorporate the client's needs and preferences in the plan of care. Assessment of the client's self-care abilities determines the amount and type of nursing assistance to provide. Clients whose hand coordination is impaired, whose cognitive function is impaired, whose illness alters energy levels and motivation, or whose therapy imposes restrictions on activities will need assistance from the nurse. Information about past or current problems alerts the nurse to specific interventions required or referrals that may be necessary. Questions to elicit this information are shown in the accompanying Assessment Interview.

Physical Assessment

For information about mouth assessment, see Chapter 29 ∞. Dental caries and periodontal disease are the two problems that most frequently affect the teeth. Both problems are commonly associated with plaque and tartar deposits. **Plaque** is an invisible soft film that adheres to the enamel surface of teeth; it consists of bacteria, molecules of saliva, and remnants of epithelial cells and leukocytes. When

ASSESSMENT INTERVIEW **Oral Hygiene**

ORAL HYGIENE PRACTICES

- What are your usual mouth care or denture care practices?
- What oral hygiene products do you routinely use (e.g., mouthwash, type of toothpaste, dental floss, denture cleaner)?
- Do you have any loose or sensitive teeth?
- Do you experience bleeding after brushing or flossing your teeth?
- When was your last dental examination, and how often do you see your dentist?

SELF-CARE ABILITIES

- Do you have any problems managing your mouth care?

PAST OR CURRENT MOUTH PROBLEMS

- Have you had or do you have any problems such as bleeding, swollen, or reddened gums, ulcerations, lumps, or tooth pain?
- Have your eating patterns changed due to mouth pain or discomfort with chewing?

plaque is unchecked, tartar (dental calculus) is formed. **Tartar** is a visible, hard deposit of plaque and dead bacteria that forms at the gum lines. Tartar buildup can alter the fibers that attach the teeth to the gum and eventually disrupt bone tissue. Periodontal disease is characterized by **gingivitis** (red, swollen gingiva), bleeding, receding gum lines, and the formation of pockets between the teeth and gums. In advanced periodontal disease (**pyorrhea**), the teeth are loose and pus is evident when the gums are pressed. Table 33.6 lists additional problems of the mouth.

Identifying Clients at Risk

Certain clients are prone to oral problems because of an inability to maintain oral hygiene. Among these are clients who are older, seriously ill, confused, comatose, depressed, or dehydrated. Effective oral hygiene requires fine motor skills, adequate vision, and motivation. Poor oral health is a common problem among older adults in general. It can be more of a problem for an older adult who has cognitive, visual, or physical impairments (Lee, Plassman, Pan, & Wu, 2016, p. 30). Critically ill clients can experience complications that may lead to ventilator-associated pneumonia, a longer hospital stay, increased cost of care, and even death if oral assessment and care are not properly performed (Robinson, Hoze, Hevener, & Nichols, 2018). A number of research studies have shown an association between pathogenic oral bacteria and the incidence of aspiration pneumonia in clients following a stroke. Furthermore, research has shown reduced respiratory infections in cardiac surgery clients who rinsed with chlorhexidine before intubation and continued to receive it postoperatively ("Oral Care," 2017). In addition, people with nasogastric tubes or who are receiving oxygen are likely to develop dry oral mucous membranes, especially if they breathe through their mouths. Clients who have had oral or jaw surgery must have meticulous oral hygiene care to prevent the development of infections.

Clinical Alert!

Clients in long-term care settings are at high risk for oral health problems. The nurse must assess the client's oral health and teach the AP about the importance of and methods for promoting oral hygiene.

Healthy-appearing individuals, too, may be at risk. High-risk variables such as lack of knowledge, inadequate nutrition, lack of money or insurance for dental care, excessive intake of refined sugars, and family history of periodontal disease also need to be identified. Some older adults may also be at risk, for example, those who choose salty and enamel-eroding sugary foods because of a decline in their number of taste buds. The decreased saliva production in older adults, which produces a dry mouth and thinning of the oral mucosa, is another factor.

Poor fluid intake, heavy smoking, alcohol use, high salt intake, anxiety, and many medications can worsen a dry mouth. Medications that can cause dryness of the mouth include diuretics; laxatives, if used excessively; and tranquilizers, such as diazepam (Valium). Some chemotherapeutic agents used to treat cancer also cause oral dryness and mucositis (inflammation of mucous membranes). A common side effect of the anticonvulsant drug phenytoin (Dilantin) is gingival hyperplasia. Optimal oral hygiene (e.g., brushing with a soft-bristle toothbrush and flossing) is needed.

Clients who are receiving or have received radiation treatments to the head and neck may have permanent damage to salivary glands. This results in a very dry mouth and can often be treated by providing a thick liquid called *artificial saliva*. Some clients prefer to just sip on liquids to moisten their mouth. Radiation can also cause damage to teeth and the jaw structure, with actual damage occurring years after the radiation.

TABLE 33.6 Common Problems of the Mouth

Problem	Description	Nursing Implications
Halitosis	Bad breath	Teach or provide regular oral hygiene.
Glossitis	Inflammation of the tongue	As above
Gingivitis	Inflammation of the gums	As above
Periodontal disease	Gums appear spongy and bleeding	As above
Reddened or excoriated mucosa		Check for ill-fitting dentures.
Excessive dryness of the buccal mucosa		Increase fluid intake as health permits.
Cheilosis	Cracking of lips	Lubricate lips; use antimicrobial ointment to prevent infection.
Dental caries	Teeth have darkened areas; may be painful	Advise client to see a dentist.
Sordes	Accumulation of foul matter (food, microorganisms, and epithelial elements) in the mouth	Teach or provide regular cleaning.
Stomatitis	Inflammation of the oral mucosa	Teach or provide regular cleaning.
Parotitis	Inflammation of the parotid salivary glands	Teach or provide regular oral hygiene.

Diagnosing

Two nursing diagnoses related to problems with oral hygiene and the oral cavity are altered oral mucous membranes and lack of knowledge. Signs and symptoms of altered oral mucous membranes can include a coated tongue; dry mouth (**xerostomia**); halitosis; gingival hyperplasia, difficulty eating, and oral pain or discomfort; and oral lesions or ulcers. These may be the result of inadequate oral hygiene, physical injury or drying effect (e.g., mouth breathing, oxygen therapy, decreased salivation, temperature extreme, NPO), mechanical factor (e.g., surgery, broken teeth or ill-fitting dentures), autoimmune disease, or infection. The diagnosis of lack of knowledge is discussed in Chapter 17 ∞.

Planning

In planning care, the nurse and, if appropriate, the client and family set outcomes for each nursing diagnosis. The nurse then performs nursing interventions and activities to achieve the client outcomes.

During the planning phase, the nurse also identifies interventions that will help the client achieve these goals. Specific, detailed nursing activities performed by the nurse may include the following:

- Monitor every shift for dryness of the oral mucosa.
- Monitor for signs and symptoms of glossitis (inflammation of the tongue) and stomatitis (inflammation of the mouth).
- Assist dependent clients with oral care.
- Provide special oral hygiene for clients who are debilitated, are unconscious, or have lesions of the mucous membranes or other oral tissues.
- Teach clients about good oral hygiene practices and other measures to prevent tooth decay.
- Reinforce the oral hygiene regimen as part of discharge teaching.

Implementing

Providing oral hygiene is an independent nursing function; yet, research has shown that oral hygiene is one of the most overlooked aspects of basic nursing care. Moreover, the oral care provided by nurses is often inadequate. Barriers to providing effective oral care include the low priority placed on oral care by primary care providers and nurses, many of whom treat it as a "comfort" measure rather than a reduction of bacteria that can cause disease; inadequate knowledge of how to assess and provide effective oral care; lack of appropriate supplies (e.g., suction toothbrush for dependent clients); and insufficient time (Sheffler, 2018). Studies have shown that when oral care is part of a written protocol, nurses document oral care consistently.

Good oral hygiene includes daily stimulation of the gums, mechanical brushing and flossing of the teeth, and rinsing of the mouth. Brushing and rinsing stimulates salivary flow and removes harmful bacteria. The nurse is often in a position to help clients maintain oral hygiene by helping or teaching them to clean the teeth and oral cavity, by inspecting whether clients (especially children) have done so, or by actually providing mouth care to clients who are ill or incapacitated. The nurse can also be helpful in identifying problems that require the intervention of a dentist or oral surgeon and arranging a referral.

Promoting Oral Health Throughout the Lifespan

A major role of the nurse in promoting oral health is to teach clients about specific oral hygienic measures.

Infants and Toddlers

Most dentists recommend that dental hygiene should begin when the first tooth erupts and be practiced after each feeding. Cleaning can be accomplished by using a wet washcloth or small gauze moistened with water.

Dental caries occur frequently during the toddler period, often as a result of the excessive intake of sweets or a prolonged use of the bottle during naps and at bedtime. The nurse should give parents the following instructions to promote and maintain dental health:

- Beginning at about 18 months of age, brush the child's teeth with a soft toothbrush. Use only a toothbrush moistened with water at first and introduce toothpaste later. Use one that contains fluoride.
- Give a fluoride supplement daily or as recommended by the primary care provider or dentist, unless the drinking water is fluoridated.
- Schedule an initial dental visit for the child at about 2 or 3 years of age, as soon as all 20 primary teeth have erupted.
- Some dentists recommend an inspection type of visit when the child is about 18 months old to provide an early pleasant introduction to the dental examination.
- Seek professional dental attention for any problems such as discoloring of the teeth, chipping, or signs of infection such as redness and swelling.

Preschoolers and School-Age Children

Because deciduous teeth guide the entrance of permanent teeth, dental care is important to keep these teeth in good repair. Abnormally placed or lost deciduous teeth can cause misalignment of permanent teeth. Fluoride remains important at this stage to prevent dental caries. Preschoolers need to be taught to brush their teeth after eating and to limit their intake of refined sugars. Parental supervision may be needed to ensure the completion of these self-care activities. Regular dental checkups are required during these years when permanent teeth appear.

Adolescents and Adults

Proper diet and tooth and mouth care should be evaluated and reinforced in adolescents and adults. Oral piercings have become increasingly popular among adolescents and adults. School nurses may be the first and perhaps the only source of information about body piercing for children and adolescents (Desai, 2018). Specific measures to prevent tooth decay and periodontal disease are listed in Client Teaching.

CLIENT TEACHING Measures to Prevent Tooth Decay

- Brush the teeth thoroughly after meals and at bedtime. Assist children or inspect their mouths to be sure the teeth are clean. If the teeth cannot be brushed after meals, vigorous rinsing of the mouth with water is recommended.
- Floss the teeth daily.
- Ensure an adequate intake of nutrients, particularly calcium; phosphorus; vitamins A, C, and D; and fluoride.
- Avoid sweet foods and drinks between meals. Take them in moderation at meals.
- Eat coarse, fibrous foods (cleansing foods), such as fresh fruits and raw vegetables.
- Have topical fluoride applications as prescribed by the dentist.
- Have a checkup by a dentist every 6 months.

Older Adults

The rate of edentulism (lack of teeth) among older adults continues to decline (Humphreys, 2016). As a result, older clients are at risk for dental cavities and periodontal disease. Older adults who have self-care deficits are at an increased risk because they cannot maintain their oral hygiene practices or may not be able to visit the dentist on a routine basis. Furthermore, those who suffer the worst oral health and hygiene include older adults residing in nursing homes and older adults with dementia. Poor oral hygiene among frail and dependent nursing home residents can place them at risk for serious illness such as pneumonia.

Along with the increasing evidence that poor oral health is a serious problem among older clients is the lack of effective oral care by health caregivers. Examples of interventions that can improve the oral health of residents in long-term care settings include consistent oral assessment by the nurses, instruction of AP on how to deliver effective oral care, providing sufficient oral hygiene supplies, and expectations of the administration that oral care should receive the same priority as other kinds of care. Nurses have an important role in promoting optimal geriatric oral health care.

Brushing and Flossing the Teeth

Thorough brushing of the teeth is important in preventing tooth decay. The mechanical action of brushing removes food particles that can harbor and incubate bacteria. It also stimulates circulation in the gums, thus maintaining their healthy firmness. One of the techniques recommended for brushing teeth is called the sulcular technique, which removes plaque and cleans under the gingival margins. Many toothpastes are marketed. Fluoride toothpaste is often recommended because of its antibacterial protection.

Caring for Artificial Dentures

Some clients have artificial teeth in the form of a plate—a complete set of teeth for one jaw. They may have a lower plate or an upper plate or both. When only a few artificial teeth are needed, the client may have a bridge rather than a plate. A bridge may be fixed or removable. Artificial teeth are fitted to the individual and usually will not fit another individual.

Clients who wear dentures or other types of oral prostheses should be encouraged to use them. Ill-fitting dentures or other oral prostheses can cause discomfort and chewing difficulties, and can contribute to oral problems as well as poor nutrition and enjoyment of food. Those who do not wear their prostheses are prone to shrinkage of the gums, which results in further tooth loss.

Like natural teeth, artificial dentures collect microorganisms and food. They need to be cleaned regularly, at least once a day. They can be removed from the mouth, scrubbed with a toothbrush, rinsed, and reinserted. Some people use a dentifrice (toothpaste) for cleaning teeth, and others use commercial cleaning compounds for dentures.

Assisting Clients with Oral Care

When providing oral care for partially or totally dependent clients, the nurse should wear gloves to guard against infections. Other required equipment includes a curved basin that fits snugly under the client's chin (e.g., a kidney basin) to receive the rinse water and a towel to protect the client and the bedclothes. See Skill 33.4.

Foam swabs are often used in healthcare agencies to clean the mouths of dependent clients (Figure 33.6 ■). These swabs are convenient and effective in removing excess debris from the teeth and mouth, but are *not* effective for removal of plaque and biofilm that hold pathogenic microorganisms. In fact, in one study that informed nurses on the benefits of tooth-brushing over the use of foam swabs it resulted in a 50% reduction in ventilator-acquired pneumonia rates (Sheffler, 2018).

Most people prefer privacy when they remove their artificial teeth to clean them. Many do not like to be seen without their teeth; one of the first requests of many postoperative clients is "May I have my teeth in, please?" The Variation section in Skill 33.4 describes how to clean artificial dentures. Special care should be taken so as not to lose the client's dentures.

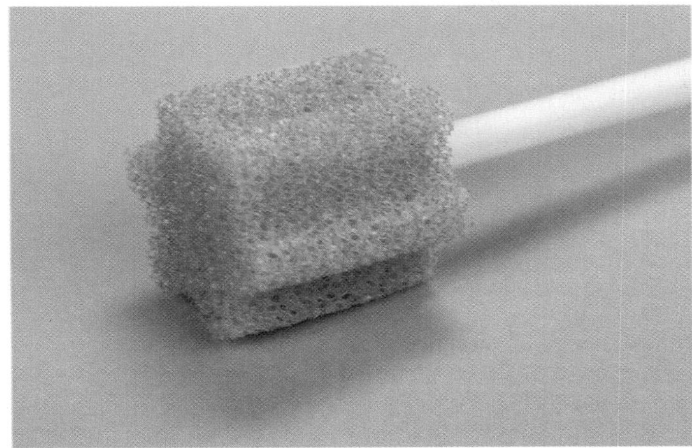

Figure 33.6 ■ Example of a foam swab used to clean the mouth of a dependent client.

SKILL 33.4

Brushing and Flossing the Teeth

PURPOSES

- To remove food particles from around and between the teeth
- To remove dental plaque
- To promote the client's feelings of well-being
- To prevent sores and infection of the oral tissues
- To prevent oral pathogenic microorganisms traveling to the lungs

ASSESSMENT

- Determine the extent of the client's self-care abilities.
- Assess the client's usual mouth care practices.
- Inspect lips, gums, oral mucosa, and tongue for deviations from normal.
- Identify presence of oral problems such as tooth caries, halitosis, gingivitis, and loose or broken teeth.
- Check if the client has bridgework or wears dentures. If the client has dentures, ask if any tenderness or soreness is present and, if so, the location of the area(s) for ongoing assessment.
- Assess safety concerns (e.g., if client requires thickened liquids, this needs to be carried out for the rinse water for oral care).
- Some clients may have oral piercings. Ask the client what hygienic measures are needed for the care of the piercings.

PLANNING

Assignment

Oral care, including brushing and flossing of teeth and denture care, can be assigned to AP. After performing the above assessment, the nurse should instruct the AP as to the type of oral care and amount of assistance needed by the client. Remind the AP to report changes in the client's oral mucosa.

Equipment

Brushing and Flossing

- Towel
- Clean gloves
- Curved basin (emesis basin)
- Toothbrush (soft bristle)
- Cup of tepid water
- Dentifrice (toothpaste)
- Mouthwash
- Dental floss, at least two pieces 20 cm (8 in.) in length
- Floss holder (optional)

Cleaning Artificial Dentures

- Clean gloves
- Tissue or piece of gauze
- Denture container
- Clean washcloth
- Toothbrush or stiff-bristled brush
- Dentifrice or denture cleaner
- Tepid water
- Container of mouthwash
- Curved basin (emesis basin)
- Towel

IMPLEMENTATION

Preparation

Assemble all the necessary equipment.

Performance

1. Prior to performing the procedure, introduce self and verify the client's identity using agency protocol. Explain to the client what you are going to do, why it is necessary, and how to participate.
2. Perform hand hygiene and observe other appropriate infection prevention procedures. **Rationale:** *Wearing gloves while providing mouth care prevents the nurse from acquiring infections. Gloves also prevent transmission of microorganisms to the client.*
3. Provide for client privacy by drawing the curtains around the bed or closing the door to the room. Some agencies provide signs indicating the need for privacy. **Rationale:** *Hygiene is a personal matter.*
4. Prepare the client.
   - Assist the client to a sitting position in bed, if health permits. If not, assist the client to a side-lying position with the head turned. **Rationale:** *This position prevents liquid from draining down the client's throat.*
5. Prepare the equipment.
   - Place the towel under the client's chin.
   - Apply clean gloves.
   - Use a soft-bristle toothbrush (a small one for a child) and the client's choice of dentifrice.
   - Moisten the bristles of the toothbrush with tepid water and apply the dentifrice to the toothbrush.
   - For the client who must remain in bed, place or hold the curved basin under the client's chin, fitting the small curve around the chin or neck.
   - Inspect the mouth and teeth.
6. Brush the teeth.
   - Hand the toothbrush to the client, or brush the client's teeth as follows:
     a. Hold the brush against the teeth with the bristles at a 45° angle. The tips of the outer bristles should rest against and penetrate under the gingival sulcus. ❶ The brush will clean under the sulcus of two or three teeth at one time. **Rationale:** *This sulcular technique removes plaque and cleans under the gingival margins.*
     b. Move the bristles up and down gently in short strokes from the sulcus to the crowns of the teeth. ❷

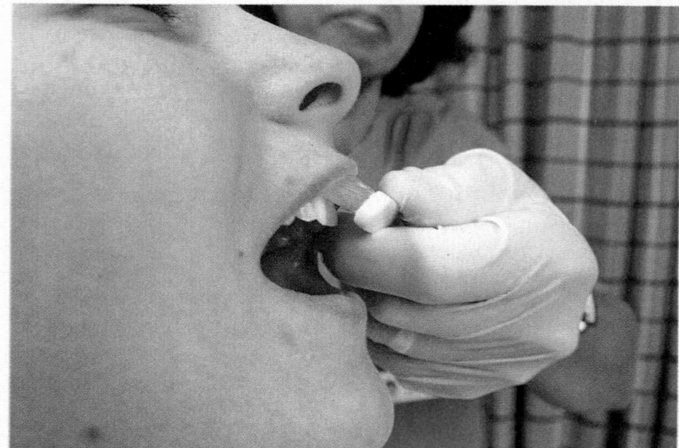

❶ The sulcular technique: Place the bristles at a 45° angle with the tips of the outer bristles under the gingival margins.

Brushing and Flossing the Teeth—*continued*

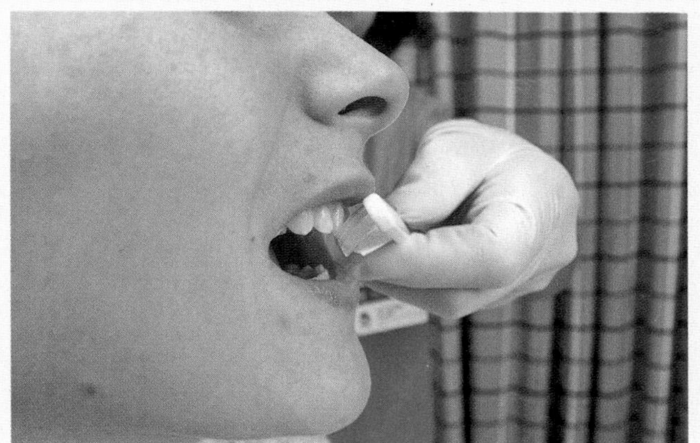

❷ Brushing from the sulcus to the crowns of the teeth.

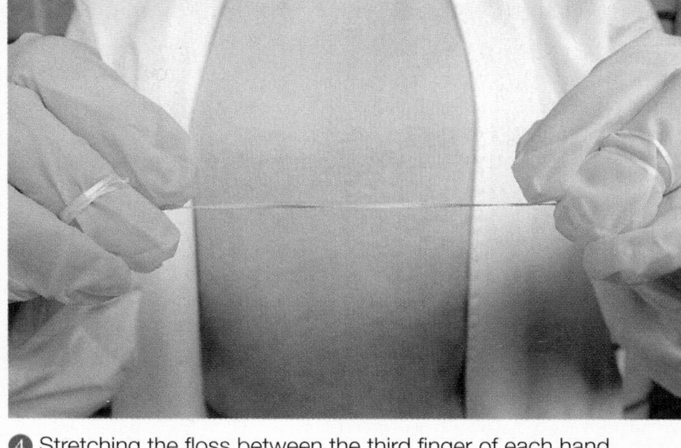

❹ Stretching the floss between the third finger of each hand.

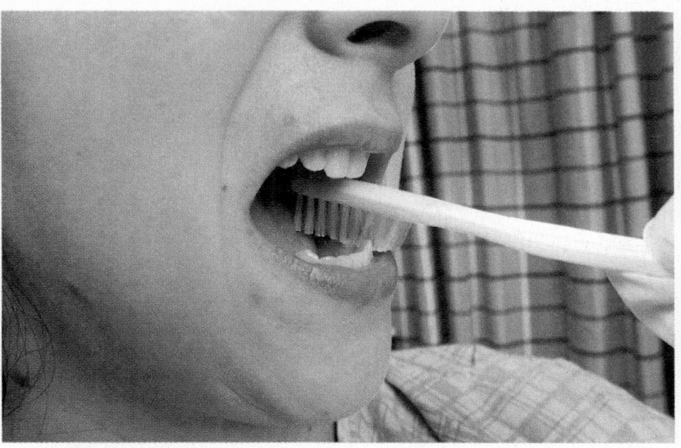

❸ Brushing the biting surfaces.

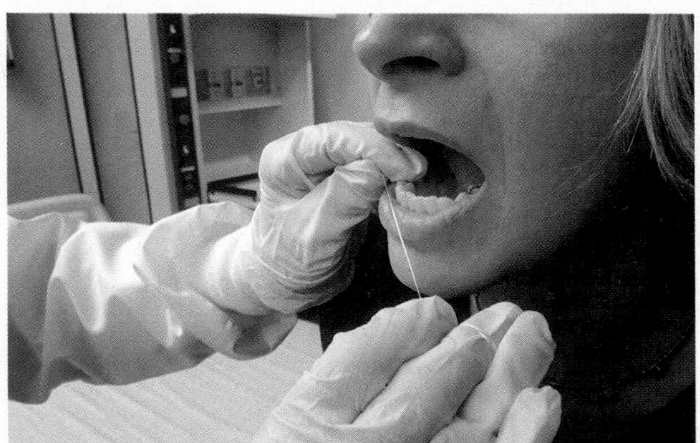

❺ Flossing the lower teeth by using the index fingers to stretch the floss.

c. Repeat until all outer and inner surfaces of the teeth and sulci of the gums have been cleaned.
d. Clean the biting surfaces by moving the brush back and forth over them in short strokes. ❸
e. Brush the tongue gently with the toothbrush. **Rationale:** *Brushing removes bacteria and freshens breath. A coated tongue may be caused by poor oral hygiene and low fluid intake. Brushing gently and carefully helps prevent gagging or vomiting*.

- Hand the client the water cup or mouthwash to rinse the mouth vigorously. Then ask the client to spit the water or mouthwash and excess dentifrice into the basin. Some agencies supply a standard mouthwash. Alternatively, a mouth rinse of normal saline can be an effective cleaner and moisturizer. **Rationale:** *Vigorous rinsing loosens and washes away food particles*.
- Repeat the preceding steps until the mouth is free of dentifrice and food particles.
- Remove the curved basin and help the client wipe the mouth.

7. Floss the teeth.

- Assist the client to floss independently, or floss the teeth of an alert and cooperative client as follows. Waxed floss is less likely to fray than unwaxed floss; however, particles between the teeth attach more readily to unwaxed floss than to waxed floss.

a. Wrap one end of the floss around the middle finger of each hand. ❹
b. To floss the upper teeth, use your thumb and index finger to stretch the floss. Move the floss up and down between the teeth. When the floss reaches the gum line, gently slide the floss into the space between the gum and the tooth. Gently move the floss away from the gum with up and down motions (American Dental Association, n.d.). Start at the back on the right side and work around to the back of the left side, or work from the center teeth to the back of the jaw on either side.
c. To floss the lower teeth, use your index fingers to stretch the floss. ❺

- Give the client tepid water or mouthwash to rinse the mouth and a curved basin in which to spit the water.
- Assist the client in wiping the mouth.

8. Remove and dispose of equipment appropriately.

- Remove and clean the curved basin.
- Remove and discard the gloves.
- Perform hand hygiene.

9. Document assessment of the teeth, tongue, gums, and oral mucosa. Include any problems such as sores or inflammation, or bleeding and swelling of the gums. Check agency protocol for documentation of brushing and flossing teeth.

Continued on page 782

SKILL 33.4

Brushing and Flossing the Teeth—*continued*

QSEN Patient-Centered Care: Home Considerations

- Assess the oral hygiene practices and attitude toward oral hygiene of family members and the client.
- Remind adults to replace their toothbrush every 3 to 4 months and a child's toothbrush more frequently.
- Clients with nasogastric tubes or who are receiving oxygen are likely to develop dry oral mucous membranes, especially if they breathe through their mouths. More frequent oral hygiene will be needed.

Variation: Artificial Dentures

1. Remove the dentures.
   - Apply gloves. **Rationale:** *Wearing gloves decreases the likelihood of spreading infection.*
   - If the client cannot remove the dentures, take a tissue or gauze, grasp the upper plate at the front teeth with your thumb and second finger, and move the denture up and down slightly. ❻ **Rationale:** *The slight movement breaks the suction that holds the plate on the roof of the mouth.*
   - Lower the upper plate, move it out of the mouth, and place it in the denture container.
   - Lift the lower plate, turning it so that the left side, for example, is slightly lower than the right, to remove the plate from the mouth without stretching the lips. Place the lower plate in the denture container.
   - Remove a partial denture by exerting equal pressure on the border of each side of the denture, not on the clasps, which can bend or break.
2. Clean the dentures.
   - Take the denture container to a sink. Take care not to drop the dentures. Place a washcloth in the bowl of the sink. **Rationale:** *This prevents damage if the dentures are dropped.*
   - Using a toothbrush or special stiff-bristled brush, scrub the dentures with the cleaning agent and tepid water.
   - Rinse the dentures with tepid running water. **Rationale:** *Rinsing removes the cleaning agent and food particles.* If the dentures are stained, soak them in a commercial cleaner. Be sure to follow the manufacturer's directions. To prevent corrosion, dentures with metal parts should not be soaked overnight.
3. Inspect the dentures and the mouth.
   - Observe the dentures for any rough, sharp, or worn areas that could irritate the tongue or mucous membranes of the mouth, lips, and gums.
   - Inspect the mouth for any redness, irritated areas, or indications of infection.
   - Assess the fit of the dentures. People who have them should see a dentist at least once a year to check the fit and the presence of any irritation to the soft tissues of the mouth. Clients who need repairs to their dentures or new dentures may need a referral for financial assistance.
4. Return the dentures to the mouth.
   - Offer some mouthwash and a curved basin to rinse the mouth. If the client cannot insert the dentures independently, insert the plates one at a time. Hold each plate at a slight angle while inserting it, to avoid injuring the lips. ❼
   - *Note:* If clients perform self-cleaning of dentures, ensure that dentures are placed in the appropriate container. **Rationale:** *Many older adult clients leave dentures on food trays and risk losing them when food trays are removed. The cost of replacement dentures may not be covered by Medicare.*
5. Assist the client as needed.
   - Wipe the client's hands and mouth with the towel.
   - If the client does not want to or cannot wear the dentures, store them in a denture container with water. Label the container with the client's name and identification number. (Do not place the container on the food tray.)
6. Remove and discard gloves.
7. Perform hand hygiene.
8. Document all assessments and include any problems such as an irritated area on the mucous membrane.

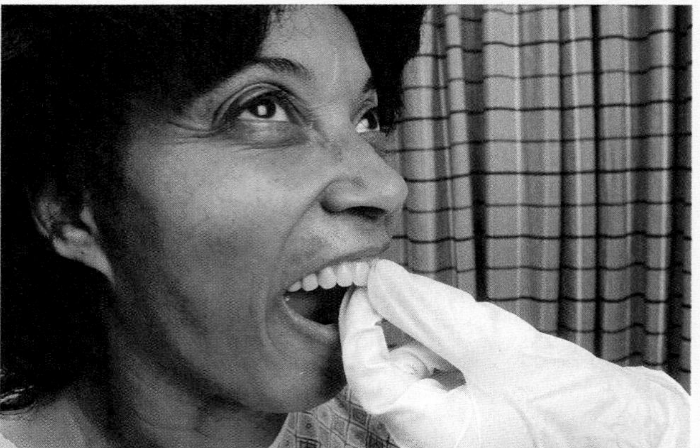

❻ Removing the top dentures by first breaking the suction.

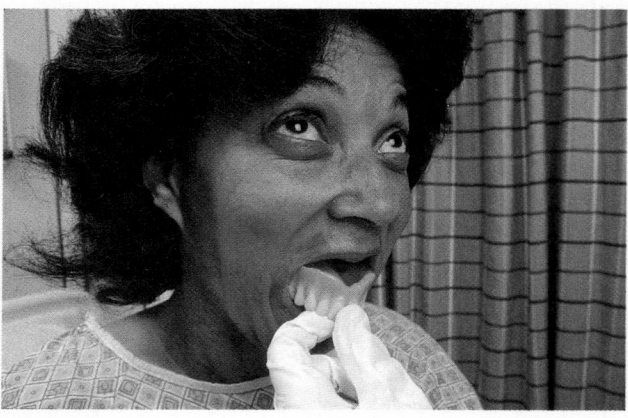

❼ Inserting the dentures at a slight angle.

Clients with Special Oral Hygiene Needs

For the client who is debilitated or unconscious or who has excessive dryness, sores, or irritations of the mouth, it may be necessary to clean the oral mucosa and tongue in addition to the teeth. Agency practices differ in regard to special mouth care and the frequency with which it is provided. Depending on the health of the client's mouth, special care may be needed every 2 to 8 hours.

Mouth care for clients who are unconscious or debilitated is important because their mouths tend to become dry and consequently predisposed to tooth decay and infections. Saliva has antiviral, antibacterial, and antifungal effects. Dry mouth—called *xerostomia*—occurs when the supply of saliva is reduced. This condition can be caused by side effects of certain medications (e.g., antihistamines, antidepressants, antihypertensives). The drying irritates the soft tissues in the mouth, which can cause inflammation and susceptibility to infection (American Dental Association, 2018). Other reasons for a client to experience xerostomia include oxygen therapy, tachypnea, and NPO status in which the client cannot take fluids by mouth.

For clients with special oral hygiene needs, the nurse focuses on removal of plaque and microorganisms as well as client comfort. If possible, a soft-bristled toothbrush should be used because it provides the best means of plaque removal. A suction toothbrush may be needed for dependent clients. If the client cannot tolerate the use of a toothbrush, the nurse can use an oral swab or a gauze wrapped around a gloved finger and soaked with saline to swab the teeth, tongue, and oral mucosa. A foam swab (see Figure 33.6) can be used to provide oral hygiene to dependent clients. Use of lemon-glycerin swabs is not recommended because they irritate and dry the oral mucosa and can decalcify teeth. Mouthwashes containing alcohol can irritate the oral mucosa and cause dryness. Mineral oil is contraindicated as a moisturizer for the lips or inside the mouth because aspiration of it can initiate an infection (lipid pneumonia). A water-soluble moisturizer, absorbed by the skin and tissue, provides important hydration. Saliva substitutes can also help moisturize the oral cavity.

Skill 33.5 focuses on oral care for a client who is unconscious but may be adapted for conscious clients who are seriously ill or have mouth problems.

Providing Special Oral Care for the Unconscious or Debilitated Client

SKILL 33.5

PURPOSES

- To maintain the intactness and health of the lips, tongue, and mucous membranes of the mouth
- To prevent oral infections and potential respiratory infections
- To clean and moisten the membranes of the mouth and lips

ASSESSMENT

- Inspect lips, gums, oral mucosa, and tongue for deviations from normal.
- Identify presence of oral problems such as tooth caries, halitosis, gingivitis, and loose or broken teeth.
- Assess for gag reflex, ability to swallow, and ability to follow commands.

PLANNING

Assignment

Special oral care may be assigned to AP; however, the nurse needs to assess for the gag reflex. Dependent on this assessment, the nurse needs to inform the AP of the correct positioning of the client and how to use the oral suction catheter or suction toothbrush, if needed. Remind the AP to report changes in the client's oral mucosa.

Equipment

- Towel
- Curved basin (emesis basin)
- Clean gloves
- Bite block to hold the mouth open and teeth apart (optional)
- Toothbrush (soft bristle); suction toothbrush if needed
- Cup of tepid water
- Dentifrice or denture cleaner
- Tissue or piece of gauze to remove dentures (optional)
- Denture container as needed
- Mouthwash
- Rubber-tipped bulb syringe
- Suction catheter with suction apparatus when aspiration is a concern
- Foam swabs and cleaning solution for cleaning the mucous membranes
- Water-soluble lip moisturizer

IMPLEMENTATION

Performance

1. Prior to performing the procedure, introduce self and verify the client's identity using agency protocol. Explain to the client and the family what you are going to do and why it is necessary.
2. Perform hand hygiene and observe other appropriate infection prevention procedures.
3. Provide for client privacy by drawing the curtains around the bed or closing the door to the room. Some agencies provide signs indicating the need for privacy. **Rationale:** *Hygiene is a personal matter*.
4. Prepare the client.
   - Position the unconscious client in a side-lying position, with the head of the bed lowered. **Rationale:** *In this position, the saliva automatically runs out by gravity rather than being aspirated into the lungs*. This position is chosen for the unconscious client receiving mouth care. If the client's head cannot be lowered, turn it to one side. **Rationale:** *The fluid will readily run out of the mouth or pool in the side of the mouth, where it can be suctioned*.
   - Place the suctioning equipment nearby. **Rationale:** *This is a safety precaution to use for suctioning the oral cavity as needed*.
   - Place the towel under the client's chin.
   - Place the curved basin against the client's chin and lower cheek to receive the fluid from the mouth. ❶
   - Apply gloves.
5. Clean the teeth and rinse the mouth.
   - If the client has natural teeth, brush the teeth as described in the first part of Skill 33.4. Brush gently and carefully to avoid injuring the gums. Use a bite block (if needed) to hold the mouth open and teeth apart. Do not put your fingers in the client's mouth. **Rationale:** *This prevents accidental closing down on the toothbrush and biting your finger*. If the client has artificial teeth, clean them as described in the Variation section of Skill 33.4.
   - Rinse the client's mouth by drawing about 10 mL of water or alcohol-free mouthwash into the syringe and injecting it

Continued on page 784

Providing Special Oral Care for the Unconscious or Debilitated Client—*continued*

SKILL 33.5

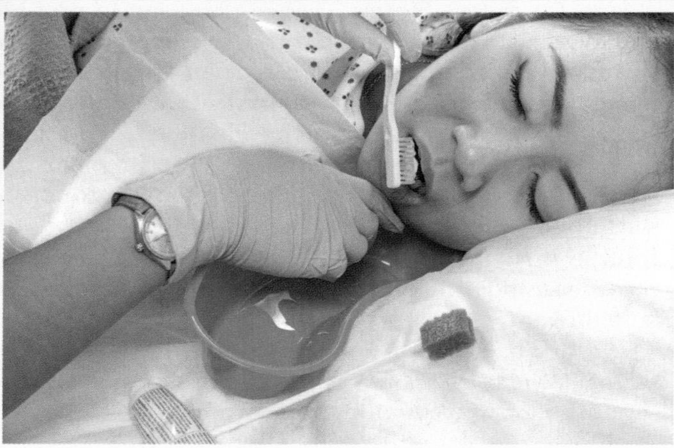

❶ Position of the client and placement of the curved basin when providing special mouth care.

gently into each side of the mouth. **Rationale:** *If the solution is injected with force, some of it may flow down the client's throat and be aspirated into the lungs.*
- Watch carefully to make sure that all the rinsing solution has run out of the mouth into the basin. If not, suction the fluid from the mouth. **Rationale:** *Fluid remaining in the mouth may be aspirated into the lungs.*
- Repeat rinsing until the mouth is free of dentifrice, if used.

6. Inspect and clean the oral tissues.
   - If the tissues appear dry or unclean, clean them with the foam swabs or gauze and cleaning solution following agency policy.
   - Use a moistened foam swab to wipe the mucous membrane of one cheek. Discard the swab in a waste container; use a fresh one to clean the next area. **Rationale:** *Using separate applicators for each area of the mouth prevents the transfer of microorganisms from one area to another.*
   - Clean all mouth tissues in an orderly progression, using separate applicators: the cheeks, roof of the mouth, base of the mouth, and tongue.
   - Observe the tissues closely for inflammation and dryness.
   - Rinse the client's mouth as described in step 5.
7. Ensure client comfort.
   - Remove the basin, and dry around the client's mouth with the towel. Replace artificial dentures, if indicated.
   - Lubricate the client's lips with water-soluble moisturizer. **Rationale:** *Lubrication prevents cracking and subsequent infection.*
   - Remove and discard gloves.
   - Perform hand hygiene.
8. Document assessment of the teeth, tongue, gums, and oral mucosa. Include any problems such as sores or inflammation and swelling of the gums.

EVALUATION

- Consider the client's medical diagnosis and treatment (e.g., chemotherapy, oxygen) and the necessary nursing interventions related to oral hygiene.
- Conduct an ongoing assessment, if appropriate, of the oral mucosa, gums, tongue, and lips.
- Report deviations from normal to the primary care provider.
- Conduct appropriate follow-up such as a referral to a dentist for dental caries.

LIFESPAN CONSIDERATIONS Oral Hygiene

INFANTS

- Most dentists recommend that dental hygiene should begin when the first tooth erupts and be practiced after each feeding. Cleaning can be accomplished by using a wet washcloth or small gauze moistened with water.

CHILDREN

- Beginning at about 18 months of age, brush the child's teeth with a soft toothbrush. Use only a toothbrush moistened with water. Introduce toothpaste later and use one that contains fluoride.
- Frequent snacking on products containing sugar increases the child's risk for developing cavities.

OLDER ADULTS

- Oral care is often difficult for certain older adults to perform due to problems with dexterity or cognitive problems with dementia.
- Most long-term healthcare facilities have dentists that come on a regular basis to see clients with special needs.
- Dryness of the oral mucosa is a common finding in older adults. Because this can lead to tooth decay, advise clients to discuss it with their dentist or primary care provider.
- Decay of the tooth root is common among older adults. When the gums recede, the tooth root is more vulnerable to decay.

Evaluating

Using data collected during care—status of oral mucosa, lips, tongue, teeth, and so on—the nurse judges whether desired outcomes have been achieved.

If outcomes have not been achieved, the nurse and client need to explore the reasons before modifying the care plan. Examples of questions to consider are as follows:

- Did the nurse overestimate the client's functional abilities?
- Is the client's hand coordination or cognitive function impaired?
- Did the client's condition change?
- Has there been a change in the client's energy level or motivation?

Hair

The appearance of the hair often reflects an individual's feelings of self-concept and sociocultural well-being. Each individual has particular ways of caring for hair. Becoming familiar with hair care needs and practices that may be different from our own is an important aspect of providing competent nursing care to all clients. People who feel ill may not groom their hair as before. A dirty scalp and hair are itchy and uncomfortable, and can have an odor. The hair may also reflect state of health (e.g., excessive coarseness and dryness may be associated with endocrine disorders such as hypothyroidism).

Developmental Variations

Newborns may have **lanugo** (the fine hair on the body of the fetus, also referred to as down or woolly hair) over their shoulders, back, and sacrum. This generally disappears, and the hair distribution on the eyebrows, head, and eyelashes of young children subsequently becomes noticeable. Some newborns have hair on their scalps; others are free of hair at birth but grow hair over the scalp during the first year of life.

Pubic hair usually appears in early puberty followed in about 6 months by the growth of axillary hair. Boys develop facial hair in later puberty.

In adolescence, the sebaceous glands increase in activity as a result of increased hormone levels. As a result, hair follicle openings enlarge to accommodate the increased amount of sebum, which can make the adolescent's hair oilier.

In older adults, the hair is generally thinner, grows more slowly, and loses its color as a result of aging tissues and diminishing circulation. Men often lose their scalp hair and may become completely bald. This phenomenon may occur even when a man is relatively young. Older individuals' hair also tends to be drier than normal. With age, axillary and pubic hair becomes finer and scanter, in contrast to the eyebrows, which become bristly and coarse. Many women develop hair on their faces, which may be a concern to them.

●○● NURSING MANAGEMENT

Assessing

Assessment of the client's hair, hair care practices, and potential problems includes a nursing health history and physical assessment.

Nursing History

During the nursing history the nurse elicits data about usual hair care, self-care abilities, history of hair or scalp problems, and conditions known to affect the hair. Chemotherapeutic agents and radiation of the head may cause **alopecia** (hair loss). Hypothyroidism may cause the hair to be thin, dry, or brittle. Use of some hair dyes and curling or straightening preparations can cause the hair to become dry and brittle. Questions to elicit these data are shown in the accompanying Assessment Interview.

Physical Assessment

Physical assessment of the hair is discussed in Chapter 29 ∞. Problems include dandruff, hair loss, ticks, pediculosis, scabies, and hirsutism.

Dandruff

Often accompanied by itching, **dandruff** appears as a diffuse scaling of the scalp. In severe cases it involves the auditory canals and the eyebrows. Dandruff can usually be treated effectively with a commercial shampoo. In severe or persistent cases, the client may need the advice of the primary care provider.

Hair Loss

Hair loss and growth are continual processes. Some permanent thinning of hair normally occurs with aging. Baldness, common in men, is thought to be a hereditary problem for which there is no known remedy other than the wearing of a hairpiece or a surgical hair transplant, in which hair is taken from the back or the sides of the scalp and surgically moved to the hairless area. Although some medications are being developed, their long-term outcomes are unknown.

Ticks

Small gray-brown parasites that bite into tissue and suck blood, **ticks** transmit several diseases to people, in particular Rocky Mountain spotted fever, Lyme disease, and tularemia. To remove a tick, use blunt tweezers or gloved fingers and grasp the tick as close to the skin as possible. Gently pull the tick away using perpendicular traction to remove the tick. Be careful to not twist or squeeze the tick's body. If the head breaks off and remains in the skin, use tweezers to remove in a manner similar to that used for removing a splinter. Wash the area with antibacterial soap. Save the tick in a bottle of rubbing alcohol in case the primary care provider wants to identify the type of tick. The following practices to remove a tick are ineffective

ASSESSMENT INTERVIEW Hair Care

HAIR CARE PRACTICES

- What are your usual hair care practices?
- What hair care products do you routinely use (e.g., hair spray, lubricant, shampoo, conditioners, hair dye, curling or straightening preparations)?

SELF-CARE ABILITIES

- Do you have any problems managing your hair?

PAST OR CURRENT HAIR PROBLEMS

- Have you had any of the following conditions or therapies: recent chemotherapy, hypothyroidism, radiation of the head, unexplained loss of hair, growth of excessive body hair?

or dangerous: applying heat with a match and applying substances such as petroleum jelly or gasoline.

Pediculosis (Lice)

Lice are parasitic insects that infest mammals. Infestation with lice is called **pediculosis**. Hundreds of varieties of lice infest humans. Three common kinds are *Pediculus capitis* (the head louse), *Pediculus corporis* (the body louse), and *Pediculus pubis* (the crab louse).

Pediculus capitis is found on the scalp and tends to stay hidden in the hairs; similarly, *Pediculus pubis* stays in pubic hair. *Pediculus corporis* tends to cling to clothing, so that when a client undresses, the lice may not be in evidence on the body; these lice suck blood from the individual and lay their eggs on the clothing. The nurse can suspect their presence in the clothing if (a) the client habitually scratches, (b) there are scratches on the skin, and (c) there are hemorrhagic spots on the skin where the lice have sucked blood.

Head and pubic lice lay their eggs on the hairs; the eggs look like oval particles, similar to dandruff, clinging to the hair. Bites and pustular eruptions may also be noticed at the hair lines and behind the ears.

Lice are very small, grayish white, and difficult to see. The crab louse in the pubic area has red legs. Lice may be contracted from infested clothes and direct contact with an infested individual.

The treatment often includes topical pediculicides. Lice have become more of a nuisance because the resistance to previous agents has increased, resulting in the development of newer products. Head lice can be treated with over-the-counter permethrin (i.e., Nix) and pyrethrins (i.e., Rid) as first-line treatments. Other options, if these treatments do not work, include prescribed medications such as malathion (Ovide), benzyl alcohol (Ulesfia), spinosad (Natroba), and topical ivermectin (Sklice) (Centers for Disease Control and Prevention [CDC], 2016). Natural products offered by health food stores are also available (e.g., Lice B Gone). However, the literature does not show evidence supporting the use of herbal treatments when used in the curative treatment of head lice. Clients need to be reminded that natural products are not required to meet U.S. Food and Drug Administration (FDA) standards. Some home remedies suggest applying an oily substance such as olive oil, mayonnaise, tea tree oil, or petroleum jelly to smother the lice. There is no clear scientific evidence to support this form of treatment.

Removal of nits (eggs) after applying the treatment is necessary. Fine-toothed "nit" combs are available. Transmission is from head-to-head (hair-to-hair) contact. The hair care items and bedding of a client who has a lice infestation should be washed with hot water.

Scabies

Scabies is a contagious skin infestation by the itch mite. The characteristic lesion is the burrow produced by the female mite as it penetrates into the upper layers of the skin. Pimple-like skin rash lesions are most commonly observed between the fingers, wrists and elbows, beneath breast tissue, and in the groin area (CDC, 2017). The mites cause intense itching that is more pronounced at night because the increased warmth of the skin has a stimulating effect on the parasites. Secondary lesions caused by scratching include vesicles, papules, pustules, excoriations, and crusts. Treatment involves thorough cleansing of the body with soap and water to remove scales and debris from crusts, and then an application of a scabicide topical cream. All bed linens and clothing should be washed in very hot or boiling water.

Hirsutism

The growth of excessive body hair is called **hirsutism**. The acceptance of body hair in the axillae and on the legs is often dictated by culture. For example, in some countries, the well-groomed woman, as depicted in magazines, has no hair on her legs or under her axillae. In many cultures, it is not expected for well-groomed women to remove this hair. Excessive facial hair on a woman is thought to be unattractive in some cultures.

The cause of excessive body hair is not always known. Older women may have some on their faces, and women in menopause may also experience the growth of facial hair. Excessive body hair may be due to the action of the endocrine system. Heredity is also thought to influence the pattern of hair distribution.

Diagnosing

Nursing diagnoses related to hair hygiene and hair and scalp problems include altered skin integrity, potential for infection, and altered body image. Examples of these nursing diagnoses with contributing factors follow:

- Altered skin integrity related to:
  a. Pruritus secondary to scabies
  b. Pruritus secondary to head lice
  c. Insect bite.
- Potential for infection related to:
  a. Scalp laceration
  b. Insect bite.
- Altered body image related to alopecia.

Planning

In planning care, the nurse and, if appropriate, the client and family set outcomes for each nursing diagnosis. The nurse then performs nursing interventions and activities to achieve the client outcomes.

The specific, detailed nursing activities provided by the nurse to assist the client should take into account the client's personal preferences, health, and energy resources as well as the time, equipment, and personnel available. Often, clients like to receive hair care after a bath, before receiving visitors, and before retiring. Nursing interventions may include instructing the client and family on alternative methods for hair care including facilitating the assistance of a barber or beautician, as necessary. At some agencies, shampoos can be given to clients only after a primary care provider's order.

Implementing

Hair needs to be brushed or combed and washed, as needed, to keep it clean. Nurses may need to provide hair care for clients who cannot meet their own self-care needs.

Brushing and Combing Hair

It is important for the nurse to ask clients about their hair care practices. For example, for some, brushing can stimulate the circulation of blood in the scalp, distribute the oil along the hair shaft, and help to arrange the hair. For others with natural, highly textured hair, brushing or combing can cause hair breakage and split ends. Some people use their fingers for removing tangles instead of a comb or brush (Matrix, n.d.; White, 2017).

Long hair may present a problem for clients confined to bed because it may become matted. Again, it is important for the nurse to ask the client or family about their hair care. Some clients are pleased to have their hair tied neatly in the back or braided until they feel better and can look after it themselves. Braiding also prevents tangling and matting for clients confined to bed.

Clinical Alert!

Excessively matted or tangled hair may be infested with lice.

Some individuals have thicker, drier, curlier hair than others. Very curly hair may stand out from the scalp. Although the shafts of curly or kinky hair look strong and wiry, they have less strength than straight hair shafts and can break easily. Dry hair and dry scalp are often concerns for people with thick, curly hair. As a result, they generally wash their hair less often because frequent shampooing could damage their hair.

Some individuals with curly hair have their hair straightened, while others may style their hair in small braids or dreadlocks (Figure 33.7 ■). Dreadlocks are ropes of hair. This style is also known as dreads, or locs. Different methods are used to form the locs such as rolling, braiding, and backcombing. In some cultures, dreadlocks are an expression of religious beliefs, whereas in other cultures, they represent ethnic pride. Individuals may also wear dreadlocks more for style than cultural or religious reasons. There are many different styles of dreadlocks (Curl Centric, n.d.). These braids or dreads do not have to be unbraided before washing. If, however, unbraiding becomes necessary, the nurse should obtain the client's permission to do so. Some clients may apply oil between the braids and massage it into the scalp. The oil prevents the hair strands from breaking and the scalp from becoming too dry.

Shampooing the Hair

Hair should be washed as often as needed to keep it clean. There are several ways to shampoo clients' hair, depending on their health, strength, and age. The client who is well enough to take a shower can shampoo while in the shower. The client who is unable to shower may be given a shampoo while sitting on a chair in front of a sink. The back-lying client who can move to a stretcher can be given a shampoo on a stretcher wheeled to a sink. The client who must remain in bed can be given a shampoo with water brought to the bedside. A commercial product, similar to the bag bath, called a "head bath" is another approach (Figure 33.8 ■). It consists of a specially designed cap (looks like a shower cap) placed over the hair. The cap contains shampoo and conditioner and gently massaging the cap cleans the hair and scalp. In some agencies, volunteer beauticians with portable shampoo chairs may be available to assist with hair care.

Individuals with thick, coarse, dry, or curly hair may co-wash their hair. This term is short for "conditioner-only washing." It means skipping the shampoo and using only conditioner on the hair (Jin, 2017). Shampooing can cause more dryness and damage due to detergents in some shampoos and the friction caused by sudsing and rubbing (Matrix, n.d.). The conditioner gently lifts oil and debris from the scalp and hair. Cowashing softens the hair and keeps the scalp moisturized. Softening the hair makes it easier to comb and less likely to cause breakage. This method of washing is particularly beneficial for natural hair care (Williams, n.d.). Jin (2017) describes a three-step process for co-washing: (1) Fully saturate the hair with water;

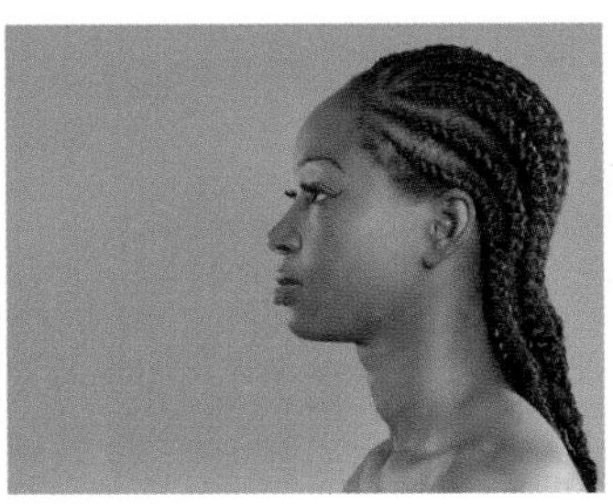

A

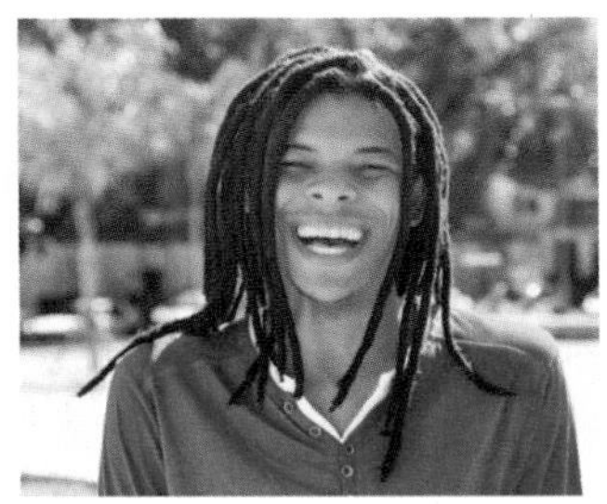

B

Figure 33.7 ■ Examples of hairstyle with *A*, braids and *B*, dreadlocks.

A, Mathias Zegler/123RF; *B*, Daniel Ernst/123RF.

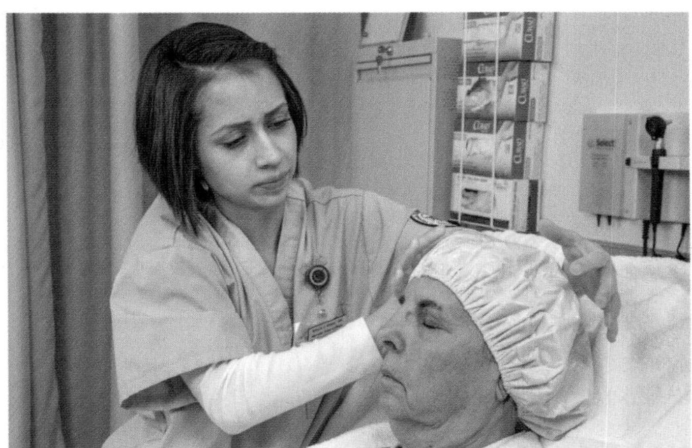

Figure 33.8 ■ Using a rinse-free shampoo cap.

(2) use enough conditioner to coat hair strands from root to tip; and (3) massage the conditioner into the scalp and distribute evenly through the ends. Allow time for the conditioner to absorb, usually 3 to 5 minutes. Rinse, dry, and style as usual. Many people who co-wash feel that it is important to shampoo with a conventional shampoo every 2 to 4 weeks to remove conditioner buildup (Matrix, n.d.).

Water used for the shampoo should be 40.5°C (105°F) for an adult or child to be comfortable and to avoid injuring the scalp. If the hair is being washed to destroy lice, a medicated shampoo should be used. Dry shampoos are also available. They will remove some of the dirt, odor, and oil. Their main disadvantage is that they dry the hair and scalp.

How often a person needs a shampoo is highly individual, depending largely on the client's activities and the amount of sebum secreted by the scalp. Oily hair tends to look stringy and dirty, and it feels unclean to the individual. Skill 33.6 describes how to provide hair care for clients.

SKILL 33.6

Providing Hair Care

PURPOSES

- To stimulate the blood circulation to the scalp
- To distribute hair oils and provide a healthy sheen
- To increase the client's comfort
- To assess or monitor hair or scalp problems (e.g., matted hair or dandruff)

ASSESSMENT

Determine

- History of the following conditions or therapies: recent chemotherapy, hypothyroidism, radiation of the head, unexplained hair loss, and growth of excessive body hair
- Usual hair care practices and routinely used hair care products (e.g., hair spray, shampoo, conditioners, hair oil preparation, hair dye, curling or straightening preparations)
- Whether wetting the hair will make it easier or difficult to comb. Kinky hair is easier to comb when wet and very difficult to comb when dry.

Assess

- Condition of the hair and scalp. Is the hair straight, curly, kinky? Is the hair matted or tangled? Is the scalp dry?
- Evenness of hair growth over the scalp, in particular, any patchy loss of hair; hair texture, oiliness, thickness, or thinness; presence of lesions, infections, or infestations on the scalp; presence of hirsutism
- Self-care abilities (e.g., any problems managing hair care)

PLANNING

Assignment

Brushing and combing hair, shampooing hair, and shaving facial hair can be assigned to AP unless the client has a condition in which the procedure would be contraindicated (e.g., cervical spinal injury or trauma). The nurse needs to assess the AP's knowledge and experience of hair care for clients of other cultures, if appropriate.

Equipment

- Clean brush and comb (A wide-toothed comb is usually used for individuals with thick, coarse, or curly hair because finer combs pull the hair into knots and may also break the hair.)
- Towel
- Hair oil preparation, if appropriate

IMPLEMENTATION

Performance

1. Prior to performing the procedure, introduce self and verify the client's identity using agency protocol. Explain to the client what you are going to do, why it is necessary, and how to participate.
2. Perform hand hygiene and observe other appropriate infection prevention procedures.
3. Provide for client privacy by drawing the curtains around the bed or closing the door to the room. Some agencies provide signs indicating the need for privacy. **Rationale:** *Hygiene is a personal matter*.
4. Position and prepare the client appropriately.
   - Assist the client who can sit to move to a chair. **Rationale:** *Hair is more easily brushed and combed when the client is in a sitting position*.
   - If health permits, assist a client confined to a bed to a sitting position by raising the head of the bed. Otherwise, assist the client to alternate side-lying positions, and do one side of the head at a time.
   - If the client remains in bed, place a clean towel over the pillow and the client's shoulders. Place it over the sitting client's shoulders. **Rationale:** *The towel collects any removed hair, dirt, and scaly material*.
   - Remove any pins or ribbons in the hair.
5. Remove any mats or tangles gradually.
   - Mats can usually be pulled apart with fingers or worked out with repeated brushings.
   - If the hair is very tangled, rub alcohol or an oil, such as mineral oil, on the strands to help loosen the tangles.
   - Comb out tangles in a small section of hair toward the ends. Stabilize the hair with one hand and comb toward the ends of the hair with the other hand. **Rationale:** *This avoids scalp trauma*.
6. Brush and comb the hair.
   - For short hair, brush and comb one side at a time. Divide long hair into two sections by parting it down the middle from the front to the back. If the hair is very thick, divide each section into front and back subsections or into several layers.
7. Arrange the hair as neatly and attractively as possible, according to the individual's desires.
   - Braiding long hair helps prevent tangles.
8. Document assessments and special nursing interventions. Daily combing and brushing of the hair are not normally recorded.

Providing Hair Care—*continued*

Variation: Hair Care for Individuals with Natural or Thick, Curly Hair

- Position and prepare the client.
  - Separate the hair into four sections, proceeding from one section to the next.
- Untangle the hair first, if appropriate.
  - Use fingers to reduce hair breakage and discomfort. Move fingers in a circular motion starting at the roots and gently moving up to the tip of the hair.
- Comb the hair.
  - Dampen the hair with water or a leave-in conditioner. **Rationale:** *This will help loosen any tangles.*
- Apply hair oil preparation as the client indicates.
  - Using a large and open-toothed comb, grasp a small section of hair and, holding the hair at the tip, start untangling at the tip and work down toward the scalp.
- Ask the client if he or she would like the hair braided. **Rationale:** *Braiding will decrease tangling; however, the choice is the client's.*

SKILL 33.6

EVALUATION

- Conduct ongoing assessments for problems such as dandruff, alopecia, pediculosis, scalp lesions, or excessive dryness or matting.
- Evaluate effectiveness of medication (e.g., for treating pediculosis), if appropriate.

LIFESPAN CONSIDERATIONS Hair Care

INFANTS

- Shampoo an infant's hair daily to prevent seborrhea.

CHILDREN

- Monitor school-age children for nits (pediculosis).

OLDER ADULTS

- Ensure adequate warmth for older adults when shampooing their hair, because they are susceptible to chilling.

Beard and Mustache Care

Beards and mustaches also require daily care. The most important aspect of the care is to keep them clean. Food particles tend to collect in beards and mustaches, and they need washing and combing periodically. Clients may also wish a beard or mustache trim to maintain a well-groomed appearance.

Clinical Alert!

A beard or mustache should not be shaved off without the client's consent.

Male clients often shave or are shaved after a bath. Frequently clients supply their own electric or safety razors. See Box 33.1 for the steps involved in shaving facial hair with a safety razor. If a client is taking an anticoagulant (e.g., Coumadin, heparin), an electric shaver should be used. Check agency policy because some facilities do not provide safety razors.

Evaluating

Using data collected during care, the nurse judges whether desired outcomes have been achieved. Examples of client outcomes that are measurable or observable include the client being able to:

- Perform hair grooming with assistance (specify).
- Exhibit clean, well-groomed, resilient hair with a healthy sheen.
- Reduce or get rid of scalp lesions or infestations.
- Describe factors, interventions, and preventive measures for a specific hair problem (e.g., dandruff).

BOX 33.1 Using a Safety Razor to Shave Facial Hair

- Wear gloves in case facial nicks occur and you come in contact with blood.
- Apply shaving cream or soap and water to soften the bristles and make the skin more pliable.
- Hold the skin taut, particularly around creases, to prevent cutting the skin.
- Hold the razor so that the blade is at a 45° angle to the skin, and shave in short, firm strokes in the direction of hair growth.
- After shaving the entire area, wipe the client's face with a wet washcloth to remove any remaining shaving cream and hair.
- Dry the face well, then apply aftershave lotion or powder as the client prefers.
- To prevent irritating the skin, pat on the lotion with the fingers and avoid rubbing the face.

Note: Check agency policy as some do not allow safety razors because of the risk of impaired skin integrity from cutting the skin. Only electric razors can be used to shave clients with bleeding tendencies. Check the electric razor for safety aspects.

Eyes

Normally eyes require no special hygiene, because lacrimal fluid continually washes the eyes, and the eyelids and lashes prevent the entrance of foreign particles. Special interventions are needed, however, for unconscious clients and for clients recovering from eye surgery or having eye injuries, irritations, or infections. In unconscious clients, the blink reflex may be absent, and excessive drainage may accumulate along eyelid margins. In clients with eye trauma or eye infections, excessive discharge or drainage is common. Excessive secretions on the lashes need to be removed before they dry on the lashes as crusts. Clients who wear eyeglasses or contact lenses also may require instruction from and care by the nurse.

ASSESSMENT INTERVIEW Eyes

FOR CLIENTS WHO WEAR EYEGLASSES

- When do you use your glasses?
- What is your vision like with and without the glasses?

FOR CLIENTS WHO WEAR CONTACT LENSES

- How often do you wear lenses? Daily? On special occasions?
- How long do you wear your lenses in a given day, including sleep time?
- Do you have any problems with the lenses (e.g., cleaning, insertion, removal, damage)?
- Do you carry an emergency identification label to alert others to remove the lenses and ensure appropriate care in an emergency? (If not, advise the client to acquire one.)
- What are your insertion and removal procedures?
- What are your cleaning and storage procedures?
- Have you had any problems with either or both eyes or eyelids, such as excessive tearing, burning, redness, sensitivity to light, swelling, or feelings of dryness? Describe them.
- Are you using any eyedrops or ointments? (These medications can combine chemically with soft lenses and cause lens damage and eye irritation.)

FOR ALL CLIENTS

- When did you last have your eyesight tested?
- Are you currently taking any eye medication? If so, provide name, dosage, and frequency.
- Do you have any of the following eye problems: difficulty reading or seeing objects, blurring of vision, tearing, spots or floaters, photophobia (sensitivity to light), burning, itching, pain, double vision, flashing lights, or halos around lights?

●○● NURSING MANAGEMENT

Assessing

Assessment of the client's eyes includes a nursing health history and physical assessment.

Nursing History

During the nursing history, the nurse obtains data about the client's eyeglasses or contact lenses, recent examination by an ophthalmologist, and any history of eye problems and related treatments. Questions to elicit these data are shown in the accompanying Assessment Interview.

Physical Assessment

In physical assessment, all external eye structures are inspected for signs of inflammation, excessive drainage, encrustations, or other obvious abnormalities. Inspection of the external eye structures is discussed in Chapter 29 ∞.

Diagnosing

Nursing diagnoses related to eye problems may include potential for infection and potential for injury. Examples of these diagnoses and possible contributing factors follow:

- potential for infection related to:
  a. Improper contact lens hygiene.
- potential for injury related to:
  a. Prolonged wearing of contact lenses
  b. Absence of blink reflex associated with unconsciousness.

Planning

In planning care, the nurse identifies nursing activities that will assist the client to maintain the integrity of the eye structures and to prevent eye injury and infection.

Implementing

Nursing activities may include teaching clients about how to insert, clean, and remove contact lenses and ways to protect the eyes from injury and strain.

Eye Care

Dried secretions that have accumulated on the lashes need to be softened and wiped away. Soften dried secretions by placing a sterile cotton ball moistened with sterile water or normal saline over the lid margins. Wipe the loosened secretions from the inner canthus of the eye to the outer canthus to prevent the particles and fluid from draining into the lacrimal sac and nasolacrimal duct.

If the client is unconscious and lacks a blink reflex or cannot close the eyelids completely, drying and irritation of the cornea must be prevented. Lubricating eyedrops may be ordered. Box 33.2 gives suggestions for providing eye care for the comatose client.

BOX 33.2 Eye Care for the Comatose Client

When a comatose client's corneal reflex is impaired, eye care is essential to keep moist the areas of the cornea that are exposed to air.

- Administer moist compresses to cover the eyes every 2 to 4 hours.
- Clean the eyes with saline solution and cotton balls. Wipe from the inner to outer canthus. This prevents debris from being washed into the nasolacrimal duct.
- Use a new cotton ball for each wipe. This prevents extending infection in one eye to the other eye.
- Instill ophthalmic ointment or artificial tears into the lower lids as ordered. This keeps the eyes moist.
- If the client's corneal reflex is absent, keep the eyes moist with artificial tears and protect the eye with a protective shield. A primary care provider should order these interventions.
- Monitor the eyes for redness, exudate, or ulceration.

Eyeglass Care

It is essential that the nurse exercise caution when cleaning eyeglasses to prevent breaking or scratching the lenses. Glass lenses can be cleaned with warm water and dried with a soft tissue that will not scratch the lenses. Plastic lenses are easily scratched and may require special cleaning solutions and drying tissues. When not being worn, all glasses should be placed in an appropriately labeled case and stored in the client's bedside table drawer.

Contact Lens Care

Contact lenses, thin curved disks of hard or soft plastic, fit on the cornea of the eye directly over the pupil. They float on the tear layer of the eye. For some people, contact lenses offer several advantages over eyeglasses: (a) They cannot be seen and thus have cosmetic value; (b) they are highly effective in correcting some astigmatisms; (c) they are safer than glasses for some physical activities; (d) they do not fog, as eyeglasses do; and (e) they provide better vision in many cases.

Contact lenses may be either hard or soft or a compromise between the two types—gas-permeable lenses. Hard contact lenses are made of a rigid, unwettable, airtight plastic that does not absorb water or saline solutions. They usually cannot be worn for more than 12 to 14 hours and are rarely recommended for first-time wearers.

Soft contact lenses cover the entire cornea. Being more pliable and soft than hard lenses, they mold to the eye for a firmer fit. The duration of extended wear varies by brand from 1 to 30 days or more. Eye specialists recommend that long-wear brands be removed and cleaned at least once a week. These lenses require scrupulous care and handling.

Gas-permeable lenses are rigid enough to provide clear vision but are more flexible than the traditional hard lens. They permit oxygen to reach the cornea, thus providing greater comfort, and will not cause serious damage to the eye if left in place for several days.

Most clients normally care for their own contact lenses. In general, each lens manufacturer provides detailed cleaning instructions. Depending on the type of lens and cleaning method used, warm tap water, normal saline, or special rinsing or soaking solutions may be used.

All users should have a special container for their lenses. Some contain a solution so that the lenses are stored wet; in others, the lenses are dry. Each lens container has a slot or cup with a label indicating whether it is for the right or left lens. It is essential the correct lens be stored in the appropriate slot so that it will be placed in the correct eye.

General Eye Care

Many clients may need to learn specific information about care of the eyes. Some examples follow:

- Avoid home remedies for eye problems. Eye irritations or injuries at any age should be treated medically and immediately.
- If dirt or dust gets into the eyes, clean them copiously with clean, tepid water as an emergency treatment.
- Take measures to guard against eyestrain and to protect vision, such as maintaining adequate lighting for reading and obtaining shatterproof lenses for glasses.
- Schedule regular eye examinations, particularly after age 40, to detect problems such as cataracts and glaucoma.

Evaluating

Using data collected during care, the nurse judges whether desired outcomes have been achieved. Examples of desired outcomes to evaluate the effectiveness of nursing interventions follow:

- Conjunctiva and sclera free of inflammation
- Eyelids free of secretions
- No tearing
- No eye discomfort
- Demonstrates appropriate methods of caring for contact lenses
- Describes interventions to prevent eye injury and infection.

Ears

Normal ears require minimal hygiene. Clients who have excessive **cerumen** (earwax) and dependent clients who have hearing aids may require assistance from the nurse. Hearing aids are usually removed before surgery.

Cleaning the Ears

The auricles of the ear are cleaned during the bed bath. The nurse or client must remove excessive cerumen that is visible or that causes discomfort or hearing difficulty. Visible cerumen may be loosened and removed by retracting the auricle up and back. If this measure is ineffective, the use of a ceruminolytic (wax-softening agents used to soften the cerumen) or irrigation may be necessary. Irrigation, however, may cause complications, including infection and tympanic membrane perforation (Hayter, 2016). Because ear irrigations have the potential to cause discomfort or even injury, the nurse must have competence in aural irrigation prior to performing the procedure.

Clients with hearing aids are at greater risk for cerumen impaction for two reasons. The hearing aid (a foreign body) causes excessive cerumen production, and the presence of the hearing aid prevents the body's normal mechanism for removal of cerumen from functioning.

It is important for nurses to advise clients to never use bobby pins, toothpicks, or cotton-tipped applicators to remove cerumen. Bobby pins and toothpicks can injure the ear canal and rupture the tympanic membrane. Cotton-tipped applicators can cause wax to become impacted within the canal.

Care of Hearing Aids

A hearing aid is a battery-powered, sound-amplifying device used by people with hearing impairments. It consists of a microphone that picks up sound and converts it

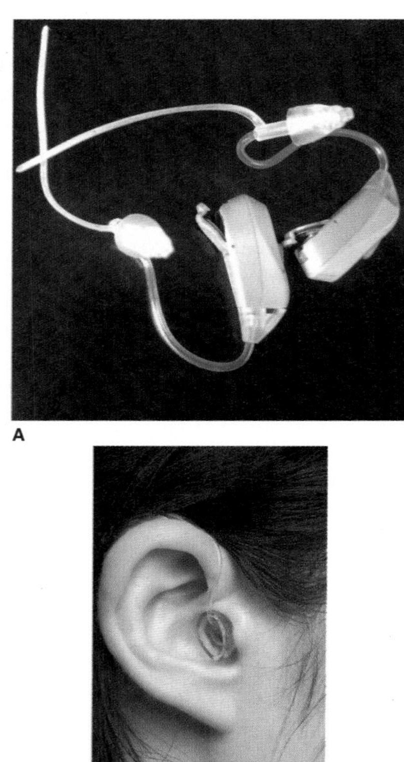

Figure 33.9 ■ *A*, A behind-the-ear (BTE) open-fit hearing aid; *B*, a BTE open-fit hearing aid in place.
A, djgunner/E+/Getty Images; *B*, Diane Macdonald/Moment Open/Getty Images.

to electric energy, an amplifier that magnifies the electric energy electronically, a receiver that converts the amplified energy back to sound energy, and an earmold that directs the sound into the ear. There are several types of hearing aids:

- *Behind-the-ear (BTE) open fit.* BTEs are the newest in hearing aid technology. A BTE has no earmold and it is barely visible with a clear tube that runs down into the ear canal. It does not occlude the ear canal (Figure 33.9 ■).
- *Behind-the-ear (BTE) with earmold.* This is a widely used type because it fits snugly behind the ear. The hearing aid case, which holds the microphone, amplifier, and receiver, is attached to the earmold by a plastic tube (Figure 33.10 ■).
- *In-the-ear (ITE) hearing aid.* This one-piece aid has all its components housed in the earmold. It is more visible than other types but has more room for features such as volume control (Figure 33.11 ■).
- *In-the-canal (ITC) hearing aid.* An ITC aid fits completely inside the ear canal. It looks like the ITE hearing aid except a smaller portion of the hearing aid shows in the outer ear. In addition to having cosmetic appeal, the ITC does not interfere with telephone use or the wearing of eyeglasses. However, it is not suitable for clients with progressive hearing loss, it requires adequate ear canal diameter and length for a good fit, and it tends to plug with cerumen more than other aids.
- *Completely-in-the-canal (CIC) aid.* Almost invisible to an observer, the CIC aid has to be custom designed to fit the individual's ear (Figure 33.12 ■).

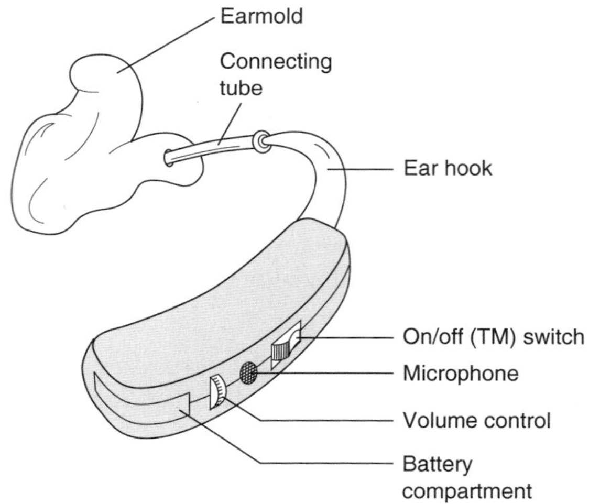

Figure 33.10 ■ A behind-the-ear hearing aid with earmold.

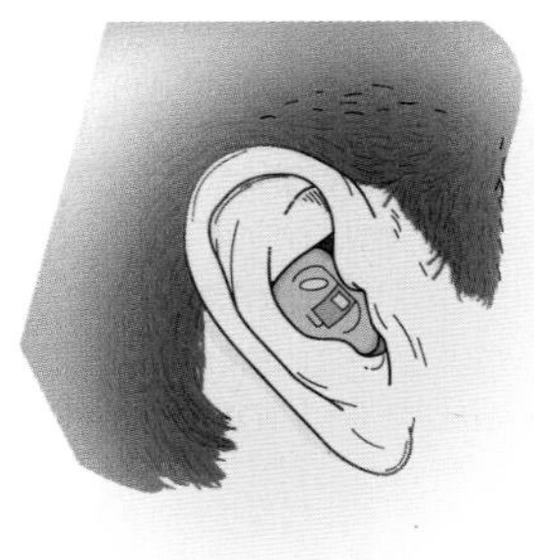

Figure 33.11 ■ An in-the-ear (ITE) hearing aid.

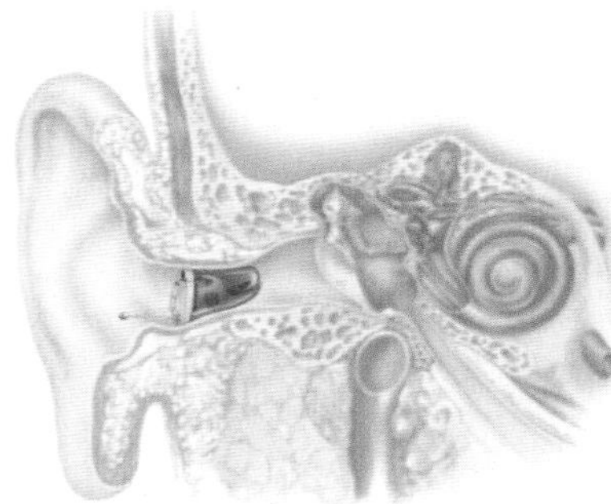

Figure 33.12 ■ A completely-in-the-canal (CIC) hearing aid in place.

QSEN Patient-Centered Care: Hearing Aids

People who need a hearing aid may not wear one because they view it as a stigma of old age. It is important for the client who just purchased a hearing aid to know that it often takes weeks or even months to adjust to it. At first, the sounds may seem shrill as they start hearing high-frequency sounds that had been forgotten. Remind them that it is a hearing aid, not a hearing cure. Encourage them to not give up. The client needs to adjust to the hearing aid gradually by increasing the amount of time each day until the aid can be worn for a full day. Encourage clients to purchase their hearing aids from a company that has a minimum warranty of a 30-day return policy. Emphasize the importance of maintaining the hearing aid, that is, having it cleaned and checked regularly.

For correct functioning, hearing aids require appropriate handling during insertion and removal, regular cleaning of the earmold, and replacement of dead batteries. With proper care, hearing aids generally last 5 to 10 years. Earmolds generally need readjustment every 2 to 3 years. Skill 33.7 describes how to remove, clean, and insert a hearing aid.

Removing, Cleaning, and Inserting a Hearing Aid

SKILL 33.7

PURPOSE

- To maintain proper hearing aid function

Assessment

Determine if the client has experienced any problems with the hearing aid and hearing aid practices. Assess for the presence of inflammation, excessive wax, drainage, or discomfort in the external ear.

PLANNING

Assignment

A nurse can assign the task of caring for a hearing aid to the AP. It is important, however, for the nurse to first determine that the AP knows the correct way to care for a hearing aid. Inform the AP to report the presence of ear inflammation, discomfort, excess wax, or drainage to the nurse.

Equipment

- Client's hearing aid
- Soap, water, and towels or a damp cloth
- Wax pick
- New battery (if needed)

IMPLEMENTATION

Performance

1. Prior to performing the procedure, introduce self and verify the client's identity using agency protocol. Explain to the client what you are going to do, why it is necessary, and how to participate.
2. Perform hand hygiene and observe other appropriate infection prevention procedures.
3. Provide for client privacy by drawing the curtains around the bed or closing the door to the room. Some agencies provide signs indicating the need for privacy. **Rationale:** *Hygiene is a personal matter*.
4. Remove the ITE hearing aid.
   - Turn the hearing aid off and lower the volume. The on/off switch may be labeled "O" (off), "M" (microphone), "T" (telephone), or "TM" (telephone/microphone). **Rationale:** *The batteries continue to run if the hearing aid is not turned off*.
   - Remove the earmold by rotating it slightly forward and pulling it outward.
   - If the hearing aid is not to be used for several days, remove the battery. **Rationale:** *Removal prevents corrosion of the hearing aid from battery leakage*.
   - Store the hearing aid in a safe place and label with client's name. Avoid exposure to heat and moisture. **Rationale:** *Proper storage prevents loss or damage*.
5. Clean the earmold.
   - Detach the earmold if possible. **Rationale:** *Removal facilitates cleaning and prevents inadvertent damage to the other parts*. Do not remove the earmold if it is glued or secured by a small metal ring.
   - If the earmold is detachable, wipe it clean daily and soak it in a mild soapy solution once a week. Rinse and dry it well. Do not use isopropyl alcohol. **Rationale:** *Alcohol can damage the hearing aid*.
   - If the earmold is not detachable, wipe it with a damp cloth.
   - Check that the earmold opening is patent. Use the hearing aid brush to clear away built-up wax. Hold the device with the opening facing downward to allow loose particles to fall out of the hearing aid. Use a wax pick to clear anything out of the holes that didn't come out with the brush.
   - Reattach the earmold if it was detached from the rest of the hearing aid.
6. Insert the hearing aid.
   - Determine from the client if the earmold is for the left or the right ear.
   - Check that the battery is inserted in the hearing aid. Turn off the hearing aid, and make sure the volume is turned all the way down. **Rationale:** *A volume that is too loud is distressing*.
   - Inspect the earmold to identify the ear canal portion. Some earmolds are fitted for only the ear canal and concha; others are fitted for all contours of the ear. The canal portion, common to all, can be used as a guide for correct insertion.
   - Line up the parts of the earmold with the corresponding parts of the client's ear.
   - Rotate the earmold slightly forward, and insert the ear canal portion.
   - Gently press the earmold into the ear while rotating it backward.
   - Check that the earmold fits snugly by asking the client if it feels secure and comfortable.
   - Adjust the other components of a behind-the-ear or body hearing aid.
   - Turn the hearing aid on, and adjust the volume according to the client's needs.
7. Correct problems associated with improper functioning.
   - If the sound is weak or there is no sound:
     a. Ensure that the volume is turned high enough.
     b. Ensure that the earmold opening is not clogged.
     c. Check the battery by turning the hearing aid on, turning up the volume, cupping your hand over the earmold, and listening. A constant whistling sound indicates the battery is functioning. If necessary, replace the battery. Be sure that the negative (−) and positive (+) signs on the battery match those where indicated on the hearing aid.
     d. Ensure that the ear canal is not blocked with wax, which can obstruct sound waves.

Continued on page 794

SKILL 33.7

Removing, Cleaning, and Inserting a Hearing Aid—*continued*

- If the client reports a whistling sound or squeal after insertion:
  a. Turn the volume down.
  b. Ensure that the earmold is properly attached to the receiver.
  c. Reinsert the earmold.

8. Document pertinent data.
- The removal and the insertion of a hearing aid are not normally recorded. If removed for a length of time, document that it was removed along with the hearing aid location.
- Report and record any problems the client has with the hearing aid.

EVALUATION
- Speak to the client in a normal conversational tone and observe client behaviors.
- Compare the client's hearing ability to previous assessments.
- Report to the primary care provider any deviations from normal for the client.

Nose

Nurses usually need not provide special care for the nose, because clients can ordinarily clear nasal secretions by blowing gently into a soft tissue. When the external nares are encrusted with dried secretions, they should be cleaned with a cotton-tipped applicator or moistened with saline or water. The applicator should not be inserted beyond the length of the cotton tip; inserting it further may cause injury to the mucosa.

Supporting a Hygienic Environment

Because people are usually confined to bed when ill, often for long periods, the bed becomes an important element in the client's life. A place that is clean, safe, and comfortable contributes to the client's ability to rest and sleep and to a sense of well-being. From a holistic perspective, bedmaking can be viewed as the preparation of a healing space. When performed with caring intention for benefit of the clients occupying the space during their healing journey, the environment will be affected in positive ways.

Basic furniture in a healthcare facility includes the bed, bedside table, overbed table, one or more chairs, and a storage space for clothing. Most bed units also have a call light, light fixtures, electric outlets, and hygienic equipment in the bedside table. Three types of equipment often installed in an acute care facility are a suction outlet for several kinds of suction, an oxygen outlet for most oxygen equipment, and a sphygmomanometer to measure the client's blood pressure. Some long-term care agencies also permit clients to have personal furniture, such as a television, a chair, and lamps, at the bedside. In the home, a client often has personal and medical equipment.

Environment

In Florence Nightingale's book *Notes on Nursing*, she discussed many concepts including ventilation and warming, light, cleanliness of rooms, noise, and beds and bedding. These concepts are just as important today and the nurse is often an influencing factor (e.g., dimming lights, controlling noise, providing a clean bed). When providing a comfortable environment, it is important to consider the client's age, severity of illness, and level of activity.

Room Temperature

A room temperature between 20°C and 23°C (68°F and 74°F) is comfortable for most clients.

People who are very young, very old, or acutely ill frequently need a room temperature higher than normal.

Ventilation

Effective ventilation is important to remove unpleasant odors and stale air. Odors caused by urine, draining wounds, or vomitus, for example, can be offensive to people. Room deodorizers can help eliminate odors. However, good hygienic practices are the best way to prevent offensive body and breath odors. Hospitals prohibit smoking in client rooms and throughout the entire hospital.

Noise

Hospital environments can be quite noisy, and special care needs to be taken to reduce noise in the hallways and nursing care units. Environmental distractions such as environmental noises and staff communication noise are particularly troublesome for hospitalized clients. For example, increased noise has been linked to stress reaction, sleep disturbance, and increased perception of pain. Environmental noises include the sound of paging systems, telephones, and call lights; doors closing; elevator chimes; industrial floor cleaners; and carts being wheeled through corridors.

Staff communication is a major source of noise, particularly at staff change of shift in the morning when staff conversations and many of the environmental noises occur simultaneously. It is important for nurses to increase their awareness of noise on their units and intervene to find solutions. Some hospitals have instituted Quiet Time in the afternoon on nursing units by announcing Quiet Time over the intercom, dimming the lights, providing comfort measures, and purposefully decreasing activity and noise so clients can rest or nap (McGough et al., 2018). The Quiet

Time is often in the afternoon because many of the required activities for client care take place in the morning.

Hospital Beds

The frame of a hospital bed is divided into three sections. This permits the head and the foot to be elevated separately. Most hospital beds have electric motors to operate the movable joints. The motor is activated by pressing a button or moving a small lever, located either at the side of the bed or on a small panel separate from the bed but attached to it by a cable, which the client can readily use. Common bed positions are shown in Table 33.7.

Hospital beds are usually 66 cm (26 in.) high and 0.9 m (3 ft) wide, narrower than the usual bed, so that the nurse can reach the client from either side of the bed without undue stretching. The length is usually 1.9 m (6.5 ft). Some beds can be extended in length to accommodate very tall clients. Long-term care facilities for ambulatory clients usually have low beds to facilitate movement in and out of bed. Most hospital beds have "high" and "low" positions that can be adjusted either mechanically or electrically by a button or lever. The high position permits the nurse to reach the client without undue stretching or stooping. The low position allows the client to step easily to the floor.

Mattresses

Mattresses are usually covered with a water-repellent material that resists soiling and can be cleaned easily. Most mattresses have handles on the sides called lugs by which the mattress can be moved.

Many special mattresses are also used in hospitals to relieve pressure on the body's bony prominences, such as the heels. They are particularly helpful for clients confined to bed for a long time. For additional information about mattresses, see Chapter 36 ∞.

Side Rails

Side rails, also referred to as bedrails, are used on both hospital beds and stretchers. They are of various shapes and sizes and are usually made of metal. A bed can have two full-length side rails or four half- or quarter-length side rails (also called split rails). Some side rails have two positions: up and down. Others have three: high, intermediate, and low. Devices to raise and lower side rails differ. Often one or two knobs are pulled to release the side and permit it to be moved. When side rails are being used, it is important that the nurse never leave the bedside while the rail is lowered.

For decades, the use of side rails has been routine practice with the rationale that the side rails serve as a safe

TABLE 33.7 Commonly Used Bed Positions

Position	Description	Uses
Flat Head of bed Foot of bed	Mattress is completely horizontal.	Client sleeping in a variety of bed positions, such as back-lying, side-lying, and prone (face down) To maintain spinal alignment for clients with spinal injuries To assist clients to move and turn in bed Bedmaking by nurse
Fowler's position	Semi-sitting position in which head of bed is raised to an angle between 45° and 60°, typically at 45°. Knees may be flexed or horizontal.	Convenient for eating, reading, visiting, watching TV Relief from lying positions To promote lung expansion for client with respiratory problem To assist a client to a sitting position on the edge of the bed
Semi-Fowler's position	Head of bed is raised between 15° and 45°, typically at 30°.	Relief from lying position To promote lung expansion
Trendelenburg's position	Head of bed is lowered and the foot raised in a straight incline.	To promote venous circulation in certain clients To provide postural drainage of basal lung lobes
Reverse Trendelenburg's position	Head of bed raised and the foot lowered. Straight tilt in direction opposite to Trendelenburg's position.	To promote stomach emptying and prevent esophageal reflux in client with hiatal hernia

and effective means of preventing clients from falling out of bed. Research, however, has not validated this assumption. In fact, studies have shown that raised side rails do not prevent clients from getting out of bed unassisted and have led to more serious falls, injuries, and even death. If all the bed's side rails are up and restrict the client's freedom to leave the bed, and the client did not voluntarily request all rails to be up, they are considered a restraint by the Centers for Medicare and Medicaid Services (CMS). If, however, one side rail is up to assist the client to get in and out of the bed, it is not a restraint.

In addition to falls because of raised side rails, side rail entrapment can occur. Deaths have occurred as a direct result of side rail entrapment in a variety of healthcare settings, including hospitals. Client entrapment occurs when a client gets caught or entangled in the openings or gaps around the hospital bed—this usually involves a side rail. Clients at highest risk for entrapment include older or frail adults and clients who are agitated, delirious, confused, and hypoxic.

The CMS mandates that nurses in both acute care and long-term care facilities decrease the routine use of side rails. Alternatives to side rails do exist and can include low-height bed, mats placed at the side of the bed, motion sensors, and bed alarms (see Chapter 32 ∞).

Safety Alert! **SAFETY**

Side rail entrapment, injuries, and death do occur. When side rails are used, the nurse must assess the client's physical and mental status and closely monitor high-risk (frail, older, or confused) clients.

Footboard or Footboot

These devices are used to support the immobilized client's foot in a normal right angle to the legs to prevent plantar flexion contractures (see Chapter 44 ∞).

Intravenous Rods

Intravenous rods (poles, stands, standards), usually made of metal, support IV infusion containers while fluid is being administered to a client. These rods were traditionally freestanding on the floor beside the bed. Now, IV rods are often attached to the hospital beds. Some hospital units have overhead hanging rods on a track for IVs.

Making Beds

Nurses need to be able to prepare hospital beds in different ways for specific purposes. In most instances, beds are made after the client receives hygienic care and when beds are unoccupied. At times, however, nurses need to make an occupied bed or prepare a bed for a client who is having surgery (an anesthetic, postoperative, or surgical bed). Regardless of what type of bed equipment is available, whether the bed is occupied or unoccupied, or the purpose for which the bed is being prepared, certain practice guidelines pertain to all bedmaking.

Unoccupied Bed

An unoccupied bed can be either closed or open. Generally the top covers of an open bed are folded back (thus the term *open bed*) to make it easier for a client to get in. Open and closed beds are made the same way, except that the top sheet, blanket, and bedspread of a closed bed are drawn up to the top of the bed and under the pillows.

Beds are often changed after bed baths. The replacement clean linen can be collected before the bath. The linens are not usually changed unless they are soiled. Check the policy at each clinical agency. Unfitted sheets, blankets, and bedspreads are mitered at the corners of the bed. The purpose of mitering is to secure the bedclothes while the bed is occupied (Figure 33.13 ■). Skill 33.8 explains how to change an unoccupied bed.

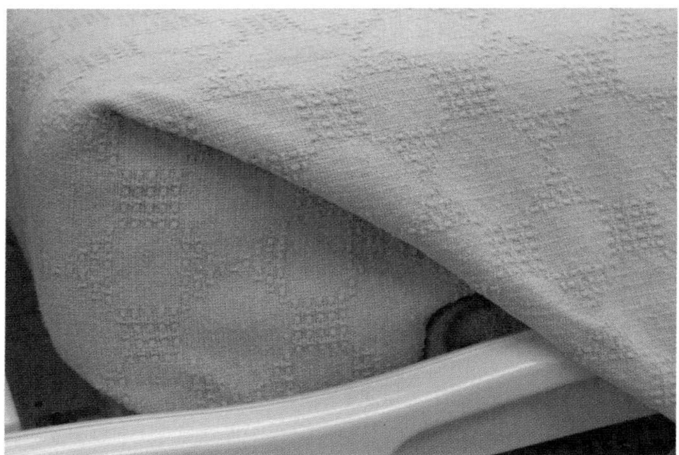

Figure 33.13 ■ Mitered corners help keep bed linens secure.

PRACTICE GUIDELINES **Bedmaking**

- Wear gloves while handling a client's used bed linen. Linens and equipment that have been soiled with secretions and excretions harbor microorganisms that can be transmitted to others directly or by the nurse's hands or uniform. Wash hands after removing gloves.
- Hold soiled linen away from uniform.
- Linen for one client is never (even momentarily) placed on another client's bed.
- Place soiled linen directly in a portable linen hamper or tucked into a pillow case at the end of the bed before it is gathered up for disposal.
- Do not shake soiled linen in the air because shaking can disseminate secretions and excretions and the microorganisms they contain.
- When stripping and making a bed, conserve time and energy by stripping and making up one side as much as possible before working on the other side.
- To avoid unnecessary trips to the linen supply area, gather all linen before starting to strip a bed.

Changing an Unoccupied Bed

PURPOSES

- To promote the client's comfort
- To provide a clean, neat environment for the client
- To provide a smooth, wrinkle-free bed foundation, thus minimizing sources of skin irritation

ASSESSMENT

Assess

- Client's health status to determine that the client can safely get out of bed. In some hospitals it is necessary to have a written order to get out of bed if the client has been in bed continuously.
- Client's blood pressure, pulse, and respirations if indicated. **Rationale:** *Client may experience orthostatic hypotension when moved from a lying position to sitting to standing, particularly if it is the first time out of bed for a while.*
- Client's mobility status. **Rationale:** *This may influence the need for additional assistance with transferring the client from the bed to a chair.*
- Tubes and equipment connected to the client. **Rationale:** *This may influence the need for additional linens or waterproof pads.*

PLANNING

Assignment

Bedmaking is usually assigned to AP. If appropriate, inform the AP of the proper disposal method of linens that contain drainage. Ask the AP to inform you immediately if any tubes or dressings become dislodged or removed. Stress the importance of the call light being readily available while the client is out of bed.

Equipment

- Clean gloves, if needed
- Two flat sheets or one fitted and one flat sheet
- Cloth drawsheet (optional)
- One blanket
- One bedspread
- Incontinent pads (optional)
- Pillowcase(s) for the head pillow(s)
- Plastic laundry bag or portable linen hamper, if available

IMPLEMENTATION

Preparation

Determine what linens the client may already have in the room. **Rationale:** *This avoids accumulation of unnecessary extra linens.*

Performance

1. If the client is in bed, prior to performing the procedure, introduce self and verify the client's identity using agency protocol. Explain to the client what you are going to do, why it is necessary, and how to participate.
2. Perform hand hygiene and observe other appropriate infection control procedures.
3. Provide for client privacy.
4. Place the fresh linen on the client's chair or overbed table; do not use another client's bed. **Rationale:** *This prevents cross-contamination via soiled linen.*
5. Assess and assist the client out of bed using assistive devices (e.g., cane, walker, safety belt) as appropriate. **Rationale:** *This ensures client safety.*
   - Make sure that this is an appropriate and convenient time for the client to be out of bed.
   - Assist the client to a comfortable chair.
6. Raise the bed to a comfortable working height.
7. Apply clean gloves if linens and equipment have been soiled with secretions or excretions.
8. Strip the bed.
   - Check bed linens for any items belonging to the client, and detach the call bell or any drainage tubes from the bed linen.
   - Loosen all bedding systematically, starting at the head of the bed on the far side and moving around the bed up to the head of the bed on the near side. **Rationale:** *Moving around the bed systematically prevents stretching and reaching and possible muscle strain.*
   - Remove the pillowcases, if soiled, and place the pillows on the bedside chair near the foot of the bed.
   - Fold reusable linens, such as the bedspread and top sheet on the bed, into fourths. First, fold the linen in half by bringing the top edge even with the bottom edge, and then grasp it at the center of the middle fold and bottom edges. ❶ **Rationale:** *Folding linens saves time and energy when reapplying the linens on the bed and keeps them clean.*
   - Remove the incontinent pad and discard it if soiled.
   - Roll all soiled linen inside the bottom sheet, hold it away from your uniform, and place it directly in the linen hamper, not on the floor. ❷ **Rationale:** *These actions are essential to prevent the transmission of microorganisms to the nurse and others.*
   - Grasp the mattress securely, using the lugs if present, and move the mattress up to the head of the bed.
   - Remove and discard gloves if used. Perform hand hygiene.
9. Apply the bottom sheet and drawsheet (optional).
   - If using a flat sheet, place the folded bottom sheet with its center fold on the center of the bed. Make sure the sheet is hem side down for a smooth foundation. Spread the sheet out over the mattress, and allow a sufficient amount of sheet at the top to tuck under the mattress **Rationale:** *The top of the sheet needs to be well tucked under to remain securely in place, especially when the head of the bed is elevated.*

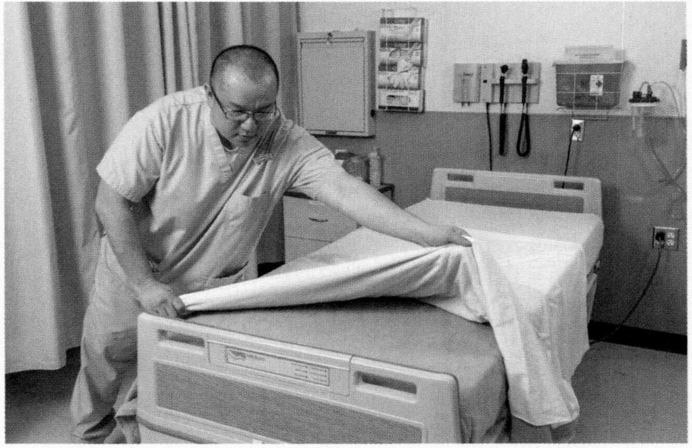

❶ Fold reusable linens into fourths when removing them from the bed.

Continued on page 798

Changing an Unoccupied Bed—*continued*

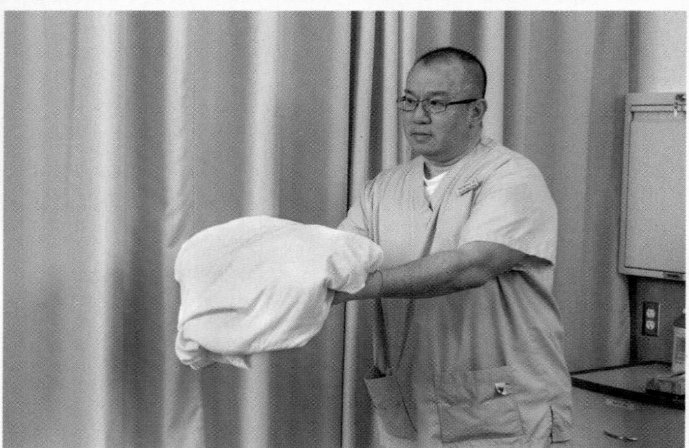

2 Roll soiled linen inside the bottom sheet and hold away from the body.

- If using a fitted sheet, pull sheet over ends of mattress. 3
- Place the flat sheet along the edge of the mattress at the foot of the bed and do not tuck it in (unless it is a contour or fitted sheet).
- Miter the sheet at the top corner on the near side and tuck the sheet under the mattress, working from the head of the bed to the foot.
- If a drawsheet is used, place it over the bottom sheet so that the center fold is at the centerline of the bed and the top and bottom edges extend from the middle of where the client's back would be on the bed to the area where the midthigh or knee would be. Fanfold the uppermost half of the folded drawsheet at the center or far edge of the bed and tuck in the near edge.
- *Optional:* Before moving to the other side of the bed, place the top linens on the bed hem side up, unfold them, tuck them in, and miter the bottom corners. **Rationale:** *Completing one entire side of the bed at a time saves time and energy*.

10. Move to the other side and secure the bottom linens.
- Tuck in the bottom sheet under the head of the mattress, pull the sheet firmly, and miter the corner of the sheet.
- Pull the remainder of the sheet firmly so that there are no wrinkles. **Rationale:** *Wrinkles can cause discomfort for the client and breakdown of skin*. Tuck the sheet in at the side.
- Tuck in the drawsheet, if appropriate.

11. Apply the top sheet, blanket, and spread.
- Place the top sheet, hem side up, on the bed so that its center fold is at the center of the bed and the top edge is even with the top edge of the mattress.
- Unfold the sheet over the bed.
- Follow the same procedure for the blanket and the spread, but place the top edges about 15 cm (6 in.) from the head of the bed to allow a cuff of sheet to be folded over them.
- Tuck in the sheet, blanket, and spread at the foot of the bed, and miter the corner, using all three layers of linen. Leave the sides of the top sheet, blanket, and spread hanging freely. Loosen the top covers around the foot of the bed to provide space for the client's feet.
- Fold the top of the top sheet down over the spread, providing a cuff. 4 **Rationale:** *A cuff on the sheet makes it easier for the client to pull the covers up*.
- Move to the other side of the bed and secure the top bedding in the same manner.

12. Put clean pillowcases on the pillows as required.
- Grasp the closed end of the pillowcase at the center with one hand.
- Gather up the sides of the pillowcase and place them over the hand grasping the case. Then grasp the center of one short side of the pillow through the pillowcase. 5
- With the free hand, pull the pillowcase over the pillow.
- Adjust the pillowcase so that the pillow fits into the corners of the case and the seams are straight. **Rationale:** *A smoothly fitting pillowcase is more comfortable than a wrinkled one*.
- Place the pillows appropriately at the head of the bed.

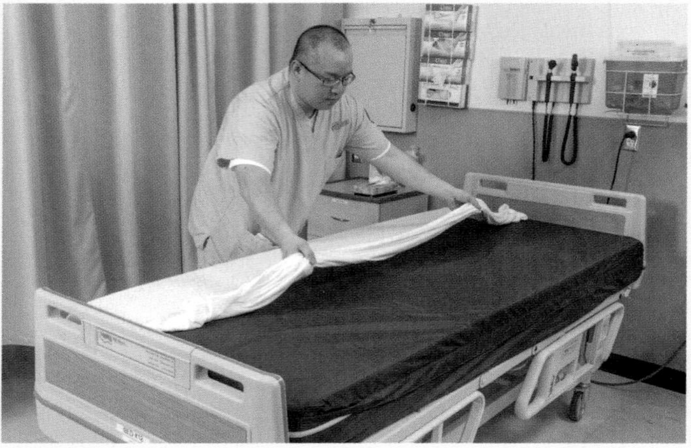

3 Placing the bottom sheet on the bed.

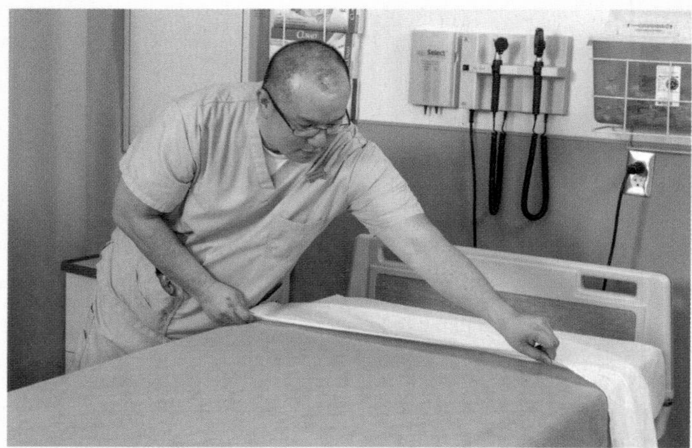

4 Making a cuff of the top linens.

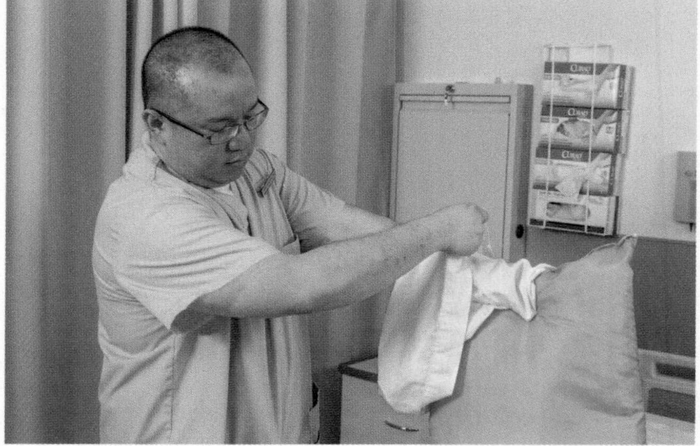

5 Method for putting a clean pillowcase on a pillow.

Changing an Unoccupied Bed—*continued*

13. Provide for client comfort and safety.
- Attach the signal cord so that the client can conveniently reach it. Most beds now have a call light button on the side rail.
- If the bed is currently being used by a client, either fold back the top covers at one side or fanfold them down to the center of the bed. **Rationale:** *This makes it easier for the client to get into the bed.*
- Place the bedside table and the overbed table so that they are available to the client.
- Leave the bed in the high position if the client is returning by stretcher, or place it in the low position if the client is returning to bed after being up.

14. Document and report pertinent data.
- Bedmaking is not normally recorded.
- Record any nursing assessments, such as the client's physical status and pulse and respiratory rates before and after being out of bed, as indicated.

Variation: Surgical Bed

A surgical bed is used for the client who is having surgery and will return to bed for the postoperative phase. When making a surgical bed, the linens are fanfolded *horizontally* to facilitate transfer of the client into the bed. In some agencies, the client is brought back to the unit on a stretcher and transferred to the bed in the room. In other agencies, the client's bed is brought to the surgery suite and the client is transferred there. In the latter situation, the bed needs to be made with clean linens as soon as the client goes to surgery so that it can be taken to the operating room when needed.

1. Strip the bed.
2. Place and leave the pillows on the bedside chair. **Rationale:** *Pillows are left on a chair to facilitate transferring the client into the bed.*
3. Apply the bottom linens as for an unoccupied bed. Place a bath blanket on the foundation of the bed if this is agency practice. **Rationale:** *A flannel bath blanket provides additional warmth.*
4. Place the top covers (sheet, blanket, and bedspread) on the bed as you would for an unoccupied bed. Do not tuck them in or miter the corners.
5. Make a cuff at the top of the bed as you would for an unoccupied bed. Fold the top linens up from the bottom.
6. On the side of the bed where the client will be transferred, fold up the two outer corners of the top linens so they meet in the middle of the bed forming a triangle. ❻
7. Pick up the apex of the triangle and fanfold the top linens lengthwise to the other side of the bed. ❼ **Rationale:** *This facilitates the client's transfer into the bed.*

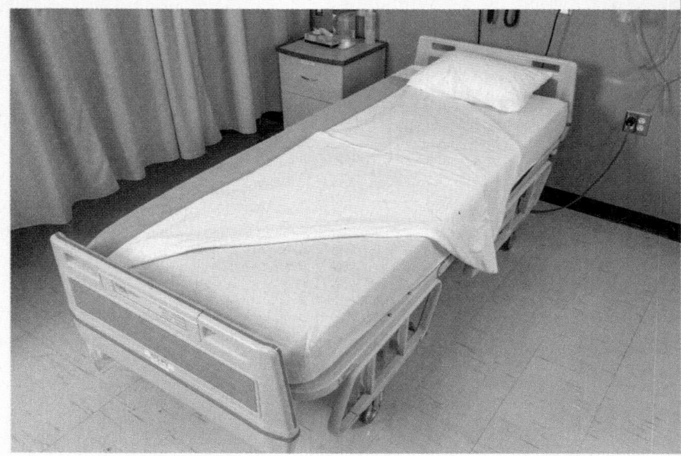

❻ Fold up the two outer corners of the top linens, forming a triangle.

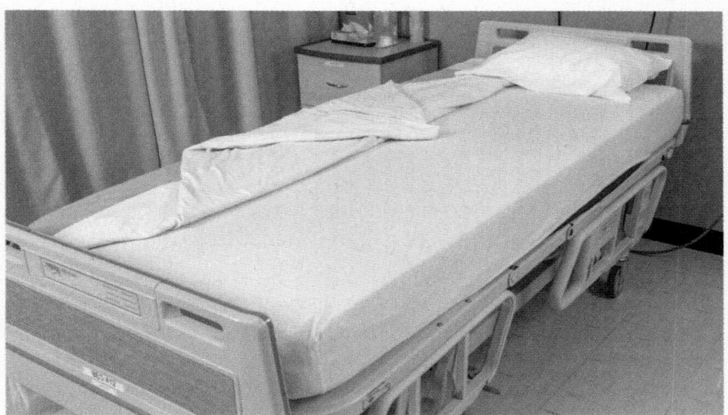

❼ Surgical bed. The linens are horizontally fanfolded to the other side of the bed to facilitate transfer of the client into the bed.

8. Leave the bed in high position with the side rails down. **Rationale:** *The high position facilitates the transfer of the client.*
9. Lock the wheels of the bed if the bed is not to be moved. **Rationale:** *Locking the wheels keeps the bed from rolling when the client is transferred from the stretcher to the bed.*

EVALUATION
- Make sure the call light is accessible to the client.
- Compare client parameters of activity (e.g., pulse and respirations) to previous assessment data particularly if the client has been on bedrest for an extended period of time or if it is the first time that the client is getting out of bed after surgery.

Changing an Occupied Bed

Some clients may be too weak to get out of bed. Either the nature of their illness may contraindicate their sitting out of bed, or they may be restricted in bed by the presence of traction or other therapies. When changing an occupied bed, the nurse works quickly and disturbs the client as little as possible to conserve the client's energy, using the following guidelines:

- Maintain the client in good body alignment. Never move or position a client in a manner that is contraindicated by the client's health. Obtain help if necessary to ensure safety.
- Move the client gently and smoothly. Rough handling can cause the client discomfort and abrade the skin.
- Explain what you plan to do throughout the procedure before you do it. Use terms that the client can understand. Encourage client participation when appropriate.
- Use the bedmaking time, like the bed bath time, to assess and meet the client's needs.

See Skill 33.9 for instructions on changing an occupied bed.

SKILL 33.9

Changing an Occupied Bed

PURPOSES

- To conserve the client's energy
- To promote client comfort
- To provide a clean, neat environment for the client
- To provide a smooth, wrinkle-free bed foundation, thus minimizing sources of skin irritation

ASSESSMENT

- Assess skin condition and need for a special mattress (e.g., an egg-crate mattress), footboard, or heel protectors.
- Assess client's ability to reposition self. **Rationale:** *This will determine if additional assistance is needed.*
- Determine presence of incontinence or excessive drainage from other sources indicating the need for protective waterproof pads.
- Note specific orders or precautions for moving and positioning the client.

PLANNING

Assignment

Bedmaking is usually assigned to AP. Inform the AP to what extent the client can assist or if another individual will be needed to assist the AP. Instruct the AP about the handling of any dressings or tubes of the client and also the need for special equipment (e.g., footboard, heel protectors), if appropriate.

Equipment

- Two flat sheets or one fitted and one flat sheet
- Cloth drawsheet (optional)
- One blanket
- One bedspread
- Incontinent pads (optional)
- Pillowcase(s) for the head pillow(s)
- Plastic laundry bag or portable linen hamper, if available

IMPLEMENTATION

Preparation

- Determine what linens the client may already have in the room. **Rationale:** *This avoids hoarding of unnecessary extra linens.*

Performance

1. Prior to performing the procedure introduce self and verify the client's identity using agency protocol. Explain to the client what you are going to do, why it is necessary, and how to participate.
2. Perform hand hygiene and observe other appropriate infection control procedures. Apply clean gloves if linen is soiled with body fluids.
3. Provide for client privacy.
4. Remove the top bedding.
   - Remove any equipment attached to the bed linen, such as a signal light.
   - Loosen all top linen at the foot of the bed, and remove the spread and the blanket.
   - Leave the top sheet over the client (the top sheet can remain over the client if it is being changed and if it will provide sufficient warmth), or replace it with a bath blanket as follows:
     a. Spread the bath blanket over the top sheet.
     b. Ask the client to hold the top edge of the blanket.
     c. Reaching under the blanket from the side, grasp the top edge of the sheet and draw it down to the foot of the bed, leaving the blanket in place. ❶
     d. Remove the sheet from the bed and place it in the soiled linen hamper.
5. Change the bottom sheet and the drawsheet.
   - Raise the side rail that the client will turn toward. **Rationale:** *This protects clients from falling and allows them to support themselves in the side-lying position*. If there is no side rail, have another nurse support the client at the edge of the bed.
   - Assist the client to turn on the side away from the nurse and toward the raised side rail.
   - Loosen the bottom linens on the side of the bed near the nurse.

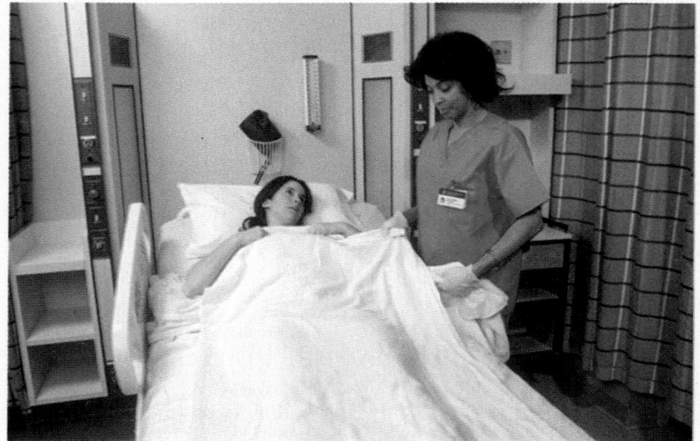

❶ Removing top linens under a bath blanket.

   - Fanfold the dirty linen (i.e., drawsheet and the bottom sheet) toward the center of the bed ❷ as close to and under the client as possible. **Rationale:** *This leaves the near half of the bed free to be changed*.
   - Place the new bottom sheet on the bed, and vertically fanfold the half to be used on the far side of the bed as close to the client as possible. ❸ Tuck the sheet under the near half of the bed and miter the corner if a contour sheet is not being used.
   - Place the clean drawsheet on the bed with the center fold at the center of the bed. Fanfold the uppermost half vertically at the center of the bed and tuck the near side edge under the side of the mattress. ❹
   - Assist the client to roll over toward you, over the fanfolded bed linens at the center of the bed, onto the clean side of the bed. Ensure that the client is not near the edge of the bed.

Changing an Occupied Bed—*continued*

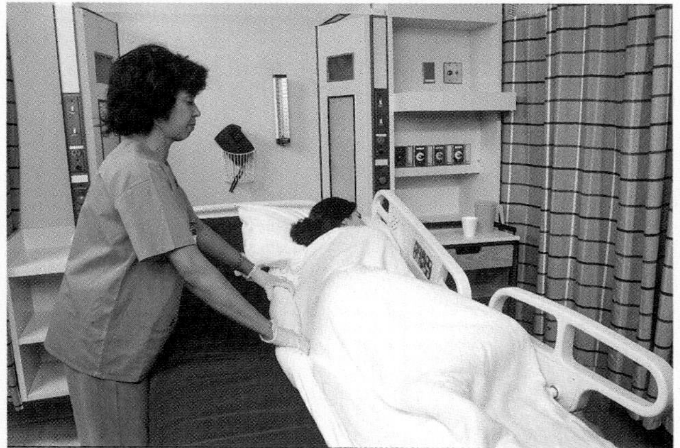
❷ Moving soiled linen as close to the client as possible.

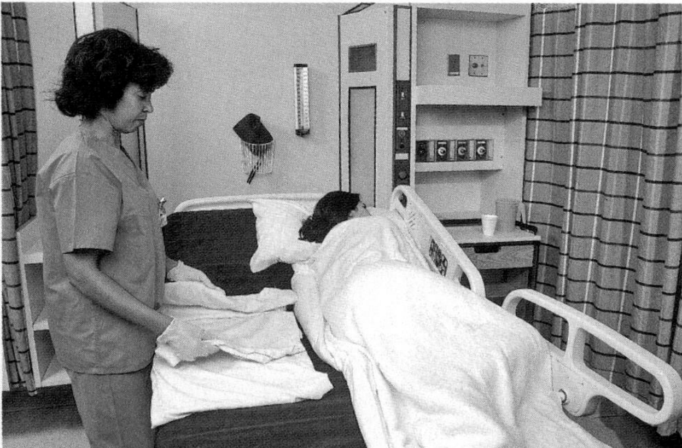
❸ Placing a new bottom sheet on half of the bed.

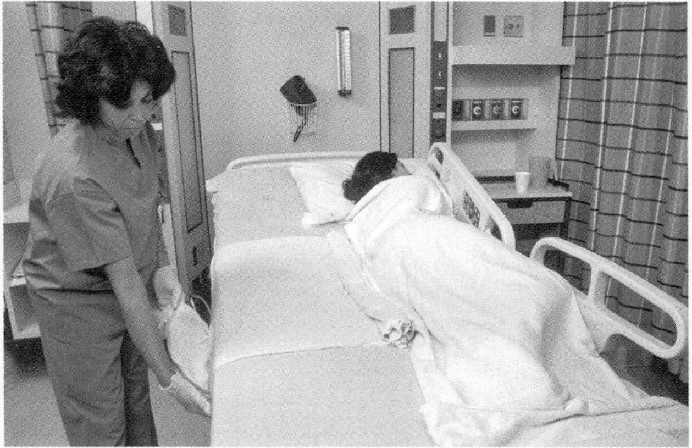
❹ Placing a clean drawsheet on the bed.

- Move the pillows to the clean side for the client's use. Raise the side rail before leaving the side of the bed.
- Move to the other side of the bed and lower the side rail.
- Remove the used linen and place it in the portable hamper.
- Unfold the fanfolded bottom sheet from the center of the bed.
- Facing the side of the bed, use both hands to pull the bottom sheet so that it is smooth and tuck the excess under the side of the mattress.
- Unfold the drawsheet fanfolded at the center of the bed and pull it tightly with both hands. Pull the sheet in three divisions: (a) Face the side of the bed to pull the middle division, (b) face the far top corner to pull the bottom division, and (c) face the far bottom corner to pull the top division.
- Tuck the excess drawsheet under the side of the mattress.

6. Reposition the client in the center of the bed.
- Reposition the pillows at the center of the bed.
- Assist the client to the center of the bed. Determine what position the client requires or prefers and assist the client to that position.

7. Apply or complete the top bedding.
- Spread the top sheet over the client and either ask the client to hold the top edge of the sheet or tuck it under the shoulders. The sheet should remain over the client when the bath blanket or used sheet is removed. ❺
- Complete the top of the bed.

8. Ensure continued safety of the client.
- Raise the side rails. Place the bed in the low position before leaving the bedside.
- Attach the call light to the bed linen within the client's reach.
- Put items used by the client within easy reach.

9. Document. Many agencies use a checklist that indicates if bed linens were changed.

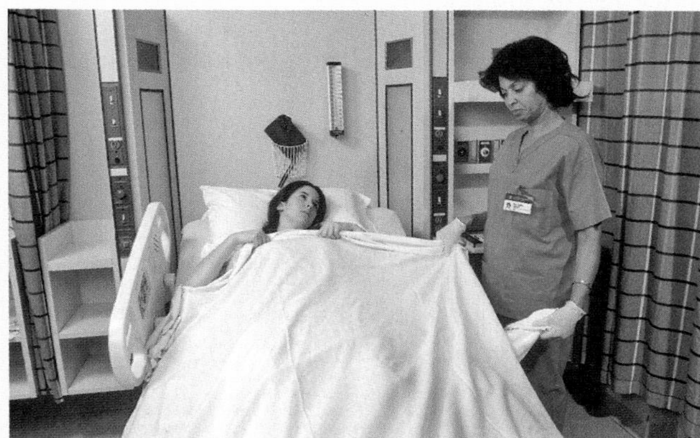
❺ Client holds the top edge of sheet while the nurse removes the bath blanket.

EVALUATION

- Conduct appropriate follow-up, such as determining client's comfort and safety, patency of all drainage tubes, and client's access to call light to summon help when needed.
- Reassess all tubing, oxygen apparatus, IV pumps, and so forth. **Rationale:** *This prevents errors in supportive devices resulting from procedure.*

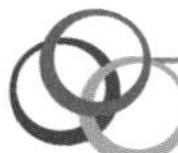

Critical Thinking Checkpoint

It is the fourth day following a female client's abdominal surgery. She is progressing well, is ambulating several times each day, has been providing for her own hygienic needs, and is planning on going home tomorrow. During your early morning assessment, you note that the client's hair is oily and matted and she has an unpleasant body odor. Her dentures in a container at the bedside are in need of cleaning. You check her abdominal incision and verify that there is no drainage, redness, or signs of infection. You inquire about her ability to take care of her own bath and personal needs, and offer to assist her with her bath. She replies that she had a bath yesterday, doesn't feel that she needs another one today, and requests to omit her personal care for the day.

1. You are considering altered self-care (bathing) as an appropriate nursing diagnosis for the client. You review the signs and symptoms and related factors and discover what?
2. What else should you ask the client?
3. Why is it important that you obtain the assessments you have already completed along with the above questions you asked?
4. What approaches might you use if you feel that the client does need her hair shampooed and needs to have her personal care attended to?
5. What advantages does performing baths and personal hygiene for clients offer to the nurse?

Answers to Critical Thinking Checkpoint questions are available on the faculty resources website. Please consult with your instructor.

Chapter 33 Review

CHAPTER HIGHLIGHTS

- Clients' hygienic practices are influenced by numerous factors including culture, religion, environment, developmental level, health and energy, and personal preferences.
- The major functions of the skin are to protect underlying tissues, regulate body temperature, secrete sebum, transmit sensations through nerve receptors for sensory perception, and produce and absorb vitamin D in conjunction with ultraviolet rays from the sun.
- When planning hygiene care, the nurse must take the client's preferences into consideration.
- Nurses provide perineal-genital care for clients who are unable to do so for themselves.
- Nurses can often teach clients how to prevent foot problems.
- Oral hygiene should include daily dental flossing and mechanical brushing of the teeth.
- Regular dental checkups and fluoride supplements are recommended to maintain healthy teeth.
- Nurses provide special oral care to clients who are unconscious or debilitated.
- Hair care varies per individual client. It is necessary for the nurse to discuss the client preferences for hair care.
- Clients with a hearing aid may require nursing assistance with the device.
- Nurses need to provide a positive and safe environment for clients.
- Nurses need to be able to prepare hospital beds in different ways for specific purposes.

TEST YOUR KNOWLEDGE

1. A client can bathe most of her body except for the back, hands, and feet. She also can walk to and from the bathroom and dress herself when given clothing. Which functional level describes this client?
   1. Totally dependent (+4)
   2. Moderately dependent (+3)
   3. Semidependent (+2)
   4. Independent (0)

2. The client is unresponsive and requires total care by nursing staff. Which assessment does the nurse check first before providing special oral care to the client?
   1. Presence of pain
   2. Condition of the skin
   3. Gag reflex
   4. Range of motion

3. Which assessment finding would be normal with a client's hair when giving a shampoo?
   1. Dry, dark, thin
   2. Smooth, taut, shiny
   3. Smooth texture and not oily or dry
   4. Tender, warm scalp

4. The client wears an in-the-ear (ITE) hearing aid and because of arthritis needs someone to insert the hearing aid. Which action does the nurse teach the assistive personnel (AP) to do before inserting the client's hearing aid?
   1. Turn the hearing aid off.
   2. Soak the hearing aid in soapy solution to clean it.
   3. Turn the volume all the way up.
   4. Remove the batteries.

5. When making a client's bed, which safety measure will the nurse implement?
   1. Begin at the head and move toward the foot, loosening bottom linens.
   2. Miter corners at the head of the bed.
   3. Place the soiled sheet in a laundry bag.
   4. Prepare the client.

6. The nurse is preparing to provide a morning bath to a client diagnosed with dementia. What can the nurse do to ensure a positive bathing experience for the client? Select all that apply.
   1. Move slowly
   2. Be flexible
   3. Help the client feel in control
   4. Avoid stopping once the bath is started
   5. Be prepared
7. The nurse is observing the assistive personnel (AP) perform perineal care for a client. Which action indicates that the nurse needs to discuss additional teaching with the AP?
   1. Uses a clean portion of the washcloth for each stroke
   2. Wipes from the pubis to the rectum
   3. Uses clean gloves
   4. Does not retract the foreskin
8. The nurse is planning a presentation on oral health at an intergenerational community center. Which statements will be important to include? Select all that apply.
   1. Using a bottle during naps and bedtime can cause dental caries in a toddler.
   2. Schedule a visit to the dentist when your child is ready to go to school.
   3. It is important for parents to supervise a child's brushing of his or her teeth.
   4. Most older adults have dentures and don't need to worry about oral care.
   5. Older adults are at risk for periodontal disease.
9. The nurse is discussing foot care with a client who was recently diagnosed with diabetes. Which statement by the client indicates a need for further teaching?
   1. "I am going to use a mirror to check my feet."
   2. "I enjoy walking barefoot around the house."
   3. "I will file my nails."
   4. "I will increase the time that I wear new shoes each day."
10. The client is complaining of shortness of breath. His respirations are 28 and labored. The bed is currently in the flat position. The nurse puts the bed in which position?
   1. Fowler's
   2. Semi-Fowler's
   3. Trendelenburg's
   4. Reverse Trendelenburg's

See Answers to Test Your Knowledge in Appendix A

READINGS AND REFERENCES

Suggested Readings

Bencosme, J. (2018). Periodontal disease: What nurses need to know. *Nursing, 48*(7), 23–27. doi:10.1097/01.NUERSE.0000534088.56615.e4

The author, a registered dental hygienist, provides a comprehensive overview of periodontal disease and practical steps nurses can take to help clients treat the disease.

Jablonski-Jaudon, R. A., Kolanowski, A. M., Winstead, V., Jones-Townsend, C., & Azuero, A. (2016). Maturation of the MOUTh intervention: From reducing threat to relationship-centered care. *Journal of Gerontological Nursing, 42*(3), 15–23. doi:10.3928/00989134-20160212-05

The authors state that mouth care is oral infection control (p. 15). This is especially important in residents of nursing homes because consistent oral hygiene reduces the incidence of pneumonia. One of the main reasons for the omission of mouth care is care resistant behavior (CRB). The article is the summary of a research study; however, the description of the various strategies to prevent and minimize CRB is very informative and includes approach, establishing rapport, avoiding elderspeak, using gestures or pantomime, cueing, and chaining.

Related Research

Bridges, E., McNeil, M., & Munroe, M. (2016). Research in review: Driving critical care practice change. *American Journal of Critical Care, 25*(1), 76–84. doi:10.4037/ajcc2016564

Dale, C. M., Angus, J. E., Sinuff, T., & Rose, L. (2016). Ethnographic investigation of oral care in the intensive care unit. *American Journal of Critical Care, 25*(3), 249–256. doi:10.4037/ajcc2016795

Lee, K. H., Plassman, B. L., Pan, W., & Wu, B. (2016). Mediation effect of oral hygiene on the relationship between cognitive function and oral health in older adults. *Journal of Gerontological Nursing, 42*(5), 30–37. doi:10.3928/00989134-20151218-03

References

Alzheimer's Association. (n.d.). *Bathing*. Retrieved from https://www.alz.org/help-support/caregiving/daily-care/bathing

American Dental Association. (n.d.). *5 steps to a flawless floss*. Retrieved from http://www.mouthhealthy.org/en/az-topics/f/Flossing%20Steps

American Dental Association. (2018). *Oral health topics: Xerostomia (dry mouth)*. Retrieved from http://www.ada.org/en/member-center/oral-health-topics/xerostomia

Ball, J. W., Bindler, R. C., Cowen, K., & Shaw, M. (2017). *Principles of pediatric nursing: Caring for children* (7th ed.). New York, NY: Pearson.

Centers for Disease Control and Prevention. (2016). *Head lice treatment*. Retrieved from https://www.cdc.gov/parasites/lice/head/treatment.html

Centers for Disease Control and Prevention. (2017). *Scabies fact sheet*. Retrieved from https://www.cdc.gov/parasites/scabies/fact_sheet.html

Curl Centric. (n.d.). *Dreadlocks: The only guide you'll ever need*. Retrieved from https://www.curlcentric.com/dreadlocks

Denny, J., & Munro, C. L. (2017). Chlorhexidine bathing effects on health-care-associated infections. *Biological Research for Nursing, 19*, 123–136. doi:10/1177/1099800416654013

Desai, N. (2018). *Body piercing in adolescents and young adults*. Retrieved from https://www.uptodate.com/contents/body-piercing-in-adolescents-and-young-adults

Hayter, K. L. (2016). Listen up for safe ear irrigation. *Nursing, 46*(6), 62–65. doi:10.1097/01.NURSE.0000481437.02178.3b

Humphreys, K. (2016). Oral health of older people living in the community. *British Journal of Community Nursing, 21*, 332–334.

Jin, J. (2017). *Do you really need shampoo?* Retrieved from http://www.realsimple.com/beauty-fashion/hair/hair-care/co-wash-natural-hair

Lee, K. H., Plassman, B. L., Pan, W., & Wu, B. (2016). Mediation effect of oral hygiene on the relationship between cognitive function and oral health in older adults. *Journal of Gerontological Nursing, 42*(5), 30–37. doi:10.3928/00989134-20151218-03

Matrix. (n.d.). *6 co-washing tips for natural and relaxed African American hair*. Retrieved from http://www.matrix.com/blog/6-co-washing-tips-for-natural-and-relaxed-aftrican-american-hair

McGough, N. H., Keane, T., Uppal, A., Dumlao, M., Rutherford, W., Kellogg, K., . . . Fields, W. (2018). Noise reduction in progressive care units. *Journal of Nursing Care Quality, 33*(2), 166–172. doi:10.1097/NCQ.0000000000000275

Oral care for acutely and critically ill patients. (2017). *Critical Care Nurse, 37*(3), e19–e21. doi:10.4037/ccn2017179

Robinson, C. , Hoze, M., Hevener, S., & Nichols, A. A. (2018). Development of an RN champion model to improve the outcomes of ventilator-associated pneumonia patients in the intensive care unit. *The Journal of Nursing Administration, 48*(2), 79–84. doi:10.1097/NNA.0000000000000578

Sheffler, K. (2018). The power of a toothbrush. *ASHA Leader, 23*(5), 50–57. doi:10.1044/leader.FTR1.23052018.50

White, L. (2017). *How to comb natural [African-American] hair without breakage*. Retrieved from https://www.dryscalp-gone.com/comb-natural-hair-without-breakage/

Wilkinson, J. M., & Barcas, L. (2017). *Pearson nursing diagnosis handbook* (11th ed.). New York, NY: Pearson.

Williams, C. (n.d.). *Cowashing African American hair*. Retrieved from http://hair.lovetoknow.com/Cowashing_African_American_Hair

Selected Bibliography

Association of Professional Piercers. (n.d.). *Suggested aftercare for oral piercings*. Retrieved from https://www.safepiercing.org/docs/APP_Oral_13-print.pdf

Flavell, T. (2016). Using soap substitutes, bath additives and leave-on emollients. *Journal of Community Nursing, 30*(3), 29–34.

Hearing aids linked to better cognitive function in elderly. (2016). *ASHA Leader, 21*(7), 15. doi:10.1044/leader.RIB2.21072016.15

Hearing loss & hearing aids. (2016). *Hearing Health, 32*(2), 4.

Hedges, C., Wolak, E., Smith-Miller, C. A., & Brown, T. (2018). The path to a quieter unit. *American Nurse Today, 13*(9), 40–46.

Oral care for acutely and critically ill patients. (2018). *Critical Care Nurse, 38*(6), 80.

While, A. (2016). Identifying hearing loss in older people. *British Journal of Community Nursing, 21*, 318. doi:10.12968/bjcn.2016.21.6.318

34 Diagnostic Testing

LEARNING OUTCOMES

After completing this chapter, you will be able to:

1. Describe the nurse's role for each of the phases involved in diagnostic testing.
2. List common blood tests.
3. Discuss the nursing responsibilities for specimen collection.
4. Explain the rationale for the collection of each type of specimen.
5. Describe how to collect and test stool specimens.
6. Compare and contrast the different types of urine specimens.
7. Describe how to collect sputum and throat specimens.
8. Describe visualization procedures that may be used for the client with gastrointestinal, urinary, and cardiopulmonary alterations.
9. Compare and contrast CT, MRI, and nuclear imaging studies.
10. Describe the nurse's role in caring for clients undergoing aspiration and biopsy procedures.
11. Verbalize the steps used in:
    a. Obtaining a capillary blood specimen to measure blood glucose.
    b. Collecting a urine specimen for culture and sensitivity by clean catch.
12. Recognize when it is appropriate to assign diagnostic testing skills to assistive personnel.
13. Demonstrate appropriate documentation and reporting of diagnostic testing information.

KEY TERMS

abdominal paracentesis, *827*
angiography, *824*
anoscopy, *823*
arterial blood gases, *808*
ascites, *827*
aspiration, *826*
biopsy, *826*
blood chemistry, *808*
blood urea nitrogen (BUN), *807*
cannula, *827*
clean-catch urine specimens, *816*
clean voided urine specimens, *816*
colonoscopy, *823*
complete blood count (CBC), *805*
computed tomography (CT), *825*
creatinine, *807*
cystoscope, *824*
cystoscopy, *824*
echocardiogram, *824*
electrocardiogram (ECG), *824*
electrocardiography, *824*
expectorate, *822*
guaiac test, *815*
hematocrit (Hct), *807*
hemoglobin (Hgb), *807*
hemoglobin A1C (HbA1C), *808*
hemoptysis, *823*
intravenous pyelography (IVP), *824*
kidneys, ureters, and bladder (KUB), *824*
leukocyte, *807*
lumbar puncture, *826*
lung scan, *824*
magnetic resonance imaging (MRI), *825*
manometer, *827*
midstream urine specimens, *816*
occult blood, *815*
peak level, *807*
phlebotomist, *805*
polycythemia, *807*
positron emission tomography (PET), *826*
proctoscopy, *823*
proctosigmoidoscopy, *823*
radiopharmaceutical, *825*
reagent, *816*
red blood cell (RBC) count, *807*
red blood cell (RBC) indices, *807*
retrograde pyelography, *824*
saliva, *822*
serum osmolality, *807*
specific gravity, *821*
sputum, *822*
steatorrhea, *814*
stress electrocardiography, *824*
thoracentesis, *828*
trocar, *827*
trough level, *807*
ultrasonography, *824*
urine osmolality, *822*
venipuncture, *805*
white blood cell (WBC) count, *807*

Introduction

Diagnostic tests are tools that provide information about clients. Tests may be used for basic screening as part of a wellness check. Frequently tests are used to help confirm a diagnosis, monitor an illness, and provide valuable information about the client's response to treatment. Nurses require knowledge of the most common laboratory and diagnostic tests because one primary role of the nurse is to teach the client and family or significant other how to prepare for the test and the care that may be required following the test. Nurses must also know the implications of the test results in order to provide the most appropriate nursing care for the client.

Diagnostic Testing Phases

Diagnostic testing occurs in many environments. The traditional sites include hospitals, clinics, and the primary care provider's office. Many test sites, however, are located in the community. Examples include the home, workplace, shopping malls, and mobile units. The more complex diagnostic tests are performed at diagnostic centers specifically built to provide those tests.

Diagnostic testing involves three phases: pretest, intratest, and posttest.

Pretest

The major focus of the pretest phase is client preparation. A thorough assessment and data collection (e.g., biologic, psychologic, sociologic, cultural, and spiritual) assist the nurse in determining communication and teaching strategies. Prior to radiologic studies it is important to ask female clients if pregnancy is possible. If pregnancy is suspected, special precautions may be necessary or the test may need to be postponed.

The nurse also needs to know what equipment and supplies are needed for the specific test. Common questions include the following: What type of sample will be needed and how will it be collected? Does the client need to stop oral intake for a certain number of hours prior to the test? Does the test include administration of dye (contrast media) and, if so, is it injected or swallowed? Are fluids restricted or forced? Are medications given or withheld? How long is the test? Is a consent form required? Answers to these types of questions can help avoid costly mistakes and reduce inconvenience to all involved. Most facilities have information about the tests available to the healthcare team. The laboratory at the facility can also act as a resource for information.

Intratest

This phase focuses on specimen collection and performing or assisting with certain diagnostic testing. The nurse uses standard precautions and sterile technique as appropriate. During the procedure the nurse provides emotional and physical support while monitoring the client as needed (e.g., vital signs, pulse oximetry, ECG). The nurse ensures correct labeling, storage, and transportation of the specimen to avoid invalid test results.

Postest

The focus of this phase is on nursing care of the client and follow-up activities and observations. As appropriate, the nurse compares the previous and current test results and modifies nursing interventions as needed. The nurse also reports the results to appropriate health team members. The National Patient Safety Goals identify the importance of reporting critical results of tests and diagnostic procedures.

Safety Alert! SAFETY

2019 The Joint Commission National Patient Safety Goals

Goal 2: Improve the Effectiveness of Communication Among Caregivers.

- Report critical results of tests and diagnostic procedures on a timely basis. **Rationale:** *Critical results of tests and diagnostic procedures fall significantly outside the normal range and may indicate a life-threatening situation*. The objective is to provide the responsible licensed caregiver these results within an established time frame so that the client can be promptly treated.

Nursing Diagnoses

Nursing diagnoses are based on client data and need. Examples of nursing diagnoses include anxiety or fear related to possible diagnosis of acute or chronic illness pending conclusion of diagnostic testing and lack of knowledge (state diagnostic test) related to insufficient information regarding the process for test.

Blood Tests

Blood tests are commonly used diagnostic tests that can provide valuable information about the hematologic system and many other body systems. Various members of the healthcare team can perform a **venipuncture** (puncture of a vein for collection of a blood specimen). A **phlebotomist**, an individual from a laboratory who performs venipuncture, usually collects the blood specimen for the tests ordered by the primary care provider. In some institutions, nurses may draw blood samples. The nurse needs to know the guidelines for drawing blood samples for the facility and also the state's nurse practice act.

Complete Blood Count

Specimens of venous blood are taken for a **complete blood count (CBC)**, which includes hemoglobin and hematocrit measurements, erythrocyte (red blood cell) count, red blood cell indices, leukocyte (white blood cell) count, and a differential white cell count. The CBC is a basic screening test and one of the most frequently ordered blood tests (Table 34.1).

CLIENT TEACHING Preparing for Diagnostic Testing

The nurse should conduct the following interventions:

- Instruct the client and family about the procedure for the diagnostic test ordered (e.g., whether food is allowed prior to or after testing, and the length of time of the test).
- Explain the purpose and procedure of the test.
- Instruct the client and family about activity restrictions related to testing, if applicable (e.g., remain supine for 1 hour after testing is completed).
- Instruct the client and family on the reaction the diagnostic test may produce (e.g., flushing if a dye is injected).
- Inform the client and family of the time frame for when the results will be available.
- Instruct the client and family to ask any questions so that the healthcare provider can clarify information and allay any fears.

TABLE 34.1 Complete Blood Count with Clinical Implications

Component	Normal Findings (Adult)	Possible Causes of Abnormal Findings: Increased	Possible Causes of Abnormal Findings: Decreased
RED BLOOD CELL (RBC) COUNT The number of RBCs.	*Men*: 4.6–6.0 million/µL *Women*: 4.0–5.0 million/µL	Dehydration Polycythemia vera High altitude Cardiovascular disease	Blood loss Anemias Leukemias Chronic renal failure Pregnancy
HEMOGLOBIN (HGB) Composed of a pigment (heme), which contains iron, and a protein (globin).	*Men*: 13.5–18 g/dL *Women*: 12–15 g/dL	Polycythemia Dehydration Chronic obstructive Pulmonary disease Heart failure	Blood loss Anemias Kidney diseases Cancers
HEMATOCRIT (HCT) The hematocrit or packed cell volume (Hct, PCV, or crit) is a fast way to determine the percentage of RBCs in the plasma. The Hct is reported as a percentage because it is the concentration of RBCs in the blood.	*Men*: 40–54% *Women*: 36–46%	Dehydration Hypovolemia Diabetic acidosis Burns	Acute blood loss Pregnancy Dietary deficiencies Anemias
RBC INDICES *Mean corpuscular volume (MCV)* The mean or average size of the individual RBC.	80–98 µm^3	Chronic liver disease Pernicious anemia	Iron deficiency anemia Lead poisoning
Mean corpuscular hemoglobin (MCH) Amount of Hgb present in one cell.	27–31 pg	Macrocytic anemias	Microcytic anemia
Mean corpuscular hemoglobin concentration (MCHC) The proportion of each cell occupied by Hgb.	32–36%	Rarely seen	Microcytic, hypochromic anemia
WHITE BLOOD CELL (WBC) COUNT Count of the total number of WBCs in a cubic millimeter of blood.	*Adult*: 4500–10,000/µL (mm^3)	Acute infections Tissue necrosis (e.g., myocardial infarction [MI]) Collagen diseases	Viral infections Hematopoietic diseases Rheumatoid arthritis
DIFFERENTIAL COUNT The proportion of each of the five types of WBCs in a sample of 100 WBCs.			
Neutrophils	50–70%	Acute infections	Viral diseases Leukemias Aplastic and iron deficiency anemia
Lymphocytes	25–35%	Viral infection Chronic infections Lymphocytic leukemia	Cancers Leukemia Multiple sclerosis Renal failure
Monocytes	4–6%	Viral infections Hodgkin's disease	Lymphocytic leukemia Aplastic anemia
Eosinophils	1–3%	Allergic reactions Phlebitis Cancer Parasitic infections	Stress (burns, shock) Adrenocortical hyperfunction
Basophils	0.4–1.0%	Leukemia Inflammatory process	Hypersensitivity reaction Stress Pregnancy

TABLE 34.1 Complete Blood Count with Clinical Implications—*continued*

Component	Normal Findings (Adult)	Possible Causes of Abnormal Findings	
		Increased	**Decreased**
PLATELET COUNT Platelets are basic elements in the blood that promote coagulation.	150,000–400,000/µL	Pulmonary embolism Polycythemia vera Acute blood loss Splenectomy	Idiopathic (unknown cause) Thrombocytopenic purpura Cancer Systemic lupus erythematosus (SLE)

From *Pearson Handbook of Laboratory and Diagnostic Tests with Nursing Implications*, 8th ed. (pp. 221, 223, 326, 350, 415, 417), by J. Kee, 2017. Reprinted and electronically reproduced by permission of Pearson Education, Inc., Hoboken, NJ.

Hemoglobin (Hgb) is the main intracellular protein of erythrocytes. It is the iron-containing protein in the red blood cells that transports oxygen through the body. The hemoglobin test is a measure of the total amount of hemoglobin in the blood. The **hematocrit (Hct)** measures the percentage of RBCs in the total blood volume. Hemoglobin and hematocrit are often ordered together and commonly referred to as "H&H" when ordering laboratory tests.

Hemoglobin and hematocrit increase with dehydration as the blood becomes more concentrated, and decrease with hypervolemia and resulting hemodilution. Both the hemoglobin and hematocrit are related to the **red blood cell (RBC) count**, which is the number of RBCs per cubic millimeter of whole blood. Low RBC counts are indicative of anemia. Clients with chronic hypoxia may develop higher than normal counts, a condition known as **polycythemia**. **Red blood cell (RBC) indices** may be performed as part of the CBC to evaluate the size, weight, and hemoglobin concentration of RBCs.

The **leukocyte** or **white blood cell (WBC) count** determines the number of circulating WBCs per cubic millimeter of whole blood. High WBC counts are often seen in the presence of a bacterial infection; by contrast, WBC counts may be low if a viral infection is present. In the WBC differential, leukocytes are identified by type, and the percentage of each type is determined. This information is useful in diagnosing certain disorders.

Serum Electrolytes

Serum electrolytes are often routinely ordered for any client admitted to a hospital as a screening test for electrolyte and acid–base imbalances. Serum electrolytes also are routinely assessed for clients at risk in the community, for example, clients who are being treated with a diuretic for hypertension or heart failure. The most commonly ordered serum tests are for sodium, potassium, chloride, and bicarbonate ions. Serum electrolytes may be ordered as a BMP (basic metabolic panel). The laboratory terminology varies depending on the laboratory. Normal values of commonly measured electrolytes are shown in Box 34.1.

Blood levels of two metabolically produced substances, urea and creatinine, are routinely used to evaluate renal function. The kidneys, through filtration and tubular secretion, normally eliminate both. Urea, the end product of protein metabolism, is measured as **blood urea nitrogen (BUN)**. **Creatinine** is produced in relatively constant quantities by the muscles and is excreted by the kidneys. Thus the amount of creatinine in the blood relates to renal excretory function.

Serum Osmolality

Serum osmolality is a measure of the solute concentration of the blood. The particles included are sodium ions, glucose, and urea (BUN). Serum osmolality can be estimated by doubling the serum sodium, because sodium and its associated chloride ions are the major determinants of serum osmolality. Serum osmolality values are used primarily to evaluate fluid balance. Normal values are 280 to 300 mOsm/kg. An increase in serum osmolality indicates a fluid volume deficit; a decrease reflects a fluid volume excess.

Drug Monitoring

Therapeutic drug monitoring is often conducted when a client is taking a medication with a narrow therapeutic range (e.g., digoxin, theophylline, aminoglycosides). This monitoring includes drawing blood samples for peak and trough levels to determine if the blood serum levels of a specific drug are at a therapeutic level and not a subtherapeutic or toxic level. The **peak level** indicates the highest concentration of the drug in the blood serum, and the **trough level** represents the lowest concentration. Ideally, a client's peak and trough levels fall within the therapeutic range.

BOX 34.1 Normal Electrolyte Values for Adults*

VENOUS BLOOD	
Sodium	135–145 mEq/L
Potassium	3.5–5.3 mEq/L
Chloride	95–105 mEq/L
Calcium (total) (ionized)	4.5–5.5 mEq/L or 8.5–10.5 mg/dL 56% of total calcium (2.5 mEq/L or 4.0–5.0 mg/dL)
Magnesium	1.5–2.5 mEq/L or 1.6–2.5 mg/dL
Phosphate	1.8–2.6 mEq/L (phosphorus)
Serum osmolality	280–300 mOsm/kg water

*Normal laboratory values vary from agency to agency.

Arterial Blood Gases

Measurement of **arterial blood gases** is another important diagnostic procedure (see Chapter 49 ∞). Specialty nurses, medical technicians, and respiratory therapists normally take specimens of arterial blood from the radial, brachial, or femoral arteries. Because of the relatively great pressure of the blood in these arteries, it is important to prevent hemorrhaging by applying pressure to the puncture side for about 5 to 10 minutes after removing the needle.

Blood Chemistry

A number of other tests may be performed on blood serum (the liquid portion of the blood). These are often referred to as a **blood chemistry**. In addition to serum electrolytes, common chemistry examinations include determining certain enzymes that may be present (including lactic dehydrogenase [LDH], creatine kinase [CK], aspartate aminotransferase [AST], and alanine aminotransferase [ALT]), serum glucose, hormones such as thyroid hormone, and other substances such as cholesterol and triglycerides. These tests provide valuable diagnostic cues. For example, cardiac markers (e.g., CPK-MB, myoglobin, troponin T, and troponin I) are released into the blood during a myocardial infarction (MI, or heart attack). Elevated levels of these markers in the venous blood can help differentiate between an MI and chest pain that is caused by angina or pleurisy.

A common laboratory test is the glycosylated hemoglobin or **hemoglobin A1C (HbA1C)** test, which is a measurement of blood glucose that is bound to hemoglobin. Hemoglobin A1C is a reflection of how well blood glucose levels have been controlled during the prior 3 to 4 months. The normal range is 4.0% to 5.5%. An elevated HbA1C reflects hyperglycemia in people with diabetes.

The first specific blood test used to detect and guide treatment for heart failure is the brain natriuretic peptide or B-type natriuretic peptide (BNP) test. The left ventricle secretes B-type natriuretic peptide in response to increased ventricular volume and pressure. BNP levels increase as heart failure becomes more severe.

See Table 34.2 for normal values of common blood chemistry tests.

TABLE 34.2 Common Blood Chemistry Tests with Clinical Implications

Test	Normal Findings (Adult)	Significance	Possible Causes of Increased Level	Possible Causes of Decreased Level
LIVER FUNCTION TESTS				
ALT (alanine aminotransferase), formerly known as serum glutamic-pyruvic transaminase (SGPT)	*Adult*: 10–35 unit/L	Marker of hepatic injury; more specific of liver damage than AST	Acute viral hepatitis, necrosis of the liver, cirrhosis, heart failure, acute alcohol intoxication	Exercise
AST (aspartate aminotransferase), formerly known as serum glutamic-oxaloacetic transaminase (SGOT)	*Adult*: 8–35 unit/L	Found in heart, liver, and skeletal muscle. Can also be used to indicate liver injury	Acute myocardial infarction, liver necrosis, hepatitis, musculoskeletal diseases and trauma, acute pancreatitis	Pregnancy; diabetic ketoacidosis, chronic hemodialysis
Albumin	*Adults*: 3.5–5.0 g/dL or 52–68% of total protein	A component of proteins produced by the liver	No pathology causes the liver to produce more albumin. An increased level reflects dehydration	Cirrhosis of the liver, acute liver failure, severe burns, severe malnutrition, renal disorders
Alkaline phosphatase	*Adults*: 4.2–13 unit/dL	Found in the tissues of the liver, bone, intestine, kidney, and placenta. Used as an index of liver and bone disease when correlated with other clinical findings	Liver disease, bone disease, hyperparathyroidism, rheumatoid arthritis (active)	Malnutrition, pernicious anemia, hypothyroidism
Ammonia	*Adults*: 15–60 mcg/dL	The liver converts ammonia, a by-product of protein metabolism, into urea, which is excreted by the kidneys	Liver disease, cirrhosis, Reye syndrome, heart failure	Renal failure, hypertension
Bilirubin	*Adults*: *Total*: 0.1–1.2 mg/dL *Direct*: 0.1–0.3 mg/dL *Indirect*: 0.1–1.2 mg/dL	Results from the breakdown of hemoglobin in the red blood cells; removed from the body by the liver, which excretes it into the bile	*Total*: hepatitis, obstruction of the common bile or hepatic ducts *Direct*: hepatitis, choledocholithiasis *Indirect*: hemolytic anemias, transfusion reaction	Iron-deficiency anemia

TABLE 34.2 Common Blood Chemistry Tests with Clinical Implications—*continued*

Test	Normal Findings (Adult)	Significance	Possible Causes of Increased Level	Possible Causes of Decreased Level
GGT (gamma-glutamyl transferase)	*Men*: 4–23 international unit/L *Women*: 3–13 international unit/L	Found primarily in the liver and kidney, with smaller amounts in the prostate, spleen, and heart muscle. Is more specific for liver diseases.	Liver disease, alcohol abuse	Not clinically significant
Prothrombin	*Adults*: 10–13 seconds	A protein produced by the liver for clotting of blood	Liver disease or damage, vitamin K deficiency, deficiency of factors II, V, VII, or X	Thrombophlebitis, pulmonary embolism
CARDIAC MARKERS CK (creatine kinase)	*Total*: *Men*: 50–170 units/L *Women*: 25–140 units/L *Isoenzymes*: MM (CK_3): 90–100% MB (CK_2): 0–6% BB (CK_1): 0%	An enzyme found in the heart and skeletal muscles. Has three isoenzymes: MM or CK_3, MB or CK_2, and BB or CK_1 Most laboratories have replaced CPK isoenzymes with CPK-MB fraction only.	*Total*: acute MI, skeletal muscle disease, cerebrovascular accident (CVA) *CK isoenzymes*: MB (CK_2): myocardial infarct, angina pectoris, cardiac surgery	Not clinically significant
Myoglobin	*Male*: 20–90 ng/mL *Female*: 12–75 ng/mL	After an MI, serum levels of myoglobin rise in 2–4 h, making it an early marker for muscle damage in MI	MI, angina, other muscle injury (e.g., trauma), renal failure, severe burns	Not clinically significant
Troponin I Troponin T	*Troponin I*: <0.1–0.5 ng/mL *Troponin T*: <0.2 ng/mL	Cardiac troponin is highly concentrated in the heart muscle. This test is used in the early diagnosis of MI. After an MI, troponin I begins to increase in 4–6 h and remains elevated for 5–7 days Troponin T begins to increase in 3–4 h and remains elevated for 10–14 days	*Troponin I*: small infarct, myocardial injury *Troponin T*: acute MI, unstable angina, myocarditis	Not clinically significant
BNP (Brain natriuretic peptide or B-Type natriuretic peptide)	<100 pg/mL or <100 ng/L	A hormone produced by the ventricles of the heart that is a marker of ventricular systolic and diastolic dysfunction. This test is useful in diagnosing and guiding treatment of heart failure	Heart failure, hypertension, acute MI	Not clinically significant
LIPOPROTEIN PROFILE Cholesterol	*Adults (desirable)*: <200 mg/dL	This test is an important screening test for heart disease	Acute MI, atherosclerosis, hypothyroidism, cholangitis	Hyperthyroidism, malnutrition, chronic anemias
HDL-C (high-density lipoprotein cholesterol)	*Adults*: 29–77 mg/dL	A class of lipoproteins produced by the liver and intestines; the "good" cholesterol	HDL excess, chronic liver disease, long-term aerobic or vigorous exercise	Familial hypolipoproteinemia, familial hypertriglyceridemia, poorly controlled diabetes mellitus, chronic kidney disease

Continued on page 810

TABLE 34.2 Common Blood Chemistry Tests with Clinical Implications—*continued*

Test	Normal Findings (Adult)	Significance	Possible Causes of Increased Level	Possible Causes of Decreased Level
LDL (low-density lipoprotein)	*Adults (desirable)*: 60–160 mg/dL	Up to 70% of the total serum cholesterol is present in LDL; the "bad" cholesterol	Type II familial hyperlipidemia. Secondary causes can include diet high in cholesterol and saturated fat, nephritic syndrome, multiple myeloma, diabetes mellitus, chronic kidney disease	Hypolipoproteinemia, hyperthyroidism, chronic anemias, severe hepatocellular disease
Triglycerides	*12–29 Years*: 10–140 mg/dL *39–39 Years*: 20–150 mg/dL *40–49 Years*: 30–160 mg/dL; *>50 Years*: 40–190 mg/dL	This test evaluates suspected atherosclerosis and measures the body's ability to metabolize fat	Hyperlipoproteinemia, acute MI, hypertension, hypothyroidism	Hyperthyroidism, hyperparathroidism, protein malnutrition, exercise

From *Pearson Handbook of Laboratory and Diagnostic Tests with Nursing Implications*, 8th ed. (pp. 18, 19, 26, 36, 77, 82, 94, 151, 200, 283, 301, 346, 387, 392), by J. L. Kee, 2017. Reprinted and electronically reproduced by permission of Pearson Education, Inc., Hoboken, NJ: Pearson.

Metabolic Screening

Newborns are routinely screened for congenital metabolic conditions. Tests for phenylketonuria (PKU) and congenital hypothyroidism are required in all states in the United States. Other conditions that are frequently screened for include sickle cell disease and galactosemia. Screening involves collecting peripheral venous blood (via a heelstick) on prepared blotting paper and sending the specimen to the state laboratory for analysis. Discovered abnormalities allow the provider and parents to plan early care (e.g., special diets for children with PKU) that can prevent long-term complications.

Capillary Blood Glucose

A capillary blood specimen is taken to measure the current blood glucose level when frequent tests are required or when a venipuncture cannot be performed. This technique is less painful than a venipuncture and easily performed. Therefore, clients can perform this technique on themselves.

The development of home glucose test kits and reagent strips has simplified the testing of blood glucose and greatly facilitated the management of home care by clients with diabetes. A number of manufacturers have developed blood glucose meters or monitors (Figure 34.1 ■).

Advances in technology have resulted in clients having greater choices for a glucose meter that meets their needs. Glucose meters can vary in the following ways: blood drop size, meter size, code versus non-code requirement, audio, wireless data transfer, lights, ability to store results, cost of the meter, and test strips (McElwee-Malloy, 2016). Future technology is exploring ways to help clients with diabetes manage their diet and medications. For example, smart contact lenses, now in development, may someday measure blood sugar values from tears (Kraft, 2019, p. 30).

It is important that clients who require glucose monitoring be comfortable and confident in the use of the meter. Once the client chooses a blood glucose meter, it is imperative for the nurse or client to review the manufacturer's

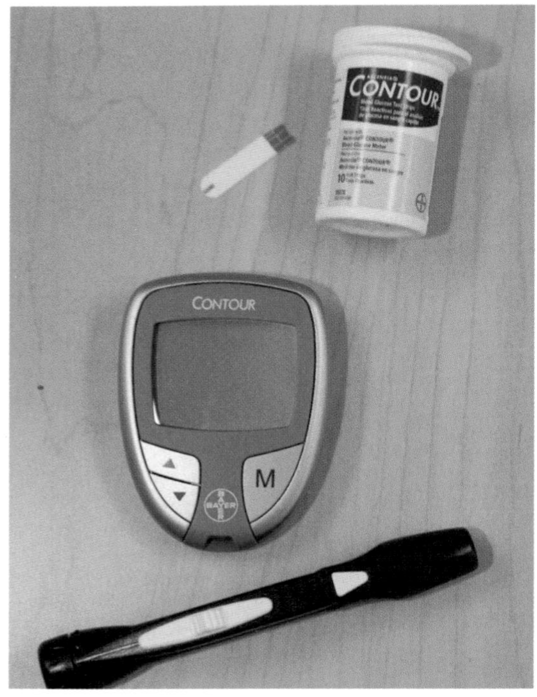

Figure 34.1 ■ Blood glucose monitor, test strips, and lancet injector.
Shirlee Snyder.

operating guidelines. Being familiar with the proper use of the equipment helps ensure accurate readings. This will assist clients in controlling their diabetes. Clients who are comfortable taking their blood glucose readings and knowledgeable about interpreting the results will feel empowered to make changes, as needed, for optimal self-management skills.

QSEN Patient-Centered Care: Capillary Blood Glucose

Nurses should consider the following aspects when caring for clients in the home setting:

- Assess the client or caregiver's ability and willingness to perform blood glucose monitoring at home.
- Teach the proper use of the lancet and glucose monitor, and provide written guidelines. Allow time for a return demonstration. The client may need several visits to completely learn the procedure.
- Ensure the client's ability to obtain supplies and purchase reagent strips. The strips are relatively expensive and may not be covered by the client's insurance.
- Stress the importance of record keeping. Instruct the client on when to do glucose monitoring, how to record the blood glucose levels, and when to notify the primary care provider.
- Children with diabetes who need to perform fingersticks should be taught about safe practices for cleaning blood from surfaces (household bleach is best) and about safe storage of equipment to prevent other children from gaining access to it. Identify a place in the school where the child can store glucose-monitoring equipment and perform the procedure in private.

Capillary blood specimens are commonly obtained from the lateral aspect or side of the finger in adults. This site avoids the nerve endings and calloused areas at the fingertip. The earlobe may be used as a safe alternative site unless the client is in a suspected hypoglycemic state (Chan, Lau, Ho, Leung, & Lee, 2016). See Evidence Based Practice. Skill 34.1 describes how to obtain a capillary blood specimen and measure blood glucose using a portable meter.

EVIDENCE-BASED PRACTICE

Evidence-Based Practice

What Is the Accuracy and Acceptability of Performing Capillary Blood Glucose Monitoring at the Earlobe?

Capillary blood glucose monitoring, in current practice, is obtained from the fingertip. In some circumstances, however, the fingertip may not be appropriate. The pricking procedure can be painful because the fingertip contains many sensory nerves and repeated pricking can lead to tissue damage. Clinicians would like to identify other body parts as alternative sites for blood glucose monitoring. It is important that other sites are as reliable as the fingertip for the safety of the client. Several studies have been conducted to compare the blood glucose concentration at alternative body sites (e.g., palm, forearm, thigh, calf, and earlobe). These studies reported that the forearm and thigh were less reliable. Evidence did show that the palm was more suitable; however, it would seem that if the fingertips were contraindicated the palm may not be a viable alternative. Findings for using the earlobe as an alternative site have been limited and inconclusive.

Chan, Lau, Ho, Leung, and Lee (2016) conducted a quantitative study to examine the accuracy and acceptability of performing capillary blood glucose monitoring at the earlobe. They recruited 120 participants from a diabetes outpatient clinic and the medical wards from an acute care hospital. The participants were divided into four groups: 30 whose glycemic state was stable; 30 receiving IV infusion; 30 diagnosed with chronic renal impairment and with a serum creatinine higher than 150 pmol/L; and 30 aged 65 or older who had been on bedrest for at least 48 hours. Data collection was standardized in the following sequence: a fingertip stick and while waiting the result, the participant rated the pain level of the fingerstick on a six-point Faces Pain Scale; then a blood sample at the lower part of the earlobe (taken on the same side as the fingertip used), followed by the participant rating the level of pain for the procedure. All blood glucose measurements were conducted before meal time or in a fasting state. The entire data collection took approximately 5 minutes.

The blood glucose measurements between the two sites were compared and the results were highly comparable. These findings were true even for the participants who had nephropathy, were immobile, or were receiving an IV infusion. The findings, however, did reveal that the difference between the two sampling sites was more obvious in the three participants who were in a hypoglycemic state, with the reading from the earlobe generally higher. The participants perceived the level of pain with the skin pricking significantly lower for the earlobe than the fingertip.

Implications

Because previous studies resulted in mixed results, the researchers used a more stringent research method and a larger sample size to examine blood glucose concentration at the earlobe compared with the fingertip. Their intent was not to replace current practice but to provide evidence that the earlobe could be used as an alternative site. The researchers suggest that performing capillary blood glucose monitoring at the earlobe is practical and acceptable to both clinicians and clients. That is, the blood glucose reading between the fingertip and the earlobe was highly comparable (except in the hypoglycemic state) and the participants reported less pain when using the earlobe.

SKILL 34.1

Obtaining a Capillary Blood Specimen to Measure Blood Glucose

PURPOSES

- To determine or monitor blood glucose levels of clients at risk for hyperglycemia or hypoglycemia
- To promote blood glucose regulation by the client
- To evaluate the effectiveness of insulin administration

ASSESSMENT

Before obtaining a capillary blood specimen, determine:

- The policies and procedures for the facility
- The frequency and type of testing
- The client's understanding of the procedure
- The client's response to previous testing.
- Assess the client's skin at the puncture site to determine if it is intact and the circulation is not compromised. Check color, warmth, and capillary refill.
- Review the client's record for medications that may prolong bleeding such as anticoagulants or medical problems that may increase the bleeding response.
- Assess the client's self-care abilities that may affect the accuracy of test results, such as visual impairment and finger dexterity.

PLANNING

Assignment

Check the applicable nurse practice act and the facility policy and procedure manual to determine who can perform this skill. It is usually considered an invasive technique and one that requires problem-solving and application of knowledge. It is the responsibility of the nurse to know the results of the test and supervise assistive personnel (AP) responsible for assisting the nurse.

Equipment

- Blood glucose meter (glucometer)
- Blood glucose reagent strip compatible with the meter
- 2×2 gauze
- Antiseptic swab
- Clean gloves
- Sterile lancet (a sharp device to puncture the skin)
- Lancet injector (a spring-loaded mechanism that holds the lancet)
- Warm cloth or other warming device (optional)

IMPLEMENTATION

Preparation

Review the type of meter and the manufacturer's instructions. Assemble the equipment at the bedside.

Performance

1. Prior to performing the procedure, introduce self and verify the client's identity using agency protocol. Explain to the client what you are going to do, why it is necessary, and how to participate. Discuss how the results will be used in planning further care or treatments.
2. Perform hand hygiene and observe other appropriate infection prevention procedures.
3. Provide for client privacy.
4. Prepare the equipment.
   - Some meters turn on when a test strip is inserted into the meter. ❶
   - Calibrate the meter and run a control sample according to the manufacturer's instructions and/or confirm the code number. The newer no-code models do not require calibration. The technology is integrated into the test strips.
5. Select and prepare the vascular puncture site.
   - Choose a vascular puncture site (e.g., the side of an adult's finger). Avoid sites beside bone. Wrap the finger first in a warm cloth *or* hold a finger in a dependent (below heart level) position. If the earlobe is used, rub it gently with a small piece of gauze. **Rationale:** *These actions increase the blood flow to the area, ensure an adequate specimen, and reduce the need for a repeat puncture.*
   - Clean the site with the antiseptic swab or soap and water and allow it to dry completely. **Rationale:** *Alcohol can affect accuracy, and the site stings when punctured if wet with alcohol.*
6. Obtain the blood specimen.
   - Apply gloves.
   - Place the injector, if used, against the site, and release the needle, thus permitting it to pierce the skin. Make sure the lancet is perpendicular to the site. **Rationale:** *The lancet is designed to pierce the skin at a specific depth when it is in a perpendicular position relative to the skin.* ❷

     or
   - Prick the site with a lancet or needle, using a darting motion.
   - Gently squeeze (but do not touch) the puncture site until a drop of blood forms. The size of the drop of blood can vary depending on the meter. Some meters require as little as 0.3 mL of blood to accurately test blood sugar.

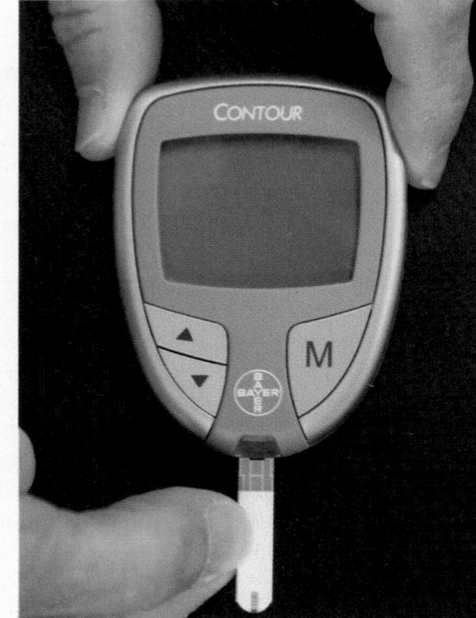

❶ Insert the test strip into the meter.
Shirlee Snyder.

Obtaining a Capillary Blood Specimen to Measure Blood Glucose—*continued*

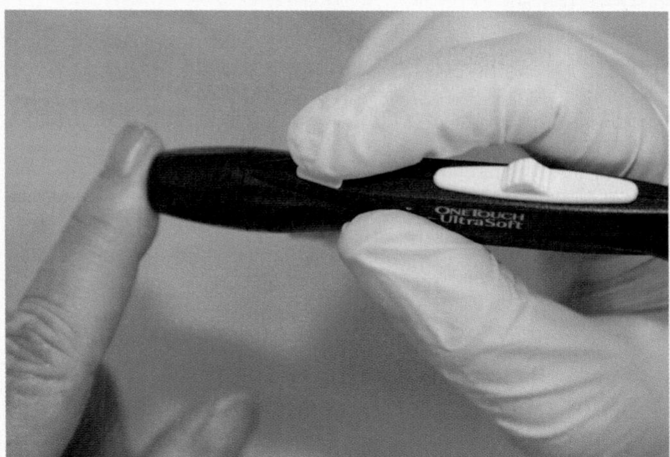

❷ Place the injector against the site.
Shirlee Snyder.

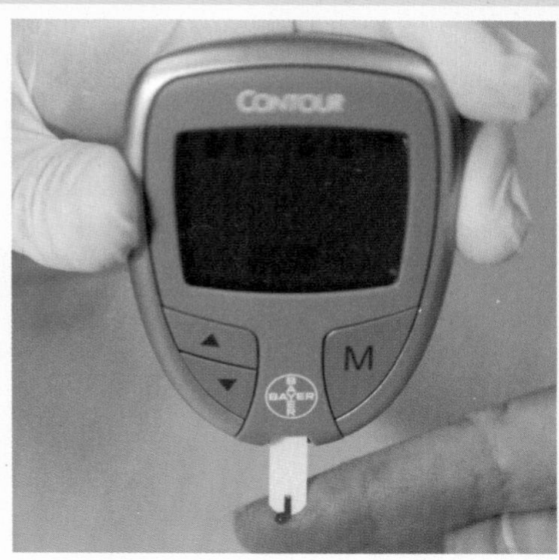

❸ Apply the blood to the test strip.
Shirlee Snyder.

- Hold the reagent strip under the puncture site until adequate blood covers the indicator square. The pad will absorb the blood and a chemical reaction will occur. Do not smear the blood. **Rationale:** *Smearing will cause an inaccurate reading*.
- Some meters wick the blood by just touching the puncture site with the strip. ❸
- Ask the client to apply pressure to the skin puncture site with a 2×2 gauze. **Rationale:** *Pressure will assist hemostasis*.

7. Expose the blood to the test strip for the period and the manner specified by the manufacturer. As soon as the blood is placed on the test strip:
- Follow the manufacturer's recommendations on the glucose meter and monitor for the amount of time indicated by the manufacturer. **Rationale:** *The blood must remain in contact with the test strip for a prescribed time to obtain accurate results*.
- Some glucose meters have the test strip placed in the machine before the specimen is obtained.

8. Measure the blood glucose.
- Place the strip into the meter according to the manufacturer's instructions. Refer to the specific manufacturer's recommendations for the specific procedure.
- After the designated time, most glucose meters will display the glucose reading automatically. Correct timing ensures accurate results. ❹
- Turn off the meter and discard the test strip and 2×2 gauze in a biohazard container. Discard the lancet into a sharps container.
- Remove and discard gloves.
- Perform hand hygiene.

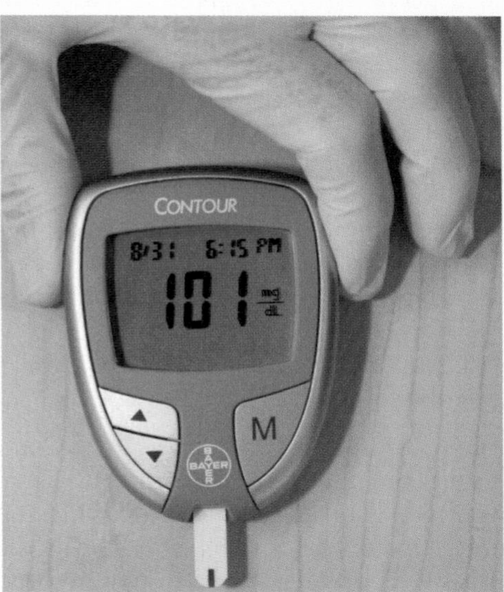

❹ Read the results.
Shirlee Snyder.

9. Document the method of testing and results on the client's record. If appropriate, record the client's understanding and ability to demonstrate the technique. The client's record may also include a flow sheet on which capillary blood glucose results and the amount, type, route, and time of insulin administration are recorded. Always check if a diabetic flow sheet is being used for the client.

10. Check for orders for sliding scale insulin based on capillary blood glucose results. Administer insulin as prescribed.

EVALUATION

- Compare glucose meter reading with normal blood glucose level, status of puncture site, and motivation of the client to perform the test independently.
- Compare blood glucose reading to previous readings and the client's current health status.
- Report abnormal results to the primary care provider. Some agencies may have a standing policy to obtain a venipuncture blood glucose level if the capillary blood glucose exceeds a certain value.
- Conduct appropriate follow-up such as asking the client to explain the meaning of the results or demonstrating the procedure at the next scheduled test.
- Prepare the client for home glucose monitoring and review frequency, record keeping, and insulin administration if appropriate.

LIFESPAN CONSIDERATIONS Capillary Blood Glucose

INFANTS

- The outer aspect of the heel is the most common site for neonates and infants. Placing a warm cloth on the infant's heel often increases the blood flow to the area.

CHILDREN

- Use the side of a fingertip for a young client older than age 2, unless contraindicated.
- Allow the child to choose the puncture site, when possible.
- Praise the young client for cooperating and assure the child that the procedure is not a punishment.

OLDER ADULTS

- Older adults may have arthritic joint changes, poor vision, or hand tremors and may need assistance using the glucose meter or obtaining a meter that accommodates their limitations.
- Older adults may have difficulty obtaining diabetic supplies due to financial concerns or homebound status.
- Older adults often have poor circulation. Warming the hands by wrapping with a warm washcloth for 3 to 5 minutes or placing the hand dependently for a few moments may help in obtaining a blood sample.

Specimen Collection and Testing

The nurse contributes to the assessment of a client's health status by collecting specimens of body fluids. All hospitalized clients have at least one laboratory specimen collected during their stay at a healthcare facility. Laboratory examination of specimens such as blood, stool, urine, sputum, and wound drainage provides important adjunct information for diagnosing healthcare problems and also provides a measure of the responses to therapy.

Nurses often assume the responsibility for specimen collection. Depending on the type of specimen and skill required, the nurse may be able to delegate this task to AP under the supervision of the nurse.

Nursing responsibilities associated with specimen collection include the following:

- Provide client comfort, privacy, and safety. Clients may experience embarrassment or discomfort when providing a specimen. The nurse should provide the client with as much privacy as possible and handle the specimen discreetly. The nurse needs to be nonjudgmental and sensitive to possible sociocultural beliefs that may affect the client's willingness to participate in the specimen collection procedure.
- Explain the purpose of the specimen collection and the procedure for obtaining the specimen. Clients may experience anxiety about the procedure, especially if it is perceived as being intrusive or if they fear an unknown test result. A clear explanation will facilitate the client's cooperation in the collection of the specimen. With proper instruction, many clients are able to collect their own specimen, which promotes independence and reduces or avoids embarrassment.
- Use the correct procedure for obtaining a specimen or ensure that the client or staff follow the correct procedure. Aseptic technique is used in specimen collection to prevent contamination that can cause inaccurate test results. A nursing procedure or laboratory manual is often available if the nurse is unfamiliar with the procedure. If there is any question about the procedure, the nurse calls the laboratory for directions before collecting the specimen.
- Note relevant information on the laboratory requisition slip, for example, medications the client is taking that may affect the results.
- Transport the specimen to the laboratory promptly. Fresh specimens provide more accurate results.
- Report abnormal laboratory findings to the healthcare provider in a timely manner consistent with the severity of the abnormal results.

QSEN Patient-Centered Care: Specimen Collection

If specimen collection is done in the home or an outpatient basis, the nurse teaches the client how to obtain the specimens. Written instructions and specimen containers are provided to ensure correct and safe performance of the procedure. The nurse also ensures that the laboratory knows where to send the test results.

Stool Specimens

Analysis of stool specimens can provide information about a client's health condition. Some reasons for testing feces include the following:

- To analyze for dietary products and digestive secretions. For example, an excessive amount of fat in the stool (**steatorrhea**) can indicate faulty absorption of fat from the small intestine. A decreased amount of bile can indicate obstruction of bile flow from the liver and gallbladder into the intestine. For these kinds of tests, the nurse needs to collect and send the total quantity of stool expelled at one time instead of a small sample.
- To detect the presence of ova and parasites. When collecting specimens for parasites, it is important that the sample be transported immediately to the laboratory while it is still warm. Usually three stool specimens, over a period of days, are evaluated to confirm the presence of and to identify the organism so that appropriate treatment can be ordered. Always check agency policies and procedures for specimen collection. For example, a stool specimen for ova and parasites may be collected in specialized containers with preservatives.

- To detect the presence of bacteria or viruses. Only a small amount of feces is required because the specimen will be cultured. Collection containers or tubes must be sterile and aseptic technique must be used during collection. Stools need to be sent immediately to the laboratory. The nurse needs to note on the laboratory requisition if the client is receiving any antibiotics.
- To determine the presence of **occult (hidden) blood**. Bleeding can occur as a result of gastrointestinal ulcers, inflammatory disease, or tumors. The fecal occult blood test (FOBT), often referred to as the **guaiac test**, can be readily performed by the nurse in the clinical area or by the client at home. There are two types of FOBTs: the traditional guaiac test (Hemoccult) and the fecal immunochemical test (FIT) (also called an immunochemical fecal occult blood test or iFOBT).

Collecting Stool Specimens

The nurse is responsible for collecting stool specimens ordered for laboratory analysis. Before obtaining a specimen, the nurse needs to determine the reason for collecting the stool specimen and the correct method of obtaining and handling it (i.e., how much stool to obtain, whether to add a preservative to the stool, and whether to send it immediately to the laboratory). It may be necessary to confirm this information by checking with the agency laboratory. In many situations only a single specimen is required; in others, timed specimens are necessary, and every stool passed is collected within a designated time period.

AP may obtain and collect stool specimen(s) in certain situations, so the nurse needs to consider the collection process before assigning this task. For example, a random stool specimen collected in a specimen container may be assigned, but the nurse should do a stool culture requiring a sterile swab in a test tube. An incorrect collection technique can cause inaccurate test results.

The task of obtaining and testing a stool specimen for occult blood may be performed by AP. It is important for the nurse to instruct the AP to inform the nurse if blood is detected or whether the test is positive. In addition, the stool specimen should be saved to allow the nurse to repeat the test.

Nurses need to give clients the following instructions:

- Defecate in a clean bedpan or bedside commode.
- If possible, do not contaminate the specimen with urine or menstrual discharge. Void before the specimen collection.
- Do not place toilet tissue in the bedpan after defecation. Contents of the paper can affect the laboratory analysis.
- Notify the nurse as soon as possible after defecation, particularly for specimens that need to be sent to the laboratory immediately.

When obtaining stool samples—that is, when handling the client's bedpan, when transferring the stool sample to a specimen container, and when disposing of the bedpan contents—the nurse follows medical aseptic technique meticulously. Wear clean gloves to prevent hand contamination and take care not to contaminate the outside of the specimen container. Use one or two clean tongue blades to transfer the specimen to the container and then wrap them in a paper towel before disposing of them in the waste container. This practice reduces the chance of contact with other articles and the spread of microorganisms. The amount of stool to be sent depends on the purpose for which the specimen is collected. Usually about 2.5 cm (1 in.) of formed stool or 15 to 30 mL of liquid stool is adequate. For some timed specimens, however, the entire stool passed may need to be sent. Visible pus, mucus, or blood should be included in sample specimens. For a stool culture, the nurse dips a sterile swab into the specimen, preferably where purulent fecal matter is present and, using sterile technique, places the swab in a sterile test tube.

Ensure that the specimen label and the laboratory requisition have the correct information on them and are securely attached to the specimen container. Inappropriate identification of the specimen risks errors of diagnosis or therapy for the client.

Because fresh specimens provide the most accurate results, the nurse sends the specimen to the laboratory immediately. If this is not possible, the nurse follows the directions on the specimen container. In some instances, refrigeration is indicated because bacteriologic changes take place in stool specimens left at room temperature. To prevent contamination, never place a stool specimen in a refrigerator that contains food or medication.

Document all relevant information. Record the collection of the specimen on the client's chart and on the nursing care plan. Include in the recording the date and time of the collection and all nursing assessments (e.g., color, odor, consistency, and amount of feces); presence of abnormal constituents, such as blood or mucus; results of test for occult blood if obtained; discomfort during or after defecation; status of perianal skin; and any bleeding from the anus after defecation.

QSEN Patient-Centered Care: Stool Specimens

Home care considerations for the nurse include the following:

- Ask the client or caregiver to call when the stool specimen is obtained. If a laboratory test is needed, the home health nurse can pick up the specimen or a family member may take it to the laboratory.
- Place the stool specimen inside a plastic biohazard bag. Carry the bag in a sealed container marked "Biohazard" and take it to the laboratory promptly. Do not expose the specimen to extreme temperatures in the car.

Fecal Occult Blood Testing

Fecal occult blood testing (FOBT) is the most frequently performed fecal analysis. There are two types of FOBT: the traditional guaiac smear (Hemoccult) and the fecal immunochemical test (FIT or iFOBT).

A commonly used test product to measure occult blood is the Hemoccult test, which uses a chemical **reagent** (substance used in a chemical reaction to detect a specific substance). This reagent detects the presence of the enzyme peroxidase in the hemoglobin molecule. To perform the test, the nurse or client uses a tongue blade to place a small amount of stool on a slide or card and then closes the card. The card is turned over and two drops of a reagent are placed onto each smear on the back of the card. The nurse then observes for a color change (Figure 34.2 ■). A blue color indicates a guaiac-positive result, that is, the presence of occult blood. No color change or any color other than blue is a negative finding, indicating the absence of blood in the stool. Because the results are color based, a nurse who is color blind should not be responsible for reading the results.

Certain foods, medications, and vitamin C produce inaccurate test results for the Hemoccult test. False-positive results can occur if the client has recently ingested (a) red meat (beef, lamb, liver, and processed meats); (b) raw vegetables or fruits, particularly radishes, turnips, horseradish, and melons; or (c) certain medications that irritate the gastric mucosa and cause bleeding, such as aspirin or other nonsteroidal anti-inflammatory drugs, steroids, iron preparations, and anticoagulants. False-negative results can occur if the client has taken more than 250 mg/day of vitamin C from all sources (dietary and supplemental) up to 3 days before the test—even if bleeding is present.

The FIT has a higher sensitivity and specificity for the detection of colon cancer (Lieberman et al., 2016). When comparing the two types of FOBTs, the FIT has the following advantages: no dietary or medication restrictions, fewer false positives, and requires only one sample as opposed to the three stool samples and dietary restrictions required for the guaiac test.

An emerging screening strategy for colorectal cancer is the FIT-DNA. This test combines a FIT with testing for altered DNA biomarkers in cells shed into the stool (U.S. Preventive Services Task Force, 2016, p. 2567).

Guidelines for instructing clients to collect their stool for occult blood are listed in Client Teaching.

Urine Specimens

The nurse is responsible for collecting urine specimens for a number of tests: **clean voided urine specimens** for routine urinalysis, **clean-catch** or **midstream urine specimens** for urine culture, and timed urine specimens for a variety of tests that depend on the client's specific health problem. Urine specimen collection may require collection via straight catheter insertion. If this is necessary, refer to Chapter 47 ∞, Skill 47.2.

Clean Voided Urine Specimen

A clean voided specimen is usually adequate for routine examination. Many clients are able to collect a clean voided specimen and provide the specimen independently with minimal instructions. Male clients generally are able to void (urinate) directly into the specimen container, and female clients usually sit or squat over the toilet, holding the container between their legs during voiding. Routine urine examination is usually done on the first voided specimen in the morning because it tends to have a higher, more uniform concentration and a more acidic pH than specimens later in the day.

At least 10 mL of urine is generally sufficient for a routine urinalysis. Clients who are seriously ill, physically

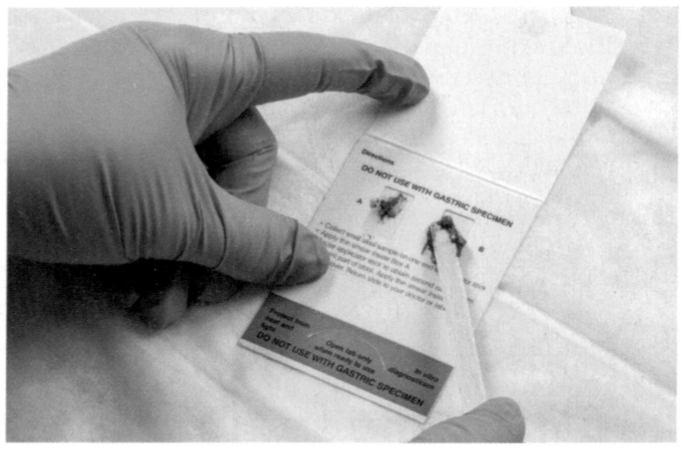

A

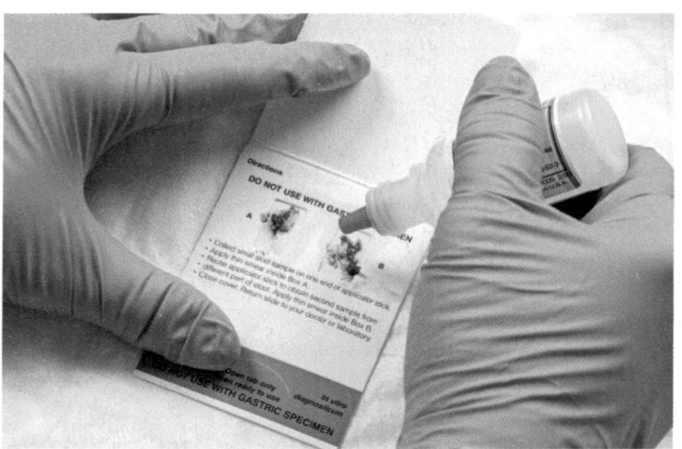

B

Figure 34.2 ■ *A*, Opening the front cover of a Hemoccult slide and applying a thin smear of feces on the slide. *B*, Opening the flap on the back of the slide and applying two drops of developing fluid over each smear.

CLIENT TEACHING Collecting Stool for Occult Blood

USING THE HEMOCCULT TEST

- Avoid restricted foods, medications, and vitamin C for the period recommended by the manufacturer and during the test. Usually specified foods and vitamin C are restricted for 3 days before the test and specified medications for 7 days before the test.
- Use a ballpoint pen to label the specimens with your name, address, age, and date of specimen. Usually three specimens are collected from consecutive and different bowel movements. Each specimen must be dated accurately.
- Avoid collecting specimens during your menstrual period and for 3 days afterward, and while you have bleeding hemorrhoids or blood in your urine.
- Remove toilet bowl cleaners from the toilet bowl. Flush the toilet twice before proceeding with the test.
- Avoid contaminating the specimen with urine or toilet tissue. Empty your bladder before the test. To facilitate specimen collection, insert a plastic "hat" backwards in the toilet or bedside commode to help obtain a stool specimen. Some recommend placing a cling wrap across the back of the toilet seat, leaving slack in it to defecate on. Apply clean gloves. Transfer the stool to a clean, dry container.
- Use the tongue blade provided to transfer the specimen to the test folder. Only a small amount of stool is required. Take the sample from the center of a formed stool to ensure a uniform sample.
- Wrap the tongue blade in a paper towel and dispose of it in the waste receptacle. Do not flush the stick. Remove and discard gloves.
- Follow the manufacturer's directions explicitly for the test product being used. Test products vary.
- Consult your healthcare provider if there is any problem understanding the instructions.
- Return completed specimens to your primary care provider or laboratory as instructed.

USING FIT

- Avoid collecting specimens during your menstrual period and for 3 days afterward, and while you have bleeding hemorrhoids or blood in your urine.
- Toilet cleaners may affect test results and should be removed before using the FIT.
- Flush the toilet.
- Put the used toilet paper in the waste bag provided. Do not put it in the toilet bowl.
- Use the brush from the kit to brush the surface of the stool for several seconds. Shake the brush once to dislodge any clumps of stool or excess water.
- Swab the brush on the space indicated on the test card for several seconds.
- Add the brush to the waste bag and throw it away.
- Send the sample to the lab for testing (Tresca, 2018).

LIFESPAN CONSIDERATIONS Stool Specimen

INFANTS

- To collect a stool specimen for an infant, the stool is scraped from the diaper, being careful not to contaminate the stool with urine.

CHILDREN

- A child who is toilet trained should be able to provide a fecal specimen, but may prefer being assisted by a parent.
- When explaining the procedure to the child, use words appropriate for the child's age rather than medical terms. Ask the parent what words the family normally uses to describe a bowel movement.
- A specimen for pinworms is collected by the parent early in the morning, after sleep and before the child has a bowel movement. Scotch tape is attached to a tongue blade and the sticky side is laid flat against the perineum and anus to pick up any eggs or small worms. The tongue blade is then examined under a microscope.

OLDER ADULTS

- Older adults may need assistance if serial stool specimens are required.

incapacitated, or disoriented may need to use a bedpan or urinal in bed; others may require supervision or assistance in the bathroom. Whatever the situation, clear and specific directions are required:

- The specimen must be free of fecal contamination, so urine must be kept separate from feces.
- Female clients should discard the toilet tissue in the toilet or in a waste bag rather than in the bedpan because tissue in the specimen makes laboratory analysis more difficult.
- Put the lid tightly on the container to prevent spillage of the urine and contamination of other objects.
- If the outside of the container has been contaminated by urine, clean it with a disinfectant.

The nurse must (a) make sure that the specimen label and the laboratory requisition carry the correct information and (b) attach them securely to the specimen. Inappropriate identification of the specimen can lead to errors of diagnosis or therapy for the client.

AP may be assigned to collect a routine urine specimen. Provide the AP with clear directions on how to instruct the client to collect his or her own urine specimen or how to correctly collect the specimen for the client who may need to use a bedpan or urinal.

Clinical Alert!

Kidney function directly relates to cardiac output. Therefore, any health problem that changes cardiac output may affect urine output.

Clean-Catch or Midstream Urine Specimen

Clean-catch or midstream voided specimens are collected when a urine culture is ordered to identify microorganisms causing a urinary tract infection. Although some contamination by skin bacteria may occur with a clean-catch specimen, the risk of introducing microorganisms into the urinary tract through catheterization is more significant. Care is taken to ensure that the specimen is as free as possible from contamination by microorganisms around the urinary meatus. Clean-catch specimens are collected in a sterile specimen container with a lid (Figure 34.3 ■). Disposable clean-catch kits are available. Skill 34.2 explains how to collect a clean-catch urine specimen for culture.

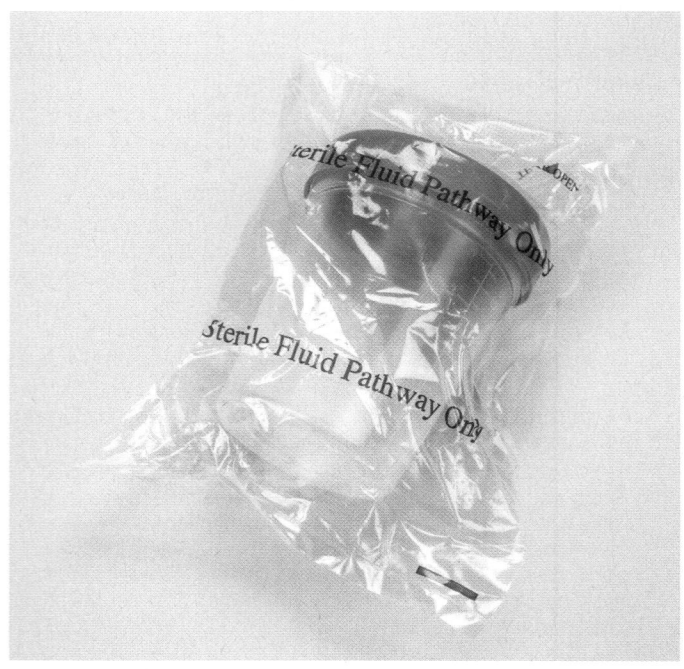

Figure 34.3 ■ Disposable clean-catch specimen equipment.

Collecting a Urine Specimen for Culture and Sensitivity by Clean Catch

SKILL 34.2

PURPOSE

- To determine the presence of microorganisms, the type of organism(s), and the antibiotics to which the organisms are sensitive

ASSESSMENT

- Determine the ability of the client to provide the specimen.
- Assess the color, odor, and consistency of the urine and the presence of clinical signs of urinary tract infection (e.g., frequency, urgency, dysuria, hematuria, flank pain, cloudy urine with foul odor).

PLANNING

Assignment

AP may perform the collection of a clean-catch or midstream urine specimen. It is important, however, for the nurse to inform the AP about how to instruct the client in the correct process for obtaining the specimen. Proper cleansing of the urethra should be emphasized to avoid contaminating the urine specimen.

Equipment

Equipment used varies from agency to agency. Some agencies use commercially prepared disposable clean-catch kits. Others use agency-prepared sterile trays. Both prepared trays and kits generally contain the following items:

- Clean gloves
- Antiseptic towelettes
- Sterile specimen container
- Specimen identification label.

In addition the nurse needs to obtain the following:

- Completed laboratory requisition form
- Urine receptacle, if the client is not ambulatory
- Basin of warm water, soap, washcloth, and towel for the non-ambulatory client.

IMPLEMENTATION

Preparation

Gather the necessary equipment needed for the collection of the specimen. Use visual aids, if available, to assist the client to understand the midstream collection technique.

Performance

1. Prior to performing the procedure, introduce self and verify the client's identity using agency protocol. Explain to the client that a urine specimen is required, give the reason, and explain the method to be used to collect it. Discuss how the results will be used in planning further care or treatments.
2. Perform hand hygiene and observe other appropriate infection prevention procedures.
3. Provide for client privacy.
4. For an ambulatory client who is able to follow directions, instruct the client on how to collect the specimen.
   - Direct or assist the client to the bathroom.
   - Ask the client to wash and dry the genitals and perineal area with soap and water. **Rationale:** *Washing the perineal area reduces the number of skin and transient bacteria, decreasing the risk of contaminating the urine specimen.*
   - Ask the client if he or she is sensitive to any antiseptic or cleansing agent. **Rationale:** *This will avoid unnecessary irritation of the genitals or perineum.*

Collecting a Urine Specimen for Culture and Sensitivity by Clean Catch—*continued*

- Instruct the client on how to clean the urinary meatus with antiseptic towelettes. **Rationale:** *The antiseptic further reduces bacterial contamination of the urinary meatus and the risk of contaminating the specimen.*

For Female Clients

- Spread the labia minora with one hand and with the other hand, use one towelette to cleanse one side of the labia minora. Use another towelette for cleaning the other side of the labia minora. Use the third towelette to clean over the urethra. Always cleanse the perineal area from front to back and discard the towelette. ❶ Use all towelettes provided. **Rationale:** *Cleaning from front to back cleans the area of least contamination to the area of greatest contamination.*

For Male Clients

- If uncircumcised, retract the foreskin slightly to expose the urinary meatus.
- Using a circular motion, clean the urinary meatus and the distal portion of the penis. ❷ Use each towelette only once, then discard. Clean several inches down the shaft of the penis. **Rationale:** *This cleans from the area of least contamination to the area of greatest contamination.*

5. For a client who requires assistance, prepare the client and equipment.
   - Apply clean gloves.
   - Wash the perineal area with soap and water, rinse, and dry.
   - Assist the client onto a clean commode or bedpan. If using a bedpan or urinal, position the client as upright as allowed or tolerated. **Rationale:** *Assuming a normal anatomic position for voiding facilitates urination.*
   - Remove and discard gloves.
   - Perform hand hygiene.
   - Open the clean-catch kit, taking care not to contaminate the inside of the specimen container or lid. **Rationale:** *It is important to maintain sterility of the specimen container to prevent contamination of the specimen.*
   - Apply clean gloves.
   - Clean the urinary meatus and perineal area as described in step 4.
6. Collect the specimen from a nonambulatory client or instruct an ambulatory client on how to collect it.
   - Instruct the client to start voiding. **Rationale:** *Bacteria in the distal urethra and at the urinary meatus are cleared by the first few milliliters of urine expelled.*
   - Place the specimen container into the midstream of urine and collect the specimen, taking care not to touch the container to the perineum or penis. **Rationale:** *It is important to avoid contaminating the interior of the specimen container and the specimen itself.*
   - Collect urine in the container.
   - Cap the container tightly, touching only the outside of the container and the cap. **Rationale:** *This prevents contamination or spilling of the specimen.*
   - If necessary, clean the outside of the specimen container with disinfectant. **Rationale:** *This prevents transfer of microorganisms to others.*
   - Remove and discard gloves.
   - Perform hand hygiene.
7. Label the specimen and transport it to the laboratory.
   - Ensure that the specimen label is attached to the specimen cup, not the lid, and that the laboratory requisition provides the correct information. Place the specimen in a plastic bag that has a biohazard label on it. Attach the requisition securely to the bag. **Rationale:** *Inaccurate identification or information on the specimen container risks errors in diagnosis or therapy.*
   - Arrange for the specimen to be sent to the laboratory immediately. **Rationale:** *Bacterial cultures must be started immediately before any contaminating organisms can grow, multiply, and produce false results.*
8. Document pertinent data.
   - Record collection of the specimen, any pertinent observations of the urine such as color, odor, or consistency, and any difficulty in voiding that the client experienced.
   - Indicate on the laboratory slip if the client is taking any current antibiotic therapy or if the client is menstruating.

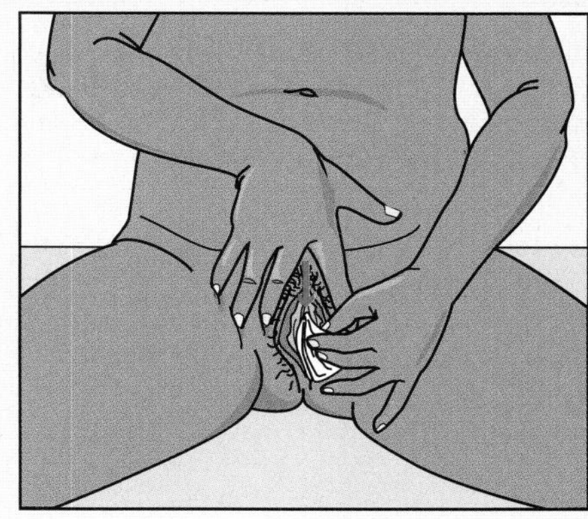

❶ Cleansing the female urinary meatus. Spread the labia minora with one hand and with the other hand, cleanse the perineal area from front to back.

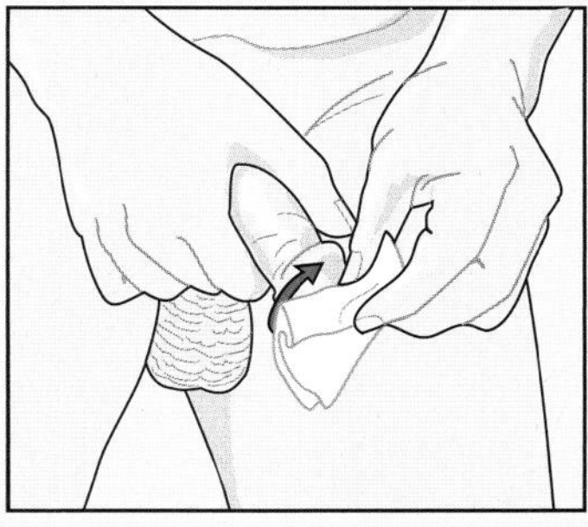

❷ Cleansing the male urinary meatus. Retract the foreskin if needed. Using a towelette, cleanse the urinary meatus by moving in a circular motion from the center of the urethral opening around the glans and down the distal portion of the shaft of the penis.

SAMPLE DOCUMENTATION

6/15/20 0800 Informed of MD order for clean-catch urine for C&S. Instructed how to perform. Stated she understood. Urine specimen cloudy. States she continues to have burning on urination. Urine specimen sent to laboratory. Antibiotic started per MD orders. T. Sanchez, RN

EVALUATION

- Report laboratory results to the primary care provider.
- Discuss findings of the laboratory test with primary care provider.
- Conduct appropriate follow-up nursing interventions as needed, such as administering ordered medications and client teaching.

LIFESPAN CONSIDERATIONS Urine Specimen

INFANTS

- Clean the perineal area and the urethral opening as you would with an adult client. Apply a specimen bag that has an adhesive backing that attaches to the skin. After the infant has voided the desired amount, gently remove the bag from the skin.

CHILDREN

- When collecting a routine urine specimen, explain the procedure in simple nonmedical terms appropriate to the child and ask the child to void using a clean collecting receptacle (e.g., specimen cup, potty chair, bedpan, toilet collection device).
- Give the child a clean specimen container to play with.
- Allow a parent to assist the child, if possible. The child may feel more comfortable with a parent present.
- For sterile urine specimens, straight catheterization may be necessary, in which a urinary catheter is inserted using sterile technique, the specimen is obtained, and the catheter is removed.

OLDER ADULTS

- For a clean-catch urine specimen, older adults may have difficulty controlling the stream of urine.
- Older women with arthritis may have difficulty holding the labia apart during the collection of clean-catch urine.

Timed Urine Specimen

Some urine examinations require collection of all urine produced and voided over a specific period of time, ranging from 1 to 2 hours to 24 hours. Timed specimens generally either are refrigerated or contain a preservative to prevent bacterial growth or decomposition of urine components. Each voiding of urine is collected in a small, clean container and then emptied immediately into the large refrigerated bottle or carton.

Timed urine specimen tests are performed for the following purposes:

- To assess the ability of the kidney to concentrate and dilute urine.
- To determine disorders of glucose metabolism, for example, diabetes mellitus.
- To determine levels of specific constituents, for example, albumin, amylase, creatinine, urobilinogen, or certain hormones (e.g., estriol or corticosteroids), in the urine.

To collect a timed urine specimen, follow these steps:

- Obtain a specimen container with preservative (if indicated) from the laboratory. Label the container with identifying information for the client, the test to be performed, time started, and time of completion.
- Provide a clean receptacle to collect urine (bedpan, commode, or toilet collection device).
- Post signs in the client's chart or electronic health record, Kardex, room, and bathroom alerting personnel to save all urine during the specified time.
- At the start of the collection period, have the client void and discard this urine.
- Save all urine produced during the timed collection period in the container, refrigerating or placing the container on ice as indicated. Avoid contaminating the urine with toilet paper or feces.
- At the end of the collection period, instruct the client to completely empty the bladder and save this voiding as part of the specimen. Take the entire amount of urine collected to the laboratory with the completed requisition.
- Record collection of the specimen, time started and completed, and any pertinent observations of the urine on appropriate records.

Clinical Alert!

If the client or staff forgets and discards the client's urine during a timed collection, the procedure must be restarted from the beginning.

QSEN Patient-Centered Care: Collecting Urine Specimens in the Home Setting

The nurse should consider the following aspects when collecting urine specimens in the home setting:

- Assess the client's ability and willingness to collect a timed urine specimen. If poor eyesight or hand tremors are a problem, suggest using a clean funnel to pour the urine into the container.
- Always wash hands well with warm, soapy water before and after collecting urine samples.
- Always wear gloves when handling another individual's urine.
- The home should have a refrigerator or other method for cooling the urine samples. Tell the client to keep the specimen container in plastic in the refrigerator, separate from other refrigerator contents. The client may also use a cooler with ice.

Indwelling Catheter Specimen

Closed drainage urinary systems now have needleless ports, which means that needles are not needed to obtain a sample. This protects the nurse from a needlestick injury and maintains the integrity and sterility of the catheter system. The needleless port accepts a Luer-Lok syringe (Figure 34.4 ■). Position the syringe perpendicular to the center of the port and insert, twist, and lock into the port. When the specimen is obtained and the syringe removed, the port seals itself.

To collect a specimen from a Foley (retention) catheter or a drainage tube, follow these steps:

- Apply clean gloves.
- If there is no urine in the catheter, clamp the drainage tubing at least 8 cm (3 in.) below the sampling port for about 30 minutes. This allows fresh urine to collect in the catheter.

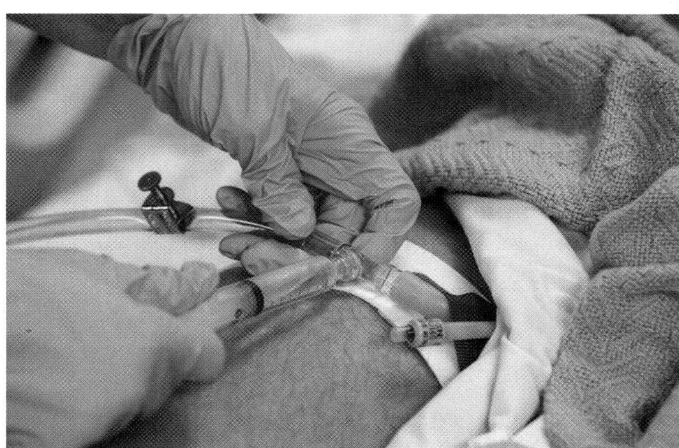

Figure 34.4 ■ Obtaining a urine specimen from a retention catheter using a needleless port.

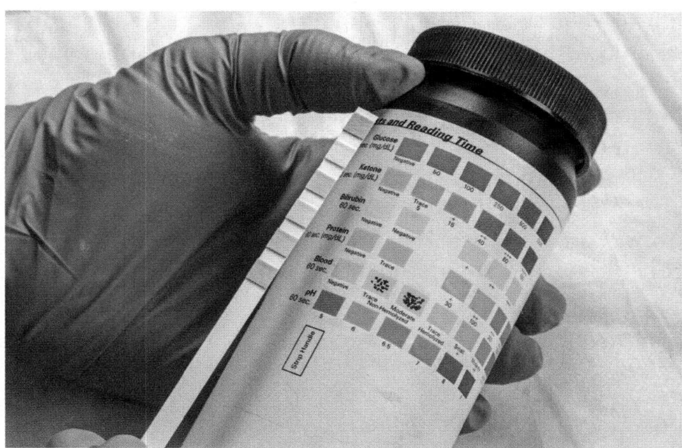

Figure 34.5 ■ After dipping the reagent strip (dipstick) into fresh urine, wait the stated time period and compare the results to the color chart.

- Wipe the area where the Luer-Lok syringe will be inserted with a disinfectant swab.
- Insert the Luer-Lok syringe at a 90-degree angle into the needleless port.
- Withdraw the required amount of urine, for example, 3 mL for a urine culture or 30 mL for a routine urinalysis.
- Transfer the urine to the specimen container. If a sterile culture tube is used, make sure the syringe does not touch the outside of the container.
- Unclamp the catheter.
- Discard the syringe in an appropriate sharps container.
- Cap the container.
- Remove gloves and discard.
- Perform hand hygiene.
- Label the container, and send the urine to the laboratory immediately for analysis or refrigeration.
- Record collection of the specimen and any pertinent observations of the urine on the appropriate records.

Urine Testing

Nurses in a healthcare facility or clients in the home setting can use commercially prepared kits to test for abnormal constituents in the urine. These include tests for specific gravity, pH, and the presence of abnormal constituents such as glucose, ketones, protein, and occult blood. These kits contain the required equipment and an appropriate reagent, which may be in the form of a tablet, fluid, or paper test strip or dipstick. When the urine contacts the reagent, a chemical reaction occurs, causing a color change that is then compared with a chart to interpret the significance of the color (Figure 34.5 ■). Specific directions for the amount of urine needed, the time required for the chemical reaction, and the meaning of the colors produced vary among manufacturers. Thus it is essential that nurses and clients read and follow directions supplied by each manufacturer. In addition, testing materials need to be checked to ascertain that they are not outdated.

Urine testing may be performed by AP. It is important for the AP to understand the specific specimen collection procedure and report the results of the test to the nurse. Inform the AP to save the urine sample to allow the nurse to repeat the test if necessary.

SPECIFIC GRAVITY

Specific gravity is an indicator of urine concentration, or the amount of solutes (metabolic wastes and electrolytes) present in the urine. The specific gravity of distilled water is 1.00; the specific gravity of urine normally ranges from 1.010 to 1.025. As urine becomes more concentrated, its specific gravity increases. Excess fluid intake or diseases affecting the ability of the kidneys to concentrate urine can result in low specific gravity readings. A high specific gravity may indicate fluid deficit or dehydration, or excess solutes such as glucose in the urine. Specific gravity can be measured with the use of a multiple-test dipstick that has a separate reagent area for specific gravity.

URINARY PH

Urinary pH is measured to determine the relative acidity or alkalinity of urine and assess the client's acid–base status. Quantitative measurements of urine pH can be performed in the laboratory, but dipsticks or litmus paper often are used on nursing units or in clinics to obtain less precise pH measurements. Urine normally is slightly acidic, with an average pH of 6 (7 is neutral, less than 7 is acidic, greater than 7 is alkaline). Because the kidneys play a critical role in regulating acid–base balance, assessment of urine pH can be useful in determining whether the kidneys are responding appropriately to acid–base imbalances. In metabolic acidosis, urine pH should decrease as the kidneys excrete hydrogen ions; in metabolic alkalosis, the pH should increase (see Chapter 51 ∞).

GLUCOSE

Urine is tested for glucose to screen clients for diabetes mellitus and to assess clients during pregnancy for abnormal glucose tolerance. Normally, the amount of glucose in the urine is negligible, although individuals who have ingested large amounts of sugar may show small amounts of glucose in their urine.

Testing urine for glucose is *not* a measure of current blood glucose level and is considered an inadequate measurement. The American Diabetes Association (ADA, 2018) states that testing urine for glucose is *only* for people who *cannot or will not* test their blood glucose levels. It is important for clients to understand that urine testing is considered an inadequate measurement of blood glucose.

KETONES

Ketone bodies, a product of the breakdown of fatty acids, normally are not present in the urine. They may, however, be found in the urine of clients with poorly controlled diabetes. Urine testing for ketone level is advised for type 1 diabetics who are at home and not feeling well, who are running a fever, or who have blood glucose consistently over 240 mg/dL (ADA, 2015).

PROTEIN

Protein molecules normally are too large to escape from glomerular capillaries into the filtrate. If the glomerular membrane has been damaged, however (e.g., because of an inflammatory process such as glomerulonephritis), it can become "leaky," allowing proteins to escape. Urine testing for the presence of protein generally is done with a reagent strip (commonly referred to as a *dipstick*).

OCCULT BLOOD

Normal urine is free from blood. When blood is present, it may be clearly visible or not visible (occult). Commercial reagent strips are used to test for occult blood in the urine.

Clinical Alert!

Blood in urine is indicative of damage to the kidney or urinary tract.

OSMOLALITY

Urine osmolality is a measure of the solute concentration of urine that is a more exact measurement of urine concentration than specific gravity. It is also used to monitor fluid and electrolyte balance. Normal values are 50 to 1200 mOsm/kg. The average urine osmolality is 200 to 800 mOsm/kg. An increased urine osmolality indicates a fluid volume deficit; a decreased urine osmolality reflects fluid volume excess. This test is sent to the laboratory rather than being evaluated at the bedside like the previous tests.

Sputum Specimens

Sputum is the mucous secretion from the lungs, bronchi, and trachea. It is important to differentiate it from **saliva**, the clear liquid secreted by the salivary glands in the mouth, sometimes referred to as "spit." Healthy individuals do not produce sputum. Clients need to cough to bring sputum up from the lungs, bronchi, and trachea into the mouth in order to expectorate it into a collecting container.

An AP can obtain a sputum specimen that is expectorated by a client. It is important to instruct the AP on when to collect the specimen, how to position the client, and how to correctly collect the specimen. A nurse should obtain a sputum specimen by use of pharyngeal suctioning, however, because it is an invasive process requiring aseptic technique and knowledge application and problem-solving. A "sputum trap" is used when the specimen is obtained by suctioning. (See Chapter 49 ∞, Skill 49.2.)

Sputum specimens are usually collected for one or more of the following reasons:

- For culture and sensitivity to identify a specific microorganism and its drug sensitivities.
- For cytology to identify the origin, structure, function, and pathology of cells. Specimens for cytology often require collection of three consecutive early-morning specimens and are tested to identify cancer in the lung and its specific cell type.
- For acid-fast bacillus (AFB), which also requires collection, often for 3 consecutive days, to identify the presence of tuberculosis (TB). Some agencies use a special glass container when the presence of AFB is suspected.
- To assess the effectiveness of therapy.

Sputum specimens are often collected in the morning. Upon awakening, the client can cough up the secretions that have accumulated during the night. Sometimes specimens are collected during postural drainage, when the client can usually produce sputum. When a client cannot cough, the nurse must sometimes use pharyngeal suctioning to obtain a specimen.

To collect a sputum specimen, the nurse follows these steps:

- Offer mouth care so that the specimen will not be contaminated with microorganisms from the mouth.
- Ask the client to breathe deeply and then cough up 1 to 2 teaspoons (4 to 10 mL) of sputum.
- Wear gloves and personal protective equipment to avoid direct contact with the sputum. Follow special precautions if tuberculosis is suspected. Obtain the specimen in a room equipped with a special airflow system or ultraviolet light, or outdoors. If these options are not available, wear a mask capable of filtering droplet nuclei.
- Ask the client to **expectorate** (cough up) the sputum into the specimen container. Make sure the sputum does not contact the outside of the container (Figure 34.6 ■). If the outside of the container does become contaminated, wash it with a disinfectant.
- Following sputum collection, offer mouthwash to remove any unpleasant taste.
- Label and transport the specimen to the laboratory. Ensure that the specimen label and the laboratory requisition contain the correct information. Arrange for the specimen to be sent to the laboratory immediately or refrigerated. Bacterial cultures must be started immediately before any contaminating organisms can grow, multiply, and produce false results.

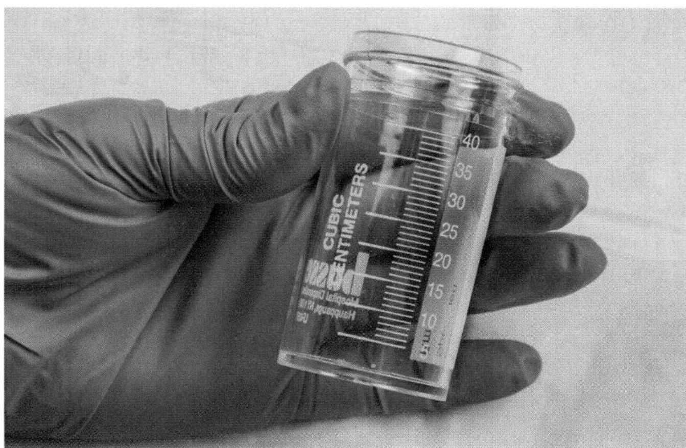

Figure 34.6 ■ Sputum specimen container.

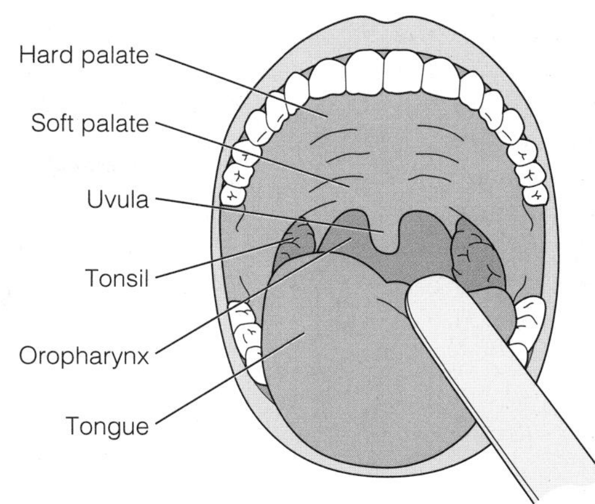

Figure 34.7 ■ Depressing the tongue to view the pharynx.

- Document the collection of the sputum specimen on the client's chart. Include the amount, color, consistency (thick, tenacious, watery), presence of **hemoptysis** (blood in the sputum), odor of the sputum, any measures needed to obtain the specimen (e.g., postural drainage), any discomfort experienced by the client, and any interventions implemented to ensure adequate air exchange postprocedure, such as O_2 saturation monitoring or administration of O_2.

Throat Culture

A throat culture sample is collected from the mucosa of the oropharynx and tonsillar regions using a culture swab. The sample is then cultured and examined for the presence of disease-producing microorganisms. Obtaining a throat culture is an invasive procedure that requires the application of scientific knowledge and potential problem-solving to ensure client safety. Thus it is best for the nurse to perform this procedure.

To obtain a throat culture specimen, the nurse applies clean gloves, then inserts the swab into the oropharynx and runs the swab along the tonsils and areas on the pharynx that are reddened or contain exudate. The gag reflex, active in some clients, may be decreased by having the client sit upright if health permits, open the mouth, extend the tongue, and say "ah," and by taking the specimen quickly. The sitting position and extension of the tongue help expose the pharynx; saying "ah" relaxes the throat muscles and helps minimize contraction of the constrictor muscle of the pharynx (the gag reflex). If the posterior pharynx cannot be seen, use a light and depress the tongue with a tongue blade (Figure 34.7 ■).

Visualization Procedures

Visualization procedures include *indirect visualization* (noninvasive) and *direct visualization* (invasive) techniques for visualizing body organ and system functions.

Clients with Gastrointestinal Alterations

Direct visualization techniques include **anoscopy**, the viewing of the anal canal; **proctoscopy**, the viewing of the rectum; **proctosigmoidoscopy**, the viewing of the rectum and sigmoid colon; and **colonoscopy**, the viewing of the large intestine. Indirect visualization of the gastrointestinal tract is achieved by roentgenography. X-rays of the gastrointestinal tract can detect strictures, obstructions, tumors, ulcers, inflammatory disease, or other structural changes such as hiatal hernias. Visualization of the tract is enhanced by the introduction of a radiopaque substance such as barium. For examination of the upper gastrointestinal tract or small bowel, the client drinks the barium sulfate. This examination

LIFESPAN CONSIDERATIONS Sputum and Throat Specimens

INFANTS

- When taking a throat swab, avoid occluding an infant's nose because infants normally breathe only through the nose.

CHILDREN

- Have a parent stand the young child between the parent's legs with the child's back to the parent and the parent's arms gently but firmly around the child. As the parent tips the child's head back, ask the child to open wide and stick the tongue out. Assure the child that the procedure will be over quickly and may "tickle" but should not hurt.

OLDER ADULTS

- Older adults may need encouragement to cough because a decreased cough reflex occurs with aging.
- Allow time for older adults to rest and recover between coughs when obtaining a sputum specimen.

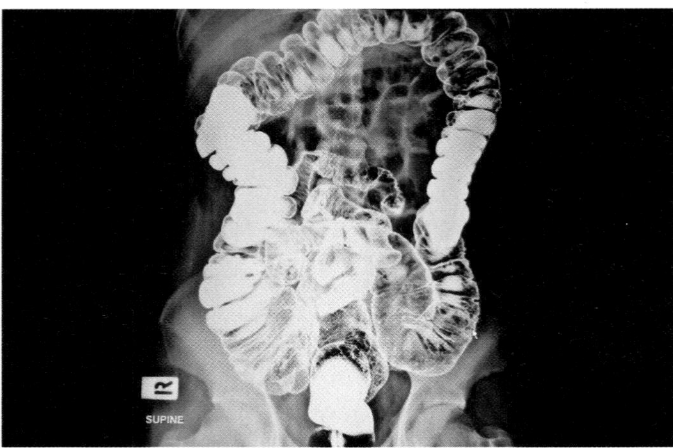

Figure 34.8 ■ X-ray of the colon during a barium enema exam.
plepraisaeng/123RF.

is often referred to as a *barium swallow*. For examination of the lower gastrointestinal tract, the client is given an enema containing the barium. This examination is commonly referred to as a *barium enema*. These x-rays usually include fluoroscopic examination; that is, projection of the x-ray films onto a screen, which permits continuous observation of the flow of barium (Figure 34.8 ■). Nurses are responsible for preparing clients before these studies and for follow-up care.

Clients with Urinary Alterations

Visualization procedures also may be used to evaluate urinary function. An x-ray of the **kidneys, ureters, and bladder** is commonly referred to as a **KUB**. **Intravenous pyelography (IVP)** and **retrograde pyelography** are also radiographic studies used to evaluate the urinary tract. In an IVP, contrast medium is injected intravenously; during retrograde pyelography, the contrast medium is instilled directly into the kidney pelvis via the urethra, bladder, and ureters. Following injection or instillation of the contrast medium, x-rays are taken to evaluate urinary tract structures. Renal **ultrasonography** is a noninvasive test that uses reflected sound waves to visualize the kidneys. During a **cystoscopy**, the bladder, ureteral orifices, and urethra can be directly visualized using a **cystoscope**, a lighted instrument inserted through the urethra. Nurses are responsible for preparing clients before these studies and for follow-up care.

Clients with Cardiopulmonary Alterations

A number of visualization procedures can be done to examine the cardiovascular system and respiratory tract.

Electrocardiography provides a graphic recording of the heart's electrical activity. Electrodes placed on the skin transmit the electrical impulses to an oscilloscope or graphic recorder. With the wave forms recorded, the **electrocardiogram (ECG)** can then be examined to detect dysrhythmias and alterations in conduction indicative of myocardial damage, enlargement of the heart, or drug effects.

Stress electrocardiography uses ECGs to assess the client's response to an increased cardiac workload during exercise. As the body's demand for oxygen increases with exercising, the cardiac workload increases, as does the oxygen demand of the heart muscle itself. Clients with coronary artery disease may develop chest pain and characteristic ECG changes during exercise.

Angiography is an invasive procedure requiring informed consent of the client. A radiopaque dye is injected into the vessels to be examined. Using fluoroscopy and x-rays, the flow through the vessels is assessed and areas of narrowing or blockage can be observed. Coronary angiography is performed to evaluate the extent of coronary artery disease; pulmonary angiography may be performed to assess the pulmonary vascular system, particularly if pulmonary emboli are suspected. Other vessels that may be studied include the carotid and cerebral arteries, the renal arteries, and the vessels of the lower extremities.

An **echocardiogram** is a noninvasive test that uses ultrasound to visualize structures of the heart and evaluate left ventricular function. Images produced as ultrasound waves are reflected back to a transducer after striking cardiac structures. The nurse should tell the client that this test causes no discomfort, although the conductive gel used may be cold.

X-ray examination of the chest is done both to diagnose disease and to assess the progress of a disease. For an x-ray examination, the nurse needs to inform the client that jewelry and clothing from the waist up must be removed.

A **lung scan**, also known as ventilation and perfusion scan, is a series of two lung scans. The ventilation quotient (VQ) scan measures how well air is flowing through the lungs. The perfusion scan shows where blood flows through the lungs. Both scans use a radioactive substance that is traced by a special type of scanner. The emissions from the radioisotopes indicate how well air and blood are traveling through the lungs. The VQ scan is frequently used to screen for a pulmonary embolism. The client needs to be informed that no radiation precautions are necessary because the amount of radioactivity is very small. The scans may take 20 to 40 minutes.

Laryngoscopy and bronchoscopy are sterile procedures that are conducted with a laryngoscope and bronchoscope, respectively. Tissue samples may also be taken for biopsy. The client is usually given a sedative before the examination resulting in the client being awake but drowsy during the procedure. A local anesthetic is sprayed on the client's pharynx to prevent gagging; alternatively, the client gargles with an anesthetic to numb the throat. The bronchoscope is then inserted to visualize the larynx or bronchi (Figure 34.9 ■). Informed consent is required for these procedures.

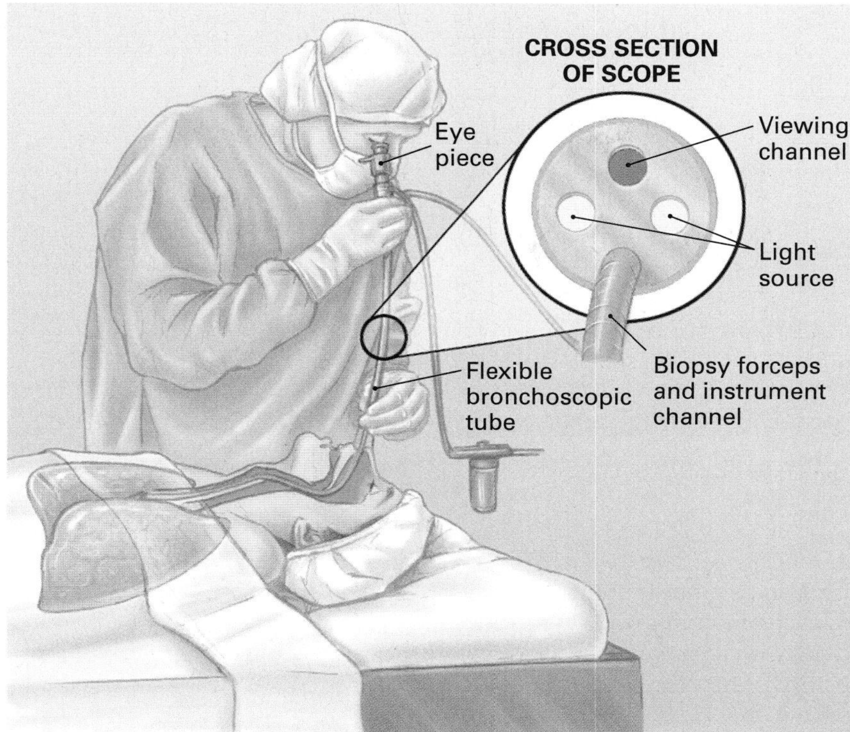

Figure 34.9 ■ Bronchoscopy.

Computed Tomography

Computed tomography (CT), also called *CT scanning, computerized tomography*, or *computerized axial tomography (CAT)*, is a painless, noninvasive x-ray procedure that has the unique capability of distinguishing minor differences in the density of tissues. The CT produces a three-dimensional image of the organ or structure, making it more sensitive than the x-ray machine.

Magnetic Resonance Imaging

Magnetic resonance imaging (MRI) is a noninvasive diagnostic scanning technique in which the client is placed in a magnetic field. Clients with implanted metal devices (e.g., pacemaker, metal hip prosthesis) cannot undergo an MRI because of the strong magnetic field. There is no exposure to radiation. If a contrast media is injected during the procedure, it is not an iodine contrast. Another advantage to the MRI is that it provides a better contrast between normal and abnormal tissue than the CT scan. It is, however, more costly.

All removable metallic objects (e.g., rings, watches, cell phones, body jewelry) should be removed before entering the area of the magnet. Body jewelry made of titanium, niobium, or surgical stainless steel, however, will not be attracted to the magnet. Recent reports have shown that in a very few instances, people with tattoos or permanent cosmetics have experienced edema or burning in the tattoo during an MRI.

Transdermal patches containing a foil backing may cause burning or injury. It is important to ask clients if they are using a transdermal patch so it can be removed before undergoing an MRI. Because the patch may lose its adhesiveness, advise the client to apply a new patch after the MRI.

Safety Alert! SAFETY

Advise clients to inform the MRI operator if they have a tattoo or permanent makeup and to let the operator know of any unusual sensations felt at the site of the tattoo during the MRI.

The MRI is commonly used for visualization of the brain, spine, limbs and joints, heart, blood vessels, abdomen, and pelvis. The procedure involves the client lying on a platform that moves into either a narrow, closed, high-magnet scanner or an open, low-magnet scanner. The client must lie very still. A two-way communication system is used to monitor the client's response and to help relieve feelings of claustrophobia. Earplugs are offered to the client to reduce the discomfort from the loud noises that occur during the test. The procedure lasts between 60 and 90 minutes (Figure 34.10 ■).

Nuclear Imaging Studies

Nuclear imaging studies involve the therapeutic use of radioactive isotopes for diagnostic purposes. A **radiopharmaceutical**, a pharmaceutical (targeted to a specific organ) with an embedded radioisotope, is administered through various routes for the test. The distribution

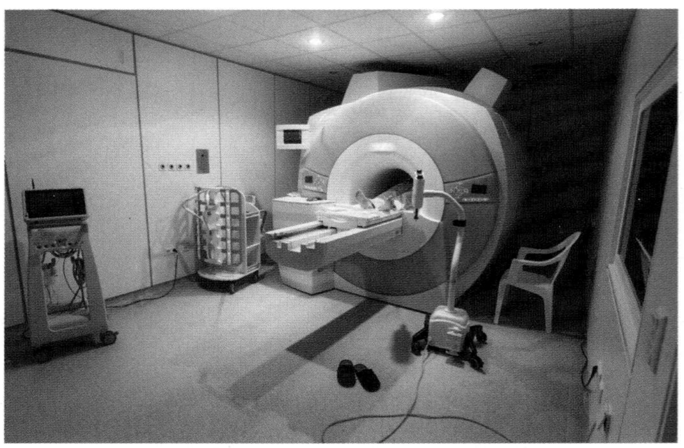

Figure 34.10 ■ Client being scanned in an MRI scanner.
zlikovec/123RF.

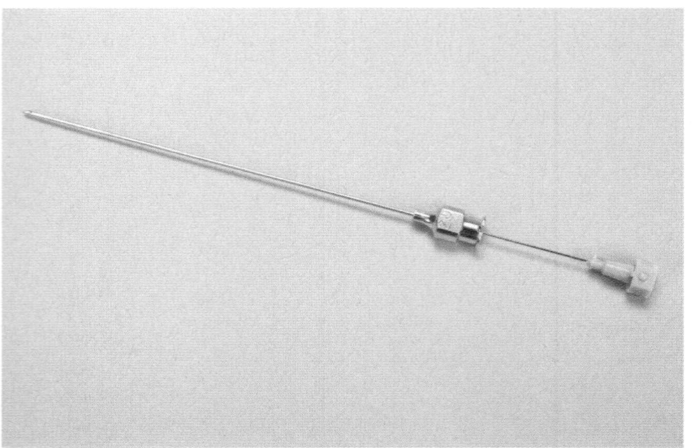

Figure 34.11 ■ A spinal needle with the stylet protruding from the hub.

of the isotope is different in normal tissue than it is in diseased tissue. For example, the distribution of the isotope in normal tissue is equal, uniform, and gray. Hyperfunction of an organ shows darker images that are referred to as "hot" spots. In contrast, hypofunctioning of an organ appears as lighter images that are called "cold" spots.

Positron emission tomography (PET) is a noninvasive radiologic study that involves the injection or inhalation of a radioisotope. Images are created as the radioisotope is distributed in the body. This allows study of various aspects of organ function and may include evaluation of blood flow and tumor growth, for example.

Aspiration and Biopsy

Aspiration is the withdrawal of fluid that has abnormally collected (e.g., pleural cavity, abdominal cavity) or the obtaining of a specimen (e.g., cerebrospinal fluid). A **biopsy** is the removal and examination of tissue. Biopsies are usually performed to determine a diagnosis or to detect malignancy. Both aspiration and biopsy are invasive procedures and require strict sterile technique.

Clinical Alert!

Determine if the facility requires a signed consent form for an aspiration or biopsy procedure.

Lumbar Puncture

In a **lumbar puncture** (LP, or spinal tap), cerebrospinal fluid (CSF) is withdrawn through a needle (Figure 34.11 ■) inserted into the subarachnoid space of the spinal canal between the third and fourth lumbar vertebrae or between the fourth and fifth lumbar vertebrae. At this level, the needle avoids damaging the spinal cord and major nerve roots (Figure 34.12 ■). The client is positioned laterally with the head bent toward the chest, the knees flexed onto the abdomen, and the back at the edge of the bed or

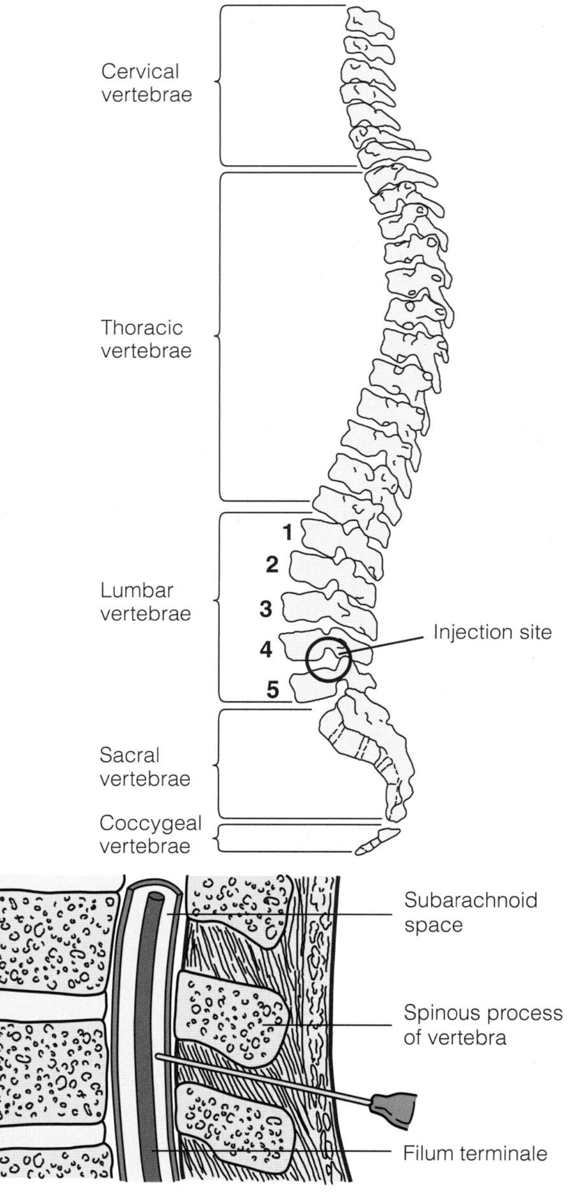

Figure 34.12 ■ A diagram of the vertebral column, indicating a site for insertion of the lumbar puncture needle into the subarachnoid space of the spinal canal.

LIFESPAN CONSIDERATIONS **Lumbar Puncture**

CHILDREN

- Briefly demonstrate the procedure on a doll or stuffed animal. Allow time to answer questions.
- One member of the healthcare team should stay in close physical contact with the child, maintain eye contact, and talk to and reassure the child during the procedure.

OLDER ADULTS

- Some clients need help maintaining the flexed position due to arthritis, weakness, or tremors.
- Provide an extra blanket to keep the client warm during the procedure. Older adults have a decreased metabolism and less subcutaneous fat.
- If the client has a hearing loss, speak slowly, distinctly, and loud enough, especially when unable to make eye contact.

examining table (Figure 34.13 ■). In this position the back is arched, increasing the spaces between the vertebrae so that the spinal needle can be inserted readily. During a lumbar puncture, the primary care provider frequently takes CSF pressure readings using a **manometer**, a glass or plastic tube calibrated in millimeters (Figure 34.14 ■).

Abdominal Paracentesis

Normally the body creates just enough peritoneal fluid for lubrication. The fluid is continuously formed and absorbed into the lymphatic system. However, in some disease processes, a large amount of fluid accumulates in the abdominal cavity; this condition is called **ascites**. Normal ascitic fluid is serous, clear, and light yellow in color. An **abdominal paracentesis** is carried out to obtain a fluid specimen for laboratory study and to relieve pressure on the abdominal organs due to the presence of excess fluid.

A primary care provider performs the procedure with the assistance of a nurse. Strict sterile technique is followed. A common site for abdominal paracentesis is midway between the umbilicus and the symphysis pubis on the midline (Figure 34.15 ■). The primary care provider makes a small incision with a scalpel, inserts the **trocar** (a sharp, pointed instrument) and **cannula** (tube), and then withdraws the trocar, which is inside the cannula (Figure 34.16 ■). Tubing is attached to the cannula and the fluid flows through the tubing into a receptacle. If the purpose of the paracentesis is to obtain a specimen, the primary care provider may use a long aspirating needle attached to a syringe rather than making an incision and using a trocar and cannula. Normally about 1500 mL is the maximum amount of fluid drained at one time to avoid hypovolemic shock. The fluid is drained very slowly for the same reason. Some fluid is placed in the specimen container before the cannula is withdrawn. The small incision may or may not be sutured; in either case, it is covered with a small sterile bandage.

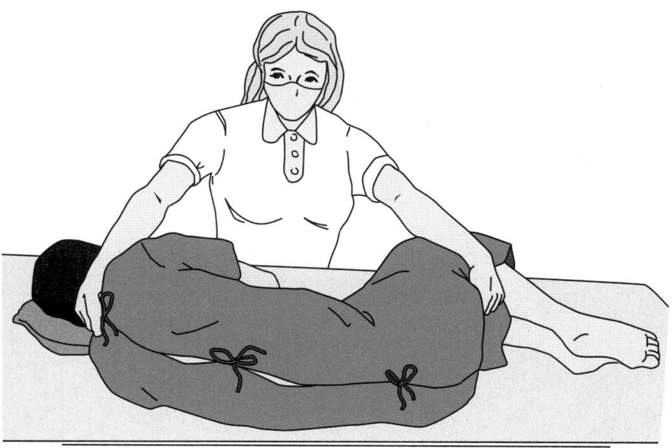

Figure 34.13 ■ Supporting the client for a lumbar puncture.

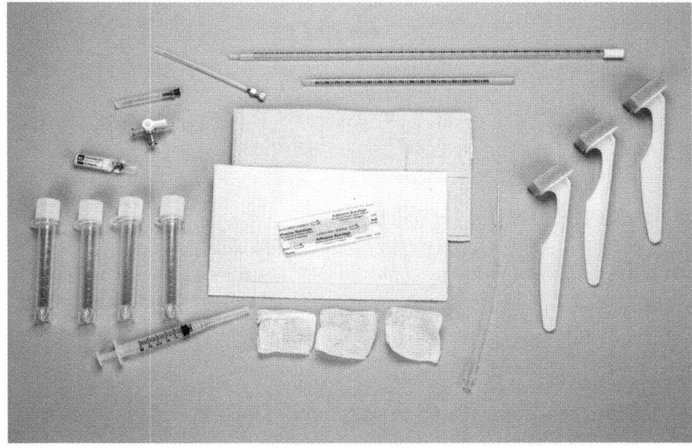

Figure 34.14 ■ A preassembled lumbar puncture set. Note the manometer at the top of the set.

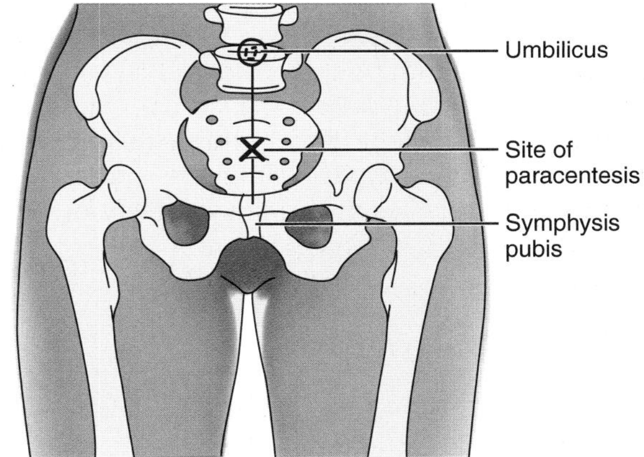

Figure 34.15 ■ A common site for an abdominal paracentesis.

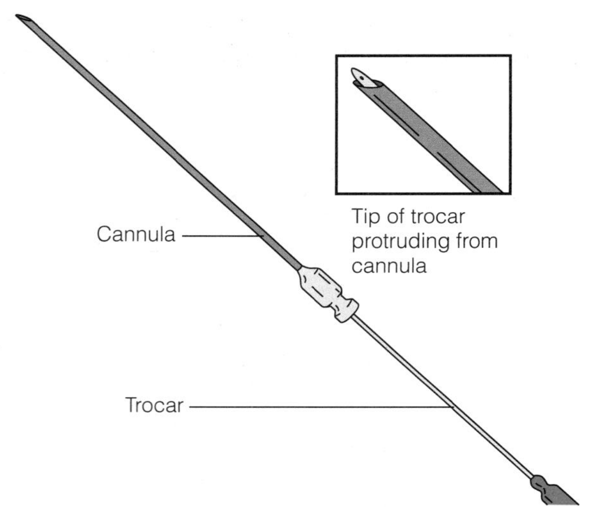

Figure 34.16 ■ A trocar and cannula may be used for an abdominal paracentesis.

LIFESPAN CONSIDERATIONS **Abdominal Paracentesis**

OLDER ADULTS

- Provide pillows and blankets to help older adults remain comfortable during the procedure.
- Ask the client to empty the bladder just before the procedure. Older adults may need to void more frequently and in smaller amounts.
- Remove ascitic fluid slowly and monitor the client for signs of hypovolemia. Older adults have less tolerance for fluid loss and may develop hypovolemia if a large volume of fluid is drained rapidly.

Thoracentesis

Normally, only sufficient fluid to lubricate the pleura is present in the pleural cavity. However, excessive fluid can accumulate as a result of injury, infection, or other pathology. In such a case or in the case of pneumothorax, a primary care provider may perform a **thoracentesis** to remove the excess fluid or air to ease breathing. Thoracentesis is also performed to introduce chemotherapeutic drugs intrapleurally.

The nurse assists the client to assume a position that allows easy access to the intercostal spaces. This is usually a sitting position with the arms above the head, which spreads the ribs and enlarges the intercostal space. Two positions commonly used are one in which the arm is elevated and stretched forward (Figure 34.17*A* ■) and one in which the client leans forward over a pillow (Figure 34.17*B*). To make sure that the needle is inserted below the fluid level when fluid is to be removed (or above any fluid if air is to be removed), the primary care provider will palpate and percuss the chest and select the exact site for insertion of the needle. A site on the lower posterior chest is often used to remove fluid, and a site on the upper anterior chest is used to remove air (Figure 34.18 ■). A chest x-ray prior to the procedure will help pinpoint the best insertion site.

The primary care provider and the assisting nurse follow strict sterile technique. The primary care provider attaches a syringe or stopcock to the aspirating needle. The stopcock must be in the closed position so that no air can enter the pleural space. The primary care provider inserts the needle through the intercostal space to the pleural cavity. In some instances, the primary care provider threads a small plastic tube through the needle and then withdraws the needle. (The tubing is less likely to puncture the pleura.)

If a syringe is used to collect the fluid, the plunger is pulled out to withdraw the pleural fluid as the stopcock is opened. If a large container is used to receive the fluid, the tubing is attached from the stopcock to the adapter on the receiving bottle. When the adapter and stopcock are opened, gravity allows fluid to drain from the pleural cavity into the container, which should be kept below the

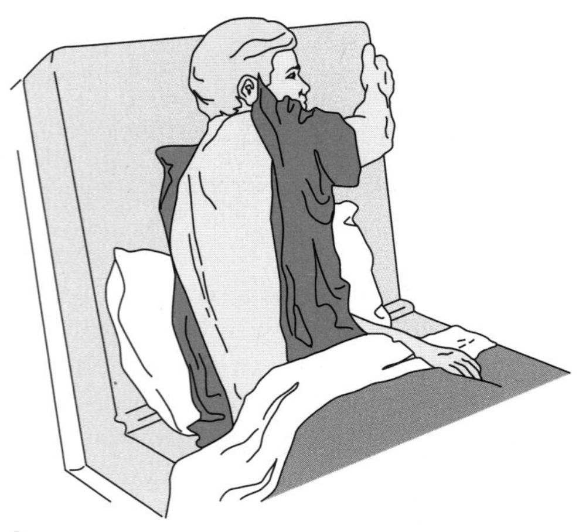

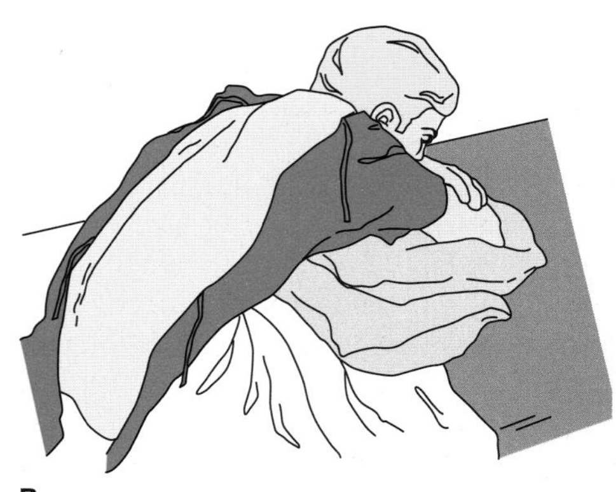

Figure 34.17 ■ Two positions commonly used for a thoracentesis: *A*, sitting on one side with arm held to the front and up; *B*, sitting and leaning forward over a pillow.

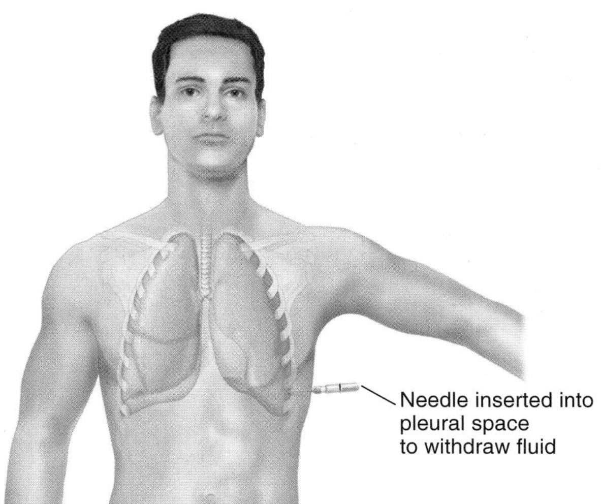

Figure 34.18 ■ Needle is inserted into the pleural space on the lower posterior chest to withdraw fluid.

From *Medical Terminology: A Living Language*, 7th ed. (p. 252), by B. Fremgen and S. Frucht, 2019. Reprinted and electronically reproduced by permission of Pearson Education, Inc., Hoboken, NJ.

LIFESPAN CONSIDERATIONS Thoracentesis

OLDER ADULTS

- Some older clients will need help maintaining the proper position due to arthritis, tremors, or weakness.
- Provide support with pillows during the procedure.
- Provide an extra blanket to keep your client warm during the procedure. Some older adults may have a decreased metabolism and less subcutaneous fat.

level of the client's lungs. After the fluid has been withdrawn, the primary care provider removes the needle or plastic tubing.

Bone Marrow Biopsy

Another type of diagnostic study is the *biopsy*. A biopsy is a procedure whereby tissue is obtained for examination. Biopsies are performed on many different types of tissues, for example, bone marrow, liver, breast, lymph nodes, and lung.

A bone marrow biopsy is the removal of a specimen of bone marrow for laboratory study. The biopsy is used to detect specific diseases of the blood, such as pernicious anemia and leukemia. The bones of the body commonly used for a bone marrow biopsy are the sternum, iliac crests, anterior or posterior iliac spines, and proximal tibia in children. The *posterior superior iliac crest* is the preferred site with the client placed prone or on the side (Figure 34.19 ■).

For most individuals, a bone marrow biopsy can be an extremely painful and distressing experience. A premedication such as an analgesic or antianxiety drug may be administered to the client. After injecting a local anesthetic, a small incision may be made with a scalpel to avoid tearing the skin or pushing skin into the bone marrow with a needle. The primary care provider then introduces a bone marrow needle with stylet into the red marrow of the spongy bone (Figure 34.20 ■).

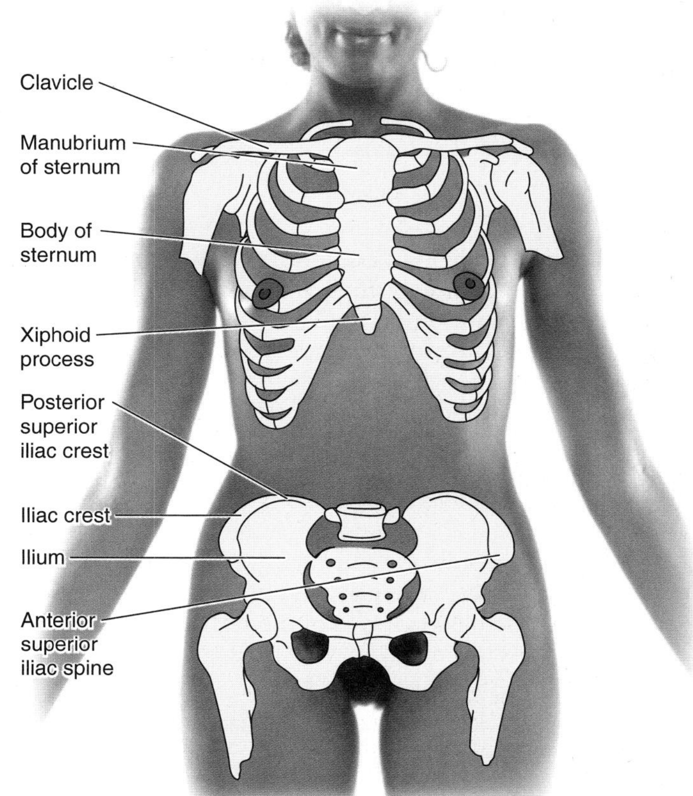

Figure 34.19 ■ The sternum and the iliac crests are common sites for a bone marrow biopsy.

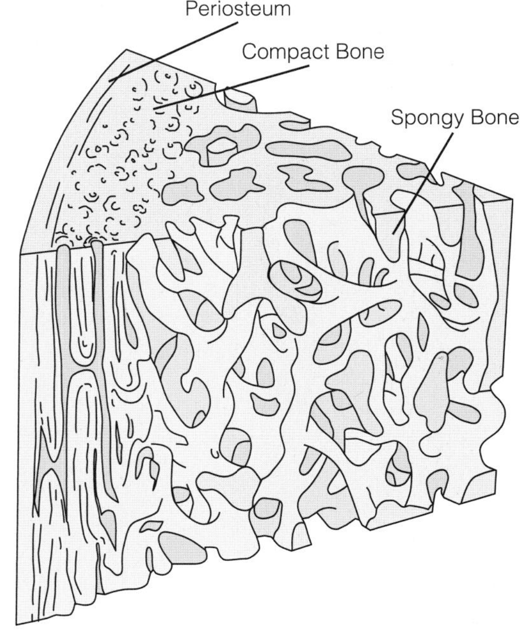

Figure 34.20 ■ A cross section of a bone.

LIFESPAN CONSIDERATIONS Bone Marrow Biopsy

CHILDREN

- Young clients need emotional support due to the pain and pressure associated with this procedure.
- Young clients may require gentle restraint to prevent movement during the procedure.

OLDER ADULTS

- Older adults with osteoporosis will experience less needle pressure.
- Ask the client to empty the bladder for comfort before the procedure.
- Provide pillows and blankets to help older adults remain comfortable during the procedure.

Once the needle is in the marrow space, the stylet is removed and a 10-mL syringe is attached to the needle. The plunger is withdrawn until 1 to 2 mL of marrow has been obtained. The primary care provider replaces the stylet in the needle, withdraws the needle, and places the specimen in test tubes or on glass slides.

Liver Biopsy

A liver biopsy is a short procedure, generally performed at the client's bedside, in which a sample of liver tissue is aspirated. A primary care provider inserts a needle in the intercostal space between two of the right lower ribs and into the liver (Figure 34.21 ■) or through the abdomen below the right rib cage (subcostally).

The client exhales and is instructed to hold his or her breath while the primary care provider inserts the biopsy needle, injects a small amount of sterile normal saline to clear the needle of blood or particles of tissue picked up during insertion, and aspirates liver tissue by drawing back on the plunger of the syringe. After the needle is withdrawn, the nurse applies pressure to the site to prevent bleeding, often by positioning the client on the biopsy site (Figure 34.22 ■).

Because many clients with liver disease have blood clotting defects and are prone to bleeding, prothrombin time and platelet count are normally taken well in advance of the test. If the test results are abnormal, the biopsy may be contraindicated.

Table 34.3 describes how the nurse assists with the above aspiration and biopsy procedures.

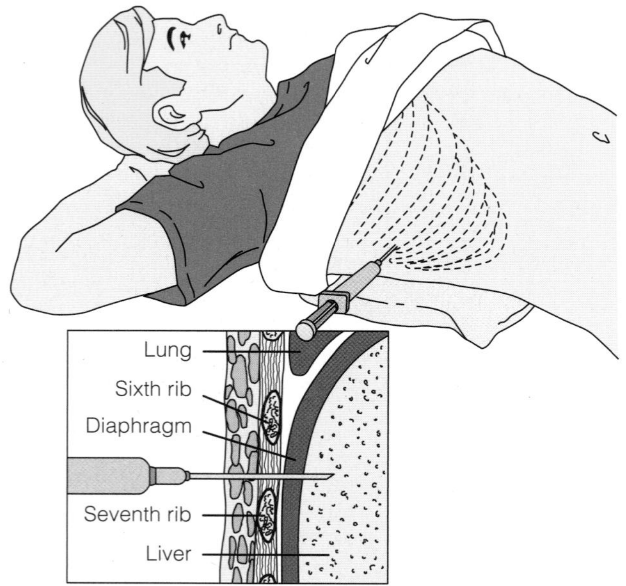

Figure 34.21 ■ A common site for a liver biopsy.

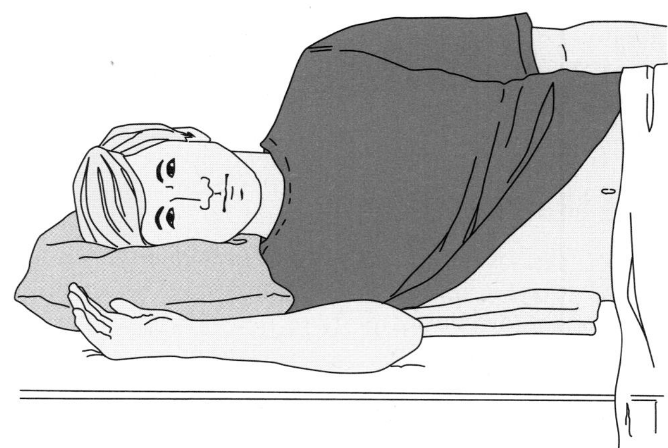

Figure 34.22 ■ The position used to provide pressure on a liver biopsy site.

TABLE 34.3 Assisting with Aspiration and Biopsy Procedures

Procedure	Preprocedure	During the Procedure	Postprocedure
Lumbar puncture	Prepare the client: • Explain the procedure to the client and support people. The primary care provider will be taking a small sample of spinal fluid from the lower spine. A local anesthetic will be given to minimize discomfort. Explain when and where the procedure will occur (e.g., the bedside or in a treatment room) and who will be present (e.g., the primary care provider and the nurse). Explain that it will be necessary to lie in a certain position without moving for about 15 min. A slight pinprick will be felt when the local anesthetic is injected and a sensation of pressure as the spinal needle is inserted. • Have the client empty the bladder and bowels prior to the procedure to prevent unnecessary discomfort. • Position and drape the client. • Open the lumbar puncture set.	Support and monitor the client throughout: • Stand in front of the client and support the back of the neck and knees if the client needs help remaining still. • Reassure the client throughout the procedure by explaining what is happening. Encourage normal breathing and relaxation. • Observe the client's color, respirations, and pulse during the procedure. Ask the client to report headache or persistent pain at the insertion site. Handle specimen tubes appropriately: • Wear gloves when handling test tubes. • Label the specimen tubes in sequence. • Send the CSF specimens to the laboratory immediately. Place a small sterile dressing over the puncture site.	Ensure the client's comfort and safety: • Assist the client to a dorsal recumbent position with only one head pillow. The client remains in this position for 1–12 h, depending on the primary care provider orders. • Determine whether analgesics are ordered and can be given for headaches. • Offer oral fluids frequently, unless contraindicated, to help restore the volume of CSF. Monitor the client: • Observe for swelling or bleeding at the puncture site. • Monitor changes in neurologic status. • Determine whether the client is experiencing any numbness, tingling, or pain radiating down the legs. Document the procedure on the client's chart: • Include date and time performed; the primary care provider's name; the color, character, and amount of CSF; and the number of specimens obtained. Also document CSF pressure and the nurse's assessments and interventions.
Abdominal paracentesis	Prepare the client: • Explain the procedure: obtaining the specimen usually takes about 15 min. Emphasize the importance of remaining still during the procedure. Tell the client when and where the procedure will occur and who will be present. • Have the client void just before the paracentesis to reduce the possibility of puncturing the urinary bladder. • Help the client assume a sitting position in bed, in a chair, or on the edge of the bed supported by pillows. • Maintain the client's privacy and provide blankets for warmth.	Assist and monitor the client: • Support the client verbally and describe the steps of the procedure as needed. • Observe the client closely for signs of distress (e.g., abnormal pulse rate, skin color, and blood pressure). • Observe for signs of hypovolemic shock induced by the loss of fluid: pallor, dyspnea, diaphoresis, drop in BP, and restlessness or increased anxiety. Place a small sterile dressing over the site of the incision after the cannula or aspirating needle is withdrawn.	Monitor the client closely: • Observe for hypovolemic shock. • Observe for scrotal edema with male clients. • Monitor VS, urine output, and drainage from the puncture site every 15 min for at least 2 h and every hour for 4 h or as the client's condition indicates. • Measure the abdominal girth at the level of the umbilicus. Document all relevant information: • Include date and time performed; the primary care provider's name; abdominal girth before and after; the color, clarity, and amount of drained fluid; and the nurse's assessments and interventions. Transport the correctly labeled specimens to the laboratory.

Continued on page 832

TABLE 34.3 Assisting with Aspiration and Biopsy Procedures—*continued*

Procedure	Preprocedure	During the Procedure	Postprocedure
Thoracentesis	Prepare the client: • Explain the procedure to the client. Normally, the client may experience some discomfort and a feeling of pressure when the needle is inserted. The procedure may bring considerable relief if breathing has been difficult. The procedure takes only a few minutes, depending primarily on the time it takes for the fluid to drain from the pleural cavity. To avoid puncturing the lungs, it is important for the client not to cough while the needle is inserted. Explain when and where the procedure will occur and who will be present. • Help position the client and cover the client as needed with a bath blanket.	Support and monitor the client throughout: • Support the client verbally and describe the steps of the procedure as needed. • Observe the client for signs of distress, such as dyspnea, pallor, and coughing. Collect drainage and laboratory specimens. Place a small sterile dressing over the site of the puncture.	Monitor the client: • Assess pulse rate, respiratory rate, and skin color. • Do not remove more than 1,000 mL of fluid from the pleural cavity within the first 30 min. • Observe changes in the client's cough, sputum, respiratory depth, and breath sounds, and note complaints of chest pain. Position the client appropriately: • Some agency protocols recommend that the client lie on the unaffected side with the head of the bed elevated 30° for at least 30 min because this position facilitates expansion of the affected lung and eases respirations. Document all relevant information: • Include date and time performed; the primary care provider's name; the amount, color, and clarity of fluid drained; and nursing assessments and interventions provided. Transport the correctly labeled specimens to the laboratory.
Bone marrow biopsy	Prepare the client: • Explain the procedure. The client may experience pain when the marrow is aspirated and hear a crunching sound as the needle is pushed through the cortex of the bone. The procedure usually takes 15–30 min. Explain when and where the procedure will occur, who will be present, and which site will be used. • Administer a premedication as ordered. • Help the client assume a supine position (with one pillow if desired) for a biopsy of the sternum (sternal puncture) or a prone position for a biopsy of either iliac crest. Fold the bedclothes back or drape the client to expose the area.	Monitor and support the client throughout: • Describe the steps of the procedure as needed and provide verbal support. • Observe the client for pallor, diaphoresis, and faintness due to bleeding or pain. Place a small dressing over the site of the puncture after the needle is withdrawn: • Some agency protocols recommend direct pressure over the site for 5–10 min to prevent bleeding. Assist with preparing specimens as needed.	Monitor the client: • Assess for discomfort and bleeding from the site. The client may experience some tenderness in the area. Bleeding and hematoma formation need to be assessed for several days. Report bleeding or pain to the nurse in charge. • Provide an analgesic as needed and ordered. Document all relevant information: • Include date and time of the procedure; the primary care provider's name; and any nursing assessments and interventions. • Document any specimens obtained. Transport the correctly labeled specimens to the laboratory.

TABLE 34.3 Assisting with Aspiration and Biopsy Procedures—*continued*

Procedure	Preprocedure	During the Procedure	Postprocedure
Liver biopsy	Prepare the client: • Give preprocedural medications as ordered. Vitamin K may be given for several days before the biopsy to reduce the risk of hemorrhage. • Explain the procedure and tell the client that the primary care provider will take a small sample of liver tissue by putting a needle into the client's side or abdomen. Explain that a sedative and local anesthetic will be given, so the client will feel no pain. Explain when and where the procedure will occur, who will be present, the time required, and what to expect as the procedure is being performed (e.g., the client may experience mild discomfort when the local anesthetic is injected and slight pressure when the biopsy needle is inserted). • Ensure that the client fasts for at least 2 h before the procedure. • Administer the appropriate premedication about 30 min beforehand or at the specified time. • Help the client assume a supine position with the upper right quadrant of the abdomen exposed. Cover the client with the bedclothes so that only the abdominal area is exposed.	Monitor and support the client throughout: • Support the client in a supine position. • Instruct the client to take a few deep inhalations and exhalations and to hold the breath after the final exhalation for up to 10 sec as the needle is inserted, the biopsy obtained, and the needle withdrawn. Holding the breath after exhalation immobilizes the chest wall and liver and keeps the diaphragm in its highest position, avoiding injury to the lung and laceration of the liver. • Instruct the client to resume breathing when the needle is withdrawn. • Apply pressure to the site of the puncture to help stop any bleeding. Apply a small dressing to the site of the puncture.	Position the client appropriately: • Assist the client to a right side-lying position with a small pillow or folded towel under the biopsy site. Instruct the client to remain in this position for several hours. Monitor the client: • Assess the client's VS every 15 min for the first hour following the test or until the signs are stable. Then monitor vital signs every hour for 24 h or as needed. • Determine whether the client is experiencing abdominal pain. Severe abdominal pain may indicate bile peritonitis. • Check the biopsy site for localized bleeding. Pressure dressings may be required if bleeding does occur. Document all relevant information: • Include date and time performed; the primary care provider's name; and all nursing assessments and interventions. Transport the correctly labeled specimens to the laboratory.

LIFESPAN CONSIDERATIONS Liver Biopsy

OLDER ADULTS

- Observe for skin irritation from tape applied to the sterile dressing. Older adults often have fragile skin.
- Ask the client to empty the bladder before the procedure. Older adults may need to void more often and in smaller amounts.

LIFESPAN CONSIDERATIONS General Considerations

CHILDREN

- Children may be frightened of even noninvasive procedures to collect specimens if they are not sure what is going to happen. Cooperation can be maximized by:
  - Demonstrating on dolls or teddy bears.
  - Allowing the child to examine and explore the collection materials being used.
  - Explaining in age-appropriate language what will be done.
  - Having parents actively involved in gently holding and comforting the child during and after the procedure.
  - Being well prepared to conduct the procedure.
  - Performing the procedure quickly, competently, and as gently as possible.

OLDER ADULTS

- In older adults, homeostatic mechanisms are not as efficient as in the younger clients. When undergoing diagnostic tests that challenge these functions, care must be taken to accurately monitor functions and note any changes. Examples:
  - Dehydration and electrolyte imbalance can occur from laxative preps given before bowel diagnostic tests, such as a colonoscopy.
  - Fluid restrictions and NPO status for a length of time can lead to hypovolemia and electrolyte imbalances.
  - Many dye contrasts used for x-rays and scans can cause renal damage (especially in clients with diabetes).
  - Sedation used for certain procedures may require a longer recovery time for older clients.
  - Having several tests at a time or for several days compounds these potential problems and increases fatigue.

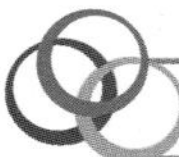

Critical Thinking Checkpoint

A 68-year-old woman is admitted with fever, nausea, vomiting, and abdominal pain. She informs you that she is a "borderline diabetic" and "only has to watch what she eats." She tells you that she has not eaten for 3 days and has had difficulty "keeping liquids down." While doing the nursing history, she describes her urine as dark and foul smelling. Upon further questions, she states she does have some burning on urination. She describes her abdominal pain as constant and generalized, and rates it as a 5 or 6 on a scale of 0 to 10. The primary care provider called in the following orders:

CBC and electrolytes STAT
Capillary blood glucose STAT and q4h
VS and TPR q4h
Urine specimen for C&S
CXR
Flat plate abdominal x-ray.

1. When measuring the client's capillary blood glucose, you do not obtain enough blood to cover the indicator square on the reagent strip. What could be possible reasons and what should you do?
2. The laboratory work returns with the following results: WBC = 17,000/mm^3 with neutrophils = 80%; Hct = 46.2. Based on these results, what are your nursing interventions?
3. The primary care provider orders IV fluids and an antibiotic with the first dose to be given STAT. You have not obtained the urine specimen yet. Which has priority (e.g., starting the IV, administrating the antibiotic, or obtaining the urine specimen) and why?
4. Three days later, the client has the following laboratory results: Hct = 39.2 and WBC = 10,000/mm^3. What do those results indicate to you?
5. The abdominal x-ray shows a possible mass. An MRI of the abdomen is ordered. The client is quite anxious because she has heard from her friend that the procedure is difficult for people who are claustrophobic. How will you respond?

Answers to Critical Thinking Checkpoint questions are available on the faculty resources site. Please consult with your instructor.

Chapter 34 Review

CHAPTER HIGHLIGHTS

- Diagnostic testing involves three phases. Client preparation is the focus during the pretest phase. During the intratest phase, the nurse performs or assists with the diagnostic test and collects the specimen. Providing nursing care of the client and follow-up activities and observations are the role of the nurse during the posttest phase.
- Blood tests are commonly used diagnostic tests. Routinely ordered blood tests can include complete blood count (CBC) and serum electrolytes.
- A capillary blood glucose is a frequent test performed by nurses and clients. This test is used to monitor glucose levels of clients at risk for hyper- and hypoglycemia. It also evaluates the effectiveness of insulin administration.
- Nursing responsibilities associated with specimen collection include (a) providing client comfort, privacy, and safety; (b) explaining the purpose of and procedure for the specimen collection; (c) using correct procedure for obtaining the specimen; (d) noting relevant information on the laboratory requisition slip; (e) transporting the specimen promptly; and (f) reporting abnormal findings.
- The nurse is responsible for obtaining stool specimens ordered for laboratory analysis.
- Nurses collect urine specimens for a number of tests. A clean voided specimen is used for routine examination. A clean-catch or midstream voided specimen is collected when a urine culture is ordered to identify microorganisms. Timed urine specimens are collected for a variety of tests, depending on the client's health problem. Nurses can complete some simple urine tests (e.g., specific gravity, pH, glucose, ketones, protein, and occult blood) by using a reagent strip.
- Sputum and throat culture specimens help determine the presence of disease-producing organisms.
- Visualization procedures include indirect visualization or noninvasive procedures such as lung scan, echocardiogram, electrocardiography, x-ray, CT, and MRI. In contrast, direct visualization or invasive techniques visualize body organs and system functions. Examples of invasive procedures include colonoscopy, barium enema, intravenous pyelography, and angiography.
- Examples of aspiration and biopsy tests include lumbar puncture, abdominal paracentesis, thoracentesis, bone marrow biopsy, and liver biopsy. These tests are invasive procedures and require strict sterile technique. After the procedure, the nurse assesses the client for possible complications and provides appropriate nursing interventions as needed.

TEST YOUR KNOWLEDGE

1. A nurse needs to collect a specimen from a client. The nurse has never collected this type of specimen in the past. What should the nurse do?
   1. Notify the physician.
   2. Ask another nurse to collect the specimen.
   3. Consult the nursing procedure manual.
   4. Delegate the collection of the specimen to an unlicensed assistive personnel.
2. A client is having a timed urine collection done. The unlicensed assistive personnel does not save one specimen. What should the nurse do?
   1. Continue with the test and document that one specimen is missing.
   2. End the test immediately and send what is collected to the laboratory.
   3. Document that the test cannot be completed.
   4. Start the test over.

3. The client has a urinary health problem. Which procedure is performed using indirect visualization?
1. Intravenous pyelography (IVP)
2. Kidneys, ureter, bladder (KUB)
3. Retrograde pyelography
4. Cystoscopy

4. Which noninvasive procedure provides information about the physiology or function of an organ?
1. Angiography
2. Computerized tomography (CT)
3. Magnetic resonance imaging (MRI)
4. Positron emission tomography (PET)

5. When assisting with a bone marrow biopsy, the nurse should take which action?
1. Assist the client to a right side-lying position after the procedure.
2. Observe for signs of dyspnea, pallor, and coughing.
3. Assess for bleeding and hematoma formation for several days after the procedure.
4. Stand in front of the client and support the back of the neck and knees.

6. During an assessment, the nurse learns that the client has a history of liver disease. Which diagnostic tests might be indicated for this client? Select all that apply.
1. Alanine aminotransferase (ALT)
2. Myoglobin
3. Cholesterol
4. Ammonia
5. Brain natriuretic peptide or B-type natriuretic peptide (BNP)

7. The nurse practitioner requests a laboratory blood test to determine how well a client has controlled her diabetes during the past 3 months. Which blood test will provide this information?
1. Fasting blood glucose
2. Capillary blood specimen
3. Glycosylated hemoglobin
4. GGT (gamma-glutamyl transferase)

8. The client is supposed to have a fecal occult blood test done on a stool sample. The nurse is going to use the Hemoccult test. Which of the following indicates that the nurse is using the correct procedure? Select all that apply.
1. Mixes the reagent with the stool sample before applying to the card.
2. Collects a sample from two different areas of the stool specimen.
3. Assesses for a blue color change.
4. Asks a colleague to verify the pink color results.
5. Asks the client if he has taken vitamin C in the past few days.

9. For a lumbar puncture, which position should the nurse place the client in?
1. Lateral with head bent toward the chest and knees flexed onto the abdomen
2. Lying prone, with the knees drawn up toward the abdomen
3. Sitting bent over from the waist with legs extended
4. Supine with knees pulled toward the chest

10. The nurse needs to collect a sputum specimen to identify the presence of tuberculosis (TB). Which nursing action(s) is/are indicated for this type of specimen? Select all that apply.
1. Collect the specimen in the evening.
2. Send the specimen immediately to the laboratory.
3. Ask the client to spit into the sputum container.
4. Offer mouth care before and after collection of the sputum specimen.
5. Collect a specimen for 3 consecutive days.

See Answers to Test Your Knowledge in Appendix A.

READINGS AND REFERENCES

Suggested Reading

Gallegos, Y., Taha, A. A., & Rutledge, D. N. (2016). Preventing contrast-induced acute kidney injury. *American Journal of Nursing*, *116*(12), 38–45. doi:10.1097/01.NAJ.0000508664.33963.20

The authors provide a comprehensive review of contrast-induced acute kidney injury (CI-AKI) and provide an evidence-based review of screening, risk assessment, and hydration protocols. This information is helpful in preventing CI-AKI, which can be caused by intravascular iodinated contrast media used in diagnostic radiographic imaging scans.

Related Research

Woodall, M., & DeLetter, M. (2018). Colorectal cancer: A collaborative approach to improve education and screening in a rural population. *Clinical Journal of Oncology Nursing*, *22*(1), 69–75. doi:10.1188/18.CJON.69-75

References

American Diabetes Association. (2015). *DKA (ketoacidosis) & ketones*. Retrieved from http://www.diabetes.org/living-with-diabetes/complications/ketoacidosis-dka.html?referrer

American Diabetes Association. (2018). *Checking your blood glucose*. Retrieved from http://www.diabetes.org/living-with-diabetes/treatment-and-care/blood-glucose-control/checking-your-blood-glucose.html

Chan, H. Y. L., Lau, T. S. L., Ho, S. Y., Leung, D. Y. P., & Lee, D. T. F. (2016). The accuracy and acceptability of performing capillary blood glucose measurements at the earlobe. *Journal of Advanced Nursing*, *72*(8), 1766–1773. doi:10.1111/jan.12944

Fremgen, B. F., & Frucht, S. S. (2019). *Medical terminology: A living language* (7th ed.). Hoboken, NJ: Pearson.

The Joint Commission. (2019). *National Patient Safety Goals effective January 2019*. Retrieved from https://www.jointcommission.org/assets/1/6/NPSG_Chapter_HAP_Jan2019.pdf

Kee, J. L. (2017). *Pearson handbook of laboratory and diagnostic tests: With nursing implications* (8th ed.). Hoboken, NJ: Pearson.

Kraft, D. (2019, January). "Connected" and high-tech: Your medical future. *National Geographic, Special Issue: Medicine*, 27–36.

Lieberman, D., Ladabaum, U., Cruz-Correa, M., Ginsburg, C., Inadomi, J. M., Kim, L. S., . . . Wender, R. C. (2016). Screening for colorectal cancer and evolving issues for physicians and patients. *JAMA*, *22*, 2135–2145. doi:10.1001/jama.2016.17418

McElwee-Malloy, M. (2016). The right meter for you. *Diabetes Forecast*, *69*(2), 50–60.

Tresca, A. J. (2018). *Fecal immunochemical test to detect hidden blood*. Retrieved from https://www.verywellhealth.com/fecal-immunochemical-test-fit-1942655

U.S. Preventive Services Task Force. (2016). Screening for colorectal cancer. U.S. preventive services task force recommendation statement. *JAMA*, *315*, 2564–2575. doi:10.1001/jama.2016.5989

Selected Bibliography

Dunning, T. (2016). How to monitor blood glucose. *Nursing Standard*, *30*(22), 36. doi:10.7748/ns.30.22.36.s45

Mariani, H. S., Layden, B. T., & Aleppo, G. (2017). Continuous glucose monitoring: A perspective on its past, present, and future applications for diabetes management. *Clinical Diabetes*, *35*(1), 60–65. doi:10.2337/cd16-0008

Pereira, K. (2017). Insights into glucose monitoring for diabetes. *American Nurse Today*, *12*(7), 6–9.

Proehl, J. A. (2016). How you can avoid laboratory errors. *American Nurse Today*, *11*(3), 14–16.

Reagh, K. (2016). Thoracentesis in a nutshell. *Nursing made Incredibly Easy!*, *14*(1), 10–12. doi:10.1097.NME.0000475214.85842.fc

Shepard, L. H. (2017). Patient teaching: CT scan essentials. *Nursing made Incredibly Easy!*, *15*(5), 19–21. doi:10.1097/01.NME.0000521813.15388.21

35 Medication Administration

LEARNING OUTCOMES

After completing this chapter, you will be able to:

1. Define selected terms related to the administration of medications.
2. Describe legal aspects of administering medications.
3. Describe actions of drugs on the body.
4. Identify factors affecting medication action.
5. Describe various routes of administration for medication, including opioids.
6. Identify essential parts of a medication order.
7. List examples of various types of medication orders.
8. State systems of measurement that are used in the administration of medications.
9. Describe four formulas for calculating drug dosages.
10. List six essential steps to follow when administering medication.
11. State the "rights" to accurate medication administration.
12. Describe the physiologic changes in older adults that alter medication administration and effectiveness.
13. Verbalize the steps used in administering oral medications safely.
14. Outline the steps required for nasogastric and gastrostomy tube medication administration.
15. Identify equipment required for parenteral medications.
16. Verbalize the steps used in:
    a. Preparing medications from ampules
    b. Preparing medications from vials
    c. Mixing medications in one syringe.
17. Identify the sites used for:
    a. Intradermal injection
    b. Subcutaneous injection
    c. Intramuscular injection.
18. Verbalize the steps used in administering parenteral medications by the following routes:
    a. Intradermal
    b. Subcutaneous
    c. Intramuscular.
19. Verbalize the steps used in administering intravenous medications using IV push.
20. Verbalize the steps used in administering the following topical medications:
    a. Dermatologic
    b. Ophthalmic
    c. Otic
    d. Nasal
    e. Vaginal
    f. Rectal
    g. Respiratory inhalation.
21. Recognize when it is appropriate to assign medication administration to assistive personnel.
22. Demonstrate appropriate documentation and reporting of medication administration skills.

KEY TERMS

absorption, *841*
adverse effects, *839*
agonist, *841*
ampule, *875*
anaphylactic reaction, *839*
antagonist, *841*
bevel, *873*
biotransformation, *842*
brand name, *837*
buccal, *853*
cannula, *873*
chemical name, *837*
cumulative effect, *840*
desired effect, *839*
detoxification, *842*
distribution, *842*
drug, *837*
drug abuse, *840*
drug allergy, *839*
drug dependence, *840*
drug habituation, *840*
drug half-life, *841*
drug interaction, *840*
drug tolerance, *840*
drug toxicity, *839*
dry powder inhaler (DPI), *908*
elimination half-life, *841*
epidural, *854*
excretion, *842*
gastrostomy tube, *868*
gauge, *873*
generic name, *837*
hub, *873*
hypodermic, *853*
hypodermic syringe, *869*
iatrogenic disease, *840*
idiosyncratic effect, *840*
illicit drugs, *840*
inhibiting effect, *840*
insulin syringe, *870*
intradermal (ID), *854*
intradermal (ID) injection, *881*
intramuscular (IM), *853*
intramuscular (IM) injections, *886*
intraspinal, *854*
intrathecal, *854*
intravenous (IV), *854*
irrigation, *911*
lavage, *911*
medication, *837*
medication reconciliation, *858*
meniscus, *865*
metabolism, *842*
metabolites, *842*
metered-dose inhaler (MDI), *908*
nasogastric tube, *868*
nebulizer, *908*
NPO, *863*
official name, *837*
onset of action, *841*
ophthalmic, *899*
oral, *852*
otic, *902*
parenteral, *853*
peak plasma level, *841*
percutaneous, *898*
pharmacist, *837*
pharmacodynamics, *841*
pharmacogenetics, *843*
pharmacogenomics, *843*
pharmacokinetics, *841*
pharmacology, *837*
pharmacopoeia, *838*
pharmacy, *837*
physiologic dependence, *840*
piggyback, *894*
plateau, *841*
potentiating effect, *840*
prefilled unit-dose systems, *870*
prescription, *837*
prn order, *845*
psychologic dependence, *840*
receptor, *841*
reconstitution, *876*
shaft, *873*
side effect, *839*
single order, *845*
standing order, *845*
stat order, *845*
subcutaneous, *853*
sublingual, *852*
synergistic effect, *840*
therapeutic effect, *839*
topical, *854*
trade name, *837*
transdermal patch, *898*
tuberculin syringe, *872*
vial, *875*
volume-control infusion set, *894*

Introduction

A **medication** is a substance administered for the diagnosis, cure, treatment, or relief of a symptom or for prevention of disease. In the healthcare context, the words *medication* and *drug* are generally used interchangeably. The term **drug** also has the connotation of an illicitly obtained substance such as heroin, cocaine, or amphetamines. Medications have been known and used since antiquity. Over the centuries the number of drugs available has increased greatly, and knowledge about these drugs has become correspondingly more accurate and detailed.

In the United States, medications are usually dispensed on the order of primary care providers and dentists. More and more, U.S. state legislatures are authorizing nurse practitioners and other advanced practice nurses to prescribe drugs. The written direction for the preparation and administration of a drug is called a **prescription**. One drug can have as many as four kinds of names: its generic name, trade name (or brand name), official name, and chemical name. The **generic name** is assigned by the United States Adopted Names (USAN) Council and is used throughout the drug's lifetime. A drug's **trade name** (sometimes called the **brand name**) is the name given by the drug manufacturer and identifies it as property of that company. The name selected is usually short and easy to remember. When the drug is under patent protection, the company markets the drug under its trade name. When the drug is no longer protected by patent, the company may market its product under either the generic or trade name. Other companies that wish to market the off-patent drug must use the same generic name but will create their own trade name. Thus, one drug may be manufactured by several companies and have several trade names. For example, the drug hydrochlorothiazide (generic name) is known by the trade names Esidrix and HydroDIURIL. The **official name** is the name under which a drug is listed in one of the official publications (e.g., the *United States Pharmacopeia*). The **chemical name** is the name by which a chemist knows it; this name describes the constituents of the drug precisely.

Medications are often available in a variety of forms (Table 35.1).

Pharmacology is the study of the effect of drugs on living organisms. **Pharmacy** is the art of preparing, compounding, and dispensing drugs. The word also refers to the place where drugs are prepared and dispensed. The licensed **pharmacist** prepares, makes, and dispenses drugs as ordered by a physician, dentist, nurse practitioner, or physician assistant. A clinical pharmacist is a

TABLE 35.1 Types of Drug Preparations

Type	Description
Aerosol spray or foam	A liquid, powder, or foam deposited in a thin layer on the skin by air pressure
Aqueous solution	One or more drugs dissolved in water
Aqueous suspension	One or more drugs finely divided in a liquid such as water
Caplet	A solid form, shaped like a capsule, coated and easily swallowed
Capsule	A gelatinous container to hold a drug in powder, liquid, or oil form
Cream	A nongreasy, semisolid preparation used on the skin
Elixir	A sweetened and aromatic solution of alcohol used as a vehicle for medicinal agents
Extract	A concentrated form of a drug made from vegetables or animals
Gel or jelly	A clear or translucent semisolid that liquefies when applied to the skin
Liniment	A medication mixed with alcohol, oil, or soapy emollient and applied to the skin
Lotion	A medication in a liquid suspension applied to the skin
Lozenge (troche)	A flat, round, or oval preparation that dissolves and releases a drug when held in the mouth
Ointment (salve, unction)	A semisolid preparation of one or more drugs used for application to the skin and mucous membrane
Paste	A preparation like an ointment, but thicker and stiff, that penetrates the skin less than an ointment
Pill	One or more drugs mixed with a cohesive material, in oval, round, or flattened shapes
Powder	A finely ground drug or drugs; some are used internally, others externally
Suppository	One or several drugs mixed with a firm base such as gelatin and shaped for insertion into the body (e.g., the rectum); the base dissolves gradually at body temperature, releasing the drug
Syrup	An aqueous solution of sugar often used to disguise unpleasant-tasting drugs
Tablet	A powdered drug compressed into a hard, small disk; some are readily broken along a scored line; others are enteric coated to prevent them from dissolving in the stomach
Tincture	An alcoholic or water-and-alcohol solution prepared from drugs derived from plants
Transdermal patch	A semipermeable membrane shaped in the form of a disk or patch that contains a drug to be absorbed through the skin over a long period of time

specialist who often guides the primary care provider in prescribing drugs. A pharmacy technician is a member of the health team who in some states administers drugs to clients.

Drug Standards

Drugs may have natural (e.g., plant, mineral, and animal) sources, or they may be synthesized in the laboratory. Drugs vary in strength and activity. Drugs must be pure and of uniform strength if dosages are to be predictable in their effect. Drug standards have therefore been developed to ensure uniform quality. In the United States, official drugs are those designated by the federal Food, Drug, and Cosmetic Act. These drugs are officially listed in the *United States Pharmacopeia* (USP) and described according to their source, physical and chemical properties, tests for purity and identity, method of storage, assay, category, and normal dosages. There is a trend for people to purchase "natural" vitamins and supplements from health food stores or over the counter (OTC) at pharmacies. An example of this is a thyroid supplement. The natural form varies in strength and is difficult to regulate, while the synthetic thyroid is much more predictable in strength and management of symptoms for clients who need to take a thyroid supplement.

A **pharmacopoeia** (also spelled *pharmacopeia*) is a book containing a list of products used in medicine, with descriptions of the product, chemical tests for determining identity and purity, and formulas and prescriptions. The United States' *National Formulary* lists drugs and their therapeutic value and can include drugs that may still be used but not listed in the USP.

Pharmacopoeias and formularies are helpful reference sources for nurses and nursing students. Nurses not only administer thousands of medications but also are responsible for assessing their effectiveness and recognizing unfavorable reactions to drugs. Medication or drug handbooks and agency formularies are also valuable resources for nurses. Because it is impossible to commit to memory all pertinent information about a very large number of drugs, nurses must have a reliable reference readily available.

Legal Aspects of Drug Administration

Within the United States, laws have been enacted to control the development and administration of drugs. Table 35.2 provides a summary of U.S. drug legislation.

Nurses need to (a) know how the nurse practice act in their state defines and limits their functions and (b) recognize the limits of their own knowledge and skills. To function beyond the limits of nursing practice acts or one's ability is to endanger clients' lives and leave oneself open to professional negligence lawsuits. Under the law, nurses are responsible for their own actions regardless of whether there is a written order. For example, if a primary care provider writes an incorrect order (e.g., morphine 100 mg instead of morphine 10 mg), *a nurse who administers the written incorrect dosage is responsible for the error as is the primary care provider*. Therefore, nurses should question any order that appears unreasonable and refuse to give the medication until the order is clarified.

Another aspect of nursing practice governed by law is the use of controlled substances. Controlled substances can be kept in a locked drawer, cupboard, medication cart, or computer-controlled dispensing system, depending on the agency. Laws require careful monitoring of controlled substances. Agencies may have special inventory forms for recording the use of controlled substances. The information required usually includes the name of the client, the date and time of administration, the name of the drug, the dosage, and the signature of the individual who prepared and gave the drug. The name of the primary care provider who ordered the drug may also be part of the record. Some agencies may require a verifying signature of another registered nurse for administration of a controlled substance. Most healthcare agencies maintain a list of high-alert medications, including controlled substances, which require the verification of two registered nurses. Before removing a controlled substance, the nurse verifies the number actually available with the number indicated on the controlled substance medication (Figure 35.1 ■) and the inventory record. If the number is not the same, the nurse must investigate and correct the discrepancy before proceeding.

TABLE 35.2 U.S. Drug Legislation

Legislation	Content
Food, Drug, and Cosmetic Act (1938)	Implemented by the U.S. Food and Drug Administration (FDA); requires that labels be accurate and that all drugs be tested for harmful effects.
Durkham-Humphrey Amendment (1952)	Clearly differentiates drugs that can be sold only with a prescription, those that can be sold without a prescription, and those that should not be refilled without a new prescription.
Kefauver-Harris Amendment (1962)	Requires proof of safety and efficacy of a drug for approval.
Comprehensive Drug Abuse Prevention and Control Act (1970) (Controlled Substances Act)	Categorizes controlled substances and limits how often a prescription can be filled; established government-funded programs to prevent and treat drug dependence.

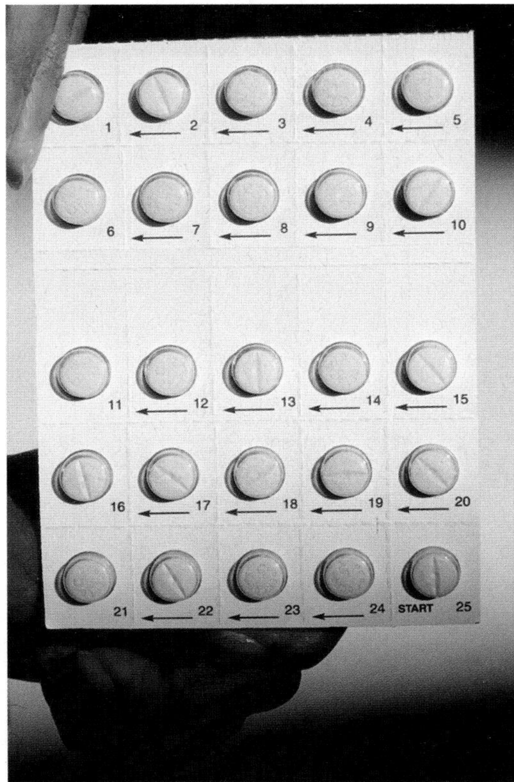

Figure 35.1 ■ Some controlled substances are kept in specially designed packages or plastic containers that are sectioned and numbered.

Included on the inventory record are the controlled substances wasted during preparation. When a portion or all of a controlled substance dose is discarded, the nurse must ask a second nurse to witness the discarding. Both nurses must sign the control inventory form.

In most agencies, counts of controlled substances are taken at the end of each shift. The count total should match with the total at the end of the last shift minus the number used. If the totals do not match and the discrepancy cannot be resolved, it must be reported immediately to the nurse manager, nursing supervisor, and pharmacy according to agency policy. In facilities that use a computerized dispensing system, manual counts are not required, because the dispensing system runs a continuous count; however, discrepancies must be reported and accounted for.

Effects of Drugs

The **therapeutic effect** of a drug, also referred to as the **desired effect**, is the primary effect intended, that is, the reason the drug is prescribed. For example, the therapeutic effect of morphine sulfate is analgesia, and the therapeutic effect of diazepam is relief of anxiety. See Table 35.3 for kinds of therapeutic actions.

A **side effect**, or secondary effect, of a drug is one that is unintended. Side effects are usually predictable and may be either harmless or potentially harmful. For example, digitalis increases the strength of myocardial contractions (desired effect), but it can have the side effect of nausea and vomiting. Some side effects are tolerated for the drug's therapeutic effect; more severe side effects, also called **adverse effects** or reactions, may justify the discontinuation of a drug. The nurse should monitor for dose-related side effects or adverse effects and report these to the healthcare provider, who may discontinue the medication or change the dosage.

Drug toxicity (harmful effects of a drug on an organism or tissue) results from overdosage, ingestion of a drug intended for external use, or buildup of the drug in the blood because of impaired metabolism or excretion (cumulative effect). Some toxic effects are apparent immediately; some are not apparent for weeks or months. Fortunately, most drug toxicity is avoidable if careful attention is paid to dosage and monitoring for toxicity. An example of a toxic effect is respiratory depression due to the cumulative effect of morphine sulfate in the body.

A **drug allergy** is an immunologic reaction to a drug. When a client is first exposed to a foreign substance (antigen), the body may react by producing antibodies. A client can react to a drug in the same manner as an antigen and thus develop symptoms of an allergic reaction.

Allergic reactions can be either mild or severe. A mild reaction has a variety of symptoms, from skin rashes to diarrhea (Table 35.4). An allergic reaction can occur anytime from a few minutes to 2 weeks after the administration of the drug. A severe allergic reaction usually occurs immediately after the administration of the drug and is called an **anaphylactic reaction**. This response can be fatal if the symptoms are not noticed immediately and treatment is not obtained promptly. The earliest symptoms

TABLE 35.3 Therapeutic Actions of Drugs

Drug Type	Description	Examples
Palliative	Relieves the symptoms of a disease but does not affect the disease itself.	Morphine sulfate, aspirin for pain
Curative	Cures a disease or condition.	Penicillin for infection
Supportive	Supports body function until other treatments or the body's response can take over.	Norepinephrine bitartrate for low blood pressure; aspirin for high body temperature
Substitutive	Replaces body fluids or substances.	Thyroxine for hypothyroidism, insulin for diabetes mellitus
Chemotherapeutic	Destroys malignant cells.	Busulfan for leukemia
Restorative	Returns the body to health.	Vitamin, mineral supplements

TABLE 35.4 Common Mild Allergic Responses

Symptom	Description
Skin rash	Either an intraepidermal vesicle rash or a rash typified by an urticarial wheal or macular eruption; rash is usually generalized over the body
Pruritus	Itching of the skin with or without a rash
Angioedema	Edema due to increased permeability of the blood capillaries
Rhinitis	Excessive watery discharge from the nose
Lacrimal tearing	Excessive tearing
Nausea, vomiting	Stimulation of these centers in the brain
Wheezing and dyspnea	Shortness of breath and wheezing on inhalation and exhalation due to accumulated fluids and swelling of the respiratory tissues
Diarrhea	Irritation of the mucosa of the large intestine

are a subjective feeling of swelling in the mouth and tongue, acute shortness of breath, acute hypotension, and tachycardia.

Drug tolerance exists in a client who exhibits an unusually low physiologic response to a drug and who requires increases in the dosage to maintain a given therapeutic effect. Drugs that commonly produce tolerance are opioids, barbiturates, and ethyl alcohol. A **cumulative effect** is the increasing response to repeated doses of a drug that occurs when the rate of administration exceeds the rate of metabolism or excretion. As a result, the amount of the drug builds up in the client's body unless the dosage is adjusted. Toxic symptoms may occur. An **idiosyncratic effect** is one that is unexpected and may be individual to a client. Underresponse and overresponse to a drug may be idiosyncratic. Also, the drug may have a completely different effect from the normal one or cause unpredictable and unexplainable symptoms in a particular client.

A **drug interaction** occurs when the administration of one drug before, at the same time as, or after another drug alters the effect of one or both drugs. Drug interactions may be beneficial or harmful. The effect of one or both drugs may be either increased (**potentiating effect**) or decreased (**inhibiting effect**). Potentiating effects may be additive or synergistic. When two of the same types of drug increase the action of *each other*, the effect is known as additive. A **synergistic effect** occurs when two different drugs increase the action of *one or another* drug. For example, probenecid, which blocks the excretion of penicillin, can be given with penicillin to increase blood levels of the penicillin for longer periods (synergistic effect). Two analgesics, such as aspirin and codeine, are often given together because together they provide greater pain relief (additive effect). In addition, certain foods may interact adversely with a medication (see Table 46.1 in Chapter 46 ∞).

Iatrogenic disease (disease caused unintentionally by medical therapy) can be a result of drug therapy. Hepatic toxicity resulting in biliary obstruction, renal damage, and malformations of the fetus as a result of specific drugs taken during pregnancy are examples.

Drug Misuse

Drug misuse is the improper use of common medications in ways that lead to acute and chronic toxicity. Both OTC drugs and prescription drugs may be misused. Laxatives, antacids, vitamins, headache remedies, and cough and cold medications are often self-prescribed and overused. Most people suffer no harmful effects from these drugs, but some do. For example, a client might use an OTC cough medicine to treat a cough that might be caused by a serious underlying problem such as throat cancer.

Drug abuse is the inappropriate intake of a substance, either continually or periodically. By definition, drug use is abusive when society considers it abusive. For example, the intake of alcohol at work may be considered alcohol abuse, but intake at a social gathering may not. Drug abuse has two main aspects, drug dependence and habituation. **Drug dependence** is the reliance on or need to take a drug or substance. The two types of dependence, physiologic and psychologic, may occur separately or together. **Physiologic dependence** is due to biochemical changes in body tissues, especially the nervous system. These tissues come to require the substance for normal functioning. A dependent individual who stops using the drug experiences withdrawal symptoms. **Psychologic dependence** is emotional reliance on a drug to maintain a sense of well-being, accompanied by feelings of need or cravings for that drug. There are varying degrees of psychologic dependence, ranging from mild desire to craving and compulsive use of the drug.

Drug habituation means a mild form of psychologic dependence. The individual develops the habit of taking the substance and feels better after taking it. The habituated individual tends to continue the habit even though it may be injurious to health.

Illicit drugs, also called *street drugs*, are those sold illegally. Illicit drugs are of two types: (a) drugs unavailable for purchase under any circumstances, such as heroin (in the United States), and (b) drugs normally available with a prescription that are being obtained through illegal channels. Illicit drugs often are taken because of their mood-altering effect; that is, they make the user feel happy or relaxed.

Actions of Drugs on the Body

The action of a drug in the body can be described in terms of its half-life, the time interval required for the body's elimination processes to reduce the concentration of the drug in the body by one-half. For example, if a drug's half-life is 8 hours, then the amount of drug in the body is as follows:

Initially: 100%
After 8 hours: 50%
After 16 hours: 25%
After 24 hours: 12.5%
After 32 hours: 6.25%

Because the purpose of most drug therapy is to maintain a constant drug level in the body, repeated doses are required to maintain that level. When an orally administered drug is absorbed from the gastrointestinal (GI) tract into the blood plasma, its concentration in the plasma increases until the elimination rate equals the rate of absorption. This point is known as the *peak plasma level* (Figure 35.2 ■). When a drug is given intravenously (IV), its level is high immediately after administration and decreases through time. Another dose is given in order to maintain therapeutic levels. If the client does not receive another dose of the drug (either orally or IV), the concentration steadily decreases. Key terms related to drug actions are as follows:

- **Onset of action**: the time after administration when the body initially responds to the drug
- **Peak plasma level**: the highest plasma level achieved by a single dose when the elimination rate of the drug equals the absorption rate
- **Drug half-life** (**elimination half-life**): the time required for the elimination process to reduce the concentration of the drug to one-half what it was at initial administration
- **Plateau**: a maintained concentration of a drug in the plasma during a series of scheduled doses.

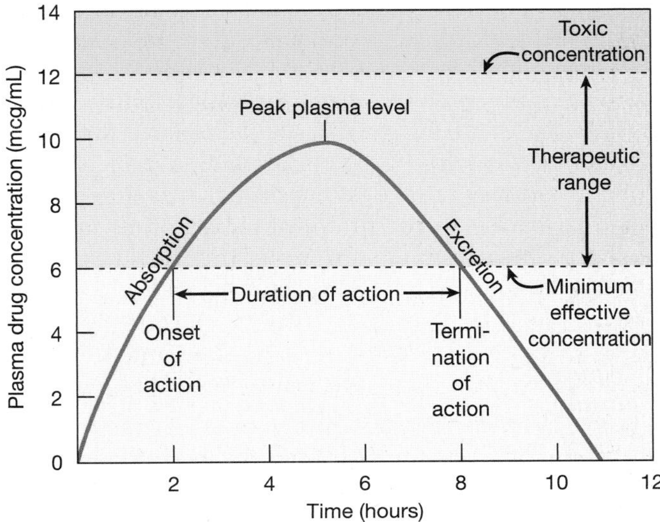

Figure 35.2 ■ A graphic plot of drug concentration in the blood plasma following a single dose.

Pharmacodynamics

Pharmacodynamics is the mechanism of drug action and the relationships between drug concentration and resulting effects in the body (Adams, Holland, & Urban, 2020, p. 49). A **receptor** is the drug's specific target, usually a protein located on the surface of a cell membrane or within the cell. As the drug binds to the receptor, it enhances or inhibits the normal cellular function. The binding is usually reversible and the action of the drug terminated once the drug leaves the receptor (Adams et al., 2020).

Most drugs exert their effects by chemically binding with receptors at the cellular level. When a drug binds to its receptor, the pharmacologic effects are either agonism or antagonism. When a drug produces the same type of response as the physiologic or endogenous substance, it is referred to as an **agonist**. For example, epinephrine-like drugs act on the heart to increase the heart rate. Conversely, a drug that inhibits cell function by occupying receptor sites is called an **antagonist**. The antagonist prevents natural body substances or other drugs from activating the functions of the cell by occupying the receptor sites. For example, naloxone (Narcan) is an opioid antagonist used as an antidote for respiratory depression caused by an opioid drug (e.g., morphine). This drug competes with opioid receptor sites in the brain and thereby prevents the opioid from binding to its receptors. By blocking the effect of the opioid, respiratory depression is reversed.

Pharmacokinetics

Pharmacokinetics is the study of the absorption, distribution, biotransformation, and excretion of drugs.

Absorption

Absorption is the process by which a drug passes into the bloodstream. Unless the drug is administered directly into the bloodstream, absorption is the first step in the movement of the drug through the body. For absorption of a drug to occur, the correct form of the drug must be administered through the correct route.

The rate of absorption of a drug in the stomach is variable. Food, for example, can delay the dissolution and absorption of some drugs as well as their passage into the small intestine, where most drug absorption occurs. Food can also combine with molecules of certain drugs, thereby changing their molecular structure and subsequently inhibiting or preventing their absorption. Another factor that affects the absorption of some drugs is the acid medium in the stomach. Acidity can vary according to the time of day, foods ingested, use of antacid medications, and the age of the client. Some drugs do not dissolve or have limited ability to dissolve in the GI fluids, decreasing their absorption into the bloodstream. Absorption of some drugs can occur in the tissues of the mouth prior to reaching the stomach. For example, nitroglycerin is administered under the tongue, where it is absorbed into the blood vessels that carry it directly to the heart, the intended site of action. If swallowed, this drug will be absorbed into the bloodstream and carried to the liver, where it will be destroyed. The first-pass effect occurs when oral drugs first pass through the liver and are partially metabolized prior to reaching the target organ. This requires higher oral doses in order to achieve the appropriate effect.

A drug administered directly into the bloodstream, that is, intravenously, is immediately in the vascular system without having to be absorbed. This, then, is the route of choice for rapid action. The intramuscular route is the next most rapid route due to the highly vascular nature of muscle tissue. Because subcutaneous tissue has a poorer blood supply than muscle tissue, absorption from subcutaneous tissue is slower. The rate of absorption of a drug can be accelerated by the application of heat, which increases blood flow to the area; conversely, absorption can be slowed by the application of cold. In addition, the injection of a vasoconstrictor drug such as epinephrine into the tissue can slow absorption of other drugs. The absorption of drugs from the rectum into the bloodstream tends to be unpredictable. Therefore, this route is normally used when other routes are unavailable or when the intended action is localized to the rectum or sigmoid colon.

Distribution

Distribution is the transportation of a drug from its site of absorption to its site of action. When a drug enters the bloodstream, it is carried to the most vascular organs—that is, liver, kidneys, and brain. Body areas with lower blood supply—that is, skin and muscles—receive the drug later. The chemical and physical properties of a drug determine the area of the body to which the drug will be attracted. For example, fat-soluble drugs will accumulate in fatty tissue, whereas other drugs may bind with plasma proteins.

Biotransformation

Biotransformation, also called **detoxification** or **metabolism**, is a process by which a drug is converted to a less active form. Most biotransformation takes place in the liver, where many drug-metabolizing enzymes in the cells detoxify the drugs. The products of this process are called **metabolites**. There are two types of metabolites: active and inactive. An *active metabolite* has a pharmacologic action itself, whereas an *inactive metabolite* does not.

Biotransformation may be altered if a client is very young, is older, or has an unhealthy liver. Nurses must be alert to the accumulation of the active drug in these clients and to subsequent toxicity.

Excretion

Excretion is the process by which metabolites and drugs are eliminated from the body. The kidneys eliminate most drug metabolites in the urine; however, some are excreted in the feces, the breath, perspiration, saliva, and breast milk. Certain drugs, such as general anesthetic agents, are excreted in an unchanged form via the respiratory tract. The efficiency with which the kidneys excrete drugs and metabolites diminishes with age. Older people may require smaller doses of a drug because the drug and its metabolites may accumulate in the body.

Factors Affecting Medication Action

A number of factors other than the drug itself can affect its action. A client may not respond in the same manner to successive doses of a drug. In addition, the identical drug and dosage may affect individual clients differently.

Developmental Factors

During pregnancy women must be very careful about taking medications. Drugs taken during pregnancy pose a risk throughout the pregnancy, but pose the highest risk during the first trimester, due to the formation of vital organs and functions of the fetus during this time. Most drugs are contraindicated because of their possible adverse effects on the fetus.

Infants usually require small dosages because of their body size and the immaturity of their organs, especially the liver and kidneys. Differences in gastric acidity and liver enzymes required for drug metabolism may require different medication choices and dosages than adults. In adolescence or adulthood, allergic reactions may occur to drugs formerly tolerated.

Older adults have different responses to medications due to physiologic changes that occur with aging. These changes include decreased liver and kidney function, which can result in the accumulation of the drug in the body. In addition, the older adult may be on multiple drugs and incompatibilities may occur.

Older adults often experience decreased gastric motility and decreased gastric acid production and blood flow, which can impair drug absorption. Increased adipose tissue and decreased total body fluid proportionate to the body mass can increase the possibility of drug toxicity. Older adults may also experience a decreased number of protein-binding sites and changes in the blood–brain barrier. The latter permits fat-soluble drugs to move readily to the brain, often resulting in dizziness and confusion. For example, this can occur with beta-blockers.

Gender

Differences in the way men and women respond to drugs are chiefly related to the distribution of body fat and fluid and hormonal differences. Because most drug research is done on men, more research on women is required to reflect the effects of hormonal changes on drug actions in women.

ANATOMY & PHYSIOLOGY REVIEW

Pharmacokinetics of an Oral Medication

GI SYSTEM: STOMACH, SMALL INTESTINE

The oral medication reaches the systemic circulation through the GI system. As a result, numerous factors can affect the absorption of the pill.

QUESTIONS

1. Which would be absorbed the fastest: pill, capsule, or liquid?
2. A client is experiencing diarrhea. How could this affect absorption of an oral drug?
3. How does the presence of food in the stomach affect the rate of absorption?

CARDIOVASCULAR SYSTEM

Once the pill is absorbed into the bloodstream, it is carried or delivered to the sites of pharmacologic action where the drug produces its effects.

QUESTION

1. How is distribution of the oral medication affected if a client has less than normal cardiac output (e.g., low BP, prolonged capillary refill)?

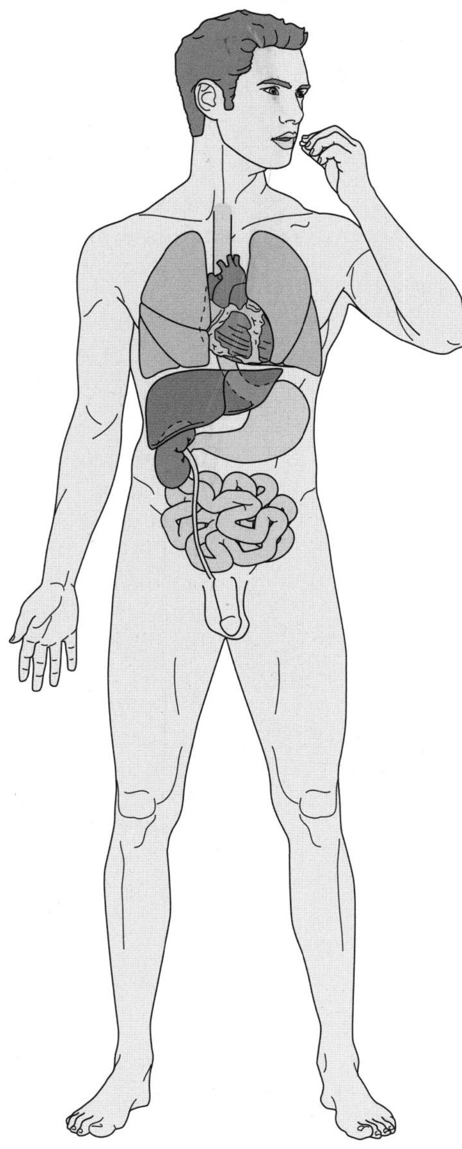

LIVER

Most biotransformation takes place in the liver. Any decrease in the ability of the liver to metabolize medication could lead to an accumulation of the active drug in the bloodstream. This could put the client at risk for toxic effects and adverse reactions.

QUESTIONS

1. What are risk factors that can affect liver function?
2. A client is suspected of having decreased liver function. What information would be essential for the nurse to know about the oral medication that is to be given?

KIDNEYS

Drug excretion occurs mainly through the kidneys into the urine. If there is any impairment in kidney function, medications may not be excreted at the anticipated speed. Subsequent medication administration may lead to accumulation and potential toxicity.

QUESTIONS

1. Why would very young and very old clients need to be closely monitored by the nurse for signs and symptoms of drug toxicity?
2. How can the nurse assess kidney function?

Answers to Anatomy & Physiology Review Questions are available on the faculty resources site. Please consult with your instructor.

Genetic and Cultural Factors

Personal genetic makeup influences a client's response to a drug. The study of how genes affect an individual's response to drugs is called **pharmacogenomics**, a combination of pharmacology and genomics, to study the role of the genome (*all* the genes) in response to drugs. This term is often used interchangeably with **pharmacogenetics**, which refers to the study of how DNA variation in a *single or few* genes influences the response to a single drug (Fulton et al., 2018, p. 699). The goal of pharmacogenomics is to develop "effective, safe medications, with doses tailored to a client's genetic makeup" (Hull, 2018, p. 10). Pharmacogenomics is increasingly becoming a component of *precision medicine*, sometimes called *precision health*, which focuses on the development of prevention and treatment strategies that include attention to an individual's variability in genes, environment, and lifestyle (Montgomery et. al., 2017, p. 15). Thus, nurses need a genetic and genomic knowledge base.

QSEN Patient-Centered Care: Drug Action

Cultural factors and practices (e.g., values and beliefs) can also affect a drug's action. For example, a herbal remedy (e.g., the herb ginseng) may speed up or slow down the metabolism of prescribed medications. Following are guidelines for nurses who care for clients from other cultures:

- Avoid profiling and stereotyping.
- Remember that there may be differences in medication responses among different ethnic groups and differences *within* ethnic groups.
- Ask about health beliefs, values, customs, and practices by conducting a cultural assessment.
- Be accepting of differences in cultural beliefs and practices.
- Learn about drug responses (including adverse effects) that are related to ancestry.
- Ask the client direct, specific questions to reveal the presence or absence of potential adverse effects of medications.
- Monitor the client and document findings carefully because it may be possible to maintain a therapeutic benefit at a lower dosage of a given drug.
- Implement a treatment plan with the client and family that is consistent with their cultural and traditional beliefs while incorporating the necessary modern treatments.
- Keep cultural context in mind when planning education for clients and families.

Diet

Nutrients can affect the action of a medication. For example, vitamin K, found in green leafy vegetables, can counteract the effect of an anticoagulant such as warfarin (Coumadin). See Table 46.1 in Chapter 46 ∞.

Environment

Environmental temperature and noise may affect drug activity. When environmental temperature is high, the peripheral blood vessels dilate, thus intensifying the action of vasodilators. In contrast, a cold environment and the consequent vasoconstriction inhibit the action of vasodilators but enhance the action of vasoconstrictors. A client who takes a sedative or analgesic in a busy, noisy environment may not benefit as fully as if the environment were quiet and peaceful.

Psychologic Factors

A client's expectations about what a drug can do can affect the response to the medication. For example, a client who believes that codeine is ineffective as an analgesic may experience minimal or no relief from pain after it is given.

Illness and Disease

Illness and disease can also affect the action of drugs. For example, aspirin can reduce the body temperature of a feverish client but has no effect on the body temperature of a client without fever. Drug action is altered in clients with circulatory, liver, or kidney dysfunction.

Time of Administration

The time of administration of oral medications affects the relative speed with which they act. Some orally administered medications are absorbed more quickly if the stomach is empty, whereas other medications have a more rapid absorption when administered with food.

Medication Orders

A physician usually determines the client's medication needs and orders medications, although in some settings nurse practitioners and physician assistants (PAs) can now order drugs. State law dictates whether the nurse practitioner and PAs have prescriptive ability and the class of drug which they may prescribe. Also, each health agency will have its own policies. Usually the order is written, although telephone and verbal orders are acceptable in some agencies. Nursing students need to know the agency policies about medication orders. In some hospitals, for example, only licensed nurses are permitted to accept telephone and verbal orders. It is strongly recommended that health agencies have solid guidelines in place to reduce or eliminate errors occurring from verbal orders. For example, for all verbal or telephone orders the nurse must first write down the order and then read it back, verbatim, to the prescribing care provider.

Safety Alert! SAFETY

Encourage the prescribing care provider to provide correct spelling of a drug, using aids such as "B as in boy." It is also important for the provider to pronounce numbers separately. For example, the number 16 should be stated as "one six" to avoid confusion with the number 60.

Policies about primary care providers' orders vary considerably from agency to agency. For example, a client's orders may be automatically canceled after surgery or an examination involving an anesthetic agent. The primary care provider must then write new orders.

Most agencies also have lists of abbreviations officially accepted for use in the agency. To prevent medication errors, The Joint Commission mandates that agencies must standardize abbreviations, acronyms, and symbols used throughout the organization and *must* list abbreviations that are never to be used. The Institute for Safe Medication Practices (ISMP) has published a comprehensive list of error-prone abbreviations, symbols, and dose designations that should not be used when communicating medical information. See Table 35.5 for the list of unacceptable abbreviations.

Types of Medication Orders

Four types of medication orders are commonly used:

1. A **stat order** indicates that the medication is to be given immediately and only once (e.g., morphine sulfate 10 milligrams IV stat).
2. The **single order** or *one-time order* is for medication to be given once at a specified time (e.g., Seconal 100 milligrams at bedtime before surgery).
3. The **standing order** may or may not have a termination date. A standing order may be carried out indefinitely (e.g., multiple vitamins daily) until an order is written to cancel it, or it may be carried out for a specified number of days (e.g., KCl twice daily × 2 days). In some agencies, standing orders are automatically canceled after a specified number of days and must be reordered.
4. A **prn order**, or *as-needed order*, permits the nurse to give a medication when, in the nurse's judgment, the client requires it (e.g., Amphojel 15 mL prn). The nurse must use good judgment about when the medication is needed and when it can be safely administered.

TABLE 35.5 Unacceptable Abbreviations—The Official "Do Not Use" List from The Joint Commission and Institute for Safe Medication Practices (ISMP)

Abbreviation	Potential Problem	Use Instead
**U, u (unit)	Mistaken for "0" (zero), the number "4" (four), or "cc"	Write "unit"
**IU (international unit)	Mistaken for IV (intravenous) or the number 10 (ten)	Write "International Unit"
**Q.D., QD, q.d., qd (daily)	Mistaken for each other	Write "daily"
**Q.O.D., QOD, q.o.d., qod (every other day)	Period after the Q mistaken for "I" and the "O" mistaken for "I"	Write "every other day"
**Trailing zero (X.0 mg)	Decimal point is missed	Write X mg
**Lack of leading zero (.X mg)	Decimal point is missed	Write 0.X mg
**MS	Can mean morphine sulfate or magnesium sulfate Confused for one another	Write "morphine sulfate"
**MSO_4 and $MgSO_4$	Can mean morphine sulfate or magnesium sulfate Confused for one another	Write "magnesium sulfate"
> (greater than) < (less than)	Opposite of intended; mistakenly use incorrect symbol	Write "more than" Write "less than"
@	Mistaken for the number "2" (two)	Write "at"
Cc	Mistaken for U (units) when poorly written	Write "mL" or "milliliters"
μg	Mistaken for mg (milligrams) resulting in one thousand-fold overdose	Write "mcg" or "micrograms"
TIW (three times a week)	Has been misinterpreted as "two times a week" or "three times a day" resulting in misdosing	Write "three times weekly"
AS (left ear) AD (right ear) AU (both ears) OD (right eye) OS (left eye) OU (each eye)	Mistaken for OS (left eye), OD (either "overdose" or "optic density"), and OU ("each eye" or "both eyes") Mistaken as AD, AS, AU (right ear, left ear, each ear)	Write "left ear," "right ear," or "both ears," as appropriate Use "right eye," "left eye," or "each eye"
HS	Has been used to indicate "half strength" and "bedtime" or "hour of sleep"	Write out "half strength" or "at bedtime," as appropriate
SC, SQ, sub q (subcutaneous)	SC mistaken as "SL" (sublingual); SQ mistaken as "5 every"; the "q" in "sub q" has been mistaken as "every"	Write "subcut" or "subcutaneously"
Apothecary units	Unfamiliar to many practitioners Confused with metric units	Use metric units
Abbreviations for drug names	Misinterpreted due to similar abbreviations for multiple drugs	Write drug names in full

**These abbreviations are from The Joint Commission's *Official "Do Not Use" List* and the others are from ISMP's *List of Error-Prone Abbreviations*.

Essential Parts of a Medication Order

The drug order has seven essential parts, as listed in Box 35.1. In addition, unless it is a standing order it should state the number of doses or the number of days the drug is to be administered.

BOX 35.1 Essential Parts of a Drug Order

- Full name of the client
- Date and time the order is written
- Name of the drug to be administered
- Dosage of the drug
- Frequency of administration
- Route of administration
- Signature of the individual writing the order

The *client's full name*, that is, the first and last names and middle initials or names, should always be used to avoid confusion between two clients who may have the same last name. In some agencies, the client's identification number and primary care provider's name are placed on the order as further identification. Some hospitals imprint the client's name, identification number, and room number on all forms; some agencies use stickers with similar information.

In addition to the *day*, the *month*, and the *year* the order was written, some agencies also require that the time of day be written. Writing the *time of day* on the order can eliminate errors when the nursing shifts change and makes clear when certain orders automatically terminate. For example, in some settings opioids can be ordered only for 48 hours after surgery. Therefore, a drug that is ordered at 1600 hours November 1, 2020, is automatically canceled at 1600 hours November 3, 2020. Many health agencies use the 24-hour clock, which eliminates confusion between morning and afternoon times. The 24-hour clock starts at midnight, which is 0000 hours (see Chapter 14 ∞).

The *name of the drug to be administered* must be clearly written. In some settings only generic names are permitted; however, trade names are widely used in hospitals and health agencies.

The *dosage of the drug* includes the amount, the times or *frequency of administration*, and in many instances the strength; for example, tetracycline 250 mg (amount) four times a day (frequency); potassium chloride 10% (strength) 5 mL (amount) three times a day with meals (time and frequency). It is strongly recommended that dosages be written in the metric system for safety reasons.

Also included in the order is the *route of administration* of the drug. This part of the order, like other parts, is frequently abbreviated. It is not unusual for a drug to have several possible routes of administration; therefore, it is important that the route be included in the order.

The *signature* of the ordering primary care provider or nurse (if receiving a verbal or telephone order) makes the drug order a legal request. *An unsigned order has no validity*, and the ordering healthcare provider needs to be notified if the order is unsigned.

When a primary care provider writes a prescription for a client, the prescription also includes information for the pharmacist. Therefore, a prescription's content differs from that of a medication order in a hospital. Compare the parts of a prescription listed in Box 35.2 with those shown in Figure 35.3 ■.

BOX 35.2 Parts of a Prescription

- Descriptive information about the client: name, address, and sometimes age
- Date on which the prescription was written
- The Rx symbol, meaning "take thou"
- Medication name, dosage, and strength
- Route of administration
- Dispensing instructions for the pharmacist, for example, "Dispense 30 capsules"
- Directions for administration to be given to the client, for example, "take on an empty stomach"
- Refill and special labeling, for example, "Refill × 1"
- Prescriber's signature

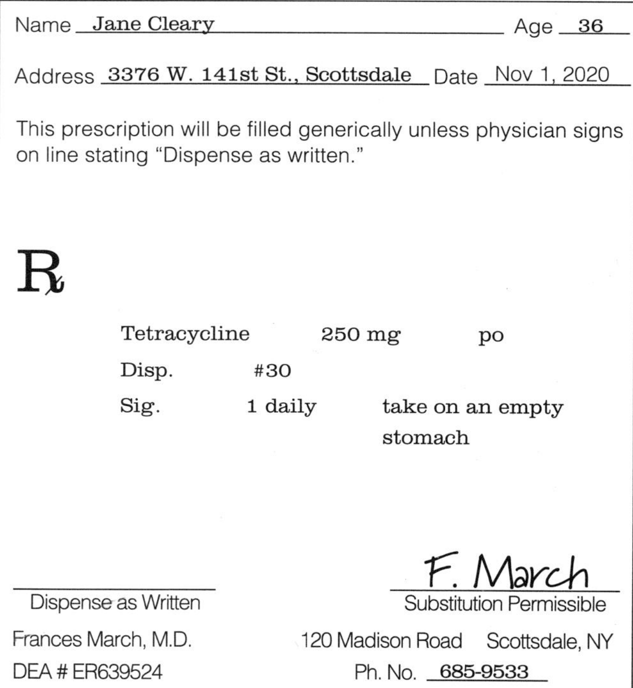
Name Jane Cleary Age 36
Address 3376 W. 141st St., Scottsdale Date Nov 1, 2020

This prescription will be filled generically unless physician signs on line stating "Dispense as written."

℞

Tetracycline 250 mg po
Disp. #30
Sig. 1 daily take on an empty stomach

F. March

Dispense as Written Substitution Permissible

Frances March, M.D. 120 Madison Road Scottsdale, NY
DEA # ER639524 Ph. No. 685-9533

Figure 35.3 ■ A prescription filled out by a primary care provider.

Communicating a Medication Order

A drug order is written on the client's chart by a primary care provider or by a nurse receiving a telephone or verbal order from a primary care provider. Most acute care agencies have a specified time frame (e.g., 24 or 48 hours) in which the primary care provider issuing the telephone or verbal order must cosign the order written by the nurse. The nurse or clerk then copies the medication order to a Kardex or medication administration record (MAR). Increasingly, nurses receive computer printouts of a client's medications instead of a copy of the primary care provider's order. This method avoids errors and saves nursing time.

Clinical Alert!

If your assigned client receives new medication orders, double-check the transcribed information with the primary care provider's order. This ensures client safety.

MARs vary in form, but all include the client's name, drug name and dose; and times and method of administration (Figure 35.4 ■). In some agencies, the date the order was prescribed and the date the order expires are also included.

The nurse should always question the primary care provider about any order that is ambiguous, unusual (e.g., an abnormally high dosage of a medication), or contraindicated by the client's condition. When the nurse judges a primary care provider–ordered medication inappropriate, the following actions are required:

- Contact the primary care provider and discuss the rationale for believing the medication or dosage to be inappropriate.
- Document in notes the following: when the primary care provider was notified, what was conveyed to the primary care provider, and how the primary care provider responded.
- If the primary care provider cannot be reached, document all attempts to contact the primary care provider and the reason for withholding the medication.
- If someone else gives the medication, document data about the client's condition before and after the medication.
- If an incident report (see Chapter 3) is indicated, clearly document factual information.

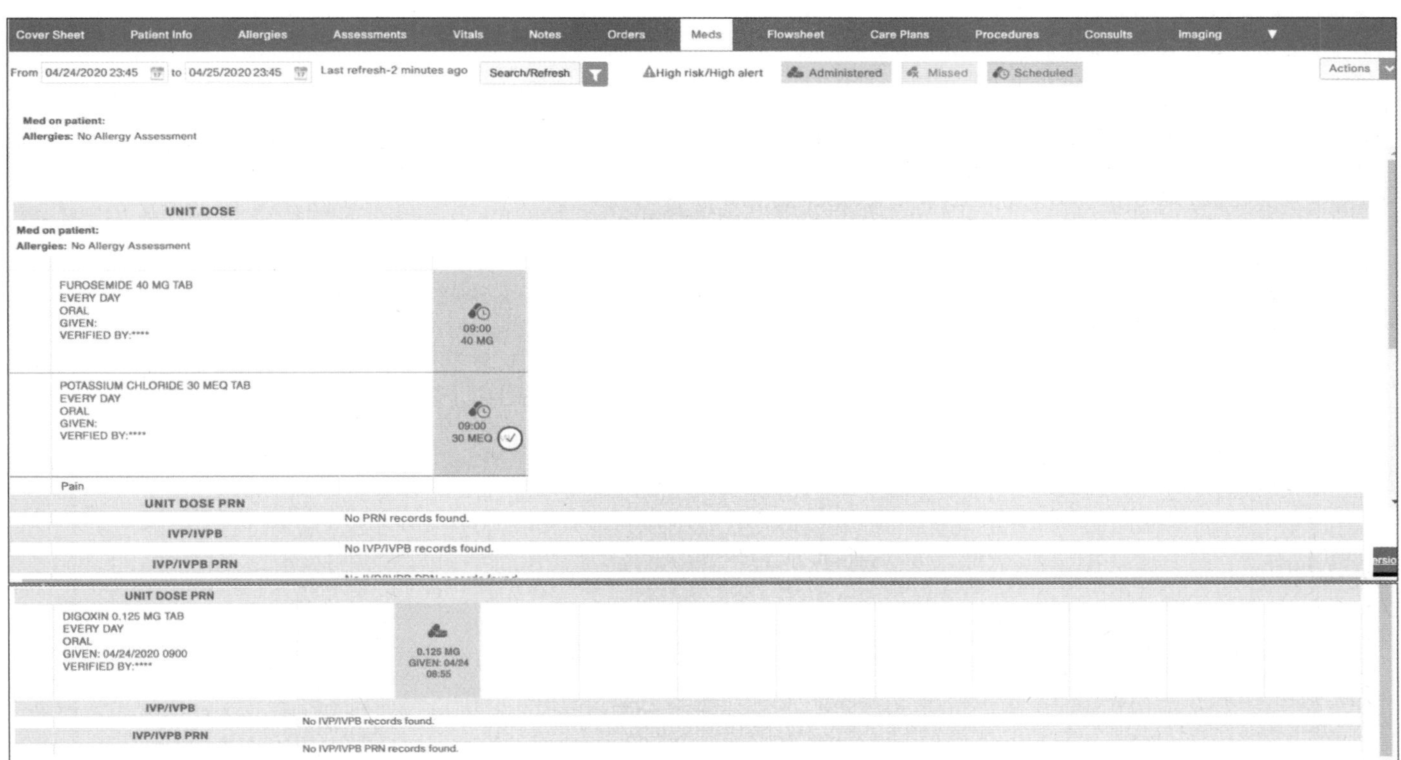

Figure 35.4 ■ Sample EHR medication administration record (MAR).

Systems of Measurement

Two common systems of measurement used in North America are the metric system and the household system.

Metric System

The metric system is prescribed by law in most European countries and in Canada. It is logically organized into units of 10; it is a decimal system. Basic units can be multiplied or divided by 10 to form secondary units. Multiples are calculated by moving the decimal point to the right, and division is accomplished by moving the decimal point to the left.

Basic units of measurement are the *meter*, the *liter*, and the *gram*. Prefixes derived from Latin designate subdivisions of the basic unit: *deci* (1/10 or 0.1), *centi* (1/100 or 0.01), and *milli* (1/1000 or 0.001). Multiples of the basic unit are designated by prefixes derived from Greek: *deka* (10), *hecto* (100), and *kilo* (1000). Only the measurements of volume (the liter) and of weight (the gram) are discussed in this chapter. These are the measures used in medication administration (Figure 35.5 ■). The *kilogram* (kg) is the only multiple of the gram used, and the *milligram* (mg) and *microgram* (mcg) are subdivisions. Fractional parts of the liter are usually expressed in *milliliters* (mL), for example, 600 mL; multiples of the liter are usually expressed as *liters* or milliliters, for example, 2.5 liters or 2500 mL. In nursing practice it is important to understand the difference between weight and volume. A drug dosage may be ordered by weight (i.e., grams, mg, mcg), but administered by volume (mL). For example, a healthcare provider prescribes 20 mg (weight) of codeine in an elixir (liquid) form. The codeine elixir bottle is labeled 10 mg per 5 mL. The nurse administers 10 mL (volume) of codeine elixir.

Household System

Household measures may be used when more accurate systems of measure are not required. Included in household measures are drops, teaspoons, and tablespoons. Approximate volume equivalents between metric and household systems include: 15 drops = 1 mL; 4 mL = 1 teaspoon, and 15 mL = 1 tablespoon.

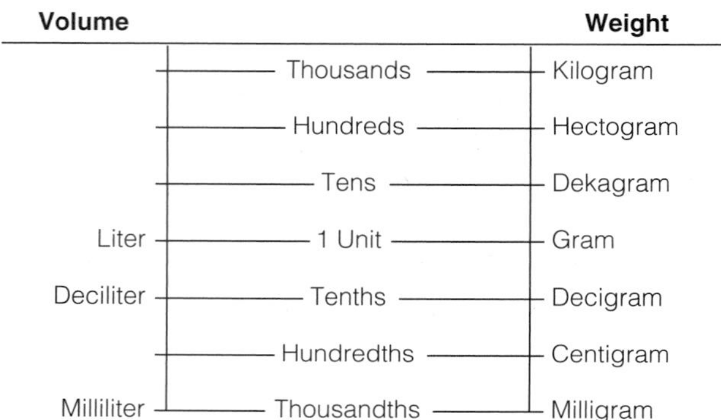

Figure 35.5 ■ Basic metric measurements of volume and weight.

Converting Units of Weight and Measure

Sometimes the nurse needs to convert weights within the metric system or convert units of volume or units of weight.

Converting Weights within the Metric System

It is relatively simple to arrive at equivalent units of weight within the metric system because the system is based on units of 10. Only three metric units of weight are used for drug dosages, the gram (g), milligram (mg), and microgram (mcg): 1000 mg or 1,000,000 mcg equals 1 gram (g). Equivalents are computed by dividing or multiplying; for example, to change milligrams to grams, the nurse divides the number of milligrams by 1000. The simplest way to divide by 1000 is to move the decimal point three places to the left:

$$500 \text{ mg} = ? \text{ g}$$

Move the decimal point three places to the *left*:

$$\text{Answer} = 0.5 \text{ g}$$

It is important to put a 0 in front of the decimal point; otherwise, the reader may miss the decimal point and administer a wrong dose of medication.

Conversely, to convert grams to milligrams, multiply the number of grams by 1000, or move the decimal point three places to the right:

$$0.006 \text{ g} = ? \text{ mg}$$

Move the decimal point three places to the *right*:

$$\text{Answer} = 6 \text{ mg}$$

Converting Units of Volume

Liters and milliliters are the volumes commonly used in preparing solutions for enemas, irrigating solutions for bladder irrigations, and solutions for cleaning open wounds. In some situations, the nurse needs to convert the volumes of such solutions.

Converting Units of Weight

The units of weight most commonly used in nursing practice are the gram, milligram, and kilogram. Learning these equivalents helps the nurse make weight conversions readily, as when converting pounds to kilograms and vice versa when determining an individual's weight. When converting pounds to kilograms, the nurse converts by dividing or multiplying by 2.2:

$$\begin{aligned} 2.2 \text{ lb} &= 1 \text{ kg} \\ 110 \text{ lb} &= x \text{ kg} \\ x &= \frac{110 \times 1}{2.2} \\ &= 50 \text{ kg} \end{aligned}$$

or

$$\begin{aligned} 50 \text{ kg} &= x \text{ lb} \\ 1 \text{ kg} &= 2.2 \text{ lb} \\ x &= \frac{2.2 \times 50}{1} \\ &= 110 \text{ lb} \end{aligned}$$

Methods of Calculating Dosages

Four common formulas are used to calculate drug dosages. Any of the formulas can be used. Nursing students are encouraged to review all four and to choose the method that works best for them. It is important to use one method consistently to avoid confusion in calculations and, thus, promote client safety. When calculating drug dosages, there are times when the nurse may need to round numbers. Box 35.3 reviews general guidelines for rounding.

Basic Formula

The basic formula for calculating drug dosages is commonly used and easy to remember:

D = desired dose (i.e., dose ordered by primary care provider)
H = dose on hand (i.e., dose on label of bottle, vial, ampule)
V = vehicle (i.e., form in which the drug comes, such as tablet or liquid).

$$\text{Formula} = \frac{D \times V}{H} = \text{amount to administer}$$

Example
Order: Erythromycin 500 mg
On hand: 250 mg in 5 mL

$$D = 500\text{ mg} \quad H = 250\text{ mg} \quad V = 5\text{ mL}$$

$$\frac{500\ \cancel{\text{mg}}}{250\ \cancel{\text{mg}}} \times 5\text{ mL} = \frac{2500}{250} = 10\text{ mL}$$

Another Example
Order: Lanoxin (digoxin) 0.5 mg daily.
On hand: Lanoxin (digoxin) 250 mcg/tab

Note: Before doing the drug calculation, the nurse needs to convert the 0.5 mg to an equivalent amount of mcg:
Move the decimal point three places to the right

$$0.5\text{ mg} = 500\text{ mcg}$$

Now, D and H match

$$D = 500\text{ mcg} \quad H = 250\text{ mcg} \quad V = \text{tablet}$$

$$\frac{500\ \cancel{\text{mcg}}}{250\ \cancel{\text{mcg}}} \times 1\text{ tablet} = 2\text{ tablets}$$

BOX 35.3 Guidelines for Rounding Numbers in Drug Calculations

GENERALLY . . .

- Quantities *greater than 1* are rounded to the nearest *tenth*.
- Quantities *less than 1* are rounded to the nearest *hundredth* (Olsen, Giangrasso, & Shrimpton, 2016, p. 10).
- To round to the nearest tenth:
  - Look at the number in the hundredths place. If this number is 5 or greater, add 1 to the tenths place number. For example, 1.67 = 1.7. If the number in the hundredths place is less than 5, leave the number in the tenths place as is. For example, 1.63 = 1.6.
- To round to the nearest hundredth:
  - Look at the number in the thousandths place. If this number is 5 or greater, add 1 to the hundredths place number. For example, 0.825 = 0.83. If the number in the thousandths place is less than 5, leave the number in the hundredths place as is. For example, 0.823 = 0.82.

ORAL MEDICATIONS

- A capsule cannot be divided.
- Tablets that are scored (a line marked on the tablet) may be divided. A tablet must be scored by the manufacturer to be divided properly.
- For tablets that are *not* scored and capsules, it may not be realistic to administer the exact amount as calculated. For example, if the calculation for *x* results in 1.9 tablets or capsules, the nurse gives 2 tablets or capsules because it is unrealistic to accurately administer 1.9 tablets or capsules.
- If the oral medication is a liquid, the nurse checks to see if it is possible to administer an accurate dosage. This often depends on the syringes used to draw up the medication. For example, a tuberculin syringe is a 1-mL syringe that includes markings for hundredths of a milliliter. These syringes are often used in pediatrics because they can measure medications given in very small amounts. The nurse needs to pay attention to the markings on the syringe. Some syringes (e.g., 3-mL) have calibrations where each line indicates one-tenth of a milliliter. In contrast, the calibration lines for larger syringes (e.g., 10-mL) indicate a 0.2-mL increment. The nurse must select the proper size syringe for the calculated volume of medication.

PARENTERAL MEDICATIONS

- Rounding depends on the amount (i.e., less than or more than 1) and the syringe used. As indicated above, a TB syringe can be used for very small amounts (e.g., to the hundredth of a mL). Larger syringes would be used for rounding to a tenth of a milliliter.

IV INFUSION

- By gravity:
  - Round to the nearest whole number. For example, if the flow rate calculation equals 37.5 drops/minute, the nurse adjusts the flow rate to 38 drops/minute.
- By IV pump:
  - If the IV pump uses only whole numbers, round to the nearest whole number.
  - Some IV pumps used in critical care units can be set to a tenth of a rate (e.g., 11.1 mL/h). Round to the nearest tenth decimal point.

ROUNDING DOWN

- Rounding down may be used in pediatrics or when administering high-alert medications to adults. This type of rounding is done to avoid the danger of an overdose (Olsen et al., 2016, p. 11).
- To round down to hundredths, drop all of the numbers after the hundredth place. For tenths, drop all of the numbers after the tenth place, and for whole numbers, all of the numbers after the decimal. For example, 6.6477 rounded down to the nearest
  - Hundredth = 6.64.
  - Tenth = 6.6.
  - Whole number = 6.

Ratio and Proportion Method

The ratio and proportion method is considered the oldest method used for calculating dosage problems. The equation is set up with the known quantities on the left side (i.e., H and V). The right side of the equation consists of the desired dose (i.e., D) and the unknown amount to administer (i.e., x). The equation looks like this:

$$H : V :: D : x$$

Once the equation is set up, multiply the extremes (i.e., H and x) and the means (i.e., V and D). Then solve for x.

Example
Order: Keflex 750 mg
On hand: Keflex 250 mg capsules

$$H = 250 \text{ mg} : V = 1 \text{ capsule} :: D = 750 \text{ mg} : x$$

$$250 : 1 :: 750 : x$$

Multiply the extremes (i.e., H and x) and the means (V and D):

$$250x = 750$$

$$x = 3 \text{ tablets}$$

Another Example
Order: Diflucan (fluconazole) 0.4 g
On hand: Diflucan (fluconazole) 200 mg tablets

Note: Before doing the drug calculation, the nurse needs to convert 0.4 gram to milligrams by moving the decimal three places to the right:

$$0.4 \text{ g} = 400 \text{ mg}$$

$$H = 200 \text{ mg} : V = \text{tablet} :: D = 400 \text{ mg} : x$$

$$200 : 1 :: 400 : x$$

Multiply the extremes (i.e., H and x) and the means (V and D):

$$\frac{\cancel{200}\, x}{\cancel{200}} = \frac{400}{200}$$

We determine that $x = 2$ tablets.

Fractional Equation Method

The fractional equation method is similar to ratio and proportion, except it is written as a fraction:

$$\frac{H}{V} = \frac{D}{x}$$

The formula consists of cross multiplying and solving for x:

$$\frac{H}{V} = \frac{D}{x}$$

$$Hx = DV$$

$$x = \frac{DV}{H}$$

Example
Order: Lanoxin 0.25 mg
On hand: Lanoxin 0.125 mg tablets

$$\frac{0.125 \text{ mg}}{1 \text{ tablets}} = \frac{0.25 \text{ mg}}{x \text{ tablets}}$$

Cross multiply:

$$0.125\, x = 0.25$$

Solve for x:

$$\frac{\cancel{0.125}x}{\cancel{0.125}} = \frac{0.25}{0.125}$$

$$x = 2 \text{ tablets}$$

Example Requiring Conversion
Order: Daypro (oxaprozin) 1.8 g PO once daily each morning
On hand: Daypro (oxaprozin) 600 mg per caplet

Note: Before doing the drug calculation, the nurse must convert 1.8 g to milligrams by moving the decimal three places to the right:

$$1.8 \text{ g} = 1800 \text{ mg}$$

$$\frac{600 \text{ mg}}{1 \textit{ caplet}} = \frac{1800 \text{ mg}}{x \textit{ caplet}}$$

Cross multiply:

$$600\, x = 1800$$

Solve for x:

$$\frac{\cancel{600}\, x}{\cancel{600}} = \frac{1800}{600}$$

$$x = 3 \textit{ caplets}$$

Dimensional Analysis

The dimensional analysis method is often used in the physical sciences when a quantity in one unit of measurement is converted to an equivalent quantity in a different unit of measurement by canceling matching units of measurement. In some of the previous examples, the nurse needed to convert units of measurement. This involved extra steps or equations. One advantage of dimensional analysis is that only one equation is needed. The three components (D, H, and V) are still needed to solve the problem. However, when the units of measurement differ for D and H, the dimensional analysis method includes the conversion factor in the equation. Six steps are suggested when using dimensional analysis:

1. Identify the dose on hand.
2. Identify the desired dose.
3. Write down the conversion factor, if needed.
4. Set up the equation.
5. Cancel units that appear in the numerator and denominator.
6. Multiply the numerator. Multiply the denominator. Divide the products.

Example
Order: Valsartan 120 mg
On hand: Valsartan 40 mg tablets

1. Identify the dose on hand: 40 mg
2. Identify the desired dose: 120 mg
3. No conversion is needed.
4. Set up the equation. Remember to put V (the form in which the drug comes) in the *numerator*:

$$\frac{1 \text{ tablet}}{40 \text{ mg}} \times \frac{120 \text{ mg}}{1}$$

5. Cancel units:

$$\frac{1 \text{ tablet}}{40 \cancel{\text{mg}}} \times \frac{120 \cancel{\text{mg}}}{1}$$

6. Multiply the numerator and denominator and then divide:

$$\frac{1 \text{ tablet}}{40} \times \frac{120}{1} = \frac{120}{40} = 3 \text{ tablets}$$

Example Using a Conversion Factor
Order: dofetilide 0.5 mg
On hand: 125 mcg capsules

1. Identify the dose on hand: 125 mcg capsule
2. Identify the desired dose: 0.5 mg
3. Write down conversion:

$$\frac{1000 \text{ mcg}}{1 \text{ mg}}$$

4. Set up the equation. Remember (a) to put the form of the drug in the numerator and (b) to set up the conversion factor so that units that need to cancel appear in both numerator and denominator:

$$\frac{1 \text{ capsule}}{125 \text{ mcg}} \times \frac{1000 \text{ mcg}}{1 \text{ mg}} \times \frac{0.5 \text{ mg}}{1}$$

5. Cancel units:

$$\frac{1 \text{ capsule}}{125 \cancel{\text{mcg}}} \times \frac{1000 \cancel{\text{mcg}}}{1 \cancel{\text{mg}}} \times \frac{0.5 \cancel{\text{mg}}}{1}$$

6. Multiply numerator and denominator and then divide:

$$\frac{1 \text{ capsule}}{125} \times \frac{1000}{1} \times \frac{0.5}{1} = \frac{500}{125} = 4 \text{ capsules}$$

Calculation for Individualized Drug Dosages

Nurses often need to individualize the dosage of a medication for pediatric clients. Other clients who may require an individualized dosage include those receiving chemotherapy and clients who are critically ill. The two methods for individualizing drug dosages are body weight and body surface area.

BODY WEIGHT

Unlike adult dosages, children's dosages are not always standard. Body weight significantly affects dosage; therefore, dosages are calculated. Dosages based on weight use kilograms of body weight and per kilogram medication recommendations to arrive at appropriate and safe doses.

The steps involved in calculating an individualized dose are as follows:

1. Convert pounds to kilograms.
2. Determine the drug dose per body weight by multiplying drug dose × body weight × frequency.
3. Choose a method of drug calculation to determine the amount of medication to administer.

Example
Order: Keflex, 20 mg/kg/day in three divided doses. The client weighs 20 pounds.
On hand: Keflex oral suspension 125 mg per 5 Ml

1. Convert pounds to kilograms:

$$20 \div 2.2 = 9 \text{ kg}$$

2. Multiply drug dose × body weight × frequency:

$$20 \text{ mg} \times 9 \text{ kg} = 1 \text{ day} = 180 \text{ mg/day}$$

$$180 \div 3 \text{ divided doses} = 60 \text{ mg per dose}$$

3. The nurse chooses his or her preferred method of calculation (e.g., basic formula, ratio and proportion, fractional, dimensional analysis) to determine how many milliliters per dose of medication. (The answer is 2.4 mL per dose.)

BODY SURFACE AREA

Sometimes the body surface calculation may be used instead of body weight to individualize the medication dosage. It is considered to be the most accurate method of calculating a child's dose. Body surface area is determined by using a nomogram and the child's height and weight. Figure 35.6 ■ shows a standard nomogram that will give a child's body surface area based on the weight and height of the child. The formula is the ratio of the child's body surface area to the surface area of an average adult (1.7 square meters, or 1.7 m^2), multiplied by the normal adult dose of the drug:

$$\frac{\text{Child's dose} = \text{surface area of child}(\text{m}^2)}{1.7 \text{ m}^2} \times \text{normal adult dose}$$

For example, a child who weighs 10 kg and is 50 cm tall has a body surface area of 0.4 m^2. Therefore, the child's dose of tetracycline corresponding to an adult dose of 250 mg would be as follows:

$$\frac{0.4 \text{ (surface area of child)}}{1.7 \text{ (surface area of average adult)}} = 0.23$$

(per rounding guidelines the number 0.23 becomes 0.2)

$$0.2 \times 250 \text{ (normal adult dose)} = 50 \text{ mg}$$

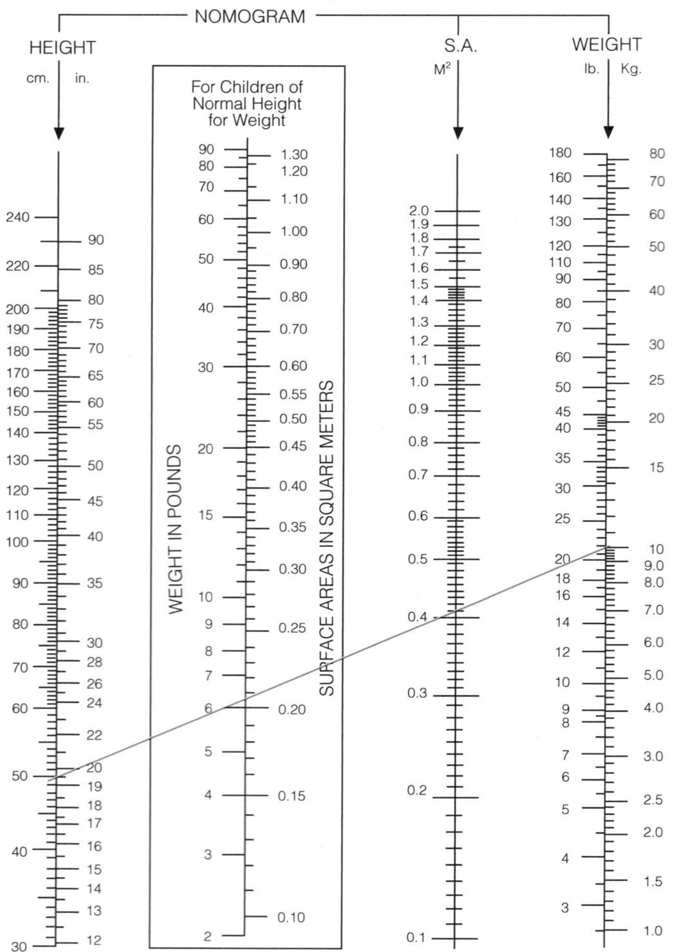

Figure 35.6 ■ Nomogram with estimated body surface area. Astraight line is drawn between the child's height (on the left) and the child's weight (on the right). The point at which the line intersects the surface area column is the estimated body surface area.

Routes of Administration

Pharmaceutical preparations are generally designed for one or two specific routes of administration (Table 35.6). The route of administration should be indicated when the drug is ordered. When administering a drug, the nurse should ensure that the pharmaceutical preparation is appropriate for the route specified. The nurse often administers opioids for pain management. The routes for opioid delivery are also discussed in this chapter.

Oral

Oral administration is the most common, least expensive, and most convenient route for most clients. In oral administration, the drug is swallowed. Because the skin is not broken as it is for an injection, oral administration is also a safe method.

The major disadvantages can include an unpleasant taste of the drugs, irritation of the gastric mucosa, irregular absorption from the GI tract, slow absorption, and, in some cases, harm to the client's teeth. For example, the liquid preparation of ferrous sulfate (iron) can stain the teeth.

Sublingual

In **sublingual** administration a drug is placed under the tongue, where it dissolves (Figure 35.7 ■). In a relatively short time, the drug is largely absorbed into the blood vessels on the underside of the tongue. The medication should not be swallowed. Nitroglycerin is one example of a drug commonly given in this manner.

TABLE 35.6 Routes of Administration

Route	Advantages	Disadvantages
Oral	Most convenient Usually least expensive Safe, does not break skin barrier Administration usually does not cause stress Some new oral medications are designed to rapidly dissolve on the tongue, allowing for faster absorption and action	Inappropriate for clients with nausea or vomiting Drug may have unpleasant taste or odor Inappropriate when GI tract has reduced motility Inappropriate if client cannot swallow or is unconscious Cannot be used before certain diagnostic tests or surgical procedures Drug may discolor teeth, harm tooth enamel Drug may irritate gastric mucosa Drug can be aspirated by seriously ill clients
Sublingual	Same as for oral, *plus*: Drug can be administered for local effect More potent than oral route because drug directly enters the blood and bypasses the liver	If swallowed, drug may be inactivated by gastric juice Drug must remain under tongue until dissolved and absorbed. May cause stinging or irritation of the mucous membranes Drug is rapidly absorbed into the bloodstream
Buccal	Same as for sublingual	Same as for sublingual
Rectal	Can be used when drug has objectionable taste or odor Drug released at slow, steady rate Provides a local therapeutic effect	Dose absorbed is unpredictable May be perceived as unpleasant by the client Limited use

TABLE 35.6 Routes of Administration—*continued*

Route	Advantages	Disadvantages
Vaginal	Provides a local effect	May be messy and may soil clothes
Topical	Few side effects	Drug can enter body through abrasions and cause systemic effects Leaves residue on the skin that may soil clothes
Transdermal	Prolonged systemic effect Few side effects Avoids GI absorption problems Onset of drug action faster than oral	Rate of delivery may be variable Verify that the previous patch has been removed and disposed of appropriately to avoid overdose
Subcutaneous	Absorption is slower (an advantage for insulin and heparin administration)	Must involve sterile technique because breaks skin barrier More expensive than oral Can administer only small volume Some drugs can irritate tissues and cause pain Can produce anxiety Breaks skin barrier
Intramuscular	Can administer larger volume than subcutaneous Drug is rapidly absorbed	Can produce anxiety Breaks skin barrier
Intradermal	Absorption is slow (this is an advantage in testing for allergies)	Amount of drug administered must be small Breaks skin barrier
Intravenous	Rapid effect	Limited to highly soluble drugs Drug distribution inhibited by poor circulation
Inhalation	Introduces drug throughout respiratory tract Rapid localized relief Drug can be administered to unconscious client	Drug intended for localized effect can have systemic effect Of use only for the respiratory system

Buccal

Buccal means "pertaining to the cheek." In buccal administration, a medication (e.g., a tablet) is held in the mouth against the mucous membranes of the cheek until the drug dissolves (Figure 35.8 ■). The drug may act locally on the mucous membranes of the mouth or systemically when it is swallowed in the saliva.

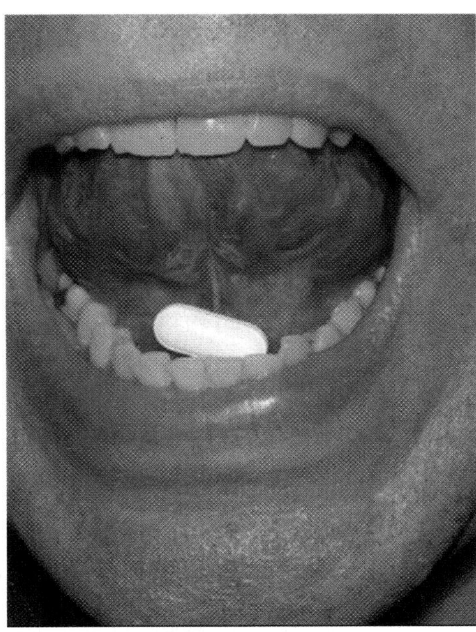

Figure 35.7 ■ Sublingual administration of a tablet.

Parenteral

The **parenteral** route is defined as other than through the alimentary or respiratory tract; that is, by needle. The following are some of the more common routes for parenteral administration:

- **Subcutaneous** (**hypodermic**)—into the subcutaneous tissue, just below the skin
- **Intramuscular (IM)**—into a muscle

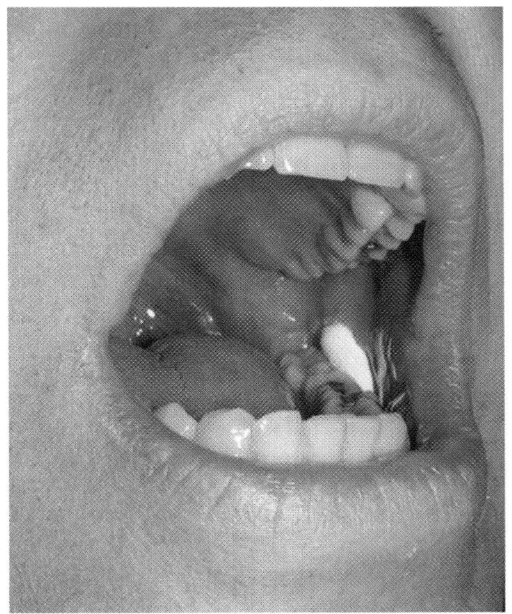

Figure 35.8 ■ Buccal administration of a tablet.

- **Intradermal (ID)**—under the epidermis (into the dermis)
- **Intravenous (IV)**—into a vein.

Some of the less commonly used routes for parenteral administration are intra-arterial (into an artery), intracardiac (into the heart muscle), intraosseous (into a bone), **intrathecal** or **intraspinal** (into the spinal canal), intrapleural (into the pleural space), **epidural** (into the epidural space), and intra-articular (into a joint). Sterile equipment and sterile drug solution are essential for all parenteral therapy. The main advantage is fast absorption.

Topical

Topical applications are those applied locally to the skin or to the mucous membranes. They affect only the area to which they are applied. Topical applications include the following:

- Dermatologic preparations—applied to the skin
- Instillations and irrigations—applied into body cavities or orifices, such as the urinary bladder, eyes, ears, nose, rectum, or vagina
- Inhalations—administered into the respiratory tract by a nebulizer or positive pressure breathing apparatus. Air, oxygen, and vapor are generally used to carry the drug into the lungs.

Routes for Opioid Delivery

Opioids can be given via the following routes: oral, transnasal, transdermal, transmucosal, rectal, topical, subcutaneous, intramuscular, IV (bolus and continuous), intraspinal (epidural and intrathecal), and as continuous local anesthetics.

Oral

The oral route is preferred for opioids because of ease of administration. Because the duration of action of most opioids is approximately 4 hours, people with chronic pain have had to awaken during the night to medicate themselves for pain. To avoid this problem, long-acting or sustained-release formulations of morphine with a duration of 8 or more hours have been developed. An example of a long-acting morphine is MS Contin, a controlled-release tablet. Clients receiving long-acting morphine may also need prn "rescue" doses of immediate-release analgesics such as Actiq, the short-acting oral transmucosal fentanyl citrate (OTFC) for acute breakthrough pain. Another method of oral opiate delivery is high-concentration liquid morphine. This formulation enables clients who can swallow only small amounts to continue taking the drug orally.

Transnasal

Transnasal administration has the advantage of rapid action of the medication because of direct absorption through the vascular nasal mucosa. A commonly used agent is butorphanol (Stadol) for acute migraines. Treating migraines via the nasal route is particularly beneficial because of the nausea, vomiting, and gastroparesis that can occur with migraines, making oral medications contraindicated.

Transdermal

Transdermal drug therapy is advantageous in that it delivers a relatively stable plasma drug level and is noninvasive. Fentanyl is a lipophilic synthetic opioid (i.e., binds to subcutaneous fat) and is available as a skin patch with various dosages (12 to 100 mcg). The nurse must remember that fentanyl is 100 times more potent than morphine and is ordered in micrograms (mcg) not milligrams (mg). It provides drug delivery for up to 72 hours. The transdermal route is distinguished from the topical route in that the effects of the medications are systemic after the medication is absorbed. Nurses must teach clients not to use heat (e.g., hot tubs, heating pads) with the fentanyl patch, because increased absorption may result. A client with a fever may absorb the medication faster because of the vasodilation from the increased skin temperature. Used patches should be disposed of in a tamper-proof container. This is especially true in the home setting because a used patch can contain enough residual medication to harm a small child or animal if ingested.

Transmucosal

Many clients with cancer-related pain experience breakthrough pain even though they are on a fixed schedule for pain control. The transmucosal route is helpful for breakthrough pain because the oral mucosa is well vascularized, which helps with rapid absorption. Two forms of fentanyl are available for transmucosal delivery: oral transmucosal fentanyl citrate (OTFC; Actiq) and a fentanyl buccal tablet (Fentora).

Rectal

Some opioid medicines are available in suppository form. The rectal route is particularly useful for clients who have dysphagia (difficulty swallowing) or nausea and vomiting. An example is the belladonna and opium suppositories, which are used to relieve moderate to severe pain caused by ureteral spasm (Mayo Clinic, 2019).

Subcutaneous

Although the subcutaneous route has been used extensively to deliver opioids, another technique uses subcutaneous catheters and infusion pumps to provide continuous subcutaneous infusion (CSCI) of opioids. CSCI is particularly helpful for clients (a) whose pain is poorly controlled by oral medications, (b) who are experiencing dysphagia or GI obstruction, or (c) who have a need for prolonged use of parenteral opioids. CSCI involves the use of a small, light, battery-operated pump that administers the drug through a 23- or 25-gauge butterfly needle. The needle can be inserted into the anterior chest, the subclavicular region, the abdominal wall, the outer aspects of the upper arms, or the thighs. Client mobility is maintained with the application of a shoulder bag or holster to hold the pump. The site is rotated every 7 days and medication infusion rates are usually 3 to 5 mL per hour (Infusion Nurses Society, 2016).

QSEN Patient-Centered Care: Home Care Considerations for CSCI

Because family caregivers must operate the pump as well as change and care for the injection site, the nurse needs to provide appropriate instruction. Caregivers need to be able to:

- Describe the basic parts and symbols of the system.
- Identify ways to determine whether the pump is working.
- Change the battery.
- Change the medication.
- Demonstrate stopping and starting the pump.
- Demonstrate tubing care, site care, and changing of the injection site.
- Identify signs indicating the need to change an injection site.
- Describe general care of the pump when the client is ambulatory, bathing, sleeping, or traveling.
- Identify actions to take to solve problems when the alarm signals.

Intramuscular

The intramuscular (IM) route should *not* be used for administration of analgesics. Disadvantages include variable absorption and unpredictable onset of action and peak effect, as well as the tissue damage that may result, even if properly administered. Regardless of precautions taken, there is pain involved with administration.

Intravenous

The IV route provides the most rapid onset for pain relief with few side effects. However, just as the onset of pain relief occurs in 5 to 10 minutes, so can adverse effects, such as respiratory depression. The analgesic can be administered by IV bolus or by continuous infusion. IV medications should be given slowly to decrease adverse effects. Caution is needed to prevent the introduction of air or bacteria into the tubing, and to prevent the introduction of medications that are incompatible with other medications dissolved in the IV solution.

Intraspinal

Another method of delivery is the infusion of opioids into the epidural or intrathecal (subarachnoid) space (Figure 35.9 ■). Intraspinal infusion may be administered to clients who require pain management in a variety of practice settings (e.g., acute care, outpatient, and home care).

Analgesics administered via the intraspinal route are delivered adjacent to the opioid receptors in the dorsal horn of the spinal cord. Two commonly used medications are morphine sulfate and fentanyl. All medicines administered via the intraspinal route need to be sterile and preservative free (preservatives are neurotoxic). The major benefit of intraspinal drug therapy is superior analgesia with less medication used. The epidural space is most commonly used because the dura mater acts as a protective barrier against infection, including

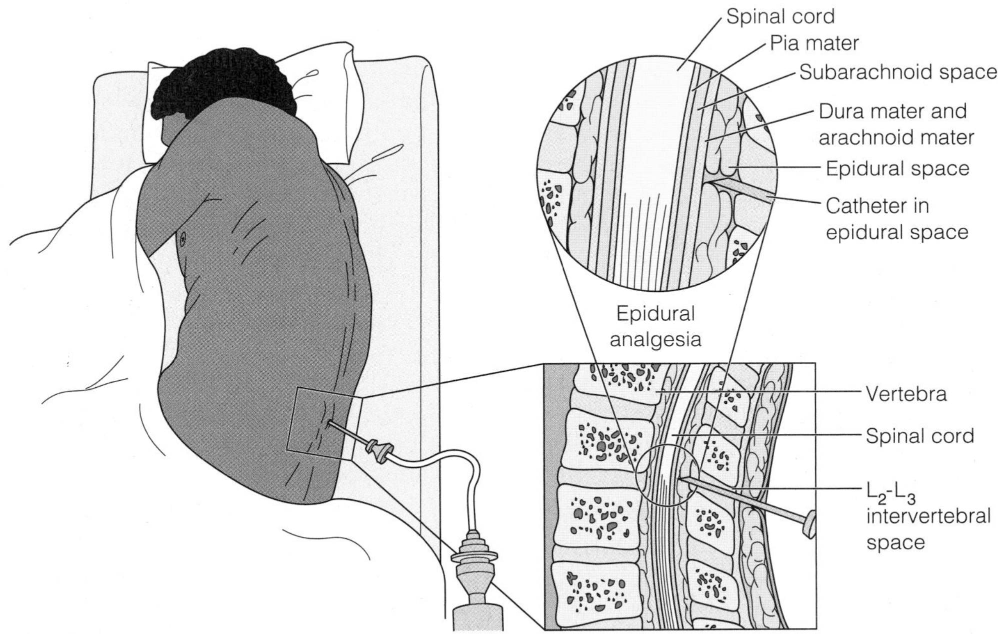

Figure 35.9 ■ Placement of an intraspinal catheter in the epidural space.

meningitis, and there is less risk of developing a "spinal headache." Intraspinal catheters are not in constant contact with blood; thus, an infusion can be stopped and restarted later without concern that the catheter is no longer patent.

Intrathecal administration delivers medication directly into the cerebrospinal fluid (CSF) that bathes and nourishes the spinal cord. Medicines quickly bind to the opioid receptor sites in the dorsal horn when administered in this fashion, speeding the onset and peak effect, while prolonging the duration of action of the analgesic. An example of how the route of administration affects the relative potency of opioids is as follows: A client who requires 300 mg of oral morphine per day to control pain will need 100 mg of parenteral morphine, 10 mg of epidural morphine, and only 1 mg of intrathecal morphine in a 24-hour period. Very little drug is absorbed by blood vessels into the systemic circulation. In fact, the drug must circulate through the CSF to be excreted. As a result, there may be a delayed onset (24 hours following the administration) of respiratory depression, because medication that has left the spinal opioid sites travels through the brain to be eliminated.

In contrast, the epidural infusion requires a higher dose of opioid to create the desired effect, which can produce adverse effects of itching, urinary retention, and respiratory depression. Often, an opioid (e.g., fentanyl) and a local anesthetic (e.g., bupivacaine) are combined to lower the dose of opioid needed. As a result, there may be an increase in fall risk for some clients who develop muscular weakness in their legs or orthostatic hypotension in response to the local anesthetic.

The anesthesiologist or nurse anesthetist inserts a needle into the intrathecal or epidural space (typically in the lumbar region) and threads a catheter through the needle to the desired level. The catheter is connected to tubing that is then positioned along the spine and over the client's shoulder for the nurse to access. The entire catheter and tubing are taped securely to prevent dislodgment. Often an occlusive, transparent dressing is placed over the insertion site for easy identification of catheter displacement or local inflammation. Temporary catheters, used for short-term acute pain management, are usually placed at the lumbar or thoracic vertebral level and usually removed after 2 to 4 days. Permanent catheters, for clients with chronic pain, may be tunneled subcutaneously through the skin and exit at the client's side or be connected to a pump implanted in the abdomen. Tunneling of the catheter reduces the risk of infection and displacement of the catheter. After the catheter is inserted, the nurse is responsible for monitoring the infusion and assessing the client per institutional policy.

Safety Alert! **SAFETY**

As a precaution, have naloxone (Narcan), sodium chloride 0.9% diluent, and injection equipment on hand for each client receiving an opioid-containing epidural infusion.

Continuous Local Anesthetics

Continuous subcutaneous administration of long-acting local anesthetics into or near a surgical site is a technique that can be used to provide postoperative pain control. This technique has been used for a variety of surgical procedures, including knee arthroplasty, abdominal hysterectomy, hernia repair, and mastectomy. Nursing interventions for the client with infusion of a continuous local anesthetic include the following:

- Conduct pain assessment and documentation every 2 to 4 hours while the client is awake.
- Check the dressing every shift to ensure it is intact. The dressing is not usually changed in order to avoid dislodging the catheter. Contact the primary care provider if the dressing becomes loose.
- Check the site of the catheter. It should be clean and dry.
- Assess the client for signs of local anesthetic toxicity (e.g., cardiac arrhythmias, dizziness; ringing in the ears; a metallic taste; tingling or numbness of the lips, gums, or tongue) or neurologic deficit distal to the catheter insertion site.
- Notify the primary care provider of signs of local anesthetic toxicity or neurologic deficit. If detected early, prompt treatment should be initiated in order to prevent serious complications.

Administering Medications Safely

The nurse should always assess a client's health status and obtain a medication history prior to giving any medication. The extent of the assessment depends on the client's illness or current condition, the intended drug, and the route of administration. For example, if a client has dyspnea, the nurse assesses respirations carefully before administering any medication that might affect breathing. It is important to determine whether the route of administration is suitable. For example, a client who is nauseated may not be able to keep down a drug taken orally. In general, the nurse assesses the client *prior* to administering any medication to obtain baseline data by which to evaluate the effectiveness of the medication.

The medication history includes information about the drugs the client is taking currently or has taken recently. This includes prescription drugs; OTC drugs such as antacids, alcohol, and tobacco; and recreational drugs such as marijuana. Sometimes an incompatibility with one or more of these drugs affects the choice of a new medication.

Clients often take vitamins, herbs, and food supplements, or use folk remedies that they do not list in their medication history. Because many of these have unknown or unpredictable actions and side effects, they need to be noted, with attention paid to possible incompatibilities with other prescribed medications.

An important part of the history is clients' knowledge of their drug allergies. Some clients can tell a nurse, "I am allergic to penicillin, adhesive tape, and curry." The nurse should clarify with the client any side effects, adverse reactions, or allergic responses due to medications. Other clients may not be sure about allergic reactions. An illness occurring after a drug was taken may not be identified as an allergy, but the client may associate the drug with an illness or unusual reaction. The client's primary care provider can often give information about allergies. During the history, the nurse tries to obtain information about drug dependencies. How often drugs are taken and the client's perceived need for them are measures of dependence.

Also included in the history are the client's normal eating habits. Sometimes the medication schedule needs to be coordinated with mealtimes or the ingestion of foods. When a medication must be taken with food on a specified schedule, clients can often adjust their mealtime or have a snack (e.g., with a bedtime medication). In addition, certain foods are incompatible with certain medications; for example, milk is incompatible with tetracycline.

It is also important for the nurse to identify any problems the client may have in self-administering a medication. A client with poor eyesight, for example, may require special labels for the medication container; clients with unsteady hands may not be able to hold a syringe or to inject themselves. Obtaining information as to how and where clients store their medications is also important. If clients have difficulty opening certain containers, they may change containers, but leave old labels on, which increases the risk of medication errors.

The nurse needs to consider socioeconomic factors for all clients, but especially for older clients. Two common problems are lack of transportation to obtain medications and inadequate finances to purchase medications. When aware of these problems, the nurse can refer the client to the proper resources to ensure that medications are purchased.

Medication Administration Errors

"Medication errors cause at least one death every day and injure approximately 1.3 million people annually in the United States alone" (World Health Organization, 2017, para. 3). Medication errors can occur at all stages of the medication administration process: prescribing, transcribing, dispensing, administering, or monitoring.

Nurses who do not follow the five rights (right drug, right client, right dose, right time, right route) of medication administration contribute to medication errors. Common reasons why nurses do not follow the five rights include poor pharmacologic knowledge, miscalculations, interruptions, increased workloads, and fatigue (Chu, 2016; Godshall & Riehl, 2018). Increased workloads may influence nurses to take shortcuts and fail to take standardized procedures. For example, one observational study of 293 nurses found that only 6.5% checked their clients' wristbands (Chu, 2016).

Nurses' thinking processes during medication administration are complex and require critical thinking and focus for client safety. Research has validated that when nurses are interrupted during any step of the medication administration process, there is a risk in both number and severity of medication administration errors. As a result, the Institute of Medicine recommends that organizations adopt strategies to reduce interruptions during medication administration as part of a safety program (Flynn, Evanish, Fernald, Hutchinson, & Lefaiver, 2016).

Clinical Alert!

During the medication administration process is *not* the time for the nurse to multitask! For client safety, the nurse must not be interrupted and must be able to focus on administering medications safely.

Of interest are studies that investigated the sources of interruption during medication administration. Sources include monitor alarms, telephone calls, and family inquiries, with the most common source being questions from nurse colleagues and other healthcare team members. As a result, many healthcare facilities have implemented the "sterile cockpit rule," which means eliminating interruptions and distractions during medication preparation to avoid medication errors. Studies have evaluated the effectiveness of interventions to reduce interruptions and distractions during medication administration. These strategies include using a medication safety checklist, placing signs outside and within medication rooms to promote a quiet environment, having others take nonurgent telephone calls for the nurse who is administering medications, and creating a "No Interruption or Quiet Zone" by placing red duct tape around the medication cart and medication-dispensing machines. The red-taped area indicates "do not disturb with nonurgent matters" to others. Another approach is where the nurse wears a bright, colorful "Do Not Disturb" sash or vest during medication administration.

Technology, when used appropriately, can help decrease medication administration errors. For example, some studies have shown that barcode medication administration (BCMA) can reduce medication errors by 54% to 87% (Godshall & Riehl, 2018). Another example is the use of "smart" IV pumps, which have error-prevention software, drug libraries, and dosing limits that give an alert when the dosing is out of range (Chu, 2016; Lapkin, Levett-Jones, Chenoweth, & Johnson, 2016).

Lapkin et al. (2016) completed a synthesis of 16 systematic reviews and focused on which interventions were most effective in reducing medication administration errors. They found that there was no one single intervention to prevent medication errors. Rather, many approaches, such as those listed above, along with education and the use of barcode technology, were more successful in reducing medication administration errors.

Nurses play an important role in medication safety because they perform the last safety checks before a medication is administered to a client. Therefore, it is important that healthcare leaders recognize the complexity of the nurse's environment and the importance of medication administration, and examine ways to reduce system factors that impact client safety, such as interruptions during medication administration. If a medication error does occur, the nurse needs to report the error and follow agency policy. See Table 35.7 for an overview of safety strategies to prevent medication errors.

Medication Reconciliation

Another safety issue that affects the nurse is the need to ensure that clients receive the appropriate medications and dosages as they move or transition through a facility. The Institute for Healthcare Improvement (IHI) (Midelfort, n.d.) defines **medication reconciliation** as "the process of identifying the most accurate list possible of all medications a patient is taking—including name, dosage, frequency, and route—and using this list to provide correct medications for patients anywhere within the healthcare system. Reconciliation involves comparing the patient's current list of medications against the physician's admission, transfer, or discharge orders" (para. 2). Preventing adverse drug events (ADEs) is the incentive behind the idea of medication reconciliation. Approximately half of hospital medication errors occur when clients transition in care both within and outside of the organization (Midelfort, n.d.; Agency for Healthcare Research and Quality, 2019).

TABLE 35.7 Safety Strategies to Prevent Medication Administration Errors

Stage	Safety Strategy
Prescribing	• Computerized provider order entry • Medication reconciliation at times of transitions in care
Transcribing	• Computerized provider order entry to eliminate handwriting errors
Dispensing	• Clinical pharmacists to manage the medication dispensing process • Use of "tall man" lettering (e.g., DOPamine and DOBUTamine) to minimize confusion between look-alike, sound-alike, or confusing medications • Automated dispensing cabinets for high-risk medications
Administering	• Follow the "five rights" of medication administration • Institute strategies to minimize interruptions while nurse is administering medications • Use BCMA to ensure medications are given to the correct client • Use smart infusion pumps for IV infusions • Keep current in pharmacology knowledge and medication calculations • Identify high-alert medication (e.g., anticoagulants, sedatives, insulin, and opioids)

From *Medication Errors and Adverse Drug Events*, by Agency for Healthcare Research and Quality (AHRQ), 2019; *Simple Steps to Reduce Medication Errors* by R. Chu, 2016; *The Effectiveness of Interventions Designed to Reduce Medication Administration Errors: A Synthesis of Findings from Systematic Reviews* by S. Lapkin, T. Levett-Jones, L. Chenoweth, & M. Johnson, 2016; *Preventing High-Alert Medication Errors in Hospital Patients* by W. Votroubek, 2018.

PRACTICE GUIDELINES Administering Medications

- Nurses who administer medications are responsible for their own actions. Question any order that is illegible or that you consider incorrect. Call the provider who prescribed the medication for clarification.
- Be knowledgeable about the medications you administer. You need to know why the client is receiving the medication. Look up the necessary information if you are not familiar with the medication.
- Federal laws govern the use of controlled substances. Keep these medications in a locked place.
- Use only medications that are in a clearly labeled container.
- Do not use liquid medications that are cloudy or have changed color. Oral suspension is an exception.
- Calculate drug doses accurately. If you are uncertain, ask another nurse to double-check your calculations.
- Administer only medications personally prepared.
- Before administering a medication, identify the client correctly using the appropriate means of identification, such as checking the identification bracelet.
- Do not leave medications at the bedside, with certain exceptions (e.g., nitroglycerin, cough syrup). Check agency policy.
- If a client vomits after taking an oral medication, report this to the nurse in charge, or the primary care provider, or both.
- Take special precautions when administering certain medications; for example, have another nurse check the dosages of anticoagulants, insulin, and certain IV preparations.
- Most hospital policies require new orders from the primary care provider for a client's postsurgery care.
- When a medication is omitted for any reason, record the fact together with the reason.
- When a medication error is made, report it immediately to the nurse in charge, the primary care provider, or both.
- Always check a medication's expiration date.
- Perform hand hygiene between clients. Antiseptic gels are appropriate to use if hands are not visibly soiled. Hand washing with soap and water is required for visibly soiled hands.

All facilities accredited by The Joint Commission must have protocols and processes in place for medication reconciliation, particularly in the following transition areas: on admission, during transfer between units, and at discharge. Box 35.4 provides an overview of the elements of medication reconciliation. The nurse needs to make a complete list of the client's medications (including prescriptions, vitamins, supplements, and OTC) on admission. This current list needs to be compared to any new medications ordered by the primary care provider on admission and during the client's hospital stay. Medications that are to be administered around the time of shift report need to be discussed at the report. For example, insulin is a common medication scheduled between night and day shifts. It is important that the oncoming nurse know if the medication was given or not. If a client is transferred to another setting, within or outside of the facility, a complete list of the client's medications must be communicated to the next provider of care. This list is also provided to clients on discharge from the facility. In addition, the client should receive, at discharge, written and oral information on each medication to be taken at home. It is important for the nurse to emphasize to clients the importance of keeping the list of their medications handy and taking it with them to their follow-up visits and to future hospitalizations, if any. Maintaining their list of current medications helps improve communication and avoid potential errors in medication administration. The U.S. Food and Drug Administration (FDA, 2019b) developed a form called "My Medicine Record" to help consumers keep track of their prescription medications, OTC drugs, and dietary supplements. This form is available online and can be downloaded. Individuals can then complete it by either writing in the information or entering the information on their computers and printing it.

BOX 35.4 Elements of Medication Reconciliation

The Joint Commission (2019a) requires medication reconciliation to occur:

- *At admission:* Collect a list of the medications the client is currently taking when he or she is admitted to the hospital or seen in an outpatient setting. Compare the medication information the client brought to the hospital with the medications ordered for the client by the hospital in order to identify and resolve discrepancies (p. 6).
- *At discharge:* Provide the client (or family as needed) with written information on the medications the client should be taking when he or she is discharged from the hospital or at the end of an outpatient encounter (p. 6). Explain the importance of managing medication information to the client.

The IHI (Midelfort, n.d.) recommends that medication reconciliation also occur when transferring the client from one care setting to another. That is, compare the medication information the client brought to the hospital with the current medications ordered for the client by the hospital and to the transfer orders to identify and resolve any discrepancies.

Safety Alert! SAFETY

2019 The Joint Commission National Patient Safety Goals

Goal 3.06.01: Maintain and Communicate Accurate Patient Medication Information.

Rationale: *There is evidence that medication discrepancies can affect patient outcomes. Medication reconciliation is intended to identify and resolve discrepancies—it is a process of comparing the medications a patient is taking (and should be taking) with newly ordered medications. The comparison addresses duplication, omissions, and interactions, and the need to continue current medications.*

Medication Dispensing Systems

Medical facilities vary in their medication dispensing systems. The systems can include the following:

- ***Medication cart.*** The medication cart is on wheels, allowing the nurse to move the cart to outside the client's room. The cart contains small numbered drawers that correlate to the room numbers on the nursing unit. The small drawer is labeled with the name of the client currently in that room and holds the client's medications for the shift or 24 hours. The medication is usually in unit-dose packaging; that is, the individual drug package states the drug name, dose, and expiration date (Figure 35.10 ■). A larger locked drawer in the cart contains the controlled substances rather than keeping them in the client's individual drawer. The cart may also include a supply drawer that contains client-labeled bulk containers, such as Metamucil, that are too large for the small individual drawer. The MAR is usually located in a binder or a computer located on top of the medication cart. The nurse either carries a key for the medication cart or enters a special code to open the cart, because it must be kept locked when not in use.
- ***Medication cabinet.*** Some facilities have a locked cabinet in the client's room. This cabinet holds the client's

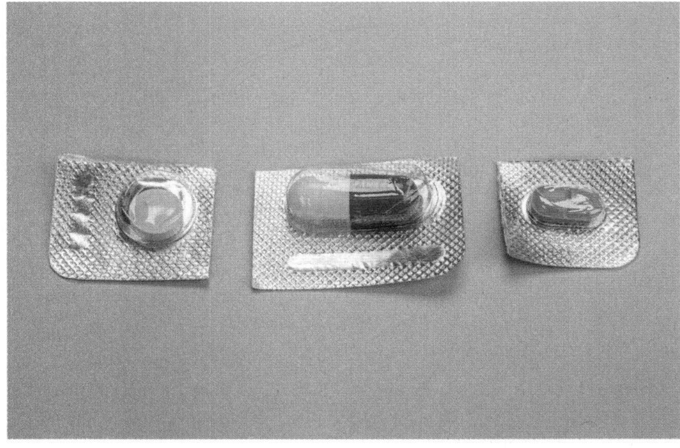

Figure 35.10 ■ Unit-dose medication packages.

unit-dose medications and MAR. Controlled substances are not kept in this cabinet but at another location on the nursing unit. The nurse uses either a key or a special code to open the client's medication cabinet, because it must be locked when not in use.

- ***Medication room.*** Depending on the facility, a medication room may be used for a variety of purposes. For example, the medication carts, when not in use, may be placed in this room. The medication room may also be the central location for stock medications, controlled medications, and drugs used for emergencies. The medication room may have a refrigerator for IV and other medications needing a cold environment. The room may also contain other medication administration supplies (e.g., syringes, needles). Nurses access the medication room by either a key or a special code as the room is often kept locked. Check agency policy.
- ***Automated dispensing cabinet (ADC).*** This computerized access system (Figure 35.11 ■) automates the distribution, management, and control of medications. The nurse uses either a biometric fingerprint or a password to access the system, selects the client's name from an on-screen list, and selects the medication(s). The benefit of using ADCs is the reduction in the risk for medication errors. These benefits include improved drug security, inventory control, computerized alerts, and the potential to limit access to certain high-alert drugs. To further promote safety, many facilities have instituted a pharmacy profiling system as part of the ADC. This means that a nurse cannot remove a medication from an ADC unless a pharmacist has reviewed the order and released the medication.

Process of Administering Medications

When administering any drug, regardless of the route of administration, the nurse must do the following:

1. ***Identify the client.*** Errors can and do occur, usually because one client gets a drug intended for another. One of The Joint Commission's National Patient Safety Goals is to improve the accuracy of client identification. This goal requires a nurse to use at least two client identifiers whenever administering medications. Acceptable identifiers may be the client's name, an assigned identification number, a telephone number, or other client-specific identifier. In most hospitals, clients wear a wristband with their name and hospital identification number. Before giving the client any drug, always check the client's identification band. Many hospitals use BCMA technology for medication administration. A nurse preparing to administer a medication using BCMA scans or enters the nurse's own ID, the client's wristband, and each package of medication to be administered. BCMA often includes two or more client-specific identifiers that meet the identifier requirement (Figure 35.12 ■). In long-term care and home care settings, the requirement for two identifiers is appropriate at the first encounter. Thereafter, and in any situation of continuing one-to-one care in which the clinician knows the resident, one identifier can be facial recognition (The Joint Commission, 2019b).
2. ***Inform the client.*** If the client is unfamiliar with the medication, the nurse should explain the intended action as well as any side effects or adverse effects that might occur. Listen to the client. It is easy to get so

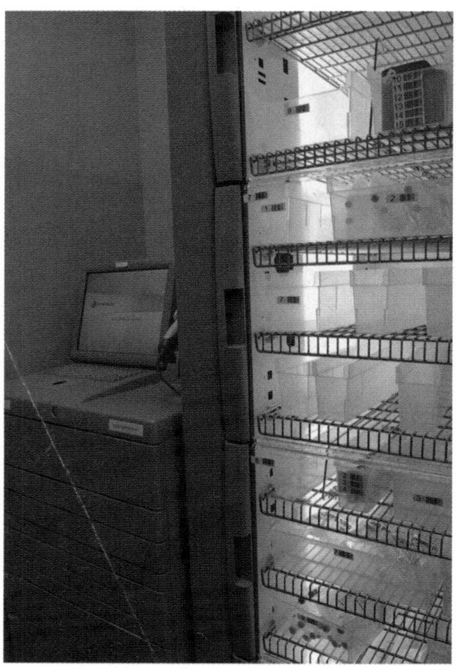

Figure 35.11 ■ Automated dispensing cabinet.

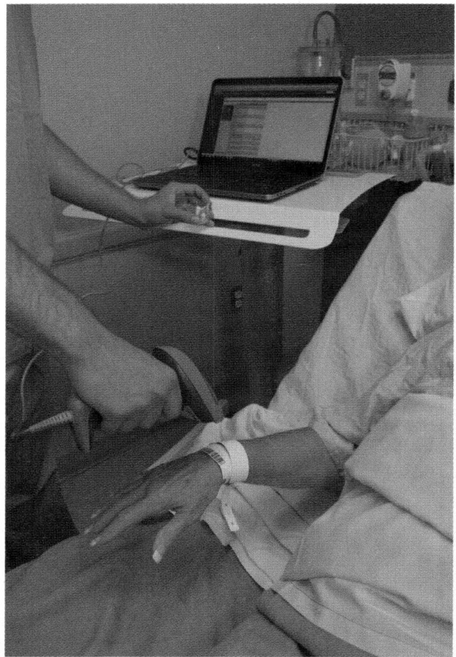

Figure 35.12 ■ The nurse scans the bar code on the client's wristband before administering the medication.

Safety Alert! SAFETY

2019 The Joint Commission National Patient Safety Goals

Goal 1: Improve the Accuracy of Patient Identification.

- Use at least two patient identifiers when providing care, treatment, and services.
  Rationale: *Wrong-patient errors occur in virtually all stages of diagnosis and treatment. The intent for this goal is two-fold: first, to reliably identify the client as the individual for whom the service or treatment is intended; second, to match the service or treatment to that individual. Acceptable identifiers may be the individual's name, an assigned identification number, telephone number, or other person-specific identifier.*

Clinical Alert!

Do not ask "Are you John Jones?" because the client may answer "yes" to the wrong name.

focused on the task of timely medication administration that the nurse may miss relevant information provided by the client. For example, if the client says that he does not take a pill for high blood pressure, this should be an "alert" for the nurse to stop and check if this is the correct medication for that client.

3. ***Administer the drug.*** Read the MAR carefully and perform three checks with the labeled medications (Box 35.5). Then administer the medication in the prescribed dosage, by the route ordered, at the correct time. There has been a change in what is considered the correct time. Historically, a "30-minute rule" (i.e., administer medications within 30 minutes before or after the scheduled time) was used. In medication error research, one-third of reported medication errors were because of the wrong time. Moreover, 18,000 nurses who responded to an extensive survey clearly stated that the "30-minute rule" was unsafe, was impossible to follow given the current complex nature of medication administration, and created pressure to take shortcuts that led to errors. Subsequently, the ISMP developed new guidelines for timely administration of scheduled medications. Hospitals are to use these guidelines as a resource as they develop their own specific guidelines for their facility through an interdisciplinary team that includes nurses. The underlying principle of the guidelines is that medication administration still has to be timely; however, hospitals can determine which medications should be on a tight time schedule and which can be administered with greater flexibility at the discretion of the nurse (ISMP, 2011). See Table 35.8 for the ISMP guidelines for timely medication administration.

BOX 35.5 Check Three Times for Safe Medication Administration

FIRST CHECK

- Read the MAR and remove the medication(s) from the client's drawer. Verify that the client's name and room number match the MAR.
- Compare the label of the medication against the MAR.
- If the dosage does not match the MAR, determine if you need to do a math calculation.
- Check the expiration date of the medication.

SECOND CHECK

While preparing the medication (e.g., pouring, drawing up, or placing unopened package in a medication cup), look at the medication label and check against the MAR.

THIRD CHECK

Recheck the label on the container (e.g., vial, bottle, or unused unit-dose medications) against the MAR before returning to its storage place *or* before giving the medication to the client.

Certain aspects of medication administration are important for the nurse to check each time a medication is administered. These are referred to as the "rights." Traditionally, there were 5 rights to medication administration. More rights have been added as seen in Box 35.6.

TABLE 35.8 Acute Care Guidelines for Timely Administration of Scheduled Medications

Type of Scheduled Medication	Goals for Timely Administration
TIME-CRITICAL SCHEDULED MEDICATIONS	
Hospital-defined time-critical medications* *Limited number of drugs where delayed or early administration of more than 30 minutes may cause harm or sub-therapeutic effect Includes but not limited to: Medications with a dosing schedule more frequent than every 4 hours	Administer at the **exact time indicated when necessary** (e.g., rapid-acting insulin), **otherwise, within 30 minutes** before or after the scheduled time
NON-TIME-CRITICAL SCHEDULED MEDICATIONS	
Daily, weekly, monthly medications	**Within 2 hours** before or after the scheduled time
Medications prescribed more frequently than daily, but no more frequently than every 4 hours	**Within 1 hour** before or after the scheduled time

From Acute Care Guidelines for Timely Administration of Scheduled Medications, by the Institute for Safe Medication Practices, © 2011. Used wtih permission of ISMP.

BOX 35.6 Ten "Rights" of Medication Administration

RIGHT MEDICATION

- The medication given was the medication ordered.

RIGHT DOSE

- The dose ordered is appropriate for the client.
- Give special attention if the calculation indicates multiple pills or tablets or a large quantity of a liquid medication. This can be an indication that the math calculation may be incorrect.
- Double-check calculations that appear questionable.
- Know the usual dosage range of the medication.
- Question a dose outside of the usual dosage range.

RIGHT TIME

- Give the medication at the right frequency and at the time ordered according to agency policy.
- Medications should be given within the agency guidelines.

RIGHT ROUTE

- Give the medication by the ordered route.
- Make certain that the route is safe and appropriate for the client.

RIGHT CLIENT

- Medication is given to the intended client.
- Check the client's identification band with each administration of a medication.
- Know the agency's name alert procedure when clients with the same or similar last names are on the nursing unit.

RIGHT CLIENT EDUCATION

- Explain information about the medication to the client (e.g., why receiving, what to expect, any precautions).

RIGHT DOCUMENTATION

- Document medication administration after giving it, not before.
- If time of administration differs from prescribed time, note the time on the MAR and explain the reason and follow-through activities (e.g., pharmacy states medication will be available in 2 hours) in nursing notes.
- If a medication is not given, follow the agency's policy for documenting the reason why.

RIGHT TO REFUSE

- Adult clients have the right to refuse any medication.
- The nurse's role is to ensure that the client is fully informed of the potential consequences of refusal and to communicate the client's refusal to the healthcare provider.

RIGHT ASSESSMENT

- Some medications require specific assessments prior to administration (e.g., apical pulse, blood pressure, laboratory results).
- Medication orders may include specific parameters for administration (e.g., do not give if pulse less than 60 or systolic blood pressure less than 100).

RIGHT EVALUATION

- Conduct appropriate follow-up (e.g., was the desired effect achieved or not? Did the client experience any side effects or adverse reactions?).

4. ***Provide assistive interventions as indicated.*** Clients may need help when receiving medications. They may require physical assistance, for instance, in assuming positions for intramuscular injections, or they may need guidance about measures to enhance drug effectiveness and prevent complications, such as drinking fluids. Some clients express fear about their medications. The nurse can relieve fears by listening carefully to clients' concerns and giving correct information.
5. ***Record the drug administered.*** The facts recorded in the chart, in ink or by computer printout, are name of the drug, dosage, method of administration, specific relevant data such as pulse rate (taken in most settings prior to the administration of digitalis), and any other pertinent information. The record should also include the exact time of administration and the signature of the nurse providing the medication. Many medication records are designed so that the nurse signs once on the page and initials each medication administered. Often, medications that are given regularly are recorded on a special flow record. PRN (as-needed) or stat (at-once) medications are recorded separately.
6. ***Evaluate the client's response to the drug.*** The kinds of behavior that reflect the action or lack of action of a drug and its untoward effects are as variable as the purposes of the drugs themselves. The anxious client may show the desired effects of a tranquilizer by behavior that reflects a lowered stress level (e.g., slower speech or fewer random movements). How well a client slept can often measure the effectiveness of a sedative, and the effectiveness of an analgesic can be measured by how much pain the client feels. In all nursing activities, nurses need to be aware of the medications that a client is taking and record their effectiveness as assessed by the client and the nurse on the client's chart. The nurse may also report the client's response directly to the nurse manager and primary care provider.

Developmental Considerations

It is important for the nurse to be aware of how growth and development affect administration of medications for all age groups, particularly the very young and the very old.

Infants and Children

Knowledge of growth and development is essential for the nurse administering medications to children. Oral medications for children are usually prepared in sweetened liquid form to make them more palatable. The parents may provide suggestions about what method is best for their child. Do not use necessary foods such as milk or orange juice to mask the taste of medications, because the child may develop unpleasant associations and refuse that food in the future.

Children tend to fear any procedure in which a needle is used because they anticipate pain or because the procedure is unfamiliar and threatening. The nurse needs to acknowledge that the child will feel some pain; denying this fact only deepens the child's distrust. After the injection, the nurse (or the parent) can cuddle and speak softly to the infant and give the child a toy to dismiss the child's association of the nurse only with pain.

Older Adults

Older adults can have special problems, most of which are related to physiologic changes, to past experiences, and to established attitudes toward medications. See Box 35.7 for a list of the physiologic changes in older adults that may affect the administration and effectiveness of medications.

BOX 35.7 Physiologic Changes Associated with Aging That Influence Medication Administration and Effectiveness

- Altered memory
- Decreased visual acuity
- Decrease in renal function, resulting in slower elimination of drugs and higher drug concentrations in the bloodstream for longer periods
- Less complete and slower absorption from the GI tract
- Increased proportion of fat to lean body mass, which facilitates retention of fat-soluble drugs and increases potential for toxicity
- Decreased liver function, which hinders biotransformation of drugs
- Decreased organ sensitivity, which means that the response to the same drug concentration in the target organ is less in older people than in the young
- Altered quality of organ responsiveness, resulting in adverse effects becoming pronounced before therapeutic effects are achieved
- Decrease in manual dexterity due to arthritis or decrease in flexibility

Many of these changes increase the possibility of cumulative effects and toxicity. For example, digoxin, which is frequently taken by older adults, can accumulate to toxic levels and be lethal. It is common for older adults to take several different medications daily. The possibility of error increases with the number of medications taken, whether self-administered at home or administered in a hospital. The greater number of medications also increases the problem of drug interactions. A general rule to follow is that older adults should take as few medications as possible.

Older adults usually require smaller dosages of drugs, especially sedatives and other central nervous system depressants. Reactions of older adults to medications, particularly sedatives, are often unpredictable. It is common to see irritability, confusion, disorientation, restlessness, and incontinence as a result of sedatives. Nurses therefore need to observe clients carefully for adverse reactions. Prescribers often follow the unwritten rule to "start low and go slow" when prescribing medications for older adults. The initial prescribed dosage will often be low and then gradually increased with careful monitoring of the actions and side effects of the drug.

Attitudes of older adults toward medical care and medications vary. Older adults tend to believe in the wisdom of the healthcare provider more willingly than younger people. Some older people may be confused by the prescription of several medications and may passively accept their medications from nurses but not swallow them, spitting out tablets or capsules after the nurse leaves the room. For this reason, the nurse is advised to stay with clients until they have swallowed the medications. Other clients may be suspicious of medications and actively refuse them.

Older adults are mature adults capable of reasoning. Therefore, the nurse needs to explain the reasons for and the effects of medications. This education can prevent clients from continuing to take a medication long after there is a need for it or discontinuing a drug too quickly. For example, clients should know that diuretics will cause them to urinate more frequently and may reduce ankle edema. All clients need instructions about medications. These instructions should include when to take the drugs, what effects to expect, and when to consult a primary care provider.

Because some clients are required to take several medications daily and because visual acuity and memory may be impaired, the nurse needs to develop simple, realistic plans for clients to follow at home. For example, remembering to take drugs can be difficult for some people, including older adults. Scheduling medications at mealtime or at bedtime helps clients to remember to take their medications. Some clients may take their medications and then an hour later may not remember whether they took them. One solution is to use a special container strictly for medications. An empty container indicates that the individual took the pills. Special containers with individual slots and markings for each day can reduce confusion. Loss of visual acuity presents problems that can be overcome by writing out the plan in block letters large enough to be read. In some situations, enlisting the help of a family member can be helpful.

Older adults may have decreased dexterity due to arthritis or stiffness of their hands and fingers due to aging. This causes difficulty in opening medication containers or in self-administration of other medications such as eyedrops, eardrops, insulin injections, and inhalers. Nurses can help clients make the necessary changes or enlist the assistance of another individual to help them administer their medications.

Oral Medications

The oral route is the most common route by which medications are given. As long as a client can swallow and retain the drug in the stomach, this is the route of choice (see Skill 35.1). Oral medications are contraindicated when a client is vomiting, has gastric or intestinal suction, or is unconscious and unable to swallow. Such clients in a hospital are usually on orders for "nothing by mouth" (the Latin is *nil per os*: **NPO**).

SKILL 35.1

Administering Oral Medications

PURPOSE

- To provide a medication that has systemic effects or local effects on the GI tract or both (see specific drug action)

ASSESSMENT

Assess

- Type of administration: oral, sublingual, or buccal
- Allergies to medication(s)
- Client's ability to swallow the medication
- Presence of vomiting or diarrhea that would interfere with the ability to absorb the medication
- Specific drug action, side effects, interactions, and adverse reactions
- Client's knowledge of and learning needs about the medication
- Perform appropriate assessments (e.g., vital signs, laboratory results) specific to the medication.
- Determine if the assessment data influence administration of the medication (i.e., is it appropriate to administer the medication or does the medication need to be held and the prescriber notified?).

PLANNING

Assignment

In acute care settings, administration of oral and enteral medications is performed by the nurse and is not assigned to assistive personnel (AP). The nurse can inform the AP of the intended therapeutic effects and specific side effects of the medication and request the AP to report specific client observations to the nurse for follow-up. In some long-term care settings, trained AP may administer certain medications to stable clients. It is important, however, for the nurse to remember that the medication knowledge of the AP is limited and *assessment and evaluation of the effectiveness of the medication remain the responsibility of the nurse*.

Equipment

- Client's MAR or computer printout
- Dispensing system
- Disposable medication cups: small paper or plastic cups for tablets and capsules, waxed or plastic calibrated medication cups for liquids
- Pill crusher or cutter
- Straws to administer medications that may discolor the teeth or to facilitate the ingestion of liquid medication for certain clients
- Drinking glass and water or juice
- Soft foods such as applesauce or pudding to use for crushed medications for clients who may choke on liquids

IMPLEMENTATION

Preparation

1. Know the reason why the client is receiving the medication, the drug classification, contraindications, usual dosage range, side effects, and nursing considerations for administering and evaluating the intended outcomes for the medication.
2. Check the MAR.
   - Check for the drug name, dosage, frequency, route of administration, and expiration date for administering the medication, if appropriate. **Rationale:** *Orders for certain medications (e.g., controlled substances, antibiotics) expire after a specified time frame and they need to be reordered by the primary care provider*.
   - If the MAR is unclear or pertinent information is missing, compare the MAR with the prescriber's most recent written order.
   - Report any discrepancies to the charge nurse or the primary care provider, as agency policy dictates.
3. Verify the client's ability to take medication orally.
   - Determine whether the client can swallow, is NPO, is nauseated or vomiting, has gastric suction, or has diminished or absent bowel sounds.
4. Organize the supplies.
   - Gather the MAR(s) for each client together so that medications can be prepared for one client at a time. **Rationale:** *Organization of supplies saves time and reduces the chance of error*.

Performance

1. Perform hand hygiene and observe other appropriate infection prevention procedures.
2. Unlock the dispensing system.
3. Obtain the appropriate medication.
   - Read the MAR and take the appropriate medication from the shelf, drawer, or refrigerator. The medication may be dispensed in a bottle, box, or unit-dose package.
   - Compare the label of the medication container or unit-dose package against the order on the MAR or computer printout. **Rationale:** *This is a safety check to ensure that the right medication is given*. If these are not identical, recheck the prescriber's written order in the client's chart. If there is still a discrepancy, check with the pharmacist. ❶
   - Check the expiration date of the medication. Return expired medications to the pharmacy. **Rationale:** *Outdated medications are not safe to administer*.
   - Use only medications that have clear, legible labels. **Rationale:** *This ensures accuracy*.
4. Prepare the medication.
   - Calculate the medication dosage accurately.
   - Prepare the correct amount of medication for the required dose, without contaminating the medication. **Rationale:** *Aseptic technique maintains drug cleanliness*.
   - While preparing the medication, recheck each prepared drug and container with the MAR again. **Rationale:** *This second safety check reduces the chance of error*.

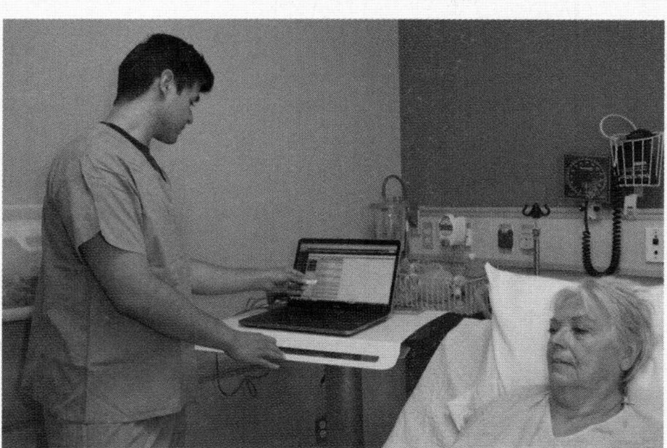

❶ Compare the medication label to the MAR.

Administering Oral Medications—*continued*

Tablets or Capsules

- Place packaged unit-dose capsules or tablets directly into the medicine cup. Do not remove the medication from the package until at the bedside. **Rationale:** *The wrapper keeps the medication clean. Not removing the medication facilitates identification of the medication in the event the client refuses the drug or assessment data indicate to hold the medication. Unopened unit-dose packages can usually be returned to the medication cart.*
- If using a stock container, pour the required number into the bottle cap, and then transfer the medication to the disposable cup without touching the tablets.
- Keep medications that require specific assessments, such as pulse measurements, respiratory rate or depth, or blood pressure, separate from the others. **Rationale:** *This reminds the nurse to complete the needed assessment(s) in order to decide whether to give the medication or to withhold the medication if indicated.*
- Break only scored tablets if necessary to obtain the correct dosage. Use a cutting or splitting device if needed. Check the agency policy as to how unused portions of a medication are to be discarded. 2
- If the client has difficulty swallowing, check if the medication can be crushed. Some drug handbooks have an appendix that lists the "Do Not Crush" medications. The ISMP (2018) website provides an updated list of medications that should not be crushed. Some medications that should not be crushed include time-released and enteric-coated medications. An example is oxycodone (OxyContin), a long-acting opioid that normally lasts 12 hours after administration. If the tablet is crushed, the client gets a surge of action in the first 2 hours, and may then start having severe pain again in 4 to 6 hours, because the opioid effect wears off too soon. The crushing of these tablets causes an uneven effect, and the long or sustained action of the medication is lost.
- If it is acceptable, crush the tablets to a fine powder with a pill crusher or between two medication cups. Then, mix the powder with a small amount of soft food (e.g., custard, applesauce).

Clinical Alert!

Check with the pharmacy before crushing tablets. Sustained-action, enteric-coated, buccal, or sublingual tablets should not be crushed.

Liquid Medication

- Thoroughly mix the medication before pouring. Discard any medication that has changed color or turned cloudy, the exception being oral suspensions.
- Remove the cap and place it upside down on the countertop. **Rationale:** *This avoids contaminating the inside of the cap.*
- Hold the bottle so the label is next to your palm and pour the medication away from the label. **Rationale:** *This prevents the label from becoming soiled and illegible as a result of spilled liquids.* 3

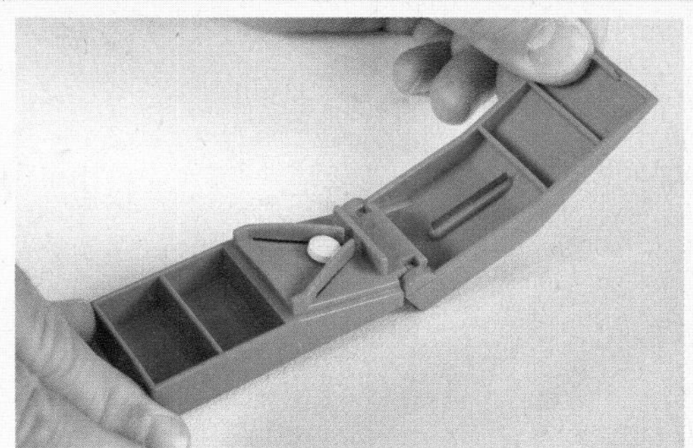

2 A cutting device can be used to divide tablets.

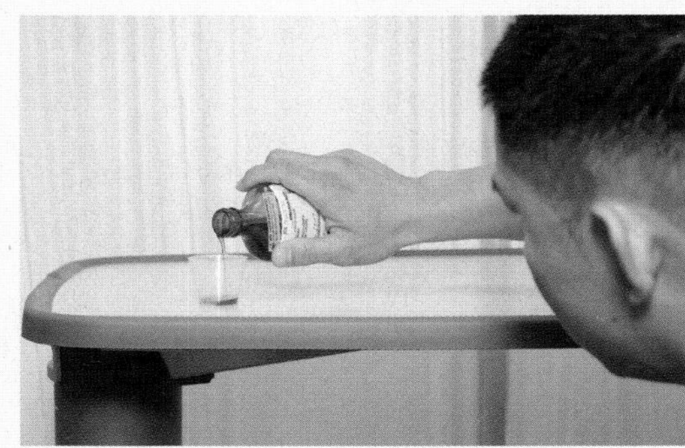

3 Pouring a liquid medication from a bottle.

- Place the medication cup on a flat surface at eye level and fill it to the desired level, using the *bottom* of the **meniscus** (crescent-shaped upper surface of a column of liquid) to align with the container scale. 4 **Rationale:** *This method ensures accuracy of measurement.*
- Before capping the bottle, wipe the lip with a paper towel. **Rationale:** *This prevents the cap from sticking.*
- When giving small amounts of liquids (e.g., less than 5 mL), prepare the medication in a specially designed oral syringe. 5

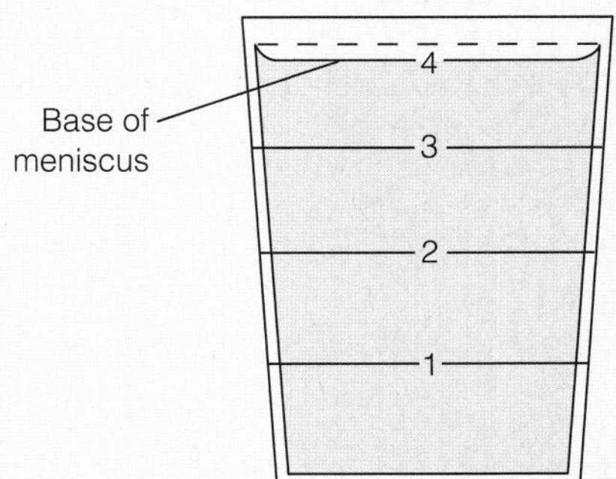

4 The *bottom* of the meniscus is the measuring guide.

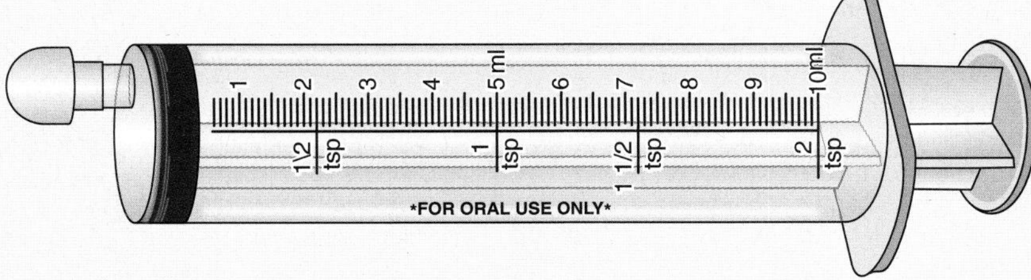

5 Oral syringe with both household and metric measurements. Note that it states "FOR ORAL USE ONLY" on the side and that the tip is to the side to help differentiate it from a syringe that would be used for parenteral administration.

Continued on page 866

Administering Oral Medications—*continued*

SKILL 35.1

Label the syringe with the name of the medication and the route (PO). **Rationale:** *Any oral solution removed from the original container and placed into a syringe should be labeled to avoid medications being given by the wrong route (e.g., IV). This practice facilitates client safety and avoids tragic errors.*

- Keep unit-dose liquids in their package and open them at the bedside.

Safety Alert! SAFETY

2019 The Joint Commission National Patient Safety Goals

Goal 3: Improve the Safety of Using Medications.

- Label all medications, medication containers, and other solutions on and off the sterile field in perioperative and other procedural settings.
  Note: Medication containers include syringes, medicine cups, and basins.
  Rationale: *Medications or other solutions in unlabeled containers are unidentifiable. Errors, sometimes tragic, have resulted from medications and other solutions being removed from their original containers and placed into unlabeled containers. This unsafe practice neglects basic principles of safe medication management, yet it is routine in many organizations. The labeling of all medications, medication containers, and other solutions is a risk-reduction activity consistent with safe medication management. This practice addresses a recognized risk point in the administration of medications in perioperative and other procedural settings.*

Oral Controlled Substances

- If an agency uses a manual recording system for controlled substances, check the record for the previous drug count and compare it with the supply available.
- Remove the next available tablet and drop it in the medicine cup.
- After removing a tablet, record the necessary information on the appropriate control record and sign it.
- Computer-controlled dispensing systems allow access only to the selected drug and automatically record its use.

All Medications

- Place the prepared medication and MAR together on the medication cart.
- Recheck the label on the container before returning the bottle, box, or envelope to its storage place. **Rationale:** *This third check further reduces the risk of error.*
- Avoid leaving prepared medications unattended. **Rationale:** *This precaution prevents potential mishandling errors.*
- Lock the medication cart before entering the client's room. **Rationale:** *This is a safety measure because medication carts are not to be left open when unattended.*
- Check the room number against the MAR if agency policy does not allow the MAR to be removed from the medication cart. **Rationale:** *This is another safety measure to ensure that the nurse is entering the correct client room.*

5. Provide for client privacy.
6. Prepare the client.
   - Introduce self and verify the client's identity using agency protocol. **Rationale:** *This ensures that the right client receives the medication.*
   - Assist the client to a sitting position or, if not possible, to a side-lying position. **Rationale:** *These positions facilitate swallowing and prevent aspiration.*
   - If not previously assessed, take the required assessment measures, such as pulse and respiratory rates or blood pressure. Take the apical pulse rate before administering digitalis preparations. Take blood pressure before giving antihypertensive drugs. Take the respiratory rate prior to administering opioids. **Rationale:** *Opioids depress the respiratory center.* If any of the findings are above or below the predetermined parameters, consult the primary care provider before administering the medication.
7. Explain the purpose of the medication and how it will help, using language that the client can understand. Include relevant information about effects; for example, tell the client receiving a diuretic to expect an increase in urine output. **Rationale:** *Information can facilitate acceptance of and compliance with the therapy.*
8. Administer the medication at the correct time.
   - Take the medication to the client within the guidelines of the agency.
   - Give the client sufficient water or preferred juice to swallow the medication. Before using juice, check for any food and medication incompatibilities. **Rationale:** *Fluids ease swallowing and facilitate absorption from the GI tract. Grapefruit juice may not be safe for clients who take certain medications.* Liquid medications other than antacids or cough preparations may be diluted with 15 mL (1/2 oz) of water to facilitate absorption.
   - If the client is unable to hold the pill cup, use the pill cup to introduce the medication into the client's mouth, and give only one tablet or capsule at a time. **Rationale:** *Putting the cup to the client's mouth maintains the cleanliness of the nurse's hands. Giving one medication at a time eases swallowing.*
   - If an older child or adult has difficulty swallowing, ask the client to place the medication on the back of the tongue before taking the water. **Rationale:** *Stimulation of the back of the tongue produces the swallowing reflex.*
   - If the medication has an objectionable taste, give the medication with juice, applesauce, or pudding if there are no contraindications. **Rationale:** *Juices, applesauce, or pudding may mask the taste of the medication.*
   - If the client says that the medication you are about to give is different from what the client has been receiving, do not give the medication without first checking the original order. **Rationale:** *Most clients are familiar with the appearance of medications taken previously. Unfamiliar medications may signal a possible error.*
   - Stay with the client until all medications have been swallowed. **Rationale:** *The nurse must see the client swallow the medication before the drug administration can be recorded.* The nurse may need to check the client's mouth to ensure that the medication was swallowed and not hidden inside the cheek. A primary care provider's order or agency policy is required for medications left at the bedside.
9. Document each medication given.
   - Record the medication given, dosage, time, any complaints or assessments of the client, and your signature.
   - If medication was refused or omitted, record this fact on the appropriate record; document the reason, when possible, and the nurse's actions according to agency policy.
10. Dispose of all supplies appropriately.
    - Replenish stock (e.g., medication cups) and return the cart to the appropriate place.
    - Discard used disposable supplies.

Administering Oral Medications—*continued*

Home Setting

The nurse should instruct the client to:

- Learn the names of the medications as well as their actions and possible adverse effects. Carry a complete list of all prescriptions, OTC medications, and home remedies at all times.
- Keep all medications out of reach of children and pets.
- If using a syringe to administer the medication to an infant or child, remove and dispose of the plastic cap that fits on the end of the syringe. Infants and small children have been known to choke on these caps.
- Take the medications only as prescribed. Know which medications need to be taken on an empty stomach and which can be taken with food. Immediately consult the nurse, pharmacist, or primary care provider about any problems with the medication.
- Always check the medication label to make sure the correct medication is being taken.
- Request labels printed with larger type on medication containers if labels are difficult to read.
- Check the expiration date and discard medications appropriately. The FDA (2019a) recommends that consumers and caregivers discard expired, unwanted, or unused medicines from their home as quickly as possible to help reduce the chance that others accidently take or intentionally misuse the unneeded medicine, and to help reduce drugs from entering the environment (para. l). The choices for disposing of unused or expired medicine include (1) medicine take-back options (this is preferred and includes the two options of periodic events and permanent collection sites); (2) disposal in the household trash by mixing the medicine with a nontoxic but bad-tasting product (e.g., cat litter or used coffee grounds), placing the mixture in a sealed plastic bag, and putting it in the trash; deleting all personal information from the prescription label or medicine packaging and disposing the container; and (3) flushing certain potentially dangerous medicines in the toilet. The FDA has a list of 14 medications (e.g., opioids) that should be immediately flushed when they are no longer needed *and* take-back options are not available. These medications are considered harmful and may be fatal with just one dose if taken by an individual other than for whom it was prescribed.
- Ask the pharmacist to substitute childproof caps with ones that are more easily opened, as necessary, for older adults.
- If a dose or more is missed, do not take two or more doses; ask the pharmacist or primary care provider for directions.
- Do not crush or cut a tablet or capsule without first checking with the primary care provider or pharmacist. Doing so may affect the medication's absorption.
- Never stop taking the medication without first discussing it with the primary care provider.
- Always check with the pharmacist before taking any nonprescription medications. Some OTC medications can interact with the prescribed medication.

Additionally, the nurse can set up a medication plan to assist clients and family members to remember a schedule. Weekly pill containers (available at pharmacies) or a written plan may be helpful.

EVALUATION

- Return to the client when the medication is expected to take effect (usually 30 minutes) to evaluate the effects of the medication on the client.
- Observe for desired effect (e.g., relief of pain or decrease in body temperature).
- Note any adverse effects or side effects (e.g., nausea, vomiting, skin rash, or change in vital signs).
- Compare to previous findings, if available.
- Report significant deviations from normal to the primary care provider.

LIFESPAN CONSIDERATIONS Administering Oral Medications

- Knowledge of growth and development is essential for the nurse administering medications to infants and children.
- Nurses must know the range of safe medication dosages for infants and children.

INFANTS

- Oral medications can be effectively administered in several ways:
  - A syringe or dropper
  - A medication nipple that allows the infant to suck the medication
  - Mixed in small amounts of food
  - A spoon or medication cup, for older children.
- Never mix medications into foods that are essential, since the infant may associate the food with an unpleasant taste and refuse that food in the future. Never mix medications with formula.
- Place a small amount of liquid medication along the inside of the baby's cheek and wait for the infant to swallow before giving more to prevent aspiration or spitting out.
- When using a spoon, retrieve and refeed medication that is thrust outward by the infant's tongue.

CHILDREN

- Whenever possible, children should be given a choice between the use of a spoon, dropper, or syringe.
- Oral medications for children are usually prepared in sweetened liquid form to make them more palatable. Crush medications that are not supplied in liquid form and mix them with substances available on most pediatric units, such as honey, flavored syrup, jam, or a fruit puree. However, present the medication to the child honestly and not as a food or a treat.
- Essential foods such as milk or orange juice should not be used to mask the taste of medications because the child may develop unpleasant associations and refuse that food in the future.
- Place the young child or toddler on your lap or a parent's lap in a sitting position.
- Administer the medication slowly with a measuring spoon, plastic syringe, or medicine cup.
- To prevent nausea, pour a carbonated beverage over finely crushed ice and give it before or immediately after the medication is administered.
- Follow medication with a drink of water, juice, a soft drink, or a Popsicle or frozen juice bar. This removes any unpleasant aftertaste.
- For children who take sweetened medications on a long-term basis, follow the medication administration with oral hygiene. These children are at high risk for dental caries.

OLDER ADULTS

- The physiologic changes associated with aging influence medication administration and effectiveness. See Box 35.7 for additional information.
- Socioeconomic factors such as lack of transportation and decreased finances may influence obtaining medications when needed.

Nasogastric and Gastrostomy Medications

Clients who are NPO for an extended time will often need enteral feedings delivered by a tube. A **nasogastric tube** or a **gastrostomy tube**, in addition to providing nutrition, is also an alternative route for administering medications through the nasogastric or gastrostomy tube. A nasogastric (NG) tube is inserted by way of the nasopharynx and is placed into the client's stomach for the purpose of feeding the client or to remove gastric secretions. A gastrostomy tube is surgically placed directly into the client's stomach and provides another route for administering medications and nutrition (see Chapter 46 ∞). Other tubes that may be used for enteral feedings are the Dobhoff tube and a jejunostomy tube. The Dobhoff tube is an NG tube that is small-bore and flexible, making it more comfortable to the client than the usual NG tube. The jejunostomy tube is surgically placed through the skin of the abdomen into the small intestine. Both the Dobhoff and jejunostomy tubes are smaller than the NG and gastrostomy tubes, and certain medications may cause clogging of the tubes. Some sources say to not administer medications that must be crushed through them because the clogging risk is greater than with an NG or gastrostomy tube (Houston & Fuldauer, 2017). Be sure to check the facility policies.

Previously, enteral ports and IVs had similar connectors, which caused severe client injury and death because of a client receiving a medication by the wrong route. For example, an error in connection could result in enteral formula being delivered intravenously. Other misconnection examples include connection of a feeding tube to an infant's tracheostomy tube or a connection of a feeding tube to an in-line ventilator suction catheter. These connector safety issues resulted in a new industry standard for enteral connectors. The new enteral connectors promote client safety by reducing the risk of misconnections between unrelated systems by implementing a unique mechanical design. The new devices are referred to as *ENFit*. The ENFit devices are not compatible with a Luer-Lok connection or any other type of medical connector and consequently prevent administration of an enteral feeding or medication by the wrong route.

The new ENFit devices have a female connector that fits around the male connector on the feeding tube, which is the *reverse* of the traditional orientation (ECRI Institute, 2017). The ENFit connector system also requires the use of a new enteral-specific syringe that can be used for medication administration, flushing, and bolus feeding (ECRI Institute, 2017). The ENFit syringes may look different depending on the manufacturer but they are all compatible with the ENFit system. There are two syringe tip sizes: the standard tip syringe to administer medicine, flush, hydrate, or bolus feed through enteral tubes, and the low-dose tip syringe to ensure small-volume dosing accuracy with syringe sizes of 5 mL or smaller (Figure 35.13 ■). Guidelines for administering medications by NG tubes and gastrostomy tubes are shown in the Practice Guidelines box.

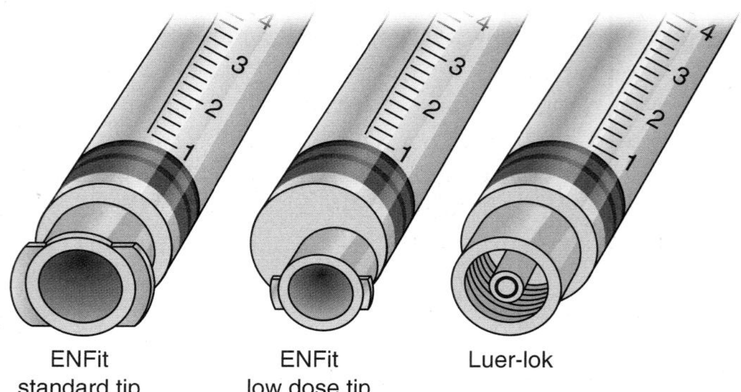

Figure 35.13 ■ Comparison of the new ENFit tip syringes to be used with enteral feeding device connectors. A Luer-Lok syringe will not work with the ENFit connector system.

PRACTICE GUIDELINES Administering Medications by Nasogastric or Gastrostomy Tube Using ENFit Connectors

- Always check with the pharmacist to see if the client's medications come in a liquid form because these are less likely to cause tube obstruction.
- If medications do not come in liquid form, check to see if they may be crushed. (Note that enteric-coated, sustained-action, buccal, and sublingual medications should never be crushed.)
- Do not add medication directly to an enteral feeding formula because of potential incompatibility.
- Do not crush two or more medications at the same time because the chemical reaction that can occur is much greater than when combining drugs orally.
- Liquid medication must be further diluted with purified water, especially if the liquid form is viscous.
- Each medication should be administered separately.
- Use only clean enteral syringes with the ENFit device to administer medication through an enteral feeding tube.
- Crush a tablet into a fine powder and dissolve in 30 to 60 mL of warm purified water. Cold liquids may cause client discomfort. Use only purified water for mixing and flushing. Some medications are mixed with other fluids, such as normal saline, in order to maximize dissolution. Nurses are encouraged to consult with a pharmacist.
- Purified water is the simplest fluid for diluting powdered or liquid medication. The *United States Pharmacopeia* requires that purified water be used for preparation of drug dosage forms. Purified water is free of chemical and biological contaminants. Drinking water (tap, bottled, and well water) may contain chemical contaminants. Sterile water for irrigation is an example of a purified water product; however, there is no need for the water to be sterile (Boullata et al., 2017, p. 80).
- Flushing the enteral feeding tube between medications decreases the incidence of enteral tube obstruction and drug interactions (Boullata et al., 2017, p. 80). Flush only with purified water (no carbonated beverages, juices, coffee, or other liquids).
- Read medication labels carefully before opening a capsule. Open hard gelatin capsules and mix the powder with sterile water.

PRACTICE GUIDELINES Administering Medications by Nasogastric—*continued*

- Do not administer whole or undissolved medications because they will clog the tube.
- Assess tube placement prior to administration of medications. (See Chapter 46 ∞ for methods to verify tube placement).
- Before giving the medication, aspirate all the stomach contents and measure the residual volume. Check agency policy if residual volume is greater than 100 mL.
- Verify that the end of the feeding tube or feeding tube extension set is an ENFit connector.
- When administering the medication(s):
  - Flush the tubing. Attach the ENFit syringe that contains the 15 to 30 mL (5 to 10 mL for children) of water to flush the tube before administering the first medication. The type of water to be used for flush is determined per agency policy.
  - Unscrew the syringe used for flushing the tube. Twist the ENFit syringe that contains the medication into the ENFit port.
  - Gently push the syringe plunger to transfer medication into the enteral access site. Twist to unlock the syringe.
  - If you are giving several medications, administer each one separately and flush with at least 15 to 30 mL (5 mL for children) of purified water between each medication.
  - When you have finished administering all medications, flush with another 15 to 30 mL (5 to 10 mL for children) of purified water to clear the tube.
- If the tube is connected to suction, disconnect the suction and keep the tube clamped for 20 to 30 minutes after giving the medication to enhance absorption.

Parenteral Medications

Parenteral administration of medications is a common nursing procedure. Nurses give parenteral medications intradermally (ID), subcutaneously, intramuscularly (IM), or intravenously (IV). Because these medications are absorbed more quickly than oral medications and are not retrievable once injected, the nurse must prepare and administer them carefully and accurately. Administering parenteral drugs requires the same nursing knowledge as for oral and topical drugs; however, because injections are invasive procedures, aseptic technique must be used to minimize the risk of infection.

Equipment

To administer parenteral medications, nurses use syringes and needles to withdraw medication from ampules and vials.

Syringes

Syringes have three parts: the tip, which connects with the needle; the barrel, or outside part, on which the scales are printed; and the plunger, which fits inside the barrel (Figure 35.14 ■). When handling a syringe, the nurse may touch the outside of the barrel and the handle of the plunger; however, the nurse must *avoid letting any unsterile object touch the tip or inside of the barrel, the shaft of the plunger, or the shaft or tip of the syringe.*

Several kinds of syringes are available in differing sizes, shapes, and materials. Syringes range in sizes from 1 to 60 mL. A nurse typically uses a syringe ranging from 1 to 3 mL in size for injections (e.g., subcutaneous or intramuscular). A **hypodermic syringe** comes in 3- and 5-mL sizes. The choice of syringe depends on many factors, such as medication, location of injection, and type of tissue. Syringes ranging from 1 to 3 mL may have two scales marked on them: the minim and the milliliter. The milliliter scale is the one normally used; the minim scale is used for very small dosages (Figure 35.15 ■). The larger sized syringes (e.g., 10, 20, and 60 mL) are not used to administer drugs directly but can be useful for adding medications to IV solutions, pushing medication through an IV line, or irrigating wounds.

The tip of a syringe varies and is classified as either a Luer-Lok (sometimes spelled Luer-Lock) or non–Luer-Lok, also known as a Slip Tip syringe. A Luer-Lok syringe has a tip that requires the needle to be twisted onto it to

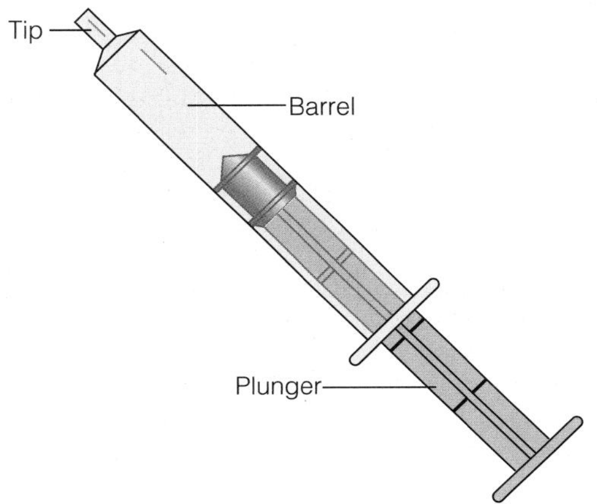

Figure 35.14 ■ The three parts of a syringe.

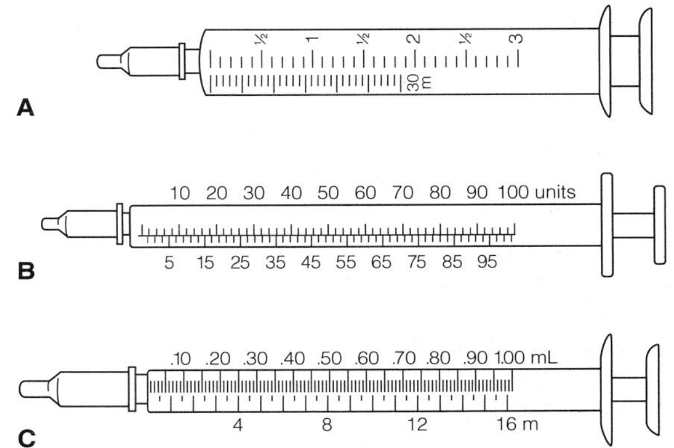

Figure 35.15 ■ Three kinds of syringes: *A*, 3-mL syringe marked in tenths (0.1) of milliliters and in minims; *B*, insulin syringe marked in 100 units; *C*, tuberculin syringe marked in tenths and hundredths (0.01) of 1 milliliter (mL) and in minims.

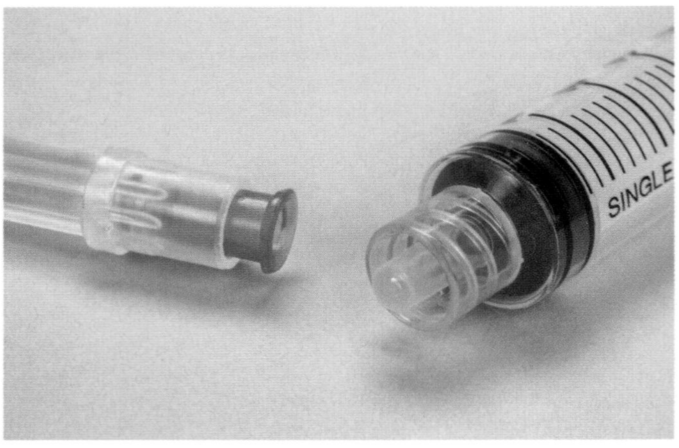

A

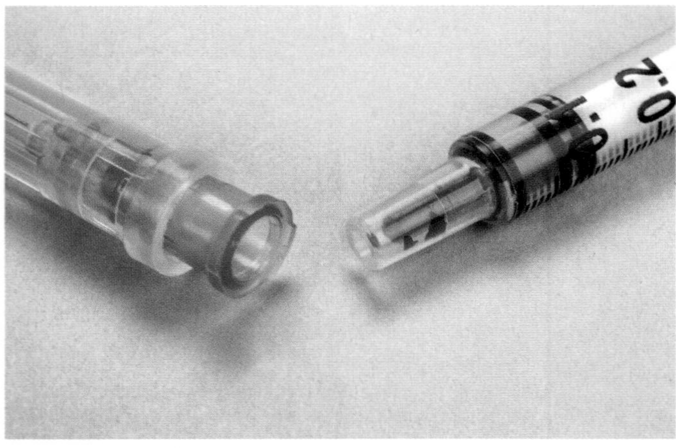

B

Figure 35.16 ■ Tips of syringes: *A*, Luer-Lok syringe (note threaded tip); *B*, non–Luer-Lok syringe (note the smooth graduated tip).

avoid accidental removal of the needle (Figure 35.16 ■). A non–Luer-Lok or Slip Tip syringe has a smooth graduated tip, and needles are slipped onto it. The larger 60-mL non–Luer-Lok syringe is often used for irrigation purposes (e.g., wounds, tubes). See Figure 35.17 ■.

Most syringes used today are made of plastic, are individually packaged for sterility in a paper wrapper or a rigid plastic container (Figure 35.18 ■), and are disposable. The syringe and needle may be packaged together or separately. Needleless systems are also available in which the needle is replaced by a plastic cannula or a more rigid blunt tip instead of a sharp tip.

Injectable medications are frequently supplied in disposable **prefilled unit-dose systems**. These are available as (a) prefilled syringes ready for use or (b) prefilled sterile cartridges and needles that require the attachment of a reusable holder (injection system) before use (Figure 35.19 ■). Examples of the latter system are the Tubex and Carpuject injection systems. The manufacturers provide specific directions for use. Because most prefilled cartridges are overfilled, excess medication must be ejected before the injection to ensure the right dosage. Because the needle is fused to the syringe, the nurse cannot change the gauge or the length of the needle. The nurse, however, can transfer the medication into a regular syringe if the assessment of the client necessitates a different needle gauge or length. The Carpuject has a removable protective cap, which allows the prefilled cartridge to become a vial so that the nurse can withdraw the medication for an injection. However, recent guidelines state to *not* withdraw IV push medications from these types of syringes. Nurses have adopted the unsafe practice of using the prefilled syringe cartridges as single-dose or multiple-dose vials by withdrawing the medication from the cartridges. That type of use of the cartridges, which was never intended, can lead to contamination (Shastay, 2016, p. 41).

An **insulin syringe** is similar to a hypodermic syringe, but the scale is specially designed for insulin: a 100-unit calibrated scale intended for use with U-100 insulin. This is the only syringe that should be used to administer insulin. Several low-dose insulin syringes are also available (e.g., 30-unit and 50-unit). These syringes frequently have a nonremovable needle. All insulin syringes are calibrated on the 100-unit

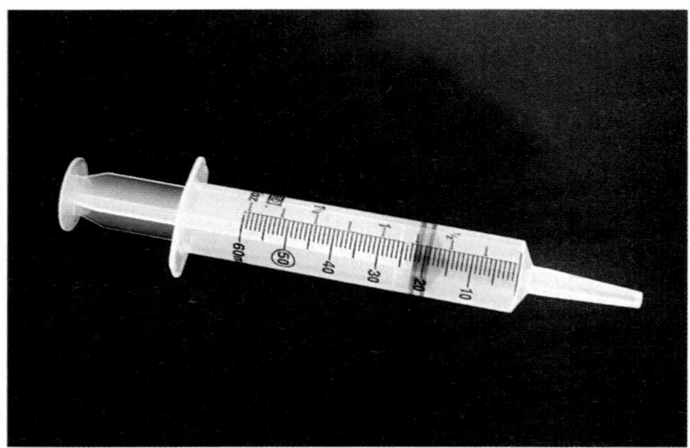

Figure 35.17 ■ A 60-mL non–Luer-Lok syringe, which can be used for irrigation of tubes or wounds.

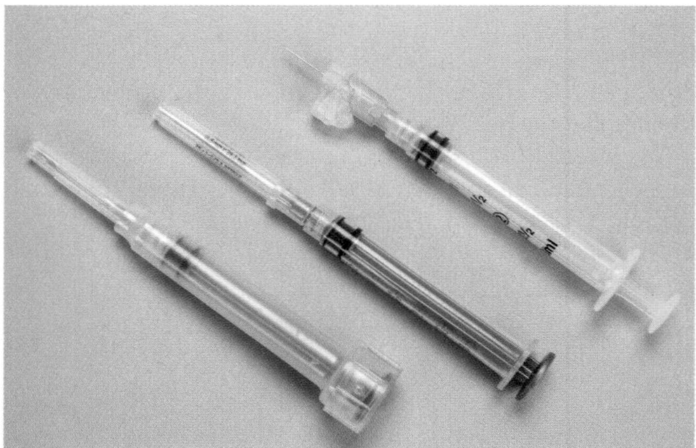

Figure 35.18 ■ Disposable plastic syringes and needles: *Top*, syringe with needle safety device; *middle*, with plastic cap over the needle; *bottom*, with plastic case over the needle and syringe.

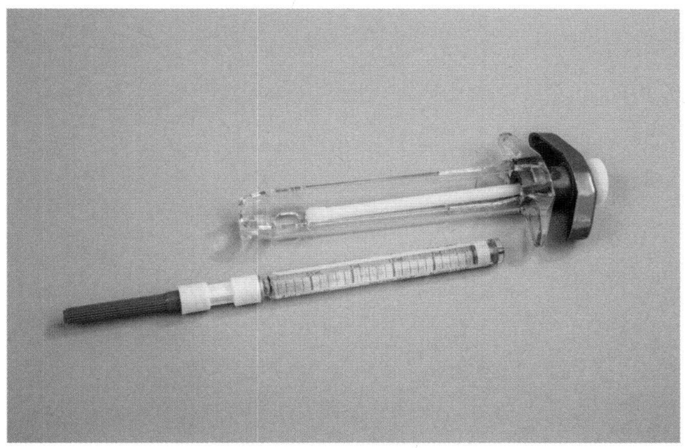

A

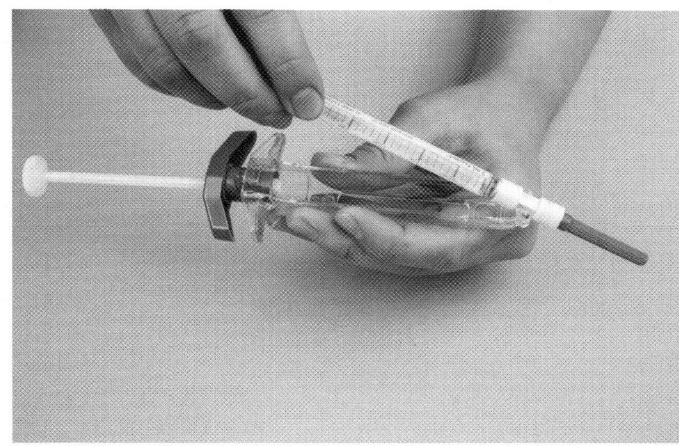

B

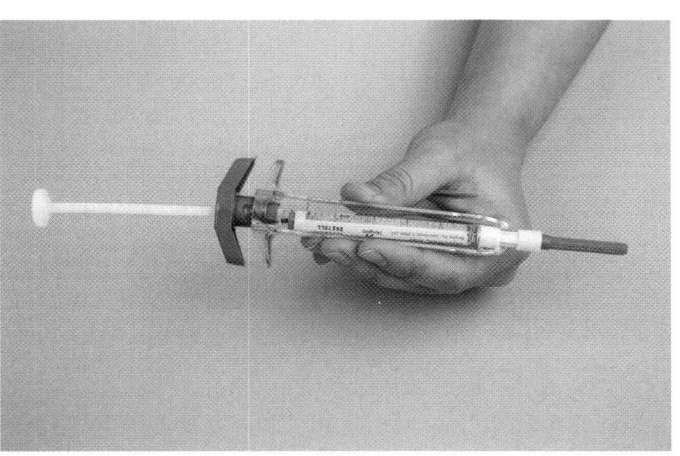

C

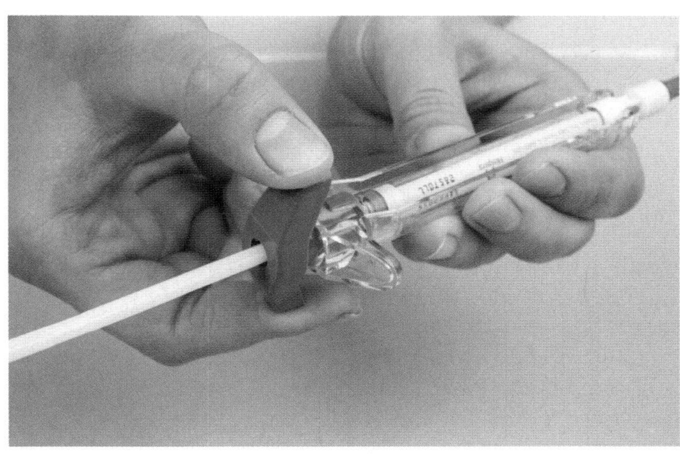

D

Figure 35.19 ■ *A*, Carpuject syringe and prefilled sterile cartridge with needle; *B*, assembling the device; *C*, the cartridge slides into the syringe barrel; *D*, the top twists securing the cartridge into the unit.

scale in North America. The correct choice of syringe is based on the amount of insulin required (Figure 35.20 ■).

An insulin pen is an insulin injector device that looks like a pen and contains an insulin cartridge. The pen is easy to use: The client attaches a new needle for each injection, primes the pen per the manufacturer's directions, dials in a dose, inserts the needle into the injection site, presses the injection button, and holds the injection button and pen against the skin for at least 5 seconds after the injection to deliver the insulin. The parts of an insulin pen are shown in Figure 35.21 ■. Many clients use the insulin pen for self-administration of insulin.

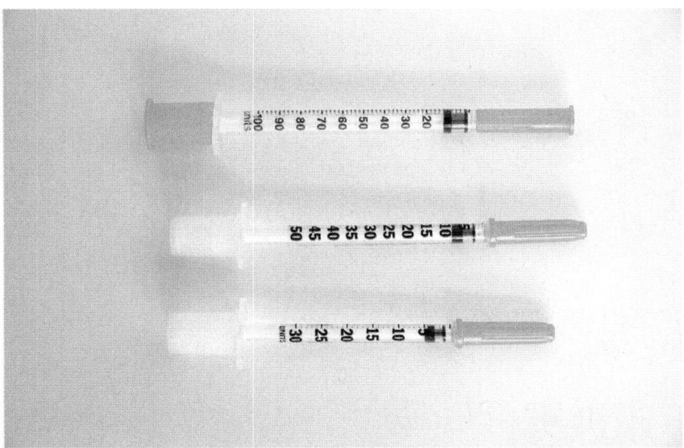

Figure 35.20 ■ Different insulin syringes based on the amount of insulin required. Note the difference in the number of units of insulin per line.

Not all pens are the same. Each pen works only with specific types of insulins. Clients have a choice between a reusable or disposable pen. Clients who use a reusable pen insert an insulin cartridge, which is purchased separately. The pen, after being loaded, is kept at room temperature until the insulin is gone and then another cartridge is loaded into the pen. A disposable pen comes prefilled with a cartridge of insulin and is stored in the refrigerator until the time of use when it is kept at room temperature after opening. When the insulin is used up, the pen is discarded. The majority of people worldwide use disposable insulin pens (Brown & Hertig, 2016). Some pens allow clients to inject half units of insulin and others only dose in whole units. Another difference among insulin pens is whether the pen has a safety needle system that is different from standard insulin pen needles. The pens look similar and

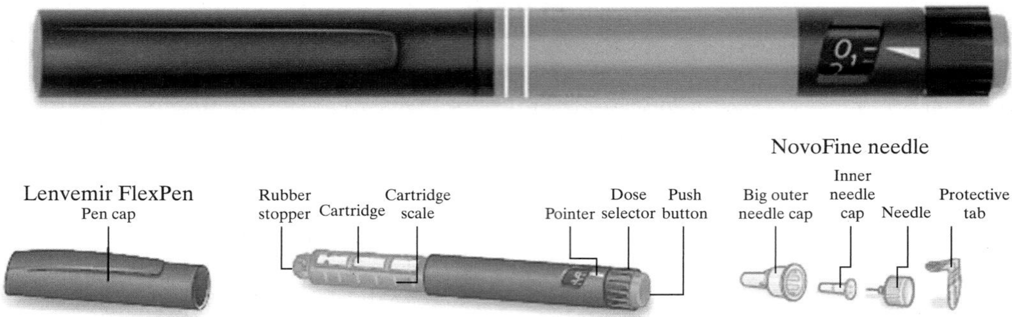

Figure 35.21 ■ Insulin pen. The dose selector knob dials the desired dose of insulin. Pressing the injection button administers the insulin.
ANTHONY GIANGRASSO; DOLORES SHRIMPTON, DOSAGE CALCULATIONS, 2nd Ed., © 2018. Reprinted and Electronically reproduced by permission of Pearson Education, Inc., New York, NY.

clients may not be aware of the differences. Both the automatic safety needle and standard needle systems have a larger outer protective cover that, when removed, exposes either a retractable needle shield (Figure 35.22*A* ■) or a plain inner needle cover (Figure 35.22*B*). The automatic safety needle shield is not intended to be removed before injection, but the inner needle cover on the standard needle system *must* be removed before injection to allow the administration of insulin (ISMP, 2017c, p. 2).

Studies have shown benefits for nurses who use the insulin pen versus vial and syringe in the acute care setting, such as the following: Nurses felt it was easier to teach clients to self-administer insulin with the insulin pen; insulin pen use decreased the risk of dosing error and unintended needlestick injury and reduced the amount of time to prepare and administer insulin; insulin pens were more convenient and easier to use than syringes and vials; and not only nurses preferred using the pens but client satisfaction was also higher (Haines, Miklich, & Rochester-Eyeguokan, 2016, p. S5).

Insulin pens, however, also have a risk: the cartridges can become contaminated and transmit bloodborne pathogens if a pen is used in multiple clients, even if the needle is changed. Only a single client is supposed to use an insulin pen. Unfortunately, there were reports of incidents on the reuse of insulin pens on thousands of clients at different facilities by healthcare professionals. This practice exposed those clients to the risk of transmission of bloodborne pathogens. As a result, organizations such as the FDA and the Centers for Disease Control and Prevention (CDC) recommended that facilities develop policies and procedures to ensure safe use of insulin pens. ISMP suggested that hospitals transition away from insulin pens and return to using insulin vials and syringes. This recommendation resulted in research being conducted. For example, one survey of almost 500 hospitals found that 74% used insulin pens and 15% were no longer using them. The majority of the hospitals used the best practice of storing the insulin pens in the pharmacy prior to administration and in a client-specific location after administration. Half used two identifiers on the pen and a label with a barcode. Unfortunately, 30% reported that insulin pens were being used on more than one client (Brown & Hertig, 2016). Studies have been conducted to recommend best practices for safe use of insulin pens and additional research is needed to evaluate the impact of these recommendations (Haines et al., 2016). It is important for the nurse to know the policies and procedure of the facility.

The **tuberculin syringe** was originally designed to administer tuberculin solution. It is a narrow syringe, calibrated in tenths and hundredths of a milliliter (up to 1 mL) on one scale and in sixteenths of a minim (up to 1 minim) on the other scale. This type of syringe can also be useful in administering other drugs, particularly when small or precise measurement is indicated (e.g., pediatric dosages).

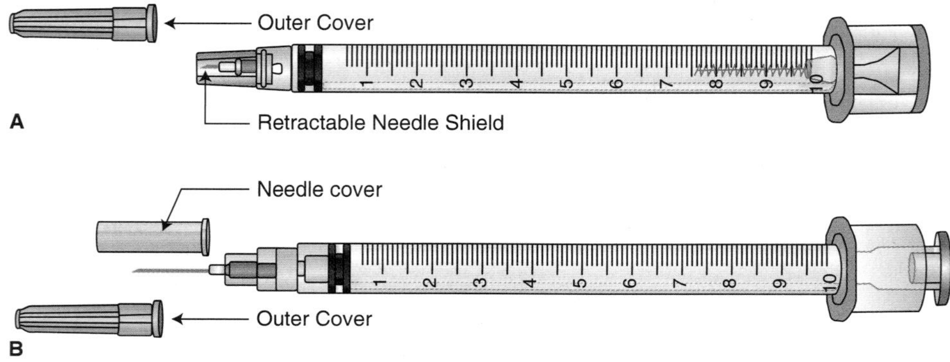

Figure 35.22 ■ *A*, Insulin pen with safety needle where the needle shield automatically retracts on injection and recovers and locks over the needle when withdrawn from the skin; *B*, Standard insulin pen needle where both the outer cover and inner needle cover need to be removed before injection.

Needles

Needles are made of stainless steel, and most are disposable. A needle has three parts: the **hub**, which fits onto the syringe; the **cannula**, or **shaft**, which is attached to the hub; and the **bevel**, which is the slanted part at the tip of the needle that helps the needle cut through the skin with minimal trauma (Figure 35.23 ■). A disposable needle has a plastic hub, which is color coded (Figure 35.24 ■). Needles used for injections have three variable characteristics:

1. *Slant or length of the bevel.* The bevel of the needle may be short or long. Longer bevels provide the sharpest needles and cause less discomfort. They are commonly used for subcutaneous and intramuscular injections. Short bevels are used for intradermal and IV injections because a long bevel can become occluded if it rests against the side of a blood vessel.
2. *Length of the shaft.* The shaft length of commonly used needles varies from 1/2 to 2 inches. The appropriate needle length is chosen according to the client's muscle development, the client's weight, and the type of injection.
3. **Gauge** *(or diameter) of the shaft.* The gauge varies from #18 to #30. The larger the gauge number, the smaller the diameter of the shaft. Smaller gauges produce less tissue trauma, but larger gauges are necessary for viscous medications, such as penicillin.

For an adult requiring a subcutaneous injection, it is appropriate to use a needle of #24 to #26 gauge and 3/8 to 5/8 inch long. Obese clients may require a 1-inch needle. For intramuscular injections, a longer needle (e.g., 1 to 1 1/2 in.) with a larger gauge (e.g., #20 to #22 gauge) is used. Slender adults and children usually require a shorter needle. The nurse must assess the client to determine the appropriate needle length.

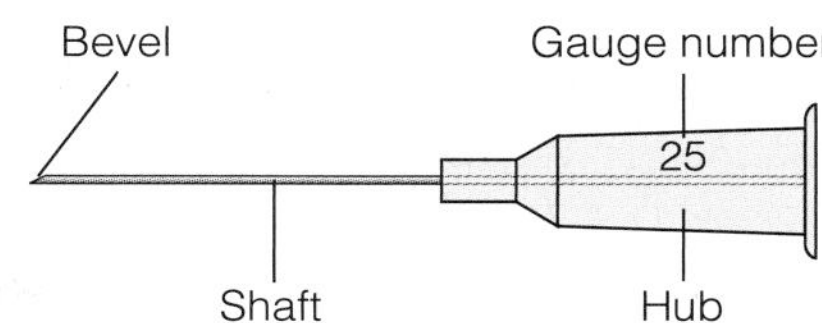

Figure 35.23 ■ The parts of a needle.

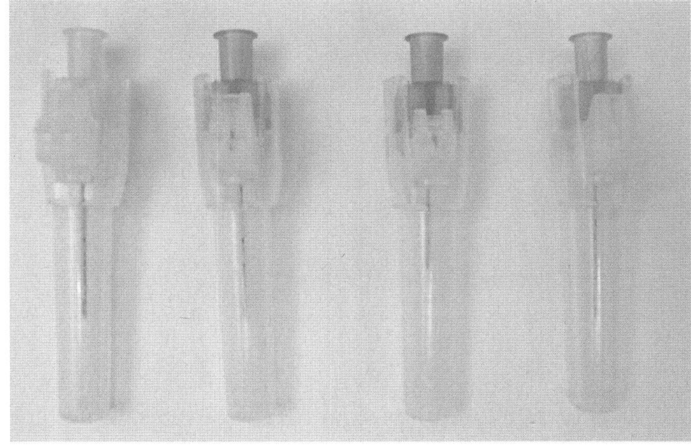

Figure 35.24 ■ Safety needles with different colored hubs to indicate gauge: yellow—20 gauge; green—21 gauge; blue—23 gauge; and orange—25 gauge.

Preventing Needlestick Injuries

One of the most potentially hazardous procedures that healthcare personnel face is using and disposing of needles and sharps. Needlestick injuries present a major risk for infection with hepatitis B virus, HIV, and many other pathogens. Standards have been set by the Occupational Safety and Health Administration (OSHA) to prevent such injuries. Some of these are summarized in Box 35.8.

BOX 35.8 Avoiding Puncture Injuries

- Use appropriate puncture-proof disposal containers to dispose of uncapped needles and sharps (Figure 35.25 ■). These are provided in all client areas. Never throw sharps in wastebaskets. Sharps include any items that can cut or puncture skin such as:
  - Needles
  - Surgical blades
  - Lancets
  - Razors
  - Broken glass
  - Broken capillary pipettes
  - Exposed dental wires
  - Reusable items (e.g., large-bore needles, hooks, rasps, drill points)
  - ANY SHARP INSTRUMENT!
- Never bend or break needles before disposal.
- Never recap *used* needles (i.e., ones that have been inserted into clients) except under specified circumstances (e.g., when

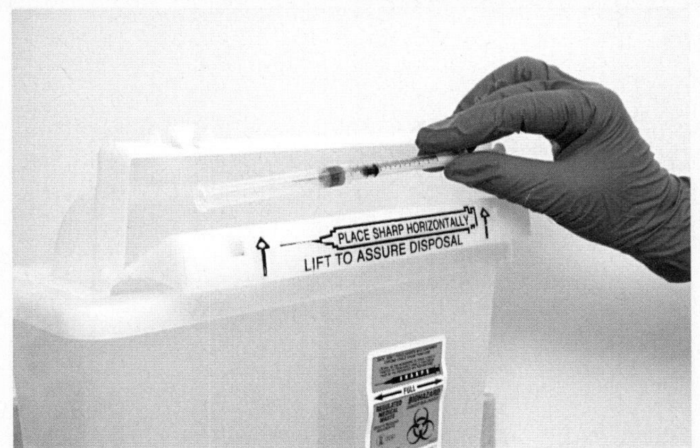

Figure 35.25 ■ Dispose of used syringe and needle in a sharps container.

Continued on page 874

BOX 35.8 Avoiding Puncture Injuries—*continued*

transporting a syringe to the laboratory for an arterial blood gas or blood culture).

- When recapping a needle (i.e., drawing up a medication into a syringe *prior* to administration):
  - Use a one-handed "scoop" method. This is performed by (a) placing the needle cap and syringe with needle horizontally on a flat surface; (b) inserting the needle into the cap, using one hand (Figure 35.26 ■); and then (c) using your other hand to pick up the cap and tighten it to the needle hub. Be careful not to contaminate the needle. If the needle becomes contaminated, replace the needle with a new one.

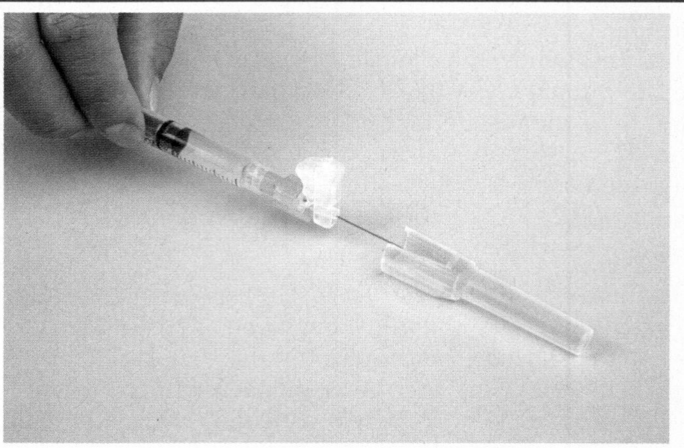

Figure 35.26 ■ Recapping a needle using the one-handed scoop method.

In addition, the Needlestick Safety and Prevention Act is a federal law that requires safer needle devices to prevent exposure to bloodborne pathogens and requires documentation of all needlestick injuries. If an unintentional needlestick injury occurs, the nurse needs to follow specific steps outlined by the agency.

Safety syringes have been designed in recent years to protect healthcare workers. Safety devices are categorized as either *passive* or *active*. The nurse does not need to activate the passive safety device. For example, for some syringes, after injection, the needle retracts immediately into the barrel (Figure 35.27 ■). In contrast, the active safety device requires the nurse to manually activate the safety feature. For example, the nurse activates a mechanism to retract the needle into the syringe barrel, or the nurse, after injection, manually pulls a plastic sheath or guard over the needle (Figure 35.28 ■).

According to International Safety Center's Exposure Prevention Information Network (EPINet) data from 2012 to 2016, injuries from disposable syringes make up most needlesticks (28.1%), and of those, 19.5% are from insulin syringes. Nearly 95% of the injuries occurred at the client's bedside or exam room (Mitchell & Parker, 2018, p. 44). Even though almost all of the disposable syringes had a safety design, sharps injuries occurred when the safety features were *not* activated.

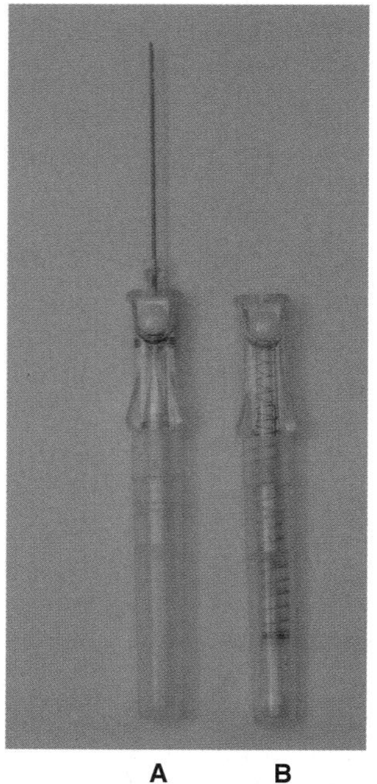

Figure 35.27 ■ Passive safety device: *A*, before injection; *B*, the needle retracts immediately into the barrel after injection.

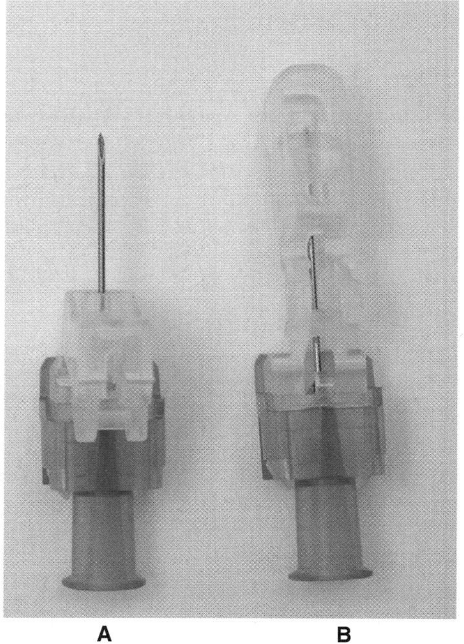

Figure 35.28 ■ Active safety device: *A*, before injection; *B*, the nurse manually pulls the sheath or guard over the needle after injection.

Preparing Injectable Medications

Injectable medications can be prepared by withdrawing the medication from an ampule or vial into a sterile syringe, using prefilled syringes, or using needleless injection systems. Figure 35.29 ■ shows an example of a needleless system used to access medication from a vial.

Ampules and Vials

Ampules and vials (Figure 35.30 ■) are frequently used to package sterile parenteral medications. An **ampule** is a glass container usually designed to hold a single dose of a drug. It is made of clear glass and has a distinctive shape with a constricted neck. Ampules vary in size from 1 to 10 mL or more. Most ampule necks have colored marks around them, indicating where they are prescored for easy opening.

To access the medication in an ampule, the ampule must be broken at its constricted neck. Traditionally, files have been used to score the ampule. Today plastic ampule openers are available that prevent injury from broken glass. The device consists of a plastic cap that fits over the top of an ampule. The head of the ampule, when broken, remains inside the cap and is placed into a sharps container (Figure 35.31 ■). If an ampule opener is not available, the nurse can clean the ampule neck with an alcohol swab and, using dry sterile gauze, snap off the top of the ampule. Once the ampule is broken, the fluid is aspirated into a syringe using a filter needle or a filter straw (Figure 35.32 ■). Both prevent aspiration of any glass particles.

A **vial** is a small glass bottle with a sealed rubber cap. Vials come in different sizes, from single-use vials to multiple-dose vials. They usually have a metal or plastic cap that protects the rubber seal and must be removed to access the medication. To access the medication in a vial, the vial must be pierced with a needle. In addition, air must be injected into a vial before the medication can be withdrawn. Failure to inject air before withdrawing the medication leaves a vacuum within the vial that makes withdrawal difficult.

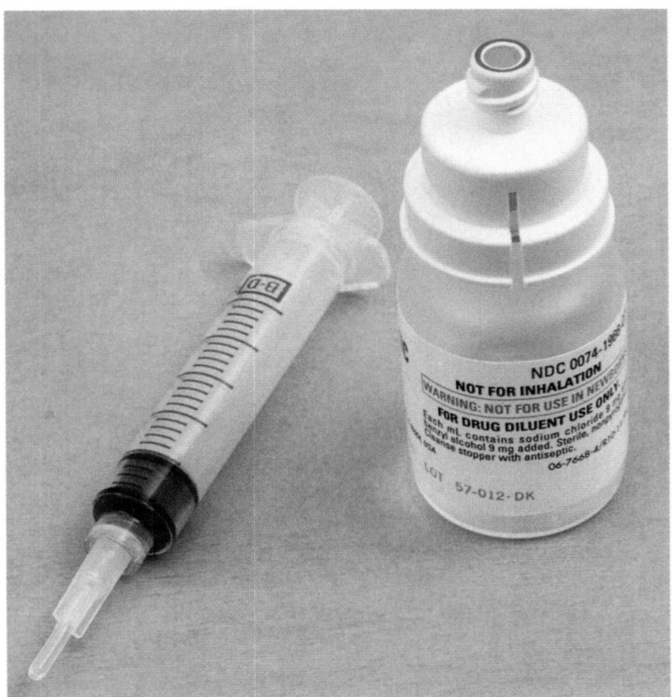

Figure 35.29 ■ A needleless system can extract medicine from a vial.

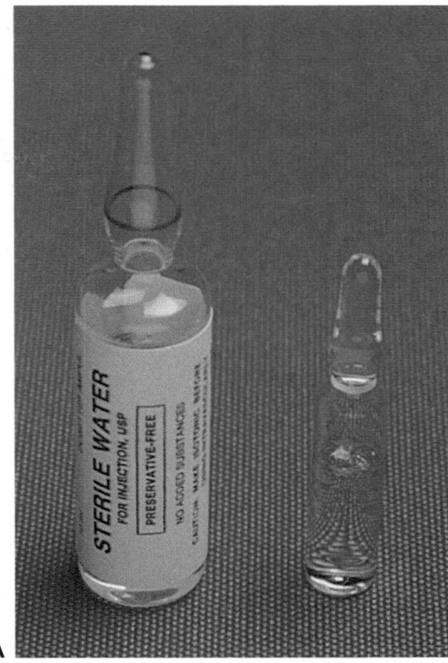

A

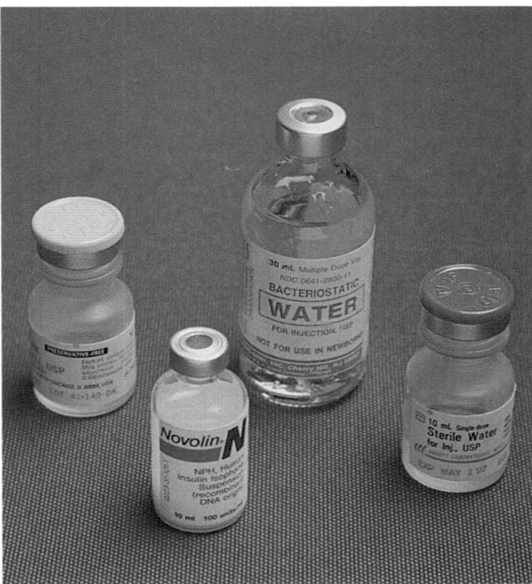

B

Figure 35.30 ■ *A*, Ampules; *B*, vials.

A single-dose vial (SDV) contains only one dose of medication and should *only* be used once. Usually an SVD contains more than the single dose. *Never* save this leftover medication because SVDs lack an antimicrobial preservative. Discard the vial after every use. Investigations by the CDC have identified improper uses of syringes, needles, and medication vials that have resulted in disease transmission, such as hepatitis B (CDC, n.d.; ISMP, 2017a). The *One and Only* health campaign is aimed at

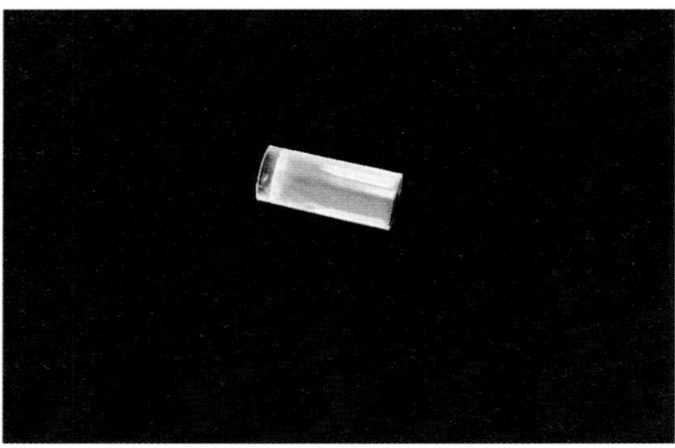

A

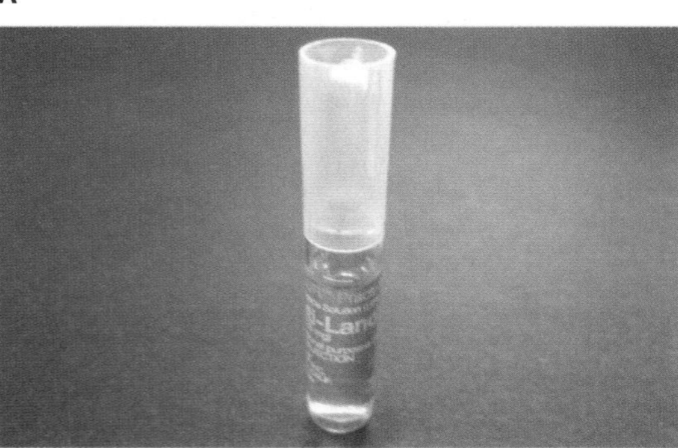

B

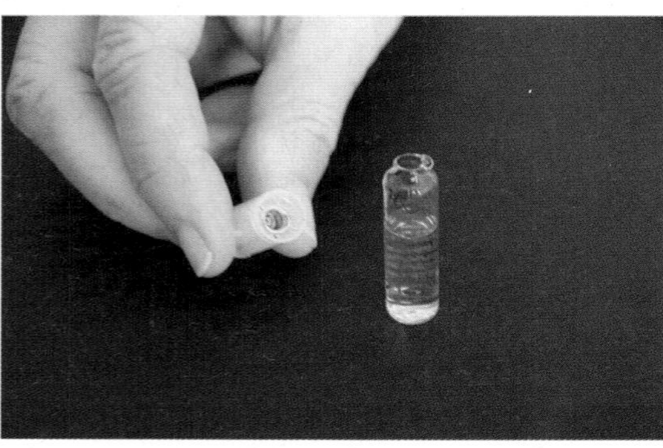

C

Figure 35.31 ■ *A*, Ampule opener: *B*, plastic opener is placed over top of ampule; *C*, top of ampule remains in opener after ampule is broken open.
A–C, Shirlee Snyder.

raising awareness about safe injection practice. The slogan is: *One needle, One syringe, Only One time.*

In contrast, a multidose vial (MDV) is a bottle of liquid medication that contains more than one dose, such as insulin or vaccination vials. Whenever possible, use of single-dose vials is preferred over multidose vials, especially when medications will be administered to multiple clients. If an MDV vial must be used, both the needle or cannula and syringe used to access the vial must be sterile. MDVs do contain an antimicrobial preservative but the preservatives have no effect on bloodborne viruses. Thus, the nurse *must* use aseptic technique.

Some drugs (e.g., penicillin) may be dispensed as powders in vials. A liquid (diluent) must be added to a powdered medication before it can be injected. The technique of adding a diluent to a powdered drug to prepare it for administration is called **reconstitution**. Powdered drugs usually have printed instructions (enclosed with each packaged vial) that describe the amount and kind of solvent to be added. Commonly used diluents are sterile water or sterile normal saline. Some preparations are supplied in SDVs; others come in MDVs. The following are two examples of the preparation of powdered drugs:

1. ***Single-dose vial:*** Instructions for preparing an SVD state that 1.5 mL of sterile water is to be added to the sterile dry powder, thus providing a single dose of 2 mL. The volume of the drug powder was 0.5 mL. Therefore, the 1.5 mL of water plus the 0.5 mL of powder results in 2 mL of solution. In other instances, the addition of a solution does not increase the volume. Therefore, it is important to follow the manufacturer's directions.
2. ***Multidose vial:*** A dose of 750 mg of a certain drug is ordered for a client. On hand is a 10-g multidose vial. The directions for preparation read: "Add 8.5 mL of sterile water, and each milliliter will contain 1.0 g or

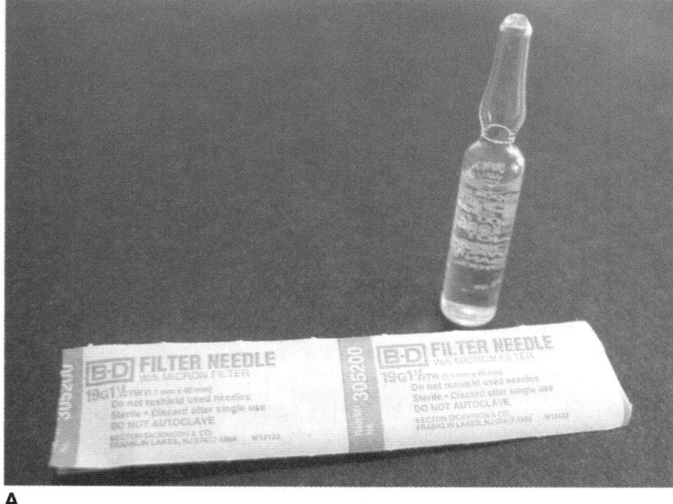

A

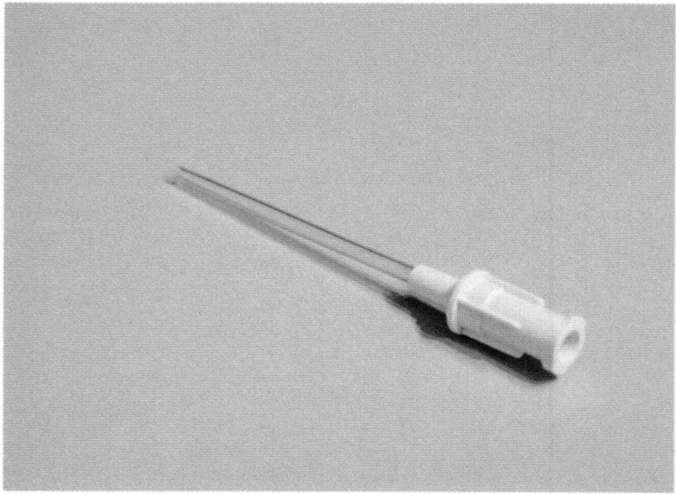

B

Figure 35.32 ■ A filter needle, *A*, or a filter straw, *B*, prevents glass from being withdrawn with the medication.
A–B, Shirlee Snyder.

1000 mg." To determine the amount to inject, the nurse does these calculations:

$$1 \text{ mL} = 1000 \text{ mg}$$
$$x \text{ mL} = 750 \text{ mg}$$
$$\text{(cross multiply)}$$
$$x = \frac{750 \times 1}{1000}$$
$$x = 0.75$$

The nurse will give 0.75 mL of the medication.

Glass and rubber particulate have been found in medications withdrawn from ampules and vials using a regular needle. As a result, it is strongly recommended that the nurse use a filter needle or a filter straw when withdrawing medications from ampules and a filter needle when withdrawing from vials to prevent withdrawing glass and rubber particles. After drawing the medication into the syringe, the filter needle or filter straw, whichever is appropriate, is replaced with the regular needle for injection. This prevents tracking of the medication through the client's tissues during the insertion of the needle, which minimizes discomfort. Using a new needle following the withdrawal of the medication from the vial also minimizes discomfort that can result from minor "dulling" of the needle tip from passing through the vial stopper. Also, if the client has a latex allergy, changing the needle would be important when using a vial with a rubber stopper or cap.

Skills 35.2 and 35.3 describe how to prepare medications from ampules and vials, respectively. Additionally, it is important to remember that when powdered drugs have been reconstituted, or an MDV is used, the date and time should be written on the label of the vial. Many of these drugs have to be used within a certain time period following reconstitution, so nurses need to check the expiration time after it has been reconstituted or the vial punctured.

Preparing Medications from Ampules

SKILL 35.2

ASSESSMENT

Assess

- Client allergies to medication
- Specific drug action, side effects, interactions, and adverse reactions
- Client's knowledge of and learning needs about the medication
- Intended route of parenteral medication to determine appropriate size of syringe and needle for the client
- Ordered medication for clarity and expiration date
- Perform appropriate assessments (e.g., vital signs, laboratory results) specific to the medication.
- Determine if the assessment data effect administration of the medication (i.e., is it appropriate to administer the medication or does the medication need to be held or the primary care provider notified?).

PLANNING

Assignment

Preparing medications from ampules involves knowledge and use of sterile skills. Therefore, these techniques are not assigned to AP.

Equipment

- Client's MAR or computer printout
- Ampule of sterile medication
- File (if ampule is not scored) and small gauze square or plastic ampule opener
- Antiseptic swabs
- Syringe
- Needle for administering the medication
- Filter needle or filter straw for withdrawing medication from the ampule

IMPLEMENTATION

Preparation

1. Check the MAR.
   - Check the label on the ampule carefully against the MAR to make sure that the correct medication is being prepared.
   - Follow the three checks for administering medications. Read the label on the medication (1) when it is taken from the medication cart, (2) before withdrawing the medication, and (3) after withdrawing the medication.
2. Organize the equipment.

Performance

1. Perform hand hygiene and observe other appropriate infection prevention procedures.
2. Prepare the medication ampule for drug withdrawal.
   - Flick the upper stem of the ampule several times with a fingernail. **Rationale:** *This will bring all medication down to the main portion of the ampule.*
   - Use an ampule opener or place a piece of sterile gauze or alcohol wipe between your thumb and the ampule neck or around the ampule neck, and break off the top by *bending* it toward you to ensure the ampule is broken away from yourself and away from others. **Rationale:** *The sterile gauze protects the fingers from the broken glass, and any glass fragments will spray away from the nurse.* ❶
   - Dispose of the top of the ampule in the sharps container.
3. Withdraw the medication.
   - Place the ampule on a flat surface.
   - Attach the filter needle or straw to the syringe. **Rationale:** *The filter needle or straw prevents glass particles from being withdrawn with the medication.*
   - Remove the cap from the filter needle or filter straw and insert the needle or straw into the center of the ampule. Do not touch the rim of the ampule with the needle or straw tip or shaft. **Rationale:** *This will keep the needle or straw sterile.* Withdraw all of the drug.

Continued on page 878

SKILL 35.2

Preparing Medications from Ampules—*continued*

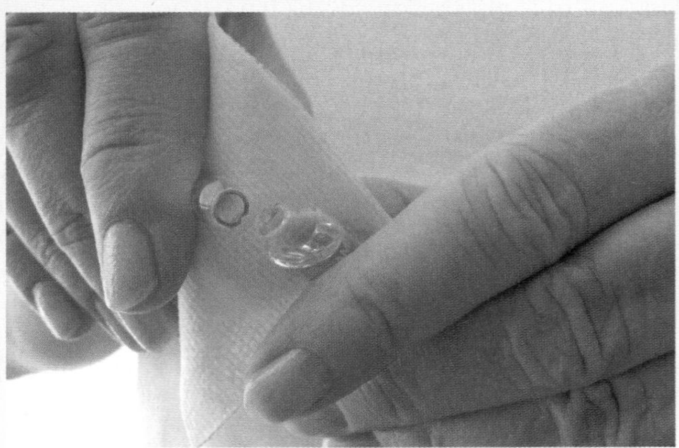

A

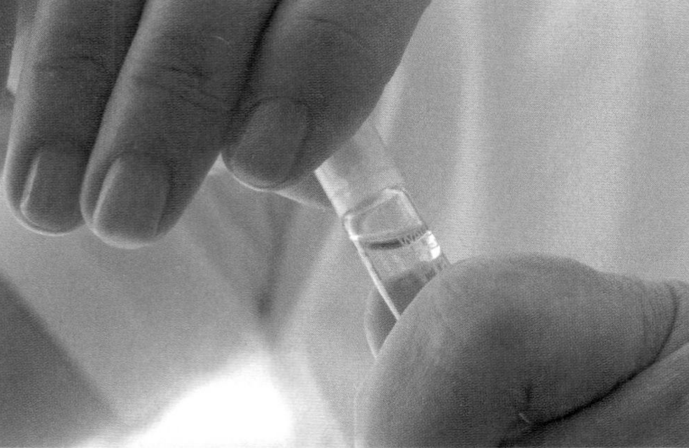

B

❶ *A*, Breaking the neck of an ampule using a gauze pad; *B*, breaking the neck of an ampule using an ampule opener.
A–B, Shirlee Snyder.

- Hold the ampule slightly on its side, if necessary, to obtain all of the medication. ❷
- Dispose of the filter needle or straw and ampule by placing them in a sharps container.
- If giving an injection replace the filter needle or filter straw with a regular needle, tighten the cap at the hub of the needle, expel bubbles, and push the prescribed amount of solution into the needle.
- Discard excess medication into an acceptable receptacle, depending on the ordered amount.

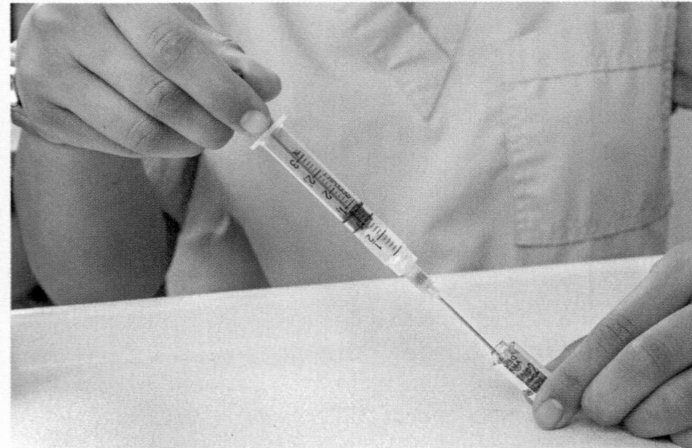

A

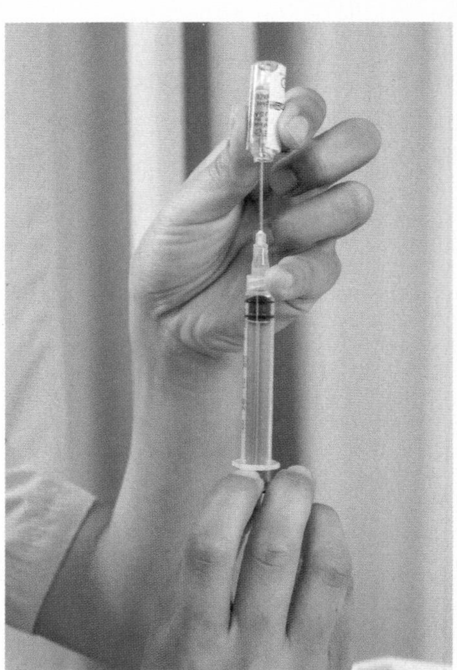

B

❷ Withdrawing a medication *A*, from an ampule on a flat surface; and *B*, from an inverted ampule.

SKILL 35.3

Preparing Medications from Vials

PLANNING

Assignment

Preparing medications from vials involves knowledge and use of sterile technique. Therefore, these techniques are not assigned to AP.

Equipment

- Client's MAR or computer printout
- Vial of sterile medication
- Antiseptic swabs
- Safety needle and syringe
- Filter needle (check agency policy)
- Sterile water or normal saline, if drug is in powdered form

Preparing Medications from Vials—*continued*

IMPLEMENTATION

Preparation

- Follow the same preparation as described in Skill 35.2.

Performance

1. Perform hand hygiene and observe other appropriate infection prevention procedures.
2. Prepare the medication vial for drug withdrawal.
   - Mix the solution, if necessary, by rotating the vial between the palms of the hands, not by shaking. **Rationale:** *Some vials contain aqueous suspensions, which settle when they stand. In some instances, shaking is contraindicated because it may cause the mixture to foam.*
   - Remove the protective cap, or clean the rubber cap of a previously opened vial with an antiseptic wipe by rubbing in a circular motion. **Rationale:** *The antiseptic cleans the cap and reduces the number of microorganisms.*
3. Withdraw the medication.
   - Attach a filter needle, as agency practice dictates, to draw up premixed liquid medications from MDVs. **Rationale:** *Using the filter needle prevents any solid particles from being drawn up through the needle.*
   - Ensure that the needle is firmly attached to the syringe.
   - Remove the cap from the needle, then draw up into the syringe the amount of air equal to the volume of the medication to be withdrawn.
   - Carefully insert the needle into the upright vial through the center of the rubber cap, maintaining the sterility of the needle.
   - Inject the air into the vial, keeping the bevel of the needle above the surface of the medication. ❶ **Rationale:** *The air will allow the medication to be drawn out easily because negative pressure will not be created inside the vial. The bevel is kept above the medication to avoid creating bubbles in the medication.*
   - Withdraw the prescribed amount of medication using either of the following methods:
     a. Hold the vial down (i.e., with the base lower than the top), move the needle tip so that it is below the fluid level, and withdraw the medication. Avoid drawing up the last drops of the vial. ❷ **Rationale:** *Proponents of this method say that keepingii the vial in the upright position while withdrawing the medication allows particulate matter to precipitate out of the solution. Leaving the last few drops reduces the chance of withdrawing foreign particles.*
     or
     b. Invert the vial, ensure the needle tip is *below* the fluid level, and gradually withdraw the medication. ❸ **Rationale:** *Keeping the tip of the needle below the fluid level prevents air from being drawn into the syringe.*
   - Hold the syringe and vial at eye level to determine that the correct dosage of drug is drawn into the syringe. Eject air remaining at the top of the syringe into the vial.
   - When the correct volume of medication plus a little more (e.g., 0.25 mL) is obtained, withdraw the needle from the vial, and replace the cap over the needle using the scoop method, thus maintaining its sterility.
   - If necessary, tap the syringe barrel to dislodge any air bubbles present in the syringe. Carefully and slowly expel the air and any excess medication from the syringe, maintaining the "needle up" position. **Rationale:** *The tapping motion will cause the air bubbles to rise to the top of the syringe where they can be ejected out of the syringe. Sometimes when ejecting the air bubbles, the resulting amount of medication is less than ordered. Drawing up a little extra medication, as in the previous step, helps avoid this.*
   - If giving an injection, replace the filter needle, if used, with a safety needle of the correct gauge and length. Eject air from the new needle and verify correct medication volume before injecting the client.

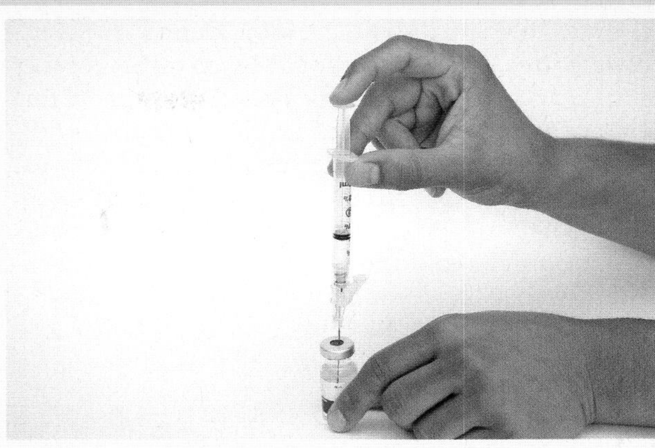

❶ Injecting air into a vial.

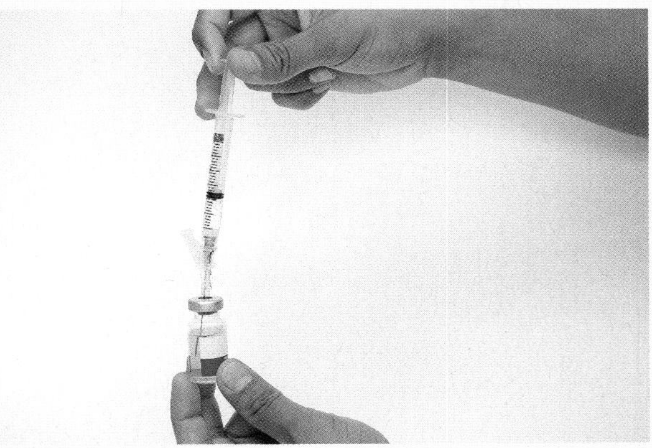

❷ Withdrawing a medication from a vial that is held with the base down.

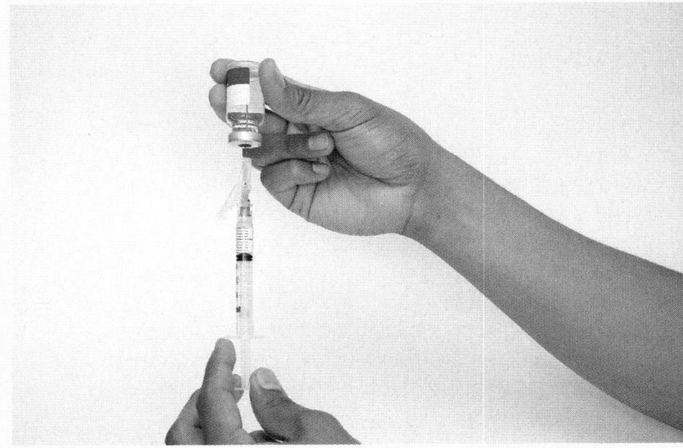

❸ Withdrawing a medication from an inverted vial.

Variation: Preparing and Using Multidose Vials

- Read the manufacturer's directions.
- Withdraw an equivalent amount of air from the vial before adding the diluent, unless otherwise indicated by the directions.
- Add the amount of sterile water or saline indicated in the directions.
- If an MDV is reconstituted, label the vial with the date and time it was prepared, the amount of drug contained in each milliliter of solution, and your initials. **Rationale:** *Time is an important factor to consider in the expiration of these medications.*
- Once the medication is reconstituted, store it in a refrigerator or as recommended by the manufacturer.
- Discard the vial if sterility is compromised or questionable.
- Remember to use a sterile syringe and needle for each access to the MDV.

Mixing Medications in One Syringe

Frequently, clients need more than one drug injected at the same time. To spare the client the experience of being injected twice, two drugs (if compatible) are often mixed in one syringe and given as one injection. It is common, for instance, to combine two types of insulin in this manner or to combine injectable preoperative medications such as morphine with atropine or scopolamine. Drugs can also be mixed in IV solutions. When uncertain about drug compatibilities, the nurse should consult a pharmacist or check a compatibility chart before mixing the drugs.

The nurse must also exercise caution when mixing short- and long-acting insulins, because they vary in content. Chemically, insulin is a protein that, when hydrolyzed in the body, yields a number of amino acids. Some insulin preparations contain an additional modifying protein, such as globulin or protamine, which slows absorption. This fact is particularly relevant when mixing two insulin preparations for injection because many insulin syringes have needles that cannot be changed. A vial of insulin that does not have the added protein (i.e., regular insulin) should *never* be contaminated with insulin that does have the added protein (i.e., Lente or NPH insulin). Skill 35.4 describes how to mix medications in one syringe.

SKILL 35.4

Mixing Medications Using One Syringe

ASSESSMENT

Assess

- Client allergies to medications
- Specific drug action, side effects, interactions, and adverse reactions
- Client's knowledge of and learning needs about the medications
- Intended route of parenteral medication to determine appropriate size of syringe and needle for the client
- Ordered medications for clarity and expiration date
- Determine that the two medications are compatible.

PLANNING

Assignment

Mixing medications in one syringe involves knowledge and use of aseptic technique. Therefore, this procedure is not assigned to AP.

Equipment

- Client's MAR or computer printout
- Two vials of medication; one vial and one ampule; two ampules; or one vial or ampule and one cartridge
- Antiseptic swabs
- Sterile syringe and safety needle or insulin syringe and needle (If insulin is being given, use a small-gauge hypodermic needle, e.g., #26 gauge.)
- Additional sterile subcutaneous or intramuscular safety needle (optional)

IMPLEMENTATION

Preparation

1. Check the MAR.
   - Check the label on the medications carefully against the MAR to make sure that the correct medication is being prepared.
   - Follow the three checks for administering medications. Read the label on the medication (1) when it is taken from the medication cart, (2) before withdrawing the medication, and (3) after withdrawing the medication.
   - Before preparing and combining the medications, ensure that the total volume of the injection is appropriate for the injection site.
2. Organize the equipment.

Performance

1. Perform hand hygiene and observe other appropriate infection prevention procedures.
2. Prepare the medication ampule or vial for drug withdrawal.
   - See Skill 35.2, Performance section, step 2, for an ampule.
   - Inspect the appearance of the medication for clarity. Note, however, that some medications are always cloudy. **Rationale:** *Preparations that have changed in appearance should be discarded.*
   - If using insulin, thoroughly mix the solution in each vial prior to administration. Rotate the vials between the palms of the hands. **Rationale:** *Mixing ensures an adequate concentration and thus an accurate dose. Shaking insulin vials can make the medication frothy, making precise measurement difficult.*
   - Clean the tops of the vials with antiseptic swabs.
3. Withdraw the medications.

Mixing Medications from Two Vials

- Take the syringe and draw up a volume of air equal to the volume of medications to be withdrawn from both vials A and B.
- Inject a volume of air equal to the volume of medication to be withdrawn into vial A. Make sure the needle does not touch the solution. **Rationale:** *This prevents cross-contamination of the medications.*
- Withdraw the needle from vial A and inject the remaining air into vial B.
- Withdraw the required amount of medication from vial B. **Rationale:** *The same needle is used to inject air into and withdraw medication from the second vial. It must not be contaminated with the medication in vial A.*
- Using a newly attached sterile needle, withdraw the required amount of medication from vial A. Avoid pushing the plunger because that will introduce medication B into vial A. If using a syringe with a fused needle, withdraw the medication from vial A. The syringe now contains a mixture of medications from vials A and B. **Rationale:** *With this method, neither vial is contaminated by microorganisms or by medication from the other vial.* Be careful to withdraw only the ordered amount and to not create air bubbles. **Rationale:** *The syringe now contains two medications and an excess amount cannot be returned to the vial.*

See also the Variation later in this skill.

Mixing Medications from One Vial and One Ampule

- First prepare and withdraw the medication from the vial. **Rationale:** *Ampules do not require the addition of air prior to withdrawal of the drug.*

SKILL 35.4

Mixing Medications Using One Syringe—*continued*

- Then withdraw the required amount of medication from the ampule.

Mixing Medications from One Cartridge and One Vial or Ampule

- First ensure that the correct dose of the medication is in the cartridge. Discard any excess medication and air.
- Draw up the required medication from a vial or ampule into the cartridge. Note that when withdrawing medication from a vial, an equal amount of air must first be injected into the vial.
- If the total volume to be injected exceeds the capacity of the cartridge, use a syringe with sufficient capacity to withdraw the desired amount of medication from the vial or ampule, and transfer the required amount from the cartridge to the syringe.

Variation: Mixing Insulins

The following is an example of mixing 10 units of regular insulin and 30 units of NPH insulin, which contains protamine.

- Inject 30 units of air into the NPH vial and withdraw the needle. (There should be no insulin in the needle.) The needle should not touch the insulin. ❶
- Inject 10 units of air into the regular insulin vial and immediately withdraw 10 units of regular insulin. ❷ and ❸ Always withdraw the regular insulin first. **Rationale:** *This minimizes the possibility of the regular insulin becoming contaminated with the additional protein in the NPH.*

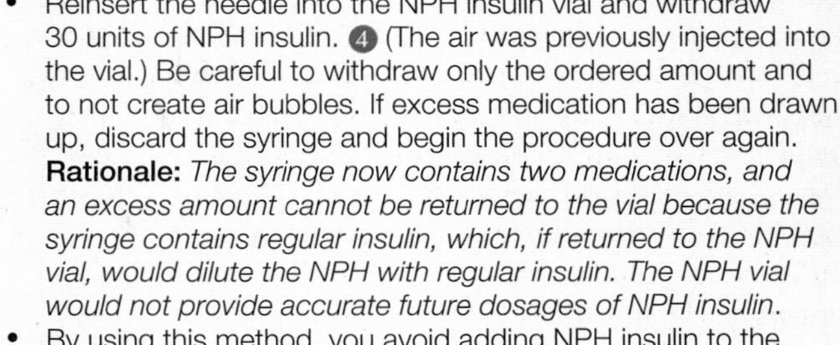

- Reinsert the needle into the NPH insulin vial and withdraw 30 units of NPH insulin. ❹ (The air was previously injected into the vial.) Be careful to withdraw only the ordered amount and to not create air bubbles. If excess medication has been drawn up, discard the syringe and begin the procedure over again. **Rationale:** *The syringe now contains two medications, and an excess amount cannot be returned to the vial because the syringe contains regular insulin, which, if returned to the NPH vial, would dilute the NPH with regular insulin. The NPH vial would not provide accurate future dosages of NPH insulin.*
- By using this method, you avoid adding NPH insulin to the regular insulin.

Clinical Alert!

One way to determine which insulin to *withdraw* first is to remember the saying "Clear before cloudy." (Regular insulin is clear and NPH is cloudy due to the proteins in the insulin.)

Safety Alert! SAFETY

Insulin is a high-alert medication, meaning that it can cause significant client harm if used in error. Check the health agency's policy regarding administration because some agencies may require insulin doses to be checked by two nurses.

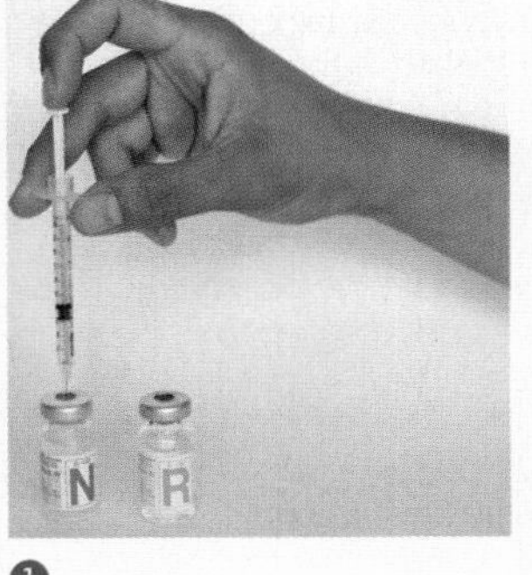

❶

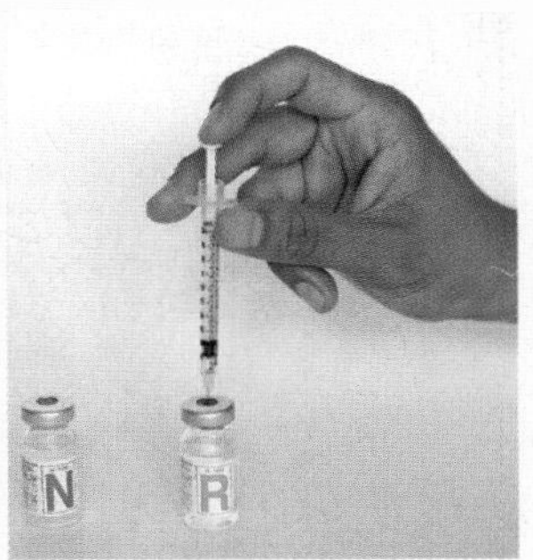

❷

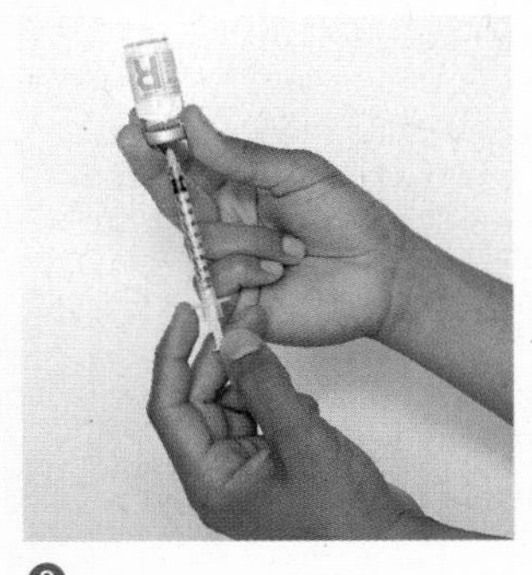

❸

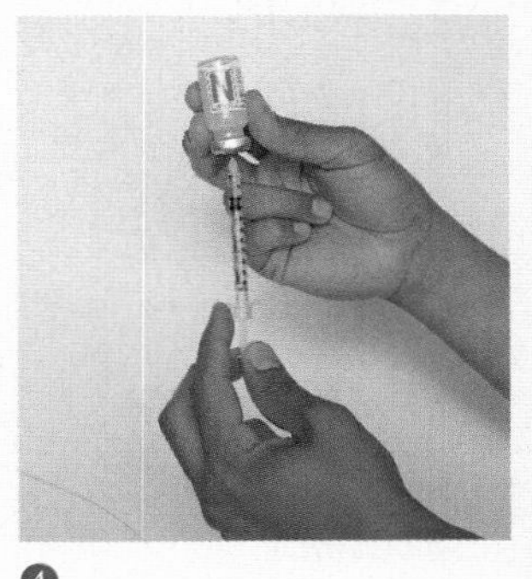

❹

Intradermal Injections

An **intradermal (ID) injection** is the administration of a drug into the dermal layer of the skin just beneath the epidermis. Usually only a small amount of liquid is used, for example, 0.1 mL. This method of administration is frequently used for allergy testing and tuberculosis (TB) screening. Common sites for ID injections are the inner lower arm, the upper chest, and the back beneath the scapulae (Figure 35.33 ■). The left arm is commonly used for TB screening and the right arm is used for all other tests.

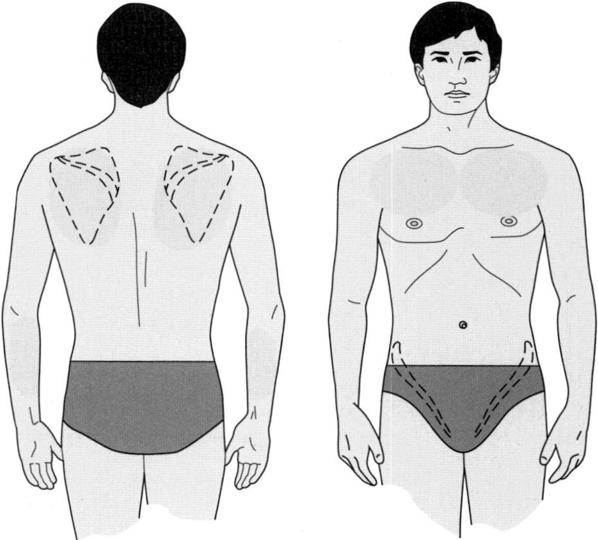

Figure 35.33 ■ Body sites commonly used for intradermal injections.

QSEN Patient-Centered Care: Administering an ID Injection

In the home setting, the nurse needs to assess the client's knowledge about the ID injection and the reason for follow-up with the healthcare professional. Set up an appointment for the visit. Instruct and explain why the injection site should not be washed, rubbed, or scratched.

The steps for administering an intradermal injection are described in Skill 35.5.

SKILL 35.5

Administering an Intradermal Injection for Skin Tests

PURPOSE

- To provide a medication that the client requires for allergy testing and TB screening

ASSESSMENT

Assess

- Appearance of injection site
- Specific drug action and expected response
- Client's knowledge of drug action and response
- Check agency protocol about sites to use for skin tests.

PLANNING

Assignment

Administering ID injections is an invasive technique that involves the application of nursing knowledge, problem-solving, and sterile technique. This skill is not assigned to AP. The nurse, however, can inform the AP about symptoms of allergic reactions and the necessity of reporting those observations immediately to the nurse.

Equipment

- Client's MAR or computer printout
- Vial or ampule of the correct medication
- Sterile 1-mL syringe calibrated into hundredths of a milliliter (i.e., tuberculin syringe) and a #25- to #27-gauge safety needle that is 1/4 to 5/8 inch long
- Alcohol swabs
- 2 × 2 sterile gauze square (optional)
- Clean gloves (according to agency protocol)
- Bandage (optional)
- Epinephrine on hand in case of allergic anaphylactic reaction

IMPLEMENTATION

Preparation

1. Check the MAR.
   - Check the label on the medication carefully against the MAR to make sure that the correct medication is being prepared.
   - Follow the three checks for administering medications. Read the label on the medication (1) when it is taken from the medication cart, (2) before withdrawing the medication, and (3) after withdrawing the medication.
2. Organize the equipment.

Performance

1. Perform hand hygiene and observe other appropriate infection prevention procedures.
2. Prepare the medication from the vial or ampule for drug withdrawal.
   - See Skills 35.2 and 35.3.
3. Prepare the client
   - Prior to performing the procedure, introduce self and verify the client's identity using agency protocol. **Rationale:** *This ensures that the right client receives the medication.*
4. Explain to the client that the medication will produce a small wheal, sometimes called a bleb. A wheal is a small raised area, like a blister. The client will feel a slight prick as the needle enters the skin. Some medications are absorbed slowly through the capillaries into the general circulation, and the bleb gradually disappears. Other drugs remain in the area and interact with the body tissues to produce redness and induration (hardening), which will need to be interpreted at a particular time (e.g., in 24 or 48 hours). This reaction will also gradually disappear. **Rationale:** *Information can facilitate acceptance of and compliance with the therapy.*
5. Provide for client privacy.
6. Select and clean the site.
   - Select a site (e.g., the forearm about a hand's width above the wrist and three or four finger widths below the antecubital space).
   - Avoid using sites that are tender, inflamed, or swollen and those that have lesions.
   - Apply gloves as indicated by agency policy.
   - Cleanse the skin at the site using a firm circular motion starting at the center and widening the circle outward. Allow the area to dry thoroughly.
7. Prepare the syringe for the injection.
   - Remove the needle cap while waiting for the antiseptic to dry.
   - Expel any air bubbles from the syringe. Small bubbles that adhere to the plunger are of no consequence. **Rationale:** *A small amount of air will not harm the tissues.*
   - Grasp the syringe in your dominant hand, close to the hub, holding it between thumb and forefinger. Hold the needle almost parallel to the skin surface, with the bevel of the needle up. **Rationale:** *The possibility of the medication entering the subcutaneous tissue increases when using an angle greater than 15°.*
8. Inject the fluid.
   - With the nondominant hand, pull the skin at the site until it is taut. For example, if using the ventral forearm, grasp the client's dorsal forearm and gently pull it to tighten the ventral skin. **Rationale:** *Taut skin allows for easier entry of the needle and less discomfort for the client.*
   - Insert the tip of the needle far enough to place the bevel through the epidermis into the dermis. The outline of the bevel should be visible under the skin surface.
   - Stabilize the syringe and needle. Inject the medication carefully and slowly so that it produces a small wheal on the skin. **Rationale:** *This verifies that the medication entered the dermis.* ❶
   - Withdraw the needle quickly at the same angle at which it was inserted. Activate the needle safety device. Apply a bandage if indicated.
   - Do not massage the area. **Rationale:** *Massage can disperse the medication into the tissue or out through the needle insertion site.*
   - Dispose of the syringe and needle into the sharps container. **Rationale:** *Do not recap the needle in order to prevent needlestick injuries.*
   - Remove and discard gloves.
   - Perform hand hygiene.
   - Circle the injection site with ink to observe for redness or induration (hardening), per agency policy.
9. Document all relevant information.
   - Record the testing material given, the time, dosage, route, site, and nursing assessments.

SKILL 35.5

Administering an Intradermal Injection for Skin Tests—*continued*

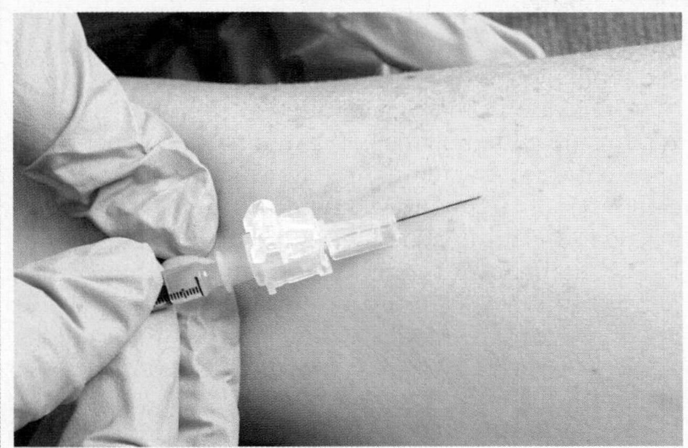

A

Epidermis
Dermis
Subcutaneous tissue

B

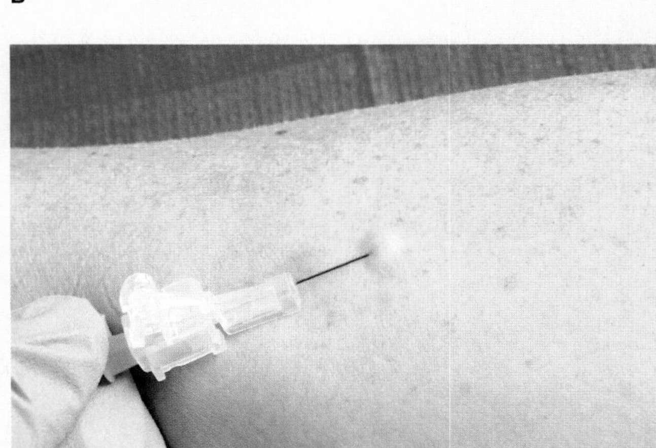

C

❶ For an intradermal injection: *A*, the needle enters the skin at a 5° to 15° angle; *B*, *C*, the medication forms a bleb or wheal under the epidermis.

EVALUATION

- Evaluate the client's response to the testing substance. **Rationale:** *Some medications used in testing may cause allergic reactions*. Epinephrine may need to be used.
- Evaluate the condition of the site in 24 or 48 hours, depending on the test. Measure the area of redness and induration in millimeters at the largest diameter and document findings.

LIFESPAN CONSIDERATIONS **Administering an Intradermal Injection**

CHILDREN

- Children should be gently restrained during the procedure in order to prevent injury from a sudden movement.
- Make sure the child understands that the injection is not a punishment.
- Ask the child not to rub or scratch the injection site. Rubbing the site can interfere with test results by irritating the underlying tissue.

Subcutaneous Injections

Among the many kinds of drugs administered subcutaneously are vaccines, insulin, and heparin. Common sites for subcutaneous injections are the outer aspect of the upper arms and the anterior aspect of the thighs. These areas are convenient and normally have good blood circulation. Other areas that can be used are the abdomen, the scapular areas of the upper back, and the upper ventrogluteal and dorsogluteal areas (Figure 35.34 ■). Only small doses (0.5 to 1 mL) of medication are usually injected via the subcutaneous route. Check agency policy.

The type of syringe used for subcutaneous injections depends on the medication being given. Generally a 1- or 2-mL syringe is used for most subcutaneous injections. However, if insulin is being administered, an insulin syringe is used; if heparin is being administered, a prefilled cartridge may be used.

Needle sizes and lengths are selected based on the client's body mass, the intended angle of insertion, and the planned site. Generally a #25-gauge, 5/8-inch needle is used for adults of normal weight and the needle is inserted at a 45° angle; a 3/8-inch needle is used at a 90° angle. A child may need a 1/2-inch needle inserted at a 45° angle.

One method nurses use to determine length of needle is to pinch the tissue at the site and select a needle length that is half the width of the skinfold. To determine the

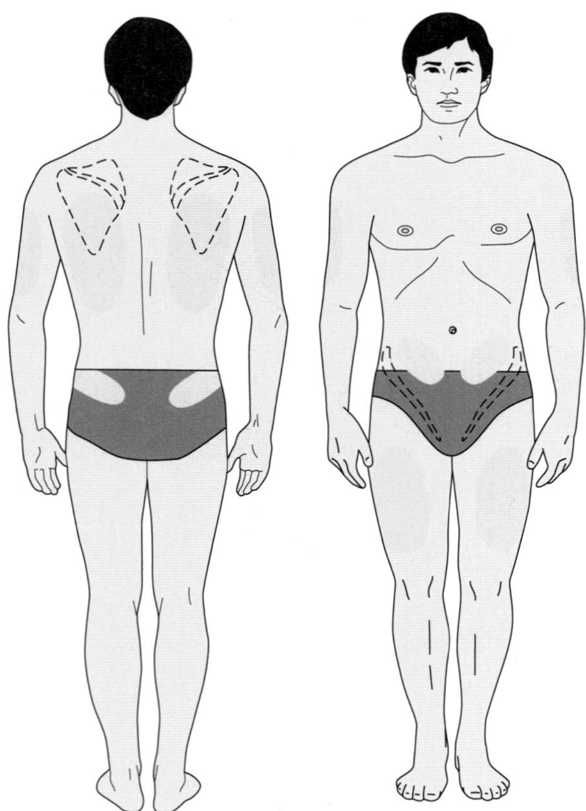

Figure 35.34 ■ Body sites commonly used for subcutaneous injections.

angle of insertion, a general rule to follow relates to the amount of tissue that can be pinched or grasped at the site. A 45° angle is used when 1 inch of tissue can be grasped at the site; a 90° angle is used when 2 inches of tissue can be grasped.

When administering insulin to adults, the current standard needle gauge is #30 gauge with a short needle (4 to 6 mm). Most clients prefer the shorter and thinner needles because they are less painful. The risk of injecting into the muscle is lessened with the shorter needle.

Subcutaneous injection sites need to be rotated in an orderly fashion to minimize tissue damage, aid absorption, and avoid discomfort. This is especially important for clients who must receive repeated injections, such as those with diabetes. Because insulin is absorbed at different rates at different parts of the body, the blood glucose levels of a client who has diabetes can vary when various sites are used. Insulin is absorbed most quickly when injected into the abdomen and then into the arms, and most slowly when injected into the thighs and buttocks. Rotate the injection sites weekly to prevent lipohypertrophy, fat pads under the surface of the skin (Sexson, Lindauer, & Harvath, 2016, p. 50).

The steps for administering a subcutaneous injection are described in Skill 35.6.

SKILL 35.6

Administering a Subcutaneous Injection

PURPOSES

- To provide a medication the client requires (see specific drug action)
- To allow slower absorption of a medication compared with either the intramuscular or intravenous route

ASSESSMENT

Assess

- Allergies to medication
- Specific drug action, side effects, and adverse reactions
- Client's knowledge and learning needs about the medication
- Status and appearance of subcutaneous site for lesions, erythema, swelling, ecchymosis, inflammation, and tissue damage from previous injections
- Ability of the client to cooperate during the injection
- Previous injection sites used

PLANNING

Assignment

Administering subcutaneous injections is an invasive technique that involves the application of nursing knowledge, problem-solving, and sterile technique. Therefore, this skill is not assigned to AP. The nurse, however, can inform the AP of the intended therapeutic effects and specific side effects of the medication and direct the AP to report specific client observations to the nurse for follow-up.

Equipment

- Client's MAR or computer printout
- Vial or ampule of the correct sterile medication
- Syringe and needle (e.g., insulin syringe, #25-gauge needle or smaller, 3/8 or 5/8 in. long)
- Antiseptic swabs
- Dry sterile gauze for opening an ampule (optional)
- Clean gloves

IMPLEMENTATION

Preparation

1. Check the MAR.
   - Check the label on the medication carefully against the MAR to make sure that the correct medication is being prepared.
   - Follow the three checks for administering medications. Read the label on the medication (1) when it is taken from the medication cart, (2) before withdrawing the medication, and (3) after withdrawing the medication.
2. Organize the equipment.

Administering a Subcutaneous Injection—*continued*

Performance

1. Perform hand hygiene and observe other appropriate infection prevention procedures (e.g., clean gloves).
2. Prepare the medication from the ampule or vial for drug withdrawal.
   - See Skill 35.2 (ampule) or 35.3 (vial).
   - If the medication is insulin or heparin, the dosage needs to be verified by another nurse. **Rationale:** *Double checking the dosage avoids medication errors.*
3. Provide for client privacy.

Clinical Alert!

When asking another nurse to verify the dosage of insulin or heparin, leave the needle and syringe in the vial and ask, "What dosage do I have in the syringe?" The other nurse needs to then check the vial medication name and concentration as well as calculate the dosage. This is a safer and more accurate method of double checking than saying to another nurse, "I have 10 units of insulin," which "presets" the other nurse's checking of the medication dosage and can lead to an error.

4. Prepare the client.
   - Prior to performing the procedure, introduce self and verify the client's identity using agency protocol. **Rationale:** *This ensures that the right client receives the right medication.*
   - Assist the client to a position in which the arm, leg, or abdomen can be relaxed, depending on the site to be used. **Rationale:** *A relaxed position of the site minimizes discomfort.*
   - Obtain assistance in holding an uncooperative client. **Rationale:** *This prevents injury due to sudden movement after needle insertion.*
5. Explain the purpose of the medication and how it will help, using language that the client can understand. Include relevant information about effects of the medication. **Rationale:** *Information can facilitate acceptance of and adherence to the therapy.*
6. Select and clean the site.
   - Select a site free of tenderness, hardness, swelling, scarring, itching, burning, or localized inflammation. Select a site that has not been used frequently. **Rationale:** *These conditions could hinder the absorption of the medication and may also increase the likelihood of injury and discomfort at the injection site.*
   - Apply clean gloves.
   - As agency protocol indicates, clean the site with an antiseptic swab. Start at the center of the site and clean in a widening circle to about 5 cm (2 in.). Allow the area to dry thoroughly. **Rationale:** *The mechanical action of swabbing removes skin secretions, which contain microorganisms.*
   - Place and hold the swab between the third and fourth fingers of the nondominant hand, or position the swab on the client's skin above the intended site. **Rationale:** *Using this technique keeps the swab readily accessible when the needle is withdrawn.*
7. Prepare the syringe for injection.
   - Remove the needle cap while waiting for the antiseptic to dry. Pull the cap straight off to avoid contaminating the needle by the outside edge of the cap. **Rationale:** *The needle will become contaminated if it touches anything but the inside of the cap, which is sterile.*
   - Dispose of the needle cap.
8. Inject the medication.
   - Grasp the syringe in your dominant hand by holding it between your thumb and fingers. With palm facing to the side or upward for a 45° angle insertion, or with the palm downward for a 90° angle insertion, prepare to inject. ❶
   - Using the nondominant hand, pinch or spread the skin at the site, and insert the needle using the dominant hand and a firm, steady push. Recommendations vary about whether to pinch or spread the skin and at what angle to administer subcutaneous injections. The most important consideration is the depth of the subcutaneous tissue in the area to be injected. If the client has more than 1/2 inch of adipose tissue in the injection site, it would be safe to administer the injection at a 90° angle with the skin spread. If the client is thin or lean and lacks adipose tissue, the subcutaneous injection should be given with the skin pinched and at a 45° to 60° angle. One way to check that the pinch of skin is subcutaneous tissue is to ask the client to flex and extend the elbow. If any muscle is being held in the pinch, you will feel it contract and relax. If so, release the pinch and try again. ❷
   - When the needle is inserted, move your nondominant hand to the end of the plunger. Some nurses find it easier to move the nondominant hand to the barrel of the syringe and the dominant hand to the end of the plunger.
   - Inject the medication by holding the syringe steady and depressing the plunger with a slow, even pressure. **Rationale:** *Holding the syringe steady and injecting the medication at an even pressure minimizes discomfort for the client.*
   - It is recommended that with many subcutaneous injections, especially insulin, the needle should be embedded within the skin for 5 seconds after complete depression of the plunger. **Rationale:** *This ensures complete delivery of the dose.*

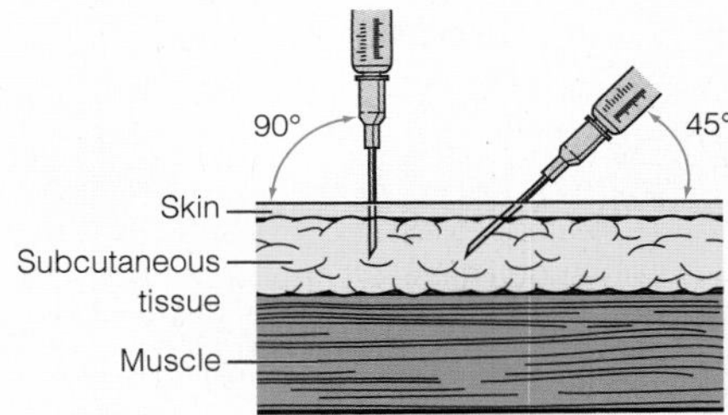

❶ Inserting a needle into the subcutaneous tissue using 90° and 45° angles.

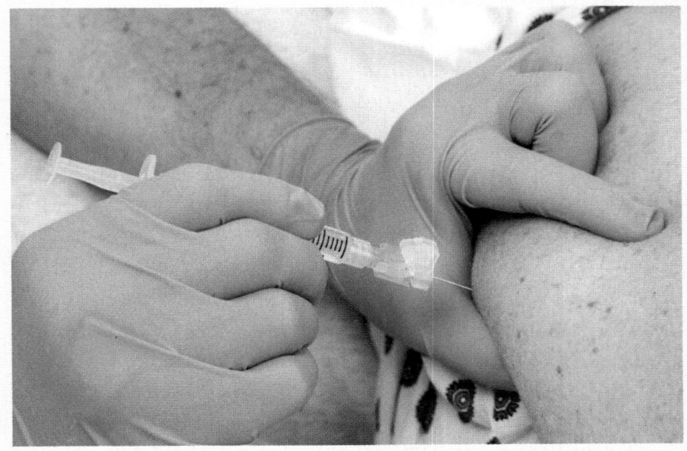

❷ Administering a subcutaneous injection into pinched tissue.

Continued on page 886

SKILL 35.6

Administering a Subcutaneous Injection—*continued*

9. Remove the needle.
- Remove the needle smoothly, pulling along the line of insertion while depressing the skin with your nondominant hand. **Rationale:** *Depressing the skin minimizes the client's discomfort when the needle is withdrawn.* If you have a passive safety syringe, the needle will be in the barrel of the syringe after administering the medication.
- If bleeding occurs, apply pressure to the site with dry sterile gauze until it stops. *Bleeding rarely occurs after subcutaneous injection.*

10. Dispose of supplies appropriately.
- Activate the needle safety device or discard the *uncapped* needle and attached syringe into designated receptacles. **Rationale:** *Proper disposal protects the nurse and others from injury and contamination. The CDC recommends not capping the needle before disposal to reduce the risk of needlestick injuries.*
- Remove and discard gloves.
- Perform hand hygiene.

11. Document all relevant information.
- Document the medication given, dosage, time, route, and any assessments.
- Many agencies prefer that medication administration be recorded on the medication record. The nurse's notes are used when prn medications are given or when there is a special problem.

12. Assess the effectiveness of the medication at the time it is expected to act and document it.

Variation: Administering a Heparin Injection

The subcutaneous administration of heparin requires special precautions because of the drug's anticoagulant properties.
- Select a site on the abdomen at least 2 inches *away* from the umbilicus and above the level of the iliac crests. Some agencies support the practice of subcutaneous injection of heparin in the thighs or arms as alternate sites to the abdomen. Avoid injecting into bruises, scars, masses, or areas of tenderness.
- Use a 3/8-inch, #25- or #26-gauge needle or smaller, and insert it at a 90° angle. If a client is very lean or emaciated, use a needle longer than 3/8 inch and insert it at a 45° angle. The arms or thighs may be used as alternate sites.
- Do *not* aspirate when giving heparin by subcutaneous injection. **Rationale:** *Aspiration can possibly damage the surrounding tissue and cause bleeding as well as ecchymoses (bruises).*
- Do not massage the site after the injection. **Rationale:** *Massaging could cause bleeding and ecchymoses and hasten drug absorption.*
- Alternate the sites of subsequent injections.

Variation: Administering Enoxaparin (Lovenox)

Lovenox is a low molecular weight heparin that is used to prevent deep vein thrombosis (DVT). Administration of Lovenox has special considerations also.
- Choose an area on the abdomen at least 2 inches from the umbilicus and above the level of the iliac crests.
- Lovenox syringes come prefilled. Check that the syringe is for the correct dosage. Every syringe comes with a small air bubble. Do *not* expel the air bubble unless you have to adjust the dose.
- Pinch an inch of the cleansed area on the abdomen to make a fold in the skin. Insert the full length of the needle at a 90° angle into the fold of the skin.
- Press the plunger with your thumb until the syringe is empty.
- Pull the needle straight out at the same angle that it was inserted and release the skinfold.
- Point the needle down and away from yourself and others and push down on the plunger to activate the safety shield (Sanofi-Aventis, n.d.).

EVALUATION
- Conduct appropriate follow-up such as desired effect (e.g., relief of pain, sedation, lowered blood sugar, a prothrombin time within pre-established limits), any adverse effects (e.g., nausea, vomiting, skin rash), and clinical signs of side effects.
- Compare to previous findings if available.
- Report deviations from normal to the primary care provider.

Intramuscular Injections

Injections into muscle tissue, or **intramuscular (IM) injections**, are absorbed more quickly than subcutaneous injections because of the greater blood supply to the body muscles. Muscles can also take a larger volume of fluid without discomfort than subcutaneous tissues can, although the amount varies among individuals, chiefly based on muscle size and condition and the site used. An adult with well-developed muscles can usually safely tolerate up to 3 mL of medication in the gluteus medius and gluteus maximus muscles (Figure 35.35 ■). A volume of 1 to 2 mL is usually recommended for adults with less developed muscles. In the deltoid muscle, volumes of 0.5 to 1 mL are recommended.

Usually a 3- to 5-mL syringe is needed. The size of syringe used depends on the amount of medication being administered. The standard prepackaged intramuscular

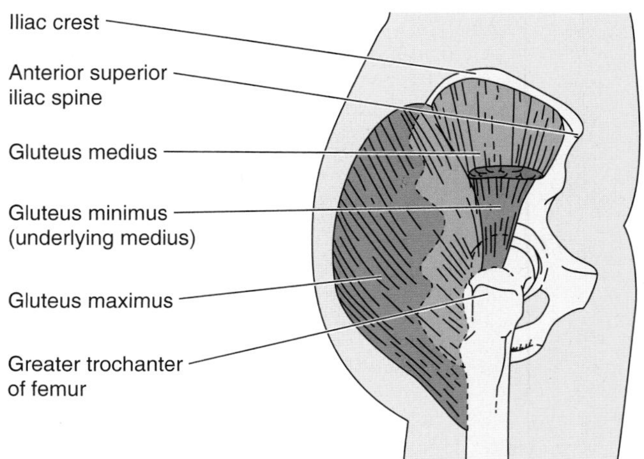

Figure 35.35 ■ Lateral view of the right buttock showing the three gluteal muscles used for intramuscular injections.

needle is 1 1/2 inches and #21 or #22 gauge. Several factors indicate the size and length of the needle to be used:

- The muscle
- The type of solution
- The amount of adipose tissue covering the muscle
- The age of the client.

For example, a smaller needle such as a #23- to #25-gauge needle 1 inch long is commonly used for the deltoid muscle. More viscous solutions require a larger gauge (e.g., #20 gauge). Clients who are obese may require a needle longer than 1 1/2 inches (e.g., 2 in.), and clients who are emaciated may require a shorter needle (e.g., 1 in.). Needle length must be long enough to penetrate the subcutaneous fat layer and be injected into the muscle. See Table 35.9 for a comparison of injection type information.

A major consideration in the administration of IM injections is the selection of a safe site located away from large blood vessels, nerves, and bone. Several body sites can be used for IM injections. These sites are discussed in detail next. Contraindications for using a specific site include tissue injury and the presence of nodules, lumps, abscesses, tenderness, or other pathology.

Ventrogluteal Site

The ventrogluteal site is in the gluteus medius muscle, which lies over the gluteus minimus (see Figure 35.35). The ventrogluteal site is the *preferred* site for IM injections because the area:

- Contains no large nerves or blood vessels.
- Provides the greatest thickness of gluteal muscle consisting of both the gluteus medius and gluteus minimus.
- Is sealed off by bone.
- Contains consistently less fat than the buttock area, thus eliminating the need to determine the depth of subcutaneous fat.

Research on the ventrogluteal site as the best site spans several decades, but the use of this site for IM injections varies in clinical practice. Studies continue to show that some nurses still use the dorsogluteal site due to what they were taught in nursing school and lack of familiarity with the ventrogluteal landmarks (Blanchard & Payette, 2016).

The client position for the injection can be a back, prone, or side-lying position. The side-lying position, however, helps locate the ventrogluteal site more easily.

TABLE 35.9 Comparison of Injection Information

	Syringe Size	Needle Size	Needle Length	Volume of Fluid	Aspiration?	Common Sites	Common Uses
Intradermal (ID)	Tuberculin Syringe	#25–#27 gauge	1/4–5/8 inch	0.1 mL	No	• Inner lower arm • Upper chest • Back beneath scapulae	• Allergy testing • TB screening
Subcutaneous	1- to 2-mL syringe Insulin Syringe	#25 gauge #30 gauge for insulin	Adult of normal weight: 5/8-inch needle inserted at 45° angle OR 3/8-inch needle inserted at 90° angle Insulin needle: 4–6 mm	0.5–1 mL	No	• Outer aspect of upper arms • Anterior aspect of thigh • Abdomen	• Vaccines • Insulin • Heparin
Intramuscular (IM)	Deltoid: 1-mL syringe Ventrogluteal: 3- to 5-mL syringes*	Deltoid: #23–#25 gauge Ventrogluteal: #21 or #22 gauge	Deltoid: 1 inch Ventrogluteal: 1.5 inches	Deltoid: 0.5–1 mL Ventrogluteal: 3 mL max for adult with well-developed gluteal muscle 1–2 mL for adults with less developed gluteal muscle	Deltoid: No Ventrogluteal: No scientific evidence confirming or rejecting aspiration	Deltoid Ventrogluteal	Deltoid: Immunizations Ventrogluteal: Medication that requires large muscle for absorption and/or volume greater than 1 Ml

*Size depends on amount of medication being administered.

Position the client on his or her side with the knee bent and raised slightly toward the chest. The trochanter will protrude, which facilitates locating the ventrogluteal site. To establish the exact site, the nurse places the heel of the hand on the client's greater trochanter, with the fingers pointing toward the client's head. The right hand is used for the left hip, and the left hand for the right hip. With the index finger on the client's anterior superior iliac spine, the nurse stretches the middle finger dorsally (toward the buttocks), palpating the crest of the ilium and then pressing below it. The triangle formed by the index finger, the third finger, and the crest of the ilium is the injection site (Figures 35.36 ■ and 35.37 ■). Figure 35.36 shows the landmarks and Figure 35.37 shows administering an IM injection into the ventrogluteal site while using the preferred Z-track method as shown in Skill 35.7.

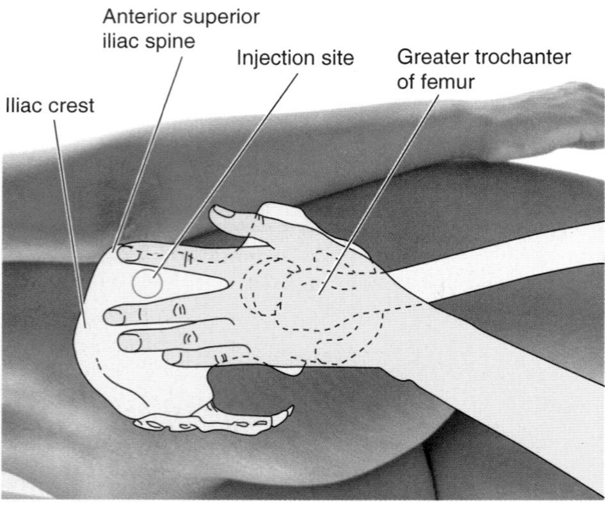

Figure 35.36 ■ Landmarks for the ventrogluteal site for an intramuscular injection.

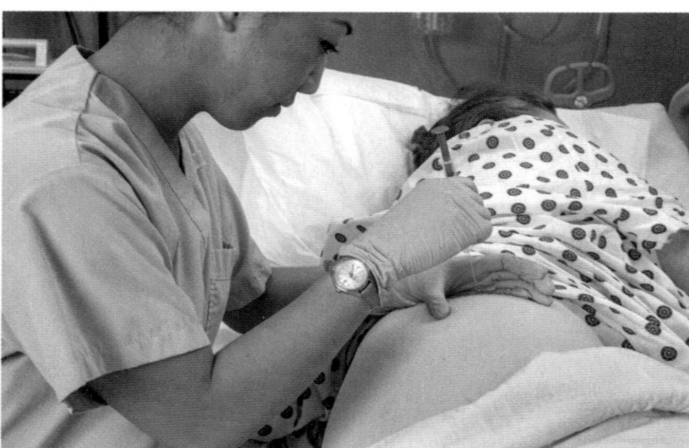

Figure 35.37 ■ Administering an intramuscular injection into the ventrogluteal site using the Z-track method.

Clinical Alert!

Do Not Use the Dorsogluteal Site for IM Injections

Nursing literature and research, over the past 20 years, provides evidence that the dorsogluteal site should be avoided for IM injection because it presents an unacceptable risk for clients. The site is close to nerves and arteries, and thick subcutaneous tissue at the site can result in the medication being injected into subcutaneous tissue instead of muscle, affecting the intended therapeutic effect.

Vastus Lateralis Site

The vastus lateralis muscle is usually thick and well developed in both adults and children. It is recommended as the site of choice for IM injections for infants and young children because it is the largest muscle mass (Bindler, Ball, London, & Davidson, 2017). Because there are no major blood vessels or nerves in the area, it is desirable for infants whose gluteal muscles are poorly developed. It is situated on the anterior lateral aspect of the infant's thigh (Figure 35.38 ■). The middle third of the muscle is suggested as the site. In the adult, the landmark is established by dividing the area between the greater trochanter of the femur and the lateral femoral condyle into thirds and selecting the middle third (Figures 35.39 ■ and 35.40 ■). The client can assume a back-lying or a sitting position for an injection into this site.

Rectus Femoris Site

The rectus femoris muscle, which belongs to the quadriceps muscle group, is used *only occasionally* for IM injections. It is situated on the anterior aspect of the thigh (Figure 35.41 ■). Its chief advantage is that clients who administer their own injections can reach this site easily. Its main disadvantage is that an injection here causes considerable discomfort.

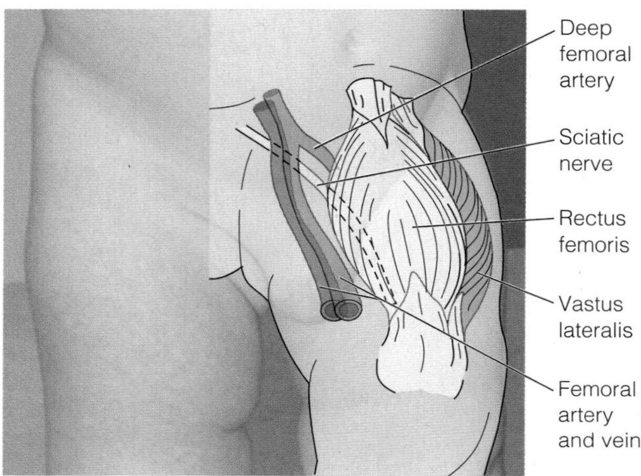

Figure 35.38 ■ The vastus lateralis muscle of an infant's upper thigh, used for intramuscular injections.

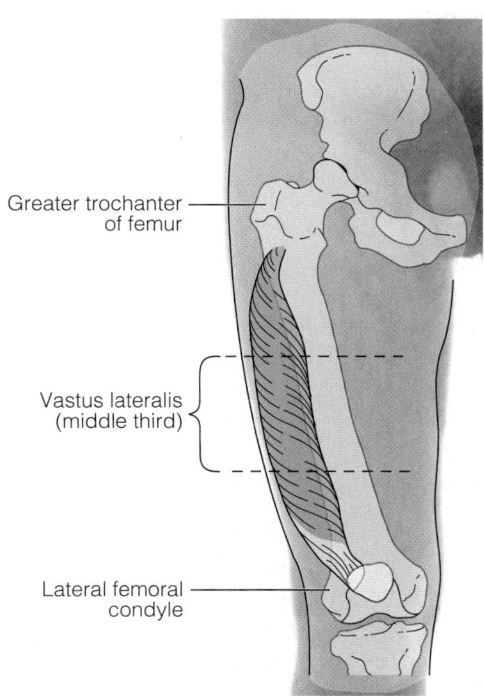

Figure 35.39 ■ Landmarks for the vastus lateralis site of an adult's right thigh, used for an intramuscular injection.

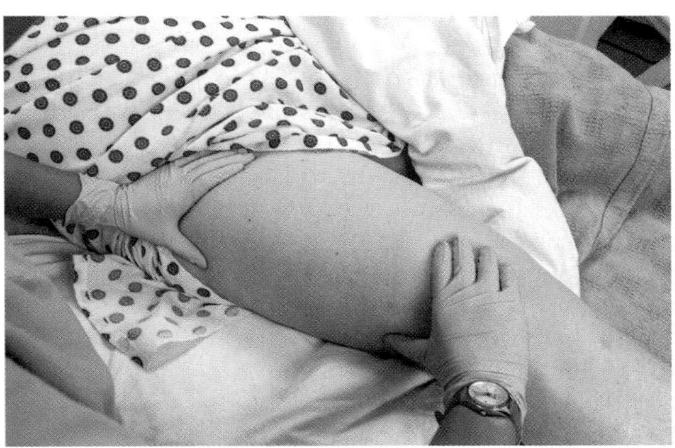

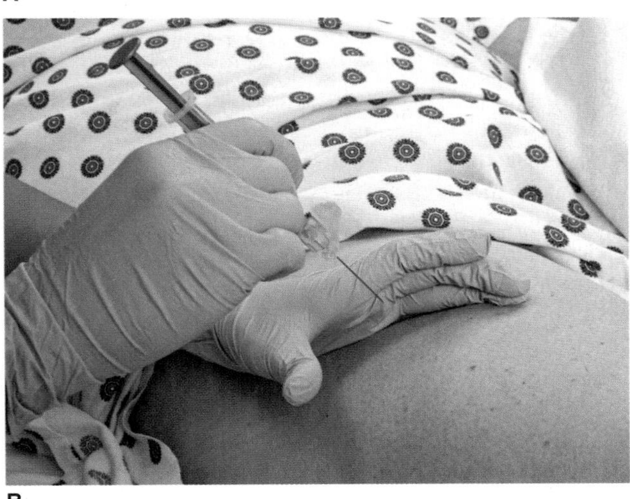

Figure 35.40 ■ *A*, Determining landmarks; *B*, administering an intramuscular injection by the Z-track method into the vastus lateralis site.

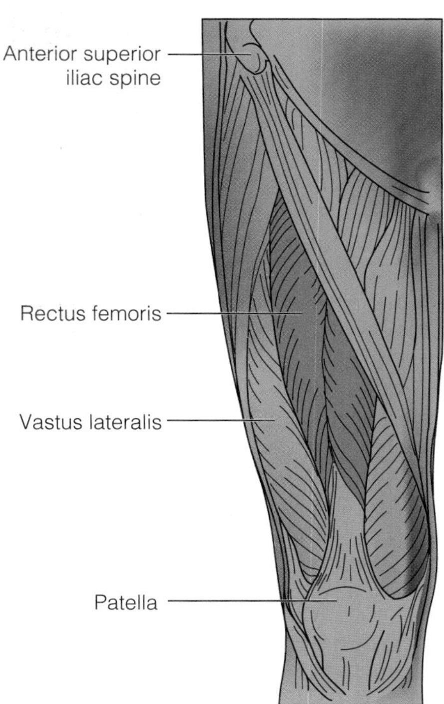

Figure 35.41 ■ Landmarks for the rectus femoris muscle of the upper right thigh, used for intramuscular injections.

Deltoid Site

The deltoid muscle is found on the uppermost part of the upper arm. It is a relatively small muscle. No more than 1 mL of solution can be administered. This site is recommended for the administration of immunizations and vaccines in adults because these medications are usually small in volume.

The nurse locates the upper landmark for the deltoid site by placing four fingers across the deltoid muscle with the first finger on the acromion process. The top of the axilla is the line that marks the lower border landmark (Figure 35.42 ■). A triangle within these boundaries indicates the deltoid muscle about 5 cm (2 in.) below the acromion process (Figures 35.43 ■ and 35.44 ■).

Firmly pressing the injection site for 10 seconds before inserting the needle is thought to reduce the sensory input from an injection, regardless of the site.

Intramuscular Injection Technique

Skill 35.7 describes how to administer an IM injection using the Z-track technique, which is recommended for IM injections. The Z-track method has been found to be a less painful technique and to decrease leakage of irritating medications into the subcutaneous tissue (Yilmaz, Khorshid, & Dedeoglu, 2016). Although the Z-track technique is not always used in practice, research evidence supports its effectiveness and recommends its routine use.

An issue with IM injection technique is the practice of aspirating for blood prior to administering the injection. Is this practice based on tradition or evidence? Historically, nurses were taught to aspirate for blood before

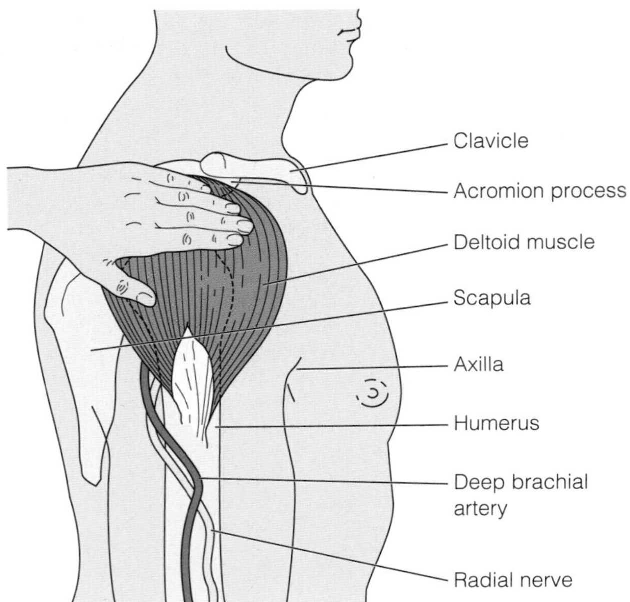

Figure 35.42 ■ A method of establishing the deltoid muscle site for an intramuscular injection.

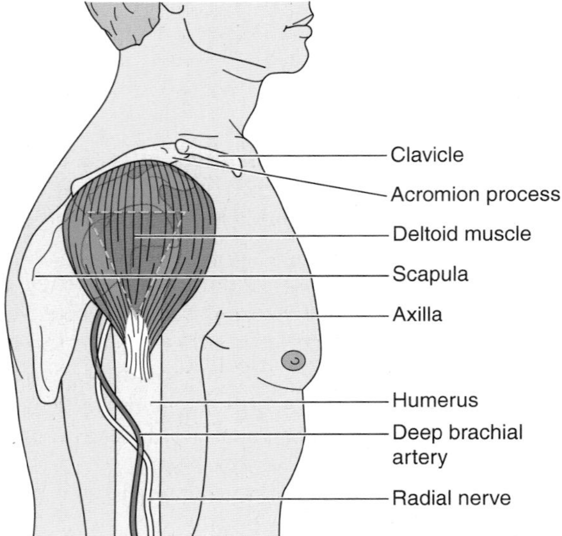

Figure 35.43 ■ Landmarks for the deltoid muscle of the upper arm, used for intramuscular injections.

all IM injections to prevent unintentionally injecting the medication into a blood vessel and it becoming an unintentional IV medication and potentially causing a serious reaction. Aspiration technique consists of pulling the syringe plunger back for 5 to 10 seconds to create negative pressure in the tissue and allowing time for the blood to appear if the needle is in a small vessel. Literature and integrative reviews of evidence indicate that the practice of aspiration before vaccination injections into the deltoid has no basis in scientific evidence. Moreover, the CDC (2018) states that the practice of aspiration is unnecessary for vaccinations because

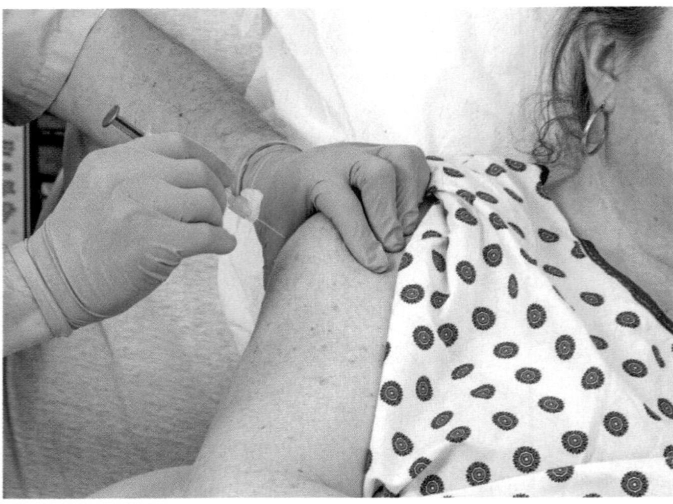

Figure 35.44 ■ Administering an intramuscular injection into the deltoid site.

there are no large vessels located at the recommended vaccination sites.

The evidence, however, is *not* clear regarding aspiration at IM sites *other* than the deltoid (i.e., ventrogluteal). Some believe that no aspiration is needed when using the ventrogluteal site because this site avoids all major nerves and blood vessels. In 2016, a study by Thomas, Mraz, and Rajcam investigated how often RNs used aspiration during an IM injection, how long the nurses spent in aspiration, and the incidence of blood aspiration. The sample size of the study consisted of 164 practicing RNs. The majority of the nurses learned their IM technique before 2000 when slow aspiration was recommended. Three percent learned IM injection technique in 2011 and later when no aspiration was recommended. When asked how often they aspirated during an IM injection, the most frequent response was every time. Approximately 60% of the sample reported never having aspirated blood during the injections, 40% aspirated blood at least once, and 4% noted blood aspiration 13 times or more. Of those who aspirated blood during injection, 31% did not remember in which muscle it occurred but the most frequently reported muscle was the dorsal gluteal. The researchers concluded that blood aspiration does occur and recommended that complete elimination of aspiration during IM injection may not be safe practice (p. 555). The researchers recommended that nurses should identify whether a medication would be harmful if given IV and could be a safety issue for the client. If so, the aspiration during the IM injection should be implemented. It is noted that this study was limited to a small sample and cannot be generalized. Based on this study, Mraz, Thomas, and Rajcan (2018) developed a clinical practice guideline for IM injection. The guideline includes the nurse assessing the client to determine if there is a safety risk to the client or the nurse, such as an emergency situation or a combative client, and if so, to not aspirate, and if there is no safety risk, to continue on the pathway of the guideline. The nurse also needs to evaluate the medication, specifically for a greater than 10% dextrose level and osmolarity of greater than 900 mOsm/liter (p. 755). Medications with these parameters are known to be irritants or vesicants to peripheral veins and need to be infused through a central vein. Thus, the researchers recommend aspiration that should be completed over 5 to 10 seconds. The researchers note that their guideline has not been tested for effectiveness. Testing the tool will be needed for more information about improving IM injection technique. What is seen in nursing practice regarding IM injection aspiration often varies and can be confusing to the nursing student. Reviewing the agency policies and procedures may help.

Administering an Intramuscular Injection

SKILL 35.7

PURPOSE

- To provide a medication the client requires (see specific drug action)

ASSESSMENT

Assess

- Client allergies to medication(s)
- Specific drug action, side effects, and adverse reactions
- Client's knowledge of and learning needs about the medication
- Tissue integrity of the selected site
- Client's age and weight to determine site and needle size
- Client's ability or willingness to participate
- Determine whether the size of the muscle is appropriate to the amount of medication to be injected. An average adult's deltoid muscle can usually absorb 0.5 mL of medication, although some authorities believe 1 mL can be absorbed by a well-developed deltoid muscle. The gluteus medius muscle can often absorb 1 to 4 mL, although 4 mL may be very painful and may be contraindicated by agency protocol.

PLANNING

Assignment

The administration of IM injections is an invasive technique that involves the application of nursing knowledge, problem-solving, and sterile technique. Assignment to AP would be inappropriate. The nurse, however, can inform the AP of the intended therapeutic effects and specific side effects of the medication and direct the AP to report specific client observations to the nurse for follow-up.

Equipment

- Client's MAR or computer printout
- Sterile medication (usually provided in an ampule or vial or pre-filled syringe)
- Syringe and needle of a size appropriate for the amount and type of solution to be administered
- Antiseptic swabs
- Clean gloves

IMPLEMENTATION

Preparation

1. Check the MAR.
   - Check the label on the medication carefully against the MAR to make sure that the correct medication is being prepared.
   - Follow the three checks for administering the medication and dose. Read the label on the medication (1) when it is taken from the medication cart, (2) before withdrawing the medication, and (3) after withdrawing the medication.
   - Confirm that the dose is correct.
2. Organize the equipment.

Performance

1. Perform hand hygiene and observe other appropriate infection prevention procedures.
2. Prepare the medication from the ampule or vial for drug withdrawal.
   - See Skill 35.2 (ampule) or 35.3 (vial).
   - Whenever feasible, change the needle on the syringe before the injection. **Rationale:** *Because the outside of a new needle is free of medication, it does not irritate subcutaneous tissues as it passes into the muscle.*
   - Invert the syringe needle uppermost and expel all excess air.
3. Provide for client privacy.
4. Prepare the client.
   - Prior to performing the procedure, introduce self and verify the client's identity using agency protocol. **Rationale:** *This ensures that the right client receives the medication.*
   - Assist the client to a supine, lateral, prone, or sitting position, depending on the chosen site. If the target muscle is the gluteus medius (ventrogluteal site), have the client in the supine position flex the knee(s); in the lateral position, flex the upper leg; and in the prone position, toe in. **Rationale:** *Appropriate positioning promotes relaxation of the target muscle.*
   - Obtain assistance in holding an uncooperative client. **Rationale:** *This prevents injury due to sudden movement after needle insertion.*
5. Explain the purpose of the medication and how it will help, using language that the client can understand. Include relevant information about effects of the medication. **Rationale:** *Information can facilitate acceptance of and adherence to the therapy.*
6. Select, locate, and clean the site.
   - Select a site free of skin lesions, tenderness, swelling, hardness, or localized inflammation and one that has not been used frequently.
   - If injections are to be frequent, alternate sites. Avoid using the same site twice in a row. **Rationale:** *This reduces the discomfort of IM injections.* If necessary, discuss with the prescribing primary care provider an alternative method of providing the medication.
   - Locate the exact site for the injection. See the discussion of sites earlier in this chapter.
   - Apply clean gloves.

Continued on page 892

Administering an Intramuscular Injection—*continued*

- Clean the site with an antiseptic swab. Using a circular motion, start at the center and move outward about 5 cm (2 in.). **Rationale:** *This prevents entry of bacteria into the injection site.*
- Transfer and hold the swab between the third and fourth fingers of your nondominant hand in readiness for needle withdrawal, or position the swab on the client's skin above the intended site. Allow skin to dry prior to injecting medication. **Rationale:** *This reduces the stinging sensation from the antiseptic upon injection.*

7. Prepare the syringe for injection.
   - Remove the needle cover and discard without contaminating the needle.
   - If using a prefilled unit-dose medication, take caution to avoid dripping medication on the needle prior to injection. If this does occur, wipe the medication off the needle with a sterile gauze. Some sources recommend changing the needle if possible. **Rationale:** *Medication left on the needle can cause pain when it is tracked through the subcutaneous tissue.*
8. Inject the medication using the Z-track technique.
   - Use the ulnar side of the nondominant hand to pull the skin approximately 2.5 cm (1 in.) to the side. Under some circumstances, such as for an emaciated client or an infant, the muscle may be pinched. **Rationale:** *Pulling the skin and subcutaneous tissue or pinching the muscle makes it firmer and facilitates needle insertion.* ❶
   - Holding the syringe between the thumb and forefinger (as if holding a pen), pierce the skin quickly and smoothly at a 90° angle (see Figure 35.40), and insert the needle into the muscle. ❷ **Rationale:** *Using a quick motion lessens the client's discomfort. Holding the syringe like a pen or pencil reduces accidental depression of the plunger and inadvertent administration of the medication while the needle is being inserted.*
   - Hold the barrel of the syringe steady with your nondominant hand and aspirate by pulling back on the plunger with your dominant hand. ❸ Aspirate for 5 to 10 seconds. **Rationale:** *If the needle is in a small blood vessel, it takes time for the blood to appear.* If blood appears in the syringe, withdraw the needle, discard the syringe, and prepare a new injection. **Rationale:** *This step determines whether the needle has been inserted into a blood vessel.* **Note**: *Current research, as stated previously, may or may not support aspiration. Thus, it is recommended that nursing students consult the policy manual at the institution where they are practicing to determine their recommended guidelines for IM injection technique.*
   - If blood does not appear, inject the medication steadily and slowly (approximately 10 seconds per milliliter) while holding the syringe steady if using the ventrogluteal site. **Rationale:** *Injecting medication slowly promotes comfort and allows time for tissue to expand and begin absorbing the medication. Holding the syringe steady minimizes discomfort.*
   - After the injection, wait 10 seconds if using the ventrogluteal site. **Rationale:** *Waiting permits the medication to disperse into the muscle tissue, thus decreasing the client's discomfort.*

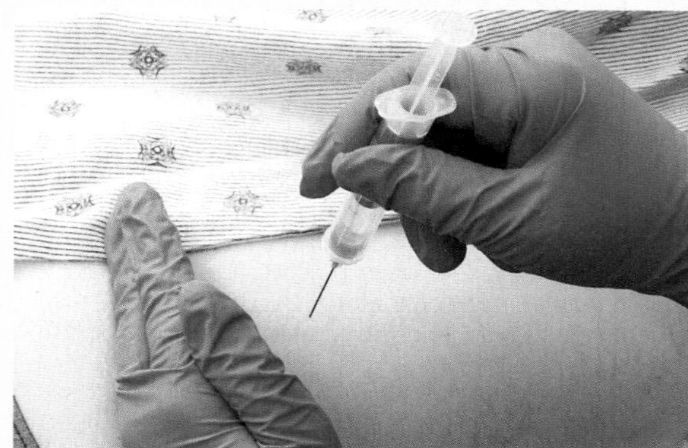

❷ Holding the syringe between the thumb and forefinger. Note that the nurse is using the Z-track technique.

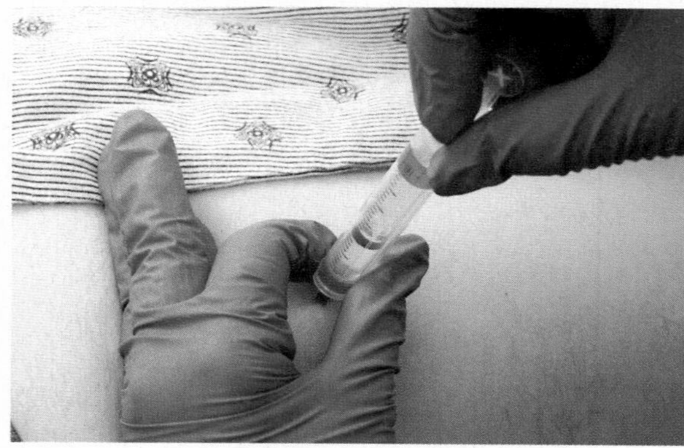

❸ In addition to pulling the skin to the side, the nondominant hand is holding the barrel of the syringe to prevent it from moving while the dominant hand aspirates by pulling back on the plunger.

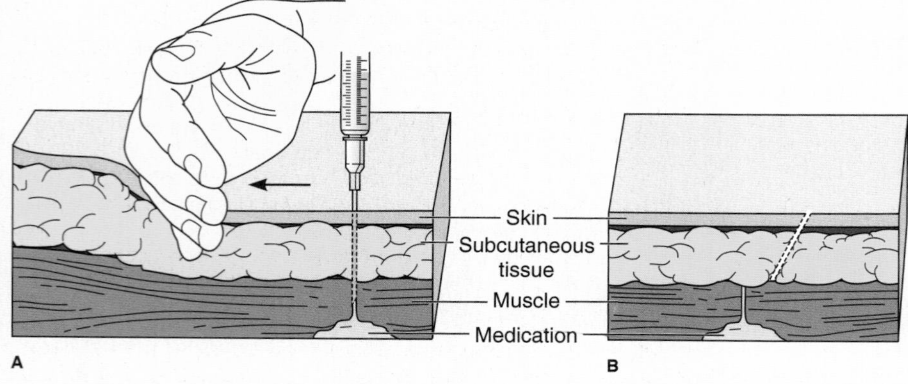

❶ Inserting an intramuscular needle at a 90° angle using the Z-track method: *A*, skin pulled to the side; *B*, skin released. *Note*: When the skin returns to its normal position after the needle is withdrawn, a seal is formed over the intramuscular site. This prevents seepage of the medication into the subcutaneous tissues and subsequent discomfort.

Administering an Intramuscular Injection—*continued*

9. Withdraw the needle.
   - Withdraw the needle smoothly at the same angle of insertion. **Rationale:** *This minimizes tissue injury.* Release the skin.
   - Apply gentle pressure at the site with a dry sponge. **Rationale:** *Use of an alcohol swab may cause pain or a burning sensation.*
   - It is not necessary to massage the area at the site of injection. **Rationale:** *Massaging the site may cause the leakage of medication from the site and result in irritation.*
   - If bleeding occurs, apply pressure with a dry sterile gauze until it stops.
10. Activate the needle safety device and discard the attached syringe into the proper receptacle.
11. Remove and discard gloves.
    - Perform hand hygiene.
12. Document all relevant information.
    - Include the time of administration, drug name, dose, route, and the client's reactions.
13. Assess the effectiveness of the medication at the time it is expected to act.

EVALUATION

- Conduct appropriate follow-up, such as desired effect (e.g., relief of pain or vomiting); any adverse reactions or side effects; local skin or tissue reactions at injection site (e.g., redness, swelling, pain, or other evidence of tissue damage).
- Compare to previous findings, if available.
- Report significant deviation from normal to the primary care provider.

LIFESPAN CONSIDERATIONS Intramuscular Injections

INFANTS

- The vastus lateralis site is recommended as the site of choice for IM injections for infants. There are no major blood vessels or nerves in this area, and it is the infant's largest muscle mass. It is situated on the anterior lateral aspect of the thigh.
- Obtain assistance to immobilize an infant or young child. The parent may hold the child. This prevents accidental injury during the procedure.

CHILDREN

- Use needles that will place medication in the main muscle mass; infants and children usually require smaller, shorter needles (#22 to #25 gauge, 5/8 to 1 in. long) for IM injections.
- The vastus lateralis is recommended as the site of choice for toddlers and children.
- For the older child and adolescent, the recommended sites are the same as for the adult: ventrogluteal or deltoid. Ask in which arm they would like the injection.

OLDER ADULTS

- Older clients may have a decreased muscle mass or muscle atrophy. A shorter needle may be needed. Assessment of an appropriate injection site is critical. Absorption of medication may occur more quickly than expected.

Intravenous Medications

Because IV medications enter the client's bloodstream directly by way of a vein, they are appropriate when a rapid effect is required. This route is also appropriate when medications are too irritating to tissues to be given by other routes. When an IV line is already established, this route is desirable because it avoids the discomfort of other parenteral routes. Methods for administering medications intravenously include the following:

- Intermittent intravenous infusion (e.g., piggyback setup)
- Volume-controlled infusion (often used for children)
- Intravenous push (IVP) or bolus
- Intermittent injection ports (devices).

In all of these methods, the client has an existing intravenous line or an IV access site such as a saline lock. Most agencies have procedures and policies about who may administer an IV medication. Chapter 51 ∞ describes the technique for performing a venipuncture and establishing an IV line.

With all IV medication administration, it is very important to observe clients closely for signs of adverse reactions. Because the drug enters the bloodstream directly and acts immediately, there is no way it can be withdrawn or its action terminated. Therefore, the nurse must take special care to avoid any errors about the preparation of the drug and the calculation of the dosage. When the administered drug is particularly potent, an antidote to the drug should be available. In addition, assess the vital signs before, during, and after infusion of the drug.

Before adding any medications to an existing IV infusion, the nurse must check for the "rights" and check compatibility of the drug and the existing IV fluid. Be aware of any incompatibilities of the drug and the fluid that is infusing. For example, the drug phenytoin (Dilantin) is incompatible with dextrose and will form a precipitate if injected through a port in an IV line with glucose or dextrose infusing.

Intermittent Intravenous Infusions

An intermittent infusion is a method of administering a medication mixed in a small amount of IV solution, such as 50 or 100 mL. It is important for the label on an IV intermittent medication to be designed to prevent medication errors. The ISMP (2010) developed recommended principles for these medication labels. See Figure 35.45 ■ for a sample label. The drug is administered at regular intervals, such as every 4 hours, with the drug being infused for a short period of time such as 30 to 60 minutes. A commonly used additive or secondary IV setup is the **piggyback**.

In the piggyback setup (Figure 35.46 ■), a second set connects the second container to the tubing of the primary container at the upper port. This setup is used solely for intermittent drug administration. Various manufacturers describe these sets differently, so the nurse must check the manufacturer's labeling and directions carefully. Needleless systems can use threaded-lock or lever-lock cannulas to connect the secondary set to the ports of the primary infusion.

Another method of intermittently administering an IV medication is by a syringe pump or mini-infuser. The medication is mixed in a syringe that is connected to the primary IV line via a mini-infuser (Figure 35.47 ■).

Volume-Control Infusions

Intermittent medications may also be administered by a **volume-control infusion set** such as Buretrol, Soluset, Volutrol, and Pediatrol (Figure 35.48 ■). Such sets are small fluid containers (100 to 150 mL in size) attached below the primary infusion container so that the medication is administered through the client's IV line. Volume-control sets are frequently used to infuse solutions into children and older clients when the volume administered is critical and must be carefully monitored. Box 35.9 provides additional information.

Intravenous Push

Intravenous push (IVP) or bolus is the IV administration of an undiluted drug directly into the systemic circulation.

Janice James (client name) Room 267 (location)
MR#6789101 (second identifier)

cefotaxime (generic name) **1 g** (client dose)
(CLAFORAN) (BRAND NAME)

In D5W (diluent) IVPB (route)

Total Volume 50 mL (total volume)

(bar code)

Exp: 5-26-2020 (expiration date) RPh Initials: *SJS* (Pharmacist initials)

St. Rose Pharmacy (Pharmacy information, if required)

Infuse medication over 20–30 minutes (comments)

Figure 35.45 ■ Sample label for an IV piggyback medication using ISMP recommendations.

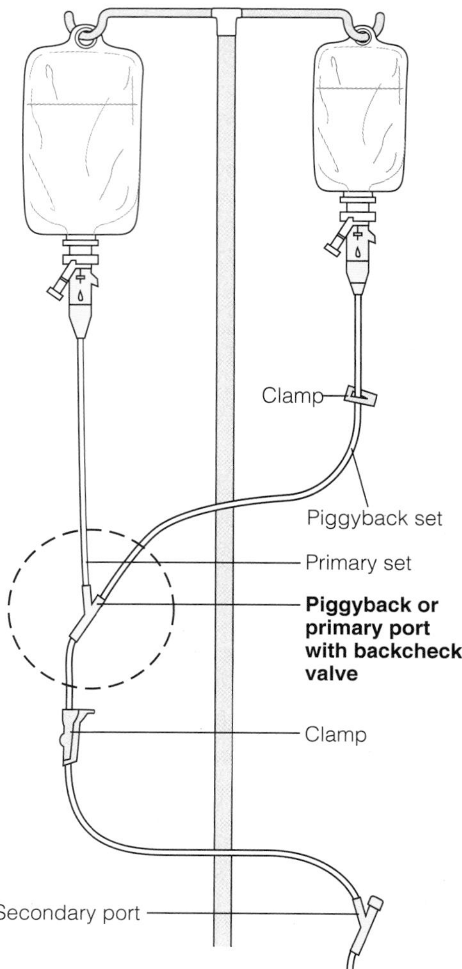

Figure 35.46 ■ Secondary intravenous line using an intravenous piggyback (IVPB) setup.

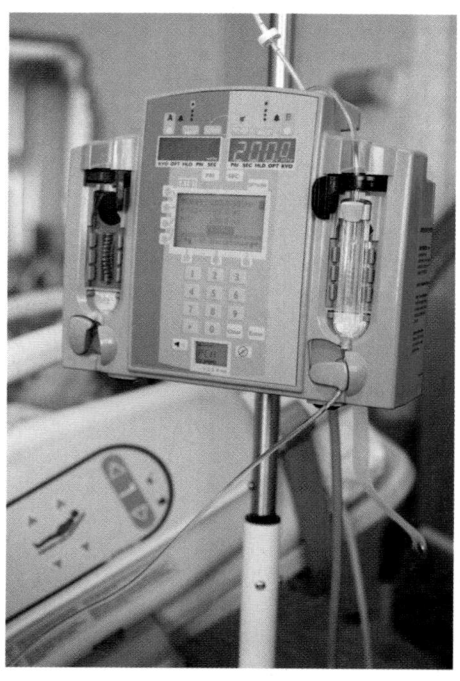

Figure 35.47 ■ Syringe pump for administration of IV medications.
nazdravie/123RF.

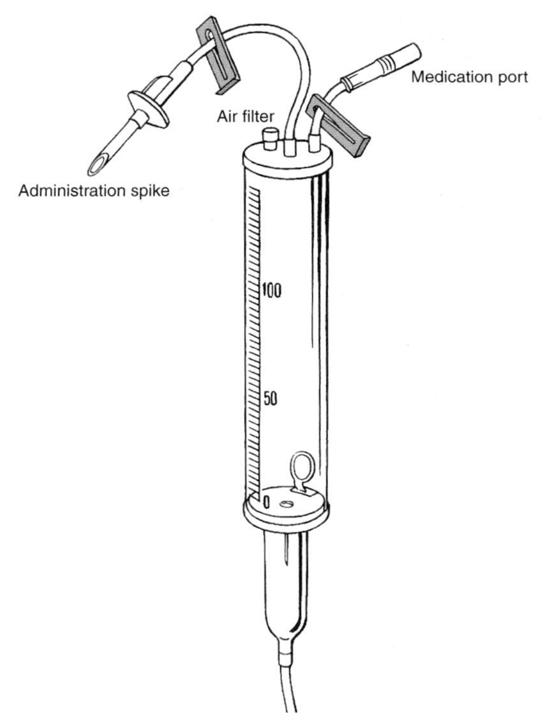

Figure 35.48 ■ A volume-control infusion set.

BOX 35.9 Adding a Medication to a Volume-Control Infusion Set

- Withdraw the required dose of the medication into a syringe.
- Ensure that there is sufficient fluid in the volume-control fluid chamber to dilute the medication. Generally, at least 50 mL of fluid is used. Check the directions from the drug manufacturer or consult the pharmacist.
- Close the inflow to the fluid chamber by adjusting the upper roller or slide clamp above the fluid chamber; also ensure that the clamp on the air vent of the chamber is open.
- Clean the medication port on the volume-control fluid chamber with an antiseptic swab.
- Inject the medication into the port of the partially filled volume-control set.
- Gently rotate the fluid chamber until the fluid is well mixed.
- Open the line's upper clamp, and regulate the flow by adjusting the lower roller or slide clamp below the fluid chamber.
- Attach a medication label to the volume-control fluid chamber.
- Document relevant data, and monitor the client and the infusion.

It is used when a medication cannot be diluted or in an emergency. An IVP can be introduced directly into a vein by venipuncture or into an existing IV line through an injection port or through an IV lock.

There are two major disadvantages to this method of drug administration: Any error in administration cannot be corrected after the drug has entered the client, and the drug may be irritating to the lining of the blood vessels.

The nurse must check if the medication to be administered IVP is compatible with the primary infusing solution. Before administering a bolus, the nurse should look up the maximum concentration recommended for the particular drug and the rate of administration. The administered medication takes effect immediately (Skill 35.8).

QSEN Patient-Centered Care: Administering IVP Antibiotics

Shortened hospital stays and the need to cut costs have led to clients or their caregivers being taught to administer IVP antibiotics at home. The antibiotic is delivered IVP directly into a venous access device with pre- and postadministration flushing.

The nurse must:

- Know which antibiotics are unsuitable for IVP administration.
- Know the adverse side effects:
  - Phlebitis (pain and tenderness over the vein, erythema, swelling, and warmth)
  - Speed shock (systemic reaction when a drug is given too rapidly)
  - Venous spasm (cramping and pain above the infusion site)
  - Infiltration.
- Assess caregiver or client's eyesight and manual dexterity. Both are needed for safe administration of the antibiotic.
- Provide thorough teaching about:
  - Venous access device
  - Administration rate (minutes/dose)
  - Schedule for medication administration
  - Flushing technique
  - Adverse reactions
  - Signs that indicate an emergency and the need to call 911
  - Proper storage of medication.
- Inspect appearance of medication and check expiration date.

Clinical Alert!

Never administer a medication IVP into an IV line that is infusing blood, blood products, or parenteral nutrition. Check the compatibility of the IV solution and what to do if it is incompatible with the IVP medication. Check if the IVP medication needs to be diluted before administration.

Intermittent Infusion Devices

Intermittent infusion devices (Figure 35.49 ■) may be attached to a peripheral IV catheter to allow medications to be administered intravenously without requiring a continuous intravenous infusion. The Infusion Nurses Society (2016) recommends considering use of an extension set between the peripheral catheter and needleless connector to reduce catheter manipulation (p. S68). This device has a port to insert into the peripheral catheter and a needleless injection cap at the other end with the extension tubing between the two ends (Figure 35.50 ■).

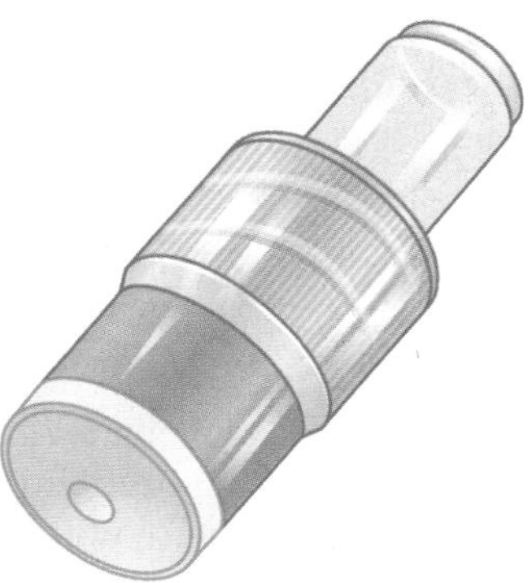

Figure 35.49 ■ Intermittent infusion device with an injection port.

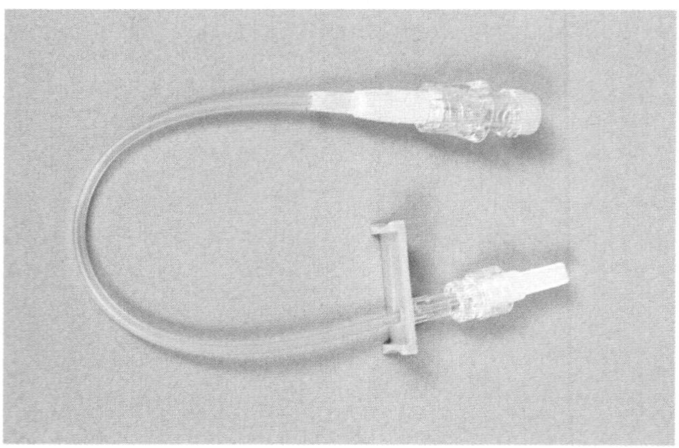

Figure 35.50 ■ Intermittent infusion device with injection port and extension tubing.

Intermittent injection ports have a port that allows a needleless adapter to be connected for administering medications. Skill 51.5 in Chapter 51 ∞ describes how to convert an IV infusion to an intermittent injection port. With the needleless system, the injection adapter may be attached at the time of IV catheter placement, allowing a closed system to be maintained.

Intermittent injection ports must be flushed prior to and after medication administration. Most agencies use saline flushes with medication administration through peripheral IV lines. When administering a medication through a central venous access device (CVAD), some agencies use the SASH (saline–administer drug–saline–heparin) flushing procedure. Flushing the port maintains patency of the IV catheter and port, and reduces the risks of mixing incompatible medications within the system (see Skill 35.8).

Clients who require long-term venous access for administering medications (e.g., people receiving chemotherapy for cancer treatment) may have a specialized catheter or port to allow central venous access. The catheter may be tunneled subcutaneously and accessed through an intermittent injection port attached to the distal end of the venous catheter. Other devices have an implantable port or vascular access port surgically inserted under the skin so that no portion of the device exits the body. To administer medications, the port is accessed using a specialized needle through the skin. See Chapter 51 ∞ for more information about central venous lines.

SKILL 35.8

Administering Intravenous Medications Using IV Push

PURPOSE

- To achieve immediate and maximum effects of a medication

ASSESSMENT

- Inspect and palpate the IV insertion site for signs of infection, infiltration, or a dislocated catheter.
- Inspect the surrounding skin for redness, pallor, or swelling.
- Palpate the surrounding tissues for coldness and the presence of edema, which could indicate leakage of the IV fluid into the tissues.
- Take vital signs for baseline data if the medication being administered is particularly potent.
- Determine if the client has allergies to the medication(s).
- Check the compatibility of the medication(s) and IV fluid.
- Determine specific drug action, side effects, normal dosage, recommended administration time, and peak action time.
- Check the patency of the IV catheter.

PLANNING

Assignment

Administering intravenous medication via IVP involves the application of nursing knowledge and critical thinking. This procedure is not assigned to AP. The nurse, however, can inform the AP of the intended therapeutic effects and specific side effects of the medication and direct the AP to report specific client observations to the nurse for follow-up. **Note**: *Administration of IVP medications varies by state nurse practice acts. For example, some states may allow the RN to assign certain medications to be given by an LPN or LVN, whereas other states may allow only the RN to administer IVP medications. The nurse needs to know the scope of practice according to the state's nurse practice act and agency policies.*

Equipment

- Client's MAR
- Medication in a prefilled syringe, vial or ampule
- Filter needle or filter straw for withdrawing medication from an ampule or vial
- Sterile syringe (3 to 5 mL) (to prepare medication)

Administering Intravenous Medications Using IV Push—*continued*

- Two 0.9% preservative-free normal saline prefilled syringes (10 mL each). **Rationale:** *These maintain the patency of the IV catheter. Saline is frequently used for peripheral locks.*
- Antiseptic swabs
- Watch with a digital readout or second hand
- Clean gloves. **Rationale:** *OSHA recommends gloves be worn when performing vascular access procedures.*

IMPLEMENTATION

Preparation

1. Check the MAR.
   - Check the label on the medication carefully against the MAR to make sure that the correct medication is being prepared.
   - Follow the three checks for correct medication and dose. Read the label on the medication (1) when it is taken from the medication cart, (2) before withdrawing the medication, and (3) after withdrawing the medication.
   - Calculate the medication dosage accurately and the recommended delivery rate (e.g., 20 mg over 1 minute).
   - Confirm that the route is correct.
   - Determine the manufacturer's or institutional guidelines for the rate of administration of the IV medication.
2. Organize the equipment.

Performance

1. Perform hand hygiene and observe other appropriate infection prevention procedures.
2. Prepare the medication.
   - Prepare the medication into a syringe according to the manufacturer's direction. **Rationale:** *It is important to have the correct dose and the correct dilution, if appropriate.* Label the syringe. **Rationale:** *It is unsafe to prepare a syringe away from the client's bedside and carry it unlabeled to the bedside, even if the intent is to administer it immediately (Shastay, 2016, p. 42). Also, the NPSGs require practitioners to label all medications on and off the sterile field (The Joint Commission, 2019a, p. 3).*
3. Perform hand hygiene and apply clean gloves. **Rationale:** *This reduces the transmission of microorganisms and reduces the likelihood of the nurse's hands contacting the client's blood.*
4. Provide for client privacy.
5. Prepare the client.
   - Prior to performing the procedure, introduce self and verify the client's identity using agency protocol. **Rationale:** *This ensures that the right client receives the right medication.*
   - If not previously assessed, take the appropriate assessment measures necessary for the medication. If any of the findings are above or below the predetermined parameters, consult the primary care provider before administering the medication.
6. Explain the purpose of the medication and how it will help, using language that the client can understand. Include relevant information about the effects of the medication. **Rationale:** *Information can facilitate acceptance of and adherence to the therapy.*
7. Administer the medication by IVP.

IV Lock (Intermittent Infusion Device)

- Clean the needleless injection port with the antiseptic swab. If using a disinfection cap, remove it and discard it. Do not reuse this cap. **Rationale:** *This prevents microorganisms from entering the circulatory system.*
- Insert the first saline needleless syringe into the injection port and flush with 1 to 2 mL, then aspirate for a blood return. **Rationale:** *The presence of blood confirms that the catheter is in the vein. In some situations, blood will not return even though the catheter is patent.*
- Flush the remaining saline into the vascular access device. **Rationale:** *This removes blood from the catheter and the intermittent infusion device.*
- Observe the area above the IV catheter for puffiness or swelling. This indicates infiltration into tissue, which would require removal of the IV catheter.
- Remove the syringe.
- Clean the needleless connector or injection port with a new antiseptic swab. **Rationale:** *This prevents the transfer of microorganisms.* Allow to dry completely.
- Insert the needleless syringe containing the prepared medication into the needleless connector or injection port.
- Inject the medication at the recommended rate of infusion. Use a watch or digital readout to time the injection by dividing the dose over time increments (e.g., 1 mL over 1 minute would be 0.25 mL each 15 seconds). ❶ **Rationale:** *Injecting the drug too rapidly can have a serious adverse reaction.*
- Observe the client closely for adverse reactions. Remove the syringe when all medication is administered.
- Clean the needleless connector or injection port with a new antiseptic swab.
- Attach the second saline syringe, and flush at the same time frame as the medication. **Rationale:** *The saline injection flushes the medication through the catheter. Administering the saline flush with the same time parameters as the medication avoids a sudden bolus of medication and potential adverse effects.*

Existing Line

- Check the medication's compatibility with the primary infusing solution. **Rationale:** *Flushing the primary infusion line will*

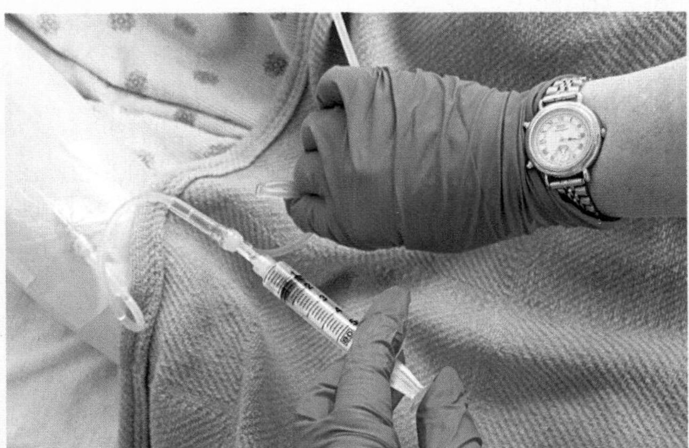

❶ Using a watch with a second hand to time the rate of a medication injection.

Continued on page 898

Administering Intravenous Medications Using IV Push—*continued*

SKILL 35.8

be mandatory before and after administering the medication if there is incompatibility.

- Identify the injection port closest to the client. **Rationale:** *Access points closest to the client allows the medication to reach the central circulation as soon as possible with a minimal amount of flushing required.*
- Clean the port with an antiseptic swab.
- Stop the IV flow by closing the clamp or pinching the tubing above the injection port. ❷
- Insert the medication syringe cannula into the injection port. ❸
- Inject the medication at the ordered rate. Use the watch or digital readout to time the medication administration. **Rationale:** *This ensures safe drug administration because a too rapid injection could be dangerous.*
- Remove the medication syringe. Disinfect the injection port with a new antiseptic swab.

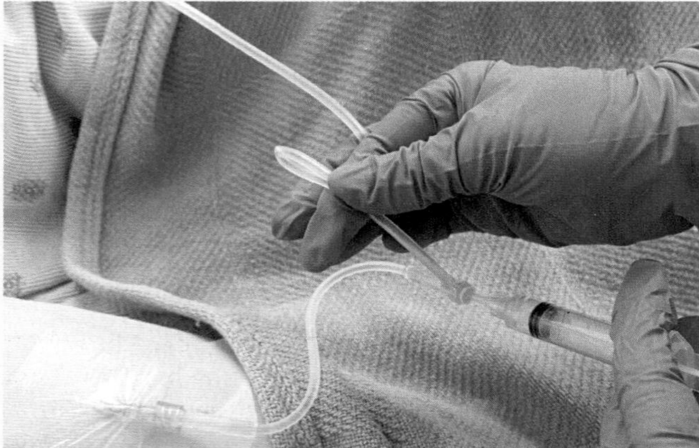

❷ Stopping the IV flow by pinching the tubing above the injection port.

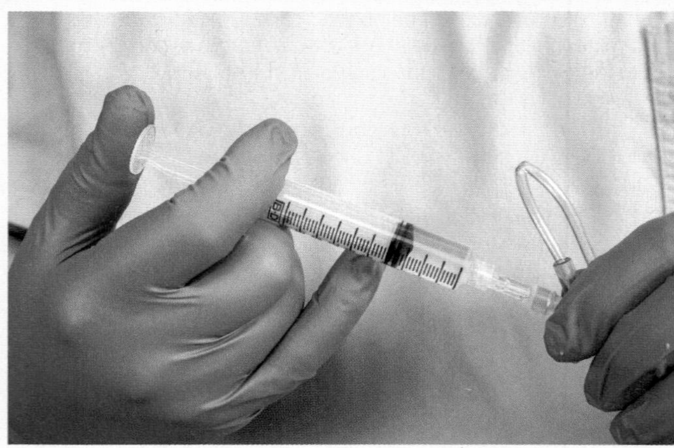

❸ Injecting a medication by IV push to an existing IV using a needleless system.

- Insert the saline syringe into the injection port and flush at the same rate as the drug was injected until the entire drug dose has been cleared from the infusion system.
- Release the clamp or tubing to resume correct flow rate.

8. Dispose of equipment according to agency practice. **Rationale:** *This reduces the spread of microorganisms.*
9. Remove and discard gloves.
   - Perform hand hygiene.
10. Observe the client closely for adverse reactions.
11. Determine agency practice about recommended times for changing the IV lock. Some agencies advocate a change every 48 to 72 hours for peripheral IV access devices.
12. Document all relevant information.
    - Record the date, time, drug, dose, and route; client response; and assessments of infusion or saline lock site if appropriate.

EVALUATION

- Conduct appropriate follow-up such as desired effect of medication, any adverse reactions or side effects, or change in vital signs.
- Reassess status of IV lock site and patency of IV infusion, if running.
- Compare to previous findings, if available.
- Report significant deviations from normal to the primary care provider.

Topical Medications

A topical medication is applied locally to the skin or to mucous membranes in areas such as the eye, external ear canal, nose, vagina, and rectum. Most topical applications used therapeutically are not absorbed well, completely, or predictably when applied to intact skin because the skin's thick outer layer serves as a natural barrier to drug diffusion. This route of absorption through the skin, called **percutaneous**, can be increased if the skin is altered by a laceration, burn, or some other problem. However, if high concentrations or large amounts of a topical medication are applied to the skin, especially if it is done repeatedly, sufficient amounts of the drug can enter the bloodstream to cause systemic effects, usually undesirable ones.

A particular type of topical or dermatologic medication delivery system is the **transdermal patch**. This system administers sustained-action medications (e.g., opioids, nitroglycerin, estrogen, and nicotine) via multilayered films containing the drug and an adhesive layer. The rate of delivery of the drug is controlled and varies with each product (e.g., from 12 hours to 1 week). Generally, the patch is applied to a hairless, clean area of skin that is not subject to excessive movement or wrinkling (i.e., the trunk or lower abdomen). It may also be applied

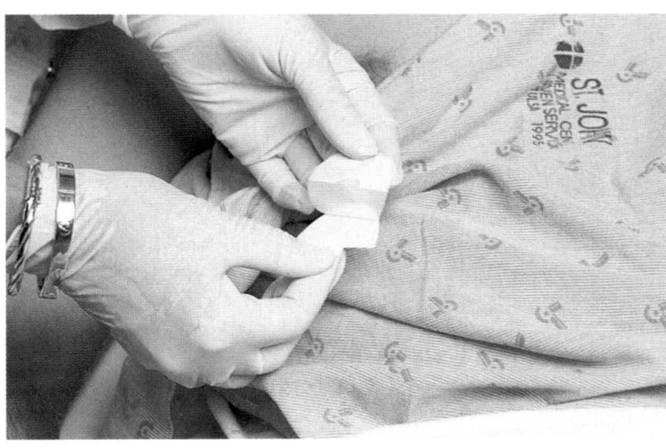

A

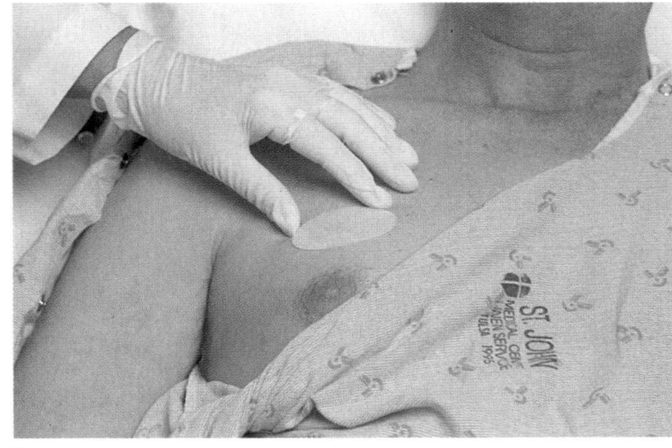

B

Figure 35.51 ■ Transdermal patch administration: *A*, protective coating removed from patch; *B*, patch immediately applied to clean, dry, hairless skin and labeled with date, time, and initials.

on the side, lower back, or buttocks. Patches should not be applied to areas with cuts, burns, or abrasions, or on distal parts of extremities (e.g., the forearms). If hair is likely to interfere with patch adhesion or removal, clipping (not shaving) may be necessary before application (Figure 35.51 ■).

Clinical Alert!

The nurse should wear gloves when applying a transdermal patch to avoid getting any of the medication on his or her skin, which can result in the nurse receiving the effect of the medication.

Reddening of the skin with or without mild local itching or burning, as well as allergic contact dermatitis, may occasionally occur. Upon removal of the patch, any slight reddening of the skin usually disappears within a few hours. All applications should be changed regularly to prevent local irritation, and each successive application should be placed on a different site. The transdermal patch should be dated, timed, and initialed by the nurse before it is applied to the client.

All clients need to be assessed for allergies to the drug and to materials in the patch before the patch is applied. If a client has a transdermal patch on and develops a fever, the medication may be absorbed and metabolize at a faster rate than normal. The client will need to be monitored for changes in effects of the medication.

When transdermal patches are removed, care needs to be taken as to how and where they are discarded. In the home environment, if they are simply discarded into a trash can, pets or children can be exposed to them, causing effects from any drug remaining on the patch. When removed, they should be folded with the medication side to the inside, put into a closed container, and kept out of reach of children and pets.

Clinical Alert!

It is important to keep track of the transdermal patches. Some patches are clear and may be difficult to see and, as a result, be overlooked. If the client is obese, patches may be difficult to find in the skinfolds. Duplication of patches may cause adverse reactions. Remove the old patch and clean the skin thoroughly before applying a new one.

Skin Applications

Topical skin or dermatologic preparations include ointments, pastes, creams, lotions, powders, sprays, and patches. See Table 35.1 earlier in this chapter. See Practice Guidelines for applying topical medications. Before applying a dermatologic preparation, thoroughly clean the area with soap and water and dry it with a patting motion. Skin encrustations harbor microorganisms and these as well as previously applied applications can prevent the medication from coming in contact with the area to be treated. Nurses should wear gloves when administering skin applications and always use surgical asepsis when an open wound is present.

Ophthalmic Medications

Medications may be administered to the eye using irrigations or instillations. An eye irrigation is administered to wash out the conjunctival sac to remove secretions or foreign bodies or to remove chemicals that may injure the eye. Medications for the eyes, called **ophthalmic** medications, are instilled in the form of liquids or ointments. Eyedrops are packaged in monodrip plastic containers that are used to administer the preparation. Ointments are usually supplied in small tubes. All containers must state that the medication is for ophthalmic use. Sterile preparations and sterile technique are indicated. Prescribed liquids are usually diluted, for example, less than 1% strength.

Skill 35.9 illustrates how to administer ophthalmic instillations.

PRACTICE GUIDELINES Applying Skin Preparations

POWDER
Make sure the skin surface is dry. Spread apart any skinfolds, and sprinkle the site until the area is covered with a fine, thin layer of powder. Cover the site with a dressing if ordered.

SUSPENSION-BASED LOTION
Shake the container before use to distribute suspended particles. Put a little lotion on a small gauze dressing or pad, and apply the lotion to the skin by stroking it evenly in the direction of the hair growth.

CREAMS, OINTMENTS, PASTES, AND OIL-BASED LOTIONS
Warm and soften the preparation in gloved hands to make it easier to apply and to prevent chilling (if a large area is to be treated). Smear it evenly over the skin using long strokes that follow the direction of the hair growth. Explain that the skin may feel somewhat greasy after application. Apply a sterile dressing if ordered by the primary care provider.

AEROSOL SPRAY
Shake the container well to mix the contents. Hold the spray container at the recommended distance from the area (usually about 15 to 30 cm [6 to 12 in.] but check the label). Cover the client's face with a towel if the upper chest or neck is to be sprayed. Spray the medication over the specified area.

TRANSDERMAL PATCHES
Select a clean, dry area that is free of hair and matches the manufacturer's recommendations. Remove the patch from its protective covering, holding it without touching the adhesive edges, and apply it by pressing firmly with the palm of the hand for about 10 seconds. Advise the client to avoid using a heating pad over the area to prevent an increase in circulation and the rate of absorption. Remove the patch at the appropriate time, folding it with the sticky, medicated sides together. Dispose of the patch per agency policy. Some patches contain nonvisible metal in their backing. This may cause burning of the skin in the area of the patch. Inform clients to tell MRI personnel that they are wearing a transdermal patch (Kantorovich, 2016).

SKILL 35.9

Administering Ophthalmic Instillations

PURPOSE

- To provide an eye medication the client requires (e.g., an antibiotic) to treat an infection or for other reasons (see specific drug action)

ASSESSMENT

In addition to the assessment performed by the nurse related to the administration of any medication, prior to applying ophthalmic medications, assess:

- Appearance of eye and surrounding structures for lesions, exudate, erythema, or swelling
- The location and nature of any discharge, lacrimation, and swelling of the eyelids or of the lacrimal gland
- Client complaints (e.g., itching, burning pain, blurred vision, and photophobia)
- Client behavior (e.g., squinting, blinking excessively, frowning, or rubbing the eyes).
- Determine if assessment data influence administration of the medication (i.e., is it appropriate to administer the medication or does the medication need to be held and the primary care provider notified?).

PLANNING

Assignment

Due to the need for assessment, interpretation of client status, and use of sterile technique, ophthalmic medication administration is not assigned to AP.

Equipment

- Client's MAR or computer printout
- Clean gloves
- Sterile absorbent sponges soaked in sterile normal saline
- Medication
- Sterile eye dressing (pad) as needed and paper tape to secure it

For irrigation, add:

- Irrigating solution (e.g., normal saline) and irrigating syringe or tubing
- Dry sterile absorbent pads
- Moisture-resistant pad
- Basin (e.g., emesis basin)

IMPLEMENTATION

Preparation

1. Check the MAR.
   - Check the MAR for the drug name, dose, and strength. Also confirm the prescribed frequency of the instillation and which eye is to be treated.
   - Check client allergy status.
   - If the MAR is unclear or pertinent information is missing, compare it with the most recent primary care provider's written order.
   - Report any discrepancies to the charge nurse or primary care provider, as agency policy dictates.
2. Know the reason why the client is receiving the medication, the drug classification, contraindications, usual dose range, side effects, and nursing considerations for administering and evaluating the intended outcomes of the medication.

Performance

1. Compare the label on the medication tube or bottle with the medication record and check the expiration date.
2. If necessary, calculate the medication dosage.
3. Introduce self and explain to the client what you are going to do, why it is necessary, and how to participate. The administration of an ophthalmic medication is not usually painful. Ointments are often soothing to the eye, but some liquid preparations may sting initially. Discuss how the results will be used in planning further care or treatments.
4. Perform hand hygiene and observe other appropriate infection prevention procedures.

Administering Ophthalmic Instillations—*continued*

5. Provide for client privacy.

6. Prepare the client.
- Prior to performing the procedure, verify the client's identity using agency protocol. **Rationale:** *This ensures that the right client receives the right medication*.
- Assist the client to a comfortable position, usually lying.

7. Clean the eyelid and the eyelashes.
- Apply clean gloves.
- Use sterile cotton balls moistened with sterile irrigating solution or sterile normal saline, and wipe from the inner canthus to the outer canthus. **Rationale:** *If not removed, material on the eyelid and lashes can be washed into the eye. Cleaning toward the outer canthus prevents contamination of the other eye and the lacrimal duct*.

8. Administer the eye medication.
- Check the ophthalmic preparation for the name, strength, and number of drops if a liquid is used. **Rationale:** *Checking medication data is essential to prevent a medication error*. Draw the correct number of drops into the shaft of the dropper if a dropper is used. If ointment is used, discard the first bead. **Rationale:** *The first bead of ointment from a tube is considered to be contaminated*.
- Instruct the client to look up to the ceiling. Give the client a dry sterile absorbent pad. **Rationale:** *The client is less likely to blink if looking up. While the client looks up, the cornea is partially protected by the upper eyelid. A pad is needed to press on the nasolacrimal duct after a liquid instillation to prevent systemic absorption or to wipe excess ointment from the eyelashes after an ointment is instilled*.
- Expose the lower conjunctival sac by placing the thumb or fingers of your nondominant hand on the client's cheekbone just below the eye and gently drawing down the skin on the cheek. If the tissues are edematous, handle the tissues carefully to avoid damaging them. **Rationale:** *Placing the fingers on the cheekbone minimizes the possibility of touching the cornea, avoids putting any pressure on the eyeball, and prevents client from blinking or squinting*.
- Holding the medication in the dominant hand, place hand on client's forehead to stabilize hand. Approach the eye from the side and instill the correct number of drops onto the outer third of the lower conjunctival sac. Hold the dropper 1 to 2 cm (0.4 to 0.8 in.) above the sac. ❶ **Rationale:** *The client is less likely to blink if a side approach is used. When instilled into the conjunctival sac, drops will not harm the cornea as they might if dropped directly on it. The dropper must not touch the sac or the cornea*.

or
- Holding the tube above the lower conjunctival sac, squeeze 2 cm (0.8 in.) of ointment from the tube into the lower conjunctival sac from the inner canthus outward. ❷
- Instruct the client to close the eyelids but not to squeeze them shut. **Rationale:** *Closing the eye spreads the medication over the eyeball. Squeezing can injure the eye and push out the medication*.
- For liquid medications, press firmly or have the client press firmly on the nasolacrimal duct for at least 30 seconds. **Rationale:** *Pressing on the nasolacrimal duct prevents the medication from running out of the eye and down the duct, preventing systemic absorption*. ❸

Variation: Irrigation
- Place moisture-resistant absorbent pads under the head, neck, and shoulders. Place an emesis basin next to the eye to catch drainage. Some eye medications cause systemic reactions such as confusion or a decrease in heart rate and

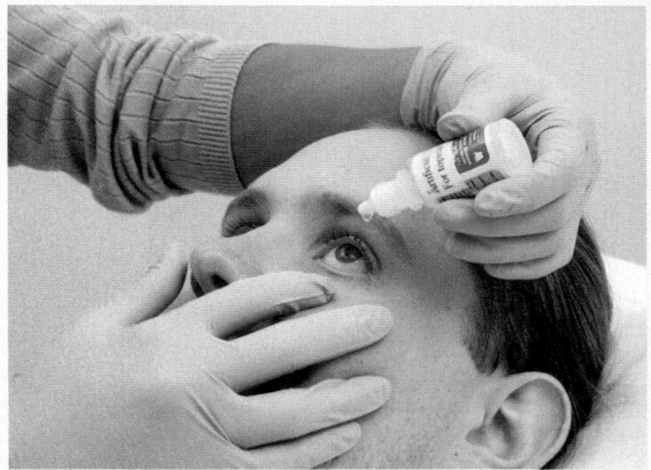

❶ Instilling an eyedrop into the lower conjunctival sac.

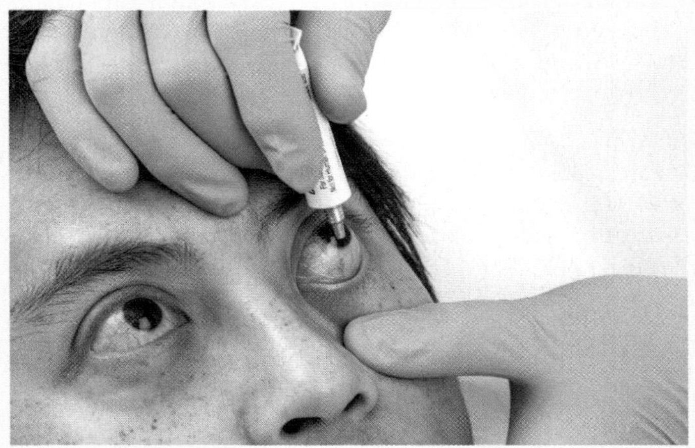

❷ Instilling an eye ointment into the lower conjunctival sac.

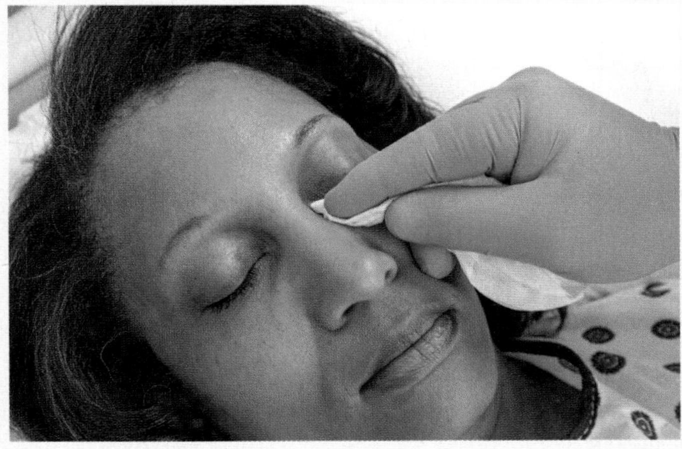

❸ Pressing on the nasolacrimal duct.

Continued on page 902

SKILL 35.9

Administering Ophthalmic Instillations—*continued*

blood pressure if the eyedrops go down the nasolacrimal duct and get into the systemic circulation.

- Expose the lower conjunctival sac. Or, to irrigate in stages, first hold the lower lid down, then hold the upper lid up. Exert pressure on the bony prominences of the cheekbone and beneath the eyebrow when holding the eyelids. **Rationale:** *Separating the lids prevents reflex blinking. Exerting pressure on the bony prominences minimizes the possibility of pressing the eyeball and causing discomfort.*
- Fill and hold the eye irrigator about 2.5 cm (1 in.) above the eye. **Rationale:** *At this height the pressure of the solution will not damage the eye tissue, and the irrigator will not touch the eye.*
- Irrigate the eye, directing the solution onto the lower conjunctival sac and from the inner canthus to the outer canthus. **Rationale:** *Directing the solution in this way prevents possible injury to the cornea and prevents fluid and contaminants from flowing down the nasolacrimal duct.*
- Irrigate until the solution leaving the eye is clear (no discharge is present) or until all the solution has been used.
- Instruct the client to close and move the eye periodically. **Rationale:** *Eye closure and movement help to move secretions from the upper to the lower conjunctival sac.*

9. Clean and dry the eyelids as needed. Wipe the eyelids gently from the inner to the outer canthus to collect excess medication.
10. Remove and discard gloves.
    - Perform hand hygiene.
11. Apply an eye pad if needed, and secure it with paper eye tape.
12. Assess the client's response immediately after the instillation or irrigation and again after the medication should have acted.
13. Document all relevant assessments and interventions. Include the name of the drug or irrigating solution, the strength, the number of drops if a liquid medication, the time, and the response of the client.

EVALUATION

- Perform follow-up based on findings of the effectiveness of the administration or outcomes that deviated from expected or normal for the client. Compare findings to previous data if available.
- Report significant deviations from normal to the primary care provider.

LIFESPAN CONSIDERATIONS Administering Ophthalmic Medications

INFANTS AND CHILDREN

- Explain the technique to the parents of an infant or child.
- For a young child or infant, obtain assistance to immobilize the arms and head. The parent may hold the infant or young child. **Rationale:** *This prevents accidental injury during medication administration.*
- For a young child, use a doll to demonstrate the procedure. **Rationale:** *This facilitates cooperation and decreases anxiety.*
- Drops may be tolerated better by children than ointment since they are less likely to cause blurred vision.
- An IV bag and tubing may be used to deliver irrigating fluid to the eye.

Otic Medications

Instillations or irrigations of the external auditory canal are referred to as **otic** and are generally carried out for cleaning purposes. Sometimes applications of heat and antiseptic solutions are prescribed. Irrigations performed in a hospital require aseptic technique so that microorganisms will not be introduced into the ear. Sterile technique is used if the eardrum is perforated. The position of the external auditory canal varies with age, which affects the administration of otic medications. For children under 3 years of age, the pinna is gently drawn down and back. For ages 4 to adulthood, the pinna is gently lifted upward and backward to straighten the ear canal.

Skill 35.10 explains how to administer otic instillations.

SKILL 35.10

Administering Otic Instillations

PURPOSE

- To soften earwax so that it can be readily removed at a later time
- To provide local therapy to reduce inflammation, destroy infective organisms in the external ear canal, or both
- To relieve pain

ASSESSMENT

In addition to the assessment performed by the nurse related to the administration of any medications, prior to applying otic medications, assess:

- Appearance of the pinna of the ear and meatus for signs of redness and abrasions
- Type and amount of any discharge.
- Determine if assessment data influence administration of the medication (i.e., is it appropriate to administer the medication or does the medication need to be held and the primary care provider notified?).

Administering Otic Instillations—*continued*

SKILL 35.10

PLANNING

Assignment

Due to the need for assessment, interpretation of client status, and use of sterile technique, otic medication administration is not assigned to AP.

Equipment

- Client's MAR or computer printout
- Clean gloves
- Clean washcloth or gauze
- Correct medication bottle with a dropper
- Flexible rubber tip (optional) for the end of the dropper, which prevents injury from sudden motion, for example, by a disoriented client
- Cotton ball

For irrigation, add:

- Moisture-resistant pad
- Basin (e.g., emesis basin)
- Irrigating solution at the appropriate temperature, about 500 mL (16 oz) or as ordered. **Rationale:** *A solution that is not at body temperature may induce dizziness.*
- Container for the irrigating solution
- Syringe (rubber bulb or Asepto syringe is frequently used)

IMPLEMENTATION

Preparation

1. Check the MAR.
   - Check the MAR for the drug name, strength, number of drops, and prescribed frequency.
   - Check client allergy status.
   - If the MAR is unclear or pertinent information is missing, compare it with the most recent primary care provider's written order.
   - Report any discrepancies to the charge nurse or primary care provider, as agency policy dictates.
2. Know the reason why the client is receiving the medication, the drug classification, contraindications, usual dose range, side effects, and nursing considerations for administering and evaluating the intended outcomes of the medication.

Performance

1. Compare the label on the medication container with the medication record and check the expiration date.
2. If necessary, calculate the medication dosage.
3. Explain to the client what you are going to do, why it is necessary, and how to participate. The administration of an otic medication is not usually painful. Discuss how the results will be used in planning further care or treatments.
4. Perform hand hygiene and observe other appropriate infection prevention procedures.
5. Provide for client privacy.
6. Prepare the client.
   - Prior to performing the procedure, introduce self and verify the client's identity using agency protocol. **Rationale:** *This ensures that the right client receives the right medication.*
   - Assist the client to a comfortable position for eardrop administration, lying with the ear being treated uppermost.
7. Clean the pinna of the ear and the meatus of the ear canal.
   - Apply gloves if infection is suspected.
   - Use a clean washcloth or gauze to wipe the pinna and auditory meatus. **Rationale:** *This removes any discharge present before the instillation so that it will not be washed into the ear canal.*
8. Administer the ear medication.
   - Warm the medication container in your hand, or place it in warm water for a short time. **Rationale:** *This promotes client comfort and prevents nerve stimulation and pain.*
   - Partially fill the ear dropper with medication.
   - Straighten the auditory canal. Pull the pinna upward and backward for clients over 4 years of age. **Rationale:** *The auditory canal is straightened so that the solution can flow the entire length of the canal.* ❶

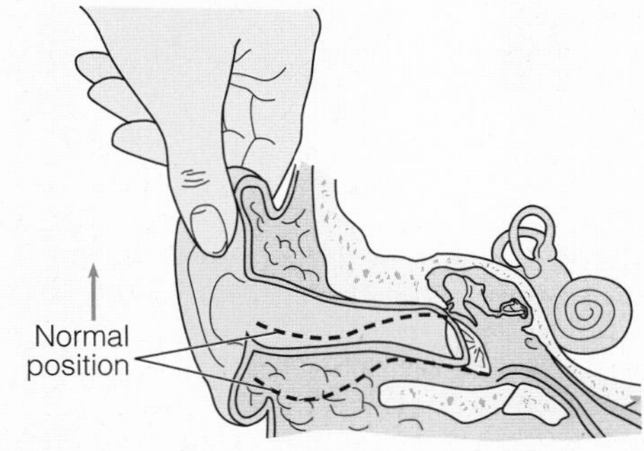

❶ Straightening the adult ear canal by pulling the pinna upward and backward.

   - Instill the correct number of drops along the side of the ear canal. ❷
   - Press gently but firmly a few times on the tragus of the ear (the cartilaginous projection in front of the exterior meatus of the ear). **Rationale:** *Pressing on the tragus assists the flow of medication into the ear canal.*
   - Ask the client to remain in the side-lying position for about 5 minutes. **Rationale:** *This prevents the drops from escaping and allows the medication to reach all sides of the canal cavity.*
   - Insert a small piece of cotton loosely at the meatus of the auditory canal for 15 to 20 minutes. Do not press it into the canal. **Rationale:** *The cotton helps retain the medication*

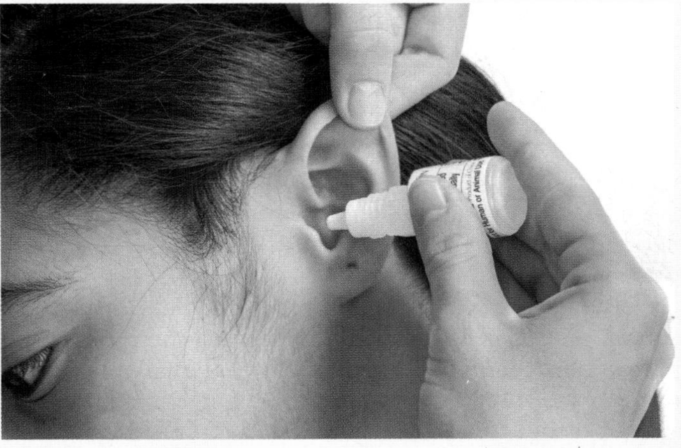

❷ Instilling eardrops.

Continued on page 904

SKILL 35.10

Administering Otic Instillations—*continued*

when the client is up. If pressed tightly into the canal, the cotton would interfere with the action of the drug and the outward movement of normal secretions.

Variation: Ear Irrigation

- Explain that the client may experience a feeling of fullness, warmth, and, occasionally, discomfort when the fluid comes in contact with the tympanic membrane.
- Assist the client to a sitting or lying position with head tilted toward the affected ear. **Rationale:** *The solution can then flow from the ear canal to a basin.* ❸
- Place the moisture-resistant pad around the client's shoulder under the ear to be irrigated, and place the basin under the ear to be irrigated.
- Fill the syringe with solution.

or

- Hang up the irrigating container, and run solution through the tubing and the nozzle. **Rationale:** *Solution is run through the tubing and nozzle to remove air from the tubing and nozzle.*
- Straighten the ear canal.
- Insert the tip of the syringe into the auditory meatus, and direct the solution gently upward against the top of the canal. **Rationale:** *The solution will flow around the entire canal and out at the bottom. The solution is instilled gently because strong pressure from the fluid can cause discomfort and damage the tympanic membrane.*
- Continue instilling the fluid until all the solution is used or until the canal is cleaned, depending on the purpose of the irrigation. Take care not to block the outward flow of the solution with the syringe.
- Assist the client to a side-lying position on the affected side. **Rationale:** *Lying with the affected side down helps drain the excess fluid by gravity.*

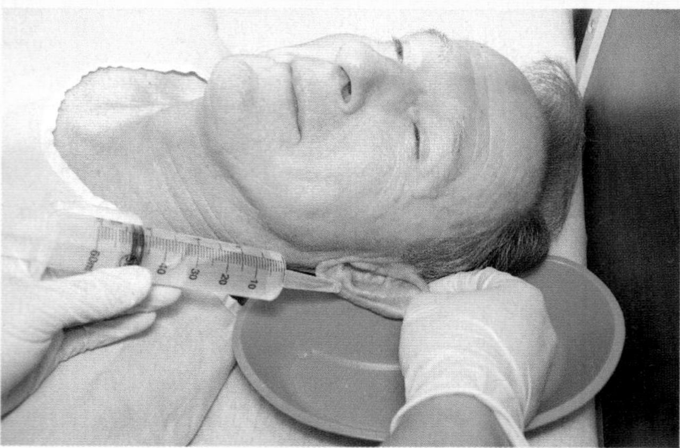

❸ Ear irrigation.

- Place a cotton ball in the auditory meatus to absorb the excess fluid.

9. Remove and discard gloves.
   - Perform hand hygiene.
10. Assess the client's response and the character and amount of discharge, appearance of the canal, discomfort, and so on, immediately after the instillation and again when the medication is expected to act. Inspect the cotton ball for any drainage.
11. Document all nursing assessments and interventions relative to the procedure. Include the name of the drug or irrigating solution, the strength, the number of drops if a liquid medication, the time, and the response of the client.

EVALUATION

- Perform follow-up based on findings of the effectiveness of the administration or outcomes that deviated from expected or normal for the client. Compare findings to previous data if available.
- Report significant deviations from normal to the primary care provider.

LIFESPAN CONSIDERATIONS Administering Otic Medications

INFANTS AND CHILDREN

- Obtain assistance to immobilize an infant or young child. This prevents accidental injury due to sudden movement during the procedure.
- Because in infants and children under 3 years of age the ear canal is directed upward, to administer medication, gently pull the pinna down and back. For a child *older* than 3 years of age, pull the pinna upward and backward.

Nasal Medications

Nasal instillations (nose drops and sprays) usually are instilled for their astringent effect (to shrink swollen mucous membranes), to loosen secretions and facilitate drainage, or to treat infections of the nasal cavity or sinuses. Nasal decongestants are the most common nasal instillations. Many of these products are available without a prescription. Clients need to be taught to use these agents with caution. Chronic use of nasal decongestants may lead to a rebound effect, that is, an increase in nasal congestion. If excess decongestant solution is swallowed, serious systemic effects may also develop, especially in children. Saline drops are safer as a decongestant for children.

Usually clients self-administer sprays. It is suggested that clients blow their noses prior to administration of nasal sprays unless contraindicated. In the seated position with the head tilted back, the client holds the tip of the container just inside the nares and inhales as the spray enters the nasal passages. For clients who use nasal sprays repeatedly, the nares need to be assessed for irritation. In children, nasal sprays are given with the head in an upright position to prevent excess spray from being swallowed.

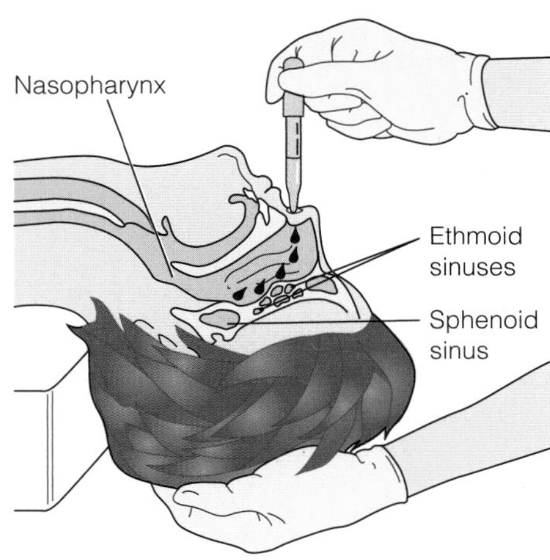

Figure 35.52 ■ Position of the head to instill drops into the ethmoid and sphenoid sinuses.

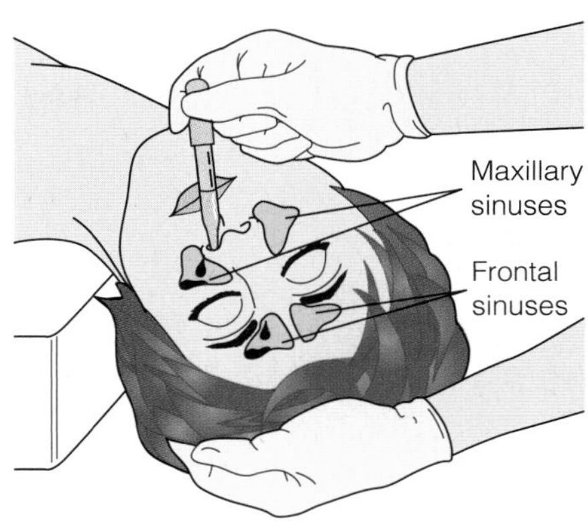

Figure 35.53 ■ Position of the head to instill drops into the maxillary and frontal sinuses.

Nasal drops may be used to treat sinus infections. Clients need to learn ways to position themselves to effectively treat the affected sinus:

- To treat the ethmoid and sphenoid sinuses, instruct the client to lie back with the head over the edge of the bed or a pillow under the shoulders so that the head is tipped backward (Figure 35.52 ■).
- To treat the maxillary and frontal sinuses, instruct the client to assume the same back-lying position, with the head turned toward the side to be treated (Figure 35.53 ■). The client should also be instructed to (a) breathe through the mouth to prevent aspiration of medication into the trachea and bronchi, (b) remain in a back-lying position for at least 1 minute so that the solution will come into contact with the entire nasal surface, and (c) avoid blowing the nose for several minutes.

Vaginal Medications

Vaginal medications are inserted as creams, jellies, foams, or suppositories to treat infection or to relieve vaginal discomfort (e.g., itching or pain). Medical aseptic technique is usually used. Vaginal creams, jellies, and foams are applied by using a tubular applicator with a plunger. Suppositories are inserted with the index finger of a gloved hand. Suppositories are designed to melt at body temperature, so they are generally stored in the refrigerator to keep them firm for insertion. See Skill 35.11 for administering vaginal instillations.

A vaginal irrigation (douche) is the washing of the vagina by a liquid at a low pressure. Vaginal irrigations are not necessary for ordinary female hygiene and are used to prevent infection by applying an antimicrobial solution that discourages the growth of microorganisms, to remove an offensive or irritating discharge, and to reduce inflammation or prevent hemorrhage by the application of heat or cold. In hospitals, sterile supplies and equipment are used; in a home, sterility is not usually necessary because people are accustomed to the microorganisms in their environments. Sterile technique, however, is indicated if there is an open wound.

Administering Vaginal Instillations

SKILL 35.11

PURPOSES

- To treat or prevent infection
- To reduce inflammation
- To relieve vaginal discomfort

ASSESSMENT

In addition to the assessment performed by the nurse related to the administration of any medications, prior to applying vaginal medications, assess:

- The vaginal orifice for inflammation; amount, character, and odor of vaginal discharge
- For complaints of vaginal discomfort (e.g., burning or itching).
- Determine if assessment data influence administration of the medication (i.e., is it appropriate to administer the medication or does the medication need to be held and the primary care provider notified?).

Continued on page 906

Administering Vaginal Instillations—*continued*

PLANNING

Assignment

Due to the need for assessments and interpretation of client status, vaginal medication administration is not assigned to AP.

Equipment

- Drape
- Correct vaginal suppository or cream
- Applicator for vaginal cream
- Clean gloves
- Lubricant for a suppository
- Disposable towel
- Clean perineal pad

For an irrigation, add:

- Moisture-proof pad
- Vaginal irrigation set (these are often disposable) containing a nozzle, tubing and a clamp, and a container for the solution
- Irrigating solution (It is recommended that the solution be warmed to a temperature of 37.8°C to 43.3°C [100°F to 110°F] if not specified, to minimize discomfort caused by cooler solutions.)

IMPLEMENTATION

Preparation

1. Check the MAR.
   - Check the MAR for the drug name, strength, and prescribed frequency.
   - Check client allergy status.
   - If the MAR is unclear or pertinent information is missing, compare it with the most recent primary care provider's written order.
   - Report any discrepancies to the charge nurse or primary care provider, as agency policy dictates.
2. Know the reason why the client is receiving the medication, the drug classification, contraindications, usual dose range, side effects, and nursing considerations for administering and evaluating the intended outcomes of the medication.

Performance

1. Compare the label on the medication container with the medication record and check the expiration date.
2. If necessary, calculate the medication dosage.
3. Explain to the client what you are going to do, why it is necessary, and how to participate. Explain to the client that a vaginal instillation is normally a painless procedure, and in fact may bring relief from itching and burning if an infection is present. Many people feel embarrassed about this procedure, and some may prefer to perform the procedure themselves if instruction is provided. Discuss how the results will be used in planning further care or treatments.
4. Perform hand hygiene and observe other appropriate infection prevention procedures.
5. Provide for client privacy.
6. Prepare the client.
   - Prior to performing the procedure, introduce self and verify the client's identity using agency protocol. **Rationale:** *This ensures that the right client receives the right medication.*
   - Ask the client to void. **Rationale:** *If the bladder is empty, the client will have less discomfort during the treatment, and the possibility of injuring the vaginal lining is decreased.*
   - Assist the client to a back-lying position with the knees flexed and the hips rotated laterally.
   - Drape the client appropriately so that only the perineal area is exposed.
7. Prepare the equipment.
   - Unwrap the suppository, and place it on the opened wrapper.

   or
   - Fill the applicator with the prescribed cream, jelly, or foam. Directions are provided with the manufacturer's applicator.
8. Assess and clean the perineal area.
   - Apply gloves. **Rationale:** *Gloves prevent contamination of the nurse's hands from vaginal and perineal microorganisms.*
   - Inspect the vaginal orifice, note any odor of discharge from the vagina, and ask about any vaginal discomfort.
   - Provide perineal care to remove microorganisms. **Rationale:** *This decreases the chance of moving microorganisms into the vagina.*
9. Administer the vaginal suppository, cream, foam, jelly, or irrigation.

Suppository

- Lubricate the rounded (smooth) end of the suppository, which is inserted first. **Rationale:** *Lubrication facilitates insertion.*
- Lubricate your gloved index finger.
- Expose the vaginal orifice by separating the labia with your nondominant hand.
- Insert the suppository about 8 to 10 cm (3 to 4 in.) along the posterior wall of the vagina, or as far as it will go. **Rationale:** *The posterior wall of the vagina is about 2.5 cm (1 in.) longer than the anterior wall because the cervix protrudes into the uppermost portion of the anterior wall.* ❶
- Ask the client to remain lying in the supine position for 5 to 10 minutes following insertion. The hips may also be elevated on a pillow. **Rationale:** *This position allows the medication to flow into the posterior fornix after it has melted.*

Vaginal Cream, Jelly, or Foam

- Gently insert the applicator about 5 cm (2 in.).
- Slowly push the plunger until the applicator is empty. ❷
- Remove the applicator and place it on the towel. **Rationale:** *The applicator is placed on the towel to prevent the spread of microorganisms.*
- Discard the applicator if disposable or clean it according to the manufacturer's directions.
- Ask the client to remain lying in the supine position for 5 to 10 minutes following the insertion.

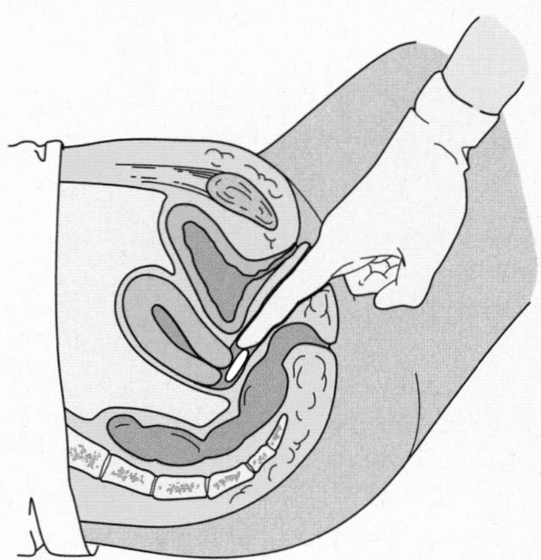

❶ Instilling a vaginal suppository.

Administering Vaginal Instillations—*continued*

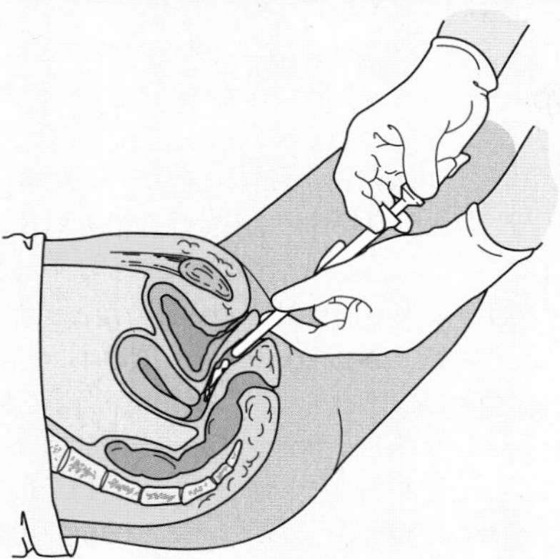

❷ Using an applicator to instill a vaginal cream.

Irrigation

- Place the client on a bedpan.
- Clamp the tubing. Hold the irrigating container about 30 cm (12 in.) above the vagina. **Rationale:** *At this height, the pressure of the solution should not be great enough to injure the vaginal lining.*
- Run fluid through the tubing and nozzle into the bedpan. **Rationale:** *Fluid is run through the tubing and nozzle to remove air and to moisten the nozzle.*
- Insert the nozzle carefully into the vagina. Direct the nozzle toward the sacrum, following the direction of the vagina.
- Insert the nozzle about 7 to 10 cm (3 to 4 in.), start the flow, and rotate the nozzle several times. **Rationale:** *Rotating the nozzle irrigates all parts of the vagina.*
- Use all of the irrigating solution, permitting it to flow out freely into the bedpan.
- Remove the nozzle from the vagina.
- Assist the client to a sitting position on the bedpan. **Rationale:** *Sitting on the bedpan will help drain the remaining fluid by gravity.*

10. Ensure client comfort.
- Dry the perineum with tissues as required.
- Apply a clean perineal pad if there is excessive drainage.

11. Remove and discard gloves.
- Perform hand hygiene.

12. Document all nursing assessments and interventions relative to the skill. Include the name of the drug or irrigating solution, the strength, the time, and the response of the client.

EVALUATION

- Perform follow-up based on findings of the effectiveness of the administration or outcomes that deviated from expected or normal for the client. Compare findings to previous data if available.
- Report significant deviations from normal to the primary care provider.

LIFESPAN CONSIDERATIONS Administering Rectal Medications

INFANTS AND CHILDREN

- Obtain assistance to immobilize an infant or young child. This prevents accidental injury due to sudden movement during the procedure.
- For a child under 3 years of age, the nurse should use the gloved fifth finger for insertion. After this age, the index finger can usually be used.
- For a child or infant, insert a suppository 5 cm (2 in.) or less.

Rectal Medications

Insertion of medications into the rectum in the form of suppositories is a frequent practice. Rectal administration is a convenient and safe method of giving certain medications. Advantages include the following:

- It avoids irritation of the upper GI tract in clients who encounter this problem (e.g., in clients who are nauseated or vomiting).
- It is advantageous when the medication has an objectionable taste or odor.
- The drug is released at a slow but steady rate.
- Rectal suppositories are thought to provide higher bloodstream levels (titers) of medication because the venous blood from the lower rectum is not transported through the liver.

It is important to assess:

- Any contraindications to the rectal route (e.g., recent rectal surgery or rectal pathology, such as bleeding).
- Any cardiac contraindications (e.g., arrhythmias, recent MI). Insertion of a rectal suppository may cause unintended vagus nerve stimulation and may trigger an arrhythmia such as bradycardia.

To insert a rectal suppository:

- Assist the client to a left lateral or left Sims' position, with the upper leg flexed.
- Fold back the top bedclothes to expose the buttocks.
- Put a glove on the hand used to insert the suppository.
- Unwrap the suppository and lubricate the smooth rounded end, or see the manufacturer's instructions. The rounded end is usually inserted first and lubricant reduces irritation of the mucosa.
- Lubricate the gloved index finger.
- Encourage the client to relax by breathing through the mouth. This usually relaxes the external anal sphincter.
- Insert the suppository gently into the anal canal, rounded end first (or according to manufacturer's instructions), along the rectal wall using the gloved index finger. For an adult, insert the suppository beyond the internal sphincter (i.e., 10 cm [4 in.]) (Figure 35.54 ■).

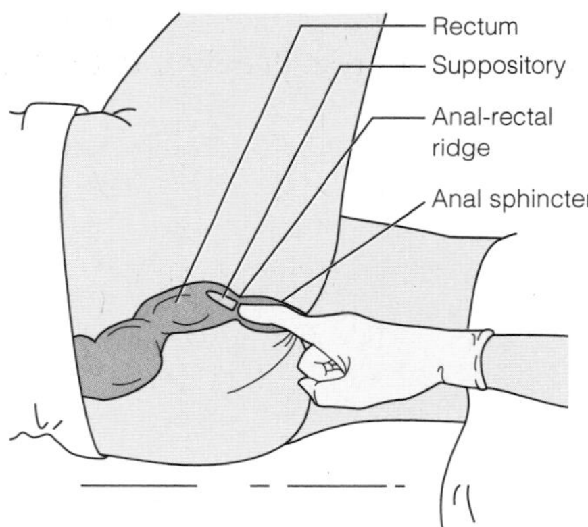

Figure 35.54 ■ Inserting a rectal suppository beyond the internal sphincter and along the rectal wall.

- Avoid embedding the suppository in feces in order for the suppository to be absorbed effectively.
- Press the client's buttocks together for a few minutes.
- Ask the client to remain in the left lateral or supine position for at least 5 minutes to help retain the suppository. The suppository should be retained for varying lengths of time according to the manufacturer's instructions.

Inhaled Medications

Medications are delivered to the respiratory system by aerosol therapy. An aerosol is a suspension of minute liquid droplets or fine solid particles suspended in a gas (Adams et al., 2020, p. 618). An advantage of aerosol therapy is that it delivers the pulmonary medication to its immediate site of action. These same drugs, however, have the potential to produce systemic effects because there is some drug absorption across the pulmonary capillaries.

Several devices are used to deliver medications via the inhalation route. A **nebulizer** is a small machine that vaporizes a liquid medication into a fine mist that is inhaled, using a face mask or handheld device (Figure 35.55*A* ■). If the drug is a solid, it may be administered using a **dry powder inhaler (DPI)**. A capsule is inserted into the center of the chamber of the inhalation device. A piercing device punctures the capsule, which allows the medication to be released upon inhalation by the client (Figure 35.55*B*).

The **metered-dose inhaler (MDI)** is the most common type of device used to deliver respiratory drugs (Figure 35.55*C*). It is a pressurized container of medication that can be used by the client to release the medication through a mouthpiece. The force with which the air moves through the nebulizer causes the large particles of medicated solution to break up into finer particles, forming a mist or fine spray. MDIs can deliver accurate doses, provide for target

A

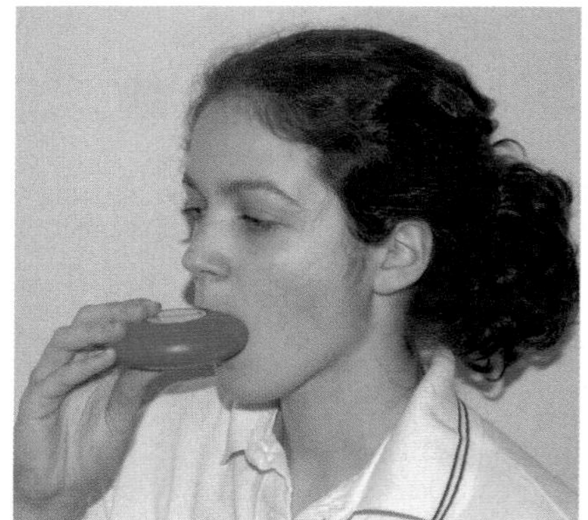

B

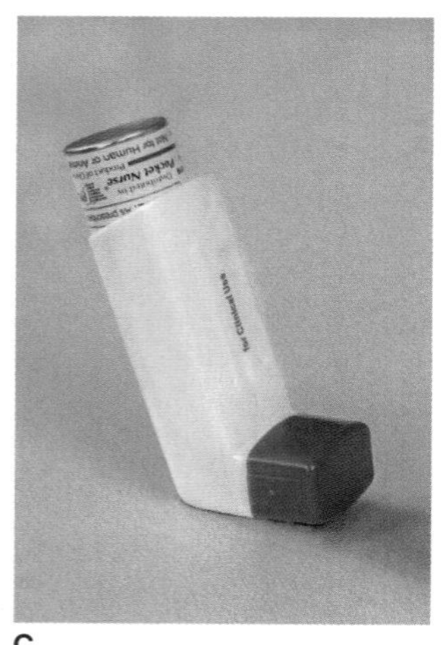

C

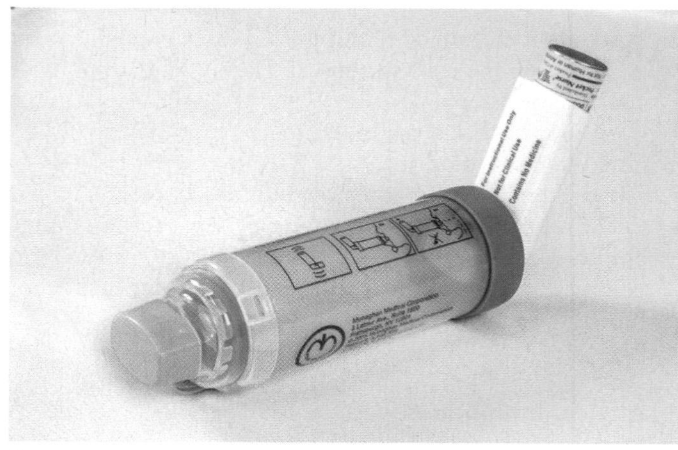

D

Figure 35.55 ■ *A*, Nebulizer with face mask; *B*, *Dry-powder inhaler (DPI)*; *C*, Metered-dose inhaler (MDI); *D*, MDI with spacer.

action at the needed sites, and sustain less systemic effects than medication delivered by other routes.

To ensure correct delivery of the prescribed medication by MDIs, nurses need to instruct clients to use aerosol inhalers correctly. The client compresses the medication canister by hand to release medication through a mouthpiece. An extender or spacer may be attached to the mouthpiece to facilitate medication absorption for better results (Figure 35.55*D*). Spacers are holding chambers into which the medication is fired and from which the client inhales, so that the dose is not lost by exhalation. The main advantage is that it decreases the problem that some clients have in coordinating the actuating (releasing) of the medication and the inhaling of the medication. Client Teaching provides instructions for clients about using an MDI.

QSEN Patient-Centered Care: Metered-Dose Inhalers

When teaching clients and family in the home setting, the nurse should include the following information:

- Review instructions and periodically assess the client's techniques for using an inhaler spacer or chamber correctly. Research shows that these devices assist in delivering the medication deeply into the lungs rather than only to the oropharynx.
- How to disinfect the MDI mouthpieces weekly by soaking for 20 minutes in 1 pint of water with 2 ounces of vinegar added.
- Teach clients how to determine the amount of medication remaining in a metered-dose inhaler canister:
    - Calculate the number of days' doses in an MDI canister. Divide the number of doses (puffs) in the canister (on the label) by the number of puffs taken per day. The previous method of floating the canister in water is not considered accurate because some of the propellant may remain (even after the medication is gone), which leads the client to incorrectly believe he or she is receiving medication.

Clinical Alert!

It is important for the nurse to assess if the client is using an MDI correctly. A client's ability to use an MDI correctly can decrease over time.

LIFESPAN CONSIDERATIONS Administering Metered-Dose Inhalers and Nebulizers

CHILDREN

- Spacers hold a medication in suspension and provide the child an opportunity to take several deep breaths in order to inhale all of the medication.
- A mask used for nebulizer treatments allows the child to breathe naturally. Some infants and children may be frightened or uncomfortable with the mask and become resistant. Use a doll or stuffed animal to demonstrate its use, and allow them to play with the equipment before putting it in place. Having the child sit in the parent's lap during the procedure can help the child relax and be more cooperative.

CLIENT TEACHING Using a Metered-Dose Inhaler

- Ensure that the canister is firmly and fully inserted into the inhaler.
- Remove the mouthpiece cap. Holding the inhaler upright, shake the inhaler vigorously for 3 to 5 seconds to mix the medication evenly.
- Exhale comfortably (as in a normal full breath).
- Hold the canister upside down.
    a. Hold the MDI 2 to 4 cm (1 to 2 in.) from the open mouth (Figure 35.56 ■).

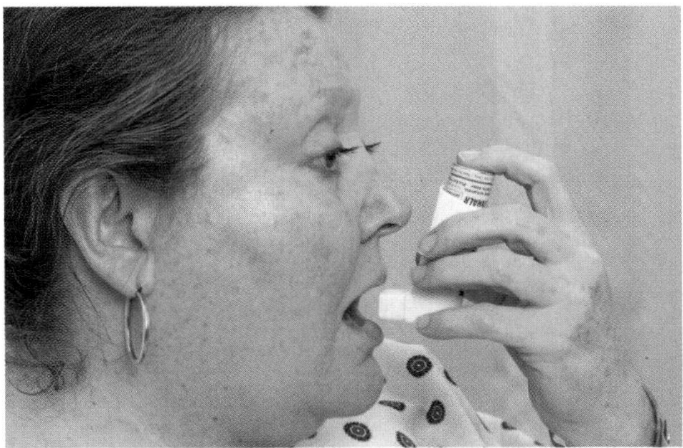

Figure 35.56 ■ Inhaler positioned 2 to 4 cm (1 to 2 in.) away from the open mouth.

or

b. Put the mouthpiece far enough into the mouth with its opening toward the throat such that the lips can tightly close around the mouthpiece (Figure 35.57 ■). An MDI with a spacer or extender is always placed in the mouth (Figure 35.58 ■).

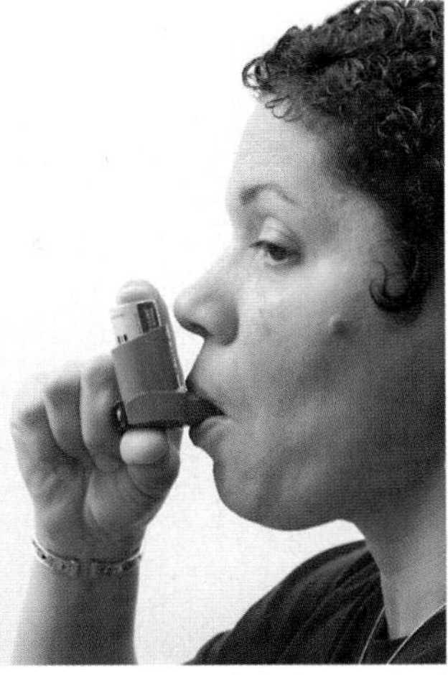

Figure 35.57 ■ Placing an MDI in mouth with lips sealed around the mouthpiece.

Continued on page 910

CLIENT TEACHING **Using a Metered-Dose Inhaler—*continued***

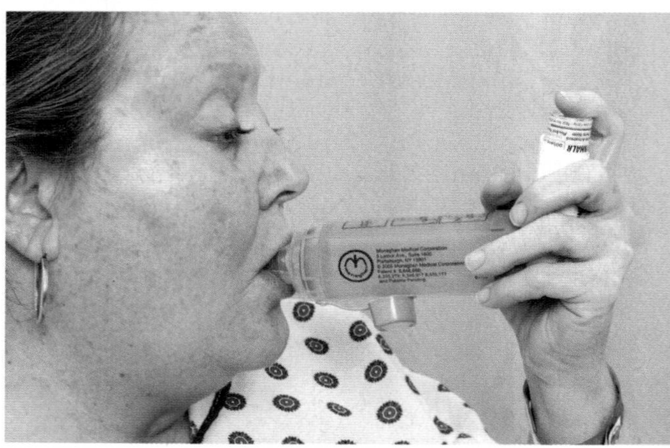

Figure 35.58 ■ An extender spacer attached to a mouthpiece placed in the mouth.

ADMINISTERING THE MEDICATION

- Press down *once* on the MDI canister (which releases the dose) and inhale slowly (for 3 to 5 seconds) and deeply through the mouth.
- Hold your breath for 10 seconds or as long as possible. **Rationale:** *This allows the aerosol to reach deeper airways*.
- Remove the inhaler from or away from the mouth.
- Exhale slowly through *pursed* lips. **Rationale:** *Controlled exhalation keeps the small airways open during exhalation*.
- Repeat the inhalation if ordered. Wait 20 to 30 seconds between inhalations of bronchodilator medications. **Rationale:** *The first inhalation has a chance to work and the subsequent dose reaches deeper into the lungs*.
- Following use of the inhaler, rinse mouth with tap water to remove any remaining medication and reduce irritation and of infection.
- Clean the MDI mouthpiece after each use. Use mild soap and water, rinse it, and let it air dry before replacing it on the device.
- Store the canister at room temperature. Avoid extremes of temperature.
- Report adverse reactions such as restlessness, palpitations, nervousness, or rash to the primary care provider.
- Many MDIs contain steroids for an anti-inflammatory effect. Prolonged use increases the risk of fungal infections in the mouth, indicating a need for attentive mouth care.

If two inhalers are to be used, the bronchodilator medication (which opens the airways) should be given prior to other medications. A mnemonic to help remember this is *B before C* (i.e., bronchodilator before corticosteroid).

Inhaled steroids may not be correctly used by clients because they do not associate these medications with immediate symptom relief. The bronchodilators act to open the airways in the short term. However, it is the inhaled steroids that keep airway inflammation under control.

EVIDENCE-BASED PRACTICE

Evidence-Based Practice

What is the Knowledge of Healthcare Providers About Different Inhaler Devices?

The number of inhaled medications given via MDI or DPI has increased and these devices have different performance requirements for the client to achieve optimal drug delivery. Many clients with asthma and COPD have recurrent exacerbations and one of the most common reasons is related to difficulty or confusion regarding how to use the inhaler properly. Healthcare professionals have a key role in teaching proper inhaler techniques to their clients. However, companies are constantly changing designs and techniques for the different inhaler devices, making it difficult for healthcare professionals to keep up with the latest information.

The literature reflects numerous studies documenting that physicians, nurses, community pharmacists, and clients lacked knowledge of how to use inhaler devices. Alismail et al. (2016) initiated a study when they observed that most of the clients in their pulmonary care clinic were not using their inhalers correctly. The purpose of their study was to investigate and compare the knowledge retention of different healthcare professionals about several different inhalation devices.

The participants included respiratory technicians (RTs), pharmacists, registered nurses (RNs), and physicians. To be a participant, the individual had to either regularly prescribe inhalation devices or educate clients about the correct use of inhalation devices. Each participant took part in two assessments: a baseline assessment and a follow-up. Five steps were included in the study: First the participants were given four different placebo inhalation devices and instructed to demonstrate the steps they would use if they were going to use the inhaler themselves. A research assistant observed the participants and used a checklist to record how many steps were performed correctly. For the second step, the participants responded to a five-question survey about the proper use of each inhaler device. In the third step, the participants watched a video explaining the correct use of each inhaler device. The answers to the survey and the practical examination were explained to the participants in the fourth step. The final step was a follow-up at 3 months after the baseline and included the same practical examination and written questionnaire as the baseline assessment.

The results showed that the baseline practical and written scores were significantly different across groups. The mean scores of RTs were significantly higher compared with RNs and physicians. The mean score of pharmacists was higher than RNs and physicians but not significantly. The practical score of all the groups improved after the intervention (i.e., the video), but the difference was not significant across the groups. There were no significant differences in the written score after the intervention.

Implications

This research reinforced other studies that also highlighted the importance of healthcare training for different inhalation devices. Proper education and refresher courses for both healthcare professionals and clients is important for improving client performance with their inhalation devices.

Irrigations

An **irrigation** (**lavage**) is the washing out of a body cavity by a stream of water or other fluid that may or may not be medicated. Irrigation is performed for one or more of the following reasons:

- To clean the area, that is, to remove a foreign object or excessive secretions or discharge
- To apply heat or cold
- To apply a medication, such as an antiseptic
- To reduce inflammation
- To relieve discomfort.

Surgical asepsis is required when there is a break in the skin (e.g., in a wound irrigation) or whenever a sterile body cavity (e.g., the bladder) is entered. Some irrigations (e.g., a vaginal, rectal, or gastric irrigation) are often safely conducted using medical asepsis.

Different kinds of syringes are used for irrigations. The most common are the Asepto and the rubber bulb (Figure 35.59 ■). The syringes are often calibrated, permitting the nurse to determine the amount of irrigant being delivered at any given time.

The Asepto syringe is a plastic (or glass) syringe with a rubber bulb. Squeezing the air out of the bulb produces negative pressure, and fluid can be sucked into the syringe. When the bulb is squeezed again, the fluid is ejected from the syringe. Asepto syringes come in several sizes ranging from 30 mL (1 oz) to 120 mL (4 oz).

The rubber bulb syringe is often used for irrigating the ears. Like the Asepto syringe, the rubber bulb syringe comes in a range of sizes.

Other syringes that can be used are the piston syringe, which has a tip to which a catheter can be attached, and the Pomeroy syringe. Catheters may be used for deep-wound irrigations and for some types of bladder irrigations. The Pomeroy syringe is a metal syringe commonly used for ear irrigations. A shield near the tip prevents the solution from spraying outward. Plastic squeezable bottles are also available for irrigations. These are commonly used for perineal irrigations and some wound irrigations.

The primary care provider orders the type, amount, temperature, and strength of the solution and the frequency of the irrigation. Generally, normal saline at body temperature (37°C [98.6°F]) is used unless specified otherwise. The amount of solution used varies with the site and purpose of the irrigation. Guidelines for administering eye and ear irrigations are given in Skills 35.9 and 35.10, respectively.

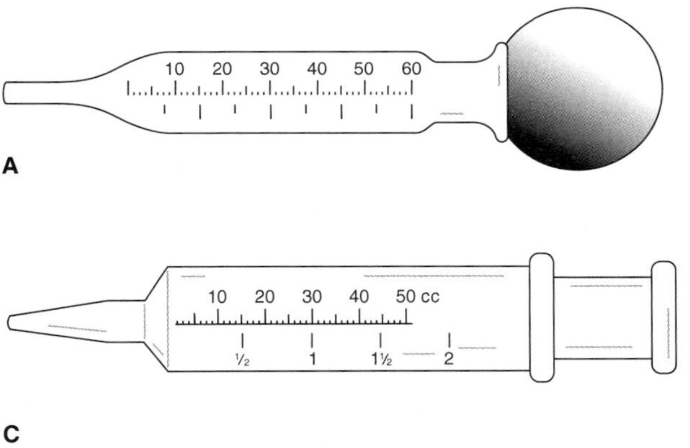

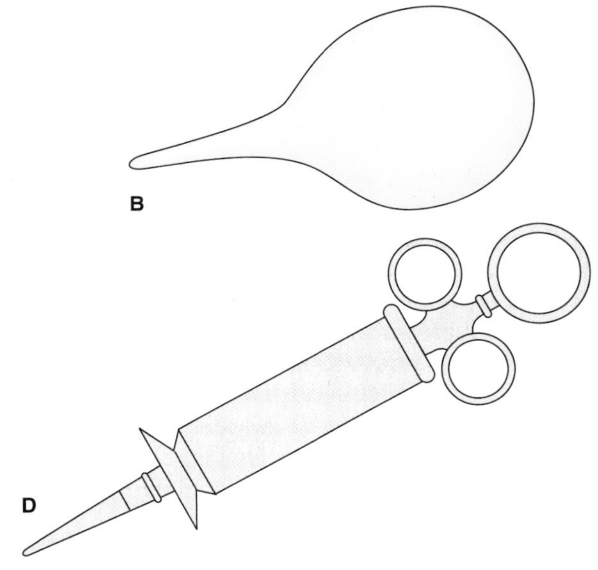

Figure 35.59 ■ Four types of syringes used for irrigations: *A*, Asepto; *B*, rubber bulb; *C*, piston syringe; *D*, Pomeroy.

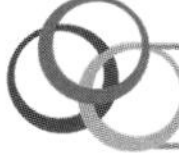

Critical Thinking Checkpoint

Mr. Ketron is a 20-year-old client who just returned to the nursing unit from surgery after undergoing an emergency appendectomy. He is awake and complaining of mild incisional pain. His dressing is dry and intact, and he has an intravenous infusion of lactated Ringer solution running at 125 mL/h. He is to receive Ancef (a cephalosporin antibiotic) 1 g intravenously every 4 hours until he is able to tolerate fluids, at which time he will be placed on oral Suprax (cefixime) 200 mg twice daily until discharged and for 1 week after returning home. He also has an order for morphine sulfate 2.5 mg to be given every 4 hours IVP as necessary for pain.

1. It is always possible that a client receiving antibiotic drugs may experience side effects or an allergic reaction. How does an allergic reaction differ from a drug side effect?
2. Predict the possible consequences of not obtaining a medication history from Mr. Ketron despite the fact that he will be receiving antibiotics and pain medication.
3. Mr. Ketron is complaining of pain and you have prepared his IVP morphine. What assessments will you make before giving the morphine?
4. What precautions should you take, if any, prior to administering Mr. Ketron's intravenous antibiotic medication?
5. Mr. Ketron will be placed on the oral antibiotic when he can tolerate food and oral fluids. What difference, if any, does it make if this drug is given before or after meals?

Answers to Critical Thinking Checkpoint questions are available on the faculty resources site. Please consult with your instructor.

Chapter 35 Review

CHAPTER HIGHLIGHTS

- Medications have several names. Nurses need to know the generic and trade names of a medication and be aware of both its therapeutic and side effects.
- Federal drug legislation regulates the production, prescription, distribution, and administration of drugs.
- Nurse practice acts define limits on the nurse's responsibilities regarding medications.
- Adverse effects of medications include drug toxicity, drug allergy, drug tolerance, idiosyncratic effect, and drug interactions.
- Several factors other than the drug itself can affect its action. These include pregnancy; age; gender; cultural, ethnic, and genetic factors; diet; client environment; psychological factors; illness and disease; and time of administration.
- Two systems of measurement are commonly used in North America: the metric system and the household system. Weights and measures may need to be converted by the nurse within these two systems.
- Several formulas can be used to calculate dosages: basic formula, ratio and proportion, fractional equation, and dimensional analysis. Pediatric dosages are calculated by the child's weight or body surface area.
- Various routes are used to administer medications: oral, sublingual, buccal, parenteral, topical, or via a nasogastric or gastrostomy tube. When administering a medication, the nurse must ensure that it is appropriate for the route specified.
- Medication orders must include the client name; date and time the order is written; name of the medication; dosage, frequency, and route of administration; and signature of the ordering primary care provider or nurse. Nurses must question any unclear orders before implementing the order.
- Telephone or verbal orders must be cosigned by the primary care provider within a time specified by agency policy (usually 24 to 48 hours).
- Nurses must always assess a client's physical status before giving any medication and obtain a medication history.
- A significant number of clients die annually due to medication errors. Most medication errors occur during the administration stage. Research shows that interruptions during medication administration create a greater risk for and severity of errors.
- Medication reconciliation is another method that the nurse uses to ensure that clients receive the appropriate medications and dosages. Three important areas for medication reconciliation to occur are (a) on admission, (b) during transfers, and (c) at discharge.
- When administering medications the nurse observes specified "rights" to ensure accurate administration. When preparing medications, the nurse checks the medication container label against the MAR three times.
- The nurse always identifies the client appropriately before administering a medication and stays with the client until the medication is taken.
- Medications, once given, are documented as soon as possible after administration.
- Parenteral medications act more quickly than those given orally or topically and must be prepared using aseptic technique.
- When preparing two insulins to be mixed in the same syringe, a vial of unmodified insulin should never be contaminated with modified insulin.
- Proper site selection is essential for an intramuscular injection to prevent tissue, bone, and nerve damage. The nurse should always palpate anatomic landmarks when selecting a site.
- The ventrogluteal site is the safest site of choice for intramuscular injections because it provides the greatest thickness of gluteal muscle and is free of penetrating nerves.
- The Z-track method for intramuscular injection is recommended because it is less painful than the traditional injection technique and decreases leakage of irritating or staining medication into subcutaneous tissues.
- Clients receiving a series of injections (e.g., insulin, low molecular weight heparin) should have injection sites rotated or alternated.
- After use, needles should *not* be recapped and must be placed in puncture-resistant containers.
- Intravenous medications can be administered by various methods: by intermittent intravenous infusion, by volume-controlled infusion, by intravenous push (IVP) or bolus, or by intermittent injection ports. In all of these methods the client has an existing IV line or an IV access site such as a saline lock.
- Topical medications are applied to the skin or mucous membranes in areas such as the eye, external ear canal, nose, vagina, and rectum.
- A metered-dose inhaler (MDI) is a handheld nebulizer that can be used by clients to self-administer measured doses of an aerosol medication. To ensure correct delivery of the prescribed medication by MDIs, nurses need to instruct clients to use aerosol inhalers correctly.
- Irrigations of body cavities may be performed (a) to remove a foreign object or excessive secretions or discharge, (b) to apply heat or cold, (c) to apply a medication, such as an antiseptic, (d) to reduce inflammation, or (e) to relieve discomfort.
- Surgical asepsis for an irrigation is required when there is a break in the skin (e.g., in a wound irrigation) or whenever a sterile body cavity (e.g., the bladder) is entered.

TEST YOUR KNOWLEDGE

1. A client tells the nurse, "This pill is a different color than the one that I usually take at home." Which is the best response by the nurse?
1. "Go ahead and take your medicine."
2. "I will recheck your medication orders."
3. "Maybe the doctor ordered a different medication."
4. "I'll leave the pill here while I check with the doctor."

2. A client is prescribed a new medication. The pharmacy notifies the nurse that the dosage is outside of route prescribing limits. The nurse is unable to reach the prescribing physician about the order. What should the nurse do?
1. Give the medication to the client as prescribed.
2. Withhold the medication.
3. Give one half of the medication dose prescribed.
4. Administer the medication through the oral route.

3. The primary care provider prescribed 5 mL of a medication to be given deep intramuscular for a 40-year-old female who is 5'7" tall and weighs 135 pounds. Which is the most appropriate equipment for the nurse to use? Select all that apply.
1. Two 3-mL syringes
2. One 5-mL syringe
3. A #20–#23 gauge needle
4. A 1-inch needle
5. A 1 1/2-inch needle

4. The nurse is to administer 0.75 mL of medication subcutaneously in the upper arm to a 300-pound adult client. The nurse can grasp approximately 2 inches of the client's tissue at the upper arm. Which is the most appropriate for the nurse to use?
1. A tuberculin syringe, #25–#27 gauge, 1/4- to 5/8-inch needle
2. Two 3-mL syringes, #20–#23 gauge, 1 1/2-inch needle
3. 3.2-mL syringe, #25 gauge, 5/8-inch needle
4. 4.2-mL syringe, #20–#23 gauge, 1-inch needle

5. The nurse is to administer a tuberculin test to a client who is 6 feet tall and weighs 180 pounds. Which is the most appropriate for the nurse to use?
1. A tuberculin syringe, #25–#27 gauge, 1/4- to 5/8-inch needle
2. Two 3-mL syringes, #20–#23 gauge, 1 1/2-inch needle
3. 2-mL syringe, #25 gauge, 5/8-inch needle
4. 2-mL syringe, #20–#23 gauge, 1-inch needle

6. The nurse is to administer 0.5 mL of a medication by intramuscular injection to an older emaciated client. Which is the most appropriate for the nurse to use?
1. A tuberculin syringe, #25–#27 gauge, 1/4- to 5/8-inch needle
2. Two 3-mL syringes, #20–#23 gauge, 1 1/2-inch needle
3. 2-mL syringe, #25 gauge, 5/8-inch needle
4. 2-mL syringe, #20–#23 gauge, 1-inch needle

7. The assigned nurse determines that an older client is experiencing an adverse effect from a prescribed medication because of which of the following?
1. Altered memory
2. Altered organ responsiveness
3. Decreased manual dexterity
4. Decreased visual acuity

8. While preparing to administer an eye ointment, the nurse inadvertently squeezes the tube, discarding the first bead of medication. What action should the nurse take at this point?
1. Administer the eye ointment as ordered, as the first bead of ointment should be discarded anyway.
2. Notify the pharmacy and request a new, unopened tube of ointment.
3. Have a second licensed nurse witness the waste and sign the chart.
4. Continue to squeeze the tube until a clear line of ointment has been discarded from the tip.

9. A primary care provider writes a prescription for 0.15 milligram of digoxin intravenously every day. The medication is available in a concentration of 400 micrograms per mL. How many mL will the nurse administer?

10. A nursing student is preparing to administer insulin to a client with diabetes. Indicate the correct order for the administration of this medication:
1. Cleanse the site with alcohol.
2. Insert the needle quickly into the subcutaneous tissue.
3. Mix the insulins.
4. Assess the skin for the injection.
5. Pinch the skin lightly.
6. Inject the medication.
7. Count to five.
8. Remove the syringe.

Correct sequence: ________

See Answers to Test Your Knowledge in Appendix A.

READINGS AND REFERENCES

Suggested Readings

Beydoun, S. (2018). The art and science of medication administration. *American Nurse Today*, *13*(9), 99–102.
Using a case study, the author illustrates the importance of using critical thinking during each step of medication administration.

Guenter, P., & Lyman, B. (2016). ENFit enteral nutrition connectors: Benefits and challenges. *Nutrition in Clinical Practice*, *31*(6), 769–772. doi:10.1177/0884533616673638
Reviews the benefits and challenges of the new enteral connectors.

Institute for Safe Medication Practices. (2018). Students have a key role in a culture of safety: Analysis of student-associated medication incidents. *Nurse AdviseERR*, *16*(9), 1–3.
The analysis identified the positive contribution students can make to medication safety and the importance of preceptor supervision.

Related Research

Lutz, M. F., Haines, S. T., Lesch, C. A., & Szumita, P. M. (2016). Facilitating the safe use of insulin pens in hospitals through a mentored quality-improvement program. *American Journal of Health-System Pharmacy*, *73*(19 Suppl. 5), S17–S31. doi:10.2146/ajhp160417

Mulhall, A. M., Zafar, M. A., Record, S., Channell, H., & Panos, R. J. (2017). A tablet-based multimedia education tool improves provider and subject knowledge of inhaler use techniques. *Respiratory Care*, *62*(2), 163–171. doi:10.4187/respcare.05008

Prentiss, A. A., Cockerel, A., & Butler, E. (2016). Nurse perceptions and safety practices of the carpuject cartridge system. *Journal of Nursing Care Quality*, *31*(4), 350–356. doi:10.1097/NCQ.0000000000000194

References

Adams, M. P., Holland, N., & Urban, C. (2020). *Pharmacology for nurses: A pathophysiologic approach* (6th ed.). Hoboken, NJ: Pearson.

Agency for Healthcare Research and Quality. (2019). *Medication errors and adverse drug events*. Retrieved from https://psnet.ahrq.gov/primers/primer/23/medication-errors

Alismail, A., Song, C. A., Terry, M. H., Daher, N., Almutairi, W. A., & Lo, T. (2016). Diverse inhaler devices: A big challenge for health-care professionals. *Respiratory Care*, *61*(5), 593–599. doi:10.4187/respcare.04293

Bindler, R. C., Ball, J. W., London, M. L., & Davidson, M. R. (2017). *Clinical skills manual for maternity and pediatric nursing* (5th ed.). Hoboken, NJ: Pearson.

Blanchard, D., & Payette, K. S. (2016). Ventrogluteal injections: It's hip! *AAACN Viewpoint*, *38*(2), 4–8.

Boullata, J. I., Carrera, A. L., Harvey, L., Escuro, A. A., Hudson, L., McGinnis, C., . . . Guenter, P. (2017). ASPEN safe practices for enteral nutrition therapy. *Journal of Parenteral and Enteral Nutrition*, *41*, 15–103. doi:10.1177/0148607116673053

Brown, K. E., & Hertig, J. B. (2016). Determining current insulin pen use practices and errors in the inpatient setting. *The Joint Commission Journal on Quality and Patient Safety*, *42*, 568–575. doi:10.1016/S1553-7250(16)30109-X

Centers for Disease Control and Prevention. (n.d.). *Single-dose or multi-dose?* Retrieved from https://www.cdc.gov/injectionsafety/PDF/SDVMDV_infographic.pdf

Centers for Disease Control and Prevention. (2018). *Vaccine administration.* Retrieved from https://www.cdc.gov/vaccines/pubs/pinkbook/vac-admin.html

Chu, R. Z. (2016). Simple steps to reduce medication errors. *Nursing*, *46*(8), 63–65. doi:10.1097/01.NURSE.0000484977.05034.9c

ECRI Institute. (2017). *Implementing the ENFit initiative for preventing enteral tubing misconnections.* Retrieved from https://www.ecri.org/components/HDJournal/Pages/ENFit-for-Preventing-Enteral-Tubing-Misconnections.aspx?tab=2#

Flynn, F., Evanish, J. Q., Fernald, J. M., Hutchinson, D. E., & Lefaiver, C. (2016). Progressive care nurses improving patient safety by limiting interruptions during medication administration. *Critical Care Nurse*, *36*(4), 19–35. doi:10.4037/ccn2016498

Fulton, C. R., Swart, M., De Luca, T., Liu, S. N., Collins, K. S., Desta, Z., . . . & Eadon, M. T. (2018). Pharmacogenetics and practice: Tailoring prescribing for safety and effectiveness. *The Journal for Nurse Practitioners*, *14*(10), 697–704. doi:10.1016/j.nurpra.2018.09.021

Godshall, M., & Riehl, M. (2018). Preventing medication errors in the information age. *Nursing*, *48*(9), 56–58. doi:10.1097/01.NURSE.0000544230.51598.38

Haines, S. T., Miklich, M. A., & Rochester-Eyeguokan, C. (2016). Best practices for safe use of insulin pen devices in hospitals: Recommendations from an expert panel Delphi consensus process. *American Journal of Health-System Pharmacy*, *73*(Suppl. 5), S4–S16. doi:10.2146/ajhp160416

Houston, A., & Fuldauer, P. (2017). Enteral feeding: Indications, complications, and nursing care. *American Nurse Today*, *12*(1), 20–24.

Hull, S. C. (2018). Are we ready for precision health? *Nursing Management*, *49*(7), 9–11. doi:10.1097/01.NUMA.0000538923.68406.3c

Infusion Nurses Society. (2016). *Infusion therapy standards of practice.* Norwood, MA: Author.

Institute for Safe Medication Practices. (2010). *Principles of designing a medication label for IV piggyback medication for patient specific, inpatient use.* Retrieved from http://www.ismp.org/tools/guidelines/labelFormats/Piggyback.asp

Institute for Safe Medication Practices. (2011). *ISMP acute care guidelines for timely administration of scheduled medications*. Retrieved from https://www.ismp.org/sites/default/files/attachments/2018-02/tasm.pdf

Institute for Safe Medication Practices. (2017a). Alarming survey results from CDC: Unsafe injection practices continue. *NurseAdviseERR*, *15*(11), 1–3.

Institute for Safe Medication Practices. (2017b). *List of error-prone abbreviations.* Retrieved from https://www.ismp.org/recommendations/error-prone-abbreviations-list

Institute for Safe Medication Practices. (2017c). *Severe hyperglycemia in patients incorrectly using insulin pens at home.* Retrieved from https://www.ismp.org/alerts/severe-hyperglycemia-patients-incorrectly-using-insulin-pens-home

Institute for Safe Medication Practices. (2018). *Oral dosage forms that should not be crushed.* Retrieved from https://www.ismp.org/recommendations/do-not-crush

The Joint Commission. (2018). *Facts about the official "do not use" list of abbreviations.* Retrieved from https://www.jointcommission.org/facts_about_do_not_use_list

The Joint Commission. (2019a). *National Patient Safety Goals effective January 2019—hospital accreditation program.* Retrieved from https://www.jointcommission.org/assets/1/6/NPSG_Chapter_HAP_Jan2019.pdf

The Joint Commission. (2019b). *National Patient Safety Goals effective January 2019—nursing care center accreditation program.* Retrieved from https://www.jointcommission.org/assets/1/6/NPSG_Chapter_NCC_Jan2019.pdf

Kantorovich, A. (2016). *Transdermal patches that must be removed before MRI.* Retrieved from https://www.pharmacytimes.com/contributor/alexander-kantorovich-pharmd-bcps/2016/08/transdermal-patches-that-must-be-removed-before-mri

Lapkin, S., Levett-Jones, T., Chenoweth, L., & Johnson, M. (2016). The effectiveness of interventions designed to reduce medication administration errors: A synthesis of findings from systematic reviews. *Journal of Nursing Management, 24,* 845–858. doi:10.1111/jonm.12390

Mayo Clinic. (2019). *Belladonna and opium (rectal route).* Retrieved from https://www.mayoclinic.org/drugs-supplements/belladonna-and-opium-rectal-route/description/drg-20075097

Midelfort, L. (n.d.). *Medication reconciliation review.* Retrieved from http://www.ihi.org/resources/Pages/Tools/MedicationReconciliationReview.aspx

Mitchell, A. H., & Parker, G. B. (2018). Changing injury trends related to diabetes and insulin injection. *American Nurse Today*, *13*(1), 44–45.

Montgomery, S., Brouwer, W. A., Everett, P. C., Hassen, E., Lowe, T., McGreal, S. B., & Eggert, J. (2017). Genetics in the clinical setting. *American Nurse Today*, *12*(10), 10–15.

Mraz, M. A. I., Thomas, C., & Rajcan, L. (2018). Intramuscular injection CLIMAT pathway: A clinical practice guideline. *British Journal of Nursing*, *27*(13), 752–756. doi:10.12968/bjon.2018.27.13.752

Olsen, J. L., Giangrasso, A. P., & Shrimpton, D. M. (2016). *Medical dosage calculations: A dimensional analysis approach* (11th ed.). Upper Saddle River, NJ: Pearson.

Sanofi-Aventis. (n.d.). *LOVENOX®: Step-by-step guide to self-injection*. Retrieved from https://nbngroup.com/Skilled%20Nurse%20Visit%20Packets/Lovenox%20Visit%20Packet/Lov_Treatment_At_Home.pdf

Sexson, K., Lindauer, A., & Harvath, T. A. (2016). Administration of subcutaneous injections. *American Journal of Nursing*, *116*(2), 49–52. doi:10.1097/01.NAJ.0000508671.49210.ba

Shastay, A. D. (2016). Evidence-based safe practice guidelines for I.V. push medications. *Nursing*, *46*(10), 38–44. doi:10.1097/01.NURSE.0000494641.31939.46

Thomas, C. M., Mraz, M., & Rajcam, L. (2016). Blood aspiration during IM injection. *Clinical Nursing Research*, *25*(5), 549–559. doi:10.1177/1054773815575074

U.S. Food and Drug Administration. (2019a). *Disposal of unused medicines: What you should know.* Retrieved from https://www.fda.gov/Drugs/ResourcesForYou/Consumers/BuyingUsingMedicineSafely/EnsuringSafeUseofMedicine/SafeDisposalofMedicines/ucm186187.htm

U.S. Food and Drug Administration. (2019b). *My medicine record.* Retrieved from https://www.fda.gov/drugs/ucm079489

Votroubek, W. (2018). *Preventing high-alert medication errors in hospital patients.* Retrieved from https://www.legalnursepdx.com/preventing-high-alert-medication-errors-in-hospital-patients

World Health Organization. (2017). *WHO launches global effort to halve medication-related errors in 5 years.* Retrieved from http://www.who.int/mediacentre/news/releases/2017/medication-related-errors/en

Yilmaz, D., Khorshid, L., & Dedeoglu, Y. (2016). The effect of the Z-track technique on pain and drug leakage in intramuscular injections. *Clinical Nurse Specialist*, *30*(6), E7–E12. doi:10.1097/NUR.0000000000000245

Selected Bibliography

Bagnasco, A., Galaverna, L., Aleo, G., Grugnetti, A. M., Rosa, F., & Sasso, L. (2016). Mathematical calculation skills required for drug administration in undergraduate nursing students to ensure patient safety: A descriptive study. *Nurse Education in Practice*, *16*(1), 33–39. doi:10.1016/j.nepr.2015.06.006

Botsford, J. A. (2016). Building on a safety culture with transparency by participating in a mentored quality-improvement program for insulin pen safety. *American Journal of Health-System Pharmacy*, *73*(19 Suppl. 5), S38–S44. doi:10.2146/ajhp160419

Cheek, D. J. (2017). Patient care in the dawn of the genomic age. *American Nurse Today*, *12*(3), 16–21.

Daley, K. A. (2017). Sharps injuries: Where we stand today. *American Nurse Today*, *12*(2), 23–24.

Farag, A., Tullai-McGuinness, S., Anthony, M. K., & Burant, C. (2017). Do leadership style, unit climate, and safety climate contribute to safe medication practices? *The Journal of Nursing Administration*, *47*, 8–15. doi:10.1097/NNA.0000000000000430

Giuliano, K. K. & Niemi, C. (2016). The urgent need for innovation in I.V. infusion devices. *Nursing*, *46*(4), 66–68. doi:10.1097/01.NURSE.0000480617.62296.d7

Goad, K. (2017). *Tips for buying an insulin pen*. Retrieved from http://www.diabetesforecast.org/2017/mar-apr/purchasing-an-insulin-pen.html?loc=ymal

Haines, S. T. (2016). Best practices in ensuring the safe use of insulin pens in the hospital: Introduction. *American Journal of Health-System Pharmacy*, *73*(19 Suppl. 5) S2–S3. doi:10.2146/ajhp160415

Halpern, L. W. (2016). Parents often give the wrong dose of medication to their children. *American Journal of Nursing*, *116*(12), 18. doi:10.1097/01.NAJ.0000508654.71188.c5

Hayter, K. L. (2016). Listen up for safe ear irrigation. *Nursing*, *46*(5), 62–65. doi:10.1097/01.NURSE.0000481437.02178.3b

Institute for Safe Medication Practices. (2018). Safety with nebulized medications requires an interdisciplinary team approach. *Nurse AdviseERR*, *16*(5), 1–4.

Koharchik, L., & Flavin, P. M. (2017). Teaching students to administer medications safely. *American Journal of Nursing*, *117*(1), 62–66. doi:10.1097/01.NAJ.0000511573.73435.72

Lindauer, A., Sexson, K., & Harvath, T. A. (2017). Teaching caregivers to administer eye drops, transdermal patches, and suppositories. *American Journal of Nursing*, *117*(1), 54–59. doi:10.1097/01.NAJ.0000511568.58187.36

Malone, B. R. (2016). Intimidating behavior among healthcare workers is still jeopardizing medication safety. *Nephrology Nursing Journal*, *43*(2), 157–159.

McCrea, D. L. (2017). A primer on insulin pump therapy for health care providers. *Nursing Clinics of North America*, *52*, 443–564. doi:10.1016/j.cnur.2017.07.005

Rich, A. (2018). Meeting the challenge of monitoring medications in older adults. *American Nurse Today*, *13*(9), 96–98.

Rosenberg, A. F. (2016). Participation in a mentored quality-improvement program for insulin pen safety: Opportunity to augment internal evaluation and share with peers. *American Journal of Health-System Pharmacy*, *73*(19 Suppl. 5), S32–S37. doi:10.2146/ajhp160418

Sawhney, M., Chambers, S., & Hysi, F. (2018). Removing epidural catheters: A guide for nurses. *Nursing*, *48*(12), 47–49. doi:10.1097/01.NURSE.0000546459.86617.2a

Smith, S. F., Duell, D. J., & Martin, B. C. (2017). *Clinical nursing skills* (9th ed.). Hoboken, NJ, Pearson.

White, S., Goodwin, J., Mgmt, D., & Behan, L. (2018). Nurses' use of appropriate needle sizes when administering intramuscular injections. *The Journal of Continuing Education in Nursing*, *49*(11), 519–525. doi:10.3928/00220124-20181017-09

Skin Integrity and Wound Care 36

LEARNING OUTCOMES

After completing this chapter, you will be able to:

1. Describe factors affecting skin integrity.
2. Identify clients at risk for pressure injuries.
3. Describe the four stages of pressure injury development.
4. Differentiate primary and secondary wound healing.
5. Describe the three phases of wound healing.
6. Identify three major types of wound exudate.
7. Identify the main complications of and factors that affect wound healing.
8. Identify assessment data pertinent to skin integrity, pressure sites, and wounds.
9. Identify nursing diagnoses associated with impaired skin integrity.
10. Identify essential aspects of planning care to maintain skin integrity and promote wound healing.
11. Describe nursing strategies to treat pressure injuries, promote wound healing, and prevent complications of wound healing.
12. Identify purposes of commonly used wound dressing materials and binders.
13. Verbalize the steps used in:
    a. Cleaning a sutured wound and dressing a drain.
    b. Obtaining wound specimens.
    c. Irrigating a wound.
    d. Applying dressings.
    e. Removing sutures and staples.
    f. Applying dry and moist heat and cold.
14. Identify physiologic responses to and the purposes of heat and cold.
15. Recognize when it is appropriate to assign aspects of skin and wound care to assistive personnel.
16. Demonstrate appropriate documentation and reporting of skin integrity and wound care.

KEY TERMS

aerobic, *941*
anaerobic, *941*
approximated, *923*
bandage, *946*
binder, *947*
closed wound drainage system, *933*
collagen, *924*
compress, *951*
debridement, *932*
dehiscence, *925*
eschar, *924*
evisceration, *925*
excoriation, *918*
exudate, *924*
fibrin, *923*
friction, *917*
granulation tissue, *924*
hematoma, *924*
hemorrhage, *924*
hemostasis, *923*
immobility, *917*
ischemia, *917*
keloid, *924*
maceration, *918*
packing, *937*
Penrose drain, *933*
phagocytosis, *923*
pressure injuries, *916*
primary intention healing, *923*
purulent exudate, *924*
pus, *924*
reactive hyperemia, *917*
regeneration, *923*
sanguineous exudate, *924*
secondary intention healing, *923*
serosanguineous, *924*
serous exudate, *924*
shearing force, *917*
sitz bath, *952*
suppuration, *924*
suture, *944*
tertiary intention healing, *923*
vasoconstriction, *949*
vasodilation, *917*

Introduction

The skin is the largest organ in the body and serves a variety of important functions in maintaining health and protecting the individual from injury. Important nursing functions are maintaining skin integrity and promoting wound healing. Impaired skin integrity is not a frequent problem for most healthy individuals but is a threat to older adults; to clients with restricted mobility, chronic illnesses, or trauma; and to those undergoing invasive healthcare procedures. To protect the skin and manage wounds effectively, the nurse must understand the factors affecting skin integrity, the physiology of wound healing, and specific measures that promote optimal skin conditions.

Skin Integrity

Intact skin refers to the presence of normal skin and skin layers uninterrupted by wounds. Chapter 29 ∞ provides details regarding physical examination of the integumentary system. The appearance of the skin and skin integrity are influenced by internal factors such as genetics, age, and the underlying health of the individual as well as external factors such as activity.

Genetics and heredity determine many aspects of an individual's skin, including skin color, sensitivity to sunlight, and allergies. Age influences skin integrity in that the skin of both the very young and the very old is more fragile and susceptible to injury than that of most adults. Wounds tend to heal more rapidly in infants and children, however.

Many chronic illnesses and their treatments affect skin integrity. Individuals with impaired peripheral arterial circulation may have skin on the legs that damages easily. Some medications, corticosteroids, for example, cause thinning of the skin and allow it to be much more readily harmed. Many medications increase sensitivity to sunlight and can predispose a client to severe sunburns. Some of the most common medications that cause this damage are certain antibiotics (e.g., tetracycline and doxycycline), chemotherapy drugs for cancer (e.g., methotrexate), and some psychotherapeutic drugs (e.g., tricyclic antidepressants). Poor nutrition alone can interfere with the appearance and function of normal skin.

Types of Wounds

Body wounds are either intentional or unintentional. *Intentional* trauma occurs during therapy. Examples are operations. Although removing a tumor, for example, is therapeutic, the surgeon must cut into body tissues, thus traumatizing them. *Unintentional* wounds are accidental; for example, a client may fracture an arm in an automobile collision. If the tissues are traumatized without a break in the skin, the wound is closed. The wound is open when the skin or mucous membrane surface is broken.

Wounds may be described according to how they are acquired (Table 36.1). They also can be described according to the likelihood and degree of wound contamination and depth:

- *Clean wounds* are uninfected wounds in which there is minimal inflammation and the gastrointestinal, genital, and urinary tracts are not entered. Clean wounds are primarily closed wounds.
- *Clean-contaminated wounds* are surgical wounds in which the gastrointestinal, genital, or urinary tract has been entered. Such wounds show no evidence of infection.
- *Contaminated wounds* include open, accidental, and surgical wounds involving a major break in sterile technique or spillage from the gastrointestinal tract. Contaminated wounds show evidence of inflammation.
- *Dirty* or *infected wounds* include wounds with evidence of a clinical infection, such as purulent drainage or necrosis.
- *Partial thickness wounds* are confined to the skin, that is, the dermis and epidermis, and heal by regeneration.
- *Full thickness wounds* involve the dermis, epidermis, subcutaneous tissue, and possibly muscle and bone, and require connective tissue repair.

Pressure Injuries

Pressure injuries consist of injury to the skin or underlying tissue, usually over a bony prominence, as a result of force alone or in combination with movement. Pressure injuries were previously called *pressure ulcers*, *decubitus ulcers*, *pressure sores*, or *bedsores*. Pressure injuries are a problem in both acute care settings and long-term care settings, including homes. A *Healthy People 2020* proposed objective is to reduce the rate of pressure injury–related hospitalizations among older adults by 10% (U.S. Department of Health and Human Services, 2017). One of the National Patient Safety Goals for long-term care settings is prevention of healthcare-associated pressure injuries (The Joint Commission, 2019), although the publication has not yet updated to the term *injury* instead of *ulcer*. Because healthcare-associated pressure injuries are substantially preventable, public health insurance—and increasing numbers of private health insurance companies—will no longer reimburse healthcare agencies for the cost of treating them. In addition, development of a stage 3 or 4 or unstageable pressure injury (see later in this chapter) is considered a serious reportable event (National Quality Forum, 2017).

TABLE 36.1 Types of Wounds

Type	Cause	Description and Characteristics
Incision	Sharp instrument (e.g., knife or scalpel)	Open wound; deep or shallow; once the edges have been sealed together as a part of treatment or healing, the incision becomes a closed wound.
Contusion	Blow from a blunt instrument	Closed wound, skin appears ecchymotic (bruised) because of damaged blood vessels.
Abrasion	Surface scrape, either unintentional (e.g., scraped knee from a fall) or intentional (e.g., dermal abrasion to remove pockmarks)	Open wound involving the skin
Puncture	Penetration of the skin and often the underlying tissues by a sharp instrument, either intentional or unintentional	Open wound
Laceration	Tissues torn apart, often from accidents (e.g., with machinery)	Open wound; edges are often jagged
Penetrating wound	Penetration of the skin and the underlying tissues, usually unintentional (e.g., from a bullet or metal fragments)	Open wound

Safety Alert! SAFETY

2019 The Joint Commission National Patient Safety Goals

Goal 14: Prevent Healthcare–Associated Pressure Ulcers (Decubitus Ulcers).

- Assess and periodically reassess each patient's and resident's risk for developing a pressure ulcer and take action to address any identified risks. **Rationale:** *Pressure ulcers (decubiti) continue to be problematic in all health care settings. Most pressure ulcers can be prevented, and deterioration at stage 1 can be halted. The use of clinical practice guidelines can effectively identify residents and define early intervention for prevention of pressure ulcers.*

Etiology of Pressure Injuries

Pressure injuries are due to localized **ischemia**, a deficiency in the blood supply to the tissue. The tissue is compressed between two surfaces, usually the surface of furniture such as the bed or chair and the bony skeleton. When blood cannot reach the tissue, the cells are deprived of oxygen and nutrients, the waste products of metabolism accumulate in the cells, and the tissue consequently dies. Prolonged, unrelieved pressure also damages the small blood vessels.

After the skin has been compressed, it appears pale (blanched), as if the blood had been squeezed out of it. When pressure is relieved, the skin takes on a bright red flush (erythema), called **reactive hyperemia**. In dark-skinned clients, both the blanch and flush may be difficult to detect. Compare the reactions of questionable areas with other parts of the client's skin. The flush is due to **vasodilation**, a process in which extra blood floods to the area to compensate for the preceding period of impeded blood flow. Reactive hyperemia usually lasts one-half to three-quarters as long as the duration of impeded blood flow to the area. If the redness disappears in that time, no tissue damage is anticipated. If, however, the redness does not disappear, then tissue damage has occurred.

Risk Factors

Several factors contribute to the formation of pressure injuries: friction and shearing, immobility, inadequate nutrition, fecal and urinary incontinence, decreased mental status, diminished sensation, excessive body heat, advanced age, and the presence of certain chronic conditions.

Friction and Shearing

Friction is a force acting parallel to the skin surface. For example, sheets rubbing against skin create friction. Friction can abrade the skin, that is, remove the superficial layers, making it more prone to breakdown.

Shearing force is a combination of friction and pressure (Figure 36.1 ■). It occurs commonly when a client assumes a sitting position in bed. In this position, the body tends to slide downward toward the foot of the bed. This downward movement is transmitted to the sacral bone and the deep tissues. At the same time, the skin over the sacrum tends not to move because of the adherence between the skin and the bed linens. The skin and superficial tissues are thus relatively unmoving in relation to the bed surface, whereas the deeper tissues are firmly attached to the skeleton and move downward. This causes a shearing force in the area where the deeper tissues and the superficial tissues meet. The force damages the blood vessels and tissues in this area.

Immobility

Immobility refers to a reduction in the amount and control of movement an individual has. Normally individuals move when they experience discomfort due to pressure

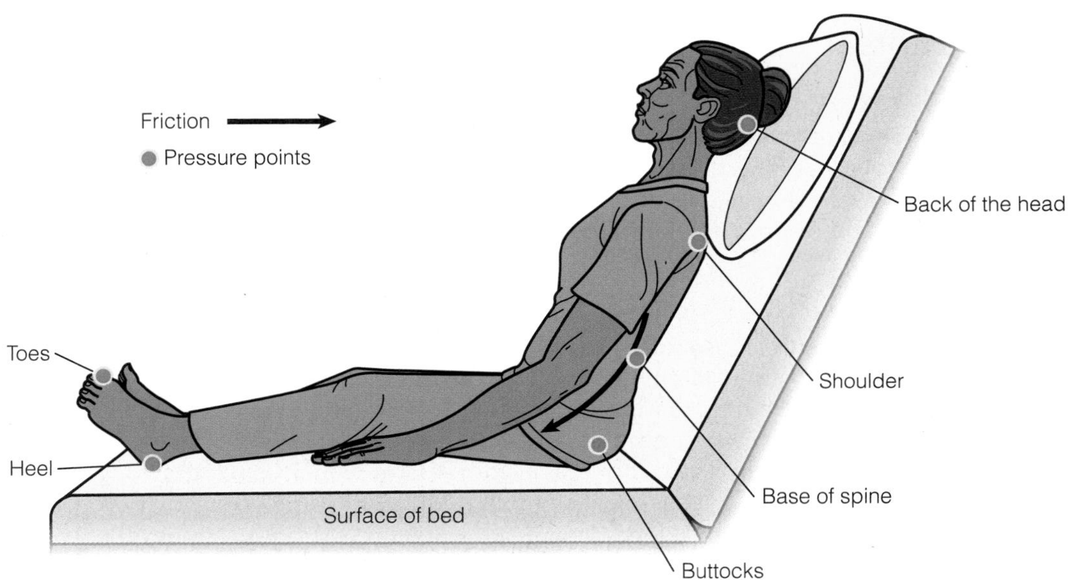

Figure 36.1 ■ Friction and pressure forces leading to shearing.

on an area of the body. Healthy individuals rarely exceed their tolerance to pressure. However, paralysis, extreme weakness, pain, or any cause of decreased activity can hinder an individual's ability to change positions independently and relieve the pressure, even if the individual can perceive the pressure.

Inadequate Nutrition

Prolonged inadequate nutrition causes weight loss, muscle atrophy, and the loss of subcutaneous tissue. These three conditions reduce the amount of padding between the skin and the bones, thus increasing the risk of pressure injury development. More specifically, inadequate intake of protein, carbohydrates, fluids, zinc, and vitamin C contributes to pressure injury formation.

Hypoproteinemia (abnormally low protein content in the blood), due either to inadequate intake or abnormal loss, predisposes the client to dependent edema. Edema (the presence of excess interstitial fluid) makes skin more prone to injury by decreasing its elasticity, resilience, and vitality. Edema increases the distance between the capillaries and the cells, thereby slowing the diffusion of oxygen to the tissue cells and of metabolites away from the cells.

Fecal and Urinary Incontinence

Moisture from incontinence promotes skin **maceration** (tissue softened by prolonged wetting or soaking) and makes the epidermis more easily eroded and susceptible to injury. Digestive enzymes in feces, urea in urine, and gastric tube drainage also contribute to skin **excoriation** (area of loss of the superficial layers of the skin; also known as *denuded* area).

Any accumulation of secretions or excretions (including sweat) is irritating to the skin, harbors microorganisms, and makes an individual prone to skin breakdown and infection. Skin or tissue injury due primarily to moisture is referred to as *moisture-related skin damage* (MASD) or *incontinence-associated dermatitis* (IAD). MASD or IAD can be considered "outside-in" damage where true pressure injuries would be considered "inside-out."

Decreased Mental Status

Individuals with a reduced level of awareness, for example, those who are unconscious, are heavily sedated, or have dementia, are at risk for pressure injuries because they are less able to recognize and respond to pain associated with prolonged pressure.

Diminished Sensation

Paralysis, stroke, or other neurologic disease may cause loss of sensation in a body area. Loss of sensation reduces an individual's ability to respond to trauma, to injurious heat and cold, and to the tingling ("pins and needles") that signals loss of circulation. Sensory loss also impairs the body's ability to recognize and provide healing mechanisms for a wound.

Excessive Body Heat

Body heat is another factor in the development of pressure injuries. An elevated body temperature increases the metabolic rate, thus increasing the cells' need for oxygen. This increased need is particularly severe in the cells of an area under pressure, which are already oxygen deficient. Severe infections with accompanying elevated body temperatures may affect the body's ability to deal with the effects of tissue compression.

Advanced Age

The aging process brings about several changes in the skin and its supporting structures, making the older adult more prone to impaired skin integrity. These changes include the following:

- Loss of lean body mass
- Generalized thinning of the epidermis
- Decreased strength and elasticity of the skin due to changes in the collagen fibers of the dermis
- Increased dryness due to a decrease in the amount of oil produced by the sebaceous glands
- Diminished pain perception due to a reduction in the number of cutaneous end organs responsible for the sensation of pressure and light touch
- Diminished venous and arterial flow due to aging vascular walls.

Chronic Medical Conditions

Certain chronic conditions such as diabetes and cardiovascular disease are risk factors for skin breakdown and delayed healing. These conditions compromise oxygen delivery to tissues by poor perfusion and thus cause poor and delayed healing and increase risk of pressure injuries.

Other Factors

Other factors contributing to the formation of pressure injuries are poor lifting and transferring techniques, incorrect positioning, hard support surfaces, and incorrect application of pressure-relieving devices.

Stages of Pressure Injuries

The recognized stages of pressure injuries related to observable tissue damage are shown in Figure 36.2 ■.

Risk Assessment Tools

Although clients may be at risk for developing a number of different alterations in skin integrity, the most common and most preventable are pressure injuries. Several risk assessment tools are available that provide the nurse with systematic means of identifying clients at high risk for pressure injury development. The tool chosen for use should include data collection in the areas of immobility, incontinence, nutrition, and level of consciousness.

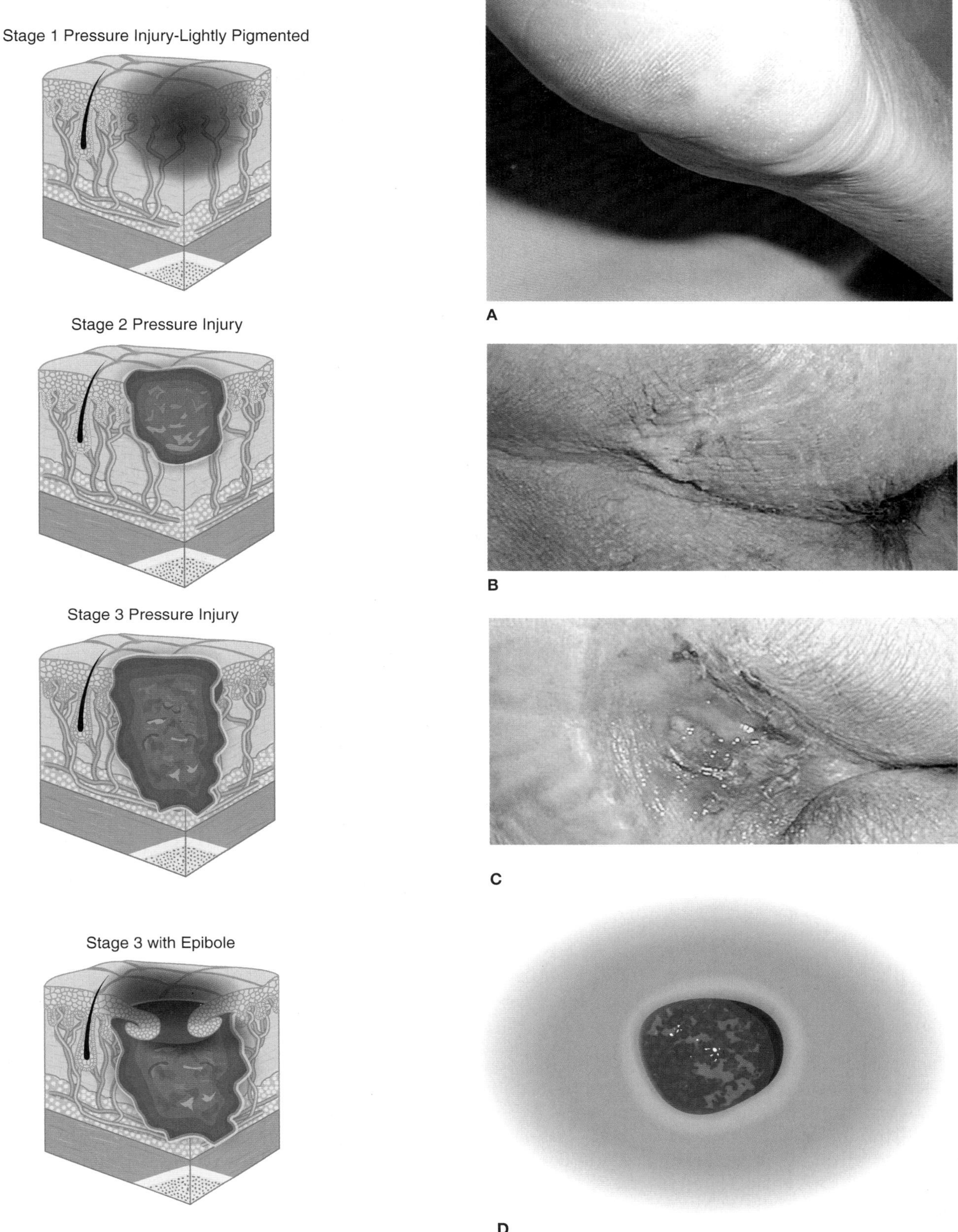

Figure 36.2 ■ Stages of pressure injuries. *A*, Stage 1: skin is unbroken and reddened, but does not blanch. *B*, Stage 2: partial-thickness skin loss. *C*, Stage 3: full-thickness skin loss and damage that may reach as deeply as the fascia. *D*, Stage 3 with epibole (the edges of the skin surrounding the injury roll under and the damage extends under the rolled tissue). *E*, Stage 4: full-thickness skin loss with tissue death or damage to underlying structures. *F*, Unstageable or unclassified: full-thickness loss. The full extent of the injury cannot be determined due to slough or eschar. *G*, Deep tissue pressure injury–depth unknown: dark area of discolored intact skin due to damage of underlying soft tissue.
Photos *A–C*, *E–G*, Cory patrick Hartley RN. WCC, OMS.

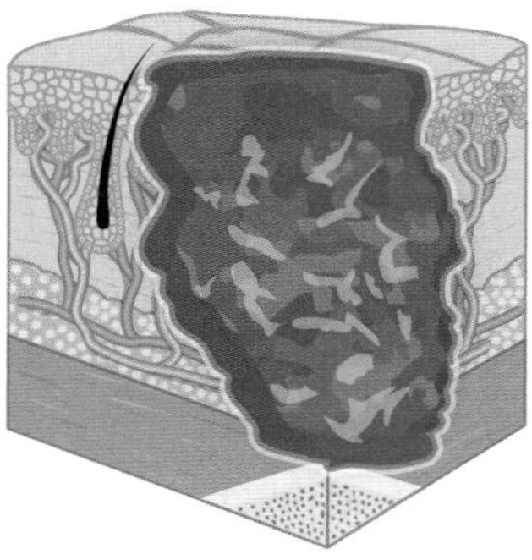

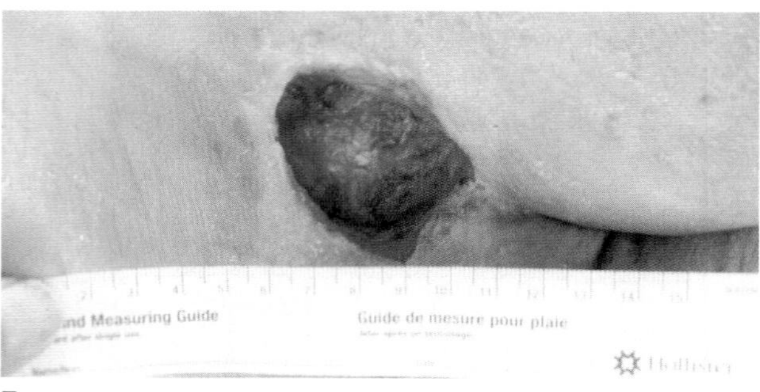

E

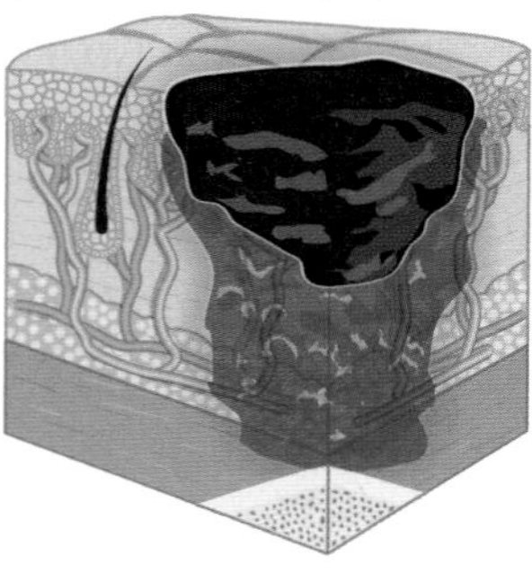

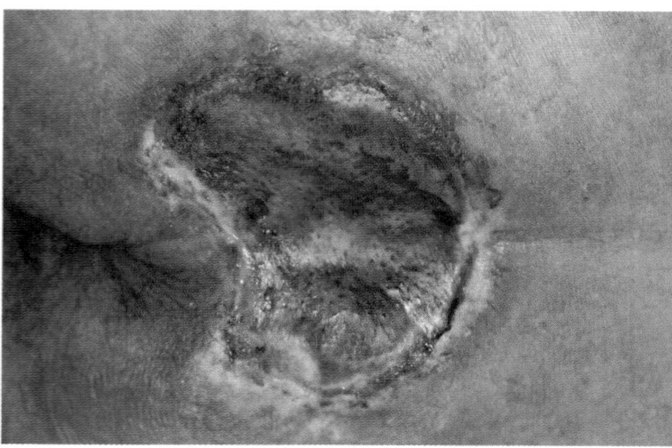

F

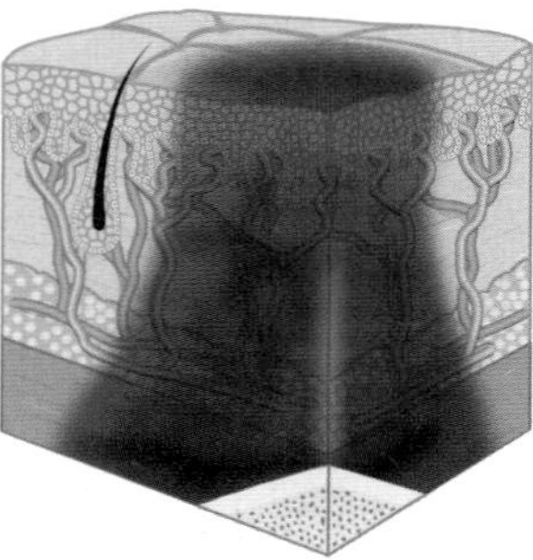

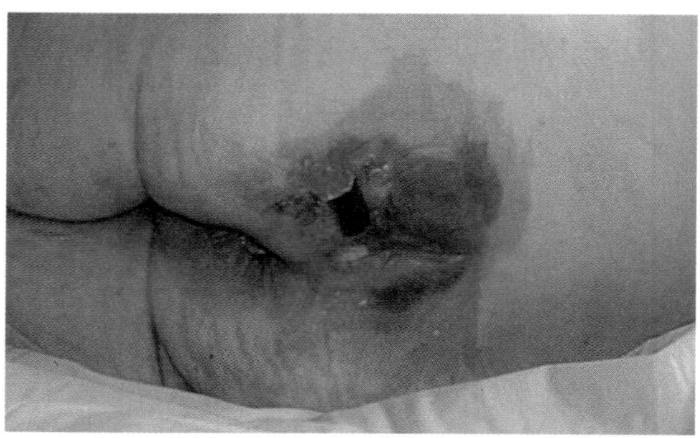

G

Figure 36.2 ■ *Continued*

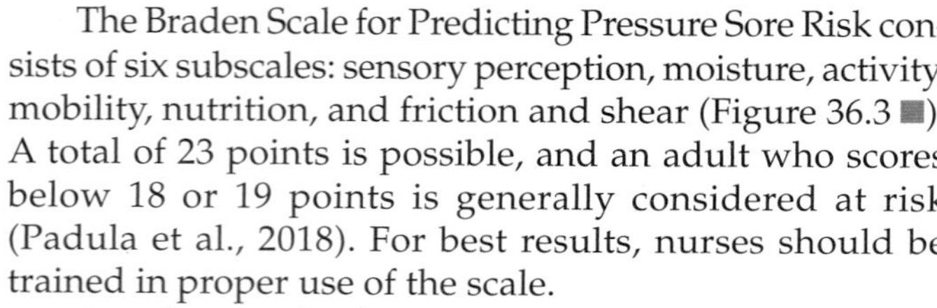

The Braden Scale for Predicting Pressure Sore Risk consists of six subscales: sensory perception, moisture, activity, mobility, nutrition, and friction and shear (Figure 36.3 ■). A total of 23 points is possible, and an adult who scores below 18 or 19 points is generally considered at risk (Padula et al., 2018). For best results, nurses should be trained in proper use of the scale.

Another tool, shown in Table 36.2, is Norton's Pressure Area Risk Assessment Scoring System (Norton, McLaren, & Exton-Smith, 1975). It includes the categories of general physical condition, mental state, activity, mobility, and incontinence. A category of medications is added by some users, resulting in a possible score of 24. Scores of 15 or 16 should be viewed as indicators, not predictors, of risk.

The Braden and Norton tools should be used when the client first enters the healthcare agency and whenever the client's condition changes. In some long-term care facilities, a risk assessment using the Braden or Norton scale is conducted on admission and then on a regular basis, usually weekly. This increases awareness of specific risk factors and serves as assessment data from which to plan goals and interventions to either maintain or improve skin integrity.

The accompanying Practice Guidelines describe the principles of assessing common pressure sites.

BRADEN SCALE FOR PREDICTING PRESSURE SORE RISK

Patient's Name ____________ Evaluator's Name ____________

	1	2	3	4	Date of Assessment			
SENSORY PERCEPTION Ability to respond meaningfully to pressure-related discomfort	**1. Completely Limited:** Unresponsive (does not moan, flinch, or grasp) to painful stimuli, due to diminished level of consciousness or sedation, OR limited ability to feel pain over most of body surface.	**2. Very Limited:** Responds only to painful stimuli. Cannot communicate discomfort except by moaning or restlessness, OR has a sensory impairment which limits the ability to feel pain or discomfort over 1/2 of body.	**3. Slightly Limited:** Responds to verbal commands but cannot always communicate discomfort or need to be turned, OR has some sensory impairment which limits ability to feel pain or discomfort in 1 or 2 extremities.	**4. No Impairment:** Responds to verbal commands. Has no sensory deficit which would limit ability to feel or voice pain or discomfort.				
MOISTURE Degree to which skin is exposed to moisture	**1. Constantly Moist:** Skin is kept moist almost constantly by perspiration, urine, etc. Dampness is detected every time patient is moved or turned.	**2. Moist:** Skin is often but not always moist. Linen must be changed at least once a shift.	**3. Occasionally Moist:** Skin is occasionally moist, requiring an extra linen change approximately once a day.	**4. Rarely Moist:** Skin is usually dry; linen requires changing only at routine intervals.				
ACTIVITY Degree of physical activity	**1. Bedfast:** Confined to bed.	**2. Chairfast:** Ability to walk severely limited or nonexistent. Cannot bear own weight and/or must be assisted into chair or wheelchair.	**3. Walks Occasionally:** Walks occasionally during day but for very short distances, with or without assistance. Spends majority of each shift in bed or chair.	**4. Walks Frequently:** Walks outside the room at least twice a day and inside room at least once every 2 hours during waking hours.				
MOBILITY Ability to change and control body position	**1. Completely Immobile:** Does not make even slight changes in body or extremity position without assistance.	**2. Very Limited:** Makes occasional slight changes in body or extremity position but unable to make frequent or significant changes independently.	**3. Slightly Limited:** Makes frequent though slight changes in body or extremity position independently.	**4. No Limitations:** Makes major and frequent changes in position without assistance.				
NUTRITION Usual food intake pattern	**1. Very Poor:** Never eats a complete meal. Rarely eats more than 1/3 of any food offered. Eats 2 servings or less of protein (meat or dairy products) per day. Takes fluids poorly. Does not take a liquid dietary supplement, OR is NPO and/or maintained on clear liquids or IV's for more than 5 days.	**2. Probably Inadequate:** Rarely eats a complete meal and generally eats only about 1/2 of any food offered. Protein intake includes only 3 servings of meat or dairy products per day. Occasionally will take a dietary supplement, OR receives less than optimum amount of liquid diet or tube feeding.	**3. Adequate:** Eats over half of most meals. Eats a total of 4 servings of protein (meat, dairy products) each day. Occasionally will refuse a meal, but will usually take a supplement if offered, OR is on a tube feeding or TPN regimen, which probably meets most of nutritional needs.	**4. Excellent:** Eats most of every meal. Never refuses a meal. Usually eats a total of 4 or more servings of meat and dairy products. Occasionally eats between meals. Does not require supplementation.				
FRICTION AND SHEAR	**1. Problem:** Requires moderate to maximum assistance in moving. Complete lifting without sliding against sheets is impossible. Frequently slides down in bed or chair, requiring frequent repositioning with maximum assistance. Spasticity, contractures, or agitation leads to almost constant friction.	**2. Potential Problem:** Moves feebly or requires minimum assistance. During a move skin probably slides to some extent against sheets, chair, restraints, or other devices. Maintains relatively good position in chair or bed most of the time but occasionally slides down.	**3. No Apparent Problem:** Moves in bed and in chair independently and has sufficient muscle strength to lift up completely during move. Maintains good position in bed or chair at all times.					
				Total Score				

Figure 36.3 ■ Braden Scale for Predicting Pressure Sore Risk.

TABLE 36.2 Norton's Pressure Area Risk Assessment Form (Scoring System)

A. General Physical Condition		B. Mental State		C. Activity		D. Mobility		E. Incontinence	
Good	4	Alert	4	Ambulatory	4	Full	4	Absent	4
Fair	3	Apathetic	3	Walks with help	3	Slightly limited	3	Occasional	3
Poor	2	Confused	2	Chairbound	2	Very limited	2	Usually urinary	2
Very bad	1	Stuporous	1	Bedfast	1	Immobile	1	Double	1

Reprinted from *An Investigation of Geriatric Nursing Problems in Hospital*, by D. Norton, R. McLaren, and A. N. Exton-Smith, 1975, Edinburgh, United Kingdom: Churchill Livingstone. Reprinted with permission.

PRACTICE GUIDELINES Assessing Common Pressure Sites

- Ensure the lighting is good, preferably natural or fluorescent, because incandescent lights can create a transilluminating effect.
- Regulate the environment before beginning the assessment so that the room is neither too hot nor too cold. Heat can cause the skin to flush; cold can cause the skin to blanch or become cyanotic.
- Inspect pressure areas (Figure 36.4 ■) for discoloration. This can be caused by impaired blood circulation to the area. The pressure areas should have brisk capillary refill when gently pressed with a finger or thumb.
- Inspect pressure areas for abrasions and excoriations. Abrasions can occur when skin rubs against a sheet. Excoriations can occur when the skin has prolonged contact with body secretions or excretions or with dampness in skinfolds.
- Palpate the surface temperature of the skin over the pressure areas (warm your hands first). Normally, the temperature is the same as that of the surrounding skin. Increased temperature is abnormal and may be due to inflammation.
- Palpate over bony prominences and dependent body areas for the presence of edema, which feels spongy or boggy.

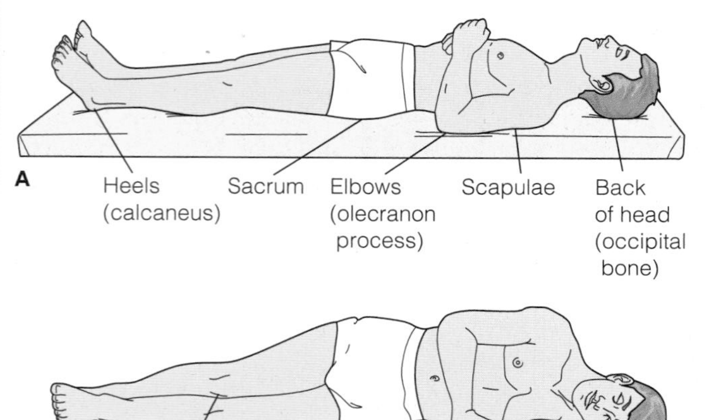

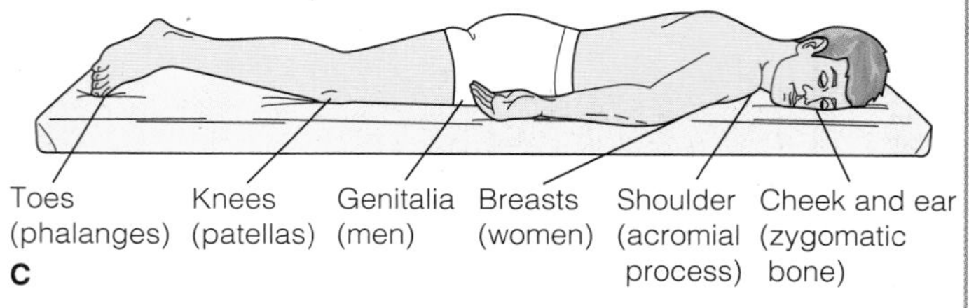

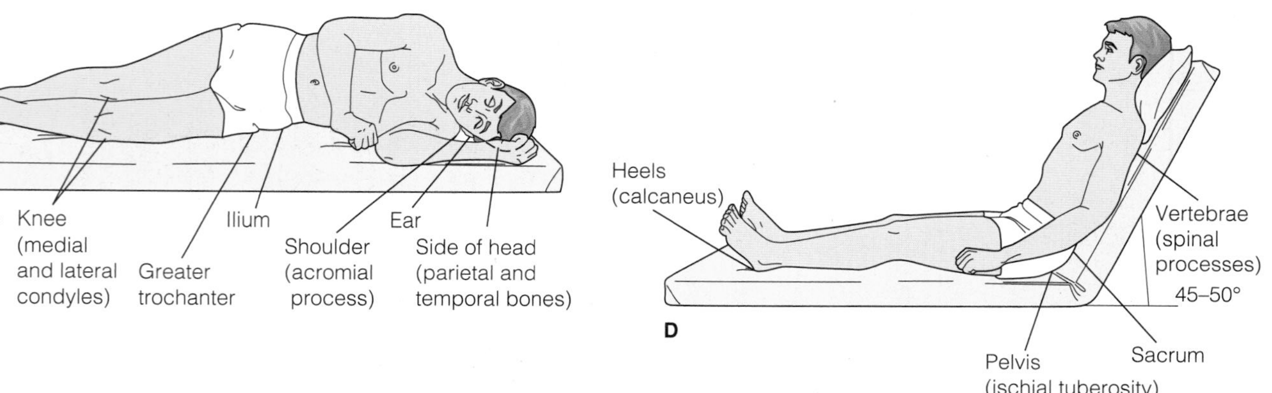

Figure 36.4 ■ Body pressure areas: *A*, supine position; *B*, lateral position; *C*, prone position; *D*, Fowler's position.

Clinical Alert!

Some nurses find the "rule of 30" a useful reminder to minimize pressure on the sacrum and coccyx by raising the head of the bed no more than 30° and turning the client laterally 30°.

Wound Healing

Healing is a quality of living tissue; it is also referred to as **regeneration** (renewal) of tissues. Healing can be considered in terms of *types of healing*, having to do with the primary care provider's decision on whether to allow the wound to seal itself or to purposefully close the wound, and *phases of healing*, which refer to the steps in the body's natural processes of tissue repair. The phases are the same for all wounds, but the rate and extent of healing depends on factors such as the type of healing, the location and size of the wound, and the health of the client.

Types of Wound Healing

The types of healing are influenced by the amount of tissue loss. **Primary intention healing** occurs where the tissue surfaces have been **approximated** (closed) and there is minimal or no tissue loss; it is characterized by the formation of minimal granulation tissue and scarring. It is also called *primary union* or *first intention healing*. An example of wound healing by primary intention is a closed surgical incision. Another example would be the use of tissue adhesive, a liquid glue that can be used to seal clean lacerations or incisions and may result in less noticeable scars.

A wound that is extensive and involves considerable tissue loss, and in which the edges cannot or should not be approximated, heals by **secondary intention healing**. An example of wound healing by secondary intention is a pressure injury. Secondary intention healing differs from primary intention healing in three ways: (1) The repair time is longer, (2) the scarring is greater, and (3) the susceptibility to infection is greater.

Wounds that are left open for 3 to 5 days to allow edema or infection to resolve or exudate to drain and are then closed with sutures, staples, or adhesive skin closures achieve **tertiary intention healing**. This is also called *delayed primary intention*.

Phases of Wound Healing

Wound healing can be broken down into three phases: inflammatory, proliferative, and maturation or remodeling.

Inflammatory Phase

The *inflammatory phase* begins immediately after injury and lasts 3 to 6 days. Two major processes occur during this phase: hemostasis and phagocytosis.

Hemostasis (the cessation of bleeding) results from vasoconstriction of the larger blood vessels in the affected area, retraction (drawing back) of injured blood vessels, the deposition of **fibrin** (connective tissue), and the formation of blood clots in the area. The blood clots provide a matrix of fibrin that becomes the framework for cell repair. A scab may also form on the surface of the wound. Consisting of clots and dead and dying tissue, this scab serves to aid hemostasis and inhibit contamination of the wound by microorganisms. Below the scab, epithelial cells migrate into the wound from the edges. The epithelial cells serve as a barrier between the body and the environment, preventing the entry of microorganisms.

In the inflammatory phase, the blood supply to the wound increases, bringing with it oxygen and nutrients needed in the healing process. The area appears reddened and edematous as a result. Exudate of fluid and cell debris is a normal accumulation and helps cleanse the wound. In surgical wounds, this lasts 1 to 3 days. Overproduction of this exudate and other factors can impair wound healing, especially in chronic wounds.

During cell migration, leukocytes (specifically, neutrophils) move into the interstitial space. These are replaced about 24 hours after injury by macrophages. These macrophages engulf microorganisms and cellular debris by a process known as **phagocytosis**. The macrophages also secrete an angiogenesis factor, which stimulates the formation of epithelial buds at the end of injured blood vessels. The microcirculatory network that results sustains

EVIDENCE-BASED PRACTICE

Evidence-Based Practice

Can a Wearable Monitor Improve Prevention of Pressure Injuries?

Although nurses know that they need to assist clients to change position regularly, Pickham et al. (2018) noted that the evidence on which repositioning protocols are based is often lacking and nurses are often unable to strictly implement the protocols. In this clinical trial, clients wore a sensor that provided data on body position and time spent in that position. Nurses caring for clients in the intervention group received a visual warning if the client was not turned according to the established protocol. More than 1300 clients in the intensive care unit were studied. Braden risk scores between the intervention and control groups were similar. After analyzing more than 100,000 hours of client care, the authors found that the intervention group showed statistically significant greater adherence to the turning protocol and fewer pressure injuries.

Implications

The authors recognize limitations of the study including that the sensor reported data only on the client's trunk and not on other parts of the body at risk for pressure injury. Data also showed that, although clients may have been repositioned, most were unable to maintain that position for the time specified in the protocol. However, the use of technology to assist the nurse in being reminded of the care protocol can improve outcomes. Further study is needed to replicate these findings and continue to determine the optimal timing and duration of the turning protocols in critical care and other care settings.

the healing process and the wound during its life. This inflammatory response is essential to healing. Measures that impair inflammation, such as steroid medications, can place the healing process at risk.

Proliferative Phase

The *proliferative phase*, the second phase in healing, extends from day 3 or 4 to about day 21 postinjury. Fibroblasts (connective tissue cells), which migrate into the wound starting about 24 hours after injury, begin to synthesize collagen. **Collagen** is a whitish protein substance that adds tensile strength to the wound. As the amount of collagen increases, so does the strength of the wound; thus the chance that the wound will remain closed progressively increases. If the wound is sutured, a raised "healing ridge" appears under the intact suture line. In a wound that is not sutured, the new collagen is often visible.

Capillaries grow across the wound, increasing the blood supply. Fibroblasts move from the bloodstream into the wound, depositing fibrin. As the capillary network develops, the tissue becomes a translucent red color. This tissue, called **granulation tissue**, is fragile and bleeds easily.

When the skin edges of a wound are not sutured, the area must be filled in with granulation tissue. When the granulation tissue matures, marginal epithelial cells migrate to it, proliferating over this connective tissue base to fill the wound. If the wound does not close by epithelialization, the area becomes covered with dried plasma proteins and dead cells. This is called **eschar**. Initially, wounds healing by secondary intention seep blood-tinged (**serosanguineous**) drainage. Later, if they are not covered by epithelial cells, they become covered with thick, gray, fibrinous tissue that is eventually converted into dense scar tissue.

Maturation Phase

The *maturation phase* begins on about day 21 and can extend 1 or 2 years after the injury. Fibroblasts continue to synthesize collagen. The wound is remodeled and contracted. The scar becomes stronger but the repaired area is never as strong as the original tissue. In some individuals, particularly dark-skinned individuals, an abnormal amount of collagen is laid down. This can result in a hypertrophic scar, or **keloid**.

Types of Wound Exudate

Exudate is material, such as fluid and cells, which has escaped from blood vessels during the inflammatory process and is deposited in tissue or on tissue surfaces. The nature and amount of exudate vary according to the tissue involved, the intensity and duration of the inflammation, and the presence of microorganisms.

The three major types of exudate are serous, purulent, and sanguineous. A **serous exudate** consists chiefly of serum (the clear portion of the blood). It looks watery and has few cells. An example is the fluid in a blister from a burn.

A **purulent exudate** is thicker than serous exudate because of the presence of **pus**, which consists of leukocytes, liquefied dead tissue debris, and dead and living bacteria. The process of pus formation is referred to as **suppuration**. Purulent exudates vary in color, some acquiring tinges of blue, green, or yellow, depending on the causative organism.

A **sanguineous exudate** consists of large amounts of red blood cells, indicating damage to capillaries that is severe enough to allow the escape of red blood cells from plasma. This type of exudate is frequently seen in open wounds.

Mixed types of exudates are often observed. A serosanguineous exudate consisting of both clear and blood-tinged drainage is commonly seen in surgical incisions. A purosanguineous discharge, consisting of pus and blood, is often seen in a new wound that is infected.

Clinical Alert!

A bright sanguineous exudate indicates fresh bleeding, whereas dark sanguineous exudate denotes older bleeding.

Complications of Wound Healing

Several events can interfere with the healing of a wound. These include hemorrhage, infection, dehiscence, and evisceration.

Hemorrhage

Some escape of blood from a wound is normal. **Hemorrhage** (massive bleeding), however, is abnormal. A dislodged clot, a slipped stitch, or erosion of a blood vessel may cause severe bleeding.

Internal hemorrhaging may be detected by swelling or distention in the area of the wound and, possibly, by sanguineous drainage from a surgical drain. Some clients will have a **hematoma**, a localized collection of blood underneath the skin that may appear as a reddish blue swelling (bruise). A large hematoma may be dangerous in that it places pressure on blood vessels and other structures and can thus obstruct flow.

The risk of hemorrhage is greatest during the first 48 hours after surgery. Hemorrhage is an emergency; the nurse should apply pressure dressings to the wound and monitor the client's vital signs. In many instances, the client must be taken to the operating room for surgical intervention.

Infection

Contamination of a wound surface with microorganisms (colonization) is an inevitable result because the surface cannot be permanently protected from contact with unsterile objects. Because the colonizing organisms compete with new cells for oxygen and nutrition, and because their by-products can interfere with a healthy surface condition, the presence of contamination can impair wound healing and lead to infection. When the microorganisms colonizing the wound multiply excessively or invade tissues, infection occurs. Infection suggested by a change in wound color, pain, odor, or drainage is confirmed by performing a culture of the wound (see Chapter 34). Severe infection causes fever and an elevated white blood cell count. Clients who are immunosuppressed, such as those with HIV or receiving myelosuppressive treatment for cancer, are especially susceptible to wound infections.

A wound can be infected with microorganisms at the time of injury, during surgery, or postoperatively. Wounds that occur as a result of injury (e.g., motor vehicle crash, bullet or knife wound) are most likely to be contaminated at the time of injury. Surgery involving the intestines can also result in infection from the microorganisms inside the intestine. Surgical infection is most likely to become apparent 2 to 11 days postoperatively.

Dehiscence with Possible Evisceration

Dehiscence is the partial or total rupturing of a sutured wound. Dehiscence usually involves an abdominal wound in which the layers below the skin also separate. **Evisceration** is the protrusion of the internal organs through an incision. A number of factors, including obesity, poor nutrition, multiple trauma, failure of suturing, excessive coughing, vomiting, and dehydration, heighten a client's risk of wound dehiscence. Wound dehiscence is more likely to occur 4 to 5 days postoperatively before extensive collagen is deposited in the wound.

Sudden straining, such as coughing or sneezing, may precede dehiscence. It is not unusual for a client to feel that "something has given way." When dehiscence or evisceration occurs, the wound should be quickly supported by large sterile dressings soaked in sterile normal saline. Place the client in bed with knees bent to decrease pull on the incision. The surgeon must be notified immediately because surgical repair of the area may be necessary.

A related complication can be the formation of a *fistula*. A fistula is a connection between any two organs or surfaces and can occur especially when surgery involves the gastrointestinal system and a pathway evolves between the internal surgical site and the wound and skin. In this situation, contents drain through the fistula to the skin surface and impair wound healing. Treatment and care of a fistula involve protection of the surrounding skin and dressings appropriate to the type and location of the fistula.

Factors Affecting Wound Healing

Characteristics of the individual such as age, nutritional status, lifestyle, and medications influence the speed of wound healing.

Developmental Considerations

Healthy children and adults often heal more quickly than older adults, who are more likely to have chronic diseases that hinder healing. For example, reduced liver function can impair the synthesis of blood clotting factors. Box 36.1 lists factors inhibiting wound healing in older adults.

BOX 36.1 Factors Inhibiting Wound Healing in Older Adults

- Vascular changes associated with aging, such as atherosclerosis and atrophy of capillaries in the skin, can impair blood flow to the wound.
- Collagen tissue is less flexible, which increases the risk of damage from pressure, friction, and shearing.
- Scar tissue is less elastic.
- Changes in the immune system may reduce the formation of the antibodies and monocytes necessary for wound healing.
- Nutritional deficiencies may reduce the numbers of red blood cells and leukocytes, thus impeding the delivery of oxygen and the inflammatory response essential for wound healing. Oxygen is needed for the synthesis of collagen and the formation of new epithelial cells.
- Having diabetes or cardiovascular disease increases the risk of delayed healing due to impaired oxygen delivery to these tissues.
- Cell renewal is slower, leading to delayed healing.

Nutrition

Wound healing places additional demands on the body. Clients require a diet rich in protein, carbohydrates, lipids, vitamins A and C, and minerals, such as iron, zinc, and copper. Malnourished clients may require time to improve their nutritional status before surgery, if this is possible. Obese clients are at increased risk of wound infection and slower healing because adipose tissue usually has a minimal blood supply.

Lifestyle

Clients who exercise regularly tend to have good circulation, and because blood brings oxygen and nourishment to the wound, they are likely to heal quickly. Smoking reduces the amount of functional hemoglobin in the blood, thus limiting the oxygen-carrying capacity of the blood, and constricts arterioles.

Medications

Anti-inflammatory drugs (e.g., steroids and aspirin) and antineoplastic agents interfere with healing. Prolonged use of antibiotics may make a client susceptible to wound infection by resistant organisms.

●○● NURSING MANAGEMENT

Assessing

Assessment of Skin Integrity

The nurse conducts an examination of the integument as part of a routine assessment and during regular care. Removing barriers to assessment is very important. Antiembolic stockings, braces, or devices must be removed to assess the skin condition underneath.

Nursing History and Physical Assessment

During the review of systems as part of the nursing history, the nurse gathers information regarding skin diseases, previous bruising, general skin condition, skin lesions, and usual healing of sores. Inspection and palpation of the skin focus on determination of skin color distribution, skin turgor, presence of edema, and characteristics of any lesions that are present. Particular attention is paid to skin condition in areas most likely to break down: in skinfolds such as under the breasts, in areas that are frequently moist such as the perineum, and in areas that receive extensive pressure such as the bony prominences. Refer to Chapter 29 ∞ for further detail regarding skin assessment.

Assessment of Wounds

Nurses commonly assess both untreated and treated wounds. Assessment for these wounds is shown in the accompanying Practice Guidelines. Although a pressure injury can be categorized as an untreated or treated wound, the specific assessment of pressure injuries is discussed separately in this chapter.

Untreated Wounds

Untreated wounds usually are seen shortly after an injury (e.g., at the scene of an accident or in an emergency center).

Treated Wounds

Treated wounds, or sutured wounds, are usually assessed to determine the progress of healing. These wounds may be inspected during changing of a dressing. If the wound itself cannot be directly inspected, the dressing is inspected and other data regarding the wound (e.g., the presence of pain) are assessed. Dressings are inspected regularly to ensure that they are clean, dry, and intact. Excessive drainage may indicate hemorrhage, infection, or an open wound.

Estimating the amount of wound drainage can be difficult. One recommendation is to describe the degree to which the dressing is saturated. Minimal drainage only stains the dressing, moderate drainage saturates the dressing without leakage prior to scheduled dressing changes, and heavy drainage overflows the dressing prior to scheduled changes. These terms, plus the description of the drainage and the amount and type of dressing material used, should be well understood by all care providers.

Sometimes, the wound extends under the skin surface (called *undermining*). The edges of the wound around an open center may be raw or appear healed, but the undermining can result in a sinus tract or tunnel that extends the wound many centimeters beyond the main wound surface. To fully assess the size of the wound, the nurse gently explores the undermined area with a sterile swab. One way to measure depth is to place a second swab parallel to the first and measure the distance from the edge of the wound to the tip of the exposed swab (Figure 36.5 ■). Sinus tracts are often caused by infection and have significant drainage. They may be treated using antibiotics, irrigation, surgical incision to open and drain the tract, or negative pressure therapy for large tracts.

PRACTICE GUIDELINES Assessing Wounds

- Assess the location and extent of tissue damage (e.g., partial thickness or full thickness). Measure the wound length, width, and depth.
- Inspect the wound for bleeding. The amount of bleeding varies according to the type of wound and location. Penetrating wounds may cause internal bleeding.
- Inspect the wound for foreign bodies (soil, broken glass, shreds of cloth, or other foreign substances).
- Assess associated injuries such as fractures, internal bleeding, spinal cord injuries, or head trauma.
- If the wound is contaminated with foreign material, determine when the client last had a tetanus toxoid injection. A tetanus immunization or booster may be necessary.
- Prevent infection by (a) cleaning or flushing abrasions or lacerations with normal saline and (b) covering the wound with a clean dressing, if possible. A sterile dressing is preferred. When applying a dressing, wrap the wound tightly enough to apply pressure and approximate the wound edges, if you are able. If the first layer of dressing becomes saturated with blood, apply a second layer. Do so without removing the first layer of dressing, because blood clots might be disturbed, resulting in more bleeding.
- Control swelling and pain by applying ice over the wound and surrounding tissues.
- If bleeding is severe or if internal bleeding is suspected, assess the client for signs of shock (rapid thready pulse, cold clammy skin, pallor, lowered blood pressure).

ASSESSING SURGICAL WOUNDS

- Inspect the color of the wound and surrounding area and approximation of wound edges.
- Note size and location of dehiscence, if present.
- Observe location, color, consistency, odor, and degree of saturation of dressings. Note number of gauzes saturated or diameter of drainage on gauze.
- Observe the amount of swelling; minimal to moderate swelling is normal in early stages of wound healing.
- Expect severe to moderate postoperative pain for 3 to 5 days; persistent severe pain or sudden onset of severe pain may indicate internal hemorrhaging or infection.
- Inspect drain security and placement, amount and character of drainage, and functioning of collecting apparatus, if present.

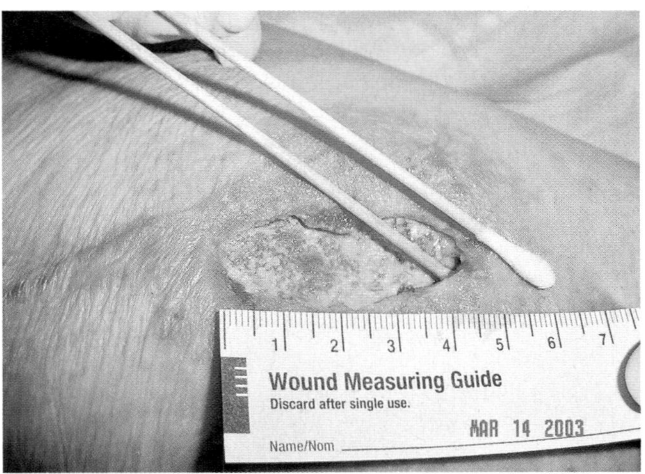

Figure 36.5 ■ Parallel swabs used to measure wound depth.
Cory patrick Hartley RN. WCC, OMS.

Pressure Injuries

When a pressure injury is present, the nurse notes the following:

- Location of the injury, related to a bony prominence.
- Size of injury in centimeters. Measure greatest length, width, and depth. To measure depth, insert a sterile applicator swab at the deepest part of the wound, and then measure it against a measuring guide.
- Presence of undermining or sinus tracts, location described by position on the face of a clock, 12 o'clock as the client's head.
- Stage of the injury (see Figure 36.2).
- Color of the wound bed and location of necrosis (dead tissue) or eschar.
- Condition of the wound margins.
- Integrity of surrounding skin.
- Clinical signs of infection, such as redness, warmth, swelling, pain, odor, and exudate (note color of exudate).

The easiest and most accurate method of documenting wound size and shape is with disposable wound-measuring guides (for example, see Figure 36.6*A* ■). For irregularly shaped wounds, the nurse can use two layers of transparent film, trace the wound margins on the top layer, and then discard the bottom layer that came in contact with the wound. To measure an area located on a curved portion of the body, use a flexible measure (Figure 36.6*B*). Electronic devices allow tracings to be digitized for improved determination of the total wound area (Landa, van Dishoeck, Steyerberg, & Hovius, 2016).

Document the status of the client's skin and wounds on a skin and wound documentation form (see Figure 36.7 ■ for an example). It is important to be able to determine how these change over time. One method of documenting the progress of healing in pressure injuries is to use the Pressure Ulcer Scale for Healing (PUSH) tool created by the National Pressure Ulcer Advisory Panel (NPUAP) (Choi, Chin, Wan, & Lam, 2016). This well-validated tool assigns scores to the injury length, width, amount of exudate, and tissue type. The change in the total score over time can be used as an indication of healing.

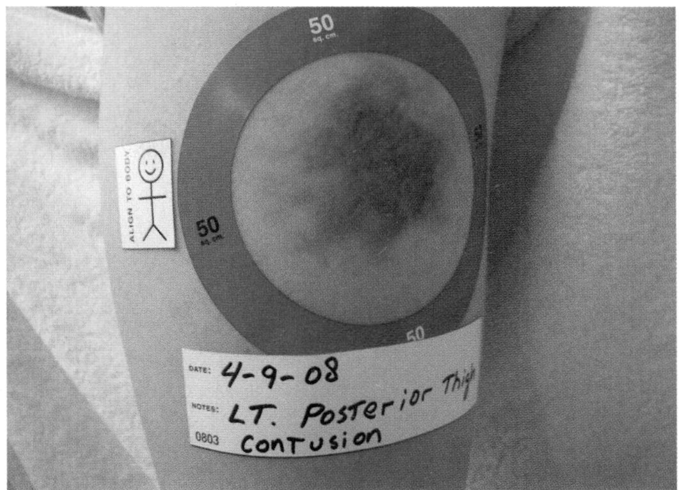

A

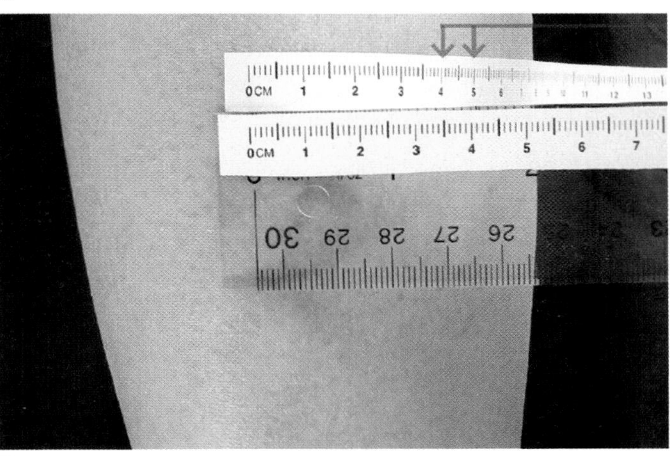

B

Figure 36.6 ■ Use of photo measuring guides provide documentation of scale and alignment with the body. *A*, This guide provides the diameter of the wound irrespective of camera distance. *B*, A flexible ruler (upper) is needed to prevent measurement error when assessing a wound on a curved part of the body. The red arrows indicate a difference of more than 0.5 cm between the two rulers.
Courtesy of KISS Healthcare, Inc.

Laboratory Data

Laboratory data can often support the nurse's clinical assessment of the wound's progress in healing. A decreased leukocyte count can delay healing and increase the possibility of infection. A hemoglobin level below the normal range indicates poor oxygen delivery to the tissues. Blood coagulation studies are also significant. Prolonged coagulation times can result in excessive blood loss and prolonged clot absorption. Hypercoagulability can lead to intravascular clotting, and result in a deficient blood supply to the wound area. Serum protein analysis provides an indication of the body's nutritional reserves for rebuilding cells. Albumin is an important indicator of nutritional status. A value below 3.5 g/dL indicates poor nutrition and may increase the risk of poor healing and infection. Wound cultures can either confirm or rule out the presence of infection. Sensitivity studies are helpful in the selection of appropriate antibiotic therapy. The nurse obtains a wound culture whenever an infection is suspected (see Skill 36.3).

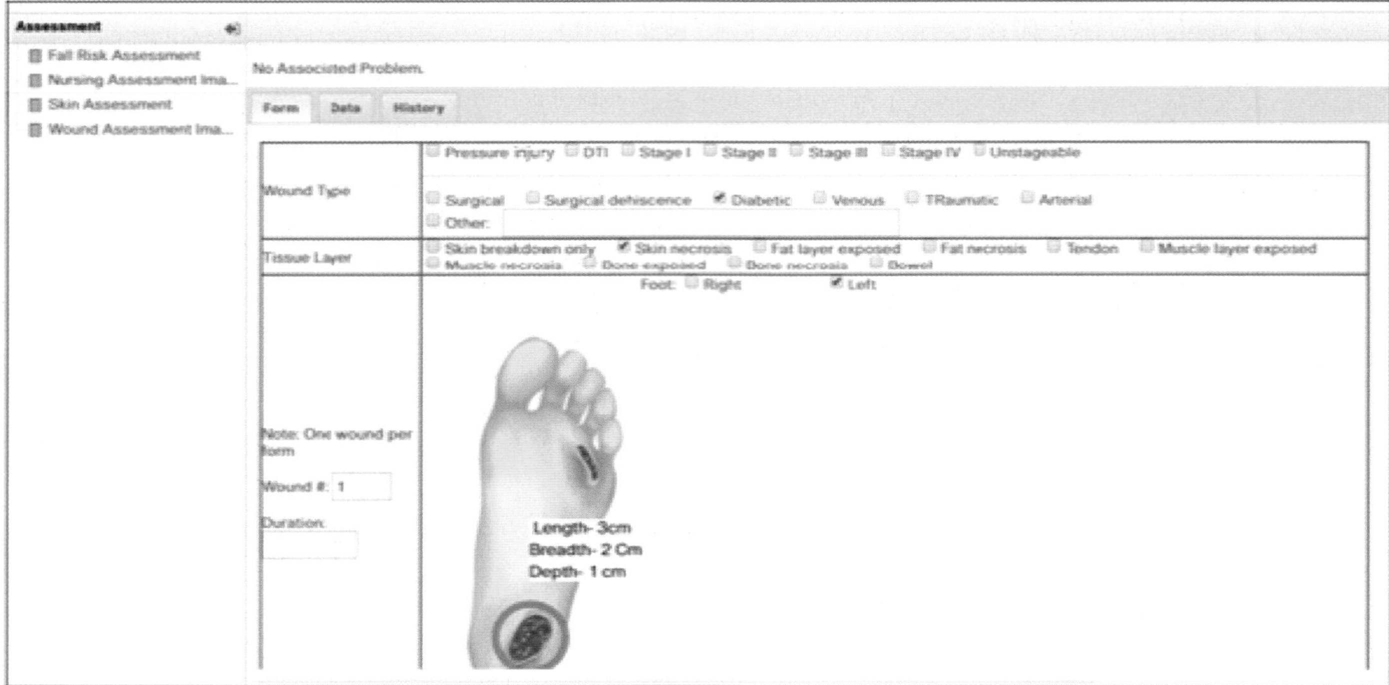

Figure 36.7 ■ Wound and skin documentation.
iCare.

Diagnosing

Examples of nursing diagnoses for a client who has skin wounds or who is at risk for skin breakdown can include potential for developing pressure injury; and actual, or potential for developing, altered skin integrity.

Planning

The major goals for clients at risk for pressure injury development are to maintain skin integrity and to avoid potential associated risks. Clients with actual wounds need goals to demonstrate progressive wound healing and regain intact skin within a specified time frame.

Planning for Home Care

Increasingly, wound care is provided in the home rather than in healthcare facilities. The client and family assume much of the responsibility for assessing and treating existing wounds and for helping to prevent pressure injuries.

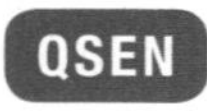

Patient-Centered Care: Assessing Readiness for Wound Care and Prevention of Pressure Injuries in the Home

When working with clients in the home, the nurse must assess the following factors in order to plan care.

CLIENT AND ENVIRONMENT

- Current level of knowledge: understanding of the cause of the wound or risk for developing a pressure injury; prevention or treatment strategies
- Self-care abilities for mobility: physical ability to change position, ambulate, and transfer including the use of assistive devices
- Self-care abilities for wound care: manual dexterity and visual acuity necessary to perform skin assessments and wound treatments
- Facilities: presence of running water, garbage, bathroom needed to perform wound care and contain potentially infectious materials
- Current level of nutrition: eating habits and preferences, laboratory values indicating need for teaching or other intervention

FAMILY

- Caregiver availability, skills, and responses: understanding of the cause of the wound or risk for developing a pressure injury; prevention or treatment strategies; willingness to assist with wound care and preventive actions
- Family role changes and coping: effect on financial status, parenting and spousal roles, sexuality, social roles
- Alternate potential primary or respite caregivers: for example, other family members, volunteers, church members, paid caregivers or housekeeping services; available community respite care (e.g., adult day care, senior centers)

COMMUNITY

- Resources: availability and familiarity with possible sources of assistance such as equipment and supply companies, organizations that offer medical supplies or financial assistance, home health agencies

In planning for client discharge, nurses are accountable for teaching the client and family wound preventive and care measures. See Client Teaching for a model. A critical pathway can also be useful for planning client care at home (see the example).

CLIENT TEACHING **Skin Integrity**

MAINTAINING INTACT SKIN

- Discuss the relationship between adequate nutrition (especially fluids, protein, vitamins B and C, iron, and calories) and healthy skin.
- Demonstrate appropriate positions for pressure relief.
- Establish a turning or repositioning schedule.
- Demonstrate the application of appropriate skin protection agents and devices.
- Instruct to report persistent reddened areas.
- Identify potential sources of skin trauma and means of avoidance.

PROMOTING WOUND HEALING

- Discuss importance of adequate nutrition (especially fluids, protein, vitamins B and C, iron, and calories).
- Instruct in wound assessment and provide mechanism for documenting.
- Emphasize principles of asepsis, especially hand hygiene and proper methods of handling used dressings.
- Provide information about signs of wound infection and other complications to report.
- Reinforce appropriate aspects of pressure injury and MASD prevention.
- Demonstrate wound care techniques such as wound cleansing and dressing changing.
- Discuss pain control measures, if indicated.

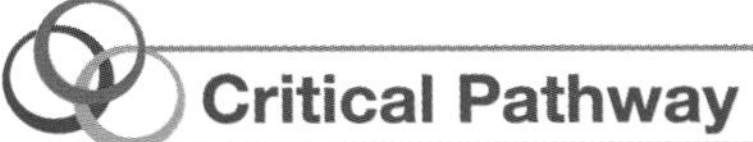

Critical Pathway **Wound Management**

Outcomes	Client verbalizes understanding of teaching, including wound care, signs and symptoms to report, follow-up care.	At time of suture removal: Client is afebrile. Client has a dry, clean wound with edges well approximated, healing by first intention.
	Date ______________	**Date** ______________
	Outpatient setting	**Daily for 10 days (Client activities)**
Knowledge	Provide simple, brief instructions regarding injury and treatment. Encourage client to ask questions and seek assistance. Assess the client's knowledge about wound care. Review written instruction sheet for wound care with client and provide copy.	Follow written discharge teaching regarding wound care and dressing change. Call primary care provider with questions or problems and return to office in 10 days for suture removal.
	Instruct client about foods high in protein and vitamin C and encourage adequate intake.	Diet high in protein and vitamin C. Cultural remedies that will not interfere with healing.
Wound Care	Irrigate and clean the wound with normal saline. Surgical consultation for wound closure. Following wound closure, apply dry sterile dressing.	Change dressing daily and prn to keep dressing dry and clean. Inspect wound daily and report any signs and symptoms of infection (redness, pain, warmth, drainage, swelling, or fever).
Medications	Tetanus toxoid if indicated.	Only if ordered.

Implementing

Nursing interventions for maintaining skin integrity and wound care involve preventing pressure injuries and MASD, treating wounds, cleaning wounds, dressing wounds, removing staples or sutures, and applying heat and cold.

Preventing Pressure Injuries and MASD

To reduce the likelihood of pressure injury or moisture damage development in all clients, the nurse employs a variety of preventive measures to maintain the skin integrity and instructs the client, support people, and caregivers in how to prevent pressure injuries. The Institute for Healthcare Improvement (2011) delineates two major steps: identifying clients at risk, and reliably implementing prevention strategies for all clients who are identified as being at risk. Specifically, the nurse conducts a pressure injury admission assessment for all clients and reassesses risk for all hospitalized clients daily. For clients at risk, the nurse also optimizes nutrition and hydration, inspects skin daily, minimizes pressure, and manages moisture by keeping the client dry and moisturizing skin.

Providing Nutrition

Because an inadequate intake of calories, protein, vitamins, and iron is believed to be a risk factor for pressure injury development, nutritional supplements should be considered for nutritionally compromised clients. The diet should be similar to that which supports wound healing, as discussed earlier. Monitor weight regularly to help assess nutritional status. Pertinent laboratory work should also be monitored including lymphocyte count, protein (especially albumin), and hemoglobin.

Maintaining Skin Hygiene

Obtain baseline data using the established tool and then reassess the skin at least daily in the hospital and weekly at home. When bathing the client, the nurse should minimize the force and friction applied to the skin, using mild cleansing agents that minimize irritation and dryness and that do not disrupt the skin's "natural barriers." Also, avoid using hot water, which increases skin dryness and irritation. Nurses can minimize dryness by avoiding exposure to cold and low humidity. Dry skin is best treated with moisturizing lotions applied while the skin is moist after bathing. The client's skin should be kept clean and dry and free of irritation and maceration by urine, feces, sweat, or incomplete drying after a bath. Apply skin protection if indicated. Dimethicone-based creams or alcohol-free barrier films are available in liquid, spray, and moist wipe format and are very effective in preventing moisture or drainage from collecting on the skin. In most cases, the nurse can apply these without a primary care provider's order.

Avoiding Skin Trauma

Providing the client with a smooth, firm, and wrinkle-free foundation on which to sit or lie helps prevent skin trauma. To prevent injury due to friction and shearing forces, clients must be positioned, transferred, and turned correctly. For bedridden clients, shearing force can be reduced by elevating the head of the bed to no more than 30°, if this position is not contraindicated by the client's condition. (For example, clients with respiratory disorders may find it easier to breathe in Fowler's position.) When the head of the bed is raised, the skin and superficial fascia stick to the bed linen while the deep fascia and skeleton slide down toward the bottom of the bed. As a result, blood vessels in the sacral area become twisted, and the tissues in the area can become ischemic and necrotic.

Baby powder and cornstarch are never used as friction or moisture prevention. These powders create harmful abrasive grit that is damaging to tissues and they are considered a respiratory hazard when airborne. Instead, use moisturizing creams and protective films, such as transparent dressings and alcohol-free barrier films.

Frequent shifts in position, even if only slight, effectively change pressure points. The client should shift weight 10° to 15° every 15 to 30 minutes and, whenever possible, exercise or ambulate to stimulate blood circulation.

When lifting a client to change position, nurses should use a lifting device rather than dragging the client across or up in bed. The friction that results from dragging the skin against a sheet can cause blisters and abrasions, which may contribute to more extensive tissue damage. Therefore, using devices or a lift team to lift the client's weight off the bed surface is the method of choice—and can help prevent back injuries to nurses.

Any at-risk client confined to bed—even when a special support mattress is used—should be repositioned at least every 2 hours, depending on the client's need, to allow another body surface to bear the weight. Six body positions can usually be used: prone, supine, right and left lateral (side-lying), and right and left Sims positions. When a lateral position is used, the nurse should avoid positioning the client directly on the trochanter and instead position the client on a 30° angle. A written schedule should be established for turning and repositioning.

In addition, massage over bony prominences should be avoided. Traditionally, nurses have used massage to stimulate blood circulation, with the intention of preventing pressure injuries. However, scientific evidence does not support this belief (Haesler, 2018).

Providing Supportive Devices

For clients confined to bed, several types of support surfaces can be used to relieve pressure. The overlay mattress is applied on top of the standard bed mattress. A replacement mattress is used instead of the standard mattress; most are made of foam and gel combinations. Specialty beds replace hospital beds. They provide pressure relief, eliminate shearing and friction, and decrease moisture. Examples are high-air-loss beds, low-air-loss beds, and beds that provide kinetic therapy. Kinetic beds provide continuous passive motion or oscillation therapy, which is intended to counteract the effects of a client's immobility. Table 36.3 lists selected mechanical devices for reducing pressure on body parts.

When a client is confined to bed or a chair, pressure-reducing devices, such as pillows made of foam, gel, air, or a combination of these, can be used. When the client is sitting, weight should be distributed over the entire seating surface so that pressure does not center on just one area. To protect a client's heels in bed, supports such as wedges or pillows can be used to raise the heels completely off the bed. Doughnut-type devices should not be used since they limit blood flow and can cause tissue damage to the areas in direct contact with the device.

Treating Wounds

Pressure injuries, MASD, and IAD are challenges for nurses because of the number of variables involved (e.g., risk factors, types of injuries, and degrees of impairment) and the numerous treatment measures advocated. Nurses should follow the agency protocols and the primary care provider's orders, if any. Prompt treatment can prevent further tissue damage and pain and facilitate wound healing. See the accompanying Practice Guidelines.

TABLE 36.3 Mechanical Devices for Reducing Pressure on Body Parts

Device	Description/Comments
Gel flotation pads	Polyvinyl, silicone, or Silastic pads filled with a gelatinous substance similar to fat.
Pillows and wedges (foam, gel, air, fluid)	Supports positioning and offloads bone-on-bone contact.
Heel protectors (sheepskin boots, padded splints, off-loading inflatable boots, foam blocks)	Can raise or "float" a body part (e.g., heels) off the surface. Prevent shearing and limit pressure on heel area.
Memory foam mattress or chair pad	Polyurethane foam mattress distributes weight over bony areas evenly. Foam molds to the body.
Alternating pressure mattress	Composed of a number of cells in which the pressure alternately increases and decreases; uses a pump.
Water bed	Support surface filled with water. Water temperature can be controlled.
Static low-air-loss (LAL) bed	Consists of many air-filled cushions divided into four or five sections. Separate controls permit each section to be inflated to a different level of firmness; thus pressure can be reduced on bony prominences but increased under other body areas for support (Figure 36.8 ■).
Active or second-generation LAL bed	Like the static LAL, but in addition gently pulsates or rotates from side to side, thus stimulating capillary blood flow and facilitating movement of pulmonary secretions.
Air-fluidized (AF) bed (static high-air-loss bed)	Forced temperature-controlled air is circulated around millions of tiny silicone-coated beads, producing a fluid-like movement. Provides uniform support to body contours. Decreases skin maceration by its drying effect. Moisture from the client penetrates the linens and soaks the beads. Airflow forces the beads away from the client and rapidly dries the sheet. A major disadvantage is that the head of the bed cannot be elevated. Some beds are a unique combination of air-fluidized therapy and low-air-loss therapy on an articulating frame. These are used with clients who require head elevation.

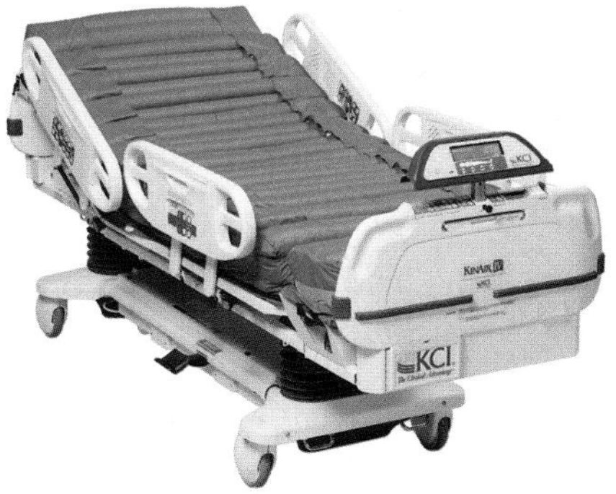

Figure 36.8 ■ Low-air-loss bed KinAir IV.
Courtesy ArjoHuntleigh Inc.

PRACTICE GUIDELINES Treating Wounds

- Minimize direct pressure on the wound. Reposition the client at least every 2 hours. Make a schedule, and record position changes on the client's chart. Provide devices to minimize or float pressure areas.
- Clean the wound with every dressing change. The method of cleaning depends on the stage of the injury, products available, and agency protocol. Skill 36.2 details the steps involved in irrigating a wound.
- Clean and dress the wound using aseptic technique. Never use alcohol or hydrogen peroxide because they are cytotoxic to tissue beds.
- If the wound is infected, obtain a sample of the drainage for culture and sensitivity to antibiotic agents (see Skill 36.3).
- Teach the client to move frequently, even if only slightly, to relieve pressure.
- Provide range-of-motion (ROM) exercises and mobility as the client's condition permits (see Chapter 44 ∞).

The RYB Color Code

To guide wound care, the nurse can use the RYB color code of wounds. This concept is based on the color of an open wound—red, yellow, or black (RYB)—rather than the depth or size of a wound. On this scheme, the goals of wound care are to protect (cover) red, cleanse yellow, and debride black.

Wounds that are red are usually in the late regeneration phase of tissue repair (i.e., developing granulation tissue). They need to be protected to avoid disturbance to regenerating tissue. The nurse protects red wounds by (a) gentle cleansing (i.e., use of a noncytotoxic wound cleanser applied without pressure); (b) protecting periwound skin with alcohol-free barrier film; (c) filling dead space with hydrogel or alginate; (d) covering with an appropriate dressing such as transparent film, hydrocolloid dressing, or a clear absorbent acrylic dressing; and (e) changing the dressing as infrequently as possible.

Yellow wounds are characterized primarily by liquid to semiliquid "slough" that is often accompanied by purulent drainage or previous infection. The nurse cleanses yellow wounds to remove nonviable tissue. Methods used may include applying damp-to-damp normal saline dressings, irrigating the wound, using absorbent dressing materials such as impregnated hydrogel or alginate dressings, and consulting with the primary care provider about the need for a topical antimicrobial to minimize bacterial growth.

Black wounds are covered with thick necrotic tissue, or eschar. A stable black wound has a firm surface that should be left in place. Blood flow in the tissue under the stable eschar is poor and the wound is susceptible to infection. The eschar acts as a natural barrier to infection by keeping the bacteria from entering the wound. An unstable black wound has a loose, spongy, soft surface that will need to be removed through **debridement** for the wound to heal. Debridement may be achieved in four different ways: sharp, mechanical, chemical, and autolytic. In *sharp debridement*, a scalpel or scissors are used to separate and remove dead tissue. In many settings, specially trained nurses (wound ostomy continence nurses [WOCNs]), physical therapists, and physician assistants are permitted to perform sharp debridement. *Mechanical debridement* is accomplished through scrubbing force or damp-to-damp dressings. *Chemical debridement* is more selective than sharp or mechanical techniques. Collagenase enzyme agents such as papain-urea are currently most recommended for this use. In *autolytic debridement*, dressings such as hydrocolloid and clear absorbent acrylic dressings trap the wound drainage against the eschar. The body's own enzymes in the drainage break down the necrotic tissue. Although this method takes longer than the other three, it is the most selective and therefore causes the least damage to healthy surrounding and healing tissues. The use of fly larvae (maggots, *Phaenicia sericata* and other species) can be extremely effective in cleansing chronic wounds because the maggots secrete enzymes that break down necrotic tissue (while leaving healthy tissue untouched), eat bacteria, and decrease bacterial growth through the rise in surface pH that results from their presence (Wilson, Nigam, Knight, & Pritchard, 2019).

Cleaning Wounds

Wound cleaning involves the removal of debris, such as foreign materials, excess slough, necrotic tissue, bacteria, and other microorganisms. The choices of cleaning agent and method depend largely on agency protocol and the primary care provider's preference. Recommended guidelines for cleaning wounds are shown in the accompanying Practice Guidelines.

PRACTICE GUIDELINES Cleaning Wounds

- Follow standard precautions for personal protection. Wear gloves, gown, goggles, and mask as indicated.
- Use solutions such as isotonic saline or wound cleansers to clean or irrigate wounds. If antimicrobial solutions are used, make sure they are well diluted.
- Microwave heating of liquids to be used on the wound is not recommended. When possible, warm the solution to body temperature before use. **Rationale:** *This prevents lowering the wound temperature, which slows the healing process. Microwave heating could cause the solution to become too hot.*
- If a wound is grossly contaminated by foreign material, bacteria, slough, or necrotic tissue, clean the wound at every dressing change. **Rationale:** *Foreign bodies and devitalized tissue act as a focus for infection and can delay healing.*
- If a wound is clean, has little exudate, and reveals healthy granulation tissue, avoid repeated cleaning. **Rationale:** *Unnecessary cleaning can delay wound healing by traumatizing newly produced, delicate tissues, reducing the surface temperature of the wound, and removing exudate, which itself may have bactericidal properties.*
- Use gauze squares or nonwoven swabs that do not shed fibers. Avoid using cotton balls and other products that shed fibers onto the wound surface. **Rationale:** *The fibers become embedded in granulation tissue and can act as foci for infection. They may also stimulate "foreign body" reactions, prolonging the inflammatory phase of healing and delaying the healing process.*
- Avoid drying a wound after cleaning it. **Rationale:** *This helps retain wound moisture.*
- Hold cleaning sponges with forceps or with a gloved hand.
- Consider not cleaning the wound at all if it appears to be clean.

Cleaning Surgical Wounds

Not all dressings on surgical wounds require changing. Sometimes surgeons in the operating room apply a dressing that remains in place until the sutures are removed, and no further dressings are required. In many situations, however, surgical dressings are changed regularly to prevent the growth of microorganisms.

Surgical drains are inserted to permit the drainage of excessive serosanguinous fluid and purulent material and to promote healing of underlying tissues. These drains may be inserted and sutured through the incision line, but they are most commonly inserted through stab wounds a few centimeters away from the incision line so that the incision itself may be kept dry. Without a drain, some wounds would heal on the surface and trap the discharge inside, and an abscess might form. These devices (e.g., the **Penrose drain**) have an open end that drains onto a dressing. The main surgical incision is considered cleaner than the surgical stab wound made for the drain insertion. The main incision is therefore cleaned first, and under no circumstances are materials that were used to clean the stab wound used subsequently to clean the main incision. In this way, the main incision is kept free of the microorganisms around the stab wound.

Wound Drainage Systems

A **closed wound drainage system** consists of a drain connected to either an electric suction or a portable drainage suction, such as a Hemovac (Figure 36.9 ■) or Jackson-Pratt (Figure 36.10 ■). The closed system reduces the potential entry of microorganisms into the wound through the drain. The drainage tubes are sutured in place and connected to a reservoir. For example, the Jackson-Pratt drainage tube is connected to a reservoir that maintains constant low suction. These portable wound suctions also provide for accurate measurement of the drainage.

The surgeon inserts the wound drainage tube during surgery. Generally the suction is discontinued 3 to 5 days postoperatively or when the drainage is minimal. When emptying the container, the nurse should wear gloves and avoid touching the drainage port (Figure 36.11 ■). To reestablish suction, the nurse places the container on a solid, flat surface with the port open, and cleanses the opening and plug with an alcohol swab. The palm of one hand then presses the top and bottom together while the other hand replaces the drainage plug before releasing hand pressure to reestablish the vacuum necessary for the closed drainage system to work (Figure 36.12 ■).

Skill 36.1 describes cleaning and dressing a surgical wound and drain.

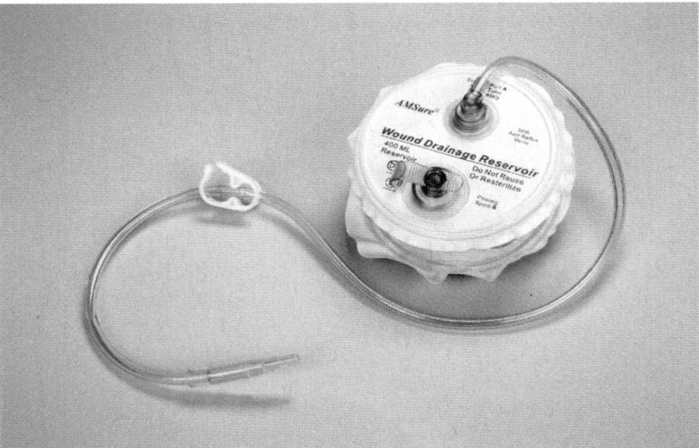

Figure 36.9 ■ Hemovac closed wound drainage system.

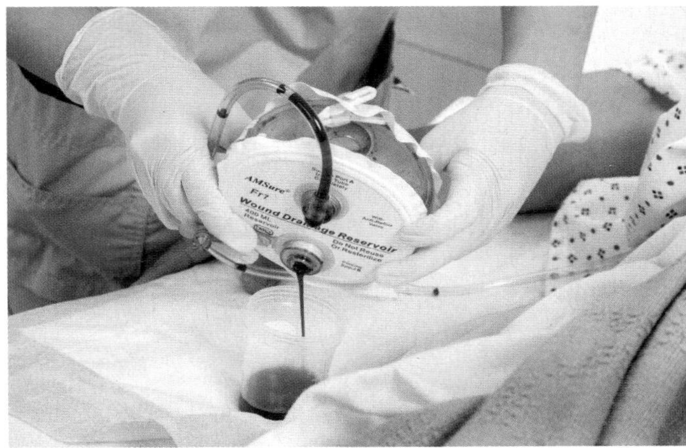

Figure 36.11 ■ Emptying drainage from Hemovac drainage system.

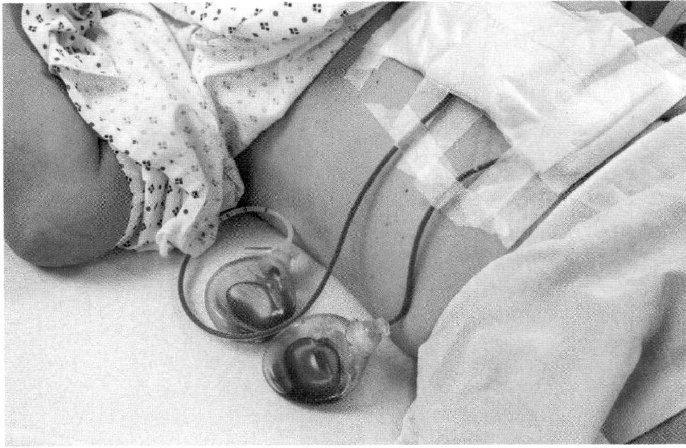

Figure 36.10 ■ Two Jackson-Pratt devices compressed to facilitate collection of exudates.

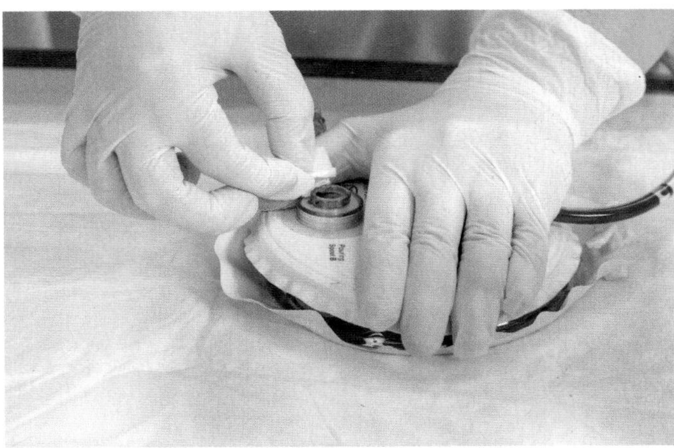

Figure 36.12 ■ With one hand, press the top and bottom together. With the other hand, replace the plug before releasing hand.

Cleaning a Sutured Wound and Dressing a Wound with a Drain

PURPOSES

- To promote wound healing by primary intention
- To prevent infection
- To assess the healing process
- To protect the wound from mechanical trauma

ASSESSMENT

Assess

- Client allergies to wound cleaning agents
- The appearance and size of the wound
- The amount and character of exudates
- Client complaints of discomfort
- The time of the last pain medication
- Signs of systemic infection (e.g., elevated body temperature, diaphoresis, malaise, leukocytosis)

PLANNING

Before changing a dressing, determine any specific orders about the wound or dressing.

Assignment

Cleaning a wound, especially one with a drain, requires application of knowledge, problem-solving, and aseptic technique. As a result, this procedure is not assigned to assistive personnel AP. The nurse can ask the AP to report soiled dressings that need to be changed or if a dressing has become loose and needs to be reinforced. The nurse is responsible for the assessment and evaluation of the wound.

Equipment

- Bath blanket (if necessary)
- Moisture-proof bag
- Mask (optional)
- Acetone or another solution (if necessary to loosen adhesive)
- Clean gloves
- Sterile gloves
- Sterile dressing set:
  - Drape or towel
  - Gauze squares
  - Container for cleaning solution
  - Cleaning solution (e.g., normal saline)
  - Two pairs of forceps
  - Gauze dressings and surgipads
- Additional supplies required for the particular dressing (e.g., extra gauze dressings and ointment, if ordered)
- Tape, tie tapes, or binder

IMPLEMENTATION

Preparation

Prepare the client and assemble the equipment.

- Obtain assistance for changing a dressing on a restless or confused client. **Rationale:** *The client might move and contaminate the sterile field or the wound.*
- Assist the client to a comfortable position in which the wound can be readily exposed. Expose only the wound area, using a bath blanket to cover the client, if necessary. **Rationale:** *Undue exposure is physically and psychologically distressing to most individuals.*
- Make a cuff on the moisture-proof bag for disposal of the soiled dressings, and place the bag within reach. **Rationale:** *Making a cuff helps keep the outside of the bag free from contamination by the soiled dressings and prevents subsequent contamination of the nurse's hands or of sterile instrument tips when discarding dressings or sponges. Placement of the bag within reach prevents the nurse from reaching across the sterile field and the wound and potentially contaminating these areas.*
- Apply a face mask, if required. **Rationale:** *Some agencies require that a mask be worn for surgical dressing changes to prevent contamination of the wound by droplet spray from the nurse's respiratory tract.*

Performance

1. Prior to performing the procedure, introduce self and verify the client's identity using agency protocol. Explain to the client what you are going to do, why it is necessary, and how to participate. Discuss how the results will be used in planning further care or treatments.
2. Perform hand hygiene and observe other appropriate prevention control procedures.
3. Provide for client privacy.
4. Remove and dispose of soiled dressings appropriately.
   - Apply clean gloves and remove the outer abdominal dressing or surgipad.
   - If adhesive tape was used, remove it by holding down the skin and pulling the tape gently but firmly toward the wound. **Rationale:** *Pressing down on the skin provides countertraction against the pulling motion. Tape is pulled toward the incision to prevent strain on the sutures or wound.*
   - Lift the outer dressing so that the underside is *away* from the client's face. **Rationale:** *The appearance and odor of the drainage may be upsetting to the client.*
   - Place the soiled dressing in the moisture-proof bag without touching the outside of the bag. **Rationale:** *Contamination of the outside of the bag is avoided to prevent the spread of microorganisms to the nurse and subsequently to others.*
   - Remove the underdressings, taking care not to dislodge any drains. If the gauze sticks to the drain, support the drain with one hand and remove the gauze with the other.
   - Assess the location, type (color, consistency), and odor of wound drainage, and the number of gauzes saturated or the diameter of drainage collected on the dressings.
   - Discard the soiled dressings in the bag as before.
   - Remove and discard gloves in the moisture-proof bag.
   - Perform hand hygiene.
5. Set up the sterile supplies.
   - Open the sterile dressing set, using aseptic technique.
   - Place the sterile drape beside the wound.
   - Open the sterile cleaning solution and pour it over the gauze sponges in the plastic container.
   - Apply sterile gloves.
6. Clean the wound, if indicated.
   - Clean the wound, using your gloved hands or forceps and gauze swabs moistened with cleaning solution.
   - If using forceps, keep the forceps tips lower than the handles at all times. **Rationale:** *This prevents their*

Cleaning a Sutured Wound and Dressing a Wound with a Drain—*continued*

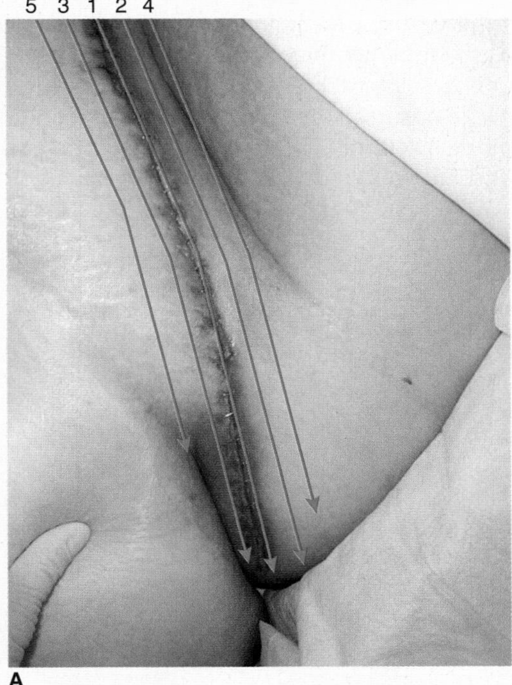

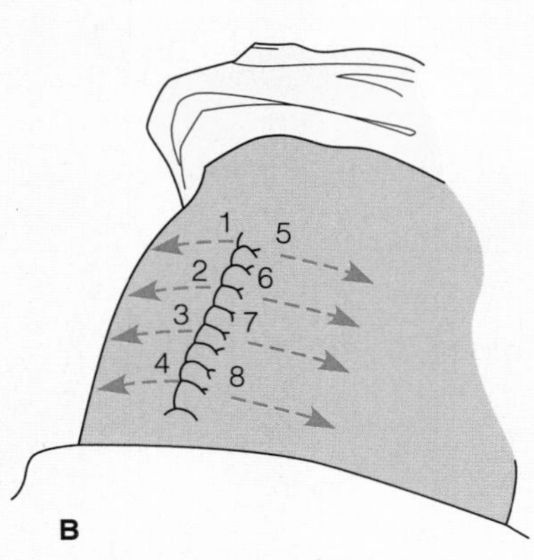

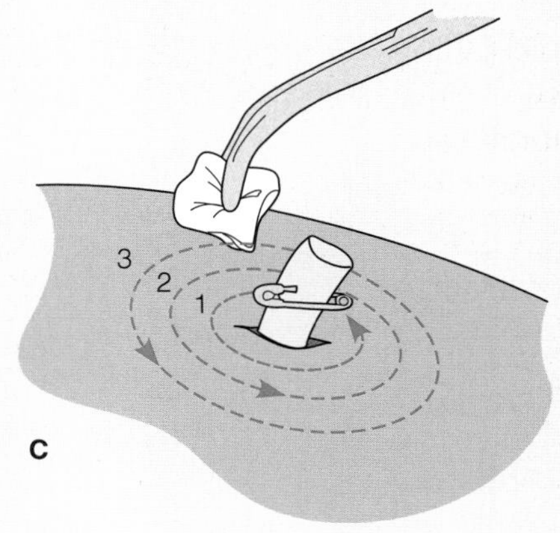

❶ Methods of cleaning surgical wounds: *A*, cleaning the wound from top to bottom, starting at the center; *B*, cleaning a wound outward from the incision; *C*, cleaning around a Penrose drain site. For all methods, a clean sterile swab is used for each stroke.
A, Cory patrick Hartley RN. WCC, OMS.

contamination by fluid traveling up to the handle and nurse's wrist and back to the tips.

- Use the cleaning methods illustrated and described in ❶ or one recommended by agency protocol.
- Use a separate swab for each stroke and discard each swab after use. **Rationale:** *This prevents the introduction of microorganisms to other wound areas.*
- If a drain is present, clean it next, taking care to avoid reaching across the cleaned incision. Clean the skin around the drain site by swabbing in half or full circles from around the drain site outward, using separate swabs for each wipe ❶ *C*.
- Support and hold the drain erect while cleaning around it. Clean as many times as necessary to remove the drainage.
- Dry the surrounding skin with dry gauze swabs as required. Do not dry the wound itself. **Rationale:** *Moisture facilitates wound healing.*

7. Apply dressings to the drain site and the incision.

- Place a precut 4×4 gauze snugly around the drain ❷, or open a 4×4 gauze to 4×8 in., fold it lengthwise to 2×8 in., and place it around the drain so that the ends overlap. **Rationale:** *This dressing absorbs the drainage and helps prevent it from excoriating the skin. Using precut gauze or folding it as described, instead of cutting the gauze, prevents any threads from coming loose and getting into the wound, where they could cause inflammation and provide a site for infection.*
- Apply the sterile dressings one at a time over the drain and the incision. Place the bulk of the dressings over the drain area and below the drain, depending on the client's usual position. **Rationale:** *Layers of dressings are placed for best absorption of drainage, which flows by gravity.*

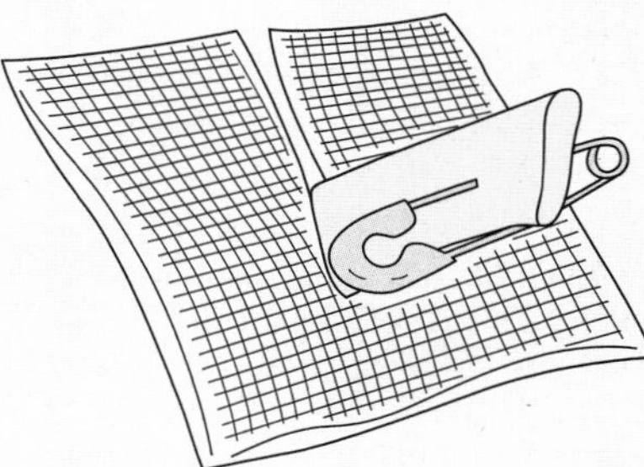

❷ Precut gauze in place around a Penrose drain.

- Apply the final surgipad. Remove and discard gloves. Secure the dressing with tape or ties.
- Perform hand hygiene.

8. Document the procedure and all nursing assessments.

SAMPLE DOCUMENTATION

3/21/2020 1100 Abdominal dressing changed. Small amount of serosanguineous drainage—size of a half dollar—in middle of dressing. Incision approximated with slight redness at edges. Sutures intact. S. Jones, RN

EVALUATION

- Conduct appropriate follow-up, such as amount of granulation tissue or degree of healing; amount of drainage and its color, consistency, and odor; presence of inflammation; and degree of discomfort associated with the incision or drain site.
- Compare to previous findings, if available.
- Report significant deviations from normal to the primary care provider.

Wound Irrigation and Packing

An irrigation (lavage) is the washing or flushing out of an area. Sterile technique is required for a wound irrigation because there is a break in the skin integrity.

Irrigation pressures should range from 4 to 15 pounds per square inch (psi). Below 4 psi, such as when using a bulb syringe, the irrigation may not be effective, and above 15 psi it may damage tissues. A 30- to 60-mL piston syringe with a 19-gauge needle or catheter provides approximately 8 psi. Using piston syringes instead of bulb syringes to irrigate a wound also reduces the risk of aspirating drainage. Commercially prepared normal saline irrigation is available in pump spray, aerosol cans, and prefilled, single-dose plastic vials called *bullets*. For deep wounds with small openings, a sterile straight catheter may also be necessary. Frequently used irrigation solutions are sterile normal saline, lactated Ringer's solution, and antibiotic solutions. Skill 36.2 details the steps involved in irrigating a wound.

SKILL 36.2

Irrigating a Wound

PURPOSES

- To clean the area
- To apply an antimicrobial solution

ASSESSMENT

Assess the client's record to determine

- Previous appearance and size of the wound
- Character of the exudate
- Presence of pain and the time of the last pain medication
- Clinical signs of systemic infection
- Allergies to the wound irrigation agent or tape.

PLANNING

- Before irrigating a wound, determine (a) the type of irrigating solution to be used, (b) the frequency of irrigations, and (c) the temperature of the solution.
- If possible, schedule the irrigation at a time convenient for the client. Some irrigations require only a few minutes and others can take much longer.
- Determine if the client requires premedication for pain or other pain management techniques prior to wound care (see Chapter 30 ∞).

Assignment

- Due to the need for aseptic technique and assessment skills, wound irrigations are not assigned to AP. However, AP may observe the wound and dressing during usual care and must report abnormal findings to the nurse. Abnormal findings must be validated and interpreted by the nurse.

Equipment

Although a wound may already be contaminated, sterile equipment is usually used during irrigation to prevent the possibility of adding new nonresident microorganisms to the site. In settings other than hospitals, some reusable supplies such as irrigating syringes or basins may be cleaned and used again for a specific wound.

- Sterile dressing equipment and dressing materials
- Sterile irrigation set or individual supplies, including:
  - Sterile syringe (e.g., a 30- to 60-mL syringe) with a catheter of an appropriate size (e.g., #18 or #19) or an irrigating (catheter) tip syringe
  - Splash shield for syringe (optional) ❶
  - Sterile graduated container for irrigating solution
  - Basin for collecting the used irrigating solution
  - Moisture-proof drape
- Moisture-proof bag
- Irrigating solution, usually 200 mL (6.5 oz) of solution room temperature or warmed to body temperature, according to the agency's or primary care provider's choice
- Goggles, gown, and mask
- Clean gloves

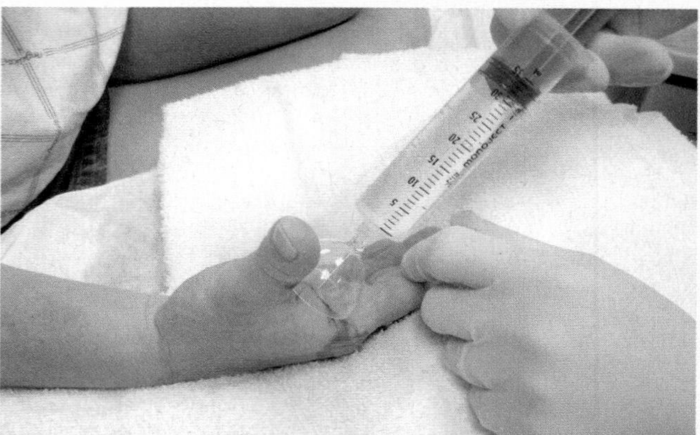

❶ A splash shield prevents contaminated fluid from spreading.
Cory patrick Hartley RN. WCC, OMS.

IMPLEMENTATION

Preparation

Check that the irrigating fluid is at the proper temperature.

Performance

1. Prior to performing the procedure, introduce self and verify the client's identity using agency protocol. Explain to the client what you are going to do, why it is necessary, and how to participate. Discuss how the results will be used in planning further care or treatments.
2. Perform hand hygiene and observe other appropriate infection prevention procedures.
3. Provide for client privacy.
4. Prepare the client.
   - Assist the client to a position in which the irrigating solution will flow by gravity from the upper end of the wound to the lower end and then into the basin.

Irrigating a Wound—*continued*

- Place the moisture-proof drape under the wound and over the bed. ❷
- Apply clean gloves and remove and discard the old dressing.
- If indicated, clean the wound from the cleanest area toward the least clean. If the wound is circular, this would be from the center of the wound outward. For a linear wound, cleanse from top to bottom, beginning in the middle and moving progressively laterally (see Skill 36.1 Figure 1).
- Assess the wound and drainage.
- Remove and discard clean gloves.
- Perform hand hygiene.

5. Prepare the equipment.
   - Open the sterile dressing set and supplies.
   - Pour the ordered solution into the solution container.
   - Position the basin below the wound to receive the irrigating fluid.
6. Irrigate the wound.
   - Apply clean gloves.
   - Instill a steady stream of irrigating solution into the wound. Make sure all areas of the wound are irrigated.
   - Use either a syringe with a catheter attached or with an irrigating tip to flush the wound. ❸
   - If you are using a catheter to reach tracks or crevices, insert the catheter into the wound until resistance is met. Do not force the catheter. **Rationale:** *Forcing the catheter can cause tissue damage*.
   - Continue irrigating until the solution becomes clear (no exudate is present).
   - Dry the area around the wound. **Rationale:** *Moisture left on the skin promotes the growth of microorganisms and can cause skin irritation and breakdown*.
   - Remove and discard gloves.
   - Perform hand hygiene.
7. Assess and dress the wound.
   - Assess the appearance of the wound again, noting in particular the type and amount of exudate still present and the presence and extent of granulation tissue.
   - Using aseptic technique, apply a dressing to the wound based on the amount of drainage expected (Table 36.4).
   - Perform hand hygiene.
8. Document the irrigation and the client's response in the client record using forms or checklists supplemented by narrative notes when appropriate. Electronic health records will use a designated wound and skin documentation sheet.

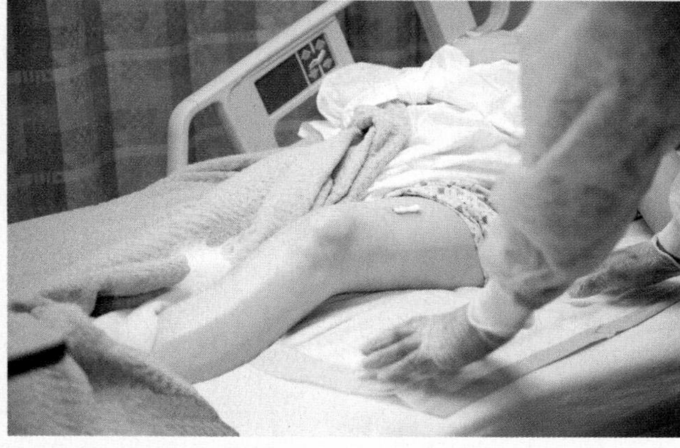

❷ Placing the moisture-proof pad under the wound.

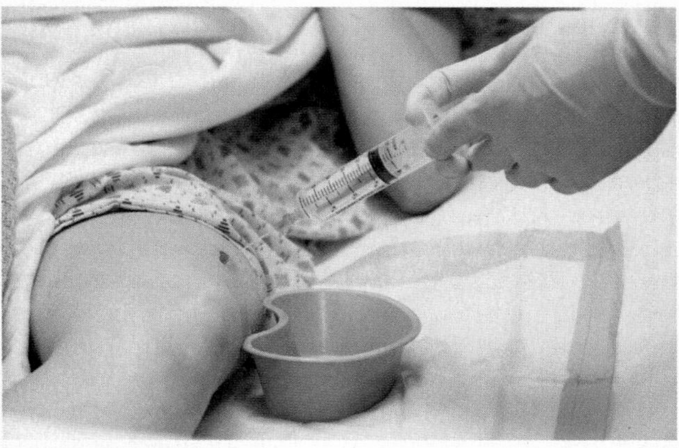

❸ Irrigating an open wound.

SAMPLE DOCUMENTATION

6/5/2020 1530 Midline abdominal wound 7 cm with intact sutures except for center 3 cm. open area with moderate amount thin serosanguineous drainage. Irrigated with NS until clear. N. Jamaghani, RN

EVALUATION

- Perform follow-up based on findings that deviate from expected or normal for the client. Relate findings to previous assessment data if available.
- Report significant deviations from normal to the primary care provider.

SKILL 36.2

Dressing Wounds

Dressings are applied for the following purposes:

- To protect the wound from mechanical injury
- To protect the wound from microbial contamination
- To provide or maintain moist wound healing
- To provide thermal insulation
- To absorb drainage or debride a wound or both
- To prevent hemorrhage (when applied as a pressure dressing or with elastic bandages)
- To splint or immobilize the wound site and thereby facilitate healing and prevent injury.

Gauze **packing** using the damp-to-damp technique has been used to pack wounds that require debridement. In this technique, moist 4×4 non–cotton-filled gauzes

PRACTICE GUIDELINES **Issues Related to the Use of Damp Gauze Versus Advanced Dressings**

- To keep the gauze damp, it must be changed or remoistened with saline frequently. **Rationale:** *If the gauze is allowed to dry out, removal results in pain and disruption of wound healing through drying of the surface and tissue adherence to the gauze.*
- A wound requires moisture and warmth for optimal healing. Evaporation of the saline causes wound cooling, vasoconstriction, and dehydration.
- Moistened gauze does not prevent introduction of bacteria into the wound.
- Gauze is easy to use and can be manipulated to fit almost any wound.
- The diversity of advanced dressings may be confusing for clients and healthcare providers.
- Although gauze is much less expensive than advanced dressings (e.g., polymers, alginates, collagens), the cost per week can be higher due to the number of dressing changes required (Kaushik et al., 2017). Including the price of the dressing, gloves, saline, and tape, the materials cost for a gauze dressing change 2 times per day versus an advanced dressing 3 times per week is very similar. However, including the cost per nurse home visit, the gauze dressing is almost 5 times as expensive.
- Wounds have been shown to heal twice as quickly with advanced dressings compared to gauze.

Conclusions: Practitioners should become familiar with the range and uses of advanced dressing materials. The selection of dressing materials must consider time, material cost, client comfort, and speed of wound healing.

are packed in the wound to absorb exudate but they are not allowed to dry before removal. However, newer advanced dressing materials have significant advantages over the use of gauze. See the accompanying Practice Guidelines for issues related to using damp-to-damp dressings.

Many of the techniques described here for dressing wounds may be combined depending on the specific type of wound. In addition, therapies are constantly being designed and evaluated. One example is negative pressure wound therapy, also termed vacuum-assisted closure (VAC), wound VAC, vacuum sealing, and topical negative pressure, which refers to the use of suction equipment to apply negative pressure to a variety of wound types. This therapy has been shown to speed tissue generation, reduce swelling around the wound, and enhance wound healing by providing a moist and protected environment (Hunt, 2016). Sterile foam sponges are placed into a clean wound and covered with a transparent adhesive drape, and then a hole is cut in the drape to allow insertion of the vacuum tubing (Figure 36.13 ■). For maximum effectiveness the vacuum is applied for almost 24 hours each day and portable systems are available for ambulatory clients.

Types of Dressings

Various dressing materials are available to cover wounds. The type of dressing used depends on (a) the location, size, and type of the wound; (b) the amount of exudate; (c) whether the wound requires debridement or is infected; and (d) such considerations as frequency of dressing change, ease or difficulty of dressing application, and cost (Table 36.4).

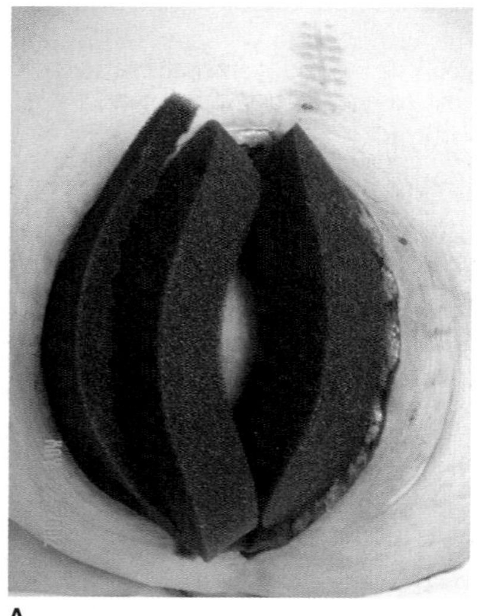
A

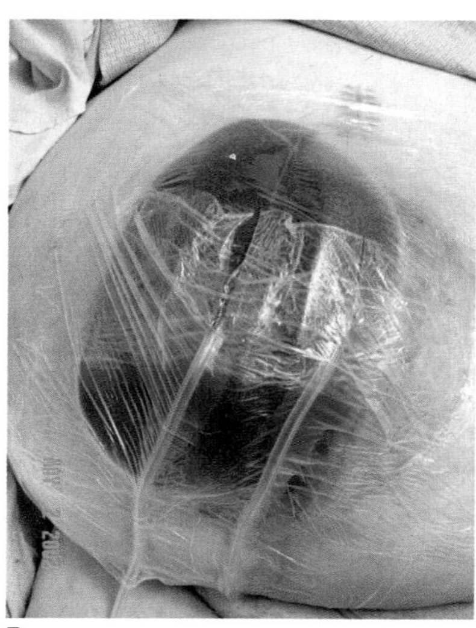
B

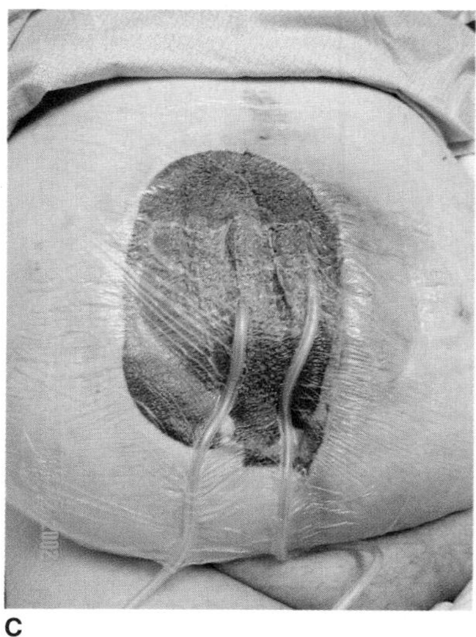
C

Figure 36.13 ■ Vacuum-assisted closure (VAC) system for wounds: *A*, foam strips laid into the wound; *B*, occlusive draping applied and suction tubing in place; *C*, finished dressing with negative pressure (suction) applied.
Photos *A, B, C*, Cory patrick Hartley RN. WCC, OMS.

TABLE 36.4 Selected Types of Wound Dressings

Dressing	Description	Purpose	Indications	Examples
Transparent film	Adhesive plastic, semipermeable, nonabsorbent dressings allow exchange of oxygen between the atmosphere and wound bed. They are impermeable to bacteria and water.	To provide protection against contamination and friction; to maintain a clean, moist surface that facilitates cellular migration; to provide insulation by preventing fluid evaporation; and to facilitate wound assessment.	IV dressing Central line dressing Superficial wounds Pressure injuries stage I	Bioclusive, Op-Site, Polyskin, Tegaderm
Impregnated nonadherent	Woven or nonwoven cotton or synthetic materials are impregnated with petrolatum, saline, zinc-saline, antimicrobials, or other agents. Require secondary dressings to secure them in place, retain moisture, and provide wound protection.	To cover, soothe, and protect partial- and full-thickness wounds without exudate.	Postoperative dressing over staples or sutures Superficial burns	Adaptic, Aquaphor gauze, Carrasyn, Xeroform dressings
Hydrocolloids	Waterproof adhesive wafers, pastes, or powders. Wafers, designed to be worn for up to 7 days, consist of two layers. The inner adhesive layer has particles that absorb exudates and form a hydrated gel over the wound; the outer film provides an occlusive seal.	To absorb exudate; to produce a moist environment that facilitates healing but does not cause maceration of surrounding skin; to protect the wound from bacterial contamination, foreign debris, and urine or feces; and to prevent shearing.	Pressure injuries stage II–IV Autolytic debridement of eschar Partial-thickness wounds	Comfeel, DuoDERM, RepliCare, Restore, Tegasorb
Clear absorbent acrylic	Transparent absorbent wafer designed to be worn 5–7 days. The acrylic layer absorbs exudates and evaporates the excess off the transparent membrane.	Maintains a transparent membrane for easy wound bed assessment, provides bacterial and shearing protection. Maintains moist wound healing. Can be used with alginates to provide packing to deeper wound beds.	Pressure injuries Skin tears Venous stasis injuries Surgical wounds Wounds undergoing chemical debridement agents	Tegaderm absorbent
Hydrogels	Glycerin or water-based nonadhesive jelly-like sheets, granules, or gels are oxygen permeable, unless covered by a plastic film. Requires secondary occlusive dressing.	To liquefy necrotic tissue or slough, rehydrate the wound bed, and fill in dead space.	Pressure injuries Skin tears Partial-thickness wounds	Carrasyn, Elasto-Gel, Nu-Gel, Purilon, Tegaderm, Vigilon
Polyurethane foams	Nonadherent hydrocolloid dressings; these need to have their edges taped down or sealed. Require secondary dressings to obtain an occlusive environment. Surrounding skin must be protected to prevent maceration. Easy to cut and fit to wound.	To absorb up to heavy amounts of exudate; to provide and maintain moist wound healing; to provide thermal insulation.	Light to highly exudating wounds Pressure injuries Skin tears Venous stasis injuries Surgical wounds Wounds undergoing chemical debridement agents	Allevyn, Curafoam, Flexzan, Lyofoam, VigiFOAM
Alginates (exudate absorbers)	Nonadherent dressings of powder, beads or granules, ropes, sheets, or paste conform to the wound surface and absorb up to 20 times their weight in exudate; require a secondary dressing.	To provide a moist wound surface by interacting with exudate to form a gelatinous mass; to absorb exudate; to eliminate dead space or pack wounds; and to support debridement.	Pressure injuries Skin tears Venous stasis injuries Surgical wounds Wounds undergoing chemical debridement agents	AlgiDerm, Curasorb, Debrisan, Kaltostat, Sorbsan
Collagen	Gels, pastes, powders, granules, sheets, sponges derived from animal sources, often cow or pig.	Assists with stopping bleeding, helps recruit cells into the wound and stimulates their proliferation to facilitate healing.	Clean, moist wounds	Biostep, Cellerate RX, NU-GEL, Promogran

Transparent Dressings

Transparent dressings are often applied to wounds including ulcerated or burned skin areas. These dressings offer several advantages:

- They act as temporary skin.
- They are nonporous, nonabsorbent, self-adhesive dressings that do not require changing as other dressings do. They are often left in place until healing has occurred or as long as they remain intact.
- Because they are transparent, the wound can be assessed through them.
- Because they are semiocclusive, the wound remains moist and can retain a small amount of serous exudate, which promotes epithelial growth, hastens healing, and reduces the risk of infection.
- Because they are elastic, they can be placed over a joint without disrupting the client's mobility.
- They adhere only to the skin area around the wound and not to the wound itself because they keep the wound moist.
- They allow the client to shower or bathe without removing the dressing.

Hydrocolloid Dressings

Hydrocolloid dressings are frequently used over pressure injuries. These dressings offer several advantages:

- They last 3 to 7 days.
- They do not need a "cover" dressing and are water resistant, so the client can shower or bathe.
- They can be molded to uneven body surfaces.
- They act as temporary skin and provide an effective bacterial barrier.
- They decrease pain and thus reduce the need for analgesics.
- They absorb moderate drainage and therefore can be used on slowly draining wounds.
- They contain wound odor.

These dressings have certain limitations, however:

- They are occlusive, are opaque, and obscure wound visibility.
- They have a limited absorption capacity.
- They can facilitate anaerobic bacterial growth.
- They can soften and wrinkle at the edges with wear and movement.
- They can be difficult to remove and may leave a residue on the skin.

Because of these limitations, hydrocolloid dressings should not be used for infected wounds or those with deep tracts or *fistulas*.

Securing Dressings

The nurse tapes the dressing over the wound, ensuring that the dressing covers the entire wound and does not become dislodged. The correct type of tape must be selected for the purpose. The nurse follows these steps:

1. Place the tape so that the dressing cannot be folded back to expose the wound. Place strips at the ends of the dressing, and space tapes evenly in the middle.
2. Ensure that the tape is long enough and wide enough to adhere to several inches of skin on each side of the dressing, but not so long or wide that the tape loosens with activity (Figure 36.14 ■).
3. Place the tape in the opposite direction from the body action, for example, across a body joint or crease, not lengthwise (Figure 36.15 ■).

Montgomery straps (tie tapes) are used for wounds requiring frequent dressing changes (Figure 36.16 ■).

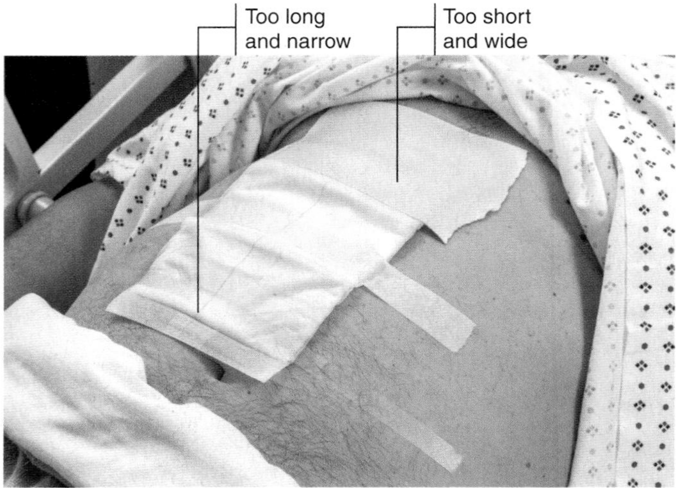

Figure 36.14 ■ The strips of tape should be placed at the ends of the dressing and must be sufficiently long and wide to secure the dressing. The tape should adhere to intact skin.

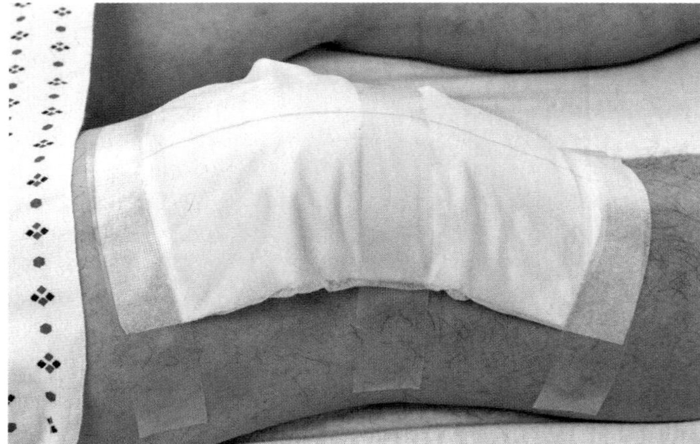

Figure 36.15 ■ Dressings over moving parts must remain secure despite the client's movement. Place the tape over a joint at a right angle to the direction the joint moves.

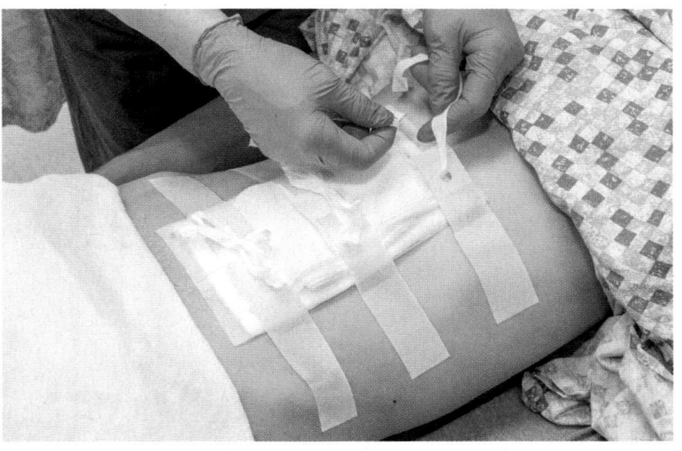

Figure 36.16 ■ Montgomery straps, or tie tapes, are used to secure large dressings that require frequent changing.

These straps prevent skin irritation and discomfort caused by removing the adhesive each time the dressing is changed.

Medical tape can cause injuries if used incorrectly. Blisters will form if too much tension is applied while placing the tape, when edema has collected after the tape was placed, and when alcohol or benzoic-based prep solutions are used under the tape. Medical tape manufacturers issue safety guidelines for specific tape products. Before using medical tapes read the safety guidelines for indications of use and safe application and removal.

Skill 36.3 provides guidelines to obtain a specimen of wound drainage.

Obtaining a Wound Drainage Specimen for Culture

SKILL 36.3

PURPOSES

- To identify the microorganisms potentially causing an infection and the antibiotics to which they are sensitive
- To evaluate the effectiveness of antibiotic therapy

ASSESSMENT

Assess

- Appearance of the wound and surrounding tissue. Check the character and amount of wound drainage
- Client complaints of pain or discomfort at the wound site
- Signs of infection such as fever, chills, or elevated white blood cell (WBC) count

PLANNING

Before obtaining a specimen of wound drainage, determine (a) whether the wound should be cleaned prior to obtaining the specimen and (b) whether the site from which to take the specimen has been specified.

Assignment

Obtaining a wound culture is an invasive procedure that requires the application of sterile technique, knowledge of wound healing, and potential problem-solving to ensure client safety; therefore, the nurse needs to perform this skill and does not assign it to AP.

Equipment

- Personal protective equipment, goggles, and gown if appropriate
- Clean gloves
- Sterile gloves if needed for aseptic technique
- Moisture-proof bag
- Sterile dressing set
- Normal saline and irrigating syringe
- Culture tube with swab and transport medium (aerobic and anaerobic tubes are available) or sterile syringe with needle for anaerobic culture
- Completed labels for each container
- Completed requisition to accompany the specimens to the laboratory

IMPLEMENTATION

Preparation

Check the medical orders to determine if the specimen is to be collected for an **aerobic** (growing only in the presence of oxygen) or **anaerobic** (growing only in the absence of oxygen) culture. Aerobic organisms are generally found on the surface of the wound, whereas anaerobic organisms would be found in deep wounds, tunnels, and cavities. Administer an analgesic 30 minutes before the procedure if the client is complaining of pain at the wound site.

Performance

1. Prior to performing the procedure, introduce self and verify the client's identity using agency protocol. Explain to the client what you are going to do, why it is necessary, and how to participate. Discuss how the results will be used in planning further care or treatments.
2. Perform hand hygiene and observe other appropriate infection prevention procedures.
3. Provide for client privacy.
4. Remove any outer dressings that cover the wound.
   - Apply clean gloves.
   - Remove the outer dressing, and observe any drainage on the dressing. Hold the dressing so that the client does not see the drainage. **Rationale:** *The appearance of the drainage could upset the client.*
   - Determine the amount, color, consistency, and odor of the drainage, for example, "one 4×4 gauze saturated with pale yellow, thick, malodorous drainage."
   - Discard the dressing in the moisture-proof bag. Handle it carefully so that the dressing does not touch the outside of the bag. **Rationale:** *Touching the outside of the bag will contaminate it.*
   - Remove and discard gloves.
   - Perform hand hygiene.

Continued on page 942

SKILL 36.3

Obtaining a Wound Drainage Specimen for Culture—*continued*

5. Open the sterile dressing set (see Skill 31.3).
6. Assess the wound.
   - Assess the appearance of the tissues in and around the wound and the drainage. Infection can cause reddened tissues with a thick discharge, which may be foul smelling, whitish, or colored.
7. Cleanse the wound using aseptic technique.
   - Apply gloves
   - If a topical antimicrobial ointment or cream is being used to treat the wound, wipe or irrigate (see Skill 36.2) to remove it. **Rationale:** *Residual antiseptic must be removed prior to culture.*
   - Cleanse the wound with normal saline until all exudate has been removed.
   - After cleansing, apply a sterile gauze pad to the wound. **Rationale:** *This absorbs excess cleansing solution.*
   - Remove and discard gloves.
   - Perform hand hygiene.
8. Obtain the aerobic culture.
   - Apply clean gloves.
   - Open a specimen tube and place the cap upside down on a firm, dry surface so that the inside will not become contaminated, or if the swab is attached to the lid, twist the cap to loosen the swab. Hold the tube in one hand and take out the swab in the other.
   - Rotate the swab back and forth over clean areas of granulation tissue from the sides or base of the wound. **Rationale:** *Microorganisms most likely to be responsible for a wound infection reside in viable tissue.* ❶
   - Do not use pus or pooled exudates to culture. **Rationale:** *These secretions contain a mixture of contaminants that are not the same as those causing the infection.*
   - Avoid touching the swab to intact skin at the wound edges. **Rationale:** *This prevents the introduction of superficial skin organisms into the culture.*
   - Return the swab to the culture tube, taking care not to touch the top or the outside of the tube. Secure the swab or lid firmly. **Rationale:** *The outside of the container must remain free of pathogenic microorganisms to prevent their spread to others.* ❷
   - Crush the barrier to the inner compartment containing the transport medium at the bottom of the tube. **Rationale:** *This ensures that the swab with the specimen is surrounded by medium, which prevents the specimen from drying out or any microorganisms from continuing to multiply.* ❸ If a specimen is required from another site, repeat the steps. Specify the exact site (e.g., inferior drain site or lower aspect of incision) on the label of each container. Be sure to put each swab in the appropriately labeled tube.

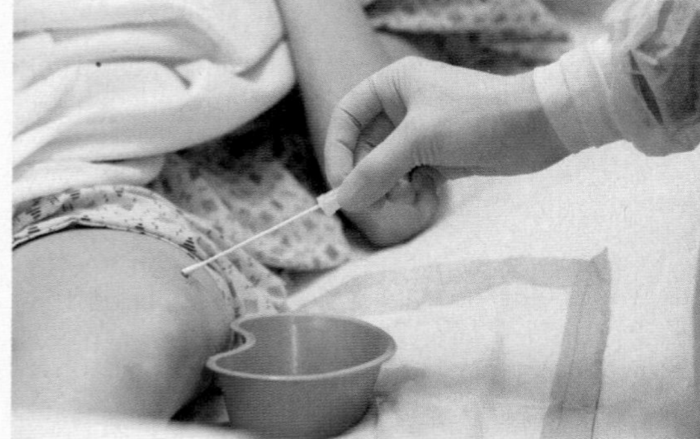

❶ Obtaining a culture specimen from the base of the wound.

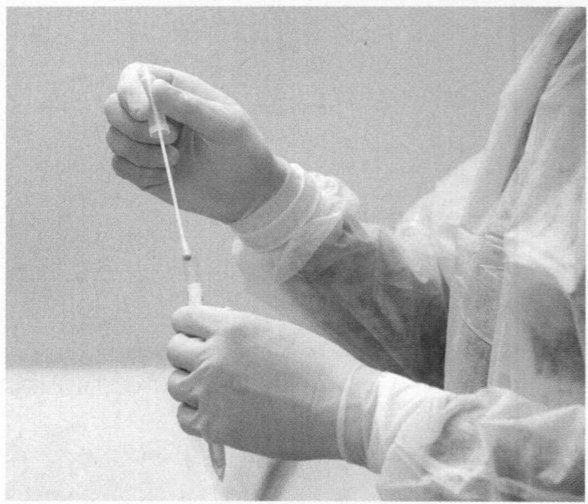

❷ Return the swab to the culturette tube.

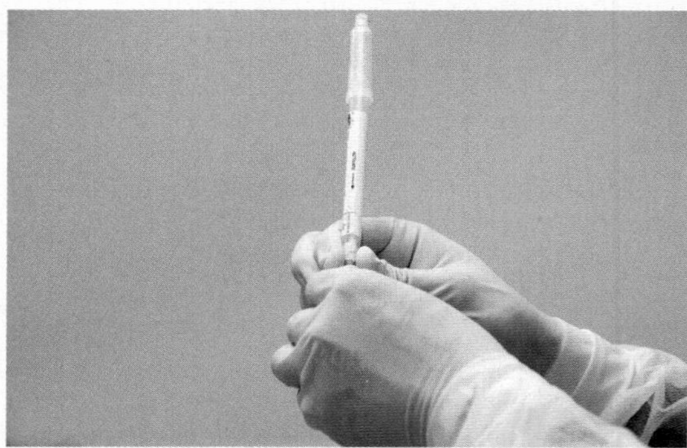

❸ Break the ampule containing the transport medium.

9. Dress the wound.
   - Apply any ordered medication to the wound.
   - Cover the wound with a sterile wound dressing. See Table 36.4 (page 939) for selecting a wound dressing.
   - Remove and discard gloves.
   - Perform hand hygiene.
10. Arrange for the specimen to be transported to the laboratory immediately. Be sure to include the completed requisition.
11. Document all relevant information.
    - Record on the client's chart the taking of the specimen and source.
    - Include the date and time; the appearance of the wound; the color, consistency, amount, and odor of any drainage; the type of culture collected; and any discomfort experienced by the client.

SAMPLE DOCUMENTATION

5/27/2020 1000 Specimen from ® hip to lab for anaerobic culture. Wound 3x3 cm, 6-mm deep, minimal amount thick yellow drainage. No odor. Skin around wound erythematous. Pain 0 on 0–10 scale. N. Jamaghani, RN

Obtaining a Wound Drainage Specimen for Culture—*continued*

Variation: Obtaining a Specimen for Anaerobic Culture

- Apply clean gloves.
- Insert a sterile 10-mL syringe (without needle) into the wound, and aspirate 1 to 5 mL of drainage into the syringe.
- Attach the needle to the syringe, and expel all air from the syringe and needle.
- Immediately inject the drainage into the anaerobic culture tube and cap the tube tightly.

or

- Use an anaerobic culture swab system in which the swab is immediately placed into a tube filled with an oxygen-free gas or gel environment.
- Label the tube or syringe appropriately.
- Remove and discard gloves.
- Perform hand hygiene.
- Send the tube or syringe of drainage to the laboratory immediately. Do not refrigerate the specimen.

EVALUATION

- Compare findings of wound assessment and drainage to previous assessments to determine any changes.
- Report the culture results to the primary care provider.
- Conduct appropriate follow-up such as administering antibiotics or modifying wound treatment as ordered.

LIFESPAN CONSIDERATIONS Pressure Injury and Wound Care

INFANTS

The skin of infants is more fragile than that of older children and adults, and more susceptible to infection, shearing from friction, and burns.

CHILDREN

- Staphylococcus and fungus are two major infectious agents affecting the skin of children. Abrasions or small lacerations, commonly experienced by children, provide an entry in the skin for these organisms. Minor wounds should be cleansed with warm, soapy water, and covered with a sterile bandage. Children should be instructed not to touch the wound.
- With more serious skin injuries, remind the child not to touch the wound, drains, or dressing. Cover with an appropriate bandage that will remain intact during the child's usual activities. Cover a transparent dressing with opaque material if viewing the site is distressing to the child. Restrain only when all alternatives have been tried and when absolutely necessary.
- For younger children, demonstrate wound care on a doll. Reassure that the wound will not be permanent and that nothing will fall out of the body.

OLDER ADULTS

- Hold wrinkled skin taut during application of a transparent dressing. Obtain assistance if needed.
- Skin is more fragile and can easily tear with removal of tape (especially adhesive tape). Use paper, clear, or foam tape and tape remover as indicated, keeping tape use to the minimum required. Use extreme caution during tape removal. If possible, use conforming gauze bandage (e.g., Elastomull, Flexicon, Kerlix Lite, or Kling) or elastic self-adherent products (e.g., Coban or Coflex) to hold a dressing in place.
- Older adults who are in long-term care facilities often have the following conditions: immobility, malnutrition, and incontinence—all of which increase the risk for development of skin breakdown.
- Skin breakdown can occur as quickly as within 2 hours, so assessments should be done with each repositioning of the client.
- A thorough assessment of a client's heels should be done every shift. The skin can break down quickly from friction of movement in bed.

QSEN Patient-Centered Care: Providing Wound Care at Home

Almost all wounds will be healing while the client is at home. Whether the nurse is performing wound care for the client or supporting the client and family in performing wound care themselves, certain principles apply.

- Perform appropriate client teaching for promoting wound healing and maintenance of healthy skin.
- Instruct family about hygiene and medical asepsis; hand cleansing before and after dressing changes; and using a clean area for storage of dressing supplies.
- Instruct the client and family on where to obtain needed supplies. Be sensitive to the cost of dressings (e.g., transparent barriers are costly) and suggest less expensive alternatives if necessary. Be creative in the use of household items for padding pressure areas.
- Instruct the client and family in proper disposal of contaminated dressings. All contaminated items should be sealed in moisture-proof containers.
- Verify how the client may bathe with the wound (i.e., does the wound need to be covered with a waterproof barrier or should it be cleansed in the shower?).
- Tap water may be used to cleanse wounds instead of normal saline (Cornish & Douglas, 2016; Edwards-Jones, Atkin, & Guttormsen, 2018).
- Provide pain medication approximately 30 minutes before the procedure if the wound care causes pain or discomfort.
- Keep pets out of the area when setting up for and performing procedures.
- Instruct the client and family to report any increasing wound drainage, pain, or redness; increasing swelling; or opening or gaping of wound edges.

Sutures and Staples

A **suture** is a thread used to sew body tissues together. Sutures used to attach tissues beneath the skin are often made of an absorbable material that disappears in several days. Skin sutures, by contrast, are made of a variety of nonabsorbable materials, such as silk, cotton, linen, wire, nylon, and Dacron (polyester fiber). Wire clips or staples are also available. Usually sutures and staples are removed 7 to 10 days after surgery.

Various suturing methods are used. Skin sutures can be broadly categorized as either interrupted (each stitch is tied and knotted separately) or continuous (one thread runs in a series of stitches and is tied only at the beginning and at the end of the run).

Retention sutures are very large sutures used in addition to skin sutures for some incisions (Figure 36.17 ■). They attach underlying tissues of fat and muscle as well as skin and are used to support incisions in individuals who are obese or when healing may be prolonged. They are frequently left in place longer than skin sutures (14 to 21 days). To prevent these large sutures from irritating the incision, the surgeon may place tubing over them or a roll of gauze under them extending down the incision line.

The primary care provider orders the removal of sutures. In some agencies, only primary care providers remove sutures; in others, registered nurses and nursing students with appropriate supervision may do so. Agency policies about removal of retention sutures vary. The nurse should verify whether they are to be removed and who may remove them.

Sterile technique and special suture scissors are used in suture removal. The scissors have a short, curved cutting tip that readily slides under the suture (Figure 36.18 ■). Wire clips or staples are removed with a special instrument that squeezes the center of the clip to remove it from the skin (Figure 36.19 ■). Guidelines for removing sutures and staples follow:

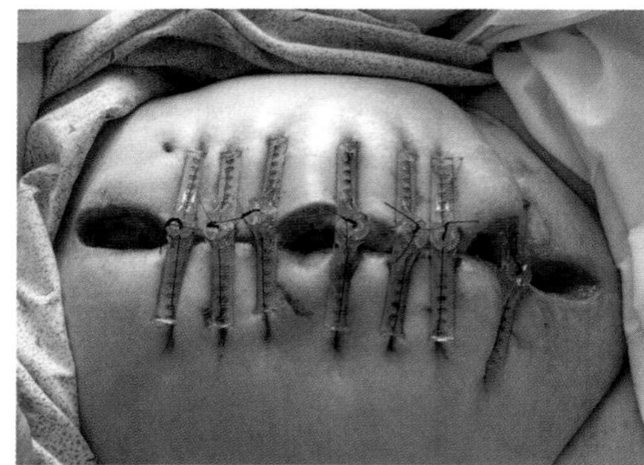

Figure 36.17 ■ A surgical incision with retention sutures.
Barry Slaven/Science Source.

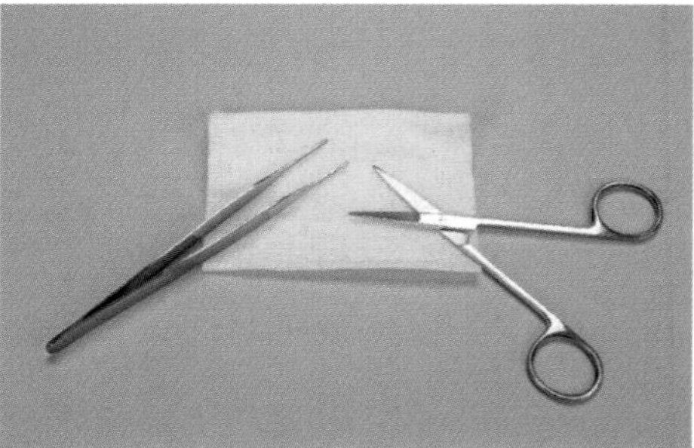

Figure 36.18 ■ Contents of a suture removal tray.

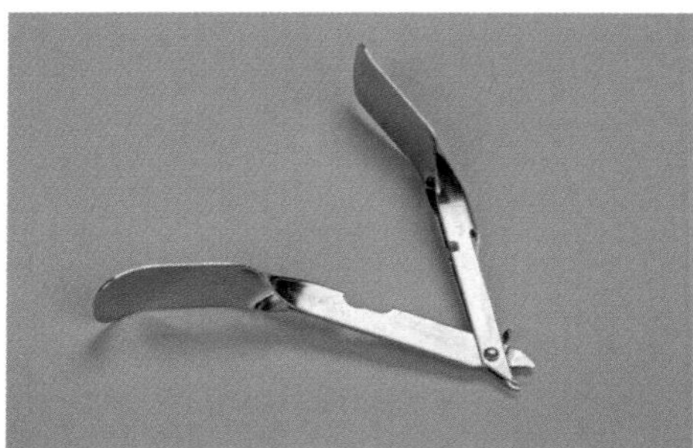

Figure 36.19 ■ Surgical staple remover.

- Before removing skin sutures, verify (a) the orders for suture removal (in many instances, only *alternate* sutures are removed one day, and the remaining sutures are removed a day or two later) and (b) whether a dressing is to be applied following the suture removal. Some primary care providers prefer no dressing; others prefer a small, light gauze dressing to prevent friction from clothing.
- Inform the client that suture removal may produce slight discomfort, such as a pulling or stinging sensation, but should not be painful.
- Remove dressings and clean the incision in accordance with agency protocol. Cleaning the suture line with an antimicrobial solution before and after suture removal may help prevent infection.
- Apply gloves.
- Remove sutures as follows:
  a. Grasp the suture at the knot with a pair of forceps or hemostat.
  b. Place the curved tip of the suture scissors under the suture as close to the skin as possible, either on the side opposite the knot (Figure 36.20 ■) or directly under the knot. Cut the suture. Sutures are cut as close to the skin as possible on one side of the visible part because the suture material that is visible to the eye is in contact with resident bacteria of the skin and must not be pulled beneath the skin during removal.
  c. Pull the suture out in one piece. Inspect the suture carefully to make sure that all suture material is removed. Suture material left beneath the skin acts as a foreign body and causes inflammation.

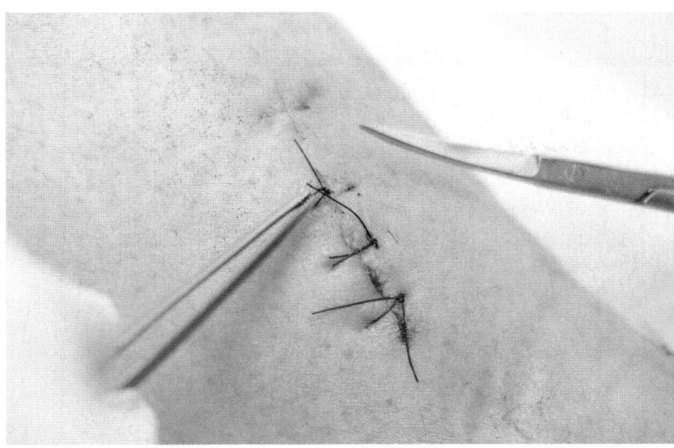

Figure 36.20 ■ Removing a skin suture.
choja/E+/Getty Images.

- Discard the suture onto a piece of sterile gauze or into the moisture-proof bag, being careful not to contaminate the instrument tips.
- Remove staples as follows:
  a. Remove dressings and clean the incision in accordance with agency protocol.
  b. Place the lower tips of a sterile surgical staple remover under the staple.
  c. Squeeze the handles together until they are completely closed (Figure 36.21 ■). Pressing the handles together causes the staple to bend in the middle and pulls the edges of the staple out of the skin. Do not lift the staple remover when squeezing the handles.
  d. When both ends of the staple are visible, gently move the staple away from the incision site.
  e. Hold the staple remover over a disposable container and release the staple remover handles, which releases the staple.
- Continue to remove every other suture or staple, that is, the third, fifth, seventh, and so forth. Alternates are removed so that remaining sutures or staples keep the skin edges in close approximation in case the wound separates.
- If no dehiscence occurs, remove the remaining sutures or staples. If dehiscence does occur, do not remove the remaining sutures, and report the dehiscence to the nurse in charge (Figure 36.22 ■).
- Some primary care providers order reinforced bandage strips (known as Steri-Strips or butterfly closures) to provide additional support to the healing wound. If ordered by the primary care provider, apply them to the wound after removing the sutures or staples.
- Reapply a dressing, if indicated.
- Document the suture or staple removal: number removed; appearance of the incision; application of a dressing, bandage, or tape (if appropriate); client teaching; and client tolerance of the procedure.

Bandaging and Binders

Bandages and binders serve various purposes:

- Supporting a wound (e.g., a fractured bone)
- Immobilizing a wound (e.g., a strained shoulder)
- Applying pressure (e.g., elastic bandages on the lower extremities to improve venous blood flow)
- Securing a dressing (e.g., for an extensive abdominal surgical wound)
- Retaining warmth (e.g., a flannel bandage on a rheumatoid joint).

There are several types of bandages and binders and several ways in which they are applied. When correctly applied, they promote healing, provide comfort, and can prevent injury (see the accompanying Practice Guidelines).

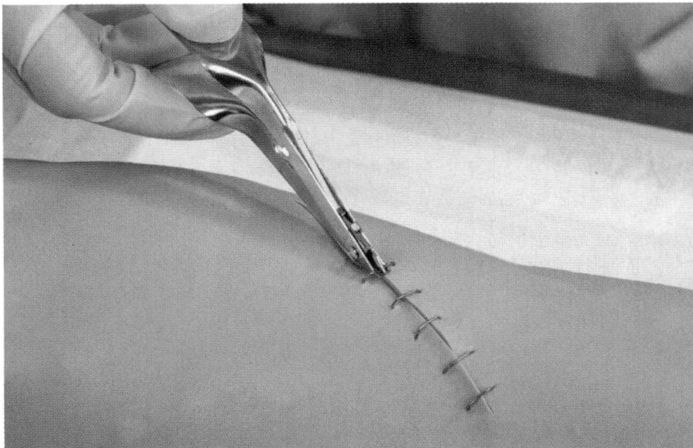

Figure 36.21 ■ Removing surgical clips or staples.

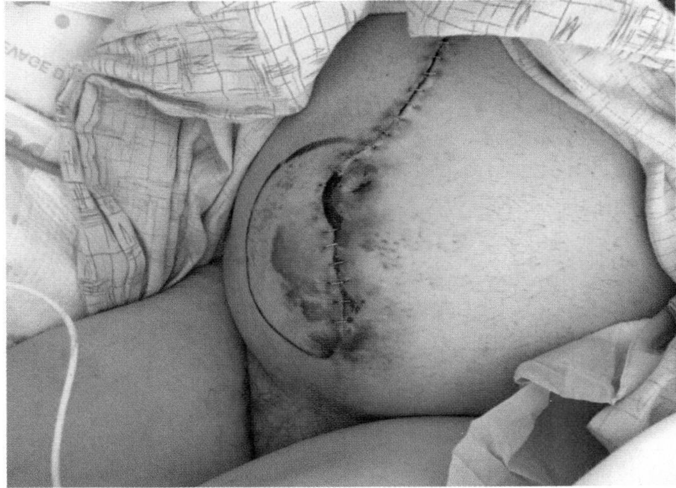

Figure 36.22 ■ Additional sutures or staples should not be removed if the wound shows dehiscence.

PRACTICE GUIDELINES **Bandaging**

- Whenever possible, bandage the part in its normal position, with the joint slightly flexed. **Rationale:** *This avoids putting strain on the ligaments and the muscles of the joint.*
- Pad between skin surfaces and over bony prominences. **Rationale:** *This prevents friction from the bandage and consequent abrasion of the skin.*
- Always bandage body parts by working from the distal to the proximal end. **Rationale:** *This aids the return flow of venous blood.*
- Bandage with even pressure. **Rationale:** *This prevents interference with blood circulation.*
- Whenever possible, leave the end of the body part (e.g., the toe) exposed. **Rationale:** *You will be able to assess the adequacy of the blood circulation to the extremity.*
- Cover dressings with bandages at least 5 cm (2 in.) beyond the edges of the dressing. **Rationale:** *This prevents the dressing and wound from becoming contaminated.*

Bandages

A **bandage** is a strip of cloth used to wrap some part of the body. Bandages are available in various widths, most commonly 1.5 to 7.5 cm (0.5 to 3 in.). They are usually supplied in rolls for easy application to a body part.

Many types of materials are used for bandages. Gauze is one of the most commonly used, because it is light and porous and readily molds to the body. It is also relatively inexpensive, so it is generally discarded when soiled. Gauze is used to retain dressings on wounds and to bandage the fingers, hands, toes, and feet. It supports dressings and at the same time permits air to circulate; it can be impregnated with petroleum jelly or other medications for application to wounds.

Elasticized bandages are applied to provide pressure to an area. They are commonly used to provide support and improve the venous circulation in the legs.

The width of the bandage used depends on the size of the body part to be bandaged. Padding (e.g., abdominal pads and gauze squares) is frequently used to cover bony prominences (e.g., the elbow) or to separate skin surfaces (e.g., the fingers) before bandaging.

Before applying a bandage, assess the area requiring support (see accompanying Practice Guidelines). When bandages are used to secure dressings, the nurse wears gloves to prevent contact with body fluids.

Basic Turns for Roller Bandages

Applying bandages to various parts of the body involves one or more of five basic bandaging turns: circular, spiral, spiral reverse, recurrent, and figure-eight. *Circular* turns are used to anchor bandages and to terminate them. Circular turns usually are not applied directly over a wound because of the discomfort the bandage would cause.

Spiral turns are used to bandage parts of the body that are fairly uniform in circumference, for example, the arm or upper leg. *Recurrent* turns are used to cover distal parts of the body, for example, the end of a finger, the skull, or the stump of an amputation. *Figure-eight* turns are used to bandage an elbow, knee, or ankle, because they permit some movement after application.

Circular Turns

- Hold the bandage in your dominant hand, keeping the roll uppermost, and unroll the bandage about 8 cm (3 in.). This length of unrolled bandage allows good control for placement and tension.
- Apply the end of the bandage to the part of the body to be bandaged. Hold the end down with the thumb of the other hand (Figure 36.23 ■).
- Encircle the body part a few times or as often as needed, making sure that each layer overlaps one-half to two-thirds of the previous layer. This provides even support to the area.
- The bandage should be firm, but not too tight. A tight bandage can interfere with blood circulation, whereas a loose bandage does not provide adequate protection.
- Secure the end of the bandage with tape or clips if there is no Velcro fastener.

Spiral Turns

- Make two circular turns to anchor the bandage.
- Continue spiral turns at about a 30° angle, each turn overlapping the preceding one by two-thirds the width of the bandage (Figure 36.24 ■).
- Secure the end as described for circular turns.

PRACTICE GUIDELINES **Assessing Before Applying Bandages or Binders**

- Inspect and palpate the area for swelling.
- Inspect for the presence of and status of wounds (open wounds will require a dressing before a bandage or binder is applied).
- Note the presence of drainage (amount, color, odor, viscosity).
- Inspect and palpate for adequacy of circulation (skin temperature, color, and sensation). **Rationale:** *Pale or cyanotic skin, cool temperature, tingling, and numbness can indicate impaired circulation.*
- Ask the client about any pain experienced (location, intensity, onset, quality).
- Assess the ability of the client to reapply the bandage or binder when needed.
- Assess the capabilities of the client regarding activities of daily living (e.g., to eat, dress, comb hair, bathe) and assess the assistance required during the convalescence period.

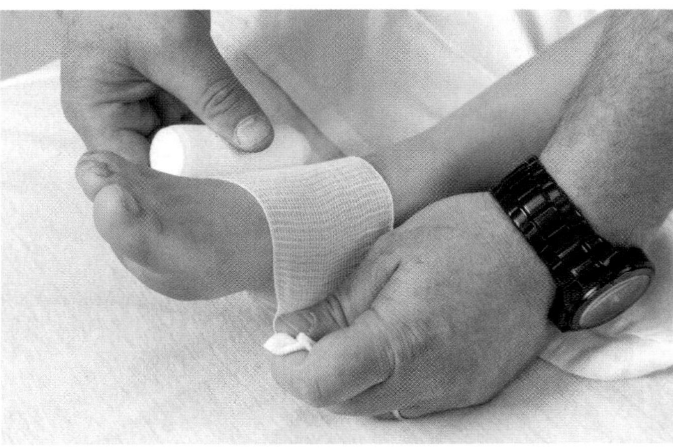

Figure 36.23 ■ Starting a bandage with circular turns.

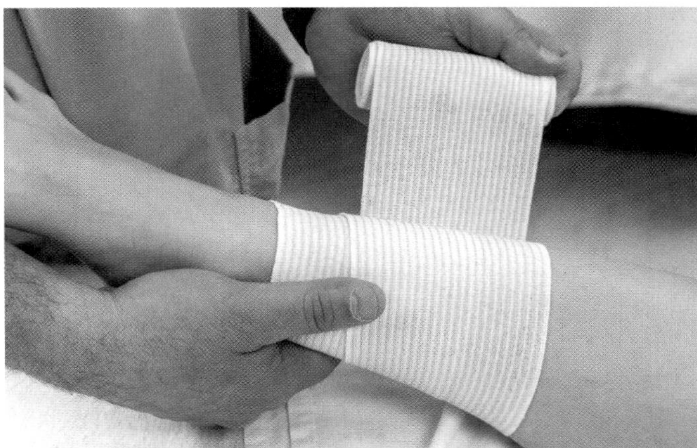

Figure 36.24 ■ Applying spiral turns.

Recurrent Turns

- Anchor the bandage with two circular turns.
- Fold the bandage back on itself, and bring it centrally over the distal end to be bandaged.
- Bring the bandage back over the end to the right of the center bandage but overlapping it by two-thirds the width of the bandage.
- Bring the bandage back on the left side, also overlapping the first turn by two-thirds the width of the bandage.
- Continue this pattern of alternating right and left until the area is covered. Overlap the preceding turn by two-thirds the bandage width each time.
- Terminate the bandage with two circular turns (Figure 36.25 ■). Secure the end appropriately.

Figure-Eight Turns

- Anchor the bandage with two circular turns.
- Carry the bandage above the joint, around it, and then below it, making a figure-eight (Figure 36.26 ■).
- Continue above and below the joint, overlapping the previous turn by two-thirds the width of the bandage.
- Terminate the bandage above the joint with two circular turns, and then secure the end appropriately.

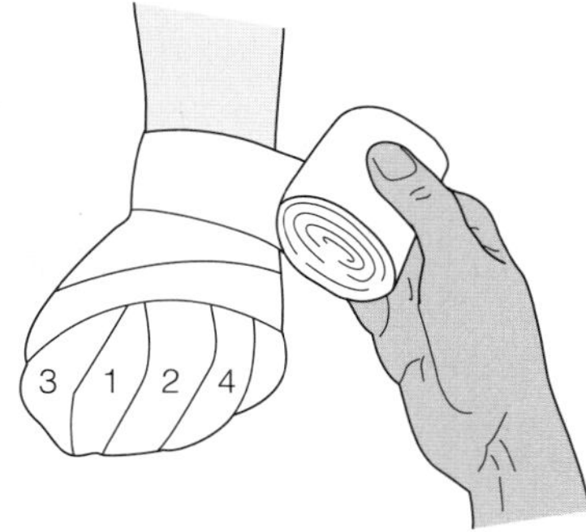

Figure 36.25 ■ Completing a recurrent bandage.

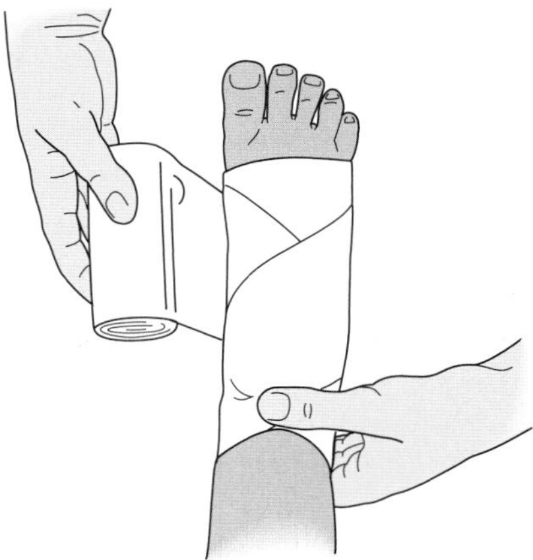

Figure 36.26 ■ Applying a figure-eight bandage.

Binders

A **binder** is a type of bandage designed for a specific body part; for example, the triangular binder (sling) fits the arm. Binders are used to support large areas of the body, such as the abdomen or chest. Binders can be simple, inexpensive, and customizable by using plain material such as the triangular sling described below, or they can be of commercial design. Commercial binders, such as the hook-and-loop (Velcro) binder, are often easier to use, more expensive, and slightly less modifiable than customized binders.

The client should have two sets of bandages or binders so that there is one to wear while the other is being washed. Teach clients and their families that bandages and binders should be washed inside a mesh laundry bag to keep them from becoming twisted and to prevent Velcro or hooks from catching on other laundry.

Arm Sling

- Ask the client to flex the elbow to an 80° angle or less, depending on the purpose. The thumb should be facing upward or inward toward the body. **Rationale:** *An 80° angle is sufficient to support the forearm, to prevent swelling of the hand, and to relieve pressure on the shoulder joint (e.g., to support the paralyzed arm of a stroke client whose shoulder might otherwise become dislocated). A more acute angle is preferred if there is swelling of the hand.*

- If a triangle sling is used, place one end of the unfolded binder over the shoulder of the uninjured side so that the binder falls down the front of the chest of the client with the point of the triangle (apex) under the elbow of the injured side.
- Take the upper corner, and carry it around the neck until it hangs over the shoulder on the injured side.
- Bring the lower corner of the binder up over the arm to the shoulder of the injured side. Using a square knot, secure this corner to the upper corner at the side of the neck on the injured side (Figure 36.27 ■). **Rationale:** *A square knot will not slip. Tying the knot at the side of the neck prevents pressure on the bony prominences of the vertebral column at the back of the neck.*
- Fold the sling neatly at the elbow, and secure it with safety pins or tape. It may be folded and fastened at the front.
- If a commercial sling is used, it may also include a second strap that goes around the back of the client's chest from the finger end of the sling to the elbow (Figure 36.28 ■). **Rationale:** *This strap holds the arm close to the body at all times, providing shoulder immobilization such as is used following a shoulder dislocation or surgery.*
- Make sure the wrist is supported, to maintain alignment.
- Remove the sling periodically to inspect the skin for indications of irritation, especially around the site of the knot.

Straight Abdominal Binder

- Place the binder smoothly around the body, commonly with the upper border of the binder at the waist and the lower border at the level of the gluteal fold. A binder placed over the waist interferes with respiration; one placed too low interferes with elimination and walking.
- Apply padding over the iliac crests if the client is thin.
- Bring the ends around the client, overlap them, and secure them with pins, clips, or Velcro (Figure 36.29 ■). If used, orient the pins horizontally to allow for comfort when bending.

Heat and Cold Applications

Heat and cold are applied to the body for local and systemic effects. Table 36.5 lists the physiologic effects of heat and cold.

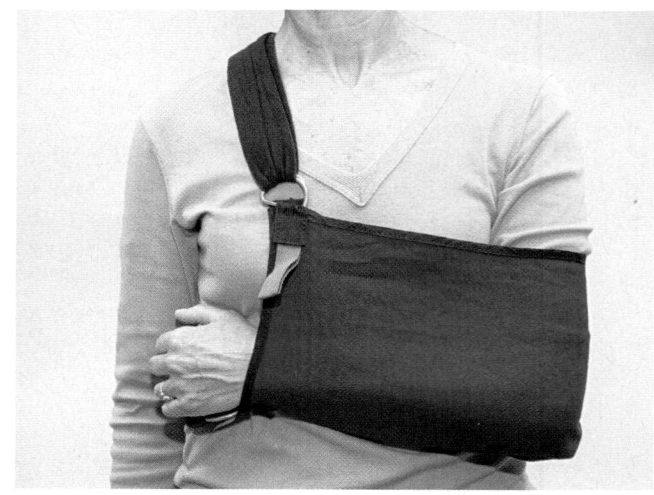

Figure 36.28 ■ A commercial arm sling.

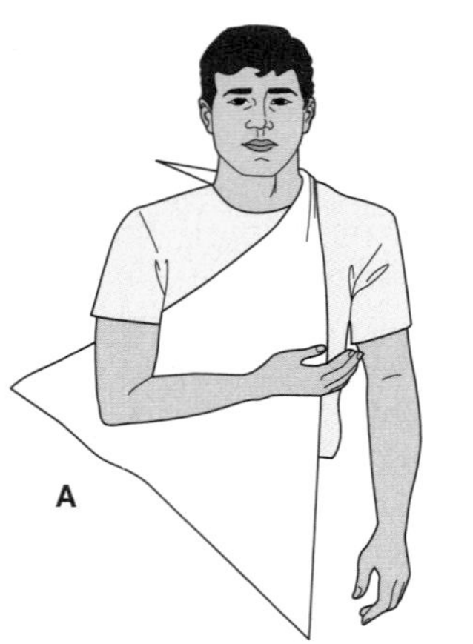

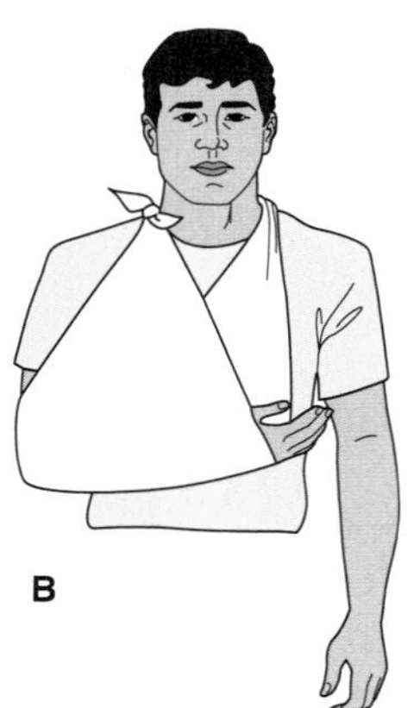

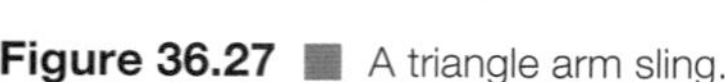

Figure 36.27 ■ A triangle arm sling.

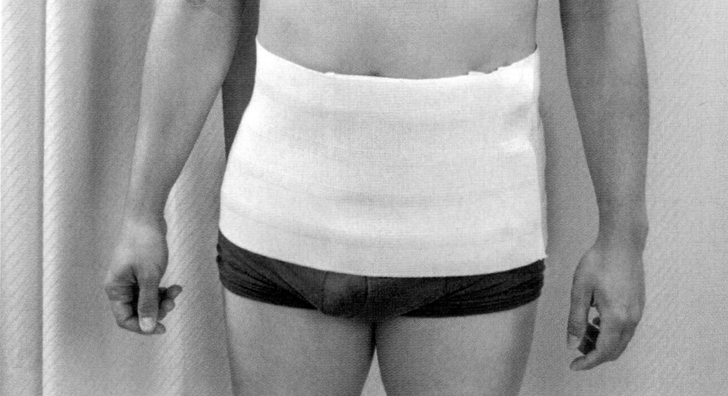

Figure 36.29 ■ A straight abdominal binder.

LIFESPAN CONSIDERATIONS Applying Bandages and Binders

CHILDREN

- Allow the child to help with the procedure by holding supplies, opening boxes, counting turns, and so on.
- If a young client is apprehensive, demonstrate the procedure on a doll or stuffed animal.
- Encourage the child to decorate the bandage.
- Teach the caregivers to apply bandages and binders safely.

OLDER ADULTS

- Older clients may need extra support during the procedure, especially if arthritis, contractures, or tremors are present.
- Avoid constricting the client's circulation with a tight bandage or binder. Observe skin and bony prominences frequently for signs of impaired circulation. The risk for skin breakdown increases with age.

TABLE 36.5 Physiologic Effects of Heat and Cold

Heat	Cold
Vasodilation	Vasoconstriction
Increases capillary permeability	Decreases capillary permeability
Increases cellular metabolism	Decreases cellular metabolism
Increases inflammation	Slows bacterial growth, decreases inflammation
Sedative effect	Local anesthetic effect

Local Effects of Heat

Heat has been a long-standing remedy for aches and pains, and individuals often equate heat with comfort and relief. Heat causes vasodilation and increases blood flow to the affected area, bringing oxygen, nutrients, antibodies, and leukocytes.

Application of heat promotes soft tissue healing and increases suppuration. A possible disadvantage of heat is that it increases capillary permeability, which allows extracellular fluid and substances such as plasma proteins to pass through the capillary walls and may result in edema or an increase in preexisting edema. Heat is often used for clients with musculoskeletal problems such as joint stiffness from arthritis, contractures, and low back pain.

Local Effects of Cold

Generally, the physiologic effects of cold are opposite to the effects of heat. Cold lowers the temperature of the skin and underlying tissues and causes **vasoconstriction**. Vasoconstriction reduces blood flow to the affected area and thus reduces the supply of oxygen and metabolites, decreases the removal of wastes, and produces skin pallor and coolness. Prolonged exposure to cold results in impaired circulation, cell deprivation, and subsequent damage to the tissues from lack of oxygen and nourishment. Cold is most often used for sports injuries (e.g., sprains, strains, fractures) to limit postinjury swelling and bleeding.

Thermal Tolerance

Various parts of the body differ in tolerance to heat and cold. The physiologic tolerance of clients also varies (Box 36.2). Specific conditions necessitate precautions in the use of hot or cold applications:

- ***Neurosensory impairment.*** Clients with sensory impairments are unable to perceive that heat is damaging the tissues and are at risk for burns or are unable to perceive discomfort from cold and prevent tissue injury.
- ***Impaired mental status.*** Clients who are confused or have an altered level of consciousness need monitoring during applications to ensure safe therapy.
- ***Impaired circulation.*** Clients with peripheral vascular disease, diabetes, or congestive heart failure lack the normal ability to dissipate heat via the blood circulation, which puts them at risk for tissue damage with heat and cold applications.

BOX 36.2 Variables Affecting Physiologic Tolerance to Heat and Cold

- *Body part.* The back of the hand and foot are not very temperature sensitive. In contrast, the inner aspect of the wrist and forearm, the neck, and the perineal area are temperature sensitive.
- *Size of the exposed body part.* The larger the area exposed to heat and cold, the lower the tolerance.
- *Individual tolerance.* The very young and the very old generally have the lowest tolerance. Individuals who have neurosensory impairments may have a high tolerance, but the risk of injury is greater.
- *Length of exposure.* Clients feel hot and cold applications most while the temperature is changing. After a period of time, tolerance increases.
- *Intactness of skin.* Injured skin areas are more sensitive to temperature variations.

- ***Immediately after injury or surgery.*** Heat increases bleeding and swelling.
- ***Open wounds.*** Cold can decrease blood flow to the wound, thereby inhibiting healing.

Adaptation of Thermal Receptors

Temperature (thermal) receptors adapt to temperature changes. When they are subjected to an abrupt change in temperature, the receptors are strongly stimulated initially. This strong stimulation declines rapidly during the first few seconds and then more slowly during the next half hour or more as the receptors adapt to the new temperature.

Nurses and clients need to understand this adaptive response when applying heat and cold. Clients may be tempted to change the temperature of a thermal application because of the change in thermal sensation following adaptation. Increasing the temperature of a hot application after adaptation can result in serious burns. Decreasing the temperature of a cold application can result in pain and serious impairment of circulation to the body part. Table 36.6 lists temperatures of hot and cold applications.

Rebound Phenomenon

The rebound phenomenon occurs at the time the maximum therapeutic effect of the hot or cold application is achieved and the opposite effect begins. For example,

TABLE 36.6 Temperatures for Hot and Cold Applications

Description	Temperature	Application
Very cold	Below 15°C (59°F)	Ice bags
Cold	15°C–18°C (59°F–65°F)	Cold pack
Cool	18°C–27°C (65°F–80°F)	Cold compresses
Tepid	27°C–37°C (80°F–98°F)	Alcohol sponge bath
Warm	37°C–40°C (98°F–104°F)	Warm bath, aquathermia pads
Hot	40°C–46°C (104°–115°F)	Hot soak, irrigations, hot compresses*

Note: The temperature of the water used to create the hot soak or compress exceeds the temperature of 43°C (110°F), which is safe to apply directly to skin (Martin & Falder, 2017).

heat produces maximum vasodilation in 20 to 30 minutes; continuation of the application beyond 30 minutes brings tissue congestion, and the blood vessels then constrict. If the heat application is continued, the client is at risk for burns because the constricted blood vessels are unable to dissipate the heat adequately via the blood circulation.

With cold applications, maximum vasoconstriction occurs when the involved skin reaches a temperature of 15°C (60°F). Below 15°C, vasodilation begins. This mechanism is protective: It helps to prevent freezing of body tissues normally exposed to cold, such as the nose and ears. Continued cold causes alternating vasodilation and vasoconstriction (called the Lewis Hunting effect).

Safety Alert! SAFETY

An understanding of the rebound phenomenon is essential for the nurse and client. Thermal applications must be halted *before* the rebound phenomenon begins.

Applying Heat and Cold

Heat can be applied to the body in both dry and moist forms. Dry heat is applied locally by means of a hot water bottle, aquathermia pad, disposable heat pack, or electric pad. Moist heat can be provided by compress, hot pack, soak, or sitz bath. Selected indications for the use of heat and cold are found in Table 36.7.

Dry cold is generally applied locally by means of a cold pack, ice bag, ice glove, or ice collar. In addition, continuous cold therapy (cryotherapy) following joint surgery or injury can be delivered by a cooling unit similar to the aquathermia pad. Moist cold can be provided by compress or a cooling sponge bath.

For all local applications of heat or cold, the nurse needs to follow these guidelines:

- Determine the client's ability to tolerate the therapy.
- Identify conditions that might contraindicate treatment (e.g., bleeding, circulatory impairment).
- Explain the application to the client.
- Assess the skin area to which the heat or cold will be applied.
- Ask the client to report any discomfort.
- Return to the client 15 minutes after starting the heat or cold therapy, and observe the local skin area for any untoward signs (e.g., redness). Stop the application if any problems occur.
- Remove the equipment at the designated time, and dispose of it appropriately.
- Examine the area to which the heat or cold was applied, and record the client's response.
- For contraindications to the use of heat or cold, see Box 36.3.

Aquathermia Pad

The aquathermia pad (also referred to as a K-pad) is constructed with tubes containing water. The pad is attached by tubing to an electrically powered control unit that has an opening for water and a temperature gauge. Some aquathermia pads have an absorbent surface through which moist heat can be applied. The other surface of the pad is waterproof. These pads are disposable.

To apply an aquathermia pad, the nurse carries out the following steps:

- Fill the reservoir of the unit two-thirds full of water as specified by the manufacturer.
- Set the desired temperature. Check the manufacturer's instructions. Most units are set at 40°C (104°F) for adults.
- Cover the pad and plug in the unit. Check for any leaks or malfunctions of the pad before use.
- Apply the pad to the body part. The treatment is usually continued for 30 minutes. Check orders and agency protocol.
- Use tape or gauze ties to hold the pad in place. Never use safety pins. They can cause leakage.
- If unusual redness or pain occurs, discontinue the treatment, and report the client's reaction.

TABLE 36.7 Selected Indications of Heat and Cold

Indication	Effect of Heat	Effect of Cold
Muscle spasm	Relaxes muscles and increases their contractility.	Relaxes muscles and decreases muscle contractility.
Inflammation	Increases blood flow, softens exudates.	Vasoconstriction decreases capillary permeability, decreases blood flow, slows cellular metabolism.
Pain	Relieves pain, possibly by promoting muscle relaxation, increasing circulation, and promoting psychologic relaxation and a feeling of comfort; acts as a counterirritant.	Decreases pain by slowing nerve conduction rate and blocking nerve impulses; produces numbness, acts as a counterirritant, increases pain threshold.
Contracture	Reduces contracture and increases joint range of motion by allowing greater distention of muscles and connective tissue.	
Joint stiffness	Reduces joint stiffness by decreasing viscosity of synovial fluid and increasing tissue distensibility.	
Traumatic injury		Decreases bleeding by constricting blood vessels; decreases edema by reducing capillary permeability.

BOX 36.3 Contraindications to the Use of Heat and Cold

Determine the presence of any conditions indicating the need for special precautions during heat and cold therapy:

- *Neurosensory impairment.* Clients with sensory impairments are unable to perceive that heat is damaging the tissues and are at risk for burns, or they are unable to perceive discomfort from cold and are unable to prevent tissue injury.
- *Impaired mental status.* Clients who are confused or have an altered level of consciousness need monitoring and supervision during applications to ensure safe therapy.
- *Impaired circulation.* Clients with peripheral vascular disease, diabetes, or congestive heart failure lack the normal ability to dissipate heat via the blood circulation, which puts them at risk for tissue damage with heat applications. Cold applications are contraindicated for these clients.
- *Open wounds.* Tissues around an open wound are more sensitive to heat and cold.

Determine the presence of any conditions contraindicating the use of heat:

- *The first 24 hours after traumatic injury.* Heat increases bleeding and swelling.
- *Active hemorrhage.* Heat causes vasodilation and increases bleeding.
- *Noninflammatory edema.* Heat increases capillary permeability and edema.
- *Skin disorder that causes redness or blisters.* Heat can burn or cause further damage to the skin.

Determine the presence of any conditions contraindicating the use of cold:

- *Open wounds.* Cold can increase tissue damage by decreasing blood flow to an open wound.
- *Impaired circulation.* Cold can further impair nourishment of the tissues and cause tissue damage. In clients with Raynaud's disease, cold increases arterial spasm.
- *Allergy or hypersensitivity to cold.* Some clients have an allergy to cold that may be manifested by an inflammatory response, for example, erythema, hives, swelling, joint pain, and occasional muscle spasm. Some react with a sudden increase in blood pressure, which can be hazardous if the client is hypersensitive.

Hot and Cold Packs

Commercially prepared hot and cold packs (Figure 36.30 ■) provide heat or cold for a designated time. Directions on the package tell how to initiate the heating or cooling process, for example, by striking, squeezing, or kneading the pack.

Electric Heating Pads

Electric pads provide a constant, even heat, are lightweight, and can be molded to a body part. They are relatively inexpensive and are often purchased by the client for home use. Electric pads, however, can burn the client if the setting is too high. Some models have waterproof covers for use when the pad is placed over a moist dressing.

In using electric pads, the nurse follows these guidelines:

- Do not insert sharp objects (e.g., pins) into the pad. The pin could damage a wire and cause an electric shock.

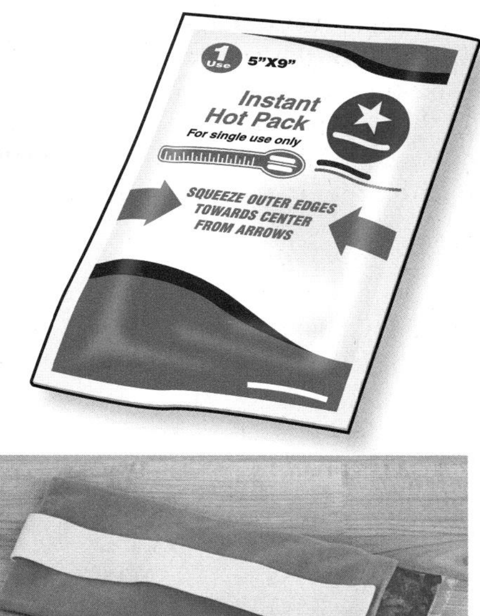

Figure 36.30 ■ Commercially prepared disposable hot and cold packs.
Cold compress, Sasimoto/Shutterstock.

- Ensure that the body area is dry unless there is a waterproof cover on the pad. Electricity in the presence of water can cause a shock.
- Do not place the pad under the client. Heat will not dissipate, and the client may be burned.

Ice Bags, Ice Gloves, and Ice Collars

Ice bags (Figure 36.31 ■), ice gloves, and ice collars are filled either with ice chips or with an alcohol-based solution. They are applied to the body to provide cold to a localized area (e.g., a collar is often applied to the throat following a tonsillectomy). Always wrap the container in a towel or cover.

Compresses

Compresses can be either warm or cold. A **compress** is a moist gauze dressing applied to a wound or injury. When hot compresses are ordered, the solution is heated to the temperature indicated by the order or according to agency protocol, for example, 40.5°C (105°F). When there is a break in the skin or when the body part (e.g., an eye) is vulnerable to microbial invasion, sterile technique is necessary; therefore, sterile gloves are needed to apply the compress and all materials must be sterile.

Soaks

A soak refers to immersing a body part (e.g., an arm) in a solution or to wrapping a part in gauze dressings and then saturating the dressing with a solution. Sterile technique is generally indicated for open wounds, such as a burn or an unhealed surgical incision. Determine agency protocol regarding the temperature of the solution. Hot soaks are frequently done to soften and remove encrusted secretions and dead tissue.

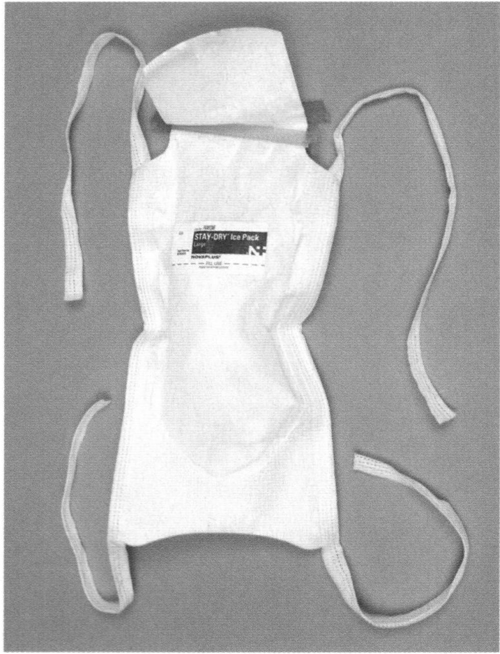

Figure 36.31 ■ Disposable ice bag.

Sitz Baths

A **sitz bath**, or hip bath, is used to soak a client's perineal or rectal area. The client sits in a special tub or chair. Disposable sitz baths are also available for home or hospital use (Figure 36.32 ■).

The temperature of the water should be from 40°C to 43°C (104°F to 110°F), unless the client is unable to tolerate the heat. Determine agency protocol. Some sitz tubs have temperature indicators attached to the water taps. The duration of the bath is generally 20 minutes, depending on the client's health. Follow these steps to provide a sitz bath:

- Assist the client into the bath. Provide support for the client's feet; a footstool can prevent pressure on the backs of the thighs.
- Provide a bath blanket for the client's shoulders, and eliminate drafts to prevent chilling.
- Observe the client closely during the bath for signs of faintness, dizziness, weakness, accelerated pulse rate, and pallor.
- Maintain the water temperature.
- Following the sitz bath, assist the client out of the bath. Help the client to dry.

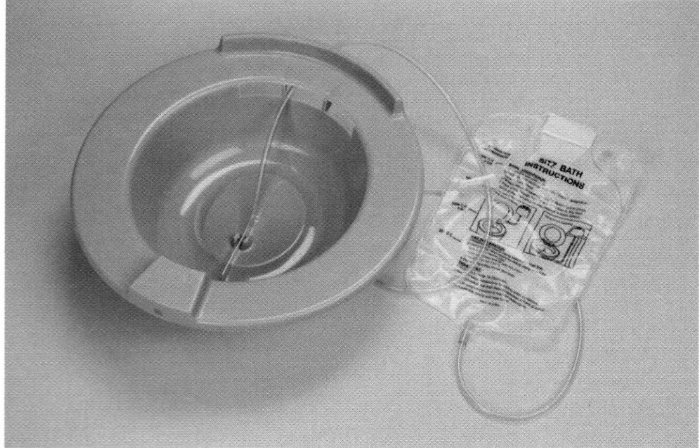

Figure 36.32 ■ A plastic single-client sitz bath.

Cooling Sponge Baths

The purpose of a cooling sponge bath is to reduce a client's fever by promoting heat loss through conduction and vaporization. Cool sponge baths are used with extreme caution, and only for clients with very high temperatures, such as over 40°C (104°F), because rapid skin temperature drop can cause chills that actually increase heat production. The bath is accompanied by antipyretic medication that acts to reset the hypothalamus set point. The temperatures for cooling sponge baths range from 27°C to 37°C (80°F to 98°F).

To provide a cooling sponge bath, the nurse should:

- Sponge the face, arms, legs, back, and buttocks. The chest and abdomen are not usually sponged. Each area is sponged slowly and gently. Rubbing may increase heat production.
- Leave each area wet and cover with a damp towel.
- Place ice bags and cold packs, if used, or a cool cloth on the forehead for comfort and in each axilla and at the groin. These areas contain large superficial blood vessels that help the transfer of heat.
- Sponge one body part and then another. The sponge bath should take about 30 minutes. A bath given more quickly tends to increase the body's heat production by causing shivering.
- Discontinue the bath if the client becomes pale or cyanotic or shivers, or if the pulse becomes rapid or irregular.
- Reassess the vital signs at 15 minutes and after completing the sponge bath.

Evaluating

The goals established during the planning phase are evaluated according to specific desired outcomes also established in that phase. To judge whether client outcomes have been achieved, the nurse uses data collected during care, such as skin status over bony prominences, nutritional and fluid intake, mental status, signs of healing if an injury is present, and so on. If outcomes are not achieved, the nurse should explore the reasons why:

- Has the client's physical condition changed?
- Were risk factors correctly identified?
- Were appropriate devices and techniques used?
- Was the client unable to comply with instructions about moving and turning? Why?
- Were appropriate pressure-relieving devices used, and were they applied correctly?
- Was the repositioning schedule adhered to?
- Are the client's nutritional and fluid intake adequate?
- Were appropriate measures used to control incontinence and protect the client's skin?
- Was the wound supported and immobilized effectively?
- Were stringent aseptic practices implemented when cleaning and changing dressings to prevent infection?
- Was the client receiving antineoplastic or anti-inflammatory medications that interfere with healing?
- Was nonviable tissue removed by autolytic, chemical, mechanical, or surgical debridement?
- Was the appropriate dressing applied to maintain moist wound healing or absorb excess drainage?

Wound and skin care, like many other aspects of nursing, is a constantly evolving area of practice. Nurses should ensure that they are using the most current and evidence-based practices available. Excellent sources of this information are the professional organizations dedicated to skin and wound practices (Box 36.4).

BOX 36.4 Wound Care Organizations

American Professional Wound Care Association (APWCA)—www.apwca.org The APWCA is a membership organization incorporating the various medical specialties involved in treating complex wounds. The mission of APWCA is to help decrease the rate of complications from all wounds, including acute, chronic, postsurgical, postradiation, reconstructive, and other problematic wounds. The association's goal is to accelerate wound healing and preserve and enhance the quality of life for these clients.

Association for the Advancement of Wound Care (AAWC)—www.aawconline.org Headquartered in the United States, the AAWC is a nonprofit, international multidisciplinary organization for wound care. This organization is open to everyone involved in wound care, including clinicians, clients and their lay caregivers, facilities, industry, students, retirees, and others interested in the care of wounds. The AAWC was founded to spread wound awareness by promoting excellence in education, clinical practice, public policy, and research. *Wound Management and Prevention* and *WOUNDS* are the official journals of the AAWC.

Dermatology Nurses' Association (DNA)—www.dnanurse.org DNA is a professional nursing organization composed of a diverse group of individuals committed to quality care through sharing knowledge and expertise. The core purpose of the DNA is to promote excellence in dermatologic care. The *Journal of the Dermatology Nurses' Association* is the official publication of the DNA.

National Alliance of Wound Care and Ostomy (NAWCO)—www.nawccb.org NAWC membership organization provides educational, research, and advocacy opportunities to members. The alliance is open to all wound care professionals and corporations doing business in the field of wound care.

Wound Ostomy and Continence Nurses Society (WOCN)—www.wocn.org WOCN is an international society of more than 5000 healthcare professionals who are experts in the care of clients with wound, ostomy, and continence problems. Membership also is open to students, corporate colleagues, and all individuals who share the mission and goals of the society. The WOCN publishes the *Journal of Wound, Ostomy and Continence Nursing*.

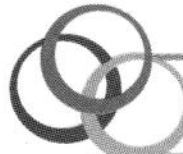

Critical Thinking Checkpoint

You have been assigned to care for Mr. Johns, a 74-year-old client being treated for a urinary tract disorder. Mr. Johns suffered a cerebrovascular accident (stroke) 6 months ago and has had difficulty ambulating and attending to his own needs because of right-sided weakness. While assessing Mr. Johns you note that he is thin for his height, is incontinent of foul-smelling urine, and has deeply reddened areas on his right hip, coccyx, and entire peritoneal area. Mr. Johns is alert and oriented to person, place, and time, but he has decreased sensation on his entire right side. He spends most of his time in bed or sitting at his bedside in a chair due to his difficulty with ambulation.

1. What data suggest that Mr. Johns is particularly vulnerable to pressure injury, MASD, or IAD development?
2. What additional information do you need in order to use the Braden scale to determine Mr. Johns' potential for pressure injury development?
3. What independent measures can you take to protect Mr. Johns' skin from further breakdown?
4. Considering that Mr. Johns does not have any areas of skin breakdown, why is it important to institute treatment for pressure injuries at this time?

Answers to Critical Thinking Checkpoint questions are available on the faculty resources site. Please consult with your instructor.

Chapter 36 Review

CHAPTER HIGHLIGHTS

- Maintaining skin integrity is an important independent function of nursing.
- Wounds are described as intentional or unintentional, closed or open, and clean, clean contaminated, contaminated, or dirty (infected).
- A pressure injury is injury caused by force that results in damage to underlying tissues. Pressure injuries usually occur over bony prominences.
- Two other factors that act in conjunction with pressure to produce a pressure injury are friction and shearing forces.
- Several factors increase the risk for the development of pressure injuries: immobility and inactivity, inadequate nutrition, fecal and urinary incontinence, decreased mental status, diminished sensation, excessive body heat, advanced age, and certain chronic medical conditions.
- There are stages of pressure injuries, which vary according to the degree of tissue damage.
- Several risk assessment tools are available to identify clients at risk for pressure injury development. They include scoring systems to evaluate a client's degree of risk.
- The types of wound healing are distinguished by the amount of tissue loss: primary intention healing and secondary intention healing.
- The wound-healing process has three phases: inflammatory, proliferative, and maturation.
- Major types of wound exudate are serous, purulent, and sanguineous. Exudate can be a combination of two or three of these types (e.g., serosanguineous). The process of pus formation is referred to as suppuration.
- The main complications of wound healing are hemorrhage, infection, dehiscence, and evisceration, each of which is identifiable by specific clinical signs and symptoms.
- Factors affecting wound healing include developmental stage, nutritional status, lifestyle, and medications.
- Meticulous skin assessment of common pressure injury sites by the nurse is an important ongoing assessment activity for clients at risk.
- Essential data for assessing wounds include wound appearance, size, drainage, swelling, pain, and the presence of tubes and drains.
- When a pressure injury is present, the nurse describes the injury in terms of location, size, depth, stage, color, condition of the wound bed and surrounding skin, and clinical signs of infection, if present.
- Laboratory data that may be used to assess the progress of wound healing include leukocyte count, hemoglobin, blood coagulation studies, serum protein analysis, and wound cultures. Nurses are usually responsible for obtaining specimens of wound drainage for culture.
- Major goals for clients at risk for developing pressure injuries are to maintain skin integrity and to avoid potential associated risks.
- Major nursing responsibilities related to wound care include assisting the client in maintaining moist wound healing, obtaining sufficient nutrition and fluids, preventing wound infections, and proper positioning.
- Nursing interventions to prevent the formation of pressure injuries include conducting ongoing assessment of risk factors and skin status, providing skin care to maintain skin integrity, ensuring adequate nutrition and hydration, implementing measures to avoid skin trauma, providing supportive devices, and client teaching.
- Treatment for pressure injuries varies according to the stage of the injury and agency protocol.
- The RYB color code of wounds can assist nurses to provide appropriate nursing interventions for wounds that heal by secondary intention. In this scheme, the nurse protects red, cleanses yellow, and debrides black wounds.
- Wound care may involve cleaning, irrigating, protecting, hydrating, and covering wounds; applying heat and cold; and applying bandages and binders.
- Surgical aseptic technique (sterile technique) is used when changing dressings on surgical wounds to promote healing and reduce the risk of infection.
- Hemovac and Jackson-Pratt drainage systems are examples of drains that may be placed in or near surgical wounds to promote drainage of excess serosanguineous or purulent exudate.
- Sutures, wire clips, or staples are used to approximate skin and underlying tissues after surgery. These are generally removed 7 to 10 days after surgery.
- Various types of dressing materials are available to protect wounds, absorb exudate, and keep the wound bed moist, thus facilitating healing.
- The type of dressing used depends on (a) location, size, and type of the wound; (b) amount of exudate; (c) whether or not the wound requires debridement, is infected, or has sinus tracts; and (d) such considerations as frequency of dressing change, ease or difficulty of dressing applications, and cost.
- Synthetic dressings have been developed for use with specific types of wounds. These include transparent adhesive films, impregnated nonadherent dressings, hydrocolloids, hydrogels, polyurethane foams, clear acrylic dressings, and alginates. The nurse must be aware of the specific purposes of each and their indications for use.
- Bandages and binders are used to hold dressings in place, apply pressure to wounds, support circulation, and immobilize joints.
- Heat and cold produce specific local physiologic and systemic responses that account for their therapeutic effects.
- Various parts of the body differ in tolerance to heat and cold. The physiologic tolerance of individuals also varies. Specific conditions such as neurosensory and circulatory impairments necessitate precautions when applying heat or cold.
- When applying heat or cold, clients and nurses need to be aware of the effects of thermal receptor adaptation and the rebound phenomenon.

TEST YOUR KNOWLEDGE

1. An adult client is incontinent and wears incontinence briefs when using the wheelchair. An irritated rash has developed in the perianal area. What care should the nurse provide?
   1. Wash the area with soap and hot water at every brief change.
   2. Apply a petroleum-based cream to the area after cleaning.
   3. Wipe the skin with an alcohol-free barrier film agent after cleaning.
   4. Keep the client in bed on absorbent pads until the area clears.

2. Proper technique for performing a wound culture includes which of the following?
   1. Cleansing the wound prior to obtaining the specimen
   2. Swabbing for the specimen in the area with the largest collection of drainage
   3. Removing crusts or scabs with sterile forceps and then culturing the site beneath
   4. Waiting 8 hours following a dose of antibiotic to obtain the specimen

3. A client has a pressure injury with a shallow, partial skin thickness, and eroded area but no necrotic areas. The nurse would treat the area with which dressing?
   1. Alginate
   2. Dry gauze
   3. Hydrocolloid
   4. No dressing is indicated

4. The nurse has applied an aquathermia pad to a client's back. After 15 minutes of treatment, the client says that the pack is no longer warm and asks the nurse to increase the temperature. How should the nurse evaluate this request?
   1. Since this client's thermal tolerance is higher than normal, increasing the temperature is necessary.
   2. This client may be experiencing a rebound effect from the application of moist heat.
   3. Adaptation of the thermal receptors often results in the decreased sensation of warmth.
   4. The aquathermia pad should be replaced with a standard hot pack.

5. Which statement, if made by the client or family member, would indicate the need for further teaching?
   1. "If a skin area gets red but then the red goes away after turning, I should report it to the nurse."
   2. "Putting foam pads under my heels or other bony areas can help decrease pressure."
   3. "If my father cannot turn himself in bed, I should help him change position every 4 hours."
   4. "The skin should be washed with only warm water (not hot) and lotion put on while it is still a little wet."

6. The nurse is writing the plan of care for a client who is confined to bed. Which intervention should be included to help reduce the effects of shearing forces on the client's skin?
   1. Keep the head of the client's bed at 30 degrees.
   2. Coat the client's back and buttocks with baby powder after bathing.
   3. Use a turn sheet lifted by two staff members to move the client in bed.
   4. Dust the linens with cornstarch each morning to allow for easier movement.

7. The nurse plans to remove the client's sutures. Which action demonstrates appropriate standard of care? Select all that apply.
   1. Use clean technique.
   2. Grasp the suture at the knot with a pair of forceps.
   3. Place the curved tip of the suture scissors under the suture as close to the skin as possible.
   4. Pull the suture material that is visible beneath the skin during removal.
   5. Remove alternate sutures first.

8. Which of the following are primary risk factors for pressure injuries? Select all that apply.
   1. Low-protein diet
   2. Insomnia
   3. Lengthy surgical procedures
   4. Fever
   5. Sleeping on a waterbed

9. Which of the following items are used to perform wound irrigation? Select all that apply.
   1. Clean gloves
   2. Mask
   3. Refrigerated irrigating solution
   4. 60-mL syringe
   5. Forceps

10. Which of the following indicates a proper principle of bandaging?
   1. Apply the bandage as tightly as possible without causing pain.
   2. Gauze bandages are used to hold absorbent dressings in place.
   3. Elastic bandages must be sterile when applied.
   4. The bandage should always cover at least one joint of the limb.

See Answers to Test Your Knowledge in Appendix A.

READINGS AND REFERENCES

Suggested Reading

Palfreyman, S. (2016). Patients at risk of pressure ulcers and moisture-related skin damage. *British Journal of Nursing*, *25*(12), S24–S28. doi:10.12968/bjon.2016.25.12.S24
It is important for the nurse to be able to differentiate pressure-related damage from that caused by moisture. The moisture damage may be described as "outside-in" because the initial breakdown is caused by substances left on the skin, whereas pressure damage may be described as "inside-out" because the damage is initially in the tissues injured by pressure between surfaces and body prominences. Prevention and treatment may differ. This article reviews the similarities and differences.

Related Research

Chen, H.-L., Cao, Y.-J., Zhang, W., Wang, J., & Huai, B.-S. (2017). Braden scale (ALB) for assessing pressure ulcer risk in hospital patients: A validity and reliability study. *Applied Nursing Research*, *33*, 169–174. doi:10.1016/j.apnr.2016.12.001

References

Choi, E. P., Chin, W. Y., Wan, E. Y., & Lam, C. L. (2016). Evaluation of the internal and external responsiveness of the Pressure Ulcer Scale for Healing (PUSH) tool for assessing acute and chronic wounds. *Journal of Advanced Nursing*, *72*(5), 1134–1143. doi:10.1111/jan.12898

Cornish, L., & Douglas, H. (2016). Cleansing of acute traumatic wounds: Tap water or normal saline? *Wounds UK*, *12*(4), 30–35.

Edwards-Jones, V., Atkin, L., & Guttormsen, K. (2018). Biofilm-based wound care: How to cleanse, debride and manage chronic wounds. *Wounds UK*, *14*(4), 10–16.

Haesler, E. (2018). Evidence summary: Skin care to reduce the risk of pressure injuries. *Wound Practice & Research*, *26*(3), 156–158.

Hunt, S. (2016). Negative pressure wound therapy: An update. *British Journal of Nursing*, *25*(20), S6–S8. doi:10.12968/bjon.2016.25.20.s6

Institute for Healthcare Improvement. (2011). *How-to guide: Prevent pressure ulcers*. Retrieved from http://www.ihi.org/knowledge/Pages/Tools/HowtoGuidePreventPressureUlcers.aspx

The Joint Commission. (2019). *2019 national patient safety goals: Nursing care center accreditation program*. Retrieved from https://www.jointcommission.org/assets/1/6/NPSG_Chapter_NCC_Jan2019.pdf

Kaushik, D., Joshi, N., Kumar, R., Gaba, S., Sapra, R., & Kumar, K. (2017). Negative pressure wound therapy versus gauze dressings for the treatment of contaminated traumatic wounds. *Journal of Wound Care*, *26*(10), 600–606. doi:10.12968/jowc.2017.26.10.600

Landa, D. L., van Dishoeck, A., Steyerberg, E. W., & Hovius, S. E. (2016). Quality of measurements of acute surgical and traumatic wounds using a digital wound-analysing tool. *International Wound Journal*, *13*, 619–624. doi:10.1111/iwj.12330

Martin, N. A., & Falder, S. (2017). A review of the evidence for threshold of burn injury. *Burns*, *43*, 1624–1639. doi:10.1016/j.burns.2017.04.003

National Quality Forum. (2017). *List of serious reportable events*. Retrieved from http://www.qualityforum.org/Topics/SREs/List_of_SREs.aspx

Norton, D., McLaren, R., & Exton-Smith, A. N. (1975). *An investigation of geriatric nursing problems in hospital*. Edinburgh, United Kingdom: Churchill Livingstone.

Padula, W. V., Pronovost, P. J., Makic, M. B. F., Wald, H. L., Moran, D., Mishra, M. K., & Meltzer, D. O. (2018). Value of hospital resources for effective pressure injury prevention: A cost-effectiveness analysis. *BMJ Quality & Safety*, *28*(2), 132–141. doi:10.1136/bmjqs-2017-007505

Pickham, D., Berte, N., Pihulic, M., Valdez, A., Mayer, B., & Desai, M. (2018). Effect of a wearable patient sensor on care delivery for preventing pressure injuries in acutely ill adults: A pragmatic randomized clinical trial (LS-HAPI study). *International Journal of Nursing Studies*, *80*, 12–19. doi:10.1016/j.ijnurstu.2017.12.012

U.S. Department of Health and Human Services. (2017). *Healthy people 2020: Topics and objectives/long-term services and supports*. Retrieved from http://www.healthypeople.gov/2020/topics-objectives/objective/oa-10

Wilson, M. R., Nigam, Y., Knight, J., & Pritchard, D. I. (2019). What is the optimal treatment time for larval therapy? A study on incubation time and tissue debridement by bagged maggots of the greenbottle fly, *Lucilia sericata*. *International Wound Journal*, *16*(1), 219–225. doi:10.1111/iwj.13015

Selected Bibliography

American Nurse Today. (May 2018). *Pressure injuries supplement*. Retrieved from https://cdn.coverstand.com/41491/492685/b14a85f4d4bc5a2a927963a02f5d3f2ed52a8405.1.pdf

Anderson, K., Davis, G., Oerter, B., Weber, A., & Roth, K. (2019). Wound cleansing: Tap water versus normal saline. *North Dakota Nurse*, *88*(1), 14.

Brown, A. (2018). When is wound cleansing necessary and what solution should be used? *Nursing Times*, *114*(9), 10.

Harries, F. J. (2016). Non-rinse skin cleansers: The way forward in preventing incontinence related moisture lesions? *Journal of Wound Care*, *25*, 268–276. doi:10.12968/jowc.2016.25.5.268

Malekian, A., Djavid, G. E., Akbarzadeh, K., Soltandallal, M., Rassi, Y., Rafinejad, J., . . . Totonchi, M. (2019). Efficacy of maggot therapy on *Staphylococcus aureus* and *Pseudomonas aeruginosa* in diabetic foot ulcers: A randomized controlled trial. *Journal of Wound, Ostomy & Continence Nursing*, *46*(1), 25–29. doi:10.1097/WON.0000000000000496

Schwartzenberger, K., Wickstrom, T., Kuntz, M., Rappuhn, H., Mendoza, A., & Pittman, M. (2018). Tap water vs. normal saline for wound care. *North Dakota Nurse*, *87*(1), 8–10.

Slachta, P. A. (Ed.). (2019). *Wound care made incredibly visual* (3rd ed.) Philadelphia, PA: Wolters Kluwer.

Spruce, L. (2017). Back to basics: Preventing perioperative pressure injuries. *AORN Journal*, *105*, 92–99. doi:10.1016/j.aorn.2016.10.018

Taroc, A.-M. (2017). A guide for adhesive removal: Principles, practice, and products. *American Nurse Today*, *12*(10), 24–26.

Voegeli, D. (2016). Incontinence-associated dermatitis: New insights into an old problem. *British Journal of Nursing*, *25*(5), 256–262. doi:10.12968/bjon.2016.25.5.256

Perioperative Nursing 37

LEARNING OUTCOMES

After completing this chapter, you will be able to:

1. Discuss various types of surgery according to the purpose, degree of urgency, and degree of risk.
2. Describe the phases of the perioperative period.
3. Identify essential aspects of preoperative assessment.
4. Give examples of pertinent nursing diagnoses for surgical clients.
5. Identify nursing responsibilities in planning perioperative nursing care.
6. Describe essential preoperative teaching, including pain assessment and management, moving, leg exercises, and deep-breathing and coughing exercises.
7. Describe essential aspects of preparing a client for surgery.
8. Compare various types of anesthesia.
9. Identify essential nursing assessments and interventions during the immediate postanesthetic phase.
10. Demonstrate ongoing nursing assessments and interventions for the postoperative client.
11. Identify potential postoperative complications and describe nursing interventions to prevent them.
12. Verbalize the steps used in:
    a. Teaching moving, leg exercises, deep breathing, and coughing
    b. Applying antiemboli stockings
    c. Managing gastrointestinal suction.
13. Evaluate the effectiveness of perioperative nursing interventions.
14. Recognize when it is appropriate to assign perioperative skills to assistive personnel.
15. Demonstrate appropriate documentation and reporting of perioperative skills.

KEY TERMS

Introduction

Surgery is a unique experience of a planned physical alteration encompassing three phases: preoperative, intraoperative, and postoperative. These three phases are together referred to as the **perioperative period**. Perioperative nursing is the delivery of nursing care through the framework of the nursing process. It also includes collaborating with members of the healthcare team, making nursing referrals, and delegating and supervising nursing care.

Perioperative nursing is practiced in hospital-based inpatient and outpatient surgical, laser, and endoscopy suites, physician office–based surgical suites (outpatient), and freestanding outpatient and ambulatory surgical centers. Outpatient procedures do not require an overnight hospital stay. The client goes to the outpatient site the day of surgery, has the procedure, and leaves the same day.

The **preoperative phase** begins when the decision to have surgery is made; it ends when the client is transferred to the operating table. The nursing activities associated with this phase include assessing the client, identifying potential or actual health problems, planning specific care based on the individual's needs, and providing preoperative teaching for the client, the family, and significant others.

The **intraoperative phase** begins when the client is transferred to the operating table and ends when the client is admitted to the postanesthesia care unit (PACU), also called the postanesthesia room (PAR). The nursing activities related to this phase include a variety of specialized procedures designed to create and maintain a safe therapeutic environment for the client and the healthcare personnel. These activities include interventions that provide for the client's safety, maintaining an aseptic environment, ensuring proper functioning of equipment, and providing the surgical team with the instruments and supplies needed during the procedure.

The **postoperative phase** begins with the admission of the client to the PACU or PAR and ends when healing is complete. During the postoperative phase, nursing activities include assessing the client's response (physiologic and psychologic) to surgery, performing interventions to facilitate healing and prevent complications, teaching and providing support to the client and support people, and planning for home care. The goal is to assist the client to achieve optimal health status.

Types of Surgery

Surgical procedures are commonly grouped according to (a) purpose, (b) degree of urgency, and (c) degree of risk.

Purpose

Surgical procedures may be categorized according to their purpose (Box 37.1).

BOX 37.1 Purposes of Surgical Procedures

Diagnostic	Confirms or establishes a diagnosis; for example, biopsy of a mass in a breast.
Palliative	Relieves or reduces pain or symptoms of a disease; it does not cure; for example, resection of nerve roots.
Ablative	Removes a diseased body part; for example, removal of a gallbladder (cholecystectomy).
Constructive	Restores function or appearance that has been lost or reduced; for example, cleft palate repair.
Transplant	Replaces malfunctioning structures; for example, kidney transplant.

Degree of Urgency

Surgery is classified by its urgency and necessity to preserve the client's life, body part, or body function. **Emergency surgery** is performed immediately to preserve function or the life of the client. Surgeries to control internal hemorrhage or repair a fracture are examples of emergency surgeries. **Elective surgery** is performed when surgical intervention is the preferred treatment for a condition that is not imminently life threatening (but may ultimately threaten life or well-being), or to improve the client's life. Examples of elective surgeries include cholecystectomy for chronic gallbladder disease, hip replacement surgery, and plastic surgery procedures such as breast reduction.

Degree of Risk

Surgery is also classified as major or minor according to the degree of risk to the client. **Major surgery** involves a high degree of risk, for a variety of reasons: It may be complicated or prolonged, large losses of blood may occur, vital organs may be involved, or postoperative complications may be likely. Examples are organ transplant, open heart surgery, and removal of a kidney. In contrast, **minor surgery** normally involves little risk, produces few complications, and is often performed in an outpatient setting. Examples are breast biopsy, removal of tonsils, and cataract extraction.

The degree of risk involved in a surgical procedure is affected by the client's age, general health, nutritional status, presence of sleep apnea, use of medications, and mental status.

Age

Neonates, infants, and older clients are greater surgical risks than children and adults. Age and developmental status affect a child's ability to cope with the physiologic and psychologic stresses of surgery. Neonates and infants have a higher metabolic rate and a different physiologic makeup than adults. These differences cause a substantially different response to a surgical procedure. For example, the blood volume in an infant is small, and fluid reserves are limited. This increases the risk of volume depletion during surgery, resulting in inadequate oxygenation of body tissues. Because of the infant's relatively large body surface area and immature temperature regulatory mechanisms, the risk of hypothermia during surgery is significant. Other organ systems, such as the kidneys, liver, and immune system, are also immature in infants, affecting their ability to metabolize and eliminate drugs and resist infection.

Toddlers and older children are better able to withstand surgery physiologically, but they often fear separation from their parents, strangers, bodily injury, mutilation, and death. The child's developmental level and age-appropriate communication are important in implementing the pediatric plan of care. The parent–child relationship, the parents' coping abilities, and the preoperative teaching and support will affect how well the child is able to deal with these surgical fears and the level of anxiety experienced.

The older adult (65 years and older) often has fewer physiologic reserves to meet the extra demands caused by surgery. The physiologic deficits of aging increase the surgical risk for the older adult. For example, because of a lower percentage of body water, decreased kidney function, and a decreased thirst response, older clients are at greater risk for fluid and electrolyte imbalances. Many older clients demonstrate changes in liver and kidney function, both of which can affect responses to anesthesia and other medications that may be administered during the perioperative period. The older client may be poorly nourished, which can impair healing. Declines in sensory function (hearing in particular) or the presence of dementia make it more difficult to understand directions and teaching. In addition, the older client is more likely to have a chronic disease, such as cardiovascular disease, lung disease, or diabetes, that affects healing and responses to medication and surgery.

General Health

Surgery is least risky when the client's general health is good. Any infection or pathophysiology increases the risk. It is important for the nurse to assess the client for an upper respiratory tract infection, which together with a general anesthetic can adversely affect respiratory function. When a client is at high risk for infection, antibiotics may be administered parenterally within 1 hour of surgery and continued for 24 to 72 hours after surgery. This practice allows time for drugs to reach therapeutic levels in the tissues but does not permit bacterial resistance to develop. Common health problems that increase surgical risk and may lead to the decision to postpone or cancel surgery are listed in Box 37.2.

BOX 37.2 Health Problems That Increase Surgical Risk

- Malnutrition can lead to delayed wound healing, infection, and reduced energy. Protein and vitamins are needed for wound healing; vitamin K is essential for blood clotting.
- Obesity leads to hypertension, impaired cardiac function, and impaired respiratory ventilation. Clients with obesity are also more likely to have delayed wound healing and wound infection because adipose tissue impedes blood circulation and its delivery of nutrients, antibodies, and enzymes required for wound healing.
- Cardiac conditions such as angina pectoris, recent myocardial infarction, hypertension, and heart failure weaken the heart. Well-controlled cardiac problems generally pose minimal operative risk.
- Blood coagulation disorders may lead to severe bleeding, hemorrhage, and subsequent shock.
- Upper respiratory tract infections or chronic obstructive pulmonary disease (COPD) adversely affect pulmonary function, especially when exacerbated by the effects of general anesthesia. They also predispose the client to postoperative lung infections.
- Renal disease impairs regulation of the body's fluids and electrolytes and excretion of drugs and other toxins.
- Diabetes mellitus predisposes the client to wound infection and delayed healing.
- Liver disease (e.g., cirrhosis) impairs the liver's abilities to detoxify medications used during surgery, produce the prothrombin necessary for blood clotting, and metabolize nutrients essential for healing.
- Uncontrolled neurologic disease such as epilepsy may result in seizures during surgery or recovery.

Nutritional Status

Adequate nutrition is required for normal tissue repair. Surgery increases the body's need for nutrients that help with the tissue healing and prevention of infection required during the postoperative period. Obesity and malnutrition increase surgical risk.

Obesity contributes to postoperative complications such as pneumonia, wound infections, and wound separation. Both clients with obesity and those who are underweight are vulnerable to perioperative pressure injuries (previously called pressure ulcers) due to the positioning required for surgery. The perioperative nurse provides padding and other measures to protect the client's skin over pressure points during surgery.

TABLE 37.1 Vitamins and Minerals Essential to Wound Healing

Vitamin or Mineral	Function
Vitamin A	Promotes epithelialization and enhances collagen synthesis
Vitamin B complex	Cofactor of the enzyme system
Vitamin C (ascorbic acid)	Essential for collagen synthesis affecting wound tensile strength
Vitamin K	Essential in the synthesis of prothrombin and thus coagulation
Iron, zinc, and copper	Involved in collagen synthesis

Many vitamins and minerals are essential in wound healing (Table 37.1). A malnourished client is at risk for delayed wound healing, wound infection, and fluid and electrolyte alterations. If a client has serious malnutrition, the surgery may be postponed to improve the nutritional status. If the surgery cannot be delayed, parenteral or enteral nutrition may be initiated.

Obstructive Sleep Apnea

Obstructive sleep apnea (OSA) is a common condition caused by partial or complete obstruction of the upper airway during sleep. Breathing is briefly interrupted during sleep with periods of apnea lasting at least 10 seconds. Unfortunately, many clients have undiagnosed OSA. Recent studies have shown that clients with OSA who undergo surgery are at increased risk for perioperative complications (Williams, Williams, Stanton, & Spence, 2017). The gold standard for diagnosis of OSA is a sleep study (polysomnography). However, sleep studies are expensive and may be difficult to obtain preoperatively because of limited resourcing and scheduling difficulties. A number of screening tools for OSA have been developed. The STOP-Bang Questionnaire is considered the most successful in identifying high-risk clients with OSA and is also considered easy to use (Harrelson & Fencl, 2016, p. 435). The STOP-Bang Questionnaire assesses whether the client **S**nores, is **T**ired during the day, if anyone has **O**bserved apnea during sleep, and has high blood **P**ressure. Additional elements include assessing the client's **B**ody mass index, **A**ge, **N**eck circumference, and **G**ender (Greenwood, 2017, p. 28; Harrelson & Fencl, 2016, p. 435). The use of a preoperative OSA screening tool increases the awareness of the healthcare team to closely monitor the previously undiagnosed surgical client who may be at high risk for OSA.

Medications

The regular use of certain medications can increase surgical risk. Consider these examples:

- *Anticoagulants* increase blood coagulation time.
- *Tranquilizers* may interact with anesthetics, increasing the risk of respiratory depression.
- *Corticosteroids* may interfere with wound healing and increase the risk of infection.
- *Diuretics* may affect fluid and electrolyte balance.

Clients may be unaware of the potential adverse interactions of medications and may fail to report the use of medications for conditions unrelated to the indication for surgery. The smart nurse interviewer should question the client and family about the use of commonly prescribed medications, over-the-counter (OTC) preparations, and any herbal remedies for specific conditions mentioned during the nursing history.

Mental Status

Disorders that affect cognitive function, such as mental illness, intellectual disability, or developmental delay, affect the client's ability to understand and cope with the stresses of surgery. These clients also may require medication such as anticonvulsants or antipsychotic drugs that can interact with anesthetic and analgesic medications used during and after surgery.

Clients with dementia may have difficulty understanding proposed surgical procedures and may respond unpredictably to anesthetics. Indicators of dementia such as confusion, disorientation, and agitation may be worsened by the change of environment in the hospital, and interfere with the client's ability to cooperate with pre- and postoperative care.

Extreme anxiety also increases surgical risk and interferes with the client's ability to process information and respond correctly to instructions. In some instances, professional counseling is indicated prior to surgery. It is also important to determine whether clients have coping skills and support systems to help them.

Preoperative Phase

Preoperative Consent

Prior to any surgical procedure, informed consent is required from the client or legal guardian. Informed consent implies that the client has been informed and involved in decisions affecting his or her health. The surgeon is responsible for obtaining the informed consent by providing the following information to the client or legal guardian:

- The nature of and the reason for the surgery
- All available options and the risks associated with each option
- The risks of the surgical procedure and its potential outcomes
- Name and qualifications of the surgeon performing the procedure
- The right to refuse consent or later withdraw consent.

The surgeon documents the informed consent conversation with the client or legal guardian in the preoperative progress note.

The surgical consent form, provided by the healthcare facility where the surgery will be performed, protects the client from incorrect or unwanted procedures and the surgeon and facility from litigation related to unauthorized surgeries or uninformed clients. This consent form becomes part of the client's medical record and goes to the operating room (OR) with the client. The RN ensures consent is in the client's chart prior to releasing the client to surgery.

Although the surgeon maintains legal responsibility for ensuring that the client has given informed consent, the nurse may witness the client's signature on the consent form. In doing so, the nurse ensures that the consent form is signed and serves as a witness to the signature, not to the fact that the client is informed. If the nurse assesses that the client does not understand the procedure to be performed, the surgeon is contacted and requested to speak with the client before surgery can proceed.

Informed consent is only possible when the client understands the provided information, that is, speaks the language and is conscious, mentally competent, and not sedated. A minor may not give informed consent. Specific guidelines regarding consent for minors vary among the states. Nurses must be aware of their responsibilities regarding consent and of the particular hospital's policies (see Chapter 3 ∞).

●○● NURSING MANAGEMENT

Assessing

Preoperative assessment includes collecting and reviewing physical, psychologic, and social client data to determine the client's needs throughout the three perioperative phases. The client's mobility and ability to function should also be assessed in the preoperative phase. The perioperative nurse collects the data by interviewing the client in the presurgical care unit or by telephone prior to the day of surgery. When data cannot be collected directly, the perioperative nurse uses other data sources such as the nursing admission assessment. Although forms vary considerably among agencies, Box 37.3 summarizes essential preoperative information that should be included.

Physical Assessment

Preoperatively, the nurse performs a brief but complete physical assessment, paying particular attention to systems that could affect the client's response to anesthesia or surgery. A brief or "mini" mental status examination provides valuable baseline data for evaluating the client's mental status and alertness after surgery. It is also important to evaluate the client's ability to understand what is happening. For example, assessment of hearing and vision help guide perioperative teaching. Respiratory and cardiovascular assessments not only provide baseline data for evaluating the client's postoperative status but also may alert care providers to a problem (e.g., a respiratory infection or irregular pulse rate) that may affect the client's response to surgery and anesthesia. Other systems (gastrointestinal, genitourinary,

BOX 37.3 Preoperative Assessment Data

- *Current health status.* Essential information includes general health status and the presence of any chronic diseases, such as diabetes or asthma, which may affect the client's response to surgery or anesthesia. Note any physical limitations that may affect the client's mobility or ability to communicate after surgery, as well as any prostheses such as hearing aids or contact lenses.
- *Allergies.* Include allergies to prescription and nonprescription drugs, food allergies, and allergies to tape, latex, soaps, or antiseptic agents. Some food allergies may indicate a potential reaction to drugs or substances used during surgery or diagnostic procedures; for example, an allergy to seafood alerts the nurse to a potential allergy to iodine-based dyes or soaps commonly used in hospitals.
- *Medications.* List all current medications (prescribed and OTC). It may be vital to maintain a blood level of some medications (e.g., anticonvulsants) throughout the surgical experience; others, such as anticoagulants or aspirin, increase the risks of surgery and anesthesia and need to be discontinued several days prior to surgery. It is important to include in the list any OTC drugs and herbal remedies the client currently takes.
- *Previous surgeries.* Previous surgical experiences may influence the client's physical and psychologic responses to surgery or may reveal unexpected responses to anesthesia.
- *Mental status.* The client's mental status and ability to understand and respond appropriately can affect the entire perioperative experience. Note any developmental disabilities, mental illness, history of dementia, or excessive anxiety related to the procedure.
- *Understanding of the surgical procedure and anesthesia.* The client should have a good understanding of the planned procedure and what to expect during and after surgery as well as the expected outcome of the procedure.
- *Smoking.* Smokers may have more difficulty clearing respiratory secretions after surgery, increasing the risk of postoperative complications such as pneumonia and atelectasis and delayed wound healing.
- *Obstructive sleep apnea (OSA).* The majority of adults do not know that they have OSA, which puts them at risk for postoperative pulmonary complications. Furthermore, when asked if they have sleep apnea, clients often state that they do not have a sleeping problem.
- *Alcohol and other mind-altering substances.* Use of substances that affect the central nervous system, liver, or other body systems can affect the client's response to anesthesia and surgery, and postoperative recovery.
- *Coping.* Clients with a healthy self-concept who have successfully employed appropriate coping mechanisms in the past are better able to deal with the stressors associated with surgery.
- *Social resources.* Determine the availability of family or other caregivers as well as the client's social support network. These resources are important to the client's recovery, particularly for the client undergoing same-day or short-stay surgery.
- *Cultural and spiritual considerations.* Culture and spirituality influence the client's response to surgery; respecting cultural and spiritual beliefs and practices can reduce preoperative anxiety and improve recovery.

and musculoskeletal) are examined to provide baseline data (see Chapter 29 ∞).

Screening Tests

The surgeon or the anesthesiologist orders preoperative diagnostic tests. Abnormalities may require treatment prior to surgery. The nurse's responsibility is to check the orders carefully, to see that they are carried out, and to ensure that the results are obtained and in the client's record prior to surgery. Table 37.2 lists routine preoperative screening tests. In addition to these routine tests, diagnostic tests directly related to the client's disease are usually appropriate (e.g., gastroscopy to clarify the pathologic condition before gastric surgery).

TABLE 37.2 Routine Preoperative Screening Tests

Test	Rationale
Complete blood count (CBC)	RBCs, hemoglobin (Hgb), and hematocrit (Hct) are important to the oxygen-carrying capacity of the blood; white blood cells (WBCs) are an indicator of immune function
Blood grouping and cross-matching	Determined in case blood transfusion is required during or after surgery
Serum electrolytes (Na^+, K^+, Ca^{2+}, Mg^{2+}, Cl^-, HCO_3^-)	To evaluate fluid and electrolyte status
Fasting blood glucose	High levels may indicate undiagnosed diabetes mellitus
Blood urea nitrogen (BUN) and creatinine	To evaluate renal function
ALT, AST, LDH, and bilirubin	To evaluate liver function
Serum albumin and total protein	To evaluate nutritional status
Urinalysis	To determine urine composition and possible abnormal components (e.g., protein or glucose) or infection
Chest x-ray	To evaluate respiratory status and heart size
Electrocardiogram (ECG) (all clients over 40 years of age and clients with pre-existing cardiac conditions)	To identify pre-existing cardiac problems or disease
Pregnancy test (all female clients of childbearing age)	To identify if the client is pregnant

Diagnosing

Examples of nursing diagnoses that may be appropriate for the preoperative client can include lack of knowledge related to no exposure to the specific perioperative experience, anxiety related to risk of death, grieving related to loss of body part (specify), and impaired coping related to previous negative experience with surgery.

Planning

The overall goal in the preoperative period is to ensure that the client is mentally and physically prepared for surgery. Examples of nursing activities to meet this goal are discussed in the Implementing section that follows.

Planning should involve the client, the family, and significant others. The perioperative nurse usually does preoperative care planning and teaching interventions on an outpatient basis either in person or via a telephone interview.

Planning for Home Care

For the perioperative client, discharge planning begins before admission for the planned procedure. Early planning to meet the discharge needs of the client is particularly important for outpatient procedures, because these clients are generally discharged within hours after the procedure is performed.

Discharge planning incorporates an assessment of the client's, family's, and significant other's abilities and resources for care, their financial resources, and the need for referrals and home health services. However, the extent of discharge planning and home care will vary significantly for clients having different types of surgery.

Implementing

The major nursing activity to ensure that the client is prepared for surgery is preoperative teaching.

Preoperative Teaching

Preoperative teaching is a vital part of nursing care. Studies have shown that preoperative teaching reduces clients' anxiety and postoperative complications and increases their satisfaction with the surgical experience. Effective preoperative teaching also facilitates the client's successful and early return to work and other activities of daily living (ADLs). Four dimensions of preoperative teaching have been identified as important to clients:

- ***Information, including what will happen to the client, when, and what the client will experience, such as expected sensations and discomfort.*** The nurse needs to listen carefully and attentively to the client to identify specific concerns and fears. Pain assessment and management are important to explain to the client because there will be discomfort after the procedure. Explain that the surgeon will order pain medication. Describe the 0-to-10 pain scale and how this is used to assess the client's level of pain. Stress the importance of working together to manage the pain because clients are able to move around easier and ambulate quicker when their pain is controlled. Research evidence shows that fewer than half of surgical clients report adequate postoperative pain relief (Manworren, Gordon, & Montgomery, 2018). The guidelines on the management of postoperative pain include a strong recommendation with high-quality evidence to offer multimodal analgesia for the treatment of perioperative pain in children and adults (Chou et al., 2016). See Chapter 30 ∞) for more information about pain assessment and management.
- ***Psychosocial support to reduce anxiety.*** The nurse provides support by actively listening and providing accurate information. It is important to correct any misunderstandings the client may have.
- ***The roles of the client and support people in preoperative preparation, the surgical procedure, and during the postoperative phase.*** Understanding his or her role during the perioperative experience increases the client's sense of control and reduces anxiety. This includes what will be expected of the client, desired behaviors, self-care activities, and what the client can do to facilitate recovery.
- ***Skills training.*** This includes moving, deep breathing, coughing, splinting incisions with the hands or a pillow, and using an incentive spirometer.

If the client is scheduled for outpatient surgery, preoperative teaching is often provided before the day of surgery using some combination of videos and verbal and written instructions. The client may have an appointment with the outpatient perioperative nurse (usually scheduled to coincide with preoperative diagnostic testing) to discuss preoperative concerns and implement the teaching plan. Written instructions are always provided to reinforce verbal teaching. Teaching is further reinforced on admission the day of surgery and before discharge from the postanesthesia unit. Preoperative instructions are summarized in Box 37.4.

When the client is a child, addressing the fears and anxieties of both the child and the family is important. Parents need to know what to expect and to be able to express their concerns. Parents should be considered members of the perioperative team and allowed to participate in providing as much care as possible.

Skill 37.1 provides guidelines for teaching clients about moving, leg exercises, and coughing.

BOX 37.4 Preoperative Instructions

PREOPERATIVE REGIMEN

- Explain the need for preoperative tests (e.g., laboratory, x-ray, ECG).
- Discuss bowel preparation, if required.
- Discuss skin preparation, including operative area and preoperative bath or shower.
- Discuss preoperative medications, if ordered.
- Explain individual therapies ordered by the primary care provider, such as IV therapy, the insertion of a urinary catheter or nasogastric tube, use of a spirometer, or antiemboli stockings.
- Discuss the visit by the anesthetist.
- Explain the need to restrict food and oral fluids before surgery.
- Provide a general timetable for perioperative events, including the time of surgery.
- Discuss the need to remove jewelry, makeup, and all prostheses (e.g., eyeglasses, hearing aids, complete or partial dentures, wig) immediately before surgery.
- Inform the client about the preoperative holding area, and give the location of the waiting room for support people.
- Teach ways to turn and move, leg exercises, deep-breathing and coughing exercises (see Skill 37.1), and splinting techniques.
- Complete the preoperative checklist.

POSTOPERATIVE REGIMEN

- Discuss the PACU's routines and emergency equipment.
- Review type and frequency of assessment activities.
- Discuss pain management.
- Explain usual activity restrictions and precautions related to getting up for the first time postoperatively.
- Describe usual dietary alterations.
- Discuss postoperative dressings and drains.
- Provide an explanation and tour of the intensive care unit if client is to be transferred there postoperatively.

OUTPATIENT SURGICAL CLIENTS

- Review all instructions in the preoperative and postoperative regimen.
- Confirm place and time of surgery, including when to arrive (e.g., 1 to 1 1/2 hours before scheduled surgery) and where to register (e.g., reception desk).
- Discuss what to wear (e.g., clients having hand surgery should wear a garment with large sleeve openings to fit over a bulky dressing; all clients need to leave valuables at home).
- Explain the need for a responsible adult to drive or accompany the client home.
- Discuss discharge criteria and how long the client should expect to stay postoperatively.
- Discuss medications, including specific preoperative medications and the client's current medication regimen.
- Communicate by telephone the evening before surgery to confirm time of surgery and arrival time.
- Communicate by telephone within 48 hours postoperatively to evaluate surgical outcomes and identify any problems or complications.

Teaching Moving, Leg Exercises, Deep Breathing, and Coughing

SKILL 37.1

PURPOSES

Moving

- To promote venous return
- To enhance lung expansion and mobilize secretions
- To stimulate gastrointestinal motility
- To facilitate early ambulation

Leg Exercises

- To promote venous return, thereby preventing thrombophlebitis and thrombus formation

Deep Breathing and Coughing

- To enhance lung expansion and mobilize secretions, thereby preventing **atelectasis** (collapse of the alveoli) and pneumonia

ASSESSMENT

Assess

- Vital signs
- Discomfort
- Temperature and color of feet and legs
- Breath sounds
- Presence of dyspnea or cough
- Learning needs of the client
- Anxiety level of the client
- Client experience with previous surgeries and anesthesia
- Incidence of postoperative nausea, vomiting, or other reaction to previous anesthesia

PLANNING

Before beginning to teach moving, leg exercises, deep-breathing exercises, and coughing, determine (a) the type of surgery, (b) the time of the surgery, (c) the name of the surgeon, (d) the preoperative orders, and (e) the agency's practices for preoperative care. Also, verify that the primary care provider has completed the medical history and physical examination and that the client or the family has signed the consent form.

Assignment

Assessment of the learning needs of the client and his or her support people and determining the teaching content and appropriate strategies for teaching require application of professional knowledge and critical thinking. Preoperative teaching is conducted by the nurse and is not assigned to assistive personnel (AP). The AP, however, can reinforce teaching, assist the client with the exercises, and report to the nurse if the client is unable to perform the exercises.

Equipment

- Pillow
- Teaching materials (e.g., audiovisual, written materials) if available at the agency

Continued on page 964

Teaching Moving, Leg Exercises, Deep Breathing, and Coughing—*continued*

IMPLEMENTATION

Preparation

Ensure that potential distracters (e.g., pain, TV, visitors) to teaching are not present. Family and significant others should be included in the teaching plan, as appropriate.

Performance

1. Prior to performing the procedure, introduce self and verify the client's identity using agency protocol. Explain to the client what you are going to teach and the importance of the client's participation in the exercises he or she is going to be taught.
2. Perform hand hygiene and observe other appropriate infection prevention procedures.
3. Provide for client privacy.
4. Show the client ways to turn in bed and to get out of bed.
   - Instruct a client who will have a right abdominal incision or a right-sided chest incision to turn to the left side of the bed and sit up as follows:
     a. Flex the knees.
     b. Splint the wound by holding the left arm and hand or a small pillow against the incision.
     c. Turn to the left while pushing with the right foot and grasping a partial side rail on the left side of the bed with the right hand.
     d. Come to a sitting position on the side of the bed by using the right arm and hand to push down against the mattress and swinging the feet over the edge of the bed.
     e. Teach a client with a left abdominal or left-sided chest incision to perform the same procedure but splint with the right arm and turn to the right.
   - For clients with orthopedic surgery (e.g., hip surgery), use special aids, such as a trapeze, to assist with movement.
5. Teach the client the following three leg exercises:
   - Alternate dorsiflexion and plantar flexion of the feet. **Rationale:** *This exercise is sometimes referred to as calf pumping, because it alternately contracts and relaxes the calf muscles, including the gastrocnemius muscles.* ❶
   - Flex and extend the knees, and press the backs of the knees into the bed while dorsiflexing the feet. ❷ Instruct clients who cannot raise their legs to do isometric exercises that contract and relax the muscles.
   - Raise and lower the legs alternately from the surface of the bed. Flex the knee of the stable leg and extend the knee of the moving leg. ❸ **Rationale:** *This exercise contracts and relaxes the quadriceps muscles.*
6. Demonstrate deep-breathing (diaphragmatic) exercises as follows:
   - Place your hands palms down on the border of your rib cage, and inhale slowly and evenly through the nose until the greatest chest expansion is achieved. ❹
   - Hold your breath for 2 to 3 seconds.
   - Then exhale slowly through the mouth.
   - Continue exhalation until maximum chest contraction has been achieved.
7. Help the client perform deep-breathing exercises.
   - Ask the client to assume a sitting position.
   - Place the palms of your hands on the border of the client's rib cage to assess respiratory depth.
   - Ask the client to perform deep breathing, as described in step 6.
8. Instruct the client to cough voluntarily after five deep inhalations.
   - Ask the client to inhale deeply, hold the breath for a few seconds, and then cough once or twice.
   - Ensure that the client coughs deeply and does not just clear the throat.

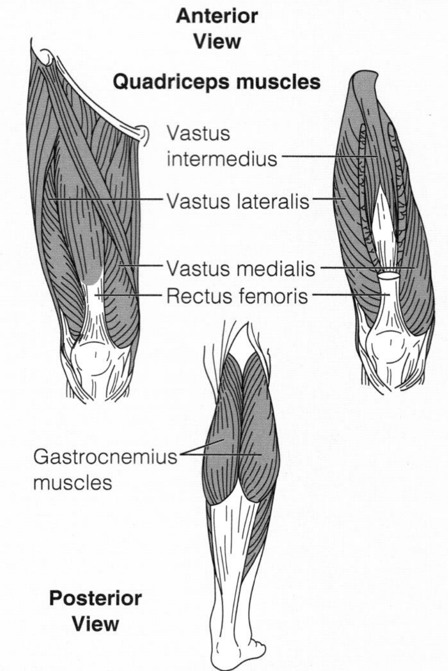

❶ Leg muscles: anterior and posterior views.

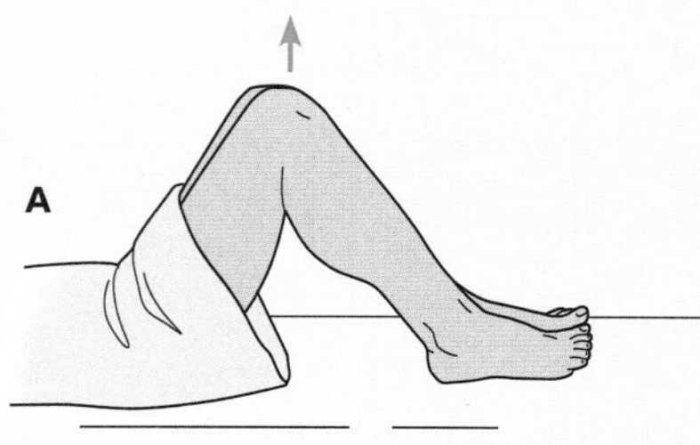

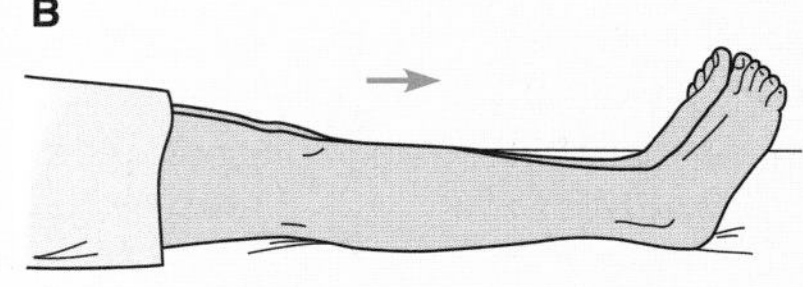

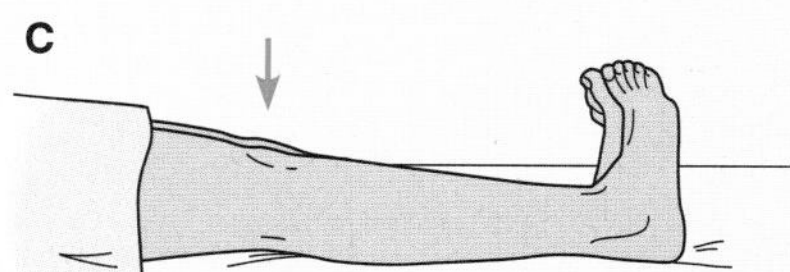

❷ Flexing and extending the knees.

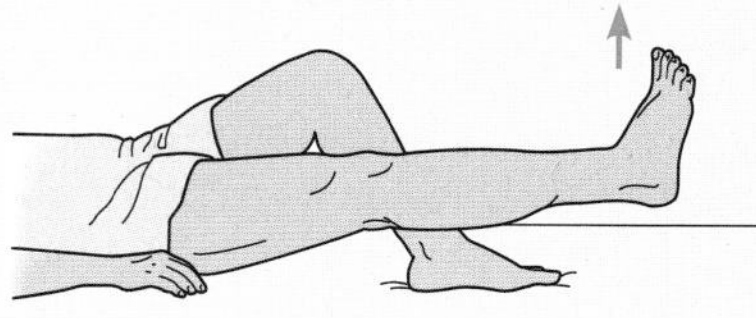

❸ Raising and lowering the legs.

SKILL 37.1

Teaching Moving, Leg Exercises, Deep Breathing, and Coughing—*continued*

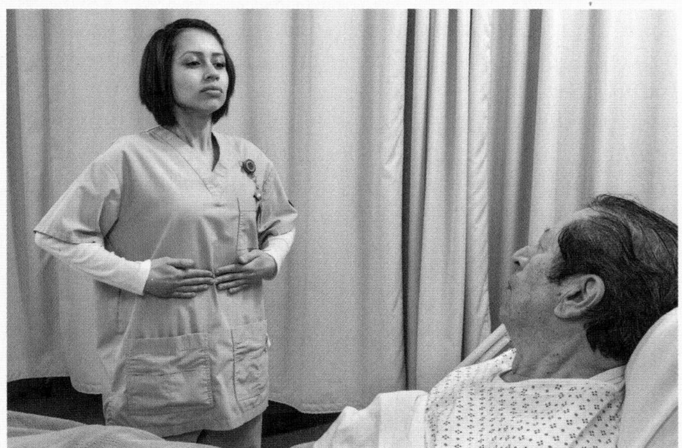

4 Demonstrating deep breathing.

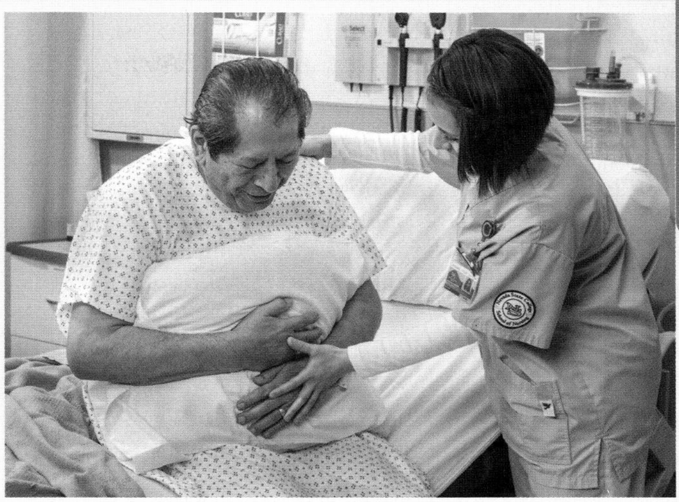

5 Splinting an incision with a pillow while coughing.

9. If the incision will be painful when the client coughs, demonstrate techniques to splint the abdomen.
   - Show the client how to support the incision by placing the palms of the hands on either side of the incision site or directly over the incision site, holding the palm of one hand over the other. **Rationale:** *Coughing uses the abdominal and other accessory respiratory muscles. Splinting the incision may reduce pain while coughing if the incision is near any of these muscles.*
   - Show the client how to splint the abdomen with clasped hands and a pillow firmly held against the client's abdomen. 5
10. Inform the client about the expected frequency of these exercises.
    - Instruct the client to start the exercises as soon after surgery as possible.
    - Encourage clients to carry out deep breathing and coughing at least every 2 hours, taking a minimum of five breaths at each session. Note, however, that the number of breaths and frequency of deep breathing vary with the client's condition. People who are susceptible to pulmonary problems may need deep-breathing exercises every hour. People with chronic respiratory disease may need special breathing exercises (e.g., pursed-lip breathing, abdominal breathing, exercises using various kinds of incentive spirometers).
11. Document the teaching and all assessments. Some agencies may have a preoperative teaching flow sheet. Check agency policy.

SAMPLE DOCUMENTATION

3/19/2020 0900 Instructed how to splint abdomen while deep breathing and coughing. Able to perform correctly. Stated that he will use this technique after surgery. A. Moore, RN

EVALUATION

Document the outcome of the teaching plan such as:

- Client's demonstrated ability to perform moving, leg exercises, and deep-breathing and coughing exercises
- Client's verbalization of key information presented.

LIFESPAN CONSIDERATIONS Preoperative Teaching

CHILDREN

- Parents need to know what to expect and be able to express their concerns.
- Separation from parents often is the child's greatest fear; the time of separation should be minimized and parents allowed to interact with the child both immediately preceding and following the surgery.
- Teaching and communicating with children (both timing and content) should be geared to the child's developmental level and cognitive abilities (e.g., "You will have a sore tummy").
- Play is an effective teaching tool with children (e.g., the child can put a bandage on an incision on a doll).

OLDER ADULTS

- Assess hearing ability to ensure the older client hears the necessary information.
- Assess short-term memory. Presenting one focused idea at a time and repeating or reinforcing information may be necessary.
- Older adults are at greater risk for postoperative complications, such as pneumonia. Reinforce moving and deep-breathing and coughing exercises.
- Assess potential postoperative needs at this time. Arrangements can be made preoperatively to obtain necessary items. Examples are medical equipment, such as walkers, raised toilet seats, and bed trapezes; Meals on Wheels; and help with transportation.
- If the older client will need to be in extended care for a period of time after surgery, this is the time to initiate these plans.
- Assess the client for risk of pressure injury development postoperatively and be extra attentive to use of proper paddings and support devices to prevent injury during positioning and transfers in the operating room. Risks include:
  - Older age
  - Poor nutritional status
  - History of diabetes or cardiovascular problems
  - History of taking steroids, which cause increased bruising and skin breakdown.

Physical Preparation

Preoperative preparation includes the following areas: nutrition and fluids, elimination, hygiene, medications, sleep, care of valuables and prostheses, special orders, surgical skin preparation, temperature, safety protocols, vital signs, antiemboli stockings, and sequential compression devices. In many agencies a preoperative checklist is used on the day of surgery. Forms may differ among agencies. Figure 37.1 ■ reflects the most common elements of a preoperative checklist. The nurse completes the agency's preoperative checklist following appropriate documenting procedures. It is essential that all pertinent records (laboratory records, x-ray films, consents) be available to perioperative personnel for reference and all physical preparation is completed to ensure client safety.

Nutrition and Fluids

Adequate hydration and nutrition promote healing. Nurses need to identify and record any signs of malnutrition or fluid imbalance. If the client is on IV fluids or on measured fluid intake, nurses must ensure that the fluid intake and output are accurately measured and recorded.

The order "NPO after midnight" has been a longstanding tradition because it was believed that anesthetics depress gastrointestinal functioning and there was a danger the client would vomit and aspirate during the administration of a general anesthetic. Re-evaluation and research, however, do not support this tradition. As a result, the American Society of Anesthesiologists (ASA) revised its practice guidelines for preoperative fasting in healthy clients undergoing elective procedures requiring general anesthesia, regional anesthesia, or sedation analgesia. According to the ASA ("Practice Guidelines," 2017, pp. 379–380), the current guidelines allow for:

- The consumption of clear liquids (no alcohol) up to 2 hours before surgery
- The consumption of breast milk up to 4 hours before surgery; infant formula may be ingested up to 6 hours before surgery

MEDICAL DOCUMENTATION	INITIALS
History and Physical completed and in chart	
Lab studies/reports in chart	
EKG report in chart	
Chest x-ray report in chart	
Operative Permit completed, signed, & witnessed in chart	
Surgical site verified	
Surgical side: _____Left _____Right _____Bilateral _____NA	
Anesthesia Permit completed, signed, & witnessed in chart	
Medication Reconciliation Form completed and signed	
PREOPERATIVE PREPARATION	
Identification bracelet accurate and affixed to wrist or ankle prior to transport	
Allergies checked, allergies bracelet on and allergy sticker on chart	
Copy of Advance Directive on chart	
Jewelry, hairpieces, hairpins, contact lenses, glasses, prosthesis, underwear, money removed	
Vital signs taken and recorded	
Time taken:_____ BP_____ Temp_____ HR_____ Resp_____ O2 Sat_____	
Dentures: □ *Full*: □ Upper □ Lower □ Partial: □ Upper □ Lower	
□ Other:	
□ Removed: □ Sent home □ Left at bedside	
□ Left in place as requested by: □ Anesthesiologist □ Client	
Client NPO□ yes since ________________ □ No	
If no: O.R. notified (Time)______________ (Whom) __________________	
Voided. Time ____________________	
Medication sheets on chart	
Most recent nursing assessment attached	

INITIALS	SIGNATURE AND TITLE

Figure 37.1 ■ Common elements of a nursing preoperative checklist.

- A light meal may be ingested up to 6 hours before the procedure
- A heavier meal (fried or fatty foods) may be eaten up to 8 hours before surgery.

Elimination

Enemas before surgery are no longer routine, but cleansing enemas may be ordered if bowel surgery is planned. The enemas help prevent postoperative constipation and contamination of the surgical area (during surgery) by feces. After surgery involving the intestines, peristalsis often does not return for 24 to 48 hours.

Prior to surgery, a straight catheterization or an indwelling Foley catheter may be ordered to ensure that the bladder remains empty. This helps prevent inadvertent injury to the bladder, particularly during pelvic surgery. If the client does not have a catheter, it is important to empty the bladder prior to receiving preoperative medications.

Hygiene

In some settings, clients are asked to bathe or shower the evening or morning of surgery (or both) with either soap or an antiseptic solution. The purpose of hygienic measures is to reduce the risk of wound infection by reducing the amount of bacteria on the client's skin. The bath includes a shampoo whenever possible.

The client's nails should be trimmed and free of polish, and all cosmetics should be removed so that the nail beds, skin, and lips are visible when circulation is assessed during the perioperative phases.

Intraoperatively the client will be required to wear a surgical cap. The surgical cap contains the client's hair and any microorganisms on the hair and scalp.

Before going into the OR the client should remove all hairpins and clips because they may cause pressure or accidental damage to the scalp when the client is unconscious. The client also removes personal clothing and puts on an OR gown.

Medications

The anesthetist or anesthesiologist may order routinely taken medications to be held the day of surgery.

In some settings, selected preoperative medications are given to the client prior to going to the OR and others are given while in the OR. Commonly used preoperative medications include the following:

- *Benzodiazepines* such as midazolam (Versed) may be administered IV prior to surgery (Adams, Holland, & Urban, 2020) to reduce anxiety and ease anesthetic induction.
- *Opioid analgesics* such as morphine provide client sedation and reduce the required amount of anesthetic.
- *Anticholinergics* such as atropine, scopolamine, and glycopyrrolate (Robinul) reduce oral and pulmonary secretions and prevent laryngospasm.
- *Dopamine blockers* such as droperidol (Inapsine) are administered parenterally to prevent nausea and vomiting; reduce anxiety, and relax muscles (Adams et al., 2020, p. 258).
- *Histamine-receptor antihistamines* such as cimetidine (Tagamet) and ranitidine (Zantac) reduce gastric fluid volume and gastric acidity.
- *Neurolept analgesic* agents such as Innovar induce general calmness and sleepiness.

Preoperative medications administered to the client before surgery are given at a scheduled time or "on call," that is, when the OR notifies the nurse to give the medication.

Sleep

Nurses should do everything to help the client sleep the night before surgery. Often a sedative is ordered. Adequate sleep helps the client manage the stress of surgery and helps healing.

Valuables

Valuables such as jewelry and money should be sent home with the client's family or significant other. If valuables and money cannot be sent home, they need to be labeled and placed in a locked storage area per the agency's policy. Removing jewelry also means removing body-piercing jewelry because there is a risk of injury from burns if an electrosurgical unit is used. If a client wishes not to remove a wedding band, the nurse can tape it in place. Wedding bands must be removed, however, if there is danger of the fingers swelling after surgery. Situations warranting removal include surgery on or cast application to an arm, or a mastectomy that involves removal of the lymph nodes. (Mastectomies may cause edema of the arm and hand.)

Prostheses

All prostheses (artificial body parts, such as partial or complete dentures, contact lenses, artificial eyes, and artificial limbs) and eyeglasses, wigs, and false eyelashes must be removed before surgery. If hearing aids are left in place, notify the OR personnel.

In some hospitals, dentures are placed in a locked storage area; in others they are placed in labeled containers and kept at the client's bedside. Partial dentures can become dislodged and obstruct an unconscious client's breathing. The nurse also checks for the presence of chewing gum or loose teeth. Loose teeth are a common problem with 5- or 6-year-olds undergoing tonsillectomy because they can become dislodged or aspirated during anesthesia.

QSEN Patient-Centered Care: Perioperative Nursing

Examples of cultural aspects of perioperative nursing include the Jehovah's Witness population and surgical clients with body art.

Jehovah's Witness is a Christian religion that believes that taking blood into the body causes loss of eternal life and that members who accept blood should be shunned by the congregation and denied the church's sacraments (called "disfellowshipped"). In 2000, this policy on blood transfusions was revised to allow the acceptance of blood products based on personal decision and conscience. Campbell, Machan, and Fisher (2016) report that "if blood is given to a Jehovah's Witness by force or coercion, or accepted by personal choice, the member can voluntarily disassociate himself or herself from the church and repent to remain in the religion thereafter" (p. 174). Based on this change in doctrine, members of this religion have medical confidentiality from the church. However, if there is a breach in the medical confidentiality, the member is "disfellowshipped" by the church. Providing culturally responsive care to this population means it is important for the healthcare provider to interview these clients privately and allow them to make informed decisions about their personal choice to accept or deny blood products. Their decisions should be private and not discussed in front of friends or family members.

Body art, a common cultural practice for thousands of years, includes body piercings, transdermal and subdermal implants, tattoos, scarification, body stretching and sculpting, dental grills, and nail art (Dunn, 2016). The most common sites for piercing are the earlobes, ear cartilage, tragus, nasal septum, eyebrow, tongue, lips, navel, breast nipples, and genitalia. Nurses need to assess the client for piercings because piercings can produce medical complications such as bleeding, skin tears, or infections. Body piercing can affect client safety in the preoperative, intraoperative, and postoperative phases.

Moving the client from the bed to the stretcher and OR table may place the client at risk for skin tears when the piercings are left in place. Dunn (2016) reports anesthetic complications with tongue piercings relating to airway management and endotracheal intubation. Body piercings can also place the client and operating room staff at risk for electrical burns if the piercings are not removed. Body art may affect positioning decisions or cause tissue trauma if not removed.

Discussion of body art with the client should begin with the preadmission process. According to the Association of periOperative Registered Nurses (AORN), all jewelry and hardware should be removed before surgery (Dunn, 2016; Smith, 2016). Clients should be instructed to remove all jewelry before the day of surgery. Dermal piercings are considered implants and the client cannot remove them. Nurses need to communicate about the client's body art with the perioperative team before the client arrives in the OR to prepare the team for delivering safe care.

Body art may have cultural or emotional significance for a client. It is important for the nurse to communicate in a nonjudgmental and culturally sensitive manner when providing nursing care to clients with unfamiliar body art. Conscious or unconscious expressions of negativity toward the client can affect the nurse-client relationship (Dunn, 2016). Likewise, Smith (2016) points out that when the role is reversed and the nurse is the one who is pierced or tattooed, it may create potential negative effects on the relationship with the client.

Special Orders

The nurse checks the surgeon's orders for special requirements (e.g., the insertion of a nasogastric tube prior to surgery; the administration of medications, such as insulin; or the application of antiemboli stockings). For the technique of inserting a nasogastric tube, see Skill 46.1 in Chapter 46 ∞).

Skin Preparation

When the appropriate skin antisepsis is implemented, the risk for a surgical site infection (SSI) may be reduced. Some clients may need to complete a full-body wash using antimicrobial soap the night before the planned surgery. In most agencies, skin preparation is carried out during the intraoperative phase. The surgical site is cleansed with an antimicrobial to remove soil and reduce the resident microbial count to subpathogenic levels. Recent evidence supports using dual-agent skin antiseptics rather than a single agent. Bashaw and Keister (2019) report that "skin preps that included a combination of CHG and alcohol are effective because the alcohol is fast-acting and the CHG provides a longer residual effect for reduction of microbes" (p. 72).

Temperature

Surgical clients are at risk of losing body heat; therefore, temperature management is an important aspect of perioperative client safety and comfort. There are many possible causes for hypothermia including minimal clothing (i.e., only a hospital gown), inactivity while in the holding area, skin exposure during insertion of IV and during surgery, and low temperatures in the OR; in addition, the administration of anesthesia impairs both thermoregulation and the ability of the body to generate and retain heat (Rightmyer & Singbartl, 2016). Complications associated with perioperative hypothermia include increased blood loss, delayed wound healing, increased risk of an SSI, and increased length of stay in the hospital.

It is important for the client's temperature to be assessed during the entire perioperative experience to prevent unintended hypothermia. Researchers recommend prewarming or warming to reduce the complications of hypothermia. One method is to use a forced-air warming system, which consists of a power unit that generates warmed air and a fan that blows the warmed air through a hose into a disposable blanket that has direct contact with the client. This method of warming can be started in the presurgical area and used throughout surgery and on into the PACU. Postoperatively, it is important to monitor temperature every hour. If the client becomes hypothermic (approximately a decrease of 2.5°F or a temperature around 35°C), warming measures should be implemented and the temperature monitored until the client reaches normothermia (Rightmyer & Singbartl, 2016).

Safety Protocols

The Joint Commission established the Universal Protocol for Preventing Wrong Site, Wrong Procedure, and Wrong Person Surgery in 2004. This protocol involves three steps. The first step requires preoperative verification. The frequency and scope of the verification process depends on the type and complexity of the procedure. Possibilities include when the procedure is scheduled, at the time of preadmission testing and assessment, at the time of admission for the procedure, and before the client leaves the preprocedure area or enters the procedure room (The Joint Commission, 2019, p. 14).

The second step involves marking of the operative site. The protocol does not specify the type of mark; however, The Joint Commission does require that the surgical site marking method be consistent throughout the facility and encourages client involvement. The facility chooses its own surgical site method (e.g., the client's initials, surgeon's initials, the word "YES"). The essential focus is that the mark must be unambiguous and a clear communication to all involved. The mark must be permanent and visible after the client has been prepped and draped for surgery. There is no clear consensus on who should mark the site. Because the mark is a communication tool about the client for members of the team, The Joint Commission (2019) suggests that the individual who knows the most about the client should mark the site. In most cases, that will be the healthcare provider performing the procedure (p. 16).

The third step is called "time-out." Before surgery begins the surgical team takes a time-out to conduct a final verification of the correct client, procedure, and site. Any questions or concerns must be resolved before the procedure can begin.

Safety Alert! SAFETY

2019 The Joint Commission National Patient Safety Goals

Universal Protocol for Preventing Wrong Site, Wrong Procedure, and Wrong Person Surgery

- Conduct a preprocedure verification process. **Rationale:** *Hospitals should always make sure that any procedure is what the client needs and is performed on the right client.*
- Mark the procedure site.
- A time-out is performed before the procedure. **Rationale:** *The purpose of the time-out is to conduct a final assessment that the correct client, site, and procedure are identified.*

Vital Signs

In the preoperative phase the nurse assesses and documents vital signs for baseline data. The nurse reports any abnormal findings, such as elevated blood pressure or elevated temperature.

Antiemboli Stockings

Antiemboli (elastic) stockings are firm elastic hose that compress the veins of the legs and thereby facilitate the return of venous blood to the heart. They also prevent edema of the legs and feet. These stockings are frequently applied to surgical clients to prevent the potential postoperative problem of venous thromboembolism (VTE).

There are several types of stockings. One type extends from the foot to the knee and another from the foot to midthigh. These stockings usually have a partial foot that exposes the heel or toes so that extremity circulation can be assessed. Elastic stockings usually come in small, medium, and large sizes.

QSEN Patient-Centered Care: Antiemboli Stockings

When caring for clients and their families in the home setting, the nurse needs to include the following information about the use of antiemboli stockings:

- Teach the client or caregiver how to apply the antiemboli stockings.
- Stress the importance of no wrinkles or rolling down of the stockings and the rationale.
- Instruct the client or caregiver to remove the stockings daily and inspect the skin on the legs.
- Provide instructions about:
  - Laundering the stockings
  - The need for two pairs of stockings to allow for one pair to be worn while the other is being laundered
  - Replacing the stockings when they lose their elasticity.

Skill 37.2 details the steps required to apply antiemboli stockings.

Applying Antiemboli Stockings

SKILL 37.2

PURPOSES

- To facilitate venous return from the lower extremities
- To prevent venous stasis and VTE
- To reduce peripheral edema

ASSESSMENT

Assess and compare both lower extremities for

- Presence and volume (e.g., strong, faint, easily obliterated) of posterior tibial and dorsalis pedis pulses
- Skin color (note pallor, cyanosis, or other pigmentation)
- Skin temperature (e.g., warm, cool)
- Presence of edema
- Skin condition (e.g., thickened, shiny, taut)

Continued on page 970

SKILL 37.2

Applying Antiemboli Stockings—*continued*

PLANNING

Before applying antiemboli stockings, determine any potential or present circulatory problems and the surgeon's orders involving the lower extremities.

Assignment

AP frequently remove and apply antiemboli stockings as part of hygiene care. The nurse should stress the importance of removing and reapplying the stockings and reporting any changes in the client's skin to the nurse. The nurse is responsible for assessment of the skin.

Equipment

- Single-use tape measure (to prevent cross-infection)
- Clean knee or thigh antiemboli stockings of appropriate size

IMPLEMENTATION

Preparation

Take measurements as needed to obtain the appropriate size stockings.

- Measure the length of both legs from the heel to the gluteal fold (for thigh-length stockings) or from the heel to the popliteal space (for knee-length stockings).
- Measure the circumference of each calf and each thigh at the widest point.
- Compare the measurements to the size chart to obtain stockings of correct size. Obtain two sizes if there is a significant difference. **Rationale:** *Stockings that are too large for the client do not place adequate pressure on the legs to facilitate venous return, and may bunch, increasing the risk of pressure and skin irritation. Stockings that are too small may impede blood flow to the feet and cause skin breakdown.*

Performance

1. Prior to performing the procedure, introduce self and verify the client's identity using agency protocol. Explain to the client what you are going to do, why it is necessary, and how to participate.
2. Perform hand hygiene and observe other appropriate infection prevention procedures.
3. Provide for client privacy.
4. Select an appropriate time to apply the stockings.
   - Apply stockings in the morning, if possible, before the client gets out of bed. **Rationale:** *In sitting and standing positions, the veins can become distended so that edema occurs; the stockings should be applied before this occurs.*
   - Assist the client who has been ambulating to lie down and elevate the legs for 15 to 30 minutes before applying the stockings. **Rationale:** *This facilitates venous return and reduces swelling.*
5. Prepare the client.
   - Assist the client to a lying position in bed.
   - Wash and dry the legs as needed.
6. Apply the stockings.
   - Reach inside the stocking from the top, and grasping the heel, turn the upper portion of the stocking inside out so the foot portion is inside the stocking leg. **Rationale:** *Firm elastic stockings are easier to fit over the foot and calf when inverted in this manner rather than bunching up the stocking.*
   - Ask the client to point the toes, then position the stocking on the client's foot. With the heel of the stocking down and stretching each side of the stocking, ease the stocking over the toes taking care to place the toe and heel portions of the stocking appropriately. ❶ **Rationale:** *Pointing the toes makes application easier.*
   - Grasp the loose portion of the stocking at the ankle and gently pull the stocking over the leg, turning it right side out in the process. ❷ and ❸ If applying thigh-length stockings, stretch them over the knee until the top is below the gluteal fold.

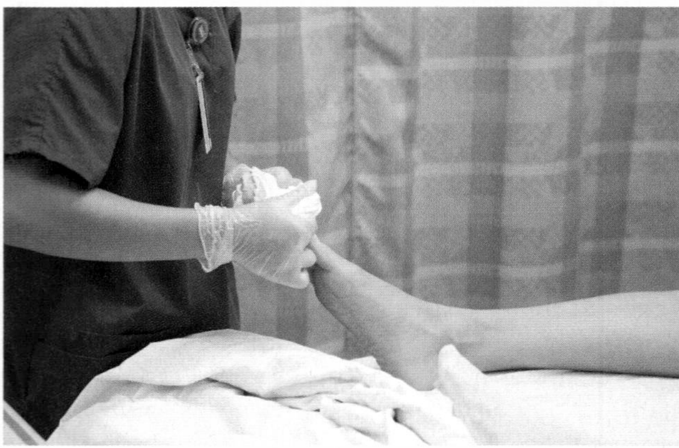

❶ Applying the stocking over the toes.

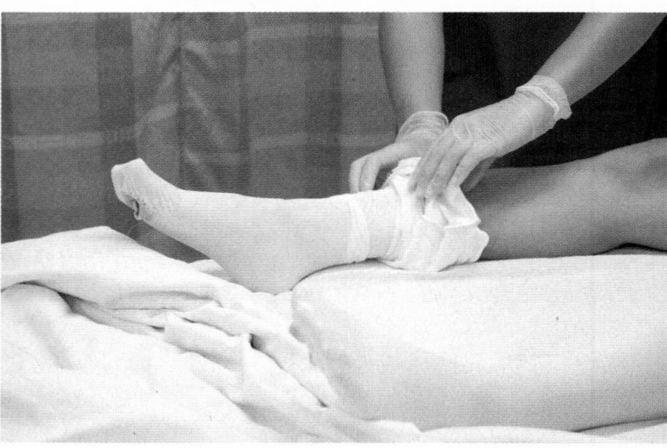

❷ Pulling the stocking snugly over the leg.

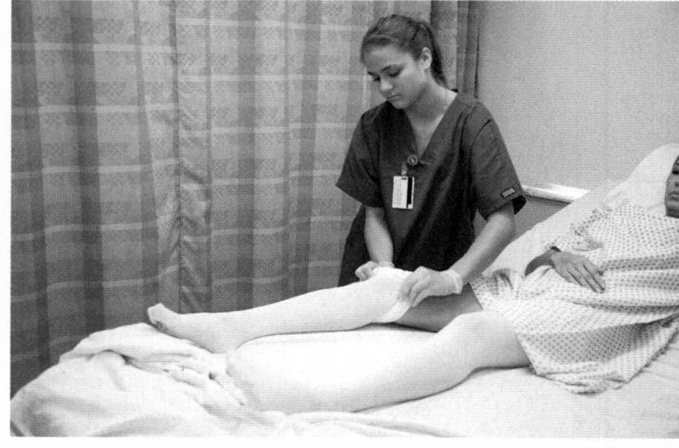

❸

Applying Antiemboli Stockings—*continued*

- Inspect the client's leg and stocking, smoothing any folds or creases. Ensure that the stocking is not rolled down or bunched at the top or ankle. Ensure that the stocking is distributed evenly and that the heel is properly centered in the heel pockets. **Rationale:** *Folds and creases can cause skin irritation under the stocking; bunching of the stocking can further impair venous return.*
- Remove the stockings per agency policy, inspecting the legs and skin while the stockings are off.
- Soiled stockings may be laundered by hand with warm water and mild soap. Hang to dry.

7. Document the procedure. Record the procedure, your assessment data, and when the stockings are removed and reapplied.

EVALUATION

- Remove antiemboli stockings per agency policy for skin care and inspection.
- Note the appearance of the legs and skin integrity, presence of edema, peripheral pulses, and skin color and temperature. Compare to previous assessment data.
- If complications occur, remove the stockings and report findings to the primary care provider.

LIFESPAN CONSIDERATIONS Antiemboli Stockings

CHILDREN

Antiemboli stockings are infrequently used on children.

OLDER ADULTS

- Because the elastic is quite strong in antiemboli stockings, the older adult may need assistance with putting on the stockings. Clients with arthritis may need to have another individual put the stockings on for them.
- Many older adults have circulation problems and wear antiemboli stockings. It is important to check for wrinkles in the stockings and to see if the stocking has rolled down or twisted. If so, correct immediately because the stockings must be evenly distributed over the limb to promote rather than hinder circulation.
- Stockings should be removed once each shift so that a thorough assessment can be made of the legs and feet. Redness and skin breakdown on the heels can occur quickly and go undetected if not thoroughly assessed on a regular basis.

Sequential Compression Devices

Clients who are undergoing surgery may benefit from a sequential compression device (SCD) to promote venous return from the legs. SCDs inflate and deflate plastic sleeves wrapped around the legs to promote venous flow. SCDs are discussed in Chapter 50 ∞ (see Skill 50.1).

Evaluating

The goals established during the planning phase are evaluated according to specific desired outcomes, also established in that phase.

Intraoperative Phase

The intraoperative nurse uses the nursing process to design, coordinate, and deliver care to meet the identified needs of clients whose protective reflexes or self-care abilities are potentially compromised because they are having operative or other invasive procedures.

Types of Anesthesia

Anesthesia is classified as *general* or *regional*. An anesthesiologist or a certified registered nurse anesthetist (CRNA) administer anesthetic agents. **General anesthesia** is the loss of all sensation and consciousness. Under general anesthesia, protective reflexes such as cough and gag reflexes are lost. A general anesthetic acts by blocking awareness centers in the brain so that amnesia (loss of memory), analgesia (insensibility to pain), hypnosis (artificial sleep), and relaxation (rendering a part of the body less tense) occur. General anesthetics are usually administered by IV infusion or by inhalation of gases through a mask or through an endotracheal tube inserted into the trachea.

General anesthesia has certain advantages. Because the client is unconscious rather than awake and anxious, respiration and cardiac function are readily regulated. Also, the anesthesia can be adjusted to the length of the operation and the client's age and physical status. Its chief disadvantage is that it depresses the respiratory and circulatory systems. Some clients become more anxious about a general anesthetic than about the surgery itself. Often this is because they fear losing the capacity to control their own bodies.

Regional anesthesia is the temporary interruption of the transmission of nerve impulses to and from a specific area or region of the body. The client loses sensation in an area of the body but remains conscious. Several techniques are used:

- **Topical (surface) anesthesia** is applied directly to the skin and mucous membranes, open skin surfaces, wounds, and burns. The most commonly used topical agents are lidocaine (Xylocaine) and benzocaine. Topical anesthetics are readily absorbed and act rapidly.
- **Local anesthesia** (infiltration) is injected into a specific area and is used for minor surgical procedures such as suturing a small wound or performing a biopsy. Lidocaine or tetracaine 0.1% may be used.

DRUG CAPSULE

Benzodiazepine: midazolam hydrochloride (Versed)

THE CLIENT UNDERGOING ANESTHESIA

IV anesthetic agent used to induce general anesthesia.

Commonly used prior to conscious sedation to produce anxiolytic, hypnotic, anticonvulsant, muscle relaxant, and amnesic effects.

NURSING RESPONSIBILITIES

- Obtain baseline vital signs and level of consciousness before administration.
- Monitor vital signs, level of consciousness, and oxygen saturation q3–5min intraoperatively and postoperatively. Notify primary care provider or CRNA if there are any changes.
- Have resuscitative equipment readily available.
- A too rapid IV administration or excessive dose increases the risk of respiratory depression or arrest.
- Dosage must be individualized based on age, underlying disease, and desired effect. Too much or too little a dosage or improper administration may result in cerebral hypoxia, agitation, involuntary movement, hyperactivity, and combativeness.

Note: Prior to administering any medication, review all aspects with a current drug handbook or other reliable source.

- A **nerve block** is a technique in which the anesthetic agent is injected into and around a nerve or small nerve group that supplies sensation to a small area of the body. Major blocks involve multiple nerves or a plexus (e.g., the brachial plexus anesthetizes the arm); minor blocks involve a single nerve (e.g., a facial nerve).
- **Spinal anesthesia** is also referred to as a **subarachnoid block (SAB)**. It requires a lumbar puncture through one of the interspaces between lumbar disk 2 (L_2) and the sacrum (S_1). An anesthetic agent is injected into the subarachnoid space surrounding the spinal cord. Spinal anesthesia is often categorized as a low, mid, or high spinal. Low spinals (saddle or caudal blocks) are primarily used for surgeries involving the perineal or rectal areas. Mid-spinals (below the level of the umbilicus—T_{10}) can be used for hernia repairs or appendectomies, and high spinals (reaching the nipple line—T_4) can be used for surgeries such as cesarean births.
- **Epidural (peridural) anesthesia** is an injection of an anesthetic agent into the epidural space, the area inside the spinal column but outside the dura mater.

Conscious sedation may be used alone or in conjunction with regional anesthesia for some diagnostic tests and surgical procedures. **Conscious sedation** refers to minimal depression of the level of consciousness such that the client retains the ability to maintain a patent airway and respond appropriately to commands. IV opioids such as morphine or fentanyl and antianxiety agents such as diazepam or midazolam are commonly used to induce and maintain conscious sedation. Conscious sedation increases the client's pain threshold and induces a degree of amnesia but allows for prompt reversal of its effects and a rapid return to normal ADLs. Procedures such as endoscopies, incision and drainage of abscesses, and even balloon angioplasty may be performed under conscious sedation.

●○● NURSING MANAGEMENT

Assessing

On the day of surgery, after the client has been admitted to the hospital, the client's family members or significant others are escorted to a surgical holding area located outside of the OR. This area is also known as a presurgical care unit (PSCU). The perioperative nurse confirms the client's identity and assesses the client's physical and emotional status. The nurse verifies the information on the preoperative checklist and evaluates the client's knowledge about the surgery and events to follow. The client's response to preoperative medications is assessed, as well as the placement and patency of tubes such as IV lines, nasogastric tubes, and urinary catheters.

Assessment continues throughout surgery, as the anesthesiologist or the CRNA continuously monitors the client's vital signs (including blood pressure, heart rate, respiratory rate, and temperature), ECG, and oxygen saturation. Fluid intake and urinary output are monitored throughout surgery, and blood loss is estimated. In addition, arterial and venous pressures, pulmonary artery pressures, and laboratory values such as blood glucose, hemoglobin, hematocrit, serum electrolytes, and arterial blood gases may be evaluated during surgery. Continual assessment is necessary to rapidly identify adverse responses to surgery or anesthesia and intervene promptly to prevent complications.

Diagnosing

Examples of nursing diagnoses that may be appropriate for the intraoperative client can include the following: potential for developing pressure injury related to perioperative positioning, potential for hypothermia related to low temperatures in the OR, and potential for surgical site infection related to altered skin integrity.

Planning

The overall goals of care in the intraoperative period are to maintain the client's safety and to maintain homeostasis. Examples of nursing activities to achieve these goals include the following:

- Position the client appropriately for surgery.
- Perform preoperative skin preparation.
- Assist in preparing and maintaining the sterile field.
- Open and dispense sterile supplies during surgery.
- Provide medications and solutions for the sterile field.
- Monitor and maintain a safe, aseptic environment.

- Manage catheters, tubes, drains, and specimens.
- Perform sponge, sharp, and instrument counts.
- Document nursing care provided and the client's response to interventions.

Implementing

Intraoperative interventions are carried out by the circulating nurse, the scrub person, and the registered nurse first assistant. The **circulating nurse** coordinates activities and manages client care by continually assessing client safety (e.g., client positioning) and by monitoring aseptic practice and the environment (e.g., temperature, humidity, and lighting). The **scrub person** is usually an RN, LPN, or certified surgical technologist (CST). They wear sterile gowns, gloves, caps, and eye protection. Their role is to assist the surgeons. Their responsibilities include draping the client with sterile drapes and handling sterile instruments and supplies. The registered nurse first assistant (RNFA) has additional education and training and functions in an expanded perioperative nursing role. The RNFA assists the surgeon by controlling bleeding, using instruments, handling and cutting tissues, and suturing during the procedure. The circulating nurse and the scrub person are responsible for accounting for all sponges, needles, and instruments at the close of surgery. This precaution prevents foreign bodies from being left inside the client.

Surgical Skin Preparation

Surgical skin preparation involves cleaning the surgical site, removing hair only if necessary, and applying an antimicrobial agent. Surgery personnel perform skin preparation near the time of surgery. The purpose of a surgical skin preparation is to reduce the risk of SSIs, the most common type of healthcare-associated infection in the surgical population and a serious complication. This is done by:

- Removing transient microbes from the skin
- Reducing the resident microbial count to subpathogenic amounts in a short time and with the least amount of tissue irritation
- Inhibiting rapid rebound growth of microbes.

Skin preparation practices to reduce the risk of SSIs include the following:

- Cleaning the surgical site and surrounding areas. This can be accomplished before the surgical prep by having the client shower and shampoo or wash the surgical site before arriving in the surgical setting, or by washing the surgical site in the surgical setting immediately before applying an antimicrobial agent.
- Remove hair from the surgical site only when necessary, for example, if it interferes with the surgical procedure. Personnel skilled in hair removal should use techniques that preserve skin integrity such as electric clippers to reduce the risk of traumatizing the skin during hair removal. Razors can disrupt skin integrity so hair removal with a razor is not recommended. Skin trauma and abrasions increase the risk of microorganisms colonizing the surgical site. If hair is to be removed, it should occur before entering the operating suite (Bashaw & Keister, 2019).
- Prepare the surgical site and surrounding area with an antimicrobial agent when indicated. A nontoxic antimicrobial agent with a broad range of germicidal action is used to inhibit the growth of microorganisms during and following the surgical procedure. Chlorhexidine gluconate is a frequently used solution. Alcohol is effective; however, its use may be restricted because of flammability.

Positioning

The position of the client during a surgical procedure is essential to the maintenance of client safety. Inadequate padding and incorrect positioning can cause serious pressure injuries. The entire operating room team is responsible for minimizing the client's risk of perioperative complications related to positioning. The client's position can affect ventilation and circulation and impair peripheral nerve function. The anesthesiologist or nurse anesthetist is responsible for directing staff to protect the client from injury.

The client's position should provide:

- Optimal visualization of and access to the surgical site
- Optimal access to IV lines and monitoring devices
- Protection of the client from harm (anatomic and physiologic considerations).

Positioning is performed after anesthesia is induced and before surgical draping of the client. The client is lifted into position to prevent shearing forces on the skin from sliding or rolling. The exact position for the client depends on the operation, that is, the surgical approach. For example, a lithotomy position is usually used for vaginal surgery.

Straps maintain positions on the operating table, and body prominences are frequently padded. The position should consider normal joint range of motion and good body alignment, thereby avoiding strain or injury to muscles, bones, and ligaments.

Pressure injuries are often not identifiable immediately. Up to 72 hours may pass before signs of an injury are visible. Nurses who care for clients postoperatively should notify the perioperative department if a pressure injury appears within 72 hours after surgery because the injury may have happened in the perioperative period (Spruce, 2017, p. 96).

Clinical Alert!

Be especially aware of the intraoperative position required for the surgery. Clients, especially older adults, are vulnerable to perioperative pressure injuries. Check the appropriate pressure points of that surgical position on the client.

ANATOMY & PHYSIOLOGY REVIEW

Client Positioning

The most common position for a client during a surgical procedure is the supine position. This position provides approaches to the cranial, thoracic, and peritoneal body cavities as well as to all four extremities and the perineum. Proper body alignment and padding of potential pressure areas are essential to preventing client risk for injury during surgery.

The potential pressure areas are the occiput, scapulae, olecranon, thoracic vertebrae, sacrum, coccyx, and calcaneus. The nursing intervention is to pad and protect bony prominences, pressure sites, and vulnerable nerves with pressure-reducing devices made of foam or gel. Proper positioning must provide optimal exposure to the surgical site as well as provide for client comfort and safety.

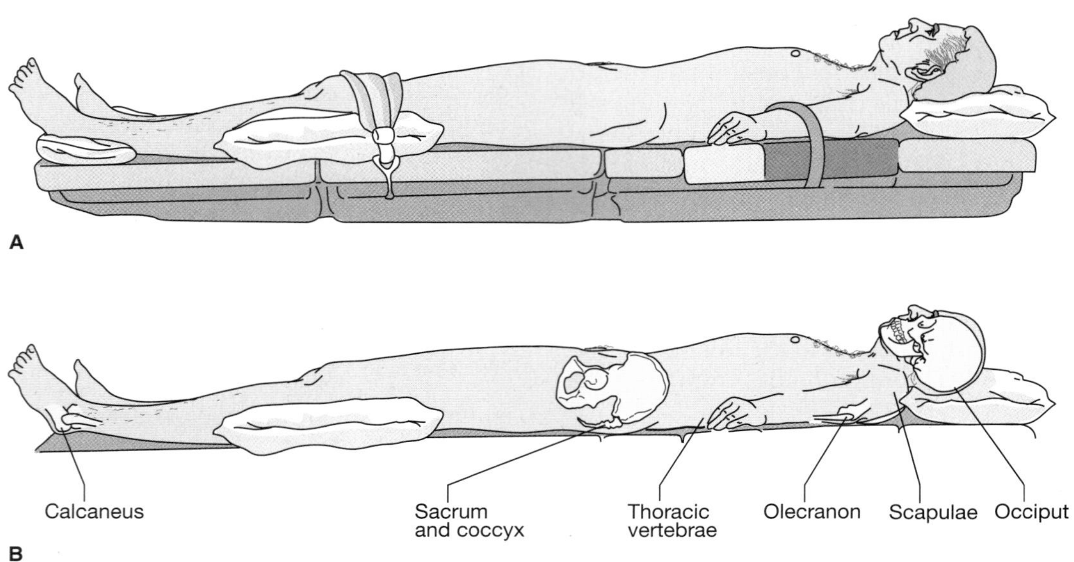

A, Supine position during a surgical procedure; *B*, potential pressure points noted.

QUESTIONS

A 78-year-old male client scheduled for a colon resection is brought to the operating room. He weighs 82 kg (180 lb), has type 2 diabetes, and has a history of arthritis in his hips and shoulders.

1. What baseline assessments would you gather before taking this client to the operating room?
2. What areas on this client are most likely to be injured as a result of poor positioning or inadequate padding?
3. What is the priority nursing diagnosis and outcome for this client?

Answers to Anatomy & Physiology Review Questions are available on the faculty resources site. Please consult with your instructor.

Evaluating

The intraoperative nurse uses the goals developed during the planning stage (e.g., maintain client safety) and collects data to evaluate whether the desired outcomes have been achieved.

Documentation

The intraoperative nurse documents the perioperative plan of care including assessment, diagnosis, outcome identification, planning, implementation, and evaluation.

Postoperative Phase

Nursing during the postoperative phase is especially important for the client's recovery because anesthesia impairs the ability of clients to respond to environmental stimuli and to help themselves, although the degree of consciousness of clients will vary. Moreover, surgery itself traumatizes the body by disrupting protective mechanisms and homeostasis.

Immediate Postanesthetic Phase

Recovery of surgical clients who required anesthesia is performed in the PACU. PACU nurses, often certified by the American Society of PeriAnesthesia Nurses (ASPAN), have specialized skills to care for clients recovering from anesthesia and surgery (Figure 37.2 ■).

During the immediate postanesthetic stage, an unconscious client is positioned on the side, with the face slightly down. A pillow is not placed under the head. In this position, gravity keeps the tongue forward, preventing occlusion of the pharynx and allowing drainage of mucus or vomitus out of the mouth rather than down the respiratory tree.

The nurse ensures maximum chest expansion by elevating the client's upper arm on a pillow. The upper arm is supported because the pressure of an arm against the chest reduces chest expansion potential. An artificial airway is maintained in place, and the client is suctioned as needed until cough and swallowing reflexes return. Generally the client spits out an oropharyngeal airway when coughing returns. Endotracheal tubes are not removed until clients are awake and able to maintain their own airway. The client is then helped to turn, cough, and take deep breaths, provided that vital signs are stable. When spinal anesthesia is used, the client may be required to remain flat for a specified period. See Chapter 49 ∞ for information about artificial airways. Assessment of the client in the immediate postanesthetic period is summarized in Box 37.5.

The return of the client's reflexes, such as swallowing and gagging, indicates that anesthesia is ending. Time of recovery from anesthesia varies with the kind of anesthetic agent used, its dosage, and the individual's response to it. Nurses should arouse clients by calling them by name and in a normal tone of voice repeatedly telling them that the surgery is over and that they are in the PACU.

The PACU nurse uses criteria developed by the anesthesia department to evaluate client readiness for discharge from the PACU. Aldrete and Kroulik (1970) were the first to introduce the Post-Anesthetic Recovery Score (PARS), also called the Aldrete Score, to provide an objective scoring system to help in the discharge decision-making process. The original Aldrete scoring system included assessment of muscle activity, respiration, circulation, consciousness, and color. In 1995, this scoring system was revised to replace the assessment of color with oxygen saturation and is called the Modified Aldrete. A rating of 0 to 2 is given to each assessment, depending on its absence or presence. The numbers given to each assessment are added up with a score of 10 indicating that the client is in the best possible condition. Many PACUs require a score of 9 for discharge.

A number of scoring systems have been developed and currently there is not one scoring system endorsed by the major organizations regulating postanesthesia care (Pusey-Reid, 2018, p. 34). Institutions need to develop assessment and discharge criteria, in conjunction with the anesthesia department, that can be used in discharging clients from the PACU. It is important for the nurse to use critical thinking and nursing judgment along with the discharge criteria.

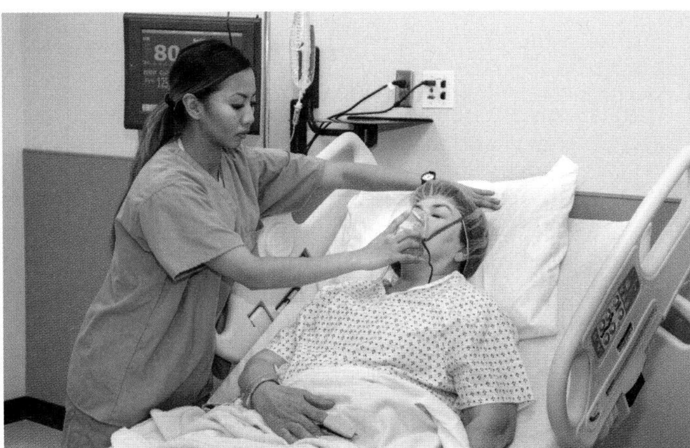

Figure 37.2 ■ PACU nurse provides constant assessment and care for clients recovering from anesthesia and surgery.

BOX 37.5 Clinical Assessment: Immediate Postanesthetic Phase

- Adequacy of airway
- Oxygen saturation
- Adequacy of ventilation:
  - Respiratory rate, rhythm, and depth
  - Use of accessory muscles
  - Breath sounds
- Cardiovascular status:
  - Heart rate and rhythm
  - Peripheral pulse amplitude and equality
  - Blood pressure
  - Capillary filling
- Level of consciousness:
  - Not responding
  - Arousable with verbal stimuli
  - Fully awake
  - Oriented to time, person, and place
- Presence of protective reflexes (e.g., gag, cough)
- Activity, ability to move extremities
- Skin color (pink, pale, dusky, blotchy, cyanotic, jaundiced)
- Fluid status:
  - Intake and output
  - Status of IV infusions (type of fluid, rate, amount in container, patency of tubing)
  - Signs of dehydration or fluid overload (see Chapter 51 ∞)
- Condition of operative site:
  - Status of dressing
  - Drainage (amount, type, and color)
- Patency of and character and amount of drainage from catheters, tubes, and drains
- Discomfort (i.e., pain) (type, location, and severity), nausea, vomiting
- Safety (i.e., necessity for side rails, call bell within reach)

Clients are usually discharged from the PACU when:

- They are conscious and oriented.
- They are able to maintain a clear airway, breathe deeply, cough, and maintain a desirable oxygen saturation level.
- Vital signs have been stable or consistent with preoperative vital signs for at least 30 minutes.
- Protective reflexes (e.g., gag, swallowing) are active.
- They are able to move all extremities.
- Intake and urinary output are adequate.
- Postanesthesia nausea and vomiting is controlled.
- Temperature is between 96.8 and 100.4°F (36–38°C).
- Dressings are dry and intact; there is no overt drainage.

Once the health status has stabilized, the client is returned to the nursing unit or the outpatient surgery discharge area.

Preparing for Ongoing Care of the Postoperative Client

While the client is in the operating room, the client's bed and room are prepared for the postoperative phase. In some agencies, the client is brought back to the unit on a stretcher and transferred to the bed in the room. In other agencies, the client's bed is brought to the surgery suite, and the client is transferred there. In the latter situation, the bed needs to be made with clean linens as soon as the client goes to surgery so that it can be taken to the OR when needed. In addition, the nurse must obtain and set up any special equipment, such as an IV pole, suction, oxygen equipment, and orthopedic appliances (e.g., traction). If these are not requested on the client's record, the nurse should consult with the perioperative nurse.

●○● NURSING MANAGEMENT

Assessing

As soon as the client returns to the nursing unit, the nurse conducts an initial assessment. The sequence of these activities varies with the situation. For example, the nurse may need to check the primary care provider's stat orders before conducting the initial assessment; in such a case, nursing interventions to implement the orders can be carried out at the same time as assessment.

The nurse consults the surgeon's postoperative orders to learn the following:

- Food and fluids permitted by mouth
- IV solutions and IV medications
- Position in bed
- Medications ordered (e.g., analgesics, antibiotics)
- Laboratory tests
- Intake and output, which in some agencies are monitored for all postoperative clients
- Activity permitted, including ambulation.

The nurse also checks the PACU record for the following data:

- Operation performed
- Presence and location of any drains
- Anesthetic used
- Postoperative diagnosis
- Estimated blood loss
- Medications administered in the PACU.

Many hospitals have postoperative protocols for regular assessment of clients. In some agencies, assessments are made every 15 minutes until vital signs stabilize, every hour for the next 4 hours, then every 4 hours for the next 2 days. It is important that the assessments be made as often as the client's condition requires. The nurse assesses the following:

- ***Level of consciousness.*** Assess orientation to time, place, and person. Most clients are fully conscious but drowsy when returned to their unit. Assess reaction to verbal stimuli and ability to move extremities.
- ***Vital signs.*** Take the client's vital signs (pulse, respiration, blood pressure, and oxygen saturation level) every 15 minutes until stable or in accordance with agency protocol. Compare initial findings with PACU data. In addition, assess the client's lung sounds and assess for signs of common circulatory problems such as postoperative hypotension, hemorrhage, or shock. Hypovolemia due to fluid losses during surgery is a common cause of postoperative hypotension. Hemorrhage can result from insecure ligation of blood vessels or disruption of sutures. Massive hemorrhage or cardiac insufficiency can lead to shock postoperatively. Common postoperative complications with their manifestations and preventive measures are listed in Table 37.3.
- ***Skin color and temperature,*** particularly that of the lips and nail beds. The color of the lips and nail beds is an indicator of **tissue perfusion** (passage of blood through the vessels). Pale, cyanotic, cool, and moist skin may be a sign of circulatory problems.

Clinical Alert!

Older adults may not show the classic signs of infection (e.g., fever, tachycardia, increased WBC count); instead there may be an abrupt change in their mental status.

- ***Comfort.*** Assess pain with the client's vital signs and as needed between vital sign measurements. Assess the location and intensity of the pain. Do not assume that reported pain is incisional; other causes may include muscle strains, flatus, and angina. Ask the client to rate pain on a scale of 0 to 10, with 0 being no pain and 10 the worst pain imaginable. Evaluate the client for objective indicators of pain: pallor, perspiration, muscle tension, and reluctance to cough, move, or ambulate. Determine when and what analgesics were last administered, and assess the client for any side effects of medication such as nausea and vomiting.

TABLE 37.3 Potential Postoperative Problems

Problem	Description	Cause	Clinical Signs	Preventive Interventions
RESPIRATORY				
Pneumonia	Inflammation of the alveoli	Infection, toxins, or irritants causing inflammatory process; immobility and impaired ventilation result in atelectasis and promote growth of pathogens	Elevated temperature, cough, expectoration of blood-tinged or purulent sputum, dyspnea, chest pain	Deep-breathing exercises and coughing, incentive spirometer, moving in bed, early ambulation
Atelectasis	A condition in which alveoli collapse and are not ventilated	Mucous plugs blocking bronchial passageways, inadequate lung expansion, analgesics, immobility	Dyspnea, tachypnea, tachycardia; diaphoresis, anxiety; pleural pain, decreased chest wall movement; dull or absent breath sounds; decreased oxygen saturation	Deep-breathing exercises and coughing, incentive spirometer, moving in bed, early ambulation
Pulmonary embolism	Blood clot that has moved to the lungs and blocks a pulmonary artery, thus obstructing blood flow to a portion of the lung	Stasis of venous blood from immobility, venous injury from fractures or during surgery, use of oral contraceptives high in estrogen, pre-existing coagulation or circulatory disorder	Sudden chest pain, shortness of breath, cyanosis, shock (tachycardia, low blood pressure)	Turning, ambulation, antiemboli stockings, sequential compression devices (SCDs)
CIRCULATORY				
Hypovolemia	Inadequate circulating blood volume	Fluid deficit, hemorrhage	Tachycardia, decreased urine output, decreased blood pressure	Early detection of signs; fluid or blood replacement
Hemorrhage	Internal or external bleeding	Disruption of sutures, insecure ligation of blood vessels	Overt bleeding (dressings saturated with bright blood; bright, free-flowing blood in drains or chest tubes), increased pain, increasing abdominal girth, swelling or bruising around incision	Early detection of signs
Hypovolemic shock	Inadequate tissue perfusion resulting from markedly reduced circulating blood volume	Severe hypovolemia from fluid deficit or hemorrhage	Rapid weak pulse, dyspnea, tachypnea; restlessness and anxiety; urine output less than 30 mL/h; decreased blood pressure; cool, clammy skin, thirst, pallor	Maintain blood volume through adequate fluid replacement, prevent hemorrhage; early detection of signs
Thrombophlebitis	Inflammation of the veins, usually of the legs and associated with a blood clot	Slowed venous blood flow due to immobility or prolonged sitting; trauma to vein, resulting in inflammation and increased blood coagulability	Aching, cramping pain; affected area is swollen, red, and hot to touch; vein feels hard	Early ambulation, leg exercises, antiemboli stockings, SCDs, adequate fluid intake
Thrombus	Blood clot attached to wall of vein or artery (most commonly the leg veins)	Thrombophlebitis for venous thrombi; disruption or inflammation of arterial wall for arterial thrombi	*Venous:* same as thrombophlebitis *Arterial:* pain and pallor of affected extremity; decreased or absent peripheral pulses	*Venous:* same as thrombophlebitis *Arterial:* maintain prescribed position; early detection of signs

Continued on page 978

TABLE 37.3 Potential Postoperative Problems—*continued*

Problem	Description	Cause	Clinical Signs	Preventive Interventions
Embolus	Foreign body or clot that has moved from its site of formation to another area of the body (e.g., the lungs, heart, or brain)	Venous or arterial thrombus; broken IV catheter, fat, or amniotic fluid	In venous system, usually becomes a pulmonary embolus (see pulmonary embolism); signs of arterial emboli may depend on the location	Turning, ambulation, leg exercises, SCDs; careful maintenance of IV catheters
URINARY				
Urinary retention	Inability to empty the bladder, with excessive accumulation of urine in the bladder	Depressed bladder muscle tone from narcotics and anesthetics; handling of tissues during surgery on adjacent organs (rectum, vagina)	Fluid intake larger than output; inability to void or frequent voiding of small amounts, bladder distention, suprapubic discomfort, restlessness	Monitoring of fluid intake and output, interventions to facilitate voiding, urinary catheterization as needed
Urinary tract infection	Inflammation of the bladder, ureters, or urethra	Immobilization and limited fluid intake, instrumentation of the urinary tract	Burning sensation when voiding, urgency, cloudy urine, lower abdominal pain	Adequate fluid intake, early ambulation, aseptic straight catheterization only as necessary, good perineal hygiene
GASTROINTESTINAL				
Nausea and vomiting		Pain, abdominal distention, ingesting food or fluids before return of peristalsis, certain medications, anxiety	Complaints of nausea, retching or gagging	IV fluids until peristalsis returns; then clear fluids, full fluids, and regular diet; antiemetic drugs if ordered; analgesics for pain
Constipation	Infrequent or no stool passage for abnormal length of time (e.g., within 48 h after solid diet started)	Lack of dietary roughage, analgesics (decreased intestinal motility), immobility	Absence of stool elimination, abdominal distention, and discomfort	Adequate fluid intake, high-fiber diet, early ambulation
Tympanites	Retention of gases within the intestines	Slowed motility of the intestines due to handling of the bowel during surgery and the effects of anesthesia	Obvious abdominal distention, abdominal discomfort (gas pains), absence of bowel sounds	Early ambulation; avoid using a straw, provide ice chips or water at room temperature
Postoperative ileus	Intestinal obstruction characterized by lack of peristaltic activity	Handling the bowel during surgery, anesthesia, electrolyte imbalance, wound infection	Abdominal pain and distention; constipation; absent bowel sounds; vomiting	Early ambulation; chewing gum; early oral intake and feeding
WOUND				
Wound infection	Inflammation and infection of incision or drain site	Poor aseptic technique; laboratory analysis of wound swab identifies causative microorganism	Purulent exudate, redness, tenderness, elevated body temperature, wound odor	Keep wound clean and dry, use surgical aseptic technique when changing dressings
Wound dehiscence	Separation of a suture line before the incision heals	Malnutrition (emaciation, obesity), poor circulation, excessive strain on suture line	Increased incision drainage, tissues underlying skin become visible along parts of the incision	Adequate nutrition, appropriate incisional support and avoidance of strain
Wound evisceration	Extrusion of internal organs and tissues through the incision	Same as for wound dehiscence	Opening of incision and visible protrusion of organs	Same as for wound dehiscence
PSYCHOLOGIC				
Postoperative depression	Mental disorder characterized by altered mood	Weakness, surprise nature of emergency surgery, news of malignancy, severely altered body image, other personal matter; may be a physiologic response to some surgeries	Anorexia, tearfulness, loss of ambition, withdrawal, rejection of others, feelings of dejection, sleep disturbances (insomnia or excessive sleeping)	Adequate rest, physical activity, opportunity to express anger and other negative feelings

- ***Fluid balance.*** Assess the type and amount of IV fluids, flow rate, and infusion site. Monitor the client's fluid intake and output. In addition to watching for shock, assess the client for signs of circulatory overload, and monitor serum electrolytes. Anesthetics and surgery affect the hormones regulating fluid and electrolyte balance (aldosterone and antidiuretic hormone in particular), placing the client at risk for decreased urine output and fluid and electrolyte imbalances.
- ***Dressing and bedclothes.*** Inspect the client's dressings and bedclothes underneath the client. Excessive bloody drainage on dressings or on bedclothes, often appearing underneath the client, can indicate hemorrhage. The amount of drainage on dressings is recorded by describing the diameter of the stains or by denoting the number and type of dressings saturated with drainage. Chapter 36 ∞ provides additional information about wound care.
- ***Drains and tubes.*** Determine color, consistency, and amount of drainage from all tubes and drains. All tubes should be patent, and tubes and suction equipment should be functioning. Drainage bags must be hanging properly. Chapter 36 ∞ provides additional information about wound drains.
- ***Any difficulties with voiding or bladder distention.***
- ***Return of peristalsis.*** Auscultate the client's abdomen to confirm the return of peristalsis. Note the passage of flatus and stool.
- ***Tolerance of food and fluids ingested.*** Document the client's time of arrival and all assessments. Many agencies have progress flow records for this purpose. Alter the frequency, parameters, and priorities to meet the individual needs of the client.

Diagnosing

Because surgery can involve many body systems both directly and indirectly and is a complex experience for the client, the nursing diagnoses focus on a wide variety of actual, potential, and collaborative problems.

Examples of actual and potential nursing diagnoses for the postoperative client can include severe pain, difficulty maintaining a clear airway, and potential for surgical site infection. Collaborative problems that may be experienced by the postoperative client are summarized in Table 37.3.

Planning

Postoperative care planning and discharge planning begin in the preoperative phase when preoperative teaching is implemented.

Planning for Home Care

To provide for continuity of care for the surgical client after discharge, the nurse needs to consider the client's needs for assistance with care in the home setting. Discharge planning for both the day surgery client and the client who has been hospitalized for several days following surgery incorporates an assessment of the client's and family's abilities for self-care, financial resources, and the need for referrals and home health services. Following is an outline of a home care assessment for a surgical client; however, it is important to remember that surgical clients have diverse needs, and additional assessment data may be required. An individualized approach to surgical discharge planning must take into account the client's age, gender, surgical procedure, and family and community support for immediate and long-term nursing care in the home.

QSEN Patient-Centered Care: Surgical Clients

The nurse should make the following home care assessments for surgical clients:

- *Self-care abilities:* ability to manage hygiene and other self-care, to perform wound care as needed, to manage tubes and stomas, and to manage prescribed medications
- *Supplies required:* wound care supplies such as dressings, hypoallergenic tape, cleansing solutions, binders or slings, elastic wraps, irrigating syringe and solution
- *Assistive devices required:* walker, cane, raised toilet seat, commode, overhead trapeze, grab bars
- *Current level of knowledge:* postoperative pain management, wound care, dressing changes, urinary catheters or other drains, activity restrictions, dietary prescriptions, prescribed exercises (e.g., range of motion, postmastectomy exercises), infection control measures such as hand washing
- *Caregiver availability, skills, and responses:* willingness and ability to assume responsibility for care as needed (e.g., wound care, catheter and tube management, meal preparation, assistance with ADLs, shopping, transportation to and from appointments), other available caregivers
- *Family role changes and coping:* effect on parenting and spousal roles, sexuality, social roles, financial status
- *Financial resources:* ability to purchase necessary supplies and equipment; other sources of funding or financial assistance (e.g., Medicare, Medicaid)—see Chapter 5 ∞
- Obtain information from the client, the family, or significant other regarding the physical environment of the home and potential issues postoperatively. This may include presence of stairs, access to the home, and accessibility of the kitchen, bathroom, and bedroom.
- Available community resources such as equipment and supply companies, support and educational organizations and groups (e.g., ostomy clubs and Reach for Recovery), home health agencies or providers, access to pharmacy services, transportation services for medical care, Meals on Wheels, and other charitable support organizations.

Implementing

Nursing interventions designed to promote client recovery and prevent complications include (a) pain management, (b) appropriate positioning, (c) deep-breathing and coughing exercises and incentive spirometry, (d) leg exercises, (e) early ambulation, (f) adequate hydration, (g) promoting urinary and gastrointestinal function, (h) diet, and (i) suction maintenance.

Pain Management

Although pain is a sensory and emotional experience that serves to alert us to harm and initiate responses to avoid or minimize harm, pain in the surgical client has little protective value. It can, in fact, have detrimental effects, leading to stimulation of the sympathetic nervous system, tachycardia, shallow breathing, atelectasis, altered gas exchange, immobility, and immunosuppression. Chapter 30 ∞ provides a more in-depth discussion of pain and pain management.

Pain is usually greatest 12 to 36 hours after surgery, decreasing after the second or third postoperative day. During the initial postoperative period, patient-controlled analgesia (PCA) or continuous analgesic administration through an IV or epidural catheter is often prescribed. The nurse monitors the infusion or amount of analgesic administered by PCA, assesses the client's pain relief, and notifies the primary care provider if the client is experiencing unacceptable side effects or inadequate pain relief. As-needed (prn) parenteral or oral analgesics should be administered on a routine basis (every 2 to 6 hours, depending on the drug, route, and dose) for the first 24 to 36 hours. When routine analgesic administration is no longer necessary, the prescribed analgesic is generally given before scheduled activities and rest periods.

An anti-inflammatory agent such as ibuprofen or ketorolac (Toradol) is often administered in conjunction with an opioid analgesic to enhance pain relief. Clients need to be reminded that analgesics are most effective when taken on a regular basis or before pain becomes severe. Because muscle tension increases pain perception and responses, nurses need to use nonpharmacologic measures in addition to prescribed analgesia. These include ensuring that the client is warm and providing back rubs, position changes, diversional activities, and adjunctive measures such as imagery.

Positioning

Position the client as ordered. Clients who have had spinal anesthetics usually lie flat for 8 to 12 hours. An unconscious or semiconscious client is placed on one side with the head slightly elevated, if possible, or in a position that allows fluids to drain from the mouth. Unless contraindicated, elevation of affected extremities (e.g., following foot surgery) with the distal extremity higher than the heart promotes venous drainage and reduces swelling.

Deep-Breathing and Coughing Exercises

Deep-breathing exercises help remove mucus, which can form and remain in the lungs due to the effects of general anesthetic and analgesics. These drugs depress the action of both the cilia of the mucous membranes lining the respiratory tract and the respiratory center in the brain. By increasing lung expansion and preventing the accumulation of secretions, deep breathing helps prevent pneumonia and atelectasis, which may result from stagnation of fluid in the lungs. Deep breathing frequently initiates the coughing reflex. Voluntary coughing in conjunction with deep breathing facilitates the movement and expectoration of respiratory tract secretions.

Encourage the client to do deep-breathing and coughing exercises hourly, or at least every 2 hours, during waking hours for the first few days. Assist the client to a sitting position in bed or on the side of the bed. The client can splint the incision with a pillow when coughing, or the nurse can splint the incision for the client to reduce discomfort.

LIFESPAN CONSIDERATIONS Postoperative Care

CHILDREN

- Infants and young children may not be able to state their level of pain postoperatively, may be physically active, and may appear not to have much pain. Use nonverbal signs such as crying, fussiness, refusal to eat, disturbed sleep, increased heart rate, increased blood pressure, and agitation to assess pain.
- Children are often undermedicated for pain postoperatively. Nurses should be alert to nonverbal signs of pain and provide medication in a timely manner. Well-controlled pain levels facilitate the healing process in children.
- Use a pediatric pain scale to assess pain.
- Some PACUs allow parents to be present when their child wakes from surgery. Having the parent at the bedside has been shown to calm the child and reduce parental anxiety.

OLDER ADULTS

- Older adults have less efficient reserves and may take longer to recover postoperatively. Be attentive to vital signs, intake and output, and mental status and note significant changes.
- Clients with dementia often experience an increase in confusion and agitation from the medications and anesthesia used during surgery. This poses a safety risk during the postoperative period and requires nursing staff to monitor these clients more frequently. It is important to maintain a calm, reassuring attitude. These changes are often long lasting, taking days or weeks to return to the preoperative level of cognition.
- Older adults may experience more fatigue and weakness after surgery. Encouraging activity is crucial, but it needs to be paced to prevent exhaustion.
- When surgery is done on an outpatient basis, nurses should follow up with phone calls that evening and the next day to check on the client's condition and make sure that postoperative instructions were understood.

Incentive Spirometry

Incentive spirometers (Figure 37.3 ■), also referred to as *sustained maximal inspiration devices (SMIs)*, measure the flow of air inhaled through the mouthpiece and are used to:

- Improve pulmonary ventilation.
- Counteract the effects of anesthesia or hypoventilation.
- Loosen respiratory secretions.
- Facilitate respiratory gaseous exchange.
- Expand collapsed alveoli.

Incentive spirometers are designed to mimic natural sighing or yawning by encouraging the client to take long, slow, deep breaths. The two general types of spirometers are the flow-oriented spirometer and the volume-oriented spirometer.

The flow-oriented spirometer consists of one or more clear plastic chambers containing freely movable colored balls or disks. The ball or disks are elevated as the client inhales. The longer the inspiratory flow is maintained, the larger the volume, so the client is encouraged to take slow, deep breaths. This type of spirometer does not measure the specific volume of air inhaled.

Volume-oriented spirometers measure the inhalation volume inspired by the client. When the client inhales, a piston-like plate or accordion-pleated cylinder rises, and markings on the side indicate the volume of inspiration achieved.

When using an incentive spirometer, the client should be assisted into a position, preferably an upright sitting position in bed or on a chair that facilitates maximum ventilation. Client Teaching lists instructions for clients in the use of incentive spirometers.

The use of incentive spirometry has been a traditional component of postoperative nursing care but there is little research evidence to support its routine use. As a result, the American Association of Respiratory Therapists no longer recommends using incentive spirometry for routine, preventive use in postop clients. However, it may be used for clients who develop atelectasis with retained airway secretions (Armstrong, 2017, p. 54).

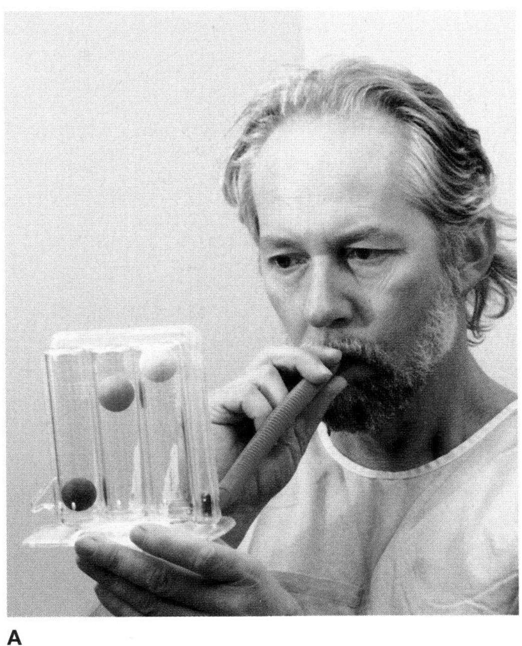

A

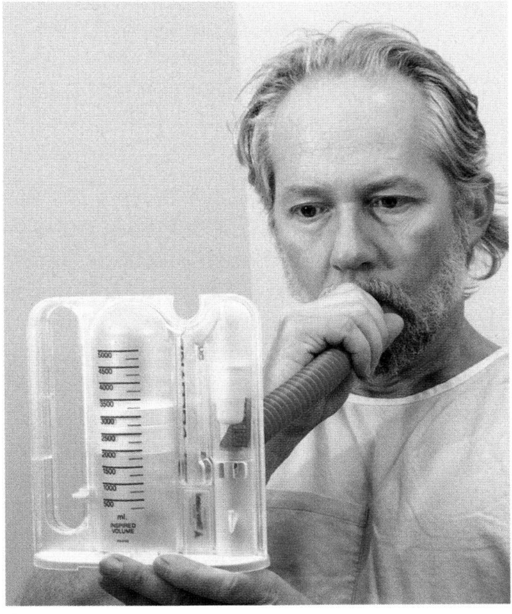

B

Figure 37.3 ■ *A*, Flow-oriented incentive spirometer; *B*, volume-oriented incentive spirometer.

CLIENT TEACHING **Using an Incentive Spirometer**

- Hold or place the spirometer in an upright position. A tilted *flow-oriented* device requires less effort to raise the balls or disks; a *volume-oriented* device will not function correctly unless upright.
- Exhale normally.
- Seal the lips tightly around the mouthpiece.
- Take in a slow, deep breath to elevate the balls or cylinder, and then hold the breath for 2 seconds initially, increasing to 6 seconds (optimal), to keep the balls or cylinder elevated if possible.
- For a flow-oriented device, avoid brisk, low-volume breaths that snap the balls to the top of the chamber. Greater lung expansion is achieved with a very slow inspiration than with a brisk, shallow breath, even though it may not elevate the balls or keep them elevated while you hold your breath. Sustained elevation of the balls or cylinder ensures adequate ventilation of the alveoli (lung air sacs).
- If you have difficulty breathing only through the mouth, a nose clip can be used.
- Remove the mouthpiece and exhale normally.
- Cough after the incentive effort. Deep ventilation may loosen secretions, and coughing can facilitate their removal.
- Relax and take several normal breaths before using the spirometer again.
- Repeat the procedure several times and then 4 or 5 times hourly. Practice increases inspiratory volume, maintains alveolar ventilation, and prevents atelectasis (collapse of the air sacs).
- Clean the mouthpiece with water and shake it dry.

EVIDENCE-BASED PRACTICE

Evidence-Based Practice

Is There a Difference in Perspectives on Incentive Spirometry Effectiveness and Use Between Nurses and Respiratory Therapists?

Incentive spirometry (IS) is ordered for clients at risk for postoperative pulmonary complications. In fact, 95% of U.S. hospitals report prescribing postop IS. There are no current guidelines or protocols for the use of IS. Of note are the numerous studies that have shown that IS alone is not adequate in reducing postoperative pulmonary complications. Additionally, there is little data indicating how IS should be used. As a result, Eltorai et al. (2018) decided to conduct an online survey of national nursing and respiratory care societies to evaluate healthcare professional viewpoints on the use of IS in their clinical practices, explore healthcare professionals' understanding of IS, determine the actual implementation of IS in client care, and explore differences between respiratory therapists and nurses.

There were 1681 respondents from four national organizations (three nursing and one respiratory care). The results of the survey indicated that the majority of healthcare professionals agreed on the following about IS: It is essential to client care, improves pulmonary function, helps to prevent and to reverse atelectasis, and helps to prevent and reverse pneumonia. It is as effective as early ambulation, deep breathing, and coughing; should be used routinely preoperatively and postoperatively; and should be used every hour, with an average of 9.6 breaths taken each session. In terms of use, 51% believed that achieving target inspiratory volume is the most important factor. Most respondents believed that they received adequate IS education and training. Finally, attitudes concerning IS indicated that the respiratory society respondents had significantly less agreement about the benefits and effectiveness of IS than the respondents from the nursing societies.

Implications

The researchers point out that the investigation has limitations. Ideally, survey responses would be collected from all nurses and respiratory therapists across the country. However, the researchers raise valid observations. For example, the respondents' strong opinions about the effectiveness of IS, in spite of supporting data, suggests that evidence is not being transferred into practice. Why is this? More investigation is needed in order to assess where these beliefs originate—in education, training, or experience. It is imperative that the clinical practice of healthcare professionals be driven by evidence and not opinion. The researchers also recommend further study to determine which specific client groups may benefit from IS, the costs of implementing IS, and optimal IS use protocols.

Leg Exercises

Encourage the client to do leg exercises taught in the preoperative period every 1 to 2 hours during waking hours. Muscle contractions compress the veins, preventing the stasis of blood in the veins, a cause of **thrombus** (stationary clot adhered to the wall of a vessel) formation and subsequent **thrombophlebitis** (inflammation of a vein followed by formation of a blood clot) and **emboli** (a blood clot that has moved). Contractions also promote arterial blood flow.

Moving and Ambulation

Encourage the client to turn from side to side at least every 2 hours. Alternate turning allows for each lung to be in the uppermost position, allowing for maximum lung expansion. Avoid placing pillows or rolls under the client's knees because pressure on the popliteal blood vessels can interfere with blood circulation to and from the lower extremities. Clients who practice turning before surgery usually find it easier to do after surgery.

The client should ambulate as soon as possible after surgery per the surgeon's orders. Generally clients begin ambulation the evening of the day of surgery or the first day after surgery, unless contraindicated. Early ambulation prevents respiratory, circulatory, urinary, and gastrointestinal complications. It also prevents general muscle weakness. Schedule ambulation for periods after the client has taken an analgesic or when the client is comfortable. Ambulation should be gradual, starting with the client sitting on the bed and dangling the feet over the side. A client who cannot ambulate is periodically assisted to a sitting position in bed, if allowed, and turned frequently. The sitting position permits the greatest lung expansion.

Hydration

Maintain IV infusions as ordered to replace body fluids lost either before or during surgery. When oral intake is permitted, initially offer only small sips of water. Large amounts of water can induce vomiting because anesthetics and narcotic analgesics temporarily inhibit the motility of the stomach. The client who cannot take fluids by mouth may be allowed by the surgeon's orders to suck ice chips. Provide mouth care and place mouthwash at the client's bedside. Postoperative clients often complain of thirst and a dry, sticky mouth. These discomforts are a result of the preoperative fasting period, preoperative medications (such as atropine), and loss of body fluid.

Measure the client's fluid intake and output for at least 2 days or until fluid balance is stable without an IV infusion. Ensuring adequate fluid balance is important. Sufficient fluids keep the respiratory mucous membranes and secretions moist, thus facilitating the expectoration of mucus during coughing. Also, an adequate fluid balance is important to maintain renal and cardiovascular function.

Urinary and Gastrointestinal Function

Anesthetic agents temporarily depress urinary bladder tone, which usually returns within 6 to 8 hours after surgery. Surgery in the pubic area, vagina, or rectum, during which the surgeon may manipulate the bladder, often causes urinary retention. Provide measures that promote urinary elimination; for example, help male clients stand at the bedside, or female clients to a bedside commode if allowed, and ensure that fluid intake is adequate. Determine whether the client has any difficulties voiding and assess the client for bladder distention. Report to the surgeon if a client does not void within 8 hours following surgery, unless another time frame is specified.

If all measures to promote voiding fail, a urinary catheterization is often ordered (see Chapter 47 ∞). Measure the fluid intake and output (I&O) of all new postoperative clients. Generally I&O records are kept for at least 2 days or until the client re-establishes fluid balance without an IV or catheter in place.

Anesthetic agents, handling of the intestines during abdominal surgery, fasting, opioids for pain management, and inactivity all inhibit bowel peristalsis. Most clients regain bowel function several hours after surgery except in pelvic or abdominal surgery where the return may be delayed for 24 to 48 hours or longer. Assess the return of peristalsis by auscultating the abdomen. Gurgling and rumbling sounds indicate peristalsis. Bowel sounds should be carefully assessed every 4 to 6 hours. Oral fluids and food are usually started after the return of peristalsis.

Diet

The surgeon orders the client's postoperative diet. Depending on the extent of surgery and the organs involved, the client may be allowed nothing by mouth for several days or may be able to resume oral intake when nausea is no longer present. When "diet as tolerated" is ordered, offer clear liquids initially. If the client tolerates these with no nausea, the diet can often progress to full liquids and then to a regular diet, provided that gastrointestinal functioning is normal. Assist very weak clients to eat. Observe the client's tolerance of the food and fluids ingested and note and report the passage of flatus or abdominal distention.

Suction

Some clients return from surgery with a gastric or intestinal tube in place and orders to connect the tube to suction. For more information about gastrointestinal tubes, see Chapter 46 ∞. The suction ordered can be continuous or intermittent. Intermittent suction is applied when a single-lumen gastric tube is used to reduce the risk of damaging the mucous membrane near the distal port of the tube. Continuous low suction (30–40 mmHg) or up to intermittent high suction (120 mmHg) may be applied if a Salem sump (double-lumen) tube is in place (Figure 37.4 ■) because the air vent lumen prevents excessive negative pressure from developing in the stomach (Smith, Duell, Martin, Aebersold, & Gonzalez, 2017, p. 656). Fluids and electrolytes must be replaced intravenously when gastric suction or continuous drainage is ordered. Nasogastric tubes may be irrigated if the lumen becomes clogged. They are generally irrigated before and after tube feedings or the instillation of medications. Nasogastric irrigation may require a primary care provider's order, particularly following gastrointestinal surgery. Skill 37.3 describes the management of gastrointestinal suction.

The surgeon orders the type and amount of suction. Most agencies have wall suction units available (Figure 37.5 ■). A suction regulator with a drainage receptacle connects to a wall outlet that provides negative pressure. Check the receptacle frequently to prevent excess drainage from interfering with the suction apparatus; empty or change the receptacle according to agency policy. Portable electric suction units or pumps (e.g., the Gomco pump) may be used in the home or when wall suction is not available.

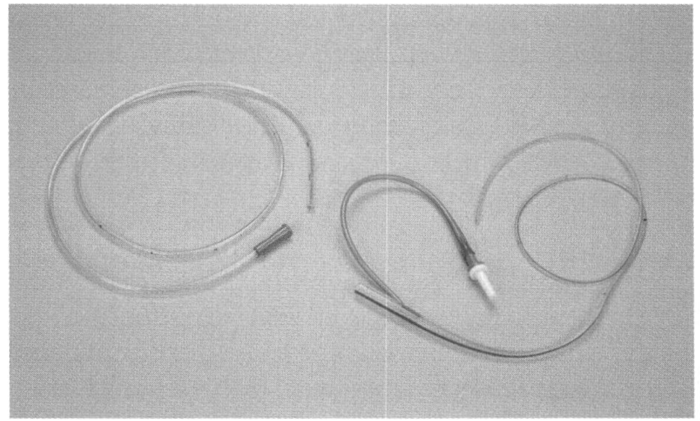

Figure 37.4 ■ Nasogastric tubes used for gastric decompression. *Left:* Levin (single-lumen) tube; *right:* Salem sump (double-lumen) tube with antireflux valve.

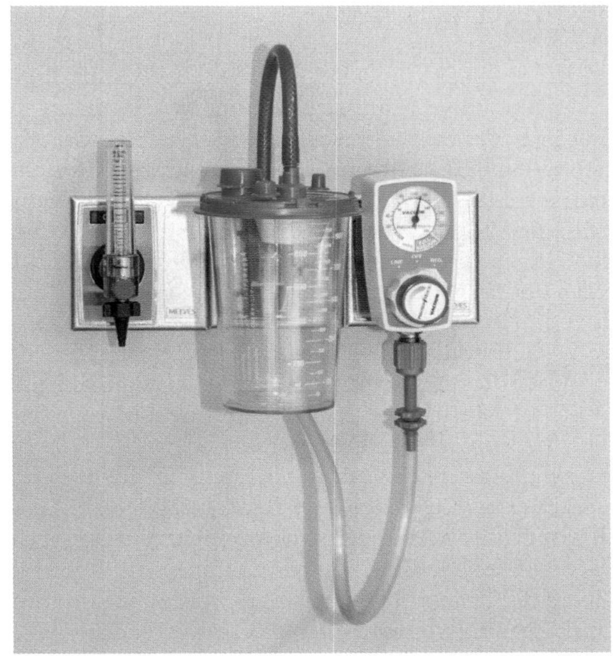

Figure 37.5 ■ Wall suction unit for generating negative pressure for nasogastric suction.

QSEN Patient-Centered Care: Gastrointestinal Suction

The nurse needs to instruct the caregiver of the client who needs gastrointestinal suction at home about the following:

- Maintain suction as ordered; do *not* increase or decrease the suction without instructions from the nurse or primary care provider.
- Offer mouth care every 2 hours.
- Avoid tension and pulling on the tube by securing it to the gown.
- Check the patency of the tube if nausea or vomiting occurs.
- Report an increasing amount of bloody drainage.

SKILL 37.3

Managing Gastrointestinal Suction

PURPOSES

- To relieve abdominal distention
- To maintain gastric decompression after surgery
- To remove blood and secretions from the gastrointestinal tract
- To relieve discomfort (e.g., when a client has a bowel obstruction)
- To maintain the patency of the nasogastric tube

ASSESSMENT

Assess

- Presence of abdominal distention on palpation
- Bowel sounds
- Abdominal discomfort
- Vital signs for baseline data
- Amount and characteristics of drainage

PLANNING

Before initiating gastric suction, determine (a) whether the suction is continuous or intermittent, (b) the ordered suction pressure, and (c) whether there is an order to irrigate the gastrointestinal tube and, if so, the type of solution to use.

Assignment

Managing gastrointestinal suction requires application of knowledge and problem-solving and is not assigned to AP. The AP, however, can assist with emptying the drainage receptacle and reporting changes in amount and color of the drainage to the nurse.

Equipment

Initiating Suction

- Gastrointestinal tube in place in the client
- Basin
- 60-mL syringe with an adapter
- Stethoscope
- Suction device for either continuous or intermittent suction
- Connector and connecting tubing
- Clean gloves

Maintaining Suction

- Graduated container as required to measure gastric drainage
- Basin of water
- Cotton-tipped applicators
- Ointment or lubricant
- Clean gloves

Irrigation

- Clean gloves
- Stethoscope
- Disposable irrigating set containing a sterile 50-mL syringe, moisture-resistant pad, basin, and graduated container
- Sterile normal saline (500 mL) or the ordered solution

IMPLEMENTATION

Performance

1. Prior to performing the procedure, introduce self and verify the client's identity using agency protocol. Explain to the client what you are going to do, why it is necessary, and how to participate. Discuss the purpose(s) of the gastrointestinal suction.
2. Perform hand hygiene and observe other appropriate infection prevention procedures.
3. Provide for client privacy.

Initiating Suction

4. Position the client appropriately.
   - Assist the client to a semi-Fowler's position if it is not contraindicated. **Rationale:** *In the semi-Fowler's position, the tube is not as likely to lie against the wall of the stomach and will therefore suction most efficiently. The semi-Fowler's position also prevents reflux of gastric contents, which could lead to aspiration.*
5. Confirm that the tube is in the stomach.
   - Apply clean gloves.
   - Check agency protocol for preferred methods to verify placement because clinical practice varies across health regions:
     a. The method of inserting air into the tube with the syringe and listening with a stethoscope over the stomach (just below the xiphoid process) for a swish of air is often used at the bedside; however, a similar gurgling sound can be heard when the tube is incorrectly placed in the lungs or esophagus and evidence does *not* support this practice.
     b. Aspirate to obtain stomach contents. Secretions from the stomach are usually greenish but can be colorless with shreds of mucus. Distinguishing between respiratory and gastric secretions is subjective.
        - Check the acidity of gastric aspirate using a pH test strip. Gastric secretions often have a pH of 5 or less. The pH of the aspirate will increase if the client is on acid-inhibiting medication.
     c. X-ray examination is considered the gold standard for determining placement, especially for high-risk clients (e.g., critically ill, dysphagic, or unconscious).
     d. Use other methods in accordance with agency protocol. See Chapter 46 ∞, Skill 46.1.
   - Remove and discard gloves.
   - Perform hand hygiene.
6. Set and check the suction.
   - Connect the appropriate suction regulator to the wall suction outlet and the collection device to the regulator. The primary care provider orders the type and setting of suction. Check the suction level by occluding the drainage tube and observing the regulator dial during a suction cycle.
   - If using a portable suction machine, turn on the machine and regulate the suction as above. The Gomco pump has two settings: low intermittent for single-lumen tubes, and high for double-lumen tubes.
7. Establish gastric suction.
   - Connect the gastrointestinal tube to the tubing from the suction by using the connector.
   - If a Salem sump tube is in place, connect the larger lumen to the suction equipment. This double-lumen tube has a smaller tube (blue pigtail) running inside the primary suction tube. **Rationale:** *The smaller tube provides a continuous flow of atmospheric air through the drainage tube at its distal end and prevents excessive suction force on the gastric mucosa at the drainage outlets. Damage to the gastric mucosa is thus avoided.*

Managing Gastrointestinal Suction—*continued*

- Always keep the air vent tube (blue pigtail) of a Salem sump tube open and above the level of the stomach when suction is applied. **Rationale:** *Closing the vent would stop the sump action and cause mucosal damage. Keeping the end of the air vent tube higher than the stomach prevents reflux of gastric contents into the air lumen of the tube.*
- After suction is applied, watch the tubing for a few minutes until the gastric contents appear to be running through the tubing into the receptacle. A Salem sump tube makes a soft, hissing sound when it is functioning correctly.
- If the suction is not working properly, check that all connections are tight and that the tubing is not kinked.
- Coil and pin the tubing to the client's gown so that it does not loop below the suction bottle. **Rationale:** *If the tubing falls below the suction bottle, the suction may be obstructed because of the pressure required to push the fluid against gravity.*

8. Assess the drainage.

- Observe the amount, color, odor, and consistency of the drainage. Normal gastric drainage has a mucoid (resembling mucus) consistency and is either colorless or yellow-green because of the presence of bile. A coffee-ground color and consistency may indicate bleeding.
- Test the gastric drainage for pH and blood when indicated. A client who has had gastrointestinal surgery can be expected to have some blood in the drainage.

Maintaining Suction

9. Assess the client and the suction system regularly.

- Assess the client every 30 minutes until the system is running effectively and then every 2 hours, or as the client's health indicates, to ensure that the suction is functioning properly. If the client complains of fullness, nausea, or epigastric pain or if the flow of gastric secretions is absent in the tubing or in the collection bottle, ineffective suctioning or blockage of the nasogastric tube is likely.
- Inspect the suction system for patency of the system (e.g., kinks or blockages in the tubing) and tightness of the connections. **Rationale:** *Loose connections can permit air to enter and thus decrease the effectiveness of the suction by decreasing the negative pressure.*

10. Relieve blockages if present.

- Perform hand hygiene.
- Apply clean gloves.
- Check the suction equipment. To do this, disconnect the nasogastric tube from the suction over a basin (to collect gastric drainage), and then, with the suction on, place the end of the suction tubing in a basin of water. If water is drawn into the drainage bottle, the suction equipment is functioning properly, but the nasogastric tube is either blocked or positioned incorrectly.
- Reposition the client (e.g., to the other side) if permitted. **Rationale:** *This may facilitate drainage.*
- Rotate the nasogastric tube and reposition it. This step is *contraindicated* for clients with gastric surgery. **Rationale:** *Moving the tube may interfere with gastric sutures.*
- Irrigate the nasogastric tube as agency protocol states or on the order of the primary care provider (see steps 14 to 16).
- Remove and discard gloves.
- Perform hand hygiene.

11. Prevent reflux into the blue pigtail vent lumen of a Salem sump tube. **Rationale:** *Reflux of gastric contents into the vent lumen may occur when stomach pressure exceeds atmospheric pressure. In this situation, gastric contents follow the path of least resistance and flow out the vent lumen rather than the drainage lumen.*

To prevent reflux:

- Place the vent tubing higher than the client's stomach to prevent gastric fluid backup into the blue lumen air vent.
- Keep the drainage lumen free of particulate matter that may obstruct the lumen (see steps 14 to 16 for irrigating a nasogastric tube).

12. Ensure client comfort.

- Clean the client's nostrils as needed, using the cotton-tipped applicators and water. Apply a water-soluble lubricant or ointment.
- Provide mouth care every 2 to 4 hours and as needed. Some postoperative clients are permitted to suck ice chips or a moist cloth to maintain the moisture of the oral mucous membranes.

13. Change the drainage receptacle according to agency policy.

- Clamp the nasogastric tube and turn off the suction.
- Apply clean gloves.
- If the receptacle is graduated, determine the amount of drainage.
- Disconnect the receptacle.
- Inspect the drainage carefully for color, consistency, and presence of substances (e.g., blood clots).
- Replace a full receptacle and attach it to the suction. Check agency policy if can reuse the same receptacle.
- Turn on the suction and unclamp the nasogastric tube.
- Observe the system for several minutes to make sure function is reestablished.
- Remove and discard gloves.
- Perform hand hygiene.
- Go to step 17.

Irrigating a Gastrointestinal Tube

14. Prepare the client and the equipment.

- Place the moisture-resistant pad under the end of the gastrointestinal tube.
- Turn off the suction.
- Apply clean gloves.
- Disconnect the gastrointestinal tube from the connector.
- Determine that the tube is in the stomach. See step 5. **Rationale:** *This ensures that the irrigating solution enters the client's stomach.*

15. Irrigate the tube.

- Draw up the ordered volume of irrigating solution in the syringe; 30 mL of solution per instillation is usual, but up to 60 mL may be given per instillation if ordered.
- Attach the syringe to the nasogastric tube and slowly inject the solution.
- Gently aspirate the solution. **Rationale:** *Forceful withdrawal could damage the gastric mucosa.*
- If you encounter difficulty in withdrawing the solution, inject 20 mL of air and aspirate again, or reposition the client or the nasogastric tube. **Rationale:** *Air and repositioning may move the end of the tube away from the stomach wall.* If aspirating difficulty continues, reattach the tube and set to intermittent low suction, and notify the nurse in charge.
- Repeat the preceding steps until the ordered amount of solution is used.
- *Note:* The blue lumen with a blue pigtail is NOT to be used for irrigation. However, if the vent lumen is blocked and requires flushing, after the flush, the pigtail should be cleared with an injection of 20 mL of air.

16. Re-establish suction.

- Reconnect the nasogastric tube to suction.
- If a Salem sump tube is used, inject the air vent lumen with 10 mL of air after reconnecting the tube to suction. **Rationale:** *This tests the patency of the vent and ensures sump functioning.*

Continued on page 986

SKILL 37.3

Managing Gastrointestinal Suction—*continued*

- Observe the system for several minutes to make sure it is functioning.
- Remove and discard gloves.
- Perform hand hygiene.

17. Document all relevant information.

- Record the time suction was started. Also record the pressure established, the color and consistency of the drainage, and nursing assessments.
- During maintenance, record assessments, supportive nursing measures, and data about the suction system.
- When irrigating the tube, record verification of tube placement; the time of the irrigation; the amount and type of irrigating solution used; the amount, color, and consistency of the returns; the patency of the system following the irrigation; and nursing assessments.

SAMPLE DOCUMENTATION

3/20/2020 1300 Returned from PACU. Salem sump tube in place and connected to low continuous suction. Checked for correct placement. Draining small to moderate amount of tannish fluid. R. Martinez, RN

EVALUATION

- Conduct appropriate follow-up such as relief of abdominal distention or discomfort, bowel sounds, character and amount of gastric drainage, integrity of nares, hydration of oral mucous membranes, patency of tube, and system functioning.
- Compare to previous findings if available.
- Report significant deviations from normal to the primary care provider.

Home Care Teaching

To ensure continuity of care and restoration of the client's health, nurses must meet the learning needs of clients and their support people. Adults want information about how their surgery and recovery period may affect activities they normally perform while recovering at home. Teaching should focus on actions to maintain comfort, to promote healing and restore wellness, and to make use of appropriate community agencies and other sources of help.

Maintaining Comfort

- Instruct the client to use pain medications as ordered, not allowing pain to become severe before taking the prescribed dose.
- If not contraindicated, discuss the use of OTC analgesics such as aspirin or acetaminophen as postoperative pain becomes less severe or if the client is reluctant to use prescription drugs due to side effects.
- Teach the client to avoid using alcohol or other central nervous system depressants while taking opioid analgesics.
- Teach the client to use nonpharmacologic measures to help manage pain, such as conscious relaxation, distraction, meditation, or visualization.
- Emphasize the importance of paying attention to increasing pain or discomfort. Instruct the client to contact the primary care provider if pain increases after a period of decreasing discomfort.
- Discuss the importance of gradually resuming activities, avoiding overexertion.
- Constipation occurs frequently as a result of decreased gastrointestinal mobility due to many causes (e.g., anesthesia, decreased activity, pain medications). Discuss strategies to prevent constipation.

Promoting Healing

- If indicated, teach the client how to change wound dressings and perform wound care. Discuss the signs and symptoms of infection and when to notify the surgeon.
- Emphasize the importance of hygiene and hand washing to prevent infections.
- Check with the surgeon regarding bathing because some prefer the wound to be kept dry. There is no evidence that water on a closed wound is harmful or interferes with wound healing. If allowed, inform the client to shower, letting the warm water wash over the incision, and to gently pat the incision dry.
- Discuss any prescribed activity restrictions such as avoiding lifting. Be specific about weight limits, if appropriate. Relate the weight limit to everyday items (e.g., a gallon of milk weighs approximately 8 pounds).
- Advise the client that he or she will tire easily and to plan short activities with frequent rest breaks.
- Intimacy such as gentle hugging and kissing is allowed for clients when they feel like it. Full sexual intercourse cannot be resumed until wound soreness and tenderness are resolved, approximately 2 to 4 weeks. Check with the surgeon for gynecologic procedures.
- Discuss the importance of keeping follow-up appointments to monitor healing and recovery after surgery.

Restoring Wellness

- Discuss the relationship of increasing activities to restoring wellness and promoting a sense of well-being.
- Teach the client that surgery and stressors can depress immune function and to avoid exposure to illness (e.g., crowded areas and people with upper respiratory illnesses) whenever possible.
- Emphasize the importance of adequate rest for healing and immune function.
- If appropriate, discuss lifestyle changes to promote wellness, such as smoking cessation, increasing activity level, reducing stress, and consuming a healthy diet high in fruits, vegetables, and whole grains with adequate protein to promote healing. Eat small portions at first because anesthesia and pain medications slow gastric emptying.

Community Agencies and Other Sources of Help

- Provide information about where durable medical equipment can be purchased, rented, or obtained free of charge; how to access home health and other services; and where to obtain supplies such as dressings or nutritional supplements.
- Suggest additional sources of information, such as the National Rehabilitation Information Center, Reach to Recovery, and United Ostomy Association.

Referrals

The nurse needs to consider appropriate referrals for the client, such as:

- Home health agencies for wound care and assessment and for assistance with ADLs if necessary
- Community social services for assistance in obtaining medical and assistive equipment
- Respiratory, physical, or occupational therapy services as indicated.

Evaluating

Using the goals developed during the planning stage, the nurse collects data to evaluate whether the identified goals and desired outcomes have been achieved. If the desired outcomes are not achieved, the nurse and client, and support people, if appropriate, need to explore the reasons before modifying the care plan. For example, if the outcome "Pain control" is not met, questions to be considered include:

- What is the client's perception of the problem?
- Does the client understand how to use PCA?
- Is the prescribed analgesic dose adequate for the client?
- Is the client allowing pain to become intense prior to requesting medication or using PCA?
- Where is the client's pain? Could it be due to a problem unrelated to surgery (e.g., chronic arthritis, anginal pain)?
- Is there evidence of a complication that could cause increased pain (an infection, abscess, or hematoma)?

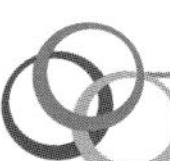

Critical Thinking Checkpoint

Mr. Teng is a 77-year-old client with a history of COPD. Currently his respiratory condition is being controlled with medications and he is free of infection. He has just been transferred to the PACU following a hernia repair performed under spinal anesthesia. His blood pressure is 132/88 mmHg, pulse 84 beats/min, respirations 28/min, and tympanic temperature 36.5°C (97.8°F). He is awake and stable.

1. What factors place Mr. Teng at increased risk for the development of complications during and after surgery?
2. Speculate about why Mr. Teng's surgeon and anesthesiologist decided to perform Mr. Teng's surgery under regional anesthesia as opposed to general anesthesia.
3. What preparations were taken during the preoperative period to protect Mr. Teng from possible complications during and after his surgery?
4. How will Mr. Teng's postoperative assessments differ from those of a client who received general anesthesia?
5. What postoperative precautions are especially important to Mr. Teng in view of his chronic lung condition?

Answers to Critical Thinking Checkpoint questions are available on the faculty resources site. Please consult with your instructor.

Chapter 37 Review

CHAPTER HIGHLIGHTS

- Surgery is a unique experience that creates stress and necessitates physical and psychologic changes.
- The perioperative period includes three phases: preoperative, intraoperative, and postoperative.
- Surgical procedures are categorized by purpose, degree of urgency, and degree of risk.
- Factors such as age, general health, nutritional status, presence of sleep apnea, medication use, and mental status affect a client's risk during surgery.
- Clients must agree to surgery via informed consent and sign a consent form.
- Nursing history and physical assessment data are important sources for planning preoperative and postoperative care.
- The overall goal of nursing care during the preoperative phase is to prepare the client mentally and physically for surgery.
- Preoperative teaching includes situational information such as expected sensations and discomfort, psychosocial support, the role of the client throughout the perioperative period, and training for the postoperative period. Many aspects of preoperative teaching are intended to prevent postoperative complications.
- Preoperative teaching should include moving, leg exercises, and deep-breathing and coughing exercises.
- Physical preparation includes the following areas: nutrition and fluids, elimination, hygiene, medications, sleep, care of valuables and prostheses, special orders, and surgical skin preparation.
- A preoperative checklist provides a guide to and documentation of a client's preparation before surgery.
- Antiemboli stockings or sequential compression devices may be ordered for some clients to facilitate venous return.
- Maintaining the client's safety and homeostasis are the overall goals of nursing care during the intraoperative phase.
- Anesthesia may be general or regional. Regional anesthesia includes topical, local, nerve block, spinal anesthesia (subarachnoid block), and epidural.

- A surgical skin preparation should be carried out as close to the time of surgery as possible and is also performed during the intraoperative phase.
- Positioning of the client during surgery is important to reduce the risk of pressure injury and nerve damage.
- Immediate postanesthetic care focuses on assessment and monitoring parameters to prevent complications from anesthesia or surgery.
- Initial and ongoing assessment of the postoperative client includes level of consciousness; vital signs, including oxygen saturation; skin color and temperature; comfort; fluid balance; and dressings, bedclothes, drains, and tubes.
- Ongoing postoperative nursing interventions include (a) managing pain, (b) appropriate positioning, (c) encouraging incentive spirometry and deep-breathing and coughing exercises, (d) promoting leg exercises and early ambulation, (e) maintaining adequate hydration and nutritional status, (f) promoting urinary elimination, and (g) continuing gastrointestinal suction.

TEST YOUR KNOWLEDGE

1. A nurse is obtaining preoperative assessment data. Which of the following should be included? Select all that apply.
   1. Current health status
   2. Allergies
   3. Current medications
   4. Mental status
   5. Previous surgeries

2. A client who is having a mastectomy expresses sadness about losing her breast. Based on this information, the nurse would identify that the client is at risk for which nursing diagnosis?
   1. Altered body image
   2. Grieving
   3. Fear
   4. Impaired coping

3. A nurse is preparing to conduct preoperative teaching. What should be included?
   1. Information related to what will happen to the client
   2. Referral of the client to the physician for any misconceptions the client may have
   3. The role of the nurse during surgery
   4. How to perform ADLs following surgery

4. The nurse assesses a postoperative client who has a rapid, weak pulse; urine output of less than 30 mL/h; and decreased blood pressure. The client's skin is cool and clammy. What complication should the nurse suspect?
   1. Thrombophlebitis
   2. Hypovolemic shock
   3. Pneumonia
   4. Wound dehiscence

5. The client is most likely to require the greatest amount of analgesia for pain during which period?
   1. Immediately after surgery
   2. 4 hours after surgery
   3. 12 to 36 hours after surgery
   4. 48 to 60 hours after surgery

6. A postop client who had abdominal surgery is holding a pillow against his abdomen during deep-breathing and coughing exercises. What term does the nurse use to describe this technique? ________

7. A nurse is caring for a client in the recovery area. Which position should the unconscious client be placed while in the immediate postanesthesia phase?
   1. Supine
   2. Prone
   3. Side-lying
   4. Supine with a pillow under the head

8. The client's postoperative orders state "diet as tolerated." The client has been NPO. The nurse will advance the client's diet to clear liquids based on which assessment? Select all that apply.
   1. Does not complain of nausea or vomiting
   2. Pain level is maintained at a rating of 2–3 out of 10
   3. States passing flatus
   4. Ambulates with minimal assistance
   5. Expresses feeling "hungry"

9. The overall goal of nursing care during the intraoperative phase is the client's ________.

10. Which of the following actions can the nurse assign to assistive personnel (AP)? Select all that apply.
   1. Teaching preoperative information
   2. Managing GI suction
   3. Reinforcing preoperative teaching
   4. Reapplying antiemboli stockings
   5. Emptying GI suction drainage

See Answers to Test Your Knowledge in Appendix A.

READINGS AND REFERENCES

Suggested Readings

Bruckenthal, P., & Simpson, M. H. (2016). The role of the perioperative nurse in improving surgical patients' clinical outcomes and satisfaction: Beyond medication. *AORN Journal*, *104*(Suppl. 6), S17–S22. doi:10.1016/j.aorn.2016.10.013

This article reviews the management of postsurgical pain and includes postsurgical pain assessment, facilitating recovery from surgery, and increasing client satisfaction during the postsurgical period.

Campbell, Y. N., Machan, M. D., & Fisher, M. (2016). The Jehovah's Witness population: Considerations for preoperative optimization of hemoglobin. *AANA Journal*, *84*, 173–178.

The purpose of this article is to clarify the current beliefs of Jehovah's Witnesses regarding receiving blood products, review ethical and legal considerations, and examine transfusion alternatives.

Related Research

Briggs, P., Hawrylack, H., & Mooney, R. (2016). Inhaled peppermint oil for postop nausea in patients undergoing cardiac surgery. *Nursing*, *46*(7), 61–67. doi:10.1097/01.NURSE.0000482882.38607.5c

George, S., Leasure, A. R., & Horstmanshof, D. (2016). Effectiveness of decolonization with chlorhexidine and mupirocin in reducing surgical site infections: A systematic review. *Dimensions of Critical Care Nursing*, *35*, 204–222. doi:10.1097/DCC.0000000000000192

Kurnat-Thoma, E. L., Roberts, M. M., & Corcoran, E. B. (2016). Perioperative heat loss prevention: A feasibility trial. *AORN Journal*, *104*, 307–319. doi:10.1016/j.aorn.2016.07.012

References

Adams, M. P., Holland, L. N., & Urban, C. Q. (2020). *Pharmacology for nurses: A pathophysiologic approach* (6th ed.). Hoboken, NJ: Pearson.

Aldrete, J. A., & Kroulik, D. (1970). A postanesthetic recovery score. *Anesthesia and Analgesia*, *49*(6), 924–934.

Armstrong, C. O. (2017). Post-op incentive spirometry: Why, when, & how. *Nursing*, *47*(6), 54–57. doi:10.1097/01.NURSE.0000516223.16649.02

Bashaw, M. A., & Keister, K. J. (2019). Perioperative strategies for surgical site infection prevention. *AORN Journal*, *109*, 68–78. doi:10.1002/aorn.12451

Campbell, Y. N., Machan, M. D., & Fisher, M. (2016). The Jehovah's Witness population: Considerations for preoperative optimization of hemoglobin. *AANA Journal*, *84*, 173–178.

Chou, R., Gordon, D. B., de Leon-Casasola, O. A., Rosenberg, J. M., Bickler, S., Brennan, T. . . . Wu, C. L. (2016). Management of postoperative pain: A clinical practice guideline from the American Pain Society, the American Society of Regional Anesthesia and Pain Medicine, and the American Society of Anesthesiologists' Committee on Regional Anesthesia, Executive Committee, and Administrative Council. *The Journal of Pain*, *17*(2), 131–157. doi:10.1016/j.jpain.2015.12.008

Dunn, D. (2016). Body art and the perioperative process. *AORN Journal*, *104*, 327–337. doi:10.1016/j.aorn.2016.07.011

Eltorai, A. E. M., Baird, G. L., Eltorai, A. S., Pangborn, J., Antoci, V., Cullen, H. A., . . . Daniels, A. H. (2018). Perspectives on incentive spirometry utility and patient protocols. *Respiratory Care*, *63*(5), 519–531. doi:10.4187/respcare.05872

Greenwood, J. (2017). Anesthetic implications of obesity and obstructive sleep apnea. *Annual Review of Nursing Research*, *35*, 17–35. doi:10.1891/0739-6686.35.17

Harrelson, B. R., & Fencl, J. L. (2016). Care of the surgical patient with obstructive sleep apnea. *AORN Journal*, *103*, 433–437. doi:10.1016/j.aorn.2016.02.004

The Joint Commission. (2019). *National Patient Safety Goals effective January 2019—hospital accreditation program.* Retrieved from https://www.jointcommission.org/assets/1/6/NPSG_Chapter_HAP_Jan2019.pdf

Manworren, R. C., Gordon, D. B., & Montgomery, R. (2018). Managing postoperative pain. *American Journal of Nursing*, *118*(1), 36–43. doi:10.1097/01.NAJ.0000529695.38192.67

Practice guidelines for preoperative fasting and the use of pharmacologic agents to reduce the risk of pulmonary aspiration: Application to healthy patients undergoing elective procedures: An updated report by the American Society of Anesthesiologists Task Force on Preoperative Fasting and the Use of Pharmacologic Agents to Reduce the Risk of Pulmonary Aspiration. (2017). *Anesthesiology*, *126*, 376–393. doi:10.1097/ALN.0000000000001452

Pusey-Reid, E. (2018). Patient readiness for PACU discharge. *Nursing Critical Care*, *13*(5), 31–34. doi:10.1097/01.CCN.0000544399.76592.be

Rightmyer, J., & Singbartl, K. (2016). Preventing perioperative hypothermia. *Nursing*, *46*(9), 57–60. doi:10.1097/01.NURSE.0000482266.09262.a9

Smith, S. F., Duell, D. J., Martin, B. C., Aebersold, M. L., & Gonzalez, L. (2017). *Clinical nursing skills* (9th ed.). Hoboken, NJ: Pearson.

Smith, F. D. (2016). Caring for surgical patients with piercings. *AORN Journal*, *103*, 584–593. doi:10.1016/j.aorn.2016.04.005

Spruce, L. (2017). Back to basics: Preventing perioperative pressure injuries. *AORN Journal*, *105*, 92–99. doi:10.1016/j.aorn.2016.10.018

Williams, R., Williams, M., Stanton, M. P., & Spence, D. (2017). Implementation of an obstructive sleep apnea screening program at an overseas military hospital. *AANA Journal*, *85*(1), 42–48.

Selected Bibliography

Dunn, N., & Ramos, R. (2017). Preventing venous thromboembolism: The role of nursing with intermittent pneumatic compression. *American Journal of Critical Care*, *26*(2), 164–167. doi:10.4037/ajcc2017504

du Plessis, M. (2016). Interventions for treating inadvertent postoperative hypothermia. *Journal of Perioperative Practice*, *26*(7–8), 158–159.

Hawker, R. J., McKillop, A., & Jacobs, S. (2017). Postanesthesia scoring methods: An integrative review of the literature. *Journal of PeriAnesthesia Nursing*, *32*(6), 557–572. doi:10.1016/j.jopan.2016.10.007

Kreutzer, L., Minami, C., & Yang, A. (2016). Preventing venous thromboembolism after surgery. *JAMA*, *315*(19), 2136. doi:10.1001/jama.2016.1457

Poulsen, M. J., & Coto, J. (2018). Nursing music protocol and postoperative pain. *Pain Management Nursing*, *19*(2), 172–176. doi:10.1016/j.pmn.2017.09.003

Powers, J. (2017). Changing guidelines for preoperative fasting. *Critical Care Nurse*, *37*(1), 76–77. doi:10.4037/ccn2017424

Rose, M., & Newman, S. D. (2016). Factors influencing patient safety during postoperative handover. *AANA Journal*, *84*(5), 329–338.

Spence, D. L., Han, T., McGuire, J., & Couture, D. (2015). Obstructive sleep apnea and the adult perioperative patient. *Journal of PeriAnesthesia Nursing*, *30*(6), 528–545. doi:10.1016/j.jopan.2014.07.014

Tocco, S., Martin, B., & Stacy, K. M. (2016). Preventing venous thromboembolism in adults. *Critical Care Nurse*, *36*(5), e20–e23. doi:10.4037/ccn2016638

Vo, H., Clayton, E., & Stolyarskaya, J. (2018). Opioid and non-opioid analgesia during surgery: Understanding how and why anesthesia providers select analgesic agents. *American Nurse Today*, *13*(5), 14–18.

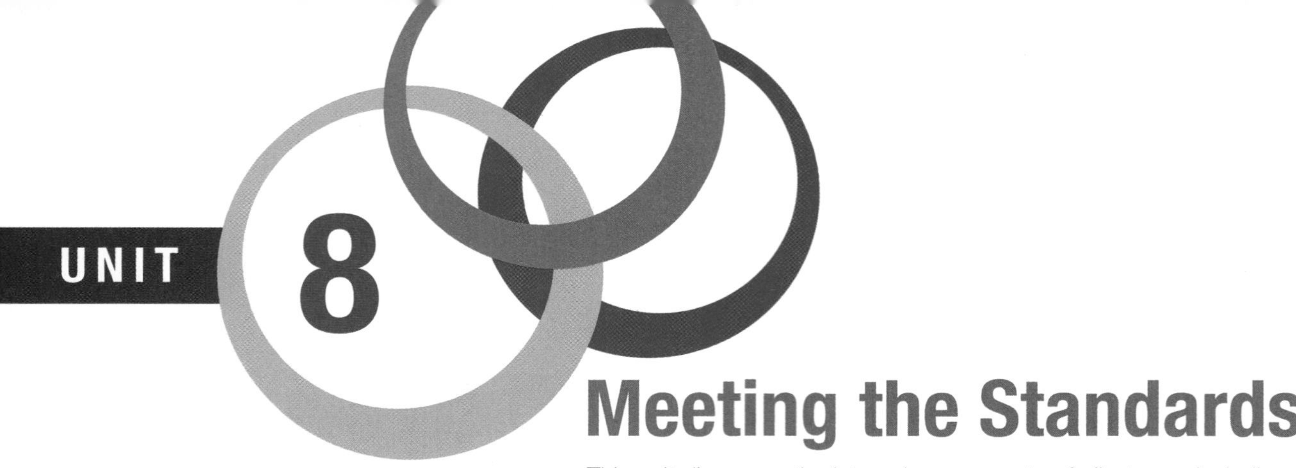

Meeting the Standards

This unit discusses the integral components of client care including asepsis, safety, hygiene, diagnostic testing, and medications, as well as skin and wound care, and care of the perioperative client. Knowledge of safety and asepsis guides every action taken by the nurse when providing client care, including administration of medications, diagnostic testing, wound care, and perioperative care.

CLIENT: Fay AGE: 36
CURRENT MEDICAL DIAGNOSES: Fractured Right Arm and Left Leg, Multiple Abrasions

Medical History: Fay was involved in a motor vehicle crash resulting in a fractured right arm, fractured left leg, and multiple abrasions and lacerations. Her right arm was set by closed reduction, and a synthetic cast was applied with a window cut over the forearm to monitor healing of a laceration requiring multiple sutures. She is taken to surgery where pins are placed in her left femur. She has no other significant health conditions. The prognosis is that she will require physical therapy to regain the ability to walk.

Personal and Social History: Fay lives alone, has no children, and her parents died more than 10 years ago. She has no siblings. She is employed as a high school mathematics teacher and lives in a third-floor walk-up apartment. She is right-hand dominant and concerned about how she will function with her right arm in a cast. She has many friends who visit throughout the day and receives many phone calls from her students and coworkers.

Questions

American Nurses Association Standard of Professional Performance #1 *is Assessment: The registered nurse collects pertinent data and information relative to the healthcare consumer's health or the situation.*

1. To assist Fay in meeting her hygiene needs, what questions will you want to ask in order to collect appropriate data for planning her care?
2. What important assessment data related to her risk for infection will be required to serve as baseline data for comparison purposes throughout her admission?
3. What are the nurse's priority assessments during the immediate postoperative period when Fay first returns to the unit after open reduction of her left leg fracture?

American Nurses Association Standard of Professional Performance #2 *is Diagnosis: The registered nurse analyzes the assessment data to determine actual or potential diagnoses, problems, and issues.*

4. Identify one actual and one potential for nursing diagnosis for Fay related to wound care, safety, and asepsis.
5. How do treatments, including medications, typically used with clients who have fractures influence your choice of diagnoses?

American Nurses Association. (2015). *Nursing: Scope and standards of practice* (3rd ed.). Silver Spring, MD: Author.

Answers to Meeting the Standards questions are available on the faculty resources site. Please consult with your instructor.

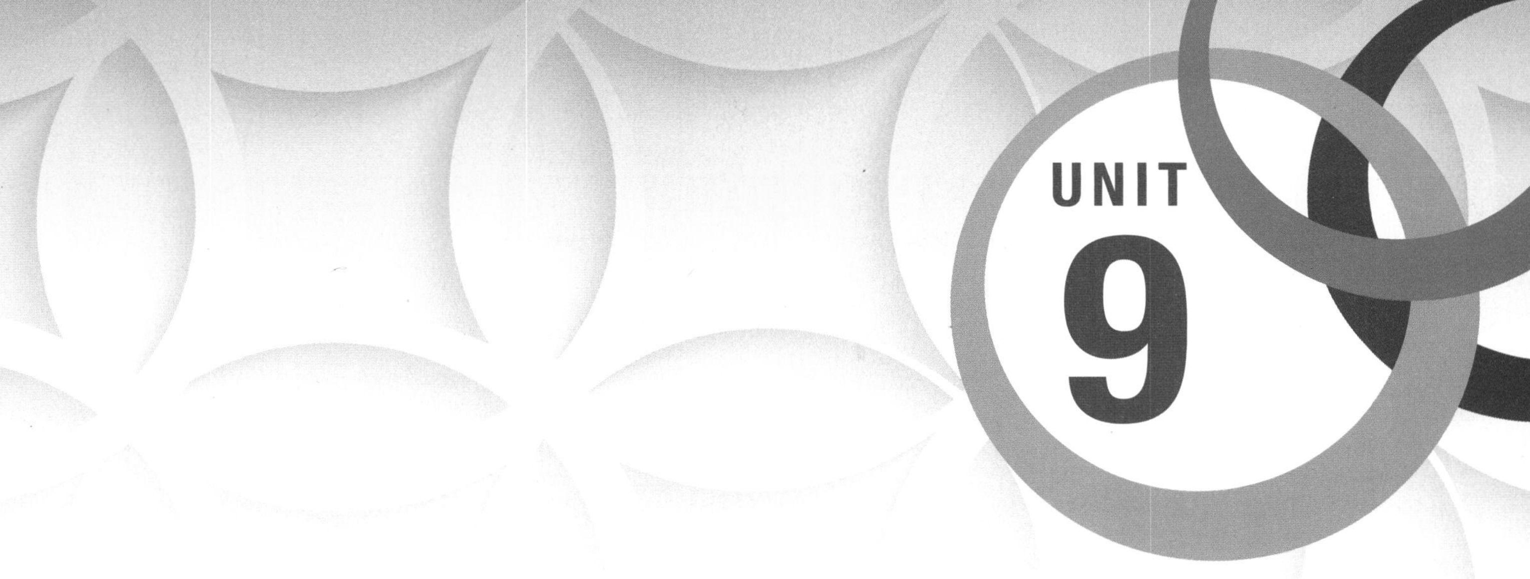

Promoting Psychosocial Health

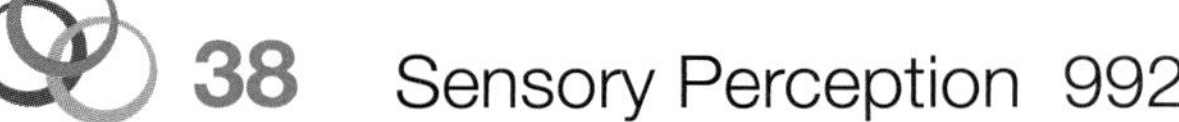

38 Sensory Perception

LEARNING OUTCOMES

After completing this chapter, you will be able to:

1. Discuss the components of the sensory-perception process.
2. Describe factors that influence sensory function.
3. Identify clinical signs and symptoms of sensory deprivation and overload.
4. Describe essential components in assessing a client's sensory-perception function.
5. Discuss factors that place a client at risk for sensory disturbances.
6. Develop nursing diagnoses and outcome criteria for clients with impaired sensory function.
7. Discuss nursing interventions to promote and maintain sensory function.
8. Identify strategies to promote a therapeutic environment for the client with acute confusion or delirium.

KEY TERMS

acute confusion, *1005*
auditory, *992*
awareness, *993*
chronic confusion, *1005*
cultural care deprivation, *994*
cultural deprivation, *994*
delirium, *1005*
dementia, *1005*
gustatory, *992*
kinesthetic, *992*
olfactory, *992*
sensoristasis, *993*
sensory deficit, *995*
sensory deprivation, *995*
sensory overload, *995*
sensory perception, *992*
sensory reception, *992*
stereognosis, *992*
tactile, *992*
visceral, *992*
visual, *992*

Introduction

An individual's senses are essential for growth, development, and survival. Sensory stimuli give meaning to events in the environment. Any alteration in individuals' sensory functions can affect their ability to function within the environment. For example, many clients have impaired sensory functions that put them at risk in the healthcare setting; nurses can help them find ways to function safely in this often confusing environment.

Components of the Sensory Experience

The sensory process involves two components: reception and perception. **Sensory reception** is the process of receiving stimuli or data. These stimuli are either external or internal to the body. External stimuli are **visual** (sight), **auditory** (hearing), **olfactory** (smell), **tactile** (touch), and **gustatory** (taste). Gustatory stimuli can be internal as well. Other types of internal stimuli are kinesthetic or visceral. **Kinesthetic** refers to awareness of the position and movement of body parts. For example, an individual walking is aware of which leg is forward. A related sense is **stereognosis**, the ability to perceive and understand an object through touch by its size, shape, and texture. For example, an individual holding a tennis ball is aware of its size, round shape, and soft surface without seeing it. **Visceral** refers to any large organ within the body. Visceral organs may produce stimuli that make an individual aware of them (e.g., a full stomach). **Sensory perception** involves the conscious organization and translation of the data or stimuli into meaningful information.

For an individual to be aware of the surroundings, four aspects of the sensory process must be present:

- ***Stimulus.*** This is an agent or act that stimulates a nerve receptor.
- ***Receptor.*** A nerve cell acts as a receptor by converting the stimulus to a nerve impulse. Most receptors are specific, that is, sensitive to only one type of stimulus, such as visual, auditory, or touch.
- ***Impulse conduction.*** The impulse travels along nerve pathways either to the spinal cord or directly to the brain (Figure 38.1 ■). For example, auditory impulses travel to the organ of Corti in the inner ear. From there the impulses travel along the eighth cranial nerve to the temporal lobe of the brain.

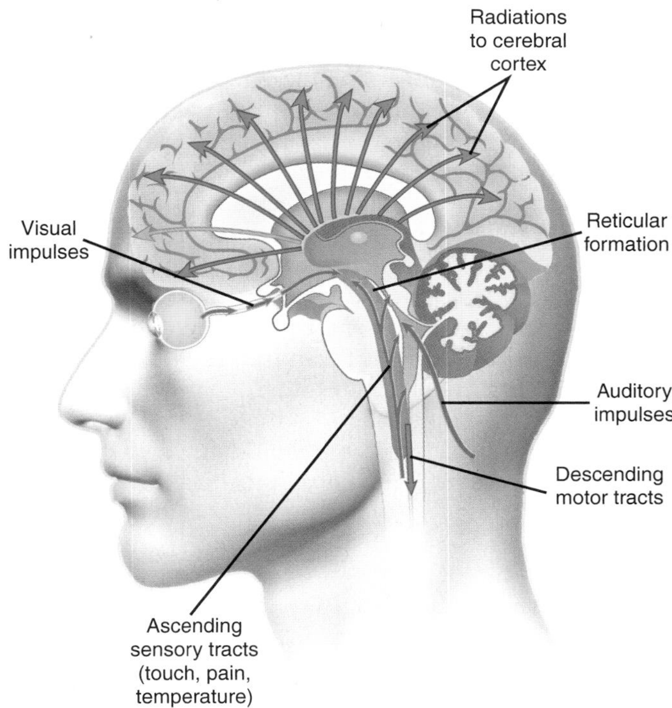

Figure 38.1 ■ The nerve impulses run along the ascending sensory tracts to reach the reticular activating system (RAS); then certain impulses reach the cerebral cortex where they are perceived.

- ***Perception.*** Perception, or awareness and interpretation of stimuli, takes place in the brain, where specialized brain cells interpret the nature and quality of the sensory stimuli. The client's level of consciousness affects the perception of the stimuli.

Arousal Mechanism

For the individual to receive and interpret stimuli, the brain must be alert, also referred to as arousal. The reticular activating system (RAS) in the brainstem is thought to mediate the arousal mechanism. The RAS has two components: the reticular excitatory area (REA) and the reticular inhibitory area (RIA). The REA is responsible for arousal and wakefulness.

People have their own zone of optimal arousal, the level at which the individual feels comfortable. **Sensoristasis** is the term used to describe the state in which an individual is in optimal arousal. Beyond this comfort zone individuals must adapt to the increase or decrease in sensory stimulation. An absence of stimuli from the RAS to the cerebrum results in the brain becoming inactive or useless. The brain has the capacity to adapt to sensory stimuli. For example, an individual living in a city may not notice traffic noise that someone from a rural area finds loud and disturbing. Not all sensory stimuli are acted on; some are stored by the memory to be used at a later date.

Awareness is the ability to perceive internal and external stimuli, and to respond appropriately through thought and action. There are several states of awareness (Table 38.1). A normal, alert individual can assimilate many kinds of stimuli at one time.

Factors Affecting Sensory Function

A number of factors affect sensory reception and perception, including an individual's developmental stage, culture, level of stress, medications, illness, lifestyle, and personality.

Developmental Stage

Perception of sensation is critical to the intellectual, social, and physical development of infants and children. Infants learn to recognize the face of their mother or caregiver and establish bonding essential to later emotional development. Young children respond to music by singing and dancing as they begin to interact with their peers in groups. As children grow, they learn to interpret visual and auditory signals when preparing to cross the street. Adults have many learned responses to sensory stimuli. The sudden loss or impairment of any sense, therefore, has a profound effect on an individual of any age.

Normal physiologic changes in older adults put them at higher risk for altered sensory function. The diminishing of sensory perception that may come with chronic disease or aging is generally gradual. Hearing loss is common in older adults. In 2010 a landmark cohort study was conducted in Beaver Dam, Wisconsin, on male veterans and nonveterans. It revealed that approximately 25% of adults age 55 to 64 and 43% age 65 to 84 have diagnosed hearing loss (Weber, 2018). Nearly half of individuals over age 75 experience loss of hearing. Age-related hearing loss is commonly in both ears equally (National Institute on Deafness and Other Communication Disorders, 2018). Smith and Gooi (2019) reported that 1 to 2 newborns per 1000 have significant hearing loss, and 2 young children per 1000 are diagnosed with significant hearing loss. In addition, many children age 11 years or younger develop hearing loss related to middle ear infections. Hearing loss is greatest in the 60 to 69 age group. Men are twice as likely to suffer hearing loss as women. Non-Hispanic Black individuals have the least prevalence of experiencing hearing loss.

TABLE 38.1 States of Awareness

State	Description
Full consciousness	Alert; oriented to time, place, person; understands verbal and written words
Disoriented	Not oriented to time, place, or person
Confused	Reduced awareness, easily bewildered; poor memory, misinterprets stimuli; impaired judgment
Somnolent	Extreme drowsiness but will respond to stimuli
Semicomatose	Can be aroused by extreme or repeated stimuli
Coma*	Will not respond to verbal stimuli

*See Glasgow Coma Scale, Table 29.10 in Chapter 29.

Culture

An individual's culture may determine the amount of sensory stimulation that he or she considers usual or normal. For example, a child reared in a big-city neighborhood where extended families share responsibilities for all the children may be accustomed to more stimulation than a child reared in a suburb of scattered single-family homes. In 2014 Christian, Muslim, and Yazidis Iraqis were displaced from Iraq to Kurdistan. Due to this displacement the normal amount of stimulation associated with ethnic origin, religious affiliation, and income level, for example, affected the amount of stimulation an individual desires and believes to be meaningful. The sudden change in cultural surroundings experienced by immigrants or visitors to a new country, especially where there are differences in language, dress, and cultural behaviors, may also result in sensory overload or cultural shock. Iraqi families were forced to leave the cities in which they were born and raised. These families experienced war and violence in their country. They were forced to relocate to other countries. This experience, together with living in a new environment, led to major depressive disorders, anxiety, posttraumatic stress disorder, and other psychosocial adverse effects due to the relocation (Khalil, Choueifaty, & Richa, 2016).

Cultural deprivation, or **cultural care deprivation**, is a lack of culturally assistive, supportive, or facilitative acts. The displacement of clients from their origin of birth can lead to a sense of isolation and loneliness. It is important that nurses be sensitive to what stimulation is culturally acceptable to a client. Bucher (2015) states that it is important to develop diversity consciousness by examining ourselves, expanding our knowledge of others and their worlds, stepping outside of ourselves, gauging the level of the playing field, checking up on ourselves, and then following through (p. 132). For example, in some cultures touching is comforting, whereas in others it is offensive. Some clients find the presence of cultural or religious symbols reassuring, and their absence a source of anxiety. Nurses should encourage clients who want to have such symbols present to do so, and to follow practices with which they are comfortable, provided that these practices do not endanger their health.

Stress

During times of increased stress, people may find their senses already overloaded and thus seek to decrease stimulation. For example, a client dealing with physical illness, pain, hospitalization, and diagnostic tests may wish to have only close support people visit. In addition, a client may need the nurse's help to decrease unnecessary stimuli (e.g., noise) as much as possible. On the other hand, clients may seek sensory stimulation during times of low stress.

Medications and Illness

Certain medications can alter an individual's awareness of environmental stimuli. Narcotics, antiepileptic agents, and sedatives, for example, can decrease awareness of stimuli. Some antidepressants can also alter perceptions of stimuli. When administering these medications the nurse is responsible for protecting the client from injury that can result from impaired sensory perception. The nurse should educate clients and their families on the effect medications produce that alter sensory perception. Anyone taking several medications concurrently may show alterations in sensory function. Older adults are at greatest risk for such alterations because they may have conditions that also alter perception and spatial orientation.

Some medications, if taken in large doses or over a long period of time, become ototoxic, injuring the auditory nerve and causing hearing loss that may be irreversible. Some of these medications are aspirin, furosemide (Lasix), the aminoglycosides, and certain drugs given for cancer chemotherapy.

Certain diseases, such as atherosclerosis, restrict blood flow to the receptor organs and the brain, thereby decreasing awareness and slowing responses. Uncontrolled diabetes mellitus can impair vision and is a leading cause of blindness in the United States; diabetic neuropathy can cause changes in the tactile sense as well. Some central nervous system diseases cause varying degrees of paralysis and sensory loss. Diseases of the inner ear can affect the kinesthetic sense.

Lifestyle and Personality

Lifestyle can influence the quality and quantity of stimulation to which a client is accustomed. A client who is employed in a large company may be accustomed to many diverse stimuli, whereas a client who is self-employed and works in the home is exposed to fewer, less diverse stimuli. Clients' personalities also differ in terms of the quantity and quality of stimuli with which they are comfortable. Some clients delight in constantly changing stimuli and excitement, whereas others prefer a more structured life with few changes.

Sensory Alterations

Individuals become accustomed to certain sensory stimuli, and when these change markedly an individual may experience discomfort. For example, when clients enter a hospital they usually experience stimuli that differ in quantity and quality from those to which they are accustomed. These changes may cause clients to become confused and disoriented (see Table 38.1). Some clients may experience excessive changes in mental alertness including delusions and hallucinations.

Nurses have become increasingly aware of the behaviors that may result from different stimuli. They now pay more attention to color, sound, privacy, and social interaction for clients so that the stimuli more closely resemble those in the home environment. Factors that contribute to alterations in behavior include sensory deprivation, sensory overload, and sensory deficits.

Sensory Deprivation

Sensory deprivation is generally thought of as a decrease in or lack of meaningful stimuli. When an individual experiences sensory deprivation, the balance in the RAS is disturbed. The RAS is unable to maintain normal stimulation to the cerebral cortex. Because of this reduced stimulation, an individual becomes more acutely aware of the remaining stimuli and often perceives them in a distorted manner. The individual often experiences alterations in perception, cognition, and emotion. Box 38.1 lists clinical signs of sensory deprivation.

BOX 38.1 Sensory Deprivation

- Excessive yawning, drowsiness, sleeping
- Decreased attention span, difficulty concentrating, decreased problem-solving ability
- Impaired memory
- Periodic disorientation, general or nocturnal confusion
- Preoccupation with somatic complaints, such as palpitations
- Hallucinations or delusions
- Crying, annoyance over small matters, depression
- Apathy, emotional lability

Sensory Overload

Sensory overload generally occurs when an individual is unable to process or manage the amount or intensity of sensory stimuli. Three factors contribute to sensory overload:

- Increased quantity or quality of internal stimuli, such as pain, dyspnea, or anxiety
- Increased quantity or quality of external stimuli, such as a noisy healthcare setting, intrusive diagnostic studies, or contacts with many strangers
- Inability to disregard stimuli selectively, perhaps as a result of nervous system disturbances or medications that stimulate the arousal mechanism.

Sensory overload can prevent the brain from ignoring or responding to specific stimuli. Because of the many stimuli, the individual has difficulty perceiving the environment in a way that makes sense. As a result the individual's thoughts race in many directions, causing restlessness and anxiety. The individual usually feels overwhelmed and does not feel in control. It is important for nurses to remember that sights and sounds that are familiar to them often represent overload to clients. Clients who have sensory overload may appear fatigued. They often cannot internalize new information and they experience cognitive overload. Factors such as pain, lack of sleep, and worry can also contribute to sensory overload. See Box 38.2 for common signs of sensory overload.

BOX 38.2 Sensory Overload

- Complaints of fatigue, sleeplessness
- Irritability, anxiety, restlessness
- Periodic or general disorientation
- Reduced problem-solving ability and task performance
- Increased muscle tension
- Scattered attention and racing thoughts

Sensory Deficits

A **sensory deficit** is impaired reception, perception, or both, of one or more of the senses. Blindness and deafness are sensory deficits. When the loss of sensory function is gradual, individuals often develop behaviors to compensate for the loss; sometimes these behaviors are unconscious. For example, an individual with gradual hearing loss in the right ear may unconsciously turn the left ear toward a speaker. However, sudden loss of one of the senses can result in disorientation, and compensatory behavior often takes days or weeks to develop.

Clients with sensory deficits are at risk for both sensory deprivation and sensory overload. For example, clients with visual problems may be unable to read, watch television, or recognize nurses by sight, which could lead to sensory deprivation. On the other hand, clients who are blind often have highly structured home environments, and the diversity and unfamiliarity of the hospital environment can create sensory overload. At the same time, impaired vision often results in an inability to move around readily or socialize with others.

Hospitalized clients are at risk for developing hospital delirium that can lead to adverse effects such as falls and injury. Kluger et al. (2018) reported hospital delirium as the most common and costly complication of hospitalized older adults. Dementia results in the alteration of memory and judgment. Standard care for older adults' admission to the hospital should include assessment for changes in memory and cognition. Providing education on the recognition of dementia and changes in mood or behavior will enhance the outcome of care and increase client safety. Discharge planning should be initiated within 24 hours of admission. Longer hospital stays can increase the risk of adverse client outcomes (Timmons et al., 2016).

●○● NURSING MANAGEMENT

Assessing

Nursing assessment of sensory-perceptual functioning includes six components: (1) nursing history, (2) mental status examination, (3) physical examination, (4) identification of clients at risk, (5) the client's environment, and (6) the client's social support network.

Nursing History

During the nursing history the nurse assesses the client's current sensory perceptions, usual functioning, sensory deficits, and potential problems. In some instances, significant others can provide data the client cannot. For example, the client's significant others may provide evidence

ASSESSMENT INTERVIEW Sensory–Perceptual Functioning

VISUAL

- How would you rate your vision (excellent, good, fair, or poor)?
- Do you wear eyeglasses or contact lenses?
- Describe any recent changes in your vision.
- Do you have any difficulty seeing near or far objects?
- Do you have any difficulty seeing at night? Have you ever experienced blurred vision, double vision, spots moving in front of your eyes, blind spots, light sensitivity, flashing lights, or halos around objects?
- When did you last visit an eye doctor?

AUDITORY

- How would you rate your hearing (excellent, good, fair, or poor)?
- Do you wear a hearing aid?
- Describe any recent changes in your hearing.
- Can you locate the direction of sounds and distinguish various voices?
- Do you experience any dizziness or vertigo? Do you experience any ringing, buzzing, humming, crackling noises, or fullness in the ears?

GUSTATORY

- Have you experienced any changes in taste (e.g., difficulty in differentiating sweet, sour, salty, and bitter tastes)?
- Do you enjoy the taste of foods as you did previously?

OLFACTORY

- Have you experienced any changes in smell?
- Do things (foods, flowers, perfumes, and so on) smell the same as previously?
- Can you distinguish foods by their odors and tell when something is burning?
- Have you experienced any changes in appetite? (Changes in appetite may be related to an impaired sense of smell.)

TACTILE

- Are you experiencing any pain or discomfort?
- Have you experienced any decrease in your ability to perceive heat, cold, or pain in your limbs?
- Do you have any numbness or tingling in your extremities?

KINESTHETIC

- Have you noticed any difficulty in perceiving the position of parts of your body?

of recent changes in the client's hearing ability, such as inattention to others, mood swings, difficulty following clear instructions, frequent requests to have something repeated, and unusually loud radio or television volumes. Examples of interview questions to elicit data about the client's sensory–perceptual functioning are shown in the accompanying Assessment Interview.

Mental Status Examination

Mental status is critical to any evaluation of the sensory-perceptual process. Data on mental status, including level of consciousness, orientation, memory, and attention span, are usually obtained during the nursing history (see Chapter 29 ∞). It is important to note that sensory alterations can cause changes in cognitive functioning and vice versa.

Physical Examination

Physical assessment determines whether the senses are impaired. During the physical examination the nurse assesses vision and hearing and the olfactory, gustatory, tactile, and kinesthetic senses. The examination should reveal the client's specific visual and hearing abilities; perception of heat, cold, light touch, and pain in the limbs; and awareness of the position of the body parts. Specific sensory tests include the following:

- Visual acuity, using a Snellen chart or other reading material such as a newspaper, and visual fields
- Hearing acuity, by observing the client's conversation with others and by performing the whisper test and the Weber and Rinne tuning fork tests
- Olfactory sense, by asking the client to identify specific aromas
- Gustatory sense, by asking the client to identify three tastes such as lemon, salt, and sugar
- Tactile sense, by testing light touch, sharp and dull sensation, two-point discrimination, hot and cold sensation, vibration sense, position sense, and stereognosis.

These tests are described in detail in Chapter 29 ∞. The nurse should also determine whether sensory adaptive devices that the client uses, such as eyeglasses or hearing aids, are adequate and functioning properly.

Clients at Risk for Sensory Deprivation or Overload

Clients at risk for sensory-perceptual alterations need to be identified to ensure that preventive measures can be initiated. Box 38.3 describes clients at risk.

Client Environment

A nurse should assess the client's environment for quantity, quality, and type of stimuli. The environment may produce insufficient stimuli, placing the client at risk for sensory deprivation, or excessive stimuli, placing the client at risk for sensory overload. Nonstimulating environments include those that (a) severely restrict physical activity and (b) limit social contact with family and friends. Because appropriate or meaningful stimuli decrease the incidence of sensory deprivation, the nurse must consider the client's healthcare environment for the presence of the following stimuli:

- Electronic devices (computers, iPADs, tablets, television, smart phones)
- Clock or calendar
- Reading material (or toys for children)
- Number and compatibility of roommates
- Number of visitors.

BOX 38.3 Clients at Risk for Sensory Deprivation and Overload

SENSORY DEPRIVATION: CLIENTS WHO

- are confined in a nonstimulating or monotonous environment in the home or healthcare agency
- have impaired vision or hearing
- have mobility restrictions such as quadriplegia or paraplegia with bedrest, traction apparatus
- are unable to process stimuli (e.g., clients who have brain damage or who are taking medications that affect the central nervous system)
- have emotional disorders (e.g., depression) and withdraw within themselves
- have limited social contact with family and friends (e.g., clients from a different culture).

SENSORY OVERLOAD: CLIENTS WHO

- have pain or discomfort
- are acutely ill and have been admitted to an acute care facility
- are being closely monitored in an intensive care unit (ICU) (Figure 38.2 ■) and have intrusive tubes such as IVs, catheters, or nasogastric or endotracheal tubes
- have decreased cognitive ability (e.g., head injury).

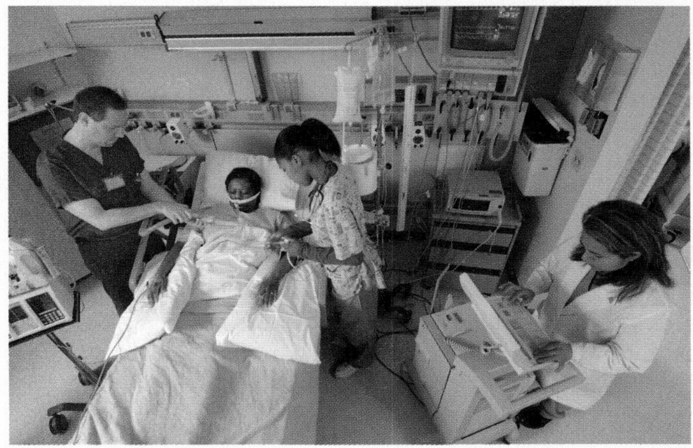

Figure 38.2 ■ A client in an ICU may experience sensory overload.
David Joel/Photographer's Choice RF/Getty Images.

To assess a healthcare environment that produces excessive stimuli, the nurse considers, for example, bright lights, noise, therapeutic measures, and frequency of assessments and procedures. In the client's home, the nurse may also note the presence of a pet, bright colors, adequate lighting, and so on.

Clinical Alert!

Are you aware of the noise level around you or the noise level you create while providing nursing care? The standard of 45 decibels (dB) for rest and sleep is often not met. For example, studies have shown that sounds in critical care units range from 60 to 83 dB, thereby suggesting sensory overload.

Social Support Network

The degree of isolation an individual feels is significantly influenced by the quality and quantity of support from family members and friends. A nurse should assess (a) whether the client lives alone, (b) who visits and when, and (c) any signs indicating social deprivation, such as withdrawal from contact with others to avoid embarrassment or dependence on others, negative self-image, reports of lack of meaningful communication with others, and absence of opportunities to discuss fears or concerns that facilitate coping mechanisms.

Diagnosing

Examples of nursing diagnoses that may be appropriate for perception and cognition can include disturbances in thinking related to confusion and inability to recall past experiences related to diminished cognitive ability.

Sensory-Perception Problem as the Etiology

Depending on the data obtained, alterations in sensory-perception function may affect other areas of human functioning and indicate other diagnoses. In these instances the sensory-perception problem becomes the etiology.

Examples of nursing diagnoses for which sensory-perception disturbances are the etiology include potential for injury related to decreased vision, hearing, or tactile stimulation, changes in consciousness, or sensory impairment; and diminished personal relationships related to decreased hearing and increased or decreased sensory perception.

Planning

Planning includes goals associated with the care of clients independent of setting and those specific to the home environment.

Planning Independent of Setting

The overall outcome criteria for clients with sensory-perception alterations are to:

- Prevent injury.
- Maintain the function of existing senses.
- Develop an effective communication mechanism.
- Prevent sensory overload or deprivation.
- Reduce social isolation.
- Perform activities of daily living (ADLs) independently and safely.

The *Nursing Interventions Classification* (NIC) publication can be a guide when planning care (Butcher, Bulechek, Dochterman, & Wagner, 2019). Appropriate nursing activities may be selected from the following nursing interventions:

- Cognitive Stimulation
- Communication Enhancement: Hearing Deficit

- Communication Enhancement: Speech Deficit
- Communication Enhancement: Visual Deficit
- Nutrition Management
- Environmental Management: Safety
- Fall Prevention
- Body Mechanics Promotion
- Peripheral Sensation Management
- Emotional Support
- Surveillance: Remote Electronic.

Planning for Home Care

To provide for continuity of care, a nurse must consider a client's needs for assistance with care in the home or residential treatment setting. Some clients with severe alterations in sensory-perception functioning may be discharged to an assisted living facility that provides the specific support the client requires. Discharge planning incorporates a reassessment of the client's abilities for self-care, the availability and skills of support people, financial resources, and the need for referrals and home health services. A major aspect of discharge planning involves the instructional needs of the client and family. The next section provides strategies to support visual and auditory function and maintain a safe environment for clients.

Implementing

Nurses can assist clients with sensory alterations by promoting healthy sensory function, helping clients manage acute sensory deficits, and adjusting environmental stimuli.

Promoting Healthy Sensory Function

Detecting sensory problems early is one step toward preventing serious problems. The arousal mechanism for sensation is normally present at birth; however, it is undifferentiated. The special senses are also present at birth, although some changes in function occur during the growth process.

In 2015 the Centers for Disease Control updated the Early Hearing Detection and Intervention (EHDI) Tracking and Surveillance System goals that were established in 2014. The guidelines were reviewed on July 18, 2017. These functional standards are intended to identify the operational, programmatic, and technical criteria that all jurisdictional EHDI programs should implement during the process of developing, using, and evaluating an EHDI Information System (EHDI-IS). The eight goals are:

- *Goal 1:* Document unduplicated individually identifiable data on the delivery of newborn hearing screening services for all infants born in the jurisdiction. (It is mandatory that the parent receive and document all individual newborn hearing procedures and results in a timely manner.)
- *Goal 2:* Support tracking and documentation of the delivery of follow-up services for every infant and child who did not receive, complete, or pass newborn hearing screening. (Receive and document information on rescreening procedures and results in a timely manner.)
- *Goal 3:* Document all cases of permanent hearing loss, including congenital, late-onset, progressive, and acquired cases for infants and children. (Provide the ability to generate and present separate lists of infants and children with presumed congenital [referred on newborn hearing screening] and late-onset, progressive, or acquired hearing loss.)
- *Goal 4:* Document the enrollment status, delivery, and outcome of early intervention services for infants and children under 3 years old with hearing loss. (Provide the ability to identify infants and children who need early intervention.)
- *Goal 5:* Maintain data quality (accurate, complete, timely data) of individual newborn hearing screening and diagnosis, early intervention, and demographic information in the EHDI-IS. (Provide the ability to regularly evaluate incoming and existing patient records to identify, prevent, and resolve duplicate and fragmented records.)
- *Goal 6:* Preserve the integrity, security, availability, and privacy of all personally identifiable health and demographic data in the EHDI-IS. (Have written confidentiality privacy practices and policies based on applicable law or regulation that protect all individuals whose data are contained in the system.)
- *Goal 7:* Enable evaluation and data analysis activities. (Provide the ability for authorized users to extract and use data to assess program progress toward achieving national and jurisdiction benchmarks.)
- *Goal 8:* Support dissemination of EHDI information to authorized stakeholders. (Provide the ability to generate, present, and transmit standard and/or custom-defined reports for authorized users without assistance from system vendor or IT personnel.)

Early screening to detect problems in vision and hearing is essential. As previously stated, infants should be screened for hearing loss by 1 month of age, and preferably before hospital discharge. In addition, children with chronic ear infections and people who live or work in an environment where there are high noise levels should receive routine auditory testing. Women who are considering pregnancy should be advised of the importance of prenatal testing for syphilis and confirmation of a positive rubella titer, because both maternal syphilis and rubella infection can cause hearing impairments in newborns. Periodic vision screening of all newborns and children is recommended to detect congenital blindness, strabismus, and refractive errors. A child's visual acuity develops during early childhood. Children often have 20/20 vision by 6 to 7 years of age (Ball, Bindler, Cowen, & Shaw, 2019, p. 728). Healthy sensory function can be promoted with environmental stimuli that provide appropriate sensory input. This input should vary and be neither excessive nor too limited. As many senses as possible should be stimulated. Different colors, sounds, textures, smells, and body positions can provide various sensations. Nurses can teach parents to stimulate infants

CLIENT TEACHING **Preventing Sensory Disturbances**

- Have regular health examinations.
- Have regular eye examinations as recommended by the primary care provider to screen for eye problems. For clients ages 40 and over, a medical eye examination is generally recommended every 3 to 5 years, or every 1 to 2 years if there is a family history of glaucoma.
- Seek early medical attention (a) if signs suggesting visual impairment arise, for example, failure to react to light, or reduced eye contact from an infant; (b) if the child complains of an earache or has an ear infection; and (c) for persistent eye redness, discharge or increased tearing, growths on or near the eye, pupil asymmetry or other irregularity, or any pain or discomfort.
- Obtain regular immunizations of children against diseases capable of causing hearing loss (e.g., rubella, mumps, and measles).
- Avoid giving infants and toddlers toys with long pointed handles and keep pointed instruments (e.g., scissors and screwdrivers) out of reach. Supervise preschoolers when they use scissors.
- Make sure that toddlers do not walk or run with a pointed object in hand; teach preschoolers to walk carefully when carrying such objects as sticks or toy weapons.
- Teach school-age children and adolescents the proper use of sports equipment (e.g., hockey sticks) and power tools.
- Wear protective eye goggles when using power tools, riding motorcycles, spraying chemicals, and so on.
- Wear ear protectors when working in an environment with high noise levels or brief loud impulse noises (e.g., blasting).
- Wear dark glasses with UV protection to avoid damage from ultraviolet rays and never look directly into the sun.

and children, and teach family members to stimulate an older adult and others in the home with sensory deficits. Social activities often help stimulate the mind and the senses.

Nurses should also teach clients at risk of sensory loss how to prevent or reduce the loss and should teach general health measures, such as getting regular eye examinations and controlling chronic diseases such as diabetes (see Client Teaching).

In the home setting clients should be assessed for their ability to adapt to the sensory impairment and to provide care safely. In addition, client safety will be enhanced by adequate lighting, diminished clutter, and removal of obstructions that may contribute to falls. If the client's home has stairs, stair lifts may be beneficial to promote independence. Other assistive devices such as flashing fire alarms or phones can be utilized by clients with hearing impairments to promote safety. The home care nurse should encourage clients with hearing impairments to use hearing aids (Figure 38.3 ■). Hearing aids require frequent changing of the small batteries. Older adults may have a diminished tactile sense or arthritic hands, making it difficult to change the batteries. The home care nurse should assess the client's ability to change the hearing aid batteries and remove ear wax to maintain optimal function.

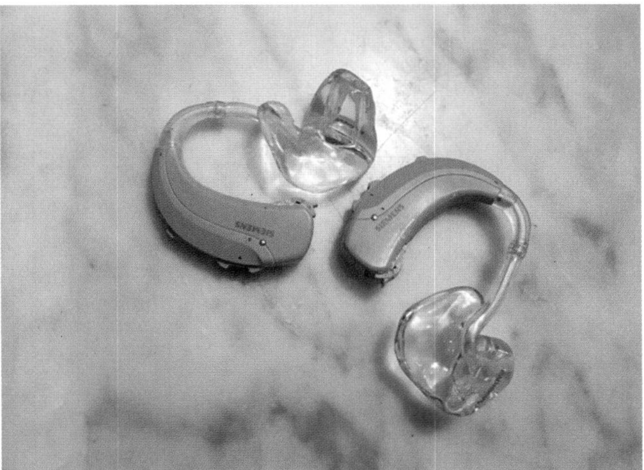

Figure 38.3 ■ Hearing aids.

For all clients with disturbances in sensory perception, provide the client and family with information on assistive devices and support organizations such as National Braille Association, Guide Dogs for the Blind, and the National Association for the Deaf.

Impaired Vision

For clients with impaired vision, nurses need to do the following in a healthcare setting:

- Orient the client to the arrangement of room furnishings and maintain an uncluttered environment.
- Keep pathways clear and do not rearrange furniture without orienting the client. Ensure that housekeeping personnel are informed about this.
- Organize self-care articles within the client's reach and orient the client to his or her location.
- Keep the call light within easy reach and place the bed in the low position.
- Assist with ambulation by standing at the client's side, walking about 1 foot ahead, and allowing the client to grasp your arm. Confirm whether the client prefers grasping your arm with the dominant or nondominant hand.

The most common vision diseases affecting older adults are macular degeneration, cataracts, glaucoma, and diabetic retinopathy. Age-related macular degeneration (ARMD) is the leading cause of blindness in adults older than age 65. Cataracts are opacities of the lenses. Development is slow and painless and may be unilateral or bilateral. They are the leading cause of blindness worldwide. Glaucoma is associated with optic nerve damage due to an increase in intraocular pressure and leads to vision loss. It is the second most common cause of blindness in the United States. Diabetic retinopathy is a microvascular disease of the eye occurring in both type 1 and type 2 diabetes (Tabloski, 2019, pp. 326–328).

Clients who have developed visual impairment related to stroke, head injury, or a disorder of the eye require the

ANATOMY & PHYSIOLOGY REVIEW

Glaucoma

Glaucoma is a group of diseases of the eye caused by increased intraocular pressure that can lead to optic nerve damage and eventual vision loss (see Figure D). Review Figure A for the normal anatomy of the eye.

A clear liquid, the aqueous humor, circulates inside the front portion of the eye, nourishing the lens and cornea. To maintain a normal level of pressure in the eye, the body constantly produces a small amount of aqueous humor and an equal amount flows out of the eye through a drainage system at the junction of the iris and the cornea. It is at this angle that the fluid passes through a trabecular meshwork, drains into the canal of Schlemm, and enters the bloodstream in the back of the eye.

In acute open-angle glaucoma, the anterior chamber angle remains open but drainage of the aqueous humor through the canal of Schlemm is impaired. This causes a slow rise of the intraocular pressure. The eye's drainage angle becomes less efficient as an individual ages and the risk of developing chronic open-angle glaucoma increases. The cause is unknown.

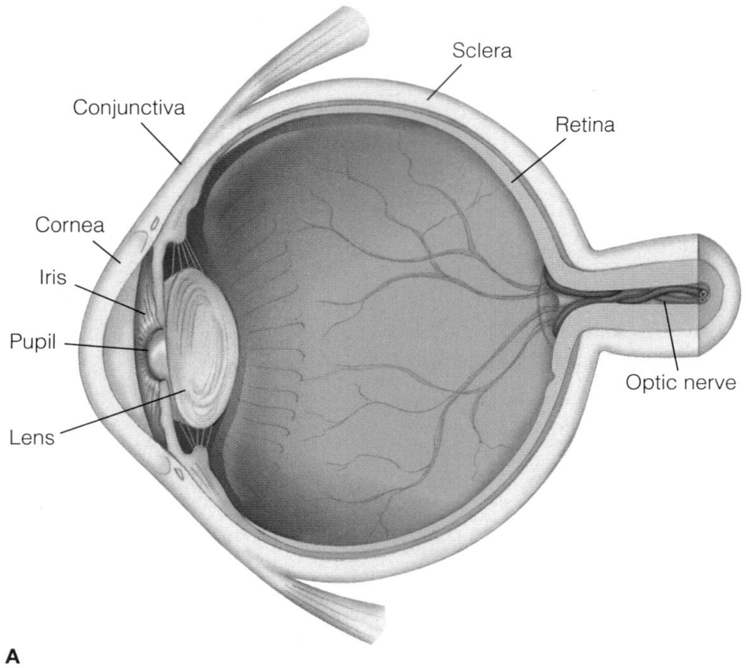

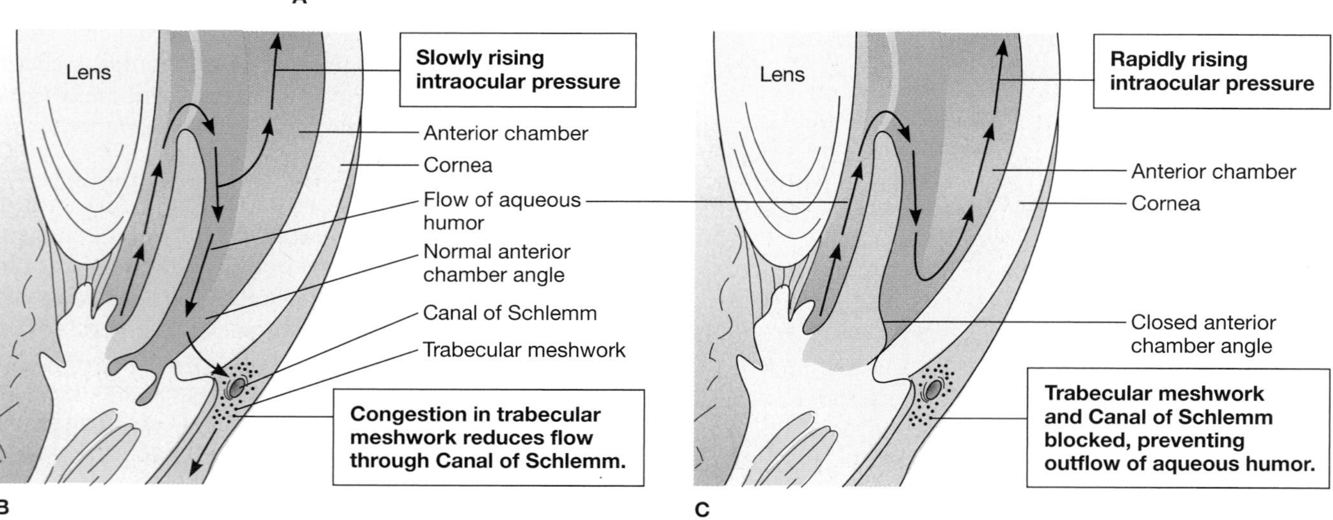

A, The normal anatomy of the eye. *B*, Open-angle (chronic) glaucoma. *C*, Closed-angle (acute) glaucoma.

ANATOMY & PHYSIOLOGY REVIEW

Glaucoma—*continued*

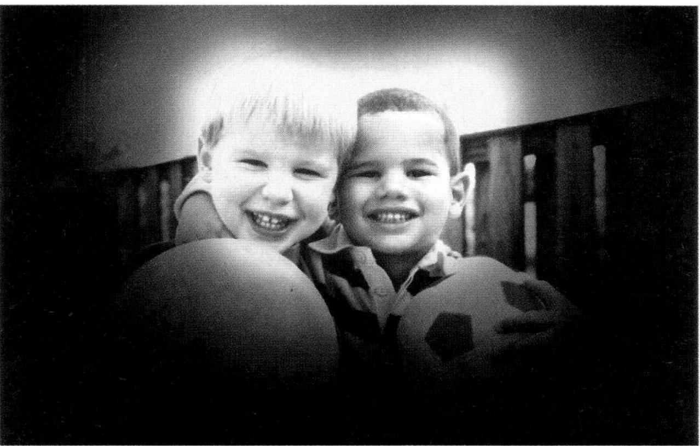

D

D, Narrowing of the optical fields is a typical symptom of untreated glaucoma.

In acute closed-angle glaucoma, the drainage angle narrows and closes or becomes blocked by the iris. The intraocular pressure can rise quickly and cause an acute attack.

QUESTIONS

1. Review Figure B. Describe the angle between the iris and the cornea:
2. Review Figure C. Describe the angle between the iris and the cornea:
3. Open-angle glaucoma is represented by which figure?
4. Closed-angle glaucoma is represented by which figure?
5. The increasing fluid pressure pushes against what important part of the eye with the resulting damage leading to vision loss?

Answers to Anatomy & Physiology Review Questions are available on the faculty resources site. Please consult with your instructor.

aid of an interdisciplinary team for rehabilitation. Norup, Guldberg, Friis, Deurell, and Forchhammer (2016) formed an interdisciplinary team on an acute and sub-acute stroke unit to assess and rehabilitate clients with visual impairment following a stroke. The visual team provided early assessment and rehabilitation. The occupational therapist focused on training the client to be safe in the hospital and outside in all environments with the use of an outdoor mobility course. The physiotherapist evaluated the client's vision during gait training. The study team determined that stroke clients have a variety of cerebral vision disorders that require rehabilitation teams to have members that specialize in the specific disorder in order to adequately care for the clients.

Research has established an association between visual impairment and greater disability in performing ADLs (e.g., bathing, dressing, eating) and instrumental tasks (e.g., shopping, housekeeping). Studies have also shown that impaired vision increases the risk of depression among older adults. Explanations for this relationship vary. One explanation is that vision loss leads to increased disability, which leads to depression. Another explanation states that loss of vision causes fear—fear of losing one's autonomy and becoming dependent on another or others. Impaired vision also affects how an individual obtains information, such as reading the newspaper. In addition, reading is often a leisure activity and its loss can affect an individual's quality of life. It is important for the nurse to be aware of and assess for signs of depression and intervene as appropriate if an older adult is experiencing depression as a result of impaired vision. Gleeson, Sherrington, Lo, Auld, and Keay (2017) conducted a study on older adults with visual loss and high rates of depression. They taught the subjects the Alexander technique, using verbal feedback and manual guidance to teach awareness of unnoticed tensions and improve coordination and balance. The study results showed that emotional distress associated with visual impairment influenced symptoms of depression. The subjects with greater visual impairment had higher rates of depressive symptoms.

Impaired Hearing

Clients with hearing impairments who are unable to hear the alarms of IV pumps and cardiac monitors need to be assessed frequently. They can be taught to use their visual sense to identify kinks in the IV tubing or a loose ECG lead, and so on. For home safety, clients with impaired

DRUG CAPSULE

Client Taking Medication for Glaucoma: travoprost (Travatan)

Norman Daniels is 68 years old and has been diagnosed with open-angle glaucoma. His intraocular pressure is 44 mmHg. The normal intraocular pressure is 10 to 21 mmHg. His ophthalmologist has prescribed travoprost (Travatan), one drop in each eye at bedtime.

Travoprost is a prostaglandin analog medication that decreases intraocular pressure in open-angle glaucoma.

NURSING RESPONSIBILITIES

- Assess eye for inflammation, exudate, and pain.
- Note iris color.

CLIENT AND FAMILY TEACHING

- Use once daily as directed.
- Do not let the tip of the dropper touch any part of the eye.
- It may be used with other eye products to lower intraocular pressure. If more than one medication is being used, administer 5 minutes apart.
- Inform of risk of darkening of the iris, eyelashes, or skin around the eye.
- Do not administer while wearing contact lenses. Remove contact lenses and wait 15 minutes after instilling one eyedrop in each eye before reinserting contact lenses.
- Discard the container within 6 weeks of removing it from the sealed pouch.
- It should not be administered by women who are pregnant or plan to become pregnant (Frandsen & Pennington, 2018).

Prior to administering any medication, review all aspects with a current drug handbook or other reliable source.

hearing need to obtain devices that either amplify sounds or respond with flashing lights to sounds such as a doorbell, phone, smoke detector, crying baby, or burglar alarm. The sounds of doorbells and alarm clocks may be amplified or changed to a lower frequency or buzzer-like sound. These devices can be obtained from hearing aid dealers, telephone companies, and appliance stores.

An important consequence of a decline in hearing as an individual ages is difficulty understanding speech. Factors that influence this difficulty are the environment, rate of speech, and presence of an accent. Environments that are noisy and reverberant (echoing, hollow sounds) can cause difficulty for the older adult. Older adults with a hearing loss have difficulty understanding fast speech. Research indicates that an older adult's ability to process verbal information is slower than that of a younger adult, and that rapid speech allows less time for the older adult to recognize acoustic or auditory cues. An individual who speaks with an accent can also affect speech understanding by an older adult. Non-native English speakers may vary their pronunciation of syllables and words, making it challenging for the older adult to understand.

Impaired Olfactory Sense

Clients with an impaired sense of smell need to be taught about the dangers of cleaning and working with chemicals. Strong chemicals such as ammonia used in confined spaces such as a bathroom may affect the client before they are smelled. Because a gas leak can go undetected, clients need to keep gas stoves and heaters in good working order. Food poisoning is a concern with clients who have difficulty detecting spoiled meat or dairy products. These clients need to carefully inspect food for freshness (check its color and texture) and check expiration dates on food packages.

Impaired Gustatory Sense

Changes in health can lead to impaired taste, which can lead to inadequate intake of required nutrition. Clients who have disease processes such as cancer or nasal impairments can experience a diminished sense of taste. Many medications, such as clarithromycin and chemotherapeutic drugs, produce a metallic taste. Alvarez-Camacho et al. (2015) reported that clients with head and neck cancer experience taste and smell alterations (TSAs). Their study aimed to determine the effect of TSAs on the overall quality of life. Clients in this study reported that the alteration in taste and smell affected their quality of life. They stated that it reduced their enjoyment of food and that eating was less rewarding. The clients also had diminished appetites and lacked the desire to eat.

Impaired Tactile Sense

Clients with an impaired sense of touch may not be aware of hot temperatures, which can cause burns, or pressure on bony prominences, which can produce pressure injuries. Clients with decreased sensation to temperature should have the temperature adjusted on their hot water heater and test water temperature with a thermometer before bathing. Clients with decreased sensation to pressure must change their position frequently.

Managing Acute Sensory Impairments

When assisting clients who have a sensory impairment, a nurse needs to (a) encourage the use of sensory aids to support residual sensory function, (b) promote the use of other senses, (c) communicate effectively, and (d) ensure client safety.

Encouraging the Use of Sensory Aids

Many sensory aids are available for clients who have visual and hearing deficits. Examples are listed in Box 38.4. Sensory aids can be used in the healthcare setting as well as in the home. In all situations, the assistance of support people needs to be enlisted whenever possible to help the client deal with the deficit.

Promoting the Use of Other Senses

When one sense is lost, a nurse can teach the client to use other senses to supplement the loss. However, the type of stimulation needs to be adapted in accordance with the client's specific deficit. For example, for the client with a visual impairment, stimulation of hearing, taste, smell, and touch can be encouraged. A radio, audiotapes of music or

BOX 38.4 Sensory Aids for Visual and Hearing Deficits

VISUAL
- Eyeglasses of the correct prescription, clean and in good repair
- Adequate room lighting, including night lights
- Sunglasses or shades on windows to reduce glare
- Bright contrasting colors in the environment
- Magnifying glass
- Phone dialer with large numbers
- Clock and wristwatch with large numbers
- Color code or texture code on stoves, washer, medicine containers, and so on
- Colored or raised rims on dishes
- Reading material with large print
- Braille or recorded books
- Service dog

HEARING
- Hearing aid in good order
- Lip reading
- Sign language
- Amplified telephones
- Telecommunication device for the deaf (TDD)
- Amplified telephone ringers and doorbells
- Flashing alarm clocks
- Flashing smoke detectors

books, clocks that chime, music boxes, and wind chimes provide auditory stimulation. Diets that include a variety of flavors, temperatures, and textures stimulate the gustatory sense. Taking sips of water between foods and eating foods separately can also emphasize the taste sensation. Fresh flowers, scented candles (safely used), room fragrances, brewing coffee, and baking can stimulate the olfactory sense. Clients can also be encouraged to remember pleasant or familiar odors such as the smell of a favorite flower or food. Measures such as providing a hug, massage, hair brushing, grooming, different textures in clothing and upholstery fabrics, and pets can stimulate tactile receptors.

Communicating Effectively

Communication with clients who have sensory impairments should convey respect, enhance the client's self-esteem, and ensure the exchange of correct information. A client with a hearing impairment has to concentrate more than other individuals do and therefore tires more readily. Fatigue compounded by an illness can further reduce the client's ability to hear. A client with a visual impairment is unable to observe most nonverbal cues during communication and relies largely on the spoken word and tone of voice. Guidelines for communicating with clients who have visual or hearing impairments are shown in Box 38.5.

Ensuring Client Safety

Nurses must implement safety precautions in healthcare settings for clients with sensory deficits. Examples of precautions include keeping the bed in the lowest position and placing the call light within reach.

Adjusting Environmental Stimuli

A hospitalized client functions best when the environment is somewhat similar to that of the individual's ordinary daily life. Sometimes nurses need to take steps to adjust the client's environment to prevent either sensory overload or sensory deprivation.

BOX 38.5 Communicating with Clients Who Have a Visual or Hearing Impairment

VISUAL IMPAIRMENT
- Always announce your presence when entering the client's room and identify yourself by name.
- Stay in the client's field of vision if the client has a partial vision loss.
- Speak in a warm and pleasant tone of voice. Some individuals tend to speak louder than necessary when talking to an individual who is blind.
- Always explain what you are about to do before touching the client.
- Explain the sounds in the environment.
- Indicate when the conversation has ended and when you are leaving the room.

HEARING IMPAIRMENT
- Before initiating conversation, convey your presence by moving to a position where you can be seen or by gently touching the client.
- Decrease background noises (e.g., television) before speaking.
- Talk at a moderate rate and in a normal tone of voice. Shouting does not make your voice more distinct and in some instances makes understanding more difficult.
- Address the client directly. Do not turn away in the middle of a remark or story. Make sure the client can see your face easily and that it is well lighted.
- Avoid talking when you have something in your mouth, such as chewing gum. Avoid covering your mouth with your hand.
- Keep your voice at about the same volume throughout each sentence, without dropping the voice at the end of each sentence.
- Always speak as clearly and accurately as possible. Articulate consonants with particular care.
- Do not "overarticulate"; mouthing or overdoing articulation is just as troublesome as mumbling. Pantomime or write ideas, or use sign language or finger spelling as appropriate.
- Use longer phrases, which tend to be easier to understand than short ones. For example, "Would you like a drink of water?" presents much less difficulty than "Would you like a drink?" Word choice is important: "Fifteen cents" and "fifty cents" may be confused, but "half a dollar" is clear.
- Pronounce every name with care. Make a reference to the name for easier understanding, for example, "Joan, the girl from the office" or "Walmart, the big downtown store."
- Introduce a new subject to the client at a slower rate, making sure that the client follows the switch to the new subject.

EVIDENCE-BASED PRACTICE

Evidence-Based Practice

What Are the Challenges That Speech-Language Pathologists Experience with Clients Who Have Aphasia and Impaired Hearing?

The speech pathologists in this study were interested in understanding whether hearing screenings are performed routinely and in accordance with the American Speech-Language-Hearing Association (ASHA) guidelines. The Silkes and Winterstein (2017) study also wanted to determine what type of follow-up was being employed when hearing loss was identified. The online survey was sent to 102 pathologists who work with adults who have aphasia. The respondents indicated that they perform some type of screening for impairments in hearing. It was determined that few of them utilize valid or reliable screening tools. The researchers determined that a need exists to develop hearing-screening tools that are accessible and validate for aphasia. They also identified the need to collaborate with other members of the healthcare team in the provision of care to these clients.

Implications

In regards to the nurse's role in caring for clients with aphasia and hearing impairments, the collaboration will allow for a totality of care to enhance communication and increase sensory perception.

LIFESPAN CONSIDERATIONS Sensory Perception

CHILDREN

Newborns should be screened for hearing loss before 1 month of age. The guidelines for collecting data on hearing loss have set a benchmark that a minimum of 90% of all children in each state will have access to early intervention including education and treatment. Infants with hearing impairment will begin treatment before 6 months of age. The development of a child with a hearing impairment should be monitored annually. Universal screening of all newborns is mandated in all states (American Academy of Pediatrics, 2018).

OLDER ADULTS

Normal changes of aging often result in varying degrees of impairments in sensory perception and the senses—hearing, vision, smell, taste, and touch. Diseases and conditions that are more common in older adults are diabetes, strokes, and other neurologic disorders such as Parkinson's disease. Each of these conditions and others will alter the client's sensory perception. Nursing interventions need to be very specific and individualized. The interventions are directed to either increase or decrease sensory stimuli.

The goals of nursing care should be focused on maintaining safety and communication with clients who have these impairments. Clients with dementia may have problems that fit more appropriately under "altered thought processes," but the goals should be similar: to maximize their potential, maintain their quality of life and dignity, and at the same time, be aware of safety and communication issues.

Preventing Sensory Overload

For clients who are at risk of overstimulation, nurses should reduce the number and type of environmental stimuli. The nurse can counteract sensory overload by blocking unnecessary stimuli and by helping the client organize and alter responses to the stimuli that cannot be blocked.

Dark glasses with UV protection can partially block lights, and a window shade or drape can reduce visual stimulation. Earplugs reduce auditory stimuli, as do soft background music and earphones. The odor from a draining wound can be minimized by keeping the dressing dry and clean.

Other methods of blocking stimuli are to reduce novelty and surprise, and to cluster care activities to provide rest intervals free of interruptions. Sometimes the number of visitors and the length of visits must be restricted.

By explaining sounds in the environment, the nurse can help the client organize them mentally, for example, a beep indicates an IV alarm. When clients understand their meaning, stimuli may be less confusing and more easily ignored. Clients can also learn through practice and feedback to alter their responses to the stimuli. They can employ relaxation techniques to reduce anxiety and stress despite continual sensory stimulation (see Chapter 42 ∞). Box 38.6 provides nursing measures for clients with sensory overload.

BOX 38.6 Preventing Sensory Overload

- Minimize unnecessary light, noise, and distraction. Provide dark glasses and earplugs as needed.
- Control pain as indicated at the level desired by the client, on a scale of 0 to 10.
- Introduce yourself by name, and address the client by name.
- Provide orienting cues, such as clocks, calendars, equipment, and furniture in the room.
- Provide a private room.
- Limit visitors.
- Plan care to allow for uninterrupted periods of rest or sleep.
- Schedule a routine of care so the client knows when and what to expect (post the schedule for the client wherever possible).
- Speak in a low tone of voice and in an unhurried manner.
- Provide new information gradually to enable the client to process the meaning. When providing information, ask the client to repeat it so that there are no misunderstandings.
- Describe any tests and procedures to the client beforehand.
- Reduce noxious odors. Empty a commode or bedpan immediately after use, keep wounds clean and covered, use a room deodorizer when indicated, and provide good ventilation.
- Take time to discuss the client's problems and to correct misinterpretations.
- Assist the client with stress-reducing techniques.

Preventing Sensory Deprivation

For clients who are at risk for sensory deprivation, nurses can increase environmental stimuli in a number of ways. For example, newspapers, books, music, and television can stimulate the visual and auditory senses. Providing objects that are pleasant to touch, such as a pet to stroke, can provide tactile and interactive stimulation. Clocks that differentiate night from day by color can help orient a client to time. The olfactory sense can be stimulated by the presence of fresh flowers or plants. When communicating with a client who has impaired hearing, it is important to speak facing the client so that the client can see the nurse's mouth. This will enhance communication with clients who read lips.

Arrangements should also be made for visitors to talk with the client regularly. Many church and community groups provide visits to individuals who are confined to their homes or who reside in nursing homes. Box 38.7 provides measures to prevent sensory deprivation.

BOX 38.7 Preventing Sensory Deprivation

- Encourage the client to use eyeglasses and hearing aids.
- Address the client by name and touch the client while speaking if this is not offensive.
- Communicate frequently with the client and maintain meaningful interactions (e.g., discuss current events).
- Provide a telephone, radio, TV, clock, and calendar.
- Provide photographs, sculptures, and wall hangings. Many libraries and museums will lend artwork free of charge, or a local school may provide art projects developed by their students.
- Have family and friends bring freshly cut flowers and plants.
- Consider having a resident pet such as fish, a cat, or a bird or make arrangements for pets to visit on a regular basis.
- Include different textured objects to feel such as a sheepskin pillow, silk scarf, soft blanket, or other inanimate object.
- Increase tactile stimulation through physical care measures such as back massages, hair care, and foot soaks.
- Encourage social interaction through activity groups or visits by family and friends.
- Encourage the use of crossword puzzles or games to stimulate mental function.
- Encourage environment changes such as a walk through a mall, or for an immobilized client, sitting near a window or at a place on the nursing unit where the client can watch local traffic.
- Encourage the use of self-stimulation techniques such as singing, humming, whistling, or reciting.

The Confused Client

Confusion can occur in clients of all ages, but it is most commonly seen in older people. Confusion often presents with subtle symptoms, and it is important for the nurse to differentiate between **acute confusion** (**delirium**) and **chronic confusion** (**dementia**). Delirium has an abrupt onset and a cause that, when treated, reverses the confusion. Dementia, often called *chronic confusion*, has symptoms that are gradual and irreversible (e.g., Alzheimer's disease). It is important to differentiate between the two (Table 38.2).

The terms *acute confusion* and *delirium* are often used interchangeably by most health professionals, with nurses tending to favor the use of *acute confusion* and physicians using the term *delirium*. Acute confusion, however, is a *nursing* diagnosis that stems from the clients' experience and behavioral response to their health condition. Acute confusion can result from drug or alcohol intoxication in all ages and is more common in young adults. The main cause of dementia is Alzheimer's disease. Caring for clients with dementia increases the complexity of care in the acute care setting. Clients with dementia have a greater likelihood of experiencing falls, developing infections, and experiencing the adverse effects of neurologic agents (Butcher, 2018). Caring for clients with dementia requires greater attention to the delivery of nursing care.

TABLE 38.2 Differentiating Between Delirium and Dementia

Characteristic	Delirium	Dementia
Distinguishing feature	Acute, fluctuating change in mental status	Memory impairment
Onset	Sudden, acute onset	Slow, insidious
Duration	Temporary; may last hours to days	Chronic, gradual, irreversible
Time of day	Worsens at night	No change with time of day
Sleep-wake cycles	Disturbed; cycles often reversed	Disturbed Fragmented Awakens often during the night
Alertness	Fluctuates; may be alert and oriented during the day but become confused and disoriented at night	Generally normal
Thinking	Disorganized, distorted; impaired attention; alterations in memory	Judgment impaired Difficulty with abstraction and word finding
Delusions, hallucinations	May have visual, auditory, and tactile hallucinations; misinterpretation of real sensory experiences	Delusions; usually no hallucinations
Causative and risk factors	Cerebral and cardiovascular disease, infections, reduced hearing and vision, environmental change, stress, sleep deprivation, polypharmacy, dehydration	Alzheimer's disease Multi-infarct dementia

Postoperative delirium occurs in older hospitalized clients following surgery. This is a very serious complication that results in increased morbidity and mortality. Factors that contribute to the development of delirium are increased age, cognitive impairment, sensory impairment, other comorbidities, and prolonged hospital stays (Tremblay & Gold, 2016). The components of delirium include the following:

- The client has a reduced ability to focus, sustain, or shift attention.
- The client exhibits a change in cognition that may include memory impairment, disorientation, or development of a perceptual disturbance. This change varies from the initial baseline assessment of the client.
- The change or disturbance develops over a short period of time and fluctuates during a 24-hour period.

There are also clinical subtypes of delirium based on psychomotor activity and levels of alertness:

- With hyperactive delirium, the client can be restless, agitated, and disoriented.
- With hypoactive delirium, the client is quiet, confused, and disoriented, and displays apathy. This may be incorrectly assessed as depression or dementia.
- In mixed delirium, the client has symptoms of both hyperactive and hypoactive delirium. The client will present with symptoms of one type of delirium that will be resolved and then present with the opposite type.

Older adults are often at risk for delirium when hospitalized for numerous reasons. Recognizing at-risk clients and the symptoms of delirium when they occur are critical steps in managing care. Unfortunately, delirium is often unrecognized or misdiagnosed by both the primary care provider and the nurse. A large number of intensive care unit clients present with symptoms of delirium. Critical care nurses are important in preventing and recognizing delirium. Clients who present with symptoms of delirium have higher mortality and morbidity rates than those who do not. Also, older adults often have other chronic medical problems (e.g., dementia, chronic obstructive pulmonary disease, hypertension, stroke) that place them at risk. Many older adults take numerous medications, with anticholinergics, narcotics, and sedatives often increasing the risk for delirium. Many older adults have a vision or hearing impairment. In addition to these predisposing factors, the nurse must also assess for *precipitating* factors that can occur while hospitalized. For example, undertreatment of pain, the unfamiliar surroundings and routine of a hospital, possible sleep deprivation, stress, and sensory overload all compound the older adult's risk for developing delirium.

Clinical Alert!

It is best to *describe* behaviors rather than use the word *confusion* or *confused* when documenting cognitive changes in older adults who may be experiencing delirium. The description of the actual behaviors provides more useful information.

Standardized tools can also be included in addition to the previously described assessments. The Confusion Assessment Method (CAM) is considered the gold standard in identifying clients with delirium. In addition, the Family CAM, or FAM-CAM, is a screening tool in which family members are interviewed to maximize the detection of delirium in clients. The tool was adapted from the CAM instrument to identify acute onset, fluctuations in the delirium course, inattention, disorganized thought processes, diminished level of consciousness, disorientation, perceptual changes, and hallucinations. Other tools include the Mini-Mental State Examination (MMSE), the Delirium Index (DI), and the NEECHAM Confusion Scale (Ball et al., 2017; Smulter, Lingehall, Gustafson, Olofsson, & Engstrom, 2015).

Older adults at risk for delirium require interventions that eliminate or decrease the effects of the previously mentioned precipitating factors. Delirium can be prevented or interventions instituted to reverse the condition. Clients who have acute confusion or delirium often know something is wrong and want help. Box 38.8 lists

BOX 38.8 Promoting a Therapeutic Environment for a Client with Acute Confusion (Delirium)

- Wear a readable name tag.
- If possible, consistent caregivers should be assigned.
- Address the client by name and introduce yourself frequently: "Good morning, Mr. Richards. I am Barbara Barcivik. I will be your nurse today."
- Identify time and place as indicated: "Today is December 5, and it is 8:00 in the morning."
- Ask the client, "Where are you?" and orient the client to place (e.g., nursing home) if indicated.
- Place a calendar and clock in the client's room. Mark holidays with ribbons, pins, or other means.
- Speak clearly and calmly to the client, allowing time for your words to be processed and for the client to give a response.
- Encourage family to visit frequently except if this activity causes the client to become hyperactive.
- Provide clear, concise explanations of each treatment procedure or task.
- Eliminate unnecessary noise.
- Reinforce reality by interpreting unfamiliar sounds, sights, and smells; correct any misconceptions of events or situations.
- Schedule activities (e.g., meals, bath, activity and rest periods, treatments) at the same time each day to provide a sense of security.
- Provide adequate sleep.
- Keep eyeglasses and hearing aid within reach.
- Ensure adequate pain management.
- Keep familiar items in the client's environment (e.g., photographs), and keep the environment uncluttered. A disorganized, cluttered environment increases confusion.
- Keep the room well lit during waking hours.
- Eliminate unnecessary medications.

nursing interventions to help promote a therapeutic environment for the client with acute confusion or delirium (Figure 38.4 ■).

Evaluating

Using the measurable and desired outcomes developed during the planning stage as a guide, the nurse collects the data needed to judge whether client goals and outcomes have been achieved. Examples of client outcomes and related indicators are shown in the Nursing Care Plan. If the desired outcomes are not achieved, the nurse and client, and support people, if appropriate, need to explore the reasons before modifying the care plan.

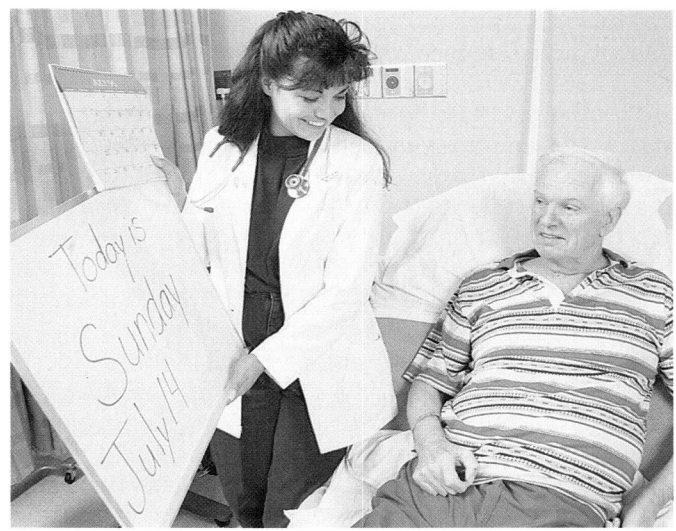

Figure 38.4 ■ Promoting orientation to time and date is essential for clients who are confused or have a memory loss.

NURSING CARE PLAN Sensory-Perception Disturbance

ASSESSMENT DATA	NURSING DIAGNOSIS	DESIRED OUTCOMES*
NURSING ASSESSMENT Julia Hagstrom is an 80-year-old widow who has recently become a resident of an extended care facility. Just prior to her admission she underwent surgery for the removal of cataracts and also experienced more difficulty with hearing. Her children were concerned about her physical safety and lack of socialization and urged her to enter a nursing home. Mrs. Hagstrom had cared for herself independently for 15 years in her own home. One day after admission the nurse finds the client somewhat confused and disoriented to place and time. She appears restless and withdrawn. She states, "I'm afraid of all of these strange creatures in this orphanage." **Physical Examination** Height: 160 cm (5′3″) Weight: 55.3 kg (122 lb) Temperature: 37°C (98.6°F) Pulse: 72 beats/min Respirations: 18/min Blood pressure: 128/74 mmHg Rinne test: negative **Diagnostic Data** Chest x-ray, CBC, and urinalysis all negative	Alterations in thinking related to change in environment and hearing loss (as evidenced by disorientation to time and place; restlessness; and altered behavior)	Cognitive Orientation [0901] as evidenced by: • Identifies significant other(s). • Identifies current place. • Identifies correct season. Hearing Compensation Behavior [1610] as evidenced by consistently demonstrated: • Positions self to advantage hearing. • Reminds others to use techniques that advantage hearing. • Eliminates background noise. • Uses hearing supportive devices.

NURSING INTERVENTIONS*/SELECTED ACTIVITIES	RATIONALE
REALITY ORIENTATION [4820]	
Provide a consistent physical environment and a daily routine.	*Routine eliminates the element of surprise, overstimulation, and further confusion.*
Provide access to familiar objects, when possible.	*Familiarity helps reduce confusion.*
Moderate human and environmental sensory stimuli for Mrs. Hagstrom because disorientation may be increased by overstimulation.	*A disruption in the quality or quantity of incoming stimuli can affect client's cognitive status. Sensory overload blocks out meaningful stimuli.*
Provide for adequate rest, sleep, and daytime naps.	*Reduces overstimulation and fatigue, which may be contributing factors to confusion.*

Continued on page 1008

NURSING CARE PLAN **Sensory-Perception Disturbance—*continued***

NURSING INTERVENTIONS*/SELECTED ACTIVITIES	RATIONALE
Use a calm and unhurried approach when interacting with Mrs. Hagstrom.	*Promotes communication that enhances the client's sense of dignity.*
Speak in a distinct manner with appropriate pace, volume, and tone.	*The client who has difficulty hearing will be better able to lip read and comprehend speech.*
Engage Mrs. Hagstrom in "here and now" activities (i.e., ADLs) that require her to focus on something other than herself that is concrete and reality oriented.	*Assists the individual to differentiate between own thoughts and reality.*

NURSING INTERVENTIONS*/SELECTED ACTIVITIES	RATIONALE
COMMUNICATION ENHANCEMENT: HEARING DEFICIT [4974]	
• Facilitate use of hearing aids, as appropriate.	*Hearing can be enhanced if the volume is appropriate and the hearing aid is consistently used.*
• Listen attentively.	*Effective listening is essential in a nurse–client relationship. Poor listening skills can undermine trust and block therapeutic communication.*
• Simplify language.	*Using simple terms and short sentences facilitates understanding and minimizes anxiety.*
• Obtain Mrs. Hagstrom's attention through touch.	*Gaining the attention of a client with a hearing impairment is an essential first step toward effective communication. However, the client's personal space should be respected and permission to touch should be obtained.*

Evaluation

Outcomes met. Mrs. Hagstrom identifies her primary nurse by sight and name on the third day. She is aware that Christmas is 3 weeks away and is anxious to go shopping with the group. Her daughter has brought new batteries for her hearing aid, which she wears during the day.

*The NOC # for desired outcomes and the NIC # for nursing interventions are listed in brackets following the appropriate outcome or intervention. Outcomes, interventions, and activities selected are only a sample of those suggested by NOC and NIC and should be further individualized for each client.

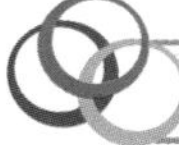

Critical Thinking Checkpoint

Mrs. Dodd is a 51-year-old client who is being cared for in the critical care unit following an automobile crash in which she suffered extensive traumatic injuries. Mrs. Dodd is connected to several monitoring devices, has an intubation tube and ventilator to assist her with respirations, and is receiving various pain and other medications.

1. Identify factors that place Mrs. Dodd at risk for the development of sensory deprivation or overload.
2. What assessment findings would alert you to Mrs. Dodd's experiencing sensory overload as opposed to sensory deprivation?
3. How can you intervene to help Mrs. Dodd during this stressful event?
4. How might the care of a client in the home setting differ from the care of a client such as Mrs. Dodd who is receiving care in a critical care unit?

Answers to Critical Thinking Checkpoint questions are available on the faculty resources site. Please consult with your instructor.

CONCEPT MAP

Sensory-Perception Disturbance

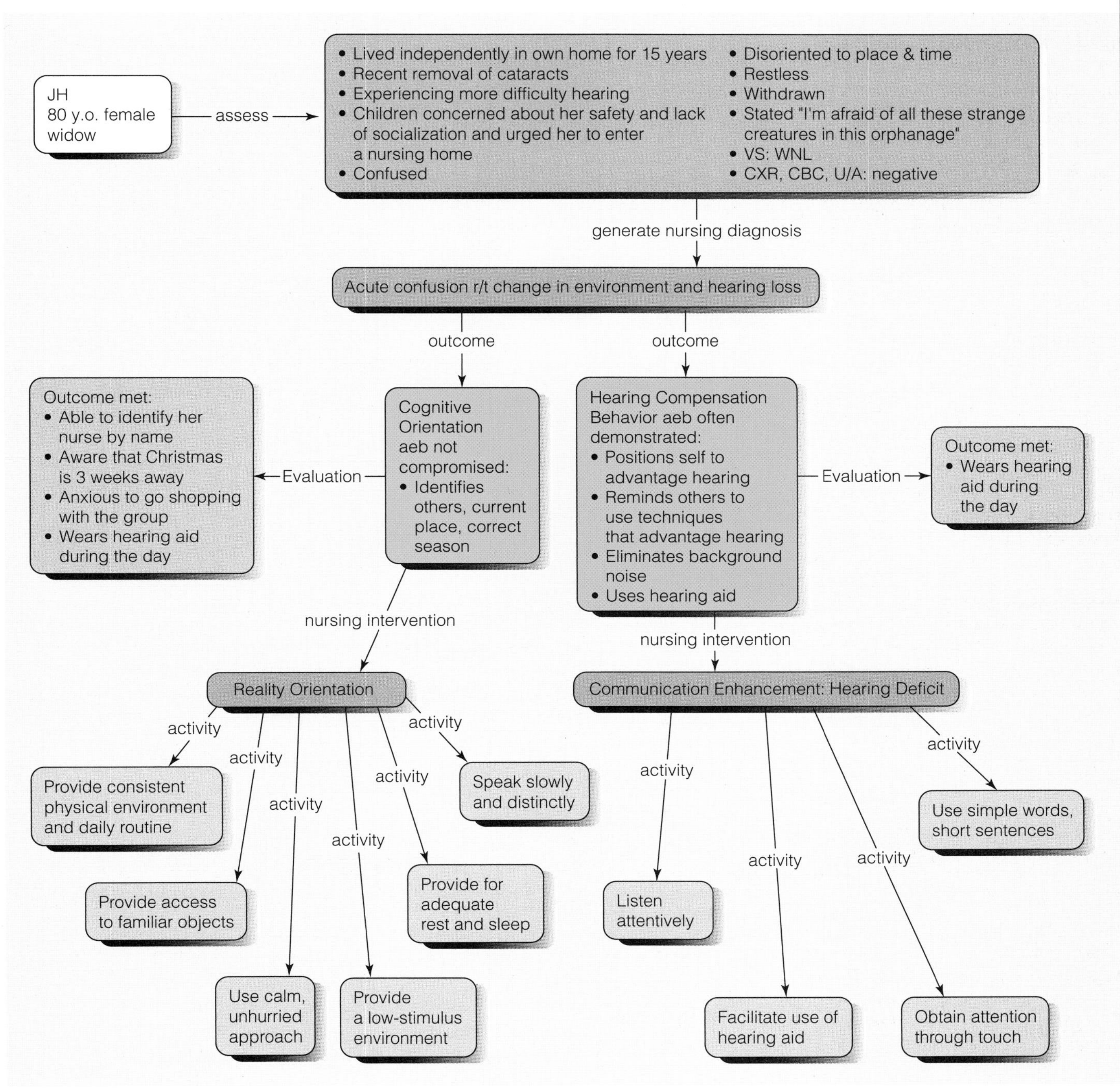

Chapter 38 Review

CHAPTER HIGHLIGHTS

- The sensory experience consists of two components: sensory reception and sensory perception.
- Sensory stimuli can be either external or internal. Visual, auditory, olfactory, tactile, and gustatory stimuli orient an individual to the external environment. Kinesthetic and visceral stimuli orient the individual to the internal environment. Kinesthetic stimuli make the individual aware of the position and movement of body parts.
- Sensory perception involves the awareness and interpretation of stimuli into meaningful information. This process occurs in the cerebral cortex.
- The reticular activating system (RAS), with its many ascending and descending connections to other areas of the brain, monitors and regulates incoming stimuli. The RAS maintains, enhances, or inhibits cortical arousal.
- The normal, alert individual can assimilate many kinds of information at one time and respond appropriately through thought and action.
- Factors affecting sensory stimulation include developmental stage, culture, stress, medications, illness, and lifestyle and personality.
- Sensory deprivation occurs when an individual receives decreased sensory input or monotonous or meaningless sensory input.
- Sensory overload occurs when an individual experiences excessive sensory input and is unable to process or manage the stimuli. The individual feels overwhelmed and not in control.
- Responses to both sensory deprivation and sensory overload include perceptual changes (e.g., mild distortions or hallucinations), cognitive changes (e.g., decreased concentration and problem-solving ability), and affective changes (e.g., apathy, anxiety, anger, depression, and rapid mood swings).
- Clients at risk for sensory deprivation include (a) those who are homebound or institutionalized, (b) those on bedrest or isolation precautions, (c) those with sensory impairments, (d) those who come from a different culture, (e) those with certain affective disorders or disturbances of the nervous system, and (f) those on certain medications that affect the central nervous system.
- Clients at risk for sensory overload include (a) those in pain, (b) those in intensive care units, (c) those with intrusive and uncomfortable monitoring or treatment equipment, and (d) those with decreased cognitive ability (e.g., head injury).
- Assessment for sensory-perception disturbances includes (a) a nursing history to identify sensory impairments, (b) mental status examination, (c) physical examination, (d) identification of clients at risk, (e) the client's environment, and (f) the client's social support network.
- Examples of nursing diagnoses related to a client's sensory-perception impairments can include disturbances in thinking, inability to recall past experiences, potential for injury, diminished ability to communicate, and diminished personal relationships.
- Goals for clients with sensory-perception disturbances include (a) preventing injury, (b) maintaining the function of existing senses, (c) developing an effective communication mechanism, (d) preventing sensory deprivation or overload, (e) reducing social isolation, and (f) performing ADLs independently and safely.
- Interventions to prevent or modify sensory deprivation, sensory overload, and sensory impairments include promoting healthy sensory function, helping clients manage sensory impairments, and adjusting environmental stimuli.
- Clients with sensory impairments need instruction about sensory aids available to support residual sensory function, ways to promote the use of other senses, and methods to ensure safety from bodily harm.
- Nurses and support people need to devise and implement effective communication mechanisms for clients who have visual and hearing impairments.
- Clients with acute confusion (delirium) need care directed toward promoting their orientation to time, place, person, and situation.

TEST YOUR KNOWLEDGE

1. The nurse suspects a client will develop sensory overload. What characteristics did the nurse observe in the client? Select all that apply.
   1. Ongoing pain
   2. Confusion at night
   3. Inability to sleep
   4. Easily angered
   5. Worrying about upcoming diagnostic tests

2. A nurse is identifying diagnoses appropriate for a client who lives alone and is recovering from cataract surgery. Which diagnosis would be the priority for this client?
   1. Social Isolation
   2. Risk for Impaired Skin Integrity
   3. Disturbed Sensory Perception
   4. Risk for Injury

3. A nursing diagnosis of potential for altered skin integrity related to sensory-perception disturbance would best fit a client who:
   1. Cut a foot by stepping on broken glass.
   2. Uses a wheelchair due to paraplegia.
   3. Wears glasses because of poor vision.
   4. Is legally blind and smokes in bed.

4. Which statement indicates the client needs a sensory aid in the home?
   1. "I tripped over that throw rug again."
   2. "I can't hear the doorbell."
   3. "My eyesight is good if I wear my glasses."
   4. "I can hear the TV if I turn it up high."

5. The odor from a hospitalized client's draining wound permeates the room; it is overwhelming and very distracting to the client and the staff. What intervention would be most helpful?
   1. Spray the room routinely with a floral room spray.
   2. Instill a vinegar solution into the wound.
   3. Keep the wound dressing dry and clean.
   4. Burn a candle in the room.

6. A client with impaired vision is admitted to the hospital. Which interventions are most appropriate to meet the client's needs? Select all that apply.
   1. Identify yourself by name.
   2. Decrease background noise before speaking.
   3. Stay in the client's field of vision.
   4. Explain the sounds in the environment.
   5. Keep your voice at the same level throughout the conversation.

7. A client is exhibiting signs and symptoms of acute confusion (delirium). Which strategy should the nurse implement to promote a therapeutic environment?
1. Keep lights in the room dimmed during the day to decrease stimulation.
2. Keep the environmental noise level high to increase stimulation.
3. Keep the room organized and clean.
4. Use restraints for client safety.

8. A client is at risk for sensory deprivation. Which of the following clinical signs would the nurse observe? Select all that apply.
1. Sleeplessness
2. Decreased attention span
3. Irritability
4. Excessive sleeping
5. Crying, depression

9. The nurse is assessing for sensory function. Match the assessment tool to the specific sense it will be testing.

Identifying taste	1. Visual
Stereognosis	2. Hearing
Snellen chart	3. Tactile
Identifying aromas	4. Olfactory
Tuning fork	5. Gustatory

10. An 85-year-old client has impaired hearing. When creating the care plan, which intervention should have the highest priority?
1. Obtaining an amplified telephone
2. Teaching the importance of changing his position
3. Providing reading material with large print
4. Checking expiration dates on food packages

See Answers to Test Your Knowledge in Appendix A.

READINGS AND REFERENCES

Suggested Readings

Broekhof, E., Bos, M. G. N., Camodeca, M., & Rieffe, C. (2018) Longitudinal associations between bullying and emotions in deaf and hard of hearing adolescents. *Journal of Deaf Studies and Deaf Education*, *1*, 17–27. doi:10.1093/deafed/enx036

This study examined the longitudinal associations of anger, fear, guilt, and shame with bullying in adolescents who are deaf or hard of hearing. Deaf and hard of hearing adolescents experienced more anger and less guilt which predicted increased bullying. More bullying predicted increased anger and decreased guilt. Thus, higher levels of anger, fear, and shame predicted increased victimization, and more victimization predicted increased anger, fear, and shame.

Ijpma, I., Timmermans, E. R., Renken, R. J., Ter Horst, G. J., & Reyners, A. K. L. (2017). Metallic taste in cancer patients treated with systemic therapy: A questionnaire-based study. *Nutrition and Cancer*, *69*(1), 140–145. doi:10.1080/01635581.2017.1250922

An adverse effect of chemotherapy is metallic taste. In this study 127 cancer clients completed a questionnaire and 46% reported taste changes. Women experienced greater metallic taste than men.

Related Research

Bourquine, E. A., Emerson, R. W., Sauerburger, D., & Barlow, J. M. (2018). Conditions that influence drivers' behaviors at roundabouts: Increasing yielding for pedestrians who are visually impaired. *Journal of Visual Impairment & Blindness*, *112*(1), 61–71.

McGinley, E. (2016). The provision of nutritional advice in patients with cancer. *Journal of Community Nursing*, *30*(5), 63–66.

References

Alvarez-Comacho, M., Gonella, S., Ghosh, S., Kubrak, C., Scimger, R. A., Chu, K. P., & Wismer, W. V. (2016). The impact of taste and smell alterations on quality of life in head and neck cancer patients. *Quality of Life Research*, *25*, 1495–1504. doi:10.1007/s11136-015-1185-2

American Academy of Pediatrics. (2018). *Newborn hearing screening FAQs*. Retrieved from https://www.healthychildren.org/English/ages-stages/baby/Pages/Purpose-of-Newborn-Hearing-Screening.aspx

Ball, J. W., Bindler, R. C., Cowen, K. J., & Shaw, M. R. (2019). *Child health nursing: Partnering with children and families* (3rd ed.). Hoboken, NJ: Pearson.

Ball, M. J., Boaz, L., Maadooliat, M., Hagle, M. E., Gettrust, L., Greene, M. T., . . . Saczynski, J. S. (2017). Preparing family caregivers to recognize delirium symptoms in older adults after elective hip or knee arthroplasty. *Journal of the American Geriatrics Society*, *65*, e13–e17. doi:10.1111/jgs.14535

Bucher, R. D. (2015). *Diversity consciousness: Opening our minds to people, cultures, and opportunities*. New York, NY: Pearson.

Butcher, L. (2018). Caring for patients with dementia in the acute care setting. *British Journal of Nursing*, *27*(7), 358–362. doi:10.12968/bjon.2018.27.7.358

Butcher, H. K., Bulechek, G. M., Dochterman, J. M., & Wagner, C. M. (Eds.). (2019). *Nursing interventions classification (NIC)* (7th ed.). St. Louis, MO: Mosby.

Centers for Disease Control. (2015). *EHDI-IS functional standards*. Retrieved from https://www.cdc.gov/ncbddd/hearingloss/ehdi-is-functional-standards-.html

Frandsen, G., & Pennington, S. (2018). *Abrams' clinical drug therapy rationales for nursing practice* (11th ed.). Philadelphia, PA: Lippincott Williams & Wilkins.

Gleeson, M., Sherrington, C., Lo, S., Auld, R., & Keay, L. (2017). Impact of the Alexander technique on well-being: A randomized controlled trial involving older adults with visual impairment. *Clinical and Experimental Optometry*, *100*, 633–641. doi:10.1111/cxo.12517

Khalil, R. B., Choueifaty, D. E., & Richa, S. (2016). Displaced Iraqi families in Kurdistan: Strangers in a strange land. *The American Journal of Psychiatry*, *173*, 16–17. doi:10.1176/appi.ajp.2015.15070990

Kluger, C., Shah, P., Maiti, S., Babalola, O. B., Mulvany, C., & Sinvani, L. (2018). Therapeutic advances in the prevention and treatment of delirium in the hospital setting. *American Journal of Therapeutics*, *25*, e3–e14.

Moorhead, S., Johnson, M., Maas, M. L., & Swanson, E. (Eds.). (2018). *Nursing outcomes classification (NOC)* (6th ed.). St. Louis, MO: Mosby.

National Institute on Deafness and Other Communication Disorders. (2018). *Age-related hearing loss*. Retrieved from https://www.nidcd.nih.gov/health/age-related-hearing-loss

Norup, A., Guldberg, A., Friis, C. R., Deurell, E. M., & Forchhammer, H. B. (2016). An interdisciplinary visual team in an acute and sub-acute stroke unit: Providing assessment and early rehabilitation. *NeuroRehabilitation*, *39*, 451–461. doi:10.3233/NRE-161376

Silkes, J. P., & Winterstein, K. (2017). Speech-language pathologists' use of hearing screening for clients with aphasia: Challenges, potential solutions, and future directions. *American Journal of Speech-Language Pathology*, *26*, 11–28. doi:10.1044/2016_AJSLP-14-0181

Smith, R. J. H., & Gooi, A. (2019). Hearing loss in children: Etiology, *UpToDate*. Waltham, MA:Wolters Kluwer.

Smulter, N., Lingehall, H. C., Gustafson, Y., Olofsson, B., & Engstrom, K. G. (2015). Validation of the Confusion Assessment Method in detecting postoperative delirium in cardiac surgery patients. *American Journal of Critical Care*, *24*(6), 480–487. doi:http://dx.doi.org/10.4037/ajcc2015551

Tabloski, P. A. (2019). *Gerontological nursing* (4th ed.). Hoboken, NJ: Pearson.

Timmons, S., O'Shea, E., O'Neill, D., Gallagher, P., de Siun, A., McArdle, D., . . . Kennelly, S. (2016). Acute hospital dementia care: Results from a national audit. *BMC Geriatrics*, *16*, 113. doi:10.1186/s12877-016-0293-3

Tremblay, P., & Gold, S. (2016). Prevention of post-operative delirium in the elderly using pharmacological agents. *Canadian Geriatrics Journal*, *19*(3), 113–126. doi:10.5770/cgj.19.226

Weber, P. C. (2018). Etiology of hearing loss. *UpToDate*. Waltham, MA: Wolters Kluwer.

Selected Bibliography

Cahill, A., Pearcy, C., Agrawal, V., Sladek, P., & Truitt, M. S. (2017). Delirium in the ICU: What about the floor? *Journal of Trauma Nursing*, *24*, 242–244. doi:10.1097/JTN.0000000000000298

Capella-McDonnall, M., & Crudden, A. (2015). Building relationships with businesses: Recommendations from employers concerning persons who are blind/visually impaired. *Journal of Rehabilitation*, *81*(3), 43–50.

Griffin-Shirley, N., Banda, D. R., Ajuwon, P. M., Cheon, J., Lee, J., Park, H. R., & Lyngdoh, S. N. (2017). A survey on the use of mobile applications for people who are visually impaired. *Journal of Visual Impairment & Blindness*, *111*(4), 307–323.

Lewerenz, D., Peter, K., & Ford, P. (2016). Prevalence of conditions causing visual impairment in students at the Oklahoma School for the Blind. *Journal of Visual Impairment & Blindness*, *110*(3), 189–194.

Loftus, C. A., & Wiesenfeld, L. A. (2017). Geriatric delirium care: Using chart audits to target improvement strategies. *Canadian Geriatrics Journal*, *20*(4), 246–252. doi:10.5770/cgj.20.276

Yang, J., Zhou, Y., Kang, Y., Xu, B., Wang, P., Lv, Y., & Wang, Z. (2017). Risk factors of delirium in sequential sedation patients in intensive care units. *BioMed Research International*, Article ID 3539872, 9 pages. doi:10.1155/2017/3539872

39 Self-Concept

LEARNING OUTCOMES

After completing this chapter, you will be able to:

1. Summarize the development of self-concept and self-esteem, including the framework described by Erikson.
2. Describe the dimensions and components of self-concept.
3. Identify common stressors affecting self-concept and coping strategies.
4. Describe the essential aspects of assessing role relationships.
5. Identify nursing diagnoses related to altered self-concept.
6. Describe nursing interventions designed to achieve identified outcomes for clients with altered self-concept.
7. Describe ways to enhance client self-esteem.

KEY TERMS

body image, *1014*
core self-concept, *1014*
global self, *1013*
global self-esteem, *1016*
ideal self, *1014*
role, *1016*
role ambiguity, *1016*
role conflicts, *1016*
role development, *1016*
role mastery, *1016*
role performance, *1016*
role strain, *1016*
self-awareness, *1012*
self-concept, *1012*
self-esteem, *1016*
specific self-esteem, *1016*

Introduction

Self-concept is one's mental image of oneself. A positive self-concept promotes an individual's mental and physical health. Individuals with a positive self-concept are better able to develop and maintain interpersonal relationships and resist psychologic and physical illness. An individual possessing a strong self-concept can better accept or adapt to changes that may occur over the lifespan. How one views oneself affects one's interaction with others.

Nurses have a responsibility to assess clients' self-concept and to identify ways to help them develop a more positive view of themselves. Individuals who have a poor self-concept may express feelings of worthlessness, self-dislike, or even self-hatred. They may feel sad or hopeless, and may state they lack energy to perform even the simplest of tasks.

Self-Concept

Self-concept involves all of the self-perceptions—appearance, values, and beliefs—that influence behavior and are referred to when using the words *I* or *me*. Self-concept influences the following:

- How one thinks, talks, and acts
- How one sees and treats another individual
- Choices one makes
- Ability to give and receive love
- Ability to take action and to change things.

There are four dimensions of self-concept:

- ***Self-knowledge:*** insight into one's own abilities, nature, and limitations
- ***Self-expectation:*** what one expects of oneself; may be realistic or unrealistic expectations
- ***Social self:*** how one is perceived by others and society
- ***Social evaluation:*** the appraisal of oneself in relationship to others, events, or situations.

Individuals who value "how I perceive me" above "how others perceive me" can be termed *me-centered*. They try hard to live up to their own expectations and compete only with themselves, not others. In contrast, strongly *other-centered* individuals have a high need for approval from others and try hard to live up to the expectations of others, comparing, competing, and evaluating themselves in relation to others. They tend to have difficulty asserting themselves, and fear disapproval. The positive self-concept, therefore, is me-centered and is formed with limited reference to others' opinions.

In addition to assessing and promoting a positive self-concept with clients, a nurse's own self-concept is important. Nurses who understand the different dimensions of themselves are better able to understand the needs, desires, feelings, and conflicts of their clients. Nurses who feel positive about themselves are more likely to help clients meet their needs.

Self-awareness refers to the relationship between an individual's own and others' perception of self. Thus, a nurse who is very self-aware has perceptions that are very congruent. Becoming more self-aware is a process that requires time and energy and is never complete. One important component of the process is introspection, which involves the nurse reflecting on personal beliefs, attitudes, motivations, strengths, and limitations. The nurse also gains insight into the self through working with other nurses who serve as mentors and by taking feedback obtained during regular performance reviews seriously and acting on it.

The nurse who has developed a clear understanding and awareness of self can respect others' beliefs and avoid projecting personal beliefs onto others. While in the caregiver role, the self-aware nurse is able to suspend judgment and focus on the needs of the client, even if they differ from those of the nurse. When conflicts arise, the nurse can analyze their own reactions through introspection and by asking these questions:

- "Why do I react this way (fear, anger, anxiety, annoyance, worry)?"
- "Can I change the way I respond to this situation to affect the client's reaction in a helpful way?"

Formation of Self-Concept

An individual is not born with a self-concept; rather, it develops as a result of social interactions with others. Chapter 23 discusses various theories of growth and development, including Erikson's stages of development, Piaget's cognitive developmental phases, and Havighurst's developmental tasks.

According to Erikson (1963), throughout life individuals face developmental tasks associated with eight psychosocial stages that provide a theoretical framework. The success with which an individual copes with these developmental tasks largely determines the development of self-concept. Difficulty coping can result in self-concept problems at the time and, often, later in life. Table 39.1 lists examples of behaviors indicating successful and unsuccessful resolution of these developmental tasks.

The development of one's self-concept consists of three broad steps:

- The infant learns that the physical self is separate and different from the environment.
- The child internalizes others' attitudes toward self.
- The child and adult internalize the standards of society.

The term **global self** refers to the collective beliefs and images one holds about oneself. It is the most complete

TABLE 39.1 Examples of Behaviors Associated with Erikson's Stages of Psychosocial Development

Stage: Developmental Tasks	Behaviors Indicating Positive Resolution	Behaviors Indicating Negative Resolution
Infancy: trust vs. mistrust	Requesting assistance and expecting to receive it Expressing belief of another individual Sharing time, opinions, and experiences	Restricting conversation to superficialities Refusing to provide an individual with personal information Being unable to accept assistance
Toddlerhood: autonomy vs. shame and doubt	Accepting the rules of a group but also expressing disagreement when it is felt Expressing one's own opinion Easily accepting deferment of a wish fulfillment	Failing to express needs Not expressing one's own opinion when opposed Overly concerned about being clean
Early childhood: initiative vs. guilt	Starting projects eagerly Expressing curiosity about many things Demonstrating original thought	Imitating others rather than developing independent ideas Apologizing and being very embarrassed over small mistakes Verbalizing fear about starting a new project
Early school years: industry vs. inferiority	Completing a task once it has been started Working well with others Using time effectively	Not completing tasks started Not assisting with the work of others Not organizing work
Adolescence: identity vs. role confusion	Asserting independence Planning realistically for future roles Establishing close interpersonal relationships	Failing to assume responsibility for directing one's own behavior Accepting the values of others without question Failing to set goals in life
Early adulthood: intimacy vs. isolation	Establishing a close, intimate relationship with another individual Making a commitment to that relationship, even in times of stress and sacrifice Accepting sexual behavior as desirable	Remaining alone Avoiding close interpersonal relationships
Middle-aged adults: generativity vs. stagnation	Being willing to share with another individual Guiding others Establishing a priority of needs, recognizing both self and others	Talking about oneself instead of listening to others Showing concern for oneself in spite of the needs of others Being unable to accept interdependence
Older adults: integrity vs. despair	Using past experience to assist others Maintaining productivity in some areas Accepting limitations	Crying and being apathetic Not accepting changes Demanding unnecessary assistance and attention from others

description that individuals can give of themselves at any one time. It is also an individual's frame of reference for experiencing and viewing the world. Some of these beliefs and images represent statements of fact, for example, "I am a woman," "I am a father," or "I am short." Others refer to less tangible aspects of self, for instance, "I am competent" or "I am shy."

Each separate image and belief one holds about oneself has a bearing on self-concept. However, self-concept is not simply a sum of its parts. The various images and beliefs individuals hold about themselves are not given equal weight and prominence. Each individual's self-concept is like a piece of art. At the center of the art are the beliefs and images that are most vital to the individual's identity. They constitute **core self-concept**. For example, "I am very smart/of average intelligence" or "I am male/female." Images and beliefs that are less important to the individual are on the periphery. For example, "I am left-/right-handed" or "I am athletic/unathletic."

Individuals are thought to base their self-concept on how they perceive and evaluate themselves in these areas:

- Vocational performance
- Intellectual functioning
- Personal appearance and physical attractiveness
- Sexual attractiveness and performance
- Being liked by others
- Ability to cope with and resolve problems
- Independence
- Particular talents.

Self-concept in these areas also extends to the choices individuals make and perceptions they have about their health. Individuals with strong positive self-concept about appearance are likely to value healthy behaviors and take action to maintain the health of their skin, hair, and body tone, for example. Individuals with negative self-concepts may be less proactive about health promotion and illness prevention activities.

Maintaining and evaluating one's self-concept is an ongoing process. Events or situations may change the level of self-concept over time. Having a basic self-concept includes how we see ourselves and how we are seen by others. There is also the **ideal self**, which is how we should be or would prefer to be. The ideal self is the individual's perception of how one should behave based on certain personal standards, aspirations, goals, and values. Sometimes this ideal self is realistic; sometimes it is not. When the perceived self is close to the ideal self, individuals do not wish to be much different from what they believe they already are. A discrepancy between the ideal self and perceived self can be an incentive to self-improvement. However, when the discrepancy is great, low self-esteem can result.

Nurses, like other adults, view themselves based on both internal and external inputs acquired over many years. The ability to appraise one's own strengths, the desire to follow in the steps of role models, and the feedback received from colleagues and clients are some of the influences on the nurse's self-concept.

Components of Self-Concept

The four components of self-concept are personal identity, body image, role performance, and self-esteem.

Personal Identity

Personal identity is the conscious sense of individuality and uniqueness that is continually evolving throughout life. Individuals often view their identity in terms of name, gender, age, race, ethnic origin or culture, occupation or roles, talents, and other situational characteristics (e.g., marital status and education).

Personal identity also includes beliefs and values, personality, and character. For instance, is the individual outgoing, friendly, reserved, generous, selfish? Personal identity thus encompasses both the tangible and factual, such as name and citizenship, and the intangible, such as values and beliefs. Identity is what distinguishes self from others.

In most Western cultures, individuals have a sexual identity, whether heterosexual, gay, lesbian, bisexual, or some other. Sexual identity is not a component of self-concept in some parts of the world where relationships and contextual behavior have a stronger role than the individual's characteristics (Hyde & DeLamater, 2017). See Chapter 40 ∞.

An individual with a strong sense of identity has integrated body image, role performance, and self-esteem into a complete self-concept. This sense of identity provides an individual with a feeling of continuity and a unity of personality. Furthermore, the individual views self as a unique individual.

Body Image

The image of physical self, or **body image**, is how an individual perceives the size, appearance, and functioning of the body and its parts. Body image has both cognitive and affective aspects. The cognitive is the knowledge of the material body; the affective includes the sensations of the body, such as pain, pleasure, fatigue, and physical movement. Body image is the sum of these attitudes, conscious and unconscious, that an individual has toward their body.

Body image includes clothing, makeup, hairstyle, jewelry, and other things intimately connected to the individual (Figure 39.1 ■). It also includes body prostheses, such as artificial limbs, dentures, and hairpieces, as well as devices required for functioning, such as wheelchairs, canes, and eyeglasses. Past as well as present perceptions and how the body has evolved over time are part of one's body image.

An individual's body image develops partly from others' attitudes and responses to that individual's body and partly from the individual's own exploration of the body. For example, body image develops in infancy as the parents or caregivers respond to the child with smiles, holding, and touching, and as the child explores their own body sensations during breastfeeding, thumb sucking, and the bath. Cultural and societal values also influence an individual's body image.

The various information and entertainment media have played a part over the years in how individuals

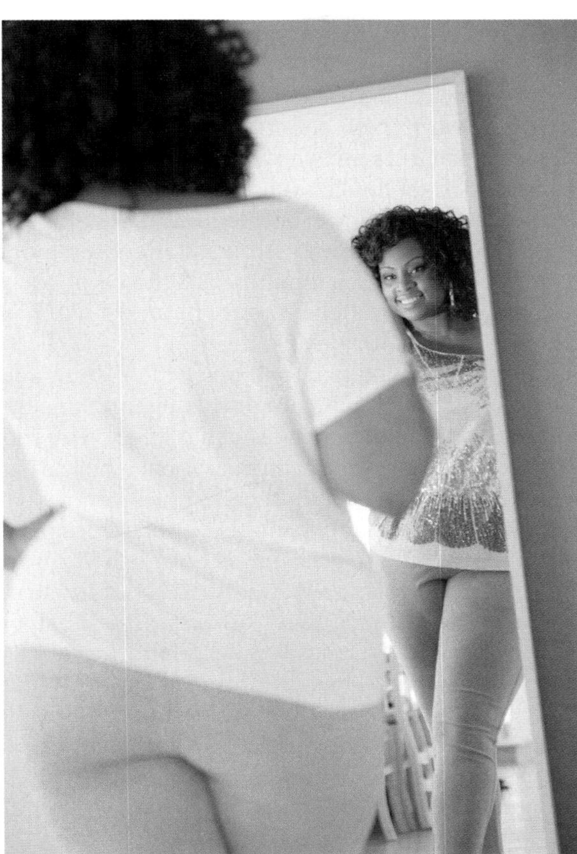

Figure 39.1 ■ Body image is the sum of an individual's conscious and unconscious attitudes about their body.
JGI/Jamie Grill/Getty Images.

view themselves and others. During adolescence, concerns related to body image are of paramount concern. The "ideal" individual portrayed by the media is really an unrealistic goal for many.

If an individual's body image closely resembles their body ideal, the individual is more likely to think positively about the physical and nonphysical components of the self. The body ideal is greatly influenced by cultural standards. For example, currently in North America the fit, well-toned body is admired.

Another aspect of body image is the understanding that different parts of the body have different values for different individuals. For example, large breasts may be highly important to one woman and unimportant to another, or the occurrence of gray hair may be traumatic to one individual and barely noticed by another.

An individual with a healthy body image will normally show concern for both health and appearance. This individual will seek help if ill and will include health-promoting practices in daily activities. An individual who has an unhealthy body image is likely to be overly concerned about minor illness and to neglect important activities like sleep and a healthy diet.

The individual who has a body image disturbance may hide or not look at or touch a body part that is significantly changed in structure by illness or trauma. Some individuals may also express feelings of helplessness, hopelessness, powerlessness, and vulnerability, and may exhibit self-destructive behavior such as over- or undereating or suicide attempts.

EVIDENCE-BASED PRACTICE

Evidence-Based Practice

Body Image in Childhood

Body image is the way in which individuals view their physical self. It can include emotions, feelings, thoughts, and perspectives on body shape, size, and weight. While several studies have examined the concept of body image in various population groups, little attention has been given to body image during childhood. Neves et al. (2017) performed an integrative review of the current body of scientific evidence relating to body image during childhood to gauge how children understand the concept of body image.

The integrative review of literature examined those studies published between January 2013 and January 2016 that evaluated the concept regarding body image in children aged 0 to 12 years. Three electronic databases including Scopus, Medline, and Virtual Health Library – BVS were searched. Studies that did not include an empirical methodology, did not evaluate a component of body image, included children with underlying diseases or conditions (e.g., cancer, burns, etc.), and included children not belonging to the age range being studied were not taken into account. After screening 7,681 studies, a total of 33 studies were included in the final analysis.

Results showed that girls had higher rates of body dissatisfaction than boys, a trend that is reflected even in older population groups such as adolescents and adults. This finding may be related to cultural influences that present a lean body as the ideal physique for females. Body mass index was shown to affect body image regardless of sex as both boys and girls who had higher body mass indices had higher body dissatisfaction. In addition, sociocultural factors such as the media, parents, and friends were found to impact health behaviors that children felt would allow them to achieve their ideal body image. For example, boys were found to admire male athletes, while girls were found to admire famous actresses and singers. Parental restrictions on eating habits and food choices were also found to contribute to how children viewed their physical selves. On the other hand, the integrative review of literature found few differences in body image perceptions based on race or ethnicity.

For all studies included in the research, it was found that there were varying concepts regarding body image in the number of children belonging to different age groups. This was found to be problematic because body image is a concept that evolves in line with distinct developmental stages that children undergo. Lastly, instruments used to measure body dissatisfaction and perception were not validated for use in the age group of interest, which may raise questions as to the validity of study results.

Implications

Understanding body image in childhood is significant because body image disturbances in childhood may contribute to psychological problems later in life. Nurses can contribute to the early identification of body image issues in children and can help parents and families in implementing early interventions that modify risk factors such as food restrictions, media usage, and eating habits.

Role Performance

Throughout life, individuals undergo numerous role changes. A **role** is a set of expectations about how the individual occupying a particular position behaves. **Role performance** is how an individual in a particular role behaves in comparison to the behaviors expected of that role. **Role mastery** means that the individual's behaviors meet role expectations. Expectations, or standards of behavior of a role, are set by society, a cultural group, or a smaller group to which an individual belongs. Each individual usually has several roles, such as husband, parent, brother, son, employee, friend, nurse, and church member. Some roles are assumed for only limited periods, such as client, student, and ill individual. **Role development** involves socialization into a particular role. For example, nursing students are socialized into nursing through exposure to their instructors, clinical experience, classes, laboratory simulations, and seminars.

Individuals need to know who they are in relation to others and what society expects for the positions they hold. **Role ambiguity** occurs when expectations are unclear, and individuals do not know what to do or how to do it and are unable to predict the reactions of others to their behavior. Failure to master a role creates frustration and feelings of inadequacy, often with consequent lowered self-esteem.

Self-concept is also affected by role strain and role conflicts. People undergoing **role strain** are frustrated because they feel or are made to feel inadequate or unsuited to a role. Role strain is often associated with sex role stereotypes. For example, women in occupations traditionally held by men might be treated as having less knowledge and competence than men in the same roles. The significance of this concept for nurses and clients is also apparent in nursing diagnoses related to the role strain experienced by caregivers.

Role conflicts arise from opposing or incompatible expectations. In an interpersonal conflict, individuals have different expectations about a particular role. For example, grandparents may have different expectations than the parents about how to care for the children. One individual's or group's role expectations may differ from the expectations of another individual or group. For example, an individual who has little flexibility in a full-time job schedule has a role conflict if the individual's spouse expects him or her to handle all the childcare problems. Sometimes role expectations violate the beliefs or values of the role occupant. For example, a nurse in a family planning clinic may be expected to advise couples about birth control methods that are not consistent with the nurse's belief system regarding prevention or management of unwanted pregnancy. Role conflict can lead to tension, a decrease in self-esteem, and embarrassment.

Self-Esteem

Self-esteem is one's judgment of one's own worth, that is, how that individual's standards and performances compare to others' standards and to one's ideal self. If an individual's self-esteem does not match the ideal self, then low self-concept results.

The two types of self-esteem are global and specific. **Global self-esteem** is how much one likes oneself as a whole. **Specific self-esteem** is how much one approves of a certain part of oneself. Global self-esteem is influenced by specific self-esteem. For example, if a man values his looks, then how he looks will strongly affect his global self-esteem. By contrast, if a man places little value on his cooking skills, then how well or badly he cooks will have little influence on his global self-esteem.

Self-esteem is derived from self and others. In infancy, self-esteem is related to the caregiver's evaluations and acceptances. Later the child's self-esteem is affected by competition with others. As an adult, an individual who has high self-esteem has feelings of significance, of competence, of the ability to cope with life, and of control over one's destiny.

The foundation for self-esteem is established during early life experiences, usually within the family structure. However, an adult's level of overall self-esteem may change markedly from day to day and moment to moment. Severe stress—for example, stress related to prolonged illness or unemployment—can substantially lower an individual's self-esteem. In healthcare, clients who believe that their condition is viewed negatively by society may have low self-esteem. Individuals frequently focus on their negative aspects and spend less time on their positive aspects. It is important for both strengths and weaknesses to be identified.

If Maslow's level of love and belonging needs are met, the needs for self-esteem are next higher on the hierarchy. When the need for self-esteem is satisfied, the individual strives for self-actualization (see Chapter 19 ∞).

Factors That Affect Self-Concept

Many factors affect an individual's self-concept. Major factors are stage of development, family and culture, stressors, resources, history of success and failure, and illness.

Stage of Development

As an individual develops, the conditions that affect the self-concept change. For example, an infant requires a supportive, caring environment, whereas a child requires freedom to explore and learn. Older adults' self-concept is based on their experiences in progressing through life's stages.

Family and Culture

A young child's values are largely influenced by the family and culture. Later on, peers influence the child and thereby affect the sense of self. When the child is confronted by differing expectations from family, culture, and peers, the child's sense of self is often confused (Figure 39.2 ■). For example, a child may realize that his parents expect he will

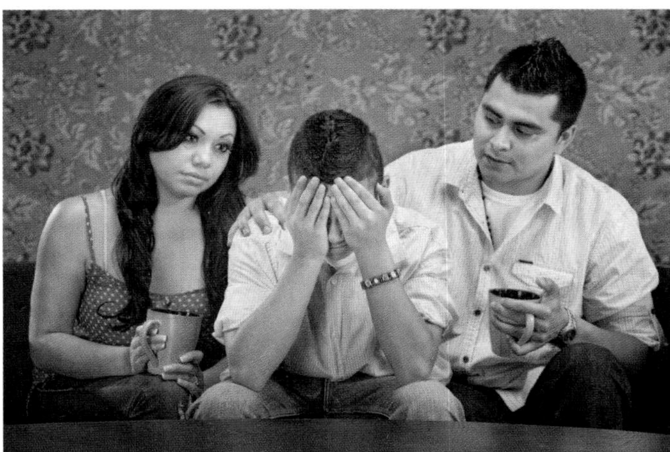

Figure 39.2 ■ A child is often pulled in opposite directions by family and peer expectations.
Scott Griessel/123RF.

not drink alcohol and that he will attend religious services each Saturday. At the same time, his peers drink beer and encourage him to spend Saturday with them.

Stressors

Stressors can strengthen the self-concept as an individual copes successfully with problems. On the other hand, overwhelming stressors can cause maladaptive responses including substance abuse, withdrawal, and anxiety. The ability of an individual to handle stressors will largely depend on personal resources. It is important for the nurse to identify any stressors that may affect aspects of the self-concept. See Box 39.1 for examples of stressors that may place a client at risk for problems with self-concept.

BOX 39.1 Stressors Affecting Self-Concept

IDENTITY STRESSORS
- Change in physical appearance (e.g., facial wrinkles)
- Declining physical, mental, or sensory abilities
- Inability to achieve goals
- Relationship concerns
- Sexuality concerns
- Unrealistic ideal self

BODY IMAGE STRESSORS
- Loss of body parts (e.g., amputation, mastectomy, hysterectomy)
- Loss of body functions (e.g., from stroke, spinal cord injury, neuromuscular disease, arthritis, declining mental or sensory abilities)
- Disfigurement (e.g., through pregnancy, severe burns, facial blemishes, colostomy, tracheostomy)
- Unrealistic body ideal (e.g., a muscular configuration that cannot be achieved)

ROLE STRESSORS
- Loss of parent, spouse, child, or close friend
- Change or loss of job or other significant role
- Divorce
- Illness of self or others that affects role performance
- Ambiguous or conflicting role expectations
- Inability to meet role expectations

SELF-ESTEEM STRESSORS
- Lack of positive feedback from significant others
- Repeated failures
- Unrealistic expectations
- Abusive relationship
- Loss of financial security

Resources

An individual's resources are internal and external. Examples of internal resources include confidence and values, whereas external resources include support network, sufficient finances, and organizations. Generally, the greater the number of resources an individual has and uses, the more positive the effect on the self-concept.

History of Success and Failure

Individuals who have a history of inability to overcome barriers come to see themselves as failures, whereas individuals with a history of successes will have a more positive self-concept. Likewise, individuals with a positive self-concept tend to find contentment in their level of success, whereas a negative self-concept can lead to viewing one's life situation as negative.

Illness

Illness and trauma can also affect an individual's self-concept. A woman who has had a mastectomy may see herself as less attractive, and the loss may affect how she acts and values herself. Individuals respond to stressors such as illness and alterations in function related to aging in a variety of ways. Acceptance, denial, withdrawal, and depression are common reactions.

●○● NURSING MANAGEMENT

Assessing

A thorough assessment includes a psychosocial assessment of the client and the family or support person because this provides clues to actual or potential problems. The nurse assessing self-concept focuses on its four components: (1) personal identity, (2) body image, (3) role performance, and (4) self-esteem.

Before conducting a psychosocial assessment, the nurse must establish trust and a working relationship with the client. Guidelines for conducting a psychosocial assessment include the following:

- Create a quiet, private environment.
- Minimize interruptions if possible.
- Maintain appropriate eye contact.
- Sit at eye level with the client.
- Demonstrate an interest in the client's concerns.

- Indicate acceptance of the client by not criticizing, frowning, or demonstrating shock.
- Ask open-ended questions to encourage the client to talk rather than close-ended questions that tend to block free sharing.
- Avoid asking more personal questions than are actually needed.
- Minimize writing detailed notes during the interview because this can create client concern that confidential material is being "recorded" as well as interfere with your ability to focus on what the client is saying.
- Determine whether the family can provide additional information.
- Maintain confidentiality.
- Be aware of your own biases and discomforts that could influence the assessment.
- Consider how the client's behavior is influenced by culture.

QSEN Patient-Centered Care: Assessing Self-Concept

It is the nurse's responsibility to use therapeutic communication and to remain sensitive to the effect that cultural influences will have on a client's behaviors and needs. Cultural background is not only assessed directly but is also considered as a factor in the areas of self-perception, role relationships, major stressors, and coping strategies. In the area of behaviors that may suggest low self-esteem, nurses need to ask themselves the following question: Is this really a behavior that would suggest low self-esteem or is it part of the cultural behavior(s) of the client? In addition, might the client be experiencing cultural dissonance, a situation in which there are conflicting beliefs and attitudes between the client's culture and the one in which the client is living?

When stressors are identified, the nurse needs to determine how the client perceives the stressor. A positive, growth-oriented perception of stressful events reinforces self-worth; a negative, hopeless, defeatist perception leads to decreased self-esteem. The nurse should also identify the client's coping style and determine whether this style is effective by asking the client such questions as these:

- When you have a problem or face a stressful situation, how do you usually deal with it?
- How effective are these methods?

Clinical Alert!

The degree to which a stressor is perceived to affect self-concept varies among individuals. For example, some individuals may respond to repeated failures by trying harder, whereas others may give up.

Personal Identity

When assessing self-concept, the information the nurse first needs is about the client's personal identity. This involves who the client believes he or she is. See the accompanying Assessment Interview for examples of questions to ask.

ASSESSMENT INTERVIEW Personal Identity

- How would you describe your personal characteristics? How do you see yourself as an individual?
- How do others describe you as an individual?
- What do you like about yourself?
- What do you do well?
- What are your personal strengths, talents, and abilities?
- What would you change about yourself if you could?
- How do you feel if you think someone does not like you?

Body Image

If there are indications of a body image disturbance (Figure 39.3 ■), the nurse should assess the client carefully for possible functional or physical problems. The disturbance may be a result of a present deformity or malfunction or an anticipated one. In addition to the stated responses about the problem, it is important to assess related behavior. See the accompanying Assessment Interview for examples of questions to ask about body image.

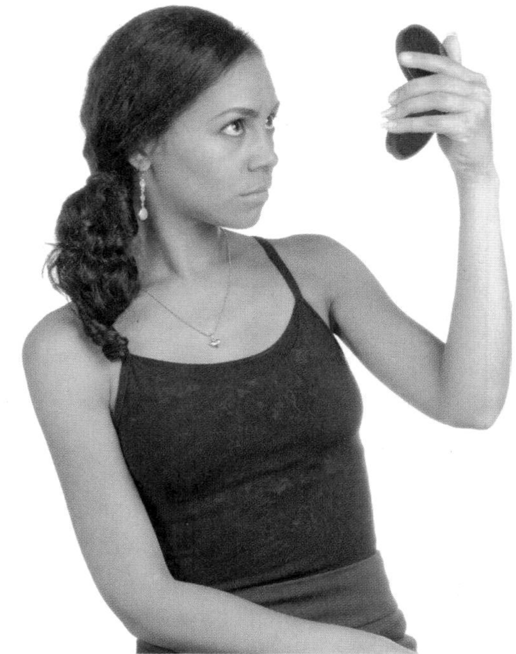

Figure 39.3 ■ Individuals do not always appear to themselves as they appear to others.
romakoma/Shutterstock.

Role Performance

The nurse assesses the client's satisfactions and dissatisfactions associated with role responsibilities and relationships: family roles, work roles, student roles, and social roles. Family roles are especially important because family relationships are particularly close. Relationships can be supportive and growth producing or, at the opposite extreme, highly stressful if there is violence or abuse. Assessment of family role relationships may begin with structural aspects such as the number in the family group, ages, and residence location. To obtain data related to the

ASSESSMENT INTERVIEW Body Image

- Is there any part of your body you would like to change?
- Do you feel different from others?
- How do you feel about your appearance?
- What changes in your body do you expect following your surgery, treatment, or illness?
- How have significant others in your life reacted to changes in your body?

client's family relationships and satisfaction or dissatisfaction with work roles and social roles, the nurse might ask some of the questions shown in the accompanying Assessment Interview. Keep in mind, however, that questions need to be tailored to the individuals and their culture, age, and situation.

Self-Esteem

A nurse can ask the following questions to determine a client's self-esteem:

- Are you satisfied with your life?
- How do you feel about yourself?
- Are you accomplishing what you want?
- What goals in life are important to you?

It is important for the nurse to determine the client's backgroundin order to not misinterpret specific behaviors. The following behaviors might reflect low self-esteem or may be misinterpreted due to the client's background:

- Avoids eye contact.
- Stoops in posture and moves slowly.
- Has an unkempt appearance.
- Is hesitant or halting in speech.
- Is overly critical of self (e.g., "I'm no good," or "People don't like me.").
- May be overly critical of others.
- Is unable to accept positive remarks about self.
- Apologizes frequently.
- Verbalizes feelings of hopelessness, helplessness, and powerlessness, such as "I really don't care what happens," "I'll do whatever anyone wants," or "Whatever is destined will happen."

Diagnosing

A positive self-concept can serve as a resource to a client when facing health challenges. Sometimes, as supported by data, the client has a problem in the area of self-perception, self-concept, self-esteem, or body image. Examples of nursing diagnoses that are appropriate for clients who have alterations in their self-concept can include impaired body image, modified role performance, and low self-esteem. Additional nursing diagnoses that may apply indirectly to clients with problems of self-concept are altered personal identity, anxiety related to changed physical appearance (e.g., amputation, mastectomy), grieving related to change in physical appearance, and challenges in parenting.

Planning

The nurse develops plans in collaboration with the client and support people when possible, according to the client's state of health, level of anxiety, resources, coping mechanisms, and sociocultural and religious affiliation. The nurse who has little experience in caring for clients with altered self-concept may wish to consult with a more experienced nurse to develop effective plans. The nurse and client set goals to enhance the client's self-concept.

The goals or desired outcomes established will vary according to the diagnoses and defining characteristics related to each individual. Specific nursing interventions can be selected to meet the individual needs of the client.

Implementing

Nursing interventions to promote or enhance a positive self-concept include helping a client to identify areas of strength. In addition, for clients who have an altered self-concept, nurses should establish a therapeutic relationship and assist clients to evaluate themselves and make behavioral changes.

ASSESSMENT INTERVIEW Role Performance

FAMILY RELATIONSHIPS

- Tell me about your family.
- What is home like?
- How is your relationship with your spouse, partner, or significant other (if appropriate)?
- What are your relationships like with your other relatives?
- Do you feel safe with your family members?
- How are important decisions made in your family?
- What are your responsibilities in the family?
- How well do you feel you accomplish what is expected of you?
- What about your role or responsibilities would you like to change?
- Are you proud of your family members?
- Do you feel your family members are proud of you?

WORK ROLES AND SOCIAL ROLES

- Do you like your work?
- How do you get along at work?
- What about your work would you like to change if you could?
- How do you spend your free time?
- Are you involved in any community groups?
- Are you most comfortable alone, with one other individual, or in a group?
- Who is most important to you?
- Whom do you seek out for help?

Identifying Areas of Strength

Individuals often perceive their problems and weaknesses more easily than their assets and strengths. Individuals with low self-esteem tend to focus even more on their limitations and to be aware of fewer strengths and many more problems. When a client has difficulty identifying personality strengths and assets, the nurse provides the client with a set of guidelines or a framework for identifying personality strengths (Box 39.2).

BOX 39.2 Framework for Identifying Personality Strengths

Note past, present, and anticipated future participation in:

- Hobbies and crafts
- Expressive arts such as writing, painting, dance, or music
- Sports and outdoor activities, including spectator sports
- Education, training, reading, technology, and related areas
- Work, vocation, job, or position

In addition, determine:

- Sense of humor and the ability to laugh at oneself and take kidding
- Health status including healthy aspects of body function and good health maintenance practices
- Special aptitudes such as sales or mechanical ability; a "green thumb"; ability to recognize and enjoy beauty; ability to solve problems; a liking for adventure or pioneering; having perseverance and the drive needed to get things done
- Relationship strengths including the ability to make people feel comfortable, the capacity to enjoy being with people, being aware of people's needs and feelings, and being able to listen
- Emotional strengths including the capacity to give and receive warmth, affection, and love; the ability to "take" anger and to feel and express a wide range of emotions; and the capacity for empathy
- Spiritual strengths such as religious faith or love of God, and membership and participation in church and related activities.

Nurses can employ the following specific strategies to reinforce strengths:

- Stress positive thinking rather than self-negation.
- Notice and verbally reinforce client strengths.
- Encourage the setting of attainable goals.
- Acknowledge goals that have been attained.
- Provide honest, positive feedback.

Enhancing Self-Esteem

Nurses assisting clients who have an altered self-concept or self-esteem must establish a therapeutic relationship. To do this the nurse must have self-awareness and effective communication skills. The following nursing techniques may help clients analyze the problem and make positive changes in their self-esteem:

- Encourage clients to appraise the situation and express their feelings.
- Encourage clients to ask questions.
- Provide accurate information.
- Become aware of distortions, inappropriate or unrealistic standards, and faulty labels in clients' speech.
- Explore clients' positive qualities and strengths.
- Encourage clients to express positive self-evaluation more than negative self-evaluation.
- Avoid criticism.
- Teach clients to substitute negative self-talk ("I can't walk to the store anymore") with positive self-talk ("I can walk half a block each morning"). Negative self-talk reinforces a negative self-concept.

Certain strategies vary depending on the age of the client (see Lifespan Considerations).

Evaluating

To determine whether client goals or desired outcomes have been achieved, the nurse uses data collected during interactions with the client and significant others. If outcomes are not achieved, the nurse should explore the reasons, considering questions such as the following:

- Have old situations recurred, triggering feelings or behaviors associated with low self-esteem?
- Have new stressful situations occurred with which the client feels unable to cope, resulting in continuing or recurrent low self-esteem (see Chapter 42 ∞)?
- Are new or additional roles causing increased stress in adapting?
- Are significant others supporting the client adequately in attempts to improve self-esteem?
- Did the client follow through on referrals to appropriate agencies? Did the agencies provide the expected services?
- Were the client's expectations too high in relation to the time needed for successful resolution of self-esteem problems?

Weaving the Tapestry of Life

The mainstays of the tapestry of life are the powers in one's life—self-esteem, love of life and humanity, and closeness to and recognition of the Godlife in oneself and others.

The weavings that form the patterns in one's life are experiences, knowledge, and dreams. Beauty can be seen throughout, but the strength of the fabric increases with age as the tapestry displays interweavings and integration of these special qualities.

As time goes on, aging is often accompanied by a fragileness of the physical body and an increased number of inevitable losses—emotional and social, as well as physical. This is when the integration of those special fibers—strengthening qualities—becomes so crucial to the overall quality of life of the individual.

When these strengths are displayed in the tapestry of life, the individual is not only given a feeling of self-worth and self-love, but the tapestry is a beautiful gift for all who behold it and are somehow touched by it.

Grace Miller

LIFESPAN CONSIDERATIONS Enhancing Self-Esteem

CHILDREN

- Children build strong self-esteem if they develop five basic attitudes: (1) security and trust, (2) identity, (3) belonging, (4) purpose, and (5) personal competence.
    - Security and trust are developed early in life; infants should learn that they can rely on their parents to meet their needs promptly and consistently. With older children, trust and security are strengthened when adults spend time with them: listening, playing, reading, or just being there. Both emotional and physical contact, such as a smile or a hug, convey warmth and caring.
    - Identity is developed when children are allowed to explore and experiment with the world around them and to express themselves as unique individuals in that world. They should be given opportunities to "practice" who they are. Preschoolers, for example, love to dress themselves and should be allowed to wear outlandish outfits (within limits of weather and safety) if they choose. Teenagers who try new hair colors and styles, some of which may "offend" their parents, are engaging in a crucial developmental step (Figure 39.4 ■).
    - Belonging is essential for all individuals, and having a sense that others in your social network care about you, want you there, and benefit by your contribution is important to healthy self-esteem. Children gain this sense of belonging by being included in activities, by being praised for their efforts and achievements, and by being valued by parents, siblings, caregivers, and other adults. Parents should make an effort to "catch their children doing well" and praise them for it (e.g., "I like the way you share with your brother."). Children should also hear that they are valued just for being themselves (e.g., "I like doing things with you. Remember when we went to the park? Wasn't that fun?").
    - Purpose and belonging are closely related. Children need opportunities to participate in the family and their community in order to discover what they can best contribute based on their strengths and skills. One mother, for example, stated "Leo (age 4) is our actor. He is wonderful with costumes and can make any of us smile when he starts his routine." Leo may never become an actor, but he knows he makes a significant contribution to his family's well-being. He brings them joy.
    - Personal competence grows as children identify and refine their skill sets. Children develop competence as they confront and solve problems, face challenges, expand their thinking, and are asked to do more than they think they can do. Adults must, however, provide children with support, guidance, appropriate assistance, and constructive feedback (including praise) in order to prevent the child from being overwhelmed. Too much frustration or uncertainty can lead to giving up, avoidance, lying, bullying, and other antisocial behaviors. If adults help children to accomplish goals that are important to them, children are more likely to develop a sense of personal competence and independence.
- Key ingredients for helping children develop high self-esteem are love, acceptance, firmness, consistency, and the establishment of expectations. Such qualities provide children with a safe, loving, supportive, and predictable world in which to live.

ADOLESCENTS

- Provide increasing levels of responsibility. Adolescents need to experience successes and failures and the consequences of their own behavior.
- Encourage discussion about issues including problems and mistakes.
- Show appreciation for effort and contributions. Emphasize the process, not just the result.
- Ask for their opinions and suggestions.
- Encourage participation in decision-making in areas that affect the adolescent. Show confidence in the teen's judgments.
- Avoid comparison with or ridicule or punishment in front of others.
- Assist in the creation of realistic goals and standards.
- Adolescents often engage in volunteer activities in their schools or communities, helping them to identify their strengths and find meaning in their activities. Knowing that they have a purpose and make a difference gives children strong self-esteem (Figure 39.5 ■).

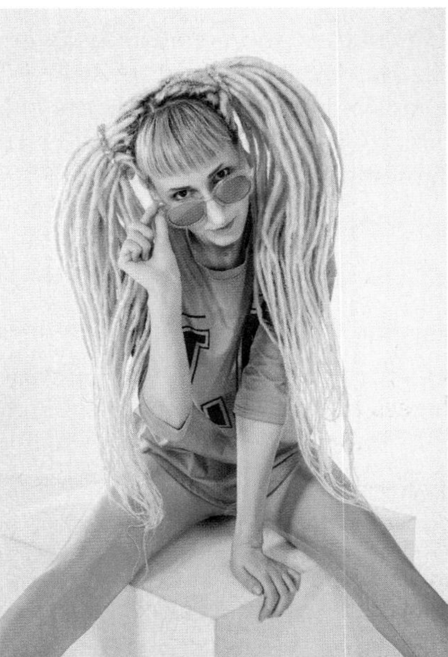

Figure 39.4 ■ Exploring different styles is a healthy and normal step in developing one's identity.
Evgeniya Litovchenko/123RF.

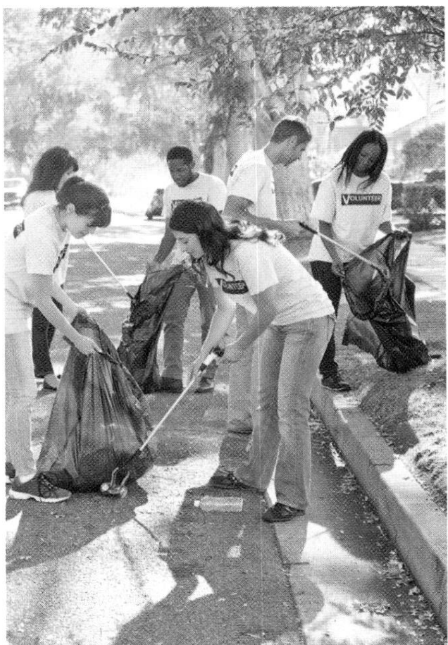

Figure 39.5 ■ Community service enhances self-esteem.
Cathy Yeulet/123RF.

Continued on page 1022

LIFESPAN CONSIDERATIONS Enhancing Self-Esteem—*continued*

ADULTS

- Explore the meaning of self-esteem and how the client's self-esteem has influenced past behaviors and actions (and can influence present and future plans and decisions).
- Assist the client in assessing the internal and external forces contributing to or detracting from their self-esteem.
- Act in ways that demonstrate belief that the client can cope with the realities and demands of life and is worthy of experiencing joy and happiness.
- Avoid comparisons with other individuals.
- Discourage statements about the self that are negative.
- Encourage the use of affirmations to enhance self-esteem, including statements such as "I like myself" or "I am a valuable individual."
- Encourage associations with positive, supportive individuals.
- Make positive statements about the client's past successes (major or minor).
- Assist the client to make a list of their positive qualities and to review this list often.
- Suggest the client do things for others. Making a contribution enhances positive feelings of self-worth.

OLDER ADULTS

Older adults who become increasingly dependent can develop low self-esteem. Old age is frequently accompanied by changes such as reduced income, decline in physical health, loss of friends and family, and retirement. In addition to those actions listed above for use with adults, nurses can use the following techniques to help older adults enhance their self-esteem:

- Encourage clients to participate in planning their own care.
- Listen carefully to their concerns.
- Assist clients to identify and use their own strengths.
- Encourage them to participate in activities in which they can be successful.
- Communicate that the client is valued. Use the client's name and ask for input.
- Encourage older adults to stay connected with their memories (Figure 39.6 ■). Reminiscing by writing or recording an autobiography or storytelling are excellent ways to do this.
- For older adults who are in hospitals or nursing homes, make sure that they are always shown respect and dignity and are provided privacy.
- Encourage creative activities to tap their resources. Examples are music, art, storytelling, quilting, and photography.
- Work with clients to establish goals in small steps that are achievable—this, in itself, can bolster self-esteem.

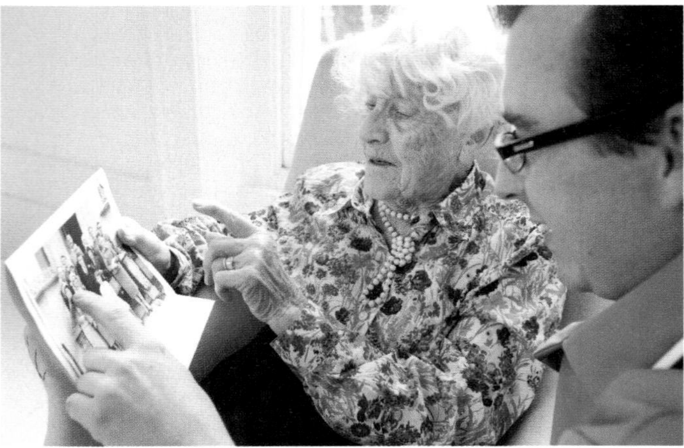

Figure 39.6 ■ Sharing memories with others can enhance seniors' self-esteem and general feelings of well-being.

The nurse, client, and significant others need to understand that to change beliefs, feelings, and behaviors affecting self-esteem requires time and ongoing effort. Unlike many physical problems (e.g., wounds) where healing can be quickly observed, improving one's self-concept can be a continuing concern and is not so easily evaluated. New crises can cause clients to doubt themselves and revert to former feelings of inadequacy. Individuals can learn from each new situation and gain new strategies for feeling satisfied with themselves.

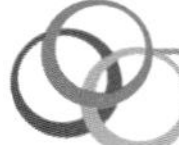

Critical Thinking Checkpoint

Craig is a 20-year-old male college student who was involved in an automobile crash 3 days ago, suffering a traumatic amputation of his left lower leg. Craig's mother has remained with him since the crash and is very supportive. His father is grief stricken and having difficulty dealing with Craig's condition because Craig was captain of his college basketball team and had aspirations of becoming a professional athlete. Craig's condition is stable and he is being placed into a rehabilitation program immediately. Soon, he will be fitted for a leg prosthesis. Usually an outgoing individual, Craig is somber and quiet. He does not look at his leg when dressings are being changed and he refuses to discuss his rehabilitation program.

1. Given Craig's age, speculate about whether Craig's self-concept is at risk for being adversely affected by his disability.
2. What data suggest that Craig's self-esteem is, or is at risk for being, negatively affected by his amputation?
3. What factors are likely to affect Craig's adaptation to his amputation and rehabilitation?
4. How would your interventions differ for a client with the same condition who was 70 years old?
5. What other groups of clients, in addition to those with amputations, are at risk for the development of altered self-esteem or body image?

Answers to Critical Thinking Checkpoint questions are available on the faculty resources site. Please consult with your instructor.

Chapter 39 Review

CHAPTER HIGHLIGHTS

- A positive self-concept is essential to an individual's mental and physical health.
- An individual's self-perception can differ from that individual's perception of how others see him or her and from the ideal self, that is, how the individual would like to be.
- Factors affecting self-concept include stage of development, family and culture, stressors, resources, history of success and failure, and illnesses that affect role performance.
- The nurse assesses four areas of self-concept: personal identity, body image, role performance and relationships, and self-esteem.
- Because a positive self-concept is basic to health, one of the nurse's major responsibilities is to assist clients whose self-concept is disturbed to develop a more positive and realistic image of themselves.
- A trusting client–nurse relationship is essential for the effective assessment of a client's self-concept, for providing help and support, and for motivating client behavior change.

TEST YOUR KNOWLEDGE

1. Sally is 170 cm (5′7″), weighs 48 kg (105 lb), and believes that she is fat. Which of the following most represents this perception?
   1. Altered body image
   2. Altered personal identity
   3. Excessive self-expectation
   4. Altered core self-concept

2. A 5-year-old girl indulges in the following activities. Select all those options that can help develop identity.
   1. Tries on her mother's lipstick and powder
   2. Wears her older sibling's shoes and clothes
   3. Acts as Cinderella in a pretend play
   4. Builds an indoor tent out of chairs and blankets
   5. Participates in arts and crafts

3. A client's spouse tells the nurse that the client is not making progress in developing a more positive self-esteem. What should the nurse's response to the spouse be?
   1. "Most clients make quicker progress."
   2. "Self-esteem work takes time and is not easily evaluated."
   3. "What have you done to help the client with this work?"
   4. "Do you think that the client is really trying?"

4. An 89-year-old client states, "I'm a lost cause. I can't even stand long enough to cook my own meals anymore." Which is the most appropriate response?
   1. "That must be difficult. What things are you still able to do?"
   2. "Well, that is to be expected at your age."
   3. "Do you have someone else who can cook for you?"
   4. "Are you a good cook?"

5. A client recovering from a lumpectomy due to breast cancer tells the nurse that she "feels ugly." For which nursing diagnosis should the nurse plan interventions?
   1. Powerlessness
   2. Social Isolation
   3. Grieving
   4. Hopelessness

6. During an annual performance review, which statement by the nurse indicates the area of self-awareness?
   1. "I rarely make any medication errors."
   2. "I am willing to mentor new nurses."
   3. "My client satisfaction reports agree that I am friendly and helpful."
   4. "All of my clients have recovered quickly from their health problems."

7. Which statement should the nurse make first when assessing a client's self-concept?
   1. Describe yourself as a person.
   2. Tell me about your family.
   3. Describe what you do when you have free time.
   4. Tell me about the work you do.

8. A 25-year-old woman who is 4 months pregnant attends an outpatient maternity clinic. She reports that her legs swell up frequently, especially in the morning, and that she is concerned of her weight gain because some of her favorite clothes no longer fit her. Which of the following responses is appropriate?
   1. "All of your experiences are perfectly normal."
   2. "Tell me more about how you feel."
   3. "You will be able to wear your favorite clothes again after you've given birth."
   4. "Do you want medication for the leg swelling?"

9. Which interventions are appropriate for a client with low or poor self-concept? Select all that apply.
   1. Encourage the client to compare self with others.
   2. Suggest the client not say negative things about self.
   3. Suggest the client say positive things about self.
   4. Recommend the client avoid situations of having to care for others.
   5. Communicate very low-level expectations of the client's behavior.

10. Self-concept may vary according to a variety of conditions affecting the individual. The nurse recognizes that even appropriate nursing interventions are least likely to alter which of the following?
   1. Resources
   2. Self-knowledge
   3. Core self-concept
   4. Social self

See Answers to Test Your Knowledge in Appendix A.

READINGS AND REFERENCES

Suggested Reading

Lowe, M. R., Marmorstein, N., Iacono, W., Rosenbaum, D., Espel-Huynh, H., Muratore, A. F., . . . Zhang, F. (2019). Body concerns and BMI as predictors of disordered eating and body mass in girls: An 18-year longitudinal investigation. *Journal of Abnormal Psychology*, *128*, 32–43. doi:10.1037/abn0000394

Overconcern with one's body is a strong predictor of the development of eating disorders. This study tested whether such findings continue when measured over follow-up starting at age 11 and ending at age 29. Findings indicated that both body dissatisfaction and weight preoccupation predicted a reduced rate of eating disorder symptom development over an 18-year follow-up period.

Related Research

Collison, D., Banbury, S., & Lusher, J. (2016). Relationships between age, sex, self-esteem and attitudes towards alcohol use amongst university students. *Journal of Alcohol & Drug Education*, *60*(2), 16–34.

References

Erikson, E. H. (1963). *Childhood and society* (2nd ed.). New York, NY: Norton.

Hyde, J. S., & DeLamater, J. D. (2017). *Understanding human sexuality* (13th ed.). New York, NY: McGraw-Hill.

Neves C. M., Cipriani F. M., Meireles J. F. F., Morgado F. F. d. R., & Ferreira M. E. C. (2017). Body image in childhood: An integrative review of literature. *Revista Paulista Pediatria*, *35*(3), 331–339.

Selected Bibliography

Demerouti, E., Sanz-Vergel, A. I., Petrou, P., & van den Heuvel, M. (2016). How work-self conflict/facilitation influences exhaustion and task performance: A three-wave study on the role of personal resources. *Journal of Occupational Health Psychology*, *21*, 391–402. doi:10.1037/ocp0000022

Demeyer, I., Romero, N., & De Raedt, R. (2018). Assessment of implicit self-esteem in older adults: The role of actual and ideal self-esteem in negative mood. *Assessment*, *25*, 302–309. doi:10.1177/1073191117691607

Gruenenfelder-Steiger, A. E., Harris, M. A., & Fend, H. A. (2016). Subjective and objective peer approval evaluations and self-esteem development: A test of reciprocal, prospective, and long-term effects. *Developmental Psychology*, *52*, 1563–1577. doi:10.1037/dev0000147

Hochgraf, A. K., McHale, S. M., & Fosco, G. M. (2018). Parent responsiveness and gender moderate bidirectional links between self-esteem and weight concerns during adolescence. *Journal of Family Psychology*, *32*, 828–834. doi:10.1037/fam0000434

Johnson, M. D., Krahn, H. J., & Galambos, N. L. (2017). Better late than early: Marital timing and subjective well-being in midlife. *Journal of Family Psychology*, *31*, 635–641. doi:10.1037/fam0000297

Lam, C. F., Wan, W. H., & Roussin, C. J. (2016). Going the extra mile and feeling energized: An enrichment perspective of organizational citizenship behaviors. *Journal of Applied Psychology*, *101*, 379–391. doi:10.1037/apl0000071

Long, T. (2016). What the mirror doesn't tell you. *American Nurse Today*, *11*(9), 38–40.

Naumann, E., Svaldi, J., Wyschka, T., Heinrichs, M., & von Dawans, B. (2018). Stress-induced body dissatisfaction in women with binge eating disorder. *Journal of Abnormal Psychology*, *127*, 548–558. doi:10.1037/abn0000371

Nelson, S. C., Kling, J., Wängqvist, M., Frisén, A., & Syed, M. (2018). Identity and the body: Trajectories of body esteem from adolescence to emerging adulthood. *Developmental Psychology*, *54*, 1159–1171. doi:10.1037/dev0000435

Nosek, M. A., Robinson-Whelen, S., Hughes, R. B., & Nosek, T. M. (2016). An internet-based virtual reality intervention for enhancing self-esteem in women with disabilities: Results of a feasibility study. *Rehabilitation Psychology*, *61*, 358–370. doi:10.1037/rep0000107

Obeid, N., Norris, M. L., Buchholz, A., Henderson, K. A., Goldfield, G., Bedford, S., & Flament, M. F. (2018). Socioemotional predictors of body esteem in adolescent males. *Psychology of Men & Masculinity*, *19*, 439–445. doi:10.1037/men0000109

Rueda Diaz, L. J., de Almeida Lopes Monteiro da Cruz, D., & de Cassia Gengo e Silva, R. (2016). Caregiver role strain: Bi-national study of content validation. *Investigacion y Educacion En Enfermeria*, *34*, 280–287. doi:10.17533/udea.iee.v34n2a07

Sexuality 40

LEARNING OUTCOMES

After completing this chapter, you will be able to:

1. Describe sexual development across the lifespan.
2. Define sexual health.
3. Discuss variations in sexual expression.
4. Give examples of how the family, culture, religion, and personal expectations and ethics influence one's sexuality.
5. Describe physiologic changes during the sexual response cycle.
6. Identify the forms of altered sexual function.
7. Identify basic sexual questions the nurse should ask during client assessment.
8. Formulate nursing diagnoses and interventions for the client experiencing sexual problems.
9. Recognize health promotion teaching related to reproductive structures.

KEY TERMS

anal stimulation, *1032*
androgyny, *1030*
body image, *1030*
coitus, *1032*
cross-dressing, *1032*
desire phase, *1034*
dysmenorrhea, *1027*
dyspareunia, *1037*
excitement phase, *1035*
female orgasmic disorder, *1037*
female sexual arousal disorder, *1036*
gender expression, *1030*
gender identity, *1030*
genital intercourse, *1032*
hypoactive sexual desire disorder, *1036*
intersex, *1031*
male erectile disorder, *1036*
male orgasmic disorder, *1037*
masturbation, *1025*
menstruation, *1025*
oral–genital sex, *1032*
orgasmic phase, *1035*
resolution phase, *1035*
sexual orientation, *1030*
sexual self-concept, *1030*
transgender, *1030*
vaginismus, *1037*
vestibulitis, *1037*
vulvodynia, *1037*

Introduction

All humans are sexual beings. Regardless of gender, age, race, socioeconomic status, religious beliefs, physical and mental health, or other demographic factors, we express our sexuality in a variety of ways throughout our lives.

Human sexuality is difficult to define. Sexuality is an individually expressed and highly personal phenomenon that evolves from life experiences. Physiologic, psychosocial, and cultural factors influence an individual's sexuality and lead to the wide range of attitudes and behaviors seen in humans. Satisfying or "normal" sexual expression can be described as whatever behaviors give pleasure and satisfaction to those adults involved, without threat of coercion or injury to self or others. What constitutes normal sexual expression, however, varies among cultures and religions.

In this chapter, *sex* refers primarily to the biology of being male, female, or some other anatomic state, and to sexual activity. *Gender* refers to the psychologic sense of being feminine or masculine and is related to the terms *woman* and *man*.

Development of Sexuality

The development of sexuality begins with conception and continues throughout the lifespan. Table 40.1 outlines characteristics of sexual development typically seen throughout the lifespan, with nursing interventions and teaching guidelines for each developmental stage.

Birth to 12 Years

The ability of the human body to experience a sexual response is present before birth. When babies find their fingers and toes, they also find their genitals. They seem to experience a pleasurable sensation from the touch but one would not call this a sexual experience. By the age of 3, more purposeful **masturbation** (excitation of one's own or another's genital organs by means other than sexual intercourse) begins, although males do not ejaculate until after puberty. By age 2 1/2 or 3, children have beginning awareness of genital differences between males and females.

Around age 9 or 10, the first physical changes of puberty begin—the development of breast buds in girls and the growth of pubic hair. As the adrenal glands mature, they produce more testosterone and estradiol, which contributes to the first experiences of sexual attraction to another individual. Girls learn about **menstruation** (monthly uterine bleeding) and related self-care.

TABLE 40.1 Sexual Development Throughout Life

Stage	Characteristics	Nursing Interventions and Teaching Guidelines
INFANCY		
Birth–18 months	Differentiates self from others gradually. External genitals are sensitive to touch. Male infants have penile erections; females, vaginal lubrication.	Self-manipulation of the genitals is normal. Caregivers need to recognize these behaviors as common in children.
TODDLER		
1–3 years	Able to identify own gender.	Body exploration and genital fondling is normal. Use names for body parts.
PRESCHOOLER		
4–5 years	Becomes increasingly aware of self. Explores own and playmates' body parts. Learns correct names for body parts. Learns to control feelings and behavior.	Answer questions about "where babies come from" honestly and simply. Parental overreaction to exploration of genitals and masturbation can lead to feelings that sex is "bad."
SCHOOL AGE		
6–12 years	Has strong identification with parent of the same gender. Tends to have friends of the same gender. Has increasing awareness of self. Increased modesty, desire for privacy. Learns the role and concepts of own gender. At about 8 or 9 years becomes concerned about specific sex behaviors and often approaches parents with explicit concerns about sexuality and reproduction.	Provide parents and children with opportunities to express their concerns and ask questions regarding sex. Answer all questions with factual data and perhaps follow up with appropriate books and other material. Advise parents to discuss basic information about sexual intercourse, menstruation, and reproduction with children at about 10 years of age. Give children reading material and then discuss it with them.
ADOLESCENCE		
12–18 years	Primary and secondary sex characteristics develop. Menarche usually takes place. Develops relationships with interested partners. Masturbation is common. May participate in heterosexual or same-sex activity. Are at risk for pregnancy and sexually transmitted infections (STIs).	Adolescents require information about body changes. Peer groups have great importance at this time and assist in forming gender roles. Dating helps adolescents prepare for adult roles. Parents influence values and beliefs regarding behavior. Teenagers require information about contraceptive measures and precautions to take with regard to STIs.
YOUNG ADULTHOOD		
18–40 years	Sexual activity is common. Establishes own lifestyle and values. Many couples share financial obligations and household tasks.	Young adults often require information about measures to prevent unwanted pregnancies (i.e., abstinence or contraceptive devices). Require information to prevent STIs. Require regular communication to understand partner's sexual needs and to work through problems and stresses.
MIDDLE ADULTHOOD		
40–65 years	Males and females experience decreased hormone production. Menopause occurs in females usually anywhere between ages 40 and 55. The climacteric occurs gradually in males. The quality rather than the number of sexual experiences becomes important. Individuals establish independent moral and ethical standards.	Females and males may need help adjusting to new roles. Clients may require counseling to help them reevaluate and direct their energies. Encourage couples to look at the positive aspects of this time of life.
LATE ADULTHOOD		
65 years and older	Interest in sexual activity often continues. Sexual activity may be less frequent. Female's vaginal secretions diminish, and breasts atrophy. Males produce fewer sperm and need more time to achieve an erection and to ejaculate.	Older adults often continue to be sexually active. Couples may require counseling about adapting their affection and sexual needs to physical limitations.

Adolescence

During early adolescence (12 to 13 years), primary and secondary sex characteristics continue to develop, necessitating more information about body changes. For boys, the testes and scrotum increase in size, the skin over the scrotum becomes darker, pubic hair grows, and axillary sweating begins. Development of the genitals to adult size takes about 5 to 6 years. For girls, the pelvis and hips broaden, the breast tissue develops, pubic hair grows (see Figure 29.25 in Chapter 29 ∞), axillary sweating begins, and vaginal secretions become milky and change from an alkaline to an acid pH.

First-time sexual activity varies dramatically according to geographical region of the world, religion, and other social conventions. In the United States, a 2017 study of more than 14,000 high school students indicated that 39.5% of students had ever had sexual intercourse, 53.8% of those had used a condom during sexual intercourse, and 9.7% had had sexual intercourse with four or more individuals during their life (Kann et al., 2018).

Teenage girls may have irregular menstruation initially, which can lead to embarrassment because of stained clothing. They can be taught to be aware of subtle signs of impending menstruation, such as tender breasts, water retention or bloating, or the appearance of skin eruptions or pimples. Girls should also be counseled regarding the variety of feminine hygiene products available (e.g., sanitary pads and tampons) so they can make intelligent choices. Parents and nurses should advise teenage girls to wash their hands thoroughly before and after inserting a tampon, to change tampons frequently, to alternate them with sanitary pads, and to use pads at night. These measures will help to decrease infection, including the risk of "toxic shock," a particular type of *Staphylococcus aureus* infection. Thorough cleaning of the genital area and wiping from front to back will also decrease infection and prevent odors.

Dysmenorrhea (painful menstruation) is prevalent among adolescent females. Cramping, lower abdominal pain radiating to the back and upper thighs, nausea, vomiting, diarrhea, and headaches may occur for a few hours up to 3 days. Dysmenorrhea results from powerful uterine contractions, which cause ischemia and cramping pain. The symptoms of dysmenorrhea are treated with administration of analgesics such as aspirin, application of heat to the abdomen, certain exercises such as abdominal muscle strengthening, biofeedback, and nonsteroidal anti-inflammatory medications, such as ibuprofen.

All adolescents want to know about sexual behaviors but are often uneasy about discussing these concerns with their parents. Nurses, the schools, and the family need to provide accurate information. During the nursing assessment, teenagers should be asked directly what they know about sex, contraception, and reproduction. Sometimes a lot of the teenager's information is based on popular myths and little, if any, on fact. The nurse should discuss factual information about sex, sexual actions and their consequences, the individual's right to decide regarding ways to express oneself sexually, and the responsibilities of each individual regarding sexual activity. See Table 40.2.

Sexually transmitted infections (STIs) are the most common bacterial infections among adolescents. Teens need education about these diseases, preventive measures, and early treatment. The common types and symptoms of STIs for which teenagers should seek medical care are listed in Box 40.1. The nurse should also inform teens about the methods of birth control: abstinence, pills, timed-release transdermal patches and implants, diaphragms, intrauterine devices, the rhythm method, and condoms to prevent an unplanned pregnancy. These are discussed later in this chapter.

TABLE 40.2 Common Sexual Misconceptions

Misconception	Fact
Nearly all males over 70 years old have erectile dysfunction.	Sexual ability is not lost due to age. Changes are commonly due to disease or medication.
Masturbation causes certain mental instabilities.	Masturbation is a common and healthy behavior.
Sexual activity weakens an individual.	There is no evidence that sexual activity weakens an individual.
Females who have experienced orgasm are more likely to become pregnant.	Conceiving is not related to experiencing orgasm.
Nice girls should not feel entitled to their own sexual satisfaction.	As women become more comfortable with their own sexuality, they advocate for their own sexual fulfillment.
A large penis provides greater sexual satisfaction than a small penis.	There is no evidence that a large penis provides greater satisfaction.
Alcohol is a sexual stimulant.	Alcohol is a relaxant and central nervous system depressant. Chronic alcoholism is associated with erectile dysfunction.
Intercourse during menstruation is dangerous (i.e., it will cause vaginal tissue damage).	There is no physiologic basis for abstinence during menses.
The face-to-face coital position is the moral or proper one.	The position that offers the most pleasure and is acceptable to both partners is the correct one.

BOX 40.1 Common Symptoms of Sexually Transmitted Infections

Infection	Male	Female
Candidiasis	Itching, irritation, discharge, plaque of cheesy material under foreskin.	Red and excoriated vulva; intense itching of vaginal and vulvar tissues; thick, white, cheesy or curd-like discharge.
Chlamydial urethritis	Urinary frequency; watery, mucoid urethral discharge.	Commonly a carrier; vaginal discharge, dysuria, urinary frequency.
Genital warts (condyloma acuminatum)	The infection is caused by the human papillomavirus (HPV). Single lesions or clusters of lesions growing beneath or on the foreskin, at the external meatus, or on the glans penis. On dry skin areas, lesions are hard and yellow-gray. On moist areas, lesions are pink or red and soft with a cauliflower-like appearance.	Certain strains of HPV have been linked to cervical cancer. Lesions appear at the bottom part of the vaginal opening and on the perineum, labia, inner walls of the vagina, and cervix.
Gonorrhea	Painful urination; urethritis with watery white discharge, which may become purulent.	May be asymptomatic; or vaginal discharge, pain, and urinary frequency may be present.
Herpes genitalis (herpes simplex of the genitals)	Primary herpes involves the presence of painful sores or large, discrete vesicles that last for weeks; vesicles rupture. Recurrent herpes is itchy rather than painful; it lasts for a few hours to 10 days.	
Human immunodeficiency virus (HIV) and acquired immunodeficiency syndrome (AIDS)	Symptoms can appear any time from several months to several years after acquiring the virus. The individual has reduced immunity to other diseases. Symptoms include any of the following for which there is no other explanation: persistent heavy night sweats; extreme fatigue; severe weight loss; enlarged lymph glands in neck, axillae, or groin; persistent diarrhea; skin rashes; blurred vision or chronic headache; harsh, dry cough; thick gray-white coating on tongue or throat.	
Syphilis	Chancre, usually on glans penis, that is painless and heals in 4–6 weeks; secondary symptoms—skin eruptions, low-grade fever, inflammation of lymph glands—in 6 weeks to 6 months after chancre heals.	Chancre on cervix or other genital areas that heals in 4–6 weeks; symptoms same as for male.
Trichomoniasis	Slight itching; moisture on top of penis; slight, early morning urethral discharge. Many males are asymptomatic.	Itching and redness of vulva and skin inside thighs; copious watery, frothy vaginal discharge.
Zika	Few if any symptoms. May include mild fever, rash, headache, joint pain, conjunctivitis (red eyes), or muscle pain. The virus can spread from mother to fetus causing severe birth defects, especially failure of normal brain development.	

Young and Middle Adulthood

In young adulthood, many individuals form intimate relationships with long-term implications. These relationships may take the form of dating, cohabitation, or marriage. Note, however, that some individuals do not form intimate relationships until late adulthood and that some never form these types of relationships.

Young adult men and women are often concerned about normal sexual response, for both themselves and their partners. In heterosexual relationships, problems may arise because of basic differences in male and female expectations and responses. Gay and lesbian couples may fare better in this respect. Couples need to communicate their needs to each other early in their courtship so a successful intimate relationship can develop and grow. Young adults should also know that because sexual needs and responses may change, each partner should listen and respond to the needs of the other.

During middle adulthood both males and females experience decreased hormone production, causing the climacteric, usually called menopause in women. These events often affect the individual's sexual self-concept, body image, and sexual identity. See Chapter 25 ∞ for further information on menopause.

Older Adulthood

Older adults may define sexuality far more broadly and include in their definition such things as touching, hugging, romantic gestures (e.g., giving or receiving flowers), comfort, warmth, dressing up, joy, spirituality, and beauty. Interest in sexual activity is not lost as individuals age. For men, however, more time is needed to achieve an erection and to ejaculate (the erection may last longer than at a younger age); more direct genital stimulation is required to achieve an erection; the volume of ejaculated fluid decreases; and the intensity of contractions with orgasm may decrease. The refractory period after orgasm is longer.

EVIDENCE-BASED PRACTICE

Evidence-Based Practice

What are the risks and rewards of adolescents becoming sexually active?

Sexual debut is the term used to describe the first experience of intercourse. In this study, Golden, Furman, and Collibee (2016) followed 174 adolescents over 10 years, gathering data 7 times. A great deal of data was collected on variables such as anxiety, depression, substance abuse, self-worth, and sexual activity. The data were analyzed to determine whether the associations of timing of sexual debut and the risk and reward variables differed by demographics.

These analyses revealed that sexual debut was related to rewards, including increases in romantic appeal and sexual satisfaction. Early sexual debut was related to risks, such as greater substance use, more internalizing and externalizing symptoms, and lower global self-worth. Rewards associated with an early debut included greater romantic appeal, dating satisfaction (males only), and sexual satisfaction (males only). Although there are some inherent risks with sexual activity, the results suggest that sexual debut at a normative or late age is also associated with a decrease in some risks and an increase in rewards.

Implications

Nurses working with teens are compelled to understand teen behavior in the context of current values of those individuals and to resist the temptation to put that behavior in the perspective of their own or earlier generations. Assessment of behavior as safe or risky will change over time as improved methods of prevention, early detection, and treatment of sex-related conditions evolve. This study reminds the nurse to consider both the risks and rewards of becoming sexually active from the adolescent's point of view.

Older women remain capable of multiple orgasms and may experience an increase in sexual desire after menopause. Vaginal lubrication and elasticity decrease with menopause and decreased estrogen, and phases of the sexual response cycle may take longer to occur. There is a possibility of pain during sexual activity and intercourse (dyspareunia) related to vaginal dryness or chronic health conditions (e.g., diabetes or arthritis). Lack of privacy may be a concern for older adults who live with family or in a rehabilitation or long-term care facility.

Many products are available to assist older adults with enhancing their sexual experiences. These range from simple lubricants to medications and surgically implanted devices that enable penile erections. Although older adults' technique may require modification, the nurse should never assume that they are less interested in or less motivated to have an active sex life.

Sexual Health

Sexual health is an individual and constantly changing phenomenon falling within the wide range of human sexual thoughts, feelings, needs, and desires. For most individuals, sexual health is not a concern until its absence or impairment is noticed. An individual's degree of sexual health is best determined by that individual, sometimes with the assistance of a qualified professional.

The Centers for Disease Control and Prevention (CDC)/Health Resources and Services Administration (HRSA) Advisory Committee on HIV, Viral Hepatitis, and STD Prevention and Treatment (2012) defines sexual health in the United States as follows:

> Sexual health is a state of well-being in relation to sexuality across the lifespan that involves physical, emotional, mental, social, and spiritual dimensions. Sexual health is an inextricable element of human health and is based on a positive, equitable, and respectful approach to sexuality, relationships, and reproduction that is free of coercion, fear, discrimination, stigma, shame, and violence. Sexual health includes: the ability to understand the benefits, risks, and responsibilities of sexual behavior; the prevention and care of disease and other adverse outcomes; and the possibility of fulfilling sexual relationships. (p. 41)

Sexual health occurs when sexual relationships are respectful, safe, and pleasurable. Sexual rights, which are essential for sexual health, are listed in Box 40.2.

BOX 40.2 Sexual Rights

1. The right to equality and non-discrimination
2. The right to life, liberty, and security of the person
3. The right to autonomy and bodily integrity
4. The right to be free from torture and cruel, inhuman, or degrading treatment or punishment
5. The right to be free from all forms of violence and coercion
6. The right to privacy
7. The right to the highest attainable standard of health, including sexual health; with the possibility of pleasurable, satisfying, and safe sexual experiences
8. The right to enjoy the benefits of scientific progress and its application
9. The right to information
10. The right to education and the right to comprehensive sexuality education
11. The right to enter, form, and dissolve marriage and other similar types of relationships based on equality and full and free consent
12. The right to decide whether to have children, the number and spacing of children, and to have the information and the means to do so
13. The right to the freedom of thought, opinion, and expression
14. The right to freedom of association and peaceful assembly
15. The right to participation in public and political life
16. The right to access to justice, remedies, and redress

From *Declaration of Sexual Rights*, by the World Association for Sexual Health, 2014. Reprinted with permission. Retrieved from http://www.worldsexology.org/wp-content/uploads/2013/08/declaration_of_sexual_rights_sep03_2014.pdf

Components of Sexual Health

Components of sexual health are sexual self-concept, body image, gender identity, and gender expression. Also see Chapter 39 ∞ for further discussion of self-concept, role, image, and identity.

One's **sexual self-concept** (how one values oneself as a sexual being) determines with whom one will have sex, the gender and kinds of individuals one is attracted to, and the values about when, where, with whom, and how one expresses sexuality. A positive sexual self-concept enables individuals to form intimate relationships throughout life. A negative sexual self-concept may impede the formation of relationships.

Body image, a central part of the sense of self, is constantly changing. Pregnancy, aging, trauma, disease, and therapies can alter an individual's appearance and function, which can affect body image. How an individual feels about their body is related to the individual's sexuality. Individuals who feel good about their bodies are likely to be comfortable with and enjoy sexual activity. Individuals who have a poor body image may respond negatively to sexual arousal. A major influence on body image for women is the media focus on physical attractiveness and breast size. Likewise, many men worry about penis size. The myth that "larger is better," particularly if it stays erect for a substantial time, is pervasive in North America. An individual's body image can suffer when the individual is unable to achieve these expectations.

Androgyny, or flexibility in gender roles, is the belief that most characteristics and behaviors are human qualities that should not be limited to one specific gender or the other. Being androgynous does not mean being sexually neutral or imply anything about one's sexual orientation. Rather, it describes the degree of flexibility an individual has regarding gender-stereotypic behaviors. Adults who can behave flexibly regarding their sexual roles may adapt better than those who adopt rigid stereotyped gender roles.

Gender identity is one's self-image as a female or male. It has a physical component and it also includes social and cultural norms. Gender identity results from developmental events that may or may not conform to an individual's apparent biological sex. Once gender identity is established, it cannot be easily changed.

Gender expression is the outward manifestation of an individual's sense of maleness or femaleness as well as what is perceived as gender-appropriate behavior. Each society defines its roles for males and females (Figure 40.1 ■).

In North America, traditional adult male roles have historically included breadwinner, lover, father, and athlete. Expected male behaviors included wearing trousers, demonstrating physical strength, and expressing feelings in a controlled fashion. Women traditionally express their emotions more freely and are gentler in their physical responses; they also have a broader choice of clothing than men do. These gender expressions are becoming much less common or expected.

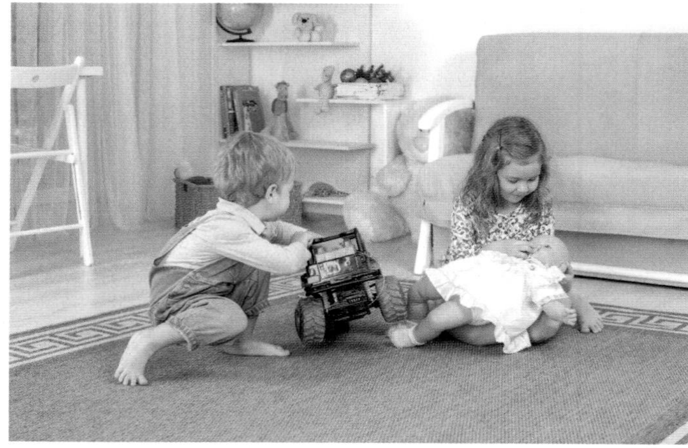

Figure 40.1 ■ Gender expression may be apparent at an early age.
Bill Aron/PhotoEdit.

Sexual health includes both freedoms and responsibilities. Sexually healthy individuals engage in activities that are freely chosen. Individuals also have freedom of their sexual thoughts, feelings, and fantasies. Sexually healthy individuals are ethically motivated to exercise behavioral, emotional, economic, and social responsibility for themselves.

Sexual Expression

There is tremendous variation in how individuals experience and express their sexuality. There are also many differences in the priority individuals place on sexuality in their lives. Sexual expression includes sexual orientation, gender identity, and performance preferences.

Sexual Orientation

One's attraction to individuals of the same sex, other sex, or both sexes is referred to as **sexual orientation.** Sexual orientation lies along a continuum with a wide range between extremes of exclusive attraction. This is one reason why the number of terms used to describe sexuality is increasing. The term LGBTQQ is frequently used. It stands for lesbian, gay, bisexual, transgender, queer, and questioning. In general, same-sex attraction has been called *homosexuality*; women attracted only to women are referred to as *lesbians*; men attracted to men are referred to as *gay* (although *gay* is also a general term for *homosexual*); individuals attracted to individuals of both genders are referred to as *bisexual*; someone who identifies with a different gender than their anatomic designation is **transgender**; someone who rejects gender stereotypes may be considered *queer*; and those who have not decided on their orientation may be *questioning*. Many other terms may also be used. The nurse should feel comfortable asking for the client's definition of a term if unsure of its meaning.

The origins of sexual orientation are still not well understood. Some biological theories describe sexual orientation in terms of the genetic composition of the individual. Psychologic theories stress the role of early learning experiences and cognitive processes. Other theories acknowledge the confluence of genetics and the environment in developing sexual orientation.

Estimates of the percentage of the population with a homosexual orientation vary. Because these individuals grow up acutely aware of the discrimination they face in North America, many do not disclose their sexual orientation. A survey of over 1.6 million Americans from 2012 to 2016 demonstrated that 4.1% of adults self-identify as lesbian, gay, bisexual, or transgender, and among those born after 1980, the number is 7.3 % (Gates, 2017).

Gender Identity

Western culture is deeply committed to the idea that there are only two sexes. Biologically speaking, however, there are many gradations running from female to male (Figure 40.2 ■). Sometimes gender is clear, in other cases there is a blending of both genders within the same individual, and in some it is unclear.

Intersex

An increasing number of babies are born with an **intersex** condition in which there are contradictions among chromosomal sex, gonadal sex, internal organs, and external genital appearance (Rich, Phipps, Tiwari, Rudraraju, & Dokpesi, 2016). The gender of such an infant is ambiguous. This means that an intersexed individual has some parts usually associated with males and some parts usually associated with females. Two of the most common syndromes leading to intersex are congenital adrenal hyperplasia and androgen-insensitivity syndrome. Intersex anatomy may not be apparent at birth. Sometimes it is undetected until puberty, until the individual is identified as an infertile adult, or until the individual dies and is autopsied.

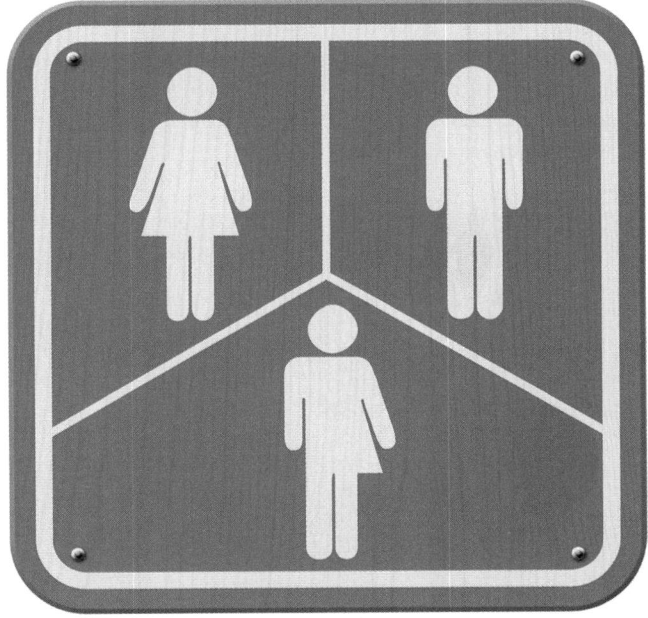

Figure 40.2 ■ Gender identity may not be a straightforward classification.
karen roach/123RF.

Transgenderism

For the transgender individual, sexual anatomy contradicts gender identity. Those who are born physically male but are emotionally and psychologically female are called male-to-female (MtF) transgender persons. Those who are born female but are emotionally and psychologically male are called female-to-male (FtM) transgender persons. Transgender and transsexual are commonly confused terms that both refer to gender identity. Transgender is a broader term that includes all individuals who do not identify with the gender that corresponds to the sex they were assigned at birth. Transsexual is a narrower term that includes individuals who desire to physically transition to the gender with which they identify.

Transgender is not considered a disorder. In the fifth edition of the *Diagnostic and Statistical Manual of Mental Disorders* (referred to as the DSM-5), transgender individuals may be viewed as having *gender dysphoria* only if they have clinically significant distress or impairment in social, school, or other important areas of functioning (Ross, 2017). Most transgender individuals report that they have felt gender dysphoria since early childhood. They often suffer for many years and try to hide the situation from family and friends. Many transgender individuals report living in poverty, psychologic trauma, attempted suicide, mistreatment in school, harassment, and sexual assault (James et al., 2016). As self-understanding and acceptance have increased, many transgender individuals have lived part or full time as members of the other sex. Their sexual orientation may be heterosexual, homosexual, or bisexual. The process of moving from one gender to another is referred to as *transition*. Some individuals decide to undergo sexual reassignment procedures, which involve varying amounts of hormone treatments and surgery. The World Professional Association for Transgender Health publishes *Standards of Care* and *Ethical Guidelines*, which describe the psychiatric, psychologic, medical, and surgical management of gender dysphoria and how professionals can offer assistance to those with this condition.

Based on nursing codes and standards, nurses have an obligation to treat transgender individuals according to the same ethical and social mandates as any other client. In 2018, the American Nurses Association authored the position statement *Nursing Advocacy for LGBTQ+ Populations*. The nurse should follow the following guidelines in care of all clients:

- Do not assume the client's gender or sexual orientation.
- Use gender-neutral language as much as possible. Do not use terms such as "sir" or "miss" without confirming the client's preference. If you make a mistake, acknowledge it.

- Reflect and seek clarification if the client expresses a concept you do not understand.
- Collaborate with all members of the healthcare team to create a welcoming and inclusive environment.
- Identify community and web-based transgender health resources.

Cross-Dressers

Cross-dressing (dressing in the clothing of the other sex) makes individuals' outward appearance consistent with their inner identity and gender role and increases their comfort with themselves. Cross-dressing is a conscious choice and may occur at home or in public settings. The frequency of the activity ranges from rarely to often. Cross-dressers may have a different name to go with the personality and wardrobe. If the social climate is one with rigid gender roles, some individuals may need to express their feminine or masculine identity by creating a separate world and persona within that social climate.

Sexual Practices

Over a lifetime, sexual fantasies and single-partner sex are the most common sexual behaviors. Male-to-female or female-to-female **oral–genital sex** is known technically as cunnilingus. This involves kissing, licking, or sucking of the female genitals including the mons pubis, vulva, clitoris, labia, and vagina. Fellatio is oral stimulation of the penis by licking and sucking. The term "sixty-nine" refers to simultaneous oral–genital stimulation by two individuals. Preconceptions and myths are a major deterrent for those who have not tried oral sex. However, like most sexual practices, oral–genital sex is not completely free of the potential for STI transmission, and safe sex practices must be used.

Anal stimulation can be a source of sexual pleasure because the anus has a rich nerve supply. Stimulation may be applied with fingers, mouth, or sex toys such as vibrators. The anus is surrounded by strong muscles, and the rectum contains no natural lubrication. Thus inserting a finger or penis in the rectum requires relaxation and water-soluble lubricant.

A common form of sexual activity for heterosexual couples is **genital intercourse**. Penile–vaginal intercourse (**coitus**) can be both physically and emotionally satisfying. Various positions are used for this kind of intercourse; the most common is lying face to face (with female or male on top). Side-lying, standing, sitting, and rear-entry positions are also used. Side-lying, female-on-top, and rear-entry positions facilitate clitoral stimulation, either by penile or manual contact. The choice of intercourse positions and activities depends on physical comfort and beliefs, values, and attitudes about different practices.

During intercourse, the man moves the penis back and forth along the vaginal walls by rhythmic thrusting movements of his hips. The woman may move her own body to match the partner's hip movements. Movements continue until orgasm is achieved by one or both partners. Simultaneous orgasm can be difficult to achieve. After coitus, caressing, hugging, and kissing can increase the shared intimacy.

The other form of genital intercourse is anal intercourse, during which the penis is inserted into the anus and rectum of the partner. Anal intercourse is commonly practiced by gay men, but heterosexual couples engage in it as well. Positions for anal intercourse are similar to those for penile–vaginal intercourse, with minor differences due to the position of the anus. Current practice dictates the use of a condom to prevent the transmission of infections. Because anorectal tissue is not self-lubricating, a lubricant must be used on the condom. Also, because normal bacterial flora from the bowel can produce infection in other parts of the body, the used condom should be removed and another applied before inserting the penis into other body orifices.

Many other varieties of sexuality are beyond the scope of this text. These include several or many partners, nudism, swinging, group sex, fetishism, sexual sadism, and sexual masochism.

Factors Influencing Sexuality

Many factors influence an individual's sexuality. Discussed here are family, culture, religion, and personal expectations and ethics.

Family

For the majority of us, the family is the earliest and most enduring social relationship. Families are the fabric of our day-to-day lives and shape the quality of our lives by influencing our outlooks on life, our motivations, our strategies for achievement, and our styles for coping with adversity. Within our families we develop our gender identity, body image, sexual self-concept, and capacity for intimacy. Through family interactions we learn about relationships and gender roles and our expectations of others and ourselves (Figure 40.3 ■).

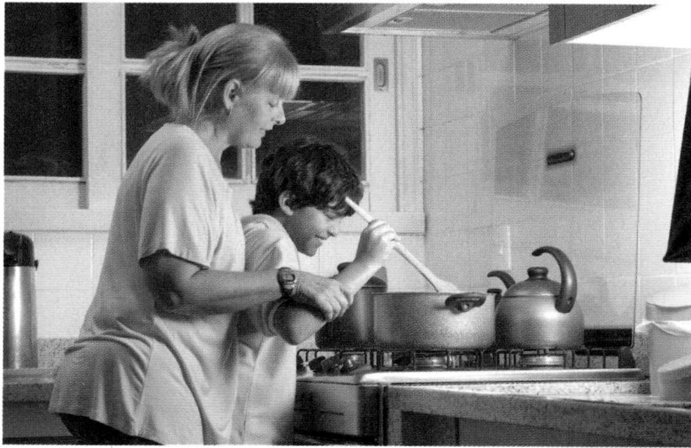

Figure 40.3 ■ Children often imitate their parents' roles.
Orange Line Media/Shutterstock.

From earliest beginnings, children observe their parents and model themselves after these role models. If parents can share affection with each other and other family members, children will most likely become adults who can give and receive affection. If parents seldom hug, hold hands, or kiss each other, their children may become adults who are very uncomfortable with romantic touch. If family expectations for gender expression is very rigid, arguments and hurt feelings will abound if an individual from this system is partnered with an individual who grew up in an androgynous family system. Family messages about sex range from "sex is so shameful it shouldn't be talked about" to "sex is a joyful part of adult relationships." The following are common sexual messages children get from their families:

- Sex is dirty.
- Premarital sex is sinful.
- Good girls don't do it.
- Masturbation is disgusting.
- Men should be the sexual experts.
- Sex is mainly for procreating.
- Bodies, including genitals, are beautiful.
- Sex should be fun for both women and men.
- Sexual thoughts and feelings are natural.
- Masturbation is a common, pleasurable activity.
- There is great variety in sexual behaviors.

Culture

Culture influences the sexual nature of dress, rules about marriage, expectations of role behavior and social responsibilities, and sex practices. Societal attitudes vary widely. Attitudes about childhood sexual play with self or children of the same gender or other gender may be restrictive or permissive. Premarital and extramarital sex and homosexuality may be culturally unacceptable or tolerated. Polygamy (several mates or marriage partners) or monogamy (one mate or marriage partner) may be the norm. Gender expression also varies from culture to culture. Culture is so much a part of everyday life that it is taken for granted. We assume that others share our own views, including those for whom we provide care. It is impossible to provide sensitive nursing care if we believe that our own culture is more important than, and preferable to, any other culture.

Cultures differ regarding which body parts they find to be erotic. In some cultures, legs are erotic and breasts are not. Body weight may also be a determinant of sexual attractiveness. There is a great deal of pressure in American culture to be very thin. Women considered obese in America are found highly attractive in other countries. Public nudity ranges from women's entire bodies and faces being covered in some Islamic societies to complete nudity in some cultures in New Guinea and Australia.

Female circumcision, also known as female genital mutilation, female ritual cutting (FRC), or female genital cutting (FGC), is a practice in parts of Africa, the Middle East, and Asia that has also spread to other regions due to immigration. Some of the cultural beliefs behind the practice include the following: Female genitals are offensive to men, if not removed the clitoris will become the size of a penis, the labia gets in the way of intercourse, the cutting enhances fertility, and it prepares the woman for childbirth. Removal of the clitoris may or may not be accompanied by removal of the labia and closure of the vaginal entrance except for a small opening. Long-term medical complications include urinary incontinence, chronic urinary tract infections, vaginal scarring, pain syndromes, infertility, and sexual dysfunctions. FGC has been banned by the United Nations and several national and international organizations (World Health Organization, 2016).

Male circumcision is controversial. Some professional groups support newborn circumcision believing it will prevent the spread of HIV and other infections (Brady, 2016). Others say there is insufficient evidence of potential medical benefits. In addition to the medical issues, there are also ethical concerns related to performing elective surgery on children too young to provide consent (Svobada, Adler, & Van Howe, 2016). In June 2013, Germany banned the circumcision of boys under the age of 18. However, circumcision is also a religious ritual among Jews and Muslims. Newborn circumcision rates vary according to geographic region in the United States.

Religion

Religion influences sexual expression. It provides guidelines for sexual behavior and acceptable circumstances for the behavior, as well as prohibited sexual behavior and the consequences of breaking the sexual rules. The guidelines or rules may be detailed and rigid or broad and flexible. Some religions view forms of sexual expression other than male–female intercourse as unnatural and hold virginity before marriage to be the rule.

Many religious values conflict with the more flexible values of society that have developed during the past few decades (often labeled the "sexual revolution"), such as the acceptance of premarital sex, unwed parenthood, homosexuality, and abortion. These conflicts create marked anxiety and potential sexual dysfunctions in some individuals. See Chapter 41 ∞ for additional information about religious values.

Personal Expectations and Ethics

Although ethics is integral to religion, ethical thought and ethical approaches to sexuality can be viewed separately from religion. Cultures have developed written or unwritten codes of conduct based on ethical principles. Personal expectations concerning sexual behavior come from these cultural norms. What one individual or culture views as bizarre, perverted, or wrong may be natural and right to another. Examples include values regarding masturbation, oral or anal intercourse, and cross-dressing. Many individuals accept a variety of sexual expressions if they are performed by consenting adults, are practiced in private, and are not harmful. Individuals need to explore and communicate clearly about various types of acceptable sexual expression to prevent domination of sexual decision-making by any individual. To assess a few of your personal values, complete the statements in Box 40.3.

BOX 40.3 Assessing Personal Sexual Values

- I believe sexual satisfaction is . . .
- When I think of my parents having sex, I . . .
- If I cared for a transgender client, I would . . .
- When I think about lesbians, gays, and bisexuals, I . . .
- Masturbation is . . .
- My beliefs about oral sex are . . .

Sexual Response Cycle

Commonly occurring phases of the human sexual response follow a similar sequence in both females and males regardless of sexual orientation. It does not matter if the motive for being sexually active is true love or passionate lust. Table 40.3 provides a summary of the physiologic changes associated with each phase of the cycle.

The response cycle starts in the brain, with conscious sexual desires called the **desire phase**. Sexually arousing stimuli, often called erotic stimuli, may be real or symbolic. Sight, hearing, smell, touch, and imagination (sexual fantasy) can all invoke sexual arousal. Sexual desire fluctuates within each individual and varies among individuals. If individuals suppress or block out conscious sexual desires, they may experience no physiologic response.

TABLE 40.3 Physiologic Changes Associated with the Sexual Response Cycle

Phase of the Sexual Response Cycle	Signs Present in Both Sexes	Signs Present in Males Only	Signs Present in Females Only
Excitement and plateau	Muscle tension increases as excitement increases. Sex flush, usually on chest. Nipple erection.	Penile erection; glans size increases as excitement increases. Appearance of a few drops of lubricant, which may contain sperm.	Erection of the clitoris. Vaginal lubrication. Labia may increase 2 to 3 times in size. Breasts enlarge. Inner two-thirds of vagina widens and lengthens; outer third swells and narrows. Uterus elevates.
Orgasmic	Respirations may increase to 40 breaths/min. Involuntary spasms of muscle groups throughout the body. Diminished sensory awareness. Involuntary contractions of the anal sphincter. Peak heart rate (110–180 beats/min), respiratory rate (40/min or greater), and blood pressure (systolic 30–80 mmHg and diastolic 20–50 mmHg above normal).	Rhythmic, expulsive contractions of the penis at 0.8-sec intervals. Emission of seminal fluid into the prostatic urethra from contraction of the vas deferens and accessory organs (stage 1 of the expulsive process). Closing of the internal bladder sphincter just before ejaculation to prevent retrograde ejaculation into bladder. Orgasm may occur without ejaculation. Ejaculation of semen through the penile urethra and expulsion from the urethral meatus. The force of ejaculation varies from man to man and at different times but diminishes after the first two to three contractions (stage 2 of the expulsive process).	Approximately 5–12 contractions in the orgasmic platform at 0.8-sec intervals. Contraction of the muscles of the pelvic floor and the uterine muscles. Varied pattern of orgasms, including minor surges and contractions, multiple orgasms, or a simple intense orgasm similar to that of the male.
Resolution	Reversal of vasocongestion in 10–30 min; disappearance of all signs of myotonia within 5 min. Genitals and breasts return to their pre-excitement states. Sex flush disappears in reverse order of appearance. Heart rate, respiratory rate, and blood pressure return to normal. Other reactions include sleepiness, relaxation, and emotional outbursts such as crying or laughing.	A refractory period during which the body will not respond to sexual stimulation; varies, depending on age and other factors, from a few moments to hours or days.	

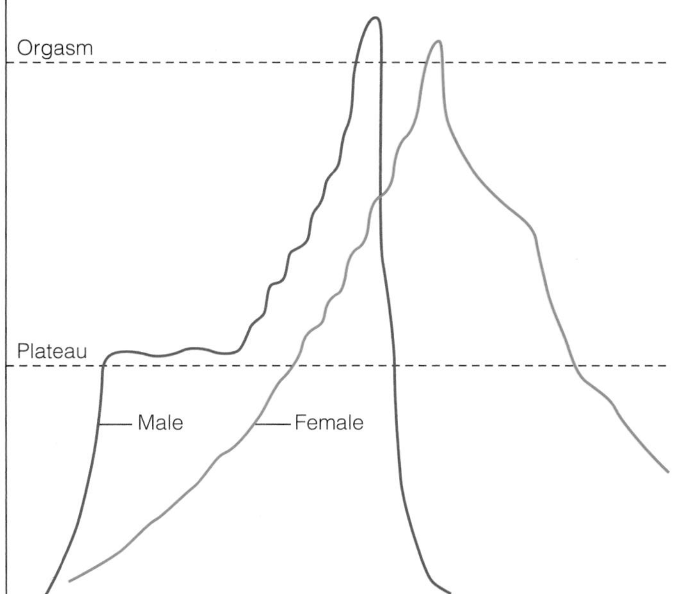

Figure 40.4 ■ Phases of the sexual response cycle.

Although psychologic issues are the more common causes of lack of sexual desire, medications, drugs, and hormone imbalances can also interfere.

The **excitement phase** involves two primary physiologic changes (Figure 40.4 ■). Vasocongestion is an increase in the blood flow to various body parts resulting in erection of the penis and clitoris and swelling of the labia, testes, and breasts. Vasocongestion stimulates sensory receptors within these body parts that transmit messages to the conscious brain, where they are usually interpreted as pleasurable sensations. When stimulation is continued, vasocongestion increases until it either is released by orgasm or fades away. Likewise, myotonia, an increase of tension in muscles, may increase until released by orgasm, or it may also fade away.

The **orgasmic phase** is the involuntary climax of sexual tension, accompanied by physiologic and psychologic release. This phase is the measurable peak of the sexual experience. Although the entire body is involved, the major focus of the orgasm is felt in the pelvic region. Male orgasms usually last 10 to 30 seconds, while female orgasms last 10 to 50 seconds. Men usually have an ejaculation and expel semen as part of their orgasm. Before puberty and in later years, males experience orgasms without ejaculation.

The **resolution phase**, the period of return to the unaroused state, may last 10 to 15 minutes after orgasm, or longer if there is no orgasm. This phase in females is varied as some women experience multiple successive orgasms followed by a longer period of resolution.

Altered Sexual Function

The ability to engage in sexual activity is of importance to most individuals. Many individuals experience transient problems with their ability to respond to sexual stimulation or to maintain the response. Fewer individuals experience problems lifelong. The problems may be generalized to all sexual interactions and settings, or they may be situational, occurring in specific circumstances or with specific types of sexual activity. It is often difficult to sort out the multiple factors contributing to an individual's or a couple's sexual problems. A number of past and current factors are involved.

Past and Current Factors

Sociocultural factors interfering in sexual function include a very strict upbringing accompanied by inadequate sex education. Rigid gender socialization may inhibit exploration of sexual activities, positions, toys, and other lovemaking behaviors. If individuals' religious affiliations lead them to believe that sex is only for procreation, they may have great difficulty in celebrating the pleasure and fun of a sexual relationship. Another factor may be parental punishment for normally exploring one's genitals or for typical childhood sex play. In our current culture, the pressures of family and work often leave mature couples with too little time and not enough energy to enjoy sex.

Psychologic factors may include negative feelings such as guilt, anxiety, or fear that interfere with the ability to experience pleasure and joy. Some individuals experience guilt when they enjoy sex or when they participate in what they label "unusual" sexual activities, or regarding their choice of partner. Adults sexually abused at any time of their lives may experience overwhelming anxiety when faced with the decision to engage in sex. Fears may include pregnancy, STIs, or pain. Because vulnerability and intimacy are inherent in most sexual relationships, fear of these may lead to an avoidance of sex. Fear of failure in sexual performance often becomes a vicious cycle; that is, fear of failure creates actual failure, which produces more fear. Individuals may worry excessively: "Am I going to lose my erection?" "Am I going to have an orgasm this time?" "My stomach is too flabby." "When did his thighs get that fat?" Depressed individuals lose interest in sexual activity and often experience a loss of sexual desire and fulfillment.

Cognitive factors include the internalization of negative expectations and beliefs. Those with low self-esteem may not understand how another individual could value and love them and also find them sexually attractive. For those who have not yet accepted their sexual orientation or gender identity, this cognitive conflict may interfere with sexual relationships.

Sexual problems may also be symptomatic of relationship problems. Conflict and anger with one's partner are not conducive to positive sexual interaction. Some individuals lose the physical attraction to another or feel more attracted to someone else.

Lack of intimacy and feeling like a sex object inhibit the feeling of communion and connection that is an important part of making love. Another factor is expecting one's partner to read one's mind about sexual needs. Failure to communicate may cause one or both partners' not knowing how to please the other. Unless the partners experiment, sex may, in time, become boring. Disagreements in sexual frequency or sexual activities may lead to further relationship conflict.

Health factors can interfere with individuals' expression of sexuality. Physical changes brought on by illness, injury, or surgery may inhibit full sexual expression. There may be sexual side effects from several conditions such as heart disease, diabetes mellitus, joint disease, cancer, and mental disorders. Surgeries such as hysterectomy, prostate surgery, and radical surgeries alter an individual's body image. Spinal cord injuries, traumatic amputations, or disfiguring accidents negatively affect sexual functioning. The presence of an STI in one partner induces fear of transmission in the other, often resulting in abstinence from sexual contact. In some situations, an STI is unknown and transmission occurs.

Many prescription medications have side effects that affect sexual functioning beyond medications intended for that purpose. Most frequently, the impact is negative, but sometimes there is a positive impact. Table 40.4 provides an overview of the effects of medications on sexual function. For example, antidepressants may slow ejaculation. This may be a problem for the man who suddenly finds himself unable to ejaculate. If the man experiences rapid ejaculation, however, the antidepressant may "cure" this problem. Some street drugs such as marijuana, amphetamines, and cocaine enhance sexual functioning. Others, such as opioids and anabolic steroids, interfere with sexual functioning.

Sexual Desire Disorders

For most individuals, sexual desire varies from day to day and over the years. Some individuals, however, report a deficiency in or absence of sexual fantasies and persistently low interest or a total lack of interest in sexual activity; these clients may have **hypoactive sexual desire disorder**. If both individuals in a relationship are similarly uninterested in sex, there really is no problem. More typically, there is a disparity of sexual needs, and the partner with the greater desire becomes dissatisfied with the sexual relationship. The key issue in the relationship is not frequency but rather the dovetailing of partners' needs.

Sexual Arousal Disorders

Sexual arousal refers to the physiologic responses and subjective sense of excitement experienced during sexual activity. Lack of lubrication and failure to attain or maintain an erection are the major disorders of the arousal phase. In **female sexual arousal disorder**, the lack of vaginal lubrication causes discomfort or pain during sexual intercourse. The diagnosis of **male erectile disorder** is usually made when the male has erection problems during 25% or more of his sexual interactions. Some males cannot attain a full erection, and others lose their erection prior to orgasm. The term commonly applied to this condition, *impotency*, implies that the male is feeble, inadequate, and incompetent. The accurate term is *erectile dysfunction* (ED), which is

TABLE 40.4 Effects of Medications on Sexual Function

Medication	Possible Effects*
Alcohol	Moderate amounts: increased sexual functioning; chronic use: decreased sexual desire, orgasmic dysfunction, and erectile dysfunction
Alpha-blockers	Inability to ejaculate
Amphetamines	Increased sex drive, delayed orgasm
Amyl nitrate	Reported enhanced orgasm; vasodilation, fainting
Anabolic steroids	Decreased sex drive, shrinking of testicles and infertility in men
Antianxiety agents	Decreased sexual desire; orgasmic dysfunction in women; delayed ejaculation
Anticonvulsants	Decreased sexual desire; reduced sexual response
Antidepressants	Decreased sexual desire; orgasmic delay or dysfunction in women; delayed or failed ejaculation; painful erection
Antihistamines	Decreased vaginal lubrication; decreased desire
Antihypertensives	Decreased sexual desire; erectile failure; ejaculation dysfunction
Antipsychotics	Decreased sexual desire; orgasmic dysfunction in women; delayed ejaculation; ejaculatory failure
Barbiturates	In low doses, increased sexual pleasure; in large doses, decreased sexual desire, orgasmic dysfunction, and erectile dysfunction
Beta-blockers	Decreased sexual desire
Cardiotonics	Decreased sexual desire
Cocaine	Increased intensity of sexual experience; with chronic use, decreased sexual desire and sexual dysfunction
Diuretics	Decreased vaginal lubrication; decreased sexual desire; erectile dysfunction
Marijuana	As for cocaine, but prolonged use reduces testosterone levels and reduces sperm production
Narcotics	Inhibited sexual desire and response; erectile and ejaculatory dysfunctions

*Nurses and clients must familiarize themselves with the specific medication prescribed or used, because effects vary in each category of drug.

objectively descriptive and nonjudgmental. The advent of medications effective in treating ED (see the Drug Capsule) can lessen the physical problem but psychologic or relationship issues may remain.

Orgasmic Disorders

The term commonly applied in the past to women who did not experience orgasm, *frigid*, implied that the woman was totally incapable of responding sexually. The more accurate and objective term is **female orgasmic disorder**, which simply means that the sexual response stops before orgasm occurs. There are variations in the disorder depending on whether the female never experiences orgasm or reaches orgasm only under certain conditions such as masturbation. *Preorgasmic* is the term used for females who have never experienced an orgasm. Compounding the orgasmic difficulty is the associated anxiety. In the preoccupation with orgasm, the real goal of being sexual—mutual pleasuring and intimacy—is lost, and the interchange becomes one of anxiety, frustration, and anger.

In **male orgasmic disorder**, the male can maintain an erection for long periods (an hour or more) but has extreme difficulty ejaculating, referred to as *delayed ejaculation*. In heterosexual intercourse, the difficulty may be limited to ejaculation in the vagina. Some males ejaculate after self-stimulation or manual or oral stimulation by the partner, whereas others have great difficulty ejaculating with any type of stimulation. This disorder is much less common than rapid ejaculation.

Rapid (premature) ejaculation is one of the most common sexual dysfunctions among males. There are many definitions, with descriptions ranging from ejaculating before being touched, ejaculating before penetration, ejaculating with one internal thrust, to ejaculating within a minute or two of penetration. The problem is best self-defined as when a man is concerned about his ejaculatory control, or the couple agrees that ejaculation is too rapid for mutual satisfaction.

Sexual Pain Disorders

Both women and men can experience **dyspareunia**, pain during or immediately after intercourse. It is associated with many physiologic causes, especially those that inhibit lubrication. Skin irritations, vaginal infections, estrogen deficiencies, and use of medications that dry vaginal secretions can cause women to experience discomfort with intercourse.

Female pelvic disorders, such as infections, lesions, endometriosis, scar tissue, or tumors, can cause painful intercourse. Similarly, in males, infection or inflammation of the glans penis or other genitourinary organs can cause pain with intercourse. Also, some contraceptive foams, creams, sponges, or latex products can irritate either the vagina or penis.

Vaginismus is the involuntary spasm of the outer one-third of the vaginal muscles, making penetration of the vagina painful and sometimes impossible. The woman often experiences desire, excitement, and orgasm with stimulation of the external sexual structures. Attempts at intercourse, however, elicit the involuntary spasm. She may have similar difficulty undergoing pelvic exams and inserting tampons or a diaphragm.

Vulvodynia is constant, unremitting burning that is localized to the vulva with an acute onset. The girl or woman has problems in sitting, standing, and sleeping related to the intensity of pain. **Vestibulitis** causes severe pain only on touch or attempted vaginal entry. Half of the women with vestibulitis report lifelong dyspareunia.

DRUG CAPSULE

Phosphodiesterase Type 5 (PDE5) Inhibitor: sildenafil citrate (Viagra); tadalafil (Cialis); vardenafil (Levitra)

THE CLIENT TAKING MEDICATION FOR ERECTILE DYSFUNCTION (ED)

In erectile dysfunction (ED), the sexually stimulated penis does not achieve or maintain an erection, often due to restricted blood flow to the penis. These medications inhibit the breakdown of the enzymes and products that allow the muscle relaxation, which facilitates adequate blood flow to the penis. The medications do not enhance sexual desire or cure the ED but allow the stimulated penis to obtain and sustain an erection.

NURSING RESPONSIBILITIES

- ED medications are contraindicated for men with uncontrolled high or low blood pressure, stroke, renal or liver problems, vision loss, or bleeding disorders.
- Men with an anatomically deformed penis should consult with the primary care provider prior to taking these medications.
- Medications come in different dose strengths and may require adjustment.

CLIENT AND FAMILY TEACHING

- General safety in using these medications is the same as for engaging in sexual activity overall. The risk of adverse outcomes of sexual activity after taking these medications is not increased.
- Explain that men who take medications that are nitrates—those that are prescribed (e.g., nitroglycerin) or those that are recreational (e.g., amyl nitrate, or "poppers")—should not take these medications.
- The client should take the medication about 1 hour prior to sexual activity. Some formulations are taken once per day and others not more than once every 3 days.
- Teach side effects to immediately report to the primary care provider: loss of vision, or an erection that lasts more than 4 hours.
- Other common side effects may include headache, muscle pain, flushing, or stuffy nose.
- These medications do not prevent pregnancy or STIs.

Note: Prior to administering any medication, review all aspects with a current drug handbook or other reliable source.

Individuals with any of these disorders report a negative impact on their sexual functioning and partner relationship, as well as their self-esteem and mental health.

Problems with Satisfaction

Some individuals experience sexual desire, arousal, and orgasm and yet feel dissatisfied with their sexual relationships. These sexual problems are more commonly related to the emotional tone of the relationship than to the physiologic response. Since giving and receiving pleasure in a mutually intimate relationship are the primary goals of sex for most individuals, dissatisfaction problems may be more disturbing than other types of sexual dysfunctions.

Satisfaction problems may be situational. For example, one partner may choose an inconvenient time, or a partner may feel anxious and therefore cannot experience much pleasure or joy. Some individuals describe their problems as related to the lack of touching and caressing in earlier lovemaking experiences. Unfortunately, individuals relating sexually for a long time often become genitally focused and neglect the rest of the body. One or both partners may feel touch starved, long for more extragenital loving, and become dissatisfied with sex.

Satisfaction problems are often related to relationship difficulties. The inability to communicate effectively in other relationship areas frequently results in sexual frustration. Partners angry with each other who make love without resolving the conflict may feel unhappy about the relationship despite having experienced arousal and orgasm. Couples who define their relationship in terms of rigid, unequal power and gender roles may have difficulty negotiating and compromising about sexual issues. Not infrequently, the individual with the least power feels helpless and dissatisfied with the sexual interchanges.

Lack of intimacy or a feeling of connectedness is understandably related to satisfaction problems. If one has sex with a stranger, the body may function well, but there is often a sense of something missing after the sexual experience. Making love to one individual while feeling more attracted to or in love with another can cause feelings of emptiness or disconnection. Even couples in a committed relationship may complain of lack of intimacy. Dissatisfaction issues include lack of romance, love, tenderness, and nurturance. Fulfillment of sexuality depends on the ability to relate with a partner in an intimate and mutually pleasing manner compatible with values and chosen lifestyle.

●○● NURSING MANAGEMENT

Assessing

Because sexuality and sexual functioning are aspects of health and well-being, they are a part of nursing care and need to be assessed. Clients are often hesitant to introduce the topic of sex with their primary healthcare providers. They may be too embarrassed, they may think that they should not have sexual problems in our liberated times, or they may think they are too old or too young to have these problems. When healthcare professionals do not introduce the topic, these clients are unrecognized and unserved.

Information about a client's sexual health status should always be an integral part of a nursing assessment. The amount and kind of data collected depend on the context of the assessment, that is, the client's reason for seeking healthcare and how the client's sexuality interacts with other problems.

Nursing History

Including a sexual history as part of the general nursing history is important for some clients and not important for others. It is critical, however, to introduce the topic of sexuality to all clients in order to give them permission to bring up any concerns or problems. All nursing histories should at least include a question such as "Have there been any changes in your sexual functioning that might be related to your illness or the medications you take?" Nurses might also facilitate communication by saying, "As a nurse, I'm concerned about all aspects of your health. Clients often have questions about sexual matters, both when they are well and when they are ill. When I take your history, sexual concerns are included to help plan a comprehensive treatment approach."

It is critical that nurses not make assumptions about clients because assumptions interfere with accurate history taking. If you start from the belief that all individuals do all things, you will be more open to clients than if you make assumptions about who is and who is not sexually active and how. Presuming that your personal beliefs are shared by others is detrimental to the nurse–client relationship.

Interviewing a client regarding sexual health may be uncomfortable for some nurses (and for the client). Nurses must be aware of their own feelings and beliefs so that they can prepare approaches for gathering data and creating the nursing care plan. The nurse sets aside personal values about sexual practices and uses a culturally sensitive, nonjudgmental, nonthreatening, and reassuring approach. It is extremely important to create an atmosphere that facilitates open communication and comfort for the client. Remind the client that all personal health information is handled in a confidential manner. Also see Chapter 4 ∞ for a review of values clarification and Chapter 10 ∞ for more information on the health history.

The accompanying Assessment Interview provides questions that nurses may ask as part of the health history. These questions typically are asked in the assessment process after a rapport has been established.

The nurse conducts a more in-depth sexual history on the following categories of clients:

- Those receiving care for pregnancy, infertility, contraception, or an STI
- Those whose illness or therapy will affect sexual functioning (e.g., clients with diabetes, gynecologic problems, or heart disease)
- Those experiencing a sexual problem.

ASSESSMENT INTERVIEW Sexual Health History

- Are you sexually active? With men, women, or both?
- Are you sexually active with one or more than one partner?
- Describe the positive and negative aspects of your sexual functioning.
- Do you have difficulty with sexual desire? Arousal? Orgasm? Satisfaction?
- Do you experience any pain during sex?
- If there are problems, how have they influenced how you feel about yourself? How have they affected your partner? How have they affected the relationship?
- Do you expect your sexual functioning to change because of your health status?
- What are your partner's concerns about your future sexual functioning?
- Do you have any other sexual questions or concerns that I have not addressed?

Physical Examination

Physical examination of the female genitals and reproductive tract and the male genitals is part of a routine physical examination in some agencies. Check agency protocol. See Chapter 29 ∞ for details of the examination. If the client has not been examined in the past year or if data from the recent nursing history indicate a need, the nurse performs a physical examination or refers the client to an appropriate member of the healthcare team. Nursing history data indicating the need for a physical examination include the following:

- Suspicion of infertility, pregnancy, or an STI
- Reports of discharge, presence of a lump or sore, or change in color, size, and shape of a genital organ
- Changes in urinary function
- Need for Papanicolaou test
- Request for birth control.

Identifying Clients at Risk

Clients at risk for altered sexual patterns include those experiencing the following:

- Altered body structure or function due to trauma, pregnancy, recent childbirth, anatomic abnormalities of the genitals, or a variety of diseases
- Physical, psychosocial, emotional, or sexual abuse; sexual assault
- Disfiguring conditions, such as burns, skin conditions, birthmarks, scars (e.g., mastectomy), and ostomies
- Specific medication therapy that causes sexual problems (see Table 40.4)
- Temporary or long-term impaired physical ability to perform grooming and maintain sexual attractiveness
- Value conflicts between personal beliefs and religious doctrine
- Loss of a partner
- Lack of knowledge or misinformation about sexual functioning and expression.

Diagnosing

Examples of nursing diagnoses that may relate specifically to sexuality or be the etiology of other nursing diagnoses can include sexual dysfunction, insufficient knowledge (e.g., about conception, STIs, contraception, or normal sexual changes over the lifespan) related to misinformation and sexual myths, unsatisfying personal relationship related to unrealistic expectations, fear related to history of sexual abuse or dyspareunia, and altered body image (e.g., from a mastectomy) related to perceived sexual rejection by partner.

Planning

Overall goals to meet clients' sexual needs include the following:

- Maintain, restore, or improve sexual health.
- Increase knowledge of sexuality and sexual health.
- Prevent the occurrence or spread of STIs.
- Prevent unwanted pregnancy.
- Increase satisfaction with the level of sexual functioning.
- Improve sexual self-concept.

Nursing interventions to promote sexual health and function focus largely on the nurse's teaching role. Clients need to be taught about sexual function, the effects of medications on sexual function, preventing STIs, and performing breast and testicular self-examinations. Besides teaching, nurses can do the following to help clients maintain a healthy sexual self-concept:

- Provide privacy during intimate body care.
- Give attention to the client's appearance and dress.
- Give clients privacy to meet their sexual needs alone or with a partner within physically safe limits.

Remember that clients' comfort in discussing sex-related topics and being examined is culturally influenced. Planning for clients must include using culturally sensitive communication techniques implemented with both clients and culturally appropriate family members.

Implementing

The interventions the nurse selects are based on the data obtained from the client and the identified nursing diagnoses. Many interventions are directed at providing information about sexual health and counseling for altered sexual function.

Nurses require six basic skills to help clients in the area of sexuality:

- Self-knowledge and comfort with their own sexuality
- Acceptance of sexuality as an important area for nursing intervention and a willingness to work with clients who express their sexuality in a variety of ways
- Knowledge of sexual growth and development throughout the life cycle
- Knowledge of basic sexuality, including how certain health problems and treatments may affect sexuality and sexual function and which interventions facilitate sexual expression and functioning
- Therapeutic communication skills
- Ability to recognize the need for all clients and family members to have the topic of sexuality introduced not only in written or audiovisual materials but also in a verbal discussion.

Clinical Alert!

As a result of culture, age, gender, and personal characteristics, not every nurse will be comfortable discussing sex with every client. However, it is the nurse's responsibility to ensure that *someone* introduces the topic for discussion with the client.

Providing Sexual Health Teaching

Educating about sexual health is an important component of nursing implementation. Many sexual problems exist because of sexual ignorance; many others can be prevented with effective sexual health teaching. Examples of important areas of teaching are sex education (including self-examination) and responsible sexual behavior.

Sex Education

Nurses can assist clients to understand their anatomy and how their body functions. Understanding the anatomy of the genitals may help women learn how their body responds to sexual stimulation. Both men and women need to learn the kind of stimulation that is pleasing and causes arousal. The importance of open communication between partners should also be encouraged. Women may also benefit from learning Kegel exercises. These exercises involve contraction and relaxation of the pubococcygeal muscle, the muscle that contracts when an individual prevents urine flow. The benefits of Kegel exercises include increased pelvic floor muscle tone; increased vaginal lubrication during sexual arousal; increased sensation during intercourse; increased genital sensitivity; stronger gripping of the base of the penis; earlier postpartum recovery of the pelvic floor muscle; and increased flexibility of episiotomy scars. Kegel exercises may also benefit males with ejaculatory control (Greenberg, Bruess, & Oswalt, 2017). The steps to perform Kegel exercises are discussed in Chapter 47 ∞ because these exercises are also used in bladder retraining.

Details about physiologic changes that occur during major developmental crises should be provided as part of general healthcare. For example, the nurse needs to discuss the effects of puberty, pregnancy, menopause, and the male climacteric on sexual function. When clients experience illness or surgery that may alter sexual function, the nurse needs to discuss effects of treatment (e.g., medications) and any changes that need to be undertaken to ensure safe sex (e.g., position changes or a safe time to resume sexual intercourse after a heart attack).

Parents often need assistance to learn ways to answer questions about sexuality and what information to provide for their children starting in the preschool years. Parents need to be the primary educators of children at an early age; however, peers, teachers, and media also teach about sexual issues.

Although there is an increasing awareness today of sexuality and sexual functioning, some individuals still hold certain myths and misconceptions about sexuality. Many of these are handed down in families and are part of the beliefs in a particular culture. Nurses must learn about the beliefs clients hold and provide up-to-date information. The website of the Sexuality Information and Education Council of the United States has a wealth of information on various aspects of sexuality.

Teaching Self-Examination

Breast self-examination (BSE) for women and testicular self-examination (TSE) for men may play a role in early detection of disease, although neither technique has medical evidence to prove its value in clients at *average* risk for breast or testicular cancer. Clients need to be assured that most lumps discovered are not cancerous, but it is essential that all lumps or other detected abnormalities be checked by the client's primary care provider for accurate diagnosis. Those clients who do wish to perform BSE should receive instruction and have their technique reviewed regularly.

Although the vast majority of breast cancers in the United States each year occur in women, men with an *increased risk* of breast cancer due to high estrogen levels or a strong family history of breast cancer should also learn BSE. For BSE a regular time is best—such as 1 week following menstruation, when breast tenderness and fullness caused by fluid retention have subsided, or on the same day of the month for men or postmenopausal women. Individuals who examine themselves regularly become familiar with the shape and texture of their breasts. The steps of BSE are very similar to those used when the nurse performs breast examination (see Skill 29.14 in Chapter 29 ∞). For techniques of breast self-examination, see Client Teaching.

Responsible Sexual Behavior

Responsible sexual behavior involves the prevention of STIs, the prevention of unwanted pregnancy, and the avoidance of sexual harassment or abuse.

STI Prevention

The prevention of STIs is an essential part of sexual health teaching (Figure 40.5 ■). Increases in these infections are due to two factors: (1) changing views of sexuality that have resulted in increased sexual activity and (2) an increase in the number of sexual partners. Because STIs elicit feelings of guilt, shame, and fear, clients frequently do

CLIENT TEACHING Breast Self-Examination

INSPECTION BEFORE A MIRROR

Look for any change in size or shape; lumps or thickenings; any rashes or other skin irritations; dimpled or puckered skin; any discharge or change in the nipples (e.g., position or asymmetry). Inspect the breasts in all of the following positions:

- Stand and face the mirror with your arms relaxed at your sides or hands resting on the hips; then turn to the right and the left for a side view (look for any flattening in the side view).
- Bend forward from the waist with arms raised over the head.
- Stand straight with the arms raised over the head and move the arms slowly up and down at the sides. (Look for free movement of the breasts over the chest wall.)
- Press your hands firmly together at chin level while the elbows are raised to shoulder level.

PALPATION: LYING POSITION

- Place a pillow under your right shoulder and place the right hand behind your head. This position distributes the right breast tissue more evenly on the chest.
- Use the finger pads (tips) of the three middle fingers (held together) on your left hand to feel for lumps in the right breast.
- Press the breast tissue against the chest wall firmly enough to know how your breast feels. A ridge of firm tissue in the lower curve of each breast is normal.
- Use small circular motions systematically all the way around the breast as many times as necessary until the entire breast has been covered. (Review Figures 5 through 7 in Skill 29.14, page 624 in Chapter 29 ∞, for patterns that the client may use.)
- Bring your arm down to your side and feel under your armpit, where breast tissue is also located.
- Repeat the exam on your left breast, using the finger pads of your right hand.

PALPATION: STANDING OR SITTING

- Repeat the examination of both breasts while upright with one arm behind your head. This position makes it easier to check the area where a large percentage of breast cancers are found, the upper outer part of the breast and toward the armpit.
- *Optional:* Do the upright BSE in the shower. Soapy hands glide more easily over wet skin. Report any changes to your healthcare provider promptly.

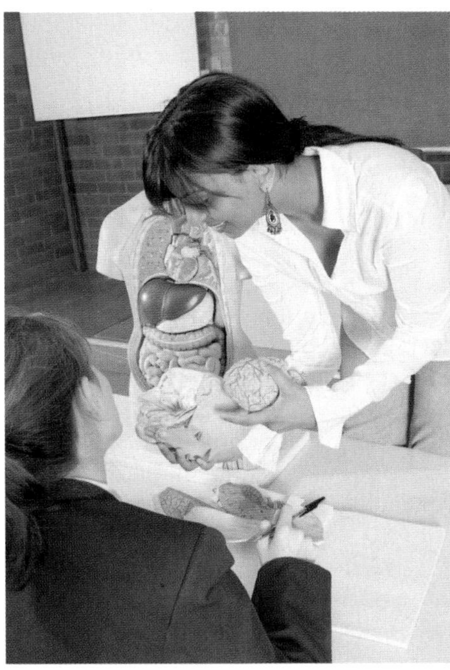

Figure 40.5 ■ Adolescents require age-appropriate teaching about sexuality and sexually transmitted infections.
Michaeljung/Shutterstock.

not seek medical help as early as they should. Clients need education about these infections, preventive measures, and early treatment. Many STIs can be treated quickly and effectively. Others may have serious consequences. Females may develop pelvic inflammatory disease (PID) resulting in damage to the reproductive structures and possible infertility. The anxiety about HIV, which may be acquired through sexual transmission, has caused many individuals to improve their safe sexual behavior, such as using a condom during genital or anal sex.

See Box 40.1 earlier in this chapter for common signs of STIs for which individuals should seek medical care. Methods for decreasing exposure to STIs are described in the Client Teaching feature.

Prevention of Unwanted Pregnancies

Prevention of unwanted pregnancies must be addressed not only with adolescents but also with couples planning the time of births to space children or limit family size. Nurses need to be familiar with various contraceptive methods and their advantages, disadvantages, contraindications, effectiveness, safety, and cost (Figure 40.6 ■). The various methods are outlined in Box 40.4. It is beyond the scope of this text to discuss contraceptives in detail.

CLIENT TEACHING Preventing Transmission of STIs

- Limit the number of sexual partners.
- Talk openly with sexual partners about how to have "safer sex," and be honest about any history of an STI.
- Abstain from high-risk sexual activity with a partner known to have or suspected of having an STI.
- Use condoms in relationships that have the potential for STI transmission.
- Follow safe sex practices during oral sex including the use of a dental dam during cunnilingus to prevent STI transmission.
- Report to a healthcare facility for examination whenever in doubt about possible exposure or when signs of an STI are evident.
- When an STI is diagnosed, notify all partners and encourage them to seek treatment.
- Discuss the use of pre-exposure prophylactic (PrEP) medications for high-risk individuals. The CDC has an HIV Risk Reduction Tool website that provides customized information about PrEP.

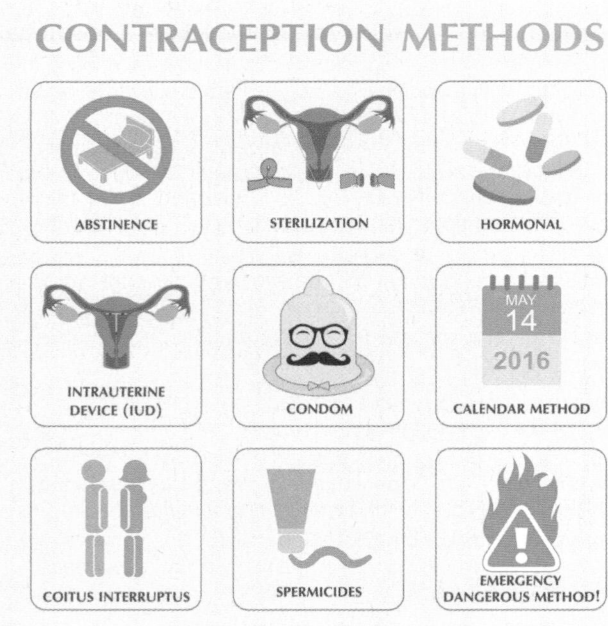

Figure 40.6 Methods of contraception.
A7880S/Shutterstock.

BOX 40.4 Methods of Contraception

- Abstinence.
- Withdrawal of the penis before ejaculation (*coitus interruptus*).
- Fertility awareness (identification of the days of the month when conception is most likely to occur and abstaining during that time). Also referred to as *natural planning*.
- Mechanical barriers: vaginal diaphragm, vaginal ring, cervical cap, condom. (*Note:* There are different types of condom materials such as latex, lambskin, polyurethane, and polyisoprene. All are equally effective at preventing pregnancy. Latex condoms are the least expensive. Lambskin pore size does not protect against STIs as well as the others. Polyurethane condoms are recommended if contact with latex should be avoided. Polyisoprene is the newest and has many of the best attributes of the other materials. Female condoms are usually made from nitrile, like that used in examination gloves.)
- Chemical barriers: insertion of spermicidal foams, creams, jellies, or suppositories into the vagina before intercourse.
- Intrauterine devices (IUDs).
- Hormonal: oral contraceptives (birth control pills), subdermal implants of synthetic progestin, transdermal patches. (*Note:* Certain antibiotics decrease the effectiveness of oral contraceptives and patches. Women on these antibiotics must use an alternative method of contraception until their antibiotic treatment is completed. Other drug interactions can occur with implants.)
- Emergency contraception: hormonal: levonorgestrel pill taken within 5 days (120 hours) of unprotected intercourse. Commonly referred to as Plan B or the morning-after pill.
- When inserted within 5 days of unprotected intercourse, a copper-bearing IUD is the most effective form of emergency contraception available (Curtis et al., 2016).
- Surgical sterilization: tubal ligation and vasectomy.
- Abortion.

Avoiding Sexual Harassment and Abuse

Sexual harassment exists when someone in a position of power threatens another individual's job or status in exchange for unwanted sexual acts. Such harassment can be severe enough to be considered abuse, but sexual abuse (also called *molestation*) is forced, unwanted sexual activity of any kind. Prevention is the most important role of the nurse and this can best be accomplished through educating adult clients and families of children about their rights and support services available if they believe sexual harassment or abuse is occurring. Assessing for, diagnosing, and intervening in possible situations of sexual harassment or abuse is a significant undertaking and not every nurse will be skilled in these roles. Sexual assault nurse examiners have specialized training in the role of assessing and treating victims of sexual assault (Valentine, 2018). However, every nurse must know of the legal requirements and proper methods of reporting suspected abuse.

Counseling for Altered Sexual Function

One technique nurses can use to help clients with altered sexual function is the PLISSIT model, developed by Annon (1976) for this purpose. The model involves four progressive levels represented by the acronym PLISSIT:

P	Permission giving
LI	Limited information
SS	Specific suggestions
IT	Intensive therapy

At each level, the nurse provides additional guidance and information to the client and therefore requires more specialized and specific knowledge and skill. All professional nurses should be able to function at the first three levels. At the levels of limited information, specific suggestions, and intensive therapy, the nurse can also refer the client to a healthcare provider more skilled to assist the client with the particular issues identified during the first level.

Permission Giving

Clients may feel that they need permission to be sexual beings, to ask questions, to show affection, and to express themselves sexually. Giving permission means that the nurse by attitude or word lets the client know that sexual thoughts, fantasies, and behaviors between informed consenting adults are allowed. Giving permission begins when the nurse acknowledges the client's spoken and unspoken sexual concerns and conveys the attitude that sexual concerns and needs are important to health and recovery.

The nurse might ask a client recuperating from a heart attack the following questions:

"Now that you're recuperating and you've had some time to sort out your feelings, have you thought about how your heart attack might alter your sex life?"

"Have you and your partner discussed how you both feel about resuming sexual activity?"

Limited Information

Clients need accurate but concise information. The nurse might explain what is common; how some medical conditions, treatments, injuries, or surgeries may affect sexuality and sexual functioning; or how aging may affect sexuality and functioning.

Continuing with the preceding example, the nurse shares information and informs the client about how the heart attack might affect the client's sex life, including the following:

"Your heart attack will not change your sexual responsiveness. Most individuals can resume intercourse in 4 to 6 weeks, but your doctor should confirm this. If you can climb a flight of stairs without having chest pain you should be able to resume having sex since it takes about the same amount of energy."

"Many clients fear sexual intercourse after a heart attack because of the physical exertion associated with it. However, your prescribed program of progressive physical activity will also increase your tolerance for sexual activity."

Many clients recuperating from childbirth or illness or disease (e.g., heart attack) need instruction about safe sexual activities and the effects that therapy may have on sexual functioning. The following topics need to be considered:

- When sexual activity is safe
- Specific sexual activities that are unsafe, and why
- Adaptations needed for resuming a satisfactory sexual life
- The side effects of prescribed medications on sexual functioning, and the need to notify the primary care provider for possible dose or medication adjustment should problems develop.

Specific Suggestions

At this level, the nurse requires specialized knowledge and skill about how sexuality and functioning may be affected by a disease process or therapy and what interventions might be effective. The nurse offers suggestions to help the client adapt sexual activity to promote optimal functioning, such as what measures might alleviate vaginal dryness, safe positions for intercourse following a total hip replacement, safe and unsafe sexual practices following a heart attack, and ways to handle ostomy appliances, urinary catheters, casts, or other devices (e.g., prostheses) during sexual activity. Similarly, nurses who work on a cardiac unit need specialized knowledge about sexual readjustment during cardiac rehabilitation, and nurses working with clients with spinal cord injuries need information about the sexual consequences of spinal injuries at various levels.

Using the example of the client recuperating from a heart attack, the nurse may offer the following suggestion:

"Many individuals express concern about the stress of certain positions for intercourse, but you may use whatever position is comfortable for you and your partner, including side-lying or partner-on-top positions."

Intensive Therapy

At this level of intervention, nurses must have specialized preparation and knowledge of sexual and gender identity disorders. Nurses who function in the sex therapist role should meet the qualifications for practice identified by the American Association of Sexuality Educators, Counselors, and Therapists (AASECT), which differentiates sex counseling from sex therapy. Sex counseling helps clients incorporate their sexual knowledge into satisfying lifestyles and socially responsible behavior. Sex therapy is a highly specialized, in-depth treatment to help clients resolve serious sexual problems. The AASECT website includes a national directory of professionals certified to provide sex education, counseling, or therapy.

Dealing with Inappropriate Sexual Behavior

Any nurse may encounter a variety of sexually inappropriate behaviors for several reasons. The behavior may be aggressive or nonaggressive. Clients may act out sexually by:

- Exposing themselves.
- Asking the nurse to provide intimate physical care, such as bathing genital areas, when they can do this themselves.
- Touching or grabbing the nurse's genitals or buttocks.
- Making blatant sexual statements to the nurse.
- Offering the nurse sex.
- Whistling; making comments about the nurse's attractiveness or desirability.
- Making sexual comments to another client in the same room or to visitors about the "hot" nurse or what they would like to do sexually with the nurse.

Possible reasons for this inappropriate behavior are:

- Fear or anxiety over future ability to function sexually.
- Unmet needs for intimacy and sexual closeness because of hospitalization, injury, illness, treatment, lack of a partner, or lack of privacy.
- Misinterpretation of the nurse's behavior as sexual or provocative.
- Need for reassurance that they are still sexual beings and still sexually attractive.
- Need for attention.
- Confusion: Neurologic impairment or trauma can lead clients to use profane sexual language, engage in masturbation, expose themselves, or inappropriately touch or grab at the nurse.
- Need to control: Clients may experience loss of control over their lives because of hospitalization, injury, or illness.
- Need for power.
- Belief that flirtatious behavior is expected due to media portrayal of nurses as sexy, available, and experienced.

Before implementing any nursing interventions, the nurse should first ensure that the behavior is inappropriate and not an attempt to communicate a physical need. Clients may expose themselves if they are febrile, pull at the penis if a catheter is uncomfortable or irritating, or reach for the nurse if unable to communicate verbally. Nursing strategies to deal with inappropriate sexual behavior are listed in Box 40.5.

Evaluating

The goals established during the planning phase are evaluated according to specific desired outcomes also established during that phase. If any outcomes have not been achieved, the nurse should explore the reasons with questions such as the following:

- Were risk factors correctly identified?
- Did the client convey all significant fears and concerns about sexuality?
- Was the client more comfortable following discussions about sexual matters?
- Did the client understand the nurse's teaching?
- Was the health teaching compatible with the client's culture and religious values?
- Was the client ready to deal with sexuality problems?

BOX 40.5 Nursing Strategies for Inappropriate Sexual Behavior

- Communicate that the behavior is not acceptable by saying, for example, "I really do not like the things you are saying," or "I see you are not dressed. I will be back in 10 minutes and will help you with breakfast when you get your clothes on."
- Tell the client how the behavior makes you feel: "When you act like that toward me, I am very uncomfortable. It embarrasses me and makes it hard for me to give you the nursing care you need."
- Identify the behavior you expect: "Please call me by my name, not 'honey'" or "I expect you to keep yourself covered when I am in the room. If you are feeling hot or something is uncomfortable, let me know, and I will try to make you more comfortable."
- Set firm limits: Take the client's hand and move it away, use direct eye contact, and say, "Don't do that!"
- Try to refocus clients from the inappropriate behavior to their real concerns and fears; offer to discuss sexuality concerns: "All morning you have been making very personal sexual comments about yourself. Sometimes clients talk like that when they are concerned about the sexual part of their life and how their illness will affect them. Are there things that you have questions about or would like to talk about?"
- Report the incident to the nurse in charge and, if appropriate, the primary care provider. Discuss the incident, your feelings, and possible interventions.
- Clarify the consequences of continued inappropriate behavior (avoidance, withdrawal of services, no chance to help resolve underlying concerns of client).

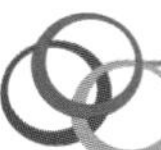

Critical Thinking Checkpoint

Mr. Curry is a 50-year-old male with diabetes who had a heart attack 3 weeks ago. He is doing well and is in a cardiac rehabilitation program. His diabetes is controlled with diet, and his only medications consist of a daily aspirin and an antihypertensive medication. During a routine checkup, you inquire how he is feeling and whether he is doing well on his medications. Reluctantly, he admits that he is having some sexual problems. You encourage further discussion of the matter by displaying interest and explaining that it is okay for him to share his concerns with you. Mr. Curry states that he is having some difficulty achieving erections, but is more concerned that he will have another heart attack if he engages in sexual activities.

1. Speculate about Mr. Curry's reluctance to discuss his sexual concerns.
2. What factors influence nurses' abilities to discuss sexual concerns with their clients?
3. What is the relationship between health and sexual function?
4. How can you best intervene to help Mr. Curry?

Answers to Critical Thinking Checkpoint questions are available on the faculty resources site. Please consult with your instructor.

Chapter 40 Review

CHAPTER HIGHLIGHTS

- Sexuality is important in developing self-identity, interpersonal relationships, intimacy, and love.
- There is a tremendous range of variation in how individuals express their sexuality including sexual orientation, gender identity, and sexual practices.
- Factors that affect sexuality include family, culture, religion, personal expectations and ethics, disease processes, medications, and relationship problems.
- Sexual problems include desire disorders, arousal disorders, orgasmic disorders, sexual pain disorders, and problems with satisfaction.
- Assessing risk for or actual sexual problems is part of the initial nursing assessment.
- Nurses assess attitudes toward sexuality, including factors that affect attitudes and behaviors.

- Before assisting clients with sexual problems, nurses must be aware of their own feelings and beliefs so they can objectively prepare approaches for gathering data and creating the nursing care plan. The nurse uses a culturally sensitive, nonjudgmental, nonthreatening, and reassuring approach.
- Nursing diagnoses for clients with sexual problems are related to altered body structure or function, lack of knowledge or misinformation about sexual matters, physical or psychologic abuse, value conflicts, and loss or lack of a partner.
- Nursing interventions focus largely on teaching clients about sexual health and function, responsible sexual behavior that includes the prevention of STIs and unwanted pregnancies, and self-examination of the breasts and testicles.
- Counseling clients with altered sexual functions can be facilitated by using the PLISSIT model: permission giving (P), limited information (LI), specific suggestions (SS), and intensive therapy (IT). Intensive therapy requires intervention by clinical nurse specialists or sex therapists.

TEST YOUR KNOWLEDGE

1. Clients may be unlikely to introduce the topic of sex with healthcare providers for which reason?
   1. They assume that healthcare providers know little about sexual functioning.
   2. Most clients have few questions or problems.
   3. Female clients prefer to discuss problems with female healthcare providers.
   4. They are too embarrassed to introduce the topic of sex.

2. A nurse is reading a research article that discusses the prevalence of androgyny in persons 20 to 30 years old. The nurse understands which of the following about androgynous persons?
   1. They do not limit behaviors to one gender over the other.
   2. They are attracted to people of the same gender.
   3. They often repress their sexual feelings.
   4. They hold rigid stereotyped gender role expectations.

3. A nurse finds an adult client masturbating on entering their room. What action should the nurse take?
   1. Tell the client that masturbation is harmful to sexual well-being.
   2. Say "excuse me" and leave the room.
   3. Request that the client stop so that care can be provided.
   4. Ask the client if there are any sexual concerns that should be discussed.

4. A nurse is preparing for pelvic physical examination of a woman who has been medically diagnosed with vaginismus. What equipment should the nurse obtain for this examination?
   1. Culture tubes to assess expected vaginal infection
   2. Extra cleaning supplies to remove thick external secretions
   3. Smaller than normal vaginal speculums
   4. Equipment for preexamination douche

5. A client who had a hysterectomy 3 days ago says to the nurse, "I no longer feel like a real woman." What is the best response?
   1. "Don't worry about that. The feeling will probably go away."
   2. "You should talk to your doctor about how you feel."
   3. "I don't blame you. I would feel like half a woman also."
   4. "I hear your concern. Tell me more about your feelings."

6. Because a client reports having dyspareunia, it is most appropriate to ask which question?
   1. "Have you talked with your partner about this discomfort?"
   2. "Have you had these spasms since you became sexually active?"
   3. "Do you have pain before your period begins?"
   4. "Do your breasts swell large enough to need a larger bra?"

7. Including at least some sexual health history questions would be most relevant for clients taking which category of drugs?
   1. Anti-inflammatories (such as aspirin or ibuprofen)
   2. Hypnotics (sleeping pills)
   3. Antihypertensives (blood pressure medications)
   4. Antihistamines (cold medications)

8. A nurse informs a client who is 8 1/2 months pregnant that it is best to abstain from intercourse until after the birth of the baby. This communication is most representative of which component of the PLISSIT model?
   1. Permission giving (P)
   2. Limited information (LI)
   3. Specific suggestions (SS)
   4. Intensive therapy (IT)

9. A 75-year-old male client reports decreased frequency of sexual intercourse although he does not express dissatisfaction or difficulty. He seems a little embarrassed by the discussion but is engaged and asks some questions. An appropriate nursing diagnosis would be which of the following?
   1. Sexual dysfunction
   2. Altered body image
   3. Inactive lifestyle
   4. Need for improved knowledge

10. Which of the following outcomes may indicate the need for referral to a more highly skilled therapist?
   1. The client verbalizes methods of modifying sexual activity according to physical limitations.
   2. The client requests the phone number of a sex education support group.
   3. Suggestions given by the nurse are ineffective in reaching the desired goals.
   4. The client reports experimenting with new sexual activities.

See Answers to Test Your Knowledge in Appendix A.

READINGS AND REFERENCES

Suggested Readings

Jarin, J., & Gomez-Lobo, V. (2016). Management of adolescents with gender dysphoria. *Contemporary OB/GYN, 61*(4), 32–38.
Definitions of terms are clearly included and descriptions of the most current diagnostic labels and guidelines for those receiving endocrine therapy are provided.

Joannides, P. (2017). *The guide to getting it on: Unzipped* (9th ed.). Waldport, OR: Goofy Foot.
A comprehensive sex education book that is both factual and fun to read.

Related Research

Yakubovich, A. R., Stöckl, H., Murray, J., Melendez-Torres, G. J., Steinert, J. I., Glavin, C. E. Y., & Humphreys, D. K. (2018). Risk and protective factors for intimate partner violence against women: Systematic review and meta-analyses of prospective-longitudinal studies. *American Journal of Public Health, 108*(7), e1–e11. doi:10.2105/AJPH.2018.304428

References

American Nurses Association. (2018). *Position statement on nursing advocacy for LGBTQ+ populations*. Retrieved from https://www.nursingworld.org/~49866e/globalassets/practiceandpolicy/ethics/nursing-advocacy-for-lgbtq-populations.pdf

Annon, J. (1976). The PLISSIT model: A proposed conceptual scheme for the behavioral treatment of sexual problems. *Journal of Sex Education and Therapy*, *2*(2), 1–15.

Brady, M. T. (2016). Newborn male circumcision with parental consent, as stated in the AAP circumcision policy statement, is both legal and ethical. *Journal of Law, Medicine & Ethics*, *44*, 256–262. doi:10.1177/1073110516654119

CDC/HRSA Advisory Committee on HIV, Viral Hepatitis and STD Prevention and Treatment. (2012). *Record of the proceedings*, May 8–9, 2012. Retrieved from http://www.cdc.gov/maso/facm/pdfs/CHACHSPT/20120508_CHAC.pdf

Curtis, K. M., Jatlaoui, T. C., Tepper, N. K., Zapata, L. B., Horton, L. G., Jamieson, D. J., & Whiteman, M. K. (2016). U.S. selected practice recommendations for contraceptive use, 2016. *MMWR Recommendations & Reports*, *65*(4), 1–66. doi:10.15585/mmwr.rr6504a1

Gates, G. J. (2017). *In US, more adults identifying as LGBT*. Retrieved from http://www.gallup.com/poll/201731/lgbt-identification-rises.aspx

Golden, R. L., Furman, W., & Collibee, C. (2016). The risks and rewards of sexual debut. *Developmental Psychology*, *52*, 1913–1925. doi:10.1037/dev0000206

Greenberg, J., Bruess, C. E., & Oswalt, S. B. (2017). *Exploring the dimensions of human sexuality* (6th ed.). Burlington, MA: Jones & Bartlett.

James, S. E., Herman, J. L., Rankin, S., Keisling, M., Mottet, L., & Anafi, M. (2016). *The report of the 2015 U.S. Transgender Survey*. Retrieved from https://transequality.org/sites/default/files/docs/usts/USTS-Full-Report-Dec17.pdf

Kann, L., McManus, T., Harris, W. A., Shanklin, S. L., Flint, K. H., Queen, B., . . . Ethier, K. A. (2018). Youth risk behavior surveillance—United States, 2017. *MMWR Surveillance Summaries*, *67*(SS-8), 1–114. doi:10.15585/mmwr.ss6708a1

Rich, A. L., Phipps, L. M., Tiwari, S., Rudraraju, H., & Dokpesi, P. O. (2016). The increasing prevalence in intersex variation from toxicological dysregulation in fetal reproductive tissue differentiation and development by endocrine-disrupting chemicals. *Environmental Health Insights*, *10*, 163–171. doi:10.4137/EHI.S39825

Ross, C. A. (2017). Response to Miccio-Fonseca (2015) and Defeo (2015) concerning commentary about DSM-5 sexual disorders section. *Journal of Child Sexual Abuse*, *26*(1), 92–95. doi:10.1080/10538712.2016.1263263

Svoboda, J. S., Adler, P. W., & Van Howe, R. S. (2016). Circumcision is unethical and unlawful. *Journal of Law, Medicine & Ethics*, *44*, 263–282. doi:10.1177/1073110516654120

Valentine, J. L. (2018). Forensic nursing: Overview of a growing profession. *American Nurse Today*, *13*(12), 42–44.

World Association for Sexual Health. (2014). *Declaration of sexual rights.* Retrieved from http://www.worldsexology.org/resources/declaration-of-sexual-rights

World Health Organization. (2016). *WHO guidelines on the management of health complications from female genital mutilation.* Retrieved from http://www.who.int/reproductivehealth/topics/fgm/management-health-complications-fgm/en

Selected Bibliography

Anwer, A. W., Samad, L., Iftikhar, S., & Baig-Ansari, N. (2017). Reported male circumcision practices in a Muslim-majority setting. *BioMed Research International*, Article ID 4957348, 8 pages. doi:10.1155/2017/4957348

Hock, R. R. (2016). *Human sexuality* (4th ed.). Boston, MA: Pearson.

Hyde, J. S., & DeLamater, J. D. (2017). *Understanding human sexuality* (13th ed.). New York, NY: McGraw-Hill.

Morgan, S. A., & Stokes, L. (2017). Overcoming marginalization in the transgender community. *American Nurse Today*, *12*(5), 34–35.

Moura da Silva, A., Ganz, J., Sousa, P., Doriqui, M., Ribeiro, M., Branco, M., . . . Soares de Britto e Alves, M. (2016). Early growth and neurologic outcomes of infants with probable congenital Zika virus syndrome. *Emerging Infectious Diseases*, *22*, 1953–1956. doi:10.3201/eid2211.160956

Rathus, S. A. Nevid, J. S., & Fichner-Rathus, L. (2016). *Human sexuality in a changing world* (10th ed.). New York, NY: Pearson.

Siddig, I. (2016). Female genital mutilation: What do we know so far? *British Journal of Nursing*, *25*(16), 912–916.

Sullivan, K., Guzman, A., & Lancellotti, D. (2017). Nursing communication and the gender identity spectrum. *American Nurse Today*, *12*(5), 6–8, 10–11.

Spirituality 41

LEARNING OUTCOMES

After completing this chapter, you will be able to:

1. Describe the interconnection of spirituality and religion concepts as they relate to health and spiritually sensitive nursing care.
2. Compare and contrast spiritual needs, spiritual disruption, and spiritual health.
3. Appreciate spiritual development by describing spiritual developmental issues of childhood and aging in particular.
4. Describe methods to assess the spiritual and religious preferences, strengths, concerns, or distress of clients and plan appropriate nursing care.
5. Describe nursing care and therapeutics to support religiosity and promote clients' spiritual health.
6. Recognize the importance of providing ethical spiritual care.
7. Describe the influence of spiritual and religious beliefs and practices that can have an impact on a client's healthcare: holy days, sacred texts, prayer and meditation, diet, healing, dress, birth, and death.
8. Describe strategies that can increase a nurse's own spiritual awareness.

KEY TERMS

agnostic, *1048*
atheist, *1048*
holy days, *1058*
meditation, *1059*
prayer, *1058*
presencing, *1053*
religion, *1048*
spiritual care, *1048*
spiritual disruption, *1048*
spiritual health, *1049*
spirituality, *1047*
spiritual or religious coping, *1049*
spiritual wellness or well-being, *1049*

Introduction

To provide holistic care, nurses need to care for the physical body and mind, and also need to care in ways that are sensitive to the client's spirit (O'Brien, 2018). Given the mounting research evidence linking spiritual health with physical and mental health (Jim et al., 2015; Koenig, 2015; Lucette, Ironson, Pargament, & Krause, 2016; Salsman et al., 2015), it is assumed that nursing care that supports clients' spiritual health will help promote other dimensions of health. Furthermore, clients often approach their health challenges, decisions, suffering, and so forth, with a worldview that reflects what are typically considered spiritual or religious beliefs (Dobratz, 2016; Mollica, Underwood, Homish, Homish, & Orom, 2016). Failure to appreciate these influential beliefs is to fail to understand what motivates, informs, comforts, and helps a client to cope. Indeed, spiritual beliefs and practices are frequently found to relieve one's suffering; unfortunately, sometimes discomforting spiritual beliefs can likewise intensify suffering (Abu-Raiya, Pargament, & Krause, 2016). Whether beliefs are comforting or discomforting, they are present at the bedside, and they require recognition and sometimes support or scrutiny.

Recognizing a client's spirituality is like standing on holy ground (O'Brien, 2018). The nurse cannot approach care for the spirit as if it were a pressure injury or even as if it were an emotional problem. Spiritual matters are not intangibles that can be fixed, cured, solved, or manipulated. Rather, the nurse's stance toward spiritually sensitive care must be one that seeks to accompany, support, and nurture. This chapter explores how the nurse can attend to the client who presents with a need to relieve spiritual disruption or to enhance spiritual health. Nurses can offer spiritually sensitive nursing care that supports spiritual health, helps with coping and adjustment, or assists a client to face a more peaceful death.

Spirituality and Related Concepts Described

Spirituality and *religion* are words that are often used interchangeably by clients and professionals alike, yet the nursing literature typically distinguishes them as separate concepts. That is, **spirituality** is generally thought to refer to the human tendency to seek meaning and purpose in life, inner peace and acceptance, forgiveness and harmony, hope, beauty, and so forth. An international study about how individuals in China, India, and the United States perceived spirituality concluded that it is a universal phenomenon (McClintock, Lau, & Miller, 2016). These researchers noted that across these diverse cultures, spirituality involved the following attributes:

love, in the fabric of relationships and as a sacred reality; unifying interconnectedness, as a sense of energetic oneness with other beings in the universe; altruism, as a commitment beyond the self with care and service; contemplative practice, such as meditation, prayer, yoga, or qigong; and religious and spiritual reflection and commitment, as a life well-examined. (p. 1600)

Another aspect of spirituality often recognized is the awareness of something transcendent—a higher power, creative force, divine being, or infinite source of energy (Weathers, McCarthy, & Coffey, 2016). For example, an individual may believe in God, Allah, the Great Spirit, or a Higher Power.

In contrast, the term **religion** is usually applied to ritualistic practices and organized beliefs. Indeed, there has been a tendency in nursing—as in psychology and other fields—to separate these two concepts. Yet trying to make religion an opposite of spirituality (e.g., institutional versus personal, objective versus subjective, narrow versus broad, cerebral versus emotional, bad versus good) is unfair to both concepts. Spirituality and religion are "inherently intertwined" (Taylor, 2012).

According to a 2012 national survey of Americans, about two-thirds view themselves as moderately to very spiritual; nearly 60% self-report that they are moderately to very religious (Hodge, 2015). Furthermore, roughly half of those who are very spiritual also see themselves as very religious. Just because individuals are spiritual does not mean that they view themselves as religious—and vice versa. Indeed, 23% of Americans are "nones"—individuals who are not affiliated with a religion (Pew Research Center, n.d.). Laird, Curtis, and Morgan (2017) observed that American healthcare professionals often think of spirituality and religion in normative ways; that is, we often think of these concepts through Western and Christian (especially Protestant) lenses. They urge awareness of and openness toward diverse spiritualties and religions.

It is important to remember that some individuals do not accept that there is an Ultimate Other or a spiritual reality. An **agnostic** is an individual who doubts the existence of God or believes the existence of God has not been proved. An **atheist** is one without belief in a deity. Atheists report that they often feel discriminated against (Brewster, Hammer, Sawyer, Eklund, & Palamar, 2016) or perceived as angry (Meier, Fetterman, Robinson, & Lappas, 2015) by those in our culture who experience and value spirituality or religion. For example, atheists perceive that others view them as immoral, not good, and needing to give up their beliefs to avoid suffering in an afterlife (Meier et al., 2015). Atheists, unsurprisingly, want to be respected for their "nonbelief" and not have nurses impose their spiritual or religious perspectives.

Spiritual Care or Spiritual Nursing Care?

Pesut and Sawatzky (2006) put forward that **spiritual care** should not be prescriptive (i.e., the following of a set guideline for intervening to resolve a client's spiritual problem). Instead it should be descriptive of ways nurses can offer spiritual support. Therefore, they suggest that:

> Spiritual nursing care is an intuitive, interpersonal, altruistic, and integrative expression that is contingent on the nurse's awareness of the transcendent dimension of life but that reflects the client's reality. At its foundational level, spiritual nursing care is an expression of self . . . . Spiritual nursing care begins from a perspective of being with the client in love and dialogue but may emerge into therapeutically oriented interventions that take direction from the client's religious or spiritual reality. (p. 23)

Although nursing terminology usually uses *spiritual care*, a few nurses use less prescriptive, and probably more appropriate, language such as *spiritually sensitive nursing care* or *spiritual nursing care*. Regardless of terminology, promising findings from recent studies indicate that such care does affect positive client outcomes such as satisfaction with care. Using data obtained from Asian Americans ($n = 805$) recently discharged from a hospital, one study found that this relationship between spiritual needs being met and client satisfaction was best explained by whether nurses provided spiritual care (Hodge, Sun, & Wolosin, 2014).

Spiritual Needs, Spiritual Disruption, Spiritual Health, and Religious Coping

If one assumes that everybody has a spiritual dimension, then it may also be assumed that all clients have spiritual needs that reflect their spirituality. Such needs are not problems to be processed, but perhaps better understood as inner movements, yearnings, or experiences. An awareness of such needs is often heightened by an illness or other health crisis. Clients may find that their beliefs are challenged by their health situation, or may cling to their beliefs more firmly and appreciatively. Or, a client may have a need to express joy or gratitude, or continue through the inwardly rewarding (yet often painful) process of spiritual transformation. Nurses need to be sensitive to indications of the client's spiritual needs and respond appropriately, as discussed later. Examples of spiritual needs are listed in Box 41.1.

Spiritual disruption or religious struggle or pain refers to the inner chaos that can occur when an individual's assumptions and beliefs are threatened or shattered. A question designed to screen for spiritual pain referred to it as "pain deep in your soul or being that is not physical" (Delgado-Guay et al., 2016). Exline, Pargament, Grubbs, and Yali (2014) identified the following as types of spiritual or religious struggle: negative emotions related to God, concerns about demonic forces, interpersonal conflicts with religious individuals or organizations, struggles to live according to moral values, doubts about religious beliefs, guilt, and worry about not finding meaningfulness in life.

BOX 41.1 Spiritual Needs

Spiritual Needs	Illustrations
Need for satisfying meaning to ascribe to illness, to life, to dying, to any loss or serious challenge	"Why would this happen to me? Having cancer is a celestial crapshoot!" "This is so unfair." "Why do bad things happen?"
Need for purpose, vocation, mission	"Now that I can't work anymore, what good is it for me to keep on living?" "What's there for me to do now with my old body?"
Need for believable beliefs, sensible worldview	"I've been told God is in control and is loving, but that doesn't make sense to me anymore."
Guilt, need to restore relationship	"I wonder if I'm being punished for something I did when I was younger." "I know I have to meet my Maker soon, so I'd better get things right with Him."
Shame, imperfection, unworthiness	"I never was good enough for . . . , but now look how sick/disabled/scarred I am!" "I am going to do whatever my family wants me to do." "I'm just using up society's resources. I'm such a burden to my family."
Need to worship, transcend self	"I am so tired/sick/befuddled/anxious, I'm beside myself . . . . I wish I could feel God was involved in this situation." "I never get to go to church because I'm always taking care of my husband."
Need for peace, composure	"I don't feel comfortable being alone or in silence." "I just wish I could make it all turn out the way I want it to."
Need to be grateful	"I know I should count my blessings; things could be worse."
Need to express love	"I keep my problems to myself, because I don't want to trouble my family any more than necessary." "You nurses do so much for me; I wish I could do nice things for you."
Isolation, abandonment, betrayal	"Why don't they come to visit anymore?" "It just seems like all my prayers bounce back to me without being heard."

When caring for clients, the following may be indicators or examples of signs and symptoms of spiritual disruption. The client may:

- Manifest a lack of enthusiasm for life, hopelessness, meaninglessness, sense of emptiness, or inadequate acceptance of self.
- Express feeling abandoned or anger toward a power greater than self or toward a spiritual community.
- Question the credibility of spiritual or religious beliefs; question the meaning of life, death, or suffering.
- Exhibit sudden changes in spiritual practices.
- Request (or refuse) to interact with a spiritual leader.
- Have no interest in religious or spiritually nurturing resources or experiences (Carpenito, 2017, p. 589).

No list could be complete, however, considering the complexity and variability of individuals and their spiritual dimensions.

Spiritual health, or **spiritual wellness or well-being**, is often portrayed as the opposite of spiritual disruption. Spiritual health is thought to not occur by chance, but by choice. That is, spiritual health results when individuals *intentionally* seek to strengthen their spiritual muscles, as it were, through various spiritual disciplines (e.g., prayer, meditation, service, fellowship with similar believers, learning from a spiritual mentor, worship, study, fasting).

Spiritual or religious coping, both positive and negative, has received considerable research attention during the past couple of decades. It refers to the spiritual beliefs or ways of thinking that help individuals cope with their challenges. Numerous studies have shown that positive religious coping helps clients adapt to illness, whereas negative religious coping is associated with maladaptation for both adolescents and adults (King et al., 2017; Reynolds, Mrug, Wolfe, Schwebel, & Wallander, 2016). For example, negative religious coping (e.g., thinking that illness is a punishment and feeling abandoned by God) were associated with depression and poorer quality of life among survivors of stem cell transplants (King et al., 2017).

Spiritual Development

Theories about human development include not just theories about physical, cognitive, and moral development, but also theories about spiritual development (Fowler, 1981). Spiritual development results from complex interactions between "nature and nurture" (Granqvist & Nkara, 2017). Thus, when assessing or supporting client spirituality, it is necessary to appreciate how spirituality and religiosity evolve with age and life experience (see Lifespan Considerations). A normal part of this development for teens

LIFESPAN CONSIDERATIONS **Spiritual Development**

CHILDREN

As with adults, children describe their spiritual health and challenges through the stories they tell and behaviors. And as with adults, they can learn spiritual principles from stories caregivers tell. Although they may not have fully developed cognitively, they can still ask questions about suffering and God and if there is an afterlife (Ferrell, Wittenberg, Battista, & Walker, 2016).

- As you respond, consider the child's cognitive and faith development stages to determine age-appropriate language. Does the child think concretely and literally about spiritual concepts like God and heaven? Or does the child think mythically and abstractly? Follow the child's cues about how to talk.
- Children's spirituality reflects or interacts with that of their authority figure(s) (e.g., parents). The spiritual beliefs and practices of the authority figure(s) will be trusted and adopted by the child. Thus, many of the cues for how to talk with a child will come from that child's parent or guardian. Generally, it is not until the teenage years and young adulthood, when children can reason abstractly, that they begin to independently construct their own spiritual beliefs and practices.

ADOLESCENTS

Teens and young adults, although likely critiquing the religion of their parents and less likely to be openly religious, often will use private religious and spiritual coping strategies (Taylor, Petersen, Oyedele, & Haase, 2015). Indeed, adolescence is a time of "forming a unique identity, gaining the ability to think critically, and differentiating self from families . . . . It is also a time of risk-taking, susceptibility to peer pressure, sensation seeking, impulsivity, and poor future orientation" (Taylor et al., 2015, p. 230). Given these developmental issues, it is important to sensitively attend to adolescents' spiritual well-being. For example, one study documented that the psychologic well-being of adolescents surviving cancer was positively correlated with their level of spiritual well-being, whereas spiritual struggle was negatively correlated with psychologic adjustment (Park & Cho, 2016). Nursing care that is sensitive to adolescent spirituality can include:

- Facilitating spiritual expression via the arts (and using art forms that are age appropriate, such as creating video montages).
- Introducing spiritually supportive resources on the internet.

MIDDLE-AGED AND OLDER ADULTS

By the time they reach middle age, most adults realize that materialism and social achievements do not meet the requirements of the soul; therefore, their focus shifts from self-centeredness towards generativity—care and concern for younger generations (Atchley, 2020).

Many older adults highly value religious coping strategies such as prayer. Evidence shows spiritual well-being to be directly correlated with mental health and less medical illness among older adults (George, Kinghorn, Koenig, Gammon, & Blazer, 2013). It is, therefore, important to address the spiritual issues of older adults. Older clients may be especially concerned about living a purposeful life, maintaining loving relationships to avoid social isolation, and preparing for a good death. Nursing care that attends to such spiritual issues includes the following:

- Supporting meaning-making activities (e.g., conducting a life review or reminiscence therapy, allowing the client to weave together the strands of lived life; encouraging the client to become dedicated to some social, political, religious, or artistic cause; supporting the client to leave a legacy or do an altruistic deed). Such activities provide older adults with a sense of purpose and assist them in making sense of the life they have lived.
- Allowing open discussions about suffering and dying, encouraging client disclosure by asking open-ended questions, and providing responses that are respectful and compassionate. Do not avoid discomforting topics and questions older clients raise by imposing positivity, giving "pat" answers, and otherwise minimizing or avoiding their spiritual pain.
- As appropriate, supporting older clients to reframe the "losses" of aging as "liberations," and confinement (e.g., to a bed or room) as monasticism. Indeed, older adults possess great wisdom and are in a season of life that promotes spiritual growth.

Older adults with dementia present special circumstances for spiritual caregiving. Nurses can help those with early stages of dementia to focus on the positives—the "haves" rather than the losses. Allowing older clients with dementia to tell their stories permits them to maintain some identity (amidst a disease that threatens the very sense of self) and allows the nurse a window into their world. Older clients with dementia can also worship and express their hope and creativity through various art forms (e.g., movement, painting, music). It is also possible for them to experience the compassion of others when they feel their caring touch or hear their soothing voice.

and young adults involves evaluating the beliefs and religiosity of authority figures to form beliefs and practices that are meaningful for them. It is not unusual, however, to find adults who have failed to complete this developmental task. Thus, when serious health challenges occur, the beliefs of childhood that have "not kept up with the times" may fail to be satisfactory for explaining such loss or change.

Spiritual Health and the Nursing Process

The nursing process, which includes assessing, diagnosing, planning, implementing, and evaluating, has often been applied to spiritual care. Although this can be a helpful approach, it is now thought to misguide spiritually sensitive nursing care (Pesut & Sawatzky, 2006). For this introductory discussion of spiritual care, content will be presented following this systematic nursing process. Recognize, however, that spiritual care is *not* about measuring the degree of spiritual health planning to fix spiritual pain, prescribing spiritual intervention, spiritual problem-solving, or manipulating, controlling, or managing spiritual outcomes or health.

●○● NURSING MANAGEMENT

Although nurses can play a pivotal role in supporting clients' spirituality, it is important to remember that the nurse is a spiritual care generalist. Spiritual care experts include chaplains, clergy, and other spiritual mentors with whom clients may identify. Likewise, although many clients view nurses as sources of spiritual support, clients often view their family and friends or community-based clergy as their primary spiritual caregivers (Daaleman, 2012).

Although there is scanty evidence directly measuring the outcomes of nurse- or even chaplain-provided spiritual care, some research findings suggest that spiritual care in a healthcare institution, especially when provided by the multidisciplinary team, is associated with positive outcomes such as improved client quality of life, decreased hospital cost, and increased use of hospice for clients with advanced cancer (Balboni et al., 2011). There is evidence that clients in a hospital or in a nursing home who have received spiritual care tend to believe they have also received overall good care at that institution (Astrow, Wexler, Texeira, He, & Sulmasy, 2007; Daaleman, 2012; Williams, Meltzer, Arora, Chung, & Curlin, 2011).

Assessing

To provide spiritually sensitive care, the nurse must first assess whether such care is needed or welcome. Data about a client's spiritual beliefs and practices can be obtained through a nursing history as well as from ongoing clinical observations of the client's behavior, verbalizations, mood, and so on. A two-tiered approach to spiritual assessment is helpful, and should include a screening and history.

Screening for Spiritual Disruption

Initially, nurses should screen clients to determine: (a) if spiritual disruption is present and (b) what spiritual support is wanted. Ideally, this screening should occur for any client entering a healthcare system for any significant health challenge. An algorithm for screening developed and tested in a Chicago hospital recommends the following process (King, Fitchett, & Berry, 2013):

- First, inquire, "Is spirituality or religion important to you as you cope with illness?"
- If the client responds with a yes, then ask, "How much strength or comfort do you get from your religion or spirituality right now?" Depending on the client's response, ask if a chaplain or other expert is wanted for discussing spiritual concerns.
- If the client responded to the initial question with a no, then ask, "Has there ever been a time when spirituality or religion was important to you?" Depending on the client's response, ask if a chaplain or other expert can discuss this with the client. (If there never was a time when spirituality was important and the client does not wish to discuss the matter further, then respect that wish.)

Other questions with the potential to screen for spiritual disruption include "How deeply at peace do you feel?" (Park & Sacco, 2016), and "How much pain that is deep in your soul or being and not physical do you have?" (Delgado-Guay et al., 2016). Depending on client responses, nurses can obtain from the client permission for making a referral to a chaplain or other spiritual care expert. See the accompanying Assessment Interview for examples of questions to ask.

Spiritual History

The nurse who has primary responsibility for coordinating a client's care ought also to conduct a spiritual history to gain a basic understanding of the spiritual or religious beliefs and practices pertinent to the client's health and healthcare. Several mnemonics are available to guide such a history. A common one is Puchalski's FICA model:

F = Faith or beliefs—for example, "What spiritual beliefs are most important to you?"
I = Implications or influence—for example, "How is your faith affecting the way you cope now?"
C = Community—for example, "Is there a group of like-minded believers with which you regularly meet?"
A = Address—for example, "How would you like your healthcare team to support you spiritually?" (Williams, Voss, Vahle. & Capp, 2016).

Additional spiritual history prompts are provided in the accompanying Assessment Interview.

Two cautions are important to remember when conducting spiritual assessment. First, a nurse-conducted spiritual assessment should limit itself to client spirituality as it relates to health (Taylor, 2015). That is, it is not the privilege of clinicians to investigate a client's spirituality unless it has a purpose related to providing healthcare. Second, a nurse should never assume that a client follows all the practices of the client's stated religion. Similarly, it is important to remember that the degree of religious

ASSESSMENT INTERVIEW Spirituality

ESSENTIAL CONTENT

- Is spirituality or religion important to you? (Or, how spiritual or religious do you think of yourself as being?)
- What spiritual or religious beliefs and practices are especially important for your healthcare team to know about?
- In what ways can I or we (nurses, healthcare team) support your spirit?

OPTIONAL FOLLOW-UP (USE AS APPROPRIATE)

- How will being sick interfere with your religious practices?
- What spiritual or religious beliefs influence you the most as you make healthcare decisions?
- How is your faith helpful to you? Is it sustaining you the way you would like it to while you are sick? In what ways is it important to you right now?
- Would you like a visit from your spiritual counselor or the hospital chaplain?
- What are your hopes and your sources of strength right now? What comforts you during hard times?

commitment and orthodoxy (i.e., how strictly one incorporates traditional religious prescriptions into daily life) is highly variable within religious traditions. How one Baptist, for example, interprets and lives his religion will be different from his Baptist neighbor. Thus, an assessment that is limited to learning with what religion the client identifies is a very limited assessment.

Although the nurse will continually be assessing, the initial spiritual assessment may best be taken at the end of the intake assessment, or following the psychosocial assessment, after the nurse has developed a relationship with the client or support person. A nurse who has demonstrated sensitivity and personal warmth, creating some rapport, will likely be more successful during a spiritual assessment.

Cues to spiritual and religious preferences, strengths, concerns, or distress may be revealed by one or more of the following:

1. ***Environment.*** Does the client have a Bible, Torah, Koran, other prayer book, devotional literature, religious medals, a rosary, a cross, a Star of David, or religious get-well cards in the room? Does a church send altar flowers or Sunday bulletins?
2. ***Behavior.*** Does the client appear to pray before meals or at other times or read religious literature? Does the client express anger at religious representatives or at a deity?
3. ***Verbalization.*** Does the client mention God or a higher power, prayer, faith, the church, synagogue, temple, a spiritual or religious leader, or religious topics? Does the client ask about a visit from the clergy? Does the client express any of the following: fear of death, concern with the meaning of life, inner conflict about religious beliefs, concern about a relationship with the deity, questions about the meaning of existence or the meaning of suffering, or concern about the moral or ethical implications of therapy?
4. ***Affect and attitude.*** Does the client appear lonely, depressed, angry, anxious, agitated, apathetic, or preoccupied?
5. ***Interpersonal relationships.*** Who visits? How does the client respond to visitors? Does a minister come? How does the client relate to other clients and nursing personnel?

Diagnosing

The prevalence of spiritual disruption varies across studies. For example, 27% of individuals surviving stem cell transplantation and over 40% of individuals with advanced cancer were observed to have spiritual struggles or pain (Delgado-Guay, et al., 2016; King et al., 2017). Nurses, as spiritual care generalists, must be extremely cautious when assessing a client's spiritual health and applying a diagnosis that could be inappropriate. In diagnosing spiritual health, the nurse may find that spiritual problems provide the diagnostic label, or that spiritual disruption is the etiology of the problem.

Spiritual Issues as the Diagnostic Label

Examples of nursing diagnoses that are appropriate for clients with spiritual issues can include spiritual disruption related to situational crises (e.g., illness, unexpected life event) or "sociocultural deprivation" (e.g., inability to attend religious services); spiritual health enhancement, a wellness diagnosis describing spiritual health that acknowledges that some clients respond to adversity with an increased sensitivity to spirituality or spiritual maturation; and potential for spiritual disruption for a client who presently shows no indication of this disruption of spirit yet may if a nurse fails to intervene.

Religious Issues as the Diagnostic Label

Examples of nursing diagnoses that are appropriate for clients with religious issues can include religious struggle, potential for religious struggle, and religious enhancement.

Spiritual or Religious Distress as the Etiology

Spiritual disruption may affect other areas of functioning and indicate other diagnoses. In these instances, spiritual disruption becomes the etiology. An example is impaired coping related to feelings of abandonment by God and loss of religious faith.

Planning

In the planning phase, the nurse identifies therapeutics to support or promote spiritual health in the context of illness.

Planning in relation to spiritual needs may involve one or more of the following:

- Helping clients to practice their religious rituals
- Supporting clients to recognize and incorporate spiritual beliefs in healthcare decision-making
- Encouraging clients to recognize positive meanings for health challenges
- Promoting a sense of hope and peace
- Providing spiritual resources when requested
- Facilitating connection with others (e.g., estranged family, clergy and faith community members).

It is important to remember that the goal of spiritual care is *not* to control clients' spiritual angst for them, tell them how to become transformed by their situation, or impose your goals for them. The plan, rather, is to gently and sensitively support, facilitate, and accompany in ways that will aid health or a good death.

Implementing

Spiritual nursing care includes actions as diverse as recognizing and validating the inner resources of an individual, such as coping methods, humor, motivation, self-determination, positive attitude, and optimism. It can also include assisting the client to leave a legacy by storytelling or recording life stories for family and friends, and encouraging creative expression through art, music, and writing. This keeps the imagination alive and serves to regenerate the body, mind, and spirit. Fostering ways for clients to keep in touch with nature and maintain a sense of wonder are also forms of spiritual care. Recognizing the seasons, the emergence of flowers in spring, the phases of the moon, the migrations of birds, and the unchanging stars provides examples of orderliness in the universe, even in the midst of chaos and loss.

Numerous nursing therapeutics are available to support and promote client spiritual health. Although diverse, some of the most common nursing therapeutics most desired by clients include (a) providing presence, (b) conversing about spirituality, (c) supporting religious practices, (d) assisting clients with prayer, and (e) referring clients for spiritual counseling (Balboni et al., 2013). One of the few studies examining what spiritual care clients perceive is appropriate for nurses to provide indicated that clients with advanced cancer are positive about such care (Balboni, et al., 2013). This study of 68 clients receiving treatment showed that over 70% reported it appropriate for a nurse to inquire about their spiritual needs, encourage them in their beliefs, or make a chaplain referral; 62% thought it appropriate for a nurse to offer prayer for a client.

Providing Presence

Presencing is a term describing the art of being present, or just being with a client during his or her suffering. To be fully present to a client, a nurse must be purposefully attentive (Fahlberg & Roush, 2016). To be comfortable being fully present to another individual, however, one must be comfortable being fully present to oneself (du Plessis, 2016). Strategies for increasing the ability to be present to a client include:

- Slow down. Calm yourself.
- Make sure that in your "heart" you are willing to be present. Take deep, slow breaths to center yourself. Nurses who listen attentively to clients yet fail to give of self (i.e., inwardly "make room") diminish their effectiveness.
- Sit down; keep your eye level at the same level as the client's.
- Allow silence.
- Smile or exude positive energy while remaining respectful of the client's emotional state (e.g., convey quiet, inner courage if the client is experiencing sorrow or despair). Follow the client's nonverbal cues.
- Focus. With whatever brief or long amount of time you have available, use it maximally by focusing completely on the client. Be physically, emotionally, and mentally present.
- Empathize with the client; actively and deeply listen (Fahlberg & Roush, 2016; Taylor, 2007b).
- Self-disclosures (e.g., telling the client about how you overcame a similar situation) are never appropriate unless the client requests it and it is shared with therapeutic intent rather than for self-serving reasons. (Ask, "Whose needs are being met here?")

Osterman and Schwartz-Barcott (1996) identified four levels or ways of being present for clients:

- Presence (when a nurse is physically present but not focused on the client)
- Partial presence (when a nurse is physically present and attending to some task on the client's behalf but not relating to the client on any but the most superficial level)
- Full presence (when a nurse is mentally, emotionally, and physically present; intentionally focusing on the client)
- Transcendent presence (when a nurse is physically, mentally, emotionally, and spiritually present for a client; involves a transpersonal and transforming experience).

Presencing is often the best and sometimes the only intervention to support a client who suffers under circumstances that medical interventions cannot address. When a client is helpless, powerless, and vulnerable, a nurse's presencing can be most beneficial. Rather than worrying about saying or doing "the right thing," nurses should focus on being fully present. In this way, nurses can promote healing, diminish client anxiety, create a sense of safety, and improve both client and their own satisfaction with the interaction (du Plessis, 2016).

Conversing About Spirituality

Initiating conversation about spiritual or religious concerns with a healthcare professional is likely hard for clients; they presumably wait for an appropriate time with a "safe" clinician. Both physicians and nurses typically find it difficult to talk with clients about this intimate and sometimes socially taboo topic (Best, Butow, & Olver, 2016; Wittenburg, Ragan, & Ferrell, 2017). Sometimes clients do not want to talk about deep inner pain, spiritual or emotional. They may instead find comfort and help from the nurse who genuinely shows interest in their life, family, and hobbies. However, sometimes clients do want to have overtly spiritual discussions with their nurse.

Taylor (2007a) proposed the goal of verbal spiritual care as being "to provide responses to clients which allow the clients to become intellectually, emotionally, and physically aware of their spirituality so that they can experience life more fully" (p. 7). Yet often when clients raise difficult spiritual concerns, clinicians avoid the topic by imposing a positive spin, minimizing the psychospiritual pain, injecting humor, or giving a pat answer. Instead of avoiding these painful and difficult conversations, nurses can provide a healing response by incorporating principles of empathic communication (Taylor, 2007a). For example, the nurse can respond to clients' comments about spirituality with a restatement of what is most central in their comments, an open question to prompt their further reflection, or a statement that tentatively names their feeling. Dimensions of a verbal response that promotes spiritual healing are identified in Table 41.1.

TABLE 41.1 Dimensions of a Spiritually Healing Response

Healing	Not Healing
Client centered *(e.g., "It seems you're feeling like no one cares.")*	Nurse centered *(e.g., "But I care about you!")*
Neutral *(e.g., "Tell me more about your thinking regarding . . . .")*	Judgmental *(e.g., "Why do you think that?")*
Immediate contributors to spiritual pain *(e.g., "Perhaps underneath all the 'why' questions you're asking, you feel abandoned.")*	Distant, tangential, or abstract contributors to spiritual pain *(e.g., "You were wondering what caused your cancer.")*
Accurately names feelings, engages emotion *(e.g., "I'm sensing that your belief makes you calm now.")*	Inaccurately or never names feelings, engages thinking *(e.g., "What do you believe about . . . ?")*

From "Spiritual Pain," by E. J. Taylor, 2007a, *Advance for Nurses*, *9*(21), pp. 15–16.

Sometimes clients ask nurses about their spiritual or religious beliefs or practices, which may provoke some nurse anxiety. However, it is likely the client wishes to get better acquainted with the nurse to determine if the nurse is safe to disclose to, or because the client wants to equalize the relationship. Occasionally, the client is collecting data, that is, he or she wants to learn a new comforting or meaningful spiritual perspective. The Practice Guidelines feature titled *Can a Nurse Self-Disclose Personal Spiritual Beliefs?* describes how a nurse can be cautious before sharing personal spiritual or religious beliefs with a client so as not to unethically impose these perspectives.

Assisting Clients with Prayer or Meditation

Many nurses pray with clients when they request it (Minton, Isaacson, & Banik, 2016; Taylor, Park, & Pfeiffer, 2014). Prayer allows individuals to connect with each other and with the divine. To pray for another is also a way for loving individuals to express care. While most clients may say that prayer makes them feel better, it is also possible that prayer could raise to awareness a spiritual struggle or a disappointment and questions about "unanswered prayers" (Taylor, 2012).

Does prayer heal clients? A recent Cochrane review of the evidence from several randomized experiments that investigated the efficacy of intercessory prayer (that is, having an individual unknown to a client pray for the client's physical healing) concluded that the findings equivocally suggest no clear positive or negative effect of intercessory prayer on health outcomes (Roberts, Ahmed, Hall, & Davison, 2009). A more helpful perspective regarding prayer is offered by Bishop (2003), who observed:

PRACTICE GUIDELINES Can a Nurse Self-Disclose Personal Spiritual Beliefs?

When self-disclosing personal spiritual perspectives, the healthcare professional can maintain a therapeutic relationship with the client by remembering the following:

- *Do not disclose to gratify your needs. Ask yourself, "Whose needs are being met when I share my beliefs?"* If you are disclosing your beliefs because you think they will benefit the client, yet the client has no desire to know your beliefs, then you are meeting your needs. Asking a client if you can share your beliefs may be inappropriate, given that clients often perceive they are "at your mercy" and may feel uncomfortable declining your offer. For example, asking, "Do you mind if I ask a personal question?" often obliges the vulnerable client to say yes, even though they wish to say no. Instead, carefully observe for when a client indicates a desire for your perspective.
- *When clients ask you about your spirituality, you may find it helpful to first assess why they are asking.* For example, "Your question about 'why?' is a tough one. What brings you to ask it now?" or "I love talking about my beliefs, but what in particular is it that you'd like to know?" Or, "Before I answer, could we explore what this means to you?" *The why behind their question should guide your response.*
- *Any time you disclose your personal beliefs, follow up the self-disclosure with an open question or reflection of feelings.* Always return the ball to the client's court. For example, "As you can see, I'm not sure of this myself, but can you tell me what would be comforting to you?" or "I wonder what is going on inside you now?"
- *Use self-disclosure infrequently and keep the disclosures short.* A request about what you believe is not a request for a religious discussion.
- *When responding to a client's query about your spiritual beliefs, try to incorporate the client's language when framing your response.* In this way, you may avoid using loaded words that could create tension. For example, if a client asks you about how they can "make things right," you can couch your response using this language, rather than talk about "repentance" and "being saved" if that is your normal language.
- *Keep your answer honest, authentic.* Sometimes this means simply saying, "I don't know."
- *If you are asked a question with which you are uncomfortable or unable to answer, you can still use the moment for healing purposes.* Healing can still occur when you use the communication skills to increase self-awareness. For example, "You know, I have to admit, I'm uncomfortable with your question. I may be uncomfortable with it because I don't like the answers I've heard others give for it. Perhaps asking the question makes you feel uncomfortable, too." [pause for response] Or, "I've been wondering that myself for a long time. Sometimes I wonder if it is . . . , but I don't know. What ideas have you considered?"
- *Make a referral to a spiritual care specialist.* Assuming the client would like to further explore the spiritual questions that are brought to the surface by health challenges, initiate a referral through the chaplain or spiritual caregiver if the client assents.

From *What Do I Say? Talking with Patients About Spirituality*, by E. J. Taylor, 2007b, Philadelphia, PA: Templeton Press.

> Prayer is a human response to existential moments, to "why" questions. Prayer is not an intervention, a technology to control the universe. It is not merely a psychologic response. It is not merely a faith response. It is not a way that unenlightened individuals delude themselves. It is a human response to serious human questions—questions that every human has likely asked, or will likely ask when faced with serious illness . . . . If it does not work as defined by science, it still works by fulfilling its role in helping a client to seek meaning in the face of existential crises and again no scientific explanation is possible. (p. 1407)

Clients may choose to participate in private prayer or want group prayer with family, friends, or clergy (Figure 41.1 ■). In such situations the nurse's responsibility is to ensure a quiet environment and privacy. Nursing care may need to be adjusted to accommodate periods for prayer. When it is assessed to be ethical and desired, the nurse who shares a belief in prayer may find praying with a client to be an inwardly powerful experience. Of course, a believing nurse can always pray privately for clients as many healthcare professionals do. Sometimes this "action" is all one can take in the presence of an otherwise powerless situation. See Practice Guidelines *Praying with Clients* for suggestions on how to pray with clients.

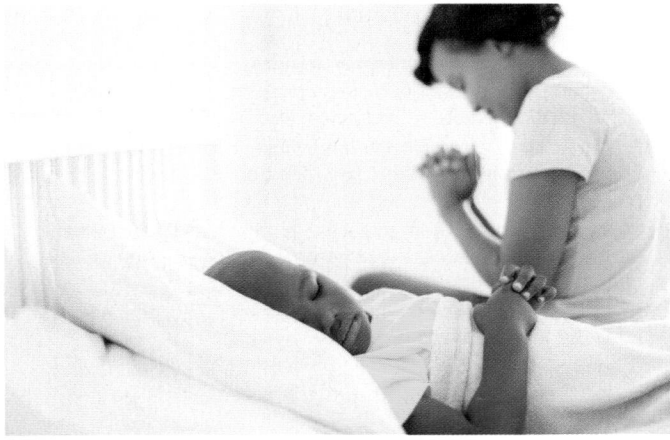

Figure 41.1 ■ Mother praying for ill child.
Hongqi Zhang/123RF.

Likewise, given the volume of evidence showing spiritually oriented meditation contributes to physical and psychologic healing (e.g., Hulett & Armer, 2016), clients will benefit when nurses support meditation. Whereas some nurses may obtain training that will allow them to teach individuals or groups various meditational techniques, most nurses can simply introduce online or recorded meditations. Nurses can also be supportive by planning uninterrupted quiet time for client meditation, and negotiate with the client prior to meditation as to how much to palliate symptoms so that the mind can remain aware.

Referring Clients to Spiritual Care Experts

There are times when spiritual care is best referred to other members of the healthcare team. Referrals can be made for hospitalized clients and their families through the hospital chaplain's office if one is available. Nurses in home and community health settings can identify spiritual resources by checking directories of community service agencies, telephone directories, or religious directories that describe available spiritual counselors and the services provided through the religious community. Many

PRACTICE GUIDELINES Praying with Clients

Sometimes a client may ask a nurse to pray. This request likely reflects the client's inner anxiety, isolation, confusion, or distress, and the yearning for comfort, peace, or understanding. When a client requests prayer, it is ethical to respond with a prayer that is mutually comfortable (Winslow & Wehtje-Winslow, 2007). However, if the client has not asked for prayer, the nurse must weigh whether an offer to pray with the client is appropriate (Taylor, 2012). Following are tips on praying with clients:

- To know if an offer of prayer is ethical, assess and follow client cues. A question that chaplains often use is: Would a prayer be helpful? Keep in mind the questions: Am I preying on a vulnerable client when I offer to pray with him or her? Am I abusing my powerful position as a nurse to impose what I think comforts?
- Assess for how and what the client would like you to pray. For example: Is there anything in particular for which you'd like me to pray? Is there a certain way of praying that you prefer? Most Protestant Americans who pray use a colloquial style of prayer that involves spontaneously expressing gratitude or needs to God. Listening to clients talk about their spirituality or religiosity will often inform you as to how to shape the prayer (e.g., to whom to address the prayer).
- Be mindful of one difference between magic and prayer. Magic invokes a greater power for personal gain. Prayer allows the greater power to do the greater good ("Thy will be done").
- Nurses who are unaccustomed to praying aloud or in public may find it helpful to have a written prayer or a scriptural passage readily available.
- Praying with the client may not involve verbalization. You may or may not hold the same religious beliefs as the client. However, if a client asks you to pray with him/her, you are duty bound to provide a conducive environment. You may remain silent and offer your presence without imposing your own beliefs on the client. This would denote respect and strengthen the nurse–client relationship.
- Because prayer can evoke deep feelings, the nurse may want to spend time with the client following a prayer to enable the client to express these feelings. Praying with a client may be a springboard for further discussion.
- Do not use prayer as a substitute for time; do not use prayer to stop a client from talking.
- Facilitate the clients' prayer practices. Schedule time for them when they will be undisturbed, palliate distressing symptoms that interfere with praying, help with articles that accompany prayers (e.g., rosaries, prayer garments, books of prayers), and so on.
- Remember that illness can interfere with some clients' ability to pray. Health challenges can also challenge one's beliefs about prayer and the power of the divine. Thus, to generically encourage a client to pray could potentially add to this sort of existing spiritual disruption. A referral to a spiritual care expert who can support the client to reconstruct meaningful beliefs and learn helpful ways to think and practice prayer would be important for such a client.

religious counselors will assist members of their faith who are not members of their specific religious community. For example, a priest may attend a client in the hospital or at home even though the client is not a member of the priest's parish. Be sure to obtain a client's approval before initiating a referral. The client often will have a preferred spiritual care provider to contact.

Referrals may be necessary when the nurse makes a diagnosis of spiritual disruption. In this situation, the nurse and religious counselor can work together to meet the client's needs. One situation the nurse may encounter is client refusal of necessary medical intervention because of religious tenets. In this case, the nurse encourages the client, primary care provider, and spiritual adviser to discuss the conflict and consider alternative methods of therapy. The nurse's major role is to provide information the client needs to make an informed decision and to support the client's decision.

Supporting Religious Practices

During the assessment of the client, the nurse will have obtained specific information about the client's religious preference and practices. Nurses need to consider specific religious practices that will affect nursing care, such as the client's beliefs about birth, death, dress, diet, prayer, sacred symbols, sacred writings, and holy days as discussed earlier in this chapter. See Practice Guidelines for ways the nurse can help clients to continue their usual spiritual practices. Box 41.2 provides health-related information about specific religions.

PRACTICE GUIDELINES Supporting Religious Practices

- Create a trusting relationship with the client so that any religious concerns or practices can be openly discussed and addressed.
- When unsure of client religious needs, ask how nurses can assist in having these needs met. Avoid relying on personal assumptions when caring for clients.
- Do not discuss personal spiritual beliefs with a client unless the client requests it. Be sure to assess whether such self-disclosure contributes to a therapeutic nurse–client relationship.
- Inform clients and family caregivers about spiritual support available at your institution (e.g., chapel or meditation room, chaplain services).
- Allow time and privacy for, and provide comfort measures prior to, private worship, prayer, meditation, reading, or other spiritual activities.
- Respect and ensure safety of the client's religious articles (e.g., icons, amulets, clothing, jewelry).
- If desired by client, facilitate clergy or spiritual care specialist visitation. Collaborate with chaplain (if available).
- Prepare client's environment for spiritual rituals or clergy visitations as needed (e.g., have chair near bedside for clergy, create private space).
- Make arrangements with a dietitian so that dietary needs can be met. If institution cannot accommodate client's needs, ask family to bring food.
- Acquaint yourself with the religions, spiritual practices, and cultures of the area in which you are working.
- Remember there can be a difference between facilitating and supporting a client's religious practice and participating in it yourself.
- Ask another nurse to assist you if a particular religious practice makes you uncomfortable.
- All spiritual therapeutics must be done within agency guidelines.

BOX 41.2 Health-Related Information About Specific Religions: A Sampler

Amish, Mennonite—Likely will not have insurance coverage; rely on religious community for support.

Anglicans, Episcopalians, Roman Catholics—Appreciate receiving Eucharist (Holy Communion), a ritual of ingesting bread and wine (or grape juice) led by clergy or lay leaders to commemorate death of Jesus. Forehead may be marked by priest with ashes on Ash Wednesday (40 days before Easter); no need to wash off. Lenten season (Ash Wednesday to Easter) may involve some degree of abstention from food.

Buddhist—May be vegetarian. Practice meditation (may desire incense, visual focal point, use breathing or chanting).

Christian Scientist—Typically oppose Western medical interventions, relying instead on lay and professional Christian Science practitioners.

Hindu—Most eat no beef; many are vegetarian. Cleanliness highly valued. Many food preferences (e.g., foods fresh or cooked in oil).

Jehovah's Witnesses—Abstain from most blood products; need to discuss alternative treatments such as blood conservation strategies, autologous techniques, hematopoietic agents, non-blood volume expanders, and so on; contact local Jehovah's Witness hospital liaison committee.

Jews—Some observe kosher diet to varying degrees (e.g., avoid pork and shellfish, do not mix dairy and meat). Sabbath observance varies (e.g., Orthodox Jews avoid traveling in vehicles, writing, turning on electric appliances and lights).

Latter-Day Saints (LDS or Mormons)—Avoid alcohol, caffeine, smoking. May prefer to wear temple undergarments. Arrange for blessing with local elders, if requested.

Muslim—Respect modesty, avoid exposing the body. Provide same-gender nurse if possible. Support prayers five times daily (may need to assist with ritual washing and positioning beforehand). Allow for family and imam (religious leader) to follow Islamic guidelines for burial when a Muslim client dies. Eat no pork, drink no alcohol. Children, pregnant women, older adults, and the ill exempt from daytime fast during month of Ramadan.

Roman Catholics—Sacrament of the Sick (previously known as Last Rites) appropriate for the ill. Be aware that some may think rite or offer of prayer means they are dying.

Seventh-Day Adventists—Avoid unnecessary treatments on Saturday (Sabbath), which begins Friday sundown, ends Saturday sundown. Adventists prefer restful, spirit-nurturing, family activities on Sabbaths. Likely to be vegetarian and abstain from caffeinated beverages. Do not smoke or drink alcohol.

EVIDENCE-BASED PRACTICE

Evidence-Based Practice

How Often Do Nurses Provide Supportive Spiritual Care?

Global research has described the spiritual needs of individuals receiving healthcare, and nursing supports spiritual well-being as a vital part of client-centered nursing care. Many nurses, however, identify barriers to providing spiritual care, such as lack of education, no time, not a priority, confusion around boundaries, and the belief that spirituality is a private topic. These barriers contribute to nurses not assessing or attending to client spiritual needs. A few studies have tried to describe the types and frequency of spiritual care, but the research has shown limitations to these studies (e.g., not measuring spiritual care therapeutics or measuring spiritual care without clarity about what it is). As a result, Mamier, Taylor, and Winslow (2019) conducted a descriptive, correlational study using a cross-sectional survey design to "describe the types and frequencies of nurse-provided therapeutics intended to support client spiritual well-being and to explore factors associated with these therapeutics" (p. 539). The two research questions were: (a) How frequently were various types of spiritual therapeutics provided by nurses? and (b) What was the relationship between nurse demographics, nurse work-related characteristics, and nurse spirituality–religiosity measures and frequency of nurse-provided spiritual care? All RNs employed by a not-for-profit, faith-based tertiary healthcare system affiliated with a health science university in the southwestern United States were invited to participate in the study. To be eligible for the study, the RN had to have provided at least 36 hours of direct client care in the 2 weeks prior to completing the survey.

The survey included the following tools: Nurse Spiritual Care Therapeutic Scale (NSCTS), which consisted of 17 nurse spiritual care therapeutics, followed by a Likert scale from 1 (never = 0 times) to 5 (very often ≥ 12 times). The items were introduced with the sentence: "During the last 72–80 hours of providing client care, how often have you . . . ?" An example of one item on the NSCTS is: "Assessed a client's spiritual or religious beliefs or practices that are pertinent to health." Spirituality and religiosity were measured in a variety of ways, such as the 5-item Duke University Religion Index and the 16-item Daily Spiritual Experiences Scale. Respondents were asked to classify themselves as "spiritual and religious," "spiritual but not religious," "neither spiritual nor religious," or "religious but not spiritual." The study also explored factors related to the work environment such as type of hospital, specific unit the RN worked on, number of hours worked, average patient load per shift, and the RN's perceptions of self and spirituality in the work environment.

Of the 554 RNs who met the inclusion criteria and completed the survey, the majority were around 39 years old with 11 years of nursing experience. They represented a variety of ethnic backgrounds with the majority being Caucasian (47.1%) and Asian (13.5%). Most held a baccalaureate or graduate degree (59.8%). The majority worked full time on the day shift and cared for an average of four clients per shift. Only 34.7% had received education about spiritual care. Almost half identified as Protestant (47.8%) and 71.5% saw themselves as "spiritual and religious." Of the total RN sample, 35.7% worked in pediatric care, 4.2% in mental health, and the remainder in adult care on medical–surgical units. Overall, nurse spirituality and religiosity scores were high.

The results of the NSCTS reflected that the most frequent spiritual practices centered on presence, listening, and spiritual assessment. The findings also showed that RNs rarely document their spiritual care. There were no differences in spiritual care therapeutics frequency between male and female RNs. There was no significant difference in NSCTS means by race or ethnicity, level of education, or workload. RN religious affiliation did not show a significant difference in frequency of spiritual care. Working the day shift and having received education in spiritual care, however, were significantly associated with spiritual care frequency. Significant differences were also found depending on where the nurse worked. The results showed that RNs providing care in psychiatric and adult medical–surgical care settings provided significantly more frequent spiritual care than RNs working in pediatric care settings.

Implications

This study, as discussed by the researchers, measured spirituality and religiousness in a variety of ways and provided a clearer perspective of the dimensions of spiritual care. It reinforces the need for educational interventions to increase RNs' knowledge and confidence in providing spiritual care. The results also indicate the need for education on how to document nurse spiritual care correctly. The information gained from this study will be useful for future comparative studies.

Religious Practices That Nurses Should Know

Many traditional religious practices and rituals are related to life events such as birth, transition from childhood to adulthood, marriage, illness, and death. Religious rules of conduct, typically influenced concurrently by culture, may also apply to matters of daily life such as dress, food, social interaction, menstruation, childrearing, and sexual relationships. When individuals get sick, they frequently rely on prayer and other spiritual practices. Decisions about health and end-of-life care are guided by spiritual or religious beliefs. Given this deep connection between spiritual or religious practices and the circumstances in which nurses often provide care, it is fitting for nurses to have some awareness and understanding of these practices (Taylor, 2012).

It is possible for nurses to unethically impose personal spiritual beliefs on clients, whose circumstances inherently leave them vulnerable. Observing guidelines for ethical conduct in spiritual caregiving is essential. The following guidelines for nurses were offered by Winslow and Wehtje-Winslow (2007):

- First seek a basic understanding of clients' spiritual needs, resources, and preferences (i.e., assess).
- Follow the client's expressed wishes regarding spiritual care.

- Do not prescribe or urge clients to adopt certain spiritual beliefs or practices, and do not pressure them to relinquish such beliefs or practices.
- Strive to understand personal spirituality and how it influences caregiving.
- Provide spiritual care in a way that is consistent with personal beliefs.

Clinical Alert!

Although some clients are eager for clinicians to offer spiritual care (and yet may feel embarrassed to ask for it), others may be uncertain about or opposed to such offers (Balboni et al., 2013; Park & Sacco, 2016). Clients often confuse religiosity with spirituality; this may contribute to their uncertainty about receiving spiritual care from nurses. Observing and using the client's language for spirituality (e.g., "being at peace" or "faith") and exhibiting large measures of sensitivity and respect will help nurses to talk therapeutically with clients to provide spiritual care.

Holy Days

Solemn religious observances and feast days throughout the year may be referred to as **holy days** and may include fasting or special foods, reflection, rituals, and prayer. Believers who are seriously ill are often exempted from such requirements. Clients may be used to spending such days with family and attending religious services. Examples of such holy days are Rosh Hashanah and Yom Kippur (Jewish); Good Friday and Christmas (Christian); Buddha's birthday (Buddhists); Mahashivratri, a celebration of Lord Shiva (Hindu); and the month-long Ramadan (Islam). Because some religions follow calendars other than the Gregorian calendar, a multifaith calendar can be used to identify the holy days of the various religious groups.

The concept of the Sabbath is common to both Christians and Jews, in response to the biblical commandment "Remember the Sabbath day to keep it holy." Most Christians observe the "Lord's Day" on Sunday, whereas Jews and sabbatarian Christians (e.g., Seventh-Day Adventists) observe Saturday as their Sabbath. Muslims traditionally gather on Friday at noon to worship and learn about their faith. Clients who are devout in their religious practices may want to avoid any special treatments or other intrusions on their day of rest and reflection.

Sacred Texts

Individuals often gain strength and hope from reading religious writings when they are ill or in crisis. Each religion has sacred and authoritative scriptures that provide guidance for its adherents' beliefs and behaviors (Taylor, 2012). In addition, sacred writings frequently tell instructive stories of the religion's leaders, kings, and heroes. In most religions, these scriptures are thought to be the word of the Supreme Being as written down by prophets or other human representatives. Christians rely on the Old and New Testaments of the Bible, Jews on the Hebrew Bible, and Muslims on the Koran; Hindus have several holy texts, or Vedas; Sikhs cherish the Adi Granth; and Buddhists value the teachings of the Tripitakas. Scriptures generally set forth religious law in the form of warnings and rules for living (e.g., the Ten Commandments). This religious law may be interpreted in various ways by subgroups of a religion's followers and may affect a client's willingness to accept treatment suggestions; for example, blood transfusions are in conflict with the biblical interpretations of Jehovah's Witnesses.

Sacred Symbols

Sacred symbols include jewelry, medals, amulets, icons, totems, or body ornamentation (e.g., tattoos) that carry religious or spiritual significance. They may be worn to pronounce one's faith, to remind the practitioner of the faith, to provide spiritual protection, or to be a source of comfort or strength (Taylor, 2012). Clients may wear religious symbols at all times, and they may wish to wear them when they are undergoing diagnostic studies, medical treatment, or surgery. For example, clients who are Roman Catholic may carry a rosary for prayer; a Muslim may carry a mala, or string of prayer beads (Figure 41.2 ■).

Individuals may have religious icons or statues in their home, car, or place of work as a personal reminder of their faith or as part of a personal place of worship or meditation. Hospitalized clients or long-term care residents may wish to have their spiritual icons or statues with them as a source of comfort.

Prayer and Meditation

Prayer involves humans experiencing the divine (however that is perceived). Some would describe prayer as an inner experience for gaining awareness of self (including Self—or the immanent manifestation of the divine). Others may view it as a conversation with the divine (e.g., to entreat or dialogue). These differing perspectives likely reflect

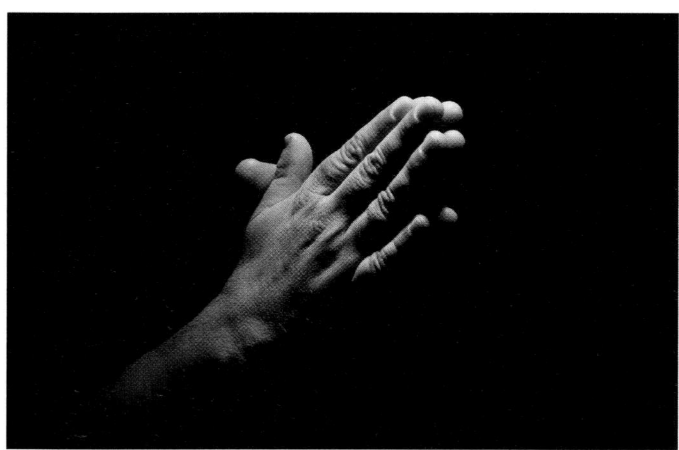

Figure 41.2 ■ Clients may bring objects to the hospital to use in prayer or other religious rituals. Caregivers should respect such objects, because they usually have great significance for clients.
Jesus Cervantes/Shutterstock.

the theological variations about how the divine relates to humanity. For example, some view the divine as transcendent (e.g., God in Heaven), while others experience the divine as immanent (e.g., the inner light or wisdom within individuals). A more complex perspective would accept that the divine engages with humanity in both—or many—ways (Borg, 1997; Taylor, 2012).

More than half of Americans (55%) pray at least daily (Pew Research Center, n.d.). However, the ways they pray vary. For example, ritual prayers (e.g., Hail Mary and memorized prayers that can be repeated) may be comforting for those who are unable or uncomfortable with a more conversational prayer (e.g., where one praises or petitions God). Other prayer experiences may be meditational, allowing for moments of silence while focused on nothing, a meaningful phrase, or a certain aspect of the divine (Fosarelli, 2008; Taylor, 2012). Although meditational and colloquial prayer experiences have been found to be associated with spiritual well-being and quality of life in healthy adults, ritual and petitionary prayer experiences may be most comforting and appropriate for those who are ill and unable to concentrate (Taylor, 2012).

Some religions have prescribed prayers that are printed in a prayer book, such as the Anglican or Episcopal Book of Common Prayer or the Catholic Missal. Some religious prayers are attributed to the source of faith; for example, the Lord's Prayer for Christians is attributed to Jesus, and the first sutra for Muslims is attributed to Mohammed.

Some religions prescribe daily prayers or dictate specific times for prayer and worship: the five daily prayers, or Salat, of Muslims (performed while facing east toward Mecca at dawn, noon, midafternoon, sunset, and evening); the daily Kaddish of Jews; or the seven canonical hours of prayer of Roman Catholics. Individuals who are ill may want to continue or increase their prayer practices. They may need uninterrupted quiet time during which they have their prayer books, rosaries, malas, or other icons available to them (Taylor, 2012).

Meditation is of Buddhist origin yet pervades Western societies. Mindfulness meditation techniques have been adapted for Christian prayer and as a nonreligious lifestyle strategy for improving health and overall well-being. Numerous studies document various physical, psychologic, and spiritual benefits for those who practice mindfulness regularly. Mindfulness techniques vary, but key elements include focused attention on the present moment or the body's experience; awareness, depth, and steadiness of breathing; and putting judgmental and intrusive thoughts "on hold." Mindfulness can be taught individually or in groups by a mindfulness expert; manualized training to nurses can prepare them to support clients to meditate (Boccia, Piccardi, & Guariglia, 2015; Buttle, 2015).

Beliefs Affecting Diet

Many religions have prescriptions regarding diet. It is important that healthcare providers prescribe diet plans with an awareness of the client's dietary and fasting beliefs. There may be rules about which foods and beverages are allowed and which are prohibited. For example, Orthodox Jews are not to eat shellfish or pork, and Muslims are not to drink alcoholic beverages or eat pork. Members of the Church of Jesus Christ of Latter-Day Saints (Mormons) are not to drink caffeinated or alcoholic beverages. Older Catholics may choose not to eat meat on Fridays because this was prescribed in years past. Buddhists and Hindus are often vegetarian, not wanting to take life to support life. Religious prescriptions may also dictate how food is prepared; for example, many Jews require kosher food, which is food prepared according to Jewish rules.

Some solemn religious observances are marked by fasting, which is the abstinence from food or certain foods for a specified period of time. Some religions also restrict beverages during a fast; others allow drinking of water or other sustaining beverages on fast days. Examples of religions that observe fasting include Islam, Judaism, and Eastern Orthodox Christians. During the month of Ramadan, devout Muslims eat no food and avoid beverages during daylight hours; the fast is broken after sunset. Members of Jewish synagogues fast on Yom Kippur, and devout Catholics may fast on Good Friday. Most religions lift the fasting requirements for seriously ill believers for whom fasting may be a detriment to health (e.g., clients with diabetes, pregnant women). Some religions may exempt nursing mothers or menstruating women from fasting requirements (Taylor, 2012).

Beliefs About Illness and Healing

Clients may have religious beliefs that attribute illness to a spiritual disease or sin. Some clients may think that disease is caused by the presence of sin and evil in this world, whereas others may believe the disease is a punishment for sin in their past. Indeed, how clients view the divine, interpret good and evil, and so forth, inevitably influences their thinking about illness and decision-making about treatment. Healing for such clients may appear to be unrelated to current treatment practices. When relevant, the nurse should assess the client's beliefs related to health and, if possible, include aspects of healing that are part of the client's belief system in the planning of care. For example, many religious traditions have rituals of healing such as anointing by a leader of the local religious community (Taylor, 2012).

Beliefs About Dress and Modesty

Many religions have traditions that dictate dress. For example, Orthodox and some conservative Jewish men believe that it is important to have their heads covered at all times and therefore wear yarmulkes. Orthodox Jewish women cover their hair with a wig or scarf as a sign of respect to God. Mormons may wear temple undergarments in compliance with religious dictates. For some individuals, it is imperative that they not shave certain hair (e.g., sideburns for Hasidic Jewish men, any hair for a Khalsa [dedicated] Sikh).

Some religions require that women dress in a conservative manner, which may include wearing sleeves and modestly cut tops, and skirts that cover the knees. Many Islamic cultures may require that the body (torso, arms, and legs) be covered, as well as the head (i.e., burkha or hijab). Hindu women accustomed to wearing saris prefer to cover all of the body except arms and feet (Figure 41.3 ■). Hospital gowns may make women wishing to comply with religious dress codes feel uneasy and uncomfortable. Clients may be especially disconcerted when undergoing diagnostic tests or treatments, such as mammography, that require body parts to be bared or shaved. Nurses need to facilitate respectful solutions at such times (Taylor, 2012).

Beliefs Related to Birth

For all religions the birth of a child is an important event giving cause for celebration. Many religions have specific ritual ceremonies that consecrate the new child to God. For example, while a baby is being born, its Muslim mother may recite a prayer. As soon as it is born, its father or someone else will recite a call to prayer into the infant's ears. Likewise, Hindus will perform a number of religious rituals when a baby is born. Most Christian parents will have their babies christened or baptized at some point; however, for some, if their infant is dying, they may want a baptism as soon as possible. In such dire circumstances, Christian parents of seriously ill infants may want baptism performed at birth by a religious nurse or primary care provider if a chaplain or clergy member is not present.

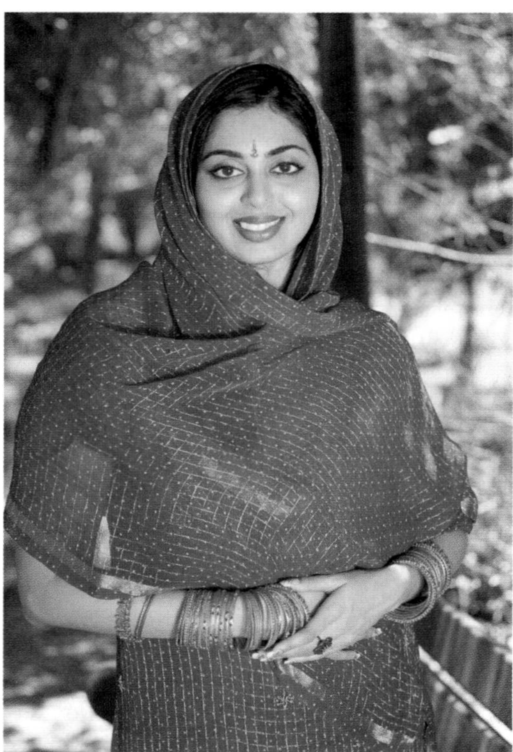

Figure 41.3 ■ Hindu woman dressed in a sari.
Hongqi Zhang/123RF.

In the Jewish and Islamic traditions, male circumcision is obligatory, whereas Hindus never practice circumcision. When nurses are aware of the religious needs of families and their infants, they can support families in fulfilling their religious obligations (Taylor, 2012).

Beliefs Related to Death

Spiritual and religious beliefs play a significant role in the believer's approach to death just as they do in other major life events. Many believe that the individual who dies transcends this life for a better place or state of being. Research findings suggest these religious beliefs may influence end-of-life care choices, such as whether to seek hospice care, have an advance care plan, or desire for resuscitation (Ohr, Jeong, & Saul, 2016; Van Norman, 2017).

Some religions have special rituals surrounding dying and death that must be observed by the faithful. Observance of these rituals provides comfort to the dying individual and loved ones. Some rituals are carried out while the individual is still alive, and can include special prayers, singing or chants, and reading of sacred scriptures. Roman Catholic priests perform the Sacrament of the Sick (previously referred to as the Last Rites) when clients are very ill or near death; Orthodox Christians have a similar ritual. Muslims who are dying want their body or head turned toward Mecca, whereas Hindus may want to face south. In the Muslim, Hindu, and Jewish traditions, a ritual bath and body preparation for burial may be done by a family member or by a ritual burial society (Taylor, 2012).

Many religious traditions also support rituals during specified periods of mourning after the death. Jews and Muslims have a tradition of burial within 24 hours following death. Hindus cremate the body within 24 hours; then the bereaved family observes a period of isolation given their defilement from living with the deceased. Jews "sit Shiva" (gather to pay respects) for several days in the home of the deceased. Buddhists perform prayers and rituals to aid the deceased to a better next life (Taylor, 2012).

During a terminal illness the client and family should be asked about end-of-life observances that could impact healthcare. The nurse can support the family of the deceased by providing an environment conducive to the performance of their traditional death rituals.

Clinical Alert!

Sharing Beliefs

Before sharing personal beliefs or practices, a nurse must consider questions such as the following:

- For what purpose am I sharing my beliefs or practices? By doing so, am I meeting my needs or my client's?
- Is my spiritual care reflecting a spiritual assessment?
- Am I preying on a vulnerable client?
- Am I offering my beliefs or practices in a manner that allows my client to refuse comfortably?
- Does my spiritual care hurt or contribute to a therapeutic relationship with the client?

Evaluating

Just as there is a question regarding the appropriateness of using the prescriptive nursing process to frame spiritual care, caution is needed when discussing the evaluation of spiritual care. Does spiritually sensitive nursing care lead to observable and measurable client outcomes? If it does not, then is it unsuccessful or unimportant? And what outcomes indicating movement toward improved spiritual health are appropriate for nurses to consider? Indeed, Taylor (2007b) suggested that clinicians' spiritually healing responses often move a client *incrementally* toward spiritual healthiness. Nurses with theistic religious beliefs might add that a client's movement toward spiritual health is evidence of God's grace, and ultimately something that is not within the purview of any clinician or individual. Given that many healthcare institutions require that spiritual care be documented in a nursing care plan, an example of how this is done is on page 1062.

Spiritual Self-Awareness for the Nurse

Nurses cannot hear, never mind respond to, a client's spiritual need unless they hear and respond to their own need and consider how countertransference can occur (Bowman, 2017; Taylor, 2007b). Indeed, the notion that effective healers are "wounded healers" has long existed. A nurse's spiritual needs, pains, or woundedness can affect how he or she cares for clients. Nurses who are unaware of, afraid of, or misunderstand their spiritual needs will be very limited in their ability to accurately identify and explore a client's spiritual needs. When clients realize the nurse does not understand them they become quiet, change the topic, give superficial responses to queries, or in other ways indicate lack of interest in continuing to talk about their spirituality.

Instead, the nurse can use his or her woundedness and spiritual self-awareness as a bridge or tool for healing communication. A healing response requires recognizing a client's innermost feelings. Awareness of one's own deeper feelings—one's own spiritual themes and inevitable woundedness—is requisite to being able to hear another's. Thus, a nurse's life story with its joys and hurts becomes a source of information for interpreting the client's story.

Healers do not need to have shared the same *experiences* as have clients, but to be compassionate they do need to recognize how they have shared similar *emotions* (Taylor, 2007b). For example, a nurse may not be able to share with a client the extreme experience of losing a limb, but can likely identify times in life when he or she felt loss, anger, or bewilderment about why tragedy happens. Recognizing and addressing the fears that are inevitable responses to caring for clients (e.g., our own fear of dying or being hurt, our fear of hurting others, or of being overwhelmed by the pain of others) is an essential requisite to spiritual care.

Beckman, Boxley-Harges, Bruick-Sorge, and Salmon (2007) offered the following strategies for nurses who wish to increase their spiritual awareness so that it can impact client care positively:

- ***Write a self-epitaph.*** Sum up in a couple of lines what is significant about your life or how you would like to be remembered.
- ***Explore personal end-of-life issues.*** Imagine having a terminal diagnosis. What feelings would you have? What would be your priorities for the time and energy you had left?
- ***Create a personal loss history.*** Answer questions such as these: What was your first experience of death? What was the most recent or difficult death in your life? How did you cope? What is your coping style at times like this? How did you feel your grief?
- ***List significant values.*** Write down what possessions, individuals, activities, roles, personal attributes, and so forth, you prize most.
- ***Conduct a spiritual self-assessment.*** Consider what gives you strength and hope. What makes you joyful or despairing? How do you explain or relate to suffering? What is your sense of purpose or mission in life? What nurtures your spirit?

You may want to test out client spiritual assessment questions on yourself! Another aspect of a spiritual self-assessment is to reflect on what has influenced your spirituality most. How does the religion of your family affect you? How would you describe your spiritual "journey"? And importantly, how does your spirituality influence your vocation—your choosing to be a nurse?

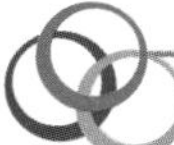

Critical Thinking Checkpoint

Terry is a 32-year-old male who received several pints of blood following an automobile crash 10 years ago. Five years ago he was diagnosed with AIDS and is now in the hospital with pneumonia and severe diarrhea. He is very ill and very discouraged. While you are caring for Terry, he comments, "I might as well die right now because I'm not going to get well. My folks were Methodist, but I guess I'm being punished because I'm not very religious."

1. Terry stated that he was "not very religious." Does that mean that he is not spiritual? Explain.
2. What data suggest that Terry may be experiencing spiritual disruption?
3. How might illness affect one's spiritual beliefs? Religious beliefs?
4. How might a spiritual assessment be of benefit to both you and Terry?
5. What questions might be helpful to ask to further understand Terry?
6. What might you say to show Terry empathy?

Answers to Critical Thinking Checkpoint questions are available on the faculty resources site. Please consult with your instructor.

NURSING CARE PLAN Spiritual Disruption

ASSESSMENT DATA	NURSING DIAGNOSIS	DESIRED OUTCOMES*
NURSING ASSESSMENT Mrs. Mandy Lee is a 51-year-old hospitalized woman who is recovering from a right radical mastectomy. Her primary care provider told her yesterday that due to metastases of the cancer, her prognosis is poor. This morning her nurse finds her tearful, stating she slept poorly and has no appetite. She asks the nurse, "Why has God allowed this to happen to me?" Throughout the course of the ensuing conversation, the nurse hears Mrs. Lee ponder aloud, "Perhaps it's because I have sinned in my life. I've not gone to church or spoken to a minister in several years . . . . Is there a chapel in the hospital where I could go and pray? . . . I'm terribly afraid of dying and what awaits me."	Spiritual disruption related to feelings of guilt and alienation from God as evidenced by questioning why "God has allowed this"; inquiries about praying in a chapel; insomnia; no appetite	Spiritual Health [2001] as evidenced by • Interacts with spiritual leader of her religion. • Participates in spiritual experience(s) that provide her comfort. • Interacts with others to share thoughts, feelings, and beliefs.

Physical Examination	Diagnostic Data
Height: 165.1 cm (5′5″)	RBC: 3.5×10^6/mL
Weight: 54.0 kg (119 lb)	Hgb: 10.5 g/L
Temperature: 36.6°C (98°F)	Hct: 35%
Pulse: 88 beats/min	
Respirations: 22/min	
Blood Pressure: 146/86 mmHg	

Large surgical dressing right chest wall and axillary region, dry and intact. Slight edema right hand and arm.

NURSING INTERVENTIONS*/SELECTED ACTIVITIES	RATIONALE
SPIRITUAL SUPPORT [5420]	
Be open to Mrs. Lee's feelings about illness and death. Listen empathically.	*Encourages expression of inner fears and concerns and teaches the client the value of confronting issues. Emotions often provide a window through which to peer at the inner workings of the human spirit.*
Assist her to properly express and relieve anger in appropriate ways.	*Anger can be a source of energy and its release a source of freedom when expressed in a constructive manner.*
Encourage the use of spiritual resources, if desired.	*Spiritual needs may sometimes be overlooked or ignored. Recognizing and respecting the client's spiritual needs is an important advocacy role for nurses.*
COPING ENHANCEMENT [5230]	
Create an accepting, nonjudgmental atmosphere.	*Establishes rapport and the therapeutic relationship, which promotes communication and open expression.*
Encourage verbalization of feelings, perceptions, and fears. Allow time for grieving.	*Being with the client who is suffering gives meaning to his or her experience.*
Acknowledge her spiritual and cultural background.	*Spiritual beliefs often provide a framework for explaining tragedy and making sense of suffering.*

Several other nursing interventions may be appropriate for Mrs. Lee, such as:

presence [5340], journaling [4740], hope inspiration [5310], meditation facilitation [5960], forgiveness facilitation [5280], guided imagery [6000], family support [7140], cultural brokerage (if, for example, her religious beliefs appeared to conflict with the healthcare system's) [7330], bibliotherapy [4680], art therapy [4330], active listening [4920], emotional support [5270], or consultation [7910].

EVALUATION

Although Mrs. Lee states she still is not satisfied with her assumptions about why tragedy has struck, she has continued to verbally express her emotions of fear and anger related to a perception of abandonment by God. She has identified a spiritual mentor with whom she plans to discuss her theological questions after discharge. She refused an offer of a chaplain visit. Conversations that used empathy and active listening while Mrs. Lee talked about her spiritual crisis demonstrated her subtle yet increased self-awareness regarding inner emotions and movements of the inner spirit. In these ways, the outcomes were achieved.

*The NOC # for desired outcomes and the NIC # for nursing interventions are listed in brackets following the appropriate outcome or intervention. Outcomes, indicators, interventions, and activities selected are only a sample of those suggested by NOC and NIC and should be further individualized for each client.

CONCEPT MAP

Spiritual Disruption

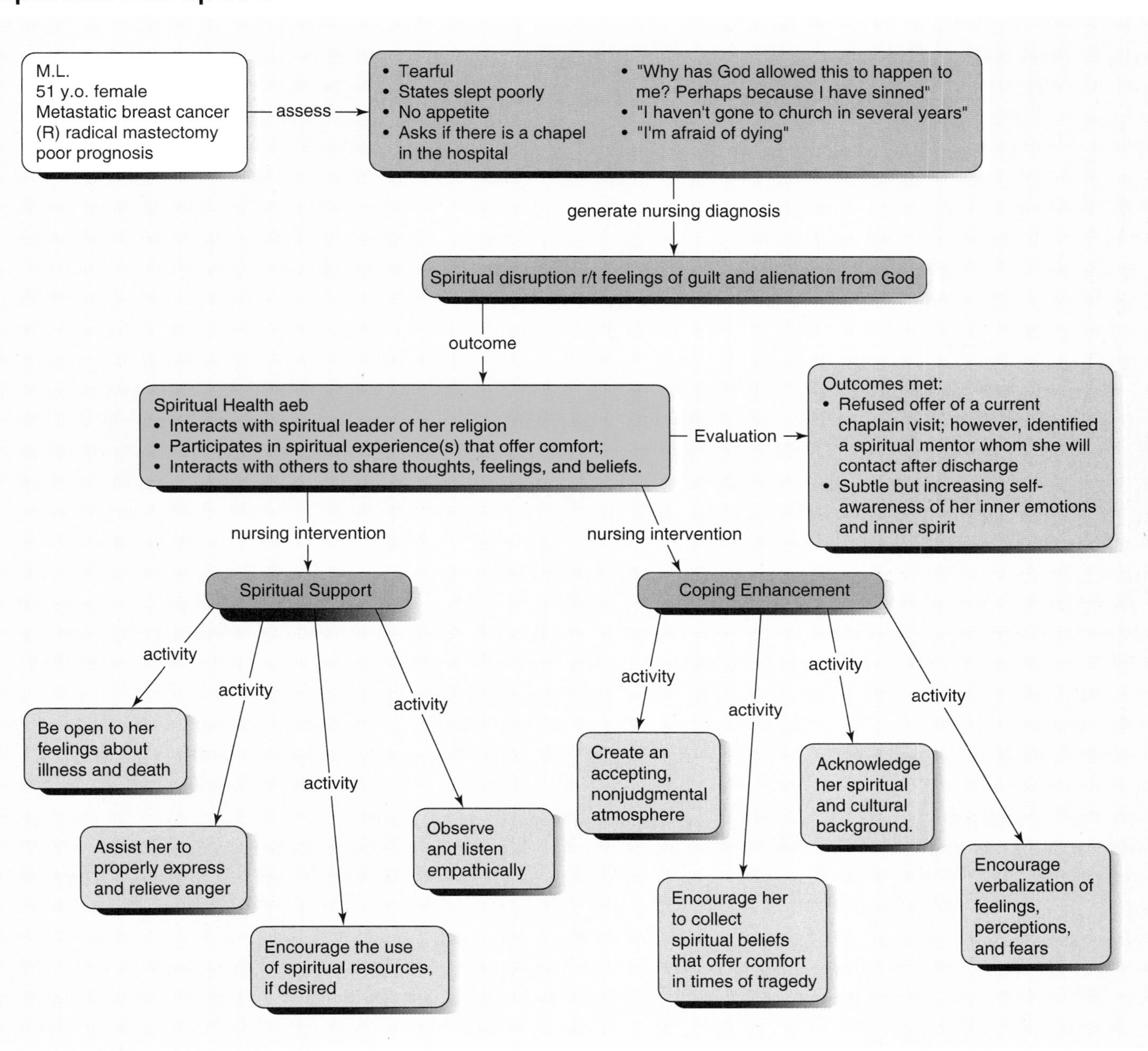

Chapter 41 Review

CHAPTER HIGHLIGHTS

- Clients have a right to receive care that respects their individual spiritual and religious values.
- The spiritual needs of clients and support people often come into focus at a time of illness. Spiritual beliefs can help individuals make sense of illness and cope with what lies ahead.
- Spiritual disruption refers to a disturbance in or a challenge to an individual's beliefs that provide strength, hope, and meaning to life. Possible factors in spiritual disruption include physiologic problems, treatment-related concerns, and situational concerns. Spiritual disruption may be reflected in a number of behaviors, including depression, anxiety, verbalizations of unworthiness, and fear of death.
- Nurses must follow ethical guidelines for providing spiritual care, and not impose personal beliefs or practices on clients.
- Spiritual assessment can follow a three-tiered approach. Initially, the nurse must determine if the client accepts a spiritual reality. For those who do, the next tier of questions should collect information not only about spiritual beliefs and practices affecting health, but also about how the client desires spiritual care from the healthcare team. Only those who manifest a spiritual need require a focused, in-depth assessment. Such an assessment may best be done by a chaplain or spiritual care expert.
- Nursing interventions that promote spiritual health include offering one's presence, conversing about spirituality, supporting the client's religious practices, empathic communication, assisting clients with prayer, and referring the client to a spiritual care expert.
- Nurses need to be aware of their own spiritual beliefs to be comfortable assisting others. When disclosing personal spiritual beliefs to a client, the nurse must first determine that the self-disclosure benefits the client rather than meeting the nurse's own personal needs.
- Nurses can support clients' religious practices if they understand needs related to holy days, sacred texts, sacred symbols, prayer and meditation, dietary practices, dress requirements or prohibitions, healing, birth rituals, and death rituals.
- It is important for nurses to increase their own spiritual awareness to understand and respond to a client's spiritual needs.

TEST YOUR KNOWLEDGE

1. Which nursing action would be most beneficial in enhancing clients' spiritual health?
   1. Discuss one's own spiritual beliefs with the client.
   2. Provide the client with privacy and a quiet room.
   3. Sit by the client's side in silence.
   4. Call a representative of the client's religion should the client wish so.

2. During assessment, a client says that it has been a long time since she has thought very much about religion. The nurse caring for this client has a strong belief in God and the healing power of prayer. What action should be taken by the nurse?
   1. Mention the nurse's belief and offer to pray with the client for forgiveness.
   2. Tell the client that the nurse will pray for her often.
   3. Ask the client if there are any spiritual needs with which the staff can assist.
   4. Refer the client for spiritual counseling.

3. A client is experiencing severe pain that cannot be controlled by analgesics. An appropriate intervention is full presencing, which involves which of the following?
   1. Physical presence
   2. Physical presence with mental awareness of the client
   3. Physical, mental, and emotional presence
   4. Physical, mental, emotional, and spiritual presence

4. A client reports, "Cancer was the best thing that happened to me! It is making me appreciate life so much more." This statement fits best with which nursing diagnosis?
   1. Spiritual disruption
   2. Potential for spiritual disruption
   3. Spiritual health enhancement
   4. Cognitive denial

5. A dying client states, "Part of what makes dying hard is that I don't know for sure where I'm going. Nurse, what do you believe happens in the hereafter?" Which ethical guideline should guide your response?
   1. Never share personal spiritual beliefs.
   2. Share all spiritual beliefs, favoring none.
   3. Share only your beliefs.
   4. First assess for what prompts the client's question.

6. A nurse enters a client's room to find him praying with his family. What action should be taken by the nurse?
   1. Stand quietly inside the room until the prayer is completed.
   2. Come to the bedside and pray with the family.
   3. Politely ask the client to allow care to proceed.
   4. Quietly shut the door and wait in the hall until asked to enter.

7. A client in the emergency department needs a transfusion of red blood cells. The client tells the nurse that, as a Jehovah's Witness, blood transfusions are not permitted. Which statement would most likely lead to a resolution for this conflict?
   1. You must accept the transfusion or else leave.
   2. Don't worry, you will be forgiven.
   3. May I please call a representative of your religion so that I can understand your position better?
   4. I understand your position; I'll be here with you as you die.

8. An 88-year-old woman has just been admitted to a skilled nursing facility. She tells the nurse that she has been a Sunday school teacher and volunteers for many of her church's projects. Which of the following nursing diagnoses is most appropriate?
   1. Potential for spiritual disruption
   2. Potential for religious struggle
   3. Spiritual health enhancement
   4. Religious struggle

9. A nurse is planning to conduct a spiritual self-assessment. What questions would the nurse include in this assessment? Select all that apply.
   1. What makes me joyful?
   2. What makes me feel despair?
   3. What possessions do I value the most?
   4. What is my purpose in life?
   5. What feeds my spirit?

10. The mother of a pediatric client states, "I can't understand why God would allow this to happen to my innocent child!" Which nursing diagnosis is most accurate?
    1. Spiritual disruption related to search for meaning of child's illness
    2. Religious struggle related to anger at God
    3. Impaired coping related to anger
    4. Potential for spiritual disruption related to threatened sense of hope

See Answers to Test Your Knowledge in Appendix A.

READINGS AND REFERENCES

Suggested Readings

Advocate Health Care. (n.d.). *Religious beliefs & healthcare decisions*. Retrieved from https://www.advocatehealth.com/about-advocate/faith/office-for-mission-and-spiritual-care/spiritual-care/religious-beliefs-and-healthcare-decisions
This series of roughly 10-page books describes the healthcare-related issues of about 20 religions. Many of these were published over 15 years ago by the now defunct Park Ridge Center in Chicago. They are now available for free online.

Clarke, J. (2013). *Everyday nursing practice: A new approach*. Hampshire, England: Macmillan.
Authored by a British nurse, this book covers a lot of ground, from what is spirituality, to what factors affect it, and how to turn personal spirituality into spiritual care (i.e., how to therapeutically use presence, touch, and so forth). The final section of the book describes how physical care of bathing, feeding, mobilizing, and comforting the sick client can be infused with spiritual care.

O'Brien, M. E. (2018). *Spirituality in nursing: Standing on holy ground* (5th ed.). Burlington, MA: Jones & Bartlett.
Authored by a Roman Catholic nurse scholar, this book considers spiritual responses to various health challenges (e.g., acute and chronic illness, childhood, aging, dying and bereavement, mass casualties) and discusses nursing spiritual care. Chapters also include discussions of servant leadership and religion in nursing history.

Puchalski, C. M., & Ferrell, B. (2010). *Making health care whole*. West Conshohocken, PA: Templeton.
This book is a repository of information about spiritual assessment and implementing spiritual care within the healthcare system. It results from a consensus conference of spiritual care scholars who discussed how to increase and improve the provision of spiritual care in palliative care settings.

Realin, A., & Ruckstuhl, M. (Ed.). (2009). *Guide to religion and culture in healthcare, Florida Hospital*. Retrieved from https://library.adu.edu/sites/default/files/guide_to_religion_and_culture_in_healthcare.pdf
This book is available online for free. It provides bulleted information about 19 religions and details a myriad of factors (e.g., whether abortion or autopsies are permissible, dietary prescriptions). Information is organized by general beliefs related to healthcare, end of life, and perinatal beliefs and practices.

Sirajjakool, S., Carr, M. F., & Bursey, E. J. (2017). *World religions for healthcare professionals* (2nd ed.). New York, NY: Routledge.
This book is authored by religionists, with a couple of chapters co-authored by a physician or nurse. The content covers 10 world religions, several of which are not commonly found in North America (5 of the 10 religions are of Asian origin). The chapters are long and not conducive to accessing clinical information readily; however, they provide rich information for the reader who is deeply curious.

Taylor, E. J. (2007). *What do I say? Talking with patients about spirituality*. Philadelphia, PA: Templeton.
After chapters discussing how to make sense of client expressions of spirituality and how to gauge personal inner responses to such client expressions, this book explores approaches to verbally communicating with clients who express spiritual need. The book is filled with exercises for practicing each of the skills introduced.

Taylor, E. J. (2012). *Religion: A clinical guide for nurses*. New York, NY: Springer.
Whereas the first 7 chapters discuss clinical aspects of caring for religious patients (e.g., assessing religiosity, legal and ethical issues, communicating about faith), the remaining 21 shorter chapters offer pertinent clinical information about the religious faith traditions most likely encountered by nurses (e.g., beliefs about suffering, health; practices related to birthing, dying, illness; how the faith community supports its sick).

Related Research

Epstein-Peterson, Z. D., Sullivan, A. J., Enzinger, A. C., Trevino, K. M., Zollfrank, A. A., Balboni, M. J., . . . Balboni, T. A. (2015). Examining forms of spiritual care provided in the advanced cancer setting. *American Journal of Hospice and Palliative Care*, *32*, 750–757. doi:10.1177/1049909114540318

Freedman, S., & Zarifkar, T. (2016). The psychology of interpersonal forgiveness and guidelines for forgiveness therapy: What therapists need to know to help their clients forgive. *Spirituality in Clinical Practice*, *3*(1), 45–58. doi:10.1037/scp0000087

Gonçalves, J. P., Lucchetti, G., Menezes, P. R., & Vallada, H. (2015). Religious and spiritual interventions in mental health care: A systematic review and meta-analysis of randomized controlled clinical trials. *Psychological Medicine*, *45*(14), 2937–2949. doi:10.1017/s0033291715001166

Ironson, G., Kremer, H., & Lucette, A. (2016). Relationship between spiritual coping and survival in patients with HIV. *Journal of General Internal Medicine*, *31*, 1068–1076. doi:10.1007/s11606-016-3668-4

Ironson, G., Stuetzle, R., Ironson, D., Balbin, E., Kremer, H., George, A., . . . Fletcher, M. A. (2011). View of God as benevolent and forgiving or punishing and judgmental predicts HIV disease progression. *Journal of Behavioral Medicine*, *34*, 414–425. doi:10.1007/s10865-011-9314-z

Park, C. L., Aldwin, C. M., Choun, S., George, L., Suresh, D. P., & Bliss, D. (2016). Spiritual peace predicts 5-year mortality in congestive heart failure patients. *Health Psychology*, *35*(3), 203–210. doi:10.1037/hea0000271

Pirutinsky, S., Carp, S., & Rosmarin, D. H. (2016). A paradigm to assess implicit attitudes towards God: The positive/negative God associations task. *Journal of Religion & Health*, *56*, 305–319. doi:10.1007/s10943-016-0303

Pujol, N., Jobin, G., & Beloucif, S. (2016). "Spiritual care is not the hospital's business": A qualitative study on the perspectives of patients about the integration of spirituality in healthcare settings. *Journal of Medical Ethics*, *42*, 733–737. doi:10.1136/medethics-2016-103565

Speed, D., & Fowler, K. (2016). What's God got to do with it? How religiosity predicts atheists' health. *Journal of Religion & Health*, *55*, 296–308. doi:10.1007/s10943-015-0083-9

Wittenberg, E., Ferrell, B., Goldsmith, J., & Buller, H. (2016). Provider difficulties with spiritual and forgiveness communication at the end of life. *American Journal of Hospice & Palliative Care*, *33*(9), 843–848. doi:10.1177/1049909115591811

References

Abu-Raiya, H., Pargament, K. I., & Krause, N. (2016). Religion as problem, religion as solution: Religious buffers of the links between religious/spiritual struggles and well-being/mental health. *Quality of Life Research*, *25*, 1265–1274. doi:10.1007/s11136-015-1163-8

Astrow, A. B., Wexler, A., Texeira, K., He, M. K., & Sulmasy, D. P. (2007). Is failure to meet spiritual needs associated with cancer patients' perceptions of quality of care and their satisfaction with care? *Journal of Clinical Oncology*, *25*, 5753–5757. doi:10.1200/JCO.2007.12.4362

Atchley, R. C. (2020). *Spirituality. Age and life stage in spiritual development*. Retrieved from https://medicine.jrank.org/pages/1634/Spirituality-Age-life-stage-in-spiritual-development.html

Balboni, T., Balboni, M., Paulk, M. E., Phelps, A., Wright, A., Peteet, J., . . . Prigerson, H. (2011). Support of cancer patients' spiritual needs and associations with medical care costs at the end of life. *Cancer*, *117*(23), 5383–5391. doi:10.1002/cncr.26221

Balboni, M. J., Sullivan, A., Amobi, A., Phelps, A. C., Gorman, D. P., Zollfrank, A., . . . Balboni, T. A. (2013). Why is spiritual care infrequent at end of life care? Spiritual care perceptions among patients, nurses, physicians, and the role of training. *Journal of Clinical Oncology*, *31*(4), 461–467. doi:10.1200/JCO.2012.44.6443

Beckman, S., Boxley-Harges, S., Bruick-Sorge, C., & Salmon, B. (2007). Five strategies that heighten nurses' awareness of spirituality to impact client care. *Holistic Nursing Practice*, *21*, 135–139. doi:10.1097/01.HNP.0000269150.80978.c3

Best, M., Butow, P., & Olver, I. (2016). Doctors discussing religion and spirituality: A systematic literature review. *Palliative Medicine*, *30*, 327–337. doi:10.1177/0269216315600912

Bishop, J. P. (2003). Prayer, science, and the moral life of medicine. *Archives of Internal Medicine*, *23*, 1405–1408. doi:10.1001/archinte.163.12.1405

Boccia, M., Piccardi, L., & Guariglia, P. (2015). The meditative mind: A comprehensive meta-analysis of MRI studies. *BioMed Research International,* Article ID 419808. doi:10.1155/2015/419808

Borg, M. (1997). *The God we never knew: Beyond dogmatic religion to a more authentic contemporary faith*. New York, NY: HarperSanFrancisco.

Bowman, T. (2017). Spirituality and countertransference: Individual and systemic considerations. *Death Studies*, *41*, 154–161. doi:10.1080/07481187.2016.1236851

Brewster, M. E., Hammer, J., Sawyer, J. S., Eklund, A., & Palamar, J. (2016). Perceived experiences of atheist discrimination: Instrument development and evaluation. *Journal of Counseling Psychology*, *63*(5), 557–570. doi:10.1037/cou0000156

Butcher, H. K., Bulechek, G. M., Dochterman, J. M., & Wagner, C. M. (Eds.). (2018). *Nursing interventions classification (NIC)* (7th ed.). St. Louis, MO: Elsevier.

Buttle, H. (2015). Measuring a journey without goal: Meditation, spirituality, and physiology. *BioMed Research International,* Article ID 891671. doi:10.1155/2015/891671

Caldeira, S., Timmins, F., de Carvalho, E. C., & Vieira, M. (2016). Nursing diagnosis of "Spiritual Distress" in women with breast cancer: Prevalence and major defining characteristics. *Cancer Nursing*, *39*(4), 321–327. doi:10.1097/ncc.0000000000000310

Carpenito, L. J. (2017). *Handbook of nursing diagnosis* (15th ed.). Philadelphia, PA: Lippincott Williams & Wilkins.

Daaleman, T. P. (2012). A health services framework of spiritual care. *Journal of Nursing Management*, *20*, 1021–1028. doi:10.1111/j.1365-2834.2012.01482.x

Delgado-Guay, M. O., Chisholm, G., Williams, J., Frisbee-Hume, S., Ferguson, A. O., & Bruera, E. (2016). Frequency, intensity, and correlates of spiritual pain in advanced cancer patients assessed in a supportive/palliative care clinic. *Palliative & Supportive Care*, *14*(4), 341–348. doi:10.1017/s147895151500108x

Dobratz, M. C. (2016). Building a middle-range theory of adaptive spirituality. *Nursing Science Quarterly*, *29*, 146–153. doi:10.1177/0894318416630090

du Plessis, E. (2016). Presence: A step closer to spiritual care in nursing. *Holistic Nursing Practice*, *30*, 47–53. doi:10.1097/hnp.0000000000000124

Exline, J. J., Pargament, K. I., Grubbs, J. B., & Yali, A. M. (2014). The religious and spiritual struggles scale: Development and initial validation. *Psychology of Religion and Spirituality*, *6*(3), 208–222. doi:10.1037/a0036465

Fahlberg, B., & Roush, T. (2016). Mindful presence: Being "with" in our nursing care. *Nursing*, *46*(3), 14–15. doi:10.1097/01.nurse.0000480605.60511.09

Ferrell, B., Wittenberg, E., Battista, V., & Walker, G. (2016). Nurses' experiences of spiritual communication with seriously ill children. *Journal of Palliative Medicine*, *19*, 1166–1170. doi:10.1089/jpm.2016.0138

Fosarelli, P. (2008). *Prayers and rituals at a time of illness and dying*. West Conshohocken, PA: Templeton.

Fowler, J. W. (1981). *Stages of faith development: The psychology of human development and the quest for meaning.* San Francisco, CA: Harper & Row.

George, L. K., Kinghorn, W. A., Koenig, H. G., Gammon, P., & Blazer, D. G. (2013). Why gerontologists should care about empirical research on religion and health: Transdisciplinary perspectives. *Gerontologist*, *53*, 898–906. doi:10.1093/geront/gnt002

Granqvist, P., & Nkara, F. (2017). Nature meets nurture in religious and spiritual development. *British Journal of Developmental Psychology, 35, 142–155.* doi:10.1111/bjdp.12170

Hodge, D. R. (2015). Spirituality and religion among the general public: Implications for social work discourse. *Social Work*, *60*, 219–227. doi:10.1093/sw/swv021

Hodge, D. R., Sun, F., & Wolosin, R. J. (2014). Hospitalized Asian patients and their spiritual needs: Developing a model of spiritual care. *Journal of Aging & Health*, *26*, 380–400. doi:10.1177/0898264313516995

Hulett, J. M., & Armer, J. M. (2016). A systematic review of spiritually based interventions and psychoneuroimmunological outcomes in breast cancer survivorship. *Integrative Cancer Therapies*, *15*(4), 405–423. doi:10.1177/1534735416636222

Jim, H. S., Pustejovsky, J. E., Park, C. L., Danhauer, S. C., Sherman, A. C., Fitchett, G., . . . Salsman, J. M. (2015). Religion, spirituality, and physical health in cancer patients: A meta-analysis. *Cancer*, *121*, 3760–3768. doi:10.1002/cncr.29353

King, S. D., Fitchett, G., & Berry, D. L. (2013). Screening for religious/spiritual struggle in blood and marrow transplant patients. *Supportive Care in Cancer*, *21*, 993–1001. doi:10.1007/s00520-012-1618-1

King, S. D., Fitchett, G., Murphy, P. E., Pargament, K. I., Martin, P. J., Johnson, R. H., . . . Loggers, E. T. (2017). Spiritual or religious struggle in hematopoietic cell transplant survivors. *Psycho-Oncology*, *26*, 270–277. doi:10.1002/pon.4029

Koenig, H. G. (2015). Religion, spirituality, and health: A review and update. *Advances in Mind-Body Medicine*, *29*(3), 19–26.

Laird, L. D., Curtis, C. E., & Morgan, J. R. (2017). Finding spirits in spirituality: What are we measuring in spirituality and health research? *Journal of Religion & Health, 56,* 1–20. doi:10.1007/s10943-016-0316-6

Lucette, A., Ironson, G., Pargament, K. I., & Krause, N. (2016). Spirituality and religiousness are associated with fewer depressive symptoms in individuals with medical conditions. *Psychosomatics*, *57*(5), 505–513. doi:10.1016/j.psym.2016.03.005

Mamier, I., Taylor, E. J., & Winslow, B. W. (2019). Nurse spiritual care: Prevalence and correlates. *Western Journal of Nursing Research*, *41*(4), 537–554. doi:10.1177/0193945918776328

McClintock, C. H., Lau, E., & Miller, L. (2016). Phenotypic dimensions of spirituality: Implications for mental health in China, India, and the United States. *Frontiers in Psychology*, *7*, Article ID 1600. doi:10.3389/fpsyg.2016.01600

Meier, B. P., Fetterman, A. K., Robinson, M. D., & Lappas, C. M. (2015). The myth of the angry atheist. *Journal of Psychology*, *149*, 219–238. doi:10.1080/00223980.2013.866929

Minton, M. E., Isaacson, M., & Banik, D. (2016). Prayer and the registered nurse (PRN): Nurses' reports of ease and dis-ease with patient-initiated prayer request. *Journal of Advanced Nursing*, *72*(9), 2185–2195. doi:10.1111/jan.12990

Mollica, M. A., Underwood, W., Homish, G. G., Homish, D. L., & Orom, H. (2016). Spirituality is associated with better prostate cancer treatment decision making experiences. *Journal of Behavioral Medicine*, *39*, 161–169. doi:10.1007/s10865-015-9662-1

Moorhead, S., Johnson, M., Maas, M. L., & Swanson, E. (Eds.). (2018). *Nursing outcomes classification (NOC)* (6th ed.). St. Louis, MO: Elsevier.

O'Brien, M. E. (2018). *Spirituality in nursing: Standing on holy ground* (5th ed.). Burlington, MA: Jones & Bartlett.

Odbehr, L. S., Hauge, S., Danbolt, L. J., & Kvigne, K. (2015). Residents' and caregivers' views on spiritual care and their understanding of spiritual needs in persons with dementia: A meta-synthesis. *Dementia*, *16*(7), 911–929. doi:10.1177/1471301215625013

Ohr, S., Jeong, S., & Saul, P. (2016). Cultural and religious beliefs and values, and their impact on preferences for end-of-life care among four ethnic groups of community dwelling older persons. *Journal of Clinical Nursing, 26,* 1681–1689. doi:10.1111/jocn.13572

Osterman, P., & Schwartz-Barcott, D. (1996). Presence: Four ways of being there. *Nursing Forum*, *31*(2), 23–30. doi:10.1111/j.1744-6198.1996.tb00490.x

Park, C. L., & Cho, D. (2016). Spiritual well-being and spiritual distress predict adjustment in adolescent and young adult cancer survivors. *Psycho-Oncology, 26,* 1293–1300. doi:10.1002/pon.4145

Park, C. L., & Sacco, S. J. (2016). Heart failure patients' desires for spiritual care, perceived constraints, and unmet spiritual needs: Relations with well-being and health-related quality of life. *Psychology of Health & Medicine*, *22,* 1011–1020. doi:10.1080/13548506.2016.1257813

Pesut, B., & Sawatzky, R. (2006). To describe or prescribe: Assumptions underlying a prescriptive nursing process approach to spiritual care. *Nursing Inquiry*, *13*, 127–134. doi:10.1111/j.1440-1800.2006.00315.x

Pew Research Center. (n.d.). *Religious landscape study*. Retrieved from http://www.pewforum.org/religious-landscape-study/

Reynolds, N., Mrug, S., Wolfe, K., Schwebel, D., & Wallander, J. (2016). Spiritual coping, psychosocial adjustment, and physical health in youth with chronic illness: A meta-analytic review. *Health Psychology Review*, *10*, 226–243. doi:10.1080/17437199.2016.1159142

Roberts, L., Ahmed, I., Hall, S., & Davison, A. (2009). Intercessory prayer for the alleviation of ill health. *Cochrane Database of Systematic Reviews*, *2009*(2), Art. No. CD000368. doi:10.1002/14651858.CD000368.pub3

Salsman, J. M., Pustejovsky, J. E., Jim, H. S., Munoz, A. R., Merluzzi, T. V., George, L., . . . Fitchett, G. (2015). A meta-analytic approach to examining the correlation between religion/spirituality and mental health in cancer. *Cancer*, *121*, 3769–3778. doi:10.1002/cncr.29350

Taylor, E. J. (2007a). Spiritual pain. *Advance for Nurses*, *9*(21), 15–16.

Taylor, E. J. (2007b). *What do I say? Talking with patients about spirituality*. Philadelphia, PA: Templeton Press.

Taylor, E. J. (2012). *Religion: A clinical guide for nurses*. New York, NY: Springer.

Taylor, E. J. (2015). Spiritual assessment. In B. R. Ferrell, N. Coyle, & J. A. Paice (Eds.), *Textbook of palliative nursing care* (4th ed., pp. 532–545). New York, NY: Oxford University.

Taylor, E. J., Park, C. G., & Pfeiffer, J. B. (2014). Nurse religiosity and spiritual care. *Journal of Advanced Nursing*, *70*(11), 2612–2621. doi:10.1111/jan.12446

Taylor, E. J., Petersen, C., Oyedele, O., & Haase, J. (2015). Spirituality and spiritual care of adolescents and young adults with cancer. *Seminars in Oncology Nursing*, *31*(3), 227–241. doi:10.1016/j.soncn.2015.06.002

Van Norman, G. A. (2017). Decisions regarding forgoing life-sustaining treatments. *Current Opinion in Anesthesiology*, *30*(2), 211–216. doi:10.1097/aco.0000000000000436

Weathers, E., McCarthy, G., & Coffey, A. (2016). Concept analysis of spirituality: An evolutionary approach. *Nursing Forum*, *51*, 79–96. doi:10.1111/nuf.12128

Williams, J. A., Meltzer, D., Arora, V., Chung, G., & Curlin, F. A. (2011). Attention to inpatients' religious and spiritual concerns: Predictors and association with patient satisfaction. *Journal of General Internal Medicine*, *26*(11), 1265–1271. doi:10.1007/s11606-011-1781-y

Williams, M. G., Voss, A., Vahle, B., & Capp, S. (2016). Clinical nursing education: Using the FICA spiritual history tool to assess patients' spirituality. *Nurse Educator*, *41*(4), E6–9. doi:10.1097/nne.0000000000000269

Winslow, G. R., & Wehtje-Winslow, B. J. (2007). Ethical boundaries of spiritual care. *Medical Journal of Australia*, *186*(10 Suppl.), S63–S66.

Wittenberg, E., Ragan, S. L., & Ferrell, B. (2017). Exploring nurse communication about spirituality. *American Journal of Hospice & Palliative Care*, *34*(6), 566–571. doi:10.1177/1049909116641630

Selected Bibliography

Hutchinson, T. A. (Ed.). (2011). *Whole person care: A new paradigm for the 21st century*. New York, NY: Springer.

Koenig, H. G. (2011). *Spirituality and health research: Methods, measurement, statistics, and resources*. West Conshohocken, PA: Templeton.

Koenig, H. G., King, D., & Carson, V. B. (2012). *Handbook of religion and health* (2nd ed.). New York, NY: Oxford University.

Stress and Coping 42

LEARNING OUTCOMES

After completing this chapter, you will be able to:

1. Differentiate the concepts of stress as a stimulus, as a response, and as a transaction.
2. Describe the three stages of Selye's general adaptation syndrome.
3. Identify physiologic, psychologic, and cognitive indicators of stress.
4. Differentiate four levels of anxiety.
5. Identify behaviors related to specific ego defense mechanisms.
6. Discuss types of coping and coping strategies.
7. Identify essential aspects of assessing a client's stress and coping patterns.
8. Identify nursing diagnoses related to stress.
9. Describe interventions to help clients minimize and manage stress.

KEY TERMS

alarm reaction, *1068*
anger, *1071*
anxiety, *1071*
burnout, *1078*
caregiver burden, *1074*
coping, *1074*
coping mechanism, *1074*
coping strategy, *1074*
countershock phase, *1069*
crisis intervention, *1078*
depression, *1072*
ego defense mechanisms, *1072*
fear, *1071*
general adaptation syndrome (GAS), *1068*
local adaptation syndrome (LAS), *1068*
shock phase, *1068*
stage of exhaustion, *1069*
stage of resistance, *1069*
stimulus-based stress models, *1068*
stress, *1067*
stressor, *1067*
transactional stress theory, *1070*

Introduction

Stress is a universal phenomenon. All individuals experience it. Parents refer to the stress of raising children, working individuals talk of the stress of their jobs, and students at all levels talk of the stress of school. Stress can result from both positive and negative experiences. A bride preparing for her wedding, a graduate preparing to start a new job, and a husband concerned about caring for his wife and family following a diagnosis of cancer all experience stress reactions.

The concept of stress is important because it provides a way of understanding the individual as a being who responds in totality (mind, body, and spirit) to a variety of changes that take place in daily life.

Concept of Stress

Stress is a condition in which an individual experiences changes in the normal balanced state. A **stressor** is any event or stimulus that causes an individual to experience stress. When an individual faces stressors, responses are referred to as *coping strategies*, *coping responses*, or *coping mechanisms*.

Sources of Stress

There are many sources of stress. They can be broadly classified as internal or external stressors, or developmental or situational stressors. *Internal stressors* originate within an individual, for example, infection or feelings of depression. *External stressors* originate outside the individual, for example, a move to another city, a death in the family, or pressure from peers. *Developmental stressors* occur at predictable times throughout an individual's life (Table 42.1). *Situational stressors* are unpredictable and may occur at any time during life. Situational stress may be positive or negative. Examples of situational stress include:

- Death of a family member
- Marriage or divorce
- Birth of a child
- New job
- Illness.

The degree to which any of these events has positive or negative effects depends to some extent on an individual's developmental stage. For example, the death of a parent may be more stressful for a 12-year-old than for a 40-year-old.

Effects of Stress

Stress can have physical, emotional, intellectual, social, and spiritual consequences. Usually the effects are mixed, because stress affects the whole individual. Physically, stress can threaten an individual's physiologic

TABLE 42.1 Selected Stressors Associated with Developmental Stages

Developmental Stage	Stressors
Child	Beginning school Establishing peer relationships Peer competition
Adolescent	Changing physique Relationships involving sexual attraction Exploring independence Choosing a career
Young adult	Marriage Leaving home Managing a home Getting started in an occupation Continuing one's education Children
Middle adult	Physical changes of aging Maintaining social status and standard of living Helping teenage children to become independent Aging parents
Older adult	Decreasing physical abilities and health Changes in residence Retirement and reduced income Death of spouse and friends

homeostasis. Emotionally, stress can produce negative or nonconstructive feelings about the self. Intellectually, stress can influence an individual's perceptual and problem-solving abilities. Socially, stress can alter an individual's relationships with others. Spiritually, stress can challenge one's beliefs and values. Many health conditions have been linked to stress (Figure 42.1 ■).

Models of Stress

Models of stress assist nurses to predict stressors in a particular situation and to understand the individual's responses. Nurses can use these models to assist clients in strengthening healthy coping responses and in adjusting unhealthy, unproductive responses. Three main models of stress are stimulus based, response based, and transaction based.

Stimulus-Based Models

In **stimulus-based stress models**, stress is defined as a stimulus, a life event, or a set of circumstances that arouses physiologic and psychologic reactions that may increase the individual's vulnerability to illness. In their classic work, Holmes and Rahe (1967) assigned a numerical value to 43 life changes or events. The scale has been modified and shortened many times. The scale of stressful life events is used to document an individual's relatively recent experiences, such as divorce, pregnancy, and retirement. In this view, both positive and negative events are stressful. Similar scales have since been developed, but all scales should be used with caution because the degree of stress an event presents is highly individual. A divorce may be highly traumatic to one individual and cause relatively little anxiety to another. In addition, many scales have not been tested for sensitivity to age, socioeconomic status, or culture.

Response-Based Models

Stress may also be considered as a response. This definition was developed and described by Selye (1956, 1976) as "the nonspecific response of the body to any kind of demand made upon it" (1976, p. 1).

Selye's stress response is characterized by a chain or pattern of physiologic events called the **general adaptation syndrome (GAS)** or *stress syndrome*. To differentiate the cause of stress from the response to stress, Selye (1976) used the term *stressor* to denote any factor that produces stress and disturbs the body's equilibrium. Stress can be observed only by the changes it produces in the body. This response of the body, the stress syndrome or GAS, occurs with the release of certain adaptive hormones and subsequent changes in the structure and chemical composition of the body. Parts of the body affected by stress are the gastrointestinal tract, the adrenal glands, and the lymphatic structures. With prolonged stress, deep ulcers appear in the lining of the stomach, the adrenal glands enlarge considerably, and the lymphatic structures, such as the thymus, spleen, and lymph nodes, atrophy (shrink).

Besides adapting globally, the body can also react locally; that is, one organ or a part of the body reacts alone. This is referred to as the **local adaptation syndrome (LAS)**. One example of the LAS is inflammation. Selye (1976) proposed that both the GAS and the LAS have three stages: alarm reaction, resistance, and exhaustion (Figure 42.2 ■).

Alarm Reaction

The initial reaction of the body is the **alarm reaction**, which alerts the body's defenses. Selye (1976) divided this stage into two parts: the shock phase and the countershock phase.

During the **shock phase** (Figure 42.2), the stressor may be perceived consciously or unconsciously by the individual. Stressors stimulate the sympathetic nervous system, which stimulates the hypothalamus. The hypothalamus releases corticotropin-releasing hormone, which stimulates the anterior pituitary gland to release adrenocorticotropic hormone. During times of stress, the adrenal medulla secretes epinephrine and norepinephrine in response to sympathetic stimulation. Significant body responses to epinephrine include the following:

1. Increased myocardial contractility, which increases cardiac output and blood flow to active muscles
2. Bronchial dilation, which allows increased oxygen intake

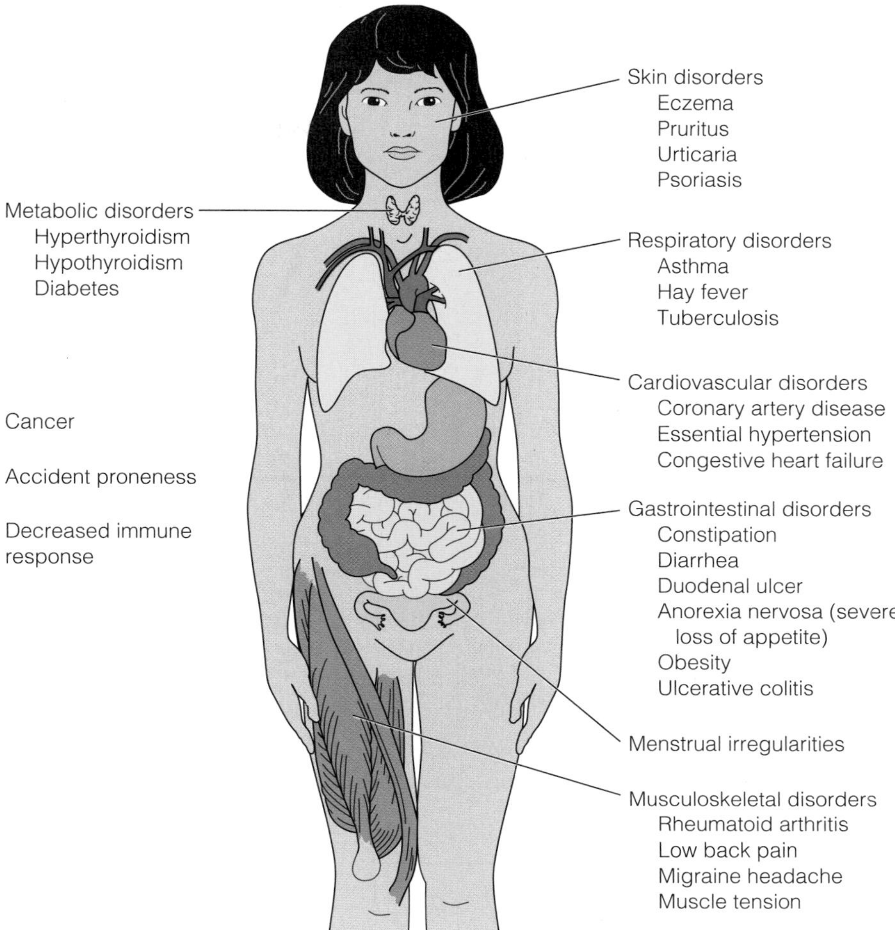

Figure 42.1 ■ Some disorders that can be caused or aggravated by stress.

3. Increased blood clotting
4. Increased cellular metabolism
5. Increased fat mobilization to provide energy and to synthesize other compounds needed by the body.

The principal effect of norepinephrine is decreased blood to the kidneys and increased secretion of renin. Renin is an enzyme that hydrolyzes one of the blood proteins to produce angiotensin. Angiotensin increases the blood pressure by constricting arterioles. All of these adrenal hormonal effects permit the individual to perform far more strenuous physical activity than would otherwise be possible. The individual is then ready for "fight or flight." This primary response is short-lived, lasting from 1 minute to 24 hours.

The second part of the alarm reaction is called the **countershock phase**. During this time, the changes produced in the body during the shock phase are reversed. An individual is best mobilized to react during the shock phase of the alarm reaction.

Stage of Resistance

The second stage in the GAS and LAS syndromes, the **stage of resistance**, is when the body's adaptation takes place. In other words, the body attempts to cope with the stressor and to limit the stressor to the smallest area of the body that can deal with it.

Stage of Exhaustion

During the third stage, the **stage of exhaustion**, the adaptation that the body made during the second stage cannot be maintained. This means that the ways used to cope with the stressor have been exhausted. If adaptation has not overcome the stressor, the stress effects may spread to the entire body. At the end of this stage, the body may either rest and return to normal, or death may be the ultimate consequence. The end of this stage depends largely on the adaptive energy resources of the individual, the severity of the stressor, and the external adaptive resources provided, such as oxygen.

Transaction-Based Models

Transactional theories of stress are based on the work of Lazarus (1966), who stated that the stimulus theory and the response theory do not consider individual differences. Neither theory explains which factors cause some individuals and not others to respond effectively nor interprets why some individuals adapt for longer periods than others.

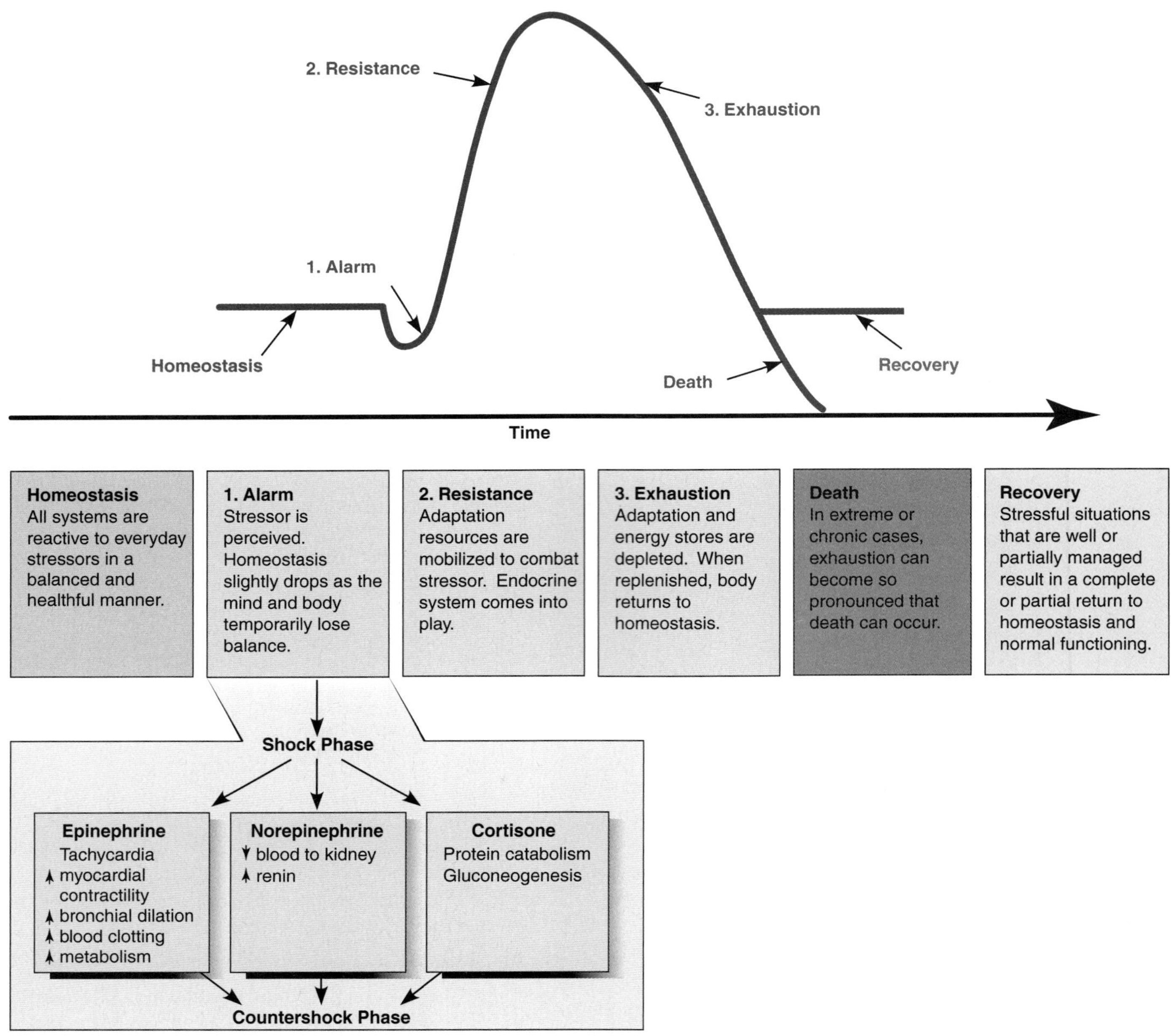

Figure 42.2 ■ The stages of adaptation to stress.

Although Lazarus (2006) recognizes that certain environmental demands and pressures produce stress in substantial numbers of individuals, he emphasizes that individuals and groups differ in their sensitivity and vulnerability to certain types of events, as well as in their interpretations and reactions. In terms of illness, one individual may respond with denial, another with anxiety, and still another with depression. To explain variations among individuals under comparable conditions, the Lazarus model considers cognitive processes that intervene between the encounter and the reaction, and the factors that affect the nature of this process. In contrast to Selye, who focuses on physiologic responses, Lazarus includes mental and psychologic components or responses as part of his concept of stress.

Lazarus's **transactional stress theory** encompasses a set of cognitive, affective, and adaptive (coping) responses that arise out of individual–environment transactions. The individual and the environment are inseparable; each affects and is affected by the other. Stress "refers to any event in which environmental demands, internal demands, or both tax or exceed the adaptive resources of an individual, social system, or tissue system" (Monat & Lazarus, 1991, p. 3). The individual responds to perceived environmental changes with adaptive or coping responses.

Indicators of Stress

Indicators of an individual's stress may be physiologic, psychologic, or cognitive.

Physiologic Indicators

Responses to stress vary depending on the individual's perception of events. The physiologic signs and symptoms of stress result from activation of the sympathetic and neuroendocrine systems of the body. Box 42.1 lists physiologic indicators of stress.

BOX 42.1 Stress

- Pupils dilate to increase visual perception when serious threats to the body arise.
- Sweat production (diaphoresis) increases to control elevated body heat due to increased metabolism.
- Heart rate and cardiac output increase to transport nutrients and by-products of metabolism more efficiently.
- Skin is pallid because of constriction of peripheral blood vessels, an effect of norepinephrine.
- Sodium and water retention increase due to release of mineralocorticoids, which increases blood volume.
- Rate and depth of respirations increase because of dilation of the bronchioles, promoting hyperventilation.
- Urinary output decreases but there may be urinary frequency or urgency.
- Mouth may be dry.
- Possible constipation and flatus or diarrhea may occur.
- For serious threats, mental alertness improves.
- Muscle tension increases to prepare for rapid motor activity or defense.
- Blood sugar increases because of release of glucocorticoids and gluconeogenesis.

Psychologic Indicators

Psychologic manifestations of stress include anxiety, fear, anger, depression, and unconscious ego defense mechanisms. Some coping patterns are helpful; others are a hindrance, depending on the situation and the length of time they are used or experienced.

Anxiety and Fear

A common reaction to stress is **anxiety**, a state of mental uneasiness, apprehension, dread, or foreboding or a feeling of helplessness related to an impending or anticipated unidentified threat to self or significant relationships. Anxiety can be experienced at the conscious, subconscious, or unconscious level. According to the National Institutes of Mental Health (2017), approximately 18% of adult Americans have anxiety disorders, although this figure may be low due to underreporting or alternative diagnoses.

Anxiety may be manifested on four levels:

1. *Mild anxiety* produces a slight arousal that enhances perception, learning, and productive abilities. Most healthy individuals experience mild anxiety, perhaps as a feeling of mild restlessness that prompts them to seek information and ask questions.
2. *Moderate anxiety* increases the arousal to a point where the individual expresses feelings of tension, nervousness, or concern. Perceptual abilities are narrowed. Attention is focused more on a particular aspect of a situation than on peripheral activities.
3. *Severe anxiety* consumes most of the individual's energies and requires intervention. Perception is further decreased. The individual, unable to focus on what is really happening, focuses on only one detail of the situation generating the anxiety.
4. *Panic* is an overpowering, frightening level of anxiety causing the individual to lose control. It is less frequently experienced than other levels of anxiety. The perception of a panicked individual can be affected to the degree that the individual distorts events.

Mild or moderate anxiety motivates goal-directed behavior. In this sense, anxiety is an effective coping strategy. For example, mild anxiety motivates students to study. Excessive anxiety, however, often has destructive effects. Table 42.2 lists indicators of these levels.

Fear is an emotion or feeling of apprehension aroused by impending or seeming danger, pain, or another perceived threat. The fear may be in response to something that has already occurred, in response to an immediate or current threat, or in response to something the individual believes will happen. The nursing student may be fearful in anticipation of the first experience in a client care setting. The student may fear that the client will not want to be cared for by the student or that the student might inadvertently harm the client. The object of fear may or may not be based in reality.

Anxiety and fear differ in four ways:

- The source of anxiety may not be identifiable; the source of fear is identifiable.
- Anxiety is related to the future, that is, to an anticipated event. Fear is related to the past, present, and future.
- Anxiety is vague, whereas fear is definite.
- Anxiety results from psychologic or emotional conflict; fear results from a specific physical or psychologic entity.

Anger

Anger is an emotional state consisting of a subjective feeling of animosity or strong displeasure. A verbal expression of anger can be a signal to others of one's internal psychologic discomfort and a call for assistance to deal with perceived stress. In contrast, hostility is usually marked by overt antagonism and harmful or destructive behavior; aggression is an unprovoked attack or a hostile, injurious, or destructive action or outlook; and violence is the exertion of physical force to injure or abuse. Verbally expressed anger differs from hostility, aggression, and violence, but it can lead to destructiveness and violence if the anger persists unabated.

A clearly expressed verbal communication of anger, when the angry individual tells the other individual about the anger and carefully identifies the source, is constructive. This clarity of communication gets the anger out into the open so the other individual can deal with it and help to alleviate it. The angry individual "gets it off the chest" and prevents an emotional buildup.

TABLE 42.2 Indicators of Levels of Anxiety

	Level of Anxiety			
Category	**Mild**	**Moderate**	**Severe**	**Panic**
Verbalization changes	Increased questioning	Voice tremors and pitch changes	Communication difficult to understand, loud speech, threats, demands	Communication may not be understandable
Motor activity changes	Mild restlessness	Tremors, facial twitches, and shakiness	Increased motor activity, inability to relax	Increased motor activity, agitation
	Sleeplessness	Increased muscle tension	Fearful facial expression	Unpredictable responses
Perception and attention changes	Feelings of increased arousal and alertness	Narrowed focus of attention	Inability to focus or concentrate	Trembling, poor motor coordination
		Able to focus but selectively inattentive	Easily distracted	Perception distorted or exaggerated
	Uses learning to adapt	Learning slightly impaired	Learning severely impaired	Unable to learn or function
Respiratory and circulatory changes	None	Slightly increased respiratory and heart rates	Tachycardia, hyperventilation	Dyspnea, palpitations, choking, chest pain, or pressure
Other changes	Easily startled, tension-relieving behavior (e.g. fidgeting)	Mild gastric symptoms (e.g., "butterflies in the stomach")	Headache, dizziness, nausea, confusion, diaphoresis (sweating)	Feeling of impending doom, paresthesia, sweating, hallucinations

Adapted from "Anxiety and Obsessive-Compulsive Disorders," by M. J. Halter in *Varcarolis' Foundations of Psychiatric-Mental Health Nursing: A Clinical Approach* (8th ed., Chapter 15), by M. J. Halter, 2018, St. Louis, MO: Elsevier; and "Disorders of Anxiety, Stress, and Trauma," by M. L. Potter in *Psychiatric Mental Health Nursing: From Suffering to Hope* (Chapter 13), by M. L. Potter and M. D. Moller, 2016, Boston, MA: Pearson.

Depression

Depression is a common reaction to events that seem overwhelming or negative. **Depression**, an extreme feeling of sadness, despair, dejection, lack of worth, or emptiness, affects millions of Americans a year. The signs and symptoms of depression and the severity of the problem vary with the client and the significance of the precipitating event. Emotional symptoms can include feelings of tiredness, sadness, emptiness, or numbness. Behavioral signs of depression include irritability, inability to concentrate, difficulty making decisions, loss of sexual desire, crying, sleep disturbance, and social withdrawal. Physical signs of depression may include loss of appetite, weight loss, constipation, headache, and dizziness. Many individuals experience short periods of depression in response to overwhelming stressful events, such as the death of a loved one or loss of a job; prolonged depression, however, is a cause for concern and may require treatment.

Ego Defense Mechanisms

Ego defense mechanisms are unconscious psychologic adaptive mechanisms or, according to Anna Freud (1967), mental mechanisms that develop as the personality attempts to defend itself, establish compromises among conflicting impulses, and calm inner tensions. Defense mechanisms are the unconscious mind working to protect the individual from anxiety. They can be precursors to conscious cognitive coping mechanisms that will ultimately solve the problem. Like some verbal and motor responses, defense mechanisms release tension. Table 42.3 describes these mechanisms and lists examples of their adaptive and maladaptive use.

Cognitive Indicators

Cognitive indicators of stress are thinking responses that include problem-solving, structuring, self-control or self-discipline, suppression, and fantasy. *Problem-solving* involves thinking through the threatening situation, using specific steps to arrive at a solution. The individual assesses the situation or problem, analyzes or defines it, chooses alternatives, carries out the selected alternative, and evaluates whether the solution succeeded.

Structuring is the arrangement or manipulation of a situation so threatening events do not occur. For example, a nurse can structure or control an interview with a client by asking only direct, closed questions so the client will not wander into areas that may be stressful. Structuring can be productive in certain situations. An individual who schedules a dental examination semiannually to prevent severe dental disease is using productive structuring.

Self-control (*discipline*) is assuming a manner and facial expression that convey a sense of being in control or in charge. When self-control prevents panic and harmful or nonproductive actions in a threatening situation, it is a helpful response that conveys strength. Self-control carried to an extreme, however, can delay problem-solving and prevent an individual from receiving the support of others, who may perceive the individual as handling the situation well, as cold, or as unconcerned.

TABLE 42.3 Defense Mechanisms

Name	Definition	Example
Altruism	Emotional conflicts and stressors dealt with by performing helpful service to others that results in satisfaction and pleasure	Serving as a volunteer to a disaster area.
Compensation	Making up for a perceived or real inability by focusing on another area and becoming proficient (may be conscious or unconscious)	A 16-year-old boy is not good at sports. He strives to get the top grades in his class and become a member of his school's honor society.
Conversion	Transfer of a mental conflict into a physical symptom	A concert pianist develops paralysis of his right hand prior to performing his first concert.
Denial	Avoiding, ignoring, or rejecting a real situation and the feelings associated with it	A man tells his wife that he wants a divorce. The wife responds by saying all couples have difficulties and that she is sure he will feel differently tomorrow.
Displacement	Transfer of emotions from one person or object onto another less threatening and more neutral person or object (sometimes called the "scapegoat" defense mechanism)	The staff nurse is yelled at by the unit supervisor at work. When she gets home, the nurse yells at her 12-year-old son for no apparent reason.
Humor	Emphasizing ironic or amusing aspects of a conflict or stressor	A nurse with cold hands comments, "Cold hands but a warm heart" before taking a patient's pulse.
Identification	Process whereby an individual takes on thoughts, mannerisms, or tastes of another individual whom the individual admires	A college student decides to become a physical therapist after spending 3 months in physical therapy due to a knee injury.
Intellectualization	Excessive reasoning or logic to transfer disturbing feelings into the intellectual sphere	A student tells her parents that no one could have done better than she did on the course exam, because the exam material was not covered well enough, and the course instructor is not a very good teacher.
Introjection	Attributing to oneself the qualities of another—intense identification in which the qualities are incorporated into the individual's own ego structure	A patient states he is "General Napoleon" and walks around the unit with his right hand over his heart.
Isolation	Separating ideas, thoughts, and actions from feelings associated with them	A nurse stops on the highway to assist in an accident. The victim's arm has been severed from the body. The nurse does not focus on feelings about the situation but focuses on applying pressure to the wound site, calling for help, and comforting the victim.
Projection	Unconsciously attributing one's thoughts or impulses to another person	Roommate A gets angry at Roommate B for being angry and not listening, when it is actually Roommate A who is angry and has not been listening.
Rationalization	Justifying illogical ideas, actions, or feelings by using acceptable explanations (most common defense mechanism—a form of self-deception)	The college student did not do well on her exam. She calls home and tells her parents that she did not get enough sleep the night before the exam.
Reaction formation	Developing the opposite behavior or emotion to unacceptable feelings or behaviors	A student does not like the teacher or the course being taught by the teacher. The student brings the teacher articles related to the course and comments how much he likes the teacher and her course.
Repression	The unconscious exclusion of unwanted experiences, ideas, emotions; repression is a first line of psychologic defense against anxiety	A 7-year-old girl displays signs of sexual abuse. Although her family is suspicious of who might have abused her and when, the girl cannot recall anything about the recent visit she had with the potential abuser.
Sublimation	The unconscious substituting of acceptable behaviors for unacceptable behaviors	An 18-year-old male who felt inadequate when compared to his brothers and was bullied in school joins the Marines.
Suppression	The conscious denial of a disturbing situation or feeling (Think of the individual as consciously "sitting on" the feelings as compared to repression, in which the individual is not aware.)	One student asks another if he is worried about the exam in their class tomorrow. The student replies, "I'd rather not think about that right now."
Undoing	Making up for an intolerable act or experience to lessen or alleviate feelings of guilt	After being caught by his mother stealing money out of her purse, the 10-year-old boy washes his hands excessively.

Suppression is consciously and willfully putting a thought or feeling out of mind: "I won't deal with that today. I'll do it tomorrow." This response relieves stress temporarily but does not solve the problem. A man who keeps ignoring a toothache, pushing it out of his mind because he fears the pain of having a filling, will not obtain relief of his symptoms.

Fantasy or *daydreaming* is likened to make-believe. Unfulfilled wishes and desires are imagined as fulfilled, or a threatening experience is reworked or replayed so it ends differently from reality. Experiences can be relived, everyday problems solved, and plans for the future made. The outcome of current problems may also be fantasized. For example, a client awaiting the results of a breast biopsy may fantasize the surgeon as saying, "You do not have cancer." Fantasy responses can be helpful if they lead to problem-solving. For example, the client awaiting breast biopsy results might say to herself, "Even if the doctor says, 'You have cancer,' as long as he also says it can be treated, I can accept that." Fantasies can be destructive and nonproductive if an individual uses them to excess and retreats from reality.

Coping

Coping may be described as dealing with change—successfully or unsuccessfully. A **coping strategy** (**coping mechanism**) is a natural or learned way of responding to a changing environment or specific problem or situation. According to Folkman and Lazarus (1991), coping is "the cognitive and behavioral effort to manage specific external and/or internal demands that are appraised as taxing or exceeding the resources of the person" (p. 210).

Two types of coping strategies have been described: problem focused and emotion focused. *Problem-focused coping* refers to efforts to improve a situation by making changes or taking action. *Emotion-focused coping* includes thoughts and actions that relieve emotional distress. Emotion-focused coping does not improve the situation, but the individual often feels better. Both types of strategies may occur together (Eatough & Chang, 2018).

Coping strategies are also viewed as long term or short term. *Long-term coping strategies* can be constructive and practical. In certain situations, talking with others and trying to find out more about the situation are long-term strategies. Other long-term strategies include a change in lifestyle patterns such as eating a healthy diet, exercising regularly, balancing leisure time with working, or using problem-solving in decision-making instead of anger or other nonconstructive responses.

Short-term coping strategies can reduce stress to a tolerable limit temporarily but are ineffective ways to permanently deal with reality. They may even have a destructive or detrimental effect on the individual. Examples of short-term strategies are using alcoholic beverages or drugs, daydreaming and fantasizing, relying on the belief that everything will work out, and giving in to others to avoid anger.

Coping strategies vary among individuals and are often related to the individual's perception of the stressful event. Three approaches to coping with stress are to alter the stressor, adapt to the stressor, or avoid the stressor. An individual's coping strategies often change with a reappraisal of a situation. There is never only one way to cope. Some individuals choose avoidance; others confront a situation to cope. Still others seek information or rely on religious beliefs.

Coping can be adaptive or maladaptive. *Adaptive coping* helps the individual to deal effectively with stressful events and minimizes distress associated with them. *Maladaptive coping* can cause unnecessary distress for the individual and others associated with the individual or stressful event. In nursing literature, effective and ineffective coping are often differentiated. *Effective coping* results in adaptation; *ineffective coping* results in maladaptation.

Although the coping behavior may not always seem appropriate, the nurse needs to remember that coping is always purposeful. The effectiveness of an individual's coping is influenced by several factors, including:

- The number, duration, and intensity of the stressors
- Past experiences of the individual
- Support systems available to the individual
- Personal qualities of the individual.

If the duration of the stressors is extended beyond the coping powers of the individual, he or she becomes exhausted and may develop increased susceptibility to health problems. Reaction to long-term stress is seen in family members who undertake the care of an individual in the home for a long period. This stress is called **caregiver burden** and produces responses such as chronic fatigue, sleeping difficulties, and high blood pressure. In the case of caregiver burden, the caregiver also becomes the nurse's client and a care plan to intervene should be created (Hartnett, Thom, & Kline, 2016). Prolonged stress can also result in mental illness. As coping strategies or

TABLE 42.4 Examples of the Negative Effects of Stress on Basic Human Needs

Needs	Effects
Physiologic	Altered elimination pattern Change in appetite Altered sleep pattern
Safety and security	Expresses nervousness and feelings of being threatened Focuses on stressors, inattention to safety measures
Love and belonging	Isolated and withdrawn Becomes overly dependent Blames others for own problems
Self-esteem	Fails to socialize with others Becomes a workaholic Draws attention to self
Self-actualization	Preoccupied with own problems Shows lack of control Unable to accept reality

defense mechanisms become ineffective, the individual may have interpersonal problems, work difficulties, and a significant decrease in the ability to meet basic human needs (Table 42.4).

NURSING MANAGEMENT

Assessing

Nursing assessment of a client's stress and coping patterns includes (a) nursing history and (b) physical examination of the client for indicators of stress (e.g., nail biting, nervousness, weight changes) or stress-related health problems (e.g., hypertension, dyspnea). When obtaining the nursing history, the nurse poses questions about client-perceived stressors or stressful incidents, manifestations of stress, and past and present coping strategies. During the physical examination, the nurse observes for verbal, motor, cognitive, or other physical manifestations of stress. Remember, however, that clinical signs and symptoms may not occur when cognitive coping is effective.

In addition, the nurse should be aware of expected developmental transitions (predictable tasks that must be accomplished if the client is to grow psychologically as well as physically; see Chapters 23 to 26 ∞). Individuals go through different developmental stages from infancy to old age when certain tasks are expected to be completed or resolved. When these tasks are carried over and not resolved, stress increases as they become older. For example, if an infant does not learn to trust those around him during infancy, this mistrust may accompany him through life, influencing his relationships and possibly being the root of dysfunction, stress, and ineffective coping. This knowledge helps the nurse identify additional stressors and the client's response to them (see Table 42.1). Questions to elicit data about the client's stress and coping patterns are shown in the accompanying Assessment Interview.

Diagnosing

Examples of nursing diagnoses that are appropriate for clients who have problems related to stress, adaptation, and coping are: anxiety; caregiver stress; denial; and difficult, altered, or impaired coping (individual or family).

ASSESSMENT INTERVIEW Stress and Coping Patterns

- On a scale of 1 to 10, where 1 is "very minor" and 10 is "extreme," how would you rate the stress you are experiencing in the following areas?
  a. Home
  b. Work or school
  c. Finance
  d. Recent illness or loss of loved one
  e. Your health
  f. Family responsibilities
  g. Relationships with friends
  h. Relationship with parents or children
  i. Relationship with partner
  j. Recent hospitalization
  k. Other (specify)
- How long have you been dealing with these stressors?
- How do you usually handle stressful situations? If the client does not adequately describe, prompt with the following:
  a. Cry
  b. Get angry
  c. Talk to someone (Who?)
  d. Withdraw from the situation
  e. Control others or situation
  f. Go for a walk or perform physical exercise
  g. Try to arrive at a solution
  h. Pray
  i. Laugh, joke, or use some other expression of humor
  j. Meditate or use some other relaxation technique such as yoga or guided imagery
- How well does your usual coping strategy work?

EVIDENCE-BASED PRACTICE

Evidence-Based Practice

Do Nurses Who Participate in Unsuccessful Resuscitations Experience Significant Stress?

Thousands of clients in critical care settings require CPR every year and about half of them do not survive. In this study, McMeekin, Hickman, Douglas, and Kelly (2017) explored stress, coping, and institutional support in critical care nurses who participated in unsuccessful hospital CPR (codes). The theoretical framework of the study was Lazarus and Folkman's Transactional Model of Stress and Coping. Almost 400 nurses across the United States completed the demographic data and three surveys. Postcode stress levels were high, as were symptoms of posttraumatic stress disorder (PTSD). Denial, self-distraction, self-blame, and behavioral disengagement were coping strategies associated with PTSD but not with the level of stress.

Implications

There are several limitations in this study including the convenience sample and self-report of remembered feelings. Although the sample size was adequate for statistical analysis, it represents a very small percentage of all the critical care nurses who experience unsuccessful codes. Thus, the study needs replication. However, the findings indicate that the problem of stress in this population is likely significant and researchers and employers should strive to identify issues and propose activities that would minimize the negative impact on nurses. In particular, the use of negative coping strategies should be addressed.

Planning

The nurse develops plans in collaboration with the client and significant support people when possible, according to the client's state of health (e.g., ability to return to work), level of anxiety, support resources, coping mechanisms, and sociocultural and religious affiliation. The nurse with little experience intervening with clients undergoing stress may wish to consult with a more experienced nurse to develop effective plans. The nurse and client set goals to change the existing client responses to the stressor or stressors.

The overall client goals for individuals experiencing stress-related responses are to:

- Decrease or resolve anxiety.
- Increase ability to manage or cope with stressful events or circumstances.
- Improve role performance.

A sample nursing care plan and a concept map are shown on pages 1080–1082.

Planning for Home Care

Clients hospitalized and experiencing stress may require ongoing nursing support or referral to community agencies that can provide support to meet client needs and enhance client coping. Determining how much and what type of planning and home care follow-up is needed is based in great part on the nurse's knowledge of how the client and family have coped with previous stressors and the nature of the present stressor.

Implementing

Although stress is part of daily life, it is also highly individual; a situation that to one individual is a major stressor may not affect another. Some methods to help reduce stress will be effective for one individual; other methods will be appropriate for a different individual. A nurse who is sensitive to clients' needs and reactions can choose those methods of intervention that will be most effective for each individual.

Encouraging Health Promotion Strategies

Several health promotion strategies are often appropriate as interventions for clients with stress-related nursing diagnoses. Among these are physical exercise, optimal nutrition, adequate rest and sleep, and time management.

Exercise

Regular exercise promotes both physical and emotional health. Physiologic benefits include improved muscle tone, increased cardiopulmonary function, and weight control. Psychologic benefits include relief of tension, a feeling of well-being, and relaxation. Federal guidelines recommend 150 minutes of moderate-intensity weekly exercise for adults (U.S. Department of Health and Human Services, 2018).

Nutrition

Optimal nutrition is essential for health and in increasing the body's resistance to stress. To minimize the negative effects of stress (e.g., irritability, hyperactivity, anxiety), people need to avoid excesses of caffeine, salt, sugar, and fat, and deficiencies in vitamins and minerals. Guidelines for a well-balanced, healthy diet are detailed in Chapter 46 ∞.

Clinical Alert!

Many clients have "comfort foods"—foods they like to eat that make them feel better emotionally. These should be allowed whenever they are not contraindicated by the client's health condition.

Sleep

Sleep restores the body's energy levels and is an essential aspect of stress management. To ensure adequate sleep, clients may need help to attain comfort (such as pain management) and to learn techniques that promote peace of mind and relaxation. (See the *Using Relaxation Techniques* section.)

Time Management

Individuals who manage their time effectively usually experience less stress because they feel more in control of their circumstances. Clients who feel overwhelmed often need help to prioritize tasks and to consider whether modifications can be made to decrease role demands. Working parents, for example, may need to consider delegating tasks to family members or hiring part-time help. Controlling the demands of others is also an important aspect of effective time management because requests made by others cannot always be met. Clients may need to learn to develop an awareness of which requests they can meet without undue stress, which ones can be negotiated, and which ones need to be declined. Feelings of control can be enhanced when clients schedule a daily or weekly period of time to deal with specific tasks. Time management must address both what is important to the client and what can realistically be achieved. For example, clients need to consider whether a clean house and time spent with the children can both be accomplished satisfactorily and, if not, which is more important. Clients feeling overwhelmed need to re-examine the "should do," "ought to do," and "must do" situations in their lives and develop realistic self-expectations.

Minimizing Anxiety

Nurses carry out measures to minimize clients' anxiety and stress. For example, nurses encourage clients to take deep breaths before an injection, explain procedures before they are implemented including sensations likely to be experienced during the procedure, administer a massage to help the client relax, and offer support to clients and families during times of illness. The nurse recognizes that quick action may be necessary to avoid the contagious nature of anxiety. That is, the anxious feeling of one individual makes others around him or her also anxious. This can include family members, other clients nearby, or healthcare providers. General guidelines for helping clients who are stressed and feeling anxious are outlined in Box 42.2.

BOX 42.2 Minimizing Stress and Anxiety

- Listen attentively; try to understand the client's perspective on the situation.
- Provide an atmosphere of warmth and trust; convey a sense of caring and empathy.
- Determine if it is appropriate to encourage clients' participation in the plan of care; give them choices about some aspects of care but do not overwhelm them with choices.
- Stay with clients as needed to promote safety and feelings of security and to reduce fear.
- Control the environment to minimize additional stressors such as reducing noise, limiting the number of individuals in the room, and providing care by the same nurse as much as possible.
- Implement suicide precautions if indicated.
- Communicate in short, clear sentences.
- Help clients to:
  a. Determine situations that precipitate anxiety and identify signs of anxiety.
  b. Verbalize feelings, perceptions, and fears as appropriate. Some cultures discourage the expression of feelings.
  c. Identify personal strengths.
  d. Recognize usual coping patterns and differentiate positive from negative coping mechanisms.
  e. Identify new strategies for managing stress (e.g., exercise, massage, progressive relaxation).
  f. Identify available support systems.
- Teach clients about:
  a. The importance of adequate exercise, a balanced diet, and rest and sleep to energize the body and enhance coping abilities.
  b. Support groups available such as Alcoholics Anonymous, Weight Watchers or Overeaters Anonymous, and parenting and child abuse support groups.
  c. Educational programs available such as time management, assertiveness training, and meditation groups.

Mediating Anger

Often nurses find clients' anger difficult to handle. Caring for the client who is angry is difficult for two reasons:

- Clients seldom state, "I feel angry or frustrated," or indicate the reason for their anger. Instead, they may refuse treatment, become verbally abusive or demanding, threaten violence, or become overly critical. Their complaints rarely reflect the cause of their anger.
- Anger from clients can elicit fear and anger in the nurse, who may respond in a manner that intensifies the client's anger, even to the point of violence. Nurses may respond in a way that reduces their own stress rather than the client's stress.

Ienacco (2016) recommends the following strategies for dealing with clients' anger:

- Remember that there is a difference between anger (a subjective feeling) and aggression (a harmful behavior).
- Approach each client with a calm, reassuring manner. This will help the client feel less threatened and more secure. Express compassion and concern.
- Involve clients in their own care as much as possible. This will increase their sense of control, which helps decrease anger.
- When a client's aggression is escalating, you must protect the safety of that client, other clients, yourself, and other staff.
- Call for help immediately if your interventions have not de-escalated the client's aggressive behavior.

Safety Alert! SAFETY

A nurse who is concerned for his or her own safety while working with an angry client should withdraw from the situation or obtain support from another individual.

Using Relaxation Techniques

Several relaxation techniques can be used to quiet the mind, release tension, and counteract the fight-or-flight responses of GAS discussed earlier in this chapter. Nurses can teach these techniques to clients. Nurses should also encourage clients to use these techniques when they encounter stressful health situations. Examples of these situations are (a) during childbirth, (b) postoperatively to cope with pain, and (c) before and during a painful procedure. Many agencies now have relaxation tapes available that the client can borrow or purchase. Some clients make their own recordings. Specific relaxation techniques are discussed in Chapter 22 ∞ and include the following:

- Breathing exercises
- Massage
- Progressive relaxation
- Imagery
- Biofeedback
- Yoga
- Meditation
- Therapeutic touch
- Music therapy
- Humor and laughter.

Crisis Intervention

A *crisis* is an acute, time-limited state of disequilibrium resulting from situational, developmental, or societal sources of stress. An individual in crisis is temporarily unable to cope with or adapt to the stressor by using previous methods of problem-solving. Individuals in crisis generally have a distorted perception of the event and do not have adequate situational support or coping mechanisms. Common characteristics of crises are shown in Box 42.3.

BOX 42.3 Common Characteristics of Crises

- All crises are experienced as sudden. The client is usually not aware of a warning signal, even if others could "see it coming." The individual or family members may feel that they had little or no preparation for the event or trauma.
- The crisis is often experienced as life threatening, whether this perception is realistic or not.
- Communication with significant others is often decreased or cut off.
- There may be perceived or real displacement from familiar surroundings or loved ones.
- All crises have an aspect of loss, whether actual or perceived. The losses can include an object, an individual, a hope, a dream, or any significant factor for that client.

Crisis intervention is a short-term helping process of assisting clients to (a) work through a crisis to its resolution and (b) restore their precrisis level of functioning. It is a process that includes not only the client in crisis but also various members of the client's support network. Crisis intervention is not the specialty of any one professional group. People who intervene in crises come from the fields of nursing, medicine, psychology, social work, and theology. Police officers, teachers, school guidance counselors, and rescue workers, among others, are often on the spot in moments of crisis.

Because a state of disequilibrium is so uncomfortable, a crisis is self-limiting. However, an individual experiencing a crisis alone is more vulnerable to unsuccessful negotiation than is an individual working through a crisis with help. Working with another individual increases the likelihood that the individual in crisis will resolve it in a positive way. Often a state of crisis offers the individual or family potential for growth and change.

The traditional steps of the nursing process correspond closely to the steps of crisis intervention. In assessment, the nurse or helper must focus on the client and the problem, collecting data about the client, the client's coping style, the precipitating event, the situational supports, the client's perception of the crisis, and the client's ability to handle the problem. This information is the basis for later decisions about how and when to intervene and whom to call. An individual's perception of the event and personal response will determine the nursing diagnoses. The most common nursing diagnoses for clients in crisis are similar to those cited earlier in this chapter.

Effective planning for crisis intervention must be based on careful assessment and developed in active collaboration with the client in crisis and the significant people in that client's life.

Implementation involves crisis counseling and home crisis visits. Crisis counseling focuses on solving immediate problems and it involves individuals, groups, or families. Crisis intervention centers rely heavily on telephone counseling by volunteers who have professional consultation available to them. Also known as hotlines and often available around the clock, they allow callers to remain anonymous. The volunteers usually work within a protocol that indicates what information they need from the client to assess the crisis. Their goal is to plan steps to provide immediate relief and then long-term follow-up if necessary.

Crisis home visits are made when telephone counseling does not suffice or when the crisis workers need to obtain additional information by direct observation or to reach a client who is unobtainable by telephone. Home visits are appropriate when crisis workers need to initiate contact rather than waiting for clients to come to them; for example, when a telephone caller is assessed to be highly suicidal or when a concerned neighbor, primary care provider, or clergy member informs the agency of clients in potential crisis.

Stress Management for Nurses

Nurses, like clients, are susceptible to experiencing anxiety and stress. Nursing practice involves many stressors related to both clients and the work environment—understaffing, increasing severity of client illnesses, adjusting to various work shifts, being expected to assume responsibilities for which one is not prepared, inadequate support from supervisors and peers, visiting homes that are depressing, caring for dying clients, and so on. Although most nurses cope effectively with the physical and emotional demands of nursing, in some situations nurses become overwhelmed and develop **burnout**, a complex syndrome of behaviors that can be likened to the exhaustion stage of the general adaptation syndrome. The nurse with burnout manifests physical and emotional depletion, a negative attitude and self-concept, and feelings of helplessness and hopelessness.

Nurses can prevent burnout by using the techniques to manage stress discussed for clients. Nurses must first recognize their stress and become attuned to such responses as feelings of being overwhelmed, fatigue, angry outbursts, physical illness, and increases in drinking alcohol, smoking, or substance abuse. Once attuned to stress and personal reactions, it is necessary to identify which situations produce the strongest

DRUG CAPSULE

Selective Serotonin Reuptake Inhibitor (SSRI): sertraline HCl (Zoloft)

CLIENT TAKING ANTIANXIETY MEDICATION

Sertraline is approved to treat depression, social anxiety disorder, posttraumatic stress disorder (PTSD), panic disorder, obsessive-compulsive disorder (OCD), and premenstrual dysphoric disorder (PMDD) in adults over age 18. It is also approved for OCD in children and adolescents ages 6 to 17 years. It prevents serotonin from being reabsorbed by the sending nerve cells so that more serotonin is available for acceptance by the receiving nerve cells.

NURSING RESPONSIBILITIES

- Sertraline may be given with or without meals but with sufficient water. It is taken once per day.
- Sertraline is available as oral concentrate or tablets. The concentrate must be diluted after measurement.
- This medication should not be taken if the client is already taking a monoamine oxidase inhibitor (MAOI) or pimozide. Use with caution in clients taking anticoagulant medications. Always check the list of client medications for possible interactions.
- Adverse effects may include dry mouth, insomnia, sexual side effects, diarrhea, nausea, and sleepiness.
- There is a warning from the U.S. Food and Drug Administration (FDA) on all materials related to antidepressants due to an increased risk of suicidal thoughts and behavior from 2% to 4% in people under age 18. This risk must be balanced with the medical need. Those starting medication should be watched closely for suicidal thoughts, worsening of depression, or unusual changes in behavior.
- This is an expensive medication. Explore insurance and other forms of the client's ability to manage this cost.

CLIENT AND FAMILY TEACHING

- This medication is not habit forming and does not cause weight gain (as do some medications prescribed for similar purposes).
- Do not stop taking this medication without consulting the primary care provider. Some symptoms might improve within 1 to 2 weeks, but it could take up to 8 weeks, depending on the individual. Treatment may last 6 months to 1 year.
- Sertraline comes in different dose strengths, and the primary care provider may need to adjust the dosage to find the correct amount.
- Avoid alcohol while taking sertraline.
- Take at the same time every day.
- Store at room temperature.
- Use caution when driving, operating machinery, or performing other hazardous activities because sertraline may cause dizziness or drowsiness.

Note: Prior to administering any medication, review all aspects with a current drug handbook or other reliable source.

reactions so steps may be taken to reduce the stress. Suggestions include:

- Plan a daily relaxation program with meaningful quiet time to reduce tension (e.g., read, listen to music, soak in a tub, or meditate).
- Establish a regular exercise program to direct energy outward.
- Study assertiveness techniques to overcome feelings of powerlessness in relationships with others. Learn to say no.
- Learn to accept failures—your own and others—and make it a constructive learning experience. Recognize that most individuals do the best they can. Learn to ask for help, to show your feelings with colleagues, and to support your colleagues in times of need.
- Accept what cannot be changed. There are certain limitations in every situation. Get involved in constructive change efforts if organizational policies and procedures cause stress.
- Develop collegial support groups to deal with feelings and anxieties generated in the work setting.
- Participate in professional organizations to address workplace issues.
- Seek counseling if indicated to help clarify and cope with concerns.

Evaluating

Using the desired outcomes developed during the planning stage as a guide, the nurse collects data needed to determine whether client goals and outcomes have been achieved. Examples of client goals and related outcomes are shown in the accompanying Nursing Care Plan.

If outcomes are not achieved, the nurse, client, and support people, if appropriate, need to explore the reasons before modifying the care plan. Questions such as the following need to be considered:

- How does the client perceive the problem?
- Is there an underlying problem not identified?
- Have new stressors occurred that interfere with successful coping?
- Were existing coping strategies sufficient to meet intended outcomes?
- How does the client perceive the effectiveness of new coping strategies?
- Did the client implement new coping strategies properly?
- Did the client access and use available resources?
- Have family members and significant others provided effective support?

LIFESPAN CONSIDERATIONS Stress and Coping

INFANTS AND CHILDREN

- Children's perceptions of and responses to stress depend on their developmental stage. Infants sense stressors in their environment and respond in a diffuse way, often crying and clinging. Toddlers and preschool-age children may be frightened and react by withdrawing or losing control. School-age children and adolescents are more capable of thinking about incidents that cause stress (e.g., a catastrophic accident) and talking about it with adults.
- Temperament influences how children respond to stress. An outgoing, low-sensitivity child is less likely than a timid, intense child to be upset by a family move to a different state.
- Anxiety disorders are common psychiatric disorders in children but may be unrecognized or misdiagnosed.
- Anxiety disorders may have physiologic causes (e.g., as a result of illness, injury, stuttering) and sociocultural causes (e.g., as a result of interactions with peers or community violence).
- As children grow, they can develop more coping skills to manage stressful situations. Nurses have an important role in teaching parents to recognize stress in their children and to help their children cope.

MIDDLE-AGED ADULTS

- Middle-aged adults are often called the "sandwich generation." They care for children and grandchildren and often care for aging parents at the same time. When these activities become time and energy consuming, there is often not enough time left for attention to self. Nurses need to be aware of this and assist in suggesting resources and effective planning to ease the strain.

OLDER ADULTS

- Older adults experience many losses and changes in their lives. They may be incremental and, over time, become stressful and possibly overwhelming. Changes in health, decreased functional ability and independence, need for relocation, loss of family and friends, and becoming a caregiver for a spouse or friend are a few of the stresses often experienced by older adults. Many have survived significant challenges in their earlier lives and have learned effective coping skills. Nurses can help them plan, evaluate their strategies, and learn new strategies, if needed. Informal and formal social supports are very important in learning to successfully live with these changes and stress.
- Some effective coping methods for older adults are exercise, learning different relaxation techniques, participation in activities, adequate nutrition and rest, and engaging in expressive creative activities, such as art, music, and journaling. Referral to community resources and supports should be done when appropriate. It is most important to see older adults as unique individuals, with unique past experiences and specific needs as they age.

NURSING CARE PLAN Impaired Coping

ASSESSMENT DATA	NURSING DIAGNOSIS	DESIRED OUTCOMES*
NURSING ASSESSMENT Ruby Smithson is a 55-year-old mother of four children who is hospitalized with breast cancer. She is scheduled for a modified radical mastectomy. Ruby was relatively healthy until she found a lump in her right breast 1 week ago. She and her husband are extremely anxious about the surgery. Ruby confides to the admitting nurse that "I can't stand the idea of having one of my breasts cut off; I don't know how I'm going to be able to even look at myself." Mr. Smithson informs the nurse that Ruby has been abusing alcohol since her diagnosis and neglecting her responsibilities as a mother. She is tearful and does not see how she will be able to continue her work as a dress designer. **Physical Examination** Height: 164 cm (5′5″) Weight: 58 kg (128 lb) Temperature: 37°C (98.6°F) Pulse rate: 88 beats/min Respirations: 16/min Blood pressure: 142/88 mmHg **Diagnostic Data** Chest x-ray negative, CBC, and urinalysis within normal limits	Impaired coping related to vulnerability secondary to mastectomy (as evidenced by verbalization of inability to cope, substance abuse, inability to meet role expectations)	Coping [1302], as evidenced by often demonstrating ability to • Identify effective and ineffective coping patterns. • Verbalize sense of control. • Report decrease in negative feelings. • Modify lifestyle as needed. Social Support [1504], as evidenced by substantially adequate • Willingness to call on others for help. • Emotional assistance provided by others.

NURSING INTERVENTIONS*/SELECTED ACTIVITIES	RATIONALE
COPING ENHANCEMENT [5230]	
Provide an atmosphere of acceptance.	Establishing rapport is essential to a therapeutic relationship and supports the client in self-reflection. Recognizing problems and sharing feelings is best brought about in an atmosphere of warmth and trust.
Provide factual information concerning the diagnosis, treatment, and prognosis.	Factual information serves as a foundation for Ruby to explore feelings and alternative coping strategies. Stressed clients often misunderstand facts and require frequent clarification so that appropriate conclusions can be drawn. Having valid information helps relieve stress.

NURSING CARE PLAN Impaired Coping—*continued*

Appraise Ruby's adjustment to changes in body image.	Alteration in body image may be a major issue for Ruby and should be explored to facilitate therapeutic intervention. Coping strategies often change with a reappraisal of the situation.
Arrange situations that encourage her autonomy. Give her as many opportunities as possible to make decisions and choices for herself.	Enhances a sense of control, personal achievement, and self-esteem.
Explore with her previous methods of dealing with life problems.	Present and past coping status assists both Ruby and her husband in capitalizing on successful methods, identifying ineffective strategies, and developing new skills more appropriate to the present situation. Also determines risk for inflicting self-harm.
Encourage verbalization of feelings, perceptions, and fears.	Open, nonthreatening discussions facilitate the identification of causative and contributing factors.
Encourage Ruby to identify her own strengths and abilities.	Assists Ruby to develop appropriate strategies for coping based on personal strengths and previous experiences. Improves self-concept and sense of ability to manage stress.
Encourage Ruby to realistically describe changes in her role.	Individuals experiencing stress may have unrealistic perceptions or reality distortions. Helping Ruby clearly describe her role would be beneficial in developing realistic goals for role achievement.
Foster constructive outlets for anger and hostility.	Assists the client in channeling potentially harmful emotions and physical energy into constructive behavior.
SUPPORT SYSTEM ENHANCEMENT [5440]	
Observe the degree of family support.	Assessing family interaction serves as a basis for identifying Ruby's support systems or lack thereof.
Determine barriers to using support systems.	Although adequate support systems may be available, Ruby may not be using them or may be using them ineffectively.
Involve husband, family, and friends in the care and planning.	Supporting Ruby in acknowledging changes in her appearance conveys acceptance and provides a foundation for her to begin to adjust.
Discuss with concerned others how they can help.	Family and friends are often willing but unsure how to help. Identifying specific strategies such as praise and encouragement during rehabilitation and healing will promote acceptance of change.
Refer Ruby to a community-based breast cancer support group.	Community support is beneficial in helping to meet unresolved needs, decreasing feelings of social isolation, and facilitating a positive self-image.

EVALUATION

The coping outcome was not met. Following surgery, Ruby was withdrawn. During bathing, she would not assist and turned her head away when the dressing was removed. She refused to learn how to manage the wound drain or to discuss her feelings or plans for the future. Because clients having a mastectomy are often only hospitalized for a few days, it may be that she requires more time to reach the desired outcome. Continue to offer information and demonstrate availability for when she is ready to verbalize feelings. Social support outcome partly met. Ruby allows her husband to provide direct care and emotional support for her. A social worker was consulted. Ruby has agreed that the social worker can contact a breast cancer support group and ask the group to call her.

*The NOC # for desired outcomes and the NIC # for nursing interventions are listed in brackets following the appropriate outcome or intervention. Outcomes, indicators, interventions, and activities selected are only a sample of those suggested by NOC and NIC and should be further individualized for each client.

APPLYING CRITICAL THINKING

1. If Ruby had been able to choose a lumpectomy rather than a mastectomy (less visible, smaller, potentially less "meaningful" tissue removal), would the nursing diagnosis and expected outcomes remain the same? Why or why not?
2. Does Ruby's situation reflect more of a stimulus-based model or a response-based model? Why?
3. While working with Ruby, she becomes very angry and says to you, "You don't understand. You've never had to go through this." How would you respond?
4. Based on the preceding evaluation, do you believe that Ruby is in crisis? What factors led to your decision? How does your view change the modifications stated in her care plan?
5. Give one example of how Ruby might use the defense mechanisms described earlier in Table 42.3. Explain whether this is adaptive or maladaptive.

Answers to Applying Critical Thinking questions are available on the faculty resources site. Please consult with your instructor.

CONCEPT MAP

Impaired Coping

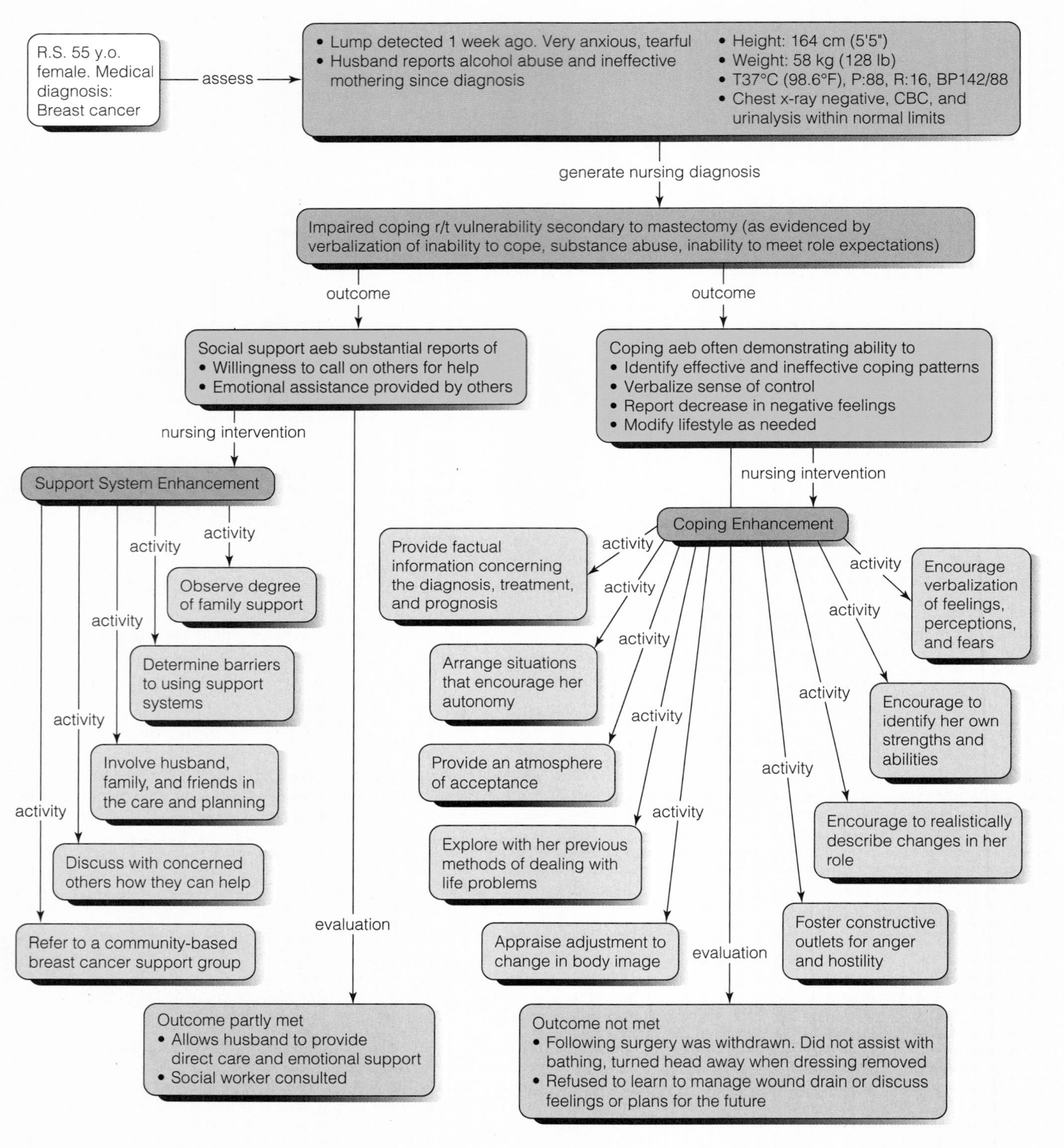

Chapter 42 Review

CHAPTER HIGHLIGHTS

- Stress is a state of physiologic and psychologic tension that affects the whole individual—physically, emotionally, intellectually, socially, and spiritually.
- Models view stress as a stimulus, as a response, or as a transaction.
- General adaptation syndrome (GAS) is a multisystem response to stress and involves three steps: alarm reaction, stage of resistance, and stage of exhaustion.
- Local adaptation syndrome (LAS) is a localized physiologic response that also expresses the three stages of GAS. An example of LAS is the inflammatory response.
- There are physiologic, psychologic, and cognitive indicators of stress. Physiologic indicators result from increased activity of the sympathetic and neuroendocrine systems.
- Common psychologic indicators of stress are anxiety, fear, anger, and depression. Anxiety, the most common response, has four levels: mild, moderate, severe, and panic. Ego defense mechanisms such as denial, rationalization, compensation, and sublimation protect individuals from anxiety.
- Cognitive indicators or thinking responses to stress include problem-solving, structuring, self-control or self-discipline, suppression, and fantasy.
- Coping strategies to deal with stress vary significantly among individuals. Strategies may be problem focused or emotion focused, long term or short term, and effective or ineffective.
- The effectiveness of individual coping depends on the number, duration, and intensity of the stressors; past experience; support systems available; and the personal qualities of the individual.
- Prolonged stress and ineffective coping interfere with the meeting of basic needs and can affect physical and mental health.
- Nursing assessment of a client experiencing stress involves a nursing history to identify perceptions of and duration of stressors and coping strategies and also a physical examination for physical indicators of stress.
- Nursing interventions for clients who are stressed are aimed at encouraging health promotion strategies (exercise, healthy diet, adequate rest, and time management), minimizing anxiety, mediating anger, teaching about specific relaxation techniques, and implementing crisis interventions as needed.
- Because nursing practice involves many stressors related to both clients and the work environment, nurses are susceptible to anxiety and burnout. Like clients, they need to implement stress reduction measures.

TEST YOUR KNOWLEDGE

1. While assessing a client's ability to cope after being diagnosed with a chronic illness, the client admits to an increase in drinking and smoking. Which type of coping strategy does the nurse recognize the client is utilizing?
   1. Short term
   2. Long term
   3. Adaptive
   4. Effective

2. A nurse manager suspects the nursing staff is experiencing burnout because of complaints and an increase in absenteeism. The nurses also appear tired and anxious. What can the manager do to help reduce this burnout?
   1. Ask the physician staff to take over some of the tasks they routinely ask the nurses to do.
   2. Make certain that the nurses are well prepared for their responsibilities.
   3. Assign each nurse to spend 30 minutes with the hospital psychologist daily.
   4. Ask administration to require 30 minutes of exercise at the end of each shift.

3. Two individuals have been in a motor vehicle crash and have similar injuries. According to the transaction-based model, their degree of stress from the crash would be
   1. Based on previous experience and personal characteristics.
   2. Extremely similar since they had the same stimulus.
   3. The identical physiologic alarm reaction.
   4. Different depending on their external resources and support levels.

4. A client informed of a cancer diagnosis assures the nurse he is fine. Which symptom is the most indicative physical evidence to the nurse of the client's stress?
   1. Constricted pupils
   2. Dilated peripheral blood vessels (flush)
   3. Hyperventilation
   4. Decreased heart rate

5. A client repeatedly tells the nurse that "all will be well" and "I'm fine" in response to learning of a health problem that requires immediate surgery. Which of the following diagnoses would the nurse find appropriate for the client at this time?
   1. *Compromised Family Coping*
   2. *Ineffective Coping*
   3. *Disabled Family Coping*
   4. *Defensive Coping*

6. The nurse has recently changed jobs to work with young adults and recognizes that sources of stress common to that population include which of the following? Select all that apply.
   1. Marriage
   2. Aging parents
   3. Starting a new job
   4. Leaving the parental home
   5. Decreased physical abilities
   6. Changing body structure

7. A middle-aged male client is experiencing job-related stress associated with the fear of being laid off, resulting in his accepting projects that require a great deal of travel. Which health promotion strategy would be the most important for this client?
   1. Exercise
   2. Sleep
   3. Nutrition
   4. Time management
8. The first time the nurse enters the client's room, the client is on the phone. Immediately, the client slams down the phone, sweeps everything off the overbed table, and demands that the nurse perform several duties "this very minute." Which of the following would be the most appropriate response for the nurse?
   1. Tell the client "I will return" and then leave the room.
   2. Tell the client no care will be given until the screaming ends.
   3. Begin providing needed care calmly and quietly.
   4. Allow the client to complete venting, then respond calmly.
9. A client newly diagnosed with a chronic condition that will significantly change the client's lifestyle must learn aspects of self-care. The client exhibits severe anxiety: increased blood pressure and pulse, headache, and nervousness. Based on this situation, how would the nurse appropriately plan the teaching?
   1. Recognize that the client's ability to learn is severely impaired and teach only the immediate, critical needs and plan to follow up and reinforce this teaching later.
   2. Recognize that the client's learning will be adaptive and begin immediately to implement the full teaching and learning plan.
   3. Recognize that the client's ability to learn will be slightly impaired and modify the usual teaching strategies to accommodate for this impairment.
   4. Recognize that the client cannot learn at this time, that the level of anxiety must first be reduced, and then teaching can be based on this new level of anxiety.
10. Which of the following defense mechanisms for coping with stress could be effective and constructive? Select all that apply.
   1. Compensation
   2. Displacement
   3. Minimization
   4. Repression
   5. Regression

See Answers to Test Your Knowledge in Appendix A.

READINGS AND REFERENCES

Suggested Reading

Staying calm in turbulent times. (2017). *Harvard Women's Health Watch*, *24*(8), 4–5.

How do you know if you are experiencing everyday anxiety or actually have a disorder? The article explains and suggests simple ways to care for self and relax.

Related Research

Lim, M. H., Rodebaugh, T. L., Gleeson, J. M., Zyphur, M. J., & Gleeson, J. F. (2016). Loneliness over time: The crucial role of social anxiety. *Journal of Abnormal Psychology*, *125*(5), 620–630. doi:10.1037/abn0000162

References

Butcher, H. K., Bulechek, G. M., Dochterman, J. M., & Wagner, C. M. (Eds.). (2018). *Nursing interventions classification (NIC)* (7th ed.). St. Louis, MO: Mosby Elsevier.

Eatough, E. M., & Chang, C. H. (2018). Effective coping with supervisor conflict depends on control: Implications for work strains. *Journal of Occupational Health Psychology*, *23*(4), 537–552. doi:10.1037/ocp0000109

Folkman, S., & Lazarus, R. S. (1991). Coping and emotion. In A. Monat & R. S. Lazarus (Eds.), *Stress and coping* (3rd ed.). New York, NY: Columbia University Press.

Freud, A. (1967). *Das Ich und die Abwehrmechanismen* [The ego and the mechanisms of defense] (Cecil Baines, Trans.) (rev. ed.). Guilford, CT: International Universities Press.

Halter, M. J. (2018). Anxiety and obsessive-compulsive disorders. In M. J. Halter (Ed.), *Varcarolis' foundations of psychiatric-mental health nursing: A clinical approach* (8th ed., Chapter 15). St. Louis, MO: Elsevier

Hartnett, J., Thom, B., & Kline, N. (2016). Caregiver burden in end-stage ovarian cancer. *Clinical Journal of Oncology Nursing*, *20*, 169–173. doi:10.1188/16.CJON.169-173

Holmes, T. H., & Rahe, R. H. (1967). The social readjustment rating scale. *Journal of Psychosomatic Research*, *11*, 213–218. doi:10.1016/0022-3999(67)90010-4

Ienacco, J. D. (2016). Aggression and violence. In M. L. Potter & M. D. Moller, *Psychiatric mental health nursing: From suffering to hope* (pp. 555–576). Boston, MA: Pearson.

Lazarus, R. S. (1966). *Psychological stress and the coping process*. New York, NY: McGraw-Hill.

Lazarus, R. S. (2006). *Stress and emotion: A new synthesis*. New York, NY: Springer.

McMeekin, D. E., Hickman, R. L., Douglas, S. L., & Kelley, C. G. (2017). Stress and coping of critical care nurses after unsuccessful cardiopulmonary resuscitation. *American Journal of Critical Care*, *26*(2), 128–135. doi:10.4037/ajcc2017916

Monat, A., & Lazarus, R. S. (Eds.). (1991). *Stress and coping* (3rd ed.). New York, NY: Columbia University.

Moorhead, S., Johnson, M., Maas, M. L., & Swanson, E. (Eds.). (2018). *Nursing outcomes classification (NOC)* (6th ed.). St. Louis, MO: Mosby Elsevier.

National Institutes of Mental Health. (2017). *Any anxiety disorder among adults*. Retrieved from https://www.nimh.nih.gov/health/statistics/prevalence/any-anxiety-disorder-among-adults.shtml

Potter, M. L. (2016). Disorders of anxiety, stress, and trauma. In M. L. Potter & M. D. Moller, *Psychiatric mental health nursing: From suffering to hope* (pp. 240–272). Boston, MA: Pearson.

Selye, H. (1956). *The stress of life*. New York, NY: McGraw-Hill.

Selye, H. (1976). *The stress of life* (rev. ed.). New York, NY: McGraw-Hill.

U.S. Department of Health and Human Services. (2018). *Physical activity guidelines: Adults*. Retrieved from https://health.gov/paguidelines/guidelines/adults.aspx

Selected Bibliography

Aydogan, U., Doganer, Y. C., Komurcu, S., Ozturk, B., Ozet, A., & Saglam, K. (2016). Coping attitudes of cancer patients and their caregivers and quality of life of caregivers. *Indian Journal of Palliative Care*, *22*, 150–156. doi:10.4103/0973-1075.179598

Bellingham, K. (2016). Chronic stress: A major driver of "disease." *Journal of the Australian Traditional-Medicine Society*, *22*(3), 177.

D'Amico, D., & Barbarito, C. (2016). *Health & physical assessment in nursing* (3rd ed.). Boston, MA: Pearson.

Jaruzel, C. B., & Gregoski, M. J. (2017). Instruments to measure preoperative acute situational anxiety: An integrative review. *AANA Journal*, *85*(1), 31–35.

Mychailyszyn, M. P. (2017). "Cool" youth: A systematic review and comprehensive meta-analytic synthesis of data from the Cool Kids family of intervention programs. *Canadian Psychology*, *58*(2), 105–115. doi:10.1037/cap0000101

Naragon-Gainey, K., Prenoveau, J. M., Brown, T. A., & Zinbarg, R. E. (2016). A comparison and integration of structural models of depression and anxiety in a clinical sample: Support for and validation of the tri-level model. *Journal of Abnormal Psychology*, *125*(7), 853–867. doi:10.1037/abn0000197

Nyatanga, B. (2016). Death anxiety and palliative nursing. *British Journal of Community Nursing*, *21*, 636. doi:10.12968/bjcn.2016.21.12.636

Stock, E. (2017). Exploring salutogenesis as a concept of health and wellbeing in nurses who thrive professionally. *British Journal of Nursing*, *26*(4), 238–241. doi:10.12968/bjon.2017.26.4.238

Williams, L. A., Wicks, M. N., Graff, J. C., Cowan, P. A., White-Means, S., Caldwell, L. D., & Tolley, E. A. (2016). Male caregivers of persons with end stage renal disease: A literature review. *Nephrology Nursing Journal*, *43*(6), 495–519.

Loss, Grieving, and Death 43

LEARNING OUTCOMES

After completing this chapter, you will be able to:

1. Describe types and sources of losses.
2. Discuss selected frameworks for identifying stages of grieving.
3. Identify clinical symptoms of grief.
4. Discuss factors affecting a grief response.
5. Identify measures that facilitate the grieving process.
6. List clinical signs of impending and actual death.
7. Describe the process of helping clients die with dignity.
8. Describe the role of the nurse in working with families or caregivers of dying clients.
9. Describe nursing measures for care of the body after death.

KEY TERMS

actual loss, *1085*
algor mortis, *1101*
anticipatory grief, *1086*
anticipatory loss, *1086*
bereavement, *1086*
cerebral death, *1094*
closed awareness, *1096*
complicated grief, *1086*
end-of-life care, *1099*
grief, *1086*
heart-lung death, *1094*
higher brain death, *1094*
hospice, *1098*
livor mortis, *1101*
loss, *1085*
mortician, *1101*
mourning, *1086*
mutual pretense, *1096*
open awareness, *1096*
palliative care, *1099*
perceived loss, *1085*
persistent vegetative state (PVS), *1094*
rigor mortis, *1100*
shroud, *1101*
undertaker, *1101*

Introduction

Everyone experiences loss, grieving, and death during his or her life. Individuals may suffer the loss of valued relationships through life changes, such as moving from one city to another; separation or divorce; or the death of a parent, spouse, or friend. Individuals may grieve changing life roles as they watch grown children leave home or they retire from their lifelong work. Losing valued material objects through theft or natural disaster can evoke feelings of grief and loss. When individuals' lives are affected by civil or national violence, they may grieve the loss of valued ideals such as safety, freedom, or democracy.

In the clinical setting, the nurse encounters clients who may experience grief related to declining health, loss of a body part, terminal illness, or the impending death of self or a significant other. The nurse may also work with clients in community settings who are grieving losses related to a personal crisis (e.g., divorce, separation, financial loss) or disaster (war, earthquakes, or terrorism). Therefore, it is important for the nurse to understand the significance of loss and develop the ability to assist clients as they work through the grieving process.

Nurses may interact with dying clients and their families or caregivers in a variety of settings, from a fetal demise (death of an unborn child), to the adolescent victim of an accident, to the older client who finally succumbs to a chronic illness. Nurses must recognize the influences on the dying process—legal, ethical, spiritual, biological, psychologic—and be prepared to provide sensitive, skilled, and supportive care to all those affected.

Loss and Grief

Loss is an actual or potential situation in which something that is valued is changed or no longer available. Individuals can experience the loss of body image, a significant other, a sense of well-being, a job, personal possessions, or beliefs. Illness and hospitalization often produce losses.

Death is a loss both for the dying individual and for those who survive. Although death is inevitable, it can stimulate individuals to grow in their understanding of themselves and others. Individuals experiencing loss often search for the meaning of the event, and it is generally accepted that finding meaning is needed in order for healing to occur. However, individuals can be well adjusted without searching for meaning, and even those who find meaning may not see it as an end point but rather as an ongoing process.

Types and Sources of Loss

There are two general types of loss, actual and perceived. An **actual loss** can be recognized by others. A **perceived loss** is experienced by an individual but cannot be verified by others. Psychologic losses are often perceived losses because they are not directly verifiable. For example, a woman who leaves her employment to care for her children at home may perceive a loss of independence and freedom. Both losses can be anticipatory. An **anticipatory loss** is experienced before the loss actually occurs. For example, a woman whose husband is dying may experience actual loss in anticipation of his death.

Loss can be viewed as situational or developmental. Losing one's job, the death of a child, and losing functional ability because of acute illness or injury are situational losses. Losses that occur in normal development—such as the departure of grown children from the home, retirement from a career, and the death of aged parents—are developmental losses that can, to some extent, be anticipated and prepared for.

There are many sources of loss: (a) loss of an aspect of oneself—a body part, a physiologic function, or a psychologic attribute; (b) loss of an object external to oneself; (c) separation from an accustomed environment; and (d) loss of a loved or valued individual.

Aspect of Self

Losing an aspect of self changes an individual's body image, even though the loss may not be obvious. A face scarred from a burn is generally obvious; loss of part of the stomach or loss of the ability to feel emotion may not be as obvious. The degree to which these losses affect an individual largely depends on the integrity of the individual's body image.

During old age, changes occur in physical and mental capabilities. Again the self-image is vulnerable. Old age is the stage when people may experience many losses: of employment, of usual activities, of independence, of health, of friends, and of family.

External Objects

Loss of external objects includes (a) loss of inanimate objects that have importance to the individual, such as losing money or the burning down of a family's house; and (b) loss of animate (live) objects such as pets that provide love and companionship.

Familiar Environment

Separation from an environment and individuals who provide security can cause a sense of loss. The 6-year-old is likely to feel loss when first leaving the home environment to attend school. Immigrants who leave their country to settle down in another also experience loss and helplessness in the form of culture shock (Arredondo-Dowd, 1981; Henry, Stiles & Biran, 2005).

Loved Ones

Losing a loved one or valued individual through illness, divorce, separation, or death can be very disturbing. In some illnesses (such as Alzheimer's disease), an individual may undergo personality changes that make friends and family feel they have lost that individual.

Grief, Bereavement, and Mourning

Grief is the total response to the emotional experience related to loss. Grief is manifested in thoughts, feelings, and behaviors associated with overwhelming distress or sorrow. **Bereavement** is the subjective response experienced by the surviving loved ones. **Mourning** is the behavioral process through which grief is eventually resolved or altered; it is often influenced by culture, spiritual beliefs, and custom. Grief and mourning are experienced not only by the individual who faces the death of a loved one but also by the individual who suffers other kinds of losses. Grieving permits the individual to cope with the loss gradually and to accept it as part of reality. Grief is a social process; it is best shared and carried out with the assistance of others.

Working through one's grief is important because bereavement may have potentially devastating effects on health. Among the symptoms that can accompany grief are anxiety, depression, weight loss, difficulties in swallowing, vomiting, fatigue, headaches, dizziness, fainting, blurred vision, skin rashes, excessive sweating, menstrual disturbances, palpitations, chest pain, and dyspnea. The grieving and the bereaved may experience alterations in libido, concentration, and patterns of eating, sleeping, activity, and communication.

Although bereavement can threaten health, a positive resolution of the grieving process can enrich the individual with new insights, values, challenges, openness, and sensitivity. For some, the pain of loss, though diminished, recurs for the rest of their lives.

Types of Grief Responses

A normal grief reaction may be abbreviated or anticipatory. Abbreviated grief is brief but genuinely felt. This can occur when the lost object is not significantly important to the grieving individual or may have been replaced immediately by another, equally esteemed object. **Anticipatory grief** is experienced in advance of the event such as the wife who grieves before her ailing husband dies. A young individual may grieve before an operation that will leave a scar. Because many of the normal symptoms of grief will have already been expressed in anticipation, the reaction when the loss actually occurs is sometimes quite abbreviated.

Disenfranchised grief occurs when an individual is unable to acknowledge the loss to others. Situations in which this may occur often relate to a socially unacceptable loss that cannot be spoken about, such as suicide, abortion, or giving a child up for adoption. Other examples include losses of relationships that are socially unsanctioned and may not be known to others (such as with extramarital relationships).

Unhealthy grief—that is, pathologic or **complicated grief**—exists when the strategies to cope with the loss are maladaptive and out of proportion or inconsistent with cultural, religious, or age-appropriate norms.

The disorder, referred to by physicians as *persistent complex bereavement disorder*, may be said to exist if the preoccupation lasts for more than 12 months and leads to reduced ability to function normally (Boelen, Lenferink, Nickerson, & Smid, 2018). Many factors can contribute to complicated grief, including a prior traumatic loss, family or cultural barriers to the emotional expression of grief, sudden death, strained relationships between the survivor and the deceased, and lack of adequate support for the survivor.

Complicated grief may take several forms. *Unresolved* or *chronic grief* is extended in length and severity. The same signs are expressed as with normal grief, but the bereaved may also have difficulty expressing the grief, may deny the loss, or may grieve beyond the expected time. With *inhibited grief*, many of the normal symptoms of grief are suppressed and other effects, including physiologic, are experienced instead. *Delayed grief* occurs when feelings are purposely or subconsciously suppressed until a much later time. A survivor who appears to be using dangerous activities as a method to lessen the pain of grieving may experience *exaggerated grief*.

Complicated grief after a death may be inferred from the following data or observations:

- The client fails to grieve; for example, a husband does not cry at, or absents himself from, his wife's funeral.
- The client avoids visiting the grave and refuses to participate in memorial services, even though these practices are a part of the client's culture.
- The client develops persistent guilt and lowered self-esteem.
- Even after a prolonged period, the client continues to search for the lost loved one. Some may consider suicide to affect reunion.
- After the normal period of grief, the client experiences physical symptoms similar to those of the individual who died.
- The client's relationships with friends and relatives worsen following the death.

Many factors contribute to unresolved grief after a death:

- Ambivalence (intense feelings, both positive and negative) toward the lost individual
- A perceived need to be brave and in control; fear of losing control in front of others
- Endurance of multiple losses, such as losing an entire family, which the bereaved finds too overwhelming to contemplate
- Extremely high emotional value invested in the dead individual; failure to grieve in this instance helps the bereaved avoid the reality of the loss
- Uncertainty about the loss—for example, when a loved one is "missing in action"
- Lack of support systems.

Stages of Grieving

Many authors have described stages or phases of grieving, perhaps the most well known of them being Kübler-Ross (1969), who described five stages: denial, anger, bargaining, depression, and acceptance (Table 43.1). Engel (1964) identified six stages of grieving: shock and disbelief,

TABLE 43.1 Client Responses and Nursing Implications in Kübler-Ross's Stages of Grieving

Stage	Behavioral Responses	Nursing Implications
Denial	Refuses to believe that loss is happening. Is unready to deal with practical problems, such as prosthesis after the loss of a leg. May assume artificial cheerfulness to prolong denial.	Verbally support client but do not reinforce denial. Examine your own behavior to ensure that you do not share in client's denial.
Anger	Client or family may direct anger at nurse or staff about matters that normally would not bother them.	Help client understand that anger is a normal response to feelings of loss and powerlessness. Avoid withdrawal or retaliation; do not take anger personally. Deal with needs underlying any angry reaction. Provide structure and continuity to promote feelings of security. Allow clients as much control as possible over their lives.
Bargaining	Seeks to bargain to avoid loss (e.g., "let me just live until [a certain time] and then I will be ready to die").	Listen attentively, and encourage client to talk to relieve guilt and irrational fear. If appropriate, offer spiritual support.
Depression	Grieves over what has happened and what cannot be. May talk freely (e.g., reviewing past losses such as money or job), or may withdraw.	Allow client to express sadness. Communicate nonverbally by sitting quietly without expecting conversation. Convey caring by touch.
Acceptance	Comes to terms with loss. May have decreased interest in surroundings and support people. May wish to begin making plans (e.g., will, prosthesis, altered living arrangements).	Help family and friends understand client's decreased need to socialize. Encourage client to participate as much as possible in the treatment program.

TABLE 43.2 Engel's Stages of Grieving

Stage	Behavioral Responses
Shock and disbelief	Refuses to accept loss. Has stunned feelings. Accepts the situation intellectually, but denies it emotionally.
Developing awareness	Reality of loss begins to penetrate consciousness. Anger may be directed at agency, nurses, or others.
Restitution	Conducts rituals of mourning (e.g., funeral).
Resolving the loss	Attempts to deal with painful void. Still unable to accept new love object to replace lost person or object. May accept more dependent relationship with support person. Thinks over and talks about memories of the lost object.
Idealization	Produces image of lost object that is almost devoid of undesirable features. Represses all negative and hostile feelings toward lost object. May feel guilty and remorseful about past inconsiderate or unkind acts to lost person. Unconsciously internalizes admired qualities of lost object. Reminders of lost object evoke fewer feelings of sadness. Reinvests feelings in others.
Outcome	Behavior influenced by several factors: importance of lost object as source of support, degree of dependence on relationship, degree of ambivalence toward lost object, number and nature of other relationships, and number and nature of previous grief experiences (which tend to be cumulative).

From "Grief and Grieving," by G. L. Engel, 1964, *American Journal of Nursing*, *64*(9), pp. 93–98. Adapted with permission.

developing awareness, restitution, resolving the loss, idealization, and outcome (Table 43.2). Sanders (1998) described five phases of bereavement: shock, awareness of loss, conservation/withdrawal, healing, and renewal (Table 43.3).

Whether an individual can integrate the loss and how this is accomplished are related to that individual's development, personality, and emotional preparedness. In addition, individuals responding to the very same loss cannot be expected to follow the same pattern or schedule in resolving their grief, even while they support each other.

Manifestations of Grief

The nurse assesses the grieving client or family members following a loss to determine the phase or stage of grieving. Physiologically, the body responds to a current or anticipated loss with a stress reaction. The nurse can assess the clinical signs of this response (see Chapter 42 ∞).

Manifestations of grief considered normal include verbalization of the loss, crying, sleep disturbance, loss of appetite, and difficulty concentrating. Complicated grieving may be characterized by extended time of denial, depression, severe physiologic symptoms, or suicidal thoughts.

Factors Influencing the Loss and Grief Responses

Several factors affect an individual's response to a loss or death. These factors include age, significance of the loss, culture, spiritual beliefs, gender, socioeconomic status, support systems, and the cause of the loss or death. Nurses can learn general concepts about the influence of these factors on the grieving experience, but the constellation of these factors and their significance will vary from client to client.

Age

Age affects an individual's understanding of and reaction to loss. With familiarity, individuals usually increase their understanding and acceptance of life, loss, and death.

Individuals rarely experience the loss of loved ones at regular intervals. As a result, preparation for these experiences is difficult. Other life losses, such as losing a pet, a friend, youth, or a job, can help individuals anticipate the more severe loss of death of loved ones by teaching them successful coping strategies.

CHILDHOOD

Children differ from adults not only in their understanding of loss and death but also in how they are affected by losing others. Losing a parent or other significant individual can threaten the child's ability to develop, and regression sometimes results. Assisting the child with the grief experience includes helping the child regain the normal continuity and pace of emotional development.

Some adults may assume that children do not have the same need as an adult to grieve the loss of others. In situations of crisis and loss, children are sometimes pushed aside or protected from the pain. They can feel afraid, abandoned, and lonely. Careful work with bereaved children is especially necessary because experiencing a loss in childhood can have serious effects later in life (Figure 43.1 ■).

EARLY AND MIDDLE ADULTHOOD

As individuals grow, they come to experience loss as part of normal development. By middle age, for example, the loss of a parent through death seems a more normal occurrence compared to the death of a younger individual. Coping with the death of an aged parent has even been viewed as an essential developmental task of the middle-aged adult.

TABLE 43.3 Sander's Phases of Bereavement

Phase	Description	Behavioral Responses
Shock	Survivors are left with feelings of confusion, unreality, and disbelief that the loss has occurred. They are often unable to process normal thought sequences. Phase may last from a few minutes to many days.	Disbelief Confusion Restlessness Feelings of unreality Regression and helplessness State of alarm Physical symptoms: dryness of mouth and throat, sighing, weeping, loss of muscular control, uncontrolled trembling, sleep disturbance, loss of appetite Psychologic symptoms: egocentric phenomenon, preoccupation with thoughts of the deceased, psychologic distancing
Awareness of loss	Friends and family resume normal activities. The bereaved experience the full significance of their loss.	Separation anxiety Conflicts Acting out emotional expectations Prolonged stress Physical symptoms: yearning, anger, guilt, frustration, shame, crying, sleep disturbance, fear of death Psychologic symptoms: oversensitivity, disbelief and denial, dreaming, sense of presence of the deceased
Conservation/withdrawal	During this phase, survivors feel a need to be alone to conserve and replenish both physical and emotional energy. The social support available to the bereaved has decreased, and they may experience despair and helplessness.	Withdrawal Despair Diminished social support Helplessness Physical symptoms: weakness, fatigue, need for more sleep, a weakened immune system Psychologic symptoms: hibernation or holding pattern, obsessional review, grief work, turning point
Healing: the turning point	During this phase, the bereaved move from distress about living without their loved one to learning to live more independently.	Assuming control Identity restructuring Relinquishing roles, such as spouse, child, or parent Physical symptoms: increased energy, sleep restoration, immune system restoration, physical healing Psychologic symptoms: forgiving, forgetting, searching for meaning, closing of the circle, hope
Renewal	In this phase, survivors move on to a new self-awareness, an acceptance of responsibility for self, and learning to live without the loved one.	New self-awareness Acceptance of responsibility Process of learning to live without Physical symptoms: functional stability, revitalization, caring for physical needs Assumption of responsibility for self-care needs Psychologic symptoms: living for oneself, loneliness, anniversary reactions, reaching out to others, time for the process of bereavement

From *Grief: The Mourning After: Dealing with Adult Bereavement*, 2nd ed., by Catherine M. Sanders, 1999, New York, NY: John Wiley & Sons, Inc.

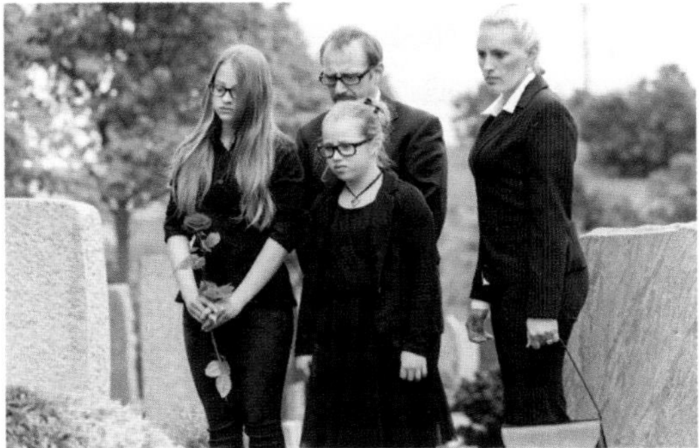

Figure 43.1 ■ Children experience the same emotions of grief as adults.
Kzenon/123RF.

The middle-aged adult can experience losses other than death. For example, losses resulting from impaired health or body function and losses of various role functions can be difficult for the middle-aged adult. How the middle-aged adult responds to such losses is influenced by previous experiences with loss, the individual's sense of self-esteem, and the strength and availability of support.

LATE ADULTHOOD

Losses experienced by older adults include loss of health, mobility, independence, and work role. Limited income and the need to change one's living accommodations can also lead to feelings of loss and grieving.

For older adults, the loss through death of a longtime mate is profound. Although individuals differ in their ability to deal with such a loss, some research suggests that health problems for widows decrease and health problems of widowers increase following the death of the spouse (Trevisan et al., 2016). This may be because the widows are relieved of the stresses of caring for their spouse while the widowers have lost the care provided by their spouse, although this would vary depending on culture and gender norms.

Because the majority of deaths occur among older adults, and because the number of older adults is increasing in North America, nurses will need to be especially alert to the potential problems of older grieving adults. These problems may intensify because the very old grieving individual may have children who, themselves, are older and possibly unwell. Some older adults no longer have living peer support people and the nurse may need to fill some of that role.

Significance of the Loss

The significance of a loss depends on the perceptions of the individual experiencing the loss. One individual may experience a great sense of loss over a divorce; another may find it only mildly disrupting. Several factors affect the significance of the loss:

- Importance of the lost individual, object, or function
- Degree of change required because of the loss
- The individual's beliefs and values.

For older adults who have already encountered many losses, an anticipated loss such as their own death may not be viewed as highly negative, and they may be apathetic about it instead of reactive. More than fearing death, some may fear loss of control or becoming a burden.

Culture

Culture influences an individual's reaction to loss. How grief is expressed is often determined by the customs of the culture. Unless an extended family structure exists, grief is handled by the nuclear family. The death of a family member in a typical nuclear family leaves a great void because the same few individuals fill most of the roles. In cultures where several generations and extended family members either reside in the same household or are physically close, the impact of a family member's death may be softened because the roles of the deceased are quickly filled by other relatives.

Some individuals believe that grief is a private matter to be endured internally. Therefore, feelings tend to be repressed and may remain unidentified. Individuals socialized to "be strong" and "make the best of the situation" may not express deep feelings or personal concerns when they experience a serious loss.

Some cultural groups value social support and the expression of loss. In some groups, expressions of grief through wailing, crying, physical prostration, and other outward demonstrations are acceptable and encouraged. Other groups may frown on this demonstration as a loss of control, favoring a more quiet and stoic expression of grief. In cultural groups where strong kinship ties are maintained, physical and emotional support and assistance are provided by family members.

Spiritual Beliefs

Spiritual beliefs and practices greatly influence both an individual's reaction to loss and subsequent behavior. Most religious groups have practices related to dying, and these are often important to the client and support people. To provide support at a time of death, nurses need to understand the client's particular beliefs and practices (see Chapter 41 ∞).

Gender

The gender roles into which many individuals are socialized in the United States affect their reactions at times of loss. Males are frequently expected to "be strong" and show very little emotion during grief, whereas it is acceptable for females to show grief by crying. When a wife dies, the husband, who is the chief mourner, may be expected to repress his own emotions and to comfort sons and daughters in their grieving.

Gender roles also affect the significance of body image changes to clients. A man might consider his facial scar to be "macho," but a woman might consider hers ugly. Thus the woman, but not the man, would see the change as a loss.

Socioeconomic Status

The socioeconomic status of an individual often affects the support system available at the time of a loss. A pension plan or insurance, for example, can offer an individual who is widowed or disabled a choice of ways to deal with a loss; an individual who is confronted with both severe loss and economic hardship may not be able to cope with either.

Support System

The individuals closest to the grieving individual are often the first to recognize and provide needed emotional, physical, and functional assistance. However, because many individuals are uncomfortable or inexperienced in dealing with losses, the usual support people may instead withdraw from the grieving individual. In addition, support may be available when the loss is first recognized, but as the support people return to their usual activities, the need for ongoing support may be unmet. Sometimes, the grieving individual is unable or unready to accept support when offered.

Cause of Loss or Death

Individual and societal views on the cause of a loss or death may significantly influence the grief response. Some diseases are considered "clean," such as cardiovascular disorders, and engender compassion, whereas others may be viewed as repulsive and less unfortunate. A loss or death beyond the control of those involved may be more acceptable than one that is preventable, such as a drunk driving incident. Injuries or deaths that occur during respected activities, such as "in the line of duty," are considered honorable, whereas those occurring during illicit activities may be considered the individual's just rewards.

●○● NURSING MANAGEMENT

Assessing

Nursing assessment of the client experiencing a loss includes three major components: (1) nursing history, (2) assessment of personal coping resources, and (3) physical assessment. During the routine health assessment of every client, the nurse poses questions regarding previous and current losses. The nature of the loss and the significance of such losses to the client must be explored.

If there is a current or recent loss, greater detail is needed in the assessment. Because clients do not always associate physical ailments with emotional responses such as grief, the nurse may need to probe to identify possible loss-related stresses. If the client reports significant losses, examine how the client usually copes with loss and what resources are available to assist the client in coping. Data regarding general health status; other personal stressors; cultural and spiritual traditions, rituals, and beliefs related to loss and grieving; and the client's support network will be needed to determine a plan of care (see the Assessment Interview). In assessing the client's response to a current loss, the nurse may identify complicated grief, which is best treated by a healthcare professional expert in assisting such clients. If the nursing assessment reveals severe physical or psychologic signs and symptoms, the client should be referred to an appropriate care provider.

Diagnosing

Examples of nursing diagnoses that may be appropriate for clients who have problems related to death, loss, and bereavement are grief and potential for complicated grief.

Planning

The overall goals for clients grieving the loss of body function or a body part are to adjust to the changed ability and to redirect both physical and emotional energy into rehabilitation. The goals for clients grieving the loss of a loved one or thing are to remember them without feeling intense pain and to redirect emotional energy into one's own life and adjust to the actual or impending loss.

Planning for Home Care

Clients who have sustained or anticipate a loss may require ongoing nursing care to assist them in adapting to the loss. Determining how much and what type of home care follow-up is needed is based in great part on the nurse's knowledge of how the client and family have coped with previous losses. To prepare for home care, the nurse reassesses the client's abilities and needs.

QSEN Patient-Centered Care: Grieving

CLIENT AND FAMILY: ASSESS

- ***Knowledge:*** understanding of the implications of the loss
- ***Self-care abilities:*** skill in caring for self and the client, based on any physical abilities that may have been altered by the loss
- ***Current coping:*** stage in the grieving or bereavement process
- ***Current manifestations of the grief response:*** adaptive or maladaptive signs and symptoms; cultural or spiritually based behaviors
- ***Role expectations:*** perception of the need to return to work or family roles
- ***Support people's availability and skills:*** sensitivity to the client's emotional and physical needs; ability to provide an accepting environment

COMMUNITY: ASSESS

- ***Resources:*** availability and familiarity with possible sources of assistance such as grief support groups, religious or spiritual centers, counseling services, physical care providers

ASSESSMENT INTERVIEW Loss and Grieving

PREVIOUS LOSS

- Have you ever lost someone or something very important to you?
- Have you or your family ever moved to a new home or location?
- What was it like for you when you first started school? Moved away from home? Got a job? Retired?
- Are you physically able to do all the things you used to do?
- Has anyone important or close to you died?
- Do you think there will be any losses in your life in the near future?

If there has been previous grieving:

- Tell me about [the loss]. What was losing like for you?
- Did you have trouble sleeping? Eating? Concentrating?
- What kinds of things did you do to make yourself feel better when something like that happened?
- Did you observe any spiritual or cultural practices when you had a loss like that?
- Whom did you turn to if you were very upset about [the loss]?
- How long did it take you to feel more like yourself again and go back to your usual activities?

CURRENT LOSS

- What have you been told about [the loss]? Is there anything else you would like to know or don't understand?
- What changes do you think this [illness, surgery, problem] will cause in your life? What do you think it will be like without [the lost object]?
- Have you ever experienced a loss like this before?
- Can you think of anything good that might come out of this?
- What kind of help do you think you will need? Who is going to be helping you with this loss?
- Are there any organizations in your community that might be able to help?

If there is current grieving:

- Are you having trouble sleeping? Eating? Concentrating? Breathing?
- Do you have any pain or other new physical problems?
- What are you doing to help you deal with this loss?
- Are you taking any drugs or medications to help you cope with this loss?

Implementing

Besides providing physical comfort, maintaining privacy and dignity, and promoting independence, the skills most relevant to situations of loss and grief are those of effective communication: attentive listening, silence, open and closed questioning, paraphrasing, clarifying and reflecting feelings, and summarizing. Less helpful to clients are responses that give advice and evaluation, those that interpret and analyze, and those that give unwarranted reassurance. Communication with grieving clients must relate to their stage of grief. Whether the client is angry or depressed affects how the client hears messages and how the nurse interprets the client's statements.

Besides using effective communication skills, the nurse implements a plan to provide client and family teaching and to help the client work through the stages of grief.

Facilitating Grief Work

- Explore and respect the client's and family's ethnic, cultural, religious, and personal values in their expressions of grief.
- Teach the client or family what to expect in the grief process, such as that certain thoughts and feelings are normal (acceptable) and that labile emotions, feelings of sadness, guilt, anger, fear, and loneliness, will stabilize or lessen over time. Knowing what to expect may lessen the intensity of some reactions.
- Encourage the client to express and share grief with support people. Sharing feelings reinforces relationships and facilitates the grief process.
- Teach family members to encourage the client's expression of grief, not to push the client to move on or enforce his or her own expectations of appropriate reactions. If the client is a child, encourage family members to be truthful and to allow the child to participate in the grieving activities of others.
- Encourage the client to resume normal activities on a schedule that promotes physical and psychologic health. Some clients may try to return to normal activities too quickly. However, a prolonged delay in return may indicate complicated grieving.

Providing Emotional Support

- Use silence and personal presence along with techniques of therapeutic communication. These techniques enhance exploration of feelings and let clients know that the nurse acknowledges their feelings.
- Acknowledge the grief of the client's family and significant others. Family support persons are part of the grieving client's world.
- Offer choices that promote client autonomy. Clients need to have a sense of some control over their own lives at a time when much control may not be possible.
- Provide information regarding how to access community resources: clergy, support groups, and counseling services.
- Suggest additional sources of information and help such as:
  a. Bereavement Network Europe
  b. Hong Kong Family Welfare Society
  c. Australian Centre for Grief and Bereavement
  d. National Hospice and Palliative Care Organization.

Examples of nursing actions appropriate for clients in various stages of the grief process are shown in the Concept Map on page 1102.

Evaluating

Evaluating the effectiveness of nursing care of the grieving client is difficult because of the long-term nature of the life transition. Criteria for evaluation must be based on goals set by the client and family.

Client goals and related desired outcomes for a grieving client will depend on the characteristics of the loss and the client. If outcomes are not achieved, the nurse needs to explore why the plan was unsuccessful. Such exploration begins with reassessing the client in case the nursing diagnoses were inappropriate. Examples of questions guiding the exploration include these:

- Do the client's grieving behaviors indicate dysfunctional grieving or another nursing diagnosis?
- Is the expected outcome unrealistic for the given time frame?
- Does the client have additional stressors previously not considered that are affecting grief resolution?
- Have nursing orders been implemented consistently, compassionately, and genuinely?

Dying and Death

The concept of death is developed over time, as the individual grows, experiences various losses, and thinks about concrete and abstract concepts. In general, humans move from a childhood belief in death as a temporary state, to adulthood in which death is accepted as very real but also very frightening, to older adulthood in which death may be viewed as more desirable than living with a poor quality of life. Table 43.4 describes some of the specific beliefs common to different age groups. The nurse's knowledge of these developmental stages helps in understanding some of the client's responses to a life-threatening situation.

Responses to Dying and Death

The reaction of any individual to another individual's impending or real death, or to the potential reality of his or her own death, depends on all the factors regarding loss and the development of the concept of death. In spite of the individual variations in clients' views about the cause of death, spiritual beliefs, availability of support systems, or any other factor, responses tend to cluster in the phases described by theorists (see Tables 43.1 to 43.3).

Both the client who is dying and the family members grieve as they recognize the loss. Signs and symptoms for the nursing diagnosis of grieving include denial, guilt,

TABLE 43.4 Development of the Concept of Death

Age	Beliefs and Attitudes
Infancy–5 years	Does not understand the concept of death. Infant's sense of separation forms basis for later understanding of loss and death. Believes death is reversible, a temporary departure, or sleep. Emphasizes immobility and inactivity as attributes of death.
5–9 years	Understands that death is final. Believes own death can be avoided. Associates death with aggression or violence. Believes wishes or unrelated actions can be responsible for death.
9–12 years	Understands death as the inevitable end of life. Begins to understand own mortality, expressed as interest in afterlife or as fear of death.
12–18 years	Fears a lingering death. May fantasize that death can be defied, acting out defiance through reckless behaviors (e.g., dangerous driving, substance abuse). Seldom thinks about death, but views it in religious and philosophic terms. May seem to reach "adult" perception of death but be emotionally unable to accept it. May still hold concepts from previous developmental stages.
18–45 years	Has attitude toward death influenced by religious and cultural beliefs.
45–65 years	Accepts own mortality. Encounters death of parents and some peers. Experiences peaks of death anxiety. Death anxiety diminishes with emotional well-being.
65+ years	Fears prolonged illness. Encounters death of family members and peers. Sees death as having multiple meanings (e.g., freedom from pain, reunion with already deceased family members).

Clinical Alert!

Individuals may use a variety of terms instead of the word *died*. Serious examples include *passed away*, *gone to a better place*, *lost*, or *free from suffering*. Humorous examples include *bought the farm*, *kicked the bucket*, or *croaked*.

anger, despair, feelings of worthlessness, crying, and inability to concentrate. They may extend to thoughts of suicide, delusions, and hallucinations. Fear, the feeling of disruption related to an identifiable source (in this case someone's death), may also be present. Many of the characteristics seen in a fearful individual are similar to those of grieving and include crying, immobility, increased pulse and respirations, dry mouth, anorexia, difficulty sleeping, and nightmares. Hopelessness occurs when the individual perceives no solutions to a problem—when the death becomes inevitable and the individual cannot see how to move beyond the death. The nurse may observe apathy, pessimism, and inability to decide. An individual who perceives a solution to the problem but does not believe that it is possible to implement the solution may be said to experience powerlessness. This loss of control may be manifested by anger, violence, acting out, or depression and passive behavior.

Caregivers, both professionals and support people, also respond to the impending death. The ongoing responsibilities for providing physical, economic, psychologic, and social support to a dying client can create extreme stress for the provider. Often, the time between a terminal diagnosis and when death will occur is unknown and those supporting the dying client become fatigued and depressed. There may be anger due to loss of time and resources for personal activities or attention to others. Within a family that usually functions effectively, death of a member may cause alterations in usual family processes. In this situation, the family may be unable to meet the physical, emotional, or spiritual needs of the members and may have difficulty communicating and problem-solving.

Professional caregivers, including nurses, may experience stress due to repeated interactions with dying clients and their families. Although most nurses who work in oncology, hospice, intensive care, emergency, or other areas where client deaths are common have chosen such assignments, there can still be a sense of failure when clients die. Just as there must be support systems for grieving clients, there must also be support systems for grieving healthcare professionals.

Some individuals may think of death as the worst occurrence in life and do their best to avoid thinking or talking about death—especially their own. Nurses are not immune to such attitudes. Nurses who are uncomfortable with dying clients tend to impede the clients' attempts to discuss dying and death in these ways:

- Change the subject (e.g., "Let's think of something more cheerful" or "You shouldn't say things like that").
- Offer false reassurance (e.g., "You are doing very well").
- Deny what is happening (e.g., "You don't really mean that" or "You're going to live until you're a hundred").
- Be fatalistic (e.g., "Everyone dies sooner or later" or "What's meant to be, will be").
- Block discussion (e.g., "I don't think things are really that bad") and convey an attitude that stops further discussion of the subject.

- Be aloof and distant or avoid the client.
- "Manage" the client's care and make the client feel increasingly dependent and powerless.

Caring for the dying and the bereaved is one of the nurse's most complex and challenging responsibilities, bringing into play all the skills needed for holistic physiologic and psychosocial care. The American Nurses Association position statement *Nurses' Roles and Responsibilities in Providing Care and Support at the End of Life* (2016) states that the nurse must demonstrate competence and compassion, communication with families, and collaboration with other members of the healthcare team to provide symptom management and support, and develop realistic plans of decision-making and care that reflect the client and family wishes. To be effective, nurses must confront their own attitudes toward loss, death, and dying, because these attitudes will directly affect their ability to provide care.

Definitions of Death

The traditional clinical signs of death were cessation of the apical pulse, respirations, and blood pressure, also referred to as **heart-lung death**. However, since the advent of artificial means to maintain respirations and blood circulation, identifying death is more difficult. Another definition of death is **cerebral death** or **higher brain death**, which occurs when the higher brain center, the cerebral cortex, is irreversibly destroyed.

Responding to requests from a number of countries to provide guidance on the formation of leading practices and health policies that determine the definition of death, the WHO and the Transplantation Society held a forum, the focus of which was to discuss death as a biological event. The legal, ethical, cultural, and religious aspects surrounding death were not considered by the members of the forum as they strictly based the debate on those scientific and medical aspects of death that could be observed and measured. After careful deliberation, the forum concluded that for death to occur, a person must have a permanent loss of the ability to use all brainstem function and a permanent incapacity for consciousness. These events may arise from the permanent ceasing of circulation or from major brain injury. In their definition of death, the WHO (2012) used the word permanent to describe a state in which the loss of function cannot be reversed on its own or restored via external intervention. This definition was not guided by terms such as brain death or cardiac death, which could incorrectly imply the death of that particular organ. Instead, participants considered the cessation of neurological and circulatory functions to determine the definition of death.

In cases where artificial life support is used, these recommendations should guide doctors on when to withdraw treatment. However, the forum agreed that their report should be the basis for further discussions in the future about this topic.

These definitions of death are differentiated from a **persistant vegetative state (PVS)** in which the client has lost cognitive function and awareness but respiration and circulation remain. Clients in a PVS may have a variety of facial, eye, and limb movements but do not interact purposefully with their environment. Depending on the cause of the PVS, some clients may recover partially or completely.

Death-Related Religious and Cultural Practices

Cultural and religious traditions and practices associated with death, dying, and the grieving process help clients cope with these experiences. Nurses are often present through the dying process and at the moment of death. Knowledge of the client's religious and cultural heritage helps nurses provide individualized care to clients and their families, even though they may not participate in the rituals associated with death.

Some individuals prefer a peaceful death at home rather than in the hospital. Members of certain ethnic groups may request that health professionals not reveal the prognosis to dying clients. They believe the individual's last days should be free of worry. Other cultures prefer that a family member (preferably a male in some cultures) be told the diagnosis so the client can be tactfully informed by a family member in gradual stages or not be told at all. Nurses also need to determine whom to call, and when, as the impending death draws near.

Beliefs and attitudes about death, its cause, and the soul also vary among cultures. Unnatural deaths, or "bad deaths," are sometimes distinguished from "good deaths." In addition, the death of an individual who has behaved well in life may be less threatening based on the belief that the individual will be reincarnated into a good life or go to heaven.

Beliefs about preparation of the body, autopsy, organ donation, cremation, and prolonging life are closely allied to the client's religion. Autopsy, for example, may be prohibited, opposed, or discouraged by Eastern Orthodox religions, Muslims, Jehovah's Witnesses, and Orthodox Jews. Some groups, such as Hindus, may oppose autopsy based on not wanting non-Hindus to touch the body. Some religions prohibit the removal of body parts or dictate that all body parts be given appropriate burial. Organ donation is prohibited by Jehovah's Witnesses, whereas Buddhists in America consider it an act of mercy and encourage it. Cremation is discouraged, opposed, or prohibited by the Baha'i, Mormon, Eastern Orthodox, Islamic, and Roman Catholic faiths. Hindus, in contrast, prefer cremation and cast the ashes in a holy river. Some religions, such as Christian Science, are unlikely to recommend medical means to prolong life, and the Jewish faith generally opposes prolonging life after irreversible brain damage. In hopeless illness, Buddhists may permit euthanasia.

Nurses also need to be knowledgeable about the client's death-related rituals, such as last rites (Figure 43.2 ■), chanting at the bedside, and other practices, such as special procedures for washing, dressing, positioning, shrouding, and attending the dead. Certain cultures retain their native customs in which family members of the same sex wash and prepare the body for burial and cremation. Muslims also customarily turn the body toward Mecca. In several religions, the body cannot be left unattended

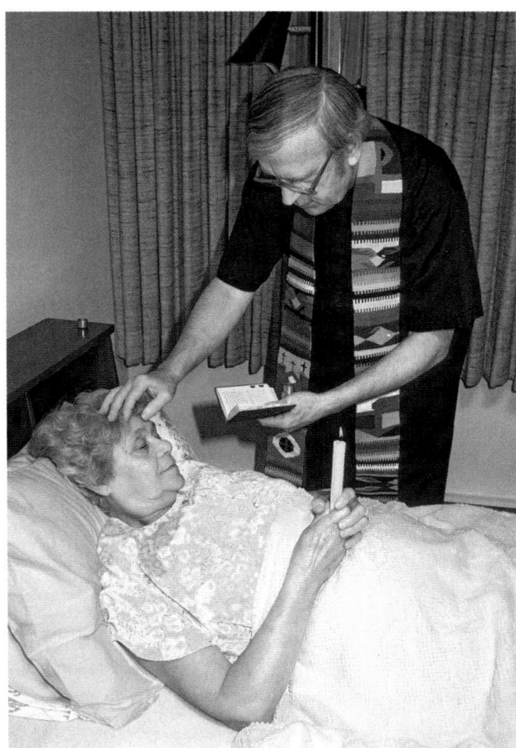

Figure 43.2 ■ Catholic clients may request last rites or the sacrament of anointing the sick.
Dennis MacDonald/Alamy Stock Photo.

while awaiting burial and individuals may be hired to sit with the body if family members do not perform this duty. Nurses need to ask family members about their preference and verify who will carry out these activities if performed at the healthcare facility. The nurse must ensure that any ritual items present in the healthcare agency are returned to the family or to the funeral home.

Death-Related Legal Issues

Laws that describe issues involving decisions about death and dying are constantly changing. These include advance directives, do not resuscitate, organ donation, and aid in dying. Nurses must remain knowledgeable about the legal issues and engage with the healthcare team to advocate for clients.

Advance Healthcare Directives

In the United States, federal law requires healthcare providers to determine clients' end-of-life care wishes by inquiring if the individual has an advance healthcare directive (see Chapter 3 ∞). This document describes preferences for future treatment, whether or not the client is currently unwell. The client specifies one or more individuals who will serve as their proxy (substitute) in making healthcare decisions should they be unable to do so. Although the majority of Americans state that it is important to have their end-of-life wishes written down, only about 27% have actually done so, and only 11% have discussed their wishes with their healthcare provider (Hamel, Wu, & Brodie, 2017b).

For individuals already diagnosed with serious, progressive, or chronic illnesses, almost every U.S. state has an additional document known as the Physician Orders for Life-Sustaining Treatment (POLST). The POLST is signed by both the client or healthcare decision maker and the primary care provider (physician, physician assistant, or nurse practitioner), and specifies current preferences for resuscitation; medical interventions such as comfort measures, intravenous medications, and noninvasive airway support; and artificial nutrition and hydration. This document remains with the client when transferred to different levels of care, including to the home, or is available in an electronic registry. The advantage of the POLST over an advance directive is that, because it is an order signed by a healthcare provider, physicians, first responders, hospitals, emergency departments, and others are compelled to follow it (Stuart, Volandes, & Moulton, 2017). However, it does not allow for a proxy to be specified. Thus, clients may wish to have both an advance directive and a POLST.

Do-Not-Resuscitate Orders

Do-not-resuscitate orders, also referred to as DNR, no code blue, no code, allow natural death (AND), and similar terms, refer to the documentation of the decision to refrain from cardiopulmonary resuscitation (CPR) should the client's heart or breathing cease from an irreversible underlying condition (also see Chapter 3 ∞). The decision should be made with the client and family, when possible, and always reflect the competent client's wishes. DNR is not the same as "do nothing" and decisions to withhold or withdraw treatment are separate from DNR decisions.

Organ Donation

Both in the U.S. and countries in the EU, the law allows competent adults to pre-authorize the donation of their organs for research, education, or transplantation. In the case of brain death, most organs continue to function normally for some time, although the client may require a ventilator to control respiratory function.

There are two main approaches to organ donation: presumed consent and explicit consent. In countries that follow the explicit consent system, such as the Netherlands, no one is considered a donor unless they voluntarily 'opt-in' to become one. However, in the presumed consent system, everyone is considered a donor unless they officially 'opt-out' of the system.

There have been debates on whether the opt-out approach is a better method than the opt-in approach (Willis & Quigley, 2014) since the former tends to yield a higher percentage of organ donors. For example, Austria, which follows the opt-out system, has a consent rate of 99.98% (Johnson & Goldstein, 2003; Thaler, 2009).

In countries such as India, organs and tissues of a person declared legally dead can be donated after permission from the family is attained. The rate of deceased organ donation is around 0.34 per million population, which is very low. To mitigate this shortage, an opt-out system for organ donation has been suggested by several medical experts (Kaushik, 2009). Nevertheless, this may not improve deceased organ donation rates because of the lack of public awareness in India. (Nagar, 2019).

Whichever approach a country decides to take, the nurse should act as an educator. In countries, where there could be resistance in consenting to organ donation, the nurse is duty bound to explain the benefits of organ donation and transplantation, clearly state what happens to the organ donor in case of death, and encourage the public to consider organ donation after their death. The nurse should also be supportive in the case where relatives of a deceased person are asked to give consent for organ donation. Here, the nurse should take into consideration the devastation and grief that the family is going through and guide them to make the best decision without pushing them to give consent.

Euthanasia, Aid in Dying

Increasing numbers of U.S. states are implementing regulations that allow for medical assistance in dying (MAID), also known as physician-assisted death, end-of-life options, or death with dignity acts. These statutes are very explicit in delineating who is eligible for this assistance and the process for applying, being approved, and implementing. MAID, in which the individual self-administers a lethal dose of medications, is not the same as active euthanasia, in which the lethal dose is administered to the individual by a physician. In some countries, both MAID and active euthanasia are illegal, while in others, one or both may be legal (ProCon.org, 2016).

Each of these death-related legal issues is complex and is best implemented by a team consisting of individuals with substantial expertise and experience with the issue. Nurses need to remain informed on changes in legislation that may affect their practice but also engage in discussions regarding the ethical aspects of the issues.

●○● NURSING MANAGEMENT

Assessing

To gather a complete database that allows accurate analysis and identification of appropriate nursing diagnoses for dying clients and their families, the nurse first needs to recognize the states of awareness manifested by the client and family members.

In cases of terminal illness, the state of awareness shared by the dying client and the family affects the nurse's ability to communicate freely with clients and other healthcare team members and to assist in the grieving process. Three types of awareness that have been described are closed awareness, mutual pretense, and open awareness (Glaser & Strauss, 1965).

In **closed awareness**, the client is not made aware of impending death. The family may choose this because they do not completely understand why the client is ill or they believe the client will recover. The primary care provider may believe it is best not to communicate a diagnosis or prognosis to the client. Nursing personnel may experience an ethical problem in this situation. See Chapter 4 ∞ for further information on ethical dilemmas.

With **mutual pretense**, the client, family, and healthcare personnel know that the prognosis is terminal but do not talk about it and make an effort not to raise the subject. Sometimes the client refrains from discussing death to protect the family from distress. The client may also sense discomfort on the part of healthcare personnel and therefore not bring up the subject. Mutual pretense permits the client a degree of privacy and dignity, but it places a heavy burden on the dying client, who then has no one in whom to confide.

With **open awareness**, the client and others know about the impending death and feel comfortable discussing it, even though it is difficult. This awareness provides the client an opportunity to finalize affairs and even participate in planning funeral arrangements.

Not all individuals are comfortable with open awareness. Some believe that terminal clients acquire knowledge of their condition even if they are not directly informed. Others believe that clients remain unaware of their condition until the end. It is difficult, however, to distinguish what clients know from what they will accept or acknowledge.

Nursing care and support for the dying client and family include making an accurate assessment of the physiologic signs of approaching death. Besides signs related to the client's specific disease, certain other physical signs indicate impending death. The four main characteristic changes are loss of muscle tone, slowing of the circulation, changes in respirations, and sensory impairment. Box 43.1 lists indications of impending clinical death.

BOX 43.1 Signs of Impending Clinical Death

LOSS OF MUSCLE TONE

- Relaxation of the facial muscles (e.g., the jaw may sag)
- Difficulty speaking
- Difficulty swallowing and gradual loss of the gag reflex
- Decreased activity of the gastrointestinal tract, with subsequent nausea, accumulation of flatus, abdominal distention, and retention of feces, especially if narcotics or tranquilizers are being administered
- Possible urinary and rectal incontinence due to decreased sphincter control
- Diminished body movement

SLOWING OF THE CIRCULATION

- Diminished sensation
- Mottling and cyanosis of the extremities
- Cold skin, first in the feet and later in the hands, ears, and nose (the client, however, may feel warm if there is a fever)
- Slower and weaker pulse
- Decreased blood pressure

CHANGES IN RESPIRATIONS

- Rapid, shallow, irregular, or abnormally slow respirations
- Noisy breathing, referred to as the death rattle, due to collecting of mucus in the throat
- Mouth breathing, dry oral mucous membranes

SENSORY IMPAIRMENT

- Blurred vision
- Impaired senses of taste and smell

Various levels of consciousness may exist just before death. Some clients are alert, whereas others are drowsy, stuporous, or comatose. Hearing is thought to be the last sense lost.

As death approaches, the nurse assists the family and other significant individuals to prepare. Depending in part on knowledge of the client's state of awareness, the nurse asks questions that help identify ways to provide support during the period before and after death. In particular, the nurse needs to know what the family expects to happen when the client dies so accurate information can be given at the appropriate depth. See the Assessment Interview for sample interview questions. When the family members know what to expect, they may better support the dying client and others who are grieving. In addition, they may make certain decisions about events surrounding the death such as whether they will want to view the body after death.

Diagnosing

A range of nursing diagnoses, addressing both physiologic and psychosocial needs, can apply to the dying client, depending on the assessment data. Diagnoses that may be particularly appropriate for the dying client are fear, hopelessness, and powerlessness. In addition, caregiver stress and alterations in family processes are common diagnoses for caregivers and family members.

Planning

Major goals for dying clients are (a) maintaining physiologic and psychologic comfort and (b) achieving a dignified and peaceful death, which includes maintaining personal control and accepting declining health status. Many clinical agencies and organizations have created documents that describe the dying client's rights. When planning care for dying clients, these guides can be useful guides.

Planning for Home Care

Clients facing death may need help accepting that they have to depend on others. Some dying clients require only minimal care; others need continuous attention and services. Clients need help, well in advance of death, in planning for the period of dependence. They need to consider what will happen and how and where they would like to die.

In a survey of 4000 Americans, Brazilians, Italians, and Japanese, 55–71% of adults stated they wished to die at home, although only about one-half of those believed that they would die there (Hamel, Wu, & Brodie, 2017a). A major factor in determining whether an individual will die in a healthcare facility or at home is the availability of willing and able caregivers. If the dying client wishes to be at home, and family or others can provide care to maintain symptom control, the nurse should facilitate a referral to outpatient hospice services. Hospice staff and nurses will then conduct a full assessment of the home and care providers' skills.

Implementing

The major nursing responsibility for clients who are dying is to assist the client to a peaceful death. More specific responsibilities include the following:

- To minimize loneliness, fear, and depression
- To maintain the client's sense of security, self-confidence, dignity, and self-worth
- To help the client accept losses
- To provide physical comfort.

Helping Clients Die with Dignity

Nurses need to ensure that the client is treated with dignity, that is, with honor and respect. Dying clients often feel they have lost control over their lives and over life itself. Helping clients die with dignity involves maintaining their humanity, consistent with their values, beliefs, and culture. By introducing options available to the client and significant others, nurses can restore and support feelings of control. Some choices that clients can make are the location of care (e.g., hospital, home, or hospice facility), times of appointments with health professionals, activity schedule, use of health resources, and times of visits from relatives and friends.

Clients want to manage the events preceding death so they can die peacefully. Nurses can help clients to determine their own physical, psychologic, and social priorities. Dying individuals often strive for self-fulfillment more than for self-preservation, and may need to find meaning in continuing to live if suffering. Part of the nurse's challenge is to support the client's will and hope.

Although it is natural for individuals to be uncomfortable discussing death, steps can be taken to make such discussions easier for both the nurse and the client. Strategies include the following:

- Identify your personal feelings about death and how they may influence interactions with clients. Acknowledge personal fears about death, and discuss them with a friend or colleague.
- Focus on the client's needs. The client's fears and beliefs may differ from the nurse's. It is important for the nurse to avoid imposing personal fears and beliefs on the client or family.
- Talk to the client or family members about how the client usually copes with stress. Clients typically use their usual coping strategies for dealing with impending death.

ASSESSMENT INTERVIEW The Family of the Dying Client

Ask the spouse, partner, or significant others:

- Have you ever been in a similar situation?
- Would you like to discuss what may happen if and when your loved one passes away?
- Would you like to ask me anything about the situation?
- Would you like me to call someone who can stay with you at this time to support you?
- Would you like to eat or drink something while waiting?
- Is there anything else I can do for you to help you at this time?

For example, if they are usually quiet and reflective, they may become more quiet and withdrawn when facing terminal illness.

- Establish a communication relationship that shows concern for and commitment to the client. Communication strategies that let the client know you are available to talk about death include the following:
  a. Describe what you see, for example, "You seem sad. Would you like to talk about what's happening to you?"
  b. Clarify your concern, for example, "I'd like to know better how you feel and how I may help you."
  c. Acknowledge the client's struggle, for example, "It must be difficult to feel so uncomfortable. I would like to help you be more comfortable."
  d. Provide a caring touch. Holding the client's hand or offering a comforting massage can encourage the client to verbalize feelings.
- Determine what the client knows about the illness and prognosis.
- Respond with honesty and directness to the client's questions about death.
- Make time to be available to the client to provide support, listen, and respond.

Hospice and Palliative Care

The hospice movement was founded by the physician Cecily Saunders in London, England, in 1967. **Hospice** care focuses on support and care of the dying client with a life expectancy of 6 months or less and the family, with the goal of facilitating a peaceful and dignified death. Hospice care is based on holistic concepts and emphasizes team-based care to improve quality of life rather than cure, support the client and family through the dying process, and support the family through bereavement. Assessing the needs of the client's family is just as important as caring for the client who is receiving hospice care (Figure 43.3 ■). The condition of the client usually deteriorates, and attention needs to be focused on the caregivers to ensure that they are receiving support and resources as these changes occur. If the hospice team meets regularly, these needs can be discussed and interventions initiated. Physical needs are usually apparent, but emotional and behavioral signs are often more subtle. A good assessment and ongoing evaluation can help indicate when modifications or changes are needed.

The principles of hospice care can be carried out in a variety of settings, the most common being the home, the hospital, or a nursing home–based unit. Services focus on symptom control and pain management. Commonly, clients are eligible for hospice care or hospice insurance benefits when certified by a physician to be likely to die within 6 months. Hospice care is always provided by a team of both health professionals and nonprofessionals to ensure a full range of care services. The National Hospice and Palliative Care Organization (2018) reports that more than 1.43 million Medicare beneficiaries access hospice services each year, representing approximately 48% of all Medicare deaths. Contrary to popular belief, only about 28% of hospice clients are diagnosed with cancer. The top noncancer primary diagnoses for those admitted to hospice are cardiac and circulatory disease, dementia, and respiratory disease.

More than 18,000 nursing personnel in the United States are nationally certified in one or more of the seven hospice and palliative care programs (Hospice and Palliative Credentialing Center, 2019).

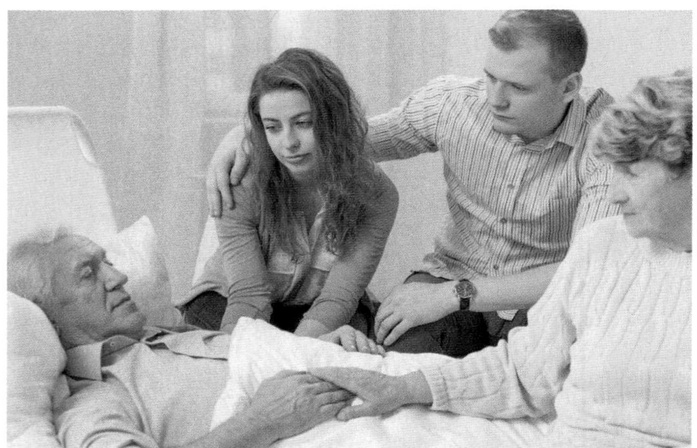

Figure 43.3 ■ Family members may be closely involved in both physical and psychologic support of the dying.
Katarzyna Białasiewicz/123RF.

EVIDENCE-BASED PRACTICE

Evidence-Based Practice

What Is the Impact of Palliative Care Consultation Services?

Evidence-Based Practice

In some geographical areas, inpatient hospice bed space is very limited. One solution to this problem is to provide palliative care consultative services (PCCS). In this study, PCCS from a team of physicians, nurses, social workers, psychologists, and chaplains was provided to 1369 hospital cancer patients in Taiwan over a 6-year period (Wu, Chu, Chen, Ho, & Pan, 2016). Of this number, about half died in the hospital, one-fourth were discharged, and one-fourth were transferred to a hospice unit. The group who died were statistically older, male, and more likely to have lung or liver cancer. Almost half of those who died already had a DNR order when PCCS began. The patients transferred to the hospice ward tended to have greater pain, constipation, dyspnea, nausea, vomiting, and delirium.

IMPLICATIONS

The authors of this report state the limitations of the study but also the benefits of heightened awareness of the characteristics of the three groups of patients and the outcomes of their care. In order to advocate for palliative and end-of-life support, nurses need to establish which groups or characteristics of clients will benefit from specific services. Studies such as these are needed because the availability of resources is limited.

Palliative care is described by the World Health Organization (n.d.) as:

> an approach that improves the quality of life of patients and their families facing the problem associated with life-threatening illness, through the prevention and relief of suffering by means of early identification and impeccable assessment and treatment of pain and other problems, physical, psychosocial and spiritual. Palliative care:
>
> - provides relief from pain and other distressing symptoms;
> - affirms life and regards dying as a normal process;
> - intends neither to hasten nor postpone death;
> - integrates the psychological and spiritual aspects of patient care;
> - offers a support system to help patients live as actively as possible until death;
> - offers a support system to help the family cope during the patient's illness and in their own bereavement;
> - uses a team approach to address the needs of patients and their families, including bereavement counselling, if indicated;
> - will enhance quality of life, and may also positively influence the course of illness;
> - is applicable early in the course of illness, in conjunction with other therapies that are intended to prolong life, such as chemotherapy or radiation therapy, and includes those investigations needed to better understand and manage distressing clinical complications. (para. 1)

Palliative care "attends to the physical, functional, psychologic, practical, and spiritual consequences of a serious illness. It is a person- and family-centered approach to care, providing seriously ill people relief from the symptoms and stress of an illness. Through early integration into the care plan of seriously ill people, palliative care improves quality of life for both the patient and the family" (National Consensus Project for Quality Palliative Care, 2018, p. i). This care may differ from hospice because the client is not necessarily believed to be imminently dying. Both hospice and palliative care can include **end-of-life care**, that is, the care provided in the final weeks before death.

Meeting the Physiologic Needs of the Dying Client

The physiologic needs of clients who are dying are related to a slowing of body processes and to homeostatic imbalances. Interventions include providing personal hygiene measures; controlling pain; relieving respiratory difficulties; assisting with movement, nutrition, hydration, and elimination; and providing measures related to sensory changes (Table 43.5).

TABLE 43.5 Physiologic Needs of Dying Clients

Problem	Nursing Care
Airway clearance	Fowler position: conscious clients Throat suctioning: conscious clients Lateral position: unconscious clients Nasal oxygen for hypoxic clients Anticholinergic medications may be indicated to help dry secretions
Air hunger	Open windows or use a fan to circulate air Morphine may be indicated in an acute episode
Bathing and hygiene	Frequent baths and linen changes if diaphoretic Mouth care as needed for dry mouth Liberal use of moisturizing creams and lotions for dry skin Moisture-barrier skin preparations for incontinent clients
Physical mobility	Assist client out of bed periodically, if able Regularly change client's position Support client's position with pillows, blanket rolls, or towels as needed Elevate client's legs when sitting up Implement pressure injury prevention program and use pressure-relieving surfaces as indicated
Nutrition	Antiemetics or a small amount of an alcoholic beverage to stimulate appetite Encourage liquid foods as tolerated
Constipation	Dietary fiber as tolerated Stool softeners or laxatives as needed
Urinary elimination	Skin care in response to incontinence of urine or feces Bedpan, urinal, or commode chair within easy reach Call light within reach for assistance onto bedpan or commode Absorbent pads placed under incontinent client; linen changed as often as needed Catheterization, if necessary Keep room as clean and odor free as possible
Sensory and perceptual changes	Check preference for light or dark room Hearing is not diminished; speak clearly and do not whisper Touch is diminished, but client will feel pressure of touch Implement pain management protocol if indicated

Pain control is essential to enable clients to maintain some quality in their life and their daily activities, including eating, moving, and sleeping. Many drugs have been used to control the pain associated with terminal illness: morphine, heroin, methadone, and alcohol. Usually the primary care provider determines the dosage, but the client's opinion should be considered; the client is the one ultimately aware of personal pain tolerance and fluctuations of internal states. Because primary care providers usually prescribe dosage ranges for pain medication, nurses use their own judgment on the amount and frequency of pain medication in providing client relief. Because of decreased blood circulation, if analgesics cannot be administered orally, they are given topically, by intravenous infusion, sublingually, or rectally, rather than subcutaneously or intramuscularly. Clients on narcotic pain medications also require implementation of a protocol to treat opioid-induced constipation. See Chapter 30 ∞ for more on pain management.

Providing Spiritual Support

Spiritual support is of great importance in dealing with death. Although not all clients identify with a specific religious faith or belief, most have a need for meaning in their lives, particularly as they experience a terminal illness.

The nurse has a responsibility to ensure that the client's spiritual needs are attended to, either through direct intervention or by arranging access to individuals who can provide spiritual care. Nurses need to be aware of their own comfort with spiritual issues and be clear about their own ability to interact supportively with the client. Nurses have an ethical and moral responsibility to not impose their own religious or spiritual beliefs on a client but to respond to the client in relation to the client's own background and needs. Communication skills are most important in helping the client articulate needs and in developing a sense of caring and trust.

Interventions may include facilitating expressions of feeling, prayer, meditation, reading, and discussion with clergy or a spiritual adviser. It is important for nurses to establish an effective interdisciplinary relationship with spiritual support specialists. For a further discussion of spiritual issues, see Chapter 41 ∞.

Supporting the Family

The most important aspects of providing support to the family members of a dying client involve using therapeutic communication to facilitate their expression of feelings. When nothing can reverse the inevitable dying process, the nurse can provide an empathetic and caring presence. The nurse also serves as a teacher, explaining what is happening and what the family can expect. Due to the stress of moving through the grieving process, family members may not absorb what they are told and may need to have information provided repeatedly. The nurse must have a calm and patient demeanor.

Clinical Alert!

Individuals who have experienced the deaths of multiple individuals in their lives, such as members of the AIDS community, those serving in war zones, or victims of natural disasters, do not necessarily feel the loss or grieve any more or less than those who have experienced fewer deaths.

Family members should be encouraged to participate in the physical care of the dying client as much as they wish to and are able. The nurse can suggest they assist with bathing, speak or read to the client, and hold hands. The nurse must not, however, have specific expectations for family members' participation. The dying and the family must be allowed as much privacy as they desire in order to meet their needs for physical and emotional intimacy. Those who feel unable to care for or be with the dying client also require support from the nurse and from other family members. They should be shown an appropriate waiting area if they wish to remain nearby.

Sometimes, it seems as if the client is "holding on," possibly out of concern for the family not being ready for the client to die. It may be therapeutic for both the client and the family for the family to verbally give permission to the client to "let go," to die when he or she is ready. This is a painful process, and the nurse must be prepared to encourage and support the family through saying their last good-byes.

After the client dies, the family should be encouraged to view the body (with or without a nurse present or after preparation by the funeral home), because this has been shown to facilitate the grieving process. They may wish to clip a lock of hair as a remembrance. Children should be included in the events surrounding the death if they wish to. If the family was not present prior to the death, they may have questions about events surrounding the final hours that the nurse should answer sensitively and honestly.

Clinical Alert!

Even when the client appears unresponsive, the nurse must always provide high-quality care. Though the client is dying, and actions may seem futile, the client deserves respect and appropriate interventions. Nurses do not provide *less* care to dying clients, just *different* care.

Postmortem Care

Rigor mortis is the stiffening of the body that occurs about 2 to 4 hours after death. Rigor mortis starts in the involuntary muscles (heart, bladder, and so on), then progresses to the head, neck, and trunk, and finally reaches the extremities.

Because the deceased's family often wants to view the body, and because it is important that the deceased appear natural and comfortable, nurses need to place the body in an anatomic position, place dentures in the mouth, and close the eyes and mouth before rigor mortis sets in. Rigor mortis usually leaves the body about 96 hours after death.

Algor mortis is the gradual decrease of the body's temperature after death. When blood circulation terminates and the hypothalamus ceases to function, body temperature falls about 1°C (1.8°F) per hour until it reaches room temperature. Simultaneously, the skin loses its elasticity and can easily be broken when removing dressings and adhesive tape.

After blood circulation has ceased, the red blood cells break down, releasing hemoglobin, which discolors the surrounding tissues. This discoloration, referred to as **livor mortis**, appears in the lowermost or dependent areas of the body.

Tissues after death become soft and eventually liquefied by bacterial fermentation. The hotter the temperature, the more rapid the change. Therefore, bodies are often stored in cool places to delay this process. Embalming prevents the process through injection of chemicals into the body to destroy the bacteria.

Nursing personnel may be responsible for care of a body after death. Postmortem care should be carried out according to the policy of the hospital or agency. Because care of the body may be influenced by religious law, the nurse should check the client's religion and make every attempt to comply. If the deceased's family or friends wish to view the body, make the environment clean and pleasant and make the body appear natural and comfortable. All equipment, soiled linen, and supplies should be removed from the bedside. Some agencies require that all tubes in the body remain in place; in other agencies, tubes may be cut to within 2.5 cm (1 in.) of the skin and taped in place; in others, all tubes may be removed.

Normally the body is placed in a supine position with the arms either at the sides, palms down, or across the abdomen. One pillow is placed under the head and shoulders to prevent blood from discoloring the face by settling in it. The eyelids are closed and held in place for a few seconds so they remain closed. Dentures are usually inserted to help give the face a natural appearance. The mouth is then closed.

Soiled areas of the body are washed; however, a complete bath is not necessary, because the body will be washed by the **mortician** (also referred to as an **undertaker**), a professional trained in care of the dead. Absorbent pads are placed under the buttocks to take up any feces and urine released because of relaxation of the sphincter muscles. A clean gown is placed on the client, and the hair is arranged. All jewelry is removed, except a wedding band in some instances, which is taped to the finger. The top bed linens are adjusted neatly to cover the client to the shoulders. Soft lighting and chairs are provided for the family.

In the hospital, after the body has been viewed by the family, the deceased's wrist identification tag is left on and additional identification tags are applied. The body is wrapped in a **shroud**, a large piece of plastic or cotton material used to enclose a body after death. Identification is then applied to the outside of the shroud. The body is taken to the morgue if arrangements have not been made to have a mortician pick it up from the client's room. Nurses have a duty to handle the deceased with dignity and to label the corpse appropriately. Mishandling can cause emotional distress to survivors. Mislabeling can create legal problems if the body is inappropriately identified and prepared incorrectly for burial or a funeral.

Evaluating

To evaluate the achievement of client goals, the nurse collects data in accordance with the desired outcomes established in the planning phase. Evaluation activities may include the following:

- Listening to the client's reports of feeling in control of the environment surrounding death, such as control over pain relief, visitation of family and support people, or treatment plans
- Observing the client's relationship with significant others
- Listening to the client's thoughts and feelings related to hopelessness or powerlessness.

Some of the special needs of older adults and their families during death and dying are found in Lifespan Considerations.

LIFESPAN CONSIDERATIONS Responses to Death

CHILDREN

- Children's response to death or loss depends on the messages they get from adults and others around them as well as their understanding of death. When adults are able to cope effectively with a death, they are more likely to be able to support children through the process.
- As children develop, they will "reprocess" their grieving around a loss or death. Preschoolers who have lost a parent, for example, often reconceptualize their understanding of that loss when they reach school age and adolescence and have greater cognitive and emotional skills. The same process occurs with parents who have lost a child to death; as the years pass and the child "would have been in first grade," for example, parents must cope with the added dimensions of the loss.

OLDER ADULTS

Older adults who are dying often have a need to know that their lives had meaning. An excellent way to assure them of this is to make recordings of them telling stories of their lives. This gives the client a sense of value and worth and also lets him or her know that family members and friends will also benefit from it. Doing this with children and grandchildren often eases communication and support during this difficult time.

Caregivers need ongoing support and teaching as the dying client's condition changes. Some of these needs are teaching:

- Ways to feed the client when swallowing becomes difficult
- Ways to transfer and reposition the client safely
- Ways to communicate if verbalization becomes more difficult
- Nonpharmacologic methods of pain control
- Comfort measures, such as frequent oral care and frequent repositioning
- When and whom to call if the client's condition changes.

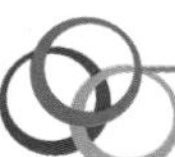

Critical Thinking Checkpoint

Mrs. Govinda, 75, was admitted to the hospital after repeated episodes of pneumonia. Despite aggressive antibiotic therapy, her condition rapidly deteriorated and she died unexpectedly 1 week after being admitted to the hospital. Mrs. Govinda's oldest son, who lived nearby and frequently cared for his mother, arranged for the funeral and visited with relatives. He misses his mother and cries occasionally but managed to return to work the following week. The youngest son had difficulty attending the funeral, has been unable to sleep or eat, cannot concentrate at work, and cannot believe that his mother is dead. The middle son did not weep at the funeral and had little to say to his brothers or other relatives. He returned home to another state but has remained distant. He is back to work but feels very fatigued and apathetic.

1. From the data provided, describe the phase of bereavement being experienced by each of the three surviving sons.
2. What factors may have affected how each of the sons reacted to the death of their mother?
3. What cues, other than physical signs, might have indicated that Mrs. Govinda was dying, even though her death was unexpected?
4. With the diagnosis of pneumonia, a respiratory infection, what physiologic (palliative) needs might she have had?
5. How might your own feelings about death affect the care you provide to the dying client?

Answers to Critical Thinking Checkpoint questions are available on the faculty resources site. Please consult with your instructor.

CONCEPT MAP

The Grieving Client

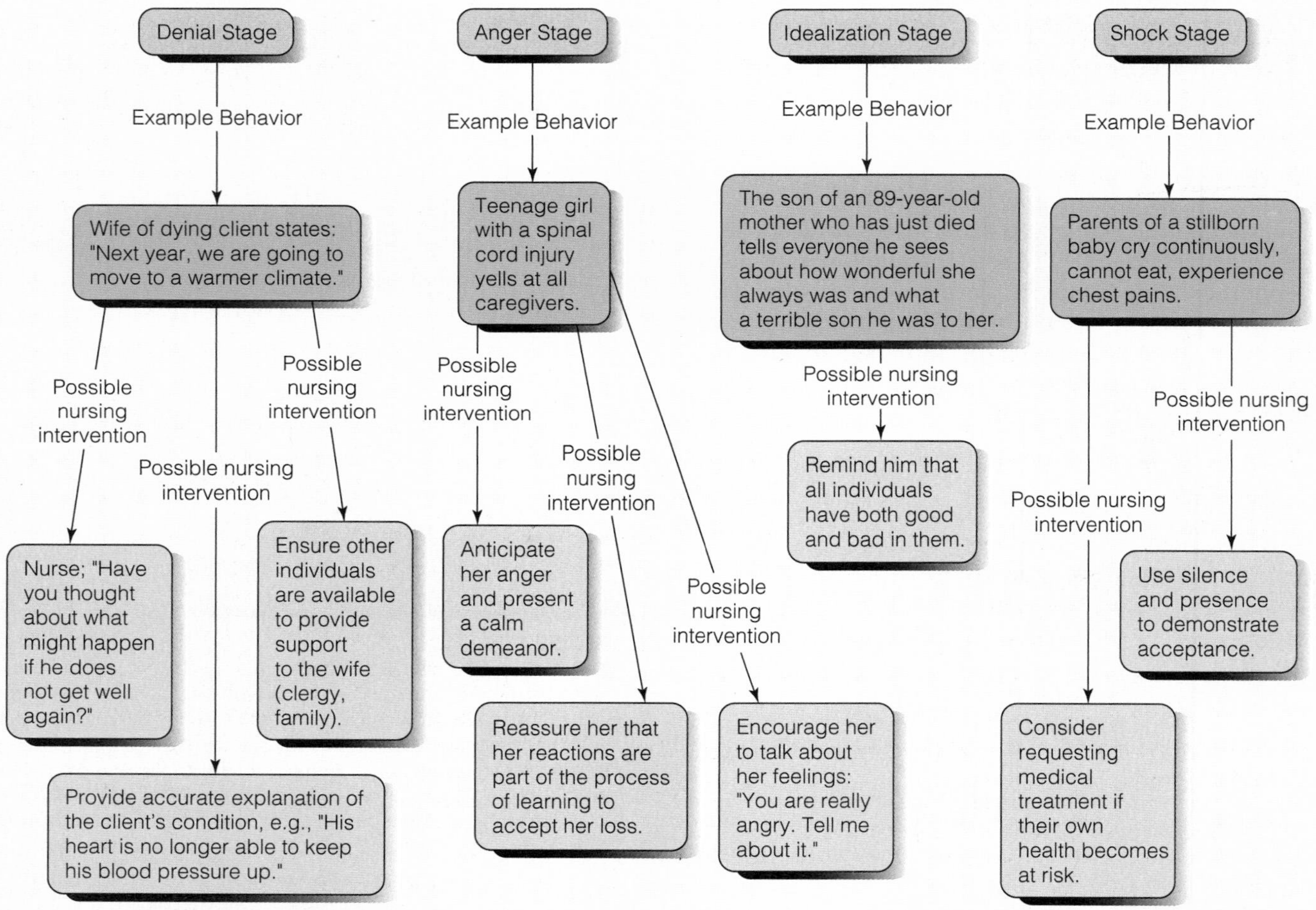

Denial Stage
- Example Behavior: Wife of dying client states: "Next year, we are going to move to a warmer climate."
  - Possible nursing intervention: Nurse; "Have you thought about what might happen if he does not get well again?"
  - Possible nursing intervention: Provide accurate explanation of the client's condition, e.g., "His heart is no longer able to keep his blood pressure up."
  - Possible nursing intervention: Ensure other individuals are available to provide support to the wife (clergy, family).

Anger Stage
- Example Behavior: Teenage girl with a spinal cord injury yells at all caregivers.
  - Possible nursing intervention: Anticipate her anger and present a calm demeanor.
  - Possible nursing intervention: Reassure her that her reactions are part of the process of learning to accept her loss.
  - Possible nursing intervention: Encourage her to talk about her feelings: "You are really angry. Tell me about it."

Idealization Stage
- Example Behavior: The son of an 89-year-old mother who has just died tells everyone he sees about how wonderful she always was and what a terrible son he was to her.
  - Possible nursing intervention: Remind him that all individuals have both good and bad in them.

Shock Stage
- Example Behavior: Parents of a stillborn baby cry continuously, cannot eat, experience chest pains.
  - Possible nursing intervention: Consider requesting medical treatment if their own health becomes at risk.
  - Possible nursing intervention: Use silence and presence to demonstrate acceptance.

Note: All nursing actions must be individualized to the client and the stage of the grieving process.

Chapter 43 Review

CHAPTER HIGHLIGHTS

- Nurses help clients deal with many losses, including loss of body image, a loved one, a sense of well-being, or a job.
- Loss, especially loss of a loved one or a valued body part, can be viewed as either a situational or a developmental loss and as either an actual or a perceived loss (both of which can be anticipatory).
- Grieving is a normal, subjective emotional response to loss; it is essential for mental and physical health. Grieving allows the bereaved individual to cope with loss gradually and to accept it as a reality.
- Knowledge of different stages or phases of grieving and factors that influence the loss reaction can help the nurse understand the responses and needs of clients.
- How an individual deals with loss is closely related to the individual's age, culture, spiritual beliefs, gender, socioeconomic status, support systems, and the significance and cause of the loss or death.
- Caring for the dying and the bereaved is one of the nurse's most complex and challenging responsibilities.
- Death-related legal issues include advance healthcare directives, do-not-resuscitate orders, organ donation, and euthanasia, aid in dying.
- Nurses' attitudes about death and dying directly affect their ability to provide care.
- Nurses must consider the entire family as requiring care in situations involving loss, especially death.
- Dying clients require open communication, physical help, and emotional and spiritual support to ensure a peaceful and dignified death. They need to maintain a sense of control in managing the events preceding death.

TEST YOUR KNOWLEDGE

1. Which of the following may be considered normal or "healthy" types of grief? Select all that apply.
   1. Abbreviated grief
   2. Anticipatory grief
   3. Disenfranchised grief
   4. Complicated grief
   5. Unresolved grief
   6. Inhibited grief

2. The family of a client who has just died wants to spend time with the client. What should the nurse do to prepare the client for the family? Select all that apply.
   1. Check the client's religion to make sure care is in compliance with religious expectations.
   2. Remove equipment from the room.
   3. Permit the family to view the client before postmortem care is done.
   4. Change the linen.
   5. Place the client in a natural body position.

3. The shift changed while the nursing staff was waiting for the adult children of a deceased client to arrive. The oncoming nurse has never met the family. Which initial greeting is most appropriate?
   1. "I'm very sorry for your loss."
   2. "I'll take you in to view the body."
   3. "I didn't know your father but I am sure he was a wonderful person."
   4. "How long will you want to stay with your father?"

4. At which age does a child begin to accept that he or she will someday die?
   1. Less than 5 years old
   2. 5–9 years old
   3. 9–12 years old
   4. 12–18 years old

5. An 82-year-old man has been told by his primary care provider that it is no longer safe for him to drive a car. Which statement by the client would indicate beginning positive adaptation to this loss?
   1. "I told the doctor I would stop driving, but I am not going to yet."
   2. "I always knew this day would come, but I hoped it wouldn't be now."
   3. "What does he know? I'm a better driver than he will ever be."
   4. "Well, at least I have friends and family who can take me places."

6. When asked to sign the permission form for surgical removal of a large but noncancerous lesion on her face, the client begins to cry. Which is the most appropriate response?
   1. "Tell me what it means to you to have this surgery."
   2. "You must be very glad to be having this lesion removed."
   3. "I cry when I am happy or relieved sometimes, too."
   4. "Isn't it wonderful that the lesion is not cancer?"

7. A nurse receives an advance health care directive to include in the medical record upon admitting a client to the hospital. The directive is witnessed by two of the client's three children. How does the nurse interpret this information?
   1. This advance directive may not be legal as children cannot witness advance directives in some states.
   2. Having the children's signatures on the advance directive is good because it indicates they agree with the client's wishes.
   3. The advance directive cannot be honored unless it is witnessed by all three children.
   4. In order to be valid, the advance directive must be witnessed by the client's physician.

8. The nurse is caring for a family in a shelter 2 days after the loss of their home due to a fire. The fire caused minor burns to several members of the family but no life-threatening conditions. Which is the *most* important assessment data for the nurse to gather at this time?
1. Availability of insurance coverage for rebuilding the house
2. Family members' understanding of the extent of their physical injuries
3. Psychologic support resources available from friends or other sources
4. Family members' grief responses and coping behaviors

9. A client who is in the terminal phases of a debilitating muscular disease tells his wife that he believes the health care team has "failed" and "given up" on him and "aren't trying as hard." What does the nurse caring for this client realize?
1. This idea of abandonment is unfounded.
2. This is a common fear in the terminally ill client.
3. When clients become terminal, physician care is no longer necessary.
4. Clients who feel this way are in denial of the facts of their care.

10. In working with a dying client, the nurse demonstrates assisting the client to die with dignity when performing which action?
1. Allows the client to make as many decisions about care as is possible
2. Shares with the client the nurse's own views about life after death
3. Avoids talking about dying and focuses on the present
4. Relieves the client of as much responsibility for self-care as is possible

See Answers to Test Your Knowledge in Appendix A.

READINGS AND REFERENCES

Suggested Readings

The American Nurses Association publishes position statements on topics of critical importance to nurses related to death and dying. Examples include *Nurses' roles and responsibilities in providing care and support at the end of life; euthanasia, assisted suicide, and aid in dying; nursing care and do not resuscitate (DNR) and allow natural death (AND) decisions*; and *nutrition and hydration at the end of life*. Retrieved from https://www.nursingworld.org/practice-policy/nursing-excellence/official-position-statements/

Related Research

Fuchs, L., Anstey, M., Feng, M., Toledano, R., Kogan, S., Howell, M. D. . . . Novack, V. (2017). Quantifying the mortality impact of do-not-resuscitate orders in the ICU. *Critical Care Medicine, 45*, 1019–1027. doi:10.1097/CCM.0000000000002312

References

American Nurses Association. (2016). *Nurses' roles and responsibilities in providing care and support at the end of life*. Retrieved from https://www.nursingworld.org/practice-policy/nursing-excellence/official-position-statements/id/nurses-roles-and-responsibilities-in-providing-care-and-support-at-the-end-of-life

Arredondo-Dowd, P. M. (1981). Personal Loss and Grief as a Result of Immigration. *Personnel and Guidance Journal*. Retrieved from https://doi.org/10.1002/j.2164-4918.1981.tb00573.x

Boelen, P. A., Lenferink, L. I. M., Nickerson, A., & Smid, G. E. (2018). Evaluation of the factor structure, prevalence, and validity of disturbed grief in DSM-5 and ICD-11. *Journal of Affective Disorders, 240*, 79–87. doi:10.1016/j.jad.2018.07.041

Citerio, G., & Murphy, P. G. (2015). Brain death the European perspective. *Seminars in Neurology, 35*(02), 139–144.

Engel, G. L. (1964). Grief and grieving. *American Journal of Nursing, 64*(9), 93–98.

European Council. (2020). More Donors and Transplantations to Save Lives. Retrieved from https://www.coe.int/en/web/human-rights-channel/organ-donation

Glaser, B., & Strauss, A. (1965). *Awareness of dying*. Chicago, IL: Aldine.

Hamel, L., Wu, B., & Brodie, M. (2017a). *Views and experiences with end-of-life medical care in Japan, Italy, the United States, and Brazil: A cross-country survey*. Retrieved from http://www.kff.org/other/report/views-and-experiences-with-end-of-life-medical-care-in-japan-italy-the-united-states-and-brazil-a-cross-country-survey

Hamel, L., Wu, B., & Brodie, M. (2017b). *Views and experiences with end-of-life medical care in the U.S.* Retrieved from http://files.kff.org/attachment/Report-Views-and-Experiences-with-End-of-Life-Medical-Care-in-the-US

Henry, H. M., Stiles, W. B., & Biran, M. W. (2005). Loss and mourning in immigration: Using the assimilation model to assess continuing bonds with native culture. *Counselling Psychology Quarterly, 18*(2): 109–119. Retrieved from https://www.researchgate.net/deref/http%3A%2F%2Fdx.doi.org%2F10.1080%2F09515070500136819

Hospice and Palliative Credentialing Center. (2019). *CHPN® candidate handbook*. Retrieved from http://documents.goamp.com/Publications/candidateHandbooks/HPCC-CHPN-Handbook.pdf

Johnson, E. J. & Goldstein, D. (2003). Do defaults save lives? Science, 302. doi:10.1126/science.1091721

Kaushik, J. (2009). Organ Transplant and Presumed Consent: Towards an "Opting-out" System. Indian Journal of Medical Ethics, 6(3), 149–152. Retrieved from https://doi.org/10.20529/ijme.2009.047

Kübler-Ross, E. (1969). *On death and dying*. New York, NY: Macmillan.

Nagar, D. (2019). An opt-out model for organ donation. *Deccan Herald*. Retrieved from https://www.deccanherald.com/opinion/panorama/an-opt-out-model-for-organ-donation-763526.html

National Consensus Project for Quality Palliative Care. (2018). *Clinical practice guidelines for quality palliative care* (4th ed.). Retrieved from https://www.nationalcoalitionhpc.org/wp-content/uploads/2018/10/NCHPC-NCPGuidelines_4thED_web_FINAL.pdf

National Hospice and Palliative Care Organization. (2018). *NHPCO facts and figures: Hospice care in America*. Retrieved from https://www.nhpco.org/sites/default/files/public/Statistics_Research/2017_Facts_Figures.pdf

ProCon.org. (2016). *Euthanasia & physician-assisted suicide (PAS) around the world: Legal status in 28 countries from Australia to Uruguay*. Retrieved from http://euthanasia.procon.org/view.resource.php?resourceID=000136

Sanders, C. M. (1998). *Grief: The mourning after: Dealing with adult bereavement* (2nd ed.). New York, NY: John Wiley & Sons.

Stuart, B., Volandes, A., & Moulton, B. W. (2017). Advance care planning: Ensuring patients' preferences govern the care they receive. *Generations, 41*(1), 31–36.

Thaler, R. (2009). Opting in vs Opting Out. *The New York Times*. September 26, 2009. Retrieved from https://www.nytimes.com/2009/09/27/business/economy/27view.html

Trevisan, C., Veronese, N., Maggi, S., Baggio, G., De Rui, M., Bolzetta, F., . . . Sergi, G. (2016). Marital status and frailty in older people: Gender differences in the Progetto Veneto Anziani longitudinal study. *Journal of Women's Health, 25*(6), 630–637. doi:10.1089/jwh.2015.5592

Willis, B. H., & Quigley, M. (2014). Opt-out Organ Donation: On evidence and Public Policy. *Journal of the Royal Society of Public Medicine, 107*(2), 56–60. Retrieved from https://dx.doi.org/10.1177%2F0141076813507707

World Health Organization. (2012). *International Guidelines for the Determination of Death – Phase 1. May 30–31, 2012*. Montreal. Canadian Blood Services. Retrieved from https://www.who.int/patientsafety/montreal-forum-report.pdf

World Health Organization. (n.d.). *WHO definition of palliative care*. Retrieved from http://www.who.int/cancer/palliative/definition/en

Wu, L., Chu, C., Chen, Y., Ho, C., & Pan, H. (2016). Relationship between palliative care consultation service and end-of-life outcomes. *Supportive Care in Cancer, 24*, 53–60. doi:10.1007/s00520-015-2741-6

Selected Bibliography

Annas, G. J., & Grodin, M. A. (2017). Frozen ethics: Melting the boundaries between medical treatment and organ procurement. *American Journal of Bioethics, 17*(5), 22–24. doi:10.1080/15265161.2017.1299252

Balch, B. (2017). Death by lethal prescription: A right for older people—or their duty? *Generations, 41*(1), 42–46.

Barbus, A. J. (1975). *The dying person's bill of rights*. Created at the Terminally Ill Patient and the Helping Person Workshop, Lansing, MI, South Western Michigan Inservice Education Council.

Carter, L. (2016). Understanding our role in bereavement. *International Journal of Childbirth Education, 31*(4), 28–30.

Chung, G., Yoon, J., Rasinski, K., & Curlin, F. (2016). US Physicians' opinions about distinctions between withdrawing and withholding life-sustaining treatment. *Journal of Religion & Health, 55*, 1596–1606. doi:10.1007/s10943-015-0171-x

Coombs Lee, B. (2017). Medical aid in dying: The cornerstone of patient-centered care. *Generations, 41*(1), 39–41.

Corr, C. A., Corr, D. M., & Doka, K. J. (2019). *Death & dying, life & living* (8th ed.). Boston, MA: Cengage.

Dalle Ave, A. L., & Bernat, J. L. (2018). Uncontrolled donation after circulatory determination of death: A systematic ethical analysis. *Journal of Intensive Care Medicine, 33*, 624–634. doi:10.1177/0885066616682200

Dickinson, G., & Leming, M. (Eds.). (2017). *Annual editions: Dying, death, and bereavement* (15th ed.). Boston, MA: McGraw-Hill.

Fahlberg, B., Foronda, C., & Baptiste, D. (2016). Cultural humility: The key to patient/family partnerships for making difficult decisions. *Nursing, 46*(9), 14–16. doi:10.1097/01.NURSE.0000490221.61685.e1

Harris, D. G., & Colombo, C. J. (2017). The road to unintended consequences is paved with good intentions. *Critical Care Medicine*, *45*, 1100–1101. doi:10.1097/CCM.0000000000002394

Iocovozzi, D. D. S. (2010). *Sooner or later: Restoring sanity to your end-of-life care*. Bloomington, IN: Pen and Publish.

Kübler-Ross, E. (1974). *Questions and answers on death and dying*. New York, NY: Macmillan.

Kübler-Ross, E. (1975). *Death: The final stage of growth*. Englewood Cliffs, NJ: Prentice Hall.

Kübler-Ross, E. (1978). *To live until we say good-bye*. Englewood Cliffs, NJ: Prentice Hall.

Malgaroli, M., Maccallum, F., & Bonanno, G. A. (2018). Symptoms of persistent complex bereavement disorder, depression, and PTSD in a conjugally bereaved sample: A network analysis. *Psychological Medicine*, *48*(14), 2439–2448. doi:10.1017/S0033291718001769

Milne, V., Doig, C., & Taylor, M. (2017). *Combining organ donation and medical assistance in death: Considering the ethical questions*. Retrieved from http://healthydebate.ca/2017/05/topic/organ-donation-medical-assistance-death

Moorlock, G., Ives, J., Bramhall, S., & Draper, H. (2016). Should we reject donated organs on moral grounds or permit allocation using non-medical criteria? A qualitative study. *Bioethics*, *30*, 282–292. doi:10.1111/bioe.12169

Murray, K. (2016). *Essentials in hospice and palliative care: A practical resource for every nurse*. Victoria, Canada: Life and Death Matters.

National Institute on Aging. (2016). *End-of-life: Helping with comfort and care*. Retrieved from http://www.elderguru.com/wp-content/uploads/2016/09/end-of-life-helping-with-comfort-and-care.pdf

Palmer, M., Saviet, M., & Tourish, J. (2016). Understanding and supporting grieving adolescents and young adults. *Pediatric Nursing*, *42*(6), 275–281.

Petrillo, L. A., Dzeng, E., Harrison, K. L., Forbes, L., Scribner, B., & Koenig, B. A. (2017). How California prepared for implementation of physician-assisted death: A primer. *American Journal of Public Health*, *107*(6), 883–888. doi:10.2105/AJPH.2017.303755

Rando, T. A. (2000). *Clinical dimensions of anticipatory mourning: Theory and practice in working with the dying, their loved ones, and their caregivers*. Champaign, IL: Research Press.

Rodríguez-Arias, D., Wilkinson, D., & Youngner, S. (2017). How can you be transparent about labeling the living as dead? *American Journal of Bioethics*, *17*(5), 24–25. doi:10.1080/15265161.2017.1299243

Sajid, M. I. (2016). Autopsy in Islam: Considerations for deceased Muslims and their families currently and in the future. *American Journal of Forensic Medicine and Pathology*, *37*, 29–31. doi:10.1097/PAF.0000000000000207

Shimizu, K., Kikuchi, S., Kobayashi, T., & Kato, S. (2017). Persistent complex bereavement disorder: Clinical utility and classification of the category proposed for Diagnostic and Statistical Manual of Mental Disorders, 5th edition. *Psychogeriatrics*, *17*(1), 17–24. doi:10.1111/psyg.12183

Squires, J. E., Coughlin, M., Dorrance, K., Linklater, S., Chassé, M., Grimshaw, J. M., . . . Knoll, G. A. (2018). Criteria to identify a potential deceased organ donor: A systematic review. *Critical Care Medicine*, *46*, 1318–1327. doi:10.1097/CCM.0000000000003200

Stroebe, M., Schut, H., & Boerner, K. (2017). Cautioning health-care professionals: Bereaved persons are misguided through the stages of grief. *Omega: Journal of Death & Dying*, *74*, 455–473. doi:10.1177/0030222817691870

Stroebe, M., Stroebe, W., Schut, H., & Boerner, K. (2017). Grief is not a disease but bereavement merits medical awareness. *Lancet*, *389*(10067), 347–349. doi:10.1016/S0140-6736(17)30189-7

Thomas, J., & Sabatino, C. (2017). Patient preferences, policy, and POLST. *Generations*, *41*(1), 102–109.

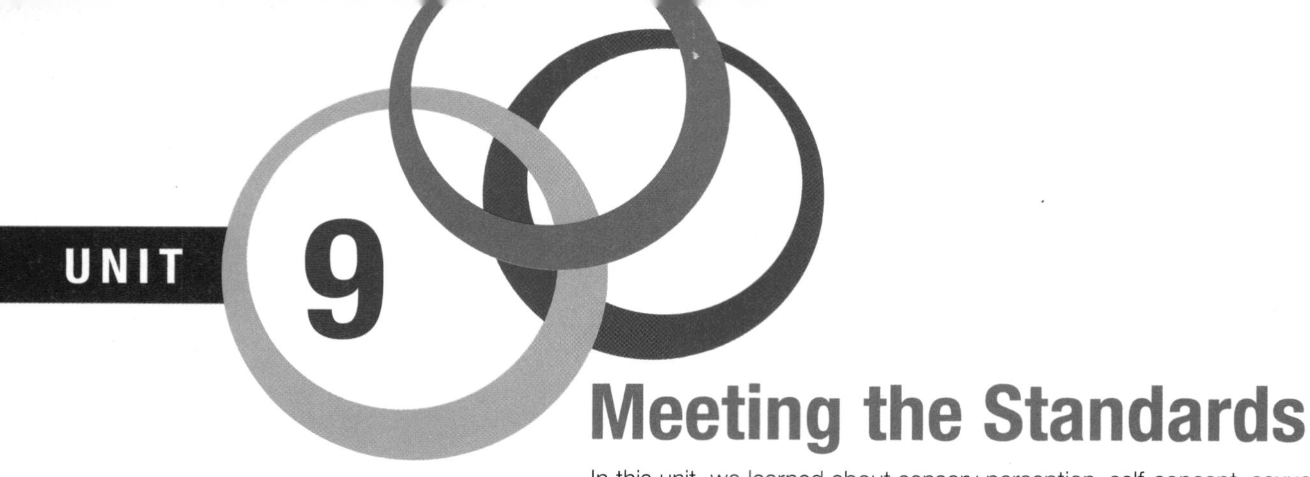

Meeting the Standards

In this unit, we learned about sensory perception, self-concept, sexuality, spirituality, stress and coping, and loss, grieving, and death. All are essential concepts that a nurse needs to consider to care properly for a client. Often, the nurse finds these topics challenging because they are somewhat abstract and involve the intangible core aspects of what makes us individuals. In the case below, you will explore how two nursing standards guide the nurse in professional practice and in providing safe, quality care.

CLIENT: Christina AGE: 72
CURRENT MEDICAL DIAGNOSIS: Breast Cancer

Medical History: Christina was diagnosed with an early-stage common form of breast cancer 4 years ago. She had removal of the lump, followed by radiation therapy and oral chemotherapy. She has no current symptoms of her cancer and is tolerating the chemotherapy without difficulty. She has no other significant health conditions. The 5-year survival projection for women with similar breast cancers is 95% and the 10-year survival rate is 82%.

Personal and Social History: Christina is retired from employment and lives with her retired husband and their cats. Their socioeconomic status is middle class. They have Social Security, Medicare, and sufficient retirement savings.

Christina is your client in the same-day surgery unit, where she is being seen for a biopsy of a new lump in her breast. During your admission interview and assessment, you identify several areas requiring nursing care planning. Christina is very anxious as shown by her elevated blood pressure and pulse, perspiration, and nervous movements. She says to you, "I just know this is cancer again. It must be that deodorant I use. Or, maybe it's the electrical wires near our house. Or, just God punishing me for bad thoughts. What do you think?"

Questions

1. How might you respond to Christina? What have you learned about stress, loss and grieving, spirituality, and other similar concepts in this unit that can assist you in providing a helpful response?

American Nurses Association Standard of Professional Performance #11 is Leadership: *The registered nurse leads within the professional practice setting and the profession. One of the many competencies is that the nurse contributes to the establishment of an environment that supports and maintains respect, trust, and dignity.*

When you examine Christina's breasts in preparing the biopsy site, she avoids meeting your eyes. She says, quietly, "I know you don't want to hear about my troubles, but I don't think my husband finds me attractive anymore."

2. What response might you make that exemplifies the competency above and your learning from this unit?

American Nurses Association Standard of Professional Performance #17 is Environmental Health: *The registered nurse practices in an environmentally safe and healthy manner. The competencies include that the registered nurse (a) participates in developing strategies to promote healthy communities and practice environments; and (b) communicates information about environmental health risks and exposure reduction strategies.*

3. Considering the standard, what categories of possible interventions might you consider for a nursing diagnosis and goal focused on Christina's need for a healing environment?

A concept found throughout the ANA Standards is that the nurse demonstrates commitment to continuous, lifelong learning and education for self and others.

4. During your care of Christina, you realize that you are insufficiently knowledgeable about breast cancer treatment effects. You wonder about the sensation in the breast after radiation therapy (for both Christina and her husband) and the support systems that would be in place for the many breast cancer survivors who might be worrying about a recurrence. Describe the various ways you might investigate answers to these questions by interacting with your colleagues.

American Nurses Association. (2015). *Nursing: Scope and standards of practice* (3rd ed.). Silver Spring, MD: Author.

Answers to Meeting the Standards questions are available on the faculty resources site. Please consult with your instructor.

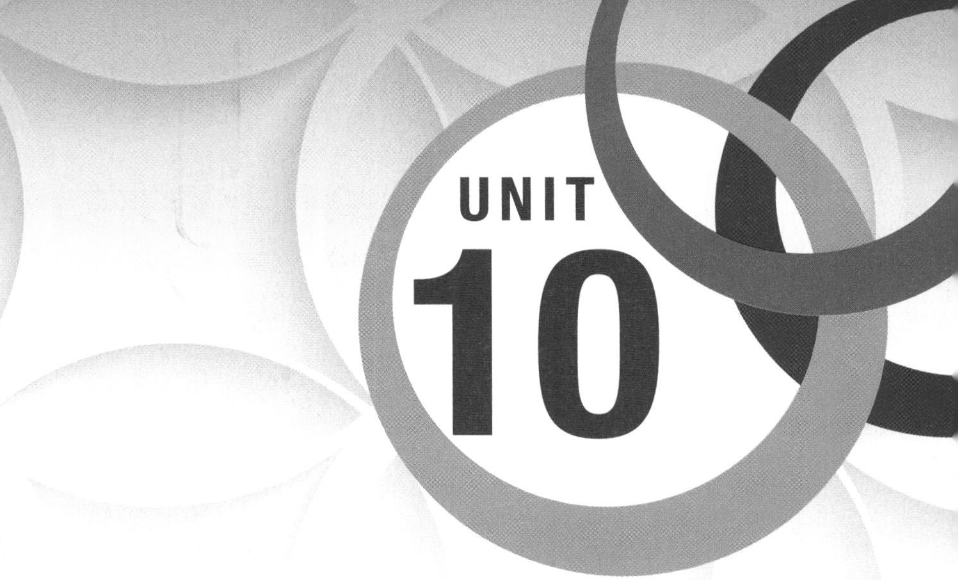

Promoting Physiologic Health

44 Activity and Exercise

LEARNING OUTCOMES

After completing this chapter, you will be able to:

1. Describe four basic elements of normal movement.
2. Differentiate isotonic, isometric, isokinetic, aerobic, and anaerobic exercise.
3. Compare the effects of exercise and immobility on body systems.
4. Identify factors influencing a client's body alignment and activity.
5. Assess activity-exercise pattern, body alignment, gait, appearance and movement of joints, mobility capabilities and limitations, muscle mass and strength, activity tolerance, and problems related to immobility.
6. Develop nursing diagnoses and outcomes related to activity, exercise, and mobility problems.
7. Use safe practices when positioning, moving, transferring, and ambulating clients.
8. Compare and contrast active, passive, and active-assistive range-of-motion (ROM) exercises.
9. Describe client teaching for clients who use mechanical aids for walking.
10. Verbalize the steps used in:
    a. Moving a client up in bed
    b. Turning a client to the lateral or prone position in bed
    c. Logrolling a client
    d. Assisting a client to sit on the side of the bed
    e. Transferring between bed and chair
    f. Transferring between bed and stretcher
    g. Assisting a client to ambulate.
11. Recognize when it is appropriate to assign aspects of moving, transferring, and ambulating a client to assistive personnel.
12. Demonstrate appropriate documentation and reporting of moving, transferring, and ambulating a client.

KEY TERMS

active ROM exercises, *1148*
activity-exercise pattern, *1109*
activity tolerance, *1115*
aerobic exercise, *1116*
ambulation, *1149*
anabolism, *1121*
anaerobic exercise, *1117*
ankylosed, *1119*
anorexia, *1121*
atelectasis, *1121*
atrophy, *1119*
basal metabolic rate (BMR), *1121*
base of support, *1109*
bedrest, *1115*
calculi, *1122*
catabolism, *1121*
center of gravity, *1109*
contracture, *1119*
crepitation, *1124*
dorsal position, *1134*
dorsal recumbent position, *1134*
embolus, *1120*
flaccid, *1119*
foot drop, *1119*
Fowler's position, *1133*
functional strength, *1115*
gait, *1124*
high-Fowler's position, *1133*
hypertrophy, *1117*
isokinetic (resistive) exercises, *1116*
isometric (static or setting) exercises, *1116*
isotonic (dynamic) exercises, *1116*
lateral position, *1135*
line of gravity, *1109*
logrolling, *1140*
lordosis, *1124*
metabolism, *1121*
mobility, *1109*
orthopneic position, *1134*
orthostatic hypotension, *1119*
osteoporosis, *1115*
pace, *1124*
paresis, *1119*
passive ROM exercises, *1148*
prone position, *1134*
proprioception, *1110*
range of motion (ROM), *1110*
relaxation response (RR), *1118*
semi-Fowler's position, *1133*
Sims' position, *1136*
spastic, *1119*
supine position, *1134*
thrombophlebitis, *1120*
thrombus, *1120*
tripod (triangle) position, *1156*
urinary incontinence, *1122*
urinary reflux, *1122*
urinary retention, *1122*
urinary stasis, *1122*
Valsalva maneuver, *1119*
vital capacity, *1120*

Introduction

Our ability to move is an essential aspect of well-being and our overall health is affected by our activities. The nursing diagnosis of inactive lifestyle emphasizes the role of exercise and activity as an essential component of health. In fact, too much sitting is emerging as a recognized health risk for a variety of chronic illnesses (Eanes, 2018).

Many *Healthy People 2020* (HealthyPeople.gov, 2019) objectives pertain to exercise and activity. Moderate exercise is identified as significant to enhancing physical fitness. The Midcourse Progress Report (Centers for Disease Control and Prevention, 2016) provides information as to the nation's progress toward the *Healthy People 2020* exercise and activity objectives. For example, the objectives relating to adults engaging in regular physical activity and meeting physical activity and muscle strengthening goals have exceeded the target. Unfortunately, the objectives for adolescents meeting the guidelines for aerobic physical activity and muscle-strengthening activity have had little or no change, as has the objective of school districts requiring regular elementary school recess for 20+ minutes.

A strong, well-developed body of research evidence supports the role of exercise in improving the health status of individuals with cardiovascular disease, pulmonary dysfunction, disabilities of aging, and depression. Integrating well-researched exercise protocols with conventional nursing and medical approaches will result in optimal treatment of these common disorders. Evidence shows that regular exercise can prevent and even reverse many of the chronic diseases experienced by aging adults.

An **activity-exercise pattern** refers to an individual's routine of exercise, activity, leisure, and recreation. It includes (a) activities of daily living (ADLs) that require energy expenditure such as hygiene, dressing, cooking, shopping, eating, working, and home maintenance, and (b) the type, quality, and quantity of exercise, including sports.

Mobility, the ability to move freely, easily, rhythmically, and purposefully in the environment, is an essential part of living. Individuals must move to protect themselves from trauma and to meet their basic needs. Mobility is vital to independence; a fully immobilized individual is as vulnerable and dependent as an infant.

Individuals often define their health and physical fitness by their activity because mental well-being and the effectiveness of body functioning depend largely on their mobility status. For example, when a client is upright, the lungs expand more easily, intestinal activity (peristalsis) is more effective, and the kidneys are able to empty completely. In addition, motion is essential for proper functioning of bones and muscles.

The ability to move without pain also influences self-esteem and body image. For most individuals, self-esteem depends on a sense of independence and a feeling of usefulness or being needed. Individuals with mobility impairments may feel helpless and burdensome to others, and their ability to work and earn a living may be compromised. Painful mobility makes coping even more difficult. Body image can be altered by paralysis, amputations, or any motor impairment. The reaction of others to impaired mobility can also alter self-esteem and body image significantly.

For those with impaired mobility, movement must be raised to the full potential to enable a satisfying life. For example, many individuals who have impairments or use wheelchairs participate in athletics to experience the joys of competition and fitness. Many individuals with paralysis can use a hand control to enter and drive adapted vans or use their mouth to manipulate a paintbrush and create art. No matter what their level of mobility, they must be encouraged to breathe fully, engage their abdominal muscles, and move as much as possible to prevent the physical and psycho-emotional hazards of immobility.

Normal Movement

Normal movement and stability are the result of an intact musculoskeletal system, an intact nervous system, and intact inner ear structures responsible for equilibrium. Body movement involves four basic elements: body alignment (posture), joint mobility, balance, and coordinated movement.

Alignment and Posture

Proper body alignment and posture bring body parts into position in a manner that promotes optimal balance and maximal body function whether the client is standing, sitting, or lying down. An individual maintains balance as long as the **line of gravity** (an imaginary vertical line drawn through the body's center of gravity) passes through the **center of gravity** (the point at which all of the body's mass is centered) and the **base of support** (the foundation on which the body rests). In humans, the usual line of gravity begins at the top of the head and falls between the shoulders, through the trunk, slightly anterior to the sacrum, and between the weight-bearing joints and base of support (Figure 44.1 ■).

When the body is well aligned, strain on the joints, muscles, tendons, or ligaments is minimized and internal structures and organs are supported. Proper body alignment enhances lung expansion and promotes efficient circulatory, renal, and gastrointestinal functions. An individual's posture is one criterion for assessing general health, physical fitness, and attractiveness. Posture reflects the mood, self-esteem, and personality of an individual, and vice versa.

Abdominal and skeletal muscles function almost continuously, making tiny adjustments that enable an erect or seated posture despite the endless downward pull of gravity.

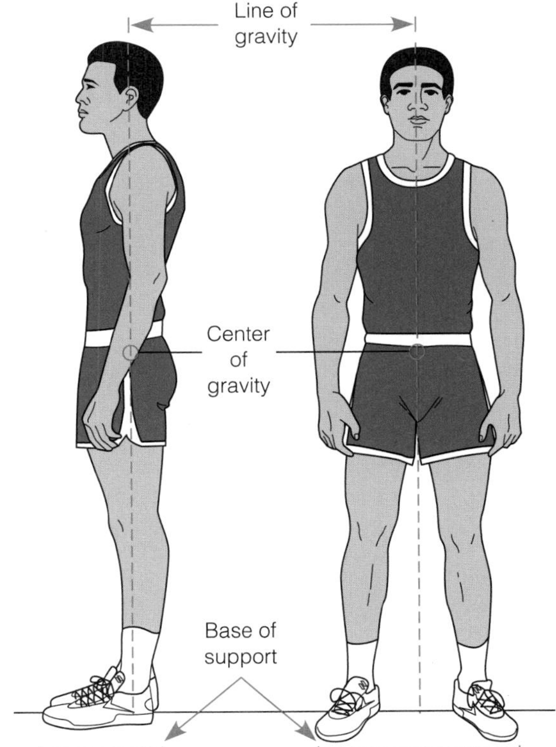

Figure 44.1 ■ The center of gravity and the line of gravity influence standing alignment.

Joint Mobility

Joints are the functional units of the musculoskeletal system. The bones of the skeleton articulate at the joints, and most of the skeletal muscles attach to the two bones at the joint. These muscles are categorized according to the type of joint movement they produce on contraction. Muscles are therefore called flexors, extensors, internal rotators, and the like. The flexor muscles are stronger than the extensor muscles. Thus, when an individual is inactive, the joints are pulled into a flexed (bent) position. If this tendency is not reduced through exercise and position changes, the muscles permanently shorten, and the joint becomes fixed in a flexed position (contracture). Types of joint movement are listed in Table 44.1.

The **range of motion (ROM)** of a joint is the maximum movement that is possible for that joint. Joint range of motion varies from individual to individual and is determined by genetic makeup, developmental patterns, the presence or absence of disease, and the amount of physical activity in which the individual normally engages. Table 44.2 shows the various joint movements and the usual ranges of motion.

Balance

The mechanisms involved in maintaining balance and posture are complex and involve informational inputs from the labyrinth (inner ear), from vision (vestibulo-ocular input), and from stretch receptors of muscles and tendons (vestibulospinal input). Mechanisms of equilibrium (sense of balance) respond, frequently without our awareness, to various head movements. **Proprioception** is the term used to describe awareness of posture, movement, and changes in equilibrium and the knowledge of position, weight, and resistance of objects in relation to the body.

TABLE 44.1 Types of Joint Movements

Movement	Action
Flexion	Decreasing the angle of the joint (e.g., bending the elbow)
Extension	Increasing the angle of the joint (e.g., straightening the arm at the elbow)
Hyperextension	Further extension or straightening of a joint (e.g., bending the head backward)
Abduction	Movement of the bone away from the midline of the body
Adduction	Movement of the bone toward the midline of the body
Rotation	Movement of the bone around its central axis
Circumduction	Movement of the distal part of the bone in a circle while the proximal end remains fixed
Eversion	Turning the sole of the foot outward by moving the ankle joint
Inversion	Turning the sole of the foot inward by moving the ankle joint
Pronation	Moving the bones of the forearm so that the palm of the hand faces downward when held in front of the body
Supination	Moving the bones of the forearm so that the palm of the hand faces upward when held in front of the body

Coordinated Movement

Balanced, smooth, purposeful movement is the result of proper functioning of the cerebral cortex, cerebellum, and basal ganglia. The cerebral cortex initiates voluntary motor activity, the cerebellum coordinates the motor activities of movement, and the basal ganglia maintain posture. When a client's cerebellum is injured, movements become clumsy, unsure, and uncoordinated.

Factors Affecting Body Alignment and Activity

A number of factors affect an individual's body alignment, mobility, and daily activity level. These include growth and development, nutrition, personal values and attitudes, certain external factors, and prescribed limitations.

Growth and Development

An individual's age and musculoskeletal and nervous system development affect posture, body proportions, body mass, body movements, and reflexes. Newborn movements are reflexive and random. All extremities are generally flexed but can be passively moved through a full range of motion. As the neurologic system matures, control over movement progresses during the first year. Gross motor development precedes fine motor skills. Gross motor development occurs in a head-to-toe fashion, that is, progression from head control, to crawling, to pulling up to a standing position, to standing, and to walking, usually after the first birthday. The contralateral motion of crawling, however brief, is an important building block for walking. Initially, walking involves a wide stance and unsteady gait, thus the term *toddler*. From ages 1 to 5 years, both gross and fine motor skills are refined. For example, preschoolers master riding a tricycle, running, jumping, using crayons to draw, fastening or using zippers, and brushing their teeth. Immobility can impair the social and motor development of young children.

From 6 to 12 years of age, refinement of motor skills continues and exercise patterns for later life are generally determined. Posture in school-age children is usually excellent. In adolescence, growth spurts and behaviors such as carrying heavy book bags on one shoulder and extended computer use may result in postural changes that often persist into adulthood.

Adults between 20 and 40 years of age generally have few physical changes affecting mobility, with the exception of pregnant women. Pregnancy alters the body's center of gravity and affects balance. The most recent

TABLE 44.2 Selected Joint Movements and Example of Corresponding Activity of Daily Living (ADL)

Body Part—Type of Joint/Movement	Normal Range and Example of Corresponding ADL	Illustration
NECK—PIVOT JOINT		
Flexion. Move the head from the upright midline position forward, so that the chin rests on the chest (Figure 44.2 ■).	45° from midline Example: nodding head "yes"	**Figure 44.2** ■ 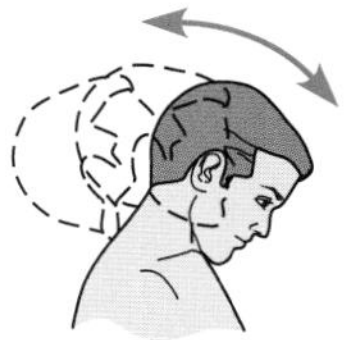
Extension. Move the head from the flexed position to the upright position (Figure 44.2).	45° from midline Example: nodding head "yes"	
Hyperextension. Move the head from the upright position back as far as possible (Figure 44.2).	45° from midline	**Figure 44.3** ■ 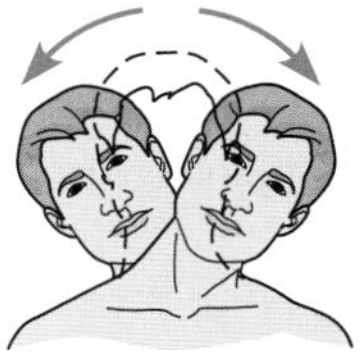
Lateral flexion. Move the head laterally to the right and left shoulders (Figure 44.3 ■).	40° from midline	
Rotation. Turn the face as far as possible to the right and left (Figure 44.4 ■).	70° from midline Example: shaking head "no"	**Figure 44.4** ■ 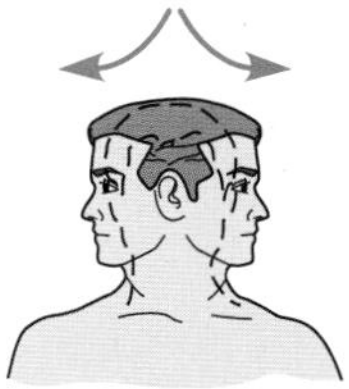
SHOULDER—BALL-AND-SOCKET JOINT		
Flexion. Raise each arm from a position by the side forward and upward to a position beside the head (Figure 44.5 ■).	180° from the side Example: reaching to turn on overhead light	**Figure 44.5** ■ 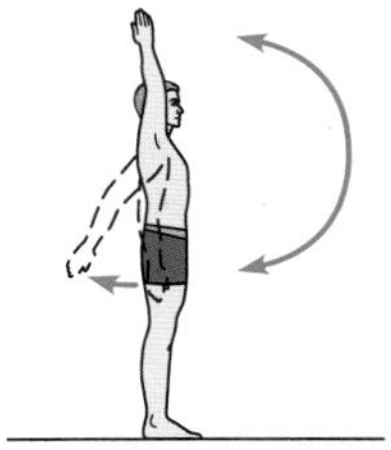
Extension. Move each arm from a vertical position beside the head forward and down to a resting position at the side of the body (Figure 44.5).	180° from vertical position beside the head	
Hyperextension. Move each arm from a resting side position to behind the body (Figure 44.5).	50° from side position	
Abduction. Move each arm laterally from a resting position at the sides to a side position above the head, palm of the hand either toward or away from the head (Figure 44.6 ■).	180° Example: reaching to bedside stand on same side of bed as arm	**Figure 44.6** ■ 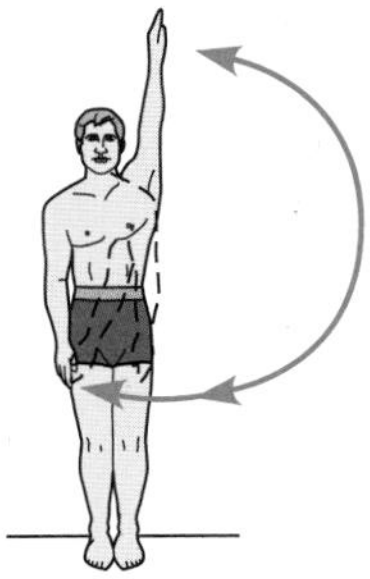
Adduction (anterior). Move each arm from a position at the sides across the front of the body as far as possible (Figure 44.6). The elbow may be straight or bent.	50° Example: reaching across body toward opposite side of bed	
Circumduction. Move each arm forward, up, back, and down in a full circle (Figure 44.7 ■).	360°	**Figure 44.7** ■ 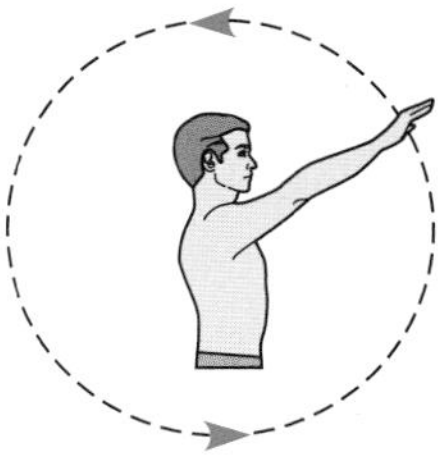
External rotation. With each arm held out to the side at shoulder level and the elbow bent to a right angle, fingers pointing down, move the arm upward so that the fingers point up (Figure 44.8 ■).	90° Example: reaching over opposite shoulder to scratch upper back	**Figure 44.8** ■ 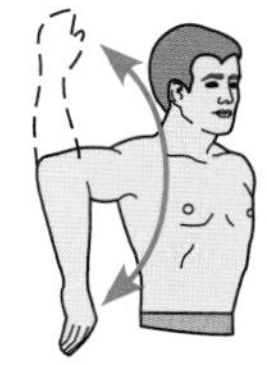
Internal rotation. With each arm held out to the side at shoulder level and the elbow bent to a right angle, fingers pointing up, bring the arm forward and down so that the fingers point down (Figure 44.8).	90° Example: reaching to scratch same side lower back	

Continued on page 1112

TABLE 44.2 Selected Joint Movements and Example of Corresponding Activity of Daily Living (ADL)—*continued*

Body Part—Type of Joint/Movement	Normal Range and Example of Corresponding ADL	Illustration
ELBOW—HINGE JOINT		
Flexion. Bring each lower arm forward and upward so that the hand is at the shoulder (Figure 44.9 ■).	150° Example: eating, bathing, shaving	**Figure 44.9 ■**
Extension. Bring each lower arm forward and downward, straightening the arm (Figure 44.9).	150° Example: eating, bathing, shaving	
Rotation for supination. Turn each hand and forearm so that the palm is facing upward (Figure 44.10 ■).	70° to 90°	**Figure 44.10 ■**
Rotation for pronation. Turn each hand and forearm so that the palm is facing downward (Figure 44.10).	70° to 90°	
WRIST—CONDYLOID JOINT		
Flexion. Bring the fingers of each hand toward the inner aspect of the forearm (Figure 44.11 ■).	80° to 90° Example: eating, bathing, shaving, writing	**Figure 44.11 ■**
Extension. Straighten each hand to the same plane as the arm (Figure 44.11).	80° to 90° Example: eating, bathing, shaving	
Hyperextension. Bend the fingers of each hand back as far as possible (Figure 44.12 ■).	70° to 90°	**Figure 44.12 ■**
Radial flexion (abduction). Bend each wrist laterally toward the thumb side with hand supinated (Figure 44.13 ■).	0° to 20°	**Figure 44.13 ■**
Ulnar flexion (adduction). Bend each wrist laterally toward the fifth finger with the hand supinated (Figure 44.13).	30° to 50°	
HAND AND FINGERS: METACARPOPHALANGEAL JOINTS—CONDYLOID; INTERPHALANGEAL JOINTS—HINGE		
Flexion. Make a fist with each hand (Figure 44.14 ■).	90° Example: squeezing, gripping, writing	**Figure 44.14 ■**
Extension. Straighten the fingers of each hand (Figure 44.14).	90°	
Hyperextension. Bend the fingers of each hand back as far as possible (Figure 44.14).	30°	
Abduction. Spread the fingers of each hand apart (Figure 44.15 ■).	20°	**Figure 44.15 ■**
Adduction. Bring the fingers of each hand together (Figure 44.15).	20° Example: writing, gripping, eating, many hobbies involving fine motor coordination (e.g., art, music)	
THUMB—SADDLE JOINT		**Figure 44.16 ■**
Flexion. Move each thumb across the palmar surface of the hand toward the fifth finger (Figure 44.16 ■).	90°	**Figure 44.17 ■**
Extension. Move each thumb away from the hand (Figure 44.16).	90°	
Abduction. Extend each thumb laterally (Figure 44.17 ■).	30°	
Adduction. Move each thumb back to the hand (Figure 44.17).	30°	

TABLE 44.2 Selected Joint Movements and Example of Corresponding Activity of Daily Living (ADL)—*continued*

Body Part—Type of Joint/Movement	Normal Range and Example of Corresponding ADL	Illustration
Opposition. Touch each thumb to the top of each finger of the same hand. The thumb joint movements involved are abduction, rotation, and flexion (Figure 44.18 ■).		Figure 44.18 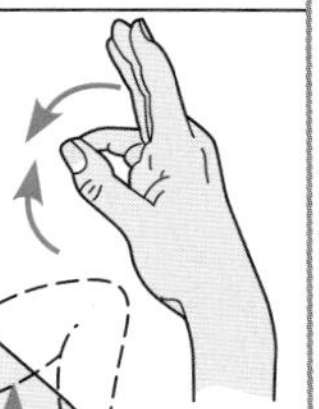 ■
HIP—BALL-AND-SOCKET JOINT **Flexion.** Move each leg forward and upward. The knee may be extended or flexed (Figure 44.19 ■).	Knee extended, 90°; knee flexed, 120° Example: walking, leg lifts in front of the body	Figure 44.19 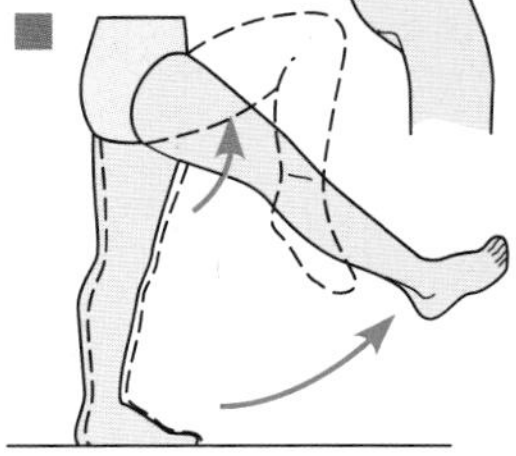 ■
Extension. Move each leg back beside the other (Figure 44.20 ■).	90° to 120° Example: walking, lining the leg up with the body	Figure 44.20 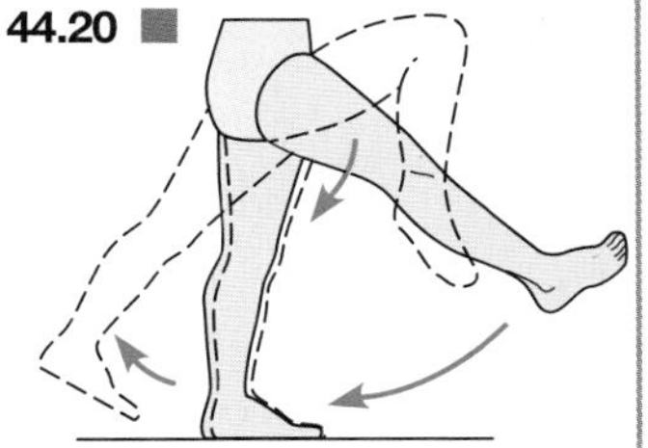 ■
Hyperextension. Move each leg back behind the body (Figure 44.20).	30° to 50° Example: walking; lying on side, reach the leg behind the body	
Abduction. Move each leg out to the side (Figure 44.21 ■).	45° to 50° Example: moving leg away from body	Figure 44.21 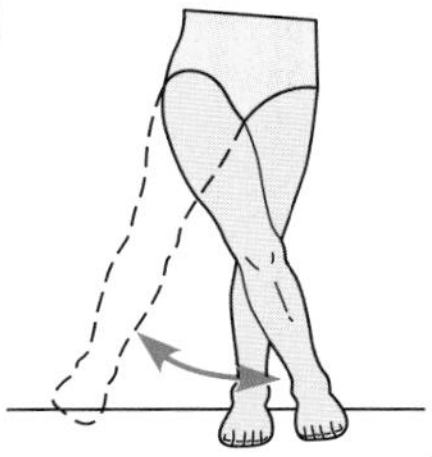 ■
Adduction. Move each leg back to the other leg and beyond in front of it (Figure 44.21).	20° to 30° beyond other leg Example: moving leg over the other leg toward the middle of the body	
Circumduction. Move each leg backward, up, to the side, and down in a circle (Figure 44.22 ■).	360° Example: leg circles clockwise and counterclockwise	Figure 44.22 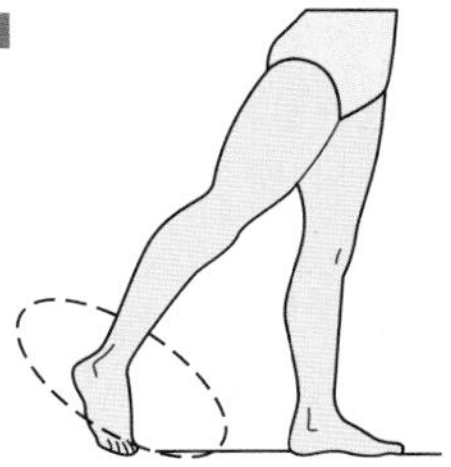 ■
Internal rotation. Flex knee and hip to 90°. Place the foot away from the midline. Move the thigh and knee *toward* the midline (Figure 44.23 ■).	40°	Figure 44.23 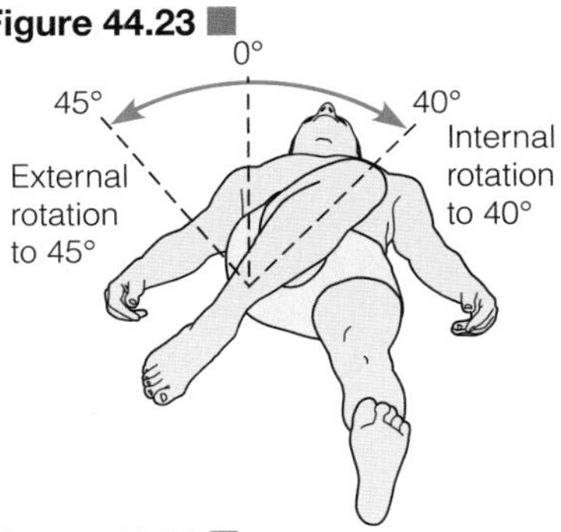 ■ 0° 45° 40° External rotation to 45° Internal rotation to 40°
External rotation. Flex knee and hip to 90°. Place the foot toward the midline. Move the thigh and knee *away* from the midline (Figure 44.23).	45°	
KNEE—HINGE JOINT **Flexion.** Bend each leg, bringing the heel toward the back of the thigh (Figure 44.24 ■).	120° to 130° Example: knee bends, walking	Figure 44.24 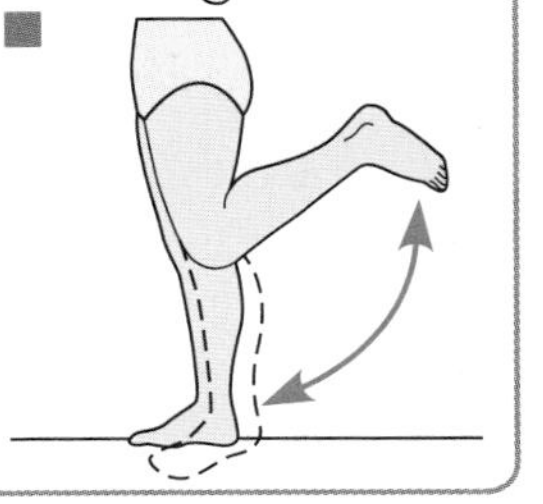 ■
Extension. Straighten each leg, returning the foot to its position beside the other foot (Figure 44.24).	120° to 130° Example: straightening leg from bent position, walking	

Continued on page 1114

TABLE 44.2 Selected Joint Movements and Example of Corresponding Activity of Daily Living (ADL)—*continued*

Body Part—Type of Joint/Movement	Normal Range and Example of Corresponding ADL	Illustration
ANKLE—HINGE JOINT **Extension (plantar flexion).** Point the toes of each foot downward (Figure 44.25 ■).	20° Example: pressing toes away from face, walking	**Figure 44.25 ■** 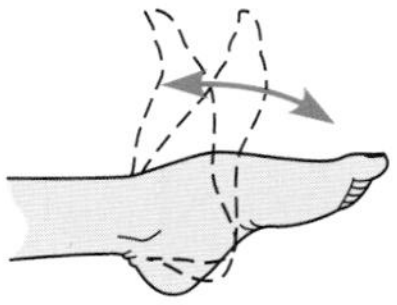
Flexion (dorsiflexion). Point the toes of each foot upward (Figure 44.25).	45° to 50° Example: pulling toes toward face, walking	
FOOT—GLIDING **Eversion.** Turn the sole of each foot laterally (Figure 44.26 ■).	5° Example: foot circles clockwise and counterclockwise	**Figure 44.26 ■** 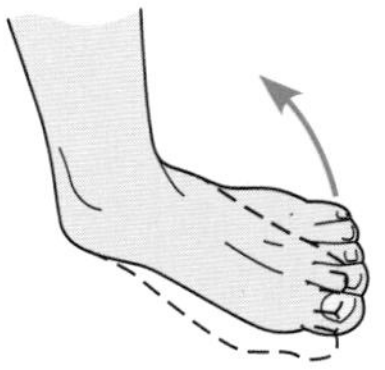
Inversion. Turn the sole of each foot medially (Figure 44.26).	5° Example: foot circles clockwise and counterclockwise Example: walking, wiggling toes	
TOES: INTERPHALANGEAL JOINTS—HINGE; METATARSOPHALANGEAL JOINTS—HINGE; INTERTARSAL JOINTS—GLIDING **Flexion.** Curl the toe joints of each foot downward (Figure 44.27 ■).	35° to 60°	**Figure 44.27 ■** 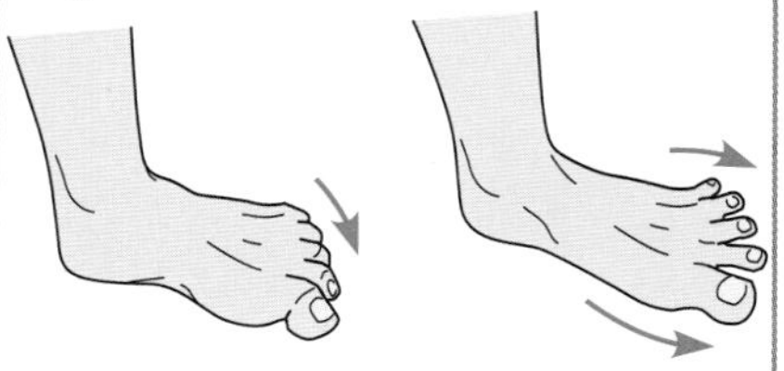
Extension. Straighten the toes of each foot (Figure 44.27).	35° to 60°	
TRUNK—GLIDING JOINT **Flexion.** Bend the trunk toward the toes (Figure 44.28 ■).	70° to 90° Example: touching toes	**Figure 44.28 ■** 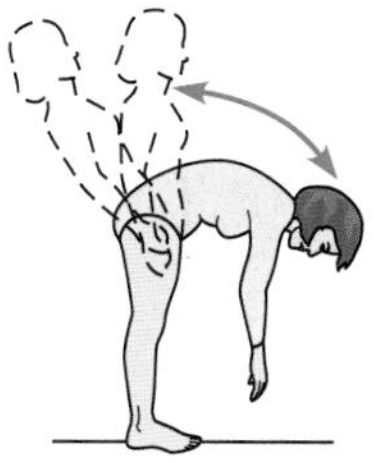
Extension. Straighten the trunk from a flexed position (Figure 44.28).		
Hyperextension. Bend the trunk backward (Figure 44.28).	20° to 30° Example: gentle supported back bend with hands on buttocks	
Lateral flexion. Bend the trunk to the right and to the left (Figure 44.29 ■).	35° on each side Example: gently allow right hand to slide down right side of thigh, repeat on left side	**Figure 44.29 ■** 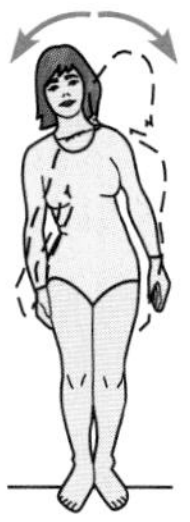
Rotation. Turn the upper part of the body from side to side (Figure 44.30 ■).	30° to 45° Example: gently swing torso right and left, maintaining forward hip alignment	**Figure 44.30 ■** 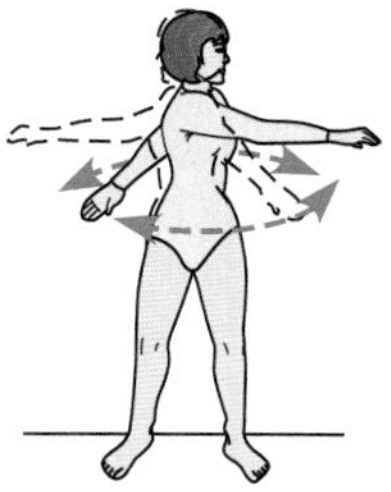

recommendations from the American College of Obstetricians and Gynecologists (2017) suggest that healthy pregnant women should exercise at least 150 minutes with moderate intensity aerobic activity every week. Thorough clinical evaluations of the client should be completed prior to recommending any exercise regimen.

As age advances, muscle tone and bone density decrease, joints lose flexibility, reaction time slows, and bone mass decreases, particularly in women who have osteoporosis. **Osteoporosis** is a condition in which the bones become brittle and fragile due to calcium depletion. Osteoporosis is common in older women and primarily affects the weight-bearing joints of the lower extremities and the anterior aspects of spinal bones, causing compression fractures of the vertebrae and hip fractures. All of these changes affect older adults' posture, gait, and balance. Posture becomes forward leaning and stooped, which shifts the center of gravity forward. To compensate for this shift, the knees flex slightly for support and the base of support is widened. Gait becomes wide based, short stepped, and shuffling.

A strong body of research supports the benefits of regular activity for older adults to maintain and regain strength, flexibility, cardiovascular fitness, and bone density. Other health benefits are well documented, including reduction in falls, mood stabilization, reduction in obesity, and diabetes management (Kraschnewski et al., 2016a).

Nutrition

Both undernutrition and overnutrition can influence body alignment and mobility. Poorly nourished people may have muscle weakness and fatigue. Vitamin D deficiency causes bone deformity during growth. Inadequate calcium intake and vitamin D synthesis and intake increase the risk of osteoporosis. Obesity can distort movement and stress joints, adversely affecting posture, balance, and joint health. See Chapter 46 ∞ for more information about nutrition.

Personal Values and Attitudes

Whether individuals value regular exercise is often the result of family influences. In families that incorporate regular exercise into their daily routine or spend time together in activities, children learn to value physical activity. Sedentary families, on the other hand, participate in sports only as spectators, and this lifestyle is often transmitted to their children. With the increase in TV, computer, and video activities, youth are increasingly sedentary with associated declines in health. Values about physical appearance also influence some individuals' participation in regular exercise. Individuals who value a muscular build or physical attractiveness may participate in regular exercise programs to produce the appearance they desire.

Choice of physical activity or type of exercise is also influenced by values. Choices may be influenced by geographic location and cultural role expectations. For many, thinking of exercise more as "recreational movement," "enhancement of well-being," and "an essential part of daily self-care" may help overcome perceptions that exercise is drudgery. Options include informal and fun activities such as dancing to music. Motivational states influence our behavior and choices, and vary widely from day to day.

External Factors

Many external factors affect an individual's mobility. Excessively high temperatures and high humidity discourage activity, whereas comfortable temperatures and low humidity are conducive to activity. Proper hydration needs vary according to the individual, health status, activity levels, and environment. Water is the best fluid to replace loss incurred through metabolic processes and exercise.

The availability of recreational facilities also influences activity; for example, lack of money may prohibit a client from joining an exercise club or gymnasium or from purchasing needed equipment. Neighborhood safety promotes outdoor activity, whereas an unsafe environment discourages individuals from going outdoors. Adolescents, in particular, may spend many hours sitting at computers, watching television, or playing video games rather than engaging in physical activities.

Prescribed Limitations

Limitations to movement may be medically prescribed for some health problems. To promote healing, devices such as casts, braces, splints, and traction are often used to immobilize body parts. Clients who are short of breath may be advised not to walk up stairs. Bedrest may be the therapeutic choice for certain clients, for example, to relieve edema, to reduce metabolic and oxygen needs, to promote tissue repair, or to decrease pain.

The term **bedrest** varies in meaning to some extent. In some agencies, bedrest means strict confinement to bed or "complete" bedrest. Others may allow the client to use a bedside commode or have bathroom privileges. Nurses need to familiarize themselves with the meaning of bedrest in their practice setting. In any case, the effects of limiting activity are immediate, and therapeutic positioning is important to prevent further complications and improve client outcomes. There is rarely a need for complete bedrest.

Exercise

Individuals participate in exercise programs to decrease risk factors for chronic diseases and to increase their health and well-being. **Functional strength** is another goal of exercise, and is defined as the ability of the body to perform work. **Activity tolerance** is the type and amount of exercise or ADLs an individual is able to perform without experiencing adverse effects.

Types of Exercise

Exercise involves the active contraction and relaxation of muscles. Exercises can be classified according to the type of muscle contraction (isotonic, isometric, or isokinetic) and according to the source of energy (aerobic or anaerobic).

Isotonic (dynamic) exercises are those in which the muscle shortens to produce muscle contraction and active movement. Most physical conditioning exercises—running, walking, swimming, cycling, and other such activities—are isotonic, as are ADLs and active ROM exercises (those initiated by the client). Examples of isotonic bed exercises are pushing or pulling against a stationary object, using a trapeze to lift the body off the bed, lifting the buttocks off the bed by pushing with the hands against the mattress, and pushing the body to a sitting position.

Isotonic exercises increase muscle tone, mass, and strength and maintain joint flexibility and circulation. During isotonic exercise, both heart rate and cardiac output quicken to increase blood flow to all parts of the body.

Isometric (static or setting) exercises are those in which muscle contraction occurs without moving the joint (muscle length does not change). These exercises involve exerting pressure against a solid object and are useful for strengthening abdominal, gluteal, and quadriceps muscles used in ambulation; for maintaining strength in immobilized muscles in casts or traction; and for endurance training. An example of an isometric bed exercise would be squeezing a towel or pillow between the knees while at the same time tightening the muscles in the fronts of the thighs by pressing the knees backwards (see Figure 44.31 ■), and holding for several seconds. These are often called "quad sets." Isometric exercises produce a mild increase in heart rate and cardiac output, but no appreciable increase in blood flow to other parts of the body.

Isokinetic (resistive) exercises involve muscle contraction or tension against resistance. During isokinetic exercises, the individual tenses (isometric) against resistance. Special machines or devices provide the resistance to the movement. These exercises are used in physical conditioning and are often done to build up certain muscle groups.

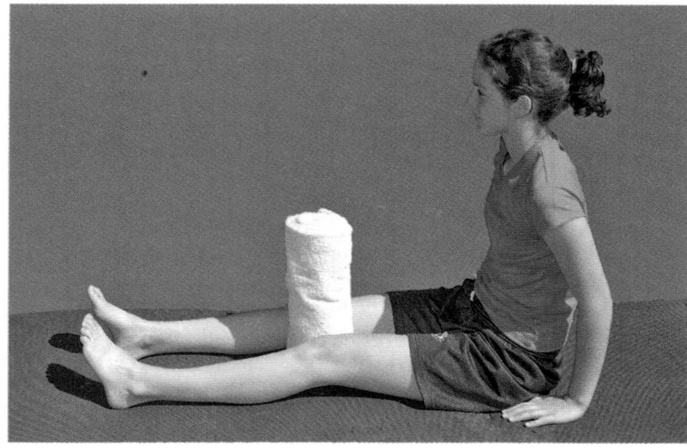

Figure 44.31 ■ Example of an isometric exercise for the knees and legs. The client sits or lies on a flat surface with the legs straight out. Using a rolled towel between the knees, the client pushes the knees together and tightens the muscles in the front of the thighs by forcing the knees downward and holding for 10 seconds.

Aerobic exercise is activity during which the amount of oxygen taken into the body is greater than that used to perform the activity. Aerobic exercises use large muscle groups that move repetitively. Aerobic exercises improve cardiovascular conditioning and physical fitness. Assessment of physical fitness is discussed in Chapter 19 ∞. The accompanying Client Teaching feature describes frequency, duration, and types of activity recommended for healthy adults.

Intensity of exercise can be measured in three ways:

1. ***Target heart rate.*** The goal is to work up to and sustain a target heart rate during exercise, based on the individual's age. To determine target heart rate, first calculate the client's maximum heart rate by subtracting his or her current age in years from 220. Then obtain the target heart rate by taking 60% to 85% of the maximum. Because heart rates vary among individuals, the tests that follow are replacing this measure.

CLIENT TEACHING **Guidelines and Minimal Requirements for Physical Activity**

FREQUENCY AND DURATION

- *Aerobic:* Cumulative 30 minutes or more daily (can be divided throughout the day) of "moderate intensity" movement as measured by talk test and perceived exertion scale.
- *Stretching:* Should be added onto that minimum requirement so that all parts of the body are stretched each day.
- *Strength training:* Should be added onto these minimum requirements so that all muscle groups are addressed at least three times a week, with a day of rest after training.

TYPE OF EXERCISE

- *Aerobic:* Elliptical exercisers, walking, biking, gardening, dancing, and swimming are recommended for all individuals, including beginners and older adults. Activities that are more strenuous include jogging, running, Spinning, power yoga, boxing, and jumping rope.
- *Stretching:* Yoga, Pilates, qigong, and many other flexibility programs are effective.
- *Strength training:* Resistance can be provided with weights, bands, balls, and body weight.

SAFETY

- Stress the importance of balance and prevention of falls, proper clothing to ensure thermal safety, checking equipment for proper function, wearing a helmet and other protective gear, using reflective devices at night, and carrying identification and emergency information.

2. *Talk test.* This test is easier to implement and keeps most people at 60% of maximum heart rate or more. When exercising, the client should experience labored breathing, yet still be able to carry on a conversation.
3. ***Borg scale of perceived exertion*** (Borg, 1998). This scale measures "how difficult" the exercise feels to the client in terms of heart and lung exertion. The scale progresses from 1 to 20 with the following markers: 7 = very, very light; 9 = very light; 11 = fairly light; 13 = somewhat hard; 15 = hard; 17 = very hard; and 19 = very, very hard.

   "Very, very hard" corresponds closely to 100% of maximum heart rate. "Very light" is close to 40%. Most people need to strive for the "somewhat hard" level (13/20), which corresponds to 75% of maximum heart rate.

Anaerobic exercise involves activity in which the muscles cannot draw out enough oxygen from the bloodstream, and anaerobic pathways are used to provide additional energy for a short time. This type of exercise is used in endurance training for athletes such as weight lifting and sprinting.

QSEN Patient-Centered Care: Therapeutic Movement Modalities

Therapeutic movement modalities from Eastern cultures are finding a place in evidence-based healthcare. In particular, Hatha yoga, qigong, and t'ai chi are receiving wide attention for improving strength and balance as well as treating a wide variety of health problems. Hatha yoga, developed in ancient Hindu culture, is a series of physical exercises, breath control, and meditation that tones and strengthens the whole individual—body, mind, and spirit (Figure 44.32 ■). The beauty of yoga is that it can be fully practiced by those who must use a wheelchair or remain in bed.

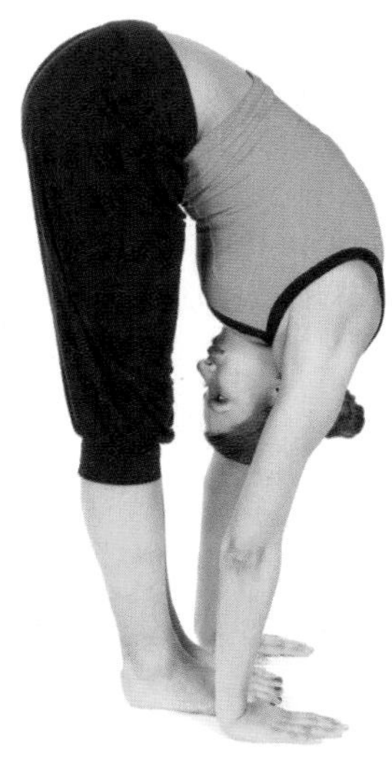

Figure 44.32 ■ Woman in a yoga stretch.
Artur Bogacki/Shutterstock.

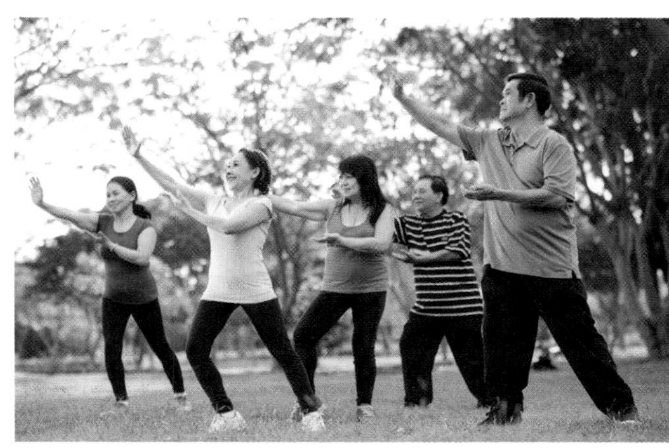

Figure 44.33 ■ Men and women practicing t'ai chi outdoors.
Dinis Tolipov/123RF.

Qigong is a Chinese discipline that involves breathing and gentle movements of mostly arms and torso. The regular practice of qigong is intended to generate as well as conserve energy to maintain health or treat illness.

Although developed as a martial art, t'ai chi is practiced today mostly for health promotion. In China, it is common to see individuals of all ages, including older adults, practicing these movement disciplines outdoors in public parks (Figure 44.33 ■).

Nurses can independently recommend that clients who are able to do so consider initiating these movement modalities. Through appropriate referrals to group classes in the community as well as the use of videotapes in homes and long-term care facilities, clients can take charge of their own health in ways that are empowering, holistic, and free of negative side effects. Nurses should assess each individual for readiness, safety issues, balance, and ability to engage in any physical activity.

Benefits of Exercise

In general, regular exercise is essential for maintaining mental and physical health.

Musculoskeletal System

The size, shape, tone, and strength of muscles (including the heart muscle) are maintained with mild exercise and increased with strenuous exercise. With strenuous exercise, muscles **hypertrophy** (enlarge), and the efficiency of muscular contraction increases. Joints lack a discrete blood supply. It is through activity that joints receive nourishment. Exercise increases joint flexibility, stability, and range of motion. Bone density and strength are maintained through weight bearing. The stress of weight-bearing and high-impact movement maintains a balance between osteoblasts (bone-building cells) and osteoclasts (bone-resorption and breakdown cells). Examples of non–weight-bearing exercise include swimming and bicycling.

Cardiovascular System

The American Heart Association (2018) places great emphasis on physical activity by recommending at least 150 minutes per week of moderate exercise or 75 minutes per week of vigorous exercise, or a combination of moderate and vigorous activity. Adequate moderate-intensity exercise increases the heart rate, the strength of heart muscle contraction, and the blood supply to the heart and muscles through increased cardiac output. Exercise also promotes heart health by reducing the harmful effects of stress. The types of exercise that will provide cardiac benefit vary. They include aerobic exercise such as walking and cycling. Research evidence supports the benefits of yoga practice on cardiovascular health.

Respiratory System

Ventilation (air circulating into and out of the lungs) and oxygen intake increase during exercise, thereby improving gas exchange. More toxins are eliminated with deeper breathing, and problem-solving and emotional stability are enhanced due to increased oxygen to the brain. Adequate exercise also prevents pooling of secretions in the bronchi and bronchioles, decreasing breathing effort and risk of infection. Attention to exercising muscles of respiration (by deep breathing) throughout an activity as well as rest enhances oxygenation (improving stamina) and circulation of lymph (improving immune function).

Gastrointestinal System

Exercise improves the appetite and increases gastrointestinal tract tone, facilitating peristalsis. Activities such as rowing, swimming, walking, and sit-ups work the abdominal muscles and can help relieve constipation.

Endocrine System and Metabolism

Exercise elevates the metabolic rate, thus increasing the production of body heat and waste products and calorie use. During strenuous exercise, the metabolic rate can increase to as much as 20 times the normal rate. This elevation lasts after exercise is completed. Exercise increases the use of triglycerides and fatty acids, resulting in a reduced level of serum triglycerides, glycosylated hemoglobin A1C (HbA1C) levels, and cholesterol. Weight loss and exercise stabilize blood sugar and make cells more responsive to insulin.

Urinary System

With adequate exercise, which promotes efficient blood flow, the body excretes wastes more effectively. In addition, stasis (stagnation) of urine in the bladder is usually prevented, which in turn decreases the risk for urinary tract infections (UTIs).

Immune System

As respiratory and musculoskeletal effort increase with exercise and as gravity is enlisted with postural changes, lymph fluid is more efficiently pumped from tissues into lymph capillaries and vessels throughout the body. Circulation through lymph nodes where destruction of pathogens and removal of foreign antigens can occur is also improved.

Psychoneurologic System

Mental or affective disorders such as depression or chronic stress may affect an individual's desire to move. The depressed client may lack enthusiasm for taking part in any activity and may even lack energy for usual hygiene practices. Lack of visible energy is often seen in a slumped posture with head bent down. Chronic stress can deplete the body's energy reserves to the point that fatigue discourages the desire to exercise, even though exercise can energize the client and facilitate coping. By contrast, clients with eating disorders may exercise excessively in an effort to prevent weight gain.

A growing body of evidence supports the role of exercise in elevating mood and relieving stress and anxiety across the lifespan. Solid data examining relationships between both aerobic and nonaerobic styles of exercise support the use of this modality to relieve symptoms of depression. The mechanism of action is thought to be a result of one or more of the following: Exercise increases levels of metabolites for neurotransmitters such as norepinephrine and serotonin; exercise releases endogenous opioids, thus increasing levels of endorphins; exercise increases levels of oxygen to the brain and other body systems, inducing euphoria; and through muscular exertion (especially with movement modalities such as yoga and t'ai chi) the body releases stored stress associated with accumulated emotional demands. Regular exercise also improves quality of sleep for most individuals.

Cognitive Function

Current research supports the positive effects of exercise on cognitive functioning, in particular decision-making and problem-solving processes, planning, and paying attention. Physical exertion induces cells in the brain to strengthen and build neuronal connections.

Spiritual Health

Yoga-style exercise improves the mind–body–spirit connection, relationship with God, and physical well-being by establishing balance in the internal and external environment. The combination of mind, body, and breath awareness is likely to have an impact on psychophysiologic functioning. The emphasis on breathing in is thought to soothe the nervous and cardiorespiratory systems, promoting relaxation and preparedness for a contemplative experience.

The **relaxation response (RR)**, first described by Dr. Herbert Benson, is beneficial for counteracting some of the harmful effects of stress on the body and mind. The RR is a healthful physiologic relaxation that can be elicited through recitation of a word or phrase or prayer while sitting quietly and relaxing your muscles.

Progressive muscle relaxation techniques involve contracting and then releasing groups of muscles throughout the body until all parts of the body feel relaxed. These movements are subtle and, along with relaxation breathing, can be done by almost anyone at any time, regardless of mobility or fitness status, providing potent stress relief and neurocardiovascular health benefits.

Effects of Immobility

Mobility and activity tolerance are affected by any disorder that impairs the ability of the nervous system, musculoskeletal system, cardiovascular system, respiratory system, and vestibular apparatus. Congenital problems such as hip dysplasia, spina bifida, cerebral palsy, and the muscular dystrophies affect motor functioning. Disorders of the nervous system such as Parkinson's disease, multiple sclerosis, central nervous system tumors, strokes, infectious processes (e.g., meningitis), and head and spinal cord injuries can leave muscle groups weakened, paralyzed (**paresis**), **spastic** (with too much muscle tone), or **flaccid** (without muscle tone). Musculoskeletal disorders affecting mobility include strains, sprains, fractures, joint dislocations, amputations, and joint replacements. Inner ear infections and dizziness can impair balance. Many other acute and chronic illnesses that limit the supply of oxygen and nutrients needed for muscle contraction and movement can seriously affect activity tolerance. Examples include chronic obstructive lung disease, anemia, congestive heart failure, and angina.

Individuals who have inactive lifestyles or who are faced with inactivity because of illness or injury are at risk for many problems that can affect major body systems. Whether immobility causes any problems often depends on the duration of the inactivity, the client's health status, and the client's sensory awareness. The most obvious signs of prolonged immobility are often manifested in the musculoskeletal system, and the deconditioning effects can be observed even after a matter of days. Clients experience a significant decrease in muscular strength and agility whenever they do not maintain a moderate amount of physical activity. In addition, immobility adversely affects the cardiovascular, respiratory, metabolic, urinary, and psychoneurologic systems. Nurses need to understand these effects and encourage client movement as much as possible. Early ambulation after illness or surgery is an essential measure to prevent complications.

Clinical Alert!

A review of studies on effects of bedrest in clients with different disorders revealed that bedrest for treatment of medical conditions is associated with worse outcomes than early mobilization. In general, there are few indications for bedrest, and bedrest may delay recovery or actually harm clients.

Musculoskeletal System

- *Disuse osteoporosis.* Without the stress of weight-bearing activity, the bones demineralize. They are depleted chiefly of calcium, which gives the bones strength and density. Regardless of the amount of calcium in an individual's diet, the demineralization process, known as *osteoporosis*, continues with immobility. The bones become spongy and may gradually deform and fracture easily.
- *Disuse atrophy.* Unused muscles **atrophy** (decrease in size), losing most of their strength and normal function.
- *Contractures.* When the muscle fibers are not able to shorten and lengthen, eventually a **contracture** (permanent shortening of the muscle) forms, limiting joint mobility. This process eventually involves the tendons, ligaments, and joint capsules; it is irreversible except by surgical intervention. Joint deformities such as **foot drop** (Figure 44.34 ■), wrist drop, and external hip rotation occur when a stronger muscle dominates the opposite muscle.
- *Stiffness and pain in the joints.* Without movement, the collagen (connective) tissues at the joint become **ankylosed** (permanently immobile). In addition, as the bones demineralize, excess calcium may deposit in the joints, contributing to stiffness and pain.

Cardiovascular System

- *Diminished cardiac reserve.* Decreased mobility creates an imbalance in the autonomic nervous system, resulting in a dominance of sympathetic activity that increases heart rate. Rapid heart rate reduces diastolic pressure, coronary blood flow, and the capacity of the heart to respond to any metabolic demands above the basal levels. Because of this diminished cardiac reserve, the immobilized client may experience tachycardia with even minimal exertion.
- *Increased use of the Valsalva maneuver.* The **Valsalva maneuver** refers to holding the breath and straining against a closed glottis. For example, clients tend to hold their breath when attempting to move up in a bed or sit on a bedpan. This builds up sufficient pressure on the large veins in the thorax to interfere with the return blood flow to the heart and coronary arteries. When the client exhales and the glottis again opens, pressure is suddenly released, and a surge of blood flows to the heart. Cardiac arrhythmias can result if the client has preexisting cardiac disease.
- *Orthostatic (postural) hypotension.* **Orthostatic hypotension** is a common result of immobilization. Under normal conditions, sympathetic nervous system activity causes automatic vasoconstriction in the blood vessels in the lower half of the body when a mobile client changes from a horizontal to a vertical posture.

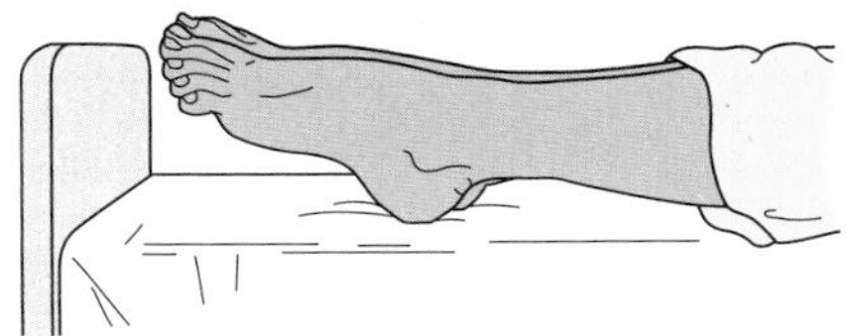

Figure 44.34 ■ Plantar flexion contracture (foot drop).

Vasoconstriction prevents pooling of the blood in the legs and effectively maintains central blood pressure to ensure adequate perfusion of the heart and brain. During any prolonged immobility, however, this reflex becomes inactive. When the immobile client attempts to sit or stand, this reconstricting mechanism fails to function properly in spite of increased adrenalin output. The blood pools in the lower extremities, and central blood pressure drops. Cerebral perfusion is seriously compromised, and the client feels dizzy or light-headed and may even faint. This sequence is usually accompanied by a sudden and marked increase in heart rate, the body's effort to protect the brain from an inadequate blood supply.

- ***Venous vasodilation and stasis.*** The skeletal muscles of an active client contract with each movement, compressing the blood vessels in those muscles and helping to pump the blood back to the heart against gravity. The tiny valves in the leg veins aid in venous return to the heart by preventing backward flow of blood and pooling. In an immobile client, the skeletal muscles do not contract sufficiently, and the muscles atrophy. The skeletal muscles can no longer assist in pumping blood back to the heart against gravity. Blood pools in the leg veins, causing vasodilation and engorgement. The valves in the veins can no longer work effectively to prevent backward flow of blood and pooling (Figure 44.35 ■). This phenomenon is known as incompetent valves. As the blood continues to pool in the veins, its greater volume increases venous blood pressure, which can become much higher than that exerted by the tissues surrounding the vessel.
- ***Dependent edema.*** When the venous pressure is sufficiently great, some of the serous part of the blood is forced out of the blood vessel into the interstitial spaces surrounding the blood vessel, causing edema. Edema is most common in parts of the body positioned below the heart. Dependent edema is most likely to occur around the sacrum or heels of a client who sits up in bed or in the feet and lower legs of a client who sits in a chair. Edema further impedes venous return of blood to the heart, causing more pooling and more edema. Edematous tissue is uncomfortable and more susceptible to injury than normal tissue.

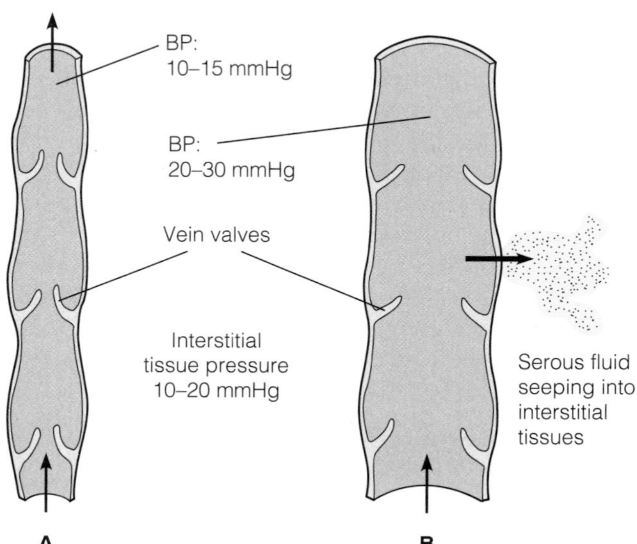

Figure 44.35 ■ Leg veins: *A*, in a mobile client; *B*, in an immobile client.

- ***Thrombus formation.*** Three factors collectively predispose a client to the formation of a **thrombophlebitis** (a clot that is loosely attached to an inflamed vein wall): impaired venous return to the heart, hypercoagulability of the blood (sometimes caused by medications such as oral contraceptives), and injury to a vessel wall.

A **thrombus** (clot) is particularly dangerous if it breaks loose from the vein wall to enter the general circulation as an **embolus** (an object that has moved from its place of origin, causing obstruction to circulation elsewhere). Large emboli that enter the pulmonary circulation may occlude the vessels that nourish the lungs to cause an infarcted (dead) area of the lung. If the infarcted area is large, pulmonary function may be seriously compromised, or death may ensue. Emboli traveling to the coronary vessels or brain can produce a similarly dangerous outcome.

Clinical Alert!

Prolonged inactivity (such as bedrest or sleeping during a long plane ride) in combination with oral contraceptive use can lead to dangerous clot formation in deep leg veins, even in otherwise healthy young women. Smoking increases this risk. Regular movement, stretching, and keeping legs uncrossed are recommended. Monitor for tenderness, redness or discoloration, warmth, and swelling in the legs.

Respiratory System

- ***Decreased respiratory movement.*** In a recumbent, immobile client, ventilation of the lungs is passively altered. The body presses against the rigid bed and decreases chest movement. The abdominal organs push against the diaphragm, restricting lung movement and making it difficult to expand the lungs fully. An immobile, recumbent client rarely sighs, partly because overall muscle atrophy also affects the respiratory muscles and partly because there is no stimulus of activity. Without these periodic stretching movements, the cartilaginous intercostal joints may become fixed in an expiratory phase of respiration, further limiting the potential for maximal ventilation. These changes produce shallow respirations and reduce **vital capacity** (the maximum amount of air that can be exhaled after a maximum inhalation).
- ***Pooling of respiratory secretions.*** Secretions of the respiratory tract are normally expelled by changing positions or posture and by coughing. Inactivity allows secretions to pool by gravity (Figure 44.36 ■), interfering with the normal diffusion of oxygen and

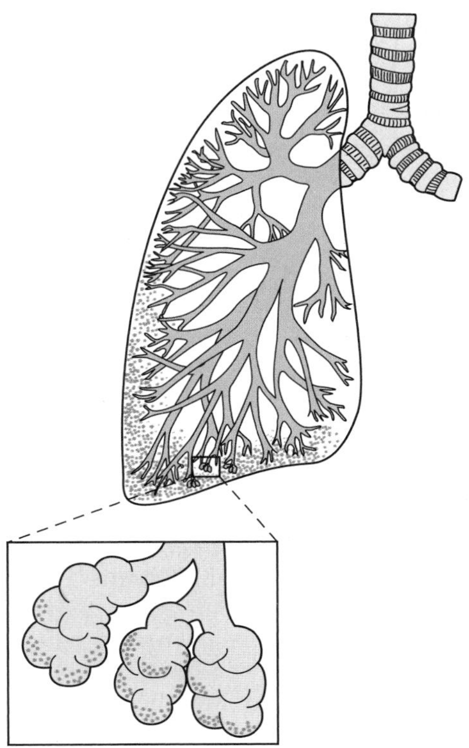

Figure 44.36 ■ Pooling of secretions in the lungs of an immobile client.

carbon dioxide in the alveoli. The ability to cough up secretions may also be hindered by loss of respiratory muscle tone, dehydration (which thickens secretions), or sedatives that depress the cough reflex. Poor oxygenation and retention of carbon dioxide in the blood can, if allowed to continue, predispose the client to respiratory acidosis, a potentially lethal disorder.

- *Atelectasis.* When ventilation is decreased, pooled secretions may accumulate in a dependent area of a bronchiole and effectively block it. Because of changes in regional blood flow, bedrest decreases the amount of surfactant produced. (Surfactant enables the alveoli to remain open.) The combination of decreased surfactant and blockage of a bronchiole with mucus can cause **atelectasis** (the collapse of a lobe or of an entire lung) distal to the mucous blockage. Immobile older, postoperative clients are at greatest risk of atelectasis.
- *Hypostatic pneumonia.* Pooled secretions provide excellent media for bacterial growth. Under these conditions, a minor upper respiratory infection can evolve rapidly into a severe infection of the lower respiratory tract. Pneumonia caused by static respiratory secretions can severely impair oxygen–carbon dioxide exchange in the alveoli and is a fairly common cause of death among weakened, immobile clients, especially heavy smokers.

Metabolism

- *Decreased metabolic rate.* **Metabolism** refers to the sum of all the physical and chemical processes by which living substance is formed and maintained and by which energy is made available for use by the body. The **basal metabolic rate (BMR)** is the minimal energy expended for the maintenance of these processes, expressed in calories per hour per square meter of body surface. In immobile clients, the basal metabolic rate and gastrointestinal motility and secretions of various digestive glands decrease as the energy requirements of the body decrease.
- *Negative nitrogen balance.* In an active client, a balance exists between protein synthesis (**anabolism**) and protein breakdown (**catabolism**). Immobility creates a marked imbalance, and the catabolic processes exceed the anabolic processes. Catabolized muscle mass releases nitrogen. Over time, more nitrogen is excreted than is ingested, producing a negative nitrogen balance. The negative nitrogen balance represents a depletion of protein stores that are essential for building muscle tissue and for wound healing.
- *Anorexia.* Loss of appetite (**anorexia**) occurs because of the decreased metabolic rate and the increased catabolism that accompany immobility. Reduced caloric intake is usually a response to the decreased energy requirements of the inactive client. If protein intake is reduced, the nitrogen imbalance may become more pronounced, sometimes so severely that malnutrition ensues.
- *Negative calcium balance.* A negative calcium balance occurs as a direct result of immobility. Greater amounts of calcium are extracted from bone than can be replaced. The absence of weight bearing and of stress on the musculoskeletal structures is the direct cause of the calcium loss from bones. Weight bearing and stress are also required for calcium to be replaced in bone.

Urinary System

- *Urinary stasis.* In a mobile client, gravity plays an important role in the emptying of the kidneys and the bladder. The shape and position of the kidneys and active kidney contractions are important in completely emptying the urine from the calyces, renal pelvis, and ureters (Figure 44.37*A* ■). The shape and position of

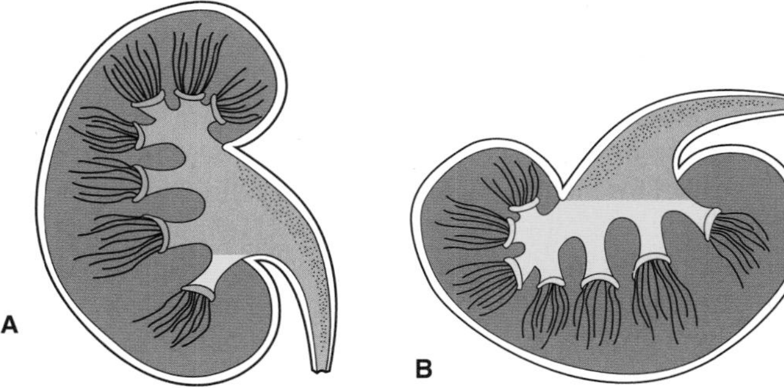

Figure 44.37 ■ Pooling of urine in the kidney: *A*, The client is in an upright position. *B*, The client is in a back-lying position.

the urinary bladder (the detrusor muscle) and active bladder contractions are also important in achieving complete emptying.

- When the client remains in a horizontal position, gravity impedes the emptying of urine from the kidneys and the urinary bladder. To urinate, the client who is supine (in a back-lying position) must push upward, against gravity (Figures 44.37*B*). The renal pelvis may fill with urine before it is pushed into the ureters. Emptying is not as complete, and **urinary stasis** (stoppage or slowdown of flow) occurs after a few days of bedrest. Because of the overall decrease in muscle tone during immobilization, including the tone of the detrusor muscle, bladder emptying is further compromised.
- ***Renal calculi.*** In a mobile client, calcium in the urine remains dissolved because calcium and citric acid are balanced in appropriately acidic urine. With immobility and the resulting excessive amounts of calcium in the urine, this balance is no longer maintained. The urine becomes more alkaline, and the calcium salts precipitate out as crystals to form renal **calculi** (stones). In an immobile client in a horizontal position, the renal pelvis filled with stagnant, alkaline urine is an ideal location for calculi to form. The stones usually develop in the renal pelvis and pass through the ureters into the bladder. As the stones pass along the long, narrow ureters, they cause extreme pain and bleeding and can sometimes obstruct the urinary tract.
- ***Urinary retention.*** The immobile client may suffer from **urinary retention** (accumulation of urine in the bladder), bladder distention, and occasionally **urinary incontinence** (involuntary urination). The decreased muscle tone of the urinary bladder inhibits its ability to empty completely. In addition, the discomfort of using a bedpan or urinal, the embarrassment and lack of privacy associated with this function, and the unnatural position for urination combine to make it difficult for the client to relax the perineal muscles sufficiently to urinate while lying in bed.
- When urination is not possible, the bladder gradually becomes distended with urine. The bladder may stretch excessively, eventually inhibiting the urge to void. When bladder distention is considerable, some involuntary urinary "dribbling" may occur (retention with overflow). This does not relieve the urinary distention, because most of the stagnant urine remains in the bladder.
- ***Urinary infection.*** Static urine provides an excellent medium for bacterial growth. The flushing action of normal, frequent urination is absent, and urinary distention often causes minute tears in the bladder mucosa, allowing infectious organisms to enter. The increased alkalinity of the urine caused by the hypercalcuria supports bacterial growth. The organism most commonly causing urinary tract infections is *Escherichia coli*, which normally resides in the colon. The normally sterile urinary tract may be contaminated by improper perineal care, the use of an indwelling urinary catheter, or occasionally **urinary reflux** (backward flow). During reflux, contaminated urine from an overly distended bladder backs up into the renal pelvis to contaminate the kidney pelvis as well.

Gastrointestinal System

Constipation is a frequent problem for immobilized clients because of decreased peristalsis and colon motility. The overall skeletal muscle weakness affects the abdominal and perineal muscles used in defecation. When the stool becomes very hard, more strength is required to expel it. The immobile client may lack this strength. This can lead to impaction.

A client's unnatural and uncomfortable position on a bedpan does not facilitate elimination. The backward-leaning posture does not promote effective use of the muscles used in defecation. Some clients are reluctant to use the bedpan in the presence of others. The embarrassment, lack of privacy, dependence on others to assist with the bedpan, and disruption of normal bowel habits may cause the client to postpone or ignore the urge for elimination. Repeated postponement eventually suppresses the urge and weakens the defecation reflex.

Some clients may make excessive use of the Valsalva maneuver by straining at stool in an attempt to expel the hard stool. This effort dangerously increases intra-abdominal and intrathoracic pressures and places undue stress on the heart and circulatory system.

Integumentary System

- ***Reduced skin turgor.*** The skin can atrophy as a result of prolonged immobility. Shifts in body fluids between the fluid compartments can affect the consistency and health of the dermis and subcutaneous tissues in dependent parts of the body, eventually causing a gradual loss in skin elasticity.
- ***Skin breakdown.*** Normal blood circulation relies on muscle activity. Immobility impedes circulation and diminishes the supply of nutrients to specific areas. As a result, skin breakdown and formation of pressure injuries can occur.

Psychoneurologic System

Due to a decline in production of mood-elevating substances such as endorphins, individuals experience negative effects on mood when unable to engage in physical activity. Clients who are unable to carry out the usual activities related to their roles (e.g., as employee, husband, mother, or athlete) become aware of an increased dependence on others. These factors lower the client's self-esteem. Frustration and the decrease in self-esteem may in turn provoke exaggerated emotional reactions. Emotional reactions vary considerably. Some clients become apathetic and withdrawn, some regress, and some become angry and aggressive.

Because the immobilized client's participation in life becomes much narrower and the variety of stimuli decreases, the client's perception of time intervals deteriorates. Problem-solving and decision-making abilities may deteriorate as a result of lack of intellectual stimulation and the stress of the illness and immobility. In addition, the loss of control over events can cause anxiety.

●○● NURSING MANAGEMENT

Assessing

Assessment of a client's activity and exercise should be routinely addressed and includes a nursing history and a physical examination of body alignment, gait, appearance and movement of joints, capabilities and limitations for movement, muscle mass and strength, activity tolerance, problems related to immobility, and physical fitness.

The nurse collects information from the client, from other nurses, and from the client's records. The examination and history are important sources of information about disabilities affecting the client's mobility and activity status, such as contractures, edema, pain in the extremities, or generalized fatigue.

Nursing History

An activity and exercise history is usually part of the comprehensive nursing history. Examples of interview questions to elicit these data are shown in the accompanying Assessment Interview. If the client indicates a recent pattern change or difficulties with mobility, a more detailed history is required. This detailed history should include the specific nature of the problem, when it first began, its frequency, its causes if known, how the problem affects daily living, what the client is doing to cope with the problem, and whether these methods have been effective.

Physical Examination

Conduct the physical examination focusing on activity and exercise patterns. The exam includes assessment of body alignment, gait, appearance and movement of joints, capabilities and limitations for movement, muscle mass and strength, activity tolerance, and problems related to immobility.

Body Alignment

Assessment of body alignment includes an inspection of the client while the client stands. The purpose of body alignment assessment is to identify:

- Normal developmental variations in posture
- Posture and learning needs to maintain good posture
- Factors contributing to poor posture, such as fatigue, pain, compression fractures, or low self-esteem
- Muscle weakness or other motor impairments.

To assess alignment, the nurse inspects the client from lateral (Figure 44.38*A* ■), anterior, and posterior perspectives. From the anterior and posterior views, the nurse should observe whether:

- The shoulders and hips are level
- The toes point forward
- The spine is straight, not curved to either side.

ASSESSMENT INTERVIEW Activity and Exercise

DAILY ACTIVITY LEVEL

- What activities do you carry out during a routine day?
- Are you able to carry out the following tasks independently?
  a. Eating
  b. Dressing and grooming
  c. Bathing
  d. Toileting
  e. Ambulating
  f. Using a wheelchair
  g. Transferring in and out of bed, bath, and car
  h. Cooking
  i. House cleaning
  j. Shopping
- Where problems exist in your ability to carry out such tasks:
  a. Would you rate yourself as partially or totally dependent?
  b. How is the task achieved (by family, friend, agency, or use of specialized equipment)?

ACTIVITY TOLERANCE

- What types of activities make you tired?
- Do you ever experience dizziness, shortness of breath, marked increase in respiratory rate, or other problems following mild or moderate activity?

EXERCISE

- What type of exercise do you carry out to enhance your physical fitness?
- What is the frequency and length of this exercise session?
- Do you believe exercise is beneficial to your health? Explain.

FACTORS AFFECTING MOBILITY

- *Environmental factors.* Do stairs, lack of railings or other assistive devices, or an unsafe neighborhood impede your mobility or exercise regimen?
- *Health problems.* Do any of the following health problems affect your muscle strength or endurance: heart disease, lung disease, stroke, cancer, neuromuscular problems, musculoskeletal problems, visual or mental impairments, trauma, or pain?
- *Financial factors.* Are your finances adequate to obtain equipment or other aids that you require to enhance your mobility?

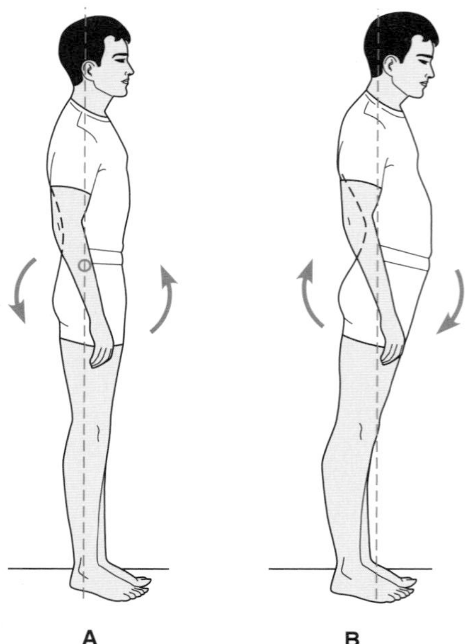

Figure 44.38 ■ A standing person with *A*, good trunk alignment; *B*, poor trunk alignment. The arrows indicate the direction in which the pelvis is tilted.

The "slumped" posture (Figure 44.38*B*) is the most common problem that occurs when people stand. The neck is flexed far forward, the abdomen protrudes, the pelvis is thrust forward to create **lordosis** (an exaggerated anterior or inward curvature of the lumbar spine), and the knees are hyperextended. Low back pain and fatigue occur quickly in people with poor posture.

Gait

The characteristic pattern of a client's **gait** (walk) is assessed to determine the client's mobility and risk for injury due to falling. Two phases of normal gait are swing and stance (Figure 44.39 ■). When one leg is in the swing phase, the other is in the stance phase. In the *stance phase*, (a) the heel of one foot strikes the ground, and (b) body weight is spread over the ball of that foot while the other heel pushes off and leaves the ground. In the *swing phase*, the leg from behind moves in front of the body.

The nurse assesses gait as the client walks into the room or asks the client to walk a distance of 10 feet down a hallway and observes for the following:

- Chin is level, gaze is straight ahead, sternum is lifted, and shoulders are down and back, relaxed away from the ears.
- Heel strikes the ground before the toe. It is here, where both feet are taking some body weight, that the spine is most rotated.
- Feet are dorsiflexed in the swing phase.
- Arm opposite the swing-through foot moves forward at the same time.
- Gait is smooth, coordinated, and rhythmic, with even weight borne on each foot. Hips gently sway with spinal rotation; the body moves forward smoothly, stopping and starting with ease.

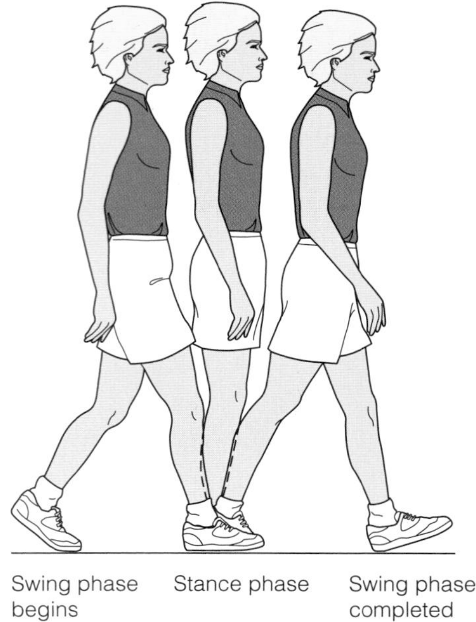

Figure 44.39 ■ The swing and stance phases of a normal gait.

The nurse may also assess **pace** (the number of steps taken per minute), which often slows with age and disability. A normal walking pace is 70 to 100 steps per minute. The pace of an older adult may slow to about 40 steps per minute.

The nurse should also note the client's need for a prosthesis or assistive device, such as a cane or walker. For a client who uses assistive aids, the nurse assesses gait without the device and compares the assisted and unassisted gaits.

Appearance and Movement of Joints

Physical examination of the joints involves inspection, palpation, assessment of range of active motion, and if active motion is not possible, assessment of range of passive motion. The nurse should assess the following:

- Any joint swelling or redness, which could indicate the presence of an injury or an inflammation
- Any deformity, such as a bony enlargement or contracture, and symmetry of involvement
- The muscle development associated with each joint and the relative size and symmetry of the muscles on each side of the body
- Any reported or palpable tenderness
- **Crepitation** (palpable or audible crackling or grating sensation produced by joint motion and frequently experienced in joints that have suffered repeated trauma over time)
- Increased temperature over the joint; palpate the joint using the backs of the fingers and compare the temperature with that of the symmetric joint
- Degree of joint movement; ask the client to move selected body parts as shown in Table 44.2.

Assessment of range of motion should not be unduly fatiguing, and the joint movements need to be performed smoothly, slowly, and rhythmically. No joint should be forced. Uneven, jerky movement and forcing can injure the joint and its surrounding muscles and ligaments.

Capabilities and Limitations for Movement

The nurse needs to obtain data that may indicate hindrances or restrictions to the client's movement and the need for assistance, including the following:

- How the client's illness influences the ability to move and whether the client's health contraindicates any exertion, position, or movement
- Limitations to movement, such as an IV line in place or a heavy cast
- Mental alertness and ability to follow directions; check whether the client is receiving medications that hinder the ability to walk safely. Narcotics, sedatives, tranquilizers, and some antihistamines cause drowsiness, dizziness, weakness, and orthostatic hypotension.
- Balance and coordination
- Presence of orthostatic hypotension before transfers; specifically, assess for any increase in pulse rate, marked fall in blood pressure, dizziness, light-headedness, and dimming of vision when the client moves from a supine to a vertical posture.
- Degree of comfort (Clients who have pain may not want to move and may require an analgesic before they are moved.)
- Vision: Is it adequate to prevent falls?

The nurse also assesses the amount of assistance the client requires for the following:

- Moving in the bed. In particular, observe for the amount of assistance the client requires for turning:
  a. From a supine position to a lateral position
  b. From a lateral position on one side to a lateral position on the other
  c. From a supine position to a sitting position in bed.
- Rising from a lying position to a sitting position on the edge of the bed. Healthy individuals can normally rise without support from the arms.
- Rising from a chair to a standing position. Normally this can be done without pushing with the arms.
- Coordination and balance. Determine the client's abilities to hold the body erect, to bear weight and keep balance in a standing position on both legs or only one, to take steps, and to push off from a chair or bed.

Muscle Mass and Strength

Before the client undertakes a change in position or attempts to ambulate, it is essential for the nurse to assess the client's strength and ability to move. Providing appropriate assistance decreases the risk of muscle strain and body injury to both the client and nurse. Assessment of upper extremity strength is especially important for clients who use ambulation aids, such as walkers and crutches. For information on how to determine muscle mass and strength in lower and upper extremities, see Chapter 29 ∞.

Physical Energy for Activities

By determining an appropriate activity level for a client, the nurse can predict whether the client has the strength and endurance to participate in activities that require similar amounts of energy. This assessment is useful in encouraging increasing independence in clients who (a) have a cardiovascular or respiratory disability, (b) have been completely immobilized for a prolonged period, (c) have decreased muscle mass or a musculoskeletal disorder, (d) have experienced inadequate sleep, (e) have experienced pain, or (f) are depressed, anxious, or unmotivated.

The most useful measures in predicting activity tolerance are heart rate, strength, and rhythm; respiratory rate, depth, and rhythm; and blood pressure. These data are obtained at the following times:

- Before the activity starts (baseline data), while the client is at rest
- During the activity
- Immediately after the activity stops
- Three minutes after the activity has stopped and the client has rested.

The activity should be stopped immediately in the event of any physiologic change indicating the activity is too strenuous or prolonged for the client. These changes include the following:

- Sudden facial paleness
- Feelings of dizziness or weakness
- Change in level of consciousness
- Heart rate or respiratory rate that significantly exceeds baseline or preestablished levels
- Change in heart or respiratory rhythm from regular to irregular
- Weakening of the pulse
- Dyspnea, shortness of breath, or chest pain
- Diastolic blood pressure change of 10 mmHg or more.

If, however, the client tolerates the activity well, and if the client's heart rate returns to baseline levels within 5 minutes after the activity ceases, the activity is considered safe. This activity, then, can serve as a standard for predicting the client's tolerance for similar activities.

Problems Related to Immobility

When collecting data pertaining to the problems of immobility, the nurse uses the assessment methods of inspection, palpation, and auscultation; checks results of laboratory tests; and takes measurements, including body weight, fluid intake, and fluid output. Specific techniques for assessing immobility problems and abnormal assessment findings related to the complications of immobility are listed in Table 44.3.

It is extremely important to obtain and record baseline assessment data soon after the client first becomes immobile. These baseline data serve as the standard against which all data collected throughout the period of immobilization are compared.

ANATOMY & PHYSIOLOGY REVIEW

Upper and Lower Body Integration and the Spine's Role in Locomotion

It is important to be aware of the connection between the upper and lower body in terms of function, comfort, and mobility. The iliopsoas muscles (hip flexors) allow us to stand upright and are crucial for spinal alignment and locomotion. Prolonged sitting and inactivity can shorten these muscles, compromising mobility, function, and comfort in the back, hips, and legs. The shoulder blades and surrounding muscles are a major part of the shoulder girdle and allow the arms to be in relationship with the back. Muscular imbalance in the shoulder girdle will cause dysfunctional movement patterns throughout the body, including the spine. Balanced strength in the pelvic muscles enhances back stability and alignment of the feet and legs. Muscular imbalance in the pelvis will also cause dysfunctional movement patterns throughout the body, including the cervical and thoracic spine. All of these considerations affect total body alignment, comfort, and gait. Proper alignment and function lead to greater efficiency of movement and conservation of energy.

It is theorized that gait originates in the spine rather than in the legs. This "spinal engine" theory (developed by S. A. Gracovetsky) rejects the notion that locomotion is a function of leg movement with the trunk being passively carried along. Rather, motion in the spine and surrounding tissues precedes that of the legs, making the spine the basic engine of locomotion. The contralateral swinging of each leg with the opposite arm (e.g., the right arm swings forward with the left leg and vice versa) constitutes the rhythm of a normal gait with free motion in the shoulders and hips. The coordinated and fluid connection between upper and lower body motion indicates overall balance, energy efficiency, and comfort in movement.

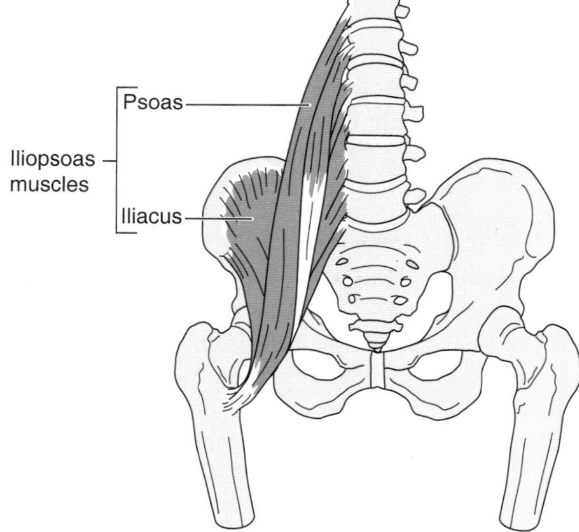

The iliopsoas muscle is frequently regarded as a single muscle because it is a blending of two muscles, the psoas and the iliacus. The psoas originates on the lumbar vertebrae and attaches to the femur. The iliacus originates on the pelvic crest and attaches to the femur. The connection between the spine and legs is evident when visualizing the iliopsoas muscles.

Nursing Implications: Nurses should keep upper–lower body connection and spinal rotation in mind when evaluating gait, and encourage clients to walk with flowing contralateral movement between upper and lower limbs and a loose, rhythmic swing in the hips.

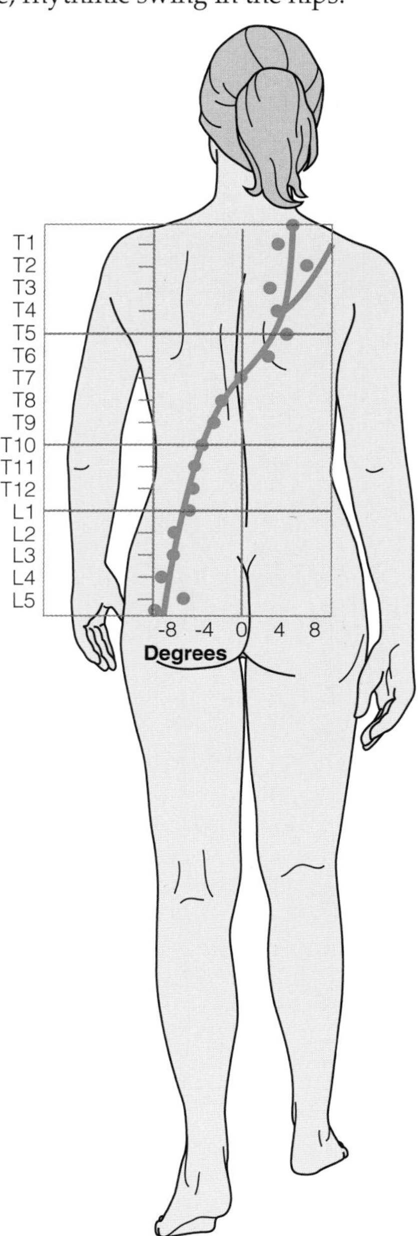

Spinal rotation precedes locomotion.

QUESTIONS

1. Why might someone with a foot or knee problem develop low back pain?
2. Why is contralateral movement of the upper and lower limbs important in a fluid, balanced gait?

Answers to Anatomy & Physiology Review Questions are available on the faculty resources site. Please consult with your instructor.

TABLE 44.3 Assessing Problems of Immobility

Assessment	Problem
MUSCULOSKELETAL SYSTEM	
Measure arm and leg circumferences.	Decreased circumference due to decreased muscle mass
Palpate and observe body joints.	Stiffness or pain in joints
Take goniometric measurements of joint ROM.	Decreased joint ROM, joint contractures
CARDIOVASCULAR SYSTEM	
Auscultate the heart.	Increased heart rate
Measure blood pressure.	Orthostatic hypotension
Palpate and observe sacrum, legs, and feet.	Peripheral dependent edema, increased peripheral vein engorgement
Palpate peripheral pulses.	Weak peripheral pulses
Measure calf muscle circumferences.	Edema
Observe calf muscles for redness, tenderness, and swelling.	Thrombophlebitis
RESPIRATORY SYSTEM	
Observe chest movements.	Asymmetric chest movements, dyspnea
Auscultate chest.	Diminished breath sounds, crackles, wheezes, and increased respiratory rate
METABOLIC SYSTEM	
Measure height and weight.	Weight loss due to muscle atrophy and loss of subcutaneous fat
Palpate skin.	Generalized edema due to low blood protein levels
URINARY SYSTEM	
Measure fluid intake and output.	Dehydration
Inspect urine.	Cloudy, dark urine; high specific gravity
Palpate urinary bladder.	Distended urinary bladder due to urinary retention
GASTROINTESTINAL SYSTEM	
Observe stool.	Hard, dry, small stool
Auscultate bowel sounds.	Decreased bowel sounds due to decreased intestinal motility
INTEGUMENTARY SYSTEM	
Inspect skin.	Break in skin integrity
PSYCHONEUROLOGIC SYSTEM	
Observe behaviors, affect, and cognition. Monitor developmental skills in children.	Anger, flat affect, crying, confusion, anxiety, decline in cognitive function, or signs such as sleep and appetite disturbances warrant further evaluation

Because a major nursing responsibility is to prevent the complications of immobility, the nurse needs to identify clients at risk of developing such complications before problems arise. Clients at risk include those who (a) are poorly nourished; (b) have decreased sensitivity to pain, temperature, or pressure; (c) have existing cardiovascular, pulmonary, or neuromuscular problems; and (d) have an altered level of consciousness.

Diagnosing

Mobility problems may be appropriate as the diagnostic label or as the etiology for other nursing diagnoses. Example of nursing diagnoses for clients with mobility problems can include inadequate physical energy for activities; potential for inadequate physical energy for activities; altered physical mobility (specify, such as with walking or transferring); inactive lifestyle; and decline in health (from inactivity).

Depending on the data obtained, problems with mobility often affect other areas of human functioning and indicate other diagnoses. In these instances, the mobility problem becomes the etiology. The etiology needs to be described more clearly in terms such as reduced ROM, neuromuscular impairment or musculoskeletal impairment of upper and lower extremities, or joint pain. Examples in which inadequate physical energy for activities is the etiology can include fear (of falling), potential for falling, and impaired self-esteem.

When problems associated with prolonged immobility arise, many other nursing diagnoses may be necessary. Examples include, but are not limited to the following: altered respiratory status, if there is stasis of pulmonary secretions; potential for infection, if there is stasis of urinary or pulmonary secretions; and potential for impaired self-esteem, if there is functional impairment or role disturbance.

Planning

When planning for desired outcomes, Nursing Outcomes Classification (NOC) labels that pertain to exercise and activity can be helpful and include the following: activity tolerance; ambulation; balance; body positioning; coordinated movement; endurance; fall prevention behavior;

fatigue level; immobility consequences, both physiologic and psycho-cognitive; joint movement; mobility; physical fitness; play participation; and self-care (Moorhead, Swanson, Johnson, & Maas, 2018).

Positioning, transferring, and ambulating clients are almost always independent nursing functions. The primary care provider usually orders specific body positions only after surgery, anesthesia, or trauma involving the nervous and musculoskeletal systems. All clients should have an activity order written by their primary care provider when they are admitted to the agency for care.

As part of planning, the nurse is responsible for identifying those clients who need assistance with body alignment and determining the degree of assistance they need. The nurse must be sensitive to the client's need to function as independently as possible yet provide assistance when the client needs it.

Most clients require some nursing guidance and assistance to learn about, achieve, and maintain proper body mechanics. The nurse should also plan to teach clients applicable skills. For example, a client with a back injury needs to learn how to get out of bed safely and comfortably, a client with an injured leg needs to learn how to transfer from bed to wheelchair safely, and a client with a newly acquired walker needs to learn how to use it safely. Nurses often teach family members or caregivers safe moving, lifting, and transfer techniques in the home setting.

The goals established for clients will vary according to the nursing diagnosis and signs and symptoms related to each individual. Examples of overall goals for clients with actual or potential problems related to mobility or activity follow.

The client will have:

- Increased tolerance for physical activity
- Restored or improved capability to ambulate and participate in ADLs
- Absence of injury from falling or improper use of body mechanics
- Absence of any complications associated with immobility.

Examples of desired outcomes, interventions, and activities are provided in the Nursing Care Plan and Concept Map on pages 1159–1161.

Planning for Home Care

Clients who have been hospitalized for activity or mobility problems often need continued care in the home. In preparation for discharge, the nurse needs to determine the client's actual and potential health problems, strengths, and resources.

QSEN Safety: Assessment Data for Discharge Plan

Following is the specific assessment data required for the nurse to address before establishing a discharge plan for clients with mobility or activity problems.

CLIENT AND ENVIRONMENT

- Capabilities or tolerance for required and desired activities: self-care (feeding, bathing, toileting, dressing, grooming, home maintenance, shopping, cooking); recreational activities
- Mobility aids required: cane, walker, crutches, wheelchair, transfer boards
- Equipment required if immobilized: special bed, side rails, pressure-reducing mattress, assistive lifting equipment
- Current level of knowledge: body mechanics for use of mobility aids; specific exercises prescribed
- Home mobility hazard appraisal: adequacy of lighting; presence of handrails; safety of pathways and stairs; congested areas; unanchored rugs, mats, or electrical cords, and any other obstacles to safe movement; structural adjustments needed for wheelchair access

FAMILY OR CAREGIVER

- Caregiver availability, skills, and willingness to assist: assess learning needs and develop appropriate teaching plan, primary people able to assist client with self-care, movement, shopping, and so on; physical and emotional status to assist with care
- Family role changes and coping: effect on financial status, parenting and spousal roles, social roles
- Availability of caregiver support: other support people available for occasional duties such as shopping, transportation, housekeeping, cooking, budgeting; refer to community agencies for respite care, where appropriate

COMMUNITY

- Resources: availability and familiarity with sources of medical equipment and assistive lifting equipment, financial assistance, homemaker services, hygienic care; Meals on Wheels; spiritual counselors and visitors; sources of respite for the caregiver

A major aspect of discharge planning involves instructional needs of the client and family. See Client Teaching features throughout this chapter.

Implementing

Nurses can initiate and apply a wide variety of exercise and activity interventions as needed to address a multitude of client concerns. Nursing Interventions Classification (NIC) labels that pertain to exercise and activity include the following: activity therapy; cardiac care; rehabilitation; constipation management; exercise promotion (strength and stretching); exercise therapy (ambulation, balance, joint mobility, muscle control); fall prevention; health education; mood management; pelvic muscle exercise; pressure ulcer prevention; progressive muscle relaxation; recreation therapy; self-care assistance; self-esteem enhancement; simple relaxation therapy; sleep enhancement; sports-injury prevention; teaching: prescribed activity and exercise; therapeutic play; weight management; and weight reduction (Butcher, Bulechek, Dochterman, & Wagner, 2018).

CLIENT TEACHING Home Care Activity and Exercise

MAINTAINING MUSCULOSKELETAL FUNCTION

- Teach the systematic performance of passive or assistive ROM exercises to maintain joint mobility.
- Demonstrate, as appropriate, the proper way to perform isotonic, isometric, or isokinetic exercises to maintain muscle mass and tone (collaborate with the physical therapist about these). Incorporate ADLs into exercise program if appropriate.
- Provide a written schedule for the type, frequency, and duration of exercises; encourage the use of a progress graph or chart to facilitate adherence with the therapy.
- Offer an ambulation schedule.
- Instruct in the availability of assistive ambulatory devices and correct use of them.
- Discuss pain control measures required before exercise.

PREVENTING INJURY

- Provide assistive devices for moving and transferring, whenever possible, and teach safe transfer and ambulation techniques.
- Discuss safety measures to avoid falls (e.g., locking wheelchairs, wearing appropriate footwear, using rubber tips on crutches, keeping the environment safe, and using mechanical aids such as raised toilet seat, grab bars, urinal, and bedpan or commode to facilitate toileting).
- Teach ways to prevent postural hypotension.

MANAGING ENERGY TO PREVENT FATIGUE

- Discuss activity and rest patterns and develop a plan as indicated; intersperse rest periods with activity periods.
- Discuss ways to minimize fatigue such as performing activities more slowly and for shorter periods, resting more often, and using more assistance as required.
- Provide information about available resources to help with ADLs and home maintenance management.
- Teach ways to increase energy (e.g., increasing intake of high-energy foods, ensuring adequate rest and sleep, controlling pain, sharing feelings with a trusted listener).
- Teach techniques to monitor activity tolerance as appropriate.

REFERRALS

- Provide appropriate information about accessing community resources: home care agencies, physical and occupational therapy agencies, local YMCAs and other agencies that provide structured exercise and movement programs, and sources of adaptive equipment.

Nursing strategies to maintain or promote body alignment and mobility involve positioning clients appropriately, moving and turning clients in bed, transferring clients, providing ROM exercises, ambulating clients with or without mechanical aids, and strategies to prevent the complications of immobility. Whenever positioning, moving, and ambulating clients, nurses must use assistive lifting or moving equipment and proper body mechanics to avoid musculoskeletal strain and injury.

Preventing Musculoskeletal Disorders (MSDs)

Nurses provide clients with the opportunity to change positions, expand their lungs, or change their environments as appropriate. It is important, however, that nurses not put their own health at risk while caring for clients. Client positioning, lifting, and transferring are significant risk factors for developing MSDs.

In the field of nursing, MSDs such as back and shoulder injuries persist as the leading and most costly U.S. occupational health problem. Manually moving and lifting clients often cause MSDs. The term *patient handling injury* (PHI) has become a recognized term for identifying nurses' injuries caused by direct client care. A literature review (Fragala et al., 2016, p. 41) resulted in the identification of four major risk factors for PHIs in nurses:

1. Exertion. The amount of exertion or effort required to lift, move, or handle a client depends on factors such as the client's size, need for assistance, cognitive status, and ability and willingness to actively participate in the move.
2. Frequency. This refers to the number of times a nurse performs client-handling tasks during a shift. Examples include pulling a client up in bed, turning a client, and performing a lateral transfer.
3. Posture or the nurse's body position when performing client-handling activities. Reaching across beds or other equipment with arms extended can lead to undesirable postures. Working in a confined space, causing nurses to assume awkward postures, and twisting the back while bending are other examples that affect posture and can increase PHI.
4. Duration of exposure or the cumulative effects of exertion, frequency, and position.

Increasingly, healthcare facilities are focusing on "no lift" policies for their employees, and 35 pounds of client weight should be the maximum a nurse should attempt. If the weight to be lifted exceeds 35 pounds or the risk factors exist, assistive devices should be used. These devices include floor-based and ceiling lifts; slings; sit-to-stand assist devices; sliding boards; friction-reducing devices; transfer sheets or power-assist, air-cushioned mattresses; and lateral transfer and transport chairs.

The American Nurses Association (ANA) has been involved in the effort to protect nurses from MSDs for many years and has taken the official position of supporting actions and policies that result in the elimination of manual handling of clients in order to establish a safe environment for nurses and clients. Evidence has shown that safe patient handling and mobility (SPHM) programs greatly reduce healthcare worker injuries (Teeple et al., 2017; Walker, Docherty, Hougendobler, Guanowsky, & Rosenthal, 2017). In 2003, the ANA launched a national Handle with Care campaign to prevent MSDs. As a result, 11 states have enacted "safe patient handling" laws or initiated rules and regulations related to the implementation of SPHM programs (Weinmeyer, 2016). However, there is not consistency among these 11 states. For example, one state requires replacing manual lifting with lifting devices and another state requires healthcare facilities to develop a comprehensive safe patient handling plan.

In 2013, the Centers for Medicare and Medicaid Services (CMS), the Institute of Medicine (IOM), the World Health Organization (WHO), the National Quality Foundation (NQF), and the ANA supported the concepts of universal standards and an interdisciplinary approach to SPHM. This resulted in the publication of *Safe Patient Handling and Mobility Interprofessional National Standards Across the Care Continuum*. These standards are voluntary performance standards to help healthcare facilities establish policies and procedures. It is the hope, however, that similar to the requirement of standard precautions, the Safe Patient Handling and Mobility Standards will become required instead of optional. To this end, the ANA worked with congressional bill sponsors in support of national legislation, which resulted in the Nurse and Health Care Worker Protection Act of 2015. Future action on this bill, however, remains to be seen (Weinmeyer, 2016).

Until all work settings provide safe environments in which nurses have the equipment they need, content pertaining to body mechanics will be included here. Readers are encouraged to support "no manual lift" and "no solo lift" policies in their workplaces, and to become involved in legislation and equipment purchase initiatives. Nurses must participate in this safety awareness, and are encouraged to support the Safe Patient Handling and Mobility Standards of the ANA and to keep informed of congressional action on bills to enforce safer client handling.

Recently, the VA produced a Safe Patient Handling app for healthcare professionals. This app provides evidence-based SPHM techniques to prevent injury of both healthcare workers and clients. The app includes comprehensive client assessments, scoring and other algorithms for specific client handling tasks, and pictures and video clips of a variety of client handling and mobility technologies.

Clinical Alert!

MSDs are caused by force, repetition, and awkward positions. The most common injuries among healthcare workers are low back pain, herniated disks, strained muscles, pulled or torn ligaments, and disk degradation.

Using Body Mechanics

Body mechanics is the term used to describe the efficient, coordinated, and safe use of the body to move objects and carry out the ADLs. When an individual moves, the center of gravity shifts continuously in the direction of the moving body parts. Balance depends on the interrelationship of the center of gravity, the line of gravity, and the base of support. The closer the line of gravity is to the center of the base of support, the greater the individual's stability (Figure 44.40*A* ■). Conversely, the closer the line of gravity is to the edge of the base of support, the more precarious the balance (Figure 44.40*B*). If the line of gravity falls outside the base of support, the individual falls (Figure 44.40*C*).

Body balance can be greatly enhanced by (a) widening the base of support and (b) lowering the center of gravity, bringing it closer to the base of support. Spreading the feet farther apart widens the base of support. Flexing the hips

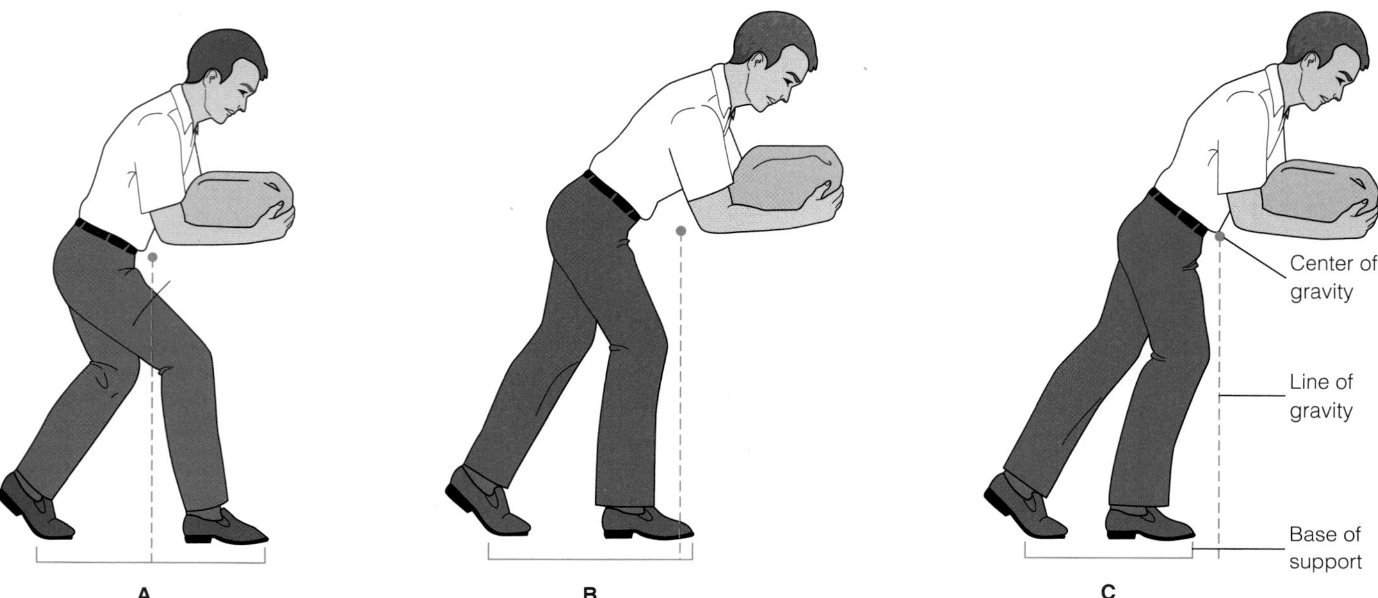

Figure 44.40 ■ *A*, Balance is maintained when the line of gravity falls close to the base of support. *B*, Balance is precarious when the line of gravity falls at the edge of the base of support. *C*, Balance cannot be maintained when the line of gravity falls outside the base of support.

and knees until achieving a squatting position lowers the center of gravity. The importance of these alterations cannot be overemphasized for nurses.

Historically, nurses believed that "correct" body mechanics would assist in the safe and efficient use of appropriate muscle groups to maintain balance, reduce the energy required, reduce fatigue, and decrease the risk of injury for both nurses and clients, especially during transferring, lifting, and repositioning. In reality, more than 30 years of evidence show that:

- Educating nurses in body mechanics alone will *not* prevent job-related injuries.
- Back belts have *not* been shown to be effective in reducing back injury.
- Nurses who are physically fit are at *no* less risk of injury.
- The formerly accepted National Institute for Occupational Safety and Health (NIOSH) "lifting equation," which recommended that workers observe a limit of 51 pounds of lifting, *cannot* be safely applied to nursing practice.
- The long-term benefits of using the proper equipment (e.g., mechanical lifts) far outweigh the costs related to injuries.
- Staff will use equipment when they have participated in the decision-making process for purchasing the equipment

Lifting

It is important to remember that nurses should ***not*** lift more than 35 pounds without assistance from proper equipment or other individuals. Types of assistive equipment include mobile-powered or mechanical lifts, ceiling-mounted lifts, sit-to-stand powered lifts, friction-reducing devices, and air transfer systems. See Figure 44.41 ■ through Figure 44.45 ■. There are also transfer chairs that can transfer the client laterally from bed to stretcher without lifting and then convert to a sitting or reclining position to transport the client through the facility.

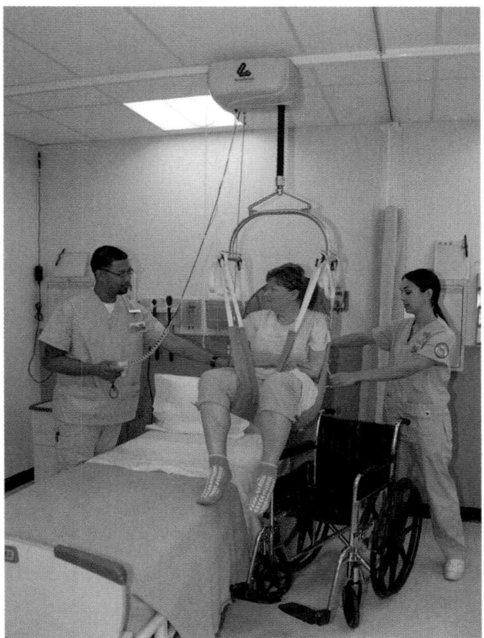

Figure 44.42 ■ A ceiling-mounted lift.
Shirlee Snyder.

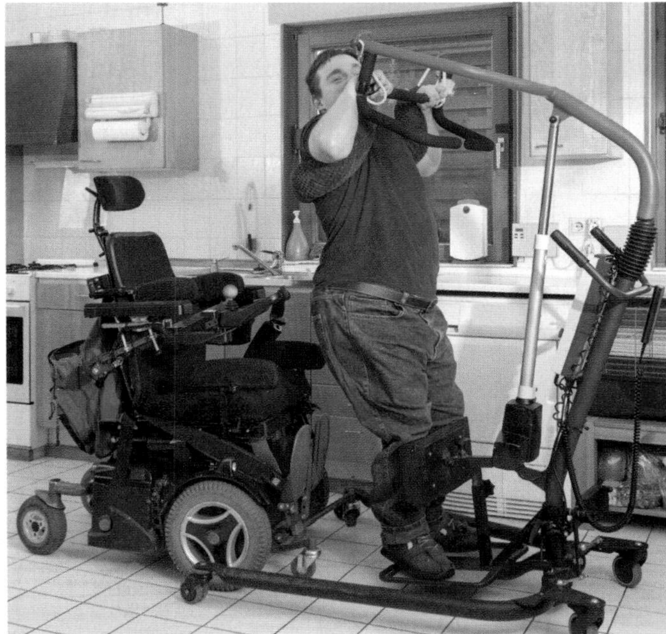

Figure 44.43 ■ A sit-to-stand power lift allows for client transfers from bed to chair. The client must be cognitive and provide some muscle tone in at least one leg and the trunk.
belushi/Shutterstock.

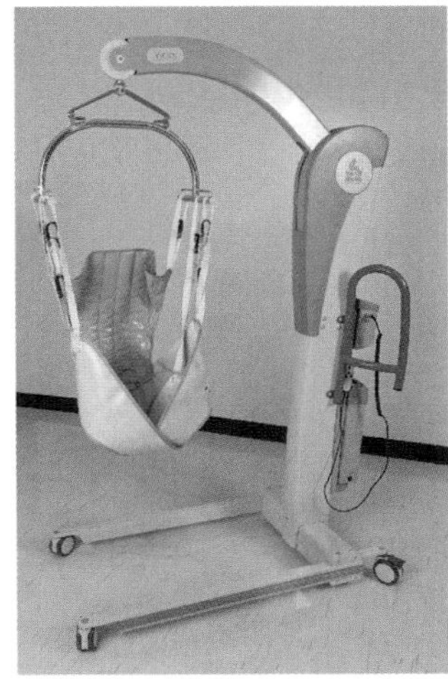

Figure 44.41 ■ A mobile electric lift functions to lift clients from bed, chair, toilet, and floor.

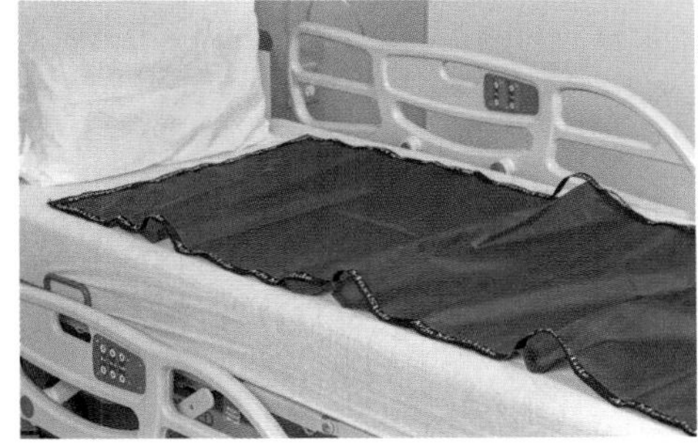

Figure 44.44 ■ Friction-reducing transfer device with handles.

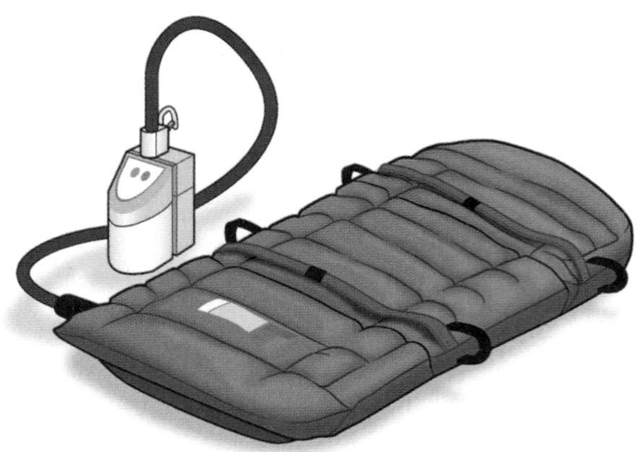

Figure 44.45 ■ An air transfer system. Once inflated, the client can be transferred laterally or repositioned on a frictionless air surface.

Pulling and Pushing

When pulling or pushing an object, an individual maintains balance with the least effort when the base of support is increased in the direction in which the movement is to be produced or opposed. For example, when pushing an object, an individual can enlarge the base of support by moving the front foot forward. When pulling an object, an individual can enlarge the base of support by (a) moving the rear leg back if facing the object or (b) moving the front foot forward if facing away from the object. It is easier and safer to pull an object toward your own center of gravity than to push it away, because you can exert more control of the object's movement when pulling it.

Clinical Alert!

Lateral-assist devices such as horizontal air transfer mattresses and transfer chairs are essential equipment for most client care areas. They help prevent acute and chronic back pain and disability. Observing principles of body mechanics is recommended even when using assistive equipment, because any lifting and forceful movement is potentially injurious, especially when repeated over time.

Pivoting

Pivoting is a technique in which the body is turned in a way that avoids twisting of the spine. To pivot, place one foot ahead of the other, raise the heels very slightly, and put the body weight on the balls of the feet. When the weight is off the heels, the frictional surface is decreased and the knees are not twisted when turning. Keeping the body aligned, turn (pivot) about 90 degrees in the desired direction. The foot that was forward will now be behind.

Positioning Clients

Positioning a client in good body alignment and changing the position regularly (every 2 hours) and systematically are essential aspects of nursing practice. Clients who can move easily automatically reposition themselves for comfort. Such clients generally require minimal positioning assistance from nurses, other than guidance about ways to maintain body alignment and to exercise their joints. However, clients who are weak, frail, in pain, paralyzed, or unconscious rely on nurses to provide or assist with position changes. For all clients, it is important to assess the skin and provide skin care before and after a position change.

Any position, correct or incorrect, can be harmful if maintained for a prolonged period. Frequent change of position helps to prevent muscle discomfort, undue pressure resulting in pressure injuries, damage to superficial nerves and blood vessels, and contractures. Position changes also maintain muscle tone and stimulate postural reflexes.

When the client is not able to move independently or assist with moving, *the preferred method is for two or more nurses to move or turn the client and use assistive equipment*. Appropriate assistance reduces the risk of muscle strain and body injury to both the client and nurse, and is likely to protect the dignity and comfort of the client.

When positioning clients in bed, the nurse can do a number of things to ensure proper alignment and promote client comfort and safety:

- Make sure the mattress is firm and level yet has enough give to fill in and support natural body curvatures.
- Ensure that the bed is clean and dry. Wrinkled or damp sheets increase the risk of pressure injury formation. Make sure extremities can move freely whenever possible. For example, the top bedclothes need to be loose enough for clients to move their feet.
- Place support devices in specified areas according to the client's position. Box 44.1 lists commonly used support devices. Use only those support devices needed to maintain alignment and to prevent stress on the client's muscles and joints. If the client is capable of movement, too many devices limit mobility and increase the potential for muscle weakness and atrophy.
- Avoid placing one body part, particularly one with bony prominences, directly on top of another body part. Excessive pressure can damage veins and predispose the client to thrombus formation. Pressure against the popliteal space may damage nerves and blood vessels in this area. Pillows can provide needed cushioning.
- Avoid friction and shearing. Friction is a force acting parallel to the skin surface. For example, sheets rubbing against skin create friction. Friction can abrade the skin (i.e., remove the superficial layers), making it more prone to breakdown. Shearing force is a combination of friction and pressure. It occurs commonly when a client assumes a sitting position in bed. In this position, the body tends to slide downward toward the foot of the bed. This downward movement is transmitted to the

sacral bone and the deep tissues. At the same time, the skin over the sacrum tends not to move because of sticking to the bed linens. The skin and superficial tissues are thus relatively unmoving in relation to the bed surface, whereas the deeper tissues are firmly attached to the skeleton and move downward. This causes a shearing force in the area where the deeper tissues and the superficial tissues meet. The force damages the tissues in this area.

- Plan a *systematic 24-hour schedule* for position changes. Frequent position changes are essential to prevent pressure injuries in immobilized clients. Such clients should be repositioned every 2 hours throughout the day and night and more frequently when there is a risk for skin breakdown. This schedule is usually outlined on the client's nursing care plan. The use of visual cues (e.g., clock sign with moveable arrows to indicate next turning time) can also serve as reminders.
- Always obtain information from the client to determine which position is most comfortable and appropriate. Seeking information from the client about what feels best is a useful guide when aligning clients and is an essential aspect of evaluating the effectiveness of an alignment intervention. Sometimes a client who appears well aligned may be experiencing real discomfort. Both appearance, in relation to alignment criteria, and comfort are important in achieving effective alignment.

BOX 44.1 Support Devices

- *Pillows.* Different sizes are available. Used for support or elevation of an arm or leg. Specially designed dense pillows can be used to elevate the upper body. Pillows can also be used as a trochanter roll by placing the pillow from the client's iliac crest to midthigh. This prevents external rotation of the leg when the client is in a supine position.
- *Mattresses.* There are two types of mattresses: ones that fit on the bed frame (e.g., standard bed mattress) and mattresses that fit on the standard bed mattress (e.g., egg-crate mattress). Mattresses should be evenly supportive.
- *Suspension or heel guard boot.* These are made of a variety of substances. They usually have a firm exterior and padding of foam to protect the skin. They prevent foot drop and relieve pressure on heels.
- *Footboard.* A flat panel often made of plastic or wood. It keeps the feet in dorsiflexion to prevent plantar flexion.
- *Hand roll.* Can be made by rolling a washcloth. Purpose is to keep hand in a functional position and prevent finger contractures.
- *Abduction pillow.* A triangular-shaped foam pillow that maintains hip abduction to prevent hip dislocation following total hip replacement.

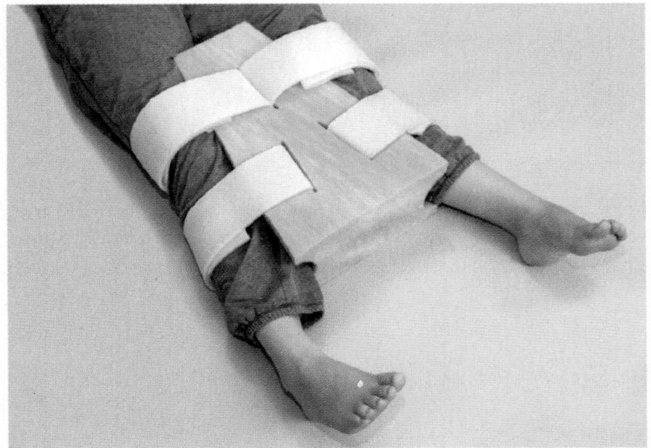

Maintaining postoperative abduction following total hip replacement.

Fowler's Position

Fowler's position, or a semisitting position, is a bed position in which the head and trunk are raised 45° to 60° relative to the bed (visualize a 90° right angle to orient your thinking) and the knees may or may not be flexed. Nurses may need to clarify the meaning of the term *Fowler's position* in their particular setting. Typically, Fowler's position refers to a 45° angle of elevation of the upper body.

Semi-Fowler's position (Figure 44.46 ■) is when the head and trunk are raised 15° to 45°. This position is sometimes called low Fowler's and typically means 30° of elevation. In **high-Fowler's position**, the head and trunk are raised 60° to 90°, and most often the client is sitting upright at a right angle to the bed (Table 44.4).

Fowler's position is the position of choice for people who have difficulty breathing and for some people with heart problems. When the client is in this position, gravity pulls the diaphragm downward, allowing greater chest expansion and lung ventilation.

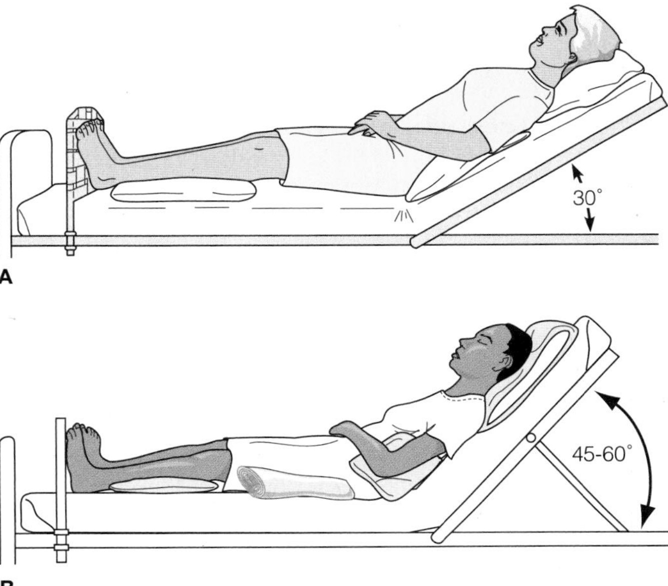

Figure 44.46 ■ *A*, Semi-Fowler's (low-Fowler's) position (supported); *B*, Fowler's position (supported). The amount of support depends on the needs of the individual client.

TABLE 44.4 Fowler's Position

Unsupported Position	Problem to Be Prevented	Corrective Measure*
Bed-sitting position with upper part of body elevated 30° to 90° commencing at hips	Posterior flexion of lumbar curvature	Pillow at lower back (lumbar region) to support lumbar region
Head rests on bed surface	Hyperextension of neck	Pillows to support head, neck, and upper back
Arms fall at sides	Shoulder muscle strain, possible dislocation of shoulders, edema of hands and arms with flaccid paralysis, flexion contracture of the wrist	Pillow under forearms to eliminate pull on shoulder and assist venous blood flow from hands and lower arms
Legs lie flat and straight on lower bed surface	Hyperextension of knees	External rotation of hips
Small pillow under thighs to flex knees	Trochanter roll lateral to femur (Figure 44.47 ■)	Heels rest on bed surface
Pressure on heels	Pillow under lower legs	Feet are in plantar flexion
Plantar flexion of feet (foot drop)	Footboard to provide support for dorsiflexion	

*The amount of correction depends on the needs of the individual client.

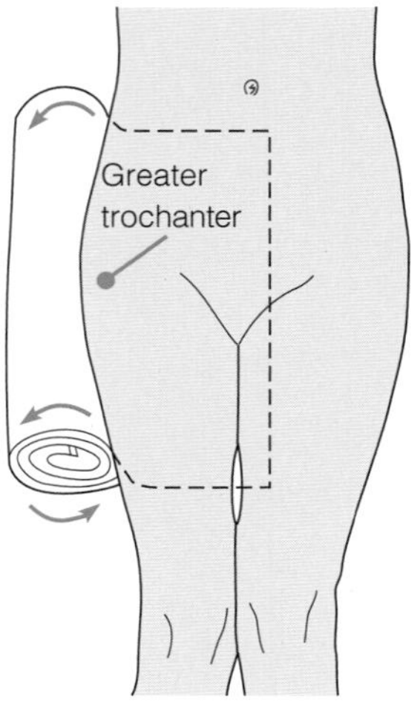

Figure 44.47 ■ Making a trochanter roll: (1) Fold the towel in half lengthwise. (2) Roll the towel tightly, starting at one narrow edge and rolling within approximately 30 cm (1 ft) of the other edge. (3) Invert the roll. Then palpate the greater trochanter of the femur and place the roll with the center at the level of the greater trochanter; place the flat part of the towel under the client; then roll the towel snugly against the hip. The amount of support depends on the needs of the individual client.

A common error nurses make when aligning clients in Fowler's position is placing an overly large pillow or more than one pillow behind the client's head. This promotes the development of neck flexion contractures. If a client desires several head pillows, the nurse should encourage the client to rest without a pillow for several hours each day to extend the neck fully and counteract the effects of poor neck alignment.

Orthopneic Position

In the **orthopneic position**, the client sits either in bed or on the side of the bed with an overbed table across the lap (Figure 44.48 ■). This position facilitates respiration by allowing maximum chest expansion. It is particularly helpful to clients who have problems exhaling, because they can press the lower part of the chest against the edge of the overbed table.

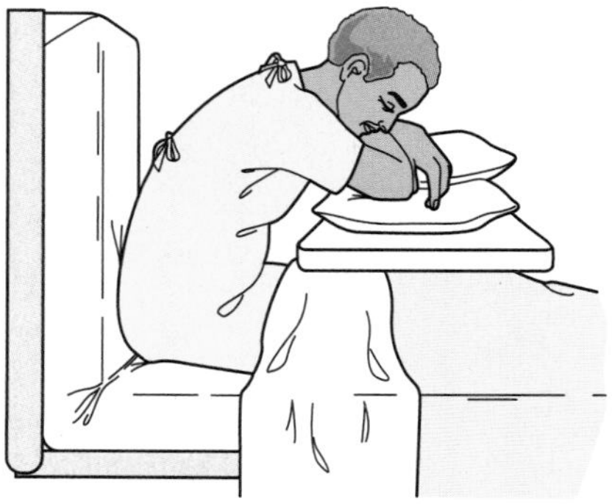

Figure 44.48 ■ Orthopneic position.

Dorsal Recumbent Position

In the **dorsal recumbent** (back-lying) **position** (Figure 44.49 ■), the client's head and shoulders are slightly elevated on a small pillow. In some agencies, the terms *dorsal recumbent* and *supine* are used interchangeably; strictly speaking, however, in the **supine** or **dorsal position** the head and shoulders are not elevated. In both positions, the client's forearms may be elevated on pillows or placed at the client's sides. Supports are similar in both positions, except for the head pillow (Table 44.5). The dorsal recumbent position is used to provide comfort and to facilitate healing following certain surgeries or anesthetics (e.g., spinal).

Prone Position

In the **prone position**, the client lies on the abdomen with the head turned to one side (Figure 44.50 ■). The hips are not flexed. Both children and adults often sleep in this

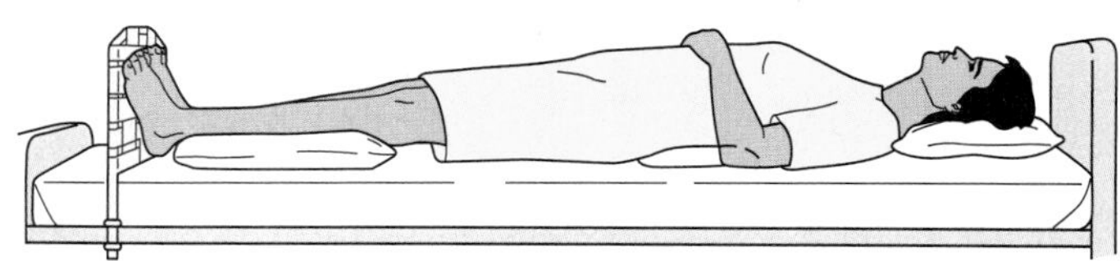

Figure 44.49 ■ Dorsal recumbent position (supported).

TABLE 44.5 Dorsal Recumbent Position

Unsupported Position	Problem to Be Prevented	Corrective Measure*
Head is flat on bed surface	Hyperextension of neck in thick-chested client	Pillow of suitable thickness under head and shoulders if necessary for alignment
Lumbar curvature of spine is apparent	Posterior flexion of lumbar curvature	Roll or small pillow under lumbar curvature
Legs may be externally rotated	External rotation of legs	Roll or sandbag placed laterally to trochanter of femur (optional)
Legs are extended	Hyperextension of knees	Small pillow under thigh to flex knee slightly
Feet assume plantar flexion position	Plantar flexion (foot drop)	Footboard or rolled pillow to support feet in dorsiflexion
Heels on bed surface	Pressure on heels	Pillow under lower legs

*The amount of correction depends on the needs of the individual client.

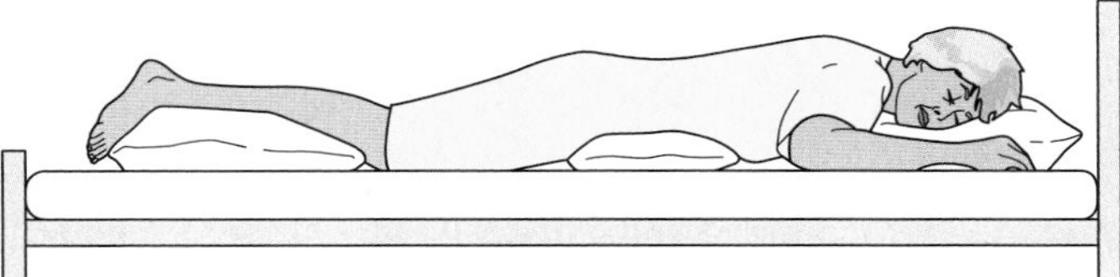

Figure 44.50 ■ Prone position (supported).

position, sometimes with one or both arms flexed over their heads. It is the only bed position that allows full extension of the hip and knee joints. When used periodically, the prone position helps to prevent flexion contractures of the hips and knees, thereby counteracting a problem caused by all other bed positions. The prone position also promotes drainage from the mouth and is especially useful for unconscious clients or those clients recovering from surgery of the mouth or throat (Table 44.6).

The prone position creates some distinct disadvantages. The pull of gravity on the trunk produces a marked lordosis in most individuals, and the neck is rotated laterally to a significant degree. For this reason, the prone position may not be recommended for clients with problems of the cervical or lumbar spine. This position also causes plantar flexion. Some clients with cardiac or respiratory problems find the prone position confining and suffocating because chest expansion is inhibited during respirations. *The prone position should be used only when the client's back is correctly aligned, only for short periods, and only for clients with no evidence of spinal abnormalities.* As a result, this position is not often used.

Lateral Position

In the **lateral** (side-lying) **position** (Figure 44.51 ■), the client lies on one side of the body. Flexing the top hip and knee and placing this leg in front of the body creates a wider, triangular base of support and achieves greater stability. The greater the flexion of the top hip and knee, the greater the stability and balance in this position. This flexion reduces lordosis and promotes good back alignment. For this reason, the lateral position is good for resting and sleeping clients. The lateral position helps to relieve pressure on the sacrum and heels in clients who sit for much

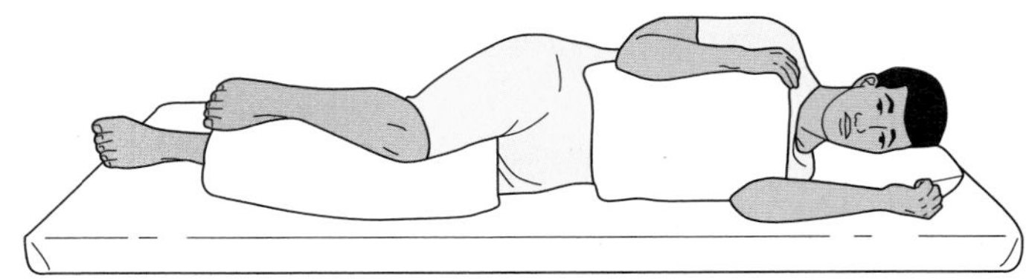

Figure 44.51 ■ Lateral position (supported).

TABLE 44.6 Prone Position

Unsupported Position	Problem to Be Prevented	Corrective Measure*
Head is turned to side and neck is slightly flexed	Flexion or hyperextension of neck	Small pillow under head unless contraindicated because of promotion of mucous drainage from mouth
Body lies flat on abdomen accentuating lumbar curvature	Hyperextension of lumbar curvature; difficulty breathing; pressure on breasts (women); pressure on genitals (men)	Small pillow or roll under abdomen just below diaphragm
Toes rest on bed surface; feet are in plantar flexion	Plantar flexion (foot drop)	Allow feet to fall naturally over end of mattress, or support lower legs on a pillow so that toes do not touch the bed

*The amount of correction depends on the needs of the individual client.

of the day or who are confined to bed and rest in Fowler's or dorsal recumbent positions much of the time. In the lateral position, most of the body's weight is borne by the lateral aspect of the lower scapula, the lateral aspect of the ilium, and the greater trochanter of the femur. Individuals who have sensory or motor deficits on one side of the body usually find that lying on the uninvolved side is more comfortable (Table 44.7).

Sims' Position

In **Sims'** (semiprone) **position** (Figure 44.52 ■), the client assumes a posture halfway between the lateral and the prone positions. The lower arm is positioned behind the client, and the upper arm is flexed at the shoulder and the elbow. Both legs are flexed in front of the client. The upper leg is more acutely flexed at both the hip and the knee than is the lower one.

Sims' position may be used for unconscious clients because it facilitates drainage from the mouth and prevents aspiration of fluids. It is also used for paralyzed clients because it reduces pressure over the sacrum and greater trochanter of the hip. It is often used for clients receiving enemas and occasionally for clients undergoing examinations or treatments of the perineal area. Many clients, especially pregnant women, find Sims' position comfortable for sleeping. Clients with sensory or motor deficits on one side of the body usually find that lying on the uninvolved side is more comfortable (Table 44.8).

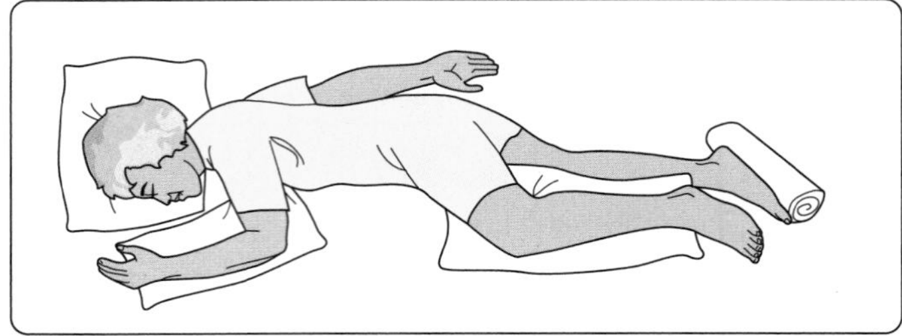

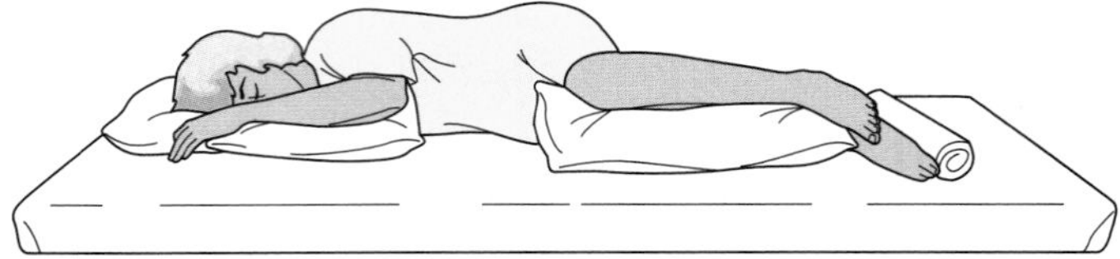

Figure 44.52 ■ Sims' position (supported).

Moving and Turning Clients in Bed

Although healthy clients usually take for granted that they can change body position and go from one place to another with little effort, ill clients may have difficulty moving, even in bed. How much assistance clients require depends on their own ability to move and their health

TABLE 44.7 Lateral Position

Unsupported Position	Problem to Be Prevented	Corrective Measure*
Body is turned to side, both arms in front of body, weight resting primarily on lateral aspects of scapula and ilium	Lateral flexion and fatigue of sternocleidomastoid muscles	Pillow under head and neck to provide good alignment
Upper arm and shoulder are rotated internally and adducted	Internal rotation and adduction of shoulder and subsequent limited function; impaired chest expansion	Pillow under upper arm to place it in good alignment; lower arm should be flexed comfortably
Upper thigh and leg are rotated internally and adducted	Internal rotation and adduction of femur; twisting of the spine	Pillow under leg and thigh to place them in good alignment; shoulders and hips should be aligned

*The amount of correction depends on the needs of the individual client.

TABLE 44.8 Sims' (Semiprone) Position

Unsupported Position	Problem to Be Prevented	Corrective Measure*
Head rests on bed surface; weight is borne by lateral aspects of cranial and facial bones	Lateral flexion of neck	Pillow supports head, maintaining it in good alignment unless drainage from the mouth is required
Upper shoulder and arm are internally rotated	Internal rotation of shoulder and arm; pressure on chest, restricting expansion during breathing	Pillow under upper arm to prevent internal rotation
Upper leg and thigh are adducted and internally rotated	Internal rotation and adduction of hip and leg	Pillow under upper leg to support it in alignment
Feet assume plantar flexion	Foot drop	Sandbags to support feet in dorsiflexion

*The amount of correction depends on the needs of the individual client.

status. Nurses should be sensitive to both the need of clients to function independently and their need for assistance to move. Correct body alignment for the client must also be maintained so that undue stress is not placed on the musculoskeletal system.

When assisting a client to move, the nurse needs to use appropriate numbers of staff and assistive devices (such as those shown in previous Figures 44.41 through 44.45) to avoid injury to self and client. Having sufficient staff and assistive devices also helps to ensure client comfort and modesty. Hydraulic lifts are examples of assistive equipment that take the place of manual lifts and transfers. A lift can be used to transfer clients between the bed and a wheelchair, the bed and the bathtub, and the bed and a stretcher. A lift consists of a base on casters, a hydraulic mechanical pump, a mast boom, and a sling. The sling may consist of a one-piece or two-piece canvas seat. The one-piece seat stretches from the client's head to the knees. The two-piece seat has one canvas strap to support the client's buttocks and thighs and a second strap extending up to the axillae to support the back. It is important to be familiar with the model used and the practices that accompany use. Before using the lift, the nurse ensures that it is in working order and that the hooks, chains, straps, and canvas seat are in good repair. Most agencies recommend that two nurses operate a lift. Check agency policy.

Actions and rationales applicable to moving and lifting clients include the following:

Clinical Alert!

Studies confirm that repositioning clients in bed, specifically pulling a client toward the head of the bed, is a significant cause of MSDs among caregivers in the healthcare industry. This risk of injury can be decreased by using friction-reducing devices.

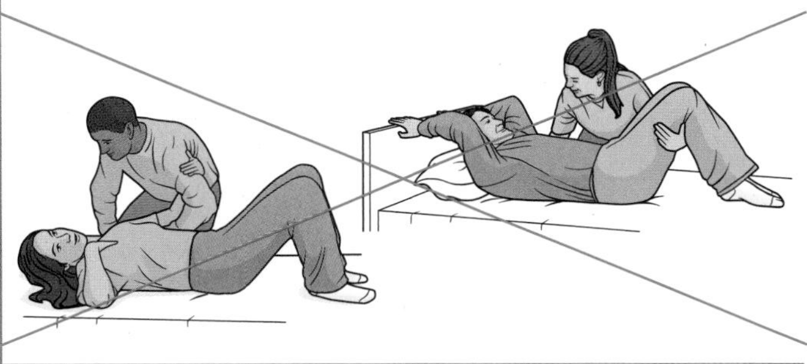

- Before moving a client, assess the degree of exertion permitted, the client's physical abilities (e.g., muscle strength, presence of paralysis) and ability to assist with the move, ability to understand instructions, degree of comfort or discomfort when moving, client's weight, presence of orthostatic hypotension (particularly important when client will be standing), and your own strength and ability to move the client.
- If indicated, use pain relief modalities or medication prior to moving the client.
- Prepare any needed assistive devices and supportive equipment (e.g., mechanical lifts, friction-reducing slide sheet, pillows, trochanter roll).
- Plan around limitations to movement such as an IV or urinary catheter.
- Be alert to the effects of any medications the client takes that may impair alertness, balance, strength, or mobility.
- Obtain required assistance from other individuals.
- Explain the procedure to the client and listen to any suggestions the client or support people have.
- Provide privacy.
- Perform hand hygiene.
- Raise the height of the bed *to bring the client close to your center of gravity.*
- Lock the wheels on the bed, and raise the rail on the side of the bed opposite you *to ensure client safety.*
- Face in the direction of the movement *to prevent spinal twisting.*
- Assume a broad stance *to increase stability and provide balance.*
- Lean your trunk forward, and flex your hips, knees, and ankles *to lower your center of gravity, increase stability, and ensure use of large muscle groups during movements.*
- Tighten your gluteal, abdominal, leg, and arm muscles *to prepare them for action and prevent injury.*
- Rock from the front leg to the back leg when pulling or from the back leg to the front leg when pushing *to overcome inertia, counteract the client's weight, and help attain a balanced, smooth motion.*
- After moving the client, determine and document the client's comfort (presence of anxiety, dizziness, or pain), body alignment, tolerance of the activity (e.g., check pulse rate, blood pressure), ability to assist, use of support devices, and safety precautions required (e.g., side rails).

QSEN Patient-Centered Care: Positioning, Moving, and Turning Clients

The nurse working in the home care setting needs to perform the following actions that relate to positioning, moving, and turning clients:

- Assess the height of the bed and the client's leg length to ensure that self-movements in and out of the bed are smooth.
- Inspect the mattress for support. A sagging mattress, a mattress that is too soft, or an underfilled waterbed used over a prolonged period can contribute to the development of hip flexion contractures and low back strain and pain. Bed boards made of plywood and placed beneath a sagging mattress are recommended for clients who have back problems or are prone to them.
- Assess the caregivers' knowledge and application of body mechanics to prevent injury.
- Demonstrate how to turn and position the client in bed. Observe the caregiver performing a return

demonstration. Reevaluate this technique periodically to reinforce correct application of body mechanics.

- Teach caregivers the basic principles of body alignment and how to check for proper alignment after the client has been changed to a new position.
- Warn caregivers of the dangers of lifting and repositioning and encourage the use of assistive devices and a "no solo lift" policy.
- Teach the caregiver to check the client's skin for redness and integrity after repositioning the client. Stress the importance of informing the nurse about the length of time skin redness remains over pressure areas after the client has been repositioned. Emphasize that reddened areas should not be massaged because doing so may lead to tissue trauma. Teach the caregiver that open areas must be inspected and treated by a healthcare professional.

Also see Skills 44.1 through 44.4 on moving and turning clients in bed and helping them sit up on the edge of the bed. *Note:* The Assessment, Planning, Assignment, and Equipment sections as listed in Skill 44.1 are the same for each of these four procedures and are not repeated. The Evaluation section at the end of Skill 44.4 is also the same for all four procedures and, thus, is not repeated.

SKILL 44.1

Moving a Client Up in Bed

PURPOSE

- To assist clients who have slid down in bed from the Fowler's position to move up in bed

ASSESSMENT

Before moving a client, assess the following:

- Client's ability to lie flat or contraindications to lie flat (e.g., respiratory status)
- Client's physical abilities to assist with the move (e.g., muscle strength, presence of paralysis)
- Client's ability to understand instructions and willingness to participate
- Client's degree of comfort or discomfort when moving; if needed, administer analgesics or perform other pain relief measures prior to the move (see Chapter 30 ∞)
- Client's weight
- The availability of equipment and other personnel to assist you.

PLANNING

Review the client record to determine if previous nurses have recorded information about the client's ability to move. Use proper assistive equipment and additional personnel whenever needed. Ensure that the client understands instructions, and provide an interpreter as needed. Determine the number of personnel and type of equipment needed to safely perform the positional change to prevent injury to staff and client.

Assignment

The skills of moving and turning clients in bed can be assigned to assistive personnel (AP). The nurse should make sure that any needed equipment and additional personnel are available to reduce risk of injury to the healthcare personnel. Emphasize the need for the AP to report changes in the client's condition that require assessment and intervention by the nurse.

Equipment

- Assistive devices such as an overhead trapeze, friction-reducing device, or a mechanical lift

IMPLEMENTATION

Preparation

Determine:

- Assistive devices that will be required
- Limitations to movement such as an IV or an indwelling urinary catheter
- Medications the client is receiving, because certain medications may hamper movement or alertness of the client
- Assistance required from other healthcare personnel.

Performance

1. Prior to performing the procedure, introduce self and verify the client's identity using agency protocol. Explain to the client what you are going to do, why it is necessary, and how to participate. Listen to any suggestions made by the client or support people.
2. Perform hand hygiene and observe other appropriate infection prevention procedures.
3. Provide for client privacy.
4. Adjust the bed and the client's position.
   - Adjust the head of the bed to a flat position or as low as the client can tolerate. **Rationale:** *Moving the client upward against gravity requires more force and can cause back strain.*
   - Raise the bed to a height appropriate for personnel safety (i.e., at the caregiver's elbows).
   - Lock the wheels on the bed and raise the rail on the side of the bed opposite you.
   - Remove all pillows, then place one against the head of the bed. **Rationale:** *This pillow protects the client's head from inadvertent injury against the top of the bed during the upward move.*
5. For the client who is able to reposition without assistance:
   - Place the bed in flat or reverse Trendelenburg's position (as tolerated by the client). Stand by and instruct the client to move self. Assess if the client is able to move without causing friction to the skin.
   - Encourage the client to reach up and grasp the upper side rails with both hands, bend knees, and push off with the feet and pull up with the arms simultaneously.
   - Ask if a positioning device is needed (e.g., pillow).

Moving a Client Up in Bed—*continued*

6. For the client who is partially able to assist:
   - *For a client who weighs less than 200 pounds:* Use a friction-reducing device and two assistants. **Rationale:** *Moving a client up in bed is not a one-person task. During any client handling, if the caregiver is required to lift more than 35 lb of a client's weight, then the client should be considered fully dependent and assistive devices should be used. This reduces risk of injury to the caregiver.*
   - *For a client who weighs between 201–300 pounds:* Use a friction-reducing slide sheet and four assistants OR an air transfer system and two assistants. **Rationale:** *Moving a client up in bed is not a one-person task. During any client handling, if the caregiver is required to lift more than 35 lb of a client's weight, then the client should be considered fully dependent and assistive devices should be used. This reduces risk of injury to the caregiver.*
   - *For a client who weighs more than 300 pounds:* Use an air transfer system and two assistants OR a total transfer lift.
   - Ask the client to flex the hips and knees and position the feet so that they can be used effectively for pushing. **Rationale:** *Flexing the hips and knees keeps the entire lower leg off the bed surface, preventing friction during movement, and ensures use of the large muscle groups in the client's legs when pushing, thus increasing the force of movement.*
   - Place the client's arms across the chest. Ask the client to flex the neck during the move and keep the head off the bed surface. **Rationale:** *This keeps the arms and head off the bed surface and minimizes friction during movement.*
   - Use the friction-reducing device and assistants to move the client up in bed. Ask the client to push on the count of three.
7. Position yourself appropriately, and move the client.
   - Face the direction of the movement, and then assume a broad stance with the foot nearest the bed behind the forward foot and weight on the forward foot. Lean your trunk forward from the hips. Flex the hips, knees, and ankles.
   - Tighten your gluteal, abdominal, leg, and arm muscles and rock from the back leg to the front leg and back again. Then, shift your weight to the front leg as the client pushes with the heels so that the client moves toward the head of the bed.
8. For the client who is unable to assist:
   - Use the ceiling lift with supine sling or mobile floor-based lift and two or more caregivers. Follow manufacturer's guidelines for using the lift. **Rationale:** *Moving a client up in bed is not a one-person task. During any client handling, if the caregiver is required to lift more than 35 lb of a client's weight, then the client should be considered to be fully dependent, and assistive devices should be used. This reduces risk of injury to the caregiver.*
9. Ensure client comfort.
   - Elevate the head of the bed and provide appropriate support devices for the client's new position.
   - See the sections on positioning clients earlier in this chapter.
10. Document all relevant information. Record:
    - Time and change of position moved from and position moved to
    - Any signs of pressure areas
    - Use of support devices
    - Ability of client to assist in moving and turning
    - Response of client to moving and turning (e.g., anxiety, discomfort, dizziness).

Turning a Client to the Lateral or Prone Position in Bed

PURPOSE

- Movement to the lateral (side-lying) position may be necessary when placing a bedpan beneath the client, when changing the client's bed linen, or when repositioning the client.

IMPLEMENTATION

Preparation

Determine:

- Assistive devices that will be required (e.g., friction-reducing device or mechanical lift)
- Limitations to movement such as an IV or an indwelling urinary catheter
- Medications the client is receiving, because certain medications may hamper movement or alertness of the client
- Assistance required from other healthcare personnel. **Rationale:** *Moving a client is not a one-person task. During any client handling, if the caregiver is required to lift more than 35 lb of a client's weight, then the client should be considered to be fully dependent and assistive devices should be used. This reduces risk of injury to the caregiver.*

Performance

1. Prior to performing the procedure, introduce self and verify the client's identity using agency protocol. Explain to the client what you are going to do, why it is necessary, and how to participate.
2. Perform hand hygiene and observe other appropriate infection prevention procedures.
3. Provide for client privacy.
4. Position yourself and the client appropriately before performing the move. Other individual(s) stands on the opposite side of the bed.
   - Adjust the head of the bed to a flat position or as low as the client can tolerate. **Rationale:** *This provides a position of comfort for the client.*
   - Raise the bed to a height appropriate for personnel safety (i.e., at the caregiver's elbows).
   - Lock the wheels on the bed.
   - Move the client closer to the side of the bed opposite the side the client will face when turned. **Rationale:** *This ensures that the client will be positioned safely in the center of the bed after turning.* Use a friction-reducing device or mechanical lift (depending on level of client assistance required) to pull the client to the side of the bed. Adjust the client's head and reposition the legs appropriately.
   - While standing on the side of the bed nearest the client, place the client's near arm across the chest. Abduct the client's far shoulder slightly from the side of the body and externally rotate the shoulder. ❶ **Rationale:** *Pulling the one arm forward facilitates the turning motion. Pulling the other arm away from the body and externally rotating the*

Continued on page 1140

SKILL 44.2

Turning a Client to the Lateral or Prone Position in Bed—*continued*

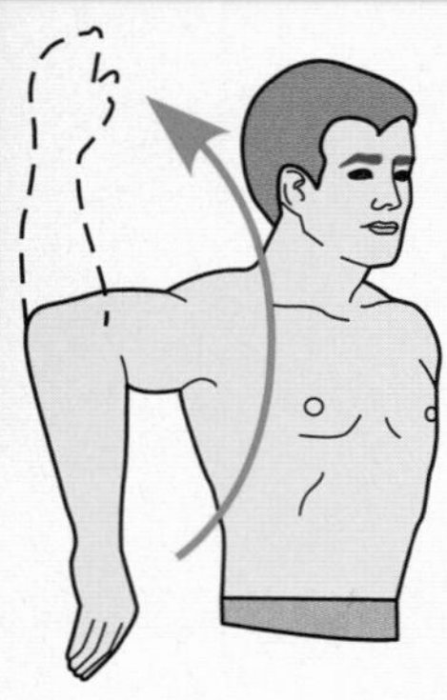

❶ External rotation of the shoulder prevents the arm from being caught beneath the client's body when the client is turned.

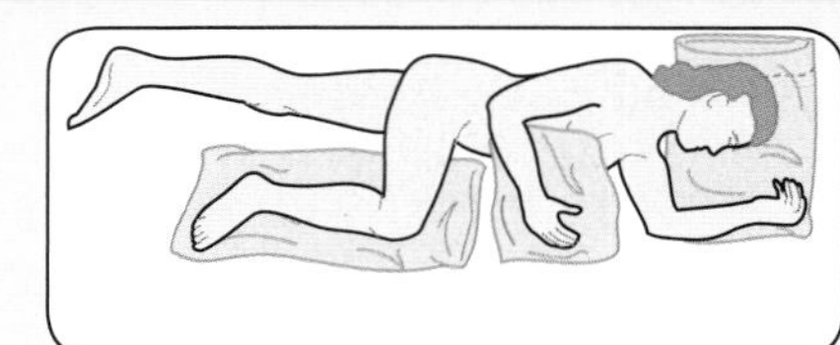

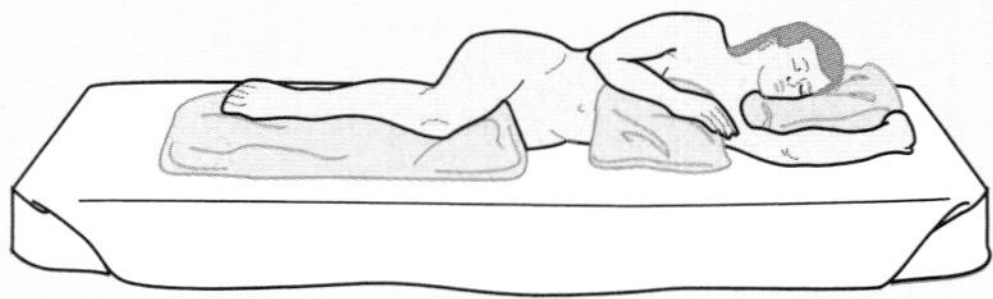

❷ Lateral position with pillows in place.

shoulder prevents that arm from being caught beneath the client's body during the roll.

- Place the client's near ankle and foot across the far ankle and foot. **Rationale:** *This facilitates the turning motion. Making these preparations on the side of the bed closest to the client helps prevent unnecessary reaching*.
- The individual on the side of the bed toward which the client will turn should be positioned directly in line with the client's waistline and as close to the bed as possible.

5. Roll the client to the lateral position. The second individual(s) standing on the opposite side of the bed helps roll the client from the other side.
   - Place one hand on the client's far hip and the other hand on the client's far shoulder. **Rationale:** *This position of the hands supports the client at the two heaviest parts of the body, providing greater control in movement during the roll*.
   - Position the client on his or her side with arms and legs positioned and supported properly. ❷

Variation: Turning the Client to a Prone Position

To turn a client to the prone position, follow the preceding steps, with two exceptions:

- Instead of abducting the far arm, keep the client's arm alongside the body for the client to roll over. **Rationale:** *Keeping the arm alongside the body prevents it from being pinned under the client when the client is rolled*.
- Roll the client completely onto the abdomen. **Rationale:** *It is essential to move the client as close as possible to the edge of the bed before the turn so that the client will be lying on the center of the bed after rolling*. Never pull a client across the bed while the client is in the prone position. **Rationale:** *Doing so can injure a woman's breasts or a man's genitals*.

6. Document all relevant information. Record:
   - Time and change of position moved from and position moved to
   - Any signs of pressure areas
   - Use of support devices
   - Ability of client to assist in moving and turning
   - Response of the client to moving and turning (e.g., anxiety, discomfort, dizziness).

SKILL 44.3

Logrolling a Client

PURPOSE

- **Logrolling** is a technique used to turn a client whose body must at all times be kept in straight alignment (like a log). An example is the client with back surgery or a spinal injury. Considerable care must be taken to prevent additional injury.

This technique requires two nurses or, if the client is large, three nurses. For the client who has a cervical injury, one nurse must maintain the client's head and neck alignment.

IMPLEMENTATION

Preparation

Determine:

- Assistive devices that will be required
- Limitations to movement such as an IV or a urinary catheter
- Medications the client is receiving, because certain medications may hamper movement or alertness of the client
- Assistance required from other healthcare personnel. At least 2–3 additional people are needed to perform this skill safely.

Performance

1. Prior to performing the procedure, introduce self and verify the client's identity using agency protocol. Explain to the client what you are going to do, why it is necessary, and how to participate.
2. Perform hand hygiene and observe other appropriate infection prevention procedures.
3. Provide for client privacy.
4. Position yourselves and the client appropriately before the move.
   - Place the client's arms across the chest. **Rationale:** *Doing so ensures that they will not be injured or become trapped under the body when the body is turned*.
5. Pull the client to the side of the bed.
   - Use a friction-reducing device to facilitate logrolling. First, stand with another nurse on the same side of the bed. Assume a broad stance with one foot forward, and grasp the rolled edge of the friction-reducing device. On a signal, pull the client toward both of you. ❶
   - One nurse counts: "One, two, three, go." Then, at the same time, all staff members pull the client to the side of the bed by shifting their weight to the back foot. **Rationale:** *Moving the client in unison maintains the client's body alignment*.
6. One nurse moves to the other side of the bed, and places supportive devices for the client when turned.

Logrolling a Client—*continued*

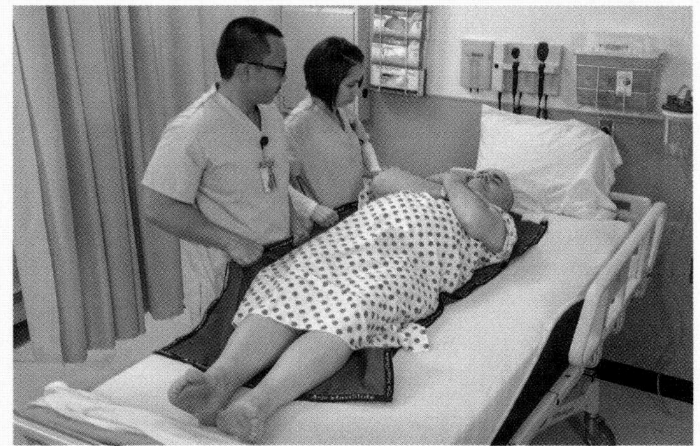

❶ Using a friction-reducing slide sheet, the nurses pull the sheet with the client on it to the edge of the bed.

- Place a pillow where it will support the client's head after the turn. **Rationale:** *The pillow prevents lateral flexion of the neck and ensures alignment of the cervical spine.*
- Place one or two pillows between the client's legs to support the upper leg when the client is turned. **Rationale:** *This pillow prevents adduction of the upper leg and keeps the legs parallel and aligned.*

7. Roll and position the client in proper alignment.
- Go to the other side of the bed (farthest from the client), and assume a stable stance.
- Reaching over the client, grasp the friction-reducing device, and roll the client toward you. ❷
- One nurse counts: "One, two, three, go." Then, at the same time, all nurses roll the client to a lateral position.
- The second nurse (behind the client) helps turn the client and provides pillow supports to ensure good alignment in the lateral position.
- Support the client's head, back, and upper and lower extremities with pillows.

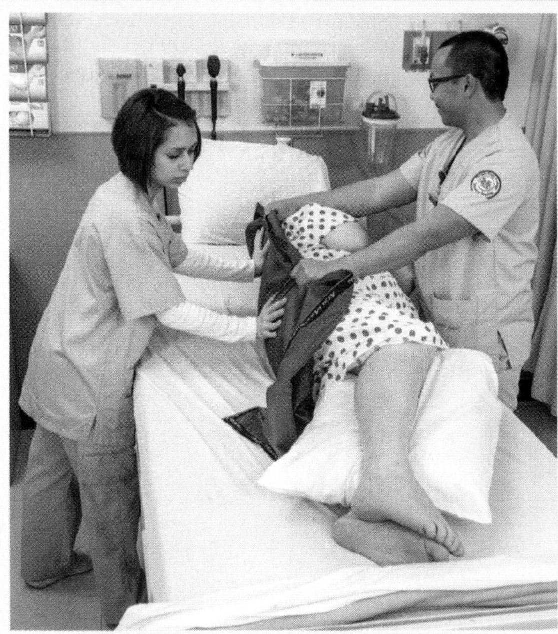

❷ The nurse on the right uses the far edge of the friction-reducing slide sheet to roll the client toward him; the nurse on the left remains behind the client and assists with turning.

- Raise the side rails and place the call bell within the client's reach.

8. Document all relevant information. Record:
- Time and change of position moved from and position moved to
- Any signs of pressure areas
- Use of support devices
- Ability of client to assist in moving and turning
- Response of client to moving and turning (e.g., anxiety, discomfort, dizziness).

Assisting a Client to Sit on the Side of the Bed (Dangling)

PURPOSE

- The client assumes a sitting position on the edge of the bed before walking, moving to a chair or wheelchair, eating, or performing other activities.

IMPLEMENTATION

Preparation

Determine:

- Assistive devices that will be required
- Limitations to movement such as an IV or a urinary catheter
- Medications the client is receiving, because certain medications may hamper movement or alertness of the client
- Assistance required from other healthcare personnel.

Performance

1. Prior to performing the procedure, introduce self and verify the client's identity using agency protocol. Explain to the client what you are going to do, why it is necessary, and how to participate.

2. Perform hand hygiene and observe other appropriate infection prevention procedures.

3. Provide for client privacy.

4. Position yourself and the client appropriately before performing the move.
- Assist the client to a lateral position facing you, using an assistive device depending on client assistance needs.
- Raise the head of the bed slowly to its highest position. **Rationale:** *This decreases the distance that the client needs to move to sit up on the side of the bed.*
- Position the client's feet and lower legs at the edge of the bed. **Rationale:** *This enables the client's feet to move easily off the bed during the movement, and the client is aided by gravity into a sitting position.*
- Stand beside the client's hips and face the far corner of the bottom of the bed (the angle in which movement will occur). Assume a broad stance, placing the foot nearest the client and head of the bed forward. Lean your trunk forward from the hips. Flex your hips, knees, and ankles.

Continued on page 1142

SKILL 44.4

Assisting a Client to Sit on the Side of the Bed (Dangling)—*continued*

5. Move the client to a sitting position, using an assistive device depending on client assistance needs.
- Place the arm nearest to the head of the bed under the client's shoulders and the other arm over both of the client's thighs near the knees. ❶ **Rationale:** *Supporting the client's shoulders prevents the client from falling backward during the movement. Supporting the client's thighs reduces friction of the thighs against the bed surface during the move and increases the force of the movement.*
- Tighten your gluteal, abdominal, leg, and arm muscles.
- Pivot on the balls of your feet in the desired direction facing the foot of the bed while pulling the client's feet and legs off the bed. **Rationale:** *Pivoting prevents twisting of the nurse's spine. The weight of the client's legs swinging downward increases downward movement of the lower body and helps make the client's upper body vertical.*
- Keep supporting the client until the client is well balanced and comfortable. ❷ **Rationale:** *This movement may cause some clients to become light-headed or dizzy.*
- Assess vital signs (e.g., pulse, respirations, and blood pressure) as indicated by the client's health status.

6. Document all relevant information. Record:
- Ability of the client to assist in moving and turning
- Type of assistive device, if one was used
- Response of the client to moving and turning (e.g., anxiety, discomfort, dizziness).

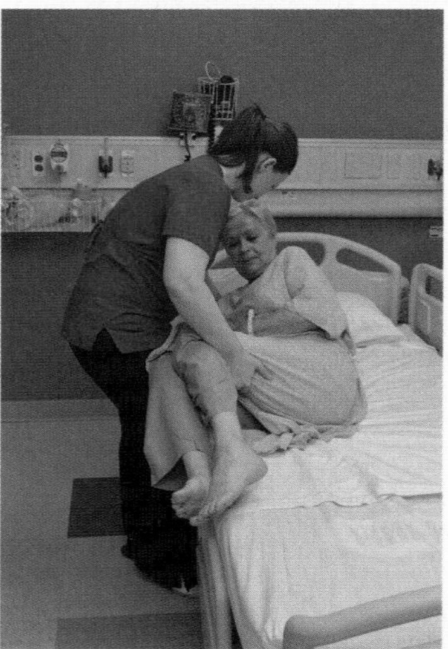

❶ Moving the client to a sitting position.

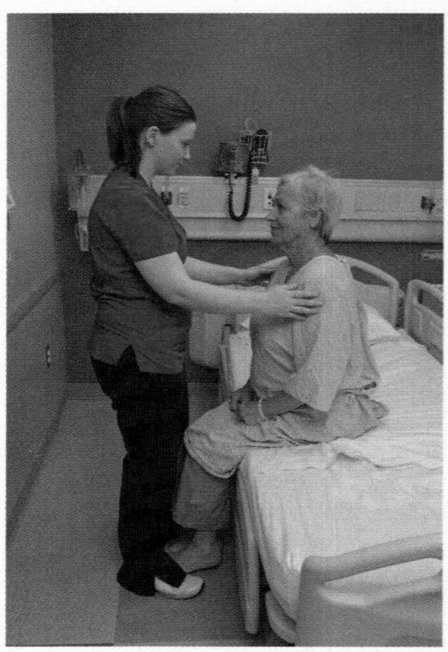

❷ Support the client until the client is well balanced and comfortable.

EVALUATION

- Check the skin integrity of the pressure areas from the previous position. Relate findings to previous assessment data if available. Conduct follow-up assessment for previous and new skin breakdown areas.
- Check for proper alignment after the position change. Do a visual check and ask the client for a comfort assessment.
- Determine that all required safety precautions (e.g., side rails) are in place.
- Determine client's tolerance of the activity (e.g., vital signs before and after dangling), particularly the first time the client changes position.
- Report significant changes to the primary care practitioner.

Note: This skill describes the process to use for a client who is able to perform the task independently and only needs standby assistance for steadying, or a client who requires minimum assistance in which the client can perform the task with or without friction-reducing assistive devices and the healthcare worker provides 25% of the work. For clients who require moderate assistance (requiring no more than 50% assistance by the caregiver) or maximum assistance (requiring more than 50% assistance by the caregiver), a lateral chair or mobile or ceiling-mounted transfer system is required.

LIFESPAN CONSIDERATIONS Positioning, Moving, and Turning Clients

INFANTS

- Position infants on their back for sleep, even after feeding. There is little risk of regurgitation and choking, and the rate of sudden infant death syndrome (SIDS) is significantly lower in infants who sleep on their backs.
- The skin of newborns can be fragile and may be abraded or torn (sheared) if the infant is pulled across a bed.

CHILDREN

- Carefully inspect the dependent skin surfaces of all infants and children confined to bed at least three times in each 24-hour period.

OLDER ADULTS

- In clients who have had strokes, there is a risk of shoulder displacement on the paralyzed side from improper moving or repositioning techniques. Use care when moving, positioning in bed, and transferring. Pillows or foam devices are helpful to support the affected arm and shoulder and prevent injury.
- Decreased subcutaneous fat and thinning of the skin place older adults at risk for skin breakdown. Repositioning approximately every 2 hours (more or less, depending on the unique needs of the individual client) helps reduce pressure on bony prominences and avoid tissue trauma.

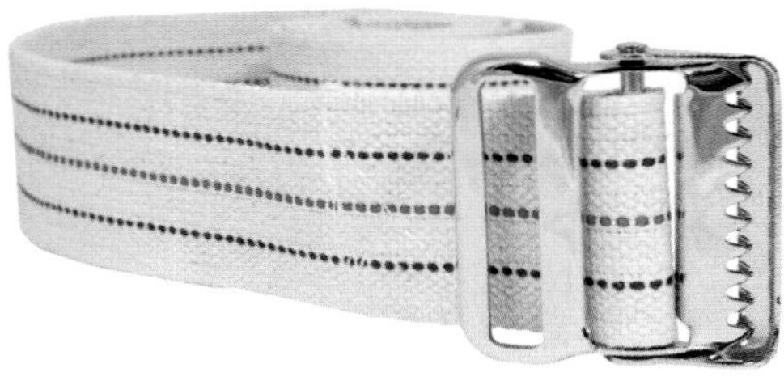

Figure 44.53 ■ Gait belt.
Noel V. Baebler/Shutterstock.

Transferring Clients

Many clients require some assistance in transferring between bed and chair or wheelchair, between wheelchair and toilet, and between bed and stretcher. Before transferring any client, however, the nurse must determine the client's physical and mental capabilities to participate in the transfer technique. In addition, the nurse must analyze and organize the activity.

A gait belt, sometimes called a transfer or walking belt, has traditionally been used to transfer a client from one position to another and for ambulation (Figure 44.53 ■). A gait belt can have handles that allow the nurse to control movement of the client during the transfer or during ambulation. The long-held belief that the use of gait belts improves safety for both clients and caregivers is based on tradition and not on evidence-based research. The few studies that have been done indicate that using a gait belt for transfer falls into either a moderate- or high-risk category for low back disorders. Gait belts are not appropriate for all clients and it is important to assess clients before using one on them. They are suitable for clients who can bear weight and require only minimal assistance. The gait belt with handles is easier to grasp. Gait belts should not be used to lift a client off the floor or for bariatric clients. In addition, they should not be relied on for use with clients who are at high risk for falls (Miller, Rockefeller, & Townsend, 2017).

A sliding board is another device that can be used to transfer a client between a bed and chair. Boards are often made of low-friction materials or with movable sliding sections. Some clients may be able to transfer themselves using a sliding transfer board. If a caregiver is needed, the client is either pushed or pulled across the transfer board using a slide sheet. Clients must have sitting balance. See Skill 44.5 for transferring a client between a bed and a chair, and Skill 44.6 for transferring a client between a bed and a stretcher. *Note:* The Evaluation section at the end of Skill 44.6 also applies to Skill 44.5.

General guidelines for transfer techniques include the following:

- Plan what to do and how to do it. Determine the space in which the transfer will take place (bathrooms, for instance, are usually cramped), the number of assistants (one or two) needed to accomplish the transfer safely, and the client's capabilities (e.g., size, weight, cognition, balance, cooperation).
- Obtain essential equipment before starting (e.g., gait or transfer belt; friction-reducing device, such as a slide sheet, slide board, or air transfer system; wheelchair; stretcher; lift) and check that all equipment is functioning correctly. The gait or transfer belt is meant only to increase control of the client's movements; if the client requires lifting, a mechanical lifting device should be used.
- Remove obstacles from the area used for the transfer.
- Explain the transfer to the client, including what the client should do.
- Explain the transfer to the nursing personnel who are helping; specify who will give directions (one staff member needs to be in charge).
- Always support or hold the client rather than the equipment and ensure the client's safety and dignity.
- During the transfer, explain step by step what the client should do, for example, "Move your right foot forward."
- Make a written plan of the transfer, including the client's tolerance (e.g., pulse and respiratory rates).

Because wheelchairs and stretchers are unstable, they can predispose the client to falls and injury. Guidelines for the safe use of wheelchairs and stretchers are shown in the accompanying Practice Guidelines.

PRACTICE GUIDELINES Wheelchair Safety

- Always lock the brakes on both wheels of the wheelchair when the client transfers in or out of it.
- Raise the footplates and move the leg rests out of the way before transferring the client into the wheelchair.
- Lower the footplates after the transfer, and place the client's feet on them.
- Ensure the client is positioned well back in the seat of the wheelchair.
- Use seat belts that fasten behind the wheelchair to protect confused clients from falls. *Note:* Seat belts are a form of restraint and must be used in accordance with policies and procedures that apply to the use of restraints (see Chapter 32 ∞).
- Back the wheelchair into or out of an elevator, rear large wheels first.
- Place your body between the wheelchair and the bottom of an incline.

Clinical Alert!

Air, foam, and gel cushions that distribute weight evenly (*not* doughnut-type cushions) are essential for clients confined to a wheelchair and must be checked frequently to ensure they are intact. Strict continence management is also important for preventing skin breakdown. Maintaining tire pressure will prevent added resistance and energy expenditure. Periodically monitor the client's upper extremities for pain and overuse syndromes.

PRACTICE GUIDELINES Safe Use of Stretchers

- Lock the wheels of the bed and stretcher before the client transfers in or out of them.
- Fasten safety straps across the client on a stretcher, and raise the side rails.
- Never leave a client unattended on a stretcher unless the wheels are locked and the side rails are raised on both sides or the safety straps are securely fastened across the client.
- Always push a stretcher from the end where the client's head is positioned. This position protects the client's head in the event of a collision.
- If the stretcher has two swivel wheels and two stationary wheels:
  a. Always position the client's head at the end with the stationary wheels and
  b. Push the stretcher from the end with the stationary wheels. The stretcher is maneuvered more easily when pushed from this end.
- Maneuver the stretcher when entering the elevator so that the client's head goes in first.

SKILL 44.5

Transferring Between Bed and Chair

PURPOSE

- A client may need to be transferred between the bed and a wheelchair or chair, the bed and the commode, or a wheelchair and the toilet. There are numerous variations in the technique. Which variation the nurse selects depends on factors related to the client and the environment that are assessed prior to beginning the transfer.

ASSESSMENT

Before transferring a client, assess the following:

- The client's body size and weight
- Ability to follow instructions
- Ability to bear weight (full, partial, or none)
- Ability to position and reposition feet on floor
- Ability to push down with arms and lean forward
- Ability to grasp
- Ability to achieve independent balance (sitting, standing, or none)
- Activity tolerance
- Muscle strength
- Joint mobility
- Presence of paralysis
- Level of comfort
- Presence of orthostatic hypotension
- The technique with which the client is familiar
- The space in which the transfer will need to be maneuvered (bathrooms, for example, are usually cramped)
- The number of assistants (one or two) needed to accomplish the transfer safely.

PLANNING

Review the client record to determine if previous nurses have recorded information about the client's ability to transfer. Implement pain relief measures so that they are effective when the transfer begins. The decision must be made at this time regarding the client's ability to participate. If the client can safely participate in the transfer, a gait or transfer belt or sliding board can be used; if not, a powered standing assist lift or full-body lift would be safer for the client and nurse.

Equipment

- Robe or appropriate clothing
- Slippers or shoes with nonskid soles
- Gait or transfer belt
- Chair, commode, wheelchair as appropriate to client need
- Slide board, if appropriate
- Lift, if appropriate

Assignment

The skill of transferring a client can be assigned to AP who have demonstrated safe transfer technique for the involved client. It is important for the nurse to assess the number of staff needed, assistive devices needed, and the client's ability to assist and to communicate specific information about what the AP should report to the nurse.

IMPLEMENTATION

Preparation

- Plan what to do and how to do it.
- Obtain essential equipment before starting (e.g., gait or transfer belt, wheelchair), and check that all equipment is functioning correctly.
- Remove obstacles from the area so clients do not trip. Make sure there are no spills or liquids on the floor on which clients could slip.
- Note any devices attached to the client (e.g., IV, urinary catheter).

Performance

1. Prior to performing the procedure, introduce self and verify the client's identity using agency protocol. Explain the transfer process to the client. During the transfer, explain step by step what the client should do, for example, "Move your right foot forward."
2. Perform hand hygiene and observe other appropriate infection prevention procedures.
3. Provide for client privacy.
4. Position the equipment appropriately.

Transferring Between Bed and Chair—*continued*

- Lower the bed to its lowest position so that the client's feet will rest flat on the floor. Lock the wheels of the bed.
- Place the wheelchair parallel to the bed and as close to the bed as possible. ❶ Put the wheelchair on the side of the bed that allows the client to move toward his or her stronger side. Lock the wheels of the wheelchair, raise the footplates, and move the leg rests out of the way.

5. Prepare and assess the client.
- Assist the client to a sitting position on the side of the bed (see Skill 44.4).
- Assess the client for orthostatic hypotension before moving the client from the bed.
- Assist the client in putting on a bathrobe and nonskid slippers or shoes.
- Place a gait or transfer belt snugly around the client's waist. Check to be certain that the belt is securely fastened.

6. Give explicit instructions to the client. Ask the client to:
- Move forward and sit on the edge of the bed (or surface on which the client is sitting) with feet placed flat on the floor. **Rationale:** *This brings the client's center of gravity closer to the nurse's.*
- Lean forward slightly from the hips. **Rationale:** *This brings the client's center of gravity more directly over the base of support and positions the head and trunk in the direction of the movement.*
- Place the foot of the stronger leg beneath the edge of the bed (or sitting surface) and put the other foot forward. **Rationale:** *In this way, the client can use the stronger leg muscles to stand and power the movement. A broader base of support makes the client more stable during the transfer.*
- Place the client's hands on the bed surface (or available stable area) so that the client can push while standing. **Rationale:** *This provides additional force for the movement and reduces the potential for strain on the nurse's back.* The client should not grasp your neck for support. **Rationale:** *Doing so can injure the nurse.*

7. Position yourself correctly.
- Stand directly in front of the client and to the side requiring the most support. Hold the gait or transfer belt with the nearest hand; the other hand supports the back of the client's shoulder. Lean your trunk forward from the hips. Flex your hips, knees, and ankles. Assume a broad stance, placing one foot forward and one back. Brace the client's feet with your feet to prevent the client from sliding forward or laterally. Mirror the placement of the client's feet, if possible. **Rationale:** *This helps prevent loss of balance during the transfer.*

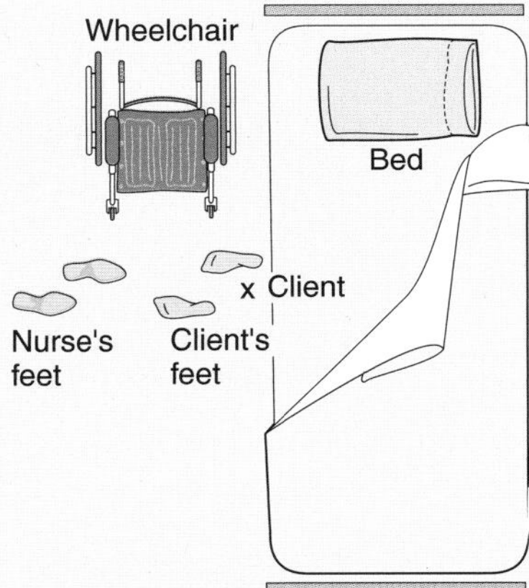

❶ The wheelchair is placed parallel to the bed and as close to the bed as possible. Note that placement of the nurse's feet mirrors that of the client's feet.

8. Assist the client to stand, and then move together toward the wheelchair or sitting area to which you wish to transfer the client.
- On the count of three or the verbal instructions of "Ready–steady–stand" and on the count of three or the word "Stand," ask the client to push down against the mattress or side of the bed while you transfer your weight from one foot to the other (while keeping your back straight) and stand upright moving the client forward (directly toward your center of gravity) into a standing position. (If the client requires more than a very small degree of pulling, even with the assistance of two nurses, a mechanical device should be obtained and used.)
- Support the client in an upright standing position for a few moments. **Rationale:** *This allows the nurse and the client to extend the joints and provides the nurse with an opportunity to ensure that the client is stable before moving away from the bed.*
- Together, pivot on your foot farthest from the chair, or take a few steps toward the wheelchair, bed, chair, commode, or car seat.

9. Assist the client to sit.
- Move the wheelchair forward or have the client back up to the wheelchair (or desired seating area) and place the legs against the seat. **Rationale:** *Having the client place the legs against the wheelchair seat minimizes the risk of the client falling when sitting down.*
- Make sure the wheelchair brakes are on.
- Have the client reach back and feel or hold the arms of the wheelchair.
- Stand directly in front of the client. Place one foot forward and one back.
- Tighten your grasp on the gait or transfer belt, and tighten your gluteal, abdominal, leg, and arm muscles.
- Have the client sit down while you bend your knees and hips and lower the client onto the wheelchair seat.

10. Ensure client safety.
- Ask the client to push back into the wheelchair seat. **Rationale:** *Sitting well back on the seat provides a broader base of support and greater stability and minimizes the risk of falling from the wheelchair. A wheelchair or bedside commode can topple forward when the client sits on the edge of the seat and leans far forward.*
- Remove the gait or transfer belt.
- Lower the leg rests and footplates, and place the client's feet on them, if applicable.

Variation: Transferring with a Belt and Two Nurses
- Even if a client is able to partially bear weight and is cooperative, it still may be safer to transfer a client with the assistance of two nurses. If so, you should position yourselves on both sides of the client, facing the same direction as the client. Flex your hips, knees, and ankles. Grasp the client's transfer belt with the hand closest to the client, and with the other hand support the client's elbows.

Continued on page 1146

SKILL 44.5

Transferring Between Bed and Chair—*continued*

- Coordinating your efforts, all three of you stand simultaneously, pivot, and move to the wheelchair. Reverse the process to lower the client onto the wheelchair seat.

Variation: Transferring a Client with an Injured Lower Extremity
When the client has an injured lower extremity, movement should always occur toward the client's unaffected (strong) side. For example, if the client's right leg is injured and the client is sitting on the edge of the bed preparing to transfer to a wheelchair, position the wheelchair on the client's left side. **Rationale:** *In this way, the client can use the unaffected leg most effectively and safely.*

Variation: Using a Slide Board
For clients who cannot stand but are able to cooperate and possess sufficient upper body strength, use a slide board to help them move without nursing assistance. ❷ **Rationale:** *This method not only promotes the client's sense of independence but also preserves your energy.*

11. Document relevant information:
- Client's ability to bear weight and pivot
- Number of staff needed for transfer and the safety measures and precautions used
- Length of time up in chair
- Client response to transfer and being up in chair or wheelchair.

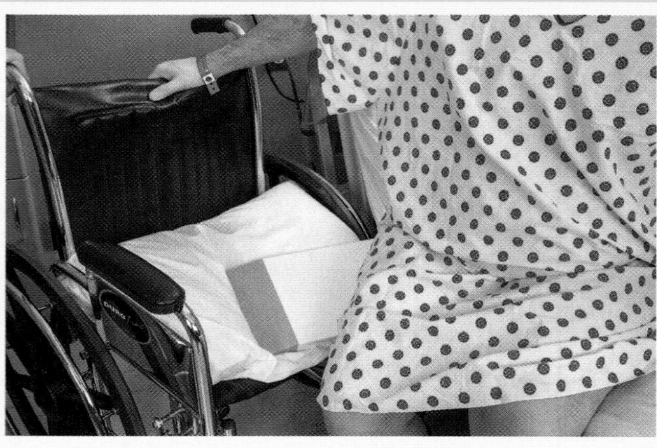
❷ Using a slide board.

Note: This skill describes the process to use for a client who is able to perform the task independently and only needs standby assistance for steadying. For clients who require moderate or maximum assistance, a lateral chair or a mobile or ceiling-mounted transfer system is required.

QSEN Patient-Centered Care: Transferring in the Home Setting

The nurse in the home care setting needs to consider the following:

- The caregiver and client should practice transfer technique(s), using appropriate equipment as needed, in the hospital or long-term care setting before being discharged.
- Assess furniture in the home. Does the client's favorite chair have arms for ease of using and sitting? Examine the fabric—is it rough? Will it cause skin abrasions? If the client will be using a wheelchair, is there enough space in the bedroom and bathroom for a safe transfer?
- Observe client and caregiver transfer technique in the home setting to reinforce prior teaching.

SKILL 44.6

Transferring Between Bed and Stretcher

PURPOSE
- The stretcher, or gurney, is used to transfer supine clients from one location to another. Whenever the client is capable of accomplishing the transfer from bed to stretcher independently, either by lifting onto it or by rolling onto it, the client should be encouraged to do so. If the client cannot move onto the stretcher independently and weighs less than 200 pounds, a friction-reducing device (i.e., slide sheet) or a lateral transfer board ❶ or an air transfer system should be used, and at least two caregivers are needed to assist with the transfer. Some friction-reducing devices have handles or long straps to avoid awkward stretching by the caregivers when pulling the client during the lateral transfer. For clients between 201 and 300 pounds, a slide sheet or transfer board and four caregivers or an air transfer system and two caregivers should be used. For clients who weigh more than 300 pounds, two caregivers and either an air transfer system or a ceiling lift with supine sling should be used.
- Depending on the client's condition (e.g., neck immobilizer, IVs, drains, chest tube), additional assistants may be needed.

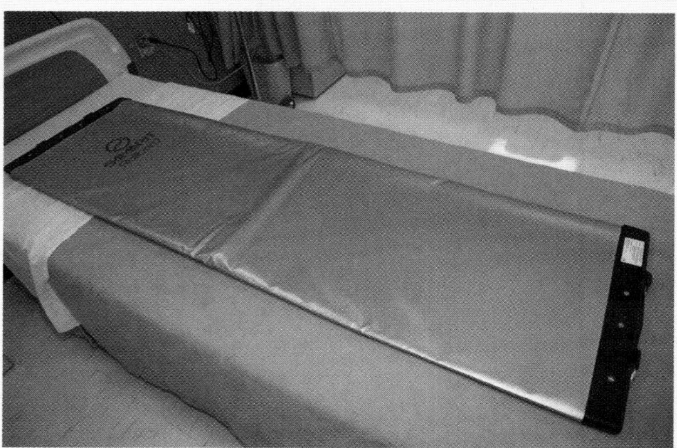
❶ A lateral transfer board. The friction-reducing material rolls when transferring clients in a supine position.
Shirlee Snyder.

Transferring Between Bed and Stretcher—*continued*

ASSESSMENT

Before transferring a client, assess the following:

- The client's body size and weight
- Ability to follow instructions
- Activity tolerance
- Level of comfort
- The space in which the transfer is maneuvered
- The number of assistants (one to four) needed to accomplish the transfer safely.

PLANNING

Review the client record to determine if previous nurses have recorded information about how the client tolerated similar transfers. If indicated, implement pain relief measures so that they are effective when the transfer begins.

Equipment

- Stretcher
- Transfer assistive devices (e.g., slide sheet, transfer board, air transfer system, lift)

Assignment

The skill of transferring a client can be assigned to AP who have demonstrated safe transfer technique for the involved client. It is important for the nurse to assess the client's capabilities and communicate specific information about what the AP should report back to the nurse.

IMPLEMENTATION

Preparation

Obtain the necessary equipment and nursing personnel to assist in the transfer.

- Note any devices attached to the client.

Performance

1. Prior to performing the procedure, introduce self and verify the client's identity using agency protocol. Explain to the client what you are going to do, why it is necessary, and how to participate. Explain the transfer to the nursing personnel who are helping and specify who will give directions (one staff member needs to be in charge).
2. Perform hand hygiene and observe other appropriate infection prevention procedures.
3. Provide for client privacy.
4. Adjust the client's bed in preparation for the transfer.
   - Lower the head of the bed until it is flat or as low as the client can tolerate.
   - Place the friction-reducing device under the client.
   - Raise the bed so that it is slightly higher (i.e., 1/2 in.) than the surface of the stretcher. **Rationale:** *It is easier for the client to move down a slant.*
   - Ensure that the wheels on the bed are locked.
   - Place the stretcher parallel to the bed next to the client and lock the stretcher wheels.
   - Fill the gap that exists between the bed and the stretcher loosely with the bath blankets (optional).
5. Transfer the client securely to the stretcher.
   - If the client can transfer independently, encourage him or her to do so and stand by for safety.
   - If the client is partially able or not able to transfer:
     - One caregiver needs to be at the side of the client's bed, between the client's shoulder and hip.
     - The second and third caregivers should be at the side of the stretcher: one positioned between the client's shoulder and hip and the other between the client's hip and lower legs.
     - All caregivers should position their feet in a walking stance.
     - Ask the client to flex the neck during the move, if possible, and place the arms across the chest. **Rationale:** *This prevents injury to those body parts.*
     - On a planned command, the caregivers at the stretcher's side pull (shifting weight to the rear foot), and the caregiver at the bedside pushes the client toward the stretcher (shifting weight to the front foot).
6. Ensure client comfort and safety.
   - Make the client comfortable, unlock the stretcher wheels, and move the stretcher away from the bed.
   - Immediately raise the stretcher side rails or fasten the safety straps across the client. **Rationale:** *Because the stretcher is high and narrow, the client is in danger of falling unless these safety precautions are taken.*

Variation: Using a Transfer Board

The transfer board is a lacquered or smooth polyethylene board measuring 45 to 55 cm (18 to 22 in.) by 182 cm (72 in.) with handholds along its edges. Transfer mattresses are also available, as are mechanical assistive devices. It is imperative to have enough staff assisting with the transfer to prevent injury to staff as well as clients. Turn the client to a lateral position away from you, position the board close to the client's back, and roll the client onto the board. Pull the client and board across the bed to the stretcher. Safety belts may be placed over the chest, abdomen, and legs.

7. Document relevant information:
   - Equipment used
   - Number of personnel needed for transfer and safety measures and precautions used
   - Destination if reason for transfer is to transport from one location to another.

EVALUATION

- Compare client capabilities such as weight bearing, pivoting ability, and strength and control during previous transfers.
- Report any significant deviations from normal to the primary care practitioner.
- Note use of appropriate safety measures (e.g., transfer belt, locking wheels of bed and stretcher) by AP during transfer process.

LIFESPAN CONSIDERATIONS Transferring Clients

INFANTS

- The infant who is lying down, on the side or supine, can be placed in either a bassinet or crib for transport. If the bassinet has a bottom shelf, it can be used for carrying the IV pump or monitor.

CHILDREN

- The toddler should be transported in a high-top crib with the side rails up and the protective top in place. Stretchers should not be used because the mobile toddler may roll or fall off.

OLDER ADULTS

- Because conditions of older adults can change from day to day, always assess the situation to ensure that you have the right equipment and enough people to assist when transferring a client.
- Use special caution with older clients to prevent skin tears or bruising during a transfer or when using a hydraulic lift.
- Write the method used to transfer each client—equipment used, best position, and number of personnel needed to assist in transfer. This can be part of the care plan and also be available in the client's room as a guide to all personnel caring for the client.
- Avoid sudden position changes. They can cause orthostatic hypotension and increase the risk of fainting and falls.

Providing ROM Exercises

Clients who experience restrictions in activity are at risk for impaired joint mobility. Promoting exercise to maintain a client's muscle tone and joint mobility is an essential function of nursing personnel. When clients are ill, they may need to perform ROM exercises until they can regain their normal activity levels.

Active ROM exercises are isotonic exercises in which the client moves each joint in the body through its complete range of movement, maximally stretching all muscle groups within each plane over the joint. These exercises maintain or increase muscle strength and endurance and help to maintain cardiorespiratory function in an immobilized client. They also prevent deterioration of joint capsules, ankylosis, and contractures (permanent shortening of the muscle).

Full ROM does not occur spontaneously in the immobilized individual who independently achieves ADLs, moves about in bed, transfers between bed and wheelchair or chair, or ambulates a short distance, because only a few muscle groups are maximally stretched during these activities. Although the client may successfully achieve some active ROM movements of the upper extremities while combing the hair, bathing, and dressing, the immobilized client is very unlikely to achieve any active ROM movements of the lower extremities when these are not used in the normal functions of standing and walking about. For this reason, most clients who use a wheelchair and many ambulatory clients need active ROM exercises until they regain their normal activity levels.

At first, the nurse may need to teach the client and family to perform the needed ROM exercises; eventually, the client may be able to accomplish these independently. Instructions for the client performing active ROM exercises are shown in the accompanying Client Teaching.

CLIENT TEACHING Active ROM Exercises

- Perform each ROM exercise as taught to the point of slight resistance, but not beyond, and never to the point of discomfort.
- Perform the movements systematically, using the same sequence during each session.
- Perform each exercise three times.
- Perform each series of exercises twice daily.

OLDER ADULTS

- For older adults, it is not essential to achieve full range of motion in all joints. Instead, emphasize achieving a sufficient range of motion to carry out ADLs, such as walking, dressing, combing hair, showering, and preparing a meal.

During **passive ROM exercises**, another individual moves each of the client's joints through its complete range of movement, maximally stretching all muscle groups within each plane over each joint. Because the client does not contract the muscles, passive ROM exercises are of no value in maintaining muscle strength but are useful in maintaining joint flexibility. For this reason, passive ROM exercises should be performed only when the client is unable to accomplish the movements actively.

Passive ROM exercises should be accomplished for each movement of the arms, legs, and neck that the client is unable to achieve actively. As with active ROM exercises, passive ROM exercises should be accomplished to the point of slight resistance, but not beyond, and never to the point of discomfort. The movements should be systematic, and the same sequence should be followed during each exercise session. Each exercise should be repeated, at the client's tolerance, from three to five times. The series of exercises should be done twice daily. Performing one series of exercises along with the bath is helpful. Passive ROM exercises are accomplished most effectively when the client lies supine in bed. General guidelines for providing passive exercises are shown in the accompanying Practice Guidelines.

During active-assistive ROM exercises, the client uses a stronger, opposite arm or leg to move each of the joints of a limb incapable of active motion. The client learns to support and move the weak arm or leg with the strong arm or leg as far as possible. Then the nurse continues the

PRACTICE GUIDELINES Providing Passive ROM Exercises

- Ensure that the client understands the reason for doing ROM exercises.
- If there is a possibility of hand swelling, make sure rings are removed.
- Clothe the client in a loose gown, and cover the body with a bath blanket.
- Use correct body mechanics when providing ROM exercises to avoid muscle strain or injury to both yourself and the client.
- Position the bed at an appropriate height.
- Expose only the limb being exercised to avoid embarrassing the client and to maintain warmth.
- Support the client's limbs above and below the joint as needed to prevent muscle strain or injury (Figure 44.54 ■). This may also be done by cupping joints in the palm of your hand or cradling limbs along your forearm (Figure 44.55 ■). If a joint is painful (e.g., arthritic), support the limb in the muscular areas above and below the joint.
- Use a firm, comfortable grip when handling the limb.
- Move the body parts smoothly, slowly, and rhythmically. Jerky movements cause discomfort and, possibly, injury. Fast movements can cause spasticity (sudden, prolonged involuntary muscle contraction) or rigidity (stiffness or inflexibility).
- Avoid moving or forcing a body part beyond the existing range of motion. Muscle strain, pain, and injury can result. This is particularly important for clients with flaccid (limp) paralysis, whose muscles can be stretched and joints dislocated without their awareness.
- If muscle spasticity occurs during movement, stop the movement temporarily, but continue to apply slow, gentle pressure on the part until the muscle relaxes; then proceed with the motion.
- If a contracture is present, apply slow, firm pressure, without causing pain, to stretch the muscle fibers.
- If rigidity occurs, apply pressure against the rigidity, and continue the exercise slowly.
- Teach client's caregiver the purposes and technique of performing passive ROM at home if appropriate.
- Avoid hypertension of joints in older adults if joints are arthritic.
- Use the exercises as an opportunity to also assess skin condition.

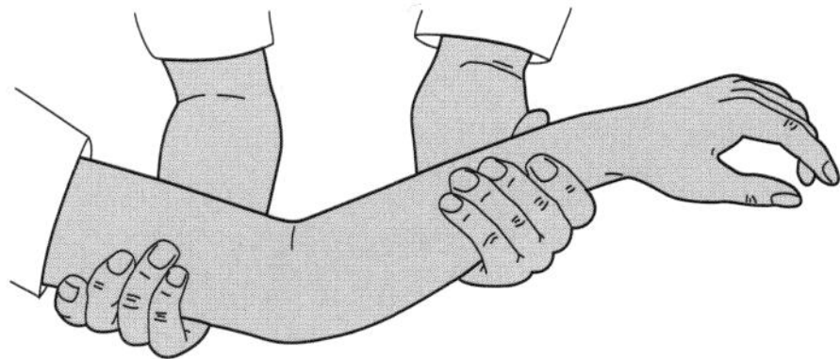

Figure 44.54 ■ Supporting a limb above and below the joint for passive exercise.

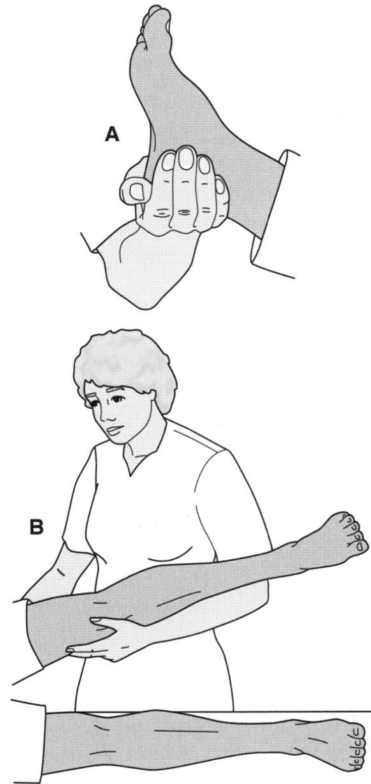

Figure 44.55 ■ Holding limbs for support during passive exercise: *A*, cupping; *B*, cradling.

movement passively to its maximal degree. This activity increases active movement on the strong side of the client's body and maintains joint flexibility on the weak side. Such exercise is especially useful for clients who have had a stroke and are hemiplegic (paralyzed on one half of the body).

Clinical Alert!

Clients who require passive ROM exercises after a disability should have a goal of progressing to active-assistive ROM exercises and, finally, to active ROM exercises.

Ambulating Clients

Ambulation (the act of walking) is a function that most people take for granted. However, when clients are ill they are often confined to bed and are thus nonambulatory. The longer clients are in bed, the more difficulty they have walking. In fact, evidence continues to support that early, routine mobilization of critically ill clients is safe, improves muscle strength and functional independence, reduces incidence of delirium, and decreases hospital length of stay (Denehy, Lanphere, & Needham, 2017; Hashem, Nelliot, & Needham, 2016; Kappel et al., 2018).

Even 1 or 2 days of bedrest can make an individual feel weak, unsteady, and shaky when first getting out of bed. A client who has had surgery, is elderly, or has been immobilized for a longer time will feel more noticeable weakness. The potential problems of immobility are far less likely to occur when clients become ambulatory as soon as possible. The nurse can assist clients to prepare for ambulation by helping them become as independent as possible while in bed. Nurses should encourage clients to perform ADLs, maintain good body alignment, and carry out active ROM exercises to the maximum degree possible yet within the limitations imposed by their illness and recovery program. Collaboration with physical therapy, when ordered, can also be very useful in strengthening the muscles needed for ambulation.

Preambulatory Exercises

Clients who have been in bed for long periods often need to perform muscle tone exercises to strengthen the muscles used for walking before attempting to walk. One of the most important muscle groups is the quadriceps femoris, which extends the knee and flexes the thigh. This group is also important for elevating the legs, for example, for walking upstairs. These exercises are frequently called quadriceps drills or sets. To strengthen these muscles, the client consciously tenses them, drawing the kneecap upward and inward. The client pushes the popliteal space of the knee against the bed surface, relaxing the heels on the bed surface (Figure 44.56 ■). On the count of 1, the muscles are tensed; they are held during the counts of 2, 3, 4; and they are relaxed at the count of 5. The exercise should be done within the client's tolerance, that is, without fatiguing the muscles. Carried out several times an hour during waking hours, this simple exercise significantly strengthens the muscles used for walking.

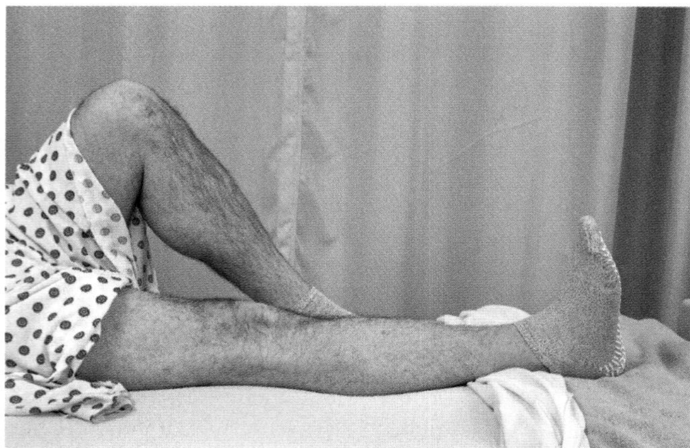

Figure 44.56 ■ Tensing the quadriceps femoris muscles before ambulation.

Assisting Clients to Ambulate

Clients who have been immobilized for even a few days may require assistance with ambulation. The amount

EVIDENCE-BASED PRACTICE

Evidence-Based Practice

Can a Formalized Ambulation Program Improve Ambulation in Hospitalized Clients?

Older adults, orthopedic clients, and clients who have had general surgery are at highest risk for immobility complications. Research clearly documents the benefits of mobilization; however, mobilization of hospitalized clients is the most commonly missed nursing care activity. Lack of personnel and time are the two common reasons given for failure to perform ambulation. Studies focused on improving ambulation in hospitalized clients have primarily focused on interventions to ambulate surgical clients earlier using a dedicated team of personnel, which is often unrealistic for most institutions. Based on these findings, Teodoro et al. (2016) conducted a pretest and posttest randomized experimental research design to determine if a formalized ambulation program could improve ambulation in hospitalized medical–surgical clients.

The research design compared a planned ambulation program with usual care. The ambulation program included daily goals for walking posted in the client's room, an education videotape about the importance of walking and what clients can do to meet their goals, and walking reminders in the client's room. The nurse assigned to care for each client directed the ambulation in the usual care group. The outcome variable was the amount of ambulation measured in steps per hour captured with a pedometer.

The study was conducted on a 30-bed medical-surgical unit of a community-based hospital. A total of 48 clients were included in the study, with 22 assigned to the ambulation program and 26 assigned to the usual care group. The study took place over 3 sequential days. On the first day (pretest period), all the clients had a pedometer attached to their gowns at 11 A.M. with instructions to wear the pedometer through the day and no instructions given about ambulation. The pedometer was removed at 6 P.M. The number of steps for the pretest period was recorded and transcribed as the average number of steps walked per hour. This monitoring was done to ensure that baseline ambulation values were similar for the two groups. The participants were then randomly assigned to either the ambulation program group or the usual care group. Between 6 and 9 P.M., the members of the ambulation program group watched a 2.5-minute video on the importance of ambulation. On day 2, the clients in the ambulation program determined their goals when a researcher asked each to estimate the distance he or she could walk outside the room on that day and then double the distance as a goal for day 3. On both days 2 and 3, all participants had the pedometer attached to their gowns at 7 A.M. and removed at 11 P.M. The researchers then recorded the number of steps for the 16-hour posttest period.

No significant differences were found between the ambulation and usual care groups for age, sex, reason for admission, or pretest amount of ambulation. However, the participants in the ambulation program had significantly higher amounts of ambulation within 2 days, while the usual care group decreased from pretest values. The ambulation intervention required little extra staff time to implement.

Implications

The intervention in this study can be easily implemented in any busy acute care setting with minimal time, effort, and cost. The use of a pedometer is an easy objective method to determine if ambulation goals for clients are being achieved and a way for clients to self-assess their progress. The researchers suggest that future research should evaluate different approaches to encouraging ambulation in hospitalized clients and consider longer evaluation periods (e.g., 3–5 days).

of assistance will depend on the client's condition, including age, health status, and length of inactivity. Assistance may mean walking alongside the client while providing standby support for safety (Skill 44.7); reinforcing instruction provided by the physical therapist to the client about the use of assistive devices such as a cane, walker, or crutches; or using a sit-to-stand lift with ambulation capability or a lift with an ambulation sling (Figure 44.57 ■).

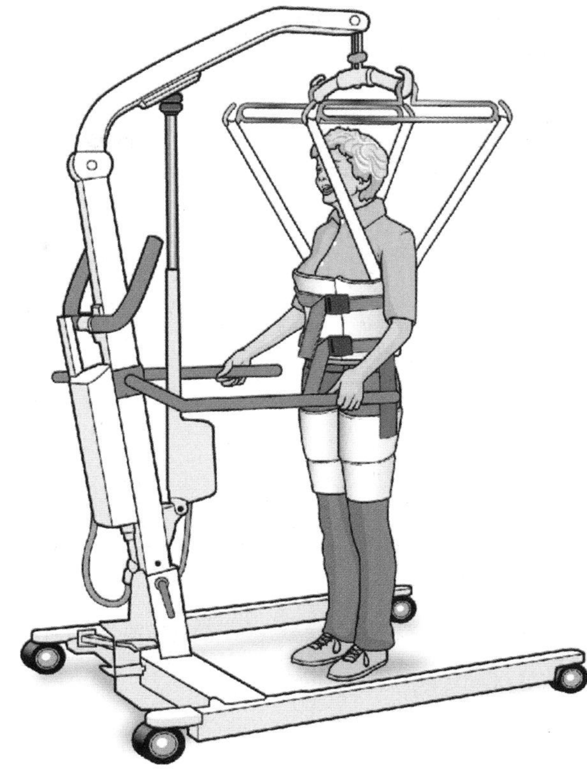

Figure 44.57 ■ Promoting ambulation by using a lift with an ambulation sling.

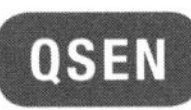

Safety: Assisting the Client to Ambulate When the nurse is assisting a client to ambulate in the home setting, the following should be considered:

- When making a home visit, assess carefully for safety issues concerning ambulation. Counsel the client and family about inadequate lighting, unfastened rugs, slippery floors, and loose objects on the floors.
- Check the surroundings for adequate supports such as railings and grab bars.
- Recommend that nonskid strips be placed on outside steps and inside stairs that are not carpeted.
- Ask to see the shoes the client intends to wear while ambulating. They should be in good repair and should support the foot.

CLIENT TEACHING **Controlling Orthostatic Hypotension**

- Rest with the head of the bed elevated 8 to 12 inches. This position makes the position change on rising less severe.
- Avoid sudden changes in position. Arise from bed in three stages:
  a. Sit up in bed for 1 minute.
  b. Sit on the side of the bed with legs dangling for 1 minute.
  c. Stand with care, holding onto the edge of the bed or another nonmovable object for 1 minute.
- Never bend down all the way to the floor or stand up too quickly after stooping.
- Postpone activities such as shaving and hair grooming for at least 1 hour after rising.
- Wear elastic stockings at night to inhibit venous pooling in the legs.
- Be aware that the symptoms of hypotension are most severe at the following times:
  a. 30 to 60 minutes after a heavy meal
  b. 1 to 2 hours after taking an antihypertension medication.
- Get out of a hot bath very slowly, because high temperatures can lead to venous pooling.
- Use a rocking chair to improve circulation in the lower extremities. Even mild leg conditioning can strengthen muscle tone and enhance circulation.
- Refrain from any strenuous activity that results in holding the breath and bearing down. This Valsalva maneuver slows the heart rate, leading to subsequent lowering of blood pressure.

Assisting a Client to Ambulate

SKILL 44.7

PURPOSE

- To provide a safe condition for the client to walk with whatever support is needed

ASSESSMENT

Assess

- Length of time in bed and the amount and type of activity the client was last able to tolerate
- Baseline vital signs
- Range of motion of joints needed for ambulating (e.g., hips, knees, ankles)
- Muscle strength of lower extremities
- Need for ambulation aids (e.g., cane, walker, crutches, lift with ambulation sling)
- Client's intake of medications (e.g., opioids, sedatives, tranquilizers, and antihistamines) that may cause drowsiness, dizziness, weakness, and orthostatic hypotension, seriously hindering the client's ability to walk safely
- Presence of joint inflammation, fractures, muscle weakness, or other conditions that impair physical mobility
- Ability to understand directions
- Level of comfort
- Weight-bearing status

Continued on page 1152

SKILL 44.7

Assisting a Client to Ambulat—*continued*

PLANNING

Implement pain relief measures so that they are effective. The amount of assistance needed while ambulating will depend on the client's condition (e.g., age, health status, length of inactivity, and emotional readiness). Review any previous experiences with ambulation and the success of such efforts. Plan the length of the walk with the client, considering the nursing or primary care practitioner's orders and the medical condition of the client. Be prepared to shorten the walk according to the client's activity tolerance.

ASSIGNMENT

Ambulation of clients is frequently assigned to AP. However, the nurse should conduct an initial assessment of the client's abilities in order to direct other personnel in providing appropriate assistance. Any unusual events that result from assisting the client in ambulation must be validated and interpreted by the nurse.

Equipment

- Assistive devices required for safe ambulation of client (e.g., gait or transfer belt, walker, cane, sit-to-stand assist device, lift with ambulation sling)
- Wheelchair for following client, or chairs along the route if the client needs to rest
- Portable oxygen tank if the client needs it

IMPLEMENTATION

Preparation

Be certain that others are available to assist you if needed. Also, plan the route of ambulation that has the fewest hazards and a clear path for ambulation.

Performance

1. Prior to performing the procedure, introduce self and verify the client's identity using agency protocol. Explain to the client how you are going to assist, why ambulation is necessary, and how to participate. Discuss how this activity relates to the overall plan of care. Stress that the client must keep the nurse informed as to how the activity is being tolerated as it progresses.
2. Perform hand hygiene and observe appropriate infection prevention procedures.
3. Ensure that the client is appropriately dressed to walk and has shoes or slippers with nonskid soles.
4. Prepare the client for ambulation.
   - Have the client sit up in bed for at least 1 minute prior to preparing to dangle legs.
   - Assist the client to sit on the edge of the bed and allow dangling for at least 1 minute.
   - Assess the client carefully for signs and symptoms of orthostatic hypotension (dizziness, light-headedness, or a sudden increase in heart rate) prior to leaving the bedside. **Rationale:** *Allowing for gradual adjustment can minimize drops in blood pressure (and fainting) that occur with shifts in position from lying to sitting, and sitting to standing.*
   - Assist the client to stand by the side of the bed for at least 1 minute until he or she feels secure.
   - Carefully attend to any IV tubing, catheters, or drainage bags. Keep urinary drainage bags below level of the client's bladder. **Rationale:** *To prevent backflow of urine into bladder and risk of infection.*
   - If the client is a high safety risk (e.g., cannot follow commands, medical instability, lack of experience with assistive device, neurologic deficits), use a lift with ambulation sling and 1 to 2 caregivers.
   - If the client is a high safety risk and has upper extremity strength and is able to grasp with at least one hand, use a lift with ambulation sling or a sit-to-stand lift with ambulation capability and 1 to 2 caregivers.
   - If the client is a low safety risk (e.g., able to follow commands, medically stable, and experienced with assistive device), use a gait or transfer belt for standby assist as needed and assistive devices as needed (e.g., crutches, walker, cane) and 1 to 2 caregivers. Make sure the belt is pulled snugly around the client's waist and fastened securely. Grasp the belt at the client's back, and walk behind and slightly to one side of the client. ❶

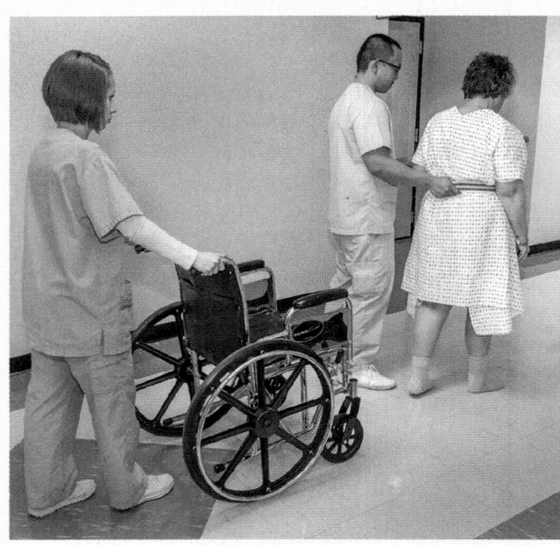

❶ Using a gait or transfer belt to support the client during ambulation.

5. Ensure client safety while assisting the client to ambulate.
   - Encourage the client to ambulate independently if he or she is able, but walk beside the client's weak side, if appropriate. If the client has a lightweight IV pole because of infusing fluids, he or she may find that holding onto the pole while ambulating helps with balance. If the pole or other equipment is cumbersome in any way, the nurse must push it to match the client's pace, securing any assistance necessary in order to move smoothly with the client.
   - Remain physically close to the client in case assistance is needed at any point.
   - If it is the client's first time out of bed following surgery, injury, or an extended period of immobility, or if the client is weak or unstable, have an assistant follow you and the client with a wheelchair in the event that it is needed quickly.
   - Encourage the client to assume a normal walking stance and gait as much as possible. Ask the client to straighten the back and raise the head so that the eyes are looking forward in a normal horizontal plane. **Rationale:** *Clients who are unsure of their ability to ambulate tend to look down at their feet, which makes them more likely to fall.*
6. Protect the client who begins to fall while ambulating.
   - If a client begins to experience the signs and symptoms of orthostatic hypotension or extreme weakness, quickly assist the client into a nearby wheelchair or other chair, and help the client to lower the head between the knees.
   - Stay with the client. **Rationale:** *A client who faints while in this position could fall head first out of the chair.*

Assisting a Client to Ambulat—*continued*

- When the weakness subsides, assist the client back to bed.
- Never catch a falling client. A caregiver probably cannot stop a client from falling. Quickly remove obstacles out of the way that may injure the client (Martin, Rogers, & Matz, n.d.; VHA Center for Engineering & Occupational Safety and Health, 2016). Do not manually lift a client from the floor; use SPHM technology.

Variation: Two Nurses

- Place a gait or transfer belt around the client's waist. Each nurse grasps the side handle with the near hand and the lower aspect of the client's upper arm with the other hand.
- Walk in unison with the client, using a smooth, even gait, at the same speed and with steps the same size as the client's. **Rationale:** *This gives the client a greater feeling of security.*

7. Document distance and duration of ambulation and assistive devices, if used, in the client record using forms or checklists supplemented by narrative notes when appropriate. Include description of the client's gait (including body alignment) when walking; pace; activity tolerance when walking (e.g., pulse rate, facial color, any shortness of breath, feelings of dizziness, or weakness); degree of support required; and respiratory rate and blood pressure after initial ambulation to compare with baseline data.

SKILL 44.7

EVALUATION

- Establish a plan for continued ambulation based on expected or normal ability for the client.

LIFESPAN CONSIDERATIONS Assisting a Client to Ambulate

CHILDREN

- Children and adolescents who have suffered a sports injury (e.g., sprained ankle) may want to be more active than they should be. A cast, splint, or boot may be put in place to limit activity and assist in healing. Teach the child the importance of appropriate activity, and the use of assistive devices (e.g., crutches) if necessary. Help children focus on what they *can* do rather than what they cannot do (e.g., "You can stand at the free-throw line and shoot baskets").

OLDER ADULTS

- Inquire how the client has ambulated previously and check any available chart notes regarding the client's abilities and modify assistance accordingly.
- Take into account a decrease in speed, strength, resistance to fatigue, reaction time, and coordination due to a decrease in nerve conduction.
- Be cautious when using a gait belt with a client with osteoporosis. Too much pressure from the belt can increase the risk of vertebral compression fractures. If a client has had abdominal surgery, it may be necessary to use a gait vest instead of a gait belt.
- If assistive devices such as a walker or cane are used, make sure clients are supervised in the beginning to learn the proper method of using them. Crutches may be much more difficult for older adults to use due to decreased upper body strength.
- Be alert to signs of activity intolerance, especially in older adults with cardiac and lung problems.
- Set small goals and increase slowly to build endurance, strength, and flexibility.
- Be aware of any fall risks the older adult may have, such as the following:
  - Effects of medications
  - Neurologic disorders
  - Orthopedic problems
  - Presence of equipment that must accompany the client when ambulating
  - Environmental hazards
  - Orthostatic hypotension
- In older adults, the body's responses return to normal more slowly. For instance, an increase in heart rate from exercise may stay elevated for hours before returning to normal.

Some clients experience orthostatic (postural) hypotension on assuming a vertical position from a lying position and may need information about ways to control this problem (see Client Teaching). The client may exhibit some or all of the following symptoms: pallor, diaphoresis, nausea, tachycardia, and dizziness. If any of these are present, the client should be assisted to a supine position in bed and closely assessed.

Using Mechanical Aids for Walking

Mechanical aids for ambulation include canes, walkers, and crutches.

Canes

Three types of canes are commonly used: the standard straight-legged cane; the tripod cane, which has three feet; and the quad cane, which has four feet and provides the most support (Figure 44.58 ■). Cane tips should have

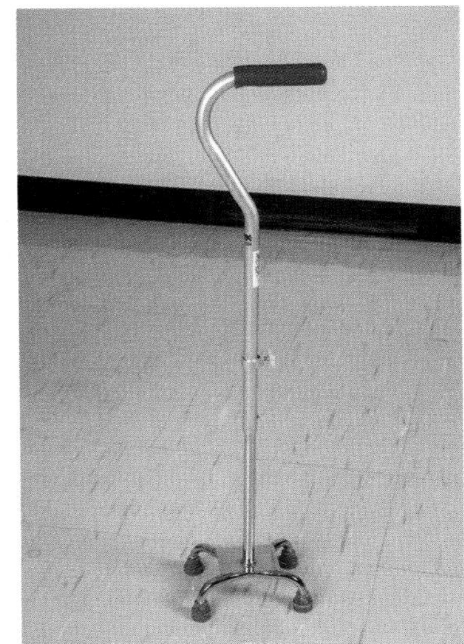

Figure 44.58 ■ A quad cane.

CLIENT TEACHING Using Canes

- Hold the cane with the hand on the stronger side of the body to provide maximum support and appropriate body alignment when walking.
- Position the tip of a standard cane (and the nearest tip of other canes) about 15 cm (6 in.) to the side and 15 cm (6 in.) in front of the near foot, so that the elbow is slightly flexed.

WHEN MAXIMUM SUPPORT IS REQUIRED

- Move the cane forward about 30 cm (1 ft), or a distance that is comfortable while the body weight is borne by both legs (Figure 44.59*A* ■).
- Then move the affected (weak) leg forward to the cane while the weight is borne by the cane and stronger leg (Figure 44.59*B*).
- Next, move the unaffected (stronger) leg forward ahead of the cane and weak leg while the weight is borne by the cane and weak leg (Figure 44.59*C*).
- Repeat the steps. This pattern of moving provides at least two points of support on the floor at all times.

AS YOU BECOME STRONGER AND REQUIRE LESS SUPPORT

- Move the cane and weak leg forward at the same time, while the weight is borne by the stronger leg (Figure 44.60*A* ■).
- Move the stronger leg forward, while the weight is borne by the cane and the weak leg (Figure 44.60*B*).

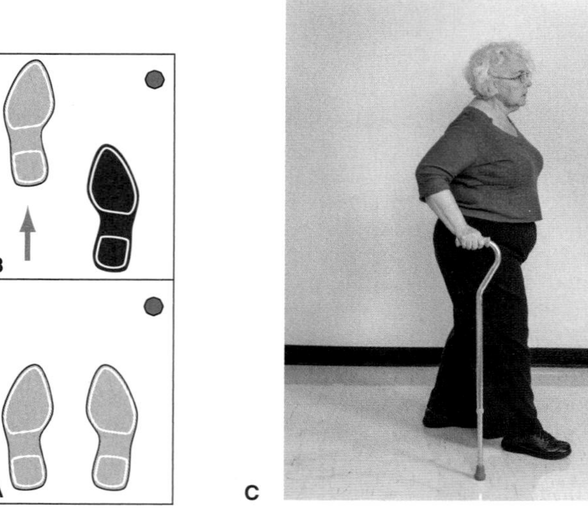

Figure 44.59 ■ Steps involved in using a cane to provide maximum support.

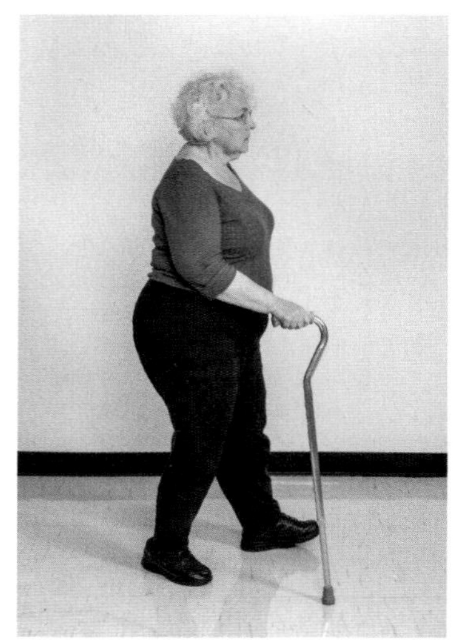

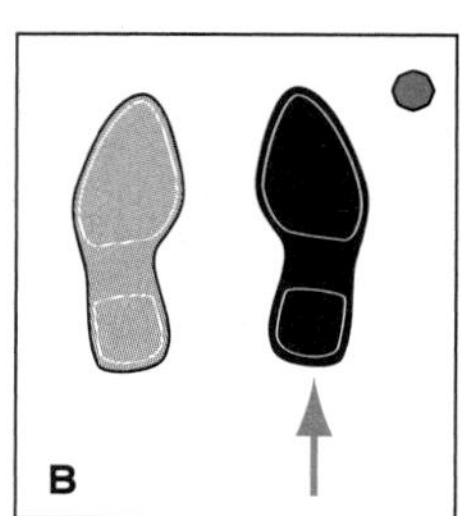

Figure 44.60 ■ Steps involved in using a cane when less than maximum support is required.

rubber caps to improve traction and prevent slipping. The standard cane is 91 cm (36 in.) long; some aluminum canes can be adjusted from 56 to 97 cm (22 to 38 in.). The length should permit the elbow to be slightly flexed. Clients may use either one or two canes, depending on how much support they require.

Walkers

Walkers are mechanical devices for ambulatory clients who need more support than a cane provides and lack the strength and balance required for crutches. Walkers come in many different shapes and sizes, with devices suited to individual needs. The standard type is made of polished aluminum. It has four legs with rubber tips and plastic handgrips (Figure 44.61*A* ■). Many walkers have adjustable legs.

The standard walker needs to be picked up to be used. The client therefore requires partial strength in both hands and wrists, strong elbow extensors, and strong shoulder depressors. The client also needs the ability to bear at least partial weight on both legs.

While four-wheeled and two-wheeled models of walkers (roller walkers) do not need to be picked up to be moved, they are less stable than the standard walker. Clients who are too weak or unstable to pick up and move the walker with each step use the roller walkers. Some roller walkers have a seat at the back so the client can sit down to rest when desired. An adaptation of the standard and four-wheeled walker is one that has two tips and two wheels (Figure 44.61*B*). This type provides more stability than the four-wheeled model yet still permits the client to keep the walker in contact with the ground all the time. The legs with wheels allow the client to easily push the walker forward, and the legs without wheels prevent the walker from rolling away as the client steps forward.

The nurse may need to adjust the height of a client's walker so that the hand bar is just below the client's waist

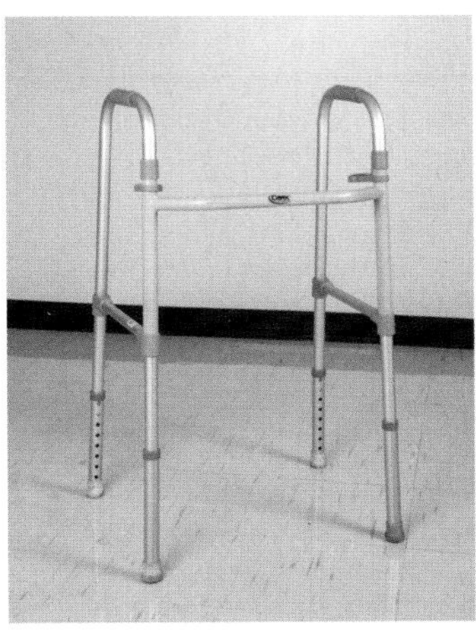

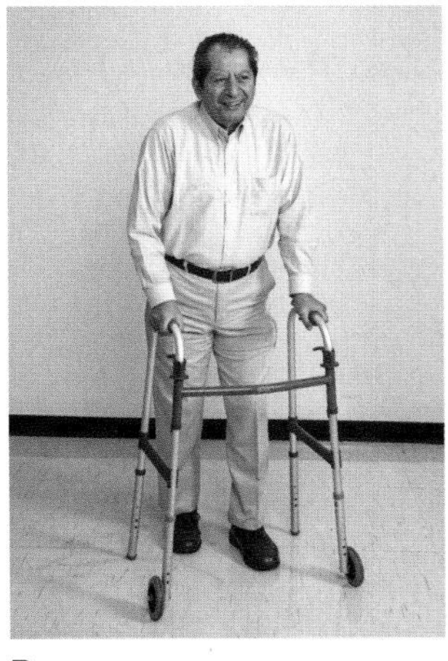

A B

Figure 44.61 ■ *A*, Standard walker; *B*, two-wheeled walker.

CLIENT TEACHING Using Walkers

WHEN MAXIMUM SUPPORT IS REQUIRED

- Move the walker ahead about 15 cm (6 in.) while your body weight is borne by both legs.
- Then move the right foot up to the walker while your body weight is borne by the left leg and both arms.
- Next, move the left foot up to the right foot while your body weight is borne by the right leg and both arms.

IF ONE LEG IS WEAKER THAN THE OTHER

- Move the walker and the weak leg ahead together about 15 cm (6 in.) while your weight is borne by the stronger leg.
- Then move the stronger leg ahead while your weight is borne by the affected leg and both arms.

and the client's elbows are slightly flexed. This position helps the client assume a more normal stance. A walker that is too low causes the client to stoop; one that is too high makes the client stretch and reach.

Crutches

Crutches may be a temporary need for some clients and a permanent one for others. Crutches should enable a client to ambulate independently; therefore, it is important to learn to use them properly. The most frequently used kinds of crutches are the underarm crutch, or axillary crutch with hand bars, and the Lofstrand crutch, which extends only to the forearm. On the Lofstrand crutch, the metal cuff around the forearm and the metal bar stabilize the wrists and thus make walking easier, especially on stairs. The platform or elbow extensor crutch also has a cuff for the upper arm to permit forearm weight bearing. All crutches require suction tips, usually made of rubber, which help to prevent slipping on a floor surface.

In crutch walking, the client's weight is borne by the muscles of the shoulder girdle and the upper extremities. Before beginning crutch walking, exercises that strengthen the upper arms and hands are recommended.

Measuring Clients for Crutches

When nurses measure clients for axillary crutches, it is most important to obtain the correct length for the crutches and the correct placement of the handpiece. There are two methods of measuring crutch length:

1. The client lies in a supine position and the nurse measures from the anterior fold of the axilla to the heel of the foot and adds 2.5 cm (1 in.).
2. The client stands erect and positions the crutch as shown in Figure 44.62 ■. The nurse makes sure the shoulder rest of the crutch is at least 3 fingerwidths, that is, 2.5 to 5 cm (1 to 2 in.), below the axilla.

To determine the correct placement of the hand bar:

1. The client stands upright and supports the body weight by the handgrips of the crutches.
2. The nurse measures the angle of elbow flexion. It should be about 30 degrees.

Crutch Gaits

The crutch gait is the gait a client assumes on crutches by alternating body weight on one or both legs and the crutches. Five standard crutch gaits are the four-point gait, three-point gait, two-point gait, swing-to gait, and swing-through gait. The gait used depends on the following individual factors: (a) the ability to take steps, (b) the ability to bear weight and keep balance in a standing position on both legs or only one, and (c) the ability to hold the body erect.

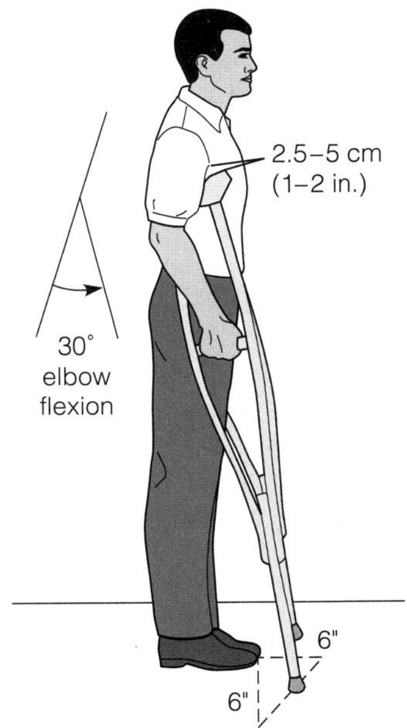

Figure 44.62 ■ The standing position for measuring the correct length for crutches.

Clients also need instruction about how to get into and out of chairs and go up and down stairs safely. All of these crutch skills are best taught before the client is discharged and preferably before the client has surgery.

Crutch Stance (Tripod Position)

Before crutch walking is attempted, the client needs to learn facts about posture and balance. The proper standing position with crutches is called the **tripod (triangle) position** (Figure 44.63 ■). The crutches are placed about 15 cm (6 in.) in front of the feet and out laterally about 15 cm (6 in.), creating a wide base of support. The feet are slightly apart. A tall client requires a wider base than does a short client. Hips and knees are extended, the back is straight, and the head is held straight and high. There should be no hunch to the shoulders and thus no weight borne by the axillae. The elbows are extended sufficiently to allow weight bearing on the hands. If the client is unsteady, the nurse places a gait or transfer belt around the client's waist and grasps the belt from above, not from below. A fall can be prevented more effectively if the belt is held from above.

Four-Point Alternate Gait

This is the most elementary and safest gait, providing at least three points of support at all times, but it requires coordination. Clients can use it when walking in crowds because it does not require much space. To use this gait, the client needs to be able to bear weight on both legs (Figure 44.64 ■, reading from bottom to top). The nurse asks the client to:

1. Move the right crutch ahead a suitable distance, such as 10 to 15 cm (4 to 6 in.).
2. Move the left front foot forward, preferably to the level of the left crutch.
3. Move the left crutch forward.
4. Move the right foot forward.

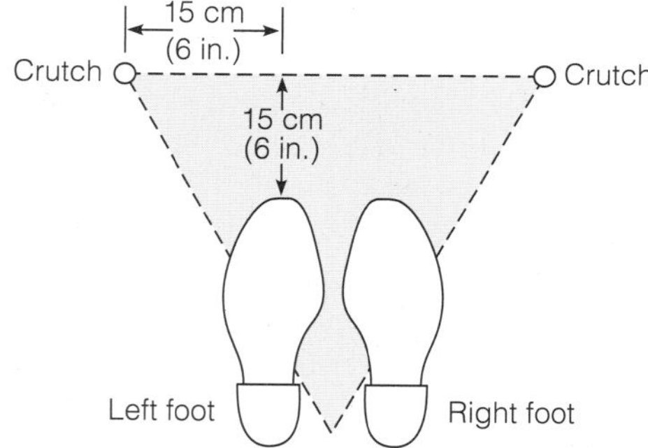

Figure 44.63 ■ The tripod position.

> **CLIENT TEACHING** Using Crutches
>
> - Follow the plan of exercises developed for you to strengthen your arm muscles before beginning crutch walking.
> - Have a healthcare professional establish the correct length for your crutches and the correct placement of the handpieces. Crutches that are too long force your shoulders upward and make it difficult for you to push your body off the ground. Crutches that are too short will make you hunch over and develop an improper body stance.
> - The weight of your body should be borne by the arms rather than the axillae (armpits). Continual pressure on the axillae can injure the radial nerve and eventually cause crutch palsy, a weakness of the muscles of the forearm, wrist, and hand.
> - Maintain an erect posture as much as possible to prevent strain on muscles and joints and to maintain balance.
> - Each step taken with crutches should be a comfortable distance for you. It is wise to start with a small rather than large step.
> - Inspect the crutch tips regularly, and replace them if worn.
> - Keep the crutch tips dry and clean to maintain their surface friction. If the tips become wet, dry them well before use.
> - Wear a shoe with a low heel that grips the floor. Rubber soles decrease the chances of slipping. Adjust shoelaces so they cannot come untied or reach the floor where they might catch on the crutches. Consider shoes with alternative forms of closure (e.g., Velcro), especially if you cannot easily bend to tie laces. Slip-on shoes are acceptable only if they are snug and the heel does not come loose when the foot is bent.

Three-Point Gait

To use this gait, the client must be able to bear the entire body weight on the unaffected leg. The two crutches and the unaffected leg bear weight alternately (Figure 44.65 ■, reading from bottom to top). The nurse asks the client to:

1. Move both crutches and the weaker leg forward.
2. Move the stronger leg forward.

Two-Point Alternate Gait

This gait is faster than the four-point gait. It requires more balance because only two points support the body at one time; it also requires at least partial weight bearing on each foot. In this gait, arm movements with the crutches are similar to the arm movements during normal walking (Figure 44.66 ■, reading from bottom to top). The nurse asks the client to:

1. Move the left crutch and the right foot forward together.
2. Move the right crutch and the left foot ahead together.

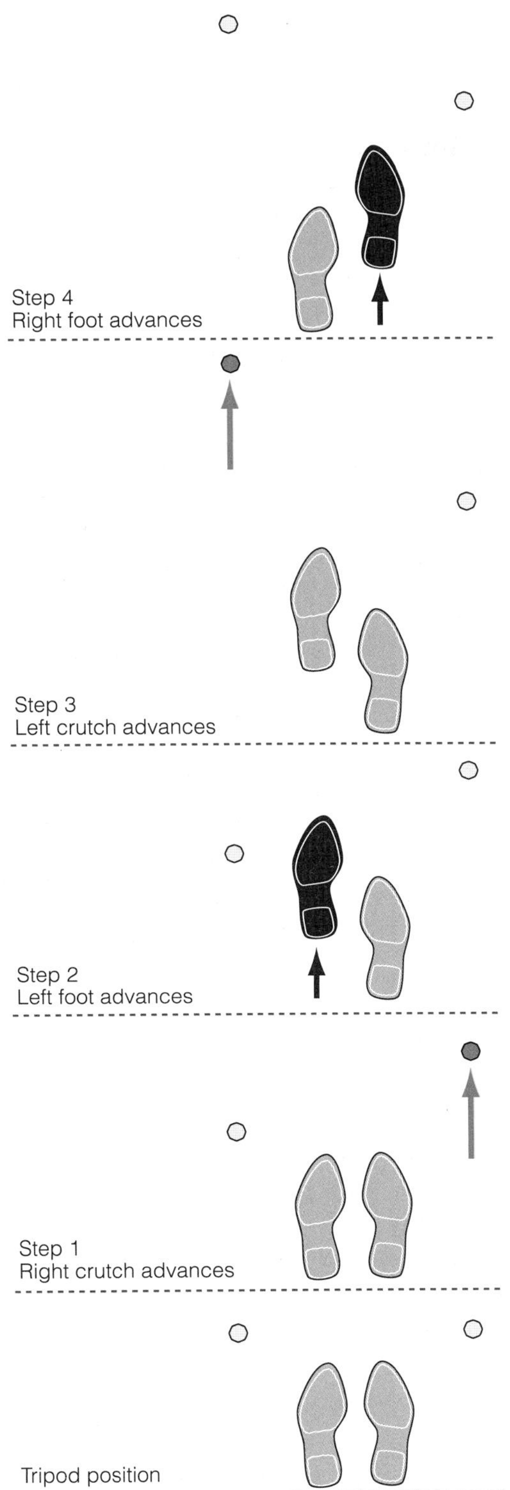

Figure 44.64 ■ The four-point alternate crutch gait.

Swing-to Gait

The swing gaits are used by clients with paralysis of the legs and hips. Prolonged use of these gaits results in atrophy of the unused muscles. The swing-to gait is the easier of these two gaits. The nurse asks the client to:

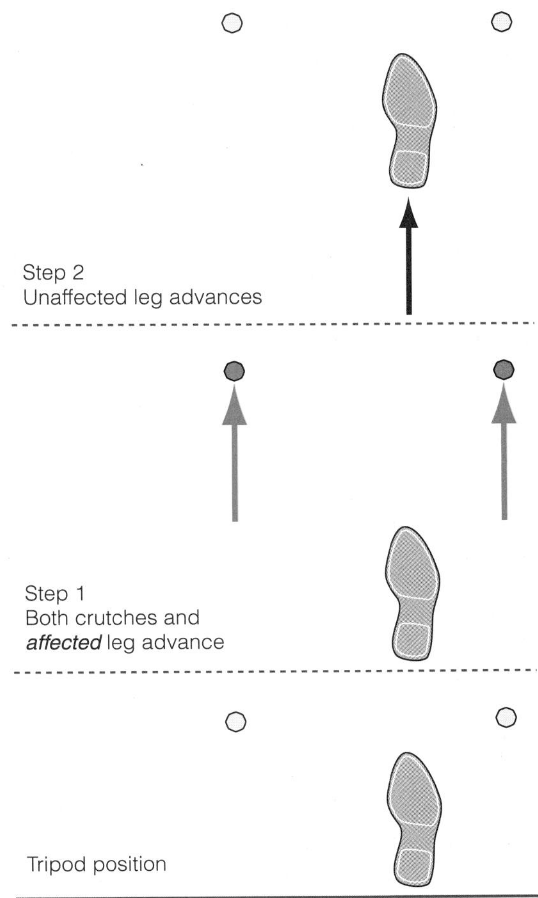

Figure 44.65 ■ The three-point crutch gait.

1. Move both crutches ahead together.
2. Lift body weight by the arms and swing to the crutches.

Swing-Through Gait

This gait requires considerable skill, strength, and coordination. The nurse asks the client to:

1. Move both crutches forward together.
2. Lift body weight by the arms and swing through and beyond the crutch.

Getting into a Chair

Chairs that have armrests and are secure or braced against a wall are essential for clients using crutches. For this procedure, the nurse instructs the client to:

1. Stand with the back of the unaffected leg centered against the chair. The chair helps support the client during the next steps.
2. Transfer the crutches to the hand on the affected side and hold the crutches by the hand bars. The client grasps the arm of the chair with the hand on the unaffected side (Figure 44.67 ■). This allows the client to support the body weight on the arms and the unaffected leg.
3. Lean forward, flex the knees and hips, and lower into the chair.

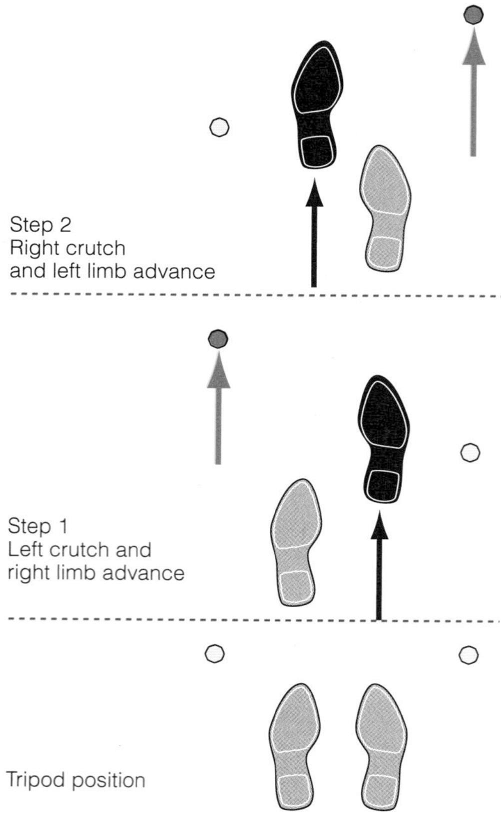

Figure 44.66 ■ The two-point alternate crutch gait.

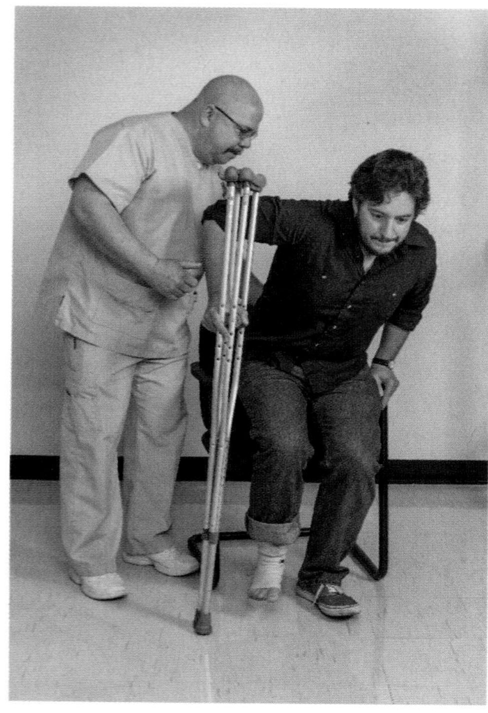

Figure 44.67 ■ A client using crutches getting into a chair.

Getting Out of a Chair

For this procedure, the nurse instructs the client to:

1. Move forward to the edge of the chair and place the unaffected leg slightly under or at the edge of the chair. This position helps the client stand up from the chair and achieve balance, because the unaffected leg is supported against the edge of the chair.
2. Grasp the crutches by the hand bars in the hand on the affected side, and grasp the arm of the chair by the hand on the unaffected side. The body weight is placed on the crutches and the hand on the armrest to support the unaffected leg when the client rises to stand.
3. Push down on the crutches and the chair armrest while elevating the body out of the chair.
4. Assume the tripod position before moving.

Going Up Stairs

For this procedure, the nurse stands behind the client and slightly to the affected side if needed. The nurse instructs the client to:

1. Assume the tripod position at the bottom of the stairs.
2. Transfer the body weight to the crutches and move the unaffected leg onto the step (Figure 44.68 ■).
3. Transfer the body weight to the unaffected leg on the step and move the crutches and affected leg up to the step. The affected leg is always supported by the crutches.
4. Repeat steps 2 and 3 until the client reaches the top of the stairs.

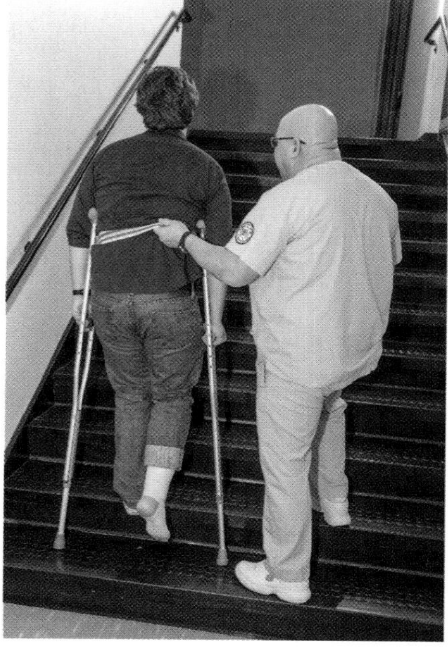

Figure 44.68 ■ Climbing stairs: placing weight on the crutches while first moving the unaffected leg onto a step.

Going Down Stairs

For this procedure, the nurse stands one step below the client on the affected side if needed. The nurse instructs the client to:

1. Assume the tripod position at the top of the stairs.
2. Shift the body weight to the unaffected leg, and move the crutches and affected leg down onto the next step (Figure 44.69 ■).

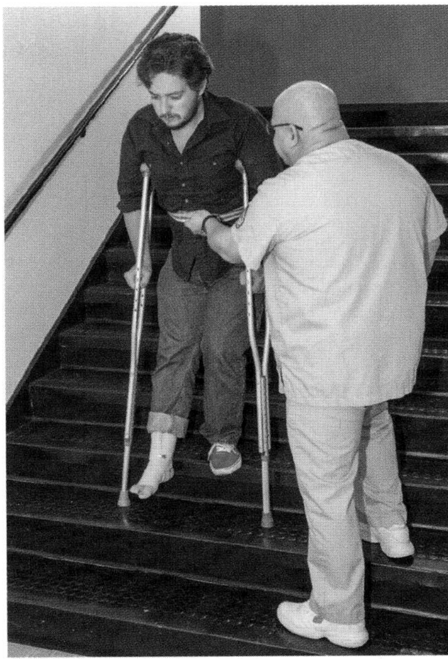

Figure 44.69 ■ Descending stairs: moving the crutches and affected leg to the next step.

3. Transfer the body weight to the crutches, and move the unaffected leg to that step. The affected leg is always supported by the crutches.
4. Repeat steps 2 and 3 until the client reaches the bottom of the stairs.

Evaluating

The goals established during the planning phase are evaluated according to specific desired outcomes, also established in that phase. Examples of these are shown in the accompanying Nursing Care Plan.

If outcomes are not achieved, the nurse, client, and support person if appropriate need to explore the reasons before modifying the care plan. For example, the following questions may be considered if an immobilized client fails to maintain muscle mass and tone and joint mobility:

- Has the client's physical or mental condition changed motivation to perform required exercise?
- Were appropriate range-of-motion exercises implemented?
- Was the client encouraged to participate in self-care activities as much as possible?
- Was the client encouraged to make as many decisions as possible when developing a daily activity plan and to express concerns?
- Did the nurse provide appropriate supervision and monitoring?
- Was the client's diet adequate to provide appropriate nourishment for energy requirements?

NURSING CARE PLAN Potential for Decline in Health

ASSESSMENT DATA	NURSING DIAGNOSIS	DESIRED OUTCOMES*
NURSING ASSESSMENT Peter Chan, a 69-year-old, unmarried accountant being treated for heart failure, states he has dyspnea with mild activity. ("I cannot climb a flight of stairs without stopping and resting and become breathless even when walking on level ground.") Prefers the orthopneic position. He works at home and sits at a table for most of the day.	Potential for decline in health related to decreased activity resulting from inadequate balance between oxygen supply and demand associated with decreased cardiac output and obesity	**Immobility Consequences:** Physiological [0204], as evidenced by • No pressure injuries • Muscle strength not compromised **Immobility Consequences:** Psycho-cognitive [0205], as evidenced by no • Apathy • Sleep disturbances • Negative body image **Mobility [0208]**, as evidenced by mildly compromised • Walking • Balance

NURSING CARE PLAN Potential for Decline in Health—*continued*

Physical Examination

Height: 178 cm (5′10″)

Weight: 102 kg (225 lb)

Temperature: 37.8°C (100.4°F)

Pulse rate: 94 beats/min

Respirations: 20/min

Blood pressure: 174/92 mmHg

Rales present in both lungs.

Respirations slightly labored. Color pale.

3+ (5 mm) edema both feet and ankles.

Diagnostic Data

CBC, and urinalysis within normal limits
CXR reveals an enlarged heart

NURSING INTERVENTIONS*/SELECTED ACTIVITIES	RATIONALE
POSITIONING [0840]	
Position to alleviate dyspnea, e.g., high Fowler's.	*Clients with increased pulmonary secretions are able to breathe better when upright because abdominal organs are lower and there is greater room for lung and diaphragmatic excursion.*
Provide support to edematous areas, e.g., elevate feet on footstool when sitting.	*Elevating the dependent area assists with decreasing tissue pressure and promoting fluid return to the venous system and the heart.*
Encourage active range-of-motion exercises.	*Active ROM helps maintain muscle strength and promote circulation. Mild activity also helps burn unneeded calories.*
EXERCISE THERAPY: MUSCLE CONTROL [0226]	
Collaborate with physical, occupational, and recreational therapists in developing and executing an individually tailored exercise program.	*This client will need a multidisciplinary approach to his care. Each member contributes from his or her area of expertise. Research supports efficacy of individually tailored exercise plans. Factors such as having an exercise partner, using music, and type of activity can motivate client and enhance adherence to the plan over time.*
Offer options, explain rationale for type of exercise and protocol to client, and allow him to make choices that appeal to him and that address his needs.	*If the client understands what the reasons are for activity, he can make good choices.*
Provide step-by-step cuing for each motor activity during exercise or ADLs.	*As-needed reminders help the client recall what to do next.*
Use visual aids to facilitate learning how to perform exercises.	*Some people have better visual memory than auditory memory.*

EVALUATION

Outcomes met. Mr. Chan did not develop any skin breakdown or other evidence of the complications of immobility to date. However, since the risk factors remain, the care plan will be ongoing.

*The NOC # for desired outcomes and the NIC # for nursing interventions are listed in brackets following the appropriate outcome or intervention. Outcomes, indicators, interventions, and activities selected are only a sample of those suggested by NOC and NIC and should be further individualized for each client.

APPLYING CRITICAL THINKING

1. What assessment findings alert you that Mr. Chan is developing problems associated with his current state of decreased mobility?
2. Mr. Chan may benefit from using a walker to assist with ambulation at home. What teaching should be done in regard to use of a walker?
3. The care plan does not address one of Mr. Chan's risk factors—obesity. Would you add this to the plan?
4. What assumptions has the nurse made in assigning the desired outcome of "Immobility Consequences: Psycho-cognitive"?
5. How are the choices of outcomes influenced by the cause of his nursing diagnosis (a chronic illness)?

Answers to Applying Critical Thinking questions are available on the faculty resources website. Please consult with your instructor.

CONCEPT MAP

Client with Potential for a Decline in Health

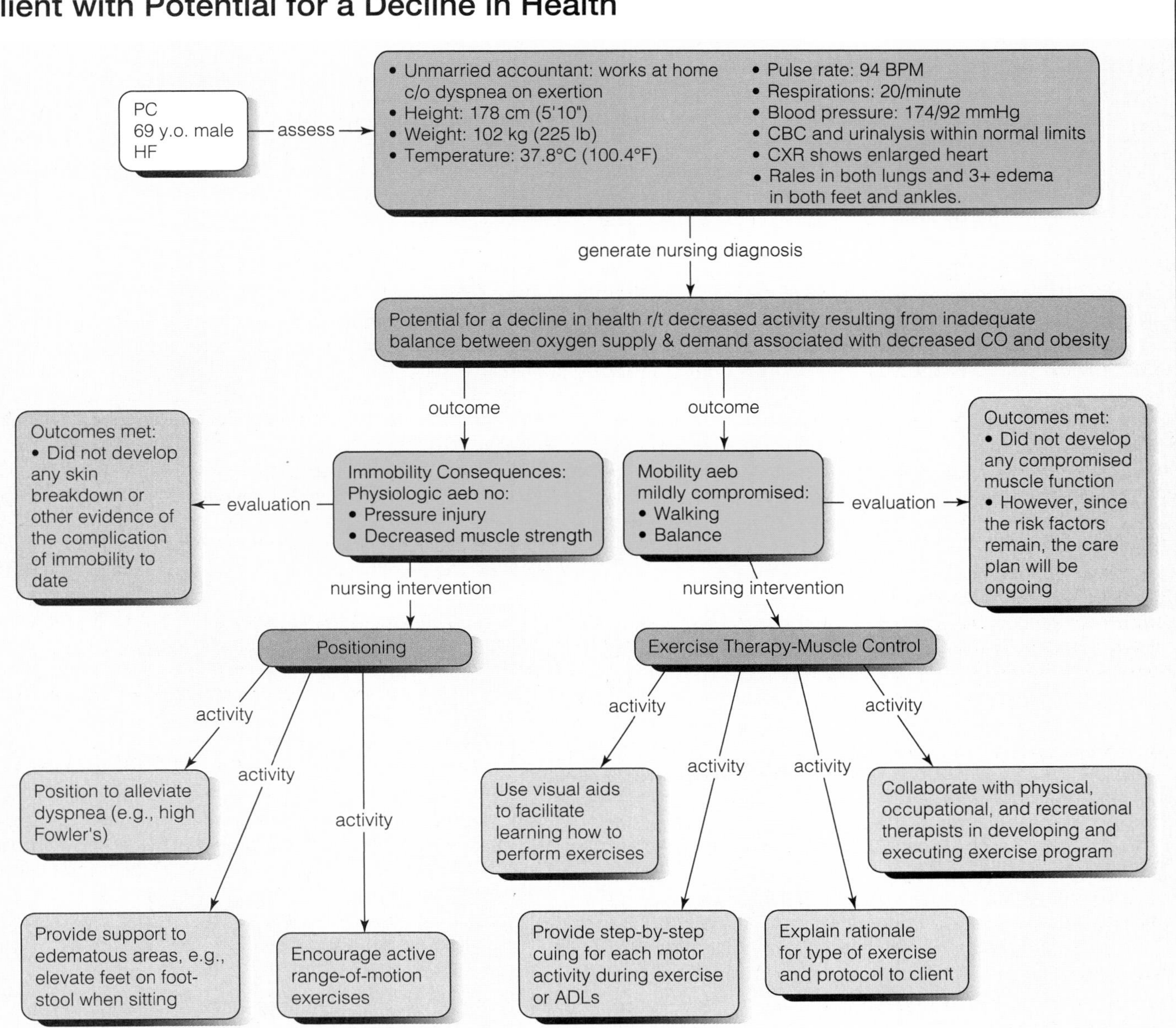
PC
69 y.o. male
HF
assess
• Unmarried accountant: works at home c/o dyspnea on exertion
• Height: 178 cm (5'10")
• Weight: 102 kg (225 lb)
• Temperature: 37.8°C (100.4°F)
• Pulse rate: 94 BPM
• Respirations: 20/minute
• Blood pressure: 174/92 mmHg
• CBC and urinalysis within normal limits
• CXR shows enlarged heart
• Rales in both lungs and 3+ edema in both feet and ankles.
generate nursing diagnosis
Potential for a decline in health r/t decreased activity resulting from inadequate balance between oxygen supply & demand associated with decreased CO and obesity
outcome
outcome
Outcomes met:
• Did not develop any skin breakdown or other evidence of the complication of immobility to date
evaluation
Immobility Consequences: Physiologic aeb no:
• Pressure injury
• Decreased muscle strength
Mobility aeb mildly compromised:
• Walking
• Balance
evaluation
Outcomes met:
• Did not develop any compromised muscle function
• However, since the risk factors remain, the care plan will be ongoing
nursing intervention
nursing intervention
Positioning
Exercise Therapy-Muscle Control
activity
activity
activity
activity
activity
activity
activity
Position to alleviate dyspnea (e.g., high Fowler's)
Provide support to edematous areas, e.g., elevate feet on foot-stool when sitting
Encourage active range-of-motion exercises
Use visual aids to facilitate learning how to perform exercises
Provide step-by-step cuing for each motor activity during exercise or ADLs
Explain rationale for type of exercise and protocol to client
Collaborate with physical, occupational, and recreational therapists in developing and executing exercise program

Chapter 44 Review

CHAPTER HIGHLIGHTS

- Exercise and activity are essential components for maintaining and regaining health and wellness.
- Research on exercise has demonstrated it to be an excellent strategy for preventing and treating some cardiovascular and pulmonary diseases, mood disorders, diseases of aging, diabetes, and immune diseases.
- The ability to move freely, easily, and purposefully in the environment is essential for individuals to meet their basic needs.
- Purposeful coordinated movement of the body relies on the integrated functioning of the musculoskeletal system, the nervous system, and the vestibular apparatus of the inner ear.
- Body movement involves four basic elements: body alignment, joint mobility, balance, and coordinated movement.
- Individuals maintain alignment and balance when the line of gravity passes through the center of gravity and the base of support.
- Exercise is physical activity performed to improve health and maintain fitness. Activity tolerance is the type and amount of exercise or daily living activities an individual is able to perform without experiencing adverse effects. Functional strength is the ability to do work.
- Exercise is classified as either isotonic, isometric, or isokinetic and as either aerobic or anaerobic.
- Many factors influence body alignment and activity. These include growth and development, nutrition, personal values and attitudes, certain external factors, and prescribed limitations to movement.
- Immobility affects almost every body organ and system adversely. Problems include disuse osteoporosis and atrophy; contractures; diminished cardiac reserve; orthostatic hypotension; venous stasis, edema, and thrombus formation; decreased respiratory movement and pooling of secretions; decreased metabolic rate and negative nitrogen balance; urinary stasis, retention, infection, and calculi; constipation; and varying emotional reactions.
- Assessment relative to a client's activity and exercise includes a nursing history and physical examination of body alignment, gait, joint appearance and movement, capabilities and limitations for movement, muscle mass and strength, activity tolerance, and problems related to immobility.
- An activity and exercise history includes daily activity level, activity tolerance, type and frequency of exercise, and factors affecting mobility.
- Nursing diagnoses that relate to activity and mobility problems can include actual and potential for inadequate physical energy for activities, and inactive lifestyle. Other relevant diagnoses are fear (of falling), impaired self-esteem, potential for falling, and, if the client is immobilized, many other potential problems such as altered repiratory status and potential for infection.
- Body mechanics is the efficient, coordinated, and safe use of the body to move objects and carry out the ADLs.
- Nurses must use good body mechanics in their daily work and especially when moving and turning clients in bed and assisting clients to make transfers. Proper body mechanics do *not* ensure protection from injury, however, and nurses and caregivers are encouraged to avoid solo manual lifting, repositioning, and transferring of clients.
- Positioning a client in good body alignment and changing the position regularly and systematically are essential aspects of nursing practice.
- Before positioning dependent clients, the nurse should plan a systematic 24-hour schedule for position changes, including positions that provide for full extension of the neck, hips, and knees. The nurse also uses appropriate supportive devices to maintain alignment and prevent strain on the client's muscles and joints.
- Before moving, turning, or transferring a client, the nurse must consider the client's health status and degree of exertion permitted, physical ability to assist, ability to comprehend instruction, degree of discomfort, and weight, and whether to use assistive devices or another caregiver to assist.
- The nurse can assist clients to prepare for ambulation by helping them become as independent as possible while in bed. Ambulating techniques that facilitate normal walking gait yet provide needed supports are most effective.
- Preambulatory exercises that strengthen the muscles for walking are essential for clients who have been immobilized for a prolonged period.
- Clients need specific instructions about appropriate use of canes, walkers, and crutches.

TEST YOUR KNOWLEDGE

1. A nurse is working on a hospital committee focused on preventing back injury in nurses. Which recommendation by this committee is most likely to result in a decrease in back injuries if followed?
   1. Nurses must wear back belts when lifting clients.
   2. All nursing personnel must attend annual body mechanics education.
   3. In order to prevent injury, nurses must strive to become physically fit.
   4. No solo lifting of clients is permitted in the facility.

2. A nurse is caring for a client diagnosed with early osteoporosis. Which intervention is most applicable for this client?
   1. Institute an exercise plan that includes weight-bearing activities.
   2. Increase the amount of calcium in the client's diet.
   3. Protect the client's bones with strict bed rest.
   4. Provide the client with assisted range-of-motion exercising twice daily.

3. Five minutes after the client's first postoperative exercise, the client's vital signs have not yet returned to baseline. Which is an appropriate nursing diagnosis?
1. Inadequate physical energy for activities
2. Potential for inadequate physical energy for activities
3. Impaired self-esteem
4. Potential for falling

4. Which statement from a client with one weak leg regarding use of crutches when using stairs indicates a need for increased teaching?
1. "Going up, the strong leg goes first, then the weaker leg with both crutches."
2. "Going down, the weaker leg goes first with both crutches, then the strong leg."
3. "The weaker leg always goes first with both crutches."
4. "A cane or single crutch may be used instead of both crutches if held on the weaker side."

5. A nurse is providing range-of-motion exercising to a client's elbow when the client complains of pain. What action should the nurse take?
1. Stop immediately and report the pain to the client's physician.
2. Discontinue the treatment and document the results in the medical record.
3. Reduce the movement of the joint just until the point of slight resistance.
4. Continue to exercise the joint as before to loosen the stiffness.

6. When assessing a client's gait, which does the nurse look for and encourage?
1. The spine rotates, initiating locomotion.
2. Gaze is slightly downward.
3. Toes strike the ground before the heel.
4. Arm on the same side as the swing-through foot moves forward at the same time.

7. Performance of activities of daily living (ADLs) and active range-of-motion (ROM) exercises can be accomplished simultaneously as illustrated by which of the following? Select all that apply.
1. Elbow flexion with eating and bathing
2. Elbow extension with shaving and eating
3. Wrist hyperextension with writing
4. Thumb ROM with eating and writing
5. Hip flexion with walking

8. A client weighs 250 pounds and needs to be transferred from the bed to a chair. Which instruction by the nurse to the assistive personnel (AP) is most appropriate?
1. "Using proper body mechanics will prevent you from injuring yourself."
2. "You are physically fit and at lesser risk for injury when transferring the client."
3. "Use the mechanical lift and another staff member to transfer the client from the bed to the chair."
4. "Use the back belt to avoid hurting your back."

9. The client is ambulating for the first time after surgery. The client tells the nurse, "I feel faint." Which is the best action by the nurse?
1. Find another nurse for help.
2. Return the client to her room as quickly as possible.
3. Tell the client to take rapid, shallow breaths.
4. Assist the client to a nearby chair.

10. The nurse is performing an assessment of an immobilized client. Which assessment causes the nurse to take action?
1. Heart rate 86 beats/min
2. Reddened area on sacrum
3. Nonproductive cough
4. Urine output of 50 mL/h

See Answers to Test Your Knowledge in Appendix A.

READINGS AND REFERENCES

Suggested Readings

Andrews, V. D., & Southard, E. P. (2017). Safe patient handling: Keeping health care workers safe. *Med-Surg Matters*, *26*(1), 4–7.
This article highlights the important role that safe patient handling and mobility programs perform in preventing employee injuries.

Crawford, A., & Harris, H. (2016). Caring for adults with impaired physical mobility. *Nursing*, *46*(12), 36–41. doi:10.1097/01.NURSE.0000504674.19099.1d
This article describes who is at risk for impaired mobility, the hazards of immobility, and nursing assessments and interventions, including client teaching, for mobility issues.

Eanes, L. (2018). Too much sitting: A newly recognized health risk. *American Journal of Nursing*, *118*(9), 26–34. doi:10.1097/01.NAJ.0000544948.27593.9b
Moderate to vigorous physical activity is an important focus of health promotion and disease prevention. The author discusses how more attention and public awareness need to be given to total daily sitting time and the need for research in the field of inactivity physiology.

Kowalski, S. L., & Anthony, M. (2017). Nursing's evolving role in patient safety. *American Journal of Nursing*, *117*(2), 34–48. doi:10.1097/01.NAJ.0000512274.79629.3c
A content analysis of AJN articles over 115 years provides a historical perspective of how client safety increased as client care became more complex.

Related Research

Choi, S. D., & Brings, K. (2016). Work-related musculoskeletal risks associated with nurses and nursing assistants handling overweight and obese patients: A literature review. *Work*, *53*, 439–448. doi:10.3233/WOR-152222

Nievera, R. A., Fick, A., & Harris, H. K. (2017). Effects of ambulation and nondependent transfers on vital signs in patients receiving norepinephrine. *American Journal of Critical Care*, *26*, 31–36. doi:10.4037/ajcc2017384

Teeple, E., Collins, J. E., Shrestha, S., Dennerlein, J. T., Losina, E., & Katz, J. N. (2017). Outcomes of safe patient handling and mobilization programs: A meta-analysis. *Work*, *58*(2), 173–184. doi:10.3233/WOR-172608

Wiggermann, N. (2016). Biomechanical evaluation of a bed feature to assist in turning and laterally repositioning patients. *Human Factors*, *58*, 748–757. doi:10.1177/0018720815612625

References

American College of Obstetricians and Gynecologists. (2017). *FAQ: Exercise during pregnancy*. Retrieved from http://www.acog.org/-/media/For%20Patients/faq119.pdf?dmc=1&ts=20130728T1630124999

American Heart Association. (2018). *American Heart Association recommendations for physical activity in adults and kids*. Retrieved from http://www.heart.org/HEARTORG/HealthyLiving/PhysicalActivity/FitnessBasics/American-Heart-Association-Recommendations-for-Physical-Activity-in-Adults_UCM_307976_Article.jsp#.WNLArxjMzwc

Borg, G. (1998). *Borg's perceived exertion and pain scales*. Champaign, IL: Human Kinetics.

Butcher, H. K., Bulechek, G. M., Dochterman, J. M., & Wagner, C. M. (Eds.). (2018). *Nursing interventions classification (NIC)* (7th ed.). St. Louis, MO: Elsevier.

Centers for Disease Control and Prevention. (2016). *Healthy People 2020 midcourse review: Physical activity*. Retrieved from https://www.cdc.gov/nchs/data/hpdata2020/HP2020MCR-C33-PA.pdf

Denehy, L., Lanphere, J., & Needham, D. M. (2017). Ten reasons why ICU patients should be mobilized early. *Intensive Care Medicine*, *43*(1), 86–90. doi:10.1007/s00134-016-4513-2

Eanes, L. (2018). Too much sitting: A newly recognized health risk. *American Journal of Nursing*, *118*(9), 26–34. doi:10.1097/01.NAJ.0000544948.27593.9b

Fragala, G., Boynton, T., Conti, M. T., Cyr, L., Enos, L., Kelly, D., . . . Vollman, K. (2016). Patient-handling injuries: Risk factors and risk-reduction strategies. *American Nurse Today*, *11*(5), 40–44.

Hashem, M. D., Nelliot, A., & Needham, D. M. (2016). Early mobilization and rehabilitation in the ICU: Moving back to the future. *Respiratory Care*, *61*(7), 971–979. doi:10.4187/respcare.04741

HealthyPeople.gov. (2019). *Healthy people 2020 topics & objectives: Physical activity*. Retrieved from https://www.healthypeople.gov/2020/topics-objectives/topic/physical-activity

Kappel, S. E., Larsen-Engelkes, J. J., Barnett, R. T., Alexander, J. W., Klinkhammer, N. L., Jones, M. J., . . . Ye, P. (2018). Creating a culture of mobility: Using real-time assessment to drive outcomes. *American Journal of Nursing*, *118*(12), 44–50. doi:10.1097/01.NAJ.0000549690.33457.bb

Kraschnewski, J. L., Sciamanna, C. N., Poger, J. M., Rovniak, L. S., Lehman, E. B., Cooper, A. B., . . . Ciccolo, J. T. (2016). Is strength training associated with mortality benefits? A 15 year cohort study of US older adults. *Preventive Medicine*, *87*, 121–127. doi:10.1016/j.ypmed.2016.02.038

Martin, M., Rogers, K. A., & Matz, M. W. (n.d.). *New and improved VA algorithms/new SPHM app!* Retrieved from https://slideplayer.com/slide/14317268

Miller, H., Rockefeller, K., & Townsend, P. (2017). International round table discussion: Do gait belts have a role in safe patient handling programs? *International Journal of Safe Patient Handling & Mobility (SPHM)*, *7*(3), 116–121.

Moorhead, S., Swanson, E., Johnson, M., & Maas, M. L. (Eds.). (2018). *Nursing outcomes classification (NOC)* (6th ed.). St. Louis, MO: Elsevier.

Teeple, E., Collins, J. E., Shrestha, S., Dennerlein, J. T., Losina, E., & Katz, J. N. (2017). Outcomes of safe patient handling and mobilization programs: A meta-analysis. *Work*, *58*(2), 173–184. doi:10.3233/WOR-172608

Teodoro, C. R., Breault, K., Garvey, C., Klick, C., O'Brien, J., Purdue, T., . . . Matney, L. (2016). STEP-UP: Study of the effectiveness of a patient ambulation protocol. *MEDSURG Nursing*, *25*(2), 111–116.

VHA Center for Engineering & Occupational Safety and Health. (2016). *Safe patient handling and mobility guidebook*. St. Louis, MO: Author.

Walker, L., Docherty, T., Hougendobler, D., Guanowsky, C., & Rosenthal, M. (2017). Sharing the lessons: The 10-year journey of a safe patient movement program. *International Journal of SPHM (Safe Patient Handling & Mobility)*, *7*(1), 20–28.

Weinmeyer, R. (2016). Safe patient handling laws and programs for health care workers. *American Medical Association Journal of Ethics*, *18*, 416–421. doi:10.1001/journalofethics.2016.18.4.hlaw1-1604

Selected Bibliography

American Nurses Association. (n.d.). *Nurse and Health Care Worker Protection Act: H.R. 4266/S.2408*. Retrieved from https://www.nursingworld.org/~4af9f9/globalassets/practiceandpolicy/work-environment/health--safety/nursehealthcareworkerprotectionact-factsheet.pdf

Bruce, R., & Forry, C. (2018). Integrating a mobility champion in the intensive care unit. *Dimensions of Critical Care Nursing*, *37*(4), 201–209. doi:10.1097/DCC.0000000000000306

Francis, R., & Dawson, J. M. (2016). Special report: Preventing patient-handling injuries in nurses. *American Nurse Today*, *11*(5), 37–44.

Link, T. (2018). Guideline implementation: Safe patient handling and movement. *AORN Journal*, *108*(6), 663–674. doi:10.1002/aorn.12423

Occupational Safety and Health Administration. (n.d.). *Safe patient handling: Busting the myths*. Retrieved from https://www.osha.gov/dsg/hospitals/documents/3.1_Myth-busters_508.pdf

Parry, A. (2016). Importance of early mobilisation in critical care patients. *British Journal of Nursing*, *25*(9), 486–488. doi:10.12968/bjon.2016.25.9.486

Powell-Cope, G., Pippins, K. M., & Young, H. M. (2017). Teaching family caregivers to assist safely with mobility. *American Journal of Nursing*, *117*(12), 49–53. doi:10.1097/01.NAJ.0000527485.94115.7e

Przybysz, L., & Levin, P. F. (2016). Initial results of an evidence-based safe patient handling and mobility program to decrease hospital worker injuries. *Workplace Health & Safety*, *65*, 83–88. doi:10.1177/2165079916670162

Reames, C. D., Price, D. M., King, E. A., & Dickinson, S. (2016). Mobilizing patients along the continuum of critical care. *Dimensions of Critical Care Nursing*, *35*, 10–15. doi:10.1097/DCC.0000000000000151

Rion, J. H. (2016). The walk to save: Benefits of inpatient cardiac rehabilitation. *MEDSURG Nursing*, *25*(3), 159–162.

Spinlife. (n.d.). *Wheelchair store: Manual wheelchairs*. Retrieved from http://www.spinlife.com/category.cfm?categoryID=2

Sleep 45

LEARNING OUTCOMES

After completing this chapter, you will be able to:

1. Explain the physiology and the functions of sleep.
2. Identify the characteristics of the NREM and REM sleep states.
3. Describe variations in sleep patterns throughout the lifespan.
4. Identify factors that affect sleep.
5. Describe common sleep disorders.
6. Identify the components of a sleep pattern assessment.
7. Develop nursing diagnoses, outcomes, and nursing interventions related to sleep problems.
8. Describe interventions that promote sleep.

KEY TERMS

biological rhythms, *1166*
electroencephalogram (EEG), *1177*
electromyogram (EMG), *1177*
electro-oculogram (EOG), *1177*
hypersomnia, *1174*
insomnia, *1173*
narcolepsy, *1174*
nocturnal emissions, *1170*
NREM sleep, *1167*
parasomnia, *1175*
polysomnography, *1177*
REM sleep, *1167*
sleep, *1165*
sleep apnea, *1174*
sleep architecture, *1167*
sleep hygiene, *1178*

Introduction

Sleep is a basic human need; it is a universal biological process common to all individuals. Humans spend about one-third of their lives asleep. We require sleep for many reasons: to cope with daily stresses, to prevent fatigue, to conserve energy, to restore the mind and body, and to enjoy life more fully. Sleep enhances daytime functioning and is vital for cognitive, physiologic, and psychosocial function. Sleeping allows the brain to restore itself. During sleep the body clears itself of adenosine. This action allows an individual to awaken feeling alert and refreshed (Sleep.org, n.d.). Sleep is an important factor in an individual's quality of life, and sleep disorders and sleep deprivation are contributing factors to the development of many chronic diseases, such as type 2 diabetes, heart disease, depression, and obesity, as reported by the Centers for Disease Control and Prevention (CDC, 2018). It is estimated that 50 million to 70 million Americans suffer from a chronic disorder of sleep and wakefulness that hinders daily functioning and adversely affects health. All ages are affected by sleep disorders. According to the CDC, the prevalence of short sleep duration, sleep-disordered breathing, and behavioral sleep problems in children ages 3 to 5 years is 20% to 50%. Sleep-disordered breathing is characterized by snoring or obstructive sleep apnea. As with adults, sleep problems in children can adversely affect cognitive and social development (Bonuck, Blank, True-Felt, & Chervin, 2016). Wheaton, Jones, Cooper, and Croft (2018) state that children and adolescents who have sleep deprivation have an increased risk of attention and behavioral problems, experience poor mental health, and have a greater likelihood of poor academic performance.

There are five health-related behaviors that lead to the development of chronic disease. Smoking, alcohol consumption, obesity, lack of exercise, and insufficient amounts of sleep contribute to an increased risk of hypertension, diabetes, obesity, depression, heart attack, and stroke (Liu et al., 2016).

Physiology of Sleep

Historically, sleep was considered a state of unconsciousness. More recently, **sleep** has come to be considered an altered state of consciousness in which the individual's perception of and reaction to the environment are decreased. Sleep is characterized by minimal physical activity, variable levels of consciousness, changes in the body's physiologic processes, and decreased responsiveness to external stimuli. Some environmental stimuli, such as a smoke detector alarm, will usually awaken a sleeper, whereas many other noises will not. It appears that individuals respond to meaningful stimuli while sleeping and selectively disregard nonmeaningful stimuli. For example, a mother may respond to her baby's crying but not to the crying of another baby.

The cyclic nature of sleep is thought to be controlled by centers located in the lower part of the brain. Neurons within the reticular formation, located in the brainstem, integrate sensory information from the peripheral nervous system and relay the information to the cerebral cortex (see Anatomy & Physiology Review). The upper part of the reticular formation consists of a network of ascending nerve fibers called the reticular activating system (RAS), which is involved with the sleep-wake cycle. An intact cerebral cortex and reticular formation are necessary for the regulation of sleep and waking states.

Neurotransmitters, located within neurons in the brain, affect the sleep-wake cycle. For example, serotonin is thought to lessen the response to sensory stimulation and gamma-aminobutyric acid (GABA) to shut off the activity in the neurons of the reticular activating system. Another key factor to sleep is exposure to darkness. Darkness and preparing for sleep (e.g., lying down, decreasing noise) cause a decrease in stimulation of the RAS. During this time, the pineal gland in the brain begins to actively secrete the natural hormone melatonin, and the individual feels less alert. During sleep, the growth hormone is secreted and cortisol is inhibited.

With the beginning of daylight, melatonin is at its lowest level in the body and the stimulating hormone, cortisol, is at its highest. Wakefulness is also associated with high levels of acetylcholine, dopamine, and noradrenaline. Acetylcholine is released in the reticular formation, dopamine in the midbrain, and noradrenaline in the pons. These neurotransmitters are localized within the reticular formation and influence cerebral cortical arousal.

Circadian Rhythms

Biological rhythms exist in plants, animals, and humans. In humans, these are controlled from within the body and synchronized with environmental factors, such as light and darkness. The most familiar biological rhythm is the circadian rhythm. It is a sort of 24-hour internal biological clock. The term *circadian* is from the Latin *circa dies*, meaning "about a day." Although sleep and waking cycles are the best known of the circadian rhythms, body temperature, blood pressure, and many other physiologic functions also follow a circadian pattern and are affected by changes in sleep patterns.

ANATOMY & PHYSIOLOGY REVIEW

Reticular Activating System

Nerve impulses from the senses reach the reticular activating system (RAS), which is in the reticular formation (located in the brainstem) with projections to the hypothalamus and cerebral cortex. The nerve fibers in the RAS relay impulses to the cerebral cortex for perception by the individual.

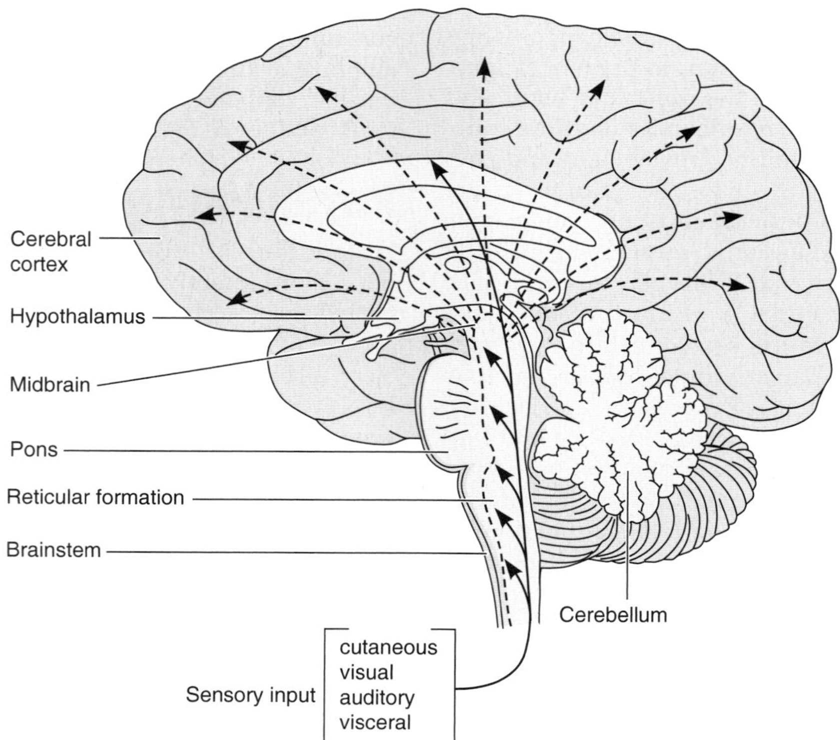

The reticular formation in the brainstem.

QUESTIONS

1. How would you describe activity of the RAS in preparation for and during sleep?
2. What happens physiologically when your alarm clock wakes you in the morning?
3. What areas of the brain are affected by head trauma or stroke and affect an individual's level of alertness?

Answers to Anatomy & Physiology Review Questions are available on the faculty resources site. Please consult with your instructor.

Chronic sleep loss can lead to cardiovascular morbidity, obesity, and metabolic dysfunction (Morgenthaler et al., 2016).

Sleep is a complex biological rhythm. When an individual's biological clock coincides with the sleep-wake cycles, the individual is said to be in circadian synchronization; that is, the individual is awake when the body temperature is highest, and asleep when the body temperature is lowest. Circadian regularity begins to develop by the 6th week of life, and by 3 to 6 months most infants have a regular sleep-wake cycle.

Types of Sleep

Sleep architecture refers to the basic organization of normal sleep. The two types of sleep are **NREM** (non–rapid-eye-movement) **sleep** and **REM** (rapid-eye-movement) sleep. During sleep, NREM and REM sleep alternate in cycles. Changes in the architecture of one's sleep can be linked to physiologic or psychosocial changes. For example, Williams syndrome is a genetic disorder of neurodevelopment that results in cognitive changes. Clients diagnosed with Williams syndrome have alterations in sleep patterns resulting in decreased sleep efficacy that affects their ability to learn, attention span, and behavior (Martens, Seyfer, Andridge, & Coury, 2017).

NREM Sleep

NREM sleep occurs when activity in the RAS is inhibited. About 75% of sleep during a night is NREM sleep. NREM sleep was previously divided into four stages. It is now divided into three stages. Each of the stages is associated with distinct brain activity and physiology. Stage 1 is the stage of very light sleep and lasts only a few minutes. During this stage, the individual feels drowsy and relaxed, the eyes roll from side to side, and the heart and respiratory rates drop slightly. The sleeper can be readily awakened and may deny that he or she was sleeping. Low-voltage brain waves are noted in stage 1 (National Sleep Foundation, 2018).

Stage 2 is the stage of sleep during which body processes continue to slow down. The eyes are generally still, the heart and respiratory rates decrease slightly, and body temperature falls. An individual in stage 2 requires more intense stimuli than in stage 1 to awaken, such as touching or shaking.

Stage 3 is the deepest stage of sleep, differing only in the percentage of delta waves recorded during a 30-second period. During *deep sleep* or *delta sleep*, the sleeper's heart and respiratory rates drop 20% to 30% below those exhibited during waking hours. The sleeper is difficult to arouse. The individual is not disturbed by sensory stimuli, the skeletal muscles are very relaxed, reflexes are diminished, and snoring is most likely to occur. This stage is essential for restoring energy and releasing important growth hormones (Box 45.1).

REM Sleep

REM sleep usually recurs about every 90 minutes and lasts 5 to 30 minutes. Most dreams take place during REM sleep but usually will not be remembered unless the individual arouses briefly at the end of the REM period.

BOX 45.1 Physiologic Changes During NREM Sleep

- Arterial blood pressure falls.
- Pulse rate decreases.
- Peripheral blood vessels dilate.
- Cardiac output decreases.
- Skeletal muscles relax.
- Basal metabolic rate decreases 10% to 30%.
- Growth hormone levels peak.
- Intracranial pressure decreases.

Clinical Alert!

Sleep deprivation in hospitalized clients contributes to delirium. Delirium initially presents as agitation, confusion, or combative behavior. Secondary delirium is hypoactive with inattention and disorganized thoughts (Miller, 2015).

During REM sleep, the brain is highly active, and brain metabolism may increase as much as 20%. For example, during REM sleep, levels of acetylcholine and dopamine increase, with the highest levels of acetylcholine release occurring during REM sleep. Because both of these neurotransmitters are associated with cortical activation, it makes sense that their levels would be high during dreaming sleep. This type of sleep is also called paradoxical sleep because electroencephalogram (EEG) activity resembles that of wakefulness. Distinctive eye movements occur, voluntary muscle tone is dramatically decreased, and deep tendon reflexes are absent. In this phase, the sleeper may be difficult to arouse or may wake spontaneously, gastric secretions increase, and heart and respiratory rates often are irregular. It is thought that the regions of the brain that are used in learning, thinking, and organizing information are stimulated during REM sleep.

Clinical Alert!

Clients who experience sleep deprivation will more commonly experience an increase in fatigue. Sleep deprivation results in a significant increase in thyroid stimulating hormone, which increases tension, anger, and hostility (Ozdemir & Atilla, 2017; Selvi, Kilic, Aydin, & Guzel Oxdemir, 2015).

Sleep Cycles

During a sleep cycle, individuals typically pass through NREM and REM sleep, the complete cycle usually lasting about 90 to 110 minutes in adults. In the first sleep cycle, a sleeper usually passes through the first two stages of NREM sleep in a total of about 20 to 30 minutes. Stage 3 lasts about 50 to 60 minutes. After stage 3 NREM, the sleep passes back through stages 2 and 1 over about 20 minutes. Thereafter, the first REM stage occurs, lasting about 10 minutes, completing the first sleep cycle. It is not unusual for the first REM period to be very brief or even skipped entirely. The healthy adult sleeper usually experiences four to six cycles of sleep during 7 to 8 hours (Figure 45.1 ■).

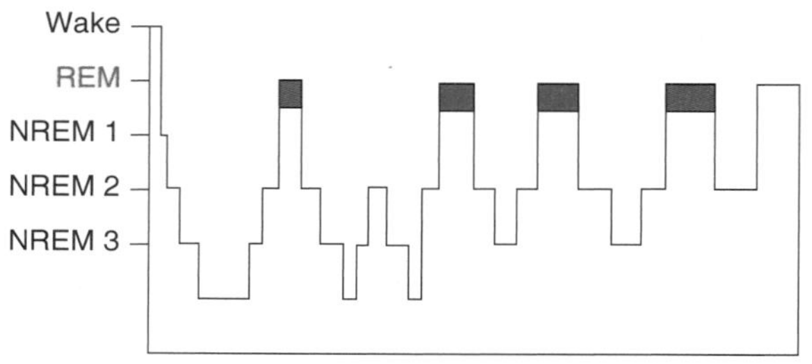

Figure 45.1 ■ Time spent in REM and non-REM stages of sleep in an adult.

The sleeper who is awakened during any stage must begin anew at stage 1 NREM sleep and proceed through all stages to REM sleep.

The duration of NREM stages and REM sleep varies throughout the sleep period. During the early part of the night, the deep sleep periods are longer. As the night progresses, the sleeper spends less time in stage 3 of NREM sleep. REM sleep increases and dreams tend to lengthen. Before sleep ends, periods of near wakefulness occur, and stages 1 and 2 NREM and REM sleep dominate.

Functions of Sleep

The effects of sleep on the body are not completely understood. Sleep exerts physiologic effects on both the nervous system and other body structures. Sleep in some way restores normal levels of activity and normal balance among parts of the nervous system. Sleep is also necessary for protein synthesis, which allows repair processes to occur.

The role of sleep in psychologic well-being is best noticed by the deterioration in mental functioning related to sleep loss. Individuals with inadequate amounts of sleep tend to become emotionally irritable, have poor concentration, and experience difficulty making decisions.

Normal Sleep Patterns and Requirements

Although it used to be believed that maintaining a regular sleep–wake rhythm is more important than the number of hours actually slept, recent research has shown that sleep deprivation is associated with significant cognitive and health problems. Although reestablishing the sleep–wake rhythm (e.g., after the disruption of surgery) is important, it is appropriate to allow and encourage daytime napping in hospitalized clients.

Newborns

Newborns sleep 12 to 18 hours a day, on an irregular schedule with periods of 1 to 3 hours spent awake. Unlike older children and adults, newborns enter REM sleep (called *active sleep* during the newborn period) immediately. Rapid eye movements are observable through closed lids, and the body movements and irregular respirations may be observed. NREM sleep (also called *quiet sleep* during the newborn period) is characterized by regular respirations, closed eyes, and the absence of body and eye movements. Newborns spend nearly 50% of their time in each of these states, and the sleep cycle is about 50 minutes.

It is best to put newborns to bed when they are sleepy but not asleep. Newborns can be encouraged to sleep less during the day by exposing them to light and by playing more with them during the day hours. As evening approaches, the environment can be less bright and quieter with less activity. Babies will even need a winding down time with no computer or tablet screen time and exposure to phones (National Sleep Foundation, n.d.c).

Infants

At first, infants awaken every 3 or 4 hours, eat, and then go back to sleep. Periods of wakefulness gradually increase during the first months. By 6 months, most infants sleep through the night (from midnight to 5 A.M.) and begin to establish a pattern of daytime naps. At the end of the first year, an infant usually takes two naps per day and should get about 14 to 15 hours of sleep in 24 hours.

About half of the infant's sleep time is spent in light sleep. During light sleep, the infant exhibits a great deal of activity, such as movement, gurgles, and coughing. Parents need to make sure that infants are truly awake before picking them up for feeding and changing. Putting infants to bed when they are drowsy but not asleep helps them to become "self-soothers." This means that they fall asleep independently and if they do awake at night, they can put themselves back to sleep. Infants who become used to parental assistance at bedtime will experience shorter sleep intervals with nighttime wakening (Cowie, Palmer, Hussain, & Alfano, 2016).

Toddlers

Between 12 and 14 hours of sleep are recommended for children 1 to 3 years of age. Most still need an afternoon nap, but the need for midmorning naps gradually decreases. The toddler may exhibit a great deal of resistance to going to bed and may awaken during the night. Nighttime fears and nightmares are also common. A security object such as a blanket or stuffed animal may help. Parents need assurance that if the child has had adequate attention from them during the day, maintaining a daily sleep schedule and consistent bedtime routine will promote good sleep habits for the entire family (National Sleep Foundation, n.d.a).

Preschoolers

The preschool-age child (3 to 5 years of age) requires 11 to 13 hours of sleep per night, particularly if the child is in preschool. Sleep needs fluctuate in relation to activity and growth spurts. Many children of this age dislike bedtime and resist by requesting another story, game, or television program. The 4- to 5-year-old may become restless and irritable if sleep requirements are not met (National Sleep Foundation, n.d.c).

Parents can help children who resist bedtime by maintaining a regular and consistent sleep schedule. It also helps to have a relaxing bedtime routine that ends in the child's room. Preschool children wake up frequently at night, and they may be afraid of the dark or experience night terrors or nightmares. Often limiting or eliminating TV will reduce the number of nightmares (National Sleep Foundation, n.d.c).

School-Age Children

The school-age child (5 to 12 years of age) needs 10 to 11 hours of sleep per night, but most receive less because of increasing demands (e.g., homework, sports, social activities). They may also be spending more time at the computer and watching TV. Some may be drinking caffeinated beverages. All of these activities can lead to difficulty falling asleep and fewer hours of sleep. Nurses can teach parents and school-age children about healthy sleep habits. A regular and consistent sleep schedule and bedtime routine need to be continued.

Clinical Alert!

Children who have a TV or computer in their bedroom are more likely to get less sleep.

Adolescents

Adolescents (12 to 18 years of age) require 8 to 10 hours of sleep each night; however, few actually get that much sleep (Figure 45.2 ■) (National Sleep Foundation, n.d.g). Teens are sleepy at times and in places where they should be fully awake—at school, at home, and on the road. This can result in lower grades, negative moods (e.g., unhappy, sad, tense), and increased potential for car crashes. Interestingly, the National Sleep Foundation (n.d.d) found that although more than half of adolescents knew they were not getting enough sleep, 90% of the parents believed their adolescent was getting enough sleep. Nurses can teach parents to recognize signs and symptoms that indicate their teen is sleep deprived (Box 45.2).

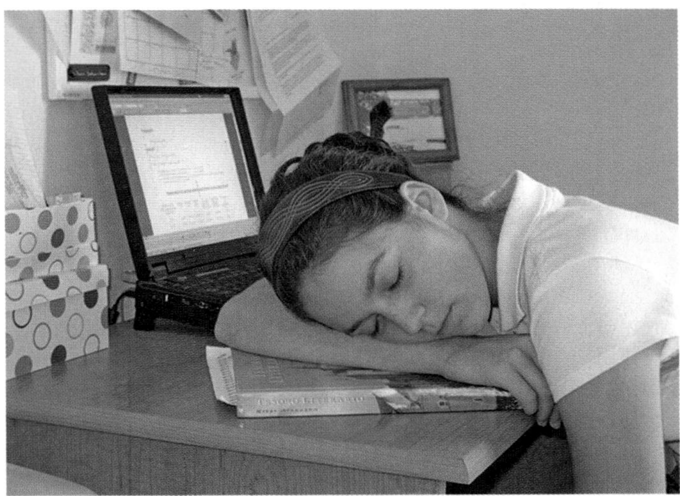

Figure 45.2 ■ Many adolescents do not get enough sleep.

As children reach adolescence, their circadian rhythms tend to shift. Research in the 1990s found that later sleep and wake patterns among adolescents are biologically determined; the natural tendency for teenagers is to stay up late at night and wake up later in the morning. A psychosocial factor affecting later bedtime in the adolescent population is the desire for greater independence. Using the internet, watching television, and cell phone usage disrupt the ability to fall asleep due to

BOX 45.2 Sleep Deprivation and Sleep Problems in Teens

The teen:

- Has difficulty waking in the morning for school.
- Falls asleep in class or during quiet times of the day.
- Increases the use of caffeinated beverages like coffee, soda, or energy drinks.
- Feels tired, making it difficult to initiate or persist in projects such as a school assignment.
- Is irritable, anxious, and angers easily on days when he or she gets less sleep.
- Is involved in many extracurricular activities, has a job, and stays up late doing homework every night, cutting into sleep time.
- Sleeps extra long periods of time on the weekend.

EVIDENCE-BASED PRACTICE

Evidence-Based Practice

Do Adolescents with Smartphones Sleep Less Than Those Without Smartphones?

Schweizer, Berchtold, Barrense-Dias, Akre, and Suris (2017) conducted a longitudinal study assessing the effect adolescent use of smartphones has on sleep duration. Five hundred and ninety-one adolescents participated in the study. The mean age of the participants was 14.3 years. The participants were divided into owners of a smartphone, new owners of a smartphone after 2 years, and nonowners. Each adolescent was asked to indicate how much sleep he or she attained nightly during school days and on weekends. In conclusion, smartphone owners experienced greater sleep problems. The disruption of sleep was most commonly associated with shorter sleep duration.

Implications

Smartphones are just like computers. Parents and adolescents should be instructed to leave the phone in another area of the home to enhance sleep outcomes.

blue-spectrum light exposure. A blue-light screen protector can reduce exposure to blue light (Kreieger, 2017).

In 2014 the American Academy of Pediatrics, the Adolescent Sleep Working Group, and the Committee on Adolescence, led by Dr. Judith Owens, reported that adolescents who do not receive adequate sleep tend to be overweight; do not engage in daily exercise; may smoke, drink, or use illicit drugs; and perform poorly in school. In 2014 the American Academy of Pediatrics released a policy statement encouraging school districts to implement later start times for middle and high school students. It is important for nurses and healthcare professionals to educate private and public schools on adolescent sleep and the importance of later start times.

During adolescence, boys begin to experience **nocturnal emissions** (orgasm and emission of semen during sleep), known as "wet dreams," several times each month. Boys need to be informed about this normal development to prevent embarrassment and fear.

Most healthy adults get 7 to 9 hours of sleep per night. This amount of sleep will assist in decreasing daytime sleepiness and contribute to health (National Sleep Foundation, n.d.b). However, individual needs do vary—some adults may be able to function well (e.g., without sleepiness or drowsiness) with 6 hours of sleep, and others may need 10 hours to function optimally. Signs that may indicate that an individual is not getting enough sleep include falling asleep or becoming drowsy during a task that is not fatiguing (e.g., listening to a presentation), not being able to concentrate or remember information, and being unreasonably irritable with others. Lack of sleep also contributes to short-term memory loss and inadequate performance on newly learned tasks. Taking a nap in the middle of the day improves mood, increases memory, reduces fatigue, and lowers blood pressure (National Sleep Foundation, n.d.h).

Adults are particularly vulnerable to sleep deprivation. Factors that contribute to diminished sleep include stress, depression, pain, shift work, travel, and lifestyle roles, such as job, student, or parenting. Adults working long hours or multiple jobs may find their sleep less refreshing. A study by Owens, Allen, and Moultrie (2017) examined the impact shift work had on nurses' quality of sleep. The descriptive study revealed that nurses are fatigued from working long consecutive shifts. Working shifts also affects their quality of life. The sleep habits of children also have an impact on the adults caring for them. A woman's sleep pattern is more commonly affected by the birth of a child. However, both parents of infants and young children experience fatigue related to interrupted sleep or sleep deprivation. This lack of sleep is associated with lower parental competence and greater stress (Corkin et al., 2017). Biological conditions such as pregnancy, menses, and the perimenopausal period can also affect a woman's sleep patterns.

Nurses need to teach adults the importance of obtaining sufficient sleep and provide tips on how to promote sleep that results in the client waking up feeling restored or refreshed. See Client Teaching later in this chapter.

Older Adults

A hallmark change with age is a tendency toward earlier bedtime and wake times. Older adults (65 to 75 years) usually awaken 1.3 hours earlier and go to bed approximately 1 hour earlier than younger adults (ages 20 to 30). Older adults may show an increase in disturbed sleep that can create a negative impact on their quality of life, mood, and alertness. They may awaken an average of six times during the night. Although the ability to sleep becomes more difficult, the need to sleep does not decrease with age. During sleep, an older adult has a flattened circadian rhythm. This is noted by the earlier bedtime and morning arousal. The circadian rhythm changes due to a decreased responsiveness of the superchiasmatic nucleus. This is what controls the internal clock to respond to cues such as light (Richards, Demartini, & Xiong, 2018). Older adults have difficulty falling back to sleep after awakening and have a diminished amount of REM sleep. Many older adults report daytime napping, which may contribute to reduced nocturnal sleep.

Medical conditions and pain are factors that interrupt sleep. Older adults who have several medical conditions and complain of having sleeping problems should discuss this with their primary care provider. The older individual may have a major sleep disorder that is complicating treatment of other conditions. It is important for the nurse to teach about the connection between sleep, health, and aging. See Client Teaching about sleep promotion later in this chapter.

Some older clients with dementia may experience *sundown syndrome*. Although not a sleep disorder directly, it refers to a pattern of symptoms (e.g., agitation, anxiety, aggression, and sometimes delusions) that occur in the late afternoon (thus the name). These symptoms can last through the night, further disrupting sleep (Graff-Radford, 2017).

Factors Affecting Sleep

Both the quality and the quantity of sleep are affected by a number of factors. *Sleep quality* is a subjective characteristic and is often determined by whether an individual wakes up feeling energetic or not. *Quantity of sleep* is the total time the individual sleeps.

Illness

Illness that causes pain or physical distress (e.g., arthritis, back pain) can result in sleep problems. Individuals who are ill require more sleep than normal, and the normal rhythm of sleep and wakefulness is often disturbed. Individuals deprived of REM sleep subsequently spend more sleep time than normal in this stage.

Respiratory conditions can disturb an individual's sleep. Shortness of breath often makes sleep difficult, and individuals who have nasal congestion or sinus drainage may have trouble breathing and hence may find it difficult to sleep.

Individuals who have gastric or duodenal ulcers may find their sleep disturbed because of pain, often a result of the increased gastric secretions that occur during REM sleep.

Certain endocrine disturbances can also affect sleep. Hyperthyroidism lengthens presleep time, making it difficult for a client to fall asleep. Hypothyroidism, conversely, decreases stage 3 sleep. Women with low levels of estrogen often report excessive fatigue. In addition, they may experience sleep disruptions due, in part, to the discomfort associated with hot flashes or night sweats that can occur with reduced estrogen levels.

Elevated body temperatures can cause some reduction in delta sleep and REM sleep. The need to urinate during the night also disrupts sleep, and individuals who awaken at night to urinate sometimes have difficulty getting back to sleep.

Environment

Environment can promote or hinder sleep. The individual must be able to achieve a state of relaxation prior to entering a period of sleep. Any change, such as noise in the environment, can inhibit sleep. The absence of usual stimuli or the presence of unfamiliar stimuli can prevent individuals from sleeping. Hospital environments can be quite noisy, and special care needs to be taken to reduce noise in the hallways and nursing care units. In fact, some hospitals have instituted "quiet times" in the afternoon on nursing units where the lights are lowered and activity and noise are purposefully decreased so clients can rest or nap.

Discomfort from environmental temperature (e.g., too hot or cold) and lack of ventilation can affect sleep. Light levels can be another factor. An individual accustomed to darkness while sleeping may find it difficult to sleep in the light. Another influence includes the comfort and size of the bed. An individual's partner who has different sleep habits, snores, or has other sleep difficulties may become a problem for the individual also.

LIFESPAN CONSIDERATIONS Sleep Disturbances

CHILDREN

Learning to sleep alone without the parent's help is a skill that all children need to master. Regular bedtime routines and rituals such as reading a book help children learn this skill and can prevent sleep disturbance. Some sleep disturbances seen in children include the following:

- *Trained night feeder.* Infants who are fed during the night, who are fed until they fall asleep and then put into bed, or who have a bottle left with them in their bed learn to expect and demand middle-of-the-night feedings. Infants who are growing well do not need night feeding after about 4 months of age. Infants should never be put to bed with a bottle. This practice increases the risk of otitis media. Infants who are diagnosed with failure to thrive may need to be fed at night.
- *Sleep refusal.* Many toddlers and young children are resistant to settling down to sleep. This sleep refusal may be due to not being tired, anxiety about separation from the parent, stress (e.g., a recent move), lack of a regular sleep routine, the child's temperament, or changes in sleep arrangements (e.g., move from a crib to a "big" bed).
- *Night terrors.* Night terrors are partial awakenings from NREM stage 3 sleep. They are usually seen in children 3 to 6 years of age. The child may sleepwalk, or may sit up in bed screaming and thrashing about. They usually cannot be wakened, but should be protected from injury, helped back to bed, and soothed back to sleep. Babysitters should be alerted to the possibility of a night terror occurring. Children do not remember the incident the next day, and there is no indication of a neurologic or emotional problem. Excessive fatigue and a full bladder may contribute to the problem. Having the child take an afternoon nap and empty the bladder before going to sleep at night may be helpful.

ADULTS

- New jobs, pregnancy, and babies are common examples that often disrupt the sleep of a young adult.
- The sleep patterns of middle-aged adults can be disrupted by the need to take care of older parents or chronically ill partners in the home.
- See Client Teaching later in this chapter for tips on promoting sleep.

OLDER ADULTS

The quality of sleep is often diminished in older adults. Some of the leading factors that often are influential in sleep disturbances include the following:

- Side effects of medications
- Gastric reflux disease
- Respiratory and circulatory disorders, which may cause breathing problems or discomfort
- Pain from arthritis, increased stiffness, or impaired mobility
- Nocturia
- Depression
- Loss of life partner or close friends
- Confusion related to delirium or dementia.

Interventions to promote sleep and rest can help enhance the rejuvenation and renewal that sleep provides. The following interventions can help promote sleep:

- Reduce or eliminate the consumption of caffeine and nicotine.
- Be sure the environment is warm and safe, especially if clients get out of bed during the night.
- Provide comfort measures, such as analgesics if indicated, and proper positioning.
- Enhance the sense of safety and security by checking on clients frequently and making sure that the call light is within reach. Answer the call light promptly.
- If lack of sleep is caused by medications or certain health conditions, interventions should focus on resolving the underlying problem.
- Evaluate the situation and find out what the rest and sleep disturbances mean to the client. The client may not perceive nighttime sleeplessness to be a serious problem, and will just do other activities and sleep when tired.

Lifestyle

Following an irregular morning and nighttime schedule can affect sleep. Moderate exercise in the morning or early afternoon is usually conducive to sleep, but exercise late in the day can delay sleep. The individual's ability to relax before retiring is an important factor affecting the ability to fall asleep. It is best, therefore, to avoid doing homework or office work before or after getting into bed.

Night shift workers frequently obtain less sleep than other workers and have difficulty falling asleep after getting off work. Wearing dark wraparound sunglasses during the drive home and light-blocking shades in the bedroom can minimize the alerting effects of exposure to daylight, thus making it easier to fall asleep when body temperature is rising.

Emotional Stress

Stress is considered by most sleep experts to be the one of the greatest causes of difficulties in falling asleep or staying asleep. Clients who are consistently exposed to stress will increase the activation of the hypothalamic–pituitary–adrenal (HPA) axis leading to sleep disorders. An individual who becomes preoccupied with personal problems (e.g., school- or job-related pressures, family or marriage problems) may be unable to relax sufficiently to get to sleep. Anxiety increases the norepinephrine blood levels through stimulation of the sympathetic nervous system. This chemical change results in less deep and REM sleep and more stage changes and awakenings.

Stimulants and Alcohol

Caffeine-containing beverages act as stimulants of the central nervous system (CNS). Drinking beverages containing caffeine in the afternoon or evening may interfere with sleep. Individuals who drink an excessive amount of alcohol often find their sleep disturbed. Alcohol disrupts REM sleep, although it may hasten the onset of sleep. While making up for lost REM sleep after some of the effects of the alcohol have worn off, individuals often experience nightmares. The alcohol-tolerant individual may be unable to sleep well and become irritable as a result.

Diet

Weight gain has been associated with reduced total sleep time as well as broken sleep and earlier awakening. Weight loss, on the other hand, seems to be associated with an increase in total sleep time and less broken sleep. Dietary L-tryptophan—found, for example, in cheese and milk—may induce sleep, a fact that might explain why warm milk helps some individuals get to sleep.

Smoking

Nicotine has a stimulating effect on the body, and smokers often have more difficulty falling asleep than nonsmokers. Smokers are usually easily aroused and often describe themselves as light sleepers. By refraining from smoking after the evening meal, the individual usually sleeps better; moreover, many former smokers report that their sleeping patterns improved once they stopped smoking.

Motivation

Motivation can increase alertness in some situations (e.g., a tired individual can probably stay alert while attending an interesting concert or surfing the web late at night). Motivation alone, however, is usually not sufficient to overcome the normal circadian drive to sleep during the night. Nor is motivation sufficient to overcome sleepiness due to insufficient sleep. A combination of boredom and lack of sleep can contribute to feeling tired.

Medications

Some medications affect the quality of sleep. Most hypnotics can interfere with deep sleep and suppress REM sleep. Beta blockers have been known to cause insomnia and nightmares. Narcotics, such as morphine, are known to suppress REM sleep and to cause frequent awakenings and drowsiness. Tranquilizers interfere with REM sleep. Although antidepressants suppress REM sleep, this effect is considered a therapeutic action. In fact, selectively depriving a depressed client of REM sleep will result in an immediate but transient improvement in mood. Clients accustomed to taking hypnotic medications and antidepressants may experience a REM rebound (increased REM sleep) when these medications are discontinued. Warning clients to expect a period of more intense dreams when these medications are discontinued may reduce their anxiety about this symptom. Boxes 45.3 and 45.4, respectively, list drugs that can disrupt sleep or cause excessive daytime sleepiness.

BOX 45.3 Drugs That Disrupt Sleep

These drugs may disrupt REM sleep, delay onset of sleep, or decrease sleep time:

- Alcohol
- Amphetamines
- Antidepressants
- Beta-blockers
- Bronchodilators
- Caffeine
- Decongestants
- Narcotics
- Steroids

BOX 45.4 Drugs That May Cause Excessive Daytime Sleepiness

These drugs may be associated with excessive daytime sleepiness:

- Antidepressants
- Antihistamines
- Beta blockers
- Narcotics

Common Sleep Disorders

A knowledge of common sleep disorders can help nurses assess the sleep complaints of their clients and, when appropriate, make a referral to a specialist in sleep disorders medicine. Although sleep disorders are typically categorized for the purpose of research as dyssomnias, parasomnias, and disorders associated with medical or psychiatric illness, it is usually more appropriate for clinicians to focus on the client's symptoms (e.g., insomnia, excessive sleepiness, and abnormal events) that occur during sleep (parasomnias).

Insomnia

Insomnia is described as the inability to fall asleep or remain asleep. Individuals with insomnia do not awaken feeling rested. Insomnia is the most common sleep complaint in America. Acute insomnia lasts one to several nights and is often caused by personal stressors or worry. If the insomnia persists for longer than a month, it is considered chronic insomnia. More often, individuals experience chronic-intermittent insomnia, which means difficulty sleeping for a few nights, followed by a few nights of adequate sleep before the problem returns (National Sleep Foundation, n.d.i). See Box 45.5 for symptoms of insomnia. The two main risk factors for insomnia are older age and female gender (National Sleep Foundation, n.d.e). Women suffer sleep loss in connection with hormonal changes (e.g., menstruation, pregnancy, and menopause). The incidence of insomnia increases with age, but it is thought that this is caused by some other medical condition.

Treatment for insomnia frequently requires the client to develop new behavior patterns that induce sleep and maintain it. Examples of behavioral treatments include the following:

- ***Stimulus control:*** creating a sleep environment that promotes sleep
- ***Cognitive therapy:*** learning to develop positive thoughts and beliefs about sleep
- ***Sleep restriction:*** limiting time in bed in order to get to sleep and stay asleep throughout the night.

BOX 45.5 Insomnia

- Difficulty falling asleep
- Waking up too early or frequently during the night
- Difficulty returning to sleep
- Waking up too early in the morning
- Unrefreshing sleep
- Daytime sleepiness
- Difficulty concentrating
- Irritability
- Non-restorative sleep
- Fatigue and irritability
- Difficulty at work or school
- Difficulty with personal relationships

From *Insomnia: Symptoms*, National Sleep Foundation, n.d.f. Retrieved from https://sleepfoundation.org/insomnia/content/symptoms

EVIDENCE-BASED PRACTICE

Evidence-Based Practice

What Are the Interventions to Promote Sleep and Rest in Hospitalized Clients?

Vincensi et al. (2016) conducted research with a threefold purpose. The first purpose of the study was to describe nursing interventions used to promote sleep. The second purpose was to determine the interventions nurses and clients identified as most effective. The study also sought to obtain feedback on the noninvasive biomedical device called the Vital Sleep headband. The Vital Sleep headband is a medical device that eliminates noise to promote sleep. It also monitors the client's vital signs and transmits the results to the nurses' station.

A cross-sectional survey design was implemented to determine if nurses and clients perceived the same sleep disturbances. The study included 87 nurses and 34 clients. Both the clients and nurses perceived that the biggest interruptions to sleep were the administration of medications, vital sign checks, and pain. The most effective nursing interventions to promote sleep reported by the clients and nurses were the administration of pharmacologic interventions and the avoidance of sleep interruptions such as the assessment of vital signs. The administration of the Vital Sleep headband with music enhanced clients' sleep.

Implications

Nurses must recognize the impact of sleep on the client's recovery. The study revealed that nursing strategies to promote sleep included the use of adequate sleep hygiene. Items and interventions to promote sleep hygiene include warm blankets, bedtime snacks, and maintaining a sleep routine. Nurses also need to develop and participate in research studies that investigate interventions to promote sleep.

The long-term efficacy of hypnotic medications is questionable. Such medications do not deal with the cause of the problem, and their prolonged use can create drug dependencies. Although antihistamines such as diphenhydramine (Benadryl) are thought to be safer for older clients than hypnotics, their side effects (i.e., atropine-like effects, dizziness, sedation, and hypotension) make them extremely hazardous. In fact, antihistamines should not be recommended for any client with a history of asthma, increased intraocular pressure, hyperthyroidism, cardiovascular disease, or hypertension.

Excessive Daytime Sleepiness

Clients may experience excessive daytime sleepiness as a result of hypersomnia, narcolepsy, sleep apnea, and insufficient sleep.

Hypersomnia

Hypersomnia refers to conditions where the affected individual obtains sufficient sleep at night but still cannot stay awake during the day. Hypersomnia can be caused by medical conditions, for example, CNS damage and certain kidney, liver, or metabolic disorders, such as diabetic acidosis and hypothyroidism. Rarely does hypersomnia have a psychologic origin.

Narcolepsy

Narcolepsy is a disorder of excessive daytime sleepiness caused by the lack of the chemical hypocretin in the area of the CNS that regulates sleep. Clients with narcolepsy have sleep attacks or excessive daytime sleepiness, and their sleep at night usually begins with a sleep-onset REM period (dreaming sleep occurs within the first 15 minutes of falling asleep). The majority of clients also have cataplexy or the sudden onset of muscle weakness or paralysis in association with strong emotion, sleep paralysis (transient paralysis when falling asleep or waking up), hypnagogic hallucinations (visual, auditory, or tactile hallucinations at sleep onset or when waking up), and/or fragmented nighttime sleep. Their fragmented nocturnal sleep is not the cause of their excessive daytime sleepiness; many clients, particularly younger clients, have sound restorative nocturnal sleep but still cannot stay awake during the daytime. Onset of symptoms tends to occur between ages 15 and 30, and symptom severity usually stabilizes within the first 5 years of onset.

CNS stimulants such as methylphenidate (Ritalin) or amphetamines have been used to reduce excessive daytime sleepiness. Xanthines, such as caffeine, stimulate the cerebral cortex to increase alertness. Antidepressants, both older monoamine oxidase inhibitors (MAOIs) and the newer serotonergic antidepressants, are usually quite effective for controlling cataplexy. Modafinil (Provigil) has psychoactive effects to alter mood, perception, and thinking to control excessive daytime sleepiness in narcoleptic clients. Although its exact mechanism of action is unknown, it has fewer side effects and a lower potential for abuse than other drugs. Modafinil is also used for sleep apnea-hypopnea syndrome (Frandsen & Pennington, 2018). Sodium oxybate (Xyrem) is approved for the treatment of cataplexy. It has been shown to reduce excessive daytime sleepiness in clients with narcolepsy, although the exact mechanism of action is unknown. Because Xyrem is difficult to administer (it is only available as a liquid and taken at bedtime and then again 2.5 to 4 hours after sleep onset) and its use is tightly controlled by the U.S. Food and Drug Administration (FDA), only those clients whose symptoms are not controlled by other medications are usually offered Xyrem. Only one pharmacy in the United States is allowed to dispense Xyrem. As a result, clients need to allow adequate time for obtaining their medications from the central pharmacy. The herbal supplement guarana can also be administered to increase mental alertness during the daytime.

Clinical Alert!

Sodium oxybate is also known as gamma hydroxybutyrate or GHB—one of the drugs frequently associated with "date rapes."

Sleep Apnea

Sleep apnea is characterized by frequent short breathing pauses during sleep. Although all individuals have occasional periods of apnea during sleep, more than five apneic episodes or five breathing pauses longer than 10 seconds per hour is considered abnormal and should be evaluated by a sleep medicine specialist. Symptoms suggestive of sleep apnea include loud snoring, frequent nocturnal awakenings, excessive daytime sleepiness, difficulties falling asleep at night, morning headaches, memory and cognitive problems, and irritability. Although sleep apnea is most frequently diagnosed in men and postmenopausal women, it may occur during childhood.

The periods of apnea, which last from 10 seconds to 2 minutes, occur during REM or NREM sleep. Frequency of episodes ranges from 50 to 600 per night. Because these apneic pauses are usually associated with an arousal, clients frequently report that their sleep is nonrestorative and that they regularly fall asleep when engaging in sedentary activities during the day.

Three common types of sleep apnea are obstructive apnea, central apnea, and mixed apnea. Obstructive apnea occurs when the structures of the pharynx or oral cavity block the flow of air. The individual continues to try to breathe; that is, the chest and abdominal muscles move. The movements of the diaphragm become stronger and stronger until the obstruction is removed. Enlarged tonsils and adenoids, a deviated nasal septum, nasal polyps, and obesity predispose the client to obstructive apnea. An episode of obstructive sleep apnea usually begins with snoring; thereafter, breathing ceases, followed by marked snorting as breathing resumes. Toward the end of each apneic episode, increased carbon dioxide levels in the blood cause the client to wake.

Central apnea is thought to involve a defect in the respiratory center of the brain. All actions involved in breathing, such as chest movement and airflow, cease. Clients who have brainstem injuries and muscular dystrophy, for example, often have central sleep apnea. At this time, there is no available treatment. Mixed apnea is a combination of central apnea and obstructive apnea.

Treatment for sleep apnea is directed at the cause of the apnea. For example, enlarged tonsils may be removed. Other surgical procedures, including laser removal of excess tissue in the pharynx, reduce or eliminate snoring and may be effective in relieving the apnea. In other cases, the use of a nasal continuous positive airway pressure (CPAP) device at night is effective in maintaining an open airway. Weight loss may also help decrease the severity of symptoms.

Sleep apnea profoundly affects an individual's work or school performance. In addition, prolonged sleep apnea can cause a sharp rise in blood pressure and may lead to cardiac arrest. Over time, apneic episodes can cause cardiac arrhythmias, pulmonary hypertension, and subsequent left-sided heart failure.

Clinical Alert!

Partners of clients with sleep apnea may become aware of the problem because they hear snoring that stops during the apneic period and then restarts. Surgical removal of tonsils or other tissue in the pharynx, if not the cause of the sleep apnea, can actually worsen the situation by removing the snoring and, thus, the warning that apnea is occurring.

Insufficient Sleep

Healthy individuals who obtain less sleep than they need will experience sleepiness and fatigue during the daytime hours. Depending on the severity and chronicity of this voluntary, albeit unintentional sleep deprivation, individuals may develop attention and concentration deficits, reduced vigilance, distractibility, reduced motivation, fatigue, malaise, and occasionally diplopia and dry mouth. The cause of these symptoms may or may not be attributed to insufficient sleep, because many Americans believe that 6.8 hours of sleep is sufficient to maintain optimal daytime performance. In fact, the sleep times of Americans have decreased dramatically during the past decade, with adults averaging only 6.8 hours of sleep on weekdays and 7.4 hours on weekends. All age groups, not just adults and adolescents, are getting less than the recommended amounts of sleep. Even 4- to 5-year-old children now average less than 9.5 hours of sleep, approximately 1.5 to 2.5 hours less than recommended.

Although the effects of obtaining less than optimal amounts of sleep are generally considered benign, there is growing evidence that insufficient sleep can have significant deleterious effects. Staying awake 19 consecutive hours produces the same impairments in reaction times and cognitive function as a blood alcohol level of 0.05, and staying awake for 24 consecutive hours has the same effects on reaction times and cognitive function as being legally drunk (with a blood alcohol level of 0.1). Nurses who report reduced hours of sleep are more likely to make an error, to have difficulty staying awake on duty, and to have difficulty staying awake while driving home from work than those who obtained more sleep.

When clients report obtaining more sleep on weekends or days off, it usually indicates that they are not obtaining sufficient sleep. Convincing clients to obtain more sleep may be difficult, but it can result in the resolution of their daytime symptoms.

Parasomnias

A **parasomnia** is behavior that may interfere with sleep and may even occur during sleep. It is characterized by physical events such as movements or experiences that are displayed as emotions, perceptions, or dreams. The *International Classification of Sleep Disorders* subdivides parasomnias into three classes: non–rapid eye movement, rapid eye movement, and miscellaneous with no specific stage of sleep (Judd & Sateia, 2019). Parasomnias with non–rapid eye movement are associated with confusion upon arousal, sleep tremors, and sleep walking. Parasomnias with rapid eye movement are associated with arousal disorders such as sleep paralysis. This may be a nightmare disorder with exaggerated features of REM sleep. Miscellaneous parasomnias are not associated with any stage of sleep and may produce nocturnal enuresis or hallucinations. The miscellaneous parasomnias are often related to a medication, substance abuse, or a medical disorder. Box 45.6 describes examples of parasomnias.

BOX 45.6 Parasomnias

- *Bruxism.* Usually occurring during stage 2 NREM sleep, this clenching and grinding of the teeth can eventually erode dental crowns, cause teeth to come loose, and lead to deterioration of the temporomandibular (TMJ) joint, which is called TMJ syndrome.
- *Enuresis.* Bed-wetting during sleep can occur in children over 3 years old. More males than females are affected. It often occurs 1 to 2 hours after falling asleep, when rousing from NREM stage 3.
- *Periodic limb movement disorder (PLMD).* In this condition, the legs jerk twice or three times per minute during sleep. It is most common among older adults. This kicking motion can wake the client and result in poor sleep. PLMD differs from restless leg syndrome (RLS), which occurs whenever the individual is at rest, not just at night when sleeping. RLS may occur during pregnancy or be due to other medical problems that can be treated. Many clients with PLMD or RLS respond well to medications such as levodopa, pramipexole, ropinirole, and gabapentin (Frandsen & Pennington, 2018).
- *Sleeptalking.* Talking during sleep occurs during NREM sleep before REM sleep. It rarely presents a problem to the individual unless it becomes troublesome to others.
- *Sleepwalking.* Sleepwalking (somnambulism) occurs during stage 3 of NREM sleep. It is episodic and usually occurs 1 to 2 hours after falling asleep. Sleepwalkers tend not to notice dangers (e.g., stairs) and often need to be protected from injury.

NURSING MANAGEMENT

Assessing

A complete assessment of a client's sleep difficulty includes a sleep history, health history, physical exam, and, if warranted, a sleep diary and diagnostic studies. All nurses, however, can take a brief sleep history and educate their clients about normal sleep.

Sleep History

A brief sleep history, which is usually part of the comprehensive nursing history, should be obtained for all clients entering a healthcare facility. It should, however, be deferred or omitted if the client is critically ill. Key questions to ask include the following:

- When do you usually go to sleep? And when do you wake up? Do you nap? If so, when? If the client is a child, it is also important to ask about bedtime rituals. This information provides the nurse with information about the client's usual sleep duration and preferred sleep times, and allows for the incorporation of the client's preferences in the plan of care.
- Do you have any problems with your sleep? Has anyone ever told you that you snore loudly or thrash around a lot at night? Are you able to stay awake at work, when driving, or engaging in your usual activities?

  These questions elicit information about sleep complaints including the possibility of excessive daytime sleepiness. Loud snoring suggests the possibility of obstructive sleep apnea, and any client replying yes to this question should be referred to a specialist in sleep disorders medicine. Referrals should also be made if clients indicate they have difficulty staying awake during the day or that their movements disturb the sleep of their bed partners.
- Do you take any prescribed medications, over-the-counter (OTC) medications, or herbal remedies to help you sleep? Or to stay awake?

  This information alerts the nurse to the use of prescription hypnotics and stimulants as well as the use of OTC sleep aids and herbal remedies.
- Is there anything else I need to know about your sleep? This allows the client to voice any concerns or bring up topics that the nurse may not have asked about.

If the client is being admitted to a long-term care facility, it is also appropriate to ask about preferred room temperature, lighting (complete darkness versus using a night light), and preferred bedtime routine.

A more detailed assessment is required if the client indicates any difficulty sleeping, difficulty remaining awake during the day, or recent changes in sleep pattern. This detailed history should explore the exact nature of the problem and its cause, when it first began and its frequency, how it affects daily living, what the client is doing to cope with the problem, and whether these methods have been effective. Questions the nurse might ask the client with a sleeping disturbance are shown in the accompanying Assessment Interview.

Health History

A health history is obtained to rule out medical or psychiatric causes of the client's difficulty sleeping. It is important to note that the presence of a medical or psychiatric illness (e.g., depression, Parkinson's disease, Alzheimer's disease, or arthritis) does not preclude the possibility that a second problem (e.g., obstructive sleep apnea) may be contributing to the difficulty sleeping. Because medications can frequently cause or exacerbate sleep disturbances, information should be obtained about all of the prescribed and nonprescription medications, including herbal remedies, that a client consumes.

Physical Examination

Rarely are sleep abnormalities noted during the physical examination unless the client has obstructive sleep apnea or some other health problem. Common findings among

ASSESSMENT INTERVIEW Sleep Disturbances

- How would you describe your sleeping problem? What changes have occurred in your sleeping pattern? How often does this happen?
- How many cups of coffee, tea, or caffeinated beverages do you drink per day? Do you drink alcohol? If so, how much?
- Do you have difficulty falling asleep?
- Do you wake up often during the night? If so, how often?
- Do you wake up earlier in the morning than you would like and have difficulty falling back to sleep?
- How do you feel when you wake up in the morning?
- Are you sleeping more than usual? If so, how often do you sleep?
- Do you have periods of overwhelming sleepiness? If so, when does this happen?
- Have you ever suddenly fallen asleep in the middle of a daytime activity? Does anything unusual happen when you laugh or get angry?
- Has anyone ever told you that you snore, walk in your sleep, or stop breathing for a while when sleeping?
- What have you been doing to deal with this sleeping problem? Does it help?
- What do you think might be causing this problem? Do you have any medical condition that might be causing you to sleep more (or less)? Are you receiving medications for an illness that might alter your sleeping pattern? Are you experiencing any stressful or upsetting events or conflicts that may be affecting your sleep?
- How is your sleeping problem affecting you?

clients with sleep apnea include an enlarged and reddened uvula and soft palate, enlarged tonsils and adenoids (in children), obesity (in adults), and in male clients a neck size greater than 17.5 inches. Occasionally a deviated septum may be noted, but it is rarely the cause of obstructive sleep apnea.

Sleep Diary

A sleep specialist may ask clients to keep a sleep diary or log for 1 to 2 weeks in order to get a more complete picture of their sleep complaints. A sleep diary may include all or selected aspects of the following information that pertain to the client's specific problem:

- Time of (a) going to bed, (b) trying to fall asleep, (c) falling asleep (approximate time), (d) any instances of waking up and duration of these periods, (e) waking up in the morning, and (f) any naps and their duration
- Activities performed 2 to 3 hours before bedtime (type, duration, and time)
- Consumption of caffeinated beverages and alcohol and amounts of those beverages
- Any prescribed medications, OTC medications, and herbal remedies taken during the day
- Bedtime rituals before sleep
- Any difficulties remaining awake during the day and times when difficulties occurred
- Any worries that the client believes may affect sleep
- Factors that the client believes have a positive or negative effect on sleep.

If the client is a child, the sleep diary or log may be completed by a parent.

Diagnostic Studies

Sleep is measured objectively in a sleep disorder laboratory by **polysomnography** in which an **electroencephalogram (EEG)**, **electromyogram (EMG)**, and **electro-oculogram (EOG)** are recorded simultaneously. Electrodes are placed on the scalp to record brain waves (EEG), on the outer canthus of each eye to record eye movement (EOG), and on the chin muscles to record the structural electromyogram (EMG). The electrodes transmit electric energy from the cerebral cortex and muscles of the face to pens that record the brain waves and muscle activity on graph paper. Respiratory effort and airflow, ECG, leg movements, and oxygen saturation are also monitored. Oxygen saturation is determined by monitoring with a pulse oximeter, a light-sensitive electric cell that attaches to the ear or a finger. Oxygen saturation and ECG assessments are of particular importance if sleep apnea is suspected. Through polysomnography, the client's activity (movements, struggling, noisy respirations) during sleep can be assessed. Such activity of which the client is unaware may be the cause of arousal during sleep.

Diagnosing

Impaired sleep, the diagnosis given to clients with sleep problems, is usually made more explicit with descriptions such as "difficulty falling asleep" or "difficulty staying asleep"; for example, impaired sleep (delayed onset of sleep) related to overstimulation prior to bedtime.

Various factors or etiologies may be involved and must be specified for the individual. These include physical discomfort or pain; anxiety about actual or anticipated loss of a loved one, loss of a job, loss of life due to serious disease process, or worry about a family member's behavior or illness; frequent changes in sleep time due to shift work or overtime; and changes in sleep environment or bedtime rituals (e.g., noisy environment, alcohol or other drug dependency, drug withdrawal, misuse of sedatives prescribed for insomnia, and effects of medications such as steroids or stimulants).

QSEN Patient-Centered Care: Sleep

When caring for a client in the home it is important to assess the client and the caregiver about their knowledge of sleep and wellness. Once the assessment is completed the nurse will develop appropriate teaching to augment the client and caregiver's knowledge. The client's sleep area should be assessed for environmental factors that can contribute to a lack of sleep. These factors include the mattress firmness, noise levels, a room that is too warm or too cold, or the use of electronics. When in the home care setting, remember to assess for the possibility of sleep disruption and deprivation in the caregiver. A sleep-deprived family member may be caring for a well-rested client. Respite care, where someone relieves the caregiver and cares for the client for a period of time, may be needed.

Sleep pattern disturbances may also be stated as the etiology of another diagnosis, in which case the nursing interventions are directed toward the sleep disturbance itself. Examples include:

Altered ability to cope related to insufficient quality and quantity of sleep, fatigue related to no restorative sleep pattern, alteration in tissue perfusion related to sleep apnea, insufficient knowledge (nonprescription remedies for sleep) related to lack of information, anxiety related to sleep apnea or the diagnosis of a sleep disorder, and impaired activity related to sleep deprivation or excessive daytime sleepiness.

Planning

The major goal for clients with sleep disturbances is to maintain (or develop) a sleeping pattern that provides sufficient energy for daily activities. Other goals may relate to enhancing the client's feeling of well-being or improving the quality and quantity of the client's sleep. The nurse plans specific nursing interventions to reach the goal based on the etiology of each nursing diagnosis. These interventions may include reducing environmental distractions, promoting bedtime rituals, providing comfort measures, scheduling nursing care to provide for uninterrupted sleep periods, and teaching stress reduction, relaxation techniques, and good sleep hygiene. Specific nursing activities associated with each of these interventions can be selected to meet the individual needs of the client. See the Nursing Care Plan and the Concept Map at the end of the chapter.

Implementing

The term **sleep hygiene** refers to interventions used to promote sleep. Nursing interventions to enhance the quantity and quality of clients' sleep involve largely nonpharmacologic measures. These involve health teaching about sleep habits, support of bedtime rituals, the provision of a restful environment, specific measures to promote comfort and relaxation, and appropriate use of hypnotic medications.

For hospitalized clients, sleep problems are often related to the hospital environment or their illness. Assisting the client to sleep in such instances can be challenging to a nurse, often involving scheduling activities, administering analgesics, and providing a supportive environment. Explanations and a supportive relationship are essential for the fearful or anxious client. Different types of hypnotics may be prescribed depending on the type of sleep problem (e.g., difficulties falling asleep or difficulties maintaining sleep). Drugs with longer half-lives are often prescribed for difficulties maintaining sleep, but must be used with caution in older adults.

Client Teaching

Healthy individuals need to learn the importance of sleep in maintaining active and productive lifestyles. They need to learn (a) the conditions that promote sleep and those that interfere with sleep, (b) safe use of sleep medications, (c) effects of other prescribed medications on sleep, (d) effects of their disease states on sleep, and (e) importance of long periods of uninterrupted sleep. Tips for promoting sleep are listed in Client Teaching.

Supporting Bedtime Rituals

Most individuals are accustomed to bedtime rituals or presleep routines that are conducive to comfort and relaxation. Altering or eliminating such routines can affect a client's sleep. Common prebedtime activities of adults include listening to music, reading, taking a soothing bath, and praying. Children need to be socialized into a presleep routine such as a bedtime story, holding onto a favorite toy or blanket, and kissing everyone goodnight. Sleep is also usually preceded by hygienic routines, such as washing the face and hands (or bathing), brushing the teeth, and voiding.

In institutional settings, nurses can provide similar bedtime rituals—assisting with a hand and face wash, providing a massage or hot drink, plumping pillows, and providing extra blankets as needed. Conversing about accomplishments of the day or enjoyable events such as visits from friends can also help to relax clients and bring peace of mind.

Creating a Restful Environment

Everyone needs a sleeping environment with minimal noise, a comfortable room temperature, appropriate ventilation, and appropriate lighting. Although most individuals prefer a darkened environment, a lowlight source may

CLIENT TEACHING Promoting Sleep

SLEEP PATTERN

- If you have difficulty falling asleep or staying asleep, it is important to establish a regular bedtime and wake-up time for all days of the week to enhance your biological rhythm. A short daytime nap (e.g., 15 to 30 minutes), particularly among older adults, can be restorative and not interfere with nighttime sleep. A younger client with insomnia should not nap.
- Establish a regular, relaxing bedtime routine before sleep such as reading, listening to soft music, taking a warm bath, or doing some other quiet activity you enjoy.
- Avoid dealing with office work or family problems before bedtime.
- Get adequate exercise during the day to reduce stress, but avoid excessive physical exertion at least 3 hours before bedtime.
- Use the bed for sleep or sexual activity, so that you associate it with sleep. Take work material, computers, and TVs out of the bedroom. Lying awake, tossing and turning, will strengthen the association between wakefulness and lying in bed (many clients with insomnia report falling asleep in a chair or in front of the TV but having trouble falling asleep in bed).
- When you are unable to sleep, get out of bed, go into another room, and pursue some relaxing activity until you feel drowsy.

ENVIRONMENT

- Create a sleep-conducive environment that is dark, quiet, comfortable, and cool.
- Keep noise to a minimum; block out extraneous noise as necessary with white noise from a fan, air conditioner, or white noise machine. Music is not recommended because studies have shown that music will promote wakefulness (it is interesting and individuals will pay attention to it).
- Sleep on a comfortable mattress and pillows.

DIET

- Avoid heavy meals 2 to 3 hours before bedtime.
- Avoid alcohol and caffeine-containing foods and beverages (e.g., coffee, tea, chocolate) at least 4 hours before bedtime. Caffeine can interfere with sleep. Both caffeine and alcohol act as diuretics, creating the need to void during sleep time.
- If a bedtime snack is necessary, consume only light carbohydrates or a milk drink. Heavy or spicy foods can cause gastrointestinal upsets that disturb sleep.

MEDICATIONS

- Use sleeping medications only as a last resort. Use OTC medications sparingly because many contain antihistamines that cause daytime drowsiness.
- Take analgesics before bedtime to relieve aches and pains.
- Consult with your healthcare provider about adjusting other medications that may cause insomnia.

provide comfort for children or those in a strange environment. Infants and children need a quiet room usually separate from the parents' room, a light or warm blanket as appropriate, and a location away from open windows or drafts.

Environmental distractions such as environmental noises and staff communication noise are particularly troublesome for hospitalized clients. Environmental noises include the sound of paging systems, telephones, and call lights; monitors beeping; doors closing; elevator chimes; furniture squeaking; and linen carts being wheeled through corridors. Staff communication is a major factor creating noise, particularly at staff change of shift.

To create a restful environment, the nurse needs to reduce environmental distractions, reduce sleep interruptions, ensure a safe environment, and provide a room temperature that is satisfactory to the client. Some interventions to reduce environmental distractions, especially noise, are listed in Box 45.7.

BOX 45.7 Reducing Environmental Distractions in Hospitals

- Close window curtains if street lights shine through.
- Close curtains between clients in semiprivate and larger rooms.
- Reduce or eliminate overhead lighting; provide a night light at the bedside or in the bathroom.
- Use a flashlight to check drainage bags, the client's identification, dressings, and IV infusions, without turning on the overhead lights.
- Ensure a clear pathway around the bed to avoid bumping the bed and jarring the client during sleeping hours.
- Close the door of the client's room.
- Adhere to agency policy about times to turn off communal televisions or radios.
- Lower the ringtone of nearby telephones.
- Discontinue use of the paging system after a certain hour (e.g., 2100 hours) or reduce its volume.
- Keep required staff conversations at low levels; conduct nursing reports or other discussions in a separate area away from client rooms.
- Wear rubber-soled shoes.
- Ensure that all cart wheels are well oiled.
- Perform only essential noisy activities during sleeping hours.
- Make sure the bed linen is smooth, clean, and dry.
- Assist or encourage the client to void before bedtime.
- Offer to provide a back massage before sleep.
- Position dependent clients appropriately to aid muscle relaxation, and provide supportive devices to protect pressure areas.
- Schedule medications, especially diuretics, to prevent nocturnal awakenings.
- For clients who have pain, administer analgesics 30 minutes before sleep.
- Listen to the client's concerns and deal with problems as they arise.

The environment must also be safe so that the client can relax. Clients who are unaccustomed to narrow hospital beds may feel more secure with side rails.

Additional safety measures include:

- Placing beds in low positions.
- Using night lights.
- Placing call bells within easy reach.

Promoting Comfort and Relaxation

Comfort measures are essential to help the client fall asleep and stay asleep, especially if the effects of the client's illness interfere with sleep. A concerned, caring attitude, along with the following interventions, can significantly promote client comfort and sleep:

- Provide loose-fitting nightwear.
- Assist clients with hygienic routines.

Individuals of any age, but especially older adults, are unable to sleep well if they feel cold. Changes in circulation, metabolism, and body tissue density reduce the older adult's ability to generate and conserve heat. To compound this problem, hospital gowns have short sleeves and are made of thin polyester. Bed sheets also are often made of polyester rather than a warm fabric, such as cotton flannel. The following interventions can be used to keep older adults warm during sleep:

- Before the client goes to bed, warm the bed with prewarmed bath blankets.
- Use 100% cotton flannel sheets or apply thermal blankets between the sheet and bedspread.
- Encourage the client to wear own clothing, such as flannel nightgown or pajamas, socks, leg warmers, long underwear, sleeping cap (if scalp hair is sparse), or sweater, or use extra blankets.

Emotional stress obviously interferes with an individual's ability to relax, rest, and sleep, and inability to sleep further aggravates feelings of tension. Sleep rarely occurs until an individual is relaxed. Relaxation techniques can be encouraged as part of the nightly routine. Slow, deep breathing for a few minutes followed by slow, rhythmic contraction and relaxation of muscles can alleviate tension and induce calm. Imagery, meditation, and yoga can also be taught. These techniques are discussed in Chapter 19 ∞.

Enhancing Sleep with Medications

Sleep medications often prescribed on a prn (as-needed) basis for clients include the sedative–hypnotics, which induce sleep, and antianxiety drugs or tranquilizers, which decrease anxiety and tension. When prn sleep medications are ordered in institutional settings, the nurse is responsible for making decisions with the client about when to administer them. These medications should be administered only with complete knowledge of their actions and effects and only when indicated.

Both nurses and clients need to be aware of the actions, effects, and risks of the specific medication prescribed. Although medications vary in their activity and effects, considerations include the following:

- Sedative-hypnotic medications produce a general CNS depression and an unnatural sleep; REM or NREM sleep is altered to some extent, and daytime drowsiness and a morning hangover effect may occur. Some of the new hypnotics, such as zolpidem (Ambien), do not alter REM sleep or produce rebound insomnia when discontinued.
- Antianxiety medications decrease levels of arousal by facilitating the action of neurons in the CNS that suppress responsiveness to stimulation. These medications are contraindicated in pregnant women because of their associated risk of congenital anomalies, and in breastfeeding mothers because the medication is excreted in breast milk.
- Sleep medications vary in their onset and duration of action and will impair waking function as long as they are chemically active. Some medication effects can last many hours beyond the time that the client's perception of daytime drowsiness and impaired psychomotor skills have disappeared. Clients need to be cautioned about such effects and about driving or handling machinery while the drug is in their system.
- Sleep medications affect REM sleep more than NREM sleep. Clients need to be informed that one or two nights of increased dreaming (REM rebound) are usual after the drug is discontinued after long-term use.
- Initial doses of medications should be low and increases added gradually, depending on the client's response. Older adults, in particular, are susceptible to side effects because of their metabolic changes; they need to be closely monitored for changes in mental alertness and coordination. Clients need to be instructed to take the smallest effective dose and then only for a few nights or intermittently as required.
- Regular use of any sleep medication can lead to tolerance over time (e.g., 4 to 6 weeks) and rebound insomnia. In some instances, this may lead clients to increase the dosage. Clients must be cautioned about developing a pattern of drug dependency.
- Abrupt cessation of barbiturate sedative-hypnotics can create withdrawal symptoms such as restlessness, tremors, weakness, insomnia, increased heart rate, seizures, convulsions, and even death. Long-term users need to taper their medications under the supervision of a specialist.

About half of the clients who seek medical intervention for sleep problems are treated with sedative–hypnotics. Sometimes the prescription of hypnotics can be appropriate. For example, women with chronic difficulties maintaining sleep or nonrestorative sleep associated with menopausal symptoms often benefit by the prescription of 10 mg of zolpidem, a low dose that was documented to be both safe and efficacious in this population. Hypnotics are not appropriate if clients have any symptoms suggestive of sleep-related breathing disorders or decreased renal or hepatic function.

Table 45.1 presents some of the common medications used for enhancing sleep and the half-life of these medications. The half-life represents how long it takes for half of the medication to be metabolized and eliminated by the body; hence, those with shorter half-lives are less likely to cause residual drowsiness after administration, but may be less effective for the treatment of sleep maintenance insomnia.

Evaluating

Using data collected during care and the desired outcomes developed during the planning stage as a guide, the nurse judges whether client goals and outcomes have been achieved. Data collection may include (a) observations of the duration of the client's sleep, (b) questions about how the client feels on awakening, or (c) observations of the client's level of alertness during the day.

If the desired outcomes are not achieved, the nurse and client should explore the reasons, which may include answers to the following questions:

- Were etiologic factors correctly identified?
- Has the client's physical condition or medication therapy changed?
- Did the client comply with instructions about establishing a regular sleep–wake pattern?
- Did the client avoid ingesting caffeine?
- Did the client participate in stimulating daytime activities to avoid excessive daytime naps?
- Were all possible measures taken to provide a restful environment for the client?
- Were the comfort and relaxation measures effective?

TABLE 45.1 Selected Sedative–Hypnotic Medications Used for Insomnia

Medication	Half-Life (Hours)
Chloral hydrate (Noctec)	8–11
Eszopiclone (Lunesta)	5–6
Flurazepam (Dalmane)	47–100
Lorazepam (Ativan)	10–20
Melatonin	1
Temazepam (Restoril)	8–24
Triazolam (Halcion)	2–3
Zaleplon (Sonata)	1
Zolpidem (Ambien)	2.5

DRUG CAPSULE

Non-Benzodiazepine Sedative-Hypnotics: zolpidem (Ambien)

THE CLIENT WITH MEDICATIONS THAT AFFECT SLEEP OR ALERTNESS

Zolpidem is used for the short-term (7- to 10-day) management of insomnia. The medication is used to reduce sleep latency and awakenings, and to lengthen sleep durations. Unlike traditional benzodiazepine sedative-hypnotics, zolpidem does not reduce REM sleep durations or cause rebound insomnia when it is discontinued. At therapeutic doses, it causes little or no respiratory depression, and it has a low potential for abuse. Clients using it for short periods have not demonstrated tolerance, physical dependence, or withdrawal symptoms. It has a rapid onset of action and a half-life of 2.5 hours.

NURSING RESPONSIBILITIES

- The drug has a rapid onset of action, so it should not be given until just prior to bedtime in order to minimize sedation while awake.
- Clients should be monitored for side effects (e.g., daytime drowsiness and dizziness). Older clients and those with hepatic insufficiency should start with a lower dose (e.g., 5 mg).
- According to the American Geriatrics Society Beers Criteria (2019), the administration of zolpidem to older adults can place the client at risk for falls; avoid the administration of zolpidem unless safer alternatives are not available.

CLIENT AND FAMILY TEACHING

- Clients should be cautioned that zolpidem can intensify the actions of other CNS depressants and warned against combining zolpidem with alcohol and all other drugs that depress CNS function.
- Clients should be cautioned not to take this medication until they are ready to go to bed because of its rapid onset of action. Some clients may engage in activities such as driving and eating with no memory of having participated in those activities.

Central Nervous System Stimulant modafinil (Provigil)

Modafinil has been approved by the FDA for the treatment of narcolepsy, excessive daytime sleepiness associated with obstructive sleep apnea, and shift-work sleep disorder. Because the drug does not alter the function of the dopamine neurotransmitter system, modafinil lacks the addictive potential of traditional stimulants. The drug alters mood, perception, and thinking. The onset of action is rapid and reaches peak plasma levels in 2 to 4 hours. It has a long half-life (approximately 15 hours) and thus can usually be administered only once a day (in the morning). It does not interfere with sleep at night.

NURSING RESPONSIBILITIES

- Monitor the client for side effects, particularly if the client is older or has hepatic dysfunction. Side effects are rare and usually consist of headache, nausea, and nervousness.
- If the client has obstructive sleep apnea, ensure that the client continues to use nasal CPAP.

CLIENT AND FAMILY TEACHING

- Explain that modafinil is not a substitute for obtaining adequate amounts of sleep. Any client with the diagnosis of narcolepsy, obstructive sleep apnea, or shift-work sleep disorder needs to obtain adequate amounts of sleep in addition to taking prescribed medications.
- Caution clients with obstructive sleep apnea that it is very important to continue using nasal CPAP and that modafinil is being prescribed only to reduce excessive daytime sleepiness and will not reduce the number of apneic episodes during sleep.
- Modafinil may accelerate the metabolism of oral contraceptives, leading to lower plasma levels. Women using low-dose birth control pills may want to consider switching birth control methods or adding a second type of birth control.

Note: Prior to administering any medication, review all aspects with a current drug handbook or other reliable source.

NURSING CARE PLAN **Sleep**

ASSESSMENT DATA	NURSING DIAGNOSIS	DESIRED OUTCOMES*
NURSING ASSESSMENT Jack Harrison is a 36-year-old police officer assigned to a high-crime police precinct. One week ago he received a surface bullet wound to his arm. Today he arrives at the outpatient clinic to have the wound redressed. While speaking with the nurse, Mr. Harrison mentions that he has recently been promoted to the rank of detective and has assumed new responsibilities. He states that since his promotion, he has experienced increasing difficulty falling asleep and sometimes staying asleep. He expresses concern over the danger of his occupation and his desire to do well in his new position. He complains of waking up feeling tired and irritable.	Impaired sleep related to anxiety (as evidenced by difficulty falling and remaining asleep, fatigue, and irritability)	**Sleep** [0004] as evidenced by: • No compromise in sleeping through the night consistently • No compromise in feeling rejuvenated after sleep • No dependence on sleep aids

Continued on page 1182

NURSING CARE PLAN Sleep—*continued*

ASSESSMENT DATA		NURSING DIAGNOSIS	DESIRED OUTCOMES*
Physical Examination Height: 185.4 cm (6′2″) Weight: 85.7 kg (189 lb) Temperature: 37.0°C (98.6°F) Pulse: 80 beats/min Respirations: 18/min Blood pressure: 144/88 mmHg	**Diagnostic Data** CBC within normal range, x-ray left arm: evidence of superficial soft tissue injury		

NURSING INTERVENTIONS*/SELECTED ACTIVITIES	RATIONALE
SLEEP ENHANCEMENT [1850]	
Determine the client's sleep and activity pattern.	*The amount of sleep an individual needs varies with lifestyle, health, and age.*
Encourage Mr. Harrison to establish a bedtime routine to facilitate transition from wakefulness to sleep.	*Rituals and routines induce comfort, relaxation, and sleep.*
Encourage him to eliminate stressful situations before bedtime.	*Stress interferes with an individual's ability to relax, rest, and sleep.*
Instruct Mr. Harrison and significant others about factors (e.g., physiologic, psychologic, lifestyle, frequent work shift changes, excessively long work hours, and other environmental factors) that contribute to sleep pattern disturbances.	*Knowledge of causative factors can enable the client to begin to control factors that inhibit sleep.*
Discuss with Mr. Harrison and his family comfort measures, sleep-promoting techniques, and lifestyle changes that can contribute to optimal sleep.	*Knowledge of factors that affect sleep enables the client to implement changes in lifestyle and prebedtime activities.*
Monitor bedtime food and beverage intake for items that facilitate or interfere with sleep.	*Milk and protein foods contain tryptophan, a precursor of serotonin, which is thought to induce and maintain sleep. Stimulants should be avoided because they inhibit sleep.*
Discuss specific situations or individuals that threaten Mr. Harrison or his family.	*Fear is reduced when the reality of a situation is confronted in a safe environment. Awareness of factors that cause intensification of fears enhances control.*
Assist him to use coping responses that have been successful in the past.	*Feelings of safety and security increase when a client identifies previously successful ways of dealing with anxiety-provoking or fearful situations.*
ANXIETY REDUCTION [5820]	
Create an atmosphere to facilitate trust.	*Trust is an essential first step in the therapeutic relationship.*
Seek to understand Mr. Harrison's perspective of a stressful situation.	*Anxiety is a feeling aroused by a vague, nonspecific threat. Identifying the client's perspective will facilitate planning for the best approach to anxiety reduction.*
Encourage verbalization of feelings, perceptions, and fears.	*Open expression of feelings facilitates identification of specific emotions such as anger or helplessness, distorted perceptions, and unrealistic fears.*
Determine the client's decision-making ability.	*Maladaptive coping mechanisms are characterized by an inability to make decisions and choices.*

EVALUATION

Outcome met. Mr. Harrison acknowledges his insomnia is a somatic expression of his anxiety regarding job promotion and fear of failing. He states that talking with the police department counselor has been helpful. He is practicing relaxation techniques each night and sleeps an average of 7 hours a night. Mr. Harrison expresses a feeling of being rested on awakening.

*The NOC # for desired outcomes and the NIC # for nursing interventions are listed in brackets following the appropriate outcome or intervention. Outcomes, interventions, and activities selected are only a sample of those suggested by NOC and NIC and should be further individualized for each client.

APPLYING CRITICAL THINKING

1. What further information would be helpful to obtain from Mr. Harrison about his sleep problem?
2. What suggestions can you make that may help him develop better sleep habits?
3. What are the most common problems that interfere with clients' ability to sleep?

Answers to Applying Critical Thinking questions are available on the faculty resources site. Please consult with your instructor.

CONCEPT MAP

Sleep

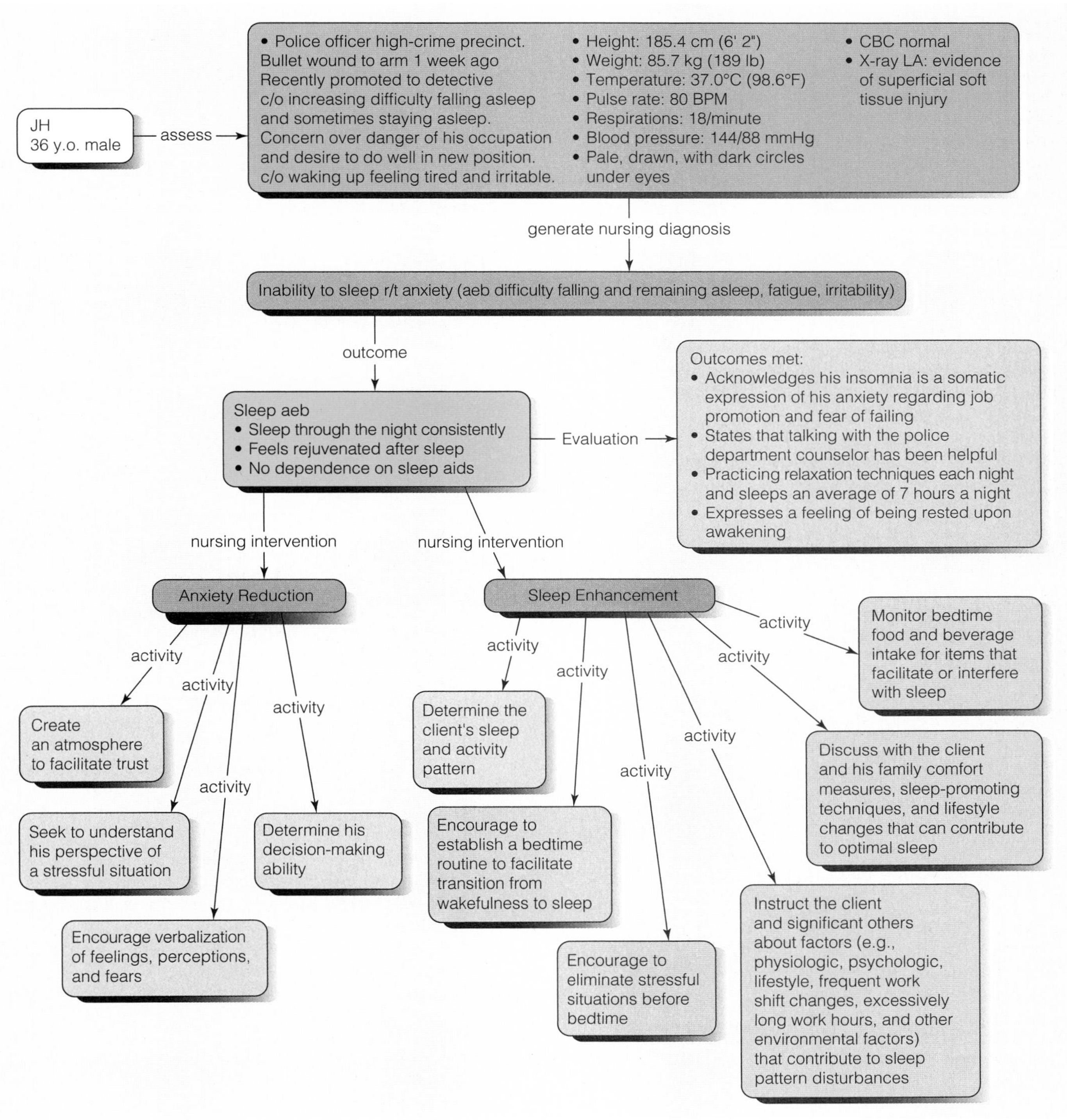

Chapter 45 Review

CHAPTER HIGHLIGHTS

- Sleep is needed for optimal psychologic and physiologic functioning.
- Insufficient sleep is widespread among all age groups in this country. Approximately 50 million to 70 million Americans suffer from a chronic disorder of sleep and wakefulness that hinders daily functioning and adversely affects health. Reports from government agencies have stated that sleep disorders and sleep deprivation are an unmet public health problem.
- Sleep is a naturally occurring altered state of consciousness in which an individual's perception and reaction to the environment are decreased.
- The sleep cycle is controlled by specialized areas in the brainstem and is affected by the individual's circadian rhythm.
- NREM sleep consists of three stages, progressing from stage 1, very light sleep, to stage 3, deep sleep. NREM sleep dominates during naps and nocturnal sleep periods. NREM sleep is essential for physiologic well-being.
- REM sleep recurs about every 90 minutes and is often associated with dreaming. REM sleep is essential for psychosocial and mental equilibrium.
- During a normal night's sleep, an adult has four to six sleep cycles, each with NREM (quiet sleep) and REM (rapid-eye-movement) sleep.
- The ratio of NREM to REM sleep varies with age.
- Many factors can affect sleep, including illness, environment, lifestyle, emotional stress, stimulants and alcohol, diet, smoking, motivation, and medications.
- Common sleep disorders include insomnia, hypersomnia, narcolepsy, parasomnias (such as somnambulism, sleeptalking, and bruxism), and sleep apnea.
- Assessment of a client's sleep includes a sleep history, a health history, and a physical examination to detect signs that may indicate the presence of sleep apnea.
- Nursing responsibilities to help clients sleep include (a) teaching clients ways to enhance sleep, (b) supporting bedtime rituals, (c) creating a restful environment, (d) promoting comfort and relaxation, and (e) enhancing sleep with medications.

TEST YOUR KNOWLEDGE

1. A client is admitted for a sleep disorder. The nurse knows that the reticular activating system (RAS) is involved in the sleep–wake cycle. In the accompanying illustration, which letter indicates the location of the RAS?

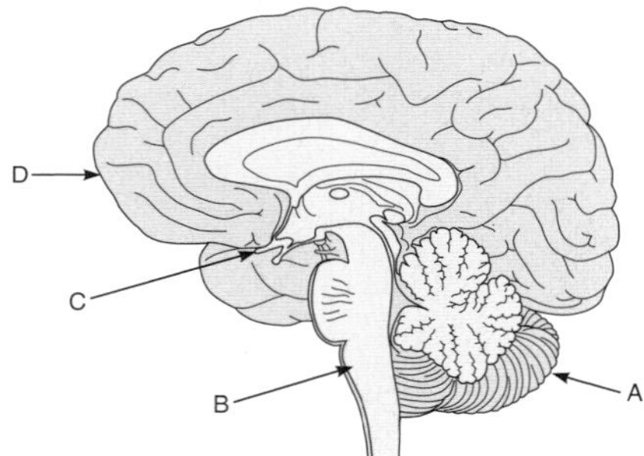

1. A
2. B
3. C
4. D

2. A nurse is admitting a critically ill client to the intensive care unit. What questions should the nurse ask regarding this client's sleep history?

1. No questions should be asked.
2. When do you usually go to sleep?
3. Do you have any problems with sleeping?
4. What are your bedtime rituals?

3. A nurse is working with a client to develop an expected outcome for the nursing diagnosis *Disturbed Sleep Pattern*, difficulty staying asleep related to anxiety secondary to multiple life stressors. Which expected outcome would be most applicable to this client's situation?

1. The client will sleep at least 8 hours each night.
2. The client will list three positive coping mechanisms for anxiety relief.
3. The client will report getting sufficient sleep to provide energy for daily activities.
4. The client will manifest less anxiety after taking prescribed medications.

4. A client reports to the nurse that she has been taking barbiturate sleeping pills every night for several months and now wishes to stop taking them. Which statement is the most appropriate advice for the nurse to provide the client?

1. Take the last pill on a Friday night so disrupted sleep can be compensated on the weekend.
2. Continue to take the pills since sleeping without them after such a long time will be difficult and perhaps impossible.
3. Discontinue taking the pills.
4. Continue taking the pills and discuss tapering the dose with the primary care provider.

5. During a well-child visit, a mother tells the nurse that her 4-year-old daughter typically goes to bed at 10:30 P.M. and awakens each morning at 7 A.M. She does not take a nap in the afternoon. Which is the best response by the nurse?
   1. Encourage the mother to consider putting her daughter to bed between 8 and 9 P.M.
   2. Reassure the mother that it is normal for 4-year-olds to resist napping, but encourage her to insist that she rest quietly each afternoon.
   3. Recommend that her daughter be allowed to sleep later in the morning.
   4. Reassure her that her daughter's sleep pattern is normal and that she has outgrown her need for an afternoon nap.
6. A client complains of being unable to stay awake during the day even after sleeping throughout the night. What should the nurse suggest to this client?
   1. Go to your physician for a physical examination.
   2. Go to a mental health professional for evaluation of possible depression.
   3. Purchase an over-the-counter sleep aid to deepen nighttime sleep.
   4. Drink more caffeinated beverages in the daytime to stay awake.
7. During a yearly physical, a 52-year-old male client mentions that his wife frequently complains about his snoring. During the physical exam, the nurse notes that his neck size is 18 inches, his soft palate and uvula are reddened and swollen, and he is overweight. What is the most appropriate nursing intervention for the nurse to recommend to this client?
   1. Recommend that he and his wife sleep in separate bedrooms so that his snoring does not disturb his wife.
   2. Refer him to a dietitian for a weight-loss program.
   3. Caution him not to drink or take sleeping pills since they may make his snoring worse.
   4. Refer him to a sleep disorders center for evaluation and treatment of his symptoms.
8. A new nursing graduate's first job requires 12-hour night shifts. Which strategy will make it easier for the graduate to sleep during the day and remain awake at night?
   1. Wear dark wraparound sunglasses when driving home in the morning, and sleep in a darkened bedroom.
   2. Exercise on the way home to avoid having to stand around waiting for equipment at the gym.
   3. Drink several cups of strong coffee or 16 oz of caffeinated soda when beginning the shift.
   4. Try to stay in a brightly lit area when working at night.
9. The nurse is answering questions after a presentation on sleep at a local seniors' center. A woman in her late 70s asks for an opinion about the advisability of allowing her husband to nap for 15 to 20 minutes each afternoon. Which is the nurse's best response?
   1. "Taking an afternoon nap will interfere with his being able to sleep at night. If he's tired in the afternoon, see if you can interest him in some type of stimulating activity to keep him awake."
   2. "He shouldn't need to take an afternoon nap if he's getting enough sleep at night."
   3. "Unless your husband has trouble falling asleep at night, a brief afternoon nap is fine."
   4. "Encourage him to consume coffee or some other caffeinated beverage at lunch to prevent drowsiness in the afternoon."
10. During admission to a hospital unit, the client tells the nurse that her sleep tends to be very light and that it is difficult for her to get back to sleep if she's awakened at night. Which interventions should the nurse implement? Select all that apply.
    1. Remind colleagues to keep their conversation to a minimum at night.
    2. Encourage the client's family members to bring in a radio to play soft music at night.
    3. Deliver necessary medications and procedures at 1.5- or 3-hour intervals between 11 P.M. and 6 A.M.
    4. Encourage the client to ask family members to bring in a fan to provide white noise.
    5. Increase the temperature in the room.

See Answers to Test Your Knowledge in Appendix A.

READINGS AND REFERENCES

Suggested Readings

Matre, D., Andersen, M. R., Knardahl, S., & Nilsen, K. B. (2016). Conditioned pain modulation is not decreased after partial sleep restriction. *European Journal of Pain*, *20*, 408–416. doi:10.1002/ejp.741

Sleep difficulties contribute to chronic pain conditions. The study determined if sleep restriction affects heat pain perception and conditioned pain response. The results of the study revealed that sleep restriction leads to increased heat pain perception.

Pallesen, S., Gundersen, H. S., Kristoffersen, M., Bjorvatn, B., Thun, E., & Harris, A. (2017). The effects of sleep deprivation on soccer skills. *Perceptual and Motor Skills*, *124*, 812–829. doi:10.1177/0031512517707412

The study examined the effects of sleep deprivation on an athlete's soccer skills. The study results revealed a negative effect of sleep deprivation on the continuous kick test.

Related Research

Louis, J., & Street, L. (2018). Obstructive sleep apnea in pregnancy—what you need to know: Sleep disordered breathing has implications for both mother and fetus. *Contemporary OB/GYN*, *63*(2), 18–22.

Taheri, M., & Irandoust, K. (2018). The exercise induced weight loss improves self-reported quality of sleep in obese elderly women with sleep disorders. *Sleep and Hypnosis*, *20*(1), 54–59. doi:10.5350/Sleep.Hypn.2017.19.0134

References

American Geriatrics Society. (2019). American Geriatics Society 2019 updated AGS Beers Criteria for potentially inappropriate medication use in older adults. *Journal of American Geriatrics Society*, *67*(4), 674–694. doi:10.1111/jgs.15767

Bonuck, K. A., Blank, A., True-Felt, B., & Chervin, R. (2016). Promoting sleep health among families of young children in Head Start: Protocol for a social-ecological approach. *Preventing Chronic Disease*, *13*, 160144. doi.org/10.5888/pcd13.160144

Butcher, H. K., Bulechek, G. M., Dochterman, J. M., & Wagner, C. M. (Eds.). (2018). *Nursing interventions classification (NIC)* (7th ed.). St. Louis, MO: Elsevier.

Centers for Disease Control and Prevention. (2018). *Sleep and sleep disorders*. Retrieved from https://www.cdc.gov/sleep/index.html

Corkin, M., Peterson, E., Andrejic, N., Waldie, K., Reese, E., & Morton, S. (2017). Predicators of mothers' self-identified challenges in parenting infants: Insights from a large, nationally diverse cohort. *Journal of Child and Family Studies*, *27*, 653–670. doi:10.1007/s10826-017-0903-5

Cowie, J., Palmer, C., Hussain, H., & Alfano, C. (2016). Parental involvement in infant sleep routines predicts differential sleep patterns in children with and without anxiety disorders. *Child Psychiatry & Human Development*, *47*, 636–646. doi:10.1007/s10578-015-0597-0

Frandsen, G., & Pennington, S. (2018). *Abrams' clinical drug therapy rationales for nursing practice* (11th ed.). Philadelphia, PA: Lippincott Williams & Wilkins.

Graff-Radford, J. (2017). *Sundowning: Late day confusion*. Retrieved from https://www.mayoclinic.org/diseases-conditions/alzheimers-disease/expert-answers/sundowning/faq-20058511

Judd, B. G., & Sateia, M. J. (2019). Classification of sleep disorders. Retrieved from https://www.uptodate.com/contents/classification-of-sleep-disorders

Krieger, L. (2017). Better sleep A to Z. *Good Housekeeping*, *264*(3), 107–112.

Liu, Y., Croft, J. B., Wheaton, A. G., Kanny, D., Cunningham, T. J., Lu, H., . . . Giles, W. H. (2016). Clustering of five health-related behaviors for chronic disease prevention among adults, United States, 2013. *Preventing Chronic Disease*, *13*, 160054. doi:10.5888/pcd13.160054

Martens, M. A., Seyfer, D. L., Andridge, R. R., & Coury, D. L. (2017). Use and effectiveness of sleep medications by parent report in individuals with Williams syndrome. *Journal of Developmental & Behavioral Pediatrics*, *38*(9), 765–771. doi:10.1097/DBP.0000000000000503

Miller, N. (2015). Sleep deprivation and delirium risk in hospitalized patients. *Nursing Made Incredibly Easy*, *13*(1), 22–28. doi:10.1097/01.NME.0000457284.31841.36

Morgenthaler, T. I., Hashmi, S., Croft, J. B., Dort, L., Heald, J., & Mullington, J. (2016). High school start times and the impact on high school students: What we know, and what we hope to learn. *Journal of Clinical Seep Medicine*, *12*(12), 1681–1689. doi:10.5664/jcsm.6358

National Sleep Foundation. (n.d.). *Stages of human sleep.* Retrieved from http://sleepdisorders.sleepfoundation.org/chapter-1-normal-sleep/stages-of-human-sleep

National Sleep Foundation. (n.d.a). *Children and sleep.* Retrieved from https://www.sleepfoundation.org/articles/children-and-sleep

National Sleep Foundation. (n.d.b). *How much sleep do adults really need?* Retrieved from https://sleep.org/articles/how-much-sleep-adults/

National Sleep Foundation. (n.d.c). *How much sleep do babies and kids need?* Retrieved from https://sleepfoundation.org/excessivesleepiness/content/how-much-sleep-do-babies-and-kids-need

National Sleep Foundation. (n.d.d). *Improve your memory with a good night's sleep.* Retrieved from https://sleepfoundation.org/excessivesleepiness/content/improve-your-memory-good-nights-sleep

National Sleep Foundation. (n.d.e). *Insomnia and women.* Retrieved from https://sleepfoundation.org/insomnia/content/insomnia-women

National Sleep Foundation. (n.d.f). *Insomnia: Symptoms.* Retrieved from https://sleepfoundation.org/insomnia/content/symptoms

National Sleep Foundation. (n.d.g). *Myths and facts about sleep.* Retrieved from https://sleepfoundation.org/how-sleep-works/myths-and-facts-about-sleep/page/0/1

National Sleep Foundation. (n.d.h). *Sleeping during the day: Is it OK?* Retrieved from http://sleep.org/articles/sleeping-during-the-day/

National Sleep Foundation. (n.d.i). *What is insomnia?* Retrieved from https://sleepfoundation.org/insomnia/content/what-is-insomnia

Owens, B., Allen, W., & Moultrie, D. (2017). The impact of shift work on nurses' quality of sleep. *ABNF Journal*, *28*(3), 59–63.

Owens, J., Adolescent Sleep Working Group, & Committee on Adolescence. (2014). Insufficient sleep in adolescents and young adults: An update on causes and consequences. *Pediatrics*, *134*(3), e921–e932. doi:10.1542/peds.2014-1696

Ozdemir, P. G., & Atilla, E. (2017). A supportive therapeutic and diagnostic modality: sleep deprivation. *Sleep and Hypnosis*, *19*(3), 78–79. doi:10.5350/Sleep.Hypn.2016.18.0121

Richards, K., Demartini, J., & Xiong, G. (2018). Understanding sleep disorders in older adults. *Psychiatric Times*, *35*(2), 17–20.

Schweizer, A., Berchtold, A., Barrense-Dias, Y., Akre, C., & Suris, J. C. (2017). Adolescents with a smartphone sleep less than their peers. *European Journal of Pediatrics*, *176*, 131–136. doi:10.1007/s00431-016-2823-6

Selvi, Y., Kilic, S., Aydin, A., & Guzel Oxdemir, G. (2015). The effects of sleep deprivation on dissociation and profiles of mood, and its association with biochemical changes. *Archives of Neuropsychiatry*, *52*(1), 83–88. doi:10.5152/npa.2015.7116

Sleep.org. (n.d.). *What is the sleep/wake cycle?* Retrieved from https://sleep.org/articles/sleepwake-cycle/

Vincensi, B., Pearce, K., Redding, J., Brandonisio, S., Tzou, S., & Meiusi, E. (2016). Sleep in the hospitalized patient: Nurse and patient perceptions. *MedSurg Nursing*, *25*(5), 351–356.

Wheaton, A. G., Jones, S. E., Cooper, A. C., & Croft, J. B. (2018). Short sleep duration among middle school and high school students—United States, 2015. *Morbidity and Mortality Weekly Report*, *67*(3), 85–90.

Selected Bibliography

Amyx, M., Xiong, X., Xie, Y., & Buekens, P. (2017). Racial/ethnic differences in sleep disorders and reporting trouble sleeping among women of childbearing age in the United States. *Maternal Child Health Journal*, *21*, 306–314. doi:10.1007/s10995-016-2115-9

Boivin, D. B. (2017). Treating delayed sleep–wake phase disorder in young adults. *Journal of Psychiatry & Neuroscience*, *42*(5), E9–E10. doi:10.1503/jpn.160243

Ozcan, E., Aydin, E. F., & Ozcan, H. (2017). Paroxysmal nocturnal sleep disorder with atypic clinical appearance and therapy with sleep hygiene: A case report. *Sleep and Hypnosis*, *19*(1), 18–20. doi:10.5350/Sleep.Hypn.2016.18.0114

Pruitt, B. (2015). PTSD's effect on sleep and sleep disorders. *The Journal of Respiratory Care Practitioners*, *28*(5), 19–22.

Tokizawa, K., Sawada, S., Tetsuo, L., & Jian, L. (2015). Effects of partial sleep restriction and subsequent daytime napping on prolonged exertional heat strain. *Occupational and Environmental Medicine*, *72*(7), 521–528. doi:10.1136/oemed-2014-102548

Nutrition 46

LEARNING OUTCOMES

After completing this chapter, you will be able to:

1. Identify essential nutrients and their dietary sources.
2. Describe normal digestion, absorption, and metabolism of carbohydrates, proteins, and lipids.
3. Identify factors influencing nutrition.
4. Identify nutritional variations throughout the lifecycle.
5. Evaluate a diet using a food guide.
6. Discuss essential components and purposes of nutritional assessment and nutritional screening.
7. Identify risk factors for and clinical signs of malnutrition.
8. Describe nursing interventions to promote optimal nutrition.
9. Discuss nursing interventions to treat clients with nutritional problems.
10. Verbalize the steps used in:
    a. Inserting a nasogastric tube.
    b. Removing a nasogastric tube.
    c. Administering a tube feeding.
    d. Administering a gastrostomy or jejunostomy tube feeding.
11. Recognize when it is appropriate to assign aspects of feeding clients to assistive personnel.
12. Plan, implement, and evaluate nursing care associated with nursing diagnoses related to nutritional problems.
13. Demonstrate appropriate documentation and reporting of nutritional therapy.

KEY TERMS

24-hour food recall, *1208*
anabolism, *1189*
anemia, *1195*
anorexia nervosa, *1197*
basal metabolic rate (BMR), *1191*
body mass index (BMI), *1191*
bottle mouth syndrome, *1196*
bulimia, *1197*
caloric value, *1191*
calorie, *1191*
catabolism, *1189*
cholesterol, *1189*
complete proteins, *1188*
demand feeding, *1195*
diet history, *1208*
disaccharides, *1188*
dysphagia, *1193*
enteral, *1213*
enzymes, *1188*
essential amino acids, *1188*
fad, *1192*
fat-soluble vitamins, *1190*
fats, *1189*
fatty acids, *1189*
food diary, *1208*
food frequency record, *1208*
gastrostomy, *1217*
glycerides, *1189*
glycogen, *1188*
ideal body weight (IBW), *1191*
incomplete proteins, *1189*
iron deficiency anemia, *1195*
jejunostomy, *1217*
kilojoule (kJ), *1191*
large calorie (Calorie, kilocalorie [Kcal]), *1191*
lipids, *1189*
lipoproteins, *1190*
macrominerals, *1190*
macronutrients, *1188*
malnutrition, *1202*
metabolism, *1191*
microminerals, *1190*
micronutrients, *1188*
mid-arm circumference (MAC), *1205*
mid-arm muscle area (MAMA), *1205*
minerals, *1190*
monosaccharides, *1188*
monounsaturated fatty acids, *1189*
nasoenteric (nasointestinal) tube, *1217*
nasogastric tube, *1213*
nitrogen balance, *1189*
nonessential amino acids, *1188*
nutrients, *1187*
nutrition, *1187*
nutritive value, *1187*
obese, *1202*
oils, *1189*
overnutrition, *1202*
overweight, *1202*
percutaneous endoscopic gastrostomy (PEG), *1217*
percutaneous endoscopic jejunostomy (PEJ), *1217*
polysaccharides, *1188*
polyunsaturated fatty acids, *1189*
protein-calorie malnutrition (PCM), *1203*
pureed diet, *1210*
refeeding syndrome, *1219*
regurgitation, *1195*
resting energy expenditure (REE), *1191*
saturated fatty acids, *1189*
skinfold measurement, *1205*
small calorie (c, cal), *1191*
triglycerides, *1189*
undernutrition, *1203*
unsaturated fatty acid, *1189*
urea, *1206*
vitamin, *1190*
water-soluble vitamins, *1190*

Introduction

Nutrition is the sum of all the interactions between an organism and the food it consumes. In other words, nutrition is what an individual eats and how the body uses it. **Nutrients** are organic and inorganic substances found in foods that are required for body functioning. Adequate food intake consists of a balance of nutrients: water, carbohydrates, proteins, fats, vitamins, and minerals. Foods differ greatly in their **nutritive value** (the nutrient content of a specified amount of food), and no one food provides all essential nutrients. Nutrients have three major functions: providing energy for body processes and movement, providing structural material for body tissues, and regulating body processes.

Essential Nutrients

The body's most basic nutrient need is water. Because every cell requires a continuous supply of fuel, the most important nutritional need, after water, is for nutrients that provide fuel, or energy. The energy-providing nutrients are carbohydrates, fats, and proteins. Hunger compels people to eat enough energy-providing nutrients to satisfy their energy needs. Carbohydrates, fats, protein, minerals, vitamins, and water are referred to as **macronutrients**, because they are needed in large amounts (e.g., hundreds of grams) to provide energy. **Micronutrients** are those vitamins and minerals that are required in small amounts (e.g., milligrams or micrograms) to metabolize the energy-providing nutrients.

Carbohydrates

Carbohydrates are composed of the elements carbon (C), hydrogen (H), and oxygen (O) and are of two basic types: simple carbohydrates (sugars) and complex carbohydrates (starches and fiber). Natural sources of carbohydrates also supply vital nutrients, such as protein, vitamins, and minerals that are not found in processed foods. Processed carbohydrate foods are relatively low in nutrients in relation to the large number of calories they contain. High-sugar-content (and solid fat) foods are referred to as "empty calories." In addition, alcoholic beverages contain significant amounts of carbohydrate, but very few nutrients and, thus, they are also empty calories.

Types of Carbohydrates

SUGARS

Sugars, the simplest of all carbohydrates, are water soluble and are produced naturally by both plants and animals. Sugars may be **monosaccharides** (single molecules) or **disaccharides** (double molecules). Of the three monosaccharides (glucose, fructose, and galactose), glucose is by far the most abundant simple sugar.

Most sugars are produced naturally by plants, especially fruits, sugar cane, and sugar beets. However, other sugars come from animal sources. For example, lactose, a combination of glucose and galactose, is found in animal milk. Processed or refined sugars (e.g., table sugar, molasses, and corn syrup) have been extracted and concentrated from natural sources.

Not all sugars have calories and not all sweeteners are sugars. Sugar substitutes are available from both natural and manufactured sources and have almost no calories. Often referred to as "artificial" sugar, noncaloric sweeteners including saccharin and aspartame are much sweeter than sugar by volume. Sugar alcohols such as erythritol and sorbitol are low in calories, do not contain ethanol (present in alcoholic beverages), and are often used in chewing gums. Some sweeteners are not easily categorized, such as the extract from the leaf of the stevia plant.

STARCHES

Starches are the insoluble, nonsweet forms of carbohydrate. They are **polysaccharides**; that is, they are composed of branched chains of dozens, sometimes hundreds, of glucose molecules. Like sugars, nearly all starches exist naturally in plants, such as grains, legumes, and potatoes. Other foods, such as cereals, breads, flour, and puddings, are processed from starches.

FIBER

Fiber, a complex carbohydrate derived from plants, supplies roughage, or bulk, to the diet. However, fiber cannot be digested by humans. This complex carbohydrate satisfies the appetite and helps the digestive tract to function effectively and eliminate waste. Fiber is present in the outer layer of grains, bran, and in the skin, seeds, and pulp of many vegetables and fruits.

Carbohydrate Digestion

Major enzymes of carbohydrate digestion include ptyalin (salivary amylase), pancreatic amylase, and the disaccharidases: maltase, sucrase, and lactase. **Enzymes** are biological catalysts that speed up chemical reactions. The desired end products of carbohydrate digestion are monosaccharides. Some simple sugars are already monosaccharides and require no digestion. Essentially, all monosaccharides are absorbed by the small intestine in healthy individuals.

Carbohydrate Metabolism

Carbohydrate metabolism is a major source of body energy. After the body breaks carbohydrates down into glucose, some glucose continues to circulate in the blood to maintain blood levels and to provide a readily available source of energy. The remainder is used as energy or stored. Insulin, a hormone secreted by the pancreas, enhances the transport of glucose into cells.

Storage and Conversion

Carbohydrates are stored either as glycogen or as fat. **Glycogen** is a large polymer (compound molecule) of glucose. Almost all body cells can store glycogen; however, most is stored in the liver and skeletal muscles, where it is available for conversion back into glucose. Glucose that cannot be stored as glycogen is converted to fat.

Proteins

Amino acids, organic molecules made up primarily of carbon, hydrogen, oxygen, and nitrogen, combine to form proteins. Every cell in the body contains some protein, and about three-quarters of body solids are proteins.

Amino acids are categorized as essential or nonessential. **Essential amino acids** are those that cannot be manufactured in the body and must be supplied as part of the protein ingested in the diet. Nine essential amino acids—histidine, isoleucine, leucine, lysine, methionine, phenylalanine, tryptophan, threonine, and valine—are necessary for tissue growth and maintenance. A tenth, arginine, appears to have a role in the immune system.

Nonessential amino acids are those that the body can manufacture. The body takes amino acids derived from the diet and reconstructs new ones from their basic elements. Nonessential amino acids include alanine, aspartic acid, cystine, glutamic acid, glycine, hydroxyproline, proline, serine, and tyrosine.

Proteins may be complete or incomplete. **Complete proteins** contain all of the essential amino acids plus many nonessential ones. Most animal proteins, including meats, poultry, fish, dairy products, and eggs, are complete proteins. Some animal proteins, however, contain less than the required amount of one or more essential amino acids and therefore cannot alone support continued growth. These proteins are sometimes referred to as *partially complete proteins*. Examples are gelatin, which has small amounts of tryptophan, and the milk protein casein, which has only a little arginine.

Incomplete proteins lack one or more essential amino acids (most commonly lysine, methionine, or tryptophan) and are usually derived from vegetables. If, however, an appropriate mixture of plant proteins is provided in the diet, a balanced ratio of essential amino acids can be achieved. For example, a combination of corn (low in tryptophan and lysine) and beans (low in methionine) is a complete protein. Such combinations of two or more vegetables are called *complementary proteins*. Another way to take full advantage of vegetable proteins is to eat them with a small amount of animal protein. Spaghetti with cheese, rice with pork, noodles with tuna, and cereal with milk are just a few examples of combining vegetable and animal proteins.

Protein Digestion

Digestion of protein foods begins in the stomach, where the enzyme *pepsin* breaks protein down into smaller units. However, most protein is digested in the small intestine. The pancreas secretes the proteolytic enzymes trypsin, chymotrypsin, and carboxypeptidase; glands in the intestinal wall secrete aminopeptidase and dipeptidase. These enzymes break protein down into smaller molecules and eventually into amino acids.

Storage

Amino acids are absorbed by active transport through the small intestine into the portal blood circulation. The liver uses amino acids to synthesize specific proteins (e.g., liver cells and the plasma proteins albumin, globulin, and fibrinogen). Plasma proteins are a storage medium that can rapidly be converted back into amino acids.

Other amino acids are transported to tissues and cells throughout the body where they are used to make protein for cell structures. In a sense, protein is stored as body tissue. The body cannot actually store excess amino acids for future use. However, a limited amount is available in the "metabolic pool" that exists because of the constant breakdown and buildup of the protein in body tissues.

Protein Metabolism

Protein metabolism includes three activities: **anabolism** (building tissue), **catabolism** (breaking down tissue), and maintaining nitrogen balance.

ANABOLISM

All body cells synthesize proteins from amino acids. The types of proteins formed depend on the characteristics of the cell and are controlled by its genes.

CATABOLISM

Because a cell can accumulate only a limited amount of protein, excess amino acids are degraded for energy or converted to fat. Protein degradation occurs primarily in the liver.

NITROGEN BALANCE

Because nitrogen is the element that distinguishes protein from lipids and carbohydrates, nitrogen balance reflects the status of protein nutrition in the body. **Nitrogen balance** is a measure of the degree of protein anabolism and catabolism; it is the net result of intake and loss of nitrogen. When nitrogen intake equals nitrogen output, a state of nitrogen balance exists.

Lipids

Lipids are organic substances that are greasy and insoluble in water but soluble in alcohol or ether. **Fats** are lipids that are solid at room temperature; **oils** are lipids that are liquid at room temperature. In common use, the terms *fats* and *lipids* are used interchangeably. Lipids have the same elements (carbon, hydrogen, and oxygen) as carbohydrates, but they contain a higher proportion of hydrogen.

Fatty acids, made up of carbon chains and hydrogen, are the basic structural units of most lipids. Fatty acids are described as saturated or unsaturated, according to the relative number of hydrogen atoms they contain. **Saturated fatty acids** are those in which all carbon atoms are filled to capacity (i.e., saturated) with hydrogen; an example is butyric acid, found in butter. An **unsaturated fatty acid** is one that could accommodate more hydrogen atoms than it currently does. It has at least two carbon atoms that are not attached to a hydrogen atom; instead, there is a double bond between the two carbon atoms. Fatty acids with one double bond are called **monounsaturated fatty acids**; those with more than one double bond (or many carbons not bonded to a hydrogen atom) are **polyunsaturated fatty acids**. An example of a polyunsaturated fatty acid is linoleic acid, found in vegetable oil.

Based on their chemical structure, lipids are classified as simple or compound. **Glycerides**, the simple lipids, are the most common form of lipids. They consist of a glycerol molecule with up to three fatty acids attached. **Triglycerides** (which have three fatty acids) account for more than 90% of the lipids in food and in the body. Triglycerides may contain saturated or unsaturated fatty acids. Saturated triglycerides are found in animal products, such as butter, and are usually solid at room temperature. Unsaturated triglycerides are usually liquid at room temperature and are found in plant products, such as olive oil and corn oil.

Cholesterol is a fatlike substance that is both produced by the body and found in foods of animal origin. Most of the body's cholesterol is synthesized in the liver; however, some is absorbed from the diet (e.g., from milk, egg yolk, and organ meats). Cholesterol is needed to create bile acids and to synthesize steroid hormones. Along with phospholipids, large quantities of cholesterol are present in cell membranes and other cell structures.

Lipid Digestion

Although chemical digestion of lipids begins in the stomach, they are digested mainly in the small intestine, primarily by bile, pancreatic lipase, and enteric lipase, an intestinal enzyme. The end products of lipid digestion are glycerol, fatty acids, and cholesterol. These are immediately reassembled inside the intestinal cells into triglycerides and cholesterol esters (cholesterol with a fatty acid attached to it), which are not water soluble. For these reassembled products to be transported and used, the small intestine and the liver must convert them into soluble compounds called lipoproteins. **Lipoproteins** are made up of various lipids and a protein.

Lipid Metabolism

Converting fat into usable energy occurs through the use of the enzyme hormone-sensitive lipase, which breaks down triglycerides in adipose cells, releasing glycerol and fatty acids into the blood. A pound of fat provides 3500 kilocalories. Fasting individuals will obtain most of their calories from fat metabolism, but some amount of carbohydrate or protein must also be used because the brain, nerves, and red blood cells require glucose. Only the glycerol molecules in fat can be converted to glucose.

Micronutrients

A **vitamin** is an organic compound that cannot be manufactured by the body and is needed in small quantities to catalyze metabolic processes. Thus, when vitamins are lacking in the diet, metabolic deficits result. Vitamins are generally classified as fat soluble or water soluble. **Water-soluble vitamins** include C and the B-complex vitamins: B_1 (thiamine), B_2 (riboflavin), B_3 (niacin or nicotinic acid), B_6 (pyridoxine), B_9 (folic acid, folate, folacin), B_{12} (cobalamin), pantothenic acid, and biotin. The body cannot store water-soluble vitamins; thus, people must get a daily supply in the diet. Water-soluble vitamins can be degraded by food processing, storage, and preparation.

Fat-soluble vitamins include A, D, E, and K. The body can store these vitamins, although there is a limit to the amounts of vitamins E and K the body can store. Therefore, a daily supply of fat-soluble vitamins is not absolutely necessary. Vitamin content is highest in fresh foods consumed soon after harvest.

Minerals are found in organic compounds, as inorganic compounds, and as free ions. Calcium and phosphorus make up 80% of all mineral elements in the body. The two categories of minerals are macrominerals and microminerals. **Macrominerals** are those that people require daily in amounts over 100 mg. They include calcium, phosphorus, sodium, potassium, magnesium, chloride, and sulfur. **Microminerals** are those that people require daily in amounts less than 100 mg. They include iron, zinc, manganese, iodine, fluoride, copper, cobalt, chromium, and selenium.

Common problems associated with the mineral nutrients are iron deficiency resulting in anemia, and osteoporosis resulting from loss of bone calcium. Additional information about major minerals associated with the body's fluid and electrolyte balance is given in Chapter 51 ∞.

ANATOMY & PHYSIOLOGY REVIEW

Digestive System

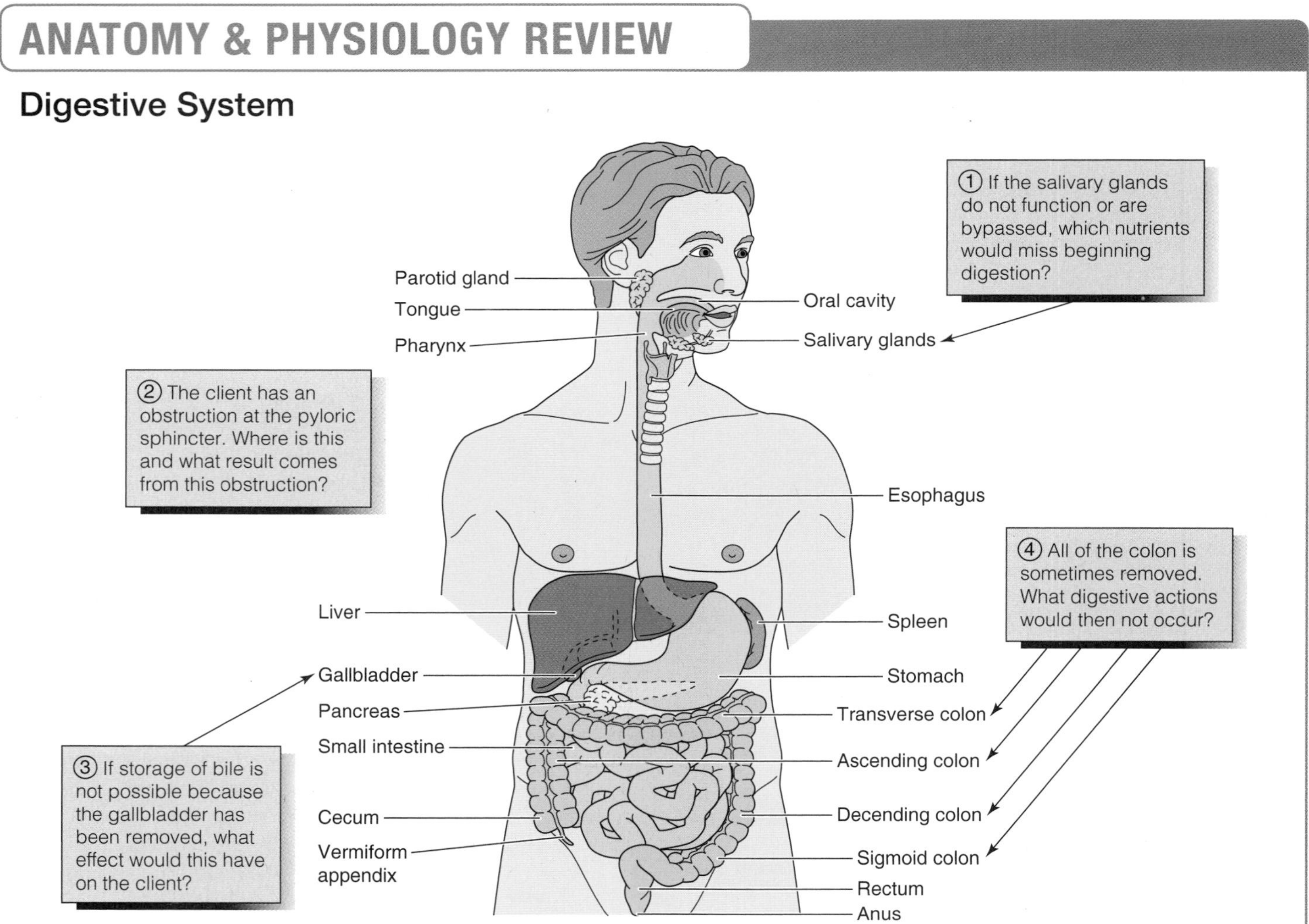
Parotid gland
Tongue
Pharynx
Oral cavity
Salivary glands
① If the salivary glands do not function or are bypassed, which nutrients would miss beginning digestion?
② The client has an obstruction at the pyloric sphincter. Where is this and what result comes from this obstruction?
Esophagus
④ All of the colon is sometimes removed. What digestive actions would then not occur?
Liver
Spleen
Gallbladder
Stomach
Pancreas
Transverse colon
Small intestine
Ascending colon
③ If storage of bile is not possible because the gallbladder has been removed, what effect would this have on the client?
Cecum
Decending colon
Vermiform appendix
Sigmoid colon
Rectum
Anus

Answers to Anatomy & Physiology Review questions are available on the faculty resources site. Please consult with your instructor.

Energy Balance

Energy balance is the relationship between the energy derived from food and the energy used by the body. The body obtains energy in the form of calories from carbohydrates, protein, fat, and alcohol. The body uses energy for voluntary activities such as walking and talking and for involuntary activities such as breathing and secreting enzymes. An individual's energy balance is determined by comparing his or her energy intake with energy output.

Energy Intake

The amount of energy that nutrients or foods supply to the body is their **caloric value**. A **calorie** is a unit of heat energy. A **small calorie (c, cal)** is the amount of heat required to raise the temperature of 1 gram of water 1 degree Celsius. This unit of measure is used in chemistry and physics. A **large calorie (Calorie, kilocalorie [Kcal])** is the amount of heat energy required to raise the temperature of 1 gram of water 15 to 16 degrees Celsius and is the unit used in nutrition (although it is not universally capitalized). In the metric system, the measure is the **kilojoule (kJ)**. One Calorie (Kcal) equals 4.18 kilojoules.

The energy liberated from the metabolism of food has been determined to be:

- 4 Calories/gram (17 kJ) of carbohydrates
- 4 Calories/gram (17 kJ) of protein
- 9 Calories/gram (38 kJ) of fat
- 7 Calories/gram (29 kJ) of alcohol.

Energy Output

Metabolism refers to all biochemical and physiologic processes by which the body grows and maintains itself. Metabolic rate is normally expressed in terms of the rate of heat liberated during these chemical reactions. The **basal metabolic rate (BMR)** is the rate at which the body metabolizes food to maintain the energy requirements of an individual who is awake and at rest. The energy in food maintains the basal metabolic rate of the body and provides energy for activities such as running and walking.

Resting energy expenditure (REE) is the amount of energy required to maintain basic body functions; in other words, the calories required to maintain life. The REE of healthy individuals is generally about 1 cal/kg of body weight/h for men and 0.9 cal/kg/h for women although there is great variation among individuals. BMR is calculated by measuring the REE in the early morning, 12 hours after eating.

The actual daily expenditure of energy depends on the degree of activity of the individual. Some activities require many times the REE. Examples of approximate real caloric expenditures compared to the REE are as follows:

Studying: 150%
Heavy housework (e.g., vacuuming): 400%
Walking steadily at 3.5 mph: 450%
Gardening: 600%
Average jogging, cycling, energetic swimming: 800%

Body Weight and Body Mass Standards

Maintaining a healthy or ideal body weight requires a balance between the expenditure of energy and the intake of nutrients. Generally, when energy requirements of an individual equate with the daily caloric intake, the body weight remains stable. **Ideal body weight (IBW)** is the optimal weight recommended for optimal health. To determine an individual's approximate IBW, the nurse can consult standardized tables or can quickly calculate a value using the Rule of 5 for females and the Rule of 6 for males (Box 46.1). Many standardized tables and formulas were developed many years ago and are based on limited samples. The nurse should use great caution in suggesting that these weights apply to all clients.

BOX 46.1 Approximating Ideal Body Weight

Rule of 5 for Females	Rule of 6 for Males
100 lb (45.5 kg) for 5 ft (152 cm) of height	106 lb (48.2 kg) for 5 ft (152 cm) of height
+5 lb (2.27 kg) for each inch (2.54 cm) over 5 ft (152 cm)	+6 lb (2.73 kg) for each inch (2.54 cm) over 5 ft (152 cm)
± 10% for body-frame size*	± 10% for body-frame size*

*Determine body-frame size by measuring the client's wrist circumference and applying to the table below. Add 10% for large body-frame size, and subtract 10% for small body-frame size.

	Female Wrist Measurements			Male Wrist Measurements
	Height Less Than 5′2″ (Less Than 155 cm)	Height 5′2″–5′5″ (155–163 cm)	Height More Than 5′5″ (More Than 163 cm)	Height More Than 5′5″ (More Than 163 cm)
Small	Less than 5.5″ (140 mm)	Less than 6.0″ (152 mm)	Less than 6.25″ (159 mm)	5.5″–6.5″ (140–165 mm)
Medium	5.5″–5.75″ (140–146 mm)	6″–6.25″ (152–159 mm)	6.25″–6.5″ (159–165 mm)	6.5″–7.5″ (165–191 mm)
Large	More than 5.75″ (146 mm)	More than 6.25″ (159 mm)	More than 6.5″ (165 mm)	More than 7.5″ (191 mm)

Many health professionals consider the body mass index to be a more reliable indicator of an individual's healthy weight. For people older than 18 years, the **body mass index (BMI)** is an indicator of changes in body fat stores and whether an individual's weight is appropriate for height, and may provide a useful estimate of malnutrition. However, the results must be used with caution in people who have fluid retention (e.g., ascites or edema), athletes, or older adults. To calculate the BMI:

Measure the individual's height in meters, e.g., 1.7 m (1 meter = 3.3 ft, or 39.6 in.)
Measure the weight in kilograms, e.g., 72 kg (1 kg = 2.2 pounds)

Calculate the BMI using the following formula:

$$\text{BMI} = \frac{\text{weight in kilograms}}{(\text{height in meters})^2}$$

or

$$\frac{72 \text{ kilograms}}{1.7 \times 1.7 \text{ meters}} = 24.9$$

Box 46.2 provides an interpretation of the results.

BOX 46.2 Classification of Overweight and Obesity by BMI, Waist Circumference, and Associated Disease Risks*

	BMI (kg/m^2)	Obesity Class	Disease Risk* Relative to Normal Weight and Waist Circumference: Men: 102 cm (40 in.) or Less; Women: 88 cm (35 in.) or Less	Men > 102 cm (40 in.); Women > 88 cm (35 in.)
Underweight	<18.5		—	—
Normal+	18.5–24.9		—	—
Overweight	25.0–29.9		Increased	High
Obesity	30.0–34.9	I	High	Very high
	35.0–39.9	II	Very high	Very high
Extreme obesity	40.0+	III	Extremely high	Extremely high

*Disease risk for type 2 diabetes, hypertension, and cardiovascular disease.

+Increased waist circumference can also be a marker for increased risk even in individuals of normal weight.

From *Aim for a Healthy Weight*, National Heart, Lung, and Blood Institute, n.d., Washington, DC: U.S. Department of Health & Human Services. Retrieved from http://www.nhlbi.nih.gov/health/public/heart/obesity/lose_wt/bmi_dis.htm

Another measure of body mass is percent body fat. Because BMI uses only height and weight, it can give misleading results for certain groups of clients such as athletes, frail older adults, and children. The most accurate percentage of body fat can be measured by underwater (hydrostatic) weighing and dual-energy x-ray absorptiometry (DEXA), but these methods are time consuming and expensive. Air displacement plethysmography (commonly referred to as the BOD POD system) is faster and much less expensive (Nelms, Sucher, & Lacey, 2016). Other indirect but more practical measures include waist circumference (see Box 46.2), skinfold testing, and bioelectrical impedance analysis.

Factors Affecting Nutrition

Although the nutritional content of food is an important consideration when planning a diet, an individual's food preferences and habits are often a major factor affecting actual food intake. Habits about eating are influenced by developmental considerations, gender, ethnicity and culture, beliefs about food, personal preferences, religious practices, lifestyle, economics, medications and therapy, health, alcohol consumption, advertising, and psychologic factors.

Development

People in rapid periods of growth (i.e., infancy and adolescence) have increased needs for nutrients. Older adults, on the other hand, may need fewer calories and also need some dietary changes in view of their risk for coronary heart disease, osteoporosis, and hypertension.

Sex

Nutrient requirements are different for males and females because of body composition and reproductive functions. The larger muscle mass of males translates into a greater need for calories and proteins. Because of menstruation, females require more iron than males do prior to menopause. Pregnant and lactating females have increased caloric and fluid needs.

Ethnicity and Culture

Ethnicity often determines food preferences. Traditional foods (e.g., rice for Asians, pasta for Italians, curry for Indians) are eaten long after other customs are abandoned.

Nurses should not use a "good food, bad food" approach, but rather should realize that variations of intake are acceptable under different circumstances. The only "universally" accepted guidelines are (a) to eat a wide variety of foods to furnish adequate nutrients and (b) to eat moderately to maintain body weight. Food preference probably differs as much among individuals of the same cultural background as it does between cultures. Not all Italians like pizza, for example, and many undoubtedly enjoy Mexican food.

Beliefs About Food

Beliefs about effects of foods on health and well-being can affect food choices. Many people acquire their beliefs about food from television, magazines, and other media. Some people are reducing their intake of animal fats in response to evidence that excessive consumption of animal fats is a major risk factor in vascular disease, including heart attack and stroke.

Food fads that involve nontraditional food practices are relatively common. A **fad** is a widespread but short-lived interest or a practice followed with considerable zeal. It may be based either on the belief that certain foods have special powers or on the notion that certain foods are harmful. Food fads appeal to the individual seeking a miracle cure for a disease, the individual who desires superior health, or someone who wants to delay aging. Some fad diets are harmless, but others are potentially dangerous. Determining the needs a fad diet fills for the client enables the nurse both to support these needs and to suggest a more nutritious diet.

Personal Preferences

People develop likes and dislikes based on associations with a typical food. A child who loves to visit his grandparents may love pickled crabapples because they are served in the grandparents' home. Another child who dislikes a very strict aunt grows up to dislike the chicken casserole she often prepared. People often carry such preferences into adulthood.

Individual likes and dislikes can also be related to familiarity. Children often say they dislike a food before they sample it. Some adults are very adventuresome and eager to try new foods. Others prefer to eat the same foods repeatedly. Preferences in the tastes, smells, flavors (blends of taste and smell), temperatures, colors, shapes, and sizes of food influence an individual's food choices. Some people may prefer sweet and sour tastes to bitter or salty tastes. Textures play a great role in food preferences. Some people prefer crisp food to limp food, firm to soft, tender to tough, smooth to lumpy, or dry to soggy.

Religious Practices

Religious practice also affects diet. Some Roman Catholics avoid meat on certain days, and some Protestant faiths prohibit meat, tea, coffee, or alcohol. Both Orthodox Judaism and Islam prohibit pork. Orthodox Jews observe kosher customs, eating certain foods only if they are inspected by a rabbi and prepared according to dietary laws. The nurse must plan care with consideration of such religious dietary practices.

Lifestyle

Certain lifestyles are linked to food-related behaviors. Individuals who are always in a hurry may buy convenience grocery items or eat restaurant meals. Those who spend many hours at home may take time to prepare more meals "from scratch." Individual differences also influence lifestyle patterns (e.g., cooking skills, concern about health). Some individuals work at different times, such as evening or night shifts. They might need to adapt their eating habits to this and also make changes in their medication schedules if they are related to food intake.

Muscular activity affects metabolic rate more than any other factor; the more strenuous the activity, the greater the stimulation of the metabolism. Mental activity, which requires only about 4 Kcal per hour, provides very little metabolic stimulation.

Economics

What, how much, and how often an individual eats are frequently affected by socioeconomic status. For example, people with limited income, including some older adults, may not be able to afford meat and fresh vegetables. In contrast, individuals with higher incomes may purchase more proteins and fats and fewer complex carbohydrates. Not all individuals have the financial resources for extensive food preparation and storage facilities. The nurse should not assume that clients have their own stove, refrigerator, or freezer. In some low-income areas, food costs at small local grocery stores can be significantly higher than at large chain stores farther away.

Medications and Therapy

The effects of drugs on nutrition vary considerably. They may alter appetite, disturb taste perception, or interfere with nutrient absorption or excretion. Nurses need to be aware of the nutritional effects of specific drugs when evaluating a client for nutritional problems. The nursing history interview should include questions about the medications the client is taking. Conversely, nutrients can affect drug utilization. Some nutrients can decrease drug absorption; others enhance absorption. For example, the calcium in milk hinders absorption of the antibiotic tetracycline but enhances the absorption of the antibiotic erythromycin. Older adults are at particular risk for drug–food interactions due to the number of medications they may take, age-related physiologic changes affecting medication actions (e.g., decrease in lean-to-fat ratio, decrease in renal or hepatic function), and disease-restricted diets. Selected drug and nutrient interactions are shown in Table 46.1.

Therapies prescribed for certain diseases (e.g., chemotherapy and radiation for cancer) may also adversely affect eating patterns and nutrition. Normal cells of the bone marrow and the gastrointestinal (GI) mucosa are naturally very active and particularly susceptible to antineoplastic agents. Oral ulcers, intestinal bleeding, or diarrhea resulting from the toxicity of the antineoplastic agents used in chemotherapy can seriously diminish an individual's nutritional status.

The effects of radiotherapy depend on the area that is treated. Radiotherapy of the head and neck may cause decreased salivation, taste distortions, and swallowing difficulties; radiotherapy of the abdomen and pelvis may cause malabsorption, nausea, vomiting, and diarrhea. Many clients undergoing radiotherapy feel profound fatigue and anorexia (loss of appetite).

Health

An individual's health status greatly affects eating habits and nutritional status. Missing teeth, ill-fitting dentures, or a sore mouth makes chewing food difficult. Difficulty swallowing (**dysphagia**) due to a painfully inflamed throat or a stricture of the esophagus can prevent an individual from obtaining adequate nourishment. Disease processes and surgery of the GI tract can affect digestion, absorption, metabolism, and excretion of essential nutrients. GI and other diseases also create nausea, vomiting, and diarrhea, all of which can adversely affect an individual's appetite and nutritional status. Gallstones, which can block the

TABLE 46.1 Selected Drug–Nutrient Interactions

Drug	Effect on Nutrition
Acetylsalicylic acid (aspirin)	Decreases folic acid absorption when taken together orally. Increases excretion of vitamin C, thiamine, potassium, amino acids, and glucose. May cause nausea and gastritis.
Antacids containing aluminum or magnesium hydroxide	Decrease absorption of phosphate and vitamin A. Inactivate thiamine. May cause deficiency of calcium and vitamin D. Increase excretion of sodium, potassium, chloride, calcium, magnesium, zinc, and riboflavin.
Thiazide diuretics	May cause anorexia, nausea, vomiting, diarrhea, or constipation. Decrease absorption of vitamin B_{12}. May cause diarrhea, nausea, or vomiting.
Potassium chloride	Increases excretion of potassium, magnesium, and calcium. May cause anorexia, nausea, or vomiting. Is incompatible with protein hydrolysates.
Laxatives	May cause calcium and potassium depletion. Mineral oil and phenolphthalein (Ex-Lax) decrease absorption of vitamins A, D, E, and K.
Antihypertensives	Hydralazine may cause anorexia, vomiting, nausea, and constipation. Methyldopa increases need for vitamin B_{12} and folate. May cause dry mouth, nausea, vomiting, diarrhea, and constipation.
Anti-inflammatory agents	Colchicine decreases absorption of vitamin B_{12}, carotene, fat, lactose, sodium, potassium, protein, and cholesterol. Prednisone decreases absorption of calcium and phosphorus.
Antidepressants	Amitriptyline increases food intake (large amounts may suppress intake).
Antineoplastics	Can cause nausea, vomiting, anorexia, malabsorption, and diarrhea.
Nutrient	**Effect on Drugs**
Grapefruit	Can cause toxicity when taken with a variety of medications including amiodarone, carbamazepine, cisapride, cyclosporine, diazepam, nifedipine, saquinavir, statins, terfenadine, verapamil.
Vitamin K	Can decrease the effectiveness of warfarin (Coumadin).
Tyramine (found in aged cheeses, tap beer, dried sausages, fermented soy, sauerkraut)	In combination with monoamine oxidase inhibitor (MAOI) medications, e.g., isocarboxazid (Marplan), isoniazid, linezolid, phenelzine, tranylcypromine, creates sudden increase in epinephrine leading to headaches, increased pulse and blood pressure, and possible death.
Milk	Interferes with absorption of tetracycline antibiotics.

flow of bile, are a common cause of impaired lipid digestion. Metabolic processes can be impaired by diseases of the liver. Diseases of the pancreas can affect glucose metabolism or fat digestion. Autoimmune and genetic disorders such as celiac disease and irritable bowel syndrome may be worsened when eating foods containing wheat or gluten.

Between 30 million and 50 million Americans have lactose intolerance (also called lactose maldigestion), a shortage of the enzyme lactase, which is needed to break down the sugar in milk. Certain populations are more widely affected, especially African Americans, American Indians, Ashkenazi Jews, Asians, and Hispanics and Latinos although they may not always show symptoms (DeBruyne & Pinna, 2017).

Alcohol Consumption

The calories in alcoholic drinks include both those of the alcohol itself and of the juices or other beverages added to the drink. These can constitute large numbers of calories, for example, 150 calories for a regular 12-ounce beer, and 160 calories for a "screwdriver" (1.5 ounces vodka plus 4 ounces orange juice). Drinking alcohol can lead to weight gain by adding these calories to the regular diet plus the effect of alcohol on fat metabolism. A small amount of the alcohol is converted directly to fat. However, the greater effect is that the remainder of the alcohol is converted into acetate by the liver. The acetate released to the bloodstream is used for energy instead of fat and the fat is then stored.

Excessive alcohol use contributes to nutritional deficiencies in several ways. Alcohol may replace food in an individual's diet, and it can depress the appetite. Excessive alcohol can have a toxic effect on the intestinal mucosa, thereby decreasing the absorption of nutrients. The need for vitamin B increases, because it is used in alcohol metabolism. Alcohol can impair the storage of nutrients and increase nutrient catabolism and excretion.

Several studies have shown health benefits of moderate alcohol consumption such as with red wine. Examples include reduced risk of cardiovascular disease, strokes, dementia, diabetes, and osteoporosis. However, any benefits of alcohol must be weighed against the many harmful effects, and the possibility of alcohol abuse.

Advertising

Food producers try to persuade consumers to change from the product they currently use to the brand of the producer. Popular actors are often used in television, radio, Internet, and print to influence consumers' choices. Advertising is thought to influence individuals' food choices and eating patterns to a certain extent. Of note is that such products as alcoholic beverages, coffee, frozen foods, and soft drinks are more heavily advertised than such products as bread, vegetables, and fruits. Convenience foods (frozen or packaged and easy to prepare) and take-out (fast) foods are heavily advertised. Children's television show commercials often promote snack foods, candy, soda, and sugared cereals over fresh, healthy foods. Australia, Canada, Sweden, and Great Britain have adopted regulations prohibiting food advertising on programs targeting audiences of young children.

There has been an increase in advertising that targets older adults in particular and encourages use of herbs and supplements. Some products are nutritionally safe, whereas others are not and can cause interactions with medications they might be taking or cause unexpected side effects. The cost of some of these supplements is also usually high, is generally not covered by health insurance, and may take money that the individual could spend for healthier food.

Psychologic Factors

Although some people overeat when stressed, depressed, or lonely, others eat very little under the same conditions. Anorexia and weight loss can indicate severe stress or depression. Anorexia nervosa and bulimia are severe psychophysiologic conditions seen most frequently in female adolescents.

Nutritional Variations Throughout the Lifecycle

Nutritional requirements vary throughout the lifecycle. Guidelines follow for the major developmental stages.

Neonate to 1 Year

The neonate's fluid and nutritional needs are met by breast milk or formula. Fluid needs of infants are proportionately greater than those of adults because of a higher metabolic rate, immature kidneys, and greater water losses through the skin and the lungs. Therefore, fluid balance is a critical factor. Under normal environmental conditions, infants do not need additional water beyond that obtained from breast or bottle formula feedings; however, neonates in very warm environments may require additional fluids.

The total daily nutritional requirement of the newborn is about 80 to 100 mL of breast milk or formula per kilogram of body weight. The newborn infant's stomach capacity is about 90 mL, and feedings are required every 2 1/2 to 4 hours.

The newborn infant is usually fed "on demand." **Demand feeding** means that the child is fed when hungry rather than on a set time schedule. This method tends to decrease the problem of overfeeding or underfeeding the infant. The newborn who is hungry usually cries and exhibits tension in the entire body. During feeding, the infant sucks readily and needs burping after each ounce of formula or after 5 minutes of breastfeeding.

Infants demonstrate satiety (fullness) by slowing their sucking activity or by falling asleep. Infants should not be coaxed into finishing the feeding. This could lead to discomfort or overfeeding. When feeding is completed, healthy infants can be placed in a supine position for sleep during the first 6 months of life to reduce the risk of sudden infant death syndrome (SIDS).

Regurgitation, or spitting up, during or after a feeding is a common occurrence during the first year. Although this may concern parents, it does not usually result in nutritional deficiency. Demonstration of adequate weight gain should reassure parents that the infant is receiving adequate nutrition.

Adding solid food to the diet usually takes place between 4 and 6 months of age. Six-month-old infants can consume solid food more readily because they can sit up, can hold a spoon, and have decreased sucking and tongue protrusion reflexes. Solid foods (strained or pureed) are generally introduced in the following order: cereals (rice before oat and wheat), fruits, vegetables (yellow before green), and strained meats. Foods are introduced one at a time, usually with only one new food introduced every 5 days to ensure that the infant tolerates the food and demonstrates no allergy to it. This sequence can vary according to cultural preferences. With the eruption of teeth at about 7 to 9 months, the infant is ready to chew and can experience different textures of food. At this time, the infant enjoys finger foods, such as skinless fruit cut into small pieces to prevent choking, dry cereal, or toast.

Because honey can contain spores of *Clostridium botulinum* and this has been a source of infection (and death) for infants, children less than 12 months old should not be fed honey. According to the Centers for Disease Control and Prevention (CDC) (2017), honey is safe for children 1 year of age and older.

At about 6 months of age, infants require iron supplementation to prevent **iron deficiency anemia**. Iron deficiency anemia is a form of **anemia** (decrease in red blood cells) caused by inadequate supply of iron for synthesis of hemoglobin. Cow's milk is low in iron and, thus, iron-fortified cereals or formulas are usually recommended by 6 months of age and are continued until the child reaches 18 months.

Weaning from the breast or bottle to the cup takes place gradually and is usually achieved by 12 to 24 months of age. It is recommended that infants be breastfed exclusively for 6 months and then until 1 year of age or longer as desired (Spatz, 2017). Some infants have difficulty giving up the bottle, particularly at naptime or bedtime. Parents should be warned that having the bottle in bed could lead to **bottle mouth syndrome**. The term describes decay of the teeth caused by constant contact with sweet liquid from the bottle. Some dentists advocate brushing or cleaning the infant's teeth to prevent bottle mouth syndrome, especially for the infant who requires a bottle only at naptime or bedtime. Weaning from the bottle can be facilitated by diluting the formula with water increasingly until the infant is drinking plain water. By the age of 1, most infants can be completely fed on table food, and milk intake is about 20 ounces per day.

Toddler

Because of a maturing GI tract, toddlers can eat most foods and adjust to three meals each day. Toddlers' fine motor skills are sufficiently well developed for them to learn how to feed themselves. Before the age of 20 months, most toddlers require help with glasses and cups because their wrist control is limited. By age 3, when most of the deciduous teeth have emerged, the toddler can bite and chew adult table food.

Developing independence may be exhibited through the toddler's refusal of certain foods. Meals should be short because of the toddler's brief attention span and environmental distractions. Often toddlers display their liking of rituals by eating foods in a certain order, cutting foods a specific way, or accompanying certain foods with a particular drink.

The toddler is less likely to have fluid imbalances than the infant. The toddler's GI function is more mature, and the percentage of fluid body weight is lower. A healthy toddler weighing 15 kg (33 lb) needs about 1250 mL of fluid per 24 hours.

During the toddler stage, the caloric requirement is 1000 to 1400 Kcal/day. From 1 to 2 years of age, the toddler may eat a combination of prepared toddler foods and some table foods. Parents should be instructed to read labels carefully and be aware that table foods offer more variety and are less expensive and more nutritious than prepared toddler foods. The need for adequate iron, calcium, and vitamins C and A, which are common toddler deficiencies, should also be discussed.

The following suggestions may help parents meet the child's nutritional needs and promote effective parent–child interactions: (a) Make mealtime a pleasant time by avoiding tensions at the table and discussions of bad behavior; (b) offer a variety of simple, attractive foods in small portions; (c) do not use food as a reward or punish a child who does not eat; (d) schedule meals, sleep, and snack times that will allow for optimal appetite and behavior; and (e) avoid routinely serving sweet desserts. Many children show dislike of particular foods. In some cases, this may be a natural mechanism to protect the child from food allergies. When in doubt, the child should be evaluated by a professional for food allergies (DeBruyne & Pinna, 2017).

Preschooler

The preschooler eats adult foods. Parents should become informed about the diet of their child in day care or preschool settings so that they can ensure that the child's total nutritional needs are being met. Children at this age are very active and may rush through meals to return to playing. Active children often require snacks between meals. Cheese, fruit, yogurt, raw vegetables, and milk are good choices. The 4-year-old still requires parents' help in cutting meat and may spill milk when pouring from a large container. Parents also need to teach the preschooler how to use utensils and should provide them with the opportunity to practice (e.g., buttering bread). However, 4- and 5-year-olds often use their fingers to pick up food. Children at this age may enjoy helping in the kitchen, and both girls and boys should be encouraged to do so.

The preschooler is even less at risk than the toddler for fluid imbalances. The average 5-year-old weighing 20 kg (45 lb) requires at least 75 mL of liquid per kilogram of body weight per day, or 1500 mL every 24 hours.

School-Age Child

School-age children require a balanced diet including approximately 1600 to 2200 Kcal/day. They can eat three meals a day and one or two nutritious snacks. Children need a protein-rich food at breakfast to sustain the prolonged physical and mental effort required at school. Children who skip breakfast become inattentive and restless by late morning and have decreased problem-solving ability. Undernourished children become fatigued easily and face a greater risk of infection, resulting in frequent absences from school.

The average healthy 8-year-old weighing 30 kg (66 lb) requires about 1750 mL of fluid per day. Many school-age children have only one meal a day with their family, at dinner. Mealtime should be a social time enjoyed by all, and parents should encourage good eating habits. Parents should be aware that children learn many of their food habits by observing their parents. Eating a balanced diet should be the norm for both parent and child.

The school-age child generally eats lunch at school. The child may bring lunch from home or get lunch at the school. Many dietary problems stem from this independence in food choices. Children may trade their food, not eat lunch at all, or buy sweets or junk food with their lunch money. Parents should discuss with the child the foods that they should eat and continue to provide a balanced diet in the home setting.

Poor eating habits may cause obesity. Childhood obesity is an increasing problem. More than 23% of American children ages 2 to 18 are at or above the

95% for BMI (Ogden et al., 2016). Obesity in school-age children tends to result in adult obesity and all the related health risks. It is both caused by and results in decreased activity and psychosocial problems. Obese children may be ridiculed and discriminated against by peers. Such behavior reinforces low self-esteem. The CDC's Division of Adolescent and School Health has established many programs to address both prevention and treatment of childhood obesity. The goal of treatment for children who are overweight is to reduce weight gain, allowing their weight to increase more slowly than their height. Counseling and teaching for parents should include the following:

- Reviewing the child's eating habits, including snacks
- Altering meal content
- Using rewards other than food
- Promoting regular exercise.

Adolescent

The adolescent's need for nutrients and calories increases, particularly during the growth spurt. In particular, the need for protein, calcium, vitamin D, iron, and B vitamins increases during adolescence. An adequate diet for an adolescent is 1 quart of milk per day and appropriate amounts of meat, vegetables, fruits, breads, and cereals. Calcium intake during adolescent years (1200 to 1500 mg/day) may help decrease osteoporosis (a decrease in bone density) in later life. Peak bone mineralization occurs on average at 12.5 years in girls and 14.0 years in boys when 40% of total adult bone mass is accumulated. The majority of adolescent females do not get enough calcium in their diets (Rolfes, Pinna, & Whitney, 2018).

Many parents observe that teenagers, particularly boys, seem to eat all the time. Teenagers have active lifestyles and irregular eating patterns. They tend to diet or snack frequently, often eating high-calorie foods such as soft drinks, ice cream, and fast foods. Parents and nurses can promote better lifelong eating habits by encouraging teenagers to eat healthy snacks. Parents can provide healthy snacks such as fruits and cheese and limit the junk food available in the home. The teenager's food choices relate to physical, social, and emotional factors and impulses and may not be influenced by teaching. Nurses need to advise parents to help adolescents take responsibility for their decisions in many areas of life, and to avoid conflicts that relate to food.

Common problems related to nutrition and self-esteem among adolescents include obesity, anorexia nervosa, and bulimia. Obesity continues to be a problem in the adolescent period. Depression is not unusual among adolescents who are obese. Treatment of obesity in this age group includes education on nutrition and assessment of psychosocial problems that may produce overeating.

Under social pressure to be slim, some adolescents severely limit their food intake to a level significantly below that required to meet the demands of normal growth. Sometimes, the adolescent may develop an eating disorder, such as anorexia or bulimia. These disorders are considered to be related to the need for control. **Anorexia nervosa** is characterized by a prolonged inability or refusal to eat, rapid weight loss, and emaciation in individuals who continue to believe they are fat. Individuals with anorexia may also induce vomiting and use laxatives and diuretics to remain thin. **Bulimia** is an uncontrollable compulsion to consume enormous amounts of food (binge) and then expel it by self-induced vomiting or by taking laxatives (purge). These illnesses are most effectively treated in the early stages by psychotherapy. Hospitalization may be necessary when the effects of starvation become life threatening.

Young Adult

Many young adults are aware of food groups but may not be knowledgeable about how many servings they need or how much a serving constitutes. The nurse should provide the young adult client with resources such as a chart or list that contains the foods and the amounts needed in each group.

Young adult females need to maintain adequate iron intake. Many do not ingest sufficient dietary iron each day. To prevent iron deficiency anemia, menstruating females should ingest 18 mg of iron daily. The nurse should instruct the female client to include iron-rich foods, such as organ meats (liver and kidneys), eggs, fish, poultry, leafy vegetables, and dried fruits, in her daily diet. In addition, the World Health Organization (WHO) recommends folate (folic acid) supplements for all women of childbearing ability. Because folate can prevent neural tube defects in the fetus but must be taken prior to and during the early portion of the pregnancy, the United States and more than 50 other countries have mandated folic acid supplementation of enriched grain products.

Calcium is needed in young adulthood to maintain bones and help decrease the chances of developing osteoporosis in later life. Along with calcium, the individual must have adequate vitamin D, necessary for the calcium to enter the bloodstream. Vitamin D is made in the skin on exposure to the sun. If the individual does not get sufficient sun exposure (15 minutes three times each week), supplements may be indicated.

Obesity may occur during the young adult years as the active teen becomes the sedentary adult but does not decrease caloric intake. The young adult who is overweight or obese is at risk for hypertension, a major health problem for this age group.

Hypertension and obesity are 2 of more than 40 risk factors identified in the development of cardiovascular (CV) disease. Preventing these risk factors and lowering the risk of CV disease are critical. Low-fat and low-cholesterol diets play a significant role in both the prevention and treatment of CV disease.

DRUG CAPSULE

Mineral: ferrous sulfate (Slow-Fe, Feosol), ferrous gluconate (Fergon)

CLIENT WITH IRON DEFICIENCY ANEMIA

Iron is required for the formation of red blood cells. When iron stores are low, the body cannot produce enough red blood cells and anemia can develop. Symptoms of iron deficiency anemia include fatigue, listlessness, anorexia, and pallor. Although iron deficiency anemia is not the only kind of anemia, it is possibly the most common and one of the easiest to treat. Immediate and timed-release forms are available.

NURSING RESPONSIBILITIES

- Administer on an empty stomach, 1 hour before or 2 hours after meals, with a full glass of water. If the client experiences gastric upset, administer with or after food. The immediate-release formulation is administered up to three times per day.
- Vitamin C increases absorption of iron from the stomach. Some preparations contain both iron and vitamin C.
- Administer at least 2 hours apart from antacids, ciprofloxacin, tetracycline, and several other medications. Consult a drug handbook for possible drug interactions.
- Liquid forms should be diluted in a glass of water or juice and sipped through a straw to prevent staining of the teeth.
- Shake suspension forms well before each use; take with a full glass of water.
- Iron comes in different dose strengths and may require adjustment for optimal effect.

CLIENT AND FAMILY TEACHING

- Take the medication on an empty stomach, 1 hour before or 2 hours after meals, with a full glass of water. If upset stomach occurs, take with or after food, but not with coffee, tea, eggs, or milk because these decrease absorption. Do not lie down for 30 minutes after taking the tablet or capsule.
- Sustained-release capsules and tablets must be swallowed whole. Do not crush or chew them because side effects may be increased.
- Common side effects may include nausea, stomach cramps, vomiting, and constipation. These should decrease within a few days even while continuing the iron.
- Stools will turn green-black, and this is normal.
- Do not stop taking the medication, even if you feel stronger.
- Do not take iron without consulting the primary care provider if you have a history of intestinal problems.
- Store at room temperature, away from moisture and sunlight. Keep away from children. Accidental overdose can be fatal.

Note: Prior to administering any medication, review all aspects with a current drug handbook or other reliable source.

Middle-Aged Adult

The middle-aged adult should continue to eat a healthy diet, following the recommended portions of the food groups, with special attention to protein and calcium intake, and limiting cholesterol and caloric intake. Two or three liters of fluid should be included in the daily diet. Postmenopausal females need to ingest sufficient calcium and vitamin D to reduce osteoporosis, and antioxidants such as vitamins A, C, and E may be helpful in reducing the risks of heart disease in women. Although iron supplements are no longer needed, the amount in a multivitamin is not harmful.

Middle-aged adults who gain weight may not be aware of some common facts about this age period. Decreased metabolic activity and decreased physical activity mean a decrease in caloric need. The nurse's role in nutritional health promotion is to counsel clients to prevent obesity by reducing caloric intake and participating in regular exercise. Clients should also be warned that being overweight is a risk factor for many chronic diseases, such as diabetes and hypertension, and for problems of mobility, such as arthritis.

For the client who requires additional resources, a variety of programs is frequently available. Most programs use behavior modification techniques and group support to assist clients in reaching their goals. Clients should seek medical advice before considering any major changes in their diets.

During late middle age, gastric juice secretions and free acid gradually decline. Some individuals may complain of "heartburn" (acid indigestion) or an increase in belching. They may determine that certain foods disagree with them. Clients should be advised to develop sensible eating habits and avoid fried or fatty foods.

Older Adults

The older adult requires the same basic nutrition as the younger adult. However, fewer calories are needed by older adults because of the lower metabolic rate and the decrease in physical activity.

Some older adults may need more carbohydrates for fiber and bulk, but most nutrient requirements remain relatively unchanged. Such physical changes as tooth loss and impaired sense of taste and smell may affect eating habits. Decreased saliva and gastric juice secretion may also affect the older adult's nutrition.

Psychosocial factors may also contribute to nutritional problems. Some older adults who live alone do not want to cook for themselves or eat alone. They may adopt poor dietary habits. Other factors, such as lack of transportation, poor access to stores, and inability to prepare the food also affect nutritional status. Loss of spouse, anxiety, depression, dependence on others, and lowered income all affect eating habits (Table 46.2). Guidelines to include high-nutrient foods compatible with the nutritional needs of older adults are summarized in Client Teaching. Also see Lifespan Considerations.

TABLE 46.2 Problems Associated with Nutrition in Older Adults

Problems	Nursing Interventions
Difficulty chewing	Encourage regular visits to the dentist to have dentures repaired, refitted, or replaced. Chop fruits and vegetables; shred green, leafy vegetables; select ground meat, poultry, or fish.
Lowered glucose tolerance	Eat more complex carbohydrates (e.g., breads, cereals, rice, pasta, potatoes, and legumes) rather than sugar-rich foods.
Decreased social interaction, loneliness	Promote appropriate social interaction at meals, when possible. Encourage the client and family to take an interest in food preparation and serving, perhaps as an activity they can do together. Encourage family or caregivers to present the food at a dining table with other people. If food preparation is not possible, suggest community resources, such as Meals on Wheels. Suggest inviting friends over for meals.
Loss of appetite and senses of smell and taste	Eat essential, nutrient-dense foods first; follow with desserts and low-nutrient-density foods. Review dietary restrictions, and find ways to make meals appealing within these guidelines. Eat small meals frequently instead of three large meals a day.
Limited income	Suggest using generic brands and coupons. Substitute milk, dairy products, and beans for meat. Avoid convenience foods if able to cook. Buy foods that are on sale and store for future use. Suggest community resources and nutrition programs.
Difficulty sleeping at night	Have the major meal at noon instead of in the evening. Avoid tea, coffee, or other stimulants in the evening.

CLIENT TEACHING Nutrition for Older Adults

- Include each food group on MyPlate. For example, a 65-year-old female of average height and weight who performs less than 30 minutes of exercise per day requires 1600 Kcal consisting of the following:

  Grains: 5 ounces

  Vegetables: 2 cups

  Fruits: 1.5 cups

  Milk, yogurt, or cheese: 3 cups

  Meat or beans: 5 ounces
- Reduce caloric intake. Caloric needs generally decrease in older adults often because of decreased activity. Older adults need to consume nutrient-dense foods and avoid foods that are high in calories but have few nutrients.
- Reduce fat consumption. Use leaner cuts of meat, and limit portions to 4 to 6 oz per day. (Be sure intake of protein is sufficient, because older adults often consume inadequate amounts of these foods.) Broil, boil, or bake foods instead of frying them. Use low-fat milk and cheese; limit intake of butter, margarine, and salad dressings.
- Reduce consumption of empty calories. Substitute fruit or puddings made with low-fat milk in place of pastry, cookies, and rich desserts.
- Reduce sodium consumption for clients who have hypertension or other cardiac problems. Avoid canned soups, ketchup, and mustard that are high in sodium (not all are). Avoid salted, smoked, cured, and pickled meats (e.g., ham and bacon), poultry, and fish. Do not add salt when cooking foods or at the table.
- Ensure adequate calcium intake (at least 800 mg) to prevent bone loss. Milk, cheese, yogurt, cream soups, puddings, and frozen milk products are good sources.
- Ensure adequate vitamin D intake. Vitamin D is essential to maintain calcium homeostasis. Include some milk, because other dairy products are not usually fortified with vitamin D. If milk cannot be tolerated because of a lactose deficiency, provide vitamin supplements.
- Ensure adequate iron intake. Iron intake in older adults may be compromised by such factors as increased incidence of GI disturbance, chronic diarrhea, regular aspirin use, and possible reduction in meat consumption.
- Consume fiber-rich foods to prevent constipation and minimize use of laxatives. Because fiber-rich foods provide bulk and a feeling of fullness, they help clients control their appetites and lose weight. Examples are bran and beans. Some clients may also require fiber supplements such as insoluble bulk-forming or soluble fiber products.

LIFESPAN CONSIDERATIONS Nutrition

CHILDREN

- Children learn eating habits from their parents. It is the parents' responsibility to be good nutritional role models, both in terms of what they eat and how they incorporate food into their lifestyle.
- During the preschool and early school-age years, children learn lifelong eating habits. It is the parents' responsibility to provide the child with adequate amounts of nutritious foods in an environment that is relaxed and comfortable for eating. It is the child's responsibility to decide what and how much of the nutritious foods to eat. Parents should be counseled that eating can become a source of conflict if the parent tries to tell the child what and how much to eat, or if the child tries to tell the parent what foods should be eaten. Children's access to "junk food" should be limited, but completely forbidding a food may also create conflict.
- Adolescents who are vegans or vegetarians are at risk for some nutritional deficits.

Continued on page 1200

LIFESPAN CONSIDERATIONS Nutrition—*continued*

OLDER ADULTS

Most older adults take several medications. Considerations for potential problems include the following:

- Some foods interact adversely or decrease the effectiveness of certain medications, such as foods high in vitamin K and the anticoagulant warfarin (Coumadin). Older adults should not change their diet significantly without consulting the healthcare provider since drug dosage may have been based on the older adult's previous dietary intake.
- Some medications increase appetite, such as glucocorticoids.
- Some medications decrease appetite by their actions or by causing an unpleasant taste.
- Certain tablets should not be crushed to be given by mouth or by gastric tubes, such as enteric-coated or slow-release medications.

Conditions such as neuromuscular disorders and dementia can make it difficult for older adults to eat or to be fed. Safety should always be a priority concern with attention paid to prevent aspiration. All healthcare personnel and family caregivers should be taught proper techniques to reduce this risk. Effective techniques include:

- Use the chin-tuck method when feeding clients with dysphagia. Have them flex the head toward the chest when swallowing to decrease the risk of aspiration into the lungs.
- Use foods of prescribed consistency. Many older adults can swallow foods with thicker consistency more easily than thin liquids.
- Try to focus on food preferences—the family can help provide this information.
- Try to maintain mealtime as a positive social occasion with conversations and extra attention to having a pleasant environment.

Economic factors may influence older adults' nutritional status if they cannot afford food, especially if a prescribed diet requires expensive supplements. Inexpensive or convenience foods such as canned soups are often high in fat and sodium.

Standards for a Healthy Diet

Various daily food guides have been developed to help healthy individuals meet the daily requirements of essential nutrients and to facilitate meal planning. Food group plans emphasize the general types or groups of foods rather than the specific foods, because related foods are similar in composition and often have similar nutrient values. For example, all grains, whether wheat or oats, are significant sources of carbohydrate, iron, and the B vitamin thiamine. Food guides currently used include *2015–2020 Dietary Guidelines for Americans* (2015) and the U.S. Department of Agriculture's (USDA's) MyPlate.

Dietary Guidelines for Americans

This guide is published by the USDA every 5 years, and the 2015–2020 edition contains recommendations for the total diet that allows food choices that result in a nutrient-rich and calorie-balanced intake. Key points of the latest dietary guidelines follow:

- Shift to more plant-based foods such as vegetables, fruits, grains, beans, and nuts.
- Significantly reduce foods with added sugars and solid fats.
- Engage in regular physical activity.
- Consume foods, including milk products, each day that increase commonly insufficient nutrients: vitamin D, calcium, potassium, and fiber.
- Keep daily total fat intake within 20% to 35% of total calories, less than 10% from saturated fatty acids and less than 300 mg cholesterol. (See also Client Teaching for ways to reduce fat intake.)
- Consume less than 2300 mg of sodium per day.
- If you drink alcohol, do so in moderation (one drink per day for women and two drinks per day for men).

These dietary recommendations are intended to help achieve the nutritional goals stated in *Healthy People 2020* (U.S. Department of Health and Human Services, 2019). Those goals include 22 specific nutritional objectives, such as the following:

- Reduce the incidence of obese adults (target = 30.5%) and children ages 2 to 19 (target = 14.5%).
- Increase the proportion of individuals ages 2 years and older who consume no more than 2300 mg of sodium daily.
- Prevent inappropriate weight gain in youth and adults.
- Reduce consumption of calories from solid fats (target = 14.2%) and added sugars in the population ages 2 years and older (target = 9.7%).

MyPlate

In May 2011, First Lady Michelle Obama introduced the MyPlate icon as a simple reminder of how to implement the dietary guidelines. This depiction and the website that

CLIENT TEACHING Reducing Dietary Fat

- Cook meat by grilling, baking, broiling, or microwaving rather than frying.
- Substitute popcorn or pretzels for such snacks as potato chips, cheese puffs, and corn chips.
- Read labels. Some crackers, for example, are high in fat; others are not.
- Limit desserts high in fat, such as ice cream, cake, and cookies.
- Substitute hard candies for chocolate bars.
- Use skim or reduced-fat milk instead of whole milk, for drinking as well as in recipes.
- Use less butter or margarine on breads.
- Remove fat from meat and skin from chicken before cooking.
- Eat less meat; eat more fish.
- Use less dressing, or use low-fat dressings, on salads.
- Eat plant sources of protein (e.g., kidney, lima, and navy beans).
- Use nuts as a source of protein, but since they are high in fat, use to replace meat rather than in addition.

accompanies it promote getting more fruits and vegetables, whole grains, and low-fat dairy foods into the diet (Figure 46.1 ■).

Using and following the guide does not guarantee that an individual will consume the necessary levels of all essential nutrients. For example, someone who chooses cooked and low-fiber fruits and vegetables might not have an adequate intake of dietary fiber even though the recommended number of servings is eaten. However, the food guide is easy to follow, and individuals who eat a variety of foods from each group, in the suggested amounts, are likely to come close to recommended nutrient levels.

Recommended Dietary Intake

The Committee on the Scientific Evaluation of Dietary Reference Intakes of the Institute of Medicine publishes dietary reference intakes (DRIs) tables, which contain four sets of reference values: estimated average requirements (EARs), recommended dietary allowances (RDAs), adequate intakes (AIs), and tolerable upper intake levels (ULs). Definitions of these terms are found in Box 46.3. The values for RDAs and AIs in the tables are modified for different age groups and according to gender. The effect of illness or injury (increasing the need for nutrients) and the variability among individuals within any given subgroup are not taken into account in the DRIs.

Consumers most commonly learn recommended dietary intake information from the U.S. Food and Drug Administration (FDA) nutrition labels. Food labeling is required for most prepared foods, such as breads, cereals, canned and frozen foods, snacks, desserts, and drinks. Nutrition labeling for raw produce (fruits and vegetables) and fish is voluntary. Everyone must learn how to read and interpret these labels.

In Figure 46.2 ■, the section at the top of the label ❶ indicates serving size and number of servings in the container. The remaining information on the label indicates the values for *each serving*. Serving sizes were updated to be more realistic in 2018. If the individual consumes a container that has more than one serving, he or she must multiply the values to determine the real nutrient content. The next section ❷ indicates the number of total

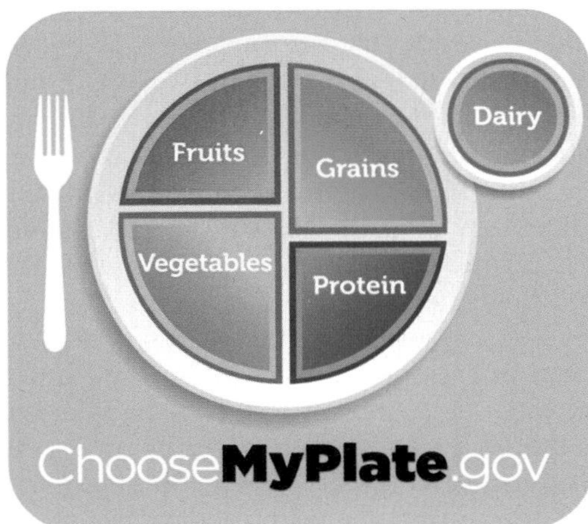

Figure 46.1 ■ MyPlate illustrates the five food groups using a familiar mealtime visual, a place setting.
From U.S. Department of Agriculture, 2013.

BOX 46.3 Definitions for Dietary Reference Value Tables

Dietary reference intakes (DRIs) are the standards for nutrient recommendations that include the following values:

- *Recommended dietary allowance (RDA):* the average daily nutrient intake level sufficient to meet the nutrient requirement of nearly all (97% to 98%) healthy individuals in a particular life stage and gender group
- *Adequate intake (AI):* used when RDA cannot be determined; a recommended average daily nutrient intake level based on observed or experimentally determined approximations or estimates of nutrient intake for a group (or groups) of healthy individuals that are assumed to be adequate
- *Tolerable upper intake level (UL):* the highest average daily nutrient intake level likely to pose no risk of adverse health effects to almost all individuals in a particular life stage and gender group. As intake increases above the UL, the potential risk of adverse health effects increases.

Source: Nutrient Recommendations: Dietary Reference Intakes, National Institutes of Health Office of Dietary Supplements, n.d. Retrieved from https://ods.od.nih.gov/Health_Information/Dietary_Reference_Intakes.aspx

Nutrition Facts

1	8 servings per container	
	Serving size	**2/3 cup (55g)**
2	**Amount per serving**	
	Calories	**230**
		% Daily Value*
3	**Total Fat** 8g	**10%**
	Saturated Fat 1g	**5%**
	Trans Fat 0g	
	Cholesterol 0mg	**0%**
	Sodium 160mg	**7%**
	Total carbohydrate 37g	**13%**
	Dietary Fiber 4g	**14%**
	Total Sugars 12g	
4	Includes 10g Added Sugars	**20%**
	Protein 3g	
5	Vitamin D 2mcg	10%
	Calcium 200mg	15%
	Iron 8mg	45%
	Potassium 235mg	6%
6	* The % Daily Value (DV) tells you how much a nutrient in a serving of food contributes to a daily diet. 2,000 calories a day is used for general nutrition advice.	

Figure 46.2 ■ The Nutrition Facts label.
From *The New and Improved Nutrition Facts Label—Key Changes*, by the U.S. Food and Drug Administration, 2018. Retrieved from https://www.fda.gov/files/food/published/The-New-and-Improved-Nutrition-Facts-Label-%E2%80%93-Key-Changes.pdf

calories per serving. Based on a 2000-calorie diet, a serving with 100 calories is considered moderate and 400 calories high. Section ❸ has nutrients that should be minimized: both saturated and *trans* fats. *Trans* fats are created when unsaturated oils are hydrogenated to create a solid form and are used in frying foods, margarine, and many snack products. They are also present in meat and dairy fats. *Trans* fats have been shown to increase cholesterol and contribute to heart disease. In section ❹, the manufacturer must list added sugar in addition to the total carbohydrates, fiber, and total sugars. It is considered difficult to stay within calorie limits consuming more than 10 percent of total daily calories from added sugar. The next section ❺ includes the actual values of the vitamins and minerals most commonly insufficient in American diets. In 2018, vitamins A and C were removed from the label, potassium and vitamin D were added, and the daily value (DV) of calcium and iron were updated. The footnote ❻ indicates that the DV shows the percent of a typical individual's daily requirement of that component contained in each serving. When adding the percent values from all foods eaten in one day, the goal is for the total DV of each of these to be at least 100%.

BOX 46.4 Combinations of Plant Proteins That Provide Complete Proteins

Grains plus legumes = complete protein.
Legumes plus nuts or seeds = complete protein.
Grains, legumes, nuts, or seeds plus milk or milk products (e.g., cheese) = complete protein.

Grains	Legumes	Nuts and Seeds
Brown rice	Black beans	Almonds
Barley	Kidney beans	Brazil nuts
Corn meal	Lima beans	Cashews
Millet	Soybeans	Pecans
Oats/oatmeal	Lentils	Walnuts
Rye	Tofu	Pumpkin seeds
Whole wheat	Black-eyed peas	Sesame seeds
	Split peas	Sunflower seeds
Examples	Black-eyed peas and rice	
	Lentil soup and whole-wheat bread	
	Beans and tortillas	
	Lima beans and sesame seeds	
	Cereal with milk	
	Macaroni with cheese	

Vegetarian Diets

Individuals may become vegetarians for economic, health, religious, ethical, or ecologic reasons. There are two basic vegetarian diets: those that use only plant foods (vegan) and those that include milk, eggs, or dairy products. Some individuals eat fish and poultry but not beef, lamb, or pork; others eat only fresh fruit, juices, and nuts; and still others eat plant foods and dairy products but not eggs.

Vegetarian diets can be nutritionally sound if they include a wide variety of foods and if proper protein and vitamin and mineral supplementation are provided. Because the proteins found in plant foods are incomplete proteins, vegetarians must eat complementary protein foods to obtain all of the essential amino acids. A plant protein can be complemented by combining it with a different plant protein. The combination produces a complete protein (Box 46.4). Obtaining complete proteins is especially important for growing children and pregnant and lactating women, whose protein needs are high. Generally, legumes (starchy beans, peas, lentils) have complementary relationships with grains, nuts, and seeds. Complementary foods must be eaten in the same meal. Diets such as the fruitarian diet do not provide sufficient amounts of essential nutrients and are not recommended for long-term use.

Foods of animal origin are the best source of vitamin B_{12}. Therefore, vegans need to obtain this vitamin from other sources: brewer's yeast, foods fortified with vitamin B_{12}, or a vitamin supplement. Because iron from plant sources is not absorbed as efficiently as iron from meat, vegans should eat iron-rich foods (e.g., green leafy vegetables, whole grains, raisins, and molasses) and iron-enriched foods. They should eat a food rich in vitamin C at each meal to enhance iron absorption. Calcium deficiency is a concern only for strict vegetarians. It can be prevented by including in the diet soybean milk and tofu (soybean curd) fortified with calcium and leafy green vegetables.

Altered Nutrition

Malnutrition is commonly defined as the lack of necessary or appropriate food substances, but in practice includes both undernutrition and overnutrition. **Overnutrition** refers to a caloric intake in excess of daily energy requirements, resulting in storage of energy in the form of adipose tissue. As the amount of stored fat increases, the individual becomes overweight or obese. An individual is said to be **overweight** when the BMI is between 25 and 29.9 kg/m^2 and **obese** when the BMI is greater than 30 kg/m^2 (National Heart, Lung, and Blood Institute, n.d.).

Excess body weight increases the stress on body organs and predisposes individuals to chronic health problems such as hypertension and diabetes mellitus. Obesity that interferes with mobility or breathing is referred to as morbid obesity. Obese individuals may also manifest undernourishment in important nutrients (e.g., essential vitamins or minerals) even though excess calories are ingested.

Undernutrition refers to an intake of nutrients insufficient to meet daily energy requirements because of inadequate food intake or improper digestion and absorption of food. An inadequate food intake may be caused by the inability to acquire and prepare food, inadequate knowledge about essential nutrients and a balanced diet, discomfort during or after eating, dysphagia, anorexia, nausea, vomiting, and so on. Improper digestion and absorption of nutrients may be caused by an inadequate production of hormones or enzymes or by medical conditions resulting in inflammation or obstruction of the GI tract.

Inadequate nutrition is associated with marked weight loss, generalized weakness, altered functional abilities, delayed wound healing, increased susceptibility to infection, decreased immunocompetence, impaired pulmonary function, and prolonged length of hospitalization. In response to undernutrition, carbohydrate reserves, stored as liver and muscle glycogen, are mobilized. However, these reserves can only meet energy requirements for a short time (e.g., 24 hours) and then body protein is mobilized.

Protein-calorie malnutrition (PCM), seen in starving children of underdeveloped countries, is now also recognized as a significant problem of clients with long-term deficiencies in caloric intake (e.g., those with cancer and chronic disease). Characteristics of PCM are depressed visceral proteins (e.g., albumin), weight loss, and visible muscle and fat wasting.

Protein stores in the body are generally divided into two compartments: somatic and visceral. Somatic protein consists largely of skeletal muscle mass; it is assessed most commonly by conducting anthropometric measurements such as the mid-arm circumference (MAC) and the mid-arm muscle area (MAMA). (See the *Anthropometric Measurements* section on page 1205.) Visceral protein includes plasma protein, hemoglobin, several clotting factors, hormones, and antibodies. It is usually assessed by measuring serum protein levels such as albumin and transferrin, discussed in the *Biochemical (Laboratory) Data* section of *Assessing*, which follows.

●○●NURSING MANAGEMENT

Assessing

A nutritional assessment identifies clients at risk for malnutrition and those with poor nutritional status. In most healthcare facilities, the responsibility for nutritional assessment and support is shared by the primary care provider, the dietitian, and the nurse. A comprehensive nutritional assessment is often performed by a nutritionist or a dietitian, and the primary care provider. Components of a nutritional assessment are shown in Table 46.3 and may be remembered as ABCD data: anthropometric, biochemical, clinical, and dietary.

Nutritional Screening

Because a comprehensive nutritional assessment is time consuming and expensive, various levels and types of assessment are available. Nurses perform a nutritional screen. A nutritional screen is an assessment performed to identify clients at risk for malnutrition or those who are malnourished. For clients who are found to be at moderate or high risk for malnutrition (Box 46.5), follow-up is provided in the form of a comprehensive assessment by a dietitian. Medicare standards for nursing homes require that any resident who experiences unplanned or undesired weight loss of 5% or more in 1 month, 7.5% or more in 3 months, or 10% or more in 6 months receive a full nutritional assessment by a nurse.

Nurses carry out nutritional screens through routine nursing histories and physical examinations. Custom-designed screens for a particular population (e.g., older adults and pregnant women) and specific disorders (e.g., cardiac disease) are available.

TABLE 46.3 Components of a Nutritional Assessment

	Screening Data	Additional In-Depth Data
Anthropometric data	• Height • Weight • Ideal body weight • Usual body weight • Body mass index	• Triceps skinfold (TSF) • Mid-arm circumference (MAC) • Mid-arm muscle area (MAMA)
Biochemical data	• Hemoglobin • Serum albumin • Total lymphocyte count	• Serum transferrin level • Urinary urea nitrogen • Urinary creatinine excretion
Clinical data	• Skin • Hair and nails • Mucous membranes • Activity level	• Hair analysis • Neurologic testing
Dietary data	• 24-hour food recall • Food frequency record	• Selective food frequency record • Food diary • Diet history

BOX 46.5 Summary of Risk Factors for Nutritional Problems

DIET HISTORY
- Chewing or swallowing difficulties (including ill-fitting dentures, dental caries, and missing teeth)
- Inadequate food budget
- Inadequate food intake
- Inadequate food preparation facilities
- Inadequate food storage facilities
- Intravenous fluids (other than total parenteral nutrition for 10 or more days)
- Living and eating alone
- Physical disabilities
- Restricted or fad diets

MEDICAL HISTORY
- Alcohol or substance abuse
- Catabolic or hypermetabolic condition: burns, trauma
- Chronic illness: end-stage renal disease, liver disease, AIDS, pulmonary disease (e.g., chronic obstructive pulmonary disease [COPD]), cancer
- Fluid and electrolyte imbalance
- GI problems: anorexia, dysphagia, nausea, vomiting, diarrhea, constipation
- Neurologic or cognitive impairment
- Oral and GI surgery
- Unintentional weight loss or gain of 10% within 6 months

MEDICATION HISTORY*
- Antacids
- Antidepressants
- Antihypertensives
- Anti-inflammatory agents
- Antineoplastic agents
- Aspirin
- Digitalis
- Diuretics (thiazides)
- Laxatives
- Potassium chloride

*The potential effects of some medications on nutrition are shown in Table 46.1 on page 1194.

Screening tools such as the Patient-Generated Subjective Global Assessment (PG-SGA) and the one created by the Nutrition Screening Initiative (NSI) can be incorporated into the nursing history. The PG-SGA is a method of classifying clients as either well nourished, moderately malnourished, or severely malnourished based on a dietary history and physical examination. It was established primarily for use with cancer clients, but has been widely tested and is appropriate for both inpatient and outpatient clients with various diagnoses.

The NSI tool is consistent with the U.S. Older Americans Act (authorized through 2018) Nutrition Programs goals. The NSI screens older adults using a nutrition checklist that contains nine warning signs of conditions that can interfere with good nutrition (Box 46.6).

Nursing History

As mentioned earlier, nurses obtain considerable nutrition-related data in the routine admission nursing history. Data include but are not limited to the following:

- Age, sex, and activity level
- Difficulty eating (e.g., impaired chewing or swallowing)
- Condition of the mouth, teeth, and presence of dentures
- Changes in appetite
- Changes in weight
- Physical disabilities that affect purchasing, preparing, and eating
- Cultural and religious beliefs that affect food choices
- Living arrangements (e.g., living alone) and economic status

BOX 46.6 Nutritional Screening Tool

Read the statement. Circle the number in the Yes column for those that apply to you. Total your nutritional assessment.

If you scored 0–2: Good! Recheck your nutritional score in 6 months.

If you scored 3–5: You are at moderate nutritional risk. See what can be done to improve your eating habits and lifestyle. Recheck your score in 3 months.

If you scored 6 or above: You are at high nutritional risk. Take this checklist to your doctor, nurse practitioner, or home health nurse. Ask for help to improve your nutritional health.

Nutritional Assessment Statements	Yes
I have an illness or condition that made me change the kind or amount of food I eat.	2
I eat fewer than two meals per day.	3
I eat few fruits, vegetables, or milk products.	2
I have three or more drinks of beer, liquor, or wine almost every day.	2
I have tooth or mouth problems that make it hard for me to eat.	2
I do not always have enough money to buy the food I need.	4
I eat alone most of the time.	1
I take three or more different prescribed or over-the-counter drugs a day.	1
Without wanting to, I have lost or gained 10 pounds in the last 6 months.	2
I am not always physically able to shop, cook, or feed myself.	2
Total	____

From "Determine Your Nutritional Health," by the Nutrition Screening Initiative, 2008, Washington, DC: National Council on Aging. Reprinted with permission by the Nutrition Screening Initiative, a project of the American Dietetic Association, funded in part by a grant from Ross Products Division, Abbott Laboratories, Inc.

- General health status and medical condition
- Medication history.

Anthropometric Measurements

Anthropometric measurements are noninvasive techniques that aim to quantify body composition. A **skinfold measurement** is performed to determine fat stores. The most common site for measurement is the triceps skinfold (TSF). The fold of skin measured includes subcutaneous tissue but not the underlying muscle. It is measured in millimeters using special calipers. To measure the TSF, locate the midpoint of the upper arm (halfway between the acromion process and the olecranon process), then grasp the skin on the back of the upper arm along the long axis of the humerus (Figure 46.3 ■). Placing the calipers 1 cm (0.4 in.) below the nurse's fingers, measure the thickness of the fold to the nearest millimeter.

The **mid-arm circumference (MAC)** is a measure of fat, muscle, and skeleton. To measure the MAC, ask the client to sit or stand with the arm hanging freely and the forearm flexed to horizontal. Measure the circumference at the midpoint of the arm, recording the measurement in centimeters, to the nearest millimeter (e.g., 24.6 cm) (Figure 46.4 ■).

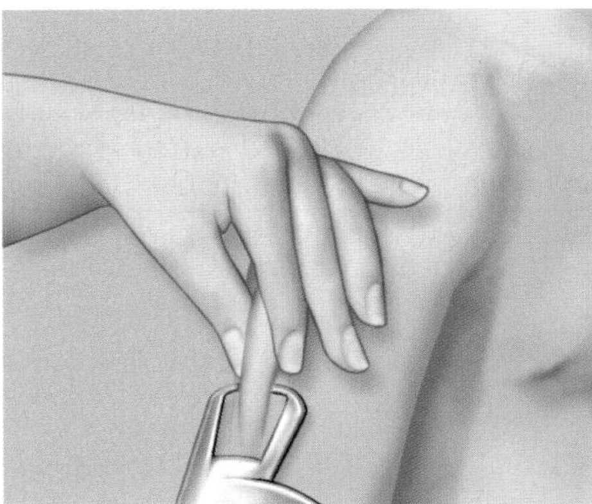

Figure 46.3 ■ Measuring the triceps skinfold.

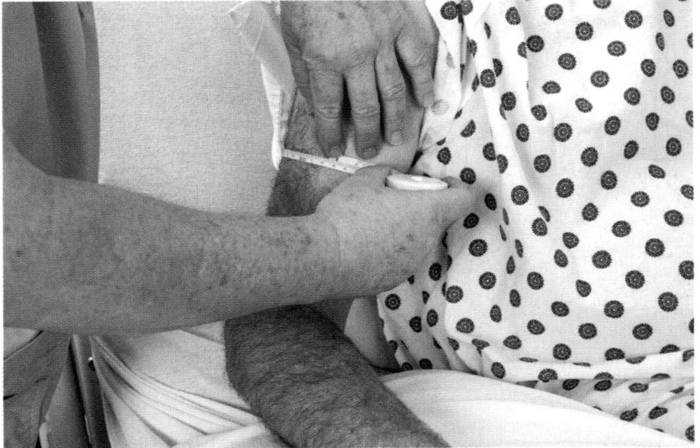

Figure 46.4 ■ Measuring the mid-arm circumference.

The **mid-arm muscle area (MAMA)** is then calculated by using reference tables or by using a formula that incorporates the TSF and the MAC. The MAMA is an estimate of lean body mass, or skeletal muscle reserves. If tables are not available, the nurse uses the following formula to calculate the MAMA from the triceps skinfold and MAC direct measurements:

$$\text{MAMA}\,(\text{cm}^2) = \frac{[\text{midarm circumference}\,(\text{cm}) - (3.14 \times \text{TSF cm})]^2}{4\pi} - 10\,(\text{males})\,\text{or} - 6.5\,(\text{females})$$

Values for anthropometric measurements for adults vary by ethnicity. Examples of variations in MAC are shown in Table 46.4.

Changes in anthropometric measurements occur slowly and reflect chronic rather than acute changes in nutritional status. They are used, therefore, to monitor the client's progress for months to years rather than days to weeks. Ideally, initial and subsequent measurements need to be taken by the same clinician. In addition, measurements obtained need to be interpreted with caution. Fluctuations in hydration status that often occur during illness can influence the accuracy of results. In addition, normal standards often do not account for normal changes in body composition such as those that occur with aging.

Biochemical (Laboratory) Data

Laboratory tests provide objective data to the nutritional assessment, but because many factors can influence these tests, no single test specifically predicts nutritional risk or measures the presence or degree of a nutritional problem. The tests most commonly used are serum proteins, urinary urea nitrogen and creatinine, and total lymphocyte count.

Serum Proteins

Serum protein levels provide an estimate of visceral protein stores. Tests commonly include hemoglobin, albumin, transferrin, and total iron-binding capacity. A low hemoglobin level may be evidence of iron deficiency anemia. However, abnormal blood loss or a pathologic process

TABLE 46.4 MAC Values for Adults

Ethnicity	Male	Female
ALL	34.3 cm	32.2 cm
Non-Hispanic White	34.3 cm	32 cm
Non-Hispanic Black	35.2 cm	34.8 cm
Non-Hispanic Asian	31.3	28.4 cm
Hispanic	34.4	32.6 cm

From "Anthropometric Reference Data for Children and Adults: United States, 2011–2014," in *Vital and Health Statistics, 3*(39), 2016, by C. D. Fryar, Q. Gu, C. L. Ogden, and K. M. Flegal, National Center for Health Statistics.

such as GI cancer must be ruled out before iron deficiency related to diet is confirmed.

Albumin, which accounts for over 50% of the total serum proteins, is one of the most common visceral proteins evaluated as part of the nutritional assessment. Because there is so much albumin in the body and because it is not broken down very quickly (i.e., it has a half-life of 18 to 20 days), albumin concentrations change slowly. A low serum albumin level is a useful indicator of prolonged protein depletion rather than acute or short-term changes in nutritional status. However, many conditions besides malnutrition can depress albumin concentration, such as altered liver function, hydration status, and losses from open wounds and burns.

Transferrin binds and carries iron from the intestine through the serum. Because it has a shorter half-life than albumin (8 to 9 days), transferrin responds more quickly to protein depletion than albumin. Serum transferrin can be measured directly or by a total iron-binding capacity (TIBC) test, which indicates the amount of iron in the blood to which transferrin can bind. Transferrin levels below normal are found with protein loss, iron deficiency anemia, pregnancy, hepatitis, or liver dysfunction.

Prealbumin, also referred to as thyroxine-binding albumin or transthyretin, has the shortest half-life and smallest body pool and is, therefore, the most responsive serum protein to rapid changes in nutritional status. Prealbumin levels of 15 to 35 mg/dL are normal, below 15 indicates clients at risk, and below 11 indicates that aggressive nutritional intervention is needed.

Urinary Tests

Urinary urea nitrogen and urinary creatinine are measures of protein catabolism and the state of nitrogen balance. **Urea**, the chief end product of amino acid metabolism, is formed from ammonia detoxified by the liver, circulated in the blood, and transported to the kidneys for excretion in urine. Urea concentrations in the blood and urine, therefore, directly reflect the intake and breakdown of dietary protein, the rate of urea production in the liver, and the rate of urea removal by the kidneys.

The state of nitrogen balance is determined by comparing the nitrogen intake (grams of protein) to the nitrogen output over a 24-hour period. A positive nitrogen balance exists when intake exceeds nitrogen output; a negative nitrogen balance occurs when output exceeds nitrogen intake. Protein intake must be accurately recorded and kidney function must be normal to ensure the validity of a urinary urea nitrogen test.

Urinary creatinine reflects an individual's total muscle mass because creatinine is the chief end product of the creatine produced when energy is released during skeletal muscle metabolism. The rate of creatinine formation is directly proportional to the total muscle mass. Creatinine is removed from the bloodstream by the kidneys and excreted in the urine at a rate that closely parallels its formation. The greater the muscle mass, the greater the excretion of creatinine. As skeletal muscle atrophies during malnutrition, creatinine excretion decreases. Urinary creatinine is influenced by protein intake, exercise, age, sex, height, renal function, and thyroid function.

Total Lymphocyte Count

Certain nutrient deficiencies and forms of PCM can depress the immune system. The total number of lymphocyte white blood cells decreases as protein depletion occurs.

Clinical Data (Physical Examination)

Physical examination reveals some nutritional deficiencies and excesses besides obvious weight changes. Assessment focuses on rapidly proliferating tissues such as skin, hair, nails, eyes, and mucosa but also includes a systematic review comparable to any routine physical examination. See Box 46.7 and Figure 46.5 ■ for signs associated with malnutrition. These signs must be viewed as suggestive of malnutrition because the signs are nonspecific. For example, red conjunctiva may indicate an infection rather than a nutritional deficit, and dry, dull hair may be related to excessive exposure to the sun rather than severe protein-energy malnutrition. To confirm malnutrition, clinical findings need to be substantiated with laboratory tests and dietary data.

BOX 46.7 Malnutrition

Area of Examination (Possible Cause)	Signs Associated with Malnutrition
General appearance and vitality	Apathetic, listless, looks tired, easily fatigued
Weight	Overweight or underweight
Skin	Dry, flaky, or scaly; pale or pigmented; presence of petechiae or bruises; lack of subcutaneous fat; edema
Nails	Brittle, pale, ridged, or spoon shaped (iron deficiency)
Hair	Dry, dull, sparse, loss of color, brittle (Figure 46.6*A*)
Eyes	Pale or red conjunctiva, dryness, soft cornea, dull cornea, night blindness (vitamin A deficiency)
Lips	Swollen, red cracks at side of mouth, vertical fissures (B vitamins deficiency) (Figure 46.6*C*)
Tongue	Swollen, beefy red or magenta colored, smooth appearance (B vitamins deficiency); decrease or increase in size
Gums	Spongy, swollen, inflamed; bleed easily (vitamin C deficiency)
Muscles	Underdeveloped, flaccid, wasted, soft
GI system	Anorexia, indigestion, diarrhea, constipation, enlarged liver, protruding abdomen
Nervous system	Decreased reflexes, sensory loss, burning and tingling of hands and feet (B vitamins deficiency), mental confusion or irritability

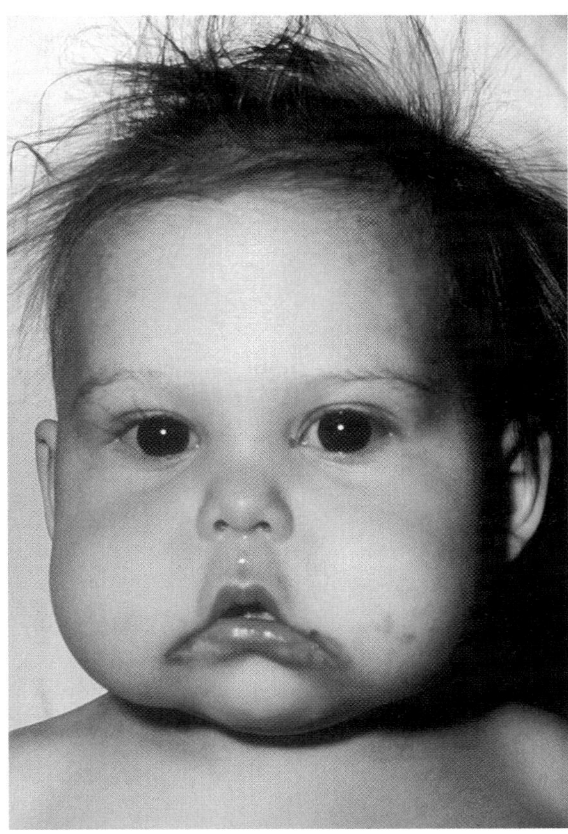

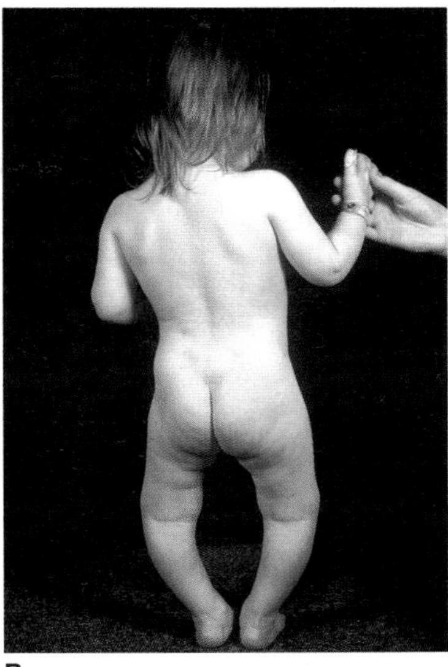

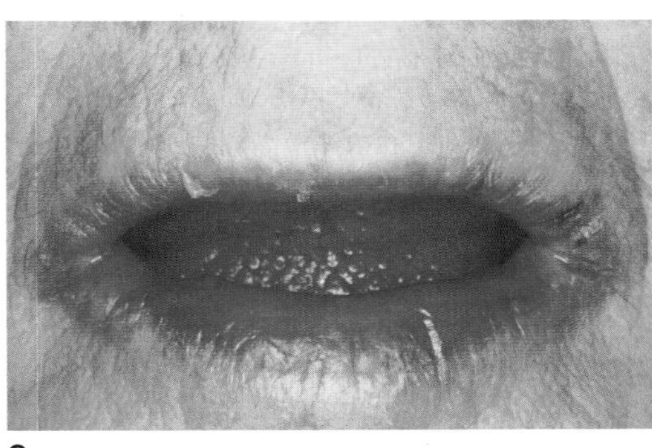

Figure 46.5 ■ Examples of nutritional deficiencies: *A*, dull, sparse hair and inflammation of the corners of the mouth from protein deficiency; *B*, rickets from vitamin D or calcium deficiency; *C*, pellagra, caused by a chronic lack of niacin (vitamin B).
A, from Centers for Disease Control and Prevention; *B*, Biophoto Associates/Science Source; *C*, Clinical Photography, Central Manchester University Hospitals NHS Foundation Trust, UK/Science Source.

Calculating Percentage of Weight Loss

Accurate assessment of the client's height, current body weight (CBW), and usual body weight (UBW) is essential. Although the client's CBW can be compared with an ideal body weight discussed earlier, the IBW is based on healthy individuals and does not account for changes in the client's body composition that accompany illness or reflect any changes in weight. The client's UBW better indicates weight change and the possibility of malnutrition. Calculation and interpretation of the percentage of deviation from UBW and the percentage of weight loss are shown in Box 46.8. An important aspect of weight assessment, obtained during the nursing history, is a description of weight change. The nurse should document any weight loss or gain, the duration of the change, and whether the weight change was intentional or unintentional.

BOX 46.8 Calculating and Interpreting the Percentage of Deviation from Usual Body Weight and the Percentage of Weight Loss

CALCULATING PERCENTAGE OF USUAL BODY WEIGHT

$$\text{\% Usual body weight} = \frac{\text{current weight}}{\text{usual body weight}} \times 100$$

Mild malnutrition	85–90%
Moderate malnutrition	75–84%
Severe malnutrition	Less than 74%

CALCULATING PERCENTAGE OF WEIGHT LOSS

$$\text{\% Weight loss} = \frac{\text{usual weight} - \text{current weight}}{\text{usual weight}} \times 100$$

Significant Weight Loss	Severe Weight Loss
5% over 1 mo	Greater than 5% over 1 mo
7.5% over 3 mo	Greater than 7.5% over 3 mo
10% over 6 mo	Greater than 10% over 6 mo

Dietary Data

Dietary data include the client's usual eating patterns and habits; food preferences, allergies, and intolerances; frequency, types, and quantities of foods consumed; and social, economic, ethnic, or religious factors influencing nutrition. Factors may include, but are not limited to, living and eating companions, ability to purchase and prepare food, availability of refrigeration and cooking facilities, income, and effect of religion and ethnicity on food choices.

Four possible methods for collecting dietary data are a 24-hour food recall, a food frequency record, a food diary, and a diet history.

For a **24-hour food recall**, the nurse asks the client to recall all of the food and beverages the client consumes during a typical 24-hour period when at home. The data obtained are then generally evaluated according to the Food Guide to judge overall adequacy.

A **food frequency record** is a checklist that indicates how often general food groups or specific foods are eaten. Frequency may be categorized as times/day, times/week, times/month, or frequently, seldom, never. This record provides information about the types of foods eaten but not the quantities. When specific foods or nutrients are suspected of being deficient or excessive, the healthcare professional may use a selective food frequency that focuses, for example, on fat, fruit, vegetable, or fiber intake.

A **food diary** is a detailed record of measured amounts (portion sizes) of all food and fluids a client consumes during a specified period, usually 3 to 7 days.

A **diet history** is a comprehensive time-consuming assessment of a client's food intake that involves an extensive interview by a nutritionist or dietitian. It includes characteristics of foods usually eaten and the frequency and amount of food consumed. It may include a 24-hour recall, a food frequency record, and a food diary. Medical and psychosocial factors are also assessed to evaluate their impact on nutritional requirements, food habits, and choices. Data obtained are analyzed by computer and translated into caloric and nutrient intake. Results are compared with the DRIs appropriate for the client's age, sex, and condition.

Diagnosing

Some nursing diagnoses for clients with nutritional problems are: obesity, excess dietary intake, insufficient dietary intake, and overweight. Many other nursing diagnoses may apply to certain individuals, because nutritional problems often affect other areas of human functioning. Examples include constipation related to inadequate fluid intake and fiber intake, and altered self-esteem related to obesity.

Planning

Major goals for clients with or at risk for nutritional problems include the following:

- Maintain or restore optimal nutritional status.
- Promote healthy nutritional practices.
- Prevent complications associated with malnutrition.
- Decrease weight.
- Regain specified weight.

Specific nursing activities associated with each of these goals can be selected to meet the individual needs of the client. See the Nursing Care Plan and Concept Map at the end of this chapter.

Planning for Home Care

To provide for continuity of care, the nurse must consider the client's need for assistance with nutrition. Some clients will need help with eating, purchasing food, and preparing meals; others will need instructions about nutrition therapy.

Home care planning incorporates an assessment of the client's and family's abilities for self-care, financial resources, and the need for referrals and home health services. A major aspect of discharge planning involves the instructional needs of the client and family (see Client Teaching).

CLIENT TEACHING Healthy Nutrition

- Instruct clients about the content of a healthy diet based on the MyPlate and *Dietary Guidelines for Americans*
- Encourage clients, particularly older clients, to reduce dietary fat (see Client Teaching on reducing dietary fat, page 1200).
- Instruct strict vegetarians about proper protein complementation and additional vitamin and mineral supplementation.
- Discuss foods high in specific nutrients required such as protein, iron, calcium, vitamin C, and fiber.
- Discuss importance of properly fitted dentures and dental care.
- Discuss safe food preparation and preservation techniques as appropriate.

DIETARY ALTERATIONS

- Explain the purpose of the diet.
- Discuss allowed and excluded foods.
- Explain the importance of reading food labels when selecting packaged foods.
- Include family or significant others.
- Reinforce information provided by the dietitian or nutritionist as appropriate.
- Discuss herbs and spices as alternatives to salt and substitutes for sugar.

FOR CLIENTS WHO ARE OVERWEIGHT

- Discuss physiologic, psychologic, and lifestyle factors that predispose to weight gain.
- Provide information about desired weight range and recommended calorie intake.
- Discuss principles of a well-balanced diet and high- and low-calorie foods.

CLIENT TEACHING Healthy Nutrition—*continued*

- Encourage intake of low-calorie, caffeine-free beverages, and plenty of water.
- Discuss ways to adapt eating practices by using smaller plates, taking smaller servings, chewing each bite a specified number of times, and putting fork down between bites.
- Discuss ways to control the desire to eat by taking a walk, drinking a glass of water, or doing slow deep-breathing exercises.
- Discuss the importance of exercise and help the client plan an exercise program.
- Discuss stress reduction techniques.
- Provide information about available community resources (e.g., weight-loss groups, dietary counseling, exercise programs, self-help groups).

FOR CLIENTS WHO ARE UNDERWEIGHT

- Discuss factors contributing to inadequate nutrition and weight loss.
- Discuss recommended calorie intake and desired weight range.
- Provide information about the content of a balanced diet.
- Provide information about ways to increase calorie intake (e.g., high-protein or high-calorie foods and supplements).
- Discuss ways to manage, minimize, or alter the factors contributing to malnourishment.
- If appropriate, discuss ways to purchase low-cost nutritious foods.
- Provide information about community agencies that can assist in providing food (e.g., Meals on Wheels).

PREVENTING FOODBORNE ILLNESS

- Reinforce hygienic handling of food and dishes:
  - Wash hands before preparing foods.
  - Wash hands and all dishes, utensils, and cutting boards with hot water and soap after contact with raw meats.
  - Defrost frozen foods in the refrigerator.
  - Cook beef, poultry, and eggs thoroughly. Use a cooking thermometer.
  - Refrigerate leftovers promptly (at 40°F [5°C] or less) and keep no more than 3 to 5 days.
  - Wash or peel raw fruits and vegetables.
  - Do not use foods from containers that have been damaged or have opened seals.
  - Follow the rules "keep hot foods hot and cold foods cold" and "when in doubt, throw it out."
- Recommend the client consider a preventive vaccination for hepatitis A.
- Instruct clients to seek medical attention for prolonged vomiting, fever, abdominal pain, or severe diarrhea following a meal.

Implementing

Nursing interventions to promote optimal nutrition for hospitalized clients are often provided in collaboration with the primary care provider who writes the diet orders and the dietitian who informs clients about special diets. The nurse reinforces this instruction and, in addition, creates an atmosphere that encourages eating, provides assistance with eating, monitors the client's appetite and food intake, administers enteral and parenteral feedings, and consults with the primary care provider and dietitian about nutritional problems that arise.

In the community setting, the nurse's role is largely educational. Nurses promote optimal nutrition at health fairs, in schools, at prenatal classes, and with well or ill clients and support people in their homes. In the home setting, nurses also initiate nutritional screens, refer clients at risk to appropriate resources, instruct clients about enteral and parenteral feedings, and offer nutrition counseling as needed. Nutrition counseling involves more than providing information. The nurse must help clients integrate diet changes into their lifestyle and provide strategies to motivate them to change their eating habits.

All dietary instructions must be individually designed to meet the client's intellectual ability, motivation level, lifestyle, culture, and economic status. Both nutritionists and dietitians help to adapt a diet to suit the client. Simple verbal instructions need to be given and reinforced with written material. Family and support persons must be included in the dietary instruction.

Assisting with Special Diets

Alterations in the client's diet are often needed to treat a disease process such as diabetes mellitus, to prepare for a special examination or surgery, to increase or decrease weight, to restore nutritional deficits, or to allow an organ to rest and promote healing. Diets are modified in one or more of the following aspects: texture, kilocalories, specific nutrients, seasonings, or consistency.

Hospitalized clients who do not have special needs eat the regular (standard or house) diet, a balanced diet that supplies the metabolic requirements of a sedentary individual (about 2000 Kcal). Most agencies offer clients a daily menu from which to select their meals for the next day; others provide standard meals to each client on the general diet.

A variation of the regular diet is the light diet, designed for postoperative and other clients who are not ready for the regular diet. Foods in the light diet are plainly cooked and fat is usually minimized, as are bran and foods containing a great deal of fiber.

Diets modified in consistency are often given to clients before and after surgery or procedures or to promote healing in clients with GI distress. These diets include clear liquid, full liquid, soft, and diet as tolerated. In some agencies, GI surgery clients are not permitted red-colored liquids or candy since, if vomited, the color may be confused with blood.

Clear Liquid Diet

This diet is limited to water, tea, coffee, clear broths, ginger ale or other carbonated beverages, strained and clear juices, and plain gelatin. Note that "clear" does not necessarily mean "colorless." This diet provides the client with fluid and carbohydrate (in the form of sugar), but does not supply adequate protein, fat, vitamins, minerals, or calories. It is a short-term diet (24 to

36 hours) provided for clients after certain surgeries or in the acute stages of infection, particularly of the GI tract. The major objectives of this diet are to relieve thirst, prevent dehydration, and minimize stimulation of the GI tract. Examples of foods allowed in clear liquid diets are shown in Box 46.9.

Full Liquid Diet

This diet contains only liquids or foods that turn to liquid at body temperature, such as ice cream (see Box 46.9). Full liquid diets are often eaten by clients who have GI disturbances or cannot tolerate solid or semisolid foods. This diet is not recommended for long-term use because it is low in iron, protein, and calories. In addition, its cholesterol content may be high because of the amount of cow's milk offered. Clients who must receive only liquids for long periods are usually given a nutritionally balanced oral supplement, such as Boost, Ensure, or Sustacal. The full liquid diet is monotonous and difficult for clients to accept. Planning six or more feedings per day may encourage a more adequate intake.

Soft Diet

The soft diet is easily chewed and digested. It is often ordered for clients who have difficulty chewing and swallowing. It is a low-residue (low-fiber) diet containing very few uncooked foods; however, restrictions vary among agencies and according to individual tolerance. Examples of foods that can be included in a soft or semisoft diet are shown in Box 46.9. The **pureed diet** is a modification of the soft diet. Liquid may be added to the food, which is then blended to a semisolid consistency.

Diet as Tolerated

"Diet as tolerated" is ordered when the client's appetite, ability to eat, and tolerance for certain foods may change. For example, on the first postoperative day a client may be given a clear liquid diet. If no nausea occurs, normal intestinal motility has returned as evidenced by active bowel sounds and client reports passing gas, and the client feels like eating, the diet may be advanced to a full liquid, light, or regular diet.

Modification for Disease

Many special diets may be prescribed to meet requirements for disease processes or altered metabolism. For example, a client with diabetes mellitus may need a diet recommended by the American Diabetes Association, an obese client may need a calorie-restricted diet, a cardiac client may need sodium and cholesterol restrictions, and a client with allergies will need a hypoallergenic diet.

Some clients must follow certain diets (e.g., the diabetic diet) for a lifetime. If the diet is long term, the client must understand the diet and also develop a healthy, positive attitude toward it. Assisting clients and support persons with special diets is a function shared by the dietitian or nutritionist and the nurse. The dietitian informs the client and support persons about the specific foods allowed and not allowed and assists the client with meal planning. The nurse reinforces this instruction, assists the client to make changes, and evaluates the client's responses.

Dysphagia

Some clients may have no difficulty with choosing a healthy diet, but be at risk for nutritional problems due to dysphagia. These clients may have inadequate solid or fluid intake, be unable to swallow their medications, or aspirate food or fluids into the lungs—causing pneumonia. Clients at risk for dysphagia include older adults, those who have experienced a stroke, clients with cancer who have had radiation therapy to the head and neck, and others with cranial nerve dysfunction. Consider dysphagia if the client exhibits the following behaviors: coughs,

BOX 46.9 Examples of Foods for Clear Liquid, Full Liquid, and Soft Diets

Clear Liquid	Full Liquid	Soft
Coffee, regular and decaffeinated	All foods on clear liquid diet plus:	All foods on clear and full liquid diets, plus:
Tea	Milk and milk drinks	Meat: all lean, tender meat, fish, or poultry (chopped, shredded); spaghetti sauce with ground meat over pasta
Carbonated beverages	Puddings, custards	Meat alternatives: scrambled eggs, omelet, poached eggs; cottage cheese and other mild cheese
Bouillon, fat-free broth	Ice cream, sherbet	Vegetables: mashed potatoes, sweet potatoes, or squash; vegetables in cream or cheese sauce; other cooked vegetables as tolerated (e.g., spinach, cauliflower, asparagus tips), chopped and mashed as needed; avocado
Clear fruit juices (apple, cranberry, grape)	Vegetable juices	Fruits: cooked or canned fruits; bananas, grapefruit and orange sections without membranes, applesauce
Other fruit juices, strained	Refined or strained cereals (e.g., cream of rice)	Breads and cereals: enriched rice, barley, pasta; all breads; cooked cereals (e.g., oatmeal)
Popsicles	Cream, butter, margarine	Desserts: soft cake, bread pudding
Gelatin	Eggs (in custard and pudding)	
Sugar, honey	Smooth peanut butter	
Hard candy	Yogurt	

chokes, or gags while eating; complains of pain when swallowing; has a gurgling voice; requires frequent oral suctioning.

Nurses may be the first individuals to detect dysphagia and are in an excellent position to recommend further evaluation; implement specialized feeding techniques and diets; and work with clients, family members, and other healthcare professionals to develop a plan to assist the client with difficulties. If the client condition suggests dysphagia, the nurse should review the history in detail; interview the client or family; assess the mouth, throat, and chest; and observe the client swallowing. Although absence of or a reduced gag reflex indicates the client will have difficulty swallowing, the presence of the gag reflex should not be interpreted to indicate that swallowing will not be impaired.

A multidisciplinary group developed the National Dysphagia Diet (NDD), which delineates standards of food textures (American Dietetic Association, 2002). The four levels of liquid foods are thin, nectar-like, honey-like, and spoon-thick liquids. The four levels of semi-solid or solid foods are pureed, mechanically altered, mechanically soft, and regular. In consultation with the dietitian, occupational therapist, swallowing specialist, speech-language pathologist, and primary care provider, these levels can be used to determine a consistent approach to a particular client's dysphagia. For example, a mechanically soft diet may result in lower pneumonia rates than a pureed diet in clients who have had a stroke and a history of aspiration pneumonia. Due to confusion regarding the terminology used to describe varying levels of food thickness, the International Dysphagia Diet Standardisation Initiative (IDDSI) developed standardized terminology and definitions to describe texture-modified foods and thickened liquids used for individuals with dysphagia of all ages, in all care settings, and all cultures (Cichero et al., 2017). See the IDDSI Framework in Figure 46.6 ■. Early detection and intervention can prevent the adverse outcomes of dysphagia in most clients.

Stimulating the Appetite

Physical illness, unfamiliar or unpalatable food, environmental and psychologic factors, and physical discomfort or pain may depress the appetites of many clients. A short-term decrease in food intake usually is not a problem

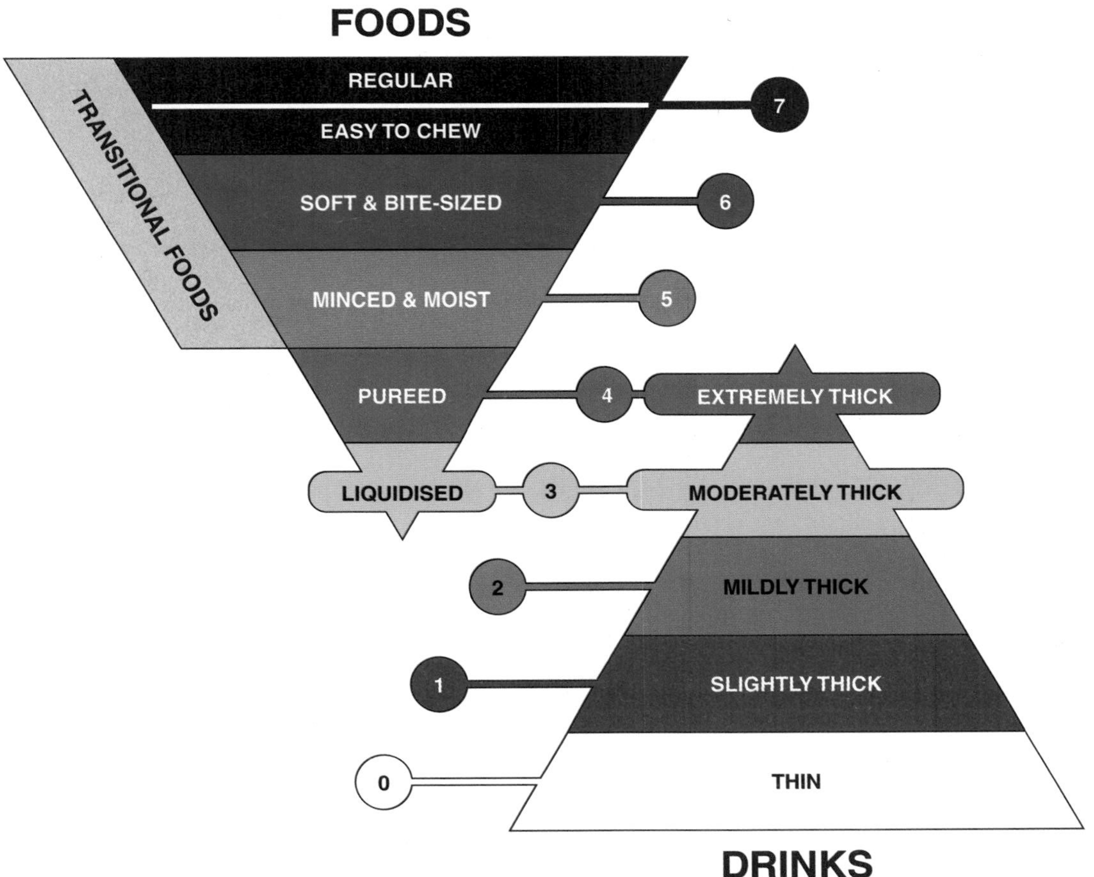

Figure 46.6 ■ The IDDSI Framework

for adults; over time, however, it leads to weight loss, decreased strength and stamina, and other nutritional problems. Decreased food intake is often accompanied by a decrease in fluid intake, which may cause fluid and electrolyte problems. Stimulating a client's appetite requires the nurse to determine the reason for the lack of appetite and then deal with the problem. Some general interventions for improving the client's appetite are summarized in Box 46.10.

BOX 46.10 Improving Appetite

- Provide familiar food that the client likes. Often the family and friends of clients are pleased to bring food from home but may need some guidance about special diet requirements.
- Select small portions so as not to discourage the client.
- Avoid unpleasant or uncomfortable treatments immediately before or after a meal.
- Provide a tidy, clean environment that is free of unpleasant sights and odors. A soiled dressing, a used bedpan, an uncovered irrigation set, or even used dishes can negatively affect the appetite.
- Encourage or provide oral hygiene before mealtime. This improves the client's ability to taste.
- Relieve illness symptoms that depress appetite before mealtime; for example, give an analgesic for pain or an antipyretic for a fever or allow rest for fatigue.
- Reduce psychologic stress. A lack of understanding of therapy, the anticipation of an operation, and fear of the unknown can cause anorexia. Often, the nurse can help by discussing feelings with the client, giving information and assistance, and allaying fears.

Assisting Clients with Meals

Because clients in healthcare agencies are frequently confined to their beds, meals are brought to the client. The client receives a tray that has been assembled in a central kitchen. Nursing personnel may be responsible for giving out and collecting the trays; however, in most settings this is done by dietary personnel. Long-term care facilities and some hospitals serve meals to mobile clients in a special dining area. Guidelines for providing meals to clients are summarized in Box 46.11.

Individuals who frequently require help with their meals include older adults who are weakened, individuals with disabilities such as visual impairment, those who must remain in a back-lying position, or those who cannot use their hands. The client's nursing care plan will indicate that assistance is required with meals.

The nurse must be sensitive to clients' feelings of embarrassment, resentment, and loss of autonomy. Whenever possible, the nurse should help clients feed themselves rather than feed them. Some clients become depressed because they require help and because they believe they are burdensome to busy nursing personnel. Although feeding a client is time consuming, nurses should try to appear unhurried and convey that they have ample time. Sitting at the bedside is one way to convey this impression. If the client is to be fed by assistive personnel, the nurse must ensure that the same standards are met.

When feeding a client, ask in which order the client would like to eat the food. If the client cannot see, tell

BOX 46.11 Providing Client Meals

- Offer the client assistance with hand washing and oral hygiene before a meal.
- If it is permitted, assist the client to a comfortable position in bed or in a chair, whichever is appropriate.
- Clear the overbed table so there is space for the tray. If the client must remain in a lying position in bed, arrange the overbed table close to the bedside so the client can see and reach the food.
- Check each tray for the client's name, the type of diet, and completeness. Do not leave an incorrect diet for a client to eat.
- Assist the client as required (e.g., remove the food covers, butter the bread, pour the tea, and cut the meat).
- For a client with a visual impairment, identify the placement of the food as you would describe the time on a clock (Figure 46.7 ■). For instance, the nurse might say, "The potatoes are at eight o'clock, the chicken at 12 o'clock, and the green beans at 4 o'clock."
- After the client has completed the meal, observe how much and what the client has eaten and the amount of fluid taken. Use a standard tool to estimate the amount eaten in relation to a typical meal. For example, if served a donut and coffee for breakfast, although the client may have consumed both of these, they certainly do not represent 100% of a nutritious breakfast.
- If the client is on a special diet or is having problems eating, record the amount of food eaten and any pain, fatigue, or nausea experienced.
- If the client is not eating, document this so that changes can be made, such as rescheduling the meals, providing smaller, more frequent meals, or obtaining special self-feeding aids.

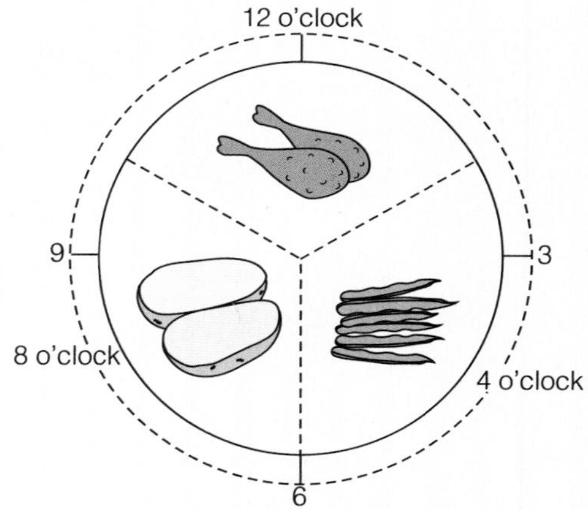

Figure 46.7 ■ For a client who is visually impaired, the nurse can use the clock system to describe the location of food on the plate.

the client which food is being given. Always allow ample time for the client to chew and swallow the food before offering more. Also, provide fluids as requested or, if the client cannot communicate, offer fluids after every three or four mouthfuls of solid food. Make the time a pleasant one, choosing topics of conversation that are of interest to clients who want to talk.

Although normal utensils should be used whenever possible, special utensils may be needed to assist a client to eat. For clients who have difficulty drinking from a cup or glass, a straw often permits them to obtain liquids with less effort and less spillage. Special drinking cups are also available. One model has a spout; another is specially designed to permit drinking with less tipping of the cup than is normally required.

Many adaptive feeding aids are available to help clients maintain independence. A standard eating utensil with a built-up or widened handle helps clients who cannot grasp objects easily. Utensils with wide handles can be purchased, or a regular eating utensil can be modified by taping foam around the handle. The foam increases friction and steadies the client's grasp. Handles may be bent or angled to compensate for limited motion. Collars or bands that prevent the utensil from being dropped can be attached to the end of the handle and fit over the client's hand. Clients requiring pureed or liquid diets are sometimes fed with a feeding syringe.

Plates with rims and plastic or metal plate guards enable the client to pick up the food by first pushing it against this raised edge. A suction cup or damp sponge or cloth may be placed under the dish to keep it from moving while the client is eating. No-spill mugs and two-handled drinking cups are especially useful for individuals with impaired hand coordination. Stretch terry cloth and knitted or crocheted glass covers enable the client to keep a secure grasp on a glass. Lidded tip-proof glasses are also available. Figures 46.8 ■ and 46.9 ■ show some of these aids.

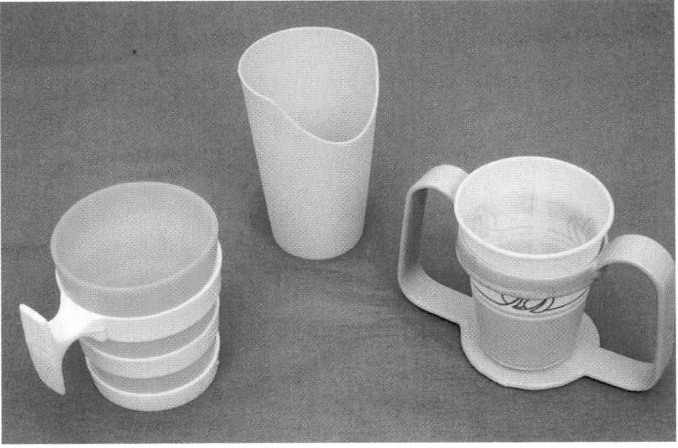

Figure 46.8 ■ Left to right: glass holder, cup with hole for nose, two-handled cup holder.

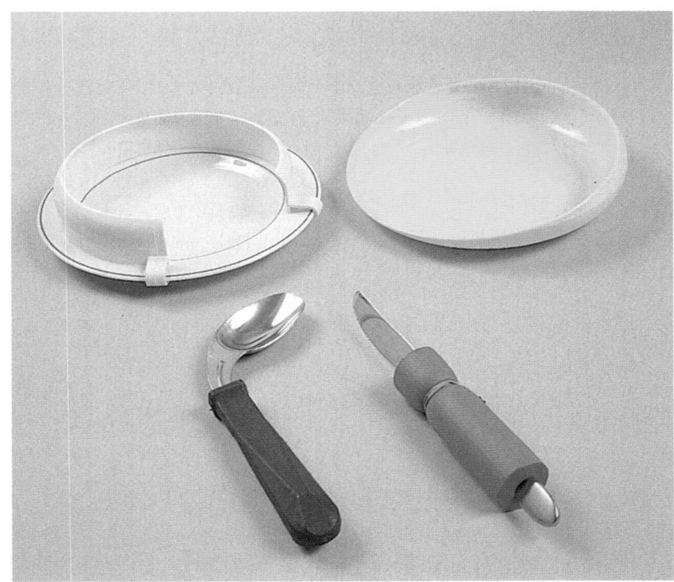

Figure 46.9 ■ Dinner plate with guard attached and lipped plate facilitates scooping; angled spoon and padded knife facilitate grip.

Special Community Nutritional Services

In many places, community programs have been developed to help special groups meet nutritional needs. For older adults who cannot prepare meals or leave their homes, ready-to-eat meals or frozen dinners are delivered to the home by local organizations. Meals on Wheels is one such well-known organization. For individuals who can prepare meals but have physical disabilities and cannot shop for groceries, grocery delivery services are available.

For low-income individuals in the United States, the USDA funds the Supplemental Nutrition Assistance Program (SNAP). Through this program, individuals and families can use an electronic benefit card (similar to a debit card) to purchase food at any approved store. The value of the benefit provided depends on the size and income of the family.

Enteral Nutrition

Alternative feeding methods that ensure adequate nutrition include **enteral** (through the GI system) methods. Enteral nutrition (EN), also referred to as total enteral nutrition (TEN), is provided when the client cannot ingest foods or the upper GI tract is impaired and the transport of food to the small intestine is interrupted. Enteral feedings are administered through nasogastric and small-bore feeding tubes, or through gastrostomy or jejunostomy tubes.

Enteral Access Devices

Enteral access is achieved by means of nasogastric or nasointestinal (nasoenteric) tubes, or gastrostomy or jejunostomy tubes.

A **nasogastric tube** is inserted through one of the nostrils, down the nasopharynx, and into the alimentary tract. Traditional firm, large-bore nasogastric tubes

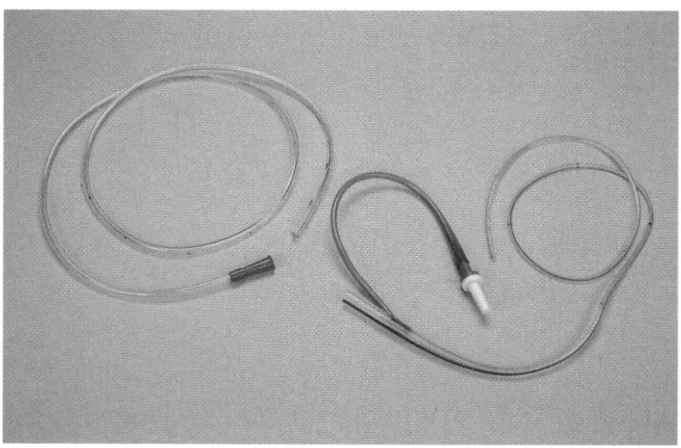

Figure 46.10 ■ *Left*, Single-lumen Levin tube. *Right*, Double-lumen Salem sump tube with filter on air vent port.

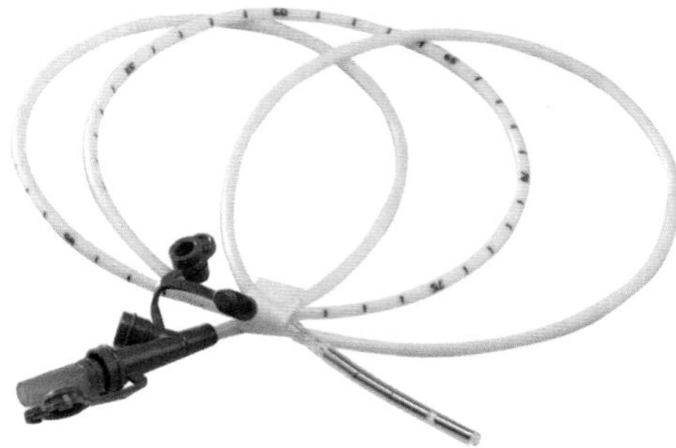

Figure 46.11 ■ A polyurethane feeding tube designed for nasogastric and nasoduodenal feeding with a weighted tip for easier insertion. The feeding port is incompatible with Luer-Lok or IV connections, reducing the risk of accidental connection or infusion. Tubes can be 8Fr–12Fr and 36"–55" long. Cardinal Health.

(i.e., those larger than 12 Fr in diameter) are placed into the stomach. Examples are the Levin tube, a flexible rubber or plastic, single-lumen tube with holes near the tip, and the Salem sump tube, with a double lumen (Figure 46.10 ■). The larger lumens allow delivery of liquids to the stomach or removal of gastric contents. When the Salem tube is used for suction of gastric contents, the smaller vent lumen (the proximal port is often referred to as the *blue pigtail*) allows for an inflow of atmospheric air, which prevents a vacuum if the gastric tube adheres to the wall of the stomach. Irritation of the gastric mucosa is thereby avoided. Softer, more flexible and less irritating small-bore feeding tubes (SBFTs), smaller than 12 Fr in diameter, are frequently used for enteral nutrition (Figure 46.11 ■).

Nasogastric tubes are used for feeding clients who have adequate gastric emptying, and who require short-term feedings. They are not advised for feeding clients without intact gag and cough reflexes since the risk of accidental placement of the tube into the lungs is much higher in those clients. Skill 46.1 provides guidelines for inserting a nasogastric tube. If the nurse is unsuccessful in placing the tube using the standard methods or the client has a particularly challenging anatomic condition, the tube may be placed by a physician endoscopically or by specially trained nurses using electromagnetic-guided bedside placement (Gerritsen et al., 2016). Skill 46.4 later in this chapter outlines the steps for removing a nasogastric tube.

SKILL 46.1

Inserting a Nasogastric Tube

PURPOSES

- To administer tube feedings and medications to clients unable to eat by mouth or swallow a sufficient diet without aspirating food or fluids into the lungs
- To establish a means for suctioning stomach contents to prevent gastric distention, nausea, and vomiting
- To remove stomach contents for laboratory analysis
- To lavage (wash) the stomach in case of poisoning or overdose of medications

ASSESSMENT

- Check for history of nasal surgery or deviated septum. Assess patency of nares.
- Determine presence of gag reflex.
- Assess mental status or ability to participate in the procedure.

PLANNING

Before inserting a nasogastric tube, determine the size of tube to be inserted and whether the tube is to be attached to suction.

Assignment

Insertion of a nasogastric tube is an invasive procedure requiring application of knowledge (e.g., anatomy and physiology, risk factors) and problem-solving. In some agencies, only healthcare providers with advanced training are permitted to insert nasogastric tubes that require use of a stylet. Assignment or delegation of this skill to assistive personnel (AP) is not appropriate. The AP, however, can assist with the oral hygiene needs of a client with a nasogastric tube.

Equipment

- Large- or small-bore tube (nonlatex preferred)
- Nonallergenic adhesive tape, 2.5 cm (1 in.) wide
- Commercial securement device, if available
- Clean gloves
- Water-soluble lubricant
- Topical lidocaine (optional)
- Facial tissues
- Glass of water and drinking straw
- 20- to 50-mL catheter-tip syringe
- Basin
- pH test strip or meter (optional)
- Bilirubin dipstick (optional)
- Stethoscope
- Disposable pad or towel
- Antireflux valve for air vent if Salem sump tube is used
- Suction apparatus
- Safety pin and elastic band
- Clamp or plug (optional)
- CO_2 detector (optional)

Inserting a Nasogastric Tube—*continued*

IMPLEMENTATION

Preparation

- Assist the client to a high-Fowler's position if the client's health condition permits, and support the head on a pillow. **Rationale:** *It is often easier to swallow in this position and gravity helps the passage of the tube.*
- Place a towel or disposable pad across the chest.

Performance

1. Prior to performing the insertion, introduce self and verify the client's identity using agency protocol. Explain to the client what you are going to do, why it is necessary, and how to participate. The passage of a gastric tube is unpleasant because the gag reflex is activated during insertion. Establish a method for the client to indicate distress and a desire for you to pause the insertion. Raising a finger or hand is often used for this.
2. Perform hand hygiene and observe other appropriate infection prevention procedures (e.g., clean gloves).
3. Provide for client privacy.
4. Assess the client's nares.
    - Apply clean gloves.
    - Ask the client to hyperextend the head, and, using a flashlight, observe the intactness of the tissues of the nostrils, including any irritations or abrasions.
    - Examine the nares for any obstructions or deformities by asking the client to breathe through one nostril while occluding the other.
    - Select the nostril that has the greater airflow.
5. Prepare the tube.
    - If a small-bore tube is being used, ensure stylet or guidewire is secured in position. **Rationale:** *An improperly positioned stylet or guidewire can traumatize the nasopharynx, esophagus, and stomach.*
    - If a large-bore tube is being used, place the tube in a basin of warm water while preparing the client. **Rationale:** *This allows the tubing to become more pliable and flexible. However, if the softened tube becomes difficult to control, it may be helpful to place the distal end in a basin of ice water to help it hold its shape.*
6. Determine how far to insert the tube.
    - Use the tube to mark off the distance from the tip of the client's nose to the tip of the earlobe and then from the tip of the earlobe to the tip of the xiphoid. ❶ **Rationale:** *This length approximates the distance from the nares to the stomach. This distance varies among individuals.*
    - Mark this length with adhesive tape if the tube does not have markings.
7. Insert the tube.
    - Lubricate the tip of the tube well with water-soluble lubricant or water to ease insertion. **Rationale:** *A water-soluble lubricant dissolves if the tube accidentally enters the lungs. An oil-based lubricant, such as petroleum jelly, will not dissolve and could cause respiratory complications if it enters the lungs.* Agency policy should permit topical lidocaine anesthetic to be used on the tube or in the client's nose to numb the area (Solomon & Jurica, 2017).
    - Insert the tube, with its natural curve downward, into the selected nostril. Ask the client to hyperextend the neck, and gently advance the tube toward the nasopharynx. **Rationale:** *Hyperextension of the neck reduces the curvature of the nasopharyngeal junction.*
    - Direct the tube along the floor of the nostril and toward the midline. **Rationale:** *Directing the tube along the floor avoids the projections (turbinates) along the lateral wall.*
    - Slight pressure and a twisting motion are sometimes required to pass the tube into the nasopharynx, and some clients' eyes may water at this point. **Rationale:** *Tears are a natural body response. Provide the client with tissues as needed.*
    - If the tube meets resistance, withdraw it, relubricate it, and insert it in the other nostril. **Rationale:** *The tube should never be forced against resistance because of the danger of injury.*
    - Once the tube reaches the oropharynx (throat), the client will feel the tube in the throat and may gag and retch. Ask the client to tilt the head forward, and encourage the client to drink and swallow. **Rationale:** *Tilting the head forward facilitates passage of the tube into the posterior pharynx and esophagus rather than into the larynx; swallowing moves the epiglottis over the opening to the larynx.* ❷
    - If the client gags, stop passing the tube momentarily. Have the client rest, take a few breaths, and take sips of water to calm the gag reflex.

❶ Measuring the appropriate length to insert a nasogastric tube.

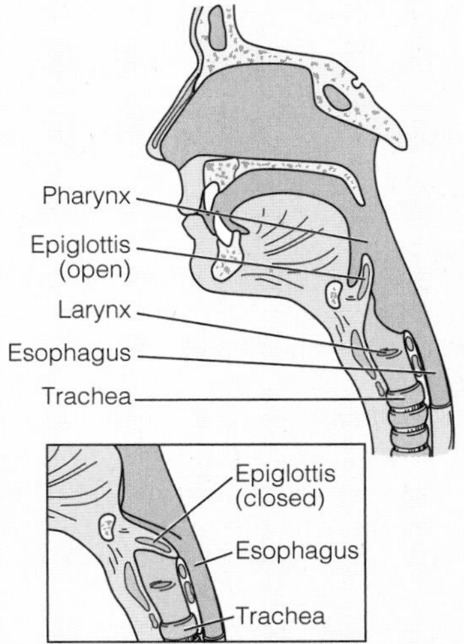

❷ Swallowing closes the epiglottis.

Continued on page 1216

Inserting a Nasogastric Tube—*continued*

- In cooperation with the client, pass the tube 5 to 10 cm (2 to 4 in.) with each swallow, until the indicated length is inserted.
- If the client continues to gag and the tube does not advance with each swallow, withdraw it slightly, and inspect the throat by looking through the mouth. **Rationale:** *The tube may be coiled in the throat. If so, withdraw it until it is straight, and try again to insert it.*
- If a CO_2 detector is used, after the tube has been advanced approximately 30 cm (12 in.), draw air through the detector. Any change in color of the detector indicates placement of the tube in the respiratory tract. Immediately withdraw the tube and reinsert.

8. Ascertain correct placement of the tube.
   - Nasogastric tubes are radiopaque, and position can be confirmed by x-ray. If an SBFT is used, leave the stylet or guidewire in place until correct position is verified by x-ray. This is the only definitive method of verifying feeding tube tip placement. If an x-ray is not feasible, at least two of the following methods should be used.
   - Aspirate stomach contents, and check the pH, which should be acidic. **Rationale:** *Testing pH is a reliable way to determine location of a feeding tube.* Gastric contents are commonly pH 1 to 5; 6 or greater would indicate the contents are from lower in the intestinal tract or in the respiratory tract. However, pH may not discriminate between gastric and esophageal placement (Morton & Fontaine, 2018).

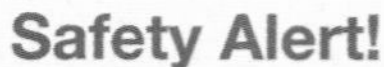

Safety Alert! SAFETY

If the stylet has been removed, never reinsert it while the tube is in place. **Rationale:** *The stylet is sharp and could pierce the tube and injure the client or cut off the tube end.*

   - Because small-bore tubes offer more resistance during aspirations than large-bore tubes and are more likely to collapse when negative pressure is applied, it may not be possible to obtain an aspirate from an SBFT. Aspirate can also be tested for bilirubin. Bilirubin levels in the lungs should be almost zero, while levels in the stomach will be approximately 1.5 mg/dL and in the intestine more than 10 mg/dL.
   - Historically, nurses placed a stethoscope over the client's epigastrium and injected 10 to 30 mL of air into the tube while listening for a whooshing sound. This method does not guarantee tube position. Even if the sound is heard, the tube could be in the stomach or the lungs (Lyman, Peyton, & Healey, 2018).
   - If the signs indicate placement in the lungs, remove the tube and begin again.
   - If the signs do not indicate placement in the lungs or stomach, advance the tube 5 cm (2 in.), and repeat the tests.
9. Secure the tube by taping it to the bridge of the client's nose.
   - If the client has oily skin, wipe the nose first with alcohol to defat the skin.
   - Apply a commercial securement device
     or
   - Cut 7.5 cm (3 in.) of tape, and split it lengthwise at one end, leaving a 2.5-cm (1-in.) tab at the end.
   - Place the tape over the bridge of the client's nose, and bring the split ends either under and around the tubing, or under the tubing and back up over the nose. ❸

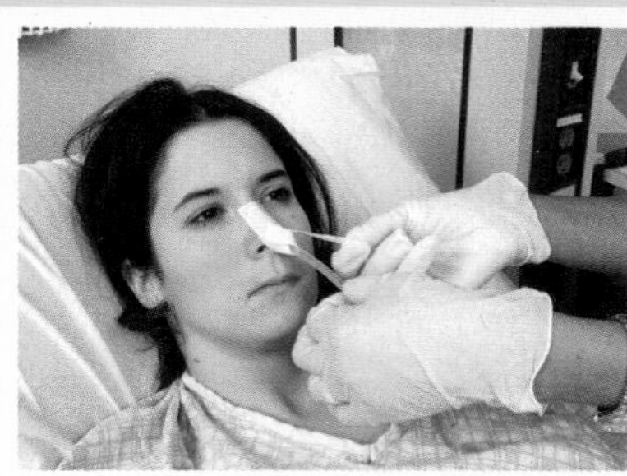

❸ Taping a nasogastric tube to the bridge of the nose.

     Ensure that the tube is centrally located prior to securing with tape to maximize airflow and prevent irritation to the side of the nares. **Rationale:** *Taping in this manner prevents the tube from pressing against and irritating the edge of the nostril.*
10. Once correct position has been determined, attach the tube to a suction source or feeding apparatus as ordered, or clamp the end of the tubing.
11. Secure the tube to the client's gown.
    - Loop an elastic band around the end of the tubing, and attach the elastic band to the gown with a safety pin.
      or
    - Attach a piece of adhesive tape to the tube, and pin the tape to the gown. **Rationale:** *The tube is attached to prevent it from dangling and pulling.*
    - If a Salem sump tube is used, attach the antireflux valve to the vent port (if used) and position the port above the client's waist. **Rationale:** *This prevents gastric contents from flowing into the vent lumen.*
    - Remove and discard gloves.
    - Perform hand hygiene.
12. Document relevant information: the insertion of the tube, the means by which correct placement was determined, and client responses (e.g., discomfort or abdominal distention).
13. Establish a plan for providing daily nasogastric tube care.
    - Inspect the nostril for discharge and irritation.
    - Clean the nostril and tube with moistened, cotton-tipped applicators.
    - Apply water-soluble lubricant to the nostril if it appears dry or encrusted.
    - Change the adhesive as required.
    - Give frequent mouth care. Due to the presence of the tube, the client may breathe through the mouth.
14. If suction is applied, ensure that the patency of both the nasogastric and suction tubes is maintained.
    - Irrigation of the tube may be required at regular intervals. In some agencies, irrigations must be ordered by the primary care provider. Prior to each irrigation, recheck tube placement.
    - If a Salem sump tube is used, follow agency policies for irrigating the vent lumen with air to maintain patency of the suctioning lumen. Often, a sucking sound can be heard from the vent port if it is patent.
    - Keep accurate records of the client's fluid intake and output, and record the amount and characteristics of the drainage.
15. Document the type of tube inserted, date and time of tube insertion, type of suction used, color and amount of gastric contents, and the client's tolerance of the procedure.

Inserting a Nasogastric Tube—*continued*

SKILL 46.1

SAMPLE DOCUMENTATION

11/5/2020 1030 #8 Fr feeding tube inserted without difficulty through R nare with stylet in place. To x-ray to check placement. Radiologist reports tube tip in stomach. Stylet removed. Aspirate pH 4. Tube secured to nose. Pt. verbalizes understanding of need to not pull on tube. L. Traynor, RN

EVALUATION

Conduct appropriate follow-up, such as degree of client comfort, client tolerance of the nasogastric tube, correct placement of nasogastric tube in stomach, client understanding of restrictions, color and amount of gastric contents if attached to suction, or stomach contents aspirated.

LIFESPAN CONSIDERATIONS Inserting a Nasogastric Tube

INFANTS AND YOUNG CHILDREN

- Restraints may be necessary during tube insertion and throughout therapy. **Rationale:** *Restraints will prevent accidental dislodging of the tube.*
- Place the infant in an infant seat or position the infant with a rolled towel or pillow under the head and shoulders.
- When assessing the nares, obstruct one of the infant's nares and feel for air passage from the other. If the nasal passageway is very small or is obstructed, an orogastric tube may be more appropriate.
- Measure appropriate nasogastric tube length from the nose to the tip of the earlobe and then to the point midway between the umbilicus and the xiphoid process.
- If an orogastric tube is used, measure from the tip of the earlobe to the corner of the mouth to the xiphoid process.
- Do not hyperextend or hyperflex an infant's neck. **Rationale:** *Hyperextension or hyperflexion of the neck could occlude the airway.*
- Tape the tube to the area between the end of the nares and the upper lip as well as to the cheek.

Although the focus of this chapter is nutrition, nasogastric tubes may be inserted for reasons other than to provide a route for feeding the client, including these:

- To prevent nausea, vomiting, and gastric distention following surgery. In this case, the tube is attached to a suction source.
- To remove stomach contents for laboratory analysis.
- To lavage (wash) the stomach in cases of poisoning or overdose of medications.

A **nasoenteric (nasointestinal) tube**, a longer tube than the nasogastric tube (at least 40 cm [15.75 in.] for an adult), is inserted through one nostril down into the upper small intestine. See Figure 46.12*A* ■. Some agencies require specially trained nurses or primary care providers to perform this procedure. Nasoenteric tubes are used for clients who are at risk for aspiration. Clients at risk for aspiration are those who manifest the following:

- Decreased level of consciousness
- Poor cough or gag reflexes
- Inability to participate in the procedure
- Restlessness or agitation.

Gastrostomy and **jejunostomy** devices are used for long-term nutritional support, generally more than 6 to 8 weeks. Tubes are placed surgically or by laparoscopy through the abdominal wall into the stomach (gastrostomy) or into the jejunum (jejunostomy). See Figure 46.12*B*. A **percutaneous endoscopic gastrostomy (PEG)** (Figure 46.13 ■) or **percutaneous endoscopic jejunostomy (PEJ)** (Figure 46.14 ■) is created by using an endoscope to visualize the inside of the stomach, making

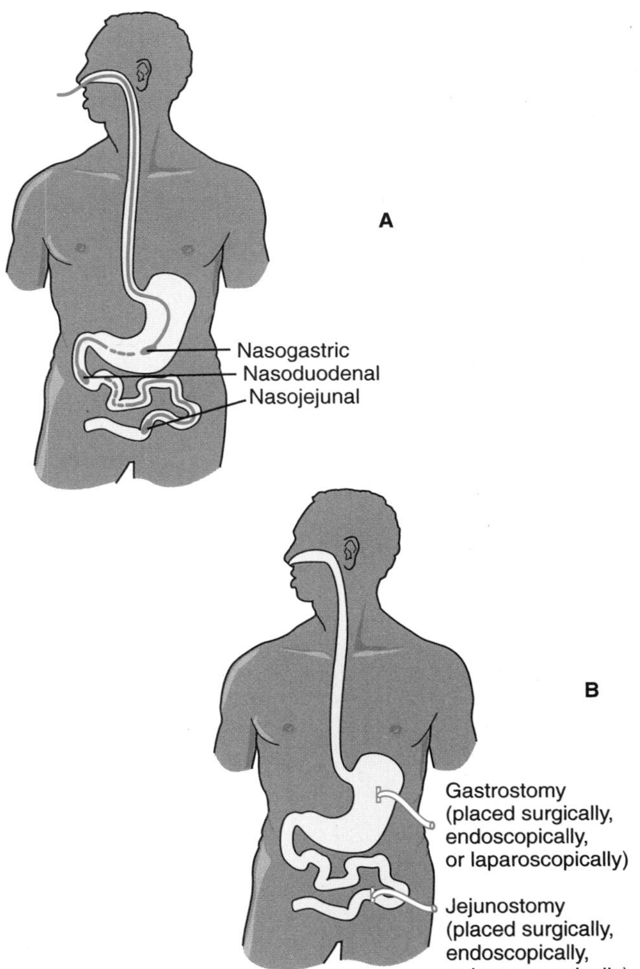

Figure 46.12 ■ Placements for enteral access: *A*, for nasoenteric and nasointestinal tubes; *B*, for gastrostomy and jejunostomy tubes.

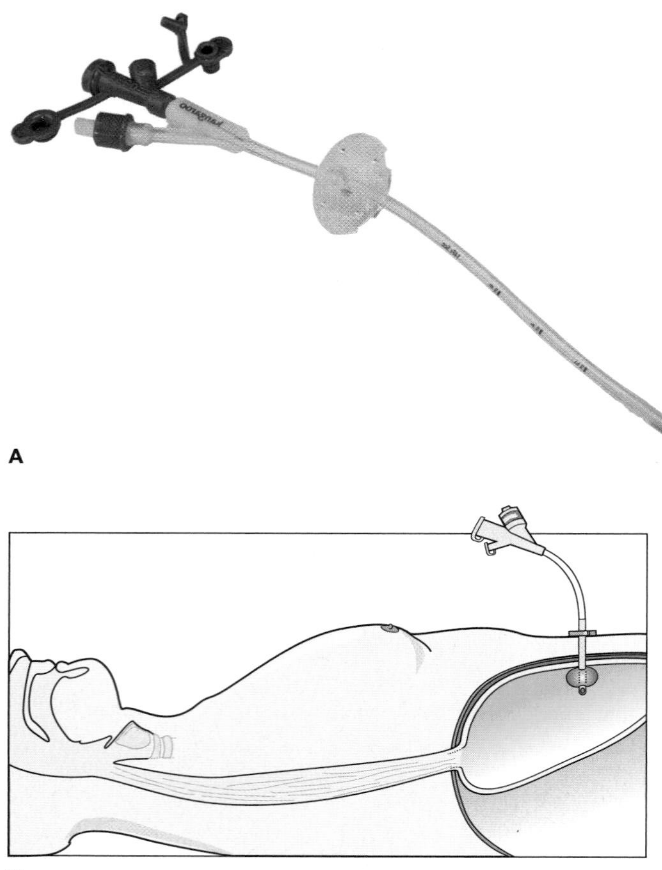

A

B

Figure 46.13 ■ Percutaneous endoscopic gastrostomy (PEG) tube.
A, Cardinal Health.

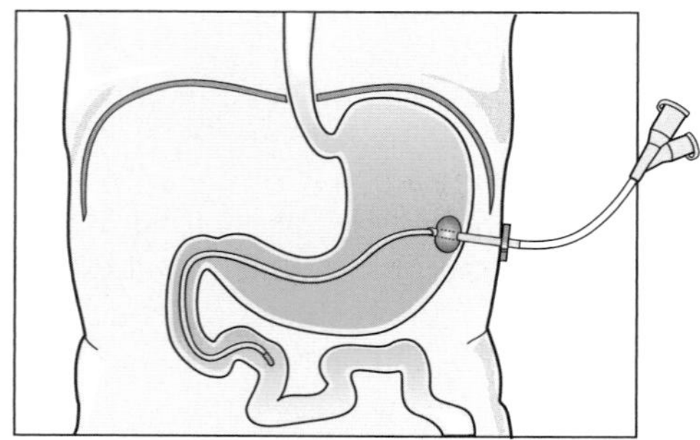

Figure 46.14 ■ Percutaneous endoscopic jejunostomy (PEJ) tube.

a puncture through the skin and subcutaneous tissues of the abdomen into the stomach, and inserting the PEG or PEJ catheter through the puncture.

The surgical opening is sutured tightly around the tube or catheter to prevent leakage. Care of this opening before it heals requires sterile technique. The catheter has an external bumper and an internal inflatable retention balloon to maintain placement. When the tract is established (about 1 month), the tube or catheter can be removed and reinserted for each feeding. Alternatively, a skin-level tube can be used that remains in place (Figure 46.15 ■). A feeding set is attached when needed.

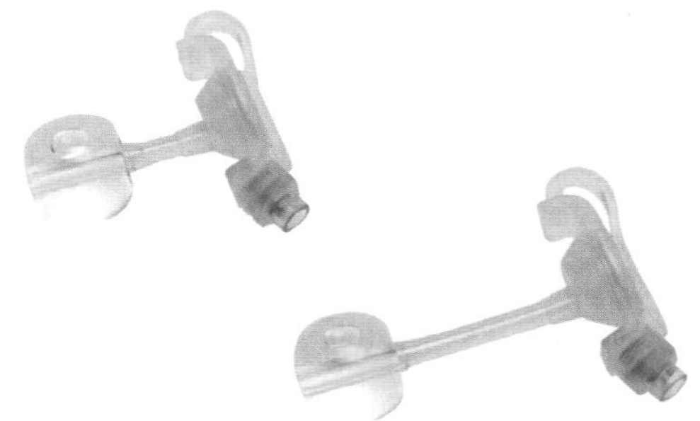

Figure 46.15 ■ Low-profile gastrostomy feeding tubes.
Cardinal Health.

Testing Feeding Tube Placement

Before feedings are introduced, tube placement is confirmed by radiography, particularly when a small-bore tube has been inserted or when the client is at risk for aspiration. After placement is confirmed, the nurse marks the tube with indelible ink or tape at its exit point from the nose and documents the length of visible tubing for baseline data. The nurse is responsible, however, for verifying tube placement (i.e., GI placement versus respiratory placement) before each intermittent feeding and at regular intervals (e.g., at least once per shift) when continuous feedings are being administered. See Skill 46.1, step 8.

Methods nurses use to check tube placement include the following:

1. Aspirate GI secretions. Gastric secretions tend to be a grassy-green, off-white, or tan color; intestinal fluid is stained with bile and has a golden yellow or brownish green color.
2. Measure the pH of aspirated fluid. Testing the pH of aspirates can help distinguish gastric from respiratory and intestinal placement as follows:
   - Gastric aspirates tend to have a pH of 1 to 5 but may be as high as 6 if the client is receiving medications that control gastric acid.
   - Small intestine aspirates generally have a pH equal to or higher than 6.
   - Respiratory secretions are more alkaline with values of 7 or higher. However, there is a slight possibility of respiratory placement when the pH reading is as low as 5.

   Therefore, when pH readings are 5 or higher, radiographic confirmation of tube location needs to be considered, especially in clients with diminished cough and gag reflexes.
3. Confirm length of tube insertion with the insertion mark. If more of the tube is now exposed, the position of the tip should be questioned.

Currently, the most effective method is radiographic verification of tube placement. Repeated x-ray studies, however, are not feasible in terms of cost. More research is required to devise effective alternatives, especially for placement of small-bore tubes. In the meantime, nurses should (a) ensure initial radiographic verification of small-bore tubes, (b) aspirate contents when possible and check their acidity, (c) closely observe the client for signs of obvious distress, and (d) consider tube dislodgment after episodes of coughing, sneezing, and vomiting.

Enteral Feedings

The type and frequency of feedings and amounts to be administered are ordered by the primary care provider. Liquid feeding mixtures are available commercially or may be prepared by the dietary department in accordance with the primary care provider's orders. A standard formula provides 1 Kcal per milliliter of solution with protein, fat, carbohydrate, minerals, and vitamins in specified proportions.

Enteral feedings can be given intermittently or continuously. Intermittent feedings are the administration of 300 to 500 mL of enteral formula several times per day. The stomach is the preferred site for these feedings, which are usually administered over at least 30 minutes. Initial intermittent feedings should be no more than 120 mL. If tolerated, increase by 120 mL each feeding until the goal is reached (Morton & Fontaine, 2018). Bolus intermittent feedings are those that use a syringe to deliver the formula into the stomach. Because the formula is delivered rapidly by this method, it is not usually recommended but may be used in long-term situations if the client tolerates it. These feedings must be given only into the stomach; the client must be monitored closely for distention and aspiration.

Continuous feedings are generally administered over a 24-hour period using an infusion pump (often referred to as a kangaroo pump) that guarantees a constant flow rate (Figure 46.16 ■). Initial continuous feedings should be no more than 40 mL per hour. If tolerated, increase by 20 mL each feeding until the goal is reached (Morton & Fontaine, 2018). Continuous feedings are essential when feedings are administered in the small bowel. Pumps are also used when smaller bore gastric tubes are in place or when gravity flow is insufficient to instill the feeding.

Cyclic feedings are continuous feedings that are administered in less than 24 hours (e.g., 12 to 16 hours). These feedings, often administered at night, allow the client to attempt to eat regular meals through the day. Because nocturnal feedings may use higher nutrient densities and higher infusion rates than the standard continuous feeding, particular attention needs to be given to monitoring fluid status and circulating volume.

Enteral feedings are administered to clients through open or closed systems. Open systems use an open-top container or a syringe for administration. Enteral feedings for use with open systems are provided in flip-top cans or powdered formulas that are reconstituted with sterile water. Sterile water, rather than tap water, reduces the risk of microbial contamination. Open systems should have no more than 8 hours of premixed formula or 4 hours of reconstituted formula poured at one time (DeBruyne, Pinna, & Whitney, 2016). At the completion of this time, remaining formula should be discarded and the container rinsed before new formula is poured. The bag and tubing should be replaced every 24 hours. Closed systems consist of a prefilled container that is spiked with enteral tubing and attached to the enteral access device. Prefilled containers can hang safely for 48 hours if sterile technique is used. Closed system materials are more expensive than open system materials, but if nursing care costs and the potential cost of infections resulting from contamination are included, closed systems are less expensive (DeBruyne et al., 2016).

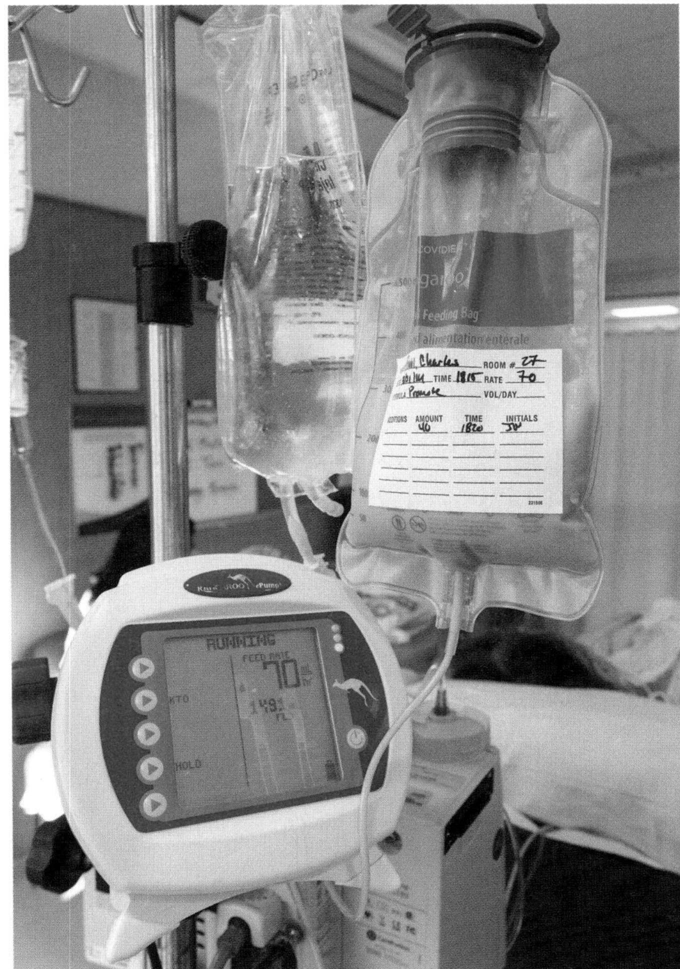

Figure 46.16 ■ An enteric feeding pump.

A somewhat rare but potentially fatal complication of tube feeding is **refeeding syndrome**—a combination of fluid and electrolyte shifts that can occur after a lengthy period of malnutrition or starvation. This syndrome can occur when the starving body converts from creating glucose from carbohydrates to creating it from protein stores since carbohydrate was unavailable. The body's reaction to the sudden presence of glucose and synthesis of protein leads to the shifts. People at high risk for developing refeeding syndrome are those with chronic alcoholism, anorexia nervosa, massive weight loss, cancer clients receiving chemotherapy, or anyone who has gone 7 to 10 days without food. The nurse takes a detailed history and examines laboratory data that can indicate malnutrition, such as albumin and prealbumin levels. Serum potassium, calcium, phosphate, and magnesium levels must be checked and supplemented until within normal levels before feeding. Experts suggest beginning feeding for at-risk clients with less than the desired amount and increasing to the full desired daily feeding slowly (Mullins, 2016).

Skill 46.2 provides the essential steps involved in administering a tube feeding, and Skill 46.3 indicates the steps involved in administering a gastrostomy or jejunostomy tube feeding.

Clinical Alert!

Enteral feedings should be started postoperatively in surgical clients without the need to wait for flatus or a bowel movement (Baird, 2016).

SKILL 46.2

Administering a Tube Feeding

PURPOSES

- To restore or maintain nutritional status
- To administer medications

ASSESSMENT

Assess

- For any clinical signs of malnutrition or dehydration.
- For allergies to any food in the feeding. If the client is lactose intolerant, check the tube feeding formula. Notify the primary care provider if any incompatibilities exist.
- For the presence of bowel sounds.
- For any problems that suggest lack of tolerance of previous feedings (e.g., delayed gastric emptying, abdominal distention, diarrhea, cramping, or constipation).

PLANNING

Before commencing a tube feeding, determine the type, amount, and frequency of feedings and tolerance of previous feedings.

Assignment

Administering a tube feeding requires application of knowledge and problem-solving and is not usually assigned to AP. Some agencies, however, may allow a trained AP to administer a feeding if allowed by law (for example, in California, APs are prohibited from performing tube feedings by the Nursing Practice Act). In any case, it is the responsibility of the nurse to assess tube placement and determine that the tube is patent; reinforce major points, such as making sure the client is sitting upright; and instruct the AP to report any difficulty administering the feeding or any complaints voiced by the client.

Equipment

- Correct type and amount of feeding solution
- 60-mL catheter-tip syringe
- Emesis basin
- Clean gloves
- pH test strip or meter
- Large syringe or calibrated plastic feeding bag with label and tubing that can be attached to the feeding tube or prefilled bottle with a drip chamber, tubing, and a flow-regulator clamp
- Measuring container from which to pour the feeding (if using open system)
- Water (60 mL unless otherwise specified) at room temperature
- Feeding pump as required

Safety Alert! SAFETY

Do not add colored food dye to tube feedings. Previously, blue dye was often added to assist in recognition of aspiration. However, the FDA reports cases of many adverse reactions to the dye, including toxicity and death.

IMPLEMENTATION

Preparation

Assist the client to a Fowler's position (at least 30° elevation) in bed or a sitting position in a chair, the normal position for eating. If a sitting position is contraindicated, a slightly elevated right side-lying position is acceptable. **Rationale:** *These positions enhance the gravitational flow of the solution and prevent aspiration of fluid into the lungs.*

Performance

1. Prior to performing the feeding, introduce self and verify the client's identity using agency protocol. Explain to the client what you are going to do, why it is necessary, and how to participate. Inform the client that the feeding should not cause any discomfort but may cause a feeling of fullness.
2. Perform hand hygiene and observe other appropriate infection prevention procedures.
3. Provide privacy for this procedure if the client desires it. Tube feedings are embarrassing to some clients.
4. Assess tube placement.
   - Apply clean gloves.
   - Attach the syringe to the open end of the tube and aspirate. Check the pH.

Administering a Tube Feeding—*continued*

- Allow 1 hour to elapse before testing the pH if the client has received a medication.
- Use a pH meter rather than pH paper if the client is receiving a continuous feeding. Follow agency policy if the pH is equal to or greater than 6.

5. Assess residual feeding contents.
   - If the tube is placed in the stomach, aspirate all contents and measure the amount before administering the feeding. **Rationale:** *This is done to evaluate absorption of the last feeding; that is, whether undigested formula from a previous feeding remains.* If the tube is in the small intestine, residual contents cannot be aspirated.
   - If 100 mL (or more than half the last feeding) is withdrawn, check with the primary care provider or refer to agency policy before proceeding. The precise amount is usually determined by the primary care provider's order or by agency policy. **Rationale:** *At some agencies, a feeding is delayed when the specified amount or more of formula remains in the stomach.* Some guidelines allow for up to 500 mL residual before holding the next feeding (Houston & Fuldauer, 2017).
   or
   - Reinstill the gastric contents into the stomach if this is the agency policy or primary care provider's order. **Rationale:** *Discarding the contents could disturb the client's electrolyte balance.*
   - If the client is on a continuous feeding, check the gastric residual every 4 to 6 hours or according to agency protocol.
6. Administer the feeding.
   - Before administering feeding:
     a. Check the expiration date of the feeding.
     b. Warm the feeding to room temperature. **Rationale:** *An excessively cold feeding may cause abdominal cramps.*
   - When an open system is used, clean the top of the feeding container with alcohol before opening it. **Rationale:** *This minimizes the risk of contaminants entering the feeding syringe or feeding bag.*

Feeding Bag (Open System)

- Apply a label that indicates the date, time of starting the feeding, and nurse's initials on the feeding bag. Hang the labeled bag from an infusion pole about 30 cm (12 in.) above the tube's point of insertion into the client.
- Clamp the tubing and add the formula to the bag.
- Open the clamp, run the formula through the tubing, and reclamp the tube. **Rationale:** *The formula will displace the air in the tubing, thus preventing the instillation of excess air into the client's stomach or intestine.*
- Attach the bag to the feeding tube ❶ and regulate the drip by adjusting the clamp to the drop factor on the bag (e.g., 20 drops/mL) if not placed on a pump.

Syringe (Open System)

- Remove the plunger from the syringe and connect the syringe to a pinched or clamped nasogastric tube. **Rationale:** *Pinching or clamping the tube prevents excess air from entering the stomach and causing distention.*
- Add the feeding to the syringe barrel. ❷
- Permit the feeding to flow in slowly at the prescribed rate. Raise or lower the syringe to adjust the flow as needed. Pinch or clamp the tubing to stop the flow for a minute if the client experiences discomfort. **Rationale:** *Quickly administered feedings can cause flatus, cramps, or vomiting.*

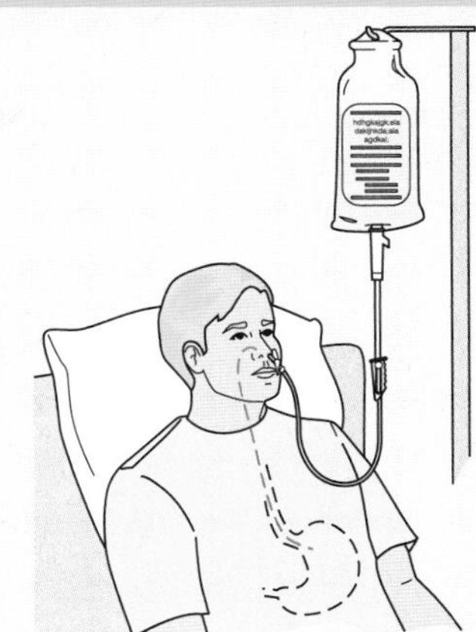

❶ Using a calibrated plastic bag to administer a tube feeding.

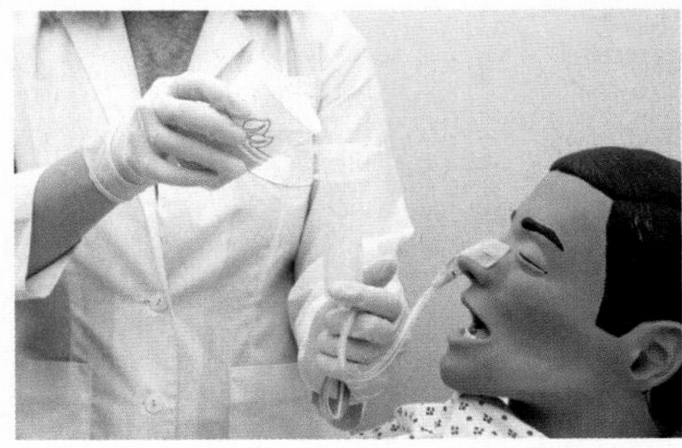

❷ Using the barrel of a syringe to administer a tube feeding.

Prefilled Bottle with Drip Chamber (Closed System)

- Remove the screw-on cap from the container and attach the administration set with tubing. ❸
- Close the clamp on the tubing.
- Hang the container on an IV pole about 30 cm (12 in.) above the tube's insertion point into the client.

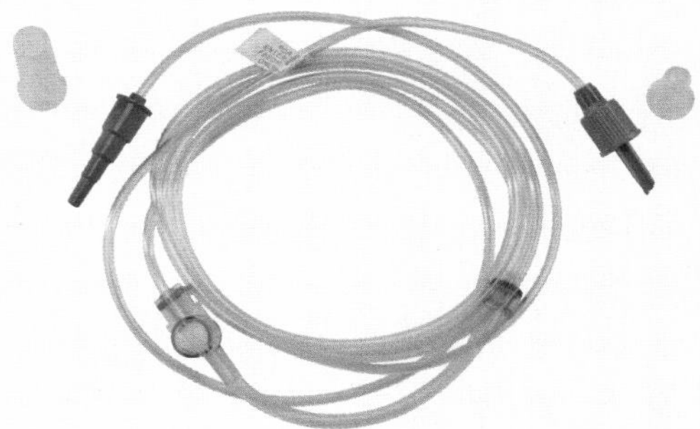

❸ Feeding set with spike and tubing. Note, the special safety screw spike and graduated connector prevent accidental connection to intravenous tubing.
Cardinal Health.

Continued on page 1222

Administering a Tube Feeding—*continued*

SKILL 46.2

- Squeeze the drip chamber to fill it to one-third to one-half of its capacity.
- Open the tubing clamp, run the formula through the tubing, and reclamp the tube. **Rationale:** *The formula will displace the air in the tubing, thus preventing the instillation of excess air*.
- Attach the feeding set tubing to the feeding tube and regulate the drip rate to deliver the feeding over the desired length of time or attach to a feeding pump.

7. If another bottle is not to be immediately hung, flush the feeding tube before all of the formula has run through the tubing.
   - Instill 50 to 100 mL of water through the feeding tube or medication port. **Rationale:** *Water flushes the lumen of the tube, preventing future blockage by formula*.
   - Be sure to add the water before the feeding solution has drained from the neck of a syringe or from the tubing of an administration set. **Rationale:** *Adding the water before the syringe or tubing is empty prevents the instillation of air into the stomach or intestine and thus prevents unnecessary distention*.
8. Clamp the feeding tube.
   - Clamp the feeding tube before all of the water is instilled. **Rationale:** *Clamping prevents air from entering the tube*.
9. Ensure client comfort and safety.
   - Secure the tubing to the client's gown. **Rationale:** *This minimizes pulling of the tube, thus preventing discomfort and dislodgment*.
   - Ask the client to remain sitting upright in Fowler's position or in a slightly elevated right lateral position for at least 30 minutes. **Rationale:** *These positions facilitate digestion and movement of the feeding from the stomach along the alimentary tract, and prevent the potential aspiration of the feeding into the lungs*.
   - Check the agency's policy on the frequency of changing the nasogastric tube and the use of smaller lumen tubes if a large-bore tube is in place. **Rationale:** *These measures prevent irritation and erosion of the pharyngeal and esophageal mucous membranes*.
10. Dispose of equipment appropriately.
    - If the equipment is to be reused, wash it thoroughly with soap and water so that it is ready for reuse.
    - Change the equipment every 24 hours or according to agency policy.
    - Remove and discard gloves.
    - Perform hand hygiene.
11. Document all relevant information.
    - Document the feeding, including amount and kinds of fluids administered (feeding plus any water used to flush the tubing), duration of the feeding, and assessments of the client.
    - Record the volume of the feeding and water administered on the client's intake and output record.
12. Monitor the client for possible problems.
    - Carefully assess clients receiving tube feedings for problems.
    - To prevent dehydration, give the client supplemental water in addition to the prescribed tube feeding as ordered.

Variation: Continuous-Drip Feeding

- Clamp the tubing at least every 4 to 6 hours, or as indicated by agency protocol or the manufacturer, and aspirate and measure the gastric contents. Then flush the tubing with 30 to 50 mL of water. **Rationale:** *This determines adequate absorption and verifies correct placement of the tube*. If placement of a small-bore tube is questionable, a repeat x-ray should be done.
- Determine agency protocol regarding withholding a feeding. Many agencies withhold the feeding if more than 75 to 100 mL of feeding is aspirated.
- To prevent spoilage or bacterial contamination, do not allow the feeding solution to hang longer than 12 hours for an open system and 48 hours for a closed system. Check agency policy or manufacturer's recommendations regarding time limits.
- Follow agency policy regarding how frequently to change the feeding bag and tubing. Changing the feeding bag and tubing every 24 hours reduces the risk of contamination.

SAMPLE DOCUMENTATION

11/5/2020 1330 Aspirated 20 mL pale yellow fluid from NG tube, pH 4.5. Client in Fowler's position. 1 L room-temperature ordered formula begun @ 60 mL/hour on pump. No nausea reported. L. Traynor, RN

EVALUATION

Perform a follow-up examination of the following:

- Tolerance of feeding (e.g., nausea, cramping)
- Bowel sounds
- Regurgitation and feelings of fullness after feedings
- Weight gain or loss
- Fecal elimination pattern (e.g., diarrhea, flatulence, constipation)
- Skin turgor
- Urine output and specific gravity
- Glucose and acetone in urine.

Relate findings to previous assessment data if available. Report significant deviations from normal to the primary care provider.

Administering an Intermittent Gastrostomy or Jejunostomy Feeding

SKILL 46.3

PURPOSES

See Skill 46.2.

ASSESSMENT

See Skill 46.2.

Planning

Before beginning a gastrostomy or jejunostomy feeding, determine the type and amount of feeding to be instilled, frequency of feedings, and any pertinent information about previous feedings (e.g., the positioning in which the client best tolerates the feeding).

Assignment

See Skill 46.2.

Equipment

- Correct amount of feeding solution
- Graduated container
- 60-mL catheter-tip syringe

For a Tube That Remains in Place

- Mild soap and water
- Clean gloves
- Petrolatum, zinc oxide ointment, or other skin protectant
- Precut 4×4 gauze squares
- Uncut 4×4 gauze squares
- Paper tape
- Extension tube with clamp for low-profile gastrostomy tube or very short tube in place

For Tube Insertion

- Clean gloves
- Moisture-proof bag
- Water-soluble lubricant
- Feeding tube

IMPLEMENTATION

Preparation

See Skill 46.2.

Performance

1. Prior to performing the feeding, introduce self and verify the client's identity using agency protocol. Explain to the client what you are going to do, why it is necessary, and how to participate. Discuss how the results will be used in planning further care or treatments.
2. Perform hand hygiene and observe other appropriate infection prevention procedures (e.g., clean gloves).
3. Provide for client privacy.
4. Insert a feeding tube, if one is not already in place.
   - Wearing gloves, remove the dressing. Then discard the dressing and gloves in the moisture-proof bag.
   - Perform hand hygiene.
   - Apply new clean gloves.
   - Lubricate the end of the tube, and insert it into the ostomy opening 10 to 15 cm (4 to 6 in.).
   - For a low-profile gastrostomy, attach extension tubing.
5. Check the location and patency of the tube.
   - Determine correct placement of the tube by aspirating secretions and checking the pH.
   - Follow agency policy for amount of residual formula. This may include withholding the feeding, rechecking in 3 to 4 hours, or notifying the primary care provider if a large residual remains.
   - For continuous feedings, check the residual every 4 to 6 hours and hold feedings according to agency policy.
   - Clamp the feeding tube. Remove the syringe plunger. Insert the syringe barrel into the tube. Pour 15 to 30 mL of water into the barrel, open the tube clamp, and allow the water to flow into the tube. **Rationale:** *This determines the patency of the tube. If water flows freely, the tube is patent*. Clamp the tubing.
   - If the water does not flow freely, notify the nurse in charge or the primary care provider.
6. Administer the feeding.
   - Hold the barrel of the syringe 7 to 15 cm (3 to 6 in.) above the ostomy opening.
   - Slowly pour the solution into the barrel, open the clamp, and allow the solution to flow through the tube by gravity.
   - Just before the syringe is empty, add 30 mL of water. **Rationale:** *Water flushes the tube and preserves its patency*.
   - If the tube is to remain in place, hold it upright, remove the syringe, and then clamp or plug the tube to prevent leakage.
   - If a tube was inserted for the feeding, remove it.
   - Remove and discard gloves.
   - Perform hand hygiene.
7. Ensure client comfort and safety.
   - After the feeding, ask the client to remain in the sitting position or a slightly elevated right lateral position for at least 30 minutes. **Rationale:** *This minimizes the risk of aspiration*.
   - Assess status of peristomal skin. **Rationale:** *Gastric or jejunal drainage contains digestive enzymes that can irritate the skin*. Document any redness and broken skin areas.
   - Check orders about cleaning the peristomal skin, applying a skin protectant, and applying appropriate dressings. Generally, the peristomal skin is washed with mild soap and water at least once daily. The tube may be rotated between thumb and forefinger to release any sticking and promote tract formation. Petrolatum, zinc oxide ointment, or other skin protectant may be applied around the stoma, and precut 4×4 gauze squares may be placed around the tube. The precut squares are then covered with regular 4×4 gauze squares, and the tube is coiled over them and taped in place.
   - Observe for common complications of enteral feedings: aspiration, hyperglycemia, abdominal distention, diarrhea, and fecal impaction. Report findings to primary care

Continued on page 1224

Administering an Intermittent Gastrostomy or Jejunostomy Feeding—*continued*

SKILL 46.3

provider. Often, a change in formula or rate of administration can correct problems.
- When appropriate, teach the client how to administer feedings and when to notify the healthcare provider concerning problems.

8. Document all assessments and interventions.

SAMPLE DOCUMENTATION

1/24/2020 2045 No fluid aspirated from gastrostomy tube. Client in Fowler's position. 30 mL water flowed freely by gravity through tube. 250 mL room-temperature Ensure formula given over 20 minutes. No complaints of discomfort. L. Traynor, RN

EVALUATION

See Skill 46.2.

LIFESPAN CONSIDERATIONS Administering a Tube Feeding

INFANTS AND YOUNG CHILDREN

- Feeding tubes may be removed after each feeding and reinserted at the next feeding to prevent irritation of the mucous membrane, nasal airway obstruction, and stomach perforation that may occur if the tube is left in place continuously. Check agency practice.
- Orogastric feeding tubes may be preferred since infants are nose-breathers (Rolfes et al., 2018).
- Formula should not be allowed to hang more than 4 hours (DeBruyne & Pinna, 2017).
- Position a small child or infant in your lap, provide a pacifier, and hold and cuddle the child during feedings. This promotes comfort, supports the normal sucking instinct of the infant, and facilitates digestion.

OLDER ADULTS

- Physiologic changes associated with aging may make the older adult more vulnerable to complications associated with enteral feedings. Decreased gastric emptying may necessitate checking frequently for gastric residual. Diarrhea from administering the feeding too fast or at too high a concentration may cause dehydration. If the feeding has a high concentration of glucose, assess for hyperglycemia because with aging, the body has a decreased ability to handle increased glucose levels.
- Conditions such as hiatal hernia and diabetes mellitus may cause the stomach to empty more slowly. This increases the risk of aspiration in a client receiving a tube feeding. Checking for gastric residual more frequently can help document this if it is an ongoing problem. Changing the formula or the rate of administration, repositioning the client, or obtaining a primary care provider's order for a medication to increase stomach emptying may resolve this problem.

EVIDENCE-BASED PRACTICE

Evidence-Based Practice

Will Increasing Nurses' Knowledge Decrease the Need for Long-Term Feeding Tube Reinsertions?

The authors of this study wanted to know if increasing nursing home nurses' knowledge of long-term gastrostomy or gastrojejunostomy feeding tube practices would decrease the frequency of the need for tube reinsertion in their hospital interventional radiology unit (Shipley, Gallo, & Fields, 2016). A 10-item pre- and posttest method was used with the 1-hour educational in-service between the tests. The in-service was based on numerous evidence-based reports of best practices in tube care. Although the number of nurses who completed both tests was small ($n = 16$), there was a statistically significant increase in their knowledge as measured on the posttest. Importantly, the number of tube replacements after the intervention was half of those prior to the study.

Implications

This was a small study using only two nursing homes and requires replication with varied and larger samples. However, the nurses' receptivity to the intervention and the significant decrease in the need for tube reinsertion suggest an effective intervention. Nurses are always learning, and techniques for preventing feeding tube clogs and displacements are relevant learning topics.

Before administering a tube feeding, the nurse must determine any food allergies of the client and assess tolerance to previous feedings. Table 46.5 lists essential assessments to conduct before administering tube feedings. The nurse must also check the expiration date on a commercially prepared formula or the preparation date and time of agency-prepared solution, discarding any formula that has passed the expiration date or that was prepared more than 24 hours previously.

Feedings are usually administered at room temperature unless the order specifies otherwise. The nurse warms the specified amount of solution in a basin of warm water or leaves it to stand for a while until it reaches room temperature. Because a formula that is warmed can grow

TABLE 46.5 Assessing Clients Receiving Tube Feedings

Assessments	Rationale
Allergies to any food in the feeding	*Common allergenic foods include milk, sugar, water, eggs, and vegetable oil.*
Bowel sounds before each feeding or, for continuous feedings, every 4 to 8 hours	*To determine intestinal activity.*
Correct placement of tube before feedings	*To prevent aspiration of feedings.*
Presence of regurgitation and feelings of fullness after feedings	*May indicate delayed gastric emptying, need to decrease quantity or rate of the feeding, or high fat content of the formula.*
Dumping syndrome: nausea, vomiting, diarrhea, cramps, pallor, sweating, heart palpitations, increased pulse rate, and fainting after a feeding	*Clients with a jejunostomy may experience these symptoms, which result when hypertonic foods and liquids suddenly distend the jejunum. To make the intestinal contents isotonic, body fluids shift rapidly from the client's vascular system.*
Abdominal distention, at least daily (Measure abdominal girth at the umbilicus.)	*Abdominal distention may indicate intolerance to a previous feeding.*
Diarrhea, constipation, or flatulence	*The lack of bulk in liquid feedings may cause constipation. The presence of hypertonic or concentrated ingredients may cause diarrhea and flatulence.*
Urine for sugar and acetone	*Hyperglycemia may occur if the sugar content of the feeding is too high.*
Hematocrit and urine specific gravity	*Both hematocrit and urine specific gravity increase as a result of dehydration.*
Serum BUN and sodium levels	*Feeding formula may have a high protein content. If a high protein intake is combined with an inadequate fluid intake, the kidneys may not be able to excrete nitrogenous wastes adequately.*

microorganisms, it should not hang longer than the manufacturer recommends. Excessively cold feedings can reduce the flow of digestive juices by causing vasoconstriction and may cause cramps. Guidelines for teaching clients and families regarding administration of tube feedings in the home are found in Client Teaching.

Managing Clogged Feeding Tubes

Even if feeding tubes are flushed with water before and after feedings and medications, tubes still may become clogged—especially SBFTs. This can occur when the feeding container runs dry, solid medication is not adequately crushed, or medications are mixed with formula. Even the important practice of aspirating to check residual volume increases the incidence of clogging. To avoid the necessity of removing the tube and reinserting a new tube, both prevention and intervention strategies must be used.

To prevent clogged feeding tubes, flush liberally (at least 30 mL water) before, between, and after each separate medication is instilled, using a 60-mL piston syringe. Too great a pressure can rupture the tube—especially small-bore feeding tubes. Do not add medications to formula or to each other because the combination could create a precipitate that clogs the tube.

CLIENT TEACHING Tube Feedings

Clients and caregivers need the following instructions to manage these feedings:

- Preparation of the formula. Include name of the formula and how much and how often it is to be given; the need to inspect the formula for expiration date and leaks and cracks in bags or cans; how to mix or prepare the formula, if needed; and aseptic techniques such as cleansing the container's top with alcohol before opening it, and changing the syringe administration set every 24 hours.
- Proper storage of the formula. Include the need to refrigerate diluted or reconstituted formula and formula that contains additives.
- Administration of the feeding. Include proper hand cleansing technique, how to fill and hang the feeding bag, operation of an infusion pump if indicated, the feeding rate, and client positioning during and after the feeding.
- Discuss strategies for hanging formula containers if an IV pole is unavailable or inconvenient.
- Plan for optimal timing of feedings to allow for daily activities. Many clients can tolerate having the majority of their feedings run during sleep so they are free from the equipment during the day.
- Management of the enteral or parenteral access device. Include site care; aseptic precautions; dressing change, as indicated; how the site should look normally; and flushing protocols (e.g., type of irrigant and schedule).
- Daily monitoring needs. Include temperature, weight, and intake and output.
- Signs and symptoms of complications to report. Include fever, increased respiratory rate, decrease in urine output, increased stool frequency or diarrhea, and altered level of consciousness.
- Whom to contact about questions or problems. Include emergency telephone numbers of home care agency, nursing clinician, primary care provider, or 24-hour on-call emergency service.

Many strategies have been used to try to unclog feeding tubes. The first strategy that should be tried is to reposition the client (this may allow a kink to straighten). Alternately flush and aspirate the tube with water using a 60-mL syringe. If the clog is in the external portion of the tube, rolling it between the thumb and fingers may help dislodge the block (Thompson, 2017). Do not flush with juice or carbonated beverages (Shipley et al., 2016). A combination of pancreatic enzymes and sodium bicarbonate has been shown to be effective at unclogging (Schallom, 2016).

If efforts to unclog a feeding tube are unsuccessful, the tube may need to be removed. Skill 46.4 describes the steps in removing a nasogastric tube.

SKILL 46.4

Removing a Nasogastric Tube

ASSESSMENT

Assess

- For the presence of bowel sounds
- For the absence of nausea or vomiting when tube is clamped

PLANNING

Assignment

Due to the need for assessment of client status, the skill of removing a nasogastric tube is not assigned to AP.

Equipment

- Disposable pad or towel
- Tissues
- Clean gloves
- 60-mL syringe (optional)
- Moisture-proof trash bag

IMPLEMENTATION

Preparation

- Confirm the primary care provider's order to remove the tube.
- Assist the client to a sitting position if health permits.
- Place the disposable pad or towel across the client's chest to collect any spillage of secretions from the tube.
- Provide tissues to the client to wipe the nose and mouth after tube removal.

PERFORMANCE

1. Prior to performing the removal, introduce self and verify the client's identity using agency protocol. Explain to the client what you are going to do, why it is necessary, and how to participate. Discuss how the results will be used in planning further care or treatments.
2. Perform hand hygiene and observe other appropriate infection prevention procedures (e.g., clean gloves).
3. Provide for client privacy.
4. Detach the tube.
   - Apply clean gloves.
   - Disconnect the nasogastric tube from the suction apparatus, if present.
   - Unpin the tube from the client's gown.
   - Remove the adhesive securing the tube to the nose.
5. Remove the nasogastric tube.
   - Optional: Instill 50 mL of air or water into the tube. **Rationale:** *This clears the tube of any contents such as feeding or gastric drainage.*
   - Ask the client to take a deep breath and to hold it. **Rationale:** *This closes the glottis, thereby preventing accidental aspiration of any gastric contents.*
   - Pinch the tube with the gloved hand. **Rationale:** *Pinching the tube prevents any contents inside the tube from draining into the client's throat.*
   - Smoothly, withdraw the tube.
   - Place the tube in the trash bag. **Rationale:** *Placing the tube immediately into the bag prevents the transference of microorganisms from the tube to other articles or individuals.*
   - Observe the intactness of the tube. **Rationale:** *This ensures that no portion of the tube has broken off in the client.*
6. Ensure client comfort.
   - Provide mouth care.
   - Assist the client as required to blow the nose. **Rationale:** *Excessive secretions may have accumulated in the nasal passages.*
7. Dispose of the equipment appropriately.
   - Place the pad, bag with tube, and gloves in the biohazard receptacle designated by the agency. **Rationale:** *Correct disposal prevents the transmission of microorganisms.*
   - Remove and discard gloves.
   - Perform hand hygiene.
8. Document all relevant information.
   - Record the removal of the tube, the amount and appearance of any drainage if connected to suction, and any relevant assessments of the client.

SAMPLE DOCUMENTATION

11/8/2020 1500 Complete NG tube removed intact without difficulty. Oral & nasal care given. No bleeding or excoriation noted. Client states is hungry & thirsty. 60 mL apple juice given. No c/o nausea. L. Traynor, RN

EVALUATION

- Perform a follow-up examination, such as presence of bowel sounds, absence of nausea or vomiting when tube is removed, and intactness of tissues of the nares.
- Relate findings to previous assessment data if available.
- Report significant deviations from normal to the primary care provider.

Parenteral Nutrition

Parenteral nutrition, also referred to as total parenteral nutrition (TPN) or intravenous hyperalimentation, is the IV infusion of dextrose, water, fat, proteins, electrolytes, vitamins, and trace elements. Because TPN solutions are hypertonic (highly concentrated in comparison to the solute concentration of blood), they are injected only into high-flow central veins, where they are diluted by the client's blood.

TPN is a means of achieving an anabolic state in clients who are unable to maintain a normal nitrogen balance. Such clients may include those with severe malnutrition, severe burns, bowel disease disorders (e.g., ulcerative colitis or enteric fistula), acute renal failure, hepatic failure, metastatic cancer, or major surgeries where nothing may be taken by mouth for more than 5 days.

TPN is not risk free. Infection prevention is of utmost importance during TPN therapy. The nurse must always observe aseptic technique when changing solutions, tubing, dressings, and filters. Clients are at increased risk of fluid, electrolyte, and glucose imbalances and require frequent evaluation and modification of the TPN mixture.

TPN solutions are 10% to 50% dextrose in water, plus a mixture of amino acids and special additives such as vitamins (e.g., B complex, C, D, K), minerals (e.g., potassium, sodium, chloride, calcium, phosphate, magnesium), and trace elements (e.g., cobalt, zinc, manganese). Additives are modified to each client's nutritional needs. Fat emulsions may be given to provide essential fatty acids to correct or prevent essential fatty acid deficiency or to supplement the calories for clients who, for example, have high calorie needs or cannot tolerate glucose as the only calorie source. Note that 1000 mL of 5% glucose or dextrose contains 50 grams of sugar. Thus, a liter of this solution provides less than 200 calories!

Because TPN solutions are high in glucose, infusions are started gradually to prevent hyperglycemia. The client needs to adapt to TPN therapy by increasing insulin output from the pancreas. For example, an adult client may be given 1 liter (40 mL/h) of TPN solution the first day; if the infusion is tolerated, the amount may be increased to 2 liters (80 mL/h) for 24 to 48 hours, and then to 3 liters (120 mL/h) within 3 to 5 days. Glucose levels are monitored during the infusion.

When TPN therapy is to be discontinued, the TPN infusion rates are decreased slowly to prevent hyperinsulinemia and hypoglycemia. Weaning a client from TPN may take up to 48 hours but can occur in 6 hours as long as the client receives adequate carbohydrates either orally or intravenously.

Peripheral parenteral nutrition (PPN) is delivered into the smaller peripheral veins. PPN cannot handle as concentrated a solution as central lines, but can accommodate lipids. For example, a 20% lipid emulsion can provide nearly 2000 Kcal/day through a peripheral vein. PPN is considered to be a safe and convenient form of therapy. One major disadvantage, however, is the frequent incidence of phlebitis (vein inflammation) associated with PPN. Peripheral parenteral nutrition is administered to clients whose needs for IV nutrition will last only a short time or in whom placement of a central IV catheter is contraindicated. It is a form of therapy used more frequently to *prevent* nutritional deficits than to correct them.

Enteral or parenteral feedings may be continued beyond hospital care in the client's home or may be initiated in the home.

Evaluating

The goals established in the planning phase are evaluated according to specific desired outcomes, also established in that phase. If the outcomes are not achieved, the nurse should explore the reasons. The nurse might consider the following questions:

- Was the cause of the problem correctly identified?
- Was the family included in the teaching plan? Are family members supportive?
- Is the client experiencing symptoms that cause loss of appetite (e.g., pain, nausea, fatigue)?
- Were the outcomes unrealistic for this client?
- Were the client's food preferences considered?
- Is anything interfering with digestion or absorption of nutrients (e.g., diarrhea)?

NURSING CARE PLAN Nutrition

ASSESSMENT DATA	NURSING DIAGNOSIS	DESIRED OUTCOMES*
NURSING ASSESSMENT Mrs. Rose Santini, a 59-year-old homemaker, attends a community hospital–sponsored health fair. She approaches the nutrition information booth, and the clinical specialist in nutritional support gathers a nutritional history. Mrs. Santini is very upset about her 9-kg (20-lb) weight gain. She relates to the nurse clinician that since the death of her husband 1 month ago she has lost interest in many of her usual physical and social activities. She no longer attends YMCA exercise and swimming sessions and has lost contact with her couple's bridge group. Mrs. Santini states she is bored, depressed, and very unhappy about her appearance. She has a small frame and has always prided herself on her petite figure. She says her eating habits have changed considerably. She snacks while watching TV and rarely prepares a complete meal. **Physical Examination** Height: 162.6 cm (5′4″) Weight: 66 kg (145 lb) Temperature: 37°C (98.6°F) Pulse: 76 beats/min Respirations: 16/min Blood pressure: 144/84 mmHg Triceps skinfold: 21 mm Small frame, weight in excess of 10% over ideal for height and frame **Diagnostic Data** CBC normal, urinalysis negative, chest x-ray negative, thyroid profile within normal limits	Overweight related to excess intake and decreased activity expenditure (as evidenced by weight gain of 9 kg [20 lb], triceps skinfold greater than normal, undesirable eating patterns)	Weight-Loss Behavior [1627] as evidenced by demonstrating: • Eats three meals each day that result in a 500-calorie reduction in intake. • Establishes a physical exercise plan that engages her in 15 to 20 minutes of exercise daily by day 5. • Identifies eating habits that contribute to weight gain by day 2.

NURSING INTERVENTIONS*/SELECTED ACTIVITIES	RATIONALE
WEIGHT REDUCTION ASSISTANCE [1280]	
Determine current eating patterns by having Mrs. Santini keep a diary of what, when, and where she eats.	*Increases awareness of activities and foods that contribute to excessive intake.*
Set a weekly goal for weight loss.	*The desirable weight-loss rate is 1/2–1 kg (1–2 lb) per week.*
Encourage use of internal reward systems when goals are accomplished.	*Goal setting provides motivation, which is essential for a successful weight-loss program.*
Set a realistic plan with Mrs. Santini to include reduced food intake and increased energy expenditure.	*A combined plan of calorie reduction and exercise can enhance weight loss since exercise increases caloric utilization.*
Assist client to identify motivation for eating and internal and external cues associated with eating.	*Awareness of factors that contribute to overeating will assist the individual in planning behavior modification techniques to avoid situations that prompt excess food consumption.*
Encourage attendance at support groups for weight loss or refer to a community weight-control program.	*Membership in a support group can enhance clients' continuation of weight-loss efforts.*
Develop a daily meal plan with a well-balanced diet, reduced calories, and reduced fat.	*Snack foods tend to be high in calories and fat and low in nutritional values.*

NURSING INTERVENTIONS*/SELECTED ACTIVITIES	RATIONALE
NUTRITIONAL COUNSELING [5246]	
Facilitate identification of eating behaviors to be changed.	*Increases individual's awareness of those actions that contribute to excessive intake.*
Use accepted nutritional standards to assist Mrs. Santini in evaluating adequacy of dietary intake.	*Comparing the individual's dietary history with nutritional standards will facilitate identification of nutritional deficiencies or excesses.*
Help Mrs. Santini to consider factors of age, past eating experiences, culture, and finances in planning ways to meet nutritional requirements.	*Social, economic, physical, and psychologic factors play a role in nutrition and malnutrition.*

NURSING CARE PLAN Nutrition—*continued*

Discuss Mrs. Santini's knowledge of the basic food groups, as well as perceptions of the needed diet modification.	*Helps to determine the client's knowledge base and identify misconceptions and gaps in understanding.*
Discuss food likes and dislikes.	*Incorporating Mrs. Santini's food preferences into the dietary plan will promote adherence to the weight-loss program.*
Assist Mrs. Santini in stating her feelings and concerns about goal achievement.	*Fear of success, failure, or other concerns may block goal achievement.*
BEHAVIOR MODIFICATION [4360]	
Assist Mrs. Santini to identify strengths and reinforce these.	*Reinforcing strengths enhances self-esteem and encourages the individual to draw on these assets during the weight-loss program.*
Encourage her to examine her own behavior.	*Involving Mrs. Santini in self-appraisal will promote identification of behaviors that may be contributing to excessive caloric intake.*
Identify the behavior to be changed in specific, concrete terms (e.g., stop snacking in front of the TV).	*Identification of specific behaviors is essential for planning behavior modification.*
Consider that it is easier to increase a behavior than to decrease a behavior (e.g., increase activities or hobbies that involve the hands such as sewing versus decreasing TV snacking).	*Habitual behaviors are difficult to change. Breaking old habits may be easier if viewed from the standpoint of increasing an enjoyable, healthy activity.*
Choose reinforcers that are meaningful to Mrs. Santini.	*Positive reinforcement is not likely to be an effective part of behavior modification if the reinforcer is meaningless to the individual.*

EVALUATION

Outcome met. Mrs. Santini kept a dietary log for 5 days and has eaten balanced meals each day, resulting in a daily deficit of 400 to 500 calories. She is aware that she eats excessively because she is bored and depressed. She has reestablished her former social contacts including her church bridge club. Mrs. Santini has purchased a stationary bicycle and exercises 20 minutes daily. She enrolled in a knitting class that meets two nights per week. She has lost 2/3 kg (1 1/2 lb) in the past week. As a reward, Mrs. Santini renewed her membership to the YMCA.

*The NOC # for desired outcomes and the NIC # for nursing interventions are listed in brackets following the appropriate outcome or intervention. Outcomes, interventions, and activities selected are only a sample of those suggested by NOC and NIC and should be further individualized for each client.

APPLYING CRITICAL THINKING

1. How do Mrs. Santini's personal characteristics influence her nutritional needs?
2. What further information do you need regarding Mrs. Santini's present diet?
3. Offer suggestions for ways to modify Mrs. Santini's tendency to snack.
4. Mrs. Santini asks what her weight should be. How do you respond?

Answers to Applying Critical Thinking questions are available on the student resources site. Please consult with your instructor.

CONCEPT MAP

Nutrition

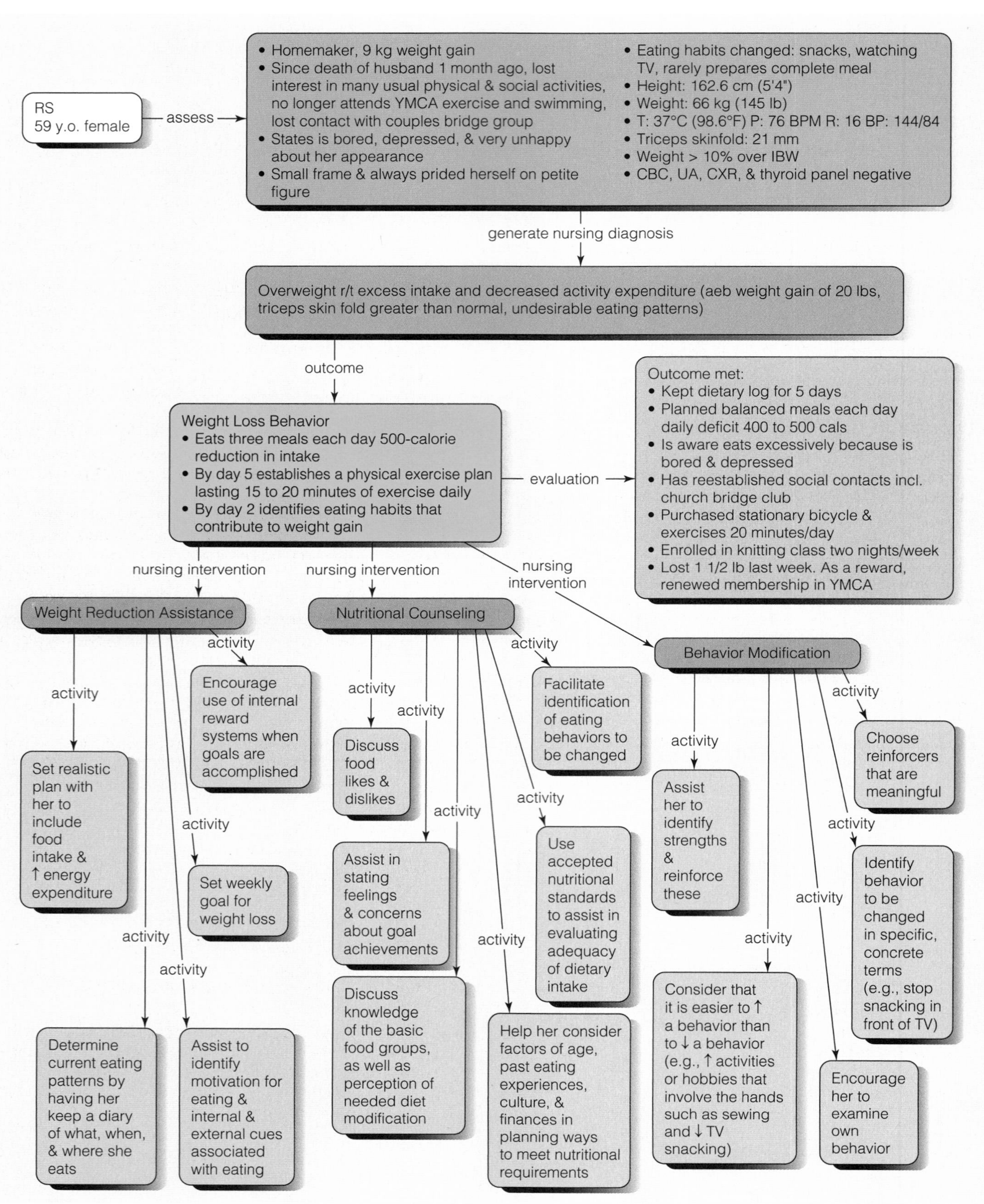
RS
59 y.o. female
assess
• Homemaker, 9 kg weight gain
• Since death of husband 1 month ago, lost interest in many usual physical & social activities, no longer attends YMCA exercise and swimming, lost contact with couples bridge group
• States is bored, depressed, & very unhappy about her appearance
• Small frame & always prided herself on petite figure
• Eating habits changed: snacks, watching TV, rarely prepares complete meal
• Height: 162.6 cm (5'4")
• Weight: 66 kg (145 lb)
• T: 37°C (98.6°F) P: 76 BPM R: 16 BP: 144/84
• Triceps skinfold: 21 mm
• Weight > 10% over IBW
• CBC, UA, CXR, & thyroid panel negative
generate nursing diagnosis
Overweight r/t excess intake and decreased activity expenditure (aeb weight gain of 20 lbs, triceps skin fold greater than normal, undesirable eating patterns)
outcome
Weight Loss Behavior
• Eats three meals each day 500-calorie reduction in intake
• By day 5 establishes a physical exercise plan lasting 15 to 20 minutes of exercise daily
• By day 2 identifies eating habits that contribute to weight gain
evaluation
Outcome met:
• Kept dietary log for 5 days
• Planned balanced meals each day daily deficit 400 to 500 cals
• Is aware eats excessively because is bored & depressed
• Has reestablished social contacts incl. church bridge club
• Purchased stationary bicycle & exercises 20 minutes/day
• Enrolled in knitting class two nights/week
• Lost 1 1/2 lb last week. As a reward, renewed membership in YMCA
nursing intervention
Weight Reduction Assistance
activity
Set realistic plan with her to include food intake & ↑ energy expenditure
Encourage use of internal reward systems when goals are accomplished
Set weekly goal for weight loss
Determine current eating patterns by having her keep a diary of what, when, & where she eats
Assist to identify motivation for eating & internal & external cues associated with eating
nursing intervention
Nutritional Counseling
Discuss food likes & dislikes
Assist in stating feelings & concerns about goal achievements
Discuss knowledge of the basic food groups, as well as perception of needed diet modification
Help her consider factors of age, past eating experiences, culture, & finances in planning ways to meet nutritional requirements
Use accepted nutritional standards to assist in evaluating adequacy of dietary intake
Facilitate identification of eating behaviors to be changed
nursing intervention
Behavior Modification
Assist her to identify strengths & reinforce these
Consider that it is easier to ↑ a behavior than to ↓ a behavior (e.g., ↑ activities or hobbies that involve the hands such as sewing and ↓ TV snacking)
Encourage her to examine own behavior
Identify behavior to be changed in specific, concrete terms (e.g., stop snacking in front of TV)
Choose reinforcers that are meaningful

Chapter 46 Review

CHAPTER HIGHLIGHTS

- Essential nutrients are grouped into categories: carbohydrates, proteins, lipids, vitamins, and minerals.
- Nutrients serve three basic purposes: forming body structures (such as bones and blood), providing energy, and helping to regulate the body's biochemical reactions.
- The amount of energy that nutrients or foods supply to the body is their caloric value. The basal metabolic rate (BMR) is the rate at which the body metabolizes food to maintain the energy and requirements of an individual who is awake and at rest. The amount of energy required to maintain basic body functions is referred to as the resting energy expenditure (REE).
- An individual's state of energy balance can be determined by comparing caloric intake with caloric expenditure.
- Ideal body weight (IBW) is the optimal weight recommended for optimal health.
- Body mass index (BMI) and percentage of body fat are indicators of changes in body fat stores. They indicate whether an individual's weight is appropriate for height and may provide a useful estimate of nutrition.
- Factors influencing an individual's nutrition include development, gender, ethnicity and culture, beliefs about foods, personal preferences, religious practices, lifestyle, economics, medications and therapy, health, alcohol consumption, advertising, and psychologic factors.
- Nutritional needs vary considerably according to age, growth, and energy requirements. Adolescents have high energy requirements due to their rapid growth; a diet plentiful in milk, meats, green and yellow vegetables, and fresh fruits is required. Middle-aged adults and older adults often need to reduce their caloric intake because of decreases in metabolic rate and activity levels.
- Various daily food guides have been developed to help healthy individuals meet the daily requirements of essential nutrients and to facilitate meal planning. These include the *Dietary Guidelines for Americans* and MyPlate.
- Both inadequate and excessive intakes of nutrients result in malnutrition. The effects of malnutrition can be general or specific, depending on which nutrients and what level of deficiency or excess are involved.
- Assessment of nutritional status may involve all or some of the following: nutritional screening, nursing history data, anthropometric measurements, biochemical (laboratory) data, clinical data (physical examination), calculation of the percentage of weight loss, and a dietary history.
- Nursing diagnoses for clients with nutritional problems may be broadly stated as insufficient dietary intake or overweight. Because nutritional problems may affect many other areas of human functioning, a nutritional problem may be the etiology of other diagnoses, such as constipation and low self-esteem.
- Major goals for clients with or at risk for nutritional problems include the following: Maintain or restore optimal nutritional status, decrease or regain specified weight, promote healthy nutritional practices, and prevent complications associated with malnutrition.
- Assisting clients and support persons with therapeutic diets is a function shared by the nurse and the dietitian. The nurse reinforces the dietitian's instructions, assists the client to make beneficial changes, and evaluates the client's response to planned changes.
- Because many hospitalized clients have poor appetites, a major responsibility of the nurse is to provide nursing interventions that stimulate their appetites.
- Whenever possible, the nurse should help incapacitated clients to feed themselves; a number of self-feeding aids help clients who have difficulty handling regular utensils.
- The nurse can refer clients to various community programs that help special subgroups of the population meet their nutritional needs.
- Enteral feedings, administered through nasogastric, nasointestinal, gastrostomy, or jejunostomy tubes, are provided when the client is unable to ingest foods or the upper GI tract is impaired.
- A nasogastric or nasointestinal tube is used to provide enteral nutrition for short-term use. A gastrostomy or jejunostomy tube can be used to supply nutrients via the enteral route for long-term use.
- The two most accurate methods of confirming GI tube placement are radiographs and pH testing of aspirate.
- Parenteral nutrition, provided when oral intake is insufficient or unadvisable, is given intravenously into a large central vein (e.g., the superior vena cava).

TEST YOUR KNOWLEDGE

1. A client receives several tube feedings each day. After documenting the client's tolerance of the feedings and assessments in the medical record, on which of the following should a nurse also document the amount fed?
   1. Graphic sheet
   2. Dietary consultation notes
   3. Vital signs record
   4. Intake and output record

2. An adult reports usually eating 3 cups dairy, 2 cups fruit, 2 cups vegetables, 5 ounces grains, and 5 ounces meat each day. The nurse would counsel the client to:
   1. Maintain the diet; the servings are adequate.
   2. Increase the number of servings of dairy.
   3. Decrease the number of servings of vegetables.
   4. Increase the number of servings of grains.

3. A nurse completes measuring the triceps skinfold of a client. In order to obtain the most meaningful data, how soon should the nurse repeat this measurement?
   1. Two days
   2. Ten days to two weeks
   3. One month
   4. One year

4. A client begins to gag and cough as a nasogastric tube is passed into his oropharynx. What is the correct nursing action?
  1. Remove the tube and attempt reinsertion.
  2. Give the client a few sips of water.
  3. Use firm pressure to pass the tube through the glottis.
  4. Have the client tilt the head back to open the passage.

5. What is the proper technique with gravity tube feeding?
  1. Hang the feeding bag 1 foot higher than the tube's insertion point into the client.
  2. Administer the next feeding only if there is less than 25 mL of residual volume from the previous feeding.
  3. Place client in the left lateral position.
  4. Administer feeding directly from the refrigerator.

6. A 55-year-old female is about 9 kg (20 lb) over her desired weight. She has been on a "low-calorie" diet with no improvement. Which statement reflects a healthy approach to the desired weight loss? "I need to:
  1. Increase my exercise to at least 30 minutes every day."
  2. Switch to a low-carbohydrate diet."
  3. Keep a list of my forbidden foods on hand at all times."
  4. Buy more organic and less processed foods."

7. An older Asian client has mild dysphagia from a recent stroke. The nurse plans the client's meals based on the need to:
  1. Have at least one serving of thick dairy (e.g., pudding, ice cream) per meal.
  2. Eliminate the beer usually ingested every evening.
  3. Include as many of the client's favorite foods as possible.
  4. Increase the calories from lipids to 40%.

8. Two months ago a client weighed 195 pounds. The current weight is 182 pounds. Calculate the client's percentage of weight loss and determine its significance.

_____ % weight loss
  1. Not significant
  2. Significant weight loss
  3. Severe weight loss
  4. Unable to determine significance

9. Which of the sites on the diagram below indicates the correct location for the tip of a small-bore nasally placed feeding tube?

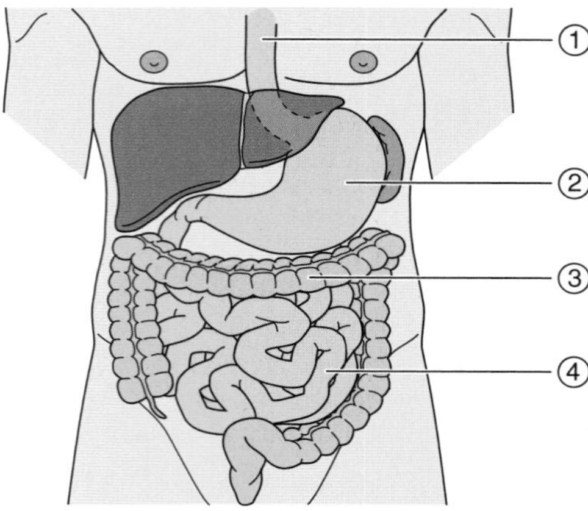

Gastrointestinal tract

10. Which meal would the nurse recommend to the client as highest in calcium, iron, and fiber?
  1. 3 ounces cottage cheese with 1/3 cup raisins and 1 banana
  2. 1/2 cup broccoli with 3 ounces chicken and 1/2 cup peanuts
  3. 1/2 cup spaghetti with 2 ounces ground beef and 1/2 cup lima beans plus 1/2 cup ice cream
  4. 3 ounces tuna plus 1 ounce cheese sandwich on whole-wheat bread plus a pear

See Answers to Test Your Knowledge in Appendix A.

READINGS AND REFERENCES

Suggested Reading

Ojo, O. (2017). Providing optimal enteral nutrition support in the community. *British Journal of Community Nursing*, *22*(5), 218–221. doi:10.12968/bjcn.2017.22.5.218

There are increasing numbers of clients receiving tube-based nutrition in the home. This article describes the role of the nurse in screening for dysphagia and malnutrition and managing feeding tubes.

Related Research

Gerritsen, A., de Rooij, T., Dijkgraaf, M. G., Busch, O. R., Bergman, J. J., Ubbink, D. T., . . . Besselink, M. G. (2016). Electromagnetic-guided bedside placement of nasoenteral feeding tubes by nurses is non-inferior to endoscopic placement by gastroenterologists: A multicenter randomized controlled trial. *American Journal of Gastroenterology*, *111*, 1123–1132. doi:10.1038/ajg.2016.224

References

American Dietetic Association. (2002). *National dysphagia diet: Standardization for optimal care*. Chicago, IL: Author.

Baird, M. S. (2016). *Manual of critical care nursing: Nursing interventions and collaborative management* (7th ed.). St. Louis, MO: Elsevier.

Butcher, H. K., Bulechek, G. M., Dochterman, J. M., & Wagner, C. M. (Eds.). (2018). Nursing interventions classification (NIC) (7th ed.). St. Louis, MO: Elsevier.

Centers for Disease Control and Prevention. (2017). *Botulism: Prevention*. Retrieved from https://www.cdc.gov/botulism/prevention.html

Cichero, J. A. Y., Lam, P., Steele, C. M., Hanson, B., Chen, J., Dantas, R. O., . . . Stanschus, S. (2017). Development of international terminology and definitions for texture-modified foods and thickened fluids used in dysphagia management: The IDDSI Framework. *Dysphagia*, *32*, 293–314. doi:10.1007/s00455-016-9758-y

DeBruyne, L. K., & Pinna, K. (2017). *Nutrition for health and healthcare* (6th ed.). Boston, MA: Cengage.

DeBruyne, L. K., Pinna, K., & Whitney, E. (2016). *Nutrition and diet therapy* (9th ed.). Boston, MA: Cengage.

Fryar, C. D., Gu, Q., Ogden, C. L., & Flegal, K. M. (2016). Anthropometric reference data for children and adults: United States, 2011–2014. National Center for Health Statistics. *Vital and Health Statistics*, *3*(39). Retrieved from https://www.cdc.gov/nchs/data/series/sr_03/sr03_039.pdf

Gerritsen, A., de Rooji, T., Mijkgraaf, M. C., Busch, O. R., Bergman, J. J., Ubbink, D. T., ... Besselink, M. J. (2016). Electromagnetic-guided bedside placement of nasoenteral feeding tubes by nurses is non-inferior to endoscopic placement by gastroenterologists: A multicenter randomized controlled trial. *American Journal of Gastroenterology*, *111*, 1123–1132. doi:10.1038/ajg.2016.224

Houston, A., & Fuldauer, P. (2017). Enteral feeding: Indications, complications, and nursing care. *American Nurse Today*, *12*(1), 20–25.

Lyman, B., Peyton, C., & Healey, F. (2018). Reducing nasogastric tube misplacement through evidence-based practice: Is your practice up-to-date? *American Nurse Today*, *13*(11), 6–11.

Moorhead, S., Johnson, M., Maas, M. L., & Swanson, E. (Eds.). (2019). *Nursing outcomes classification (NOC)* (6th ed.). St. Louis, MO: Mosby Elsevier.

Morton, P. G., & Fontaine, D. K. (2018). *Critical care nursing: A holistic approach* (11th ed.). Philadelphia, PA: Wolters Kluwer.

Mullins, A. (2016). Refeeding syndrome: Clinical guidelines for safe prevention and treatment. *Support Line*, *38*(1), 10–13.

National Heart, Lung, and Blood Institute. (n.d.). *Aim for a healthy weight: Classification of overweight and obesity by BMI, waist circumference, and associated disease risks*. Washington, DC: U.S. Department of Health & Human Services. Retrieved from http://www.nhlbi.nih.gov/health/public/heart/obesity/lose_wt/bmi_dis.htm

National Institutes of Health Office of Dietary Supplements. (n.d.). *Nutrient recommendations: Dietary reference intakes*. Retrieved from https://ods.od.nih.gov/Health_Information/Dietary_Reference_Intakes.aspx

Nelms, M. N., Sucher, K. P., & Lacey, K. (2016). *Nutrition therapy and pathophysiology* (3rd ed.). Boston, MA: Cengage.

Nutrition Screening Initiative. (2008). *Determine your nutritional health*. Washington, DC: National Council on Aging.

Ogden, C. L., Carroll, M. D., Lawman, H. G., Fryar, C. D., Kruszon-Moran, D., Kit, B. K., & Flegal, K. M. (2016). Trends in obesity prevalence among children and adolescents in the United States, 1988–1994 through 2013–2014. *JAMA*, *315*, 2292–2299. doi:10.1001/jama.2016.6361

Rolfes, S. R., Pinna, K., & Whitney, E. (2018). *Understanding normal and clinical nutrition* (11th ed.). Stamford, CT: Cengage.

Schallom, M. (2016). How to recognize, prevent, and troubleshoot mechanical complications of enteral feeding tubes. *American Nurse Today*, *11*(2), 1–7.

Shipley, K., Gallo, A.-M., & Fields, W. (2016). Is your feeding tube clogged? Maintenance of gastrostomy and gastrojejunostomy tubes. *MEDSURG Nursing*, *25*(4), 224–228.

Solomon, R., & Jurica, K. (2017). Closing the research-practice gap: Increasing evidence-based practice for nasogastric tube insertion using education and an electronic order set. *Journal of Emergency Nursing*, *43*, 133–137. doi:10.1016/j.jen.2016.09.001

Spatz, D. L. (2017). SPN position statement: The role of pediatric nurses in the promotion and protection of human milk and breastfeeding. *Journal of Pediatric Nursing*, *37*, 136–139. doi:10.1016/j.pedn.2017.08.031

Thompson, R. (2017). Troubleshooting PEG feeding tubes in the community setting. *Journal of Community Nursing*, *31*(2), 61–66.

U.S. Department of Health and Human Services & U.S. Department of Agriculture. (2015). *2015–2020 dietary guidelines for Americans* (8th ed.). Retrieved from http://health.gov/dietaryguidelines/2015/guidelines/

U.S. Department of Health and Human Services. (2019). *Healthy People 2020 nutrition and weight status: Objectives*. Retrieved from http://www.healthypeople.gov/2020/topics-objectives/topic/nutrition-and-weight-status

U.S. Food and Drug Administration. (2018). *New and improved nutrition facts label—key changes*. Retrieved from https://www.fda.gov/files/food/published/The-New-and-Improved-Nutrition-Facts-Label-%E2%80%93-Key-Changes.pdf

Selected Bibliography

Lyman, B. (2019). *Challenge 15: Nasogastric feeding and drainage tube placement and verification*. Retrieved from https://patientsafetymovement.org/actionable-solutions/challenge-solutions/nasogastric-tube-ngt-placement-and-verification

National Academies of Sciences, Engineering, and Medicine. (2017). *Nutrition across the lifespan for healthy aging: Proceedings of a workshop*. Washington, DC: National Academies Press. doi:10.17226/24735

Peterson, C. M., Thomas, D. M., Blackburn, G. L., & Heymsfield, S. B. (2016). Universal equation for estimating ideal body weight and body weight at any BMI. *American Journal of Clinical Nutrition*, *103*, 1197–1203. doi:10.3945/ajcn.115.121178

Roth, R. A. (2018). *Nutrition and diet therapy* (12th ed.). Clifton Park, NY: Cengage. doi:10.12968/bjcn.2015.20.Sup6a.S24

Wyer, N. (2017). Parenteral nutrition: Indications and safe management. *British Journal of Community Nursing*, *22*(Suppl. 7), S22–S28. doi:10.12968/bjcn.2017.22.Sup7.S22

47 Urinary Elimination

LEARNING OUTCOMES

After completing this chapter, you will be able to:

1. Describe the process of urination, from urine formation through micturition.
2. Identify factors that influence urinary elimination.
3. Identify common causes of selected urinary problems.
4. Describe nursing assessment of urinary function, including subjective and objective data.
5. Identify normal and abnormal characteristics and constituents of urine.
6. Develop nursing diagnoses and desired outcomes related to urinary elimination.
7. Describe nursing interventions to maintain normal urinary elimination, prevent urinary tract infection, and manage urinary incontinence.
8. Delineate ways to prevent urinary infection.
9. Explain the care of clients with indwelling catheters or urinary diversions.
10. Verbalize the steps used in:
    a. Applying an external urinary device
    b. Performing urinary catheterization
    c. Performing bladder irrigation.
11. Recognize when it is appropriate to assign aspects of urinary elimination to assistive personnel.
12. Demonstrate appropriate documentation and reporting of applying an external catheter, performing urethral urinary catheterization, and performing bladder irrigation.

KEY TERMS

anuria, *1239*
bladder retraining, *1247*
blood urea nitrogen (BUN), *1243*
CAUTI, *1250*
creatinine clearance, *1243*
Credé's maneuver, *1250*
detrusor muscle, *1235*
diuresis, *1238*
diuretics, *1238*
dysuria, *1240*
enuresis, *1240*
flaccid, *1250*
habit training, *1247*
ileal conduit, *1264*
irrigation, *1259*
meatus, *1235*
micturition, *1236*
nephrostomy, *1263*
neurogenic bladder, *1240*
nocturia, *1239*
nocturnal enuresis, *1240*
oliguria, *1239*
polydipsia, *1239*
polyuria, *1238*
postvoid residual (PVR), *1243*
reflux, *1235*
suprapubic catheter, *1262*
trigone, *1235*
ureterostomy, *1263*
urgency, *1239*
urinary frequency, *1239*
urinary hesitancy, *1240*
urinary incontinence (UI), *1240*
urinary retention, *1240*
urination, *1236*
vesicostomy, *1263*
voiding, *1236*

Introduction

Elimination from the urinary tract is usually taken for granted. Only when a problem arises do most individuals become aware of their urinary habits and any associated symptoms.

An individual's urinary habits depend on social culture, personal habits, and physical abilities. In North America, most individuals are accustomed to privacy and clean (even decorative) surroundings while they urinate.

Personal habits regarding urination are affected by the social politeness of leaving to urinate, the availability of a private clean facility, and initial bladder training. Urinary elimination is essential to health, and voiding can be postponed for only so long before the urge normally becomes too great to control.

Physiology of Urinary Elimination

Urinary elimination depends on the effective functioning of the upper urinary tract's kidneys and ureters and the lower urinary tract's urinary bladder, urethra, and pelvic floor (Figure 47.1 ■).

Kidneys

The paired kidneys are situated on either side of the spinal column, behind the peritoneal cavity. The right kidney is slightly lower than the left due to the position of the liver. They are the primary regulators of fluid and acid–base balance in the body. The functional units of the kidneys, the nephrons, filter the blood and remove metabolic wastes.

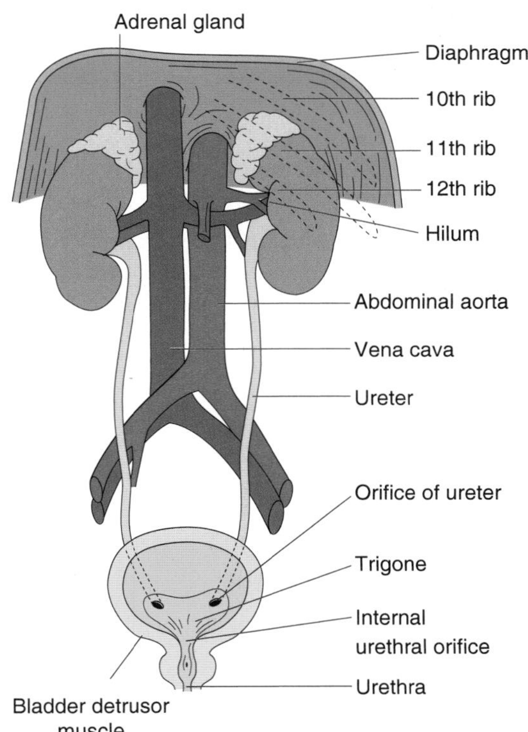

Figure 47.1 ■ Anatomic structures of the urinary tract.

In the average adult 1200 mL of blood, or about 21% of the cardiac output, passes through the kidneys every minute. Each kidney contains approximately 1 million nephrons.

Ureters

Once the urine is formed in the kidneys, it moves through the collecting ducts into the calyces of the renal pelvis and from there into the ureters. In adults the ureters are from 25 to 30 cm (10 to 12 in.) long and about 1.25 cm (0.5 in.) in diameter. The upper end of each ureter is funnel shaped as it enters the kidney. The lower ends of the ureters enter the bladder at the posterior corners of the floor of the bladder (see Figure 47.1). At the junction between the ureter and the bladder, a flaplike fold of mucous membrane acts as a valve to prevent **reflux** (backflow) of urine up the ureters.

Bladder

The urinary bladder is a hollow, muscular organ that serves as a reservoir for urine and as the organ of excretion. When empty, it lies behind the symphysis pubis. In men, the bladder lies in front of the rectum and above the prostate gland (Figure 47.2 ■); in women it lies in front of the uterus and vagina (Figure 47.3 ■).

The wall of the bladder is made up of smooth muscle layers called the **detrusor muscle**. The detrusor muscle allows the bladder to expand as it fills with urine, and to contract to release urine to the outside of the body during voiding. The **trigone** at the base of the bladder is a triangular area marked by the ureter openings at the posterior corners and the opening of the urethra at the anterior inferior corner (see Figure 47.1).

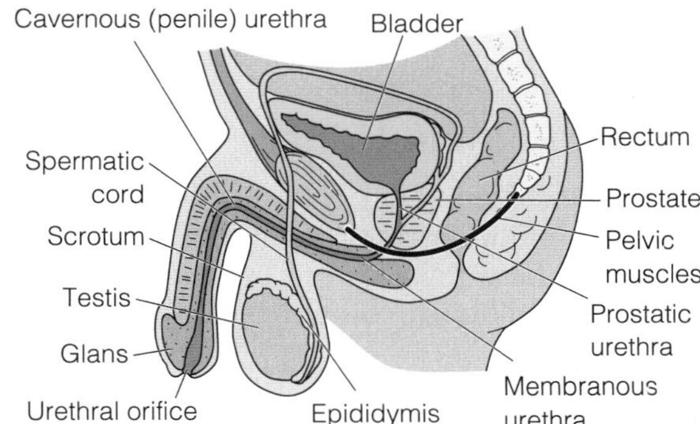

Figure 47.2 ■ The male urogenital system.

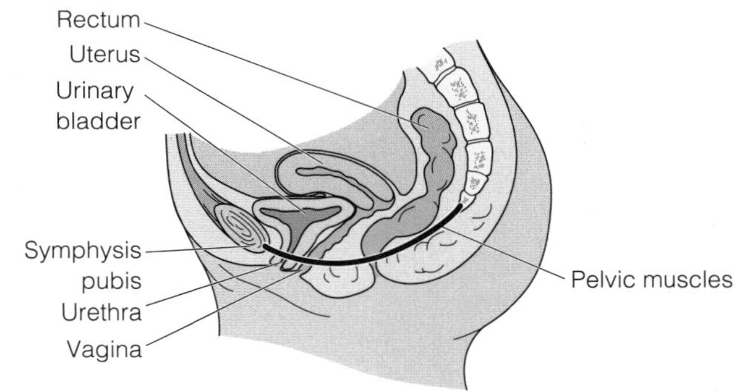

Figure 47.3 ■ The female urogenital system.

The bladder is capable of considerable distention because of rugae (folds) in the mucous membrane lining and because of the elasticity of its walls. When full, the dome of the bladder may extend above the symphysis pubis; in extreme situations, it may extend as high as the umbilicus. Normal bladder capacity is between 300 and 600 mL of urine.

Urethra

The urethra extends from the bladder to the urinary **meatus** (opening). The male urethra is approximately 20 cm (8 in.) long and serves as a passageway for semen as well as urine (see Figure 47.2). The meatus is located at the distal end of the penis. In the adult woman, the urethra lies directly behind the symphysis pubis, anterior to the vagina, and is between 3 and 4 cm (1.5 in.) long (see Figure 47.3). The urethra serves only as a passageway for the elimination of urine. The urinary meatus is located between the labia minora, in front of the vagina and below the clitoris.

In both men and women, the urethra has a mucous membrane lining that is continuous with the bladder and the ureters. Thus, an infection of the urethra can extend through the urinary tract to the kidneys. Women are particularly prone to urinary tract infections (UTIs) because of their short urethra and the proximity of the urinary meatus to the vagina and anus.

Pelvic Floor

The vagina, urethra, and rectum pass through the pelvic floor, which consists of sheets of muscles and ligaments that

ANATOMY & PHYSIOLOGY REVIEW

Female and Male Urinary Bladders and Urethras

The pelvic floor muscles (PFM) are under voluntary control and are important in controlling urination (continence). These muscles can become weakened by pregnancy and childbirth, chronic constipation, a decrease in estrogen (menopause), being overweight, aging, and lack of general fitness.

Review the figures and find the pelvic floor muscles.

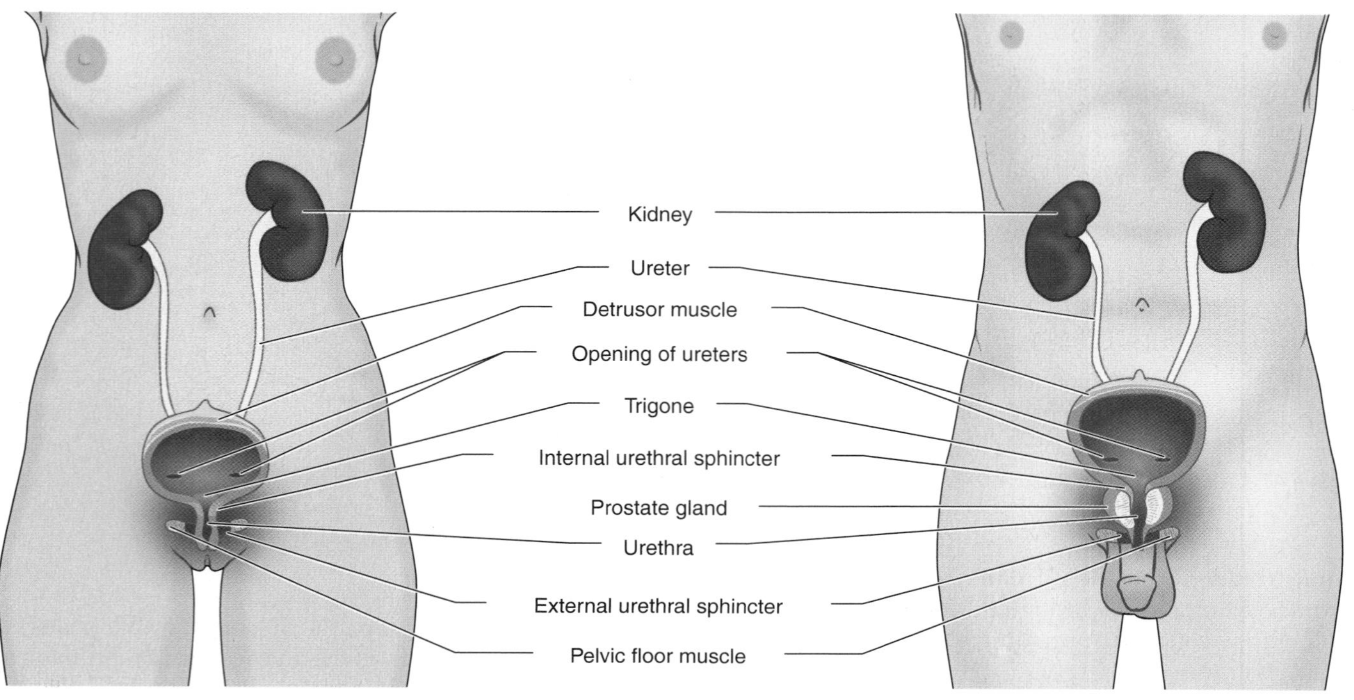

QUESTIONS

1. Do you think pelvic floor muscles can be strengthened? Provide your rationale.
2. Explain how exercising the pelvic floor muscles helps to control urination.

Answers to Anatomy & Physiology Review questions are available on the faculty resources site. Please consult with your instructor.

provide support to the viscera of the pelvis (see Figures 47.2 and 47.3). These muscles and ligaments extend from the symphysis pubis to the coccyx forming a sling. Specific sphincter muscles contribute to the continence mechanism (see the Anatomy & Physiology Review). The internal sphincter muscle situated in the proximal urethra and the bladder neck is composed of smooth muscle under *involuntary* control. It provides active tension designed to close the urethral lumen. The external sphincter muscle is composed of skeletal muscle under *voluntary* control, allowing the individual to choose when urine is eliminated.

Urination

Micturition, **voiding**, and **urination** all refer to the process of emptying the urinary bladder. Urine collects in the bladder until pressure stimulates special sensory nerve endings in the bladder wall called *stretch receptors*. This occurs when the adult bladder contains between 250 and 450 mL of urine. In children, a considerably smaller volume, 50 to 200 mL, stimulates these nerves.

The stretch receptors transmit impulses to the spinal cord, specifically to the voiding reflex center located at the level of the second to fourth sacral vertebrae, causing the internal sphincter to relax and stimulating the urge to void. If the time and place are appropriate for urination, the conscious portion of the brain relaxes the external urethral sphincter muscle and urination takes place. If the time and place are inappropriate, the micturition reflex usually subsides until the bladder becomes more filled and the reflex is stimulated again.

Voluntary control of urination is possible only if the nerves supplying the bladder and urethra, the neural tracts of the cord and brain, and the motor area of the cerebrum are all intact. The individual must be able to sense that the bladder is full. Injury to any of these parts of the nervous system—for example, by a cerebral hemorrhage or spinal cord injury above the level of the sacral region—results in intermittent involuntary emptying of the bladder. Older adults whose cognition is impaired may not be aware of the need to urinate or able to respond to this urge by seeking toilet facilities.

Factors Affecting Voiding

Numerous factors affect the volume and characteristics of the urine produced and the manner in which it is excreted.

Developmental Factors

See Table 47.1 and the Lifespan Considerations feature for summaries of the developmental changes affecting urinary output.

Psychosocial Factors

For many individuals, a set of conditions helps stimulate the micturition reflex. These conditions include privacy, normal position, sufficient time, and, occasionally, running water. Circumstances that do not allow for the client's accustomed conditions may produce anxiety and muscle tension. As a result, the client is unable to relax abdominal and perineal muscles and the external urethral sphincter; thus, voiding is inhibited. Clients also may voluntarily suppress urination

TABLE 47.1 Changes in Urinary Elimination Throughout the Lifespan

Stage	Variations
Fetuses	The fetal kidney begins to excrete urine between the 11th and 12th week of development.
Infants	Ability to concentrate urine is minimal because of immature kidneys; therefore, urine is colorless and odorless and has a specific gravity of 1.008.
	Because of neuromuscular immaturity, voluntary urinary control is absent and an infant may urinate as often as 20 times a day.
Children	Most renal growth occurs during the first 5 years of life.
	The kidneys' efficiency (i.e., regulation of electrolyte and acid–base balance) greatly increases after age 2.
	At approximately 2 1/2 to 3 years of age, the child can perceive bladder fullness, hold urine after the urge to void, and communicate the need to urinate.
	Full urinary control usually occurs at age 4 or 5 years; daytime control is usually achieved by age 3 years.
Adults	The kidneys reach maximum size between 35 and 40 years of age.
	After 50 years, the kidneys begin to diminish in size and function. Most shrinkage occurs in the cortex of the kidney as individual nephrons are lost.
Older Adults	An estimated 30% of nephrons are lost by age 80.
	Renal blood flow decreases because of vascular changes and a decrease in cardiac output.
	The ability to concentrate urine declines.
	Bladder muscle tone diminishes, causing increased frequency of urination and nocturia (awakening to urinate at night).
	Diminished bladder muscle tone and contractibility may lead to residual urine in the bladder after voiding, increasing the risk of bacterial growth and infection.
	Urinary incontinence may occur due to mobility problems or neurologic impairments.

LIFESPAN CONSIDERATIONS Factors Affecting Voiding

INFANTS AND CHILDREN

- UTIs are the second most common infection in children, after respiratory infections. They are seen more frequently in newborn and young infant boys than girls and are most often due to obstructions or malformations of the urinary system (Ball, Bindler, Cowen, & Shaw, 2017). In older infants and children, girls have more UTIs than boys, usually due to contamination of the urethra with stool.
- Children often forget to wash their hands. Teaching proper perineal hygiene can reduce infection. Girls should learn to wipe from front to back and wear cotton underwear.
- Teach children and parents that they should go to the bathroom as soon as the sensation to void is felt and not try to hold the urine in.

OLDER ADULTS

Many changes of aging cause specific problems in urinary elimination. Many conditions can be treated to lessen symptoms. Some of the following conditions are etiologic factors in problems with urinary elimination:

- Many older men have enlarged prostate glands, which can inhibit complete emptying of the bladder, resulting in urinary retention and urgency that can cause incontinence.
- After menopause women have decreased estrogen levels, which results in a decrease in perineal tone and support of bladder, vagina, and supporting tissues. This often results in urgency and stress incontinence and can even increase the incidence of UTIs.
- Increased stiffness and joint pain, previous joint surgery, and neuromuscular problems can impair mobility, making it difficult to get to the bathroom.
- Cognitive impairment, such as in dementia, often prevents the individual from understanding the need to urinate and the actions needed to perform the activity.

Interventions that may improve these conditions include:

- Medications or surgery to relieve obstructions in men and strengthen support in the urogenital area in women.
- Behavioral training for better bladder control.
- Providing safe, easy access to the bathroom or bedside commode, whether at home or in an institution. Make sure the room is well lit, the environment is safe, and the proper assistive devices are within reach (such as walkers, canes).
- Habit training, such as taking the client to the bathroom at a regular, scheduled time. This can often work very well with clients who have cognitive impairments.

because of perceived time pressures; for example, nurses often ignore the urge to void until they are able to take a break. This behavior can increase the risk of UTIs.

Fluid and Food Intake

The healthy body maintains a balance between the amount of fluid ingested and the amount of fluid eliminated. When the amount of fluid intake increases, therefore, the output normally increases. Certain fluids, such as alcohol, increase fluid output by inhibiting the production of antidiuretic hormone. Fluids that contain caffeine (e.g., coffee, tea, and cola drinks) also increase urine production. By contrast, food and fluids high in sodium can cause fluid retention because water is retained to maintain the normal concentration of electrolytes.

Medications

Many medications, particularly those affecting the autonomic nervous system, interfere with the normal urination process and may cause retention (Box 47.1). **Diuretics** (e.g., chlorothiazide and furosemide) increase urine formation by preventing the reabsorption of water and electrolytes from the tubules of the kidney into the bloodstream. Some medications may alter the color of the urine.

Muscle Tone

Good muscle tone is important to maintain the stretch and contractility of the detrusor muscle so the bladder can fill adequately and empty completely. Clients who require a retention catheter for a long period may have poor bladder muscle tone because continuous drainage of urine prevents the bladder from filling and emptying normally. Pelvic floor muscle tone also contributes to the ability to store and empty urine.

Pathologic Conditions

Some diseases and pathologies can affect the formation and excretion of urine. Diseases of the kidneys may affect the ability of the nephrons to produce urine. Abnormal amounts of protein or blood cells may be present in the urine, or the kidneys may virtually stop producing urine altogether, a condition known as renal failure. Heart and circulatory disorders such as heart failure, shock, or hypertension can affect blood flow to the kidneys, interfering with urine production. If abnormal amounts of fluid are lost through another route (e.g., vomiting or high fever), the kidneys retain water and urinary output falls.

Processes that interfere with the flow of urine from the kidneys to the urethra affect urinary excretion. A urinary stone (calculus) may obstruct a ureter, blocking urine flow from the kidney to the bladder. Hyperplasia (enlargement) of the prostate gland, a common condition affecting older men, may obstruct the urethra, impairing urination and bladder emptying.

Surgical and Diagnostic Procedures

Some surgical and diagnostic procedures affect the passage of urine and the urine itself. The urethra may swell following a cystoscopy, and surgical procedures on any part of the urinary tract may result in some postoperative bleeding; as a result, the urine may be red or pink tinged for a time.

Spinal anesthetics can affect the passage of urine because they decrease the client's awareness of the need to void. Surgery on structures adjacent to the urinary tract (e.g., the uterus) can also affect voiding because of swelling in the lower abdomen.

Altered Urine Production

Although patterns of urination are highly individual, most individuals void about 5 to 6 times a day. Individuals usually void when they first awaken in the morning, before they go to bed, and around mealtimes. Table 47.2 shows the average urinary output per day at different ages.

Polyuria

Polyuria (or **diuresis**) refers to the production of abnormally large amounts of urine by the kidneys, often several liters more than the client's usual daily output. Polyuria can follow excessive fluid intake, a condition known as

BOX 47.1 Medications That May Cause Urinary Retention

- Anticholinergic medications, such as Atropine, Robinul, and Pro-Banthine
- Antidepressant and antipsychotic agents, such as tricyclic antidepressants and monoamine oxidase inhibitors (MAOIs)
- Antihistamine preparations, such as pseudoephedrine (Actifed and Sudafed)
- Antihypertensives, such as hydralazine (Apresoline) and methyldopa (Aldomet)
- Antiparkinsonism drugs, such as levodopa, trihexyphenidyl (Artane), and benztropine mesylate (Cogentin)
- Beta-adrenergic blockers, such as propranolol (Inderal)
- Opioids, such as hydrocodone (Vicodin)

TABLE 47.2 Average Daily Urine Output by Age

Age	Amount (mL)
1–2 days	15–60
3–10 days	100–300
10 days–2 months	250–450
2 months–1 year	400–500
1–3 years	500–600
3–5 years	600–700
5–8 years	700–1000
8–14 years	800–1400
14 years through adulthood	1500
Older adulthood	1500 or less

polydipsia, or may be associated with diseases such as diabetes mellitus, diabetes insipidus, and chronic nephritis. Polyuria can cause excessive fluid loss, leading to intense thirst, dehydration, and weight loss.

Oliguria and Anuria

The terms *oliguria* and *anuria* are used to describe decreased urinary output. **Oliguria** is low urine output, usually less than 500 mL a day or 30 mL an hour for an adult. Although oliguria may occur because of abnormal fluid losses or a lack of fluid intake, it often indicates impaired blood flow to the kidneys or impending renal failure and should be promptly reported to the primary care provider. Restoring renal blood flow and urinary output promptly can prevent renal failure and its complications. **Anuria** refers to a lack of urine production.

Altered Urinary Elimination

Despite normal urine production, a number of factors or conditions can affect urinary elimination. Frequency, nocturia, urgency, and dysuria often are manifestations of underlying conditions such as a UTI. Enuresis, incontinence, retention, and neurogenic bladder may be either a manifestation or the primary problem affecting urinary elimination. Selected factors associated with altered patterns of urine elimination are identified in Table 47.3.

Frequency and Nocturia

Urinary frequency is voiding at frequent intervals, that is, more than 4 to 6 times per day. An increased intake of fluid causes some increase in the frequency of voiding. Conditions such as UTI, stress, and pregnancy can cause frequent voiding of small quantities (50 to 100 mL) of urine. Total fluid intake and output may be normal.

Nocturia is voiding 2 or more times at night. Like frequency, it is usually expressed in terms of the number of times the individual gets out of bed to void, for example, "nocturia × 4."

Urgency

Urgency is the sudden, strong desire to void. There may or may not be a great deal of urine in the bladder, but the individual feels a need to void immediately. Urgency accompanies psychologic stress and irritation of the trigone and urethra. It is also common in individuals who have poor external sphincter control and unstable bladder contractions. It is not a normal finding.

TABLE 47.3 Selected Factors Associated with Altered Urinary Elimination

Pattern	Selected Associated Factors
Polyuria	Ingestion of fluids containing caffeine or alcohol Prescribed diuretic Presence of thirst, dehydration, and weight loss History of diabetes mellitus, diabetes insipidus, or kidney disease
Oliguria, anuria	Decrease in fluid intake Signs of dehydration Presence of hypotension, shock, or heart failure History of kidney disease Signs of renal failure such as elevated blood urea nitrogen (BUN) and serum creatinine, edema, hypertension
Frequency or nocturia	Pregnancy Increase in fluid intake UTI
Urgency	Presence of psychologic stress UTI
Dysuria	Urinary tract inflammation, infection, or injury Hesitancy, hematuria, pyuria (pus in the urine), and frequency
Enuresis	Family history of enuresis Difficult access to toilet facilities Home stresses
Incontinence	Bladder inflammation, stroke (cerebrovascular accident [CVA]), spinal cord injury, or other disease Difficulties in independent toileting (mobility impairment) Leakage when coughing, laughing, sneezing Cognitive impairment Retention Distended bladder on palpation and percussion Associated signs, such as pubic discomfort, restlessness, frequency, and small urine volume Recent anesthesia Recent perineal surgery Presence of perineal swelling Medications prescribed Lack of privacy or other factors inhibiting micturition

Dysuria

Dysuria means voiding that is either painful or difficult. It can accompany a stricture (decrease in diameter) of the urethra, urinary infections, and injury to the bladder and urethra. Often clients will say they have to push to void or that burning accompanies or follows voiding. The burning may be described as severe, like a hot poker, or more subdued, like a sunburn. Often, **urinary hesitancy** (a delay and difficulty in initiating voiding) is associated with dysuria.

Enuresis

Enuresis is involuntary urination in children beyond the age when voluntary bladder control is normally acquired, usually 4 or 5 years of age. **Nocturnal enuresis** often is irregular in occurrence and affects boys more often than girls. Diurnal (daytime) enuresis may be persistent and pathologic in origin. It affects women and girls more frequently.

Urinary Incontinence

Urinary incontinence (UI), is any involuntary urine leakage. UI is a widespread problem internationally, peaking in the geriatric population (Searcy, 2017, p. 447). About 16% to 18% of postmenopausal women develop UI (Tso & Lee, 2018). UI can lead to depression, feelings of shame and embarrassment, and isolation, and can prevent individuals from traveling far from home (Kehinde, 2016; Nazarko, 2017). Kehinde (2016) reports that UI increases admission to long-term care facilities. Older adults have the highest incidence of UI, which puts them at risk for skin breakdown, recurrent UTIs, and falls related to symptoms of urgency. In spite of the high numbers of adults with UI, it is underreported and undertreated and can lead to a decreased quality of life. Many individuals do not seek help because they think nothing can be done or they think they are too old for treatment (Leaver, 2017). It is important to remember that UI is *not* a normal part of aging and often is treatable.

The types of UI can be classified based on symptoms: stress, urgency, mixed, overflow, and transient and functional.

Stress Urinary Incontinence

Stress urinary incontinence (SUI), the most common type of UI, occurs because of weak pelvic floor muscles or urethral hypermobility, causing urine leakage with such activities as laughing, coughing, sneezing, or any body movement that puts pressure on the bladder. Facts that make women more likely to experience SUI include shorter urethras, the trauma to the pelvic floor associated with childbirth, and changes related to menopause. For men, SUI may result after a prostatectomy. It is important for clients to understand that SUI is not related to emotional stress but is caused by increased intra-abdominal pressure on the bladder, as well as anatomic changes to the urethra and pelvic floor muscle weakness.

Urgency Urinary Incontinence

Urgency urinary incontinence (UUI) is also called overactive bladder (Palmer & Willis-Gray, 2017; Tso & Lee, 2018). It is described as an urgent need to void and the inability to stop urine leakage, which can range from a few drops to soaking of undergarments. Normally the bladder contracts on urination. Individuals with an overactive bladder experience contractions while the bladder is filling, leading to an urgency to void, which can lead to UI (Nazarko, 2017).

Mixed Urinary Incontinence

Mixed incontinence is diagnosed when symptoms of both SUI and UUI are present. The SUI and UUI symptoms do not occur at the same time; usually the individual experiences episodes of isolated SUI and isolated UUI. It is very common among older women (Searcy, 2017). Treatment is usually based on which type of UI is the most bothersome to the client.

Overflow Urinary Incontinence

This is when the bladder overfills and urine leaks out due to pressure on the urinary sphincter. It occurs in men with an enlarged prostate and clients with a neurologic disorder (e.g., multiple sclerosis, Parkinson's disease, spinal cord injury). An impaired neurologic function can interfere with the normal mechanisms of urine elimination, resulting in a **neurogenic bladder**. The client with a neurogenic bladder does not perceive bladder fullness and is therefore unable to control the urinary sphincters.

Transient and Functional Urinary Incontinence

Transient urinary incontinence results from factors outside of the urinary tract (e.g., medications, delirium, infection, constipation). Functional urinary incontinence (FUI) is a subcategory of transient urinary incontinence. FUI is connected with a cognitive or physical impairment, for example, unavailable toileting facilities or the inability to reach a toilet due to physical limitations. An individual with cognitive impairment may recognize the need to void but be unable to communicate the need.

Urinary Retention

When emptying of the bladder is impaired, urine accumulates and the bladder becomes overdistended, a condition known as **urinary retention**. Overdistention of the bladder causes poor contractility of the detrusor muscle, further impairing urination. Common causes of urinary retention include benign prostatic hyperplasia (BPH), surgery, and some medications (see Box 47.1). Acute urinary retention is the most common complication postoperatively (Hoke & Bradway, 2016). Clients with urinary retention may experience overflow incontinence, eliminating 25 to 50 mL of urine at frequent intervals. The bladder is firm and distended on palpation and may be displaced to one side of the midline.

EVIDENCE-BASED PRACTICE

Evidence-Based Practice

What Are the Outcomes of the Application of Nonpharmacologic and Nonsurgical Resources to Treat Female Urinary Incontinence?

Women are at greater risk for UI than men and the risk increases with age. UI affects the quality of life as well as the social, physical, psychologic, occupational, and sexual aspects of women's lives. Unfortunately, most women never seek or receive UI treatments. Believing that healthcare providers should use evidence-based practice in UI health services, Mendes, Rodolpho, and Hoga (2016) conducted an integrative review (IR) of literature to answer the question posed in the title. The IR resulted in an initial 1592 empirical studies with 198 potentially relevant papers identified. Further analysis resulted in 14 studies that met the eligibility criteria of the IR. Studies were conducted in 10 countries, indicating the international relevance of UI.

The types of treatments used in the studies included electrical stimulation, transvaginal electrical stimulation, vaginal cone, global postural reeducation, biofeedback for pelvic floor muscle (PFM) training, cognitive behavioral therapy, extracorporeal magnetic stimulation therapy, multidimensional exercise treatment, interferential therapy, interpersonal support, and digital vaginal palpation. PFM training was the main resource used to treat UI. All the UI treatments focused on improving the skills required to perform PFM exercises. The researchers found that all the treatments and equipment that were used resulted in the improvement of UI or its cure. The effectiveness of adding PFM training to other active treatments as compared with the same active treatment alone increased the effectiveness in reducing all types of UI.

Implications

UI treatment requires multiprofessional involvement and close relationships among healthcare providers. For example, the studies that included interpersonal support and nurse monitoring in addition to PFM exercises improved the effectiveness of UI treatment.

●○● NURSING MANAGEMENT

Assessing

A complete assessment of a client's urinary function includes the following:

- Nursing history
- Physical assessment of the genitourinary system, hydration status, and examination of the urine
- Relating the data obtained to the results of any diagnostic tests and procedures.

Nursing History

The nurse determines the client's normal voiding pattern and frequency, appearance of the urine and any recent changes, any past or current problems with urination, the presence of an ostomy, and factors influencing the elimination pattern.

Examples of interview questions to elicit this information are shown in the Assessment Interview. The number of questions asked depends on the individual and the responses to the first three categories.

Physical Assessment

Complete physical assessment of the urinary tract usually includes percussion of the kidneys to detect areas of tenderness. Palpation and percussion of the bladder are also performed. If the client's history or current problems indicate a need for it, the urethral meatus of both male and female clients is inspected for swelling, discharge, and inflammation.

ASSESSMENT INTERVIEW Urinary Elimination

VOIDING PATTERN

- How many times do you urinate during a 24-hour period?
- Has this pattern changed recently?
- Do you need to get out of bed to void at night? How often?

DESCRIPTION OF URINE AND ANY CHANGES

- How would you describe your urine in terms of color, clarity (clear, transparent, or cloudy), and odor (faint or strong)?

URINARY ELIMINATION PROBLEMS

- What problems have you had or do you now have with passing your urine?
- Passage of small amounts of urine?
- Voiding at more frequent intervals?
- Trouble getting to the bathroom in time, or feeling an urgent need to void?
- Painful voiding?
- Difficulty starting urine stream?
- Frequent dribbling of urine or feeling of bladder fullness associated with voiding small amounts of urine?
- Reduced force of stream?
- Accidental leakage of urine? If so, when does this occur (e.g., when coughing, laughing, or sneezing; at night; during the day)?
- Past urinary tract illness such as infection of the kidney, bladder, or urethra? History of renal, ureteral, or bladder surgery?

FACTORS INFLUENCING URINARY ELIMINATION

- *Medications.* What medications are you taking? Do you know if any of your medications increase urinary output or cause retention of urine? Note specific medication and dosage.
- *Fluid intake.* How much and what kind of fluid do you drink each day (e.g., six glasses of water, two cups of coffee, three cola drinks with or without caffeine)?
- *Environmental factors.* Do you have any problems with toileting (mobility, removing clothing, toilet seat too low, facility without grab bar)?
- *Stress.* Are you experiencing any major stress? If so, what are the stressors? Do you think these affect your urinary pattern?
- *Disease.* Have you had or do you have any illnesses that may affect urinary function, such as hypertension, heart disease, neurologic disease, cancer, prostatic enlargement, or diabetes?
- *Diagnostic procedures and surgery.* Have you recently had a cystoscopy or anesthetic?

TABLE 47.4 Characteristics of Normal and Abnormal Urine

Characteristic	Normal	Abnormal	Nursing Considerations
Amount in 24 hours (adult)	1200–1500 mL	Under 1200 mL A large amount over intake	Urinary output normally is approximately equal to fluid intake. Output of less than 30 mL/h may indicate decreased blood flow to the kidneys and should be immediately reported.
Color, clarity	Straw, amber Transparent	Dark amber Cloudy Dark orange Red or dark brown Mucous plugs, viscid, thick	Concentrated urine is darker in color. Dilute urine may appear almost clear, or very pale yellow. Some foods and drugs may color urine. Red blood cells in the urine (hematuria) may be evident as pink, bright red, or rusty brown urine. Menstrual bleeding can also color urine but should not be confused with hematuria. White blood cells, bacteria, pus, or contaminants such as prostatic fluid, sperm, or vaginal drainage may cause cloudy urine.
Odor	Faint aromatic	Offensive	Some foods (e.g., asparagus) cause a musty odor; infected urine can have a fetid odor; urine high in glucose has a sweet odor.
Sterility	No microorganisms present	Microorganisms present	Urine in the bladder is sterile. Urine specimens, however, may be contaminated by bacteria from the perineum during collection.
pH	4.5–8	Over 8 Under 4.5	Freshly voided urine is normally somewhat acidic. Alkaline urine may indicate a state of alkalosis, UTI, or a diet high in fruits and vegetables. More acidic urine (low pH) is found in starvation, with diarrhea, or with a diet high in protein foods or cranberries.
Specific gravity	1.010–1.025	Over 1.025 Under 1.010	Concentrated urine has a higher specific gravity; diluted urine has a lower specific gravity.
Glucose	Not present	Present	Glucose in the urine indicates high blood glucose levels (greater than 180 mg/dL) and may be indicative of undiagnosed or uncontrolled diabetes mellitus.
Ketone bodies (acetone)	Not present	Present	Ketones, the end product of the breakdown of fatty acids, are not normally present in urine. They may be present in the urine of clients who have uncontrolled diabetes mellitus, who are in a state of starvation, or who have ingested excessive amounts of aspirin.
Blood	Not present	Occult (microscopic) Bright red	Blood may be present in the urine of clients who have UTI, kidney disease, or bleeding from the urinary tract.

Because problems with urination can affect the elimination of wastes from the body, it is important for the nurse to assess the skin for color, texture, and tissue turgor as well as the presence of edema. If incontinence, dribbling, or dysuria is noted in the history, the skin of the perineum should be inspected for irritation because contact with urine can excoriate the skin.

Assessing Urine

Normal urine consists of 96% water and 4% solutes. Organic solutes include urea, ammonia, creatinine, and uric acid. Variations in color can occur. Characteristics of normal and abnormal urine are shown in Table 47.4.

Measuring Urinary Output

Normally, the kidneys produce urine at a rate of approximately 60 mL/h or about 1500 mL/day. Urine output is affected by many factors, including fluid intake, body fluid losses through other routes such as perspiration and breathing or diarrhea, and the cardiovascular and renal status of the individual.

Urine outputs below 30 mL/h may indicate low blood volume or kidney malfunction and must be reported. To measure fluid output the nurse follows these steps:

- Wear clean gloves to prevent contact with microorganisms or blood in urine.
- Ask the client to void in a clean urinal, bedpan, commode, or toilet collection device ("hat") (Figure 47.4 ■).
- Instruct the client to keep urine separate from feces and to avoid putting toilet paper in the urine collection container.
- Pour the voided urine into a calibrated container.
- Hold the container at eye level and read the amount in the container. Containers usually have a measuring scale on the inside.
- Record the amount on the fluid intake and output (I&O) sheet, which may be at the bedside or in the bathroom.
- Rinse the urine collection and measuring containers with cool water and store appropriately.

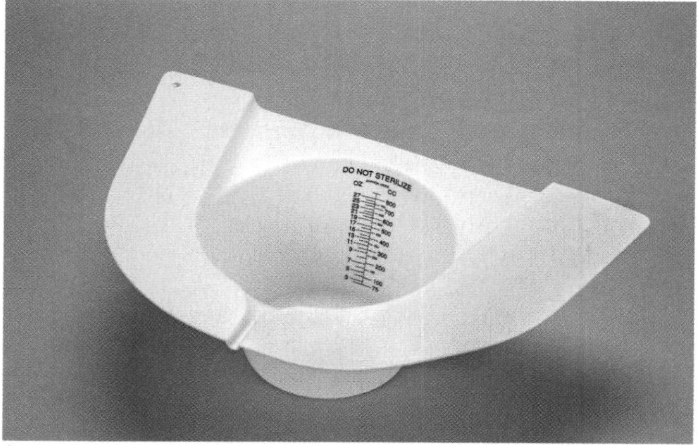

Figure 47.4 ■ A urine "hat"—a urine collection device for the toilet.

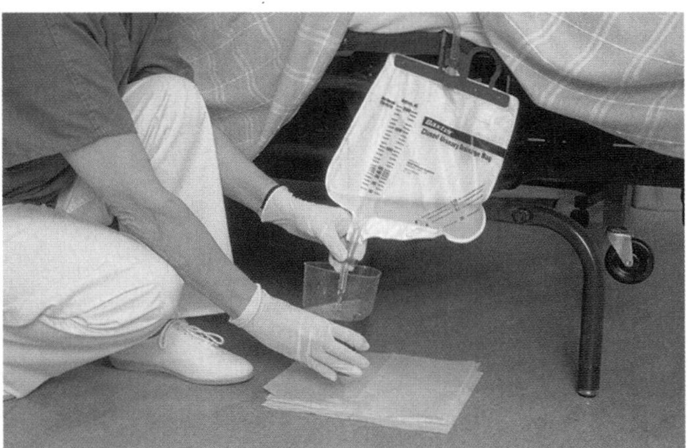

Figure 47.5 ■ Urine being measured from a urine collection bag.

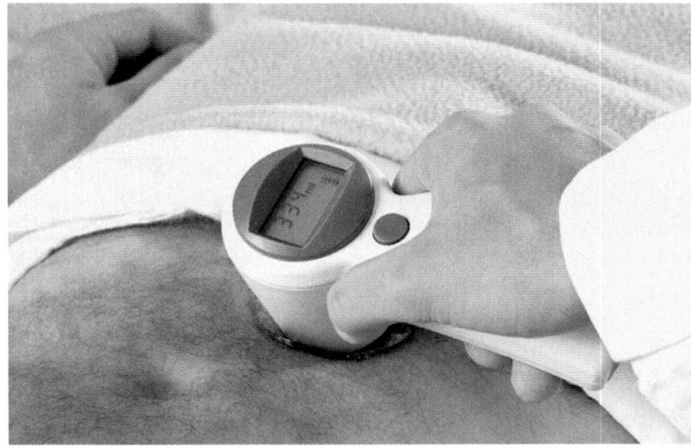

Figure 47.6 ■ A handheld, portable ultrasound device can measure bladder urine volume noninvasively. It is placed 1–1.5 inch above the symphysis pubis and tilted toward the bladder.

- Remove gloves and perform hand hygiene.
- Calculate and document the total output at the end of each shift and at the end of 24 h on the client's chart.

Many clients can measure and record their own urine output when the procedure is explained to them.

When measuring urine from a client who has a urinary catheter, the nurse follows these steps:

- Apply clean gloves.
- Take the calibrated container to the bedside.
- Place the container under the urine collection bag so that the spout of the bag is above the container but not touching it. The calibrated container is not sterile, but the inside of the collection bag is sterile (Figure 47.5 ■).
- Open the spout and permit the urine to flow into the container.
- Close the spout, then proceed as described in the previous list.

Measuring Residual Urine

Postvoid residual (PVR) (urine remaining in the bladder following voiding) is normally 50 to 100 mL. However, a bladder outlet obstruction (e.g., enlargement of the prostate gland) or loss of bladder muscle tone may interfere with complete emptying of the bladder during urination. Manifestations of urine retention may include frequent voiding of small amounts (e.g., less than 100 mL in an adult), urinary stasis, and UTI. PVR is measured to assess the amount of retained urine after voiding and determine the need for interventions (e.g., medications to promote detrusor muscle contraction).

To measure PVR, the nurse catheterizes or bladder scans the client after voiding (Figure 47.6 ■). The amount of urine voided and the amount obtained by catheterization or bladder scan are measured and recorded. An indwelling catheter may be inserted if the PVR exceeds a specified amount.

Diagnostic Tests

Blood levels of two metabolically produced substances, urea and creatinine, are routinely used to evaluate renal function. The kidneys through filtration and tubular secretion normally eliminate both urea and creatinine. Urea, the end product of protein metabolism, is measured as **blood urea nitrogen (BUN)**. Creatinine is produced in relatively constant quantities by the muscles. The **creatinine clearance** test uses 24-hour urine and serum creatinine levels to determine the glomerular filtration rate, a sensitive indicator of renal function. Other tests related to urinary functions such as collecting urine specimens, measuring specific gravity, and visualization procedures are described in Chapter 34 ∞.

Diagnosing

An example of a nursing diagnosis for clients with urinary elimination problems is altered urinary elimination, and to help make it more specific, identify the problem. An example is altered urinary elimination (urinary retention). Another example of a nursing diagnosis is urinary incontinence and specifying the type (i.e., functional, overflow, reflex, stress, or urge). Other examples of nursing diagnoses include potential for incontinence (specify type) and potential altered urinary elimination (urinary retention).

Clinical examples of assessment data clusters and related nursing diagnoses, outcomes, and interventions are shown in the Nursing Care Plan and Concept Map at the end of this chapter.

Problems of urinary elimination also may become the etiology for other problems experienced by the client. Examples include the following:

- Potential for infection if the client has urinary retention or undergoes an invasive procedure such as catheterization or cystoscopic examination.
- Impaired self-esteem or social seclusion if the client is incontinent. Incontinence can be physically and emotionally distressing to clients because it is considered socially unacceptable. Often the client is embarrassed about dribbling or having an accident and may restrict normal activities for this reason.
- Potential for developing altered skin integrity if the client is incontinent. Bed linens and clothes saturated with urine irritate and macerate the skin. Prolonged skin dampness leads to dermatitis (inflammation of the skin) and subsequent formation of dermal ulcers.
- Lack of knowledge if the client requires self-care skills to manage (e.g., a new urinary diversion ostomy).

Planning

The goals established will vary according to the diagnosis and signs and symptoms. Examples of overall goals for clients with urinary elimination problems may include the following:

- Maintain or restore a normal voiding pattern.
- Regain normal urine output.
- Prevent associated risks such as infection, skin breakdown, fluid and electrolyte imbalance, and lowered self-esteem.
- Perform toileting activities independently with or without assistive devices.
- Contain urine with the appropriate device, catheter, ostomy appliance, or absorbent product.

Appropriate preventive and corrective nursing interventions that relate to these must be identified. Specific nursing activities associated with each of these interventions can be selected to meet the client's individual needs. Examples of clinical applications of these using nursing diagnoses, NIC, and NOC designations are shown in the Nursing Care Plan and Concept Map at the end of the chapter.

Planning for Home Care

To provide for continuity of care, the nurse needs to consider the client's needs for teaching and assistance with care in the home. Discharge planning includes assessment of the client and family's resources and abilities for self-care, available financial resources, and the need for referrals and home health services.

QSEN Patient-Centered Care: Urinary Elimination

The nurse needs to complete an assessment of the following home care capabilities related to urinary elimination problems and needs:

CLIENT AND ENVIRONMENT

- ***Self-care abilities:*** ability to consume adequate fluids, to perceive bladder fullness, to ambulate and get to the toilet, to manipulate clothing for toileting, and to perform hygiene measures after toileting
- ***Current level of knowledge:*** fluid and dietary intake modifications to promote normal patterns of urinary elimination, bladder training methods, and specific techniques to promote voiding care for indwelling catheter or ostomy (if appropriate)
- ***Assistive devices required:*** ambulatory aids such as walker, cane, or wheelchair; safety devices such as grab bars; toileting aids such as raised toilet seat, urinal, commode, or bedpan; presence of a urinary catheter
- ***Physical layout of the toileting facilities:*** presence of mobility aids; toilet at correct height to enable older clients to get up after voiding
- ***Home environment factors that interfere with toileting:*** distance to the bathroom from living areas or bedrooms; barriers such as stairways, scatter rugs, clutter, or narrow doorways that interfere with bathroom access; lighting (including night lighting)
- ***Urinary elimination problems:*** type of incontinence and precipitating factors; manifestations of UTI such as dysuria, frequency, urgency; evidence of benign prostatic hyperplasia and effect on urination; ability to perform self-catheterization and care for other urinary elimination devices such as indwelling catheter, urinary diversion ostomy, or condom drainage.

FAMILY

- ***Caregiver availability, skills, and responses:*** ability and willingness to assume responsibilities for care, including assisting with toileting, intermittent catheterization, indwelling catheter care, urinary drainage devices or ostomy care; ready access to laundry facilities; access to and willingness to use respite or relief caregivers
- ***Family role changes and coping:*** effect on spousal and family roles, sleep and rest patterns, sexuality, and social interactions

DRUG CAPSULE

Anticholinergic Agent: oxybutynin ER (Ditropan XL)

THE CLIENT WITH MEDICATIONS FOR URGENCY URINARY INCONTINENCE

Anticholinergic agents reduce urgency and frequency by blocking muscarinic receptors in the detrusor muscle of the bladder, thereby inhibiting contractions and increasing storage capacity. They are useful in relieving symptoms associated with voiding problems in clients with neurogenic bladder and reflex neurogenic bladder, and UUI.

NURSING RESPONSIBILITIES

- Monitor for constipation, dry mouth, urinary retention, blurred vision, and mental confusion in older adults; symptoms may be dose related.
- Keep primary care provider informed of expected responses to therapy (e.g., effect on urinary frequency, urge incontinence, nocturia, and bladder emptying).
- Start with small doses in clients over the age of 75.
- Try using intermittently.
- Oxybutynin is contraindicated in clients with urinary retention, GI motility problems (partial or complete GI obstruction, paralytic ileus), or uncontrolled narrow-angle glaucoma.

CLIENT AND FAMILY TEACHING

- Explain the reason for taking oxybutynin.
- Explain the side effects and the importance of reporting them to the healthcare provider.
- Exercise caution in hot environments. By suppressing sweating, oxybutynin can cause fever and heat stroke.
- Provide strategies for managing dry mouth.
- Instruct and advise regarding behavioral therapies for urge suppression.

Note: Prior to administering any medication, review all aspects with a current drug handbook or other reliable source.

- ***Financial resources:*** ability to purchase protective pads and garments, supplies for catheterization or ostomy care.

COMMUNITY

- ***Environment:*** access to public restrooms and sanitary facilities
- ***Current knowledge of and experience with community resources:*** medical and assistive equipment and supply companies, home health agencies, local pharmacies, available financial assistance, support and educational organizations

Client Teaching addresses the learning needs of the client and family.

CLIENT TEACHING Urinary Elimination in the Home Setting

FACILITATING URINARY ELIMINATION SELF-CARE

- Teach the client and family to maintain easy access to toilet facilities, including removing scatter rugs and ensuring that halls and doorways are free of clutter.
- Suggest graduated lighting for night-time voiding: a dim night light in the bedroom and low-wattage hallway lighting.
- Advise the client and family to install grab bars and elevated toilet seats as needed.
- Provide for instruction in safe transfer techniques. Contact physical therapy to provide training as needed.
- Suggest clothing that is easily removed for toileting, such as elastic waist pants or Velcro closures.

PROMOTING URINARY ELIMINATION

- Instruct the client to respond to the urge to void as soon as possible; avoid voluntary urinary retention.
- Teach the client to empty the bladder completely at each voiding.
- Emphasize the importance of drinking eight to ten 8-ounce glasses of water daily.
- Teach female clients about PFM exercises to strengthen perineal muscles.
- Inform the client about the relationship between tobacco use and bladder cancer and provide information about smoking cessation programs as indicated.
- Teach the client to promptly report any of the following to the primary care provider: pain or burning on urination, changes in urine color or clarity, foul-smelling urine, or changes in voiding patterns (e.g., nocturia, frequency, dribbling).

ASEPSIS

- Teach the client to maintain perineal-genital cleanliness, washing with soap and water daily and cleansing the anal and perineal area after defecating.
- Instruct female clients to wipe from front to back (from the urinary meatus toward the anus) after voiding, and to discard toilet paper after each swipe.
- Provide information about products to protect the skin, clothing, and furniture for clients who are incontinent. Emphasize the importance of cleaning and drying the perineal area after incontinence episodes. Instruct in the use of protective skin barrier products as needed.
- Teach clients with an indwelling catheter and their family about care measures such as cleaning the urinary meatus, managing and emptying the collection device, maintaining a closed system, and bladder irrigation or flushing if ordered.
- For clients with a urinary diversion, teach about care of the stoma, drainage devices, and surrounding skin. For continent diversions, teach the client how to catheterize the stoma to drain urine.
- For clients with an indwelling catheter or urinary diversion, emphasize the importance of maintaining a generous fluid intake (2.5 to 3 quarts daily) and of promptly reporting changes in urinary output, signs of urinary retention such as abdominal pain, and manifestations of UTI such as malodorous urine, abdominal discomfort, fever, or confusion.

MEDICATIONS

- Emphasize the importance of taking medications as prescribed. Instruct the client to take the full course of antibiotics ordered to treat a UTI, even though symptoms are relieved.
- Inform the client and family about any expected changes in urine color or odor associated with prescribed medications.
- For clients with urinary retention, emphasize the need to contact the primary care provider before taking any medication (even over-the-counter medications such as antihistamines) that may exacerbate symptoms.
- For clients taking medications that may damage the kidneys (e.g., aminoglycoside antibiotics), stress the importance of maintaining a generous fluid intake while taking the medication.
- Suggest measures to reduce anticipated side effects of prescribed medications, such as increasing intake of potassium-rich foods when taking a potassium-depleting diuretic such as furosemide.

DIETARY ALTERATIONS

- Teach the client about dietary changes to promote urinary function, such as consuming cranberry juice and foods that acidify the urine to reduce the risk of repeated UTIs or forming calcium-based urinary stones. See the *Dietary Measures* section on page 1259.
- Instruct clients with stress or urge incontinence to limit their intake of caffeine, alcohol, citrus juices, and artificial sweeteners because these are bladder irritants that may increase incontinence. Also, teach clients to limit their evening fluid intake to reduce the risk of night-time incontinence episodes.

MEASURES SPECIFIC TO URINARY PROBLEMS

- Provide instructions for clients with specific urinary problems or treatments such as these:
  a. Timed urine specimens (see Chapter 34 ∞)
  b. Urinary incontinence
  c. Urinary retention
  d. Retention catheters.

REFERRALS

- Make appropriate referrals to home health agencies, community agencies, or social services for assistance with resources such as installing grab bars and raised toilet seats; providing wheelchair access to bathrooms; obtaining toileting aids such as commodes, urinals, or bedpans; and services such as home health aides for assistance with activities of daily living (ADLs).

COMMUNITY AGENCIES AND OTHER RESOURCES

- Provide information about resources for durable medical equipment such as commodes or raised toilet seats, possible financial assistance, and medical supplies such as drainage bags, incontinence briefs, or protective pads.
- Suggest additional sources of information and help such as the National Council of Independent Living, United Ostomy Association, National Association for Continence, and Simon Foundation for Continence.

Implementing

Maintaining Normal Urinary Elimination

Most interventions to maintain normal urinary elimination are independent nursing functions. These include promoting adequate fluid intake, maintaining normal voiding habits, and assisting with toileting.

Promoting Fluid Intake

Increasing fluid intake increases urine production, which in turn stimulates the voiding reflex. A normal daily intake averaging 1500 mL of measurable fluids is adequate for most adult clients.

Many clients have increased fluid requirements, necessitating a higher daily fluid intake. For example, clients who are perspiring excessively (have diaphoresis) or who are experiencing abnormal fluid losses through vomiting, gastric suction, diarrhea, or wound drainage require fluid to replace these losses in addition to their normal daily intake requirements.

Clients who are at risk for UTI or urinary calculi (stones) should consume 2000 to 3000 mL of fluid daily. Dilute urine and frequent urination reduce the risk of UTI as well as stone formation.

Increased fluid intake may be contraindicated for some clients such as individuals with kidney failure or heart failure. For these clients, a fluid restriction may be necessary to prevent fluid overload and edema.

Maintaining Normal Voiding Habits

Prescribed medical therapies often interfere with a client's normal voiding habits. When a client's urinary elimination pattern is adequate, the nurse helps the client adhere to normal voiding habits as much as possible (see Practice Guidelines).

Assisting with Toileting

Clients who are weakened by a disease process or impaired physically may require assistance with toileting. The nurse should assist these clients to the bathroom and remain with them if they are at risk for falling. The bathroom should contain an easily accessible call signal to summon help if needed. Clients also need to be encouraged to use handrails placed near the toilet.

For clients unable to use bathroom facilities, the nurse provides urinary equipment close to the bedside (e.g., urinal, bedpan, commode) and provides the necessary assistance to use them.

Preventing Urinary Tract Infections

The rate of UTI is greater in women than men because of the short urethra and its proximity to the anal and vaginal areas. Most UTIs are caused by bacteria common to the intestinal environment (e.g., *Escherichia coli*). These gastrointestinal (GI) bacteria can colonize the perineal area and move into the urethra, especially when there is urethral trauma, irritation, or manipulation.

For women who have experienced a UTI, nurses need to provide instructions about ways to prevent a recurrence. The following guidelines are useful for anyone:

- Drink eight 8-ounce glasses of water per day to flush bacteria out of the urinary system.
- Practice frequent voiding (every 2 to 4 hours) to flush bacteria out of the urethra and prevent organisms from ascending into the bladder. Void immediately after intercourse.
- Avoid use of harsh soaps, bubble bath, powder, or sprays in the perineal area. These substances can be irritating to the urethra and encourage inflammation and bacterial infection.

PRACTICE GUIDELINES Maintaining Normal Voiding Habits

POSITIONING

- Assist the client to a normal position for voiding: standing for male clients; for female clients, squatting or leaning slightly forward when sitting. These positions enhance movement of urine through the tract by gravity.
- If the client is unable to ambulate to the lavatory, use a bedside commode for females and a urinal for males standing at the bedside.
- If necessary, encourage the client to push over the pubic area with the hands or to lean forward to increase intra-abdominal pressure and external pressure on the bladder.

RELAXATION

- Provide privacy for the client. Many clients cannot void in the presence of another individual.
- Allow the client sufficient time to void.
- Suggest the client read or listen to music.
- Provide sensory stimuli that may help the client relax. Pour warm water over the perineum of a female or have the client sit in a warm bath to promote muscle relaxation. Applying a hot water bottle to the lower abdomen of both men and women may also foster muscle relaxation.
- Turn on running water within hearing distance of the client to stimulate the voiding reflex and to mask the sound of voiding for clients who find this embarrassing.
- Provide ordered analgesics and emotional support to relieve physical and emotional discomfort to decrease muscle tension.

TIMING

- Assist clients who have the urge to void immediately. Delays only increase the difficulty in starting to void, and the desire to void may pass.
- Offer toileting assistance to the client at usual times of voiding, for example, on awakening, before or after meals, and at bedtime.

FOR CLIENTS WHO ARE CONFINED TO BED

- Warm the bedpan. A cold bedpan may prompt contraction of the perineal muscles and inhibit voiding.
- Elevate the head of the client's bed to Fowler's position, place a small pillow or rolled towel at the small of the back to increase physical support and comfort, and have the client flex the hips and knees. This position simulates the normal voiding position as closely as possible.

- Avoid tight-fitting pants or other clothing that creates irritation to the urethra and prevents ventilation of the perineal area.
- Wear cotton rather than nylon underclothes. Accumulation of perineal moisture facilitates bacterial growth. Cotton enhances ventilation of the perineal area.
- Girls and women should always wipe the perineal area from front to back following urination or defecation in order to prevent introduction of GI bacteria into the urethra.
- If recurrent urinary infections are a problem, take showers rather than baths. Bacteria present in bath water can readily enter the urethra.

Managing Urinary Incontinence

It is important to remember that UI is *not* a normal part of aging and often is treatable. The preliminary assessment and identification of the symptoms of UI are truly within the scope of nursing practice. All clients should be asked about their voiding patterns. Older adults who are incontinent while in their home or who manage to contain or conceal their incontinence from others do not consider themselves incontinent. Therefore, if asked if they are incontinent, they may deny it. However, asking if they lose urine when they cough, sneeze, or laugh or if they need to use some type of incontinence product may provide more accurate information. Independent nursing interventions for clients with UI include (a) a behavior-oriented continence training program that may consist of bladder retraining, habit training, and pelvic floor muscle exercises; (b) meticulous skin care; and (c) for males, application of an external drainage device (condom-type catheter device).

Clinical Alert!

If the client has any type of incontinence, recommend the use of incontinence pads because they are designed to absorb urine as opposed to feminine hygiene pads.

Continence (Bladder) Retraining

A continence retraining program requires the involvement of the nurse, the client, and support people. Clients must be alert and physically able to participate in the training protocol. A bladder retraining program may include the following:

- Education of the client and support people.
- **Bladder retraining** promotes complete bladder contraction and emptying and requires that the client postpone voiding, resist or inhibit the sensation of urgency, and void according to a timetable rather than according to the urge to void. The goals are to gradually lengthen the intervals between urination to correct the client's frequent urination, to stabilize the bladder, and to diminish urgency. This form of training may be used for clients who have bladder instability and urge incontinence. Delayed voiding provides larger voided volumes and longer intervals between voiding. Initially, voiding may be encouraged every 2 to 3 hours except during sleep and then every 4 to 6 hours. A vital component of bladder training is inhibiting the urge-to-void sensation. To do this, the nurse instructs the client to practice deep, slow breathing until the urge diminishes or disappears. This is performed every time the client has a premature urge to void. Guidelines for bladder retraining are in the Practice Guidelines.
- **Habit training**, also referred to as timed or prompted voiding and scheduled toileting, attempts to keep clients dry by having them void at regular intervals, such as every 2 to 4 hours. The goal is to keep the client dry and is a common therapy for frail older clients and clients with dementia.
- Lifestyle modification can greatly influence the incidence of UI. For example, weight loss in overweight clients can reduce UI because the abdominal weight places extra force on the bladder. Eliminating beverages containing caffeine, citrus drinks, and alcohol and balancing fluid intake where there is sufficient fluid intake during the day and limited fluids before bedtime can decrease UI (Stewart, 2018).

PRACTICE GUIDELINES Bladder Retraining

- Determine the client's voiding pattern and encourage voiding at those times, or establish a regular voiding schedule and help the client to maintain it, whether the client feels the urge or not (e.g., on awakening, every 1 or 2 hours during the day and evening, before retiring at night, every 4 hours at night). The stretching–relaxing sequence of such a schedule tends to increase bladder muscle tone and promote more voluntary control. Consider a double-voiding technique to promote complete bladder contraction and emptying. This technique promotes urinary drainage through position changes or a brief period of standing prior to a second void (Stewart, 2018). Encourage the client to inhibit the urge-to-void sensation when a premature urge to void is experienced. Instruct the client to practice slow, deep breathing until the urge diminishes or disappears.
- When the client finds that voiding can be controlled, the intervals between voiding can be lengthened slightly without loss of continence.
- Regulate fluid intake, particularly during evening hours, to help reduce the need to void during the night.
- Encourage fluids between the hours of 0600 and 1800.
- Avoid excessive consumption of citrus juices, carbonated beverages (especially those containing artificial sweeteners), alcohol, and drinks containing caffeine because these irritate the bladder, increasing the risk of incontinence.
- Schedule diuretics early in the morning.
- Explain to clients that adequate fluid intake is required to ensure adequate urine production that stimulates the micturition reflex.
- Apply protector pads to keep the bed linen dry and provide specially made waterproof underwear to contain the urine and decrease the client's embarrassment. Avoid using diapers, which are demeaning and also suggest that incontinence is permissible.
- Assist the client with a PFM exercise program to increase the general muscle tone and a program aimed at strengthening the pelvic floor muscles.
- Provide positive reinforcements to encourage continence. Praise clients for attempting to toilet and for maintaining continence.

Pelvic Floor Muscle Exercises

Pelvic floor muscle (PFM), or Kegel, exercises help to strengthen pelvic floor muscles (see Figures 47.2 and 47.3) and can reduce or eliminate episodes of incontinence. The client can identify the perineal muscles by tightening the anal sphincter as if to control the passing of gas, around the vagina and the urethra as if trying to stop urine mid flow. When the exercise is properly performed, contraction of the muscles of the buttocks and thighs is avoided. PFM exercises can be performed anytime, anywhere, sitting or standing. Specific client instructions are summarized in Client Teaching.

Maintaining Skin Integrity

Skin that is continually moist becomes macerated (softened). Urine that accumulates on the skin is converted to ammonia, which is very irritating to the skin. Because both skin irritation and maceration can cause skin breakdown and ulceration, the incontinent client requires meticulous skin care. To maintain skin integrity, the nurse gently cleanses the client's perineal area with mild soap and water or a commercially prepared no-rinse cleanser after episodes of incontinence. The nurse then rinses the area thoroughly if soap and water were used, and dries it gently and thoroughly. Clean, dry clothing or bed linen should be provided. The nurse applies barrier ointments or creams to protect the skin from contact with urine. If it is necessary to pad the client's clothes for protection, the nurse should use products that absorb wetness and leave a dry surface in contact with the skin.

Specially designed incontinence drawsheets provide significant advantages over standard drawsheets for incontinent clients confined to bed. These sheets are like a drawsheet but are double layered, with a quilted upper nylon or polyester surface and an absorbent viscose rayon layer below. The rayon soaker layer generally has a waterproof backing on its underside. Fluid (i.e., urine) passes through the upper quilted layer and is absorbed and dispersed by the viscose rayon, leaving the quilted surface dry to the touch. This absorbent sheet helps maintain skin integrity; it does not stick to the skin when wet, decreases the risk of bedsores, and reduces odor.

Applying External Urinary Devices

To prevent the complications and inconveniences associated with incontinence in males, an external urinary device, also referred to as a penile sheath or condom catheter, attached to a urinary drainage system may be used. External urinary devices may be more comfortable than an indwelling catheter and cause fewer UTIs. Latex or silicone devices are available. The silicone penile sheath has two advantages in that it allows the client or his caregivers to assess the skin without removing the sheath and it has oxygen and water vapor transmission properties, allowing the skin to breathe (Nazarko, 2018, p. 112).

Methods of applying external urinary devices vary. The nurse needs to follow the manufacturer's instructions when applying a condom. First the nurse determines when the client experiences incontinence. Some clients may require an external urinary device at night only, others continuously with daily changes. Skill 47.1 describes how to apply and remove an external device.

CLIENT TEACHING Pelvic Floor Muscle Exercises (Kegel Exercises)

- Contract your PFMs where you pull your rectum, urethra, and vagina up inside, followed by relaxation. Do *not* hold your breath or tighten your thighs, buttocks, or abdomen while doing PFM exercises.
- Hold each contraction for several seconds. It is suggested that at least eight contractions should be performed three times a day (Ostle, 2016; Stewart, 2018).
- Make the exercises part of your daily life, for example, before getting out of bed in the morning, when working at the kitchen sink, or on your way to the bathroom. The exercises can be done anywhere, anytime, and in any position.
- To control episodes of stress incontinence, perform a pelvic floor muscle contraction when initiating any activity that increases intra-abdominal pressure, such as coughing, laughing, sneezing, or lifting.

SKILL 47.1 Applying an External Urinary Device

PURPOSES

- To collect urine and control urinary incontinence
- To permit the client physical activity while controlling UI
- To prevent skin irritation as a result of UI

ASSESSMENT

- Review the client record to determine a voiding pattern and other pertinent data, such as latex sensitivity or allergy.
- Apply clean gloves to examine the client's penis for swelling or excoriation that would contraindicate use of the condom catheter.

PLANNING

- Discuss the use of external urinary devices with the client and family or caregiver.
- Determine if the client has had an external catheter previously and any difficulties with it.
- Perform any procedures that are best completed without the catheter in place; for example, weighing the client would be easier without the tubing and bag.

Applying an External Urinary Device—*continued*

SKILL 47.1

Assignment

Applying an external urinary device may be assigned to assistive personnel (AP). However, the nurse must determine if the specific client has unique conditions such as impaired circulation or latex allergy that would require special training of the AP in the use of the device. Abnormal findings must be validated and interpreted by the nurse.

Equipment

- Penile sheath of appropriate size. Use the manufacturer's size guide as indicated. Use latex-free silicone for clients with latex allergies. Use self-adhering condom devices, or those with Velcro, tape, or other external securing device. ❶
- Leg drainage bag if ambulatory or urinary drainage bag with tubing
- Clean gloves
- Basin of warm water and soap
- Washcloth and towel
- External fixation device (e.g., flexible, self-adhesive tape or Velcro strap, if needed)

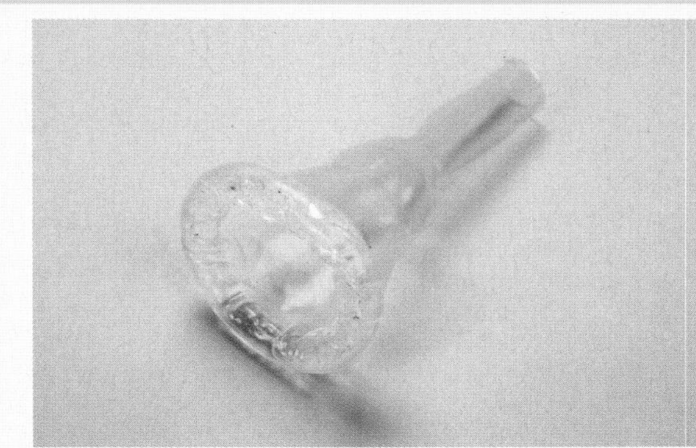

❶ An external urinary device.

IMPLEMENTATION

Preparation

- Assemble the leg drainage bag or urinary drainage bag for attachment to the condom sheath.
- If the condom supplied is not rolled onto itself, roll the condom outward onto itself to facilitate easier application.

Performance

1. Prior to performing the procedure, introduce self and verify the client's identity using agency protocol. Explain to the client what you are going to do, why it is necessary, and how to participate.
2. Perform hand hygiene and observe other appropriate infection prevention procedures.
3. Position the client in either a supine or a sitting position. Provide for client privacy.
   - Drape the client appropriately with the bath blanket, exposing only the penis.
4. Apply clean gloves.
5. Inspect and clean the penis.
   - Clean the genital area and dry it thoroughly. **Rationale:** *This minimizes skin irritation and excoriation after the condom is applied.*
6. Apply and secure the condom.
   - Roll the condom smoothly over the penis, leaving 2.5 cm (1 in.) between the end of the penis and the rubber or plastic connecting tube. ❷ **Rationale:** *This space prevents irritation of the tip of the penis and provides for full drainage of urine.*
   - Secure the condom firmly, but not too tightly, to the penis. Some condoms have an adhesive inside the proximal end that adheres to the skin of the base of the penis. Many condoms are packaged with special tape. If neither is present, use a strip of elastic tape or Velcro around the base of the penis over the condom. Ordinary tape is *contraindicated* because it is not flexible and can stop blood flow.
7. Securely attach the urinary drainage system.
   - Make sure that the tip of the penis is not touching the condom and that the condom is not twisted, which can occur if there is too much space between the tip of the penis and the funnel of the sheath. **Rationale:** *A twisted condom could obstruct the flow of urine.*
   - Attach the urinary drainage system to the condom device.
   - Remove and discard gloves.
   - Perform hand hygiene.

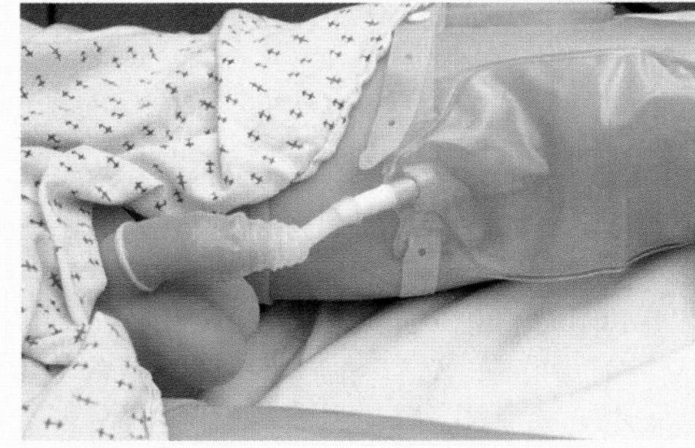

❷ A self-adhering external urinary device rolled over the penis.

   - If the client is to remain in bed, attach the urinary drainage bag to the bed frame.
   - If the client is ambulatory, attach the bag to the client's leg using both straps. ❸ **Rationale:** *Attaching the drainage bag to the leg using both straps helps control the movement of the tubing and reduces traction on the sheath and the risk of it becoming dislodged.*
8. Teach the client about the drainage system.
   - Instruct the client to keep the drainage bag below the level of the condom device and to avoid loops or kinks in the tubing. Instruct the client to report pain, irritation, swelling, wetness, or leaking around the penis to the primary care provider.

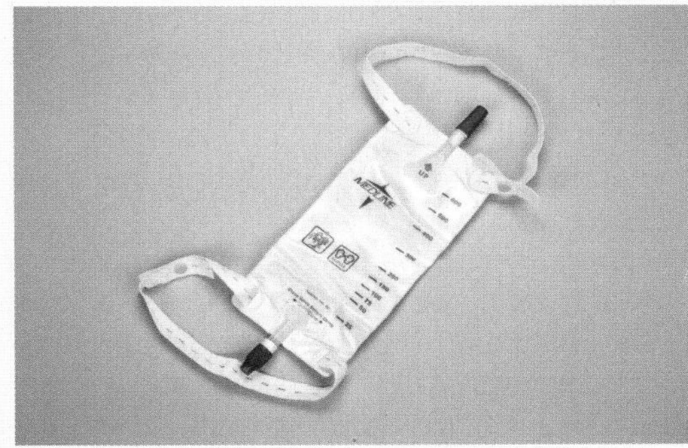

❸ Urinary drainage leg bag.

Continued on page 1250

SKILL 47.1

Applying an External Urinary Device—*continued*

9. Inspect the penis 30 minutes following device application and at least every 4 hours. Check urine flow. Document these findings.
   - Assess the penis for swelling and discoloration. **Rationale:** *This indicates that the condom is too tight.*
   - Assess urine flow if the client has voided. Normally, some urine is present in the tube if the flow is not obstructed.
   - Assess for redness or skin blistering the first few days. **Rationale:** *This could indicate a latex allergy*.
10. Change the external urinary device as indicated and provide skin care. In most settings, the condom is changed daily.
    - Remove the elastic or Velcro strip, apply clean gloves, and roll off the condom.
    - Wash the penis with soapy water, rinse, and dry it thoroughly.
    - Assess the foreskin for signs of irritation, swelling, and discoloration.
    - Reapply a new external urinary device.
    - Remove and discard gloves.
    - Perform hand hygiene.
11. Document in the client record using forms or checklists supplemented by narrative notes when appropriate. Record the application of the external urinary device, the time, and pertinent observations, such as irritated areas on the penis.

SAMPLE DOCUMENTATION

4/22/2020 2145 Condom catheter applied for the night per client request. Glans clean, skin intact. Catheter attached to bedside collection bag. Instructed to notify staff if pain, irritation, swelling, wetness, or leaking occurs. Verbalized that he would. L. Chan, RN

EVALUATION

- Perform a detailed follow-up based on findings that deviated from expected or normal for the client. Relate findings to previous assessment data if available.
- Report significant deviations from normal to the primary care provider.

Managing Urinary Retention

Interventions that assist the client to maintain a normal voiding pattern, discussed earlier, also apply when dealing with urinary retention. If these actions are unsuccessful, the primary care provider may order a cholinergic drug such as bethanechol chloride (Urecholine) to stimulate bladder contraction and help voiding. Clients who have a **flaccid** bladder (weak, soft, and lax bladder muscles) may use manual pressure on the bladder to promote bladder emptying. This is known as **Credé's maneuver** or Credé's method. It is not advised without a primary care provider or nurse practitioner's order and is used only for clients who have lost and are not expected to regain voluntary bladder control. When all measures fail to initiate voiding, urinary catheterization may be necessary to empty the bladder completely. An indwelling Foley catheter may be inserted until the underlying cause is treated. Alternatively, intermittent straight catheterization (every 3 to 4 hours) may be performed because the risk of UTI may be less than with an indwelling catheter.

Urinary Catheterization

Urinary catheterization is the introduction of a catheter through the urethra into the urinary bladder. This is usually performed only when absolutely necessary, because the danger exists of introducing microorganisms into the bladder. The Centers for Disease Control and Prevention [CDC] developed criteria for indwelling urinary catheter (IUC) insertion as listed in Box 47.2.

The most frequent healthcare-associated infection (HAI) is a UTI, and IUCs cause 80% of these UTIs (Institute for Healthcare Improvement [IHI], n.d.). A catheter-associated urinary tract infection (**CAUTI**) is a UTI associated with an IUC that has been in place for more than 2 calendar days when the day of placement was day one (CDC, 2019). Clients with a CAUTI remain in the hospital longer and need to be placed on antibiotic therapy, which increases healthcare costs. The high incidence and high costs related to CAUTI, in addition to the fact that most are preventable, resulted in the Centers for Medicare and Medicaid Services (CMS) not reimbursing hospitals unless the CAUTI was documented as present on admission (McNeill, 2017). It is well known that the risk to the client of developing a CAUTI correlates to the length of time the catheter is in place. According to the IHI (n.d.), the risk of infection increases by 3% to 7% for *each day* that a catheter remains in place. Best practice is to remove a urinary catheter that is not necessary.

BOX 47.2 CDC Criteria for IUC Insertion

- Acute urinary retention or bladder outlet obstruction
- Critically ill and needs accurate measurements of urine output
- Selected surgical procedures (e.g., urologic surgery)
- Assist in healing of open sacral or perineal wounds in incontinent clients.
- Client requires prolonged immobilization (e.g., multiple trauma injuries)
- To improve comfort for end-of-life care if needed.

From *Guidelines for Prevention of Catheter-Associated Urinary Tract Infections* (2009) by CDC, 2017, p. 11. Retrieved from https://www.cdc.gov/hicpac/pdf/CAUTI/CAUTIguideline2009final.pdf

Although most HAIs are decreasing, the rates for CAUTI are rising. The American Nurses Association (ANA, n.d.) states that there is no universally accepted evidence-based tool to reduce CAUTI as there are for other HAIs. The ANA, together with the CMS Partnership for Patients (PfP), made CAUTI reduction a priority. Their actions resulted in an evidence-based, user-friendly tool to help nurses prevent CAUTI in hospitals. Box 47.3 provides evidence-based guidelines for preventing CAUTIs.

Another hazard is trauma with urethral catheterization, particularly in the male client, whose urethra is longer and more tortuous. It is important to insert a catheter along the normal contour of the urethra. Damage to the urethra can occur if the catheter is forced through

BOX 47.3 Preventing or Reducing the Risk of CAUTI

AVOID UNNECESSARY USE OF AN INDWELLING URINARY CATHETER (IUC)

- Develop criteria for appropriate catheter insertion (see Box 47.2).
- Consider alternatives to an IUC (e.g., external condom catheter, toileting protocols).
- Use a bladder scanner to assess for urinary retention.

NURSE PREPARATION FOR INSERTION OF IUC

- Perform hand hygiene.
- Perform pericare, then re-perform hand hygiene.

INSERT IUC USING ASEPTIC TECHNIQUE

- Catheter kit should include a catheter and all necessary items.
- Use the smallest catheter possible that allows for proper drainage and decreases urethral trauma.
- Catheters should only be inserted by trained individuals.
- Use aseptic technique and sterile equipment.
- Obtain assistance prn (e.g., two-person insertion) to help position the client, improve visualization, and help prevent breaks in aseptic technique.
- Insert the IUC to appropriate length and check urine flow *before* inflating the balloon.
- Inflate the IUC balloon per manufacturer's instructions.
- Secure the IUC.

MAINTAIN THE IUC

- Use hand hygiene and standard precautions during any manipulation of the catheter or collecting system.
- Maintain a sterile, closed drainage system.
- Maintain unobstructed urine flow; keep catheter and tubing from kinking.
- Keep the collection bag below the level of the bladder at all times, but do *not* rest the bag on the floor.
- Empty the collection bag regularly with a separate, clean collecting container for each client; and prevent contact of the drainage spigot with the nonsterile collecting container.

PRACTICES TO AVOID

- Irrigation of catheters, except in cases of catheter obstruction
- Disconnecting the catheter from the drainage tubing
- Replacing catheters routinely
- Cleaning the periurethral area with antiseptics. Routine hygiene (cleaning the meatus during daily bathing) is appropriate.

REVIEW URINARY CATHETER NECESSITY DAILY AND REMOVE PROMPTLY

- Assess the need for catheter in daily nursing assessments; contact the primary care provider if criteria not met.
- Develop nursing protocols that allow nurses to remove urinary catheters if criteria for necessity are not met and there are no contraindications for removal.

From "Back to Basics: How Evidence-Based Nursing Practice Can Prevent Catheter-Associated Urinary Tract Infections," by L. McNeill, 2017, *Urologic Nursing, 37*(4), pp. 204–206; *Streamlined Evidence-Based RN Tool: Catheter Associated Urinary Tract Infection (CAUTI) Prevention*, by American Nurses Association, n.d. Retrieved from http://nursingworld.org/CAUTI-Tool; and "Improving Outcomes with the ANA CAUTI Prevention Tool," by T. L. Panchisin, 2016, *Nursing, 46*(3), pp. 55–59.

Safety Alert! SAFETY

2019 The Joint Commission National Patient Safety Goals

Goal 7: Reduce the Risk of Healthcare-Associated Infections

NPSG.07.06.01 Implement evidence-based practices to prevent indwelling catheter-associated urinary tract infections (CAUTI).

- Educate staff and licensed independent practitioners involved in the use of indwelling urinary catheters about CAUTI and the importance of infection prevention.
- Educate patients who will have an indwelling catheter, and their families as needed, on CAUTI prevention and the symptoms of a urinary tract infection.
- Develop written criteria, using established evidence-based guidelines, for placement of an indwelling urinary catheter.
- Follow written procedures based on established evidence-based guidelines for inserting and maintaining an indwelling urinary catheter.
- Measure and monitor CAUTI-prevention processes and outcomes in high-volume areas.

strictures or at an incorrect angle. In males, the urethra is normally curved, but it can be straightened by elevating the penis to a position perpendicular to the body.

Catheters are commonly made of rubber or plastics although they may be made from latex, silicone, or Teflon. Latex catheters are inexpensive and the most commonly used. Silicone catheters may be used if the client has a latex allergy or prolonged catheterization is required (Schaeffer, 2017). There are also antimicrobial catheters, coated with an antimicrobial agent; however, they are more expensive and studies have been inconsistent as to whether they reduce the occurrence of CAUTI. Catheters are sized by the diameter of the lumen using the French (Fr) scale: the larger the number, the larger the lumen. Box 47.4 provides guidelines for catheter selection.

The straight catheter is a single-lumen tube with a small eye or opening about 1.25 cm (0.5 in.) from the insertion tip (Figure 47.7 ■).

The indwelling, or Foley, catheter is a double-lumen catheter. The outside end of this two-way indwelling catheter

BOX 47.4 Selecting a Urinary Catheter

- Check if client has a latex allergy.
- Determine the appropriate catheter length by the client's gender. For adult female clients use a 22-cm catheter; for adult male clients, a 40-cm catheter.
- Determine appropriate catheter size by the size of the urethral canal. Use sizes such as #8 or #10 for children, #14 or #16 for adults. Men frequently require a larger size than women, for example, #18. The lumen of a silicone catheter is slightly larger than that of a same-sized latex catheter.
- Select the appropriate balloon size. For adults, use a 5-mL balloon to facilitate optimal urine drainage. The smaller balloons allow more complete bladder emptying because the catheter tip is closer to the urethral opening in the bladder. However, a 30-mL balloon is commonly used to achieve hemostasis of the prostatic area following a prostatectomy. Use 3-mL balloons for children.

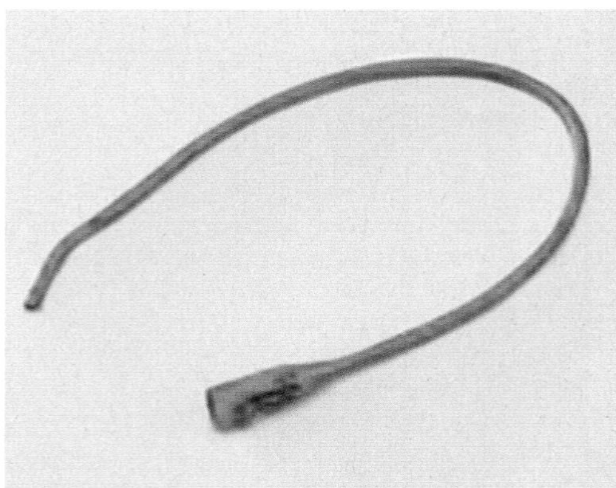

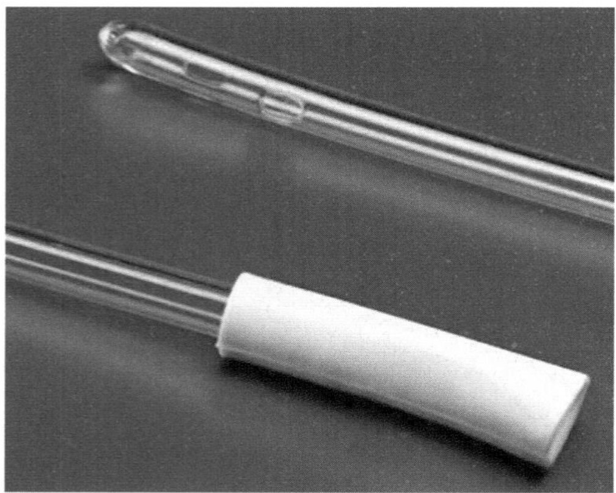

Figure 47.7 ■ Red-rubber or plastic Robinson straight catheters.
Cardinal Health.

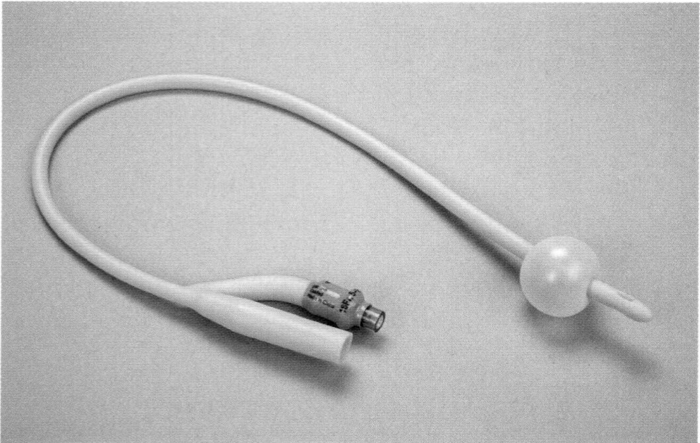

Figure 47.8 ■ An indwelling (Foley) catheter with the balloon inflated.

is bifurcated; that is, it has two openings, one to drain the urine, the other to inflate the balloon (Figure 47.8 ■). The larger lumen drains urine from the bladder and the second smaller lumen is used to inflate the balloon near the tip of the catheter to hold the catheter in place within the bladder.

A variation of the indwelling catheter is the coudé (elbowed) catheter, which has a curved tip (Figure 47.9 ■). This is sometimes used for men who have an enlarged prostate (benign prostatic hyperplasia), because its tip is somewhat stiffer than a regular catheter and thus it can be better controlled during insertion, and passage is often less traumatic.

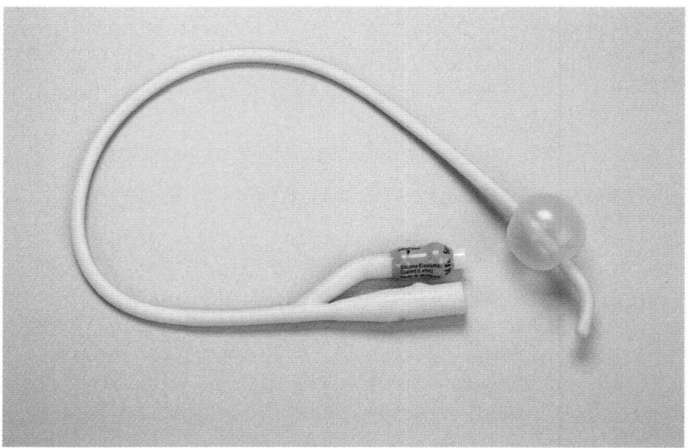

Figure 47.9 ■ A coudé catheter.

Clients who require continuous or intermittent bladder irrigation may have a three-way Foley catheter (Figure 47.10 ■). The three-way catheter has a third lumen through which sterile irrigating fluid can flow into the bladder. The fluid then exits the bladder through the drainage lumen, along with the urine.

The size of the indwelling catheter balloon is indicated on the catheter along with the diameter, for example, "#16 Fr—5 mL balloon." The purpose of the catheter balloon is to secure the catheter in the bladder. Historically, nurses pretested the catheter balloon to prevent insertion of a defective catheter. Panchisin (2016) states that manufacturers no longer recommend inflating the IUC balloon before insertion as it may cause microtears, increasing the risk of infection (p. 56). Pretesting of *silicone* balloons is *not* recommended because the silicone can form a cuff or crease at the balloon area that can cause trauma to the urethra

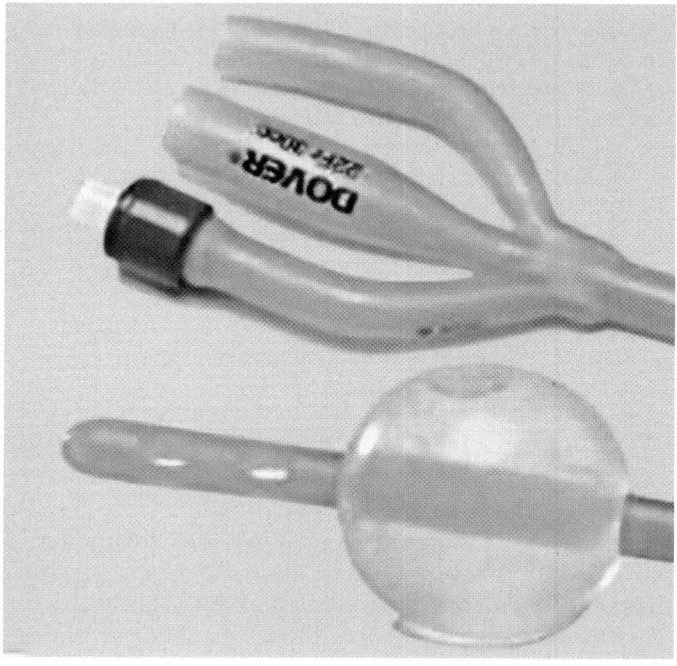

Figure 47.10 ■ A three-way Foley catheter often used for continuous bladder irrigation.
Cardinal Health.

during catheter insertion. It is important to follow the manufacturer's instructions for the proper volume to use for balloon inflation. Improperly inflated catheter balloons may cause drainage and deflation difficulties.

Indwelling catheters are usually connected to a closed gravity drainage system. This system consists of the catheter, drainage tubing, and a collecting bag for the urine. A closed system cannot be opened anywhere along the system, from catheter to collecting bag. It is the standard of care because it reduces the risk of microorganisms entering the system and infecting the urinary tract. Urinary drainage systems typically depend on the force of gravity to drain urine from the bladder to the collecting bag.

Skill 47.2 describes catheterization of females and males, using straight and indwelling catheters.

Nursing Interventions for Clients with Indwelling Catheters

Nursing care of the client with an indwelling catheter and continuous drainage is mostly directed toward preventing infection of the urinary tract and encouraging urinary flow through the drainage system. It includes encouraging large amounts of fluid intake, accurately recording

Performing Indwelling Urinary Catheterization

SKILL 47.2

PURPOSES

Straight catheter:

- To relieve discomfort due to bladder distention
- To assess the amount of residual urine if the bladder empties incompletely
- To obtain a sterile urine specimen
- To empty the bladder completely prior to surgery.

Indwelling catheter:

- To relieve urinary retention or bladder outlet obstruction
- For selected surgical procedures
- To facilitate accurate measurement of urinary output for critically ill clients whose output needs to be monitored hourly
- To provide for intermittent or continuous bladder drainage and/or irrigation
- To prevent urine from contacting an incision after perineal surgery if needed
- To assist in healing of open sacral or perineal wounds in incontinent clients
- To improve comfort for end-of-life care if needed.

ASSESSMENT

- Determine the most appropriate method of catheterization based on the purpose and any criteria specified in the order such as total amount of urine to be removed or size of catheter to be used.
- Use a straight catheter if only a one-time urine specimen is needed, if amount of residual urine is being measured, or if temporary emptying of the bladder is required.
- Use an indwelling catheter if the bladder must remain empty, intermittent catheterization is contraindicated, or continuous urine measurement or collection is needed.
- Assess the client's overall condition. Determine if the client is able to participate and hold still during the procedure and if the client can be positioned supine with head relatively flat. For female clients, determine if she can have knees bent and hips externally rotated.
- Determine when the client last voided or was last catheterized.
- If catheterization is being performed because the client has been unable to void, when possible, complete a bladder scan to assess the amount of urine present in the bladder. **Rationale:** *This prevents catheterizing the bladder when insufficient urine is present. Often, a minimum of 500 to 800 mL of urine indicates urinary retention and the client should be reassessed until that amount is present.*

PLANNING

- Allow adequate time to perform the catheterization. Although the entire procedure can require as little as 15 minutes, several sources of difficulty could result in a much longer period of time. If possible, it should not be performed just prior to or after a meal.
- Some agencies require two nurses to be present for the procedure: one to perform the catheterization and the other to assist with positioning and ensure there is no break in aseptic technique.
- Some clients may feel uncomfortable being catheterized by nurses of the opposite gender. If this is the case, obtain the client's permission. Also consider whether agency policy requires or encourages having an individual of the client's same gender present for the procedure.

Assignment

Due to the need for sterile technique and detailed knowledge of anatomy, insertion of a urinary catheter is not assigned to AP.

Equipment

For a straight catheterization:

- Straight catheterization kit:
  - Sterile straight catheter of appropriate size
  - Sterile gloves
  - Waterproof drape(s)
  - Antiseptic solution
  - Cleansing balls
  - Forceps
  - Water-soluble lubricant
  - Urine receptacle
  - Specimen container.

(An extra catheter should also be at hand in case of a break in aseptic technique.)

For an indwelling catheter:

- Closed catheterization kit ❶:
  - Sterile indwelling catheter of appropriate size

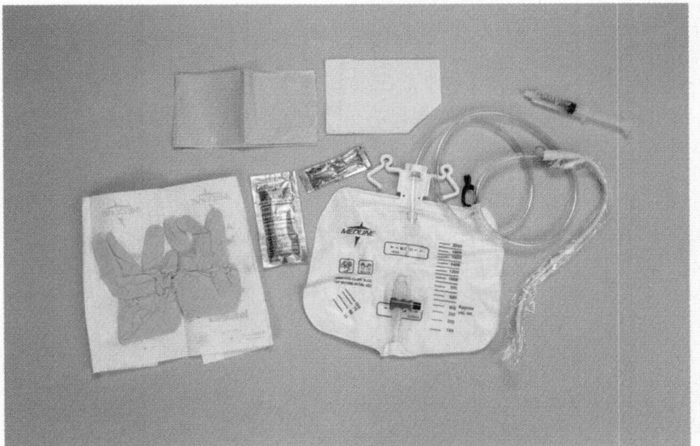

❶ A closed indwelling urinary catheter insertion kit.

Continued on page 1254

Performing Indwelling Urinary Catheterization—*continued*

- Sterile gloves
- Waterproof drape(s)
- Antiseptic solution
- Cleansing balls
- Forceps
- Water-soluble lubricant
- Syringe prefilled with sterile water in amount specified by catheter manufacturer
- Collection bag and tubing
- 5–10 mL 2% Xylocaine gel or water-soluble lubricant for male urethral injection (if agency permits)
- Clean gloves
- Supplies for performing perineal cleansing
- Bath blanket or sheet for draping the client
- Adequate lighting (Obtain a flashlight or lamp if necessary.)

(An extra catheter should also be at hand in case of a break in aseptic technique.)

IMPLEMENTATION

Preparation

- If using a catheterization kit, read the label carefully to ensure that all necessary items are included.
- Apply clean gloves and perform routine perineal care to cleanse the meatus from gross contamination. ❷ For women, use this time to locate the urinary meatus relative to surrounding structures. ❸
- Remove and discard gloves.
  - Perform hand hygiene.

Performance

1. Prior to performing the procedure, introduce self and verify the client's identity using agency protocol. Explain to the client what you are going to do, why it is necessary, and how to participate.

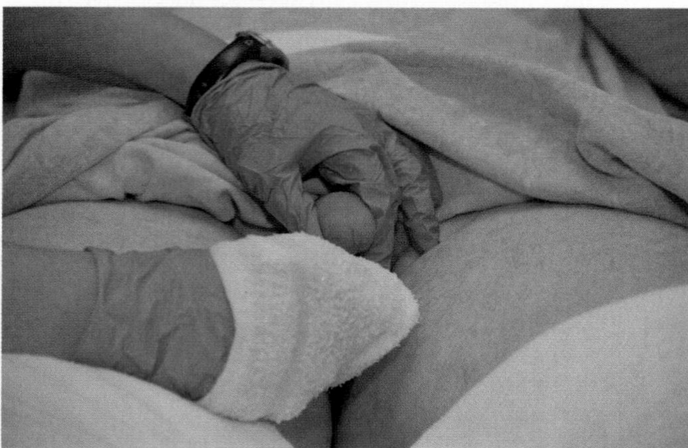

A

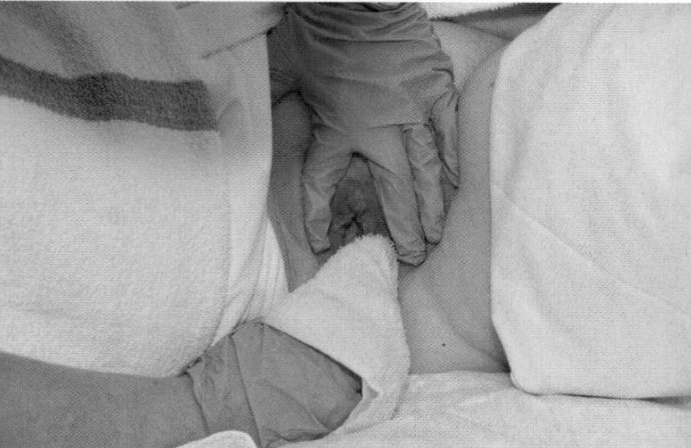

B

❷ *A*, Male and *B*, female pericare in preparation for catheterization.

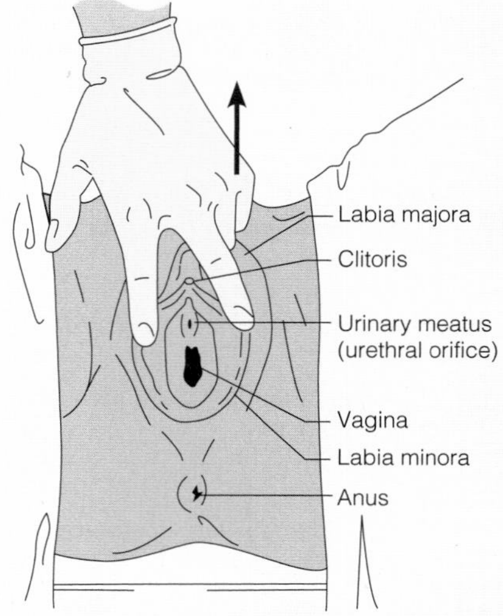

❸ To expose the urinary meatus, separate the labia minora and retract the tissue upward.

2. Perform hand hygiene and observe other appropriate infection prevention procedures.
3. Provide for client privacy.
4. Place the client in the appropriate position and drape all areas except the perineum.
   - *Female:* supine with knees flexed, feet about 2 feet apart, and hips slightly externally rotated, if possible
   - *Male:* supine, thighs slightly abducted or apart
5. Establish adequate lighting. Stand on the client's right if you are right-handed, on the client's left if you are left-handed.
6. If using a collecting bag and it is not contained within the catheterization kit, open the drainage package and place the end of the tubing within reach. **Rationale:** *Because one hand is needed to hold the catheter once it is in place, open the package while two hands are still available.*
7. If agency policy permits, apply clean gloves and inject 10 to 15 mL Xylocaine gel into the urethra of the male client. Wipe the underside of the penile shaft to distribute the gel up the urethra. Wait at least 5 minutes for the gel to take effect before inserting the catheter.
8. Remove and discard gloves.
   - Perform hand hygiene.
9. Open the catheterization kit. Place a waterproof drape under the buttocks (female) or penis (male) without contaminating the center of the drape with your hands.
10. Apply sterile gloves.
11. Organize the remaining supplies:
    - Saturate the cleansing balls with the antiseptic solution. ❹
    - Open the lubricant package. ❺
    - Remove the specimen container and place it nearby with the lid loosely on top.
    - Remove plastic covering of indwelling catheter. 

Performing Indwelling Urinary Catheterization—*continued*

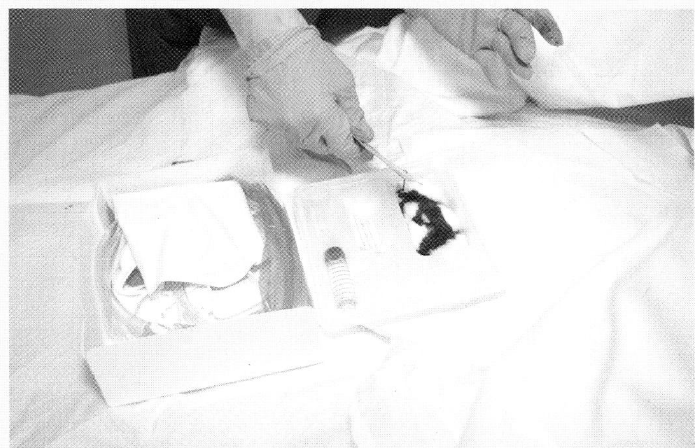

④ Saturating the cleansing balls with the antiseptic solution.

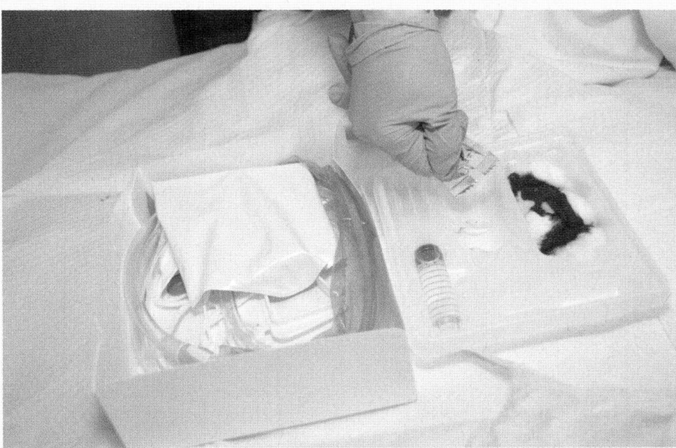

⑤ Putting lubricant on the tray.

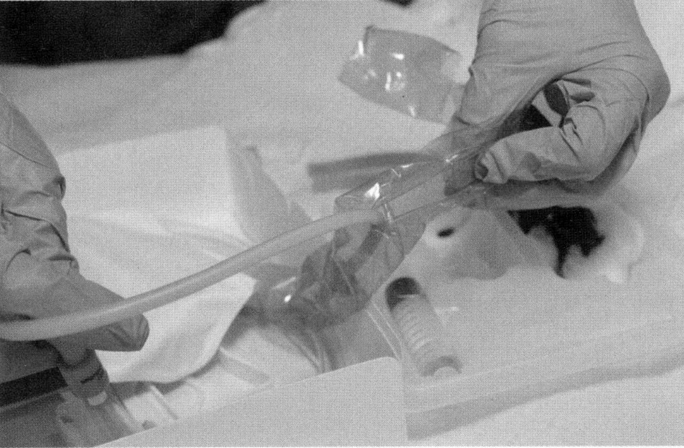

⑥ Removing the wrapping of the IUC.

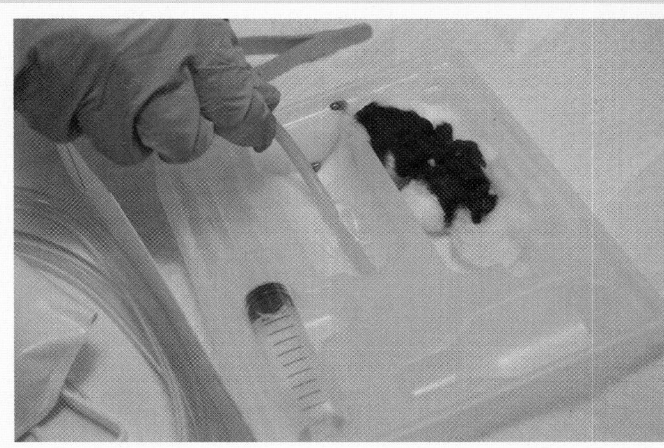

⑦ Lubricating the catheter.

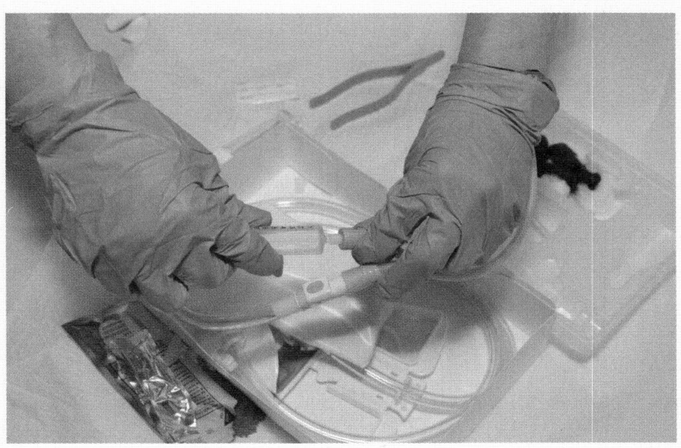

⑧ Attaching the prefilled syringe to the IUC.

12. Lubricate the catheter 2.5 to 5 cm (1 to 2 in.) for females, 15 to 17.5 cm (6 to 7 in.) for males, and place it with the drainage end inside the collection container. ⑦
13. Attach the prefilled syringe to the indwelling catheter inflation hub. ⑧ Do not pre-inflate the balloon. **Rationale:** *Pre-inflation is no longer recommended and may cause microtears, risking infection.*
14. If desired, place the fenestrated drape over the perineum, exposing the urinary meatus. ⑨
15. Cleanse the meatus. Note: *The nondominant hand is considered contaminated once it touches the client's skin.*
    - *Females:* Use your nondominant hand to spread the labia so that the meatus is visible. Establish firm but gentle pressure on the labia. The antiseptic may make the tissues slippery but the labia must not be allowed to return over the cleaned meatus. Note: *Location of the urethral meatus is best identified during the cleansing process. Pick up a cleansing ball with the forceps in your dominant hand and wipe one side of the labia majora in an anteroposterior direction.* ⑩ Use great care that wiping the client does not contaminate this

Continued on page 1256

Performing Indwelling Urinary Catheterization—*continued*

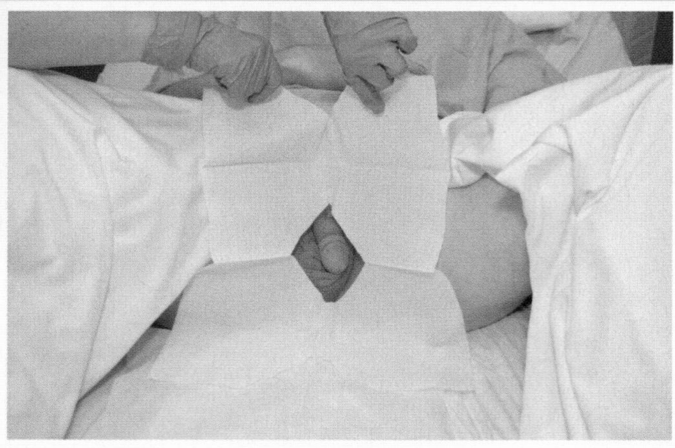

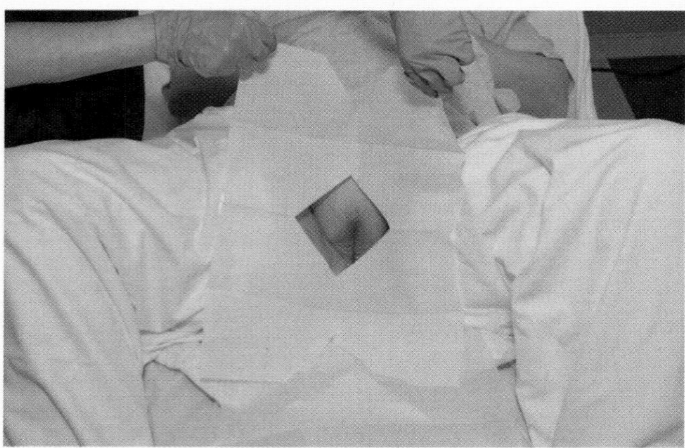

⑨ Drape over the perineum of male and female.

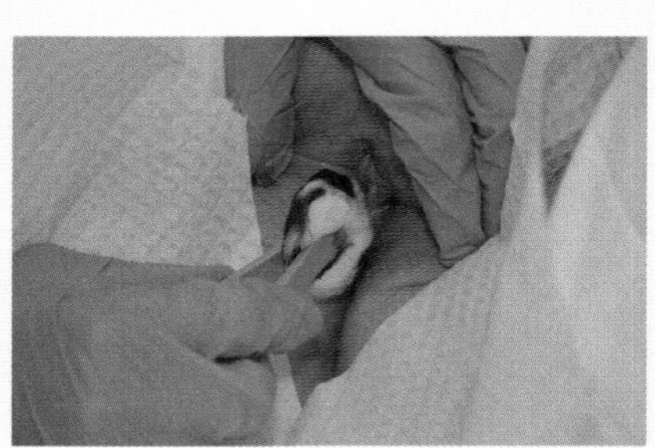

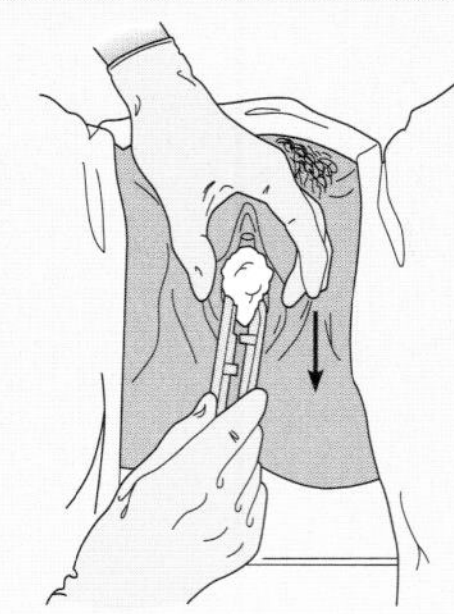

⑩ When cleaning the urinary meatus, move the swab downward.

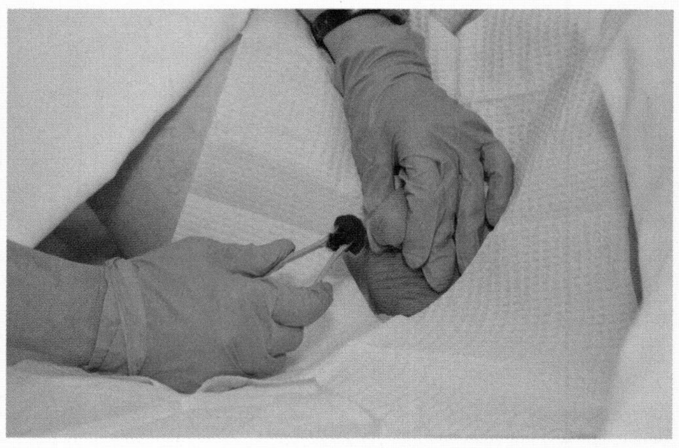

⑪ Cleanse center of male meatus in a circular motion around the glans.

sterile hand. Use a new ball for the opposite side. Repeat for the labia minora. Use the last ball to cleanse directly over the meatus.

- *Males:* Use your nondominant hand to grasp the penis just below the glans. If necessary, retract the foreskin. Hold the penis firmly upright, with slight tension. **Rationale:** *Lifting the penis in this manner helps straighten the urethra.* Pick up a cleansing ball with the forceps in your dominant hand and wipe from the center of the meatus in a circular motion around the glans. ⑪ Use great care that wiping the client does not contaminate the sterile hand. Use a new ball and repeat 3 more times. The antiseptic may make the tissues slippery but the foreskin must not be allowed to return over the cleaned meatus nor the penis be dropped.

16. Insert the catheter.

- Grasp the catheter firmly 5 to 7.5 cm (2 to 3 in.) from the tip. Ask the client to take a slow deep breath and insert the catheter as the client exhales. ⑫ Slight resistance is expected as the catheter passes through the sphincter. If necessary, twist the catheter or hold pressure on the catheter until the sphincter relaxes.
- Advance the catheter 5 cm (2 in.) farther after the urine begins to flow through it. **Rationale:** *This is to be sure it is fully in the bladder, will not easily fall out, and the balloon is in the bladder completely.* For male clients, advance the catheter to the "Y" bifurcation of the catheter.
- If the catheter accidentally contacts the labia or slips into the vagina, it is considered contaminated and a new, sterile catheter must be used. The contaminated catheter may be left in the vagina until the new catheter is inserted to help avoid mistaking the vaginal opening for the urethral meatus.

17. Hold the catheter with the nondominant hand.

18. For an indwelling catheter, inflate the IUC balloon with the designated volume. ⑬

- *Without* releasing the catheter (and, for females, without releasing the labia), hold the inflation valve between two fingers of your nondominant hand while you attach the syringe (if not left attached earlier) and inflate with your dominant hand. If the client complains of discomfort, immediately withdraw the instilled fluid, advance the catheter farther, and attempt to inflate the balloon again.
- Pull gently on the catheter until resistance is felt to ensure that the balloon has inflated and to place it in the trigone of the bladder.

19. Collect a urine specimen if needed. For a straight catheter, allow 20 to 30 mL to flow into the bottle without touching the catheter to the bottle. For an indwelling catheter preattached to a drainage bag, a specimen may be taken from the bag this initial time only.

Performing Indwelling Urinary Catheterization—*continued*

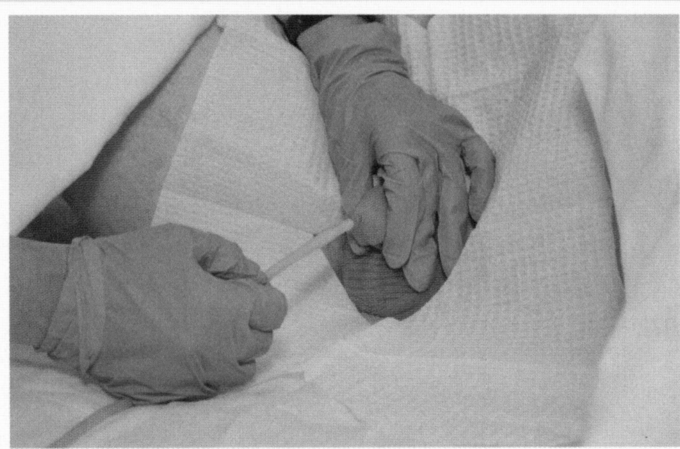

20. Allow the straight catheter to continue draining into the urine receptacle. If necessary (e.g., open system), attach the drainage end of an indwelling catheter to the collecting tubing and bag.
21. Examine and measure the urine. In some cases, only 750 to 1000 mL of urine are to be drained from the bladder at one time. Check agency policy for further instructions if this should occur.
22. Remove the straight catheter when urine flow stops. For an indwelling catheter, secure the catheter tubing to the thigh for female clients or the upper thigh or lower abdomen for male clients to prevent movement on the urethra or excessive tension or pulling on the indwelling balloon. Adhesive and nonadhesive catheter-securing devices are available and should be used to secure the catheter tubing to the client. ⓮ **Rationale:** *This prevents unnecessary trauma to the urethra.*

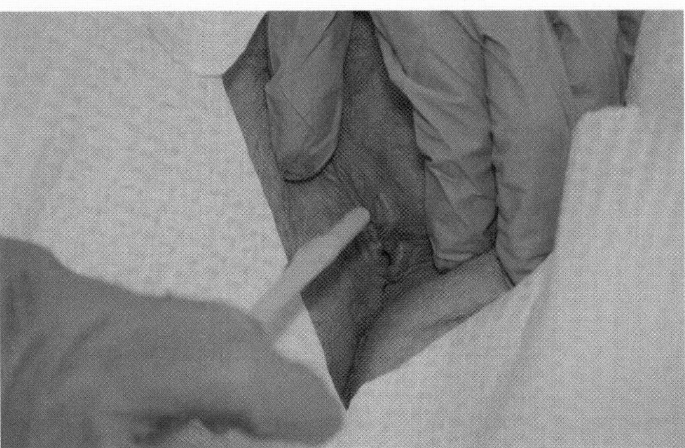

⓬ Insert the catheter.

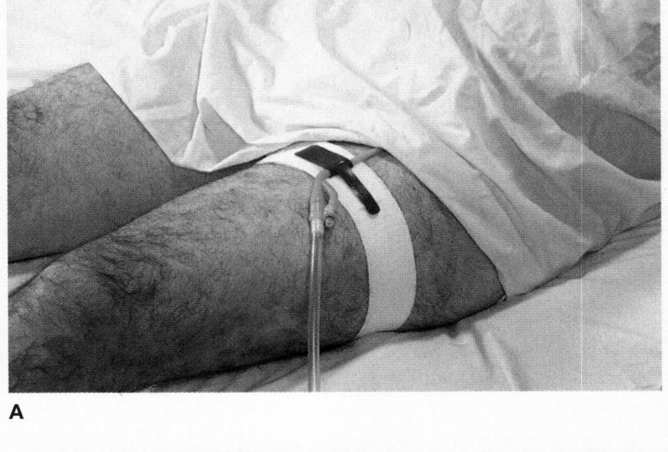

A

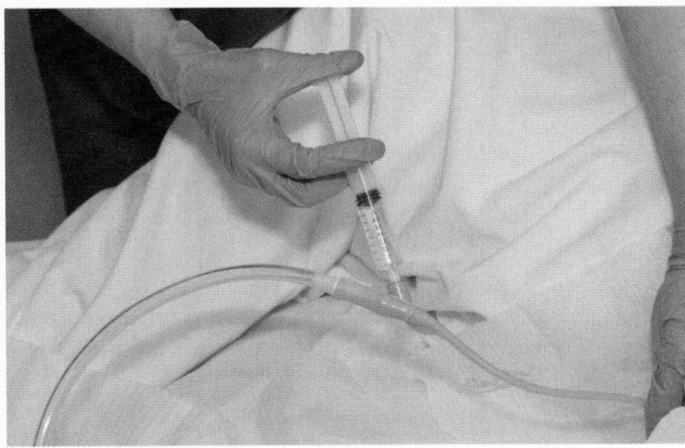

⓭ Inflating the IUC balloon.

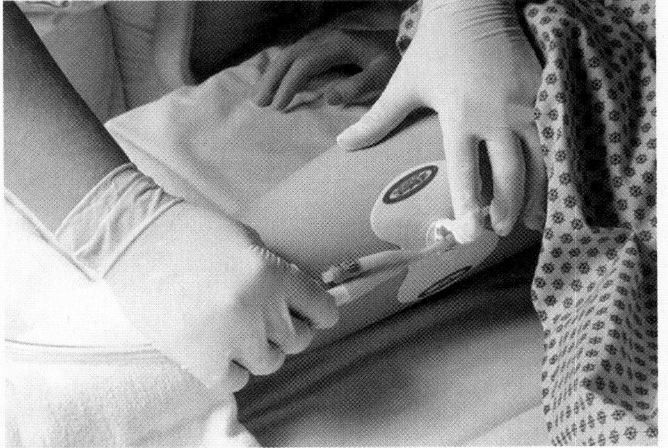

B

⓮ Catheter securement devices: *A*, nonadhesive device (Velcro strap); *B*, adhesive device.

Continued on page 1258

SKILL 47.2

Performing Indwelling Urinary Catheterization—*continued*

23. Next, hang the bag below the level of the bladder. No tubing should fall below the top of the bag. ⓯
24. Wipe any remaining antiseptic or lubricant from the perineal area. Replace the foreskin if retracted earlier. Return the client to a comfortable position. Instruct the client on positioning and moving with the catheter in place.
25. Discard all used supplies in appropriate receptacles.
26. Remove and discard gloves.
    - Perform hand hygiene.
27. Document the catheterization procedure including catheter size and results in the client record using forms or checklists supplemented by narrative notes when appropriate.

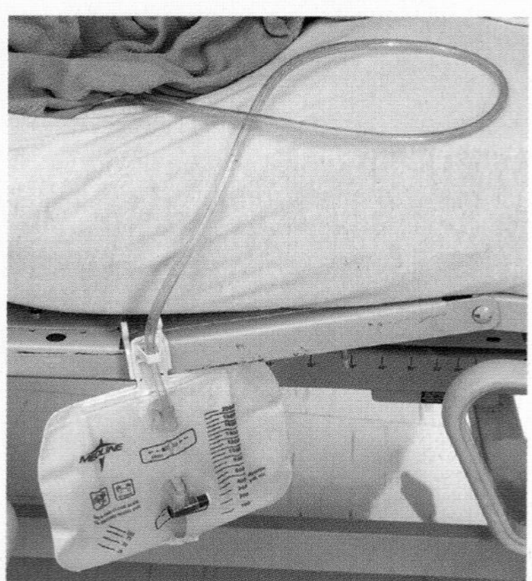

⓯ Correct position for urine drainage bag and tubing.

SAMPLE DOCUMENTATION

2/24/2020 0530 Client agreed to insertion of pre-op catheter as per order. #16 Fr Foley with 5-mL balloon inserted without difficulty, secured to thigh, connected to continuous drainage. Immediate return of 300 mL pale, clear, yellow urine. G. Hampton, RN

EVALUATION

- Notify the primary care provider of the catheterization results.
- Perform a detailed follow-up based on findings that deviated from expected or normal for the client. Compare findings to previous assessment data if available.
- Teach the client how to care for the indwelling catheter, to drink more fluids, and provide other appropriate instructions.

LIFESPAN CONSIDERATIONS Urinary Catheterization

INFANTS AND CHILDREN

- Adapt the size of the catheter for pediatric clients.
- Ask a family member to assist in holding the child during catheterization, if appropriate.

OLDER ADULTS

When catheterizing older clients, be very attentive to problems of limited movement, especially in the hips. Arthritis, or previous hip or knee surgery, may limit their movement and cause discomfort. Modify the position (e.g., side-lying) as needed to perform the procedure safely and comfortably. For women, obtain the assistance of another nurse to flex and hold the client's knees and hips as necessary or place her in a modified Sims' position.

the fluid I&O, maintaining the patency of the drainage system, preventing contamination of the drainage system, and teaching these measures to the client.

Fluids

The client with an indwelling catheter should drink up to 3000 mL/day if permitted. Large amounts of fluid ensure a large urine output, which keeps the bladder flushed out and decreases the likelihood of urinary stasis and subsequent infection. Large volumes of urine also minimize the risk of sediment or other particles obstructing the drainage tubing.

Dietary Measures

Acidifying the urine of clients with an indwelling catheter may reduce the risk of UTI and calculus formation. Foods such as eggs, cheese, meat and poultry, whole grains, cranberries, plums and prunes, and tomatoes tend to increase the acidity of urine. Conversely, most fruits and vegetables, legumes, and milk and milk products result in alkaline urine.

Perineal Care

No special cleaning other than routine daily hygienic care with soap and water is necessary for clients with an indwelling catheter, nor is special meatal care recommended. The nurse should check agency practice in this regard.

Changing the Catheter and Tubing

Routine changing of catheter and tubing is *not* recommended. Collection of sediment in the catheter or tubing and impaired urine drainage are indicators for changing the catheter and drainage system. When this occurs the catheter and drainage system are removed and discarded, and a new sterile catheter with a closed drainage system is inserted using aseptic technique.

Removing Indwelling Catheters

Indwelling catheters are removed after their purpose has been achieved, usually on the order of the primary care provider. Unfortunately, not all primary care providers know which of their clients has an indwelling catheter. As a result, some facilities have incorporated an alert system that requires the provider to take an action after a specified time frame. Increasingly, healthcare facilities are allowing the nurse to remove an indwelling catheter through the use of a nurse-driven protocol with specific criteria.

If the catheter has been in place for a short time (e.g., 48 to 72 hours), the client usually has little difficulty regaining normal urinary elimination patterns. Swelling of the urethra, however, may initially interfere with voiding, so the nurse should regularly assess the client for urinary retention until voiding is reestablished.

Clients who have had an indwelling catheter for a prolonged period may require bladder retraining to regain bladder muscle tone. With an indwelling catheter in place, the bladder muscle does not stretch and contract regularly as it does when the bladder fills and empties by voiding. A few days before removal, the catheter may be clamped for specified periods of time (e.g., 2 to 4 hours), then released to allow the bladder to empty. This allows the bladder to distend and stimulates its musculature. Check agency policy regarding bladder training procedures.

To remove an indwelling catheter the nurse follows these steps:

- Obtain a receptacle for the catheter (e.g., a disposable basin); a clean, disposable towel; clean gloves; and a sterile syringe to deflate the balloon. The syringe should be large enough to withdraw all the solution in the catheter balloon. The size of the balloon is indicated on the label at the end of the catheter.
- Ask the client to assume a supine position as for a catheterization.
- *Optional:* Obtain a sterile specimen before removing the catheter. Check agency protocol.
- Remove the catheter-securing device attaching the catheter to the client, apply gloves, and then place the towel between the legs of the female client or over the thighs of the male.
- Insert the syringe into the injection port of the catheter, and withdraw the fluid from the balloon. After the fluid has been aspirated, the walls of the balloon do *not* deflate to their original shape but collapse into uneven ridges, forming a "cuff" around the catheter. This cuff is more pronounced with a silicone catheter. This cuff may cause discomfort to the client as the catheter is removed.
- Do not pull the catheter while the balloon is inflated; doing so will injure the urethra.
- After all of the fluid is removed from the balloon, gently withdraw the catheter and place it in the waste receptacle.
- Dry the perineal area with a towel.
  - Measure the urine in the drainage bag.
- Remove and discard gloves.
  - Perform hand hygiene.
- Record the removal of the catheter. Include in the recording (a) the time the catheter was removed; (b) the amount, color, and clarity of the urine; (c) the intactness of the catheter; and (d) instructions given to the client.
- Provide the client with either a urinal (men), bedpan, commode, or toilet collection device ("hat") to be used with each subsequent unassisted void.
- Following removal of the catheter, determine the time of the first voiding and the amount voided during the first 8 hours. Compare this output to the client's intake.
- Observe for dysfunctional voiding behaviors (i.e., <100 mL per void), which might indicate urinary retention. If this occurs, perform an assessment of PVR using a bladder scanner if available. Generally a PVR greater than 200 mL will require straight catheterization as needed.

Clean Intermittent Catheterization

Clean intermittent catheterization (CIC) is performed by many clients who have some form of neurogenic bladder dysfunction such as that caused by spinal cord injury and multiple sclerosis. Clean or medical aseptic technique is used. CIC has these benefits:

- Enables the client to retain independence and gain control of the bladder
- Reduces incidence of UTI
- Protects the upper urinary tract from reflux
- Allows normal sexual relations without incontinence
- Reduces the use of aids and appliances
- Frees the client from embarrassing dribbling.

The procedure for self-catheterization is similar to that used by the nurse to catheterize a client. Essential steps are outlined in the accompanying Client Teaching. Because the procedure requires physical and mental preparation, client assessment is important. The client should have:

- Sufficient manual dexterity to manipulate a catheter
- Sufficient mental ability
- Motivation and acceptance of the procedure
- For women, reasonable agility to access the urethra
- Bladder capacity greater than 100 mL.

Before teaching CIC, the nurse should establish the client's voiding patterns, the volume voided, fluid intake, and residual amounts. CIC is easier for males to learn because of the visibility of the urinary meatus. Females need to learn initially with the aid of a mirror but eventually should perform the procedure by using only the sense of touch (as described in Client Teaching).

Urinary Irrigations

An **irrigation** is a flushing or washing-out with a specified solution. Bladder irrigation is carried out on a primary care provider's order, usually to wash out the bladder and sometimes to apply a medication to the bladder lining. Catheter irrigations may also be performed to maintain or restore the

CLIENT TEACHING Clean Intermittent Catheterization (CIC)

- Catheterize as often as needed to maintain. At first, catheterization may be necessary every 2 to 3 hours, increasing to 4 to 6 hours.
- Attempt to void before catheterization; insert the catheter to remove residual urine if unable to void or if amount voided is insufficient (e.g., less than 100 mL).
- Assemble all needed supplies ahead of time. Good lighting is essential, especially for women.
- Wash your hands.
- Clean the urinary meatus with either a towelette or soapy washcloth, then rinse with a wet washcloth. Women should clean the area from front to back.
- Assume a position that is comfortable and that facilitates passage of the catheter, such as a semireclining position in bed or sitting on a chair or the toilet. Men may prefer to stand over the toilet; women may prefer to stand with one foot on the side of the toilet.
- Apply lubricant to the catheter tip (1 in. [2.5 cm] for women; 2 to 6 in. [5 to 15 cm] for men). Some catheters are coated with a slippery surface that may require activation of a wetting solution and eliminating the need for a lubricant.
- Insert the catheter until urine flows through.
  a. If a woman, locate the meatus using a mirror or other aid, or use the "touch" technique as follows:
     - Place the index finger of your nondominant hand on your clitoris.
     - Place the third and fourth fingers at the vagina.
     - Locate the meatus between the index and third fingers.
     - Direct the catheter through the meatus and then upward and forward.
  b. If a man, hold the penis with a slight upward tension at a 60° to 90° angle to insert the catheter. Return the penis to its natural position when urine starts to flow.
- Hold the catheter in place until all urine is drained.
- Withdraw the catheter slowly *to ensure complete drainage of urine.*
- Discard the catheter. Evidence does not endorse catheter reuse (Beauchemin, Newman, LeDanseur, Jackson, & Ritmiller, 2018).
- Contact your care provider if your urine becomes cloudy or contains sediment; if you have bleeding, difficulty, or pain when passing the catheter; or if you have a fever.
- Drink at least 2000 to 2500 mL of fluid a day *to ensure adequate bladder filling and flushing.* To keep your urine acidic and reduce the risk of bladder infections, drink cranberry and prune juices.

patency of a catheter, for example, to remove pus or blood clots blocking the catheter. Sterile technique is used.

The closed method is the preferred technique for catheter or bladder irrigation because it is associated with a lower risk of UTI. Closed catheter irrigations may be either continuous or intermittent. This method is most often used for clients who have had genitourinary surgery. The continuous irrigation helps prevent blood clots from occluding the catheter. A three-way, or triple lumen, catheter (see Figure 47.10) is generally used for closed irrigations. The irrigating solution flows into the bladder through the irrigation port of the catheter and out through the urinary drainage lumen of the catheter.

Occasionally an open irrigation may be necessary to restore catheter patency. The risk of injecting microorganisms into the urinary tract is greater with open irrigations, because the connection between the indwelling catheter and the drainage tubing is broken. Strict precautions must be taken to maintain the sterility of both the drainage tubing connector and the interior of the indwelling catheter.

The open method of catheter or bladder irrigation is performed with double-lumen indwelling catheters. It may be necessary for clients who develop blood clots and mucous fragments that occlude the catheter or when it is undesirable to change the catheter. Techniques for bladder irrigation are outlined in Skill 47.3.

SKILL 47.3 Performing Bladder Irrigation

PURPOSES

- To maintain the patency of a urinary catheter and tubing (closed continuous irrigation)
- To free a blockage in a urinary catheter or tubing (open intermittent irrigation)

ASSESSMENT

- Determine the client's current urinary drainage system. Review the client record for recent I&O and any difficulties the client has been experiencing with the system. Review the results of previous irrigations.
- Assess the client for any discomfort, bladder spasms, or distended bladder.

PLANNING

Before irrigating a catheter or bladder, check (a) the reason for the irrigation; (b) the order authorizing the continuous or intermittent irrigation (in most agencies, a primary care provider's order is required); (c) the type of sterile solution, the amount and strength to be used, and the rate (if continuous); and (d) the type of catheter in place. If these are not specified on the client's chart, check agency protocol.

Assignment

Due to the need for sterile technique, urinary irrigation is generally not assigned to AP. If the client has continuous irrigation, the AP may care for the client and note abnormal findings. These must be validated and interpreted by the nurse.

Performing Bladder Irrigation—*continued*

Equipment

- Clean gloves (two pairs)
- Indwelling catheter in place
- Drainage tubing and bag (if not in place)
- Drainage tubing clamp
- Antiseptic swabs
- Sterile receptacle
- Sterile irrigating solution warmed or at room temperature (Label the irrigant clearly with the words *Bladder Irrigation*, including the information about any medications that have been added to the original solution, and the date, time, and nurse's initials.)
- Infusion tubing
- IV pole

IMPLEMENTATION

Performance

1. Prior to performing the procedure, introduce self and verify the client's identity using agency protocol. Explain to the client what you are going to do, why it is necessary, and how to participate. The irrigation should not be painful or uncomfortable. Discuss how the results will be used in planning further care or treatments.
2. Perform hand hygiene and observe other appropriate infection prevention procedures.
3. Provide for client privacy.
4. Apply clean gloves.
5. Empty, measure, and record the amount and appearance of urine present in the drainage bag. **Rationale:** *Emptying the drainage bag allows more accurate measurement of urinary output after the irrigation is in place or completed. Assessing the character of the urine provides baseline data for later comparison.*
6. Discard urine and gloves.
7. Prepare the equipment.
   - Perform hand hygiene.
   - Connect the irrigation infusion tubing to the irrigating solution and flush the tubing with solution, keeping the tip sterile. **Rationale:** *Flushing the tubing removes air and prevents it from being instilled into the bladder.*
   - Apply clean gloves and cleanse the port with antiseptic swabs.
   - Connect the irrigation tubing to the input port of the three-way indwelling catheter.
   - Connect the drainage bag and tubing to the urinary drainage port if not already in place.
   - Remove and discard gloves.
   - Perform hand hygiene.
8. Irrigate the bladder.
   - For closed continuous irrigation using a three-way catheter, open the clamp on the urinary drainage tubing (if present). ❶ **Rationale:** *This allows the irrigating solution to flow out of the bladder continuously.*
     a. Apply clean gloves.
     b. Open the regulating clamp on the irrigating fluid infusion tubing and adjust the flow rate as prescribed by the primary care provider or to 40 to 60 drops per minute if not specified.
     c. Assess the drainage for amount, color, and clarity. The amount of drainage should equal the amount of irrigant entering the bladder plus expected urine output. Empty the bag frequently so that it does not exceed half full.
   - For closed intermittent irrigation, determine whether the solution is to remain in the bladder for a specified time.
     a. If the solution is to remain in the bladder (a bladder irrigation or instillation), close the clamp to the urinary drainage tubing. **Rationale:** *Closing the flow clamp allows the solution to be retained in the bladder and in contact with bladder walls.*

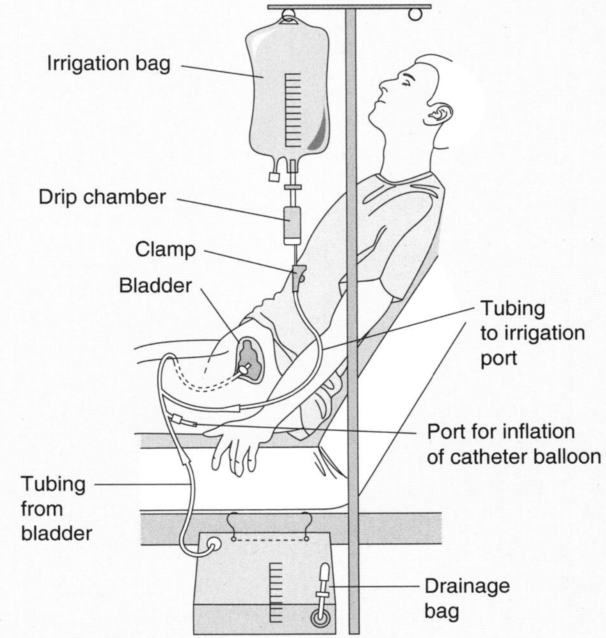

❶ A continuous bladder irrigation (CBI) setup.

     b. If the solution is being instilled to irrigate the catheter, open the flow clamp on the urinary drainage tubing. **Rationale:** *Irrigating solution will flow through the urinary drainage port and tubing, removing mucous shreds or clots.*
     c. If a three-way catheter is used, open the flow clamp to the irrigating fluid infusion tubing, allowing the specified amount of solution to infuse. Then close the clamp on the infusion tubing.

     or

     d. If a two-way catheter is used, connect an irrigating syringe with a needleless adapter to the injection port on the drainage tubing and instill the solution.
     e. After the specified period the solution is to be retained has passed, open the drainage tubing flow clamp and allow the bladder to empty.
     f. Assess the drainage for amount, color, and clarity. The amount of drainage should equal the amount of irrigant entering the bladder plus expected urine output.
     g. Remove and discard gloves.
        - Perform hand hygiene.
9. Assess the client and the urinary output.
   - Assess the client's comfort.
   - Apply clean gloves.

Continued on page 1262

Performing Bladder Irrigation—*continued*

SKILL 47.3

- Empty the drainage bag and measure the contents. Subtract the amount of irrigant instilled from the total volume of drainage to obtain the volume of urine output.
- Remove and discard gloves.
  - Perform hand hygiene.

10. Document findings in the client record using forms or checklists supplemented by narrative notes when appropriate.
    - Note any abnormal constituents such as blood clots, pus, or mucous shreds.

Variation: Open Irrigation Using a Two-Way Indwelling Catheter

1. Assemble the equipment. Use an irrigation tray ❷ or assemble individual items, including:
   - Clean gloves
   - Disposable water-resistant towel
   - Sterile irrigating solution
   - Sterile irrigation set
   - Sterile basin
   - Sterile 30- to 50-mL irrigating syringe
   - Antiseptic swabs
   - Sterile protective cap for catheter drainage tubing.
2. Prepare the client (see steps 1–5 of main procedure for catheter irrigation).

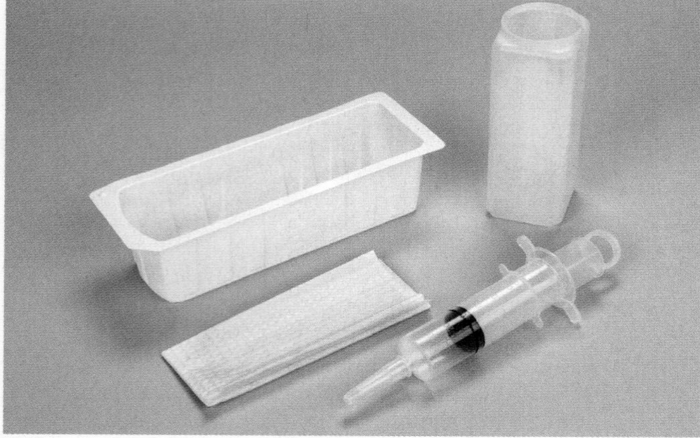

❷ An irrigation set.

3. Prepare the equipment.
   - Perform hand hygiene.
   - Using aseptic technique, open supplies and pour the irrigating solution into the sterile basin or receptacle. **Rationale:** *Aseptic technique is vital to reduce the risk of instilling microorganisms into the urinary tract during the irrigation.*
   - Place the disposable water-resistant towel under the catheter.
   - Apply clean gloves.
   - Disconnect catheter from drainage tubing and place the catheter end in the sterile basin. Place sterile protective cap over end of drainage tubing. **Rationale:** *The end of the drainage tubing will be considered contaminated if it touches bed linens or skin surfaces.*
   - Draw the prescribed amount of irrigating solution into the syringe, maintaining the sterility of the syringe and solution.
4. Irrigate the bladder.
   - Insert the tip of the syringe into the catheter opening.
   - Gently and slowly inject the solution into the catheter at approximately 3 mL per second. In adults, about 30 to 40 mL generally is instilled for catheter irrigations; 100 to 200 mL may be instilled for bladder irrigation or instillation. **Rationale:** *Gentle instillation reduces the risks of injury to bladder mucosa and of bladder spasms.*
   - Remove the syringe and allow the solution to drain back into the basin.
   - Continue to irrigate the client's bladder until the total amount to be instilled has been injected or when fluid returns are clear and clots are removed.
   - Remove the protective cap from the drainage tube and wipe with antiseptic swab.
   - Reconnect the catheter to drainage tubing.
   - Remove and discard gloves.
   - Perform hand hygiene.
   - Assess the drainage for amount, color, and clarity. The amount of drainage should equal the amount of irrigant entering the bladder plus any urine that may have been dwelling in the bladder. Determine the amount of fluid used for the irrigation and subtract from total output on the client's I&O record.
5. Assess the client and the urinary output and document the procedure as in steps 8 and 9.

EVALUATION

- Perform detailed follow-up based on findings that deviated from expected or normal for the client. Relate findings to previous assessment data if available.
- Report significant deviations from normal to the primary care provider.

Suprapubic Catheter Care

A **suprapubic catheter** is inserted surgically through the abdominal wall above the symphysis pubis into the urinary bladder. The suprapubic catheter may have a balloon or pigtail that holds it in the bladder depending on the manufacturer (Figure 47.11 ■). The healthcare provider inserts the catheter using local anesthesia or during bladder or vaginal surgery. The catheter may be secured in place with sutures to reinforce the security of the catheter and is then attached to a closed drainage system. The suprapubic catheter may be placed for temporary bladder drainage until the client is able to resume normal voiding (e.g., after urethral, bladder, or vaginal surgery) or it may become a permanent device (e.g., urethral or pelvic trauma).

Care of clients with a suprapubic catheter includes regular assessments of the client's urine, fluid intake, and comfort; maintenance of a patent drainage system; skin care around the insertion site; and periodic clamping of the catheter prior to removing it if it is not a permanent appliance. If the catheter is temporary, orders generally include leaving the catheter open to drainage for 48 to 72 hours, then clamping the catheter for 3- to 4-hour periods during the day until the client can void satisfactory amounts. Satisfactory voiding is determined by measuring the client's residual urine after voiding.

Care of the catheter insertion site involves sterile technique. Dressings around the newly placed suprapubic catheter are changed whenever they are soiled with

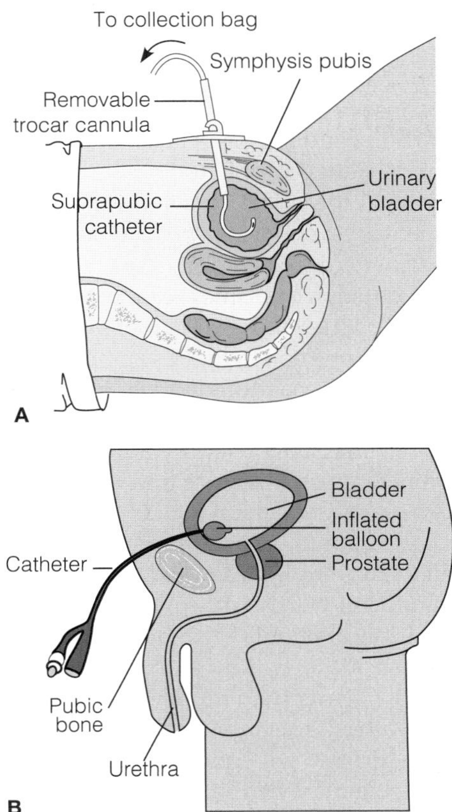

Figure 47.11 ■ A suprapubic catheter in place: *A*, using a pigtail loop; *B*, using a balloon to keep the catheter in place.

drainage to prevent bacterial growth around the insertion site and reduce the potential for infection. Cleanse with 4×4s with chlorhexidine gluconate and warm water. The area is dressed with a 4×4 and taped in an occlusive fashion. Securing the catheter tube to the abdomen helps to reduce tension at the insertion site. For catheters that have been in place for an extended period, no dressing may be needed and the healed insertion tract enables removal and replacement of the catheter as needed. Formation, however, of a healed insertion tract takes approximately 6 weeks to 6 months to develop. Before that time, the catheter needs to be replaced within 30 minutes if it falls out to prevent the opening from closing over. The nurse assesses the insertion area at regular intervals. If pubic hair invades the insertion site, it may be carefully trimmed with scissors. Any redness or discharge at the skin around the insertion site must be reported.

Urinary Diversions

A urinary diversion is the surgical rerouting of urine from the kidneys to a site other than the bladder. Clients with bladder cancer often need a urinary diversion when the bladder must be removed or bypassed. There are two categories of diversions: incontinent and continent.

Incontinent

With incontinent diversions clients have no control over the passage of urine and require the use of an external ostomy appliance to contain the urine. Urinary diversions may or may not involve the removal of the bladder (cystectomy). Examples of incontinent diversions include ureterostomy, nephrostomy, vesicostomy, and ileal conduits. A **ureterostomy** is when one or both of the ureters may be brought directly to the side of the abdomen to form small stomas. This procedure, however, has some disadvantages in that the stomas provide direct access for microorganisms from the skin to the kidneys, the small stomas are difficult to fit with an appliance to collect the urine, and they may narrow, impairing urine drainage. A **nephrostomy** diverts urine from the kidney via a catheter inserted into the renal pelvis to a nephrostomy tube and bag (Figure 47.12 ■).

A **vesicostomy** may be formed when the bladder is left intact but voiding through the urethra is not possible (e.g., due to an obstruction or a neurogenic bladder). The ureters

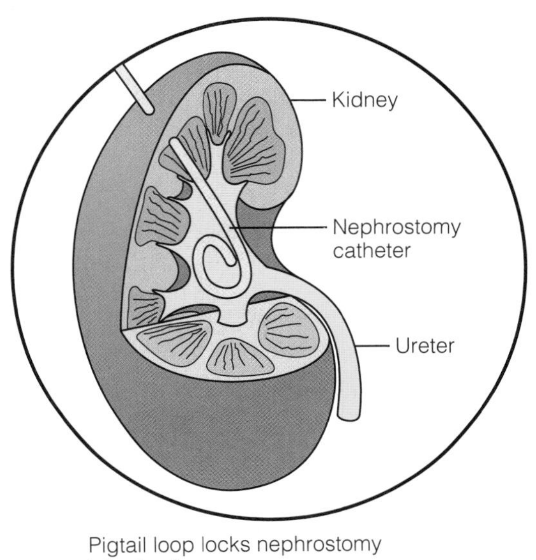

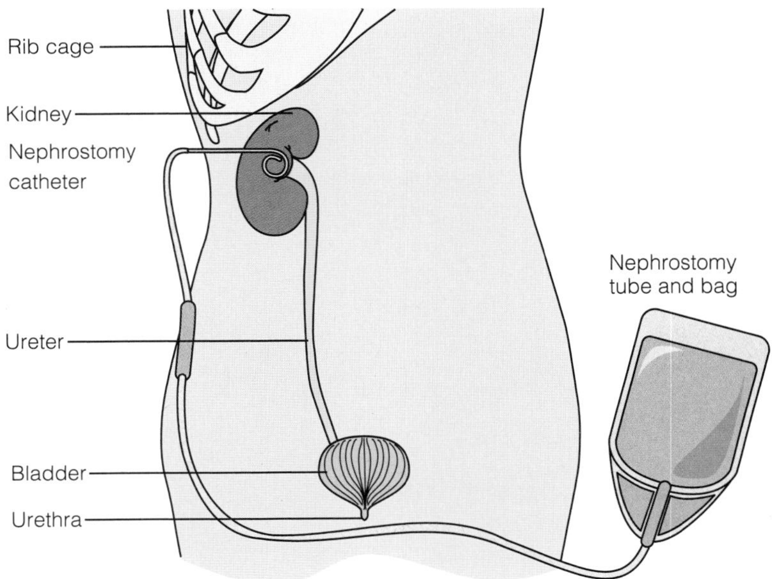

Figure 47.12 ■ A nephrostomy.

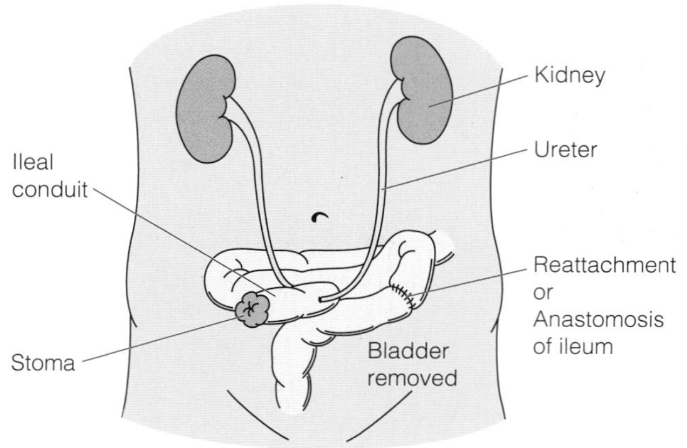

Figure 47.13 ■ An incontinent urinary diversion (ileal conduit).

remain connected to the bladder, and the bladder wall is surgically attached to an opening in the skin below the navel, forming an opening (stoma) for urinary drainage.

The most common incontinent urinary diversion is the **ileal conduit** or ileal loop (Figure 47.13 ■). In this procedure, a segment of the ileum is removed and the intestinal ends are reattached. One end of the portion removed is closed with sutures to create a pouch, and the other end is brought out through the abdominal wall to create a stoma. The ureters are implanted into the ileal pouch. The ileal stoma is more readily fitted with an appliance than ureterostomies because of its larger size. The mucous membrane lining of the ileum also provides some protection from ascending infection. Urine drains continuously from the ileal pouch.

Continent

Continent urinary diversion involves creation of a mechanism that allows the client to control the passage of urine, either by intermittent catheterization of the internal reservoir (e.g., Kock pouch) or by creating a neobladder or internal pouch.

The Kock (pronounced "coke") pouch, or continent ileal bladder conduit, also uses a portion of the ileum to form a reservoir for urine (Figure 47.14 ■). In this procedure, nipple valves are formed by doubling the tissue backward into the reservoir where the pouch connects to the skin and the ureters connect to the pouch. These valves close as the pouch fills with urine, preventing leakage and reflux of urine back toward the kidneys. The client empties the pouch by inserting a clean catheter approximately every 2 to 3 hours at first and increases to every 5 to 6 hours as the pouch expands. Between catheterizations, a small dressing is worn to protect the stoma and clothing.

A continent diversion with a neobladder involves replacing a diseased or damaged bladder with a piece of ileum and colon that is located in the same location as the bladder that was removed. A pouch or new bladder is created. The ureters are sutured to one end of the new pouch or bladder and this new bladder is then sutured to the functional urethra to facilitate client voiding control (Figure 47.15 ■). The client will need to relearn how to void. Voiding occurs when the urethral sphincter muscle relaxes and abdominal straining occurs to put pressure on the pouch.

When caring for clients with a urinary diversion, the nurse must accurately assess I&O; note any changes in urine color, odor, or clarity (mucous shreds are commonly seen in the urine of clients with an ileal diversion); and frequently assess the condition of the stoma and surrounding skin. Clients who must wear a urine collection appliance are at risk for impaired skin integrity because of irritation by urine. Well-fitting appliances are vital. The nurse should consult with the wound ostomy continence nurse (WOCN) to identify strategies for management of stoma and peristomal problems when selecting the most appropriate appliance for the client's needs. The steps of changing a urostomy appliance are similar to those described in the procedure for changing a bowel diversion appliance (see Chapter 48 ∞). However, there are some differences, including the following: Incontinent urinary diversions drain continually. As a result, some type of wicking material (e.g., rolled dry gauze pad or tampon) can be placed over the stoma to absorb the urine and keep the skin dry throughout the measurement and change of the ostomy appliance. Immediately following surgery, ureteral stents may be present and protruding from the stoma. These remain in place for 10 to 14 days postop and are removed by either the surgeon or the WOCN, depending on institutional protocol. Ureteral

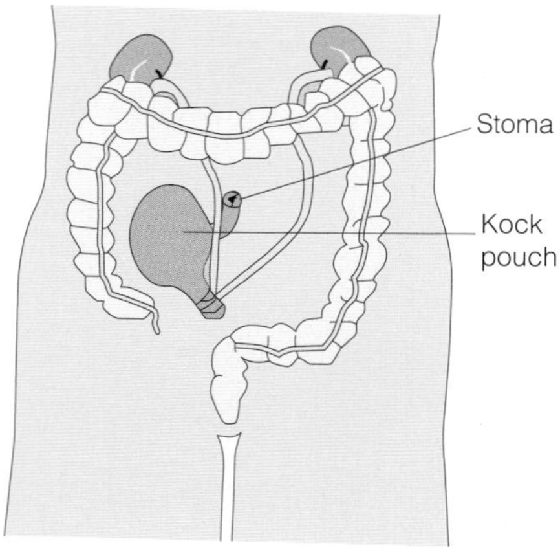

Figure 47.14 ■ The Kock pouch—a continent urinary diversion.

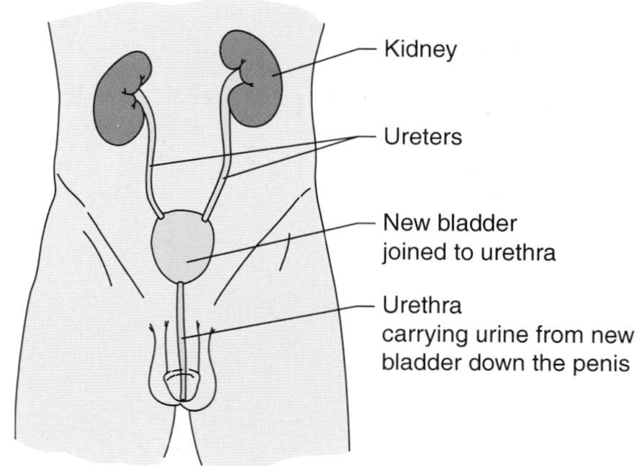

Figure 47.15 ■ A neobladder.

stents are used to maintain the patency of ureters at the anastomotic sites.

Clients with urinary diversions may experience body image and sexuality problems and may require assistance in coping with these changes and managing the stoma. Most clients are able to resume their normal activities and lifestyle.

Evaluating

Using the overall goals and desired outcomes identified in the planning stage, the nurse collects data to evaluate the effectiveness of nursing activities. If the desired outcomes are not achieved, explore the reasons before modifying the care plan. For example, if the outcome "Remains dry between voidings and at night" is not met, examples of questions that need to be considered include:

- What is the client's perception of the problem?
- Does the client understand and comply with the health-care instructions provided?
- Is access to toilet facilities a problem?
- Can the client manipulate clothing for toileting? Can adjustments be made to allow easier disrobing?
- Are scheduled toileting times appropriate?
- Is there adequate transition lighting for night-time toileting?
- Are mobility aids such as a walker, elevated toilet seat, or grab bar needed? If currently used, are they appropriate or adequate?
- Is the client performing PFM exercises appropriately as scheduled?
- Is the client's fluid intake adequate? Does the timing of fluid intake need to be adjusted (e.g., restricted after dinner)?
- Is the client restricting caffeine, citrus juice, carbonated beverages, and artificial sweetener intake?
- Is the client taking a diuretic? If so, when is the medication taken? Do the times need to be adjusted (e.g., taking second dose no later than 4 p.m.)?
- Should continence aids such as a condom catheter or absorbent pads be used?

NURSING CARE PLAN Urinary Elimination

ASSESSMENT DATA	NURSING DIAGNOSIS	DESIRED OUTCOMES*
NURSING ASSESSMENT Mr. John Baker, 68 years old, was admitted to the hospital with urinary retention, hematuria, and fever. The admitting nurse gathers the following information when taking a nursing history. Mr. Baker states he has noticed urinary frequency during the day for the past 2 weeks, and that he doesn't feel he has emptied his bladder after urinating. He also has to get up two or three times during the night to urinate. During the past few days, he has had difficulty starting urination and dribbles afterward. He verbalizes the embarrassment his urinary problems cause in his interactions with others. Mr. Baker is concerned about the cause of this urinary problem. He is diagnosed with benign prostatic hyperplasia (BPH) and referred to a urologist who suggests a transurethral resection of the prostate (TURP). He is placed on antibiotic therapy. **Physical Examination** Height: 185.4 cm (6′2″) Weight: 85.7 kg (189 lb) Temperature: 38.1°C (100.6°F) Pulse: 88 beats/min Respirations: 20/min Blood pressure: 146/86 mmHg Bladder scan for urinary retention indicated 400 mL urine. Straight catheterization performed. **Diagnostic Data** CBC normal; urinalysis: amber, clear, pH 6.5, specific gravity 1.025, negative for glucose, protein, ketone, RBCs, and bacteria; IVP: evidence of enlarged prostate gland	Altered urinary elimination (urinary retention) related to bladder neck obstruction by enlarged prostate gland (as evidenced by dysuria, frequency, nocturia, dribbling, hesitancy, and bladder distention)	**Urinary Continence [0502]** sometimes demonstrated as evidenced by: • Able to start and stop stream • Empties bladder completely **Knowledge: Treatment Regimen [1813]** as evidenced by substantial knowledge of: • Self-care responsibilities for ongoing treatment • Self-monitoring techniques

NURSING INTERVENTIONS*/SELECTED ACTIVITIES	RATIONALE
URINARY INCONTINENCE CARE [0610] Monitor urinary elimination, including consistency, odor, volume, and color.	*These parameters help determine adequacy of urinary tract function.*
Help the client select appropriate incontinence garment or pad for short-term management while more definitive treatment is designed.	*Appropriate undergarments can help diminish the embarrassing aspects of urinary incontinence.*

NURSING CARE PLAN Urinary Elimination—*continued*

URINARY INCONTINENCE CARE [0610]	
Instruct Mr. Baker to limit fluids for 2 to 3 hours before bedtime.	*Decreased fluid intake several hours before bedtime will decrease the incidence of urinary retention and overflow incontinence, and promote rest.*
Instruct him to drink a minimum of 1500 mL (six 8-ounce glasses) of fluids per day.	*Increased fluids during the day will increase urinary output and discourage bacterial growth.*
Limit ingestion of bladder irritants (e.g., colas, coffee, tea, alcohol, and chocolate).	*Alcohol, coffee, and tea have a natural diuretic effect and are bladder irritants.*
URINARY RETENTION CARE [0620]	
Instruct Mr. Baker or a family member to record urinary output.	*Serves as an indicator of urinary tract and renal function and of fluid balance.*
Monitor degree of bladder distention by palpation and percussion or bladder scanner.	*An enlarged prostate compresses the urethra so that urine is retained. Checking for bladder distention provides information about bladder emptying and potential residual urine.*
Implement intermittent catheterization, as appropriate.	*Helps maintain tonicity of the bladder muscle by preventing overdistention and providing for complete emptying.*
Provide enough time for bladder emptying (10 minutes).	*In addition to the effect of an enlarged prostate on the bladder, stress or anxiety can inhibit relaxation of the urinary sphincter. Sufficient time should be allowed for micturition.*
Instruct the client in ways to avoid constipation or stool impaction.	*Impacted stool may place pressure on the bladder outlet, causing urinary retention.*
TEACHING: DISEASE PROCESS [5602]	
Appraise Mr. Baker's current level of knowledge about benign prostatic hyperplasia.	*Assessing the client's knowledge will provide a foundation for building a teaching plan based on his present understanding of his condition.*
Explain the pathophysiology of the disease and how it relates to urinary anatomy and function.	*In this case, urinary retention and overflow incontinence are caused by obstruction of the bladder neck by an enlarged prostate gland.*
Describe the rationale behind management, therapy, and treatment recommendations.	*Adequate information about treatment options is important to diminish anxiety, promote compliance, and enhance decision-making.*
Instruct Mr. Baker on which signs and symptoms to report to the healthcare provider (e.g., burning on urination, hematuria, oliguria).	*In the individual with prostatic hyperplasia, urinary retention and an overdistended bladder reduce blood flow to the bladder wall, making it more susceptible to infection from bacterial growth. Monitoring for these manifestations of UTI is essential to prevent urosepsis.*

EVALUATION

Outcomes partially met. Following straight catheterization, Mr. Baker reported continued difficulty initiating a urinary stream but experienced less dribbling and nocturia. He and his wife selected an undergarment that was acceptable to Mr. Baker and he reports that he feels more confident. Intermittent catheterization not indicated. Intake is approximately 200 mL in excess of output. He is able to discuss the correlation between his enlarged prostate and urinary difficulties. A transurethral resection of the prostate is scheduled in 2 weeks.

*The NOC # for desired outcomes and the NIC # for nursing interventions are listed in brackets following the appropriate outcome or intervention. Outcomes, interventions, and activities selected are only a sample of those suggested by NOC and NIC and should be further individualized for each client.

APPLYING CRITICAL THINKING

1. Considering Mr. Baker's history and assessment data, what other physical conditions could explain his symptoms?
2. The primary care provider has recommended surgery. What assumptions will the nurse need to validate in helping prepare Mr. and Mrs. Baker for this surgery?
3. It does not appear that other alternatives have been considered. Why might this be so?
4. Incontinence can lead to client decisions to limit social interactions. What would be an appropriate response if Mr. Baker states that he will just stay home until he has his surgery?

Answers to Applying Critical Thinking questions are available on the faculty resources site. Please consult with your instructor.

CONCEPT MAP

Urinary Elimination

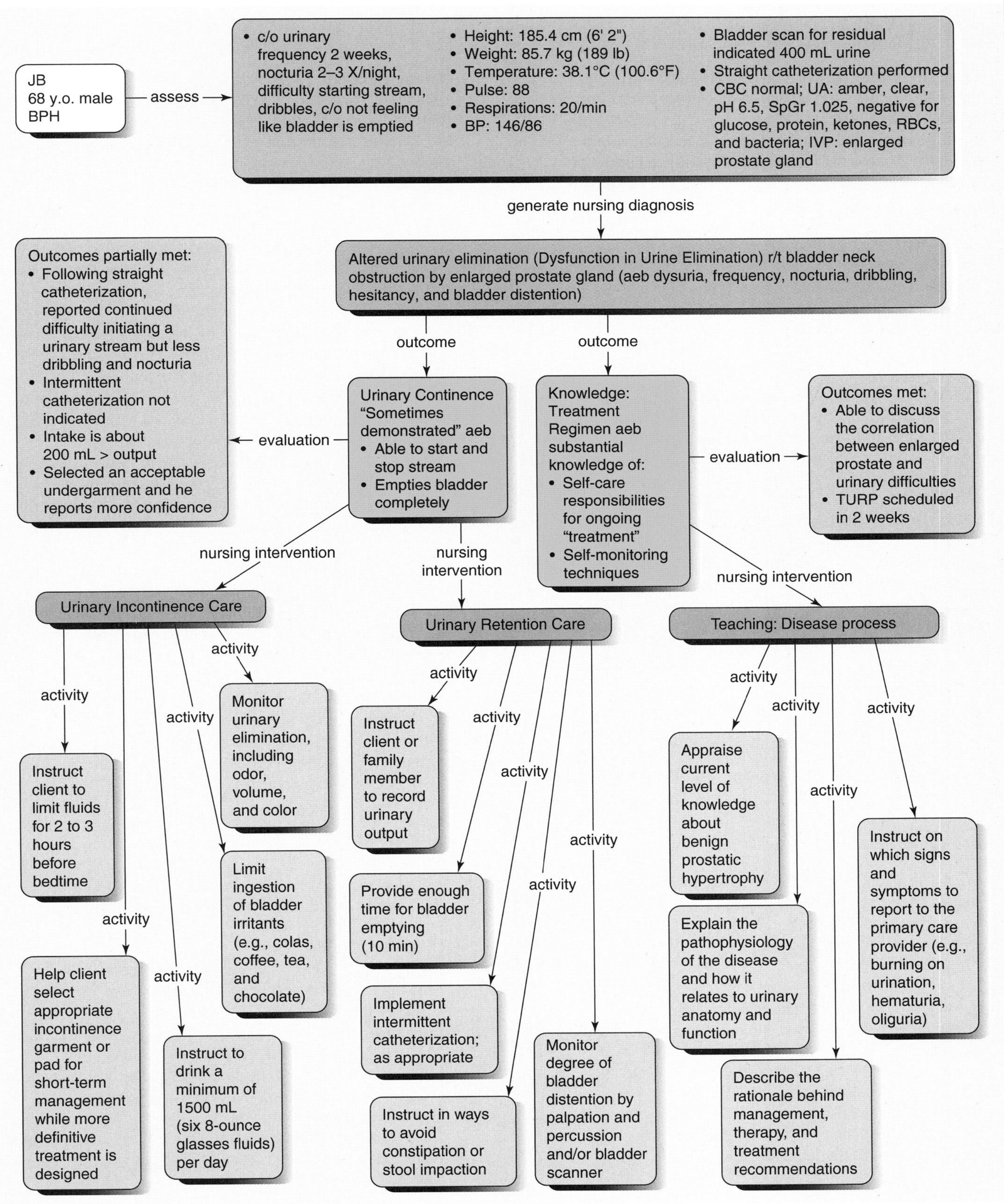

Chapter 47 Review

CHAPTER HIGHLIGHTS

- Urinary elimination depends on normal functioning of the upper urinary tract's kidneys and ureters and the lower urinary tract's urinary bladder, urethra, and pelvic floor.
- Urine is formed in the nephron, the functional unit of the kidney, through a process of filtration, reabsorption, and secretion.
- The normal process of urination is stimulated when sufficient urine collects in the bladder to stimulate stretch receptors. Impulses from stretch receptors are transmitted to the spinal cord and the brain, causing relaxation of the internal sphincter (unconscious control) and, if appropriate, relaxation of the external sphincter (conscious control).
- In the adult, urination generally occurs after 250 to 450 mL of urine has collected in the bladder.
- Many factors influence an individual's urinary elimination, including growth and development, psychosocial factors, fluid intake, medications, muscle tone, various diseases and conditions, and surgical and diagnostic procedures.
- Alterations in urine production and elimination include polyuria, oliguria, anuria, frequency, nocturia, urgency, dysuria, enuresis, incontinence, and retention. Each may have various influencing and associated factors that need to be identified.
- Millions of Americans, mostly women, suffer from urinary incontinence (UI). UI can have a significant impact on the client's quality of life, creating physical problems, such as skin breakdown, and also psychosocial problems, such as social isolation and withdrawal, less positive relationships with others, poorer perceived health, negative effect on sexual function and intimacy, depression, and a barrier to physical and everyday activities.
- The five main types of UI are stress, urge, mixed, overflow, and transient and functional incontinence.
- Nurses, as part of their clinical practice, should assess all clients for UI. Assessment of a client's urinary function includes (a) a nursing history that identifies voiding patterns, recent changes, past and current problems with urination, and factors influencing the elimination pattern; (b) a physical assessment of the genitourinary system; (c) inspection of the urine for amount, color, clarity, and odor; and, if indicated, (d) testing of urine for specific gravity, pH, and the presence of glucose, ketone bodies, protein, and occult blood.
- Examples of nursing diagnoses that may apply to clients with urinary elimination problems can include altered urinary elimination (specify specific problem, e.g., urinary retention), urinary incontinence (specify type) and related diagnoses such as potential for infection.
- Goals for the client with problems with urinary elimination include maintaining or restoring normal voiding patterns and preventing associated risks such as skin breakdown.
- In planning for home care, the nurse considers the client's needs for teaching and assistance in the home.
- Interventions include assisting the client to maintain adequate fluid intake and normal voiding patterns, and assisting with toileting.
- The most common cause of UTI is bacteria. Women in particular are prone to UTIs because of their short urethras.
- Urinary catheterization may be needed for clients with urinary retention but is only performed when all other measures to facilitate voiding fail. Sterile technique is essential to prevent urinary infections.
- It is well documented that the risk to the client of developing a CAUTI correlates to the length of time the catheter is kept in place.
- Care of clients with indwelling catheters is directed toward assessing the necessity for the catheter, preventing infection of the urinary tract, and encouraging urinary flow through the drainage system.
- Clients with urinary retention may be taught to perform clean intermittent catheterization to enhance their independence, reduce the risk of infection, and eliminate incontinence.
- Bladder or catheter irrigations may be used to apply medication to bladder walls or maintain catheter patency.
- A urinary diversion is the surgical rerouting of urine from the kidneys to a site other than the bladder. There are two categories of diversions: incontinent and continent.

TEST YOUR KNOWLEDGE

1. A client is diagnosed with an elevated aldosterone level. Which aspect of urinary elimination will this finding affect?
   1. Increased urine output
   2. Urinary incontinence
   3. Decreased urine output
   4. Urinary retention

2. A client needs a test to determine the amount of residual urine. Which of the following would the nurse use this assessment for? Select all that apply.
   1. To evaluate glomerular filtration rate
   2. To determine the extent of renal failure
   3. To determine the amount of retained urine after voiding
   4. To determine the need for medications
   5. To evaluate fluid volume status

3. A nurse is applying an external urinary device to a client. Before attaching the device to the drainage bag, what should the nurse do?
   1. Wash her hands.
   2. Document the client's tolerance of the procedure.
   3. Instruct the client about the drainage system.
   4. Ensure that the condom is not twisted.

4. The catheter slips into the vagina during a straight catheterization of a female client. The nurse does which action?
   1. Leaves the catheter in place and gets a new sterile catheter.
   2. Leaves the catheter in place and asks another nurse to attempt the procedure.
   3. Removes the catheter and redirects it to the urinary meatus.
   4. Removes the catheter, wipes it with a sterile gauze, and redirects it to the urinary meatus.

5. You have explained to the client the reason for and steps involved for insertion of an indwelling urinary catheter. List the following actions in the correct sequence:
   1. Apply sterile gloves
   2. Attach prefilled syringe
   3. Secure IUC appropriately to prevent urethural irritation
   4. Perform pericare
   5. Insert catheter to appropriate length and check urine flow
   6. Lubricate catheter
   7. Inflate balloon
   8. Perform hand hygiene
   9. Clean urinary meatus with antiseptic solution
   10. Open catheter kit
   1. 8, 10, 4, 1, 2, 6, 9, 5, 7, 3
   2. 2, 4, 8, 10, 1, 6, 2, 9, 5, 7, 3
   3. 4, 8, 1, 10, 6, 2, 9, 5, 7, 3
   4. 10, 4, 8, 1, 7, 2, 6, 9, 5, 3
6. During shift report, the nurse learns that an older female client is unable to maintain continence after she senses the urge to void and becomes incontinent on the way to the bathroom. Which specific type of urinary incontinence is the most appropriate for the nursing diagnosis?
   1. Stress
   2. Reflex
   3. Functional
   4. Urge
7. A female client has a urinary tract infection (UTI). Which teaching points by the nurse would be helpful to the client? Select all that apply.
   1. Limit fluids to avoid the burning sensation on urination.
   2. Review symptoms of UTI with the client.
   3. Wipe the perineal area from back to front.
   4. Wear cotton underclothes.
   5. Take baths rather than showers.
8. The nurse will need to assess the client's performance of clean intermittent catheterization (CIC) for a client with which urinary diversion?
   1. Ileal conduit
   2. Kock pouch
   3. Neobladder
   4. Vesicostomy
9. Which focus is the nurse most likely to teach for a client with a flaccid bladder?
   1. Habit training: Attempt voiding at specific time periods.
   2. Bladder retraining: Delay voiding according to a preschedule timetable.
   3. Credé's maneuver: Apply gentle manual pressure to the lower abdomen.
   4. Kegel exercises: Contract the pelvic floor muscles.
10. Which of the following behaviors indicates that the client on a bladder retraining program has met the expected outcomes? Select all that apply.
   1. Voids each time there is an urge.
   2. Practices slow, deep breathing until the urge decreases.
   3. Uses adult diapers, for "just in case."
   4. Drinks citrus juices and carbonated beverages.
   5. Performs pelvic floor muscle exercises.

See Answers to Test Your Knowledge in Appendix A.

READINGS AND REFERENCES

Suggested Readings

Beauchemin, L., Newman, D. K., LeDanseur, M., Jackson, A., & Ritmiller, M. (2018). Best practices for clean intermittent catheterization. *Nursing*, *48*(9), 49–54. doi:10.1097/01.NURSE.0000544216.23783.bc

CIC is not taught in many undergraduate nursing programs. This article provides a synopsis of best practices for CIC.

Francis, K. (2018). Damage control: Differentiating incontinence-associated dermatitis from pressure injury. *Nursing*, *48*(6), 18–25. doi:10.1097/01.NURSE.0000532739.93967.20

The author discusses how to differentiate, classify, and document incontinence-associated dermatitis and pressure injuries with an emphasis on assessing clients with dark skin.

Related Research

Ferguson, A. (2018). Implementing a CAUTI prevention program in an acute care hospital setting. *Urologic Nursing*, *38*(6), 273–302. doi:10.7257/1053-816X.2018.38.6.273

Rhone, C., Breiter, Y., Benson, L., Petri, H., Thompson, P., & Murphy, C. (2017). The impact of two-person indwelling urinary catheter insertion in the emergency department using technical and socioadaptive interventions. *Journal of Clinical Outcomes Management*, *24*(10), 451–456.

Schlittenhardt, M., Smith, S. C., & Ward-Smith, P. (2016). Tele-continence care: A novel approach for providers. *Urologic Nursing*, *36*(5), 217–223. doi:10.7257/1053-816X.2016.36.5.217

References

American Nurses Association. (n.d.). *Streamlined evidence-based RN tool: Catheter associated urinary tract infection (CAUTI) prevention.* Retrieved from https://www.nursingworld.org/~4aede8/globalassets/practiceandpolicy/innovation--evidence/clinical-practice-material/cauti-prevention-tool/anacautipreventiontool-final-19dec2014.pdf

Ball, J., Bindler, R., Cowen, K., & Shaw, M. (2017). *Principles of pediatric nursing* (7th ed.). Hoboken, NJ: Pearson.

Beauchemin, L., Newman, D. K., LeDanseur, M., Jackson, A., & Ritmiller, M. (2018). Best practices for clean intermittent catheterization. *Nursing*, *48*(9), 49–54. doi:10.1097/01.NURSE.0000544216.23783.bc

Butcher, H. K., Bulechek, G. M., Dochterman, J. M., & Wagner, C. M. (Eds.). (2018). *Nursing interventions classification (NIC)* (7th ed.). St. Louis, MO: Elsevier.

Centers for Disease Control and Prevention. (2017). *Guidelines for prevention of catheter-associated urinary tract infections (2009).* Retrieved from https://www.cdc.gov/hicpac/pdf/CAUTI/CAUTIguideline2009final.pdf

Centers for Disease Control and Prevention. (2019). *Urinary tract infection (catheter-associated urinary tract infection (CAUTI) and non-catheter-associated urinary tract infection (UTI) and other urinary system infection (USI) events.* Retrieved from https://www.cdc.gov/nhsn/pdfs/pscmanual/7psccauticurrent.pdf

Hoke, N., & Bradway, C. (2016). A clinical nurse specialist-directed initiative to reduce postoperative urinary retention in spinal surgery patients. *American Journal of Nursing*, *116*(8), 47–52. doi:10.1097/01.NAJ.0000490176.22393.69

Institute for Healthcare Improvement. (n.d.). *Catheter-associated urinary tract infection.* Retrieved from http://www.ihi.org/Topics/CAUTI/Pages/default.aspx

The Joint Commission. (2019). *National Patient Safety Goals effective January 2019—hospital accreditation program.* Retrieved from https://www.jointcommission.org/assets/1/6/NPSG_Chapter_HAP_Jan2019.pdf

Kehinde, O. (2016). Common incontinence problems seen by community nurses. *Journal of Community Nursing*, *30*(4), 46–55.

Leaver, R. (2017). Assessing patients with urinary incontinence: The basics. *Journal of Community Nursing*, *31*(1), 40–46.

McNeill, L. (2017). Back to basics: How evidence-based nursing practice can prevent catheter-associated urinary tract infections. *Urologic Nursing*, *37*(4), 204–206. doi:10.7257/1053-816X.2017.37.4.204

Mendes, A., Rodolpho, J. R. C., & Hoga, L. A. (2016). Non-pharmacological and non-surgical treatments for female urinary incontinence: An integrative review. *Applied Nursing Research*, *31*, 146–153. doi:10.1016/j.apnr.2016.02.005

Moorhead, S., Swanson, E., Johnson, M., & Maas, M. L. (Eds.). (2018). *Nursing outcomes classification (NOC)* (6th ed.). St. Louis, MO: Elsevier.

Nazarko, L. (2017). Beyond the bladder: Holistic care when urinary incontinence develops. *British Journal of Community Nursing*, *22*(1), 662–666. doi:10.12968/bjcn.2017.22.1.662

Nazarko, L. (2018). Male urinary incontinence management: Penile sheaths. *British Journal of Community Nursing*, *23*(3), 110–116. doi:10.12968/bjcn.2018.23.3.110

Ostle, Z. (2016). Assessment, diagnosis and treatment of urinary incontinence in women. *British Journal of Nursing*, *25*(2), 84–91. doi:10.12968/bjon.2016.25.2.84

Palmer, M. H., & Willis-Gray, M. (2017). Overactive bladder in women. *American Journal of Nursing*, *117*(4), 34–41. doi:10.1097/01.NAJ.0000515207.69721.94

Panchisin, T. L. (2016). Improving outcomes with the ANA CAUTI prevention tool. *Nursing*, *46*(3), 55–59. doi:10.1097/01.NURSE.0000480603.14769.d6

Schaeffer, A. J. (2017). *Placement and management of urinary bladder catheters in adults*. Retrieved from https://www.uptodate.com/contents/placement-and-management-of-urinary-bladder-catheters-in-adults

Searcy, J. A. R. (2017). Geriatric urinary incontinence. *Nursing Clinics of North America*, *52*(3), 447–455. doi:10.1016/j.cnur.2017.04.002

Stewart, E. (2018). Assessment and management of urinary incontinence in women. *Nursing Standard*, *33*(2), 75–81. doi:10.7748/ns.2018.e11148

Tso, C., & Lee, W. (2018). Postmenopausal women and urinary incontinence. *American Nurse Today*, *13*(1), 18–21.

Selected Bibliography

Ballard, J. P., Parsons, S., Rodgers, J., Mosack, V., & Starks, B. (2018). HOUDINI impacts on utilization and infection rates—A retrospective quality improvement initiative. *Urologic Nursing*, *38*(4), 184–191. doi:10.7257/1053-816X.2018.38.4.184

Cadet, M. J. (2018). Diagnosis, treatment, and prevention of cystitis. *American Nurse Today*, *13*(7), 24–27.

Collins, L. (2019). Diagnosis and management of a urinary tract infection. *British Journal of Nursing*, *28*(2), 84–88. doi:10.12968/bjon.2019.28.2.84

Culbertson, S., & Davis, A. M. (2017). Nonsurgical management of urinary incontinence in women. *JAMA*, *317*(1), 79–80. doi:10.1001/jama.2016.18433

Davis, C. (2019). Catheter-associated urinary tract infection: Signs, diagnosis, prevention. *British Journal of Nursing*, *28*(2), 96–100. doi:10.12968/bjon.2019.28.2.96

Hill, B., & Mitchell, M. (2018). Urinary catheters PART 1. *British Journal of Nursing*, *27*(21), 1234–1236. doi:10.12968/bjon.2018.27.21.1234

Knill, L., Maduro, R., & Payne, J. E. (2018). Targeting zero CAUTIs. *American Nurse Today*, *13*(11), 54–57.

Schreiber, M. L. (2016). Ostomies: Nursing care and management. *MEDSURG Nursing*, *25*(2), 127–130.

Yates, A. (2016). The risks and benefits of suprapubic catheters. *Nursing Times 11*(6/7), 19–22.

Fecal Elimination 48

LEARNING OUTCOMES

After completing this chapter, you will be able to:

1. Describe the physiology of defecation.
2. Distinguish normal from abnormal characteristics and constituents of feces.
3. Identify factors that influence fecal elimination and patterns of defecation.
4. Identify common causes and effects of selected fecal elimination problems.
5. Describe methods used to assess fecal elimination.
6. Identify examples of nursing diagnoses, outcomes, and interventions for clients with elimination problems.
7. Identify measures that maintain normal fecal elimination patterns.
8. Describe the purpose and action of commonly used enema solutions.
9. Describe essentials of fecal stoma care for clients with an ostomy.
10. Recognize when it is appropriate to assign assistance with fecal elimination to assistive personnel.
11. Verbalize the steps used in:
    a. Administering an enema
    b. Changing a bowel diversion ostomy appliance.
12. Demonstrate appropriate documentation and reporting related to fecal elimination.

KEY TERMS

bedpan, *1282*
bowel incontinence, *1277*
carminatives, *1283*
cathartics, *1283*
chyme, *1271*
colostomy, *1290*
commode, *1282*
constipation, *1275*
defecation, *1272*
diarrhea, *1277*
enema, *1284*
fecal impaction, *1276*
fecal incontinence, *1277*
feces, *1271*
flatulence, *1278*
flatus, *1272*
gastrocolic reflex, *1274*
gastrostomy, *1290*
hemorrhoids, *1272*
ileostomy, *1290*
jejunostomy, *1290*
laxatives, *1275*
meconium, *1274*
ostomy, *1290*
peristalsis, *1272*
stoma, *1290*
stool, *1271*
suppositories, *1283*

Introduction

Nurses frequently are consulted or involved in assisting clients with elimination problems. These problems can be embarrassing to clients and can cause considerable discomfort. The elimination of feces is a recognizable public topic in North America. For example, laxative advertisements, describing such feelings as tiredness due to irregularity, keep the subject in the public consciousness. Some older adults are preoccupied with their bowels. Individuals who have had a bowel movement once a day for many years can view missing one day as a serious problem.

Physiology of Defecation

Elimination of the waste products of digestion from the body is essential to health. The excreted waste products are referred to as **feces** or **stool**.

Large Intestine

The large intestine extends from the ileocecal (ileocolic) valve, which lies between the small and large intestines, to the anus. The colon (large intestine) in the adult is generally about 125 to 150 cm (50 to 60 in.) long. It has seven parts: the cecum; ascending, transverse, and descending colons; sigmoid colon; rectum; and anus (Figure 48.1 ■).

The large intestine is a muscular tube lined with mucous membrane. The muscle fibers are both circular and longitudinal, permitting the intestine to enlarge and contract in both width and length.

The colon's main functions are the absorption of water and nutrients, the mucoid protection of the intestinal wall, and fecal elimination. The waste products leaving the stomach through the small intestine and then passing through the ileocecal valve are called **chyme**. The ileocecal valve regulates the flow of chyme into the large intestine and prevents backflow into the ileum. As much as 1500 mL of chyme passes into the large intestine daily, and all but about 100 mL is reabsorbed in the proximal half of the colon. The 100 mL of fluid is excreted in the feces.

The colon also serves a protective function in that it secretes mucus. This mucus contains large amounts of bicarbonate ions. The mucous secretion is stimulated by excitation of parasympathetic nerves. During extreme stimulation—for example, as a result of emotions—large amounts of mucus are secreted, resulting in the passage of stringy mucus with little or no feces. Mucus serves to

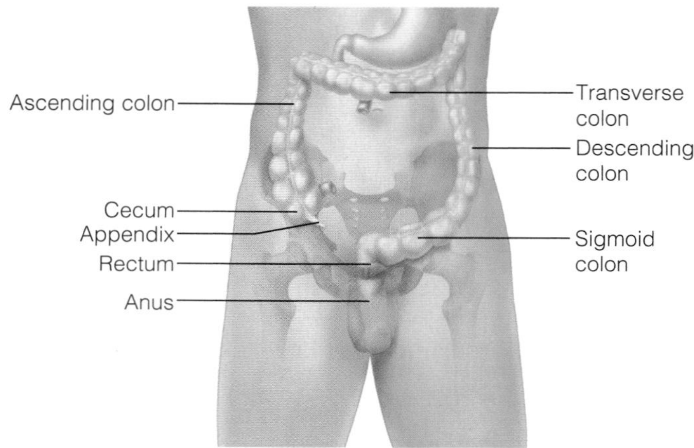

Figure 48.1 ■ The large intestine.
B. F. FREMGEN, and S. S. FRUCHT, MEDICAL TERMINOLOGY: A LIVING LANGUAGE, 6th Ed.,© 2016. Reprinted and Electronically reproduced by permission of Pearson Education, Inc., New York, NY.

protect the wall of the large intestine from trauma by the acids formed in the feces, and it serves as an adherent for holding the fecal material together. Mucus also protects the intestinal wall from bacterial activity.

The colon acts to transport along its lumen the products of digestion, which are eventually eliminated through the anal canal. These products are flatus and feces. **Flatus** is largely air and the by-products of the digestion of carbohydrates. **Peristalsis** is wavelike movement produced by the circular and longitudinal muscle fibers of the intestinal walls; it propels the intestinal contents forward.

Rectum and Anal Canal

The rectum in the adult is usually 10 to 15 cm (4 to 6 in.) long; the most distal portion, 2.5 to 5 cm (1 to 2 in.) long, is the anal canal. The rectum has folds that extend vertically. Each of the vertical folds contains a vein and an artery. It is believed that these folds help retain feces within the rectum. When the veins become distended, as can occur with repeated pressure, a condition known as **hemorrhoids** occurs (Figure 48.2 ■).

The anal canal is bounded by an internal and an external sphincter muscle (Figure 48.3 ■). The internal sphincter is under involuntary control, and the external sphincter normally is voluntarily controlled. The internal sphincter muscle is innervated by the autonomic nervous system; the external sphincter is innervated by the somatic nervous system.

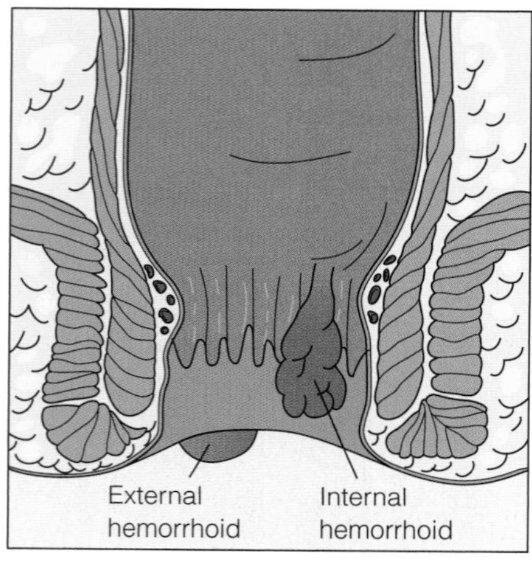

Figure 48.2 ■ Internal and external hemorrhoids.

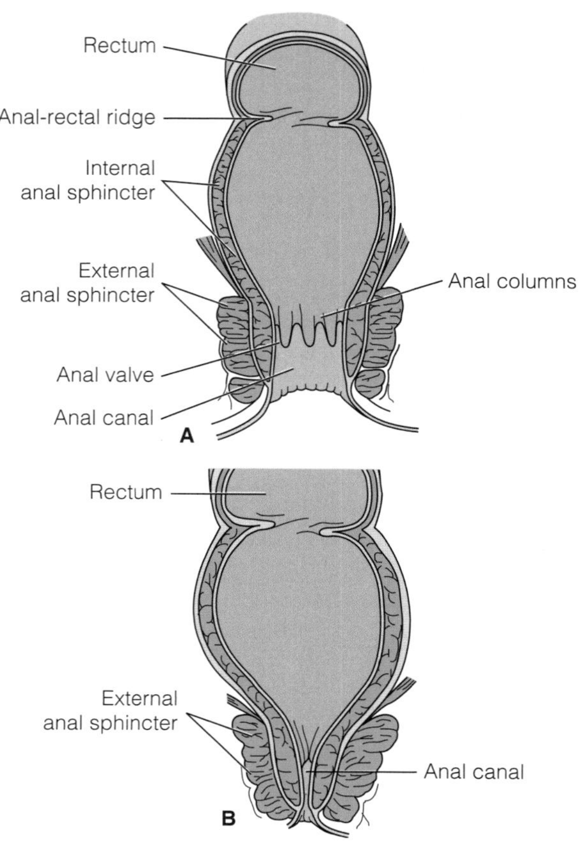

Figure 48.3 ■ The rectum, anal canal, and anal sphincters: *A*, open; *B*, closed.

Defecation

Defecation is the expulsion of feces from the anus and rectum. It is also called a *bowel movement*. The frequency of defecation is highly individual, varying from several times per day to two or three times per week. The amount defecated also varies among individuals. When peristaltic waves move the feces into the sigmoid colon and the rectum, the sensory nerves in the rectum are stimulated and the individual becomes aware of the need to defecate.

Clinical Alert!

Individuals (especially children) may use very different terms for a bowel movement. The nurse may need to try several different common words before finding one the client understands.

When the internal anal sphincter relaxes, feces move into the anal canal. After the individual is seated on a toilet or bedpan, the external anal sphincter is relaxed voluntarily. Expulsion of the feces is assisted by contraction of the abdominal muscles and the diaphragm, which increases abdominal pressure, and by contraction of the muscles of the pelvic floor, which moves the feces through

TABLE 48.1 Characteristics of Normal and Abnormal Feces

Characteristic	Normal	Abnormal	Possible Cause
Color	Adult: brown	Clay or white	Absence of bile pigment (bile obstruction); diagnostic study using barium
	Infant: yellow	Black or tarry	Drug (e.g., iron); bleeding from upper gastrointestinal tract (e.g., stomach, small intestine); diet high in red meat and dark green vegetables (e.g., spinach)
		Red	Bleeding from lower gastrointestinal tract (e.g., rectum); some foods (e.g., beets)
		Pale	Malabsorption of fats; diet high in milk and milk products and low in meat
		Orange or green	Intestinal infection
Consistency	Formed, soft, semisolid, moist	Hard, dry	Dehydration; decreased intestinal motility resulting from lack of fiber in diet, lack of exercise, emotional upset, laxative abuse
		Diarrhea	Increased intestinal motility (e.g., due to irritation of the colon by bacteria)
Shape	Cylindrical (contour of rectum) about 2.5 cm (1 in.) in diameter in adults	Narrow, pencil-shaped, or stringlike stool	Obstructive condition of the rectum
Amount	Varies with diet (about 100–400 g/day)		
Odor	Aromatic: affected by ingested food and individual's own bacterial flora	Pungent	Infection, blood
Constituents	Small amounts of undigested roughage, sloughed dead bacteria and epithelial cells, fat, protein, dried constituents of digestive juices (e.g., bile pigments, inorganic matter)	Pus Parasites Blood Large quantities of fat Foreign objects	Mucus Bacterial infection Inflammatory condition Gastrointestinal bleeding Malabsorption Accidental ingestion

the anal canal. Normal defecation is facilitated by (a) thigh flexion, which increases the pressure within the abdomen, and (b) a sitting position, which increases the downward pressure on the rectum.

If the defecation reflex is ignored, or if defecation is consciously inhibited by contracting the external sphincter muscle, the urge to defecate normally disappears for a few hours before occurring again. Repeated inhibition of the urge to defecate can result in expansion of the rectum to accommodate accumulated feces and eventual loss of sensitivity to the need to defecate. Constipation can be the ultimate result.

Feces

Normal feces are made of about 75% water and 25% solid materials. They are soft but formed. If the feces are propelled very quickly along the large intestine, there is not time for most of the water in the chyme to be reabsorbed and the feces will be more fluid, containing perhaps 95% water. Normal feces require a normal fluid intake; feces that contain less water may be hard and difficult to expel.

Feces are normally brown, chiefly due to the presence of stercobilin and urobilin, which are derived from bilirubin (a red pigment in bile). Another factor that affects fecal color is the action of bacteria such as *Escherichia coli* or staphylococci, which are normally present in the large intestine. The action of microorganisms on the chyme is also responsible for the odor of feces. Table 48.1 lists the characteristics of normal and abnormal feces.

Factors That Affect Defecation

Defecation patterns vary at different stages of life. Circumstances of diet, fluid intake and output, activity, psychologic factors, defecation habits, medications, diagnostic and medical procedures, pathologic conditions, and pain also affect defecation.

Development

See Table 48.2 for a summary of the developmental changes affecting defecation.

Diet

Sufficient bulk (cellulose, fiber) in the diet is necessary to provide fecal volume. Inadequate intake of dietary fiber contributes to the risk of developing obesity, type 2 diabetes, coronary artery disease, and colon cancer. Fiber is classified into two categories: insoluble fiber and soluble fiber. Insoluble fiber promotes the movement of material through the digestive system and increases stool bulk. Sources of insoluble fiber include whole-wheat flour, wheat bran, nuts, and many vegetables. Soluble fiber dissolves in water to form a gel-like material. It can help lower blood cholesterol

TABLE 48.2 Changes in Defecation Throughout the Lifespan

Stage	Variations
Newborns and Infants	• **Meconium** is the first fecal material passed by the newborn, normally up to 24 hours after birth. It is dark green, tarry, odorless, and sticky. Transitional stools, which follow for about a week, are generally greenish yellow; they contain mucus and are loose. • Infants pass stool frequently, often after each feeding. The intestine is immature, causing water to not be well absorbed and frequent soft, liquid stools. Stool becomes less frequent and firmer after solid foods are started. • Breastfed infants have light yellow to golden feces. Infants who take formula have dark yellow or tan, more formed stool.
Toddlers	• Some control of defecation starts at 1½ to 2 years of age. Daytime control is typically achieved by age 2½, after toilet training.
School-Age Children and Adolescents	• Bowel habits are similar to those of adults. Patterns of defecation vary in frequency, quantity, and consistency. • Some school-age children may delay defecation because of an activity such as play.
Older Adults	• Many suffer from constipation because of reduced activity levels, inadequate fluid and fiber intake, and muscle weakness. • Many believe that "regularity" means a bowel movement every day and may use over-the-counter (OTC) medications to relieve what they consider constipation. May need to be advised that normal patterns of bowel elimination vary considerably.

and glucose levels (Mayo Clinic, 2018). Sources of soluble fiber include oats, peas, beans, apples, citrus fruits, carrots, barley, and psyllium. The Mayo Clinic recommends the following daily amount of fiber:

- Men ages 50 and younger: 38 grams
- Men ages 51 and older: 30 grams
- Women ages 50 and younger: 25 grams
- Women ages 51 and older: 21 grams.

It is important to drink plenty of water because fiber works best when it absorbs water.

Bland diets and low-fiber diets are lacking in bulk and therefore create insufficient residue of waste products to stimulate the reflex for defecation. Low-residue foods, such as rice, eggs, and lean meats, move more slowly through the intestinal tract. Increasing fluid intake with such foods increases their rate of movement.

Certain foods are difficult or impossible for some individuals to digest. This inability results in digestive upsets and, in some instances, the passage of watery stools. Irregular eating can also impair regular defecation. Individuals who eat at the same times every day usually have a regularly timed, physiologic response to the food intake and a regular pattern of peristaltic activity in the colon.

Spicy foods can produce diarrhea and flatus in some individuals. Excessive sugar can also cause diarrhea. Other foods that may influence bowel elimination include the following:

- Gas-producing foods, such as cabbage, onions, cauliflower, bananas, and apples
- Laxative-producing foods, such as bran, prunes, figs, chocolate, and alcohol
- Constipation-producing foods, such as cheese, pasta, eggs, and lean meat.

Fluid Intake and Output

Even when fluid intake is inadequate or output (e.g., urine or vomitus) is excessive for some reason, the body continues to reabsorb fluid from the chyme as it passes along the colon. The chyme becomes drier than normal, resulting in hard feces. In addition, reduced fluid intake slows the chyme's passage along the intestines, further increasing the reabsorption of fluid from the chyme. Healthy fecal elimination usually requires a daily fluid intake of 2000 to 3000 mL. If chyme moves abnormally quickly through the large intestine, however, there is less time for fluid to be absorbed into the blood; as a result, the feces are soft or even watery.

Activity

Activity stimulates peristalsis, thus facilitating the movement of chyme along the colon. Weak abdominal and pelvic muscles are often ineffective in increasing the intra-abdominal pressure during defecation or in controlling defecation. Weak muscles can result from lack of exercise, immobility, or impaired neurologic functioning. Clients confined to bed are often constipated.

Psychologic Factors

Some individuals who are anxious or angry experience increased peristaltic activity and subsequent nausea or diarrhea. In contrast, individuals who are depressed may experience slowed intestinal motility, resulting in constipation. How someone responds to these emotional states is the result of individual differences in the response of the enteric nervous system to vagal stimulation from the brain.

Defecation Habits

Early bowel training may establish the habit of defecating at a regular time. Many individuals defecate after breakfast due to the **gastrocolic reflex** (increased peristalsis of the colon after food has entered the stomach). If an individual ignores this urge to defecate, water continues to be reabsorbed, making the feces hard and difficult to expel. When the normal defecation reflexes are inhibited or ignored, these conditioned reflexes tend to be progressively weakened. When habitually ignored, the urge to defecate is ultimately lost. Adults may ignore these reflexes because of the pressures of time or work. Hospitalized clients may suppress the urge because of embarrassment about using a bedpan, because of lack of privacy, or because defecation is too uncomfortable.

Medications

Some drugs have side effects that can interfere with normal elimination. Some cause diarrhea; others, such as large doses of certain tranquilizers and repeated administration of opioids, cause constipation because they decrease gastrointestinal activity through their action on the central nervous system. Iron supplements act more locally on the bowel mucosa and can cause constipation or diarrhea.

Some medications directly affect elimination. **Laxatives** are medications that stimulate bowel activity and so assist fecal elimination. Other medications soften stool, facilitating defecation. Certain medications suppress peristaltic activity and may be used to treat diarrhea.

Medications can also affect the appearance of the feces. Any drug that causes gastrointestinal bleeding (e.g., aspirin products) can cause the stool to be red or black. Iron salts lead to black stool because of the oxidation of the iron; antibiotics may cause a gray-green discoloration; and antacids can cause a whitish discoloration or white specks in the stool. Pepto-Bismol, a common OTC drug, causes stools to be black.

Diagnostic Procedures

Before certain diagnostic procedures, such as visualization of the colon (colonoscopy or sigmoidoscopy), the client is restricted from ingesting food or fluid. The client may also be given a cleansing enema prior to the examination. In these instances normal defecation usually will not occur until eating resumes.

Anesthesia and Surgery

General anesthetics cause the normal colonic movements to cease or slow by blocking parasympathetic stimulation to the muscles of the colon. Clients who have regional or spinal anesthesia are less likely to experience this problem.

Surgery that involves direct handling of the intestines can cause temporary stoppage of intestinal movement. This condition, called ileus, usually lasts 24 to 48 hours. Listening for bowel sounds that reflect intestinal motility is an important nursing assessment following surgery.

Pathologic Conditions

Spinal cord injuries and head injuries can decrease the sensory stimulation for defecation. Impaired mobility may limit the client's ability to respond to the urge to defecate and the client may experience constipation. Or, a client may experience fecal incontinence because of poorly functioning anal sphincters.

Pain

Clients who experience discomfort when defecating (e.g., following hemorrhoid surgery) often suppress the urge to defecate to avoid the pain. Such clients can experience constipation as a result. Clients taking opioid analgesics for pain may also experience constipation as a side effect of the medication.

Fecal Elimination Problems

Four common problems are related to fecal elimination: constipation, diarrhea, bowel incontinence, and flatulence.

Constipation

Constipation may be defined as fewer than three bowel movements per week. This infers the passage of dry, hard stool or the passage of no stool. It occurs when the movement of feces through the large intestine is slow, thus allowing time for additional reabsorption of fluid from the large intestine. Associated with constipation are difficult evacuation of stool and increased effort or straining of the voluntary muscles of defecation. The individual may also have a feeling of incomplete stool evacuation after defecation. However, it is important to define constipation in relation to the individual's regular elimination pattern. Some individuals normally defecate only a few times a week; others defecate more than once a day. Careful assessment of the client's habits is necessary before a diagnosis of constipation is made. Box 48.1 lists the common characteristics of constipation.

BOX 48.1 Common Characteristics of Constipation

- Decreased frequency of defecation
- Hard, formed stools
- Straining at stool; painful defecation
- Reports of rectal fullness or pressure or incomplete bowel evacuation
- Abdominal pain, cramps, or distention
- Anorexia, nausea
- Headache

Many causes and factors contribute to constipation. Among them are the following:

- Insufficient fiber intake
- Insufficient fluid intake
- Insufficient activity or immobility
- Irregular defecation habits
- Change in daily routine
- Lack of privacy
- Chronic use of laxatives or enemas
- Irritable bowel syndrome (IBS)
- Pelvic floor dysfunction or muscle damage
- Poor motility or slow transit
- Neurologic conditions (e.g., Parkinson's disease), stroke, or paralysis
- Emotional disturbances such as depression or mental confusion

- Medications such as opioids, iron supplements, antihistamines, antacids, and antidepressants
- Habitual denial and ignoring the urge to defecate.

Constipation can cause health problems for some clients. In children constipation is often associated with changes in activity, diet, and toileting habits (Ball, Bindler, Cowen, & Shaw, 2017). Straining associated with constipation is often accompanied by holding the breath. This Valsalva maneuver can present serious problems to people with heart disease, brain injuries, or respiratory disease. Holding the breath while bearing down increases intrathoracic pressure and vagal tone, slowing the pulse rate.

The reasons for constipation can range from lifestyle habits (e.g., lack of exercise) to serious malignant disorders (e.g., colorectal cancer). The nurse should evaluate any complaints of constipation carefully for each individual. A change in bowel habits over several weeks with or without weight loss, pain, or fever should be referred to a primary care provider for a complete medical evaluation. See Box 48.2 for risk factors and symptoms of colorectal cancer.

Fecal Impaction

Fecal impaction is a mass or collection of hardened feces in the folds of the rectum. Impaction results from prolonged retention and accumulation of fecal material. In severe impactions the feces accumulate and extend well up into the sigmoid colon and beyond. A client who has a fecal impaction will experience the passage of liquid fecal seepage (diarrhea) and no normal stool. The liquid portion of the feces seeps out around the impacted mass. Impaction can also be assessed by digital examination of the rectum, during which the hardened mass can often be palpated.

Along with fecal seepage and constipation, symptoms include frequent but nonproductive desire to defecate and rectal pain. A generalized feeling of illness results; the client becomes anorexic, the abdomen becomes distended, and nausea and vomiting may occur.

The causes of fecal impaction are usually poor defecation habits and constipation. Also, the administration of medications such as anticholinergics and antihistamines will

BOX 48.2 Colorectal Cancer

RISK FACTORS

Nonmodifiable

- Age (risk increases after age 50; leading cause of death in women aged 75 and older)
- Race (incidence and mortality rates are highest in non-Hispanic Black individuals)
- Personal or family history of colorectal polyps
- Personal history of inflammatory bowel disease

Modifiable

- Cigarette smoking
- Poor diet (e.g., low in fiber and high in fat; high amounts of red or processed meats)
- Lack of physical activity
- Obesity
- Heavy consumption of alcohol

SYMPTOMS

Early colorectal cancer often has no symptoms. Screening is important and includes using high-sensitivity fecal occult blood testing, sigmoidoscopy, or colonoscopy beginning at age 45 and continuing until age 75.

Inform clients to see their primary care provider if they have any of the following:

- A change in bowel habits such as diarrhea, constipation, or narrowing of the stool that lasts for more than a few days
- A feeling of needing to have a bowel movement that is not relieved by doing so
- Rectal bleeding or blood in the stool (often, though, the stool will look normal)
- Cramping or steady abdominal pain
- Weakness and fatigue
- Unexpected weight loss

From *Colorectal Cancer Facts & Figures 2017–2019*, by American Cancer Society, 2017. Retrieved from https://www.cancer.org/content/dam/cancer-org/research/cancer-facts-and-statistics/colorectal-cancer-facts-and-figures/colorectal-cancer-facts-and-figures-2017-2019.pdf; *Colorectal Cancer Risk Factors*, by American Cancer Society, 2018. Retrieved from https://www.cancer.org/cancer/colon-rectal-cancer/causes-risks-prevention/risk-factors.html; and "The Big 3: An Updated Overview of Colorectal, Breast, and Prostate Cancers," by J. Gordon, E. Fischer-Cartlidge, and M. Barton-Burke, 2017, *Nursing Clinics of North America*, *52*, 27–52.

DRUG CAPSULE

Emollient or Surfactant: docusate calcium (Surfak), docusate sodium (Colace)

CLIENT WITH DRUGS FOR TREATING THE LOWER GASTROINTESTINAL TRACT

Docusates lower the surface tension of fecal material, which allows water and lipids to penetrate the stool, resulting in a softer fecal mass. They do not stimulate peristalsis.

Docusates are commonly used for prevention of constipation and to decrease the strain of defecation in individuals who should avoid straining during bowel movements (e.g., cardiac disease [prevent Valsalva maneuver], eye surgery, rectal surgery).

NURSING RESPONSIBILITIES

- Assess the client for abdominal distention, bowel sounds, and usual bowel movement frequency.
- Evaluate the effectiveness of the medication.

CLIENT AND FAMILY TEACHING

- Advise the client to drink a glass of fluid (e.g., water, juice, milk) with each dose.
- Explain that it may take 1 to 3 days to soften fecal material.
- Advise the client not to take docusate within 2 hours of other laxatives, especially mineral oil, because it may cause increased absorption of the mineral oil.
- Discuss other forms of bowel regulation (e.g., increasing fiber intake, fluid intake, and activity).

Note: Prior to administering any medication, review all aspects with a current drug handbook or other reliable source.

increase the client's risk in the development of a fecal impaction. The barium used in radiologic examinations of the upper and lower gastrointestinal tracts can also be a causative factor. Therefore, after these examinations, laxatives or enemas are usually given to ensure removal of the barium.

Clinical Alert!

An older adult with a fecal impaction may show symptoms of delirium. Assess for fecal impaction if the client with constipation problems has a sudden change in mental status.

Digital examination of the impaction through the rectum should be done gently and carefully. Although digital rectal examination is within the scope of nursing practice, some agency policies require a primary care provider's order for digital manipulation and removal of a fecal impaction.

Although fecal impaction can generally be prevented, treatment of impacted feces is sometimes necessary. When fecal impaction is suspected, the client is often given an oil retention enema, a cleansing enema 2 to 4 hours later, and daily additional cleansing enemas, suppositories, or stool softeners. If these measures fail, manual removal is often necessary.

Diarrhea

Diarrhea refers to the passage of liquid feces and an increased frequency of defecation. It is the opposite of constipation and results from rapid movement of fecal contents through the large intestine. Rapid passage of chyme reduces the time available for the large intestine to reabsorb water and electrolytes. Some individuals pass stool with increased frequency, but diarrhea is not present unless the stool is relatively unformed and excessively liquid. The individual with diarrhea finds it difficult or impossible to control the urge to defecate. Diarrhea and the threat of incontinence are sources of concern and embarrassment. Often, spasmodic cramps are associated with diarrhea. Bowel sounds are increased. With persistent diarrhea, irritation of the anal region extending to the perineum and buttocks generally results. Fatigue, weakness, malaise, and emaciation are the results of prolonged diarrhea.

When the cause of diarrhea is irritants in the intestinal tract, diarrhea is thought to be a protective flushing mechanism. It can create serious fluid and electrolyte losses in the body, however, that can develop within frighteningly short periods of time, particularly in infants, small children, and older adults.

The prevalence of *Clostridium difficile* infection (CDI), which produces mucoid and foul-smelling diarrhea, has been increasing in recent years. Clients at the highest risk for the development of CDI include immunosuppressed individuals, clients of advanced age, and those who have recently used antimicrobial agents, usually fluoroquinolones (Sams & Kennedy-Malone, 2017). Older adults are at the greatest risk due to underlying disease(s) and greater exposure in hospitals and extended care facilities. Infection control against CDI includes hand hygiene, contact precautions, and cleaning of surfaces with a bleach solution. All individuals involved in the care of the client need to be reminded to wash their hands with soap and water because alcohol-based hand gels are not effective against *C. difficile*. Also, wearing gloves when coming into contact with soiled linens is needed to prevent the spread of the bacteria and spores that exist with *C. difficile* (Smith & Taylor, 2016). Table 48.3 lists some of the major causes of diarrhea and the physiologic responses of the body.

The irritating effects of diarrhea stool increase the risk for skin breakdown. Therefore, the area around the anal region should be kept clean and dry and be protected with zinc oxide or other ointment. In addition, a fecal collector can be used (see page 1289).

Bowel Incontinence

Bowel incontinence, also called **fecal incontinence**, refers to the loss of voluntary ability to control fecal and gaseous discharges through the anal sphincter. The incontinence may occur at specific times, such as after meals, or it may occur irregularly. Fecal incontinence is generally associated with impaired functioning of the anal sphincter or its nerve supply, such as in some neuromuscular diseases, spinal cord trauma, and tumors of the external anal sphincter muscle.

The prevalence of bowel incontinence increases with age. Bowel incontinence is an emotionally distressing problem that can ultimately lead to social isolation. Afflicted individuals withdraw into their homes or, if in the hospital, the confines of their room, to minimize the embarrassment associated with soiling. Treatment depends on the cause of the fecal incontinence. Many help manage their situation

TABLE 48.3 Major Causes of Diarrhea

Cause	Physiologic Effect
Psychologic stress (e.g., anxiety)	Increased intestinal motility and mucous secretion
Medications	Inflammation and infection of mucosa due to overgrowth of pathogenic intestinal microorganisms
Antibiotics	Irritation of intestinal mucosa
Iron	Irritation of intestinal mucosa
Cathartics	Incomplete digestion of food or fluid
Allergy to food, fluid, drugs	Increased intestinal motility and mucous secretion
Intolerance of food or fluid	Reduced absorption of fluids
Diseases of the colon (e.g., malabsorption syndrome, Crohn's disease)	Inflammation of the mucosa often leading to ulcer formation

by modifying their diet (e.g., decreasing alcohol, caffeine, greasy or spicy food, gas-producing vegetables). Weight loss improves continence by removing weight on the pelvic muscles. Pelvic muscle function is also enhanced by exercises. A regular defecation schedule can also help (Gump & Schmelzer, 2016). Several surgical procedures are used for the treatment of fecal incontinence. These include repair of the sphincter and bowel diversion or colostomy.

Flatulence

The three primary sources of flatus are (1) action of bacteria on the chyme in the large intestine, (2) swallowed air, and (3) gas that diffuses between the bloodstream and the intestine.

Most gases that are swallowed are expelled through the mouth by eructation (belching). However, large amounts of gas can accumulate in the stomach, resulting in gastric distention. The gases formed in the large intestine are chiefly absorbed through the intestinal capillaries into the circulation. **Flatulence** is the presence of excessive flatus in the intestines and leads to stretching and inflation of the intestines (intestinal distention). Flatulence can occur in the colon from a variety of causes, such as foods (e.g., cabbage, onions), abdominal surgery, or opioids. If the gas is propelled by increased colon activity before it can be absorbed, it may be expelled through the anus. If excessive gas cannot be expelled through the anus, it may be necessary to insert a rectal tube to remove it.

LIFESPAN CONSIDERATIONS Factors in Potential Bowel Elimination Problems

CHILDREN

- Successful toilet training can prevent many problems with elimination. The family should be assessed for "readiness to train." Assess the child's physical, cognitive, and interpersonal skills, and parental readiness. Does the child have sphincter control (usually by 18 to 24 months)? Does the child understand the meaning of toileting? Is the child able to express him- or herself and does the child demonstrate interest in learning? Are parents ready to work with the child?
- Encourage a regular toileting routine for children. When toilet training, ensure that toddlers can rest their feet comfortably on the floor or a footstool, and are not frightened or pressured while toileting.
- An acute episode of dehydration and constipation (often related to an illness) can lead to chronic stool problems. Constipation can cause painful defecation, which causes the child to withhold stool, leading to more severe constipation, more pain on defecation, more withholding, and so on. Breaking the cycle by helping ease defecation is important to prevent long-term problems.

OLDER ADULTS

- Poor fluid intake and inability to eat a high-fiber diet, due to swallowing or chewing difficulties, are often causes of constipation.
- Medications that are commonly taken by older adults such as antacids, many antihypertensives, antidepressants, diuretics, and narcotics for pain also contribute to constipation.
- Clients receiving tube feedings can experience diarrhea. To alleviate it, they require a change of formula, a change in its strength, or a change in the speed or temperature of tube feeding administration.
- Clients receiving laxative preparation for x-rays or other procedures may experience fluid and electrolyte imbalances due to diarrhea.
- Clients with cognitive impairment, such as Alzheimer's disease, may be unaware of what and when they eat or drink or of their bowel habits. It is important that caregivers monitor the client's bowel elimination patterns.
- Individuals with impaired mobility may have difficulty getting to the bathroom or using a regular toilet. A raised toilet seat and other devices, such as bars to assist in ambulation, may be very helpful. The decrease in activity may also contribute to constipation.

ANATOMY & PHYSIOLOGY REVIEW

Small and Large Intestines

Review the figure and reflect back on your anatomy and physiology courses.

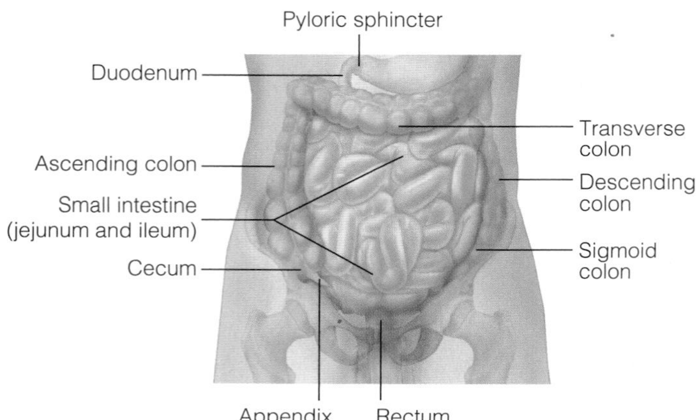

Small and large intestines.
B. F. FREMGEN, and S. S. FRUCHT, MEDICAL TERMINOLOGY: A LIVING LANGUAGE, 6th Ed.,© 2016. Reprinted and Electronically reproduced by permission of Pearson Education, Inc., New York, NY.

QUESTIONS

1. What are the primary functions of the small intestine?
2. What are the primary functions of the large intestine?
3. What part of the small intestine connects to the colon?
4. What consistency would the stool be in a client with an ileostomy and why?
5. Compare and contrast the consistency of stool in a transverse colostomy and a descending colostomy.
6. How would you describe the stool discharged from a sigmoidostomy?

Answers to Anatomy & Physiology Review questions are available on the faculty resources site. Please consult with your instructor.

NURSING MANAGEMENT

Assessing

Assessment of fecal elimination includes taking a nursing history; performing a physical examination of the abdomen, rectum, and anus; and inspecting the feces. The nurse also should review any data obtained from relevant diagnostic tests.

Nursing History

A nursing history for fecal elimination helps the nurse learn the client's normal pattern. The nurse obtains a description of usual feces and any recent changes and collects information about any past or current problems with elimination, the presence of an ostomy, and factors influencing the elimination pattern.

Examples of questions to obtain this information are shown in the Assessment Interview. The number of questions to ask is adapted to the individual client, according to the client's responses in the first three categories. For example, questions about factors influencing elimination might be addressed only to clients who are experiencing problems.

When obtaining data about the client's defecation pattern, the nurse needs to understand that the time of defecation and the amount of feces expelled are as individual as the frequency of defecation. Often, the patterns individuals follow depend largely on early training and on convenience.

Physical Examination

Physical examination of the abdomen in relation to fecal elimination problems includes inspection, auscultation, percussion, and palpation with specific reference to the intestinal tract. Auscultation precedes palpation because palpation can alter peristalsis. Examination of the rectum and anus includes inspection and palpation. Physical examination of the abdomen, rectum, and anus is discussed in Chapter 29 ∞.

Inspecting the Feces

Observe the client's stool for color, consistency, shape, amount, odor, and the presence of abnormal constituents. Table 48.1, earlier in this chapter, summarizes normal and abnormal characteristics of stool and possible causes.

Diagnostic Studies

Diagnostic studies of the gastrointestinal tract include direct visualization techniques, indirect visualization techniques, and laboratory tests for abnormal constituents (see Chapter 34 ∞).

Diagnosing

Examples of nursing diagnoses for clients with fecal eliminal problems can include bowel incontinence, constipation, and diarrhea. Clinical application of selected diagnoses is shown at the end of the chapter in the Nursing Care Plan and Concept Map.

Fecal elimination problems may affect many other areas of human functioning and as a consequence may be the etiology of other nursing diagnoses. Examples include: Potential for decreased fluid volume or potential for altered electrolytes related to prolonged diarrhea, potential for developing altered skin integrity related to prolonged diarrhea or bowel incontinence, impaired self-esteem related to fecal incontinence, lack of knowledge (bowel training, ostomy management) related to lack of previous experience.

ASSESSMENT INTERVIEW Fecal Elimination

DEFECATION PATTERN

- When do you usually have a bowel movement?
- Has this pattern changed recently?

DESCRIPTION OF FECES AND ANY CHANGES

- Have you noticed any changes in the color, texture (hard, soft, watery), shape, or odor of your stool recently?

FECAL ELIMINATION PROBLEMS

- What problems have you had or do you now have with your bowel movements (constipation, diarrhea, excessive flatulence, seepage, or incontinence)?
- When and how often does it occur?
- What do you think causes it (food, fluids, exercise, emotions, medications, disease, surgery)?
- What have you tried to solve the problem, and how effective was it?

FACTORS INFLUENCING ELIMINATION

- *Use of elimination aids.* What routines do you follow to maintain your usual defecation pattern? Do you use natural aids such as specific foods or fluids (e.g., a glass of hot lemon juice before breakfast), laxatives, or enemas to maintain elimination?
- *Diet.* What foods do you believe affect defecation? What foods do you typically eat? What foods do you avoid? Do you take meals at regular times?
- *Fluid.* What amount and kind of fluid do you take each day (e.g., 6 glasses of water, 2 cups of coffee)?
- *Exercise.* What is your usual daily exercise pattern? (Obtain specifics about exercise rather than asking whether it is sufficient; ideas of what is sufficient vary among individuals.)
- *Medications.* Have you taken any medications that could affect the intestinal tract (e.g., iron, antibiotics)?
- *Stress.* Are you experiencing any stress? Do you think this affects your defecation pattern? How?

PRESENCE AND MANAGEMENT OF OSTOMY

- What is your usual routine with your colostomy or ileostomy?
- What type of appliance do you wear and did you bring a spare with you?
- What problems, if any, do you have with it?
- How can the nurses help you manage your colostomy or ileostomy?

Planning

The major goals for clients with fecal elimination problems are to:

- Maintain or restore normal bowel elimination pattern.
- Maintain or regain normal stool consistency.
- Prevent associated risks such as fluid and electrolyte imbalance, skin breakdown, abdominal distention, and pain.

Appropriate preventive and corrective nursing interventions that relate to these must be identified. Specific nursing activities associated with each of these interventions can be selected to meet the client's individual needs. Examples of clinical applications of these using nursing diagnoses, Nursing Interventions Classifications (NIC), and Nursing Outcomes Classifications (NOC) designations are shown in the Nursing Care Plan at the end of the chapter.

Planning for Home Care

Clients who have ongoing elimination problems will need continuing care in the home setting. In preparation for discharge, the nurse needs to assess the client's and family's ability to meet specific care needs.

QSEN Patient-Centered Care Fecal Elimination

The following specific home care assessment data are required before developing a home care plan.

CLIENT AND ENVIRONMENT

- *Self-care abilities for toileting:* ability to get to the toilet, to adjust clothing for toileting, to perform toileting hygiene, and to flush the toilet
- *Mechanical aids required:* walker, cane, wheelchair, raised toilet seat, grab bars, bedpan, commode
- *Mechanical barriers that limit access to the toilet or are unsafe:* poor lighting, cluttered pathway to bathroom, narrow doorway for wheelchair, and so on
- *Bowel elimination problem:* alterations in characteristics of feces, diarrhea, constipation, incontinence, presence of ostomy, and methods of handling these
- *Level of knowledge:* planned bowel management or training program, prescribed medications, ostomy care, dietary alterations, and fluid and exercise requirements or restrictions
- *Facilities:* adequacy of bathroom facilities to assist toileting hygiene and ostomy care and to contain potentially infectious fecal effluent or stool

FAMILY

- *Caregiver availability and skills:* caregivers able to assist with toileting, medications, ostomy care, or other prescribed therapeutic measures
- *Family role changes and coping:* effect on financial status, parenting and spousal roles, sexuality, social roles
- *Alternate potential primary or respite caregivers:* for example, other family members, volunteers, church members, paid caregivers or housekeeping services; available community respite care (adult day care, seniors' centers)

COMMUNITY

- Availability of and familiarity with possible sources of assistance: equipment and supply companies, financial assistance, home health agencies

Using the assessment data, the nurse designs a teaching plan for the client and family (see Client Teaching).

CLIENT TEACHING Fecal Elimination

FACILITATING TOILETING

- Ensure safe and easy access to the toilet. Make sure lighting is appropriate, scatter rugs are removed or securely fastened, and so on.
- Facilitate instruction as needed about transfer techniques.
- Suggest ways that garments can be adjusted to make disrobing easier for toileting (e.g., Velcro closing on clothing).

MONITORING BOWEL ELIMINATION PATTERN

- Instruct the client, if appropriate, to keep a record of time and frequency of stool passage, any associated pain, and color and consistency of the stool.

DIETARY ALTERATIONS

- Provide information about required food and fluid alterations to promote defecation or to manage diarrhea.

MEDICATIONS

- Discuss problems associated with overuse of laxatives, if appropriate, and the use of alternatives to laxatives, suppositories, and enemas.
- Discuss the addition of a fiber supplement if the client is taking a constipating medication.

MEASURES SPECIFIC TO ELIMINATION PROBLEM

- Provide instructions associated with specific elimination problems and treatment, such as constipation, diarrhea, and ostomy care.

COMMUNITY AGENCIES AND OTHER SOURCES OF HELP

- Make appropriate referrals to home care or community care for assistance with resources such as installation of grab bars and raised toilet seats, structural alterations for wheelchair access, homemaker or home health aide services to assist with activities of daily living, and an enterostomal therapy nurse for assistance with stoma care and selection of ostomy appliances.
- Provide information about companies where durable medical equipment (e.g., raised toilet seats, commodes, bedpans, urinals) can be purchased, rented, or obtained free of charge, and where medical supplies such as incontinence pads or ostomy irrigating supplies and appliances can be obtained.
- Suggest additional sources of information and help such as ostomy self-help and support groups or clubs.

Implementing

Promoting Regular Defecation

The nurse can help clients achieve regular defecation by attending to (a) the provision of privacy, (b) timing, (c) nutrition and fluids, (d) exercise, and (e) positioning. See Client Teaching for healthy habits related to bowel elimination.

Privacy

Privacy during defecation is extremely important to many clients. The nurse should therefore provide as much privacy as possible for such clients but may need to stay with those who are too weak to be left alone. Some clients also prefer to wipe, wash, and dry themselves after defecating. A nurse may need to provide water, washcloth, and towel or wipes for this purpose.

Timing

A client should be encouraged to defecate when the urge is recognized. To establish regular bowel elimination, the client and nurse can discuss when peristalsis normally occurs and provide time for defecation. Many clients have well-established routines. Other activities, such as bathing and ambulating, should not interfere with the defecation time.

Nutrition and Fluids

The diet a client needs for regular normal elimination varies, depending on the kind of feces the client currently has, the frequency of defecation, and the types of foods that the client finds assist with normal defecation.

CLIENT TEACHING Healthy Defecation

- Establish a regular exercise regimen.
- Include high-fiber foods, such as vegetables, fruits, and whole grains, in the diet.
- Maintain fluid intake of 2000 to 3000 mL/day.
- Do not ignore the urge to defecate.
- Allow time to defecate, preferably at the same time each day.
- Avoid OTC medications to treat constipation and diarrhea.

For Constipation

Increase daily fluid intake, and instruct the client to drink hot liquids, warm water with a squirt of fresh lemon, and fruit juices, especially prune juice. Include fiber in the diet, that is, foods such as raw fruit, bran products, and whole-grain cereals and bread.

For Diarrhea

Encourage oral intake of fluids and bland food. Eating small amounts can be helpful because small amounts are more easily absorbed. Excessively hot or cold fluids should be avoided because they stimulate peristalsis. In addition, highly spiced foods and high-fiber foods can aggravate diarrhea. See Client Teaching for details about managing diarrhea.

For Flatulence

Limit carbonated beverages, the use of drinking straws, and chewing gum—all of which increase the ingestion of air. Gas-forming foods, such as cabbage, beans, onions, and cauliflower, should also be avoided.

Exercise

Regular exercise helps clients develop a regular defecation pattern. A client with weak abdominal and pelvic muscles (which delay normal defecation) may be able to strengthen them with the following isometric exercises:

- In a supine position, the client tightens the abdominal muscles as though pulling them inward, holding them for about 10 seconds and then relaxing them. This should be repeated 5 to 10 times, four times a day, depending on the client's health.
- Again in a supine position, the client can contract the thigh muscles and hold them contracted for about 10 seconds, repeating the exercise 5 to 10 times, four times a day. This helps the client confined to bed gain strength in the thigh muscles, thereby making it easier to use a bedpan.

Positioning

Although the squatting position best facilitates defecation, on a toilet seat the best position for most individuals seems to be leaning forward.

CLIENT TEACHING Managing Diarrhea

- Drink at least 8 glasses of water per day to prevent dehydration. Consider drinking a few glasses of electrolyte replacement fluids a day.
- Eat foods with sodium and potassium. Most foods contain sodium. Potassium is found in meats and many vegetables and fruits, especially purple grape juice, tomatoes, potatoes, bananas, cooked peaches, and apricots.
- Increase foods containing soluble fiber, such as rice, oatmeal, and skinless fruits and potatoes.
- Avoid alcohol and beverages with caffeine, which aggravate the problem.
- Limit foods containing insoluble fiber, such as high-fiber whole-wheat and whole-grain breads and cereals, and raw fruits and vegetables.
- Limit fatty foods.
- Thoroughly clean and dry the perianal area after passing stool to prevent skin irritation and breakdown. Use soft toilet tissue to clean and dry the area. Apply a dimethicone-based cream or alcohol-free barrier film as needed.
- If possible, discontinue medications that cause diarrhea.
- When diarrhea has stopped, reestablish normal bowel flora by eating fermented dairy products, such as yogurt or buttermilk.
- Seek a primary care provider consultation right away if weakness, dizziness, or loose stools persist more than 48 hours.

For clients who have difficulty sitting down and getting up from the toilet, an elevated toilet seat can be attached to a regular toilet. Clients then do not have to lower themselves as far onto the seat and do not have to lift as far off the seat. Elevated toilet seats can be purchased for use in the home.

A bedside **commode**, a portable chair with a toilet seat and a receptacle beneath that can be emptied, is often used for the adult client who can get out of bed but is unable to walk to the bathroom (Figure 48.4 ■). Some commodes have wheels and can slide over the base of a regular toilet when the waste receptacle is removed, thus providing clients the privacy of a bathroom. Potty chairs are available for children.

Clients restricted to bed may need to use a **bedpan**, a receptacle for urine and feces. Female clients use a bedpan for both urine and feces; male clients use a bedpan for feces and a urinal for urine. The two main types of bedpans are the regular high-back pan and the slipper, or fracture, pan (Figure 48.5 ■). The slipper pan has a low back and is used for clients unable to raise their buttocks because of physical problems or therapy that contraindicates such movement. Many older adults benefit from the use of a slipper pan. See Practice Guidelines for the techniques of giving and removing a bedpan.

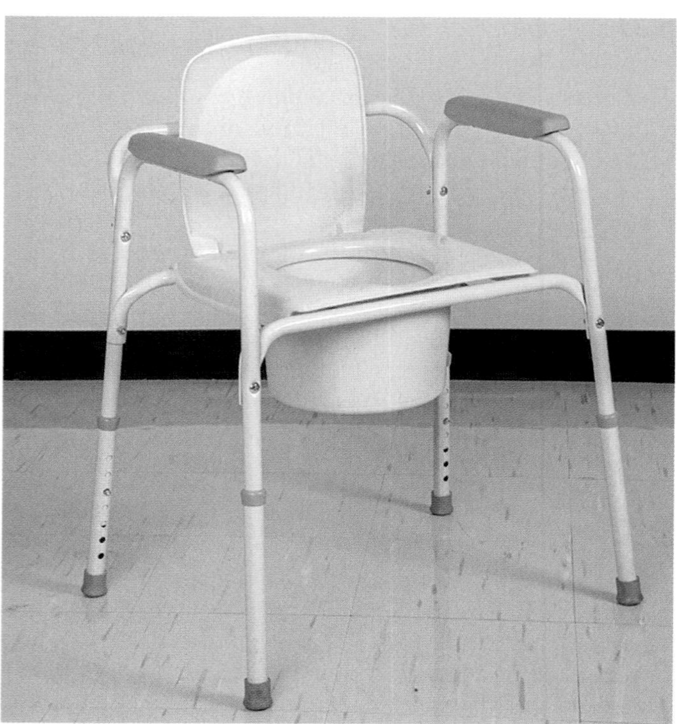

Figure 48.4 ■ A commode with overlying seat.

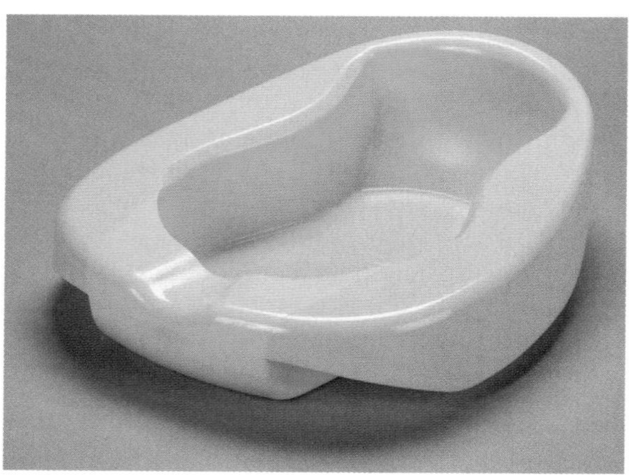

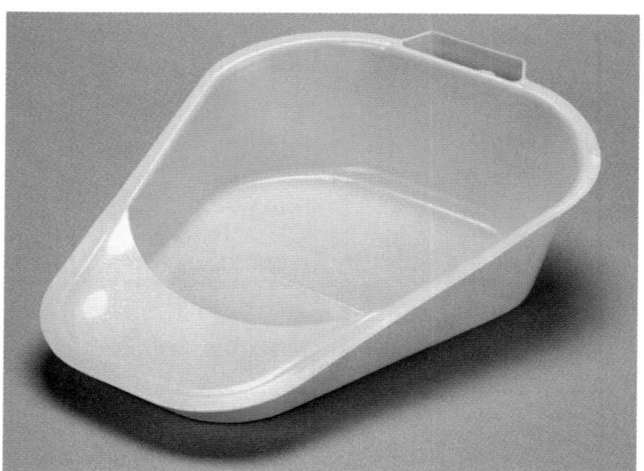

Figure 48.5 ■ *Left*, The high-back or regular bedpan; *right*, the slipper or fracture pan.

PRACTICE GUIDELINES Giving and Removing a Bedpan

- Provide privacy.
- Wear clean gloves.
- If the bedpan is metal, warm it by rinsing it with warm water.
- Adjust the bed to a height appropriate to prevent back strain.
- Elevate the side rail on the opposite side to prevent the client from falling out of bed.
- Ask the client to assist by flexing the knees, resting the weight on the back and heels, and raising the buttocks, or by using a trapeze bar, if present.
- Help lift the client as needed by placing one hand under the lower back, resting your elbow on the mattress, and using your forearm as a lever.
- Lubricate the back of the bedpan with a small amount of hand lotion or liquid soap to reduce tissue friction and shearing.
- Place a regular bedpan so that the client's buttocks rest on the smooth, rounded rim. Place a slipper pan with the flat, low end under the client's buttocks (Figure 48.6 ■).

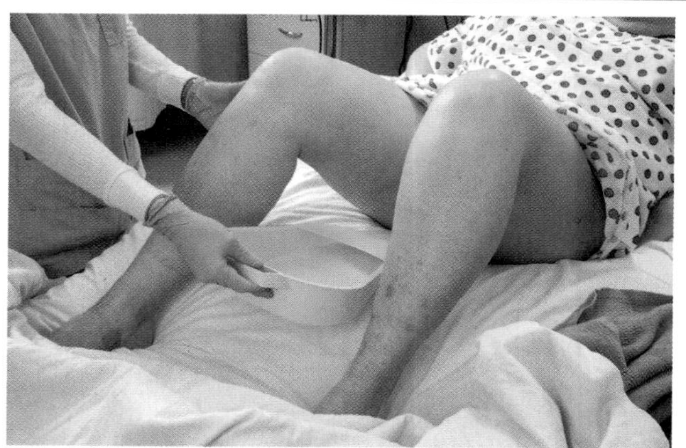

Figure 48.6 ■ Placing a slipper pan under the buttocks.

PRACTICE GUIDELINES Giving and Removing a Bedpan—*continued*

- For the client who cannot assist, obtain the assistance of another nurse to help lift the client onto the bedpan or place the client on his or her side, place the bedpan against the buttocks (Figure 48.7 ■), and roll the client back onto the bedpan.
- Provide a more normal position for the client's lower back by elevating the client's bed to a semi-Fowler's position, if permitted. If elevation is contraindicated, support the client's back with pillows as needed to prevent hyperextension of the back.
- Cover the client with bed linen to maintain comfort and dignity.

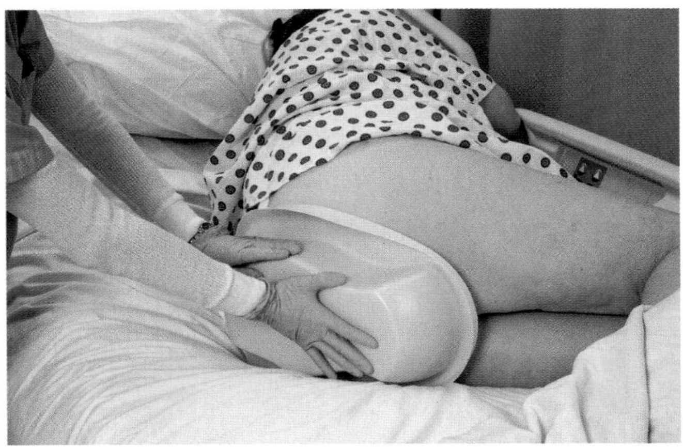

Figure 48.7 ■ Placing a regular bedpan against the client's buttocks.

- Provide toilet tissue, place the call light within reach, lower the bed to the low position, elevate the side rail if indicated, and leave the client alone.
- Answer the call light promptly.
- Do not leave clients on a bedpan longer than 15 minutes unless they are able to remove the pan themselves. Lengthy stays on a bedpan can cause skin breakdown.
- When removing the bedpan, return the bed to the position used when giving the bedpan, hold the bedpan steady to prevent spillage of its contents, cover the bedpan, and place it on the adjacent chair.
- If the client needs assistance, apply gloves and wipe the client's perineal area with several layers of toilet tissue. If a specimen is to be collected, discard the soiled tissue into a moisture-proof receptacle other than the bedpan. For female clients, clean from the urethra toward the anus to prevent transferring rectal microorganisms into the urinary meatus.
- Wash the perineal area of dependent clients with soap and water as indicated and thoroughly dry the area.
- For all clients, offer warm water, soap, a washcloth, and a towel to wash the hands.
- Assist the client to a comfortable position, empty and clean the bedpan, and return it to the bedside.
- Remove and discard your gloves and wash your hands.
- Spray the room with air freshener as needed to control odor unless contraindicated because of respiratory problems or allergies.
- Document color, odor, amount, and consistency of urine and feces, and the condition of the perineal area.

Teaching About Medications

The most common categories of medications affecting fecal elimination are cathartics and laxatives, antidiarrheals, and antiflatulents.

Cathartics and Laxatives

Cathartics are drugs that induce defecation. They can have a strong, emptying effect. A laxative is mild in comparison to a cathartic, and it produces soft or liquid stools that are sometimes accompanied by abdominal cramps. Examples of cathartics are castor oil, cascara, phenolphthalein, and bisacodyl. Table 48.4 describes the different types of laxatives.

Laxatives are contraindicated in the client who has nausea, cramps, colic, vomiting, or undiagnosed abdominal pain. Clients need to be informed about the dangers of laxative use. Continual use of laxatives to encourage bowel evacuation weakens the bowel's natural responses to fecal distention, resulting in chronic constipation. To eliminate chronic laxative use, it is usually necessary to teach the client about dietary fiber, regular exercise, taking sufficient fluids, and establishing regular defecation habits. In addition, any medication regimen should be examined to see whether it could cause constipation.

Some laxatives are given in the form of **suppositories**. These act in various ways: by softening the feces, by releasing gases such as carbon dioxide to distend the rectum, or by stimulating the nerve endings in the rectal mucosa. The best results can be obtained by inserting the suppository 30 minutes before the client's usual defecation time or when the peristaltic action is greatest, such as after breakfast.

Antidiarrheal Medications

These medications slow the motility of the intestine or absorb excess fluid in the intestine. Guidelines for using antidiarrheals are shown in Box 48.3.

Antiflatulent Medications

Antiflatulent agents such as simethicone do not decrease the formation of flatus but they do coalesce the gas bubbles and facilitate their passage by belching through the mouth or expulsion through the anus. A combination of simethicone and loperamide (Imodium Advanced) is effective in relieving abdominal bloating and gas associated with acute diarrhea; however, no convincing evidence has been shown for common flatulence. **Carminatives** are herbal oils known to act as agents that help expel gas from the stomach and intestines. Suppositories can also be given to relieve flatus by increasing intestinal motility.

Decreasing Flatulence

There are a number of ways to reduce or expel flatus, including exercise, moving in bed, ambulation, and avoiding gas-producing foods. Movement stimulates peristalsis and the escape of flatus and reabsorption of gases in the intestinal capillaries. Certain medications can decrease flatulence. Bismuth subsalicylate

TABLE 48.4 Types of Laxatives

Type	Action	Examples	Pertinent Teaching Information
Bulk forming	Increases the fluid, gaseous, or solid bulk in the intestines.	Psyllium hydrophilic mucilloid (Metamucil), methylcellulose (Citrucel)	May take 12 or more hours to act: Sufficient fluid must be taken. Safe for long-term use.
Osmotic	Draws water into the intestine by osmosis, and works by holding water in the stool to soften the stool. The active ingredient is polyethylene glycol (PEG).	MiraLax, GoLYTELY, NuLYTELY	A laxative that is helpful in the treatment of constipation. It is a powder that is tasteless when mixed in a flavored liquid such as juice. Used for cleaning of the colon before colonoscopy. Requires drinking a large volume (4 L), which may be difficult for clients to tolerate. Has an unpleasant taste.
Saline	The active ingredients are usually magnesium, sulfate, citrate, and phosphate ions, which draw water into the intestines. The additional water softens the stool and stimulates peristalsis.	Fleet Phospho-Soda, milk of magnesia, and magnesium citrate	Should be taken with one to two 8-ounce glasses of water. May be rapid acting. Can cause fluid and electrolyte imbalance, particularly in older people and children with cardiac and renal disease. Use caution when giving to older adults.
Stimulant or irritant	Irritates the intestinal mucosa or stimulates nerve endings in the wall of the intestine, causing rapid propulsion of the contents.	Bisacodyl (Dulcolax, Correctol), senna (Senokot, Ex-Lax), cascara, castor oil	Acts more quickly than bulk-forming agents. Fluid is passed with the feces. May cause cramps. Use only for short periods of time. Prolonged use may cause fluid and electrolyte imbalance.
Stool softener or surfactant	Softens and delays the drying of the stool; causes more water and fat to be absorbed into the stool.	Docusate sodium (Colace) Docusate calcium (Surfak)	Slow-acting; may take several days.
Lubricant	Lubricates the stool and colon mucosa.	Mineral oil (Haley's M-O)	Prolonged use inhibits the absorption of some fat-soluble vitamins.

BOX 48.3 Guidelines for Using Antidiarrheal Medications

- If the diarrhea persists for more than 3 or 4 days, determine the underlying cause. Using a medication such as an opiate when the cause is an infection, toxin, or poison may prolong diarrhea.
- Long-term use of OTC medications (e.g., loperamide hydrochloride [Imodium]) can produce dependence.
- Some antidiarrheal agents can cause drowsiness (e.g., diphenoxylate hydrochloride [Lomotil]) and should not be used when driving an automobile or running machinery.
- Kaolin-pectin preparations (e.g., Kaopectate) may absorb nutrients.
- Bulk laxatives and other absorbents may be used to help bind toxins and absorb excess bowel liquid.
- Bismuth preparations (e.g., Pepto-Bismol), often used to treat "traveler's diarrhea," may contain aspirin and should not be given to children and teenagers with chickenpox, influenza, and other viral infections.

(Pepto-Bismol) can be effective; however, it should not be used as a continuous treatment because it contains aspirin and could cause salicylate toxicity. Alpha-galactosidase (Beano) is effective for reducing flatulence caused by eating fermentable carbohydrates (e.g., beans, bran, fruit).

Administering Enemas

An **enema** is a solution introduced into the rectum and large intestine. The action of an enema is to distend the intestine and sometimes to irritate the intestinal mucosa, thereby increasing peristalsis and the excretion of feces and flatus. The enema solution should be at 37.7°C (100°F) because a solution that is too cold or too hot is uncomfortable and causes cramping. Enemas are classified into groups: cleansing, retention, and distention reduction, which includes carminative and return-flow enemas.

Cleansing Enema

Cleansing enemas are intended to remove feces. They are given chiefly to:

- Prevent the escape of feces during surgery.
- Prepare the intestine for certain diagnostic tests such as x-ray or visualization tests (e.g., colonoscopy).
- Remove feces in instances of constipation or impaction.

Cleansing enemas use a variety of solutions. Table 48.5 lists commonly used solutions.

Hypertonic solutions exert osmotic pressure, which draws fluid from the interstitial space into the colon. The increased volume in the colon stimulates peristalsis and thus defecation. A commonly used hypertonic enema is the commercially prepared Fleet phosphate enema. Hypotonic

TABLE 48.5 Commonly Used Enema Solutions

Solution	Constituents	Action	Time to Take Effect	Adverse Effects
Hypertonic	90–120 mL of solution (e.g., sodium phosphate [Fleet])	Draws water into the colon.	5–10 min	Retention of sodium
Hypotonic	500–1000 mL of tap water	Distends colon, stimulates peristalsis, and softens feces.	15–20 min	Fluid and electrolyte imbalance; water intoxication
Isotonic	500–1000 mL of normal saline	Distends colon, stimulates peristalsis, and softens feces.	15–20 min	Possible sodium retention
Soapsuds	500–1000 mL (3–5 mL soap to 1000 mL water)	Irritates mucosa, distends colon.	10–15 min	Irritates and may damage mucosa
Oil (mineral, olive, cottonseed)	90–120 mL	Lubricates the feces and the colonic mucosa.	0.5–3 h	

solutions (e.g., tap water) exert a lower osmotic pressure than the surrounding interstitial fluid, causing water to move from the colon into the interstitial space. Before the water moves from the colon, it stimulates peristalsis and defecation. Because the water moves out of the colon, the tap water enema should not be repeated because of the danger of circulatory overload when the water moves from the interstitial space into the circulatory system.

Safety Alert! SAFETY

Special precautions must be used to alert nurses to possible contraindications when Fleet enemas are prescribed for clients with renal failure. The label on the Fleet enema warns that using more than one enema every 24 hours can be harmful. Clients and family may underestimate the risks for a client with decreased renal function because a Fleet enema can be obtained over the counter in stores.

Isotonic solutions, such as physiologic (normal) saline, are considered the safest enema solutions to use. They exert the same osmotic pressure as the interstitial fluid surrounding the colon. Therefore, there is no fluid movement into or out of the colon. The instilled volume of saline in the colon stimulates peristalsis. Soapsuds enemas stimulate peristalsis by increasing the volume in the colon and irritating the mucosa. Only pure soap (i.e., Castile soap) should be used in order to minimize mucosa irritation.

Some enemas are large volume (i.e., 500 to 1000 mL) for an adult and others are small volume (90 to 120 mL), including hypertonic solutions. The amount of solution administered for a high-volume enema will depend on the age and medical condition of the individual. For example, clients with certain cardiac or renal diseases would be adversely affected by significant fluid retention that might result from large-volume hypotonic enemas.

Cleansing enemas may also be described as high or low. A high enema is given to cleanse as much of the colon as possible. The client changes from the left lateral position to the dorsal recumbent position and then to the right lateral position during administration so that the solution can follow the large intestine. The low enema is used to clean the rectum and sigmoid colon only. The client maintains a left lateral position during administration.

The force of flow of the solution is governed by (a) the height of the solution container, (b) size of the tubing, (c) viscosity of the fluid, and (d) resistance of the rectum. The higher the solution container is held above the rectum, the faster the flow and the greater the force (pressure) in the rectum. During most adult enemas, the solution container should be no higher than 30 cm (12 in.) above the rectum. During a high cleansing enema, the solution container is usually held 30 to 48 cm (12 to 18 in.) above the rectum because the fluid is instilled farther to clean the entire bowel.

Retention Enema

A retention enema introduces oil or medication into the rectum and sigmoid colon. The liquid is retained for a relatively long period (e.g., 1 to 3 hours). An oil retention enema acts to soften the feces and to lubricate the rectum and anal canal, thus facilitating passage of the feces. Antibiotic enemas are used to treat infections locally, anthelmintic enemas to kill helminths such as worms and intestinal parasites, and nutritive enemas to administer fluids and nutrients to the rectum.

Carminative Enema

A carminative enema is given primarily to expel flatus. The solution instilled into the rectum releases gas, which in turn distends the rectum and the colon, thus stimulating peristalsis. For an adult, 60 to 80 mL of fluid is instilled.

Return-Flow Enema

A return-flow enema, also called a Harris flush, is occasionally used to expel flatus. Alternating flow of 100 to 200 mL of fluid into and out of the rectum and sigmoid colon stimulates peristalsis. This process is repeated five or six times until the flatus is expelled and abdominal distention is relieved.

From a holistic perspective, it is important for the nurse to remember that clients may perceive this type of procedure as a significant violation of personal space. The nurse needs to consider personal space, gender of the caregiver, and the potential meaning of the structures and fluids found in this private area of the body. Keep in mind the client's potential discomfort with the gender of the caregiver and try to accommodate the client's preferences whenever possible. When it is not possible to honor the client's wishes, respectfully explain the circumstances. A gentle, matter-of-fact approach is often most helpful. Also, insertion of anything foreign into an orifice of a client's body may trigger memories of past abuse. Monitor the client for emotional responses to the procedure (both subtle and extreme) because this could indicate a history of trauma and require appropriate referral for counseling. Simply asking the client to describe the experience will give the nurse more information for possible referral.

Skill 48.1 describes how to administer an enema.

Clinical Alert!

Some clients may wish to administer their own enemas. If this is appropriate, the nurse validates the client's knowledge of correct technique and assists as needed.

SKILL 48.1

Administering an Enema

PURPOSE

- To achieve one or more of the following actions: cleansing, retention, carminative, or return-flow

ASSESSMENT

Assess

- When the client last had a bowel movement and the amount, color, and consistency of the feces
- Presence of abdominal distention
- Whether the client has sphincter control
- Whether the client can use a toilet or commode or must remain in bed and use a bedpan

PLANNING

Before administering an enema, determine that there is a primary care provider's order. At some agencies, a primary care provider must order the type of enema and the time to give it, for example, the morning of an examination. At other agencies, enemas are given at the nurse's discretion (i.e., as necessary on a prn order). In addition, determine the presence of kidney or cardiac disease that contraindicates the use of a hypotonic or hypertonic solution.

Assignment

Administration of some enemas may be assigned to assistive personnel (AP). However, the nurse must ensure the personnel are competent in the use of standard precautions. Abnormal findings such as inability to insert the rectal tip, client inability to retain the solution, or unusual return from the enema must be validated and interpreted by the nurse.

Equipment

- Disposable linen-saver pad
- Bath blanket
- Bedpan or commode
- Clean gloves
- Water-soluble lubricant if tubing not prelubricated
- Paper towel

Large-Volume Enema

- Solution container with tubing of correct size and tubing clamp
- Correct solution, amount, and temperature

Small-Volume Enema

- Prepackaged container of enema solution with lubricated tip

IMPLEMENTATION

Preparation

- Lubricate about 5 cm (2 in.) of the rectal tube (some commercially prepared enema sets already have lubricated nozzles). **Rationale:** *Lubrication facilitates insertion through the sphincter and minimizes trauma.*
- Run some solution through the connecting tubing of a large-volume enema set and the rectal tube to expel any air in the tubing, then close the clamp. **Rationale:** *Air instilled into the rectum, although not harmful, causes unnecessary distention.*

Performance

1. Prior to performing the procedure, introduce self and verify the client's identity using agency protocol. Explain to the client what you are going to do, why it is necessary, and how to participate. Discuss how the results will be used in planning further care or treatment. Indicate that the client may experience a feeling of fullness while the solution is being administered. Explain the need to hold the solution as long as possible.
2. Perform hand hygiene and observe other appropriate infection prevention procedures.
3. Apply clean gloves.
4. Provide for client privacy.
5. Assist the adult client to a left lateral position, with the right leg as acutely flexed as possible ❶, with the linen-saver pad under the buttocks. **Rationale:** *This position facilitates the flow of solution by gravity into the sigmoid and descending colon, which are on the left side. Having the right leg acutely flexed provides for adequate exposure of the anus.*
6. Insert the enema tube.
   - For clients in the left lateral position, lift the upper buttock. ❷ **Rationale:** *This ensures good visualization of the anus.*

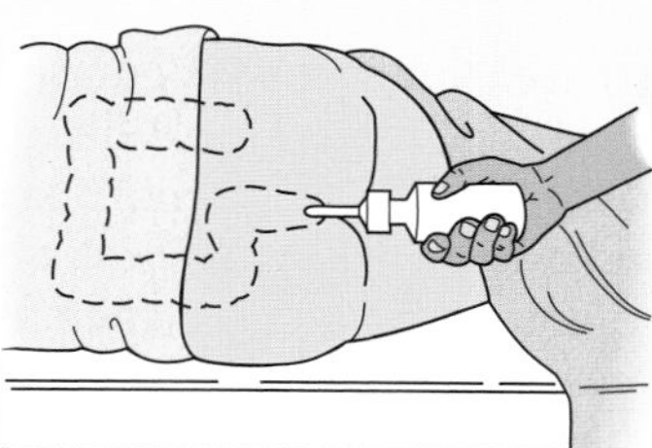

❶ Assuming a left lateral position for an enema. Note the commercially prepared enema.

Administering an Enema—*continued*

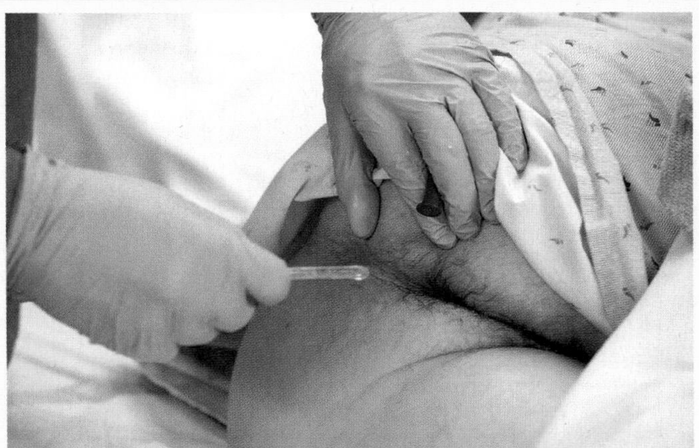

❷ Inserting the enema tube.

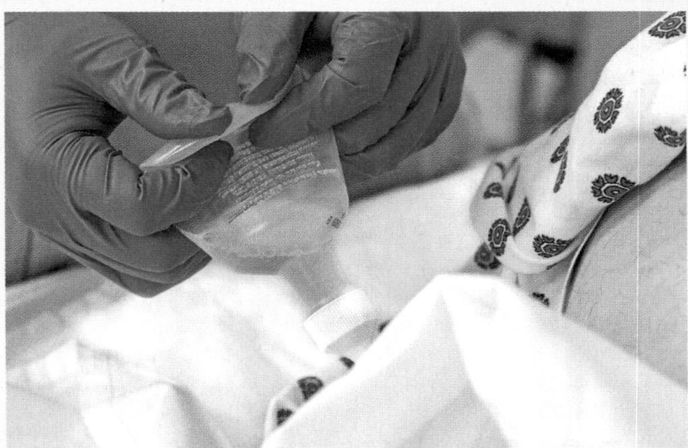

❹ Rolling up a commercial enema container.

- Insert the tube smoothly and slowly into the rectum, directing it toward the umbilicus. ❸ **Rationale:** *The angle follows the normal contour of the rectum. Slow insertion prevents spasm of the sphincter.*
- Insert the tube 7 to 10 cm (3 to 4 in.). **Rationale:** *Because the anal canal is about 2.5 to 5 cm (1 to 2 in.) long in the adult, insertion to this point places the tip of the tube beyond the anal sphincter into the rectum.*
- If resistance is encountered at the internal sphincter, ask the client to take a deep breath, then run a small amount of solution through the tube. **Rationale:** *This relaxes the internal anal sphincter.*
- Never force tube or solution entry. If instilling a small amount of solution does not permit the tube to be advanced or the solution to freely flow, withdraw the tube. Check for any stool that may have blocked the tube during insertion. If present, flush it and retry the procedure. You may also perform a digital rectal examination to determine if there is an impaction or other mechanical blockage. If resistance persists, end the procedure and report the resistance to the primary care provider and nurse in charge.

7. Slowly administer the enema solution.

- Raise the solution container, and open the clamp to allow fluid flow.
  or
- Compress a pliable container by hand.
- During most low enemas, hold or hang the solution container no higher than 30 cm (12 in.) above the rectum. **Rationale:** *The higher the solution container is held above the rectum, the faster the flow and the greater the force (pressure) in the rectum.* During a high enema, hang the solution container about 30 to 49 cm (12 to18 in.). **Rationale:** *Fluid must be instilled farther for a high enema to clean the entire bowel.* See agency protocol.
- Administer the fluid slowly. If the client complains of fullness or pain, lower the container or use the clamp to stop the flow for 30 seconds, and then restart the flow at a slower rate. **Rationale:** *Administering the enema slowly and stopping the flow momentarily decreases the likelihood of intestinal spasm and premature ejection of the solution.*
- If you are using a plastic commercial container, roll it up as the fluid is instilled. This prevents subsequent suctioning of the solution. ❹
- After all the solution has been instilled or when the client cannot hold any more and feels the desire to defecate (the urge to defecate usually indicates that sufficient fluid has been administered), close the clamp, and remove the enema tube from the anus.
- Place the enema tube in a disposable towel as you withdraw it.

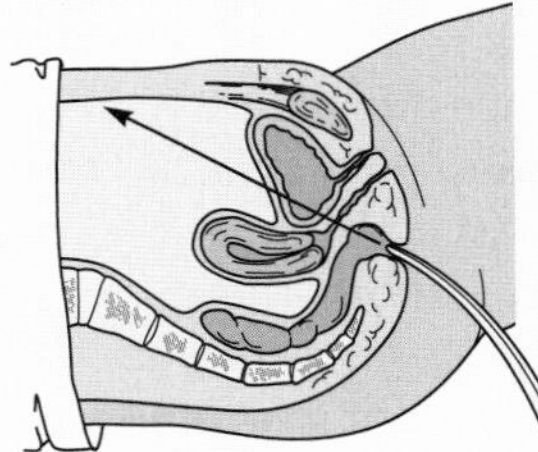

❸ Inserting the enema tube following the direction of the rectum.

8. Encourage the client to retain the enema.

- Ask the client to remain lying down. **Rationale:** *It is easier for the client to retain the enema when lying down than when sitting or standing, because gravity promotes drainage and peristalsis.*
- Request that the client retain the solution for the appropriate amount of time, for example, 5 to 10 minutes for a cleansing enema or at least 30 minutes for a retention enema.

9. Assist the client to defecate.

- Assist the client to a sitting position on the bedpan, commode, or toilet. A sitting position facilitates the act of defecation.
- Ask the client who is using the toilet not to flush it. The nurse needs to observe the feces.
- If a specimen of feces is required, ask the client to use a bedpan or commode.
- Remove and discard gloves.
- Perform hand hygiene.

10. Document the type and volume, if appropriate, of enema given. Describe the results.

SAMPLE DOCUMENTATION

8/2/2020 1000. States last BM five days ago. Abdomen distended and firm. Bowel sounds hypoactive. Fleet enema, given per order, resulted in large amount of firm brown stool. States he "feels better." M. Lopez, RN

VARIATION: ADMINISTERING AN ENEMA TO AN INCONTINENT CLIENT

Occasionally a nurse needs to administer an enema to a client who is unable to control the external sphincter muscle and thus cannot retain the enema solution for even a few minutes. In that case, after the enema

Continued on page 1288

Administering an Enema—*continued*

SKILL 48.1

tube is inserted, the client assumes a supine position on a bedpan. The head of the bed can be elevated slightly, to 30 degrees if necessary for easier breathing, and pillows used to support the client's head and back.

VARIATION: ADMINISTERING A RETURN-FLOW ENEMA

For a return-flow enema, the solution (100 to 200 mL for an adult) is instilled into the client's rectum and sigmoid colon. Then the solution container is lowered so that the fluid flows back out through the rectal tube into the container, pulling the flatus with it. The inflow–outflow process is repeated five or six times (to stimulate peristalsis and the expulsion of flatus), and the solution is replaced several times during the procedure if it becomes thick with feces.

Document the type of solution; length of time the solution was retained; the amount, color, and consistency of the returns; and the relief of flatus and abdominal distention in the client record using forms or checklists supplemented by narrative notes when appropriate.

EVALUATION

- Perform a detailed follow-up based on findings that deviated from expected or normal for the client. Compare findings to previous assessment data if available. Report significant deviations from expected to the primary care provider.

LIFESPAN CONSIDERATIONS Administering an Enema

INFANTS AND CHILDREN

- Provide a careful explanation to the parents and child before the procedure. An enema is an intrusive procedure and therefore threatening to the child.
- The enema solution should be isotonic (usually normal saline). Some hypertonic commercial solutions (e.g., Fleet phosphate enema) can lead to hypovolemia and electrolyte imbalances. In addition, the osmotic effect of the enema may produce diarrhea and subsequent metabolic acidosis.
- Infants and small children who do not have sphincter control need to be assisted in retaining the enema. The nurse administers the enema while the infant or child is lying with the buttocks over the bedpan, and the nurse firmly presses the buttocks together to prevent the immediate expulsion of the solution. Older children can usually hold the solution if they understand what to do and are not required to hold it for too long a period. It may be necessary to ensure that the bathroom is available for an ambulatory child before starting the procedure or to have a bedpan ready.
- Enema temperature should be 37.7°C (100°F) unless otherwise ordered.
- Large-volume enemas consist of 50 to 200 mL in children less than 18 months old; 200 to 300 mL in children 18 months to 5 years; and 300 to 500 mL in children 5 to 12 years old.
- For infants and small children, the dorsal recumbent position is frequently used. Position them on a small padded bedpan with support for the back and head. Secure the legs by placing a diaper under the bedpan and then over and around the thighs. Place the underpad under the client's buttocks to protect the bed linen, and drape the client with the bath blanket.
- Insert the tube 5 to 7.5 cm (2 to 3 in.) in the child and only 2.5 to 3.75 cm (1 to 1.5 in.) in the infant.
- For children, lower the height of the solution container appropriately for the age of the child. See agency protocol.
- To assist a small child in retaining the solution, apply firm pressure over the anus with tissue wipes, or firmly press the buttocks together.

OLDER ADULTS

- Older adults may fatigue easily.
- Older adults may be more susceptible to fluid and electrolyte imbalances. Use tap water enemas with great caution.
- Monitor the client's tolerance during the procedure, watching for vagal episodes (e.g., slow pulse) and dysrhythmias.
- Protect older adults' skin from prolonged exposure to moisture.
- Assist older clients with perineal care as indicated.

Digital Removal of a Fecal Impaction

Digital removal involves breaking up the fecal mass digitally and removing it in portions. Because the bowel mucosa can be injured during this procedure, some agencies restrict and specify the personnel permitted to conduct digital disimpactions. Rectal stimulation is also contraindicated for some clients because it may cause an excessive vagal response resulting in cardiac arrhythmia. Before disimpaction it is suggested an oil retention enema be given and held for 30 minutes. After a disimpaction, the nurse can use various interventions to remove remaining feces, such as a cleansing enema or the insertion of a suppository.

Clinical Alert!

Clients with a history of cardiac disease or dysrhythmias may be at risk with digital stimulation to remove an impaction. Digital examination of the rectum can cause stimulation of the vagal nerve, which can slow the heart rate. If in doubt, the nurse should check with the primary care provider before performing the procedure.

Because manual removal of an impaction can be painful, the nurse may use, if the agency permits, 1 to 2 mL of lidocaine (Xylocaine) gel on a gloved finger inserted into the anal canal as far as the nurse can reach. The lidocaine will anesthetize the anal canal and rectum and should be inserted 5 minutes before the disimpaction.

Disimpacting the client requires great sensitivity and a caring, yet matter-of-fact, approach. Be aware of personal facial expressions or anything that may convey distaste or disgust to the client. When dealing with fecal matter, many clients feel a sense of shame that relates to childhood experiences that may have been traumatic in some way. Control issues may also be triggered, and can manifest in many ways. Confusion and negative feelings are easily triggered in both client and nurse. Awareness and an ability to discuss these issues with a client, when appropriate, are important to providing appropriate care. Self-awareness will help the nurse be more therapeutically present to the client.

For digital removal of a fecal impaction:

1. If indicated, obtain assistance from a second individual who can comfort the client during the procedure.
2. Ask the client to assume a right or left side-lying position, with the knees flexed and the back toward the nurse. When the client lies on the right side, the sigmoid colon is uppermost; thus, gravity can aid removal of the feces. Positioning on the left side allows easier access to the sigmoid colon.
3. Place a disposable absorbent pad under the client's buttocks and a bedpan nearby to receive stool.
4. Drape the client for comfort and to avoid unnecessary exposure of the body.
5. Apply clean gloves and liberally lubricate the gloved index finger.
6. Gently insert the index finger into the rectum and move the finger along the length of the rectum.
7. Loosen and dislodge stool by gently massaging around it. Break up stool by working the finger into the hardened mass, taking care to avoid injury to the mucosa of the rectum.
8. Carefully work stool downward to the end of the rectum and remove it in small pieces. Continue to remove as much fecal material as possible. Periodically assess the client for signs of fatigue, such as facial pallor, diaphoresis, or change in pulse rate. Manual stimulation should be minimal.
9. Following disimpaction, assist the client to clean the anal area and buttocks. Then assist the client onto a bedpan or commode for a short time because digital stimulation of the rectum often induces the urge to defecate.

Bowel Training Programs

For clients who have chronic constipation, frequent impactions, or fecal incontinence, bowel training programs may be helpful. The program is based on factors within the client's control and is designed to help the client establish normal defecation. Such matters as food and fluid intake, exercise, and defecation habits are all considered. Before beginning such a program, clients must understand it and want to be involved. The major phases of the program are as follows:

- Determine the client's usual bowel habits and factors that help and hinder normal defecation.
- Design a plan with the client that includes the following:
  a. Fluid intake of about 2500 to 3000 mL/day
  b. Increase in fiber in the diet
  c. Intake of hot drinks, especially just before the usual defecation time
  d. Increase in exercise.
- Maintain the following daily routine for 2 to 3 weeks:
  a. Administer a cathartic suppository (e.g., Dulcolax) 30 minutes before the client's defecation time to stimulate peristalsis.
  b. When the client experiences the urge to defecate, assist the client to the toilet or commode or onto a bedpan. Note the length of time between the insertion of the suppository and the urge to defecate.
  c. Provide the client with privacy for defecation and a time limit; 30 to 40 minutes is usually sufficient.
  d. Teach the client to lean forward at the hips, to apply pressure on the abdomen with the hands, and to bear down for defecation. These measures increase pressure on the colon. Straining should be avoided because it can cause hemorrhoids.
- Provide positive feedback when the client successfully defecates. Refrain from negative feedback if the client fails to defecate.
- Offer encouragement to the client and convey that patience is often required. Many clients require weeks or months of training to achieve success.

Fecal Incontinence Pouch

To collect and contain large volumes of liquid feces, the nurse may place a fecal incontinence collector pouch around the anal area (Figure 48.8 ■). The purpose of the pouch is to prevent progressive perianal skin irritation and breakdown and frequent linen changes necessitated by incontinence. In many agencies, the pouch is replacing the traditional approach to this problem; that is, inserting a large Foley catheter into the client's rectum and inflating the balloon to keep it in place—a practice that may damage the rectal sphincter and rectal mucosa. A rectal catheter also increases peristalsis and incontinence by stimulating sensory nerve fibers in the rectum.

A fecal collector is secured around the anal opening and may or may not be attached to drainage. Pouches are best applied before the perianal skin becomes excoriated. If perianal skin excoriation is present, the nurse either (a) applies a dimethicone-based moisture-barrier cream or alcohol-free barrier film to the skin to protect it from feces until it heals and then applies the pouch, or (b) applies a skin barrier or hydrocolloid barrier underneath the pouch to achieve the best possible seal.

Nursing responsibilities for clients with a rectal pouch include (a) regular assessment and documentation of the perianal skin status, (b) changing the bag every 72 hours or sooner if there is leakage, (c) maintaining the drainage

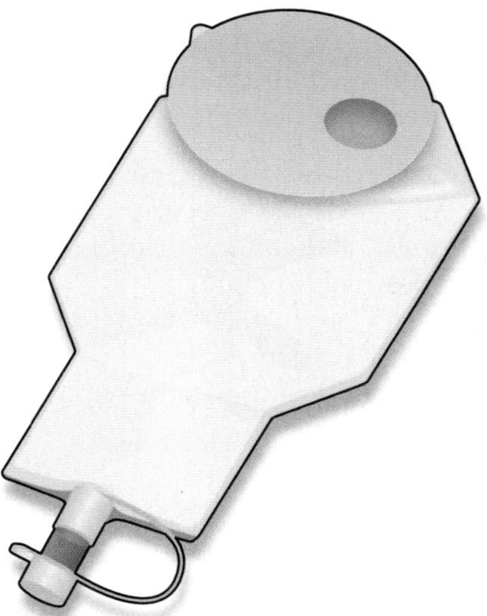

Figure 48.8 ■ A drainable fecal collector pouch.

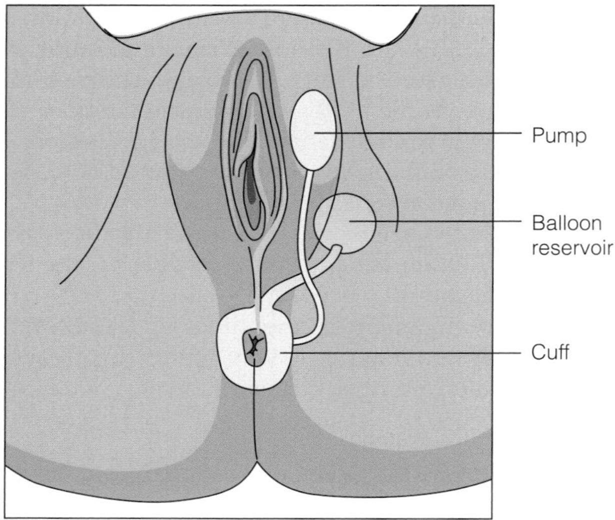

Figure 48.9 ■ Inflatable artificial sphincter.

system, and (d) providing explanations and support to the client and support people.

Some clients (e.g., post-stroke, post-trauma, quadriplegia, or paraplegia) may be treated for fecal incontinence with surgical repair of a damaged sphincter or an artificial bowel sphincter. The artificial sphincter consists of three parts: a cuff around the anal canal, a pressure-regulating balloon, and a pump that inflates the cuff (Figure 48.9 ■). The cuff is inflated to close the sphincter, maintaining continence. To have a bowel movement, the client deflates the cuff. The cuff automatically reinflates in 10 minutes. Management of this device is usually specific to the device; contact the manufacturing company for details.

Administering enemas and rectal medications may be harmful with this device in place. Ensure safety of these practices with the device instruction guide provided by the device manufacturer.

Evaluating

The goals established during the planning phase are evaluated according to specific desired outcomes, also established in that phase. If outcomes are not achieved, the nurse should explore the reasons. The nurse might consider some or all of the following questions:

- Were the client's fluid intake and diet appropriate?
- Was the client's activity level appropriate?
- Are prescribed medications or other factors affecting the gastrointestinal function?
- Do the client and family understand the provided instructions well enough to comply with the required therapy?
- Were sufficient physical and emotional support provided?

Bowel Diversion Ostomies

An **ostomy** is an opening for the gastrointestinal, urinary, or respiratory tract onto the skin. There are many types of intestinal ostomies. A **gastrostomy** is an opening through the abdominal wall into the stomach. A **jejunostomy** opens through the abdominal wall into the jejunum, an **ileostomy** opens into the ileum (small bowel), and a **colostomy** opens into the colon (large bowel). Gastrostomies and jejunostomies are generally performed to provide an alternate feeding route. The purpose of bowel ostomies is to divert and drain fecal material. Bowel diversion ostomies are often classified according to (a) their status as permanent or temporary, (b) their anatomic location, and (c) the construction of the **stoma**, the opening created in the abdominal wall by the ostomy. A stoma is generally red in color and moist. Initially, slight bleeding may occur when the stoma is touched and this is considered normal. The client does not feel the stoma because there are no nerve endings in the stoma.

Permanence

Colostomies can be either temporary or permanent. Temporary colostomies are generally performed for traumatic injuries or inflammatory conditions of the bowel. They allow the distal diseased portion of the bowel to rest and heal. Permanent colostomies are performed to provide a means of elimination when the rectum or anus is nonfunctional as a result of a birth defect or a disease such as cancer of the bowel.

Clinical Alert!

Surgery to reconnect the ends of the bowel of a temporary ostomy may be called a take-down.

Anatomic Location

An ileostomy generally empties from the distal end of the small intestine. A cecostomy empties from the cecum (the first part of the ascending colon). An ascending colostomy empties from the ascending colon, a transverse colostomy from the transverse colon, a descending colostomy from the descending colon, and a sigmoidostomy from the sigmoid colon (Figure 48.10 ■).

The location of the ostomy influences the character and management of the fecal drainage. The farther along the bowel, the more formed the stool (because the large bowel reabsorbs water from the fecal mass) and the more

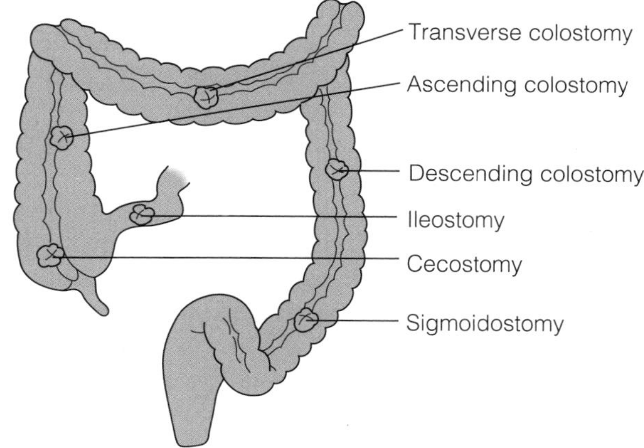

Figure 48.10 ■ The locations of bowel diversion ostomies.

control over the frequency of stomal discharge can be established. For example:

- An ileostomy produces liquid fecal drainage. Drainage is constant and cannot be regulated. Ileostomy drainage contains some digestive enzymes, which are damaging to the skin. For this reason, ileostomy clients must wear an appliance continuously and take special precautions to prevent skin breakdown. Compared to colostomies, however, odor is minimal because fewer bacteria are present.
- An ascending colostomy is similar to an ileostomy in that the drainage is liquid and cannot be regulated, and digestive enzymes are present. Odor, however, is a problem requiring control.
- A transverse colostomy produces a malodorous, mushy drainage because some of the liquid has been reabsorbed. There is usually no control.
- A descending colostomy produces increasingly solid fecal drainage. Stools from a sigmoidostomy are of normal or formed consistency, and the frequency of discharge can be regulated. Clients with a sigmoidostomy may not have to wear an appliance at all times, and odors can usually be controlled.

The length of time that an ostomy is in place also helps to determine the consistency of the stool, particularly with transverse and descending colostomies. Over time, the stool becomes more formed because the remaining functioning portions of the colon tend to compensate by increasing water reabsorption.

Surgical Construction of the Stoma

Stoma constructions are described as single, loop, divided, or double-barreled colostomies. The *single* stoma is created when one end of bowel is brought out through an opening onto the anterior abdominal wall. This is referred to as an *end* or *terminal colostomy*; the stoma is permanent (Figure 48.11 ■).

In the *loop colostomy*, a loop of bowel is brought out onto the abdominal wall and supported by a plastic bridge or by a piece of rubber tubing (Figure 48.12 ■). A loop stoma has two openings: the proximal or afferent end, which is active, and the distal or efferent end, which is inactive. The loop colostomy is usually performed in an emergency procedure and is often situated on the right transverse colon. It is a bulky stoma that is more difficult to manage than a single stoma.

The *divided colostomy* consists of two edges of bowel brought out onto the abdomen but separated from each other (Figure 48.13 ■). The opening from the digestive or proximal end is the colostomy. The distal end in this situation is often referred to as a *mucous fistula*, since this section of bowel continues to secrete mucus. The divided colostomy is often used in situations where spillage of feces into the distal end of the bowel needs to be avoided.

The *double-barreled colostomy* resembles a double-barreled shotgun (Figure 48.14 ■). In this type of colostomy, the proximal and distal loops of bowel are sutured

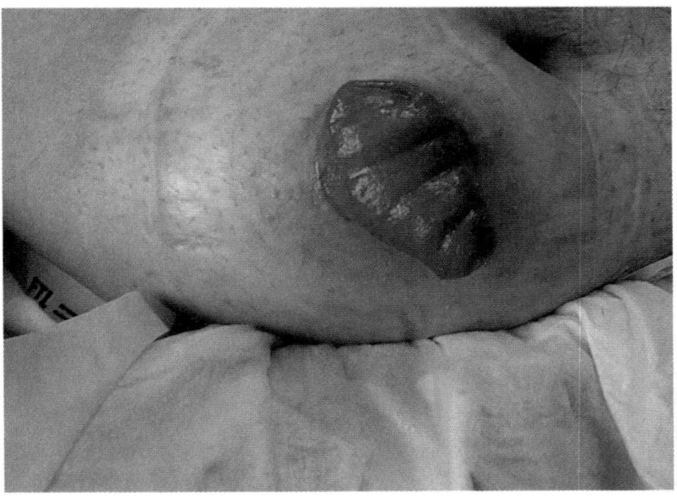

Figure 48.12 ■ Loop colostomy.
Cory patrick Hartley RN. WCC, OMS.

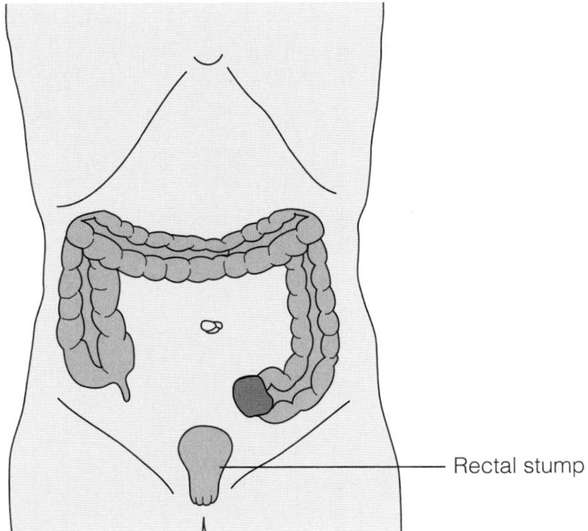

Figure 48.11 ■ End colostomy. The diseased portion of bowel is removed and a rectal pouch remains.

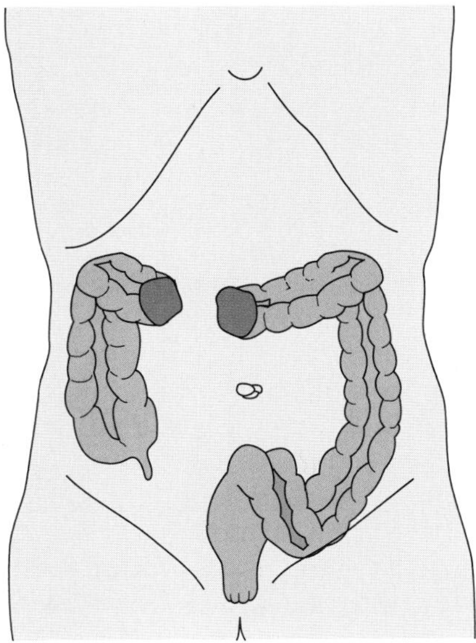

Figure 48.13 ■ Divided colostomy with two separated stomas.

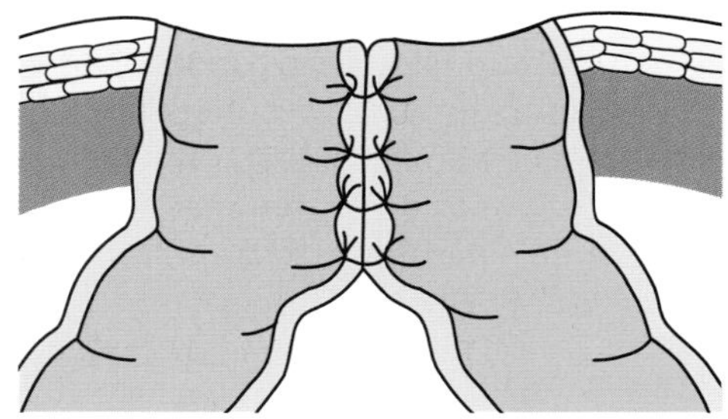

Figure 48.14 ■ Double-barreled colostomy.

together for about 10 cm (4 in.) and both ends are brought up onto the abdominal wall.

Ostomy Management

Clients with fecal diversions need considerable psychologic support, instruction, and physical care. This section is limited to the nurse's physical interventions of stoma assessment, application of an appliance to collect feces and protect skin, and promotion of self-care. Many agencies have access to a wound ostomy continence nurse (WOCN) to assist these clients. If possible, clients should meet with the WOCN prior to the surgery to assist in marking the stoma site, also termed *siting*. Burch (2018) states that "preoperative stoma siting is likely to result in a well-placed stoma, in a position that best suits the client's lifestyle, resulting in fewer problems with the appliance, including leakage, and a better quality of life for the client" (p. S10). Additionally, national organizations (e.g., United Ostomy Associations of America) have support groups whose mission is to improve the quality of life of individuals who have, or will have, an ostomy. Members of local chapters of such an organization have been known to meet and visit with a client who has a new ostomy. It is common for a client with a new ostomy to feel frightened and alone. Talking with another individual who has gone through a similar experience may help the client realize that he or she is not alone and others are willing to listen and help.

Dietary Considerations

An ileostomy or colostomy usually begins functioning by the 4th or 5th postoperative day. Clients with an ileostomy or colostomy have few dietary restrictions. Nutritional deficiencies, however, can result from ileostomies. In addition to poor absorption of vitamin B_{12}, iron, magnesium, fat, and folic acid, excess water and sodium can be lost through the ileostomy's liquid waste (Schreiber, 2016, p. 129). Over time, the bowel can compensate for some of the absorption losses, but it is important to monitor the client and provide supplements as needed.

Stomal blockages can be avoided by informing clients to chew well and increase their hydration. The usual changes in diet are focused on minimizing gas and odor. Foods that produce gas include broccoli, cruciferous vegetables, carbonated liquids, and alcohol. Odor-producing foods include onions, asparagus, cruciferous vegetables, eggs, and fish. Foods that provide a natural deodorizer include yogurt, parsley, and buttermilk (Hollister, 2017; Schreiber, 2016, p. 129).

Stoma and Skin Care

Care of the stoma and skin is important for all clients who have ostomies. The fecal material (effluent) from a colostomy or ileostomy is irritating to the peristomal skin, with the resulting moisture-associated skin damage being the most common cause of peristomal skin problems. This is particularly true of stool from an ileostomy, which contains digestive enzymes. In addition to pain and discomfort, the peristomal skin damage can cause difficulty in obtaining an adequate seal from the appliance, which causes the client embarrassment and stress from the leakage. It is important to assess the peristomal skin for irritation each time the appliance is changed. Any irritation or skin breakdown needs to be treated immediately. The skin is kept clean by washing off any excretion with water and drying thoroughly. If soap is used, it should not contain cream or lotion that may leave a residue, which can interfere with the skin barrier adhesive (Hollister, 2017).

Different materials can be used to treat and manage moisture-associated skin damage. Metcalf (2018) suggests the proactive approach of using the materials to anticipate and manage the causes of skin damage to *prevent* peristomal skin breakdown from occurring in the first place. Examples of materials include stoma powder, which absorbs moisture and also creates a dry coating, increasing adhesion of the stoma appliance. Protective films, available as wipes or spray, act as a barrier against the fecal material and are applied prior to attaching the appliance. Sealant pastes can be applied directly onto unbroken skin or to the opening of the appliance to provide a better seal. Because the paste can be difficult to remove, it should be used primarily in the area(s) that have been assessed to be at risk for potential leakage.

An ostomy appliance should protect the skin, collect stool, and control odor. The appliance consists of a skin barrier and a pouch. Some clients may prefer to also wear an adjustable ostomy belt, which attaches to an ostomy pouch to hold the pouch firmly in place (Figure 48.15 ■).

Skin barriers are important because they protect the peristomal skin. They come in two shapes: flat or convex. The flat barrier is used when the skin around the stoma is smooth with no wrinkles, creases, folds, or gullies. A convex ostomy skin barrier has some degree of protrusion (curved or rounded shape) on the adhesive side, which can better adapt to skin around the stoma that is not smooth (Hoeflok & Purnell, 2017; Metcalf, 2018). In addition, skin barriers can have either a cut-to-fit opening or a stretch-back opening to accommodate the stoma. A stretch-back opening eliminates

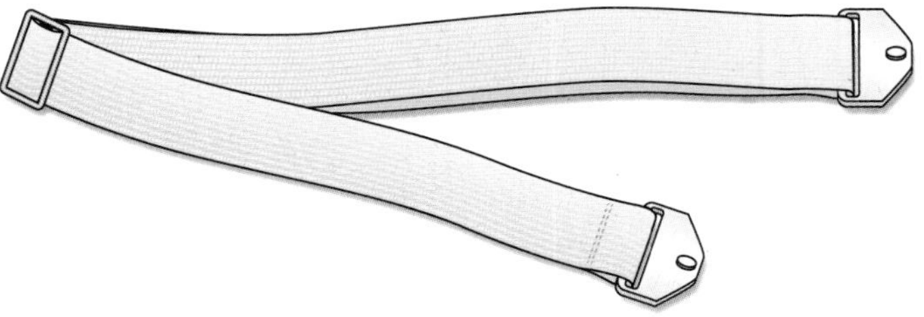

Figure 48.15 ■ Adjustable ostomy belt.

the need to measure, cut, or rely on a pattern. No matter how much or how little the opening is stretched, it conforms snugly around the stoma (Zeigler & Min, 2017, p. 8).

Appliances can be one piece where the skin barrier is already attached to the pouch (Figure 48.16*A* ■), or an appliance can consist of two pieces: a separate pouch with a flange and a separate skin barrier with a flange where the pouch fastens to the barrier at the flange (Figure 48.16*B*). The pouch can be removed without removing the skin barrier when using a two-piece appliance. Pouches can be closed or drainable (Figure 48.17 ■). A drainable pouch usually has a clip where the end of the pouch is folded over the clamp and clipped (Figure 48.18 ■). Newer drainable pouches have an integrated closure system instead of a clamp. With the integrated closure system, the client folds up the end of the pouch three times and presses firmly to seal the pouch.

Drainable pouches are usually used by clients who need to empty the pouch more than twice a day. Closed pouches are often used by clients who have a regular stoma discharge (e.g., sigmoid colostomy) and only have to empty the pouch one or two times a day. Some clients find it easier to change a closed pouch than emptying a drainable pouch, which requires some dexterity.

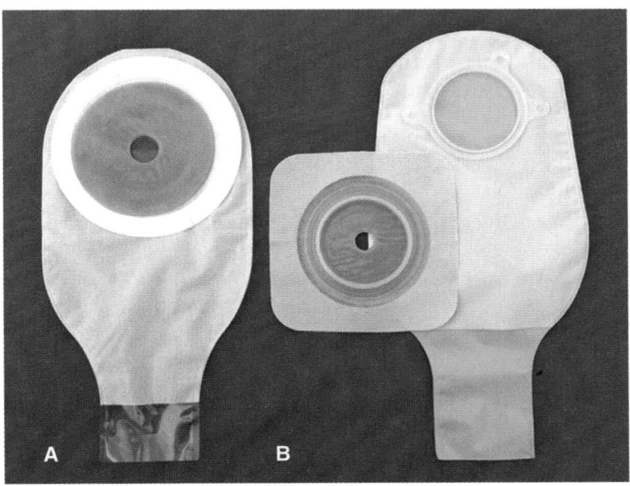

Figure 48.16 ■ *A*, A one-piece ostomy appliance or pouching system; *B*, a two-piece ostomy appliance or pouching system.
Shirlee Snyder.

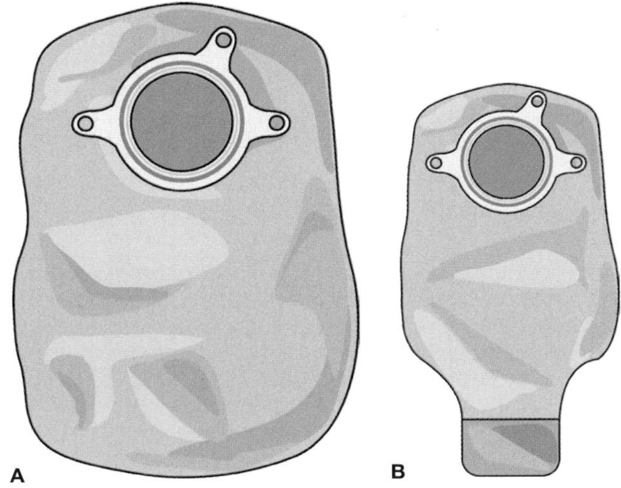

Figure 48.17 ■ *A*, A closed pouch; *B*, a drainable pouch.

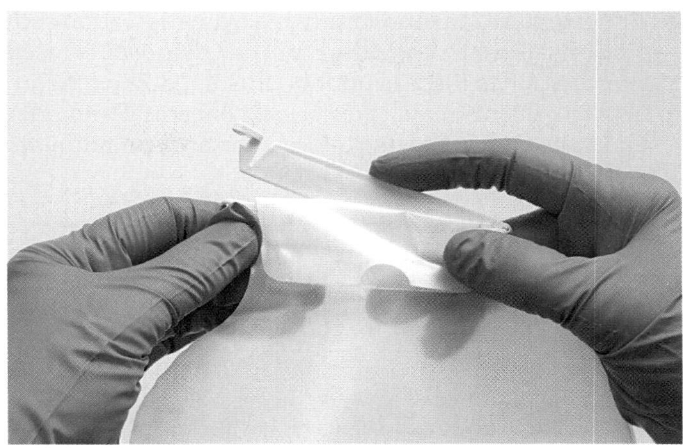

Figure 48.18 ■ Applying a pouch clamp.
Shirlee Snyder.

Odor control is essential to clients' self-esteem. As soon as clients are ambulatory, they can learn to work with the ostomy in the bathroom to avoid odors at the bedside. Selecting the appropriate kind of appliance promotes odor control. An intact appliance contains odors. Most pouches contain odor-barrier material. Some pouches also have a pouch filter that allows gas out of the pouch but not the odor.

The pouch should be changed on a routine basis, before leakage occurs. The most common routine for changing the appliance is every 2 to 3 days (Hollister, 2017). Some manufacturers recommend removing the pouch and skin barrier twice a week to clean and inspect the peristomal skin unless stool leaks onto the peristomal skin, necessitating a change. If the skin is erythematous, eroded, or ulcerated, the pouch should be changed every 24 to 48 hours to allow appropriate treatment of the skin. More frequent changes are recommended if the client complains of pain or discomfort.

The type of ostomy and amount of output influence how often the pouch is emptied. The pouch is emptied when it is one-third to one-half full of discharge or gas. If the pouch overfills, it can cause separation of the skin barrier from the skin and allow stool to come in contact with the skin. This results in the entire appliance needing to be removed and a new one applied.

QSEN Patient-Centered Care Ostomy Care

When providing nursing care for the client with an ostomy, the nurse should consider the following:

- Provide the client with the names and phone numbers of a WOCN, supply vendor, and other resource people to contact when needed. Provide pertinent internet resources for information and support.
- Inform the client of signs to report to a healthcare provider (e.g., peristomal redness, skin breakdown, and changes in stomal color).
- Provide client and family education regarding care of the ostomy and appliance when traveling.

- Educate the client and family regarding infection control precautions, including proper disposal of used pouches since these cannot be flushed down a toilet.
- Younger clients may have special concerns about odor and appearance. Provide information about community support groups. A visit from someone who has had an ostomy under similar circumstances may be helpful.

Skill 48.2 explains how to change a bowel diversion ostomy appliance.

EVIDENCE-BASED PRACTICE

Evidence-Based Practice

Can Nursing Students Develop Empathy for Clients with an Ostomy?

Approximately 750,000 people in the United States are living with an ostomy. In addition to providing and teaching ostomy care, nurses need to be able to empathize with their clients. Empathy communicates appreciation and comprehension of the client's experience and is a major part of the therapeutic nurse–client relationship. Literature shows that empathy can be developed through education. Hood, Haskins, and Roberson (2018) developed and implemented an ostomy simulation for 30 first-year nursing students enrolled in their second clinical course in an associate degree program within a university setting. The experience included a guided reflection booklet for the students to record their reflections before, during, and after the wearing of an ostomy appliance. Participation in the study was voluntary.

The students were provided brief ostomy education about placement, purpose, and nursing care in the traditional classroom setting in preparation for the following day. Students were told to complete the preactivity reflection questions. On the following day, students were assigned a partner and a "My Ostomy Story" card, which presented a simulated client identity, including medical and social history relevant to the client's ostomy journey. During this laboratory experience, students were asked to take on both a nurse and a client role. Using the "My Ostomy Story" card, students determined the anatomical placement of the ostomy and fitted their partner with an ostomy appliance. Students were informed to go about with their usual routines with the appliance in place for 24 hours. They were asked to complete the reflection-in-action portion of the reflection booklet before returning the next day. The next morning the students were encouraged to create a simulated stool appropriate to their ostomy and place the simulated stool in the ostomy bag. The student pairs worked together to empty and remove the appliance under faculty direction. Students were asked to complete the final reflection-on-action and return the booklet the following day.

The researchers conducted an analysis of the student reflections, which resulted in the identification of three distinct themes. "Encountering emotions" was the first theme. The students expressed a range of emotions before beginning the project, with apprehension and hesitation being the strongest. They considered the potential implications and inconvenience on their physical comfort and their social life. The impact on their body image began *before* the ostomy bag was first applied. The second theme, "becoming aware," occurred as a result of the students placing, wearing, and removing an ostomy appliance. The students became aware of the physical challenges faced by their future clients. Again, the students became aware of body image issues brought on by wearing an ostomy bag. They also became mindful of the need for their clients to be treated with dignity and respect. The third theme, "impacting personal practice," came about through the hands-on experiences of placing and removing the bag with a student partner. Students also recognized the need to provide clients with nonjudgmental, emotional support.

Implications

The analysis of the themes of the student reflections before, during, and after the ostomy experience demonstrated the ability of students to become self-aware of their emotions. As the authors stated, the experience of accepting another individual and helping him or her feel understood is an important part of empathy. This ostomy learning experience was an effective strategy that helped nursing students identify with the feelings and reality of others as well as acquire needed nursing skills. This study can provide helpful information for nurse educators to provide similar learning activities for students to learn about other types of client experiences.

SKILL 48.2

Changing a Bowel Diversion Ostomy Appliance

PURPOSES

- To assess and care for the peristomal skin
- To collect stool for assessment of the amount and type of output
- To minimize odors for the client's comfort and self-esteem

ASSESSMENT

Determine the following:

- The type of ostomy and its placement on the abdomen. Surgeons often draw diagrams when there are two stomas. If there is more than one stoma, it is important to confirm which is the functioning stoma.
- The type and size of appliance currently used and the special barrier substance applied to the skin, according to the nursing care plan.

Assess

- *Stoma color:* The stoma should appear red, similar in color to the mucosal lining of the inner cheek, and slightly moist. Very pale or darker-colored stomas with a dusky bluish or purplish hue indicate impaired blood circulation to the area. Notify the surgeon immediately.
- *Stoma size and shape:* Most stomas protrude slightly from the abdomen. New stomas normally appear swollen, but swelling generally decreases over 2 or 3 weeks or for as

Changing a Bowel Diversion Ostomy Appliance—*continued*

long as 6 weeks. Failure of swelling to recede may indicate a problem, for example, blockage.

- *Stomal bleeding:* Slight bleeding initially when the stoma is touched is normal, but other bleeding should be reported.
- *Status of peristomal skin:* Any redness and irritation of the peristomal skin—the 5 to 13 cm (2 to 5 in.) of skin surrounding the stoma—should be noted. Temporary redness after removal of adhesive is normal.
- *Amount and type of feces:* Assess the amount, color, odor, and consistency. Inspect for abnormalities, such as pus or blood.
- *Complaints:* Complaints of burning sensation under the skin barrier may indicate skin breakdown. The presence of abdominal discomfort or distention also needs to be determined.
- Learning needs of the client and family members regarding the ostomy and self-care.
- The client's emotional status, especially strategies used to cope with the body image changes and the ostomy.

PLANNING

Review features of the appliance to ensure that all parts are present and functioning correctly.

Assignment

Care of a *new* ostomy is not assigned to AP. However, aspects of ostomy function are observed during usual care and may be recorded by a WOCN in addition to the unit nurse. Abnormal findings must be validated and interpreted by the nurse. In some agencies, AP may be assigned to remove and replace *well-established* ostomy appliances.

Equipment

- Clean gloves
- Bedpan
- Moisture-proof bag (for disposable pouches)
- Cleaning materials, including warm water, mild soap (optional), washcloth, towel
- Tissue or gauze pad
- Skin barrier (optional)
- Stoma measuring guide
- Pen or pencil and scissors
- New ostomy pouch with optional belt
- Tail closure clamp
- Deodorant for pouch (optional)

IMPLEMENTATION

Preparation

1. Determine the need for an appliance change.
   - Assess the used appliance for leakage of stool. **Rationale:** *Stool can irritate the peristomal skin.*
   - Ask the client about any discomfort at or around the stoma. **Rationale:** *A burning sensation may indicate breakdown beneath the faceplate of the pouch.*
   - Assess the fullness of the pouch. **Rationale:** *The weight of an overly full bag may loosen the skin barrier and separate it from the skin, causing the stool to leak and irritate the peristomal skin.*
2. If there is pouch leakage or discomfort at or around the stoma, change the appliance.
3. Select an appropriate time to change the appliance.
   - Avoid times close to meal or visiting hours. **Rationale:** *Ostomy odor and stool may reduce appetite or embarrass the client.*
   - Avoid times immediately after meals or the administration of any medications that may stimulate bowel evacuation. **Rationale:** *It is best to change the pouch when drainage is least likely to occur.*
   - The best time to change a pouching system is first thing in the morning when the bowel is least active (Hollister, 2017).

Performance

1. Prior to performing the procedure, introduce self and verify the client's identity using agency protocol. Explain to the client what you are going to do, why it is necessary, and how to participate. Discuss how the results will be used in planning further care or treatments. Changing an ostomy appliance should not cause discomfort, but it may be distasteful to the client. Communicate acceptance and support to the client. It is important to change the appliance competently and quickly. Include support people as appropriate.
2. Perform hand hygiene and observe other appropriate infection prevention procedures.
3. Apply clean gloves.
4. Provide for client privacy preferably in the bathroom, where clients can learn to deal with the ostomy as they would at home.
5. Assist the client to a comfortable sitting or lying position in bed or preferably a sitting or standing position in the bathroom. **Rationale:** *Lying or standing positions may facilitate smoother pouch application, that is, avoid wrinkles.*
6. Unfasten the belt if the client is wearing one.
7. Empty the pouch and remove the ostomy skin barrier.
   - Empty the contents of a drainable pouch through the bottom opening into a bedpan or toilet. **Rationale:** *Emptying before removing the pouch prevents spillage of stool onto the client's skin.*
   - If the pouch uses a clamp, do not throw it away because it can be reused.
   - Assess the consistency, color, and amount of stool.
   - Peel the skin barrier off slowly, beginning at the top and working downward, while holding the client's skin taut. **Rationale:** *Holding the skin taut minimizes client discomfort and prevents abrasion of the skin.*
   - Discard the disposable pouch in a moisture-proof bag.
8. Clean and dry the peristomal skin and stoma.
   - Use toilet tissue to remove excess stool.
   - Use warm water and a washcloth to clean the skin and stoma. ❶ Check agency practice on the use of soap. **Rationale:** *Soap is sometimes not advised because it can be irritating to the skin.* If soap is allowed, do not use deodorant or moisturizing soaps. **Rationale:** *They may interfere with the adhesives in the skin barrier.*
   - Dry the area thoroughly by patting with a towel. **Rationale:** *Excess rubbing can abrade the skin.*

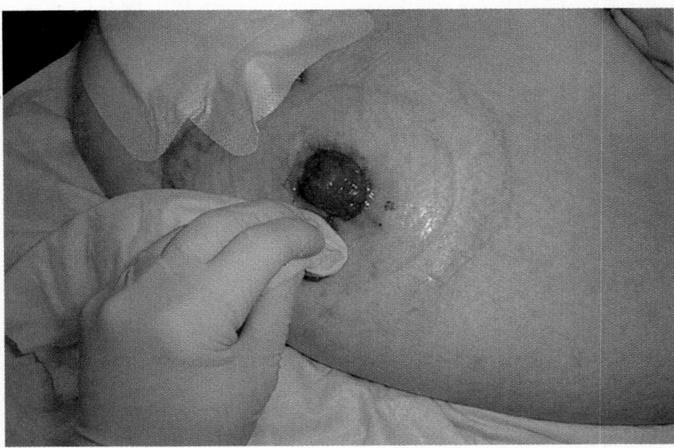

❶ Cleaning the skin.
Cory patrick Hartley RN. WCC, OMS.

Continued on page 1296

SKILL 48.2

Changing a Bowel Diversion Ostomy Appliance—*continued*

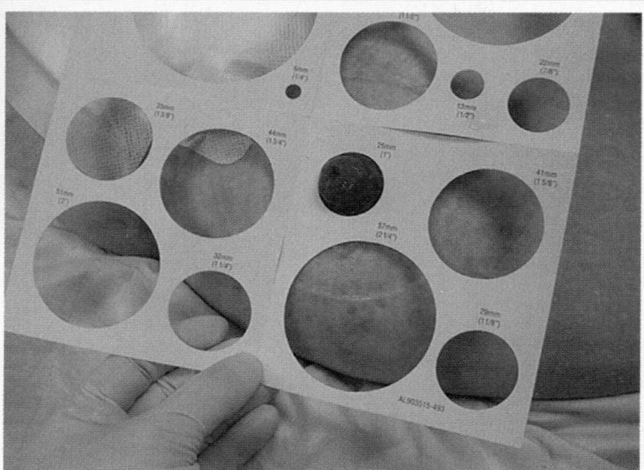

❷ A guide for measuring the stoma.
Cory patrick Hartley RN. WCC, OMS.

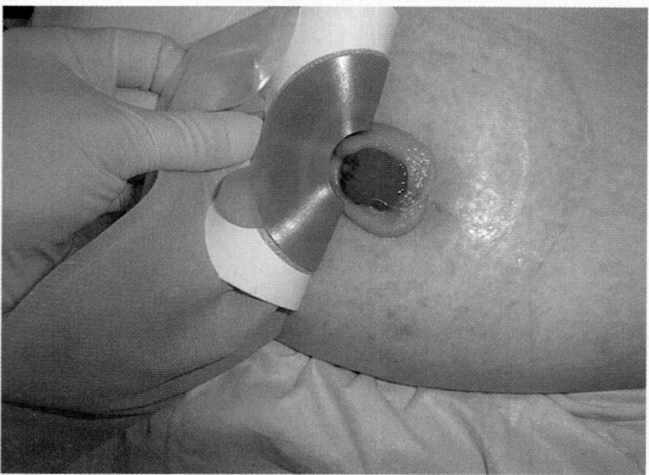

❹ Centering the skin barrier over the stoma.
Cory patrick Hartley RN. WCC, OMS.

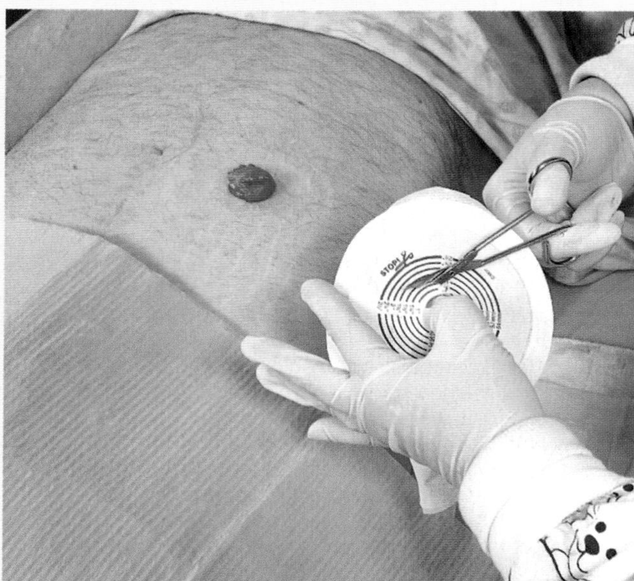

❸ The nurse is making a stoma opening on a disposable one-piece pouch.

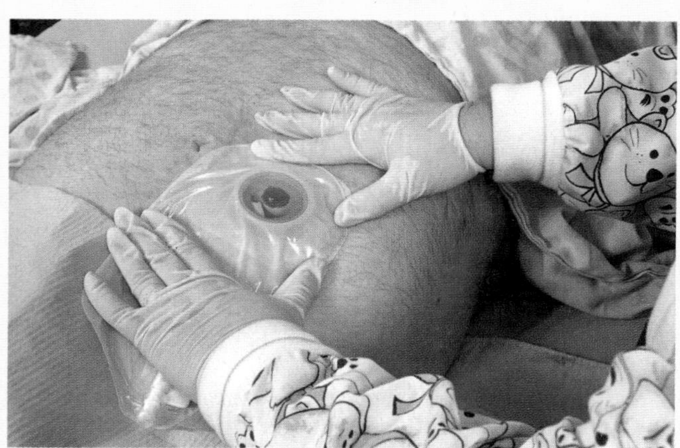

❺ Pressing the skin barrier of a disposable one-piece pouch for 30 seconds to activate the adhesives in the skin barrier.

9. Assess the stoma and peristomal skin.
   - Inspect the stoma for color, size, shape, and bleeding.
   - Inspect the peristomal skin for any redness, ulceration, or irritation. Transient redness after the removal of adhesive is normal.
10. Place a piece of tissue or gauze over the stoma, and change it as needed. **Rationale:** *This absorbs any seepage from the stoma while the ostomy appliance is being changed.*
11. Prepare and apply the skin barrier (peristomal seal).
    - Use the guide ❷ to measure the size of the stoma.
    - On the backing of the skin barrier, trace a circle the same size as the stomal opening.
    - Cut out the traced stoma pattern to make an opening in the skin barrier. ❸ Make the opening no more than 1/8 inch (2–3 mm) larger than the stoma. **Rationale:** *This allows space for the stoma to expand slightly when functioning and minimizes the risk of stool contacting peristomal skin.*
    - Remove the backing to expose the sticky adhesive side. The backing can be saved and used as a pattern when making an opening for future skin barriers.

For a One-Piece Pouching System

- Center the one-piece skin barrier and pouch over the stoma, and gently press it onto the client's skin for 30 seconds. ❹, ❺ **Rationale:** *The heat and pressure help activate the adhesives in the skin barrier.*

For a Two-Piece Pouching System

- Center the skin barrier over the stoma and gently press it onto the client's skin for 30 seconds.
- Remove the tissue over the stoma before applying the pouch.
- Snap the pouch onto the flange or skin barrier wafer.
- For drainable pouches, close the pouch according to the manufacturer's directions.
- Remove and discard gloves. Perform hand hygiene.

12. Document the procedure in the client record using forms or checklists supplemented by narrative notes when appropriate. Record pertinent assessments and interventions. Report any increase in stoma size, change in color indicative of circulatory impairment, and presence of skin irritation or erosion. Record on the client's chart discoloration of the stoma, the appearance of the peristomal skin, the amount and type of drainage, the client's reaction to the procedure, the client's experience with the ostomy, and skills learned by the client.

Changing a Bowel Diversion Ostomy Appliance—*continued*

SKILL 48.2

SAMPLE DOCUMENTATION

8/3/2020 0900 Colostomy bag changed. Moderate to large amount of semi-formed brown stool. Stoma reddish color. No redness or irritation around stoma. Client looked at stoma today and started asking questions as to how she will be able to change the pouch when she is home. Asked if she would like to do the next changing of the pouch. Stated "yes." G. Hsu, RN

VARIATION: EMPTYING A DRAINABLE POUCH

- Empty the pouch when it is one-third to one-half full of stool or gas. **Rationale:** *Emptying before it is overfull helps avoid breaking the seal with the skin and stool then coming in contact with the skin.*
- While wearing gloves, hold the pouch outlet over a bedpan or toilet. Lift the lower edge up.
- Unclamp or unseal the pouch.
- Drain the pouch. Loosen feces from sides by moving fingers down the pouch.
- Clean the inside of the tail of the pouch with a tissue or a premoistened towelette.
- Apply the clamp or seal the pouch.
- Dispose of used supplies.
- Remove and discard gloves.
- Perform hand hygiene.
- Document the amount, consistency, and color of stool.

EVALUATION

- Relate findings to previous data if available. Adjust the teaching plan and nursing care plan as needed. Reinforce the teaching each time the care is performed. Encourage and support self-care as soon as possible because clients should be able to perform self-care by discharge. **Rationale:** *Client learning is facilitated by consistent nursing interventions.*
- Perform detailed follow-up based on findings that deviated from expected or normal for the client. Report significant deviations from normal to the primary care provider.

Colostomy Irrigation

A colostomy irrigation (CI), similar to an enema, is a form of stoma management used only for clients who have a sigmoid or descending colostomy. The purpose of irrigation is to distend the bowel sufficiently to stimulate peristalsis, which stimulates evacuation. CI has many potential benefits. For example, CI makes the wearing of a colostomy pouch unnecessary; decreases odor and flatus; facilitates sleeping, eating, and traveling; and has been shown to improve quality of life (Bauer, Arnold-Long, & Kent, 2016, p. 69). Currently, colostomy irrigations are not routinely taught to most clients; however, best evidence indicates clients with a descending or sigmoid colostomy should be given the option to learn CI (Bauer et al., 2016). CI may be taught in the home or the ostomy clinic.

Routine irrigations (e.g., every 24 to 48 hours) for control of elimination is the client's decision. Some clients prefer to control the time of elimination through rigid dietary regulation and not be bothered with CI, which can take up 30to 90 minutes to complete. When CI is chosen, it should be done at the same time each day.

Bauer, Arnold-Long, and Kent (2016) explain the following process for CI: The client fills the irrigation bag with usually 500 to 750 mL of lukewarm tap water. An irrigation cone is attached to the irrigation tubing. After priming the irrigation tubing, the client attaches the irrigation sleeve to the ostomy wafer or the client's body. The client lubricates the stoma cone and gently places it into the stoma and opens the clamp on the tubing. After the volume is infused, the cone is held in place for about 5 minutes or when cramping begins. The cone is removed and the client waits for the initial return of the irrigation fluid and stool. A secondary return of fluid and stool occurs and can take 30 to 90 minutes to complete. After stool evacuation is complete, the pouch is replaced or the stoma is covered.

NURSING CARE PLAN Altered Bowel Elimination

ASSESSMENT DATA	NURSING DIAGNOSIS	DESIRED OUTCOMES
NURSING ASSESSMENT Mrs. Emma Brown is a 78-year-old widow of 9 months. She lives alone in a low-income housing complex for older adults. Her two children live with their families in a city approximately 150 miles away. She has always enjoyed cooking for her family; however, now that she is alone, she does not cook for herself. As a result, she has developed irregular eating patterns and tends to prepare soup-and-toast meals. She gets little exercise and has had bouts of insomnia since her husband's death. For the past month, Mrs. Brown has been having a problem with constipation. She states she has a bowel movement about every 3 to 4 days and her stools are hard and painful to excrete. Mrs. Brown decides to attend the health fair sponsored by the housing complex and seeks assistance from the county public health nurse.	Constipation related to low-fiber diet and inactivity (as evidenced by infrequent, hard stools; painful defecation; abdominal distention)	**Bowel Elimination [0501]**, not compromised as evidenced by: • Ease of stool passage • Stool soft and formed • Passage of stool without aids

Continued on page 1298

NURSING CARE PLAN Altered Bowel Elimination—*continued*

Physical Examination

Height: 162 cm (5′4″)
Weight: 65 kg (143 lb)
Temperature: 36.2°C (97.2°F)
Pulse: 82 beats/min
Respirations: 20/min
Blood pressure: 128/74 mmHg
Active bowel sounds, abdomen slightly distended

Diagnostic Data

CBC: Hgb 10.8
Urinalysis negative

NURSING INTERVENTIONS*/SELECTED ACTIVITIES	RATIONALE
CONSTIPATION/IMPACTION MANAGEMENT [0450]	
Identify factors (e.g., medications, bedrest, diet) that may cause or contribute to constipation.	*Assessing causative factors is an essential first step in teaching and planning for improved bowel elimination.*
Encourage increased fluid intake, unless contraindicated.	*Sufficient fluid intake is necessary for the bowel to absorb sufficient amounts of liquid to promote proper stool consistency.*
Evaluate medication profile for gastrointestinal side effects.	*Constipation is a common side effect of many drugs including narcotics and antacids.*
Teach Mrs. Brown how to keep a food diary.	*An appraisal of food intake will help identify if Mrs. Brown is eating a well-balanced diet and consuming adequate amounts of fluid and fiber. Excessive meat or refined food intake will produce small, hard stools.*
Instruct Mrs. Brown on a high-fiber diet, as appropriate.	*Fiber absorbs water, which adds bulk and softness to the stool and speeds up passage through the intestines.*
Instruct her on the relationship of diet, exercise, and fluid intake to constipation and impaction.	*Fiber without adequate fluid can aggravate, not facilitate, bowel function.*
Exercise Promotion [0200]	
Encourage verbalization of feelings about exercise or need for exercise.	*Perceptions of the need for exercise may be influenced by misconceptions, cultural and social beliefs, fears, or age.*
Determine Mrs. Brown's motivation to begin or continue an exercise program.	*Individuals who have been successful in an exercise program can assist Mrs. Brown by providing incentive and enhancing motivation. For example, a walking partner may be beneficial.*
Inform Mrs. Brown about the health benefits and physiologic effects of exercise.	*Activity influences bowel elimination by improving muscle tone and stimulating peristalsis.*
Instruct her about appropriate types of exercise for her level of health, in collaboration with a primary care provider.	*Any individual beginning an exercise program should consult a primary care provider primarily for a cardiac evaluation. Mrs. Brown's age and lack of activity should be considered in planning the level of activity.*
Assist Mrs. Brown to set short-term and long-term goals for the exercise program.	*Realistic goal setting provides direction and motivation.*

Evaluation

Outcome not met. Mrs. Brown has kept a food diary and is able to identify the need for more fluid and fiber, but has not consistently included fiber in her diet. She has started a walking program with a neighbor but is only able to walk for 10 minutes at a time twice a week. She states her last bowel movement was 3 days ago.

*The NOC # for desired outcomes and the NIC # for nursing interventions are listed in brackets following the appropriate outcome or intervention. Outcomes, interventions, and activities selected are only a sample of those suggested by NOC and NIC and should be further individualized for each client.

APPLYING CRITICAL THINKING

1. You learn that Mrs. Brown's stools have been liquid, in very small amounts, and at infrequent intervals, generally occurring when she feels the urge to defecate. What additional data are important to obtain from her?
2. What nursing intervention is most appropriate before making suggestions to correct or prevent the problem she is experiencing?
3. What suggestions can you give her about maintaining a regular bowel pattern?
4. Explain why cathartics and laxatives are generally contraindicated for individuals in Mrs. Brown's situation.

Answers to Applying Critical Thinking questions are available on the faculty resources site. Please consult with your instructor.

CONCEPT MAP

Altered Bowel Elimination

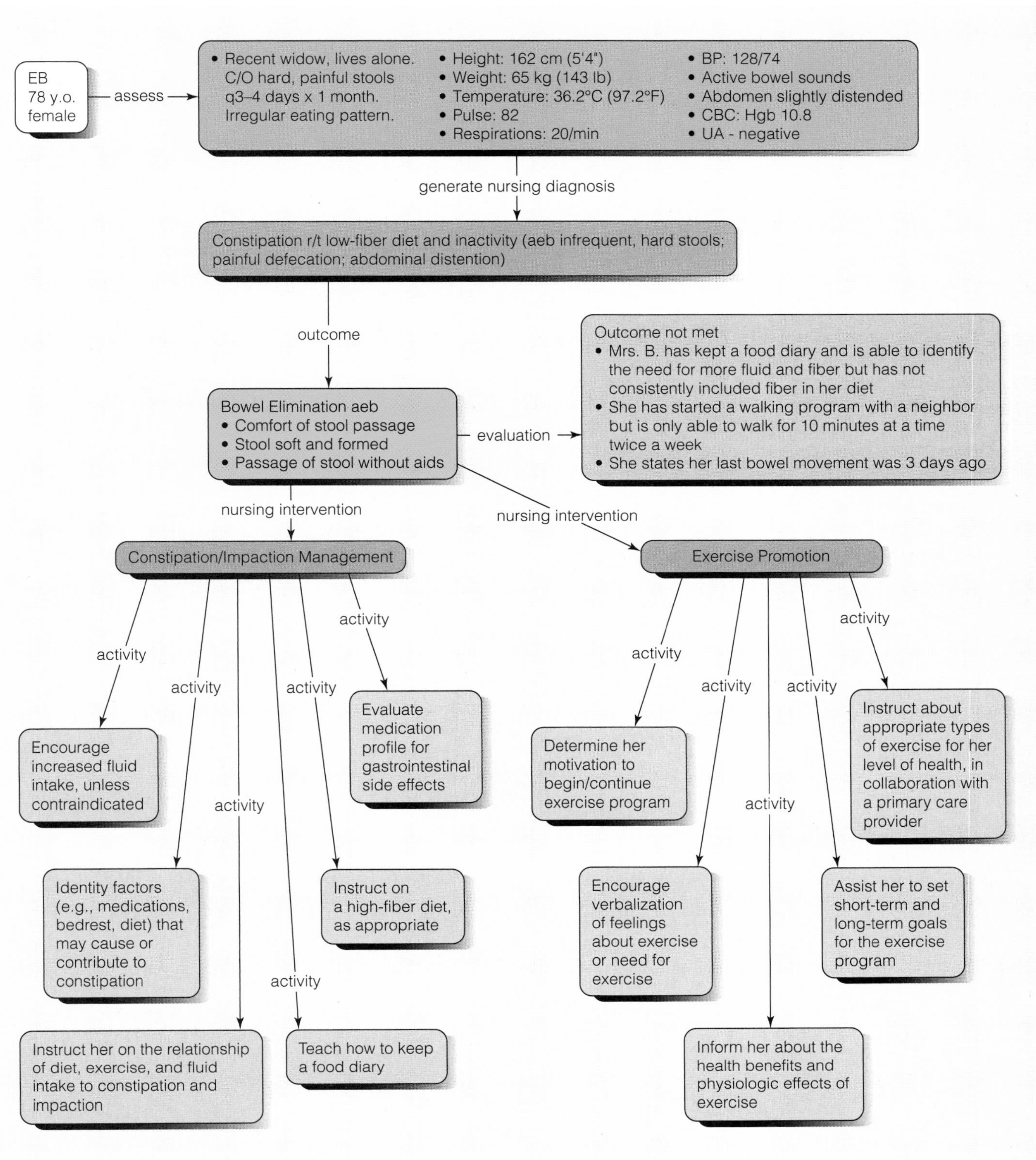

Chapter 48 Review

CHAPTER HIGHLIGHTS

- Primary functions of the large intestine are the absorption of water and nutrients, the mucoid protection of the intestinal wall, and fecal elimination.
- Patterns of fecal elimination vary greatly among individuals, but a regular pattern of fecal elimination with formed, soft stools is essential to health and a sense of well-being.
- Various factors affect defecation: developmental level, diet, fluid intake, activity and exercise, psychologic factors, defecation habits, medications, diagnostic and medical procedures, pathologic conditions, and pain.
- Common fecal elimination problems include constipation, diarrhea, bowel incontinence, and flatulence. Each has specific defining characteristics and contributing causes that often relate to or are identical to the factors that affect defecation.
- Lack of exercise, irregular defecation habits, and overuse of laxatives are all thought to contribute to constipation. Sufficient fluid and fiber intake are required to keep feces soft.
- An adverse effect of constipation is straining during defecation, during which the Valsalva maneuver may be used. Cardiac problems may ensue.
- An adverse effect of prolonged diarrhea is fluid and electrolyte imbalance.
- Assessment relative to fecal elimination includes a nursing history; physical examination of the abdomen, rectum, and anus; and in some situations, visualization studies and inspection and analysis of stool for abnormal constituents such as blood.
- A nursing history includes data about the client's defecating pattern, description of feces and any changes, problems associated with elimination, and data about possible factors altering bowel elimination.
- When inspecting the client's stool, the nurse must observe its color, consistency, shape, amount, and odor, and the presence of abnormal constituents.
- A function of the nurse is to assist clients with diet and bowel preparation before endoscopic and radiographic studies of the large intestine.
- Nursing diagnoses that relate specifically to altered bowel elimination can include bowel incontinence. However, because altered elimination patterns affect several areas of human functioning, diagnoses such as potential for decreased fluid volume, potential for altered electrolytes, potential for developing altered skin integrity, impaired self-esteem, and lack of knowledge may also apply.
- Normal defecation is often facilitated in both well and ill clients by providing privacy, teaching clients to attend to defecation urges promptly, assisting clients to normal sitting positions whenever possible, encouraging appropriate food and fluid intake, and scheduling regular exercise.
- Nursing strategies include administering cathartics and antidiarrheals; administering cleansing, carminative, retention, or return-flow enemas; applying protective skin agents; monitoring fluid and electrolyte balance; and instructing clients in ways to promote normal defecation.
- The purpose of an enema is to increase peristalsis and the excretion of feces and flatus. Enemas are classified into groups: cleansing, retention, and distention reduction, which includes carminative and return-flow enemas.
- Digital removal of an impaction should be carried out gently because of vagal nerve stimulation and subsequent depressed cardiac rate. A primary care provider's order is often necessary.
- Clients who have bowel diversion ostomies require special care, with attention to psychologic adjustment, diet, and stoma and skin care. A variety of stoma management methods is available to these clients, depending on the type and position of the ostomy.

TEST YOUR KNOWLEDGE

1. A client asks an RN why it is more difficult to use a bedpan than a toilet for defecating. Which of the following is the best response?
   1. The sitting position decreases the contractions of the muscles of the pelvic floor.
   2. The sitting position increases the downward pressure on the rectum, making it easier to pass stool.
   3. The sitting position increases the pressure within the abdomen.
   4. The sitting position inhibits the urge to urinate, allowing one to defecate.

2. An older client tells a nurse that in order to achieve a daily bowel movement, the client uses laxatives most days of the week. What should the nurse tell this client? Select all that apply.
   1. Normal patterns of elimination are different for everyone.
   2. Increase fiber intake to 20–35 grams a day.
   3. Engage in enjoyable exercise.
   4. Ignore the urge to have a bowel movement.
   5. Have 6–8 glasses of fluid daily.

3. A client has received an oil retention enema. What time frame should the nurse provide the client for the enema to take effect?
   1. 1–3 hours
   2. 10–20 minutes
   3. 5–10 minutes
   4. 10–15 minutes

4. The nurse is most likely to report which finding to the primary care provider for a client who has an established colostomy?
   1. The stoma extends 1/2 in. above the abdomen.
   2. The skin under the appliance looks red briefly after removing the appliance.
   3. The stoma color is a deep red-purple.
   4. The ascending colostomy delivers liquid feces.

5. Which goal is the most appropriate for clients with diarrhea related to ingestion of an antibiotic for an upper respiratory infection?
1. The client will wear a medical alert bracelet for antibiotic allergy.
2. The client will return to his or her previous fecal elimination pattern.
3. The client will verbalize the need to take an antidiarrheal medication prn.
4. The client will increase intake of insoluble fiber such as grains, rice, and cereals.

6. A client with a new stoma who has not had a bowel movement since surgery last week reports feeling nauseous. What is the appropriate nursing action?
1. Prepare to irrigate the colostomy.
2. After assessing the stoma and surrounding skin, notify the surgeon.
3. Assess bowel sounds and administer antiemetic.
4. Administer a bulk-forming laxative, and encourage increased fluids and exercise.

7. The nurse assesses a client's abdomen several days after abdominal surgery. It is firm, distended, and painful to palpate. The client reports feeling "bloated." The nurse consults with the surgeon, who orders an enema. The nurse prepares to give what kind of enema?
1. Soapsuds
2. Retention
3. Return flow
4. Oil retention

8. Which of the following is most likely to validate that a client is experiencing intestinal bleeding?
1. Large quantities of fat mixed with pale yellow liquid stool
2. Brown, formed stools
3. Semisoft black-colored stools
4. Narrow, pencil-shaped stool

9. Which nursing diagnoses is/are most applicable to a client with fecal incontinence? Select all that apply.
1. Bowel incontinence
2. Potential for decreased fluid volume
3. Altered body image
4. Social seclusion
5. Potential for developing altered skin integrity

10. A student nurse is assigned to care for a client with a sigmoidostomy. The student will assess which ostomy site?

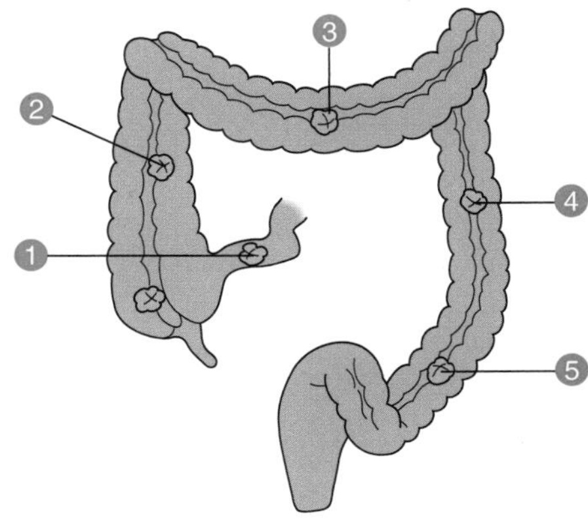

See Answers to Test Your Knowledge in Appendix A.

READINGS AND REFERENCES

Suggested Readings

Hoeflok, J., & Purnell, P. (2017). Understanding the role of convex skin barriers in ostomy care. *Nursing*, *47*(9), 51–56. doi:10.1097/01.NURSE.0000516224.24273.88
This article reviews the advantages of convex skin barriers and their role in ostomy care.

Metcalf, C. (2018). Managing moisture-associated skin damage in stoma care. *British Journal of Nursing*, *27*(22), S6–S14. doi:10.12968/bjon.2018.27.22.S6
This article provides helpful information about the different types of appliances and accessories that can be used to treat moisture-associated skin damage in stoma care.

Related Research

Cutting, K. (2016). Comparing ostomates' perceptions of hydrocolloid and silicone seals: A survey. *British Journal of Nursing*, *25*(22), S24–S29. doi:10.12968/bjon.2016.25.22.S30

Oliver, J. S., Ewell, P., Nicholls, K., Chapman, K., & Ford, S. (2016). Differences in colorectal cancer risk knowledge among Alabamians: Screening implications. *Oncology Nursing Forum*, *43*(1), 77–85. doi:10.1188/16.ONF.77-85

Saraiva de Aguiar, F. A., Pinheiro de Jesus, B., Cardoso Rocha, F., Barbosa Cruz, I., de Andrade Neto, G. R., Meira Rios, B. R., . . . Batista Andrade, D. L. (2019). Colostomy and self-care: Meanings for ostomized patients. *Journal of Nursing UFPE Online*, *13*(1), 105–110. doi:10.5205/1981-8963-v13i01a236771p105-110-2019

References

American Cancer Society. (2017). *Colorectal cancer facts & figures 2017–2019*. Retrieved from https://www.cancer.org/content/dam/cancer-org/research/cancer-facts-and-statistics/colorectal-cancer-facts-and-figures/colorectal-cancer-facts-and-figures-2017-2019.pdf

American Cancer Society. (2018). *Colorectal cancer risk factors*. Retrieved from https://www.cancer.org/cancer/colon-rectal-cancer/causes-risks-prevention/risk-factors.html

Ball, J. W., Bindler, R., Cowen, K., & Shaw, M. (2017). *Principles of pediatric nursing* (7th ed.). Hoboken, NJ: Pearson.

Bauer, C., Arnold-Long, M., & Kent, D. J. (2016). Colostomy irrigation to maintain continence: An old method revived. *Nursing*, *46*(8), 59–62. doi:10.1097/01.NURSE.0000484963.00982.b5

Burch, J. (2018). Research and expert opinion on siting a stoma: A review of the literature. *British Journal of Nursing*, *27*(16), S4–S12. doi:10.12968/bjon.2018.27.16.S4

Fremgen, B. F., & Frucht, S. S. (2016). *Medical terminology* (6th ed.). Hoboken, NJ: Pearson.

Gordon, J., Fischer-Cartlidge, E., & Barton-Burke, M. (2017). The big 3: An updated overview of colorectal, breast, and prostate cancers. *Nursing Clinics of North America*, *52*, 27–52. doi:10.1016/j.cnur.2016.11.004

Gump, K., & Schmelzer, M. (2016). Gaining control over fecal incontinence. *MEDSURG Nursing*, *25*(2), 97–102.

Hollister. (2017). *Understanding your colostomy*. Retrieved from http://www.hollister.com/~/media/files/pdfs%E2%80%93for%E2%80%93download/ostomy%E2%80%93care/understanding%E2%80%93your%E2%80%93colostomy_923054-0917.pdf

Hood, D. G., Haskins, T. L., & Roberson, S. C. (2018). Stepping into their shoes: The ostomy experience. *Journal of Nursing Education*, *57*(4), 233–236. doi:10.3928/01484834-20180322-08

Mayo Clinic. (2018). *Dietary fiber: Essential for a healthy diet*. Retrieved from http://www.mayoclinic.org/healthy-lifestyle/nutrition-and-healthy-eating/in-depth/fiber/art-20043983

Moorhead, S., Swanson, E., Johnson, M., & Maas, M. L. (Eds.). (2018). *Nursing outcomes classification (NOC)* (6th ed.). St. Louis, MO: Elsevier.

Sams, A. W., & Kennedy-Malone, L. (2017). Recognition and management of *Clostridium difficile* in older adults. *The Nurse Practitioner*, *42*(5), 50–55. doi:10.1097/01.NPR.0000512254.47992.8e

Schreiber, M. L. (2016). Evidence-based practice. Ostomies: Nursing care and management. *MEDSURG Nursing*, *25*(2), 127–130.

Smith, S., & Taylor, J. (2016). Best practices in caring for patients infected with *Clostridium difficile. Critical Care Nurse*, *36*(3), 71–72. doi:10.4037/ccn2016696

Zeigler, M. H., & Min, A. (2017). Ostomy management: Nuts and bolts for every nurse's toolbox. *American Nurse Today*, *12*(9), 6–11.

Selected Bibliography

Burch, J. (2016). Making maintaining dignity a top priority: Caring for older people with a stoma in the community. *British Journal of Community Nursing*, *21*(6), 280–282. doi:10.12968/bjcn.2016.21.6.280

Burch, J. (2017). Stoma care: An update on current guidelines for community nurses. *British Journal of Community Nursing*, *22*(4), 162–166. doi:10.12968/bjcn.2017.22.4.162

Peate, I. (2016). How to perform digital removal of faeces. *Nursing Standard*, *30*(40), 36–39. doi:10.7748/ns.30.40.36.s43

Perrin, A. (2016). Convex stoma appliances: An audit of stoma care nurses. *British Journal of Nursing*, *25*(22), S10–S15. doi:10.12968/bjon.2016.25.22.S10

Walls, P. (2018). Seeking a consensus for a glossary of terms for peristomal skin complications. *Journal of Stomal Therapy Australia*, *38*(4), 8–12.

Williams, J. (2017). The importance of choosing the correct stoma appliance to meet patient needs. *British Journal of Community Nursing*, *22*(2), 58–60. doi:10.12968/bjcn.2017.22.2.58

Oxygenation 49

LEARNING OUTCOMES

After completing this chapter, you will be able to:

1. Outline the structure and function of the respiratory system.
2. Describe the processes of breathing (ventilation) and gas exchange (respiration).
3. Explain the role and function of the respiratory system in transporting oxygen and carbon dioxide to and from body tissues.
4. Describe the mechanisms for respiratory regulation.
5. Identify factors influencing respiratory function.
6. Identify four major types of conditions that can alter respiratory function.
7. Describe nursing assessments for oxygenation status.
8. Describe nursing measures to promote respiratory function and oxygenation.
9. Explain the use of therapeutic measures such as medications, inhalation therapy, oxygen therapy, artificial airways, airway suctioning, and chest tubes to promote respiratory function.
10. State outcome criteria for evaluating client responses to measures that promote adequate oxygenation.
11. Verbalize the steps used in:
    a. Administering oxygen by cannula, face mask, or face tent
    b. Oropharyngeal, nasopharyngeal, and nasotracheal suctioning
    c. Suctioning a tracheostomy or endotracheal tube
    d. Providing tracheostomy care.
12. Recognize when it is appropriate to assign aspects of oxygen therapy, suctioning, and tracheostomy care to assistive personnel.
13. Demonstrate appropriate documentation and reporting of oxygen therapy, suctioning, and tracheostomy care.

KEY TERMS

adventitious breath sounds, *1309*
apnea, *1309*
atelectasis, *1305*
bradypnea, *1309*
cyanosis, *1309*
diffusion, *1307*
dyspnea, *1309*
emphysema, *1307*
erythrocytes, *1307*
eupnea, *1309*
expectorate, *1314*
hematocrit, *1307*
hemoglobin, *1307*
hemothorax, *1341*
humidifiers, *1315*
hypercapnia, *1309*
hypercarbia, *1309*
hyperinflation, *1333*
hyperoxygenation, *1333*
hyperventilation, *1333*
hypoxemia, *1309*
hypoxia, *1309*
lung compliance, *1305*
lung recoil, *1305*
mucus clearance device (MCD), *1317*
noninvasive positive pressure ventilation (NPPV), *1324*
orthopnea, *1309*
oxyhemoglobin, *1307*
pleural effusion, *1341*
pneumothorax, *1341*
postural drainage, *1317*
respiratory membrane, *1305*
sputum, *1309*
stridor, *1309*
suctioning, *1329*
surfactant, *1305*
tachypnea, *1309*
tidal volume, *1305*
vibration, *1317*

Introduction

Oxygen, a clear, odorless gas that constitutes approximately 21% of the air we breathe, is necessary for proper functioning of all living cells. The absence of oxygen can lead to cellular, tissue, and organism death. Cellular metabolism produces carbon dioxide, which must be eliminated from the body to maintain normal acid–base balance. Delivery of oxygen and removal of carbon dioxide require the integration of several systems including the hematologic, cardiovascular, and respiratory systems. The respiratory system provides the movement and transfer of gases between the atmosphere and the blood. Impaired function of the system can significantly affect our ability to breathe, transport gases, and participate in everyday activities.

Respiration is the process of gas exchange between the individual and the environment and involves four components:

1. Ventilation or breathing, the movement of air in and out of the lungs as we inhale and exhale
2. Alveolar-capillary gas exchange, which involves the diffusion of oxygen and carbon dioxide between the alveoli and the pulmonary capillaries
3. Transport of oxygen and carbon dioxide between the tissues and the lungs
4. Movement of oxygen and carbon dioxide between the systemic capillaries and the tissues.

Structure and Processes of the Respiratory System

The structure of the respiratory system facilitates gas exchange and protects the body from foreign matter such as particulates and pathogens. The four processes of the respiratory system include pulmonary ventilation, alveolar gas exchange, transport of oxygen and carbon dioxide, and systemic diffusion.

Structure of the Respiratory System

The respiratory system (Figure 49.1 ■) is divided structurally into the upper respiratory system and the lower respiratory system. The mouth, nose, pharynx, and larynx compose the upper respiratory system. The lower respiratory system includes the trachea and lungs, with the bronchi, bronchioles, alveoli, pulmonary capillary network, and pleural membranes.

Air enters through the nose, where it is warmed, humidified, and filtered. Hairs at the entrance of the nares trap large particles in the air, and smaller particles are filtered and trapped as air changes direction on contact with the nasal turbinates and septum. Irritants in the nasal passages initiate the sneeze reflex. A large volume of air rapidly exits through the nose and mouth during a sneeze, helping to clear nasal passages.

Inspired air passes from the nose through the pharynx. The pharynx is a shared pathway for air and food. It includes both the nasopharynx and the oropharynx, which are richly supplied with lymphoid tissue that traps and destroys pathogens entering with the air.

The larynx is important for maintaining airway patency and protecting the lower airways from swallowed food and fluids. During swallowing, the inlet to the larynx (the epiglottis) closes, routing food to the esophagus. The epiglottis is open during breathing, allowing air to move freely into the lower airways. Below the larynx, the trachea

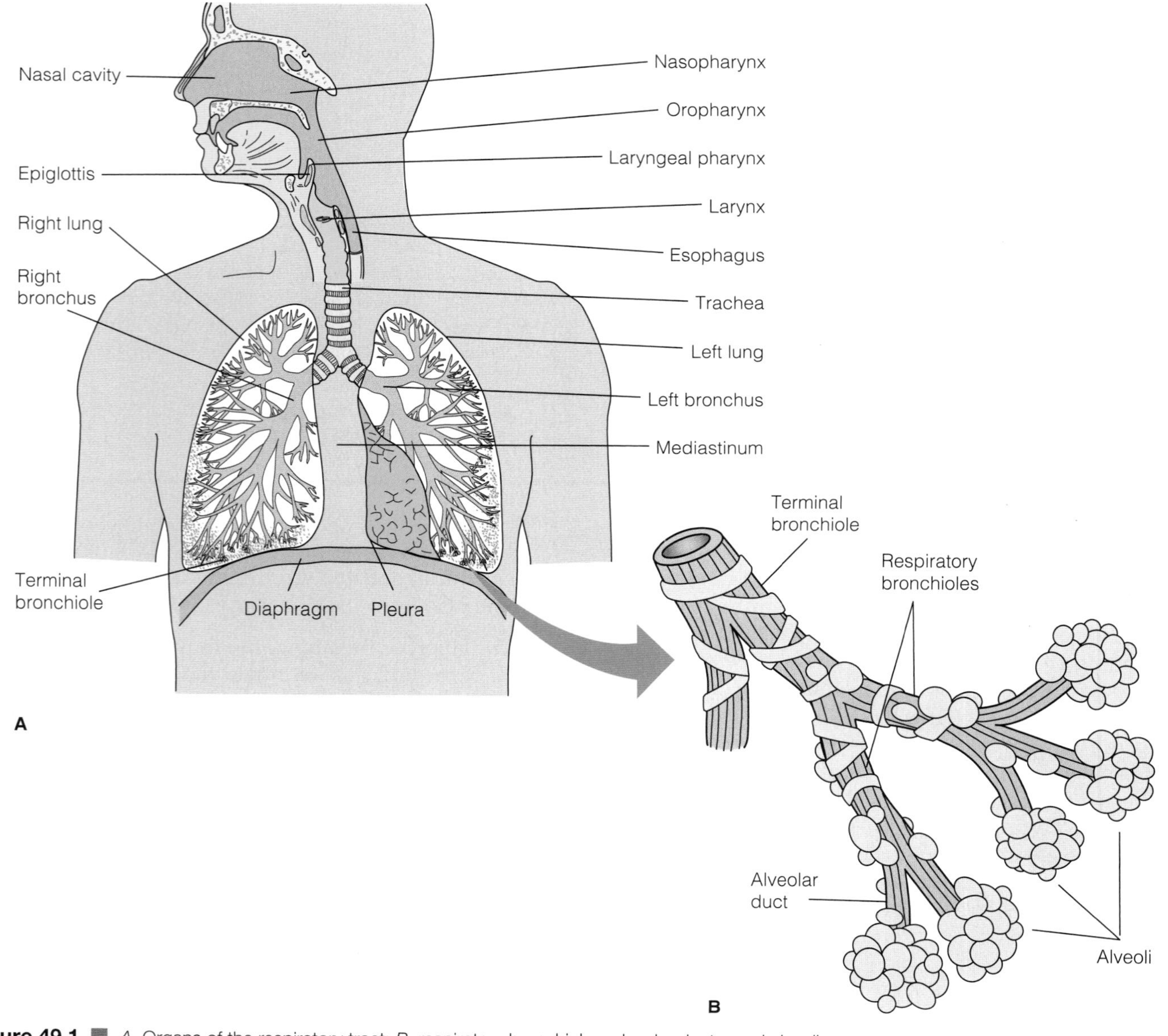

Figure 49.1 ■ *A*, Organs of the respiratory tract; *B*, respiratory bronchioles, alveolar ducts, and alveoli.

leads to the right and left main bronchi (primary bronchi) and the other conducting airways of the lungs. Within the lungs, the primary bronchi divide repeatedly into smaller and smaller bronchi, ending with the terminal bronchioles. Together these airways are known as the bronchial tree. The trachea and bronchi are lined with mucosal epithelium. These cells produce a thin layer of mucus, the "mucous blanket," that traps pathogens and microscopic particulate matter. These foreign particles are then swept upward toward the larynx and throat by cilia, tiny hairlike projections on the epithelial cells. The cough reflex is triggered by irritants in the larynx, trachea, or bronchi.

After air passes through the trachea and bronchi, it enters the respiratory bronchioles and alveoli where all gas exchange occurs. This gas exchange or respiratory zone of the lungs includes the respiratory bronchioles (which have scattered air sacs in their walls), the alveolar ducts, and the alveoli (see Figure 49.1). Alveoli have very thin walls, composed of a single layer of epithelial cells covered by a thick mesh of pulmonary capillaries. The alveolar and capillary walls form the **respiratory membrane** (also known as the *alveolar–capillary membrane*), where gas exchange occurs between the air on the alveolar side and the blood on the capillary side. The airways move air to and from the alveoli; the right ventricle and pulmonary vascular system transport blood to the capillary side of the membrane. For example, deoxygenated blood leaves the right heart through the pulmonary artery and enters the lungs and capillaries. Oxygenated blood returns via capillaries to the pulmonary vein to the heart (Figure 49.2 ■). The thin, highly permeable membrane of the respiratory membrane (estimated to be not more than 0.0004 mm thick) is essential to normal gas exchange. Thus, fluid or other materials in the alveoli interfere with the respiratory process.

The outer surface of the lungs is covered by a thin, double layer of tissue known as the pleura. The parietal pleura lines the thorax and surface of the diaphragm. It doubles back to form the visceral pleura, covering the external surface of the lungs. Between these pleural layers is a potential space that contains a small amount of pleural fluid, a serous lubricating solution. This fluid prevents friction during the movements of breathing and serves to keep the layers adherent through its surface tension.

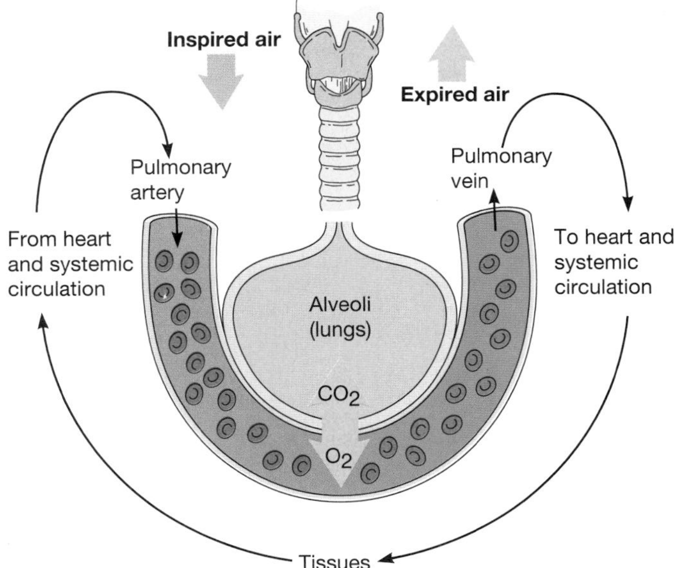

Figure 49.2 ■ Gas exchange occurs between the air on the alveolar side and the blood on the capillary side.

Pulmonary Ventilation

The first process of the respiratory system, ventilation of the lungs, is accomplished through the act of breathing: inspiration (inhalation) as air flows into the lungs, and expiration (exhalation) as air moves out of the lungs. Adequate ventilation depends on several factors:

- Clear airways
- An intact central nervous system (CNS) and respiratory center (medulla and pons in the brainstem)
- An intact thoracic cavity capable of expanding and contracting
- Adequate pulmonary compliance and recoil.

A number of mechanisms, including ciliary action and the cough reflex, work to keep airways open and clear. In some cases, however, these defenses may be overwhelmed. The inflammation, edema, and excess mucous production that occur with some types of pneumonia may clog small airways, impairing ventilation of distal alveoli.

The degree of chest expansion during normal breathing is minimal, requiring little energy expenditure. In adults, approximately 500 mL of air is inspired and expired with each breath. This is known as **tidal volume**. Breathing during strenuous exercise or some types of heart disease requires greater chest expansion and effort. At this time, more than 1500 mL of air may be moved with each breath. Accessory muscles of respiration, including the anterior neck muscles, intercostal muscles, and muscles of the abdomen, are used. Active use of these muscles and noticeable effort in breathing are seen in clients with obstructive pulmonary disease.

Lung compliance, the expansibility or stretchability of lung tissue, plays a significant role in the ease of ventilation. At birth, the fluid-filled lungs are stiff and resistant to expansion, much as a new balloon is difficult to inflate. With each subsequent breath, the alveoli become more compliant and easier to inflate, just as a balloon becomes easier to inflate after several tries. Lung compliance tends to decrease with aging, making it more difficult to expand alveoli and increasing the risk for **atelectasis**, or collapse of a portion of the lung.

In contrast to lung compliance is **lung recoil**, the continual tendency of the lungs to collapse away from the chest wall. Just as lung compliance is necessary for normal inspiration, lung recoil is necessary for normal expiration. The surface tension of fluid lining the alveoli has the greatest effect on recoil. **Surfactant**, a lipoprotein produced by specialized alveolar cells, reduces the surface tension of alveolar fluid. Without surfactant, lung expansion is exceedingly difficult and the lungs collapse. Premature infants whose lungs are not yet capable of producing adequate surfactant often develop respiratory distress syndrome.

ANATOMY & PHYSIOLOGY REVIEW

The Respiratory System

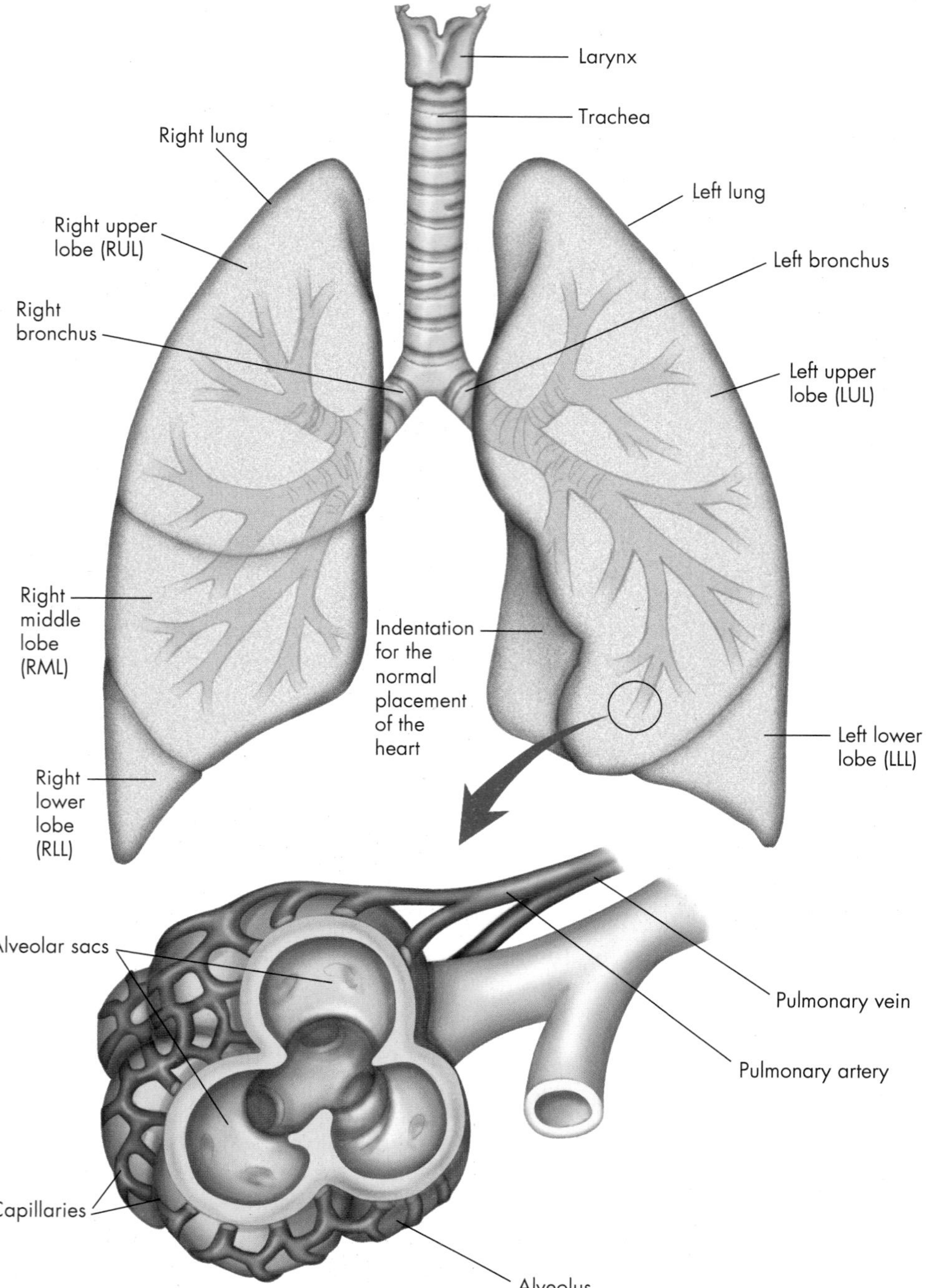

The larynx, trachea, bronchi, and lungs with an expanded view showing the structures of an alveolus and the pulmonary blood vessels.

QUESTIONS

1. Pneumonia occurs when microorganisms get into the lower respiratory tract and overwhelm the body's defenses. Name at least two normal defense mechanisms present in the *upper* airway that help prevent microorganisms getting into the lower respiratory tract.
2. Microorganisms can travel past the upper respiratory tract defense mechanisms. What defense mechanisms are present in the *lower* respiratory tract that may help the client?
3. The microorganisms have quickly multiplied and overpowered the client's defense mechanisms. The client has pneumonia and the alveoli are filled with infectious fluid. How will this affect gas exchange at the respiratory or alveolar–capillary membrane?

Answers to Anatomy & Physiology Review questions are available on the faculty resources site. Please consult with your instructor.

Alveolar Gas Exchange

After the alveoli are ventilated, the second phase of the respiratory process—the diffusion of oxygen from the alveoli and into the pulmonary blood vessels—begins. **Diffusion** is the movement of gases or other particles from an area of greater pressure or concentration to an area of lower pressure or concentration. Pressure differences in the gases on each side of the respiratory membrane affect diffusion. Carbon dioxide diffuses from the blood into the alveoli, where it can be eliminated with expired air.

Transport of Oxygen and Carbon Dioxide

The third part of the respiratory process involves the transport of respiratory gases. Oxygen needs to be transported from the lungs to the tissues, and carbon dioxide must be transported from the tissues back to the lungs. Normally most of the oxygen (97%) combines loosely with **hemoglobin** (oxygen-carrying red pigment) in the red blood cells (RBCs) and is carried to the tissues as **oxyhemoglobin** (the compound of oxygen and hemoglobin).

Several factors affect the rate of oxygen transport from the lungs to the tissues:

1. Cardiac output
2. Number of erythrocytes and blood hematocrit
3. Exercise.

Any pathologic condition that decreases cardiac output (e.g., damage to the heart muscle, blood loss, or pooling of blood in the peripheral blood vessels) diminishes the amount of oxygen delivered to the tissues. The heart compensates for inadequate output by increasing its pumping rate or heart rate; however, with severe damage or blood loss, this compensatory mechanism may not restore adequate blood flow and oxygen to the tissues.

The second factor influencing oxygen transport is the number of **erythrocytes** or red blood cells (RBCs) and the hematocrit. The **hematocrit** is the percentage of the blood that is erythrocytes. Normally the hematocrit is about 40% to 54% in men and 37% to 50% in women. Excessive increases in the blood hematocrit raise the blood viscosity, reducing the cardiac output and therefore reducing oxygen transport. Excessive reductions in the blood hematocrit, such as occur in anemia, reduce oxygen transport.

Exercise also has a direct influence on oxygen transport. In well-trained athletes, oxygen transport can be increased up to 20 times the normal rate, due in part to an increased cardiac output and to increased use of oxygen by the cells.

Systemic Diffusion

The fourth process of respiration is diffusion of oxygen and carbon dioxide between the capillaries and the tissues and cells down to a concentration gradient similar to diffusion at the alveolar–capillary level. As cells consume oxygen, the partial pressure of oxygen in the tissues decreases, causing the oxygen at the arterial end of the capillary to diffuse into the cells. When cells consume more oxygen during exercise or stress, the pressure gradient increases and diffusion is enhanced, allowing the cells to regulate their own flow of oxygen. Carbon dioxide from metabolic processes accumulates in the tissues and diffuses into the capillaries where the partial pressure of carbon dioxide is lower. In reduced blood flow states such as shock, capillary blood flow may decrease, interfering with tissue oxygen delivery.

Respiratory Regulation

Respiratory regulation includes both neural and chemical controls to maintain the correct concentrations of oxygen, carbon dioxide, and hydrogen ions in body fluids. The nervous system of the body adjusts the rate of alveolar ventilations to meet the needs of the body so that PO_2 and PCO_2 remain relatively constant. The body's "respiratory center" is actually a number of groups of neurons located in the medulla oblongata and pons of the brain.

A chemosensitive center in the medulla oblongata is highly responsive to increases in blood CO_2 or hydrogen ion concentration. By influencing other respiratory centers, this center can increase the activity of the inspiratory center and the rate and depth of respirations. In addition to this direct chemical stimulation of the respiratory center in the brain, special neural receptors sensitive to decreases in oxygen (O_2) concentration are located outside the central nervous system in the carotid bodies (just above the bifurcation of the common carotid arteries) and aortic bodies located above and below the aortic arch. Decreases in arterial oxygen concentrations stimulate these chemoreceptors, and they in turn stimulate the respiratory center to increase ventilation. Of the three blood gases (hydrogen, oxygen, and carbon dioxide) that can trigger chemoreceptors, increased carbon dioxide concentration normally has the strongest effect on stimulating respiration.

However, in clients with certain chronic lung ailments such as **emphysema**, oxygen concentrations, not carbon dioxide concentrations, play a major role in regulating respiration. For some clients, decreased oxygen concentrations are the main stimuli for respiration because the chronically elevated carbon dioxide levels that occur with emphysema "desensitize" the central chemoreceptors. This is sometimes called the *hypoxic drive*. Increasing the concentration of oxygen depresses the respiratory rate. Thus, oxygen must be administered cautiously to these clients and often at low flow rates.

Clinical Alert!

Oxygen is considered a drug and must be carefully prescribed based on individual client conditions.

Factors Affecting Respiratory Function

Factors that influence oxygenation affect the cardiovascular system as well as the respiratory system. These factors include age, environment, lifestyle, health status, medications, and stress.

Age

Developmental factors have important influences on respiratory function. At birth, profound changes occur in the respiratory systems. The fluid-filled lungs drain, the PCO_2 rises, and the neonate takes a first breath. The lungs gradually expand with each subsequent breath, reaching full inflation by 2 weeks of age.

Changes of aging that affect the respiratory system of older adults become especially important if the system is compromised by changes such as infection, physical or emotional stress, surgery, anesthesia, or other procedures. These types of changes are seen:

- Chest wall and airways become more rigid and less elastic.
- The amount of exchanged air is decreased.
- The cough reflex and cilia action are decreased.
- Mucous membranes become drier and more fragile.
- Decreases in muscle strength and endurance occur.
- If osteoporosis is present, adequate lung expansion may be compromised.
- A decrease in efficiency of the immune system occurs.
- Gastroesophageal reflux disease is more common in older adults and increases the risk of aspiration. The aspiration of stomach contents into the lungs often causes bronchospasm by setting up an inflammatory response.

Environment

Altitude, heat, cold, and air pollution affect oxygenation. The higher the altitude, the lower the PO_2 an individual breathes. As a result, the individual at high altitudes has increased respiratory and cardiac rates and increased respiratory depth, which usually become most apparent when the individual exercises.

Healthy individuals exposed to air pollution, such as smog or secondhand tobacco smoke, may experience stinging of the eyes, headache, dizziness, and coughing. Individuals who have a history of existing lung disease and altered respiratory function experience varying degrees of respiratory difficulty in a polluted environment. Some are unable to perform self-care in such an environment.

Lifestyle

Physical exercise or activity increases the rate and depth of respirations and hence the supply of oxygen in the body. Sedentary individuals, by contrast, lack the alveolar expansion and deep-breathing patterns of individuals with regular activity and are less able to respond effectively to respiratory stressors.

Certain occupations predispose an individual to lung disease. For example, silicosis is seen more often in sandstone blasters and potters than in the rest of the population; anthracosis in coal miners; and organic dust disease in farmers and agricultural employees who work with moldy hay.

Health Status

In the healthy individual, the respiratory system can provide sufficient oxygen to meet the body's needs. Diseases of the respiratory system, however, can adversely affect the oxygenation of the blood.

Medications

A variety of medications can decrease the rate and depth of respirations. The most common medications having this effect are the benzodiazepine sedative–hypnotics and antianxiety drugs (e.g., diazepam [Valium], lorazepam [Ativan], midazolam [Versed]), barbiturates (e.g., phenobarbital), and opioids such as morphine. When administering these, the nurse must carefully monitor respiratory status, especially when the medication is begun or when the dose is increased. Older clients are at high risk of respiratory depression and usually require reduced dosages.

Stress

When stress and stressors are encountered, both psychologic and physiologic responses can affect oxygenation. Some individuals may hyperventilate in response to stress. When this occurs, arterial PO_2 rises and PCO_2 falls. The individual may experience light-headedness and numbness and tingling of the fingers, toes, and around the mouth as a result.

Physiologically, the sympathetic nervous system is stimulated and epinephrine is released during stress. Epinephrine causes the bronchioles to dilate, increasing blood flow and oxygen delivery to active muscles. Although these responses are adaptive in the short term, when stress continues they can be destructive, increasing the risk of cardiovascular disease.

Alterations in Respiratory Function

Respiratory function can be altered by conditions that affect:

- Patency (open airway)
- The movement of air into or out of the lungs
- The diffusion of oxygen and carbon dioxide between the alveoli and the pulmonary capillaries
- The transport of oxygen and carbon dioxide via the blood to and from the tissue cells.

Conditions Affecting the Airway

A completely or partially obstructed airway can occur anywhere along the upper or lower respiratory passageways. An upper airway obstruction—that is, in the nose, pharynx, or larynx—can occur when a foreign object such as food is present, when the tongue falls back into the oropharynx when an individual is unconscious, or when secretions collect in the passageways. Lower airway obstruction involves partial or complete occlusion of the passageways in the bronchi and lungs most often due to increased accumulation of mucus or inflammatory exudate.

Assessing for and maintaining a patent airway is a nursing responsibility, one that often requires immediate action. Partial obstruction of the upper airway passages is indicated by a low-pitched snoring sound during inhalation. Complete obstruction is indicated by extreme inspiratory effort that produces no chest movement and an inability to cough or speak. Such a client, in an effort to obtain air, may also exhibit marked sternal and intercostal retractions. Lower airway obstruction is not always as easy to observe. **Stridor**, a harsh, high-pitched sound, may be heard during inspiration. The client may have altered arterial blood gas levels, restlessness, dyspnea, and **adventitious breath sounds** (abnormal breath sounds). See Table 29.8, page 610.

Conditions Affecting Movement of Air

The term *breathing patterns* refers to the rate, volume, rhythm, and relative ease or effort of respiration. Normal respiration (**eupnea**) is quiet, rhythmic, and effortless. **Tachypnea** (rapid respirations) is seen with fevers, metabolic acidosis, pain, and hypoxemia. **Bradypnea** is an abnormally slow respiratory rate, which may be seen in clients who have taken drugs such as morphine or sedatives, who have metabolic alkalosis, or who have increased intracranial pressure (e.g., from brain injuries). **Apnea** is the absence of any breathing.

Hypoventilation, that is, inadequate alveolar ventilation, may be caused by either slow or shallow breathing, or both. Hypoventilation may occur because of diseases of the respiratory muscles, drugs, or anesthesia. Hypoventilation may lead to increased levels of carbon dioxide (**hypercarbia** or **hypercapnia**) or low levels of oxygen (hypoxemia).

Hyperventilation is the increased movement of air into and out of the lungs. During hyperventilation, the rate and depth of respirations increase and more CO_2 is eliminated than is produced. Hyperventilation can also occur in response to stress or anxiety.

Orthopnea is the inability to breathe easily unless sitting upright or standing. Difficulty breathing or the feeling of being short of breath (SOB) is called **dyspnea**. Dyspnea may occur with varying levels of exertion or at rest. The client with dyspnea will generally have observable (objective) signs such as flaring of the nostrils, labored-appearing breathing, increased heart rate, cyanosis, and diaphoresis. Dyspnea has many causes, most of which stem from cardiac or respiratory disorders.

Conditions Affecting Diffusion

Impaired diffusion may affect levels of gases in the blood, particularly oxygen, which does not diffuse as readily as carbon dioxide. **Hypoxemia**, or reduced oxygen levels in the blood, may be caused by conditions that impair diffusion at the alveolar–capillary level such as pulmonary edema or atelectasis (collapsed alveoli) or by low hemoglobin levels. The cardiovascular system compensates for hypoxemia by increasing the heart rate and cardiac output, to attempt to move adequate oxygen to the tissues. If the cardiovascular system is unable to compensate or hypoxemia is severe, tissue **hypoxia** (insufficient oxygen anywhere in the body) results, potentially causing cellular injury or death. Box 49.1 lists signs of hypoxia. **Cyanosis** (bluish discoloration of the skin, nail beds, and mucous membranes due to reduced hemoglobin and decreased oxygen saturation) may be present with hypoxemia or hypoxia.

BOX 49.1 Hypoxia

- Rapid pulse
- Rapid, shallow respirations and dyspnea
- Increased restlessness or light-headedness
- Flaring of the nares
- Substernal or intercostal retractions
- Cyanosis

Adequate oxygenation is essential for cerebral functioning. The cerebral cortex can tolerate hypoxia for only 3 to 5 minutes before permanent damage occurs. The face of the acutely hypoxic individual usually appears anxious, tired, and drawn. The individual usually assumes a sitting position, often leaning forward slightly to permit greater expansion of the thoracic cavity.

Conditions Affecting Transport

Once oxygen moves into the lungs and diffuses into the capillaries, the cardiovascular system carries the oxygen to all body tissues, and moves CO_2 from the cells back to the lungs where it can be exhaled from the body. Conditions that decrease cardiac output, such as heart failure or hypovolemia, affect tissue oxygenation and also the body's ability to compensate for hypoxemia.

●○● NURSING MANAGEMENT

Assessing

Nursing assessment of oxygenation status includes a history, physical examination, and review of relevant diagnostic data.

Nursing History

A comprehensive nursing history relevant to oxygenation status should include data about current and past respiratory problems; lifestyle; presence of cough, **sputum** (coughed-up material), or pain; medications for breathing; and presence of risk factors for impaired oxygenation status. Examples of interview questions to elicit this information are shown in the Assessment Interview.

LIFESPAN CONSIDERATIONS Respiratory Development

INFANTS

- Respiratory rates are highest and most variable in newborns. The respiratory rate of a neonate is 40 to 80 breaths per minute.
- Infant respiratory rates average about 30 per minute.
- Because of rib cage structure, infants rely almost exclusively on diaphragmatic movement for breathing. This is seen as abdominal breathing, as the abdomen rises and falls with each breath.

CHILDREN

- The respiratory rate gradually decreases, averaging around 25 per minute in the preschooler and reaching the adult rate of 12 to 18 per minute by late adolescence.
- During infancy and childhood, viral upper respiratory infections (e.g., colds) are common and, fortunately, usually not serious. Infants and preschoolers also are at risk for airway obstruction by foreign objects such as coins and small toys. Cystic fibrosis is a congenital disorder that affects the lungs, causing them to become congested with thick, tenacious (sticky) mucus. Asthma is another chronic disease often identified in childhood. The airways of the asthmatic child react to stimuli such as allergens, exercise, or cold air by constricting, becoming edematous, and producing excessive mucus. Airflow is impaired, and the child may wheeze as air moves through narrowed air passages.

OLDER ADULTS

- Older adults are at increased risk for acute respiratory diseases such as pneumonia and chronic diseases such as emphysema and chronic bronchitis. Chronic obstructive pulmonary disease (COPD) may affect older adults, particularly after years of exposure to cigarette smoke or industrial pollutants. Obstructive airway changes are accelerated with the genetic deficiency of the enzyme alpha$_1$-antitrypsin.
- Pneumonia may not present with the usual symptoms of a fever, but will present with atypical symptoms, such as confusion, weakness, loss of appetite, and increase in heart rate and respirations.

Nursing interventions should be directed toward achieving optimal respiratory effort, gas exchange, self-care habits, and wellness. Additionally, nurses play an important role in chronic disease management by assisting clients to cope with and minimize the effects of illnesses such as COPD.

- Always encourage wellness and prevention of disease by reinforcing the need for good nutrition, exercise, and immunizations, such as for influenza and pneumonia.
- Increase fluid intake, if not contraindicated by other problems, such as cardiac or renal impairment.
- In hospitalized and immobile clients, encourage ambulation and frequent changing of positions to allow for better lung expansion and air and fluid movement.
- Teach the client to use deep-breathing and coughing techniques for better lung expansion and airway clearance. (See Client Teaching throughout this chapter.)
- Pace activities to conserve energy.
- Encourage the client to eat more frequent, smaller meals to decrease gastric distention, which can cause pressure on the diaphragm.
- Teach the client to avoid extreme hot or cold temperatures, which can further tax the respiratory system.
- Teach actions and side effects of drugs, inhalers, and treatments.

ASSESSMENT INTERVIEW Oxygenation

CURRENT RESPIRATORY PROBLEMS

- Have you noticed any changes in your breathing pattern (e.g., shortness of breath, difficulty breathing, need to be in upright position to breathe, or rapid and shallow breathing)?
- If so, which of your activities might cause these symptom(s) to occur?
- How many pillows do you use to sleep at night?

HISTORY OF RESPIRATORY DISEASE

- Have you had colds, allergies, asthma, tuberculosis, bronchitis, pneumonia, or emphysema?
- How frequently have these occurred? How long did they last? And how were they treated?
- Have you been exposed to any pollutants?

LIFESTYLE

- Do you smoke? If so, how much? If not, did you smoke previously, and when did you stop?
- Does any member of your family smoke?
- Is there cigarette smoke or other pollutants (e.g., fumes, dust, coal, asbestos) in your workplace?
- Do you use alcohol? If so, how many drinks (mixed drinks, glasses of wine, or beers) do you usually have per day or per week?
- Describe your exercise patterns. How often do you exercise and for how long?

PRESENCE OF COUGH

- How often and how much do you cough?
- Is it productive, that is, accompanied by sputum, or nonproductive, that is, dry?
- Does the cough occur during certain activity or at certain times of the day?

DESCRIPTION OF SPUTUM

- When is the sputum produced?
- What is the amount, color, thickness, odor?
- Is it ever tinged with blood?

PRESENCE OF CHEST PAIN

- How does going outside in the heat or the cold affect you?
- Do you experience any pain with breathing or activity?
- If so, where is the pain located?
- Describe the pain. How does it feel?
- Does it occur when you breathe in or out?
- How long does it last, and how does it affect your breathing?
- Do you experience any other symptoms when the pain occurs (e.g., nausea, shortness of breath or difficulty breathing, lightheadedness, palpitations)?
- What activities precede your pain?
- What do you do to relieve the pain?

PRESENCE OF RISK FACTORS

- Do you have a family history of lung cancer, cardiovascular disease (including strokes), or tuberculosis?
- The nurse should also note the client's weight, activity pattern, and dietary assessment. Risk factors include obesity, sedentary lifestyle, and diet high in saturated fats.

MEDICATION HISTORY

- Have you taken or do you take any over-the-counter or prescription medications for breathing (e.g., bronchodilator, inhalant, narcotic)?
- If so, which ones? What are the dosages, times taken, and results, including side effects?

Physical Examination

In assessing a client's oxygenation status, the nurse uses all four physical examination techniques: inspection, palpation, percussion, and auscultation. The nurse first observes the rate, depth, rhythm, and quality of respirations, noting the position the client assumes for breathing. The nurse also inspects for variations in the shape of the thorax that may indicate adaptation to chronic respiratory conditions. For example, clients with emphysema frequently develop a *barrel chest*.

The nurse palpates the thorax for bulges, tenderness, or abnormal movements. Palpation is also used to detect vocal (tactile) fremitus. The thorax can be percussed for diaphragmatic excursion (the movement of the diaphragm during maximal inspiration and expiration). However, this is not commonly done in acute care and long-term care settings. The nurse frequently auscultates the chest to assess if the client's breath sounds are normal or abnormal. See Chapter 29 ∞, Skill 29.11 on page 611 for more information.

Diagnostic Studies

The primary care provider may order various diagnostic tests to assess respiratory status, function, and oxygenation. Included are sputum specimens, throat cultures, visualization procedures (see Chapter 34 ∞), venous and arterial blood specimens, and pulmonary function tests.

Measurement of arterial blood gases is an important diagnostic procedure (see Chapter 51 ∞). Specimens of arterial blood are normally taken by specialty nurses, respiratory therapists, or medical technicians. Blood for these tests is taken directly from the radial, brachial, or femoral arteries or from catheters placed in these arteries. Because of the relatively high pressure of the blood in these arteries, it is important to prevent hemorrhaging by applying pressure to the puncture site for about 5 minutes after removing the needle. Frequently the noninvasive measurement of oxygen saturation (using a device placed on the fingertip) is sufficient for attaining a measurement of oxygenation of the arterial blood.

Pulmonary Function Tests

Pulmonary function tests measure lung volume and capacity. Clients undergoing pulmonary function tests, which are usually carried out by a respiratory therapist, do not require an anesthetic. The client breathes into a machine. The tests are painless, but the client's cooperation is essential. It requires the ability to follow directions and some hand–eye coordination. Nurses need to explain the tests to clients beforehand and help them to rest afterward because the tests are often tiring. Table 49.1 describes the measurements taken, and Figure 49.3 ■ shows their relationships and normal adult values.

Diagnosing

Examples of nursing diagnoses for clients with oxygenation problems can include altered respiratory status, altered breathing pattern, altered gas exchange, and inadequate physical energy for activities. The preceding nursing diagnoses may also be the etiology of several other nursing diagnoses, such as fatigue related to altered breathing pattern, insomnia related to orthopnea and required oxygen therapy, and social seclusion related to inadequate physical energy for activities and inability to travel to usual social activities.

Planning

The overall outcomes or goals for a client with oxygenation problems are to:

- Maintain a patent airway.
- Improve comfort and ease of breathing.
- Maintain or improve pulmonary ventilation and oxygenation.
- Improve the ability to participate in physical activities.
- Prevent risks associated with oxygenation problems such as skin and tissue breakdown, syncope, acid–base imbalances, and feelings of hopelessness and social isolation.

TABLE 49.1 Pulmonary Volumes and Capacities

Measurement	Description
Tidal volume (V_T)	Volume inhaled and exhaled during normal quiet breathing
Inspiratory reserve volume (IRV)	Maximum amount of air that can be inhaled over and above a normal breath
Expiratory reserve volume (ERV)	Maximum amount of air that can be exhaled following a normal exhalation
Residual volume (RV)	The amount of air remaining in the lungs after maximal exhalation
Total lung capacity (TLC)	The total volume of the lungs at maximum inflation; calculated by adding the V_T, IRV, ERV, and RV
Vital capacity (VC)	Total amount of air that can be exhaled after a maximal inspiration; calculated by adding the V_T, IRV, and ERV
Inspiratory capacity	Total amount of air that can be inhaled following normal quiet exhalation; calculated by adding the V_T and IRV
Functional residual capacity (FRC)	The volume left in the lungs after normal exhalation; calculated by adding the ERV and RV
Minute volume (MV)	The total volume or amount of air breathed in 1 minute

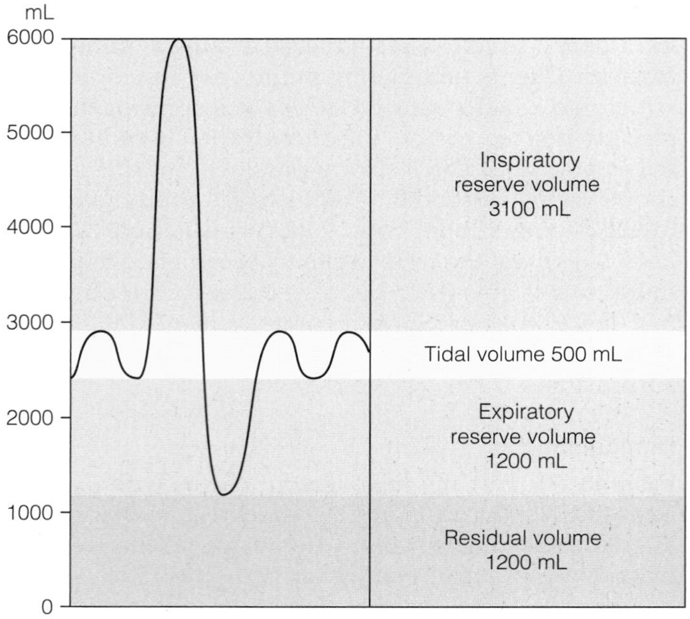

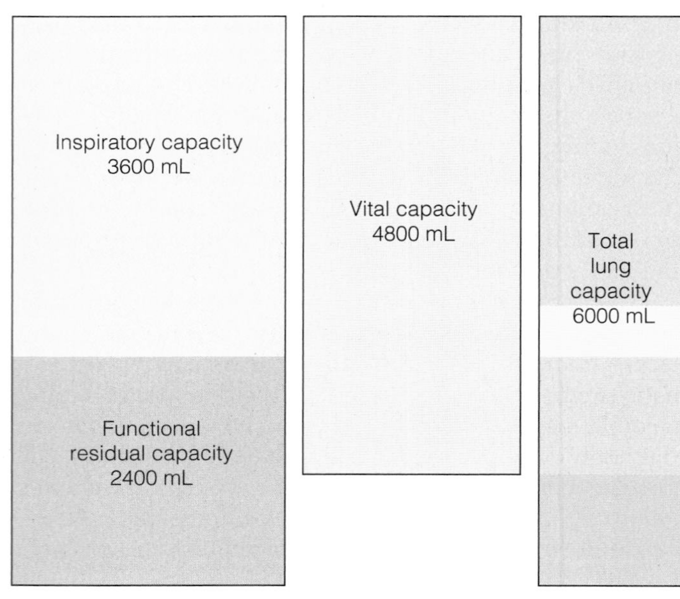

Figure 49.3 ■ The relationship of lung volumes and capacities. Volumes (mL) shown are for an average adult male; female volumes are 20% to 25% smaller.

These outcomes provide direction for planning interventions and as criteria for evaluating client progress.

A clinical example of desired outcomes, interventions, and activities is provided in the Nursing Care Plan and Concept Map at the end of the chapter.

Planning for Home Care

To provide for continuity of care, the nurse needs to consider the client's learning needs and needs for assistance with care in the home. *Client Teaching: Home Care Oxygenation* addresses the learning needs of the client and family. Planning incorporates an assessment of the client's and family's knowledge and abilities for self-care, financial resources, and evaluation of the need for referrals and for home health services.

QSEN Patient-Centered Care: Oxygenation

When conducting a home care assessment for a client with oxygenation problems and needs, the nurse includes the following assessments:

CLIENT

- *Self-care abilities:* ability to ambulate and perform activities of daily living (ADLs) independently
- *Exercise and activity pattern:* type and regularity of usual exercise, perceived and actual energy for desired and required leisure activities
- *Assistive devices required:* supplemental oxygen, humidifier, nebulizer treatments, or inhalers; walker, cane, or wheelchair; grab bars, shower chair, and other devices to promote safety and minimize energy expenditure; scale to monitor weight on a regular basis
- *Home environment for factors that impair airway clearance, gas exchange, or activity tolerance:* indoor pollutants such as cigarette smoke, dust, and allergens such as pets; lack of humidity in the air; and barriers such as stairs
- *Current level of knowledge:* importance of avoiding smoking and other pollutants; dietary salt and other restrictions (if appropriate); recommended activities; medications; need to limit exposure to respiratory infections; use of prescribed nebulizer, multidose inhaler, powdered dose inhaler, or home oxygen; activity level

FAMILY

- *Caregiver availability, skills, and responses:* ability and willingness to provide care as needed (help with ADLs, providing meals, assisting with transportation and shopping, caring for dependents; performing treatments such as percussion and postural drainage)
- *Family role changes and coping:* effect on financial status, parenting and spousal roles, sexuality, social roles
- *Alternate potential primary or respite caregivers:* for example, other family members, volunteers, church members, paid caregivers, or housekeeping services; available community respite care (e.g., adult day care, senior centers)

COMMUNITY

- *Environment:* usual temperature and humidity; presence of air pollutants such as automobile exhaust, industrial smoke and pollutants, smoke from field burning
- *Current knowledge of and experience with community resources:* medical and assistive equipment and supply companies, respiratory and physical therapy services, home health agencies, local pharmacies, available financial assistance, support and educational organizations such as the local lung association, COPD support groups

CLIENT TEACHING Home Care Oxygenation

MAINTAINING AIRWAY CLEARANCE AND EFFECTIVE GAS EXCHANGE

- Emphasize to the client and family the importance of not smoking or lighting any flammable materials (e.g., candles) in the same room. Refer them to smoking cessation programs as needed. For family members resistant to not smoking, emphasize the need to avoid smoking inside the home.
- Instruct the client in effective coughing techniques such as controlled coughing or "huff" coughing (see *Client Teaching: Forced Expiratory Technique (Huff Coughing)* in the *Implementing* section).
- Discuss the significance of changes in sputum, including the amount and characteristics such as color, viscosity, and odor. Instruct the client when to contact a healthcare provider.
- Teach the client to maintain a fluid intake of 2500 to 3000 mL (2.5 to 3 qt) per day if not contraindicated due to other health conditions such as heart failure or renal disease.
- Instruct the client of the rationale for using and how to use nebulizers or inhalers if prescribed; see Chapter 35 ∞, pages 908–911.
- Teach the client and family how to use home oxygen delivery systems, emphasizing safety considerations.

PROMOTING EFFECTIVE BREATHING

- Teach relaxation techniques such as progressive muscle relaxation, meditation, and visualization. Use DVDs or phone apps as needed.
- Help the client identify specific factors that affect breathing such as stress, exposure to allergens or air pollution, and exposure to cold. Assist with identifying possible interventions and measures to avoid these factors.

MEDICATIONS

- Teach the client about prescribed medications, including the rationale for the medications, the dose, the desired and possible adverse effects, and any precautions about using a medication with food, beverages, or other medications.

SPECIFIC MEASURES FOR OXYGENATION PROBLEMS

- Provide instructions and rationale for specific procedures and problems such as:
  a. Suctioning oropharyngeal and nasopharyngeal cavities
  b. Caring for a temporary or permanent tracheostomy
  c. Preventing the spread of tuberculosis and other respiratory infections to family members and others.

REFERRALS

- Make appropriate referrals to home health agencies or community social services for assistance in obtaining medical and assistive equipment such as grab bars, respiratory and physical therapy services, and home health or housekeeping services to assist with ADLs.

COMMUNITY AGENCIES AND OTHER SOURCES OF HELP

- Provide information about where durable medical equipment can be purchased, rented, or obtained free of charge; how to access home oxygen equipment and support services and physical and occupational therapy services; and where to obtain supplies such as tracheostomy supplies or nutritional supplements.
- Suggest additional sources of information such as the American Lung Association and the Asthma and Allergy Foundation of America.

Implementing

Examples of nursing interventions to facilitate pulmonary ventilation may include ensuring a patent airway, positioning, encouraging deep breathing and coughing, and ensuring adequate hydration. Other nursing interventions helpful to ventilation are suctioning, lung inflation techniques, administration of analgesics before deep breathing and coughing, postural drainage, and percussion and vibration. Nursing strategies to facilitate the diffusion of gases through the alveolar membrane include encouraging coughing, deep breathing, and suitable activity. A client's nursing care plan should also include appropriate dependent nursing interventions such as oxygen therapy, tracheostomy care, and maintenance of a chest tube.

Promoting Oxygenation

Most individuals in good health give little thought to their respiratory function. Changing position frequently, ambulating, and exercising usually maintain adequate ventilation and gas exchange.

Client Teaching lists other ways to promote healthy breathing.

When individuals become ill, however, their respiratory functions may be inhibited for such reasons as pain and immobility. Shallow respirations inhibit both diaphragmatic excursion and lung distensibility. The result of inadequate chest expansion is pooling of respiratory secretions, which ultimately harbor microorganisms and promote infection. Additionally, shallow respirations may potentiate alveolar collapse, which may cause decreased diffusion of gases and subsequent hypoxemia.

CLIENT TEACHING Promoting Healthy Breathing

- Sit straight and stand erect to permit full lung expansion.
- Exercise regularly.
- Breathe through the nose.
- Breathe in to expand the chest fully.
- Do not smoke cigarettes, cigars, or pipes.
- Eliminate or reduce the use of household pesticides and irritating chemical substances.
- Do not incinerate garbage in the house.
- Avoid exposure to secondhand smoke.
- Use building materials that do not emit vapors.
- Make sure furnaces, ovens, and wood stoves are correctly ventilated.
- Support a pollution-free environment.

Interventions by the nurse to maintain the normal respirations of clients include:

- Positioning the client to allow for maximum chest expansion
- Encouraging or providing frequent changes in position
- Encouraging deep breathing and coughing

- Encouraging ambulation
- Implementing measures that promote comfort, such as giving pain medications.

The semi-Fowler's or high-Fowler's position allows maximum chest expansion in clients who are confined to bed, particularly those with dyspnea. The nurse also encourages clients to turn from side to side frequently, so that alternate sides of the chest are permitted maximum expansion. Clients with severe pneumonia or other pulmonary disease in one lung, if positioned laterally, should be generally positioned with the "good lung down" to improve diffusion of oxygen to the blood from functioning alveoli. Dyspneic clients often sit in bed and lean over their overbed tables (which are raised to a suitable height), usually with a pillow for support. This orthopneic position is an adaptation of the high-Fowler's position. Some clients also sit upright and lean on their arms or elbows, which is called the tripod position. The advantage to these positions is that each one forces the diaphragm down and forward and stabilizes the chest, which reduces the work of breathing. Also, a client in the orthopneic position can press the lower part of the chest against the table to help in exhaling (Figure 49.4 ■).

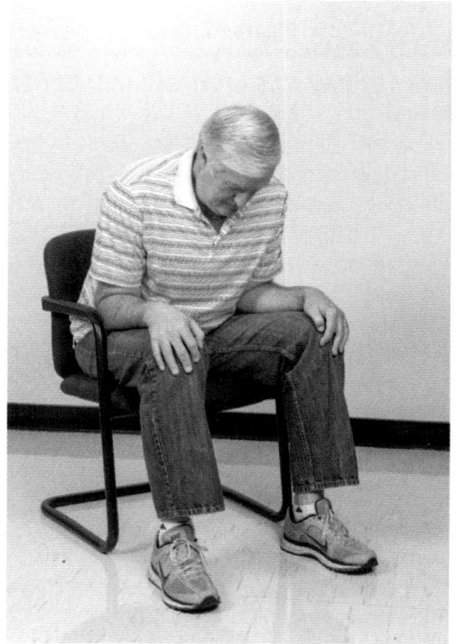

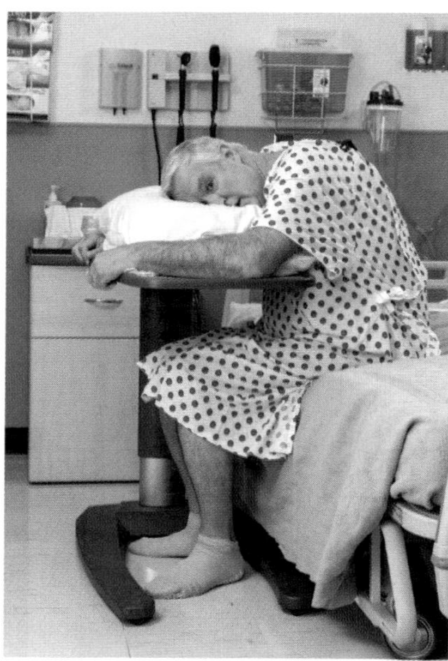

Figure 49.4 ■ Two sitting tripod positions that help assist with breathing.

Deep Breathing and Coughing

The nurse can facilitate respiratory functioning by encouraging deep-breathing exercises and coughing to remove secretions from the airways. When coughing raises secretions high enough, the client may either **expectorate** (spit out) or swallow them. Swallowing the secretions is not harmful but does not allow the nurse to view the secretions for documentation purposes or to obtain a specimen for testing.

Clients with conditions that increase secretions or impair mobilization of secretions such as chest surgery, COPD, or cystic fibrosis often require encouragement to cough and breathe deeply. Specialized breathing exercises may be prescribed for clients with chronic obstructive diseases as part of their pulmonary rehabilitation. These generally require collaboration with other healthcare providers. One technique, pursed-lip breathing, may help alleviate dyspnea. The client is taught to breathe in normally through the nose and exhale through pursed lips as if about to whistle, and blow slowly and purposefully, tightening the abdominal muscles to assist with exhalation. Clients may practice by slowly blowing a ping-pong ball across a table or visualizing that they are trying to make a candle flame waver.

Normal forceful coughing is highly effective, but some clients may lack the strength or ability to cough normally. Normal forceful coughing involves the client inhaling deeply and then coughing twice while exhaling. Alternative cough techniques such as forced expiratory technique, or huff coughing, may be taught as alternatives for those clients who are unable to perform a normal forceful cough. A client with a pulmonary condition (e.g., COPD) is instructed to exhale through pursed lips and to exhale with a "huff" sound in mid-exhalation. The huff cough helps prevent the high expiratory pressures that collapse diseased airways. This cough technique is described in Client Teaching.

Hydration

Adequate hydration maintains the moisture of the respiratory mucous membranes. Normally, respiratory tract secretions are thin and are therefore moved readily by ciliary action. However, when the client is dehydrated or when the environment has a low humidity, the respiratory secretions can become thick and tenacious. Fluid intake should be as great as the client can tolerate. See Chapter 51 ∞ for normal daily fluid intake.

CLIENT TEACHING Forced Expiratory Technique (Huff Coughing)

- After using a bronchodilator treatment (if prescribed), inhale deeply and hold your breath for a few seconds.
- Cough twice while exhaling. The first cough loosens the mucus; the second expels secretions.
- For huff coughing, lean forward and exhale sharply with a "huff" sound mid-exhalation. This technique helps keep your airways open while moving secretions up and out of the lungs.
- Inhale by taking rapid short breaths in succession ("sniffing") to prevent mucus from moving back into smaller airways.
- Rest and breathe slowly between coughs.
- Try to avoid prolonged episodes of coughing because these may cause fatigue and hypoxia.

Humidifiers are devices that add water vapor to inspired air. Room humidifiers provide cool mist to room air. Nebulizers are used to deliver humidity and medications. They may be used with oxygen delivery systems to provide moistened air directly to the client. Their purposes are to prevent mucous membranes from drying and becoming irritated and to loosen secretions for easier expectoration.

Medications

A number of types of medications can be used for clients with oxygenation problems.

Bronchodilators, anti-inflammatory drugs, leukotriene modifiers, expectorants, and cough suppressants are some medications that may be used to treat respiratory problems. *Bronchodilators,* including sympathomimetic drugs and xanthines, reduce bronchospasm, opening tight or congested airways and facilitating ventilation. These drugs may be administered orally or intravenously, but the preferred route is by inhalation to prevent many systemic side effects.

Because drugs used to dilate the bronchioles and improve breathing are usually drugs that enhance the sympathetic nervous system, clients must be monitored for side effects of increased heart rate, blood pressure, anxiety, and restlessness. This is especially important in older adults, who may also have cardiac problems. Some over-the-counter drugs for respiratory problems have these same effects, so clients should be cautioned about taking them without checking with their primary care provider.

Another class of drugs used is the *anti-inflammatory drugs,* such as glucocorticoids. They can be given orally, intravenously, or by inhaler. They work by decreasing the edema and inflammation in the airways and allowing a better air exchange. If both bronchodilators and anti-inflammatory drugs are ordered by inhaler, the client should be instructed to use the bronchodilator inhaler first and then the anti-inflammatory inhaler. If the bronchioles are dilated first, more tissue is exposed on which the anti-inflammatory drugs can act. Newer formulations may combine a long-acting bronchodilator with an inhaled corticosteroid to improve client compliance with therapy because they require less time and less frequent dosing.

Another class of drugs is the *leukotriene modifiers.* These medications decrease the effects of leukotrienes on the smooth muscle of the respiratory tract. Leukotrienes cause bronchoconstriction, mucous production, and edema of the respiratory tract.

Expectorants help "break up" mucus, making it more liquid and easier to expectorate. Guaifenesin is a common expectorant found in many prescription and nonprescription cough syrups. When frequent or prolonged coughing interrupts sleep, *cough suppressants* such as codeine may be prescribed.

Other medications can be used to improve oxygenation by improving cardiovascular function. The *digitalis glycosides* act directly on the heart to improve the strength of contraction and slow the heart rate. *Beta-adrenergic stimulating agents* such as dobutamine similarly increase cardiac output, thus improving oxygen transport. *Beta-adrenergic blocking agents* such as propranolol affect the sympathetic nervous system to reduce the workload of the heart. These drugs, however, can negatively affect people with asthma or COPD because they may constrict airways by blocking beta-2 adrenergic receptors.

Percussion, Vibration, and Postural Drainage

Percussion, vibration, and postural drainage (PVD) are performed according to a primary care provider's order by nurses, respiratory therapists, physical therapists, or an interdisciplinary team of these healthcare team members. Percussion, sometimes called *clapping,* is forceful striking of the skin with cupped hands. Mechanical percussion cups and vibrators are also available. When the hands are used, the fingers and thumb are held together and flexed slightly to form a cup, as one would to scoop up water. Percussion over congested lung areas can mechanically dislodge tenacious secretions from the bronchial walls. Cupped hands trap the air against the chest. The trapped air then sets up vibrations through the chest wall to the secretions.

To percuss a client's chest, follow these steps:

- Cover the area with a towel or gown to reduce discomfort.
- Ask the client to breathe slowly and deeply to promote relaxation.
- Alternately flex and extend the wrists rapidly to slap the chest (Figure 49.5 ■).
- Percuss each affected lung segment for 1 to 2 minutes.

When done correctly, the percussion action should produce a hollow, popping sound. Percussion is avoided over the breasts, sternum, spinal column, and kidneys.

CLIENT TEACHING Using Cough Medications

- Do not take cough medications in excessive amounts because of adverse side effects.
- If you have diabetes mellitus, avoid cough syrups that contain sugar or alcohol; these can disturb metabolism.
- When a cough medicine does not act as expected, consult a healthcare professional.
- Be aware of side effects (e.g., drowsiness) that can make the operation of machinery dangerous.

DRUG CAPSULE

Sympathomimetics: albuterol (Proventil, Ventolin)

CLIENT WITH RESPIRATORY MEDICATIONS THAT CAUSE BRONCHODILATION BY STIMULATING BETA-2 ADRENERGIC RECEPTORS IN THE LUNG

The beta-2 adrenergic agonists are called *sympathomimetic drugs* because they "mimic" the action of sympathetic stimulation to the beta-2 receptors in the smooth muscle of the lung. At therapeutic levels these drugs promote bronchodilation and so relieve bronchospasm.

Sympathomimetic agents are useful in the treatment of bronchospasm in reversible obstructive airway diseases such as asthma and bronchitis. They are also useful in preventing exercise-induced bronchospasm.

Drugs that block the parasympathetic nervous system (anticholinergics) such as ipratropium (Atrovent) may be used alone or in combination (Combivent) with sympathomimetic agents to provide additional bronchodilation.

NURSING RESPONSIBILITIES

- Most inhaled sympathomimetics have a very rapid onset and short duration of action, so they are useful for relief of acute attacks but not for prophylaxis.
- Monitor the client's respiratory status while administering sympathomimetics. This includes respiratory rate, lung sounds, oxygen saturation, and subjective symptoms.
- These medications should be used with caution in clients with conditions such as cardiac disease, vascular disease, hypertension, hyperthyroidism, and pregnancy.
- Monitor the client for common side effects including increased heart rate (due to sympathetic stimulation of the heart) and tremors.
- Monitor for other side effects that occur with excessive dosing, which may include CNS stimulation, gastrointestinal upset, hypertension, and sweating.

CLIENT AND FAMILY TEACHING

- Caution the client to use the least amount of medication needed to get relief for the shortest time period necessary. This will help prevent adverse effects.
- Counsel the client to report immediately any chest pain or changes in heart rate or rhythm.
- Teach the client and family how to use the delivery system. This will most often be a metered-dose inhaler (MDI) or dry powder inhaler (DPI) or nebulizer.
- Teach the client to record the frequency and intensity of symptoms.

Note: Prior to administering any medication, review all aspects with a current drug handbook or other reliable source.

DRUG CAPSULE

Glucocorticosteroids Inhaled: fluticasone (Flovent)

CLIENT WITH RESPIRATORY MEDICATIONS THAT SUPPRESS INFLAMMATION

Glucocorticosteroids are administered to clients with oxygenation problems to suppress inflammation. They can be administered either by inhalation, orally, or intravenously. The route of administration depends on the severity of the client's disorder and the individual's response. Glucocorticosteroids (steroids) are well absorbed from the respiratory tract so giving them by inhalation is often effective. Steroids suppress the inflammatory response in the airways by decreasing synthesis and release of inflammatory mediators, decreasing activity of inflammatory cells, and decreasing edema.

NURSING RESPONSIBILITIES

- Glucocorticosteroids are intended for preventive therapy. They will not be useful in an acute attack.
- If the client is also taking a sympathomimetic medication, delivery of inhaled corticosteroids to the respiratory tract may be enhanced by administering the sympathomimetic first (and waiting 3 to 5 minutes).
- It is important to monitor the client's respiratory status while administering steroids. This includes respiratory rate, lung sounds, oxygen saturation, and subjective symptoms.
- These medications should be used with caution or not at all in clients with conditions such as allergy, pregnancy, lactation, and systemic infections.
- Monitor the client for side effects of the medications. Most commonly this could be an increase in heart rate (due to sympathetic stimulation of the heart) and tremors.
- The client should be monitored for other side effects, which will usually only occur with excessive dosing and may include CNS stimulation, gastrointestinal upset, hypertension, and sweating.

CLIENT AND FAMILY TEACHING

- Caution the client to use the least amount needed to get relief for the shortest time period necessary. This will help prevent adverse effects. Alternate-day therapy may be recommended to decrease adrenal suppression.
- Make sure the client understands that these drugs are *not* for acute attacks. They are intended to be preventive therapy.
- Teach the client and family how to use the delivery system. This will most often be a metered-dose inhaler (MDI) or dry powder inhaler (DPI) or nebulizer.
- Counsel the client to rinse the mouth after using inhaled corticosteroids to decrease the risk of oropharyngeal or esophageal fungal infections (thrush).
- Counsel the client to report adverse effects such as sore throat, hoarseness, and pharyngeal and laryngeal fungal infections.
- Teach the client to record the frequency and intensity of symptoms.

Note: Prior to administering any medication, review all aspects with a current drug handbook or other reliable source.

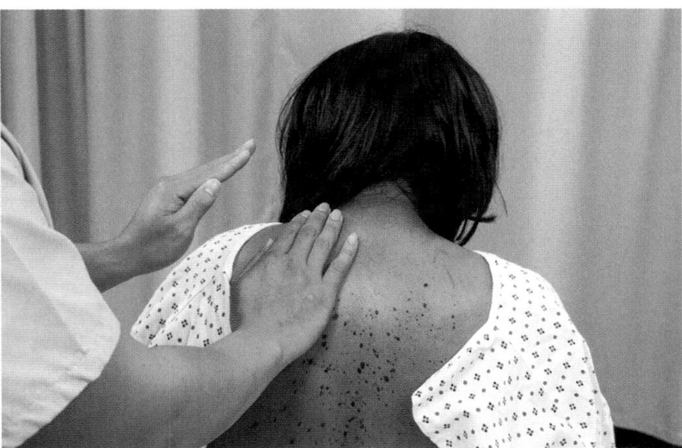

Figure 49.5 ■ Percussing the upper posterior chest.

Vibration is a series of vigorous quiverings produced by hands that are placed flat against the client's chest wall. Vibration is used after percussion to increase the turbulence of the exhaled air and thus loosen thick secretions. It is often done alternately with percussion.

To vibrate the client's chest, the nurse follows these steps:

- Place hands, palms down, on the chest area to be drained, one hand over the other with the fingers together and extended (Figure 49.6 ■). Alternatively, the hands may be placed side by side.
- Ask the client to inhale deeply and exhale slowly through the nose or pursed lips.
- During the exhalation, tense all the hand and arm muscles, and using mostly the heel of the hand, vibrate (shake) the hands, moving them downward. Stop the vibrating when the client inhales.
- Vibrate during five exhalations over one affected lung segment.
- After each vibration, encourage the client to cough and expectorate secretions into the sputum container.

Postural drainage is the drainage by gravity of secretions from various lung segments. Secretions that remain in the lungs or respiratory airways promote bacterial growth and subsequent infection. They also can obstruct the smaller airways and cause atelectasis. Secretions in the major airways, such as the trachea and the right and left main bronchi, are usually coughed into the pharynx, where they can be expectorated, swallowed, or effectively removed by suctioning.

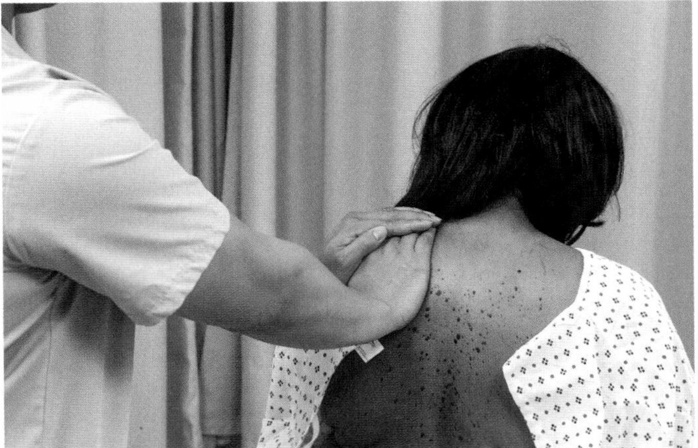

Figure 49.6 ■ Vibrating the upper posterior chest.

A wide variety of positions is necessary to drain all segments of the lungs, but not all positions are required for every client. Only those positions that drain specific affected areas are used. The lower lobes require drainage most frequently because the upper lobes drain by gravity. Before postural drainage, the client may be given a bronchodilator medication or nebulization therapy to loosen secretions. Postural drainage treatments are scheduled two or three times daily, depending on the degree of lung congestion. The best times include before breakfast, before lunch, in the late afternoon, and before bedtime. It is best to avoid hours shortly after meals because postural drainage at these times can be tiring and can induce vomiting.

The nurse needs to evaluate the client's tolerance of postural drainage by assessing the stability of the client's vital signs, particularly the pulse and respiratory rates, and by noting signs of intolerance, such as pallor, diaphoresis, dyspnea, nausea, and fatigue. Some clients do not react well to certain drainage positions, and the nurse must make appropriate adjustments. For example, some become dyspneic in Trendelenburg's position and require only a moderate tilt or a shorter time in that position.

The sequence for PVD is usually as follows: positioning, percussion, vibration, and removal of secretions by coughing or suction. Each position is usually assumed for 10 to 15 minutes, although beginning treatments may start with shorter times and gradually increase.

Following PVD, the nurse should auscultate the client's lungs, compare the findings to the baseline data, and document the amount, color, and character of expectorated secretions.

Today, kinetic therapy beds with modalities such as vibration and percussion therapy are available. These beds provide continuous lateral rotational therapy (CLRT) along with vibration and percussion modules that are programmed to perform for a specific amount of time.

Mucus Clearance Devices

A **mucus clearance device (MCD)** is used for clients with excessive secretions such as with cystic fibrosis, COPD, and bronchiectasis. The Flutter MCD is an example of one of these devices. It is a small, handheld device with a hard plastic mouthpiece at one end and a perforated cover at the other end. Inside the device is a steel ball that sits in a circular cone shape (Figure 49.7 ■). The client inhales slowly and then, keeping the cheeks firm, exhales fast through the device, causing the steel ball to move up and down. This movement causes vibrations that loosen mucus from the airways and assist its movement up the airways to be expectorated.

Oxygen Therapy

The medical administration of supplemental oxygen is considered to be a process similar to that of administering

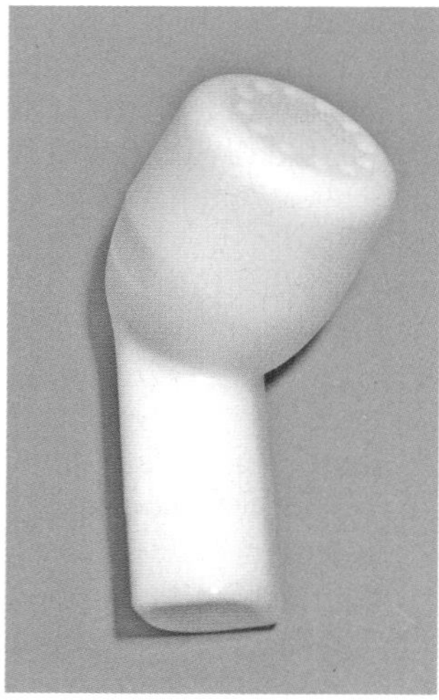

Figure 49.7 ■ Flutter mucus clearance device.
Shirlee Snyder.

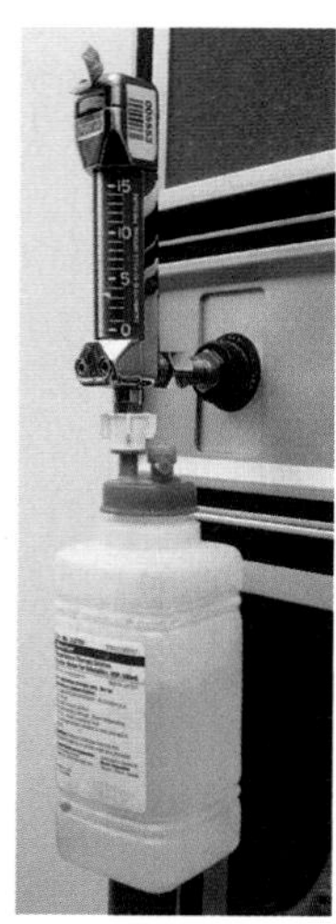

Figure 49.8 ■ An oxygen humidifier attached to a wall outlet oxygen flow meter.

medications and requires similar nursing actions. Determining the effectiveness of oxygen therapy involves several measures, including checking vital signs and peripheral blood oxygen saturation (pulse oximetry). Supplemental oxygen is indicated for clients who have hypoxemia due to the reduced ability for diffusion of oxygen through the respiratory membrane, hyperventilation, or substantial loss of lung tissue due to tumors or surgery. Others who may require oxygen are those with severe anemia or blood loss, or similar conditions in which there are inadequate numbers of RBCs or hemoglobin to carry the oxygen.

Oxygen therapy is prescribed by the healthcare provider, who orders the concentration, method of delivery, and depending on the method, liter flow per minute (L/min). The order may also call for the nurse to titrate the oxygen to achieve a desired saturation level as measured by pulse oximetry. When administering oxygen as an *emergency measure*, the nurse may initiate the therapy, and then contact the healthcare provider for an order.

Oxygen is supplied in two ways in healthcare facilities: by portable systems (cylinders or tanks) and from wall outlets. Long-term care or assisted living facilities may use similar oxygen supplies or those used more commonly in the home.

Clients who require oxygen therapy in the home may use small cylinders of oxygen, oxygen in liquid form, or an oxygen concentrator. Portable oxygen delivery systems are available to increase the client's independence. Home oxygen therapy services are available in most communities. These services generally supply the oxygen and delivery devices, training for the client and family, equipment maintenance, and emergency services should a problem occur.

Oxygen administered from a cylinder or wall-outlet system is dry. Dry gases dehydrate the respiratory mucous membranes. Humidifying devices that add water vapor to inspired air are an essential accessory of oxygen therapy, particularly for liter flows over 4 L/min (Figure 49.8 ■). These devices provide 20% to 40% humidity. A humidifier bottle is attached below the flow meter gauge so that the oxygen passes through water and then through the specific oxygen tubing and equipment prescribed for the client (e.g., nasal cannula or mask).

Humidifiers prevent mucous membranes from drying and becoming irritated and loosen secretions for easier expectoration. Oxygen passing through water picks up water vapor before it reaches the client. The more bubbles created during this process, the more water vapor is produced. Very low liter flows (e.g., 1 to 2 L/min by nasal cannula) do not require humidification. When a client is breathing very low flow oxygen, enough atmospheric air is inhaled (which naturally has water vapor in it) to prevent mucosal drying.

Oxygen cylinders need to be handled and stored with caution and strapped securely in wheeled transport devices or stands to prevent possible falls and outlet breakages. They should be placed away from traffic areas and heaters.

A regulator that releases oxygen at a safe level and at a desirable rate must be attached before the oxygen supply is used. On a cylinder, the contents gauge indicates the pressure or amount of oxygen remaining in the tank and the flow meter or flow indicator indicates the gas flow in liters per minute. A flow meter is also required for wall-outlet systems.

To use an oxygen wall-outlet system, carry out these steps:

- Attach the flow meter to the wall outlet, exerting firm pressure. The flow meter should be in the off position (Figure 49.9 ■).
- Fill the humidifier bottle with distilled or tap water per agency protocol. This can be done before coming to the bedside. Some humidifier bottles come prefilled by the manufacturer.
- Attach the humidifier bottle to the base of the flow meter (if indicated).
- Attach the prescribed oxygen tubing and delivery device to the humidifier.
- Regulate the flow meter to the prescribed level. The line for the prescribed flow rate (e.g., 2 L/min) should be in the middle of the ball of the flow meter (Figure 49.10 ■).

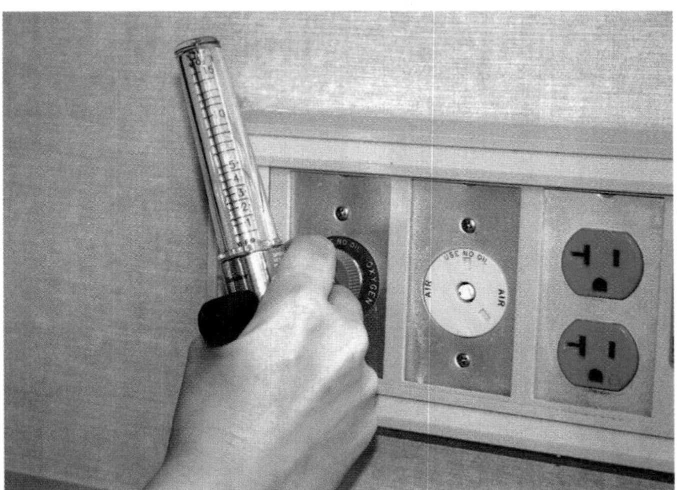

Figure 49.9 ■ Insert flow meter into the wall unit.
Shirlee Snyder.

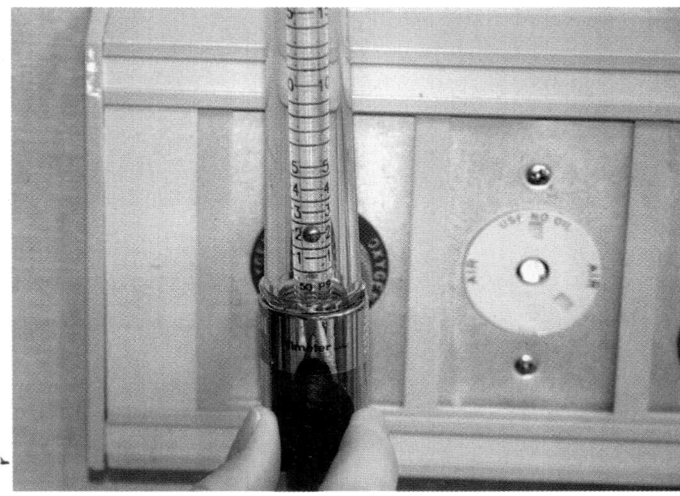

Figure 49.10 ■ This flow meter is set to deliver 2 L/min.
Shirlee Snyder.

Safety precautions are essential during oxygen therapy (Box 49.2). Although oxygen by itself will not burn or explode, it does facilitate combustion. For example, a bed sheet ordinarily burns slowly when ignited in the atmosphere; however, if saturated with free-flowing oxygen and ignited by a spark, it will burn rapidly and explosively. The greater the concentration of oxygen, the more rapidly fires start and burn, and such fires are difficult to extinguish. Because oxygen is colorless, odorless, and tasteless, individuals are often unaware of its presence. It is important to teach clients about this aspect of oxygen therapy.

BOX 49.2 Oxygen Therapy Safety Precautions

- For home oxygen use or when the facility permits smoking, teach family members and roommates to smoke only outside or in provided smoking rooms away from the client and oxygen equipment.
- Place cautionary signs reading "No Smoking: Oxygen in Use" on the client's door, at the foot or head of the bed, and on the oxygen equipment.
- Instruct the client and visitors about the hazard of smoking with oxygen in use.
- Make sure that electric devices (such as razors, hearing aids, radios, televisions, and heating pads) are in good working order to prevent the occurrence of short-circuit sparks.
- Avoid materials that generate static electricity, such as woolen blankets and synthetic fabrics. Cotton blankets should be used, and clients and caregivers should be advised to wear cotton fabrics.
- Avoid the use of volatile, flammable materials, such as oils, greases, alcohol, ether, and acetone (e.g., nail polish remover), near clients receiving oxygen.
- Be sure that electric monitoring equipment, suction machines, and portable diagnostic machines are all electrically grounded.
- Make known the location of fire extinguishers, and make sure personnel are trained in their use.

Like any medication, oxygen is not completely harmless to the client. Clients can receive an inadequate amount or an excessive amount of oxygen and both can lead to a decline in the client's condition. An inadequate amount of oxygen (hypoxia) will lead to cell death, and if left untreated can ultimately lead to death. Pulmonary oxygen toxicity, now called *hyperoxic acute lung injury*, can lead initially to pulmonary tissue damage and also damage other internal organs. Hyperoxic acute lung injury can develop from prolonged exposure to toxic levels of oxygen ($FiO_2 \geq 0.70$) (Kallet & Branson, 2016, p. 809). The lowest concentration needed to achieve the desired blood oxygen saturation (e.g., greater than 90% or a level prescribed by the healthcare provider) should be used.

Oxygen Delivery Systems

Low-flow and high-flow systems are available to deliver oxygen to the client. The choice of system depends on the client's oxygen needs, comfort, and developmental considerations. Low-flow systems deliver oxygen via small-bore tubing. Low-flow administration devices include nasal cannulas, face masks, oxygen tents, and transtracheal catheters. With these types of devices, room air is also inhaled along with the supplemental oxygen. As a result, the fraction of inspired oxygen (FiO_2) will vary depending on the respiratory rate, tidal volume, and liter flow.

High-flow systems supply all the oxygen required during ventilation in precise amounts, regardless of the client's respirations. The high-flow system used to deliver a precise and consistent FiO_2 is the Venturi mask with large-bore tubing.

Cannula

The nasal cannula (nasal prongs) is the most common and inexpensive device used to administer oxygen (Figure 49.11*A* ■). The nasal cannula is easy to apply and does not interfere with the client's ability to eat or talk. It also is relatively comfortable, permits some freedom of movement, and is well tolerated by the client. It delivers a relatively low concentration of oxygen (24% to 45%) at flow rates of 2 to 6 L/min. Above 6 L/min, the client tends to swallow air and the FiO_2 is not increased. Limitations of the plain nasal cannula include inability to deliver higher concentrations of oxygen, and that it can be drying and irritating to mucous membranes.

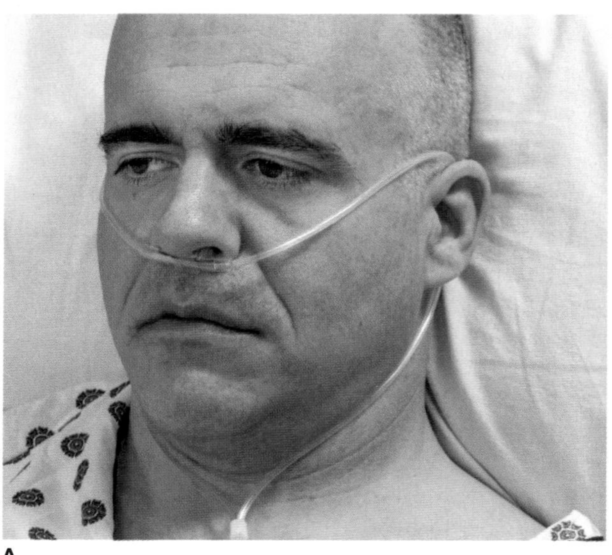

A

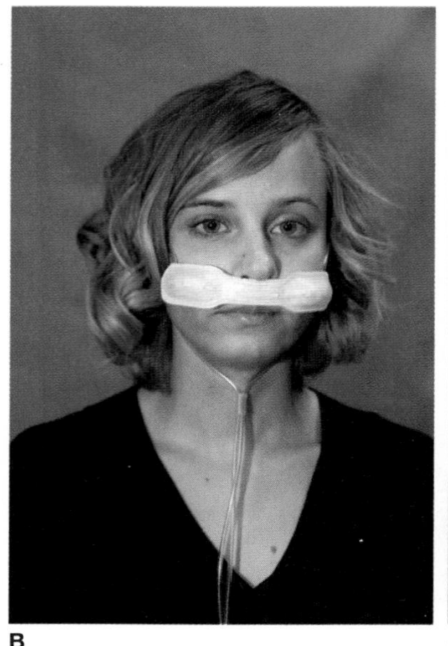

B

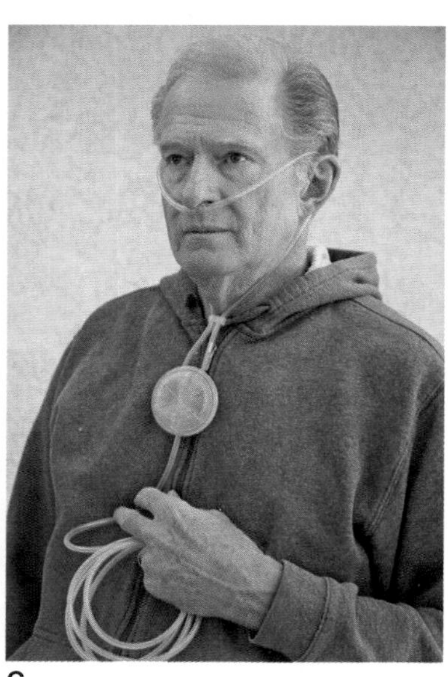

C

Figure 49.11 ■ *A*, Nasal cannula; *B*, mustache reservoir nasal cannula; *C*, pendant reservoir nasal cannula.
B–C, Shirlee Snyder.

Reservoir nasal cannulas are oxygen-conserving devices and are also called Oxymizer oxygen-conserving devices. They are used primarily in the home setting. The reservoir nasal cannula stores oxygen in the reservoir while the client breathes out and then delivers a 100% oxygen bolus when the client breathes in. As a result it delivers a higher oxygen concentration at a lower flow rate than the plain nasal cannula because it conserves oxygen. It can deliver FiO_2 of 0.5 or greater, while providing the same benefits of a plain nasal cannula. The two styles of reservoir nasal cannulas (Oxymizers) are the mustache and pendant styles (see Figure 49.11*B* and *C*). Humidification is not necessary with the reservoir nasal cannula, because it collects water vapor while the client breathes out and returns it when the client breathes in.

Administering oxygen by cannula is detailed in Skill 49.1.

SKILL 49.1

Administering Oxygen by Cannula, Face Mask, or Face Tent

Before administering oxygen, check (a) the order for oxygen, including the administering device and the liter flow rate (L/min) or the percentage of oxygen; (b) the levels of oxygen (PaO_2) and carbon dioxide ($PaCO_2$) in the client's arterial blood (PaO_2 is normally 80 to 100 mmHg; $PaCO_2$ is normally 35 to 45 mmHg); and (c) whether the client has COPD. *Note:* If the client has not had arterial blood gases ordered, oxygen saturation should be checked using a noninvasive oximeter.

PURPOSES

Cannula

- To deliver a relatively low concentration of oxygen when only minimal oxygen support is required
- To allow uninterrupted delivery of oxygen while the client ingests food or fluids

Face Mask

- To provide moderate oxygen support and a higher concentration of oxygen or humidity than is provided by cannula
- To provide a high flow of oxygen when attached to a Venturi system

Face Tent

- To provide high humidity
- To provide oxygen when a mask is poorly tolerated

ASSESSMENT

See also Skill 29.11, Assessing the Thorax and Lungs, on pages 611–614.

Assess

- Skin and mucous membrane color: Note whether cyanosis is present, presence of mucus, sputum production, and impedance of airflow.
- Breathing patterns: Note depth of respirations and presence of tachypnea, bradypnea, or orthopnea.
- Chest movements: Note whether there are any intercostal, substernal, suprasternal, supraclavicular, or tracheal retractions during inspiration or expiration.
- Chest wall configuration (e.g., kyphosis, unequal chest expansion, barrel chest).
- Lung sounds audible by ear and auscultating the chest.
- Presence of clinical signs of hypoxemia: tachycardia, tachypnea, restlessness, dyspnea, cyanosis, and confusion. Tachycardia and tachypnea are often early signs. Confusion is a later sign of severe oxygen deprivation.
- Presence of clinical signs of hypercarbia (hypercapnia): restlessness, hypertension, headache, lethargy, tremor, or elevated carbon dioxide levels in the blood.

Administering Oxygen by Cannula, Face Mask, or Face Tent—*continued*

- Presence of clinical signs of hyperoxic acute lung injury: tracheal irritation and cough, dyspnea, and decreased pulmonary ventilation.

Determine

- Vital signs, including pulse rate and quality, and respiratory rate, rhythm, and depth.
- Whether the client has COPD. A high carbon dioxide level in the blood is the normal stimulus to breathe. However, people with COPD may have a chronically high carbon dioxide level, and their stimulus to breathe is hypoxemia. During continuous oxygen administration, arterial blood gas levels of oxygen (PaO_2) and carbon dioxide ($PaCO_2$) are measured periodically to monitor hypoxemia.
- Results of diagnostic studies such as chest x-ray.
- Hemoglobin, hematocrit, and complete blood count.
- Oxygen saturation levels.
- Pulmonary function tests, if available.

PLANNING

Consult with a respiratory therapist as needed in the beginning and during ongoing care of clients receiving ordered oxygen therapy. In many agencies, the respiratory therapist establishes the initial equipment and client teaching. However, it is important for the nurse to continually assess the client's need for oxygenation and oxygen therapy.

ASSIGNMENT

Initiating the administration of oxygen is considered similar to administering a medication and is not assigned to assistive personnel (AP). However, reapplying the oxygen delivery device may be performed by the AP, and many aspects of the client's response to oxygen therapy are observed during usual care and may be recorded by individuals other than the nurse. Abnormal findings must be validated and interpreted by the nurse. The nurse is also responsible for ensuring that the correct delivery method is being used.

Equipment

Cannula

- Oxygen supply with a flow meter and adapter
- Humidifier with distilled water or tap water according to agency protocol
- Nasal cannula and tubing
- Tape (optional)
- Padding for the elastic band (optional)

Face Mask

- Oxygen supply with a flow meter and adapter
- Humidifier with distilled water or tap water according to agency protocol
- Prescribed face mask of the appropriate size
- Padding for the elastic band (optional)

Face Tent

- Oxygen supply with a flow meter and adapter
- Humidifier with distilled water or tap water according to agency protocol
- Face tent of the appropriate size

IMPLEMENTATION

Preparation

1. Determine the need for oxygen therapy, and verify the order for the therapy.
   - Perform a respiratory assessment to develop baseline data if not already available.
2. Prepare the client and support individual(s).
   - Assist the client to a semi-Fowler's position if possible. **Rationale:** *This position permits easier chest expansion and hence easier breathing*.
   - Explain that oxygen is not dangerous when safety precautions are observed. Inform the client and support individual(s) about the safety precautions connected with oxygen use.

Performance

1. Prior to performing the procedure, introduce self and verify the client's identity using agency protocol. Explain to the client what you are going to do, why it is necessary, and how to participate. Discuss how the effects of the oxygen therapy will be used in planning further care or treatments.
2. Perform hand hygiene and observe other appropriate infection prevention procedures.
3. Provide for client privacy, if appropriate.
4. Set up the oxygen equipment and the humidifier.
   - Attach the flow meter to the wall outlet or tank. The flow meter should be in the off position.
   - If needed, fill the humidifier bottle. (This can be done before coming to the bedside.)
   - Attach the humidifier bottle to the base of the flow meter.
   - Attach the prescribed oxygen tubing and delivery device to the humidifier.
5. Turn on the oxygen at the prescribed rate and ensure proper functioning.
   - Check that the oxygen is flowing freely through the tubing. There should be no kinks in the tubing, and the connections should be airtight. There should be bubbles in the humidifier as the oxygen flows through. You should feel the oxygen at the outlets of the cannula, mask, or tent.
   - Set the oxygen at the flow rate ordered.
6. Apply the appropriate oxygen delivery device.

Cannula

- Put the cannula over the client's face, with the outlet prongs fitting into the nares and the tubing hooked around the ears (see Figure 49.11*A*).
- If the cannula will not stay in place, tape it at the sides of the face.
- Pad the tubing and band over the ears and cheekbones as needed.

Face Mask

- Guide the mask toward the client's face, and apply it from the nose downward.
- Fit the mask to the contours of the client's face (see Figure 49.12*A*). **Rationale:** *The mask should mold to the face so that very little oxygen escapes into the eyes or around the cheeks and chin*.
- Secure the elastic band around the client's head so that the mask is comfortable but snug.
- Pad the band behind the ears and over bony prominences. **Rationale:** *Padding will prevent irritation from the mask*.

Face Tent

- Place the tent over the client's face, and secure the ties around the head (see Figure 49.13).

Continued on page 1322

SKILL 49.1

Administering Oxygen by Cannula, Face Mask, or Face Tent—*continued*

7. Assess the client regularly.
- Assess the client's vital signs, level of anxiety, color, and ease of respirations, and provide support while the client adjusts to the device. Some clients may complain of claustrophobia.
- Assess the client in 15 to 30 minutes, depending on the client's condition, and regularly thereafter.
- Assess the client regularly for clinical signs of hypoxia, tachycardia, confusion, dyspnea, restlessness, and cyanosis. Review oxygen saturation or arterial blood gas results if they are available.

Nasal Cannula
- Assess the client's nares for encrustations and irritation. Apply a water-soluble lubricant as required to soothe the mucous membranes.
- Assess the top of the client's ears for any signs of irritation from the cannula tubing. If present, padding with a gauze pad may help relieve the discomfort.

Face Mask or Tent
- Inspect the facial skin frequently for dampness or chafing, and dry and treat it as needed.

8. Inspect the equipment on a regular basis.
- Check the liter flow and the level of water in the humidifier in 30 minutes and whenever providing care to the client.
- Be sure that water is not collecting in dependent loops of the tubing.
- Make sure that safety precautions are being followed.

9. Document findings in the client record using forms or checklists supplemented by narrative notes when appropriate.

SAMPLE DOCUMENTATION

9/16/2020 0930 Returned from physical therapy with c/o dyspnea. Resp. 26/min, shallow. P-92, BP 160/98, SpO_2 92%. Skin warm, no cyanosis. Lung sounds clear, no retractions. Oxygen per nasal cannula applied @ 2 L/min. P. Isola, RN

9/16/2020 1000 No further c/o of dyspnea. Resp. 20/min, P 88, BP 152/92, SpO_2 96%. oxygen per nasal cannula continues @ 2 L/min. P. Isola, RN

EVALUATION
- Perform follow-up based on findings that deviated from expected or normal for the client. Relate findings to previous data if available (e.g., check oxygen saturation to evaluate adequate oxygenation).
- Report significant deviations from normal to the primary care provider.

LIFESPAN CONSIDERATIONS Oxygen Delivery Equipment

INFANTS

Oxygen Hood
- An oxygen hood is a rigid plastic dome that encloses an infant's head. It provides precise oxygen levels and high humidity.
- The gas should not be allowed to blow directly into the infant's face, and the hood should not rub against the infant's neck, chin, or shoulder.

CHILDREN

Oxygen Tent
- The tent consists of a rectangular, clear, plastic canopy with outlets that connect to an oxygen or compressed air source and to a humidifier that moisturizes the air or oxygen.
- Because the enclosed tent becomes very warm, some type of cooling mechanism is provided to maintain the temperature at 20°C to 21°C (68°F to 70°F).
- Cover the child with a gown or a cotton blanket. Some agencies provide gowns with hoods, or a small towel may be wrapped around the head. *The child needs protection from chilling and from the dampness and condensation in the tent.*
- Flood the tent with oxygen by setting the flow meter at 15 L/min for about 5 minutes. Then, adjust the flow meter according to orders. *Flooding the tent quickly increases the oxygen to the desired level.*
- The tent can deliver approximately 30% oxygen.
- Children may fight having a mask placed on their faces. They are often fearful when placed in oxygen tents or hoods. These are normal responses that vary based on experience, developmental stage, degree of threat to body image, and attachment or abandonment issues. Providing safe toys and a beloved blanket or pillow to hold can help, as can fostering the parent–child bond even though separated by the plastic. Encourage parents to interact with their child around and through the tubing and tent.

Face Mask

Face masks that cover the client's nose and mouth may be used for oxygen inhalation. Most masks are made of clear, pliable plastic that can be molded to fit the face. They are held to the client's head with elastic bands. Some have a metal clip that can be bent over the bridge of the nose for a snug fit. Exhalation ports on the sides of the mask allow exhaled carbon dioxide to escape.

Some masks have reservoir bags, which provide higher oxygen concentrations to the client. A portion of the client's expired air is directed into the bag. Because this air comes from the upper respiratory passages (e.g., the trachea and bronchi), where it does not take part in gaseous exchange, its oxygen concentration remains the same as that of inspired air.

A variety of oxygen masks are marketed:

- The simple face mask delivers oxygen concentrations from 35% to 65% at liter flows of 8 to 12 L/min, respectively (Smith, Duell, Martin, Aebersold, & Gonzalez, 2017, p. 1189) (Figure 49.12*A* ■).
- The partial rebreather mask delivers oxygen concentrations of 40% to 60% at liter flows of 6 to 10 L/min, respectively (Smith et al., 2017, p. 1189). The oxygen reservoir bag that is attached allows the client to rebreathe about the first third of the exhaled air in conjunction with oxygen (Figure 49.12*B*). Thus, it increases the FiO_2 by recycling expired oxygen. The partial rebreather bag must not totally deflate during inspiration to avoid carbon dioxide buildup. If this problem occurs, the nurse increases the liter flow of oxygen so that the bag remains one-third to one-half full.
- The nonrebreather mask delivers the highest oxygen concentration possible—60% to 100%—by means other than intubation or mechanical ventilation, at liter flows of 6 to 15 L/min (Smith et al., 2017, p. 1189). One-way valves on the mask and between the reservoir bag and the mask prevent the room air and the client's exhaled air from entering the bag so only the oxygen in the bag is inspired (Figure 49.12*C*). In some cases, one of the side valves is removed so that the client can still inhale room air if the oxygen supply is accidentally cut off. To prevent carbon dioxide buildup, the nonrebreather bag must not totally deflate during inspiration. If it does, the nurse can correct this problem by increasing the liter flow of oxygen.
- The Venturi mask delivers oxygen concentrations varying from 24% to 40% or 50% at liter flows of 4 to 10 L/min (Figure 49.12*D*). The Venturi mask has wide-bore tubing and color-coded jet adapters that correspond to a precise oxygen concentration and liter flow. For example, in some cases, a blue adapter delivers a 24% concentration of oxygen at 4 L/min, and a green adapter delivers a 35% concentration of oxygen at 8 L/min. However, colors and

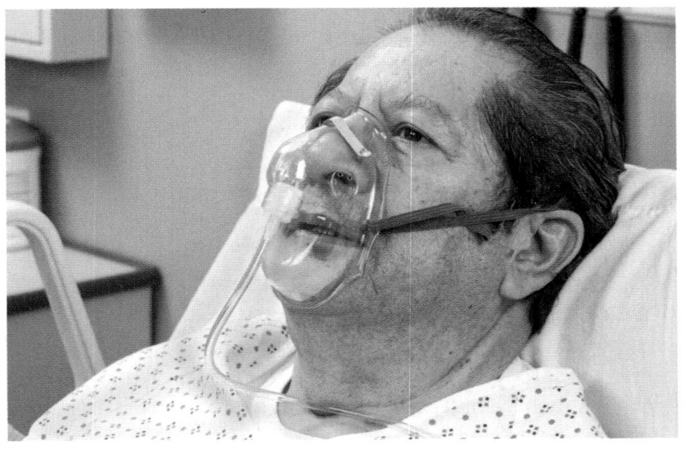

A

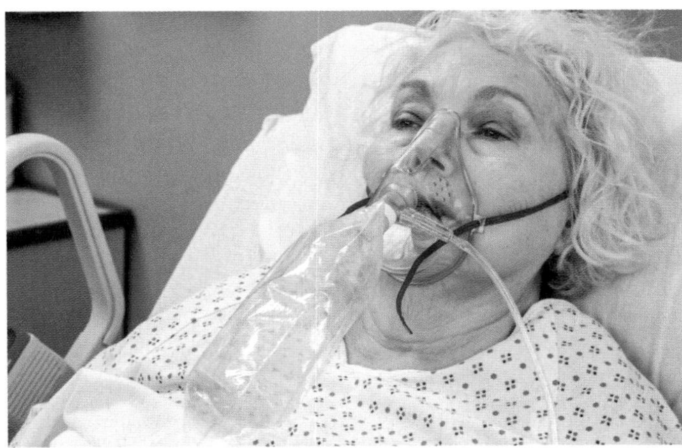

B

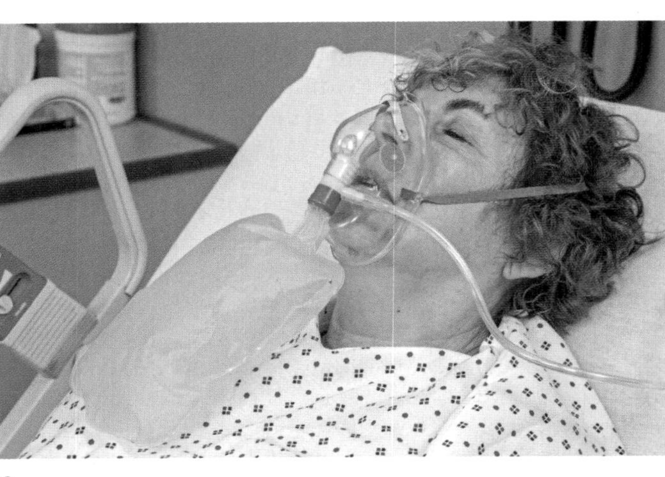

C

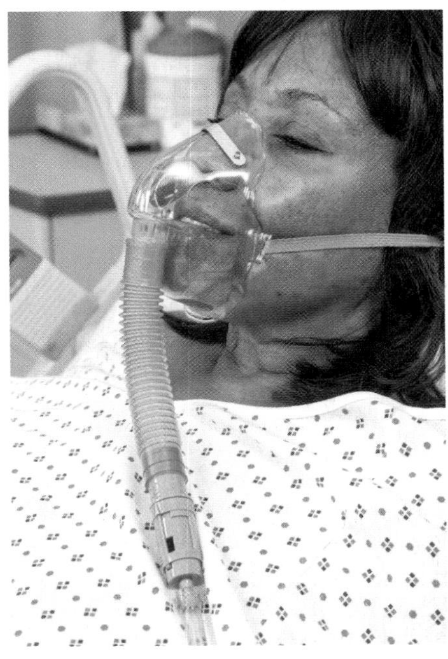

D

Figure 49.12 ■ *A*, A simple face mask; *B*, a partial rebreather mask; *C*, a nonrebreather mask; *D*, a Venturi mask.

concentrations may vary by manufacturers so the equipment must be examined carefully. Other manufacturers use a dial or setting for the desired concentration. Turning the oxygen source flow rate higher than specified by the equipment manufacturer will not increase the concentration delivered to the client.

Initiating oxygen by mask is much the same as initiating oxygen by cannula, except that the nurse must find a mask of appropriate size. Smaller sizes are available for children. Administering oxygen by mask or face tent is detailed in Skill 49.1. Limitations of masks include difficulty in achieving a proper fit and poor tolerance by some clients who may complain of feeling hot or "smothered."

Face Tent

Face tents (Figure 49.13 ■) can replace oxygen masks when masks are poorly tolerated by clients. Face tents provide varying concentrations of oxygen, for example, 28% to 100% concentration of oxygen at 8 to 12 L/min. It is convenient for providing humidification and oxygenation; however, oxygen concentration cannot be controlled (Smith et al., 2017, p. 1190). Frequently inspect the client's facial skin for dampness or chafing, and dry and treat as needed. As with face masks, the client's facial skin must be kept dry.

Transtracheal Catheter

A transtracheal catheter is placed through a surgically created tract in the lower neck directly into the trachea. Once the tract has matured (healed), the client removes and cleans the catheter two to four times per day. Oxygen applied to the catheter at greater than 1 L/min should be humidified, and high flow rates, as much as 15 to 20 L/min, can be administered (Figure 49.14 ■).

Noninvasive Positive Pressure Ventilation (NPPV)

In certain circumstances clients require mechanical assistance to maintain adequate breathing. This assistance may be accomplished by the use of **noninvasive positive pressure ventilation (NPPV)**, delivery of air or oxygen under pressure without the need for an invasive tube such

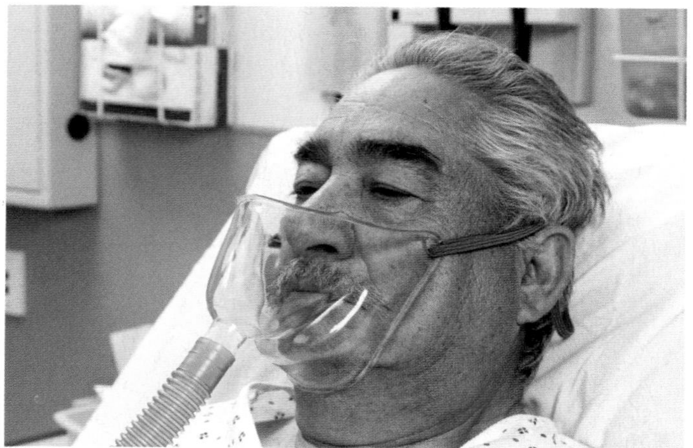

Figure 49.13 ■ An oxygen face tent.

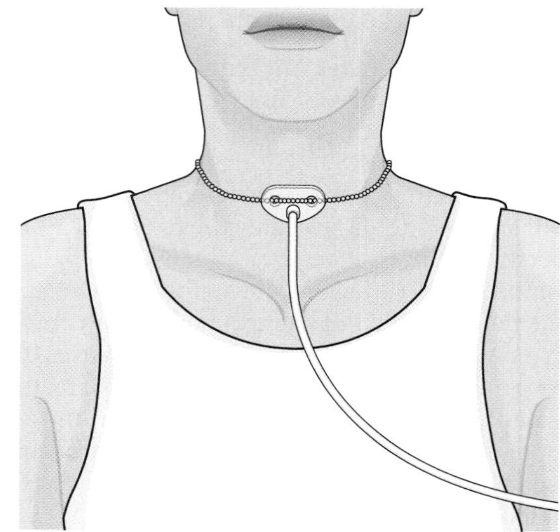

Figure 49.14 ■ Transtracheal catheter.

as an endotracheal tube or tracheostomy tube. Conditions requiring noninvasive ventilation include acute and chronic respiratory failure, pulmonary edema, COPD, and obstructive sleep apnea (OSA).

This discussion focuses on the use of noninvasive ventilation devices in the treatment of sleep apnea due to the prevalence of this condition. Sleep apnea affects millions of Americans. When breathing stops (apnea), the individual's carbon dioxide level rises, breathing is stimulated, and then it resumes. There are different types of sleep apnea but OSA is the most common. Clients with OSA experience frequent episodes of partial or complete upper airway obstruction for at least 10 seconds during sleep (Harrelson & Fencl, 2016). Risk factors include male gender, obesity, and age over 40; however, it can affect anyone at any age, including children. OSA can lead to a number of health problems including hypertension, fatigue, memory problems, cardiovascular disease, and increased perioperative complications (Williams, Williams, Stanton, & Spence, 2017). If an underlying cause can be treated, OSA may be reduced or eliminated.

The most common and least invasive treatment for OSA is positive pressure ventilation. A mask fitted over the client's nose during sleep provides air under pressure during inhalation and exhalation so that the airway is kept open and cannot collapse. This mask and pump system is called continuous positive airway pressure (CPAP) (Figure 49.15 ■). A variation of CPAP is bilevel positive airway pressure (BiPap) in which the pressure delivered during exhalation is less than the pressure delivered during inhalation.

The nurse's primary role in caring for clients using CPAP or BiPAP devices is to ensure optimal functioning and use of the device since it may need to be used nightly for the remainder of their lives. There may be significant issues with adherence to CPAP therapy due to discomfort or other barriers, so the nurse should provide client education and support and also collaborate with the respiratory therapist and other involved healthcare providers.

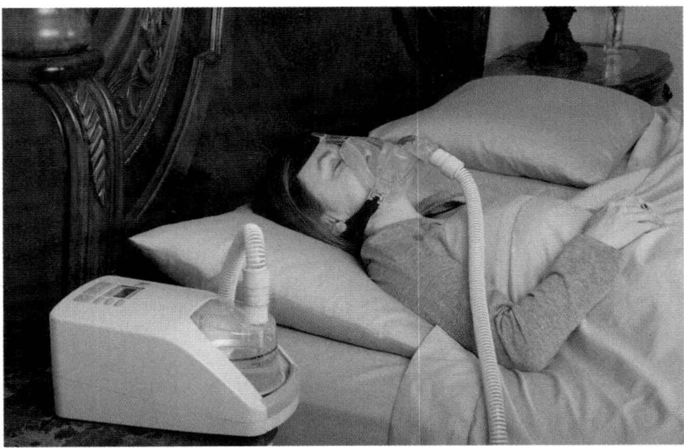

Figure 49.15 ■ A CPAP machine in use in the client's home.
Brian Chase/123RF.

QSEN Patient-Centered Care: Home Oxygen Delivery

Three major oxygen systems for home care use are available in most communities: cylinders or tanks of compressed gas, liquid (cryogenic) oxygen, and oxygen concentrators.

1. *Cylinders ("green tanks"):* These are the system of choice for clients who need oxygen on a prn basis. Advantages are that cylinders deliver all liter flows (1 to 15 L/min), and oxygen evaporation does not occur during storage. Disadvantages are that the cylinders are heavy and awkward to move, the supply company must be notified when a refill is needed, and they are costly for the high-use client.
2. *Liquid oxygen:* Liquid systems have two parts—a large stationary container and a portable unit with a small lightweight tank that is refilled from the stationary unit. Liquid reservoirs store oxygen at –212°C (–350°F) in a smaller amount of space than compressed gas. Advantages are that these reservoirs are lighter in weight and cleaner in appearance than cylinders and they are not as difficult to operate. Disadvantages of liquid oxygen are that many home care medical supply and service companies are not able to handle it, oxygen evaporation occurs when the unit is not used, only low flows (1 to 4 L/min) can be used or freezing occurs, and the portable unit designed to be carried over the shoulder weighs 8 to 10 pounds, a possible burden to the typical COPD client. A wheeled cart can be used to carry the unit but may be awkward.
3. *Oxygen concentrators:* Concentrators are electrically powered systems that manufacture oxygen from room air. At 1 L/min, such a system can deliver a concentration of about 95% oxygen, but the concentration drops when the flow rate increases (e.g., 75% concentration at 4 L/min). The oxygen can be delivered by pulse dose or continuous flow. Pulse dose is based on breathing, that is, oxygen is delivered each time the client takes a breath.

Advantages of oxygen concentrators are that they are more attractive in appearance, resembling furniture rather than medical equipment; they eliminate the need for regular delivery of oxygen or refilling of cylinders; because the supply of oxygen is constant, they alleviate the client's anxiety about running out of oxygen; and they are the most economical system when continuous use is required. Major disadvantages of a concentrator are that it is expensive; it lacks real portability (small units weigh 28 pounds); it tends to be noisy; it is powered by electricity (an emergency backup unit, for example, an oxygen tank, must be provided for clients for whom a power failure could be life threatening); and heat produced by the concentrator motor is a problem for those who live in trailers, small houses, or warm climates, where air conditioners are required. The oxygen concentrator must also be checked periodically with an oxygen analyzer to ensure that it is providing an adequate delivery of oxygen.

Another type of oxygen concentrator is the *oxygen enricher*. It uses a plastic membrane that allows water vapor to pass through with the oxygen, thus eliminating the need for a humidifying device. It is also thought to filter out bacteria present in the air. The enricher provides an oxygen concentration of 40% at all flow rates, it tends to be quieter than the concentrator, there is less chance of combustion (since the gas is only 40% oxygen), it has only two moving parts (thus decreasing the risk of something going wrong), and a nebulizer can be operated off the enricher because of the high flow rate.

Social services or the case manager needs to ensure that the client has appropriate help in choosing a reputable home oxygen vendor. Services furnished should include:

- A 24-hour emergency service
- Trained personnel to make the initial delivery and instruct the client in safe, appropriate use of the oxygen and maintenance of the equipment
- At least monthly follow-up visits to check the equipment and reinstruct the client as necessary
- A regular cost review to ensure that the system is the most cost effective one for that client, with routine notification of the primary care provider or home care professional if it seems that another system is more appropriate.

The nurse needs to also ensure that the client knows about the financial reimbursements available from Medicare and Medicaid or other insurance agencies.

Artificial Airways

Artificial airways are inserted to maintain a patent air passage for clients whose airways have become or may become obstructed. A patent airway is necessary so that air can flow to and from the lungs. Four of the more common types of airways are oropharyngeal, nasopharyngeal, endotracheal, and tracheostomy.

Oropharyngeal and Nasopharyngeal Airways

Oropharyngeal and nasopharyngeal airways are used to keep the upper air passages open when secretions or the tongue may obstruct them (e.g., in a client who is sedated, is semicomatose, or has an altered level of consciousness). These airways are easy to insert and have a low risk of complications. Sizes vary and should be appropriate to the size and age of the client. The nasopharyngeal airway should be well lubricated with water-soluble gel prior to inserting. The oropharyngeal airway may be lubricated with water or saline, if necessary.

Oropharyngeal airways (Figure 49.16 ■) stimulate the gag reflex and are only used for clients with altered levels of consciousness with no gag reflex (e.g., because of general anesthesia, overdose, or head injury). To insert the airway:

- Place the client in a supine or semi-Fowler's position.
- Apply clean gloves.
- Hold the lubricated airway by the outer flange, with the distal end pointing up or curved upward.
- Open the client's mouth and insert the airway along the top of the tongue.
- When the distal end of the airway reaches the soft palate at the back of the mouth, rotate the airway 180 degrees downward, and slip it past the uvula into the oral pharynx.
- If not contraindicated, place the client in a side-lying position or with the head turned to the side to allow secretions to drain out of the mouth.
- The oropharynx may be suctioned as needed by inserting the suction catheter alongside the airway.
- Remove and discard gloves.
- Perform hand hygiene.
- Do not tape the airway in place; remove it when the client begins to cough or gag.
- Provide mouth care at least every 2 to 4 hours, keeping suction available at the bedside.
- As appropriate for the client's condition, remove the airway every 8 hours to assess the mouth and provide oral care. Reinsert the airway immediately.

Nasopharyngeal airways are tolerated better by alert clients because the nasal airway does not cause the client to gag. They are inserted through the nares, terminating in the oropharynx (Figure 49.17 ■). When inserting, use the largest nostril, use a water-soluble lubricant, and insert with the curve of the tube toward the mouth. Advance the tube gently, straight in, following the floor of the nose. When caring for a client with a nasopharyngeal airway, provide frequent oral and nares care, reinserting the airway in the other naris every 8 hours or as ordered to prevent necrosis of the mucosa.

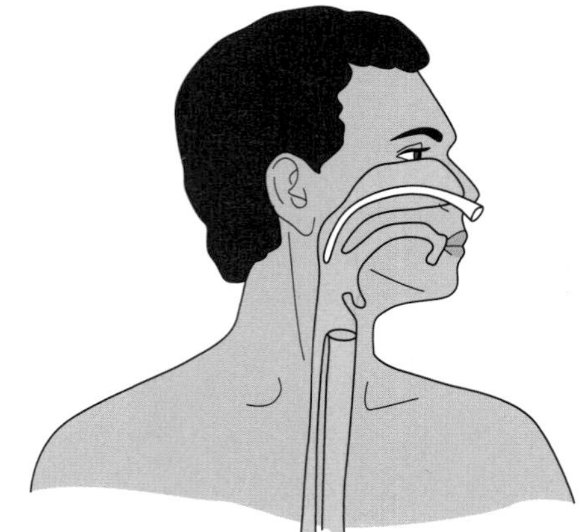

Figure 49.17 ■ A nasopharyngeal airway in place.

Endotracheal Tubes

Endotracheal tubes (ETTs) are most commonly inserted in clients who have had general anesthetics or for those in emergency situations where mechanical ventilation is required. An ETT is inserted by an anesthesiologist, primary care provider, certified registered nurse anesthetist (CRNA), or respiratory therapist with specialized education. It is inserted through the mouth or the nose and into the trachea, using a laryngoscope as a guide (Figure 49.18 ■). The tube terminates just superior to (above) the bifurcation of the trachea into the bronchi. The tube may have an air-filled cuff to prevent air leakage around it. Because an ETT passes through the epiglottis and glottis, the client is unable to speak while it is in place. Nursing interventions for clients with ETTs are shown in Box 49.3.

Tracheostomy

Clients who need airway support due to a temporary or permanent condition may have a tracheostomy. A tracheostomy is an opening into the trachea through the neck.

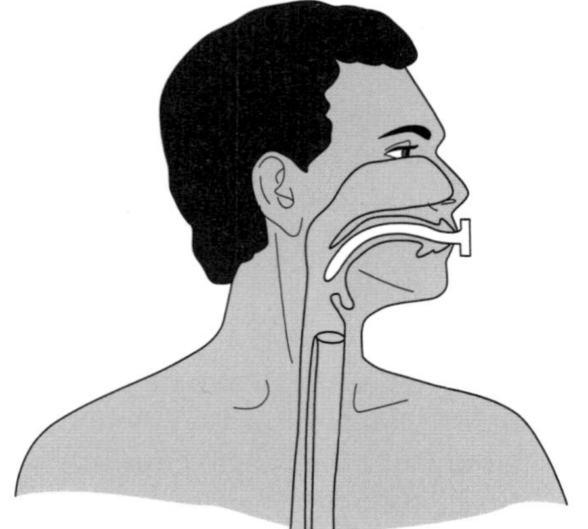

Figure 49.16 ■ An oropharyngeal airway in place.

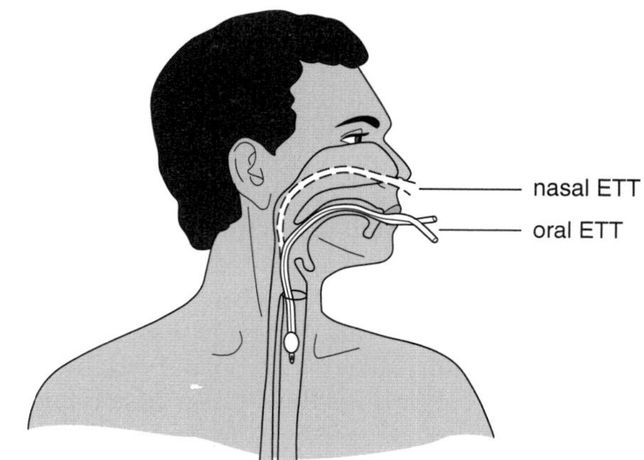

Figure 49.18 ■ An endotracheal tube (ETT).

BOX 49.3 Nursing Interventions for Clients with Endotracheal Tubes

- Perform hand hygiene before and after contact with the client. Wear gloves when handling respiratory secretions or objects contaminated with respiratory secretions.
- Assess the client's respiratory status at least every 2 hours, or more frequently if indicated. Include respiratory rate, rhythm, depth, equality of chest excursion, and lung sounds; level of consciousness; oxygen saturation, percentage of oxygen used, and by what means (e.g., ventilator); and skin color in your assessment.
- Frequently assess nasal and oral mucosa for redness and irritation. Report any abnormal findings to the primary care provider.
- Secure the endotracheal tube with tape or a commercially prepared holder to prevent movement of the tube farther into or out of the trachea. Assess the position of the tube frequently. Notify the healthcare provider immediately if the tube is dislodged out of the airway. If the tube advances into a main bronchus, it will need to be repositioned to ensure ventilation of both lungs.
- Unless contraindicated, elevate the head of the bed 30° to 45°.
- Using sterile technique, suction the endotracheal tube as needed to remove excessive secretions. Perform subglottic suctioning before deflating the cuff of the endotracheal tube or before moving the tube. Wear goggles when performing suctioning.
- Closely monitor cuff pressure, maintaining a pressure of 20 to 25 mmHg (or as recommended by the tube manufacturer) to minimize the risk of tracheal tissue necrosis. If recommended, deflate the cuff periodically.
- Provide oral hygiene and nasal care every 2 to 4 hours. Use an oropharyngeal airway to prevent the client from biting down on an oral endotracheal tube. Move oral endotracheal tubes to the opposite side of the mouth every 8 hours or per agency protocol, taking care to maintain the position of the tube in the trachea. **Rationale:** *This prevents irritation to the oral mucosa.*
- Provide humidified air or oxygen because the endotracheal tube bypasses the upper airways, which normally moisten the air.
- If the client is on mechanical ventilation, ensure that all alarms are enabled at all times because the client cannot call for help should an emergency occur.
- Communicate frequently with the client, providing a note pad or picture board for the client to use in communicating.
- Inform the client and family that an endotracheal tube is usually used as a short-term artificial airway. Instruct the client and family not to manipulate the tube and to call for the nurse if the client is uncomfortable.

A tube is usually inserted through this opening and an artificial airway is created. A tracheostomy is performed using one of two techniques: the traditional open surgical method or via a percutaneous insertion. The percutaneous method can be done at the bedside in a critical care unit. The open technique is done in an operating room where a surgical incision is made in the trachea just below the larynx. A curved tracheostomy tube is inserted to extend through the stoma into the trachea (Figure 49.19 ■). Tracheostomy tubes are available in different sizes and may be plastic, silicone, or metal, and cuffed, uncuffed, or fenestrated. A fenestrated tracheostomy tube has an opening that allows air to pass through to the vocal cords, thus allowing the client to communicate.

Tracheostomy tubes have an outer cannula that is inserted into the trachea and a flange that rests against the neck. The flange allows the tube to be secured in place with tracheostomy tapes or twill ties, or Velcro collars (Figure 49.20 ■). All tubes also have an obturator, which is used to insert the outer cannula and is then removed. The obturator, along with a spare tracheostomy tube of the same size and smaller, is kept at the client's bedside in case the tube becomes dislodged and needs to be reinserted. Some tracheostomy tubes have an inner cannula that is inserted and locked into place inside the outer cannula. The purpose of the inner cannula is to prevent tube obstruction by allowing regular cleaning or replacement. Many plastic inner cannulas are cleaned with a solution of full or half-strength hydrogen peroxide and sterile water. Some facilities, however, recommend using normal saline only. It is important to check the manufacturer's instructions for cleaning tracheostomy tubes because silicone tubes and metal tubes can be damaged by using hydrogen peroxide. The outer cannula of the tracheostomy tube remains in place to maintain a patent airway.

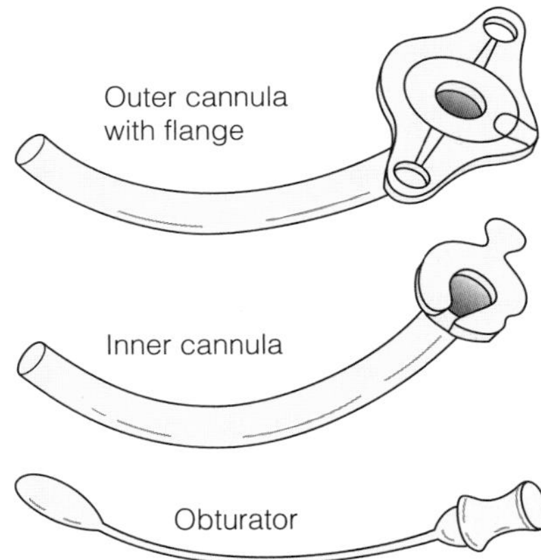

Figure 49.20 ■ Components of a tracheostomy tube.

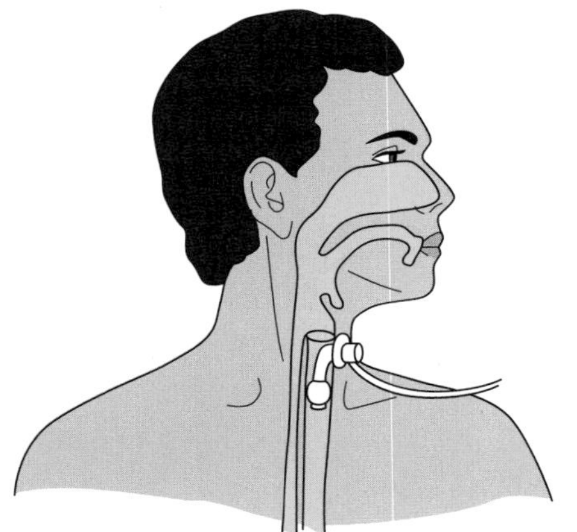

Figure 49.19 ■ A tracheostomy tube in place.

Clinical Alert!

Some inner cannulas are disposable. These cannulas have a different method of attachment than the nondisposable tubes. Also, the different types of disposable tubes are not interchangeable.

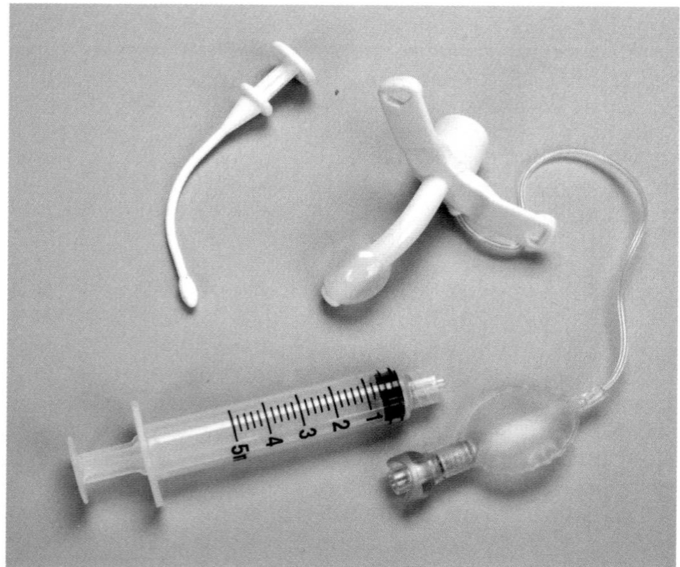

Figure 49.21 ■ A tracheostomy tube with a low-pressure cuff.

Cuffed tracheostomy tubes are surrounded by an inflatable cuff that produces an airtight seal between the tube and the trachea. This seal prevents aspiration of oropharyngeal secretions and air leakage between the tube and the trachea. Cuffed tubes are often used immediately after a tracheostomy and are essential when ventilating a tracheostomy client with a mechanical ventilator. Children do not require cuffed tubes, because their tracheas are elastic enough to seal the air space around the tube.

Low-pressure cuffs (Figure 49.21 ■) are commonly used to distribute a low, even pressure against the trachea, thus decreasing the risk of tracheal tissue necrosis. They do not need to be deflated periodically to reduce pressure on the tracheal wall. Foam cuffed tracheostomy tubes (Figure 49.22 ■) do not require injected air; instead, when the port is opened, ambient air enters the balloon, which then conforms to the client's trachea. Air is removed from the cuff prior to insertion or removal of the tube.

The nurse provides tracheostomy care for the client with a new or recent tracheostomy to maintain patency of the tube and reduce the risk of infection. Initially a tracheostomy may need to be suctioned (see the section on suctioning that follows) and cleaned as often as every 1 to 2 hours. After the initial inflammatory response subsides, tracheostomy care may only need to be done once or twice a day, depending on the client. For a client with a new tracheostomy, sterile technique should be used when providing tracheostomy care in order to prevent infection. It is recommended that two staff members be present when changing tracheostomy tube ties because it is safer to have someone hold the tracheostomy tube in place when changing the ties. After the stoma has healed, clean gloves can be used while changing the dressing and tie tapes.

Skill 49.4 later in this chapter describes tracheostomy care. Unfortunately, research related to tracheostomy care is limited. As a result, little evidence guides the procedure, and there is no defined standard technique or sequence of steps for the process. The procedure varies across reference texts, procedure manuals, and clinical practice guidelines. Bolsega and Sole (2018) conducted an exploratory study of tracheostomy care practices of nurses and respiratory therapists using a simulated setting. They found a wide discrepancy in both equipment selected and the steps performed during tracheostomy care. They point out that written tracheostomy care protocols are important to reduce variations in practice and the need for establishing an evidence-based approach for performing tracheostomy care to prevent complications.

When the client breathes through a tracheostomy, air is no longer heated, humidified, and filtered as it is when passing through the upper airways; therefore, special precautions are necessary. Humidity may be provided with a mist collar (Figure 49.23 ■). Clients with long-term tracheostomies may use a heat and moisture exchanger device, also known as artificial noses, that fit onto the connector of the inner cannula (Figure 49.24 ■). They collect heat and moisture from the client's breath during expiration and

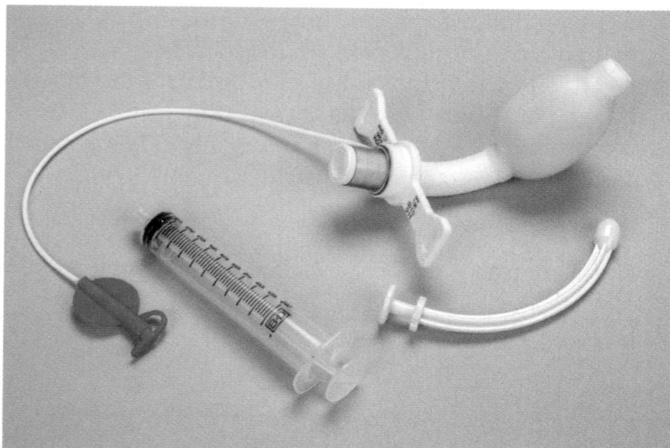

Figure 49.22 ■ A tracheostomy tube with a foam cuff.

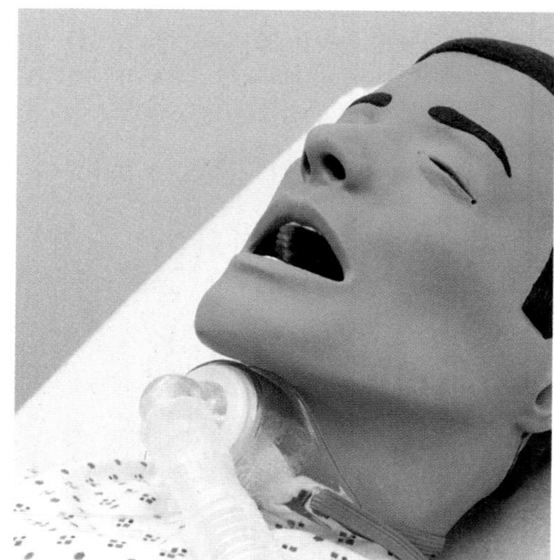

Figure 49.23 ■ A tracheostomy mist collar.

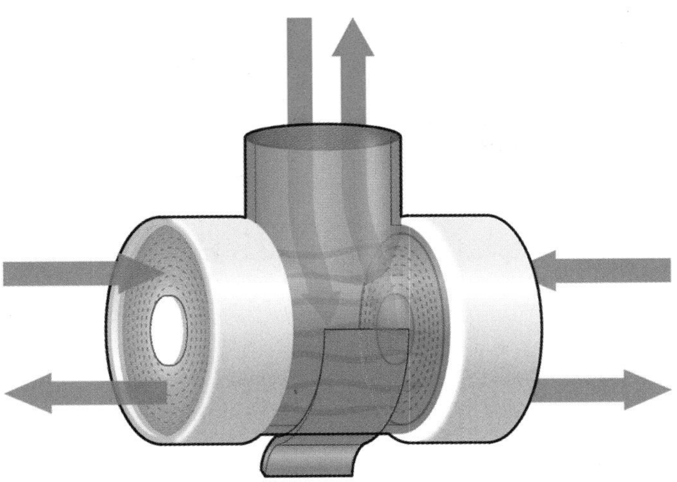

Figure 49.24 ■ Heat and moisture exchanger device.

use it to warm and humidify the next inspired breath (Ari, Alwadeai, & Fink, 2017). Clients may also wear a stoma protector such as a 4×4 gauze held in place with a cotton tie over the stoma or a light scarf to filter air as it enters the tracheostomy.

Suctioning

When clients have difficulty handling their secretions or an artificial airway is in place, suctioning may be necessary to clear air passages. **Suctioning** is the aspiration of secretions through a catheter connected to a suction machine or wall suction outlet. Even though the upper airways (the oropharynx and nasopharynx) are not sterile, sterile technique is recommended for all suctioning to avoid introducing pathogens into the airways. It is best to check the agency's policy because some facilities may use clean rather than sterile technique for nasopharyngeal and oropharyngeal suctioning with the rationale that the catheter does not extend down to the lower airway.

Oropharyngeal and nasopharyngeal suctioning removes secretions from the upper respiratory tract. Nasotracheal suctioning provides closer access to the trachea and requires sterile technique. Skill 49.2 outlines oral, oropharyngeal, nasopharyngeal, and nasotracheal suctioning.

Suction catheters are flexible, made of plastic, and may be either open tipped or whistle tipped (Figure 49.25 ■). The whistle-tipped catheter is less irritating to respiratory tissues, although the open-tipped catheter may be more effective for removing thick mucous plugs. An oral suction tube, or Yankauer suction tube, is used to suction the oral cavity (Figure 49.26 ■). Alert clients can be taught how to use this method of oral suctioning themselves. Most suction catheters have a thumb port on the side to control the suction. The catheter is connected to suction tubing, which in turn is connected to a collection chamber and suction control gauge (Figure 49.27 ■).

The nurse decides when suctioning is needed by assessing the client for signs of respiratory distress or evidence that the client is unable to cough up and expectorate secretions. Dyspnea, bubbling or rattling (adventitious) breath sounds, poor skin color (pallor,

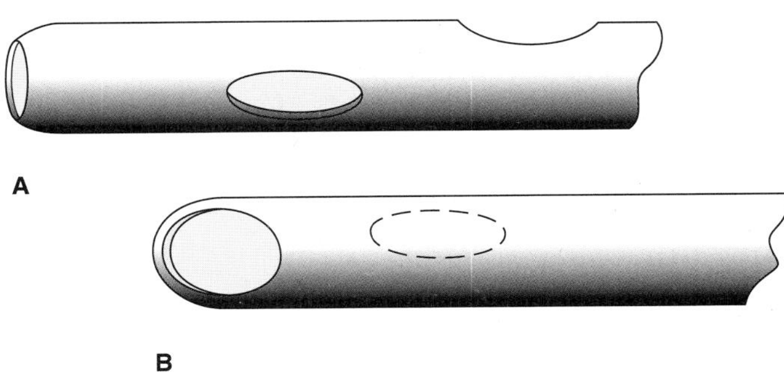

Figure 49.25 ■ Types of suction catheters: *A*, open tipped; *B*, whistle tipped.

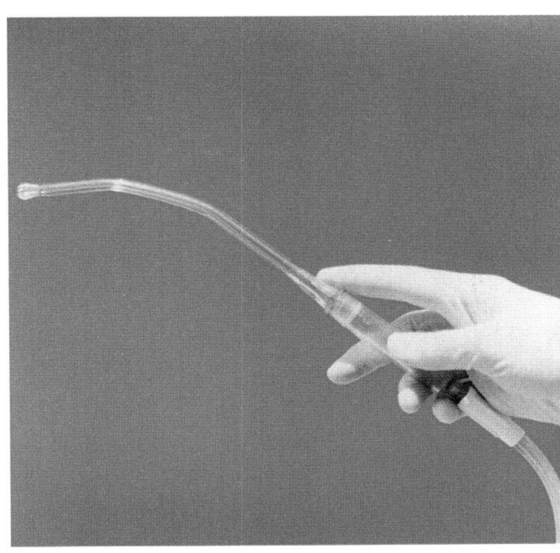

Figure 49.26 ■ Oral (Yankauer) suction tube.
Shirlee Snyder.

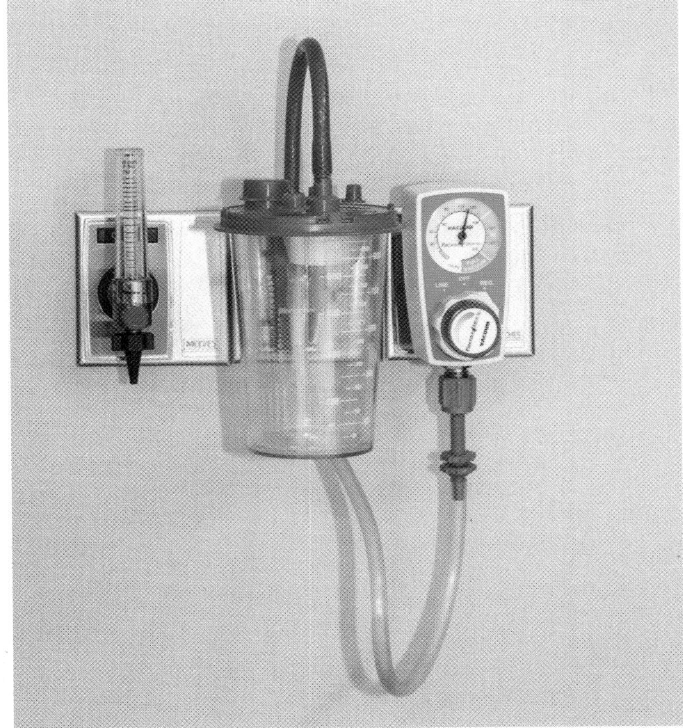

Figure 49.27 ■ A wall suction unit.

SKILL 49.2

Oral, Oropharyngeal, Nasopharyngeal, and Nasotracheal Suctioning

PURPOSES

- To remove secretions that obstruct the airway
- To facilitate ventilation
- To obtain secretions for diagnostic purposes
- To prevent infection that may result from accumulated secretions

ASSESSMENT

Assess for clinical signs indicating the need for suctioning:

- Restlessness, anxiety
- Noisy respirations
- Adventitious (abnormal) breath sounds when the chest is auscultated
- Change in mental status
- Skin color
- Rate and pattern of respirations
- Pulse rate and rhythm
- Decreased oxygen saturation

PLANNING

Assignment

Oral suctioning using a Yankauer suction tube can be assigned to AP and to the client or family, if appropriate, since this is not a sterile procedure. The nurse needs to review the procedure and important points such as not applying suction during insertion of the tube to avoid trauma to the mucous membrane. Oropharyngeal suctioning uses a suction catheter and, although not a sterile procedure, should be performed by a nurse or respiratory therapist. Suctioning can stimulate the gag reflex, hypoxia, and dysrhythmias that may require problem-solving. In contrast, nasopharyngeal and nasotracheal suctioning use sterile technique and require application of knowledge and problem-solving and should be performed by the nurse or respiratory therapist.

Equipment

Oropharyngeal, Nasopharyngeal, and Nasotracheal Suctioning (Using Sterile Technique)

- Towel or moisture-resistant pad
- Portable or wall suction machine with tubing, collection receptacle, and suction pressure gauge
- Sterile disposable container for fluids
- Sterile normal saline or water
- Goggles or face shield, if appropriate
- Moisture-resistant disposal bag
- Sterile gloves
- Sterile suction catheter kit (#12 to #18 Fr for adults, #8 to #10 Fr for children, and #5 to #8 Fr for infants)
- Water-soluble lubricant
- Y-connector
- Sputum trap, if specimen is to be collected

Oral and Oropharyngeal Suctioning (Using Clean Technique)

- Yankauer suction catheter or suction catheter kit
- Clean gloves

IMPLEMENTATION

Performance

1. Prior to performing the procedure, introduce self and verify the client's identity using agency protocol. Explain to the client what you are going to do, why it is necessary, and how to participate. Inform the client that suctioning will relieve breathing difficulty and that the procedure is painless but may be uncomfortable and stimulate the cough, gag, or sneeze reflex. **Rationale:** *Knowing that the procedure will relieve breathing problems is often reassuring and enlists the client's cooperation.*
2. Perform hand hygiene and observe other appropriate infection prevention procedures.
3. Provide for client privacy.
4. Prepare the client.
   - Position a conscious client who has a functional gag reflex in the semi-Fowler's position with the head turned to one side for oral suctioning or with the neck hyperextended for nasal suctioning. **Rationale:** *These positions facilitate the insertion of the catheter and help prevent aspiration of secretions.*
   - Position an unconscious client in the lateral position, facing you. **Rationale:** *This position allows the tongue to fall forward, so that it will not obstruct the catheter on insertion. The lateral position also facilitates drainage of secretions from the pharynx and prevents the possibility of aspiration.*
   - Place the towel or moisture-resistant pad over the pillow or under the chin.
5. Prepare the equipment.
   - Turn the suction device on and set to appropriate negative pressure on the suction gauge. The amount of negative pressure should be high enough to clear secretions but not too high. **Rationale:** *Too high of a pressure can cause the catheter to adhere to the tracheal wall and cause irritation or trauma.* A rule of thumb is to use the lowest amount of suction pressure needed to clear the secretions.

For Oral and Oropharyngeal Suction

- Apply clean gloves.
- Moisten the tip of the Yankauer or suction catheter with sterile water or saline. **Rationale:** *This reduces friction and eases insertion.*
- Pull the tongue forward, if necessary, using gauze.
- Do not apply suction (that is, leave your finger off the port) during insertion. **Rationale:** *Applying suction during insertion causes trauma to the mucous membrane.*
- Advance the catheter about 10 to 15 cm (4 to 6 in.) along one side of the mouth into the oropharynx. **Rationale:** *Directing the catheter along the side prevents gagging.*
- It may be necessary during oropharyngeal suctioning to apply suction to secretions that collect in the mouth and beneath the tongue.
- Remove and discard gloves.
- Perform hand hygiene.

For Nasopharyngeal and Nasotracheal Suction

- Open the lubricant.
- Open the sterile suction package.
  a. Set up the cup or container, touching only the outside.
  b. Pour sterile water or saline into the container.

Oral, Oropharyngeal, Nasopharyngeal, and Nasotracheal Suctioning—*continued*

c. Apply the sterile gloves, or apply an unsterile glove on the nondominant hand and then a sterile glove on the dominant hand. **Rationale:** *The sterile gloved hand maintains the sterility of the suction catheter, and the unsterile glove prevents the transmission of the microorganisms to the nurse.*

- With your sterile gloved hand, pick up the catheter and attach it to the suction unit. ❶

6. Test the pressure of the suction and the patency of the catheter by applying your sterile gloved finger or thumb to the port or open branch of the Y-connector (the suction control) to create suction.
   - If needed, apply or increase supplemental oxygen.
7. Lubricate and introduce the catheter.
   - Lubricate the catheter tip with sterile water, saline, or water-soluble lubricant. **Rationale:** *This reduces friction and eases insertion.*
   - Remove oxygen with the nondominant hand, if appropriate.
   - *Without applying suction*, insert the catheter into either naris and advance it along the floor of the nasal cavity. **Rationale:** *This avoids the nasal turbinates.*
   - Never force the catheter against an obstruction. If one nostril is obstructed, try the other.
8. Perform suctioning.
   - Apply your finger to the suction control port to start suction, and gently rotate the catheter. **Rationale:** *Gentle rotation of the catheter ensures that all surfaces are reached and prevents trauma to any one area of the respiratory mucosa due to prolonged suction.*
   - Apply suction for 5 to 10 seconds while slowly withdrawing the catheter, then remove your finger from the control and remove the catheter. **Rationale:** *Intermittent suction reduces the occurrence of trauma or irritation to the trachea and nasopharynx.*
   - A suction attempt should last only 10 to 15 seconds. During this time, the catheter is inserted, the suction applied and discontinued, and the catheter removed.
9. Rinse the catheter and repeat suctioning as above if necessary.
   - Rinse and flush the catheter and tubing with sterile water or saline.
   - Relubricate the catheter, and repeat suctioning until the air passage is clear.
   - Allow sufficient time between each suction for ventilation and oxygenation. Limit suctioning to 5 minutes in total.

   Rationale: *Applying suction for too long may cause secretions to increase or may decrease the client's oxygen supply.*
   - Encourage the client to breathe deeply and to cough between suctions. Use supplemental oxygen, if appropriate. **Rationale:** *Coughing and deep breathing help carry secretions from the trachea and bronchi into the pharynx, where they can be reached with the suction catheter. Deep breathing and supplemental oxygen replenish the oxygen supply that was decreased during the suctioning process.*
10. Obtain a specimen if required.
    - Use a sputum trap ❷ as follows:
      a. Attach the suction catheter to the tubing of the sputum trap.
      b. Attach the suction tubing to the sputum trap air vent.
      c. Suction the client. The sputum trap will collect the mucus during suctioning.
      d. Remove the catheter from the client. Disconnect the sputum trap tubing from the suction catheter. Remove the suction tubing from the trap air vent.
      e. Connect the tubing of the sputum trap to the air vent. **Rationale:** *This retains any microorganisms in the sputum trap.*
    - Connect the suction catheter to the tubing.
    - Flush the catheter to remove secretions from the tubing.
11. Promote client comfort.
    - Offer to assist the client with oral or nasal hygiene.
    - Assist the client to a position that facilitates breathing.
12. Dispose of equipment and ensure availability for the next suction.
    - Dispose of the catheter, gloves, water, and waste container.
      a. Rinse the suction tubing as needed by inserting the end of the tubing into the used water container.
      b. Wrap the catheter around your sterile gloved hand and hold the catheter as the glove is removed over it for disposal.
    - Perform hand hygiene.

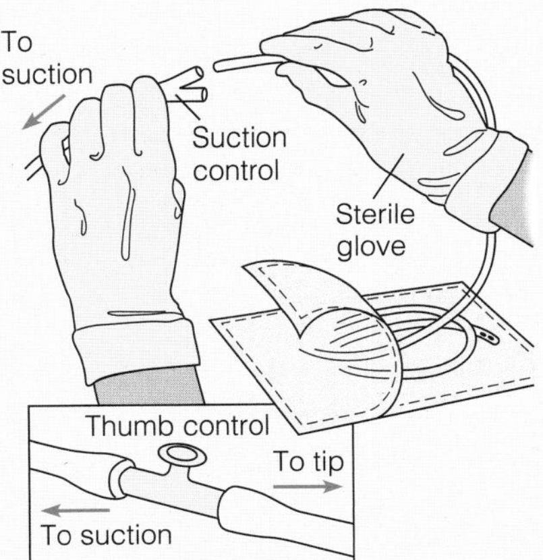

❶ Attaching the catheter to the suction unit.

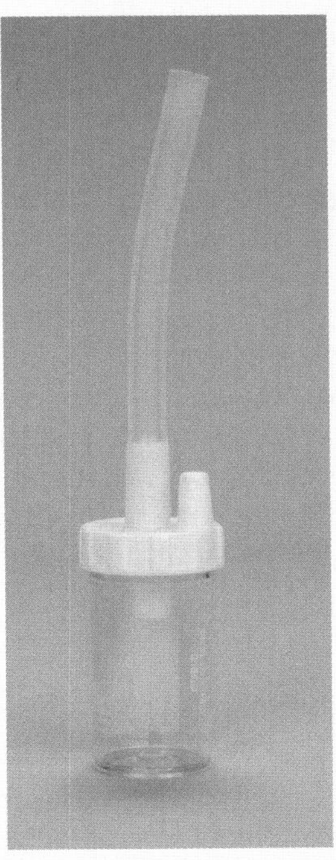

❷ A sputum collection trap.

Continued on page 1332

Oral, Oropharyngeal, Nasopharyngeal, and Nasotracheal Suctioning—*continued*

SKILL 49.2

- Empty and rinse the suction collection container as needed or indicated by protocol. Change the suction tubing and container daily.
- Ensure that supplies are available for the next suctioning (suction kit, gloves, water or normal saline).

13. Assess the effectiveness of suctioning.
- Auscultate the client's breath sounds to ensure they are clear of secretions. Observe skin color, dyspnea, level of anxiety, and oxygen saturation levels.

14. Document relevant data.
- Record the procedure: the amount, consistency, color, and odor of sputum (e.g., foamy, white mucus; thick, green-tinged mucus; or blood-flecked mucus) and the client's respiratory status before and after the procedure. This may include lung sounds, rate and character of breathing, and oxygen saturation.
- If the procedure is carried out frequently (e.g., every hour), it may be appropriate to record only once, at the end of the shift; however, the frequency of the suctioning must be recorded.

SAMPLE DOCUMENTATION

12/12/2020 0830 Producing large amounts of thick, tenacious white mucus to back of oral pharynx but unable to expectorate into tissue. Client uses Yankauer suction tube as needed. O_2 sat increased from 89% before suctioning to 93% after suctioning. RR also decreased from 26 to 18–20 after suctioning. Lungs clear to auscultation throughout all lobes. Continuous O_2 at 2 L/min via n/c. Will continue to reassess every hour. L. Webb, RN

EVALUATION

- Conduct appropriate follow-up, such as appearance of secretions suctioned; breath sounds; respiratory rate, rhythm, and depth; pulse rate and rhythm; and skin color.
- Compare findings to previous assessment data if available.
- Report significant deviations from normal to the primary care provider.

LIFESPAN CONSIDERATIONS Suctioning

INFANTS

- A bulb syringe is used to remove secretions from an infant's nose or mouth. Care needs to be taken to avoid stimulating the gag reflex.

CHILDREN

- A catheter is used to remove secretions from an older child's mouth or nose.

OLDER ADULTS

- Older adults often have cardiac or pulmonary disease, thus increasing their susceptibility to hypoxemia related to suctioning. Watch closely for signs of hypoxemia. If noted, stop suctioning and hyperoxygenate.

duskiness, or cyanosis), restlessness, tachycardia, or decreased oxygen saturation (SpO_2) levels (also called O_2 sat) may indicate the need for suctioning. Good nursing judgment and critical thinking are necessary. Suctioning irritates mucous membranes, can increase secretions if performed too frequently, and can cause the client's oxygen saturation to drop further, put the client in bronchospasm, and if the client has a head injury, cause the intracranial pressure to increase. In other words, suctioning is based on *clinical need* versus a fixed schedule.

In addition to removing secretions that obstruct the airway and facilitating ventilation, suctioning can be performed to obtain secretions for diagnostic purposes and to prevent infection that may result from accumulated secretions.

QSEN Patient-Centered Care: Suctioning

The nurse who is providing care in the home setting for a client who requires suctioning needs to consider the following:

- Teach clients and families that the most important aspect of infection control is frequent hand washing.
- Airway suctioning in the home is considered a clean procedure.
- The catheter or Yankauer should be flushed by suctioning recently boiled or distilled water to rinse away mucus, followed by the suctioning of air through the device to dry the internal surface and, thus, discourage bacterial growth. The outer surface of the device may be wiped with alcohol or hydrogen peroxide. The suction catheter or Yankauer should be allowed to dry and then be stored in a clean, dry area.
- Suction catheters treated in the manner described above may be reused. It is recommended that catheters be discarded after 24 hours. Yankauer suction tubes may be cleaned, boiled, and reused.

Following endotracheal intubation or a tracheostomy, the trachea and surrounding respiratory tissues are irritated and react by producing excessive secretions. Sterile suctioning is necessary to remove these secretions from the trachea and bronchi to maintain a patent airway. The frequency of suctioning depends on the client's health and how recently the intubation was done. Suctioning may be necessary in clients who have increased secretions because of pneumonia or inability to clear secretions because of altered level of consciousness. Some clients have a cough that brings secretions to the opening of the tracheostomy or endotracheal tube. They will only need suctioning at the opening of the tube and not deep suctioning.

Suctioning is associated with several complications: hypoxemia, trauma to the airway, healthcare-associated infection, and cardiac dysrhythmia, which is related to the hypoxemia. The following techniques are used to minimize or decrease these complications:

- ***Suction only as needed.*** Because suctioning the client with an ETT or tracheostomy is uncomfortable for the client and potentially hazardous because of hypoxemia, it should be performed only when indicated and *not* on a fixed schedule.
- ***Sterile technique.*** Infection of the lower respiratory tract can occur during tracheal suctioning. The nurse using sterile technique during the suctioning process can prevent this complication.
- ***No saline instillation.*** Instilling normal saline into the airway has been a common practice and a routine part of the suctioning procedure. It was thought that the saline would facilitate removal of secretions and improve the client's oxygenation status. Research, however, has shown that saline instillation does *not* facilitate removal of secretions and causes adverse effects such as hypoxemia and increased risk of pneumonia (Restrepo, Mathai, Luna, Ramirez, & Olaniyi-Adegbola, 2016).
- **Hyperinflation**. This involves giving the client breaths that are greater than the tidal volume set on the ventilator through the ventilator circuit or via a manual resuscitation bag. Three to five breaths are delivered before and after each pass of the suction catheter.
- **Hyperventilation**. This involves increasing the number of breaths the client is receiving. This can be done through the ventilator or using a manual resuscitation bag.

  Both hyperinflation and hyperventilation help prevent suction hypoxemia; however, they should be used with caution because they can cause injury as a result of overdistention of the lungs.
- **Hyperoxygenation**. This can be done with a manual resuscitation bag or through the ventilator and is performed by increasing the oxygen flow (usually to 100%) before suctioning and between suction attempts. This is the best technique to avoid suction-related hypoxemia.
- ***Safe catheter size.*** To prevent hypoxia when tracheostomy and endotracheal suctioning are administered, the outer diameter of the suction catheter should not exceed one-half the internal diameter of the artificial airway. A formula to determine suction catheter size is to multiply the artificial airway's diameter times 2. For example, an artificial airway (e.g., tracheostomy) diameter of 8 mm $\times$ 2 = 16. A size 16 French suction catheter would be safe to use (Smith et al., 2017, p. 1207).

The nurse uses sterile techniques to prevent infection of the respiratory tract (Skill 49.3). The traditional method of suctioning an ETT or tracheostomy is sometimes referred to as the *open suction system*. If a client is connected to a ventilator, the nurse disconnects the client from the ventilator, suctions the airway, reconnects the client to the ventilator, and discards the suction catheter. Other drawbacks to the open suction system include the nurse needing to wear personal protective equipment (e.g., goggles or face shield, gown) to avoid exposure to the client's sputum and the potential cost of one-time catheter use, especially if the client requires frequent suctioning.

With the *closed suction system* (Figure 49.28 ■), the suction catheter attaches to the ventilator tubing and the client does not need to be disconnected from the ventilator. The nurse is not exposed to any secretions because the suction catheter is enclosed in a plastic sheath. The catheter can be reused as many times as

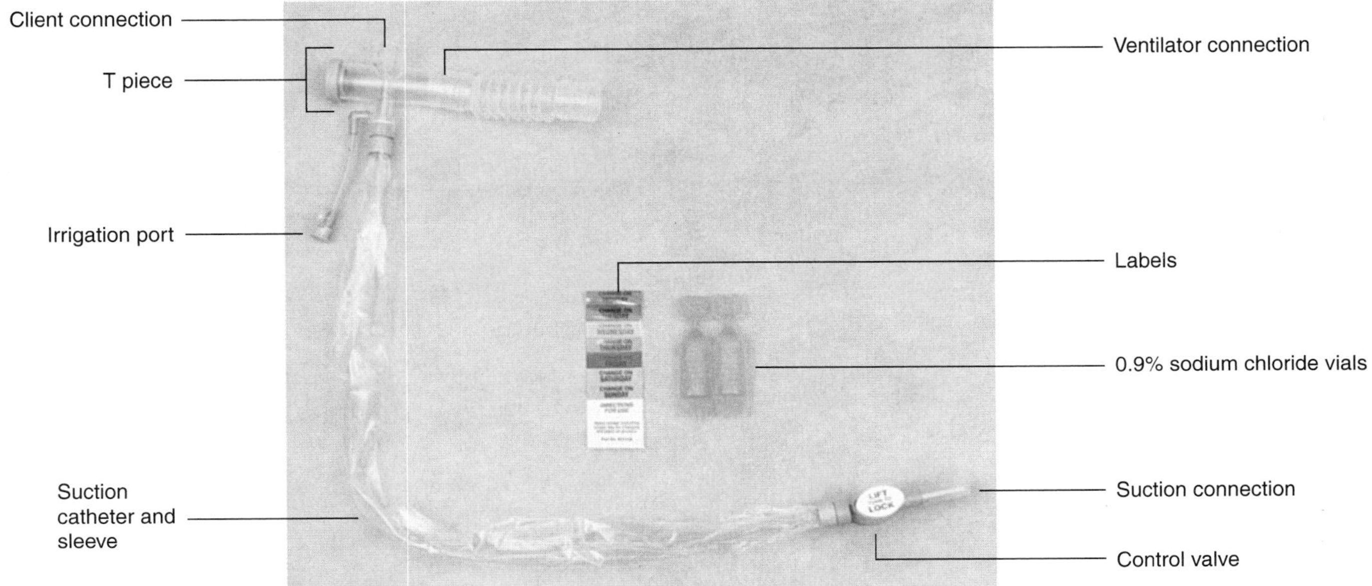

Figure 49.28 ■ A closed suction system.

necessary until the system is changed. The nurse needs to inquire about the agency's policy for changing the closed suction system.

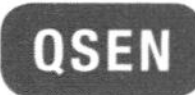

Patient-Centered Care: Suctioning a Tracheostomy or Endotracheal Tube

In the home care setting, the nurse needs to consider the following for clients requiring suctioning of a tracheostomy or endotracheal tube:

- Whenever possible, the client should be encouraged to clear the airway by coughing.
- Clients may need to learn to suction their secretions if they cannot cough effectively.
- Clean gloves should be used when endotracheal suctioning is performed in the home environment.
- The nurse needs to instruct the caregiver on how to determine the need for suctioning and the correct process and rationale underlying the practice of suctioning to avoid potential complications of suctioning.
- Stress the importance of adequate hydration as it thins secretions, which can aid in the removal of secretions by coughing or suctioning.

SKILL 49.3

Suctioning a Tracheostomy or Endotracheal Tube

PURPOSES

- To maintain a patent airway and prevent airway obstructions
- To promote respiratory function (optimal exchange of oxygen and carbon dioxide into and out of the lungs)
- To prevent pneumonia that may result from accumulated secretions

ASSESSMENT

Assess the client for the presence of adventitious (abnormal) breath sounds. Assess the client's cough reflex and note the client's ability or inability to remove the secretions by coughing.

PLANNING

Assignment

Suctioning a tracheostomy or endotracheal tube is a sterile, invasive technique requiring application of scientific knowledge and problem-solving. This skill is performed by a nurse or respiratory therapist and is not assigned to AP.

Equipment

- Resuscitation bag (bag valve mask) connected to 100% oxygen
- Sterile towel (optional)
- Equipment for suctioning (see Skill 49.2)
- Goggles and mask (if necessary)
- Gown (if necessary)
- Sterile gloves
- Moisture-resistant bag

IMPLEMENTATION

Preparation

Determine if the client has been suctioned previously and, if so, review the documentation of the procedure. This information can be very helpful in preparing the nurse for both the physiologic and psychologic impact of suctioning on the client.

Performance

1. Prior to performing the procedure, introduce self and verify the client's identity using agency protocol. Explain to the client what you are going to do, why it is necessary, and how to participate. Inform the client that suctioning usually causes some intermittent coughing and that this assists in removing the secretions.
2. Perform hand hygiene and observe other appropriate infection prevention procedures.
3. Provide for client privacy.
4. Prepare the client.
   - If not contraindicated, place the client in the semi-Fowler's position to promote deep breathing, maximum lung expansion, and productive coughing. **Rationale:** *Deep breathing oxygenates the lungs, counteracts the hypoxic effects of suctioning, and may induce coughing. Coughing helps to loosen and move secretions.*
5. Prepare the equipment for an open suction system—see *Variation* section for a closed suction system.
   - Attach the resuscitation apparatus to the oxygen source. ❶ Adjust the oxygen flow to 100%.

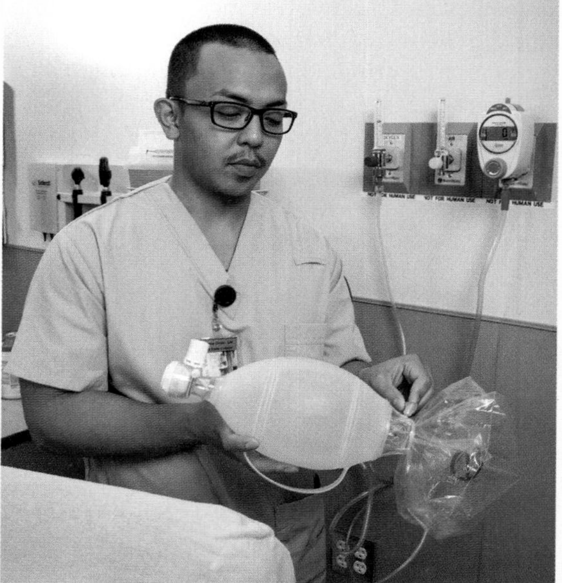

❶ Attaching the resuscitation apparatus to the oxygen source.

   - Open the sterile supplies:
     a. Suction kit or catheter
     b. Sterile basin or container.

Suctioning a Tracheostomy or Endotracheal Tube—*continued*

- Pour sterile normal saline or water into sterile basin or container.
- Place the sterile towel, if used, across the client's chest below the tracheostomy or on a workspace.
- Turn on the suction, and set the pressure in accordance with agency policy. The suction pressure should be set at what is needed to adequately remove secretions. The recommended suction pressure for the open suction system is 100–120 mm Hg vacuum (Smith et al., 2017, p. 1207).
- Apply goggles, mask, and gown if necessary.
- Apply sterile gloves. Some agencies recommend putting a sterile glove on the dominant hand and an unsterile glove on the nondominant hand. **Rationale:** *The sterile gloved hand maintains the sterility of the suction catheter, and the unsterile glove holds the suction connecting tubing and prevents transmission of the microorganisms to the nurse.*
- Holding the catheter in the dominant hand and the connector in the nondominant hand, attach the suction catheter to the suction tubing (see Figure ❶ in Skill 49.2).

6. Flush and lubricate the catheter.
- Using the dominant hand, place the catheter tip in the sterile saline solution.
- Using the thumb of the nondominant hand, occlude the thumb control and suction a small amount of the sterile solution through the catheter. **Rationale:** *This determines that the suction equipment is working properly and lubricates the outside and the lumen of the catheter. Lubrication eases insertion and reduces tissue trauma during insertion. Lubricating the lumen also helps prevent secretions from sticking to the inside of the catheter.*

7. If the client does not have copious secretions, hyperventilate the lungs with a resuscitation bag before suctioning.
- Summon an assistant, if one is available, for this step.
- Using your nondominant hand, turn on the oxygen to 12 to 15 L/min.
- If the client is receiving oxygen, disconnect the oxygen source from the tracheostomy tube using your nondominant hand.
- Attach the resuscitator to the tracheostomy or ETT. ❷
- Compress the resuscitation bag three to five times, as the client inhales. This is best done by a second staff member who can use both hands to compress the bag.
- Observe the rise and fall of the client's chest to assess the adequacy of each ventilation.
- Remove the resuscitation device and place it on the bed or the client's chest with the connector facing up.

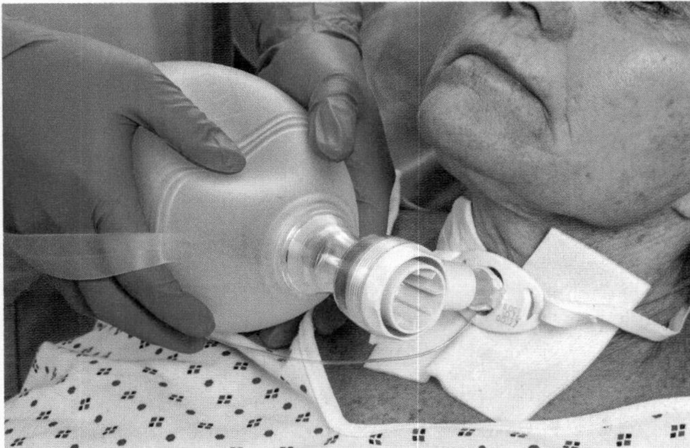
❷ Attaching the resuscitator to the tracheostomy tube.

Variation: Using a Ventilator to Provide Hyperventilation
If the client is on a ventilator, use the ventilator for hyperventilation and hyperoxygenation. Newer models have a mode that provides 100% oxygen for 2 minutes and then switches back to the previous oxygen setting as well as a manual breath or sigh button. **Rationale:** *The use of ventilator settings provides more consistent delivery of oxygenation and hyperinflation than a resuscitation device.*

8. If the client has copious secretions, do not hyperventilate with a resuscitator. *Instead:*
- Keep the regular oxygen delivery device on and increase the liter flow or adjust the FiO_2 to 100% for several breaths before suctioning. **Rationale:** *Hyperventilating a client who has copious secretions can force the secretions deeper into the respiratory tract.*

9. Quickly but gently insert the catheter *without* applying any suction.
- With your nondominant thumb off the suction port, quickly but gently insert the catheter into the trachea through the tracheostomy tube. ❸ **Rationale:** *To prevent tissue trauma and oxygen loss, suction is not applied during insertion of the catheter.*
- Insert the catheter about 1 to 2 cm (1/2 to 1 in.) past the distal end of the tube until resistance is felt, even if the client coughs (Smith et al., 2017, p. 1208).

10. Perform suctioning.
- Apply suction for 5 to 10 seconds by placing the nondominant thumb over the thumb port. **Rationale:** *Suction time is restricted to 10 seconds or less to minimize oxygen loss.*
- Rotate the catheter by rolling it between your thumb and forefinger while slowly withdrawing it. **Rationale:** *This prevents tissue trauma by minimizing the suction time against any part of the trachea.*
- Withdraw the catheter completely, and release the suction.
- Hyperventilate the client.
- Suction again, if needed.

11. Reassess the client's oxygenation status and repeat suctioning.
- Observe the client's respirations and skin color. Check the client's pulse if necessary, using your nondominant hand. If the client is on a cardiac monitor, assess the rate and rhythm.
- Encourage the client to breathe deeply and to cough between suctions.

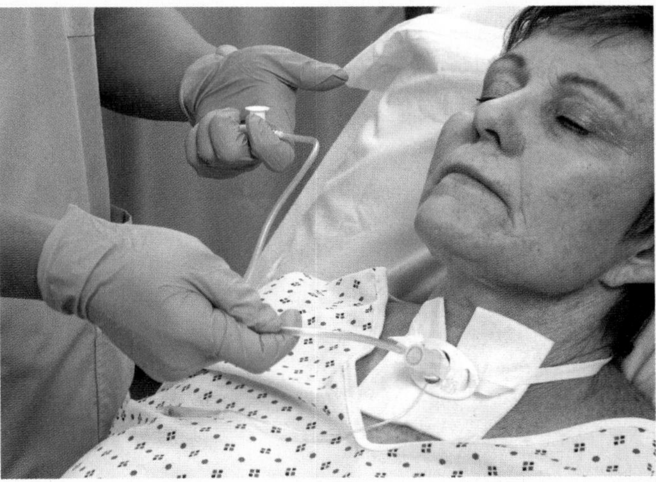
❸ Inserting the catheter into the trachea through the tracheostomy tube. *Note:* Suction is not applied while inserting the catheter.

Continued on page 1336

SKILL 49.3

Suctioning a Tracheostomy or Endotracheal Tube—*continued*

- Allow 2 to 3 minutes with oxygen, as appropriate between suctions when possible. **Rationale:** *This provides an opportunity for reoxygenation of the lungs.*
- Flush the catheter and repeat suctioning until the air passage is clear and the breathing is relatively effortless and quiet.
- After each suction, pick up the resuscitation bag with your nondominant hand and ventilate the client with no more than three breaths.

12. Dispose of equipment and ensure availability for the next suction.
- Flush the catheter and suction tubing.
- Turn off the suction and disconnect the catheter from the suction tubing.
- Wrap the catheter around your sterile hand and peel the glove off so that it turns inside out over the catheter. Remove the other glove.
- Discard the gloves and the catheter in the moisture-resistant bag.
- Perform hand hygiene.
- Replenish the sterile fluid and supplies so that the suction is ready for use again. **Rationale:** *Clients who require suctioning often require it quickly, so it is essential to leave the equipment at the bedside ready for use.*
- Be sure that the ventilator and oxygen settings are returned to presuctioning settings. **Rationale:** *On some ventilators this is automatic, but always check. It is very dangerous for clients to be left on 100% oxygen.*

13. Provide for client comfort and safety.
- Assist the client to a comfortable, safe position that aids breathing. If the client is conscious, a semi-Fowler's position is frequently indicated. If the client is unconscious, Sims' position aids in the drainage of secretions from the mouth.

14. Document relevant data.
- Record the suctioning, including the amount and description of suction returns and any other relevant assessments.

Variation: Closed Suction System

- If a catheter is not already attached, apply clean gloves, aseptically open a new closed suction system catheter set, and attach the ventilator connection on the T piece to the ventilator tubing. Attach the client connection to the ETT or tracheostomy.
- Attach one end of the suction connecting tubing to the suction connection port of the closed system and the other end of the connecting tubing to the suction device.
- Turn suction on, occlude or kink tubing, and depress the suction control valve (on the closed catheter system) to set suction to the appropriate level. Release the suction control valve.
- Use the ventilator to hyperoxygenate and hyperinflate the client's lungs.
- Unlock the suction control mechanism if required by the manufacturer.
- Advance the suction catheter enclosed in its plastic sheath with the dominant hand. Steady the T piece with the nondominant hand.
- Depress the suction control valve and apply continuous suction for no more than 10 seconds and gently withdraw the catheter.
- Repeat as needed remembering to provide hyperoxygenation and hyperinflation as needed.
- When suctioning is completed, withdraw the catheter into its sleeve and close the access valve, if appropriate. **Rationale:** *If the system does not have an access valve on the client connector, the nurse needs to observe for the potential of the catheter migrating into and partially obstructing the artificial airway.*
- Flush the catheter by instilling normal saline into the irrigation port and applying suction. Repeat until the catheter is clear.
- Close the irrigation port and close the suction valve.
- Remove and discard gloves.
- Perform hand hygiene.

SAMPLE DOCUMENTATION

12/13/2020 1000 Coarse crackles in RLL and LLL. Requires suctioning about every 1–2 h. Obtained large amount of pinkish-tinged, white thin mucus via ETT. Breath sounds clearer after suctioning. SpO_2 increased from 90% before suctioning to 95% after suctioning. Client signals when he wants to be suctioned. C. Holmes, RN

EVALUATION

- Perform a follow-up examination of the client to determine the effectiveness of the suctioning (e.g., respiratory rate, depth, and character; breath sounds; color of skin and nail beds; character and amount of secretions suctioned; changes in vital signs [e.g., heart rate, oxygen saturation]).
- Compare findings to previous assessment data if available.
- Report significant deviations from normal to the primary care provider.

LIFESPAN CONSIDERATIONS Suctioning a Tracheostomy or Endotracheal Tube

INFANTS AND CHILDREN

- Have an assistant gently restrain the child to keep the child's hands out of the way. The assistant should maintain the child's head in the midline position.

OLDER ADULTS

- Healthcare-associated pneumonia and ventilator-associated pneumonia (VAP) can occur because of infected secretions in the upper airway. Oral antiseptic rinses (e.g., chlorhexidine gluconate) reduce the rate of healthcare-associated pneumonia in critically ill clients ("Prevention," 2017).
- Do a thorough lung assessment before and after suctioning to determine effectiveness of suctioning and to be aware of any special problems.

Providing Tracheostomy Care

PURPOSES

- To maintain airway patency
- To maintain cleanliness and prevent infection at the tracheostomy site
- To facilitate healing and prevent skin excoriation around the tracheostomy incision
- To promote comfort

ASSESSMENT

Assess

- Respiratory status including ease of breathing, rate, rhythm, depth, lung sounds, and oxygen saturation level
- Pulse rate
- Character and amount of secretions from tracheostomy site
- Presence of drainage on tracheostomy dressing or ties
- Appearance of incision (note any redness, swelling, purulent discharge, or odor)

PLANNING

Assignment

Tracheostomy care involves application of scientific knowledge, sterile technique, and problem-solving, and therefore needs to be performed by a nurse or respiratory therapist.

Equipment

- Sterile disposable tracheostomy cleaning kit or supplies including sterile containers, sterile nylon brush or pipe cleaners, sterile applicators, gauze squares
- Disposable inner cannula if applicable
- Towel or drape to protect bed linens
- Sterile suction catheter kit (suction catheter and sterile container for solution)
- Sterile normal saline (Some agencies may use a mixture of hydrogen peroxide and sterile normal saline. Check agency protocol for soaking solution.)
- Sterile gloves (two pairs—one pair is for suctioning if needed)
- Clean gloves
- Moisture-proof bag
- Commercially prepared sterile tracheostomy dressing or sterile 4×4 gauze dressing
- Cotton twill ties or Velcro collar
- Clean scissors

IMPLEMENTATION

Performance

1. Prior to performing the procedure, introduce self and verify the client's identity using agency protocol. Explain to the client what you are going to do, why it is necessary, and how to participate. Provide for a means of communication, such as eye blinking or raising a finger, to indicate pain or distress. Follow through by carefully observing the client throughout the procedure, and offering periodic eye contact, caring touch, and verbal reassurance.
2. Perform hand hygiene and observe other appropriate infection prevention procedures.
3. Provide for client privacy.
4. Prepare the client and the equipment.
   - Assist the client to a semi-Fowler's or Fowler's position *to promote lung expansion*.
   - Suction the tracheostomy tube, if needed. (See Skill 49.3.)
   - If suctioning was required, allow the client to rest and restore oxygenation.
   - Open the tracheostomy kit or sterile basins.
   - Establish a sterile field.
   - Open other sterile supplies as needed including sterile applicators, suction kit, tracheostomy dressing, and disposable inner cannula, if applicable.
   - Pour the soaking solution and sterile normal saline into separate containers.
   - Apply clean gloves.
   - Remove the oxygen source.
   - Unlock the inner cannula (if present) and remove it by gently pulling it out toward you in line with its curvature. Place the inner cannula in the soaking solution, if not a disposable inner cannula. **Rationale:** *This moistens and loosens dried secretions*.
   - Based on the client's respiratory assessments, place oxygen source over or near the outer cannula. **Rationale:** *This prevents oxygen desaturation by maintaining oxygen to the client*.
   - Remove the soiled tracheostomy dressing. Place the soiled dressing in your gloved hand and peel the glove off so that it turns inside out over the dressing. Remove and discard the gloves and the dressing.
   - Perform hand hygiene.
   - Apply sterile gloves. Keep your dominant hand sterile during the procedure.
5. Clean the inner cannula. (See the *Variation* section for using a disposable inner cannula.)
   - Remove the inner cannula from the soaking solution.
   - Clean the lumen and entire inner cannula thoroughly using the brush or pipe cleaners moistened with sterile normal saline. ❶ Inspect the cannula for cleanliness by holding it at eye level and looking through it into the light.
   - Rinse the inner cannula thoroughly in the sterile normal saline.
   - After rinsing, gently tap the cannula against the inside edge of the sterile saline container. Use a pipe cleaner folded in half to dry only the inside of the cannula; do not dry the outside. **Rationale:** *This removes excess liquid from the cannula and prevents possible aspiration by the client, while leaving a film of moisture on the outer surface to lubricate the cannula for reinsertion*.
6. Replace the inner cannula, securing it in place.
   - Insert the inner cannula by grasping the outer flange and inserting the cannula in the direction of its curvature.
   - Lock the cannula in place by turning the lock (if present) into position to secure the flange of the inner cannula to the outer cannula.

Continued on page 1338

Providing Tracheostomy Care—*continued*

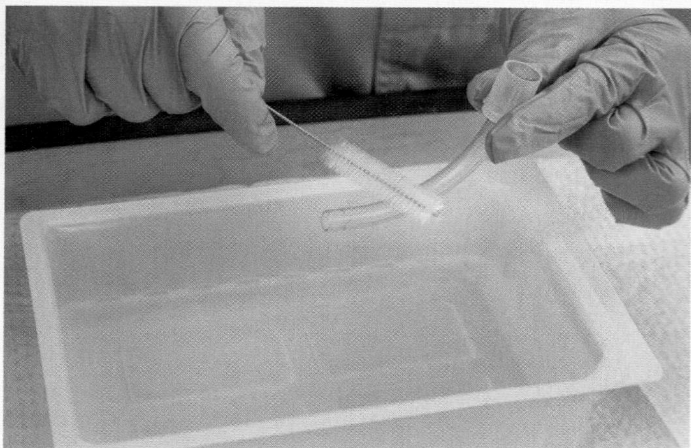

❶ Cleaning the inner cannula with a brush.

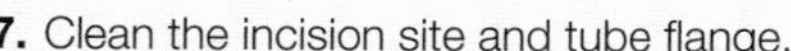

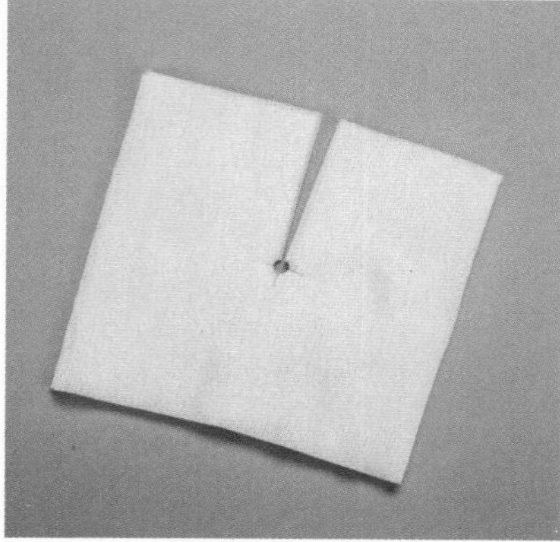

❸ A commercially prepared tracheostomy dressing of nonraveling material.

7. Clean the incision site and tube flange.
   - Using sterile applicators or gauze dressings moistened with normal saline, clean the incision site. ❷ Handle the sterile supplies with your dominant hand. Use each applicator or gauze dressing only once and then discard. **Rationale:** *This avoids contaminating a clean area with a soiled gauze dressing or applicator*.
   - Hydrogen peroxide may be used (usually in a half-strength solution mixed with sterile normal saline; use a separate sterile container if this is necessary) to remove crusty secretions around the tracheostomy site. Do not use directly on the site. Check agency policy. Thoroughly rinse the cleaned area using gauze squares moistened with sterile normal saline. **Rationale:** *Hydrogen peroxide can be irritating to the skin and inhibit healing if not thoroughly removed*.
   - Clean the flange of the tube in the same manner.
   - Thoroughly dry the client's skin and tube flanges with dry gauze squares.
8. Apply a sterile dressing.
   - Use a commercially prepared split-gauze tracheostomy dressing of nonraveling material. ❸ Never use cotton-filled gauze squares or cut the 4×4 gauze. **Rationale:** *Cotton lint or gauze fibers can be aspirated by the client, potentially creating a tracheal abscess*. Newer products include a nonadhesive hydrocellular dressing, which is a cushioned pad that absorbs large amounts of secretions.
   - Place the dressing under the flange of the tracheostomy tube.
   - While applying the dressing, ensure that the tracheostomy tube is securely supported. **Rationale:** *Excessive movement of the tracheostomy tube irritates the trachea*.
9. Change the tracheostomy ties or Velcro collar.
   - Change as needed to keep the skin clean and dry.
   - Twill tape and specially manufactured Velcro ties are available. Twill tape is inexpensive and readily available; however, it is easily soiled and can trap moisture, which leads to irritation of the skin of the neck. Velcro ties are becoming more commonly used. ❹ They are wider, are more comfortable, and cause less skin abrasion.
   - For client safety, the literature recommends a two-person technique when changing the securing device to prevent tube dislodgement. This involves one staff member holding the tracheostomy tube in place while the other changes the securing device.

Two-Strip Method (Twill Tape)

- Cut two unequal strips of twill tape, one approximately 25 cm (10 in.) long and the other about 50 cm (20 in.) long. **Rationale:** *Cutting one tape longer than the other allows them to be fastened at the side of the neck for easy access and to avoid the pressure of a knot on the skin at the back of the neck*.

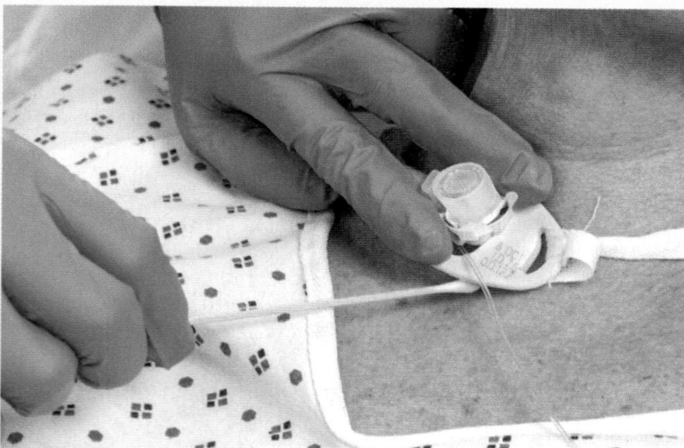

❷ Using an applicator stick to clean the tracheostomy site.

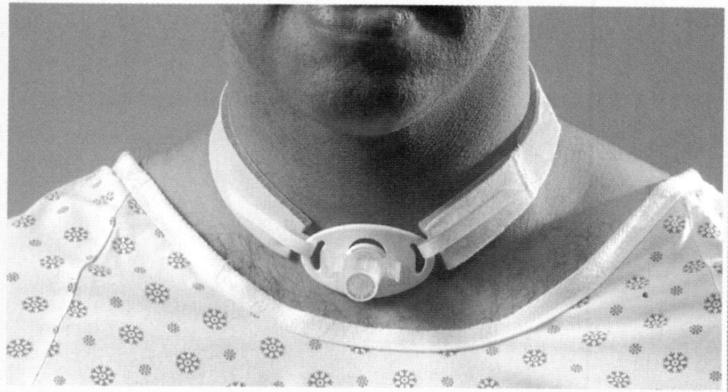

❹ A Velcro tracheostomy tie.

Providing Tracheostomy Care—*continued*

- Cut a 1-cm (0.5-in.) lengthwise slit approximately 2.5 cm (1 in.) from one end of each strip. To do this, fold the end of the tape back onto itself about 2.5 cm (1 in.), then cut a slit in the middle of the tape from its folded edge.
- Leaving the old ties in place, thread the slit end of one clean tape through the eye of the tracheostomy flange from the bottom side; then thread the long end of the tape through the slit, pulling it tight until it is securely fastened to the flange. **Rationale:** *Leaving the old ties in place while securing the clean ties prevents inadvertent dislodging of the tracheostomy tube. Securing tapes in this manner avoids the use of knots, which can come untied or cause pressure and irritation.*
- If old ties are very soiled or it is difficult to thread new ties onto the tracheostomy flange with old ties in place, have an assistant apply a sterile glove and hold the tracheostomy in place while you replace the ties. **Rationale:** *This is very important because movement of the tube during this procedure may cause irritation and stimulate coughing. Coughing can dislodge the tube if the ties are undone.*
- Repeat the process for the second tie.
- Ask the client to flex the neck. Slip the longer tape under the client's neck, place a finger between the tape and the client's neck, ❺ and tie the tapes together at the side of the neck. **Rationale:** *Flexing the neck increases its circumference the way coughing does. Placing a finger under the tie prevents making the tie too tight, which could interfere with coughing or place pressure on the jugular veins.*
- Tie the ends of the tapes using square knots. Cut off any long ends, leaving approximately 1 to 2 cm (0.5 in.). **Rationale:** *Square knots prevent slippage and loosening. Adequate ends beyond the knot prevent the knot from inadvertently untying.*
- Once the clean ties are secured, remove the soiled ties and discard.

One-Strip Method (Twill Tape)

- Cut a length of twill tape 2.5 times the length needed to go around the client's neck from one tube flange to the other.

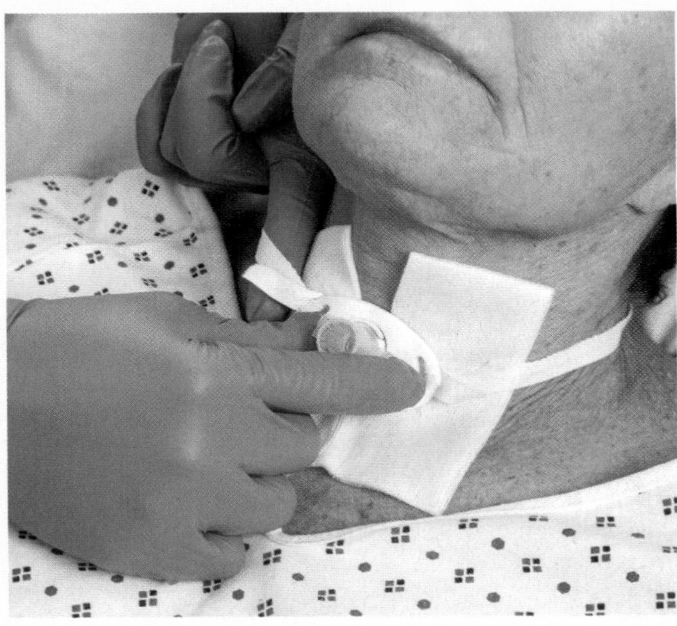

❺ Placing a finger underneath the tie tape before tying it.

- Thread one end of the tape into the slot on one side of the flange.
- Bring both ends of the tape together. Take them around the client's neck, keeping them flat and untwisted.
- Thread the end of the tape next to the client's neck through the slot from the back to the front.
- Have the client flex the neck. Tie the loose ends with a square knot at the side of the client's neck, allowing for slack by placing one finger under the ties as with the two-strip method. Cut off long ends.
- Tape and pad the tie knot.
- Place a folded 4×4 gauze square under the tie knot, and apply tape over the knot. **Rationale:** *This reduces skin irritation from the knot and prevents confusing the knot with the client's gown ties.*
- Check the tightness of the ties.
- Frequently check the tightness of the tracheostomy ties and position of the tracheostomy tube. **Rationale:** *Swelling of the neck may cause the ties to become too tight, interfering with coughing and circulation. Ties can loosen in restless clients, allowing the tracheostomy tube to extrude from the stoma.*

Velcro Collar Method

- Thread one piece of the collar with the Velcro end into the slot on one side of the flange.
- Take the collar around the back of the client's neck, keeping it flat.
- Thread the other piece of the collar with the Velcro end into the slot on the other side of the flange.
- Take the second piece of the collar around the back of the client's neck, keeping it flat.
- Have the client flex the neck and secure the two pieces of the collar together with the Velcro, allowing space for one to two fingers between the collar and the client's neck.
- Check the tightness of the collar as with the tie method.

10. Remove and discard sterile gloves.
- Perform hand hygiene.

11. Document all relevant information.
- Record suctioning, tracheostomy care, and the dressing change, noting your assessments.

Variation: Using a Disposable Inner Cannula

- Check policy for frequency of changing inner cannula because standards vary among institutions.
- Open a new cannula package.
- Using a gloved hand, unlock the current inner cannula (if present) and remove it by gently pulling it out toward you in line with its curvature.
- Check the cannula for amount and type of secretions and discard properly.
- Pick up the new inner cannula touching only the outer locking portion.
- Insert the new inner cannula into the tracheostomy.
- Lock the cannula in place by turning the lock (if present) or clipping in place.

SAMPLE DOCUMENTATION

12/11/2020 0900 Respirations 18–20/min. Lung sounds clear. Able to cough up secretions requiring little suctioning. Inner cannula changed. Trach dressing changed. Minimal amount of serosanguineous drainage present. Trach incision area pink to reddish in color 0.2 cm around entire opening. No broken skin noted in the reddened area. J. Garcia, RN

Continued on page 1340

SKILL 49.4

Providing Tracheostomy Care—*continued*

EVALUATION

- Perform appropriate follow-up such as determining character and amount of secretions, drainage from the tracheostomy, appearance of the tracheostomy incision, pulse rate and respiratory status compared to baseline data, and complaints of pain or discomfort at the tracheostomy site.
- Compare findings to previous assessment data if available.
- Report significant deviations from normal to the primary care provider.

QSEN **Patient-Centered Care: Tracheostomy Care**

In the home care setting, the nurse needs to consider the following for clients requiring tracheostomy care:

- For tracheostomies older than 1 month, clean technique (rather than sterile technique) is used for tracheostomy care.
- Stress the importance of good hand hygiene to the caregiver.
- Tap water may be used for rinsing the inner cannula.
- Teach the caregiver the tracheostomy care procedure and observe a return demonstration. Periodically reassess caregiver knowledge and tracheostomy care technique.
- Inform the caregiver of the signs and symptoms that may indicate an infection of the stoma site or lower airway.
- Names and telephone numbers of healthcare personnel who can be reached for emergencies or advice must be available to the client or caregiver.
- If the tracheostomy is permanent, provide contact information for available support groups.

LIFESPAN CONSIDERATIONS **Tracheostomy Care**

INFANTS AND CHILDREN

- An assistant should always be present while tracheostomy care is performed.
- Always keep a sterile, packaged tracheostomy tube taped to the child's bed so that if the tube dislodges, a new one is available for immediate reintubation.

OLDER ADULTS

- Older adult skin is fragile and prone to breakdown. Care of the skin at the tracheostomy stoma is very important.

EVIDENCE-BASED PRACTICE

Evidence-Based Practice

How Important Is Communication to a Client with a Tracheostomy?

It is unknown how many tracheostomies are performed each year; however, this procedure has become common practice. Few studies have explored the communication experience of tracheostomy clients in the intensive care unit (ICU). As a result, Tolotti et al. (2018) conducted a study to explore the actual experiences of adult clients with tracheostomies, who were not under sedation or mechanically ventilated, in their communication with nurses during their stay in the ICU. The researchers used interpretive phenomenology methodology to gain a deeper understanding of the clients' subjective experiences when they communicated with nurses. The methods for data collection included: (1) Observation during the clients' stay in the ICU. Observational data were used to gain a better understanding of the problems the clients reported in their interviews and during data analysis to provide a clearer context in which the communication occurred. (2) In-depth interviews with the clients after they left the ICU. The purpose was to explore the communication difficulties experienced by the clients during their communication experience with the nurses and to identify what facilitated and hindered their communication. The researchers asked the clients which nurses they particularly remembered. (3) Interviews with the nurses whom the clients remembered best in relation to their communication experiences. The study included a total of eight clients. Between three and five participant observations were conducted per client. Seven interviews were conducted with the nurses.

The data analysis resulted in two themes to the actual experience of communication, four factors relating to discomfort during communication and three to comfort. The first theme was *feeling powerless and frustrated*. The clients found it difficult to communicate, which was frustrating, and not being able to speak caused a feeling of powerlessness. As one client stated, "not being able to speak blocked all other human activities." The second theme was *facing continual misunderstanding, resignation, and anger*. The clients tried to use different strategies such as saying words softly, using their eyes, and moving their head. Communication boards required a lot of concentration and attention and often clients were too weak to write legibly. Clients took for granted that the nurses would be able to understand them. When this did not happen, the clients developed feelings of anger or resignation and they just gave up trying to communicate.

The four sources of discomfort included: (1) *Struggling with not knowing what is happening*. The clients often reported they were not aware of their clinical condition and the therapeutic decisions. Some did not remember receiving any information, whereas others reported that the reason they did not receive information was due to the lack of time or because the nurses had other more urgent situations. (2) *Feeling as if other people have given up on me*. Because of the difficulty in communicating and perceiving that there was little hope that their condition would improve, some clients gave up. What gave strength to some of the clients to not give up was the presence of their loved ones. (3) *Living in isolation*. Not being able to speak made it difficult to interact with others, causing a sense of isolation that was linked to a feeling of worthlessness. Sleeping was a way of reducing this suffering, and clients became angry when their sleep was interrupted. (4) *Feeling invisible*. The clients reported that because they could not speak and relate to others they were not involved in the care plan and felt as though they did not exist. Some did not like it when the physicians would not speak directly to them but only to the nurses. Clients felt that decisions were being made and they were not informed or involved in the process.

The three sources of comfort included: (1) *Comforted by being with significant people*. The presence of family was very important and was a source of comfort, encouragement, hope, and protection. The family members also acted as intermediaries as they helped the nurses understand what the clients needed. (2) *Reassured by having my call bell nearby*. Having a safe and quick way to call for help was a source of great reassurance. (3) *Feeling comforted by the nurses' presence*. The clients acknowledged the nurses' specialized competence and their trustworthiness. They were comforted when the nurses showed interest in them, which they perceived through the nurses' gestures, words, smiles, and time they spent with them.

The study also analyzed those themes that were similar and different for both the clients and the nurses. *Frustration because of difficulty with communication* occurred among both groups. The anger and frustration reported by the clients was also reported by the nurses. The nurses reported that repeatedly having to say "I don't understand" was very difficult and sometimes led them to use avoidance strategies such as doing other things. The *comfort factors* for both groups included the presence of caring, as expressed previously by the clients. The nurses reported that showing that they cared for the clients was important to them. Another important comfort factor for both was the presence of family members. Some nurses, however, were ambivalent about the presence of family members. While they recognized the importance for the clients, the family members were sometimes perceived as causing interference with the nurse's work. The *discomfort factors* for both included the lack of information, as previously reported by the clients. For nurses, the information problems were due mainly to communication difficulties; that is, not being able to easily talk with the client could impact the ability to provide correct and complete information. The nurses also reported a feeling of isolation. Specifically, they were not able to provide the amount of one-on-one time that they desired with the clients because there was not enough time.

Implications

Communication is a key element of an effective and therapeutic nurse-client relationship. This study reflected the importance of communication for tracheostomy clients and showed how communication is linked to many aspects of the client's experience. The results of this study can help nurses to become aware of tracheostomy clients' sources of comfort and discomfort during communication with nurses and to use strategies to reduce tracheostomy clients' feelings of frustration and powerlessness due to their inability to use their voice.

Chest Tubes and Drainage Systems

If the thin, double-layered pleural membrane is disrupted by lung disease, surgery, or trauma, the negative pressure between the pleural layers may be lost. The lung then collapses because it is no longer drawn outward as the diaphragm and intercostal muscles contract during inhalation. When air collects in the pleural space, it is known as a **pneumothorax**. A **hemothorax** is the accumulation of blood in the pleural space, and a **pleural effusion** exists when there is excessive fluid in the pleural space. The air, blood, or fluid in the pleural space places pressure on lung tissue and interferes with lung expansion. Chest tubes may be inserted into the pleural cavity to restore negative pressure and drain collected fluid or blood. Because air rises, chest tubes for pneumothorax often are placed in the upper anterior thorax, whereas chest tubes used to drain blood and fluid generally are placed in the lower lateral chest wall.

When chest tubes are inserted, they must be connected to a sealed drainage system or a one-way valve that allows air and fluid to be removed from the chest cavity but prevents air from entering from the outside. Sterile disposable drainage systems are used to prevent outside air from entering the chest tube. These systems typically have a suction control chamber, a water-seal chamber, and a closed collection chamber, for drainage (Figure 49.29 ■). With the water-seal system, when the client inhales, the water prevents air from entering the system from the

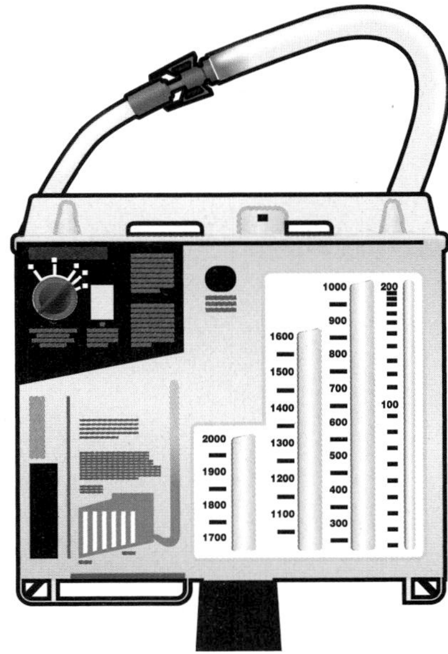

Figure 49.29 ■ A disposable chest drainage system.

atmosphere. During exhalation, however, air can exit the chest cavity, bubbling up through the water. Suction can be added to the system to facilitate removing air and secretions from the chest cavity. The drainage system should always be kept below the level of the client's chest to prevent fluid and drainage from being drawn back into the chest cavity.

A Heimlich valve may be used for ambulatory clients (Figure 49.30 ■). The Heimlich valve is a one-way flutter valve that allows air to escape from the chest cavity, but prevents air from reentering. The arrow on the cover of the valve should always point away from the client. At each assessment, observe the inner valve carefully for movement during exhalation, indicating airflow through the device. The Heimlich valve is not designed to collect fluid. Another device, attached to the chest tube and called the Pneumostat, also has a one-way valve and, unlike the Heimlich valve, a small built-in collection chamber. It is used exclusively for clients with a pneumothorax who usually have small amounts of fluid (Figure 49.31 ■).

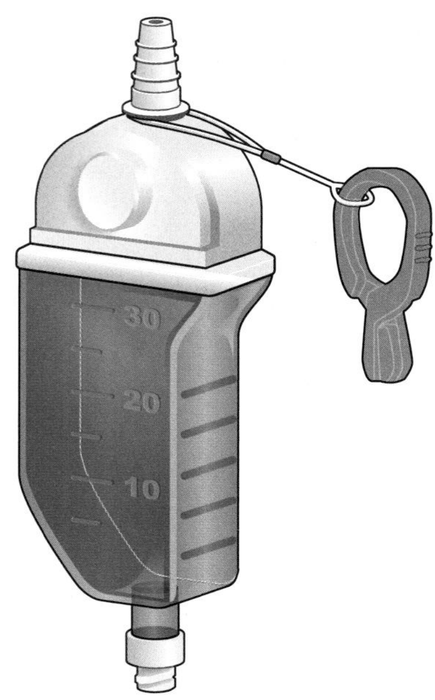

Figure 49.31 ■ The Pneumostat is an example of a device often used for clients with a pneumothorax. It has a one-way valve and a small collection chamber.

Nursing responsibilities regarding drainage systems include the following:

- Monitor and maintain the patency and integrity of the drainage system.
- Assess the client's vital signs, oxygen saturation, cardiovascular status, and respiratory status. Check the breath sounds bilaterally and check for symmetry of breath sounds.
- Observe the dressing site at least every 4 hours. Inspect the dressing for excessive and abnormal drainage, such as bleeding or foul-smelling discharge. Palpate around the dressing site, and listen for a crackling sound indicative of subcutaneous emphysema. *Subcutaneous emphysema, which is air in the subcutaneous tissues, can result from a poor seal at the chest tube insertion site.*
- Determine level of discomfort with and without activity and medicate the client for pain if indicated.
- Encourage deep-breathing exercises and coughing every 2 hours (this may be contraindicated in clients who have had a lung removed). Have the client sit upright to perform the exercises, and splint the chest around the tube insertion site with a pillow or with a hand to minimize discomfort.
- Reposition the client every 2 hours. When the client is lying on the affected side, place rolled towels beside the tubing. *Frequent position changes promote drainage, prevent complications, and provide comfort. Rolled towels prevent occlusion of the chest tube by the client's weight.*
- Assist the client with range-of-motion exercises of the affected shoulder three times per day to maintain joint mobility.
- Ensure that the connections are securely taped and that the chest tube is secured to the client's chest wall.
- Keep the collection device below the client's chest level.
- Frequently check the water-seal and suction control chambers. The water can evaporate and water may need to be added to the chamber. The water-seal level should fluctuate with respiratory effort.
- Assess the drainage in the tubing and collection chamber. The drainage is measured at regularly scheduled times (check agency policy). Mark the date and time at the fluid level on the drainage chamber. The unit is not replaced until almost full.
- Avoid aggressive chest tube manipulation (e.g., milking or stripping the tube). Milking requires a healthcare provider's order. Stripping is no longer considered an acceptable practice (Smith et al., 2017, p. 1217).
- Avoid clamping the chest tube because this increases the risk of a tension pneumothorax. You can clamp the tube for a moment to replace the drainage unit or to locate the source of an air leak, but never when transporting a client or for any extended period of time.

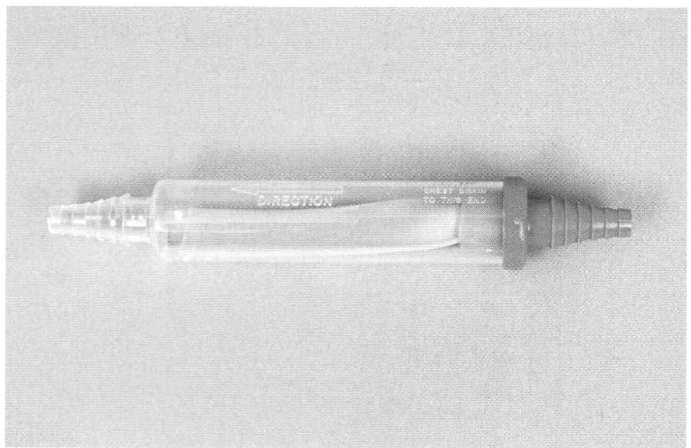

Figure 49.30 ■ Heimlich chest drain valve.

- If the tube becomes disconnected from the collecting system, submerge the end in 2.5 cm (1 in.) of sterile saline or water *to maintain the seal*. If the chest tube is inadvertently pulled out, the wound should be immediately covered with a dry sterile dressing. If you can hear air leaking out of the site, ensure that the dressing is not occlusive. *If the air cannot escape, this would lead to a tension pneumothorax. A tension pneumothorax occurs when there is buildup of air in the pleural space and it cannot escape, causing increased pressure. This pressure can eventually compromise cardiovascular function.*
- When transporting and ambulating the client:
  a. Keep the water-seal unit below chest level and upright.
  b. Disconnect the drainage system from the suction apparatus before moving the client and make sure the air vent is open.
- Use standard precautions and personal protective equipment while manipulating the system and assisting with insertion or removal.

Chest tube insertion and removal require sterile technique and must be done without introducing air or microorganisms into the pleural cavity. Removal of a chest tube is a brief but quite painful procedure. Medicate the client before the removal. Remove the dressing around the tube and prepare the dressing that will cover the insertion site. This will be an occlusive dressing if there is no purse-string suture around the insertion site to prevent air from entering the chest. Generally, the healthcare provider performs the removal but, in some areas, specially trained nurses may be permitted to do so.

Evaluating

Using the goals and desired outcomes identified in the planning stage of the nursing process, the nurse collects data to evaluate the effectiveness of interventions. If outcomes are not achieved, the nurse, client, and support person if appropriate need to explore the reasons before modifying the care plan. For example, if the outcome "Respirations unlabored and rate is within expected range" is not met, examples of questions that need to be considered include the following:

- What is the client's perception of the problem?
- Is the client complaining of shortness of breath or difficulty breathing?
- Is the client taking medications or performing treatments such as percussion, vibration, and postural drainage as prescribed?
- Has the client been exposed to an upper respiratory infection that is affecting breathing?
- Do other factors need to be considered, such as the client's psychologic stress level?

Examples of questions to consider if the outcome "Able to complete ADLs without fatigue" is not met include the following:

- What other factors may be affecting the client's ability to complete ADLs?
- Is the client getting adequate sleep? If not, what is interfering with the client's rest?
- Are there assistive devices (e.g., a shower chair, clothing that is easy to put on) that could help the client achieve this goal?
- Does the client need help with housework and other ADLs?
- Is the client's diet adequate to meet nutritional needs?

NURSING CARE PLAN Altered Respiratory Status

ASSESSMENT DATA	NURSING DIAGNOSIS	DESIRED OUTCOMES*
NURSING ASSESSMENT Julie Singh, a 39-year-old secretary, was admitted to the hospital with an elevated temperature; fatigue; rapid, labored respirations; and mild dehydration. The nursing history reveals that she has had a "bad cold" for several weeks that just wouldn't go away. She has been dieting for several months and skipping meals. Ms. Singh mentions that in addition to her full-time job as a secretary she is attending college classes two evenings a week. She has smoked one package of cigarettes per day since she was 18 years old. Chest x-ray confirms pneumonia. **Physical Examination** Height: 167.6 cm (5′6″) Weight: 54.4 kg (120 lb) Temperature: 39.4°C (103°F) Pulse: 68 beats/min **Diagnostic Data** Chest x-ray: right lobar infiltration WBC: 14,000 pH: 7.49	Altered respiratory status related to thick sputum, secondary to pneumonia (as evidenced by rapid respirations, diminished and adventitious breath sounds, thick yellow sputum)	**Respiratory Status: Airway Patency [0410]** as evidenced by: • No deviation from normal range for respiratory rate • No accumulation of sputum • No adventitious breath sounds

Continued on page 1344

NURSING CARE PLAN Altered Respiratory Status—*continued*

Respirations: 24/min	$PaCO_2$: 33 mmHg
Blood pressure: 118/70 mmHg	HCO_3^-: 20 mEq/L
Skin pale; cheeks flushed	PaO_2: 80 mmHg
Chills; use of accessory muscles; inspiratory crackles with diminished breath sounds right base; expectorating thick, yellow sputum	O_2 sat: 88%

NURSING INTERVENTIONS*/SELECTED ACTIVITIES	RATIONALE
COUGH ENHANCEMENT [3250]	
Assist Ms. Singh to a sitting position with head slightly flexed, shoulders relaxed, and knees flexed.	*Lying flat causes the abdominal organs to shift toward the chest, crowding the lungs and making it more difficult to breathe.*
Encourage her to take several deep breaths.	*Deep breathing promotes oxygenation before controlled coughing.*
Encourage her to take a deep breath, hold for 2 seconds, and cough two or three times in succession.	*Controlled coughing is accomplished by closure of the glottis and the explosive expulsion of air from the lungs by the work of abdominal and chest muscles.*
Promote systemic fluid hydration, as appropriate.	*Adequate fluid intake enhances liquefaction of pulmonary secretions and facilitates expectoration of mucus.*
Respiratory Monitoring [3350]	
Monitor rate, rhythm, depth, and effort of respirations.	*Provides a basis for evaluating adequacy of ventilation.*
Note chest movement, watching for symmetry, use of accessory muscles, and supraclavicular and intercostal muscle retractions.	*Presence of nasal flaring and use of accessory muscles during respirations may occur in response to ineffective ventilation.*
Auscultate breath sounds, noting areas of decreased or absent ventilation and presence of adventitious sounds.	*As fluid and mucus accumulate, abnormal breath sounds can be heard including crackles and diminished breath sounds resulting from fluid-filled air spaces and diminished lung volume.*
Auscultate lung sounds after treatments to note results.	*Assists in evaluating prescribed treatments and client outcomes.*
Monitor client's ability to cough effectively.	*Respiratory tract infections alter the amount and character of secretions. An ineffective cough compromises airway clearance and prevents mucus from being expelled.*
Monitor client's respiratory secretions.	*People with pneumonia commonly produce rust-colored, purulent sputum.*
Institute respiratory therapy treatments (e.g., nebulizer) as needed.	*A variety of respiratory therapy treatments may be used to open constricted airways and liquefy secretions.*
Monitor for increased restlessness, anxiety, and air hunger.	*These clinical manifestations would be early indicators of hypoxia.*
Note changes in SpO_2, tidal volume, and arterial blood gas values, as appropriate.	*Evaluates the status of oxygenation, ventilation, and acid–base balance.*

Evaluation

Outcome partially met. Ms. Singh coughs and deep breathes purposefully q1–2h during the day. Her fluid intake is approximately 1500 mL each day. Cough continues to be productive of moderately thick, rusty-colored sputum. Inspiratory crackles remain present in right lower lobe.

*The NOC # for desired outcomes and the NIC # for nursing interventions are listed in brackets following the appropriate outcome or intervention. Outcomes, interventions, and activities selected are only a sample of those by NOC and NIC and should be further individualized for each client.

APPLYING CRITICAL THINKING

1. What factors may have led the medical staff to suspect that Ms. Singh had more than a very bad cold? Would you have come to the same conclusion?
2. The care plan appropriately focuses on the acute care of this client. Once she is significantly improved, the nurse will perform discharge teaching. What areas should be included?
3. The client already has some signs of respiratory distress. What signs might indicate that her condition was deteriorating into a more emergency situation? How would you handle this?
4. It appears that the client's sputum has not been cultured. In caring for this client, what infection control guidelines would be needed?
5. The oxygen order is for a face mask at 6 L/min. She repeatedly pulls it off and you find it lying in the sheets. How might you intervene?

Answers to Applying Critical Thinking questions are available on the faculty resources site. Please consult with your instructor.

CONCEPT MAP

Altered Respiratory Status

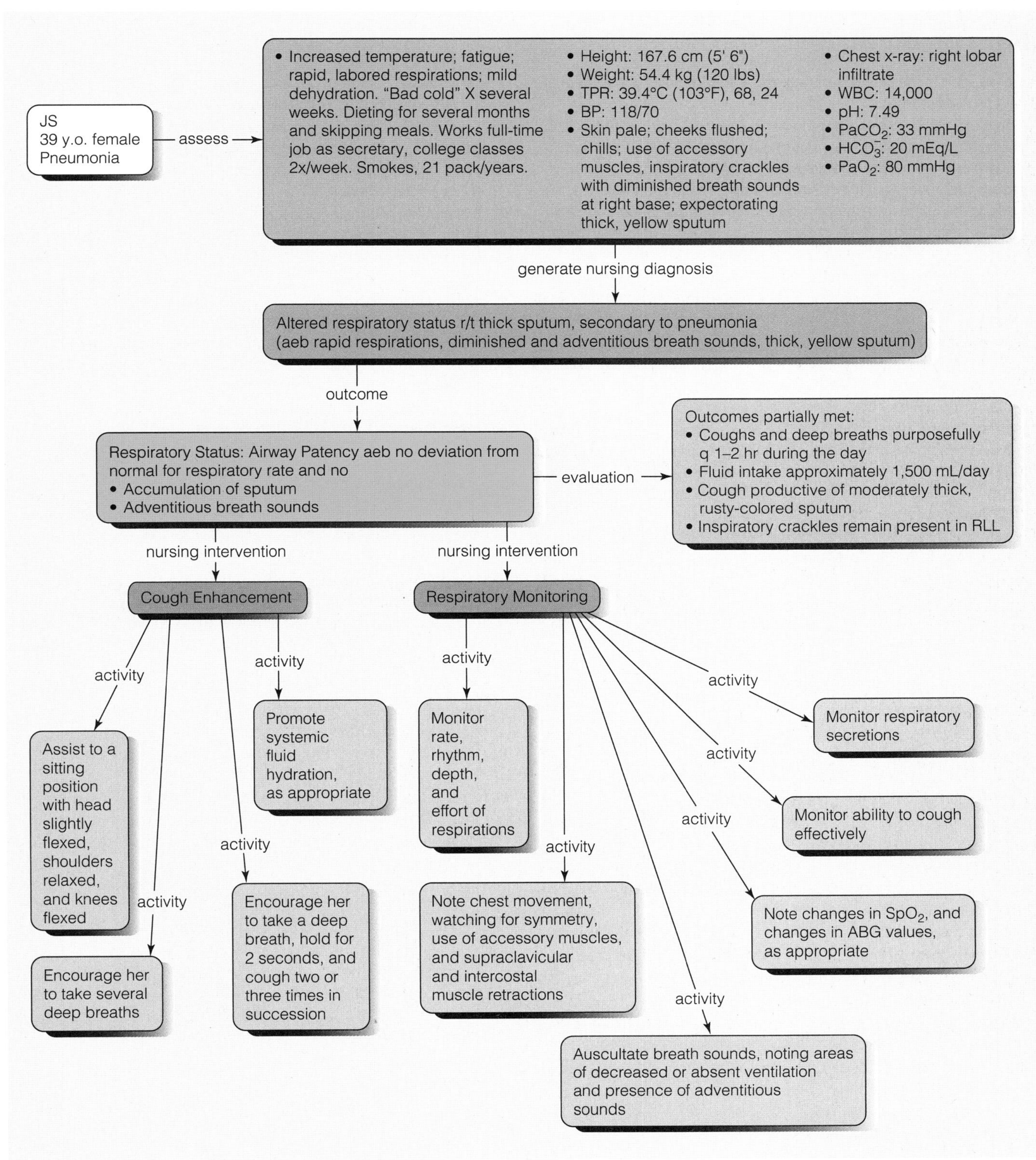

Chapter 49 Review

CHAPTER HIGHLIGHTS

- Respiration is the process of gas exchange between the individual and the environment.
- The respiratory system contributes to effective respiration through pulmonary ventilation (the movement of air between the atmosphere and the lungs), the diffusion of oxygen and carbon dioxide across the pulmonary membrane, transport of oxygen from the tissues to the lungs and carbon dioxide from the tissues to the lungs, and transport of oxygen and carbon dioxide between the systemic capillaries and the tissues.
- Alveoli and the capillaries that surround them form the respiratory membrane, where gas exchange between the lungs and the blood occurs.
- Effective pulmonary ventilation, or breathing, requires clear airways, an intact central nervous system and respiratory center, an intact thoracic cavity and musculature, and adequate pulmonary compliance (stretch) and recoil.
- Gas exchange occurs by diffusion, as gas molecules move from an area of higher concentration to an area of lower concentration. At the respiratory membrane, oxygen moves from the alveolus into the blood, while carbon dioxide moves from the blood into the alveolus.
- Most oxygen (97%) is carried to the tissues loosely combined with hemoglobin in RBCs. Anemia, which is too few RBCs or low hemoglobin levels, impairs oxygen transportation.
- Respiratory regulation includes both neural and chemical controls to maintain the correct concentrations of oxygen, carbon dioxide, and hydrogen ions in body fluids. The body's respiratory center is located in the medulla oblongata and pons of the brain.
- Respiratory rates normally are highest in neonates and infants, gradually slowing to adult ranges.
- Aging affects the respiratory system: The chest wall becomes more rigid and lungs less elastic.
- Other factors affecting oxygenation include the environment, lifestyle, health status, medications, and stress.
- Respiratory function can be altered by conditions that affect the patency of the airway, movement of air into or out of the lungs, diffusion of oxygen and carbon dioxide between the alveoli and the pulmonary capillaries, and the transport of oxygen and carbon dioxide via the blood to and from the tissue cells.
- Hypoxia, insufficient oxygen in the tissues, can result from impaired ventilation (hypoventilation) or impaired diffusion, or from impaired oxygen transportation to the tissues because of anemia or decreased cardiac output.
- Airway obstruction interferes with ventilation. A low-pitched snoring sound, stridor, and abnormal breath sounds may accompany partial airway obstruction. Extreme inspiratory effort with no chest movement indicates complete upper airway obstruction.
- Normal respirations are quiet and unlabored; altered respiratory patterns include tachypnea, bradypnea, hyperventilation, hypoventilation, and dyspnea. Shortness of breath is a subjective sensation of not getting enough air.
- The nursing history includes questions about current or past respiratory problems and about lifestyle, presence of symptoms such as cough or shortness of breath, smoking and other risk factors, and medications.
- Diagnostic tests that may be performed to assess oxygenation include sputum and throat culture specimens; blood tests such as arterial blood gases; pulmonary function tests; and visualization procedures such as x-rays, lung scans, laryngoscopy, and bronchoscopy.
- Nursing diagnoses for the client with problems of oxygenation include altered respiratory status, altered breathing pattern, altered gas exchange, and inadequate physical energy for activities. These problems also may be the etiology for several other nursing diagnoses, including fatigue, insomnia, *and* social isolation.
- In discharge and home care planning, the nurse assesses the client's self-care abilities and need for assistive devices, home environment, compliance with medical regimen, and knowledge level. The ability of the family or support people to provide assistance and financial support and to cope with the changes is also assessed, as are community factors such as the environment and resources.
- The nurse teaches the client about home care activities to maintain a patent airway and gas exchange and to promote healthy breathing. Dietary modifications, prescribed medications, and specific procedures also are taught, and the nurse makes referrals to community agencies as needed.
- Nursing interventions to promote oxygenation include promoting healthy breathing, deep breathing and coughing, and hydration; administering medications; implementing measures to clear secretions (e.g., percussion, vibration, postural drainage, and mucus clearing devices); initiating and monitoring oxygen therapy; initiating or assisting with procedures to maintain the airway (e.g., artificial airways and suctioning); providing tracheostomy care; and monitoring chest drainage systems.
- The effectiveness of nursing interventions is evaluated by using the goals and desired outcomes identified in the planning stage of the nursing process. If a goal is not met, the nurse asks pertinent questions to assess the reason for not meeting the goal.

TEST YOUR KNOWLEDGE

1. When planning care, for which client would the nurse include close observation for a decreased or absent cough reflex?
   1. The client with a nasal fracture
   2. The client with impairment of vagus nerve conduction
   3. The client with a sinus infection
   4. The client with reduction in respiratory membrane conduction
2. A client diagnosed with chronic obstructive lung disease receiving oxygen at 1.5 liters per minute via nasal cannula is complaining of shortness of breath. What action should the nurse take?
   1. Increase the oxygen to 3 liters per minute via nasal cannula.
   2. Lower the head of the client's bed to semi-Fowler's position.
   3. Have the client breathe through pursed lips.
   4. Encourage the client to breathe more rapidly.
3. The nurse is preparing to perform tracheostomy care. Prior to beginning the procedure the nurse performs which action?
   1. Tells the client to raise two fingers to indicate pain or distress.
   2. Changes the twill tape holding the tracheostomy in place.
   3. Cleans the incision site.
   4. Checks the tightness of the ties and knot.
4. A nurse has placed an oropharyngeal airway in a client. What action should the nurse take at this time?
   1. Tape the airway in place.
   2. Suction the client.
   3. Turn the client's head to the side.
   4. Insert a nasal trumpet.
5. Which of the following client conditions can alter respiratory function? Select all that apply.
   1. A client who has increasing thick secretions.
   2. A client with eupnea.
   3. A client with GI bleeding resulting in a large blood loss.
   4. A client with heart failure.
   5. A client with a temperature of 103.6°F (39.7°C) and experiencing severe pain.
6. While a client with chest tubes is ambulating, the connection between the tube and the water seal dislodges. Which action by the nurse is most appropriate?
   1. Assist the client to ambulate back to bed.
   2. Reconnect the tube to the water seal.
   3. Assess the client's lung sounds with a stethoscope.
   4. Have the client cough forcibly several times.
7. The nurse makes the assessment that which client has the greatest risk for a problem with the transport of oxygen from the lungs to the tissues? A client who has
   1. Anemia.
   2. An infection.
   3. A fractured rib.
   4. A tumor of the medulla.
8. Which term does the nurse document to best describe a client experiencing shortness of breath when lying down who must assume an upright or sitting position to breathe more comfortably and effectively?
   1. Dyspnea
   2. Hyperpnea
   3. Orthopnea
   4. Acapnea
9. A client with emphysema is prescribed corticosteroid therapy on a short-term basis for acute bronchitis. The client asks the nurse how the steroids will help him. The nurse responds by saying that the corticosteroids will do which of the following?
   1. Promote bronchodilation.
   2. Help the client to cough.
   3. Prevent respiratory infection.
   4. Decrease inflammation in the airways.
10. The nurse is planning to perform percussion and postural drainage. Which is an important aspect of planning the client's care?
    1. Percussion and postural drainage should be done before lunch.
    2. The order should be coughing, percussion, positioning, and then suctioning.
    3. A good time to perform percussion and postural drainage is in the morning after breakfast when the client is well rested.
    4. Percussion and postural drainage should always be preceded by 3 minutes of 100% oxygen.

See Answers to Test Your Knowledge in Appendix A.

READINGS AND REFERENCES

Suggested Readings

Higginson, R., Parry, A., & Williams, M. (2016). Airway management in the hospital environment. *British Journal of Nursing, 25*(2), 94–100. doi:10.12968/bjon.2016.25.2.94
This is a review of airway management, including both acute and chronic. It includes airway assessment, airways, oxygen delivery, and suctioning.

O-Dell, A., Diegel-Vacek, L., Burt, L., & Corbridge, S. (2018). Managing stable COPD: An evidence-based approach. *American Journal of Nursing, 118*(9), 36–47. doi:10.1097/01.NAJ.0000544950.73334.58
This article provides information about the latest revisions of evidence-based changes relating to COPD classification and pharmacologic, nonpharmacologic, and comorbidity management.

Related Research

Cui, L., Ying-hui, J., Weijie, G., Yue-xian, S., Xinhua, X., Wen-xi, S., . . . Jinhua, S. (2017). Variation in nurse self-reported practice of managing chest tubes: A cross-sectional study. *Journal of Clinical Nursing, 27,* e1013–e1021. doi:10.1111.jocn.14127

Gross, S. L., Jennings, C. D., & Clark, R. C. (2016). Comparison of three practices for dressing chest tube insertion sites: A randomized controlled trial. *MEDSURG Nursing, 25*(4), 229–231, 250.

Harjot, K., Kumar, S. H., & Krishan, G. K. (2016). Effectiveness of teaching intervention on knowledge and practices regarding endotracheal tube suctioning among staff nurses. *International Journal of Nursing Education, 8*(2), 8–11. doi:10.5958/0974-9357.2016.00038.6

McDonough, K., Crimlisk, J., Nicholas, P., Cabral, H., Quinn, E. K., & Jalisi, S. (2016). Standardizing nurse training strategies to improve knowledge and self-efficacy with tracheostomy and laryngectomy care. *Applied Nursing Research, 32,* 212–216. doi:10.1016/j.apnr.2016.08.003

References

Ari, A., Alwadeai, K. S., & Fink, J. B. (2017). Effects of heat and moisture exchangers and exhaled humidity on aerosol deposition in a simulated ventilator-dependent adult lung model. *Respiratory Care, 62*(5), 538–543. doi:10.4187/respcare.05015

Bolsega, T. J., & Sole, M. L. (2018). Tracheostomy care practices in a simulated setting. *Clinical Nurse Specialist, 32*(4), 182–188. doi:10.1097/NUR.0000000000000385

Butcher, H. K., Bulechek, G. M., Dochterman, J. M., & Wagner, C. M. (Eds.). (2018). *Nursing interventions classification (NIC)* (7th ed.). St. Louis, MO: Elsevier.

Harrelson, B. R., & Fencl, J. L. (2016). Care of the surgical patient with obstructive sleep apnea. *AORN Journal, 103,* 433–437. doi:10.1016/j.aorn.2016.02.004

Kallet, R. H., & Branson, R. D. (2016). Should oxygen therapy be tightly regulated to minimize hyperoxia in critically ill patients? *Respiratory Care, 61*(6), 801–817. doi:10.4187/respcare.04933

Moorhead, S., Swanson, E., Johnson, M., & Maas, M. L. (Eds.). (2018). *Nursing outcomes classification (NOC)* (6th ed.). St. Louis, MO: Elsevier.

Prevention of ventilator-associated pneumonia in adults. (2017). *Critical Care Nurse, 37*(3), e22–e25. doi:10.4037/ccn2017460

Restrepo, R. D., Mathai, A. A., Luna, A. A., Ramirez, C., & Olaniyi-Adegbola, O. (2016). How deep can we go? Following the endotracheal suctioning clinical practice guidelines. *Respiratory Care, 61*(10), OF-36.

Rice, J. (2018). *Medical terminology for health care professionals* (9th ed.). Hoboken, NJ: Pearson.

Smith, S. F., Duell, D. J., Martin, B.C., Aebersold, M. L., & Gonzalez, L. (2017). *Clinical nursing skills: Basic to advanced skills* (9th ed.). Hoboken, NJ: Pearson.

Tolotti, A., Bagnasco, A., Catania, G., Aleo, G., Pagnucci, N., Cadorin, L., . . . Sasso, L. (2018). The communication experience of tracheostomy patients with nurses in the intensive care unit: A phenomenological study. *Intensive and Critical Care Nursing, 46*, 24–31. doi:10.1016/j.iccn.2018.01.001

Williams, R., Williams, M., Stanton, M. P., & Spence, D. (2017). Implementation of an obstructive sleep apnea screening program at an overseas military hospital. *AANA Journal, 85*(1), 42–48.

Selected Bibliography

Bonvento, B., Wallace, S., Lynch, J., Coe, B., & McGrath, B. A. (2017). Role of the multidisciplinary team in the care of the tracheostomy patient. *Journal of Multidisciplinary Healthcare, 10*, 391–398. doi:10.2147/JMDH.S118419

Chike-Harris, K., & Kinyon-Munch, K. (2019). Asthma 101: Teaching children to use metered dose inhalers. *Nursing, 49*(3), 56–60. doi:10.1097/01.NURSE.0000552703.80996.43

Hood, K., Lewis, B., & Bowens, C. D. (2017). Reducing fresh tracheostomy decannulations following implementation of a fresh tracheostomy guideline. *Critical Care Nursing Clinics of North America, 29*, 131–141. doi:10.1016/j.cnc.2017.01.001

Institute for Safe Medication Practices. (2018). Ongoing risk: Misconnections of tracheostomy pilot balloon ports with IV infusions can result in fatal outcomes. *NurseAdviseERR, 16*(10), 1–3.

Memorial Sloan Kettering Cancer Center. (2017). *Caring for your Heimlich valve and chest tube.* Retrieved from https://www.mskcc.org/cancer-care/patient-education/care-heimlich-valve

Siela, D., & Kidd, M. (2017). Oxygen requirements for acutely and critically ill patients. *Critical Care Nurse, 37*(4), 58–70. doi:10.4037/ccn2017627

Circulation 50

LEARNING OUTCOMES

After completing this chapter, you will be able to:

1. Outline the structure and physiology of the cardiovascular system.
2. Identify major risk factors for the development of cardiovascular disease and related health promotion objectives from *Healthy People 2020.*
3. Describe three major alterations in cardiovascular function.
4. Outline the nursing management of a client with cardiovascular disease.
5. Describe the critical nature of cardiopulmonary resuscitation.
6. Verbalize the steps used in
   a. Applying a sequential compression device.
7. Recognize when it is appropriate to assign aspects of applying a sequential compression device to assistive personnel.
8. Demonstrate appropriate documentation and reporting when applying a sequential compression device.

KEY TERMS

afterload, *1352*
atherosclerosis, *1354*
atria, *1349*
atrioventricular (AV) node, *1351*
atrioventricular (AV) valves, *1349*
automaticity, *1350*
blood pressure (BP), *1352*
bundle of His, *1351*
cardiac output (CO), *1351*
contractility, *1352*
coronary arteries, *1350*
C-reactive protein (CRP), *1357*
creatine kinase (CK), *1361*
diastole, *1350*
endocardium, *1349*
epicardium, *1349*
heart failure, *1358*
hemoglobin, *1354*
homocysteine, *1357*
ischemia, *1358*
metabolic syndrome (Met-S), *1357*
myocardial infarction (MI), *1358*
myocardium, *1349*
pericardium, *1349*
peripheral vascular resistance (PVR), *1352*
preload, *1351*
Purkinje fibers, *1351*
semilunar valves, *1349*
septum, *1349*
sinoatrial (SA or sinus) node, *1350*
stroke volume (SV), *1351*
systole, *1350*
troponin, *1361*
ventricles, *1349*

Introduction

The circulatory, or cardiovascular, system is responsible for the transport of oxygen, fluids, electrolytes, and products of metabolism via the blood to and from tissues.

Physiology of the Cardiovascular System

The respiratory and cardiovascular systems are closely linked and dependent on one another to deliver oxygen to the tissues of the body. Alterations in function of either system can affect the other and lead to tissue hypoxia (lack of oxygen).

The heart and the blood vessels make up the cardiovascular system. Together with blood, it is the major transport system of the body, bringing oxygen and nutrients to the cells and removing wastes for disposal. The heart serves as the system's pump, moving blood through the vessels to the tissues.

The Heart

The heart, a hollow, cone-shaped organ about the size of a fist, is located in the mediastinum, which is between the lungs and beneath the sternum. It is enclosed by a double layer of fibroserous membrane known as the **pericardium**. The parietal, or outermost, pericardium serves to protect the heart and anchor it to surrounding structures. The visceral pericardium adheres to the surface of the heart, forming the heart's outermost layer, the **epicardium**. The heart wall contains two additional layers: the **myocardium**, cardiac muscle cells that form the bulk of the heart and contract with each beat, and the **endocardium**, which lines the inside of the heart's chambers and great vessels.

Four hollow chambers within the heart, two upper **atria** and two lower **ventricles**, are separated longitudinally by the interventricular **septum**, forming two parallel pumps. The atria and ventricles are separated from one another by the **atrioventricular (AV) valves**: the tricuspid valve on the right and the bicuspid or mitral valve on the left. The valves are named for the number of cusps (or leaflets) present on the valve. The ventricles, in turn, are separated from the great vessels (the pulmonary arteries and aorta) by the **semilunar valves** (named for their crescent moon shape): the pulmonary (also called the pulmonic) valve on the right and the aortic valve on the left. The valves serve to direct the flow of blood, allowing it to move from the atria to the ventricles, and the ventricles to the great vessels, but preventing backflow.

Deoxygenated blood from the veins enters the right side of the heart through the superior and inferior venae cavae (singular is vena cava). From there, it flows into the right ventricle, which pumps it through the pulmonary artery into the lungs for gas exchange across the alveolar–capillary membrane. Freshly oxygenated blood returns to the left atrium via the pulmonary veins. From here, the blood enters the left ventricle to be pumped out for systemic circulation through the aorta (Figure 50.1 ■).

Coronary Circulation

The heart muscle does not receive oxygen or nourishment from the blood within its chambers. Instead, it is supplied by the **coronary arteries**. The coronary arteries originate at the base of the aorta, branching out to encircle and penetrate the myocardium. These arteries fill during ventricular relaxation, bringing oxygen-rich blood to the myocardium (Figure 50.2 ■). If these arteries become clogged with atherosclerotic plaques or are obstructed by a blood clot, the myocardium is deprived of oxygen, and the client may develop chest pain (angina) or experience a myocardial infarction (heart attack). The cardiac veins drain the deoxygenated blood from the myocardium into the coronary sinus, which empties into the right atrium.

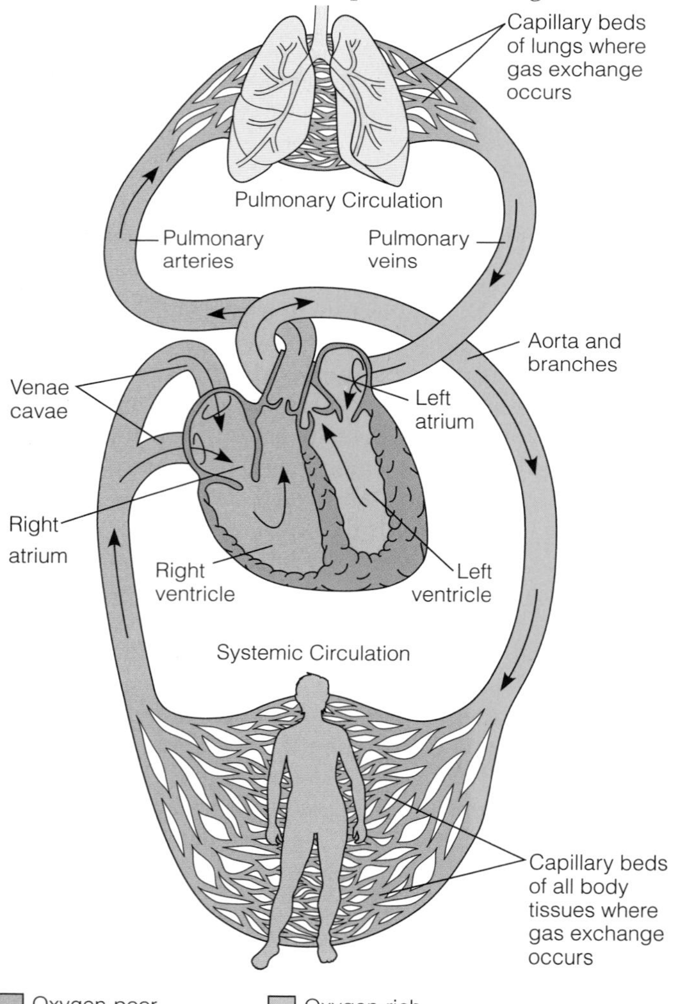

Figure 50.1 ■ The heart and blood vessels. The left side of the heart pumps oxygenated blood into the arteries. Deoxygenated blood returns via the venous system into the right side of the heart.

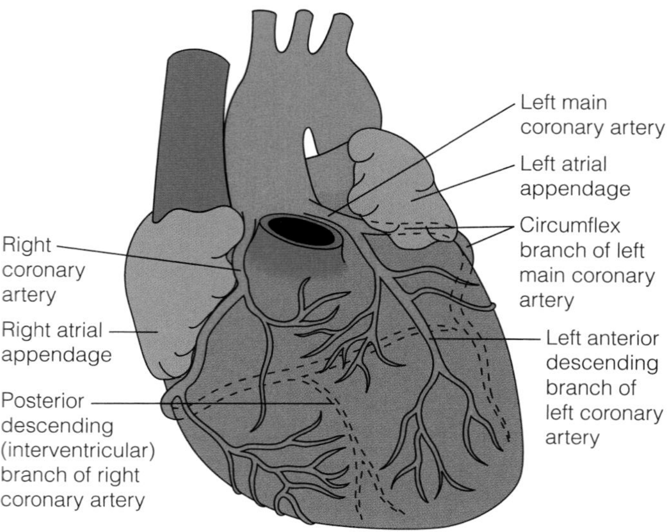

Figure 50.2 ■ The coronary arteries supply the heart muscle with oxygenated blood.

Cardiac Cycle

With each heartbeat, the myocardium goes through a cycle of contraction (systole) and relaxation (diastole). **Systole** is when the heart ejects (propels) the blood into pulmonary and systemic circulation. **Diastole** is when the ventricles fill with blood. The diastolic phase of the cardiac cycle is twice as long as the systolic phase. This is important because diastole (or ventricular filling) is largely a passive process. The longer diastolic phase allows this filling to occur. At the end of the diastolic phase, the atria contract, adding additional volume to the ventricles. This volume is sometimes called *atrial kick.* The relationship between the phases of the cardiac cycle and normal heart sounds is described in Table 50.1.

Cardiac Conduction System

Cardiac muscle contraction is a mechanical event that occurs in response to electrical stimulation. Cardiac muscle is unique in that, unlike skeletal muscle, it can generate electrical impulses and contractions independently of the nervous system. This unique property of heart muscle is called **automaticity**. A network of specialized cells and pathways known as the cardiac conduction system normally controls the electrical activity and contractions of the heart.

The primary pacemaker of the heart is the **sinoatrial (SA or sinus) node**, located where the superior vena cava enters the right atrium. The SA node normally initiates

TABLE 50.1 Cardiac Cycle and Heart Sounds

Sound	Phase of Cardiac Cycle
S_1—first sound	Beginning of ventricular systole; the sound is caused by closure of the atrioventricular valves—the tricuspid and the mitral.
S_2—second sound	Beginning of ventricular diastole; the sound is caused by closure of the semilunar valves—the aortic and pulmonic.

electrical impulses that are conducted throughout the heart and result in ventricular contraction. In adults, it usually discharges impulses at a regular rate of 60 to 100 times per minute, the "normal" heart rate. The impulse then spreads throughout the atria via the interatrial pathways. These conduction pathways converge and narrow through the **atrioventricular (AV) node**, slightly delaying transmission of the impulse to the ventricles. This delay allows the atria to contract slightly before ventricular contraction occurs. From the AV node, the impulse then progresses down through the intraventricular septum to the ventricular conduction pathways: the **bundle of His**, the right and left bundle branches, and the **Purkinje fibers**. These fibers terminate in ventricular muscle, stimulating contraction (Figure 50.3 ■).

Cardiac Output

As the ventricles contract during systole, blood flows out of the ventricles through the aorta and pulmonary artery into systemic and pulmonary circulation. The heart muscle then relaxes (the diastolic phase), allowing the ventricles to refill and cardiac muscle to be perfused. This repeated contraction and relaxation of the heart is known as the cardiac cycle. The cycle is repeated 60 to 100 times a minute in an adult, stimulated by impulses generated by the SA node.

With each contraction, a certain amount of blood, known as the stroke volume, is ejected from the ventricles into circulation. In adults, the average stroke volume is about 70 mL per beat. **Cardiac output (CO)** is the amount of blood pumped by the ventricles in 1 minute. Cardiac output is calculated by multiplying the **stroke volume (SV)**, the amount of blood ejected with each contraction, times the heart rate (HR). Thus, $SV \times HR = CO$. Normal cardiac output is 4 to 8 L/min. Cardiac output is an important indicator of how well the heart is functioning as a pump. If CO is poor, oxygen and nutrients do not reach cells as needed, impairing tissue perfusion. Cardiac output is affected by several factors, as discussed next.

HEART RATE

An increased heart rate increases CO, even if the stroke volume does not change. In contrast, CO decreases when the heart rate falls if stroke volume remains constant. There are physiologic limits to the increase in CO that occurs with increased heart rate. Very rapid heart rates, more than 150 beats per minute in an adult, may not allow adequate time for the ventricles to fill, causing CO to fall. Heart rate is influenced by many factors including the autonomic nervous system, blood pressure, hormones such as thyroid hormone, and some medications.

PRELOAD

Preload is the degree to which muscle fibers in the ventricle are stretched at the end of the relaxation period (diastole). Preload largely depends on the amount of blood returning to the heart from venous circulation; increased volume causes increased stretch, leading to more forceful contraction of cardiac muscle fibers. This physiologic relationship is referred to as the Frank-Starling law of the heart, which states that the length of ventricular muscle fibers (stretch) at the end of diastole directly affects the strength (force) of contraction. For example, exercise increases venous return and therefore increases preload; in response, the heart contracts more forcefully, causing stroke volume and CO to increase during exercise.

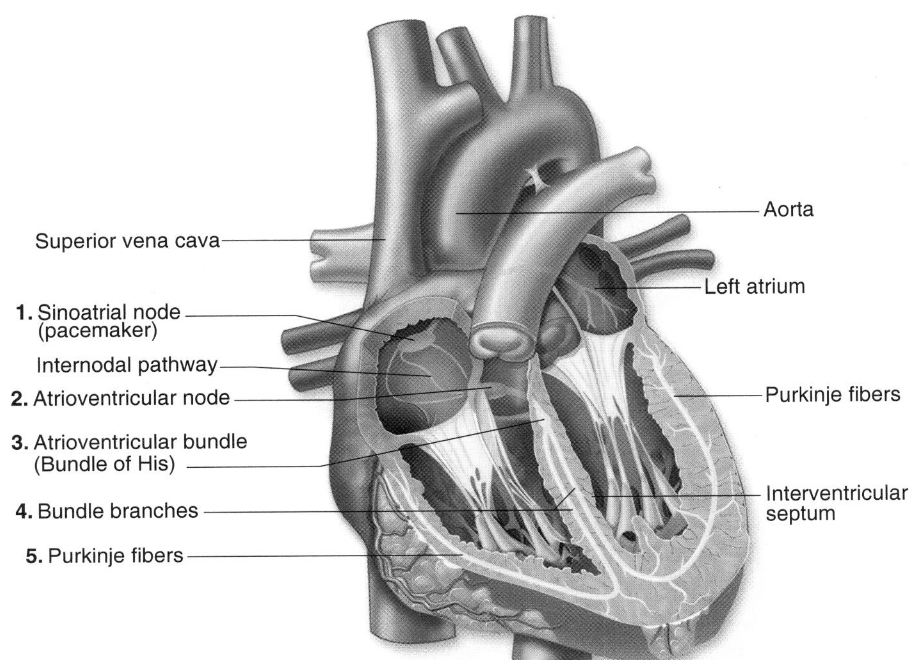

Figure 50.3 ■ The conduction system of the heart. The impulse is initiated by the SA node (1), then travels to the AV node (2), the bundle of His (3), bundle branches (4), and finally to the Purkinje fibers (5).
From *Medical Terminology for Health Care Professionals* (9th ed., p. 261), by J. Rice, 2018. Reproduced by permission of Pearson Education, Inc., Hoboken, NJ.

CONTRACTILITY

Contractility is the natural ability of cardiac muscle fibers to shorten or contract. Stroke volume decreases if contractility is poor, reducing cardiac output. Contractility is affected by the autonomic nervous system and certain drugs. Drugs that affect contractility are called inotropic drugs; positive inotropic drugs increase contractility, and negative inotropic drugs decrease contractility.

AFTERLOAD

Afterload is the resistance that the ventricle must overcome during systole to eject blood into circulation. The right ventricle ejects blood into the pulmonary circulation, and the left ventricle ejects blood through the aortic valve to the systemic circulation. Blood flows from an area of higher pressure to an area of lower pressure. To move blood into the circulatory system, the ventricles must generate sufficient pressure to overcome vascular resistance or the pressure within the arteries, known as *afterload*. The right ventricle pumps blood into the low-pressure, low-resistance pulmonary vascular system; therefore, the pressures generated by the right ventricle are fairly low. The left ventricle, by contrast, pumps blood into the higher pressure systemic arterial system, generating much higher pressures and requiring more work. The higher the afterload, the harder the heart has to work to eject its contents, resulting in increased myocardial oxygen demand. For example, systemic vasoconstriction increases the arterial blood pressure and afterload, increasing the cardiac workload; vasodilation, on the other hand, reduces arterial pressure and the workload of the heart. Table 50.2 summarizes the factors related to cardiac function.

TABLE 50.2 Factors Related to Cardiac Function

Indicator	Definition
Cardiac output (CO)	Amount of blood ejected from the heart each minute; CO = SV × HR
Stroke volume (SV)	Amount of blood ejected from the heart with each beat
Heart rate (HR)	Number of beats each minute
Contractility	Inotropic state of the myocardium, strength of contraction
Preload	Left ventricular end diastolic volume, stretch of the myocardium
Afterload	Resistance against which the heart must pump

Blood Vessels

With each cardiac contraction, blood is ejected into a closed system of blood vessels that transport blood to the tissues and return it to the heart. The heart supports two circulatory systems: the low-pressure pulmonary system and the higher pressure systemic system.

Deoxygenated blood from the right ventricle enters the pulmonary system through the pulmonary arteries, which eventually branch out to form arterioles and the dense capillary networks that encompass the alveoli. Oxygen diffuses into the blood from the alveoli, and carbon dioxide diffuses into the alveoli from the blood. This diffusion occurs across the alveolar–capillary membrane. The blood then returns to the left side of the heart via venules and the pulmonary veins. Note that the pulmonary vascular system is the only part of the circulatory system in which arteries (which transport blood away from the heart) carry deoxygenated blood, and veins (which transport blood toward the heart) contain oxygenated blood.

The muscular left ventricle of the heart pumps oxygenated blood into the aorta. The blood then moves into major arteries that branch from the aorta and into successively smaller arteries, arterioles, and finally into the thin-walled capillary beds of organs and tissues. It is in the capillary beds that oxygen and nutrients are exchanged for metabolic waste products. The deoxygenated blood then returns to the heart through a series of venules and veins that become progressively larger until they empty into the superior and inferior venae cavae.

With the exception of capillaries, blood vessel walls have three distinct layers, or tunics. The innermost layer, the tunica intima, is smooth endothelium that facilitates blood flow. The tunica media is made up of elastic fibers and smooth muscle cells innervated by the autonomic nervous system. This allows vessels to constrict or dilate, depending on the needs of the body. The tunica media of arteries is thicker and more muscular than that of veins, a feature that helps maintain blood pressure and continuous circulation to the tissues. The outermost layer of blood vessels is the tunica adventitia, a layer of connective tissue that supports, protects, and anchors the vessel to surrounding tissues. Capillaries contain only one thin layer of tunica intima, allowing gases and molecules to diffuse between the blood and the tissues.

Arterial Circulation

Arterial circulation moves blood from the heart to the tissues, maintaining a constant flow to the capillary beds despite the intermittent pumping action of the heart.

Blood flow, the volume of blood flowing through a given vessel, organ, or the entire circulatory system over a specific period, is determined by pressure differences and resistance. Blood always moves from an area of higher pressure to an area of lower pressure. The greater the difference between pressures, the greater the blood flow. **Blood pressure (BP)** is the force exerted on arterial walls by the blood flowing within the vessel. See Chapter 28 ∞ for a further explanation of blood pressure. Mean arterial pressure (MAP) maintains blood flow to the tissues throughout the cardiac cycle. It is a product of cardiac output times **peripheral vascular resistance (PVR)**, or CO × PVR = MAP.

ANATOMY & PHYSIOLOGY REVIEW

Preload and Afterload

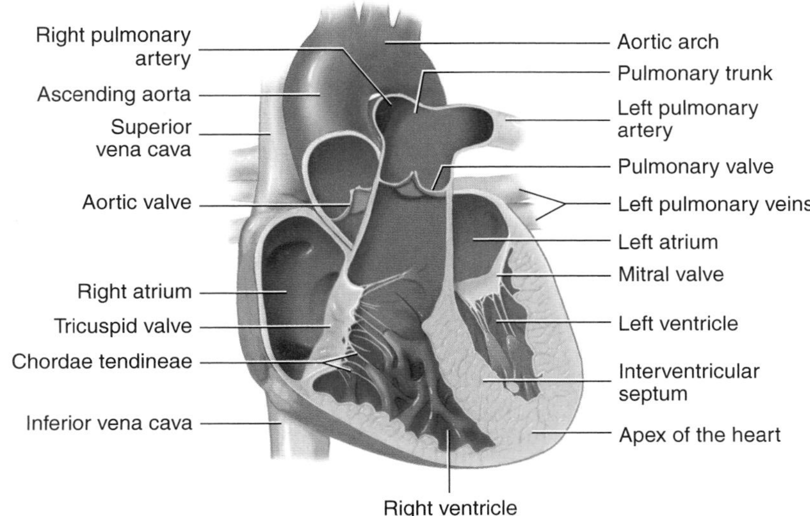

QUESTIONS

Preload is affected by the amount of blood returning to the heart from the venous circulation. Review the figure.

1. Which side of the heart is primarily affected by preload?
2. What could cause an *increase* of venous blood return to the heart?
3. When would an increase in preload have a positive effect or outcome for the client?
4. When does an increase in preload have a negative effect or outcome for the client?
5. What medication classification decreases preload? (*Hint:* Think about what could cause a decrease in venous return of volume to the heart.)

Afterload is the resistance against which the heart must pump. Review the figure.

6. Which side of the heart is primarily affected by afterload?
7. What can cause an increase in afterload (e.g., what can cause the left side of the heart to work harder)?
8. Based on the physiology, afterload can be decreased by medications that would have what physiologic result or outcome?

Answers to Anatomy & Physiology Review questions are available on the faculty resources site. Please consult with your instructor.

Resistance is the opposite of flow; peripheral vascular resistance opposes blood flow to the tissues. PVR is determined by:

- The viscosity, or thickness, of the blood
- Blood vessel length
- Blood vessel diameter.

Venous Return

In contrast to the high-pressure arterial system, venous pressure is too low to adequately return blood from peripheral tissues to the heart without assistance. The fall in intrathoracic pressure that occurs with breathing draws blood upward toward the heart, an adaptation known as the respiratory pump. Skeletal muscle activity contributes to the muscular pump, as muscle contractions move blood toward the heart. Venous valves are vital in making these pumps work; once blood passes a valve, it cannot flow backward away from the heart. See Figure 50.1 earlier in this chapter for an illustration of the relationship between arteries and veins and the entire circulatory system.

Blood

Blood serves as the transport medium within the cardiovascular system, bringing oxygen and nutrients from the environment (via the lungs and gastrointestinal system) to the cells. Blood is a complex mixture of living elements (the blood cells) suspended in fluid (the plasma). Its primary functions are:

- Transporting oxygen, nutrients, and hormones to the cells, and metabolic wastes from the cells for elimination
- Regulating body temperature, pH, and fluid volume
- Preventing infection and blood loss.

As previously noted in Chapter 49 ∞, most oxygen is transported bound to hemoglobin. **Hemoglobin** is a major component of red blood cells (erythrocytes), the predominant cell present in blood. Because of hemoglobin's importance in oxygen transportation, anemia (too few red blood cells [RBCs] that contain too little or abnormal hemoglobin) interferes with oxygen delivery to the tissues, leading to fatigue and activity intolerance.

Lifespan Considerations

At birth, major changes occur in the cardiovascular system. As the lungs expand, pressure in the pulmonary vascular system falls, changing pressure relationships within the heart. The foramen ovale (an opening between the two atria of the fetal heart) closes as pressure on the right side of the heart falls and pressure on the left side increases. Arterial PO_2 rises and arterial PCO_2 falls, prompting closure of the ductus arteriosus (a short vessel between the pulmonary artery and aorta of the fetus).

Pulse rates are highest and most variable in newborns. The resting heart rate for a neonate ranges from 100 to 170 beats/min immediately after birth and then the average heart rate is 120 beats/min (Ball, Bindler, Cowen, & Shaw, 2017, p. 125). The heart rate decreases to 80 to 130 in infants up to 2 years of age, and continues to decrease throughout early childhood until reaching the adult rate of 60 to 100 by about age 10 years. Irregular heart rates are common in infants and young children, often increasing and decreasing with each breath. This pattern of irregularity is known as sinus arrhythmia, a normal variation in heart rate.

Congenital heart disease occurs in approximately 1% of all live births (Ball et al., 2017, p. 518). Deaths, however, from congenital heart disease have significantly decreased due to diagnostic advances and new surgical techniques. Acquired heart diseases, though rare in childhood, include rheumatic fever, an inflammatory disorder that may occur following streptococcal infection (e.g., strep throat) and lead to heart valve damage. For most individuals, however, the heart continues to function effectively well into older adulthood unless the blood supply to the heart muscle is impaired by blood vessel disease. **Atherosclerosis**, the buildup of fatty plaque within the arteries, is the primary contributor to cardiovascular disease (CVD), which is the leading cause of death in North America.

Children are rarely affected by diseases of the blood vessels, although the increase in childhood obesity has increased the incidence in this age group. Hypertension or elevated BP may be associated with obesity, sedentary lifestyle, and stress in children and adolescents. During middle adulthood, the incidence of hypertension increases significantly. Hypertension, known as the silent killer because of its lack of symptoms, is a major risk factor for sudden cardiac death in middle adulthood.

Factors Affecting Cardiovascular Function

Many factors affect cardiovascular function. Some of these factors are called risk factors, because, if present, they increase the risk of CVD. Risk factors have been identified for CVD, hypertension, and peripheral vascular disease, and the majority of these factors are the same for all three disorders.

Risk Factors

Major traditional risk factors for CVD in general are classified as either *nonmodifiable* (cannot be reduced) or *modifiable* (can be reduced). Newer, nontraditional

LIFESPAN CONSIDERATIONS Circulation

CHILDREN

- Blood pressure should be taken routinely on children after age 3 years, but is not typically evaluated before that age.
- Heart murmurs, extra sounds detected when listening to the heart, are common in children, especially in the preschool years. The vast majority are not associated with a pathology, but are due to normal blood flow or transitional physiologic processes that increase cardiac output (e.g., anemia, fever, exercise).

OLDER ADULTS

Normal changes of aging may contribute to problems of circulation in older adults, even when there is no actual pathology:

- Blood vessels become less elastic and have an increase in calcification. This results in restricted blood flow and a decrease of oxygen and nutrients delivered to tissues (heart, peripheral, and cerebral).
- Impaired valve function in the heart is often the result of increased stiffness and calcification and results in a decrease in cardiac output.
- A decrease of muscle tone in the heart results in a decrease in cardiac output.
- There is a decrease in baroreceptor response to blood pressure changes, making the heart and blood vessels less responsive to exercise and stress. This often results in dizziness, falls, orthostatic hypotension, and mental changes.
- A decrease in conduction ability in the heart also makes the heart less responsive to changes and stresses. This can also result in dizziness, falls, orthostatic hypotension, and mental changes.

All of these factors become important if the individual is challenged by stressors, such as exercise, stress, fever, surgery, or other changes. If challenged, the circulatory system of older adults is not as effective or as quick to return to normal. Individuals living with normal changes of aging and pathologic conditions of the circulatory system need to learn to balance diet, medications, and exercise. Nurses have a major role in working with these clients to develop appropriate interventions and provide teaching to help them maintain optimal functioning. Teaching clients to recognize any changes or worsening of their condition is very important. They need to know when to contact their primary care provider to make any needed changes. Changing lifestyles and fine-tuning medications can be critical, and nurses can be a part of this in every phase of the nursing process.

cardiovascular risk factors have also been identified (Box 50.1). It is important to remember that most CVD is preventable. Research has shown that individuals with low cardiovascular risk factors have a substantially reduced risk of developing CVD. Unfortunately, the processes that lead to CVD begin early in life. Research has shown that the major lifestyle behaviors associated with CVD (e.g., patterns of diet, physical activity, and tobacco use) do influence the development of CVD risk factors in childhood, adolescence, and adulthood.

BOX 50.1 Risk Factors for Cardiovascular Disease

HIGH RISK FACTORS

- Nonmodifiable
  - Heredity
  - Age
  - Gender
- Modifiable
  - Elevated serum lipid level
  - Hypertension
  - Cigarette smoking
  - Diabetes
  - Obesity
  - Sedentary lifestyle

OTHER RISK FACTORS

- Stress
- Alcohol
- Diet and nutrition

NONTRADITIONAL RISK FACTORS

- Metabolic syndrome (Met-S)
- C-reactive protein (CRP)
- Elevated homocysteine level

Nonmodifiable Risk Factors

The first nonmodifiable risk factor is *heredity*. There is a genetic influence on the development of CVD. That is, if a client has a parent with heart disease, he or she is at higher risk. In addition, members of certain racial and ethnic groups, such as African Americans, have a higher risk of developing CVD (Ferdinand, 2016). The second is *age*. Cardiovascular disorders primarily affect individuals over age 65. The third nonmodifiable risk factor is *gender*. Until menopause, estrogen has a protective effect in women, slowing the progression of atherosclerosis and reducing the risk of CVD. This effect is lost at menopause, when women's death rate from heart disease increases; however, it's not as great as men's (American Heart Association [AHA], 2016). Nurses need to assess and teach both men and women about cardiovascular risk factors.

Modifiable Risk Factors

Modifiable risk factors include elevated serum lipid levels, hypertension, cigarette smoking, diabetes, obesity, and sedentary lifestyle. Many of the *Healthy People 2020* objectives relate to these modifiable risk factors.

ELEVATED SERUM LIPID LEVELS

A strong link exists between elevated serum lipid levels and the development of CVD. Lipid disorders, also called dyslipidemias, are abnormalities of lipoprotein metabolism and include elevations of total cholesterol, low-density lipoprotein (LDL) cholesterol, or triglycerides, or deficiencies of high-density lipoprotein (HDL) cholesterol. A high dietary intake of saturated fats *increases* the total LDL levels, and intake of polyunsaturated fatty acids *decreases* total LDL in most individuals. Studies have also shown that *trans*-fatty acids (e.g., stick margarine, deep-fried foods) raise LDL levels and lower HDL levels, resulting in an increase in total cholesterol.

Older adults, just like all other age groups, have become more obese, which leads to high cholesterol levels. It is this kind of data that accounts for *Healthy People 2020* (Office of Disease Prevention and Health Promotion [DPHP], 2019b) promoting the following objectives: Increase the proportion of adults who have had their blood cholesterol checked within the preceding 5 years; reduce the proportion of adults with high total blood cholesterol levels; reduce the mean total blood cholesterol levels among adults; and increase the proportion of adults with elevated LDL cholesterol who have been advised by a healthcare provider regarding cholesterol-lowering management, including lifestyle changes and, if indicated, medication.

HYPERTENSION

Hypertension increases the risk of CVD in several ways. First, it increases the workload of the heart, increasing oxygen demand and coronary blood flow. The increased workload also causes hypertrophy of the ventricles. Over time this can contribute to heart failure. Second, hypertension causes endothelial damage to the blood vessels, which stimulates the development of atherosclerosis. Atherosclerotic plaques cause a worsening of hypertension by narrowing the vessel lumens and decreasing vessel elasticity. Therefore, there is a cyclical relationship between these two conditions that raises an affected individual's risk for CVD.

High sodium intake can affect blood pressure and contribute to the development of hypertension. First, it may increase the release of natriuretic hormone, which indirectly contributes to hypertension. Additionally, sodium stimulates vasopressor mechanisms, which cause vasoconstriction. There is also evidence that other factors such as low potassium, calcium, and magnesium intake may contribute to vasoconstriction and the development of hypertension.

Healthy People 2020 (DPHP, 2019b) includes the following objectives relating to hypertension: Reduce the proportion of adults, children, and adolescents with hypertension; increase the proportion of adults with prehypertension and hypertension who meet the recommended guidelines for body mass index (BMI), saturated fat consumption, sodium intake, physical activity, and moderate alcohol consumption; increase the proportion of adults with hypertension who are taking the prescribed medications to lower their blood pressure; and increase the proportion of adults with hypertension whose blood pressure is under control.

CIGARETTE SMOKING

The cardiovascular system is affected by cigarette smoking. Nicotine increases heart rate, blood pressure, and peripheral vascular resistance, increasing the heart's workload. Smoking causes vasoconstriction, and in areas where vessels already are narrowed by atherosclerosis, tissue oxygenation can be impaired.

Healthy People 2020 (DPHP, 2019e) includes many objectives relating to tobacco use, including, but not limited to: Reduce cigarette smoking by adolescents and adults; increase smoking cessation attempts by adolescent and adult smokers and during pregnancy; increase tobacco cessation counseling in healthcare settings; and establish laws that prohibit smoking in public places and worksites.

DIABETES

Diabetes mellitus increases the risk of CVD and myocardial infarction (MI). High blood glucose levels are associated with accelerated development of atherosclerosis as well as high levels of serum lipids and triglycerides. Closely monitoring blood glucose levels in clients with diabetes and checking blood glucose levels in all clients for the development of increased levels are important nursing functions. Control of blood glucose levels can greatly reduce risk and slow development of atherosclerosis. Examples of objectives in *Healthy People 2020* (DPHP, 2019a) that pertain to diabetes include the following: Reduce the annual number of new cases of diagnosed diabetes in the population; reduce the death rate among individuals with diabetes; reduce the rate of lower extremity amputations in individuals with diagnosed diabetes; improve glycemic control among individuals with diabetes; and increase the proportion of individuals with diagnosed diabetes who receive formal diabetes education.

OBESITY

Obesity and diabetes are major health problems that are rapidly getting worse in the United States. In addition, individuals with obesity have an increased risk for the development of CVD because obesity is often accompanied by elevated serum lipid levels and is associated with hypertension. Thus, adults who are obese are at risk for diabetes and hypertension. Additionally, obesity places an increased workload on the heart, which increases oxygen demand. Research has shown that obese individuals have an increased risk for heart failure and death, and that risk increases in proportion to the degree of obesity.

Examples of objectives in *Healthy People 2020* (DPHP, 2019c) that pertain to weight include: Increase the proportion of adults who are at a healthy weight; reduce the proportion of children and adolescents who are considered obese; and increase the proportion of physician office visits that include counseling or education related to nutrition or weight.

SEDENTARY LIFESTYLE

Regular physical activity is associated with a reduction in the risk of death due to CVD, whereas a sedentary lifestyle is associated with increased risk. Physical exercise or activity increases the heart rate and, hence, the supply of oxygen in the body. With regular vigorous exercise, the heart muscle becomes more powerful and efficient. Aerobic exercise slows the atherosclerotic process, directly reducing the risk of CVD, and decreases the risks of obesity and diabetes mellitus, therefore indirectly reducing risk of CVD as well.

A healthy lifestyle that includes a heart-healthy diet and physical activity promotes cardiovascular health. This is true throughout the lifespan. Because children and adolescents spend a great deal of time in school, one of the *Healthy People 2020* (DPHP, 2019d) objectives is to increase the number of states with licensing regulations for physical activity in child care that require activity programs providing large muscle or gross motor activity, development, and/or equipment. The *Healthy People 2020* objectives also include increasing the proportion of adolescents and adults who meet current federal physical activity guidelines for aerobic physical activity and for muscle-strengthening activity.

Other Risk Factors

The American Heart Association (2016) includes other risk factors that contribute to heart disease risk: stress, alcohol, and diet and nutrition.

STRESS

How one responds to stress may be a contributing factor. For example, some individuals may react to stress by developing or increasing other major risk factors such as overeating, start smoking, or increase the amount of their smoking. It is important for nurses to share stress management tools.

ALCOHOL

Drinking too much alcohol can increase blood pressure, increase risk of cardiomyopathy, contribute to high triglycerides, produce irregular heartbeats, and contribute to obesity (AHA, 2016). There is a cardioprotective effect of *moderate* alcohol consumption. This effect, however, is based on a limit of one drink per day. One drink can equal any one of the following: 12 oz. of regular beer, 5 oz. of wine, 1.5 oz of 80-proof spirits, or 1 oz. of 100-proof spirits (Harvard Health Publishing, 2018).

DIET AND NUTRITION

The food and amount of food one eats can also affect the modifiable risk factors: cholesterol, blood pressure, diabetes, and obesity. A healthy diet (see Chapter 46 ∞) and lifestyle are the best weapons in the fight against cardiovascular disease.

Nontraditional Risk Factors

Other emerging modifiable risk factors that may influence cardiovascular function include the presence of metabolic syndrome or C-reactive protein or an elevated homocysteine level.

METABOLIC SYNDROME

Metabolic syndrome (Met-S) is a cluster of cardiovascular risk factors that increase the risk for cardiovascular disease, diabetes, and death. Five risk factors are included in Met-S: central obesity (e.g., increased waist circumference), increased triglycerides, decreased HDL cholesterol, hypertension, and elevated fasting glucose. An individual is considered to have metabolic syndrome when at least three of the five risk factors are present. Each risk factor is usually treated individually. Overall, lifestyle activities and behaviors, such as nutrition and physical activity, are the best preventions for the development of Met-S risk factors.

C-REACTIVE PROTEIN

Many studies have shown that acute myocardial infarction (AMI) involves an inflammatory process. A useful screening test for this inflammatory process is the **C-reactive protein (CRP)** assay. However, a CRP can be elevated in other inflammatory conditions (e.g., trauma, infections, rheumatoid arthritis). Currently a more highly sensitive measurement to detect CRP is used for cardiovascular risk assessment and is called hs-CRP. An hs-CRP level of 1 mg/L is considered low risk for CVD. Moderate risk is an hs-CRP between 1 and 3 mg/L, and greater than 3 mg/L is considered high risk for CVD (Stöppler, 2018). Usually, CRP screening is completed along with cholesterol screening to determine cardiovascular risk assessment. If the results are high, smoking cessation, diet, and exercise are recommended guidelines to reduce the CRP and cholesterol levels.

ELEVATED HOMOCYSTEINE LEVEL

Homocysteine is an amino acid that has been shown to be increased in many individuals with atherosclerosis. Clients with elevated homocysteine levels may have an increased risk of MI, CVD, stroke, and peripheral vascular disease. It is thought that individuals can reduce their homocysteine level by taking a multivitamin that provides folate, vitamin B_6, vitamin B_{12}, and riboflavin. However, clinical trials that attempted to lower homocysteine levels through B-vitamin treatment have varied in their results. As a result, there is controversy regarding the significance of homocysteine as a risk factor for CVD and stroke (Chrysant & Chrysant, 2018).

QSEN Patient-Centered Care: Gender Disparities in Clients with Cardiovascular Disease

Once considered a man's disease, more women than men are now living and dying with CVD (Banman & Sawatzky, 2017; [CDC], 2017). Women's risk factors are different from men's. For example, women with diabetes and those who smoke are at higher risk than men who have diabetes or smoke. Other risk factors for women include pregnancy complications such as preeclampsia, gestational diabetes, and pregnancy-induced hypertension (Kalman & Wells, 2018, p. 22). The Association of Women's Health, Obstetric and Neonatal Nurses (AWHONN, 2018) reports that risk factor trends for women are of concern. For example, more women than men have metabolic syndrome; 2 out of 3 women older than 20 are overweight or obese, which contributes to the development of diabetes; and more women over 65 years old have hypertension than men of similar age. Additionally, in the past 40 years, mortality rates from CVD have decreased for men but have not improved for women age 25 to 34 (AWHONN, 2018). Researchers are asking why this is, especially if estrogen is considered to be cardioprotective in younger women.

Many women are not aware that their MI symptoms may be different from men's. For example, men often describe chest pain as "an elephant sitting on my chest," whereas women may feel it as pressure or discomfort or have pain in the neck, jaw, throat, abdomen, or back (CDC, 2017). Other symptoms that women may experience (e.g., shortness of breath, indigestion, unusual fatigue, insomnia, anxiety) are vague and easily missed by healthcare providers (Kalman & Wells, 2018).

Prevention strategies have helped reduce mortality rates for men but the rates have not decreased as rapidly for women. One possible reason for this difference is that women may not be aware of their risk for heart disease and, therefore, have minimal concern for adopting more health promotion activities. Nurses are often a woman's first and most consistent point of contact with the healthcare system. Thus, it is important for nurses to assess for and discuss CVD risk factors with their female clients.

Alterations in Cardiovascular Function

Cardiovascular function can be altered by conditions that affect:

1. The function of the heart as a pump
2. Blood flow to organs and peripheral tissues
3. The composition of the blood and its ability to transport oxygen and carbon dioxide.

Three major alterations in cardiovascular function are decreased cardiac output, impaired tissue perfusion, and disorders that affect the composition or amount of blood available for transport of gases.

Decreased Cardiac Output

Although the heart is normally able to increase its rate and force of contraction to increase cardiac output during exercise, fever, or other times of need, some conditions interfere with these mechanisms.

The vessels that supply blood to the heart muscle may become occluded by atherosclerosis or a blood clot, shutting off the blood supply to a portion of the myocardium. When this happens, the tissue becomes necrotic and dies, a condition known as a **myocardial infarction (MI)** or *heart attack.* If a large portion of the heart muscle is affected, particularly in the left ventricle, cardiac output falls because the affected muscle no longer contracts. Signs and symptoms of MI are variable and may include the following:

- Chest pain; substernal or radiating to the left arm, jaw
- Nausea
- Shortness of breath
- Diaphoresis.

Heart failure may develop if the heart is unable to keep up with the body's need for oxygen and nutrients to the tissues. Heart failure usually occurs because of MI, but it may also result from chronic overwork of the heart, such as in clients with uncontrolled hypertension or extensive arteriosclerosis. In left-sided heart failure, the vessels of the pulmonary system become congested or engorged with blood. This may cause fluid to escape into the alveoli and interfere with gas exchange, a condition known as *pulmonary edema.* Signs of heart failure may include the following:

- Pulmonary congestion; adventitious lung sounds
- Shortness of breath
- Dyspnea on exertion (DOE)
- Increased heart rate
- S_3 heart sound
- Increased respiratory rate
- Nocturia
- Orthopnea
- Distended neck veins.

Other diseases such as myocarditis and cardiomyopathy also can affect the heart muscle, impairing its ability to contract and pump. Box 50.2 gives examples of conditions that may precipitate heart failure.

BOX 50.2 Examples of Conditions That May Precipitate Heart Failure

CONDITIONS THAT INCREASE PRELOAD
- Hypervolemia
- Valvular disorders such as mitral regurgitation
- Congenital defects such as patent ductus arteriosus

CONDITIONS THAT INCREASE AFTERLOAD
- Hypertension
- Atherosclerosis

CONDITIONS THAT AFFECT MYOCARDIAL FUNCTION
- Myocardial infarction
- Cardiomyopathy
- Coronary artery disease

Very irregular or excessively rapid or slow heart rates can also decrease cardiac output. With irregular or very rapid heart rates, the ventricles may not fill adequately between beats, so stroke volume (amount pumped with each beat) falls. If the heart rate is too slow, the heart may not be able to increase its stroke volume enough to maintain the cardiac output. Abnormalities of heart rate and rhythm are known as dysrhythmias and can be identified on an electrocardiogram (ECG).

Alterations in the structure of the heart can affect cardiac output. Congenital heart defects result in abnormal blood flow and may even allow venous and arterial blood to mix. Oxygen supply to body tissues is affected in this case. Acquired heart diseases such as bacterial endocarditis and rheumatic fever may damage the heart valves, affecting the flow of blood within the heart and to the great vessels. For example, if the mitral (bicuspid) valve becomes scarred and stenotic (constricted), it may not open fully, impairing filling of the left ventricle. Or, if the mitral valve does not fully close (mitral insufficiency), blood may escape back or regurgitate into the left atrium instead of entering the aorta each time the ventricle contracts.

Impaired Tissue Perfusion

Atherosclerosis is by far the most common cause of impaired blood flow to organs and tissues. As vessels narrow and become obstructed, distal tissues receive less blood, oxygen, and nutrients. **Ischemia** is a lack of blood supply due to obstructed circulation. Any artery in the body may be affected by atherosclerosis, although the effects are most often associated with coronary arteries, vessels supplying blood to the brain, and arteries in peripheral tissues. Partial obstruction of coronary arteries causes myocardial ischemia, often resulting in angina pectoris; if the obstruction is complete a heart attack (MI) occurs. Partial obstruction of cerebral vessels may cause a transient ischemic attack (TIA); if the obstruction is complete, a stroke occurs. Peripheral vascular disease leads to ischemia of distal tissues such as the legs and feet. Gangrene and amputation may result. Signs of impaired peripheral arterial circulation in the legs and feet may include the following:

- Decreased peripheral pulses
- Pain or paresthesias
- Pale skin color
- Cool extremities
- Decreased hair distribution.

The risk factors for peripheral atherosclerosis are similar to those for CVD and include cigarette smoking, high fat intake, obesity, and a sedentary lifestyle. Hypertension and diabetes also increase the risk for atherosclerosis, particularly if the blood pressure or blood glucose levels are not maintained at near-normal levels.

Although much less common, other disorders such as vessel inflammation, arterial spasm, and blood clots also can occlude blood vessels, leading to ischemia. Tissue edema can impair flow through vessels and can increase the distance oxygen and nutrients must diffuse across to reach cells.

On the venous side, incompetent valves may allow blood to pool in veins, causing edema and decreasing venous return to the heart (Figure 50.4 ■). Veins also can become inflamed, reducing blood flow and increasing the risk of thrombus (clot) formation. Thrombi may then break loose, becoming emboli. These emboli tend to travel as far as the pulmonary circulation where they become trapped in small vessels (pulmonary emboli), occluding blood supply to the capillary side of the alveolar–capillary membrane. Although alveolar ventilation to the affected area often remains adequate, no gas exchange occurs there because of impaired blood flow. Signs of acute pulmonary embolism (PE) can be nonspecific and variable but may include the following:

- Sudden onset of shortness of breath
- Pleuritic chest pain.

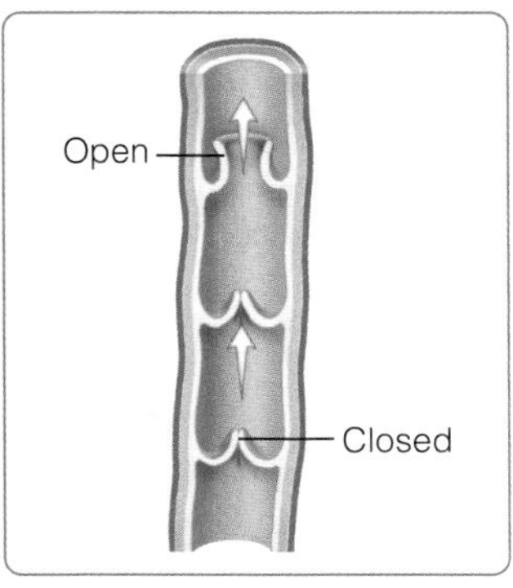

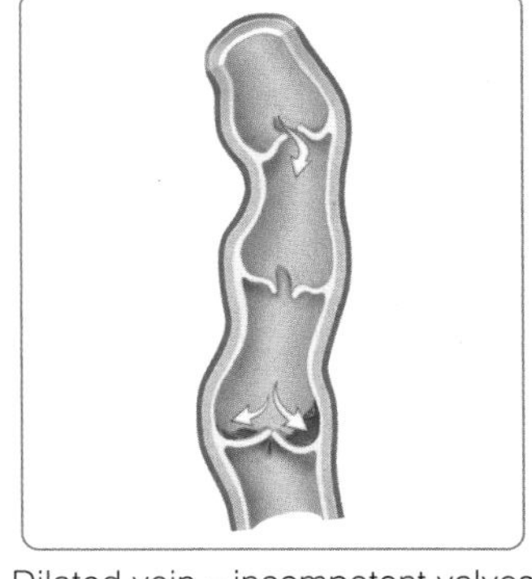

Figure 50.4 ■ *Left:* Vein with competent valve; *right*, vein with incompetent valve that allows blood to pool in the veins.
From *Medical Terminology for Health Care Professionals* (9th ed., p. 293), by J. Rice, 2018. Reproduced by permission of Pearson Education, Inc., Hoboken, NJ.

Blood Alterations

Because most oxygen is transported to the tissues in combination with hemoglobin, the problems of inadequate RBCs, low hemoglobin levels, or abnormal hemoglobin structure can affect tissue oxygenation. Anemia has several different causes: RBCs are lost along with other components because of acute or chronic bleeding; if diet is deficient in iron or folic acid, hemoglobin and RBCs are not formed adequately; and some disorders cause RBCs to break down excessively. Clients with sickle cell disease produce an abnormal form of hemoglobin and may experience tissue ischemia during exacerbations of the disease. Signs of anemia may include the following:

- Chronic fatigue
- Pallor
- Shortness of breath
- Hypotension.

Blood volume also affects tissue oxygenation. If the blood volume is inadequate, as in hemorrhage or severe dehydration, blood pressure and cardiac output fall, and tissues may become ischemic. Conversely, clients with hypervolemia (excess blood volume), which can result from fluid retention or kidney failure, may develop heart failure and peripheral edema, also leading to tissue ischemia.

●○● NURSING MANAGEMENT

Assessing

Nursing assessment of the cardiovascular system status includes a history, physical examination, and a review of relevant diagnostic data, including cardiac monitoring.

Nursing History

A comprehensive nursing history should include data regarding:

- Current and past cardiovascular problems
- Family history of cardiovascular problems such as high blood pressure, increased cholesterol level, heart attack, and stroke
- Other medical history including diabetes and respiratory disorders
- Exercise and activity level
- History of tobacco use
- Diet, including fat and salt intake, alcohol intake, caffeine intake including soft drinks and chocolate

ASSESSMENT INTERVIEW Circulation

CURRENT OR PAST CARDIOVASCULAR PROBLEMS

- Do you have high blood pressure?
- Do you have any history of heart disease such as angina, heart attack, or heart failure? Have you ever had a cardiac catheterization, angiogram, or angioplasty? Have you ever been diagnosed with rheumatic fever, endocarditis, pericarditis, or other diseases of the heart? If so, when? Have you had cardiac surgery or stent placement?
- Have you ever been told that you have peripheral vascular disease? Do you ever develop pain in the calves of your legs when walking? How far can you walk before it occurs? What do you do to relieve it? Have you had surgery on your blood vessels?
- Do your feet and ankles ever swell or feel very cold, numb, or tingling? Do you experience pain in your feet? Is the pain changed by position?
- Do you become extremely fatigued with activity? Have you ever been told that you are anemic?

MEDICATION HISTORY

- Have you taken or do you take any over-the-counter or prescription medications for your heart or blood pressure or to increase blood flow?
- Do you take any anticoagulants or other medications to “thin” your blood?

LIFESTYLE

- Do you use tobacco? If so, what kind?
- Do you exercise? What kind of exercise and how often?
- How often do you drink alcoholic beverages such as beer, wine, or liquor? How much do you usually drink at a time?

- Presence of any symptoms such as pain, shortness of breath, dizziness, fatigue, palpitations, cough, and fainting
- Medications for heart, blood pressure, circulation, and cholesterol
- Lifestyle, including social support, stressors, and methods of coping.

Physical Assessment

To examine the cardiovascular system, a nurse first evaluates blood pressure in both arms (the results should be within 10 mmHg of each other) and palpates peripheral pulses for their strength and equality. The apical pulse is auscultated for rate, rhythm, and the quality of heart sounds. Apical pulse rate and peripheral pulse rates should not vary more than a few beats per minute from one another. Carotid arteries are auscultated for bruits (a sound of turbulence), which may indicate atherosclerosis and narrowing (see Chapter 29 ∞). Also important as an indicator of cardiac function is lung sounds. By auscultating the lungs for adventitious sounds, the nurse assesses for increased pulmonary vessel pressure secondary to decreased cardiac output.

Much information about the cardiovascular system is obtained by assessing the skin for color, temperature, hair distribution, lesions, and edema. Clients with extensive peripheral vascular disease may have cool feet with weak pulses and shiny, nearly hairless shins and feet. Pitting edema of the feet and ankles may be noted in clients with heart failure. See Chapter 29 ∞ for specific techniques for assessing the respiratory and cardiovascular systems.

One noninvasive measure used to assess for peripheral vascular disease is the ankle brachial index (ABI). This is the ratio of arterial pressure in the ankle compared with that in the arm. The ABI is a simple, reliable means for diagnosing peripheral arterial disease (PAD) (Park, 2016). The ABI has been traditionally determined using a conventional sphygmomanometer and a Doppler instrument. Aneroid BP cuffs, however, are being replaced by automated blood pressure equipment. To perform an ABI, the client has to be supine for 5 to 10 minutes while the nurse gathers BP cuffs, a handheld Doppler instrument, and ultrasound gel. Place a BP cuff on the client's right arm and right ankle. After applying the gel, use the Doppler to determine the client's systolic pressure in the right arm and right ankle using the right dorsalis pedis and posterior tibial arteries. Repeat this procedure for the client's left arm and ankle. Use the higher ankle pressure (dorsalis pedis or posterior tibial) for each lower extremity and the higher arm pressure. Box 50.3 explains how to measure the ABI.

Diagnostic Studies

Many diagnostic studies are available that can help to identify the presence of CVD. Diagnostic studies may also be used as screening tools to identify increased risk so that modifications can be made to reduce the risk of development of CVD. An example of this is the serum lipid level. If a client has an elevated serum lipid level, he or she should be educated about the effects of diet and the importance of reducing lipids to reduce the risk of CVD.

BOX 50.3 Measurement of an Ankle Brachial Index (ABI)

The ABI measurement compares the systolic blood pressure of the lower extremity with the systolic blood pressure of the brachial artery. A ratio is calculated based on the results.

$$\text{ABI} = \frac{\text{systolic pressure of the ankle}}{\text{systolic pressure of the arm}}$$

Example

$$\text{ABI} = \frac{\text{132 systolic pressure of ankle}}{\text{124 systolic pressure of arm}} = 1.06$$

Interpretation of ABI:

- 1.00–1.40: normal
- 0.9–1.0: acceptable
- 0.8–0.90: some arterial disease
- 0.5 – 0.8: moderate arterial disease
- Less than 0.5: severe arterial disease

From *Measuring and Understanding the Ankle-Brachial Index (ABI)*, by Stanford Medicine, n.d.

Cardiac Monitoring

Cardiac monitoring allows for continuous observation of the client's cardiac rhythm. Cardiac monitoring is a recording of the heart's electrical activity. It is used in many instances: for clients who have known or suspected CVD, during and after surgery, to monitor responses to drug therapy, and to monitor clients at risk for serious complications such as shock. Electrodes placed on the client's chest are attached to a monitor cable and bedside monitor (Figure 50.5 ■). The monitor is equipped with alarms used to warn of potential problems such as very fast, very slow, or irregular heart rates. The alarm limits are usually set for 20 beats higher and lower than the client's baseline rate, often at 100 to 110 and 50 to 55, respectively, for adults. For ambulatory clients (in the hospital or at home), the electrodes connect to a transmitter unit (also called telemetry). This unit electronically sends the signal to a central monitor for display or may store the information to be retrieved later in the primary care provider's office. Another name for this type of ambulatory monitoring is a Holter monitor. Electrodes are attached and the client wears the monitor for 24 hours. A continuous ECG is recorded and later analyzed for irregularities.

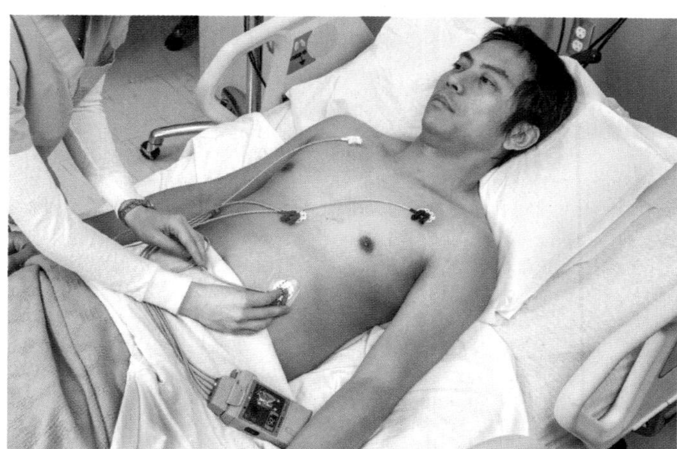

Figure 50.5 ■ A client with cardiac monitoring.

Electrocardiography most commonly uses 12 "leads" or 12 different views of the heart. In contrast, cardiac monitoring uses 2 or 3 leads at any given time.

Clinical Alert!

It is important to remember that ECG monitoring is a recording of the electrical activity of the heart; it does not reflect mechanical contraction and cardiac output. *Always* remember to check the client to assess for cardiac function. Just looking at the ECG does not give an assessment of the client's status.

Blood Tests

Specimens of venous blood can be used for several tests that may reflect some aspect of cardiovascular functioning.

Because hemoglobin is the molecule to which oxygen attaches, an individual's hemoglobin level gives an indication of the oxygen-carrying capacity of the blood. A decreased hemoglobin level increases the risk of oxygen deficit in body tissues, especially when CVD is present.

Measurement of serum electrolytes is important for clients with cardiovascular problems because electrolyte abnormalities such as hyperkalemia (higher than normal potassium) and hypokalemia (lower than normal potassium) can have a critical effect on the heart. Serum levels of magnesium, calcium, sodium, and phosphorus are also important to assess.

Measurement of certain enzyme levels in the blood is an important part of the diagnostic evaluation of clients with chest pain. Enzymes such as **creatine kinase (CK)** and **troponin** are released into the blood during an MI, as a result of cell membrane damage. Elevated levels of these enzymes can help differentiate between an MI (when myocardial cells actually die) and chest pain from a different cause such as angina or pleuritic pain.

Hemodynamic Studies

Hemodynamics is the study of the forces or pressures involved in blood circulation. Hemodynamic studies or monitoring procedures may be performed to evaluate fluid status and cardiovascular function. Parameters evaluated in hemodynamic studies include heart rate, arterial blood pressure, central venous pressure, pressures in the pulmonary vascular system, and CO. Some of these parameters—for example, heart rate, arterial blood pressure, and venous pressure—are measured directly using an arterial, central venous, or pulmonary artery catheter; others, such as stroke volume and cardiac output, are calculated. Hemodynamic studies are performed in a diagnostic cardiac laboratory and require informed consent. Clients in intensive and cardiac care units may undergo continuous hemodynamic monitoring to evaluate cardiovascular status and the effect of interventions. Nurses in these units are responsible for obtaining accurate readings and maintaining the integrity of the system.

Diagnosing

Examples of diagnoses for clients with circulation problems can include inadequate cardiac output, impaired tissue perfusion, and blood alterations (e.g., decreased RBCs, low hemoglobin level, anemia).

Planning

When planning care the nurse identifies nursing interventions that will assist the client to achieve these broad goals:

- Maintain or restore an adequate cardiac output.
- Maintain or improve tissue perfusion.

Obviously, goals will vary according to the diagnosis and the signs and symptoms for each individual. Appropriate preventive and corrective nursing interventions that relate to these must be identified. Specific nursing activities can be selected to meet the client's individual needs. Examples of NIC interventions related to decreased cardiac output and tissue perfusion include the following:

- Circulatory Care: Arterial Insufficiency
- Cardiac Care
- Hemodynamic Regulation.

To promote the transport of oxygen and carbon dioxide, the nurse can optimize CO by reducing stress, planning appropriate activities, and positioning the client for improved vascular blood flow.

Implementing

Promoting Circulation

Most individuals in good health give little thought to their cardiovascular function. Changing position frequently, ambulating, and exercising usually maintain adequate cardiovascular functioning. See Client Teaching for other ways to promote a healthy heart.

Immobility is harmful to cardiovascular function. Without activity of the calf and leg muscles, blood pools in the veins of the lower extremities. This stagnant (sluggish) blood flow may allow clots to develop (venous thrombosis). With time, these clots can break loose and become emboli, eventually lodging in the small vessels of the pulmonary vascular system. Blood flow and gas exchange in the lungs are then impaired.

Many nursing interventions can help clients maintain cardiac and vascular function. They may be classified as vascular and cardiac.

CLIENT TEACHING Promoting a Healthy Heart

- Exercise regularly, participating in at least 30 minutes of moderate-intensity aerobic exercise 5 times a week.
- Do not smoke.
- Maintain your ideal weight.
- Use the DASH eating plan (Dietary Approaches to Stop Hypertension) by eating foods low in saturated fat, total fat, and cholesterol, and high in fruits, vegetables, and low-fat dairy foods.
- Drink alcohol in moderation, if at all, consuming no more than 1 cocktail or 1 glass of wine or beer daily.
- Reduce stress and manage anger.
- Effectively manage diabetes and hypertension, maintaining blood glucose and blood pressure levels within normal limits.
- If female, discuss with your healthcare provider the advantages and risks of hormone replacement therapy after menopause (or after a total hysterectomy).
- Consult your primary care provider about the advisability of low-dose aspirin therapy to further reduce the risk of CVD.

CLIENT TEACHING **Home Care and Circulation**

MAINTAINING CARDIAC OUTPUT AND TISSUE PERFUSION

- Teach the symptoms of heart failure to the client and family and emphasize when to contact the primary care provider.
- Teach the client about the importance of maintaining regular physical activity to promote circulation and vascular health. Emphasize the need to increase activity levels gradually with the goal of exercising (walking, swimming, weight training, or aerobic exercise as recommended by the care provider) for at least 30 minutes 5 times per week.
- Instruct the client to avoid exposure to cold, wearing warm clothing as needed.
- Teach cardiopulmonary resuscitation or refer for instruction.

DIETARY ALTERATIONS

- Instruct the client and family about prescribed dietary restrictions such as a low-sodium diet. Refer to a dietitian as needed for further instruction.
- Discuss dietary measures to reduce the risk of atherosclerosis, including reducing total and saturated fats in the diet, reducing weight if obese, and increasing the intake of dietary fiber.

MEDICATIONS

- Instruct the client and family about prescribed medications, including effects, side effects, and administration.

Vascular

- Position with the legs elevated to promote venous return to the heart. This is particularly important for clients with venous dysfunction. Care should be taken, however, to avoid this position in clients with cardiac dysfunction because it will increase preload and may increase stress on the heart.
- Avoid pillows under the knees or more than 15 degrees of knee flexion to improve blood flow to the lower extremities and reduce venous stagnation.
- Encourage leg exercises (such as flexion and extension of the feet, active contraction and relaxation of calf muscles) for a client on bedrest, and promote ambulation as soon as possible.
- Encourage or provide frequent position changes.

Cardiac

- Position the client in a high-Fowler's position to decrease preload and reduce pulmonary congestion.
- Monitor intake and output. Fluid restriction is usually not required for clients with mild to moderate cardiac dysfunction. With severe heart failure, a fluid restriction may be ordered.

Medications

Many classes of medications are administered to clients with cardiovascular disorders. Drugs such as nitrates, calcium channel blockers, and angiotensin-converting enzyme (ACE) inhibitors reduce the workload of the heart and prevent vasoconstriction. Various drugs are used to treat cardiac dysrhythmias. Positive inotropic drugs such as digoxin are used to increase the contractile strength of the heart. (See the Drug Capsule feature on digoxin in Chapter 28 ∞.) Beta-adrenergic blocking agents such as propranolol or metoprolol may be given to block the sympathetic nervous system action on the heart and decrease oxygen consumption. Direct vasodilators may be used for clients with peripheral vascular disease and sometimes hypertension. Often clients are on numerous medications, and it is an important role of the nurse to help the client understand the purposes, effects, and side effects of the different medications.

Administering medications is an important nursing function. Nurses are responsible for assessing for the effects of medications and also for potential complications. Examples include:

- When diuretics are administered, the nurse assesses intake, output, and serum potassium level (because many diuretics can lower potassium level).
- When positive inotropic medications are administered, the nurse should assess blood pressure, heart rate, peripheral pulses, and lung sounds as indicators of cardiac output.
- When antihypertensive medications are administered, it is critical for the nurse to monitor blood pressure. Additionally, many antihypertensive medications can cause orthostatic hypotension.

Preventing Venous Stasis

When clients have limited mobility or are confined to bed, venous return to the heart is impaired and the risk of venous stasis increases. Immobility is a problem not only for ill or debilitated clients but also for some travelers who sit with legs dependent for long periods in a motor vehicle or an airplane.

Venous stasis may allow clots (venous thrombosis) to develop in a deep vein, often in the thigh or calf. This is called deep venous thrombosis or deep vein thrombosis (DVT). If the thrombus breaks free, it can travel and become a PE where it blocks a pulmonary artery or one of its branches. Blood flow and gas exchange in the lungs are then impaired. If the clot is large enough, sudden death can occur. DVT in the popliteal vein and those above it are strongly associated with the development of PEs (Roberts & Lawrence, 2017, p. 39). The term *venous thromboembolism* (VTE) incorporates both DVT and PE. VTE is one of the most common preventable causes of hospital-related death, especially among older adults because advancing age is a major risk for VTE (Dunn & Ramos, 2017).

Preventing venous stasis is an important nursing intervention to reduce the risk of complications following surgery, trauma, or major medical problems. Positioning and leg exercises are discussed in Chapter 44 ∞ and antiemboli stockings in Chapter 37 ∞. Sequential compression devices are an additional mechanical measure to help prevent venous stasis.

Sequential Compression Devices

Clients who are undergoing surgery or who are immobilized because of illness or injury or are in a critical care unit may benefit from sequential compression devices (SCDs) to promote venous return from the legs. Another term used in the literature is intermittent pneumatic compression devices (IPCDs), and because there are different types of IPCDs, they are often collectively referred to as SCDs. SCDs are useful in preventing thrombi and edema, which may result from venous stasis, but they are not used for clients who have arterial insufficiency, cellulitis, infection of the extremity, active DVT, or preexisting venous thrombosis. SCDs inflate and deflate plastic sleeves to promote venous flow. The plastic sleeves are attached by tubing to an air pump that alternately inflates and deflates portions of the sleeve to a specified pressure.

SCDs are available in foot (sometimes called a foot pump or foot impulse device), knee-length, or thigh-length sleeves. The foot pump artificially stimulates the venous plantar plexus (a large vein located in the foot) to increase blood circulation in the foot. The inflation and deflation of the pump simulate the blood flow that results from walking. For the knee-length or thigh-length SCDs, the ankle area inflates first, followed by the calf region, and then the thigh area. This sequential inflation and deflation process assists the leg muscles in moving blood toward the heart (Figure 50.6 ■).

Foot, knee-high, and thigh-high SCDs are effective mechanical prophylaxis against VTEs if they are continuously worn. Unfortunately, research evidence shows that SCD therapy has either not been applied when it should have been, or has been incorrectly applied (Dunn & Ramos, 2017). This is problematic when it is the nurse's role to apply, maintain, and monitor SCD therapy. One barrier for nonadherance is that clients did not want to wear them because of discomfort, warmth, or sleep disruption. One study found that products that used "breathable" material were tolerated better by clients. It is important for the nurse to educate the client about the purpose and importance of the SCDs and to problem solve how to make them more comfortable (e.g., selecting SCD sleeves that fit properly).

Nurses must be attentive in their practice of applying and reapplying SCD devices after procedures, baths, and during chair activities (Dunn & Ramos, 2017, p. 166). The SCD is only removed for ambulation and is usually discontinued when the client resumes normal activity or is discharged.

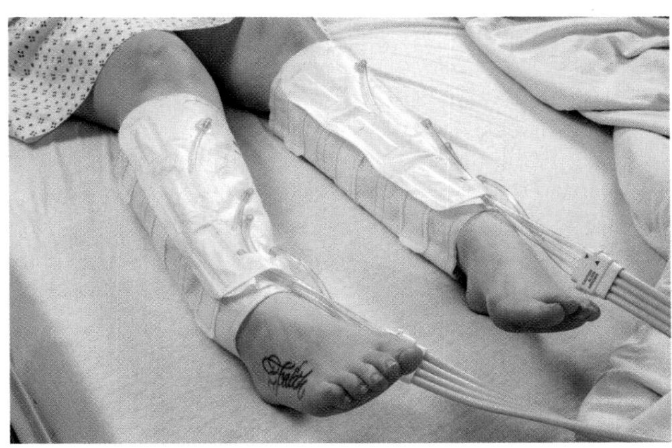

Figure 50.6 ■ Sequential compression devices enhance venous return. They are available in foot, knee-high, or thigh-high versions.

Sequential compression therapy often goes together with other preventive measures. The client's risk level for DVT or PE often determines the preventive measures used. For example, clients at low risk may require only antiemboli stockings or ambulation. Clients at moderate risk may have both antiemboli stockings and sequential therapy, or low molecular weight heparin (LMWH) prophylaxis as part of their treatment (Crumley, 2018). The primary care provider may order antiemboli stockings, sequential therapy, and anticoagulation therapy for the high-risk client.

QSEN **Patient-Centered Care: Sequential Compression Devices**

A sequential compression device may be used in the home. Inform the client or caregiver how to apply the device correctly and how to operate the system, including how to respond to the alarm.

Skill 50.1 outlines how to apply a sequential compression device.

EVIDENCE-BASED PRACTICE

Evidence-Based Practice

Is There a Difference in Effectiveness and Safety of Different Intermittent Pneumatic Compression Devices (IPCDs) in the Prevention of VTE in Clients After Total Hip Replacement (THR)?

VTE is a common complication after a THR. Preventive measures commonly include prophylactic anticoagulation and IPCDs, or a combination of both. The IPCDs have a major advantage over anticoagulation in that they do not increase the risk of bleeding. A wide range of IPCDs are available. As a result, Andrews (2016) evaluated the effectiveness of different IPCDs after THR in order to inform clinical decision-making.

Andrews reviewed randomized controlled trials (RCTs) and quasi-randomized designs comparing different IPCDs for clients after THR for the prevention of VTE. One quasi-randomized trial met the inclusion criteria. This study consisted of 121 participants from a single medical center who had a THR. The participants were either in the calf–thigh pump intervention group or a plantar pump intervention group. All participants had the IPCD in place immediately after the THR for 4 hours per day for 21 days. A D-dimer blood level (for thrombogenesis) was measured before and after the THR. Postoperative swelling was measured by thigh and lower leg circumferences at 6 a.m. on the day of surgery and again at the same time on days 3, 7, 14, and 21. These measurements were compared to the preoperative measurements.

The results showed no cases of DVT or PE in either group during the first 3 weeks after the THR. The calf–thigh IPCD was more effective for reducing thigh swelling.

Implications

The author concluded that there was insufficient evidence for an informed choice of specific IPC device to use to prevent VTE after THR and that more research needs to be conducted. Andrews (2016) stressed the importance of nurses focusing on the risk–benefit ratio of the IPCD, applying the device correctly, and monitoring client adherence.

SKILL 50.1

Applying Sequential Compression Devices

PURPOSES

- To promote venous return from the legs
- To decrease risk of DVT and PE

ASSESSMENT

Assess for baseline data:

- Cardiovascular status, including heart rate and rhythm, peripheral pulses, and capillary refill
- Color and temperature of extremities
- Movement and sensation of feet and lower extremities

PLANNING

Check the primary care provider's order for type of SCD sleeve. **Rationale:** *Foot, knee- and thigh-length sleeves are available.*

- Read the manufacturer's directions for connecting and operating the compression controller.

Assignment

Assistive personnel (AP) often remove and reapply the SCD when performing hygiene care. The nurse should check that the AP knows the correct application process for the SCD. Remind the AP that the client should not have the SCD removed for long periods of time because the purpose of the SCD is to promote circulation. Remind AP to inspect the SCD sleeve and tubing each time prior to applying the sleeves.

Equipment

- Measuring tape
- SCD, including disposable sleeves, air pump, and tubing

IMPLEMENTATION

Performance

1. Prior to performing the procedure, introduce self and verify the client's identity using agency protocol. Explain to the client what you are going to do, why it is necessary, and the procedure for applying the sequential compression device. **Rationale:** *The client's participation and comfort will be increased by understanding the rationale for applying the SCD.*
2. Perform hand hygiene and observe other appropriate infection prevention procedures.
3. Provide for client privacy and drape the client appropriately.
4. Prepare the client.
   - Place the client in a dorsal recumbent or semi-Fowler's position.
   - Measure the client's calf to determine sleeve size: medium (less than 21 in.), large (less than 26 in.), or extra-large (less than 32 in.) (Bartzak, 2018). Depending on the manufacturer, the thigh circumference may be needed to determine the size needed for a thigh-length sleeve.
5. Apply the sequential compression sleeves.
   - Place a sleeve under each leg with the opening at the knee.
   - Wrap the sleeve securely around the leg, securing the Velcro tabs. ❶ Allow two fingers to fit between the leg and the sleeve. **Rationale:** *This amount of space ensures that the sleeve does not impair circulation when inflated.*

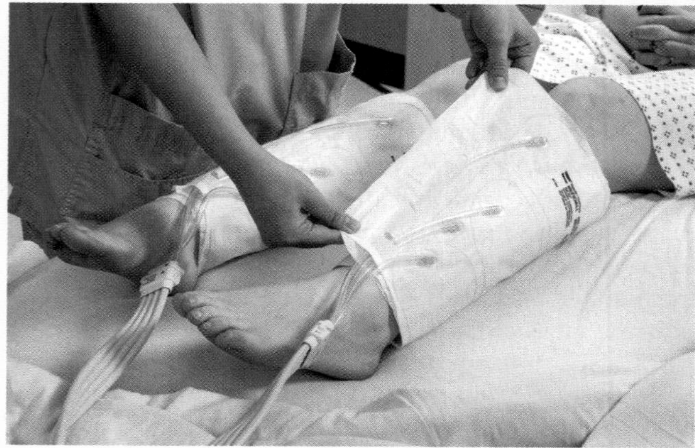

❶ Applying a sequential compression device to the leg.

6. Connect the sleeves to the control unit and adjust the pressure as needed.
   - Connect the tubing to the sleeves and control unit, ensuring that arrows on the plug and the connector are in alignment and that the tubing is not kinked or twisted. **Rationale:** *Improper alignment or obstruction of the tubing by kinks or twists will interfere with operation of the SCD.*
   - Turn on the control unit and adjust the alarms and pressures as needed. The sleeve cooling control and alarm should be on; ankle pressure is usually set at 35 to 55 mmHg. **Rationale:** *It is important to have the sleeve cooling control on for comfort and to reduce the risk of skin irritation from moisture under the sleeve. Proper pressure settings prevent injury to the client. Alarms warn of possible control unit malfunctions.*
7. Document the procedure.
   - Record baseline assessment data and application of the SCD. Note control unit settings.
   - Assess and document skin integrity and neurovascular and peripheral vascular status per agency policy while the SCD is in place. Remove the unit and notify the primary care provider if the client complains of numbness and tingling or leg pain. These may be symptoms of nerve compression.

EVALUATION

- Perform appropriate follow-up assessments, such as peripheral vascular status including pedal pulses, skin color and temperature, skin integrity, and neurovascular status, including movement and sensation.
- Compare to the baseline data, if available.
- Report significant deviations from normal to the primary care provider.

LIFESPAN CONSIDERATIONS Sequential Compression Devices

CHILDREN

- Because young children tend to be more active, the SCD is rarely necessary unless the child is immobile (e.g., comatose).

OLDER ADULTS

- SCD sleeves may become loose as clients move around in bed. Check that the sleeves are secure and properly positioned.

DRUG CAPSULE

Low Molecular Weight Heparin: enoxaparin (Lovenox)

PREVENTION OF DEEP VEIN THROMBOSIS

The low molecular weight heparins are anticoagulants used to prevent deep vein thrombosis after hip, knee, or abdominal surgery. They are also used for clients at risk for thromboembolus secondary to prolonged bedrest due to acute illness. These heparins are given subcutaneously either once a day or every 12 hours. They have a predictable dose response and do not require daily laboratory test monitoring.

NURSING RESPONSIBILITIES

- Administration:
  - Administer deep subcutaneous. Do not give intramuscular.
  - Client should be lying down during administration.
  - Do not expel the air bubble from the prefilled syringe. This avoids loss of the drug.
  - The manufacturer recommends injection into the right or left anterior lateral or posterior lateral aspect of the abdominal wall for best absorption.
  - Alternate between right and left abdomen sites.
  - Insert the entire length of the needle into a skinfold created by the thumb and forefinger; hold the skinfold until the needle is withdrawn.
  - Do not massage the injection site to minimize bruising.
- Do not mix with other injections.
- Lovenox and regular heparin cannot be used interchangeably.
- Assess baseline lab data (e.g., CBC, liver function, coagulation) and monitor periodically.
- Observe for early signs and symptoms of bleeding.

CLIENT AND FAMILY TEACHING

- Review how to administer (see previous section).
- Administer at the same time each day.
- Report any unusual bleeding or bruising.
- Avoid aspirin or nonsteroidal anti-inflammatory drugs (NSAIDs).

Note: Prior to administering any medications, review all aspects with a current drug handbook or other reliable source.

Cardiopulmonary Resuscitation

Cardiopulmonary resuscitation (CPR) is a combination of oral resuscitation (mouth-to-mouth breathing or use of a mask), which supplies oxygen to the lungs, and external cardiac massage (chest compression), which is intended to reestablish cardiac function and blood circulation. CPR is also referred to as *basic life support (BLS).*

The AHA issues revised standards for CPR every 5 years (e.g., 2010, 2015). It covers all aspects of emergency cardiac care and simplifies CPR procedures so more healthcare professionals and lay rescuers might learn and perform them correctly. The complete guidelines are available online.

A cardiac arrest is the cessation of cardiac function; the heart stops beating. Often a cardiac arrest is unexpected and sudden. When it occurs, the heart no longer pumps blood to any of the organs of the body. Breathing then stops, and the individual becomes unconscious and limp. Within 20 to 40 seconds of a cardiac arrest, the victim is clinically dead. After 4 to 6 minutes, the lack of oxygen supply to the brain causes permanent and extensive damage.

The three cardinal signs of a cardiac arrest are apnea, absence of a carotid or femoral pulse, and dilated pupils. The individual's skin appears pale or grayish and feels cool. Cyanosis is evident when respiratory function fails before heart failure.

A respiratory arrest (pulmonary arrest) is the cessation of breathing. It often occurs because of a blocked airway, but it can occur following a cardiac arrest and for other reasons. A respiratory arrest may occur abruptly or be preceded by short, shallow breathing that becomes increasingly labored.

It is vital that all nurses be trained to perform CPR so resuscitation measures can be initiated immediately when a cardiac or respiratory arrest occurs. Nurses also can be instrumental in increasing community awareness of the need for CPR training and ensuring its availability.

Each healthcare facility has policies and procedures for announcing cardiac or respiratory arrest and initiating interventions, as well as a name by which this emergency is referred. Such emergencies are often referred to as a "code." There may be a button at the head of each bed for calling a code, an extension dialed on the phone, or a special phone used to announce the emergency. It is critical that each member of the client care team know the procedure for announcing this emergency. Calling the code summons the code team to the location of the emergency. The code team is made up of specially trained staff who can handle the emergency. Individuals are needed to perform rescue breathing, deliver chest compressions, administer medications, and make a record of the code activities. One staff member must be designated as the code leader—the individual who directs the activities of the other team members.

Some clients have requested via an advance directive that, should they arrest, they not be resuscitated. It is every individual's right to make an advance directive of his or her wishes, and a client's code status should always be documented, per agency policy, in the medical record (e.g., do not resuscitate [DNR]). Under most circumstances, if there is no DNR order in the record, all clients who arrest will have resuscitation efforts begun. *Both legally and ethically, there is no such thing as a "partial code," "slow code," or "mini code."*

Throughout any emergency situation, the nurse must remember the individual behind all of the technology. There is a client with spiritual and emotional needs who requires a personal connection. Holding a hand, making eye contact, talking directly to them—brief, seemingly small things make a huge difference to clients. To humanize healthcare is always a goal. Nursing *therapeutic presence* is the key. This should be extended to family members as well.

Evaluating

Using the overall goals identified in the planning stage, the nurse collects data to evaluate the effectiveness of interventions.

If desired outcomes are not achieved, the nurse, client, and support people if appropriate need to explore the reasons before modifying the care plan. For example, if the outcome "cardiac pump effectiveness" is not achieved, questions to be considered might include the following:

- Have other outcome measures for the goal of maintaining adequate cardiac output been met?
- Are prescribed medications being administered or taken as ordered?
- Are any additional factors placing stress on the heart?
- Is there a balance between factors that affect cardiac output, such as preload and afterload?
- Are there signs of fluid overload such as weight gain?

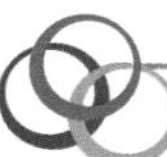

Critical Thinking Checkpoint

Mrs. Gloria Peterson reports that she is having increasing difficulty because she experiences severe pain in her calf muscles after walking for more than a city block. The pain subsides if she rests for a few minutes, but returns with activity. Her feet are cool and pale; pedal and posterior tibial pulses are not palpable, and femoral pulses are difficult to palpate. She lives in a downtown apartment and uses public transportation to travel across town to visit her husband's grave weekly.

1. What are the circulatory causes of her leg pain? Which risk factors would you expect to find in her history to support this conclusion?
2. Name two nursing diagnoses appropriate for Mrs. Peterson. Which would have the highest priority and why?
3. The primary care provider suggests that Mrs. Peterson cease her visits to the cemetery since she has to walk a long way there to reach the grave site. Would you agree with this plan? Why or why not? What considerations or viewpoints influence your choice?
4. Mrs. Peterson says that she wears antiemboli stockings because her friend told her they help the circulation in her legs. How would you respond to this information?

Answers to Critical Thinking Checkpoint questions are available on the faculty resources site. Please consult with your instructor.

Chapter 50 Review

CHAPTER HIGHLIGHTS

- The cardiovascular system transports gases in the blood to and from the tissues and facilitates the diffusion of gases between the capillaries and body tissues.
- The heart and the blood vessels make up the cardiovascular system. Together with blood, it is the major system for transporting oxygen and nutrients to the cells and removing wastes for disposal.
- The right side of the heart receives deoxygenated blood from the body and pumps it to the lungs via the pulmonary arteries; the left side receives oxygenated blood from the lungs and pumps it out to the body via the aorta.
- Coronary arteries supply oxygen and nutrients to the heart muscle.
- The cardiac cycle is made up of systolic and diastolic periods.
- The cardiac conduction system controls the electrical activity of the heart and the cardiac cycle: systole, contraction of the heart muscle and ejection of blood, and diastole, the relaxation period during which the heart fills with blood.
- Cardiac output depends on stroke volume, or the amount of blood ejected during systole, and heart rate.
- Systemic blood vessels carry blood to the tissues through a system of arteries, arterioles, and capillaries and return it to the heart through the venules, veins, and the venae cavae.
- Blood pressure rises gradually from birth to reach the adult range during adolescence.
- Atherosclerosis causes fatty plaque to develop within arteries.
- Decreased cardiac output, impaired tissue perfusion, and disorders affecting the blood are the major cardiovascular problems that affect oxygenation.
- Cardiac output may fall with a myocardial infarction (MI), heart failure, dysrhythmias, and structural alterations of the heart (e.g., valve deformities).
- The most common cause of impaired blood flow to organs and tissues is atherosclerosis; this can lead to tissue ischemia and pain.
- Cardiac monitoring is used for continuous observation of the heart rate and rhythm.
- Nursing interventions to promote circulation include using sequential compression devices to promote venous return from the legs, which prevents venous stasis.
- Cardiopulmonary resuscitation (CPR) is used during cardiopulmonary arrest. Each nurse needs to be aware of the hospital's policies and procedures regarding emergencies.

TEST YOUR KNOWLEDGE

1. A post-myocardial infarction client asks the nurse about return to exercise. What information should the nurse give this client?
   1. It is better to exercise when it is cold.
   2. Environmental temperatures have little impact on cardiac function.
   3. Avoid exercise when the weather is hot or cold.
   4. Hot temperatures increase peripheral blood vessel contraction.

2. The client's electrocardiogram (ECG) monitor reflects normal electrical activity through the heart's conduction system. The nurse knows that the electrical impulse travels in which sequence?
   1. Atrioventricular node
   2. Bundle branches
   3. Sinoatrial node
   4. Bundle of His
   5. Purkinje fibers

   Place the numbers in the correct sequence: ___________

3. Which would most likely be included in the evaluation of the client goal of "Demonstrate adequate tissue perfusion"?
   1. Symmetrical chest expansion
   2. Use of pursed-lip breathing
   3. Brisk capillary refill
   4. Activity intolerance

4. A client has complaints of being tired, listless, and unable to tolerate activity at usual levels. Which laboratory value would the nurse review first while assessing this complaint?
   1. Blood urea nitrogen
   2. Hemoglobin and hematocrit
   3. Blood sugar
   4. Serum potassium

5. A client has a heart rate of 170 beats per minute. For what will the nurse assess next in this client?
   1. Increased cardiac output
   2. Increased preload
   3. Decreased afterload
   4. Decreased cardiac output

6. The nurse is assigned to three clients with the following diagnoses: myocardial infarction (MI), heart failure (HF), and anemia. In planning for their nursing care, the nurse knows that all three clients will have which sign or symptom?
   1. Pain
   2. Distended neck veins
   3. Shortness of breath
   4. Nausea

7. Which set of assessment data best validates that the nurse should initiate cardiopulmonary resuscitation on a comatose client?
   1. Cool, pale skin; unconsciousness; absence of radial pulse
   2. Cyanosis, slow pulse, dilated pupils
   3. Absent pulses, flushed skin, pinpoint pupils
   4. Apnea, absence of carotid or femoral pulses, dilated pupils

8. Which diagnoses would be most appropriate for clients with cardiovascular disease? Select all that apply.
   1. Impaired tissue perfusion
   2. Confusion
   3. Inadequate cardiac output
   4. Impaired sleep
   5. Inadequate physical energy for activities

9. The surgeon ordered sequential compression devices (SCDs) to be applied postoperatively. The client asks why the SCDs are needed. Which is the best response by the nurse when teaching the client about the purpose of SCDs?
   1. They promote arterial circulation.
   2. They promote venous return from the legs.
   3. They decrease afterload.
   4. They decrease postoperative pain.

10. A client with severe mitral stenosis is having surgery tomorrow. While teaching the client, the nurse shows the client a diagram of the heart. Identify with an "X" which valve the client will have replaced.

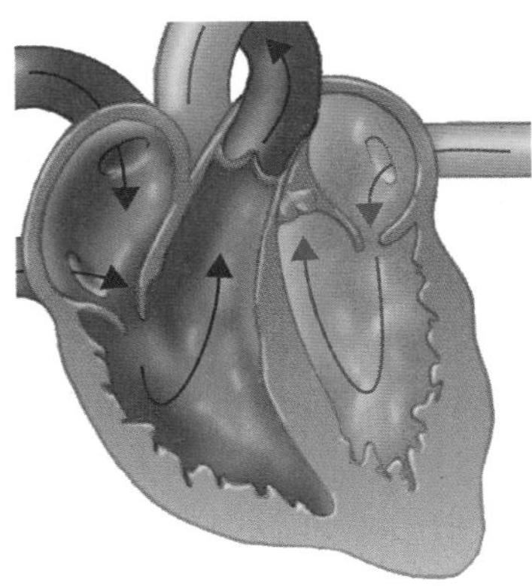

See Answers to Test Your Knowledge in Appendix A.

READINGS AND REFERENCES

Suggested Readings

Bowers, M. T. (2019). Chronic heart failure: Impact of the current guidelines. *The Journal for Nurse Practitioners*, *15*(1), 125–131. doi:10.1016/j.nurpra.2018.10.016

This article provides the recommendations from the updated 2017 guideline for the management of chronic heart failure.

Campo, D. L. (2016). Recognizing myocardial infarction in women: A case study. *American Journal of Nursing*, *116*(9), 46–49. doi:10.1097/01.NAJ.0000494694.48122.46

The author discusses the signs and symptoms of MI in women and highlights how failure to recognize them may lead to misdiagnosis and even death.

Shoulders, B., & Powell, L. (2019). Reaching for goal: Incorporating the latest hypertension guidelines into practice. *The Journal for Nurse Practitioners*, *15*(1), 102–109. doi:10.1016/j.nurpra.2018.09.011

The purpose of this article is to present the key highlights in the updated hypertension guidelines and how nurses can incorporate the best available evidence when providing care to clients with hypertension.

Related Research

Reeder, M., Childs, D. B., Gibson, I. J., Williams, C., & Williams, J. (2017). Cardiovascular disease in African-American women: An assessment of awareness. *ABNF Journal*, *28*(3), 76–80.

Wade, R., Paton, F., & Woolacott, N. (2017). Systematic review of patient preference and adherence to the correct use of graduated compression stockings to prevent deep vein thrombosis in surgical patients. *Journal of Advanced Nursing*, *73*(2), 336–348. doi:10.1111/jan.13148

References

American Heart Association. (2016). *Understand your risks to prevent a heart attack*. Retrieved from http://www.heart.org/HEARTORG/Conditions/HeartAttack/UnderstandYourRiskstoPreventaHeartAttack/Understand-Your-Risks-to-Prevent-a-Heart-Attack_UCM_002040_Article.jsp#.WTXUpsbMxn4

Andrews, L. (2016). Different types of intermittent pneumatic compression devices for preventing venous thromboembolism in patients after total hip replacement. *Orthopaedic Nursing*, *35*, 424–425. doi:10.1097/NOR.0000000000000302

Association of Women's Health, Obstetric and Neonatal Nurses. (2018). Women's cardiovascular health. *Journal of Obstetric, Gynecologic, & Neonatal Nursing*, *47*(5), 722–723. doi:10.1016/j.jogn.2018.07.002

Ball, J., Bindler, R., Cowen, K., & Shaw, M. (2017). *Principles of pediatric nursing* (7th ed.). New York, NY: Pearson.

Banman, L., & Sawatzky, J. V. (2017). The role of self-efficacy in cardiovascular disease prevention in women. *Canadian Journal of Cardiovascular Nursing*, *27*(3), 11–19.

Bartzak, P. J. (2018). A renewed respect for sequential compression devices. *Med-Surg Matters*, *27*(3), 1–3.

Centers for Disease Control and Prevention. (2017). *Women and heart disease fact sheet*. Retrieved from https://www.cdc.gov/dhdsp/data_statistics/fact_sheets/fs_women_heart.htm

Chrysant, S. G., & Chrysant, G. S. (2018). The current status of homocysteine as a risk factor for cardiovascular disease: A mini review. *Expert Review of Cardiovascular Therapy*, *16*(8), 559–565. doi:10.1080/14779072.2018.1497974

Crumley, C. E. (2018). Venous thromboembolism: Very troubling events. *American Nurse Today*, *13*(8), 16–20.

Dunn, N., & Ramos, R. (2017). Preventing venous thromboembolism: The role of nursing with intermittent pneumatic compression. *American Journal of Critical Care*, *26*(2), 164–167. doi:10.4037/ajcc2017504

Ferdinand, K. C. (2016). Cardiovascular risk reduction in African Americans: Current concepts and controversies. *Global Cardiology Science & Practice*, *2*, 1–13. doi:10.21542/gcsp.2016.2

Harvard Health Publishing. (2018). *Facts about alcohol and heart health*. Retrieved from https://www.health.harvard.edu/heart-health/facts-about-alcohol-and-heart-health

Kalman, M., & Wells, M. (2018). Women and cardiovascular disease. *American Nurse Today*, *13*(6), 22–26.

Office of Disease Prevention and Health Promotion. (2019a). *Diabetes*. Retrieved from https://www.healthypeople.gov/node/3514/objectives

Office of Disease Prevention and Health Promotion. (2019b). *Heart disease and stroke data details*. Retrieved from https://www.healthypeople.gov/node/3516/data-details

Office of Disease Prevention and Health Promotion. (2019c). *Nutrition and weight status*. Retrieved from https://www.healthypeople.gov/2020/topics-objectives/topic/nutrition-and-weight-status/objectives

Office of Disease Prevention and Health Promotion. (2019d). *Physical activity*. Retrieved from https://www.healthypeople.gov/2020/topics-objectives/topic/physical-activity/objectives

Office of Disease Prevention and Health Promotion. (2019e). *Tobacco use*. Retrieved from https://www.healthypeople.gov/2020/topics-objectives/topic/tobacco-use/objectives

Park, C. W. (2016). *Ankle-brachial index measurement*. Retrieved from http://emedicine.medscape.com/article/1839449-overview#a3

Rice, J. (2018). *Medical terminology for health care professionals* (9th ed.). Hoboken, NJ: Pearson.

Rice, J. (2018). *Medical terminology for health care professionals* (9th ed.). Hoboken, NJ: Pearson.

Roberts, S. H., & Lawrence, S. M. (2017). Venous thromboembolism: Updated management guidelines. *American Journal of Nursing*, *117*(5), 38–47. doi:10.1097/01.NAJ.0000516249.54064.53

Stanford Medicine. (n.d.). *Measuring and understanding the ankle brachial index (ABI)*. Retrieved from https://stanfordmedicine25.stanford.edu/the25/ankle.html

Stöppler, M. C. (2018). *C-reactive protein CRP test, ranges, symptoms, and treatment*. Retrieved from http://www.medicinenet.com/c-reactive_protein_test_crp/page2.htm

Turley, S. (2017). *Medical language* (4th ed.). New York, NY: Pearson.

Selected Bibliography

American Heart Association. (2016). *Managing blood pressure with a heart-healthy diet*. Retrieved from http://www.heart.org/HEARTORG/Conditions/HighBloodPressure/MakeChangesThatMatter/Managing-Blood-Pressure-with-a-Heart-Healthy-Diet_UCM_301879_Article.jsp#.WTRSM8bMw5s

Compression stockings. (2017). *Mayo Clinic Health Letter*, *35*(2), 7.

Corbett, K., Dugan, A., Vitale, C., & Gravel, T. (2019). Long-term effects of opioids on the cardiovascular system: Examine the evidence. *Nursing*, *49*(4), 47–49. doi:10.1097/01.NURSE.0000554247.12754.28

Gilmore, L. (2018). The ethics of slow codes and the implications for nurses. *American Journal of Nursing*, *118*(12), 11.

Kreutzer, L., Minami, C., & Yang, A. (2016). Preventing venous thromboembolism after surgery. *JAMA*, *315*(19), 2136. doi:10.1001/jama.2016.1457

Pattison, K. H. (2019). Medications for heart failure management: What nurses need to know. *American Nurse Today*, *14*(2), 20–23.

Simmons, K. (2017). Sequential compression devices in the pediatric patient population. *AORN Journal*, *106*(2), 13–14. doi:10.1016/S0001-2092(17)30658-0

Thomas, N., & Bennett, N. (2017). Introducing a device to assist in the application of anti-embolism stockings. *British Journal of Nursing*, *26*(9), 510–513. doi:10.12968/bjon.2017.26.9.510

Tocco, S., Martin, B., & Stacy, K. M. (2016). Preventing venous thromboembolism in adults. *Critical Care Nurse*, *36*(5), e20–e23. doi:10.4037/ccn2016638

Twibell, R., May, A., & May, P. (2018). When the heart stops: Life-giving updates on cardiac arrest. *American Nurse Today*, *13*(2), 6–10.

Fluid, Electrolyte, and Acid–Base Balance 51

LEARNING OUTCOMES

After completing this chapter, you will be able to:

1. Discuss the function, distribution, composition, movement, and regulation of fluids and electrolytes in the body.
2. Describe the regulation of acid–base balance in the body, including the roles of buffers, the lungs, and the kidneys.
3. Identify factors affecting normal body fluid, electrolyte, and acid–base balance.
4. Discuss risk factors for, and causes and effects of, fluid, electrolyte, and acid–base imbalances.
5. Collect assessment data related to clients' fluid, electrolyte, and acid–base balances.
6. Identify examples of nursing diagnoses, outcomes, and interventions for clients with altered fluid, electrolyte, or acid–base balance.
7. Teach clients measures to maintain fluid and electrolyte balance.
8. Implement measures to correct imbalances of fluids, electrolytes, acids, and bases, such as enteral or parenteral replacements and blood transfusions.
9. Evaluate the effect of nursing and collaborative interventions on clients' fluid, electrolyte, or acid–base balance.
10. Verbalize the steps used in:
    a. Inserting a short peripheral catheter
    b. Monitoring an intravenous infusion
    c. Changing an intravenous container and tubing
    d. Discontinuing an intravenous infusion and removing a short peripheral catheter
    e. Changing a short peripheral catheter access to an intermittent infusion device
    f. Initiating, maintaining, and terminating a blood transfusion using a Y-set.
11. Recognize when it is appropriate to assign aspects of fluid, electrolyte, and acid–base balance to assistive personnel.
12. Demonstrate appropriate documentation and reporting of fluid, electrolyte, and acid–base balance activities.

KEY TERMS

acid, *1376*
acidosis, *1377*
active transport, *1372*
acute hemolytic transfusion reaction (AHTR), *1422*
agglutinins, *1420*
agglutinogens, *1420*
alkalosis, *1377*
anions, *1370*
antibodies, *1420*
antigens, *1420*
arterial blood gases (ABGs), *1392*
bases, *1376*
buffers, *1377*
cations, *1370*
central vascular access device (CVAD), *1400*
colloid osmotic pressure, *1371*
colloids, *1371*
compensation, *1385*
crystalloids, *1371*
dehydration, *1380*
diffusion, *1372*
drop factor, *1410*
electrolytes, *1370*
extracellular fluid (ECF), *1370*
extravasation, *1414*
filtration, *1372*
filtration pressure, *1372*
fluid volume deficit (FVD), *1379*
fluid volume excess (FVE), *1380*
hematocrit (Hct), *1392*
homeostasis, *1369*
hydrostatic pressure, *1372*
hypercalcemia, *1384*
hyperchloremia, *1385*
hyperkalemia, *1384*
hypermagnesemia, *1385*
hypernatremia, *1381*
hyperphosphatemia, *1385*
hypertonic, *1371*
hypervolemia, *1380*
hypocalcemia, *1384*
hypochloremia, *1385*
hypokalemia, *1381*
hypomagnesemia, *1384*
hyponatremia, *1381*
hypophosphatemia, *1385*
hypotonic, *1371*
hypovolemia, *1379*
infiltration, *1409*
insensible fluid loss, *1373*
interstitial fluid, *1370*
intracellular fluid (ICF), *1370*
intravascular fluid, *1370*
ions, *1370*
isotonic, *1371*
metabolic acidosis, *1386*
metabolic alkalosis, *1386*
milliequivalent, *1370*
oncotic pressure, *1371*
osmolality, *1371*
osmosis, *1372*
osmotic pressure, *1371*
overhydration, *1380*
peripherally inserted central venous catheter (PICC), *1400*
pH, *1376*
pitting edema, *1380*
plasma, *1370*
renin-angiotensin-aldosterone system, *1373*
respiratory acidosis, *1385*
respiratory alkalosis, *1386*
selectively permeable, *1371*
solutes, *1371*
solvent, *1371*
specific gravity, *1392*
third space syndrome, *1379*
vesicant, *1414*
volume expanders, *1398*

Introduction

In good health, a delicate balance of fluids, electrolytes, acids, and bases maintains the body. This balance, or **homeostasis**, depends on multiple physiologic processes that regulate fluid intake and output, as well as the movement of water and the substances dissolved in it between body compartments.

Almost every illness has the potential to threaten this balance. Even in daily living, factors such as excessive temperatures or vigorous activity can affect homeostasis if adequate water and salt intake are not maintained. Therapeutic measures, such as the use of diuretics or nasogastric suction, can also disturb the body's homeostasis unless water and electrolytes are replaced.

Body Fluids and Electrolytes

The proportion of the human body composed of fluid is surprisingly large. Approximately 60% of the average healthy adult's weight is water, the primary body fluid. In good health this volume remains relatively constant, and an individual's weight varies by less than 0.2 kg (0.5 lb) in 24 hours, regardless of the amount of fluid ingested.

Age, sex, and body fat affect total body water. Infants have the highest proportion of water, accounting for 70% to 80% of their body weight. The proportion of body water decreases with age. In adults older than 60 years of age, it represents only about 50% of total body weight. Women generally have a lower percentage of body water than men. In both women and older adults, this is due to lower levels of muscle mass and a greater percentage of fat tissue. Fat tissue is essentially free of water, whereas lean tissue contains a significant amount of water. Therefore, water makes up a greater percentage of a lean individual's body weight than of an individual who is obese.

Distribution of Body Fluids

The body's fluid is divided into two major compartments, intracellular and extracellular. **Intracellular fluid (ICF)** is found within the cells of the body. It constitutes approximately two-thirds of the total body fluid in adults. **Extracellular fluid (ECF)** is found outside the cells and accounts for about one-third of total body fluid. ECF is further subdivided into compartments. The two main compartments of ECF are intravascular and interstitial. **Intravascular fluid**, or **plasma**, accounts for approximately 20% of ECF and is found within the vascular system. **Interstitial fluid**, accounting for approximately 75% of ECF, surrounds the cells (Figure 51.1 ■).

Intracellular fluid is vital to normal cell functioning. It contains solutes such as oxygen, electrolytes, and glucose, and it provides a medium in which metabolic processes of the cell take place.

Composition of Body Fluid

Extracellular and intracellular fluids contain oxygen from the lungs, dissolved nutrients from the gastrointestinal tract, excretory products of metabolism such as carbon dioxide, and charged particles called **ions**.

Many salts dissociate in water; that is, they break up into electrically charged ions. The salt called sodium chloride breaks up into one ion of sodium (Na^+) and one ion of chloride (Cl^-). These charged particles are called **electrolytes** because they are capable of conducting electricity. The number of ions that carry a positive charge,

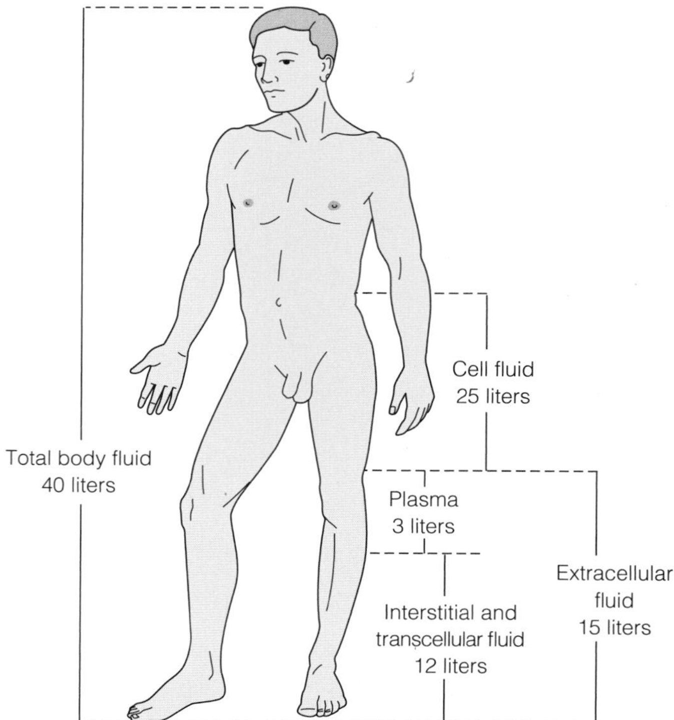

Figure 51.1 ■ Total body fluid represents 40 L in an adult male weighing 70 kg (154 lb).

called **cations**, and ions that carry a negative charge, called **anions**, should be equal.

Electrolytes generally are measured in milliequivalents per liter (mEq/L) or milligrams per 100 milliliters (mg/100 mL). The term **milliequivalent** refers to the chemical combining power of the ion, or the capacity of cations to combine with anions to form molecules, whereas the term *milligram* refers to the weight of the ion. Therefore, 1 mEq of any anion equals 1 mEq of any cation in terms of their capacity to combine into molecules. For example, sodium and chloride combine equally, so 1 mEq of Na^+ equals 1 mEq of Cl^-; however, a molecule of sodium is not equal in weight to a molecule of chloride.

Clinically, the milliequivalent system is most often used. However, nurses need to be aware that different systems of measurement may be found when interpreting laboratory results. For example, calcium levels frequently are reported in milligrams per deciliter (1 dL = 100 mL) instead of milliequivalents per liter.

The composition of fluids varies from one body compartment to another. In ECF, the principal electrolytes are sodium, chloride, and bicarbonate. Other electrolytes such as potassium, calcium, and magnesium are present, but in much smaller quantities. Plasma and interstitial fluid, the two primary components of ECF, contain essentially the same electrolytes and solutes, with the exception of protein. Plasma is a protein-rich fluid, containing large amounts of albumin, but interstitial fluid contains little or no protein.

The composition of ICF differs significantly from that of ECF. Potassium and magnesium are the primary cations present in ICF, and phosphate and sulfate are the major anions. As in ECF, other electrolytes are present within the cell, but in much smaller concentrations (Figure 51.2 ■).

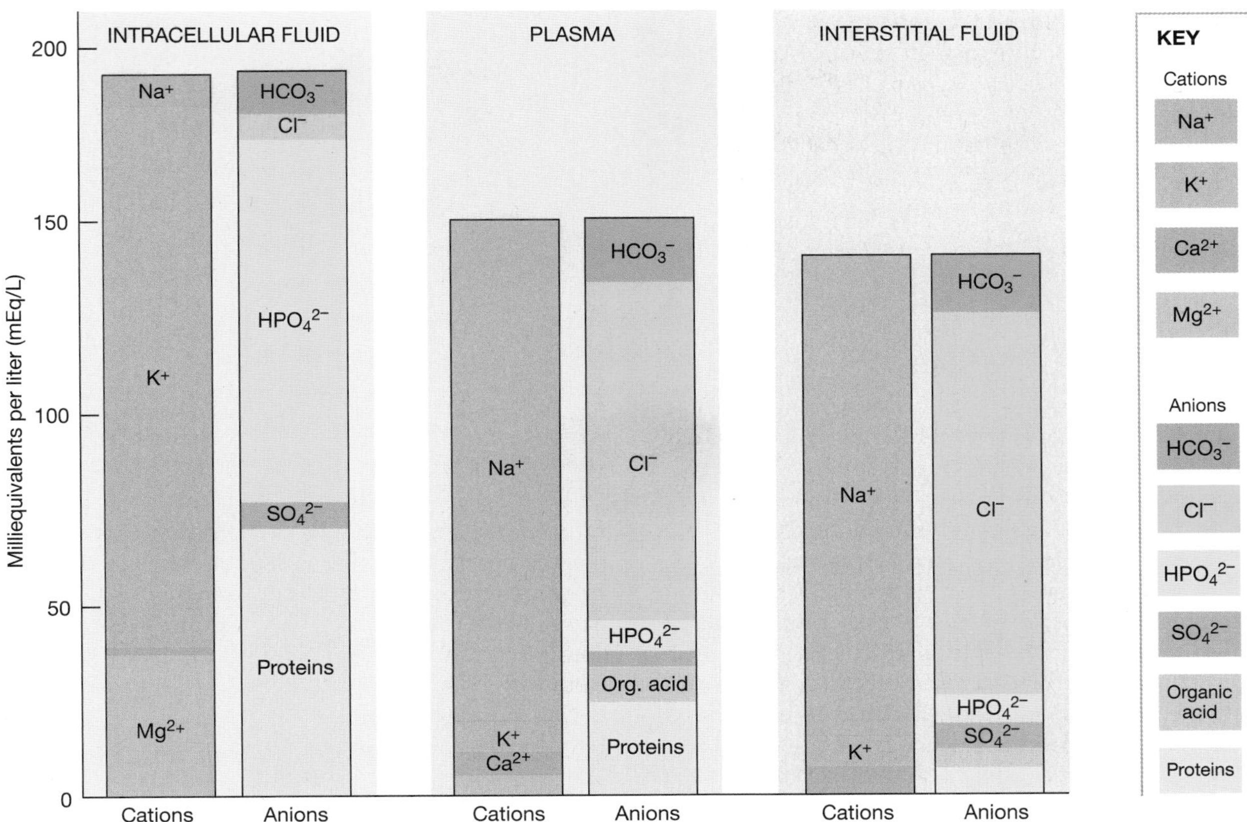

Figure 51.2 ■ Electrolyte composition (cations and anions) of body fluid compartments.

F. H. MARTINI , J. L. NATH, and E. F. BARTHOLOMEW, FUNDAMENTALS OF ANATOMY & PHYSIOLOGY, 11th Ed., © 2018. Reprinted and Electronically reproduced by permission of Pearson Education, Inc., New York, NY.

Other body fluids such as gastric and intestinal secretions also contain electrolytes. This is of particular concern when these fluids are lost from the body (for example, in severe vomiting or diarrhea, or when gastric suction removes gastric secretions). Fluid and electrolyte imbalances can result from excessive losses through these routes.

Movement of Body Fluids and Electrolytes

The body fluid compartments are separated from one another by cell membranes and the capillary membrane. Although these membranes are completely permeable to water, they are considered to be **selectively permeable** to solutes, because substances other than water move across them with varying degrees of ease. Small particles such as ions, oxygen, and carbon dioxide move easily across these membranes, but larger molecules such as glucose and proteins have more difficulty moving between fluid compartments.

Solutes are substances dissolved in a liquid. Solutes may be **crystalloids** (salts that dissolve readily into true solutions) or **colloids** (substances such as large protein molecules that do not readily dissolve into true solutions). A **solvent** is the component of a solution that can dissolve a solute. In the body, water is the solvent; the solutes include electrolytes, gases such as oxygen and carbon dioxide, glucose, urea, amino acids, and proteins.

The concentration of solutes in body fluids is usually expressed as the **osmolality**. Osmolality is determined by the total solute concentration within a fluid compartment and is measured as parts of solute per kilogram of water.

Osmolality is reported as milliosmoles per kilogram (mOsm/kg). Sodium is by far the greatest determinant of the osmolality of plasma, or serum osmolality. The term *tonicity* may also be used to refer to the osmolality of one solution in relation to another solution. Solutions may be termed isotonic, hypertonic, or hypotonic. In relation to body fluids, an **isotonic** solution has the same osmolality as ECF. Normal saline, 0.9% sodium chloride, is an example of an isotonic solution. **Hypertonic** solutions, such as 3% sodium chloride, have a higher osmolality than ECF. **Hypotonic** solutions, such as 0.45% sodium chloride, have a lower osmolality than ECF. See Table 51.11 later in this chapter for additional information about intravenous (IV) solutions.

Osmotic pressure is the power of a solution to pull water across a semipermeable membrane. When two solutions of different concentrations are separated by a semipermeable membrane, the solution with the higher solute concentration exerts a higher osmotic pressure, pulling water across the membrane to equalize the concentrations of the solutions. In the body, plasma proteins also exert osmotic pressure called **colloid osmotic pressure** or **oncotic pressure**, holding water in plasma, and when necessary pulling water from the interstitial space into the vascular compartment. This is an important mechanism for maintaining vascular volume.

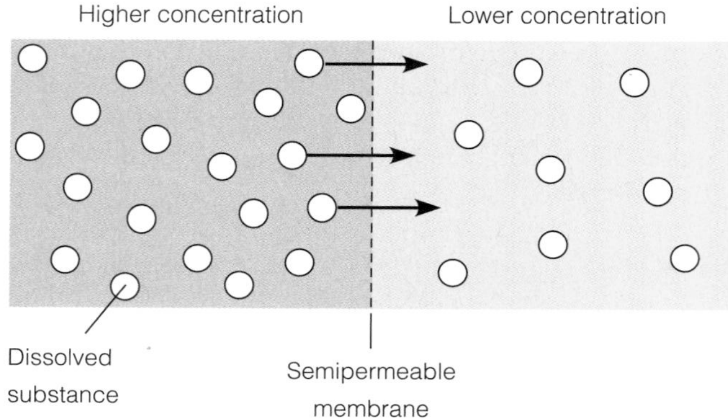

Figure 51.3 ■ Diffusion: the movement of molecules through a semipermeable membrane from an area of higher concentration to an area of lower concentration.

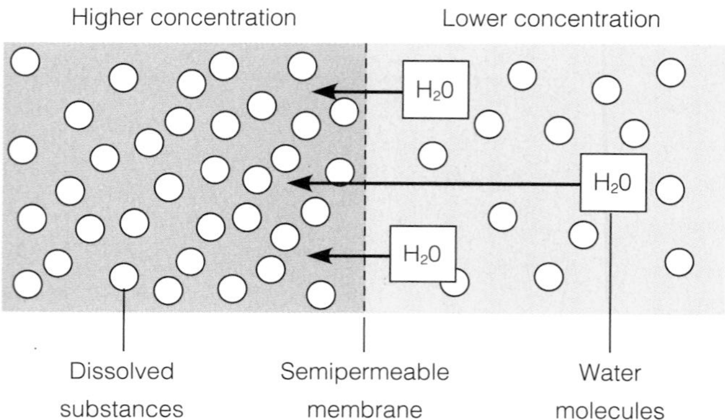

Figure 51.4 ■ Osmosis: the movement of water molecules from a less concentrated area to a more concentrated area in an attempt to equalize the concentration of solutions on two sides of a membrane.

The methods by which water and solutes move in the body are called diffusion, osmosis, filtration, and active transport. **Diffusion** occurs when two solutes of different concentrations are separated by a semipermeable membrane (Figure 51.3 ■). The rate of diffusion of a solute varies according to the size of the molecules, the concentration of the solution, and the temperature of the solution. **Osmosis** is a specific kind of diffusion in which *water* moves across cell membranes, from the less concentrated solution (the solution with less solute and more water) to the more concentrated solution (the solution with more solute and less water) (Figure 51.4 ■). In other words, water moves toward the higher concentration of solute in an attempt to equalize the concentrations of both water and solute.

Filtration is a process whereby fluid and solutes move together across a membrane from an area of higher pressure to an area of lower pressure. **Filtration pressure** is the pressure that results in the movement of the fluid and solutes out of a compartment. **Hydrostatic pressure** is the pressure exerted by a fluid within a closed system on the walls of the container in which it is held. The hydrostatic pressure of blood is the force exerted by blood against blood vessel walls. Osmotic pressure opposes and balances the force of hydrostatic pressure, and holds fluid in the vascular compartment to maintain the vascular volume. However, when hydrostatic pressure is greater than osmotic pressure, fluid filters out of the blood vessels. Filtration pressure is the difference between the hydrostatic pressure and the osmotic pressure (Figure 51.5 ■). **Active transport** is the movement of solutes across cell membranes from a less concentrated solution to a more concentrated one. This process differs from diffusion and osmosis, which are passive processes, in that metabolic energy is expended.

Regulating Body Fluids

In a healthy individual, the volumes and chemical composition of the fluid compartments stay within specific and narrow limits. Normally, fluid intake and fluid loss are balanced. Illness can upset this balance so that the body has too little or too much fluid.

Fluid Intake

During periods of normal activity at moderate temperature, the average adult drinks about 1200 to 1500 mL/day, despite the fact that adults need 2500 mL/day for normal functioning. The additional 1000-mL volume is acquired from foods and from the oxidation of these foods during metabolic processes. The water content of food is relatively large, contributing about 1000 mL/day. Water as a by-product of food metabolism accounts for most of the remaining fluid volume required. This quantity is approximately 200 mL/day for the average adult (Table 51.1).

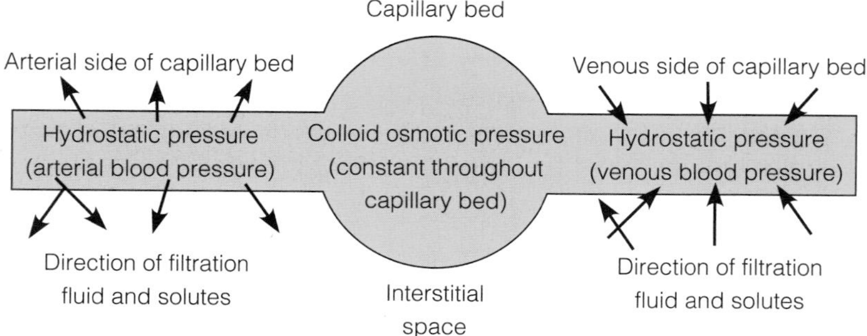

Figure 51.5 ■ Schematic of filtration pressure changes within a capillary bed. On the arterial side, arterial blood pressure exceeds colloid osmotic pressure, so that water and dissolved substances move out of the capillary into the interstitial space. On the venous side, venous blood pressure is less than colloid osmotic pressure, so that water and dissolved substances move into the capillary.

TABLE 51.1 Average Daily Fluid Intake for an Adult

Source	Amount (mL)
Oral fluids	1200–1500
Water in foods	1000
Water as by-product of food metabolism	200
Total	2400–2700

The thirst mechanism is the primary regulator of fluid intake. The thirst center is located in the hypothalamus of the brain. A number of stimuli trigger the thirst center, including the osmotic pressure of body fluids, vascular volume, and angiotensin (a hormone released in response to decreased blood flow to the kidneys), causing the sensation of thirst and the desire to drink fluids.

Thirst is normally relieved immediately after drinking a small amount of fluid, when the ingested fluid distends the upper gastrointestinal tract, but before the fluid is actually absorbed from the gastrointestinal tract. However, this relief is only temporary, and thirst returns in about 15 minutes. The thirst is again temporarily relieved by drinking a small amount of fluid. This mechanism protects the individual from drinking too much, because it takes between 30 minutes and 1 hour for fluid to be absorbed and distributed throughout the body.

Fluid Output

Fluid losses from the body counterbalance the intake of fluid, as shown in Table 51.2. Urine is formed by the kidneys and excreted from the urinary bladder, and is the major route of fluid output. Normal urine output for an adult is 1400 to 1500 mL per 24 hours, or at least 0.5 mL per kilogram per hour.

The chyme that passes from the small intestine into the large intestine contains both water and electrolytes. The volume of chyme entering the large intestine in an adult is normally about 1500 mL/day. Of this amount, all but about 100 mL is reabsorbed in the proximal half of the large intestine. The reabsorbed volume contains primarily water and electrolytes.

Insensible fluid losses occur through the skin and the lungs. They are called insensible because it is usually not noticeable and cannot be measured. Insensible fluid loss through the skin occurs in two ways, diffusion and perspiration. Water loss through the skin is not noticeable but normally accounts for 350 to 400 mL/day. Another type of insensible loss is the water in exhaled air. In an adult, this is normally 350 to 400 mL/day.

TABLE 51.2 Average Daily Fluid Output for an Adult

Route	Amount (mL)
Urine	1400–1500
Insensible losses	
Lungs	350–400
Skin	350–400
Sweat	100
Feces	100–200
Total	2300–2600

Maintaining Homeostasis

The volume and composition of body fluids are regulated through several homeostatic mechanisms. A number of organs and systems contribute to this regulation, including the kidneys, lungs, and the cardiovascular and gastrointestinal systems. Hormones such as antidiuretic hormone, the renin-angiotensin-aldosterone system, and atrial natriuretic factor are also involved, as are mechanisms to monitor and maintain vascular volume.

The kidneys are the primary regulator of body fluids and electrolyte balance. They regulate the volume and osmolality of ECF by regulating water and electrolyte excretion. The kidneys control the reabsorption of water from plasma filtrate and ultimately the amount excreted as urine. Electrolyte balance is maintained by selective retention and excretion by the kidneys. The kidneys also play a significant role in acid–base regulation, excreting hydrogen ion (H^+) and retaining bicarbonate.

Several neuroendocrine control mechanisms help control fluid and electrolyte balance. The antidiuretic hormone (ADH) regulates water excretion from the kidney, is synthesized in the anterior portion of the hypothalamus, and acts on the collecting ducts of the nephrons. When serum osmolality rises, ADH is produced, causing the collecting ducts to become more permeable to water. This increased permeability allows more water to be reabsorbed into the blood. As more water is reabsorbed, urine output falls and serum osmolality decreases because the water dilutes body fluids. Conversely, if serum osmolality decreases, ADH is suppressed, the collecting ducts become less permeable to water, and urine output increases. Excess water is excreted, and serum osmolality returns to normal (Figure 51.6 ■).

Specialized receptors in the kidneys respond to changes in renal perfusion, stimulating the **renin-angiotensin-aldosterone system**. If blood flow or pressure to the kidney decreases, renin is released. Renin causes the conversion of angiotensinogen to angiotensin I, which is then converted to angiotensin II by angiotensin-converting enzyme. Angiotensin II acts directly on the nephrons to promote sodium and water retention. In addition, it stimulates the release of aldosterone from the adrenal cortex. Aldosterone also promotes sodium retention in the distal nephron. The net effect of the renin-angiotensin-aldosterone system is to increase blood volume (and renal perfusion) through sodium and water retention.

The atrial natriuretic factor (ANF) is released from cells in the atrium of the heart in response to excess blood volume and stretching of the atrial walls. Acting on the nephrons, ANF promotes sodium wasting and acts as a

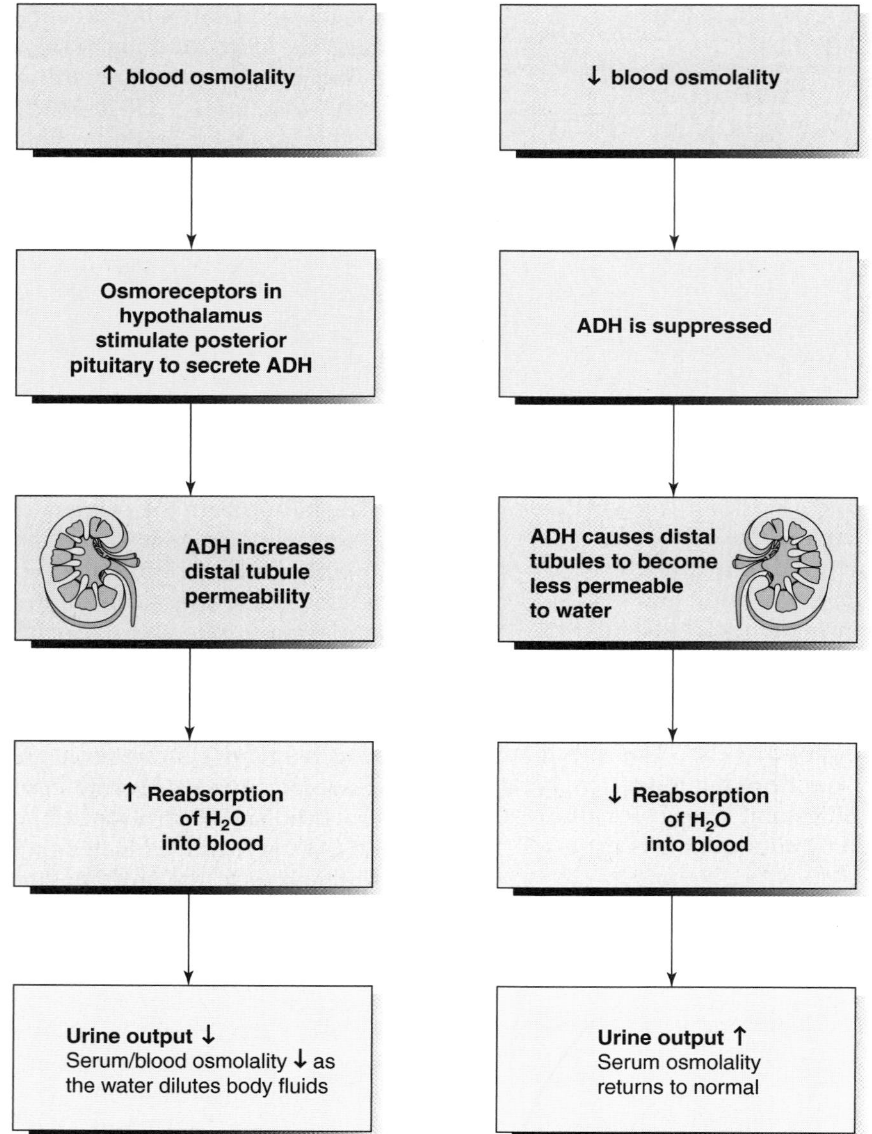

Figure 51.6 ■ Antidiuretic hormone (ADH) regulates water excretion from the kidneys.

potent diuretic, thus decreasing blood volume. ANF also inhibits thirst, reducing fluid intake.

Regulating Electrolytes

Electrolytes, charged ions capable of conducting electricity, are present in all body fluids and fluid compartments. Just as maintaining fluid balance is vital to normal body functioning, so is maintaining electrolyte balance. Although the concentration of specific electrolytes differs between fluid compartments, a balance of cations (positively charged ions) and anions (negatively charged ions) always exists. Electrolytes are important for:

- Maintaining fluid balance
- Contributing to acid–base regulation
- Facilitating enzyme reactions
- Transmitting neuromuscular reactions.

Most electrolytes enter the body through dietary intake and are excreted in the urine. Some electrolytes, such as sodium chloride and potassium, are not stored by the body and must be consumed daily to maintain normal levels. Other electrolytes, such as calcium, are stored in the body; when serum levels drop, ions can shift out of storage into the blood to maintain adequate serum levels for normal functioning, at least in the short term. The regulatory mechanisms and functions of the major electrolytes are summarized in Table 51.3.

Sodium

Sodium (Na^+) is the most abundant cation in ECF and a major contributor to serum osmolality. Normal serum sodium levels are 135 to 145 mEq/L. Sodium functions largely in controlling and regulating water balance. Sodium is found in many foods (Table 51.4).

TABLE 51.3 Regulation and Functions of Electrolytes

Electrolyte	Regulation	Function
Sodium (Na^+)	• Renal reabsorption or excretion • Aldosterone increases Na^+ reabsorption in collecting duct of nephrons	• Regulating ECF volume and distribution • Maintaining blood volume • Transmitting nerve impulses and contracting muscles
Potassium (K^+)	• Renal excretion • Aldosterone increases K^+ excretion • Movement into and out of cells • Insulin helps move K^+ into cells; tissue damage and acidosis shift K^+ out of cells into ECF	• Maintaining ICF osmolality • Transmitting nerve and other electrical impulses • Regulating cardiac impulse transmission and muscle contraction • Skeletal and smooth muscle function • Regulating acid–base balance
Calcium (Ca^{2+})	• Redistribution between bones and ECF • Parathyroid hormone and calcitriol increase serum Ca^{2+} levels; calcitonin decreases serum levels	• Forming bones and teeth • Transmitting nerve impulses • Regulating muscle contractions • Maintaining cardiac pacemaker (automaticity) • Blood clotting
Magnesium (Mg^{2+})	• Conservation and excretion by kidneys • Intestinal absorption increased by vitamin D and parathyroid hormone	• Intracellular metabolism • Operating sodium–potassium pump • Relaxing muscle contractions • Transmitting nerve impulses • Regulating cardiac function
Chloride (Cl^-)	• Excreted and reabsorbed along with sodium in the kidneys • Aldosterone increases chloride reabsorption with sodium	• HCl production • Regulating ECF balance and vascular volume • Regulating acid–base balance • Buffer in oxygen–carbon dioxide exchange in RBCs
Phosphate (PO_4^{3-})	• Excretion and reabsorption along with sodium in the kidneys • Parathyroid hormone decreases serum levels by increasing renal excretion • Reciprocal relationship with calcium: increasing serum calcium decreases phosphate levels; decreasing serum calcium increases phosphate	• Forming bones and teeth • Metabolizing carbohydrate, protein, and fat • Cellular metabolism; producing ATP and DNA • Muscle, nerve, and RBC function • Regulating acid–base balance • Regulating calcium levels
Bicarbonate (HCO_3^-)	• Excretion and reabsorption by the kidneys • Regeneration by kidneys	• Major body buffer involved in acid–base regulation

TABLE 51.4 Electrolyte-Rich Foods

Electrolyte	Vegetables	Fruits	Meats and Fish	Beverages	Other
Sodium	Dried, canned, pickled or brined vegetables, seaweeds	Dried, canned, pickled, or brined	Bacon, cold cuts, cured meats	Chocolate milk	Canned soups, processed cheese, cereal, table salt
Potassium	Raw carrots, baked potatoes, spinach, raw tomatoes	Avocados, bananas, dried fruits, apricots, cantaloupe, oranges	Beef, cod, pork, veal	Milk, orange juice, coconut water	Nuts
Calcium	Kale, broccoli, watercress, bok choy, okra	Oranges, dried apricots, dates, rhubarb, kiwi	Sardines, salmon	Milk	Yogurt, kefir, almonds, tofu
Magnesium	Dark leafy greens, beans and lentils	Avocados, bananas, dried fruits	Mackerel, tuna, turbot	Coffee, chocolate syrup prepared with milk	Nuts, seeds, whole grains, dark chocolate
Phosphate	Legumes	Spinach, butternut squash, okra	Fish, beef, turkey, chicken	Milk	Nuts, yogurt, whole grains

Potassium

Potassium (K^+) is the major cation in ICF, with only a small amount found in the ECF. ICF levels of potassium are usually 125 to 140 mEq/L, while normal serum potassium levels are 3.5 to 5.0 mEq/L. The ratio of intracellular to extracellular potassium must be maintained for neuromuscular response to stimuli. Potassium is a vital electrolyte for skeletal, cardiac, and smooth muscle activity. It is also involved in maintaining acid–base balance, and it contributes to intracellular enzyme reactions. Potassium must be ingested daily because the body cannot conserve it. See Table 51.4 for foods containing potassium.

Calcium

The vast majority (99%) of calcium (Ca^{2+}) in the body is stored in the skeletal system, with a relatively small amount in extracellular fluid. Although the calcium outside the bones and teeth amounts to only about 1% of the total calcium in the body, it is vital in regulating neuromuscular function, including muscle contraction and relaxation, as well as cardiac function. ECF calcium is regulated by a complex interaction of parathyroid hormone, calcitonin (a hormone produced by the thyroid), and calcitriol (a metabolite of vitamin D). When calcium levels in the ECF fall, parathyroid hormone and calcitriol cause calcium to be released from bones into ECF and increase the absorption of calcium in the intestines, thus raising serum calcium levels. Conversely, calcitonin stimulates the deposition of calcium in bone, reducing the concentration of calcium ions in the blood.

With increasing age, the intestines absorb calcium less effectively, and more calcium is excreted by the kidneys. Calcium shifts out of the bone to replace these ECF losses, increasing the risk of osteoporosis and fractures of the wrists, vertebrae, and hips. Lack of weight-bearing exercise (which helps keep calcium in the bones) and a vitamin D deficiency contribute to this risk, as do genetics and lifestyle factors. See Table 51.4 for foods containing calcium.

Serum calcium levels are often reported in two ways, based on the way it is circulating in the plasma. Approximately 50% of serum calcium circulates in a free, or unbound, form. The other 50% circulates bound to either plasma proteins or other nonprotein ions. The total serum calcium level (normal range: 8.5 to 10.5 mg/dL) represents both bound and unbound calcium. The ionized serum calcium level (normal range: 4.0 to 5.0 mg/dL) represents free, or unbound, calcium.

Magnesium

Magnesium (Mg^{2+}) is found primarily in the skeleton and ICF, where it is the second most abundant intracellular cation. It is important for intracellular metabolism, and for protein and DNA synthesis within the cells. Only about 1% of the body's magnesium is in ECF, and it has a normal serum level of 1.5 to 2.5 mEq/L. In ECF it is involved in regulating neuromuscular and cardiac function. Maintaining and ensuring adequate magnesium levels is an important part of the care of clients with cardiac disorders. See Table 51.4 for foods high in magnesium.

Chloride

Chloride (Cl^-) is the major anion of ECF, and normal serum levels are 95 to 108 mEq/L. Chloride functions with sodium to regulate serum osmolality and blood volume. The concentration of chloride in ECF is regulated secondarily to sodium; when sodium is reabsorbed in the kidney, chloride usually follows. Chloride is a major component of gastric juice as hydrochloric acid (HCl) and is involved in regulating acid–base balance. It also acts as a buffer in the exchange of oxygen and carbon dioxide in red blood cells (RBCs). Chloride is found in the same foods as sodium.

Phosphate

Phosphate (PO_4^{3-}) is the major anion of ICF. It also is found in ECF, bone, skeletal muscle, and nerve tissue. Normal serum levels of phosphate in adults range from 2.5 to 4.5 mg/dL. Phosphate is involved in many chemical actions of cells, and is essential for functioning of muscles, nerves, and RBCs. It is also involved in the metabolism of protein, fat, and carbohydrate. Phosphate is absorbed from the intestine and is found in many foods (see Table 51.4).

Bicarbonate

Bicarbonate (HCO_3^-) is present in both ICF and ECF. Its primary function is regulating acid–base balance as an essential component of the body's buffering system. The kidneys regulate extracellular bicarbonate levels. Bicarbonate is excreted when too much is present; if more is needed, the kidneys both regenerate and reabsorb bicarbonate ions. Unlike electrolytes that must be consumed in the diet, adequate amounts of bicarbonate are produced through metabolic processes.

Acid–Base Balance

An important part of regulating the homeostasis of body fluids is regulating their acidity and alkalinity. An **acid** is a substance that releases hydrogen ions (H^+) in solution. **Bases**, or alkalis, have a low hydrogen ion concentration and can accept hydrogen ions in solution. The relative acidity or alkalinity of a solution is measured by its **pH**, which is an inverse reflection of the hydrogen ion concentration of the solution. The higher the hydrogen ion concentration, the lower the pH; the lower the hydrogen ion concentration, the higher the pH. Water has a pH of 7 and is neutral. Solutions with a pH lower than 7 are acidic; those with a pH higher than 7 are alkaline.

Regulation of Acid–Base Balance

Body fluids are normally maintained within a narrow range that is slightly alkaline. The normal pH of arterial blood is between 7.35 and 7.45 (Figure 51.7 ■). Acids are continually produced during metabolism. Several body systems, including the respiratory and renal systems, and buffers are actively involved in maintaining the narrow pH range necessary for optimal functioning. Buffers help maintain acid–base balance by neutralizing excess acids or bases.

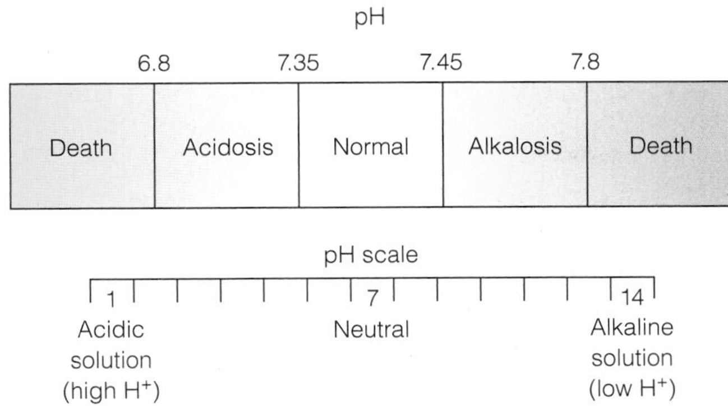

Figure 51.7 ■ Body fluids are normally slightly alkaline, between a pH of 7.35 and 7.45.

The lungs and the kidneys help maintain a normal pH by either excreting or retaining acids and bases as needed.

Buffers

Buffers prevent excessive changes in pH by binding with or releasing hydrogen ions. If body fluids become too acidic, meaning excess hydrogen ions are present in body fluids, buffers bind with the hydrogen ions. If body fluids become too alkaline, meaning not enough hydrogen ions are present in body fluids, buffers can release hydrogen ions. The action of a buffer is immediate, but limited in its capacity to maintain or restore normal acid–base balance.

The major buffer in ECF is the bicarbonate (HCO_3^-) and carbonic acid (H_2CO_3) system. The amounts of bicarbonate and carbonic acid in the body vary; however, as long as a ratio of 20 parts of bicarbonate to 1 part of carbonic acid is maintained, the pH remains within its normal range of 7.35 to 7.45. However, adding a strong acid to ECF can change this ratio because bicarbonate is depleted in neutralizing the acid. When this happens, the pH drops, and the client has a condition called **acidosis**. The ratio can also be upset by adding a strong base to ECF, depleting carbonic acid as it combines with the base. In this case the pH rises and the client has **alkalosis**.

Respiratory Regulation

The lungs help regulate acid–base balance by eliminating or retaining carbon dioxide (CO_2). When combined with water, carbon dioxide forms carbonic acid ($CO_2 + H_2O = H_2CO_3$). This chemical reaction is reversible; carbonic acid breaks down into carbon dioxide and water. The lungs help regulate acid–base balance by altering the rate and depth of respirations. The response of the respiratory system to changes in pH is rapid, occurring within minutes. Carbon dioxide levels in the blood are measured as PCO_2, the partial pressure of the dissolved CO_2 in venous blood, and $PaCO_2$, the partial pressure of the dissolved CO_2 in arterial blood. Normal $PaCO_2$ is 35 to 45 mmHg.

Renal Regulation

Although buffers and the respiratory system can compensate for changes in pH, the kidneys are the ultimate long-term regulator of acid–base balance. They are slower to respond to changes, requiring hours to days to correct imbalances, but their response is more permanent and selective than that of the other systems. The kidneys maintain acid–base balance by selectively excreting or conserving bicarbonate and hydrogen ions. The normal serum bicarbonate level is 22 to 26 mEq/L. The relationship between respiratory and renal regulation of acid–base balance is further explained in Box 51.1.

BOX 51.1 Physiologic Regulation of Acid–Base Balance

Lungs				Kidneys
$CO_2 + H_2O$	↔	H_2CO_3	↔	$H + HCO_3$
Carbon dioxide + Water		Carbonic acid		Hydrogen + bicarbonate

The lungs and kidneys are the two major systems that work on a continuous basis to help regulate the acid–base balance in the body. In the aforementioned biochemical reactions, the processes are all reversible and go back and forth as the body's needs change. The lungs can work very quickly and do their part by either retaining or getting rid of carbon dioxide by changing the rate and depth of respirations. The kidneys work much more slowly; they may take hours to days to regulate the balance by either excreting or conserving hydrogen and bicarbonate ions. Under normal conditions, the two systems work together to maintain homeostasis.

Factors Affecting Body Fluid, Electrolytes, and Acid–Base Balance

The ability of the body to adjust fluids, electrolytes, and acid–base balance is influenced by age, sex and body size, environmental temperature, and lifestyle.

Age

Infants and growing children have much greater fluid turnover than adults because their higher metabolic rate increases fluid loss. Infants lose more fluid through the kidneys because immature kidneys are less able to conserve water than adult kidneys. In addition, infants' respiratory rate is much higher than that of adults, and their body surface area is proportionately greater than that of adults, both of which increases insensible fluid losses. This higher turnover of fluid, combined with the losses produced by disease, can create critical fluid imbalances in children much more rapidly than in adults.

In older individuals, the normal aging process may affect fluid balance. The thirst response is often diminished. Antidiuretic hormone levels remain normal or may even be elevated, but the nephrons become less able to conserve water in response to ADH. Higher levels of

LIFESPAN CONSIDERATIONS **Fluid and Electrolyte Imbalance**

INFANTS AND CHILDREN

Infants are at high risk for fluid and electrolyte imbalance because:

- Their immature kidneys cannot concentrate urine.
- They have a rapid respiratory rate and proportionately larger body surface area than adults, leading to greater insensible losses through the skin and respirations.
- They cannot express thirst, nor actively seek fluids.

Vomiting and diarrhea in infants and young children can lead quickly to electrolyte imbalance. Oral rehydration therapy (ORT) with electrolyte solutions such as Pedialyte should be used to restore fluid and electrolyte balance in mild to moderate dehydration. Prompt treatment with ORT can prevent the need for IV therapy and hospitalization. Even if the child is vomiting, small sips of an ORT solution can be helpful.

OLDER ADULTS

Older adults are at high risk for fluid and electrolyte imbalance because of *decreases* in:

- Thirst sensation
- Ability of the kidneys to concentrate urine
- Intracellular fluid and total body water
- Response to body hormones that help regulate fluid and electrolytes.

Other factors that may influence fluid and electrolyte balance in older adults are:

- Use of diuretics for hypertension and heart disease
- Decreased intake of food and water, especially in older adults with dementia or who are dependent on others to feed them and offer them fluids
- Preparations for diagnostic tests that include being NPO for long periods of time, laxatives, or contrast dyes
- Impaired renal function, for example, in older adults with diabetes.

All of these conditions increase older adults' risk for fluid and electrolyte imbalance, particularly under conditions that challenge the normal compensatory mechanisms, such as a fever, influenza, surgery, or heat exposure. The change can happen quickly and become serious in a short time. Smart observations and quick actions by the nurse can help prevent serious consequences. A change in mental status may be the first symptom of impairment and must be further evaluated to determine the cause.

atrial natriuretic factor in older adults may also contribute to this impaired ability to conserve water. These normal changes of aging increase the risk of dehydration. When combined with the increased likelihood of heart diseases, impaired renal function, and multiple drug regimens, the older adult's risk for fluid and electrolyte imbalance is significant.

Sex and Body Size

Total body water also is affected by sex and body size. Fat cells contain little or no water, but lean muscle tissue has a high water content; therefore, individuals with a higher percentage of body fat have less body water than individuals with a higher percentage of lean muscle. Women generally have proportionately more body fat and, therefore, less body water than men.

Environmental Temperature

Individuals with an illness and those participating in strenuous activity are at increased risk for fluid and electrolyte imbalances when the environmental temperature is high. Fluid losses through sweating are increased in hot environments as the body attempts to disperse heat. These losses are even greater in individuals who are not accustomed to a hot environment.

Both electrolytes and water are lost through sweating. When only water is replaced, electrolyte depletion is a risk. An individual who is electrolyte depleted may experience fatigue, weakness, headache, and gastrointestinal symptoms such as anorexia and nausea. The risk of adverse effects is even greater if lost water is not replaced. Body temperature rises, and the individual is at risk for heat exhaustion or heatstroke; this happens when an individual's heat production exceeds the body's ability to dissipate heat. Consuming adequate amounts of cool liquids, particularly during strenuous activity, reduces the risk of adverse effects from heat. Balanced electrolyte solutions and carbohydrate-electrolyte solutions such as sports drinks are recommended because they replace both water and electrolytes lost through perspiration.

Lifestyle

Lifestyle factors such as diet, exercise, stress, and alcohol consumption affect fluid, electrolyte, and acid–base balance.

Intake of fluids and electrolytes is affected by diet. Individuals with anorexia nervosa or bulimia are at risk for severe fluid and electrolyte imbalances because of inadequate intake or purging regimens (e.g., induced vomiting, use of diuretics and laxatives). Seriously malnourished individuals have decreased serum protein levels, and may develop edema because serum osmotic pressure is reduced. When calorie intake is not adequate to meet the body's needs, fat stores are broken down and fatty acids are released, increasing the risk of acidosis.

Regular weight-bearing exercise such as walking or running has a beneficial effect on calcium balance. The rate of bone loss that occurs in postmenopausal women and older men is slowed with weight-bearing exercise, reducing the risk of osteoporosis.

Stress can increase cellular metabolism, blood glucose concentration, and catecholamine levels. In addition, stress can increase production of ADH and stimulate the renin-angiotensin-aldosterone system, both of which decrease urine production. The overall response of the body to stress is to increase blood volume.

Heavy alcohol consumption increases the risk of low calcium, magnesium, and phosphate levels. Individuals who drink large amounts of alcohol are also at risk for acidosis associated with breakdown of fat tissue.

Disturbances in Fluid Volume, Electrolyte, and Acid–Base Balances

A number of factors such as illness, trauma, surgery, and medications can affect the body's ability to maintain fluid, electrolyte, and acid–base balance. The kidneys play a major role in maintaining fluid, electrolyte, and acid–base balances, and renal disease is a significant cause of imbalances. In addition, decreased blood flow to the kidneys due to cardiovascular disease stimulates the renin-angiotensin-aldosterone system, causing sodium and water retention. Diseases such as diabetes mellitus, cancer, and chronic obstructive lung disease may affect acid–base balance. Clients who are confused or unable to communicate their needs are at risk for inadequate fluid intake. Vomiting, diarrhea, or nasogastric suction can cause significant fluid losses. Tissue trauma, such as burns, causes fluid and electrolytes to be lost from damaged cells. Medications such as diuretics or corticosteroids can result in abnormal losses of electrolytes and fluid loss or retention.

Fluid Imbalances

Fluid imbalances are of two basic types: isotonic and osmolar. Isotonic imbalances occur when water and electrolytes are lost or gained in equal proportions, so that the osmolality of body fluids remains constant. Osmolar imbalances involve the loss or gain of only water, so that the osmolality of the serum is altered. Thus, four categories of fluid imbalances may occur: (1) an isotonic loss of water and electrolytes, (2) an isotonic gain of water and electrolytes, (3) a hyperosmolar loss of only water, and (4) a hypo-osmolar gain of only water. These are referred to, respectively, as fluid volume deficit, fluid volume excess, dehydration (hyperosmolar imbalance), and overhydration (hypo-osmolar imbalance).

Fluid Volume Deficit

Isotonic **fluid volume deficit (FVD)** occurs when the body loses both water and electrolytes from the ECF in similar proportions. Thus, the decreased volume of fluid remains isotonic. In FVD, fluid is initially lost from the intravascular compartment, so it often is called **hypovolemia**.

FVD generally occurs as a result of (a) abnormal losses through the skin, gastrointestinal tract, or kidney; (b) decreased intake of fluid; (c) bleeding; or (d) movement of fluid into a third space. See the section on third space syndrome that follows.

For the risk factors and clinical signs related to FVD, see Table 51.5.

THIRD SPACE SYNDROME

In **third space syndrome**, fluid shifts from the vascular space into an area where it is not readily accessible as extracellular fluid. This fluid remains in the body but is essentially unavailable for use, causing an isotonic fluid volume deficit. Fluid may be isolated in the bowel, in injured tissue (e.g., severe burns), or in potential spaces such as the peritoneal or pleural cavities.

Third spacing has two distinct phases: loss and reabsorption. The client with third space syndrome during the loss phase has an isotonic fluid deficit. During the reabsorption phase, tissues begin to heal and fluid moves back into the intravascular space. Careful nursing assessment is vital to effectively identify and intervene for clients experiencing third spacing. Because fluid shifts from the vascular compartment (loss phase) and then back into the vascular compartment after time (reabsorption phase), assessment for manifestations of fluid volume deficit and excess is vital.

TABLE 51.5 Isotonic Fluid Volume Deficit

Risk Factors	Clinical Manifestations	Nursing Interventions
Loss of water and electrolytes from: • Vomiting • Diarrhea • Excessive sweating • Polyuria • Fever • Nasogastric suction • Abnormal drainage or wound losses Insufficient intake due to: • Anorexia • Nausea • Inability to access fluids • Impaired swallowing • Confusion, depression	Complaints of weakness and thirst Weight loss: • 2% loss = mild FVD • 5% loss = moderate • 8% loss = severe Fluid intake less than output Decreased tissue turgor Dry mucous membranes, sunken eyeballs, decreased tearing Subnormal temperature Weak pulse; tachycardia Decreased blood pressure Postural (orthostatic) hypotension (significant drop in BP when moving from lying to sitting or standing position) Decreased capillary refill Decreased central venous pressure Decreased urine volume (<30 mL/hr) Increased specific gravity of urine (>1.030) Increased hematocrit Increased blood urea nitrogen (BUN)	Assess for clinical manifestations of FVD. Monitor weight and vital signs, including temperature. Assess tissue turgor. Monitor fluid intake and output. Monitor laboratory findings. Administer oral and IV fluids as indicated. Provide frequent mouth care. Implement measures to prevent skin breakdown. Provide for safety (e.g., provide assistance for a client rising from bed or chair).

Fluid Volume Excess

Fluid volume excess (FVE) occurs when the body retains both water and sodium in similar proportions to normal ECF. This is commonly referred to as **hypervolemia** (increased blood volume). FVE is always secondary to an increase in the total body sodium content, which leads to an increase in total body water. Because both water and sodium are retained, the serum sodium concentration remains essentially normal and the excess volume of fluid is isotonic. Specific causes of FVE include (a) excessive intake of sodium chloride; (b) administering sodium-containing infusions too rapidly, particularly to clients with impaired regulatory mechanisms; and (c) disease processes that alter regulatory mechanisms, such as heart failure, renal failure, cirrhosis of the liver, and Cushing's syndrome.

The risk factors and clinical manifestations for FVE are summarized in Table 51.6.

EDEMA

In fluid volume excess, both intravascular and interstitial spaces have an increased water and sodium content. Excess interstitial fluid is known as edema. Edema typically is most apparent in areas where the tissue pressure is low, such as around the eyes, and in dependent tissues (known as dependent edema), where hydrostatic capillary pressure is high (Figure 51.8 ■).

Pitting edema is edema that leaves a small depression or pit after finger pressure is applied to the swollen area. The pit is caused by movement of fluid to adjacent tissue, away from the point of pressure (Figure 51.9 ■). Within 10 to 30 seconds the pit normally disappears as fluid returns to the area.

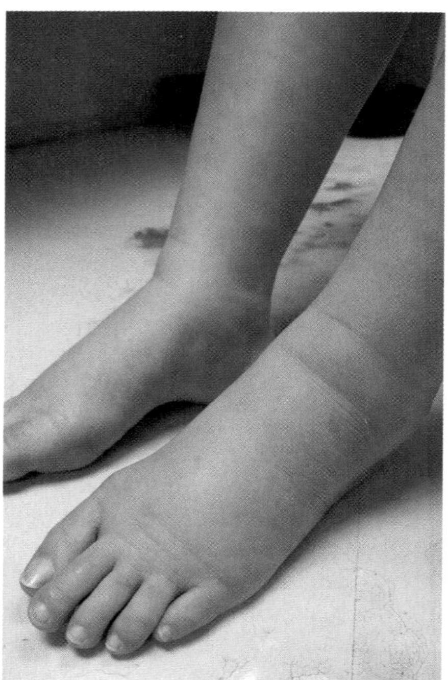

Figure 51.8 ■ Dependent pedal edema.
Amawasri Pakdara/123RF.

Dehydration

Dehydration, or a hyperosmolar fluid imbalance, occurs when water is lost from the body, leaving the client with excess sodium. Because water is lost while electrolytes, particularly sodium, are retained, serum osmolality and serum sodium levels increase. Water is drawn into the vascular compartment from the interstitial space and cells, resulting in cellular dehydration. Older adults are at particular risk for dehydration because of decreased thirst sensation. Dehydration can also affect clients who are hyperventilating, have a prolonged fever, are in diabetic ketoacidosis, or are receiving enteral feedings with insufficient water intake.

Overhydration

Overhydration, or a hypo-osmolar fluid imbalance, occurs when water is gained in excess of electrolytes, resulting in low serum osmolality and low serum sodium levels. Water is drawn into the cells, causing them to swell. In the brain, this can lead to cerebral edema and impaired neurologic function. Overhydration, sometimes called water intoxication, often occurs when both fluid and electrolytes are lost, for example, through excessive sweating, but only water is replaced. It can also result from the syndrome of inappropriate antidiuretic hormone (SIADH), a disorder that can occur with some malignant tumors, AIDS, head injury, or administration of certain drugs such as barbiturates or anesthetics.

Electrolyte Imbalances

The most common and clinically significant electrolyte imbalances involve sodium, potassium, calcium, magnesium, chloride, and phosphate.

TABLE 51.6 Isotonic Fluid Volume Excess

Risk Factors	Clinical Manifestations	Nursing Interventions
Excess intake of sodium-containing IV fluids Excess ingestion of sodium in diet or medications (e.g., sodium bicarbonate antacids such as Alka-Seltzer or hypertonic enema solutions such as Fleet's) Impaired fluid balance regulation related to: • Heart failure • Renal failure • Cirrhosis of the liver	Weight gain: • 2% gain = mild FVE • 5% gain = moderate • 8% gain = severe Fluid intake greater than output Full, bounding pulse; tachycardia Increased blood pressure and central venous pressure Distended neck veins Moist crackles (rales) in lungs; dyspnea, shortness of breath Mental confusion	Assess for clinical manifestations of FVE. Monitor weight and vital signs. Assess for edema. Assess breath sounds. Monitor fluid intake and output. Monitor laboratory findings. Place in Fowler's position. Administer diuretics as ordered. Restrict fluid intake as indicated. Restrict dietary sodium as ordered. Implement measures to prevent skin breakdown.

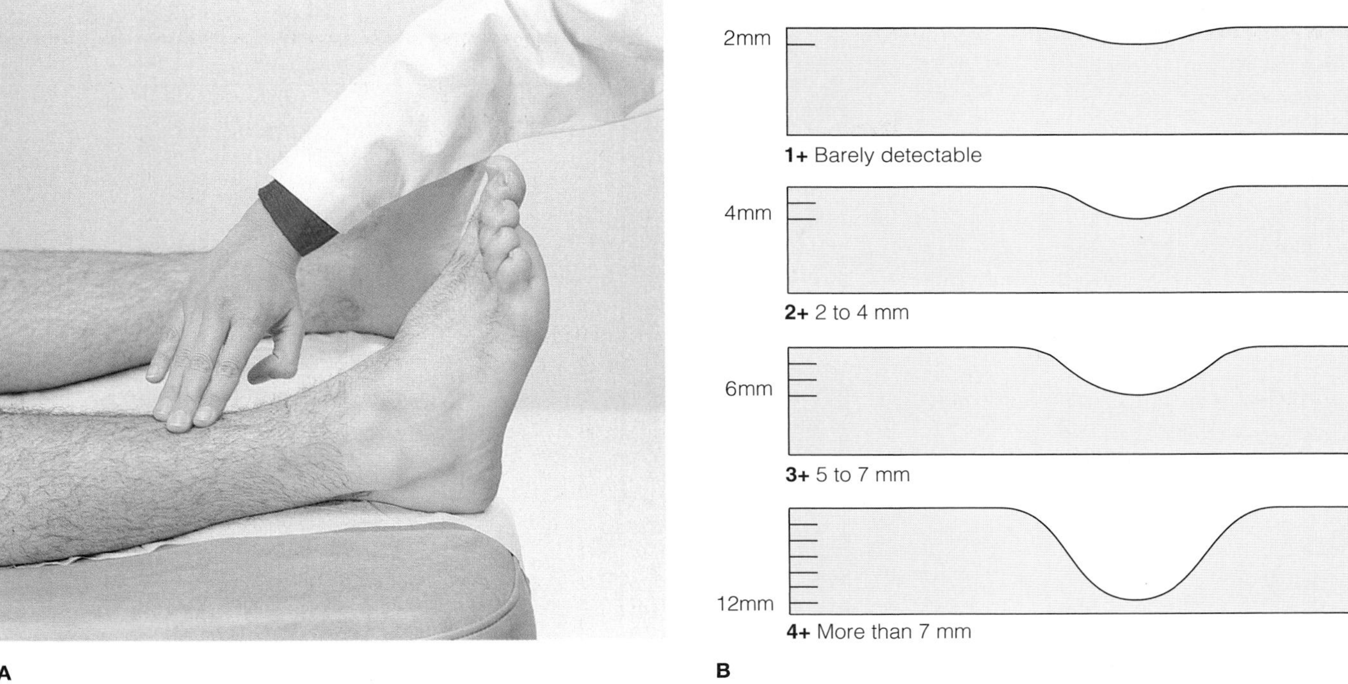

Figure 51.9 ■ Evaluation of edema. *A*, Palpate for edema over the tibia as shown here and behind the medial malleolus, and over the dorsum of each foot. *B*, Four-point scale for grading edema.

Sodium

Sodium (Na^+), the most abundant cation in the extracellular fluid, not only moves into and out of the body but also moves in careful balance among the three fluid compartments. It is found in most body secretions, for example, saliva, gastric and intestinal secretions, bile, and pancreatic fluid. Therefore, continuous or excessive excretion of any of these fluids can result in a sodium deficit. Because of its role in regulating water balance, sodium imbalances usually are accompanied by water imbalances.

Hyponatremia is a sodium deficit, or serum sodium level of less than 135 mEq/L, and is, in acute care settings, a common electrolyte imbalance. Because of sodium's role in determining the osmolality of ECF, hyponatremia typically results in a low serum osmolality. Water is drawn out of the vascular compartment into interstitial tissues and the cells (Figure 51.10*A* ■), causing the clinical manifestations associated with this disorder. As sodium levels decrease, the brain and nervous system are affected by cellular edema. Severe hyponatremia, serum levels below 115 mEq/L, is a medical emergency and can cause permanent neurologic dysfunction (Walker, 2016).

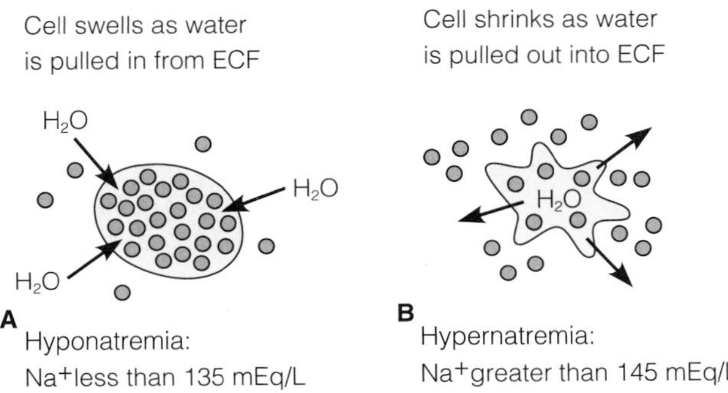

Figure 51.10 ■ The extracellular sodium level affects cell size. *A*, In hyponatremia, cells swell; *B*, in hypernatremia, cells shrink in size.

Hypernatremia is excess sodium in ECF, or a serum sodium of greater than 145 mEq/L. Because the osmotic pressure of extracellular fluid is increased, fluid moves out of the cells into the ECF (Figure 51.10*B*). As a result, the cells become dehydrated. Like hyponatremia, the primary manifestations of hypernatremia are neurologic in nature.

It is important to note that normally an individual's thirst mechanism protects against hypernatremia. When an individual becomes thirsty, the body is stimulated to drink water, which helps correct the hypernatremia. Clients at highest risk for hypernatremia are those who are unable to access water, such as clients who are unconscious, clients who are unable to request fluids such as infants or older adults with dementia, or ill clients with an impaired thirst mechanism. Table 51.7 lists risk factors and clinical signs for hyponatremia and hypernatremia.

Potassium

Although the amount of potassium (K^+) in extracellular fluid is small, it is vital to normal neuromuscular and cardiac function. Normal renal function is important for maintenance of potassium balance, because 80% of potassium is excreted by the kidneys. Potassium must be replaced daily to maintain its balance, which normally happens through food intake.

Hypokalemia is a potassium deficit, defined as a serum potassium level of less than 3.5 mEq/L. Gastrointestinal losses of potassium through vomiting and gastric suction

TABLE 51.7 Electrolyte Imbalances

Risk Factors	Clinical Manifestations	Nursing Interventions
HYPONATREMIA Loss of Sodium • Gastrointestinal fluid loss • Sweating • Use of diuretics Gain of Water • Hypotonic tube feedings • Excessive drinking of water • Excess IV D_5W (dextrose in water) administration Syndrome of Inappropriate ADH (SIADH) • Head injury • AIDS • Malignant tumors	Lethargy, confusion, apprehension Muscle twitching Abdominal cramps Anorexia, nausea, vomiting Headache Seizures, coma *Laboratory findings*: Serum sodium < 135 mEq/L Serum osmolality < 280 mOsm/kg	Assess clinical manifestations. Monitor fluid intake and output. Monitor laboratory data (e.g., serum sodium). Assess client closely if administering hypertonic saline solutions. Encourage food and fluid high in sodium if permitted (e.g., table salt, bacon, ham, processed cheese). Limit water intake as indicated.
HYPERNATREMIA Loss of Water • Insensible water loss (hyperventilation or fever) • Diarrhea • Water deprivation Gain of Sodium • Parenteral administration of saline solutions • Hypertonic tube feedings without adequate water • Excessive use of table salt (1 tsp contains 2300 mg of sodium) Conditions such as: • Diabetes insipidus • Heat stroke	Thirst Dry, sticky mucous membranes Tongue red, dry, swollen Weakness Severe hypernatremia: • Fatigue, restlessness • Decreasing level of consciousness • Disorientation • Convulsions *Laboratory findings*: Serum sodium > 145 mEq/L Serum osmolality > 300 mOsm/kg	Monitor fluid intake and output. Monitor behavior changes (e.g., restlessness, disorientation). Monitor laboratory findings (e.g., serum sodium). Encourage fluids as ordered. Monitor diet as ordered (e.g., restrict intake of salt and foods high in sodium).
HYPOKALEMIA Loss of Potassium • Vomiting and gastric suction • Diarrhea • Heavy perspiration • Use of potassium-wasting drugs (e.g., diuretics) • Poor intake of potassium (as with debilitated clients, alcoholics, anorexia nervosa) • Hyperaldosteronism	Muscle weakness, leg cramps Fatigue, lethargy Anorexia, nausea, vomiting Decreased bowel motility Cardiac dysrhythmias Depressed deep-tendon reflexes Weak, irregular pulses *Laboratory findings*: Serum potassium < 3.5 mEq/L Arterial blood gases (ABGs) may show alkalosis T-wave flattening and ST-segment depression on ECG	Monitor heart rate and rhythm. Monitor clients receiving digitalis (e.g., digoxin) closely, because hypokalemia increases risk of digitalis toxicity. Administer oral potassium as ordered with food or fluid to prevent gastric irritation. Administer IV potassium solutions at a rate no faster than 10–20 mEq/h; never administer undiluted potassium intravenously. For clients receiving IV potassium, monitor for pain and inflammation at the injection site. Teach clients about potassium-rich foods. Teach clients how to prevent excessive loss of potassium (e.g., through abuse of diuretics and laxatives).
HYPERKALEMIA Decreased Potassium Excretion • Renal failure • Hypoaldosteronism • Potassium-conserving diuretics High Potassium Intake • Excessive use of K^+-containing salt substitutes • Excessive or rapid IV infusion of potassium • Potassium shift out of the tissue cells into the plasma (e.g., infections, burns, acidosis)	Increased bowel mobility Irritability, apathy, confusion Cardiac dysrhythmias or arrest Muscle weakness, areflexia (absence of reflexes) Decreased heart rate Irregular pulse Paresthesias and numbness in extremities *Laboratory findings*: Serum potassium > 5.0 mEq/L Peaked T wave, widened QRS on ECG	Closely monitor cardiac status and ECG. Administer diuretics and other medications such as glucose and insulin as ordered. Hold potassium supplements and K^+-conserving diuretics. Monitor serum K^+ levels carefully; a rapid drop may occur as potassium shifts into the cells. Teach clients to avoid foods high in potassium and salt substitutes.

TABLE 51.7 Electrolyte Imbalances—*continued*

Risk Factors	Clinical Manifestations	Nursing Interventions
HYPOCALCEMIA Surgical Removal of the Parathyroid Glands Conditions such as: • Hypoparathyroidism • Acute pancreatitis • Hyperphosphatemia • Thyroid carcinoma Inadequate Vitamin D Intake • Malabsorption • Hypomagnesemia • Alkalosis • Sepsis • Alcohol abuse	Numbness, tingling of the extremities and around the mouth Muscle tremors, cramps; if severe can progress to tetany and convulsions Cardiac dysrhythmias; decreased cardiac output Positive Trousseau's and Chvostek's signs (see Table 51.9 and Figure 51.11) Confusion, anxiety, possible psychoses Hyperactive deep-tendon reflexes *Laboratory findings*: Serum calcium $<$ 8.5 mg/dL (total) or 4.5 mEq/L (ionized) Lengthened QT intervals Prolonged ST segments	Closely monitor respiratory and cardiovascular status. Take precautions to protect a confused client. Administer oral or parenteral calcium supplements as ordered. When administering intravenously, closely monitor cardiac status and ECG during infusion. Teach clients at high risk for osteoporosis about: • Dietary sources rich in calcium. • Recommendation for 1000–1500 mg of calcium per day. • Calcium supplements. • Regular exercise. • Estrogen replacement therapy for postmenopausal women.
HYPERCALCEMIA • Prolonged immobilization Conditions such as • Hyperparathyroidism • Malignancy of the bone • Paget's disease	Lethargy, weakness Depressed deep-tendon reflexes Bone pain Anorexia, nausea, vomiting Constipation Polyuria, hypercalciuria Flank pain secondary to urinary calculi Dysrhythmias, possible heart block *Laboratory findings*: Serum calcium $>$ 10.5 mg/dL (total) or 5.5 mEq/L (ionized) Shortened QT intervals Shortened ST segments	Increase client movement and exercise. Encourage oral fluids as permitted to maintain a dilute urine. Teach clients to limit intake of food and fluid high in calcium. Encourage ingestion of fiber to prevent constipation. Protect a confused client; monitor for pathologic fractures in clients with long-term hypercalcemia. Encourage intake of acid–ash fluids (e.g., prune or cranberry juice) to counteract deposits of calcium salts in the urine.
HYPOMAGNESEMIA • Excessive loss from the gastrointestinal tract (e.g., from nasogastric suction, diarrhea, fistula drainage) • Long-term use of certain drugs (e.g., diuretics, aminoglycoside antibiotics) Conditions such as: • Chronic alcoholism • Pancreatitis • Burns	Neuromuscular irritability with tremors Increased reflexes, tremors, convulsions Positive Chvostek's and Trousseau's signs (see Table 51.9 and Figure 51.11) Tachycardia, elevated blood pressure, dysrhythmias Disorientation and confusion Vertigo Anorexia, dysphagia Respiratory difficulties *Laboratory findings*: Serum magnesium $<$ 1.5 mEq/L Prolonged PR intervals, widened QRS complexes, prolonged QT intervals, depressed ST segments, broad flattened T waves, prominent U waves	Assess clients receiving digitalis for digitalis toxicity. Hypomagnesemia increases the risk of toxicity. Take protective measures when there is a possibility of seizures: • Assess the client's ability to swallow water prior to initiating oral feeding. • Initiate safety measures to prevent injury during seizure activity. • Carefully administer magnesium salts as ordered. Encourage clients to eat magnesium-rich foods if permitted (e.g., whole grains, meat, seafood, and green leafy vegetables). Refer clients to alcohol treatment programs as indicated.
HYPERMAGNESEMIA Abnormal retention of magnesium, as in: • Renal failure • Adrenal insufficiency • Treatment with magnesium salts	Peripheral vasodilation, flushing Nausea, vomiting Muscle weakness, paralysis Hypotension, bradycardia Depressed deep-tendon reflexes Lethargy, drowsiness Respiratory depression, coma Respiratory and cardiac arrest if hypermagnesemia is severe *Laboratory findings*: Serum magnesium $>$ 2.5 mEq/L Electrocardiogram showing prolonged QT interval, prolonged PR interval, widened QRS complexes, tall T waves	Monitor vital signs and level of consciousness when clients are at risk. If patellar reflexes are absent, notify the primary care provider. Advise clients who have renal disease to contact their primary care provider before taking over-the-counter drugs.

DRUG CAPSULE

Diuretic Agent: furosemide (Lasix)

THE CLIENT WITH FLUID VOLUME EXCESS

Furosemide, which is a loop diuretic, inhibits sodium and chloride reabsorption in the loop of Henle and the distal renal tubule. This results in significant diuresis, with renal excretion of water, sodium chloride, potassium, magnesium, hydrogen, and calcium.

Furosemide is commonly used for the clinical management of edema secondary to heart failure, treatment of hypertension, and treatment of hepatic or renal disease. Therapeutic effects include diuresis and lowering of blood pressure.

NURSING RESPONSIBILITIES

- Assess the client's fluid status regularly. Assessment should include daily weight, close monitoring of intake and output, vital signs, skin turgor, edema, lung sounds, and mucous membranes.
- Monitor the client's potassium levels. Furosemide is a loop diuretic, which excretes potassium and may result in hypokalemia.
- Administer in the morning to avoid increased urination during hours of sleep.
- If the client is also taking digitalis glycosides, he or she should be assessed for anorexia, nausea, vomiting, muscle cramps, paresthesia, and confusion. The potassium-depleting effect of furosemide places the client at increased risk for digitalis toxicity.

CLIENT AND FAMILY TEACHING

- Medication should be taken exactly as directed. If a dose is missed, take it as soon as possible; however, if a day has been missed, do not double the dose the next day.
- Weigh yourself daily, and report weight gain or loss of more than 3 pounds in 1 day to your primary care provider.
- Contact your primary care provider immediately if you begin to experience muscle weakness, cramps, nausea, dizziness, numbness, or tingling of the extremities.
- Some form of potassium supplementation may be needed. Your primary care provider may order oral potassium supplements for you; if not, you may need to consume a diet high in potassium.
- Make position changes from lying to sitting and sitting to standing slowly in order to minimize dizziness.

Note: Prior to administering any medication, review all aspects in a current drug handbook or other reliable source.

are common causes of hypokalemia, as is the use of potassium-wasting diuretics, such as thiazide or loop diuretics. Symptoms of hypokalemia are usually mild until the level drops below 3 mEq/L, unless the decrease in potassium is rapid. When the decrease is gradual, the body compensates by shifting potassium from the intracellular environment into the serum.

Hyperkalemia is a potassium excess, defined as a serum potassium level greater than 5.0 mEq/L. Hyperkalemia is less common than hypokalemia, and rarely occurs in clients with normal renal function. It is, however, more dangerous than hypokalemia and can lead to cardiac arrest. As with hypokalemia, symptoms are more severe and occur at lower levels when the increase in potassium is rapid. Table 51.7 lists risk factors and clinical signs for hypokalemia and hyperkalemia.

Clinical Alert!

Potassium may be given intravenously for severe hypokalemia. It must **always** be diluted appropriately and **never** be given IV push. Potassium that is to be given IV should be mixed in the pharmacy and double-checked prior to administration by two nurses. The usual concentration of IV potassium is 20 to 40 mEq/L.

Calcium

Regulating the level of calcium (Ca^{2+}) in the body is more complex than the other major electrolytes, so calcium balance can be affected by many factors. Imbalances of this electrolyte are relatively common.

Hypocalcemia is a calcium deficit, defined as a total serum calcium level of less than 8.5 mg/dL or an ionized calcium level of less than 4.5 mEq/L. Severe depletion of calcium can cause tetany with muscle spasms and paresthesias (numbness and tingling around the mouth, hands, and feet), and can lead to seizures. Two signs indicate hypocalcemia: Chvostek's sign is a contraction of the facial muscles in response to tapping the facial nerve in front of the ear (Figure 51.11*A* ■); Trousseau's sign is a carpal spasm in response to inflating a blood pressure cuff on the upper arm to 20 mmHg greater than the systolic pressure for 2 to 5 minutes (Figure 51.11*B*). Clients at greatest risk for hypocalcemia are those whose parathyroid glands have been removed. This is frequently associated with thyroidectomy or other neck surgery, which can result in unintentional removal or damage to the parathyroid glands. Low serum magnesium levels (hypomagnesemia) and chronic alcoholism also increase the risk of hypocalcemia.

Hypercalcemia is a calcium excess, defined as a total serum calcium level greater than 10.5 mg/dL, or an ionized calcium level of greater than 5.5 mEq/L. It most often occurs when calcium is released in excess from the bony skeleton. This is usually due to malignancy or prolonged immobilization. The risk factors and clinical manifestations related to calcium imbalances are found in Table 51.7.

Magnesium

Magnesium (Mg^{2+}) imbalances are relatively common in hospitalized clients, although they may be unrecognized.

Hypomagnesemia is a magnesium deficiency, defined as a serum magnesium level of less than 1.5 mEq/L. It occurs more frequently than hypermagnesemia. Chronic alcoholism is the most common cause of hypomagnesemia. Magnesium deficiency also may aggravate the manifestations of alcohol withdrawal, such as delirium tremens (DTs).

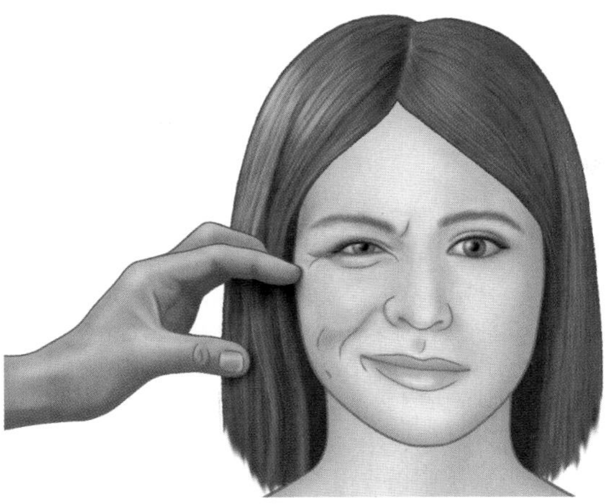

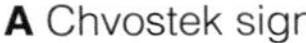

A Chvostek sign

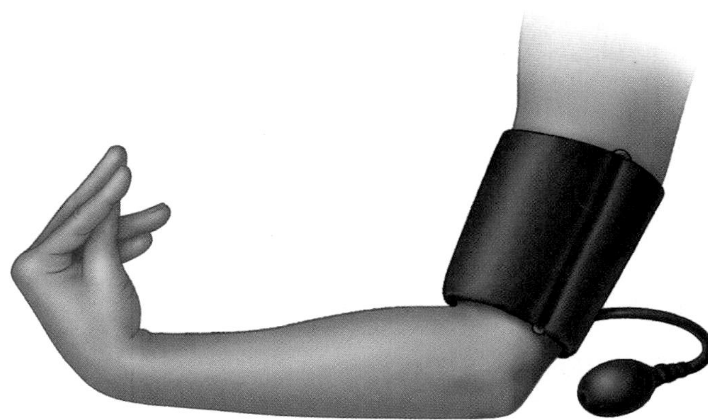

B Trousseau sign

Figure 51.11 ■ *A*, Positive Chvostek sign; *B*, positive Trousseau sign.

Hypermagnesemia is a magnesium excess, defined as a serum magnesium level above 2.5 mEq/L, due to increased intake or decreased excretion. It is often iatrogenic, meaning caused by medical treatment; usually the cause is oversupplementation with magnesium. Table 51.7 lists risk factors and manifestations for clients with altered magnesium balance.

Chloride

Because of the relationship between sodium ions and chloride ions (Cl^-), imbalances of chloride commonly occur in conjunction with sodium imbalances.

Hypochloremia is a chloride deficit, defined as a serum chloride level below 95 mEq/L, and is usually related to excess loss of chloride through the GI tract, kidneys, or sweating. Hypochloremic clients are at risk for alkalosis, and may experience muscle twitching, tremors, or tetany.

Hyperchloremia is a chloride excess, defined as a serum chloride level above 108 mEq/L. Excess replacement of sodium chloride or potassium chloride is a risk factor for high serum chloride levels, as are conditions that lead to hypernatremia. The manifestations of hyperchloremia include acidosis, weakness, and lethargy, with the risk of dysrhythmias or coma.

Phosphate

Phosphate (PO_4^{3-}) is found in both intracellular and extracellular fluid. Most of the phosphorus (P^+) in the body exists as PO_4^{3-}. Phosphate imbalances frequently are related to therapeutic interventions for other disorders.

Hypophosphatemia is a phosphate deficit, defined as a serum phosphate level of less than 2.5 mg/dL. Glucose and insulin administration and total parenteral nutrition can cause phosphate to shift into the cells from extracellular fluid compartments, leading to hypophosphatemia. Alcohol withdrawal, acid–base imbalances, and the use of antacids that bind with phosphate in the GI tract are other possible causes. Manifestations of hypophosphatemia include paresthesias, muscle weakness and pain, mental changes, and possibly seizures.

Hyperphosphatemia is a phosphate excess, defined as a serum phosphate level greater than 4.5 mg/dL. It occurs when phosphate shifts out of the cells into extracellular fluids (e.g., due to tissue trauma or chemotherapy), in renal failure, or when excess phosphate is administered or ingested. Infants who are fed cow's milk are at risk for hyperphosphatemia, as are individuals who use phosphate-containing enemas or laxatives. Manifestations of hyperphosphatemia include numbness and tingling around the mouth and in the fingertips, muscle spasms, and tetany.

Acid–Base Imbalances

Acid–base imbalances are usually classified as respiratory or metabolic by the cause of the disorder. Carbonic acid levels are normally regulated by the lungs through the retention or excretion of carbon dioxide, and problems lead to respiratory acidosis or alkalosis. Bicarbonate and hydrogen ion levels are regulated by the kidneys, and problems lead to metabolic acidosis or alkalosis. Healthy regulatory systems will attempt to correct acid–base imbalances, a process called **compensation**.

Respiratory Acidosis

Any condition that causes carbon dioxide retention, either due to hypoventilation or impaired lung function, causes carbonic acid levels to increase and pH to fall below 7.35, a condition known as **respiratory acidosis**. Serious lung diseases such as asthma and chronic obstructive pulmonary disease (COPD) are common causes of respiratory acidosis. Central nervous system depression due to anesthesia or a narcotic overdose can slow the respiratory rate enough to cause carbon dioxide retention. When respiratory acidosis occurs, the kidneys retain bicarbonate to restore the normal carbonic acid to bicarbonate ratio. The kidneys are relatively slow to respond to changes in acid–base balance, however, so this compensatory response may require hours to days to restore normal pH.

Respiratory Alkalosis

When an individual hyperventilates, more carbon dioxide than normal is exhaled, carbonic acid levels fall, and the pH rises to greater than 7.45. This condition is called **respiratory alkalosis**. Psychogenic or anxiety-related hyperventilation is a common cause of respiratory alkalosis. Other causes include fever and respiratory infections. In respiratory alkalosis, the kidneys will excrete bicarbonate to return pH to within the normal range. Often, however, the cause of the hyperventilation is eliminated and pH returns to normal before renal compensation occurs.

Metabolic Acidosis

When bicarbonate levels are low in relation to the amount of carbonic acid in the body, pH falls and **metabolic acidosis** develops. This may occur because of renal failure and the inability of the kidneys to excrete hydrogen ions and produce bicarbonate. It also may occur when too much acid is produced in the body, for example, in diabetic ketoacidosis or starvation when fat tissue is broken down for energy. Metabolic acidosis stimulates the respiratory center, and the rate and depth of respirations increase. Carbon dioxide is eliminated and carbonic acid levels fall, minimizing the change in pH. This respiratory compensation occurs within minutes of the onset of the pH imbalance.

Metabolic Alkalosis

In **metabolic alkalosis**, the amount of bicarbonate in the body exceeds the normal 20-to-1 ratio. Ingestion of bicarbonate of soda as an antacid is one cause of metabolic alkalosis, as is prolonged vomiting with loss of hydrochloric acid from the stomach. The respiratory center is depressed in metabolic alkalosis, and respirations slow and become shallower. Carbon dioxide is retained and carbonic acid levels increase, helping balance the excess bicarbonate. The risk factors and manifestations for acid–base imbalances are listed in Table 51.8.

●○● NURSING MANAGEMENT

Assessing

Assessing clients for fluid, electrolyte, and acid–base balance and imbalances is an important nursing responsibility. Components of the assessment include (a) the nursing

ANATOMY & PHYSIOLOGY REVIEW

Gas Exchange

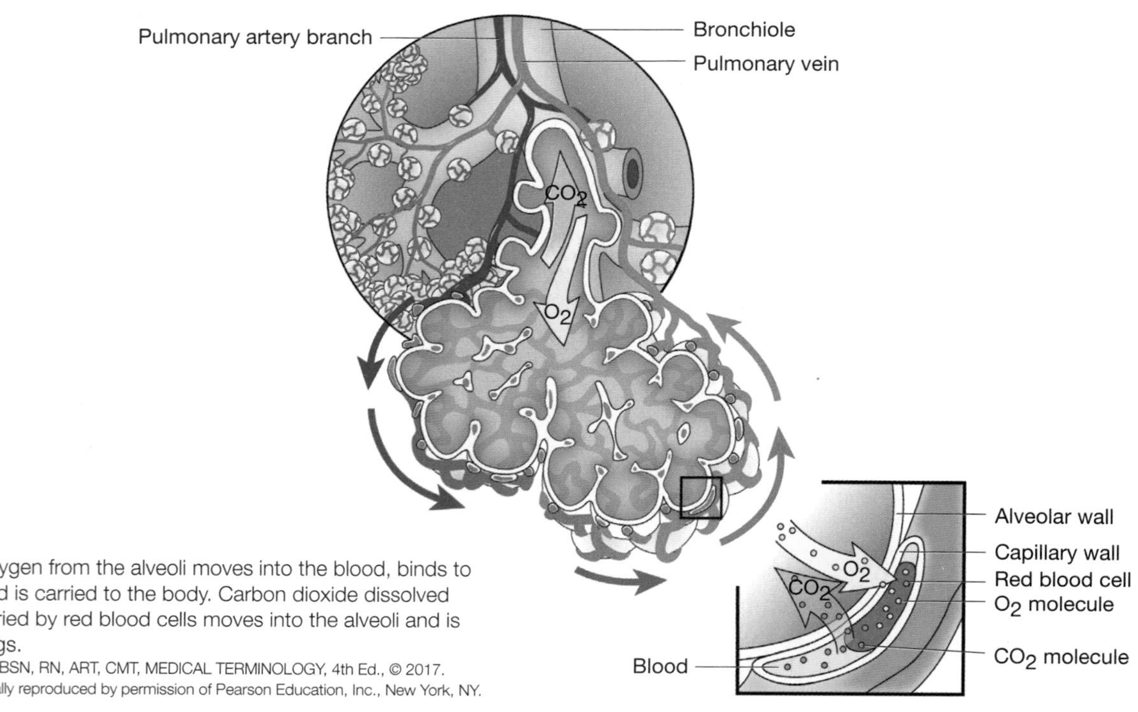

Gas exchange. Oxygen from the alveoli moves into the blood, binds to red blood cells, and is carried to the body. Carbon dioxide dissolved in the blood or carried by red blood cells moves into the alveoli and is exhaled by the lungs.

QUESTIONS

1. Hypoventilation can affect gas exchange. What are some causes of hypoventilation?
2. How does shallow breathing and hypoventilation cause $PaCO_2$ to increase and pH to decrease?
3. ABGs that indicate an increased $PaCO_2$ and a decreased pH reflect which acid–base imbalance?
4. Hyperventilation can also affect gas exchange. What are some causes of hyperventilation?
5. How does hyperventilation cause a decreased $PaCO_2$ and increased pH?
6. ABGs that indicate a decreased $PaCO_2$ and an increased pH reflect which acid–base imbalance?

Answers to Anatomy & Physiology Review Questions are available on the faculty resources site. Please consult with your instructor.

TABLE 51.8 Acid–Base Imbalances

Risk Factors	Clinical Manifestations	Nursing Interventions
RESPIRATORY ACIDOSIS Acute lung conditions that impair alveolar gas exchange (e.g., pneumonia, acute pulmonary edema, aspiration of foreign body, near-drowning) Chronic lung disease (e.g., asthma, cystic fibrosis, or emphysema) Overdose of narcotics or sedatives that depress respiratory rate and depth Brain injury that affects the respiratory center Airway obstruction	Increased pulse and respiratory rates Headache, dizziness Confusion, decreased level of consciousness (LOC) Convulsions Warm, flushed skin Chronic: Weakness Headache *Laboratory findings*: Arterial blood pH < 7.35 $PaCO_2 > 45$ mmHg HCO_3^- normal or slightly elevated in acute; >26 mEq/L in chronic	Frequently assess respiratory status and lung sounds. Monitor airway and ventilation; insert artificial airway and prepare for mechanical ventilation as necessary. Administer pulmonary therapy measures such as inhalation therapy, percussion and postural drainage, bronchodilators, and antibiotics as ordered. Monitor fluid intake and output, vital signs, and arterial blood gases. Administer narcotic antagonists as indicated. Maintain adequate hydration (2–3 L of fluid per day).
RESPIRATORY ALKALOSIS Hyperventilation due to: • Extreme anxiety • Elevated body temperature • Overventilation with a mechanical ventilator • Hypoxia • Salicylate overdose Brainstem injury Fever Increased basal metabolic rate	Complaints of shortness of breath, chest tightness Light-headedness with circumoral paresthesias and numbness and tingling of the extremities Difficulty concentrating Tremulousness, blurred vision *Laboratory findings (in uncompensated respiratory alkalosis)*: Arterial blood pH > 7.45 $PaCO_2 < 35$ mmHg	Monitor vital signs and ABGs. Assist client to breathe more slowly. Help client breathe in a paper bag or apply a rebreather mask (to inhale CO_2).
METABOLIC ACIDOSIS Conditions that increase nonvolatile acids in the blood (e.g., renal impairment, diabetes mellitus, starvation) Conditions that decrease bicarbonate (e.g., prolonged diarrhea) Excessive infusion of chloride-containing IV fluids (e.g., NaCl) Excessive ingestion of acids such as salicylates Cardiac arrest	Kussmaul's respirations (deep, rapid respirations) Lethargy, confusion Headache Weakness Nausea and vomiting *Laboratory findings*: Arterial blood pH < 7.35 Serum bicarbonate less than 22 mEq/L $PaCO_2 < 38$ mmHg with respiratory compensation	Monitor ABG values, intake and output, and LOC. Administer IV sodium bicarbonate carefully if ordered. Treat underlying problem as ordered.
METABOLIC ALKALOSIS Excessive acid losses due to: • Vomiting • Gastric suction Excessive use of potassium-losing diuretics Excessive adrenal corticoid hormones due to: • Cushing's syndrome • Hyperaldosteronism Excessive bicarbonate intake from: • Antacids • Parenteral $NaHCO_3$	Decreased respiratory rate and depth Dizziness Circumoral paresthesias, numbness and tingling of the extremities Hypertonic muscles, tetany *Laboratory findings*: Arterial blood pH > 7.45 Serum bicarbonate > 26 mEq/L $PaCO_2 > 45$ mmHg with respiratory compensation	Monitor intake and output closely. Monitor vital signs, especially respirations, and LOC. Administer ordered IV fluids carefully. Treat underlying problem.

history, (b) physical assessment of the client, (c) clinical measurements, and (d) review of laboratory test results.

Nursing History

The nursing history is particularly important for identifying clients who are at risk for fluid, electrolyte, and acid–base imbalances. A client's current and past medical history reveals conditions such as chronic lung disease or diabetes mellitus that can disrupt normal balances. Medications prescribed to treat acute or chronic conditions (e.g., diuretic therapy for hypertension) also may place a client at risk for altered homeostasis. Functional, developmental, and socioeconomic factors must also be considered in assessing a client's risk. Older adults and very young children, clients who must depend on others to meet their nutrition and hydration needs, and individuals who cannot afford or do not have the means to cook food for a balanced diet (e.g., homeless individuals) are at greater risk for fluid and electrolyte imbalances. Common risk factors are listed in Box 51.2.

BOX 51.2 Common Risk Factors for Fluid, Electrolyte, and Acid–Base Imbalances

CHRONIC DISEASES AND CONDITIONS
- Chronic lung disease (COPD, asthma, cystic fibrosis)
- Heart failure
- Kidney disease
- Diabetes mellitus
- Cushing's syndrome or Addison's disease
- Cancer
- Malnutrition, anorexia nervosa, bulimia
- Ileostomy

ACUTE CONDITIONS
- Acute gastroenteritis
- Bowel obstruction
- Head injury or decreased level of consciousness
- Trauma such as burns or crushing injuries
- Surgery
- Fever, draining wounds, fistulas

MEDICATIONS
- Diuretics
- Corticosteroids
- Nonsteroidal anti-inflammatory drugs

TREATMENTS
- Chemotherapy
- IV therapy and total parenteral nutrition
- Nasogastric suction
- Enteral feedings
- Mechanical ventilation

OTHER FACTORS
- Age: Very old or very young
- Inability to access food and fluids independently

When obtaining a nursing history, the nurse needs to not only recognize risk factors but also gather data about the client's food and fluid intake, fluid output, and the presence of signs or symptoms suggestive of altered fluid and electrolyte balance. The Assessment Interview provides examples of questions to elicit information regarding fluid, electrolyte, and acid–base balance.

Physical Assessment

Physical assessment to evaluate a client's fluid, electrolyte, and acid–base status focuses on the skin, the oral cavity and mucous membranes, the eyes, the cardiovascular and respiratory systems, and neurologic and muscular status. Data from this physical assessment are used to expand and verify information obtained in the nursing history. Refer to Tables 51.5 through 51.9 for possible abnormal findings related to specific imbalances.

Clinical Measurements

Three simple clinical measurements that the nurse can initiate without a primary care provider's order are daily weights, vital signs, and fluid intake and output.

Daily Weights

Daily weights provide a relatively accurate assessment of a client's fluid status. Significant changes in weight over a short time, for example, more than 2.3 kg (5 lb) in a week or more than 1 kg (2.2 lb) in 24 hours, are indicative of acute fluid changes. Each kilogram (2.2 lb) of weight gained or lost corresponds to 1 L of fluid gained or lost. Such fluid gains or losses indicate changes in total body fluid volume rather than in any specific compartment, such as the intravascular compartment. Rapid losses or gains of 5% to 8% of total body weight indicate moderate to severe fluid volume deficits or excesses.

To obtain accurate weight measurements, the scale should be balanced before each use, and the client should be weighed (a) at the same time each day (e.g., before breakfast and after the first void), (b) wearing the same or similar clothing, and (c) on the same scale. The type of scale (i.e., standing, bed, or chair) should be documented.

Regular assessment of weight is particularly important for clients in the community and extended care facilities who are at risk for fluid imbalance. For these clients, measuring intake and output may be impractical because of lifestyle or problems with incontinence. Regular weight measurement, either daily, every other day, or weekly, provides valuable information about the client's fluid status.

Vital Signs

Changes in vital signs may indicate, or in some cases precede, fluid, electrolyte, and acid–base imbalances. For example, elevated body temperature may be a result of dehydration or a cause of increased body fluid losses.

Tachycardia is an early sign of hypovolemia. Pulse *volume* will decrease in FVD and increase in FVE. Irregular pulse rhythms may occur with electrolyte imbalances. Changes in respiratory rate and depth may cause respiratory acid–base imbalances or indicate a compensatory mechanism in metabolic acidosis or alkalosis.

Blood pressure (BP), a sensitive measure for detecting blood volume changes, may fall significantly with FVD and hypovolemia or increase with FVE. Postural, or orthostatic, hypotension may also occur with FVD and hypovolemia. To assess for orthostatic hypotension, measure the client's BP and pulse in a supine position. Allow the client to remain in that position for 3 to 5 minutes, leaving the blood pressure cuff on the arm. Ask the client to stand up and immediately reassess the BP and pulse. A drop of 10 to 15 mmHg in the systolic BP with a corresponding drop in diastolic pressure and an increased pulse rate (by 10 or more beats per minute) is indicative of orthostatic or postural hypotension.

Fluid Intake and Output

Measurement and recording of all fluid intake and output (I&O) during a 24-hour period provides important data

TABLE 51.9 Focused Physical Assessment for Fluid, Electrolyte, or Acid–Base Imbalances

System	Assessment Focus	Technique	Possible Abnormal Findings
Skin	Color, temperature, moisture Turgor Edema	Inspection, palpation Gently pinch up a fold of skin over sternum for adults, on the abdomen or medial thigh for children Inspect for visible swelling around eyes, in fingers, and in lower extremities Compress the skin over the dorsum of the foot, around the ankles, over the tibia, in the sacral area	Flushed, warm, very dry Moist or diaphoretic Cool and pale Poor turgor: Skin remains tented for several seconds instead of immediately returning to normal position Skin around eyes is puffy, lids appear swollen; rings are tight; shoes leave impressions on feet Depression remains (pitting): See scale for describing edema in Figure 51.9.
Mucous membranes	Color, moisture	Inspection	Mucous membranes dry, dull in appearance; tongue dry and cracked
Eyes	Firmness	Gently palpate eyeball with lid closed	Eyeball feels soft to palpation
Fontanels (infant)	Firmness, level	Inspect and gently palpate anterior fontanel	Fontanel bulging, firm Fontanel sunken, soft
Cardiovascular system	Heart rate Peripheral pulses Blood pressure Capillary refill Venous filling	Auscultation, cardiac monitor Palpation Auscultation of Korotkoff's sounds BP assessment lying and standing Palpation Inspection of jugular veins and hand veins	Tachycardia, bradycardia; irregular; dysrhythmias Weak and thready; bounding Hypotension Postural hypotension Slowed capillary refill Jugular venous distention; flat jugular veins, poor venous refill
Respiratory system	Respiratory rate and pattern	Inspection	Increased or decreased rate and depth of respirations
	Lung sounds	Auscultation	Crackles or moist rales
Neurologic	Level of consciousness (LOC) Orientation, cognition Motor function Reflexes Abnormal reflexes	Observation, stimulation Questioning Strength testing Deep-tendon reflex (DTR) testing *Chvostek's sign*: Tap over facial nerve about 2 cm anterior to tragus of ear *Trousseau's sign*: Inflate a blood pressure cuff on the upper arm to 20 mmHg greater than the systolic pressure, leave in place for 2–5 min	Decreased LOC, lethargy, stupor, or coma Disoriented, confused; difficulty concentrating Weakness, decreased motor strength Hyperactive or depressed DTRs Facial muscle twitching including eyelids and lips on side of stimulus Carpal spasm: contraction of hand and fingers on affected side

ASSESSMENT INTERVIEW Fluid, Electrolyte, and Acid–Base Balance

CURRENT AND PAST MEDICAL HISTORY

- Are you currently seeing a healthcare provider for treatment of any chronic diseases such as kidney disease, heart disease, lung disease, high blood pressure, diabetes mellitus, diabetes insipidus, or thyroid, parathyroid, or adrenal disorders?
- Have you recently experienced any acute conditions such as gastroenteritis, severe trauma, head injury, or surgery?

MEDICATIONS AND TREATMENTS

- Are you currently taking any medications on a regular basis such as diuretics, steroids, potassium supplements, calcium supplements, hormones, salt substitutes, or antacids?
- Have you recently undergone any treatments such as dialysis, parenteral nutrition, tube feedings, or been on a ventilator?

FOOD AND FLUID INTAKE

- How much and what type of fluids do you drink each day?
- Describe your diet for a typical day. (Pay particular attention to the client's intake of foods high in sodium, and of protein, whole grains, fruits, and vegetables.)
- Have there been any recent changes in your food or fluid intake, for example, as a result of following a weight-loss program?
- Are you on any type of restricted diet?
- Has your food or fluid intake recently been affected by changes in appetite, nausea, or other factors such as pain or difficulty breathing?

FLUID OUTPUT

- Have you noticed any recent changes in the frequency or amount of urine output?

Continued on page 1390

ASSESSMENT INTERVIEW Fluid, Electrolyte, and Acid–Base Balance—*continued*

- Have you recently experienced any problems with vomiting, diarrhea, or constipation?
- Have you noticed any other unusual fluid losses such as excessive sweating?

FLUID, ELECTROLYTE, AND ACID–BASE IMBALANCES

- Have you gained or lost weight in recent weeks?
- Have you recently experienced any symptoms such as excessive thirst, dry skin or mucous membranes, dark or concentrated urine, or low urine output?
- Do you have problems with swelling of your hands, feet, or ankles? Do you ever have difficulty breathing, especially when lying down or at night? How many pillows do you use to sleep?
- Have you recently experienced any of the following symptoms: difficulty concentrating or confusion; dizziness or feeling faint; muscle weakness, twitching, cramping, or spasm; excessive fatigue; abnormal sensations such as numbness, tingling, burning, or prickling; abdominal cramping or distention; heart palpitations?

about a client's fluid and electrolyte balance. Generally, I&O are measured for hospitalized clients, particularly those at increased risk for fluid and electrolyte imbalance.

The unit used to measure I&O is the milliliter (mL). In household measures, 30 mL is roughly equivalent to 1 fluid ounce, 500 mL to 1 pint, and 1000 mL to 1 quart. To measure fluid intake, nurses convert household measures such as a cup or soup bowl to metric units. Most agencies have a form for recording I&O, usually a bedside or computer record on which the nurse lists all items measured and the quantities per shift (Figure 51.12 ■).

Usually these forms provide conversion tables, since the sizes of dishes vary from agency to agency. Examples of equivalents are given in Box 51.3. Some agencies have a different form for recording the specifics of IV fluids, such as the type of solution, additives, time started, amount absorbed, and amount remaining per shift.

It is important to inform clients, family members, and all caregivers that accurate measurements of the client's fluid I&O are required, explaining why and emphasizing

BOX 51.3 Commonly Used Fluid Containers and Their Volumes

Water glass	200 mL
Juice glass	120 mL
Cup	180 mL
Soup bowl	
Adult	180 mL
Child	100 mL
Teapot	240 mL
Creamer	
Large	90 mL
Small	30 mL
Water pitcher	1000 mL
Jell-O, custard dish	100 mL
Ice cream dish	120 mL
Paper cup	
Large	200 mL
Small	120 mL

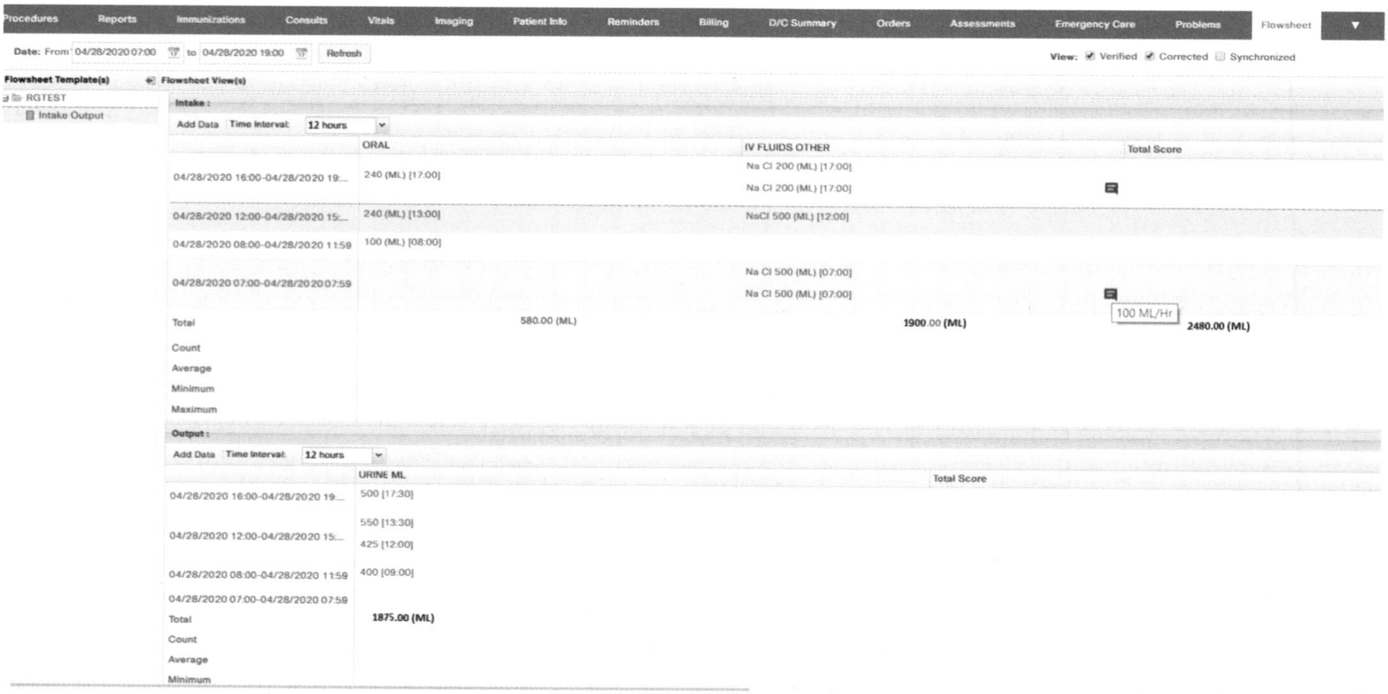

Procedures | Reports | Immunizations | Consults | Vitals | Imaging | Patient Info | Reminders | Billing | D/C Summary | Orders | Assessments | Emergency Care | Problems | Flowsheet

Date: From 04/28/2020 07:00 to 04/28/2020 19:00 Refresh

View: Verified Corrected Synchronized

Flowsheet Template(s): RGTEST — Intake Output

Flowsheet View(s)

Intake:

Add Data Time Interval: 12 hours

	ORAL	IV FLUIDS OTHER	Total Score
04/28/2020 16:00-04/28/2020 19:...	240 (ML) [17:00]	Na Cl 200 (ML) [17:00] Na Cl 200 (ML) [17:00]	
04/28/2020 12:00-04/28/2020 15:...	240 (ML) [13:00]	NaCl 500 (ML) [12:00]	
04/28/2020 08:00-04/28/2020 11:59	100 (ML) [08:00]		
04/28/2020 07:00-04/28/2020 07:59		Na Cl 500 (ML) [07:00] Na Cl 500 (ML) [07:00]	100 ML/Hr
Total	580.00 (ML)	1900.00 (ML)	2480.00 (ML)
Count			
Average			
Minimum			
Maximum			

Output:

Add Data Time Interval: 12 hours

	URINE ML	Total Score
04/28/2020 16:00-04/28/2020 19:...	500 [17:30]	
04/28/2020 12:00-04/28/2020 15:...	550 [13:30] 425 [12:00]	
04/28/2020 08:00-04/28/2020 11:59	400 [09:00]	
04/28/2020 07:00-04/28/2020 07:59		
Total	1875.00 (ML)	
Count		
Average		
Minimum		

Figure 51.12 ■ A sample EHR 24-hour fluid intake and output record.

the need to use a bedpan, urinal, commode, or in-toilet collection device (unless a urinary drainage system is in place). Instruct the client not to put toilet tissue into the container with urine. Clients who wish to be involved in recording fluid intake measurements need to be taught how to compute the values and what foods are considered fluids.

To measure fluid intake, each item of fluid consumed or administered is recorded, specifying the time and type of fluid. All of the following fluids need to be recorded:

- ***Oral fluids:*** Water, milk, juice, soft drinks, coffee, tea, cream, soup, and any other beverages. Include water taken with medications. To measure the amount of water consumed from a water pitcher, measure how much water remains in the pitcher and subtract this amount from the volume of the full pitcher.
- ***Ice chips:*** Record the fluid volume as approximately one-half the volume of the ice chips. For example, if the ice chips fill a cup holding 200 mL and the client consumed all of the ice chips, the volume consumed would be recorded as 100 mL.
- ***Foods that are or become liquid at room temperature:*** These include ice cream, sherbet, custard, and gelatin. Do not measure foods that are pureed, because purees are simply solid foods prepared in a different form.
- ***Tube feedings:*** Remember to include the volume of water used for flushes before and after medication administration, intermittent feedings, residual checks, or any other water given via a feeding tube.
- ***Parenteral fluids:*** The exact amount of IV fluid administered must be recorded, since some fluid containers may be overfilled. Blood transfusions are included in the total.
- ***IV medications:*** IV medications that are administered as an intermittent or continuous infusion must also be included (e.g., ceftazidime 1 g in 50 mL of sterile water). Most IV medications are mixed in 50 to 100 mL of solution.
- ***Catheter or tube irrigants:*** Fluid used to irrigate urinary catheters, nasogastric tubes, and intestinal tubes must be recorded if not immediately withdrawn as part of the irrigation.

To measure fluid output, measure the following fluids (remember to observe appropriate infection control precautions):

- ***Urinary output:*** Following each voiding, pour the urine into a measuring container, note the amount, and record the amount and time on the I&O form. For clients with retention catheters, empty the drainage bag into a measuring container at the end of the shift (or at prescribed times if output is to be measured more often). Note and record the amount of urine output. In intensive care areas, urine output often is measured hourly. If a client is incontinent of urine, estimate and record these outputs. For example, for an incontinent client the nurse might record "Incontinent × 3" or "Drawsheet soaked in 12-in. diameter." A more accurate estimate of the urine output of infants and incontinent clients may be obtained by first weighing diapers or incontinence pads that are dry, and then subtracting this weight from the weight of the soiled items. Each gram of weight left after subtracting is equal to 1 mL of urine. If urine is frequently soiled with feces, the number of voidings may be recorded rather than the volume of urine.
- ***Vomitus and liquid feces:*** The amount and type of fluid and the time need to be specified.
- ***Tube drainage:*** This includes gastric or intestinal drainage.
- ***Wound and fistula drainage:*** Drainage may be recorded by documenting the type and number of dressings or linen saturated with drainage, or by measuring the exact amount of drainage collected in a vacuum drainage (e.g., Hemovac) or gravity drainage system.

Fluid I&O measurements are totaled at the end of the shift (every 8 to 12 hours), and the totals are recorded in a client's chart. In intensive care areas, nurses may record I&O hourly. Usually the staff on the night shift totals the amounts of I&O recorded for each shift and records the 24-hour total.

To determine whether fluid output is proportional to fluid intake, or whether there are any changes in a client's fluid status, (a) compare the total 24-hour fluid output measurement with the total 24-hour fluid intake measurement and (b) compare both to previous measurements. Urinary output is normally equivalent to the amount of fluid intake; the usual range is 1500 to 2000 mL in 24 hours, or 40 to 80 mL in 1 hour (0.5 mL/kg per hour). Clients whose output substantially exceeds intake are at risk for fluid volume deficit, whereas clients whose intake substantially exceeds output are at risk for fluid volume excess. In assessing a client's fluid balance it is important to consider additional factors that may affect I&O. For example, a client who is extremely diaphoretic or has rapid, deep respirations has fluid losses that cannot be measured but must still be considered in evaluating fluid status.

When there is a significant discrepancy between intake and output or when fluid intake or output is inadequate (for example, a urine output of less than 30 mL/h in an adult), this information should be reported to the primary care provider.

Laboratory Tests

Many laboratory studies are conducted to determine a client's fluid, electrolyte, and acid–base status. Some of the more common tests are discussed here.

Serum Electrolytes

Serum electrolyte levels are often ordered for clients admitted to the hospital as a screening test for electrolyte and acid–base imbalances. Serum electrolytes also are routinely assessed for clients at risk in the community, for example, clients who are being treated with a diuretic for hypertension or heart failure. The most commonly ordered serum tests are for sodium, potassium, chloride, magnesium, and bicarbonate ions. Normal values of commonly measured electrolytes are shown in Box 51.4. Some primary care providers use a diagram format for keeping track of the client's electrolytes when documenting in their progress notes (Figure 51.13 ■).

BOX 51.4 Normal Electrolyte Values for Adults*

Venous Blood	
Sodium	135–145 mEq/L
Potassium	3.5–5.0 mEq/L
Chloride	95–108 mEq/L
Calcium, total	4.5–5.5 mEq/L or 8.5–10.5 mg/dL
Calcium, ionized	56% of total calcium (2.5 mEq/L or 4.0–5.0 mg/dL)
Magnesium	1.5–2.5 mEq/L or 1.6–2.5 mg/dL
Phosphate (phosphorus)	1.8–2.6 mEq/L or 2.5–4.5 mg/dL
Serum osmolality	280–300 mOsm/kg water

*Normal laboratory values vary from agency to agency.

Complete Blood Count

A complete blood count (CBC), another basic screening test, includes information about **hematocrit (Hct)**, which measures the percentage of the volume of whole blood that is composed of RBCs. Hematocrit is a measure of the volume of cells in relation to plasma and is, therefore, affected by changes in plasma volume; hematocrit increases with dehydration and decreases with overhydration. Normal hematocrit values are 40% to 54% in men and 37% to 47% in women.

Osmolality

Serum osmolality is a measure of the solute concentration of blood. The particles included are sodium ions, glucose, and urea (blood urea nitrogen, or BUN). Serum osmolality can be estimated by doubling the serum sodium value, because sodium and its associated chloride ions are the major determinants of serum osmolality. Serum osmolality is used primarily to evaluate fluid balance. Normal values are 280 to 300 mOsm/kg. An increase in serum osmolality indicates a fluid volume deficit; a decrease reflects a fluid volume excess.

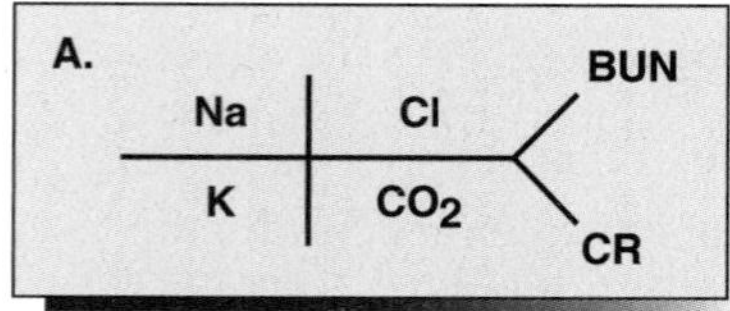

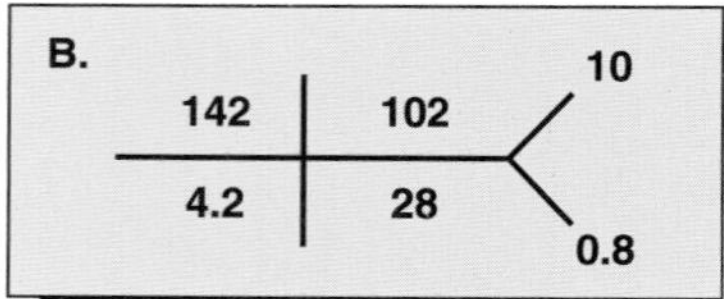

Figure 51.13 ■ *A*, Format for a diagram of serum electrolyte results; *B*, example that may be seen in a primary care provider's documentation notes.

Urine osmolality is a measure of the solute concentration of urine. The particles included are nitrogenous wastes, such as creatinine, urea, and uric acid. Normal values are 500 to 800 mOsm/kg. An increased urine osmolality indicates a fluid volume deficit; a decreased urine osmolality reflects a fluid volume excess.

Urine Specific Gravity

Specific gravity is an indicator of urine concentration that correlates with urine osmolality, and it can be measured quickly and easily by nursing personnel. Normal specific gravity ranges from 1.005 to 1.030 (usually 1.010 to 1.025). When urine osmolality is high, in fluid volume deficit, the specific gravity rises; when urine osmolality is low, in fluid volume excess, the specific gravity is low.

Urine pH

Measurement of urine pH may be obtained by laboratory analysis or by using a dipstick on a freshly voided specimen. Because the kidneys play a critical role in regulating acid–base balance, assessment of urine pH can be useful in determining whether the kidneys are responding appropriately to acid–base imbalances. Normally the pH of the urine is relatively acidic, averaging about 6.0, but a range of 4.6 to 8.0 is considered normal. In metabolic acidosis, urine pH should decrease as the kidneys retain bicarbonate and excrete hydrogen ions; in metabolic alkalosis, the pH should increase as the kidneys retain hydrogen ions and excrete bicarbonate.

Arterial Blood Gases

Arterial blood gases (ABGs) are performed to evaluate a client's acid–base balance and oxygenation. Arterial blood is used because it provides a more accurate reflection of gas exchange in the pulmonary system than venous blood. Blood gases may be drawn by laboratory technicians, respiratory therapy personnel, or nurses with specialized skills. Because a high-pressure artery is used to obtain blood, it is important to apply pressure to the puncture site for at least 5 minutes after the procedure to reduce the risk of bleeding or bruising.

Six measurements are commonly used to interpret arterial blood gas tests:

- pH is a measure of the relative acidity or alkalinity of the blood, and is an inverse measure of the number of hydrogen ions in a solution. The normal range for arterial pH is narrow, and death may ensue with pH values below 6.8 or above 7.8.
- PaO_2 is the partial pressure of oxygen dissolved in arterial plasma, and is an indirect measure of blood oxygen content. PaO_2 represents one of the two forms in which oxygen is transported in blood, and accounts for only about 3% of the oxygen content of the blood.
- $PaCO_2$ is the partial pressure of carbon dioxide in arterial plasma, and is the respiratory component of acid–base determination. Because carbon dioxide is regulated by the lungs, $PaCO_2$ is used to determine if an acid–base imbalance is respiratory in origin.
- HCO_3^- is a measure of the bicarbonate dissolved in arterial plasma, and represents the metabolic component of acid–base balance.

- Base excess (BE) is a calculated value of bicarbonate levels, also reflective of the metabolic component of acid–base balance. If the number is preceded by a plus sign, it represents a base excess; a BE above +2 indicates alkalosis. If the number is preceded by a minus sign, it represents a base deficit; a BE below −2 indicates acidosis.
- SpO_2 is oxygen saturation, which represents the percentage of hemoglobin that is combined (saturated) with oxygen. SpO_2 is the other form in which oxygen is transported in the blood and accounts for about 97% of the oxygen in the blood.

Normal ABG values are listed in Table 51.10 along with changes associated with common acid–base imbalances. Note that although the PaO_2 and SpO_2 are important for assessing respiratory status, they generally do not provide useful information for assessing acid–base balance and so are not included in this table.

When evaluating ABG results to determine acid–base balance, it is important to use a systematic approach such as the one outlined in Box 51.5. Nurses need to assess each measurement individually, and then look at the interrelationships to determine what type of acid–base imbalance may be present.

TABLE 51.10 Arterial Blood Gas Values

NORMAL VALUES OF ARTERIAL BLOOD GASES*

pH	7.35–7.45
PaO_2	80–100 mmHg
$PaCO_2$	35–45 mmHg
HCO_3^-	22–26 mEq/L
Base excess	−2 to +2 mEq/L
O_2 saturation	95–98%

ARTERIAL BLOOD GAS VALUES IN COMMON ACID–BASE DISORDERS

Disorder		ABG Values
Respiratory acidosis	pH	<7.35
	$PaCO_2$	>45 mmHg (excess CO_2 and carbonic acid)
	HCO_3^-	Normal (or >26 mEq/L with renal compensation)
Respiratory alkalosis	pH	>7.45
	$PaCO_2$	<35 mmHg (inadequate CO_2 and carbonic acid)
	HCO_3^-	Normal (or <22 mEq/L with renal compensation)
Metabolic acidosis	pH	<7.35
	$PaCO_2$	Normal (or <35 mmHg with respiratory compensation)
	HCO_3^-	<22 mEq/L (inadequate bicarbonate)
Metabolic alkalosis	pH	>7.45
	$PaCO_2$	Normal (or >45 mmHg with respiratory compensation)
	HCO_3^-	>26 mEq/L (excess bicarbonate)

*Some normal values will vary according to the kind of test carried out in the laboratory. Nurses are advised to use the normal values issued by the agency when interpreting laboratory results.

BOX 51.5 Interpreting ABGs—Do You Have a Match?

1. Look at each number separately.
   - Label the pH:
     - If the pH is less than 7.35, the problem is acidosis.
     - If the pH is greater than 7.45, the problem is alkalosis.
   - Label the $PaCO_2$:
     - If the $PaCO_2$ is less than 35 mmHg, more carbon dioxide is being exhaled than normal and indicates respiratory alkalosis or compensation for a metabolic imbalance.
     - If the $PaCO_2$ is greater than 45 mmHg, less carbon dioxide is being exhaled than normal and indicates respiratory acidosis or compensation for a metabolic imbalance.
   - Label the bicarbonate:
     - If the HCO_3^- is less than 22 mEq/L, bicarbonate levels are lower than normal, indicating metabolic acidosis or compensation for a respiratory imbalance.
     - If the HCO_3^- is greater than 26 mEq/L, bicarbonate levels are higher than normal, indicating metabolic alkalosis or compensation for a respiratory imbalance.
2. Determine the cause of the acid–base imbalance.
   - Look at the pH—is it acidosis, alkalosis, or within the normal range?
3. Determine if the origin of the imbalance is respiratory or metabolic.
   - Check the $PaCO_2$ and HCO_3^-. Which one corresponds with the same acid–base status as the pH?

     EXAMPLE

     pH = 7.33 (acidosis)

     $PaCO_2$ = 55 (acidosis)

     HCO_3 = 29 (alkalosis)

     $PaCO_2$ (acidosis) MATCHES the pH (acidosis) = respiratory problem

     Client has respiratory acidosis.
4. Look for evidence of compensation.
   - Look at the value that does **not** match the pH:

     EXAMPLES

     a. In respiratory acidosis (pH $<$ 7.35, $PaCO_2$ $>$ 45 mmHg), if the HCO_3^- is greater than 26 mEq/L, the kidneys are retaining bicarbonate to minimize the acidosis: renal compensation.

     b. In respiratory alkalosis (pH $>$ 7.45, $PaCO_2$ $<$35 mmHg), if the HCO_3^- is less than 22 mEq/L, the kidneys are excreting bicarbonate to minimize the alkalosis: renal compensation.

     c. In metabolic acidosis (pH $<$ 7.35, HCO_3^- $<$ 22 mEq/L), if the $PaCO_2$ is less than 35 mmHg, carbon dioxide is being eliminated to minimize the acidosis: respiratory compensation.

     d. In metabolic alkalosis (pH $>$ 7.45, HCO_3^- $>$26 mEq/L), if the $PaCO_2$ is greater than 45 mmHg, carbon dioxide is being retained to compensate for excess base: respiratory compensation.

Note: If the pH is within normal range, the body has completely compensated. Complete metabolic compensation takes time to develop and is the result of a chronic condition (e.g., chronic respiratory acidosis with COPD). If the pH is not within the normal range, compensation is partial.

Diagnosing

Examples of diagnoses for clients with fluid and acid–base imbalances can include actual or potential for: decreased fluid volume, increased fluid volume, and altered gas exchange. Clinical applications of selected diagnoses are shown in the Nursing Care Plan and the Concept Map at the end of this chapter.

Fluid, electrolyte, and acid–base imbalances affect many other body areas and as a consequence may be the etiology of other nursing diagnoses, such as dry mucous membranes related to fluid volume deficit; skin breakdown related to dehydration or edema; inadequate cardiac output related to hypovolemia or cardiac dysrhythmias secondary to electrolyte imbalance (K^+ or Mg^{2+}); risk for injury (e.g., dizziness, orthostatic hypotension) related to hypovolemia; confusion related to electrolyte imbalance.

Planning

When planning care a nurse identifies nursing interventions that will assist the client to achieve these broad goals:

- Maintain or restore normal fluid balance.
- Maintain or restore normal balance of electrolytes in the intracellular and extracellular compartments.
- Maintain or restore gas exchange and oxygenation.
- Prevent associated risks (e.g., tissue breakdown, decreased cardiac output, confusion, other neurologic signs).

Goals will vary according to the diagnosis and defining characteristics for each client. Appropriate preventive and corrective nursing interventions that relate to these must be identified. Specific nursing activities can be selected to meet a client's individual needs. Examples of application of these using NIC and NOC designations are shown in the Nursing Care Plan and the Concept Map at the end of this chapter. Examples of NIC interventions related to fluid, electrolyte, and acid–base balance include the following:

- Acid–base management
- Electrolyte management
- Fluid monitoring
- Hypovolemia management
- Intravenous (IV) therapy.

Specific nursing activities associated with each of these interventions can be selected to meet the individual needs of the client.

Nursing activities to meet goals and outcomes related to fluid, electrolyte, and acid–base imbalances are discussed in the next section. These include (a) monitoring fluid intake and output, cardiovascular and respiratory status, and results of laboratory tests; (b) assessing the client's weight, location and extent of edema if present, skin turgor and skin status, specific gravity of urine, and level of consciousness and mental status; (c) fluid intake modifications; (d) dietary changes; (e) parenteral fluid, electrolyte, and blood replacement; and (f) other appropriate measures such as administering prescribed medications and oxygen, providing skin care and oral hygiene, positioning the client appropriately, and scheduling rest periods.

Planning for Home Care

To provide for continuity of care, a client's needs for assistance with care in the home need to be considered. Home care planning includes assessment of a client's and family's resources and abilities for care, and the need for referrals and home health services.

QSEN Patient-Centered Care: Assessing Fluid, Electrolyte, and Acid–Base Balance

To establish a home care plan, the nurse needs to assess specific data such as the following:

CLIENT

- *Risk factors for imbalances:* the client's age, medications such as diuretic therapy or corticosteroids, and presence of chronic diseases such as diabetes mellitus, heart disease, lung disease, or dementia (see Box 51.2 on page 1388)
- *Self-care abilities for maintaining food and fluid intake:* mobility; ability to chew and swallow; ability to access fluids and respond to thirst, to purchase food, and prepare a balanced diet
- *Current level of knowledge (as appropriate):* prescribed diet, any fluid restrictions, activity restrictions, actions and side effects of prescribed medications, regular weight monitoring, gastric tube care and enteral feedings, central line or PICC catheter care, and parenteral fluids and nutrition

FAMILY

- *Caregiver availability, skills, and responses:* availability and willingness to assume responsibility for care, knowledge and ability to provide assistance with preparing food and maintaining adequate intake of food and fluids, knowledge of risk factors and early warning signs of problems
- *Family role changes and coping:* effect on financial status, parenting and spousal roles, social roles
- *Alternate potential primary or respite caregivers:* other family members, friends, volunteers, church members, paid caregivers or housekeeping services; available community respite care (e.g., adult day care, senior centers)

COMMUNITY

- *Current knowledge of and experience with community resources:* home health agencies, organizations that offer financial assistance or assistance with food preparation, Meals on Wheels or meal services (e.g., at senior centers, homeless shelters), pharmacies, home IV services, and respiratory care services

Based on the data gathered in assessment of the home situation, the nurse tailors the teaching plan for the client and family (see Client Teaching).

CLIENT TEACHING Promoting Fluid and Electrolyte Balance

- Consume six to eight glasses of water daily.
- Avoid excess amounts of foods or fluids high in salt, sugar, and caffeine.
- Eat a well-balanced diet. Include adequate amounts of milk, milk products, or calcium-enriched alternatives to maintain bone calcium levels.
- Limit alcohol intake because it has a diuretic effect.
- Increase fluid intake before, during, and after strenuous exercise, particularly when the environmental temperature is high, and replace lost electrolytes from excessive perspiration as needed with commercial electrolyte solutions.
- Maintain normal body weight and body mass index for age and gender.
- Learn about and monitor side effects of medications that affect fluid and electrolyte balance (e.g., diuretics) and ways to handle side effects.
- Recognize possible risk factors for fluid and electrolyte imbalance such as prolonged or repeated vomiting, frequent watery stools, or inability to consume fluids because of illness.
- Seek prompt professional healthcare for notable signs of fluid imbalance such as sudden weight gain or loss, decreased urine volume, swollen ankles, shortness of breath, dizziness, or confusion.

CLIENT TEACHING Home Care and Fluid, Electrolyte, and Acid–Base Balance

MONITORING FLUID INTAKE AND OUTPUT

- Teach and provide the rationale for monitoring fluid intake and output to the client and family as appropriate, for example, how to use a commode or collection device ("hat") in the toilet, how to empty and measure urinary catheter drainage, or how to count or weigh diapers.
- Instruct and provide the rationale for regular weight monitoring to the client and family, including weighing at the same time every day, using the same scale, and with the client wearing the same amount of clothing.
- Educate and provide the rationale to the client and family on when to contact a healthcare professional, such as in the cases of a significant change in urine output; any change of 2.2 kilograms (5 pounds) or more in a 1- to 2-week period or 1 kilogram (2 pounds) or more in 24 hours; prolonged episodes of vomiting, diarrhea, or inability to eat or drink; dry, sticky mucous membranes; extreme thirst; swollen fingers, feet, ankles, or legs; difficulty breathing, shortness of breath, need for an increased number of pillows to sleep on, or rapid heartbeat; and changes in behavior or mental status.

MAINTAINING FOOD AND FLUID INTAKE

- Instruct the client and family about any diet or fluid restrictions, such as a low-sodium diet.
- Teach family members the rationale for the importance of offering fluids regularly to clients who are unable to meet their own needs because of age, impaired mobility or cognition, or other conditions such as impaired swallowing due to a stroke.
- If the client is on enteral or IV fluids and feeding at home, teach and provide rationales to caregivers about proper administration and care. Contact a home health or home IV service to provide services and teaching.

SAFETY

- Instruct and provide the rationale to the client for changing positions slowly if appropriate, especially when moving from a supine to a sitting or standing position.
- Inform and provide the rationale to the client and family about the importance of good mouth and skin care. Teach the client to change positions frequently and to elevate the feet when sitting for a long period.
- Teach the client and family how to care for IV access sites or gastric tubes. Include what to do if tubes become dislodged.

MEDICATIONS

- Emphasize the importance of and rationale for taking medications as prescribed.
- Instruct clients taking diuretics to take the medication in the morning. If a second daily dose is prescribed, they should take it in the late afternoon to avoid disrupting sleep to urinate.
- Inform clients about any expected side effects of prescribed medications and how to handle them (e.g., if a potassium-depleting diuretic is prescribed, increase intake of potassium-rich foods; if taking a potassium-sparing diuretic, avoid excess potassium intake such as using a salt substitute).
- Teach clients when to contact their primary care provider, for example, if they are unable to take a prescribed medication or have signs of an allergic or toxic reaction to a medication.

MEASURES SPECIFIC TO CLIENT'S PROBLEM

- Provide instructions and rationales specific to the client's fluid, electrolyte, or acid–base imbalance, such as:
  a. Fluid volume deficit
  b. Risk for fluid volume deficit
  c. Fluid volume excess
  d. Risk for fluid volume excess.

REFERRALS

- Make appropriate referrals to home health or community social services for assistance with resources such as meals, meal preparation and food delivery, IV infusions and access, enteral feedings, and homemaker or home health aide services to help with ADLs.

COMMUNITY AGENCIES AND OTHER SOURCES OF HELP

- Provide information about companies or agencies that can provide durable medical equipment such as commodes, lift chairs, or hospital beds for purchase, rental, or free of charge.
- Provide a list of sources for supplies such as catheters and drainage bags, measuring devices, tube feeding formulas, and electrolyte replacement drinks.
- Suggest additional sources of information and help such as the American Dietetic Association, the American Heart Association, and the American Lung Association.

PRACTICE GUIDELINES Facilitating Fluid Intake

- Explain to the client the reason for the required intake and the specific amount needed. This provides a rationale for the requirement and promotes compliance.
- Establish a 24-hour plan for ingesting the fluids. For a hospitalized or long-term care client, half of the total volume is given during the day shift, and the other half is divided between the evening and night shifts, with most of that ingested during the evening shift. For example, if 2500 mL is to be ingested in 24 hours, the plan may specify 7–3 (1500 mL); 3–11 (700 mL); and 11–7 (300 mL). Try to avoid the ingestion of large amounts of fluid immediately before bedtime to prevent the need to urinate during sleeping hours.
- Set short-term outcomes that the client can realistically meet. Examples include ingesting a glass of fluid every hour while awake or a pitcher of water by lunchtime.
- Identify fluids the client likes and make available a variety of those items, including fruit juices, noncaffeinated soft drinks, and milk (if allowed). Remember that beverages such as coffee, tea, and other caffeinated beverages have a diuretic effect, so their consumption should be limited.
- Help the client to select foods that tend to become liquid at room temperature (e.g., gelatin, ice cream, sherbet, custard), if these are allowed.
- For clients who are confined to bed, supply appropriate cups, glasses, and straws to facilitate adequate fluid intake, and keep fluids within easy reach.
- Make sure fluids are served at the appropriate temperature (i.e., hot fluids hot and cold fluids cold) and according to client preference.
- Encourage clients to participate in maintaining the fluid intake record if possible. This assists them to evaluate the achievement of desired outcomes.
- Be alert to any cultural implications of food and fluids. Some cultures may restrict certain foods and fluids, or temperatures of foods and fluids, and view others as having healing properties.

Implementing

Promoting Wellness

Most individuals rarely think about their fluid, electrolyte, or acid–base balance. They know it is important to drink adequate fluids and consume a balanced diet, but they may not understand the potential effects when this is not done. Nurses can promote clients' health by providing wellness teaching that will help them maintain fluid and electrolyte balance.

Enteral Fluid and Electrolyte Replacement

Fluids and electrolytes can be provided orally in the home or hospital if a client's health permits, meaning that the client is not vomiting, has not experienced an excessive fluid loss, and has an intact gastrointestinal tract and gag and swallow reflexes. Clients who are unable to ingest solid foods may be able to ingest fluids.

Fluid Intake Modifications

Increased fluids (ordered as "push fluids") are often prescribed for clients with actual or potential decreased fluid volume arising, for example, from mild diarrhea or mild to moderate fevers. Guidelines for helping clients increase fluid intake are shown in Practice Guidelines.

Restricted fluids may be necessary for clients who have fluid retention (increased fluid volume) as a result of kidney failure, heart failure, SIADH, or other disease processes. Fluid restrictions vary from "nothing by mouth" to a precise amount ordered by a primary care provider. The restriction of fluids can be difficult for some clients, particularly if they are experiencing thirst. Guidelines for helping clients restrict fluid intake are shown in Practice Guidelines.

Dietary Changes

Specific fluid and electrolyte imbalances may require simple dietary changes. For example, clients receiving potassium-depleting diuretics need to be informed about foods with high potassium content (e.g., bananas, oranges, and leafy greens). Some clients with fluid retention need to avoid foods high in sodium. Most healthy clients can benefit from foods rich in calcium.

PRACTICE GUIDELINES Helping Clients Restrict Fluid Intake

- Explain the reason for the restricted intake and how much and what types of fluids are permitted orally. Many clients need to be informed that ice chips, gelatin, and ice cream, for example, are considered fluid.
- Help the client decide the amount of fluid to be taken with each meal, between meals, before bedtime, and with medications. For a hospitalized or long-term care client, half the total volume is usually scheduled during the day shift, when the client is most active, receives two meals, and takes most oral medications. A large part of the remainder is scheduled for the evening shift to permit fluids with meals and evening visitors.
- Identify fluids or fluid-like substances the client likes and make sure that these are provided, unless contraindicated. A client who is allowed only 200 mL of fluid for breakfast, for example, should receive the type of fluid he or she prefers.
- Set short-term goals that make the fluid restriction more tolerable. For example, schedule a specified amount of fluid at one or two hourly intervals between meals. Some clients may prefer fluids only between meals if the food provided at mealtime helps relieve thirst.
- Place allowed fluids in small containers such as a 4-ounce juice glass to allow the perception of a full container.
- Periodically offer the client ice chips as an alternative to water, because ice chips are approximately half of the frozen volume after they melt.
- Provide frequent mouth care and rinses to reduce the thirst sensation.
- Instruct the client to avoid ingesting or chewing salty or sweet foods (hard candy or gum), because these foods tend to produce thirst. Sugarless gum or candy may be an alternative for some clients.
- Encourage the client to participate in maintaining the fluid intake record if possible.

Oral Electrolyte Supplements

Some clients can benefit from oral electrolyte supplements, particularly when a medication is prescribed that affects electrolyte balance, when dietary intake is inadequate for a specific electrolyte, or when fluid and electrolyte losses are excessive, for example, as a result of excessive perspiration.

Corticosteroids and many diuretics can cause too much potassium to be eliminated through the kidneys. For clients taking these medications, potassium supplements may be prescribed. Instruct clients taking oral potassium supplements to take the medication with juice to mask the unpleasant taste and reduce the possibility of gastric distress. Emphasize the importance of taking the medication as prescribed and seeing their primary care provider on a regular basis. Because hyperkalemia can have serious cardiac effects, clients should never increase the amount of potassium being taken without an order to do so. In addition, inform clients that most salt substitutes contain potassium, so it is important to consult with their primary care provider before using salt substitutes.

Individuals who ingest insufficient milk and milk products benefit from calcium supplements. The recommended daily allowance for calcium is 1000 to 1500 mg. It is generally recommended that postmenopausal women take 1500 mg of calcium per day to reduce the risk of osteoporosis. Long-term use of corticosteroid drugs can also cause calcium loss from the bone, and calcium supplements may help reduce this loss. Clients who take supplemental calcium need to maintain a fluid intake of at least 2500 mL per day (unless contraindicated) to reduce the risk of kidney stones, which are commonly composed of calcium salts.

Although routine supplements for other electrolytes generally are not recommended, clients who have poor dietary habits, who are malnourished, or who have difficulty accessing or eating fresh fruits and vegetables may benefit from electrolyte supplements. A daily multiple vitamin with minerals may achieve the desired goal. Individuals who engage in strenuous activity in a warm environment need to be encouraged to replace water and electrolytes lost through excessive perspiration by consuming a sports drink through available commercial fluid and electrolyte solutions.

Liquid nutritional supplements are often given to clients who are malnourished or have poor eating habits. They are used with frequency in older adults to bolster nutritional status and caloric intake. It is very important that clients read product labels accurately to be aware of the contents of the supplement. Some of them are very high in protein and high in potassium, which may be contraindicated in an individual with impaired kidney function.

Parenteral Fluid and Electrolyte Replacement

IV fluid therapy is essential when clients are unable to take sufficient food and fluids orally. It is an efficient and effective method of supplying fluids directly into the intravascular fluid compartment and replacing electrolyte losses. The primary care provider usually orders the IV fluid therapy. The nurse is responsible for administering and maintaining the therapy and for teaching the client and significant others how to continue the therapy at home if necessary.

Intravenous Solutions

IV solutions can be classified as isotonic, hypotonic, or hypertonic. Most IV solutions are isotonic, having the same concentration of solutes as blood plasma. Isotonic solutions are often used to restore vascular volume. Hypertonic solutions have a greater concentration of solutes than plasma; hypotonic solutions have a lesser concentration of solutes. Table 51.11 provides examples of IV solutions and nursing implications.

IV solutions can also be categorized according to their purpose. Nutrient solutions contain some form of carbohydrate (e.g., dextrose, glucose, or levulose) and water. Water is supplied for fluid requirements and carbohydrate for calories and energy. For example, 1 L of 5% dextrose provides 170 calories. Nutrient solutions are useful in

TABLE 51.11 Selected Intravenous Solutions

Type/Examples	Comments/Nursing Implications
ISOTONIC SOLUTIONS 0.9% NACL (normal saline) Lactated Ringer's (a balanced electrolyte solution) 5% dextrose in water (D_5W)	Isotonic solutions such as normal saline (NS) and lactated Ringer's initially remain in the vascular compartment, expanding vascular volume. Assess clients carefully for signs of hypervolemia such as bounding pulse and shortness of breath. D_5W is isotonic on initial administration but provides free water when dextrose is metabolized, expanding intracellular and extracellular fluid volumes. D_5W is avoided in clients at risk for increased intracranial pressure (IICP) because it can increase cerebral edema.
HYPOTONIC SOLUTIONS 0.45% NaCl (half normal saline) 0.33% NaCl (one-third normal saline)	Hypotonic solutions are used to provide free water and treat cellular dehydration. These solutions promote waste elimination by the kidneys. Do not administer to clients at risk for IICP or third-space fluid shift.
HYPERTONIC SOLUTIONS 5% dextrose in normal saline (D_5NS) 5% dextrose in 0.45% NaCl (D_5 1/2NS) 5% dextrose in lactated Ringer's (D_5LR)	Hypertonic solutions draw fluid out of the intracellular and interstitial compartments into the vascular compartment, expanding vascular volume. Do not administer to clients with kidney or heart disease or clients who are dehydrated. Watch for signs of hypervolemia.

preventing dehydration and ketosis but do not provide sufficient calories to promote wound healing, weight gain, or normal growth in children. Common nutrient solutions are 5% dextrose in water (D_5W) and 5% dextrose in 0.45% sodium chloride (dextrose in half-normal saline).

Electrolyte solutions contain varying amounts of cations and anions. Commonly used solutions are normal saline (0.9% sodium chloride solution), Ringer's solution (which contains sodium, chloride, potassium, and calcium), and lactated Ringer's solution (which contains sodium, chloride, potassium, calcium, and lactate). Lactate is metabolized in the liver to form bicarbonate. Saline and balanced electrolyte solutions are commonly used to restore vascular volume, particularly after trauma or surgery. They also may be used to replace fluid and electrolytes for clients with continuing losses, for example, those experiencing gastric suction or wound drainage. Lactated Ringer's solution is an alkalizing solution that may be given to treat metabolic acidosis. Acidifying solutions, in contrast, are administered to counteract metabolic alkalosis. Examples of acidifying solutions are 5% dextrose in 0.45% sodium chloride and 0.9% sodium chloride solution.

Volume expanders are used to increase the blood volume following severe loss of blood (e.g., from hemorrhage) or loss of plasma (e.g., from severe burns, which draw large amounts of plasma from the bloodstream to the burn site). Examples of volume expanders are dextran, plasma, albumin, and Hespan (a synthetic plasma expander).

Peripheral Venous Access Site Selection

The site chosen for peripheral venous access (venipuncture) varies with the client's age, length of time an infusion is to run, the type of solution used, and the condition of veins. For adults, veins in the arm are commonly used; for infants, veins in the scalp and dorsal foot veins are often used. The larger veins of the adult's forearm are preferred over the metacarpal veins of the hand for infusions that need to be given rapidly and for solutions that are hypertonic, are highly acidic or alkaline, or contain irritating medications. The loss of subcutaneous tissue, thinning of the skin, and fragile veins in the older adult can be a challenge for the nurse when performing a venipuncture. It is common practice for the initial venipuncture to be in the most distal portion of the arm because this allows for subsequent venipunctures to move upward. The veins of the hands of the older adult, however, are not the best initial sites for venipuncture because of the loss of subcutaneous tissue and thinning of the skin (Gorski, 2018; Infusion Nurses Society [INS], 2016a).

The metacarpal, basilic, and cephalic veins are common venipuncture sites (Figure 51.14 ■). The ulna and radius act as natural splints at these sites, and the client has greater freedom of arm movement for activities such as eating. Although the antecubital basilic and median cubital veins are convenient, they are usually kept for blood draws, bolus injections of medication, and insertion sites for a peripherally inserted central catheter (PICC) line (Figure 51.14*A*). See Practice Guidelines for vein selection and general tips for easier IV starts.

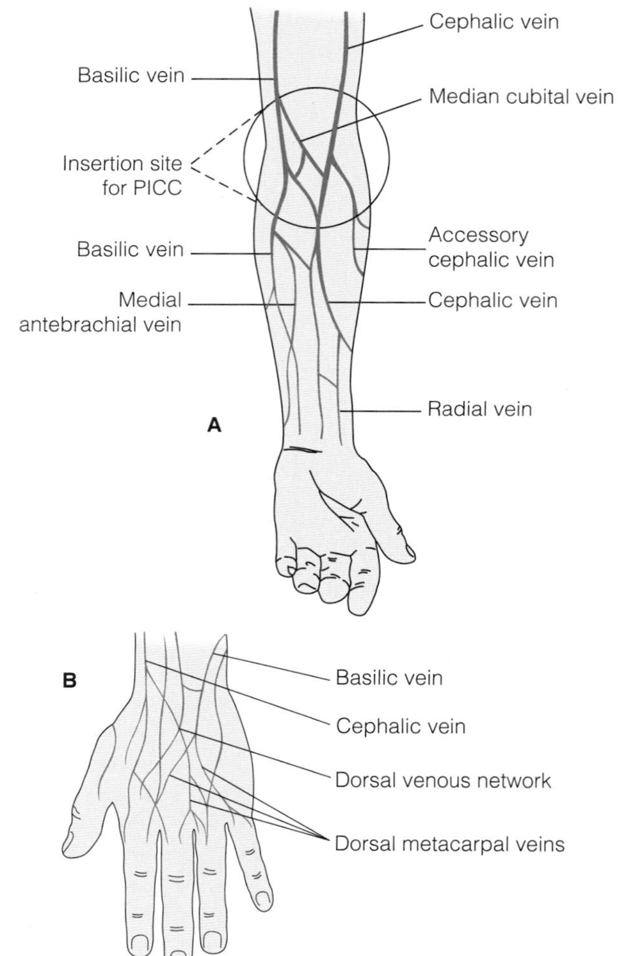

Figure 51.14 ■ Commonly used venipuncture sites: *A*, arm; *B*, hand. *A* also shows the site used for a peripherally inserted central catheter (PICC).

PRACTICE GUIDELINES Vein Selection

- Traditionally, nurses used distal veins of the arm first with subsequent venous access starts to be proximal to the previous site. Current INS recommendations are to "use the venous site most likely to last the full length of the prescribed therapy using the forearm to increase dwell time, decrease pain during dwell time, promote self-care, and prevent accidental removal and occlusions" (Gorski, 2018, p. 276; INS, 2016a, p. S54).
- Use the client's nondominant arm whenever possible.
- Select a vein that is:
  a. Easily palpated and feels soft and full
  b. Naturally splinted by bone
  c. Large enough to allow adequate circulation around the catheter.
- Avoid using veins that are:
  a. In areas of flexion (e.g., the antecubital fossa)
  b. Highly visible, because they tend to roll away from the needle
  c. Damaged by previous use, phlebitis, infiltration, or sclerosis
  d. Continually distended with blood, or knotted or tortuous
  e. In a surgically compromised or injured extremity (e.g., following a mastectomy), because of possible impaired circulation and discomfort for the client.

Historically, nurses used their eyes and hands to locate a suitable vein for a venipuncture. This could be especially challenging in some clients such as older adults, dark-skinned clients whose veins may not be visible, or clients with obesity, because their veins may not be visible or palpable. The use of visualization technology has improved the practice of IV access. The *Infusion Therapy Standards of Practice* (INS, 2016a) state that nurses should "use vascular visualization technology to increase success for patients with difficult venous access" (p. S51). Transillumination devices are available that use light to allow for the location and identification of blood vessels. The client's skin color does not affect the ability to highlight veins. Technology also includes near-infrared (nIR) light technology and ultrasonography for short peripheral catheter placement in adult and pediatric clients with difficult venous access (Gorski, 2018; INS, 2016a, pp. S44–S45).

Intravenous Infusion Equipment

Because equipment varies according to the manufacturer, nurses must become familiar with the equipment used in each particular agency. IV equipment consists of vascular access devices, catheter stabilization devices, site protection devices, solution containers, infusion administration sets, IV filters, and IV poles.

Vascular Access Devices

The *Infusion Therapy Standards of Practice* (INS, 2016a) states that the type of vascular access device (VAD) depends on the client's vascular or venous access needs, which are based on the prescribed therapy, length of treatment, vascular integrity, client preference, and ability and resources available to care for the device (p. S51). All catheters must be radiopaque.

A *short peripheral catheter* is used for usually less than 1 week (check agency policy). It comes in a variety of gauge sizes (a #20 to #24 gauge is used for most infusion therapies) and types (e.g., winged or nonwinged, and over-the-needle) and the tip of the catheter ends in a peripheral vein (INS, 2016a). Over-the-needle catheters (ONCs), also known as angiocatheters, are commonly used for adult clients. The plastic catheter fits over a needle (stylet) used to pierce the skin and vein wall (Figure 51.15 ■). Once inserted into the vein, the needle (stylet) is withdrawn and discarded, leaving the catheter in place. The nurse should use short peripheral catheters equipped with a passive or active safety mechanism to prevent sharps injury. The active safety device requires activation by the nurse, and the passive safety device automatically activates after the stylet is removed from the catheter. Use of the passive safety device is recommended for the prevention of a needlestick injury.

A butterfly or wing-tipped needle with plastic flaps attached to the shaft is sometimes used (Figure 51.16 ■). The flaps are held tightly together to hold the needle securely during insertion; after insertion, they are flattened against the skin and secured with tape. The butterfly

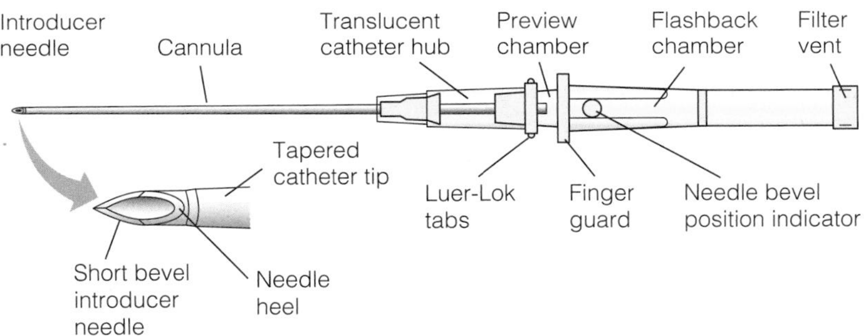

Figure 51.15 ■ Schematic of an over-the-needle short peripheral catheter.

PRACTICE GUIDELINES General Tips for Easier Insertion of a Short Peripheral Catheter

- Review the client's medical history. Avoid using an arm affected by hemiplegia or with a dialysis access, on the same side as a mastectomy, or near infections, below previous infiltrations or extravasations, and veins affected by phlebitis.
- Dilate the vein. Ways to do this include (a) dangle the client's arm over the side of the bed to encourage dependent vein filling, (b) ask the client to open and close his or her fist, (c) stroke the vein downward or lightly tap the vein, or (d) apply warm compresses to the site for 10 minutes.
- Make sure the client is positioned comfortably and has been medicated for pain if appropriate. Pain and anxiety stimulate the sympathetic nervous system and trigger vasoconstriction.
- Because of the risk of nerve injuries, as well as discomfort and restriction of movement, hand veins should be a last choice.
- If the ordered IV medication is irritating to veins and therapy is expected to last more than a few days, consult with the IV nurse or medical team to determine whether the client is a candidate for a midline catheter, a peripherally inserted central catheter, or another type of central venous access device.
- Use the smallest gauge catheter that will accommodate the therapy and allow good venous flow around the catheter tip. Use #20- to #24-gauge catheters for routine hydration or intermittent therapy and for transfusion therapy, use #22- to #24-gauge catheters for neonates, pediatric clients, and older adults to minimize insertion-related trauma (INS, 2016a, p. S51).
- Raise the bed or stretcher to a comfortable working height, and keep all equipment within reach. Stabilize the client's hand or arm with your nondominant arm, tucking it under your forearm if necessary to prevent movement.
- Limit your attempts to two. If you are not successful after two tries, ask another nurse to try. Limit total attempts to no more than four (INS, 2016a). If venous sites are not found, use a vascular visualization method.

Clinical Alert!

A short peripheral catheter placed in an emergency situation where aseptic technique has been compromised shall be replaced as soon as possible, preferably within 24 to 48 hours (INS, 2016a, p. S91).

needle is most frequently used for short-term therapy such as with a single-dose IV push medication, or blood sample retrieval. It is not left in place (Gorski, 2018).

A *midline catheter* is 7.6 to 20.3 cm (3 to 8 in.) in length and inserted near the antecubital area into the basilic, cephalic, or brachial veins, with the preference being the basilica vein because of its larger diameter. The catheter tip is advanced no farther than the distal axillary vein in the upper arm; the tip does not enter the central vasculature. The INS classifies the midline catheter as a peripheral catheter. The duration of infusion therapy, however, does differ. For example, a short peripheral catheter is used when the duration of infusion therapy is for less than 1 week; the duration of therapy using a midline catheter can last from 1 to 4 weeks.

A **peripherally inserted central venous catheter (PICC)** is inserted in the basilic or cephalic vein just above or below the antecubital space of the right arm. The tip of the catheter rests in the superior vena cava. These catheters frequently are used for long-term IV access when the client will be managing IV therapy at home.

When long-term IV therapy or parenteral nutrition is anticipated, or a client is receiving IV medications that are damaging to vessels (e.g., chemotherapy), a **central vascular access device (CVAD)** may be inserted. A CVAD is defined by the location of the catheter tip in a *central vein*. The CVAD catheter tip should reside in the lower one-third of the superior vena cava, above the right atrium (Figure 51.17 ■). CVADs may be inserted at a client's bedside or, for longer term access, surgically inserted. They permit freedom of movement for ambulation; however, there is greater risk of complications, including hemothorax or pneumothorax, cardiac perforation, thrombosis, and infection. Assess the client closely for signs and symptoms such as shortness of breath, chest pain, cough, hypotension, tachycardia, and anxiety after the insertion procedure.

Implanted vascular access devices (IVADs) (Figures 51.18 ■ and 51.19 ■) are used for clients with chronic

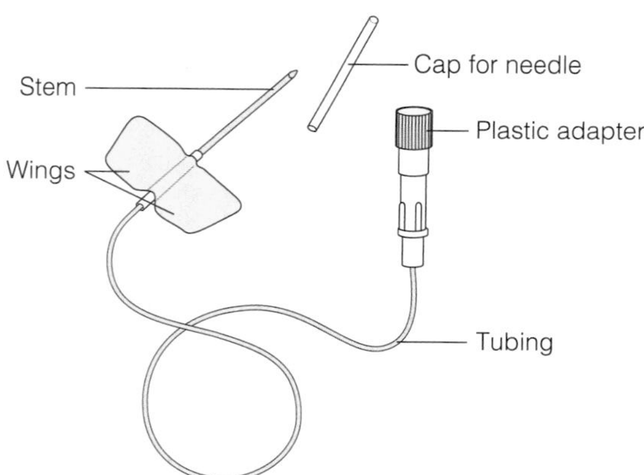

Figure 51.16 ■ Schematic of a butterfly needle with adapter.

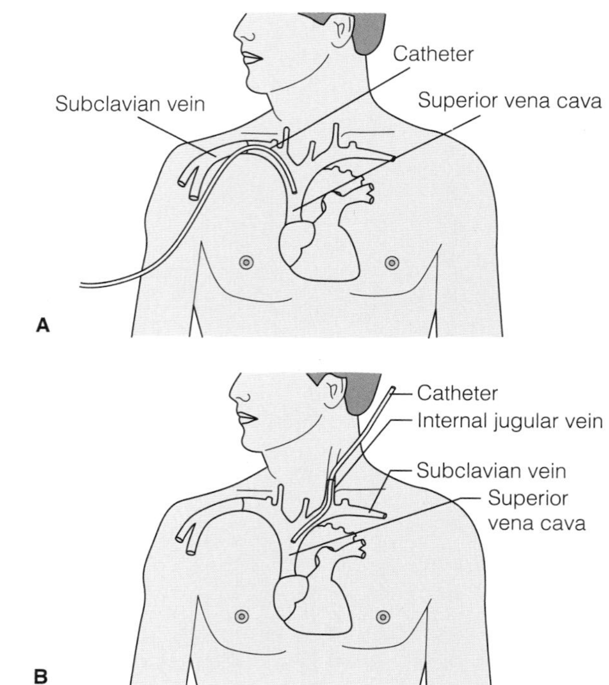

Figure 51.17 ■ Central vascular access devices with *A*, subclavian vein insertion, and *B*, left jugular insertion.

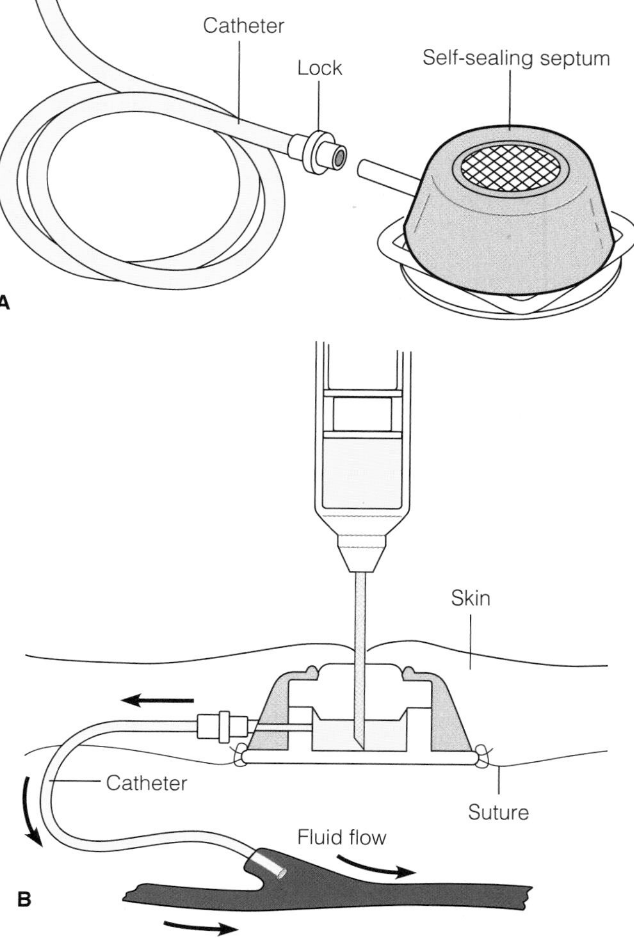

Figure 51.18 ■ An implanted vascular access device: *A*, components; *B*, the device in place.

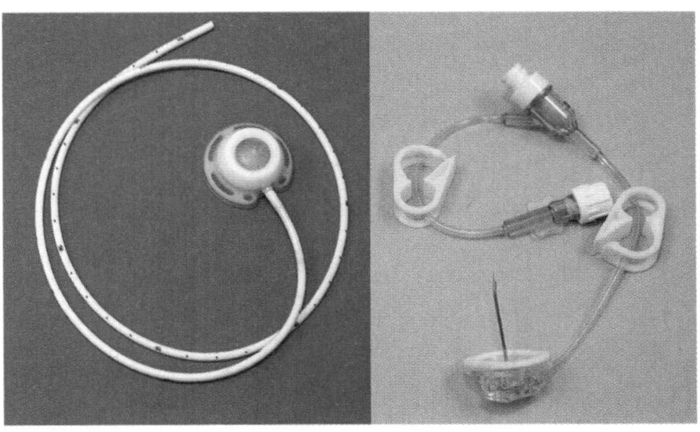

Figure 51.19 ■ *Left*, An implanted vascular access device; *Right*, a Huber needle with extension tubing.

illness who require long-term IV therapy (e.g., intermittent medications such as chemotherapy, total parenteral nutrition, and frequent blood samples). This type of device is designed to provide repeated access to the central venous system, avoiding the trauma and complications of multiple venipunctures. Using local anesthesia, implantable ports are surgically placed into a small subcutaneous pocket under the skin, usually on the anterior chest near the clavicle, and no part of the port is exposed. The distal end of the catheter is placed in the subclavian or jugular vein.

Special precautions need to be taken with all central lines and venous access ports to ensure asepsis and catheter patency. Nursing care of clients with these devices is outlined in Practice Guidelines.

PRACTICE GUIDELINES Caring for Clients with a Central Vascular Access Device

- After insertion, document the date; the insertion site; the brand, gauge, and catheter length; the location of the catheter tip (verified by x-ray); the length of the external segment; and client teaching. Do not use the access device until correct placement has been verified by x-ray.

SITE CARE

- Use strict aseptic technique (including the use of sterile gloves and mask) when caring for CVADs.
- The frequency of dressing changes is dependent on the dressing material. Transparent semipermeable membrane (TSM) dressings or tape and gauze are acceptable; however, gauze dressings do not allow for visualization of the insertion site and need to be changed every 48 hours or if the site requires visual inspection (Gorski, 2018, p. 404). In contrast, TSM dressings allow for visualization and can be left in place for 5 to 7 days if they remain clean, dry, and intact (INS, 2016b, p. 114). A recent innovation is a TSM dressing that has an integrated gel pad containing chlorhexidine gluconate 2% (CHG). This dressing provides a clear sterile covering for the CVAD, helps secure the device, and provides a continuous application of chlorhexidine at the insertion site. See Figure ❶. All dressings should be changed when loose or soiled.
- Assess the site for any redness, swelling, tenderness, or drainage. Compare the length of the external portion of the catheter with its documented length to assess for possible displacement. Report and document any position changes or signs of infection.
- Follow agency protocol for cleaning solutions and types of dressings. Chlorhexidine gluconate is the preferred agent to clean the insertion site.
- Clean the skin around the site with chlorhexidine solution, using a back-and-forth motion for at least 30 seconds (INS, 2016b). Allow the site to air dry.
- Apply a new stabilization device.
- Apply a sterile dressing.

CATHETER CARE AND FLUSHING

- Change the catheter cap as indicated by agency protocol. The catheter hub can be a source of infection. The INS (2016b) states that if using manual disinfection, vigorously scrub with antiseptic wipe using friction and allow to dry completely (p. 111). See agency protocol for length of scrub (e.g., 5 to 60 seconds). Also available are commercial single-use Luer access valve disinfection caps (port protectors). This cap contains isopropyl alcohol, which cleans the needleless connector before access and also protects it from contamination between uses. The cap is twisted onto the needleless connector and left in place until the next access to the connector is needed. The nurse removes and discards the old cap and the connector is ready for use without further wiping. If using a disinfection cap, remove it and discard. Do not reuse this cap. According to INS (2016a), "use of passive disinfection caps containing disinfecting agents has been shown to reduce intraluminal microbial contamination and reduce the rates of central line-associated blood stream infection (CLABSI)" (p. S69). See Figures ❷ to ❺.
- The solution used and frequency of flushing are determined by agency protocol for the specific type of port being used. If heparin is used as part of the flushing protocol, the concentration should not be in amounts that cause systemic anticoagulation but in the lowest possible concentration to maintain patency (e.g., 10 units/mL).

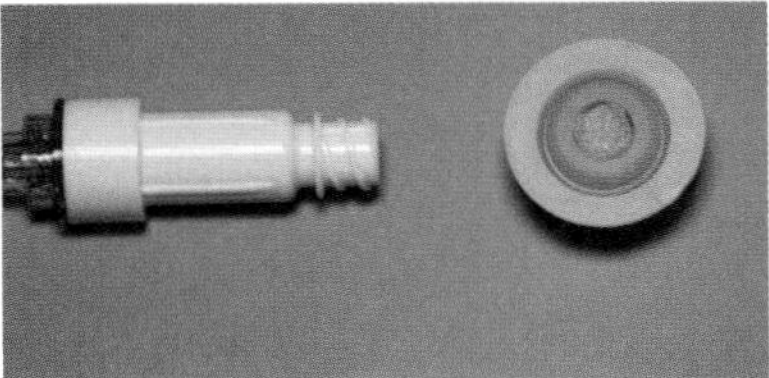

❸ Cap contains disinfecting solution.
Shirlee Snyder.

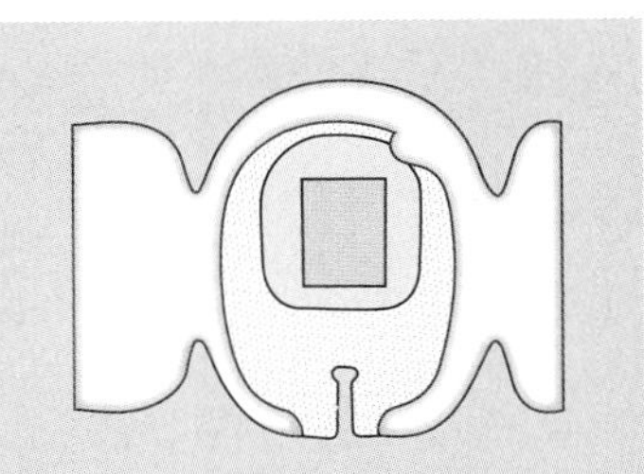

❶ Tegaderm™ CHG dressing that can be used on a CVAD.

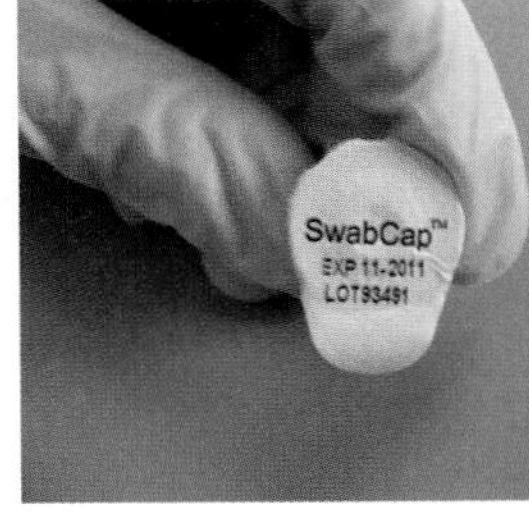

❷ Disinfecting cap (SwabCap™).
Shirlee Snyder.

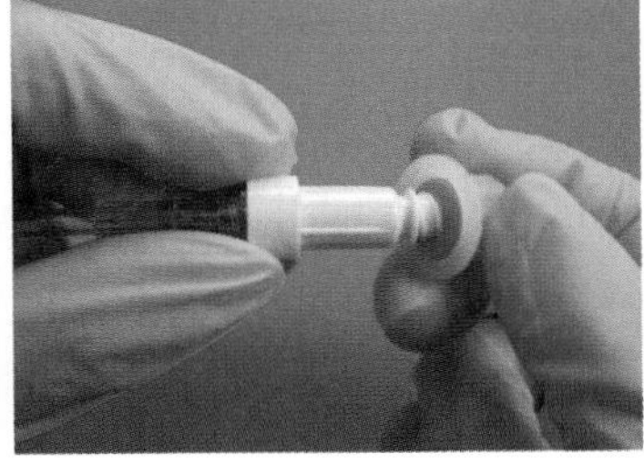

❹ Twist cap onto needleless connector.
Shirlee Snyder.

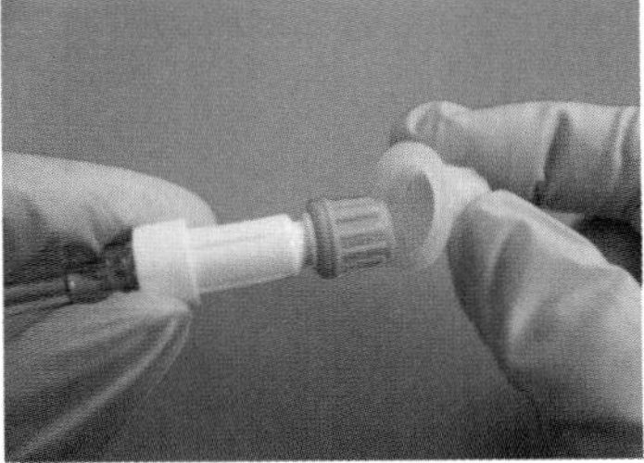

❺ Remove outer packaging and leave cap in place.
Shirlee Snyder.

Continued on page 1402

PRACTICE GUIDELINES Caring for Clients with a Central Vascular Access Device—*continued*

- Flush the catheter before and after each dose of medication. The initial flush is to assess patency of the catheter, and the flush after administration of the medication is to ensure that the complete dose has entered the bloodstream and to prevent contact between incompatible medications.
- Use a 10-mL syringe to flush the catheter. Never apply force if you feel resistance.
- CVADs need to be locked after the final flush solution to decrease the risk of occlusion (INS, 2016b). Locking a catheter creates a column of fluid inside the lumen to maintain patency. The process for locking a catheter varies depending on the manufacturer of the needleless connector.
- Blood reflux into the catheter lumen after flushing increases the risk of infection. Thus, it is important for the nurse to know the type of needleless connector being used: positive-pressure, negative-pressure, or neutral-displacement needleless connector.

TEACHING

Provide clients with the following instructions:

- Do not allow anyone to take a blood pressure on the arm in which a PICC line is inserted.
- Wear a medical alert tag or bracelet if the device will be in place for a long period of time.
- For a PICC line, activity does not need to be restricted, except that the arm should not be immersed in water. Showering is allowed if the site and catheter are covered by a TSM dressing.
- For an implanted central venous access port, there are no activity restrictions, but the port or catheter tip can become dislodged. Signs of a dislodged catheter tip include pain in the neck or ear on the affected side, swishing or gurgling sounds, or palpitations; signs of a dislodged port include free movement of the port, swelling, or difficulty accessing the port. If any of these occur, or if symptoms of infection develop, notify the primary care provider immediately.

Safety Alert! SAFETY

2019 The Joint Commission National Patient Safety Goals

Goal 7: Reduce the risk of healthcare-associated infections.

Goal 7.04.01: Implement evidence-based practices to prevent central line–associated bloodstream infections. This requirement covers short- and long-term central venous catheters and peripherally inserted central catheter (PICC) lines.

- Implement policies and practices aimed at reducing the risk of central line–associated bloodstream infections.
- Perform hand hygiene prior to catheter insertion or manipulation.
- Use a standardized protocol to disinfect catheter hubs and injection ports before accessing the ports.

Catheter Stabilization Devices

Securing or stabilizing an IV catheter helps decrease movement of the catheter at the insertion site, which helps prevent the catheter from being dislodged and other complications such as infiltration, phlebitis, and infection (Gorski, 2018). The INS standards (2016a) recommend the use of manufactured catheter stabilization devices (Figure 51.20 ■) over other methods such as sterile tapes and surgical strips.

Site Protection Devices

Site protection refers to the use of methods or products that protect the catheter site (Gorski, 2018, p. 233). For example, a clear plastic protector placed over the site can prevent accidental snagging of the catheter hub or the IV line (Figure 51.21 ■). It may be needed for clients who are confused or have cognitive deficits.

EVIDENCE-BASED PRACTICE

Evidence-Based Practice

Is There a Difference in Rate of Infection Among Types of CVAD Dressings?

The use of dressing and securement products is important in the prevention of CVAD complications (e.g., infection, dislodgement). There are many CVAD dressings and securements available to clinicians. The diversity of available dressings and securements makes evidence-based decision-making difficult. The ideal CVAD dressing should provide barrier protection from infection, provide securement to prevent accidental removal or dislodgement, be comfortable for the client, be easy to use, and be cost effective. There is no consensus on the best type of dressing to use with CVADs in spite of more than 2 decades of research. As a result, Ullman et al. (2016) conducted a study to compare available dressings and securement devices for CVADs in terms of infection, skin irritation, failed catheter securement, dressing condition, and mortality (p. 180).

The researchers conducted a Cochrane systematic review that included all randomized controlled trials that evaluated the effects of CVAD dressings and securement devices. The results included 22 studies for meta-analysis. The review found no clear evidence linking gauze and tape and standard polyurethane with skin irritation, failed catheter securement, dressing condition or durability, and mortality. The review did find that there is high-quality evidence that the use of medication-impregnated dressing products (e.g., patch or whole dressing) reduces the incidence of CVAD-related bloodstream infection in comparison with all other dressing types (p. 192). There was not enough research for the authors to make recommendations about CVAD security using the different dressing and securement products.

Implications

The evidence of the effectiveness of chlorhexidine gluconate–impregnated dressing in reducing infection mainly came from studies in intensive care unit (ICU) settings. The authors point to the need for more high-quality research especially as new products become available. More evidence is needed to support effective clinical decision-making.

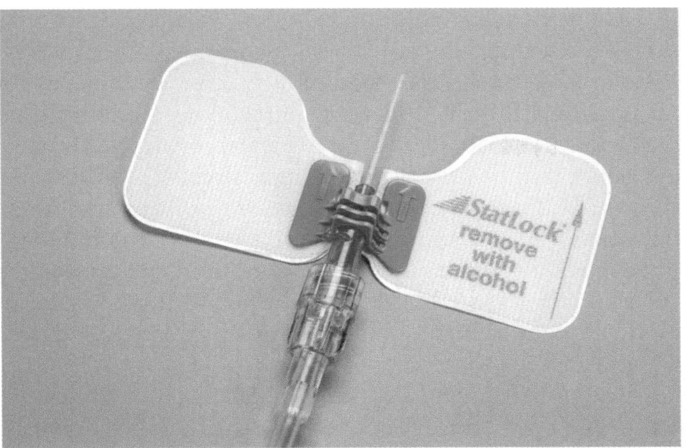

Figure 51.20 ■ Manufactured catheter stabilization device.

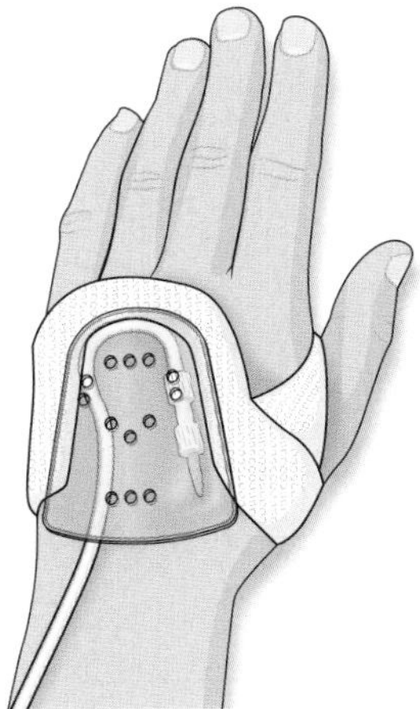

Figure 51.21 ■ IV site protection device.

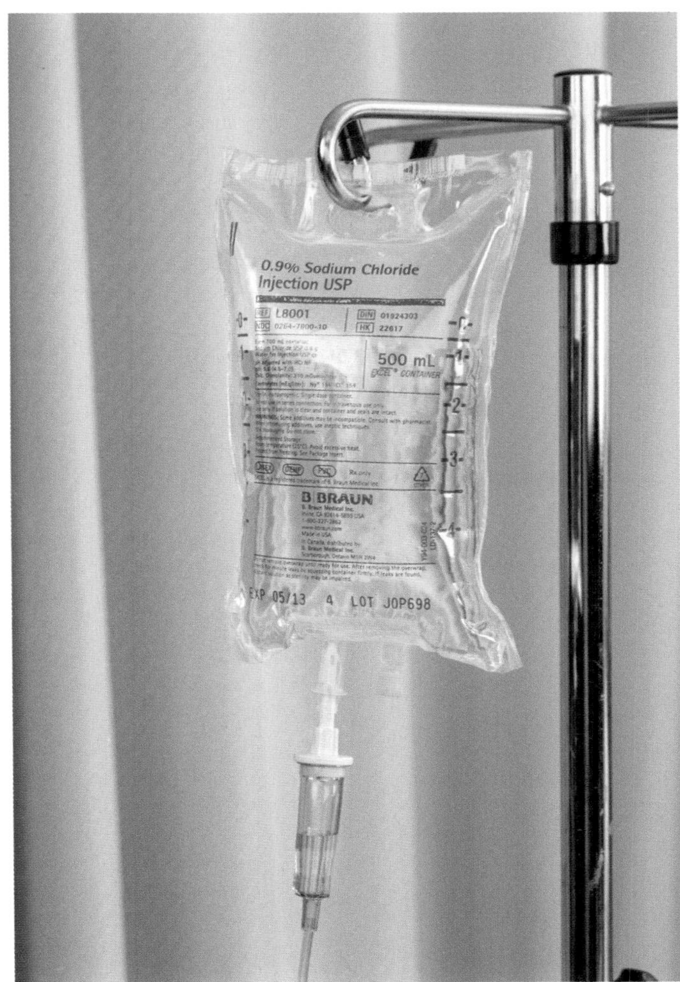

Figure 51.22 ■ A plastic intravenous solution container.

Solution Containers

Solution containers are available in various sizes (50, 100, 250, 500, or 1000 mL); the smaller containers are often used to administer medications. Most solutions are currently dispensed in plastic containers (Figure 51.22 ■). However, glass bottles may need to be used if the administered medications are incompatible with plastic. Glass bottles require an air vent so that air can enter the bottle and replace the fluid that enters the client's vein. Some bottles contain a tube that serves as a vent; other containers require a vent on the administration set. Air vents usually have filters to prevent contamination from the air that enters the container. Air vents are not required for plastic solution bags, because the bags collapse under atmospheric pressure when the solution enters the vein.

It is essential that the solution be sterile and in good condition, that is, clear. Cloudiness, evidence that the container has been opened previously, or leaks indicate possible contamination. Always check the expiration date on the label. Return any questionable or contaminated solutions to the pharmacy or IV therapy department.

Clinical Alert!

Do not write directly on a plastic IV bag with a ballpoint pen (may puncture the bag) or indelible marker (may absorb through the bag into the solution).

Infusion Administration Sets

Infusion administration sets (also called administration infusion sets) consist of an insertion spike, a drip chamber, a roller valve or screw clamp, tubing with secondary ports, and a protective cap over the connecter to the IV catheter (Figure 51.23 ■). The insertion spike is kept sterile and inserted into the solution container when the equipment is set up and ready to start. The drip chamber permits a predictable amount of fluid to be delivered. A macrodrip drip chamber delivers between 10 and 20 drops (abbreviated gtts) per milliliter of solution. The specific amount is written on the package. Microdrip sets deliver 60 drops per milliliter of solution (Figure 51.24 ■). Many infusion sets include an in-line filter to trap air, particulate matter, and microbes. A special infusion set may be required if the IV flow rate will be regulated by an infusion pump.

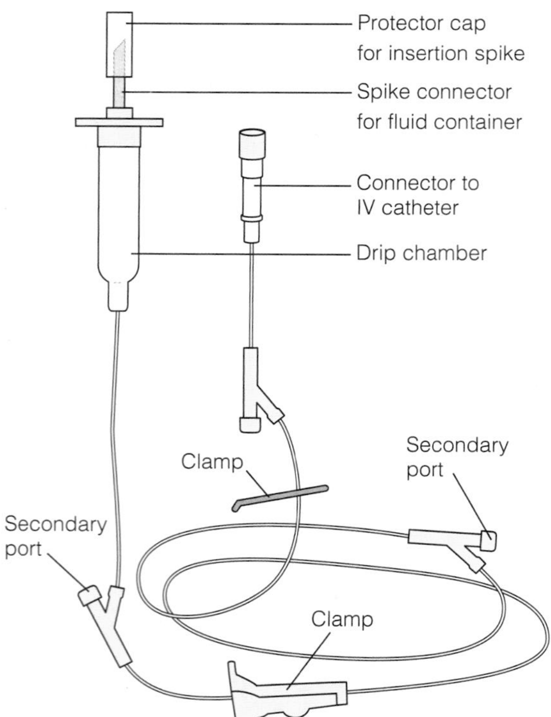

Figure 51.23 ■ A standard IV infusion administration set.

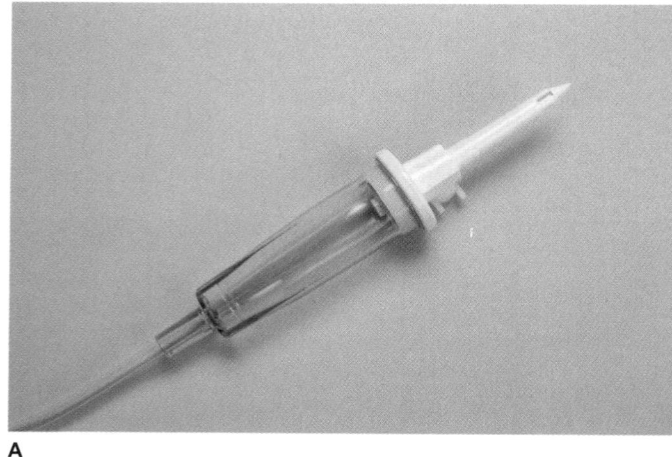

A

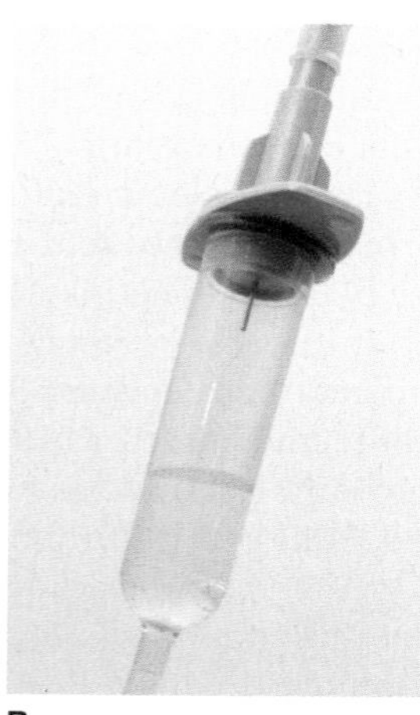

B

Figure 51.24 ■ Infusion set spikes and drip chambers: *A*, nonvented macrodrip and *B*, nonvented microdrip.

Most infusion sets include one or more injection ports for administering IV medications or secondary infusions. Needleless systems are used because they reduce the risk of needlestick injury and contamination of the IV line. The needleless ports can be accessed with a syringe that has a Luer-Lok to administer medications (Figure 51.25 ■). When more than one solution needs to be infused at the same time, *secondary sets* such as the piggyback IV setups are used. Another variation is a *volume-control set*, which is used if the volume of fluid or medication administered is to be carefully controlled (see Chapter 35 ∞).

Rather than using a continuous infusion, an intermittent infusion lock may be created by attaching a sterile needleless connector (also called an injection cap or port) (Figure 51.26 ■) to an existing IV catheter hub. This keeps the venous vascular access available for the administration of intermittent or emergency medications. The device is commonly referred to as a saline lock because periodic

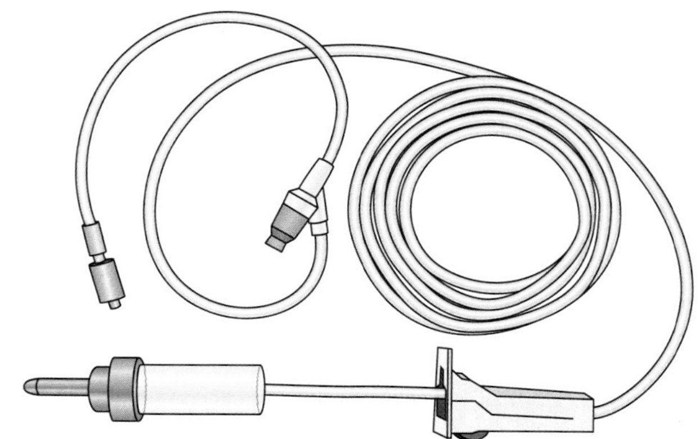

Figure 51.25 ■ Needleless injection port on an IV infusion administration set.

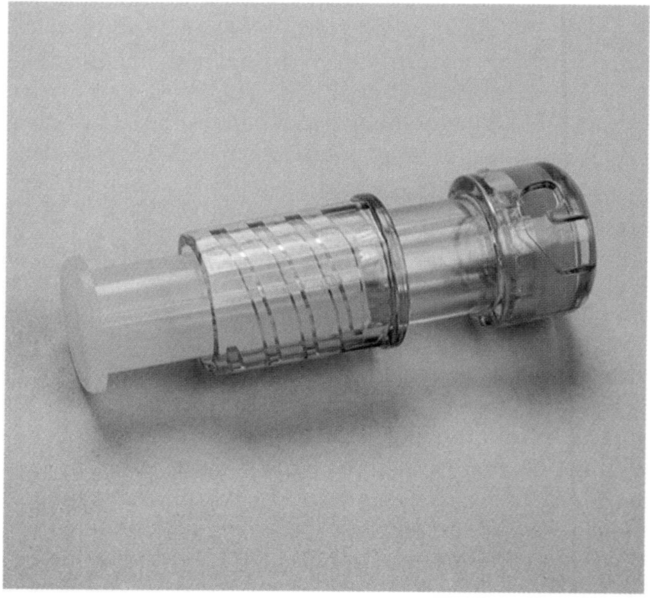

Figure 51.26 ■ A needleless connector.

injection with saline is used to keep blood from coagulating within the tubing.

Intravenous Filters

IV filters are used to remove air and particulate matter from IV infusions and to reduce the risk of complications (e.g., infusion-related phlebitis) associated with routine IV therapies (Figure 51.27 ■). Use filters according to the manufacturer's directions for use and the filtration requirements of the infusion therapy solution or medication (INS, 2016a). When using filters, the nurse must remember that the filter should never be considered a substitute for quality care and meticulous technique.

Intravenous Poles

IV poles (rods) are used to hang the solution container. Some poles are attached to hospital beds; others stand on the floor or hang from the ceiling. Still others are floor models with casters that can be pushed along when a client is up and walking. In the home, plant hangers or robe hooks (even kitchen cabinet knobs or an S-hook over the top of a door) may be used to hang solution containers. The height of most poles is adjustable. The higher the solution container, the greater the force of the solution as it enters the client and the faster the rate of flow.

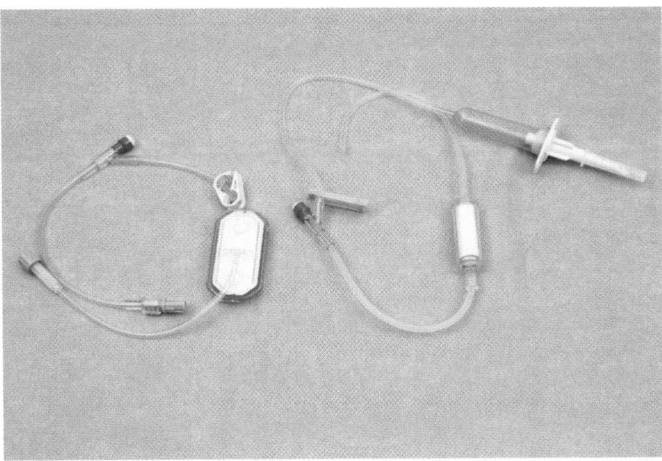

Figure 51.27 ■ Two types of IV filters.

Starting an Intravenous Infusion

Although the primary care provider is responsible for ordering IV therapy for clients, nurses initiate, monitor, and maintain the prescribed IV infusion. This is true not only in hospitals and long-term care facilities but increasingly in community-based settings such as clinics and clients' homes.

Before starting an infusion, the nurse determines the following:

- The type and amount of solution to be infused
- The exact amount (dose) of any medications to be added to a compatible solution
- The rate of flow or the time over which the infusion is to be completed.

If solutions are prepared by the pharmacy or another department, the nurse must verify that the solution supplied exactly matches that which the primary care provider ordered.

Understanding the purpose for the infusion is as important as assessing the client. For example, a nurse should question an order for 5% dextrose in water at 150 mL/h if the client has peripheral edema and other signs of fluid overload.

To start an IV infusion and insert a short peripheral catheter, see Skill 51.1.

Starting an Intravenous Infusion and Inserting a Short Peripheral Catheter

SKILL 51.1

Before preparing the infusion, the nurse first verifies the primary care provider's order indicating the type of solution, the amount to be administered, the rate of flow or time over which the infusion is to be completed, and any client allergies (e.g., to tape or povidone-iodine).

PURPOSES

- To supply fluid when clients are unable to take in an adequate volume of fluids by mouth
- To provide salts and other electrolytes needed to maintain electrolyte balance
- To provide glucose (dextrose), the main fuel for metabolism
- To provide water-soluble vitamins and medications
- To establish a lifeline for rapidly needed medications

ASSESSMENT

Assess

- Vital signs (pulse, respiratory rate, and BP) for baseline data.
- Allergy to latex (e.g., tourniquet), tape, or iodine.
- Bleeding tendencies.
- Disease or injury to extremities.
- Status of veins to determine appropriate vascular access site. Avoid sites that have been used recently. **Rationale:** *Recently used sites will be more prone to complications and discomfort.* Determine if the client is right- or left-handed. **Rationale:** *Do not use the dominant hand if possible.* If venous sites are not found, avoid blind venipuncture and use a vascular visualization method (INS, 2016b, p. 53).
- The agency policy about clipping hair in the area before a venipuncture. Shaving is not recommended because of the possibility of nicking the skin and subsequent infection.

Continued on page 1406

SKILL 51.1

Starting an Intravenous Infusion and Inserting a Short Peripheral Catheter—*continued*

PLANNING

Prior to initiating the IV infusion, consider how long the client is likely to have the IV, what kinds of fluids will be infused, and what medications the client will be receiving or is likely to receive. These factors may affect the choice of vein and catheter size. Review the client record regarding previous infusions. Note any complications and how they were managed. Consider using local anesthetic agents to reduce the pain and discomfort of catheter insertion.

Assignment

Due to the need for knowledge of anatomy and use of sterile technique, IV infusion therapy is not assigned to AP. AP may care for clients receiving IV therapy, and the nurse must ensure that the AP knows how to perform routine tasks such as bathing and positioning without disturbing the IV. The AP should also know what complications or adverse signs, such as leakage, should be reported to the nurse.

In many states, a licensed practical nurse or licensed vocational nurse with special IV therapy training may start IV infusions. Check the state's nurse practice act.

Equipment

Substitute appropriate supplies if the client has tape, antiseptic, or latex allergies.

- Infusion set
- Extension tubing (optional)
- Sterile parenteral solution
- IV pole
- Nonallergenic tape
- Clean gloves (sterile gloves are needed for site palpation after skin antisepsis)
- Single-use and latex-free tourniquet
- Antiseptic swabs such as 10% povidone-iodine or 2% chlorhexidine gluconate with alcohol or 70% isopropyl alcohol. The preferred antiseptic is alcoholic chlorhexidine solution as it has a residual effect on the skin for up to 48 hours (Gorski, 2018, p. 287).
- IV catheter with passive safety mechanism. **Rationale:** *The passive design automatically retracts the needle avoiding needlestick injury*. Choose an IV catheter of the appropriate type and size based on the size of the vein and the purpose of the IV. A #20- to #24-gauge catheter is indicated for most adults. Use the *smallest* gauge that can be used for the prescribed IV infusion. Always have an extra catheter and ones of different sizes available.
- Vein visualization device, if needed
- Sterile gauze dressing or transparent semipermeable membrane (TSM) dressing (preferred)
- Stabilization device
- IV protection device
- Splint, if required
- Towel or bed protector
- Local anesthetic (optional and per agency policy)
- Electronic infusion device or pump (The nurse decides what device is needed as appropriate to the client's condition.)

IMPLEMENTATION

Preparation

- If possible, select a time to perform the venipuncture that is convenient for the client. Unless initiating IV therapy is urgent, provide any scheduled care before establishing the infusion to minimize excessive movement of the affected limb. **Rationale:** *Moving the limb after the infusion has been established could dislodge the catheter*.
- Make sure that the client's clothing or gown can be removed over the IV apparatus if necessary. Many agencies provide special gowns that open over the shoulder and down the sleeve for easy removal.
- Visitors or family members may be asked to leave the room if desired by the nurse or the client.

Performance

1. Prior to performing the procedure, introduce self and verify the client's identity using agency protocol. Explain to the client what you are going to do, why it is necessary, and how to participate. Venipuncture can cause discomfort for a few seconds, but there should be no ongoing pain after insertion. If possible, explain how long the IV will need to remain in place and how it will be used.
2. Perform hand hygiene and observe other appropriate infection prevention procedures.
3. Position the client appropriately.
   - Assist the client to a comfortable position, either sitting or lying. Expose the limb to be used but provide for client privacy.

   (*Note*: Steps 4 through 10 may be performed outside of the client's room and then the system transported to the client's bedside.)
4. Apply a medication label to the solution container if a medication is added.
   - In most agencies, medications are added and labels are applied to IV containers in the pharmacy; if they are not, apply the label upside down on the container. **Rationale:** *The label is applied upside down so it can be read easily when the container is hanging up*.
5. Open and prepare the infusion set.
   - Remove tubing from the package and straighten it out.
   - Slide the tubing clamp along the tubing until it is just below the drip chamber to facilitate its access.
   - Close the clamp.
   - Leave the ends of the tubing covered with the plastic caps until the infusion is started. **Rationale:** *This will maintain the sterility of the ends of the tubing*.
   - Consider using extension tubing between the peripheral catheter and needleless connector. **Rationale:** *This reduces catheter manipulation, which can cause phlebitis*. Flush the extension tubing also.
6. Spike the solution container.
   - Expose the insertion site of the bag or bottle by removing the protective cover.
   - Remove the cap from the spike and insert the spike into the insertion site of the bag or bottle. ❶
7. Hang the solution container on the pole.
   - Adjust the pole so that the container is suspended about 1 m (3 ft) above the client's head. **Rationale:** *This height is needed to enable gravity to overcome venous pressure and facilitate flow of the solution into the vein*.
8. Partially fill the drip chamber with solution.
   - Squeeze the chamber gently until it is half full of solution. ❷ **Rationale:** *The drip chamber is partially filled with solution to prevent air from moving down the tubing*.
9. Prime the tubing as described next. The term *prime* means "to make ready" but in common use refers to flushing the tubing to remove air.
   - Remove the protective cap and hold the tubing over a container. Maintain the sterility of the end of the tubing and the cap.

Starting an Intravenous Infusion and Inserting a Short Peripheral Catheter—*continued*

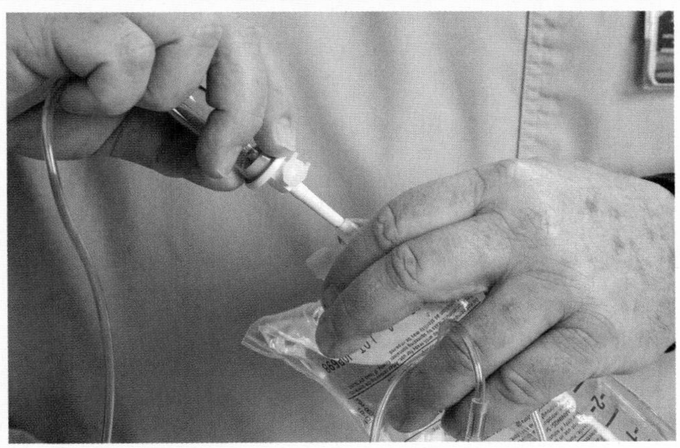

❶ Inserting the spike.

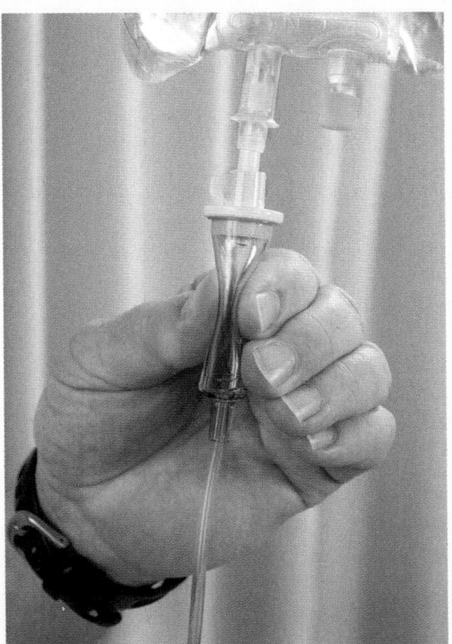

❷ Squeezing the drip chamber.

- Release the clamp and let the fluid run through the tubing until all bubbles are removed. Tap the tubing if necessary with your fingers to help the bubbles move. **Rationale:** *The tubing is primed to prevent the introduction of air into the client. Air bubbles smaller than 0.5 mL usually do not cause problems in peripheral lines.*
- Reclamp the tubing and replace the tubing cap, maintaining sterile technique.
- If an infusion control pump, electronic device, or controller is being used, follow the manufacturer's directions for inserting the tubing and setting the infusion rate.

10. Perform hand hygiene again just prior to client contact.

11. Select the venipuncture site.

- Use the client's nondominant arm, unless contraindicated (e.g., mastectomy, fistula for dialysis). Identify possible venipuncture sites by looking for veins that are relatively straight. The vein should be palpable, but may not be visible, especially in clients with dark skin. Consider the catheter length; look for a site sufficiently distal to the wrist or elbow such that the tip of the catheter will not be at a point of flexion. **Rationale:** *Sclerotic veins may make initiating and maintaining the IV difficult. Joint flexion increases the risk of irritation of vein walls by the catheter.* Choose the site most likely to last the full length of the IV therapy, which most likely will be using a vein in the forearm (Gorski, 2018, p. 176).
- Check agency protocol about shaving if the site is very hairy. Shaving is not recommended. **Rationale:** *Shaving can cause microabrasions that can increase the risk of infection.*
- Place a towel or bed protector under the extremity to protect linens (or furniture if in the home).

12. Dilate the vein.

- Place the extremity in a dependent position (lower than the client's heart). **Rationale:** *Gravity slows venous return and distends the veins. Distending the veins makes it easier to insert the needle properly.*
- Apply a tourniquet 15 to 20 cm (6 to 8 in.) above the venipuncture site. ❸ Explain that the tourniquet will feel tight. **Rationale:** *The tourniquet must be tight enough to obstruct venous flow but not so tight that it occludes*

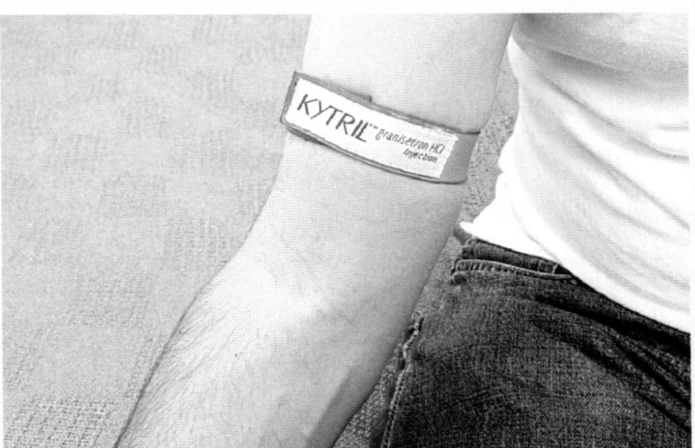

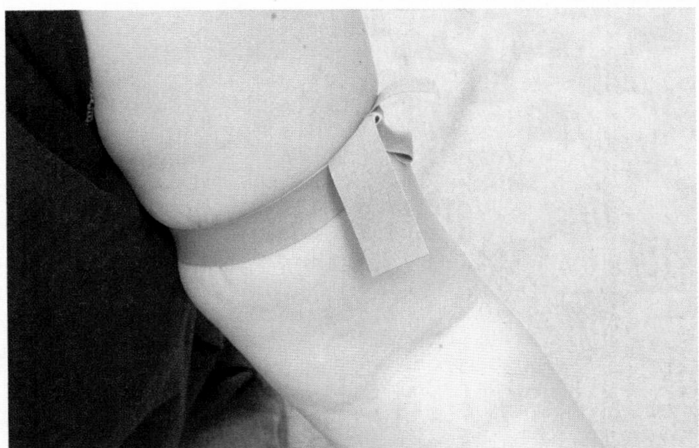

❸ Two types of tourniquets.

Continued on page 1408

Starting an Intravenous Infusion and Inserting a Short Peripheral Catheter—*continued*

arterial flow. Obstructing arterial flow inhibits venous filling. If a radial pulse can be palpated, the arterial flow is not obstructed.

- Use the tourniquet on only one client. **Rationale:** *This avoids cross-contamination to other clients.* Be sure to ask if the client has a latex allergy.
- For older adults with fragile skin, instead of applying a tourniquet, place the arm in a dependent position to allow the veins to engorge. **Rationale:** *The tourniquet can cause tissue damage and may not be needed to allow the vein to dilate.*
- If the vein is not sufficiently dilated:
  a. Massage or stroke the vein distal to the site and in the direction of venous flow toward the heart. **Rationale:** *This action helps fill the vein.*
  b. Encourage the client to clench and unclench the fist. **Rationale:** *Contracting the muscles compresses the distal veins, forcing blood along the veins and distending them.*
  c. Lightly tap the vein with your fingertips. **Rationale:** *Tapping may distend the vein.*
- If the preceding steps fail to distend the vein so that it is palpable, remove the tourniquet and wrap the extremity in a warm towel for 10 to 15 minutes. **Rationale:** *Heat dilates superficial blood vessels, causing them to fill.* Then repeat steps to dilate the vein.
- If no venous sites are visible or easily palpated, use vein visualization technology to improve insertion success (INS, 2016b).

13. Remove the tourniquet while preparing the insertion site.

14. Minimize insertion pain as much as possible.

- Although the pain of insertion should be brief, prevention can and should be offered. Transdermal analgesic creams (e.g., EMLA, Synera) may be used, depending on policy. The length of time for the topical analgesic to take effect will vary depending on the agent used (Gorski, 2018).
- If desired and permitted by policy, inject 0.3 mL of 1% lidocaine (without epinephrine) intradermally over the site where you plan to insert the IV catheter. (Be sure to first apply gloves and clean the skin site as described in step 15.) Allow 15 to 30 seconds for the anesthetic to take effect (Gorski, 2018, p. 284).

15. Apply clean gloves and clean the venipuncture site. **Rationale:** *Gloves protect the nurse from contamination by the client's blood.*

- Clean the skin with soap and water if visibly soiled. Remove excess hair if necessary using scissor or surgical clippers.
- Clean the skin at the site of entry with a topical single-use antiseptic swab. The preferred antiseptic is chlorhexidine gluconate-alcohol solution; if there is a contraindication, 70% alcohol, tincture of iodine, or an iodophor may be used (Gorski, 2018, p. 287). Check for allergies to iodine or shellfish before cleansing skin with Betadine or iodine products.
- When using chlorhexidine solution (preferred), use a back-and-forth motion for a minimum of 30 seconds to scrub the insertion site and surrounding area (INS, 2016b, p. 59). Allow the site to completely air dry before inserting the catheter. Do *not* fan, blow on, or wipe the skin.
- If using povidone-iodine, apply using applicator and allow to remain on the skin for 1.5 to 2 minutes or longer to completely dry for adequate antisepsis. The use of concentric circles or a back-and forth motion for this skin preparation has not been studied (INS, 2016b, p. 59). Alcohol should not be applied after the application of povidone-iodine preparation because it counteracts the effects of povidone-iodine (Gorski, 2018, p. 288).

16. Reapply a tourniquet above the intended venipuncture site or use vein visualization technology, if needed.

- If vein palpation is necessary after application of skin antiseptic, apply sterile gloves.

17. Insert the catheter and initiate the infusion.

- Remove the catheter assembly from its sterile packaging. Review instructions for using the catheter because a variety of needle safety devices are manufactured. Remove the cover of the needle (stylet).
- Use the nondominant hand to pull the skin taut below the entry site. **Rationale:** *This stabilizes the vein and makes the skin taut for needle entry. It can also make initial tissue penetration less painful.*
- Holding the over-the-needle catheter at a 15- to 30-degree angle with needle (stylet) bevel up, insert the catheter through the skin and into the vein. A sudden lack of resistance is felt as the needle (stylet) enters the vein. Use a slow, steady insertion technique and avoid jabbing or stabbing motions.
- Once blood appears in the lumen or clear "flashback" chamber of the needle, lower the angle of the catheter until it is almost parallel with the skin, and advance the needle (stylet) and catheter approximately 0.5 to 1 cm (about 1/4 in.) farther into the vein. ❹ Holding the needle assembly steady, advance the catheter forward off the stylet until the hub is at the venipuncture site. The exact technique depends on the type of device used. **Rationale:** *The catheter is advanced to ensure that it, and not just the stylet, is in the vein.*
- If there is no blood return, try redirecting the catheter assembly again toward the vein. If the stylet has been withdrawn from the catheter even a small distance, or the catheter tip has been pulled out of the skin, the catheter must be discarded and a new one used. **Rationale:** *Reinserting the stylet into the catheter can result in damage or slicing of the catheter. A catheter that has been removed from the skin is considered contaminated and cannot be reused.*
- If blood begins to flow out of the vein into the tissues as the catheter is inserted, creating a hematoma, the insertion has not been successful. This is sometimes referred to as a blown vein. Immediately release the tourniquet and remove the catheter, applying pressure over the insertion site with dry gauze. Attempt the venipuncture in another site, in the opposite arm if possible. **Rationale:** *Placing the tourniquet back on the same arm above the unsuccessful site may cause it to bleed. Placing the IV below the unsuccessful site could result in infusing fluid into the already punctured vein, causing it to leak.*

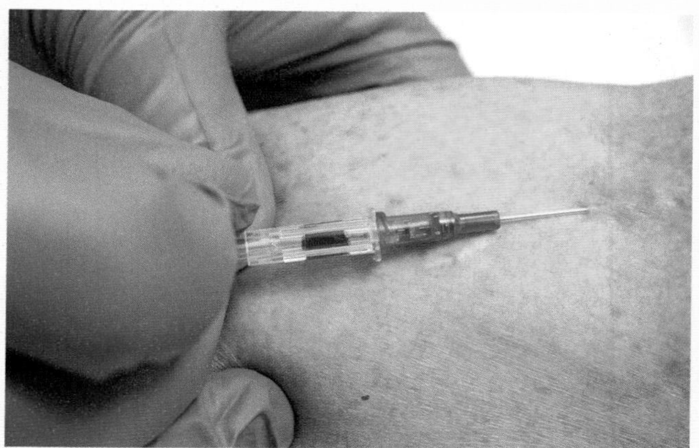

❹ Blood is noted in the flashback chamber once the stylet has entered the vein.

Starting an Intravenous Infusion and Inserting a Short Peripheral Catheter—*continued*

- Release the tourniquet.
- Put pressure on the vein proximal to the catheter to eliminate or reduce blood oozing out of the catheter. Stabilize the hub with thumb and index finger of the nondominant hand.
- Remove the protective cap from the distal end of the tubing and hold it ready to attach to the catheter, maintaining the sterility of the end.
- Stabilize the catheter hub and apply pressure distal to the catheter with your finger. ❺ **Rationale:** *This prevents excessive blood flow through the catheter.*
- Carefully remove the stylet, engage the needle safety device if it does not engage automatically, and attach the end of the infusion tubing to the catheter hub. Place the stylet directly into a sharps container. If this is not within reach, place the stylet into its original package and dispose in a sharps container as soon as possible. Consider use of an extension set to reduce catheter manipulation. If used, prime the extension set prior to inserting the short peripheral catheter.
- Initiate the infusion or flush the catheter with sterile normal saline. ❻ **Rationale:** *Blood must be removed from the catheter lumen and tubing immediately. Otherwise, the blood will clot inside the lumen.* Watch closely for any signs that the catheter is infiltrated. **Infiltration** is when the tip of the IV catheter is outside the vein and the fluid is entering the tissues instead of the intended vascular route. It is manifested by localized swelling, coolness, pallor, and discomfort at the IV site. **Rationale:** *Inflammation or infiltration necessitates removal of the IV needle or catheter to avoid further trauma to the tissue.*

18. Stabilize the catheter and apply a dressing.
- Secure the catheter according to the manufacturer's instructions and agency policy. Several methods are used to stabilize the catheter including the use of a dressing and securement device. If tape is used, it must be sterile tape or surgical strips and they should be applied only to the catheter adapter and not placed directly on the catheter–skin junction site. Use of a manufactured stabilization device is preferred (INS, 2016a).
- Apply a TSM dressing over the insertion site. ❼ The TSM allows for continuous assessment of the site. Do not use ointment of any kind under a TSM dressing. Additional tape may be used to secure the IV catheter below the TSM, if necessary. Do not place tape on the TSM dressing.
- Label the dressing with the date and time of insertion, gauge, and your initials. ❽
- Apply an IV site protection device, if available. Protection devices are available that help prevent dislodgement of the IV catheter and still provide easy assessment of the IV site.
- Loop the tubing and secure it with tape. **Rationale:** *Looping and securing the tubing prevent the weight of the tubing or any movement from pulling on the needle or catheter.*

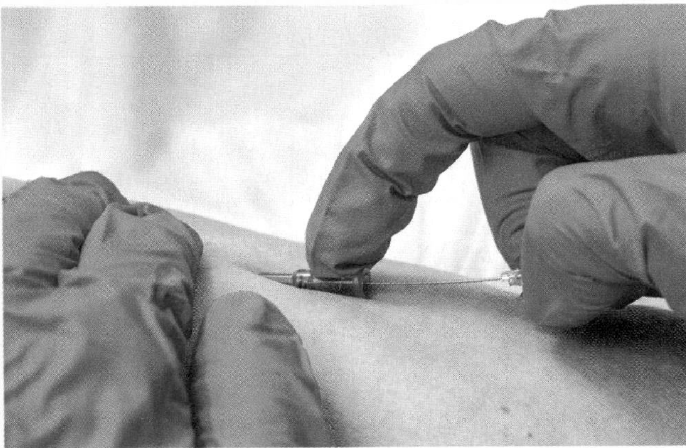

❺ Stabilize the catheter hub and occlude the vein with finger(s) while removing the stylet.

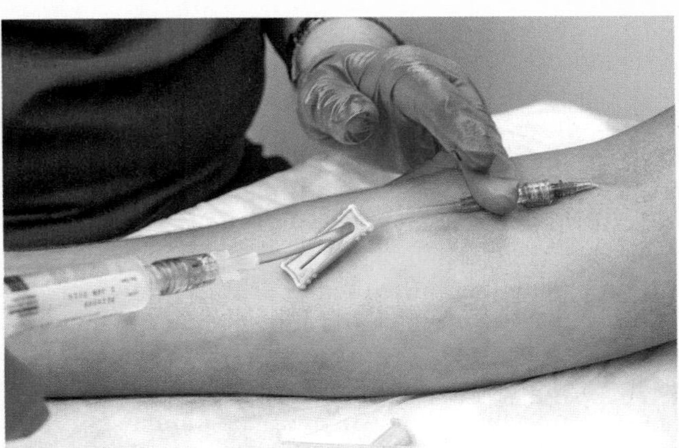

❻ The catheter is stabilized while gently flushing it to determine patency.

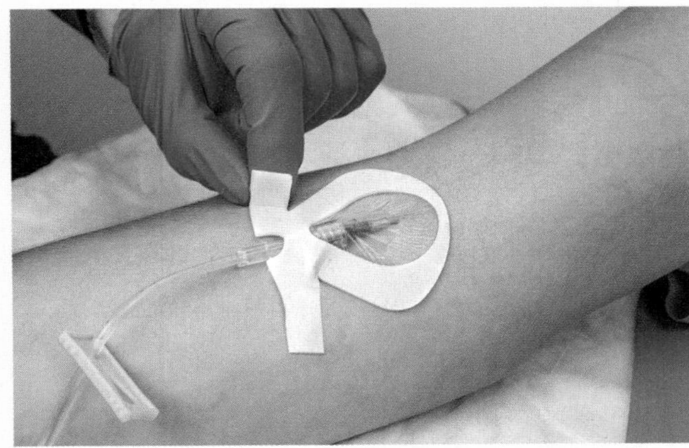

❼ Applying a sterile one-piece IV stabilization and TSM dressing device.

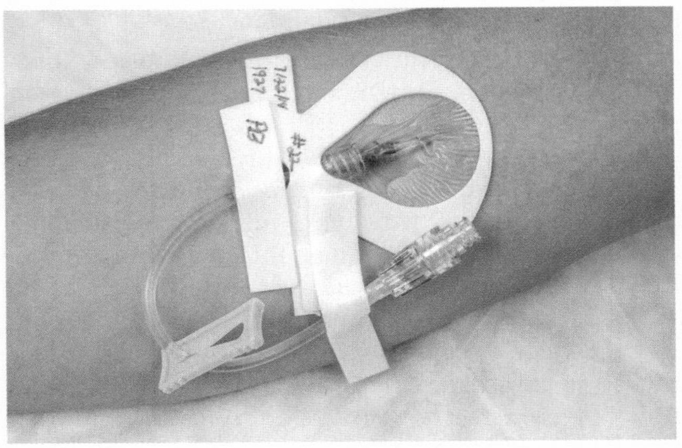

❽ IV site is labeled with date, time, size of catheter, and initials.

Continued on page 1410

SKILL 51.1

Starting an Intravenous Infusion and Inserting a Short Peripheral Catheter—*continued*

19. Discard the tourniquet.
    - Remove and discard gloves.
    - Perform hand hygiene.
20. Ensure appropriate infusion flow.
    - Apply a padded arm board to splint the joint if needed.
    - Adjust the infusion rate of flow according to the order.
21. Label the IV tubing.
    - Label the tubing with the date and time of attachment and your initials. ⑨ This labeling may also be done when the infusion is started. **Rationale:** *The tubing is labeled to ensure that it is changed at regular intervals (i.e., according to agency policy).*

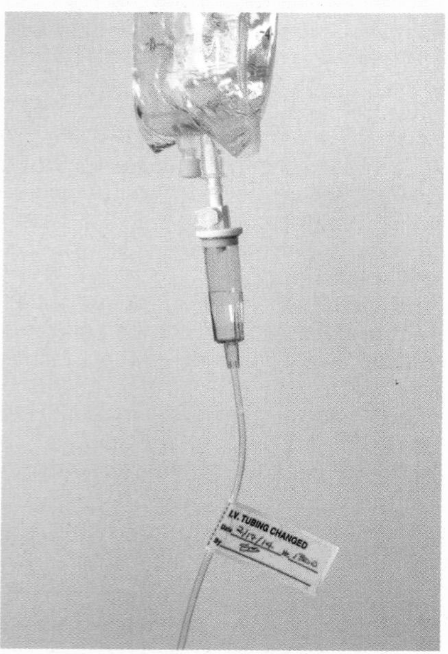

⑨ Tubing labeled with date, time, and nurse's initials.

22. After IV insertion, complete the following client teaching:
    - Any limitations as to movement or mobility and protection of the site
    - Signs and symptoms to report to the nurse
    - Alarms if an electronic infusion device is being used
    - Infection prevention precautions, including hand hygiene by all healthcare providers who provide care (Gorski, 2018, p. 296).
23. Document all assessments and interventions.
    - Record the venipuncture on the client's chart. Some agencies provide a special form for this purpose. Include the date and time of the venipuncture; use of visualization technology as appropriate; type, length, and gauge of the needle or catheter; venipuncture site, how many attempts were made, amount and type of solution used, including any additives (e.g., kind and amount of medications); flow rate; the type of dressing applied; the client's general response; and client education.

SAMPLE DOCUMENTATION

1/15/2020 0600 Inserted 20-gauge, 1-inch angiocath in the right cephalic vein 4 inches above the (L) wrist on first attempt. StatLock used to stabilize catheter and TSM dressing applied. IV infusing at 125 mL/h. Explained reason for IV. Verbalized understanding. A. Luis, RN

EVALUATION

- Regularly check the client for intended and adverse effects of the infusion.
- Perform follow-up based on findings or outcomes that deviated from expected or normal for the client. Compare findings to previous data if available.
- At least every 4 hours, check the skin status at IV site (warm temperature and absence of pain, redness, or swelling), status of the dressing, the client's ability to perform self-care activities, and the client's understanding of any mobility limitations.
- Report significant deviations from normal to the primary care provider.

Regulating and Monitoring Intravenous Infusions

An important nursing function is to regulate the flow rate of an IV infusion. Orders for IV infusions may take several forms, for example "3000 mL over 24 hours," "1000 mL every 8 hours × 3 bags," or "125 mL/h until oral intake is adequate." The nurse initiating the IV calculates the correct flow rate, regulates the infusion, and monitors the client's responses. Unless an infusion control device is used, the nurse manually regulates the drops per minute of flow using the roller clamp to ensure that the prescribed amount of solution will be infused in the correct time span. Problems that can result from incorrectly regulated infusions include hypervolemia, hypovolemia, electrolyte imbalances, and medication complications.

The number of drops delivered per milliliter of solution varies with different brands and types of infusion sets. This rate, called the **drop factor**, is printed on the package of the infusion set. Macrodrops commonly have drop factors of 10, 12, 15, or 20 drops/mL; the drop factor for microdrip sets is always 60 drops/mL (see Figure 51.24 earlier).

To calculate flow rates, the nurse must know the volume of fluid to be infused and the specific time for the infusion. Two commonly used methods of indicating flow rates are designating (1) the number of milliliters to be administered in 1 hour (mL/h) or (2) the number of drops to be given in 1 minute (gtt/min).

Occasionally, the IV rate order will read "keep vein open" (KVO) or "to keep open" (TKO). This order does not provide adequate direction for the nurse unless agency policy specifies the milliliters per hour equivalent for this order. Generally, the KVO rate is less than 50 mL/h. Some IV pumps have a keep-open rate choice built in. If the IV is not on this type of pump and no policy exists, contact the primary care provider for clarification.

Milliliters per Hour

Hourly rates of infusion can be calculated by dividing the total infusion volume by the total infusion time in hours. For example, if 3000 mL is infused in 24 hours, the number of milliliters per hour is

$$\frac{3000 \text{ mL (total infusion volume)}}{24 \text{ h (total infusion time)}} = 125 \text{ mL/h}$$

Nurses need to check infusions at least every hour to ensure that the indicated milliliters per hour have infused and that IV patency is maintained.

Drops per Minute

The nurse who begins an infusion must regulate the drops per minute to ensure that the prescribed amount of solution will infuse. Drops per minute are calculated by the following formula:

$$\text{Drops per minute} = \frac{\text{Total infusion volume} \times \text{drop factor}}{\text{Total time of infusion in minutes}}$$

If the requirements are 1000 mL in 8 hours and the drip factor is 20 drops/mL, the drops per minute should be

$$\frac{1000 \text{ mL} \times 20}{8 \times 60 \text{ min (480 min)}} = 41 \text{ drops/min}$$

The nurse regulates the drops per minute by tightening or releasing the IV tubing clamp and counting the drops for 15 seconds, then multiplying that number by 4.

A number of factors influence flow rate (Box 51.6).

Devices to Control Infusions

Historically, the nurse manually regulated the IV rate with the roller clamp on the administration set. Although a roller clamp can still be used, a number of other devices are available to control the rate of an infusion. The term *flow-control device* refers to any manual, mechanical, or electronic infusion device used to regulate the IV flow rate. The *Infusion Therapy Standards of Practice* (INS, 2016a) state that the choice of a flow-control device (e.g., manual flow regulator, elastomeric balloon pump, electronic infusion device) should consider the age and mobility of the client, severity of illness, type of therapy, and healthcare setting (p. S48).

In the acute healthcare setting, electronic infusion devices (EIDs) are predominantly used to regulate the infusion rate at preset limits. They are used for IV infusions that require precise flow control and for client safety. EIDs are powered by electricity or battery and are programmed to regulate the IV flow rate in either drops per minute or milliliters per hour (Figure 51.28 ■). They use positive pressure to deliver the IV solution, provide an accurate flow rate, are easy to use, and have alarms that signal problems with the infusion (e.g., when the solution in the IV bag is low, when there is air in the tubing, or when flow is impeded by an occlusion). The alarms are helpful; however, the nurse must still conduct regular assessment and evaluation of the IV site to ensure safe infusion.

Clinical Alert!

Many EIDs use low infusion pressures, often lower than the pressure of a gravity delivery. As a result, they do not detect infiltration. When an infiltration occurs, the inline pressure may drop and not trigger an alarm. Thus, it is important for the nurse to assess for infiltration for clients with EIDs (Gorski, 2018, p. 252).

Another type of flow-control device is the multichannel pump. This type of pump can deliver several medications and fluids at the same time, at multiple rates, from bags, bottles, or syringes (Gorski, 2018, p. 249). The multichannel pump usually has two to four

BOX 51.6 Factors Influencing Flow Rates

- *The position of the forearm.* Sometimes a change in the position of the client's arm decreases flow. Slight pronation, supination, extension, or elevation of the forearm on a pillow can increase flow.
- *The position and patency of the tubing.* Tubing can be obstructed by the client's weight, a kink, or a clamp closed too tightly. The flow rate also diminishes when part of the tubing dangles below the puncture site.
- *The height of the infusion bottle.* Elevating the height of the infusion bottle a few inches can speed the flow by creating more pressure.
- *Possible infiltration or fluid leakage.* Swelling, a feeling of coldness, and tenderness at the venipuncture site may indicate infiltration.
- *Relationship of the size of the angiocath to the vein.* A catheter that is too large may impede the infusion flow.

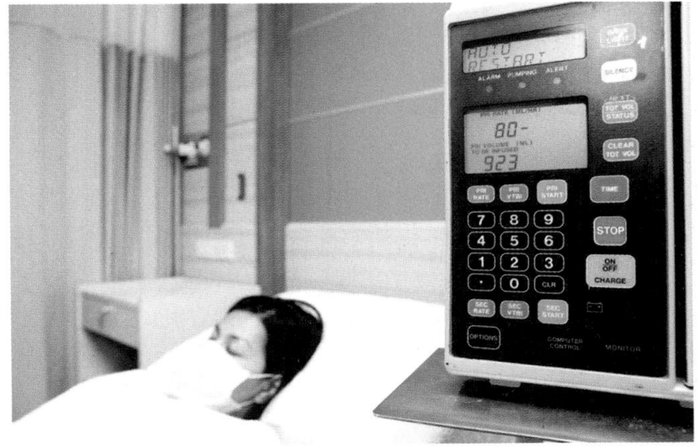

Figure 51.28 ■ An EID.
Jatuporn Amorntangsati/123RF.

channels with each channel being programmed independently (Figure 51.29 ■).

Newer systems, called smart pumps, are EIDs with a computer system. They are programmable and include drug libraries with dose rate calculators, automatic flushing between medications, dual or triple simultaneous line control, memory, multiple alarm settings, air in line, pressure and resistance, battery, schedule reminders, volume settings down to 0.1 mL, panel locks, and digital displays (Giuliano & Ruppel, 2017, p. 64). Smart pumps have advanced complex IV medication and client safety. However, safety issues still exist. It is important that nurses who use this technology work closely with vendors to make suggestions on how to improve the technology.

Mechanical flow-control devices are often used to regulate infusion rates in home care and ambulatory settings. Examples of these nonelectric methods include use of a Dial-A-Flo in-line gravity control device and the elastomeric pump. The Dial-A-Flo in-line device (Figure 51.30 ■) is a manual regulator that controls the amount of fluid to be administered. The Dial-A-Flo may be used in situations where a pump is not available or required, but prevention of fluid overload is important. The nurse presets the volume to be infused by rotating the dial to the desired rate. It is important for the nurse to remember to verify the flow rate by counting the drops.

The elastomeric infusion pump (Figure 51.31 ■), a nonelectric portable disposable pump, is prefilled with a medication and connects to the client's needleless connector. It is a lightweight, disposable pump that delivers medications at a controlled rate. The medication is held in a reservoir (balloon) that is inside a rigid, transparent container. The balloon exerts positive pressure to administer the medication into the tubing that is attached to the client's vascular access device. It has

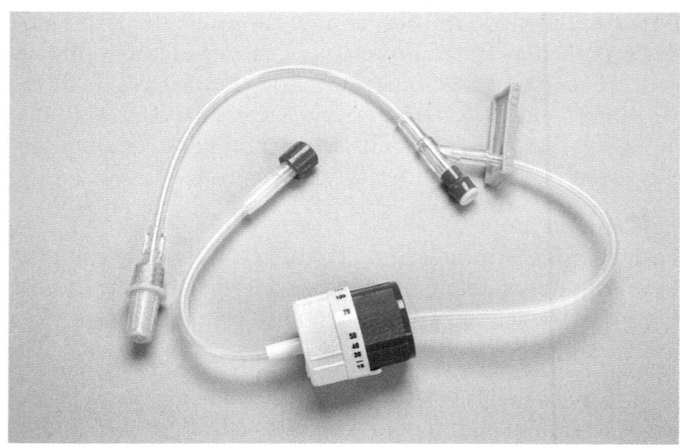

A

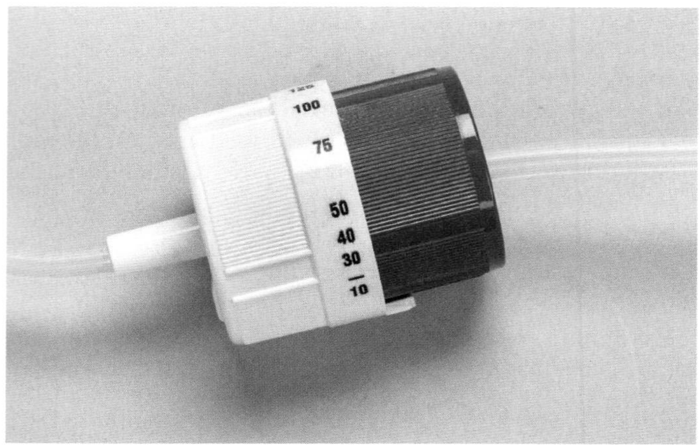

B

Figure 51.30 ■ *A*, The Dial-A-Flo in-line gravity control device; *B*, the manual rate-flow regulator.

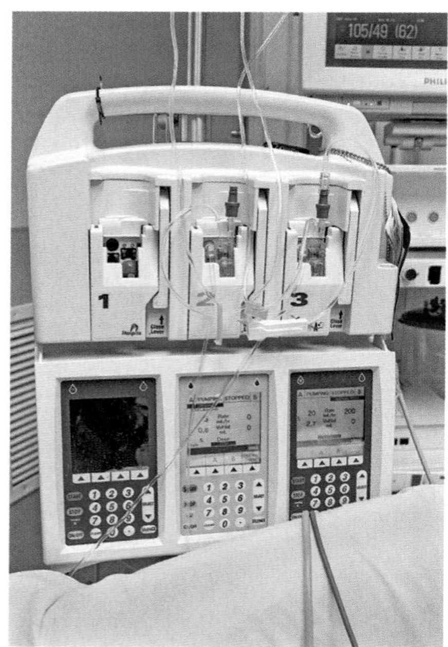

Figure 51.29 ■ Programmable multichannel infusion pump.

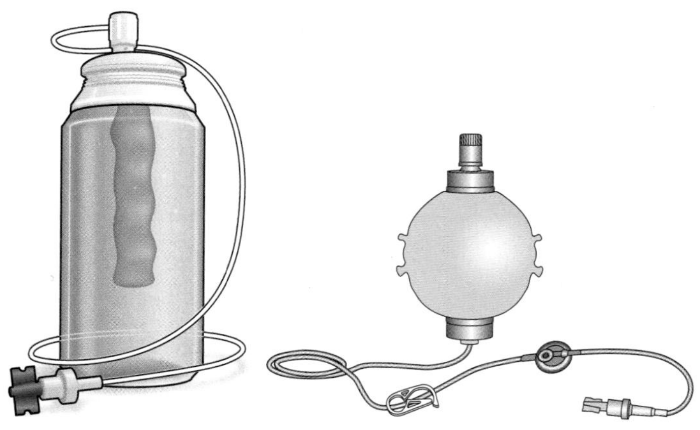

Figure 51.31 ■ Examples of elastomeric infusion pumps often used in home settings.

an integrated flow restrictor that controls the flow rate (Gorski, 2018, p. 241). The elastomeric infusion pump is portable and can be put in a loose pocket or bag while infusing, allowing the client to be mobile. When the infusion is finished, the entire device is discarded. The elastomeric pump provides ease of use in the home care setting.

Clinical Alert!

A flow-rate-control device should be used when administering IV fluid to older adults or pediatric clients. Both of these age groups are especially at risk for complications of fluid overload, which can occur with rapid infusion of IV fluids.

Skill 51.2 outlines the steps involved in monitoring an IV infusion.

Monitoring an Intravenous Infusion

SKILL 51.2

PURPOSES

- To maintain the prescribed flow rate
- To prevent complications associated with IV therapy

ASSESSMENT

Assess

- Appearance of infusion site; patency of system
- Type of fluid being infused and rate of flow
- Response of the client

PLANNING

Review the client record regarding previous infusions and use of infusion devices. Note any complications and how they were managed. Gather the pertinent data.

- From the order, determine the type and sequence of solutions to be infused.
- Determine the rate of flow and infusion schedule.

Assignment

Due to the need for sterile technique and technical complexity, inspection of IV sites and regulation of IV rates is not assigned to AP. AP may care for clients with such devices, and the nurse must ensure that the AP knows what complications or adverse signs should be reported to the nurse.

In many states, a licensed practical nurse or licensed vocational nurse with special IV therapy training may manage infusions. Check the state's nurse practice act.

Equipment

None

IMPLEMENTATION

Performance

1. Prior to performing the procedure, introduce self and verify the client's identity using agency protocol. Explain to the client what you are going to do, why it is necessary, and how to participate.
2. Perform hand hygiene and observe other appropriate infection prevention procedures.
3. Position the client appropriately.
   - Assist the client to a comfortable position, either sitting or lying.
   - Expose the IV site but provide for client privacy.
4. Ensure that the correct solution is being infused.
   - Compare the label on the container (including added medications) to the order. If the solution is incorrect, slow the rate of flow to a minimum to maintain the patency of the catheter. If the infusing solution is contraindicated for the client, stop the infusion and saline-lock the catheter. **Rationale:** *Just stopping the infusion may allow a thrombus to form in the IV catheter. If this occurs, the catheter must be removed and another venipuncture performed before the infusion can be resumed. Because IV tubing contains approximately 12 to 15 mL, it may be desirable to prevent even this much additional incorrect solution to infuse when the correct IV solution container is hung on existing tubing. In this case, all tubing should be removed until new tubing, primed with the correct solution, can be started.*
   - Change the solution to the correct one, using new tubing if indicated.
   - Document and report the error according to agency protocol.
5. Observe the rate of flow every hour.
   - Compare the rate of flow regularly, for example, every hour, against the infusion schedule. **Rationale:** *Infusions that are off schedule can be harmful to a client*. To read the volume in an IV bag, pull the edges of the bag apart at the level of the fluid and read the volume remaining. **Rationale:** *Stretching the bag allows the fluid meniscus to fall to the proper level*.
   - Observe the position of the solution container. If it is less than 1 m (3 ft) above the IV site, readjust it to the correct height of the pole. **Rationale:** *If the container is too low with a gravity IV infusion, the solution may not flow into the vein because there is insufficient gravitational pressure to overcome the pressure of the blood within the vein*.
   - If too much fluid has infused in the time interval, check agency policy. The primary care provider may need to be notified.

Continued on page 1414

SKILL 51.2

Monitoring an Intravenous Infusion—*continued*

- In some agencies, you will slow the infusion to less than the ordered rate so that it will be completed at the planned time. **Rationale:** *Solution administered too quickly may cause a significant increase in circulating blood volume (which is about 6 L in an adult). Hypervolemia may result in pulmonary edema and cardiac failure*. Assess the client for manifestations of hypervolemia and its complications, including dyspnea; rapid, labored breathing; cough; crackles; tachycardia; and bounding pulses.
- In other agencies, if the order is for a specified amount of fluid per hour, the IV may be adjusted to the correct rate and the client monitored for signs of fluid overload.
- If the rate is too slow, adjust the IV to the prescribed rate. Also, check agency policy. Some agencies permit nursing personnel to adjust an IV that is behind time by a specified percentage. Adjustments above this amount may require a primary care provider's order. **Rationale:** *Solution that is administered too slowly can supply insufficient fluid, electrolytes, or medication for a client's needs*.
- If the prescribed rate of flow is 150 mL/h or more, check the rate of flow more frequently, for example, every 15 to 30 minutes.

6. Inspect the patency of the IV tubing and catheter.
- Observe the drip chamber. If it is less than half full, squeeze the chamber to allow the correct amount of fluid to flow in.
- Inspect the tubing for kinks or obstructions to flow. Arrange the tubing so that it is lightly coiled and under no pressure. Sometimes the tubing becomes caught under the client's body and the weight blocks the flow.
- Observe the position of the tubing. If it is dangling below the venipuncture, coil it carefully on the surface of the bed. **Rationale:** *The solution may not flow upward into the vein against the force of gravity*.
- Determine catheter position. Some methods include:
  a. Aspirate the catheter for a blood return. Do this slowly and gently.
  b. Lower the solution container below the level of the infusion site and observe for a return flow of blood from the vein. **Rationale:** *A return flow of blood indicates that the needle is patent and in the vein. Blood returns in this instance because venous pressure is greater than the fluid pressure in the IV tubing. Absence of blood return may indicate that the needle is no longer in the vein or that the tip of the catheter is partially obstructed by a thrombus, the vein wall, or a valve in the vein. (Note: With some catheters, no blood may appear even with patency because the soft catheter walls collapse during siphoning.)*
  c. If there is leakage, locate the source. If the leak is at the catheter connection, tighten the tubing into the catheter. If the leak is elsewhere in the tubing, slow the infusion and replace the tubing. Estimate the amount of solution lost, if it was substantial. If the IV insertion site is leaking, the catheter will have to be removed and IV vascular access reestablished at a new site.

7. Inspect the insertion site for fluid infiltration.
- If infiltration is present, stop the infusion and remove the catheter. Restart the infusion at another site.
- Start supportive treatment (e.g., elevate extremity or apply heat to the site [INS, 2016a]). **Rationale:** *Warmth promotes comfort and vasodilation, facilitating absorption of the fluid from interstitial tissues*.
- If the infiltration involves a **vesicant**, a medication or fluid that causes blisters, severe tissue injury, or necrosis if it escapes from the vein (Mattox, 2017, p. e2), it is called **extravasation** and other measures are indicated. The extravasation of a vesicant drug should be considered an emergency. Usually, vesicants are administered only through CVADs and by specially certified nurses. Most nurses relate vesicants to chemotherapy medications, such as paclitaxel; however, there are a number of non-chemotherapeutic medications (e.g., vancomycin, dopamine, diazepam, phenytoin).
- For an extravasation:
  a. Stop the infusion immediately.
  b. For a short peripheral catheter, disconnect the tubing from the catheter hub and attach a 3- or 5-mL syringe. Aspirate any fluid remaining in the hub and catheter. Do *not* flush the catheter.
  c. Remove the catheter. Use a dry gauze pad to control bleeding.
  d. Apply a new dry dressing. Do not apply excessive pressure to the area. **Rationale:** *Applying pressure will disperse fluid farther into surrounding tissue* (Gorski, 2018, p. 446).
  e. For a CVAD, do not remove the catheter. Clamp and cap the catheter hub. Follow agency procedure for flushing when extravasation is suspected.
  f. Assess motion, sensation, and capillary refill distal to the injury. Measure the circumference of the extremity and compare it with the opposite extremity. Using a skin marker, outline the area with visible signs of extravasation to assess for changes.
  g. Notify the primary care provider.
  h. Photograph the site if that is agency policy.
  i. The affected arm should be elevated and, depending on the drug, heat or cold therapy should be implemented.
  j. Pharmacologic treatment may be instituted depending on the type of vesicant that has caused the damage. Two such medications to lessen tissue injury are phentolamine for extravasation of vasopressors and hyaluronidase, which can be used in extravasation of some hyperosmolar solutions (e.g., calcium chloride), radiographic contrast media, and plant alkaloids (e.g., vincristine) (Gorski, 2018, p. 446). The best results occur when administered immediately after an extravasation (INS, 2016a, p. S100).

8. Inspect the insertion site for phlebitis (inflammation of a vein).
- Inspect and palpate the site at least every 8 hours. Phlebitis can occur as a result of injury to a vein, for example, because of mechanical trauma or chemical irritation. Chemical injury to a vein can occur from IV electrolytes (especially potassium and magnesium) and medications. The clinical signs can include redness, warmth, swelling at the IV site, burning pain along the course of a vein, tenderness, palpable venous cord, and purulent drainage.
- If phlebitis is detected, discontinue the infusion, and apply warm or cold compresses to the venipuncture site. Do not use this injured vein for further infusions.

9. Inspect the IV site for bleeding.
- Oozing or bleeding into the surrounding tissues can occur while the infusion is freely flowing, but is more likely to occur after the catheter has been removed from the vein.
- Observation of the vascular access site is extremely important for clients who bleed readily, such as those receiving anticoagulants.

Monitoring an Intravenous Infusion—*continued*

10. Teach the client ways to maintain the infusion system, for example:
    - Inform of any limitations on movement or mobility.
    - Explain alarms if an electronic control device is used.
    - Instruct to notify a nurse if:
      a. The flow rate suddenly changes or the solution stops dripping.
      b. The solution container is nearly empty.
      c. There is blood in the IV tubing.
      d. Discomfort or swelling is experienced at the IV site.
    - Inform that the nurse will be checking the venipuncture site.
11. Document relevant information (often on a specified form).
    - Record the status of the IV insertion site and any adverse responses of the client.
    - Document the client's IV fluid intake at least every 8 hours according to agency policy. Include the date and time; amount and type of solution used; container number; flow rate; and the client's general response. In most agencies, the amount remaining in each IV container is also recorded at the end of the shift.

SKILL 51.2

EVALUATION

- Perform follow-up based on findings or outcomes that deviated from expected or normal for the client. Consider urinary output compared to intake, tissue turgor, specific gravity of urine, vital signs, and lung sounds compared to baseline data.
- Regularly check the client for intended and adverse effects of the infusion. Report significant deviations from normal to the primary care provider.

Changing Intravenous Containers and Tubing

IV solution containers are changed when only a small amount of fluid remains in the neck of the container and fluid still remains in the drip chamber. However, all IV bags should be changed every 24 hours, regardless of how much solution remains, to minimize the risk of contamination. Change primary administration sets and secondary tubing that remains continuously attached to them "no more frequently than every 96 hours" (INS, 2016a, p. S84). Change intermittent infusion sets without a primary infusion every 24 hours or whenever their sterility is in question (INS, 2016a). Add-on devices (e.g., extension sets, filters, stopcocks) should be changed at the same time the administration set is changed. The INS *Infusion Therapy Standards* (2016a) state to "perform dressing changes on short peripheral catheters if the dressing becomes damp, loosened, or visibly soiled and at least every 5 to 7 days" (p. S82). Skill 51.3 provides guidelines for changing an IV solution container and tubing.

Changing an Intravenous Container and Tubing

SKILL 51.3

PURPOSES

- To maintain the flow of required fluids
- To maintain sterility of the IV system and decrease the incidence of phlebitis and infection
- To maintain patency of the IV tubing

ASSESSMENT

Assess

- Presence of fluid infiltration, leakage, bleeding, or phlebitis at IV site
- Allergy to tape or iodine
- Infusion rate and amount absorbed
- Blockages in IV system
- Appearance of the dressing for integrity, moisture, and need for change

PLANNING

Review primary care provider's orders for changes in fluid administration.

Assignment

This procedure includes assessment of the IV site and should be completed by a registered nurse. In many states, licensed vocational nurses with IV certification may complete the procedure.

Equipment

- Container with the correct kind and amount of sterile solution
- Administration set, including sterile tubing and drip chamber

IMPLEMENTATION

Preparation

- Obtain the correct solution container.
- Read the label of the new container.
- Verify that you have the correct solution, correct client, correct additives (if any), and correct dose (number of bags or total volume ordered).

Performance

1. Prior to performing the procedure, introduce self and verify the client's identity using agency protocol. Explain to the client what you are going to do, why it is necessary, and how to participate.
2. Perform hand hygiene and observe other appropriate infection prevention procedures.

Continued on page 1416

Changing an Intravenous Container and Tubing—*continued*

SKILL 51.3

3. Set up the IV equipment with the new container and label. See Skill 51.1, steps 1 to 9.
   - Label the tubing as shown in Figure 9 in Skill 51.1.
4. Assess the IV site.
   - Inspect the IV site for the presence of infiltration or inflammation. **Rationale:** *Inflammation or infiltration necessitates removal of the IV catheter to avoid further trauma to the tissues.*
   - Go to step 5 or discontinue and relocate the IV site if indicated. See Skills 51.1 and 51.4.
5. Disconnect the used tubing or remove the cap on an intermittent infusion device (i.e., needleless connector).
   - Apply clean gloves.
   - Place a sterile swab under the hub of the catheter. **Rationale:** *This absorbs any leakage that might occur when the tubing is disconnected.*
   - Clamp the tubing. With the fourth or fifth finger of the nondominant hand, apply pressure to the vein above the end of the catheter. **Rationale:** *This helps prevent blood from coming out of the needle during the change of tubing.*
   - Holding the hub of the catheter with the thumb and index finger of the nondominant hand, remove the tubing or cap with the dominant hand, using a twisting and pulling motion. **Rationale:** *Holding the catheter firmly but gently maintains its position in the vein.*
   - Remove the used IV tubing.
   - Place the end of the used tubing in the basin or other receptacle.
6. Connect the new tubing or cap and reestablish the infusion.
   - Continue to hold the catheter and grasp the new tubing with the dominant hand.
   - Remove the protective tubing cap and, maintaining sterility, insert the tubing end securely into the needle hub. Twist it to secure it.
   - Open the clamp to start the solution flowing.
7. Secure IV tubing with additional tape as required.
8. Regulate the rate of flow of the solution according to the order on the chart.
9. Document all relevant information.
   - Record the change of the solution container and tubing in the appropriate place on the client's chart. Also record the fluid intake according to agency practice. Record the number of the container if the containers are numbered at the agency. Also record your assessments.

EVALUATION

Evaluate the following:

- Status of IV site
- Patency of IV system
- Accuracy of flow

When an IV infusion is no longer necessary to maintain the client's fluid intake or to provide a route for medication administration, the infusion is either discontinued and the catheter removed or the catheter is left in place and converted to a saline lock. Guidelines for discontinuing an IV infusion or converting the catheter to a lock are outlined in Skills 51.4 and 51.5, respectively.

Discontinuing an Intravenous Infusion and Removing a Short Peripheral Catheter

SKILL 51.4

PURPOSE

- To discontinue an IV infusion when the therapy is complete or when the IV site needs to be changed

ASSESSMENT

Assess

- Appearance of the venipuncture site
- Any bleeding from the infusion site
- Amount of fluid infused
- Appearance of short peripheral catheter

PLANNING

Review the client record regarding the primary care provider's orders. Note if there were any previous infusions and if there were any complications and how they were managed.

ASSIGNMENT

In some states and agencies, removal of a peripheral IV catheter may be assigned to AP. In others, removal of IV infusions or devices is not assigned to AP. In any case, the nurse must ensure that the AP knows what complications or adverse signs following removal should be reported to the nurse.

In many states, a licensed practical nurse or licensed vocational nurse with special IV therapy training may discontinue IV infusions. Check the state's nurse practice act.

Equipment

- Clean gloves
- Linen-saver pad
- Small sterile dressing and tape

Discontinuing an Intravenous Infusion—*continued*

IMPLEMENTATION

Performance

1. Prior to performing the procedure, introduce self and verify the client's identity using agency protocol. Explain to the client what you are going to do, why it is necessary, and how to participate. Explain the reason for discontinuing the IV and that the procedure should cause no discomfort other than that associated with removing the tape.
2. Perform hand hygiene and observe other appropriate infection prevention procedures.
3. Assist the client to a comfortable position, either sitting or lying. Expose the IV site but provide for client privacy. Place a linen-saver pad under the extremity that has the IV.
4. Prepare the equipment.
   - Clamp the infusion tubing. **Rationale:** *Clamping the tubing prevents the fluid from flowing out of the needle onto the client or bed*.
   - Apply clean gloves.
   - Remove the dressing, stabilization device, and tape at the venipuncture site while holding the needle firmly and applying countertraction to the skin. ❶ **Rationale:** *Movement of the catheter can injure the vein and cause discomfort to the client. Countertraction prevents pulling the skin and causing discomfort*. Use appropriate solution (e.g., alcohol) as indicated to loosen the dressing and securement device adhesive.
   - Assess the vascular access site. **Rationale:** *Assess for signs of infection or phlebitis*.
   - Apply the sterile gauze above the vascular access site with the nondominant hand. Only touch the upper portion of the gauze pad and maintain sterility of the lower portion that is in contact with the venipuncture site.
5. Withdraw the catheter from the vein with the dominant hand.
   - Withdraw the catheter by pulling it out along the line of the vein using gentle, even pressure. **Rationale:** *Pulling it out in line with the vein avoids injury to the vein*. Do not press down on the sterile gauze pad while removing the catheter. ❷
   - Immediately apply firm pressure to the site, using sterile gauze, for a minimum of 30 seconds or until hemostasis is achieved. **Rationale:** *Pressure helps stop the bleeding and prevents hematoma formation*.
   - Hold the client's arm above heart level if any bleeding persists. **Rationale:** *Raising the limb decreases blood flow to the area*.
   - Teach the client to inform the nurse if the site begins to bleed at any time or the client notes any other abnormalities in the area.

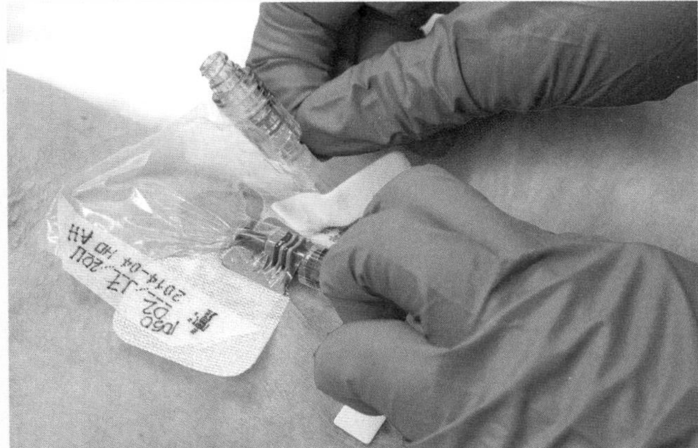

❶ Remove the dressing, stabilization device, and tape while holding the IV catheter firmly.

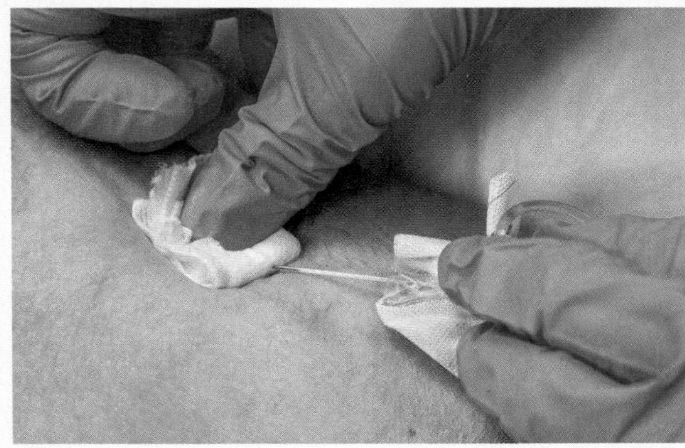

❷ Withdraw the IV catheter from the vein. Do not apply pressure on the sterile gauze pad until the catheter is completely removed.

6. Examine the catheter removed from the client.
   - Check the catheter to make sure it is intact. **Rationale:** *If a piece of tubing remains in the client's vein it could move centrally (toward the heart or lungs)*.
   - Report a broken catheter to the nurse in charge or the primary care provider immediately.
   - If a broken piece can be palpated, apply a tourniquet above the insertion site. **Rationale:** *Application of a tourniquet decreases the possibility of the piece moving until a primary care provider is notified*.
7. Cover the venipuncture site.
   - Apply new sterile dressing to the site with tape. ❸ **Rationale:** *The dressing continues the pressure and covers the open area in the skin, preventing infection*.
   - Discard used supplies appropriately.
   - Remove and discard gloves.
   - Perform hand hygiene.
8. Read the amount remaining in the IV solution container.
9. Apply a black-out label (❹*A*) over the existing IV solution label prior to discarding the IV solution into a biohazard container (❹*B*). **Rationale:** *The existing IV label contains client information. The black-out label conceals client information and ensures client confidentiality*. These labels are called IV HIPAA-compliant labels.
10. Document all relevant information.
    - Record the amount of fluid infused on the intake and output record and in the record, according to agency policy. Include the container number, type of solution used, time of discontinuing the infusion, and the client's response.

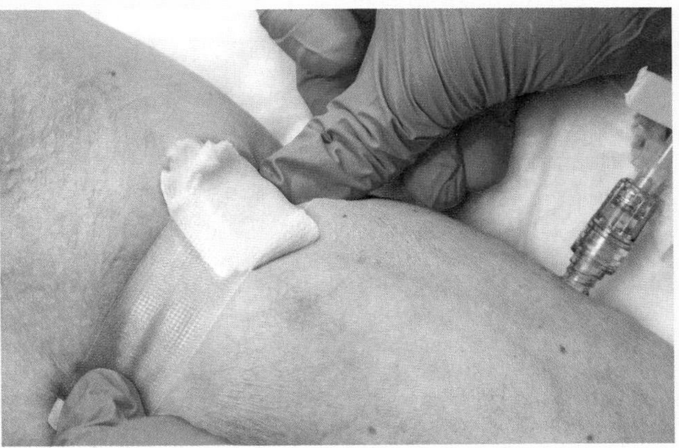

❸ Apply new sterile dressing to the site with tape.

Continued on page 1418

SKILL 51.4

Discontinuing an Intravenous Infusion—*continued*

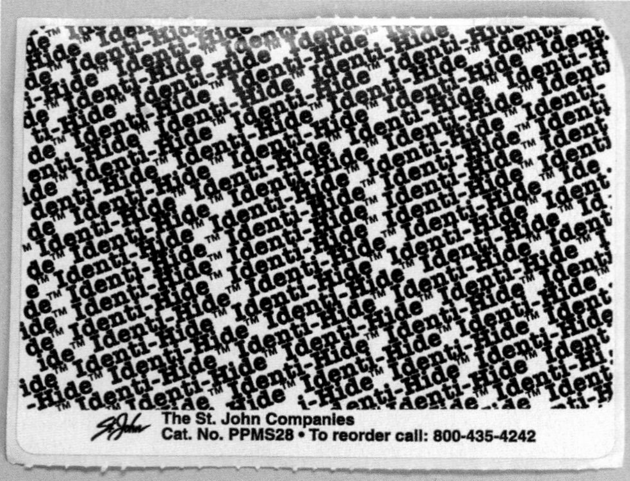

A

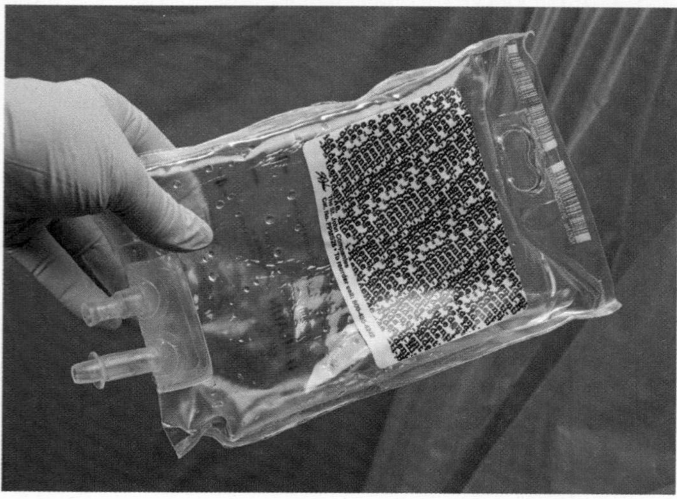

B

4 *A*, An IV black-out label; *B*, discarding an IV bag into a biohazard container after applying a black-out label to ensure client confidentiality.

EVALUATION

- Perform follow-up based on findings or outcomes that deviated from expected or normal for the client. Relate findings to previous data if available.
- Report significant deviations from normal to the primary care provider.

SKILL 51.5

Changing a Short Peripheral Catheter to an Intermittent Infusion Device

PURPOSE

- To permit IV administration of medications or fluids on an intermittent basis

ASSESSMENT

Assess

- Patency of the IV catheter
- Appearance of the site (evidence of inflammation or infiltration)

PLANNING

Review the primary care provider's order.

- A specific order may be written to insert or convert peripheral vascular access to a saline lock. The order also may be implied; for example, IV fluids are to be discontinued but the client has orders for an IV antibiotic every 6 hours or is receiving analgesics intravenously.
- From the primary care provider's order, determine the type and sequence of intermittent infusions.
- Review the client record regarding previous infusions and use of infusion devices. Note any complications and how they were managed.

Assignment

Due to the need for sterile technique and technical complexity, this procedure is not assigned to AP. AP may care for clients with such devices, and the nurse must ensure that the AP knows what complications or adverse signs should be reported to the nurse.

In many states, a licensed practical nurse or licensed vocational nurse with special IV therapy training may manage intermittent infusion devices. Check the state's nurse practice act.

Equipment

- Needleless connector
- Extension tubing (optional)
- Clean gloves
- TSM dressing
- Sterile 2×2 or 4×4 gauze
- Sterile saline for injection (without preservative) in a prefilled syringe
- Isopropyl alcohol wipes
- Tape
- Clean emesis basin

Changing a Short Peripheral Catheter to an Intermittent Infusion Device—*continued*

IMPLEMENTATION

Preparation

- Obtain the needed equipment and take to the client's bedside.

Performance

1. Prior to performing the procedure, introduce self and verify the client's identity using agency protocol. Explain to the client what you are going to do, why it is necessary, and how to participate. Explain the reason for the intermittent infusion device and that changing an IV to a saline lock should cause no discomfort other than that associated with removing tape from the IV tubing.
2. Perform hand hygiene and observe other appropriate infection prevention procedures.
3. Assist the client to a comfortable position, either sitting or lying. Expose the IV site but provide for client privacy.
4. Assess the IV site and determine the patency of the catheter (see Skill 51.2). If the catheter is not fully patent or there is evidence of phlebitis or infiltration, discontinue the catheter and establish a new vascular access site.
   - Expose the IV catheter hub and loosen any tape or dressing that is holding the IV tubing in place or that will interfere with insertion of the needleless connector with extension tubing into the catheter.
   - Clamp the IV tubing to stop the flow of IV fluid.
   - Open the gauze pad and place it under the IV catheter hub. **Rationale:** *This absorbs any leakage that might occur when the tubing is disconnected.*
   - Open the alcohol wipe and needleless connector, leaving the needleless connector in its sterile package.
   - Consider use of an extension tubing between the peripheral catheter and needleless connector. **Rationale:** *This reduces catheter manipulation, which can cause phlebitis*. Prime the extension tubing.
5. Remove the IV tubing and insert the needleless connector and extension tubing into the short peripheral catheter.
   - Apply clean gloves.
   - Stabilize the IV catheter with your nondominant hand and use the little finger to place slight pressure on the vein above the end of the catheter. Twist the IV tubing connection to loosen it from the IV catheter and remove it, placing the end of the tubing in a clean emesis basin.
   - Pick up the needleless connector from its package and remove the protective sleeve from the male adapter maintaining its sterility. Insert the connector into the IV catheter or extension tubing, twisting it to engage the Luer-Lok. Do not allow the male luer of the extension set to touch the skin.
6. Instill saline per agency policy. **Rationale:** *Saline is used to maintain patency of the IV catheter when fluids are not infusing through the catheter*. The intermittent lock will need to be flushed with a prescribed solution after each intermittent infusion or at least every 24 hours if not in use, according to agency policy (Gorski, 2018). The INS recommends the smallest volume for flushing with most organizations using 3 mL. Nurses may use different methods of flushing. Some recommend flushing the lock by injecting saline using the push–pause method (a rapid succession of push–pause–push–pause movements exerted on the plunger of the syringe barrel) with the rationale that this creates a turbulence within the catheter lumen that causes a swirling effect to remove any debris (e.g., blood or medication) attached to the catheter lumen. However, no research supports this method of flushing. There are differences of opinion and practice regarding this type of flushing versus a smooth injection of the flush solution. Research is needed to provide evidence of which is the most effective (Gorski, 2018, p. 303).
7. Cover the site with a TSM dressing. **Rationale:** *The TSM dressing provides protection from infection, allows for ease of assessment of the venipuncture site, and also promotes comfort, preventing the plug from catching on clothing or bedding*.
8. Remove and discard gloves.
   - Perform hand hygiene.
9. Teach the client how to maintain the lock.
   - Notify the nurse or primary care provider if the needleless connector or IV catheter comes out; if the site becomes red, inflamed, or painful; or if any drainage or bleeding occurs at the site.
10. Document all relevant information.
    - Record the date and time when the infusion device was converted, the status of the IV insertion site, and any adverse responses of the client.

EVALUATION

- Perform follow-up based on findings or outcomes that deviated from expected or normal for the client. Relate findings to previous data if available.
- Examine the IV site at regular intervals. Note patency and ease of flushing.
- Report significant deviations from normal to the primary care provider.

Complications of Infusion Therapy

Local complications of infusion therapy occur as adverse reactions or trauma to the venipuncture site. Correct venipuncture technique is a primary factor in prevention along with frequent assessments and monitoring of the venipuncture site. Common local complications include infiltration, extravasation, and phlebitis.

Infiltration can be caused by puncture of the vein during venipuncture, dislodgement of the catheter, or a poorly secured infusion device (Gorski, 2018).

Extravasation is similar to infiltration with the difference between the two being the solution. That is, extravasation is the unintended administration of *vesicant* drugs or fluids into the subcutaneous tissue. Five measures can help prevent infiltration and extravasation. The first measure is the selection of the venipuncture site. Areas of joint flexion such as the hand, wrist, and antecubital fossa should be avoided. The gauge of the catheter should be the smallest that can deliver the prescribed therapy in an appropriate size vein. Knowing the osmolality and pH of medications and fluids is also important. For example, hypertonic fluids and medications should not be infused through a peripheral vein. Using a manufactured catheter stabilization device to prevent unnecessary movement of the catheter in the vein is the fourth measure. Finally, the last measure is assessing patency of the catheter and vein frequently.

Phlebitis is an inflammation of the vein of which there are three types. *Mechanical phlebitis* can be caused by too large of a catheter in a small vein or catheter movement causing irritation of the vein. *Chemical phlebitis* occurs when a vein becomes inflamed by irritating or vesicant solutions or medications. *Bacterial phlebitis* is inflammation of the vein and a bacterial infection, which can be caused by poor aseptic technique during insertion of the IV catheter or breaks in the integrity of the IV equipment. See Box 51.7 for common signs and symptoms of infiltration, extravasation, and phlebitis.

It is important for the nurse to regularly assess all clients with an IV access for signs of phlebitis. One of the INS *Standards* directs nurses to document symptoms of phlebitis using a standardized scale (INS, 2016a). While recent evidence recommends a need for a phlebitis scale that has strong measurement properties for use in clinical practice, there are two commonly used assessment scales that are also recommended by the INS: the INS Phlebitis Scale and the Visual Infusion Phlebitis (VIP) Scale. The INS Phlebitis Scale progresses from Grade 0 (no symptoms) to Grade 4 (includes all symptoms: pain, erythema, streak formation, palpable venous cord, purulent drainage). The VIP Scale progresses from Score 0 (no symptoms) to Score 5 (all symptoms) (INS, 2016a, p. S96)

Prevention strategies for phlebitis include practicing good hand hygiene, assessing the length of time needed for the infusion therapy, and considering alternatives (e.g., midline catheter or PICC) for long-term therapy, choosing the smallest catheter, stabilizing the catheter, infusing solutions at the prescribed rate, avoiding insertion of a peripheral IV catheter in an area of flexion, and assessing the IV site at least every 4 hours (Gorski, 2018, p. 443).

BOX 51.7 Signs and Symptoms of Common Local Complications of Infusion Therapy

INFILTRATION

- Coolness of skin around site
- Skin blanching, tautness (i.e., client states it feels "tight")
- Edema at, above, or below the insertion site
- Leakage at insertion site
- Absence of or "pinkish" blood return
- Difference in size of opposite hand or arm

EXTRAVASATION

Same as infiltration and can also include:

- Burning, stinging pain
- Redness followed by blistering, tissue necrosis, and ulceration

PHLEBITIS

- Redness at the site
- Skin warm
- Swelling
- Palpable cord along the vein
- Increase in temperature

From "Complications of Peripheral Venous Access Devices: Prevention, Detection, and Recovery Strategies," by E. Mattox, 2017, *Critical Care Nurse, 37*(2), pp. e1–e14; *Phillips's Manual of I.V. Therapeutics* (7th ed.), by L. A. Gorski, 2018, Philadelphia, PA: F.A. Davis; and *Infusion Therapy Standards of Practice* (5th ed.), by Infusion Nurses Society, 2016a, Norwood, MA: Author.

Blood Transfusions

IV fluids can be effective in restoring intravascular (blood) volume; however, they do not affect the oxygen-carrying capacity of the blood. When red or white blood cells, platelets, or blood proteins are lost because of hemorrhage or disease, it may be necessary to replace these components to restore the blood's ability to transport oxygen and carbon dioxide, clot, fight infection, and keep extracellular fluid within the intravascular compartment. A blood transfusion is the introduction of whole blood or blood components into venous circulation.

Blood Groups

Human blood is commonly classified into four main groups: A, B, AB, and O. The surface of an individual's RBCs contains a number of proteins known as **antigens** that are unique for each individual. Many blood antigens have been identified, but the A, B, and Rh antigens are the most important in determining blood group or type. Because antigens promote agglutination or clumping of blood cells, they are also known as **agglutinogens**. The A antigen is present on the RBCs of individuals with blood group A, the B antigen is present on the RBCs of individuals with blood group B, and A and B antigens are both present on the RBCs in individuals with group AB blood. Neither antigen is present on the RBCs of individuals with group O blood.

Preformed **antibodies** to RBC antigens are present in the plasma; these antibodies are often called **agglutinins**. Individuals with blood group A have B antibodies (agglutinins); A antibodies are present in individuals with blood group B; and individuals with blood group O have antibodies to both A and B antigens. Individuals with group AB blood do not have antibodies to either A or B antigens (Table 51.12). These naturally occurring antibodies are responsible for the rapid and severe reaction that occurs when ABO-incompatible blood is administered (Gorski, 2018).

Rhesus (Rh) Factor

The Rh factor antigen is present on the RBCs of approximately 85% of the people in the United States. Blood

TABLE 51.12 The Blood Groups with Their Constituent Agglutinogens and Agglutinins

Blood Types	RBC Antigens (Agglutinogens)	Plasma Antibodies (Agglutinins)
A	A	B
B	B	A
AB	A and B	—
O	—	A and B

that contains the Rh factor is known as Rh positive (Rh^+); blood that does not contain the Rh factor is known as Rh negative (Rh^-). In contrast to the ABO blood groups, Rh^- blood does not naturally contain Rh antibodies. However, after exposure to blood containing Rh factor (e.g., an Rh^- mother carrying a fetus with Rh^+ blood, or transfusion of Rh^+ blood into a client who is Rh^-), Rh antibodies develop. Subsequent exposure to Rh^+ blood places the client at risk for an antigen–antibody reaction and hemolysis of RBCs.

Blood Typing and Crossmatching

To avoid transfusing incompatible RBCs, blood from the donor and from the recipient is tested for compatibility. This is referred to as a *type and crossmatch*. Blood typing is done to determine the ABO blood group and Rh factor status. This test is also performed on pregnant women and neonates to assess for incompatibility between their blood types (particularly Rh factor incompatibilities).

Because blood typing only determines the presence of the ABO and Rh antigens, crossmatching is also necessary prior to transfusion to identify possible interactions of minor antigens with their corresponding antibodies. RBCs from the donor blood are mixed with serum from the recipient; a reagent (Coombs' serum) is added, and the mixture is examined for visible agglutination. If no antibodies to the donated RBCs are present in the recipient's serum, agglutination does not occur and the risk of a transfusion reaction is small.

QSEN Patient-Centered Care: Blood and Blood Products

Jehovah's Witness is a Christian religion that believes that taking blood into the body causes loss of eternal life; thus the church decided that members who accepted blood would be shunned by the congregation and denied the church's sacraments (called "disfellowshipped"). In 2000, this policy on blood transfusions was revised to allow the acceptance of blood products based on personal decision and conscience. Based on this change in doctrine, members of this religion have medical confidentiality from the church. However, if there is a breach in the medical confidentiality, the member is "disfellowshipped" by the church. Providing culturally responsive care to this population means it is important for the healthcare provider to interview these clients privately and allow them to make informed decisions about their personal choice to accept or deny blood products. Their decisions should be private and not discussed in front of friends or family members (Campbell, Machan, & Fisher, 2016).

Selection of Blood Donors

Screening of blood donors is rigorous. Criteria have been established to protect the donor from possible ill effects of donation and to protect the recipient from exposure to diseases transmitted through the blood. Blood donors are unpaid volunteers. Potential donors are eliminated by a history of hepatitis B or C, HIV infection (or risk factors for HIV infection), heart disease, most cancers, severe asthma, bleeding disorders, or seizures. Donation may be deferred for individuals who have malaria, have been exposed to malaria or hepatitis, are anemic, have high or low BP, have low body weight, or who are pregnant, have had recent surgery, or take certain medications. Receiving tattoos or piercings in unlicensed facilities results in a 12-month deferral period by the Red Cross (MacIntyre, 2017, p. 46).

Blood and Blood Products for Transfusion

Most clients do not require transfusion of whole blood. It is much more common for clients to receive a transfusion of a particular blood component specific to their individual needs. Table 51.13 lists some of the common blood products that may be transfused.

TABLE 51.13 Blood Products for Transfusion

Product	Use
Whole blood	Not commonly used except for extreme cases of acute hemorrhage. Replaces blood volume and all blood products: RBCs, plasma, plasma proteins, fresh platelets, and other clotting factors.
Packed red blood cells (PRBCs)	Used to increase the oxygen-carrying capacity of blood in anemias, surgery, and disorders with slow bleeding. One unit of PRBCs has the same amount of oxygen-carrying RBCs as a unit of whole blood. One unit raises hematocrit by approximately 2% to 3%.
Autologous RBCs	Used for blood replacement following planned elective surgery. Client donates blood for autologous transfusion 4–5 weeks prior to surgery.
Platelets	Replaces platelets in clients with bleeding disorders or platelet deficiency. Fresh platelets are most effective. Each unit should increase the average adult client's platelet count by about 5000 platelets per microliter.
Fresh frozen plasma	Provides clotting factors. Does not need to be typed and crossmatched (contains no RBCs).
Albumin and plasma protein fraction	Blood volume expander; provides plasma proteins.
Clotting factors and cryoprecipitate	Used for clients with clotting factor deficiencies. Each provides different factors involved in the clotting pathway; cryoprecipitate also contains fibrinogen.

Transfusion Reactions

Transfusion of ABO- or Rh- incompatible blood can result in an **acute hemolytic transfusion reaction (AHTR)**, which causes destruction of the transfused RBCs and subsequent risk of kidney damage or failure. Other forms of acute transfusion reactions may also occur, including febrile or allergic reactions, transfusion-associated circulatory overload (TACO) , and transfusion-related acute lung injury (TRALI). Because the risk of an adverse reaction is high when blood is transfused, clients must be frequently and carefully assessed before and during transfusion. Many reactions become evident within 5 to 15 minutes of initiating the transfusion, but reactions can develop any time during a transfusion; for this reason, clients are most closely monitored during the initial period of the transfusion. Stop the transfusion immediately if signs of a reaction develop. Keep the line open with normal saline. Do not use the saline attached to the Y-set tubing because the filter contains blood and you do not want to give the client who is experiencing an acute transfusion reaction another drop of blood. Instead, use new IV tubing. Disconnect the infusion tubing from the hub of the IV catheter and replace with the new IV tubing. Do not piggyback the new tubing into the access port of the transfusion tubing, because it is possible that some of the blood product could be administered to the client. Hydrate the client with normal saline and notify the primary care provider. Continue to monitor vital signs (Gorski, 2018). Possible transfusion reactions, their clinical signs and symptoms, and nursing implications are listed in Table 51.14.

TABLE 51.14 Transfusion Reactions

Reaction: Cause	Clinical Signs	Nursing Intervention*
Acute hemolytic transfusion reaction (AHTR): incompatibility between client's blood and donor's blood	Fever or chills, flank pain, and reddish or brown urine, tachycardia, hypotension	1. Discontinue the transfusion immediately. *Note*: When the transfusion is discontinued, the blood tubing must be removed as well. Use *new* tubing for the normal saline infusion. 2. Maintain vascular access with normal saline, or according to agency protocol. 3. Notify the primary care provider immediately. 4. Monitor vital signs. 5. Monitor fluid intake and output. 6. Send the remaining blood, bag, filter, tubing, a sample of the client's blood, and a urine sample to the laboratory.
Nonhemolytic febrile reaction: sensitivity of the client's blood to white blood cells, platelets, or plasma proteins; does not cause hemolysis	Fever; chills; warm, flushed skin; headache; anxiety; nausea, vomiting	1. Discontinue the transfusion immediately. 2. Keep the vein open with a normal saline infusion. 3. Notify the primary care provider. 4. Give antipyretics as ordered.
Allergic reaction (mild): sensitivity to infused plasma proteins	Flushing, urticaria, with or without itching	1. Stop the transfusion immediately. Keep vein open with normal saline. 2. Notify the primary care provider. 3. Administer medication (antihistamines, steroids) as ordered.
Allergic reaction (severe): antibody–antigen reaction	Dyspnea, stridor, decreased oxygen saturation, hypotension, shock	1. Stop the transfusion immediately. 2. Keep the vein open with a normal saline solution. 3. Notify the primary care provider immediately. 4. Monitor vital signs. Administer cardiopulmonary resuscitation if needed. 5. Administer medications and/or oxygen as ordered.
Transfusion-associated circulatory overload (TACO): blood administered faster than the circulation can accommodate or client has underlying cardiovascular or renal dysfunction	Dyspnea, orthopnea, crackles (rales), distended neck veins, tachycardia, hypertension	1. Stop the transfusion immediately. 2. Place the client upright. 3. Notify the primary care provider. 4. Administer diuretics and oxygen as ordered.
Transfusion-related acute lung injury (TRALI); occurs in response to infused donor leukocyte antibodies	Acute respiratory distress, hypotension, hypoxemia, fever, chills	1. Stop the transfusion. 2. Keep the vein open with a normal saline infusion. 3. Notify the primary care provider. 4. Oxygen therapy with or without mechanical ventilation 5. Hypotension often corrected by fluid resuscitation. Vasopressor therapy may be needed. 6. Send the remaining blood and tubing to the laboratory.

* Nurses should follow the agency's protocol regarding interventions. These may vary among agencies.

From "A Review of Current Practice in Transfusion Therapy" by M. Carman, J. Uhlenbrock, & S. McClintock, 2018, *American Journal of Nursing, 118*(5), pp. 36–44; "Early Identification of Acute Hemolytic Transfusion Reactions: Realistic Implications for Best Practice in Patient Monitoring" by J. B. Menendez & B. Edwards, 2016, *MEDSURG Nursing, 25*(2), pp. 88–90; and *Phillips's Manual of I.V. Therapeutics* (7th ed.), by L. A. Gorski, 2018, Philadelphia, PA: F.A. Davis.

The hospital must have a protocol relating to transfusion reactions. Common measures include:

- Notify the blood bank.
- Examine the label on the blood container to check for errors in identifying the client, blood, or blood component.
- Obtain laboratory specimens (e.g., blood work, urine sample).
- Send blood container (whether or not it contains any blood), attached infusion set, and IV solution to the blood bank.

Administering Blood

Special precautions are necessary when administering blood. When a transfusion is ordered, the nurse or other personnel obtain blood in plastic bags from the blood bank just before starting the transfusion. One unit of whole blood is 500 mL; a unit of packed red blood cells (PRBCs) is 200 to 250 mL. Do not store the blood in the refrigerator on the nursing unit; lack of temperature control may damage the blood. Once blood or a blood product is removed from the blood bank refrigerator, it must be administered within a limited amount of time (e.g., PRBCs should not hang for more than 4 hours after being removed from the blood bank refrigerator). Follow agency policies for verifying that the unit is correct for the client. The U.S. Food and Drug Administration ([FDA], 2018) requires blood products to have bar codes to allow for scanning and machine-readable information on blood and blood component container labels to help reduce medication errors and increase client safety.

Traditionally, blood has usually been administered through an #18- to #20-gauge IV needle or catheter with the belief being that using smaller needles may slow the infusion and damage blood cells (hemolysis). However, studies have shown that blood infusions through smaller gauge catheters can be completed within 4 hours without hemolysis. Current practice guidelines established by the INS recommend that a #20- to #24-gauge short peripheral catheter is acceptable for transfusion of cellular blood components in adults (INS, 2016b, p. 225). When rapid transfusion is required a #14 to #18-gauge is recommended (INS, 2016a, p. S135). Blood administration sets (Y-sets) are used to keep the vein open while starting the transfusion and to flush the line with normal saline before the blood enters the tubing (Figure 51.32 ■). The infusion tubing has a filter inside the drip chamber. A transfusion should be completed within 4 hours of initiation. The maximum time for use of a blood filter is 4 hours (Gorski, 2018). The INS (2016a) states: "Administer blood or blood components with 0.9% sodium chloride. No other solutions or medications should be added to or infused through the same administration set with blood or blood components unless they have been approved by the FDA for this use" (p. S136). If an additional unit needs to be transfused, follow agency guidelines. A new blood administration set is to be used with each component, or

Safety Alert! SAFETY

2019 The Joint Commission National Patient Safety Goals

Goal 1: Improve the accuracy of patient identification.
Goal 01.03.01: Eliminate transfusion errors related to patient misidentification.

- Before initiating a blood or blood component transfusion:
  - Match the blood or blood component to the order.
  - Match the patient to the blood or blood component.
  - Use a two-person verification process or a one-person verification process accompanied by automated identification technology, such as bar coding.

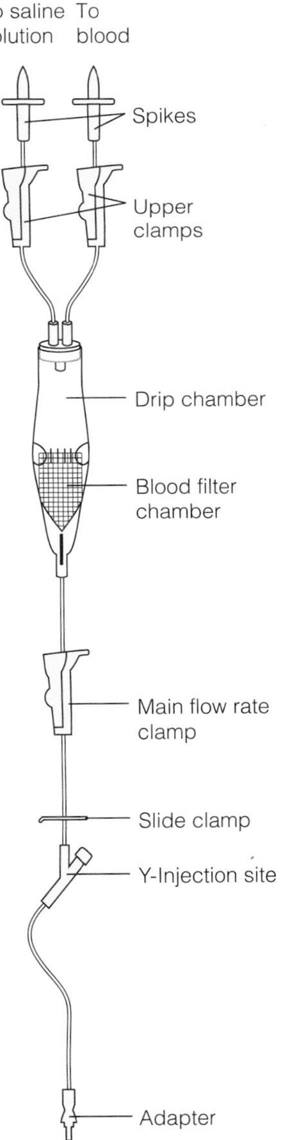

Figure 51.32 ■ Schematic of a Y-set for blood administration.

if more than 1 unit can be infused in 4 hours, the transfusion set can be used for a 4-hour period (Gorski, 2018, p. 580). New IV tubing is used for administering other IV fluids following a transfusion.

To initiate, maintain, and terminate a blood transfusion, see Skill 51.6.

Clinical Alert!

Normal saline must always be used when giving a blood transfusion. If the client has an infusion of any other IV solution, stop that infusion and flush the line with saline prior to initiating the transfusion, or establish IV access through an additional site. Solutions other than saline can cause damage to the blood components.

SKILL 51.6

Initiating, Maintaining, and Terminating a Blood Transfusion Using a Y-Set

PURPOSES

- To restore blood volume after severe hemorrhage
- To restore the oxygen-carrying capacity of the blood
- To provide plasma factors, such as antihemophilic factor (AHF) or factor VIII, or platelet concentrates, which prevent or treat bleeding

ASSESSMENT

Assess

- Vital signs; oxygen saturation is often included
- Physical examination including fluid balance and heart and lung sounds as manifestations of hypo- or hypervolemia
- Status of infusion site and patency of vascular access device
- Blood test results such as hemoglobin value or platelet count
- Any unusual symptoms

PLANNING

- Review the client record regarding previous transfusions. Note any complications and how they were managed (e.g., allergies or previous adverse reactions to blood).
- Confirm the primary care provider's order for the number and type of units and the desired speed of infusion.
- In some agencies, written consent for transfusion is required. Check policy and obtain as indicated.
- Know the purpose of the transfusion.
- Plan to begin the transfusion as soon as the component is ready. Typing and crossmatching can take several hours.
- Note any premedication ordered by the primary care provider (e.g., acetaminophen or diphenhydramine). Schedule their administration (usually 30 minutes prior to the transfusion).

Assignment

Due to the need for sterile technique and technical complexity, blood transfusion is not assigned to AP. The nurse must ensure that the AP knows what complications or adverse signs can occur and should be reported to the nurse. In some states only registered nurses (RNs) can administer blood or blood products.

Equipment

- Unit of whole blood, PRBCs, or other component
- Blood administration set
- IV pump, if needed (use EIDs that have a labeled indication for blood transfusion)
- 250 mL normal saline for infusion
- IV pole
- Venipuncture set containing a #20- to #24-gauge catheter (if one is not already in place)
- Alcohol swabs
- Tape
- Clean gloves

IMPLEMENTATION

Preparation

- If the client has an IV solution infusing, check whether the IV catheter and solution are appropriate to administer blood. The IV catheter size ranges between #20 and #24 gauge, and the solution *must* be normal saline. Dextrose (which causes lysis of RBCs), Ringer's solution, medications and other additives, and hyperalimentation solutions are incompatible. Refer to step 6 if the infusing solution is not compatible.
- If the client does not have an IV solution infusing, check agency policies. In some agencies an infusion must be running before the blood is obtained from the blood bank. In this case, you will need to perform a venipuncture on a suitable vein (see Skill 51.1) and start an IV infusion of normal saline.
- Obtain assistance of another RN to perform client and blood identification process.

Performance

1. Prior to performing the procedure, introduce self and verify the client's identity using agency protocol. Explain to the client what you are going to do, why it is necessary, and how to participate. Instruct the client to report promptly any sudden chills, nausea, itching, rash, dyspnea, back pain, or other unusual symptoms.
2. Provide for client privacy and prepare the client.
   - Assist the client to a comfortable position, either sitting or lying. Expose the IV site but provide for client privacy.
3. Perform hand hygiene and observe other appropriate infection prevention procedures.
4. Prepare the infusion equipment.
   - Ensure that the blood filter inside the drip chamber is suitable for the blood components to be transfused.

Initiating, Maintaining, and Terminating a Blood Transfusion Using a Y-Set—*continued*

SKILL 51.6

Attach the blood tubing to the blood filter, if necessary. **Rationale:** *Blood filters have a surface area large enough to allow the blood components through easily but are designed to trap clots*.

- Apply gloves.
- Close all the clamps on the Y-set: the main flow rate clamp and both Y-line clamps.
- Insert the piercing pin (spike) into the saline solution.
- Hang the container on the IV pole about 1 m (39 in.) above the venipuncture site.

5. Prime the tubing.

- Open the upper clamp on the normal saline tubing, and squeeze the drip chamber until it covers the filter and one-third of the drip chamber above the filter.
- Tap the filter chamber to expel any residual air in the filter.
- Open the main flow rate clamp, and prime the tubing with saline.
- Close both clamps.

6. Start the saline solution.

- If an IV solution incompatible with blood is infusing, stop the infusion and discard the solution and tubing according to agency policy.
- Attach the blood tubing primed with normal saline to the IV catheter.
- Open the saline and main flow rate clamps and adjust the flow rate. Use only the main flow rate clamp to adjust the rate.
- Allow a small amount of solution to infuse to make sure there are no problems with the flow or with the venipuncture site. **Rationale:** *Infusing normal saline before initiating the transfusion also clears the IV catheter of incompatible solutions or medications*.

7. Obtain the correct blood component for the client.

- Check the primary care provider's order with the requisition.
- Check the requisition form and the blood bag label with a laboratory technician or according to agency policy. Specifically, check the client's name, identification number, blood type (A, B, AB, or O) and Rh group, the blood donor number, and the expiration date of the blood. Observe the blood for abnormal color, RBC clumping, gas bubbles, and extraneous material. Return outdated or abnormal blood to the blood bank.
- With another nurse (most agencies require an RN) and in the presence of the client, verify the following before initiating the transfusion (Gorski, 2018, p. 584; INS, 2016b, p. 229):
  a. *Order:* Check the blood or component against the primary care provider's written order.
  b. *Transfusion consent form:* Ensure the form is completed per facility policy.
  c. *Client identification:* The name and identification number on the client's identification band must be identical to the name and number attached to the unit of blood.
  d. *Unit identification:* The unit identification number on the blood container, the transfusion form, and the tag attached to the unit must agree.
  e. *Blood type:* The ABO group and Rh type on the primary label of the donor unit must agree with those recorded on the transfusion form.
  f. *Expiration:* The expiration date and time of the donor unit should be verified as acceptable.
  g. *Compatibility:* The interpretation of compatibility testing must be recorded on the transfusion form and on the tag attached to the unit.
  h. *Appearance:* There should be no discoloration, foaming, bubbles, cloudiness, clots or clumps, or loss of integrity of the container.

Clinical Alert!

It is safer to have one nurse read the information for verification to the other nurse; this avoids errors that can be made if both nurses look at the tags together.

- If any of the information does not match *exactly*, notify the charge nurse and the blood bank. Do not administer blood until discrepancies are corrected or clarified.
- Sign the appropriate form with the other nurse according to agency policy.
- Make sure that the blood is left at room temperature for no more than 30 minutes before starting the transfusion. Agencies may designate different times at which the blood must be returned to the blood bank if it has not been started. **Rationale:** *As blood components warm, the risk of bacterial growth also increases*. If the start of the transfusion is unexpectedly delayed, return the blood to the blood bank after 30 minutes. Do *not* store blood in the unit refrigerator. **Rationale:** *The temperature of unit refrigerators is not precisely regulated and the blood may be damaged*.

8. Prepare the blood bag.

- Invert the blood bag gently several times to mix the cells with the plasma. **Rationale:** *Rough handling can damage the cells*.
- Expose the port on the blood bag by pulling back the tabs.
- Insert the remaining Y-set spike into the blood bag.
- Suspend the blood bag.

9. Establish the blood transfusion.

- Close the upper clamp below the IV saline solution container.
- Open the upper clamp below the blood bag. The blood will run into the saline-filled drip chamber. If necessary, squeeze the drip chamber to reestablish the liquid level with the drip chamber one-third full. (Tap the filter to expel any residual air within the filter.)
- Readjust the flow rate with the main clamp.
- Remove and discard gloves.
- Perform hand hygiene.

10. Observe the client closely for the first 15 minutes.

- INS (2016b) states to "start the transfusion slowly at approximately 2 mL per minute for the first 15 minutes, and remain near the patient; increase the transfusion rate if there are no signs of a reaction" (p. 230). **Rationale:** *This small amount is enough to produce a severe reaction but small enough that the reaction could be treated successfully*.

Continued on page 1426

SKILL 51.6

Initiating, Maintaining, and Terminating a Blood Transfusion Using a Y-Set—*continued*

- Note adverse reactions, such as chills, nausea, vomiting, skin rash, dyspnea, back pain, or tachycardia. **Rationale:** *The earlier a transfusion reaction occurs, the more severe it tends to be. Promptly identifying such reactions helps to minimize the consequences.*
- Remind the client to call a nurse immediately if any unusual symptoms are felt during the transfusion such as chills, nausea, itching, rash, dyspnea, or back pain.
- If any of these reactions occur, report them to the nurse in charge, and take appropriate nursing action. See Table 51.14 on page 1422.

11. Document relevant data.

- Record starting the blood, including vital signs, type of blood, blood unit number, sequence number (e.g., #1 of three ordered units), site of the venipuncture, size of the catheter, and drip rate.

SAMPLE DOCUMENTATION

1/21/2020 1400 1 unit of PRBCs (#65234) hung to be infused over 3 hours. IV site in (L) forearm with 20 guage angiocath. VS taken (see transfusion record). Informed to contact nurse if begins to experience any discomfort during transfusion. Stated he would use the call light. C. Jones, RN

12. Monitor the client.

- 15 minutes after initiating the transfusion (or according to agency policy), check the vital signs. If there are no signs of a reaction, establish the required flow rate. Most adults can tolerate receiving 1 unit of blood in 1.5 to 2 hours. Do not transfuse a unit of blood for longer than 4 hours.
- Assess the client, including vital signs, per agency policy. If the client has a reaction and the blood is discontinued, send the blood bag and tubing to the laboratory for investigation of the blood.

13. Terminate the transfusion.

- Apply clean gloves.
- If no infusion is to follow, clamp the blood tubing. Check agency protocol to determine if the blood component bag needs to be returned or if the blood bag and tubing can be disposed of in a biohazard container. The IV line can be discontinued or capped with an adapter or a new infusion line and solution container may be added. If another transfusion is to follow, clamp the blood tubing and open the saline infusion arm. Check agency protocol. A new blood administration set is to be used with each component, or if more than 1 unit can be infused in 4 hours, the transfusion set can be used for a 4-hour period (Gorski, 2018, p. 580).
- If the primary IV is to be continued, flush the maintenance line with saline solution. Disconnect the blood tubing system and reestablish the IV infusion using new tubing. Adjust the drip to the desired rate. Often a normal saline or other solution is kept running in case of delayed reaction to the blood.
- Measure vital signs.

14. Follow agency protocol for appropriate disposition of the used supplies.

- Discard the administration set according to agency practice.
- Dispose of blood bags and administration sets.
  a. On the requisition attached to the blood unit, fill in the time the transfusion was completed and the amount transfused.
  b. Attach one copy of the requisition to the client's record and another to the empty blood bag if required by agency policy.
  c. Agency policy generally involves returning the bag to the blood bank for reference in case of subsequent or delayed adverse reaction.
- Remove and discard gloves.
- Perform hand hygiene.

15. Document relevant data.

- Record completion of the transfusion, the amount of blood absorbed, the blood unit number, and the vital signs. If the primary IV infusion was continued, record connecting it. Also record the transfusion on the IV flow sheet and intake and output record.

SAMPLE DOCUMENTATION

4/21/2020 1415 c/o feeling warm, headache, & backache. Skin flushed. T 102.6°F, BP 140/90, P 112, R 28. Approximately 50 mL PRBCs (#65234) infused over past 15 minutes. Infusion stopped. IV tubing changed, NS infusing at 15 mL/hr. Blood & attached tubing sent to blood bank. Dr. Riley notified. Will continue to monitor. C. Jones, RN

EVALUATION

- Perform follow-up based on findings or outcomes that deviated from expected or normal for the client. Compare findings to previous data if available.
- Report significant deviations from normal to the primary care provider.

Evaluating

Using the overall goals identified in the planning stage of maintaining or restoring fluid balance, maintaining or restoring pulmonary ventilation and oxygenation, maintaining or restoring normal balance of electrolytes, and preventing associated risks of fluid, electrolyte, and acid–base imbalances, the nurse collects data to evaluate the effectiveness of interventions.

If desired outcomes are not achieved, the nurse, client, and support person if appropriate need to explore the reasons before modifying the care plan. For example, if the outcome "Urine output is greater than 1300 mL per day and within 500 mL of intake" is not achieved, questions to be considered might include the following:

- Have other outcome measures for the goal of achieving fluid balance been met?

- Does the client understand and comply with planned fluid intake?
- Is all urinary output being measured?
- Are unusual or excessive amounts of fluid being lost by another route (e.g., gastric suction, excessive perspiration, fever, rapid respiratory rate, wound drainage)?
- Are prescribed medications being taken or administered as ordered?

NURSING CARE PLAN Decreased Fluid Volume

ASSESSMENT DATA	NURSING DIAGNOSIS	DESIRED OUTCOMES*
NURSING ASSESSMENT Merlyn Chapman, a 27-year-old sales clerk, reports weakness, malaise, and flu-like symptoms for 3–4 days. Although thirsty, she is unable to tolerate fluids because of nausea and vomiting, and she has liquid stools 2–4 times per day.	Decreased fluid volume related to nausea, vomiting, and diarrhea as evidenced by decreased urine output, increased urine concentration, weakness, fever, decreased skin or tongue turgor, dry mucous membranes, increased pulse rate, and decreased blood pressure	**Fluid Balance [0601]** as evidenced by not compromised: • 24-hour intake and output balance • Urine specific gravity • Blood pressure • Pulse rate • Temperature • Skin turgor • Moist mucous membranes

Physical Examination	Diagnostic Data
Height: 160 cm (5′3′′)	Urine specific gravity: 1.035
Weight: 66.2 kg (146 lb)	Serum sodium 145 mEq/L
Mild fever: 38.6°C (101.5°F)	Serum potassium 3.2 mEq/L
Pulse: 96 beats/min	Chest x-ray negative
Respirations: 24/min	
Scant urine output	
BP: 102/84 mmHg	
Dry oral mucosa, furrowed tongue, cracked lips	

NURSING INTERVENTIONS*/SELECTED ACTIVITIES	RATIONALE
Fluid Management [4120]	
Weigh daily and monitor trends.	*Weight helps to assess fluid balance.*
Maintain accurate I&O record.	*Accurate records are critical in assessing the client's fluid balance.*
Monitor vital signs as appropriate.	*Vital sign changes such as increased heart rate, decreased blood pressure, and increased temperature indicate hypovolemia.*
Give fluids as appropriate.	*As her nausea decreases encourage oral intake of fluids as tolerated, again to replace lost volume.*
Administer IV therapy as prescribed.	*Mrs. Chapman will probably require IV replacement of fluid. This is especially true because her oral intake is limited because of nausea and vomiting.*

Evaluation
Outcomes met. Ms. Chapman required fluid replacement of a total of 5 liters. Her blood pressure increased to 122/74 mmHg, pulse rate decreased to a resting level of 74 beats/min, and respirations decreased to 12/min. Her urine output increased as the fluid was replaced and was adequate at > 0.5 mL/kg per hour by the time of discharge. The urine specific gravity was 1.015. Lab work on the day of discharge was K^+: 3.8 and Na^+: 140. She had elastic skin turgor and moist mucous membranes. She was taking oral fluids and was able to discuss symptoms of decreased fluid volume that would necessitate her calling her healthcare provider.

*The NOC # for desired outcomes and the NIC # for nursing interventions and selected activities are listed in brackets following the appropriate outcome or intervention. Outcomes, interventions, and activities selected are only a sample of those suggested by NOC and NIC and should be further individualized for each client.

APPLYING CRITICAL THINKING

1. Offer suggestions for ways to help Mrs. Chapman increase her oral intake.
2. Mrs. Chapman asks why you weigh her every morning. How do you respond?

Answers to Applying Critical Thinking questions are available on the faculty resources website. Please consult with your instructor.

CONCEPT MAP

Decreased Fluid Volume

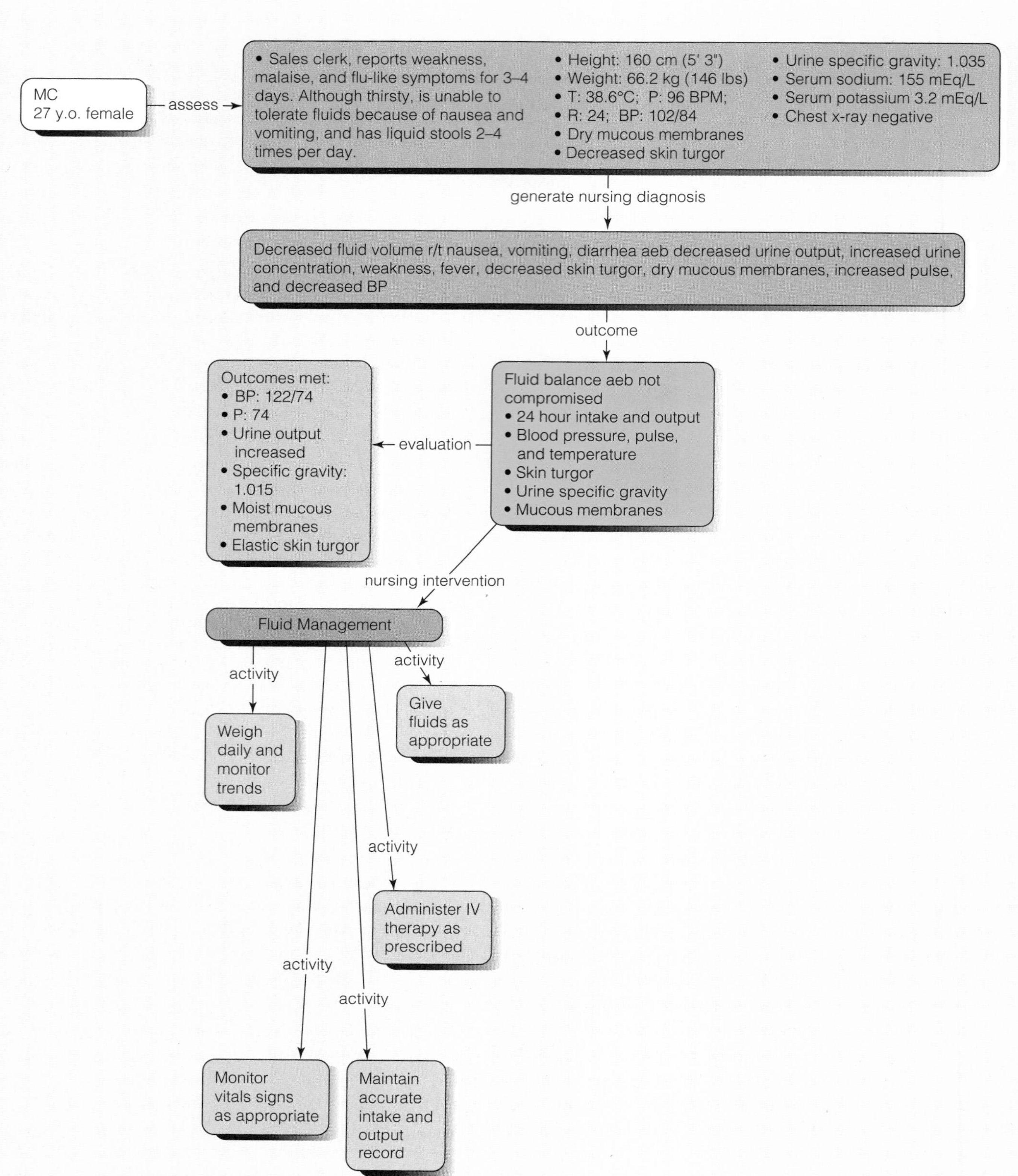

Chapter 51 Review

CHAPTER HIGHLIGHTS

- A balance of fluids, electrolytes, acids, and bases in the body is necessary for good health.
- Body fluid is divided into two major compartments: intracellular fluid (ICF) inside the cells and extracellular fluid (ECF) outside the cells.
- ECF is subdivided into two compartments: intravascular (plasma) and interstitial. It constitutes about one-third of total body fluid.
- ECF is in constant motion throughout the body. It is the transport system that carries nutrients to and waste products from the cells.
- The percentage of total body fluid varies according to an individual's age, body fat, and gender. The younger an individual is, and the less body fat present, the greater the proportion of body fluid; post-adolescent females have a smaller percentage of fluid in relation to total body weight than men.
- There are two types of body electrolytes (ions): positively charged ions (cations) and negatively charged ions (anions).
- The principal ions of ECF are sodium (cation), chloride (anion), and bicarbonate (anion); the principal ions of ICF are potassium and magnesium (cations), and phosphate and sulfate (anions).
- Fluids and electrolytes move among the body compartments by osmosis, diffusion, filtration, and active transport.
- The major fluid pressures exerted as part of the movement of fluid and electrolytes from one compartment to another are osmotic pressure and hydrostatic pressure.
- The three sources of body fluid are liquids and food, which are ingested, and the oxidation of food. Fluid intake is regulated by the thirst mechanism.
- Fluid output occurs chiefly through excretion of urine, although body fluid is also lost through sweat, feces, and respiration.
- In healthy adults, measurable fluid intake and output should balance (about 1500 mL per day). The output of urine normally approximates the oral intake of fluids. Water from food and oxidation is balanced by fluid loss through urine, feces, and insensible losses, such as losses through the skin as perspiration.
- A number of body systems and organs are involved in regulating the volume and composition of body fluids: the kidneys, lungs, the cardiovascular and gastrointestinal systems, and the endocrine system. The kidneys are the primary regulator of fluid and electrolyte balance.
- Substances such as antidiuretic hormone, the renin-angiotensin-aldosterone system, and atrial natriuretic factor are also involved in maintaining fluid balance.
- The acid–base balance (pH range) of body fluids is maintained within a precise range of 7.35 to 7.45.
- Acid–base balance is regulated by buffers, which neutralize excess acids or bases; the lungs, which eliminate or retain carbon dioxide, a potential acid; and the kidneys, which excrete or conserve bicarbonate and hydrogen ions.
- Factors that influence an individual's fluid, electrolyte, and acid–base balance include age, sex, body size, environmental temperature, and lifestyle. Illness, trauma, surgery, and certain medications can place individuals at risk for fluid, electrolyte, and acid–base imbalances.
- Fluid imbalances include fluid volume deficit (FVD), also referred to as hypovolemia; fluid volume excess (FVE), also referred to as hypervolemia; dehydration, a deficit in water and an increase in serum sodium level; and overhydration, an excess of water and decrease in serum sodium level.
- Acid–base imbalance occurs when the normal 20-to-1 ratio of bicarbonate to carbonic acid is upset. Imbalances may be either respiratory or metabolic in origin; either can result in acidosis or alkalosis.
- Fluid, electrolyte, and acid–base imbalances are most accurately determined through laboratory examination of blood plasma.
- Assessment relative to fluid, electrolyte, and acid–base balances includes (a) a nursing history; (b) physical examination of the skin, oral cavity, eyes, jugular vein, veins of the hand, and the neurologic system; (c) measurement of body weight, vital signs, and fluid intake and output; and (d) diagnostic studies of blood and urine.
- A nursing history includes data about the client's fluid and food intake; fluid output; signs of fluid, electrolyte, and acid–base imbalances; and medications, therapies, or disease processes that may disrupt these balances.
- Nursing diagnoses that relate specifically to fluid, electrolyte, and acid–base imbalances include decreased fluid volume, increased fluid volume, potential for fluid volume imbalance, and altered gas exchange. Other diagnoses that may be relevant are altered skin integrity, inadequate cardiac output, impaired tissue perfusion, and inadequate physical energy.
- In many instances, fluids and electrolytes can be provided orally to clients who are experiencing or at risk of developing decreased fluid volume. The nurse needs to establish with the client a 24-hour plan for ingesting the necessary fluids and to respect the client's fluid preferences.
- For clients with fluid retention, fluids may need to be restricted; a schedule and short-term goals that make the fluid restriction more tolerable need to be developed.
- For clients experiencing excessive fluid losses, the administration of fluids and electrolytes intravenously is necessary. Meticulous aseptic technique is required when caring for clients with IV infusions.
- Preventing complications such as infiltration, extravasation, and phlebitis is an important aspect of IV therapy.
- The administration of blood transfusions involves accurately matching and identifying the blood for the individual, correctly identifying the recipient, and monitoring the client throughout the procedure for transfusion reactions.

TEST YOUR KNOWLEDGE

1. A client tells the nurse about passing out after following a fasting diet for 5 days. Which acid–base imbalance would the nurse expect to assess in this client?
   1. Respiratory acidosis
   2. Respiratory alkalosis
   3. Metabolic acidosis
   4. Metabolic alkalosis

2. A client complains of a headache 10 minutes after the transfusion of a unit of packed red blood cells was initiated. The nurse assesses that the client has slight shortness of breath and feels warm to the touch. What action by the nurse is priority?
   1. Notify the client's physician.
   2. Discontinue the transfusion.
   3. Slow the rate of the transfusion.
   4. Prepare to resuscitate the client.

3. The nurse administers an IV solution of D_5 1/2NS to a post-operative client. This is classified as what type of intravenous solution?

4. An older client comes to the emergency department experiencing chest pain and shortness of breath. An arterial blood gas is ordered. Which ABG results indicate respiratory acidosis?
   1. pH 7.54; $PaCO_2$ 28 mmHg; HCO_3 22 mEq/L
   2. pH 7.32; $PaCO_2$ 46 mmHg; HCO_3 24 mEq/L
   3. pH 7.31; $PaCO_2$ 35 mmHg; HCO_3 20 mEq/L
   4. pH 7.50; $PaCO_2$ 37 mmHg; HCO_3 28 mEq/L

5. The intake and output (I&O) record of a client with a nasogastric tube who has been attached to suction for 2 days shows greater output than input. Which nursing diagnoses are most applicable? Select all that apply.
   1. Decreased fluid volume
   2. Potential for decreased fluid volume
   3. Dry oral mucous membranes
   4. Altered gas exchange
   5. Inadequate cardiac output

6. Which client statement indicates a need for further teaching regarding treatment for hypokalemia?
   1. "I will use avocado in my salads."
   2. "I will be sure to check my heart rate before I take my digoxin."
   3. "I will take my potassium in the morning after eating breakfast."
   4. "I will stop using my salt substitute."

7. A client has had a subclavian central venous catheter inserted. What should the nurse assess as a priority for this client's care?
   1. Presence of bibasilar crackles
   2. Tachycardia
   3. Decreased pedal pulses
   4. Headache

8. The client's arterial blood gas results are pH 7.32; $PaCO_2$ 58; HCO_3 32. The nurse knows that the client is experiencing which acid–base imbalance?
   1. Metabolic acidosis
   2. Respiratory acidosis
   3. Metabolic alkalosis
   4. Respiratory alkalosis

9. A client is admitted to the hospital for hypocalcemia. Nursing interventions relating to which system would have the highest priority?
   1. Renal
   2. Cardiac
   3. Gastrointestinal
   4. Neuromuscular

10. The nurse would assess for signs of hypomagnesemia in which of the following clients? Select all that apply.
   1. A client with renal failure
   2. A client with pancreatitis
   3. A client taking magnesium-containing antacids
   4. A client with excessive nasogastric drainage
   5. A client with chronic alcoholism

See Answers to Test Your Knowledge in Appendix A.

READINGS AND REFERENCES

Suggested Readings

Carman, M., Uhlenbrock, J. S., & McClintock, S. M. (2018). A review of current practice in transfusion therapy. *American Journal of Nursing, 118*(5), 36–44. doi:10.1097/01.NAJ.0000532808.81713.fc

The authors provide an excellent review of blood products commonly transfused, potential complications of blood transfusions, and the role of nursing in transfusion.

MacIntyre, L. M. (2017). The growing need for diverse blood donors. *American Journal of Nursing, 117*(7), 44–48. doi:10.1097/01.NAJ.0000520945.31600.3f

A well-written article about how the changing demographics in the United States impact the growing need for closer phenotype matching for individuals who require frequent blood transfusions.

Mattox, E. A. (2017). Complication of peripheral venous access devices: Prevention, detection, and recovery strategies. *Critical Care Nurse, 37*(2), e1–e14. doi:10.4037/ccn2017657

A comprehensive focus on strategies for prevention, detection, and recovery for selected complications of short peripheral catheters and PICCs.

Related Research

Conley, S. B., Buckley, P., Magarace, L., & Pedulla, L. V. (2017). Standardizing best nursing practice for implanted ports: Applying evidence-based professional guidelines to prevent central line-associated bloodstream infections. *Journal of Infusion Nursing, 40*(3), 165–174. doi:10.1097/NAN.0000000000000217

Ehrhardt, B. S., Givens, K. E., & Lee, R. C. (2018). Making it stick: Developing and testing the difficult intravenous access (DIVA) tool. *American Journal of Nursing, 118*(7), 56–62. doi:10.1097/01.NAJ.0000541440.91369.00

Fowler, S. B., Penoyer, D. A., & Bourgault, A. (2018). Insertion and removal of PIVCs: Exploring best practices. *Nursing, 48*(7), 65–67. doi:10.1097/01.NURSE.0000534108.88895.e2

References

American Nurses Association. (2015). *Nursing: Scope and standards of practice* (3rd ed.). Silver Spring, MD: Author.

Bauldoff, G., Gubrud, P., & Carno, M. (2020). *LeMone & Burke's medical-surgical nursing: Clinical reasoning in patient care* (7th ed.). Hoboken, NJ: Pearson.

Butcher, H. K., Bulechek, G. M., Dochterman, J. M., & Wagner, C. M. (Eds.). (2018). *Nursing interventions classifications (NIC)* (7th ed.). St. Louis, MO: Elsevier.

Campbell, Y. N., Machan, M. D., & Fisher, M. D. (2016). The Jehovah's Witness population: Considerations for preoperative optimization of hemoglobin. *AANA Journal, 84*(3), 173–178.

Giuliano, K. K., & Ruppel, H. (2017). Are smart pumps smart enough? *Nursing, 47*(3), 64–66. doi:10.1097/01.NURSE.0000512888.75246.88

Gorski, L. A. (2018). *Phillip's manual of I.V. therapeutics: Evidence-based practice for infusion therapy* (7th ed.). Philadelphia, PA: F.A. Davis.

Infusion Nurses Society. (2016a). *Infusion therapy standards of practice* (5th ed.). Norwood, MA: Author.

Infusion Nurses Society. (2016b). *Policies and procedures for infusion therapy* (5th ed.). Norwood, MA: Author.

The Joint Commission. (2019). *National Patient Safety Goals effective January, 2019*. Retrieved from https://www.jointcommission.org/assets/1/6/NPSG_Chapter_HAP_Jan2019.pdf

Martini, F. H., Nath, J. L., & Bartholomew, E. F. (2018). *Fundamentals of anatomy & physiology* (11th ed.). New York, NY: Pearson.

Menendez, J. B., & Edwards, B. (2016). Early identification of acute hemolytic transfusion reactions: Realistic implications for best practice in patient monitoring. *MEDSURG Nursing, 25*(2), 88–90, 109.

Moorhead, S., Johnson, M., Maas, M. L., & Swanson, E. (Eds.). (2018). *Nursing outcomes classification (NOC): Measurement of health outcomes* (6th ed.). St. Louis, MO: Elsevier.

Turley, S. M. (2017). *Medical language* (4th ed.). New York, NY: Pearson.

Ullman, A., Cooke, M., Mitchell, M., Lin, F., New, K., Long, D., . . . Rickard, C. (2016). Dressing and securement for central venous access devices (CVADs): A Cochrane systematic review. *International Journal of Nursing Studies*, *59*, 177–196. doi:10.1016/j.ijnurstu.2016.04.003

U.S. Food and Drug Administration. (2018). *Bar code label requirements for blood and blood components questions and answers*. Retrieved from http://www.fda.gov/BiologicsBloodVaccines/DevelopmentApprovalProcess/AdvertisingLabelingPromotionalMaterials/BarCodeLabelRequirements/ucm133136.htm

Walker, M. D. (2016). Fluid and electrolyte imbalances: Interpretation and assessment. *Journal of Infusion Nursing*, *39*(6), 382–386. doi:10.1097/NAN.0000000000000193

Selected Bibliography

American Heart Association. (2017). *Top 25 foods that add the most sodium to your diet*. Retrieved from https://sodiumbreakup.heart.org/top_25_foods_that_add_the_most_sodium_to_your_diet

Barnhart, E., Alway, A., & Halm, M. (2019). Rotating peripheral IV catheters based on clinical indication. *American Nurse Today*, *14*(1), 46–48.

Cameron-Watson, C. (2016). Port protectors in clinical practice: An audit. *British Journal of Nursing*, *25*(8), S25–S31. doi:10.12968/bjon.2016.25.8.S25

Conley, S. B. (2016). Central line-associated bloodstream infection prevention: Standardizing practice focused on evidence-based guidelines. *Clinical Journal of Oncology Nursing*, *20*(1), 23–26. doi:10.1188/16.CJON.23-26

Cortez-Gann, J., Gilmore, K. D., Foley, K. W., Kennedy, M. B., McGee, T., & Kring, D. (2017). Blood transfusion vital sign frequency: What does the evidence say? *MEDSURG Nursing*, *26*(2), 89–92.

Harrison, L. T. (2016). Safely managing smart pumps in the clinical setting. *Nursing Management*, *47*(6), 20–21. doi:10.1097/01.NUMA.0000483128.55731.5e

Helton, J., Hines, A., & Best, J. (2016). Peripheral IV site rotation based on clinical assessment vs. length of time since insertion. *MEDSURG Nursing*, *25*(1), 44–49.

Oliver, G., & Jones, M. (2016). The importance of adequate CVC securement to prevent infection. *British Journal of Nursing*, *25*(8), S32–S33. doi:10.12968/bjon.2016.25.8.S32

Pompey, J., & Abraham-Settles, B. (2019). Clarifying the confusion of arterial blood gas analysis: Is it compensation or combination? *American Journal of Nursing*, *119*(3), 52–56. doi:10.1097/01.NAJ.0000554035.74335.59

Rickard, C., Ullman, A., Kleidon, T., & Marsh, N. (2017). Clinical update: Ten tips for dressing and securement of IV device wounds. *Australian Nursing & Midwifery Journal*, *24*(10), 32–34.

Spencer, T. R. (2018). Securing vascular access devices. *American Nurse Today*, *13*(9), 29–31.

Thomas, S. B. (2017). Acute hypervolemic hyponatremia: A case report. *Nursing*, *47*(10), 53–57. doi:10.1097/01.NURSE.0000522006.83149.20

Tweed, V. (2017). Magnesium: Superstar rising. *Better Nutrition*, *79*(4), 24–26.

Ullman, A., Marsh, N., & Rickard, C. (2017). Securement for vascular access devices: Looking to the future. *British Journal of Nursing*, *26*(8), S24–S26. doi:10.12968/bjon.2017.26.8.S24

Williamson, K., Gonzalez, L., Neusbaum, A., & Messing, J. (2017). Reducing the risk of central line-associated bloodstream infections. *American Nurse Today*, *12*(5), 42, 44, 46.

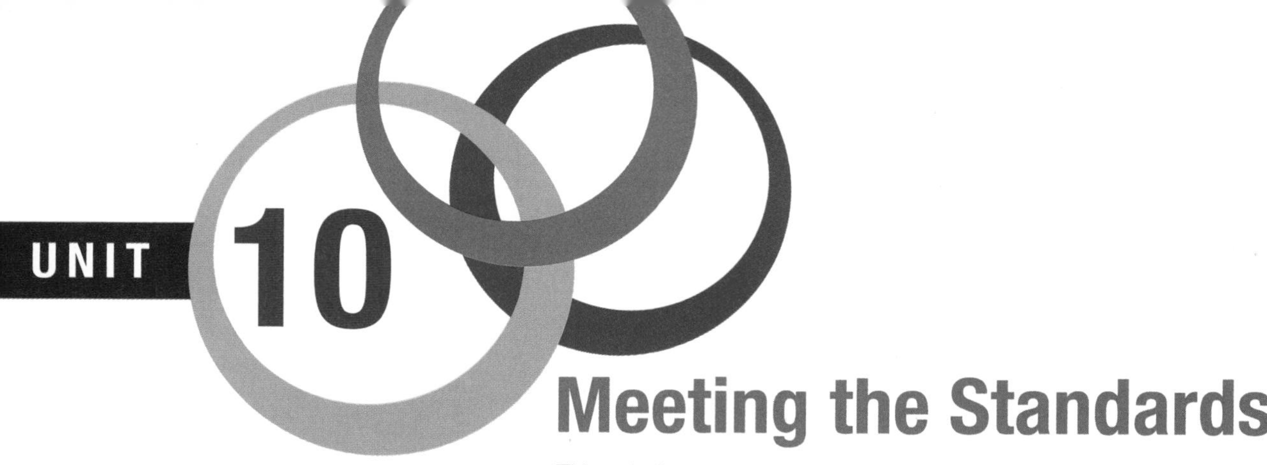

Meeting the Standards

This unit discusses the fundamentals of physiologic health including activity and exercise, sleep, pain management, nutrition, urinary and fecal elimination, oxygenation, circulation, fluid and electrolyte balance, and acid–base balance. Most clients in the acute care setting will have one or more issues related to these physiologic requirements and the nurse must be alert to the client's needs to prevent complications from developing.

CLIENT: Agnes AGE: 71
CURRENT MEDICAL DIAGNOSES: Fractured left hip

Medical History: Agnes is a healthy and active woman who lives alone. Agnes and her sisters decided it would be fun to go roller skating, and she fell and fractured her left hip. The fracture was diagnosed by x-ray in the emergency department. She underwent open reduction of the fracture and was admitted to the orthopedic unit of the hospital. She will be transferred to a rehabilitation facility once her condition has stabilized. Agnes has a 30-year history of hypertension that she controls with diet and atenolol 50 mg once daily and hydrochlorothiazide 25 mg once per day.

Personal and Social History: Agnes is single and has no children, but she has many friends as well as two sisters and a brother who live nearby. Even in the emergency department after hearing the diagnosis, she and her sisters have been laughing about what fun it will be telling people she broke her hip roller skating. She has a wonderful sense of humor and is often heard laughing. She retired 6 years ago after having worked for 45 years as a pediatric nurse.

Questions

American Nurses Association Standard of Practice #3 is Outcomes Identification: *The registered nurse identifies expected outcomes for a plan individualized to the healthcare consumer or the situation.*

1. Develop an expected outcome for this client related to chapters in this unit including activity and exercise, pain management, fecal elimination, and circulation.
2. What risks can you identify for this client related to activity and exercise, sleep, nutrition, and oxygenation?

American Nurses Association Standard of Practice #4 is Planning: *The registered nurse develops a plan that prescribes strategies to attain expected, measurable outcomes for consumer, family, and others as appropriate.*

3. When planning care with Agnes related to activity and exercise, pain management, nutrition, fecal elimination, oxygenation, and circulation, establish the priorities of care.

American Nurses Association Standard of Practice #5A is Coordination of Care: *The registered nurse coordinates care delivery.*

4. Of activity and exercise, sleep, pain management, nutrition, urinary elimination, fecal elimination, oxygenation, circulation, and fluid, electrolyte, and acid–base balance, which one carries the greatest risk to Agnes's independence and quality of life?
5. What actions can the nurse take to promote and maximize Agnes's independence?

American Nurses Association. (2015). *Nursing: Scope and standards of practice* (3rd ed.). Silver Spring, MD: Author.

Answers to Meeting the Standards Questions are available on the faculty resources site. Please consult with your instructor.

APPENDIX A

Answers to Test Your Knowledge

CHAPTER 1 Historical and Contemporary Nursing Practice

1. **Answer:** 4. **Rationale:** Option 1, Clara Barton is noted for establishing the American Red Cross. Lillian Wald and Mary Brewster, Options 2 and 3, are considered the founder of public health nursing. **Cognitive Level:** Analyzing. **Client Need:** Safe, Effective Care Environment. **Nursing Process:** Implementation. **Learning Outcome:** 1-1.
2. **Answer:** 2. **Rationale:** A clinical nurse specialist has an advanced degree or expertise and is considered to be an expert in a specialized area of practice (oncology in this case). The nurse provides direct client care, educates others, consults, conducts research, and manages care. A nurse practitioner usually deals with nonemergency acute or chronic illness and provides primary ambulatory care. The nurse educator is responsible for classroom and often clinical teaching. A nurse entrepreneur usually has an advanced degree, manages a health-related business, and may be involved in education, consultation, or research. **Cognitive Level:** Understanding. **Client Need:** N/A. **Nursing Process:** N/A. **Learning Outcome:** 1-3.
3. **Answer:** 2. **Rationale:** Person (individual or client), environment, health, and nursing are relevant when providing care for any client whether in the hospital, at home, in the community, or in elementary school systems. These elements can be used to understand diseases, conduct and apply research, and develop nursing theories, as well as implement the nursing process. **Cognitive Level:** Applying. **Client Need:** N/A. **Nursing Process:** N/A. **Learning Outcome:** 1-5.
4. **Answer:** 2. **Rationale:** Continuing education refers to formalized experiences designed to enhance the knowledge or skill of practitioners. The other answers are examples of in-service education, which is designed to upgrade the knowledge or skills of current employees with regard to the specific setting, and is usually less formal in presentation. **Cognitive Level:** Analyzing. **Client Need:** Safe, Effective Care Environment. **Nursing Process:** N/A. **Learning Outcome:** 1-7.
5. **Answer:** 3. **Rationale:** Health promotion focuses on maintaining normal status without consideration of diseases. Option 1 is an example of illness prevention. Option 2 is aesthetic (i.e., not needed for health promotion or disease prevention). Option 4 focuses on disease detection. **Cognitive Level:** Remembering. **Client Need:** N/A. **Nursing Process:** N/A. **Learning Outcome:** 1-9.
6. **Answer:** 3. **Rationale:** All are noted nurses. Linda Richards was America's first trained nurse, and Mary Mahoney was America's first African American trained nurse. **Cognitive Level:** Remembering. **Client Need:** N/A. **Nursing Process:** N/A. **Learning Outcome:** 1-1.
7. **Answer:** 2. **Rationale:** Option 1, the advanced beginner, demonstrates marginally acceptable performance. Option 3, the proficient practitioner, has 3 to 5 years of experience and has developed a holistic understanding of the client. Option 4, the expert practitioner, demonstrates highly skilled intuitive and analytic ability in new situations. **Cognitive Level:** Remembering. **Client Need:** N/A. **Nursing Process:** N/A. **Learning Outcome:** 1-14.
8. **Answer:** 4. **Rationale:** The National Student Nurses' Association developed the *Code of Academic and Clinical Conduct* for nursing students in 2001. Option 1, ANA, developed *Standards of Nursing Practices*. Option 2, NLN, focuses on nursing education. Option 3, the American Association of Colleges of Nursing (AACN), is the national organization that focuses on the advancement and maintenance of America's baccalaureate and higher degree nursing education programs. **Cognitive Level:** Remembering. **Client Need:** N/A. **Nursing Process:** N/A. **Learning Outcome:** 1-16.
9. **Answer:** 1. **Rationale:** All will impact nursing but not necessarily the supply and demand issue. The aging population contributes to more older adults needing specialized care because of chronic illnesses (increasing the demand). Fewer nursing faculty to educate students and fewer nurses practicing because of retirement contribute to the decreasing supply. **Cognitive Level:** Analyzing. **Client Need:** N/A. **Nursing Process:** N/A. **Learning Outcome:** 1-15.
10. **Answer:** 2. **Rationale:** All of the expanded roles function as healthcare advocates and all could work with individuals affected by violence. However, the forensic nurse specifically integrates forensic skills into nursing practice. **Cognitive Level:** Remembering. **Client Need:** N/A. **Nursing Process:** N/A. **Learning Outcome:** 1-12.

CHAPTER 2 Evidence-Based Practice and Research in Nursing

1. **Answer:** 4. **Rationale:** Trial and error is not considered valid evidence, and may even be harmful to clients. Clinical experience (option 1), the opinions of experts (option 2), and client values and preferences (option 3) are all considered valid evidence in EBP. **Cognitive Level:** Remembering. **Client Need:** N/A. **Nursing Process:** N/A. **Learning Outcome:** 2-3.
2. **Answer:** 2. **Rationale:** In experimental design, the investigator manipulates the independent variable by administering an experimental treatment to some participants while withholding it from others. In a nonexperimental design, the investigator does not manipulate the independent variable. A pilot study is a test study before the actual one begins and is not a type of research design. **Cognitive Level:** Understanding. **Client Need:** N/A. **Nursing Process:** N/A. **Learning Outcome:** 2-4.
3. **Answer:** 3. **Rationale:** This study investigates the subjective experience of stress, through the collection of narrative data. Options 1, 2, and 4 are examples of quantitative research using numbers and values. **Cognitive Level:** Applying. **Client Need:** N/A. **Nursing Process:** N/A. **Learning Outcome:** 2-4.
4. **Answer:** 2. **Rationale:** The key purpose of a study's methodology is to generate data that are reliable and valid; thus controlling extraneous variables is a major function. The hypotheses

that are tested are formed during the problem identification phase of a study (option 1). Grants and funding sources are not related to methodology (option 3). Protecting participants' rights (option 4) is an important consideration, but not the key purpose of a methodology. **Cognitive Level:** Understanding. **Client Need:** N/A. **Nursing Process:** N/A. **Learning Outcome:** 2-5.

5. **Answer:** 2. **Rationale:** PICO stands for patient or client, population, or problem; intervention; comparison; and outcome. These are helpful components of a research question and help to identify key terms for a literature search. Options 1, 3, and 4 are incorrect. **Cognitive Level:** Remembering. **Client Need:** N/A. **Nursing Process:** N/A. **Learning Outcome:** 2-5.
6. **Answer:** 3. **Rationale:** All nurses, including new graduates, could help to identify clinical problems in direct client care (option 1). Nurse managers would most likely use research findings to develop policies and procedures and may not necessarily have an advanced degree (option 2). All nurses, including new graduates, could participate in data collection (option 4). **Cognitive Level:** Applying. **Client Need:** N/A. **Nursing Process:** N/A. **Learning Outcome:** 2-6.
7. **Answer:** 1. **Rationale:** The research problem has significance if it has the potential to contribute to nursing science by enhancing client care, testing or generating a theory, or resolving a day-to-day clinical problem. If the adolescents are showing improved behavior, then these techniques have significance in enhancing client care. **Cognitive Level:** Understanding. **Client Need:** N/A. **Nursing Process:** N/A. **Learning Outcome:** 2-5.
8. **Answer:** 4. **Rationale:** The right to self-determination means that participants feel free of constraints, coercion, or any undue influence to participate in a study. There is not enough information given to indicate if any of the other rights in options 1, 2, and 3 have been violated. **Cognitive Level:** Applying. **Client Need:** N/A. **Nursing Process:** N/A. **Learning Outcome:** 2-7.
9. **Answer:** 3, 2, 1, 5, 4, 6. **Cognitive Level:** Remembering. **Client Need:** N/A. **Nursing Process:** N/A. **Learning Outcome:** 2-2.
10. **Answer:** 3. **Rationale:** There may have been unique aspects to this research that would not be applicable in a different setting or with different clients. Not all research is flawed (option 1) and it may or may not have taken cost into consideration (option 2). Research is not limited to the study of physiologic problems (option 4). **Cognitive Level:** Understanding. **Client Need:** N/A. **Nursing Process:** N/A. **Learning Outcome:** 2-1.

CHAPTER 3 Legal Aspects of Nursing

1. **Answer:** 4. **Rationale:** Obtaining informed consent for specific medical treatment is the responsibility of the person who is going to perform the procedure, in this case the physician. Informed consent suggests that the client has been given complete information, including benefits, risks, and alternatives if the treatment is not given. It is the physician's responsibility to make sure the client's understanding is clear. It is important that the person obtaining the consent (the physician in this case) answer the client's questions. If the client has questions, he should not sign the form, and it is not the nurse's responsibility to answer the questions (options 1 and 2). Telling the client what he "should have" done is demeaning and not an appropriate therapeutic response (option 3). **Cognitive Level:** Applying. **Client Need:** Safe, Effective Care Environment. **Nursing Process:** Assessment. **Learning Outcome:** 3-4.
2. **Answer:** 4. **Rationale:** Battery is the willful touching of an individual without permission. Another name for an unintentional tort is malpractice or professional negligence. This situation is an *intentional* tort because the nurse executed the act on purpose. Assault is the attempt or threat to touch another individual unjustifiably or without permission. Invasion of privacy injures the feelings of the individual and does not take into consideration how revealing information or exposing the client will affect the client's feelings. **Cognitive Level:** Analyzing. **Client Need:** Safe, Effective Care Environment. **Nursing Process:** N/A. **Learning Outcome:** 3-10.
3. **Answer:** 2. **Rationale:** The nurse should call the individual who wrote the order for clarification. Administering the medication is incorrect because knowing the dose is outside the normal range and not questioning the order could lead to client harm and liability for the nurse. Calling the pharmacist is not the best answer because it will not solve the problem, and the nurse needs to seek clarification from the individual who wrote the order. The nurse should suspend administration but not refuse to administer the medication until the issue is resolved. **Cognitive Level:** Applying. **Client Need:** Safe, Effective Care Environment. **Nursing Process:** Implementation. **Learning Outcome:** 3-7.
4. **Answer:** 1. **Rationale:** Foreseeability is the link between the nurse's act and the injury suffered. The client did not use the call light and got out of bed unassisted. Nighttime confusion occurs with some clients, but unless the nurse had knowledge or awareness that this would happen, there was no link between the nurse's action and the client's fall. Damages and injury may well be present, but these probably are not due to any action or inaction on the nurse's part (options 2 and 3). Duty was addressed as the call light was within reach (option 4). **Cognitive Level:** Understanding. **Client Need:** Safe, Effective Care Environment. **Nursing Process:** Evaluation. **Learning Outcome:** 3-9.
5. **Answer:** 2. **Rationale:** While taking vital signs was an appropriate task to delegate to the UAP, the responsibility of the action—in this case, the inaction since the vitals were recorded inaccurately—is not fully assumed by the UAP and remains with the nurse. Delegating this task was not the responsibility of the nurse manager and so the responsibility of the action is not his/hers (option 4). **Cognitive Level:** Understanding. **Client Need:** Safe, Effective Care Environment. **Nursing Process:** Implementation. **Learning Outcome:** 3-7.
6. **Answer:** 3. **Rationale:** A DNR order only controls CPR and similar lifesaving treatments. All other care continues as previously ordered. Competent clients can still decide about their own care (including the DNR order). Nothing about the DNR order is related to when the client may die. Because clients' medical conditions and their views of their lives can change, a new DNR order is required for each admission to a healthcare agency. Once admitted, that order stands until changed or until it expires according to agency policy. **Cognitive Level:** Applying. **Client Need:** Psychosocial Integrity. **Nursing Process:** Planning. **Learning Outcome:** 3-7.
7. **Answer:** 3. **Rationale:** The only individual entitled to information without written consent is the client and those providing direct care. The nurse has open access to information regarding assigned clients only. **Cognitive Level:** Applying. **Client Need:** Safe, Effective Care Environment. **Nursing Process:** Implementation. **Learning Outcome:** 3-11.
8. **Answer:** 1, 2, and 5. **Rationale:** The nurse is subject to the limitation of the state law and should be familiar with the Good Samaritan laws in the specific state. Gross negligence would be described by the individual state law. Unless there is another equally or more qualified individual present, the nurse needs to stay until the injured individual leaves. The nurse should ask someone else to call or go for additional help. Since there was no prior agreement, the nurse cannot accept compensation. Also, the nurse is not employed by the accident victim. The same client rights apply at the scene of an accident as those in the workplace. **Cognitive Level:** Applying. **Client Need:** Safe, Effective Care Environment. **Nursing Process:** Planning. **Learning Outcome:** 3-13.

9. **Answer:** 1, 3, and 4. **Rationale:** Interacting with others (versus isolating self from others) and setting limits on the number of hours working are positive behaviors and not indicative of possible impairment. The other options are warning signs for impairment. **Cognitive Level:** Analyzing. **Client Need:** Safe, Effective Care Environment. **Nursing Process:** Evaluation. **Learning Outcome:** 3-6.
10. **Answer:** 2 and 3. **Rationale:** Standards of practice require a complete assessment. A nurse needs to be sure the client's needs have been met. They both can impact client safety and do not follow standards of care. The other options meet the standards of practice. **Cognitive Level:** Analyzing. **Client Need:** Safe, Effective Care Environment. **Nursing Process:** Implementation. **Learning Outcome:** 3-7.

CHAPTER 4 Values, Ethics and Advocacy

1. **Answer:** 1. **Rationale:** A nurse's actions in an ethical dilemma must be defensible according to moral and ethical standards. The nurse may have strong personal beliefs but distancing oneself from the situation does not serve the client (option 2). A team is not always required to reach decisions (option 3), and the nurse is not obligated to follow the client's wishes automatically when they may have negative consequences for self or others (option 4). **Cognitive Level:** Applying. **Client Need:** Safe, Effective Care Environment. **Nursing Process:** Planning. **Learning Outcome:** 4-2.
2. **Answer:** 2. **Rationale:** The nurse has an ethical responsibility to act only when actions are safe or risks minimized. This nurse is putting the client at unnecessary risk for a medication error. Many medical practices are controversial but not necessarily unethical (option 1). The nurse should follow agency policy. Although some may view nurses' strikes as unethical, supporting others who are striking is a personal decision (option 3). Although a client statement in confidence to a nurse may have ethical overtones, it does not automatically constitute an ethical dilemma. Since the assigned healthcare provider is a member of the team, principles of confidentiality do not include him or her (option 4). **Cognitive Level:** Analyzing. **Client Need:** Safe, Effective Care Environment. **Nursing Process:** N/A. **Learning Outcome:** 4-4.
3. **Answer:** 1. **Rationale:** Autonomy is the client's (or surrogate's) right to make his or her own decision. The nurse is obliged to respect a client's or significant other's informed decision. These parents may modify their decision as time goes on and the child's condition, or their feelings, change. This situation is not clearly one of nonmaleficence (do no harm) in option 2 or beneficence (do good) in option 3 since there are many aspects of both. If the child appeared to be suffering or an effective treatment was being denied, these principles might apply. Justice (fairness) generally applies when the rights of one client are being balanced against those of another client (option 4). **Cognitive Level:** Applying. **Client Need:** Safe, Effective Care Environment. **Nursing Process:** N/A. **Learning Outcome:** 4-3.
4. **Answer:** 3. **Rationale:** In values clarification, clients are assisted to think about the factors that influence their beliefs and decisions. Any judgmental statement that reflects the rightness or wrongness of the client's thoughts or actions will impede this process (options 1, 2, and 4). **Cognitive Level:** Applying. **Client Need:** Safe, Effective Care Environment. **Nursing Process:** Implementation. **Learning Outcome:** 4-2.
5. **Answer:** 1. **Rationale:** Resource allocation and financial considerations are major issues in home health care. When clients are in their own home, they operate from their own values and client autonomy must be respected. Community resources may be of benefit for this client to be able to afford the proper supplement at the correct dose or to provide assistance in other financial areas, so the client has the treatment needs met. The client already knows she should take the prescribed amount (option 2). Telling the physician will not help to solve the situation (option 3). Weighing the client merely assesses the need, which has already been established (option 4). **Cognitive Level:** Analyzing. **Client Need:** Safe, Effective Care Environment. **Nursing Process:** Implementation. **Learning Outcome:** 4-5.
6. **Answer:** 4. **Rationale:** Altruism is a concern for the welfare and well-being of others. A professional behavior of this value is demonstrating the understanding of cultures, beliefs, and perspectives of others. Human dignity, social justice, and autonomy are not the values described here. **Cognitive Level:** Applying. **Client Need:** Safe, Effective Care Environment. **Nursing Process:** Planning. **Learning Outcome:** 4-1.

CHAPTER 5 Healthcare Delivery Systems

1. **Answer:** 3. **Rationale:** Actions such as diet modification that help to prevent an illness or detect it in its early stages are primary preventions. Treatment of a disease such as with antibiotic therapy (option 1) or surgery (option 4) is secondary prevention, while rehabilitation efforts following an illness (option 2) are considered tertiary prevention. **Cognitive Level:** Analyzing. **Client Need:** Health Promotion and Maintenance. **Nursing Process:** N/A. **Learning Outcome:** 5-1.
2. **Answer:** 3. **Rationale:** Patient-focused care is a delivery model that brings all services and care providers to the client. Activities provided by auxiliary personnel (physical therapy, respiratory therapy, ECG testing, and phlebotomy) are moved close to the client, thereby decreasing the number of personnel involved and the number of steps needed to get the work done. **Cognitive Level:** Understanding. **Client Need:** Health Promotion and Maintenance. **Nursing Process:** Assessment. **Learning Outcome:** 5-2.
3. **Answer:** 3. **Rationale:** Differentiated practice is a system in which the best possible use of nursing personnel is based on their educational preparation and resultant skill sets. This model consists of specific job descriptions for nurses according to their education or training. Patient-focused care, shared governance, and managed care are not the models described in the stem. **Cognitive Level:** Understanding. **Client Need:** Safe, Effective Care Environment. **Nursing Process:** Planning. **Learning Outcome:** 5-3.
4. **Answer:** 2, 3, 5, 6. **Rationale:** Though there is an increase in complementary and alternative medicine use, this does not affect how health care is delivered (option 1). Chronic illness is prevalent in this group (option 4). **Cognitive Level:** Understanding. **Client Need:** N/A. **Nursing Process:** Diagnosis. **Learning Outcome:** 5-4.
5. **Answer:** 4. **Rationale:** A health maintenance organization involves a set monthly membership fee and predictable visit or deductible costs. Medicare covers a minimal number of preventive and outpatient services so the cost cannot be anticipated (option 1). Individual fee-for-service insurance is perhaps the most costly to the client, with potentially large differences between the amount of coverage the insurance company pays and the provider's charges (option 2). PPOs are less costly than fee-for-service entities, but more expensive than HMOs (option 3). **Cognitive Level:** Analyzing. **Client Need:** Safe, Effective Care Management. **Nursing Process:** Planning. **Learning Outcome:** 5-6.

CHAPTER 6 Community Nursing and Care Continuity

1. **Answer:** 2. **Rationale:** PHC involves issues of the environment, agriculture, and housing. It also involves other social, economic, and political issues such as poverty, transportation, unemployment, and economic development to sustain the population. Distribution and participation are two of the

five principles incorporated in PHC. Consumerism and governmental subsidies are not part of the PHC makeup. Low life expectancies and high mortality rates among children are two concerns about health care that led to the global health strategy of primary health care. **Cognitive Level:** Applying. **Client Need:** N/A. **Nursing Process:** N/A. **Learning Outcome:** 6-1.

2. **Answer:** 2. **Rationale:** In community-based healthcare, clients are cared for according to their geographic locations such as where they live or work, rather than at a major medical center or similar provider setting, which facilitates access. The other options are incorrect because emphasis is more on client wellness and prevention than on illness and may be paid for through any of the usual forms of insurance or payment (including managed care, private pay, or welfare). **Cognitive Level:** Analyzing. **Client Need:** Safe, Effective Care Environment. **Nursing Process:** N/A. **Learning Outcome:** 6-4.
3. **Answer:** 3. **Rationale:** Social interparticipation refers to community activities that are designed to meet people's needs for companionship. Socialization refers to the process of transmitting values, knowledge, culture, and skills to others. Social control refers to the way in which order is maintained in a community. Mutual support refers to the community's ability to provide resources at a time of illness or disaster. **Cognitive Level:** Applying. **Client Need:** Safe, Effective Care Environment. **Nursing Process:** N/A. **Learning Outcome:** 6-4.
4. **Answer:** 4. **Rationale:** Effective discharge planning would have included an assessment of home care needs prior to the client leaving the hospital. The kind of care is determined before the client leaves the current setting. That is why it is called discharge "planning." Following a thorough assessment, the client would be taught self-care strategies and a basic plan of care for the coming days (option 3). Obtaining medications and a ride home does not indicate the client possesses the knowledge and skills needed to manage care after discharge (option 2). If the client will need care at home, those referrals would be made by the discharge planner and communicated to the client. Option 4 indicates the client knows and accepts these referrals. **Cognitive Level:** Analyzing. **Client Need:** Safe, Effective Care Environment. **Nursing Process:** Evaluation. **Learning Outcome:** 6-7.
5. **Answer:** 4. **Rationale:** Production, distribution, and consumption of goods and services are the means by which the community provides for the economic needs of its members. It includes supplying food and clothing as well as providing water, electricity, police and fire protection, and the disposal of refuse. **Cognitive Level:** Applying. **Client Need:** N/A. **Nursing Process:** N/A. **Learning Outcome:** 6-5.

CHAPTER 7 Home Health Nursing Care

1. **Answer:** 3. **Rationale:** Although hospitals have recently become more welcoming to families, a major strength of home care is the involvement and proximity of loved ones. Curative and lifesaving approaches may be used both at home and in the hospital (option 1). An asset of home care nurses is their ability to manage complex symptoms (option 2). This includes expertise in pain management, but the same legal strategies are available in either in-home care or hospitals (option 4). **Cognitive Level:** Applying. **Client Need:** N/A. **Nursing Process:** N/A. **Learning Outcome:** 7-2.
2. **Answer:** 4. **Rationale:** Indirect care is provided by the home health nurse to the client each time the nurse consults with other health care providers about ways to improve nursing care for the client. Hands-on care, direct care, and client advocacy are not described in the stem (options 1, 2, and 3). **Cognitive Level:** Understanding. **Client Need:** Safe and Effective Care Environment. **Nursing Process:** Planning. **Learning Outcome:** 7-4.
3. **Answer:** 4. **Rationale:** Home health nurses can express concern when a situation suggests the possibility for injury. They must document information they provide and the family's response to instruction as well as make ongoing assessments about the family's use of safety precautions. While not inappropriate, the client is not likely to act upon the information the nurse provides in option 1. Nurses cannot expect to change a family's living space and lifestyle and such an intervention may be resented by the client (option 2). The nurse has an obligation to bring safety issues to the client's attention (option 3). **Cognitive Level:** Applying. **Client Need:** Safe, Effective Care Environment. **Nursing Process:** Implementation. **Learning Outcome:** 7-6.
4. **Answer:** 1. **Rationale:** If the caregiver's own health is becoming threatened, it may be a sign of overload. It would be appropriate for the caregiver to ask for assistance from others (option 2), or to ask for clarification of ways he or she can assist the client (option 3). Sadness related to a poor prognosis would be a normal and expected response as long as it does not evolve into depression (option 4). **Cognitive Level:** Applying. **Client Need:** Psychosocial Integrity. **Nursing Process:** Diagnosis. **Learning Outcome:** 7-7.
5. **Answer:** 4. **Rationale:** A physician's authorization of the plan of care is needed before home healthcare by a nurse can be initiated. Insurance coverage is not required, although the agency may need proof of the client's ability to pay if insurance is not available or adequate (option 1). Many clients benefit from home healthcare even if there is no in-home caregiver present or needed (option 2). The health problem for which home care is needed may be chronic or acute and may necessitate preventive, curative, or palliative therapy (option 3). **Cognitive Level:** Applying. **Client Need:** Safe, Effective Care Environment. **Nursing Process:** Planning. **Learning Outcome:** 7-3.
6. **Answer:** 1, 3, and 6. **Rationale:** Nurses may work with hospice clients as a subset of home health. In home healthcare, nurses care for both client and family and perform physical, psychosocial, and emotional interventions. Skilled nursing facilities are not considered locations for home health nursing care (option 2). Home healthcare can include high-tech equipment and procedures (option 4). Clients may have home care whether or not they can afford other healthcare (option 5). **Cognitive Level:** Remembering. **Client Need:** Safe, Effective Care Environment. **Nursing Process:** Planning. **Learning Outcome:** 7-4.
7. **Answer:** 4. **Rationale:** The emergency response necklace only works within the client's home in proximity to the base station. It will not activate away from home. The client needs to wear it at all times when home. It can be worn when away from home but the client must understand that activating it when away will not summon assistance. It is appropriate for the client to wear a medical alert bracelet at all times (option 1) and have a list of medications posted on the refrigerator (option 2). Area rugs should be removed if clients could trip on them (option 3). **Cognitive Level:** Applying. **Client Need:** Safe, Effective Care Environment. **Nursing Process:** Evaluation. **Learning Outcome:** 7-6.

CHAPTER 8 Electronic Health Records and Information Technology

1. **Answer:** 2. **Rationale:** Maintaining privacy and security of data is a significant issue. One way in which data can be protect in computers is by password-protecting it. Only those persons who have a legitimate need to access the data receive the password. Information in a computer data system may not always be safe, and it would be inappropriate for the nurse to say this (option 1). A nurse's involvement does not ensure security (option 3). Reminding the client that there is indeed cause for privacy concerns is not therapeutic (option 4). **Cognitive Level:** Applying. **Client Need:** Safe Effective Care

Environment. **Nursing Process:** Implementation. **Learning Outcome:** 8-2, 8-4.

2. **Answer:** 3. **Rationale:** Control over who has access to confidential computerized data is the greatest concern. Computer hackers can bypass codes and gain access to personal information, which could result in identity theft. The benefits often outweigh the cost (option 1). Computerized data can be much more accurate than paper-and-pencil data (option 2). Due to ease of making copies and backups, electronic data can last forever (option 4). **Cognitive Level:** Analyzing. **Client Need:** Safe, Effective Care Environment. **Nursing Process:** N/A. **Learning Outcome:** 8-2.
3. **Answer:** 4. **Rationale:** Since learners may do their online work at different times and do much of their work offline, it may be harder for them to feel and act like a class group. The courses are often self-paced and, thus, may take a longer or shorter time to complete than on-campus courses (option 1). Interpersonal communication is possible through email and chat, plus audio and video file sharing allow learners to see and hear the faculty as well as one another (option 2). For most web-based courses, learners may log on at their convenience (option 3). **Cognitive Level:** Understanding. **Client Need:** N/A. **Nursing Process:** N/A. **Learning Outcome:** 8-1.
4. **Answer:** 1. **Rationale:** The Cumulative Index to Nursing and Allied Health Literature (CINAHL) focuses on nursing and allied health articles, including research. The user can search systematically for articles that are related to nursing research, peer reviewed, published, and so on. The Google search engine gives a variety of sites, both health-related and non-health-related, but there are no restrictions for accuracy with this database. Educational Resources Information Center (ERIC) would include all areas of academia, not just nursing. PsychINFO includes only psychological abstracts. **Cognitive Level:** Applying. **Client Need:** N/A. **Nursing Process:** N/A. **Learning Outcome:** 8-5.
5. **Answer:** 4. **Rationale:** Spreadsheets are programs that can manipulate numbers. Data are arranged in columns and rows. Spreadsheets are used for budgets and are useful for working with staffing, scheduling, invoicing, research, and other analyses. A database is used to manage detailed information (option 1). In Word processing, documents are checked for spelling and grammar, and individualized to include pictures, charts, and designs (option 2). Graphics programs have become popular with their ability to create charts, tables, and pictures (option 3). **Cognitive Level:** Applying. **Client Need:** Health Promotion and Maintenance. **Nursing Process:** Implementation. **Learning Outcome:** 8-3.

CHAPTER 9 Critical Thinking and Clinical Reasoning

1. **Answer:** 2. **Rationale:** Nurses who utilize good critical-thinking skills are able to think and act in areas where there are neither clear answers nor standard procedures. Treatment options, especially for the home health client, can be extensive. There are many points to consider (good and bad), and choosing between treatment options can cause conflict among family members. The nurse in this case must use creativity, analysis based on science, and problem-solving skills, all of which contribute to critical-thinking skills. Options 1, 3, and 4 do not require much reasoning. **Cognitive Level:** Applying. **Client Need:** Health Promotion and Maintenance. **Nursing Process:** Evaluation. **Learning Outcome:** 9-1.
2. **Answer:** 1. **Rationale:** The nurse recognizes that many assumptions (beliefs) could interfere with the client eating—such as that the food presented is not culturally appropriate. These assumptions must be clarified with the process of clinical reasoning. Options 2 and 3 reach conclusions not supported by the facts. In option 4, the nurse has made a judgment or has an opinion that may not be accurate. Also, the nurse is acting without assessment. Implementation should be preceded by assessment. **Cognitive Level:** Applying. **Client Need:** Physiological Integrity. **Nursing Process:** Assessment. **Learning Outcome:** 9-2.
3. **Answer:** 2. **Rationale:** Reviewing evidence-based literature and identifying similarities in the clinical manifestations of symptoms is an act of clinical reasoning. Past experiences in care enhance the nurse's ability to recognize and respond in the delivery of client-centered care. Clinical judgment in nursing is a decision-making process to ascertain the right action to implement at the appropriate time during client care (option 1). Reflection is the nurse's review of the care provided to determine strategies to improve future care (option 3). Intuition is a problem-solving approach that relies on a nurse's inner sense (option 4). **Cognitive Level:** Applying. **Client Need:** Physiological Integrity. **Nursing Process:** N/A. **Learning Outcome:** 9-2.
4. **Answer:** 1. **Rationale:** The research method uses a research study-based approach to problem-solving. Trial and error (option 2) and intuition (option 3) would involve unstructured approaches resulting in less predictable results. The nursing process generally uses application of known interventions, previously determined by the scientific (research) process (option 4). **Cognitive Level:** Applying. **Client Need:** N/A. **Nursing Process:** N/A. **Learning Outcome:** 9-5.
5. **Answer:** 2. **Rationale:** Intuition is the understanding or learning of things without the conscious use of reasoning. It is also known as sixth sense, hunch, instinct, feeling, or suspicion. Clinical experience allows the nurse to recognize cues and patterns and begin to reach correct conclusions using intuition. Finding no cause for concern in the physical assessment of the client, the nurse is not satisfied and continues to assess the client's surroundings, finding the error. Trial and error is solving problems through a number of approaches until a solution is found (option 1). Judgment is not part of problem solving (option 3). The scientific method requires that the nurse evaluate potential solutions to a given problem in an organized, formal, and systematic approach (option 4). **Cognitive Level:** Applying. **Client Need:** N/A. **Nursing Process:** Planning. **Learning Outcome:** 9-4.
6. **Answer:** 2. **Rationale:** The nurse's intuition is like a sixth sense that allows the nurse to recognize cues and patterns to reach correct conclusions. The nurse appropriately obtains vital signs and an oxygen saturation to assess the client's clinical picture more fully. Option 1 supports appropriate nursing actions, but the client's respiratory status should be assessed first. Usually, a physician must order a chest x-ray (option 3). The rapid response team (option 4) may be needed if the client's condition becomes more critical. **Cognitive Level:** Applying. **Client Need:** Physiological Integrity. **Nursing Process:** Implementing. **Learning Outcome:** 9-2.
7. **Answer:** 1. **Rationale:** By reconsidering the type of dressing used based on research, the nurse is using integrity. Options 2 and 3 are critical thinking attitudes characterized by an awareness of the limits of one's own knowledge, and being trustworthy. Option 4 indicates an attitude of not being easily swayed by the opinions of others. **Cognitive Level:** Applying. **Client Need:** Health Promotion and Maintenance. **Nursing Process:** Planning. **Learning Outcome:** 9-4.
8. **Answer:** 1, 2, 4, 5. **Rationale:** While option 3 might be true, medicine and nursing have evolved tremendously, and so has the need for nurses to be critical thinkers. According to R. Alfaro LeFevre's *Top 10 Reasons to Improve Thinking*, patients are sicker, with multiple problems, and so nursing care requires a more critical form of thinking in order to meet their nursing needs; redesigning care delivery is useless if nurses don't have

the thinking skills required to deal with today's world; consumers and payers demand to see evidence of benefits, efficiency, and results; and today's progress often creates new problems that can't be solved by old ways of thinking. **Cognitive Level:** Applying. **Client Need:** Physiological Integrity. **Nursing Process:** Assessment. **Learning Outcome:** 9-1.

9. **Answer:** 2. **Rationale:** The nurse recognizes the need to obtain further information from the client in order to respond directly to the client's statement. Option 1 passes off the client's educational needs to another practitioner. Options 3 and 4 are nontherapeutic. **Cognitive Level:** Applying. **Client Need:** Physiological Integrity. **Nursing Process:** Planning. **Learning Outcome:** 9-5.
10. **Answer:** 4. **Rationale:** A nurse thinks critically, evaluates possible solutions, and uses problem-solving. Intuition (option 1) is not a sufficient basis for implementing wound care when significant data on alternative care strategies are available. Research (option 2) is a more comprehensive rigorous process and not typically implemented while caring for an infected wound. Trial and error (option 3) is unsafe and inappropriate for care of an infected wound. **Cognitive Level:** Understanding. **Client Need:** Physiological Integrity. **Nursing Process:** Planning. **Learning Outcome:** 9-5.

CHAPTER 10 Assessing

1. **Answer:** 3. **Rationale:** Delivery or organized care is not part of the nursing process, though each phase is interrelated (option 1). The nursing process is not part of the medical model as nurses treat the client's response to the disease or problem (option 2). The nursing process is individualized for each client's care plan. It is not about standardizing care (option 4). **Cognitive Level:** Applying. **Client Need:** N/A. **Nursing Process:** Diagnosis. **Learning Outcome:** 10-1.
2. **Answer:** 1, 2, 5. **Rationale:** Diagnosing is analyzing and synthesizing data in order to identify client strengths and health problems that can be prevented or resolved by collaborative and independent nursing interventions as well as developing a list of nursing and collaborative problems. Developing a plan and specifying goals and outcomes is part of the planning phase. **Cognitive Level:** Applying. **Client Need:** N/A. **Nursing Process:** Assessment. **Learning Outcome:** 10-1.
3. **Answer:** 2. **Rationale:** Primary data come from the client (option 4), whereas secondary data come from any other source (chart, family). Subjective data are covert (reported or an opinion), whereas objective data can be measured or validated (weight—option 1, edema—option 3). If the spouse had stated that the client had eaten only toast and tea, this would be secondary objective (measured) data. **Cognitive Level:** Applying. **Client Need:** N/A. **Nursing Process:** Assessment. **Learning Outcome:** 10-5.
4. **Answer:** 2. **Rationale:** The nurse should use a combination of directive and nondirective approaches during the interview to determine areas of concern for the client. Simply noting the concern, without dealing with it, or passing the questions off to the doctor can leave the impression that the nurse does not care about the client's concerns or dismisses them as unimportant (options 1 and 3). A closed question (option 4) does not allow the client to offer much information, besides yes/no or one-word answers. **Cognitive Level:** Applying. **Client Need:** N/A. **Nursing Process:** Assessment. **Learning Outcome:** 10-8.
5. **Answer:** 4. **Rationale:** Frameworks help the nurse be systematic in data collection. Other members of the healthcare team may use very different conceptual organizing frameworks so data may not correlate (option 1). Cost-effective care (option 2) is more likely to occur with systematic application of the nursing process, but use of a framework for assessment alone may not accomplish this goal. Because the framework is structured and because of the nature of client needs and problems, creativity and intuition in care planning are not assured (option 3). **Cognitive Level:** Applying. **Client Need:** N/A. **Nursing Process:** Assessment. **Learning Outcome:** 10-10.
6. **Answer:** 1. **Rationale:** Assessing provides a database of the client's physiologic and psychosocial responses to his or her health status. Client strengths and problems (option 2) are identified in the diagnosing phase of the nursing process; a care plan is established (option 3) in the planning phase; and care, prevention, and wellness promotion (option 4) are part of the implementing phase. **Cognitive Level:** Remembering. **Client Need:** N/A. **Nursing Process:** Assessment. **Learning Outcome:** 10-3.
7. **Answer:** 3. **Rationale:** In validating, the nurse confirms that data are complete and accurate. Subjective data are collected in the collecting activity (option 1), a framework is applied to the data in the organizing activity (option 2), and data are recorded in the documenting activity (option 4). **Cognitive Level:** Understanding. **Client Need:** N/A. **Nursing Process:** Assessment. **Learning Outcome:** 10-4.
8. **Answer:** 1. **Rationale:** The nursing process focuses on client needs. It is dynamic rather than static (option 2), emphasizes client responses rather than physiology and illness (option 3), and is collaborative rather than used exclusively by nurses (option 4). **Cognitive Level:** Understanding. **Client Need:** N/A. **Nursing Process:** Assessment. **Learning Outcome:** 10-4.
9. **Answer:** 4. **Rationale:** Interpreting collected data is necessary to help validate their accuracy. Observing includes the senses of smell, hearing, and touch in addition to vision (option 1). Observing must often be performed simultaneously with other activities (option 2). A systematic approach to observing data helps ensure nothing is missed and the nurse pays attention to the most important data first (option 3). **Cognitive Level:** Understanding. **Client Need:** N/A. **Nursing Process:** Assessment. **Learning Outcome:** 10-6.
10. **Answer:** 2, 4, and 5. **Rationale:** The nurse plans the interview so that privacy is observed. A comfortable distance between nurse and client to respect the client's personal space is about 3 feet. Using a standard form will help ensure the nurse doesn't omit gathering any vital information. Lighting should be at a normal level—neither bright nor dim (option 1). The nurse should be at the same height as the client, usually sitting, at approximately a 45° angle facing the client. The nurse standing over the client creates an uncomfortable atmosphere for an interview (option 3). **Cognitive Level:** Applying. **Client Need:** N/A. **Nursing Process:** Planning. **Learning Outcome:** 10-9.

CHAPTER 11 Diagnosing

1. **Answer:** 3. **Rationale:** Learning from peers and seasoned nurses is helpful but does not take the place of didactic information (options 1 and 2). Experience teaches much information, but it never takes the place of concrete, scientific theory (option 4). **Cognitive Level:** Applying. **Client Need:** N/A. **Nursing Process:** Diagnosis. **Learning Outcome:** 11-4.
2. **Answer:** 2. **Rationale:** Because the venous return is impaired, fluid is static, resulting in swelling. Therefore, decreased venous return is the cause (etiology) of the problem. Increased fluid volume is the nursing diagnosis, and edema of the lower extremity is the sign, symptom, or critical attribute. The cause is known. **Cognitive Level:** Application. **Client Need:** N/A. **Nursing Process:** Diagnosis. **Learning Outcome:** 11-6.
3. **Answer:** 1. **Rationale:** States the relationship between the stem (impairment in caregiver role) and the cause of the problem. Option 2: The diagnostic statement says the same thing as the related factor (falls and collapse). Option 3: It is inappropriate to use medical diagnoses such as stroke within a nursing diagnosis statement. Option 4 is vague. The statement must be specific and guide the plan of care (fatigue may be a

result of sleep deprivation and does not direct intervention). **Cognitive Level:** Applying. **Client Need:** N/A. **Nursing Process:** Diagnosis. **Learning Outcome:** 11-2.

4. **Answer:** 4. **Rationale:** The PES format assists with comprehensive and accurate organization of client data. More efficient planning may or may not reduce healthcare costs. Nursing diagnostic statements should be confirmed with the client but using PES does not ensure this. PES statements can be wellness or illness focused. **Cognitive Level:** Applying. **Client Need:** N/A. **Nursing Process:** Diagnosis. **Learning Outcome:** 11-5.
5. **Answer:** 1. **Rationale:** A collaborative (multidisciplinary) problem is indicated when both medical and nursing interventions are needed to prevent or treat the problem. If nursing care alone (whether that care involves independent or dependent nursing actions) can treat the problem, a nursing diagnosis is indicated. If medical care alone can treat the problem, a medical diagnosis is indicated. **Cognitive Level:** Applying. **Client Need:** N/A. **Nursing Process:** Diagnosis. **Learning Outcome:** 11-3.
6. **Answer:** 1. **Rationale:** A syndrome diagnosis is associated with a cluster of other diagnoses (in this situation, urinary elimination alteration, impaired skin integrity, and powerlessness). Currently, there are six syndrome diagnoses on the NANDA International list. The others are incorrect options. **Cognitive Level:** Understanding. **Client Need:** N/A. **Nursing Process:** Diagnosis. **Learning Outcome:** 11-2.
7. **Answer:** 3. **Rationale:** Diagnostic labels are continuously reviewed and revised as indicated by research—much more of which is needed. The original taxonomy has been replaced by Taxonomy II and is no longer based on a nurse theorist (options 1 and 2). New diagnoses are approved by NANDA International's Diagnostic Review Committee, not by a vote of nurses (option 4). **Cognitive Level:** Remembering. **Client Need:** N/A. **Nursing Process:** Diagnosis. **Learning Outcome:** 11-7.
8. **Answer:** 1, 4, and 5. **Rationale:** A client's movement toward a goal (option 1) or whose behavior is inconsistent with population norms (options 4 and 5) represents a cue that further analysis toward creating a nursing diagnosis is required. Corrected vision (option 2) and bladder and bowel control at age 18 months (option 3) are consistent with population norms. **Cognitive Level:** Analyzing. **Client Need:** N/A. **Nursing Process:** Diagnosis. **Learning Outcome:** 11-4.

CHAPTER 12 Planning

1. **Answer:** 4. **Rationale:** Strategic planning is an ongoing process focused on organizational change rather than individual clients so it is least useful and not relevant in this case. The client requires initial planning because he has just arrived on the orthopedic unit for the first time (option 1). Of the three types of planning that need to be done at this time, initial is the highest priority since he has just had surgery. The client also requires the ongoing type of planning necessary to determine the care appropriate for this shift (option 2). Discharge planning needs to start on admission to ensure adequate client preparation for management of health needs outside the health agency (option 3). **Cognitive Level:** Applying. **Client Need:** Safe, Effective Care Environment. **Nursing Process:** Planning. **Learning Outcome:** 12-2.
2. **Answer:** 2. **Rationale:** The nurse must consider a variety of factors when assigning priorities, including resources available to the nurse and client. Factors in this case include the distance between the client's home and the hospital and the fact that therapy is ordered on a twice daily basis. Driving 80 miles two times a day may not be feasible, but perhaps there are other alternatives that could be considered (e.g., a neighbor who might be willing to drive the client, or someone in the area who may be able to assist with the therapy). **Cognitive Level:** Applying. **Client Need:** Psychosocial Integrity. **Nursing Process:** Planning. **Learning Outcome:** 12-5.
3. **Answer:** 2. **Rationale:** More detailed assessment data and consultation with the client would be needed to absolutely confirm the priority. Postoperative nausea to the level of inhibiting oral intake has the greatest likelihood of leading to complications and requires nursing intervention now. The client's pain level is not extreme considering the recency of the surgery, and pain intervention can be assumed to be effective (option 1). Although the constipation is probably bordering on abnormal, a nursing intervention would most likely begin with oral treatment, which is not possible due to the nausea. More invasive interventions such as an enema or suppository would not be commonly administered the first day postoperative (option 3). Wound infection can occur, but there are no data to indicate that this requires a change in the current plan (option 4). **Cognitive Level:** Applying. **Client Need:** Physiological Integrity. **Nursing Process:** Planning. **Learning Outcome:** 12-5.
4. **Answer:** 1. **Rationale:** Desired outcomes are the more specific, observable criteria used to evaluate whether the goals have been met. Ambulating without a walker by a certain date is specific as well as measurable. **Cognitive Level:** Applying. **Client Need:** Physiological Integrity. **Nursing Process:** Planning. **Learning Outcome:** 12-8.
5. **Answer:** 3. **Rationale:** Although there may be standard policies or routines for measuring intake and output, the nursing intervention should specify if this is to be done "routinely" or at specific intervals (e.g., q4h). The nurse is also aware, however, that critical thinking indicates that the intake and output should be monitored more frequently than ordered if assessment reveals abnormal findings. **Cognitive Level:** Understanding. **Client Need:** Physiological Integrity. **Nursing Process:** Planning. **Learning Outcome:** 12-9.
6. **Answer:** 3, 1, 4, and 2. **Rationale:** In planning, first the nurse sets priorities and then writes goals or outcomes, selects interventions, and then writes the nursing care plan. **Cognitive Level:** Understanding. **Client Need:** N/A. **Nursing Process:** Planning. **Learning Outcome:** 12-1.
7. **Answer:** 4. **Rationale:** An individualized care plan is tailored to meet the unique needs of a specific client, needs that are not addressed by the standardized care plan. In this situation, the client had complications following a relatively routine procedure, something that is unplanned and a rare occurrence and must fit with the needs of the client. **Cognitive Level:** Understanding. **Client Need:** N/A. **Nursing Process:** Planning. **Learning Outcome:** 12-3.
8. **Answer:** 1. **Rationale:** Goal statements provide the standard against which outcomes are measured. Nursing diagnoses are prioritized before goals are written (option 2). Both independent and dependent interventions may be appropriate for any goal (option 3). Clarity of the goal does not influence delegation of the intervention (option 4). **Cognitive Level:** Analyzing. **Client Need:** N/A. **Nursing Process:** Planning. **Learning Outcome:** 12-6.
9. **Answer:** 4. **Rationale:** NOC outcomes should reflect both the nurse's and the client's values of what is trying to be achieved. The outcomes still must be customized (option 1), but address only one nursing diagnosis at a time (option 2). Outcomes are narrow or specific end points, not broad (option 3). **Cognitive Level:** Applying. **Client Need:** N/A. **Nursing Process:** Planning. **Learning Outcome:** 12-7.
10. **Answer:** 1. **Rationale:** Interventions should address the etiology of the nursing diagnosis. Both independent and dependent interventions should be selected if appropriate (option 2) and several interventions may be needed for a single outcome (option 3). Both action and assessment-type interventions can be used (option 4). **Cognitive Level:** Applying. **Client Need:** N/A. **Nursing Process:** Planning. **Learning Outcome:** 12-10.

CHAPTER 13 Implementing and Evaluating

1. **Answer:** 3. **Rationale:** The first step of implementing is reassessing the client to determine that the activity is still indicated and safe. The next action would be to determine if assistance is required (option 2), then implement the intervention (delegating if appropriate) (option 1), and last document the intervention (option 4). **Cognitive Level:** Understanding. **Client Need:** N/A. **Nursing Process:** Implementation. **Learning Outcome:** 13-3.
2. **Answer:** 4. **Rationale:** It is never acceptable practice for the nurse to document a nursing activity before it is carried out. This would be very unsafe because many things can cause an activity to be postponed or canceled and prior charting would be inaccurate, misleading, and potentially dangerous. In a few situations, it may be permissible to chart frequent or routine activities some time following the activities such as at the end of a shift or after a particular interval (e.g., every 4 hours) rather than immediately following the activity. **Cognitive Level:** Applying. **Client Need:** N/A. **Nursing Process:** Implementation. **Learning Outcome:** 13-4.
3. **Answer:** 4. **Rationale:** Though assessment is the first phase of the nursing process it is carried out during all phases (option 1). Evaluation is carried out at the end of the process (option 2). Though the two processes overlap, there is a difference between the data collected (option 3). Assessment data are collected for the nurse to make a diagnosis and evaluate desired outcomes. Evaluation data are collected for the purpose of comparing them to prescribed goals and judging the effectiveness of the nursing care. **Cognitive Level:** Understanding. **Client Need:** N/A. **Nursing Process:** Evaluation. **Learning Outcome:** 13-5.
4. **Answer:** 2. **Rationale:** There is no reason to delete (option 1) or modify the nursing diagnosis (option 3) or demote its priority (option 4) because the risk factors that prompted it are still present. **Cognitive Level:** Analyzing. **Client Need:** Safe, Effective Care Environment. **Nursing Process:** Evaluation. **Learning Outcome:** 13-7.
5. **Answer:** 2. **Rationale:** Because this assessment focuses on how care is provided, it is a process evaluation. A structure evaluation (option 1) would focus on the setting (e.g., how well equipment functions), and outcome evaluations (option 3) focus on changes in client status (e.g., whether reported satisfaction levels vary with type of individual who answers the call light). An audit (option 4) would be a chart or document review. **Cognitive Level:** Analyzing. **Client Need:** N/A. **Nursing Process:** Evaluation. **Learning Outcome:** 13-8.
6. **Answer:** 1, 2, 3, 4. **Rationale:** Successful evaluation depends on the effectiveness of the steps that precede it. During the evaluation step, the nurse collects data for the purpose of comparing it with preselected goals/outcomes and judging the effectiveness of the nursing care. During the assessment phase, the nurse collects data for the purpose of making diagnoses. **Cognitive Level:** Applying. **Client Need:** N/A. **Nursing Process:** Evaluation. **Learning Outcome:** 13-1.
7. **Answer:** 3. **Rationale:** This client needs psychosocial support rather than skills related to knowledge (options 1 and 2) or hands-on activity (option 4). **Cognitive Level:** Understanding. **Client Need:** N/A. **Nursing Process:** Evaluation. **Learning Outcome:** 13-2.
8. **Answer:** 1, 4, and 5. **Rationale:** Nurses should always have clear rationales for their actions, clients should be given options whenever possible, and client teaching is a constant, integral part of implementing. Primary care provider orders must be critically evaluated and modified to meet individual client needs (option 2). Clients may have nurses provide needed care but should take care of themselves whenever possible since dependency has its own complications (option 3). **Cognitive Level:** Analyzing. **Client Need:** N/A. **Nursing Process:** Evaluation. **Learning Outcome:** 13-4.
9. **Answer:** 2. **Rationale:** Evaluating requires that client behavior be compared to expected outcomes. Goals may be partially met in addition to completely met or unmet (option 1). An outcome may be achieved but not be a direct result of the plan or interventions (option 3). A care plan should be continued, modified, or terminated based on achievement of outcomes (option 4). **Cognitive Level:** Analyzing. **Client Need:** N/A. **Nursing Process:** Evaluation. **Learning Outcome:** 13-6.
10. **Answer:** 4. **Rationale:** Quality improvement (QI) plans corrective actions for problems. QI focuses on process rather than outcomes (option 1) and client care rather than structure (option 2), and aims for improvement rather than confirmation of quality (option 3). **Cognitive Level:** Understanding. **Client Need:** N/A. **Nursing Process:** Evaluation. **Learning Outcome:** 13-9.

CHAPTER 14 Documenting and Reporting

1. **Answer:** 3. **Rationale:** All of the other answers endanger the client's confidentiality. **Cognitive Level:** Applying. **Client Need:** Safe, Effective Care Environment. **Nursing Process:** Implementation. **Learning Outcome:** 14-1.
2. **Answer:** 1. **Rationale:** Subjective data consist of information obtained from what the client says. When possible, the nurse quotes the client's words; otherwise, they are summarized. Objective data consist of information that is measured or observed. Assessment is the interpretation or conclusion drawn about the subjective and objective data. This is the area where the problems are documented initially. The client's condition and level of progress are subsequently described. Planning is the care designed to resolve the problem. **Cognitive Level:** Applying. **Client Need:** Safe, Effective Care Environment. **Nursing Process:** Assessment. **Learning Outcome:** 14-3.
3. **Answer:** 4. **Rationale:** When a mistake is recorded, a line should be drawn through it and the words "mistaken entry" should be written above or next to the original entry, then initial or signature–whichever is agency policy—should be placed. The original entry must remain visible. Erasure, blotting out, or correction fluid should not be used (options 1 and 2). When a mistake is recorded the correction applies to only the erroneous information not the entire page (option 3). **Cognitive Level:** Applying. **Client Need:** Safe, Effective Care Environment. **Nursing Process:** Evaluation. **Learning Outcome:** 14-6.
4. **Answer:** 4. **Rationale:** Option 4 is the "best" answer although it could be more complete by adding the response of the primary care provider. Option 1 is too vague because it is not clear if the nurse found the client or was present when the client fell. Also, there is no need to write the word *client* because it is the client's chart. Option 2 is judgmental, revealing a negative attitude toward the client. It would be better to describe specific signs and symptoms such as staggering, slurred speech, and smell of alcohol on breath. Option 3 is too general and can be more specific by charting "2 cm × 3 cm purplish bruise on mid-inner thigh along with color." **Cognitive Level:** Analyzing. **Client Need:** Safe, Effective Care Environment. **Nursing Process:** Evaluation. **Learning Outcome:** 14-6.
5. **Answer:** 1. Within normal limits; 2. Bathroom privileges; 3. As needed; 4. Diet as tolerated. **Cognitive Level:** Remembering. **Client Need:** Safe, Effective Care Environment. **Nursing Process:** Implementation. **Learning Outcome:** 14-6.
6. **Answer:** 2. **Rationale:** The graphic record provides the trend of the vital signs. Option 1, verbal information, is not appropriate for validation assessment that is measurable. This is more appropriate for pain or dizziness. The medication record would not include documentation of blood pressure ranges (option 3). The progress notes (option 4) provide information about how the client is progressing. It may have information about the client's BP if it was a problem. The best answer is option 2. **Cognitive Level:** Applying. **Client Need:** Safe,

Effective Care Environment. **Nursing Process:** Assessment. **Learning Outcome:** 14-4.

7. **Answer:** 1, 2, and 4. **Rationale:** Option 3 is incorrect because it could be a HIPAA violation if others hear protected health information. Option 5 is not needed unless it is a concern and it would not be done for every client. **Cognitive Level:** Analyzing. **Client Need:** Safe, Effective Care Environment. **Nursing Process:** Implementation. **Learning Outcome:** 14-8.
8. **Answer:** 2, 3, and 5. **Rationale:** Option 1: "MS" is on the "Do Not Use" list—the nurse needs to write out morphine sulfate. Option 4 has three errors—should not have a trailing zero after the decimal point; "u" and "SQ" are on the "Do Not Use" list. **Cognitive Level:** Analyzing. **Client Need:** Safe, Effective Care Environment. **Nursing Process:** Implementation. **Learning Outcome:** 14-7.
9. **Answer:** 3. **Rationale:** It should never be assumed that the client fell out of bed, became tangled in bedding, or anything else (options 1, 2, and 4). Accurate notations consist of facts or observations rather than opinions or interpretations. The client was found on the floor, and the call light was activated. Those are the only things known until the nurse gets further information from questioning the client. **Cognitive Level:** Applying. **Client Need:** Safe, Effective Care Environment. **Nursing Process:** Evaluation. **Learning Outcome:** 14-6.
10. **Answer:** 1, 2, and 4. **Rationale:** Military time is commonly used; documenting worries or concerns provides clues to other nurses; gossip, unprofessional comments or thoughts, or personnel issues should not be recorded in the client's chart. Option 3 is incorrect because charting should be done as events occur. Waiting until the end of the shift increases the chance of forgetting something. **Cognitive Level:** Applying. **Client Need:** Safe, Effective Care Environment. **Nursing Process:** Implementation. **Learning Outcome:** 14-6.

CHAPTER 15 Caring

1. **Answer:** 1. **Rationale:** *Knowing* means understanding the other's needs and how to respond to those needs. Sensing that a client is withdrawn and sullen, the nurse knows that spending extra time can sometimes allow the client to feel comfortable in talking about what might be bothering him. **Cognitive Level:** Analyzing. **Client Need:** Psychosocial Integrity. **Nursing Process:** Assessment. **Learning Outcome:** 15-2.
2. **Answer:** 1. **Rationale:** Teaching the client to make self-care decisions at home empowers him to care for his illness. Empowerment is not the primary goal for options 2, 3, and 4. **Cognitive Level:** Applying. **Client Need:** Health Promotion and Maintenance. **Nursing Process:** Implementation. **Learning Outcome:** 15-4.
3. **Answer:** 3. **Rationale:** Roach uses the Six C's of caring in nursing. Swanson's theory includes five caring processes (option 1). Mayeroff was a philosopher who saw caring as "helping the other grow" (option 2). Watson developed the Theory of Human Care, which is the basis for nursing's role in society (option 4). **Cognitive Level:** Remembering. **Client Need:** Psychosocial Integrity. **Nursing Process:** Planning. **Learning Outcome:** 15-3.
4. **Answer:** 1. **Rationale:** This situation reflects personal knowing, which is developed through critical reflection on one's own actions and feelings. Aesthetic knowing arises from a deep appreciation of the uniqueness of each individual (option 2). Empirical knowing includes objective observation and scientific theories (option 3). Ethical knowing involves confronting and resolving conflicting values and beliefs (option 4). **Cognitive Level:** Analyzing. **Client Need:** Psychosocial Integrity. **Nursing Process:** Evaluation. **Learning Outcome:** 15-2.
5. **Answer:** 4. **Rationale:** Ethical knowing focuses on matters of obligation or what ought to be done and goes beyond simply following the ethical codes of the discipline. **Cognitive Level:** Applying. **Client Need:** N/A. **Nursing Process:** N/A. **Learning Outcome:** 15-2.
6. **Answer:** 4. **Rationale:** Caring practice involves connection, mutual recognition, and involvement. It is more than just performing skills adequately or even efficiently. It's a sense that the nurse has made a difference to someone else. Caring means that people, relationships, and things matter. Explaining a procedure, then seeking permission to begin lets the client know that the nurse respects the client as an individual. All other options are examples of appropriate and professional nursing care, but do not address a caring aspect. **Cognitive Level:** Applying. **Client Need:** Psychosocial Integrity. **Nursing Process:** Implementation. **Learning Outcome:** 15-4.
7. **Answer:** 1, 3, and 4. **Rationale:** Options 1, 3, and 4 are healthy options for self-care. Use of alcohol as a way to destress can be unhealthy (option 2). Gossiping is negative energy and should be avoided (option 5). **Cognitive Level:** Applying. **Client Need:** Psychosocial Integrity. **Nursing Process:** Evaluation. **Learning Outcome:** 15-5.
8. **Answer:** 1. **Rationale:** Empirical knowing is gained from studying scientific models and theories. Aesthetic knowing arises from application in practice (option 2). Personal knowing arises from self-examination (option 3). Ethical knowing arises from confronting conflicting values (option 4). **Cognitive Level:** Applying. **Client Need:** N/A. **Nursing Process:** N/A. **Learning Outcome:** 15-2.
9. **Answer:** 4. **Rationale:** Meditation involves the described behaviors. Storytelling involves communication with others (option 1). Yoga combines various postures with breathing practices (option 2). Music therapy involves listening to music (option 3). **Cognitive Level:** Analyzing. **Client Need:** N/A. **Nursing Process:** N/A. **Learning Outcome:** 15-5.
10. **Answer:** 3. **Rationale:** Twenty-five minutes of vigorous activity 3 days a week is the recommendation for a healthy lifestyle. Ten minutes is an insufficient amount of time for moderate exercise (option 1), as is 20 minutes (option 2). Daily vigorous activity for 30 minutes may be too strenuous (option 4), depending on the client's level of conditioning. **Cognitive Level:** Applying. **Client Need:** Health Promotion and Maintenance. **Nursing Process:** Implementation. **Learning Outcome:** 15-6.

CHAPTER 16 Communicating

1. **Answer:** 3. **Rationale:** Nonverbal, gentle touch is an important tool; overstimulation may affect the client in a negative way. Option 1: Written communication requires a higher level of consciousness than verbal. Option 2: The client does not have a hearing problem but lacks the ability to interpret and understand communication. Option 4: Lack of facial expression may increase fear. **Cognitive Level:** Applying. **Client Need:** Psychosocial Integrity. **Nursing Process:** Implementation. **Learning Outcome:** 16-7.
2. **Answer:** 3, 1, 2, 4. **Rationale:** During the preinteraction phase (option 3), the nurse gathers information about the client before meeting the client. During the introductory phase (option 1), the nurse usually engages in some social interaction to put the client at ease. During the working phase (option 2), the nurse helps the client to explore feelings and plan a program. During the termination phase (option 4), the nurse summarizes or reviews the process that took place. **Cognitive Level:** Analyzing. **Client Need:** Psychosocial Integrity. **Nursing Process:** Planning. **Learning Outcome:** 16-6.
3. **Answer:** 1. **Rationale:** The client is nonverbal, so speaking when facing the client, using an interpreter, or using the client's dominant language does not address the client's ability to communicate. **Cognitive Level:** Applying. **Client Need:** Psychosocial Integrity. **Nursing Process:** Implementation. **Learning Outcome:** 16-4.

4. **Answer:** 1. **Rationale:** Respect is correct because the nurse is validating the client's feeling. It is not genuineness (option 2) because the nurse is giving information versus being genuine. Concreteness (option 3) is giving a specific example. The nurse is not confronting (option 4) but supporting through respect for the client's feelings. **Cognitive Level:** Applying. **Client Need:** Psychosocial Integrity. **Nursing Process:** Implementation. **Learning Outcome:** 16-6.
5. **Answer:** 1, 3, 5. **Rationale:** These options reflect impairments to communication. Option 1 is a sensory deficit of deafness. Option 3 is a possible cognitive impairment, and option 5 is an example of a structural deficit. The nursing diagnosis altered verbal communication may *not* be useful when an individual's communication problems are caused by a psychiatric illness (option 2). If the communication issue is due to a problem coping, the diagnosis of fear or anxiety may be more appropriate (option 4). **Cognitive Level:** Applying. **Client Need:** N/A. **Nursing Process:** Diagnosis. **Learning Outcome:** 16-7.
6. **Answer:** 2 and 3. **Rationale:** Assessing possible visual or hearing problems allows the nurse to provide appropriate interventions (e.g., inserting hearing aid). Communicating what will be occurring at a stressful time helps the client feel more secure and can reduce anxiety. Option 1 is not the best answer as the client could say yes or no or nod the head and the nurse will not know if the client fully understands. It would be better to ask the client to tell you where he or she is. Option 4 is important to do; however, immediately after surgery is not the best time as the client may be in pain or groggy from the anesthesia. Option 5 is false reassurance because the nurse does not know if the client is going to feel better. **Cognitive Level:** Applying. **Client Need:** Psychosocial Integrity. **Nursing Process:** Implementation. **Learning Outcome:** 16-4.
7. **Answer:** 4. **Rationale:** Nonverbal communication, or body language, often tells the nurse more about what a person is feeling than what is actually said. The interpretation of such observations requires validation with the client. **Cognitive Level:** Applying. **Client Need:** Psychosocial Integrity. **Nursing Process:** Implementation. **Learning Outcome:** 16-3.
8. **Answer:** 4. **Rationale:** Option 4 is a therapeutic technique using an open-ended question that allows the client to elaborate. The other options are barriers to communication. Option 1 is incorrect because the client did not ask about the abilities of the surgeon and the response does not focus on the client. Option 2 is changing the subject, and option 3 is giving advice. **Cognitive Level:** Analyzing. **Client Need:** Psychosocial Integrity. **Nursing Process:** Implementation. **Learning Outcome:** 16-7.
9. **Answer:** 4. **Rationale:** An important characteristic of assertive communication includes the use of "I" statements versus "you" statements. "You" statements place blame and put the listener in a defensive position. "I" statements encourage discussion. **Cognitive Level:** Analyzing. **Client Need:** Psychosocial Integrity. **Nursing Process:** Assessment. **Learning Outcome:** 16-4.
10. **Answer:** 1. **Rationale:** It encourages the client to verbalize and choose the topic of the conversation. Option 2 is used when the nurse is unsure of the message and asks the client to repeat or restate the message. Option 3 is used to help a client differentiate the real from the unreal, and there is no information available to indicate this is a concern in this situation. Option 4 is used at the end of an interview or teaching session. **Cognitive Level:** Applying. **Client Need:** Psychosocial Integrity. **Nursing Process:** Assessment. **Learning Outcome:** 16-4.

CHAPTER 17 Teaching

1. **Answer:** 2. **Rationale:** Options 1 and 3 are psychomotor, and 4 is under the cognitive domain. **Cognitive Level:** Understanding. **Client Need:** Health Promotion and Maintenance. **Nursing Process:** Implementation. **Learning Outcome:** 17-3.
2. **Answer:** 3. **Rationale:** Options 1 and 2 are passive learning strategies. Learning is faster and retention better when the learner is actively involved. Option 4 promotes affective learning about adapting to a chronic health condition and is important. However, the question asks about learning diet information. **Cognitive Level:** Applying. **Client Need:** Physiological Integrity. **Nursing Process:** Implementation. **Learning Outcome:** 17-9.
3. **Answer:** 3. **Rationale:** Motivation is the desire to learn and influences how quickly and to what extent a person learns. It is generally greatest when a person recognizes a need and believes the need will be met through learning. Clients who struggle with rules or following prescribed courses of treatment are not motivated to learn the best reason for their particular plan of action (option 1). The client who is already waiting to go home may be motivated for that, but not to the extent of being ready to learn how to achieve this end (option 2). Motivation must be experienced by the client, not by someone else, as in being a "coach" for newcomers (option 4). **Cognitive Level:** Applying. **Client Need:** Psychosocial Integrity. **Nursing Process:** Assessment. **Learning Outcome:** 17-5.
4. **Answer:** 1. **Rationale:** Individuals learn in various ways, such as visually, group learning, auditory, and participatory. The individual knows how learning has occurred in the past. Option 2 is a component of the implementation phase of teaching, and the question is asking how to assess a client's style of learning. Options 3 and 4 involve others and it is best to ask the client. **Cognitive Level:** Remembering. **Client Need:** Health Promotion and Maintenance. **Nursing Process:** Assessment. **Learning Outcome:** 17-7.
5. **Answer:** 3. **Rationale:** Options 1 and 4 are not specific enough because they do not include the specific learning need. Option 2 is a wellness nursing diagnosis; the data would need to address that the client is seeking health information and why in order to be the correct answer. **Cognitive Level:** Remembering. **Client Need:** Physiological Integrity. **Nursing Process:** Diagnosis. **Learning Outcome:** 17-9.
6. **Answer:** 2, 3, and 5. **Rationale:** Options 2, 3, and 5 are open-ended questions that will give the client the opportunity to provide information that will help the nurse assess level of knowledge and subsequently provide and discuss needed information with the client. Options 1 and 4 are closed-ended (yes or no) questions. A "no" answer may cause a discussion but it will be difficult for the nurse to assess if it is the information the client really wants to know. **Cognitive Level:** Applying. **Client Need:** Psychosocial Integrity. **Nursing Process:** Assessment. **Learning Outcome:** 17-7.
7. **Answer:** 1, 2. **Rationale:** The inability to identify changes in the skin around the stoma would indicate that instruction has not been effective. The client's stating he does not want to perform self-care to the ostomy or the client's asking his wife to learn the care would indicate that effective learning did not occur. **Cognitive Level:** Analyzing. **Client Need:** Health Promotion and Maintenance. **Nursing Process:** Evaluation. **Learning Outcome:** 17-13.
8. **Answer:** 3. **Rationale:** All are important factors to assess. The priority, however, would be the potential economic factor because the medications can be very expensive and the client may not take them if he or she cannot afford them. **Cognitive Level:** Applying. **Client Need:** Physiological Integrity. **Nursing Process:** Assessment. **Learning Outcome:** 17-7.
9. **Answer:** 3. **Rationale:** This option is the easiest for the nurse to evaluate. Option 1 is difficult to evaluate because "understand" is too vague. Option 2 refers more to an affective outcome and the question is asking about a cognitive outcome. Option 4 is telling more about the husband than the client. **Cognitive Level:** Analyzing. **Client Need:** Health Promotion and Maintenance. **Nursing Process:** Evaluation. **Learning Outcome:** 17-13.

10. **Answer:** 2. **Rationale:** This is the only option that clearly reflects the teaching process, the evaluation method, and the response of the client indicating evidence of learning. **Cognitive Level:** Analyzing. **Client Need:** Physiological Integrity. **Nursing Process:** Evaluation. **Learning Outcome:** 17-14.

CHAPTER 18 Leading, Managing, and Delegating

1. **Answer:** 1. **Rationale:** This is a situation in which urgent decisions are needed, and one staff member provides instructions without input from others (autocratic). This is especially appropriate if the rest of the group is not functioning at an appropriate level. Option 2 would be found in shared governance structures when the risks are low and there is time for collaboration. Option 3 is most effective in groups with high levels of professional and personal maturity and where cooperation and coordination are not significant. Option 4 involves the rigid use of rules. Because managing casualties is a highly unpredictable activity, enforcement of rules is not appropriate. **Cognitive Level:** Analyzing. **Client Need:** Safe, Effective Care Environment. **Nursing Process:** N/A. **Learning Outcome:** 18-2.
2. **Answer:** 1. **Rationale:** In this situation, the manager needs to verify and clarify the client's statement with the assigned nurse before taking any direct action. Assigning another nurse to administer the client's medications (option 2) could be dangerous because it assumes the client is accurate in his statement. It is premature to review proper medication procedures with the nurse before knowing for certain that the procedure has not been followed (option 3). If the manager determines that there is disagreement about whether or not the medications have been given, it might be appropriate for the manager, nurse, and client to discuss the situation together (option 4) but certainly not before the manager has a private conversation about the situation with the nurse. **Cognitive Level:** Applying. **Client Need:** Safe, Effective Care Environment. **Nursing Process:** Planning. **Learning Outcome:** 18-7.
3. **Answer:** 4. **Rationale:** The RN is ultimately responsible for the action, reporting it, and following through on any action. Part of delegation is supervision and evaluation, ultimate responsibilities that belong to the RN. The nurse manager, aide, or client did not delegate the task of vital signs so therefore are not responsible for the time lapse between discovery and action. **Cognitive Level:** Applying. **Client Need:** Safe, Effective Care Environment. **Nursing Process:** Planning. **Learning Outcome:** 18-6.
4. **Answer:** 1, 2, 3, 4. **Rationale:** Enough time is not one of the five rights of delegation. **Cognitive Level:** Analyzing. **Client Need:** Safe, Effective Care Environment. **Nursing Process:** Planning. **Learning Outcome:** 18-8.
5. **Answer:** 4. **Rationale:** Interaction between the two groups may lead to a compromise. Option 1: Although explaining the reasons for the desired change is useful, overemphasis on the rationale may not be useful since resistance is often more emotional than rational. Option 2: This situation does not meet the criteria for an autocratic leadership style. There is no urgency and the task primarily involves the staff. Option 3: If the manager is not solidly committed to the new proposal, it should not be introduced, because it will result in unnecessary disturbance. Option 4: The manager should be open to modification of the proposal if justified. **Cognitive Level:** Applying. **Client Need:** Safe, Effective Care Planning. **Nursing Process:** Implementation. **Learning Outcome:** 18-10.
6. **Answer:** 2. **Rationale:** Managers are employees and have been given authority by the institution for which they work. The other options are characteristic of leaders more than managers. **Cognitive Level:** Understanding. **Client Need:** Safe, Effective Care Planning. **Nursing Process:** N/A. **Learning Outcome:** 18-1.
7. **Answer:** 1, 2, 3, 4. **Rationale:** The nurse as manager is focused on systems. **Cognitive Level:** Applying. **Client Need:** Safe, Effective Care Planning. **Nursing Process:** Evaluation. **Learning Outcome:** 18-3.
8. **Answer:** 3. **Rationale:** Middle managers supervise first-level managers and serve as liaison between first- and upper-level managers. First-level managers supervise nonmanagerial staff (option 1) and report institutional changes to direct-care staff (option 2). Creating institutional goals and strategic plans is the responsibility of upper-level managers (option 4). **Cognitive Level:** Understanding. **Client Need:** Safe, Effective Care Planning. **Nursing Process:** Evaluation. **Learning Outcome:** 18-4.
9. **Answer:** 4. **Rationale:** Evaluating outcomes and effectiveness is part of the coordinating function of management. **Cognitive Level:** Remembering. **Client Need:** Safe, Effective Care Planning. **Nursing Process:** N/A. **Learning Outcome:** 18-5.
10. **Answer:** 3. **Rationale:** In this situation, the AP was not given the right direction and communication—that the client was not permitted to be out of bed. AP commonly weigh clients so it was the right task and right person (options 1 and 2). Although supervision might have prevented the error, it was the nurse's responsibility to tell the AP of the client's mobility status and, if necessary, the proper way to weigh such a client (option 4). **Cognitive Level:** Analyzing. **Client Need:** Safe, Effective Care Planning. **Nursing Process:** Evaluation. **Learning Outcome:** 18-9.

CHAPTER 19 Health Promotion

1. **Answer:** 1. **Rationale:** The concept of holism emphasizes that nurses must keep the whole person in mind and strive to understand how one area of concern relates to the whole person. In this situation, the stress from a job loss will affect the person's chronic condition. The nurse must also consider the relationship of the individual to the external environment and to others. Options 2, 3, and 4 only focus on the physiology of the person's condition. **Cognitive Level:** Understanding. **Client Need:** Psychosocial Integrity. **Nursing Process:** Implementation. **Learning Outcome:** 19-1.
2. **Answer:** 3. **Rationale:** Learning about sleep will increase the older adult's well-being, which is the focus of health promotion. Prevention of falls (option 1) is health protection because the focus is avoiding injury. Learning about cardiovascular risk factors (option 2) relates to health protection and disease prevention. How to stop smoking (option 4) focuses on health protection and avoiding illness. **Cognitive Level:** Applying. **Client Need:** Health Promotion/Maintenance and Psychosocial Integrity. **Nursing Process:** Planning. **Learning Outcome:** 19-5.
3. **Answer:** 2. **Rationale:** Choices are often related to learned experiences, lifestyle, and values. The client obviously values the business more than physical health. When an individual feels strongly enough, a lower level need (rest) can be postponed until a higher level need (success, safety) is met. It is very likely that no one else can meet that need for him and the lower need must still be met eventually. **Cognitive Level:** Applying. **Client Need:** Health Promotion and Maintenance. **Nursing Process:** Assessment. **Learning Outcome:** 19-3.
4. **Answer:** 3. **Rationale:** A client in this stage recognizes there is a problem, is seriously considering changing, actively gathers information, and verbalizes plans to change in the near future. Option 1 reflects the precontemplation stage in which the client denies there is a problem. Option 2 reflects the planning stage in which the client makes final plans to accomplish the change, and option 4 is the maintenance stage in which the client made the change and demonstrates the appropriate behavioral change. **Cognitive Level:** Analyzing. **Client Need:** Health Promotion and Maintenance. **Nursing Process:** Assessment. **Learning Outcome:** 19-8.

5. **Answer:** 2. **Rationale:** In the elderly population, health promotion and illness prevention are important, but the focus is often on learning to adapt to and live with increasing changes and limitations. Maximizing strengths continues to be of prime importance in maintaining optimal function and quality of life. Rest and exercise, and high obesity percentages are life span considerations of children (options 1 and 3). Safety promotion and injury prevention are life span considerations for adolescents. **Cognitive Level:** Applying. **Client Need:** Health Promotion and Maintenance. **Nursing Process:** Planning. **Learning Outcome:** 19-8.
6. **Answer:** 2, 3, and 5. **Rationale:** The *Healthy People 2020* goals are broad based. Options 1 and 4 are specific methods to promote healthy behaviors and would be seen in the objectives for a *Healthy People 2020* topic area. **Cognitive Level:** Comprehending. **Client Need:** Health Promotion and Maintenance. **Nursing Process:** N/A. **Learning Outcome:** 19-4.
7. **Answer:** 1. **Rationale:** Option 2 is a strategy for the contemplation stage, option 3 is a strategy for the preparation stage, and option 4 is a strategy for the maintenance stage. **Cognitive Level:** Applying. **Client Need:** Health Promotion and Maintenance. **Nursing Process:** Implementation. **Learning Outcome:** 19-9.
8. **Answer:** 4. **Rationale:** Change is a complex process and a nurse should not give up or assume that the client does not want to change (option 1). Individuals often resist a tough approach because it can make them feel cornered. This approach may work for some individuals but not for everyone (option 2). The goal of teaching is to try to help the client become the expert as well (option 3). **Cognitive Level:** Applying. **Client Need:** Health Promotion and Maintenance. **Nursing Process:** Implementation. **Learning Outcome:** 19-11.
9. **Answer:** 1, 2, 4. **Rationale:** Options 3 and 5 are not examples of a homeostatic mechanism. Self-regulation, compensation, negative feedback, and utilizations of multiple mechanisms to correct a physiological imbalance are homeostatic mechanisms. **Cognitive Level:** Applying. **Client Need:** Health Promotion and Maintenance. **Nursing Process:** Assessment. **Learning Outcome:** 19-2.
10. **Answer:** 3. **Rationale:** Option 1 is a physiologic need. Option 2 is a love and belonging need, and option 4 is a safety and security need. **Cognitive Level:** Analyzing. **Client Need:** Health Promotion and Maintenance. **Nursing Process:** Assessment. **Learning Outcome:** 19-3.

CHAPTER 20 Health, Wellness, and Illness

1. **Answer:** 2. **Rationale:** The social component of wellness focuses on the ability to interact successfully with people and within the environment of which each person is a part, to develop and maintain intimacy with significant others, and to develop respect and tolerance for those with different opinions and beliefs. **Cognitive Level:** Understanding. **Client Need:** Health Promotion and Maintenance. **Nursing Process:** Assessment. **Learning Outcome:** 20-2.
2. **Answer:** 2. **Rationale:** The mother has taken on the sick role by expecting to be excused from her usual role responsibilities. The sick role states that individuals are not answerable for their illness, contrary to the obese client's perspective (option 1). In the sick role, the client tries to get better as opposed to the man who misses his physical therapy appointments (option 3). The older adult is not following the sick role expectation to rely on competent help (option 4). **Cognitive Level:** Applying. **Client Need:** Health Promotion/Maintenance and Physiological Integrity. **Nursing Process:** Assessment. **Learning Outcome:** 20-7.
3. **Answer:** 1. **Rationale:** Locus of control (LOC) is a concept from social learning theory. People who exercise internal control are more likely than others to take the initiative on their own health care and to be more knowledgeable about their health. They are also more likely to adhere to prescribed health care regimens such as taking medication, making and keeping appointments with physicians, maintaining diets, and giving up smoking. People who believe their health is largely controlled by outside forces (chance or others) are referred to as externals. **Cognitive Level:** Analyzing. **Client Need:** Health Promotion and Maintenance. **Nursing Process:** Analysis. **Learning Outcome:** 20-3.
4. **Answer:** 2, 3, and 4. **Rationale:** Significant evidence exists that a trusting relationship with the provider, effectiveness of the medication, and simple dosing regimen are important predictors of adherence to a medical regimen. Neither education nor sex has been shown to be a predictive factor (options 1 and 5). **Cognitive Level:** Applying. **Client Need:** Health Promotion and Maintenance. **Nursing Process:** Planning. **Learning Outcome:** 20-5.
5. **Answer:** 1. **Rationale:** Although not always practical, direct observation is the best method to measure adherence (for example, watching clients who are addicted to heroin actually take their methadone dose). Because lack of adherence may be life threatening or damaging to the client as well as others, waiting until the client displays illness and waiting until laboratory values reflect a lack of adherence are not the best methods (options 2 and 3). Client report or recall is not always accurate, even if the client believes he or she is telling the truth (option 4). **Cognitive Level:** Analyzing. **Client Need:** Health Promotion and Maintenance. **Nursing Process:** Evaluation. **Learning Outcome:** 20-5.
6. **Answer:** 4. **Rationale:** The actual term used to describe the diagnosis is less important because the client may have no frame of reference for it. That is not to say that the diagnosis is unimportant because clients may be familiar with common diagnoses such as heart disease or cancer and ascribe historical meaning to them. Ability to perform usual activities, culture, and availability of healthcare will all be strong influences on the client's definition of health or wellness (options 1, 2, and 3). **Cognitive Level:** Analyzing. **Client Need:** Health Promotion and Maintenance. **Nursing Process:** Assessment. **Learning Outcome:** 20-1.
7. **Answer:** 4. **Rationale:** Genetics is an internal variable affecting health. Options 1, 2, and 3 are all external variables. **Cognitive Level:** Remembering. **Client Need:** Health Promotion and Maintenance. **Nursing Process:** Assessment. **Learning Outcome:** 20-4.
8. **Answer:** 2. **Rationale:** By definition, a chronic illness has no known cure, so the individual will always have it to some degree. Although acute illnesses may have severe symptoms, many chronic illnesses also have severe symptoms (option 1). Although signs and symptoms of chronic illnesses may never go completely away, they can get better and worse at different times (option 3). Chronic illnesses can be treated, just not cured (option 4). **Cognitive Level:** Understanding. **Client Need:** Health Promotion and Maintenance. **Nursing Process:** Planning. **Learning Outcome:** 20-6.
9. **Answer:** 3, 5, 1, 4, and 2. **Rationale:** The proper sequence of Suchman's stages of illness are signs and symptoms appear, the client takes on the sick role, the client makes contact with medical care, the client takes on a dependent role, and the client goes into rehabilitation and recovery. **Cognitive Level:** Remembering. **Client Need:** Health Promotion and Maintenance. **Nursing Process:** Evaluation. **Learning Outcome:** 20-8.
10. **Answer:** 1, 2, 3, and 5. **Rationale:** In the sick role, the woman would likely feel guilt and some anger but give up usual roles and accept help from others, and decrease social interactions. The only reaction that would be unlikely is that she would take on a job to pay expenses. This would be inconsistent with the sick role. **Cognitive Level:** Applying. **Client Need:** Health Promotion and Maintenance. **Nursing Process:** Planning. **Learning Outcome:** 20-9.

CHAPTER 21 Culturally Responsive Nursing Care

1. **Answer:** 1, 2, 5. **Rationale:** REACH: Racial and Ethnic Approaches to Community Health is an initiative of the Centers for Disease Control and Prevention. Six core health areas that are the focus of this initiative include infant mortality, deficits in breast and cervical cancer screening and management, cardiovascular diseases, diabetes, HIV infections/AIDS, and child and adult immunizations. This initiative was congruent with the identification of the leading causes of death in the United States, which include chronic lower respiratory disease and stroke, along with heart disease, cancer, unintentional injuries, and diabetes. **Cognitive Level:** Understanding. **Client Need:** Psychosocial Integrity. **Nursing Process:** N/A. **Learning Outcome:** 21-3.
2. **Answer:** 4. **Rationale:** "Right" and "wrong" terms should be avoided in culturally sensitive areas and where differing views are present (option 1). The nurse, not the physician, is the caregiver in this situation, so it is the nurse's responsibility to teach and see that the plan of care is carried out (option 2). If the client's views can lead to harmful behavior or outcomes, then an attempt is made to shift the client's perspectives to the scientific view (option 3). **Cognitive Level:** Applying. **Client Need:** Psychosocial Integrity. **Nursing Process:** N/A. **Learning Outcome:** 21-10.
3. **Answer:** 3. **Rationale:** The nurse should indicate that he or she is open to diverse views and practices. Option 1 assumes the client follows this particular cultural practice, which may not be the case. The nurse should assess before intervening. It may be good to learn more about the culture (option 2), but that is not the best starting place to care for the client. Subcultures exist among all cultures. Reading books is helpful, but assessment of individual situations is the best approach. Option 4 reflects an incorrect approach to culturally appropriate care. The nurse needs to assess which customs and practices the individual client performs before drawing conclusions. **Cognitive Level:** Applying. **Client Need:** Psychosocial Integrity. **Nursing Process:** N/A. **Learning Outcome:** 21-10.
4. **Answer:** 4, 5. **Rationale:** Race has been a term used to refer to groupings of people according to common origin or background and associated with perceived biological markers (option 1). Diversity occurs not only *between* cultural groups but also within cultural groups (option 2). A subculture is usually composed of people who have a distinct identity and yet are related to a larger cultural group (option 3). **Cognitive Level:** Applying. **Client Need:** Psychosocial Integrity. **Nursing Process:** N/A. **Learning Outcome:** 21-4.
5. **Answer:** 3. **Rationale:** National cultural health goals include providing equal access to quality healthcare for everyone. It would be inappropriate for all cultures to receive the same care; care should be customized (option 1). The same life expectancy for all U.S. citizens is not realistic (option 2). Assimilation (option 4) is not an appropriate health goal because assimilation is a conscious effect. Therefore, it is not always possible and this may cause severe stress and anxiety. **Cognitive Level:** Applying. **Client Need:** Psychosocial Integrity. **Nursing Process:** Evaluation. **Learning Outcome:** 21-3.
6. **Answer:** 1. **Rationale:** Herbal teas are an example of a restoring health action. Prayer (option 2) and exercise (option 4) would be examples of maintaining actions, whereas wearing symbolic objects (option 3) is a protective action. **Cognitive Level:** Understanding. **Client Need:** Psychosocial Integrity. **Nursing Process:** Implementation. **Learning Outcome:** 21-6.
7. **Answer:** 2. **Rationale:** Steam is a natural substance and would be compatible with folk healing preferences. Hospitalization and medications are typical Western medical strategies (options 1 and 3). A watch-and-wait approach (option 4) is not particularly associated with a folk healing perspective. **Cognitive Level:** Applying. **Client Need:** Psychosocial Integrity. **Nursing Process:** Planning. **Learning Outcome:** 21-5.
8. **Answer:** 1, 2, 3, and 6. **Rationale:** Technology skills (option 4) and intelligence (option 5) are individual, personal characteristics and less influenced by one's culture than valuing of older adults (option 1), gender roles (option 2), nonverbal communication (option 3), or diet (option 6). Culture may, however, influence how technologic skills (option 4) and intelligence (option 5) are viewed and valued. **Cognitive Level:** Understanding. **Client Need:** Psychosocial Integrity. **Nursing Process:** Assessment. **Learning Outcome:** 21-5.
9. **Answer:** 3. **Rationale:** People who migrate and settle in another country often find themselves making changes to their lifestyles in order to match the culture of the host country. They might have to speak a language different from their native language, eat food that is different from what they usually eat, and dress differently. It is a time-consuming process and can be very stressful. Acculturation is also a two-way process, where the host country eventually adapts and attunes itself to the migrants. Options 2 and 4 do not require acculturation, since they are not long-lasting, permanent events. Option 1 may be related to acculturation, only if one thinks of a place of work as a culture in its own right. Thus, changing careers, moving from one place of work to another, may require a change in the way of doing things and getting used to the new "culture" one is working in. **Cognitive level:** Understanding. **Client Need:** N/A. **Nursing Process:** N/A. **Learning Outcome:** 21-1.
10. **Answer:** 2. **Rationale:** A nurse should not make assumptions about the client and be humble enough to admit that they don't know everything. Thus, if there is anything which the nurse cannot understand, they must check with the client. In that way, the nurse would be able to administer care that is culturally competent. Options 1 and 3 are not compatible with culturally competent care. While a nurse should be able to converse with the client and answer his/her questions about the host country, the nurse should never impose and try to convince the client to submit to the culture of the new country. **Cognitive level:** Applying. **Client need:** Psychosociocultural wellbeing. **Nursing Process:** Assessment. **Learning outcomes:** 21-4.

CHAPTER 22 Complementary and Alternative Healing Modalities

1. **Answer:** 3. **Rationale:** Although the effectiveness of alternative therapies is sometimes not scientifically established, many individuals report significant benefit from them for a wide variety of conditions. Alternative therapies often cost less, but this is not a primary consideration (option 1). Clients often seek alternative therapies because traditional therapies are ineffective, but this is not the primary difference (option 2). Both traditional and alternative therapies utilize products from nature (option 4). **Cognitive Level:** Applying. **Client Need:** Physiological Integrity. **Nursing Process:** N/A. **Learning Outcome:** 22-1.
2. **Answer:** 1. **Rationale:** Therapeutic horseback riding, or animal-assisted therapy is the use of the rhythmic movement of the horse to increase sensory processing and improve posture, balance, and mobility in people with movement dysfunctions. **Cognitive Level:** Applying. **Client Need:** Psychological Integrity. **Nursing Process:** N/A. **Learning Outcome:** 22-9.
3. **Answer:** 2. **Rationale:** Grounding relates to one's connection with reality. Being grounded suggests stability, security, independence, having a solid foundation, and living in the present. Energy, centering, and sadness or depression (options 1, 3, and 4) does not relate to groundedness. **Cognitive Level:** Applying. **Client Need:** Health Promotion/Maintenance and Psychosocial Integrity. **Nursing Process:** Implementation. **Learning Outcome:** 22-2.
4. **Answer:** 4. **Rationale:** Naturopathy focuses on the total individual. The primary focus is disease prevention. Naturopathy may be the best choice in decreasing disease rates by empowering and educating individuals about ways to stay healthy. Belief in a higher being is not a core principle. **Cognitive Level:** Analyzing. **Client Need:** Health Promotion and Maintenance. **Nursing Process:** N/A. **Learning Outcome:** 22-5.

5. **Answer:** 2. **Rationale:** Colonics is the procedure for washing the inner wall of the colon by filling it with water or herbal solutions and then draining it. Colon cleansing is a controversial method of detoxification and the issue requires further discussion. Establishing a baseline regarding the client's knowledge regarding the process is most appropriate. **Cognitive Level:** Applying. **Client Need:** Health Promotion and Maintenance. **Nursing Process:** N/A. **Learning Outcome:** 22-7.
6. **Answer:** 2. **Rationale:** Thirty percent of current prescription drugs are derived from plants. Herbs and medications are similar in structure and therapeutic value (option 1). Some medications may be more powerful than herbs but not all are (option 3), and herbs tend to be less dangerous than medications (option 4). **Cognitive Level:** Remembering. **Client Need:** Physiological Integrity. **Nursing Process:** Implementation. **Learning Outcome:** 22-4.
7. **Answer:** 1. **Rationale:** Serious interactions can occur between herbs and medications. It is acceptable that individuals choose herbs as a way to maintain health and treat minor disorders (option 2). Although the knowledge the nurse gains may be helpful, contributing to research is not the primary reason for assessing herb use (option 3). While we hope clients share important information with us, they also have free will about what they choose to share (option 4). **Cognitive Level:** Applying. **Client Need:** Physiological Integrity. **Nursing Process:** Assessment. **Learning Outcome:** 22-10.
8. **Answer:** 4. **Rationale:** The oils in options 1, 2, and 3 will burn the skin if they are not diluted in a carrier oil. **Cognitive Level:** Understanding. **Client Need:** Physiological Integrity. **Nursing Process:** Planning. **Learning Outcome:** 22-10.
9. **Answer:** 1, 2, 4, and 5. **Rationale:** Massage is a way of communicating without words, including the caring intent of the provider. It provides mental and physical relaxation. Massage speeds the removal of metabolic waste products, allowing more oxygen and nutrients to reach the cells and tissues. It lowers blood pressure and slows the heart rate. Passive exercise from massage cannot strengthen muscles (option 3). **Cognitive Level:** Remembering. **Client Need:** Physiological Integrity. **Nursing Process:** Planning. **Learning Outcome:** 22-6.
10. **Answer:** 1. **Rationale:** There is no evidence that massage (option 2), herbs (option 3), or yoga (option 4) improves pregnancy rates, although relaxation and good physical conditioning are generally encouraged. **Cognitive Level:** Remembering. **Client Need:** Physiological Integrity. **Nursing Process:** Implementation. **Learning Outcome:** 22-10.

CHAPTER 23 Concepts of Growth and Development

1. **Answer:** 1, 3, 5. **Rationale:** Options 2 and 4 are related to development. Development is an increase in the complexity of function and skill progression, and development skills include the ability to adapt to one's environment. **Cognitive Level:** Applying. **Client Need:** Health Promotion and Maintenance. **Nursing Process:** Assessment. **Learning Outcome:** 23-1.
2. **Answer:** 4. **Rationale:** The study of growth (physical) and development (function and skills) is correct because the answer needs to have both components to be complete. Option 1 addresses only the growth aspects. Option 2 addresses only developmental aspects, and option 3 addresses only the environmental factors that might influence growth and development. **Cognitive Level:** Remembering. **Client Need:** Health Promotion and Maintenance. **Nursing Process:** Assessment. **Learning Outcome:** 23-1.
3. **Answer:** 3. **Rationale:** Toddlers typically demonstrate negative behavior and are hesitant around strangers, resisting close contact with those they do not know well. They do not have sophisticated language skills and often use crying or fussing to communicate. Older school-age children and adolescents are likely to cooperate without complaint in many health procedures (option 1). School-age children, engaged in the task of industry versus inferiority, display curiosity about how things work, asking many questions of nurses (option 2). Preschool-age children, who are in the fantasy, curiosity, and exploration stage, like to manipulate objects and play "pretend" (option 4). **Cognitive Level:** Analyzing. **Client Need:** Health Promotion and Maintenance. **Nursing Process:** Planning. **Learning Outcome:** 23-7.
4. **Answer:** 4. **Rationale:** Adolescents need to establish identity, which involves developing a more mature sense of independence and responsibility. Providing adolescents with schoolwork keeps them connected to peer groups and gives a sense of accomplishment. Also, it prevents clients from "worrying" about getting behind in school assignments. Interaction with peers is very important during this stage, but they are likely to be attending school during the day (option 1); an infant's sense of trust is reinforced if parents room-in, and older infants and toddlers experience less separation anxiety if parents are nearby (option 2); and preschool and school-age children would benefit from the distraction and social interaction of others in the recreation room (option 3). **Cognitive Level:** Applying. **Client Need:** Health Promotion and Maintenance. **Nursing Process:** Implementation. **Learning Outcome:** 23-5.
5. **Answer:** 2. **Rationale:** The client is in Erikson's stage of integrity versus despair. Finding meaning and purpose in his life after retirement is a sign of achievement. His comments regarding visits to his family and being asked by friends to help with their projects indicate that he is actively involved and purposeful (options 1 and 4). His comment regarding needing medication for knee pain can be expected in many older adults, especially those who have been laborers or suffered injury when younger (option 3). **Cognitive Level:** Analyzing. **Client Need:** Health Promotion and Maintenance. **Nursing Process:** Evaluation. **Learning Outcome:** 23-5.
6. **Answer:** 1. **Rationale:** School-age children (6-12 years) are in the preadolescent period where the peer group begins to increasingly influence behavior. The nurse must allow time and energy for the school-age child to pursue hobbies and school activities and should recognize and support the child's achievement. **Cognitive Level:** Applying. **Client Need:** Health Promotion and Maintenance. **Nursing Process:** Implementation. **Learning Outcome:** 23-2.
7. **Answer:** 2. **Rationale:** Erikson's late childhood stage focuses on initiative versus guilt. During this stage, the children are beginning to have the ability to evaluate their own behavior and are learning the degree to which assertiveness and purpose influence the environment. Option 1 is incorrect because Fowler's focus is spiritual development. Both options 3 and 4 are names of adult theorists. **Cognitive Level:** Applying. **Client Need:** Health Promotion and Maintenance. **Nursing Process:** Planning. **Learning Outcome:** 23-7.
8. **Answer:** 1. **Rationale:** Piaget identifies this phase as the intuitive thought phase with significant behaviors as follows: egocentric thinking diminishes, thinks of one idea at a time, includes others in the environment, words express thoughts. Erikson identifies this developmental stage as industry versus inferiority, and the children are learning the degree to which assertiveness and purpose influence the environment. They begin to have the ability to evaluate their own behavior. Fowler identifies this stage as intuitive-projective, a combination of images and beliefs given by trusted others, mixed with the child's own experience and imagination. Therefore, the nurse knows that this child has a normal imagination and needs to explore and learn about this new piece of equipment in language appropriate to his age. For option 2, imagination is normal for this age group, and stating that he needs to be "a big boy" is counterproductive. Option 3 is incorrect because his language skills are developing and he needs to understand

the world around him. Option 4 is incorrect because adding to his fears will only increase his anxiety level and decrease his trust in you as a nurse. **Cognitive Level:** Applying. **Client Need:** Health Promotion and Maintenance. **Nursing Process:** Implementation. **Learning Outcome:** 23-11.

9. **Answer:** 1. **Rationale:** All the nursing actions listed here are appropriate, but attachment theory emphasizes the importance of parents being available to their child when the child is experiencing stress. The best action would be to encourage the mother to stay with her child as much as possible. Putting a picture of the mother in the crib (option 2) may provide some comfort, since by 15 months of age, children demonstrate object permanence and people permanence, so the child "knows" the mother will return. Holding and cuddling the child (option 3) may also provide comfort, but the child must trust the caregiver, and the nurse's other responsibilities may restrict the amount of time and when he or she can be with the child. Distraction (option 4) can temporarily refocus the child's attention, but it does not address the need for emotional and physical contact with the parent. **Cognitive Level:** Applying. **Client Need:** Health Promotion and Maintenance. **Nursing Process:** Implementation. **Learning Outcome:** 23-10.
10. **Answer:** 4. **Rationale:** Adulthood, age 25 to 65 years, is characterized by the central task of generativity versus stagnation. Positive resolution is indicated by creativity, productivity, and concern for others. Negative resolution is characterized by self-indulgence, self-concern, and lack of interests and communication. **Cognitive Level:** Understanding. **Client Need:** Health Promotion and Maintenance. **Nursing Process:** Planning. **Learning Outcome:** 23-7.

CHAPTER 24 Promoting Health from Conception Through Adolescence

1. **Answer:** 4. **Rationale:** Providing opportunities for the parent to express worries and discuss facts about SIDS gives more control over the situation. The nurse can also provide the parent with information about the Back to Sleep campaign. Option 1: The highest incidence of SIDS occurs between 2 and 4 months of age, but it does occur in older infants. It is not the best response because it provides facts but does not address the parent's immediate concerns. Option 2: SIDS affects boys more than girls. However, this information is likely to increase anxiety and does not address the concerns of the parent. Option 3: There is no known cause of SIDS, although respiratory problems may be present in some infants. This response is insensitive to the needs of the parent. **Cognitive Level:** Applying. **Client Need:** Psychosocial Integrity. **Nursing Process:** Implementation. **Learning Outcome:** 24-8.
2. **Answer:** 3. **Rationale:** Preschool-age children use fantasy and make-believe to learn about, understand, and master their environment, including their concepts of death. The child's conceptualization of death is consistent with her cognitive development. The response in option 1 negates the child's understanding and limits her ability to develop fuller understanding and adapt to the loss. Option 2 negates the child's attempts to understand and deal with the loss. Option 4 is incorrect because at 4 years of age, children can hear explanations such as "when people get old they will die," but these children do not have a firm grasp of the meaning of time and age, and probably will not understand. **Cognitive Level:** Applying. **Client Need:** Health Promotion/Maintenance and Psychosocial Integrity. **Nursing Process:** Implementation. **Learning Outcome:** 24-6.
3. **Answer:** 1. **Rationale:** It is the responsibility of adults to supervise children constantly and closely when around water. Option 2, learning water safety and how to swim, is important and should be encouraged at an early age, but that still does not ensure a child's safety. Option 3 is incorrect because young children are at risk near any amount of water that can cover the nose and mouth. Option 4: Infants and toddlers can drown in a very small amount of water, even several inches in a bathtub or "kiddie pool." **Cognitive Level:** Applying. **Client Need:** Safe, Effective Care Environment and Health Promotion/Maintenance. **Nursing Process:** Planning. **Learning Outcome:** 24-8.
4. **Answer:** 2. **Rationale:** School-age children acquire stereognosis, the ability to identify an unseen object simply by touch. Option 1: Birth weight triples by about 12 months. Children enter school age weighing about 45 pounds and gain about 5 to 7 pounds per year. Option 3: Significant physical change occurs during the school-age years. Option 4: Fat deposits do not normally appear until puberty. **Cognitive Level:** Understanding. **Client Need:** Health Promotion and Maintenance. **Nursing Process:** Assessment. **Learning Outcome:** 24-1.
5. **Answer:** 2. **Rationale:** The nurse must present an open, accepting attitude to the adolescent's questions while encouraging the adolescent to find relationships that promote discussion of feelings, concerns, and fears. Giving directions and suggesting counseling may turn the student from seeking help (options 1 and 3). Just giving written information on a particular topic will not address the complete situation the student comes seeking assistance with (option 4). **Cognitive Level:** Applying. **Client Need:** Psychosocial Integrity. **Nursing Process:** Implementation. **Learning Outcome:** 24-8.
6. **Answer:** 2. **Rationale:** Molding of the head is made possible by the fontanels and occurs during vaginal deliveries as the head comes through the birth canal. Within a week, the newborn's head usually regains its symmetry. It is normal with vaginal deliveries. Babies born via cesarean section do not experience molding. Molding is not permanent—a fact that makes parents feel more reassured. Option 1 dismisses the parent's concerns. This condition is not abnormal and does not need to be referred to the doctor but rather the nurse needs to reassure the parents that nothing is wrong (option 3). Option 4 is not necessarily true nor does it adequately answer the parents' concerns. **Cognitive Level:** Applying. **Client Need:** Psychosocial Integrity. **Nursing Process:** Implementation. **Learning Outcome:** 24-1.
7. **Answer:** 1. **Rationale:** Although toddlers like to explore the environment, they always need to have a significant individual nearby. Parents need to know that young children experience acute separation anxiety and that abandonment is their greatest fear. Option 2: This is normal toddler development. Option 3: The child is probably not old enough to perform manipulative-type strategies. Option 4: This is normal behavior for this age group. **Cognitive Level:** Applying. **Client Need:** Health Promotion and Maintenance. **Nursing Process:** Assessment. **Learning Outcome:** 24-3.
8. **Answer:** 2. **Rationale:** Regression is reverting to an earlier development stage (bed-wetting, using baby talk, etc.) as part of the child's experiences with separation anxiety. Nurses can assist parents by helping them understand that this behavior is normal and will pass as the child reestablishes herself as part of the family and works through her own frustration with the situation. Regressive behavior is not based on physiology and, unless it lasts, would not have to be further investigated (option 1). Strict discipline may not be the better solution over understanding and caring (option 3). Option 4 does not provide the parents with an understanding of the root of the problem. **Cognitive Level:** Applying. **Client Need:** Health Promotion and Maintenance. **Nursing Process:** Implementation. **Learning Outcome:** 24-2.
9. **Answer:** 1. **Rationale:** During the phase of concrete operations, children change from egocentric interactions to cooperative interactions. They also develop an increased understanding of concepts that are associated with specific objects. They learn to add and subtract and understand cause-and-effect relationships. Option 2 action is indicative of the preconceptual phase—an egocentric approach that uses magical thinking. Option 3 action is indicative of the formal operations phase—reasoning is deductive and futuristic.

Option 4 is indicative of physical growth. **Cognitive Level:** Applying. **Client Need:** Health Promotion and Maintenance. **Nursing Process:** Assessment. **Learning Outcome:** 24-4.

10. **Answer:** 1. **Rationale:** Often the first noticeable sign of puberty in females is the appearance of the breast bud, although the appearance of hair along the labia may precede this. Option 2: The growth spurt in girls is between ages 10 and 14, but is too vague to be noticeable. Option 3: The eccrine glands are found over most of the body and produce sweat. The apocrine glands develop in the axillae, anal and genital areas, external auditory canals, and around the umbilicus and the areola of the breasts. Option 4: Mood swings are not as definitive as physical changes. **Cognitive Level:** Analyzing. **Client Need:** Health Promotion and Maintenance. **Nursing Process:** Assessment. **Learning Outcome:** 24-2.

CHAPTER 25 Promoting Health in Young and Middle-Aged Adults

1. **Answer:** 3. **Rationale:** The average age for the onset of menopause in American women is 47 years. Therefore, there is nothing abnormal about ongoing menses in a 45-year-old woman, and gynecologic care is not warranted (option 1). As a woman nears menopause, ovulation may become irregular and difficult to predict. Conception remains a possibility, and the lack of predictable ovulation may actually increase the likelihood of unintended pregnancy (option 2). Many women have no negative symptoms during menopause, and the experience of menopause is highly culturally determined (option 4). **Cognitive Level:** Analyzing. **Client Need:** Health Promotion and Maintenance. **Nursing Process:** Implementation. **Learning Outcome:** 25-2.
2. **Answer:** 2. **Rationale:** Generation X includes individuals born in years 1965 to 1978. The Baby Boomers were born in the years 1945 to 1964 (option 1). Generation Y includes people born between the years 1979 and 2000 (option 3). Millennials were born between the years 1979 and 2000 (option 4). **Cognitive Level:** Remembering. **Client Need:** Health Promotion and Maintenance. **Nursing Process:** Assessment. **Learning Outcome:** 25-1.
3. **Answer:** 3. **Rationale:** Lung cancer is the most common cause of cancer death in women age 24 to 65 years. Breast cancer is common, but deaths related to breast cancer have declined (option 1). Lymphoma and colon cancer are significant diseases for both men and women (options 2 and 4). **Cognitive Level:** Analyzing. **Client Need:** Health Promotion and Maintenance. **Nursing Process:** Assessment. **Learning Outcome:** 25-7.
4. **Answer:** 1, 2, 3, 5. **Rationale:** Other factors indicating problems include a variety of physical complaints, digestive disorders, increase in isolation, problems with close relationships, and financial failure. Brain tumors are not an indicator for suicide. **Cognitive Level:** Applying. **Client Need:** Psychosocial Integrity. **Nursing Process:** Assessment. **Learning Outcome:** 25-7.
5. **Answer:** 2. **Rationale:** Kohlberg's initial work indicated that moral development was completed by adulthood, but more recent research has demonstrated that moral development continues throughout adulthood. Moral development refers to a decision-making process of right and wrong, and proceeds in a series of predictable stages (option 3). Moral development and spirituality are unrelated, and represent very different spheres of human thought and behavior (option 4). **Cognitive Level:** Analyzing. **Client Need:** Psychosocial Integrity. **Nursing Process:** Assessment. **Learning Outcome:** 25-5.
6. **Answer:** 2. **Rationale:** The middle-aged individual is generally attempting to relate to adult children and grandchildren as well as assisting aging parents. Hence, continuous efforts to meet the needs of others occur. Selecting a life partner is the developmental task for young adults. Reviewing one's life course is the task for older adulthood (option 3). Establishing a sense of self is usually achieved during adolescence (option 4). **Cognitive Level:** Analyzing. **Client Need:** Health Promotion and Maintenance. **Nursing Process:** Assessment. **Learning Outcome:** 25-3.
7. **Answer:** 2. **Rationale:** Hypertension is a major problem for young African American adults, particularly men. The causes for this are unknown. Options 1, 3, and 4 are not evidence-based statements. **Cognitive Level:** Analyzing. **Client Need:** Safe, Effective Care Environment. **Nursing Process:** Assessment. **Learning Outcome:** 25-7.
8. **Answer:** 1, 2, 3, and 5. **Rationale:** Hypertension (elevated blood pressure) forces the heart to work harder, resulting in decreased function of the heart; the electrocardiogram assesses cardiac rhythm and rate; high cholesterol levels are directly related to a decrease in arterial size, which decreases circulation blood to the cardiac tissue; activity level (e.g., dyspnea on exertion) can indicate cardiovascular disease. While cardiac impairment may decrease sexual performance, which is important to assess, the others would have priority given the limitations for the screening program (option 4). **Cognitive Level:** Analyzing. **Client Need:** Health Promotion and Maintenance. **Nursing Process:** Assessment. **Learning Outcome:** 25-9.
9. **Answer:** 1. **Rationale:** Asking the individual if they are afraid of someone at home, or if someone hurt them, is a critical step in a comprehensive assessment. Intimate partner violence is a serious problem for women and men of all ages, cultures, and socioeconomic levels. The nurse should suspect it in clients whose injuries are not consistent with the history they give. Referring the client to a shelter without completing a thorough assessment may lead to inappropriate care (option 2); the nursing process requires assessment before intervention. Collaboration with other healthcare professionals may be very helpful but an assessment needs to be done first (option 3). Documentation of the assessment does not directly address, reduce, or solve the concern (option 4). **Cognitive Level:** Analyzing. **Client Need:** Safe, Effective Care Environment. **Nursing Process:** Assessment. **Learning Outcome:** 25-7.
10. **Answer:** 3. **Rationale:** Each of these activities indicates achievement of a developmental task, but the nurse must know which task is appropriate for the client's chronological age. Obtaining and decorating a place to live is an activity that establishes independence from parents, a task for young adults. Creating a scrapbook is an important strategy to enhance ego integrity, a developmental task for older adults (option 1). Working with philanthropic groups is a hallmark of generativity, a developmental task for those in midlife (option 2). Considering career paths is more appropriate to the identity task of adolescence (option 4). **Cognitive Level:** Applying. **Client Need:** Health Promotion and Maintenance. **Nursing Process:** Assessment. **Learning Outcome:** 25-3.

CHAPTER 26 Promoting Health in Older Adults

1. **Answer:** 2. **Rationale:** Independence established prior to the loss of a mate makes adjustment easier. A person who had meaningful relationships and friendships or economic security, ongoing interests in the community or private hobbies, and a peaceful philosophy of life copes more easily with bereavement. **Cognitive Level:** Applying. **Client Need:** Psychosocial Integrity. **Nursing Process:** Assessment. **Learning Outcome:** 26-11.
2. **Answer:** 3. **Rationale:** Because the hearing loss occurs in the ability to distinguish high-pitched tones, speaking in a low and distinctive voice tone is the most appropriate method of communicating with the clients. Hearing loss in the older adult includes a loss of the ability to discern higher frequencies, and speaking slowly at a particular volume is not the best way to communicate with the clients (option 1). The stem indicates the

clients have noticeable hearing loss, but does not indicate the clients are deaf; large lettering is appropriate if the client has a visual problem (option 2); hearing aids are not usually effective when the problem is related to neural damage (option 4). **Cognitive Level:** Analyzing. **Client Need:** Health Promotion and Maintenance. **Nursing Process:** Assessment. **Learning Outcome:** 26-8.

3. **Answer:** 2. **Rationale:** This type of conversation is a necessary part of successful aging, and the nurse should support the reminiscence. There is no need for a psychological consult as this is not abnormal behavior for this age group (option 1). It is not necessary to redirect the client to other topics of conversation since reminiscing is not an unhealthy behavior (option 3). Elders generally respond better to familiar caregivers (option 4). **Cognitive Level:** Applying. **Client Need:** Health Promotion and Maintenance. **Nursing Process:** Assessment. **Learning Outcome:** 26-12.
4. **Answer:** 4. **Rationale:** It is a myth regarding the aging process that most older adults are depressed. By relating that depression is not a normal part of aging, the nurse can further dialogue with the daughter. The older client's number of losses is less important than how she copes (option 1). A depressed affect may be the older adult's usual look (option 2). It is yet to be determined if in fact she is depressed (option 3). **Cognitive Level:** Remembering. **Client Need:** Safe and Effective Care Environment. **Nursing Process:** Implementation. **Learning Outcome:** 26-15.
5. **Answer:** 3. **Rationale:** With the normal aging process, there is a decrease in muscle tone, digestive juices, and intestinal activity. These together may lead to indigestion and constipation in the older adult. It would be premature, as well as outside the scope of nursing practice, for the nurse to consider any other pathology (options 1 and 4) or to tell the client that there is a need for invasive testing (option 2). **Cognitive Level:** Applying. **Client Need:** Safe, Effective Care Environment. **Nursing Process:** Implementation. **Learning Outcome:** 26-8.
6. **Answer:** 1. **Rationale:** The client has lost muscle strength. Strengthening exercises will improve his mobility and lessen the possibility of a fall. Option 2: Information indicates the client has difficulty rising from a seating position, not standing after he reaches the position; further assessment is needed before implementing this intervention. Option 3: Praise should come after the proper intervention is implemented and a plan is in place so that the praise is focused toward a goal to resolve the problem. Option 4 resolves the problem immediately but does nothing to resolve the underlying problem. **Cognitive Level:** Applying. **Client Need:** Safe, Effective Care Environment. **Nursing Process:** Implementation. **Learning Outcome:** 26-8.
7. **Answer:** 4. **Rationale:** Sexual activity is possible for older adults although the responses are slower. The clients would need a health history and physical assessment of the cardiovascular system before drawing this conclusion (option 1). With the introduction of Viagra, older men are more able to perform than in the past (option 2). Older men's interest tends to decline, but it is not known whether it is related to impotence; apparently this older client is interested in sexual activity (option 3). **Cognitive Level:** Analyzing. **Client Need:** Health Promotion and Maintenance. **Nursing Process:** Implementation. **Learning Outcome:** 26-16.
8. **Answer:** 3. **Rationale:** Presbyopia is loss of near vision related to aging. Option 1 is loss of hearing ability related to aging. Option 2 is dry mouth related to a decrease in saliva, and option 4 is a decrease in the motility of the esophagus related to aging. **Cognitive Level:** Remembering. **Client Need:** Health Promotion and Maintenance. **Nursing Process:** Assessment. **Learning Outcome:** 26-8.
9. **Answer:** 4. **Rationale:** This response reflects an understanding of the different stages of independence and control an older adult experiences when admitted to the hospital and the need for the nurse to assess the client's need for control and autonomy. After admission, the client willingly gives up autonomy to the hospital routine because the client wants to get better (option 4). As the client's health improves and progresses, he or she wants to increase autonomy (option 1). Before discharge the client is thinking about if he or she can go home (option 2). Option 3 is not realistic given the usual hospital routine. **Cognitive Level:** Analyzing. **Client Need:** Psychosocial Integrity. **Nursing Process:** Planning. **Learning Outcome:** 26-6.
10. **Answer:** 3. **Rationale:** The nurse treats the older woman with empathy. Saying the sister is dead may trigger agitation or an argument. It may start the grieving process all over again and be distressing for the woman (option 1). These responses should be avoided. It is more compassionate to focus on the woman's feelings, and encourage her to talk about her sister and remembered events. Long-term memory remains functional in many clients with dementia compared to short-term memory. By having her reminisce, the nurse can stimulate the woman's recall of events from a long time ago (option 3). It is deceptive to say the sister won't visit today or that the woman should wait to see if she does visit today (option 4). **Cognitive Level:** Applying. **Client Need:** Psychosocial Integrity. **Nursing Process:** Implementation. **Learning Outcome:** 26-12.

CHAPTER 27 Promoting Family Health

1. **Answer:** 1. **Rationale:** Grandparents, aunts, and uncles are considered extended family members. Parents and spouse are considered immediate family members. Children who no longer live at home are considered immediate family members. Roommates and close family friends may be considered extended family members if grandparents, aunts, and uncles do not exist. **Cognitive Level:** Analyzing. **Client Need:** Health Promotion and Maintenance. **Nursing Process:** Assessment. **Learning Outcome:** 27-2.
2. **Answer:** 3. **Rationale:** Tay-Sachs is a neurodegenerative disease that occurs primarily in descendants of Eastern European Jews. Simply because of this family's race, they are at risk for developing this health problem. The elderly couple is active and so is not at as high of risk simply because of age (option 1). Just because the family is led by a teenage mother, even though maturity is one of the factors the nurse will assess in this situation, does not necessarily indicate that a health risk exists (option 2). Although poverty is a major problem that affects the family, the fact that there is health insurance is a positive sociologic factor (option 4). **Cognitive Level:** Applying. **Client Need:** Health Promotion and Maintenance. **Nursing Process:** Assessment. **Learning Outcome:** 27-4.
3. **Answer:** 1. **Rationale:** The health history of the client's current living partners is critical information since many illnesses are communicable or environmental. Giving this advice, the nurse also validates that family are whoever the client says they are. History of illness data of blood relatives is also extremely valuable and should always be included, whether or not the client lives with them. Neither the history nor the physical exam is more important than the other—both are necessary for a complete plan of care. **Cognitive Level:** Applying. **Client Need:** Health Promotion and Maintenance. **Nursing Process:** Assessment. **Learning Outcome:** 27-4.
4. **Answer:** A visual representation of family members by gender, age, health status, and lines of relationships through the generations is referred to as a genogram. **Cognitive Level:** Remembering. **Client Need:** Health Promotion and Maintenance. **Nursing Process:** Assessment. **Learning Outcome:** 27-4.
5. **Answer:** 1, 2, and 4. **Rationale:** It is essential for the nurse to determine the duration of the illness, the meaning of the illness to the family and its significance to family systems, and the

financial impact of the illness in order to completely assess the impact of the illness on the family as a whole. Duration of the illness will determine the degree of disruption and adaptation required. These factors affect the members of the family in addition to the ill client. Option 3: Coping mechanisms used by other families with similar illnesses may not be relevant because families vary greatly in their makeup and function patterns. Option 5: Knowing the incidence of the illness in the community at large is an important factor for the community health nurse in exploring epidemiologic issues such as prevention strategies and public health policies but is not as relevant for assisting the particular family. **Cognitive Level:** Understanding. **Client Need:** Psychosocial Integrity. **Nursing Process:** Assessment. **Learning Outcome:** 27-6.

6. **Answer:** 1. **Rationale:** Presenting to the clinic indicates the family is probably ready to face the health challenges caused by the previous activities. There is no evidence that the adult child or parent is experiencing impaired coping (option 2). Alteration in parenting applies when the parent is unable to care for a child rather than the reverse. Although some strain must be experienced by the child, evidence does not indicate that impairment in caregiver role is the most important aspect of the situation. **Cognitive Level:** Analyzing. **Client Need:** Health Promotion and Maintenance. **Nursing Process:** Diagnosis. **Learning Outcome:** 27-6.
7. **Answer:** 1. **Rationale:** This describes a state in which a family with previous normal functioning experiences a dysfunction. The communication patterns have affected how the family works as a unit. Impaired Verbal Communication means that the members are not able to communicate because of complications with speaking or saying the words, which is not the case in this situation (option 2). Ineffective Family Coping must be related to an etiology, so option 3 is incorrect. Option 4 is incorrect as the family does recognize the problem as members of the family seek assistance from outside sources. **Cognitive Level:** Analyzing. **Client Need:** Health Promotion and Maintenance. **Nursing Process:** Diagnosis. **Learning Outcome:** 27-6.
8. **Answer:** 4. **Rationale:** The focus of activity on personal purposes does not promote effective family functioning. A family system that functions efficiently focuses primarily on purposes involving the total system, allows input from the outside, has personal boundaries that are well defined, and has interdependent family members. **Cognitive Level:** Analyzing. **Client Need:** Health Promotion and Maintenance. **Nursing Process:** Evaluation. **Learning Outcome:** 27-3.
9. **Answer:** 2. **Rationale:** A family should provide an environment that supports the growth of the individual members. It is neither possible nor appropriate for the family to try to provide everything each member wants (option 1), nor that members are accepted into society (option 3). Although the family protects its members, a healthy family will share and use appropriate resources with the broader community (option 4). **Cognitive Level:** Applying. **Client Need:** Health Promotion and Maintenance. **Nursing Process:** Planning. **Learning Outcome:** 27-1.
10. **Answer:** 2. **Rationale:** A child who doesn't speak and is watchful when parents are near would be a significant indicator of a possible abuse situation. The baby may have an untreated condition, but chronic cold symptoms are not evidence of abuse (option 1). Dirty clothes or clothes not meeting the nurse's standards are not signs of abuse (option 3). Not having a regular physician would be a concern for health promotion and maintenance, but not for abuse (option 4). **Cognitive Level:** Analyzing. **Client Need:** Health promotion and maintenance. **Nursing Process:** Planning. **Learning Outcome:** 27-5.

CHAPTER 28 Vital Signs

1. **Answer:** 2. **Rationale:** Body temperature is frequently measured orally even if the client has eaten or drank something cold or hot. One only needs to wait 30 minutes, and then this site can be used. Axilla is the preferred site for newborns, not adults (option 1). The popliteal site would not be used given the history of heart disease. There could be circulatory issues that might affect accurate reading since this site is much farther away from the heart (option 3). Rectal would be contraindicated in this client given the history of heart disease. With the diagnosis of heart disease, the nurse would need to assess for the presence of hemorrhoids (option 4). **Cognitive Level:** Analyzing. **Client Need:** Health Promotion and Maintenance. **Nursing Process:** Planning. **Learning Outcome:** 28-5.
2. **Answer:** 3. **Rationale:** The apical rate would confirm the rate and determine the actual cardiac rhythm for a client with an abnormal rhythm; a radial pulse would reveal only the heart rate and suggest an arrhythmia. For clients in shock, use the carotid or femoral pulse (option 1). The radial pulse is adequate for determining a change in the orthostatic heart rate (option 2). The radial pulse is appropriate for routine postoperative vital sign checks for clients with regular pulses (option 4). **Cognitive Level:** Understanding. **Client Need:** Health Promotion and Maintenance. **Nursing Process:** Planning. **Learning Outcome:** 28-5.
3. **Answer:** 2. **Rationale:** Persons in a semi-Fowler's position will better aid themselves and the nurse to assess their respiratory status. The prone, side-lying, and supine positions increase the volume of blood inside the thoracic cavity and compress the chest, compromising the client's respirations. **Cognitive Level:** Understanding. **Client Need:** Health Promotion and Maintenance. **Nursing Process:** Planning. **Learning Outcome:** 28-3d.
4. **Answer:** 2. **Rationale:** If the cuff is inflated to about 30 mmHg over previous systolic pressure, that would be 168. To ensure that the diastolic has been determined, the cuff should be released slowly until the mid-60s mmHg (and then completely) for someone with a previous reading of 74. The cuff should be deflated at a rate of 2 to 3 mm per second. Thus, a range of 90 mmHg will require 30 to 45 seconds. **Cognitive Level:** Analyzing. **Client Need:** Health Promotion and Maintenance. **Nursing Process:** Implementation. **Learning Outcome:** 28-3e.
5. **Answer:** 1. **Rationale:** The cardiac catheterization client will need a thorough assessment since she is just returning to the nursing unit. Invasive procedures, such as a catheterization, will need to be closely assessed. More than likely a Doppler will be needed to ensure the pedal pulse is present and stable in the extremity used during the procedure. Unlicensed personnel are not usually delegated Doppler ultrasound device use. **Cognitive Level:** Applying. **Client Need:** Health Promotion and Maintenance. **Nursing Process:** Planning. **Learning Outcome:** 28-8.
6. **Answer:** 3, 4, and 5. **Rationale:** For this client, the nurse could take an axillary, tympanic, or temporal artery temperature. Due to the facial drooping and difficulty swallowing, the oral route is not recommended (option 1). Although the rectal route could be used, it would require unnecessary moving and positioning of a client who cannot assist, and it would not provide a significant advantage over the other routes (option 2). **Cognitive Level:** Applying. **Client Need:** Health Promotion and Maintenance. **Nursing Process:** Assessment. **Learning Outcome:** 28-1.
7. **Answer:** 4. **Rationale:** The posterior tibial and pedal pulses in the foot are considered peripheral and at least one of them should be palpable in normal individuals. Option 1: A bounding radial pulse is more indicative that perfusion exists. Options 2 and 3: Apical and carotid pulses are central and not peripheral.

Cognitive Level: Analyzing. Client Need: Health Promotion and Maintenance. Nursing Process: Diagnosing. Learning Outcome: 28-9.

8. **Answer:** 3. **Rationale:** Dyspnea, difficult or labored breathing, is commonly related to inadequate oxygenation. Therefore, the client is likely to experience shortness of breath, that is, a sense that none of the breaths provide enough oxygen and an immediate second breath is needed. Option 1: Shallow respirations are seen in tachypnea (rapid breathing). Option 2: Wheezing is a high-pitched breathing sound that may or may not occur with dyspnea. Option 4: The medical term for coughing up blood is hemoptysis and is unrelated to dyspnea. **Cognitive Level:** Applying. **Client Need:** Health Promotion and Maintenance. **Nursing Process:** Evaluation. **Learning Outcome:** 28-7.
9. **Answer:** This blood pressure should be recorded as 180/105/95 mmHg using the systolic/1st diastolic/2nd diastolic convention. **Rationale:** Phase 1 first sound is a clear tapping when deflation of the cuff begins. Phase 2 has a muffled, swishing sound. In phase 3, blood is flowing freely via an increasingly open artery; sounds are more crisp and more intense but softer than phase 1. Phase 4 sounds become muffled and have a soft blowing quality. In phase 5 the last sound is heard followed by silence. **Cognitive Level:** Analyzing. **Client Need:** Health Promotion and Maintenance. **Nursing Process:** Assessment. **Learning Outcome:** 28-9.
10. **Answer:** 4. **Rationale:** The SpO2 in this case is 97%. Option 1 indicates the systolic blood pressure of 121 mmHg, option 2 the mean arterial pressure of 95 mmHg, option 3 the pulse of 87 beats/min, and option 5 the diastolic blood pressure of 84 mmHg. In addition, the client's temperature is shown. **Cognitive Level:** Understanding. **Client Need:** Health Promotion and Maintenance. **Nursing Process:** Assessment. **Learning Outcome:** 28-3f.

CHAPTER 29 Health Assessment

1. **Answer:** 2. **Rationale:** Resonance is a normal sound over the lung. Tympany would be heard over the stomach (air filled) (option 1), hyperresonance is never a normal finding (option 3), and dullness would be heard below (not above) the 10th intercostal space (option 4). **Cognitive Level:** Remembering. **Client Need:** Health Promotion and Maintenance. **Nursing Process:** Evaluation. **Learning Outcomes:** 29-3; 29-4k.
2. **Answer:** 1, 2, 3. **Rationale:** Examining the body through use of touch describes palpation (option 4). Striking the body to elicit a sound from a body part describes percussion (option 5). **Cognitive Level:** Applying. **Client Need:** Health Promotion and Maintenance. **Nursing Process:** Planning. **Learning Outcome:** 29-2.
3. **Answer:** 1. **Rationale:** A bruit suggests abnormal turbulence in the aorta, and the primary care provider must be notified. For absence of bowel sounds to be considered abnormal, they must be silent for 3 to 5 minutes (option 2). Continuous bowel sounds are normally heard over the ileocecal valve following meals (option 3). Bowel sounds are more commonly irregular than they are regular (option 4). **Cognitive Level:** Understanding. **Client Need:** Health Promotion and Maintenance. **Nursing Process:** Evaluation. **Learning Outcomes:** 29-3; 29-4o; 29-8.
4. **Answer:** 1. **Rationale:** If a pedal pulse, which is more distal than the popliteal, is present, then adequate arterial circulation to the leg is present even though the popliteal artery has not been located. Presence of a femoral pulse would not provide confirmation that arterial flow exists below that point (option 2). Taking a thigh BP requires locating the popliteal pulse (option 3). Because the purpose of finding the popliteal pulse is to provide information about arterial circulation to the leg, checking the distal pulse before requesting assistance from another nurse is appropriate (option 4). **Cognitive Level:** Analyzing. **Client Need:** Health Promotion and Maintenance. **Nursing Process:** Planning. **Learning Outcomes:** 29-3; 29-4m.
5. **Answer:** 2. **Rationale:** Visual acuity often lessens with age. Facial hair is likely to become coarser, not finer (option 1). The sense of smell becomes less, rather than more acute (option 3). The respiratory rate and rhythm is regular at rest (option 4). However, both may change quickly with activity and be slow to return to the resting level. **Cognitive Level:** Analyzing. **Client Need:** Health Promotion and Maintenance. **Nursing Process:** Evaluating. **Learning Outcome:** 29-3.
6. Answers include color, turgor, temperature, moisture, lesions, odor, and edema. **Cognitive Level:** Remembering. **Client Need:** Health Promotion and Maintenance. **Nursing Process:** Assessment. **Learning Outcome:** 29-4b.
7. **Answer:** 3. **Rationale:** Recent memory includes events of the current day. Recalling a series of numbers tests immediate recall (option 1). Recalling childhood events tests remote (long-term) memory (option 2), and subtracting backward from 100 tests attention span and calculation skills (option 4). **Cognitive Level:** Applying. **Client Need:** Health Promotion and Maintenance. **Nursing Process:** Planning. **Learning Outcomes:** 29-3; 29-4q.
8. **Answer:** 4. **Rationale:** If the client can only read the first three lines, vision is impaired and could lead to falls or other injuries. This impaired vision is not related to ability to read (option 1) or memory (option 2). Myopia (option 3) is a medical diagnosis. **Cognitive Level:** Analyzing. **Client Need:** Health Promotion and Maintenance. **Nursing Process:** Diagnosing. **Learning Outcomes:** 29-3; 29-8.
9. **Answer:** 1, 2, 3, 4. **Rationale:** Using a stethoscope to transmit sounds to the ears is done during auscultation, not indirect percussion. **Cognitive Level:** Applying. **Client Need:** Health Promotion and Maintenance. **Nursing Process:** Implementation. **Learning Outcome:** 29-2.
10. **Answer**: Of the terms listed, only equal, symmetrical, and firm are normal findings. Atrophied, flaccid, contractured, hypertrophied, crepitation, spastic, and tremor are abnormal findings. Review the terms in the glossary to go over their meanings. **Cognitive Level:** Understanding. **Client Need:** Health Promotion and Maintenance. **Nursing Process:** Evaluation. **Learning Outcomes:** 29-4p; 29-8.

CHAPTER 30 Pain Assessment and Management

1. **Answer:** 1. **Rationale:** During the transduction phase, noxious stimuli trigger the release of biochemical mediators, such as prostaglandins, bradykinin, serotonin, histamine, and substance P, which sensitize nociceptors. Noxious or painful stimulation also causes movement of ions across cell membranes, which excites nociceptors. Pain medications such as ibuprofen or aspirin can work during this phase by blocking the production of prostaglandin or by decreasing the movement of ions across the cell membrane. **Cognitive Level:** Analyzing. **Client Need:** Physiological Integrity. **Nursing Process:** Assessment. **Learning Outcome:** 30-2.
2. **Answer:** 2. **Rationale:** In a postoperative client, it is important to assess pain intensity frequently to manage the acute pain experience. Option 1: The most pain a client is willing to tolerate before taking action can be discussed with the client after the pain intensity has been assessed. Option 3, location of pain, is important, but it is not the priority. Option 4: Pain history is important but not for a client in acute pain. **Cognitive Level:** Analyzing. **Client Need:** Safe, Effective Care Environment. **Nursing Process:** Assessment. **Learning Outcome:** 30-4.

3. **Answer:** 4. **Rationale:** Pain Assessment in Advanced Dementia (PAINAD) is designed specifically for older adults with advanced dementia and looks at specific indicators (breathing, vocalisation, facial expression, body language, and consolability). Options 2 and 3 are self-report measures of pain intensity developed for children (4-16years). **Cognitive level:** Applying; **Client need:** Physiological integrity; **Nursing process:** Assessment; **Learning Outcome:** 30-4.
4. **Answer:** 1 and 2 **Rationale:** The client is at risk of developing Opioid Induced Respiratory Depression (OIRD). The nurse should assess the client's alertness by using the sedation scale and respiratory rate. Early recognition will enable appropriate management and ensure patient safety. Options 3 and 4 can be assessed at a later stage. **Cognitive level:** Applying. **Client need:** Safe, Effective care environment. **Nursing process:** Implementation. **Learning Outcome:** 30-6.
5. **Answer:** 3. **Rationale:** Opioids may depress the respiratory system, so the nurse should assess the respiratory rate before administering opioids. Options 1 and 2 are subjective data. Option 4 is not applicable to assess prior to administering an opioid medication to a client. **Cognitive Level:** Applying. **Client Need:** Safe, Effective Care Environment. **Nursing Process:** Assessment. **Learning Outcome:** 30-5.
6. **Answer:** 3. **Rationale:** Pain post below-knee amputation is associated with damage to neural tissue and the description of 'electric shock-type' pain is characteristic of neuropathic pain. The management of neuropathic pain is distinct from other types of pain and it includes the use of adjuvants such as anticonvulsants. **Cognitive level:** Analysing. **Client need:** Physiological Integrity. **Nursing process:** Assessment. **Learning Outcome:** 30-1.
7. **Answer:** 1, 4, and 5. **Rationale:** NSAIDs can cause the side effect of GI bleeding. Clients should be taught to take NSAIDs with food and a full glass of water. Finding out how often the client takes the NSAID can help assess the likelihood of side effects occurring. Options 2 and 3 do not relate to NSAIDs. **Cognitive Level:** Applying. **Client Need:** Physiological Integrity. **Nursing Process:** Implementation. **Learning Outcome:** 30-10.
8. **Answer:** 2. **Rationale:** The words *pain* and *complain* may have emotional or sociocultural meanings (options 1 and 4). It is better to ask clients if they are having any discomfort—they can then elaborate in their own words. Option 3 is too general and expects clients to report their pain without being asked. **Cognitive Level:** Applying. **Client Need:** Safe, Effective Care Environment. **Nursing Process:** Assessment. **Learning Outcome:** 30-4.
9. **Answer:** 3 and 5. **Rationale:** Older clients may deny pain because it may indicate a worsening of their condition that may threaten their independence. Older adults may use words other than *pain*. Although many perceive pain as a natural outcome of aging, it is not a natural part of aging (option 1). Pain perception may decrease (option 2) and opioids can be used with careful monitoring by the nurse (option 4). **Cognitive Level:** Understanding. **Client Need:** Physiological Integrity. **Nursing Process:** Planning. **Learning Outcome:** 30-6.
10. **Answer:** 1. **Rationale:** Based on the information provided, the nurse needs to determine the client's understanding of the effects of pain on recovery and if the client has misconceptions about pain. The signs and symptoms do not support option 2. Options 3 and 4 could be true, but the priority is option 1. Movement enhances respiratory, cardiovascular, and GI recovery from general anesthesia and the outcomes associated with a surgical procedure. **Cognitive Level:** Analyzing. **Client Need:** Physiological Integrity. **Nursing Process:** Diagnosis. **Learning Outcome:** 30-5.

CHAPTER 31 Asepsis and Infection Prevention

1. **Answer:** 1. **Rationale:** When a client has an airborne disease and must go elsewhere in the hospital, the client must wear a mask. **Cognitive Level:** Analyzing. **Client Need:** Safe, Effective Care Environment. **Nursing Process:** Planning. **Learning Outcome:** 31-9.
2. **Answer:** 1, 2, 3. **Rationale:** The nurse should instruct the client to minimize exposure to others when recovering from surgery to reduce the risk of infection (option 4). The nurse should instruct the client to get adequate rest and sleep when recovering from surgery to reduce the risk of infection (option 5). **Cognitive Level:** Applying. **Client Need:** Safe, Effective Care Environment. **Nursing Process:** Implementation. **Learning Outcome:** 31-8.
3. **Answer:** 3. **Rationale:** Paper towels and a sink for hand washing should be in the client's room so they can be used before the staff leave the room. A blood pressure cuff is needed in the client's room to prevent cross contamination. A cabinet stocked with gloves and gowns would be outside the room (option 1). Cards and records should never be taken into an isolation room (option 2). The sign explaining the kind of isolation should be on the outside of the door to alert the staff of what is needed to enter (option 4). **Cognitive Level:** Applying. **Client Need:** Safe, Effective Care Environment. **Nursing Process:** Implementation. **Learning Outcome:** 31-10.
4. **Answer:** 1. **Rationale:** Unless overly contaminated by material that has splashed in the nurse's face and cannot be effectively rinsed off, goggles may be worn repeatedly (option 1). Since gowns are at high risk for contamination, they should be used only once and then discarded or washed (option 2). Surgical masks (option 3) and gloves (option 4) are never washed or reused. **Cognitive Level:** Understanding. **Client Need:** Safe, Effective Care Environment. **Nursing Process:** Implementation. **Learning Outcome:** 31-11b.
5. **Answer:** 4. **Rationale:** It should not be necessary to unroll this small edge of the cuff. The most important consideration is the sterility of the fingers and hand that will be used to perform the sterile procedure. The rolled-under portion is now contaminated and should not be unrolled by the nurse or colleague since it would then touch the remaining sterile portion of the glove (option 3). **Cognitive Level:** Applying. **Client Need:** Safe, Effective Care Environment. **Nursing Process:** Implementation. **Learning Outcome:** 31-11d.
6. **Answer:** 1, 2, 3, 4, and 5. **Rationale:** Proper use of alcohol-based products includes following these steps: Apply a palmful of product into a cupped hand—enough to cover all surfaces of both hands (option 1); rub palms together (option 2); interlace fingers palm to palm (option 3); rub palms against back of hands (option 4); and rub all surfaces of each finger with opposite hand (option 5); continue until product is dry—about 20 to 30 seconds, not 10 to 15 seconds as stated incorrectly in option 6. **Cognitive Level:** Applying. **Client Need:** Safe, Effective Care Environment. **Nursing Process:** Implementation. **Learning Outcome:** 31-11a.
7. **Answer:** Because a malnourished client with a wound is less able to resist an infection, potential for infection is the most likely nursing diagnosis. Others may include pain or altered nutrition but they are less focused on the immediate health risk. **Cognitive Level:** Applying. **Client Need:** Safe, Effective Care Environment. **Nursing Process:** Diagnosing. **Learning Outcome:** 31-7.
8. **Answer:** 2. **Rationale:** Raw foods touched by human hands can carry significant infectious organisms and must be washed or peeled. Antimicrobial soap is not indicated for regular use

and may lead to resistant organisms. Hand hygiene should occur as needed. Hot water can dry and harm skin, increasing the risk of infection (option 1). Clients should learn all the signs of inflammation and infection (e.g., redness, swelling, pain, heat) and not rely on the presence of pus to indicate this (option 3). Individuals should not share washcloths or towels (option 4). **Cognitive Level:** Analyzing. **Client Need:** Safe, Effective Care Environment. **Nursing Process:** Evaluation. **Learning Outcomes:** 31-8; 31-5.

9. **Answer:** 1. **Rationale:** Sterile objects are considered unsterile if placed lower than the waist. Only area 1 in this situation would be considered sterile. Above the neck, higher than 2 inches above the elbow, below the waist or table, and the back are all considered unsterile. **Cognitive Level:** Applying. **Client Need:** Physiological Integrity. **Nursing Process:** Planning. **Learning Outcomes:** 31-1; 31-11c.
10. **Answer:** 3. **Rationale:** All items within 1 inch of the edge of the sterile field are considered contaminated because the edge of the field is in contact with unsterile areas. When hands are ungloved, forceps tips are to be held downward to prevent fluid from becoming contaminated by the hands and then returned to the sterile field (option 1). Fields should be established immediately before use to prevent accidental contamination when not observed closely (option 2). Reaching over a sterile field increases the chances of dropping an unsterile item onto or touching the sterile field (option 4). **Cognitive Level:** Applying. **Client Need:** Safe, Effective Care Environment. **Nursing Process:** Evaluation. **Learning Outcome:** 31-11c.

CHAPTER 32 Safety

1. **Answer:** 3. **Rationale:** In the event of a fire, the nurse's priority responsibility is to rescue or protect the clients under his or her care. The next priorities are to report or alert the fire department, contain or confine the fire, and extinguish the fire. **Cognitive Level:** Understanding. **Client Need:** Safe, Effective Care Environment. **Nursing Process:** Implementation. **Learning Outcome:** 32-5.
2. **Answer:** 4. **Rationale:** Exposure to x-rays in the first trimester could cause harm to the developing fetus. Banging into objects is what a toddler would be likely to do, not an expectant mother (option 1). Bicycle rides and recreational activities would be good for the developing fetus; the mother should stay as active as possible during the pregnancy. Physical activity promotes good health (options 2 and 3). **Cognitive Level:** Understanding. **Client Need:** Safe, Effective Care Environment. **Nursing Process:** Implementation. **Learning Outcome:** 32-4.
3. **Answer:** 1, 2, 3. **Rationale:** The ability to stand in place for a minute before ambulating would be applicable if the client were demonstrating signs of orthostatic hypotension (option 4). The use of alcohol with prescribed medications would be beneficial if the client were prescribed sedatives or hypnotics (option 5). **Cognitive Level:** Applying. **Client Need:** Safe, Effective Care Environment. **Nursing Process:** Implementation. **Learning Outcome:** 32-7.
4. **Answer:** 3. **Rationale:** A home that was built prior to 1978 has lead-based paint. The ingestion of lead-based paint chips places that child at risk for elevated serum lead levels and neurologic deficits. The most appropriate nursing diagnosis for this child is potential for poisoning. Option 1: The risk for suffocation is greater in infants and is not related to a home with lead-based paint. Options 2 and 4 are not related to lead-based paint. **Cognitive Level:** Applying. **Client Need:** Safe, Effective Care Environment. **Nursing Process:** Nursing Diagnosis. **Learning Outcome:** 32-5.
5. **Answer:** 4. **Rationale:** Option 4 is an intervention that can allow the client to feel independent and also alert the nursing staff when the client needs assistance. It is the most realistic answer that promotes client safety. Option 1 can increase agitation and confusion and removes the client's independence. Option 2 would help but transfers the responsibility to the family member. Option 3 is inappropriate because the client could fall during the unobserved interval and it is not a realistic answer for the nurse. **Cognitive Level:** Analyzing. **Client Need:** Safe, Effective Care Environment. **Nursing Process:** Implementation. **Learning Outcomes:** 32-6; 32-11a.
6. **Answer:** 2 and 5. **Rationale:** Options 2 and 5 are measures needed to keep the client safe in the event of another seizure. Option 1 is incorrect because the current nursing literature states to not put anything in the client's mouth during a seizure. Options 3 and 4 are more relevant after the cause of the seizure is known. Seizures are not all classified as epilepsy. **Cognitive Level:** Applying. **Client Need:** Safe, Effective Care Environment. **Nursing Process:** Planning. **Learning Outcomes:** 32-7; 32-11b.
7. **Answer:** 3. **Rationale:** Providing adequate lighting will help prevent the client from falling. The environment should be clutter-free because any clutter can cause the client to fall (option 1). Wearing terry cloth slippers would allow the client to fall. The client should have rubber skid-resistant slippers (option 2). Noise should be kept to a minimum but turning off alarms would endanger a client (option 4). **Cognitive Level:** Understanding. **Client Need:** Safe, Effective Care Environment. **Nursing Process:** Implementation. **Learning Outcome:** 32-6.
8. **Answer:** 1, 2, 3, and 5. **Rationale:** These four options are alternatives to restraints and it is necessary for the nurse to attempt alternative options before making the decision to call the healthcare provider for an order for restraints (option 4). Orienting the client and explaining the IV device may help depending on the level of confusion and is an intervention for confused clients. Covering up or disguising the device may help by eliminating the strange distraction, and a mitt is considered an alternative as long as it is not tied to the bed and the client can remove it if desired. **Cognitive Level:** Applying. **Client Need:** Safe, Effective Care Environment. **Nursing Process:** Planning. **Learning Outcomes:** 32-8; 32-11c.
9. **Answer:** 3. **Rationale:** Suicide and homicide are two leading causes of death among teenagers. Adolescent males commit suicide at a higher rate than adolescent females. Options 1 and 2 are true; however, neither would be as high a priority as preventing suicide. Option 4 is not true. A driver's education course does not ensure safe practice. **Cognitive Level:** Analysis. **Client Need:** Safe, Effective Care Environment. **Nursing Process:** Planning. **Learning Outcome:** 32-5.
10. **Answer:** 1, 3, 4, and 5. **Rationale:** Standards require documentation of the necessity for restraints. The implementation of range-of-motion exercises prevents joint stiffness and pain from disuse. Orienting the client helps the nurse determine the necessity of the restraint. Option 2 is inappropriate because it may cause injury if the side rail is lowered without untying the restraint. **Cognitive Level:** Applying. **Client Need:** Safe, Effective Care Environment. **Nursing Process:** Implementation. **Learning Outcomes:** 32-8; 32-11c.

CHAPTER 33 Hygiene

1. **Answer:** 3. **Rationale:** The client fits the descriptors for a semidependent functional level (see Table 33.2). **Cognitive Level:** Applying. **Client Need:** Physiological Integrity. **Nursing Process:** Assessment. **Learning Outcome:** 33-3.
2. **Answer:** 3. **Rationale:** The client will be positioned in a side-lying position with the head of the bed lowered because the client is at risk for aspiration. The absence of the gag reflex

lets the nurse know that the client has no natural defense (cough) and is at a higher risk for aspiration. All other answers are assessments more appropriate prior to bathing the client. **Cognitive Level:** Applying. **Client Need:** Physiological Integrity. **Nursing Process:** Assessment. **Learning Outcome:** 33-4.

3. **Answer:** 3. **Rationale:** The hair should be smooth in texture and neither oily nor dry. Dry or thin hair could be a sign of alopecia, and darkness would depend on hair color through the gene pool (option 1). Skin is assessed as being smooth, taut, or shiny, not hair (option 2). A tender, warm scalp could indicate a problem, so this would not be normal (option 4). **Cognitive Level:** Analyzing. **Client Need:** Physiological Integrity. **Nursing Process:** Assessment. **Learning Outcome:** 33-3.
4. **Answer:** 1. **Rationale:** Turn off the hearing aid. Option 2 is incorrect because an in-the-ear hearing aid is cleaned with a damp cloth. Option 3 is incorrect; make sure the volume is turned all the way down because a too loud volume is distressing. Check that the battery is in the hearing aid; do not remove the batteries (option 4). **Cognitive Level:** Applying. **Client Need:** Physiological Integrity. **Nursing Process:** Implementation. **Learning Outcome:** 33-13g.
5. **Answer:** 3. **Rationale:** Placing the soiled sheet in the laundry bag reduces the spread of microorganisms, which is a safety measure for both the nurse and client. Beginning at the head and moving toward the foot, loosening the bottom linens, provides maximum workspace. Mitering the corners at the head of the bed prevents linens from becoming easily loosened. Preparing the client readies the client for the procedure. **Cognitive Level:** Applying. **Client Need:** Physiological Integrity. **Nursing Process:** Implementation. **Learning Outcome:** 33-14.
6. **Answer:** 1, 2, 3, 5. **Rationale:** When bathing a client with dementia, the nurse should stop if the client begins to feel distressed (option 4). **Cognitive Level:** Applying. **Client Need:** Physiological Integrity. **Nursing Process:** Implementation. **Learning Outcome:** 33-8.
7. **Answer:** 4. **Rationale:** It is important to retract the foreskin to remove the smegma that collects under the foreskin and can cause bacterial growth. **Cognitive Level:** Analyzing. **Client Need:** Physiological Integrity. **Nursing Process:** Evaluation. **Learning Outcome:** 33-1.
8. **Answer:** 1, 3, and 5. **Rationale:** The developmental level warrants supervision. If the bottle is given during naps or bedtime, the solution has continuous contact with the toddler's teeth. The first visit to the dentist should occur between the ages of 2 and 3 (option 2). More than 50% of older adults have their own teeth (option 4). **Cognitive Level:** Applying. **Client Need:** Health Promotion and Maintenance. **Nursing Process:** Planning. **Learning Outcome:** 33-4.
9. **Answer:** 2. **Rationale:** The client needs to avoid walking barefoot because that could cause injury that may result in an infection. Also, neurologic impairment is likely as a result of the diabetes, which may result in decreased sensation. The client would be unaware of an injury. **Cognitive Level:** Analyzing. **Client Need:** Health Promotion and Maintenance. **Nursing Process:** Evaluation. **Learning Outcome:** 33-4.
10. **Answer:** 1. **Rationale:** Fowler's is a semi-sitting position that should ease the client's breathing. The head of the bed (HOB) in semi-Fowler's is lower (option 2). The HOB is lowered in the Trendelenburg position (option 3). Although the HOB is raised in the reverse Trendelenburg position, it is a straight tilt and may not be as comfortable as Fowler's (option 4). **Cognitive Level:** Applying. **Client Need:** Safe, Effective Care Environment. **Nursing Process:** Implementation. **Learning Outcome:** 33-11.

CHAPTER 34 Diagnostic Testing

1. **Answer:** 3. **Rationale:** A nursing procedure or laboratory manual is often available if the nurse is unfamiliar with the procedure. If there is any question about the procedure, the nurse should call the laboratory for directions before collecting the specimen. **Cognitive Level:** Applying. **Client Need:** Physiological Integrity. **Nursing Process:** Assessment. **Learning Outcome:** 34-3.
2. **Answer:** 4. **Rationale:** The test cannot be continued, and it should not be documented that one specimen is missing (option 1). The test is not to be ended immediately, and the specimen should not be sent to the laboratory (option 2). The test is not complete. The nurse should not document that the test cannot be completed. It needs to be restarted (option 3). **Cognitive Level:** Analyzing. **Client Need:** Physiological Integrity. **Nursing Process:** Implementation. **Learning Outcome:** 34-6.
3. **Answer:** 2. **Rationale:** A KUB is an x-ray of the kidneys, ureters, and bladder. This does not require direct visualization. Option 1 is an IVP, an intravenous pyelogram, which requires the injection of a contrast media. Option 3 is a retrograde pyelography, which requires the injection of a contrast media. Option 4 is a cystoscopy, which uses a lighted instrument (cystoscope) inserted through the urethra, resulting in direct visualization. **Cognitive Level:** Remembering. **Client Need:** Physiological Integrity. **Nursing Process:** Assessment. **Learning Outcome:** 34-8.
4. **Answer:** 4. **Rationale:** This type of nuclear scan demonstrates the ability of tissues to absorb the chemical to indicate the physiology and function of an organ. Option 1 is an invasive procedure that focuses on blood flow through an organ. Options 2 and 3 provide information about density of tissue to help distinguish between normal and abnormal tissue of an organ. **Cognitive Level:** Remembering. **Client Need:** Physiological Integrity. **Nursing Process:** Assessment. **Learning Outcome:** 34-9.
5. **Answer:** 3. **Rationale:** Bone marrow aspiration includes deep penetration into soft tissue and large bones such as the sternum and iliac crest. This penetration can result in bleeding. The client should be observed for bleeding in the days following the procedure. Option 1 is a nursing action during a liver biopsy. Option 2 is a nursing action for a thoracentesis, and option 4 is a nursing action for a lumbar puncture. **Cognitive Level:** Applying. **Client Need:** Physiological Integrity. **Nursing Process:** Implementation. **Learning Outcome:** 34-10.
6. **Answer:** 1 and 4. **Rationale:** ALT is an enzyme that contributes to protein and carbohydrate metabolism. An increase in the enzyme indicates damage to the liver. The liver contributes to the metabolism of protein, which results in the production of ammonia. If the liver is damaged, the ammonia level is increased. Options 2, 3, and 5 (myoglobin, cholesterol, and BNP) are relevant for heart disease. **Cognitive Level:** Applying. **Client Need:** Physiological Integrity. **Nursing Process:** Assessment. **Learning Outcome:** 34-2.
7. **Answer:** 3. **Rationale:** A glycosylated hemoglobin will indicate the glucose levels for a period of time, which is indicated by the nurse practitioner. Options 1 and 2 will provide information about the current blood glucose, not the past history. Option 4 is used to assess for liver disease. **Cognitive Level:** Remembering. **Client Need:** Physiological Integrity. **Nursing Process:** Planning. **Learning Outcome:** 34-2.
8. **Answer:** 2, 3, and 5. **Rationale:** The nurse should obtain the stool specimen from two different areas of the stool. The nurse should observe for a blue color change, which is indicative of a positive result. The nurse should assess for the ingestion of vitamin C by the client because it is contraindicated for 3 days prior to taking the specimen. Option 1 is incorrect since the reagent is placed on the specimen after it is applied to the

testing card. Option 4 is incorrect because a pink color would be considered negative and does not require verification. **Cognitive Level:** Applying. **Client Need:** Physiological Integrity. **Nursing Process:** Planning. **Learning Outcome:** 34-5.

9. **Answer:** 1. **Rationale:** Lying in the lateral position with the head bent toward the chest and knees flexed onto the abdomen is the correct position for a lumbar puncture. In this position the back is arched, increasing the spaces between the vertebrae so that the spinal needle can be readily inserted. Lying prone with knees down toward the abdomen would position the client too high for the physician and could lead to increased intracranial pressure (option 2). Sitting would not arch the back enough to increase the space between the vertebrae for puncture (option 3). Supine with knees pulled toward the chest does not expose the vertebrae to be punctured (option 4). **Cognitive Level:** Applying. **Client Need:** Physiological Integrity. **Nursing Process:** Implementation. **Learning Outcome:** 34-10.
10. **Answer:** 2, 4, and 5. **Rationale:** The sputum specimen should be sent immediately to the laboratory. The client should be provided mouth care before and after the specimen is collected. The sputum specimen should be collected for three consecutive days. Option 1 is incorrect because the sputum specimen is collected in the morning not in the evening. Option 3 is incorrect because the term *spit* indicates that saliva is being examined. The client needs to cough up or expectorate mucus or sputum. **Cognitive Level:** Analyzing. **Client Need:** Physiological Integrity. **Nursing Process:** Implementation. **Learning Outcome:** 34-7.

CHAPTER 35 Medication Administration

1. **Answer:** 2. **Rationale:** If there is any doubt, the medication administration process should be interrupted until the question is clarified. Listen to the client. Find out any other information the client may have about that certain medication. For example, does he know the dosage of the medication taken at home? Do not administer the medication (option 1). Inform the client that you will check the chart first. Review the chart to make sure there is no discrepancy between the physician's order and the MAR. Review the physician's progress notes because the medication may have been increased or reduced as part of the treatment plan (option 3). Check with the pharmacist because sometimes a pill may be a different color or shape based on the pharmaceutical company. Do not leave medications at the bedside. Medications should never be left unattended (option 4). Inform the client of your findings. The client will appreciate that you took the time to make sure that he received the correct medication. While it takes time to check out the client's statement, you will be glad that you avoided a potential medication error. **Cognitive Level:** Applying. **Client Need:** Physiological Integrity. **Nursing Process:** Implementation. **Learning Outcome:** 35-11.
2. **Answer:** 2. **Rationale:** If the primary care provider cannot be reached, all attempts to contact the primary care provider and the reason for withholding the medication are documented. The nurse should not give the medication as prescribed, since the pharmacy has identified that the dose prescribed is outside of dosing limits (option 1). Giving one half of the medication prescribed is outside the nurse's licensure (option 3). Administering the medicine through the oral route might not be the best for the medication and changing the route is outside of the nurse's licensure (option 4). **Cognitive Level:** Applying. **Client Need:** Physiological Integrity. **Nursing Process:** Evaluation. **Learning Outcome:** 35-6.
3. **Answer:** 1, 3, and 5. **Rationale:** Five milliliters is too large an amount to inject into one site. The nurse needs to divide the amount into two 2.5-mL injections. A 3-mL syringe could be used (option 1). The length of the needle will depend on the muscle development of the client. The nurse needs to assess the client. The presumption, based on the information provided, is that this client's muscle mass is within normal limits. The needle length would need to be 1 1/2 inches because the medication is be given "deep IM" (option 5). This also suggests that the medication should be given in the preferred site for IM injections—the ventrogluteal site—because it provides the greatest thickness of gluteal muscle. The gauge of the needle for an IM injection into the ventrogluteal muscle can range between #20 and #23 (option 3). The nurse needs to assess the viscosity of the medication. Smaller gauges (e.g., #23) produce less tissue trauma; however, viscous solutions may require a larger gauge (e.g., #20–#21). **Cognitive Level:** Analyzing. **Client Need:** Physiological Integrity. **Nursing Process:** Implementation. **Learning Outcome:** 35-5.
4. **Answer:** 3. **Rationale:** The type of syringe for subcutaneous injections depends on the medication to be given. This situation does not indicate that the medication is insulin and, thus, another syringe is needed. Generally a 2-mL syringe is used for most subcutaneous injections. Generally, a #20- to #23-gauge needle is used for IM injections. Needle size and length are based on the client's body mass, the intended angle of insertion, and the site of the injection. Generally, a #25-gauge, 5/8-inch needle is used for adults of normal weight and the needle is inserted at a 45° angle. Because 2 inches of tissue can be grasped or pinched at the site of the injection, the nurse should administer the medication at a 90° angle to ensure the medication reaches subcutaneous tissue. **Cognitive Level:** Analyzing. **Client Need:** Physiological Integrity. **Nursing Process:** Implementation. **Learning Outcome:** 35-18b.
5. **Answer:** 1. **Rationale:** A tuberculin test is given by intradermal injection. A tuberculin syringe is used because the dosage will most likely be 0.1 mL. A short, fine needle is needed to avoid entering the subcutaneous tissue. The needle should have a short bevel and usually be between #25 and #27 gauge. The needle should be between 1/4 to 5/8 inch long. **Cognitive Level:** Analyzing. **Client Need:** Physiological Integrity. **Nursing Process:** Implementation. **Learning Outcome:** 35-18a.
6. **Answer:** 4. **Rationale:** If the nurse goes by the amount of the medication (0.5 mL) only, the deltoid muscle would be the site. However, knowing and assessing the client is critical. The muscles of an older, emaciated client will most likely be diminished or atrophied. The nurse should consider the ventrogluteal site because that site will have the most muscle mass. **Cognitive Level:** Analyzing. **Client Need:** Physiological Integrity. **Nursing Process:** Implementation. **Learning Outcomes:** 35-17c; 35-12.
7. **Answer:** 2. **Rationale:** Altered quality of organ responsiveness, resulting in adverse effects becoming pronounced before therapeutic effects are achieved, is one effect of medications on the older client. **Cognitive Level:** Applying. **Client Need:** Physiological Integrity. **Nursing Process:** Assessment. **Learning Outcome:** 35-12.
8. **Answer:** 1. **Rationale:** There is no need to notify the pharmacy for a new tube of ointment or to have the wastage witnessed by another nurse. **Cognitive Level:** Applying. **Client Need:** Physiological Integrity. **Nursing Process:** Implementation. **Learning Outcome:** 35-20c.
9. **Answer:** 0.375 or rounded to 0.38 mL. **Rationale:** After converting to like numbers, the formula would be set up as follows:

   400 micrograms = 1 mL

   150 micrograms = X mL

   Cross multiply $(400X = 150)$

   Divide by 400

   $X = 0.375$

   Cognitive Level: Applying. **Client Need:** Physiological Integrity. **Nursing Process:** Implementation. **Learning Outcome:** 35-9.

10. Answer: 3, 4, 1, 5, 2, 6, 7, and 8. **Rationale:** This is the correct order for this skill—first the nurse mixes the insulin, assesses the skin, and cleanses the skin. The nurse would then pinch the skin, insert the needle, inject the medication, count to five, and remove the syringe. **Cognitive Level:** Applying. **Client Need:** Physiological Integrity. **Nursing Process:** Implementation. **Learning Outcome:** 35-18b.

CHAPTER 36 Skin Integrity and Wound Care

1. **Answer:** 3. **Rationale:** Cleansing should be done with a mild cleansing agent and warm water, so option 1 is not appropriate. Petroleum-based creams are now thought to offer poor overall skin protection and to interfere with incontinence brief absorption (option 2). Keeping the client in bed to treat this area is not necessary and may lead to problems with immobility (option 4). **Cognitive Level:** Applying. **Client Need:** Safe, Effective Care Management. **Nursing Process:** Implementation. **Learning Outcome:** 36-2.
2. **Answer:** 1. **Rationale:** Wound culture specimens should be obtained from a cleaned area of the wound. Microbes responsible for the infection are more likely to be found in viable tissue. Collected drainage contains old and mixed organisms. An appropriate specimen can be obtained without causing the client the discomfort of debriding. The nurse does not generally debride the wound to obtain a specimen. Once systemic antibiotics have been begun, the interval following a dose will not significantly affect the concentration of wound organisms. **Cognitive Level:** Applying. **Client Need:** Physiological Integrity. **Nursing Process:** Implementation. **Learning Outcome:** 36-13b.
3. **Answer:** 3. **Rationale:** Hydrocolloid dressings protect shallow injuries and maintain an appropriate healing environment. Alginates (option 1) are used for wounds with significant drainage; dry gauze (option 2) will stick to new granulation tissue, causing more damage. A dressing is needed to protect the wound and enhance healing. **Cognitive Level:** Applying. **Client Need:** Physiological Integrity. **Nursing Process:** Implementation. **Learning Outcome:** 36-12.
4. **Answer:** 3. **Rationale:** After about 15 minutes of heat application, the thermal receptors adapt to the temperature increase and the sensation of warmth is diminished. Clients often request that the temperature be increased because they do not feel the same amount of heat. This can lead to burns. There is no evidence that this client has increased thermal tolerance or that the rebound effect is occurring. **Cognitive Level:** Analyzing. **Client Need:** Physiological Integrity. **Nursing Process:** Planning. **Learning Outcome:** 36-14.
5. **Answer:** 3. **Rationale:** Immobile and dependent clients should be repositioned at least every 2 hours, not every 4, so this client or family member requires further teaching. Warm water and moisturizing damp skin are correct techniques for skin care. Red areas that do not return to normal skin color should be reported. It would also be correct to use a foam pad to help relieve pressure. **Cognitive Level:** Analyzing. **Client Need:** Physiological Integrity. **Nursing Process:** Evaluation. **Learning Outcome:** 36-10.
6. **Answer:** 3. **Rationale:** The head of the client's bed should be kept at less than 30 degrees elevation as much as possible (option 1). Baby powder and cornstarch should not be used because they cause abrasive grit damage to tissues (options 2 and 4). **Cognitive Level:** Applying. **Client Need:** Physiological Integrity. **Nursing Process:** Implementation. **Learning Outcome:** 36-10.
7. **Answer:** 1, 2, 3, and 5. **Rationale:** Option 4 is not correct. The suture material that is visible is in contact with bacteria and must not be pulled beneath the skin during removal. **Cognitive Level:** Applying. **Client Need:** Physiological Integrity. **Nursing Process:** Implementation. **Learning Outcome:** 36-13e.
8. **Answer:** 1, 3, and 4. **Rationale:** Risk factors for pressure injuries include low-protein diet, lengthy surgical procedures, and fever. Protein is needed for adequate skin health and healing. During surgery, the client is on a hard surface and may not be well protected from pressure on bony prominences. Fever increases skin moisture, which can lead to skin breakdown, plus the stress on the body from the cause of the fever could impair circulation and skin integrity. Insomnia (option 2) would generally involve restless sleeping, which transfers pressure to different parts of the body and would reduce the chances of skin breakdown. A waterbed (option 5) distributes pressure more evenly than a regular mattress and, thus, actually reduces the chances of skin breakdown. **Cognitive Level:** Remembering. **Client Need:** Health Promotion and Maintenance. **Nursing Process:** Assessment. **Learning Outcome:** 36-1.
9. **Answer:** 1, 2, and 4. **Rationale:** To irrigate a wound, the nurse uses clean gloves to remove the old dressing and to hold the basin collecting the irrigating fluid. A mask should be worn when splashing can occur such as when irrigating a wound. A 60-mL syringe is the correct size to hold the volume of irrigating solution plus deliver safe irrigating pressure. The irrigation fluid should be room or body temperature—certainly not refrigerated. Forceps may be used to remove or apply a dressing but are not required for irrigation. **Cognitive Level:** Remembering. **Client Need:** Physiological Integrity. **Nursing Process:** Planning. **Learning Outcome:** 36-13c.
10. **Answer:** 2. **Rationale:** Gauze bandages are used to hold absorbent dressings in place. How tight the bandage is applied depends on the purpose (option 1). Elastic bandages are generally not sterile because they are used to support a body part and not cover a wound (option 3). The bandage may or may not cover at least one joint of the limb (option 4).

    Cognitive Level: Applying. **Client Need:** Physiological Integrity. **Nursing Process:** Evaluation. **Learning Outcome:** 36-13d.

CHAPTER 37 Perioperative Nursing

1. **Answer:** 1, 2, 3, 4, 5. **Rationale:** All options should be obtained when completing a preoperative assessment. **Cognitive Level:** Analyzing. **Client Need:** Physiological Integrity. **Nursing Process:** Assessment. **Learning Outcome:** 37-3.
2. **Answer:** 2. **Rationale:** Grieving is the state in which an individual experiences reactions in response to an expected significant loss and is often characterized by negative responses such as shame, embarrassment, guilt, or revulsion. Option 3, fear, is usually characterized by feelings of dread, fright, apprehension, or alarm. Impaired coping, option 4, is usually characterized by verbalization of inability to cope or ask for help, inappropriate use of defense mechanisms, or inability to meet role expectations. **Cognitive Level:** Applying. **Client Need:** Psychologic Integrity. **Nursing Process:** Diagnosis. **Learning Outcome:** 37-4.
3. **Answer:** 1. **Rationale:** The nurse should provide information including what will happen to the client, when, and what the client will experience. The nurse should clarify any misconceptions the client may have. The nurse should also explain the roles of the client and support people in preoperative preparation, the surgical procedure, and during the postoperative phase. How to perform activities of daily living following surgery is not a part of preoperative teaching. **Cognitive Level:** Applying. **Client Need:** Physiological Integrity. **Nursing Process:** Evaluation. **Learning Outcome:** 37-6.
4. **Answer:** 2. **Rationale:** The symptoms describe decreased cardiac output and not any of the other listed complications. **Cognitive Level:** Applying. **Client Need:** Physiological Integrity. **Nursing Process:** Assessment. **Learning Outcome:** 37-10.
5. **Answer:** 3. **Rationale:** Options 1 and 2 are incorrect because the client is still recovering from the anesthesia used during surgery. Option 4 is incorrect because pain usually decreases

after the second or third postoperative day. **Cognitive Level:** Applying. **Client Need:** Physiological Integrity. **Nursing Process:** Implementation. **Learning Outcome:** 37-10.

6. **Answer:** Splinting. **Rationale:** If the incision is painful when the client coughs, splinting the abdomen may reduce the pain. **Cognitive Level:** Remembering. **Client Need:** Physiological Integrity. **Nursing Process:** Implementation. **Learning Outcome:** 37-6.
7. **Answer:** 3. **Rationale:** The unconscious client should be positioned on the side, with the face slightly down. In the supine position, the client could occlude the airway. In the prone position, the client's operative site may not be readily assessed. A pillow under the head could cause the client's airway to become obstructed. **Cognitive Level:** Applying. **Client Need:** Physiological Integrity. **Nursing Process:** Implementation. **Learning Outcome:** 37-9.
8. **Answer:** 1 and 3. **Rationale:** The absence of nausea and vomiting indicates that the client may be ready for clear liquids. Anesthetics, narcotics, fasting, and inactivity all inhibit peristalsis. Oral fluids and food are started after the return of peristalsis. The client may feel hungry but peristalsis may not be present (option 5). Options 2 and 4 are important but not related specifically to advancing the client's diet. **Cognitive Level:** Applying. **Client Need:** Physiological Integrity. **Nursing Process:** Assessment. **Learning Outcome:** 37-9.
9. **Answer:** Safety. **Rationale:** The client's protective reflexes are compromised, especially with general anesthesia. Thus, the perioperative nurse needs to maintain the client's safety during surgery. **Cognitive Level:** Analyzing. **Client Need:** Safe, Effective Care Environment. **Nursing Process:** Planning. **Learning Outcome:** 37-5.
10. **Answer:** 3, 4, and 5. **Rationale:** Preoperative teaching (option 1) includes assessment of the client's learning needs and determining the teaching content and strategies that require professional knowledge and cannot be assigned. However, the AP can reinforce what the nurse has taught the client (option 3). Managing GI suction (option 2) requires application of knowledge and problem-solving and is not assigned to AP. The AP, however, can assist with emptying the drainage receptacle and reporting changes in amount and color of the drainage to the nurse (option 5). AP frequently remove and reapply antiemboli stockings (option 4). **Cognitive Level:** Applying. **Client Need:** Safe, Effective Care Environment. **Nursing Process**: Implementation **Learning Outcome:** 37-14.

CHAPTER 38 Sensory Perception

1. **Answer:** 1, 3, 5. **Rationale:** Pain, sleeplessness, and worry can contribute to sensory overload. Nocturnal confusion and being easily annoyed are manifestations of sensory deprivation (options 2 and 4). **Cognitive Level:** Analyzing. **Client Need:** Psychosocial Integrity. **Nursing Process:** Evaluation. **Learning Outcome:** 38-3.
2. **Answer:** 4. **Rationale:** Since the client lives alone and is recovering from cataract surgery, the client's risk for injury is great. Social Isolation would be appropriate for the client with long-term vision changes but not one with an acute change as in cataract surgery. Risk for Impaired Skin Integrity is used to describe clients who have altered tactile sensation. Disturbed Sensory Perception is used to describe clients whose perception has been altered by physiological factors such as pain, sleep deprivation, immobility, disease states such as CVA, or brain trauma. **Cognitive Level:** Applying. **Client Need:** Psychosocial Integrity. **Nursing Process:** Diagnosis. **Learning Outcome:** 38-6.
3. **Answer:** 2. **Rationale:** Because of the paraplegia (paralysis of lower body), the client is unable to feel discomfort. The client will be taught to lift self using chair arms every 10 minutes if possible. Option 1 is an actual problem versus a potential problem. In option 3, the client wears glasses that help correct the poor vision. Option 4 is more of a potential for injury diagnosis. **Cognitive Level:** Applying. **Client Need:** Psychosocial Integrity. **Nursing Process:** Diagnosis. **Learning Outcome:** 38-6.
4. **Answer:** 2. **Rationale:** This client could use an assistive device that flashes a light when the doorbell rings. Option 1 relates to safety of the environment rather than sensory alteration. Options 3 and 4 reflect how the client adapts to the sensory alteration. **Cognitive Level:** Analyzing. **Client Need:** Safe, Effective Care Environment. **Nursing Process:** Evaluation. **Learning Outcome:** 38-7.
5. **Answer:** 3. **Rationale:** Spraying the room with a floral spray will add to the sensory overload (option 1). Vinegar is not instilled into wounds (option 2). Burning a candle will add to the sensory overload and burning candles is not safe in the hospital environment (option 4). **Cognitive Level:** Applying. **Client Need:** Psychosocial Integrity. **Nursing Process:** Implementation. **Learning Outcome:** 38-7.
6. **Answer:** 1, 3, and 4. **Rationale:** Options 2 and 5 relate to interventions for a client with a hearing impairment. **Cognitive Level:** Applying. **Client Need:** Psychosocial Integrity. **Nursing Process:** Implementation. **Learning Outcome:** 38-7.
7. **Answer:** 3. **Rationale:** A disorganized, cluttered environment increases confusion. Option 1: Keeping the room well lit during waking hours promotes adequate sleep at night. It is important to eliminate unnecessary noise (option 2). The client does not meet the standard criteria for restraint application (option 4). **Cognitive Level:** Applying. **Client Need:** Safe, Effective Care Environment. **Nursing Process:** Implementation. **Learning Outcome:** 38-8.
8. **Answer:** 2, 4, and 5. **Rationale:** Options 1 and 3 are clinical signs of sensory overload. **Cognitive Level:** Remembering. **Client Need:** Psychosocial Integrity. **Nursing Process:** Assessment. **Learning Outcome:** 38-3.
9. **Answer:** Identifying taste: 5; Stereognosis: 3; Snellen chart: 1; Identifying aromas: 4; Tuning fork: 2. **Cognitive Level:** Remembering. **Client Need:** Health Promotion and Maintenance. **Nursing Process:** Assessment. **Learning Outcome:** 38-4.
10. **Answer:** 1. **Rationale:** The amplified telephone helps with hearing and provides a means for communicating with others. Option 2 refers to a tactile impairment. Option 3 relates to a visual impairment, and option 4 an olfactory impairment. **Cognitive Level:** Applying. **Client Need:** Psychosocial Integrity. **Nursing Process:** Planning. **Learning Outcome:** 38-7.

CHAPTER 39 Self-Concept

1. **Answer:** 1. **Rationale:** Sally has an inappropriate view of her physical self, which is body image. Personal identity is a sense of uniqueness (option 2); self-expectation consists of those things one believes the self should be able to do (option 3); and core self-concept includes the most vital central beliefs about one's identity (option 4). **Cognitive Level:** Applying. **Client Need:** Psychosocial Integrity. **Nursing Process:** Diagnosing. **Learning Outcome:** 39-2.
2. **Answer:** All the above. **Rationale:** Identity development in childhood is not restricted to gender-based activities and includes those activities that promote imagination, exploration, and independence. **Cognitive Level:** Analyzing. **Client Need:** Psychosocial integrity. **Nursing Process:** Assessment. **Learning Outcome:** 39-2.
3. **Answer:** 2. **Rationale:** It is not appropriate to reinforce her feelings by comparing the client to other clients (option 1), or to blame the spouse for the slowness (option 3), or to instill doubt by asking if the client is really trying (option 4). **Cognitive Level:** Applying. **Client Need:** Psychosocial Integrity. **Nursing Process:** Implementation. **Learning Outcome:** 39-2.
4. **Answer:** 1. **Rationale:** This response encourages the client to say more and focuses on the positive. Option 2 is

condescending and closes the discussion. Both options 3 and 4 ignore the emotional component of the client's statement and do not address the client's feelings of worthlessness. **Cognitive Level:** Applying. **Client Need:** Psychosocial Integrity. **Nursing Process:** Implementation. **Learning Outcomes:** 39-6; 39-7.

5. **Answer:** 3. **Rationale:** The diagnosis *Grieving* is appropriate, since the client is expressing a feeling related to a change in physical appearance. The client's feelings of being ugly do not support the diagnosis of *Powerlessness, Social Isolation,* and *Hopelessness*. **Cognitive Level:** Analyzing. **Client Need:** Psychosocial Integrity. **Nursing Process:** Diagnosis. **Learning Outcome:** 39-1.
6. **Answer:** 3. **Rationale:** Self-awareness consists of the relationship between own and others' perceptions of the individual. The other options reflect only how the nurse sees himself or herself. **Cognitive Level:** Analyzing. **Client Need:** Psychosocial Integrity. **Nursing Process:** Evaluation. **Learning Outcome:** 39-2.
7. **Answer:** 1. **Rationale:** The first information the nurse gathers when assessing self-concept should focus on the client's personal identity. Option 2 assesses role performance. Option 3 assesses social role and option 4 assesses work role. **Cognitive Level:** Applying. **Client Need:** Psychosocial Integrity. **Nursing Process:** Assessment. **Learning Outcome:** 39-6.
8. **Answer:** 2. **Rationale:** Options 1 and 3 are dismissive of the client's concerns. Medication for leg swelling is usually not needed in pregnancy. By asking the client to talk more about her concerns, the nurse can explore the client's feelings and views regarding the changes she is experiencing in her body and can find ways on how to appropriately address such concerns. **Cognitive Level:** Analyzing. **Client Need:** Psychosocial Integrity. **Nursing Process:** Assessment. **Learning Outcome:** 39-4.
9. **Answer:** 2 and 3. **Rationale:** The client with poor self-concept should be encouraged to say positive self-statements and minimize negative ones. Such clients should not be encouraged to compare themselves with others (option 1). Having them care for others can be a very therapeutic intervention for such individuals (option 4). They should be given realistic and normal levels of expectations for their behavior. **Cognitive Level:** Applying. **Client Need:** Psychosocial Integrity. **Nursing Process:** Implementation. **Learning Outcome:** 39-6.
10. **Answer:** 4. **Rationale:** The social self is how one is perceived by others and is difficult, if not impossible, to influence since the client does not control the viewpoints of others. With planning, the number of the client's resources can be increased, self-knowledge improved, and core self-concept broadened since these are within the client's control. **Cognitive Level:** Analyzing. **Client Need:** Psychosocial Integrity. **Nursing Process:** Planning. **Learning Outcome:** 39-3.

CHAPTER 40 Sexuality

1. **Answer:** 4. **Rationale:** Clients still may feel shame and discomfort regarding sexuality. Most clients assume that providers have a great deal of information (option 1). Many clients have questions and concerns (option 2). Although talking with someone of the same gender may make it easier for some women, it is not a requirement for assessment and intervention (option 3). **Cognitive Level:** Analyzing. **Client Need:** Health Promotion and Maintenance. **Nursing Process:** Planning. **Learning Outcome:** 40-1.
2. **Answer:** 1. **Rationale:** Androgyny has nothing to do with gender attraction or with repression of sexual feelings (options 2 and 3). Androgynous individuals do not hold rigid stereotyped gender role expectations since androgyny means flexibility in gender roles (option 4). **Cognitive Level:** Analyzing. **Client Need:** Health Promotion and Maintenance. **Nursing Process:** Assessment. **Learning Outcome:** 40-3.
3. **Answer:** 2. **Rationale:** In this situation, the nurse should quickly and politely leave the room. Masturbation is not harmful to sexual well-being (option 1). It is inappropriate to ask the client to stop so that care can be provided (option 3). Masturbation does not indicate sexual concerns that should be discussed (option 4). **Cognitive Level:** Applying. **Client Need:** Health Promotion and Maintenance. **Nursing Process:** Implementation. **Learning Outcome:** 40-5.
4. **Answer:** 3. **Rationale:** Clients with vaginismus experience involuntary spasm of the outer one-third of the vaginal muscles. This spasm makes internal examination, tampon use, and intercourse difficult. Use of smaller than normal vaginal speculums may make examination easier. **Cognitive Level:** Applying. **Client Need:** Health Promotion and Maintenance. **Nursing Process:** Planning. **Learning Outcome:** 40-8.
5. **Answer:** 4. **Rationale:** More information is needed before intervening. Also, the client needs the opportunity to express her feelings. Option 1 is an unprofessional response and false reassurance. The ANA *Code of Ethics* indicates that clients are entitled to a timely and appropriate response to their needs. Option 2 suggests postponing the discussion and that the primary care provider is the better healthcare provider to deal with her concerns, which is untrue. Option 3 represents feeding into her negative self-concept and inappropriate self-disclosure. **Cognitive Level:** Applying. **Client Need:** Health Promotion and Maintenance. **Nursing Process:** Implementation. **Learning Outcome:** 40-4.
6. **Answer:** 1. **Rationale:** Dyspareunia is painful intercourse. Knowledge of the partner's awareness will contribute to resolution. Involuntary vaginal spasms are called vaginismus (option 2). Painful menstruation is called dysmenorrhea (option 3). Breast swelling can occur during portions of the menstrual cycle but is unrelated to painful intercourse (option 4). **Cognitive Level:** Analyzing. **Client Need:** Health Promotion and Maintenance. **Nursing Process:** Assessment. **Learning Outcomes:** 40-6; 40-7.
7. **Answer:** 3. **Rationale:** Antihypertensive medications are known to affect sexual functioning in several different ways, so some focused history questions would be indicated. There is no evidence of a relationship between sexual functioning and anti-inflammatories, hypnotics, or antihistamines (options 1, 2, and 4). However, the underlying condition that leads the client to take other medications could be important. Side effects of any medication could impact sexual interest or energy level, which reinforces the importance of including taking a sexual health history for all clients. **Cognitive Level:** Applying. **Client Need:** Health Promotion and Maintenance. **Nursing Process:** Assessment. **Learning Outcomes**: 40-6; 40-7; 40-8.
8. **Answer:** 2. **Rationale:** LI includes instructing clients regarding when sexual activity is safe or unsafe. P involves giving permission to be sexual beings and to discuss issues (option 1). SS includes specific suggestions that help clients promote optimal functioning (option 3). Intensive therapy (IT) requires special skills offered by a nurse specialist or sex therapist (option 4). **Cognitive Level:** Analyzing. **Client Need:** Health Promotion and Maintenance. **Nursing Process:** Implementation. **Learning Outcomes:** 40-1; 40-9.
9. **Answer:** 4. **Rationale:** A change in sexual frequency is not abnormal but may suggest an opportunity to improve his knowledge. It does not suggest pathology or altered body image (options 1 and 2). It would be incorrect to assume his lifestyle is inactive merely because the frequency of his sexual activity has decreased (option 3). Further assessment of the reason for the decrease in sexual activity is indicated. **Cognitive Level:** Applying. **Client Need:** Health Promotion and Maintenance. **Nursing Process:** Diagnosing. **Learning Outcomes:** 40-1; 40-2; 40-4; 40-8.

10. **Answer:** 3. **Rationale:** The key term is *ineffective*. If the suggestions given by the nurse are ineffective in reaching the desired goals, the client may require intervention from someone with more specialized skills. Verbalizing constructive methods of modifying sexual activity are healthy responses and do not require a more skilled therapist (option 1). The generalist nurse can refer the client to education and support groups (option 2). Experimenting with new sexual activities is probably a healthy direction and does not suggest the need for referral (option 4). **Cognitive Level:** Understanding. **Client Need:** Health Promotion and Maintenance. **Nursing Process:** Evaluation. **Learning Outcome:** 40-8.

CHAPTER 41 Spirituality

1. **Answer:** 2, 3 and 4. **Rationale:** A nurse should not impose her religious beliefs on her clients, who might be vulnerable. The nurse's role in the spiritual care of a client is to help the latter find strength and solace in their own beliefs. Therefore, Option 1 is not acceptable. Option 2 is correct as a private and quiet environment is conducive for praying. Options 3 and 4 denote offering support and facilitating the client's spiritual needs. However, the nurse should leave the room if the client wishes to pray alone. If it is requested by the client, the nurse should arrange a meeting between the client and his/her religious representative.
2. **Answer:** 3. **Rationale:** The client can be asked general questions to elicit information about what beliefs and practices are important to the present health care situation, and what, if anything, the client would like from the health care team to support spiritual health. Offering to pray with the client is over the boundary of professional practice unless the client requests such intervention and the nurse is comfortable with the arrangement (options 1 and 2). At this point, there is no information that indicates the client is in need of referral for counseling. This would occur only if the client demonstrates spiritual distress at the level best handled by a specialist (option 4). **Cognitive Level:** Applying. **Client Need:** Psychosocial Integrity. **Nursing Process:** Implementation. **Learning Outcomes:** 41-5; 41-6.
3. **Answer:** 3. **Rationale:** The key term is *full*. Option 1 would be inadequate, option 2 is only partial presencing, and option 4 is transcendent presencing. **Cognitive Level:** Remembering. **Client Need:** Psychosocial Integrity. **Nursing Process:** Implementation. **Learning Outcome:** 41-5.
4. **Answer:** 3. **Rationale:** This client portrays no disruption (option 1) or potential for disruption (option 2), but rather the potential for enhanced spiritual health as a result of the transformative illness experience. Option 4 is not a valid diagnosis. **Cognitive Level:** Applying. **Client Need:** Psychosocial Integrity. **Nursing Process:** Diagnosis. **Learning Outcomes:** 41-1; 41-2.
5. **Answer:** 4. **Rationale:** Assessment is always the first step of the process of spiritual caregiving or any nursing activity. Options 1, 2, and 3 may not respect the spiritual beliefs of either the nurse or the client. While an assessment may lead the nurse to share personal beliefs, these are never urged on the client. **Cognitive Level:** Applying. **Client Need:** Psychosocial Integrity. **Nursing Process:** Implementation. **Learning Outcomes:** 41-1; 41-6; 41-7.
6. **Answer:** 4. **Rationale:** The nurse should wait in the hall until the prayer is over and the client or family give permission to enter the room. **Cognitive Level:** Applying. **Client Need:** Psychosocial Integrity. **Nursing Process:** Implementation. **Learning Outcome:** 41-6.
7. **Answer:** 3. **Rationale:** Options 1, 2, and 4 are potentially uncaring or unethical. Jehovah's Witnesses have a well-developed network of representatives who can be called to explain and explore medical options with their fellow believers and medical staff. **Cognitive Level:** Analyzing. **Client Need:** Psychosocial Integrity. **Nursing Process:** Evaluation. **Learning Outcomes:** 41-1; 41-5; 41-7.
8. **Answer:** 2. **Rationale:** Residing in the skilled nursing facility likely will curb the client's participation in her church. Options 1, 3, and 4 are incorrect because it is not known if the relocation or an alteration in religious practice will affect her spiritual health in either a negative or positive way. **Cognitive Level:** Applying. **Client Need:** Psychosocial Integrity. **Nursing Process:** Diagnosis. **Learning Outcomes:** 41-1; 41-2; 41-4.
9. **Answer:** 1, 2, 4, 5. **Rationale:** Option 3 is a question used for identifying significant values. **Cognitive Level:** Applying. **Client Need:** Psychosocial Integrity. **Nursing Process:** Assessment. **Learning Outcome:** 41-8.
10. **Answer:** 1. **Rationale:** Although the mother is arguably angry, it is unknown whether this anger is impairing her religiosity or her coping. More data are needed before determining that either option 2 or 3 is the best diagnosis. The mother is experiencing distress versus being at risk for it (option 4). **Cognitive Level:** Applying. **Client Need:** Psychosocial Integrity. **Nursing Process:** Diagnosis. **Learning Outcomes:** 41-2; 41-4.

CHAPTER 42 Stress and Coping

1. **Answer:** 1. **Rationale:** Short-term coping strategies can reduce stress to a tolerable limit temporarily but are ineffective ways to deal with reality permanently. They can even have a destructive or detrimental effect on the person. An example of short-term strategies is using alcoholic beverages or drugs. **Cognitive Level:** Analyzing. **Client Need:** Psychosocial Integrity. **Nursing Process:** Assessment. **Learning Outcome:** 42-6.
2. **Answer:** 2. **Rationale:** In this situation, the best alternative is to be certain that the nurses are well prepared for the responsibilities of their jobs, as the frustration of being unprepared leads to burnout. Asking physicians to assume nursing tasks is not appropriate. Counseling and exercise cannot be made requirements for the staff. **Cognitive Level:** Applying. **Client Need:** Psychosocial Integrity. **Nursing Process:** Planning. **Learning Outcome:** 42-9.
3. **Answer:** 1. **Rationale:** In the transaction model, stress is a very personal experience and varies widely among individuals. Option 2 represents the stimulus model, and option 3 represents the response model of stress. In option 4, external resources and support are a factor in determining stress levels but omit the key aspects of internal personal influences. **Cognitive Level:** Applying. **Client Need:** Psychosocial Integrity. **Nursing Process:** Assessment. **Learning Outcome:** 42-1.
4. **Answer:** 3. **Rationale:** With stress, respirations increase, pupils dilate, peripheral blood vessels constrict, and the heart rate increases. **Cognitive Level:** Applying. **Client Need:** Psychosocial Integrity. **Nursing Process:** Assessment. **Learning Outcome:** 42-3.
5. **Answer:** 4. **Rationale:** *Defensive Coping* is the repeated projection of falsely positive self-evaluation based on a self-protective pattern that defends against underlying perceived threats to positive self-regard. **Cognitive Level:** Analyzing. **Client Need:** Psychosocial Integrity. **Nursing Process:** Diagnosing. **Learning Outcome:** 42-8.
6. **Answer:** 1, 3, and 4. **Rationale:** Common stressors among young adults include marriage, starting a new job, and leaving the parental home. Stressors from aging parents are more common among middle-aged adults (option 2); decreased physical abilities is a stressor in older adults (option 5); and changing body structure serves as a stressor in both children and older adults (option 6). **Cognitive Level:** Understanding. **Client Need:** Psychosocial Integrity. **Nursing Process:** Planning. **Learning Outcome:** 42-7.

7. **Answer:** 2. **Rationale:** All four areas of health promotion strategies may be important, but for this client sleep is likely to be the most adversely affected by travel in which changing time zones and unfamiliar sleeping quarters are common. It is easier for clients to adapt to modifying exercise (option 1), nutrition (option 3), and time management (option 4) during travel than it is to control sleep. Thus, it becomes the most important area requiring intervention to avoid worsening the existing stress. **Cognitive Level:** Applying. **Client Need:** Psychosocial Integrity. **Nursing Process:** Implementation. **Learning Outcome:** 42-9.
8. **Answer:** 4. **Rationale:** Unless the nurse feels in physical danger, it is important to remain with the client, allow the anger to dissipate, and then begin assessing the cause. Leaving the room provides no therapeutic action (option 1). Option 2 may be considered setting limits, which can be helpful, but cannot occur until the client is calmer. All behavior is meaningful; it is inappropriate to ignore the client's behavior (option 3). **Cognitive Level:** Applying. **Client Need:** Psychosocial Integrity. **Nursing Process:** Implementation. **Learning Outcome:** 42-9.
9. **Answer:** 1. **Rationale:** This client is exhibiting severe anxiety and, therefore, learning is impaired but not impossible (see Table 42.2). Therefore, it is most appropriate for the nurse to teach only those things that are critical for the client to learn at this time. The nurse also recognizes that learning may not be retained at this level of anxiety and plans to reinforce the teaching when the client is less anxious. **Cognitive Level:** Applying. **Client Need:** Psychosocial Integrity. **Nursing Process:** Planning. **Learning Outcome:** 42-4.
10. **Answer:** 1, 2, and 4. **Rationale:** Compensation (option 1) may allow the client to overcome a weakness. Displacement (option 2) allows the client to express feelings safely. Repression (option 4) protects the client from further emotional trauma until able to cope. Minimization (option 3) prevents the client from accepting responsibility for actions. Regression (option 5) returns the client to a lower or previous developmental level. *Note:* Each of these may be more or less effective defenses depending on the exact context of the situation. **Cognitive Level:** Understanding. **Client Need:** Psychosocial Integrity. **Nursing Process:** Assessment. **Learning Outcome:** 42-5.

CHAPTER 43 Loss, Grieving, and Death

1. **Answer:** 1, 2, and 3. **Rationale:** Correct answers include abbreviated (normal grief that is briefly experienced), anticipatory grief (experienced before the loss or death but appropriate), and disenfranchised grief (the emotions are felt privately, just not expressed in public). Unhealthy abnormal types of grief include complicated grief (option 4) in several different forms: Unresolved grief is extended in length and severity (option 5). With inhibited grief, symptoms are suppressed, and other effects, including somatic, are experienced instead (option 6). **Cognitive Level:** Remembering. **Client Need:** Psychosocial Integrity. **Nursing Process:** Diagnosing. **Learning Outcome:** 43-2.
2. **Answer:** 1, 2, 4, 5. **Rationale:** The nurse should not permit the family to view the client before cleaning and care are provided. **Cognitive Level:** Applying. **Client Need:** Psychosocial Integrity. **Nursing Process:** Implementation. **Learning Outcome:** 43-8.
3. **Answer:** 1. **Rationale:** This statement acknowledges the family's grief simply. Avoid statements that may be interpreted as overly impersonal (option 2), false support (option 3), or harsh (option 4). **Cognitive Level:** Application. **Client Need:** Psychosocial Integrity. **Nursing Process:** Implementation. **Learning Outcome:** 43-8.
4. **Answer:** 3. **Rationale:** Until children are about 5 years old, they believe that death is reversible. Between ages 5 and 9, the child knows death is irreversible but believes it can be avoided (option 2). Between 9 and 12 years of age, the child recognizes that he or she, too, will someday die (option 3). At 12 to 18 years old, the child builds on previous beliefs and may fear death, but often pretends not to care about it (option 4). **Cognitive Level:** Remembering. **Client Need:** Psychosocial Integrity. **Nursing Process:** Assessment. **Learning Outcome:** 43-4.
5. **Answer:** 4. **Rationale:** Adaptive responses indicate the client can put the loss into perspective and begin to develop strategies for coping with the loss. Although the other options are responses the client might likely give and feel, and are not pathologic, they do not demonstrate movement toward a goal of adaptation or problem-solving. **Cognitive Level:** Application. **Client Need:** Psychosocial Integrity. **Nursing Process:** Evaluation. **Learning Outcome:** 43-3.
6. **Answer:** 1. **Rationale:** The nurse needs to assess and explore the meaning of the client's crying. Options 2 and 4 leap to assumptions about the meaning of the tears and ignore the possibility of the client's distress. Option 3 suggests that the client has the same feelings as the nurse, which may not be correct. **Cognitive Level:** Application. **Client Need:** Psychosocial Integrity. **Nursing Process:** Implementation. **Learning Outcome:** 43-3.
7. **Answer:** 1. **Rationale:** The nurse must be certain that the advance directive is a legal document. In some states, relatives, heirs, and physicians cannot witness an advance directive. This is to prevent potential abuse of power. **Cognitive Level:** Analyzing. **Client Need:** Psychosocial Integrity. **Nursing Process:** Planning. **Learning Outcome:** 43-5.
8. **Answer:** 4. **Rationale:** To plan with and assist the family, the nurse needs more data regarding the family's reactions to their loss. Information on issues such as insurance coverage (option 1) can wait until later and may be more appropriately the responsibility of social services rather than the nurse. It is important for the nurse to determine their understanding of their injuries but they are stated as not life-threatening (option 2). Once the nurse has assessed the family's responses it will be important to determine availability of outside resources to assist them (option 3). **Cognitive Level:** Analyzing. **Client Need:** Psychosocial Integrity. **Nursing Process:** Assessment. **Learning Outcome:** 43-1.
9. **Answer:** 2. **Rationale:** If the client feels that his terminal state is a reflection of failure of the medical system, this fear of abandonment is common. It may not be totally unfounded because failing to cure a client is frustrating and may reflect in the care provided to the client. While nurses do provide much of the care given to terminal clients, physicians continue to be an integral part of care. **Cognitive Level:** Application. **Client Need:** Psychosocial Integrity. **Nursing Process:** Assessment. **Learning Outcome:** 43-3.
10. **Answer:** 1. **Rationale:** Assisting the client to die with dignity involves allowing the client to participate in and choose the direction of the remainder of his or her life. Sharing the nurse's own views about life after death (option 2) does not enhance client dignity. The nurse should not assume that avoiding talking about dying and emphasizing the present (option 3) is therapeutic for the client. Only if the client wishes to have someone else perform care is doing so supporting death with dignity (option 4). Otherwise, it may have the opposite effect. **Cognitive Level:** Application. **Client Need:** Psychological Integrity. **Nursing Process:** Planning. **Learning Outcome:** 43-7.

CHAPTER 44 Activity and Exercise

1. **Answer:** 4. **Rationale:** Research has shown that the only option that has any influence on frequency of back injury is a policy prohibiting solo lifting. Body mechanisms training, physical fitness, and wearing a back belt do not prevent injury.

Cognitive Level: Applying. **Client Need:** Health Promotion and Maintenance. **Nursing Process:** Planning. **Learning Outcome:** 44-7.

2. **Answer:** 1. **Rationale:** Weight bearing helps to move calcium back into the bone, thereby strengthening them. A standard intervention for those attempting to prevent or reverse osteoporosis is beginning an exercise plan that includes weight-bearing activities. Additional calcium in the diet after osteoporosis has begun is not thought to be effective (option 2). Strict bed rest may well make the osteoporosis worse because there is no weight-bearing activity (option 3). Assisted range-of-motion exercises are not weight-bearing and do not help delay or reverse osteoporosis (option 4). **Cognitive Level:** Applying. **Client Need:** Physiological Integrity. **Nursing Process:** Planning. **Learning Outcome:** 44-2.
3. **Answer:** 1. **Rationale:** Vital signs that do not return to baseline 5 minutes after exercising indicate intolerance of exercise at that time. This is a real problem, not "potential for," as in option 2. There is no evidence that the client has self-esteem problems (option 3), or is in danger of falling (option 4). **Cognitive Level:** Analyzing. **Client Need:** Physiological Integrity. **Nursing Process:** Diagnosis. **Learning Outcome:** 44-6.
4. **Answer:** 3. **Rationale:** Although the crutches (or cane) are always used along with the weaker leg, the weaker leg should go down the stairs first. The stronger leg can support the body as the weaker leg moves forward. All of the other statements are correct. **Cognitive Level:** Analyzing. **Client Need:** Physiological Integrity. **Nursing Process:** Evaluation. **Learning Outcome:** 44-9.
5. **Answer:** 3. **Rationale:** Range-of-motion exercising should never cause discomfort. In this case, the best action is to reduce the movement of the joint just until the point of slight resistance is felt and evaluate the pain response at that level. If there is no pain, the exercise can be continued. Stopping the treatment is not justified until an assessment occurs (options 1 and 2). Continuing at the same level of intensity may cause damage to the joint as well as cause the client pain (option 4). **Cognitive Level:** Applying. **Client Need:** Physiological Integrity. **Nursing Process:** Implementation. **Learning Outcome:** 44-8.
6. **Answer:** 1. **Rationale:** Normal gait involves a level gaze, an initial rotation beginning in the spine, heel strike with follow-through to the toes, and opposite arm and leg swinging forward. **Cognitive Level:** Applying. **Client Need:** Physiological Integrity. **Nursing Process:** Assessment. **Learning Outcome:** 44-5.
7. **Answer:** 1, 4, and 5. **Rationale:** Eating and bathing will flex the elbow joint, and grasping and manipulating utensils to eat and write will take the thumb through its normal ROM. Walking flexes the hip. Shaving and eating require elbow flexion, not extension (option 2). Writing brings the fingers toward the inner aspect of the forearm, thus flexing the wrist joint (option 3). **Cognitive Level:** Applying. **Client Need:** Health Promotion and Maintenance. **Nursing Process:** Implementation. **Learning Outcome:** 44-1.
8. **Answer:** 3. **Rationale:** It is prudent for nurses to understand and use proper body mechanics at all times to decrease risk, while keeping in mind the importance of assistive devices and help from other staff. While it is generally accepted that proper body mechanics alone will not prevent injury, many work settings do not yet have "no manual lift" and "no solo lift" policies and resources in place. **Cognitive Level:** Analyzing. **Client Need:** Safe, Effective Care Environment. **Nursing Process:** Implementation. **Learning Outcome:** 44-7.
9. **Answer:** 4. **Rationale:** Placing the client in a safe position is the best maneuver. Leaving the client creates unsafe conditions because the client may faint before being able to return to her room (options 1 and 2). Rapid, shallow breathing (hyperventilation) may increase the dizziness (option 3). **Cognitive Level:** Applying. **Client Need:** Safe, Effective Care Environment. **Nursing Process:** Implementation. **Learning Outcome:** 44-10g.
10. **Answer:** 2. **Rationale:** The reddened area of the skin can lead to skin breakdown. The other options are within normal limits. **Cognitive Level:** Applying. **Client Need:** Physiological Integrity. **Nursing Process:** Assessment. **Learning Outcome:** 44-3g.

CHAPTER 45 Sleep

1. **Answer:** 2. **Rationale:** This is the brainstem where the reticular formation (and RAS) is located and which integrates sensory information from the peripheral nervous system and relays the information to the cerebral cortex. An intact cerebral cortex and reticular formation are necessary for the regulation of sleep and waking states. **Cognitive Level:** Remembering. **Client Need:** Physiological Integrity. **Nursing Process:** Assessment. **Learning Outcome:** 45-1.
2. **Answer:** 1. **Rationale:** When a client is critically ill or being admitted for an outpatient procedure, sleep history can be omitted or deferred. **Cognitive Level:** Applying. **Client Need:** Physiological Integrity. **Nursing Process:** Assessment. **Learning Outcome:** 45-6.
3. **Answer:** 3. **Rationale:** The best outcome statement for this client is to report getting sufficient sleep to provide energy for daily activities. The client may require more than 8 hours of sleep to feel rested and have sufficient energy (option 1). Simply listing coping mechanisms for anxiety relief is not as helpful as actually getting sleep (option 2). Antianxiety medications are probably not the most important factor for this client (option 4). **Cognitive Level:** Applying. **Client Need:** Physiological Integrity. **Nursing Process:** Planning. **Learning Outcome:** 45-7.
4. **Answer:** 4. **Rationale:** Suddenly stopping barbiturate sleeping pills can precipitate a dangerous withdrawal. Doses should be tapered gradually and the tapering process supervised by the client's primary care provider. **Cognitive Level:** Analyzing. **Client Need:** Physiological Integrity. **Nursing Process:** Implementation. **Learning Outcome:** 45-4.
5. **Answer:** 1. **Rationale:** Preschool children require 10 to 12 hours of sleep per night. Young children often rise early, so it is more appropriate to put the child to bed earlier in the evening. **Cognitive Level:** Analyzing. **Client Need:** Health Promotion and Maintenance. **Nursing Process:** Implementation. **Learning Outcome:** 45-3.
6. **Answer:** 1. **Rationale:** Daytime hypersomnia is often due to medical conditions such as kidney, liver, or metabolic disturbances. The nurse should suggest that the client be evaluated by a physician. Daytime hypersomnia is rarely caused by psychologic issues. An over-the-counter sleep aid is not a good choice as the man already sleeps well at night and sleep aids can sometimes cause future sleep disturbances. Caffeinated beverages may increase daytime wakefulness but will not help any underlying problem that may be present. **Cognitive Level:** Applying. **Client Need:** Health Promotion and Maintenance. **Nursing Process:** Implementation. **Learning Outcome:** 45-6.
7. **Answer:** 4. **Rationale:** The client's symptoms, combined with his weight, suggest that he has obstructive sleep apnea and should be referred to a sleep disorders specialist for further evaluation. It would not be wrong to refer him to a dietitian for weight-loss counseling (option 2), but being evaluated by a sleep disorders specialist is more critical. Drinking alcohol or taking sleeping pills is not advised in clients with sleep apnea because they disrupt the client's sleep patterns (option 3). **Cognitive Level:** Analyzing. **Client Need:** Physiological Integrity. **Nursing Process:** Implementation. **Learning Outcome:** 45-5.

8. Answer: 1. **Rationale:** Reducing exposure to bright light in the morning, when driving home, and when going to sleep will make it easier to fall asleep after work. Exercising before going to bed will increase arousal (option 2). Caffeine consumed at the beginning of a 12-hour shift will not assist the nurse in remaining awake during the latter part of the shift (option 3). Although working in a brightly lit area will reduce drowsiness, this strategy is rarely available to nurses working the night shift; lights are often dimmed in hospital corridors and client rooms (option 4). **Cognitive Level:** Analyzing. **Client Need:** Health Promotion and Maintenance. **Nursing Process:** Implementation. **Learning Outcome:** 45-7.

9. Answer: 3. **Rationale:** Napping frequently reappears in older adults. Unless the client has difficulty falling asleep at night, there is no reason he should not be allowed to take a 15- to 20-minute nap in the early afternoon. **Cognitive Level:** Analyzing. **Client Need:** Health Promotion and Maintenance. **Nursing Process:** Implementation. **Learning Outcome:** 45-3.

10. Answer: 1, 3, and 4. **Rationale:** Reducing environmental noise, as well as the number of times she is disturbed for medications and vital signs, will reduce the likelihood that she will awaken during the night. Delivering necessary care at 1.5- or 3-hour intervals is consistent with multiples of the 90-minute sleep cycle. Since it is unlikely that all of the noise in the environment can be eliminated, using a fan to generate a steady background noise may help mask sounds of individuals talking, carts being moved through the halls, and other noise. Music is not usually recommended because it can be interesting to listen to, thus encouraging wakefulness (option 2). The room temperature needs to be satisfactory for the client. A room that is too warm is not usually conducive for sleep (option 5). **Cognitive Level:** Analyzing. **Client Need:** Physiological Integrity. **Nursing Process:** Implementation. **Learning Outcome:** 45-8.

CHAPTER 46 Nutrition

1. Answer: 4. **Rationale:** Fluid intake for each feeding is not entered on the graphic sheet. The amount of fluid for a 24-hour period would be documented on this sheet (option 1). Fluid intake for tube feedings is not documented in the dietary consultation notes or the vital signs record (options 3 and 4). **Cognitive Level:** Applying. **Client Need:** Health Promotion and Maintenance. **Nursing Process:** Implementation. **Learning Outcome:** 46-13.

2. Answer: 4. **Rationale:** This client needs more grains in the diet. The client should have 6 to 7 oz grains per day, 3 cups/week dark green vegetables, 2 cups/week orange vegetables, 3 cups/week legumes, 3 cups/week starchy vegetables, 1.5 to 2 cups fruit per day, 5 to 6 oz meat and beans per day, and 3 cups milk, yogurt, and cheese per day. **Cognitive Level:** Applying. **Client Need:** Health Promotion and Maintenance. **Nursing Process:** Planning. **Learning Outcome:** 46-5.

3. Answer: 4. **Rationale:** Anthropometric measurements, such as triceps skinfold measurement, provide the most meaningful data when monitored over longer periods of time, such as several months to years. The changes in this measurement occur so slowly that remeasuring in 2 days to one month would not provide significant data. **Cognitive Level:** Applying. **Client Need:** Physiological Integrity. **Nursing Process:** Implementation. **Learning Outcome:** 46-9.

4. Answer: 2. **Rationale:** Swallowing ice or water may help calm the gag reflex and also facilitate the "swallowing" of the tube. This is a common response to the presence of a tube in the oropharynx, so removal of the tube is not necessary (option 1). The nurse should not use pressure to pass the tube (option 3). The client's head should be tilted forward at this point. Tilting the head back will open the airway, not the esophagus (option 4). **Cognitive Level:** Analyzing. **Client Need:** Physiological Integrity. **Nursing Process:** Evaluation. **Learning Outcome:** 46-10a.

5. Answer: 1. **Rationale:** For proper flow, the feeding container hangs 1 foot above the tube insertion. Feedings may be administered if there is less than 90 to 100 mL of residual volume (unless agency policy specifies otherwise) (option 2). To prevent or reduce the risk of aspiration, the client should be placed in Fowler's position during feeding (option 3). The feeding should be warmed to room temperature before administration to decrease cramping and diarrhea (option 4). **Cognitive Level:** Applying. **Client Need:** Physiological Integrity. **Nursing Process:** Implementation. **Learning Outcome:** 46-10c.

6. Answer: 1. **Rationale:** The Dietary Guidelines recommend 30 minutes of physical activity on most days of the week to achieve optimal weight. Some individuals benefit from a low-carbohydrate diet, but no particular diet is the solution for all individuals (option 2). A reasonable diet emphasizes balance and portion control rather than forbidding or requiring any specific foods (option 3). Fresh and chemical-free foods may be healthier than preserved foods but do not automatically assist with weight loss (option 4). **Cognitive Level:** Analyzing. **Client Need:** Health Promotion and Maintenance. **Nursing Process:** Evaluation. **Learning Outcome:** 46-8.

7. Answer: 3. **Rationale:** Always inquire into the client's favorite foods when planning a diet. Dairy may not be indicated for this client due to the high incidence of lactose intolerance in individuals of Asian heritage (option 1). Beer can be a source of calories and, in moderation, is not harmful, and may maintain the client's satisfaction with the dietary changes. The nurse will need to assess the ability to swallow beer safely, however (option 2). Calories from lipid sources should be kept below 35% and, when enhanced wound healing is indicated (not so with a stroke), increased protein and carbohydrates are needed rather than fats (option 4). **Cognitive Level:** Applying. **Client Need:** Health Promotion and Maintenance. **Nursing Process:** Planning. **Learning Outcome:** 46-9.

8. Answer: This client has lost 13 pounds, which is 6.7%: (195 − 182)/195 over the 2 months. If the weight loss was steady during the past 2 months, that would indicate a 3.3% loss per month. Less than 5% loss in 1 month is not significant (option 1). However, if this loss continues, the client will exceed 7.5 % over 3 months (option 2) and reach a 10% loss in 3 months, which is a severe loss (option 3). A more detailed assessment is indicated to determine the client's nutritional status. **Cognitive Level:** Applying. **Client Need:** Health Promotion and Maintenance. **Nursing Process:** Assessment. **Learning Outcome:** 46-6; 46-7; 46-8.

9. Answer: 2. **Rationale:** A small-bore nasal feeding tube tip is most commonly placed in the stomach. Option 1 indicates the esophagus. A tube tip placed there can lead to aspiration. Option 3 indicates the postpyloric duodenum. Small-bore nasal tubes can be advanced to this location if desired but such a placement is less common than gastric placement. Option 4 indicates the jejunum, where feeding tubes can be placed but usually not from a nasally placed tube. **Cognitive Level:** Understanding. **Client Need:** Physiological Integrity. **Nursing Process:** Evaluation. **Learning Outcome:** 46-10a.

10. Answer: 4. **Rationale:** 3 ounces tuna + 2 slices whole wheat bread = 3.1 mg Fe; 1 ounce cheese = ~200 mg Ca^{2+}; pear = 4.2 g fiber. Option 1: 1/3 cup raisins = 1.75 mg Fe; 3 ounces 3 ounces cottage cheese = 90 mg Ca^{2+}; 1 banana = 2.1 g fiber. Option 3: 1/2 cup spaghetti + 2 ounces ground beef = 2.3 mg Fe; 1/2 cup ice cream = 97 mg Ca^{2+}; 1/2 cup lima beans = 3.2 g fiber. Option 2: 3 ounces chicken + 1/2 cup peanuts = 2.9 mg Fe; 1/2 cup broccoli = ~158 mg Ca^{2+}; 1/2 cup broccoli = 2.4 g fiber. **Cognitive Level:** Applying. **Client Need:** Health Promotion and Maintenance. **Nursing Process:** Implementation. **Learning Outcome:** 46-1.

CHAPTER 47 Urinary Elimination

1. **Answer:** 3. **Rationale 1:** When aldosterone is released from the adrenal cortex, sodium and water are reabsorbed in greater quantities, increasing blood volume and decreasing urinary output. Elevated aldosterone levels will not increase urine output, urinary incontinence, or urinary retention (options 1, 2, and 4). **Cognitive Level:** Analyzing. **Client Need:** Physiological Integrity. **Nursing Process:** Assessment. **Learning Outcome:** 47-2.
2. **Answer:** 3, 4. **Rationale:** Residual urine is not measured to evaluate glomerular filtration rate, to determine the extent of renal failure, or to evaluate fluid volume status. **Cognitive Level:** Analyzing. **Client Need:** Physiological Integrity. **Nursing Process:** Assessment. **Learning Outcome:** 47-4.
3. **Answer:** 4. **Rationale:** The nurse should make sure that the tip of the penis is not touching the condom and that the condom is not twisted, because a twisted condom could obstruct the flow of urine. The nurse should wash her hands before and after the procedure (option 1). The nurse should document after the procedure is completed (option 2). The nurse should instruct the client about the drainage system after attaching the bag to the device (option 3). **Cognitive Level:** Applying. **Client Need:** Safe, Effective Care Environment. **Nursing Process:** Implementation. **Learning Outcome:** 47-10a.
4. **Answer:** 1. **Rationale:** The catheter in the vagina is contaminated and cannot be reused. If left in place, it may help avoid mistaking the vaginal opening for the urinary meatus. A single failure to catheterize the meatus does not indicate that another nurse is needed although sometimes a second nurse can assist in visualizing the meatus (option 2). **Cognitive Level:** Applying. **Client Need:** Safe, Effective Care Environment. **Nursing Process:** Implementation. **Learning Outcome:** 47-10b.
5. **Answer:** 2. **Rationale:** Option 2 is the correct sequence. Option 1 is incorrect because the nurse needs to perform hand hygiene after providing pericare. Option 3 is incorrect because the outside of the kit is not sterile and the nurse would not open the kit with sterile gloves. The current best practice is to not pre-inflate the balloon (option 4). **Cognitive Level:** Analyzing. **Client Need:** Health Promotion and Maintenance. **Nursing Process:** Evaluation. **Learning Outcome:** 47-10b.
6. **Answer:** 4. **Rationale:** The key phrase is "the urge to void." Option 1 occurs when the client coughs, sneezes, or jars the body, resulting in accidental loss of urine. Option 2 occurs with involuntary loss of urine at somewhat predictable intervals when a specific bladder volume is reached. Option 3 is involuntary loss of urine related to impaired function. **Cognitive Level:** Applying. **Client Need:** Physiological Integrity. **Nursing Process:** Diagnosis. **Learning Outcome:** 47-6.
7. **Answer:** 2 and 4. **Rationale:** Option 2 validates the diagnosis. Cotton underwear promotes appropriate exposure to air, resulting in decreased bacterial growth (option 4). Increased fluids decrease concentration and irritation (option 1). The client should wipe the perineal area from front to back to prevent spread of bacteria from the rectal area to the urethra (option 3). Showers reduce exposure of the area to bacteria (option 5). **Cognitive Level:** Applying. **Client Need:** Health Promotion and Maintenance. **Nursing Process:** Implementation. **Learning Outcome:** 47-7.
8. **Answer:** 2. **Rationale:** The ileal conduit and vesicostomy (options 1 and 4) are incontinent urinary diversions, and clients are required to use an external ostomy appliance to contain the urine. Clients with a neobladder can control their voiding (option 3). **Cognitive Level:** Analyzing. **Client Need:** Health Promotion and Maintenance. **Nursing Process:** Assessment. **Learning Outcome:** 47-9.
9. **Answer:** 3. **Rationale:** Because the bladder muscles will not contract to increase the intrabladder pressure to promote urination, the process is initiated manually. Options 1, 2, and 4: To promote continence, bladder contractions are required for habit training, bladder training, and increasing the tone of the pelvic floor muscles. **Cognitive Level:** Applying. **Client Need:** Physiological Integrity. **Nursing Process:** Implementation. **Learning Outcome:** 47-9.
10. **Answer:** 2 and 5. **Rationale:** It is important for the client to inhibit the urge-to-void sensation when a premature urge is experienced. Some clients may need diapers; this is not the best indicator of a successful program (option 3). Citrus juices may irritate the bladder (option 4). Carbonated beverages increase diuresis and the risk of incontinence (option 4). **Cognitive Level:** Applying. **Client Need:** Health Promotion and Maintenance. **Nursing Process:** Evaluation. **Learning Outcome:** 47-6.

CHAPTER 48 Fecal Elimination

1. **Answer:** 2. **Rationale:** Normal defecation is facilitated by thigh flexion, which increases the pressure within the abdomen, and a sitting position, which increases the downward pressure on the rectum. Expulsion of the feces is assisted by contraction of the abdominal muscles and the diaphragm, which increases abdominal pressure, and by contraction of the muscles of the pelvic floor, which moves the feces through the anal canal. **Cognitive Level:** Applying. **Client Need:** Physiological Integrity. **Nursing Process:** Implementation. **Learning Outcome:** 48-1.
2. **Answer:** 1, 2, 3, 5. **Rationale:** Older adults should be advised that normal patterns of bowel elimination vary considerably. For some, a normal pattern might be every other day; for others, twice a day. Constipation can be relieved by increasing the fiber intake to 20–35 grams per day. Adequate exercise is a preventative measure for constipation. Daily fluid intake of 6–8 glasses is an essential preventive measure for constipation. Responding to the gastrocolic reflex, and not ignoring it, also helps with constipation. **Cognitive Level:** Applying. **Client Need:** Physiological Integrity. **Nursing Process:** Implementation. **Learning Outcome:** 48-3.
3. **Answer:** 1. **Rationale:** Oil retention enemas take effect within 1–3 hours. Enemas using a hypertonic solution take effect in 5–10 minutes. Soapsuds enemas take effect in 10–15 minutes. Enemas using hypotonic or isotonic solutions take effect in 10–20 minutes. **Cognitive Level:** Applying. **Client Need:** Health Promotion and Maintenance. **Nursing Process:** Implementation. **Learning Outcome:** 48-8.
4. **Answer:** 3. **Rationale:** An established stoma should be dark pink like the color of the buccal mucosa and is slightly raised above the abdomen. The skin under the appliance may remain pink or red for a while after the adhesive is pulled off. Feces from an ascending ostomy are very liquid, less so from a transverse ostomy, and more solid from a descending or sigmoid stoma. **Cognitive Level:** Applying. **Client Need:** Physiological Integrity. **Nursing Process:** Assessment. **Learning Outcome:** 48-9.
5. **Answer:** 2. **Rationale:** Once the cause of diarrhea has been identified and corrected, the client should return to his or her previous elimination pattern. This is not an example of an allergy to the antibiotic but a common consequence of overgrowth of bowel organisms not killed by the drug (option 1). Antidiarrheal medications are usually prescribed according to the number of stools, not routinely around the clock (option 3). Increasing intake of soluble fiber such as oatmeal or potatoes may help absorb excess liquid and decrease the diarrhea, but insoluble fiber will not (option 4). **Cognitive Level:** Analyzing. **Client Need:** Physiological Integrity. **Nursing Process:** Planning. **Learning Outcome:** 48-6.
6. **Answer:** 2. **Rationale:** The client has assessment findings consistent with complications of surgery. Option 1: Irrigating

the stoma is a dependent nursing action, and is also intervention without appropriate assessment. Option 3: Assessing the peristomal skin area is an independent action, but administering an antiemetic is an intervention without appropriate assessment. Antiemetics are generally ordered to treat immediate postoperative nausea, not several days postoperative. Option 4: Administering a bulk-forming laxative to a nauseated postoperative client is contraindicated. **Cognitive Level:** Analyzing. **Client Need:** Physiological Integrity. **Nursing Process:** Implementation. **Learning Outcome:** 48-6.

7. **Answer:** 3. **Rationale:** This provides relief of postoperative flatus, stimulating bowel motility. Options 1, 2, and 4 manage constipation and do not provide flatus relief. **Cognitive Level:** Applying. **Client Need:** Physiological Integrity. **Nursing Process:** Implementation. **Learning Outcome:** 48-8.
8. **Answer:** 3. **Rationale:** Blood in the upper GI tract is black and tarry. Option 1 can be a sign of malabsorption in an infant, option 2 is normal stool, and option 4 is characteristic of an obstructive condition of the rectum. **Cognitive Level:** Analyzing. **Client Need:** Health Promotion and Maintenance. **Nursing Process:** Assessment. **Learning Outcome:** 48-2.
9. **Answer:** 1, 3, 4, and 5. **Rationale:** Option 1 is the most appropriate. The client is unable to decide when stool evacuation will occur. In option 3, client thoughts about self may be altered if unable to control stool evacuation. In option 4, the client may not feel as comfortable around others. In option 5, increased tissue contact with fecal material may result in impairment. Option 2 is more appropriate for a client with diarrhea. Incontinence is the inability to control feces of normal consistency. **Cognitive Level:** Analyzing. **Client Need:** Physiological Integrity. **Nursing Process:** Diagnosis. **Learning Outcome:** 48-6.
10. **Answer:** 5. **Rationale:** Option 5 is a sigmoidostomy site. Option 1 is an ileostomy site, option 2 is ascending colostomy, option 3 is transverse colostomy, and option 4 is descending colostomy. **Cognitive Level:** Applying. **Client Need:** Physiological Integrity. **Nursing Process:** Assessment. **Learning Outcome:** 48-9.

CHAPTER 49 Oxygenation

1. **Answer:** 2. **Rationale:** The cough reflex depends upon nerve impulse transmission via the vagus nerve to the medulla. The nurse must monitor clients with vagus nerve impairment (through spinal cord injury, trauma, CNS depression, or other means) for a decreased or absent cough reflex. This decreased or absent reflex places the client at high risk for aspiration or development of pneumonia or other respiratory infections. **Cognitive Level:** Applying. **Client Need:** Physiological Integrity. **Nursing Process:** Planning. **Learning Outcome:** 49-5.
2. **Answer:** 3. **Rationale 1:** In a client with chronic obstructive lung disease, the drive to breathe is often dependent upon low oxygen concentration. Increasing oxygen delivery by increasing the oxygen from 1.5 Lpm to 3 Lpm may be dangerous to this client (option 1). Lowering the head of the bed makes it more difficult to breathe (option 2). This client should have the head of the bed elevated to Fowler's position or should be assisted to lean over the overbed table to increase chest excursion. Chronic obstructive lung disease makes it difficult for the client to breathe out, so increasing rate of respirations will not be helpful (option 4). **Cognitive Level:** Applying. **Client Need:** Health Promotion and Maintenance. **Nursing Process:** Planning. **Learning Outcome:** 49-8.
3. **Answer:** 1. **Rationale:** Prior to starting the procedure, it is important to develop a means of communication by which the client can express pain or discomfort. The twill tape is not changed until after performing tracheostomy care (option 2). Cleaning the incision should be done after cleaning the inner cannula (option 3). Checking the tightness of the ties and knot is done after applying new twill tape (option 4). **Cognitive Level:** Applying. **Client Need:** Physiological Integrity. **Nursing Process:** Implementation. **Learning Outcome:** 49-11d.
4. **Answer:** 3. **Rationale:** The nurse should turn the client's head to the side to allow drainage of oral secretions. The airway should not be taped in place as it would then act as an airway obstruction if dislodged (option 1). Although suctioning the client is possible with the airway in place, the client should be suctioned only when it is necessary (option 2). Insertion of a nasal trumpet or nasopharyngeal airway is not necessary when the oropharyngeal airway is in place (option 4). **Cognitive Level:** Analyzing. **Client Need:** Safe, Effective Care Environment. **Nursing Process:** Implementation. **Learning Outcome:** 49-9.
5. **Answer:** 1, 3, 4, and 5. **Rationale:** Respiratory function can be altered by conditions that affect a patent airway (option 1), the movement of air into or out of the lungs (option 5—a high temperature and pain can cause tachypnea), diffusion of oxygen and carbon dioxide between the alveoli and the pulmonary capillaries (option 3 where the blood loss causes decrease in hemoglobin, which carries oxygen), and the transport of oxygen and carbon dioxide via the blood to and from the tissue cells (option 4—heart failure decreases cardiac output). Option 2 is the definition of normal respiration. **Cognitive Level:** Analyzing. **Client Need:** Physiological Integrity. **Nursing Process:** Evaluation. **Learning Outcome:** 49-6.
6. **Answer:** 2. **Rationale:** The tube should be reconnected to the water seal as quickly as possible. Assisting the client back to bed (option 1) and assessing the client's lung sounds (option 3) are possible actions after the system is reconnected. **Cognitive Level:** Applying. **Client Need:** Safe, Effective Care Environment. **Nursing Process:** Implementation. **Learning Outcome:** 49-9.
7. **Answer:** 1. **Rationale:** Anemia is a condition of decreased red blood cells and decreased hemoglobin. Hemoglobin is how the oxygen molecules are transported to the tissues. Option 2 would depend on where the infection is located. Option 3: A fractured rib would interrupt transport of oxygen from the atmosphere to the airways. Option 4: Damage to the medulla would interfere with neural stimulation of the respiratory system. **Cognitive Level:** Applying. **Client Need:** Safe, Effective Care Environment. **Nursing Process:** Assessment. **Learning Outcome:** 49-7.
8. **Answer:** 3. **Rationale:** Respiratory difficulty related to a reclining position without other physical alterations is defined as orthopnea. **Cognitive Level:** Remembering. **Client Need:** Safe, Effective Care Environment. **Nursing Process:** Diagnosis. **Learning Outcome:** 49-5.
9. **Answer:** 4. **Rationale:** Glucocorticoids are prescribed because of their anti-inflammatory effect. Options 1, 2, and 3 are not achieved with glucocorticoids. **Cognitive Level:** Analyzing. **Client Need:** Physiological Integrity. **Nursing Process:** Implementation. **Learning Outcome:** 49-9.
10. **Answer:** 1. **Rationale:** Postural drainage results in expectoration of large amounts of mucus. Clients sometimes ingest part of the secretions. The secretions may also produce an unpleasant taste in the oral cavity, which could result in nausea and vomiting. This procedure should be done on an empty stomach to decrease client discomfort. **Cognitive Level:** Applying. **Client Need:** Safe, Effective Care Environment. **Nursing Process:** Planning. **Learning Outcome:** 49-8.

CHAPTER 50 Circulation

1. **Answer:** 3. **Rationale:** The nurse should advise the client to avoid exercise in hot or cold weather as these extremes of temperature increase the workload on the heart. Cold

temperatures increase peripheral blood vessel contraction and therefore peripheral vascular resistance, making it more difficult for the heart to circulate blood. Hot temperatures decrease systemic vascular resistance by dilating peripheral vessels. This decrease makes the heart rate increase, thereby increasing the heart's workload. **Cognitive Level:** Applying. **Client Need:** Health Promotion and Maintenance. **Nursing Process:** Implementation. **Learning Outcome:** 50-4.

2. **Answer:** 3, 1, 4, 2, and 5. **Rationale:** See sequence described on pages 1350–1351. **Cognitive Level:** Remembering. **Client Need:** Health Promotion and Maintenance. **Nursing Process:** Assessment. **Learning Outcome:** 50-1.
3. **Answer:** 3. **Rationale:** Capillary refill is an assessment of capillary blood flow and thus tissue perfusion. Symmetrical chest expansion (option 1) is an assessment of respiratory function; pursed-lip breathing (option 2) is a technique used to assist clients with obstructive lung diseases to keep alveoli open during respirations. Activity intolerance (option 4) can occur because of low cardiac output (e.g., heart failure). Activity tolerance would indicate adequate tissue perfusion. **Cognitive Level:** Applying. **Client Need:** Physiological Integrity. **Nursing Process:** Planning. **Learning Outcome:** 50-4.
4. **Answer:** 2. **Rationale:** Hemoglobin is the oxygen-carrying portion of the blood, and anemia (decrease in hemoglobin and hematocrit) is often associated with client complaint of being tired, listless, and unable to tolerate normal activities. The client's symptoms may or may not be associated with the blood urea nitrogen level, an alteration in the blood sugar level, or an altered serum potassium level. **Cognitive Level:** Applying. **Client Need:** Physiological Integrity. **Nursing Process:** Assessment. **Learning Outcome:** 50-4.
5. **Answer:** 4. **Rationale:** Cardiac output equals stroke volume heart rate. Since this client has a sustained rapid heart rate, the ventricles are most likely not having sufficient time to relax and refill between contractions, so the stroke volume will decrease. At the rate of 170, the compensatory increase in heart rate is no longer helpful in increasing cardiac output. This leads to a decrease in cardiac output. **Cognitive Level:** Applying. **Client Need:** Physiological Integrity. **Nursing Process:** Assessment. **Learning Outcome:** 50-4.
6. **Answer:** 3. **Rationale:** Because the clients would experience impaired tissue perfusion resulting in respiratory compensation, they are most likely to experience the sign or symptom of shortness of breath. The client with the MI will experience cardiac impairment resulting in decreased cardiac output as well as severe chest pain resulting in increased oxygen demand with decreased availability. Clients with heart failure will have decreased pumping ability of the cardiac muscle resulting in pulmonary congestion and decreased cardiac output. Clients with anemia have fewer RBCs to carry the oxygen to the tissues, resulting in hypoxia. Options 1 and 4 would be signs for the client with the MI. Option 2 is seen in heart failure. **Cognitive Level:** Analyzing. **Client Need:** Physiological Integrity. **Nursing Process:** Planning. **Learning Outcome:** 50-3.
7. **Answer:** 4. **Rationale:** The three cardinal signs of cardiac arrest are apnea, absence of a carotid or femoral pulse, and dilated pupils. **Cognitive Level:** Applying. **Client Need:** Health Promotion and Maintenance. **Nursing Process:** Implementation. **Learning Outcome:** 50-5.
8. **Answer:** 1, 3, and 5. **Rationale:** Option 1: An example of impaired tissue perfusion is a decrease in arterial circulation in the legs related to atherosclerosis. Option 3: Examples of inadequate cardiac output are clients with MI, heart failure, or tachycardia. Option 5: Not enough blood is being pumped by the heart to meet the demands of the body. *Activity Intolerance* is when the client does not have physiologic energy for ADLs. Common reasons can be anemias and heart failure. Options 2 and 4: Confusion and impaired sleep are not directly related to cardiovascular disease. **Cognitive Level:** Applying. **Client Need:** Physiological Integrity. **Nursing Process:** Diagnosing. **Learning Outcome:** 50-4.
9. **Answer:** 2. **Rationale:** SCDs promote venous return from the legs to the heart. They inflate and deflate plastic sleeves wrapped around the legs to promote venous flow. The sequential inflation and deflation counteract blood stasis in the lower extremities. Option 1: Arterial flow is from the heart to the general circulation. Option 3: Afterload is related to the ventricles' ability to eject blood forward. These devices affect peripheral circulation. Option 4: There is no relationship between pain and the purpose of the devices. **Cognitive Level:** Applying. **Client Need:** Health Promotion and Maintenance. **Nursing Process:** Implementation. **Learning Outcome:** 50-6.
10. **Answer:**

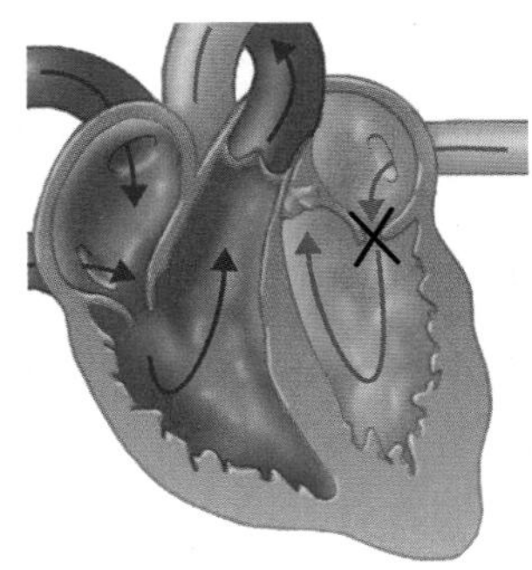

Cognitive Level: Remembering. **Client Need:** Physiological Integrity. **Nursing Process:** Implementation. **Learning Outcome:** 50-1.

CHAPTER 51 Fluid, Electrolyte, and Acid–Base Balance

1. **Answer:** 3. **Rationale:** A client who is fasting is at risk for development of metabolic acidosis. The body recognizes fasting as starvation and begins to metabolize its own proteins into ketones, which are metabolic acids. **Cognitive Level:** Analyzing. **Client Need:** Physiological Integrity. **Nursing Process:** Assessment. **Learning Outcomes:** 51-4; 51-5.
2. **Answer:** 2. **Rationale:** The priority intervention is to discontinue the transfusion. If this client is having a transfusion reaction, it will be better to limit the amount of blood transfused. The nurse would also contact the physician to collaborate on further treatment, but this action should be after the transfusion is discontinued. **Cognitive Level:** Analyzing. **Client Need:** Physiological Integrity. **Nursing Process:** Assessment. **Learning Outcome:** 51-8.
3. **Answer:** Hypertonic. **Cognitive Level:** Remembering. **Client Need:** Physiological Integrity. **Nursing Process:** Implementation. **Learning Outcome:** 51-1.
4. **Answer:** 2. **Rationale:** Because of the retention of CO_2, the clinical profile of respiratory acidosis includes decreased pH < 7.35, $PaCO_2 > 42$ mmHg, with varying levels of HCO_3 related to hypoventilation. Option 1 is respiratory alkalosis, which occurs because of blowing off of CO_2 resulting in a decreased level of acid and retention or production of bicarbonate, which in turn results in pH > 7.45, $PaCO_2 < 38$ mmHg, $HCO_3 > 26$ mEq/L related to hyperventilation. Option 3: Metabolic acidosis occurs because of a gain of hydrogen ions or a loss of HCO_3 with a pH < 7.35, normal $PaCO_2$ of 35–45 mmHg, and $HCO_3 < 22$ mEq/L, often caused by diarrhea, bicarbonate infusion, or retention related to kidney failure. Option 4: Metabolic alkalosis is caused by gain of bicarbonate or loss of hydrogen ions related to vomiting, gastric suction, or loss of upper gastrointestinal secretions by various other methods. **Cognitive Level:** Applying. **Client Need:** Physiological Integrity. **Nursing Process:** Assessment. **Learning Outcomes:** 51-2; 51-5.

5. **Answer:** 1, 3, and 5. **Rationale:** Options 1, 3, and 5 relate to decreased fluid volume. The data indicate an actual problem, which excludes option 2. Option 4 relates more to increased fluid volume. **Cognitive Level:** Analyzing. **Client Need:** Physiological Integrity. **Nursing Process:** Diagnosis. **Learning Outcome:** 51-6.
6. **Answer:** 4. **Rationale:** Salt substitutes contain potassium. The client can still use it within reason. Option 1: Avocado is higher in potassium than most foods. Option 2: Hypokalemia can potentiate digoxin toxicity and checking the pulse will help the client avoid this. Option 3: It is important to take potassium with food to avoid gastric upset. **Cognitive Level:** Applying. **Client Need:** Physiological Integrity. **Nursing Process:** Evaluation. **Learning Outcomes:** 51-7; 51-8.
7. **Answer:** 2. **Rationale:** Because insertion of a subclavian central venous catheter may result in hemothorax, pneumothorax, cardiac perforation, thrombosis, or infection, the priority finding for planning care is tachycardia. Bibasilar crackles may develop secondary to fluid overload or to the disease process but would not be particularly evident just after placement of the subclavian catheter (option 1). Decrease in pedal pulses and headache would not be associated with the placement of a subclavian catheter (options 3 and 4). **Cognitive Level:** Analyzing. **Client Need:** Physiological Integrity. **Nursing Process:** Assessment. **Learning Outcome:** 51-5.
8. **Answer:** 2. **Rationale:** Because of CO_2 retention the $PaCO_2$ is elevated. CO_2 is involved in production of acid, which will result in a decreased pH. HCO_3 will vary. Option 1: Metabolic acidosis involves a loss of bicarbonate, but no retention of CO_2. Option 3: Metabolic alkalosis involves a loss of acid or retention of HCO_3, but no retention of CO_2. Option 4: Respiratory alkalosis involves a loss of CO_2 resulting in an increased pH. **Cognitive Level:** Applying. **Client Need:** Physiological Integrity. **Nursing Process:** Assessment. **Learning Outcome:** 51-5.
9. **Answer:** 4. **Rationale:** The major clinical signs and symptoms of hypocalcemia are due to increased neuromuscular activity and not the renal, cardiac, or GI systems. **Cognitive Level:** Analyzing. **Client Need:** Physiological Integrity. **Nursing Process:** Implementation. **Learning Outcome:** 51-8.
10. **Answer:** 2, 4, and 5. **Rationale:** Options 1 and 3 relate to hypermagnesemia. **Cognitive Level:** Analyzing. **Client Need:** Physiological Integrity. **Nursing Process:** Assessment. **Learning Outcomes:** 51-4; 51-5.

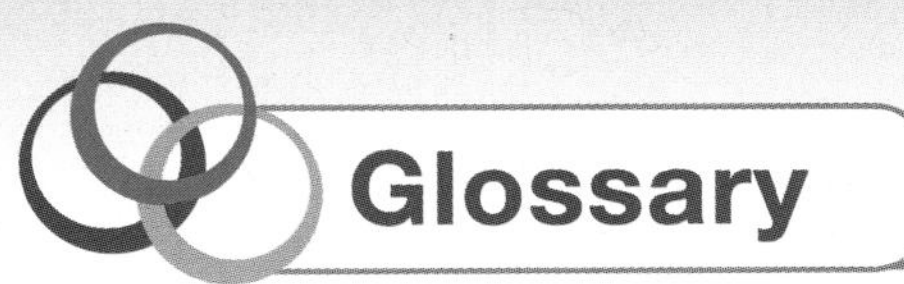

Glossary

24-hour food recall client recall of all the food and beverages consumed during a typical 24-hour period

Abdominal paracentesis a procedure to obtain a specimen of ascetic fluid for laboratory study and to relieve pressure on the abdominal organs due to the presence of excess fluid

Absorption the process by which a drug passes into the bloodstream

Abusive head trauma classified as injuries caused by violent shaking of the infant that causes whiplash and results in brain injury

Accommodation a process of change whereby cognitive processes mature sufficiently to allow an individual to solve problems that were previously unsolvable

Accountability the ability and willingness to assume responsibility for one's actions and to accept the consequences of one's behavior

Accountable care organizations (ACOs) characterized by a payment and care delivery model that ties provider reimbursements to quality metrics and reductions in the total cost of care for an assigned population of clients

Acculturation the involuntary process that occurs when individuals adapt to or borrow traits from another culture

Acid a substance that releases hydrogen ions (H^{+}) in solution

Acidosis a condition that occurs with increases in blood carbonic acid or with decreases in blood bicarbonate; blood pH below 7.35

Acquired immunity *see* Passive immunity

Action stage occurs when an individual actively implements behavioral and cognitive strategies to interrupt previous behavior patterns and adopt new ones; this stage requires a great commitment of time and energy

Active euthanasia actions that directly bring about the client's death with or without consent

Active immunity a resistance of the body to infection in which the host produces its own antibodies in response to natural or artificial antigens

Active ROM (range-of-motion) exercises isotonic exercises in which the client independently moves each joint in the body through its complete range of movement, maximally stretching all muscle groups within each plane, over the joint

Active transport the movement of solutes across cell membranes from a less concentrated solution to a more concentrated one

Activity-exercise pattern refers to an individual's pattern of exercise, activity, leisure, and recreation

Activity theory the best way to age is to stay active physically and mentally

Activity tolerance the type and amount of exercise or daily activities an individual is able to perform

Actual loss can be recognized by others

Acupressure a technique that uses the fingers to apply pressure to specific points along meridians throughout the body

Acupuncture a form of healing in which the therapist applies needles to stimulate specific sites of the body

Acute confusion abrupt onset of confusion that has a reversible cause; also called *delirium*

Acute hemolytic transfusion reaction condition caused by the transfusion of ABO- or Rh- incompatible blood, which causes destruction of the transfused RBCs and subsequent risk of kidney damage or failure

Acute illness typically characterized by severe symptoms of relatively short duration

Acute infections those that generally appear suddenly or last a short time

Acute pain pain that lasts only through the expected recovery period (as opposed to chronic)

Adaptation the process of modifying to meet new, changing, or different conditions

Adaptive mechanisms *see* Defense mechanisms

Addiction chronic, relapsing, treatable disease influenced by genetic, developmental, and environmental factors

Adherence the extent to which an individual's behavior (for example, taking medications, following diets, or making lifestyle changes) coincides with medical or health advice; commitment or attachment to a regimen

Adjuvant medication that is not classified as a pain medication and that may reduce pain alone or in combination with other analgesics, relieve other discomforts, potentiate the effect of pain medications, or reduce the pain medication's side effects

Adolescence the period during which an individual becomes physically and psychologically mature and acquires a personal identity

Adolescent growth spurt the period during puberty when sudden and dramatic physical changes occur

Adult day care a day care center that provides health and social services to older adults

Advance healthcare directives a variety of legal and lay documents that allow individuals to specify aspects of care they wish to receive should they become unable to make or communicate their preferences

Adventitious breath sounds abnormal breath sounds that occur when air passes through narrowed airways or airways filled with fluid or mucus, or when pleural linings are inflamed

Adverse effects severe side effects that may justify the discontinuation of a drug

Advocate individual who pleads the cause of another or argues or pleads for a cause or proposal

Aerobic growing only in the presence of oxygen

Aerobic exercise any activity during which the body takes in more or an equal amount of oxygen than it expends

Aesthetic knowing providing care and meeting the needs of clients through creativity and style

Afebrile absence of a fever

Affective domain known as the "feeling" domain, relates to the client's attitudes, interests, attention, awareness, and values

Afterload the resistance against which the heart must pump to eject blood into the circulation

Ageism deep and profound prejudice in American society against older adults

Ages & Stages Questionnaires (ASQ) includes 19 age-specific surveys in which parents are asked about the developmental skills observed in ages 1 month to 5 1/2 years to assist healthcare professionals in identifying children who are at risk for social and emotional developmental delays

Agglutinins specific antibodies formed in the blood

Agglutinogens a substance that acts as an antigen and stimulates the production of agglutinins

Agnostic an individual who doubts the existence of God or a supreme being or believes the existence of God has not been proved

Agonist a drug that interacts with a receptor to produce a response

Airborne precautions used for clients known to have or suspected of having serious illnesses transmitted by airborne droplet nuclei smaller than 5 microns

Alarm reaction the initial reaction of the body to stress, which alerts the body's defenses

Alexian Brothers religious order that organized care for victims of the Black Plague in the 14th century in Germany and established hospitals and provided nursing care in the 19th century

Algor mortis the gradual decrease of the body's temperature after death

Alkalosis a condition that occurs with increases in blood bicarbonate or decreases in blood carbonic acid; blood pH above 7.45

Allopathic medicine term used to describe Western medical practice

Alopecia the loss of scalp hair (baldness) or body hair

Alternative medicine an unrelated group of nonorthodox practices, often with explanatory systems that do not follow conventional biomedical explanations

Alzheimer's disease disease that involves progressive dementia, memory loss, and inability to care for self

Amblyopia reduced visual acuity in one eye

Ambulation the act of walking

Ampule a glass container usually designed to hold a single dose of a drug

Anabolism a process in which simple substances are converted by the body's cells into more complex substances (e.g., building tissue, positive nitrogen balance)

Anaerobic growing only in the absence of oxygen

Anaerobic exercise involves activity in which the muscles cannot draw out enough oxygen from the bloodstream; used in endurance training

Anal stimulation stimulation applied to anus for sexual pleasure

Anaphylactic reaction a severe allergic reaction that usually occurs immediately after the administration of a drug

Andragogy the art and science of helping adults learn

Androgyny belief that most characteristics and behaviors are human qualities and not limited to a gender

Anemia a condition in which the blood is deficient in red blood cells or hemoglobin

Anger an emotional state consisting of a subjective feeling of animosity or strong displeasure

Angiography a diagnostic procedure enabling x-ray visual examination of the vascular system after injection of a radiopaque dye

Angle of Louis the junction between the body of the sternum and the manubrium; the starting point for locating the ribs anteriorly

Animal-assisted therapy the use of specifically selected animals as a treatment modality in health and human service settings

Anions ions that carry a negative charge; includes chlorine (Cl^-), bicarbonate (HCO_3^-), phosphate (HPO_4^{2-}), and sulfate (SO_4^-)

Ankylosed permanently immobile joints

Anorexia loss of appetite

Anorexia nervosa a disease characterized by a prolonged inability or refusal to eat, rapid weight loss, and emaciation in individuals who continue to believe they are fat

Anoscopy visual examination of the anal canal using an anoscope (a lighted instrument)

Answer (legal) a written response made by a defendant

Antagonist drug that inhibits cell function by occupying the drug's receptor sites

Antibodies part of the body's plasma proteins that defend primarily against the extracellular phases of bacterial and viral infections; also called *immunoglobulins*

Anticipatory grief grief experienced in advance of an event

Anticipatory loss the experience of loss before the loss actually occurs

Antigen a substance capable of inducing the formation of antibodies

Antihelix the anterior curve of the auricle's upper aspect

Antiseptics an agent that inhibits the growth of some microorganisms

Anuria the failure of the kidneys to produce urine, resulting in a total lack of urination or output of less than 100 mL/day in an adult

Anxiety a state of mental uneasiness, apprehension, or dread producing an increased level of arousal caused by an impending or anticipated threat to self or significant relationships

Apgar scoring system a scoring system to assess newborn babies

Aphasia any defects in or loss of the power to express oneself by speech, writing, or signs, or to comprehend spoken or written language due to disease or injury of the cerebral cortex

Apical pulse a central pulse located at the apex of the heart

Apical–radial pulse measurement of the apical and radial pulse simultaneously

Apnea a complete absence of respirations

Apocrine glands sweat glands located largely in the axillae and anogenital areas; they begin to function at puberty under the influence of androgens

Approximated closed tissue surfaces

Aromatherapy therapeutic use of essential oils of plants in which odor or fragrance plays an important part

Arrhythmia an irregular heart rhythm

Arterial blood gases specimen of arterial blood that assesses oxygenation, ventilation, and acid–base status

Arterial blood pressure the measure of the pressure exerted by the blood as it pulsates through the arteries

Arteriosclerosis a condition in which the elastic and muscular tissues of the arteries are replaced with fibrous tissue

Ascites a large amount of fluid accumulation in the abdominal cavity

Asepsis freedom from infection or infectious material

Asphyxiation lack of oxygen due to interrupted breathing

Aspiration withdrawal of fluid that has abnormally collected (e.g., pleural cavity, abdominal cavity) or to obtain a specimen (e.g., cerebrospinal fluid)

Assault an attempt or threat to touch another individual unjustifiably

Assessing the process of collecting, organizing, validating, and recording data (information) about a client's health status

Assimilation the process by which an individual develops a new cultural identity and becomes like the members of the dominant culture

Assisted living facility with various degrees of personal care assistance designed to meet the needs of an older adult

Assisted suicide a form of active euthanasia in which clients are given the means to kill themselves

Astigmatism an uneven curvature of the cornea that prevents horizontal and vertical light rays from focusing on the retina

Atelectasis collapse of the air sacs

Atheist one without belief in a deity

Atherosclerosis buildup of fatty plaque within the arteries

Atria two upper hollow chambers of the heart

Atrioventricular (AV) node conduction pathways that slightly delay transmission of the impulse from the atria to the ventricles of the heart

Atrioventricular (AV) valves between the atria and ventricles of the heart, the tricuspid valve on the right and the bicuspid or mitral valve on the left

Atrophy wasting away; decrease in size of organ or tissue (e.g., muscle)

Attachment an essential human need for lasting, strong, emotional bonds with others

Attentive listening listening actively, using all senses, as opposed to listening passively with just the ear

Attitudes mental stance that is composed of many different beliefs; usually involving a positive or negative judgment toward an individual, object, or idea

Audit examination or review of records

Auditory related to or experienced through hearing

Auricle flap of the ear; also called *pinna*

Auscultation the process of listening to sounds produced within the body, such as with the use of a stethoscope that amplifies sounds and conveys them to the nurse's ears

Auscultatory gap the temporary disappearance of sounds normally heard over the brachial artery when the sphygmomanometer cuff pressure is high, followed by the reappearance of sounds at a lower level

Authoritarian leader the individual who makes decisions for the group

Authority the power given by an organization to direct the work of others; the right to act

Autoantigen an antigen that originates in an individual's own body

Autocratic leader *see* Authoritarian leader

Automaticity an electrical impulse and contraction independent of the nervous system and generated by the cardiac muscle

Autonomy the state of being independent and self-directed, without outside control, to make one's own decisions

Autopsy an examination of the body after death to determine the cause of death and to learn more about a disease process; also called *postmortem examination*

Awareness the ability to perceive environmental stimuli and body reactions and to respond appropriately through thought and action

Ayurveda Indian system of medicine where illness is viewed as a state of imbalance among the body's systems

Baby boomers generation that includes those born in years 1945–1964

Bacteremia bacteria in the blood

Bacteria the most common infection-causing microorganisms

Balance a state of equilibrium in which opposing forces counteract each other

Bandage a strip of cloth used to wrap some part of the body

Basal metabolic rate (BMR) the rate of energy utilization in the body required to maintain essential activities such as breathing

Base of support the foundation on which an object rests

Bases (alkalis) have low hydrogen ion concentration and can accept hydrogen ions in solution

Battery (legal) the willful or negligent touching of an individual (or the individual's clothes or even something the individual is carrying), which may or may not cause harm

Bedpan a receptacle for urine and feces

Bedrest strict confinement to bed (complete bedrest), or the client may be allowed to use a bedside commode or have bathroom privileges

Behaviorist theory includes the identification of what is to be taught and the shaping of behavior through positive and negative reinforcement

Beliefs interpretations or conclusions that one accepts as true

Beneficence the moral obligation to do good or to implement actions that benefit clients and their support people

Bereavement a subjective response of an individual who has experienced the loss of a significant other through death

Bevel the slanted part at the tip of a needle

Binder a type of bandage applied to large body areas (abdomen or chest) that is designed for a specific body part (e.g., arm sling); used to provide support

Bioelectromagnetics science that studies how living organisms interact with electromagnetic fields

Bioethics ethical rules or principles that govern right conduct concerning life

Biofeedback a stress management technique that brings under conscious control bodily processes normally thought to be beyond voluntary command

Biological rhythms in humans, these rhythms, such as the circadian rhythm, are controlled from within the body and synchronized with environmental factors, such as light and darkness

Biomedical health belief *see* Scientific health belief

Biomedicine term used to describe Western medical practice

Biopsy removal and examination of tissue

Biotransformation process by which a drug is converted to a less active form; also called *detoxification* or *metabolism*

Bladder retraining client postpones voiding, resists or inhibits the sensation of urgency, and voids according to a timetable rather than according to the urge to void

Blanch test a test during which the client's fingertip is temporarily pinched to assess capillary refill and peripheral circulation

Bloodborne pathogens potentially infectious organisms that are carried in and transmitted through blood or materials containing blood

Blood chemistry a number of tests performed on blood serum (the liquid portion of the blood)

Blood pressure (BP) the force exerted on arterial walls by blood flowing within the vessel

Blood urea nitrogen (BUN) a measure of blood level of urea, the end product of protein metabolism

Body image how an individual perceives the size, appearance, and functioning of his or her body and its parts

Body mass index (BMI) indicates whether weight is appropriate for height

Body temperature the balance between the heat produced by the body and the heat lost from the body

Boomerang kids slang term used for young adults who move back into their parents' homes after an initial period of independent living

Bottle mouth syndrome describes the decay of an infant's teeth caused by constant contact with sweet liquid from a bottle

Boundary the real or imaginary lines that differentiate one system from another system or a system from its environment

Bowel incontinence loss of voluntary ability to control fecal and gaseous discharges through the anal sphincter; also called *fecal incontinence*

Bradycardia abnormally slow pulse rate, less than 60 beats per minute

Bradypnea abnormally slow respiratory rate, usually less than 10 respirations per minute

Brand name name of the drug given by the drug manufacturer; also called the *trade name*

Breach of duty a standard of care that is expected in the specific situation but that the nurse did not observe; this is the failure to act as a reasonable, prudent nurse under the circumstances

Bruit a blowing or swishing sound created by turbulence of blood flow

Buccal a medication (e.g., a tablet) that is held in the mouth against the mucous membranes of the cheek until the drug dissolves

Buffers prevent excessive changes in pH by removing or releasing hydrogen ions

Bulimia an uncontrollable compulsion to eat large amounts of food and then expel it by self-induced vomiting or by taking laxatives

Bullying repeated, health-harming mistreatment of one or more individuals by one or more perpetrators

Bundle of His the right and left bundle branches of the ventricular conduction pathways

Burden of proof the duty of proving an assertion

Bureaucratic leader does not trust self or others to make decisions and instead relies on the organization's rules, policies, and procedures to direct the group's work efforts

Burn results from excessive exposure to thermal, chemical, electric, or radioactive agents

Burnout a complex syndrome of behaviors that can be likened to the exhaustion stage of the general adaptation syndrome; an overwhelming feeling that can lead to physical and emotional depletion, a negative attitude and self-concept, and feelings of helplessness and hopelessness

Calculi renal stones

Callus a thickened portion of the skin

Caloric value the amount of energy that nutrients or foods supply to the body

Calorie a unit of heat energy

Cancer-related pain may result from the direct effects of the disease and its treatment, such as radiation or chemotherapy

Cannula a tube with a lumen (channel) that is inserted into a cavity or duct and is often fitted with a trocar during insertion for abdominal paracentesis; the part of the needle that is attached to the hub; also called a *shaft*

Carbon monoxide an odorless, colorless, tasteless gas that is very toxic

Cardiac output (CO) the amount of blood ejected by the heart with each ventricular contraction

Caregiver a role that has traditionally included those activities that assist the client physically and psychologically

Caregiver burden responses to long-term stress, such as chronic fatigue, sleeping difficulties, and high blood pressure, in family members who undertake the care of an individual in the home for a long period

Caregiver role strain physical, emotional, social, and financial burdens that can seriously jeopardize the caregiver's own health and well-being

Caries tooth cavities

Caring intentional action that conveys physical and emotional security and genuine connectedness with another individual or group of individuals

Caring practice nursing care that includes connection, mutual recognition, and involvement

Carminative an agent that promotes the passage of flatus from the colon

Carrier an individual or animal that harbors a specific infectious agent and serves as a potential source of infection, yet does not manifest any clinical signs of disease

Case management a method for delivering nursing care in which the nurse is responsible for a caseload of clients across the healthcare continuum

Case manager a nurse who works with the multidisciplinary healthcare team to measure the effectiveness of the case management plan and monitor outcomes

Catabolism a process in which complex substances are broken down into simpler substances (e.g., breakdown of tissue)

Cataract an opacity of the eye lens or its capsule that blocks light rays

Cathartics drugs that induce defecation

Cations ions that carry a positive charge; includes sodium (Na^+), potassium (K^+), calcium (Ca^{2+}), and magnesium (Mg^{2+})

Causation a fact that must be proven that the harm occurred as a direct result of the nurse's failure to follow the standard of care and the nurse could have (or should have) known that failure to follow the standard of care could result in such harm

CAUTI (catheter-associated urinary tract infection) a urinary tract infection that is associated with an indwelling urinary catheter that has been in place for more than 2 calendar days

Cell-mediated defenses *see* Cellular immunity

Cellular immunity occurs through the T-cell system; also known as *cell-mediated defenses*

Center of gravity the point at which all of the mass (weight) of an object is centered

Central vascular access device defined by the location of the catheter tip in a central vein, in the lower one-third of the superios vena cava, above the right atrium

Cephalocaudal proceeding in the direction from head to toe

Cerebral death occurs when the cerebral cortex is irreversibly destroyed; also called *higher brain death*

Cerumen earwax

Change process of making something different from what it was

Change agent individual (or group) who initiates change or who assists others in making modifications in themselves or in the system

Change-of-shift report a report given to nurses on the next shift

Charismatic leader characterized by an emotional relationship between the leader and the group members; personality of the leader evokes strong feelings of commitment to both the leader and the leader's cause and beliefs

Chart a formal, legal document that provides evidence of a client's care

Charting the process of making an entry on a client record

Charting by exception (CBE) a documentation system in which only significant findings or exceptions to norms are recorded

Chemical name the name by which a chemist knows a drug; describes the constituents of the drug precisely

Chemical restraints medications used to control socially disruptive behavior

Chiropractic from the Greek meaning "done by hand"; involves adjustments of the spine and joints and is grounded in the assumption that maintaining the alignment of the spine and joints facilitates the flow of energy throughout the body, including the nervous, circulatory, respiratory, gastrointestinal, and limbic systems

Cholesterol a fatlike substance that is both produced by the body and found in foods of animal origin

Chronic confusion progressive loss of cognitive function that has symptoms that are gradual and irreversible; also called *dementia*

Chronic illness illness that lasts for an extended period of time, usually longer than 6 months

Chronic infection infection that occurs slowly, over a very long period, and may last months or years

Chronic pain prolonged pain, usually recurring or persisting over 6 months or longer, that interferes with functioning

Chyme contents of the colon

Circulating immunity *see* Humoral immunity

Circulating nurse coordinates activities and manages client care by continually assessing client safety, aseptic practice, and the environment (e.g., temperature, humidity, and lighting); with the scrub nurse, is responsible for accounting for all sponges, needles, and instruments at the close of surgery

Civil actions deals with the relationship between individuals in society

Civil law the body of law that deals with relationships among private individuals; also known as *private law*

Clara Barton a schoolteacher who volunteered as a nurse during the Civil War. Most notably, she organized the American Red Cross, which linked with the International Red Cross when the U.S. Congress ratified the Geneva Convention in 1882

Clean free of potentially infectious agents

Clean-catch specimen urine specimens for urine culture; also called *midstream urine specimen*

Clean voided specimen urine specimens for routine urinalysis

Cleansing bath a bath given for hygienic purposes

Client an individual who engages the advice or services of another who is qualified to provide this service

Client advocate an individual who acts to protect the client

Client record *see* Chart

Climacteric the point in development when reproduction capacity in the female terminates (menopause) and the sexual activity of the male decreases (andropause)

Clinical decision support systems electronic forms of nursing tools such as charts, templates, algorithms, and others, which incorporate evidence from the literature into particular client situations in order to guide care planning

Clinical judgment decision-making process to ascertain the right nursing action to be implemented at the appropriate time in the client's care

Clinical reasoning cognitive process that uses thinking strategies to gather, analyze, and evaluate the relevance of client information, and decide on possible nursing actions to improve the client's physiologic and psychosocial outcomes

Closed awareness a type of awareness in which the client is unaware of impending death

Closed questions restrictive question requiring only a short answer

Closed system does not exchange energy, matter, or information with its environment; it receives no input from the environment and gives no output to the environment

Closed wound drainage system consists of a drain connected to either an electric suction or a portable drainage suction

Clubbing elevation of the proximal aspect of the nail and softening of the nail bed

Coanalgesic a medication that is not classified as a pain medication but has properties that may reduce pain alone or in combination with other analgesics, relieve other discomforts, potentiate the effect of pain medication, or reduce the pain medication's side effects

Cochlea a seashell-shaped structure found in the inner ear; essential for sound transmission and hearing

Code of ethics a formal statement of a group's ideals and values; a set of ethical principles shared by members of a group, reflecting their moral judgments and serving as a standard for professional actions

Cognitive development refers to the manner in which individuals learn to think, reason, and use language

Cognitive domain the "thinking" domain, includes six intellectual abilities and thinking processes beginning with remembering, understanding, and applying to analyzing, evaluating, and creating

Cognitive processes the thinking processes based on the knowledge of aspects of client care

Cognitive skills intellectual skills that include problem solving, decision making, critical thinking, and creativity

Cognitive theory recognition of developmental levels of learners, and acknowledgments of the learner's motivation and environment

Coinsurance an insurance plan in which the client pays a percentage of the payment and some other group (e.g., employer, government) pays the remaining percentage

Coitus penile–vaginal intercourse

Collaboration a collegial working relationship with another healthcare provider in the provision of client care

Collaborative care plans *see* Critical pathways

Collaborative interventions actions the nurse carries out in collaboration with other health team members, such as physical therapists, social workers, dietitians, and physicians

Collagen a protein found in connective tissue; a whitish protein substance that adds tensile strength to a wound

Colloid osmotic pressure holds water in plasma, and when necessary pulls water from the interstitial space into the vascular compartment to maintain vascular volume; also called *oncotic pressure*

Colloids substances such as large protein molecules that do not readily dissolve into true solutions

Colonization the presence of organisms in body secretions or excretions in which strains of bacteria become resident flora but do not cause illness

Colonoscopy visual examination of the interior of the colon with a colonoscope

Colostomy a temporary or permanent opening into the colon (large bowel) to divert and drain fecal material

Commode a portable chair with a toilet seat and a receptacle underneath that can be emptied; often used for the adult client who is able to get out of bed but is unable to walk to the bathroom

Common law the body of principles that evolves from court decisions

Communicable disease a disease that can spread from one individual to another

Communication a two-way process involving the sending and receiving of messages

Communicator a nurse identifies client problems and then communicates them verbally or in writing to other members of the health team

Community a collection of individuals who share some attribute of their lives

Community-based healthcare (CBHC) a system that provides health-related services within the context of individuals' daily lives; that is, in places where individuals spend their time in the community

Community-based nursing (CBN) nursing care directed toward a specific population or group within the community; primary, secondary, or tertiary care may be provided to individuals or groups

Community health nursing the synthesis of nursing and public health practice as applied to promoting and preserving the health of populations

Community nursing centers (CNCs) provide primary care to specific populations and are staffed by nurse practitioners and community health nurses

Comparative analysis involves assessing study findings for their implementation potential

Compensation defense mechanism in which an individual substitutes an activity for one that he or she would prefer doing or cannot do

Compensatory counterbalancing

Complaint (legal) a document filed by a plaintiff

Complementary medicine *see* Alternative medicine

Complete blood count (CBC) specimens of venous blood; includes hemoglobin and hematocrit measurements, erythrocyte (RBC) count, leukocyte (WBC) count, red blood cell indices, and a differential white cell count

Complete proteins proteins that contain all of the essential amino acids as well as many nonessential ones

Compliance in reference to the arteries, their ability to contract and expand

Complicated grief pathologic grief; exists when coping strategies are maladaptive

Compress a moist gauze dressing applied frequently to an open wound, sometimes medicated

Compromised host any individual at increased risk for an infection

Computed tomography (CT) a painless, noninvasive x-ray procedure that has the unique capability of distinguishing minor differences in the density of tissues

Computer-based patient records (CPRs) electronic client data retrievable by caregivers, administrators, accreditors, and other individuals who require the data

Computer literacy the knowledge and ability to use computers or technology

Concept map a visual tool in which ideas or data are enclosed in circles or boxes of some shape and relationships between these are indicated by connecting lines or arrows

Concept mapping technique that uses a graphic depiction of nonlinear and linear relationships to represent critical thinking

Concurrent audit evaluation of a client's healthcare while the client is still receiving care from the agency

Conduction the transfer of heat from one molecule to another in direct contact

Conductive hearing loss the result of interrupted transmission of sound waves through the outer and middle ear structures

Confidentiality any information a participant relates will not be made public or available to others without the participant's consent

Congruent communication occurs when the verbal and nonverbal aspects of the message match

Conjunctivitis inflammation of the bulbar and palpebral conjunctiva

Conscious sedation a minimal depression of level of consciousness during which the client retains the ability to consciously maintain a patent airway and respond appropriately to verbal and physical stimuli

Consequence-based (teleological) theories the ethics of judging whether an action is moral

Constant fever a state in which the body temperature fluctuates minimally but always remains above normal

Constipation passage of small, dry, hard stool or passage of no stool for a period of time

Consumer an individual, a group of individuals, or a community that uses a service or commodity

Contact precautions used for clients known or suspected to have serious illnesses easily transmitted by direct client contact or by contact with items in the client's environment (GI, respiratory, skin or wound infections, etc.)

Contemplation stage stage in which an individual acknowledges having a problem, seriously considers changing a specific behavior, actively gathers information, and verbalizes plans to change the behavior in the near future

Content analysis data analysis that involves searching for themes and patterns in a research study that uses a qualitative approach

Continuing education (CE) formalized experiences designed to enlarge the knowledge or skills of practitioners

Continuity of care the coordination of healthcare services by healthcare providers for clients moving from one healthcare setting to another and between and among healthcare professionals

Continuity theory individuals maintain their values, habits, and behavior in old age

Contract a written or verbal agreement between two or more individuals to do or not do some lawful act

Contractility the inherent ability of cardiac muscle fibers to shorten or contract

Contract law the enforcement of agreements among private individuals or the payment of compensation for failure to fulfill the agreement

Contractual obligations duty of care established by the presence of an expressed or implied contract

Contractual relationships vary among practice settings; may be as an independent or employer–employee relationship

Contracture permanent shortening of a muscle

Convection the dispersion of heat by air currents

Conventional medicine term used to describe Western medical practice

Coordinating the process of ensuring that plans are carried out and evaluating outcomes

Coping dealing with change

Coping mechanism *see* Coping strategy

Coping strategy a natural or learned way of responding to a changing environment or specific problem or situation

Core self-concept the beliefs and images that are most vital to an individual's identity

Core temperature the temperature of the deep tissues of the body (e.g., abdominal cavity, pelvic cavity). When measured orally, the average body temperature of an adult is between 36.7°C and 37°C (98°F and 98.6°F)

Corn a conical, circular, painful, raised area on the toe or foot

Coronary arteries a network of vessels known as the coronary circulation

Coroner a physician who is authorized by the county or other government agency to determine causes of deaths under unusual circumstances

Costal (thoracic) breathing movement of the chest upward and outward

Cost–benefit analysis involves consideration of the potential risks and benefits of both implementing a change based on a study's findings and not implementing a change

Counseling the process of helping a client to recognize and cope with stressful psychologic or social problems, to develop improved interpersonal relationships, and to promote personal growth

Countershock phase second part of the alarm reaction in which the changes the body experienced during the shock phase are reversed

C-reactive protein (CRP) screening test for the inflammatory process of acute myocardial infarction (AMI)

Creatine kinase (CK) enzyme that is released into the blood during a myocardial infarction

Creatinine a nitrogenous waste that is excreted in the urine

Creatinine clearance test that uses 24-hour urine and serum creatinine levels to determine the glomerular filtration rate, a sensitive indicator of renal function

Creativity thinking that results in the development of new ideas and products

Credentialing the process of determining and maintaining competence in practice; includes licensure, registration, certification, and accreditation

Credé's maneuver manual exertion of pressure on the bladder to force urine out

Crepitation palpable or audible crackling or grating sensation produced by joint motion and frequently experienced in joints that have suffered repeated trauma over time

Crime an act committed in violation of public (criminal) law and punishable by a fine and/or imprisonment

Criminal actions deal with disputes between an individual and the society as a whole

Criminal law deals with actions against the safety and welfare of the public

Crisis intervention a short-term helping process of assisting clients to work through a crisis to its resolution and restore their precrisis level of functioning

Critical analysis a set of questions one can apply to a particular situation or idea to determine essential information and ideas and discard superfluous information and ideas

Critical pathways multidisciplinary guidelines for client care based on specific medical diagnoses designed to achieve predetermined outcomes

Critical thinking a cognitive process that includes creativity, problem solving, and decision making

Critique to critically read and evaluate research articles

Cross-contamination the movement of microorganisms from one client to another

Cross-dressing dressing in clothing of the opposite sex

Crystalloids salts that dissolve readily into true solutions

Cues any piece of information or data that influences decisions

Cultural broker an individual, such as an interpreter, who engages both healthcare provider and client effectively and efficiently in accessing the nuances and hidden sociocultural assumptions embedded in each other's language

Cultural care deprivation lack of culturally assistive, supportive, or facilitative acts

Cultural competence provision of healthcare across cultural boundaries that takes into account the context in which the client lives, as well as the situations in which the client's health problems arise

Cultural deprivation *see* Cultural care deprivation

Culturally responsive care care that is centered on the client's cultural point of view and integrates the client's values and beliefs into the plan of care

Culture a worldview and set of traditions used and transmitted from generation to generation by a particular group; includes related attitudes and institutions

Cultures laboratory cultivations of microorganisms in a special growth medium

Cumulative effect the increasing response to repeated doses of a drug that occurs when the rate of administration exceeds the rate of metabolism or excretion

Curanderismo cultural healing tradition found in Latin America that uses Western medicine beliefs, treatments, and practices at three levels of care: material level, spiritual level, and mental level

Cyanosis a bluish tinge of skin color

Cystoscope a lighted instrument used to visualize the interior of the urinary bladder

Cystoscopy visual examination of the urinary bladder with a cystoscope

Dacryocystitis inflammation of the lacrimal sac

Damages if professional negligence caused an injury, the nurse is held liable for compensation in the form of damages

Dandruff a diffuse scaling of the scalp, often accompanied by itching

Data information

Database all information about a client, includes nursing health history and physical assessment, physician's history, physical examination, and laboratory and diagnostic test results

Data warehousing the accumulation of large amounts of data that are stored over time

Debridement removal of necrotic material

Decision (legal) outcome made by a judge

Decode to relate the message perceived to the receiver's storehouse of knowledge and experience and to sort out the meaning of the message

Deductive reasoning making specific observations from a generalization

Defamation (legal) a communication that is false, or made with careless disregard for the truth, and results in injury to the reputation of another

Defecation expulsion of feces from the anus and rectum

Defendant (legal) individual against whom a plaintiff files a complaint

Defense mechanisms methods the ego uses to fulfill the needs of the id in a socially acceptable manner; also called *adaptive mechanism*

Defining characteristics client signs and symptoms that must be present to validate a nursing diagnosis

Dehiscence the partial or total rupturing of a sutured wound; usually involves an abdominal wound in which the layers below the skin also separate

Dehydration insufficient fluid in the body

Delegation "allowing a delegate to perform a specific nursing activity, skill, or procedure that is beyond the delagatee's traditional role and not routinely performed. This applies to licensed nurses as well as UAP" (NCSBN, 2016, p.6).

Delirium abrupt onset of confusion that has a reversible cause; also called *acute confusion*

Demand feeding the feeding of a child when the child is hungry

Dementia progressive loss of cognitive function that has symptoms that are gradual and irreversible; also called *chronic confusion*

Democratic leader encourages group discussion and decision making

Denver Developmental Screening Test (DDST-II) a screening test used to assess children from birth to 6 years of age

Dependent functions with regard to medical diagnoses, physician-prescribed therapies and treatments nurses are obligated to carry out

Dependent interventions activities carried out on the orders or supervision of a licensed physician or other healthcare provider authorized to write orders for nurses

Dependent variable the behavior, characteristic, or outcome that the researcher wishes to explain or predict

Depression an extreme feeling of sadness, despair, dejection, lack of worth, or emptiness

Descriptive statistics procedures that summarize large volumes of data; used to describe and synthesize data, showing patterns and trends

Desired effect *see* Therapeutic effect

Desire phase part of the response cycle, which starts in the brain, with conscious sexual desires

Detoxification the belief that physical impurities and toxins must be cleared from the body to achieve better health

Detrusor muscle the smooth muscle layers of the bladder

Development an individual's increasing capacity and skill in functioning, related to growth

Developmental stage level of achievement for a particular segment of an individual's life

Developmental task skill or behavior pattern learned during stages of development

Diagnosis a statement or conclusion concerning the nature of some phenomenon

Diagnosis-related groups (DRGs) a Medicare payment system to hospitals and physicians that establishes fees according to diagnosis

Diaphragmatic (abdominal) breathing breathing that involves the contraction and relaxation of the diaphragm, as observed by the movement of the abdomen

Diarrhea defecation of liquid feces and increased frequency of defecation

Diastole in measuring blood pressure, the period during which the ventricles relax

Diastolic pressure the pressure of the blood against the arterial walls when the ventricles of the heart are at rest

Diet history a comprehensive assessment of a client's food intake that involves an extensive interview by a nutritionist or dietitian

Differentiated practice a system in which the best possible use of nursing personnel is based on their educational preparation and resultant skill sets

Diffusion the mixing of molecules or ions of two or more substances as a result of random motion

Directing a management function that involves communicating the task to be completed and providing guidance and supervision

Directive interview a highly structured interview that uses closed questions to elicit specific information

Dirty denotes the likely presence of microorganisms, some of which may be capable of causing infection

Disaccharides sugars that are composed of double molecules

Discharge planning the process of anticipating and planning for client needs after discharge

Discovery (legal) pretrial activities to gain all the facts of a situation

Discrimination the differential treatment of individuals or groups

Discussion an informal oral consideration of a subject by two or more healthcare personnel to identify a problem or establish strategies to resolve a problem

Disease an alteration in body function resulting in a reduction of capacities or shortening of the normal lifespan

Disengagement theory aging involves mutual withdrawal (disengagement) between an older individual and others in that individual's environment

Disinfectant agent that destroys microorganisms other than spores

Distance learning learning in which individuals communicate effectively across long distances

Distribution the transportation of a drug from its site of absorption to its site of action

Diuresis *see* Polyuria

Diuretics agents that increase urine secretion

Diversity the fact or state of being different

Documenting the process of making an entry on a client record; charting, recording

Do not resuscitate (DNR) order given by a primary care provider that is generally written when the client or proxy has expressed the wish for no resuscitation in the event of a respiratory or cardiac arrest

Dorothea Dix woman leader who provided nursing care during the Civil War

Dorsal position *see* Supine position

Dorsal recumbent (back-lying) position a supine position with the head and shoulders slightly elevated

Drop factor the number of drops that equal 1 mL as specified on the package of IV tubing

Droplet nuclei residue of evaporated droplets emitted by an infected host, such as someone with tuberculosis, that can remain in the air for long periods of time

Droplet precautions used for clients known or suspected to have serious illnesses transmitted by particle droplets larger than 5 microns (diphtheria, mycoplasma, pneumonia)

Drug a chemical compound taken for disease prevention, diagnosis, cure, or relief or to affect the structure or function of the body

Drug abuse excessive intake of a substance either continually or periodically

Drug allergy an immunologic reaction to a drug

Drug dependence inability to keep the intake of a drug or substance under control

Drug habituation a mild form of psychologic dependence on a drug

Drug half-life the time required for the elimination process to reduce the concentration of a drug to one-half of what it was at initial administration; also called *elimination half-life*

Drug interaction the beneficial or harmful interaction of one drug with another drug

Drug tolerance a condition in which successive increases in the dosage of a drug are required to maintain a given therapeutic effect

Drug toxicity the quality of a drug that exerts a deleterious effect on an organism or tissue

dry powder inhaler (DPI) An inhalation device for administering a solid drug to be released upon inhalation by the client

Dullness (of sound) a thudlike sound produced by dense tissue such as the liver, spleen, or heart

Durable medical equipment (DME) company a company that provides healthcare equipment for clients at home

Duration (of sound) its length (long or short) during auscultation

Duty (legal) the nurse must have (or should have had) a relationship with the client that involves providing care and following an acceptable standard of care

Dysesthesia an unpleasant abnormal sensation that mimics the pathology of central neuropathic pain disorder, such as pain that follows a stroke or spinal cord injury

Dysmenorrhea painful menstruation

Dyspareunia pain during or immediately after intercourse

Dysphagia difficulty swallowing

Dyspnea difficult or labored breathing

Dysrhythmia a pulse with an irregular rhythm

Dysuria painful or difficult voiding

Eastern medicine an approach to health that emphasizes prevention and natural healing

Eccrine glands glands that produce sweat; found over most of the body

Echocardiogram a noninvasive test that uses ultrasound to visualize structures of the heart and evaluate left ventricular function

Ecomap a visualization of how the family unit interacts with the external community environment, such as schools, religious commitments, occupational duties, and recreational pursuits

Ectoderm the outer layer of tissue formed in the second week of life

Edema the presence of excess interstitial fluid in the body that makes skin appear swollen, shiny, and taut, and tends to blanch color

Effectiveness a measure of the quality or quantity of services provided

Efficiency a measure of the resources used in the provision of nursing services

Effleurage a stroking massage technique

Ego the realistic part of the individual that balances the gratification demands of the id with the limitations of social and physical circumstances

Ego defense mechanisms unconscious psychologic adaptive mechanisms that work to protect the individual from anxiety

E-Health use of technology in the delivery of healthcare and health information

Ejaculation expulsion of seminal fluid and sperm

Elderspeak speech style similar to babytalk; gives the message of dependence and incompetence to older adults

Elective surgery performed when surgical intervention is the preferred treatment for a condition that is not imminently life threatening or to improve the client's life

Electric shock occurs when a current travels through the body to the ground rather than through electric wiring, or from static electricity that builds up on the body

Electrocardiogram (ECG, EKG) a graph of the electrical activity of the heart

Electrocardiography provides a graphic recording of the heart's electrical activity

Electroencephalogram (EEG) a graph of the electrical activity of the brain

Electrolytes chemical substances that develop an electric charge and are able to conduct an electric current when placed in water; ions

Electromyogram (EMG) a graph of the electrical activity of muscles

Electronic communication communication involving computers and technology (i.e., email)

Electronic health records (EHRs) *see* Computer-based patient records (CPRs)

Electro-oculogram (EOG) a graph of the electrical activity of eye-to-eye movement

Elimination half-life *see* Drug half-life

Email the most common form of electronic communication

Embolus a blood clot (or a substance such as air) that has moved from its place of origin and is causing obstruction to circulation elsewhere (plural: *emboli*)

Embryonic phase the phase during which the fertilized ovum develops into an organism with most of the features of a human

Emergency surgery surgery that is performed immediately to preserve function or the life of the client

Emmetropic normal refraction so that the eyes focus images on the retina

Emotional intelligence (EI) the ability to form work relationships with colleagues, display maturity in a variety of situations, and resolve conflicts while taking into consideration the emotions of others

Empathy the ability to discriminate what the other individual's world is like and to communicate to the other this understanding in a way that shows that the helper understands the client's feelings and the behavior and experience underlying these feelings

Emphysema a chronic pulmonary condition in which the alveoli are dilated and distended

Empirical knowing knowledge that comes from science; ranges from factual, observable phenomena to theoretical analysis

Encoding involves the selection of specific signs or symbols (codes) to transmit the message, such as which language and words to use, how to arrange the words, and what tone of voice and gestures to use

Endocardium a layer of the heart wall lining the inside of the heart's chambers and great vessels

Endoderm the inner layer of tissue formed in the second week of life

End-of-life care the care provided in the final weeks before death

Endogenous developing from within

Enema used most often as a treatment for constipation, it distends the intestine and sometimes irritates the intestinal mucosa, thereby increasing peristalsis and the excretion of feces and flatus

Energy the force that integrates the body, mind, and spirit

Enhanced Nurse Licensure Compact (ENLC) allows all RNs and LPNs to have one multistate license, with the ability to practice in both their home state and all other compact states

Enteral through the gastrointestinal system

Entoderm *see* Endoderm

Enuresis bedwetting; involuntary urination in children beyond the age when voluntary bladder control is normally acquired

Environment all of the conditions, circumstances, and influences surrounding and affecting the development of an organism or individual

Enzymes biological catalysts that speed up chemical reactions

Epicardium the visceral pericardium adhering to the surface of the heart, forming the heart's outermost layer

Epidural the injection of an anesthetic agent into the epidural or intrathecal (subarachnoid) space

Epidural anesthesia the injection of an anesthetic agent into the epidural space; also known as *peridural anesthesia*

Equianalgesia refers to the relative potency of various opioid analgesics compared to a standard dose of parenteral morphine

Equilibrium a state of balance

Ernest Grant first male president of the American Nurses Association

Erythema a redness tinge of skin color associated with a variety of skin rashes

Erythrocytes red blood cells (RBCs)

Eschar necrotic tissue

Essential amino acids amino acids that cannot be manufactured in the body and must be supplied as part of the protein ingested in the diet

Ethical knowing knowledge that focuses on matters of obligation or what ought to be done

Ethics the rules or principles that govern right conduct

Ethnicity a relationship among individuals who believe that they have distinctive characteristics that make them a group

Ethnocentrism the belief that one's own culture or way of life is better than that of others

Ethnography research that provides a framework to focus on the culture of a group of individuals

Ethnopharmacology study of the effect of ethnicity on responses to prescribed medicines

Etiology the causation of a disease or condition

Eupnea normal, quiet breathing

Eustachian tube the part of the middle ear that connects the middle ear to the nasopharynx; stabilizes air pressure between the external atmosphere and the middle ear

Euthanasia the act of painlessly putting to death individuals suffering from incurable or distressing disease

Evaluating a planned ongoing, purposeful activity in which clients and healthcare professionals compare expected outcomes with actual outcomes

Evaluation statement a statement that consists of two parts: a conclusion and supporting data

Evaporation continuous vaporization of moisture from the respiratory tract and from the mucosa of the mouth and from the skin

Evidence-based practice (EBP) the use of some form of substantiation in making clinical decisions

Evisceration extrusion of the internal organs

Exacerbation the period during a chronic illness when symptoms reappear after remission

Excitement phase part of the response cycle, involves vasocongestion and myotonia

Excoriation loss of the superficial layers of the skin

Excretion elimination of a waste product produced by the body cells from the body

Exhalation (expiration) breathing out, or the movement of gases from the lungs to the atmosphere

Exogenous developing from outside sources

Exophthalmos a protrusion of the eyeballs with elevation of the upper eyelids, resulting in a startled or staring expression

Expectorate spit out

Expert witness one who has special training, experience, or skill in a relevant area and is allowed by the court to offer an opinion on some issue within that area of expertise

Expiration (exhalation) the outflow of air from the lungs to the atmosphere

Express consent an oral or written agreement

Extended family family that includes the relatives of the nuclear family (e.g., grandparents, aunts, uncles)

External auditory meatus the entrance to the ear canal

Extinction the failure to perceive touch on one side of the body when two symmetric areas of the body are touched simultaneously

Extracellular fluid (ECF) fluid found outside the body cells

Extraneous variables any variables that could influence the results of the study other than the specific variable[s] being studied for their influence

Extravasation infiltration that involves a *vesicant*, a medication or fluid that causes blisters, severe tissue injury, or necrosis if it escapes from the vein

Exudate purulent drainage

Fabiola a wealthy Roman matron; viewed by some as the patron saint of early nursing who used her position and wealth to establish hospitals for the sick

Fad a widespread but short-lived interest, or a practice followed with considerable zeal

Failure to thrive (FTT) a unique syndrome in which an infant falls below the fifth percentile for weight and height on a standard growth chart or is falling in percentiles on a growth chart

Faith refers to our beliefs and expectations about life, ourselves, and others

False imprisonment the unlawful restraint or detention of another individual against his or her wishes

Family the basic unit of society that consists of those individuals, male or female, youth or adult, legally or not legally related, genetically or not genetically related, who are considered by others to represent their significant individuals

Family-centered nursing nursing that considers the health of the family as a unit in addition to the health of individual family members

Fasciculation an abnormal contraction of a bundle of muscle fibers that appears as a twitch

Fats lipids that are solid at room temperature

Fat-soluble vitamins A, D, E, and K vitamins that the body can store

Fatty acids the basic structural units of most lipids made up of carbon chains and hydrogen

Fear an emotion or feeling of apprehension aroused by impending or seeming danger, pain, or another perceived threat

Febrile pertaining to a fever; feverish

Fecal impaction a mass or collection of hardened, putty-like feces in the folds of the rectum

Fecal incontinence *see* Bowel incontinence

Feces excreted waste products; also called *stool*

Feedback the response or message that the receiver returns to the sender during communication; the mechanism by which some of the output of a system is returned to the system as input

Felony a crime of a serious nature, such as murder, punishable by a term in prison

Female orgasmic disorder when the female sexual response stops before orgasm occurs

Female sexual arousal disorder when lack of vaginal lubrication causes discomfort or pain during sexual activity

Fetal phase characterized by a period of rapid growth in the size of the fetus; both genetic and environmental factors affect its growth

Fever elevated body temperature

Fever spike a temperature that rises to fever level rapidly following a normal temperature and then returns to normal within a few hours

Fibrin an insoluble protein formed from fibrinogen during the clotting of blood

Fidelity a moral principle that obligates the individual to be faithful to agreements and responsibilities he or she has undertaken

Filtration process whereby fluid and solutes move together across a membrane from one compartment to another

Filtration pressure the pressure in a compartment that results in the movement of fluid and substances dissolved in fluid out of the compartment

First-level manager a manager responsible for managing the work of nonmanagerial personnel and the day-to-day activities of a specific work group or groups

Fissures deep grooves that occur as a result of dryness and cracking of the skin

Fixation immobilization or the inability of the personality to proceed to the next developmental stage because of anxiety

Flaccid weak or lax

Flatness (of sound) an extremely dull sound produced, during percussion, by very dense tissue, such as muscle or bone

Flatulence the presence of excessive amounts of gas in the stomach or intestines

Flatus gas or air normally present in the stomach or intestines

Florence Nightingale considered the founder of modern nursing, she was influential in developing nursing education, practice, and administration

Flow sheet a record of the progress of specific or specialized data such as vital signs, fluid balance, or routine medications; often charted in graph form

Fluid volume deficit (FVD) (hypovolemia) loss of both water and electrolytes in similar proportions from the extracellular fluid

Fluid volume excess (FVE) (hypervolemia) retention of both water and sodium in similar proportions to normal extracellular fluid (ECF)

Focus charting a method of charting that uses key words or foci to describe what is happening to the client

Focused interview an interview in which the nurse asks the client specific questions to collect information related to the client's problem

Folk medicine beliefs and practices relating to illness prevention and healing that derive from cultural traditions rather than from modern medicine's scientific base

Fontanels unossified membranous gaps in the bone structure of the skull of a newborn that make molding of the head possible

Food diary a detailed record of measured amounts (portion sizes) of all food and fluids a client consumes during a specified period, usually 3 to 7 days

Food frequency record a checklist that indicates how often general food groups or specific foods are eaten

Foot drop plantar flexion contracture

Foreseeability a link that must exist between the nurse's act and the injury suffered

Formal leader an appointed leader selected by an organization and given official authority to make decisions and act

Formal nursing care plan a written or computerized guide that organizes information about the client's care

Fowler's position a semisitting position in which the head and trunk are raised 45° and 60° relative to the bed (typically at 45°) and the knees may be bent or may not be flexed

Fremitus the faintly perceptible vibration felt through the chest wall when the client speaks (tactile fremitus)

Friction rubbing; the force that opposes motion

Functional strength ability of the body to perform work

Fungi infection-causing microorganisms that include yeasts and molds

Gait the way an individual walks

Gastrocolic reflex increased peristalsis of the colon after food has entered the stomach

Gastrostomy an opening through the abdominal wall into the stomach

Gastrostomy tube a tube that is surgically placed directly into the client's stomach and provides another route for administering nutrition and medications

Gauge the diameter of the shaft of a needle; the larger the gauge number, the smaller the diameter of the shaft

Gender expression the outward manifestation of an individual's sense of maleness or femaleness as well as what is perceived as gender-appropriate behavior

Gender identity an individual's self-image as a female or male

General adaptation syndrome (GAS) (Selye) a general arousal response of the body to a stressor characterized by certain physiologic events and dominated by the sympathetic nervous system

General anesthesia the induced loss of all sensation and consciousness

Generalizations statements about common cultural patterns that may not hold true at the individual level

Generation X generation that includes those born in years 1965–1978

Generation Y generation that includes those born in years 1979–2000

Generativity concern for establishing and guiding the next generation

Generic name (of drug) given before a drug officially becomes an approved medication; generally used throughout the drug's lifetime

Genital intercourse penile–vaginal intercourse (coitus)

Genogram composed of visual representations of gender and lines of birth descent through the generations

Geragogy the term used to describe the process involved in stimulating and helping older adults to learn

Geriatrics medical care of older adults

Gerontology the study of aging and older adults

Gingiva the gum

Gingivitis red, swollen gingivae (gums)

Glaucoma a disturbance in the circulation of aqueous fluid that causes an increase in intraocular pressure

Global self refers to the collective beliefs and images one holds about oneself; the most complete description that individuals can give of themselves at any one time

Global self-esteem how much one likes one's perceived self as a whole

Glossitis inflammation of the tongue

Glycerides the most common form of lipids consisting of a glycerol molecule with up to three fatty acids

Glycogen the chief carbohydrate stored in the body, particularly in the liver and muscles

Goals or desired outcomes a part of a care plan that describes, in terms of observable client responses, what the nurse hopes to achieve by implementing the nursing interventions

Governance the establishment and maintenance of social, political, and economic arrangements by which practitioners control their practice, self-discipline, working conditions, and professional affairs

Granulation tissue young connective tissue with new capillaries formed in the wound healing process

Grief emotional suffering often caused by bereavement

Gross negligence involves extreme lack of knowledge, skill, or decision making that the individual clearly should have known would put others at risk for harm

Grounded theory research to understand social structures and social processes; this method focuses on the generation of categories or hypotheses that explain patterns of behavior of individuals in the study

Growth physical change and increase in size

Guaiac test performed for occult (hidden) blood in the stool to detect gastrointestinal bleeding not visible to the eye

Guided imagery state of focused attention that encourages changes in attitudes, behavior, and physiologic reactions

Gustatory referring to the sense of taste

Habit training attempts to keep clients dry by having them void at regular intervals; also referred to as *timed voiding* or *scheduled toileting*

Hand-mediated biofield therapies using the hands to alter the biofield, or energy field

Handoff communication process in which information about client care is communicated

Harm (injury) the client or plaintiff must demonstrate some type of harm or injury (physical, financial, or emotional) as a result of the breach of duty owed the client; the plaintiff will be asked to document physical injury, medical costs, loss of wages, "pain and suffering," and any other damages

Harriet Tubman African American woman known as "the Moses of Her People" for her work with the Underground Railroad; during the Civil War she nursed the sick and suffering of her own race

Health degree of wellness or well-being that the client experiences

Health behaviors the actions an individual takes to understand his or her health state, maintain an optimal state of health, prevent illness and injury, and reach his or her maximum physical and mental potential

Health beliefs concepts about health that an individual believes are true

Healthcare-associated infections (HAIs) those that originate in any healthcare setting

Healthcare proxy a legal statement that appoints a proxy to make medical decisions for the client in the event the client is unable to do so

Healthcare system the totality of services offered by all health disciplines

Health disparities differences in care experienced by one population compared with another population

Health equity the highest possible standard of health for all individuals, especially those at greatest risk for poor health

Health informatics the management of healthcare information, using computers; also called *health information technology*

Health literacy ability to read, understand, and act on provided health information

Health maintenance organization (HMO) a group healthcare agency that provides basic and supplemental health maintenance and treatment services to voluntary enrollees

Health promotion a process to facilitate movement toward accomplishment of health goals by supporting individuals to make lifestyle changes and create an environment conducive to health

Health promotion diagnosis relates to clients' preparedness to implement behaviors to improve their health condition

Health risk assessment (HRA) an assessment and educational tool that indicates a client's risk for disease or injury during the next 10 years by comparing the client's risk with the mortality risk of the corresponding age, sex, and racial group

Health status the health of an individual at a given time

Heart failure a condition that develops if the heart cannot keep up with the body's need for oxygen and nutrients to the tissues; usually occurs because of myocardial infarction, but it may also result from chronic overwork of the heart

Heart-lung death the traditional clinical signs of death: cessation of the apical pulse, respirations, and blood pressure

Heat balance the state an individual is in when the amount of heat produced by the body exactly equals the amount of heat lost

Heat exhaustion condition that is the result of excessive heat and dehydration

Heat stroke life-threatening condition with body temperature greater than 41°C (106°F)

Heimlich maneuver abdominal thrusts used to clear an obstructed airway

Helix the posterior curve of the auricle's upper aspect

Helping relationships the nurse–client relationship

Hematocrit (Hct) the proportion of red blood cells (erythrocytes) to the total blood volume

Hematoma a contusion or "black eye" resulting from injury

Hemoglobin (Hgb) the red pigment in red blood cells that carries oxygen

Hemoglobin A1C (HbA1C) measurement of blood glucose that is bound to hemoglobin

Hemolytic transfusion reaction destruction of red blood cells as a result of transfusion of incompatible blood

Hemoptysis the presence of blood in the sputum

Hemorrhage excessive loss of blood from the vascular system

Hemorrhoids distended veins in the rectum

Hemostasis cessation of bleeding

Hemothorax the accumulation of blood in the pleural cavity

Herbal medicine treating illness with herbs

Heritage things passed down from previous generations

Heritage consistent identifying with one's traditional cultural heritage

Heritage inconsistent acculturated into the local culture in which one resides

Hernia a protrusion of an organ or tissue through an opening such as the abdominal or inguinal muscles

Higher brain death *see* Cerebral death

High-Fowler's position position in which the head and trunk are raised 60° to 90°, and most often the client is sitting upright at a right angle to the bed

Hirsutism the growth of excessive body hair

Holism combined mental, emotional, spiritual, relationship, and environmental components that are considered to play crucial and equal roles in an individual's state of health

Holistic health belief holds that the forces of nature must be maintained in balance or harmony

Holy days solemn religious observances and feast days throughout the year

Home healthcare healthcare professionals providing services in the home setting to clients recovering from an acute illness or injury or those with a disability or a chronic condition

Home health nursing care services and products provided to clients in their homes that are needed to maintain, restore, or promote their physical, psychologic, and social well-being

Homeopathy an alternative therapy based on the theory that the cure for the disease lies in the disease itself; thus, treatment is with highly diluted amounts of substances that at a higher concentration would produce the same symptoms as the disease

Homeostasis the tendency of the body to maintain a state of balance or equilibrium while continually changing; a mechanism in which deviations from normal are sensed and counteracted

Homocysteine an amino acid that has been shown to be increased in many individuals with atherosclerosis

Hordeolum redness, swelling, and tenderness of the hair follicle and glands that empty at the edge of the eyelids; also called a *sty*

Horticultural therapy adjunct therapy to occupational and physical therapy that may involve viewing nature, visiting a healing garden or wander garden, or actively gardening; also called *gardening* or *healing garden*

Hospice care that focuses on support and care for the dying individual and family, with the goal of facilitating a peaceful and dignified death

Hospice nursing focuses on caring and supportive nursing and medical interventions to promote a good death

Hospital information system (HIS) computer software program suite used to manage client, financial, and administrative data

Hub the part of the needle that fits onto the syringe

Humanist a perspective that includes propositions such as the mind and body are indivisible, people have the power to solve their own problems, and people are responsible for their lives and well-being

Humanistic learning theory focuses on both the cognitive and affective qualities of the learner

Humidifier a device that adds water vapor to inspired air

Humoral immunity antibody-mediated defense; resides ultimately in the B lymphocytes and is mediated by the antibodies produced by B cells

Hydrostatic pressure the pressure a liquid exerts on the sides of the container that holds it

Hygiene the science of health and its maintenance

Hypercalcemia an excess of calcium in the blood plasma

Hypercapnia a condition in which carbon dioxide accumulates in the blood

Hypercarbia (hypercapnia) accumulation of carbon dioxide in the blood

Hyperchloremia an excess of chloride in the blood plasma

Hyperinflation giving the client breaths that are greater than the client's normal tidal volume set on the ventilator through the ventilator circuit or via a manual resuscitation bag

Hyperkalemia an excess of potassium in the blood plasma

Hypermagnesemia an excess of magnesium in the blood plasma

Hypernatremia an excess of sodium in the blood plasma

Hyperopia farsightedness

Hyperoxygenation increasing the oxygen flow before suctioning and between suction attempts to avoid suction-related hypoxemia

Hyperphosphatemia an excess of phosphate in the blood plasma

Hyperpyrexia an extremely high body temperature (e.g., 41°C [105.8°F])

Hyperresonance an abnormal booming sound produced during percussion of the lungs

Hypersomnia condition where the affected individual obtains sufficient sleep at night but still cannot stay awake during the day

Hypertension an abnormally high blood pressure; over 140 mmHg systolic and/or 90 mmHg diastolic

Hyperthermia a body temperature above the usual range

Hypertonic solutions that have a higher osmolality than body fluids

Hypertrophy enlargement of a muscle or organ

Hyperventilation very deep, rapid respirations

Hypervolemia increased blood volume

Hypnotherapy application of hypnosis (trance state or altered state of consciousness) to a medical or psychologic disorder

Hypoactive sexual desire disorder a deficiency in or absence of sexual fantasies and persistently low interest or a total lack of interest in sexual activity

Hypocalcemia deficiency of calcium in the blood plasma

Hypochloremia deficiency of chloride in the blood plasma

Hypodermic under the skin

Hypodermic syringe a type of syringe that comes in 2-, 2.5-, and 3-mL sizes; the syringe usually has two scales marked on it: the minim and the milliliter

Hypokalemia deficiency of potassium in the blood plasma

Hypomagnesemia deficiency of magnesium in the blood plasma

Hyponatremia deficiency of sodium in the blood plasma

Hypophosphatemia deficiency of phosphate in the blood plasma

Hypotension an abnormally low blood pressure; less than 100 mmHg systolic in an adult

Hypothermia a core body temperature below the lower limit of normal

Hypothesis a prediction of the relationships among two or more variables

Hypotonic solutions that have a lower osmolality than body fluids

Hypoventilation very shallow respirations

Hypovolemia an abnormal reduction in blood volume

Hypoxemia low partial pressure of oxygen or low saturation of oxyhemoglobin in the arterial blood

Hypoxia insufficient oxygen anywhere in the body

Iatrogenic disease disease caused unintentionally by medical therapy

Iatrogenic infections infections that are the direct result of diagnostic or therapeutic procedures

Id the source of instinctive and unconscious psychologic urges

Ideal body weight (IBW) the optimal weight recommended for optimal health

Ideal self how we would prefer to be; the individual's perception of how one should behave based on certain personal standards, aspirations, goals, or values

Identification perceiving one's self as similar to and behaving like another individual

Idiosyncratic effect a different, unexpected, or individual effect from the normal one usually expected from a medication; the occurrence of unpredictable and unexplainable symptoms

iGeneration generation that includes those born in the years 1995–2012

Ileal conduit urinary diversion in which the client must wear an external pouch over the stoma to collect the continuous flow of urine; also known as *ileal loop*

Ileostomy a colostomy that generally empties from the distal end of the small intestine

Illicit drugs drugs that are sold illegally; street drugs

Illness a highly personal state in which an individual feels unhealthy or ill; may or may not be related to disease

Illness behavior the course of action an individual takes to define the state of his or her health and pursue a remedy

Imagery a two-way communication between the conscious and unconscious mind involving the whole body and all its senses

Imagination an important part of preschoolers' life (the preschooler has an active imagination and fantasizes in play)

Imitation copying the behaviors and attitudes of another individual

Immobility prescribed or unavoidable restriction of movement in any area of an individual's life

Immune defenses *see* Specific defenses

Immunity a specific resistance of the body to infection; it may be natural, or resistance may develop after exposure to a disease agent

Immunoglobulins *see* Antibodies

Implementing the phase of the nursing process in which the nursing care plan is put into action

Implied consent consent that is assumed in an emergency when consent cannot be obtained from the client or a relative

Implied contract a contract that has not been explicitly agreed to by the parties but that the law nevertheless considers to exist

Incentive spirometer a device that measures the flow of air inhaled through a mouthpiece; also called a *sustained maximal inspiration device (SMI)*

Incivility behaviors that are disrespectful, rude, and impolite, and promote conflict while increasing stress

Incomplete proteins proteins that lack one or more essential amino acids; usually derived from vegetables

Incus the anvil bone of the middle ear

Independent functions areas of healthcare unique to nursing, separate and distinct from medical management

Independent interventions activities that the nurse is licensed to initiate as a result of the nurse's own knowledge and skills

Independent practice associations (IPAs) provide care in offices; clients pay a fixed prospective payment and the IPA pays the provider; earnings or losses are assumed by the IPA

Independent variable the presumed cause or influence on a dependent variable

Indicator an observable client state, behavior, or self-reported perception or evaluation; similar to desired outcomes in traditional language

Individualized care plan a plan tailored to meet the unique needs of a specific client—needs that are not addressed by the standardized plan

Inductive reasoning making generalizations from specific data

Infection the disease process produced by microorganisms

Inferences interpretations or conclusions made based on cues or observed data

Inferential statistics allows researchers to test hypotheses about relationships between variables or differences between groups

Infiltration occurs when the tip of an IV is outside the vein and the fluid is entering the tissues instead; manifested by local swelling, coolness, pallor, and discomfort at the IV site

Inflammation local and nonspecific defensive tissue response to injury or destruction of cells

Influence an informal strategy used to gain the cooperation of others without exercising formal authority

Inflicted traumatic brain injury *see* Abusive head trauma

Informal leader an individual selected by a group as its leader because of seniority, age, special abilities, or charisma

Informal nursing care plan a strategy for action that exists in the nurse's mind

Informatics the science of computer information systems

Information technology (IT) use of computers to systematically solve problems

Informed consent a client's agreement to accept a course of treatment or a procedure after receiving complete information, including the risks of treatment and facts relating to it, from the healthcare provider

Ingrown toenail the growing inward of a nail into the soft tissues around it; most often results from improper nail trimming

Inhalation the intake of air into the lungs; also called *inspiration*

Inhibiting effect the decreased effect of one or both drugs

Injury *see* Harm

Input consists of information, material, or energy that enters a system

Inquest a legal inquiry into the cause or manner of a death

Insensible fluid loss fluid loss that is not perceptible to an individual

Insensible heat loss heat loss that occurs from evaporation (vaporization) of moisture from the respiratory tract, mucosa of the mouth, and the skin

Insensible water loss continuous and unnoticed water loss

In-service education education that is designed to upgrade the knowledge or skills of employees

Insomnia inability to fall asleep or remain asleep

Inspection visual examination, which is assessing by using the sense of sight

Inspiration *see* Inhalation

Insulin syringe syringe that has a scale specially designed for insulin and is the only type of syringe that should be used to administer insulin

Integrated delivery system (IDS) a system that incorporates acute care services, home healthcare, extended and skilled care facilities, and outpatient services

Integrated healthcare system one that makes all levels of care available in an integrated form—primary care, secondary care, and tertiary care

Integrative medicine combines treatments from conventional medicine and complementary and alternative medicine for which there is high-quality evidence of safety and effectiveness

Intensity the loudness or softness of auscultated sound

Intention tremor involuntary trembling when an individual attempts a voluntary movement

Intermittent fever a body temperature that alternates at regular intervals between periods of fever and periods of normal or subnormal temperatures

Internet a worldwide computer network

Interpersonal skills all verbal and nonverbal activities individuals use when communicating directly with one another

Interpreter an individual who mediates spoken communication between individuals speaking different languages without adding, omitting, or distorting meaning or editorializing

Intersex a condition in which there are contradictions among chromosomal sex, gonadal sex, internal organs, and external genital appearance that result in ambiguous gender

Interstitial fluid fluid that surrounds the cells; includes lymph

Interview a planned communication; a conversation with a purpose

Intimacy a close friendship

Intracellular fluid (ICF) fluid found within the body cells; also called *cellular fluid*

Intradermal under the epidermis (into the dermis)

Intradermal (ID) injection the administration of a drug into the dermal layer of the skin just beneath the epidermis

Intramuscular into the muscle

Intramuscular (IM) injection the administration of a drug into the muscle tissue

Intraoperative phase the phase of surgery that begins when the client is transferred to the operating room and ends when the client is admitted to the postanesthesia care unit (PACU), also called the postanesthesia room (PAR)

Intraspinal (intrathecal) into the spinal canal

Intrathecal *see* Intraspinal

Intravascular fluid plasma

Intravenous within a vein

Intravenous pyelography (IVP) x-ray filming of the kidney and ureters after injection of a radiopaque material into the vein

Introjection the assimilation of the attributes of others

Intuition the understanding or learning of things without the conscious use of reasoning

Invasion of privacy a direct wrong of a personal nature, it injures the feelings of the individual and does not take into account the effect of revealed information on the standing of the individual in the community

Ions atoms or group of atoms that carry a positive or negative electric charge; electrolytes

Iron deficiency anemia a form of anemia caused by inadequate supply of iron for synthesis of hemoglobin

Irrigation a flushing or washing out with a specified solution; administration of a solution to wash out the conjunctival sac to remove secretions or foreign bodies or to remove chemicals that may injure the eye

Ischemia deficiency of blood supply caused by obstruction of circulation to the body part

Isokinetic (resistive) exercises muscle contraction or tension against resistance

Isolation practices that prevent the spread of infection and communicable diseases

Isometric (static or setting) exercise muscle contraction without moving the joint (muscle length does not change), which involves exerting pressure against a solid object

Isotonic solutions that have the same osmolality as body fluids

Isotonic (dynamic) exercise exercise in which muscle tension is constant and the muscle shortens to produce muscle contraction and active movement

Jaundice a yellowish tinge to skin color

Jejunostomy a tube that is placed surgically or by laparoscopy through the abdominal wall into the jejunum for long-term nutritional support

Justice fairness

Kardex the trade name for a method that makes use of a series of cards to concisely organize and record client data and instructions for daily nursing care—especially care that changes frequently and must be kept up to date

Keloid a hypertrophic scar containing an abnormal amount of collagen

Kidneys, ureters, and bladder (KUB) x-ray of the kidneys, ureters, and bladder

Kilojoule (kJ) a metric measurement referring to the amount of energy required when a force of 1 newton (N) moves 1 kg of weight 1 m of distance

Kinesthetic refers to awareness of the position and movement of body parts

Knights of Saint Lazarus an order of knights that dedicated themselves to the care of individuals with leprosy, syphilis, and chronic skin conditions

Korotkoff sounds the five phases of blood pressure sounds

Kyphosis excessive convex curvature of the thoracic spine

Laissez-faire (permissive) leader recognizes a group's need for autonomy and self-regulation

Lanugo the fine hair on the body of the fetus, also referred to as down or woolly hair

Large calorie (Calorie, kilocalorie [Kcal]) the amount of heat energy required to raise the temperature of 1 gram of water 15°C to 16°C; the unit used in nutrition

Lateral (side-lying) position position in which an individual lies on one side of the body

Lavage an irrigation or washing of a body organ, such as the stomach

Lavinia L. Dock a nursing leader and suffragist who was active in the protest movement for women's rights that resulted in the U.S. Constitution amendment allowing women to vote in 1920

Law a rule made by humans that regulates social conduct in a formally prescribed and binding manner

Laxatives medications that stimulate bowel activity and assist fecal elimination

Leader an individual who influences others to work together to accomplish a specific goal

Leadership style describes traits, behaviors, motivations, and choices used by individuals to effectively influence others

Leading question a question that influences the client to give a particular answer

Learning a change in human disposition or capability that persists over a period of time and cannot be solely accounted for by growth

Learning need a desire or a requirement to know something that is currently unknown to the learner

Leukocytes white blood cells

Leukocytosis an increase in the number of white blood cells

Liability the quality or state of being legally responsible for one's obligations and action and to make financial restitution for wrongful acts

Libel defamation by means of print, writing, or pictures

Libido urge or desire for sexual activity

License a legal permit granted to individuals to engage in the practice of a profession and to use a particular title

Licensed practical nurse (LPN) provides direct client care under the direction of an RN, physician, or other licensed practitioner

Licensed vocational (practical) nurse (LVN/LPN) a nurse who practices under the supervision of a registered nurse, providing basic direct technical care to clients

Lifestyle the values and behaviors adopted by an individual in daily life

Lift an abnormal anterior movement of the chest related to enlargement of the right ventricle

Lillian Wald founder of the Henry Street Settlement and Visiting Nurse Service, which provided nursing and social services and organized educational and cultural activities; considered the founder of public health nursing

Linda Richards America's first formally trained nurse

Line of gravity an imaginary vertical line drawn through an object's center of gravity

Lipids organic substances that are greasy and insoluble in water but soluble in alcohol or ether

Lipoproteins soluble compounds made up of various lipids

Litigation the action of a lawsuit

Living will a document that states medical treatments(s) the client chooses to omit or refuse in the event that the client is unable to make these decisions

Livor mortis discoloration of the skin caused by breakdown of the red blood cells, which occurs after blood circulation has ceased and appears in the lowermost or dependent areas of the body

Lobule earlobe

Local adaptation syndrome (LAS) the reaction of one organ or body part to stress

Local anesthesia an anesthetic agent used for minor surgical procedures that is injected into a specific area

Local infection an infection that is limited to the specific part of the body where the microorganisms remain

Locus of control (LOC) a concept about whether clients believe their health status is under their own or others' control

Logical positivism maintains that "truth" is absolute and can be discovered by careful measurement

Logrolling a technique used to turn a client whose body must at all times be kept in straight alignment

Long-term memory the repository for information stored for periods longer than 72 hours and usually weeks and years

Lordosis an exaggerated concavity in the lumbar region of the vertebral column

Loss an actual or potential situation in which something that is valued is changed or no longer available

Lumbar puncture procedure in which cerebrospinal fluid is withdrawn through a needle inserted into the subarachnoid space of the spinal canal between the third and fourth lumbar vertebrae, or between the fourth and fifth lumbar vertebrae; also called a *spinal tap*

Lung compliance expansibility of the lung

Lung recoil the tendency of lungs to collapse away from the chest wall

Lung scan records the emissions from radioisotopes that indicate how well gas and blood are traveling through the lungs; also known as a *V/Q* (ventilation/perfusion) *scan*

Luther Christman one of the founders of the American Assembly for Men in Nursing and the first male dean

Maceration the wasting away or softening of a solid as if by the action of soaking; often used to describe degenerative changes and eventual disintegration

Macrominerals any of the minerals that individuals require daily in amounts over 100 mg

Macronutrients carbohydrates, fats, and protein that are needed in large amounts to provide energy

Magico-religious health belief a belief system in which individuals attribute the fate of the world and those in it to the actions of God, the gods, or other supernatural forces for good or evil

Magnetic resonance imaging (MRI) a noninvasive diagnostic scanning technique in which the client is placed in a magnetic field

Maintenance stage stage at which an individual integrates newly adopted behavior patterns into his or her lifestyle

Major surgery surgery that involves a high degree of risk for a variety of reasons; it may be complicated or prolonged; large losses of blood may occur; vital organs may be involved; postoperative complications may occur

Male erectile disorder when a man has erection problems during 25% or more of his sexual interactions

Male orgasmic disorder disorder where a man can maintain an erection but has difficulty ejaculating

Malleus hammer bone of the middle ear

Malnutrition the lack of necessary or appropriate food substances that includes both undernutrition and overnutrition

Malpractice the negligent acts of individuals engaged in professions or occupations in which highly technical or professional skills are employed

Managed care a method of organizing care delivery that emphasizes communication and coordination of care among all healthcare team members

Management information system (MIS) software designed to facilitate the organization and application of data used to manage an organization or department

Manager one who is appointed to a position in an organization that gives the power to guide and direct the work of others

Mandated reporters a role of the nurse in which he or she identifies and assesses cases of violence against others, and in every case the situation must be reported to the proper authorities

Manometer a glass or plastic tube calibrated in millimeters that is used to take cerebrospinal pressure readings

Manslaughter second-degree murder

Manubrium the handle-like superior part of the sternum that joins with the clavicles

Margaret Higgins Sanger considered the founder of Planned Parenthood, was imprisoned for opening the first birth control information clinic in Baltimore in 1916

Mary Breckinridge a nurse who practiced midwifery in England, Australia, and New Zealand; founded the Frontier Nursing Service in Kentucky in 1925 to provide family-centered primary healthcare to rural populations

Mary Mahoney first African American professional nurse

Massage therapy the scientific manipulation of the soft tissues of the body

Mastoid a bony prominence behind the ear

Masturbation sexual self-stimulation

Maturation theory that children achieve milestone abilities and skills, such as rolling over, sitting, and walking at specific times, based on an in-born timetable

Maturity the state of maximal function and integration; the state of being fully developed

Mean arterial pressure (MAP) represents the pulse pressure actually delivered to the body's organs

Measures of central tendency measures that describe the center of a distribution of data, denoting where most of the participants lie; include the mean, median, and mode

Measures of variability measures that indicate the degree of dispersion or spread of the data; include range, variance, and standard deviation

Meatus referring to the urinary meatus, which is the external opening from the urethra to the surface of the body

Meconium the first fecal material passed by a newborn, normally up to 24 hours after birth

Medicaid a U.S. federal public assistance program paid out of general taxes and administered through the individual states to provide healthcare for those who require financial assistance

Medical asepsis all practices intended to confine a specific microorganism to a specific area, limiting the number, growth, and spread of microorganisms

Medical examiner a physician who usually has advanced education in pathology or forensic medicine who determines causes of death

Medicare a national and state health insurance program for U.S. residents older than 65 years of age

Medication a substance administered for the diagnosis, cure, treatment, or relief of a symptom or for prevention of disease

Medication reconciliation process of identifying the most accurate list possible of all medications a client is taking—including drug name, dosage, frequency, and route—and using this list to provide correct medications for clients anywhere within the healthcare system

Meditation various mindfulness techniques with key elements that include focused attention on the present moment or the body's experience; awareness, depth, and steadiness of breathing; and avoiding judgmental and intrusive thoughts

Menarche onset of menstruation

Meniscus the crescent-shaped upper surface of a column of liquid

Menopause cessation of menstruation

Menstruation the monthly discharge of blood through the vagina occurring in nonpregnant women from puberty to menopause

Mentor an individual who serves as an experienced guide, adviser, or advocate and assumes responsibility for promoting the growth and professional advancement of a less experienced individual

Mesoderm middle layer of the embryonic tissue that forms during the first 3 weeks of life

Metabolic acidosis a condition characterized by a deficiency of bicarbonate ions in the body in relation to the amount of carbonic acid in the body; the pH falls to less than 7.35

Metabolic alkalosis a condition characterized by an excess of bicarbonate ions in the body in relation to the amount of carbonic acid in the body; the pH rises to greater than 7.45

Metabolic syndrome (Met-S) a cluster of cardiovascular risk factors that increase the risk for cardiovascular disease, diabetes, and death

Metabolism the sum of all physical and chemical processes by which a living substance is formed and maintained and by which energy is made available for use by the organism; also called *biotransformation*

Metabolites end products or enzymes

Metacognitive processes include reflective thinking and awareness of the skills learned by the nurse in caring for the client. The nurse reflects on the client's status, and through the use of critical thinking skills determines the most effective plan of care.

Metaparadigm originates from the Greek *meta*, meaning "with," and *paradigm*, meaning "pattern"; based on four theoretical concepts of nursing: individual or client, environment, health, and nursing

Metered-dose inhaler (MDI) a handheld nebulizer that is a pressurized container of medication used by the client to release the medication through a mouthpiece

Methodology elements of the research process that deal with how the study is organized, who or what will be the sources of information for the study, and data collection details such as what and how data will be collected and the timing of data collection

Microminerals a vitamin or mineral

Micronutrients those vitamins and minerals required in small amounts to metabolize the energy-providing nutrients

Micturition *see* Urination

Mid-arm circumference (MAC) a measure of fat, muscle, and skeleton

Mid-arm muscle area (MAMA) calculated by using reference tables or by using a formula that incorporates the triceps skinfold and the MAC

Middle-level manager a manager who supervises a number of first-level managers and is responsible for the activities in the departments supervised

Midstream urine specimen *see* Clean-catch specimen

Mild pain pain in the 1 to 3 range on a numeric scale of 0 (no pain) to 10 (worst pain imaginable)

Milliequivalent one-thousandth of an equivalent, which is the chemical combining power of a substance

Minerals a substance found in organic compounds, as inorganic compounds and as free ions

Minor surgery surgery that involves little risk, produces few complications, and is often performed in a "day surgery" facility

Miosis constricted pupils

Misdemeanor a legal offense usually punishable by a fine or a short-term jail sentence, or both

Mixed hearing loss a combination of conduction and sensorineural loss

Mobility ability to move about freely, easily, and purposefully in the environment

Modeling observing the behavior of individuals who have successfully achieved a goal that one has set for oneself and, through observing, acquiring ideas for behavior and coping strategies

Moderate pain pain in the 4 to 6 range on a numeric scale of 0 (no pain) to 10 (worst pain imaginable)

Monosaccharides sugars that are composed of single molecules

Monounsaturated fatty acids a fatty acid with one double bond

Moral relating to right and wrong

Moral behavior the way an individual perceives the requirements necessary for individuals to live together and how he or she responds to them

Moral development process of learning to tell the difference between right and wrong and of learning what ought and ought not to be done

Moral distress when what is in the client's best interest may be contrary to the nurse's personal belief system

Morality a doctrine or system denoting what is right and wrong in conduct, character, or attitude

Moral rules specific prescriptions for actions

Mortician an individual trained in care of the dead; also called an *undertaker*

Motivation the desire to learn

Mourning the process through which grief is eventually resolved or altered

Mucus clearance device (MCD) a small, handheld device that loosens mucus from the airways and assists its movement up the airways to be expectorated; used for clients with excessive secretions such as with cystic fibrosis, COPD, and bronchiectasis

Multicultural describes an individual who has multiple patterns of identification or crosses several cultures, lifestyles, and sets of values

Multidisciplinary care plan a standardized plan that outlines the care required for clients with common, predictable—usually medical—conditions

Multimodal pain management incorporates both pharmacologic and nonpharmacologic approaches to achieve the best possible outcomes for the client

Music therapy the behavioral science concerned with the systematic application of music to produce relaxation and desired changes in emotions, behavior, and physiology

Mutual pretense a type of awareness in which the client, family, and health personnel know that the prognosis is terminal but do not talk about it and make an effort not to raise the subject

Mutual recognition model a regulatory model developed by the National Council of State Boards of Nursing, which allows for multistate licensure

Mydriasis enlarged pupils

Myocardial infarction (MI) heart attack; cardiac tissue necrosis owing to obstruction of blood flow to the heart

Myocardium a layer of the heart wall; cardiac muscle cells that form the bulk of the heart and contract with each beat

Myopia nearsightedness

Narcolepsy an uncontrollable desire for sleep or attacks of sleep during the day

Narrative charting a descriptive record of client data and nursing interventions, written in sentences and paragraphs

Nasoenteric (nasointestinal) tube a tube inserted through one of the nostrils, down the nasopharynx, and into the alimentary tract

Nasogastric tube a tube inserted by way of the nasopharynx or the oropharynx; it is placed into the stomach for the temporary purpose of feeding the client or to remove gastric secretions

Nationality refers to the sovereign state or country where an individual has membership, which may be through birth, through inheritance (parents), or through naturalization

Naturalism maintains that reality is relative or contextual and constructed by individuals who are experiencing a phenomenon; sometimes referred to as *constructivism*

Naturopathic medicine practice that focuses on nutrition, herbs, physical therapy, spinal manipulation, acupuncture, lifestyle counseling, stress management, exercise therapy, homeopathy, and hydrotherapy

Nebulizer small machine that vaporizes a liquid medication into a fine mist that is inhaled, using a face mask or handheld device

Negative feedback feedback that inhibits change

Negligence failure to behave in a reasonable and prudent manner; an unintentional tort

Nephrostomy diversion of urine from a kidney to a stoma

Nerve block chemical interruption of a nerve pathway effected by injecting a local anesthetic

Networking a process by which individuals develop linkages throughout a profession to communicate, share ideas and information, and offer support and direction to each other

Neurogenic bladder interference with the normal mechanisms of urine elimination in which the client does not perceive bladder fullness and is unable to control the urinary sphincters; the result of impaired neurologic function

Neuropathic pain experienced by individuals who have damaged or malfunctioning nerves as a result of illness, injury, or undetermined reasons

Neutral question a question that does not direct or pressure a client to answer in a certain way

Nitrogen balance a measure of the degree of protein anabolism and catabolism; net result of intake and loss of nitrogen

Nociception the physiologic processes related to pain perception

Nociceptive pain experienced when an intact, properly functioning nervous system sends signals that tissues are damaged, requiring attention and proper care

Nociceptor a pain receptor

Nocturia voiding two or more times at night

Nocturnal emissions orgasm and emission of semen during sleep

Nocturnal enuresis involuntary urination at night

Nondirective interview an interview using open-ended questions and empathetic responses to build rapport and learn client concerns

Nonessential amino acids an amino acid that the body can manufacture

Noninvasive positive pressure ventilation (NPPV) delivery of air or oxygen under pressure without the need for an invasive tube such as an endotracheal tube or tracheostomy tube for clients who require mechanical assistance to maintain adequate breathing

Nonmaleficence the duty to do no harm

Nonspecific defenses bodily defenses that protect an individual against all microorganisms, regardless of prior exposure

Nonsteroidal anti-inflammatory drugs (NSAIDs) drugs such as aspirin and ibuprofen that have anti-inflammatory, analgesic, and antipyretic effects

Nonverbal communication communication other than words, including gestures, posture, and facial expressions

Norm an ideal or fixed standard; an expected standard of behavior of group members

Normocephalic normal head size

Normocephaly normal head circumference at birth; usually 35 cm (14 in.)

Nosocomial infections infections that originate in the hospital

NPO nothing by mouth; literally, "nil per os"

NREM (non-REM) sleep sleep during which the individual experiences non–rapid eye movement

Nuclear family a family of parents and their offspring

Nurse informaticist an expert who combines computer, information, and nursing science to develop policies and procedures that promote effective use of computerized records by nurses and other healthcare professionals

Nurse Licensure Compact (NLC) an agreement between two or more states that is the mechanism used to create mutual recognition among states

Nursing the attributes, characteristics, and actions of a nurse providing care on behalf of, or in conjunction with, a client

Nursing diagnosis the nurse's clinical judgment about individual, family, or community responses to actual and potential health problems and life processes to provide the basis for selecting nursing interventions to achieve outcomes for which the nurse is accountable

Nursing ethics ethical issues that occur in nursing practice

Nursing informatics the science of using computer information systems in the practice of nursing

Nursing intervention any treatment, based on clinical judgment and knowledge, that a nurse performs to enhance client outcomes

Nursing Interventions Classification (NIC) a taxonomy of nursing actions, each of which includes a label, a definition, and a list of activities

Nursing Outcomes Classification (NOC) a taxonomy for describing client outcomes that respond to nursing interventions

Nursing process a systematic, rational method of planning and providing nursing care

Nutrients organic, inorganic, energy-producing substances found in foods and required for body functioning

Nutrition the sum of all interactions between an organism and the food it consumes

Nutritive value the nutrient content of a specified amount of food

Nystagmus rapid involuntary rhythmic eye movement

Obese when body mass index (BMI) is greater than 30 kg/m^2

Objective data information (data) that is detectable by an observer or can be tested against an accepted standard; can be seen, heard, felt, or smelled; also called *signs*

Obligatory losses essential fluid losses required to maintain body functioning

Occult blood hidden blood

Occupational exposure skin, eye, mucous membrane, or parenteral contact with blood or other potentially infectious materials that may result from the performance of an employee's duties

Official name (of drug) the name under which a drug is listed in one of the official publications (e.g., the *United States Pharmacopeia*)

Oils lipids that are liquid at room temperature

Olfactory related to smell

Oliguria production of abnormally small amounts of urine by the kidney

Oncotic pressure *see* Colloid osmotic pressure

One-point discrimination the ability to sense whether one or two areas of the skin are being stimulated by pressure

Onset of action the time after drug administration when the body initially responds to the drug

Open awareness a type of awareness in which a client and individuals around know about an impending death

Open-ended questions questions that specify only a broad topic to be discussed and invite clients to discover and explore their thoughts and feelings about the topic

Open system system in which energy, matter, and information move into and out of the system through the system's boundary

Ophthalmic pertaining to medications for the eye

Opportunistic pathogen a microorganism causing disease only in a susceptible individual

Oral a method of administration in which the drug is swallowed

Oral–genital sex oral stimulation of either female or male genitals

Organizing determining responsibilities, communicating expectations, and establishing the chain of command for authority and communication

Orgasmic phase part of the response cycle, the involuntary climax of sexual tension, accompanied by physiologic and psychologic release

Orthopnea ability to breathe only when in an upright position (sitting or standing)

Orthopneic position a sitting position to relieve respiratory difficulty in which the client sits either in bed or on the side of the bed, leaning over an overbed table across the lap

Orthostatic hypotension decrease in blood pressure related to positional or postural changes from lying to sitting or standing positions

Osmolality the concentration of solutes in body fluids

Osmosis passage of a solvent through a semipermeable membrane from an area of lesser solute concentration to one of greater solute concentration

Osmotic pressure pressure exerted by the number of nondiffusible particles in a solution; the amount of pressure needed to stop the flow of water across a membrane

Ossicles the three middle ear bones of sound transmission

Osteoporosis demineralization of the bone

Ostomy an opening on the abdominal wall for the elimination of feces or urine

Otic refers to instillations or irrigations of the external auditory canal

Otoscope an instrument used to view the ear

Outcome evaluation focuses on demonstrable changes in a client's health status as a result of nursing care

Output energy, matter, or information from a system given out by the system as a result of its processes

Overhydration occurs when water is gained in excess of electrolytes, resulting in low serum osmolality and low serum sodium levels, also known as *hypo-osmolar imbalance* or *water intoxication*

Overnutrition refers to a caloric intake in excess of daily energy requirements, resulting in storage of energy in the form of increased adipose tissue

Overweight a BMI of 25 to 29.9 kg/m^2

Oxygen saturation (SpO_2) the percentage of all hemoglobin binding sites that are occupied by oxygen

Oxyhemoglobin the compound of oxygen and hemoglobin

Pace number of steps taken per minute or the distance taken in one step when walking

Packing filling an open wound or cavity with a material such as gauze

Pain whatever the experiencing individual says it is, existing whenever he or she says it does

Pain management alleviation of pain or a reduction in pain to a level of comfort that is acceptable to the client

Pain threshold the least amount of stimuli that is needed for an individual to label a sensation as pain

Pain tolerance the maximum amount of painful stimuli that an individual is willing to withstand without seeking avoidance of the pain or relief

Palliative care the prevention and relief of suffering by means of early identification and impeccable assessment and treatment of pain and other problems, physical, psychosocial, and spiritual

Pallor paleness

Palpation the examination of the body using the sense of touch

Papanicolaou (Pap) test a method of taking a sample of cervical cells for microscopic examination to detect malignancy

Parasites microorganisms that live in or on another organism from which they obtain nourishment

Parasomnia a cluster or pattern of waking behavior that appears during sleep, such as somnambulism (sleepwalking), sleeptalking, and enuresis (bedwetting)

Parenteral drug administration using a medication route other than the alimentary or digestive tract; injected into the body intradermally, subcutaneously, intramuscularly, or intravenously

Paresis slight or incomplete paralysis

Parotitis inflammation of the parotid salivary gland

Passive (acquired) immunity a resistance of the body to infection in which the host receives natural or artificial antibodies produced by another source

Passive euthanasia allowing an individual to die by withholding or withdrawing measures to maintain life

Passive ROM exercises range-of-motion exercises in which another individual moves each of the client's joints through their complete range of movement, maximally stretching all muscle groups within each plane over each joint

Pathogenicity the ability to produce disease; a pathogen is a microorganism that causes disease

Pathologic fractures spontaneous fractures to which older adults are prone

Patient an individual who is waiting for or undergoing medical treatment and care

Patient-controlled analgesia (PCA) an interactive method of pain management that permits clients to treat their pain by self-administering doses of analgesics

Patient Self-Determination Act (PSDA) legislation requiring that every competent adult be informed in writing on admission to a healthcare institution about his or her rights to accept or refuse medical care and to use advance directives

Peak level indicates the highest concentration of the drug in the blood serum

Peak plasma level the concentration of a drug in the blood plasma that occurs when the elimination rate equals the rate of absorption

Pedagogy the discipline concerned with helping children learn

Pediculosis (lice) infestation with head lice, *Pediculus capitis*; body lice, *Pediculus corporis*; or crab lice, *Pediculus pubis*

Peer groups assume great importance and have a number of functions: provide a sense of belonging, pride, social learning, and sexual roles; most peer groups have well-defined, gender-specific modes of acceptable behavior and in adolescence, the peer groups change with age

Penrose drain a flat, thin rubber tube inserted into a wound to allow for fluid to flow from the wound; it has an open end that drains onto a dressing

Perceived loss the loss experienced by an individual that cannot be verified by others

Perception the ability to interpret the environment through the senses

Percussion (in assessment) a method in which the body surface is struck to elicit sounds that can be heard or vibrations that can be felt

Percutaneous route of absorption of a topical medication through the skin

Percutaneous endoscopic gastrostomy (PEG) a procedure in which a PEG catheter is inserted into the stomach through the skin and subcutaneous tissues of the abdomen; used as a feeding tube

Percutaneous endoscopic jejunostomy (PEJ) a procedure in which a PEJ catheter is inserted into the jejunum through the skin and subcutaneous tissues of the abdomen; used as a feeding tube

Perfusion passage of blood constituents through the vessels of the circulatory system

Pericardium double layer of fibroserous membrane of the heart; the parietal, or outermost, pericardium serves to protect the heart and anchor it to surrounding structures

Peridural anesthesia *see* Epidural anesthesia

Periodontal disease disorder of the supporting structures of the teeth

Perioperative period refers to the three phases of surgery: preoperative, intraoperative, and postoperative

Peripheral pulse a pulse located in the periphery of the body (e.g., foot, hand, or neck)

Peripherally inserted central venous catheter (PICC) a long venous catheter inserted in an arm vein and extending into the distal third of the superior vena cava

Peripheral vascular resistance (PVR) impedance or opposition to blood flow to the tissues; determined by viscosity, or thickness, of the blood; blood vessel length; blood vessel diameter

Peristalsis wavelike movements produced by circular and longitudinal muscle fibers of the intestinal walls; the movement propels the intestinal contents onward

Permissive leader *see* Laissez-faire leader

PERRLA abbreviation used to record normal assessment of the pupils (*pupils equally round* and *react* to *light* and *accommodation*)

Persistent vegetative state (PVS) loss of cognitive function and awareness but respiration and circulation remain

Personality the outward expression of the inner self

Personal knowing promotes wholeness and integrity in the personal encounter to achieve engagement

Personal protective equipment (PPE) barriers such as gloves, mask, and gown used to protect individuals from contact with potentially infective materials

Personal space the distance individuals prefer in interactions with others

Personal values values internalized from the society or culture in which one lives

PES format the three essential components of nursing diagnostic statements including the terms describing the *problem*, the *etiology* of the problem, and the defining characteristics or cluster of *signs* and *symptoms*

pH a measure of the relative alkalinity or acidity of a solution; a measure of the concentration of hydrogen ions

Phagocytosis the process by which macrophages engulf microorganisms and cellular debris

Pharmacist an individual licensed to prepare and dispense drugs and prescriptions

Pharmacodynamics the mechanism of drug action and the relationships between drug concentration and resulting effects in the body

Pharmacogenetics the study of how DNA variation in a *single or few* genes influences the response to a single drug

Pharmacogenomics the study of how genes affect an individual's response to drugs

Pharmacokinetics the study of the absorption, distribution, biotransformation, and excretion of drugs

Pharmacology the scientific study of the actions of drugs on living animals and humans

Pharmacopoeia a book containing a list of drug products used in medicine, including their descriptions and formulas

Pharmacy the art of preparing, compounding, and dispensing drugs; also refers to the place where drugs are prepared and dispensed

Phenomenology research that investigates individuals' life experiences and how they interpret those experiences

Phlebotomist an individual from a laboratory who performs venipuncture, collecting the blood specimen for the tests ordered by the primary care provider

Physical dependence an expected physical response when a client who is on long-term opioid therapy has the opioid significantly reduced or withdrawn

Physical restraints any manual method or physical or mechanical device, material, or equipment attached to a client's body that cannot be removed easily and that restricts the client's movement

Physiologic dependence biochemical changes occurring in the body as a result of excessive use of a drug

PIE an acronym for a charting model that follows a recording sequence of *problems*, *interventions*, and *evaluation* of the effectiveness of the interventions

Piggyback a secondary IV setup that connects a second container to the tubing of a primary container at the upper port; used solely for intermittent drug administration

Pilates method of physical movement and exercise designed to stretch, strengthen, and balance the body, in particular the core of the body

Pilot study a "rehearsal" before the actual study begins, consisting of testing the study with a small sample or over a short period of time

Pinna *see* Auricle

Pitch the frequency (number of the vibrations per second) heard during auscultation

Pitting edema edema in which firm finger pressure on the skin produces an indentation (pit) that remains for several seconds

Placebo any medication or procedure that produces an effect in a client because of its implicit or explicit intent, and not because of its specific physical or chemical properties

Placenta a flat, disc-shaped organ that is highly vascular and normally forms in the upper segment of the endometrium of the uterus; exchanges nutrients and gases between the fetus and the mother

Plaintiff an individual claiming infringement of legal rights by one or more individuals

Planned change an intended, purposive attempt by an individual, group, organization, or larger social system to influence its own status quo or that of another organism or situation

Planning an ongoing process that involves (a) assessing a situation, (b) establishing goals and objectives based on assessment of a situation or future trends, and (c) developing a plan of action that identifies priorities, delineates who is responsible, determines deadlines, and describes how the intended outcome is to be achieved and evaluated

Plantar wart a wart on the sole of the foot

Plaque an invisible soft film consisting of bacteria, molecules of saliva, and remnants of epithelial cells and leukocytes that adheres to the enamel surface of teeth

Plasma the fluid portion of the blood in which the blood cells are suspended

Plateau a maintained concentration of a drug in the plasma during a series of scheduled doses

Pleural effusion exists when there is excessive fluid in the pleural space

Pleximeter in percussion, the middle finger of the dominant hand that is placed firmly on the client's skin

Plexor in percussion, the middle finger of the nondominant hand or a percussion hammer used to strike the pleximeter

Pneumothorax accumulation of air in the pleural space

Point of maximal impulse (PMI) the point where the apex of the heart touches the anterior chest wall and heart movements are most easily observed and palpated

Policies rules developed to govern the handling of frequently occurring situations

Polycythemia a condition in which clients with chronic hypoxia may develop higher than normal counts of red blood cells

Polydipsia excessive thirst

Polypnea abnormally fast respirations

Polysaccharides a branched chain of dozens, sometimes hundreds, of glucose molecules; starches

Polysomnography method for measuring sleep in which an electroencephalogram (EEG), electromyogram (EMG), and electro-oculogram (EOG) are recorded simultaneously for the purpose of assessing a client's activity during sleep

Polyunsaturated fatty acids fatty acid with more than one double bond (or many carbons not bonded to a hydrogen atom)

Polyuria refers to the production of abnormally large amounts of urine by the kidneys; also known as *diuresis*

Population includes all possible members of a group who meet the criteria for a study

Positive feedback feedback that stimulates change

Positive reinforcement giving rewards such as praise for a learner's achievements

Positron emission tomography (PET) a noninvasive radiologic study that involves the injection or inhalation of a radioisotope

Postmortem examination *see* Autopsy

Postoperative phase the period of surgery that begins with the admission of a client to the postanesthesia area and ends when healing is complete

Postural drainage positioning of a client to allow the drainage, by gravity, of secretions from the lungs

Postvoid residual (PVR) urine remaining in the bladder following voiding

Potentiating effect the increased effect of one or both drugs

Practice discipline field of study in which the central focus is performance of a professional role (nursing, teaching, management, making music)

Prayer human experience and communication with the divine

Preceptor an experienced nurse who assists the novice nurse in improving nursing skill and judgment

Precontemplation stage an individual typically denies having a problem and instead views others as having a problem and therefore wants to change the other individual's behavior

Precordium an area of the chest overlying the heart

Preemptive analgesia the administration of analgesics prior to an invasive or operative procedure in order to treat pain before it occurs

Preferred provider arrangements (PPAs) similar to preferred provider organizations, but PPAs can contract with individual healthcare providers; the plan can be limited or unlimited

Preferred provider organization (PPO) a group of physicians or a hospital that provides companies with health services at a discounted rate

Prefilled unit-dose system disposable units that provide injectable medications that are available as prefilled syringes ready for use, or as prefilled sterile cartridges and needles that require the attachment of a reusable holder before use

Prejudice preconceived notion or judgment that is not based on sufficient knowledge; it may be favorable or unfavorable

Preload the degree to which muscle fibers in the ventricle are stretched at the end of diastole

Preoperative phase the period of surgery that begins when the decision for surgery has been made and ends when the client is transferred to the operating room bed

Preparation stage occurs when the individual undertakes cognitive and behavioral activities that prepare him or her for change

Presbycusis generalized loss of hearing related to aging

Presbyopia loss of elasticity of the lens and thus loss of ability to see close objects as a result of the aging process

Prescription the written direction for the preparation and administration of a drug

Presencing a term describing the art of being present, or just being with a client during his or her suffering

Pressure injuries consist of injury to the skin or underlying tissue, usually over a bony prominence, as a result of force alone or in combination with movement; previously called *pressure ulcers*, *decubitus ulcers*, *pressure sores*, or *bedsores*

Primary care (PC) the point of entry into the healthcare system at which initial healthcare is given

Primary healthcare (PHC) essential healthcare based on practical, scientifically sound, and socially acceptable methods and technology made universally accessible to individuals and families in the community through their full participation and at a cost that the community and country can afford to maintain at every stage of their development in the spirit of self-reliance and self-determination

Primary intention healing tissue surfaces are approximated (closed) and there is minimal or no tissue loss, formation of minimal granulation tissue and scarring

Primary prevention activities directed toward the protection from or avoidance of potential health risks

Primary sexual characteristics relate to the organs necessary for reproduction, such as the testes, penis, vagina, and uterus

Principles-based (deontological) theories emphasize individual rights, duties, and obligations

Priority setting the process of establishing a preferential order for nursing strategies

Private law the body of law that deals with relationships between private individuals

Prn order "as needed order"; permits the nurse to give a medication when, in the nurse's judgment, the client requires it

Problem-oriented medical record (POMR) data about the client are recorded and arranged according to the client's problems, rather than according to the source of the information

Problem-oriented record (POR) *see* Problem-oriented medical record (POMR)

Problem solving obtaining information that clarifies the nature of the problem and suggests possible solutions

Procedures steps used in carrying out policies or activities

Process evaluation a component of quality assurance that focuses on how care was given

Process recording the verbatim (word-for-word) account of a conversation

Proctoscopy the viewing of the rectum

Proctosigmoidoscopy the viewing of the rectum and sigmoid colon

Profession an occupation that requires extensive education or a calling that requires special knowledge, skill, and preparation

Professional identity sense of oneself that is influenced by characteristics, norms, and values of the nursing discipline, resulting in an individual thinking, acting, and feeling like a nurse

Professional values values acquired during socialization into nursing from codes of ethics, nursing experiences, teachers, and peers

Progress notes chart entries made by a variety of methods and by all health professionals involved in a client's care for the purpose of describing a client's problems, treatments, and progress toward desired outcomes

Prone position position in which a client lies on his or her abdomen with the head turned to one side

Proprioception awareness of posture, movement, and changes in equilibrium; knowledge of position, weight, and resistance of objects in relation to the body

Proprioceptors sensory receptors that are sensitive to movement and the position of the body

Protein-calorie malnutrition (PCM) an imbalance between nutritional intake and the body's protein requirements

Protocols a predetermined and preprinted plan specifying the procedure to be followed in a particular situation

Proxemics distances that individuals allow between themselves and objects or other individuals

Psychologic dependence a state of emotional reliance on a drug to maintain one's well-being; a feeling of need or craving for a drug

Psychologic homeostasis emotional or psychologic balance or state of mental well-being

Psychomotor domain the "skill" domain; includes motor skills such as giving an injection

Puberty the first stage of adolescence in which sexual organs begin to grow and mature

Public law refers to the body of law that deals with relationships between individuals and the government and governmental agencies

Pulse the wave of blood within an artery that is created by contraction of the left ventricle of the heart

Pulse deficit the difference between the apical pulse and the radial pulse

Pulse oximeter a noninvasive device that measures the arterial blood oxygen saturation by means of a sensor attached to the finger or other location

Pulse pressure the difference between the systolic and the diastolic blood pressure

Pulse rhythm the pattern of the beats and intervals between the beats

Pulse volume the strength or amplitude of the pulse, the force of blood exerted with each heartbeat

Pureed diet a modification of the soft diet wherein liquid may be added to the food, which is then blended to a semisolid consistency

Purkinje fibers fibers of the ventricular conduction pathways that terminate in ventricular muscle, stimulating contraction

Purulent exudate an exudate consisting of leukocytes, liquefied dead tissue debris, and dead and living bacteria

Pus pooled exudates

Pyorrhea advanced periodontal disease in which teeth are loose and pus is evident when the gums are pressed

Pyrexia a body temperature above the normal range; fever

Qi body's vital energy

Qigong breathing and mental exercises combined with body movements

Qualifiers words that have been added to some NANDA labels to give additional meaning to the diagnostic statement

Qualitative research the systematic collection and thematic analysis of narrative data

Quality a subjective description of an auscultated sound (e.g., whistling, gurgling, or snapping)

Quality assurance (QA) program an ongoing systematic process designed to evaluate and promote excellence in the healthcare provided to clients

Quality improvement (QI) follows client care rather than organizational structure, focuses on process rather than individuals, and uses a systematic approach with the intention of improving the quality of care rather than ensuring the quality of care; also known as *continuous quality improvement* (CQI), *total quality management* (TQM), *performance improvement* (PI), or *persistent quality improvement* (PQI)

Quantitative research the systematic collection, statistical analysis, and interpretation of numerical data

Race classification of individuals according to shared biological characteristics and physical features

Racism refers to assumptions held about racial groups

Radiation the transfer of heat from the surface of one object to the surface of another without contact between the two objects

Radiopharmaceutical a pharmaceutical (targeted to a specific organ) labeled with a radioisotope, administered through various routes, to determine hyperfunction or hypofunction of the organ

Range of motion (ROM) the maximum degree of movement possible for each joint

Range orders medication orders in which the selected dose varies over a prescribed range according to the client's situation and status

Rapport a relationship between two or more individuals of mutual trust and understanding

Rationale the scientific reason for selecting a specific action

Reactive hyperemia a bright red flush on the skin occurring after pressure is relieved

Readiness behaviors or cues that reflect a learner's motivation to learn at a specific time

Reagent a substance used to produce a chemical reaction to detect or measure other substances

Recent memory deals with activities of the recent past of minutes to a few hours

Receptor a location on the surface of a cell membrane or within a cell (usually a protein) to which a drug chemically binds

Reconstitution the technique of adding a diluent to a powdered drug to prepare it for administration

Record a written communication providing formal, legal documentation of a client's progress

Recording the process of making written entries about a client on the medical record

Red blood cell (RBC) count number of red blood cells per cubic millimeter of whole blood

Red blood cell (RBC) indices evaluate size, weight, and hemoglobin concentrations of RBCs

Refeeding syndrome a combination of fluid and electrolyte shifts that can occur after a lengthy period of malnutrition or starvation that is a rare but potentially fatal complication of tube feeding

Referred pain pain perceived to be in one area but whose source is another area

Reflection thinking from a critical point of view, analyzing why one acted in a certain way, and assessing the results of one's actions

Reflex an automatic response of the body to a stimulus

Reflexology a treatment based on massage of the feet to relieve symptoms in other parts of the body

Reflux backward flow

Regeneration renewal, regrowth, the replacement of destroyed tissue cells by cells that are identical or similar in structure and function

Regional anesthesia the temporary interruption of the transmission of nerve impulses to and from a specific area or region of the body; the client loses sensation in an area of the body but remains conscious

Registry private duty agency that contracts with individual practitioners

Regression a defense mechanism in which one adapts behavior that was comforting earlier in life to overcome the discomfort and insecurity of the present situation

Regurgitation the spitting up or backward flow of undigested food

Relapsing fever the occurrence of short febrile periods of a few days interspersed with periods of 1 or 2 days of normal temperature

Relationships-based (caring) theories emphasize courage, generosity, commitment, and the need to nurture and maintain relationships

Relaxation response (RR) physiologic state achieved through deep relaxation breathing

Reliability the degree to which an instrument produces consistent results on repeated use

Religion an organized system of worship

REM sleep sleep during which the individual experiences *rapid eye movements*

Remission a period during a chronic illness when there is a lessening of severity or cessation of symptoms

Remittent fever the occurrence of a wide range of temperature fluctuations, more than 2°C (3.6°F) over a 24-hour period, all of which are above normal

Renin-angiotensin-aldosterone system system initiated by specialized receptors in the juxtaglomerular cells of the kidney nephrons that respond to changes in renal perfusion

Report oral, written, or computer-based communication intended to convey information to others

Repression a defense mechanism in which painful thoughts, experiences, and impulses are removed from awareness

Research entails using formal and systematic processes to solve problems and answer questions

Research design overall structure or blueprint or the general layout of a study

Research process method in which decisions are made that result in a detailed plan or proposal for a study, as well as the actual implementation of the plan

Reservoir a source of microorganisms

Resident flora microorganisms that normally reside on the skin and mucous membranes, and inside the respiratory and gastrointestinal tracts

Res ipsa loquitur "the thing that speaks for itself"; a legal doctrine that relates to negligence in which the harm cannot be traced to a specific healthcare provider or standard but does not normally occur unless there has been a negligent act

Resolution phase the part of the response cycle period of return to the unaroused state, which may last 10 to 15 minutes after orgasm, or longer if there is no orgasm

Resonance a hollow sound as produced by lungs filled with air during percussion

Respiration the act of breathing; includes the intake of oxygen and the output of carbon dioxide from the cells to the atmosphere

Respiratory acidosis (hypercapnia) a state of excess carbon dioxide in the body

Respiratory alkalosis a state of excessive loss of carbon dioxide from the body

Respiratory character *see* Respiratory quality

Respiratory hygiene or cough etiquette calls for covering the mouth and nose when sneezing or coughing, proper disposal of tissues, and separating potentially infected individuals from others by at least 1 m (3 ft) or having them wear a surgical mask

Respiratory membrane where gas exchange occurs between the air on the alveolar side and the blood on the capillary side; the alveolar and capillary walls form the respiratory membrane

Respiratory quality refers to those aspects of breathing that are different from normal, effortless breathing; includes the amount of effort exerted to breathe and the sounds produced by breathing

Respiratory rhythm refers to the regularity of expirations and inspirations

Respondeat superior a legal term meaning "let the master answer"; an employer assumes responsibility for the conduct of its employees and can also be held responsible for malpractice by employees

Responsibility the specific accountability or liability associated with the performance of duties of a particular role

Resting energy expenditure (REE) the amount of energy required to maintain basic body functions

Resting tremor a tremor that is apparent when the client is at rest and diminishes with activity

Restraints devices used to reduce or prevent physical activity of a client or a part of the body when the client is unable to remove the device

Retrograde pyelography a radiographic study used to evaluate the urinary tract

Retrospective audit evaluation of a client's record after discharge from an agency

Review of systems *see* Screening examination

Right (legal) a privilege or fundamental power to which an individual is entitled unless it is revoked by law or given up voluntarily

Rigor mortis stiffening of the body that occurs 2 to 4 hours after death

Risk factors factors that cause a client to be vulnerable to developing a health problem

Risk management having in place a system to reduce danger to clients and staff

Risk nursing diagnosis clinical judgment that a problem does not exist, but the presence of risk factors indicates that a problem is likely to develop unless nurses intervene

Role the set of expectations about how an individual occupying a specific position behaves

Role ambiguity unclear role expectations; individuals do not know what to do or how to do it and are unable to predict the reactions of others to their behavior

Role conflict a clash between the beliefs or behaviors imposed by two or more roles fulfilled by an individual

Role development involves socialization into a particular role

Role mastery performance of role behaviors that meet social expectations

Role model providing an example of acceptable behavior(s) through demonstration

Role performance what an individual does in a particular role in relation to the behaviors expected of that role

Role strain a generalized state of frustration or anxiety experienced with the stress of role conflict and ambiguity

Root cause analysis process for identifying factors that bring about deviations in practices that lead to an event

S_1 the first heart sound; occurs when the atrioventricular valves (mitral and tricuspid) close

S_2 the second heart sound; occurs when the semilunar valves (aortic and pulmonic) close

Safety monitoring device an electronic sensor or monitor that detects when clients are attempting to get out of a bed or chair and triggers an alarm

Safety-net hospitals hospitals that provide a significant level of care to low-income, uninsured, and vulnerable populations

Sairy Gamp a character in the Charles Dickens book *Martin Chizzlewit* who represented the negative image of nurses in the early 1800s

Saliva the clear liquid secreted by the salivary glands in the mouth

Sample (statistics) segment of the population from whom data will be collected

Sanguineous exudate an exudate containing large amounts of red blood cells

Sarcopenia steady decrease in muscle fibers

Saturated fatty acids those in which all carbon atoms are filled to capacity (i.e., saturated) with hydrogen

Scabies a contagious skin infestation by the itch mite that produces intense itching, especially at night

Scald a burn from a hot liquid or vapor, such as steam

Scientific health belief based on the belief that life and life processes are controlled by physical and biochemical processes that can be manipulated by humans

Scientific validation thorough critique of a study for its conceptual and methodological integrity

Screening examination a brief review of essential functioning of various body parts or systems; also called *review of systems*

Scrub person usually UAP but can be an RN or LPN; assists the surgeons by draping the client with sterile drapes and handling sterile instruments and supplies; with the circulating nurse, is responsible for accounting for all sponges, needles, and instruments at the close of surgery

Sebaceous glands active under the influence of androgens in both males and females, which secrete sebum and become most active on the face, neck, shoulder, upper back, and chest; are often the cause of an increased incidence of acne

Sebum the oily, lubricating secretion of sebaceous glands in the skin

Seclusion the involuntary confinement of a client alone in a room or area from which the client is physically prevented from leaving

Secondary intention healing wound in which the tissue surfaces are not approximated and there is extensive tissue loss; formation of excessive granulation tissue and scarring

Secondary prevention activities designed for early diagnosis and treatment of disease or illness

Secondary sexual characteristics physical characteristics that differentiate the male from the female but do not relate directly to reproduction

Seizure a sudden onset of excessive electrical discharges in one or more areas of the brain

Seizure precautions safety measures taken to protect clients from injury should they have a seizure

Selectively permeable cell membranes that allow substances to move across them with varying degrees of ease

Self-awareness the relationship between an individual's own and others' perception of self

Self-concept the collection of ideas, feelings, and beliefs one has about oneself

Self-esteem the value one has for oneself; self-confidence

Self-regulation homeostatic mechanisms that come into play automatically in the healthy individual

Semicircular canals in the inner ear; contain the organs of equilibrium

Semi-Fowler's position a bed-sitting position in which the head and trunk are raised 15° to 45°, typically at a 30° angle of elevation; sometimes called *low Fowler's position*

Semilunar valves crescent moon-shaped valves between the cardiac ventricles and the pulmonary artery (pulmonic valve) and the aorta (aortic valve)

Sensorineural hearing loss the result of damage to the inner ear, the auditory nerve, or the hearing center in the brain

Sensoristasis the need for sensory stimulation

Sensory deficit partial or complete impairment of any sensory organ

Sensory deprivation insufficient sensory stimulation for an individual to function

Sensory memory momentary perception of stimuli by the senses

Sensory overload an overabundance of sensory stimulation

Sensory perception the organization and translation of stimuli into meaningful information

Sensory reception process of receiving environmental stimuli

Sentinel event an unexpected occurrence that results in death, permanent harm or severe temporary harm, and intervention required to sustain life

Separation anxiety the fear and frustration experienced by young children that comes with parental absences

Sepsis the presence of pathogenic organisms or their toxins in the blood or body tissues

Septicemia occurs when bacteremia results in systemic infection

Septum a dividing structure such as that between the cardiac chambers or between the two sides of the nose

Serosanguineous blood-tinged drainage seeped from wounds healing by secondary intention

Serous exudate consists chiefly of serum (the clear portion of the blood)

Serum osmolality a measure of the solute concentration of the blood

Severe pain pain in the 7 to 10 range on a numeric scale of 0 (no pain) to 10 (worst pain imaginable)

Sexual orientation the preference of an individual for one gender or the other

Sexual self-concept how one values oneself as a sexual being

Shaft the part of the needle that is attached to the hub; also called the *cannula*

Shaken baby syndrome (SBS) *see* Abusive head trauma

Shared governance a method that aims to distribute decision making among a group of individuals

Shared leadership a contemporary theory of leadership that recognizes the leadership capabilities of each member in a professional group and assumes that appropriate leadership will emerge in relation to the challenges that confront the group

Shared medical decision making a process whereby the primary healthcare provider gives the client the relevant information for all treatment alternatives, and the client provides the primary healthcare provider relevant personal information that might make one treatment or therapy more appropriate for the individual client

Shearing force a combination of friction and pressure that, when applied to the skin, results in damage to the blood vessels and tissues

Shock phase first part of the alarm reaction in which the stressor may be perceived consciously or unconsciously by the individual

Short-term memory information held in the brain for immediate use or what one has in mind at a given moment

Shroud a large piece of plastic or cotton material used to enclose a body after death

Side effect the secondary effect of a drug that is unintended; usually predictable and may be either harmless or potentially harmful

Signs detectable by an observer or can be measured or tested against an accepted standard; can be seen, heard, felt, or smelled; also called *objective data*

Sims' position side-lying position with lowermost arm behind the body and the upper arm at the shoulder and the elbow, with the client's legs flexed in front

Single order an order that is to be carried out one time only at a specified time

Sinoatrial (SA or sinus) node the primary pacemaker of the heart located where the superior vena cava enters the right atrium

Situational leader adapts style according to consideration of the staff members' abilities, knowledge of the nature of the task to be done, and sensitivity to the context or environment in which the task takes place

Situation, background, assessment, and recommendation (SBAR) process a structured approach to documentation used when nurses communicate with primary care providers and other nurses about client status

Sitz bath a bath in which the client sits in warm water to help soothe and heal the perineum

Skinfold measurement an indicator of the amount of body fat, the main form of stored energy

Slander defamation by the spoken word, stating unprivileged (not legally protected) or false words by which a reputation is damaged

Sleep an altered state of consciousness in which the individual's perception of and reaction to the environment are decreased

Sleep apnea frequent short breathing pauses during sleep

Sleep architecture basic organization of normal sleep

Sleep hygiene refers to interventions used to promote sleep

Small calorie (c, cal) the amount of heat required to raise the temperature of 1 g of water 1°C

SOAP an acronym for a charting method that follows a recording sequence of *subjective* data, *objective* data, *assessment*, and *planning*

Socratic questioning a technique one can use to look beneath the surface, recognize and examine assumptions, search for inconsistencies, examine multiple points of view, and differentiate what one knows from what one merely believes

Sojourner Truth an abolitionist, Underground Railroad agent, preacher, and women's rights advocate, she was a nurse for more than 4 years during the Civil War and worked as a nurse and counselor for the Freedman's Relief Association after the war

Solutes substances dissolved in a liquid

Solvent the liquid in which a solute is dissolved

Somatic pain originates in the skin, muscles, bone, or connective tissue

Sordes accumulation of foul matter (food, microorganisms, and epithelial elements) on the teeth and gums

Source-oriented record a record in which each healthcare provider or department makes notations in a separate section or sections of the client's chart

Spastic describing the sudden, prolonged involuntary muscle contractions of clients with damage to the central nervous system

Specific defenses immune functions directed against identifiable bacteria, viruses, fungi, or other infectious agents; also called *immune defenses*

Specific gravity the weight or degree of concentration of a substance compared with that of an equal volume of another, such as distilled water, taken as a standard

Specific self-esteem how much one approves of a certain part of oneself

Sphygmomanometer a device used to measure blood pressure

Spinal anesthesia anesthesia produced by injecting an anesthetic agent into the subarachnoid space surrounding the spinal cord; also referred to as a *subarachnoid block (SAB)*

Spiritual care describes ways in which nurses can offer spiritual support to clients

Spiritual disruption refers to the inner chaos that can occur when an individual's religious assumptions and beliefs are threatened or shattered

Spiritual health *see* Spiritual wellness or well-being

Spirituality the human tendency to seek meaning and purpose in life, inner peace and acceptance, forgiveness and harmony, hope, beauty, and so forth; includes the drive to become all that one can be and is bound to intuition, creativity, and motivation

Spiritual or religious coping refers to the spiritual beliefs or ways of thinking that help individuals cope with their challenges; can be both positive and negative

Spiritual wellness or well-being results when individuals intentionally seek to strengthen their spiritual muscles, as it were, through various spiritual disciplines (e.g., prayer, meditation, service, fellowship with similar believers, learning from a spiritual mentor, worship, study, fasting)

Sputum the mucous secretion from the lungs, bronchi, and trachea

Stage of exhaustion the third stage in the adaptation syndromes that occurs when the adaptation that the body made during the second stage cannot be maintained

Stage of resistance the second stage in the adaptation syndromes when the body's adaptation takes place

Standard a generally accepted rule, model, pattern, or measure

Standardized care plan formal plan that specifies the nursing care for groups of clients with common needs (e.g., all clients with myocardial infarction)

Standard precautions (SP) the risk of caregiver exposure to client body tissues and fluids rather than the suspected presence or absence of infectious organisms determines the use of clean gloves, gowns, masks, and eye protection

Standards of care the skills and learning commonly possessed by members of a profession

Standards of practice descriptions of the responsibilities for which nurses are accountable

Standards of professional performance as set by the American Nurses Association (ANA), describe behaviors expected in the professional nursing role

Standing order an order that may be carried out indefinitely until another order is written to cancel it, or that may be carried out for a specified number of days

Stapes stirrups bone of the middle ear

Statistically significant term applied after data have been analyzed to determine whether the results had a probability less than 0.05, which is considered the acceptable level of significance

Stat order indicates an order that is to be carried out immediately and only once

Statutory laws laws enacted by any legislative body

Steatorrhea excessive amount of fat in the stool due to a malabsorption syndrome or pancreatic enzyme deficiency

Stereognosis the ability to recognize objects by touching and manipulating them

Stereotyping refers to making the assumption that an individual reflects all characteristics associated with being a member of a group

Sterile field a microorganism-free area

Sterile technique practices that keep an area or object free of all microorganisms; also called *surgical asepsis*

Sterilization a process that destroys all microorganisms, including spores and viruses

Sternum the breastbone

Stimulus-based stress model stress is defined as a stimulus, life event, or set of circumstances that arouses physiologic or psychologic reactions that may increase the individual's vulnerability to illness

Stoma an opening created in the abdominal wall by an ostomy

Stool *see* Feces

Strabismus cross-eye

Stress a condition in which an individual experiences changes in the normal balanced state

Stress electrocardiography uses ECGs to assess a client's response to an increased cardiac workload during exercise

Stressor any event or stimulus that causes an individual to experience stress

Stridor a harsh, crowing sound made on inhalation caused by constriction of the upper airway

Strike an organized work stoppage by a group of employees to express a grievance, enforce a demand for changes in condition of employment, or solve a dispute with management

Stroke volume (SV) the amount of blood ejected with each cardiac contraction

Structure evaluation focuses on the setting in which care is given

Subarachnoid block (SAB) *see* Spinal anesthesia

Subculture usually composed of individuals who have a distinct identity and yet are related to a larger cultural group

Subcutaneous beneath the layers of the skin; hypodermic

Subjective data data that are apparent only to the individual affected; can be described or verified only by that individual; also referred to as *symptoms*

Sublingual a method of drug administration in which the drug is placed under the tongue

Substance abuse disorder (SUD) a pattern of behaviors that range from misuse to dependency or addiction to alcohol or drugs

Suctioning the aspiration of secretions through a catheter connected to a suction machine or wall suction outlet

Sudden infant death syndrome (SIDS) the sudden and unexpected death of an infant

Superego the conscience of personality; the source of feelings of guilt, shame, and inhibition

Supine position position in which the head and shoulders are not elevated; also called the *dorsal position*

Supplemental Security Income (SSI) special payments for individuals with disabilities, those who are blind, and those who are not eligible for Social Security; these payments are not restricted to healthcare costs

Suppositories solid, cone-shaped, medicated substances inserted into the rectum, vagina, or urethra

Suppuration the formation of pus

Suprapubic catheter an indwelling catheter that has been surgically placed in the bladder through the abdominal wall, either with or without a urethrally placed catheter

Surface anesthesia *see* Topical anesthesia

Surface temperature the temperature of tissue, the subcutaneous tissue, and fat

Surfactant a surface-active agent (e.g., soap or a synthetic detergent); in pulmonary physiology, a mixture of phospholipids secreted by alveolar cells into the alveoli and respiratory air passages that reduces the surface tension of pulmonary fluids and thus contributes to the elastic properties of pulmonary tissue

Surgical asepsis practices that keep an area or object free of all microorganisms; also called *sterile technique*

Suture a thread used to sew body tissues together

Sutures junction lines of the skull bones

Symptoms *see* Subjective data

Syndrome diagnosis a diagnosis that is associated with a cluster of other diagnoses

Synergistic effect when two different drugs increase the action of one or another drug

System a set of interacting identifiable parts or components

Systemic infection occurs when pathogens spread and damage different parts of the body

Systole the period during which the ventricles contract

Systolic pressure the pressure of the blood against the arterial walls when the ventricles of the heart contract

Tachycardia an abnormally rapid pulse rate; greater than 100 beats per minute

Tachypnea abnormally fast respirations; usually more than 24 respirations per minute

Tactile related to touch

T'ai chi discipline that combines physical fitness, meditation, and self-defense

Target population the universe of elements to which the researcher wishes to be able to apply the study's findings

Tartar a visible, hard deposit of plaque and dead bacteria that forms at the gum lines

Taxonomy a classification system or set of categories, such as nursing diagnoses, arranged on the basis of a single principle or consistent set of principles

Teacher a nurse who helps clients learn about their health and the healthcare procedures they need to perform to restore or maintain their health

Teaching system of activities intended to produce learning

Team nursing the delivery of individualized nursing care to clients by a team led by a professional nurse

Technical skills "hands-on" skills such as those required to manipulate equipment, administer injections, and move or reposition clients

Telehealth delivery of health-related services and information via telecommunication technologies

Telemedicine technology used to transmit electronic medical data about clients to individuals at distant locations

Telenursing use of technology to provide nursing practice at a distance

Temperament the way individuals respond to their external and internal environment

Teratogen anything that adversely affects normal cellular development in the embryo or fetus

Termination stage the ultimate goal where the individual has complete confidence that the problem is no longer a temptation or threat

Territoriality a concept of the space and things that individuals consider their own

Tertiary intention healing healing that occurs in wounds left open for 3 to 5 days and then closed with sutures, staples, or adhesive skin closures

Tertiary prevention activities designed to restore individuals with disabilities to their optimal level of functioning

Theory a system of ideas that is proposed to explain a given phenomenon (e.g., theory of gravity)

Therapeutic bath a bath given for physical effects, such as to soothe irritated skin or to promote healing of an area (e.g., the perineum); two common types are the sitz bath and the medicated bath

Therapeutic communication an interactive process between nurse and client that helps the client overcome temporary stress, get along with other people, adjust to the unalterable, and overcome psychologic blocks that stand in the way of self-realization

Therapeutic effect the primary effect intended of a drug; reason the drug is prescribed

Third space syndrome fluid shifts from the vascular space into an area where it is not readily accessible as extracellular fluid

Thoracentesis a procedure to remove excess fluid or air from the pleural cavity to ease breathing or to introduce chemotherapeutic drugs intrapleurally

Thrill a vibrating sensation over a blood vessel that indicates turbulent blood flow

Thrombophlebitis inflammation of a vein followed by formation of a blood clot

Thrombus a solid mass of blood constituents in the circulatory system; a clot (plural: *thrombi*)

Throughput a transformation that occurs after input is absorbed by the system and is then processed in a way that is useful to the system

Ticks small gray-brown parasites that bite into tissue and suck blood and transmit several diseases to individuals, in particular Rocky Mountain spotted fever, Lyme disease, and tularemia

Tidal volume the volume of air that is normally inhaled and exhaled

Tinea pedis athlete's foot (ringworm of the foot), which is caused by a fungus

Tissue perfusion passage of fluid (e.g., blood) through a specific organ or body part

Tolerance occurs when the client's opioid dose, over time, leads to a decreased sensitivity to the drug's analgesic effect and increasing doses of the opioid are needed to provide the same level of pain relief

Topical applied externally (e.g., to the skin or mucous membranes)

Topical anesthesia applied directly to the skin and mucous membranes, open skin surfaces, wounds, and burns; also called *surface anesthesia*

Top-level managers organizational executives primarily responsible for establishing goals and developing strategic plans

Tort a civil wrong committed against an individual or an individual's property

Tort law law that defines and enforces duties and rights among private individuals that are not based on contractual agreements

Trade name name of the drug given by the drug manufacturer; also known as a *brand name*

Traditional refers to those customs, beliefs, or practices that have existed for many generations without changing

Traditional Chinese medicine (TCM) based on the premise that the body's vital energy circulates through pathways or meridians and can be accessed and manipulated through specific anatomic points along the surface of the body

Tragus the cartilaginous protrusion at the entrance to the ear canal

Transactional leader a contemporary theory of leadership in which resources are exchanged as an incentive for loyalty and performance

Transactional stress theory a theory that encompasses a set of cognitive, affective, and adaptive (coping) responses that arise out of person–environment transactions; the person and the environment are inseparable and affect each other

Transcultural nursing providing care within the differences and similarities of the beliefs, values, and patterns of cultures

Transcutaneous electrical nerve stimulation (TENS) a method of applying low-voltage electrical stimulation directly over pain areas

Transdermal patch a dermatologic medication delivery system that administers sustained-action medications via multilayered films containing the drug and an adhesive layer

Transformational leader leader who fosters creativity, risk taking, commitment, and collaboration by empowering the group to share in the organization's vision

Transgender someone who identifies with a different gender than his or her anatomic designation

Translator an individual who converts written material (such as client education pamphlets) from one language into another

Tremor an involuntary trembling of a limb or body part

Trial the period during which all relevant facts are presented to a jury or judge

Trial and error way to solve problems in which a number of approaches are tried until a solution is found

Triangular fossa a depression of the antihelix

Triglycerides substances that have three fatty acids; they account for more than 90% of the lipids in food and in the body

Trigone a triangular area at the base of the bladder marked by the ureter openings at the posterior corners and the opening of the urethra at the anterior corner

Trimesters the 3-month periods during pregnancy marking certain landmarks for developmental changes in mother and the fetus; three trimesters occur during a pregnancy

Tripod (triangle) position the proper standing position with crutches; crutches are placed about 15 cm (6 in.) in front of the feet and out laterally about 15 cm (6 in.), creating a wide base of support

Trocar a sharp, pointed instrument

Troponin enzyme that is released into the blood during a myocardial infarction

Trough level represents the lowest concentration of a drug in the blood serum

Tuberculin syringe a narrow syringe, calibrated in tenths and hundredths of a milliliter on one scale and in sixteenths of a minim on the other scale that can be useful in administering other drugs, particularly when small or precise measurement is indicated

Two-point discrimination *see* One-point discrimination

Tympanic membrane the eardrum

Tympany a musical or drumlike sound produced during percussion over an air-filled stomach

Ultrasonography the use of ultrasound to produce an image of an organ or tissue

Unconscious mind the mental life of an individual of which the individual is unaware

Undernutrition intake of nutrients insufficient to meet daily energy requirements as a result of inadequate food intake or improper digestion and absorption of food

Undertaker *see* Mortician

Universal precautions (UP) An earlier term for standard precautions that some agencies may use, reflecting their applicability in all client care situations

Unplanned change haphazard change that occurs without control by any individual or group

Unprofessional conduct one of the grounds for action against a nurse's license; includes incompetence or gross negligence, conviction of practicing without a license, falsification of client records, and illegally obtaining, using, or possessing controlled substances

Unsaturated fatty acid a fatty acid that could accommodate more hydrogen atoms than it currently does

Upper-level managers organizational executives who are primarily responsible for establishing goals and developing strategic plans

Urea a substance found in urine, blood, and lymph; the main nitrogenous substance in blood

Ureterostomy type of urinary diversion that involves surgery of the ureters

Urgency the feeling that one must urinate

Urinary frequency the need to urinate often

Urinary hesitancy a delay and difficulty in initiating voiding; often associated with dysuria

Urinary incontinence a temporary or permanent inability of the external sphincter muscles to control the flow of urine from the bladder

Urinary reflux backward flow of urine

Urinary retention the accumulation of urine in the bladder and inability of the bladder to empty itself

Urinary stasis stagnation of urinary flow

Urination the process of emptying the bladder; also called *micturition* or *voiding*

Urine osmolality a measure of the solute concentration of urine, a more exact measurement of urine concentration than specific gravity

Utilitarianism a specific, consequence-based, ethical theory that judges as right the action that does the most good and least amount of harm for the greatest number of individuals; often used in making decisions about the funding and delivery of healthcare

Utility *see* Utilitarianism

Vaginismus involuntary spasm of outer one-third of vaginal muscles, making penetration of the vagina painful

Validation the determination that the diagnosis accurately reflects the problem of the client, that the methods used for data gathering were appropriate, and that the conclusion or diagnosis is justified by the data

Validity the degree to which an instrument measures what it is intended to measure

Valsalva maneuver forceful exhalation against a closed glottis, which increases intrathoracic pressure and thus interferes with venous blood return to the heart

Values something of worth; a belief held dearly by an individual

Values clarification a process by which individuals define their own value

Value system the organization of an individual's values along a continuum of relative importance

Variance a variation or deviation from a critical pathway; goals not met or interventions not performed according to the time frame

Vasoconstriction constricted blood vessels

Vasodilation an increase in the diameter of blood vessels

Vector-borne transmission transport of an infectious agent from an animal or flying or crawling insect that serves as an intermediate means via biting or depositing feces or other materials on the skin

Vehicle-borne transmission transport of an infectious agent into a susceptible host via any intermediate substance (e.g., fomites or food)

Venipuncture puncture of a vein for collection of a blood specimen or for infusion of therapeutic solutions

Ventilation the movement of air in and out of the lungs; the process of inhalation and exhalation

Ventricles two lower chambers of the heart

Veracity a moral principle that holds that one should tell the truth and not lie

Verbal communication use of verbal language to send and receive messages

Verdict the outcome made by a jury

Vernix caseosa a protective covering that develops over the unborn fetus's skin; a white, cheese-like substance that adheres to the skin and can become 1/8 inch thick by birth

Vesicant a medication or fluid that causes blisters, severe tissue injury, or necrosis if it escapes from the vein

Vesicostomy surgical production of an opening into the bladder

Vestibule contains the organs of equilibrium; found in the inner ear

Vestibulitis severe pain on touch or attempted vaginal entry

Vial a small glass medication container with a sealed rubber cap; used for single or multiple doses

Vibration a series of vigorous quiverings produced by hands that are placed flat against the chest wall to loosen thick secretions

Virulence ability to produce disease

Viruses nucleic acid–based infectious agents

Visceral internal organs

Visceral pain pain arising from organs or hollow viscera

Vision the mental image of a possible and desirable future state

Visiting nursing *ee* Home health nursing care

Visual related to sight

Visual acuity the degree of detail the eye can discern in an image

Visual fields the area an individual can see when looking straight ahead

Vital capacity the maximum amount of air that can be exhaled after a maximum inhalation

Vital signs body temperature, pulse, respiration, and blood pressure. Many agencies have designated pain as the fifth vial sign

Vitamin an organic compound that cannot be manufactured by the body and is needed in small quantities to catalyze metabolic processes

Vitiligo patches of hypopigmented skin, caused by the destruction of melanocytes in the area

Voiding *see* urination

Volume control infusion set small fluid containers (100 to 150 mL in size) attached below a primary infusion container so that a medication can be administered through the client's IV line

Volume expanders used to increase the blood volume following severe loss of blood, or loss of plasma

Vulvodynia constant and unremitting burning of the vulva

Water-soluble vitamins vitamins that the body cannot store, so individuals must get a daily supply in the diet; include C and B-complex vitamins

Well-being reflection of the objective conditions in which choices are made and that shape individuals' abilities to transform resources into given ends, such as health

Wellness a state of well-being; engaging in attitudes and behaviors that enhance quality of life and maximize personal potential

Western medicine approach to health that focuses on the use of science in the diagnosis and treatment of health problems

White blood cell (WBC) count determines the number of circulating WBCs per cubic millimeter of whole blood

Xerostomia dry mouth as a result of a reduced supply of saliva

Yoga a type of meditation that is a system of exercises for attaining bodily or mental control and well-being

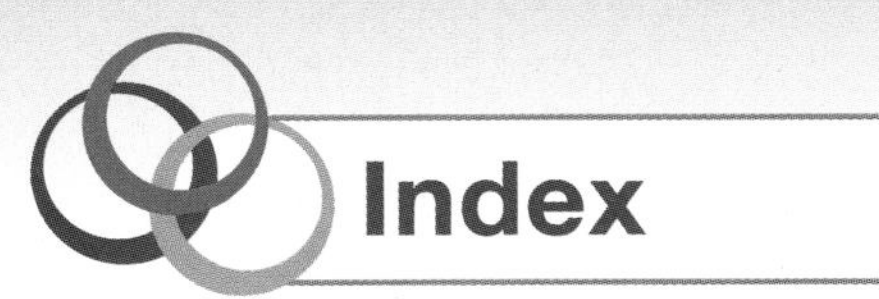

Index

Note: Page numbers followed by *f* indicate figures; those followed by *t* indicate tables, boxes, or special features

B

C

D

E

F

G

H

O

Q

R

S

U

V

W

X

Y

Z

SPECIAL FEATURES

ANATOMY & PHYSIOLOGY REVIEW

ASSESSMENT INTERVIEW

CLIENT TEACHING

CONCEPT MAP

CRITICAL PATHWAY

CRITICAL THINKING CHECKPOINT

DRUG CAPSULE

EVIDENCE-BASED PRACTICE

LIFESPAN CONSIDERATIONS

NURSING CARE PLAN

PRACTICE GUIDELINES

SKILLS